Clinical Disorders of

FLUID AND ELECTROLYTE METABOLISM

NOTICE

MAXWELL & KLEEMAN'S

Clinical Disorders of FLUID AND ELECTROLYTE METABOLISM

Fifth Edition

Edited by

ROBERT G. NARINS, M.D.

Professor of Medicine
Henry Ford Hospital
Division of Nephrology
Detroit, Michigan

McGraw-Hill, Inc.
Health Professions Division
New York St. Louis San Francisco Auckland Bogotá Caracas Lisbon London Madrid Mexico City Milan
Montreal New Delhi Paris San Juan Singapore Sydney Tokyo Toronto

MAXWELL AND KLEEMAN'S
CLINICAL DISORDERS OF FLUID AND ELECTROLYTE METABOLISM

1234567890 KGPKGP 9876543

INTERNATIONAL EDITION

Copyright 1994

Exclusive rights by McGraw-Hill, Inc., for manufacture and export. This book cannot be re-exported from the country to which it is consigned by McGraw-Hill.

When ordering this title, use ISBN 0-07-112733-X.

This book was set in Sabon by Better Graphics, Inc.
The editors were J. Dereck Jeffers and Lester A. Sheinis.
The production supervisor was Richard C. Ruzycka.
The text designer was José Fonfrias.
The cover designer was Marsha Cohen/Parallelogram.
The indexer was Tony Greenberg, M.D.
Arcata Graphics/Kingsport was printer and binder.

Library of Congress Cataloging-in-Publication Data

Maxwell & Kleeman's clinical disorders of fluid and electrolyte metabolism—5th ed. / edited by Robert G. Narins.
p. cm.
Rev. ed of: Clinical disorders of fluid and electrolyte metabolism. 4th ed. c1987.
Includes bibliographical references and index.
ISBN 0-07-041008-9
1. Body fluid disorders. 2. Water-electrolyte imbalances.
I. Maxwell, Morton H. (Morton Harrison), date. II. Kleeman, Charles R. (Charles Richard), date. III. Narins, Robert G.
IV. Title: Clinical disorders of fluid and electrolyte metabolism.
V. Title: Maxwell and Kleeman's clinical disorders of fluid and electrolyte metabolism.
[DNLM: 1. Water-Electrolyte Imbalance. WD 220 M4645 1994]
RC630.C57 1994
616.3'99—dc20
DNLM/DLC 94-14084
for Library of Congress CIP

Dedicated to That Endangered Species That Remains Charmed by the Transmembrane Traffic in Ions and the Ebb-and-Flow of Body Fluids

CONTENTS

CONTRIBUTORS

Zalman S. Agus, M.D. [34]*
Professor of Medicine
University of Pennsylvania
Philadelphia, Pennsylvania

Edward A. Alexander, M.D. [6]
Professor of Medicine and Physiology
Boston University School of Medicine
Chief of Nephrology
Boston City Hospital
Boston, Massachusetts

Robert J. Alpern, M.D. [10]
Professor of Medicine
Chief of Nephrology
Division of Nephrology
University of Texas
Southwestern Medical Center at Dallas
Dallas, Texas

Robert J. Anderson, M.D. [37]
Associate Professor of Medicine
Division of Renal Diseases
University of Colorado Health Sciences Center
Denver, Colorado

Allen I. Arieff, M.D. [46]
Professor of Medicine
Chief, Geriatic Nephrology
University of California, San Francisco School of Medicine
Veterans Administration Medical Center
Geriatrics Division
San Francisco, California

Maurice F. Attie, M.D. [11]†
Associate Professor of Medicine
Endocrinology Section, Department of Medicine
Hospital of the University of Pennsylvania
Philadelphia, Pennsylvania

John Badalamenti, M.D. [42]
Assistant Professor of Medicine
Division of Nephrology
University of Texas Medical Branch
Galveston, Texas

Kamal F. Badr, M.D. [15]
Chief of Nephrology
Division of Nephrology
Veterans Administration Medical Center
Decatur, Georgia

Kim E. Barrett, M.D. [17]
Assistant Professor of Medicine
Division of Gastroenterology
University of California, San Diego School of Medicine
San Diego, California

Robert A. Bear, M.D. [43]
Professor of Medicine
University of Toronto
Division of Nephrology
St. Michael's Hospital
Toronto, Ontario, Canada

Julio E. Benabe, M.D. [32]
Chief of Hypertension
Veterans Administration Medical Center
Decatur, Georgia

William M. Bennett, M.D. [42]
Professor of Medicine
Division of Nephrology
University of Oregon Health Sciences Center
Portland, Oregon

Tomas Berl, M.D. [5]
Professor of Medicine
University of Colorado School of Medicine
Denver, Colorado

Robert W. Berliner, M.D. [7]
Professor Emeritus of Physiology
Yale University School of Medicine
New Haven, Connecticut

Jeffrey S. Berns, M.D. [40]
Clinical Assistant Professor of Medicine
University of Pennsylvania School of Medicine
Attending Physician
Graduate Hospital
Philadelphia, Pennsylvania

James E. Bourdeau, M.D. [11]
Associate Professor of Medicine
Nephrology Section, Department of Medicine
University of Oklahoma
University of Oklahoma Health Sciences Center
Veterans Administration Medical Center
Oklahoma City, Oklahoma

Barry M. Brenner, M.D. [15]
Samuel A. Levine Professor of Medicine
Harvard Medical School;
Director, Renal Division
Department of Medicine
Brigham and Women's Hospital
Boston, Massachusetts

Euan J. F. Carlisle, M.D. [27]
Assistant Professor of Medicine
St. Joseph's Hospital
Hamilton, Ontario, Canada

Richard W. Carlson, M.D., Ph.D. [45]
Professor and Chairman
Department of Medicine
University of Illinois College of Medicine at Peoria
Peoria, Illinois

Surinder Cheema-Dhadli, Ph.D. [28]
Department of Medicine
Division of Nephrology
University of Toronto
St. Michael's Hospital
Toronto, Ontario, Canada

Arnold M. Chonko, M.D. [19]
Professor of Medicine
Division of Nephrology
University of Kansas Medical Center
Kansas City, Kansas

Jack W. Coburn, M.D. [41]
Adjunct Professor of Medicine
UCLA School of Medicine;
Staff Physician
Veterans Administration Medical Center, Wadsworth Division
West Los Angeles, California

* The numbers in brackets following the contributors' names indicate the chapters written or co-written by the contributors.

† Deceased.

Raphael M. Cohen, M.D. [40]
Clinical Assistant Professor of Medicine
University of Pennsylvania School of Medicine
Director, Peritoneal Dialysis Program and Attending Physician
Graduate Hospital
Philadelphia, Pennsylvania

Delila B. Corry, M.D. [48]
Assistant Professor in Residency
Division of Nephrology
Sepulveda Veterans Administration Medical Center
Sepulveda, California

Gabriel M. Danovitch, M.D. [39]
Clinical Professor of Medicine
UCLA School of Medicine
Los Angeles, California

Ralph A. DeFronzo, M.D. [23]
Professor of Medicine
Chief, Diabetes Center
University of Texas Health Science Center
San Antonio, Texas

Tusar K. Desai, M.D. [45]
Assistant Professor of Medicine
Wayne State University
Division of Gastroenterology
Harper Hospital and Detroit Receiving Hospitals
Detroit Medical Center
Detroit, Michigan

Kiertisin Dharmsathaphorn, M.D. [17]†
Associate Professor of Medicine
Division of Gastroenterology
University of California, San Diego School of Medicine
San Diego, California

John H. Dirks, M.D. [13]
Professor of Medicine
Department of Medicine
University of Toronto
Toronto, Ontario, Canada

Robert G. Dluhy, M.D. [49]
Associate Professor of Medicine
Harvard Medical School;
Physician, Division of Endocrinology and Hypertension
Brigham and Women's Hospital
Boston, Massachusetts

Sandra Donnelly, M.D. [27]
Assistant Professor of Medicine
University of Toronto
Mount Sinai Hospital
Toronto, Ontario, Canada

Thomas P. Dunfee, M.D. [26]
Coordinator, ESRD Training Program
Division of Nephrology and Hypertension
Henry Ford Hospital
Detroit, Michigan

Victor J. Dzau, M.D. [16]
Professor of Medicine
Chief of Cardiology
Falk Cardiovascular Research Center
Stanford, University
Stanford, California

Michael Emmett, M.D. [31]
Professor of Medicine
Chief, Nephrology Department
Baylor Hospital
Dallas, Texas

Murray Epstein, M.D., F.A.C.P. [18]
Professor of Medicine
Director, Nephrology Department
Veterans Administration Medical Center
Miami, Florida

Mark D. Faber, M.D. [43]
Senior Staff Physician
Co-Director Home Dialysis
Henry Ford Hospital
Detroit, Michigan
Clinical Instruction, Department of Medicine
University of Michigan
Ann Arbor, Michigan

Darrell D. Fanestil, M.D. [1]
Professor of Medicine
Head, Division of Nephrology
University of California, San Diego
La Jolla, California

Thomas F. Ferris, M.D. [35]
Nesbitt Professor and Chairman
Department of Medicine
University of Minnesota Medical School
Minneapolis, Minnesota

Michael J. Field, M.B., B.S., Bsc (hons), F.R.A.C.P. [7]
Lecturer in Medicine
University of Sydney;
Department of Medicine
Repatriation General Hospital
Concord, N.S.W., Australia

Stanley S. Franklin, M.D. [38]
Adjunct Professor of Medicine
Director of Hypertension
Division of Nephrology
UCLA School of Medicine
Los Angeles, California

Cosmo L. Fraser, M.D. [46]
Associate Professor of Medicine
University of California, San Francisco School of Medicine
Chief, Inpatient Dialysis
Veterans Administration Medical Center
Geriatrics Division
San Francisco, California

Michael A. Geheb, M.D. [45]
Professor of Medicine and Associate Dean for Clinical Affairs
State University of New York at Stony Brook—School of Medicine
Stony Brook, New York

F. John Gennari, M.D. [30]
Professor of Medicine
Department of Medicine
University of Vermont
Burlington, Vermont

Gerhard H. Giebisch, M.D. [7]
Sterling Professor of Cellular and Molecular Biology
Yale University School of Medicine
Department of Cellular and Molecular Physiology
New Haven, Connecticut

Jared J. Grantham, M.D. [19]
Professor of Medicine
Director of Nephrology
University of Kansas Medical Center School of Medicine
Kansas City, Kansas

Mitchell L. Halperin, M.D. [27, 28]
Professor of Medicine
St. Michael's Hospital
Renal Division
Toronto, Ontario, Canada

Marilyn T. Haupt, M.D. [45]
Associate Professor of Medicine
Chief, Division of Critical Care Medicine
Wayne State University School of Medicine
Chief, Section of Critical Care Medicine
Detroit Receiving Hospital, Detroit Medical Center
Detroit, Michigan

Bernard Hitzig, Ph.D. [8]
Assistant Professor Physiology in Medicine
Harvard Medical School;
Assistant Biologist
Massachusetts General Hospital
Boston, Massachusetts

Norman K. Hollenberg, M.D. [16]
Director and Professor of Physiologic Medicine
Brigham and Women's Hospital
Boston, Massachusetts

Henry Hulter, M.D. [14]
Associate Professor of Medicine
Division of Nephrology
San Francisco General Hospital
San Francisco, California

Daniel Ikemiyashiro, M.D. [25]
Fellow
Division of Nephrology and Hypertension
Henry Ford Hospital
Detroit, Michigan

Donald W. Inadomi, M.D. [44]
Assistant Clinical Professor of Medicine
UCLA School of Medicine;
Attending Physician
Harbor-UCLA Medical Center
Torrance, California

Julie R. Ingelfinger, M.D. [16]
Associate Professor of Pediatrics
Harvard Medical School
Co-Chief, Pediatric Nephrology Unit
Massachusetts General Hospital
Boston, Massachusetts

Kamel S. Kamel, M.D. [27, 28]
Division of Nephrology
St. Michael's Hospital
Toronto, Ontario, Canada

Rajat Kaul, M.D. [22]
Physician
Veterans Administration Medical Center
Salt Lake City, Utah

Homayoun Kazemi, M.D. [8]
Professor of Medicine
Havard Medical School
Chief of Pulmonary Medicine and Critical Care Medicine
Massachusetts General Hospital
Boston, Massachusetts

Kent A. Kirchner, M.D. [3]
Professor of Medicine
Associate Professor of Physiology and Biophysics
Associate Chairman for Academic Affairs
Department of Medicine
University of Mississippi Medical Center
Jackson, Mississippi

Charles R. Kleeman, M.D. [5, 25, 26, 33]
Professor of Medicine
Division of Nephrology
UCLA School of Medicine
Senior Advisor to the Research Committee of the Board
Cedars-Sinai Medical Center
Los Angeles, California

Keith L. Klein, M.D. [38]
Associate Clinical Professor of Medicine
UCLA School of Medicine
Los Angeles, California

Jack G. Kleinman, M.D. [9]
Associate Professor of Medicine
Nephrology Section
Medical College of Wisconsin;
Zablocki Veterans Administration Medical Center
Milwaukee, Wisconsin

James P. Knochel, M.D. [47]
Chairman, Department of Internal Medicine
Presbyterian Hospital
Dallas, Texas

Joel D. Kopple, M.D. [44]
Professor of Medicine
Chief, Neurology
Harbor-UCLA Medical Center
Torrance, California

Nelson P. Kopyt, D.O. [26]
Clinical Assistant Professor of Medicine
Temple University Health Sciences Center
Philadelphia, Pennsylvania;
Chief, Nephrology Section
Allentown Osteopathic Medical Center
Allentown, Pennsylvania

Robert A. Kreisberg [26]
Professor of Medicine
Vice Chairman, Department of Medicine
University of Alabama School of Medicine
Birmingham, Alabama

G. Gopal Krishna, M.D. [22, 25, 48]
Physician
Central Coast Nephrology
Salinas, California

James A. Kruse, M.D. [45]
Associate Professor of Medicine
Wayne State University
Director, Respiratory Care Unit
Associate Director, Medical Intensive Care Unit
Detroit Receiving Hospital, The Detroit Medical Center
Detroit, Michigan

Robert T. Kunau, M.D. [22]
Physician
Dallas Nephrology Associates
Dallas, Texas

Kiyoshi Kurokawa, M.D. [12]
Associate Professor of Medicine
University of Tokyo Faculty of Medicine
Bunkyo-Ku, Tokyo, Japan

Neil A. Kurtzman, M.D. [29]
Arnett Professor of Medicine
Professor of Physiology
Chairman, Department of Internal Medicine
Texas Tech University Health Sciences Center
School of Medicine
Lubbock, Texas

David B.N. Lee, M.D. [12]
Chief, Nephrology Department
Sepulveda V.A. Hospital
Sepulveda, California

Jacob Lemann, Jr., M.D. [9]
Professor of Medicine
Medical College of Wisconsin
Froedtert Memorial Lutheran Hospital
Milwaukee, Wisconsin

Barton S. Levine, M.D. [33]
Assistant Chief, Nephrology
Veterans Administration
Wadsworth Medical Center
Los Angeles, California

Francisco Llach, M.D. [41]
Chief, Nephrology Section
Wadsworth Veterans Administration Medical Center
Department of Nephrology
West Los Angeles, California

Manuel Martínez-Maldonado, M.D. [32]
Professor of Medicine and Vice Chairman, Department of Medicine
Emory University Medical School
Decatur, Georgia

Shaul G. Massry, M.D. [34]
Professor of Medicine
Chief of Nephrology
University of Southern California
School of Medicine
Los Angeles, California

Morton H. Maxwell, M.D. [48]
Clinical Professor of Medicine
UCLA School of Medicine
Santa Monica, California

Orson W. Moe, M.D. [10]
Department of Internal Medicine
Division of Nephrology
University of Texas
Southwestern Medical Center at Dallas
Dallas, Texas

Francis D. Moore, M.D. [1]
Moseley Professor of Surgery, Emeritus
Harvard Medical School
Surgeon-in-Chief, Emeritus
Peter Bent Brigham Hospital
Boston, Massachusetts

Gail Morrison, M.D. [21]
Associate Chairman of Medicine
Department of Medicine
Hospital of the University of Pennsylvania
Philadelphia, Pennsylvania

Farid Nakhoul, M.D. [12]
Research Fellow
UCLA School of Medicine
Sepulveda Veterans Administration Medical Center
Sepulveda, California

Robert G. Narins, M.D. [20, 22, 24, 25, 26, 31, 43]
Division Head, Nephrology
Chief, Renal-Hypertension Section
Henry Ford Hospital
Detroit, Michigan

Allen R. Nissenson, M.D. [39]
Professor of Medicine
Director, Dialysis Program
UCLA Medical School
Los Angeles, California

Helen Ocdol, M.D. [20]
Fellow, Renal-Hypertension Section
Henry Ford Hospital
Detroit, Michigan

James R. Oster, M.D. [26]
Associate Chief
Medical Service
Veterans Administration Medical Center
Miami, Florida

Mark S. Paller, M.D. [35]
Assistant Professor of Medicine
Department of Medicine—Renal
Medical School—Minneapolis;
University of Minnesota
Physician, University of Minnesota Hospital
Minneapolis, Minnesota

Guido O. Perez, M.D. [18]
Professor of Medicine
University of Miami School of Medicine;
Chief, Dialysis Unit
Veterans Administration Medical Center
Miami, Florida

Ronald D. Perrone, M.D. [6]
Associate Professor of Medicine
Tufts University School of Medicine
Assistant Physician, New England Medical Center
Boston, Massachusetts

Sidney F. Phillips, M.D. [36]
Professor of Medicine
Mayo Medical School
Rochester, Minnesota

Russel Pikus, M.D. [22]
Physician
Columbus Internal Medicine Associates
Columbus, Indiana

Gary A. Quamme, M.D. [13]
Professor of Medicine
Director of Experimental Medicine
Department of Medicine
University of British Columbia
Vancouver, British Columbia

Kent H. Raymond, M.D. [22]
Physician
Metrolina Nephrology Associate, P.A.
Charlotte, North Carolina

Floyd C. Rector, Jr., M.D. [10]
Chairman, Department of Medicine
University of California, San Francisco
School of Medicine
San Francisco, California

Gary Reed, M.D. [47]
Associate Professor
Department of Internal Medicine
University of Texas Health Science Center;
Medical Director of Emergency Suites
Parkland Memorial Hospital
Dallas, Texas

Louis J. Riley, Jr., M.D. [40]
Associate Professor of Medicine
Deputy Chief of Nephrology
Director of Clinical Medicine
Temple University
Philadelphia, Pennsylvania

Gary L. Robertson, M.D. [4]
Professor of Medicine and Neurology
Director Clinical Research Center
Northwestern University Medical School
Chicago, Illinois

Mario F. Rubin, M.D. [42]
Assistant Professor of Medicine
Division of Nephrology
University of Texas Medical School at Houston
Houston, Texas

Michael R. Rudnick, M.D. [40]
Clinical Professor of Medicine
University of Pennsylvania
The Graduate Hospital
Division of Nephrology and Hypertension
Philadelphia, Pennsylvania

Sandra Sabatini, Ph.D., M.D. [29]
Professor of Internal Medicine and Physiology
Division of Nephrology
Texas Tech University Health Sciences Center
Lubbock, Texas

Rebecca J. Schmidt, D.O. [25, 43]
Physician
Division of Nephrology
West Virginia University
Morgantown, West Virginia

Robert W. Schrier, M.D. [20]
Professor and Chairman
University of Colorado
Boulder, Colorado

Irwin Singer, M.D. [21]
Chief, Outpatient Clinic
Riviera Beach Veterans Administration Medical Center
Riviera Beach, Florida

J. Douglas Smith, M.D. [23]
Clinical Associate Professor of Medicine
Yale Medical School
New Haven, Connecticut

Susan P. Steigerwalt, M.D. [22]
Acting Section Head
Division of Nephrology and Hypertension
Henry Ford Hospital
Detroit, Michigan

Jay Stein, M.D. [3]
Provost and Senior Vice President for Health Sciences
University of Oklahoma
Oklahoma City, Oklahoma

Richard H. Sterns, M.D. [20]
Associate Professor of Medicine
University of Rochester
Rochester, New York

John B. Stokes, M.D. [2]
Professor of Medicine
Chief, Nephrology Division
University of Iowa
Iowa City, Iowa

Isaac Teitelbaum, M.D. [5]
Assistant Professor of Medicine
University of Colorado Health Sciences Center
Denver, Colorado

Michael L. Tuck, M.D. [48]
Associate Professor of Medicine
Chief, Endocrinology and Metabolism
UCLA San Fernando Valley Program
Sepulveda VA Medical Center
Sepulveda, California

Philip J. Tuso, M.D. [39]
Research Fellow, Dept. of Surgery
Senior Nephrology Fellow, Dept. of Medicine
Cedars-Sinai Medical Center
Beverly Hills, California

Somkiat Vasuvattakul, M.D. [27]
Fellow
Department of Medicine
St. Michael's Hospital
Toronto, Ontario, Canada

Abraham U. Waks, M.D. [48]
Associate Clinical Professor of Medicine
UCLA School of Medicine
Los Angeles, California

Gordon H. Williams, M.D. [49]
Professor of Medicine
Harvard Medical School;
Chief, Endocrinology-Hypertension Division
Brigham and Women's Hospital
Boston, Massachusetts

Norimoto Yanagawa, M.D. [12]
Professor of Medicine
UCLA School of Medicine
Sepulveda Veterans Administration Medical Center
Sepulveda, California

Jerry Yee, M.D. [25]
Department of Medicine
Division of Nephrology
University of Texas Health Science Center
San Antonio, Texas

Robert L. Zerbe, M.D. [4]
Associate Professor of Medicine
Lilly Laboratory of Clinical Research
Wishard Memorial Hospital
Indianapolis, Indiana

PREFACE TO THE FIFTH EDITION

A textbook is a living thing! It grows and matures by concomitantly shedding nonfunctional components, adding new topics and reshaping, updating, and, more carefully and thoughtfully, rearticulating retained features. In the preface to the fourth edition of *Clinical Disorders . . .* we defined the reasons that prompted our restructuring of the book. Shorter, more concise chapters that made facts and concepts more accessible to the readership were major goals. Each chapter stressed those relevant pathophysiologic principles that we thought would facilitate the translation of science to the bedside. This fifth edition retains the same format and is committed to the same principles.

Fluid-electrolyte and acid-base abnormalities color the clinical pictures of patients from all the specialties of internal medicine, pediatrics, surgery, and obstetrics and gynecology. The book's design was a natural creation spawned by the ubiquitous nature of these disorders. Defining the physiologic basis for electrolyte traffic across membranes and identifying the mechanisms underlying the excretion and conservation of ions and water became the natural format for Part I. Principles elaborated in Part I, in turn, became the skeleton giving structure to the first section of Part II, wherein the primary disruptions of normal ion and fluid metabolism are identified and dissected. In the second section of Part II, the principles of physiology, pathophysiology, and the clinical aspects of the primary electrolyte and fluid disorders give defining substance to those clinical settings and syndromes in which these disorders play critical roles.

A philosophical imperative integrated into each chapter is the notion that the principles of physiology and those of clinical medicine must be interwoven. Unless ultimately proving to be of clinical value, the solving of physiologic enigmas becomes a far less exciting exercise. Conversely, plying the art of medicine divorced from its physiologic underpinnings becomes a well-meaning but simply descriptive and static activity. Diseases may be viewed as perverse experiments of nature that provoke scientists to explore the mechanisms and forces that have caused normal physiology to go awry and thereby simultaneously expand the disciplines of both science and medicine. The science of medicine is the physician's ladder enabling him or her to reach beyond simple descriptions of disease and so create newer approaches to diagnosis and management. Confronted with new or unusual presentations of disease, those physicians uncomfortable with physiologic principles can only "round-up the usual suspects," missing the true nature of the process and its most rational therapy. By relying on and elaborating these principles, the authors of the chapters in this fifth edition provide the fundamentals for better patient care and for the growth of those caring for the patients. We hope you agree.

Robert G. Narins, M.D.

PREFACE TO THE FOURTH EDITION

Over more than 20 years, the first three editions of *Clinical Disorders of Fluid and Electrolyte Metabolism* have served our readership well. We take great pride and satisfaction in the sustained worldwide acceptance of our book.

The 1980s have spawned the explosive appearance of progressively greater amounts of information, while the time available for its absorption is continuously evaporating. Accordingly, we have redesigned our book to cope with this flood of medical information more effectively. As in previous editions, we continue to present in-depth, lucid descriptions of the physiology, pathophysiology, and clinical appearance of water and electrolyte disturbances. Scientific principles, interwoven with clinical observations, provide rational substance for the differential diagnosis and therapy of these ubiquitous disorders.

This fourth edition enables readers at all levels of sophistication to locate specific areas of interest rapidly, and to read and digest a given subject quickly. Purposely, we have condensed and more sharply focused our chapters. These briefer presentations are provided by a large number of authors, chosen for their depth of understanding and experience, but most importantly, for their ability to simplify and crisply present their areas of expertise. More circumscribed, up-to-date, and lucid presentations allow readers to obtain a broad overview of their topic, as well as to satisfy their specific factual needs quickly.

Part One presents the physiological basis for the scientific approach to clinical disorders of fluid and electrolyte metabolism. Up-to-date, well-referenced chapters provide detailed insight into the normal regulation of water and electrolyte metabolism. Highlighted are the specific roles of the endocrine system and the gastrointestinal tract in the normal physiologic control of fluid and electrolyte metabolism. Concise chapters on adrenal hormones, prostaglandins and kinins, and the renin-angiotensin system should add to and update the reader's understanding of modern fluid and electrolyte physiology.

Part Two, the clinical portion, has been subdivided into two parts. The first subsection treats each of the primary disturbances of water and electrolyte metabolism, while the second portion discusses a variety of complex medical and surgical conditions commonly associated with disordered mineral and water metabolism. Rather than lumping together many disparate but clinically important areas into a single chapter, we have chosen to separate them into more concentrated smaller chapters. This is most dramatically represented by the sections on disordered sodium and acid-base metabolism. Four separate chapters comprise the section on disordered sodium content and concentration: The edematous states are described in terms of pathophysiology and diagnosis, while separate chapters are presented on the treatment of edema and the approach to hypotonic and to hypertonic syndromes. The acid-base disorders are introduced with a separate chapter dealing with critical and fundamental concepts that allow one to understand and rationally approach the simple and mixed metabolic and respiratory perturbations. This chapter is then followed by additional separate sections on metabolic acidosis, a specific chapter on diabetic ketoacidosis, and an additional chapter on renal tubular acidosis. Metabolic alkalosis and the approach to respiratory acidosis and alkalosis are separately dealt with in terms of pathophysiology, diagnosis, and therapy. Finally, mixed acid-base disorders consolidate the approach developed in the previous chapters. These separate, sharply focused chapters allow one to digest the material at hand more quickly and come away with a practical understanding of and appreciation for the application of this information to the clinical setting.

Special attention has been paid to the approach to fluid and electrolyte disorders in the surgical setting. The pathophysiology and practical treatment of fluid and electrolyte disturbances in the preoperative and postoperative setting are well outlined in separate chapters. Total parenteral nutrition and its complications in the surgical setting are dealt with in two separate chapters.

We are most excited by this new edition and enthusiastically submit it as a most effective instrument of learning. We have strived to craft this edition to the needs of the 1980s. We hope that you agree that it meets these goals.

Morton H. Maxwell, M.D.
Charles R. Kleeman, M.D.
Robert G. Narins, M.D.

PART I

PHYSIOLOGIC BASIS FOR WATER AND ELECTROLYTE METABOLISM

SECTION I-1

DYNAMICS OF BODY WATER AND ELECTROLYTE DISTRIBUTION AND TRANSPORT

CHAPTER • 1

Compartmentation of body water

Darrell D. Fanestil • with a Historical Introduction by Francis D. Moore

HISTORICAL INTRODUCTION

Much of the early work in body composition was done in our laboratories at Harvard Medical School, Massachusetts General Hospital, and Peter Bent Brigham Hospital. For the seeming focus on our own work, I apologize.

During the years 1940–1941, I was appointed a research fellow of the National Research Council and studied in the laboratory of Joseph Aub at the Huntington Memorial Hospital, particularly under the direction of Waldo E. Cohn, who was a pioneer in the study of human phosphorus metabolism using ^{32}P. The first cyclotron-produced radioisotopes for medical research had become available only three years previously. In conjunction with work on a radioactive brominated dye,[55,79] we began to study very severe burns, using the volume of dilution of radiosodium (^{24}Na) as a measurement of the extracellular fluid (later shifting to radiobromide) and the dye as a tracer for lymphatic pathways. The bromide method of measuring ECF was based on the work of the late A. Baird Hastings[44] (our professor of biochemistry), using chemical bromide as a histochemical tracer for extracellular fluid in his classical studies on tissue aging. The methods of measuring plasma volume[24] and red blood cell volume[78] had been worked out by other laboratories with whom we stayed closely in touch.

At the end of the war the details of the Manhattan Project (on the production of an atomic bomb) became widely known and with them the mass production of heavy hydrogen (deuterium). I wrote to Harold Urey (who had been awarded the Nobel Prize for discovering the existence of deuterium) and told him of my idea on the use of deuterium oxide dilution for the measurement of total body water (TBW). He promptly sent me a test tube filled with 95 percent pure DHO. He said that the method "couldn't help but work." (I still have the test tube!) At that time I was unaware of the tea party in Ernest Rutherford's laboratory some years before and Georg von Hevesy's daydream about TBW measurements in humans based on putting some heavy water in the tea!

So we went to work. Using rabbits and a Lindstrom-Lang gradient tube (a difficult and fussy method), we turned out the data for the first paper on measurement of total body composition by isotope dilution.[56] Soon the falling drop was the method of choice for heavy water analysis. These values were validated by carcass desiccation to constant weight.[50,51]

From that time on it was but a step further to measurement of total body solids by isotope dilution.[12,13,16] This had never been done before or, to the best of our knowledge, even considered as a possibility. To measure total body potassium (using ^{42}K) the conventional dilution equation is used, but the equilibrium ratio has as its denominator, not the concentration of the solute in aqueous solution, but rather the concentration of the isotope in its sister or naturally occurring isotope (specific activity).[7] By this method an actual weight (in grams or milligrams) of body solids in solution can be gained by simple injection, stabilization, and equilibrium measurement.

The measurement of disappearance curves, the establishment of true equilibrium, and analytic validation were at the heart of all our work.[27,70] Working with Arthur Solomon, Isidore Edelman of our group adapted the mass spectrometer to deuterium measurement; we soon moved to tritium for the TBW measurements. With the help of Margaret Ball and Caryl Magnus Boyden, we used carcass desiccation and total carcass analysis for these validations, and finally went on to analysis of an entire human cadaver in whom the body composition had been assessed prior to death.[60] To the best of my knowledge this had not been done before (or since).

Our group then proceeded to measure total body composition by multiple isotope and tracer dilution in normal people in various age groups in both sexes, in acute and chronic illness, in obesity and heart disease.[14,15,35,52,57,88] Finally, in 1963, we published a book entitled *The Body Cell Mass and Its Supporting Environment*, which set forth the data gained and the lessons learned from those many studies, and gave credit to Georg von Hevesy for early recognition of the potential of the TBW method.[59] Some years later, in 1977, because of questions being raised about nonexchangeable hydrogen, we repeated the validation in the two Culebras articles referred to in this chapter.[9,10] By then Elkan Blout, professor of biochemistry at Harvard, had described the "hard to exchange hydrogen."[3] We also had identified some patients, particularly those with widespread ascites and edema, in whom very long times (4 to 8 h) were required for the achievement of deuterium or tritium equilibration.[58] In such patients the attainment of equilibrium distribution of the isotope must be demonstrated before calculating the volume of dilution and thence the TBW.

Our group included many brilliant people to whom I am deeply indebted, including those from other fields; young people who were later professors of biochemistry, of medicine, of pediatrics, and of veterinary medicine all have worked with us, as have several professors of surgery. Their names are listed in our coauthorship. I would be happy to send anyone who wishes an up-to-date, complete bibliography of our laboratory in this field. I started out as a junior instructor in surgery injecting rabbits, sampling them, dissecting them, taking them to dryness in a vacuum desiccator, and ended up with an extremely active, broadly based interdisciplinary research group. To my coworkers I give full credit for the wonderful work done, but it is a source of price that I started the work personally and remained closely in touch with it throughout.

Many things have happened since then in this field. Darrell Fanestil does a superb job of setting forth some of the variations that have been used. It is interesting that many of these methods have been validated by isotope dilution. In several cases, one searches the literature in vain for any effort at actual chemical or gravimetric validation to set them on a firm footing.

We never felt that these methods would become "bedside necessities." Instead, we regarded them as contributing to the fund of knowledge that practitioners of surgery, medicine, and pediatrics need in dealing with ill patients. I believe that prediction has turned out to be the case.

Francis D. Moore

WATER, THE BODY'S SOLVENT

Water is the sole solvent and the most abundant compound in the human body, constituting 40 to 80 percent of body weight. Indeed, the body is essentially an aqueous solution in which a vast complex of solutes are distributed in compartments that vary in size and that are bounded by lipid membranes. Water has a key role in the transport of nutrients, the removal of waste products, the regulation of cellular volume, and thermal control. Water, then, is the environment in which the reactions of life occur.

STRUCTURE OF WATER

The physical properties of water enable life as we know it to exist. Water, or H_2O, is a V-shaped molecule with an effective radius of less than 0.15 nm (1.5Å)[38] in which each oxygen atom is covalently bonded to the two hydrogen atoms (Fig. 1-1). In ice each oxygen atom also forms hydrogen bonds to two hydrogen atoms in other water molecules. The hydrogen bonds form with other H_2O molecules, rather than intramolecularly, as a result of the spatial separation within the molecule between the positively charged hydrogen atoms and the negatively charged electrons of the oxygen atom. The extensive hydrogen bonding between molecules in ice produces a latticelike three-dimensional, rigid array. Ice is unusual in structure in that the molecules do not assume closest packing in the crystal but form an open structure, accounting for the fact that the density of ice is less than that of water. The "hole" through the middle of the hexagon, and on through the hexagons lying below it in ice, is approximately 0.06 nm in diameter.[53] The nature of liquid water is not completely understood, but one notion holds that small icelike clusters of hydrogen-bonded H_2O molecules are continuously forming and breaking in what has been called a "flickering cluster" structure. A more recent proposal holds that ordered clusters of hydrogen-bonded water do not just randomly flicker on and off and that water does not fill the interior

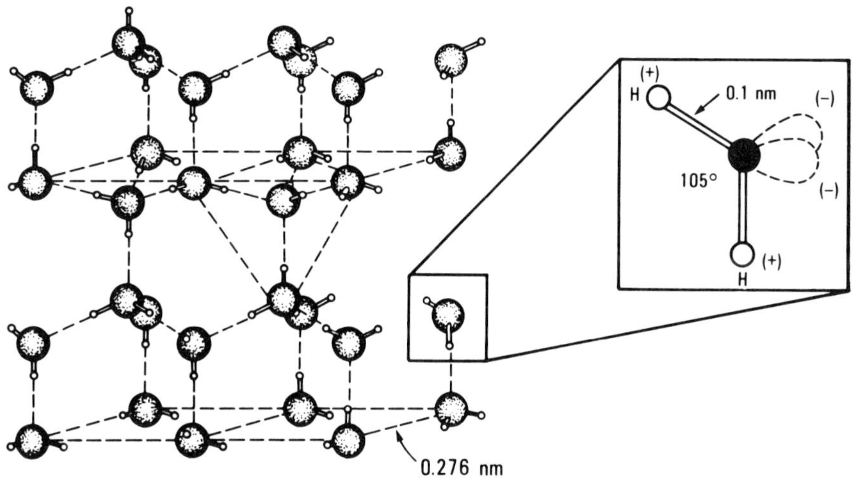

FIGURE 1-1 • The structure of ice and the water molecule. The expanded diagram on the right shows the spatial relationship in the water molecule between the oxygen atom, with its pair of orbital electrons, and the two weakly positive hydrogen atoms. The diagram on the left shows the hydrogen bonding (dashed lines) between adjacent molecules in the crystalline structure of water or ice.

of our cells in a fashion analogous to the manner in which air fills the rooms and corridors of buildings. Rather, clusters that contain up to 1000 molecules of water may travel as waves or cubic clusters.[86] Moreover, it is suggested that the properties of a large fraction of intracellular water are altered by interactions with cellular membranes such that the cubic clusters are associated with or coat all cellular membranes (intracellular organellar membranes as well as plasma membranes). If water is structured for 0.6 nm from each surface (four water molecules deep), 4 to 8 percent of cytoplasmic water is structured. If it is structured for 5 nm from each surface, 33 to 66 percent of cytoplastmic water is structured.[4]

The ability of water to form hydrogen bonds is extremely important to biology, since water molecules may attach to other compounds and to each other with these bonds. Molecules that might ordinarily stick together as precipitates in the absence of water may form hydrogen bonds with water so that the solute molecules are dissolved in water as single molecules. Thus, hydrogen bonding with water is important for the solvation of both ions and uncharged molecules, making them available for the chemical reactions that constitute life. These reactions occur in water in the various compartments of the human body that are described later in this chapter.

GIBBS-DONNAN EQUILIBRIUM

Water distribution into the various body compartments is dependent upon the permeability of the barrier between compartments to water and on the quantity of solute in each compartment. Almost all compartmental barriers in humans are highly permeable to water, the major exceptions being the distal nephron and ducts of sweat glands. Therefore, with these physiologically important but quantitatively minor exceptions, water distribution into various body compartments is determined by the solute content of the compartments. Solute distribution is principally determined by transport mechanisms and forces at compartmental barriers. The concentration of potassium and sodium into predominantly intracellular and extracellular compartments, respectively, requires the active transport of sodium out of and potassium into cells via the Na^+-K^+ ATPase. However, the Gibbs-Donnan equilibrium is an important additional force that influences distribution of solutes, including that of Na^+ and K^+. A primitive understanding of the Gibbs-Donnan effect may be made apparent by considering a hypothetical situation in which two arbitrary compartments of equal volume, A and B, are separated by a barrier that has the permeability characteristics of the wall of capillaries in the body; that is, it is permeable to water and small ions (e.g., Na^+ and Cl^-) but impermeable to larger ionized molecules (e.g., serum albumin; Fig. 1-2). Initially, we construct compartments A and B so that each contains 180 sodium ions and 180 chloride ions. We now add to compartment A ten molecules of serum albumin (each of which carries a net negative charge of −18 at pH 7.4). This must be accompanied by 180 cations (we use sodium ions in this example) to function as the counterions to the negative charge on the protein, since electrical neutrality must always be maintained. The Na^+ concentration in A now exceeds that in B by 360 to 180; this will result in the diffusion of Na^+ from A to B, accompanied by Cl^- to maintain electrical neutrality. However, this movement will increase the concentration of Cl^- in B and lower the concentration of Cl^- in A, thereby generating a concentration difference that opposes the further diffusion of Cl^- from A to B. When an equilibrium between the forces favoring movement of Na^+ (with accompanying Cl^-) from A to B and the forces favoring the movement of Cl^- (with accompanying Na^+) from B to A is reached, the distribution of Na^+ and Cl^- between the two compartments is given by the Gibbs-Donnan relationship:

$$[Na^+]_A \cdot [Cl^-]_A = [Na^+]_B \cdot [Cl^-]_B \qquad (1)$$

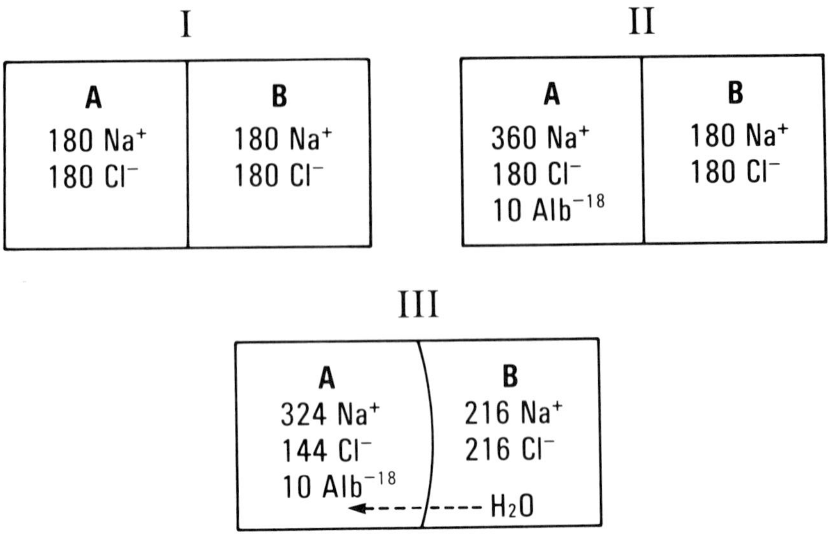

FIGURE 1-2 • Hypothetical Example of Gibbs-Donnan Effect. In I, compartments A and B are separated by a semipermeable membrane and are of equal volume and composition. In II, ten molecules of albumin (each with a net anionic charge of 18) and the accompanying cations (180 Na^+) have been added, creating a concentration gradient down which Na^+ diffuses from A to B. To maintain charge neutrality, Cl^- also diffuses from A to B. In III, an equilibrium has been achieved such that the Na^+ (and Cl^-) diffusion from A to B is equal to the Cl^- (and Na^+) diffusion from B to A. Note that because of the greater solute content in A, H_2O has moved from B to A.

where the subscripts A and B refer to the respective compartments. Since the number of Na^+ ions (X) that migrate from A to B must equal the number of Cl^- ions that migrate from A to B (to maintain electrical neutrality),

$$(360 - X) \cdot (180 - X) = (180 + X) \cdot (180 + X)$$
$$X = 36 \qquad (2)$$

In other words, at equilibrium the numbers of Na^+ and Cl^- molecules in compartment A are 324 and 144 (the difference, or "anion gap," of 180 is due to the anionic charge on the albumin), and the numbers of Na^+ and Cl^- molecules in compartment B are 216 and 216. Note that the concentration of the cation (Na^+) is greater on the side with the protein, while the concentration of the small anion (Cl^-) is greater on the side opposite the protein. There are several important consequences of this equilibrium: (1) the concentrations of the diffusible ions are different in the two compartments; (2) the total concentration of charge is greater in the compartment with protein; and (3) the total *number* of molecules is greater in the compartment with protein. In this hypothetical example the protein-containing compartment (A) has 324 Na^+ ions, 144 Cl^- ions, and 10 protein molecules (the total number of particles is 478), while the compartment opposite the protein has 216 Na^+ ions and 216 Cl^- ions (the total number of particles is 432). The important consequence of such an unequal concentration of particles on two sides of a membrane permeable to water is that the resultant difference is osmolality will exert an osmotic force that moves water across the semipermeable membrane from compartment B to A. That is, the compartment containing protein will increase in volume at the expense of the compartment lacking protein. Note that this osmotic pressure difference, which developed solely because protein was placed on one side of the membrane, is the oncotic pressure, or colloid osmotic pressure, of the protein-containing solution. In biological terms, compartment B resembles interstitial fluid and compartment A resembles blood plasma.

STARLING FORCES

The colloid osmotic pressure generated by the Gibbs-Donnan relationship favors the movement of water from interstitial fluid, which has a relatively low concentration of protein, into the intravascular (plasma) and intracellular spaces, both of which are relatively rich in protein. However, plasma volume and cell volume do not continually swell as a result of Gibbs-Donnan forces because other forces are generated to oppose the colloid osmotic force. In the case of plasma, the colloid osmotic pressure favoring the movement of water across the capillary endothelium into plasma is opposed by the hydrostatic pressure in the capillaries (imparted by the cardiac output). The case of cellular volume is considered in the next section. The movement of water across capillary walls, then, is determined by four parameters known as the Starling forces: (1) hydrostatic pressure in the capillary (P_C); (2) hydrostatic pressure in the interstitial space (P_{IS}); (3) colloid osmotic pressure in capillary plasma (π_C); and (4) colloid osmotic pressure in the interstitial space (π_{IS}).[77] P_C and π_{IS} act to move water from capillary to interstitium; P_{IS} and π_C act to move water into capillary from interstitium. When $(P_C + \pi_{IS}) > (P_{IS} + \pi_C)$, as at the arterial end of a capillary, there is net movement of water out of the capillary. Most of this filtered water is returned at the venous end of the capillary when the rise in π_C (due to removal of water from the capillary) and a fall in P_C along the length of the capillary result in a situation such that $(P_C + \pi_{IS}) < (P_{IS} + \pi_C)$. The remainder of the water filtered into the interstitium at the arterial end of the capillary is returned to the central circulation via lymphatics.

REGULATION OF CELL VOLUME

The colloid osmotic force generated by the high concentration of protein (and other anionic impermeant molecules, e.g., phosphorylated intermediates of metabolism) in cells acts to move water into cells. Cells do not normally swell until they rupture, however, because three sodium ions are actively transported out of cells for each two potassium ions transported into cells by the $Na^+ - K^+$ ATPase. This 3:2 ratio reduces the number of cations (and hence the osmolality) of intracellular fluid below that which would have been predicted from the Gibbs-Donnan relationship; therefore, cells normally attain a static volume. Another important consequence of the action of the $Na^+ - K^+$ ATPase is that the concentration of Na^+ in cells is far below that predicted by the Gibbs-Donnan relationship, while the concentration of K^+ in cells may be slightly greater than predicted. The regulation of cellular volume is considered further in a later section.

METHODS FOR DETERMINATION OF COMPARTMENTATION OF BODY WATER

DESICCATION

Early methods for determination of water in the body and in various tissues were based on desiccation. The water content of a variety of tissues, as surveyed by Skelton in 1927, is shown in Table 1-1.[74] The low water content of adipose tissue (~10 percent of tissue weight) accounts for the variation in the percent of soft tissue mass that is water, while the low water content of bone is attributable to the large crystallized mineral mass. The variation in total body fat found in normal people also accounts for the variation in the percent of total body weight that is attributable to body water, since the percentage of body weight that is water will vary inversely with the body's fat content (Fig. 1-3). This will be considered further in this chapter.

THE DILUTION TECHNIQUE

The study of body water content in living humans required the successful application of the dilution technique. Development, verification, and application of dilution techniques to the study of body water and its distribution in normal and pathological conditions blossomed in the late 1940s and 1950s. A brief account of this important era is provided in the "Historical Introduction" to this chapter, by Francis D. Moore, whose laboratory created an environment in which many of these seminal observations were made.

Briefly, in the dilution technique, a known amount of a marker substance that distributes in a given body fluid compartment is administered, and time is allowed for the marker to distribute throughout the compartment. The volume of the compartment can then be determined from the concentration of the marker in a sample of fluid from that compartment:

$$C_1V_1 = C_2V_2 \quad (3)$$

TABLE 1-1 • Content and distribution of water in various tissues in humans

Tissue	Percentage of water in organs in relation to their weight	Percentage of TBW contained various tissues
Skin	72.0	20.6
Muscle	75.7	43.4
Skeleton	22.0	5.5
Brain	74.8	2.3
Liver	68.3	2.4
Heart	79.2	0.58
Lungs	79.0	0.86
Kidneys	82.7	0.48
Spleen	75.8	0.21
Blood	83.0	6.47
Intestine	74.5	2.14
Rest of body	63.0	14.9

SOURCE: Data from Skelton,[74] who compiled and calculated earlier data.

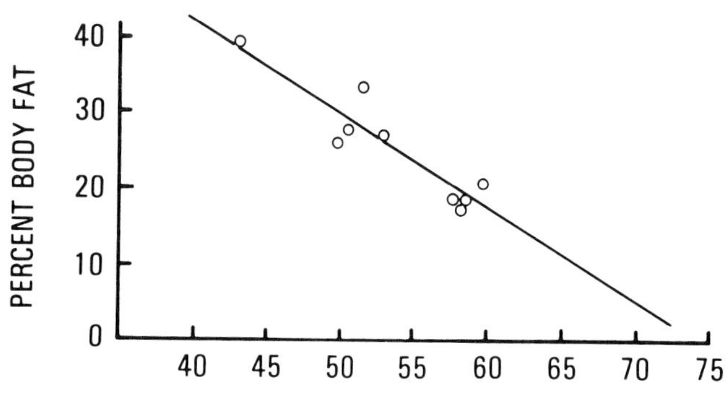

FIGURE 1-3 • Relationship of body water to body fat in human subjects. TBW was determined with antipyrine, and body fat was determined from the measurement of specific gravity. (Modified from Soberman R et al: *J Biol Chem* 179:31, 1947.)

where C represents the concentration of the marker substance and V the volume in which the marker is contained, and where the subscripts 1 and 2 represent the administered solution and the body compartment, respectively. Therefore, in the simplest case,

$$V_2 = \frac{C_1 V_1}{C_2} \tag{4}$$

Since C_1, V_1, and C_2 can all be determined, V_2 is calculated. If some of the marker is lost from the compartment (e.g., by metabolism, leakage into another compartment, or renal or hepatic excretion) during the time required for equilibration, a correction must be applied. Two types of corrections may be employed. If virtually the sole loss of the marker is in the urine, the quantity of marker remaining in the compartment can be calculated by subtraction of the amount excreted in the urine from the amount administered, and

$$V_2 = \frac{C_1 V_1 - C_E V_E}{C_2} \tag{5}$$

where C_E represents the concentration of the marker excreted in urine, and V_E is the volume of urine. A second method for correction for the loss of a marker (by slow leakage into another compartment, excretion, or metabolism) involves determination of the concentration of the marker in the compartment at several times after administration of the marker so that the rate of disappearance of the marker can be determined. The theoretical concentration of the marker at zero time (the time of administration of the marker) can then be estimated by extrapolation back to zero time. In this case,

$$V_2 = \frac{C_1 V_1}{C_0} \tag{6}$$

where C_0 is the concentration at which the marker would have been had instantaneous uniform mixing of the marker in the desired compartment occurred at time zero.

All of these techniques enable calculation of the volume of distribution (V_2) of the marker substance. This volume of distribution will approximate a compartment of body water only if the marker is not bound to protein or lipid and is (approximately) confined to and equally distributed in the compartment being measured.

TYPES OF MARKER SUBSTANCES

Marker substances useful in the determination of the compartmentation of body water (Table 1-2) may be either nonisotopic or isotopic (generally radioactive). The markers have traditionally been administered intravenously or intraperitoneally in animals. Oral administration to humans has proved acceptable in the cases of ethanol, isotopic water, and radiosulfate. On the other hand, several studies on the total body content of inorganic ions have been accomplished by use of total body neutron activation analysis, which does not require administration of a marker. In this method the subject receives a neutron exposure for 5 min (typically), and the whole body radioactivity that is generated is then analyzed in a whole body counter. In essence, the neutron activation generates endogenous "markers."[85] This method enables the simultaneous determination of the quantity of several ions. Neutron activation does not provide an endogenous marker for TBW, but an approximation of TBW can be made from estimates of the volumes of extracellular water and intracellular water, as considered in another section. The rather formidable technology required for neutron activation has limited its application to a few centers in the world.

TABLE 1-2 • Markers useful in the determination of the compartmentation of body water

Compartment	Nonisotopic	Isotopic
TBW	Antipyrine Ethanol	^{2}HHO* ^{3}HHO $H_2{}^{18}O$
ECW†	Nonmetabolized saccharides (inulin, mannitol) Thiocyanate Bromide	Chloride Sodium Bromide Sulfate
Blood (plasma)	Evans blue (T-1824) Indocyanin green	Radioalbumin Radio-erythrocytes

* HHO, or deuterated water, is not radioactive.
† Extracellular water.

NORMAL COMPARTMENTATION OF BODY WATER

TOTAL BODY WATER

Estimation of TBW by dilution of isotopic water (^{2}HHO or ^{3}HHO) is subject to over-estimation of actual TBW by exchange with hydrogen atoms that are in compounds other than H_2O. Examples of such exchangeable hydrogens in organic molecules include hydrogen atoms in amino, carboxyl, hydroxyl, and sulfhydryl positions.[66] The theoretical maximum for such an overestimation in humans has been calculated at 5.2 percent.[9] However, since the isotopes of hydrogen in water are 98-percent equilibrated in 1 h,[66] the short time for exchange with organic hydrogens probably means that TBW is usually overestimated by no more than 2 percent when determined by tritium dilution.[10] However, the rate of exchange of tritium with organic hydrogens may not be constant when metabolic activity varies or in varied environments. Oxygen 18 in water ($H_2{}^{18}O$) does not exchange with labile hydrogen atoms, and therefore its volume of distribution more closely approximates TBW.[71]

Simultaneous application of two methods for the estimation of TBW have found that values with (1) ^{2}HHO are greater than those with antipyrine (55.7 versus 54.5 percent of body weight);[76] (2) ^{3}HHO are greater than those with ethanol (61.3 versus 59.9 percent of body weight);[43] and (3) ^{3}HHO are greater than those with *N*-acetyl-amino-antipyrine (54.9 versus 52.6 percent of body weight).[18] TBW estimated in adults with $H_2{}^{18}O$ averages 3 percent less than with ^{2}HHO.[71] Lesser and Markofsky[40] concluded that ^{3}HHO overestimates TBW by about 2 percent and that antipyrine underestimates TBW by about 2 percent.

Three newer methods for estimation of TBW have been investigated. Two are based on electrical properties and one on the nuclear magnetic resonance (NMR) properties of the hydrogens in water.

Total body electrical conductivity (TOBEC) and bioelectrical impedance plethysmography (BIP), based on electrical properties, require empirical standardization of data to a population upon whom TBW has been determined by an isotopic dilution method. TOBEC involves placing the subject on a motorized platform that then passes through a large solenoidal coil. The coil is powered by a high-frequency source to generate a magnetic field that has the approximate dimensions of the human body: 31 inches in diameter by 78 inches in length. Movement of the body (with its integral solutions of electrolytes) through the magnetic field creates electrical disturbances, which are detected and analyzed to generate the Fourier coefficients. Multiple regression analysis is used to construct equations incorporating the Fourier coefficients (and, in some instances, height and body weight) that yield lean body mass (determined independently by hydrodensitometry) and TBW (determined independently by isotope dilution). Van Loan and Mayclin[82] studied 40 men and women aged nineteen to thirty-five years who ranged from 6 to 36 percent body fat and derived equations that predicted lean body mass (correlation coefficient squared, or $r^2 = 0.983$) and TBW ($r^2 = 0.961$). Use of TOBEC in normal infants has also been proposed.[20] The formidable and expensive technology required for TOBEC will limit its application.

BIP is based upon the principle that an applied electrical current is conducted by electrolyte-containing body fluids and that the volume (liters) of an electrolyte solution is determined by the resistivity (r), the height or length (L), and the impedance (Z):

$$V = rL^2/Z \tag{7}$$

If one assumes that r is constant and that the resistance (R) approximates the impedance,

$$V = rL^2/R \tag{8}$$

In tetrapolar BIP, four spot electrodes are placed in the middle of the dorsal surfaces of the hands and feet between the metacarpal- or metatarsal-phalangeal joints, and four additional electrodes are placed medially between the distal promincences of the ulna or radius and the medial or lateral malleoli. A constant frequency current (e.g., 50 kHz, 800 μA, alternating current) is applied to distal electrodes, and the impedance is estimated by the resistive voltage drop detected at the proximal electrodes.

Kushner and Schoeller[39] compared TBW by BIP and ^{2}HHO in 58 subjects. Height^2/impedance, when combined with body weight, could predict TBW:

$$\text{TBW}_{(^2\text{HHO})} = 0.5561(\text{height}^2/R) + 0.0955(\text{weight}) \tag{9}$$

where height is in centimeters, weight is in kilograms, and $r^2 = 0.986$.

Van Loan and Mayclin[81] and Lukaski and Bolonchuk[45] developed variations on this formula but confirmed the basic understanding of a close correlation between BIP and TBW. The Lukaski and Bolonchuk formula, developed from data on 110 subjects, includes gender and age:

$$\text{TBW}_{(^2\text{HHO})} = 0.377(\text{height}^2/R) + 0.14(\text{weight}) - 0.08(\text{age}) + 2.9(\text{gender}) + 4.65 \tag{10}$$

where age is in years, gender: male = 1 and female = 0, and $r^2 = 0.975$.

The utility of BIP in quantitation of TBW in normal[11] and malnourished children[21] has been validated. The technology required for BIP, unlike that for TOBEC, is not expensive. Both methods yield data that enable close approximation of TBW based on constants that had to be empirically determined.

The third method recently proposed for use in quantitation of TBW is NMR of the hydrogen atoms in water molecules. An NMR-related voltage peak is multiplied by an experimentally determined constant (obtained by NMR analysis of a known water volume). In one study in several baboons, there was close correspondence between gravimetrically determined TBW and TBW determined by NMR.[41] Application to humans has not been reported.

TBW exists in two major compartments: intracellular and extracellular. By definition, extracellular water includes all body water that is external to all cells, including erythrocytes. Thus, extracellular water includes water inside and outside blood vessels as well as water that is in the interstitium between cells and water that has crossed epithelial cells (e.g., in the gastrointestinal fluids).

EXTRACELLULAR WATER

Markers for measurement of extracellular water

Since extracellular fluid is not a homogenous compartment with precisely defined borders, measurement of the volume of extracellular fluid has been approached indirectly by distribution of markers. However, different markers do not distribute identically in the various subcompartments of extracellular water. In addition, some markers (e.g., Na^+, Cl^-, and Br^-) penetrate various cells to an extent that cannot be determined precisely or are bound to some degree.[31] Therefore, the apparent volume of extracellular fluid determined by the several markers varies over a considerable range. Table 1-3 lists mean values for extracellular fluid volume in men and women, expressed as a percent of body weight. In general, saccharides give smaller values (~16 percent), monovalent ions larger values (~27 percent), and divalent ions intermediate values (~18 percent).

This variation in the estimates of extracellular water raises two important issues. First, comparisons of extracellular water volumes from one study to another are critically dependent upon the methods and markers utilized. (Nevertheless, it is believed to be possible to employ any one technique to measure *changes* in extracellular volume.) Second, the calculated percentage of TBW that is extracellular will depend critically upon the extracellular marker employed.

Some workers apply a correction for the overestimation of extracellular water by markers known to penetrate cells. For example, Yasumura and coworkers[89] reduced by 10 percent their value for total body chloride (determined by neutron activation) before calculating extracellular water (ECW) by use of the relationship shown in equation 11:

$$\text{ECW (liters)} = 0.9\ [\text{total body Cl}^-(\text{meq})] \div \text{plasma Cl}^-(\text{meq/liter}) \quad (11)$$

After this correction was applied, extracellular water was about 45 percent of TBW (measured by ^{3}HHO dilution) in men and 50 percent in women (Table 1-4).

TABLE 1-3 • Mean values for extracellular fluid as percentage of body weight

Marker	Men	Women
Inulin	15.6	
Mannitol	16.6	
Thiosulfate	16.3	16.0
[^{35}S]sulfate	18.0	
Bromide	28.4	25.1
[^{36}Cl]	26.8	
[^{24}Na]	26.2	

SOURCE: Data compiled by Hays.[30]

TABLE 1-4 • Extracellular water as a percentage of TBW in normal humans

n	Males (ECW/TBW, %)	Age (years)	*n*	Females (ECW/TBW, %)
10	44.5 ± 4.2	20–29	10	48.6 ± 6.3
10	43.6 ± 3.7	30–39	10	51.3 ± 5.4
9	41.7 ± 2.4	40–49	10	50.4 ± 3.7
9	43.6 ± 2.7	50–59	7	49.4 ± 5.2
8	48.1 ± 4.8	60–69	12	52.5 ± 5.5
12	50.2 ± 3.3	70+	8	52.6 ± 6.4

NOTE: Values are means ± SD.
SOURCE: Data from Yasumura et al.[89]

The estimation of extracellular water by total body chloride (neutron activation) was compared by Yasumura and associates[89] with estimation of extracellular water by isotope dilution using ^{77}Br. The near identity of these independently determined values confirms the validity of use of a radiohalide generated by neutron activation in the estimation of total body chloride. Attempts are being made to estimate extracellular water by BIP (see above). An empirical formula was developed that correlated extracellular water determined by BIP and extracellular water determined by the volume of distribution of bromide ($r^2 = 0.884$).[45] However, because of the strong influence of TBW on extracellular water, the rigor with which this association holds in pathophysiological states needs to be determined.

Compartments of extracellular water

Extracellular water, as indicated previously, consists of several types of compartments: plasma water, interstitial fluid and lymph, transcellular water, and inaccessible bone water.

Plasma water

Normal plasma is about 93 to 94 percent water.[23] The remaining 6 to 7 percent of plasma volume is contributed predominantly by proteins and lipids. Thus, measurement of plasma volume provides a close measure of plasma water in normal subjects. Methods for measurement of plasma volume take advantage of the (predominantly) intravascular location of plasma albumin and erythrocytes.

Measurement of plasma volume via dilution of an albumin label must be accomplished by extrapolation to "zero time," since albumin is not confined to the intravascular space.[69] In addition, pathological states, including burns, trauma, and hepatic disease, may make plasma volume measurements with labeled albumin even more subject to error.

Plasma volume (PV) has also been estimated from a determination of total blood volume (TBV) using the dilution of labeled erythrocytes and the packed red blood cell volume, or hematocrit, as shown in equation 12:

$$PV = TBV(1.00 - \text{hematocrit}) \quad (12)$$

A potential source of error in this estimation is the validity of the hematocrit. In practice, the hematocrit is determined on blood obtained from peripheral, large veins, which do not necessarily yield the mean hematocrit for the whole body, since the hematocrit in small capillaries may be considerably smaller than in large vessels. The "whole body hematocrit" may be 85 to 92 percent of large venous hematocrit. Thus, true plasma volume may be slightly underestimated when calculated from blood volume measurements and peripheral vein hematocrit.

Hays[30] compiled plasma volume measurements obtained by a number of investigators using Evans blue and found that plasma volume averaged 4.5 percent of body weight (range 4.1 to 4.8) in both men and women.

Other compartments of extracellular water

No direct method exists for the measurement of the total volume of water in any of the other compartments of extracellular water. Obviously, their aggregate volume is equal to the difference between extracellular water and plasma water. However, the difficulty in accurately defining the volume of extracellular water makes such a calculation open to assumptions and errors. Edelman and Liebman[17] proposed that the saccharides (e.g., inulin and mannitol) are in rapid equilibrium with plasma volume and interstitial fluid and lymph, are in slow equilibrium with water in connective tissue, but not accessible to water in bone. Based on this analysis, Edelman and Liebman[17] designated: (1) interstitial and lymph water equal to 20 percent of TBW (or about 12 percent of body weight); (2) the slowly exchanging volume of extracellular water in connective tissue equal to 4.5 percent body weight (about 7 percent of TBW); and (3) the water in bone that is inaccessible to saccharides equal to 4.5 percent of body weight. This formulation means that three compartments of extracellular water—plasma water, connective tissue water, and bone water—are equal in volume, each being about 7 percent of TBW or 4.5 percent of body weight.

Transcellular water constitutes the final compartment of extracellular water. This was defined by Edelman and Liebman[17] as the several fluids in the body that have the common property of being formed by the transport activity of cells. These fluids include secretions in the salivary glands, pancreas, liver, and bilary tract as well as fluid in the gastrointestinal and respiratory tracts, thyroid follicles, sweat gland ducts, cavities of the eyes, cerebrospinal fluid, and kidneys. Markers used to measure extracellular fluid volume penetrate these fluids at widely different rates and concentrations. Therefore, this is a further factor that renders measurement of the volume of extracellular water inexact. Transcellular water, as used by some authors, also includes fluid in the pleural, pericardial, peritoneal, synovial, and joint "spaces." Although normally small, the volume of extracellular water in these spaces can become a significant fraction of TBW in disease states.

INTRACELLULAR WATER

No direct dilution method exists for the measurement of intracellular water. Therefore, intracellular water (ICW) volume has traditionally been calculated as the difference between TBW and extracellular water (ECW), as shown in equation 13:

$$ICW = TBW - ECW \quad (13)$$

This formulation obviously means that the marker used to define extracellular water will dramatically alter the calculated volume of intracellular water. The problem of accurately measuring extracellular water has been discussed previously.

An alternative method for the indirect estimation of intracellular water is based on the expectation that ~97 percent of total body potassium (TBK) is in intracellular water. If the mean concentration of potassium in intracellular water, $[K]_{cell}$, were known, the volume of intracellular water could be estimated from the relationship shown in equation 14:

$$ICW = \frac{0.97 \cdot TBK}{[K]_{cell}} \quad (14)$$

Unfortunately, there is no method that will measure concentration of K^+ in all cells. Data are available, however, to provide an indirect test of equation 14. Yasumura and coworkers[89] calculated ICW as the difference between TBW (measured by dilution of ^{3}HHO) and ECW (calculated from total body chloride measured by neutron activation analysis, as shown in equation 11). A comparison of this ICW with TBK, as measured by neutron activation analysis, is shown in Fig. 1-4. This relationship is described by equation 15:

$$ICW = 0.007\ TBK - 0.62 \quad (15)$$

Equation 15, when combined with equation 14, enables calculation of the mean potassium concentration in cell water, $[K]_{cell}$ for their data:

$$[K]_{cell} = \frac{0.97\ TBK}{0.007\ TBK - 0.62} \quad (16)$$

As shown in Table 1-5, $[K]_{cell}$ calculated by equation 16 is 141 to 144 meq/liter. $[K]_{cell}$ from equation 16 may then be used to estimate ICW using equation 14. Intracellular water calculated in this manner is also shown in Table 1-5. Thus, it may now be possible to approximate ICW from estimates of TBK by use of the approximations expressed in equations 14 and 16.

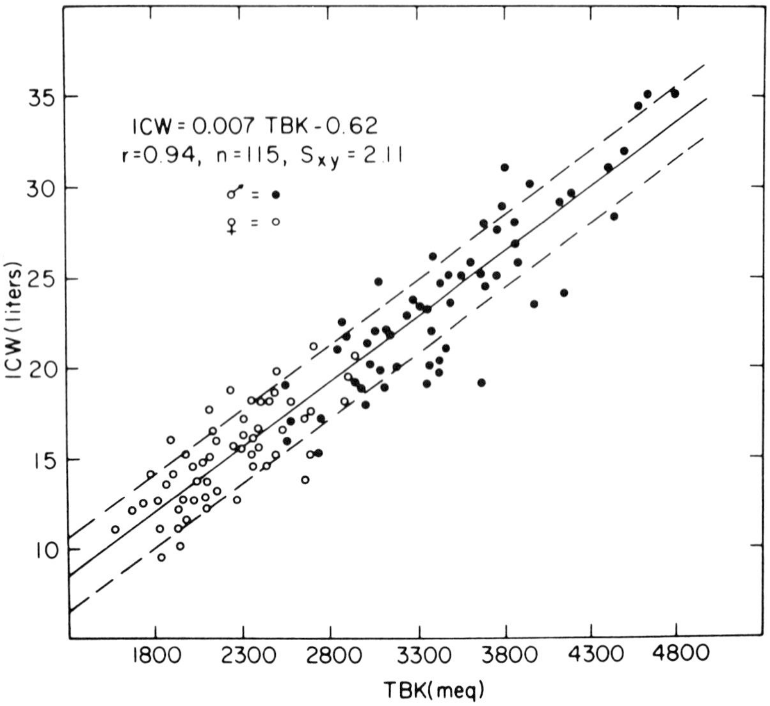

FIGURE 1-4 • Correlation between total body potassium (TBK) and intracellular water (ICW) in 115 normal male and female subjects. ICW was calculated as the difference between TBW measured by ^{3}HHO dilution and extracellular water. Extracellular water was calculated as total body choloride ÷ plasma [Cl$^-$], where total body chloride was estimated by neutron activation and equation 11.

REGULATION OF CELLULAR VOLUME

The proportion of TBW that is intracellular must be related to the factors that regulate the volume of individual cells. These factors are briefly considered in this section.

THE "DOUBLE DONNAN" EFFECT

Impermeant anionic molecules inside cells, which are predominantly proteins and organic phosphates, exert an osmotic force via the Gibbs-Donnan effect, such that water tends to move into cells. Obviously, cells do not continuously swell. Therefore, the Gibbs-Donnan osmotic force must be offset either by a high intracellular hydrostatic pressure or by some mechanism whereby the concentration of solutes in the extracellular fluid is maintained above that expected from the Gibbs-Donnan equilibrium. Plant cells with relatively rigid cell walls may be able to raise intracellular hydrostatic pressure sufficiently to prevent cellular swelling. However, mammalian cellular membranes are generally not rigid. Indeed, pliability of the cell membrane is required for many cellular functions, including phagocytosis by leukocytes, capillary passage by erythrocytes, motility of cilia, and endocytosis by most (if not all) cells. Thus, mammalian cells are believed to offset the Gibbs-Donnan force favoring cellular swelling mainly by actively extruding sodium from the cell interior to the interstitial space (Fig. 1-5). This results in fewer solute particles in the cell than predicted from the Gibbs-Donnan equilibrium, thereby lowering the osmotic force inside the cell. Sufficient sodium, with its attendant anion (chloride), is maintained in the interstitial fluid in excess of the expected Gibbs-Donnan distribution to provide the balancing osmotic activity. In effect, sodium functions as an impermeant molecule in the extracellular fluid. This situation, in which there are apparent impermeant molecules both inside cells (proteins and organic phosphates) and outside cells (sodium and chloride), has been referred to as a "Double Donnan" system. In actuality, sodium is not a truly impermeant cation, but sodium entry into the cell via passive forces and sodium extrusion from the cell by active transport result in an osmotic effect equivalent to that of apparent impermeability. This active transport of sodium

TABLE 1-5 • Calculation of mean intracellular potassium concentration

Total body potassium (meq)	$[K]_{cell}$ (meq/liter)	ICW (liters)
4800	141.2	33.0
4200	141.5	28.8
3600	142.0	24.6
3000	142.8	20.4
2400	143.9	16.2

SOURCE: Calculated from data of Yasumura et al.[89] using equation 14.

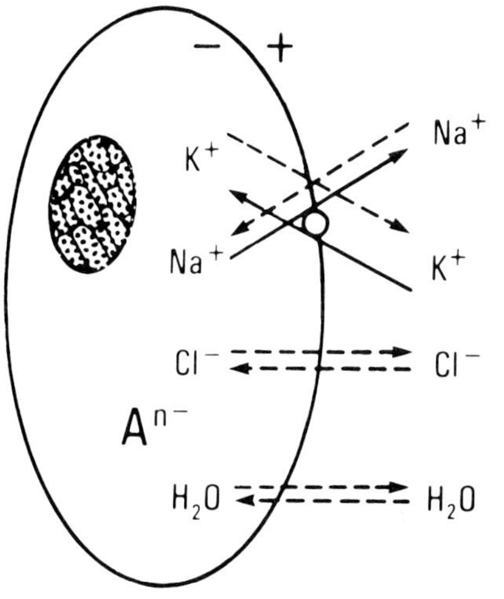

FIGURE 1-5 • The "Double-Donnan" model for regulation of cellular volume. Solid arrows indicate active transport (via the Na^+-K^+ ATPase), dashed arrows indicate passive movements. The net negative (anionic) charge on proteins and other impermeant molecules (An^-) is maintained by cellular metabolic integrity. Water and chloride are at equilibrium distributions. The active transport of Na^+ makes the cellular plasma membrane effectively impermeable to Na^+, despite the passive permeability of the membrane to this ion. This "exclusion" of Na^+ from the cell interior serves to counteract the oncotic effect of the cellular An^-, which tend to produce swelling of the cell because of the Gibbs-Donnan forces. In a metabolically intact cell, total cellular solute and hence, cellular volume are constant. (Adapted from MacKnight ADC: *Mol Physiol* 4:17, 1983.)

out of the cell is believed to occur predominantly by the ouabain-inhibitable, sodium-potassium-activated adenosine triphosphatase.

OTHER POSTULATED MECHANISMS

Other mechanisms for the maintenance of cellular volume have not been conclusively eliminated. First, another active sodium transport mechanism, dependent upon a supply of energy but not on the ouabain-sensitive ATPase, has been proposed.[67,87] Conclusive evidence for such a sodium pump has yet to be provided. Second, it has been proposed that intracellular water is more structured (i.e., more icelike, see above), thereby reducing the "activity" of water.[42] This effective change in the structure of water would result in a low affinity for sodium ion in intracellular water, thereby excluding sodium from the interior of the cell. Third, the intracellular Gibbs-Donnan forces may be offset in some circumstances by increased hydrostatic pressure inside cells. Elements that might contribute to the maintenance of a specific cellular volume under increased hydrostatic pressure in the cell could include both intracellular (cytoskeletal) and extracellular (collagen network and basement membrane) structures. The bulk of current evidence, nevertheless, favors the "Double-Donnan" situation, in which sodium is predominantly an apparent extracellular impermeant molecule due to the extrusion of sodium from the cell by the ouabain-inhibitable, $Na^+ - K^+$ ATPase.

REGULATION OF CELLULAR VOLUME IN ANISOOMOLAR CONDITIONS

Dilution of extracellular solute produces an osmotic force favoring entry of water into cells. Simultaneously, a concentration gradient is developed favoring exit of solute from cells. The opposite situations exist if extracellular solute concentration is increased. It is beyond the scope of this chapter to review knowledge about events that occur under these abnormal conditions.[19,37,68,85] In general, cells tend to swell when initially placed in a hypoosmolar solution. This apparently results from movement of water along the osmotic gradient. This initial swelling may be followed by a decrease in cell volume despite the continued hypoosmolality of the extracellular solution. This secondary adjustment in cell volume—sometimes termed regulatory volume decrease—presumably occurs because of solute loss from the cell. Thus, both possible effects of dilution of the extracellular solution—gain of water and loss of solute by cells—may occur. The transport mechanisms whereby such loss of solutes occur are complex and under current investigation.[48,62,84]

NONPATHOLOGICAL CONDITIONS AFFECTING BODY WATER AND ITS COMPARTMENTS

AGE

TBW varies from 45 to 65 percent of body weight in adults. The primary factor responsible for this large variation is the inverse reciprocal relationship between body water and body fat content (Fig. 1-2). Age is another possible factor responsible for some of this variation. Changes in total body mass attributable to bone may be responsible, in part, for the effect of age. Changes in total body fat and total body skeletal muscle mass may also contribute to an unknown extent. Table 1-6 provides

TABLE 1-6 • Mean values for TBW in normal humans in percentage of body weight

Age (years)	Men	Women
10–16	58.9	57.3
17–39	60.6	50.2
40–59	54.7	46.7
60+	51.5	45.5

SOURCE: Data compiled by Hays.[30]

TABLE 1-7 • Mean values of extracellular (ECW) and intracellular water (ICW) in normal humans in percentage of body weight

Age (years)	TBW* (% body weight)	ECW†/TBW (%)	ECW (% body weight)	ICW (% body weight)
MALES				
20–39	60.6	44.0	26.7	33.9
40–59	54.7	42.6	23.3	31.4
60+	51.5	49.1	25.3	26.2
FEMALES				
20–39	50.2	50.0	25.1	25.1
40–59	46.7	49.9	23.3	23.4
60+	45.5	52.5	23.9	21.6

* Data from Table 1-6.
† Data from Table 1-4.

TBW values by age and sex. The distribution of TBW between intra- and extracellular compartments at various ages is shown in Table 1-4. The ratio ECW/TBW was significantly lower in males over the age of 60 when compared with males between ages 20 and 59. However, there were no age-related changes in the ECW/TBW of female subjects over the age range tested. Table 1-7 combines the data in Tables 1-4 and 1-6, enabling calculation of ECW and ICW as a percentage of body weight for different ages and sexes. Since the TBW measurements and the ratio of ECW to TBW were not measured in the same subjects, the apparent 4- to 13-percent decline in ICW with age must be taken as only a tentative approximation. Indeed, Lesser and Markofsky[40] measured total body fat (by inert gas uptake) and concluded that, while ICW as a percentage of total body weight declined with age, ICW as a percentage of fat-free body mass did not decline with age. In summary, most evidence indicates that TBW decreases with age. However, it is not clear whether this change is due to a decrease in ICW, ECW, or both.

The percentage of body weight attributable to water also changes in infancy and childhood. Figure 1-6[22] shows a decline in TBW from nearly 75 percent of body weight in the newborn to approximately 60 percent of body weight by one year, with most of the decrease occurring in ECW.

The changes occurring in the first few days of life were studied in greater detail by MacLaurin,[47] who found that TBW was 71 percent of body weight in the first two weeks (Table 1-8). When infants of different birth weight and less than 72 h old were analyzed, TBW and ICW (as percentage of body weight) were inversely correlated with body weight, whereas ECW and plasma volume (as percentage of body weight) were a constant percent of body weight over the range of body weight

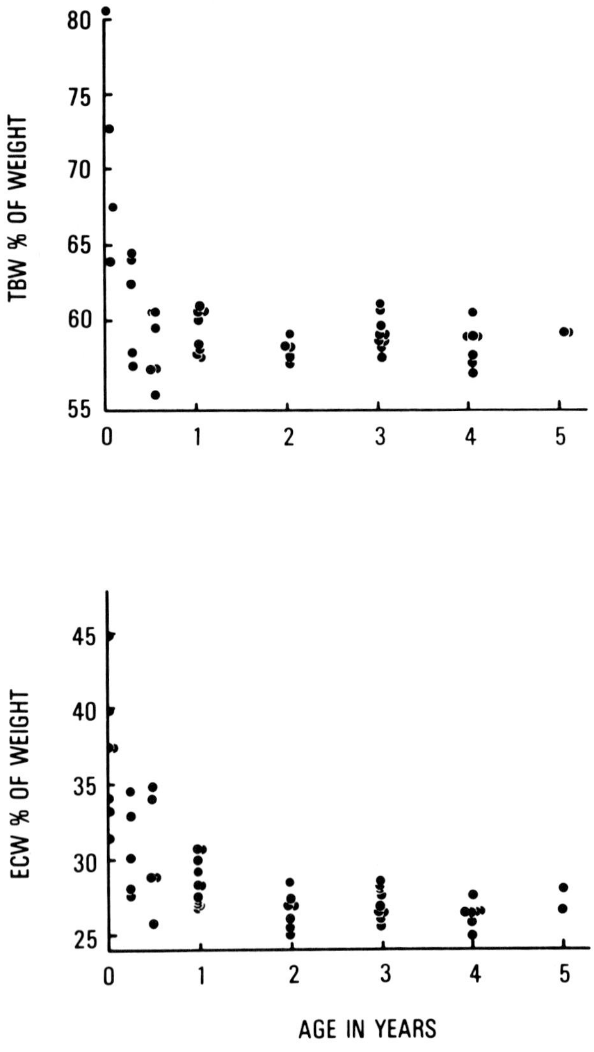

FIGURE 1-6 • TBW and ECW as percent of body weight and age in normal children. (From Flynn MA et al: *Am J Clin Nutr* 20:1125, 1967.)

TABLE 1-8 • Body water composition in the neonatal period

Age (days)	n	Weight (kg)	TBW* (ml/kg)	ECW* (ml/kg)	ICW (ml/kg)	PV† (ml/kg)
⅙–3	26	2.46	715	360	356	45.1
4–5	13	2.00	719	358	366	48.5
6–13	7	2.33	692	359	339	52.2
Total	46	2.31	713	359	356	47.2

* TBW and ECW were measured with antipyrine and thiocyanate, respectively.
† Plasma volume was measured with Evans blue.
SOURCE: Data from MacLaurin.[47]

measured (1.5 to 3.6 kg). Adolescent growth is associated with changes in the relationship between TBW (^{2}HHO dilution) and weight. Ninety-nine boys (59 aged twelve years and 40 aged fifteen years) were studied yearly for three consecutive years. Body size in the boys was 159.1 cm in height and 49.44 kg in weight at ages twelve to thirteen years versus 177.7 cm and 66.1 kg at ages sixteen to seventeen, while TBW changed from 62.1 percent of body weight at twelve to thirteen years to a high of 65.9 percent at ages fifteen to sixteen. One hundred four similarly aged girls (59 aged twelve years and 45 aged fifteen years) were also studied yearly for three consecutive years. Their size was 158.5 cm in height and 49.0 kg in weight at twelve to thirteen years versus 165.7 cm and 58.3 kg at ages sixteen to seventeen, while TBW decreased from 60.3 percent of body weight at twelve to thirteen years to 53.6 percent at sixteen to seventeen.[63] Thus, the previously known differences in TBW (as a percent of body weight) between adult males and females was demonstrated to occur during the adolescent growth spurt.

OBESITY

The inverse relationship between body fat and the percentage of body weight that is composed of TBW has been mentioned previously (Fig. 1-2). In addition, an influence of extreme obesity on the distribution of TBW between ECW and ICW has been reported. Pierson and coworkers[65] studied five subjects weighing 118 to 174 kg before and after seven weeks of dietary restriction at an average energy intake of 802 kcal/day (range 0 to 1200). TBW (^{3}HHO distribution) was from 46 to 57 percent (mean 50.2 percent) of body weight prior to and 47.5 to 58 percent (mean 52.2 percent) after weight reduction. The mean weight loss was 17.4 kg, 6.3 kg of which were from TBW. Ninety percent of the decrease in TBW was attributable to a decrease in ECW (measured by [$^{35}SO_4$] distribution). A striking finding was that the ratio of ECW/TBW (SO_4/^{3}HHO) was 0.456, a marked increase above the value of 0.33 determined in their nonobese normal controls. Unfortunately, plasma volume was not measured in this study.

MALNUTRITION AND CHRONIC ILLNESS

Malnutrition secondary to starvation or chronic illness results in apparent expansion of ECW. In 11 adults with a variety of chronic diseases causing nutritional depletion, the TBW was 61.1 percent of body weight, a finding consistent with less body fat (i.e., a larger percentage of body weight was lean body mass) than in the normal population.[18] Moreover, ECW (bromide space) was 59.3 percent of TBW, significantly greater than their expected normal of 48.1 percent. Expanded ECW had also been reported in malnourished World War II prisoners of war.[49]

Both TBW and ECW are also above normal in malnourished children. Figure 1-7 shows that ECW, as percentage of body weight, in ten malnourished children returned to or toward normal as the nutritional status was repleted.[23] Edema was not present in these particular children. There may be even more profound increases in ECW when edema is present, since Smith found a mean TBW of 84.5 percent of body weight in severely malnourished children with edema.[75]

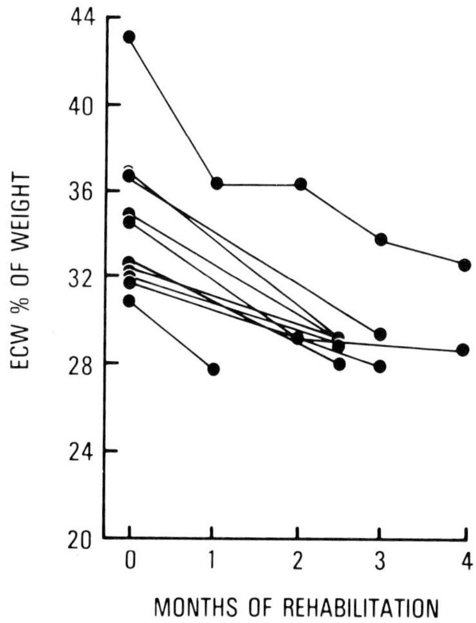

FIGURE 1-7 • Decrease in ECW during nutritional repletion of previously undernourished children. (From Flynn MA et al: *Am J Clin Nutr* 20:129, 1967.)

EXERCISE

Exercise training, with resultant adaptation to exertion, as well as acute exertion might be expected to produce alterations in body water. However, quantitation of these changes has proved difficult.

Exercise training appears to produce an increase in plasma renin and plasma aldosterone, which is presumed to result in some retention of sodium and expansion of ECW.[54] This is accompanied by expansion of plasma volume. Oscai and coworkers[64] measured blood volume by [^{131}I]albumin dilution in fourteen sedentary males (aged twenty-six to sixty-four years) before and after a sixteen-week program of running three times per week. All but two of the subjects were able to run at least 30 min and 3 miles (4.8 km) per session after 10 of the 47 training sessions. Blood volume increased 358 ± 130 ml ($p < .05$); this represented an increase of 6.2 percent. The changes in muscle mass (and hence ICW), body fat (and hence percentage of weight that is lean body mass), and ECW that occur with exercise conditioning combine to complicate accurate definition of the effects of exercise training on distribution of body water.

Definition of the effects of acute exercise on body water is also imprecise. Environmental temperature and humidity and extent of prior exercise training are among the variables that may complicate measurements and their interpretation. Moreover, acute exercise may invalidate use of ^{3}HHO as an accurate measure of TBW. Colt and coworkers[5] measured TBW with ^{3}HHO and ECW with [$^{35}SO_4$] before and after ten male runners ran 10 miles (16.1 km). Despite a 2.3-percent (1.6-kg) decrease in body weight, TBW measured by ^{3}H-dilution increased 2.4 percent (1.2 liter). This indicates that acute exercise is associated with an increase in the exchange of tritium from ^{3}HHO with either a pool of bound water or with hydrogen present in fat, protein, or carbohydrate. Thus, after acute exercise, ^{3}HHO may overestimate TBW more than the usually expected 2 percent (see above).

Acute exercise is associated with a decrease in plasma volume during exercise, and the decrease is proportional to the intensity of the exercise. Figure 1-8 shows the percent change in plasma volume with increasing workloads in four 19- to 29-year-old males before and after an 8-day training period.[6] The plasma volume was 12.3 percent greater in these subjects after the 8-day training period. Since the fractional decrease in plasma volume with acute exercise was the same before and after the 8-day training period, the absolute (milliliter) decrease in plasma volume may also have been about 12 percent greater after training. The decrease in plasma volume may be related to net flux of water out of the vascular bed into the extracellular space of exercising muscles.[73]

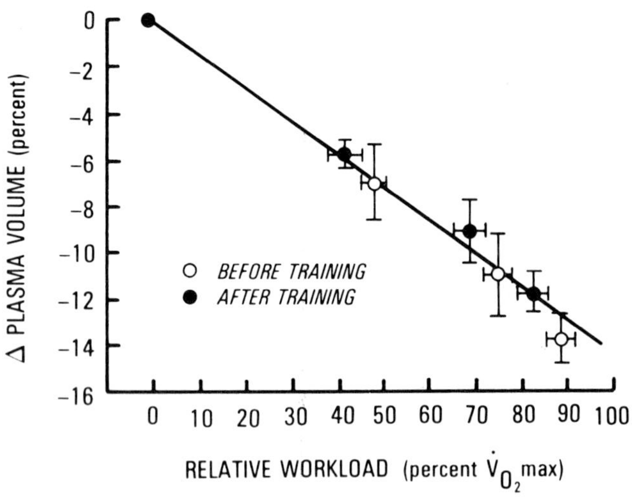

FIGURE 1-8 • Percent change in plasma volume in response to relative workload (as percent of maximal oxygen consumption, $\dot{V}_{O_2max}$) before and after exercise training. The percent change in plasma volume was calculated from antecubital vein blood hemoglobin concentrations and hematocrits. The absolute value for plasma volume was determined with Evans blue. (From Convertino VA et al: *J Appl Physiol* 54:508, 1983.)

Endurance performers in running marathons[61] and cross-country skiing[2] average a 3- to 5-percent loss of body weight during the course of the event. However, as much as an 8-percent loss of body weight has been recorded in Olympic marathon runners.[8]

HIGH ALTITUDE

Acute exposure to hypoxia at either sea level or reduced atmospheric pressure results in an increase in hematocrit that begins within minutes.[25] This acute response results from reduction in plasma volume. This reduction amounts to a 20- to 30-percent decrease in plasma volume after several days and persists for at least two months.[28,29,34] Whether this represents dehydration, redistribution of body water, or both is not convincingly established.

Hannon and associates[29] studied nine young men at an altitude of 650 ft and again while living at 14,100 ft. Except for altitude and humidity, experimental conditions and diet were "quite similar." Measurements were made of TBW (by three methods: ^{2}HHO, 4-amino-antipyrine, and body weight/body density); ECW (thiocyanate); and plasma volume (PV; Evans blue). The three methods for estimation of TBW showed that ^{2}HHO was probably not reliable under these circumstances, since after 3 days at high altitude ^{2}HHO space increased about 5 liters despite a small decrease in body weight. The other two methods for determining TBW were unchanged, ex-

TABLE 1-9 • Water and electrolyte loss in sweat

Level of dehydration* (% body weight)	Volume (liters)	Sodium		Potassium		Chloride	
		(meq)†	*(mM)*‡	*(meq)*†	*(mM)*‡	*(meq)*†	*(mM)*‡
−2.2	1.38	60.5	43.8	5.4	3.9	53.3	38.6
−4.1	1.61	57.2	35.5	6.1	3.8	51.1	31.7
−5.8	1.12	37.1	33.1	4.4	3.9	32.2	28.8
Total	4.11	155	37.7	15.9	3.9	137	33.3

* Values decrease in body weight from mean weight of 72.56 kg ($n = 8$).
† Values are quantities.
‡ Values are concentrations.
SOURCE: Calculated from data of Costill et al.[8]

cept for a small but statistically significant increase after 14 days. Hannon and associates[29] measured in these same subjects a decrease in both PV and ECW and therefore calculated a decrease in "interstitial space" (calculated as ECW − PV) and ICW. The results of these careful studies by Hannon coworkers have not been confirmed by some workers. For example, Jain and colleagues[34] measured decreases in TBW (^{3}HHO), ECW (sulfate space), and ICW.

DEHYDRATION

Analysis of loss of TBW with acute dehydration is easily assessed by change in body weight. However, assessment of distribution of water into the various compartments by markers depends upon the assumption that dehydration does not alter the distribution of the marker. VanBeaumont and coworkers[80] assumed that circulating red blood cell mass remained constant and that peripheral vein hematocrit reflected changes in total body hematocrit to calculate changes in plasma volume during 3 h of dehydration in seven men. Some subjects showed an initial (30 to 90 min) increase in plasma volume (up to 4 percent), but there was a mean decrease of 5.9 percent in the plasma volume by the end of 3 h. This may be compared with a 1.9-percent (1.6-kg) mean decrease in body weight after 3 h. This finding of a larger fractional change in plasma volume than in TBW is consistent with earlier observations by others.[36,72]

The combination of exercise and dehydration was employed by Costill and associates[8] to produce graded degrees of reduction in body weight. They also measured chloride content in muscle biopsies and calculated intracellular water volume in the biopsy, assuming the ratio of extracellular to intracellular chloride was 26:1 at both rest and after exercise and dehydration. Their findings show that about half of the water loss was from the intracellular compartment but that the greatest fractional decrease in volume occurred in the extracellular compartments.

Costill and colleagues[8] also collected and analyzed sweat during these experiments by a "total body washdown" method.[83] The results are compiled in Table 1-9.

PREGNANCY

TBW increases during pregnancy as a result of water in the amniotic fluid, fetus, placenta, enlarged organs of reproduction, and an expanded blood volume. The distribution of this water at 20, 30, and 40 weeks of pregnancy is shown in Table 1-10. The blood volume increase of about 1 liter is 85-percent due to an increase in plasma volume. Clinically detectable edema is frequently observed. Hytten and colleagues,[32] noting that the behavior of antipyrine may be altered during pregnancy, estimated TBW by ^{2}HHO distribution in 93 normal human pregnancies. The subjects were divided on clinical grounds into three groups: no edema ($n = 47$), leg edema only

TABLE 1-10 • Increase in water content of various tissues and compartments in pregnancy

Site	Water content (g)		
	20 weeks	*30 weeks*	*40 weeks*
Fetus	264	1185	2343
Placenta	153	366	540
Amniotic fluid	247	594	792
Added uterine muscle	483	668	473
Added breast tissue	135	270	304
Added plasma	506	1058	920
Added red cells	32	98	163
Total	1820	4239	5805

SOURCE: Data of Hytten and Leitch, as tabulated by Hytten.[33]

TABLE 1-11 • **Increase in total body water during pregnancy**

	Increase in TBW (liters) up to:		
Edema group (*n*)	*20 weeks*	*30 weeks*	*40 weeks*
None (47)	1.74	4.30	7.50
Leg edema (20)	1.81	4.29	7.80
"Generalized" edema (26)	2.23	5.79	10.83
Total (93)	1.88	4.68	8.50

SOURCE: Data from Hytten, Thompson, and Taggart.[32]

(n = 20), and "generalized" edema (n = 26). Body water, as shown in Table 1-11, increased with duration of pregnancy and increased more in those with "generalized edema" than in the other two groups, which were comparable. Hytten concluded that, "at least in normotensive cases, oedema is not associated with any increased liability to perinatal death" and that "all evidence suggests that oedema in pregnancy may be physiological and not in itself an ominous physical sign."[33]

REFERENCES

1. Albrink MJ et al: The displacement of serum water by the lipids of hyperlipemic serum: A new method for the rapid determination of serum water. *J Clin Invest* 34:1483, 1955.
2. Astrand PO, Saltin B: Plasma and red cell volume after prolonged severe exercise. *J Appl Physiol* 9:829, 1964.
3. Blout ER et al: The deuterium exchange of water soluble polypeptide and protein as measured by infrared spectroscopy. *J Am Chem Soc* 83:1895, 1961.
4. Clegg JS: Intracellular water and the cytomatrix: Some methods of study and current views. *J Cell Biol* 99:167S, 1984.
5. Colt EDW et al: Effect on body water of running 10 miles. *J Appl Physiol* 45:999, 1978.
6. Convertino VA et al: Plasma volume, renin and vasopressin responses to graded exercise after training. *J Appl Physiol* 54:508, 1983.
7. Corsa L Jr et al: The measurement of exchangeable potassium in man by isotope dilution. *J Clin Invest* 29:1289, 1950.
8. Costill DL et al: Muscle water and electrolytes following varied levels of dehydration in man. *J Appl Physiol* 40:6, 1976.
9. Culebras JM, Moore FD: Total body water and exchangeable hydrogen: 1. Theoretical calculation of non-aqueous exchangeable hydrogen in man. *Am J Physiol* 232:R54, 1977.
10. Culebras JM et al: Total body water and the exchangeable hydrogen: 2. A review of comparative data from animals based on isotope dilution and dessication, with a report of new data from the rat. *Am J Physiol* 232:R60, 1977.
11. Davies PSW et al: The prediction of total body water using bioelectrical impedance in children and adolescents. *Ann Hum Biol* 15:237, 1988.
12. Edelman IS, Moore FD: Body water, water distribution and water kinetics as revealed by the use of deuterium oxide. *J Clin Invest* 30:627, 1951.
13. Edelman IS et al: Body composition: Studies in the human being by the dilution principle—a progress report. *Science* 115:447, 1952.
14. Edelman IS et al: The location and turnover of the sodium of the bone, in Reifenstein EC (ed): *Metabolic Interrelations: Transactions Fourth Conference.* New York, Josiah Macy, Jr., Foundation, 1952, p 240.
15. Edelman IS et al: Further observations on total body water: 1. Normal values throughout the life span. *Surg Gynecol Obstet* 95:1, 1952.
16. Edelman IS et al: Body sodium and potassium: 4. The normal total exchangeable sodium: Its measurement and magnitude. *Metabolism* 3:530, 1954.
17. Edelman IS, Liebman J: Anatomy of body water and electrolytes. *Am J Med* 27:256, 1959.
18. Elwyn DH et al: Nutritional aspects of body water dislocations in postoperative and depleted patients. *Ann Surg* 182:76, 1975.
19. Eveloff JL, Warnock DG: Activation of ion transport systems during cell volume regulation. *Am J Physiol* 252: F1, 1987.
20. Fiorotto ML et al: Fat-free mass and total body water of infants estimated from total body electrical conductivity measurements. *Pediatr Res* 22: 417, 1987.
21. Fjeld CR et al: Total body water measured by ^{18}O dilution and bioelectrical impedance in well and malnourished children. *Pediatr Res* 27:98, 1990.
22. Flynn MA et al: Estimation of body water compartments of preschool children: 1. Normal children. *Am J Clin Nutr* 20:1125, 1967.
23. Flynn MA et al: Estimation of body water compartments of preschool children: 2. Undernourished children. *Am J Clin Nutr* 20:129, 1967.
24. Gregerson MI et al: Plasma volume determinations with dyes: Errors in colorimetry, use of the blue dye T-1824. *Am J Physiol* 113:54, 1935.
25. Gregg HW et al: The changes in the content of hemoglobin and erythrocytes of the blood in man during short exposures to low oxygen. *Am J Physiol* 50:216, 1919.
26. Gruner O, Salmen A: Vergleichende Korperwasser-bestimmungen mit hilfe von *N*-acetyl-4-aminoanti-pyrin und Alkohol. *Klin Wochenschr* 39:92, 1961.
27. Haley HB et al: The turnover rate of body water in the human, in American College of Surgeons, *Surgical Forum, 1951.* Philadelphia, Saunders, 1952, p 595.
28. Hannon JP et al: Effects of altitude acclimatization on blood composition of women. *J Appl Physiol* 26:540, 1969.
29. Hannon JP et al: Effects of acute high-altitude exposure on body fluids. *Fed Proc* 28:1178, 1969.
30. Hays RM: Dynamics of body water and electrolytes, in Maxwell MH, Kleeman CR (eds): *Clinical Disorders of Fluid and Electrolyte Metabolism*, 3d ed. New York, McGraw-Hill, 1980.
31. Headings VE et al: Bound sodium in artery wall. *Am J Physiol* 199:783, 1960.

32. Hytten FE et al: Total body water in normal pregnancy. *Br J Obstet Gynaecol* 73:553, 1966.
33. Hytten FE: Body water in human pregnancy. *J Reprod Fertil* 9(suppl):1, 1969.
34. Jain SC et al: Body fluid compartments in humans during acute high-altitude exposure. *Aviat Space Environ Med* 51:234, 1980.
35. Kinney JM et al: Relationship of energy expenditure to total exchangeable potassium. *Ann Ny Acad Sci* 110:711, 1963.
36. Kozlowski S, Saltin B: Effect of sweat loss on body fluids. *J Appl Physiol* 19:1119, 1964.
37. Kregenow FM: Osmoregulatory salt transporting mechanisms: Control of cell volume in anisotonic media. *Annu Rev Physiol* 43:493, 1981.
38. Kuntz ID, Zipp A: Water in biological systems. *N Engl J Med* 297:262, 1977.
39. Kushner RF, Schoeller DA: Estimation of total body water by bioelectrical impedance analysis. *Am J Clin Nutr* 44:417, 1986.
40. Lesser GT, Markofsky J: Body water compartments with human aging using fat-free mass as the reference standard. *Am J Physiol* 236:R215, 1979.
41. Lewis DS et al: Use of NMR for measurement of total body water and estimation of body fat. *J Appl Physiol* 60:836, 1986.
42. Ling GN, Walton CL: What retains water in living cells? *Science* 191:293, 1976.
43. Loeppky JA et al: Total body water and lean body mass estimated by ethanol dilution. *J Appl Physiol* 42:803, 1977.
44. Lowry OH, Hastings AB: Histochemical changes associated with aging. *J Biol Chem* 143:257, 1942.
45. Lukaski HC, Bolonchuk WW: Estimation of body fluid volumes using tetrapolar bioelectrical impedance measurements. *Aviat Space Environ Med* 59:1163, 1988.
46. MacKnight ADC: Volume regulation in mammalian kidney cells. *Mol Physiol* 4:17, 1983.
47. MacLaurin JC: Changes in body water distribution during the first two weeks of life. *Arch Dis Child* 41:286, 1966.
48. McCarty NA, O'Neil RG: Dihydropyridine-sensitive cell volume regulation in proximal tubule: The calcium window. *Am J Physiol* 259:F950, 1990.
49. McChance RA, Widdowson EM: A method of breaking down the weights of living persons into terms of extracellular fluid, cell mass, and fat, and some applications of it to physiology and medicine. *Proc R Soc Lond* 138:115, 1951.
50. McMurrey JD et al: The evaluation of body composition in surgical disease processes utilizing a method for the simultaneous determination of red blood cell volume, total body water, extracellular water and total exchangeable chloride, sodium, and potassium. *Surg Forum* 6:14, 1955.
51. McMurrey JD et al: Body composition: Simultaneous determination of several aspects by the dilution principle. *Metabolism* 7:651, 1958.
52. McNeill IF et al: The effects of hemorrhage and hormones on the partition of body water: 1. A method for measuring small sequential increases in the volume of the extracellular fluid. *J Surg Res* 3:322, 1963.
53. Metzler DE: *Biochemistry*. New York, Academic Press, 1977, p. 185.
54. Milledge JS et al: Sodium balance, fluid homeostasis and the renin-aldosterone system during the prolonged exercise of hill walking. *Clin Sci* 62:595, 1982.
55. Moore FD, Tobin LH: Studies with radioactive di-azo dyes: 1. Localization of radioactive di-brom trypan blue in inflammatory lesions. *J Clin Invest* 21:471, 1942.
56. Moore FD: Determination of total body water and solids with isotopes. *Science* 104:157, 1946.
57. Moore FD et al: Further observations on total body water: 2. Changes in body composition in disease. *Surg Gynecol Obstet* 95:155, 1952.
58. Moore FD et al: Body sodium and potassium: 3. Interrelated trends in alimentary, renal, and cardiovascular disease: Lack of correlation between body stores and plasma concentration. *Metabolism* 3:334, 1954.
59. Moore FD et al: *The Body Cell Mass and Its Supporting Environment: Body Composition in Health and Disease.* Philadelphia, Saunders, 1963.
60. Moore FD et al: The skeleton as a feature of body composition: Values predicted by the isotope dilution and observed by cadaver dissection in an adult female. *Hum Biol* 40:135, 1968.
61. Myhre LG et al: Plasma volume and blood metabolites in middle-aged runners during a warm-weather marathon. *Eur J Appl Physiol Occup Physiol* 48:227, 1982.
62. Natke N Jr: Cell volume regulation of rabbit cortical collecting tubule in anisotonic media. *Am J Physiol* 258: F1657, 1990.
63. Novak LP: Changes in total body water during adolescent growth. *Hum Biol* 61:407, 1989.
64. Oscai LB et al: Effect of exercise on blood volume. *J Appl Physiol* 24:622, 1968.
65. Pierson RN et al: The assessment of human body composition during weight reduction: Evaluation of a new model for clinical studies. *J Nutr* 106:1694, 1976.
66. Pinson EA: Water exchanges and barriers as studied by the use of hydrogen isotopes. *Physiol Rev* 32:123, 1952.
67. Proverbio F et al: Ouabain-insensitive Na^+-stimulated ATPase activity of basolateral plasma membranes from guinea-pig-kidney cortex cells: 2. Effect of Ca^{2+}. *Biochim Biophys Acta* 668:757, 1982.
68. Reus L: Cell volume regulation in nonrenal epithelia. *Renal Physiol Biochem* 11:187, 1988.
69. Rothschild MA et al: Tissue distribution of ^{131}I labelled human serum albumin following intravenous administration. *J Clin Invest* 34:1354, 1955.
70. Schloerb PR et al: The measurement of total body water in the human subject by deuterium oxide dilution: With a consideration of the dynamics of deuterium distribution. *J Clin Invest* 29:1296, 1950.
71. Schoeller GW et al: Total body water measurements in humans with ^{18}O and ^{2}H labeled water. *Am J Clin Nutr* 33:2686, 1980.
72. Senay LC, Jr. Christensen ML: Changes in blood plasma during progressive dehydration. *J Appl Physiol* 20:1136, 1965.
73. Sjogaard G, Saltin B: Extra- and intracellular water spaces in muscles of man at rest and with dynamic exercise. *Am J Physiol* 243:R271, 1982.
74. Skelton H: The storage of water by various tissues of the body. *Arch Intern Med* 40:140, 1927.

75. Smith R: Total body water in malnourished infants. *Clin Sci* 19:275, 1960.
76. Soberman R et al: The use of antipyrine in the measurement of total body water in man. *J Biol Chem* 179:31, 1947.
77. Starling EH: On the absorption of fluids from the connective tissue spaces. *J Physiol* 19:312, 1896.
78. Sterling K, Gray SI: Determination of the red cell volume using radiochromated erythrocytes. *J Clin Invest* 29:1614, 1950.
79. Tobin LH, Moore FD: Studies with radioactive di-azo dyes: 2. Synthesis and properties of radioactive di-brom trypan blue and radioactive di-brom evans blue. *J Clin Invest* 22:155, 1943.
80. vanBeaumont W et al: Plasma fluid and blood constituent shifts during heat exposure in resting men. *Aerospace Med* 45:176, 1974.
81. Van Loan M, Mayclin P: Bioelectrical impedance analysis: Is it a reliable estimator of lean body mass and total body water? *Hum Biol* 59:299, 1987.
82. Van Loan M, Mayclin P: A new TOBEC instrument and procedure for the assessment of body composition: Use of Fourier coefficients to predict lean body mass and total body water. *Am J Clin Nutr* 45:131, 1987.
83. Vellar OD: Studies on sweat losses of nutrients. *Scand J Clin Lab Invest* 21:157, 1968.
84. Volkl H, Lang F: Effect of potassium on cell volume regulation in renal straight proximal tubules. *J Membr Biol* 117:113, 1990.
85. Volkl, H et al: Cell volume regulation in renal cortical cells. *Renal Physiol Biochem* 11:158, 1988.
86. Watterson JG: A role for water in cell structure. *Biochem J* 248:615, 1987.
87. Whittembury G, Proverbio F: Two modes of Na extrusion in cells from guinea pig kidney cortex slices. *Pfluegers Arch* 316:1, 1970.
88. Wilson G et al: Sodium maldistribution in acute and chronic disease: Proceedings of the 45th Annual Meeting, American Society for Clinical Investigation, 1953 (abstract). *J Clin Invest* 32:612, 1953.
89. Yasumura S et al: Measurement of extracellular space by total body neutron activation. *Am J Physiol* 244:R36, 1983.

CHAPTER • 2

Principles of epithelial transport

John B. Stokes

Regulation of the volume and ionic composition of the body fluids is a monumental feat intricately orchestrated with great precision by the concerted action of the individual units of the kidney, the nephrons. Following ultrafiltration of the plasma, the filtrate undergoes selective modification by the epithelial cells that form the individual nephrons. Of the approximately 180 liters of plasma that are filtered daily, approximately 178 liters are reabsorbed; of the 22,500 m*M* of NaCl that is filtered, 22,300 m*M* is reabsorbed. The renal tubular epithelial cells are also capable of reabsorbing virtually all of the filtered $NaHCO_3$ (4500 m*M*) and glucose (1000 m*M*) as well as all of the filtered amino acids, short-chain fatty acids, and ketone bodies. Other key substances, such as K^+ and uric acid, are reabsorbed and secreted by special transport systems. How the kidney regulates the excretion of these solutes and water to precisely match the intake or the production by the organism has been the subject of investigation by renal physiologists for over a century.

The objective of this chapter is to review the principles governing transport of solute and water across epithelial cells and across cell membranes. Detailed discussion of specific transport processes by each segment of the nephron can be found in other sections of this volume. Table 2-1 is a glossary of some abbreviations and symbols used in this chapter.

TABLE 2-1 • Glossary

C	concentration
E	electromotive force (volt)
F	Faraday
G	conductance (siemens)
I	current (ampere)
J	flux
J_{max}	constant indicaing the maximum flux through a transport system
J_v	volume flow (flux)
kDa	kilodalton, unit of apparent molecular weight
K_m	constant indicating the concentration at which flux is half maximal
L_p	hydraulic conductivity
mV	millivolt (10^{-3} volt)
nm	nanometer (10^{-1} angstrom)
P	permeability
p	pressure (atmospheres or equivalent)
pA	picoampere (10^{-12} ampere)
R	gas constant
T	temperature (K)
$\overline{V}$	partial molar volume
x	distance
z	valence
Greek symbols	
$\tilde{\mu}$	electrochemical potential
$\Delta\pi$	osmotic or oncotic pressure gradient
ρ	resistance (ohm)
σ	reflection coefficient
$1-\sigma$	sieving coefficient
ψ	electrical potential (volt)
ω	mobility
Ω	ohm, unit of resistance (volt/ampere)
Subscripts	
i	any solute
w	water

ORGANIZATION OF EPITHELIA

The renal epithelial cells are a single layer of columnar, cuboidal, or thin cells that rest on a basement membrane (Fig. 2-1). In the kidney, the basement membrane provides important structural support because the epithelial cells are arranged in small tubes. The outer diameter of

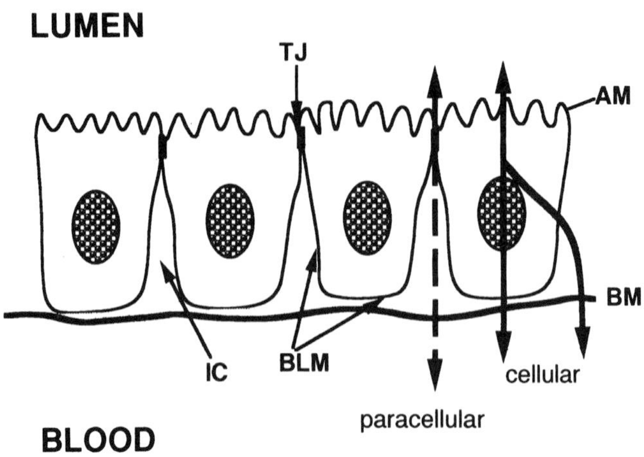

FIGURE 2-1 • Pathways for solute and water permeation across epithelia. Schematized in this figure are the features of all epithelial tissues, such as intestine, kidney tubules, sweat glands, gallbladder, and urinary bladder. The epithelial cells are a single layer resting on a basement membrane (BM). Each epithelial cell has a membrane made up of two distinct domains. The apical membrane (AM) is that portion which faces the lumen, and the basolateral membrane (BLM) faces the blood side of the epithelium. The boundary between the apical membrane and the basolateral membrane is the tight junction (TJ), which forms a ring around each epithelial cell. Solutes and water can traverse the epithelium through either the cellular pathway or the paracellular pathway. The paracellular pathway consists of the intercellular space (IC) and the tight junction. The cellular pathway includes the apical and basolateral membranes and the cell cytoplasm.

most nephron segments is 20 to 60 μm. The height of the epithelial cells varies considerably from segment to segment but ranges from 2 to 15 μm. The general features shared by all epithelial cells are (1) specific cell-to-cell connections, (2) different composition of cell membranes that face the lumen (apical membrane) compared to those that face the blood (basolateral membranes), and (3) a cell cytoskeletal system that helps keep order between and within the apical and basolateral membranes.

The connecting structure found in all epithelial cells is the tight junction. The electron photomicrograph in Figure 2-2 shows this structure at the attachment of the cells near the apical membrane. The three-dimensional structure of the tight junction is best envisioned as if the cells were a six-pack of beverage cans. The plastic that encircles the neck of each can and holds the cans together functions as the tight junction of a sheet of epithelial cells. The nature of these tight junctions is rather variable from nephron to nephron and from epithelium to epithelium. In the proximal tubule the tight junctions are shallow, while in the more distal segments they can be long, with several components. For this reason the structure is sometimes called the junctional complex. Tight junctions are connected to the cytoskeletal system. There is good evidence that in the intestine their function can change dramatically in response to intracellular events or signals.[16] These functional changes are probably mediated by the cytoskeleton. Whether such events occur in kidney epithelial cells is not known. It is clear that junctional complexes from various parts of the nephron can have different functional properties (see below). By using freeze fracture, a technique that opens cell membranes between their inner and outer leaflets, one can determine that the tight junction is composed of strands or fibrils. The number of these strands is variable from one to ten, with the actual number bearing a relationship to the function of the junctional complex; the more strands, the more restrictive is the complex to solute movement.

In addition to the tight junctions, there are two other types of structures that connect epithelial cells. *Desmosomes* serve as strong intercellular attaching structures. The type referred to as *spot desmosomes*, illustrated in Fig. 2-3, act as rivets to keep epithelial cells from coming apart. Another form, *belt desmosomes*, encircle the cell in the region of the tight junction and, when present, are a part of the junctional complex. Desmosomes are not found in all nephron segments; in fact, most segments in the human kidney do not have desmosomes. The other intercellular structure of importance to epithelial cells is the *gap junction*. These structures form communicating pores between cells that are large enough to allow proteins to pass. Gap junctions are composed of six polypeptide chains, each of which consists of a 28,000-dalton protein. The pore is about 1.5 nm in diameter.[15] To date, there have been no gap junctions de-

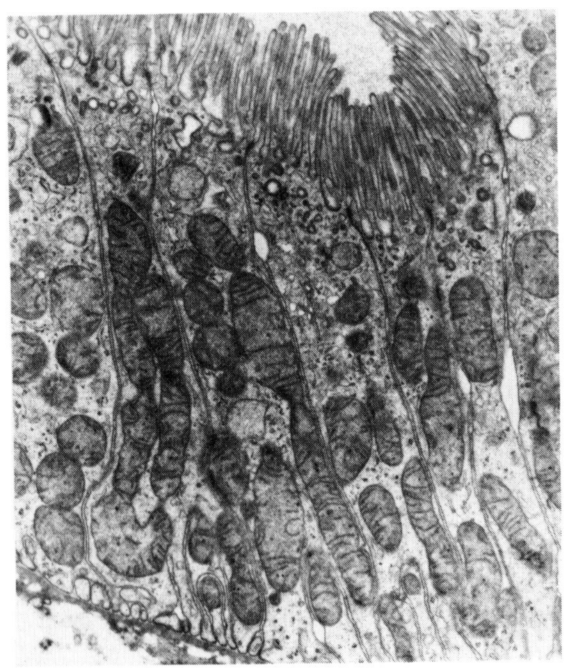

FIGURE 2-2 • Low-power electron micrograph of human proximal tubule. The apical membrane consists of microvilli sometimes called a brush border, seen in the upper region of the micrograph. Infoldings of the basolateral membrane are seen in the lower left corner. The intercellular spaces are distinguishable between the mitochondria-packed columnar cells. (Micrograph provided by Dr. C. Craig Tisher.)

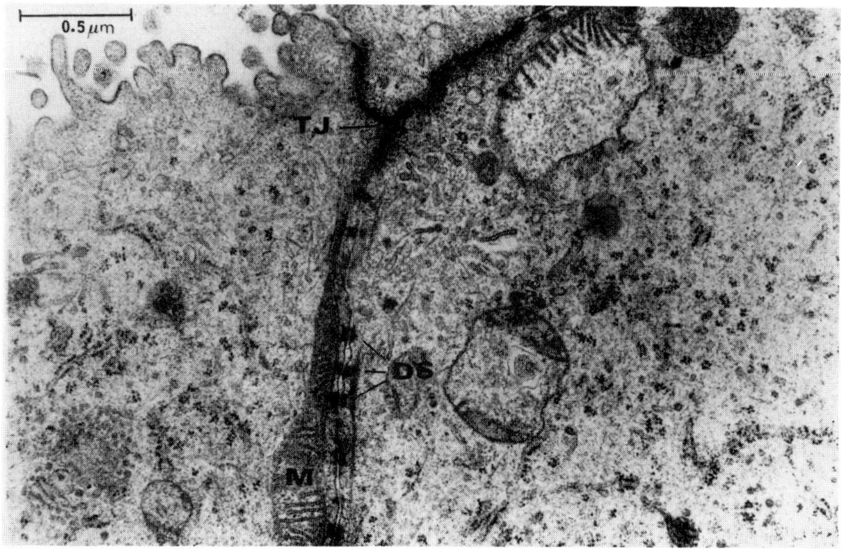

FIGURE 2-3 • High-power electron micrograph demonstrating the tight junction (TJ) and desmosomes (DS) of the rat inner medullary collecting duct. The apical membrane and the lumen are toward the upper left corner, and the tight junction can be seen where three epithelial cells have come together. Tight junctions of the collecting duct are usually long and provide high resistance. Along the intercellular space one can see a mitochondrion (M). Most renal tubular epithelial cells do not contain desmosomes. An exception is the rat inner medullary collecting duct. The reason that desmosomes are present in the collecting duct may be related to its ability to withstand large changes in hydrostatic pressure. (From Stokes et al: *Am J Physiol* 253:F251, 1987. Used by permission.)

scribed in renal epithelial cells, but they are important in some epithelia to allow the cells to communicate and act in concert.

PATHWAYS OF SOLUTE AND WATER TRANSPORT ACROSS EPITHELIA

As shown in Fig. 2.1, there are two general routes that solutes and water can take in order to traverse the epithelium: the *cellular* and the *paracellular* pathways.

PARACELLULAR PATHWAY

The paracellular pathway includes the routes around and between the cells.[3] Molecules moving from the lumen to the blood through this route must traverse first the junctional complex, then the intercellular space (lateral to the cell), and finally the basement membrane. The basement membrane provides little barrier to the movement of molecules. The lateral intercellular space is best considered as an extension of the interstitium. An important feature of the intercellular space is that it can be long and tortuous; thus, the geometry can provide resistance to movement of molecules. This space is capable of changing its volume. In general, epithelia that are absorbing large quantities of solute and water have larger intercellular spaces than do nontransporting epithelia. That the size of the space is dictated by the magnitude of the transport can be readily demonstrated by using inhibitors of transport. Inhibitors collapse the intercellular space.

Careful morphometric measurements have documented that the intercellular space of renal tubules increases as a function of distance from the tight junction to the basement membrane. Such a deduction might not be obvious at first if one sees a constant cell-to-cell distance in a transverse histologic section. However, the fact that renal epithelial cells are arranged in a tube requires that the planar area of the basal area of the cell (the part resting on the basement membrane) must be larger than the planar area of the luminal membrane. Each cell is thus shaped more or less like a cone. In fact, the size of the intercellular space increases to an even greater extent than would be predicted from simple geometric considerations. This result provides strong evidence that some of the solute and water present in the intercellular space got there by traversing the lateral cell membrane. Clearly, this space is not just a simple conduit for molecules that have crossed the tight junction.

The tight junction in most cells provides the major portion of resistance to molecular movement through the paracellular pathway. It has been somewhat difficult to obtain precise information on the nature of its transport properties, but some generalizations are well supported. The first generalization is that some tight junctions have a high permeability to ions and water, while others have a low permeability. Such characteristics of the tight junction characterize the cell as "leaky" or "tight." Because of the difficulty in making absolute measurements of the magnitude of this pathway, these terms are usually used to denote the conductive permeabilities of the paracellular pathway compared to the cellular pathway. However, it is most reasonable to think of leaky epithelia as having a highly conductive (permeable) junctional complex and tight epithelia as having a low-conductance junctional complex. The tight junctional complexes are usually longer and more complex.

The second general feature of tight junctions of particular importance to epithelial transport relates to their ionic selectivity. These selectivities favor either anions or cations on the order of 2:1. The junctional complex is too simple a structure to provide a high degree of selectivity for specific cations or specific anions. Such selectivity is best accomplished by specialized proteins in cell membranes. Nevertheless, having a junctional complex that is anion selective can represent an advantage if the cellular pathway has a transport system that primarily transports cations. Likewise, a cation selective paracellular pathway is an advantage if the cellular pathway primarily transports anions.

The demonstration that the paracellular pathway could represent a major route for the translocation of ions was made by Frömter,[7,8] who showed that, when a current was passed across the gallbladder, 95 percent of the current came between the cells. The magnitude of the paracellular resistance of the gallbladder is 30 to 50 $\Omega \cdot cm^2$, a value similar to that of the proximal tubule. The paracellular resistance of tight epithelia is commonly more than 1000 $\Omega \cdot cm^2$.

CELLULAR PATHWAYS

The majority of the transport of solutes and water occurs through the cell. This statement can be made despite the fact that the paracellular pathway might be over 100-fold more conductive than the cell. A host of specialized transport proteins are responsible for the cell's ability to transfer solute and water across the epithelium, and many of these transporters are nonconductive.

Transcellular transport occurs in two steps: the molecules must traverse both the apical membrane and the basolateral membrane. It is not surprising that the nature of the apical and basolateral membranes and the transport proteins contained within them are very different. In order to appreciate the importance and significance of these differences, we should recall the differences in the composition of the cytoplasm and the interstitial (extracellular) fluid. The largest differences are in Na^+, K^+, and Ca^{2+}. Cell Na^+concentration is 10 to 15 m*M*, cell K^+ concentration is 120 to 130 m*M*, and cell Ca^{2+} concentration is 100 to 200 n*M*. Thus, the chemical concentration gradient across the cell membrane is 10 to 20 for Na^+ and K^+ and 5,000 to 10,000 for Ca^{2+}. There should be no surprise that the apical and basolateral membranes must be very different in order to carry out vectoral transport of these and other molecules.

An example of the physical differences between the apical and basolateral membranes can be seen in Fig. 2-2. The apical membrane of these proximal tubule cells is a brush border with many villi. The brush border structure increases the effective surface area of the apical membrane by a factor of 30 to 50. In contrast to the apical membrane, the basal and lateral membranes have few infoldings and amplifications. In almost all epithelial cells, the basal and lateral membranes are quantitatively similar, with no clear division between them. Hence, they are considered a single structure called the basolateral membrane. The physical separation of the apical and basolateral membranes is maintained by the tight junction. If the tight junction is disrupted, the composition of the two membranes can become intermixed. This loss of cell polarity has been particularly well demonstrated following renal ischemia. This insult disrupts the cytoskeleton and the junctional complexes. As a result, membrane proteins that are localized and anchored to one membrane are able to migrate around the cell. This loss of polarity renders the epithelial cell incapable of performing vectoral transport.[17]

Successful vectoral transport of solute and water across the epithelium requires a coordinated effort between the apical and basolateral membranes. This organization must be accomplished at several levels: there must be appropriate transport proteins expressed; they must be sorted to the correct membrane; and the apical and basolateral transporters must be able to communicate with each other to effect integration of transport. Before discussing these issues, let us first consider some of the better-studied transporters that operate in the kidney.

MEMBRANE TRANSPORT PROTEINS

Membrane transporters fall into two major groups: those that are not directly coupled to metabolic energy and those that are directly coupled. Of course, no net transport can occur without energy; the classification simply relies on the source of the energy. Transporters that utilize the potential energy of existing electrical or chemical gradients are *channels, carriers, exchangers,* or *cotransporters.* Transporters that use the energy derived from the hydrolysis of ATP are called *pumps.* Each type of transport unit plays an integral role in the translocation of solute from one side of the epithelial cell to the other. The detailed understanding of the structure, function, and regulation of these transport proteins is the subject of intense investigation. We will begin by examining the basic principles under which each of these transport proteins functions. All pumps are ATPases and have a portion (or subunit) of the molecule devoted to binding and hydrolyzing ATP. The pump is thus phosphorylated, and a conformational change occurs. The energy from the ATP is transferred to the pump such that subsequent (or prior) binding of the solute will cause another conformational change, resulting in translocation to the opposite side of the membrane. Of the best understood pumps, those that are important for renal function are Na^+-K^+ ATPase, Ca^{2+}ATPase, and H^+ATPase.

GENERAL MODELS OF TRANSPORT PROTEINS

The understanding of channels, carriers, and cotransporters has been greatly aided by the study of simple molecules that can insert in lipid bilayers to make channels or carriers. A particularly relevant example is the antifungal agent amphotericin B. It is used clinically to treat fungal infections because the higher sterol content of the fungal cell membrane makes fungi more sensitive than are mammalian cell membranes to its action. It is well known that the renal distal nephron is the site of major toxicity because the agent is concentrated in the tubular fluid along the nephron.

Amphotericin B produces 0.4-nm pores in cell membranes. About eight molecules arrange themselves into a cylinder that spans half the lipid bilayer. Two such cylinders align themselves to span the entire membrane.[6] The resulting pore allows molecules smaller than glucose, such as Na^+, K^+, Cl^-, H^+, and water, to pass readily. Thus, cells exposed to this agent are unable to maintain their pH, Na^+, and K^+ gradients. Excessive K^+ loss into the urine of patients receiving this drug is directly attributable to this property. The inability to maintain the pH gradient because of back diffusion of H^+ ions from the lumen to the collecting duct cell is responsible for the metabolic acidosis.

The kind of transport induced by amphotericin B is depicted in Fig. 2-4A. The molecules insert themselves into the membrane to form a pore or channel that allows relatively unrestricted movement of small solutes. A second type of transport process is depicted in Fig. 2-4B. This type of molecule is a carrier because it does not completely span the membrane and must move from one side of the bilayer to the other in order to effect solute transport. One of the best-studied examples of this kind of transporter is valinomycin. It is like amphotericin B in that it is a naturally occurring substance and has a low molecular weight. However, it acts differently from amphotericin B in that it moves through the membrane, doing so with equal facility whether or not it has bound any solute. Valinomycin also differs from pore-forming agents in that it is highly selective for K^+ over other ions, including Na^+. For this reason it is frequently used in K^+-selective electrodes.

Although these two modes of transport are useful for characterizing mechanisms of solute translocation across membranes, there are limitations in their applicability to transport systems of real cells. All mammalian cell transporters are large-protein molecules that span the membrane several times. There are no examples of mobile carriers such as valinomycin. Therefore, in considering how transport proteins function, it is important to realize that they are highly ordered structures. They do not float through the cell membrane but are anchored to the cytoskeleton. In this way endogenous transporters resemble pore-forming molecules like amphotericin B. How-

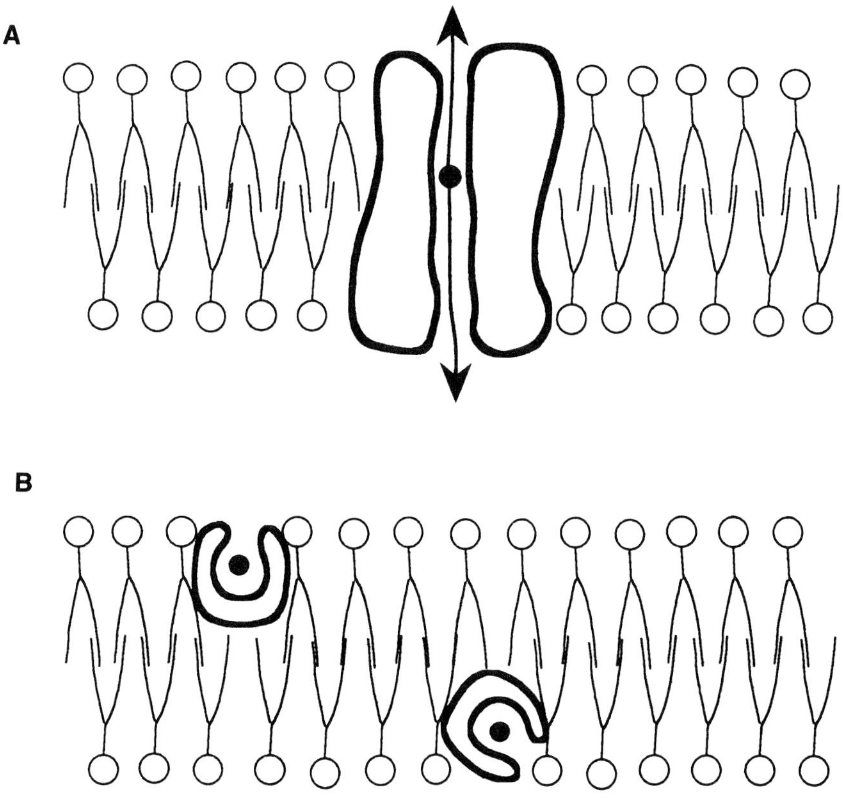

FIGURE 2-4 • General ways in which solutes can traverse cell membranes via transporters. (A) Example of a pore or channel. Such a transporter spans the entire lipid bilayer, allowing selected solutes to traverse the membrane. The polyene antibiotic amphotericin B behaves in such a way and allows permeation of univalent cations and anions as well as water and small molecules. Channels manufactured by cells work on the same principle but almost always are highly selective for a single species. (B) Example of a mobile carrier. This type of transporter does not span the cell membrane but, rather, is free to dissolve in and move within the cell membrane. Such carriers can bind a solute at one surface and carry it across the membrane, where it can dissociate from the carrier. There are no examples in which a cell manufactures this kind of carrier for its own purposes. However, valinomycin, an antibiotic not available for human use, acts as a mobile carrier for K^+ and is often used in K^+-selective electrodes.

ever, they differ from amphotericin B in that they are more selective for a particular solute and can be regulated by a variety of mediators. We shall consider a few examples of important membrane transporters that behave like channels, carriers, exchangers, cotransporters, and pumps.

TABLE 2-2 • Representative permeability coefficients of molecules through lipid bilayers

Molecule	Permeability (cm/s)
Water	5×10^{-3}
Urea	5×10^{-6}
Glucose	8×10^{-8}
Na^+	1×10^{-12}

CHANNELS

A channel (or pore) is a molecule or group of molecules that span a cell membrane and allow other molecules to pass through it. Ion channels are the most frequently studied type of channels; the term channel has come to be associated with structures that allow passage of ions. There are two major reasons for this relationship. First, there is an extraordinary number of ion channels; every physiologically relevant ion probably has at least one channel devoted to its transport. In addition, there is a large number of different types of channels for each ion species.

The second reason for the strong association of the term channel with structures that pass ions is that when ions are translocated in this fashion one can measure an electrical current. The measurement of a current produced by ion translocation was first accomplished over 40 years ago. Investigators found that, in some epithelia, clamping the voltage to 0 produced a current that was equal to the magnitude of active Na^+ transport. This way of measuring ion transport became known as the short-circuit current method and is still widely used to measure various aspects of active transport. The most recent development is the patch clamp technique, whereby one measures the current carried by ions traversing a single channel. This method has produced an explosion of information about the biophysical characteristics of ion channels, their heterogeneity and diversity, and the molecular interactions regulating their activity.

Channels can also act as conduits for uncharged solutes, the most important examples of which are water and urea. The argument that these molecules move through channels is somewhat less certain than is the case for ions because single-channel activity cannot be measured electrically. A further complicating feature is the fact that uncharged molecules are soluble, to a variable degree, in the lipid milieu of cell membranes. Table 2-2 lists the permeability of representative solutes in lipid bilayers. It is clear that water, urea, and, to some extent, glucose can cross cell membranes without the aid of specific transporters. Having specific channels or transporters, however, can increase the rate of transfer by 10- to 1000-fold.

Na^+ channel

One of the most relevant ion channels in the kidney is the Na^+ channel. It is located on the luminal (apical) membrane of the distal nephron and the collecting duct and plays a central role in the regulation of Na^+ absorption. Its activity is increased by stimulation with aldosterone. The mechanism responsible for this increase in activity or permeability is not clear, but new proteins must be synthesized. These new proteins are probably not Na^+ channels per se, because it appears that they are already present in the apical membrane. Rather, it seems most likely that aldosterone induces a protein or proteins that change the existing channel such that its activity is increased.

An example of this channel's activity is depicted in Fig. 2-5. The tracing was obtained using the patch clamp method to record Na^+ channels in the apical membrane of the rat cortical collecting duct. The membrane is oriented so that the outside of the cell is facing the bath. There are two levels of current, reflecting the presence of at least two channels. The amount of current passed by one channel is less than 1 pA (10^{-12} A). The biophysical characteristics of this channel are that it is highly selective for Na^+ over K^+; it has a low unitary conductance (5 pS); it is able to pass Na^+equally in either direction (i.e., the channel does not rectify); and the open-state probability is reduced by lowering the pH of the cytoplasmic solution. Two other characteristics of this channel can be seen in Figure 2-5. The amount of time the channel spends open or closed (without a transition) is much longer than for other channels. Many channels have mean open times of 10 ms or less. The second feature is that amiloride interacts with the channel from the outside surface and blocks the channel. The short open and closed times represent the "flickering" state of the channel as amiloride molecules bind to and then are released from the channel.[18] Higher concentrations of amiloride cause the channel to remain blocked so that no current can be identified.

The ability of the epithelial Na^+ channel to bind amiloride has enabled investigators to begin to identify the molecular structure. Having a high-affinity ligand, such as amiloride or even higher-affinity analogues, allows one to track the location of the protein through purification steps. Results to date indicate that the channel is part of a large complex of proteins with a total molecular mass of 700 to 800 kDa.[2] This complex re-

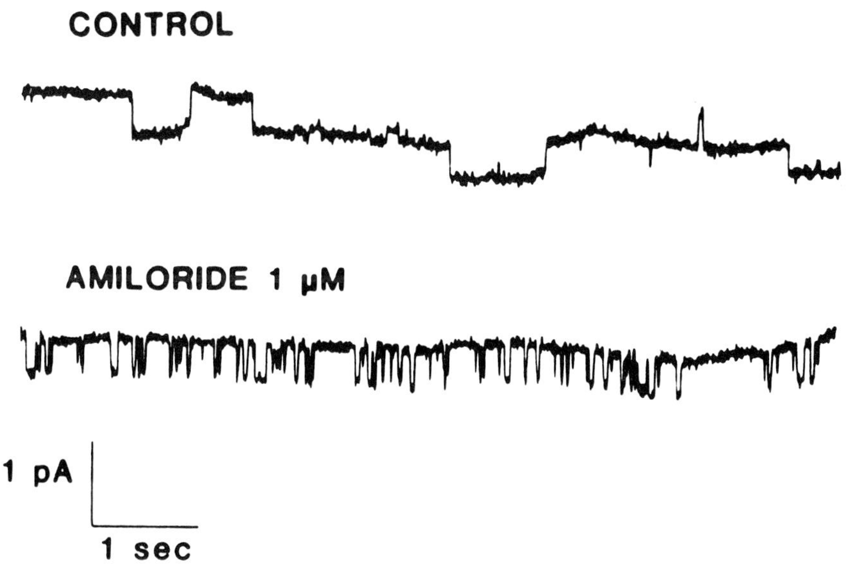

FIGURE 2-5 • Single-channel patch clamp recording from the apical membrane of a rat cortical collecting duct. The configuration of the patch is that the bath solution represents the outside of the cell, and the solution in the pipette represents the cytoplasm (an "outside-out" configuration). In the control condition, the channels open for periods often greater than 1 s, and there are at least two channels in the patch. Upon adding amiloride to the bath, the channel exhibits more rapid opening and closings, and more time is spent in the closed state than in the open state. Higher concentrations of amiloride reduce channel activity completely. In this tracing, channel openings are represented by downward deflections. Amiloride thus acts as a plug that can fit into the Na^+ channel from the outside of the cell and therefore inhibit the passage of Na^+ ions. (From Palmer LG, Frindt G: *Fed Proc* 45:2708, 1986. Used by permission.)

duces to six or more subunits, one of which binds amiloride and appears to be the actual channel protein.[1] The functions of the other subunits are not known, but some are probably involved in regulating the channel's probability of being open or closed. An extensive array of compounds appear to be involved in this regulation, including arachidonic acid metabolites, cyclic GMP, and GTP-binding proteins that may be part of the Na^+ channel complex.[4]

The epithelial Na^+ channel thus represents a kind of a pore, like amphotericin B. However, the analogy is limited, since the Na^+ channel is highly selective and is associated with proteins that can modulate its function.

CARRIERS AND EXCHANGERS

The idea that carriers are different from pores or channels has its roots in the kinetic studies of how sugars cross cell membranes. The red blood cell is an excellent model for kinetic studies because both the inside and outside concentrations can be readily manipulated. If one loads a red blood cell with glucose (or a nonmetabolizable analogue) and removes all glucose from the outside, glucose moves from inside the cell to outside down its concentration gradient. This behavior provides no particular insight into how the glucose moves. A key observation occurs when one uses tracers to measure the unidirectional flux. The addition of glucose to the outside of the cell *increases* the rate of unidirectional efflux. This behavior cannot be explained by a simple pore model. Such a model predicts that, when there is an increase in concentration of the solute on the opposite side of the membrane (trans side), the efflux rate would be reduced, not increased. The only way to explain the phenomenon of transacceleration is to invoke specific binding sites on both sides of the membrane.[14] This process is often described as "exchange diffusion." Transacceleration of unidirectional flux is a property that removes the transport function from the pore category and places it squarely into the category of carrier.

Some of the best examples of exchange diffusion are the anion exchangers, a family of transport proteins found in most cell types and particularly well studied in red blood cells. The major purpose of the red blood cell anion exchangers (often called band 3) is to assist in the rapid exchange of HCO_3^- that occurs as CO_2 enters and leaves the cell. The process works as follows. As the red blood cell enters a peripheral capillary and an environment where the P_{CO_2} is high, CO_2 gas enters the cell. CO_2 diffuses rapidly across cell membranes, and thus equilibrium is achieved quickly. The red blood cell contains large amounts of carbonic anhydrase, an enzyme that accelerates the hydration of CO_2 to H_2CO_3. The newly formed H_2CO_3 spontaneously dissociates into H^+ and HCO_3^-, whereupon the H^+ is rapidly buffered by hemoglobin and other intracellular proteins. The resulting increase in the HCO_3^- concentration in the red blood cell shifts the anion equilibrium so that HCO_3^- leaves the cell in exchange for Cl^-. This process greatly increases the amount of CO_2 that can be removed from the tissues in the relatively short transit time through the peripheral capillaries. Upon reaching the pulmonary capillary system, the process is reversed; as CO_2 leaves the red blood cell, HCO_3^- enters via the anion exchanger to combine with protons and generate more CO_2. The magnitude of anion exchange is fast enough to allow complete equilibration of CO_2 loading or unloading in less than 1 s.

The stoichiometry of this anion exchange is one Cl^- for one HCO_3^- ion; hence, there is no net charge transfer, and the process is electroneutral. An important feature of anion exchangers is the nearly absolute requirement for an anion on the trans side of the membrane to effect translocation. In the absence of an anion on the trans side, there is little or no transport; addition of the trans anion greatly increases the unidirectional anion flux.

The need for a trans anion to mediate flux raises two important issues: (1) What is the specificity of the inside and outside binding sites?, and (2) How does the exchange occur? In the case of anion exchangers, it appears that the specificity for binding Cl^- or HCO_3^- is not very great. This might be expected in the red blood cell, since the system must operate in one direction in peripheral tissues and the opposite direction in the lung. Although the anion specificity is not great, the nature of the inside and outside binding sites shows different binding affinities for anions. It seems likely that these affinities can be changed by "modifiers." One important modifier from the cytoplasmic surface is pH. Anion exchangers in many cells are activated by an increase in cell pH. The teleologic advantage of this kind of activation is to more rapidly return the cell pH to normal by accelerating the influx of Cl^- in exchange for HCO_3^-.

There are two physical models that can describe exchange transport or countertransport: the *simultaneous model* and the *alternating model*. As depicted in Fig. 2-6, the simultaneous model would require that anions bind to both the inside and outside before a conformational change occurrs. The conformation would translocate both ions simultaneously before they could be released to the opposite side. Such a process might occur like a revolving door that could only rotate if both sides were occupied. As it turns out, such a model does not describe anion exchange, and most exchangers apparently do not work in this fashion. Rather, the exchanger works like an alternating, or "ping-pong," model (Fig. 2-7). In this model the binding of one molecule causes a conformational change in the protein so that the bound ion can leave the transporter to the other side. The unoccupied binding site is thus able to bind a molecule and once again change its conformation to the original configuration. For anion exchangers in many types of cells, the anion exchange operates in a Cl^--Cl^- exchange mode (self-exchange) more often than in a Cl^--HCO_3^- mode. This type of transport at first might appear to be inefficient, but this is really not the case. Self-exchange accomplishes no net work, uses no metabolic energy, and would not even be detectable were it not for radiolabeled tracers. The detailed study of self-exchange has allowed considerable insight into the operation of many kinds of transporters.

The distinction between a carrier and an exchanger can be simply the likelihood that the conformation of the protein can change from the inside form to the outside form without binding a transported species. Whereas exchangers (like the anion exchanger) rarely change conformation without a species being bound, carriers can change conformation readily without the need for a bound solute. The glucose transporter is a good example. If translocation of glucose into the cell required an oppositely transported glucose, the net movement of glucose would be zero (self-exchange), and the cell would have to rely on other metabolic fuels.

In addition to the anion exchanger family, one of the most important and well-studied is the Na^+-H^+ exchanger. As its name implies, it is substantially more specific than the anion exchanger. In its normal mode of operation, Na^+ binds to the outside face and is translocated inside the cell. A proton can then bind to the inside face, the conformation changes to the outside face, H^+ can be released, and the cycle repeats itself. Because the Na^+ gradient normally approximates 10:1 (140 m*M* outside and 14 m*M* inside) and because the exchange involves 1 Na^+ for 1 H^+, the maximum pH gradient that can be established across the cell membrane is 10 (or 1 pH unit). This gradient is approached (but never achieved) in the late proximal tubule, where the lumen pH reaches ~6.7 to 6.8, while the cell pH is ~7.2 to 7.3.

The Na^+-H^+ exchanger is not a single molecule. There are at least two types; one type is located on the

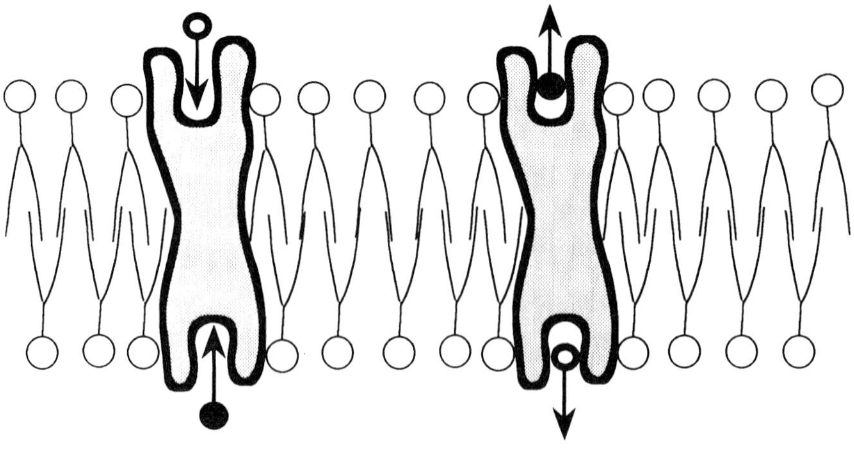

FIGURE 2-6 • "Simultaneous" model for exchange transport. In this model, which attempts to explain the process of countertransport or exchange transport, the first step (shown on the left) involves the binding of two species to the outer and inner binding sites of the transport protein. When both binding sites are occupied, the transporter undergoes a conformational change that results in reversal of the positions of the bound substrates. As shown on the right, after the conformational change these substrates are free to dissociate from the transporter and enter the other side of the membrane.

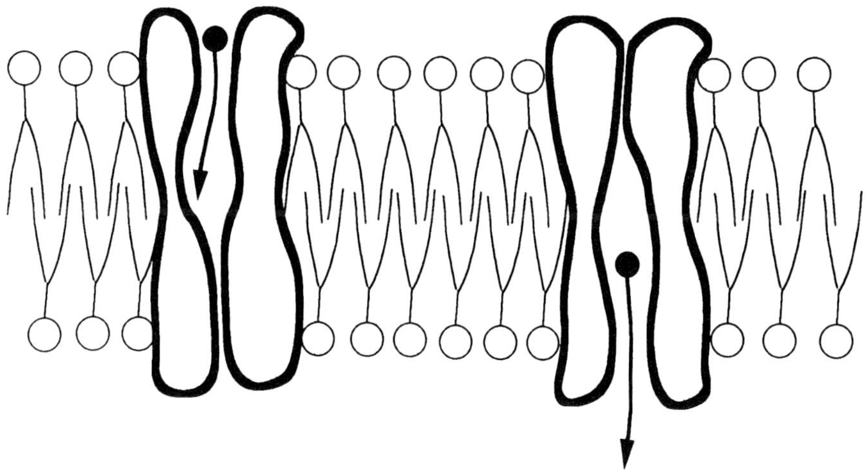

FIGURE 2-7 • "Ping-pong" model of exchange transport. In this model the transporter binds one species, after which it undergoes a conformational change exposing the opposite side of the cell membrane and allowing the unbinding of the solute and its exit from the transporter to the opposite side of the membrane. Upon binding species from the opposite side of the membrane, the protein undergoes a conformational change once again, allowing the exit of the solute to the original side. There is considerable experimental evidence indicating that exchange transport occurs by this process rather than by the simultaneous process. An attractive feature of this model is that it does not require the transport protein to rotate within the cell membrane. Furthermore, it gives the exchange transporters the general structure of pores or channels that happen to operate in a slightly different fashion than classic pores.

apical membrane of epithelial cells, such as in the proximal tubule and intestine, and another type on the basolateral membrane. The apical membrane exchanger is critical for transepithelial movements of Na^+ and H^+. The basolateral membrane exchanger helps to regulate cell pH. The idea that a single function (like Cl^--HCO_3^- exchange or Na^+-H^+ exchange) can be carried out by more than one type of molecule is becoming increasingly apparent as molecular cloning provides abundant detail on the primary structure of transport proteins.

COTRANSPORT

Thus far we have considered the translocation of a single solute across a cell membrane. The examples of transport through a channel or via a carrier have focused on the movement of one molecule at a time. Sometimes the movements involve alternating species, as in the case of exchangers. In contrast to transporters that only move one species, there are those that translocate more than one species in the same direction simultaneously. These molecules are called *cotransporters.*

From a teleologic perspective, one of the major reasons cotransporters evolved was because of the need for transporting important solutes that exist only in low concentrations or have small concentration gradients across the cell membrane. One of the richest and varied sources of cotransporters is the proximal tubule. This nephron segment has the responsibility of absorbing all of the nutrients filtered by the glomerulus. If even 10 percent of these molecules were lost into the urine, considerable energy would have to be directed toward synthesizing or obtaining additional nutrients. Clearly, it is more efficient to prevent their loss.

The Na^+ gradient across the cell membrane provides a convenient driving force for coupling to the transport of other species. We have already mentioned that the chemical gradient is 10:1. In addition, the cell membrane voltage is about 60 mV inside negative. This voltage is also a driving force for charged species. As it turns out, 60 mV provides about the same driving force for an ion with one positive charge as does a chemical gradient of 10:1. The Na^+ ion thus has twice the force favoring entry because it carries with it a positive charge.

Some important examples of solutes that are cotransported with Na^+ include glucose, amino acids, phosphate, and organic acids. We shall examine the Na^+-glucose cotransport system because it is well studied and provides a good example of the general principles of cotransport. We shall also examine the cotransport of Na^+, K^+, and Cl^-.

Na^+-glucose cotransport

Found on the apical membranes of epithelial cells of the proximal tubule and small intestine, this transporter is responsible for removing glucose from the lumen. There are actually two types of Na^+-glucose cotransporters. The most abundant form transports one Na^+ with one glucose; the other, less abundant form has a stoichiometry of two Na^+ to one glucose. The latter protein is located in the more distal portions of the proximal tubule, where the positive luminal charge of +2 greatly increases the force favoring reabsorption of Na^+ and thereby promotes removal of the remaining small amounts of glucose from the lumen.[20]

The molecular interactions involved in the 75 kDa Na^+-glucose cotransporter are schematized in Fig. 2-8. Na^+ binding occurs first. It binds to a site near a tyrosyl residue and in so doing produces a conformational

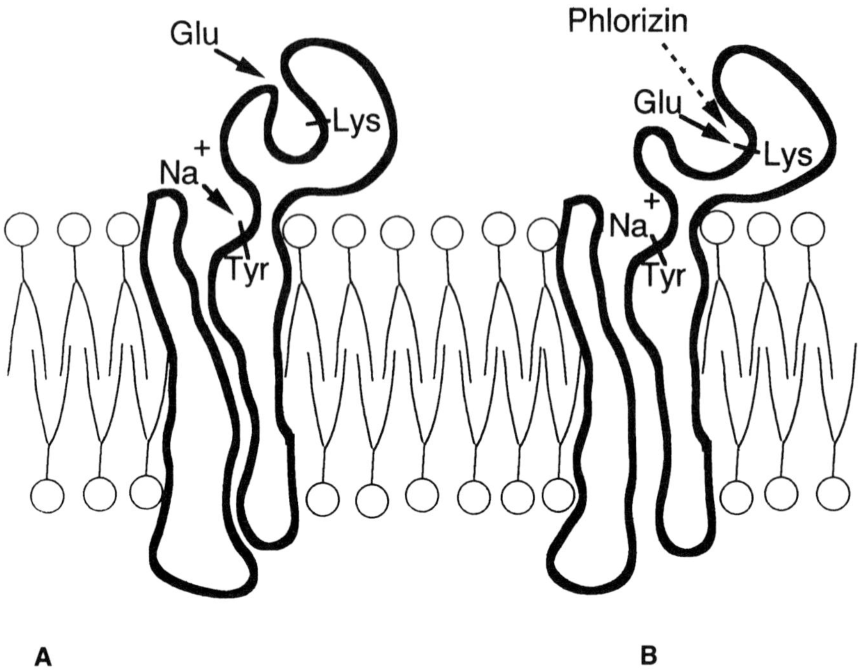

FIGURE 2-8 • Schematic representation of the Na^+-glucose cotransporter. Shown (A) are Na^+ and glucose binding sequentially to the outside of the cell membrane on the transport protein. Na^+ binds first to a site on the transport molecule on or near tyrosine (Tyr) residue. The binding of Na^+ causes a change in the conformation (B), exposing a glucose binding site near a lysine (Lys) residue. The binding of glucose produces a second conformational change that allows the translocation of Na^+ and glucose into the cell across the cell membrane. Phlorizin can compete with glucose for its binding site. The binding of phlorizin does not produce the conformational change necessary to translocate the bound species across the cell membrane. In this way phlorizin acts as an inhibitor of Na^+-glucose cotransport. The conformational shift that produces translocation of glucose and Na^+ into the cell can be reversed in the absence of binding of either species. This behavior is distinctly different from exchangers. The exact location of the binding sites and their relation to the channel through which they travel to reach the opposite side is not known. It is possible that there is more than one binding site for each species. It is also possible that there is one binding site for each species located deep within the pore of the transporter.

change in the protein that exposes the glucose binding site. Glucose then binds on or near a lysyl residue. Glucose binding produces another conformational change, allowing both species to translocate across the cell membrane. The protein can be chemically modified at either the Na^+ or glucose binding site to prevent the binding and subsequent conformational change. Phlorizin, a well-known inhibitor of this transporter, binds to the glucose site but does not produce a conformational change. Like glucose binding, phlorizin binding does not occur unless Na^+ is bound.[29]

Once the Na^+ and glucose are cotransported into the cell, the protein can change its conformation to the outward face ready to bind Na^+ and repeat the cycle. This return of the "unloaded" protein to the outward conformation displays kinetics typical of a carrier. As is the case for the glucose carrier, the rate of entry of Na^+ and glucose is increased as the cell concentration of these species is increased. This "trans activation" behavior implies that the rate-limiting step in the reaction sequence is the return of the unloaded carrier.

Na^+-K^+-$2Cl^-$ cotransport

The discovery of this cotransporter was made possible by the existence of a relatively specific family of inhibitors we now call "loop diuretics." For years, members of this family have been known to exert their diuretic effect on the thick ascending limb of Henle's loop. It was reasonably clear that they produced their action by inhibiting the entry of Cl^- (or NaCl) across the apical membrane. However, the major advance in understanding the molecular nature of the inhibition did not come from the study of kidney cells but, surprisingly, from Ehrlich ascites tumor cells.[10] Geck and coworkers discovered that furosemide inhibited a transporter that translocated four ions simultaneously. Two cations (Na^+ and K^+) are translocated with two Cl^- ions. There is no net charge transfer, and thus the transport is not sensitive to membrane voltage.

From the perspective of the clinician and nephrologist, the most important location for this protein is the apical membrane of epithelial cells of the thick ascending limb of Henle's loop.[12] However, it is quite clear that this transporter is present in a large number of cell types. It is present on the basolateral membrane of many epithelial cells that secrete fluid, such as intestine, trachea, sweat glands, and salivary glands. It is also present on many nonepithelial cells to assist with regulation of cell volume. When cells shrink following exposure to a hypertonic solution, many adapt by activating the Na^+-K^+-$2Cl^-$ cotransporter. This activation causes an increase in cell solute content, thus allowing return of volume to near normal.

Two general features of the Na^+-K^+-$2Cl^-$ cotransporter are important to the understanding of its function. First, the normal concentration gradients for Na^+, K^+, and Cl^- across the cell membrane are such that the net movement favors entry into the cell. The second feature is that the transport process is highly regulated. In many cells, the transporter operates slowly but can rapidly increase its activity in response to cell shrinkage or hormonal stimulation. Recent evidence suggests that part of this regulation is associated with phosphorylation of the transporter.

The detailed understanding of this transporter has proven to be rather difficult. It is not surprising that the kinetics of the system are complex. There appears to be a specific order of binding. Na^+ binds first, a Cl^- ion second, K^+ third, and the second Cl^- last. It seems likely that each successive binding produces a conformational change that permits binding of the next species. Loop diuretics bind to the second Cl^- binding site. This deduction derives from the observation that all three species must be present for the diuretic to bind to the transporter. However, in higher concentrations Cl^- competes with diuretic binding; this biphasic behavior is not seen with Na^+ or K^+.

Loop diuretics are not specific for the Na^+-K^+-$2Cl^-$ cotransporter. Bumetanide and furosemide both inhibit other less complex cotransporters. Although the extent to which these systems are important in the kidney is not clear, these diuretics can inhibit NaCl cotransport and KCl cotransport. There is speculation that these transporters are modifications of the parent Na^+-K^+-$2Cl^-$ transporter. Whether this hypothesis is correct will require information on the primary structure.

There is one *NaCl cotransporter* that is clearly different by pharmacologic criteria. It is present in the apical membrane of epithelial cells of the distal nephron and is not inhibited by bumetanide. (It is only slightly inhibited by furosemide at high concentrations.) This transporter, however, is inhibited by thiazide diuretics.[24] The discovery of this cotransporter and its localization explains the frequently observed additive effects of loop diuretics and thiazide diuretics in patients.

PUMPS

This class of transporter differs from channels, carriers, exchangers, and cotransporters in that pumps translocate ions by using energy derived from the hydrolysis of ATP. In this way, pumps move ions against steep chemical and/or electrical gradients. All pumps have a portion (or subunit) of the molecule devoted to binding and hydrolyzing ATP. Concomitant with ATP hydrolysis, a conformational change occurs, often accompanied by phosphorylation of the protein. The energy from the ATP is transferred to the pump so that subsequent (or prior) binding of the solute will effect a conformational change resulting in translocation to the opposite side of the membrane. Of the best understood pumps, those that are important for renal function are Na^+-K^+ ATPase, Ca^{2+} ATPase, and H^+ ATPase.

Na^+-K^+ ATPase

This protein is one of the best studied transporters in biology. It is present in almost every mammalian cell and is responsible for the generation and maintenance of the Na^+ and K^+ gradients across the cell membrane. Often called the Na^+ pump, its major function is dedicated to the translocation of Na^+ out of, and K^+ into, the cell.[26]

The kinetics of this pump have occupied the imagination of investigators for over 30 years. As depicted in Fig. 2-9, the process appears as a cycle, with the normal direction being in the clockwise direction; the essential features are as follows. One ATP and three Na^+ ions bind to the inside "face" of the pump. ATP is hydrolyzed, the pump is phosphorylated, and the protein changes confor-

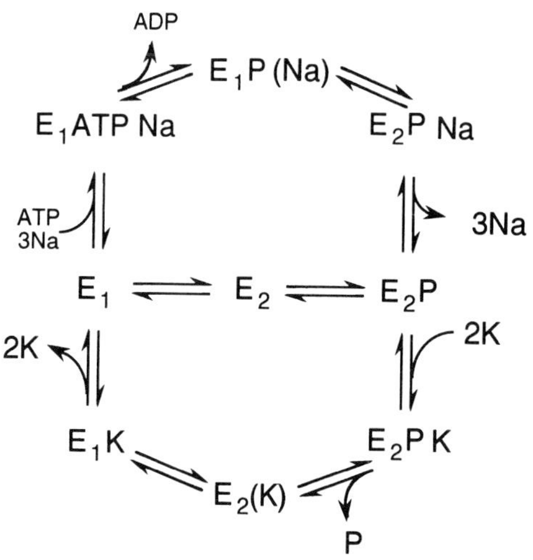

FIGURE 2-9 • Schematic representation of the cycle through which the Na^+-K^+ pump operates. The normal operation of this pump is in the clockwise direction. One ATP molecule and three Na^+ molecules bind to a conformation of the pump called E_1, a designation indicating that the enzyme (Na^+-K^+ ATPase) is in a position to accept molecules from the cytoplasmic side of the membrane. After ATP and Na^+ are bound, ATP is hydrolyzed, and the enzyme is phosphorylated. It then undergoes a series of at least two conformational changes that result in the phosphorylated enzyme releasing Na^+ to the extracellular side of the membrane. The phosphorylated enzyme now exposed to the outside of the cell is designated E_2P and can now bind two K^+ ions. Upon binding K^+, the enzyme is dephosphorylated and undergoes two conformational changes, resulting in the release of K^+ to the cytoplasmic side of the cell membrane. Note that all of the reaction steps are reversible, so that in principle the pump can work backwards and, by so doing, produce ATP. Backwards operation of the Na^+ pump occurs very rarely under normal physiologic circumstances. This pump can also undergo partial cycles (see text).

mation so that Na^+ is able to unbind and leave on the outside "face." This sequence is depicted in the top half of the cycle. The protein does not turn around in the cell membrane but, rather, undergoes a subtle conformational change following phosphorylation. The inside conformation (no Na^+ or ATP bound) is called E_1 and can be identified by a characteristic fluorescence that changes when the conformation shifts to the outside, or E_2, form. This outside conformation permits dissociation of Na^+ ions and acceptance of two K^+ ions. Upon binding K^+, the pump becomes dephosphorylated. The protein then changes its conformation, reverts to the inside (E_1) form and the K^+ ions leave on the inside of the cell. Mg^{2+} is required for several of these partial reactions.[13,23]

Several aspects of the operation of the Na^+-K^+ ATPase pump are general features of pumps. The first feature is that all of the steps are reversible. That the normal process of Na^+ extrusion and hydrolysis of ATP can be reversed has been shown in the squid axon.[5] When the appropriate gradients are imposed, ATP can be generated from ADP and inorganic P. Although such a reversal of the Na^+ pump rarely occurs under physiologic conditions, proton pumps in the mitochondria regularly operate in the "reverse" direction to generate ATP.

The second feature is that there are intermediate states of the cycle where Na^+ or K^+ ions are "occluded." These states are transitional and are represented in Fig. 2-9 by (Na) or (K). They were discovered when investigators working with the pure protein discovered that Na^+ or K^+ tracers could be hidden (or tightly bound), only later to be released. The physical interpretation of these results is that the ions in the transition state are deeply buried in the protein and can only be released by a further conformational change.

The third general feature of this pump is its electrogenic nature. By translocating three Na^+ ions for two K^+ ions, one positive charge is translocated across the membrane for each complete pump cycle. This charge translocation produces an electrical current and is responsible for a portion of the voltage across the cell membrane. It turns out that under most conditions the pump current contributes only ~10 percent to the membrane voltage. However, when the Na^+ concentration in the cell increases, the activity of the pump also increases, and more current is generated. In this way the Na^+-K^+ ATPase can participate in altering membrane voltage.

An interesting exception to this generality about ion pumps being electrogenic is the H^+-K^+ ATPase pump. This pump is found in greatest abundance in the stomach, where it is responsible for acidification of the lumen. It is also found in certain cells of the collecting duct. The stoichiometry appears to be one K^+ exchanged for one H^+, thus rendering the process electroneutral. The H^+-K^+ ATPase and the Na^+-K^+ ATPase pumps are probably genetically related, albeit distantly. Converting a Na^+ binding site to one that binds H^+ ions requires surprisingly few changes in key amino acids.

The fourth feature of the Na^+-K^+ ATPase pump is that it can undergo partial cycles. For example, in the absence of Na^+, one can observe an exchange of K^+ across the membrane. The pathway taken by K^+-K^+ exchange is depicted in the lower portion of the cycle in Fig. 2-9. Na^+-Na^+ exchange can also occur (most clearly observed in the absence of K^+) and takes the path in the upper portion of Fig. 2-9. It is also possible to detect net Na^+ or K^+ transport in the absence of the other ion. This process can occur because the protein can change its conformation from the E_1 form to the E_2 form without any ion binding, a pathway depicted in the middle of Fig. 2-9. Such transformations are detectable only under special conditions and occur relatively rarely. These kinetic features underscore the cyclic nature of the Na^+ pump and illustrate that the requirements for conformational change are not absolute.

There are now considerable data regarding the structure of Na^+-K^+ ATPase. The enzyme has been purified, crystalized, cloned, and sequenced. Figure 2-10 shows a simple schematic of how this protein is thought to aggregate in the cell membrane.[19,26] There are two subunits. The 112-kDa α subunit contains virtually all of the active sites necessary for function of the pump: Na^+ binding, K^+ binding, ATP binding, phosphorylation, and ouabain binding. The β subunit is smaller (~50 kDa), and its function is unclear. In contrast to the α subunit, it is heavily glycosylated and has a major portion of its mass on the extracellular surface. Although there is no known specific function for the β subunit, it is necessary for translocation of Na^+ and K^+ ions.

The primary structure of the Na^+-K^+ ATPase, as shown in Figure 2-10, illustrates two features that are commonly found in membrane transport proteins. One feature is that there are several regions of the protein that contain uncharged (hydrophobic) amino acids that align themselves into α helical structures. These regions insert into and span the cell membrane. The protein α helix is about 0.7 nm in diameter and must be long enough to span the lipid bilayer of the cell membrane, about 48 to 50 nm. These membrane-spanning domains thus must be thirty-two to thirty-three amino acids in length. There are eight such domains in the α subunit but only one in the β subunit of the Na^+-K^+ ATPase pump (Fig. 2-10).

These eight domains of the α subunit arrange themselves in such a way as to form a pore, or channel, through the lipid bilayer. It is through this pore that the Na^+ or K^+ ions pass in the process of being translocated. The ions do not traverse the membrane through a single α helix, since the internal diameter is too small. The precise arrangement of the amino acids lining the pore is probably of critical importance in determining the rate and

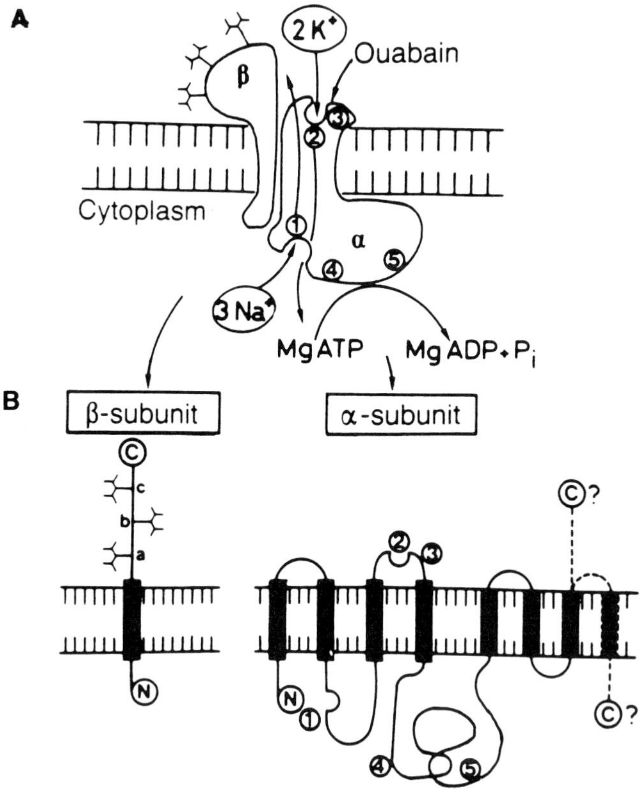

FIGURE 2-10 • Structure of the Na^+-K^+ ATPase. (A) The pump may be an α, β heterodimer. The α subunit contains the binding site for Na^+ (1), the binding site for ATP (4) the phosphorylation site (5), and the binding sites for K^+ (2) and ouabain (3). (B) In the lower panel the α subunit is shown to span the membrane seven to eight times. The β subunit, which is glycosylated in the extracellular domain, spans the membrane only once. The function of the β subunit is not known, but it is necessary for complete function of the Na^+-K^+ ATPase activity. (From Rossier BC et al: *TIBS* 12:483, 1987. Used by permission.)

nature of ions that are translocated. The arrangement of eight α helical peptide chains within the membrane to form a pore is reminiscent of the way in which amphotericin B inserts into cell membranes. It is not surprising, however, that the process of inserting transport proteins at specific locations is exceedingly more complex.

The second structural feature of transport proteins illustrated by the Na^+-K^+ ATPase is the presence of peptide sequences that loop into the cytoplasm or into the extracellular space. Located between membrane-spanning domains, some of the cytoplasmic loops contain domains required for operation or regulation of the transport protein. The cytoplasmic loop between membrane-spanning domains 4 and 5 of the Na^+-K^+ ATPase contains the ATP binding site. Also on this loop is the major phosphorylation site. Although these two sites appear to be some distance from each other in the primary sequence, the tertiary structure almost certainly places them in close proximity.

Other important sites on the cytoplasmic side include the Na^+ binding site, which is present on another cytoplasmic loop. An extracellular loop contains the K^+ binding site and the ouabain (digitalis) binding site. A major area of investigation involves understanding the consequences of modifying or elminating specific sites on transport proteins.

Isoforms of the Na^+-K^+ pump

The cloning and sequencing of the Na^+-K^+ ATPase has revealed that there is more than one type. Not only are there α and β subunits, there are also at least three forms of the α subunit and two forms of the β subunit. Each of these isoforms is the product of a different gene; they are not posttranscriptional or posttranslational modifications of the same gene. It is clear that various organs and tissues express different isoforms and that the levels of expression can change with development of the organ or following hormonal stimulus. The reason that the cell would have such an array of possibilities is not entirely clear. There are indications that the α isoforms function somewhat differently. In the rat, the α_1 isoform has a low affinity for ouabain and a high affinity for Na^+; the α_2 isoform has the opposite properties. These functional differences suggest that the expression of different isoforms is part of an overall program to meet specific needs of cells under different conditions.

The predominant Na^+-K^+ ATPase isoform in the kidney is $\alpha_1\beta_1$; to date, there is no clear evidence that other forms exist. However, the complexity of the kidney and the central importance of the Na^+-K^+ ATPase in its overall function raise the possibility that different isoforms might be distributed in different nephron segments to accomplish specific tasks.

Other ATPases: Ca^{2+} ATPase and H^+ ATPase

These two pumps also play critical roles in the overall operation of cells. Each represents a family of proteins the details of which are only now beginning to emerge. Their physiologic importance should be considered in light of the requirements to generate and maintain steep chemical gradients for Ca^{2+} and H^+.

The free Ca^{2+} concentration in the cell is normally about 100 to 150 n*M*, while free Ca^{2+} in the interstitium is about 1 m*M*. The maintenance of a chemical gradient of 1000:1 is impressive enough; when one considers the effect of the cell membrane voltage of ~60 mV (inside negative) and the fact that Ca^{2+} has two positive charges, the work necessary to keep the cell Ca^{2+} this low becomes even more impressive.

Ca^{2+} pumps are most abundant in muscle cells, where they act to sequester Ca^{2+} in the sarcoplasmic reticulum. They are also important in the distal nephron of the kidney, where their presence on the basolateral membrane provides the energy for transepithelial absorption of Ca^{2+}. The principles of operation are similar to those of the Na^+-K^+ ATPase: Mg^{2+} is necessary, the protein is phosphorylated by ATP, and the translocation of Ca^{2+} produces an electrical current. Its structure consists of multiple membrane-spanning domains and regulatory sites.

Proton pumps are also found in virtually every cell and play a critical role in the maintenance of pH across cell membranes. Like Ca^{2+} ATPase, H^+ ATPase is present in subcellular organelles, such as Golgi membranes and endoplasmic reticulum. One of the major physiologic roles the H^+ ATPase plays in renal function is in the acidification of the urine. The collecting duct contains specialized cells, termed α intercalated cells, that have the H^+ ATPase on their apical membrane (Fig. 11A). These cells play a major role in lowering urine pH.

The maximum chemical gradient for H^+ that can be established by this pump can be readily appreciated by knowing the minimum urinary pH. Most normal subjects can produce a urine with a pH of 4.4. This value is 3 pH units lower than blood. Thus, we can conclude that the H^+ pump can establish a gradient of about 1000:1. As this pump translocates ions and thus generates current, its operation is influenced by the voltage across the cell membrane. The influence of the electrical and chemical gradient has been clearly established in the turtle urinary bladder, an epithelium with a robust H^+ secretory system that functions like the collecting duct. The juxtaposition of H^+-secreting cells with Na^+-absorbing cells creates oppositely directed currents and voltages. Thus, although the process of Na^+ absorption is controlled by

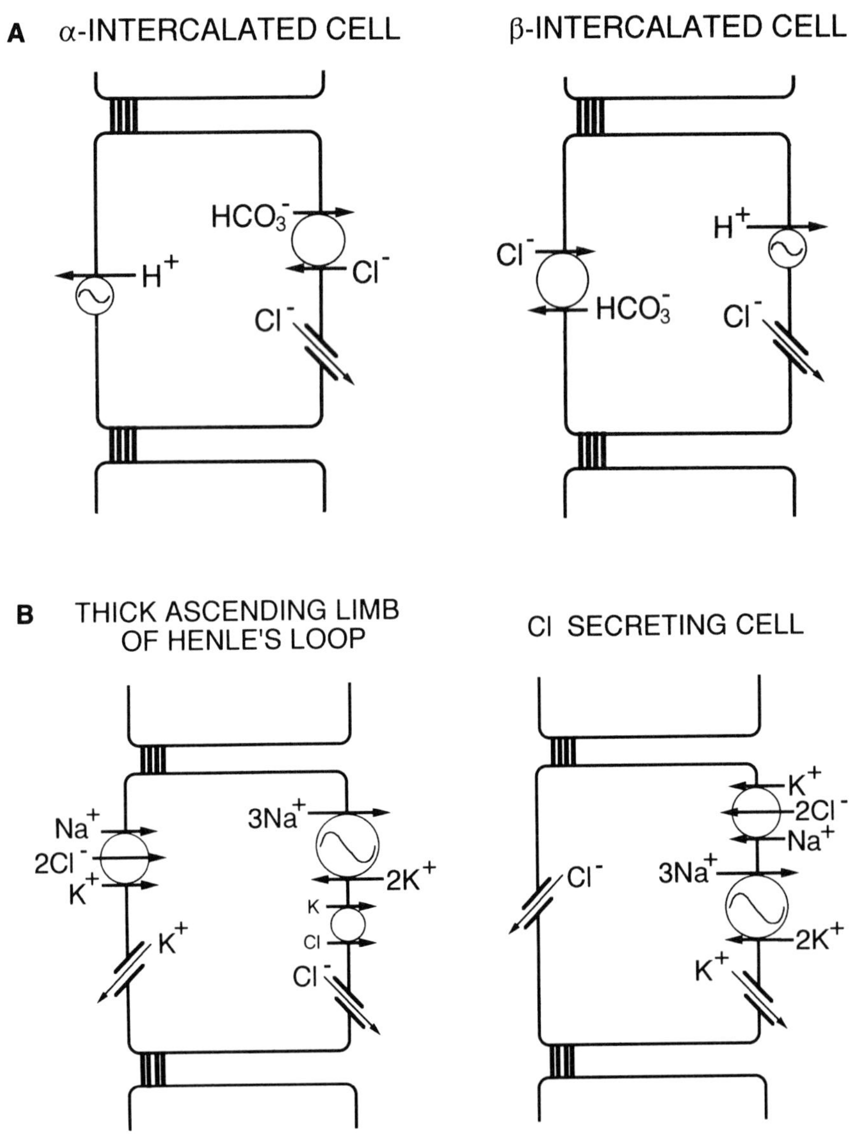

FIGURE 2-11 • Epithelial polarity and the direction of solute transport. (A) Examples of HCO_3^- absorption and secretion by collecting duct intercalated cells. Alpha-intercalated cells secrete H^+ by a pump located on the apical membrane. The HCO_3^- generated by H^+ extrusion exits the basolateral membrane by an anion exchanger. Beta-intercalated cells secrete HCO_3^- across the apical membrane in exchange for Cl^-. The HCO_3^- for secretion is generated by virtue of hydrogen ion extrusion by a H^+ pump located on the basolateral membrane. It is possible that an α-intercalated cell could turn into a β-intercalated cell by exchanging the location of the H^+ pump and the anion exchanger. As attractive as this hypothesis may seem, it is probably incorrect as the anion exchanger and H^+ pumps expressed in the α- and β-intercalated cells appear to be different proteins. (B) Epithelial polarity in Cl^--transporting cells. The thick ascending limb of Henle's loop is a good example of an epithelium that absorbs NaCl using the Na^+-K^+-$2Cl^-$ cotransporter and the Na^+-K^+ pump. Na^+, K^+, and Cl^- enter the cell on the same carrier, and K^+ is recycled back to the lumen via a K^+ channel. Na^+ is pumped out of the cell by the Na^+ pump, and Cl^- exits the cell across the basolateral membrane either via a Cl^- channel or via a KCl cotransporter. Cells that secrete NaCl into the lumen use the same types of transporters. Na^+, K^+, and Cl^- enter the cell across the basolateral membrane, and K^+ recycles to the blood via a K^+ channel. Cl^- leaves the cell across the apical membrane through a Cl^- channel. The Na^+-K^+ pump is located on the basolateral membrane and causes recycling of Na^+. To maintain electroneutrality, Na^+ is transported through the paracellular pathway across the tight junction.

one cell type, the principal cell, the voltage produced by Na^+ transport can influence the rate at which H^+ can be secreted.

INTEGRATED ASPECTS OF EPITHELIAL TRANSPORT

To effect net transport of solute, the epithelial cell must put a transport protein on one membrane that facilitates entry and another transporter on the opposite membrane that facilitates exit. Sometimes the protein responsible for exit is a pump. However, as there are more solutes to be transported than there are pumps to transport them, there obviously has to be some way to utilize the energy established by a pump to move another, unrelated solute. How the proximal tubule cell can move glucose from the lumen to the blood serves as an excellent example of how such systems work.

ACTIVE TRANSPORT

From a thermodynamic perspective, the translocation of glucose from the lumen to the blood requires energy; glucose is transported "against" its chemical gradient. Thus, glucose is *actively transported.* However, there are no transport proteins that hydrolyze ATP to translocate glucose; that is, there are no glucose pumps. The best clue regarding the nature of the source of energy for glucose absorption comes from the observation that when the Na^+-K^+ ATPase is inhibited (with ouabain), glucose transport stops. Clearly, the translocation of glucose across the proximal tubule (or intestinal) cell must be coupled in some way to the transport of Na^+. Figure 2-12 shows how the system works.

Glucose enters the cell across the apical membrane with Na^+ via the Na^+-glucose cotransporter. The gradient for Na^+ entry is sufficiently steep that glucose concentration in the cell can be increased well above its concentration in the lumen. Because the glucose concentration in the cell is higher than in blood, glucose can be transported out of the cell (across the basolateral membrane) using the chemical gradient that was created by virtue of its coupling to the Na^+ gradient on entry. The facilitated glucose carrier is all that is necessary to allow movement of glucose from the cell to the blood.

The Na^+ that enters the cell with glucose is pumped out of the cell by the Na^+-K^+ ATPase on the basolateral membrane. This pump maintains the low cell Na^+ and the gradient for Na^+-glucose entry. The K^+ that enters the cell via the basolateral Na^+-K^+ ATPase recycles across the basolateral membrane. This K^+ exit does not require direct coupling to metabolic energy, since the K^+ concentration in the cell is high. From this scheme,

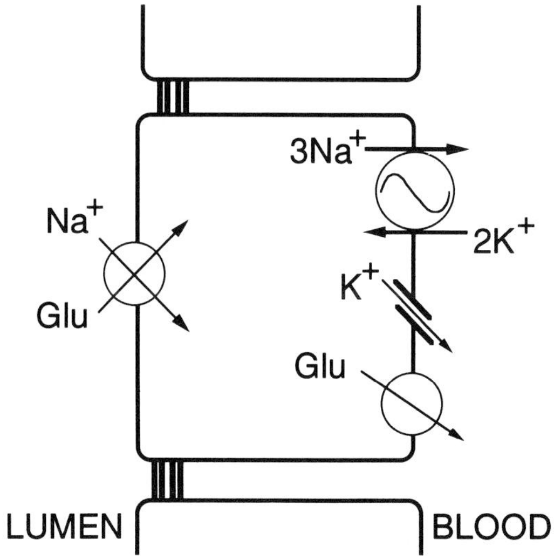

FIGURE 2-12 • Schematic of transepithelial Na^+-glucose cotransport. Examples of primary and secondary active transport. Glucose enters the cell with Na^+ and can reach a concentration in the cell higher than that in the lumen. The energy permitting this elevated concentration of glucose in the cell derives from the electrochemical potential for Na^+ across the apical membrane. Na^+-glucose cotransport is responsive to membrane voltage because of the charge carried by Na^+. The chemical concentration for Na^+ across the membrane is held constant by virtue of the activity of the Na^+-K^+ pump on the basolateral membrane, which keeps cell Na^+ low. Since the Na^+ pump uses energy in the form of ATP, Na^+ transport is considered to be primary active transport. The active transport of Na^+ creates the chemical gradients that, in turn, allow active transport of glucose across the epithelium. Glucose transport is thus secondarily active. In contrast to the entry of glucose across the apical membrane, the exit of glucose across the basolateral membrane is by a glucose carrier. The transport of glucose from the cell to the blood is influenced only by the direction of the chemical gradient for glucose.

one can readily see why inhibiting the Na^+-K^+ ATPase stops active transport of both Na^+ and glucose. Because Na^+ transport is directly coupled to ATP hydrolysis, it is called *primary active transport.* The active transport of glucose, on the other hand, is coupled to Na^+ transport and is therefore called *secondary active transport.*

EPITHELIAL POLARITY

We have seen how net solute transport by epithelial cells requires different transporters on the apical and basolateral membranes. This requirement poses a novel problem for the epithelial cell that other nonpolar cells do not face. The problem is how to get the apical membrane proteins on the apical membrane and not on the basolateral membrane; of course, the same problem exists for the basolateral membrane proteins.

How epithelial cells solve this dilemma of protein sorting is far from clear. There appear to be two general schemes.[22] One scheme would have the synthesized protein contain a peptide sequence that would signal the cell machinery to locate it in the appropriate membrane. Such a signal would be recognized by the trans-Golgi apparatus, which would direct the vesicle containing the protein to the apical or basolateral membrane, as appropriate. The second scheme would not require any particular trans-Golgi sorting but would have newly synthesized proteins inserted into either membrane at random. The polarity would be established by a process of retrieval and redirecting the transport protein to its appropriate location. This redirecting process might also be accompanied by an activating process. It would be counterproductive to insert operational transporters into membranes at random. It is likely that epithelial cell polarity is the product of a combination of these processes operating at different times and to varying degrees.

The complete understanding of the creation and maintenance of epithelial cell polarity will probably take years of intensive investigation. Its applicability to our understanding of normal and abnormal cell function is just beginning to be appreciated. Let us consider three examples.

The first example is that of recovery of an epithelial cell from ischemic injury. As mentioned earlier, ischemia produces dissolution of polarity owing to disruption of the tight junctions and the cytoskeletal system.[17] Recovery of function requires that the cell reestablish polarization. Almost certainly, this process occurs by retrieval of proteins from the "wrong" membrane and reinsertion into the "right" membrane.

The second example involves the possibility that missorting a critical protein is responsible for some specific diseases. One such possibility is polycystic kidney disease. There is now clear evidence that epithelial cells derived from some cysts have Na^+-K^+ ATPase predominantly on the apical membrane, rather than on the basolateral membrane. Such a distribution occurs normally only in the choroid plexus; all other epithelial cells have the Na^+ pump on the basolateral membrane. The process of inappropriate sorting of the Na^+ pump in polycystic kidneys seems to be a real phenomenon. Whether this process is a primary problem causing cyst formation or secondary to the production of some types of cysts remains to be determined.

The third example of the importance of protein sorting in epithelial cell polarity can be seen using comparative physiology; some epithelial cells absorb (move solute from lumen to blood) while others secrete (move solute from blood to lumen). Within the collecting duct there are cells that absorb HCO_3^-, while their neighbors secrete HCO_3^-. The current models for how this process occurs are depicted in Fig. 2-11A. Alpha-intercalated cells absorb HCO_3^- by secreting H^+ into the lumen, a process dependent on a functioning H^+ ATPase in the apical membrane. The translocation of a H^+ into the lumen leaves a OH^- behind, which (in the presence of carbonic anhydrase) rapidly combines with CO_2 gas to produce a HCO_3^-. The buildup of HCO_3^- in the cell creates a favorable chemical gradient for its exit across the basolateral membrane. The mechanism for this exit step happens to be via a Cl^--HCO_3^- exchanger, a transport protein related to the red blood cell anion exchanger. The Cl^- that enters the cell in exchange for HCO_3^- recycles across the basolateral membrane through a Cl^- channel.

In contrast to the α-intercalated cell, the β-intercalated cell secretes HCO_3^-. As shown in Fig. 2-11A, the apical membrane contains the anion exchanger, and the basolateral membrane contains the H^+ ATPase. The Cl^- channel is located on the basolateral membrane of both cell types. It is obvious that an α cell could be converted to a β cell "simply" by reversing the location of the H^+ ATPase and the anion exchanger. The importance of protein sorting becomes clear from this simple example.

This example oversimplifies the process of epithelial polarity in acid-transporting cells. It may be attractive to speculate that one type of cell could convert to another by rearranging its anion exchangers and H^+ ATPases; however, there is reason to be believe that it does not happen that way. The two anion exchangers are immunologically different, and conversion of a population of one type of cell to the other has not been unambiguously demonstrated.[21] Nevertheless, this example demonstrates the principle that cells can take existing transporters and arrange them in such a way as to either secrete or absorb, depending on the requirements of the organ.

Another example of arranging transporters is shown in Fig. 2-11B. These epithelia represent the thick ascending limb of Henle's loop as the epithelium that absorbs NaCl. The secreting epithelium could be intestine, trachea, or one of several other secretory epithelia. In this example, the Na^+-K^+ ATPase stays on the basolateral membrane, while the entry pathway, the Na^+-K^+-$2Cl^-$ cotransporter, and the exit pathways—the Cl^- and K^+ channels—insert on opposite membranes. In contrast to the intercalated cells, there is no hint that one cell type could convert to the other. Whether the seemingly identical individual transport molecules are from the same gene will not be known until the proteins are cloned and sequenced.

REGULATION OF EPITHELIAL TRANSPORT

The process of how epithelial cells regulate their solute transport is a subject worthy of many chapters. A complete review of the subject is beyond the scope of this chapter, but there are four general methods whereby the rate of solute transport can be altered. Three of these regulatory processes occur rapidly; the fourth category occurs over hours or days. The rapidly acting system can be divided into kinetic factors, endocytosis and exocytosis, and second messengers.

RAPIDLY ACTING FACTORS

Kinetic factors involve the process of increasing or decreasing the transport rate by changing the solute concentration. The example of Na^+-glucose cotransport (Fig. 2-12) illustrates the principles. As Na^+ and glucose enter the cell together, their intracellular concentrations increase, and the amount of solute available to exit across the basloateral membrane increases. Any maneuver that increases the entry of Na^+ into the cell will increase the rate of Na^+ extrusion by the Na^+-K^+ ATPase by this kinetic mechanism. This example also demonstrates that the entry of Na^+ is dependent on the concentration of glucose in the lumen. In the proximal tubule, the lumen glucose concentration falls as a function of the distance from the glomerulus. If the filtration rate increases, the length of proximal tubule exposed to luminal glucose increases, and thus Na^+ absorption is increased. This principle is one reason that proximal tubular absorption exhibits flow dependency.

The process of *endocytosis and exocytosis* as a regulatory phenomenon for transport is best understood for H^+ secretion and for vasopressin-sensitive water flow. In the resting state, where only low rates of transport are needed, transporters that might be in the apical membrane are actually sequestered in vesicles just below the surface. Upon appropriate stimulation, the subapical vesicles are inserted into the apical membrane, where they fuse to expose the transport proteins to the lumen. The increase in the number of available transporters increases the rate at which the molecule of interest can be transported. A stimulus for the insertion of vesicles containing H^+ ATPase is cell acidification; a stimulus for the insertion of vesicles containing water channels is vasopressin via the generation of cyclic AMP. Exocytosis requires the integrated action of the cytoskeleton. An important feature of this type of regulation is that stimuli activate both exocytosis and endocytosis so that the cycling of vesicles increases. Withdrawal of the stimulus reduces the exocytosis so that the vesicles reside in a quiescent state beneath the apical membrane ready for the next stimulus.

The largest and most diverse category of transport regulation involves the action of *second messengers*. The full range of second messengers has been implicated. Calcium can directly affect ion channel activity; cyclic AMP and cyclic GMP can directly regulate transporters or, more commonly, activate protein kinases that modify transporters. Second messengers can also alter cell pH and render the transporter more or less sensitive to regulation by other agents. An important feature of regulation by second messengers is that many phenomena involve the concordant regulation of both apical and basolateral transporters. For example, when a stimulus arrives to an epithelial cell causing the entry of Na^+ across the apical membrane to increase, the resulting increase in cell Na^+ will increase Na^+-K^+ ATPase activity by a kinetic effect. However, if the cell Na^+ increases too much, another set of mechanisms interact to decrease the entry of Na^+. The mechanisms used by the cell to maintain a nearly constant intracellular environment are not well understood. It is clear, however, that major changes in cell content do not normally occur despite large variations in the rate of net transport.

The final category of transport regulation is brought about by the need for *long-term adaptation*. The best-studied process is that of aldosterone's stimulation of Na^+ absorption by the collecting duct. Aldosterone, like most steroid hormones, produces its major effects by inducing or increasing the production of proteins. A model of the cell on which aldosterone produces its effect is diagramed in Fig. 2-13. The increased Na^+ transport is accompanied by an increase in three processes, all of which are critical to sustain enhanced rates.[9] One of the first events to occur is an increase in the apical membrane Na^+ permeability. Aldosterone induces a protein that increases the number of functioning Na^+ channels. The channels are already in the membrane but are not capable of being activated. The increased transport is also accom-

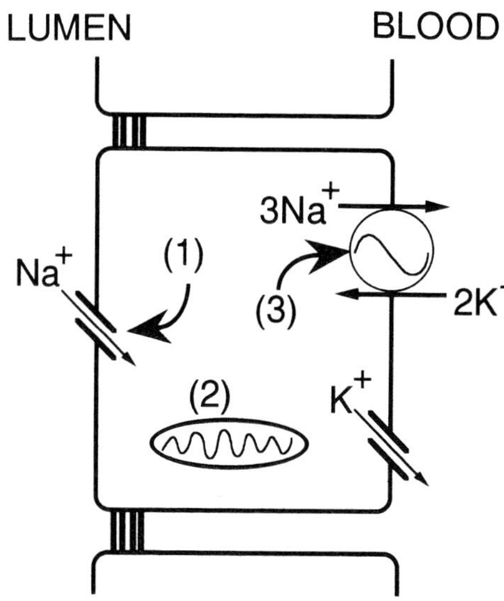

FIGURE 2-13 • Actions of aldosterone on Na^+ transport. Aldosterone produces at least three effects on collecting duct epithelial cells and other cells that are mineralocorticoid-hormone-responsive. Most mineralocorticoid-responsive tissues have electrogenic Na^+ transport, as modeled by this cell. Aldosterone (1) increases the permeability of Na^+ across the apical membrane by causing activation of Na^+ channels; (2) increases the metabolic rate and therefore ATP production by mitochondria; and (3) increases the number of Na^+-K^+ pumps on the basolateral membrane so that the increased entry of Na^+ across the apical membrane can be more effectively pumped out to the blood. Aldosterone may also increase K^+ permeability, which in this model is shown on the basolateral membrane. In the cortical collecting duct, K^+ channels are present in the apical membrane.

panied by an increased synthesis of Na^+-K^+ ATPase and an increase in their activation or insertion into the basolateral membrane. Finally, aldosterone increases the metabolic capacity of the cell. In concert, these three actions of aldosterone serve to produce a sustained increase in the ability to absorb Na^+.

BASIC TRANSPORT PROCESSES

The focus of the discussion thus far has been on the delineation of the bits and pieces of the epithelium and the pathways involved in transport. The description has been qualitative and the explanations largely intuitive. One of the features of transport physiology that has attracted the attention of many (while discouraging others) is the ability to apply quantitative physical principals. The fundamental theoretical work of Einstein, Onsager, Teorell, and others has provided the framework whereby investigators can compare the transport properties of epithelia to the predictions made from simple, nonbiological systems. Differences in performance between epithelia and inert membranes have provided powerful insights into the mechanisms of solute and water transport.

The most important of these basic processes are *diffusive flow* and *convective flow*. We will first consider diffusion. Flow produced by diffusion results from brownian motion of solute in the presence of a driving force. The net flow or flux across a membrane is best understood in the formulation of Teorell,[27] where

$$\text{Flux} = \text{permeability} \times \text{concentration} \times \text{driving force} \quad (1)$$

Thus, the net movement is directly proportional to three parameters. The permeability of a solute is related to many factors and is an intrinsic property of the membrane. It cannot be measured directly but must always be calculated. It is often useful to think of permeability as analagous to the electrical conductance of a wire. Conductance (G), the reciprocal of resistance (ρ), is related to the force (voltage, E) and the flow (current, I) by the familiar relationship $E = I\rho$. Rearranged,

$$I = GE \quad (2)$$

The similarities between the permeability of a membrane and the conductivity of a wire are that they both must be calculated by measuring (or imposing) a force and a flow. The permeability of a membrane for a solute is related to the amount of solute able to interact with or partition into the membrane.

The force acting on a solute across a membrane consists of three components: chemical, electrical, and hydrostatic. This force ($\tilde{\mu}$) varies with distance within the membrane and is therefore expressed as a differential equation:

$$\frac{d\tilde{\mu}_i}{dx} = RT\frac{d\ln C_i}{dx} + z_iF\frac{d\psi}{dx} + \overline{V}_i\frac{dp}{dx} \quad (3)$$

where $d\tilde{\mu}_i/dx$ is the force on solute i, and the three components indicate the respective chemical, electrical, and hydrostatic components. R, F, and V are constants and are given in Table 2-3. C_i is the concentration of i, ψ is the electrical potential difference (voltage) across the membrane, p is the hydrostatic pressure, x is the thickness of the membrane, T is the absolute temperature (K), and z is the valence of the ion. This differential equation has practical utility only if one knows the exact profile of the concentration and electrical gradients within the membrane. Because such information is seldom available, one can assume linear changes and thus approximate the electrochemical potential by

$$\Delta\tilde{\mu} = RT\Delta\ln C_i + z_iF\Delta\psi + \overline{V}_i\Delta P \quad (4)$$

Now we can calculate the forces involved for a physiologically relevant situation. Figure 2-14 depicts a chamber with two compartments separated by a membrane that is permeable only to K^+. The chamber is also equipped with a voltage clamp so that we can set the membrane voltage to any value we wish. We now fill the left side with a 100 m*M* KCl solution and the right side with a 10 m*M* KCl solution. It is obvious that the chemical gradient will favor movement of K^+ from left to right. The actual chemical force (calculated from equation 4) is 5800 J/mol. One can appreciate this value if we

TABLE 2-3 • Constants and conversion factors

R	=	universal gas constant
	=	82.06 cm^3 atm/mol K
	=	8.31 J/mol K
	=	1.98 cal/mol K
	=	8.3 × 10^7 dyn cm/mol K
F	=	Faraday
	=	96,500 C/mol
$\overline{V}_w$	=	partial molar volume of water
	=	~18 cm^3/mol
$\overline{V}_{Na}$	=	partial molar volume Na
	=	~24 cm^3/mol
$\overline{V}_K$	=	partial molar volume of K
	=	~39 cm^3/mol
Coulomb (C)	=	ampere second (As)
Volt (V)	=	J/C
Farad	=	C/V
Atm	=	760 mmHg
	=	1030 cmH_2O
	=	10^6 dyn/cm^2
	=	0.10 J/cm^3

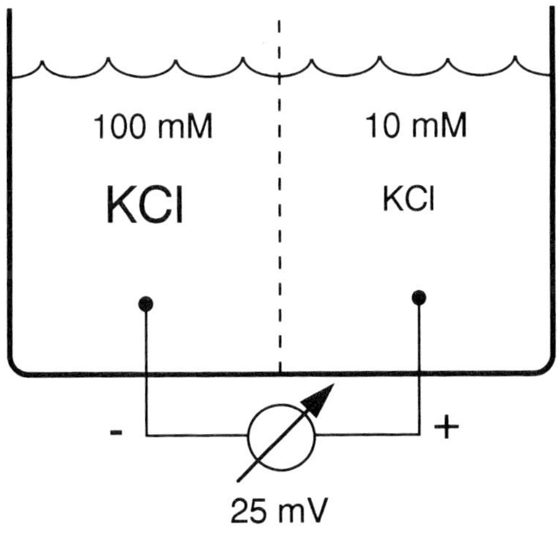

FIGURE 2-14 • Chamber containing two solutions of different concentrations of KCl separated by a membrane that is permeable only to K^+ and not to Cl^-. The chamber is also equipped with a voltage clamp that can set the voltage across the membrane to any desired value. The chemical gradient for K^+ is equivalent to about 59 mV, and, when the voltage across the membrane is set to 25 mV (right side positive), that voltage opposes the flow of K^+ from left to right down its chemical gradient. Because the chemical gradient is larger than the voltage gradient opposing it, there will be net flow of K^+ from left to right.

divide by Faraday's constant and express it as 59 mV. The 25 mV we imposed across the membrane is oppositely directed and is equal to 2400 J/mol. From the sum of the electrical and the chemical gradients, the net force on K^+ would be 3400 J/mol, favoring flow of K^+ from left to right.

The influence of pressure can be appreciated if we now impose 100 mmHg on the left side. The force on K^+ from this amount of hydrostatic pressure is only 0.4 J/mol. From these calculations, one can see that the driving forces for diffusional solute flow are dominated by electrical and chemical factors. Pressure has an insignificant effect. Such a statement is not true for the hydrostatic effects on water flow. We shall return to this special condition later.

EXPRESSIONS OF FLUX

Now that we have seen how chemical and electrical forces are expressed, we can begin to incorporate them into equations describing flux across a membrane. From equation 1 we can write

$$J_i = -\omega_i C_i\left(RT\frac{d\ln C_i}{dx} + z_i F\frac{d\psi}{dx}\right) \quad (5)$$

where J_i is the flux of solute i, ω_i the mobility of the solute in the membrane, C_i the concentration of i, and the expression in parentheses is the electrochemical force. The sign convention indicates that the flux occurs in the direction of the force. We now rearrange the equation to incorporate C_i into the force term. Recalling that $d\ln C_i = dC_i/C_i$, the expression becomes

$$J_i = -P_i\frac{dC_i}{dx} + \frac{C_i zF}{RT}\frac{d\psi}{dx} \quad (6)$$

where P_i is the permeability and is proportional to $\omega_i RT$. This expression is the famous Nernst-Planck equation and indicates that the flow of i is linearly related to both the concentration gradient and the electrical gradient.

Two important principals become apparent from this relationship when one simplifies the conditions. The first condition occurs if the solute is a nonelectrolyte, such as urea or glucose. In such a case, $z = 0$, and the expression reduces to

$$J_i = -P_i\frac{dC_i}{dx} \quad (7)$$

which is Fick's first law of diffusion applied to diffusion across a membrane.

The second condition occurs when the system is at equilibrium. By definition, equilibrium exists when $d\tilde{\mu}_i/dx = 0$. In such a case, equation 3 (neglecting the hydrostatic pressure term) reduces to

$$\Delta\psi = \psi_2 - \psi_1 = \frac{-RT}{zF}\ln\frac{C_2}{C_1} \quad (8)$$

where the subscripts refer to the two sides of the membrane. This expression requires integration of equation 3 and assumes that the chemical and electrical gradients across the membrane are linear. Such an assumption has never been proven, but the expressions resulting from this assumption have been extremely useful in dissecting diffusional from non-diffusional flows.

Equation 8 is the famous Nernst equation and relates the electrical force to the chemical force under conditions of equilibrium. From the example in Fig. 2-14 we see that a tenfold concentration gradient will produce 59 mV.

Integration of the Nernst-Planck Equation

In its differential form, equation 3 has limited practical utility. The experimentalist usually wants to make measurements in order to calculate permeability. In order to do so, one must make certain assumptions about the shape of the electrical and chemical gradients across the membrane. The Nernst equation (equation 8) assumes linear gradients at equilibrium conditions. Goldman[11] derived a particularly useful form assuming a linear electrical gradient:

$$J_i = \frac{-zF\, P_i\Delta\psi}{RT}\left[\frac{(C_2 - C_1\xi)}{1-\xi}\right] \quad (9)$$

where $\xi = \exp(-zF\Delta\psi/RT)$. This expression relates the flow of i to the permeability of the membrane to i, the voltage across the membrane, and the concentration of i on both sides. (Note that ξ is only a function of voltage.)

Another useful integration of the Nernst-Planck equation is derived for a system where there is no external current source; that is, there are no pumps in the membrane. For the situation where only Na^+, K^+, and Cl^- are present in the solutions, the voltage across the membrane is

$$\Delta\psi = \frac{-RT}{zF}\ln\left[\frac{P_K[K]_2 + P_{Na}[Na]_2 + P_{Cl}[Cl]_1}{P_K[K]_1 + P_{Na}[Na]_1 + P_{Cl}[Cl]_2}\right] \quad (10)$$

where P is the permeability of the membrane to the ion indicated by the subscript, and subscripts 1 and 2 represent the two sides of the membrane. It is important to note that if the permeability to an ion is 0, the concentration of the impermeant species has no bearing on the voltage across the membrane. In the case where there is only one permeant species, the expression reduces to the Nernst equation (equation 8).

Let us now consider what happens to our solution containing 100 mM KCl on one side and 10 mM KCl on the other. Let us take away the voltage clamp but keep the membrane that is only permeable to K^+. The situation is illustrated in Fig. 2-15, where one can see that K^+ will have a tendency to flow from left to right down its concentration gradient. At equilibrium, the voltage across the membrane will be 59 mV, with the right side positive with respect to the left. There is no net flow of either K^+ or Cl^-. The voltage is developed by virtue of the fact that a few K^+ ions cross the membrane and produce a separation of positive and negative charges. This separation, which produces an unmeasurable change in ion concentration, generates the voltage which opposes further flow of K^+ ions.

If we were to make the membrane equally permeable to K^+ and Cl^-, there would be no charge separation and no voltage generated. If Cl^- permeability were half that of K^+, the tendency for K^+ to diffuse faster than Cl^- would produce a voltage that could be calculated from equation 10. This voltage would be positive on the right and would produce opposite effects on the flow of K^+ and Cl^-. K^+ flux would be opposed by the voltage, and Cl^- flux would be enhanced. The net flux of K^+ and Cl^- would be the same so that eventually an equilibrium would be achieved where $\Delta\psi = 0$.

These principles provide the major explanation for the origin of the cell membrane voltage. A small fraction of the voltage is produced by the Na^+-K^+ ATPase as it extrudes Na^+. However, the majority of the voltage results from the K^+ concentration gradient produced by the Na^+-K^+ ATPase. As might be deduced from the situation in Fig. 2-15, most cell membranes are highly permeable to K^+ and substantially less to Cl^- or Na^+. Because of this situation, cell K^+ concentration is often close to electrochemical equilibrium.

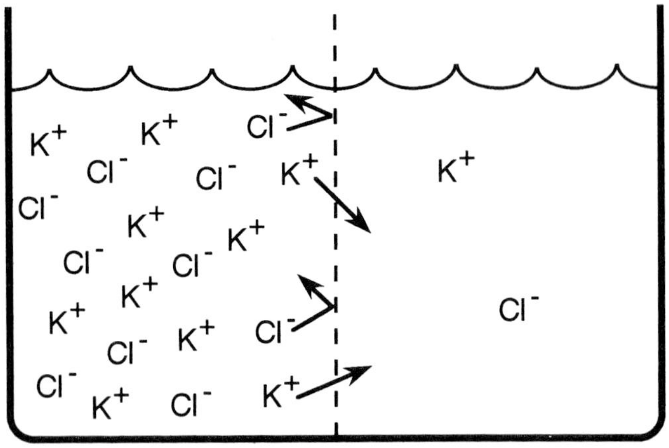

FIGURE 2-15 • Generation of a membrane potential. The situation in this figure is the same as for Figure 2-14, with 100 m*M* KCl in the left side of the chamber and 10 m*M* KCl on the right side of the chamber, separated by a membrane permeable only to K^+. In this example, we take away the voltage clamp. Almost immediately upon adding the KCl, K^+ tends to *diffuse* across the membrane from left to right. After very few of K^+ ions cross the semipermeable membrane, a voltage of sufficient magnitude is generated, which then prevents the further diffusion of K^+ ions. Therefore, a voltage across the membrane of 59 mV will be rapidly achieved well before any changes in K^+ concentrations can be measured. It is the separation of charge between K^+ and Cl^- ions that is responsible for generating this voltage. If one were to replace this membrane with one that had equal permeabilities to K^+ and Cl^-, there would be no membrane voltage generated because there would be no separation of charge between K^+ and Cl^- ions. This principle is used by cells to generate their membrane voltage. Cell membranes are, in general, highly permeable to K^+ and poorly permeable to other ions.

Let us consider one final comment about the relationship between cell membrane permeability and voltage. The ion concentration gradient will influence and be influenced by the membrane voltage only if its mode of permeation is conductive. In practical terms, the flux of an ion will be affected by voltage if it permeates via channels but not if its mode of transport is via electroneutral exchangers or cotransporters.

WATER FLOW

The diffusion of a solute across a membrane can be described quantitatively by the above formulas largely because physiologic solutions are sufficiently dilute that the solutes behave much the same as ideal gases. The formulas developed for the behavior of gases have thus been directly applied to the behavior of dilute solutions. However, water presents a different set of challenges. For example, the concentration of water in physiologic solutions is near 55.5 M.

The movement of water across a cell membrane can proceed via two types of routes. Because water can dissolve in and thus permeate through lipid (Table 2-2), water can move across cell membranes by diffusion. It can also cross cell membranes via specific channels.[28] The high mole fraction of water (compared to solutes) permits pressure to play an important role as a driving force for water flow. The expression describing this relationship is

$$J_v = -L_p \Delta P \qquad (11)$$

where J_v is the flow of water (volume), L_p is the hydraulic conductivity of the membrane (analogous to permeability), and ΔP is the pressure gradient. The driving force, pressure, can take one of two forms: hydrostatic or osmotic. Hydrostatic pressure is largely responsible for the movement of water across the glomerular basement membrane. Osmotic pressure, one form of which is oncotic pressure, is the pressure exerted across a membrane when there is a concentration difference across that membrane.

The amount of pressure exerted by an osmotic gradient ($\Delta\pi$) was developed by van't Hoff and is expressed

$$\Delta\pi = RT\Delta C_s \qquad (12)$$

where ΔC_s is the difference in osmolality. This expression is true for a membrane that is permeable to water but not solute. An example would be a lipid bilayer with a NaCl concentration gradient (Table 2-2). In this case, 1 mosm of pressure produces 19 mmHg of pressure. It is often surprising to realize that a 5-mosm difference will produce the pressure equivalent to the normal mean blood pressure. Because hydrostatic and osmotic pressures are indistinguishable (by cell membranes), we can write equation 11 as

$$J_v = -L_p(\Delta p + \Delta\pi) \qquad (13)$$

This relationship was first formulated by Starling, who noted the opposing nature of the hydrostatic and osmotic (oncotic) forces in blood vessels.

Despite the equivalence of the hydrostatic and osmotic forces, in many epithelia and membranes an osmotic gradient does not produce the same amount of water flow that is produced by a hydrostatic pressure gradient. The reason for this discrepancy is that not all membranes are impermeant to the solute producing the osmotic gradient. To understand this phenomenon, we need to understand the process of convective flow.

COUPLING OF SOLUTE AND WATER FLOW

Convective flow is the process whereby solute can be transported as a result of water flow. We know that glucose is transported along blood vessels, but we also know that the force responsible for that flow is not a concentration gradient. Rather, glucose (and all other solutes) is carried along with the flow of water that is driven by pressure. Other examples of convective flow are the ultrafiltration of solutes across a glomerular basement membrane or across a dialysis membrane. There is no difference in glucose, urea, and small ion concentration between the blood and the fluid in the earliest portion of the proximal tubule; therefore, we know that the permeability of the glomerulus to those solutes is high. Thus, small solutes not bound to albumin are completely *entrained* by the water flow. This convective flow is expressed as follows:

$$J_i^{\text{conv}} = C_i J_v \qquad (14)$$

where C_i is the concentration of solute i in the blood.

If, on the other hand, we take a membrane that is permeable to water and not to solutes, we would get no convective flow. An example of this situation is the "reverse osmosis" process often used in water purification systems in dialysis units. Clearly, in this condition, equation 14 does not describe the magnitude of the convective flow. To correct this problem, we can introduce a term that will indicate the extent to which a solute will be entrained in the water flow. It is called the *sieving coefficient* and is usually symbolized by $(1-\sigma)$. Equation 14 thus becomes

$$J_i^{\text{conv}} = (1-\sigma)C_i J_v \qquad (15)$$

The value of the sieving coefficient is between 0 and 1. The σ term is called the *reflection coefficient* and indicates the extent to which a solute acts as an ideal osmotic agent. In the example given in Fig. 2-16, the membrane with a sieving coefficient of 1 (example A) would have a reflection coefficient of 0; the membrane (example B) that allows no solute to permeate would have a sieving coefficient of 0 and a reflection coefficient of 1. The point is that solutes that are highly permeable exert little or no osmotic force.

A clinically useful example of this principal is the effect of urea or ethanol on osmotic water flow across cell membranes. Patients with high plasma concentrations of urea or ethanol will have plasma osmolalities 20 to 40 mosm or more above normal. However, their cell water is normal, indicating that there has been no effective osmotic pressure across the cell membrane. In contrast, diabetics with hyperglycemia may have substantial shifts in cell water despite measured plasma osmolalities of less than 20 mosm above normal. The clinical manifestation of this shift in water is hyponatremia. The major difference in the action of these solutes on water flow can be attributed to differences in their reflection coefficient.

MEDIATED SOLUTE TRANSPORT

Until now, our discussion of transport mechanisms has focused on diffusion and convection. However, most transport across cell membranes does not occur by these relatively simple processes. Rather, most solutes have

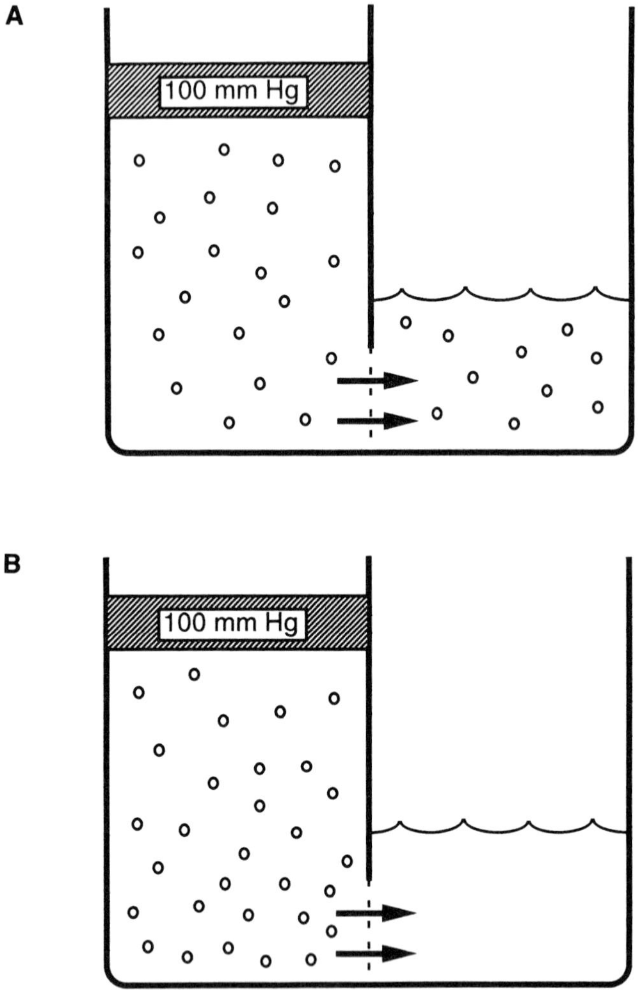

FIGURE 2-16 • Example of how the sieving coefficient affects solute flow. (A) A chamber in which one can apply hydrostatic pressure to one of two compartments that are separated by a membrane (indicated by the dashed line). This membrane is a nonselective membrane (such as cellophane) that does not discriminate between the passage of water and solutes. After filling the left side of the chamber with the solution and applying pressure, the right side of the chamber begins to fill with the solution, the composition of which is identical to the original solution. The sieving coefficient of this membrane is therefore 1 (on a scale of 0 to 1). (B) We now repeat the experiment with a membrane that is permeable to water but impermeable to the solute. After applying pressure for the same amount of time, one gets the same amount of water in the right-hand chamber but no solute. The solute becomes concentrated in the left-hand chamber. The sieving coefficient of this membrane is 0. This kind of membrane is used in "reverse osmosis" water purification systems. A solute applied to one side of a membrane in example B would be able to exert an osmotic pressure because the solute is impermeable. Solutes would not be able to exert an osmotic pressure across the membrane in example A because they are so highly permeable.

some interaction with the cell membrane usually with a protein molecule. Examples of channels, carriers, cotransporters, and exchangers were discussed in the earlier part of this chapter. The quantitative description of these processes is somewhat more complicated than is the case for diffusion, but we can make a straightforward example for a nonionized solute.

Let us consider a situation where a cellophane membrane separates two compartments, both of which contain water. Now we add glucose to one side and measure the appearance of glucose on the opposite side. The flux of glucose (J_{glu}) is given by the simple expression

$$J_{glu} = P \times [glu] \qquad (16)$$

where P is the permeability of the membrane to glucose and is independent of concentration. This expression is a simplification of equation 7 and is the same for an ion if there is no voltage across the membrane. However, if the mechanism of transport is by a carrier and not by diffusion, the magnitude of flux can usually be described by the following expression:

$$J_{glu} = \frac{J_{glu}^{max} \times [glu]}{K_m + [glu]} \qquad (17)$$

where we introduce two constants. J^{max} is the maximum rate of transport possible when the concentration is infinitely high. K_m is the concentration of glucose at which transport is half maximal. Figure 2-17 displays the characteristic changes in flux as a function of concentration for both diffusion and for carrier mediated transport. The values for J^{max} and K_m are depicted on the curve representing carrier-mediated flux.

Across an intact epithelium both mechanisms are usually present: solutes traverse the paracellular path-

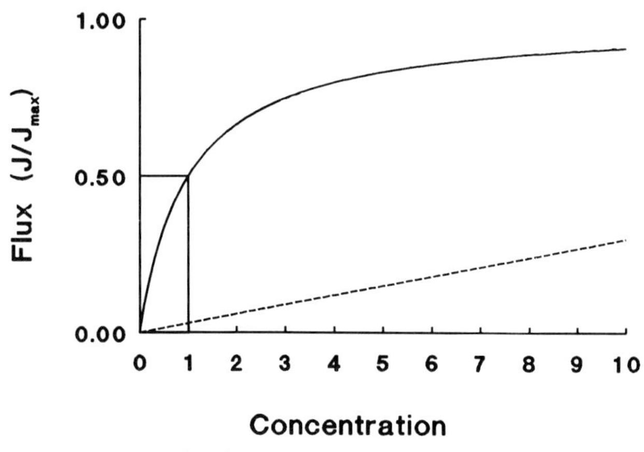

FIGURE 2-17 • Solute flux as a function of concentration. The dashed line represents the flux of a solute across a membrane if the transport is only by simple diffusion. As the concentration on one side of the membrane increases, the flux increases linearly. The solid line represents the flux of the solute as a function of concentration if the mechanism of permeation is by a carrier-mediated process. This process is usually well described by Michaelis-Menten kinetics, which includes a term (J_{max}) indicating the maximum rate of transport at an infinitely high concentration. In addition, there is a term indicating the concentration at which the rate of transport is half maximal. This concentration is called the K_m and in this example is equal to 1. The units for the K_m are units of concentration. The J_{max} in this example is also equal to 1. The units for J_{max} are the units of flux.

way by diffusion and the cellular pathway by a carrier-mediated pathway. The actual measured flux is thus the sum of the values for any concentration. It is important to note that a solute can traverse a membrane via a channel and display kinetic behavior like that of a carrier. Cotransporters, exchangers, and pumps can exhibit similar behavior but the shape of the curve is usually different. For example, the rate of glucose transport by the Na^+-glucose cotransporter takes the form

$$J_{glu} = \frac{J^{max}_{glu} \times [glu]}{K_G\left(1 + \frac{K_{Na}}{[Na]}\right) + [glu]} \quad (18)$$

where K_G is the K_m for glucose and K_{Na} is the K_m for Na^+. It is obvious that the concentration of Na^+ will have an important effect on the shape of the relationship of glucose concentration to its flux.

For a transporter that binds more than one ion and species, the relationship is somewhat more complex. An example is the description of the rate of Na^+ transport by the Na^+-K^+ ATPase where

$$J_{Na} = \frac{J^{max}_{Na}}{\left[1 + \frac{K_K}{[K]}\right]^2 \left[1 + \frac{K_{Na}}{[Na]}\right]^3} \quad (19)$$

and K_K and K_{Na} are the respective K_m values for K^+ and Na^+. Note that the terms in the denominator are raised to the power reflecting the number of ions translocated.

ACTIVE TRANSPORT

The decision as to whether a solute crosses a membrane because of a favorable electrochemical gradient or whether another energy source must be implicated is not always simple. For the case of collecting duct Na^+ absorption, the situation is straightforward. The concentration of Na^+ in the lumen can be much lower than blood; therefore, Na^+ is transported against a chemical gradient. Furthermore, the voltage across the cortical collecting duct is negative (lumen with respect to blood). This situation provides an unambiguous example of active transport. The case for the collecting duct is even clearer because we know that Na^+ is transported across the basolateral membrane by the Na^+-K^+ ATPase. Thus, Na^+ transport is via primary active transport.

The distinction between primary and secondary active transport became the focus of considerable discussion when it was discovered that the thick ascending limb of Henle's loop asborbed NaCl against a chemical gradient but that the voltage across the epithelium was lumen positive, not lumen negative, as is the case for most epithelia absorbing Na actively. Furthermore, both the NaCl absorption and the voltage were completely inhibited by ouabain, a specific inhibitor of the Na^+-K^+ ATPase. Clearly Cl^- was absorbed actively because it was transported against an electrochemical gradient. However, as shown in Fig. 2-11B, Cl^- transport is secondarily active because it is dependent on the Na^+-K^+ ATPase. The demonstration that Na^+ transport is active is not so obvious as for Cl^- because, while it is transported against its chemical gradient, it is transported down its electrical gradient. The understanding of whether or not there is active transport is a critical point in further understanding of the specific transport pathways.

One of the most useful tests of active or passive transport was developed by Ussing. He derived an expression from the Nernst-Planck equation that requires no assumptions about how the concentration and voltage gradients vary within the membrane. Rather, it relies on the measurement of unidirectional fluxes (J_{12} or J_{21}) conducted using tracers and relates the ratio of the fluxes to the electrochemical gradients:

$$\frac{J_{12}}{J_{21}} = \frac{C_1}{C_2} \exp \frac{-zF\Delta\psi}{RT} \quad (20)$$

If the measured flux ratio exceeds that predicted by this expression, a strong case can be made for active transport. In the problem of the thick ascending limb of Henle's loop, both Na^+ and Cl^- transport were shown to exceed the predicted flux ratio. Subsequent investigation of the mechanisms involved have confirmed that both species are indeed actively transported.

REFERENCES

1. Benos DJ et al: The epithelial sodium channel: Subunit number and location of the amiloride binding site. *J Biol Chem* 262:10613, 1987.
2. Benos DJ et al: Purification and characterization of the amiloride-sensitive sodium channel from A6 cultured cells and bovine renal papilla. *Proc Natl Acad Sci* 83:8525, 1986.
3. Bradley SE, Purcell EF (eds): *The Paracellular Pathway*. New York, Josiah Macy, Jr., Foundation, 1982.
4. Cantiello HF et al: G protein subunit, α_i-3, activates a pertussis toxin-sensitive Na^+ channel from the epithelial cell line, A6. *J Biol Chem* 264:20867, 1989.
5. DeWeer P, Rakowski RF: Current generated by backward-running electrogenic Na pump in squid giant axons. *Nature* 309:450, 1984.
6. Finkelstein A, Holz R: Aqueous pores created in thin lipid membranes by the polyene antibiotics nystatin and amphotericin B, in Eisenman G (ed): *Membranes*, vol 2, *Lipid Bilayers and Antibiotics*, New York, Dekker, 1973, pp. 377–408.
7. Frömter E: The route of passive ion movement across the epithelium of *Necturus* gall bladder. *J Membr Biol* 8:259, 1972.

8. Frömter E, Diamond JM: Route of passive ion permeation in epithelia. *Nature* 53:9, 1972.
9. Garty H: Mechanisms of aldosterone action in tight epithelia. *J Membr Biol* 90:193, 1986.
10. Geck P, Heinz E: The Na-K-2Cl cotransport system. *J Membr Biol* 91:97, 1986.
11. Goldman DE: Potential impedance and rectification in membranes. *J Gen Physiol* 27:37, 1943.
12. Greger R et al: Evidence for electroneutral sodium chloride cotransport in cortical thick ascending limb of Henle's loop of rabbit kidney. *Pflugers Arch* 396:308, 1983.
13. Jørgensen PL: Structure, function and regulation of Na,K-ATPase in the kidney. *Kidney Int* 29:10, 1986.
14. Lieb WR: A kinetic approach to transport studies, in Ellory JC, Young JD (eds): *Red Cell Membranes: A Methodological Approach*. New York, Academic Press, 1982, pp 135–164.
15. Loewenstein WR: Channels in junctions between cells, in Stein WD (ed): *Current Topics in Membranes and Transport*. Orlando, Academic Press, 1984, vol 21 p 221.
16. Madara JL: Loosening tight junctions: Lessons from the intestine. *J Clin Invest* 83:1089, 1989.
17. Molitoris BA, Nelson WJ: Alterations in the establishment and maintenance of epithelial cell polarity as a basis for disease processes. *J Clin Invest* 85:3, 1990.
18. Palmer LG, Frindt G: Epithelial sodium channels: Characterization by using the patch-clamp technique. *Fed Proc* 45:2708, 1986.
19. Rossier BC et al: Regulation of the sodium pump: How and why? *Trends Biol Sci* 12:483, 1987.
20. Sactor B: Sodium-coupled hexose transport. *Kidney Int* 36:342, 1989.
21. Schuster VL, Stokes JB: Chloride transport by the cortical and outer medullary collecting duct. *Am J Physiol* 253:F203, 1987.
22. Simons K, Wandinger-Ness A: Polarized sorting in epithelia. *Cell* 62:207, 1990.
23. Stein WD: *Transport and Diffusion across Cell Membranes*. New York, Academic Press, 1986, pp 477–571.
24. Stokes JB: Electroneutral NaCl transport in the distal tubule. *Kidney Int* 36:427, 1989.
25. Stokes JB et al: Purification of rat papillary collecting duct cells: Functional and metabolic assessment. *Am J Physiol* 253:F251, 1987.
26. Sweadner KJ, Goldin SM: Active transport of sodium and potassium ions: Mechanism, function, and regulation. *N Engl J Med* 302:777, 1980.
27. Teorell T: Transport processes and electrical phenomena in ionic membranes. *Prog Biophys* 20:305, 1953.
28. Verkman AS: Mechanisms and regulation of water permeability in renal epithelia. *Am J Physiol* 257:C837, 1989.
29. Wright EM, Peerce BE: Sodium-dependent conformational changes in the intestinal glucose carrier. *Ann NY Acad Sci* 456:108, 1985.

CHAPTER • 3

Sodium metabolism

Kent A. Kirchner • Jay H. Stein

Approximately one-third of total body water is contained within the extracellular fluid (ECF) space. Because this space provides the cell with essential nutrients and contains the intravascular volume that continually renews the supply of cell nutrients, it is apparent that the ECF must be of sufficient volume to maintain the very existence of the organism. The volume of this essential fluid space is directly dependent upon the quantity of total body sodium. This relationship occurs because sodium salts are virtually restricted to ECF space and are the principal osmotically active components of that compartment. An increase in ECF osmolality is a potent stimulus to thirst and, therefore, water intake. Moreover, an increase in the osmolality of the ECF also stimulates the release of antidiuretic hormone (ADH), which causes renal retention of the ingested water. From these considerations, it is obvious that maintenance of a normal body sodium is essential for maintaining a normal ECF and intravascular volume. In mammals, the responsibility for providing a normal and adequate total body sodium belongs to the kidney.

In view of the fact that dietary intake of sodium may vary widely, it follows that the kidney must have the capability to adjust urinary sodium excretion over the same range. That capability is illustrated in Fig. 3-1. If a normal 70-kg individual is ingesting a low-sodium diet of 10 meq/day, urinary sodium excretion will also equal that amount, and total body sodium and the volume of the ECF space will remain constant. If dietary sodium is abruptly increased to 150 meq/day, a 3- to 5-day period

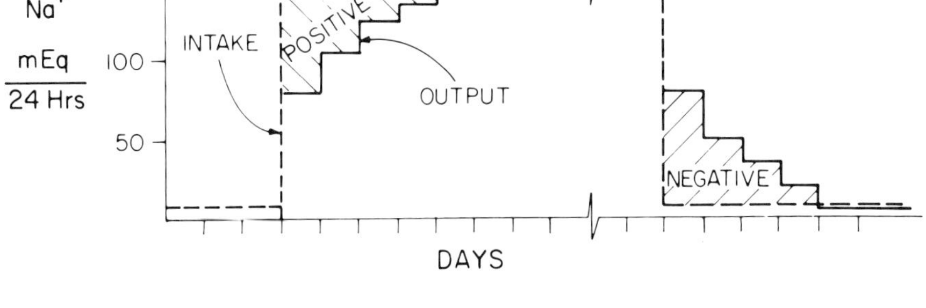

FIGURE 3-1 • Normal sodium balance. An abrupt increase in dietary sodium intake results in a 3- to 5-day period of positive sodium balance and concomitant weight gain. Thereafter, urinary sodium equals sodium intake and weight gain. Thereafter, urinary sodium equals sodium intake and weight stabilizes. When dietary sodium is decreased, negative sodium balance occurs and body weight decreases. After 3 to 5 days, however, a new steady state is again established.

of positive sodium balance occurs, and the resulting ECF expansion is reflected in a small weight gain of approximately 2 kg. Thereafter, however, urinary sodium will again equal dietary intake, and a new steady state will be achieved in which no further increase in ECF volume or body weight occurs. If dietary sodium is returned to the low level of 10 meq/day, a similar period of negative salt balance ensues, with urinary sodium excretion temporarily exceeding dietary intake. However, as the ECF approaches its original volume, the organism in some manner perceives the need for the kidney to further reduce urinary sodium to a level equal to sodium intake, preventing further depletion of the ECF space. The purpose of this chapter is to consider the mechanisms by which the state of expansion of the ECF space and/or intravascular space is perceived and how the kidney responds to that perception and adjusts urinary sodium excretion to its appropriate level.

At the outset of this discussion, a brief note of caution is warranted. In the example of maintaining sodium balance just described, it is apparent that the changes in ECF space that occur with changes in dietary sodium are relatively small. While this phenomenon emphasizes the remarkable sophistication of the homeostatic mechanism, it also makes quantitation of changes in potential determinants of urinary sodium excretion difficult. For this reason, experiments designed to dissect the mechanisms of sodium homeostasis have often utilized acute and relatively large changes in ECF volume. While these maneuvers have yielded measurable changes in a number of potential determinants of urinary sodium excretion, it is important to point out that the interpretation of data so obtained assumes that the organism's response to large changes in ECF space are qualitatively the same as those occurring with more subtle changes in volume.

THE AFFERENT LIMB: PERCEPTION OF VOLUME EXCESS OR DEFICIT

The ECF space is composed of the interstitial compartment and the intravascular compartment. Before considering possible sites whereby the volume of these compartments might be perceived, it should be pointed out that in all likelihood the organism does not perceive absolute volume but, rather, senses the relative volume, or the "fullness," of one or both components of the ECF. Perception of the fullness is perhaps best considered as the ratio of the volume of the ECF or intravascular fluid to the holding capacity of their respective spaces. This ratio determines the "effectiveness" of the volume, and the volume status of the organism is often expressed in terms of "effective ECF volume" or "effective blood volume." The necessity of considering volume in these terms is dictated by the observation that urinary sodium excretion does not necessarily respond to changes in absolute ECF or blood volume. For example, assumption of the upright position with quiet standing results in the sharp decrease in urinary sodium excretion despite the fact that no change in absolute volume occurs.[110] Normal pregnancy is also associated with avid urinary retention of sodium despite the fact that both the ECF and blood volumes are increased.[124] Perhaps one of the best examples of increasing the effectiveness of the blood volume is that demonstrated by thermoneutral, neck-out water immersion.[112] This maneuver involves quiet sitting in a tank of water filled to the individuals' neck and, as shown in Fig. 3-2, results in a marked and sustained increment in urinary sodium excretion. This natriuretic response occurs in the absence of any change in absolute blood volume but is associated with increases in cardiac preload, thoracic blood volume, cardiac output, and left atrial pressure.[137] These phenomena have led to the suggestion that the "effectiveness" of ECF volume is perceived by some receptor or receptors located within the vasculature. Before considering where such receptors might reside, it is appropriate to consider first whether the perception of volume status may also occur in the extravascular or interstitial space.

The intravenous infusion of saline, whether administered in the form of hypotonic,[157] isotonic, or hypertonic[336] solutions, results in a natriuretic response by the kidney. These solutions obviously result in expansion of the entire ECF space, including both the intravascular and extravascular compartments. A considerable body of data has now accumulated that clearly indicates that the "fullness" of the latter compartment, as well as the former, is important in determining urinary sodium excretion.

Early studies of normal humans by Goodyer and coworkers[152] and Welt and Orloff[361] found that intravenous infusions of hyperoncotic albumin resulted in a decrease rather than an increase in urinary sodium excretion. Sonnenberg and Pearce expanded the blood volume of normal, salt-depleted, and salt-loaded dogs by infusing red blood cells suspended in saline solution.[321] Utilizing dye dilution techniques, they were unable to detect any difference in the postinfusion blood volumes among these groups, and the magnitude of the natriuretic response correlated directly with preinfusion state of sodium balance. These investigators therefore concluded that the degree of extravascular volume expansion was the primary determinant of urinary sodium excretion. This conclusion is supported by studies by a number of other investigators. Wright and associates compared the natriuretic response to the infusion of equivalent amounts of saline solution and whole blood.[366] Despite a much greater increment in blood volume in the latter group, the natriuresis was greater in animals infused with saline. Coehlo and Bradley expanded the ECF space of dogs with saline and then produced hypotension by controlled hem-

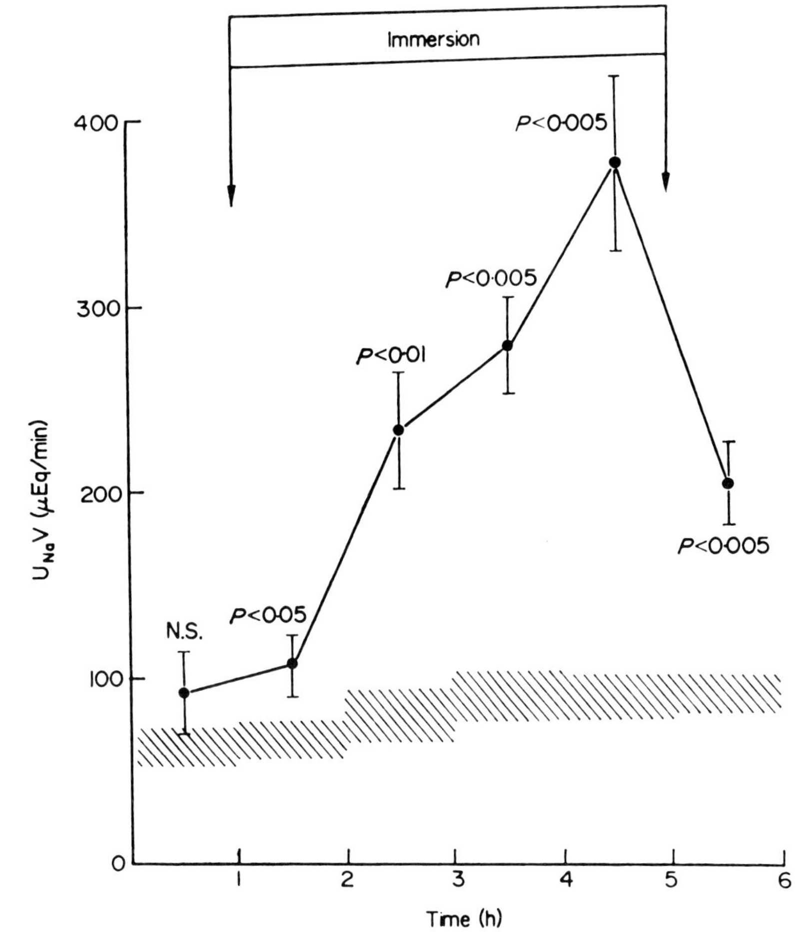

FIGURE 3-2 • Effect of neck-out water immersion on sodium excretion. The immersion to the neck of normal humans in a tank of thermo-indifferent water results in a prompt and sustained increment in sodium excretion ($U_{Na}V$). After exiting the tank, sodium excretion falls abruptly. The shaded area depicts the range of sodium excretion in nonimmersed individuals (From Epstein M et al: *Clin Sci* 43:275, 1972.)

orrhage.[69] Despite lowering mean arterial pressures to levels as low as 50 mmHg, the natriuretic response to the saline infusions persisted. Finally, more recent studies in rats have reported that the natriuretic response to saline infusion exceeds that observed when a comparable degree of plasma volume expansion is attained by the infusion of hyperoncotic albumin.[213,327,328] Thus, although the natriuretic response to neck-out water immersion and the antinatriuretic response to quiet standing support the concept of an intravascular site of volume perception, the possibility that the interstitial compartment also contributes to this phenomenon is difficult to dismiss.

PRESSURE AND VOLUME RECEPTORS

INTRATHORACIC LOW-PRESSURE VOLUME RECEPTORS

These observations of the effect of water immersion on cardiac preload, intrathoracic blood volume, and left atrial pressure are consistent with the concept that the "effectiveness" of the ECF volume is perceived by some volume receptor located on the low-pressure side of the circulation within the thorax. Also consistent with this possibility is the antinatriuretic response to ligation of the superior or inferior vena cava,[81,82,224,228] assumption of the upright posture,[110] orthostasis,[7] and the application of tourniquets to the extremities,[130] all of which decrease cardiac preload.

Anatomical observations present circumstantial evidence that volume perception may reside in some low-pressure intrathoracic location. Extensive innervation of the thoracic vena cava and pulmonary veins has been recognized for over five decades.[250] Further, innervation of all chambers of the heart and the pulmonary interstitial space has also been well documented.[98,193,273] These observations do not, however, necessarily indicate that these "receptors" are involved in the control of sodium excretion. In fact, Gauer and Henry have argued very persuasively that intrathoracic volume receptors are intimately involved in the control of ADH release.[137] On the other hand, a number of studies suggest that they may also modulate renal handling of sodium. Numerous investigators have demonstrated that when left atrial pressure is increased by inflating a small balloon catheter within the chamber, a natriuretic as well as a diuretic response is elicited.[64,87,139,224,237,286] Goetz and colleagues reported similar findings, in that a reduction in left atrial pressure, induced by surgical creation of an atrial pouch, resulted in a fall in urinary sodium excretion.[147] Kappagoda reported that increases in right as well as left atrial pressure also evoked an increase in sodium excretion.[201] Studies by Kaczmarczyk and coworkers are also consistent with an intracardiac mechanoreceptor influencing sodium excretion.[197] The latter investigators chronically monitored left atrial pressure in conscious dogs and found an impressive direct relationship between postprandial left atrial pressure and urinary sodium excretion.

Many of these observations could now be reinterpreted as reflecting the effects of atrial stretch on the release of atrial natriuretic peptide (ANP). However, several studies suggest the existence of intrathoracic low-pressure volume receptors working through a neuronal mechanism. Wennergren and associates showed that direct stimulation of right ventricular afferent fibers induced a natriuretic response.[362] Gilmore[141] and Gilmore and Doggett[12] have reported that chronic cardiac denervation attenuates the natriuretic response of the dog to acute volume expansion. Goetz and associates have shown that increasing left atrial pressure in conscious dogs with denervated hearts results in an increase in plasma ANP, which is similar to the results in normal dogs, but no natriuresis occurs.[148] They concluded that the natriuresis induced by atrial distension in the dog is mediated entirely by reflex effects from cardiac nerves. Thus, studies from a number of investigators provide persuasive evidence that left atrial pressure and possibly pressures within other intrathoracic structures are capable of influencing sodium excretion.

Despite these data, several other observations raise questions about the importance of these volume receptors. The common clinical problem of congestive heart failure, for instance, is associated with increased intrathoracic pressure, and this is accompanied by avid renal retention of sodium; several studies have offered possible explanations for this seeming paradox. Studying different models of heart failure in the dog, Zehr and associates[372] and Zucker and colleagues[374] noted anatomic abnormalities of the cardiac endothelium, including fibrosis and calcification involving the neuroreceptor endings. In addition, in the former study, it was noted that these anatomic abnormalities were associated with a failure of hemorrhagic hypotension to stimulate the release of ADH. Further, Greenberg and coworkers reported that chronic heart failure induced by tricuspid insufficiency and pulmonic stenosis attenuated the normal pressure-induced rise in the rate of atrial receptor discharge.[158] From these observations, it seems likely that chronic elevation in intracardiac pressures decreases the sensitivity of the volume receptors to alterations in that pressure, and that the inverse relationship between intracardiac pressures and urinary sodium excretion under these conditions does not preclude a role for these receptors under more physiologic conditions.

Other observations, however, continue to cast some doubt on the importance of these receptors. As noted above, vagal afferent innervation of a variety of intrathoracic structures, including the heart, has been documented. If one assumes that this afferent innervation is involved in transmitting the perception of volume, one would expect vagotomy and/or cardiac denervation to alter the natriuretic response to increases in volume. Unfortunately, there is not good agreement on this issue. Although some investigators have reported that total interruption of the cervical vagi decreases the natriuretic response to acute volume expansion,[5,137] others have been unable to confirm that finding.[140,143,277] Similarly, cardiac denervation has been reported to diminish the increment in sodium excretion in response to acute volume expansion.[141,142] However, Knox and associates found this effect to be small and relatively trivial.[210] Perhaps of most importance, however, is the question of whether intrathoracic volume receptors play any role in renal sodium handling in humans. Gilmore and Zucker found that the left atrial receptor in the dog is much more responsive to pressure changes than that of the nonhuman primate.[144,145] More recently, Cornish and Gilmore examined the renal response to acute increases in left atrial pressure in *Macaca fascicularis* monkeys and found that, despite the induction of marked increases in pressure, no increment in sodium excretion occurred.[72] Thus, it seems fair to conclude that, while a convincing body of evidence is consistent with a role for low-pressure intrathoracic receptors in the control of sodium excretion, their role in humans remains to be demonstrated.

ARTERIAL BARORECEPTORS

The initial observation suggesting the "effective" blood volume is perceived at some location within the arterial side of the circulation was reported by Epstein and colleagues in 1953 and is illustrated in Fig. 3-3.[111] Studying Korean war veterans with arteriovenous (AV) fistulas, they found that closure of the fistula was associated with a prompt increment in urinary sodium excretion and that reopening of the fistula caused a marked antinatriuresis. In view of the fact that fistula closure decreases cardiac preload and intracardiac pressures, this finding was difficult to reconcile with an important role for the above-mentioned low-pressure intrathoracic receptors in the control of urinary sodium excretion. Furthermore, closure of a fistula causes an increase in arterial diastolic blood pressure, an observation that led to the suggestion that the "effectiveness" of the circulation might be perceived by some receptor on the arterial side of the circulation. This concept has recently been reviewed by Schrier,

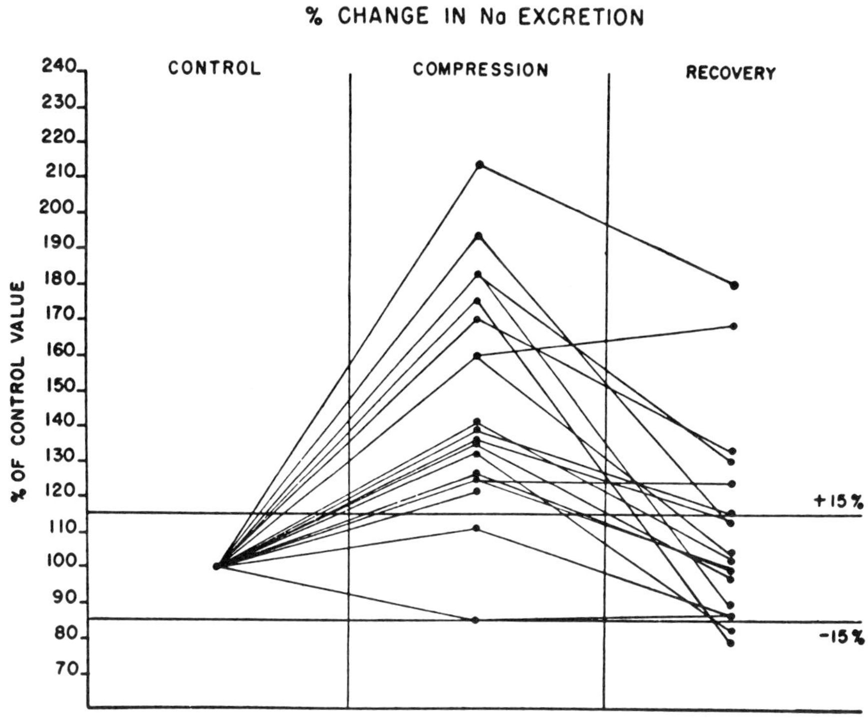

FIGURE 3-3 • Effect of arteriovenous fistula closure on sodium excretion. Compression of an arteriovenous fistula resulted in a significant and reversible increase in urinary sodium excretion in 16 of 18 humans. (From Epstein FH et al: *J Clin Invest* 32:233, 1953.)

who has argued that the adequacy of the arterial circulation, as evidenced by the interaction between cardiac output and peripheral resistance in the arterial tree, is the primary determinant of body fluid volume regulation.[301]

CAROTID SINUS RECEPTOR

A considerable body of evidence has accumulated implicating the carotid sinus in the nonosmotic control of ADH release.[137] By analogy, it is therefore reasonable to speculate that this arterial structure might participate in volume perception in terms of controlling urinary sodium excretion as well. Several observations suggest that this is in fact the case. Zambraski and colleagues demonstrated that acutely increasing carotid sinus pressure without increasing renal perfusion pressure results in a natriuretic response.[369] Conversely, Barger and coworkers[17] and Pronsnitz and colleagues[286] reported that bilateral carotid ligation is a sodium-retaining maneuver if renal perfusion pressure is kept constant.

A series of intriguing studies by Humphreys and Ayus are also of interest in this regard. These investigators studied the mechanism of the natriuresis that immediately follows unilateral nephrectomy and found that the systemic hemodynamic response was very similar to that observed following closure of an AV fistula; that is, cardiac output falls and total peripheral resistance rises.[183] Studying the mechanism of this phenomenon, these authors reported that, when unilateral nephrectomy was performed after either bilateral carotid ligation or bilateral carotid sinus denervation, the natriuresis was abolished.[185] Further, they found that if carotid artery perfusion pressure was maintained constant before and after unilateral nephrectomy, the natriuretic response was similarly prevented.[6]

These observations clearly suggest that the baroreceptor function of the carotid sinus is not only involved in controlling ADH release but at least under some circumstances modulates urinary sodium excretion as well. The studies of Gilmore and Weisfeldt, which demonstrated that carotid sinus denervation fails to influence the increment in sodium excretion that follows acute volume expansion,[143] do not necessarily exclude an important role for the carotid sinus in control of the ECF volume. Rather, their results simply indicate that factors other than carotid sinus perception of volume must also be involved in the regulation of urinary sodium excretion following acute volume expansion, and these factors are capable of eliciting a natriuretic response in this setting.

INTRARENAL BARORECEPTOR

In addition to its obvious role in the effector limb of sodium homeostasis, the kidney may also participate in the perception of effectiveness of the blood volume. In 1959, Tobian reported an inverse relationship between renal perfusion pressure and renin release.[344] Eleven years later, Blaine and coworkers demonstrated that this relationship was maintained in the nonfiltering kidney and thus confirmed a baroreceptor function of the juxtaglomerular apparatus.[36] As discussed in more detail below, this baroreceptor function has important implications in view of the role of renin in ultimately modulating the adrenal release of the salt-retaining hormone aldosterone. Experimental evidence suggesting that this baroreceptor function may be important in the maintenance of sodium balance was demonstrated by Fitzgibbons and colleagues[129] and later confirmed by Osgood and associates.[269] Both groups of investigators demonstrated that when renal perfusion pressure was reduced prior to the administration of an acute saline load, the natriuretic response to the ECF volume expansion was markedly attenuated. When renal perfusion pressure was reduced to a comparable level after giving the saline infusion, however, the increment in sodium excretion persisted. Although these findings do not necessarily implicate the juxtaglomerular apparatus baroreceptor function in this phenomenon, they clearly point out the necessity that the kidney perceive some effect of ECF volume expansion in order to appropriately excrete the saline load.

INTRACRANIAL VOLUME RECEPTOR

The fact that the central nervous system is capable of influencing urinary sodium excretion is now well established. Intracarotid infusion of hypertonic saline solution results in an increment in urinary sodium excretion that exceeds that observed when the same solution is administered systemically.[37,343] Further, the intraventricular instillation of hypertonic saline also results in an increase in sodium excretion,[99,276] and that of hypotonic saline decreases sodium excretion.[254] These results clearly demonstrate that an intracranial osmoreceptor is capable of modulating urinary sodium excretion. The potential relevance of this finding to alterations in ECF volume was provided by the important observation of Mouw and colleagues, who found that volume-depleted animals have a lower cerebrospinal fluid sodium concentration.[255] Kaloyanides and coworkers have also offered experimental findings, summarized in Fig. 3-4, implicating the central nervous system in the control of urinary sodium excretion.[199] These investigators acutely expanded either control or decapitated dogs and compared the natriuretic response of isolated kidneys perfused with blood from these dogs. The kidneys perfused by the circulation of decapitated animals had a markedly blunted natriuretic response. While these findings are consistent with an intracranial receptor of blood volume, they also may be explained by the necessity for an intact central nervous system in the effector limb of volume homeostasis. Further studies are needed to differentiate these possibilities and to better define the manner in which the central nervous system participates in the control of urinary sodium excretion.

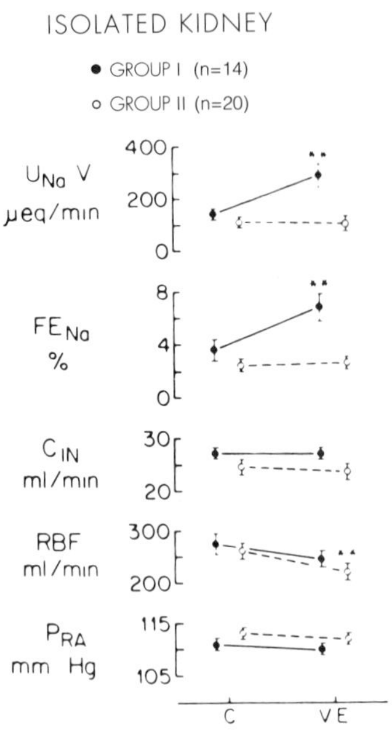

FIGURE 3-4 • Effect of decapitation on the renal response to acute ECF volume expansion. Acute expansion of the ECF space in normal dogs (Group I) results in an increase in absolute ($U_{Na}V$) and fractional (FE_{Na}) sodium excretion without altering insulin clearance (C_{in}), renal blood flow (RBF), or renal perfusion pressure (P_{RA}). In decapitated dogs (Group II), the changes in sodium excretion are abolished. (From Kaloyanides GJ et al: *J Clin Invest* 62:1288, 1978.)

INTRAHEPATIC VOLUME RECEPTOR

By virtue of its anatomic location in the portal circulation, the liver serves as a gateway for dietary sodium to gain access to the ECF. Teleologically, therefore, it would be reasonable to locate a sensor of dietary sodium within the liver and thereby provide an efficient mechanism by which dietary sodium excess could be rapidly excreted. In addition, the avid salt retention in severe liver disease is consistent with a role for the organ in perceiving ECF volume. Indeed, some investigators have reported that orally administered saline solution elicits a greater natriuretic response than does the same quantity of saline given intravenously.[61,62,226,227] Similarly, others have found that saline infused via the portal vein is more readily excreted than that given systemically.[78,275,334] Unfortunately, these results have not been uniformly observed. Schneider and colleagues[298] and Potkay and Gilmore[284] were unable to distinguish differences in urinary sodium excretion between animals receiving a hypertonic saline load intravenously and those given the same solution directly into the portal vein. In addition, Obika and colleagues found no difference in the renal response to administration of hypertonic saline by peripheral vein and by gastric gavage.[263] Thus, despite the ideal location of the liver for monitoring changes in dietary sodium and the observation that patients with severe liver disease are unable to excrete sodium normally, the evidence that this organ participates in the perception of ECF volume remains equivocal.

BLOOD COMPOSITIONAL CHANGES

Up to this point in the discussion of sensors of changes in effective ECF volume, we have considered anatomic receptors localized in various organs or organ systems. It is also possible, however, that at least a part of the perception of volume status lies in the physical chemical changes in the blood that occur as a consequence of expansion or depletion of the ECF volume. In fact, as early as 1925, Starling and Verney found that when blood perfusing an isolated heart-lung-kidney preparation was diluted with saline solution, an increment in sodium excretion occurred.[325] This finding was later confirmed by Craig and coworkers using an isolated kidney preparation.[74] Martino and Earley found that the natriuretic response to saline infusion was accompanied by a fall in serum protein concentration, and when this compositional change in the blood was reversed by the infusion of hyperoncotic albumin, the natriuresis was also reversed.[242] As discussed in more detail later, a number of studies have clearly shown that the serum protein concentration and resultant plasma oncotic pressure profoundly influence proximal reabsorption.

Schrier and Earley have also reported an important effect of hematocrit on urinary sodium excretion.[302] These investigators selectively lowered hematocrit by dilution of whole blood with plasma previously obtained from the same animals, thus preventing any change in the plasma protein concentration. This maneuver resulted in a prompt increase in sodium excretion that was accompanied by an increase in renal blood flow and a fall in renal vascular resistance. The authors attributed the change in sodium excretion to these renal hemodynamic changes. Their results, however, were in conflict with the reports of Bahlman and associates, who found no influence of hematocrit on sodium excretion when the decrease in hematocrit occurred in the absence of changes in blood volume.[8,9] The studies by Knox and associates offer a potential explanation for this apparent discrepancy.[211] These investigators employed micropuncture techniques and found that lowering hematocrit alone resulted in deceased proximal tubular sodium reabsorption. An increase in sodium excretion occurred only if the hemodilution was accompanied by volume expansion. Thus, it seems fair to conclude that the hemodynamic effects of lowering hematocrit may influence proximal reabsorption but other factors attendant to volume expansion are operative in determining whether the proximally rejected sodium reaches the final urine.

Finally, it should be emphasized that all of these studies examined the effects of hemodilution in an acute setting. The observations that patients with chronic hypoproteinemia either maintain normal volume homeostasis or retain sodium and that chronically anemic patients have no difficulty maintaining normal sodium balance indicate that other factors are ultimately responsible for perceiving the need to excrete or retain sodium.

THE EFFERENT LIMB-RENAL RESPONSE TO VOLUME EXCESS OR DEFICIT

Regardless of the mechanism by which the organism perceives changes in the ECF volume, the maintenance of a relatively constant volume requires that the kidneys excrete excess administered or dietary sodium, and, under conditions of ECF volume depletion, that they effectively conserve sodium and excrete a relatively sodium-free urine. The remainder of this chapter considers the mechanism by which the kidney defends the organism against volume excess or deficit.

REGULATORY FACTORS

GLOMERULAR FILTRATION AND GLOMERULAR-TUBULAR BALANCE

Prior to 1961, glomerular filtration was generally accepted as a major determinant of urinary sodium excretion. In that year, however, deWardener and colleagues published the classic findings depicted in Fig. 3-5, indicating that acute expansion of the ECF volume by saline loading was accompanied by a brisk natriuresis even when dogs were pretreated with supraphysiologic doses of mineralocorticoid and glomerular filtration rate (GFR) was reduced by inflation of a balloon catheter located in the aorta proximal to the renal arteries.[86] Thus, these studies unequivocally demonstrated that the natriuresis of acute volume expansion was at least in part independent of changes in GRF and suppression of aldosterone. This important observation led investigators in the field to largely ignore the effects of ECF volume on the process of glomerular filtration. It was not until ten years later, when Brenner and colleagues[50] introduced a new technology that permitted careful experimental scrutiny of the determinants of glomerular filtration, that interest in this process as it is related to sodium excretion was resurrected.

Before detailing the observations of a number of authorities who have examined the effect of volume on GFR, it is appropriate to review briefly the process and the various factors determining the rate of filtration. Glomerular filtration rate may be expressed as

$$GFR = L_P A(P_{GC} - P_T - \pi_{GC})$$

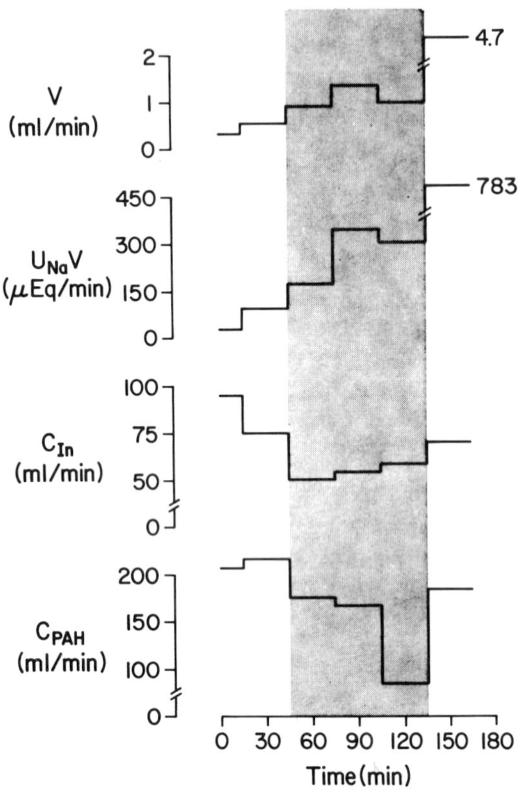

FIGURE 3-5 • The deWardener experiment. A dog receiving pharmacologic doses of mineralocorticoid was volume-expanded with isotonic saline. During the saline infusion, depicted by the shaded area, renal perfusion pressure was reduced by inflation of an intra-aortic suprarenal balloon catheter. Despite a fall in inulin clearance (C_{in}) and renal plasma flow (C_{PAH}) achieved by inflating an intra-aortic balloon, a large increase in sodium excretion and urine volume occurred. (From deWardener HE et al: *Clin Sci* 21:249, 1961.)

where L_P is the glomerular capillary hydraulic conductivity, A is the glomerular capillary surface area, P_{GC} is the hydrostatic pressure within the glomerular capillary, P_T is the hydrostatic pressure opposing filtration within Bowman's space, and π_{GC} is the mean colloid osmotic pressure (conferred by plasma protein) along the glomerular capillary length. The hydrostatic pressure gradient across the glomerular capillary ($P_{GC} - P_T$) may be termed ΔP and, accordingly, the above equation may be rewritten as

$$\text{GFR} = L_pA(\Delta P - \pi_{GC})$$

From consideration of this formula, it is apparent that four factors are responsible for determining the GFR: (1) changes in either L_p or glomerular capillary surface area (A) can modulate GFR; (2) changes in ΔP, which may result from alterations in P_{GC} or P_T, influence GFR; (3) the rate of filtrate formation may be affected by changes in the plasma protein concentration as this parameter is largely responsible for π_{GC}; and (4) though not obviously important from the above formula, the rate of glomerular plasma flow can influence GFR by determining the rate of rise in π_{GC} and, thus, the mean value for intraglomerular capillary colloid osmotic pressure.

With this brief background, we can now consider several recent studies that have examined the effect of alterations in dietary sodium on the determinants of GFR. Steiner and coworkers reported that, in the rat, chronic sodium deprivation resulted in a fall in GFR that was explained by decreases in both L_pA and glomerular plasma flow.[318] Subsequent studies by Tucker and Blantz[346] and Schor and coworkers[300] confirmed these findings, although in the latter study GFR was normal due to an offsetting increase in ΔP. The latter authors also reported certain insights into the physiologic basis for the decrease in L_pA and glomerular plasma flow. Steiner and colleagues administered saralasin to their sodium-deprived animals and found that this competitive antagonist of angiotensin II restored glomerular plasma flow to normal levels but failed to correct their defect in L_pA.[329] In the study of Tucker and Blantz, short-term administration of an angiotensin-converting enzyme inhibitor had the same effect as saralasin: restoration of glomerular plasma flow.[346] The long-term administration of the same agent, however, reversed not only the decrement in glomerular plasma flow, but also the depression of L_pA, suggesting that angiotensin II is solely responsible for the diminished GFR of chronic sodium depletion. Schor and associates reached a similar conclusion.[300] When these investigators administered angiotensin II to animals on a high-sodium diet, L_pA and glomerular plasma flow fell to values virtually indistinguishable from those seen in animals ingesting a low-sodium diet. In addition, they found that indomethacin, an inhibitor of prostaglandin synthesis, resulted in a profound diminution of GFR in sodium-depleted animals, suggesting that the deleterious effects of angiotensin II on GFR under these conditions are partially antagonized by vasodilatory prostaglandins.

The degree to which changes in GFR contribute to the overall control of urinary sodium excretion is still not certain. Under normal conditions with a GFR of 100 ml/min, the filtered load of sodium amounts to approximately 20,000 meq/day. This amount is enormous when compared to the normal urinary sodium excretion of 200 meq/day. In view of this large difference, it is apparent that very small changes in GFR could result in major alterations in sodium excretion if tubular reabsorption remained unaltered. Fortunately, the organism is endowed with a remarkably efficient mechanism that prevents this from occurring. This phenomenon, termed glomerular-tubular balance, provides that as GFR rises or falls, absolute tubular reabsorption changes in a similar direction. The mechanism by which this important process occurs has been clarified at least in the proximal tubule. Several studies have now demonstrated that the phenomenon is not due to some intrinsic property of the tubule, since net reabsorptive rate in the in vitro perfused proximal tubule is independent of flow rate when studied within a physiologic range.[58,190]

Most evidence points to changes in postglomerular hemodynamics and peritubular composition as the most likely explanation for proximal glomerular-tubular balance. According to this view, which is discussed in greater detail later in this chapter, peritubular capillary Starling forces are important in modulating absolute proximal reabsorption. As it relates to glomerular-tubular balance, it is important to note that a rise in filtration fraction (GFR/renal plasma flow) will result in an increase in the postglomerular protein concentration and thus a rise in peritubular colloid osmotic pressure. In addition, at any given renal perfusion pressure, an increment in filtration fraction will also result in a fall in peritubular capillary hydrostatic pressure. Both of these alterations in the postglomerular circulation will enhance absolute proximal reabsorption and thus contribute significantly to proximal glomerular-tubular balance. It should also be pointed out that under circumstances in which GFR and renal plasma flow increase in parallel so that no change in filtration fraction occurs, glomerular tubular balance will be maintained due to the higher rate of peritubular capillary plasma flow. This effect stems from the fact that a greater amount of reabsorbate will be required to establish equilibrium of Starling forces across the peritubular capillary when flow rate is increased. Finally, it should be noted that a direct relationship between tubular flow rate and sodium reabsorption along more distal nephron segments has also been well documented.[97,219,221,315,327] Thus, glomerular-tubular balance is not limited to the proximal tubule but, rather, is contributed to by nearly the entire nephron.

Despite the importance of glomerular-tubular balance, it should be stressed that the phenomenon does not exclude a role for alterations in GFR in the control of urinary sodium excretion. Even if glomerular-tubular balance is perfect, a change in GFR will affect sodium excretion. For example, if the normal filtered load of sodium of 20,000 meq/day is increased by 25 percent and the normal tubular reabsorptive rate of 19,800 meq/day increases similarly, the filtered load and reabsorption will be 25,000 and 24,750 meq/day, respectively. Urinary sodium excretion will therefore still increase by 50 meq/day. Thus, the consideration of glomerular-tubular balance does not exclude a potentially important role for GFR in the determination of urinary sodium excretion.

ALDOSTERONE

The importance of aldosterone in the control of urinary sodium excretion and the maintenance of normal sodium homeostasis is suggested by numerous clinical and experimental observations. First, in the absence of hormone replacement, individuals with adrenal insufficiency experience profound urinary sodium wasting when ingesting a low-sodium diet. Second, an impressive inverse relationship exists between both dietary sodium intake and aldosterone levels[70] and ECF volume and secretion of the hormone.[80] Third, adrenalectomized animals respond to the acute administration of aldosterone with an abrupt decrement in urinary sodium excretion.[252] These findings convinced early authors of the importance of aldosterone; and, in fact, until 1961, the prevalent view held that this hormone, together with GFR, was responsible for the ultimate control of urinary sodium excretion. In that year, however, deWardener and colleagues published the results of their classic experiment indicating that other factors were clearly involved in regulating the rate of tubular reabsorption of sodium.[86] In those studies, dogs were pretreated with large amounts of aldosterone prior to administration of a saline load. As noted above, a balloon catheter was also inflated in the aorta, and GFR was decreased. Despite the reduction of GFR and the presence of pharmacologic amounts of the salt-retaining hormone, a significant natriuretic response to the volume expansion was observed. This important finding raised considerable doubt as to the relative importance of aldosterone in maintaining sodium balance. In addition, the fact that chronic administration of aldosterone causes only transient retention of sodium also casts doubt on the contribution of salt-retaining steroids to the control of sodium excretion. This phenomenon, termed deoxycorticosterone acetate, (DOCA), or mineralocorticoid escape, is illustrated in Fig. 3-6. As can be seen, when a normal individual is given the salt-retaining steroid DOCA, a 4- to 5-day period of positive sodium balance occurs, which is accompanied by a weight gain of 1 to 2 kg, reflecting the expansion of the ECF volume. Thereafter, however, a new steady state of sodium balance is established, with sodium excretion again equaling sodium intake, and the body weight stabilizes. Finally, it has been noted that changes in effective arterial blood volume, such as occur with quiet standing, are immediately followed by a sharp decrement in urinary sodium excretion. This phenomenon occurs immediately despite the fact that aldosterone requires several hours for its salt-retaining effects to occur.[252]

Thus, a number of observations tended to minimize the importance of aldosterone in the control of urinary sodium excretion and the maintenance of a relatively constant ECF volume. It should also be pointed out, however, that these studies merely emphasize that, in the absence of aldosterone or in the presence of excessive amounts of it, other factors may be called into play that aid in the restoration or maintenance of sodium balance. These studies do not necessarily indicate that aldosterone is of only minimal importance in the control of urinary

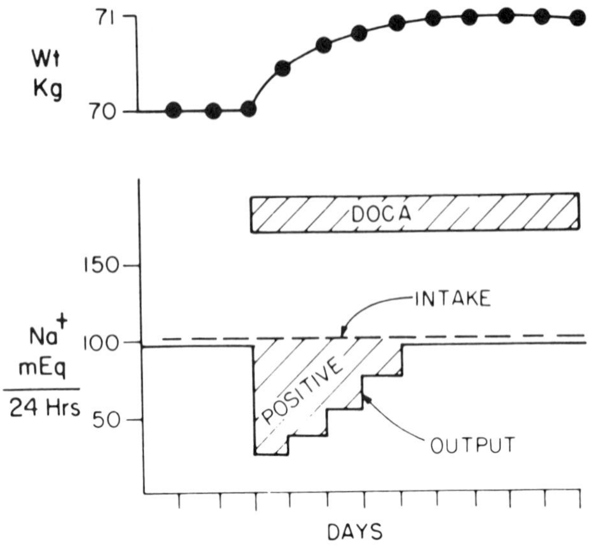

FIGURE 3-6 • The "DOCA escape" phenomenon. When a normal individual with a constant sodium intake is given the salt-retaining mineralocorticoid, DOCA, a transient period of positive sodium balance and weight gain occur. After 3 to 5 days, however, a new steady state is established with sodium excretion equal to sodium intake and no further weight gain occurs.

sodium excretion under more physiologic circumstances. Indeed, as reviewed by Seely and Levy,[308] aldosterone under normal circumstances may play an important role in the renal response to alterations in dietary sodium intake. Young and coworkers compared the effect of increasing dietary sodium in normal dogs and adrenalectomized animals on a fixed replacement dosage of mineralocorticoid.[367] They found that the weight gain and increment in ECF volume was much greater in the latter group of animals, presumably due to their inability to lower aldosterone levels. Conceptually consistent results were reported by Samuels and colleagues.[295] These investigators examined the change in ECF volume in adrenalectomized dogs maintained on low-dose mineralocorticoid replacement and a low-sodium intake and normal animals ingesting the same diet. The degree of ECF volume depletion was much greater in the former group of animals, again, most likely due to their inability to modulate appropriately the release of adrenal sodium-retaining steroids.

In view of these findings, it seems fair to conclude that aldosterone plays an important role in the control of sodium excretion under conditions of alterations in dietary sodium. However, under conditions in which aldosterone levels cannot be altered or when more abrupt changes in sodium excretion are necessary, other factors can be marshaled to protect the organism from life-threatening alterations in volume homeostasis.

The nephron site responsive to aldosterone has been partially clarified in recent years. Early micropuncture studies in the rat by Hierholzer and associates demonstrated an effect of the hormone along the surface distal tubule, and this observation led to the assumption that the distal convoluted tubule was the primary target of the aldosterone.[173] Since that time, it has become apparent that, at least in the rat, the surface distal tubule is a heterogenous structure composed of epithelia with characteristics of the loop of Henle, the distal convoluted tubule, and the early portion of the cortical collecting tubule. This finding reconciles the seeming conflict between the micropuncture studies of Hierholzer and colleagues[173] and the more recent findings of Gross and coworkers.[160,161] The latter investigators studied isolated perfused rabbit tubules and, as shown in Fig. 3-7, found that the distal convoluted tubule of the rabbit was unresponsive to aldosterone, at least in terms of an effect of transepithelial electrical potential difference, while the rabbit cortical collecting tubule developed a more negative luminal potential upon exposure to aldosterone. Since that time, a number of additional studies using similar techniques have confirmed that the hormone influences transport along this nephron segment,[2,267,305,332] and others have identified aldosterone receptors along the cortical collecting duct.[100,244,352] Whether the hormone influences transport by more distal nephron segments remains controversial, however. Doucet and Katz found receptor sites along the outer medullary collecting duct,[100] but Stokes and coworkers were unable to detect

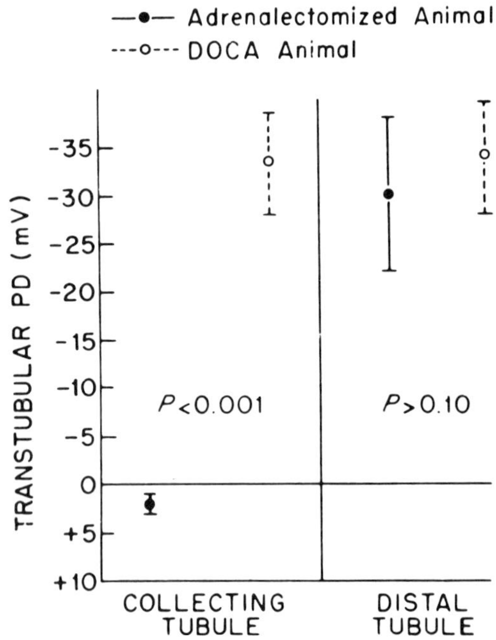

FIGURE 3-7 • Effect of mineralocorticoid on distal nephron transepithelial potential difference (PD). The PD across the collecting tubule of adrenalectomized rabbits is slightly positive while that from mineralocorticoid (DOCA)-treated rabbits is markedly negative. In contrast, mineralocorticoid treatment does not influence the PD across the distal convoluted tubule. (From Gross JB and Kokko JP: *J Clin Invest* 59:82, 1977.)

any effect on transport in this segment in vitro.[332] Using in vivo micropuncture or microcatheterization techniques, Uhlich and colleagues reported that aldosterone stimulated sodium transport by the papillary collecting duct,[347] and Ullrich and Papavasiliou reported that adrenalectomy diminished transport by this segment.[348] Unfortunately, Sonnenberg has been unable to find an effect of mineralocorticoid on transport in this most terminal nephron segment.[318,319]

The mechanism by which aldosterone affects sodium transport remains a subject of intensive investigation. It is now clear that the hormone binds to cytoplasmic receptors and the hormone-receptor complex is in some manner translocated into the cell nucleus, where it is bound to a specific receptor and initiates transcription of RNA, which eventually leads to synthesis of a unique protein. It is postulated that this protein mediates the physiologic action of the hormone, but the manner in which this occurs is not entirely clear.[107,205,223] One theory holds that the aldosterone-induced protein somehow increases cellular adenosine triphosphate (ATP) stores and thereby provides the increased energy necessary for enhanced sodium transport.[108,125] A second theory, supported by the work of Schmidt and associates contends that aldosterone stimulates basolateral membrane-bound Na^+-K^+ ATPase and thereby stimulates sodium transport.[178,297] A final theory postulates that the aldosterone-induced transport protein causes changes in cell membrane phospholipid synthesis and thus changes the membrane permeability to sodium.[150,151,307] A recent study by Petty and colleagues is of particular interest with regard to the last two theories.[281] These authors studied the effect of aldosterone on cortical collecting tubules obtained from adrenalectomized rabbits. As shown in Fig. 3-8, they found that adrenalectomy markedly decreased Na^+-K^+ ATPase activity and treatment with aldosterone 3 h prior to sacrifice restored enzyme activity to normal. When animals were also treated with amiloride, an agent known to block the apical membrane entry of sodium, however, the effect of aldosterone on the enzyme was significantly blunted. From these observations, the authors suggested that aldosterone acts ultimately by enhancing the entry of sodium into the cell across the apical membrane and that this increase in intracellular sodium is responsible for the secondary increase in Na^+-K^+ATPase activity that occurs along the basolateral cell membrane.

PHYSICAL FACTORS

Following the landmark studies of deWardener and coworkers in 1961,[86] which clearly demonstrated that factors other than GFR and aldosterone significantly influenced urinary sodium excretion, at least in response to acute expansion of the ECF volume by saline loading, a new era in renal physiology was born, in which numerous investigators sought the identity of those factors. Among the areas most intensely studied was that of the so-called physical factors. The consideration of these factors was not entirely new; exactly 100 years before the publication of the deWardener experiment, Ludwigh postulated that renal tubular reabsorption was an entirely passive process controlled by alterations in the peritubular environ-

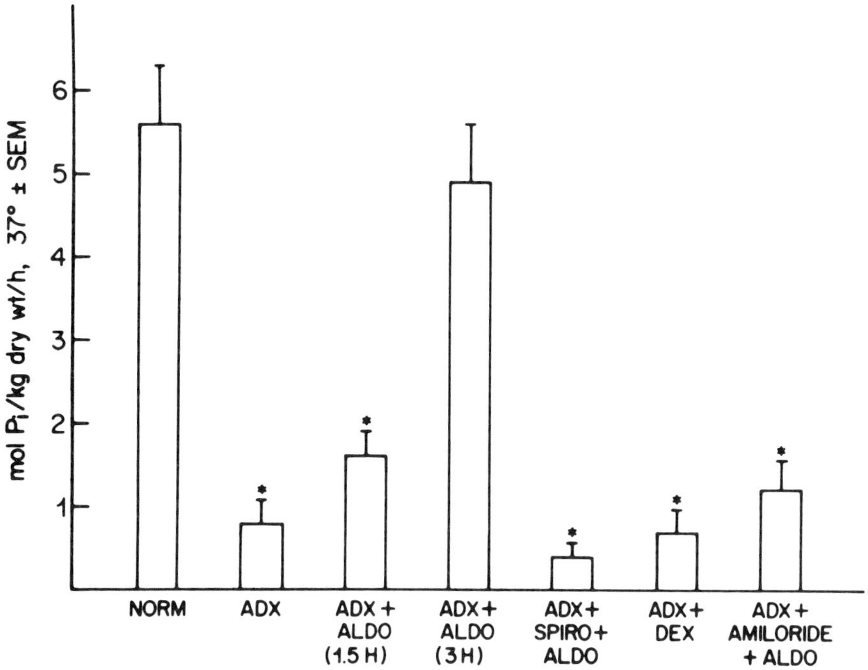

FIGURE 3-8 • Effect of mineralocorticoid on cortical collecting tubule Na^+-K^+ ATPase activity. Adrenalectomy (ADX) markedly decreases enzyme activity, which is restored to normal 3 h after mineralocorticoid (Aldo) administration but not at 1.5 h. Spironolactone (Spiro) abolishes this effect of mineralocorticoid, and glucocorticoid (Dex) fails to restore enzyme activity. Amiloride, an agent that blocks luminal membrane sodium entry, abolishes the effect of mineralocorticoid on Na^+-K^+ ATPase activity. Asterisks indicate $p < 0.001$ compared to normal (norm). (From Petty KJ et al: *J Clin Invest* 68:1514, 1981.)

ment.[236] Nevertheless, the technology of the 1960s allowed for a more intensive and accurate assessment of the possibility that these factors influence urinary sodium excretion. Before examining the evidence that this is the case, it is important to review briefly the manner in which the peritubular environment is thought to potentially modulate tubular reabsorption. At the outset, it should be emphasized that the theory and experimental data to be examined are exclusively limited to the proximal tubule. As will be readily apparent, the unique "leakiness" of that epithelia is essential to the effect of the physical factors on net sodium reabsorption.

The theoretical model for this mechanism is schematically represented in Fig. 3-9. According to this model, filtered sodium passively diffuses down its concentration gradient from tubular lumen into the proximal tubular epithelial cell. Sodium is then actively transported across the basolateral membrane from the cell into the peritubular interstitial space. Water either moves passively through the same transcellular route as sodium or is drawn across the paracellular "tight junction" by the osmotic gradient created by the transport of the cations. The interstitial solute and water content is then governed by the rate of their removal by the peritubular capillary, and this rate is determined by the balance of Starling forces between the interstitial space and the capillary plasma. These factors may be mathematically expressed as

$$J_v = K_f(\pi_C - \pi_i) - (P_C - P_i)$$

where J_v is net water reabsorption, K_f is the effective capillary hydraulic permeability coefficient, π_C and π_i are the respective oncotic pressures in the capillary plasma and the interstitial fluid, and P_C and P_i are the respective hydrostatic pressures in the capillary and interstitium. According to this formula, if peritubular capillary oncotic pressure is low and/or hydrostatic pressure is elevated, the rate of uptake of the interstitial fluid will be reduced. As a result, actively transported solute and osmotically attracted water will accumulate in the interstitial space. This accumulation will increase the P_i and lead to "backleak" of reabsorbed sodium and water from the interstitium into the tubular lumen across the relatively leaky tight junctions of the proximal epithelium. Conversely, under circumstances in which peritubular capillary oncotic pressure is high and/or hydrostatic pressure is reduced, the removal of interstitial fluid will be enhanced, P_i will consequently fall, and less backleak will occur. This series of events will lead to an increase in the net reabsorptive rate.

If this model is correct, it is apparent that a number of factors should be capable of modulating Starling forces and, therefore, proximal reabsorption. Renal perfusion pressure has been recognized for some time to influence urinary sodium excretion.[309,325] This effect is at least partially explicable by its effect on peritubular capillary hydrostatic pressure. Perfusion pressure may alter sodium excretion through influences on renal interstitial hydrostatic pressure as well. Similarly, changes in the composition of the blood also influence sodium excretion. As noted above, as early as 1925, Starling and Verney found that when the blood perfusing an isolated heart-lung-kidney preparation was diluted with normal saline, there was a substantial increase in urinary sodium excretion.[325] Since that time, numerous investigators have

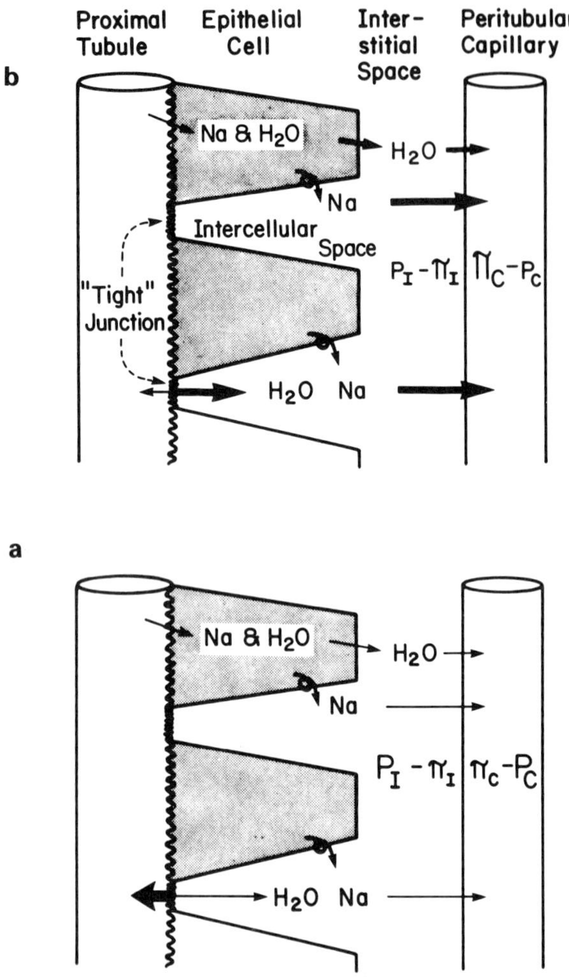

FIGURE 3-9 • Schematic representation of the "pumpleak" model of proximal tubular sodium reabsorption. Filtered sodium is passively reabsorbed from the tubular lumen into the epithelial cell down a concentration gradient. It is then actively transported into the lateral intercellular channel, which communicates directly with the interstitial space, and water moves passively via either a transcellular or paracellular pathway. The uptake of reabsorbate from the interstitium into the peritubular capillary is determined by the Starling forces across the capillary wall. Under circumstances depicted in (*a*) with a relatively high filtration fraction, peritubular oncotic pressure (π_C) is high and hydrostatic pressure (P_C) is low and peritubular capillary uptake is enhanced. As a result, relatively little "backleak" of reabsorbate across the "tight" junction occurs. When filtration fraction is relative low (*b*), π_C is decreased, P_C is increased, and peritubular capillary uptake is decreased. As a result, interstitial hydrostatic pressure (P_i) rises and backleak increases, thereby decreasing net reabsorption.

shown that selective lowering of the plasma protein concentration is associated with an increment in sodium excretion that is at least partially due to decreased proximal reabsorption, presumably due to altered peritubular oncotic pressure.[261,264,355] Finally, it should be stressed that the so-called physical factors may alter proximal reabsorption without measurable changes in either plasma protein concentration or renal perfusion pressure. For instance, if either afferent or efferent arteriolar tone is decreased, a greater portion of the renal perfusion pressure will reach the postglomerular peritubular capillary, where it will tend to decrease reabsorption. Similarly, if selective efferent arteriolar dilation occurs, not only will peritubular capillary hydrostatic pressure rise, but oncotic pressure will fall due to a lower intraglomerular capillary pressure, causing a fall in GFR and filtration fraction (GFR/renal plasma flow). These perturbations would also tend to decrease proximal reabsorption. Conversely, selective vasoconstriction of the efferent arteriole would cause an increase in GFR and filtration fraction, raise peritubular capillary oncotic pressure, and lower hydrostatic pressure. Both alterations would lead to enhanced proximal reabsorption.

The initial evidence suggesting that the processes just discussed modulate proximal reabsorption came from a series of ingenious clearance studies by Earley and coworkers, who examined the effect of acute volume expansion and renal vasodilatation on sodium excretion.[104-106,242,243] Subsequently, a number of micropuncture studies by Brenner and colleagues[46-51,116] and Windhager and coworkers [229,323] seemed to establish firmly the potential for alterations in peritubular oncotic pressure to influence the magnitude of proximal reabsorption. Despite the convincing nature of all of these studies, not all investigators in the area were able to detect an effect of peritubular oncotic pressure on proximal reabsorption. Rumrich and Ullrich,[293] Lowitz and colleagues,[235] and Bank and coworkers[13] examined this issue and, despite experimental protocols that caused marked changes in peritubular oncotic pressure, none of these authors was able to find changes in proximal reabsorption. Moreover, Conger and colleagues directly perfused peritubular capillaries with either a protein-free or protein-rich solution and found that neither perfusate influenced the rate of proximal reabsorption.[71] Thus, these studies raised some serious doubt about the importance of the so-called physical factors, in particular oncotic forces, on proximal reabsorption. In 1975, however, studies by Ott and associates shed light on these seemingly irreconcilable findings.[272] These investigators examined the effect of intrarenal infusions of hyperoncotic albumin on efferent arteriolar protein concentration and proximal reabsorption. They found that, in hydropenic dogs, increasing the former had no effect on proximal reabsorption. In animals volume-expanded by the intravenous infusion of Ringer's solution, however, the albumin infusion resulted in a marked increase in proximal reabsorption. From this observation, they suggested that expansion of ECF volume resulted in increased passive backleak, which could be reversed by raising the peritubular oncotic pressure; during hydropenia, on the other hand, when passive backleak was relatively less, raising the peritubular capillary oncotic pressure had no influence on proximal reabsorption.

Fitzgibbons and colleagues have presented data noted earlier in this chapter that also initially raised questions about the role of physical factors in the natriuretic response to acute volume expansion.[129] These investigators administered an acute saline load to animals in which renal perfusion pressure was reduced either before or after the volume load. Only in the latter circumstance did they find a natriuretic response to ECF volume expansion. Osgood and colleagues confirmed this finding and found that proximal reabsorption was decreased only when renal perfusion pressure was lowered after volume expansion.[269] Since the timing of the volume load relative to that of reducing renal perfusion pressure should have no effect on the degree to which peritubular oncotic pressure falls, these findings were difficult to reconcile with the view that physical factors played an important role in the depressed proximal reabsorption of volume expansion. Studies by Ichikawa and Brenner have clarified this issue, however.[186] Using direct micropuncture techniques to measure Starling forces across the proximal tubule and peritubular capillary, they found that when perfusion pressure was lowered after administration of the acute saline load, peritubular capillary oncotic pressure was virtually identical to that observed when the volume load was given after reducing perfusion pressure. In the former circumstance, however, peritubular hydrostatic pressure rose markedly with volume expansion and remained elevated, and in the latter condition, this parameter did not increase.

The significance of changes in renal interstitial hydrostatic pressure in the control of urinary sodium excretion has been further emphasized in a number of recent investigations. In these studies, increases in renal interstitial hydrostatic pressure, induced by increasing renal perfusion pressure, saline loading, ligation of hilar lymph ducts, or injections of albumin directly into the renal interstitium, reduced proximal reabsorption and increased urinary sodium excretion.[156,204,363] Haas and associates developed a technique for directly increasing renal interstitial hydrostatic pressure by injecting an isoncotic saline-albumin solution into a polyethylene matrix chronically implanted in the renal interstitium.[166] With this technique, increases in renal interstitial hydrostatic pressure produce marked increases in sodium excretion without inducing changes in renal blood flow (RBF) or GFR. Burnett and coworkers have observed that renal interstitial hydrostatic pressure is chronically elevated during sodium retention induced by long-term mineralocorticoid administration and have proposed that this may be an important mechanism in the mineralocorticoid escape phenomena.[59] Reductions in interstitial pressure produced by renal decapsulation, on the other hand, significantly attenuate the response to acute saline volume expansion.[135] Thus, renal interstitial hydrostatic pressure appears to be an important determinant of the natriuretic response to saline loading.

Finally, alterations in renal perfusion pressure markedly alter sodium excretion through mechanisms that are independent of changes in RBF or GFR.[260,309,311] The importance of this mechanism for modulating sodium excretion in pathologic conditions is well established. Reductions in renal perfusion pressure to below normal values have been shown to attenuate the natriuresis induced by acute saline volume expansion or by administration of natriuretic substances such as the prostaglandins and ANP.[129,164,240] However, the importance of renal perfusion pressure in the control of renal sodium excretion is best demonstrated during the physiologic escape from the sodium retaining effects of antinatriuretic substances. As noted previously, chronic administration of a mineralocorticoid produces only a short period of sodium retention followed by a return of sodium excretion to baseline levels. This escape prevents massive sodium retention despite continued mineralocorticoid administration. Increased renal perfusion pressure induced by the sodium-retaining effects of mineralocorticoids appears to be responsible for the escape phenomenon. Using an electronically servo-controlled aortic occluder to maintain renal perfusion pressure constant at its baseline value, Hall and associates found that aldosterone administration induced a sustained reduction in urinary sodium excretion and a persistently positive sodium balance of 70 to 80 meq/day for the entire 7-day period of aldosterone administration.[169] Sodium excretion greatly increased, and sodium balance was restored despite continued aldosterone infusion as renal perfusion pressure increased when the occluder was turned off. In control dogs, sodium excretion decreased during the first day of aldosterone administration but returned to baseline values as arterial pressure increased approximately 15 to 19 mmHg. Similar observations have been reported by this group during escape from the sodium-retaining effects of low doses of angiotensin II.[168] Thus, a central role for renal perfusion pressure in control of sodium excretion during pathophysiologic conditions seems clear.

The role of renal perfusion pressure in the regulation of sodium excretion under normal physiological conditions has been more difficult to demonstrate, since the kidney has so many systems regulating sodium balance that measurable changes in renal perfusion do not occur during the small alterations in sodium intake that occur in normal circumstances. Nonetheless, renal perfusion pressure critically determines the effectiveness of other systems governing sodium balance.

As mentioned above, the observation that renal perfusion pressure alters sodium excretion independently of changes in the filtered load of sodium suggest that its primary effect is on tubular reabsorption. The sites responsible for the increases in sodium excretion continue to be investigated. Most studies suggest that increases in renal perfusion pressure do not alter sodium reabsorption in the proximal tubule. Kunau and associates have found that sodium reabsorption was not altered by segments up to the end of the superficial distal tubule during increases in renal perfusion pressure.[218] They concluded that either reabsorption in the collecting ducts or deep nephrons were responsible for this effect.[218] Increases in sodium delivery from deep but not superficial nephrons have been observed in response to increases in renal perfusion pressure.[165] The loop of Henle has also been suggested as a site that is responsive to renal perfusion pressure. Decreased sodium reabsorption at this location has been observed in humans and animals with hypertension and following increases in arterial pressure induced by infusions of epinephrine.[57,206,259,337]

From the foregoing considerations, it is clear that physical factors play a significant role in control of renal sodium excretion in both health and disease.

ANGIOTENSIN II

Angiotensin II has the capability of influencing urinary sodium excretion in a number of ways. First, this polypeptide hormone has the capacity to stimulate directly the adrenal synthesis and release of the salt-retaining steroid aldosterone. Second, the hormone profoundly influences systemic vascular resistance and thereby has the capacity to modulate effective ECF volume. Third, angiotensin II has the capability of specifically altering efferent arteriolar resistance.[109,187,188] For reasons obvious from the consideration of the effect of this resistance on postglomerular hemodynamics and Starling forces, angiotensin II may alter proximal reabsorption by this mechanism. Fourth, a growing body of data has implied that the hormone may directly modulate proximal tubular reabsorption.

Studies in which angiotensin II is infused systemically have suggested a biphasic response in urinary sodium excretion.[18,19,159,172,234] At relatively low doses, angiotensin II infusion is associated with a decrease in sodium excretion, while higher doses elicit a natriuretic response. The interpretation of these observations is confused by effects of systemic angiotensin II on GFR, renal perfusion pressure, RBF, and filtration fraction. However, Olsen and associates have suggested that the natriuretic effects of systemic angiotensin II may be mediated through increases in renal perfusion pressure.[266] In her study, even very large doses of angiotensin II were antinatriuretic when renal arterial pressure was prevented from increasing. On the other hand, it should be noted that studies employing the intrarenal infusion of angiotensin II have also demonstrated a biphasic response.[351,358] Similarly, in vivo studies in nonrenal transporting epithelia have also shown a biphasic response in net sodium and water movement,[75,79] while microperfusion of peritubular capillaries with high doses of angiotensin II result in decreased proximal reabsorption.[170,330] In view of these findings, it seems certain that high doses of the hormone inhibit sodium reabsorption. Unfortunately, such an effect seems to be, at least teleologically, counterproductive in view of the reciprocal relationship between ECF volume and circulating levels of angiotensin II. In this regard, the studies of Johnson and Malvin are particularly pertinent.[195] These authors pointed out that the doses of angiotensin II utilized to elicit a natriuretic response result in plasma levels of the hormone that exceed those attained by physiologic perturbations. With this in mind, they administered angiotensin II directly into the renal artery of the dogs in a dose range designed to span the levels achieved by physiologic manipulations. With this limitation on the amount of the hormone given, they found decreased urinary sodium excretion at all levels of infusion. Further, they found that this antinatriuretic effect could be observed without any detectable change in GFR, RBF, or filtration fraction. These findings are consistent with the observations of Schuster and coworkers that physiologic doses of angiotensin II directly stimulate sodium transport in the proximal tubule through a mechanism that is receptor mediated and electroneutral.[303] In addition, several investigators have suggested that alterations in medullary blood flow may induce alterations in urinary sodium excretion by altering the medullary solute gradient.[117,287] These effects occur independently of changes in total RBF and provide another potential mechanism for angiotensin II to alter sodium excretion. However, the view that alterations in medullary blood flow induced by angiotensin II results in changes in urinary sodium excretion has been challenged by others.[292] The observation that angiotensin II is capable of increasing sodium reabsorption has been given further physiologic meaning by the studies of Hall and associates.[167] These investigators found that, when a competitive antagonist of the hormone is infused directly into the renal artery of a sodium-depleted dog, a significant increment in sodium excretion is observed. That this phenomenon is of significant importance in the long-term control of sodium homeostasis is suggested by the observations of McCaa and colleagues, illustrated in Fig. 3-10.[245] They administered an angiotensin-converting enzyme inhibitor to dogs maintained on a low-sodium diet and found that over the entire two weeks of the study animals receiving the inhibitor had higher urinary sodium excretion than animals not receiving the drug but ingesting the same diet. This inappropriate loss of sodium occurred despite a fall in both GFR and blood pressure and was not reversed by the administration of exogenous aldosterone but was attenuated by the provision of angiotensin II. Thus, while the contributions of the various mechanisms by which physiologic concentrations of angiotensin II may promote sodium reabsorption are unclear, it seems certain that the hormone is of physiologic significance in the control of urinary sodium excretion.

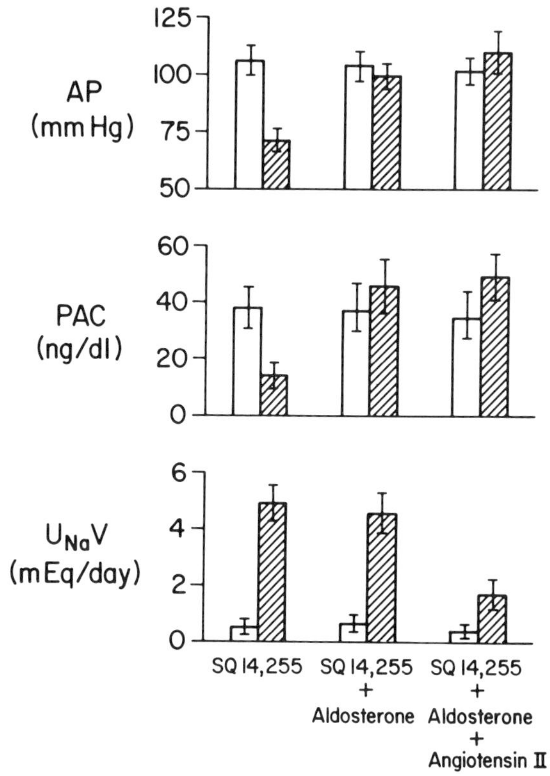

FIGURE 3-10 • Effect of an angiotensin I converting enzyme inhibitor (SQ-14,225) on dogs ingesting a low sodium diet. Administration of SQ-14,225 results in increased urinary sodium excretion ($U_{Na}V$), and decreased arterial pressure (AP) and plasma aldosterone concentration. The higher $U_{Na}V$ is not abolished by aldosterone but is partially corrected by angiotensin II administration. (From McCaa RE et al: *Circ Res* 43:132, 1978.)

RENAL NERVE ACTIVITY

The concept that the renal nerves influence renal handling of sodium and water gained initial attention in 1859, when Bernard reported that transection of the greater splanchnic nerve resulted in a diuresis that was reversible by electrical stimulation of the sectioned nerve.[32] Since that time, an abundant literature has accumulated that confirms and extends this early finding.[88,154] Renal denervation has provided a fundamental approach to examining the role of renal nerves in the control of sodium excretion. Pharmacologic "denervation" accomplished by administration of the alpha-adrenergic antagonist phenoxybenzamine has been reported to increase ipsilateral sodium excretion in anesthetized, euvolemic dogs.[335] Similar effects have been reported by a large number of investigators in anatomically denervated kidneys of anesthetized animals.[23,27,28,33,38,39,41,54,200,261a,365] The significance of these observations has been questioned, however, on the basis of the anesthetized state of the animals. Appropriately, a number of authors have therefore addressed this issue. In 1966, Gill and Bartter reported that pharmocologic sympathectomy by the administration of guanethidine resulted in an inability of normal human subjects to conserve sodium appropriately when maintained on a low dietary sodium intake.[138] Similar results were reported by Schneider and colleagues in dogs with chronic bilateral anatomic renal denervation.[299] Subsequently, the inability of denervated kidneys to adapt to dietary sodium restriction has been documented in the rabbit[153] and the rat.[92]

Unfortunately, not all investigators have confirmed this effect of renal denervation in the unanesthetized state. Lifshitz found no difference in either the renal response to acute volume expansion or the antinatriuretic response to hemorrhage between the innervated and denervated kidney of conscious dogs.[231] This report was consistent with earlier studies by Grabfield and Swanson[155] and Berne[33] and more recent reports by Sadowski and coworkers, who also studied conscious dogs.[294] The explanation for these differences remains unclear. Rogenes and Gottschalk have recently studied the effect of renal denervation in rats before and after the induction of anesthesia.[291] Although they observed a natriuretic effect of denervation, the magnitude of the increment conferred by denervation was significantly greater after anesthesia. Thus, although their studies argue for a role of the renal nerves in the control of basal sodium excretion, they also indicate that studies performed during anesthesia tend to exaggerate the quantitative contribution of renal nerve activity to the total control of urinary sodium excretion. In an editorial, Moss speculated that the failure of some investigators to find an effect of denervation in conscious animals may be due to denervation-induced hypersensitivity to endogenous circulating catecholamines.[253] According to his postulate, catecholamines may be released by the stress of the experimental procedure and thereby overcome the effect of denervation.

In addition to denervation studies, another approach used to examine the role of efferent renal nerve traffic on sodium handling has been the use of renal nerve stimulation by either direct or reflex methods. More than thirty years ago, direct electrical stimulation of the renal nerves was noted to result in an ipsilateral decrement in urinary sodium excretion.[40,179] In those studies, however, marked decreases in renal blood flow and GFR accompanied the antinatriuresis. Using graded increases in renal nerve stimulation, Kopp and DiBona have demonstrated that the renal nerves are capable of influencing sodium excretion through several mechanisms.[214] The lowest level of renal nerve activity does not by itself alter basal renin release, sodium excretion, or GFR, but does magnify the renin response to other simultaneously occurring nonneuronal stimuli. Increasing the frequency of stimulation selectively increases renin secretion and then reduces urinary sodium excretion. GFR and RBF are reduced only at the highest frequencies of renal nerve stimulation.

Indirect reflex stimulation of the renal nerves has also been examined. Maneuvers that modulate renal nerve activity include mechanical left atrial distension, stellate ganglion stimulation, carotid sinus perfusion, and bilateral carotid ligation. As noted earlier in this chapter, many authorities have reported that left atrial distension is associated with an increment in urinary sodium excretion.[145,237,288,289] Although some of this response may result from release of ANP, studies by Karim and colleagues[202] and by Prosnitz and DiBona indicate that this effect is partially due to a decrease in efferent renal nerve activity.[285] Results from the latter studies demonstrated that an approximately 15-mmHg increase in left atrial pressure reduced renal nerve activity by nearly 40 percent and increased urinary sodium excretion by approximately 80 percent. These changes occurred in the absence of measurable changes in GFR and under conditions in which renal perfusion pressure was kept constant by manipulating an aortic clamp proximal to the renal arteries. Further, they noted that bilateral cervical vagotomy totally abolished both the decrease in renal nerve activity and the increase in urinary sodium excretion. Finally, they reported that the constant infusion of vasopressin abolished the diuretic effect of left atrial distension, but the natriuretic effect was unaffected. The physiologic importance of these observations is underlined by a recent observation of Thames and colleagues, who monitored pulmonary artery wedge pressure and renal nerve activity during extracellular fluid volume expansion with a dextran saline solution.[342] Although they unfortunately did not measure urinary sodium excretion, they found a highly significant inverse correlation between pulmonary artery wedge pressure and renal nerve activity. Studies by Gilmore,[141] Takeuchi and associates,[340] and Prosnitz and DiBona[285] demonstrated that stellate ganglion stimulation results in a reduction in efferent renal nerve activity. This effect is thought to be due to carotid sinus reflex, since denervation of that structure abolished both the natriuretic effect and the reduction in renal nerve traffic.[285] Zambraski and associates performed studies that provided consistent results.[370] While perfusing isolated carotid sinuses, they observed a decrease in renal nerve activity in response to increasing perfusion pressure that was accompanied by an increase in sodium excretion. Again, these changes were observed in the absence of changes in renal perfusion pressure, GFR, or RBF. Finally, bilateral carotid ligation increases efferent renal nerve activity, and, when renal perfusion pressure is held constant, urinary sodium excretion falls.[17,286] The significance of these studies using reflex modulation of renal nerve activity is twofold. First, they provide some insight into the afferent arc of volume perception. Second, they assure that the alterations of nerve activity that occur are within a physiologic range and that within this range they are capable of influencing urinary sodium excretion.

The primary nephron site influenced by catecholamines appears to be the proximal tubule. The results of clearance studies[28,38,200] have been confirmed by direct micropuncture in denervated kidneys[22,24] and by micropuncture performed before and during renal nerve stimulation.[26] Similarly, as illustrated in Fig. 3-11, Bello-Reuss has reported that the addition of norepinephrine to the bathing media of the isolated perfused rabbit proximal convoluted tubule results in a reversible increase in the reabsorption rate in that nephron segment but not in the proximal straight tubule or pars recta.[25]

The mechanism of this effect may be multifactorial, in that catecholamines can influence proximal reabsorption in several ways. First, they have the ability to influence RBF and GFR and can thereby importantly alter the physical factors of the proximal peritubular environment. In addition, a direct relationship between renal nerve activity and activation of the renin-angiotensin system[338] and renal prostaglandin production has also been documented.[101] Since these hormones may modulate sodium transport, it is possible that they indirectly mediate the effect of renal nerve traffic. However, Zambraski and DiBona have demonstrated that angiotensin blockade

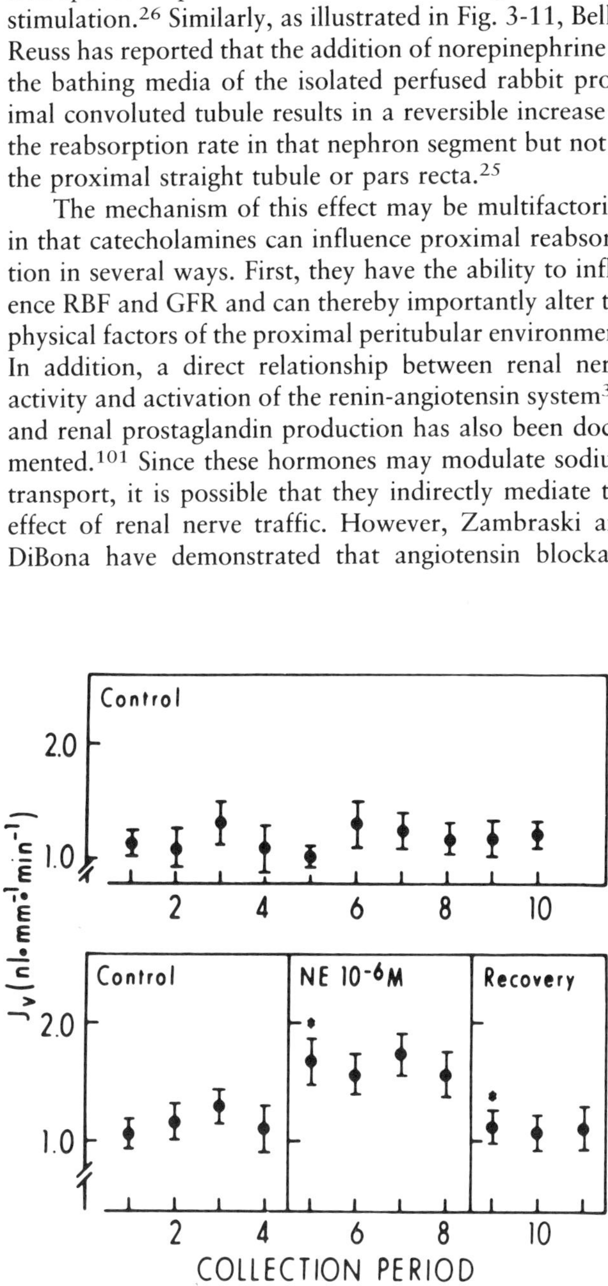

FIGURE 3-11 • Effect of norepinephrine (NE) on net fluid reabsorption (J_v) in the isolated perfused rabbit proximal convoluted tubule. The addition of 10^{-6} *M* NE to the bath causes a reversible increase in J_v. The top panel represents time control experiments without NE. (From Bello-Reuss E: *Am J Physiol* 238:F347, 1980.)

fails to blunt the antinatriuretic effect of renal nerve stimulation,[368] and DiBona has reported that inhibition of prostaglandin synthesis with indomethacin also failed to alter this effect.[88] A growing body of data indicates that the effect may be direct. The first suggestion that this is the case evolved from the studies of Barajas and Muller that provided evidence of tubular sympathetic innervation.[15] Physiologic data also support a direct effect. Numerous studies have found that renal denervation and either direct or indirect renal nerve stimulation influence urinary sodium excretion without measurably altering RBF or GFR.[23,87,88] In addition, studies by Bello-Reuss and coworkers in the rat demonstrated that the denervation-associated fall in proximal tubular reabsorption occurred in the absence of changes in single nephron GFR and in the face of an increase in the hydrostatic pressure gradient across the proximal tubular epithelium.[22] Pelayo and coworkers have confirmed that the denervation-induced reduction in proximal reabsorption occurs in the absence of changes in the physical factors that influence proximal reabsorption.[279] From these observations, it seems unlikely that altered physical factors are required for mediating the proximal effect of denervation. The in vitro microperfusion studies of Bello-Reuss[25] demonstrating a stimulatory effect of norepinephrine on proximal tubular sodium transport also argue for direct effects of the renal nerves on epithelial transport. Finally, Insel and colleagues have observed that stimulation of alpha-2 receptors increases sodium influx in isolated proximal tubule cells.[191]

Increasing evidence suggests that catecholamines may be important regulators of sodium reabsorption in distal nephron segments as well. Barajas and colleagues observed that adrenergic nerve terminals were in direct contact with tubular basement membranes of the cortical and medullary thick ascending limb of Henle's loop.[16] That this finding has physiologic significance for the control of sodium reabsorption has been demonstrated by DiBona and Sawin.[91] Using the technique of in vivo microperfusion to precisely control sodium chloride and water delivery to the rat's loop segment, they observed that low-frequency renal nerve stimulation increased tubular sodium and chloride reabsorption in the nephron segment located between the late proximal convoluted tubule and early distal convoluted tubule. Since fluid reabsorption was not increased, this effect probably occurred in the thin ascending limb, medullary or cortical thick ascending limb, or distal convoluted tubule segments, which reabsorb sodium chloride but have minimal water permeability. Stimulation of net chloride reabsorption from isolated perfused mouse medullary thick ascending limbs of Henle's loop has also been observed following addition of micromolar concentrations of isoproterenol or norepinephrine to the peritubular bathing solution.[282] Catecholamines may also alter sodium transport in the collecting duct. Acute renal denervation decreases recovery of ^{22}Na microinjected into the late distal convoluted tubule, while adrenoreceptor stimulation with epinephrine reverses the effects of vasopressin on sodium excretion in the isolated perfused kidney.[22,314] The precise role of the various neurotransmitters and classes of adrenoreceptors involved in mediating the effect of catecholamines on urinary sodium excretion continues to be investigated. Bello-Reuss found that the beta-adrenergic antagonist propranolol reversed the stimulatory effect of norepinephrine on proximal reabsorption in vitro.[25] Based on this observation, she concluded that beta-adrenergic stimulation mediated the proximal effects. Propranolol also blocks the stimulatory effects of isoproterenol or norepinephrine in the isolated perfused mouse mTALH but has no direct effects when added in the absence of the beta agonist.[282] DiBona and associates, on the other hand, have provided convincing evidence that alpha-adrenergic stimulation is antinatriuretic.[89,90,370,371] They have shown that alphaadrenergic blockade with phentolamine, phenoxybenzamine, or prazosin inhibits the antinatriuretic response to low-level renal nerve stimulation in the dog. The antinatriuretic response to low-level renal nerve stimulation was unaffected by the beta-adrenoreceptor antagonists propranolol or atenolol in their studies. Chan has also observed that phenoxybenzamine blocks proximal tubule reabsorption induced by addition of norepinephrine to the peritubular circulation.[66]

The role of alpha-2 adrenoreceptors in the regulation of renal sodium excretion has also been examined. Initial studies suggested that low-dose intrarenal infusion of the alpha-2 antagonists yohimbine or rauwolscine had no effect on sodium excretion.[268] Fildes and coworkers, on the other hand, reported that intrarenal infusion of yohimbine increased renal sodium excretion.[124a] The dose of yohimbine used in the latter study was 20- to 200-fold greater than that used in the former study and may account for the disparate results. Pettinger and associates have observed that, in isolated perfused kidneys, activation of alpha-2 adrenoreceptors reversed both vasopressin-induced sodium retention and arachidonic acid or furosemide-induced sodium excretion under conditions of alpha-1 and beta-receptor blockade.[280,313,349] As activation of alpha-2 adrenoreceptors can inhibit cAMP formation in isolated single-nephron segments, they have suggested that alpha-2 adrenoreceptors act to inhibit hormone-stimulated transport processes that depend on activation of adenylate cyclase.[280]

The contribution of the renal nerves to the long-term maintenance of sodium balance remains to be clarified. Lifschitz reported that the response to 2 percent body weight hemorrhage or 5 percent body weight volume expansion was similar between denervated and innervated kidneys in conscious dogs.[231] Bencsath and associates demonstrated that renal denervation did not interfere with sodium conservation during dietary sodium restriction in conscious rats.[29] Similar conclusions have also been reported in conscious rats by Fernandez-Ropollet and colleagues.[122] Using dogs with split bladders, Mizelle and colleagues were unable to demonstrate differences in urinary sodium excretion between innervated and denervated kidneys in the same animal during adaption to a low sodium diet.[249] Other investigators have reported that animals on sodium-restricted diets cannot maintain sodium balance following renal denervation.[92,153] Sympathetic blockade has also been reported to interfere with maintenance of sodium balance during dietary sodium restriction in humans.[138] DiBona and Sawin have observed that renal nerve activity is greater in rats maintained on a low-sodium intake than on a high sodium intake and that inhibition of renal nerve activity provides a greater contribution to the natriuretic response induced by acute saline administration in rats maintained on the low-salt diet.[93] They concluded that the contribution of the renal nerves to the regulation of urinary sodium excretion is greater during dietary sodium restriction and proposed that renal tubular sodium reabsorption mediated by increased renal nerve activity is necessary to establish maximal renal sodium conservation. The explanation for these discrepant findings will need to be clarified before the role of the renal nerves in the regulation of sodium balance can be established with certainty.

Finally, data continue to accumulate suggesting that dopamine is an important modulator of renal sodium excretion. Dopamine is synthesized and stored within the kidney, and two classes of dopamine receptors have been identified in renal tissue.[121] DA_1 receptors are localized in the renal artery, the juxtaglomerular cells, and the basolateral and brush border membranes of proximal convoluted and proximal straight tubules, as well as in the cortical collecting duct. DA_2 receptors have been identified in the renal vasculature and in membranes derived from proximal tubules.[120,121] Thus, dopamine may influence renal sodium handling through both hemodynamic and tubular mechanisms.

Many studies suggest dopamine is important in the natriuresis induced by sodium loading. There appears to be a direct relationship among renal tissue levels of dopamine, dopamine excretion, and urinary sodium excretion during acute volume expansion with saline solution and during chronic salt loading.[11,76,118] Inhibitors of dopamine production or antagonists to dopamine receptors attenuate the natriuretic response to acute saline loading in dogs,[312] in rats,[196,278] and in humans.[217] Dopamine blockade also abolishes the natriuretic response to lower-body positive pressure in humans.[31] Not all studies, however, support a role for dopamine in the natriuresis induced by sodium loading. Bradley and associates found no effect of intrarenal dopamine antagonists on the natriuresis induced by either saline loading or renal nerve stimulation in dogs.[44] Siragy and colleagues observed that a DA_1-receptor antagonist failed to attenuate natriuresis in dogs ingesting 150 to 200 meq/day of sodium but was antinatriuretic in dogs maintained on a lower sodium intake.[312] They proposed that the effect of dopamine on sodium excretion depends on the magnitude of the sodium load. During greater degrees of sodium loading, tubular sodium reabsorption is inhibited through changes in physical factors that render other stimuli for sodium excretion ineffective.

Whether dopamine plays a role in the regulation of sodium balance in euvolemic or sodium-restricted states is uncertain. Pelayo and associates found that dopamine blockade attenuated the natriuresis of Ringer's solution loading but had no effect on euvolemic rats.[278] Frederickson and colleagues demonstrated that selective DA_1-receptor blockade had no effect on baseline electrolyte excretion in the dog but did inhibit the response to exogenous dopamine.[132] On the other hand, Ball and Lee have found that inhibition of dopamine synthesis lowered urinary sodium excretion in euvolemic humans,[10] and a potent DA_1 antagonist has been shown to reduce sodium excretion in dogs maintained on a 40-meq sodium intake.[312]

Although dopamine may influence RBF and potentially GFR, its primary effect on sodium excretion appears to be mediated through direct tubular effects. Bello-Reuss and coworkers observed that dopamine added to the bath solution increased sodium reabsorption in the proximal straight tubule but not the proximal convoluted tubule of the rabbit.[26] Felder and coworkers, using rat renal cortical brush border membranes, observed that dopamine or DA_1 agonists decreased sodium uptake by inhibiting Na^+-H^+ antiport activity.[121] This response was prevented by administration of DA_1 antagonists but not by DA_2 antagonists.[121] Laradi and associates have also reported that dopamine activates the Na^+-H^+ antiport in isolated proximal tubular cells from the rabbit and have observed that the antiport was inhibited by the nonselective dopamine blocker metoclopramide.[222] However, the direction of transport was out of the lumen in this study. Whether the differences in the direction of transport are due to differences in the subtype of receptor inhibited or the experimental design are unclear. Finally, dopamine may reduce sodium reabsorption in distal nephron segments as well. Dopamine has recently been reported to antagonize the effects of ADH and mineralocorticoids in the cortical collecting duct.[256] Thus, dopamine could function as an autacoid hormone to control sodium excretion in certain circumstances. However, the exact conditions wherein dopamine plays an important role remain to be elucidated.

In summary, a large body of evidence suggests the renal nerves exert important effects on the control of sodium excretion under conditions of volume depletion or in states of increased renal nerve activity, while dopamine may be important during sodium excess. The quantitative contribution of these systems to the regulation of sodium homeostasis under normal physiologic circumstances remains undefined and requires further study.

MEDULLARY TONICITY

Numerous studies have shown that alterations in tubular reabsorption beyond the proximal tubule are operative in mediating the natriuretic response to acute volume expansion.[45,180,209,212] In 1951, Ladd reported that the prior induction of a water diuresis enhanced the ability of normal individuals to excrete a saline load.[220] In 1964, Earley and Friedler suggested that medullary tonicity influenced the rate of sodium absorption by the loop of Henle.[104] Later studies by Humphreys and associates presented additional data consistent with that hypothesis.[184] Studies reported by Stein and colleagues,[328] Higashihara and coworkers,[174] and Haas and associates demonstrated that acute saline loading resulted in preferential inhibition of sodium reabsorption in juxtamedullary nephrons.[165] Pharmacologic manipulation suggests this inhibition occurred primarily along the thin ascending limb of the loop of Henle.[270] Studies by Reineck and Parma demonstrated that induction of a water diuresis alone failed to increase sodium excretion.[287] However, when water diuresis was superimposed upon mild volume expansion, which under hydropenic conditions decreased proximal reabsorption without increasing sodium excretion, a substantial natriuretic response was observed. Micropuncture data confirmed that this effect was limited to juxtamedullary nephrons. Thus, these findings are consistent with the view that medullary tonicity is capable of altering sodium excretion only when delivery out of the proximal tubule is increased.

PROSTAGLANDINS

It should be stated at the outset that the evidence that prostaglandins (PGs; see Chap. 15) play a regulatory role in the control of urinary sodium excretion is conflicting. Thus, this section presents data regarding the concept that PGs directly modulate renal tubular sodium reabsorption. The initial enthusiasm for an effect of these substances on sodium transport was generated by clearance studies in which a marked natriuretic response was observed when either PGA_1 or PGE_1 was infused directly into the renal artery of the dog.[166,194,257] Since that time, PGD_2 and PGI_2 have also been shown to be natriuretic when given under the same conditions.[131,133] Two major problems have prevented the unequivocal acceptance of a regulatory role for PGs in sodium homeostasis. First, all of the PGs studied caused renal vasodilation. Since other vasodilator substances are also natriuretic, the observed increase in sodium excretion could be nonspecific and simply mediated by the nonspecific increase in RBF. Second, it is uncertain whether administration of PGs directly into the renal artery mimicked either the physiologic concentration or anatomical location of endogenously produced PGs. Three experimental approaches have been employed to circumvent these problems. First, attempts have been made to quantitate renal PG production and determine whether there is a consistent relationship between their synthesis and sodium excretion. Second, inhibitors of endogenous PG synthesis have been utilized to examine their effect on sodium excretion. Third, PGs have been directly applied in vitro to a variety of sodium-transporting epithelia. Despite these approaches, the role of PGs in the control of sodium excretion remains highly controversial.

Studies designed to examine the relationship between renal PG production and urinary sodium excretion have utilized the measurement of either renal venous PGE concentration or urinary PGE excretion. Using the former determination, several groups of investigators have reported an increase in the renal production of PGE in response to acute volume expansion with intravenous saline administration.[274,310,341] On the other hand, Oliver and coworkers have reported that dietary sodium deprivation is also associated with an increase in renal venous PGE_2 concentration.[265] Furthermore, Lifschitz and colleagues have found that increasing dietary sodium intake in the rabbit is associated with an increase in urinary sodium excretion but no change in urinary PGE excretion.[232] This finding seemingly dissociates renal PGE production from urinary sodium excretion and PGE excretion. Epstein and coworkers examined the effect of neck-out water immersion on sodium excretion in normal humans.[114] They found that this maneuver increased both urinary sodium and PGE excretion. However, pretreatment with indomethacin, an inhibitor of PG synthesis, had no effect on the natriuretic response to immersion but markedly diminished PGE excretion in sodium-depleted subjects. From these studies, it seems fair to conclude that, if renal PGE production plays a role in modulating urinary sodium excretion during ECF volume expansion, other factors must be able to override that influence.

The effect of inhibitors of PG synthesis on sodium excretion has been examined by numerous investigators. Dusing and associates found that these agents blunted the natriuretic response to acute saline loading in conscious rats,[103] and Altsheler and coworkers confirmed that report studying conscious dogs. In addition, Altsheler and colleagues found that PG inhibition had no effect on basal sodium excretion.[3] The latter finding was similar to that of Zambraski and Dunn, who also administered the inhibitors to conscious dogs.[369] Finally, Higashihara and coworkers found that inhibitors of PG synthesis decreased urinary chloride excretion both before and after acute volume expansion in anesthetized rats.[175]

Although these studies would suggest that endogenous PGs either fail to influence sodium excretion or tend to increase it, studies by others using similar protocols have suggested that PGs are, in fact, salt retaining. Vanherwegman and colleagues found that indomethacin inhibited sodium reabsorption in the isolated perfused dog kidney.[353] Kirschenbaum and Stein, on the other hand, reported a natriuretic response to indomethacin in the conscious dog.[207] In concert with these reports is the earlier work of Lipson and Sharp, which demonstrated that, when applied to the toad bladder, an epithelium thought to have transport characteristics similar to those of the mammalian distal nephron, PGE increased short-circuit current and sodium transport.[233]

Unfortunately, as with the clearance studies, controversy also surrounds the effects of PGs on sodium transport in vitro. Stokes and Kokko[333] and Iino and Imai,[189] studying isolated perfused rabbit tubules, reported an inhibitory effect of PGE on sodium reabsorption in the cortical collecting tubule and outer medullary collecting ducts. Stokes also found that PGE decreased chloride transport in the medullary, but not cortical, thick ascending limb of the loop of Henle.[331] This finding was consistent with the finding of Ganguli and associates that inhibitors of PG synthesis resulted in an increase in renal medullary sodium chloride concentration.[134] They also seemed to confirm the conclusion of Higashihara and colleagues, who employed micropuncture techniques in the rat and found that PG inhibition increased chloride reabsorption in the superficial loop of Henle.[175] These findings are consistent with the view that PGs inhibit tubular reabsorption of sodium. As stated above, this conclusion remains controversial. Fine and Trizna applied a variety of PGs to both the luminal and peritubular side of the isolated perfused medullary thick ascending limb of the loop of Henle and the medullary collecting duct and were unable to detect an effect of any of these agents on sodium reabsorption.[128] Similarly, they were unable to influence sodium transport in these nephron segments by the addition of any of three inhibitors of PG synthesis. Fine and Kirschenbaum subsequently reported that they found no effect of PGE on sodium reabsorption in the cortical collecting tubule.[127]

While a direct effect of PGs on sodium balance has not been established, they have been shown to modify other direct stimuli for sodium reabsorption. This interaction has been most convincingly shown by its interactions with ADH. Culpepper and Andreoli demonstrated that PGE_2 reduces ADH-stimulated chloride reabsorption in isolated perfused mouse medullary thick ascending limbs of Henle's loop.[77] PGE_2 had no effect on chloride reabsorption in that segment in the absence of ADH and had no effect on the ADH-insensitive cortical thick ascending limb. PGE_2 also antagonizes ADH antinatriuresis in the isolated erythrocyte-perfused rat kidney but has no effect on urinary sodium excretion in that preparation in the absence of ADH.[230]

Other products of arachidonic acid metabolism derived from the NADPH-dependent cytochrome P450 epoxygenase pathway may also alter renal sodium handling. Both the pars recta and the thick ascending limb of Henle's loop, with its adjacent collecting tubule, produce large amounts of epoxyeicosatrienoic acids (EETs) but only small amounts of PGs.[123] Jacobson and associates have shown that EETs inhibit sodium reabsorption in the isolated cortical collecting duct.[192] EETs also inhibit Na^+-K^+ ATPase activity in cells from the thick ascending limb of Henle's loop.[306] From the considerations outlined above, it is clear that, while products of arachidonic acid metabolism have the potential to modulate renal sodium metabolism, their role remains to be determined.

NATRIURETIC HORMONES

Following publication of the classic studies of de Wardener and coworkers,[86] numerous laboratories have pursued the identification and isolation of a humoral substance that would be released in response to ECF volume expansion and suppress tubular reabsorption of sodium. In 1979, de Bold demonstrated that administration of an extract of atrial tissue induced a profound diuresis and natriuresis in the rat (Fig. 3-12). This response was not observed when extracts of ventricular tissue were administered.[83] The activity was quickly localized to the secretory-type granules originally described in atrial tissue in 1955.[208] In short order the protein was extracted, purified, and sequenced and the gene for its production cloned. The circulating hormone derived from these secretory granules is the 28-amino-acid protein ANP, which, in addition to natriuretic and diuretic properties, produces vasorelaxation, shifts fluid from the vascular to the interstitial space, and directly and separately suppresses both aldosterone and renin production. Release of ANP is regulated primarily by changes in atrial stretch or pressure, although release can also be stimulated by vasopressin, alpha-1 agonists, and angiotensin II. Increases in plasma ANP levels are induced by saline loading; chronic high sodium intake; maneuvers that increase stretch of the cardiac atria, such as physical exercise; and pathologic conditions such as paroxysmal atrial tachycardia, inappropriate secretion of ADH, primary aldosteronism, congestive heart failure, and chronic renal insufficiency. Decreases in vascular volume and other maneuvers that decrease atrial stretch reduce plasma ANP levels.

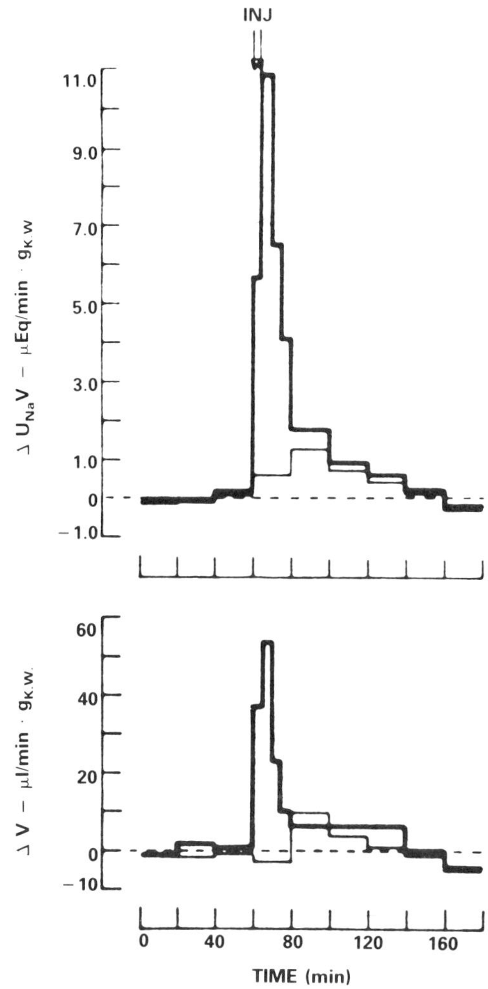

FIGURE 3-12 • Effect of atrial myocardial extract on urinary sodium excretion ($U_{Na}V$) and urine volume (*V*). Dark lines represent the increment in $U_{Na}V$ and *V* in response to an injection of atrial extract. Light lines represent changes in response to an identically prepared injection of a ventrical extract. (From DeBold AJ: *Life Sci* 28:89, 1981.)

ANP may influence renal sodium reabsorption through both direct and indirect mechanisms at a number of nephron sites. Direct effects occur at the glomerulus and in the inner medullary collecting ducts. These effects are initiated by the binding of ANP to specific ANP receptors (beta receptors) and result in the stimulation of GMP.[12,60,65] Administration of a permeable cGMP analogue in vivo reproduces the effects of ANP both at the glomerulus and in the inner medullary collecting duct.[182,373] At the glomerulus, ANP increases the GFR in both superficial and deep nephrons by increasing capillary hydrostatic pressure.[102,354] This occurs primarily through afferent arteriolar dilatation, although increases in glomerular permeability coefficient (*Kf*) and efferent arteriolar constriction have also been described. As tubuloglomerular feedback is attenuated by ANP, the glomerular hyperfiltration is sustained.[181] At the inner medullary collecting duct, Zeidel has shown that ANP reduces the rate of sodium entry through luminal amiloride inhibitable sodium channels at ANP concentrations similar to those found in plasma under basal and volume-expanded conditions.[373] It remains controversial whether changes in the GFR or direct tubular effects are the dominant direct mechanism for the natriuretic activity of ANP.

ANP may also mediate sodium excretion through a number of indirect mechanisms. In these circumstances, the renal structures involved lack specific ANP receptors, the responses are not associated with generation of GMP, and ANP does not alter transport when added to isolated tubule segments or representative cell cultures. In addition, some of these ANP responses require prestimulation of the tubule segment by some other hormone. In the proximal tubule, for example, no binding sites for ANP have been identified, and ANP has no effect on transport in perfused proximal tubules in vitro,[21,215] yet ANP inhibits angiotensin-II-stimulated sodium reabsorption at this location.[171] ANP also increases hydrostatic pressure in Henle's loop, the collecting duct, and vasa recta[246] and interstitial hydrostatic pressure in deep nephrons.[136] These events would result in unfavorable pressure gradients for sodium reabsorption along the collecting duct and in deep nephrons. The significance of this mechanism has been shown by Mendez and colleagues, who demonstrated that infusion of hyperoncotic albumin to increase peritubular oncotic pressure attenuates ANP-induced natriuresis.[246]

Despite the large body of work on the effects of ANP on renal function, the role of this peptide in the regulation of sodium balance remains unclear. A large number of studies have shown that infusions of exogenous ANP at rates that produce plasma levels within the physiologic range increase urinary sodium excretion.[1,14,34,290] However, the time course of the changes in plasma ANP and urinary sodium excretion do not always coincide. Furthermore, infusion of exogenous ANP to achieve plasma levels similar to those measured during stimuli such as volume loading do not reproduce the natriuresis quantitatively. Richards and associates found that, while 2 h of saline loading in human subjects increased plasma ANP levels approximately twofold, the natriuresis induced by saline loading could not be reproduced quantitatively by even an eightfold elevation in plasma ANP levels produced by an intravenous ANP infusion.[290] Cotter and coworkers observed that infusion of ANP at 4, 8, and 16 ng/kg per minute over successive 30-min intervals progressively increased urinary sodium excretion but that the magnitude was quite modest.[73] A 12.9-fold increase in plasma ANP levels resulted in only a 42 percent increase in sodium excretion. From these types of studies, Goetz has estimated that doubling the circulating ANP levels in normal subjects increases sodium excretion by less than 10 percent.[146] In addition, several investigators have reported that, when low doses of ANP are infused to produce plasma concentrations of ANP within the physiologic or pathologic range, the natriuresis may be delayed for up to 3 to 4 h.[1,34,35] As mentioned previously, Goetz and associates observed that increasing left atrial pressure in conscious dogs with surgically denervated hearts increased plasma ANP to levels equivalent to those found in dogs with innervated hearts but that natriuresis occurred only in the innervated group.[148] On the other hand, several studies have shown that the natriuretic response to volume expansion is markedly attenuated when the ANP response is prevented. Veress and Sonnenberg have shown that removal of the right atrial appendage reduced the natriuretic response to acute volume expansion by 50 percent compared to sham-operated rats.[345] Similar findings have been subsequently reported by Schwab and coworkers.[304] Studies employing antibodies to ANP have also suggested that ANP contributes significantly to the natriuresis induced by volume expansion. Naruse and coworkers found that urine flow and sodium excretion decreased and plasma renin activity increased in anesthetized rats followed administration of serum containing antibodies against ANP.[258] Hirth and associates have shown that rats immunized with monoclonal antibodies against ANP are unable to increase sodium excretion for 20 to 40 min following volume expansion with whole blood.[176] Finally, Mizelle and associates have shown that ANP administered continuously into the renal artery of dogs to produce levels in the physiologic range result in a sustained natriuresis.[249a]

While continued investigation is necessary to clarify the role of ANP in the regulation of sodium balance, the available data suggest it can significantly amplify the response to other natriuretic stimuli.

It should be pointed out that ANP is probably different from the natriuretic substance described by Gonick and associates.[149] This substance has been postulated to work through inhibition of Na^+-K^+ ATPase, an effect not produced by ANP. Gruber, Whitaker, and Buckalew have extracted a substance from saline-loaded normal dogs that cross reacts with antidigoxin antibodies and inhibits Na^+-K^+ ATPase.[163]

Much work remains to be done in this interesting area of sodium hemostasis.

KALLIKREIN-KININ SYSTEM AND OTHER PEPTIDES THAT POTENTIALLY MODIFY SODIUM EXCRETION

All components of the kallikrein-kinin system (see Chap. 15) are present within the kidney and have been proposed to increase sodium excretion in response to increases in ECF volume.[63] Activation of this system leads to release of glandular kallikrein, a protease that acts on the substrate kininogen to release kallidin, the renal kinin. Kallidin is subsequently converted to bradykinin by aminopeptidases. Kinins are degraded into inactive peptides by kinases I and II. The latter is also the converting enzyme responsible for activation of angiotensin I. Kinase II is located in the proximal tubule in high concentrations, thus preventing delivery of circulating kinins to the distal nephron, the primary site of endogenous kinin activity.

Using the urinary excretion of kallikrein as an indicator of activity of the renal kallikrein-kinin system, numerous studies have demonstrated a correlation between urinary kallikrein excretion and urinary sodium excretion in humans following saline administration or after several days of mineralocorticoid administration.[241,248,357] Infusion of kinins intravenously or intraarterially increases sodium excretion in experimental animals.[20,359] The natriuresis induced by kinin administration occurs both through alterations in RBF or renal perfusion pressure and through direct effects on tubular transport in the distal nephron. Willis and associates have observed that preventing the increase in RBF induced by bradykinin abolishes its natriuretic activity.[364] Mertz and colleagues have found that bradykinin administered into the aorta significantly increases renal interstitial hydrostatic pressure, thus providing another potential mechanism for humans to increase sodium excretion.[247] Kinins have also been noted to increase medullary blood flow.[115,292] Finally, Tomita and associates have reported that $10^{-9}M$ bradykinin inhibits sodium reabsorption from isolated perfused rat cortical collecting ducts.[345]

Despite these findings, a role for the kallikrein-kinin system in the regulation of sodium balance has been difficult to unequivocally demonstrate due to problems similar to those outlined in the section of PGs. Thus, correlations between urinary kallikrein and urinary sodium excretion do not establish a cause-and-effect relationship, while increases in sodium excretion induced by intravenous kinin infusion may not be representative of alterations in kinin activity in the distal nephron. Several studies have attempted to evaluate the role of endogenous kinins in sodium excretion by inhibiting their action with aprotinin, a nonspecific protease inhibitor or, recently, with a kinin-receptor antagonist. Neither aprotinin nor kinin-receptor antagonists alter sodium excretion in conscious rats maintained on normal sodium intakes.[216,238,283] Whether inhibition of kinin activity during sodium loading attenuates the natriuresis is controversial. Kauker reported that aprotinin significantly decreased urinary sodium excretion without altering the GFR in anesthetized saline-loaded rats.[203] Pollock and associates, on the other hand, found that, while aprotinin significantly decreased urinary kallikrein excretion, it had no effect on urinary sodium excretion in either conscious or anesthetized volume-expanded rats.[283] Thus, while the elements of the kallikrein-kinin system appear to have the ability to act as regulators of sodium balance, their importance remains to be elucidated.

A number of other peptides with primary function in the gastrointestinal tract or brain have also been reported to influence renal sodium handling (see Chap. 17). Vasoactive intestinal peptide, substance P, secretin, neuropeptide Y, and cholecystokinin octapeptide have all been reported to increase sodium excretion, while calcitonin gene-related peptide, insulin, neurotensin, somatostatin, and endothelin have been reported to reduce renal sodium excretion.[350] The physiologic significance of these findings remains to be elucidated.

SEGMENTAL ANALYSIS OF SODIUM TRANSPORT

PROXIMAL TUBULE

Under normal circumstances, the proximal tubule reabsorbs 50 to 75 percent of the filtered sodium load. In view of this very large reabsorptive capacity, it is reasonable to suspect that this nephron segment would participate to a major extent in the regulation of urinary sodium excretion. That this is indeed the case was first demonstrated by Dirks, Cirksena, and Berliner in 1965.[96] These investigators applied direct micropuncture techniques to the dog and found that acute volume expansion with saline solution resulted in a dramatic decrease in proximal reabsorption. Since that time, innumerable studies have confirmed this effect, not only in the dog, but in the rat as well. It was subsequently documented that the proximal tubule of juxtamedullary nephrons, as well as superficial nephrons, responds to expansion with saline by decreasing both the fractional and the absolute reabsorptive rate.[270] It is interesting, however, that these two nephron populations do not respond similarly to vascular volume expansion with intravenous hyperoncotic albumin.[271] Studies by Osgood and colleagues have demonstrated that the proximal tubule of superficial nephrons decreases fractional reabsorption in this setting but that juxtamedullary proximal reabsorption is unchanged. The reason for this difference is not clear but suggests that the mechanisms of reabsorption may differ or that deep nephrons possess a proximal tubule that is unresponsive to stimuli that diminish reabsorption when intravascular volume is selectively expanded. Conversely, Haas and associates have shown that increases in renal perfusion pressure do not change sodium reabsorption in superficial nephrons but increase sodium delivery to the descending limb of Henle's loop of deep nephrons.[165] This suggests that renal perfusion pressure may preferentially reduce sodium reabsorption in the proximal tubule of deep nephrons.

Just as the proximal tubule decreases its reabsorptive rate in response to saline-induced volume expansion, Weiner and coworkers[360] and Stein and associates[338] demonstrated that severe volume depletion causes an increase in proximal reabsorption. Thus, it appears that the proximal tubule responds in an appropriate fashion to changes in ECF volume. The mechanisms involved in this response were discussed in detail above and probably include alterations in the peritubular capillary Starling forces, renal nerve activity, and circulating or intrarenal angiotensin II levels.

Despite the evidence that proximal reabsorption decreases in response to acute ECF volume expansion and increases when that volume is decreased, a large body of evidence indicates that nephron segments beyond the proximal tubule are also important in modulating the renal response to salt excess or deficit. Numerous studies have been reported in which proximal reabsorption is significantly decreased with only trivial or no changes in sodium excretion.[45,180,209] Conversely, Knox and colleagues demonstrated that the reduction in proximal reabsorption seen with acute saline loading can be prevented by the intrarenal administration of hyperoncotic albumin; but, despite this "clamping" of proximal reabsorption, a marked increase in sodium excretion occurs.[212] These observations have led to a major investigative effort to characterize the response of nephron segments beyond the high-capacity proximal tubule to changes in ECF volume.

LOOP OF HENLE

In considering the role of the loop of Henle in the control of urinary sodium excretion, it is essential to distinguish clearly between superficial and juxtamedullary nephrons. This distinction in the rat, at least, is necessitated by anatomical differences between the loops of nephrons with glomeruli located in the superficial cortex and those arising from glomeruli located deeper in the cortex near the corticomedullary junction. The loops of Henle of the former nephrons are composed of a thin descending limb that extends to the junction of the inner and outer medulla, where it turns, giving rise to the thick ascending limb. Among nephrons so composed are those with proximal and distal tubules located on the surface of the kidney and therefore directly accessible to in vivo micropuncture. Juxtamedullary nephrons, in contrast, possess loops of Henle with descending limbs that extend deeper into the inner medulla and also contain a thin ascending limb that spans the inner medulla between the bend of Henle's loop and the junction of the inner and outer medulla, where the thick ascending limb begins. The thick ascending limb of both superficial and juxtamedullary nephrons is responsible for the active sodium reabsorption that occurs in this segment. Due to the very low water permeability of the thick ascending limb, this location is essential for both urinary concentration and urinary dilution. As discussed previously, this segment demonstrates a direct relationship between tubular delivery and sodium reabsorption.[219,251] Thus, as delivery to the thick ascending limb increases, sodium reabsorption increases, allowing this segment to buffer effects that reduce sodium reabsorption in the proximal tubule. The primary transport mechanism for sodium reabsorption in this location occurs through the $1Na^+$-$1K^+$-$2Cl^-$ cotransport system located on the luminal membrane and powered by the basolateral extrusion of intracellular sodium by Na^+-K^+ ATPase. It is this cotransport system which is selectively inhibited by furosemide and other loop diuretics. Some sodium reabsorption may also occur paracellularly through the tight junctions. In addition to sodium delivery, sodium reabsorption in the thick ascending limb is regulated by hormones and sympathetic nerve stimulation.[77,88,91,282,331] Together these influences result in a very sensitive mechanism for controlling sodium delivery to more distal nephron segments. The anatomical differences in loops of superficial and juxtamedullary nephrons may further allow these distinct nephron populations to respond differently to acute expansion of ECF volume.

Superficial loops of Henle

The effect of acute volume expansion with saline solution on sodium reabsorption in the superficial loop of Henle has been examined in the rat with both free-flow micropuncture and in vivo microperfusion. Utilizing the former method, several authors have reported that absolute reabsorption by this segment increases in response to volume expansion and have concluded that reabsorption is in part a direct function of load or sodium delivery.[219,221,326] Thus, as proximal reabsorption is decreased, the delivery of sodium to the loop is increased and, as predicted by glomerular tubular balance, reabsorption also increases. In terms of fractional reabsorption—the percentage of delivered sodium that is reabsorbed—the available data are less clear. Landwehr and associates found that fractional as well as absolute reabsorption increased in response to saline-induced volume expansion.[221] Kunau and associates, on the other hand, reported a decrease in fractional reabsorption under the same circumstances.[219] Perhaps the most definitive study of the response of the superficial loop of Henle to acute volume expansion was that of Morgan and Berliner.[251] These investigators perfused this nephron segment in vivo at a constant rate before and after acute volume expansion and found no change in reabsorptive rate. From these considerations it appears that the superficial loop of Henle does not participate to any significant degree in the natriuretic response to acute expansion of the ECF space and in fact demonstrates increased absolute rates of sodium reabsorption in this setting.

Juxtamedullary loop of Henle

As discussed earlier in this chapter, several studies have suggested that acute volume expansion preferentially inhibit sodium reabsorption in juxtamedullary nephrons, at least in the rat.[174,270,328] Further, using pharmacologic manipulation and direct measurement of the loop of

Henle to vasa recta sodium concentration gradients, Osgood and coworkers suggested that the thin ascending limb of the loop of Henle, a nephron segment that transports sodium chloride only by passive means, was the likely site for this preferential inhibition.[270] Subsequent studies indicate that this decreased reabsorption is probably due to "washout" of the normally hypertonic medullary interstitium secondary to volume expansion.[287]

DISTAL TUBULE

Early micropuncture studies considered the surface distal tubule of superficial nephrons to be the "distal-convoluted tubule." More recently, however, it has become apparent that this nephron segment, which is accessible for micropuncture, is actually quite heterogeneous and consists of cell types characteristic of the thick ascending limb, the distal convoluted tubule, and the early portion of the cortical collecting tubule. Consequently, this segment has been subdivided into the distal tubule, connecting segment (previously included as part of the late distal tubule), and early portion of the cortical collecting tubule. Although studies using in vivo microperfusion techniques are beginning to examine these segments individually, most data from micropuncture studies have examined these segments as a unit termed "distal tubule."

Micropuncture studies examining the response of this segment to acute saline infusion have found that sodium transport is comparable to that of the superficial loop of Henle in that reabsorption varies directly with delivery.[219,251] In vivo microperfusion studies have shown that when delivery is maintained constant, the reabsorptive rate is unchanged.[251] Thus, it seems fair to conclude that this nephron segment does not participate in the natriuretic response to acute volume expansion. On the other hand, the distal tubule may be important in blunting natriuretic responses. As early as 1974, Kunau and colleagues demonstrated that distal sodium reabsorption increased directly with sodium delivery, an effect that appears to depend primarily on changes in tubular sodium concentration.[159] Kaissling and coworkers have shown that a chronic high sodium delivery increases the surface area of the basolateral membrane and increases Na^+-K^+ ATPase activity in the distal convoluted tubule, connecting tubule, and cortical collecting duct.[198,225] These effects are independent of mineralocorticoids and are associated with increased transport capacity as well.[314] Thus, changes in distal nephron transport capacity may serve to maintain sodium homeostasis in the face of chronic stimuli for sodium excretion. This adaptation may explain the clinical observation that the response to chronic administration of loop diuretics becomes diminished with time. The conclusion that the distal tubule does not participate in the natriuretic response to acute volume expansion seems at odds with the previous conclusions that aldosterone is an important component of normal volume homeostasis and that the distal tubule is generally considered the site of its action. It will be recalled, however, that in vitro microperfusion studies have firmly established that aldosterone primarily influences cortical collecting tubule transport, and the greater portion of that segment lies beyond the surface distal tubule. Furthermore, it is possible, and in fact likely, that suppression of aldosterone is relatively unimportant in the natriuretic response to acute volume expansion. The major evidence of its importance is derived from more chronic studies utilizing manipulation of dietary sodium.

CORTICAL COLLECTING TUBULE

The cortical collecting tubule is inaccessible to direct micropuncture, and it is therefore impossible to directly evaluate the effect of changes in ECF volume on sodium reabsorption along this segment. Nevertheless, circumstantial considerations suggest that this nephron segment may well play a role in the determination of sodium excretion. First, aldosterone has been conclusively shown to play a central role in alterations in sodium transport in this segment, initially by increasing apical membrane sodium conductance and later by increasing Na^+-K^+ ATPase[296] activity. Second, the natriuretic substance of uremia, described by Fine and associates, has been demonstrated in vitro to decrease sodium reabsorption in this nephron segment.[125] If the same natriuretic factor is secreted in response to ECF volume expansion, it would be expected to exert a similar effect under those conditions. In addition, ANP has been shown to reduce sodium reabsorption in cortical collecting tubules isolated from rats pretreated with mineralocorticoid.[262] Thus, this location may be an important site for regulation of sodium excretion under conditions that stimulate ANP release.

Finally, it may be recalled that some investigators have reported that PGE_2 and kinins inhibit sodium reabsorption along this segment of the nephron. Although there is controversy regarding these findings and the relationship between these substances and ECF volume is still unsettled, these effects afford another potential mechanism by which the cortical collecting tubule might respond to volume changes.

MEDULLARY COLLECTING DUCT

The ability of the medullary collecting duct to reabsorb sodium has been demonstrated by both microcatheterization[30,316-318] and micropuncture techniques.[94,174,328] Further, application of these techniques in euvolemic rats has shown that this terminal nephron segment is responsible for the ability of the organism to excrete a urine that is virtually free of sodium. Although this finding suggests that the medullary collecting duct adjusts its sodium reabsorptive rate in response to salt excess or deficit, the experimental evidence remains equivocal. Utilizing the microcatheterization technique, Sonnenberg[317] and Bengele and associates[30] have reported decreased sodium reabsorption by the medullary collecting duct after saline loading. Similarly, Sonnenberg described no net reabsorption in response to blood volume expansion.[319] In addition, the same investigator found that when the ECF volume was massively expanded by the infusion of saline solution and the reinfusion of urine, net secretion of sodium occurred along the inner medullary collecting duct.[318] These findings clearly suggest that the terminal portion of the nephron plays an important regulatory role in the determination of urinary sodium excretion.

Unfortunately, not all studies of this nephron segment have reached conclusions similar to those of Sonnenberg and of Bengele and colleagues. For the most part, studies employing direct micropuncture have described reabsorption along the inner medullary collecting duct regardless of the volume status of the animal.[94,174,270,271,328] Furthermore, these studies have found that, within the ranges studied, the reabsorptive rate is a direct function of the rate of sodium delivery. The reason for these contrasting findings is unclear, but the problem may reside in the techniques being utilized to evaluate reabsorption. Sonnenberg and Chong have recently examined that issue by quantitating reabsorption in the same collecting duct after acute volume expansion using both direct micropuncture and microcatheterization.[320] They found no net reabsorption with either technique. Thus, the reason for the divergent results from different laboratories remains unclear. Further work is needed to define clearly the role of the medullary collecting duct in the final determination of urinary sodium.

SUMMARY

The maintenance of a nearly constant volume of extracellular fluid requires that the kidneys regulate urinary sodium excretion so that total body sodium remains constant. Under most circumstances, and in the absence of nonrenal losses of sodium, this is dependent upon the daily excretion of an amount of salt equal to that in the diet. Presumably, ingestion of additional sodium provokes retention of water via ADH release. Enough water is retained to ensure preservation of isotonicity, which simultaneously causes a finite increase in ECF volume. Possible mechanisms by which the individual perceives that increase in volume and the manner in which the kidney responds to that perception are schematically depicted in Fig. 3-13.

An increase in the volume of the ECF space may result in some degree of hemodilution, decreasing plasma protein concentration, and increasing in renal perfusion pressure. These changes, along with alterations in afferent and efferent arteriolar resistances, may result in increases in GFR and decreases in the reabsorptive forces across the peritubular capillaries. Thus, the filtered load

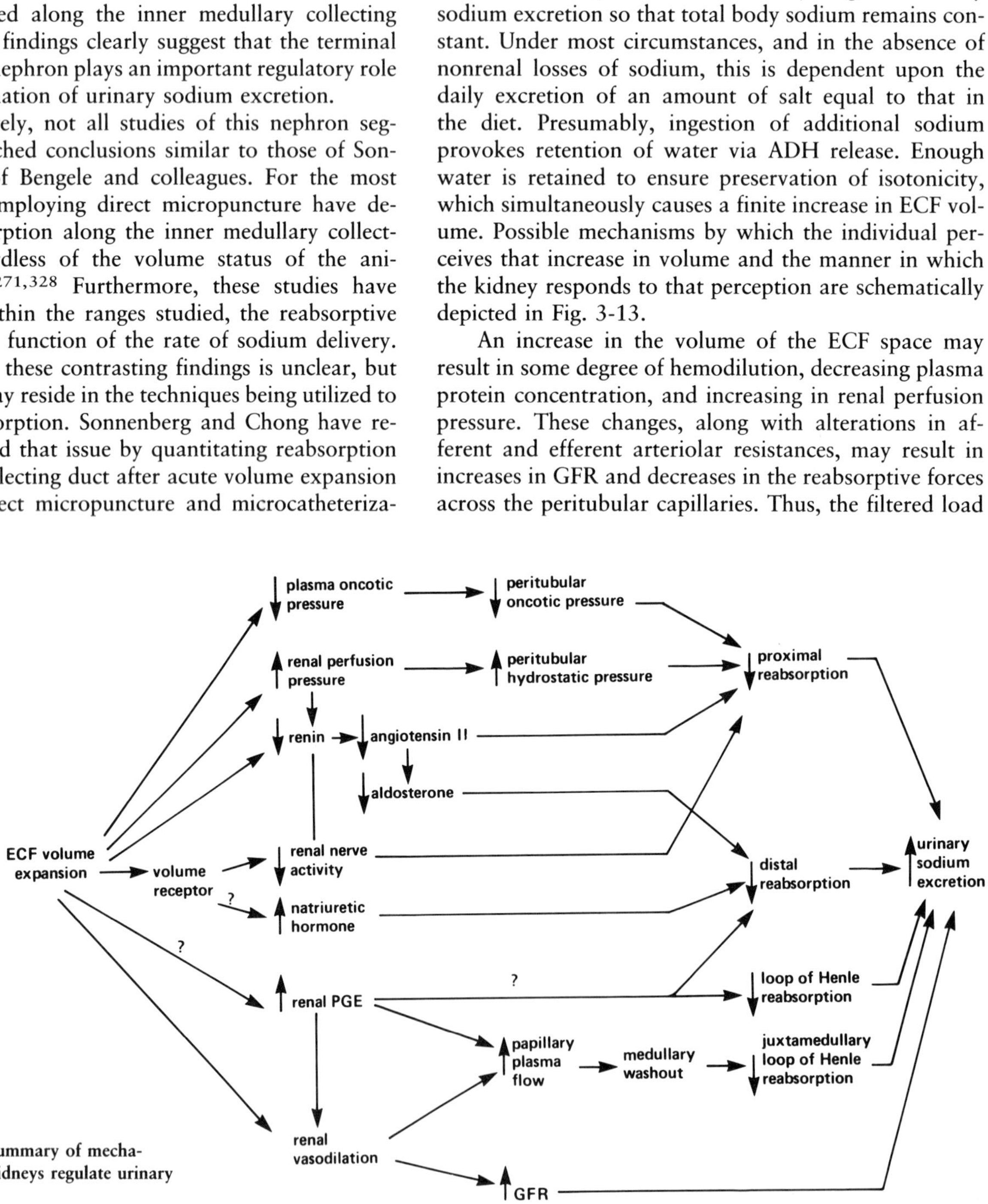

FIGURE 3-13 • Summary of mechanisms by which kidneys regulate urinary sodium excretion.

of sodium increases, while the proximal tubular sodium reabsorption decreases. In addition, perception of volume expansion by the kidney results in decreased renal release of renin, which consequently reduces the generation of angiotensin II. The decreased levels of this hormone may also diminish proximal reabsorption. The fall in angiotensin II activity also decreases the adrenal release of aldosterone and thereby decreases distal reabsorption. It is also possible that some nonrenal volume receptor perceives the increase in ECF volume. The best evidence points to the cardiac atria and/or the carotid sinuses as the sites of such a receptor. It is likely that these receptors alter renal nerve traffic and thereby lead to decreased proximal sodium reabsorption. In addition, these and/or other volume receptors mediate the release of a hormonal substance that decreases sodium reabsorption at some nephron sites. Finally, renal vasodilatation occurs with volume expansion, a phenomenon that may be partially due to elaboration of vasodilator PGs. These substances may influence reabsorption directly or modify juxtamedullary nephron reabsorption by washout of the normally hypertonic medullary interstitium.

It should be stressed that the experimental evidence leading to this schema is for the most part derived from studies involving acute and often massive expansion of the ECF space. It is possible, therefore, that some of the mechanisms outlined are not operative in the normal physiologic excretion of sodium.

REFERENCES

1. Alexander RW et al: Effects of dietary sodium and of acute saline infusion on the interrelationship between dopamine excretion and adrenergic activity in man. *J Clin Invest* 54:194, 1974.
2. Allen GG, Barratt LJ: Effect of aldosterone on the transepithelial potential difference of the rat distal tubule. *Kidney Int* 19:678, 1981.
3. Altsheler P et al: Effects of inhibitors of prostaglandin synthesis on renal sodium excretion in normal dogs and dogs with decreased renal mass. *Am J Physiol* 235:338, 1978.
4. Anderson JV et al: Atrial natriuretic peptide: Evidence of action as a natriuretic hormone at physiological plasma concentrations in man. *Clin Sci (Lond)* 72:305, 1987.
5. Atkins EI, Pearce JW: Mechanisms of the renal response to plasma volume expansion. *Can J Biochem Physiol* 37:91, 1959.
6. Ayus JC, Humphreys MH: Hemodynamic and renal functional changes after acute unilateral nephrectomy in the dog: Role of carotid sinus baroreceptors. *Am J Physiol* 242:F181, 1982.
7. Bachman DM, Youmans WB: Effects of posture on renal excretion of sodium and chloride on orthostatic hypotension. *Circulation* 7:413, 1953.
8. Bahlman J et al: The effect on urinary sodium excretion of altering the packed cell volume with albumin solutions without changing the blood volume in the dog. *Clin Sci* 32:395, 1967.
9. Bahlman J et al: The effect on urinary sodium excretion of blood volume expansion with changing the composition of blood in the dog. *Clin Sci* 32:403, 1967.
10. Ball SG, Lee MR: The effect of carbidopa administration on urinary sodium excretion in man. *Br J Clin Pharmacol* 4:115, 1977.
11. Ball SG et al: Urinary dopamine in man and rat: Effects of inorganic salts on dopamine excretion. *Clin Sci Mol Med* 55:167, 1978.
12. Ballermann BJ et al: Physiologic regulation of atrial natriuretic peptide receptors in rat renal glomeruli. *J Clin Invest* 76:2049, 1985.
13. Bank N et al: Effect of peritubular capillary perfusion rate on proximal sodium reabsorption. *Kidney Int* 1:397, 1972.
14. Banks RO: Effects of physiological dose of ANP on renal function in dogs. *Am J Physiol* 255:F907, 1988.
15. Barajas L, Muller J: The innervation of the juxtaglomerular apparatus and surrounding tubules: A quantitative analysis by serial section electron microscopy. *J Ultrastruct Res* 43:107, 1973.
16. Barajas L et al: Identification of renal neuroeffector junctions by electron microscopy of reembedded light microscopic autoradiograms of semithin sections. *J Ultrastruct Res* 77:379, 1981.
17. Barger AC et al: Role of the kidney in the pathogenesis of congestive heart failure. *Circulation* 20:273, 1959.
18. Barraclough MA: Dose-dependent opposite effects of angiotensin on renal sodium excretion. *Lancet* 2:987, 1965.
19. Barraclough MA et al: Effects of angiotensin on renal function in the rat. *Am J Physiol* 212:1153, 1967.
20. Barraclough MA, Mills IH: Effect of bradykinin on renal function. *Clin Sci* 28:69, 1965.
21. Baum M, Toto RD: Lack of direct effect on atrial natriuretic factor in the rabbit proximal tubule. *Am J Physiol* 250:F66, 1986.
22. Bello-Reuss E et al: Effects of acute unilateral denervation in the rat. *J Clin Invest* 56:208, 1975.
23. Bello-Reuss E et al: Effect of renal sympathetic nerve stimulation on proximal water and sodium reabsorption. *J Clin Invest* 57:1104, 1976.
24. Bello-Reuss E et al: Acute unilateral renal denervation in rats with extracellular volume expansion. *Am J Physiol* 232:F26, 1977.
25. Bello-Reuss E et al: Effect of catecholamines on fluid reabsorption by the isolated proximal convoluted tubule. *Am J Physiol* 238:F347, 1980.
26. Bello-Reuss E et al: Dopamine decreases fluid reabsorption in straight portions of rabbit proximal tubule. *Am J Physiol* 242:F634, 1982.
27. Bencsath P et al: Effects of chlorothiazide and furosemide on sodium and water excretion after unilateral splanchnicotomy in the dog. *Nephron* 8:329, 1971.
28. Bencsath P et al: Renal handling of sodium after chronic renal sympathectomy in the anesthetized rat. *Am J Physiol* 236:F513, 1979.
29. Bencsath P et al: Renal excretion of sodium after bilat-

eral renal sympathectomy in the anesthetized and conscious rat. *J Physiol (Lond)* 331:443, 1982.
30. Bengele HH et al: Sodium and chloride transport along the inner medullary collecting duct: Effect of saline expansion. *Am J Physiol* 238:F504, 1980.
31. Bennett ED et al: Abolition, by dopamine blockade, of the natriuretic response produced by lower body positive pressure. *Clin Sci* 63:361, 1982.
32. Bernard C: *Lecons sur les proprietes physiologiques des dequedes de Porganisme.* Paris, Ballier, 1859, p 172.
33. Berne RM: Hemodynamics and sodium excretion of denervated kidney in anesthetized and unanesthetized dog. *Am J Physiol* 171:148, 1952.
34. Bie P et al: Hemodynamic and renal effects of low-dose infusions of atrial peptide in awake dogs. *Am J Physiol* 254:R161, 1988.
35. Biollaz J et al: Atrial natriuretic peptides: Reproducibility of renal effects and response of liver blood flow. *Eur J Clin Pharmacol* 31:1, 1986.
36. Blaine EH et al: Renin release after hemorrhage and after suprarenal aortic constriction in dogs without sodium delivery to the macula densa. *Circ Res* 27:1081, 1970.
37. Blaine EH et al: A central osmosensitive receptor for renal sodium excretion. *J Physiol* 244:497, 1975.
38. Blake WD: Relative roles of glomerular filtration and tubular reabsorption in denervation diuresis. *Am J Physiol* 202:777, 1962.
39. Blake WD, Jurf AN: Renal sodium reabsorption after acute renal denervation in the rabbit. *J Physiol* 196:65, 1968.
40. Block MA et al: Renal function during stimulation of renal nerves. *Am J Physiol* 169:670, 1952.
41. Bonjour JP et al: Change of tubular reabsorption of sodium and water after renal denervation in the dog. *J Physiol* 204:571, 1969.
42. Bourgoignie JJ et al: A natriuretic factor in serum of patients with chronic uremia. *J Clin Invest* 51:1514, 1972.
43. Bourgoignie JJ et al: The presence of a natriuretic factor in urine in patients with chronic uremia: The absence of the factor in nephrotic uremic patients. *J Clin Invest* 53:1559, 1974.
44. Bradley T et al: Dopamine receptor blockade does not affect the natriuresis accompanying sodium chloride infusion in dogs. *J Lab Clin Med* 107:525, 1986.
45. Brenner BM, Berliner RW: Relationship between extracellular volume and fluid reabsorption by the rat nephron. *Am J Physiol* 217:6, 1968.
46. Brenner BM, Galla JH: Influence of postglomerular hematocrit and protein concentration on rat nephron fluid transfer. *Am J Physiol* 220:148, 1971.
47. Brenner BM, Troy JL: Postglomerular vascular protein concentration: Evidence for causal role in governing fluid reabsorption in glomerular tubular balance by the renal proximal tubule. *J Clin Invest* 50:336, 1971.
48. Brenner BM et al: The relationship between peritubular capillary protein concentration and fluid reabsorption by the renal proximal tubule. *J Clin Invest* 48:1519, 1969.
49. Brenner BM et al: The dynamics of glomerular ultrafiltration in the rat. *J Clin Invest* 50:1776, 1971.
50. Brenner BM et al: On the mechanism of inhibition of fluid reabsorption by the renal proximal tubule of the volume expanded rat. *J Clin Invest* 50:1596, 1971.
51. Brenner BM et al: Quantitative importance of changes in postglomerular colloid osmotic pressure in mediating glomerular tubular balance in the rat. *J Clin Invest* 52:190, 1973.
52. Bricker NS, Licht A: Natriuretic hormone: Biologic effects and progress in identification and isolation, in Lichardus B et al (eds): *Proceedings of a Symposium on Hormonal Regulation of Sodium Excretion.* Amsterdam, Elsevier/North-Holland, 1980, p 399.
53. Bricker NS, Licht A: Natriuretic hormone: Current status, in Massry SG, Glassock RJ (eds): *Textbook of Nephrology.* Amsterdam, Elsevier/North-Holland, 1983, p 245.
54. Bricker NS et al: The functional capacity of the kidney denervated by autotransplantation in the dog. *J Clin Invest* 37:185, 1982.
55. Briggs JP et al: Micropuncture studies of the renal effects of atrial natriuretic substance. *Pfluegers Arch* 395:271, 1982.
56. Brown PR et al: Effect of urinary extracts from salt-loaded man on urinary sodium excretion by the rat. *Kidney Int* 2:1, 1972.
57. Buckalew VM et al: Mechanism of exaggerated natriuresis in hypertensive man: Impaired sodium transport in the loop of Henle. *J Clin Invest* 48:1007, 1969.
58. Burg MB, Orloff J: Control of fluid absorption in renal proximal tubules. *J Clin Invest* 47:2016, 1968.
59. Burnett J et al: Renal interstitial pressure in mineralocorticoid escape. *Am J Physiol* 249:F396, 1985.
60. Butlen D et al: Atrial natriuretic peptide receptors along rat and rabbit nephrons: Rat atrial natriuretic peptide binding in microdissected glomeruli and tubules. *Pfluegers Arch* 408:356, 1987.
61. Carey RM: Evidence for a splanchnic sodium input monitor regulating renal sodium excretion in man: Lack of dependence upon aldosterone. *Circ Res* 43:19, 1978.
62. Carey RM et al: Gastrointestinal control of sodium excretion in sodium-depleted conscious rabbits. *Am J Physiol* 230:1504, 1976.
63. Carretero OA, Scicli AG: The renal kallikrein-kinin system. *Am J Physiol* 238:F247, 1980.
64. Carswell F et al: The effects of left atrial distension upon urine flow from the isolated perfused kidney. *J Exp Physiol* 55:173, 1970.
65. Chambardes D et al: Atrial natriuretic peptide effect on cGMP and cAMP contents in microdissected glomeruli and segments of the rat and rabbit nephrons. *Pfluegers Arch* 408:366, 1987.
66. Chan YL: Adrenergic control of bicarbonate absorption in the proximal convoluted tubule of the rat kidney. *Pfluegers Arch* 388:159, 1980.
67. Chan YL: The role of norepinephrine in the regulation of fluid absorption in the rat proximal tubule. *J Pharmacol Exp Ther* 215:65, 1980.
68. Cirksena WJ et al: Effect of thoracic cava obstruction on response of proximal tubule sodium reabsorption to saline infusion. *J Clin Invest* 45:179, 1966.

69. Coehlo JD, Bradley SE: Persistence of the natriuretic response to isotonic saline load during hemorrhagic hypotension in the dog. *Proc Soc Exp Biol Med* 131:265, 1969.
70. Coghlan JP et al: The control of aldosterone secretion. *Postgrad Med* 36:76, 1960.
71. Conger JD et al: A study of in vivo peritubular oncotic pressure and proximal tubular reabsorption in the rat. *Clin Sci* 51:379, 1976.
72. Cornish KG, Gilmore JP: Increased left atrial pressure does not alter renal function in the conscious primate. *Am J Physiol* 243:R119, 1982.
73. Cottier C et al: Renal response to low-dose infusion of atrial natriuretic peptide in normal man. *Kidney Int* 34(suppl 25):S72, 1988.
74. Craig GN et al: The effect of change in perfusion pressure and haematocrit in the isolated perfused dog kidney. *J Physiol* 186:113P, 1966.
75. Crocker AD, Munday KA: The effect of renin angiotensin system on mucosal water and sodium transfer in everted sacs of rat jejunum. *J Physiol (Lond)* 206:323, 1970.
76. Cuche JL et al: Is dopamine a physiological natriuretic hormone in the dog? *Clin Sci (Lond)* 65:479, 1983.
77. Culpepper RM, Andreoli TE: Interactions among prostaglandin E_2, antidiuretic hormone, and cyclic adenosine monophosphate in modulating Cl^- absorption in single mouse medullary thick ascending limbs of Henle. *J Clin Invest* 71:1588, 1983.
78. Daly JJ et al: A comparison of sodium excretion following the infusion of saline into systemic and portal veins in the dog: Evidence for a hepatic role in the control of sodium excretion. *Clin Sci* 33:481, 1967.
79. Davies NT et al: The effect of angiotensin on the rat intestinal fluid transfer. *J Endocrinol* 48:39, 1970.
80. Davis JO: A critical evaluation of the role of receptors in the control of aldosterone secretion and sodium excretion. *Prog Cardiovasc Dis* 4:27, 1961.
81. Davis JO et al: An extra-adrenal factor essential for chronic renal sodium retention in presence of increased sodium-retaining hormone. *Circ Res* 14:17, 1964.
82. Davis JO, Howell DS: Mechanisms of fluid and electrolyte retention in experimental preparation in dogs: 2. Thoracic inferior vena cava obstruction. *Circ Res* 1:71, 1953.
83. DeBold AJ: Heart atria granularity: Effects of changes in water-electrolyte balance. *Proc Soc Exp Biol Med* 161:508, 1979.
84. DeBold AJ: Atrial natriuretic factor of the rat heart: Studies on isolation and properties. *Proc Soc Exp Biol Med* 170:133, 1982.
85. DeBold AJ et al: A rapid and potent natriuretic response to intravenous injection of atrial myocardial extract in rats. *Life Sci* 28:89, 1981.
86. deWardener HE et al: Studies on the efferent mechanism of the sodium diuresis which follows the intravenous administration of saline in the dog. *Clin Sci* 21:249, 1961.
87. DiBona GF: Neural control of renal tubular sodium reabsorption in the dog. *Fed Proc* 37:1214, 1978.
88. DiBona GF: The functions of the renal nerves. *Rev Physiol Biochem Pharmacol* 94:76, 1982.
89. DiBona GF, Johns FJ: A study of the role of renal nerves in the renal responses to 60° head-up tilt in the anesthetized dog. *J Physiol (Lond)* 299:117, 1980.
90. DiBona GF, Osbourn JL: Nature of renal tubular adrenoceptor mediating neural regulation of sodium reabsorption. *Fed Proc* 40:553, 1981.
91. DiBona GF, Sawin LL: Effect of renal nerve stimulation on NaCl and H_2O transport in Henle's loop of the rat. *Am J Physiol* 243:F576, 1982.
92. DiBona GF, Sawin LL: Renal nerves in renal adaptation to dietary sodium restriction. *Am J Physiol* 245:F322, 1983.
93. DiBona GF, Sawin LL: Renal nerve activity in conscious rats during volume expansion and depletion. *Am J Physiol* 248:F15, 1985.
94. Diezi J et al: Micropuncture study of electrolyte transport across papillary collecting duct of the rat. *Am J Physiol* 224:623, 1973.
95. Dinerstein RJ et al: Histofluorescence techniques provide evidence for dopamine-containing neuronal elements in canine kidney. *Science* 205:497, 1979.
96. Dirks JH et al: The effect of saline infusion on sodium reabsorption by the proximal tubule of the dog. *J Clin Invest* 44:1160, 1965.
97. Dirks JH, Seely J: Effect of saline infusion and furosemide on the dog distal nephron. *Am J Physiol* 219:114, 1970.
98. Donald DE, Shepherd JF: Reflexes from the heart and lungs: Physiological curiosities or important regulatory mechanisms. *Cardiovasc Res* 12:449, 1978.
99. Dorn J, Porter JC: Diencephalic involvement in sodium excretion in the rat. *Endocrinology* 86:1112, 1970.
100. Doucet A, Katz AI: Mineralocorticoid receptors along the nephron: ^3H aldosterone binding in rabbit tubules. *Am J Physiol* 241:F605, 1981.
101. Dunham EW, Zimmerman BG: Release of prostaglandin-like material from dog kidney during nerve stimulation. *Am J Physiol* 219:1279, 1970.
102. Dunn BR et al: Renal and systemic hemodynamic effects of synthetic atrial natriuretic peptide in the anesthetized rat. *Circ Res* 59:237, 1986.
103. Dusing R et al: The role of prostaglandins in the natriuresis of acutely salt-loaded rats. *Nephron* 18:212, 1977.
104. Earley LE, Friedler RM: Observations on the mechanism of decreased tubular reabsorption of sodium and water during saline loading. *J Clin Invest* 43:1928, 1964.
105. Earley LE, Friedler RM: The effects of combined renal vasodilation and pressor agents on renal hemodynamics in the tubular reabsorption of sodium. *J Clin Invest* 45:542, 1965.
106. Earley LE et al: Factors affecting sodium reabsorption by proximal tubule as determined during blockade of distal sodium reabsorption. *J Clin Invest* 45:1668, 1966.
107. Edelman IS et al: On the mechanism of action of aldosterone on sodium transport: The role of protein synthesis. *Proc Natl Acad Sci U S A* 50:1169, 1963.
108. Edelman IS, Fimognari GM: On the biochemical mecha-

nism of action of aldosterone: 1. Modes of hormone action. *Recent Prog Horm Res* 24:1, 1968.
109. Edwards RM: Segmental effects of norepinephrine and angiotensin II in isolated renal microvessels. *Am J Physiol* 244:F526, 1983.
110. Epstein FH et al: Studies of the antidiuresis of quiet standing: The importance of charges in plasma volume in glomerular filtration rate. *J Clin Invest* 30:63, 1951.
111. Epstein FH et al: Effects of arteriovenous fistula on renal hemodynamics and electrolyte excretion. *J Clin Invest* 32:233, 1953.
112. Epstein M et al: Characterization of the natriuresis caused in normal man by immersion in water. *Clin Sci* 43:275, 1972.
113. Epstein M et al: The presence of a natriuretic factor in urine of normal men undergoing water immersion. *Kidney Int* 13:152, 1978.
114. Epstein M et al: Relationship between renal prostaglandin E and renal sodium handling during water immersion in normal man. *Circ Res* 45:71, 1979.
115. Fadem et al: Studies on the mechanism of sodium excretion during drug-induced vasodilatation in the dog. *J Clin Invest* 69:604, 1982.
116. Falchuk KH et al: Oncotic and hydrostatic pressure in peritubular capillaries and fluid reabsorption of proximal tubule. *Am J Physiol* 220:1427, 1971.
117. Faubert PF et al: Regulation of papillary plasma flow by angiotensin II. *Kidney Int* 32:472, 1987.
118. Faucheux B et al: Effects of saline and albumin on plasma and urinary catecholamines in dogs. *Am J Physiol* 232:F123, 1977.
119. Favre HJ et al: An inhibitor of sodium transport in the urine of dogs with normal renal function. *J Clin Invest* 56:1302, 1975.
120. Felder RA et al: Cortical tubular and glomerular dopamine receptors in the rat. *Am J Physiol* 246:F557, 1984.
121. Felder RA et al: The dopamine receptor in adult and maturing kidney. *Am J Physiol* 257:F315, 1989.
122. Fernandez-Repollet E et al: Role of renal nerves in maintaining sodium balance in unrestrained conscious rats. *Am J Physiol* 249:F819, 1985.
123. Ferreri NR et al: Arachidonic acid metabolism in a cell suspension isolated from rabbit renal outer medulla. *J Pharmacol Exp Ther* 231:F441, 1984.
124. Ferris TF: Renal disease, in Burrow GN, Ferris TF (eds): *Medical Complications of Pregnancy*. Philadelphia, Saunders, 1975, p 1.
124a. Fildes RD et al: Renal α-adrenoceptors and sodium excretion in the dog. *Am J Physiol* 248:F128, 1985.
125. Fimognari GM et al: Induction of RNA and protein synthesis in the action of aldosterone in the rat. *Am J Physiol* 213:954, 1967.
126. Fine LG et al: On the influence of the natriuretic factor from patients with chronic uremia on the bioelectric properties and sodium transport of the isolated mammalian collecting tubule. *J Clin Invest* 58:590, 1976.
127. Fine LG, Kirschenbaum MA: Absence of direct effects of prostaglandins on sodium chloride transport in the mammalian nephron. *Kidney Int* 19:797, 1981.
128. Fine LG, Trizna W: Influence of prostaglandins on sodium transport of isolated medullary nephron segments. *Am J Physiol* 232:F383, 1977.
129. Fitzgibbons JP et al: Dependence of saline-induced natriuresis upon exposure of the kidney to the physical effects of extracellular fluid volume expansion. *J Clin Invest* 54:1428, 1974.
130. Fitzhugh FW et al: The effect of application of tourniquets to the legs on cardiac output and renal function in normal human subjects. *J Clin Invest* 32:1163, 1953.
131. Fitzpatrick TM et al: Cardiovascular responses to PGI_2 (prostacyclin) in the dog. *Circ Res* 42:192, 1978.
132. Frederickson ED et al: Blockade of renal effects of dopamine in the dog by the DA_1 antagonist SCH23390. *Am J Physiol* 249:F236, 1985.
133. Fresinger GC et al: Prostaglandin D_2: Another renal prostaglandin? *Prostaglandins* 15:696, 1978.
134. Ganguli M et al: Evidence that prostaglandin synthesis inhibitors increase the concentration of sodium and chloride in rat renal medulla. *Circ Res* 40(suppl 1):135, 1977.
135. Garcia-Estan J et al: Role of renal interstitial hydrostatic pressure in the pressure diuresis response. *Am J Physiol* 256:F63, 1989.
136. Garcia-Estan J, Roman RJ: Role of interstitial hydrostatic pressure in natriuretic response to ANP. *Am J Physiol* 258:R1333, 1990.
137. Gauer OH, Henry JP: Neurohormonal control of plasma volume, in Guyton AC, Cowley AW (eds): *Cardiovascular Physiology II: Internationl Review of Physiology*. Baltimore, University Park Press, 1976, vol 9, p 146.
138. Gill JR Jr, Bartter FC: Adrenergic nervous system in sodium metabolism: 2. Effects of guanethidine on the renal response to sodium deprivation in normal man. *N Engl J Med* 275:1466, 1966.
139. Gillespie DJ et al: Dual effect of left atrial receptors on excretion of sodium and water in the dog. *Am J Physiol* 225:706, 1973.
140. Gilmore JP: Contribution of baroreceptors to the control of renal function. *Circ Res* 14:301, 1964.
141. Gilmore JP: Contributions of cardiac nerves to the control of body salt and water. *Fed Proc* 27:1156, 1968.
142. Gilmore JP, Daggett WM: Response of the chronic cardiac denervated to acute volume expansion. *Am J Physiol* 210:509, 1966.
143. Gilmore JP, Westfeltd ML: Contribution of intravascular receptors to the renal responses following intravascular volume expansion. *Circ Res* 17:144, 1965.
144. Gilmore JP, Zucker IH: Contribution of vagal pathways to the renal responses to head out immersion in the nonhuman primate. *Circ Res* 42:263, 1978.
145. Gilmore JP, Zucker IH: The contributions of neural pathways to blood volume homeostasis in the subhuman primate. *Basic Res Cardiol* 75:281, 1980.
146. Goetz KL: Evidence that atriopeptin is not a physiological regulator of sodium excretion. *Hypertension* 15:9, 1990.
147. Goetz KL et al: Atrial receptors and renal function in conscious dogs. *Am J Physiol* 219:1417, 1970.
148. Goetz KL et al: Atrial stretch increases sodium excretion

independently of release of atrial peptides. *Am J Physiol* 250:R946, 1986.
149. Gonick HC et al: Circulating inhibitor of sodium-potassium-activated adenosine triphosphatase after expansion of extracellular fluid volume in rats. *Clin Sci Mol Med* 53:329, 1977.
150. Goodman DBP et al: Studies on the mechanism of action of aldosterone: Hormone-induced changes in lipid metabolism. *Biochemistry* 10:3825, 1971.
151. Goodman DBP et al: Aldosterone-induced membrane phospholipid fatty acid metabolism in the toad urinary bladder. *Biochemistry* 14:2302, 1975.
152. Goodyer AVN et al: Some effects of albumin infusion on renal function in the electrolyte excretion in normal man. *J Appl Physiol* 1:671, 1949.
153. Gordon D et al: Requirement of the adrenergic nervous system for conservation of sodium by the rabbit kidney. *J Physiol (Lond)* 293:24P, 1979.
154. Gottschalk CW: Renal nerves and sodium excretion. *Annu Rev Physiol* 41:229, 1979.
155. Grabfield GP, Swanson D: Studies on denervated kidney: Effects of unilateral denervation in acute experiments on sodium chloride excretion. *Arch Int Pharmacodyn Ther* 61:92, 1939.
156. Granger JP et al: Effect of direct increases in renal interstitial hydrostatic pressure on sodium excretion. *Am J Physiol* 254:F527, 1988.
157. Green DM, Farah A: Influence of sodium load on sodium secretion. *Am J Physiol* 158:444, 1949.
158. Greenberg TT et al: Impaired atrial receptor response in dogs with heart failure due to tricuspid insufficiency and pulmonary artery stenosis. *Circ Res* 32:424, 1973.
159. Gross F, Turrian H: Pharmacology of hypertension and synthetic analogues, in Schachter M (ed): *Polypeptides which Affect Smooth Muscles and Blood Vessels.* New York, Pergamon, 1960, p 137.
160. Gross JB et al: A functional comparison of the cortical collecting tubule and the distal convoluted tubule. *J Clin Invest* 55:1284, 1975.
161. Gross JB, Kokko JP: Effects of aldosterone and potassium sparing diuretics on electrical potential differences across the distal nephron. *J Clin Invest* 59:82, 1977.
162. Gross JB, Bartter FC: Effects of prostaglandin E_1, A_1, and $F_{2\alpha}$ on renal handling of salt and water. *Am J Physiol* 225:218, 1973.
163. Gruber KA et al: Endogenous digitalis-like substance in plasma of volume-expanded dogs. *Nature* 287:743, 1980.
164. Haas JA et al: Mechanism of natriuresis during intrarenal infusion of prostaglandins. *Am J Physiol* 247:F475, 1984.
165. Haas JA et al: Effect of renal perfusion pressure on sodium reabsorption from proximal tubules of superficial and deep nephrons. *Am J Physiol* 250:F425, 1986.
166. Haas JA et al: Effect of intrarenal volume expansion on proximal sodium reabsorption. *Am J Physiol* 255:F1178, 1988.
167. Hall JE et al: Intrarenal control of electrolyte excretion by angiotensin II. *Am J Physiol* 232:F538, 1977.
168. Hall JE et al: Mechanisms of escape from sodium retention during angiotensin II hypertension. *Am J Physiol* 246:F627, 1984.
169. Hall JE et al: Role of renal hemodynamics and arterial pressure in aldosterone "escape." *Hypertension* 6(suppl 1):I-183, 1984.
170. Harris PJ, Young JA: Dose dependent stimulation and inhibition of proximal tubular sodium reabsorption by angiotensin II in the rat kidney. *Pfluegers Arch* 367:295, 1977.
171. Harris PJ et al: Atrial natriuretic peptide inhibits angiotensin-stimulated proximal tubular sodium and water reabsorption. *Nature (Lond)* 326:697, 1987.
172. Healy JK et al: Renal and pressor action of angiotensin in the normal dog. *Am J Physiol* 208:1093, 1965.
173. Hierholzer K et al: Micropuncture study of renal transtubular concentration gradient of sodium and potassium. *Pfluegers Arch* 285:193, 1965.
174. Higashihara E et al: Direct examination of chloride transport across papillary collecting duct of the rat. *Am J Physiol* 235:F219, 1978.
175. Higashihara E et al: Cortical and papillary micropuncture examination of chloride transport in segments of the rat kidney during inhibition of prostaglandin production. *J Clin Invest* 64:1277, 1979.
176. Hirth C et al: Blockade of the response to volume expansion by monoclonal antibodies against atrial natriuretic peptides. *Klin Wochenschr,* 65(suppl 8):87, 1987.
177. Hollingshead P, Willis LR: Beta adrenergic receptor mediated renal tubular sodium reabsorption. *Fed Proc* 39:521, 1980.
178. Horster M et al: Aldosterone in vitro restores nephron Na-K-ATPase of distal segments from adrenalectomized rabbits. *Pfluegers Arch* 384:203, 1980.
179. Houck CR: Alterations in renal hemodynamics and function in separate kidneys during stimulation of renal artery nerves in dogs. *Am J Physiol* 167:523, 1951.
180. Howards S et al: Depression of fractional sodium reabsorption by the proximal tubule of the dog without sodium diuresis. *J Clin Invest* 47:1561, 1968.
181. Huang CL, Cogan MG: Atrial natriuretic factor inhibits maximal tubuloglomerular feedback response. *Am J Physiol* 252:F825, 1987.
182. Huang CL et al: In vivo evidence that cGMP is the second messenger for atrial natriuretic factor. *Proc Natl Acad Sci U S A* 83:8015, 1986.
183. Humphreys MH, Ayus JC: Role of hemodynamic changes in the increased cation excretion after acute unilateral nephrectomy in the anesthetized dog. *J Clin Invest* 61:590, 1978.
184. Humphreys MH et al: Natriuresis produced by vasopressin or hemorrhage during water diuresis in the dog. *Am J Physiol* 219:658, 1970.
185. Humphreys MH et al: Prevention by vagotomy or atropine administration of the hemodynamic changes occurring after acute unilateral nephrectomy in the dog. *Circ Res* 46:575, 1980.
186. Ichikawa I, Brenner BM: Mechanism of inhibition of proximal tubule reabsorption after exposure of the rat

kidney to the physical effects of expansion of extracellular fluid volume. *J Clin Invest* 64:1466, 1979.

187. Ichikawa I, Brenner BM: Importance of efferent arteriolar tone in regulation of proximal tubule fluid reabsorption and glomerulo-tubular balance in the rat. *J Clin Invest* 65:1192, 1980.
188. Ichikawa I et al: Reversal of renal cortical actions of angiotensin II by verapamil and manganese. *Kidney Int* 16:137, 1979.
189. Iino Y, Imai M: Effects of prostaglandins on Na transport in isolated collecting tubules. *Pfluegers Arch* 373:125, 1978.
190. Imai M et al: Effects of perfusion rate on the fluxes of water, sodium chloride and urea across the proximal tubule. *Kidney Int* 11:18, 1977.
191. Insel PA et al: Radioligand binding and functional assays demonstrate post synaptic alpha$_2$ receptors on proximal tubules of rat and rabbit kidney. *J Cardiovasc Pharm 7:* (suppl 8):S9, 1985.
192. Jacobson HR et al: Effects of epoxyeicosatrienoic acids on ion transport in the rabbit cortical collecting tubule, in Baquet P et al (eds): *Prostaglandins and Membrane Ion Transport.* New York, Raven, 1984, p 311.
193. Johnston BC: Nerve endings in the human endocardium. *Am J Anat* 122:621, 1978.
194. Johnston HH et al: Effects of prostaglandin E_1 on renal hemodynamics, sodium and water excretion. *Am J Physiol* 213:939, 1968.
195. Johnson MD, Malvin RL: Stimulation of renal sodium reabsorption by angiotensin II. *Am J Physiol* 232:F298, 1977.
196. Jose PA et al: Dopamine receptors modulate sodium excretion in denervated kidney. *Am J Physiol* 250:F1033, 1986.
197. Kaczmarczyk G et al: Left atrial pressure and postprandial diuresis in conscious dogs on a high sodium intake. *Pfluegers Arch* 368:181, 1977.
198. Kaissling B, Stanton BA: Adaptation of distal tubule and collecting duct to increased sodium delivery. *Am J Physiol* 255:F1256, 1988.
199. Kaloyanides GJ et al: Evidence that the brain participates in humoral natriuretic mechanism of blood volume expansion in the dog. *J Clin Invest* 62:1288, 1978.
200. Kaplan SA, Rapaport S: Urinary excretion of sodium and chloride after splanchnicotomy: Effect on the proximal tubule. *Am J Physiol* 164:175, 1951.
201. Kappagoda CT et al: Effect of stimulating right atrial receptors on urine flow in the dog. *J Physiol (Lond)* 235:493, 1973.
202. Karim F et al: Effects of stimulation of the left atrial receptors on sympathetic efferent nerve activity. *J Physiol (Lond)* 227:243, 1972.
203. Kauker ML: Renal effects of aprotinin: A kallikrein inhibitor in saline diuresis. *Proc Soc Exp Biol Med* 178:222, 1985.
204. Khraibi AA et al: Effect of renal perfusion pressure on renal interstitial hydrostatic pressure in rats. *Am J Physiol* 256:F165, 1989.
205. Kinne R, Kirsten R: Der einfluss von Aldosteron auf die Aktivitat Mitochondrialer und Cyloplasmatischer Enzyme en der Rattenier. *Pfluegers Arch* 300:244, 1968.
206. Kirchner KA: Greater loop chloride uptake contributes to blunted pressure natriuresis in Dahl salt sensitive rats. *J Am Soc Nephrol* 1:180, 1990.
207. Kirschenbaum MA, Stein JH: The effect of inhibition of prostaglandin synthesis on urinary sodium excretion in the conscious dog. *J Clin Invest* 57:517, 1976.
208. Kisch B: Studies in comparative electron microscopy of the heart: II. Guinea pig and rat. *Exp Med Surg* 13:404, 1955.
209. Knight TF, Weinman EJ: Renal sodium reabsorption following induction of and recovery from volume expansion. *Am J Physiol* 233:F416, 1977.
210. Knox FG et al: Effect of chronic cardiac denervation on renal response to saline infusion. *Am J Physiol* 213:174, 1967.
211. Knox FG et al: The effect of dilution and expansion of blood volume on proximal sodium reabsorption. *Am J Physiol* 215:1041, 1968.
212. Knox FG et al: Effect of volume expansion on sodium excretion in the presence and absence of increased delivery from superficial proximal tubules. *J Clin Invest* 52:1642, 1973.
213. Knox FG et al: Proximal tubular reabsorption after hyperoncotic albumin infusion. *J Clin Invest* 52:1642, 1973.
214. Kopp UC, DiBona GF: The functions of the renal nerves. *The Kidney* 15:17, 1984.
215. Koscki C et al: Localization of binding sites for α-rat atrial natriuretic polypeptide in rat kidney. *Am J Physiol* 250:F210, 1986.
216. Kramer HJ et al: Effects of aprotinin on renal function and urinary prostaglandin excretion in conscious rats after acute salt loading. *Clin Sci* 56:547, 1979.
217. Krishna GG et al: Dopaminergic mediation of the natriuretic response to volume expansion. *J Lab Clin Med* 105:214, 1985.
218. Kunau RT, Lameire NH: The effect of an acute increase in renal perfusion pressure on sodium transport in the rat kidney. *Circ Res* 39:689, 1976.
219. Kunau RT et al: Characteristics of sodium reabsorption in the loop of Henle and distal tubule. *Am J Physiol* 227:1181, 1974.
220. Ladd M: Effect of prehydration upon renal excretion of sodium in man. *J Appl Physiol* 3:603, 1951.
221. Landwehr D et al: Renal tubular sodium and water reabsorption in the isotonic sodium chloride loaded rat. *Am J Physiol* 212:1327, 1967.
222. Laradi A et al: Effect of dopamine on sodium uptake by renal proximal tubule cells on rabbit. *Miner Electrolyte Metab* 12:303, 1986.
223. Law PY, Edelman IS: Induction of citrate synthase by aldosterone in the rat kidney. *J Membr Biol* 41:41, 1978.
224. Ledsone JR et al: The mechanisms by which distension of the left atrium produces diuresis in anaesthetized dogs. *J Physiol (Lond)* 159:87, 1961.
225. Le Hir M et al: Distal tubular segments of the rabbit kidney after adaptation to altered Na and K intake: 2. Changes in Na^+-K^+-ATPase activity. *Cell Tissue Res* 224:493, 1982.
226. Lennane RJ et al: A comparison of natriuresis after oral and intravenous sodium loading in sodium-depleted rab-

bits: Evidence for a gastrointestinal or portal monitor of sodium intake. *Clin Sci* 49:433, 1975.

227. Lennane RJ et al: A comparison of the natriuresis after oral and intravenous sodium loading in sodium-depleted man: Evidence for a gastrointestinal or portal monitor of sodium intake. *Clin Sci* 49:437, 1975.
228. Levinsky NG, Lalone RC: Sodium excretion during acute saline loading in dogs with vena caval constriction. *J Clin Invest* 44:565, 1965.
229. Lewy JE, Windhager EE: Peritubular control of proximal tubular fluid reabsorption in the rat kidney. *Am J Physiol* 214:943, 1968.
230. Lieberthal W et al: Interactions between ADH and prostaglandins in isolated erythrocyte-perfused rat kidney. *Am J Physiol* 252:F331, 1987.
231. Lifschitz MD: Lack of a role for the renal nerves in renal sodium reabsorption in conscious dogs. *Clin Sci* 54:567, 1978.
232. Lifschitz MD et al: Urinary prostaglandin E excretion: Effect of chronic alterations in sodium intake and inhibition of prostaglandin synthesis in the rabbit. *Prostaglandins* 16:607, 1978.
233. Lipson LC, Sharp GWG: Effect of prostaglandin E_1 on sodium transport and osmotic water flow in the toad bladder. *Am J Physiol* 220:1046, 1971.
234. Louis WJ, Doyle AE: The effects of varying doses of angiotensin on renal function and blood pressure in man and dogs. *Clin Sci* 29:489, 1965.
235. Lowitz HD et al: Micropuncture study of the action of angiotensin II on tubular sodium and water reabsorption in the rat. *Nephron* 6:173, 1969.
236. Ludwig C: *Lehrbuch der Physiologie des Menschen.* Heidelberg, CF Winker, 1861.
237. Lydtin H, Hamilton WF: Effect of acute changes in left atrial pressure on urine flow in unanesthetized dogs. *Am J Physiol* 207:530, 1964.
238. Madeddu P et al: Effect of a kinin antagonist on renal function and haemodynamics during alterations in sodium balance in conscious normotensive rats. *Clin Sci* 78:165, 1990.
239. Malvin RI, Vander AJ: Effects of angiotensin infusion on renal function in the unanesthetized rat. *Am J Physiol* 213:1205, 1967.
240. Marchand GR: Interstitial pressure during volume expansion at reduced renal artery pressure. *Am J Physiol* 235:F209, 1978.
241. Margolius HS et al: Urinary kallikrein excretion in normal man: Relationship to sodium intake and sodium-retaining steroids. *Circ Res* 35:812, 1974.
242. Martino JA, Earley LE: Demonstration of a role of physical factors as determinants of the natriuretic response to volume expansion. *J Clin Invest* 46:1963, 1967.
243. Martino JA, Earley LE: Relationship between intrarenal hydrostatic pressure and hemodynamically induced changes in sodium excretion. *Circ Res* 23:371, 1968.
244. Marver D, Schwartz MJ: Identification of mineralocorticoid target sites in the isolated rabbit cortical nephron. *Proc Natl Acad Sci U S A* 77:3672, 1980.
245. McCaa RE et al: The effects of angiotensin I-converting enzyme inhibitors on arterial blood pressure and urinary sodium excretion: Role of the renal renin-angiotensin and kallikrein-kinin systems. *Circ Res* 43:132, 1978.
246. Mendez RE et al: Modulation of the natriuretic response to atrial natriuretic peptide by alterations in peritubular Starling forces in the rat. *Circ Res* 59:605, 1986.
247. Mertz JI et al: Effects of bradykinin on renal interstitial pressures and proximal tubule reabsorption. *Am J Physiol* 247:F82, 1984.
248. Mills et al: The renal kallikrein-kinin system and the regulation of salt and water excretion. *Fed Proc* 35:181, 1976.
249. Mizelle HL et al: Role of renal nerves in compensatory adaptation of chronic reductions in sodium intake. *Am J Physiol* 252:F291, 1987.
249a. Mizelle HL et al: Renal hemodynamics and electrolyte excretion during chronic intrarenal infusion of atrial natriuretic peptide (ANP). *FASEB J* 3:A697, 1989.
250. Monidez JS: Identification of the receptor areas in the venae cavae and pulmonary veins which initiate reflex cardiac acceleration (Bainbridge reflex). *Am J Anat* 61:203, 1937.
251. Morgan T, Berliner RW: A study by continuous microperfusion of water and electrolyte movements in the loop of Henle and distal tubule of the rat. *Nephron* 6:388, 1969.
252. Morriss DJ et al: The physiologic response to aldosterone in adrenalectomized and intact rats. *Endocrinology* 92:989, 1973.
253. Moss NG: Renal function and afferent and efferent nerve activity. *Am J Physiol* 243:F425, 1982.
254. Mouw DR, Vander AJ: Evidence for brain Na receptors controlling renal Na excretion and plasma renin activity. *Am J Physiol* 219:822, 1970.
255. Mouw DR et al: Brain receptors, renin secretion and renal sodium retention in conscious sheep. *Am J Physiol* 226:56, 1974.
256. Muto S et al: Dopaminergic inhibition of the action of vasopressin on the cortical collecting tubule. *Eur J Pharmacol* 114:393, 1985.
257. Nakano J, McCurdy JR: Hemodynamic effects of prostaglandin E_1, A_1, and $F_{2\alpha}$ in dogs. *Proc Soc Exp Biol Med* 128:39, 1968.
258. Naruse M et al: Antisera to atrial natriuretic factor reduces urinary sodium excretion and increases plasma renin activity in rats. *Biochem Biophys Res Commun* 132:954, 1985.
259. Navar LG: Distal nephron diluting segment responses to altered arterial pressure and solute loading. *Am J Physiol* 222:945, 1971.
260. Navar LG et al: Autoregulatory responses of superficial nephrons and their association with sodium excretion during arterial pressure alterations in the dog. *Circ Res* 41:487, 1977.
261. Nizet A: Influence of serum albumin and dextran on sodium and water excretion by the isolated dog kidney. *Pfluegers Arch* 301:7, 1977.
261a. Nomura G et al: Effect of acute unilateral renal denervation on tubular sodium reabsorption in the dog. *Am J Physiol* 232:F16, 1977.
262. Nonoguchi H et al: Atrial natriuretic factor inhibits vasopressin-stimulated osmotic water permeability in rat

inner medullary collecting duct. *J Clin Invest* 82:1383, 1988.
263. Obika LFO et al: Lack of evidence for gastrointestinal control of sodium excretion in unanesthetized rabbits. *Am J Physiol* 240:F94, 1981.
264. O'Conner WJ: Normal sodium balance in dogs and in man. *Cardiovasc Res* 11:375, 1977.
265. Oliver JA et al: Increased renal secretion of norepinephrine and prostaglandin E_2 during sodium depletion in the dog. *J Clin Invest* 66:748, 1980.
266. Olsen ME et al: Mechanisms of angiotensin II natriuresis and antinatriuresis. *Am J Physiol* 249:F299, 1985.
267. O'Neil RG, Helman SI: Transport characteristics of renal collecting tubules: Influence of DOCA and diet. *Am J Physiol* 233:F544, 1977.
268. Osborn JL et al: Renal adrenoceptor mediation of antinatriuretic and renin secretion responses to low frequency renal nerve stimulation in the dog. *Circ Res* 53:295, 1983.
269. Osgood RW et al: Effect of aortic clamping on proximal reabsorption and sodium excretion in the rat. *Am J Physiol* 232:F92, 1977.
270. Osgood RW et al: Further studies on segmental sodium transport in the rat kidney during expansion of the extracellular fluid volume. *J Clin Invest* 64:311, 1978.
271. Osgood RW et al: Effect of hemodynamic albumin on superficial and juxtamedullary nephron sodium transport. *Am J Physiol* 237:F34, 1979.
272. Ott CE et al: Effect of increased peritubular protein concentration on proximal tubule reabsorption in the presence and absence of extracellular volume expansion. *J Clin Invest* 55:612, 1975.
273. Paintal AS: Vagal sensory receptors and their reflex effects. *Physiol Rev* 53:159, 1973.
274. Papanicolaou N et al: The release of renal prostaglandin during saline infusion in normal and hypertensive subjects. *Clin Sci* 49:459, 1975.
275. Passo SS et al: Hepatic receptors in control of sodium excretion in anesthetized cats. *Am J Physiol* 224:373, 1975.
276. Passo SS et al: Natriuresis following fourth ventrical perfusion with high-sodium artificial CSF. *Can J Physiol Pharmacol* 53:363, 1975.
277. Pearce JW: The effect of vagotomy and denervation of the choroid sinus on diuresis following plasma volume expansion. *Can J Biochem Physiol* 37:81, 1959.
278. Pelayo JC et al: Effects of dopamine blockade on renal sodium excretion. *Am J Physiol* 245:F247, 1983.
279. Pelayo JC et al: Renal denervation in the rat: Analysis of glomerular and proximal tubular function. *Am J Physiol* 244:F70, 1983.
280. Pettinger WA et al: Renal α_2 adrenoceptors and the adenylate cyclase-cAMP system: Biochemical and physiological interactions. *Am J Physiol* 252:F199, 1987.
281. Petty KJ et al: Secondary effect of aldosterone on Na-K-ATPase activity in the rabbit cortical collecting tubule. *J Clin Invest* 68:1514, 1981.
282. Polhemus RE, Hall DA: Effect of catecholamines on the potential difference and chloride effects in the mouse thick ascending limb of Henle's loop. *Kidney Int* 19:253, 1981.
283. Pollock DM et al: Dissociation of urinary kallikrein activity and salt and water excretion in the rat. *Am J Physiol* 250:F1082, 1986.
284. Potkay S, Gilmore JP: Renal response to vena caval and portal venous infusions of sodium chloride in unanesthetized dogs. *Clin Sci* 39:13, 1970.
285. Prosnitz EH, DiBona GF: Effect of decreased renal sympathetic nerve activity on renal tubular sodium reabsorption. *Am J Physiol* 235:F557, 1978.
286. Prosnitz EH et al: Mechanism of intrarenal blood flow distribution after carotid artery occlusion. *Am J Physiol* 232:F167, 1977.
287. Reineck HJ, Parma R: Effect of medullary tonicity on urinary sodium excretion in the rat. *J Clin Invest* 69:971, 1982.
288. Reinhardt HW et al: The control of sodium excretion by reflexes from the low pressure system independent of adrenal activity-experiments in conscious dogs. *Pfluegers Arch* 384:171, 1980.
289. Reinhardt HW et al: Atrial natriuresis under the condition of a constant renal perfusion pressure. *Pfluegers Arch* 389:9, 1980.
290. Richards AM et al: Contrasting plasma atrial natriuretic factor concentrations during comparable natriuresis with infusions of atrial natriuretic factor and saline in normal man. *Clin Sci* 75:455, 1988.
291. Rogenes PR, Gottschalk CW: Renal function in conscious rats with chronic unilateral denervation. *Am J Physiol* 242:F140, 1982.
292. Roman RJ et al: Influence of kinins and angiotensin II on the regulation of papillary blood flow. *Am J Physiol* 255:F690, 1988.
293. Rumrich G, Ullrich KH: The minimum requirements for the maintenance of sodium chloride reabsorption in the proximal convolution of the mammalian kidney. *J Physiol (Lond)* 197:69, 1968.
294. Sadowski J et al: Denervated and intact kidney responses to saline load in awake and anesthetized dogs. *Am J Physiol* 237:F262, 1979.
295. Samuels AI et al: Renin-angiotensin antagonists and the regulation of blood pressure. *Fed Proc* 35:2512, 1976.
296. Sansom S et al: Na^+-dependent effects of DOCA on cellular transport properties of CCDs from ADX rabbits. *Am J Physiol* 253:F753, 1987.
297. Schmidt U et al: Sodium and potassium-activated ATPase: A possible target of aldosterone. *J Clin Invest* 55:655, 1975.
298. Schneider EG et al: Lack of evidence for a hepatic osmoreceptor in conscious dogs. *Am J Physiol* 218:42, 1970.
299. Schneider E et al: Effect of chronic bilateral renal denervation on daily sodium excretion in the conscious dog. *Fed Proc* 37:645, 1978.
300. Schor N et al: Glomerular adaptations to chronic dietary salt restriction or excess. *Am J Physiol* 238:F428, 1980.
301. Schrier RW: Body fluid volume regulation in health and disease: A unifying hypothesis. *Ann Intern Med* 113:155, 1990.
302. Schrier RW, Earley LE: Effects of hematocrit on renal hemodynamics and sodium excretion in hydropenic and volume-expanded dogs. *J Clin Invest* 49:1656, 1970.

303. Schuster VL et al: Angiotensin II directly stimulates sodium transport in rabbit proximal convoluted tubules. *J Clin Invest* 73:507, 1984.
304. Schwab TR et al: Role of atrial natriuretic peptide in volume-expansion natriuresis. *Am J Physiol* 251:R310, 1986.
305. Schwartz FT, Burg MB: Mineralocorticoid effects on cation transport by cortical collecting tubules in vitro. *Am J Physiol* 235:F576, 1978.
306. Schwartzman et al: Renal cytochrome P450-related arachidonate metabolite inhibits Na^+ and K^+ ATPase. *Nature (Lond) 314:620, 1985.*
307. Scott WN et al: Inhibition of fatty acid synthesis prevents the incorporation of aldosterone-induced proteins into membranes. *J Biol Chem* 254:4957, 1979.
308. Seely JF, Levy M: Control of extracellular fluid volume, in Brenner BM, Rector FC Jr (eds): *The Kidney*. Philadelphia, Saunders, 1981, p 371.
309. Selkurt EE et al: Influence of graded arterial pressure decrement on renal clearance of creatinine, *p*-aminohippurate and sodium. *Am J Physiol* 159:369, 1949.
310. Shimizu K et al: Effects of saline infusion on prostaglandin-like materials in renal venous blood and medulla of canine kidney. *Jpn Heart J* 14:140, 1973.
311. Shipley RE, Study RS: Changes in renal blood extraction of inulin, GFR, tissue pressure and urine flow with acute alterations of renal artery blood pressure. *Am J Physiol* 167:676, 1951.
312. Siragy HM et al: Evidence that intrarenal dopamine acts as a paracrine substance at the renal tubule. *Am J Physiol* 257:F469, 1989.
313. Smyth DD et al: α_2 adrenoceptors and sodium reabsorption in the isolated perfused rat kidney. *Am J Physiol* 247:F680, 1984.
314. Smyth DD et al: α_2 adrenoceptor antagonism of vasopressin-induced changes in sodium excretion. *Am J Physiol* 248:F767, 1985.
315. Sonnenberg H: Proximal and distal tubular function in salt-deprived and salt-loaded deoxycorticosterone acetate escaped rats. *J Clin Invest* 52:263, 1973.
316. Sonnenberg H: Medullary collecting duct function in antidiuretic and in salt or water diuretic rats. *Am J Physiol* 226:501, 1974.
317. Sonnenberg H: Secretion of salt and water into the medullary collecting duct of Ringer infused rats. *Am J Physiol* 228:565, 1975.
318. Sonnenberg H: Collecting duct function in deoxycorticosterone acetate escaped, normal, and salt deprived rats: Response to hypervolemia. *Circ Res* 39:282, 1976.
319. Sonnenberg H: Effect of adrenalectomy on medullary collecting duct function in rats before and during blood volume expansion. *Pfluegers Arch* 368:55, 1977.
320. Sonnenberg H, Chong C: Comparison of micropuncture and microcatheterization in papillary collecting duct. *Am J Physiol* 239:F92, 1980.
321. Sonnenberg H, Pearce JW: Renal response to measured blood volume expansion in differently hydrated dogs. *Am J Physiol* 203:344, 1962.
322. Sowers JR et al: Relationship between urinary dopamine production and natriuresis after acute intravascular volume expansion with sodium chloride in dogs. *Endocrinology* 115:2085, 1984.
323. Spitzer A, Windhager EE: Effect of peritubular oncotic pressure changes on proximal fluid reabsorption. *Am J Physiol* 218:1188, 1970.
324. Stanton BA, Kaissling B: Adaptation of distal tubule and collecting duct to increased Na delivery: II. Na^+ and K^+ transport. *Am J Physiol* 255:F1269, 1988.
325. Starling EH, Verney EB: The secretion of urine as studied on the isolated kidney. *Proc R Soc Lond* 97:321, 1925.
326. Stein JH et al: A comparison of the segmental analysis of sodium reabsorption during Ringer's and hyperoncotic albumin infusion in the rat. *J Clin Invest* 52:2313, 1973.
327. Stein JH et al: Segmental sodium reabsorption in rats with mild and severe volume depletion. *Am J Physiol* 227:351, 1974.
328. Stein JH et al: Direct measurement of papillary collecting duct sodium transport in the rat. *J Clin Invest* 58:763, 1976.
329. Steiner RW et al: Glomerular hemodynamics in rats with chronic sodium depletion: Effect of saralasin. *J Clin Invest* 64:503, 1979.
330. Steven K: Effect of peritubular infusion on angiotensin II on the proximal nephron function. *Kidney Int* 6:73, 1974.
331. Stokes JB: Effect of prostaglandin E_2 on chloride transport across the rabbit thick ascending limb of Henle. *J Clin Invest* 64:495, 1979.
332. Stokes JB et al: Heterogeneity of the rabbit collecting tubule: Localization of mineralocorticoid hormone action to the cortical portion. *Kidney Int* 20:340, 1981.
333. Stokes JB, Kokko JP: Inhibition of sodium transport by prostaglandin E_2 across the isolated perfused rabbit collecting tubule. *J Clin Invest* 59:1099, 1977.
334. Strandhoy JW, Williamson HE: Evidence for a hepatic role in the control of sodium excretion. *Proc Soc Exp Biol Med* 133:419, 1970.
335. Strandhoy JW et al: Intrarenal effects of phenoxybenzamine on sodium reabsorption. *J Lab Clin Med* 83:263, 1974.
336. Strauss MB et al: Water diuresis produced during recumbency by the intravenous infusion of isotonic saline solution. *J Clin Invest* 30:862, 869, 1951.
337. Stumpe KD et al: Fluid reabsorption in Henle's loop and urinary excretion of sodium and water in normal rats and rats with hypertension. *J Clin Invest* 49:1200, 1970.
338. Taher MS et al: Effect of beta-adrenergic blockade on renin response to renal nerve stimulation. *J Clin Invest* 57:459, 1976.
339. Takacs L et al: Decreased proximal tubular transport capacity after renal sympathectomy. *Proc Int Cong Nephrol* 8:553, 1978.
340. Takeuchi J et al: Nervous control of the renal tubular function. *Jpn Heart J* 9:654, 1968.
341. Terashima R et al: Prostaglandin E release in the dog: Effect of sodium. *Am J Physiol* 231:1429, 1976.
342. Thames MD et al: Baroreflex stimulation of renal nerve activity during volume expansion. *Am J Physiol* 243:11810, 1982.
343. Thornborough JR et al: Receptors in cerebral circulation

affecting sodium excretion in the cat. *Am J Physiol* 225:138, 1973.
344. Tobian L et al: The effect of high perfusion pressure on the granulation of juxtaglomerular cells in an isolated kidney. *J Clin Invest* 38:605, 1959.
345. Tomita et al: Control of sodium and potassium transport in the cortical collecting duct of the rat: Effects of bradykinin, vasopressin, and deoxycorticosterone. *J Clin Invest* 76:132, 1985.
346. Tucker BJ, Blantz RC: Mechanism of altered glomerular hemodynamics during chronic sodium depletion. *Am J Physiol* 244:F11, 1983.
347. Uhlich E et al: Einfluss von Aldosteron auf den Natrium Transport in den Sammelrohren der Sangetyiernier. *Pfluegers Arch* 308:111, 1969.
348. Ullrich JJ, Papavasiliou F: Sodium reabsorption in the papillary collecting duct of rats. *Pfluegers Arch* 279:49, 1979.
349. Umemura S et al: α_2 adrenoceptors and cellular cAMP levels in single nephron segments from the rat. *Am J Physiol* 249:F28, 1985.
350. Unwin RJ et al: Brain-gut peptides, renal function and cell growth. *Kidney Int* 37:1031, 1990.
351. Vander AJ: Inhibition of distal tubular sodium reabsorption by angiotensin II. *Am J Physiol* 205:133, 1963.
352. Vandewalle A et al: Aldosterone binding along the rabbit nephron: An autoradiographic study on isolated tubules. *Am J Physiol* 240:F172, 1981.
353. Vanherwegman JL et al: Effect of indomethacin on renal hemodynamics and on water and sodium excretion by the isolated dog kidney. *Pfluegers Arch* 357:232, 1975.
354. Veldkamp PJ et al: Direct evaluation of the microvascular actions of ANP in juxtamedullary nephrons. *Am J Physiol* 254:F440, 1988.
355. Verderstraeten P, Toussaint C: Effects of plasmapheresis on renal hemodynamics and sodium excretion in dogs. *Pfluegers Arch* 306:92, 1969.
356. Veress AT, Sonnenberg H: Right atrial appendectomy reduces the renal response to acute hypervolemia in the rat. *Am J Physiol* 247:R610, 1984.
357. Watson ML et al: Urinary kallikrein and systemic prostaglandin synthesis during sodium chloride infusion in normal man. *Clin Sci* 68:537, 1985.
358. Waugh WH: Angiotensin II: Local renal effects of physiological increments in concentration. *Can J Physiol Pharmacol* 51:711, 1972.
359. Webster ME, Gilmore JP: Influence of kallidin-10 on renal function. *Am J Physiol* 206:714, 1964.
360. Weiner M et al: Accelerated reabsorption in the proximal tubule produced by volume depletion. *J Clin Invest* 50:1379, 1971.
361. Welt LG, Orloff J: The effects of an increase in plasma volume on the metabolism and the excretion of water in the electrolytes of normal subjects. *J Clin Invest* 30:751, 1951.
362. Wennergren G et al: Effects of stimulation of nonmedullated cardiac afferents on renal water and sodium excretion. *Acta Physiol Scand* 97:261, 1976.
363. Wilcox CS et al: Renal interstitial pressure and sodium excretion during hilar lymphatic ligation. *Am J Physiol* 247:F344, 1984.
364. Willis LR et al: Mechanism of natriuretic action on bradykinin. *Am J Physiol* 217:1, 1969.
365. Wilson DR et al: Effect of acute and chronic denervation on renal function after release of unilateral ureteral obstruction in the rat. *Can J Physiol Pharmacol* 57:731, 1979.
366. Wright FS et al: Renal sodium excretion after volume expansion with saline and blood. *Proc Soc Exp Biol Med* 128:1044, 1968.
367. Young DB et al: Effectiveness of the aldosterone, sodium and potassium feedback control system. *Am J Physiol* 231:945, 1976.
368. Zambraski EJ, DiBona GF: Role of angiotensin II in the antinatriuresis of low level renal nerve stimulation. *Am J Physiol* 231:1105, 1976.
369. Zambraski EJ, Dunn MJ: Renal prostaglandin E_2 secretion and excretion in conscious dogs. *Am J Physiol* 236:F552, 1979.
370. Zambraski EJ et al: Effect of sympathetic blocking agents on the antinatriuresis of reflex renal nerve stimulation. *J Pharmacol Exp Ther* 198:464, 1976.
371. Zambraski EJ et al: Specificity of neural effect on renal tubular sodium reabsorption. *Proc Soc Exp Biol Med* 151:543, 1976.
372. Zehr JE et al: ADH levels following nonhypotensive hemorrhage in dogs with chronic mitral stenosis. *Am J Physiol* 21:312, 1971.
373. Zeidel ML et al: cGMP mediates effects of atrial peptides on medullary collecting duct cells. *Am J Physiol* 252:F551, 1987.
374. Zucker IH et al: The mechanism of adaptation of left atrial stretch receptors in dogs with chronic congestive heart failure. *J Clin Invest* 60:323, 1971.

CHAPTER 4

Osmotic and nonosmotic regulation of thirst and vasopressin secretion

Robert L. Zerbe • Gary L. Robertson

ANTIDIURETIC HORMONE

The antidiuretic hormone, arginine vasopressin (AVP), is the only recognized hormone participating in the regulation of body fluid osmolality. The precision with which its secretion is osmotically regulated, the potency of its antidiuretic effects, and the rapid rate of its clearance from the circulation make vasopressin ideally suited for this role. Osmotically regulated vasopressin release "fine tunes" the rate of free-water excretion. Wide fluctuations in osmolality are prevented by the large renal capacity for free-water excretion and the essentially unlimited capacity for water intake when thirst is osmotically stimulated. Thus, under normal circumstances, this system maintains body fluid tonicity within the relatively narrow range that preserves efficient cellular function.

BACKGROUND

Vasopressin has potent pressor effects, which provided the basis for its initial recognition.[122] Over a decade later, its importance as an antidiuretic hormone was appreciated.[162] It is now generally accepted that the primary physiologic role of vasopressin is that associated with conservation of water, since normal plasma levels of vasopressin are well below those necessary to appreciably affect blood pressure.[109,133] Only in unusual situations, such as severe hypotension,[210] do vasopressin levels rise sufficiently to produce a pressor effect.

Vasopressin, like closely related oxytocin (see below), is stored and secreted from the posterior pituitary. The first significant success in the isolation of these posterior pituitary hormones was achieved by Van Dyke, who in 1942 described what was considered to be a pure protein with both vasopressin and oxytocic properties in bioassay.[189] Better purification techniques later demonstrated that the "Van Dyke protein" actually contained both vasopressin and oxytocin, which were distinctly different peptides. In 1949, the first highly purified peptide, oxytocin, was isolated from the posterior pituitary extracts.[106] This purified material enabled the elucidation of the general structure of the neurohypophyseal hormones[51] and the synthesis of oxytocin.[53] Using a similar approach, arginine vasopressin was isolated, characterized,[1,52,187] and synthesized.[54]

STRUCTURE OF NEUROHYPOPHYSEAL HORMONES

AVP is a nonapeptide containing two cysteine residues, which form a disulfide bridge between positions 1 and 6. This general structure is shared by the other mammalian neurohypophyseal hormones, lysine vasopressin, oxytocin, and vasotocin (Fig. 4-1). Lysine vasopressin differs only in that a lysine is substituted for arginine at position 8. It is presumed to have evolved from arginine vasopressin and is found only in members of the suborder Suina.[129] Retention of the antidiuretic activity following lysine substitution reflects the importance of a basic amino acid in position 8 for this action.[156] This is further supported by the observation that oxytocin, which has a leucine in place of arginine at position 8 and isoleucine in

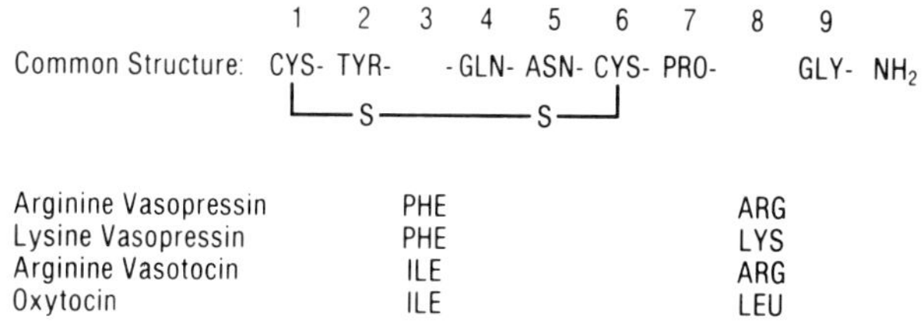

FIGURE 4-1 • Structure of neurohypophyseal hormones. Differing amino acids at positions 3 and 8 are indicated for the known mammalian hormones.

place of phenylalanine in position 3, has little antidiuretic activity,[196] whereas arginine vasotocin, which has the ring structure of oxytocin and the tripeptide side chain of AVP, has antidiuretic activity. The latter is found in all vertebrates[157] and, because of its wide phyletic distribution and close relationship to all known neurohypophyseal peptides, is thought to be the evolutionary ancestor of this class of hormones.[157] Vasotocin has been found in the neurohypophyses of mammals only during fetal and possibly early neonatal life.[167,179,193] Most but not all researchers agree that vasotocin is present in the adult mammalian pineal.[33,58,59,103,113,120,125] Though vasotocin has oxytocic, antidiuretic, and pressor activities,[196] its function in mammalian physiology is unknown.[208]

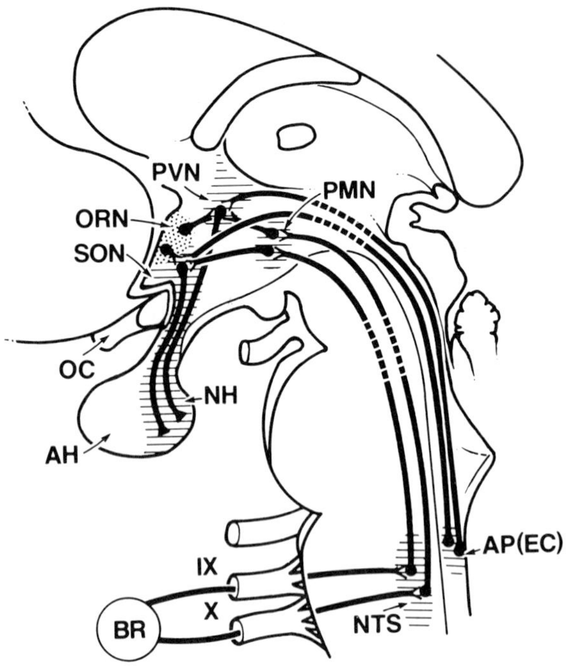

FIGURE 4-2 • Schematic representation of the neurohypophysis and its principal regulatory afferents. AH, adenohypophysis; NH, neurohypophysis; OC, optic chiasm; SON, supraoptic nucleus; PVN, paraventricular nucleus; PMN, posteromedial nucleus; ORN, osmoreceptor neurons; BR, baroreceptors; NTS, nucleus tractus solitarius; AP(EC), area postrema (emetic center). (From Robertson GL: *Vasopressin and Water Metabolism*, in Ingbar SH (ed), *The Year in Endocrinology 1977*, New York, Plenum Publishing Company, 1978, p. 205.)

SYNTHESIS AND RELEASE

Vasopressin is synthesized in neurons of the hypothalamus and then transported through axons to the posterior pituitary, where it is stored and released.[9] Three hypothalamic nuclei are known to synthesize vasopressin, but the posterior pituitary receives vasopressin-containing axons only from the magnocellular neurons of the *paraventricular* and *supraoptic* nuclei (Fig. 4-2.) Parvocellular neurons of the suprachiasmatic nucleus also synthesize vasopressin[176] but do not project to the posterior pituitary.[176] All neurons from the suprachiasmatic nucleus and a portion of the neurons from the paraventricular and suprachiasmatic nuclei send vasopressinergic axons to a number of areas within the central nervous system.[107,176,215] The role of these vasopressinergic pathways is unknown.

Like many peptide hormones, vasopressin is synthesized as a prohormone that requires further processing before release. This prohormone, which has been called *propressophysin,* has a molecular weight of 20,000 and is known to contain vasopressin, vasopressin-associated neurophysin, and a glycopeptide.[149] Oxytocin is also synthesized via a prohormone, known as prooxyphysin, which is similar to propressophysin but lacks the glycoprotein moiety. Their structures are shown in Fig. 4-3. The genes that code for propressophysin and prooxyphysin have been sequenced[154,158] and tentatively localized to chromosome 20.[132] The structure of the propressophysin gene is shown in Fig. 4-4. It is composed of three exons, which code, respectively, for (1) the signal peptide, vasopressin, and the variable N-terminal portion of neurophysin; (2) the highly conserved central region of neurophysin; and (3) the variable C-terminal portion of neurophysin and the glycopeptides.

Following synthesis, propressophysin is packaged in secretory vesicles within the cell bodies of the hypothalamic neurons. The vesicles themselves are rapidly transported down axons and stored in enlarged termini within the posterior pituitary. During transport, the propressophysin is processed by as yet unidentified enzymes believed to be contained within the secretory vesicles. This processing is accelerated by osmotic stimulation.[150]

Vasopressin is released from nerve terminals in the posterior pituitary following depolarization of the neurons. Electromicroscopic studies have shown that the neurosecretory granules discharge their contents directly into the extracellular space by exocytosis. The membrane of the secretory vesicle actually fuses with the cellular membrane, allowing unobstructed passage of the vesicular contents.[119] This method of neurohypophyseal secretion explains the apparent corelease of the neurohypophyseal hormones and their neurophysins, which aided in the identification of the latter.[142] Intracellular calcium appears to be involved in this exocytotic process, since stimulation of vasopressin release in vitro[45] and in vivo[7] is calcium-ion-dependent, and physiologic stimulation of vasopressin release in vivo causes a rise in the intracellular calcium ion concentration of neurohypophyseal nerve endings.[92]

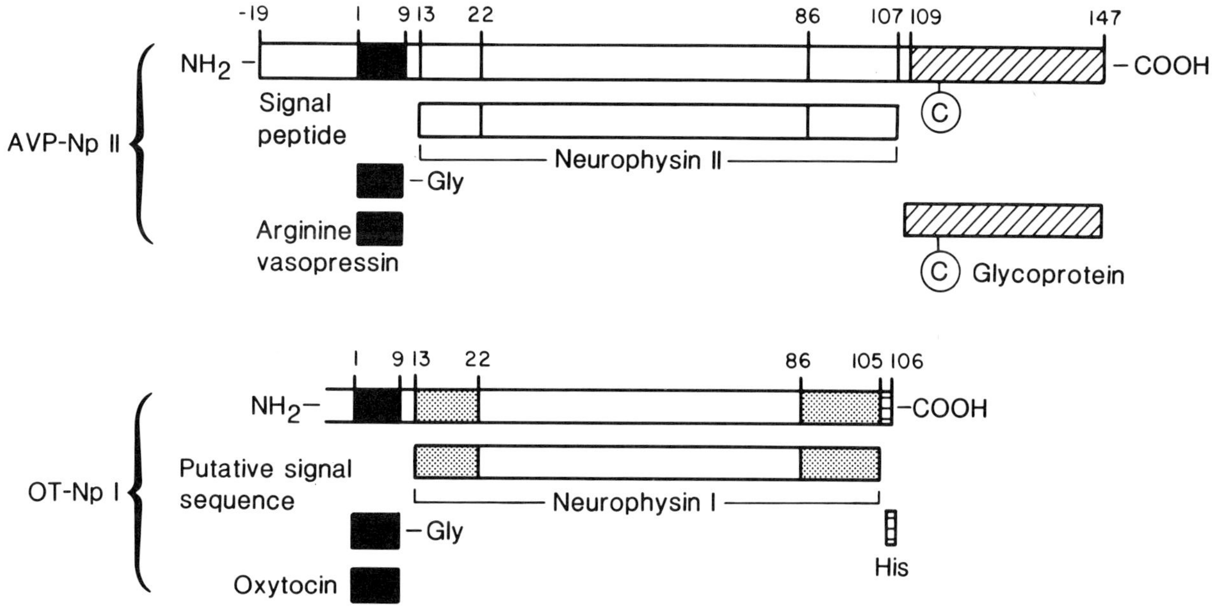

FIGURE 4-3 • The structure of propressophysin and prooxyphysin. (Redrawn from Ivell R et al: *Neuroendocrinology* 37:235, 1983. Used by permission.)

METABOLISM

Vasopressin is distributed in a fluid volume roughly equal to the extracellular space. It is not appreciably bound to plasma proteins.[101] Clearance from the circulation is rapid, with an estimated half-life in humans of between 10 and 25 min.[37,136] In humans, approximately 10 percent of administered vasopressin appears in urine.[57,136] Animal studies indicate that the remaining clearance results from approximately equal degradation by the liver and kidney.[68] There is sufficient reserve capacity for degradation, however, since disease or loss of either organ does not appreciably affect the overall clearance rate.[44] Enzymatic cleavage resulting in degradation of the vasopressin molecule takes place at four sites: in the acyclic portion of the peptides between positions 7 and 8; at the cysteinyl-tyrosyl peptide bond; in the acyclic portion of the peptide between positions 8 and 9; and at the disulfide bond.[198] Of these sites, the first two appear to be the most important for enzymatic degradation of vasopressin.[198]

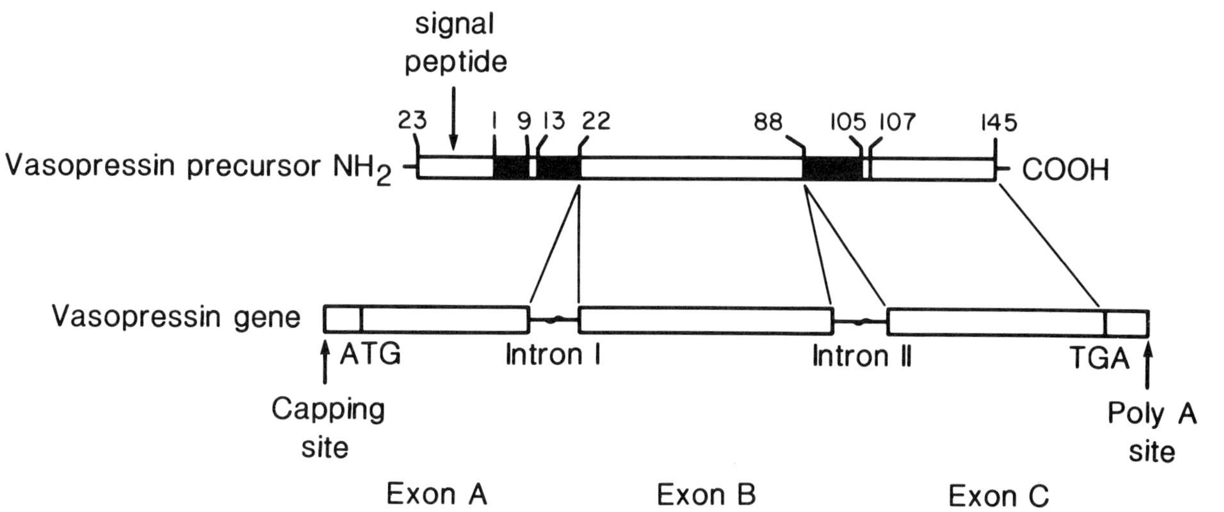

FIGURE 4-4 • The structure of the gene that codes for propressophysin. (Redrawn from Schmale H et al: *Kidney Int* 32(suppl 21):S8, 1987. Used by permission.)

In pregnancy, the metabolic clearance of vasopressin increases three- to fourfold due to placental production of vasopressinase.[40]

OSMOTIC REGULATION

Since the pioneering studies of Verney,[192] plasma osmolality has been recognized as an important factor in the regulation of vasopressin secretion. These studies, the results of which were reported over 40 years ago, continue to serve as the basis for our understanding of the functional and anatomical aspects of the osmoregulation of vasopressin secretion. Verney's experiments, which were done in conscious, water-loaded dogs, demonstrated that intracarotid infusions of hypertonic sodium chloride and certain other hypertonic solutions produced a decrease in urine output that was similar to that which occurred after injection of a posterior pituitary extract. On the basis of these experiments, he hypothesized that an *osmoreceptor* was responsible for regulation of antidiuretic hormone release from the posterior pituitary. Verney hypothesized that the osmoreceptor detected changes in tonicity by becoming osmotically dehydrated when exposed to solutes that failed to equilibrate across the osmoreceptor membrane. Additional studies following selective ligation of the vascular supply to regions of the central nervous system indicated that the osmoreceptor was located in the anterior hypothalamus near the cells of the neurohypophysis. The development of more reliable methods for assessment of hypothalamoneurohypophyseal function has led to refinements but rarely to contradiction of Verney's theories.

Quantitative characterization of osmotic regulation

The functional properties of this osmoregulatory system can be described quantitatively by analyzing the relationship between plasma vasopressin, as determined by sensitive and specific radioimmunoassay systems, and the simultaneous plasma osmolality. This approach has proved to be useful in understanding both normal and abnormal states of water balance.[133-135,205,206,208,213] In normal adults, the "osmostat" that controls vasopressin secretion appears to be set so that secretion of the hormone is very low or undetectable when plasma osmolality falls below a "threshold" of approximately 280 mosm/kg (Fig. 4-5). In the absence of vasopressin, the rate of free-water excretion is markedly increased, allowing rapid correction of the hypotonic state. The capacity of the normal kidney to excrete free water in the absence of vasopressin is so great that for practical purposes the set point of the osmoreceptor defines the lower limit for plasma osmolality in normal humans. As plasma osmolality rises above this osmotic threshold, vasopressin

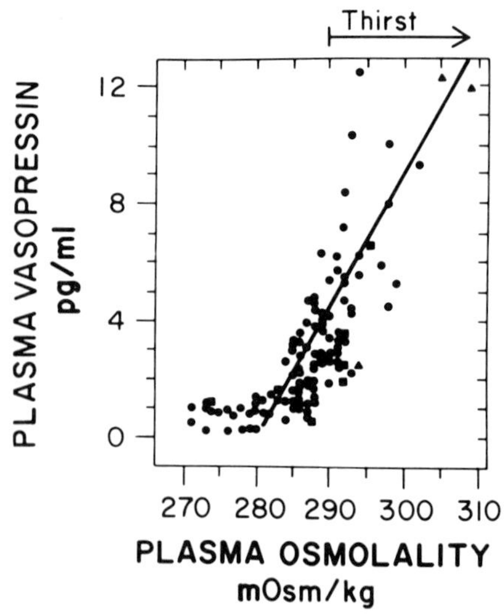

FIGURE 4-5 • Relationship between plasma osmolality and vasopressin in healthy recumbent adults under various conditions of hydration. The line represents the regression function obtained by least squares analysis of the individual data points. The normal thirst threshold is indicated at the top. (From Robertson GL et al: *Am J Med* 72:339, 1982.)

secretion increases by an amount that closely correlates with the level of plasma osmolality. This relationship can be described by a linear regression function,[135]

$$\text{Plasma vasopressin} = m\,(\text{plasma osmolality}) + b \quad (1)$$

in which the slope (m) is an index of sensitivity of the osmoreceptor mechanism, and the x intercept ($-b/m$) provides an estimate of the osmotic threshold for vasopressin secretion. Although it has been proposed that an exponential function better describes the relationship between plasma osmolality and vasopression,[200] the differences that would be expected with the two models are in fact too small to be resolved with current methods. Moreover, the linear function accurately characterizes this relationship with the physiologic range[74,143] and lends itself better to quantitative comparisons.[135]

The high linear correlation between plasma vasopressin and osmolality is most evident when the scatter due to population variation of this relationship is excluded by repeated measurements of plasma vasopressin at different levels of plasma osmolality in the same subject. Such analysis reveals that, within a normal population, the "set" or threshold of the osmostat varies by less than 3 percent, but its sensitivity varies over a wide range. When this relationship is reexamined in the same subjects under the same conditions months to years later, nearly identical estimates of the osmoreceptor threshold and sensitivity are observed.[214] Thus, despite wide individual variation, the functional properties of the osmoreceptor remain quite reproducible within individuals when examined under the same conditions of hydration and posture. Furthermore, similar studies done in monozygotic and dizygotic twin pairs demonstrate significant evidence of genetic variance in both the sensitivity and the threshold of the osmoreceptor that controls vasopressin secretion,[214] indicating that both characteristics are, at least in part, genetically determined. Neither the neurophysiologic basis for this genetically determined functional characteristic nor its effects on regulation of water balance have been fully elucidated.

Factors affecting osmotic regulation

Although quite reproducible when studied under the same conditions, the osmoregulation of vasopressin secretion is subject to a number of physiological or pathological alterations. For one thing, the sensitivity of the osmoreceptor is dependent on the *rate of rise in plasma osmolality*.[135,138] Thus, the secretion of vasopressin is enhanced significantly when the same osmotic stimulus is delivered over a short period of time (Fig. 4-6). Such potentiation of vasopressin secretion is observed only when the rise in tonicity exceeds 2 percent per hour. The importance of this potentiation in physiologic regulation of vasopressin secretion is doubtful, since such rapid changes in plasma osmolality rarely, if ever, occur in nature. This rate-dependent effect, however, must be considered in clinical studies where plasma osmolality is increased artificially by the infusion of hypertonic solutions.

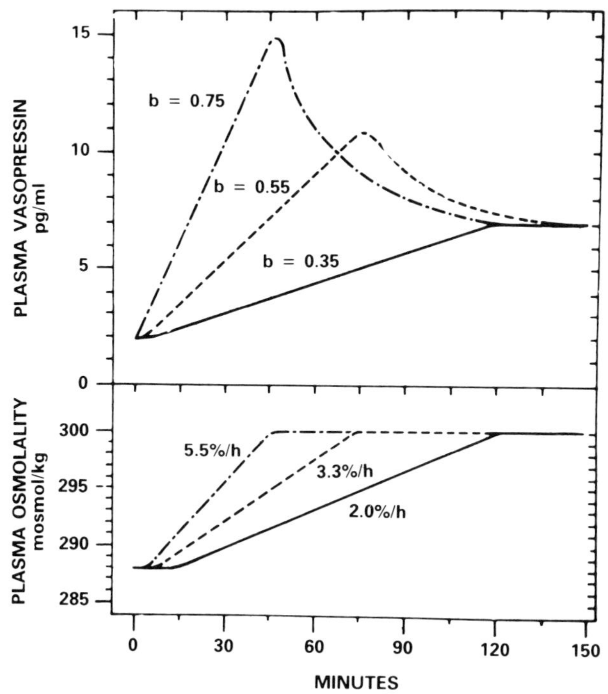

FIGURE 4-6 • The effect of varying the rate of hypertonic saline infusion on the change in plasma vasopressin concentration in healthy adults. At each rate (0.06, 0.1, and 0.16 ml/kg/min), the total volume of saline infused was constant. The rate of change in osmolality expressed as percent per hour is indicated next to each line in the bottom panel. The slope of the lines describing the relationship between plasma vasopressin and osmolality during each infusion is indicated by the values next to the lines in the upper panel. (From Robertson GL et al: *Kidney Int* 10:25, 1976.)

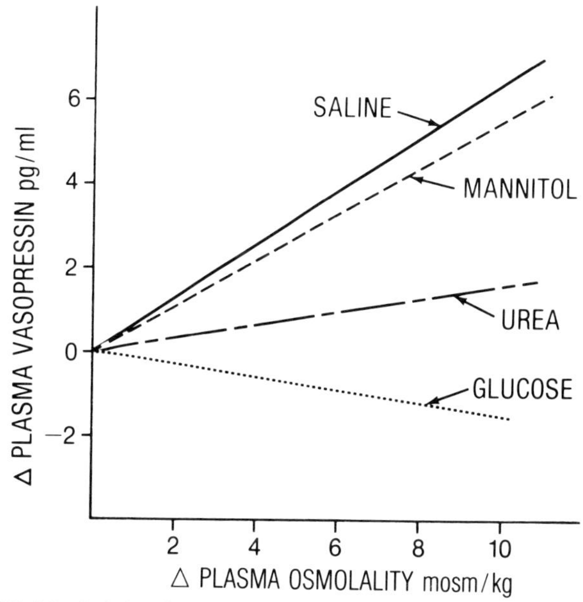

FIGURE 4-7 • Relationships between plasma vasopressin and plasma osmolality during infusions of various solutes.

The *type of solute* producing the rise in plasma osmolality is also an important factor in determining the sensitivity of the osmoreceptor.[213] Normally, sodium and its anions account for 95 percent of the osmotic pressure of plasma and extracellular fluid. Therefore, in most situations, changes in sodium concentration are responsible for the osmoregulation of vasopressin. However, as demonstrated by Verney's early studies (see above), sodium is not the only solute capable of stimulating vasopressin secretion. Mannitol, a solute that is similar to sodium in that it produces a transcellular osmotic gradient, is equipotent to sodium in osmotic stimulation of vasopressin release (Fig. 4-7).[213] The effects of urea and glucose on osmotic stimulation of vasopressin are more controversial. Verney originally described antidiuresis following bolus injection of hypertonic glucose into the carotid artery of dogs.[192] However, most animal studies have found that glucose is an ineffective osmotic stimulus both in vivo and in vitro.[111,112,169,183] The latter findings are entirely compatible with the detailed observations in normal human subjects in which a rise in osmolality produced by the infusion of hypertonic glucose resulted in a fall of immunoreactive vasopressin in plasma (Fig. 4-7).[213] In contrast, hyperglycemia produces a rise in plasma vasopressin in patients with insulin-deficient diabetes mellitus.[195] These findings are consistent with the theory that the osmoreceptors are sensitive to transcellular osmotic gradients generated by a rise in the extracellular concentration of impermeable solutes (see below) if glucose uptake by the osmoreceptors is insulin-dependent.

The effect of urea also seems to be variable. In animals, it has been reported either to have no effect[183,193] or to stimulate[112,216] vasopressin secretion. In humans, an acute increase in plasma urea produces a slight but clearly significant rise in plasma vasopressin levels.[213] Quantitatively, however, it is only about one-fourth as potent as saline solution (Fig. 4-7).[213]

Age may also be an important determinant of the sensitivity of the osmoreceptor to osmotic stimulation. When the vasopressin response to hypertonic saline solution was examined in young (mean age 35 years) and old (mean age 50 years) healthy human subjects, the older group was found to have a greater rise in vasopressin for the same degree of osmotic stimulus.[77] The osmotic threshold for vasopressin secretion did not differ, however. The cause of the apparent change in osmoreceptor sensitivity is unknown but may be linked to an alteration in the baroreceptor mechanism that also occurs with aging (see below).[147] These observations are not necessarily incompatible with the previously noted reproducibility of osmoregulatory function in normal subjects, since the aging studies represent a much longer span of time than that examined in the reproducibility studies. Moreover, the young and old groups in the aging study may not be entirely comparable, since selective factors contributing to longevity may affect the osmotic or hemodynamic stimulation of vasopressin. It also should be noted that, contrary to the human studies, aged rats undergoing prolonged fluid deprivation are unable to attain plasma vasopressin levels comparable to those found in younger controls.[172]

The effect of *sex hormones* on osmoregulation is unclear. Castration of adult male rats leads to stimulation of vasopressin that is reversible by replacement of androgen, and vasopressin levels during the estrous cycle of female rats parallel the changes in estrogen levels.[168] Furthermore, administration of estrogens to normal human males leads to an increase in urinary vasopressin excretion.[102] Nevertheless, detailed studies of the osmoregulation of plasma vasopressin in humans revealed no difference between normal males and females.[214] In healthy females, the osmoregulation of vasopressin does change slightly during the follicular and luteal phases of the menstrual cycle, but this change is due to a shift in the threshold and not in the sensitivity to osmotic stimuli.[194]

Pregnancy also affects osmoreceptor function. It has been known for many years that plasma osmolality falls by 2 to 4 percent early in gestation and remains decreased until delivery.[83] In this situation, osmotic regulation of vasopressin secretion is preserved, but secretion is initiated at a lower level of plasma osmolality.[50,39] This "resetting" of the osmostat occurs too early in pregnancy to be ascribed to reduction in blood pressure, is associated with an increase in total blood volume, and cannot be reproduced by the administration of either estrogen or progesterone. The etiology of this change in osmoregulatory function has not been determined, but its early occurrence suggests that it may be mediated, at least in part, by some humoral substance derived from the products of conception.

NEUROANATOMY OF VASOPRESSIN OSMOREGULATION

Although considerable progress has been made in describing the functional characteristics of the osmoregulatory system for vasopressin secretion, a definite anatomical description of Verney's osmoreceptor remains elusive. Jewell and Verney were the first to localize the osmoreceptor to the anterior hypothalamus. By examining the antidiuretic effect of hypertonic saline solution following selective ligation of branches of the internal carotid artery, they concluded that the osmoreceptor was very near or identical to the cell bodies of the neurohypophysis.[86] Subsequent animal studies that examined the antidiuretic effect of microinjections of hypertonic solutions in and around the anterior hypothalamus confirm the presence of osmotically sensitive areas in this region.[5,24,111,126,127] In experimental animals, lesions of the anterior hypothalamus have also been shown to interfere with osmotically stimulated vasopressin secretion and thirst and are able to do so without damaging neurosecretory cells that project to the neurohypophysis.[2,22,28,148,190] These observations support the existence of discrete osmotically sensitive cells in this area, which are important in both vasopressin secretion and thirst.

There is still controversy about whether the osmoreceptor is located inside or outside the blood-brain barrier.[113] This question not only has relevance in predicting and understanding pharmacological manipulations of osmoreceptor function but also bears directly on the issue of solute specificity. If the osmoreceptors are outside of the blood-brain barrier, their solute specificity would be determined by the permeability characteristics of their cell membranes. However, if they are located within the blood-brain barrier, the permeability characteristics of the barrier in the region of the osmoreceptors would determine their solute specificity. This distinction has some importance in understanding the true nature of the osmoreceptor mechanism, since one theory proposes that the osmoreceptor is really a sodium receptor that lies within the blood-brain barrier.[123] According to this theory, which is based on data from intracerebroventricular injections of hypertonic solutions in animals,[123] the solute specificity of the osmoreceptor mechanism is dependent on the penetration of these solutes across the blood-brain barrier. Solutes that fail to cross the blood-brain barrier stimulate vasopressin release by osmotically extracting water from the brain and raising the sodium concentration within the central nervous system. Studies in humans suggest that the blood-brain barrier has relatively little importance in osmotic stimulation of vasopressin release, since hypertonic saline solution is a much more potent stimulus for vasopressin release than is hypertonic urea,[213] even though both solutes are excluded by the blood-brain barrier.[25]

HEMODYNAMIC REGULATION

Hemodynamic factors are also known to affect vasopressin secretion. Both hypotension and hypovolemia (without hypotension) may, if sufficiently severe, produce marked elevations in plasma vasopressin.

Quantitative characterization of hemodynamic regulation

The pressure threshold for initiation of vasopressin secretion and the shape of the stimulus-response curve have been determined in humans by lowering blood pressure pharmacologically or by upright posture following phlebotomy (Fig. 4-8). Unlike the relationship between plasma vasopressin and osmolality, which is described well by a linear function (see above), the stimulus-response relationship for acute hypotension clearly conforms to an exponential function.[136] Examination of this stimulus-response curve shows that significant increases in plasma vasopressin may occur after a decline in mean arterial pressure of as little as 5 percent. However, this response does not occur consistently until blood pressure has fallen by 15 percent. Further reduction in blood pressure produced vasopressin levels that were much higher than those seen with even a substantial osmotic stimulus (see above).

The stimulus-response relationship for hypovolemic stimulation of vasopressin release in humans has been more difficult to quantitate because of technical problems with the induction and quantitation of hypovolemia. Early studies using indirect or bioassay methods showed that reducing blood volume by approximately 10 percent in animals[88] produced a significant increase in antidiuretic activity. These results were compatible with the hypothesis that ordinary changes in blood volume may

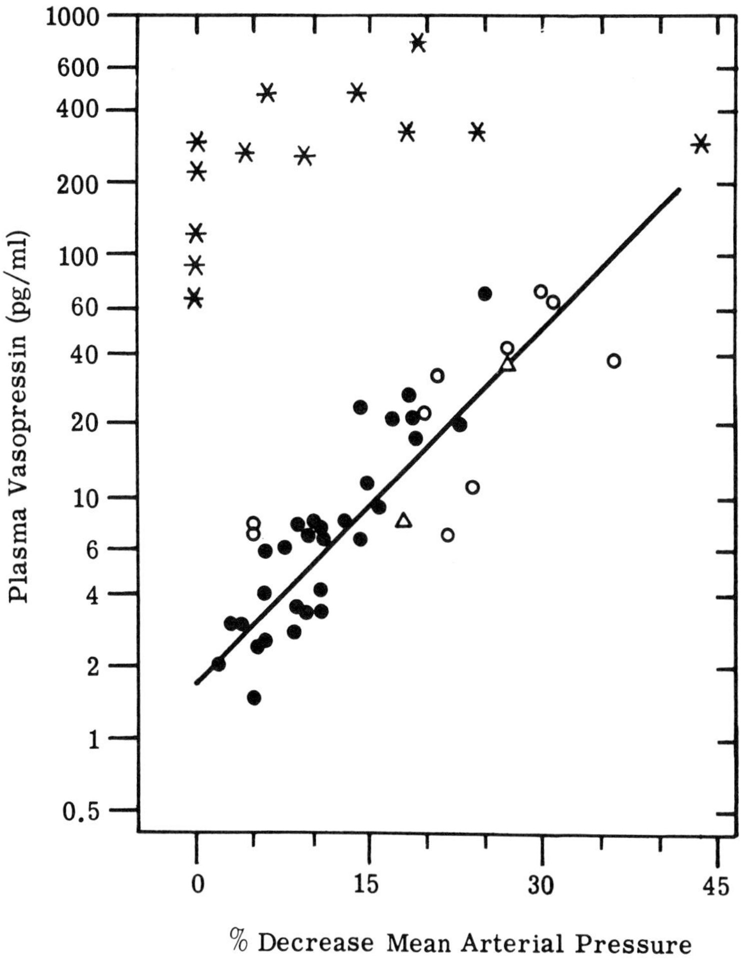

FIGURE 4-8 • Plasma vasopressin as a function of percent decrease in mean arterial pressure in healthy adults. Open circles (○) = phlebotomy and orthostasis; closed circles (●) = infusion of trimethaphan; asterisks (*) = subjects who developed nausea in association with hypotension. The oblique line indicates the regression line obtained by least squares analysis of the individual data points from all subjects who did not experience nausea. Note the log scale for plasma vasopressin. (From Rowe JW et al: *Kidney Int* 16:729, 1979.)

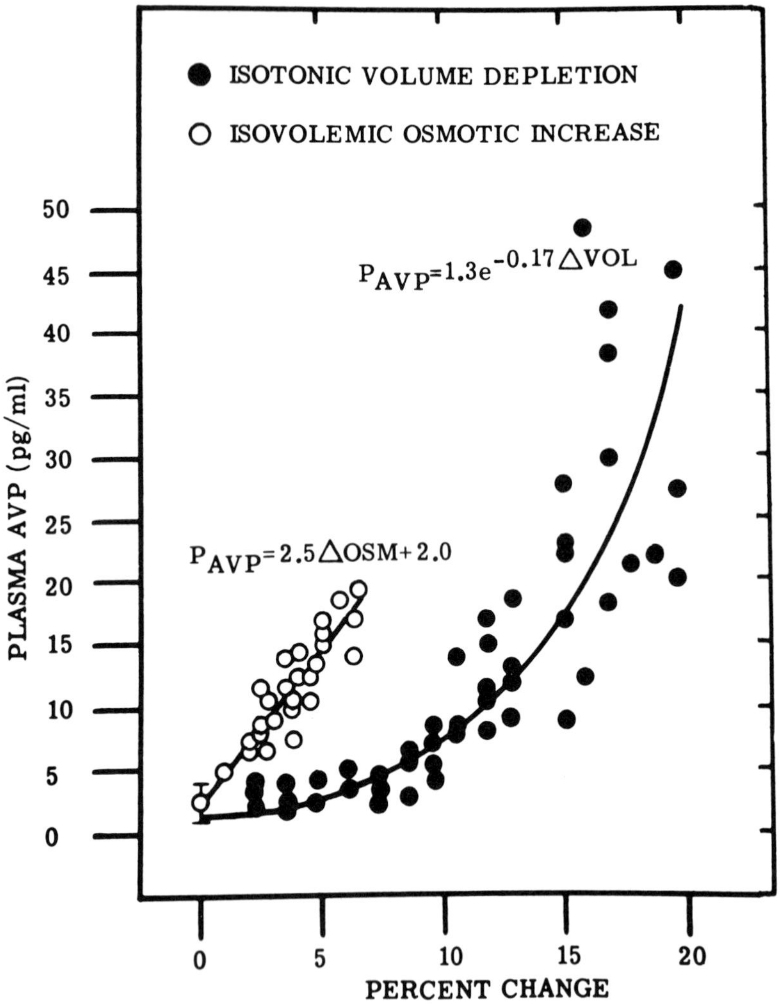

FIGURE 4-9 • The relationship between plasma vasopressin and either the percent increase in plasma osmolality (○; PAVP = 2.5 Δ osm + 2.0) or decrease in blood volume [●; PAVP = 1.3 exp(1.7 Δ vol.)] in conscious rats. (From Dunn FL et al: *J Clin Invest* 52:3212, 1973.)

contribute significantly to the physiologic regulation of circulating vasopression levels. More detailed studies indicate that small changes in blood volume may not be as important in vasopressin regulation as previously believed (Fig. 4-9). When blood volume was reduced isotonically in rats, plasma vasopressin did not increase significantly until hypovolemia exceeded 10 percent.[49] However, the stimulus-response relationship was again nonlinear. Thus, plasma vasopressin increases exponentially as the degree of hypovolemia increases. The stimulus-response relationship in humans has not been so thoroughly defined but appears to be similar quantitatively and qualitatively to that found in rats. Thus, phlebotomy sufficient to acutely lower total blood volume by 7 to 9 percent has no detectable effect on bioassayable[69] or immunoassayable[137] AVP in healthy recumbent adults. However, upright posture, which reduces effective blood volume by 10 to 15 percent, produces small but significant increases in plasma AVP,[134,161] while much larger degrees of hypovolemia induced by the combination of orthostasis and phlebotomy generally result in marked increases in hormone secretion.[137]

The difference between the stimulus-response relationships of osmotic and hemodynamic stimulation of vasopressin probably reflects a difference in the primary physiologic purpose of these two regulatory systems. Consideration of the dose-response relationships for the antidiuretic and pressor effects of vasopressin makes this difference in stimulus-response relationships more understandable. Some degree of antidiuresis is evident at vasopressin levels, which are at or even below the levels of detectability for even the most sensitive assay systems, and maximum antidiuresis occurs at plasma vasopressin levels as low as 5 pg/ml.[135] Thus, for a system to regulate vasopressin secretion in a way that makes the hormone effective in the control of water balance, it must tightly control low circulating levels, but it need not produce high levels under any circumstance. This is in contrast to the pressor effects of vasopressin, which are not evident in normal animals until plasma levels exceed 30 pg/ml.[109] The high levels of vasopressin observed during significant hypotension have been clearly shown to contribute to hemodynamic recovery and thus probably play a physiological role.[211] A system responsible for appropriately initiating the pressor effects of vasopressin would not need to regulate vasopressin secretion at low levels, but when a sufficient hemodynamic stimulus arose, it must be prepared to release large amounts of the hormone. Based on these factors, the osmoreceptor system and the baroreceptor system seem to be well suited to the control of vasopressin secretion for the purpose of water balance and, when necessary, assistance in the maintenance of blood pressure, respectively.

The ability of hemodynamic factors to affect vasopression secretion raises questions about their interaction with the osmoregulatory system. In both animals[49] and humans,[134] moderate decreases in intravascular volume or blood pressure do not interfere with the stimulatory or inhibitory effects of osmolality on vasopressin secretion. However, they do alter the relationship between plasma osmolality and vasopressin in such a way that the osmotic threshold is shifted to the left (Fig. 4-10). This kind of interaction helps to clarify the way in which the body reconciles its sometimes competing needs to preserve both intravascular volume and plasma tonicity. At relatively mild-to-moderate degrees of hypovolemia or hypotension, modest increases in plasma vasopressin and body water can be achieved without significantly altering the ability to regulate plasma osmolality. However, as the hemodynamic stimulus becomes more severe, the osmoregulatory system is increasingly compromised, since plasma vasopressin levels increase far above those necessary for maximum antidiuresis (Figs. 4-5 and 4-8). Under these conditions, the capacity to regulate osmolality may be effectively lost.

Analysis of the interaction between the osmotic and the hemodynamic control systems also provides insight into the organization of the neurohypophyseal unit. Most important in this regard is the observation that hypotonicity, if sufficiently great in magnitude, will completely suppress the stimulatory effects of moderate hypotension or hypovolemia.[49,134] This observation indicates that these two kinds of stimuli must interact in some way upon the same set of neurosecretory cells. This conclusion is supported by electrophysiologic studies in rats, which

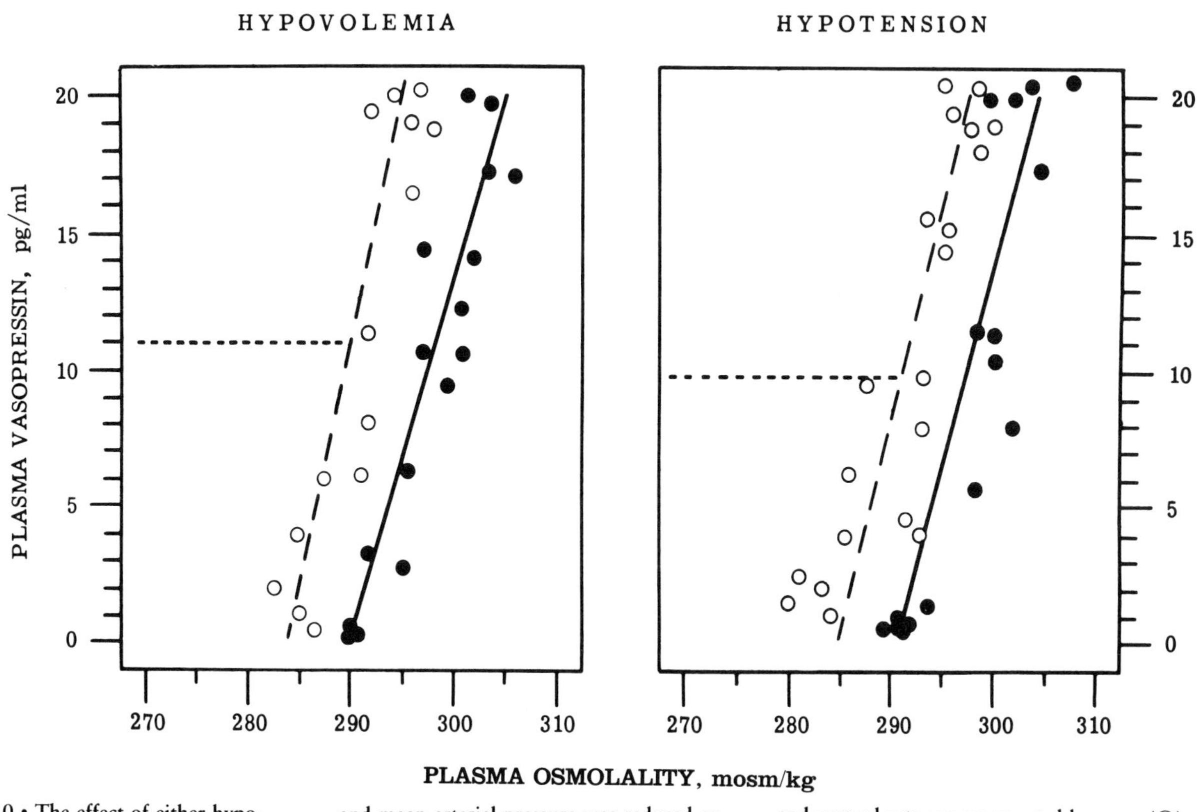

FIGURE 4-10 • The effect of either hypovolemia (panel to left) or hypotension (panel to right) on the osmotic regulation of vasopressin levels in conscious rats. Blood volume was reduced approximately 15 percent by intraperitoneal injection of polyethylene glycol and mean arterial pressure was reduced approximately 15 percent by subcutaneous injection of isoproterenol hydrochloride. Changes in plasma osmolality were induced by intraperitoneal injection of hypotonic, isotonic, or hypertonic saline. Experimental and normal rats are represented by open (○) and closed (●) circles, respectively. (From Robertson GL et al: Osmotic control of vasopressin function, in Andreoli TE et al (eds), *Disturbances in Body Fluid Osmolality*, Bethesda, American Physiological Society, 1977.)

have identified single neurons in the supraoptic nucleus that respond to both osmotic and hemodynamic stimuli.[91]

Neuroanatomy of vasopressin baroregulation

Since the early studies demonstrating hemodynamic stimulation of vasopressin secretion, efforts have been made to identify the anatomical pathways responsible for this effect. Although large gaps remain, many components of this baroregulatory reflex have been defined (Fig. 4-2). The receptors and afferent neural pathways appear to be part of a reflex arc that participates in the hemodynamic control of a number of neuroendocrine systems.[99] Hemodynamic changes are detected by stretch receptors in the wall of the left atrium and baroreceptors in the aortic arch and carotid sinuses. Atrial receptors are thought to detect small-to-moderate changes in blood volume, while baroreceptors detect changes in blood pressure, but the simplicity of this concept probably belies the true complexity of this system. Impulses from these pressure-sensitive receptors are carried to the central nervous system via the vagal and glossopharyngeal nerves.[163] The first synapse occurs in the nucleus of the tractus solitarius, an important brain stem baroregulatory center. Recent immunohistochemical and transport studies have traced ascending pathways that arise from noradrenergic cells in the nucleus of the tractus solitarius, the ventral medulla, and the locus ceruleus and project to the paraventricular and supraoptic nuclei.[155] These pathways probably mediate the ascending hemodynamic signals for vasopressin release by a tonic inhibitory influence. The pathways that mediate the effect of hypovolemia on vasopressin release appear to involve opioidergic neurons that project to the dorsolateral parabrachial nucleii, since the response to this stimulus is selectively eliminated when this area is microinjected with the broad-spectrum opioid antagonist diprenorphine (see "Opiates" below).

OTHER FACTORS AFFECTING VASOPRESSIN SECRETION

Nausea

Nausea produces a marked increase in vasopressin levels, and this increase occurs independently of changes in osmotic or hemodynamic stimuli (Fig. 4-11). The release of vasopressin appears to be mediated by the emetic center (Fig. 4-2), since it occurs when nausea is induced by either vestibular mechanisms[56] or the chemoreceptor trigger zone.[145] Emesis is not necessary for the production of this

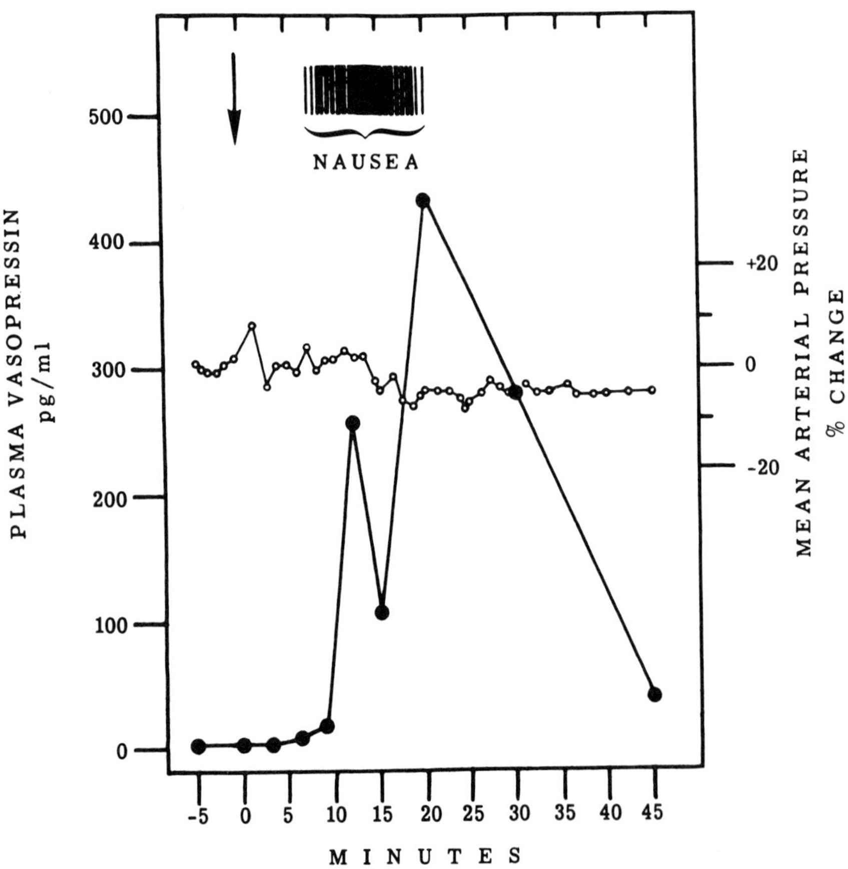

FIGURE 4-11 • The effect of apomorphine on plasma vasopressin (●) and mean arterial pressure (○) in a healthy adult. The recumbent subject was injected subcutaneously with apomorphine, 14 μg/kg at time zero (arrow). The duration and intensity of nausea is represented by vertical, spaced lines. (From Robertson GL: *Rec Prog Hormone Res* 33:333, 1976.)

effect. Stimulation by nausea can be blocked by pretreatment with antiemetics and is attenuated by water loading. The physiological importance of the response remains unknown; however, the circulating levels thus produced are sufficiently high to have peripheral pressor effects (see above). Furthermore, high levels of vasopressin markedly increase gastrointestinal peristalsis, which may contribute in some way to the initiation or recovery from the emetic process. The potent effect of nausea on vasopressin secretion may have clinical implications, since it probably contributes to the free-water retention and hyponatremia observed in clinical disorders associated with prolonged nausea. The emetic reflex can also complicate studies of vasopressin secretion in many animals, since the presence or absence of nausea is difficult to detect except by verbal report. Rats, however, appear to be unique in that they secrete oxytocin but relatively little vasopressin in response to emetic stimuli.[191]

Glucopenia

Insulin-induced hypoglycemia increases plasma vasopressin in both humans[13] and rats.[11] This effect is not due to any other recognized stimulus for vasopressin release and is correlated with the degree of hypoglycemia.[13] Hypoglycemia is much less potent than nausea or hypotension in producing vasopressin secretion (Fig. 4-12), and its effects are totally reversed by water loading.[11] Production of intracellular hypoglycemia by administration of 2-deoxyglucose also increases vasopressin secretion,[12,181] suggesting that it is not hypoglycemia per se that initiates this response but, rather, a deficiency of glucose metabolism in one or more parts of the brain. The physiologic significance of this effect is unknown. Exogenous vasopressin has been shown to increase blood glucose by increasing hepatic glycogenolysis[78] and gluconeogenesis,[203] but its importance as an insulin counterregulatory hormone has not been established.

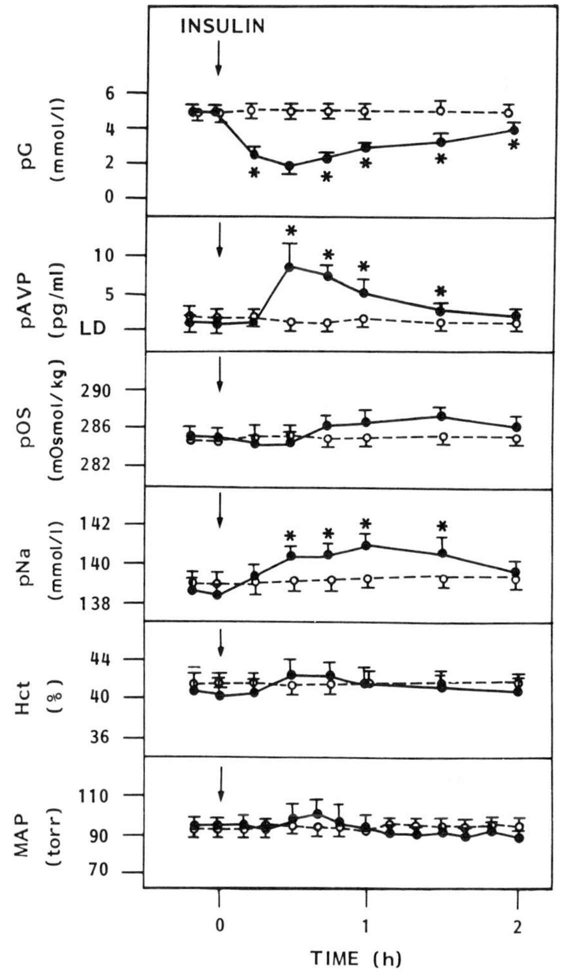

FIGURE 4-12 • Effect of insulin-induced hypoglycemia on plasma vasopressin levels. Shown are plasma glucose (pG), plasma vasopressin (pAVP), plasma osmolality (pOS), plasma sodium (pNA), hematocrit (Hct), and mean arterial pressure (MAP). Results are shown during both insulin (●—●) and sham (○——○) injections. Statistical differences ($p < 0.05$) from baseline are indicated (*). (From Baylis PH et al: *J Clin Endocrin Metals* 53:935 1981.)

Hypoxia

The effect of hypoxia on vasopressin secretion in humans remains to be clearly determined. Studies in anesthetized animals indicate that acute hypoxia without hypobaria produces marked increases in plasma vasopressin that cannot be accounted for by osmotic or hemodynamic stimuli.[6,63] In conscious humans, similar levels of acute normobaric hypoxia produce a rise only occasionally[12] and may in fact produce a fall[35] in plasma vasopressin levels. More detailed studies in humans have shown that the rise in vasopressin occurs only when the hypoxia is accompanied by nausea and/or a fall in blood pressure.[79] Thus, evidence in humans suggests that hypoxia per se is not a stimulus for vasopressin secretion but in some people may trigger release of the hormones secondary to hemodynamic or emetic stimuli.

Nociceptive stimuli

The concept that emotional stress, pain, or other nonspecific noxious stimuli increase secretion of antidiuretic hormone dates to very early studies of osmoregulation.[192] As more has been learned about other stimuli for vasopressin secretion and these factors have been taken into consideration when assessing the effects of stress on antidiuresis, it has become evident that this concept is a misleading oversimplification. Direct measurements of plasma vasopressin in conscious rats have shown that a variety of stresses, such as pain, etherization, centrifugation, and water immersion, fail to increase plasma vasopressin in the absence of hemodynamic stimuli.[93,136] In humans, stimulation of vasopressin secretion by stress is equally uncertain. Although vasopressin levels are reported to be elevated in some stressful states,[43,96] the data provided in these studies are insufficient to exclude effects of hemodynamic or other nonosmotic stimuli. For example, pain or intense emotion[112] can cause vasovagal reactions that, given the stimulatory potency of the associated hypotension and/or nausea, could account for high circulating levels of vasopressin that persist for some time. Therefore, a search for clearly established stimuli for vasopressin secretion must be made before elevations in vasopressin levels can be attributed to "stress" per se.

Vasopressin secretion may also be influenced by oropharyngeal receptors sensitive to the ingestion of fluids.[66,153,160,180,184] However, the inhibitory effect of these receptors appears to be only transient unless the ingestion of fluid results in a prompt reduction in plasma osmolality. Hence, these receptors probably function as an early warning system and not as the primary physiologic determinant of vasopressin secretion.

HORMONES AFFECTING VASOPRESSIN SECRETION

Angiotensin

Among the most intensively studied of the hormonal factors affecting vasopressin secretion is angiotensin. This intense interest stems from the closely related physiologic roles of the two hormones in the regulation of salt and water balance. Bonjour and Malvin showed that relatively small doses of infused renin or angiotensin significantly increased circulating levels of vasopressin in conscious, normally hydrated dogs.[24] This effect of peripherally infused angiotensin has been confirmed by some,[130,188] but not all,[30,34] investigators. The reason for these inconsistencies may be explained by the two opposing effects of circulating angiotensin on vasopressin secretion. Circulating angiotensin is a potent pressor that, like other pressor substances, activates baroreceptors that tend to suppress vasopressin release. Within the central nervous system, however, angiotensin has been shown both by in vivo[94,118] and in vitro[170] methods to stimulate vasopressin secretion. This central nervous system secretory effect of angiotensin seems to be mediated by anterior hypothalamic and circumventricular structures[87] and is dependent on concomitant osmotic stimulation.[164] The role of endogenous angiotensin in normal regulation of vasopressin secretion has not been determined. Pharmacological blockade of angiotensin II does not decrease the vasopressin response to hypovolemic hypotension in rats[209] or to orthostasis in humans.[38] Thus, though exogenous angiotensin has effects on vasopressin secretion, the role, if any, of endogenous angiotensin is dubious.

Norepinephrine

Catecholamines are also known to affect water balance. Some of these effects are mediated by direct renal actions,[75] but there is substantial evidence that alterations in vasopressin secretion may also be responsible. Norepinephrine has both systemic and central nervous system effects on vasopressin secretion. When given intravenously, norepinephrine causes a water diuresis[173] that is dependent on baroreceptor-mediated suppression of vasopressin release.[15] This effect appears to be due to alpha-adrenergic stimulation, since alpha blockers prevent the diuresis.[105] Systemic administration of the beta-adrenergic agonist isoproterenol causes the opposite effect,[16] a baroreceptor-mediated,[17] vasopressin-dependent[16] antidiuresis. Thus, the peripheral effects of adrenergic compounds on vasopressin secretion depend on the net effect on blood pressure as determined by their preferential binding to adrenergic receptor subtypes.

The central nervous system effects of norepinephrine differ from those observed systemically. Central injections of norepinephrine cause release of vasopressin,[55,81,99] which can be blocked by the alpha blocker phentolamine.[81] These results suggest a stimulatory role for alpha-adrenergic neurotransmitters in the regulation of vasopressin secretion. This hypothesis is supported by more rapid metabolism of brain norepinephrine following dehydration[109] and by decreased responsiveness to hemodynamic and osmotic stimulation when central nervous system catecholamines are depleted by treatment with 6-hydroxy-dopamine.[114] However, no effect on the osmotic stimulation of vasopressin is observed when catecholamines are depleted by treatment with α-methyl-paratyrosine.[90] Moreover, in vitro studies suggest that norepinephrine inhibits the release of vasopressin[166] and the firing rate of individual neurons.[9,110,117] These apparently contradictory results could be due to secondary effects of the drugs used in the in vivo studies or to methodologic artifacts associated with the in vitro studies. Thus, the central effects of norepinephrine on vasopressin secretion require additional study.

Dopamine

Neuroanatomical studies have identified dopaminergic neurons that originate in the arcuate and periventricular nuclei and innervate the posterior pituitary.[115] Though less thoroughly studied, this set of neurons shares some functional characteristics of the tuberoinfundibular and nigrostriatal dopamine systems[115] and implicates dopamine in vasopressin regulation. Certain clinical observations also suggest a role for dopamine. Psychosis, which has been considered a disorder of excessive central dopamine activity,[174] is associated with inappropriate increased vasopressin levels.[47,131] Despite these observations, it has not been possible to reach a consensus about the role, if any, of dopamine in vasopressin regulation. Studies addressing the question in humans and animals have concluded that dopamine has a stimulatory effect,[116] an inhibitory effect,[64,124] or no effect[36,95] on vasopressin secretion. Additional studies in humans that take into account the secondary cardiovascular and emetic effects of dopamine agonists and antagonists are needed to assess properly the role of dopamine in human neurohypophyseal regulation.

Opiates

For a number of reasons, there is currently a great deal of interest in the role of opiates in regulation of vasopressin secretion. Studies performed by de Bodo[41] nearly 40 years ago showed that large doses of morphine inhibited water diuresis in dogs by stimulating vasopressin secretion. This observation was confirmed by others[48,67] and served as a basis for the long-held belief that opiates stimulate vasopressin release. Careful review of these studies, however, demonstrates that in many instances the antidiuresis was associated with nausea or hypotension,[84,159] which are well-recognized side effects of morphine-like drugs and may serve as indirect stimuli for vasopressin secretion. At lower doses, morphine was shown in some studies to produce a modest increase in urine flow.[76] Despite these observations, the concept that opiates stimulate vasopressin secretion became well established.

The discovery of endogenous opiate peptides led to a reexamination of this issue in an attempt to define the role of enkephalinergic neurons and receptors in the posterior pituitary.[70,144] Early studies using beta endorphin and leu-enkephalin seemed to support a stimulatory role for opiates.[21,201] Studies that were more carefully controlled for cardiovascular effects, however, showed that opiates inhibit the rise in vasopressin produced by osmotic stimulation.[71,90] Subsequent studies using a number of synthetic peptide analogues demonstrated an inhibitory effect on basal or stimulated vasopressin secretion in humans.[26,72,212] Thus, nearly all recent studies of the effect of exogenous opiates on vasopressin secretion indicate that they are inhibitory when given in subemetic and subhypotensive doses.

The role of endogenous opioids in the regulation of vasopressin has also been investigated using a variety of opioid antagonists. Naloxone, which acts predominantly to block mu receptors, either has no effect or slightly potentiates the plasma vasopressin response to osmotic and/or nonosmotic stimuli in rats,[65,98,141,178] sheep,[182] and dogs.[197] This suggests that endogenous opioids act via mu receptors to restrain vasopressin release. However, diprenorphine, an antagonist that acts more effectively at *kappa* and *delta* as well as mu opioid receptors, selectively inhibits the vasopressin response to hypovolemic stimuli.[141] This inhibition seems to occur at least in part in the lateral parabrachial nucleus, indicating that it contains delta or kappa opioidergic synapses that are somehow involved in the volume control of vasopressin secretion.

Cholinergic agonists

Early studies of the control of vasopressin release strongly implicated cholinergic mechanisms.[128] More detailed studies using various experimental designs have confirmed that vasopressin is stimulated by cholinergic agents.[9,18,46,99,171] It has been difficult to determine the character of the receptor subtype responsible for this effect, but in vitro work[171] suggests that activation of a nicotinic receptor is responsible for the stimulation of vasopressin secretion. Nicotine, which is reported to stimulate vasopressin secretion, may act at least in part via these hypothalamic cholinergic receptors. Some believe that the effects of nicotine are mediated, not by such receptors, but by peripheral[29] or ventral brain stem[20] cholinergic receptors as well as by stimulation of the emetic center.

It is still unclear how these observations are related to the observed effects of nicotine in humans. Previous studies have demonstrated consistent antidiuresis when nicotine is given intravenously, but the doses required for this effect almost always produce nausea or hypotension.[32,105] Cigarette smoking may stimulate vasopressin release in the absence of nausea or vomiting, but there is evidence that this effect is not due to absorbed nicotine.[146] Thus, in the clinical as well as the laboratory setting, the effect of cholinergic agents has not been fully characterized.

Histamine

A number of lines of circumstantial evidence implicate histamine in the regulation of vasopressin secretion. Histamine is present in relatively high concentrations in the posterior pituitary[152] and in hypothalamic nuclei responsible for vasopressin synthesis.[27] Furthermore, there is a close temporal relationship between the increase of hypothalamic histamine concentration[185] and the appearance of vasopressin neurosecretory granules.[165] When applied microelectrophoretically to single neurons within the supraoptic nucleus, histamine produces activation.[73] Intraventricular or systemic administration of histamine produces antidiuresis in a number of species,[14,19,80,186] but interpretation of these results is hampered by its cardiovascular effects. The only evidence for a physiologic link between histamine and vasopressin secretion is the observation that histamine is depleted in the posterior pituitary of Brattleboro rats,[82] but these observations require confirmation.

Other hormones

The effects on vasopressin secretion of at least three other groups of hormones have been studied, but no consensus has been reached regarding their effects. Thyrotropin-releasing hormone (TRH) has been reported to both stimulate[202] and suppress[177] vasopressin release. Further exploration of this effect seems warranted in light of the large amount of TRH in the posterior pituitary.[85,121] Sex steroids may also affect vasopressin levels (see above). Prostaglandins[31,59,60,205] have also been reported to affect vasopressin secretion, but it is difficult to determine if these effects are direct or secondary to hemodynamic changes induced by the compounds.

THIRST

No understanding of normal water balance would be complete without consideration of thirst. It is appropriate to consider this topic in conjunction with that of vasopressin secretion because the regulation of the two systems shares many anatomical and functional features. For the purpose of this discussion, thirst is defined as a conscious desire for water. In humans, the majority of normal water needs are satisfied by anticipatory or habitual drinking. Although the factors that lead to this type of water consumption are not entirely clear, thirst, as we have defined it, appears to contribute relatively little. Thirst in healthy adults is regulated largely, if not exclusively, by plasma tonicity. This control appears to be mediated by a collection of osmosensitive neurons located in the ventromedial and anterior hypothalamus in an area very close, but not identical to,[3,4] that which mediates vasopressin secretion (Fig. 4-13). The close anatomical relationship suggests that these osmoreceptor areas may be simultaneously damaged by the same pathological process. This possibility is realized in the clinical syndrome of adipsic hypernatremia (see Chap. 21), which confirms a similar anatomical relationship between these two centers in humans.[42,139] These patients have lesions in areas of the anterior hypothalamus corresponding to those areas in animals that are known to subserve osmoregulation of vasopressin and thirst. When the dynamics of thirst and vasopressin secretion are examined, osmotic stimulation fails to produce either vasopressin release or thirst. This is not a defect in the neurohypophysis itself, since hemodynamic stimulation of vasopressin secretion is normal. At present, virtually nothing is known about the afferent pathways that innervate other areas of the brain responsible for the recognition of thirst or the acquisition of water.

The functional properties of the osmoreceptors that control thirst are also quite similar to those that control vasopressin secretion. Like the osmoreceptor for vasopressin secretion, the thirst receptor behaves as though it had a threshold or set point. Thirst is absent below this level of osmolality, but as osmolality rises above this level, thirst progressively increases. The thirst and vasopressin osmoregulatory systems differ significantly, however, in that the threshold for the former appears to be substantially higher than that for the latter.[213] Initiation

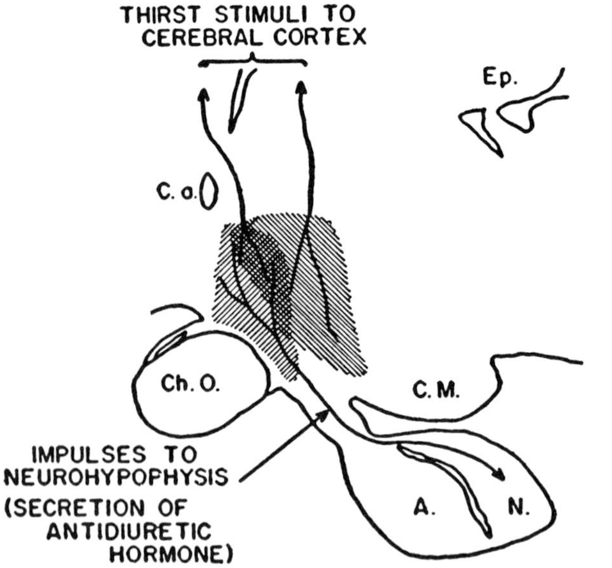

FIGURE 4-13 • Anatomical location of hypothalamic osmoreceptors that regulate thirst (hatched to right) and vasopressin secretion (hatched to left) in the goat. A. = adenohypophysis; C.a. = anterior commisure; C.M. = mamillary body; Ch.O. = optic chiasm; Ep. = epiphysis; N = neurohypophysis. (From Anderson B: *Experentia* 8:156, 1952.)

of vasopressin secretion generally begins when plasma osmolality reaches 280 mosm/kg. Thirst is generally not stimulated until osmolality exceeds 290 mosm/kg. This level of plasma osmolality is very close to that at which plasma vasopressin levels are sufficiently high to produce maximum antidiuresis. Therefore, thirst normally contributes to osmoregulation only when the ability to maximize water conservation is surpassed. This system is ideal, since it permits maximum use of the antidiuretic mechanism before subjecting the individual to the discomfort of thirst.

When the access to water is unrestricted, stimulation of thirst is an extremely effective method for the prevention of hypertonic dehydration. When fully stimulated, thirst-induced drinking can fully replace any water loss. The effectiveness of this mechanism is exemplified by patients with diabetes insipidus, who may excrete up to 20 liters of hypotonic urine daily but do not develop significant hypertonicity if a source of water is available and the thirst mechanism is intact. These simple clinical observations show that the antidiuretic system, by preventing polyuria, lessens the dependence on the thirst mechanism and eliminates the need for constant availability of fresh water. Furthermore, it prevents polyuria but is not essential for maintaining plasma tonicity.

The similarities of the osmoreceptors for thirst and vasopressin secretion extend to the type of plasma solutes to which they are sensitive. As noted previously, hypertonic saline solution and mannitol are quite effective in stimulating vasopressin secretion, while urea and glucose have little effect. The same rank order of potency is observed for thirst. Thus, when the osmotic threshold for thirst is exceeded by the infusion of hypertonic saline solution or mannitol, thirst is almost invariably stimulated, whereas comparable levels of plasma hypertonicity induced with urea or glucose cause little or no stimulation of thirst.[213]

Thirst can also result from nonosmotic stimuli, such as hypovolemia and/or hypotension, which also stimulate vasopressin secretion. This has been recognized clinically in cases of severe hemorrhage or profuse diarrhea, in which blood volume is substantially diminished without changes in osmolality. Experimentally induced sodium depletion in animals accompanied by hypovolemia stimulates thirst despite the presence of hypotonicity.[61] Substantial volume depletion (one-fifth of the total blood volume) must be present before the thirst mechanism is activated in animals.[100,151] In humans, the degree of hypovolemia required has not been precisely determined but appears to be even larger. Hemodynamic stimulation of thirst, like that for vasopressin release, interacts with osmotic stimuli. Thus, hypovolemia appears to lower the osmotic threshold for drinking in dogs[175] and humans.[140] Two systems have been implicated as mediators of hemodynamic stimulation of thirst. The first is the neural baroregulatory system, which consists of left atrial and arterial baroreceptors. All indications are that this system for thirst stimulation is quite similar to that responsible for hemodynamic stimulation of vasopressin secretion.[61] The second is the renin-angiotensin system. Hypovolemia activates this system sufficiently to produce levels of angiotensin II that have been shown by infusion studies to increase water intake in animals.[61,62] In humans, studies suggest that the renin-angiotensin system may contribute to increased water intake in some extreme pathologic states,[61] but its role in producing thirst in less severe pathologic or physiologic states is questionable.

Like vasopressin, thirst also appears to be affected by oropharyngeal receptors.[160,180,184] However, the inhibitory effect of these receptors appears to be only transient unless the ingestion of water is followed promptly by a fall in plasma osmolality. Hence, the oropharyngeal receptors probably function as an early warning system rather than as the primary determinant of thirst.

REFERENCES

1. Acher R, Chauvet J: La structure de la vasopressine de boeuf. *Biochim Biophys Acta* 12:487, 1953.
2. Almli CR, Weiss CS: Drinking behaviors, effects of lateral preoptic and lateral hypothalamic destruction. *Physiol Behav* 13:527, 1974.
3. Anderson B: Polydipsia caused by intrahypothalamic injections of hypertonic NaCl solutions. *Experientia* 8:157, 1952.
4. Anderson B, McCann SM: A further study of polydipsia evoked by hypothalamic stimulation in the goat. *Acta Physiol Scand* 33:333, 1955.
5. Anderson B, McCann SM: The effect of hypothalamic lesions on the water intake of the dog. *Acta Physiol Scand* 35:312, 1965.
6. Anderson RJ et al: Mechanism of effect of hypoxia on renal water excretion. *J Clin Invest* 62:769, 1978.
7. Aycinena P, Robertson GL: Effects of hypercalcemia on secretion of the antidiuretic hormone, arginine vasopressin. *Endocrinology* 112(suppl):142, 1983.
8. Bargmann W, Scharrer E: The site of origin of the hormones of the posterior pituitary. *Am Sci* 38:255, 1951.
9. Barker JL et al: Supraoptic neurosecretory cells: Adrenergic and cholinergic sensitivity. *Science* 171:208, 1971.
10. Baylis PH, Robertson GL: Vasopressin response to 2-deoxy-D-glucose in the rat. *Endrocrinology* 107:1970, 1980.
11. Baylis PH, Robertson GL: Rat vasopressin response to insulin-induced hypoglycemia. *Endocrinology* 107:1975.
12. Baylis PH et al: Effects of acute hypoxaemia on plasma arginine vasopressin in conscious man. *Clin Sci* 53:401, 1977.
13. Baylis PH et al: Arginine vasopressin response to insulin induced hypoglycemia in man. *J Clin Endocrinol Metab* 53:935, 1981.
14. Bennett CT, Pert A: Antidiuresis produced by injections of histamine into the cat supraoptic nucleus. *Brain Res* 78:151, 1974.
15. Berl T et al: Mechanism of suppression of vasopressin during alpha-adrenergic stimulation with norepinephrine. *J Clin Invest* 53:219, 1974.
16. Berl T et al: Effect of alpha- and beta-adrenergic stimulation on renal water excretion in normal subjects and patients with diabetes insipidus. *Kidney Int* 6:247, 1974.
17. Berl T et al: Mechanism of stimulation of vasopressin release during beta-adrenergic stimulation with isoproterenol. *J Clin Invest* 53:857, 1974.
18. Bhargava KP et al: Central cholinergic and adrenergic mechanisms in the release of antidiuretic hormone. *Br J Pharmacol* 44:617, 1972.
19. Bhargava KP et al: Mechanism of histamine induced antidiuretic response. *Br J Pharmacol* 44:617, 1972.
20. Bisset GW et al: Vasopressin release by nicotine: The site of action. *Br J Pharmacol* 54:463, 1975.
21. Bisset GW et al: Release of vasopressin by enkephalin. *Br J Pharmacol* 62:370, 1978.
22. Blass EM: Evidence for basal forebrain thirst osmoreceptors versus rat. *Brain Res* 82:69, 1974.
23. Blass EM, Epstein AN: A lateral preoptic osmosensitive zone for thirst in the rat. *J Comp Physiol Psychol* 76:378, 1971.
24. Bonjour JP, Malvin RL: Stimulation of ADH release by the renin angiotensin system. *Am J Physiol* 218:1555, 1970.
25. Bradbury M: *The Concept of a Blood Brain Barrier*. New York, Wiley, 1979, pp. 84–115.
26. Brownell J et al: Inhibition of vasopressin secretion by a met-enkephalin (FK 33-824) in humans. *Acta Endocrinol* 94:304, 1980.
27. Brownstein MJ et al: Histamine content of hypothalamic nuclei of the rat. *Brain Res* 77:151, 1976.
28. Buggy J, Johnson AK: Preoptic-hypothalamic periventricular lesions: Thirst deficits and hypernatremia. *Am J Physiol* 233:R44, 1977.

29. Cadnapaphornchai P et al: Mechanism of effect of nicotine on renal water excretion. *Am J Physiol* 227:1216, 1974.
30. Cadnapaphornchai P et al: Effect of angiotensin II on renal water excretion. *Am J Physiol* 228:155, 1975.
31. Casals-Stenzel J, Morton JJ: The vasodepressor action of prostacyclin (PGI_2) and its effect on plasma angiotensin II and vasopressin in unanesthetized normotensive and hypertensive rats. *Clin Exp Hypertens* 1:577, 1979.
32. Cates JE, Garrod O: The effect of nicotine on urinary flow in diabetes insipidus. *Clin Sci* 10:145, 1951.
33. Cheesman DW: Structural elucidation of a gonadotrophin inhibiting substance from the bovine pineal gland. *Biochim Biophys Acta* 207:247, 1970.
34. Claybaugh JR et al: The inability of infusions of angiotensin to elevate the plasma vasopressin concentration in the anesthetized dog. *Endocrinology* 90:1647, 1972.
35. Claybaugh JR et al: Response of antidiuretic hormone to acute exposure to mild and severe hypoxia in man. *J Endocrinol* 77:157, 1978.
36. Cohen M et al: In normal young men acute dopaminergic blockade does not impair free water excretion following a standard water load. *Commun Psychopharmacol* 4:323, 1980.
37. Czaczkes JW et al: Physiologic studies of antidiuretic hormone by its direct measurement in human plasma. *J Clin Invest* 43:1625, 1964.
38. Davies R et al: The interrelationship between the release of renin and vasopressin as defined by orthostasis and propranolol. *J Clin Invest* 60:1438, 1977.
39. Davison JM et al: Altered osmotic thresholds for vasopressin secretion and thirst in human pregnancy. *Am J Physiol* 246:F105, 1984.
40. Davison JM et al: Changes in the metabolic clearance of vasopressin and in plasma vasopressinase throughout human pregnancy. *J Clin Invest* 83:1313, 1989.
41. de Bodo RC: The antidiuretic action of morphine and its mechanism. *J Pharmacol Exp Ther* 82:74, 1944.
42. DeRubertis FR et al: Essential hypernatremia. *Arch Intern Med* 134:889, 1974.
43. DeWane GW, Porter JC: An apparent stress-induced release of arginine vasopressin by human neonates. *J Clin Endocrinol Metab* 51:1412, 1980.
44. Dicker SE, Nunn J: Fate and excretion of the pressor activity of vasopressin in rats. *J Physiol* 138:11, 1957.
45. Douglas WW, Poisner AM: Stimulus secretion coupling in a neurosecretory organ: The role of calcium in the release of vasopressin from the neurohypophysis. *J Physiol* 172:1, 1964.
46. Dreiffus JJ, Kelly JS: Excitation of identified supraoptic neurons by the iontophoretic application of acetylcholine. *J Physiol* 212:170P, 1970.
47. Dubovski SL et al: Syndrome of inappropriate secretion of antidiuretic hormone with exacerbated psychosis. *Clin Intern Med* 79:551, 1973.
48. Duke HN et al: The antidiuretic action of morphine: Its site and mode of action in the hypothalamus of the dog. *J Exp Physiol* 36:149, 1951.
49. Dunn FL et al: The role of blood osmolality and volume in regulating vasopressin secretion in the rat. *J Clin Invest* 52:3212, 1973.
50. Durr JA et al: Osmoregulation during pregnancy in the rat: Evidence for resetting of the threshold for vasopressin secretion during gestation. *J Clin Invest* 68:337, 1981.
51. DuVigneaud V et al: The sequence of amino acids in oxytocin with a proposal for the structure of oxytocin. *J Biol Chem* 205:949, 1953.
52. DuVigneaud V et al: Enzymatic cleavage of glycinamide from vasopressin and a proposed structure for this pressor-antidiuretic hormone of the posterior pituitary. *J Am Chem Soc* 75:4880, 1953.
53. DuVigneaud V et al: The synthesis of oxytocin. *J Am Chem* 76:3115, 1954.
54. DuVigneaud V et al: Synthesis of the pressor-antidiuretic hormone, arginine vasopressin. *J Am Chem Soc* 80:3355, 1958.
55. Dyball RE: The effects of drugs on the release of vasopressin. *Br J Pharmacol* 33:329, 1968.
56. Eversmann T et al: Increased secretion of growth hormone, prolactin, antidiuretic hormone and cortisol induced by the stress of motion sickness. *Aviat Space Environ Med* 49:53, 1978.
57. Fabian M et al: The clearance and antidiuretic potency of neurohypophysial hormones in man, and their plasma binding and stability. *J Physiol* 204:653, 1969.
58. Fernstrom JD et al: Radioimmunologic detection and measurement of nonapeptides in the pineal gland. *Endocrinology* 106:243, 1980.
59. Feuerstein G et al: Mechanisms involved in central cardiovascular effects of prostaglandin $F_{2\alpha}$. *Am J Physiol* 242:R545, 1982.
60. Feuerstein G et al: Alteration of cardiovascular neurogenic and humoral responses to acute hypovolemic hypotension by administered prostacyclin. *J Cardiovasc Pharmacol* 4:246, 1982.
61. Fitzsimons JT: The physiology of thirst and sodium appetite. *Monogr Physiol Soc* 35, 1979.
62. Fitzsimons JT, Moore-Gillon MJ: Drinking and antidiuresis in response to reductions in venous return in the dog: Neural and endocrine mechanisms. *J Physiol* 308:403, 1980.
63. Forsling ML, Rees M: Effects of hypoxia and hypercapnia on plasma vasopressin concentration. *J Endocrinol* 67:62P, 1972.
64. Forsling ML, Lightman SL: Effect of L-dopa on vasopressin secretion in man. *J Physiol* 292:64P, 1979.
65. Forsling ML et al: A comparison of the vasopressin response of rats to intraperitoneal and intravenous administration of hypertonic saline, and the effect of opioid and aminergic antagonists. *J Endocrinol* 116:217, 1988.
66. Geelen G et al: Inhibition of plasma vasopressin after drinking in dehydrated humans. *Am J Physiol* 247:R968, 1984.
67. Giarman NJ et al: Studies on the antidiuretic action of morphine. *Science* 117:225, 1953.
68. Ginsberg M, Heller H: The clearance of injected vasopressin from the circulation and its fate in the body. *J Endocrinol* 9:283, 1953.
69. Goetz KL et al: Effect of moderate hemorrhage in humans on plasma AVP and renin. *Proc Soc Exp Biol Med* 145:277, 1974.
70. Goldstein A: Opiate peptides (endorphins) in pituitary and brain. *Science* 193:1081, 1976.
71. Greidanus TB et al: Effects of morphine and beta-en-

dorphin on basal and elevated plasma levels of MSH and vasopressin. *Life Sci* 24:579, 1979.
72. Grossman A et al: Inhibition of vasopressin release in man by an opiate peptide. *Lancet* 21108, 1980.
73. Haas HL et al: Histamine: action on supraoptic and other hypothalamic neurones of the cat. *Brain Res* 88:166, 1975.
74. Hammer M et al: Relationship between plasma osmolality and plasma vasopressin in human subjects. *Am J Physiol* 238:E313, 1979.
75. Handler JS et al: Effect of adrenergic agents on toad bladder response to ADH, 3′, 5′-AMP, and theophylline. *Am J Physiol* 215:1024, 1968.
76. Handley CA, Keller AD: Changes in renal function produced by morphine in normal dogs and dogs with diabetes insipidus. *J Pharmacol Exp Ther* 99:33, 1950.
77. Helderman JH et al: The response of arginine vasopressin to intravenous ethanol and hypertonic saline in man: The impact of aging. *J Gerontol* 33:39, 1978.
78. Hems DA et al: Metabolic activities of vasopressin, glucagon and adrenaline in the intact rat. *Biochim Biophys Acta* 411:155, 1975.
79. Heyes MP et al: Acute effects of hypoxia on renal and endocrine function in normal man. *Am J Physiol* 243:R265, 1982.
80. Hisada S et al: Antidiuresis of centrally administered amines and peptides and release of antidiuretic hormone from isolated rat neurohypophysis. *Jpn J Pharmacol* 27:153, 1977.
81. Hoffman WE: Central cardiovascular and antidiuretic action of adrenergic drugs. *Neuropharmacology* 18:7, 1979.
82. Holcomb HH et al: Histamine levels are selectively decreased in the posterior pituitary lobe of Brattleboro rats lacking vasopressin. *Soc Neurosci Abstr* 8:55, 1982.
83. Hytten FE: Physiological changes in early pregnancy. *Br J Obstet Gynaecol* 75:1193, 1968.
84. Inturrisi CE, Fujimoto JM: Studies on the antidiuretic action of morphine in the rat. *Eur J Pharmacol* 2:301, 1968.
85. Jackson IMD, Reichlin S: Thyrotropin-releasing hormone (TRH): Distribution in hypothalamic and extrahypothalamic brain tissues of mammalian and submammalian chordates. *Endocrinology* 95:854, 1974.
86. Jewell PA, Verney EB: An experimental attempt to determine the site of neurohypophyseal osmoreceptors in the dog. *Philos Trans R Soc London* 240:197, 1957.
87. Johnson AK et al: Attenuated pressor responses to intracranially injected stimuli and altered antidiuretic activity following preoptic-hypothalamic periventricular ablation. *Brain Res* 157:161, 1978.
88. Johnson JA et al: Effects of separate and concurrent osmotic and volume stimuli on plasma ADH in sheep. *Am J Physiol* 218:1273, 1970.
89. Kamoi K et al: Opiates elevate the osmotic threshold for vasopressin release in rats. *Clin Res* 27:254A, 1979.
90. Kamoi K et al: Depletion of hypothalamic norepinephrine does not alter the osmoregulation of vasopressin in rats. *Endocrinology* 114:2123, 1984.
91. Kannan H, Yagi R: Supraoptic neurosecretory neurons: Evidence for the existence of converging inputs both from carotid baroreceptors and osmoreceptors. *Brain Res* 145:385, 1978.
92. Karcsu S et al: Morphological evidence of the involvement of calcium in neurohypophyseal hormone release. *Brain Res* 238:278, 1982.
93. Keil LC, Severs WB: Reduction in plasma vasopressin levels of dehydrated rat following acute stress. *Endocrinology* 100:30, 1977.
94. Keil LC et al: Release of vasopressin by angiotensin II. *Endocrinology* 96:1063, 1975.
95. Kendler KS et al: Lack of arginine vasopressin response to central dopamine blockade in normal adults. *J Clin Endocrinol Metab* 47:204, 1978.
96. Kendler KS et al: The effect of pain on plasma arginine vasopressin concentrations in man. *Clin Endocrinol* 8:80, 1978.
97. Kirchheim HR: Systemic arterial baroreceptor reflexes. *Physiol Rev* 56:100, 1976.
98. Knepel W et al: Vasopressin and β-endorphin release after osmotic and non-osmotic stimuli: Effect of naloxone and dexamethasone. *Eur J Pharmacol* 77:299, 1982.
99. Kuhn ER: Cholinergic and adrenergic release mechanism for vasopressin in the male rat: A study with injections of neurotransmitters and blocking agents into the third ventricle. *Neuroendocrinology* 16:255, 1974.
100. Larsson B et al: Vasopressin release induced by hemorrhage in the goat. *Acta Physiol Scand* 104:309, 1978.
101. Lauson HD: Metabolism of neurohypophyseal hormones, in Greep RO, Astwood EB (eds): *Handbook of Physiology*, Section 7: Endocrinology. Washington, DC, American Physiological Society, 1974, vol 4, part I, p 287.
102. Legros JJ et al: Interactions entre un derive progestalif et l'ethinyl oestradiol sur l'elimination urinaire de neurophysine, d'ocytocine et de vasopressine immunoreactives et sur le taux de neurophysine serique I et II chez l'homme normal. *C R Soc Biol* 167:1668, 1973.
103. Legros JJ et al: Immunoreactive neurophysins and vasotocin in human foetal pineal glands. *J Endocrinol* 69:289, 1976.
104. Lewis AAG, Chalmers TM: A nicotine test for the investigation of diabetes insipidus. *Clin Sci* 10:137, 1951.
105. Lieberman B et al: Effect of adrenergic blocking agents on the vasopressin inhibiting action of norepinephrine. *Proc Soc Exp Biol Med* 133:131, 1970.
106. Livermore AH, DuVigneaud V: Preparation of high potency oxytocic material by the use of countercurrent distribution. *J Biol Chem* 180:365, 1949.
107. Luerssen TG, Robertson GL: Cerebrospinal fluid vasopressin and vasotocin in health and disease, in Wood JH (ed): *Neurobiology of Cerebrospinal fluid.* New York, Plenum, 1980, vol 1, p 613.
108. Luttinger D, Seiden LS: Increased hypothalamic norepinephrine metabolism after water deprivation in the rat. *Brain Res* 208:147, 1981.
109. Malayan S et al: Effects of increases in plasma vasopressin concentration on plasma renin activity, blood pressure, heart rate and plasma corticosteroid concentration in conscious dogs. *Endocrinology* 107:1899, 1980.
110. Marks BH et al: A new technique for studying neuroendocrine systems, in Zimmerman E, George R (eds): *Narcotics and the Hypothalamus.* New York, Raven Press, 1974, p. 95.
111. Mason WT: Supraoptic neurones of rat hypothalamus are osmosensitive. *Nature* 287:154, 1980.

112. McKinley MJ et al: Sensors for antidiuresis and thirst osmoreceptors or CSF sodium detectors? *Brain Res* 141:89, 1978.
113. Milen SM et al: Biological and chromatographic characterization of a polypeptide with pressor and oxytocic activities isolated from bovine pineal gland. *Endocrinology* 72:563, 1963.
114. Miller TR et al: Effect of central catecholamine depletion on the osmotic and nonosmotic stimulation of vasopressin (antidiuretic hormone) in the rat. *J Clin Invest* 64:1599, 1979.
115. Moore KE, Demarest KT: Tuberoinfundicular and tuberohypophyseal dopaminergic neurons, in Ganong WF, Martini L: *Frontiers in Neuroendocrinology*. New York, Raven Press, 1982, vol 7, p 161.
116. Moos R, Richard P: Excitatory effect of dopamine on oxytocin and vasopressin reflex releases in the rat. *Brain Res* 241:249, 1982.
117. Moss RL et al: Responses of antidromically identified supraoptic and paraventricular units to acetycholine, noradrenaline and glutamate applied iontophoretically. *Brain Res* 35573, 1971.
118. Mouw D et al: Central action of angiotensin in stimulating ADH release. *Am J Physiol* 220:239, 1971.
119. Nagasawa J et al: Ultrastructural evidence of secretion by exocytosis and of "synaptic vesicle" formation in posterior pituitary gland. *Nature* 227:407, 1970.
120. Negro-Vilar A et al: Failure to detect radioimmunossayable arginine vasotocin in mammalian pineals. *Brain Res Bull* 4:789, 1979.
121. Oliver C et al: Distribution and concentration of TRH in the rat brain. *Endocrinology* 95:540, 1974.
122. Oliver G, Shafer EA: On the physiological action of extracts of pituitary body. *J Physiol* 18:227, 1895.
123. Olsson K: Further evidence for the importance of CSF Na^+ concentration in central control of fluid balance. *Acta Physiol Scand* 88:183, 1973.
124. Passo SS et al: A functional analysis of dopaminergic innervation of the neurohypophysis. *Am J Physiol* 241:186, 1981.
125. Pavel S et al: Vasotocin content in the pineal gland of foetal, newborn and adult male rats. *J Endocrinol* 66:283, 1975.
126. Peck JW, Blass EM: Localization of thirst and antidiuretic osmoreceptors by intracranial injections in rats. *Am J Physiol* 228:1501, 1975.
127. Peck JW, Novin D: Evidence that osmoreceptors mediating drinking in rabbits are in the lateral preoptic area. *J Comp Physiol Psychol* 74:134, 1971.
128. Pickford M: The action of acetycholine in the supraoptic nucleus of the chloralosed dog. *J Physiol* 106:264, 1947.
129. Popenoe EA et al: Partial purification and amino acid content of vasopressin from hog posterior pituitary glands. *J Am Chem Soc* 74:3713, 1952.
130. Ramsay DJ et al: Angiotensin II infusion increases vasopressin, ACTH and 11-hydroxycorticosteroid secretion. *Am J Physiol* 234:R66, 1978.
131. Raskin MA et al: Acute psychoses, increased water ingestion and inappropriate antidiuretic hormone secretion. *Am J Psychiatry* 132:907, 1975.
132. Riddell DC et al: Chromosomal assignment of human sequences encoding arginine vasopressin-neurophysin II and growth hormone releasing factor. *Som Cell Mol Genet* 11:189, 1985.
133. Robertson GL: The regulation of vasopressin function in health and disease. *Recent Prog Horm Res* 33:333, 1976.
134. Robertson GL: The role of osmotic and hemodynamic variables in regulation vasopressin, in James VHT (ed): *Proceedings of the Fifth International Congress of Endocrinology, Hamburg, July 1976*, Excerpta Medica Congress Series no. 402. Amsterdam, Excerpta Medica, 1977, p 126.
135. Robertson GL: The physiopathology of ADH secretion, in Tolis G et al (eds): *Clinical Neuroendocrinology: A Pathophysiological Approach*. New York: Raven, 1979, p 247.
136. Robertson GL, Athar S: The interaction of blood osmolality and blood volume in regulating plasma vasopressin in man. *J Clin Endocrinol Metab* 42:613, 1976.
137. Robertson GL et al: Development and clinical application of a new method for the radioimmunoassay of arginine vasopressin in human plasma. *J Clin Invest* 52:2340, 1973.
138. Robertson GL et al: The osmoregulation of vasopressin. *Kidney Int* 10:25, 1976.
139. Robertson GL et al: Osmotic control of vasopressin function, in Andreoli TE et al (eds): *Disturbances in Body Fluid Osmolality*. Bethesda, American Physiological Society, 1977, p 125.
140. Robertson GL et al: Neurogenic disorders of osmoregulation. *Am J Med* 72:339, 1982.
141. Robertson GL et al: Diprenorphrine inhibits selectively the vasopressin response to hypovolemic stimuli. *Trans Assoc Am Physicians* 98:322, 1985.
142. Robinson AG: Isolation, assay and secretion of individual human neurophysins. *J Clin Invest* 55:360, 1975.
143. Rodbard D, Munson PJ: Editorial comment. *Am J Physiol* 234:E340, 1978.
144. Rossier J et al: Hypothalamic enkephalin neurones may regulate the neurohypophysis. *Nature* 277:653, 1979.
145. Rowe JW et al: Influence of the emetic reflex on vasopressin release in man. *Kidney Int* 16:729, 1979.
146. Rowe JW et al: Evidence in man that cigarette smoking induces vasopressin release via an airway-specific mechanism. *J Clin Endocrinol Metab* 51:170, 1980.
147. Rowe JW et al: Age-related failure of volume-pressure-mediated vasopressin release. *J Clin Endocrinol Metab* 54:661, 1982.
148. Rundgren M, Fyhrquist F: A study of permanent adipsia induced by medial forebrain lesions. *Acta Physiol Scand* 103:463, 1978.
149. Russell JT et al: Biosynthesis of vasopressin, oxytocin and neurophysins: isolation and characterization of two common precursors (propressophysin and prooxyphysin). *Endocrinology* 107:1880, 1980.
150. Russell JT et al: Time course of appearance and release of (35S) cysteine labeled neurophysins and peptides in the neurohypophysis. *Brain Res* 205:299, 1981.
151. Russell PJD et al: Graded levels of hemorrhage, thirst and angiotensin II in rat. *Physiol Behav* 15:117, 1975.
152. Saavedra JM et al: Distribution of biogenic amines and related enzymes in the rat pituitary gland. *J Neurochem* 25:257, 1975.

153. Salata RA et al: Cold water stimulation of oropharyngeal receptors in man inhibits release of vasopressin. *J Clin Endocrinol Metab* 65:561, 1987.
154. Sausville E et al: The human vasopressin gene is linked to the oxytocin gene and is selectively expressed in a cultured lung cancer cell line. *J Biol Chem* 260:10236, 1985.
155. Sawchenko PE, Swanson LW: Central noradrenergic pathways for the integration of hypothalamic neuroendocrine and autonomic responses. *Science* 214:685, 1981.
156. Sawyer WH: Evolution of antidiuretic hormones and their functions. *Am J Med* 42:678, 1967.
157. Sawyer WH: Evolution of neurohypophyseal hormones and their receptors. *Fed Proc* 36:1842, 1977.
158. Schmale H et al: Vasopressin biosynthesis: From gene to peptide hormone. *Kidney Int* 32(suppl 21):S8, 1987.
159. Schneiden H, Blackmore EK: The effect of nalorphine on the antidiuretic action of morphine in rats and man. *Br J Pharmacol* 10:45, 1955.
160. Seckl JR et al: Oral hypertonic saline causes transient fall of vasopressin in humans. *Am J Physiol* 251:R214, 1986.
161. Segar WE, Moore WW: The regulation of antidiuretic hormone release in man: 1. The effects of change in position and ambient temperature on blood ADH levels. *J Clin Invest* 47:2143, 1968.
162. Shafer EA: Cronian lecture: Functions of the pituitary body. *Proc R Soc London* 81:442, 1909.
163. Share L: Extracellular fluid volume and vasopressin secretion, in Ganong WF, Martini L. (eds): *Frontiers in Neuroendocrinology*. New York, Oxford University Press, 1969, p. 183.
164. Shimizu R et al: Potentiation by angiotensin II of the vasopressin response to increasing plasma osmolality. *Endocrinology* 93:42, 1973.
165. Silverman AJ: The hypothalamic magnocellular neurosecretory system of the guinea pig: 2. Immunohistochemical localization of neurophysin and vasopressin in the fetus. *Am J Anat* 144:445, 1975.
166. Skowsky R et al: Effect of norepinephrine and isoproterenol on arginine vasopressin secretion from perfused rat pituitary glands, in *Program of the 57th Annual Meeting of the Endocrine Society*, 1975, p 186.
167. Skowsky WR, Fisher DA: Fetal nemohypophyseal arginine vasopressin and arginine vasotocin in man and sheep. *Pediatr Res* 11:627, 1977.
168. Skowsky WR et al: Effects of sex steroid hormones on arginine vasopressin in intact and castrated male and female rats. *Endocrinology* 104:105, 1979.
169. Sladek CD, Knigge KM: Osmotic control of vasopressin release by rat hypothalamoneurohypophyseal explants in organ culture. *Endocrinology* 101:1834, 1977.
170. Sladek CD, Joynt RJ: Angiotensin stimulation of vasopressin release from the rat hypothalamoneurohypophyseal system in organ culture. *Endocrinology* 104:148, 1979.
171. Sladek CD, Joynt RJ: Characterization of cholinergic control of vasopressin release by the organ-cultured rat hypothalamo-neurohypophyseal system. *Endocrinology* 104:659, 1979.
172. Sladek CD et al: Vasopressin and renin response to dehydration in aged rats. *Neurobiol Aging* 2:293, 1981.
173. Smythe CM et al: The effect of epinephrine (USP), 1-epinephrine and 1-norepinephrine on glomerular filtration rate, renal plasma flow and urinary excretion of sodium, potassium and water in normal man. *J Clin Invest* 31:400, 1952.
174. Snyder SH et al: Drugs, neurotransmitters and schizophrenia. *Science* 184:1243, 1974.
175. Sobocinska J: Effects of cervical vagosympathectomy on osmotic reactivity of the thirst mechanism in dogs. *Bull Acad Pol Sci* 17:265, 1969.
176. Sofroniew MV, Weindl A: Projections from the parvocellular vasopressin and neurophysin containing neurons of the suprachiasmatic nucleus. *Am J Anat* 153:391, 1978.
177. Sowers JR et al: Effect of TRH on serum arginine vasopressin in euthyroid and hypothyroid subjects. *Horm Res* 7:232, 1976.
178. Summy-Long JY et al: Naloxone effects on plasma vasopressin and oxytocin concentrations elevated by histamine, nicotine, isoproterenol and an acute increase in [NaCl] in cerebrospinal fluid. *Neuroendocrinology* 44:157, 1986.
179. Swaab DF et al: Arginine vasotocin in the foetal rat pituitary gland. *J Endocrinol* 72:4P, 1977.
180. Thompson CJ et al: Acute suppression of plasma vasopressin and thirst after drinking in hypernatremic humans. *Am J Physiol* 252:R1138, 1987.
181. Thompson DA et al: Increased thirst and plasma arginine vasopressin levels during 2-deoxy-D-glucose induced glucoprivation in humans. *J Clin Invest* 67:1083, 1981.
182. Thornton SN, Parrott RF: Naloxone affects the release of cortisol, but not of vasopressin or oxytocin, in dehydrated sheep. *Acta Endocrinologica (Copenhagen)* 120:50, 1989.
183. Thrasher TM et al: Thirst and vasopressin release in the dog: An osmoreceptor or sodium receptor mechanism. *Am J Physiol* 238:R333, 1980.
184. Thrasher TN et al: Satiety and inhibition of vasopressin secretion after drinking in dehydrated dogs. *Am J Physiol* 240:E394, 1981.
185. Tuomisto L: Ontogenesis and regional distribution of histamine and histamine-*N*-methyl transferase in the guinea pig brain. *J Neurochem* 28:271, 1977.
186. Tuomisto L, Eriksson L: Central antidiuretic effect of histamine in the unanesthetized goat: Effects of H_1 and H_2 antagonists. *J Pharmacol* 5(suppl 2):101, 1974.
187. Turner RA et al: The purification and the amino acid content of vasopressin in preparations. *J Biol Chem* 191:21, 1951.
188. Uhlich EP et al: Angiotensin stimulated AVP-release in humans. *Klin Wochenschr* 53:177, 1975.
189. Van Dyke HB et al: The isolation of a protein from the pars neuralis of the ox pituitary with oxytocic, pressor and diuresis inhibiting activities. *J Pharmacol* 74:177, 1975.
190. Van Germert M et al: Polyuria and impaired ADH release following medial preoptic lesioning in the rat. *Am J Physiol* 228:1293, 1974.
191. Verbalis JG et al: Oxytocin and vasopressin secretion in response to stimuli producing learned taste aversions in rats. *Behavioral Neurosci* 100:466, 1986.
192. Verney EB: The antidiuretic hormone and the factors which determine its release. *Proc R Soc London* 135:25, 1947.

193. Vizsolyi E et al: Neurohypophyseal hormones in fetal life and pregnancy: 2. Chromatographic studies in the sheep. *Gen Comp Endocrinol* 29:41, 1976.
194. Vokes TP et al: Osmoregulation of thirst and vasopressin during normal menstrual cycle. *Am J Physiol* 23:R641, 1988.
195. Vokes TP et al: Effect of insulin on osmoregulation of vasopressin. *Am J Physiol* 252:E538, 1987.
196. Walter R, Simmons WH: Metabolism of neurohypophyseal hormones: Considerations from a molecular viewpoint, in Moss A, Shares L (eds): *Neurohypophysis*, 1977, p 167.
197. Wade CE: Pituitary and adrenal hormone responses to naloxone in euhydrated and dehydrated dogs. *Am J Physiol* 249:E634, 1985.
198. Walter R et al: Chemistry and structure activity relations of the antidiuretic hormones. *Am J Med* 42:653, 1967.
199. Weissler AM, Warren JV: Vasodepressor syncope. *Am Heart J* 57:786, 1959.
200. Weitzman RE, Fisher DA: Log linear relationship between plasma arginine vasopressin and plasma osmolality. *Am J Physiol* 233:E37, 1977.
201. Weitzman RE et al: B endorphin stimulates secretion of arginine vasopressin in vivo. *Endocrinology* 101:1643, 1977.
202. Weitzman RE et al: Thyrotropin-releasing hormone stimulates release of arginine vasopressin and oxytocin in vivo. *Endocrinology* 104:904, 1979.
203. Whilton PA et al: Stimulation by vasopressin, angiotensin and oxytocin of gluconeogenesis in hepatocyte suspensions. *Biochem J* 176:893, 1978.
204. Yamamoto M et al: Vasopressin release during ventriculocisternal perfusion with prostaglandin E_2 in the dog. *J Endocrinol* 71:325, 1976.
205. Zerbe RL et al: Plasma vasopressin in uncontrolled diabetes mellitus. *Diabetes* 28:503, 1979.
206. Zerbe RL et al: Vasopressin function in the syndrome of inappropriate antidiuresis. *Annu Rev Med* 31:315, 1980.
207. Zerbe RL, Robertson GL: A comparison of plasma vasopressin measurements with a standard indirect test in the differential diagnosis of polyuria. *N Engl M Med* 305:1539, 1981.
208. Zerbe RL, Robertson GL: Arginine vasotocin: Identification and biological actions in mammals, in Fatherby K, Pal SB (eds): *Hormones in Normal and Abnormal Human Tissues*. New York, Walter de Gruyten, vol 2, 1981, p 165.
209. Zerbe RL et al: Effect of captopril on cardiovascular, sympathetic and vasopressin responses to hemorrhage. *Eur J Pharmacol* 72:391, 1981.
210. Zerbe RL et al: Cardiovascular, sympathetic and renin-angiotensin system responses to hemorrhage in vasopressin deficient rats. *Endocrinology* 111:608, 1982.
211. Zerbe RL et al: Vasopressin: An essential pressor factor for blood pressure recovery following hemorrhage. *Peptides* 3:509, 1982.
212. Zerbe RL et al: A new met-enkephalin analogue suppresses plasma vasopressin in man. *Peptides* 3:199, 1982.
213. Zerbe RL, Robertson GL: Osmoregulation of thirst and vasopressin secretion in man: The effect of various solutes. *Am J Physiol* 244:E607, 1983.
214. Zerbe RL et al: The reproducibility and heritability of individual differences in osmoregulatory function in normal human subjects. *J Lab Clin Med* 117:51, 1991.
215. Zimmerman EA: The organization of oxytocin and vasopressin pathways, in Martin JB et al (eds): *Neurosecretion and Brain Peptides*. New York, Raven Press, 1981, p 63.
216. Zuidema GD et al: Osmotic regulation of body fluids. *Am J Physiol* 187:85, 1956.

CHAPTER • 5

The physiology of the renal concentrating and diluting mechanisms

Isaac Teitelbaum • Charles R. Kleeman • Tomas Berl

In all vertebrates and invertebrates there exists an organ for the regulated excretion of water and solutes. This organ is designed to protect the body fluids from life-threatening deviations in volume, osmolality, and hydrogen ion and electrolyte concentrations. In terms of anatomy and function, the mammalian kidney is the most sophisticated and highly differentiated of these regulatory organs. However, only mammals (and to a limited extent birds) among the vertebrates possess the unique ability to excrete a urine hypertonic to plasma and thus to conserve water when the available supply is limited. Smith[211] suggested that the ability to concentrate urine may have played an important role in our ultimate domination of the dinosaur and other reptiles at the end of the Mesozoic era. In Chap. 4, there is an in-depth discussion of the regulation of total body water, with emphasis on mechanisms controlling water intake, and the release and metabolism of antidiuretic hormone (ADH). This chapter is devoted to the renal regulation of water excretion. It discusses the various hormonal and nonhormonal forces that influence renal concentration and dilution. A brief introduction to the comparative physiology of water excretion in invertebrates and lower vertebrates precedes that discussion.

COMPARATIVE PHYSIOLOGY OF WATER EXCRETION

Insects inhabit the same terrestrial and aquatic environment as do vertebrates, and they therefore face the same wide range of osmoregulatory problems. Despite their smaller size and hence larger ratios of body surface area to volume, they are capable of maintaining the osmotic pressure of their body fluids within relatively narrow limits in the face of extreme fluctuations in extrarenal conditions. For example, blood-feeding species, such as the mosquito, may consume a meal that is 2 to 12 times their unfed body weight and will excrete 50 percent of the ingested fluid during a diuresis lasting 0.5 to 5 h. Even a continuous feeder such as the locust consumes its own body weight in succulent foliage every day and excretes all or almost all the ingested water.

The ability to excrete these massive volumes of fluid appears to be related to the formation and secretion of a diuretic hormone after feeding, which acts on the ultimate excretory tubular segment of these insects, the rectum. These diuretic hormones appear to come from neurosecretory cells located in the brain. It is of interest that externally applied cyclic adenosine monophosphate (cAMP) mimics the action of the insects' diuretic hormones and that diuretic hormone stimulation causes a transient increase in tissue levels of cAMP. The insect diuretic hormone has been partially purified and categorized in several insects. It has been suggested that the hormones are peptides; in fact, Phillips[175] refers to studies indicating that insect diuretic hormones may be immunologically indistinguishable from vertebrate vasopressin (radioimmunoassay), but their comparative biological activities suggest that the two molecules are not identical. The insect hormones modulate the osmotic permeability of the rectal wall, and diuretic hormone and ADH may thereby determine the volume[175] and osmotic concentration of the rectal absorbate and final urine.

Freshwater fish are always exposed to the danger of overhydration as water moves from the animals' external environment to their interior along osmotic gradients. The primary function of their kidney is to excrete water while retaining most of the filtered solute. Glomerular filtration rates (GFR) in these freshwater fish are high, about 4 ml/kg per hour. More than half, and sometimes as much as 95 percent, of the filtered water is excreted as a copious dilute urine with very low osmolality. This implies that a low permeability to water must prevail in a large part of the ultimate segments of the renal tubule. Marine teleosts, on the other hand, are exposed to salt loading, water loss to the surrounding environment, and dehydration. They drink salt water to compensate for the osmotic water loss, absorb both water and minerals through the gut, and subsequently extrude excess sodium chloride and divalent ions through the gills and the kidneys. Filtration function is not as important as in freshwater fish, and various degrees of glomerular degeneration occur, including the extreme form of the aglomerular kidney. GFR and renal blood flow are much lower than those in freshwater teleosts. Marine teleosts usually lack a distal nephron in the mammalian sense.[167]

GFR in the freshwater teleost,[1] such as the freshwater eel, is highly variable. It appears that the number of functioning glomeruli changes under various conditions, so-called *glomerular intermittency*. Urine flow and GFR are related in linear fashion; fractional water reabsorption remains constant as both GFR and urine flow show wide variation with relatively stable urinary electrolyte concentration. Several hormones (AVT, isotocin, and prolactin) are known to alter GFR in freshwater teleosts. Hypophysectomy decreases GFR and/or urine flow, as does removal of the interrenal or adrenal cortical cells. Treatment with adrenocortical hormones restores them. The naturally occurring neurohypophyseal hormone in teleosts is *arginine vasotocin* (AVT); injection of vasopressor doses of AVT in freshwater teleosts causes glomerular diuresis primarily due to increased renal perfusion pressure. A most interesting example of salt water to fresh water adaptation is seen in the common eel (*Anguilla*). The adult female breeds in the sea. The offspring return to fresh water, where they stay until maturity, and then return to the sea to spawn. In both the sea and fresh water, this eel maintains an extracellular osmolality of about 325 to 370. Adaptive changes in the gills and kidneys allow the eel to stabilize the osmolality of body fluids when moving from the sea to fresh water. The gills excrete or retain salt. The kidneys increase urine volume about fivefold when moving from the salinity of the sea to the freshwater environment.[6a,96a] Masashi and Nishimuri[167] have studied the properties of water and ion transport in isolated perfused distal tubules from freshwater rainbow trout. They have demonstrated low water permeability similar to that reported in the mammalian thick ascending limb. The addition of arginine vasopressin to the bathing solution causes no increase in water permeability. Thus, the distal tubule is indeed nearly water-impermeable, and most likely whole distal nephrons act as the diluting segment. In freshwater teleosts, GFR is the major determinant of urine flow. AVT alters GFR through its influence on systemic and renal blood pressures and flows. In marine teleosts, GFR and urine flow are considerably lower than in freshwater teleosts.

Amphibians in fresh water must be able to produce a large volume of dilute urine in order to conserve electrolytes and eliminate excess water. On land, they must produce a small volume of more concentrated urine in order to conserve water. Therefore, the amphibians must have efficient diuretic and antidiuretic mechanisms to maintain water balance in these two environments. Amphibians are the first surviving vertebrates to venture from water to land during evolution. Their renal functions reflect, therefore, some of the evolutionary changes that occurred during the transition to this habitat. It is clear that in amphibians AVT, and of course vasopressin in much larger doses, is antidiuretic. Thus, the same molecule increases urine volume in some vertebrates while producing opposite effects in others. AVT is predominantly diuretic, but in amphibians, reptiles, and birds it is antidiuretic. The antidiuretic action is an adaptation to conserve water in the terrestrial environment. AVT first appeared as a vascular hormone with little or no direct renal action. In freshwater fish, urine volume is usually directly related to GFR, and tubular free-water reabsorption does not appear to be physiologically controlled. In these species, AVT is mainly a vasoconstrictor hormone with receptors located in the peripheral vasculature. Its diuretic effect is mediated by increased renal perfusion pressure. AVT possibly changed from a diuretic peptide in fish to an antidiuretic peptide in the early amphibians simply by an increase in the density or responsiveness of receptors in the renal preglomerular vasculature. Afferent arterial preglomerular vasoconstriction could produce graded reductions in GFR or glomerular intermittency without necessarily causing a rise in systemic pressure and thus any rise in GFR.[172]

In the *reptile,* whole-kidney GFR varies markedly depending on the state of hydration. During dehydration GFR may drop to as little as 40 percent of normal, and it may increase to 170 to 180 percent of normal during water loading. These changes in GFR appear to result primarily from changes in the number of filtering nephrons. This type of regulation is particularly appropriate for nephrons in the reptilian kidney, which lack loops of Henle running parallel to collecting ducts, and do not function in concert to produce a urine hypertonic to plasma. The naturally occurring antidiuretic hormone, AVT, appears to play the most fundamental and important role in regulating the GFR of reptiles. Physiologic amounts of AVT lead to a significant depression in GFR, and measurements of the hormone in plasma indicate a close relationship among dehydration, falling GFR, and parallel increases in AVT.

Studies of tubular function in reptiles indicate that 35 to 75 percent of the glomerular filtrate is reabsorbed isosmotically in the proximal tubule. The reptilian kidney is incapable of producing urine hyperosmotic to plasma.

However, the kidneys of many reptiles are capable of producing urine with an osmolality varying from as low as one-tenth of that of plasma to isosmotic with the plasma. Urinary dilution presumably occurs through the reabsorption of filtered solute, primarily sodium chloride, in excess of water somewhere along the nephron. A few micropuncture studies have been done indicating that this process occurs somewhere between the end of the proximal and the end of the distal tubule.[47]

The *avian* kidney commonly displays three divisions, each of which is served by its own renal artery. The avian kidney is also supplied with afferent venous blood or a functional renal portal system. The cortical nephrons, because their simple structure resembles the nephrons of reptilian kidneys, are referred to as reptilian type. The peritubular capillary network about these nephrons has both arterial and renal portal components. The contraluminal surface of each cortical nephron is exposed to afferent arterial blood along one segment and to a mixture of arteriolar and venous blood along the remainder of its length. The renal tubules vary structurally, from those resembling the reptilian nephron to those resembling the nephrons of mammalian kidneys with loops of Henle of varying length, vasa rectae, and collecting ducts. The avian glomerulus appears to be much simpler in capillary structure than that of the mammalian kidney. Glomerular capillaries of the small superficial cortical nephron can consist of a single unbranched capillary looped about the periphery of Bowman's capsule. Even the capillaries of the large juxtamedullary nephrons are not highly branched. They have only two orders of branching, or a total of four capillaries, before reuniting to form the efferent arteriole. Total kidney GFR in birds is less variable than in lesser vertebrates; however, it is much less stable than that of the mammalian kidney. The moderate decreases in GFR during dehydration appear to be an AVT-induced mechanism for assisting in the conservation of body water, and the data suggest that with most birds the maximum conservation of water occurs when the ureteral urine is close to being isosmotic to plasma. It is also possible that AVT does slightly increase the permeability of the distal portion of the nephron. This can lead to a concentrated urine, which may reach a maximum urine-to-plasma osmolar ratio of 2.0.[28]

The daily fluctuations in total body water in adult humans are very small, amounting to approximately 0.2 percent of body weight per 24 h. The average daily water turnover of a normal individual is shown in Table 5-1. Even with maximal renal conservation of water, the body is unable to prevent the continuous loss of insensible fluid through the skin, lungs, and gastrointestinal tract. For the replacement of this extrarenal loss, the individual must rely on adequate water ingestion. Humans and other mammals vary considerably in their need for an exogenous source of water during maximal renal conservation. Of all mammals, only certain *desert rodents* can so minimize their renal and extrarenal water losses that they are able to maintain water balance from that available in the preformed and oxidative water of the desert plants they ingest. These rodents can concentrate their urine to a level four to five times that of humans, and, by living in underground burrows, they reduce to a minimum their insensible pulmonary and cutaneous water losses. Humans, in contrast, even when forming maximally concentrated urine, require some exogenous source of free water to replace continued insensible and renal water losses.

The day-to-day regulation of body water is dependent, therefore, on the kidneys and on a receptor system (thirst) for signaling the relative need for water ingestion. Thirst also plays an essential role in the regulation of the volume and tonicity of the body fluids.

The maximal limits of the human kidney's ability to conserve and excrete water is realized by subjecting the individual to a period of rigid water restriction (24 h) followed by the ingestion of a large water load and the maintenance of a sustained water diuresis. At the end of the period of dehydration, urinary flow will have decreased to 0.3 to 0.5 ml/min, depending on the rate of solute excretion, urine osmolality will have increased to a high of 1200 to 1400 mosm/liter (specific gravity, 1.037 to 1.040). Then, as the subject replaces the fluid deficit by the ingestion of a large volume of water and maintains a

TABLE 5-1 • Average daily water turnover of a normal individual

	Water intake, g			Water output, g	
Source of water	*Obligatory*	*Facultative*		*Obligatory*	*Facultative*
Drink	650	1000	Urine	700	1000
Preformed	750		Skin	500	
Oxidative	350		Lungs	400	
			Feces	150	
Subtotals	1750	1000	Subtotals	1750	1000
Total	2750		Total	2750	

SOURCE: From Wolf AV: *Thirst*, Springfield, IL, Charles C Thomas, 1958. Used by permission.

positive water balance of 1000 to 1500 ml, urinary flow will gradually increase over approximately 90 min to attain a maximal rate of 10 to 15 ml/min, or approximately 10 to 15 percent of the glomerular filtrate. A minimal urinary osmolality of 30 to 60 mosm/liter will be attained, somewhat higher at higher rates of solute excretion. This state of "physiologic diabetes insipidus" will prevail as long as the sustained positive water balance is maintained. The physiologic events involved in maximal water diuresis and antidiuresis in humans are outlined in Tables 5-2 and 5-3, respectively. Tables 5-4 and 5-5 summarize osmoregulation in vertebrates[196a] and the structure of the natural neurohypophysial principles.[173a]

TABLE 5-2 • Sequence of events in water diuresis

1. Ingestion of water load to correct any water deficit and to maintain a positive water balance of 1000 to 1500 ml.
2. Dilution of all body fluids, hydration of cells of the supraoptic nuclei, inhibition of the secretion of ADH (AVP) from the neurohypophysis.
3. Destruction of circulating AVP (half-life approximately 9 to 16 min); 60 to 90 min required to reach peak water diuresis.
4. Absence of AVP at the distal nephron (cortical and medullary collecting ducts) results in maximal impermeability of these segments to water, causing almost all the water delivered to this tubular segment to appear in the urine (approximately 10 to 15% of the filtered water).
5. Continued normal resorption of salts; therefore, the emerging urine is characterized by minimal solute concentration and maximal volume.

TABLE 5-3 • Sequence of events in maximal antidiuresis

1. Moderate negative water balance, i.e., rigid water restriction of 24 h.
2. Negative water balance of approximately 1500 ml or 1 to 2% of body weight.
3. Hyperosmolality of all body cells with dehydration of the cells of the supraoptic nuclei.
4. Release of neural impulses down the neurohypophyseal stalk to the posterior pituitary gland, causing AVP release into the circulation on a sustained basis.
5. AVP acts on cortical and medullary collecting ducts to make these segments freely permeable to water; water flows along concentration gradients established by continued solute reabsorption.
6. Approximately 80 to 90% of the solute reaching the distal convoluted tubule is actively reabsorbed, and 80 to 90% or more of the water is reabsorbed, leaving small volumes of isotonic fluid for delivery into the medullary collecting duct.
7. In the medullary collecting duct, water continues to passively back-diffuse into the hypertonic medullary interstitium until urine and medulla reach maximal and equal concentrations. The small volume of filtrate reaching the collecting duct is further reduced by one-third to one-fourth its volume and is maximally concentrated (1200 to 1400 mosm/liter; specific gravity 1.037 to 1.040).

STRUCTURAL AND FUNCTIONAL ORGANIZATION OF THE RENAL MEDULLA

A description of the renal concentrating and diluting mechanisms requires some understanding of the characteristics of the nephron segments involved in these processes. We will therefore first describe the structural, biochemical, and permeability properties of these nephron segments and then describe the overall process of regulated water excretion.

DESCENDING THIN LIMB OF HENLE'S LOOP (DTLH)

The first nephron segment directly involved in urinary concentration is the DTLH. Two types of DTLH have been described (Fig. 5-1). The short loops originate in superficial and midcortical glomeruli and turn in the outer medulla, while the long loops originate in deep cortical and juxtamedullary glomeruli and penetrate variable distances into the inner medulla. Short DTLH are lined by a flat noninterdigitating epithelium in which cells are joined together by relatively deep multiple-stranded tight junctions.[133] They are of similar structure in all species studied.[113] Long DTLH, however, display greater structural heterogeneity, especially in the upper segments, and there is considerable interspecies variability. Some species (cat, golden hamster, mouse, *Octodan degus*, *Psammomys*, and rat) have a very heavily interdigitating epithelium with prominent paracellular pathways, while other species (guinea pig, humans, and rabbit) exhibit a much tighter epithelium.[132] The transition from upper to lower segments is a gradual one and occurs at a variable depth in the medulla.[133] The epithelium lining the lower segment is relatively undifferentiated, with no interspecies variability.[132] It is of interest that no correlation is apparent between a species' maximal concentrating ability and the ratio of short and long loops. In fact, in rodents capable of the highest urinary concentration, the short loops are considerably more abundant than the long loops. Overall, the structural organization of the thin limbs of the human kidney appears to resemble that of the rabbit more closely than that of any other experimental animal studied.

The DTLH exhibits no increase in adenylyl cyclase activity in response to parathyroid hormone, calcitonin, glucagon, isoproterenol, or vasopressin (Fig. 5-2).[111,159] In terms of its permeability characteristics, it is clear that

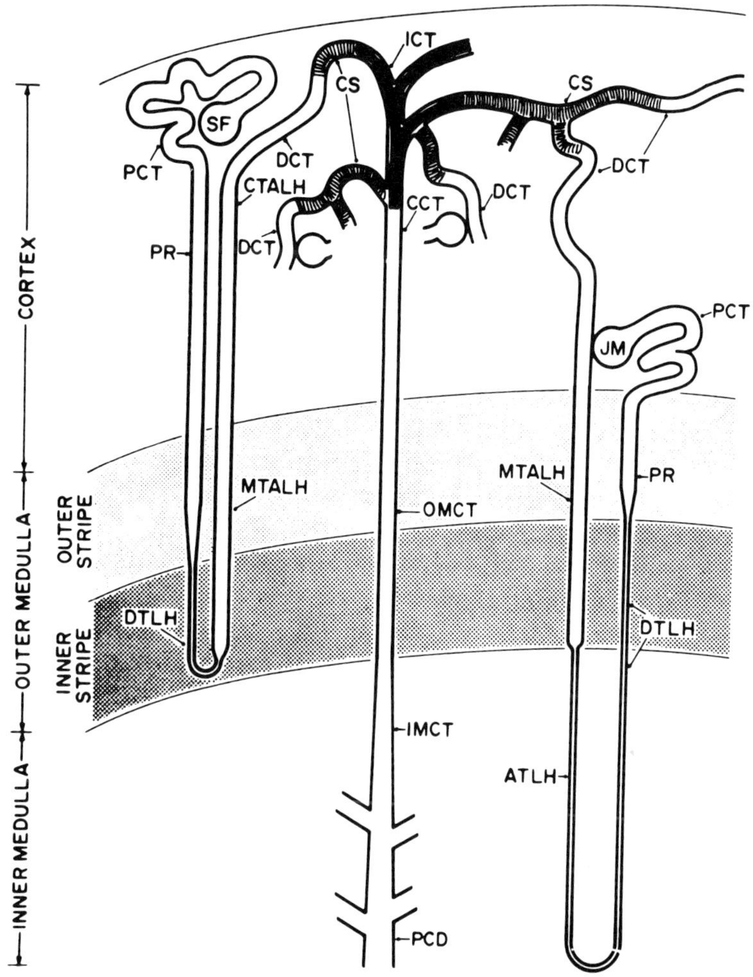

FIGURE 5-1 • Two nephron populations, superficial (SF) and juxtamedullary (JM), are depicted. The major nephron segments are labeled as follows: PCT, proximal convoluted tubule; PR, pars recta; DTLH, descending thin limb of Henle; ATLH, ascending thin limb of Henle; MTALH, medullary thick ascending limb of Henle; CTALH, cortical thick ascending limb of Henle; DCT, distal convoluted tubule; CS, connecting segment; CCT, cortical-collecting tubule; OMCT, outer medullary collecting tubule; IMCT, inner medullary collecting tubule; and PCD, papillary collecting duct. (From Jacobson, HR: *Am J Physiol* 241:F203, 1981. Used by permission.)

the DTLH is very permeable to water (Table 5-4);[111] however, determinations of its permeability to solute have yielded variable results that have been the focus of considerable controversy.[3] The significance of the controversy will be discussed in the description of the concentrating mechanism itself.

ASCENDING THIN LIMB OF HENLE'S LOOP (ATLH)

The transition from DTLH-like epithelium to that of the ATLH actually occurs somewhat proximal to the hairpin turn.[133] Functionally, therefore, the tip of Henle's loop is part of the ATLH. The ATLH is lined by a leaky epithelium with shallow tight junctions and prominent paracellular pathways; it is of uniform structure in various species.[133]

Though its functional significance is not known, vasopressin-sensitive adenylate cyclase activity has been demonstrated in the ATLH of rabbit and rat and remains untested in mouse and humans (Fig. 5-2).[159] The enzyme has not been shown to respond to any other hormone. The ATLH is virtually impermeable to water but highly permeable to solute.[105,112,150] Whether the movement of solute out of this segment occurs by passive or active processes will be discussed during our examination of the concentrating mechanism.

THICK ASCENDING LIMB OF HENLE'S LOOP (TALH)

The structure of the TALH is remarkably uniform. There is no significant interspecies variation, and it is similar in short and long loops as well. The epithelium is composed of tall, heavily interdigitated cells with large mitochondria. As the tubule ascends toward the cortex, the epithelium decreases in height and has fewer interdigitations. This transition defines the medullary (MTALH) and cortical (CTALH) sections.[116] Short loops actually have a longer TALH than do long loops because of the longer cortical section required to reach the macula densa of more superficial glomeruli (Fig. 5-1).[133]

Despite morphological homogeneity, the TALH exhibits considerable interspecies variability in its pattern of

TABLE 5-4 • Permeability characteristics of nephron segments involved in urinary concentration in the absence (−AVP) and presence (+AVP) of vasopressin

	Hydraulic conductance ($\mu M\ s^{-1}$)	P_{Urea} ($\times 10^{-5}$ cm s^{-1})	P_{Na} ($\times 10^{-5}$ cm s^{-1})	P_{Cl} ($\times 10^{-5}$ cm s^{-1})
DTLH	2000	1.23–5.3	0.17–1.94	
ATLH	12	6.7	25.5	44–117
MTALH				
−AVP	0	0.86	6.27	1.0
+AVP		0.63		
CTALH				
−AVP	8.5		2.8	1.4
+AVP				
DCT				
−AVP	0			
+AVP	0			
CS				
−AVP	0			
+AVP	0			
CCT				
−AVP	6–19	0–1	0.08	4.7
+AVP	165–375	0–1	0.15	2.1
MCT				
−AVP		0.31	0.39	
+AVP	200	0.34		
PCD				
−AVP		2.19		
+AVP	67	2.36		

ABBREVIATIONS: See legend for Fig. 5-1.
SOURCE: Adapted from Jacobson, H: *Am J Physiol* 241:F203, 1981. Used by permission.

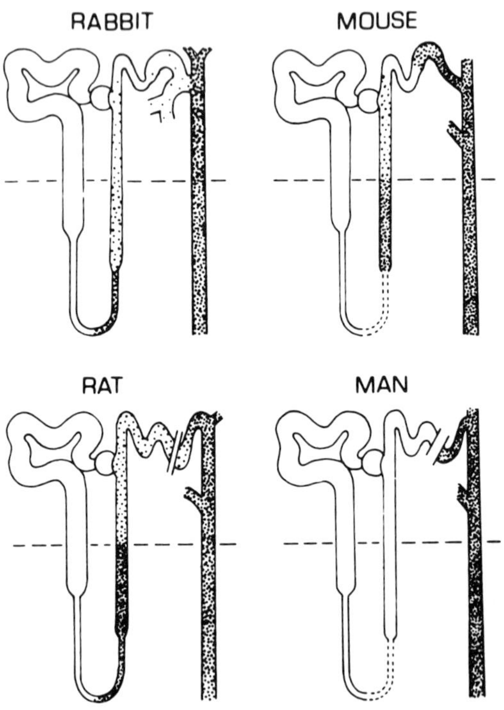

FIGURE 5-2 • Pattern of vasopressin-stimulated adenylate cyclase activity in various nephron segments. Activity is proportional to dot density. Dotted lines reflect segments in which the effect of vasopressin has not been tested. (From Morel F: *Am J Physiol* 240:F159, 1981. Used by permission.)

hormone responsiveness. In general, however, MTALH is unresponsive to parathyroid hormone and is responsive to calcitonin. Vasopressin-responsive adenylyl cyclase is present in the mouse and the rat, intermediate in the rabbit, but absent in humans (Fig. 5-2). CTALH is very responsive to parathyroid hormone but only mildly sensitive to calcitonin.[111,159] Vasopressin responsiveness is less marked than in the MTALH but clearly measurable both in the rat and mouse. Again, no such activity is noted in humans, with the rabbit displaying an intermediate response.

The hydraulic conductivity of the TALH is very low and is not altered by arginine vasopressin (AVP), even in species (e.g., mouse) with vasopressin-sensitive adenylyl cyclase in this segment.[90] While the passive permeabilities to sodium and chloride are very low, they are actively transported out of the TALH. The possibility that vasopressin is involved in the control of sodium chloride reabsorption in this nephron segment and particularly in the MTALH has been suggested in studies of tubular microperfusion in the mouse.[46,90] It has long been thought that chloride is the primary actively transported ion, with sodium following passively.[35,182] Recently, however, a number of observations have suggested that sodium may indeed be the primarily transported ion.[111]

DISTAL CONVOLUTED TUBULE (DCT) AND CONNECTING SEGMENT (CS)

The portion of the nephron between the macula densa and the first junction of two tubules (into cortical collecting ducts) is the DCT. For a short but variable distance beyond the macula densa, the cells are identical to those of the CTALH.[111,132] At this point significant interspecies differences are observed. In the rabbit there follow two clearly distinct segments: (1) an early segment composed of a single type of heavily interdigitating cells, referred to as DCT_b because of its bright appearance under the dissection microscope, changing abruptly to (2) a segment composed of two cell types having a more granular appearance and therefore referred to as DCT_g.[159] The latter portion, in conjunction with an early granular portion of the cortical collecting tubule, is termed the connecting segment.[111] The connecting segments form arcades that ascend in the cortex before draining into a cortical collecting tubule (Fig. 5-1). This arrangement probably serves to maximize the exposure of hyposmotic tubular fluid to vasopressin-sensitive tissue[132] and to ensure that tubular fluid delivered to the medulla is isotonic. In other species (e.g., rat, mouse, *Psammomys*, and humans), the DCT blends with the cortical collecting tubule with no clear demarcation; no connecting segment is identifiable.[113]

The distal tubule varies in its pattern of hormonal responsiveness as well. The rat displays varying degrees of adenylyl cyclase activity in response to parathyroid hormone, calcitonin, glucagon, and isoproterenol. In the rabbit, the DCT_b responds to calcitonin but the connecting segment does not; the opposite pattern is observed in response to isoproterenol and parathyroid hormone.[159] In regard to vasopressin, the DCT appears to be unresponsive to the hormone in mouse, rabbit, and humans. In contrast, in the rat all portions of the DCT respond to vasopressin, probably reflecting the great cellular heterogeneity of this nephron segment in this species. The connecting segment of the rabbit is also unresponsive to vasopressin, but the terminal DCT of the mouse is responsive (Fig. 5-2).

The hydraulic conductivity throughout the distal tubule and the connecting segment is essentially zero both in the absence and in the presence of AVP.[111] Permeabilities to solutes have yet to be accurately measured in these segments of the nephron.

COLLECTING DUCTS

The collecting ducts are formed in the cortex by the confluence of several distal tubules. They descend through the cortex and outer medulla individually, but upon entering the inner medulla they successively fuse together. Thus, a terminal inner medullary collecting duct (IMCD) drains from 1500 (in the rat and rabbit) to 2800 nephrons (in humans).[132]

The collecting duct epithelium is composed of two cell types: *principal cells* and *intercalated cells*.[113] Both are simple polygonal cells joined together by deep tight junctions without significant interdigitation. The ratio of principal cells to intercalated cells is approximately 2:1 in the cortical collecting tubule and increases as the tubule descends into the medulla.[111] It is now recognized that the inner medullary collecting duct itself consists of two subsegments that are morphologically, as well as functionally, distinct.[128] Whereas the initial segment of the inner medullary collecting duct consists of principal and some intercalated cells, the terminal inner medullary collecting duct possesses a cell that is morphologically different. This cell, designated the *inner medullary collecting duct cell*, has a more complex microvillar structure and is devoid of the central cilium that characterizes principal cells.[44]

The collecting tubules have been found to possess vasopressin-stimulatable adenylyl cyclase activity in all species studied. The cortical collecting tubules of the rabbit and rat also display some response to isoproterenol, while the medullary collecting tubules are unresponsive to parathyroid hormone, calcitonin, and isoproterenol.[159] The collecting tubules are virtually impermeable to water in the absence of vasopressin; the mechanism whereby vasopressin dramatically increases the hydraulic conductivity of the tubule is discussed in detail later in this chapter. Passive permeabilities to sodium and potassium are low throughout the collecting system, although in the cortical collecting tubule the permeability of potassium is approximately ten times that of sodium.[110] The cortical collecting tubule and outer medullary collecting tubule (OMCT) are essentially impermeable to urea. The aforementioned morphologic heterogeneity of the inner medullary collecting tubule is reflected in its urea permeability. Whereas the initial portion of the inner medullary collecting duct has a low basal urea permeability that is unaffected by vasopressin, the urea permeability of the terminal inner medullary collecting duct is higher in the basal state and is greatly enhanced by vasopressin.[128,192]

VASCULAR ARCHITECTURE OF THE RENAL MEDULLA

To comprehend the urinary concentrating mechanism better, a basic understanding of the medullary vasculature is needed. The efferent arterioles of juxtamedullary glomeruli give rise to the descending vasa recta, which penetrate into the medulla in discrete vascular bundles. They terminate in a dense capillary plexus investing the tubular elements of the medulla and then rejoin to form the ascending vasa recta. These vessels may then ascend toward the cortex either within or independently of the vascular bundles ultimately draining into interlobular and arcuate veins.[133]

The vascular bundles exhibit significant interspecies heterogeneity, with two general patterns described: simple and complex. Simple vascular bundles contain only descending and ascending vasa recta with no tubular elements; complex vascular bundles include the DTL of short loops of Henle. As will be discussed later, this latter arrangement may enhance urinary concentrating ability by recycling solute into the inner medulla.[133]

MECHANISMS OF URINARY CONCENTRATION AND DILUTION

By analogy with heat exchangers, Kuhn and Ryffel in 1942 recognized that small transverse differences in solute concentration between fluids in the ascending and descending limbs of Henle's loop could generate a large axial gradient for solute increasing from the corticomedullary junction to the papillary tip.[136] The existence of this so-called countercurrent multiplier was confirmed by the demonstration that osmotic pressure did indeed increase with increasing medullary depth.[238] Furthermore, in 1959 Gottschalk and Mylle, in an elegant micropuncture study, demonstrated that in antidiuretic rats tubular fluid from the bend of loops of Henle and from collecting ducts and vasa recta at the same level were equally hyperosmotic, as would be predicted by the countercurrent hypothesis.[83]

The basic requirements for the operation of this countercurrent multiplier are threefold: (1) countercurrent flow, supplied by the loop of Henle; (2) differences in permeability such that the descending limb is much more permeable to water than is the ascending limb; and (3) a source of energy, provided by the active transport of sodium chloride from the ascending limb to the surrounding interstitium. The transport of sodium chloride provides the so-called single effect, which simultaneously dilutes ascending limb fluid while raising the tonicity of the interstitium.

While there is little controversy that the single effect takes place in the ascending limb of Henle's loop, there is considerable debate as to whether both the thick and the thin segments partake in the process. In the thick ascending limb, chloride was considered to be the ion that was primarily transported, with sodium following passively.[35,182] It is now widely accepted that the primary mechanism of chloride absorption in this segment is mediated by an electroneutral Na^+-K^+-$2Cl^-$ cotransporter.*[87,158] This process begins in the outer medulla, whereas the greatest interstitial tonicity is to be found in

* Note that whether chloride or sodium is the primarily transported ion is not germane to this discussion. For purposes of urinary concentration, it is necessary only that the TALH transport *salt* into the interstitium.

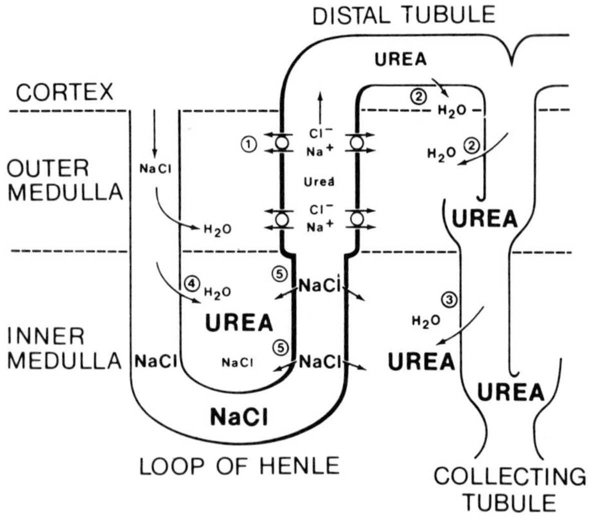

FIGURE 5-3 • Schematic representation of the passive urinary concentrating mechanism. See text for description of steps 1 through 5. (From Jamison RL, Maffly RH: *N Engl J Med* 295:1059, 1976. Used by permission.)

the inner medulla. Though one laboratory has reported a lumen-positive potential difference that can be abolished by ouabain in the ascending thin limb, suggesting that this segment actively transports chloride,[151] other investigators have been unable to detect any evidence for active transport.[104,160] How, then, does the ascending thin limb dilute its contents, and how is the inner medullary interstitium rendered hypertonic?

In 1972 Stephenson[217] and Kokko and Rector[129] simultaneously, yet independently, proposed what has become known as the "passive urinary concentrating mechanism." (Since the latter formulation stipulating the absence of active transport by the ATLH is but a special case of the former, which operates in the presence or absence of active transport, they will be treated as one.) The details of this mechanism are as follows (Fig. 5-3):

1. The thick ascending limb actively transports sodium chloride, increasing the tonicity of the surrounding interstitium. As the TALH is poorly permeable to water and urea, the tubular fluid is diluted and urea is retained.
2. Under the action of AVP in the late distal tubule (in some species) and in the cortical and outer medullary collecting ducts (in most species), hypotonic tubular fluid equilibrates with the isotonic and hypertonic cortical and outer medullary interstitium, resulting in water removal. These segments are poorly permeable to urea, and therefore its concentration increases.
3. Tubular fluid then arrives at the inner medullary collecting duct, which, in its terminal portion, is highly permeable to urea, particularly in the presence of vasopressin.[128] Urea enters the inner medulla,

doing down its concentration gradient, and in the process preserves interstitial hypertonicity.

4. The hypertonic interstitium causes the abstraction of water from the DTLH, which is relatively impermeable to sodium chloride and urea. The sodium chloride concentration in the tubule thereby increases above that of the interstitium. The tubular fluid arriving at the bend of the loop of Henle thus contains a relatively high concentration of sodium and a low concentration of urea.
5. The fluid then enters the thin ascending limb. This nephron segment is water-impermeable and has a greater permeability to sodium chloride than to urea. Sodium chloride moves passively down its concentration gradient into the interstitium, rendering tubular fluid more dilute and the interstitium more concentrated.

Let us now examine in stepwise fashion the mechanism whereby the "single effect" in the TALH is multiplied by the loop of Henle, producing a large corticomedullary osmotic gradient and markedly hypertonic medullary interstitium. This is most easily accomplished if we dissociate flow through the loop from the transtubular movements of water and solute (Fig. 5-4). In reality, of course, these two processes occur simultaneously.

We begin in the no-flow state with the active transport of sodium chloride from the TALH into the interstitium. Although the passive permeabilities of the TALH to sodium chloride and urea are small, the backleak of solute from the interstitium into the TALH is sufficient to limit the osmotic gradient that the TALH can establish to approximately 200 mosm/kg water. The TALH actively pumps sodium chloride into the interstitium until the

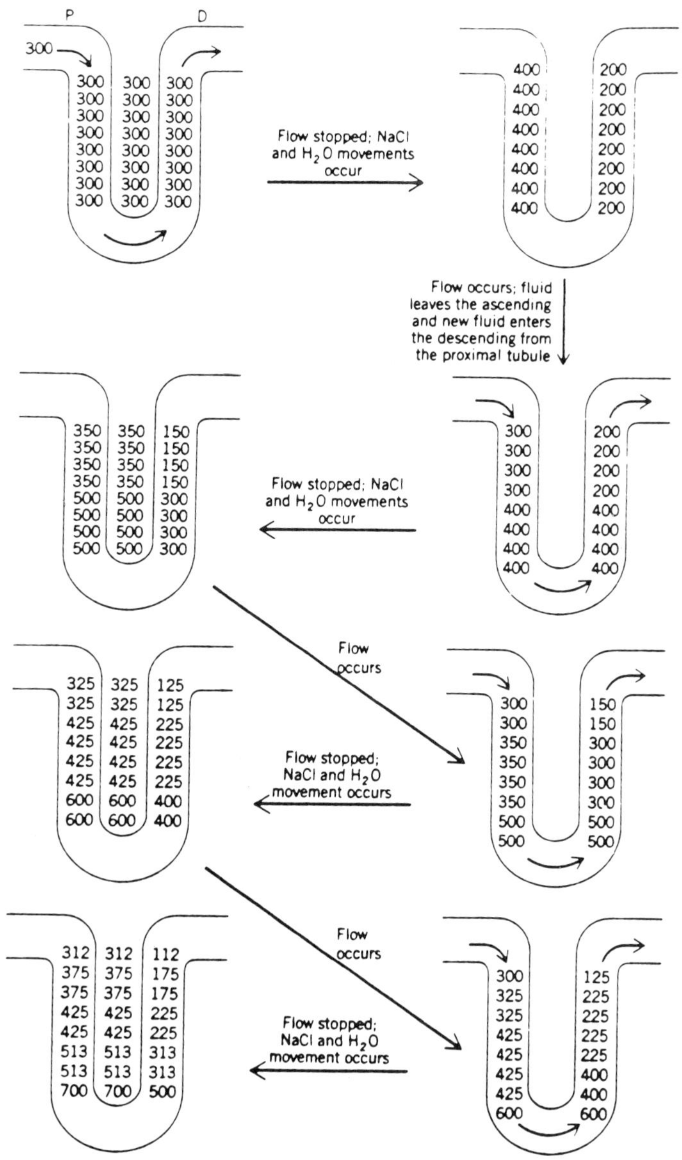

FIGURE 5-4 • Mechanism of countercurrent multiplication. See text for details. (From Vander A: *Renal Physiology,* New York, McGraw-Hill, 1980, p 84. Used by permission.)

limiting gradient is reached. Water moves down its concentration gradient from the very water-permeable DTLH into the interstitium so that DTLH fluid is now in osmotic equilibrium with the interstitium. Interstitial tonicity is preserved by the ongoing active transport of salt out of the TALH.

When flow occurs, hypotonic fluid exits the TALH to the distal tubule, and isotonic fluid enters the DTLH from the proximal tubule. Transtubular movement of water and solutes then takes place as described above, and the cycle is repeated. In this manner fluid in the DTLH becomes increasingly more concentrated as it approaches the tip of the loop. At any given level in the medulla, DTLH fluid is in equilibrium with the interstitium; fluid in the TALH has a concentration of approximately 200 mosm/kg less than that of the interstitium. Thus, fluid exiting from the TALH is approximately 200 mosm/kg less concentrated than plasma. (As solute reabsorption from the proximal tubule is isotonic, fluid entering the DTLH is isosmotic with the glomerular filtrate, i.e., plasma.) This allows for the elaboration of hypotonic urine in the absence of antidiuretic hormone (ADH). During antidiuresis, collecting tubular fluid becomes increasingly concentrated as AVP allows for equilibration with the progressively more hypertonic medullary interstitium.

Thus, the kidney functions brilliantly. As stated by Jamison and Maffly,[115] "One of the most compelling features of the countercurrent mechanism is its biologic economy. When the urine is hyperosmotic, at no point along the renal tubule does the transepithelial osmotic gradient exceed 200 mosm/kg of water. . . . Moreover, the same process that drives the multiplier also accounts for urinary dilution; in the absence of antidiuretic hormone . . . fluid coming from the ascending limb remains dilute throughout the remainder of the distal and collecting tubule."

Two issues must now be addressed. First, how is the tonicity of the inner medullary interstitium maintained? What prevents dissipation of the large corticomedullary osmotic gradient? Furthermore, as vessels containing isotonic plasma course through the hypertonic medulla, there should occur massive fluxes of solute into and water out of the vessels, further tending to diminish interstitial tonicity. Second, by what mechanism is water returned to the circulation following its reabsorption from the collecting ducts? The answers lie in an understanding of the operation of the vasa recta (Fig. 5-5).

The geometry of the medullary vasculature is analogous to that of the loop of Henle. Descending vasa recta penetrate into the medulla, running parallel to collecting tubules. As the vessels descend, they indeed lose solute and gain water as they equilibrate with the interstitium. At various levels, as the papillary tip is approached, they form a capillary plexus investing the tubular elements of the medulla. The vessels then rejoin and *abruptly turn* to form ascending vasa recta. As the vessels ascend through the progressively less concentrated medulla, solute exits and water enters the vessels. Thus, by functioning as countercurrent exchangers (not multipliers, since these processes are strictly passive), the vasa recta trap urea in the inner medulla and return reabsorbed water to the circulation.

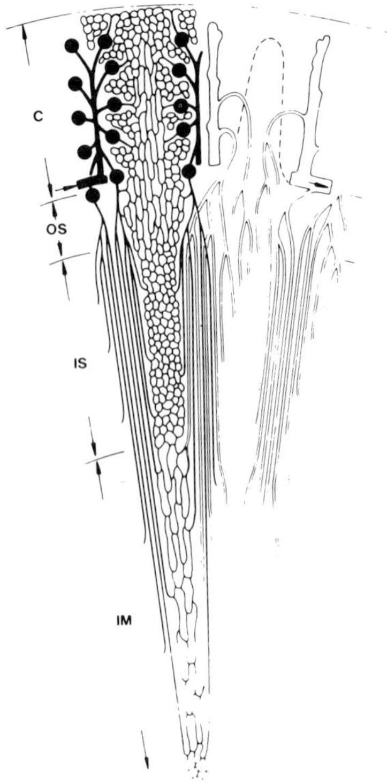

FIGURE 5-5 • Schematic representation of the microvasculature of the mammalian kidney (rat). Arterial vessels, glomeruli, and capillaries are drawn in black and shown on the left side; venous vessels are white and demonstrated on the right side. Both sides should be imagined superimposed upon each other. The dashed line separates the medullary ray from the cortical labyrinth. An arcuate artery (arrow) gives rise to interlobular arteries from which afferent arterioles originate at angles typical for their intracortical location. Efferent arterioles of superficial glomeruli, before splitting off into capillaries, ascend to the renal surface; those of midcortical glomeruli frequently split into capillaries at the border with the medullary rays, and efferent arterioles of juxtamedullary glomeruli divide into descending vasa recta. The interlobular veins are formed in the superficial cortex. Together with arcuate veins they accept blood from medullary venous vessels. Vascular bundles in the inner stripe contain descending vasa recta and all ascending vasa recta originating from the inner medulla; most ascending vasa recta from the inner stripe ascend separately from the bundles. C, cortex; OS, outer stripe; IS, inner stripe; IM, inner medulla. (From Jamison RL, Kriz W: *Urinary Concentrating Mechanism, Structure and Function,* New York, Oxford University Press, 1982, p 133. Used by permission.)

In those species with complex vascular bundles, which incorporate the DTL of short loops of Henle, the ascending vasa recta may deposit urea into the adjacent DTL of a short loop of Henle, thereby recycling it to the IMCD.[133] Note that since the DTL of short loops do not enter the inner medulla (Fig. 5-1), the addition of solute to these loops in no way interfers with the removal of water from the DTLH that is so crucial to the concentrating process.

In order for this elegant model to operate as described, a number of requirements must be met.[118] Many aspects of this model have, in fact, been experimentally supported.[193] These include:

1. The DTLH must be virtually impermeable to sodium chloride and urea and highly permeable to water. Conversely, the ATLH must be impermeable to water, with considerable permeability to sodium chloride. Furthermore, the permeability to urea must be significantly less than that to sodium chloride, because if it were not, the gradient for sodium chloride movement from lumen to interstitium would be dissipated by the entry of urea into the lumen, and the inner medullary interstitium would not be hypertonic. In vitro studies have found the descending thin limb of the rabbit to have a high hydraulic conductivity and very low permeabilities to sodium and urea (reflection coefficients 0.96 and 0.95, respectively), from which it has been concluded that solute concentration in the DTLH occurs almost entirely (96 percent) by removal of water.[106] However, it must be noted that Morgan and Berliner perfused DTLH of the rat and found much higher permeabilities to both salt and urea.[160] Likewise, in *Psammomys,* de Rouffignac and Morel have shown that approximately 85 percent of the osmotic equilibration in the DTL is accomplished by solute, largely salt, addition.[185,186] The hydraulic conductivity of the ATLH has been determined to be extremely low in both the rabbit[104] and the rat,[160] as anticipated from the "passive mechanism." However, data regarding the requisite high permeability to sodium chloride are conflicting. In the rabbit and the hamster, the permeability to sodium chloride is indeed high,[104] and, most important, much higher than that to urea.[104,130] However, in the rat, sodium chloride permeability has been reported to be too low to allow for significant passive movement of salt across this nephron segment.[160]
2. Water must be extracted from the descending limb. That this occurs is supported by the observation that administration of urea to protein-deprived rats enhances their urinary concentration often to a degree greater than can be accounted for by the increase in urinary urea alone; that is, nonurea solute is concentrated as well.[75,176] By virtue of its contribution to interstitial tonicity, the administration of urea will enhance the removal of water from the DTLH and the collecting tubules, thereby increasing the concentrations of all urinary solutes.
3. There must be a transtubular difference in sodium chloride concentration favoring outward movement of sodium chloride from the thin loop. Direct measurements of the sodium chloride concentrations in the end DTL and vasa recta at the same level (reflecting medullary interstitium) have yielded gradients for sodium chloride.[118,171] However, these gradients are not large, and it could be questioned whether they are sufficient to drive the system by purely passive means.
4. The concentration of urea entering the thin limb must be low compared with its concentration in the interstitium. Direct measurements performed at the tip of the loop and the collecting duct reveal that the urea concentration in loop fluid is too high to be compatible with a purely passive model.[173] In fact, urea addition to the descending limb clearly occurs in the rat and accounts for 35 percent of the increment in fluid osmolality in the DTLH. Furthermore, the concentrations of urea in the collecting duct and the end DTLH were measured and the gradient was found to be far smaller than would be predicted from the passive models.[173] In view of the shortcomings of this model, Bonventre and Lechene have suggested a model for urinary concentration in which fluid enters the DTLH hypertonic to the surrounding interstitium and wherein the DTLH secretes urea while reabsorbing sodium chloride.[24] The experimental evidence to support the model is, at this time, lacking.

On the other hand, and in keeping with the passive model, the requisite low permeability to urea in the thick ascending limb, cortical collecting duct, and initial inner medullary collecting duct has been well demonstrated in the rat.[127,192] Urea is thus reabsorbed in the highly urea-permeable terminal inner medullary collecting duct and from there is recycled into the adjacent thin ascending limb.[140] However, since the entry of urea might rapidly dissipate the gradient needed for passive sodium reabsorption, Layton has proposed that the passive system operates only at the very top of the loop, but that the loops of Henle turn at multiple levels within the inner medulla.[139]

In summary, the passive model on balance best satisfies current experimental evidence regarding the concentration process. There are, however, a disturbing number of conflicting experimental observations that limit total acceptance of this model.

Finally, it has been reported that ureteral excision and exposure of the renal papilla impair maximal urinary concentration.[25,200] The role of the ureter appears to be independent of ureteral peristalsis, and it has been suggested that its presence is important in preventing solute losses from the papilla.[169] The loss of urinary concentration that occurs with papillary exposure was postulated to be due to a prostaglandin-mediated increase in inner medullary plasma flow.[42] However, others have not found a salutary effect of prostaglandin inhibition,[184] and the noted defect may reflect the need for pelvic urine to bathe the papillae in order to add urea into the papillary interstitium.[25]

CONCEPT OF OSMOLAR AND FREE-WATER CLEARANCES

To describe the processes of urinary concentration and dilution quantitatively, Wesson and Anslow[236] formulated the concepts of *osmolar clearance* (Cosm), *free-water clearance* (CH_2O), and *negative free-water clearance* (T^cH_2O). This terminology was quickly adopted by their teacher and mentor, Homer Smith,[207] and has since gained widespread acceptance as a technique for quantitatively describing the processes of urinary concentration and dilution. They subdivided the total urinary volume into three virtual volumes, an isosmotic portion (Cosm), a portion that was "freed" of urinary solute during the dilution process (CH_2O), and that volume of solute-free water abstracted or resorbed from the isosmotic urine during the concentrating process (T^cH_2O).

Osmolar clearance (Cosm) is defined by the standard clearance formula as

$$\text{Cosm} = \frac{Uosm \cdot V}{Posm}$$

where *Uosm* and *Posm* in milliosmols per liter are urine and plasma osmolality, respectively, and *V* is the urinary flow rate in milliliters per minute. Thus, $Uosm \cdot V$ equals the rate of solute excretion in milliosmols per minute.

Therefore, osmolar clearance in milliliters per minute is the rate at which osmotically active solutes are removed from the plasma with sufficient water to excrete them in an isosmotic solution. At usual rates of solute excretion in a 70-kg human, Cosm varies from 2 to 4 ml/min.[112] Urinary water over and above this volume, or "solute-free" water, is the free-water clearance, or CH_2O; that is,

$$V = \text{Cosm} + CH_2O$$

or, expressed as flow rate in milliliters per minute,

$$CH_2O - V\left(1 - \frac{Uosm}{Posm}\right)$$

It is apparent that CH_2O is always derived from the measurement of the osmolar clearance, Cosm. Parenthetically, as Cosm in humans and most mammals is not affected by ADH (AVP), a change in CH_2O is under most circumstances a sensitive index of the action of AVP on the concentrating segments of the nephron (cortical and medullary collecting ducts). However, a number of physiologic factors capable of altering CH_2O, independent of AVP, are depicted in Table 5-5.

An example of the calculation of osmolar clearance and positive and negative free-water clearances, using the numbers in Fig. 5-6, will assist in clarifying these terms. Assume that 100 ml of glomerular filtrate is being formed per minute and that 70 percent of this filtrate is resorbed in isosmotic proportions up to the beginning of the descending limb of the loop of Henle. In the descending limb, an additional 10 ml of water is resorbed. Assuming no water resorption occurs in the ascending limb, 20 ml of hypotonic (150 mosm/liter) fluid is delivered into the distal convoluted tubule. If during maximal AVP activity 90 percent of the remaining water were resorbed, with enough solute to bring the urine to isotonicity by the end of the cortical collecting duct, 2 ml of isotonic fluid would be delivered to the medullary collecting duct. Here fluid would be withdrawn and urea added until 0.3 ml of maximally concentrated (1400 mosm/liter) urine is

TABLE 5-5 • Physiologic factors that alter free-water clearance (CH_2O) independent of AVP

1. Rigid sodium restriction with decrease in extracellular fluid volume impairs water diuresis through:
   a. Decreased filtered load of sodium and water
   b. Enhanced proximal tubular resorption of sodium and water
   c. Decreased velocity of flow in the loop of Henle
   d. Decreased delivery of sodium and water to the diluting segments of the nephron
   e. Decreased medullary blood flow
2. Glomerular filtration rate (GFR):
   Decrease in the GFR may impair maximal urinary dilution and water diuresis by a combination of the above mechanisms. Increase in GFR, as caused by aminophylline, dopamine, high protein intake, etc., enhances maximal urinary dilution and water diuresis.
3. Medullary blood flow:
   Decreased medullary blood flow impairs maximal water diuresis by increasing hypertonicity of the medulla, which allows increased back-diffusion of water in the descending limb of Henle's loop and collecting duct in the absence of AVP. Increased medullary blood flow would have the opposite effect.
4. Osmotic diuresis:
   Increases water diuresis but causes a modest increase (less dilute) in the minimal urinary osmolality because of increased delivery of solute and water to diluting segments with less solute resorption in these segments.
5. Diuretics:
   Impair maximal urinary dilution and water diuresis.
   a. Induce sodium depletion with resultant changes noted above (see 1).
   b. The azides selectively block sodium resorption by the cortical diluting segment. However, in the thick ascending limb of Henle's loop, furosemide, ethacrynic acid, and other loop diuretics may actually enhance water diuresis with or without change in urinary dilution if number 1 is prevented.
6. Inhibitors of prostaglandin (PGE_2) synthesis inhibit urinary dilution and maximal water diuresis by increasing sodium resorption in the ascending limb and enhancing the antidiuretic action of any residual circulating AVP.

FIGURE 5-6 • Changes in the volume and osmolality of tubular fluid along the nephron in diuresis and antidiuresis. (Adapted from Vander A: *Renal Physiology,* New York, McGraw-Hill, 1980, p 89. Used by permission.)

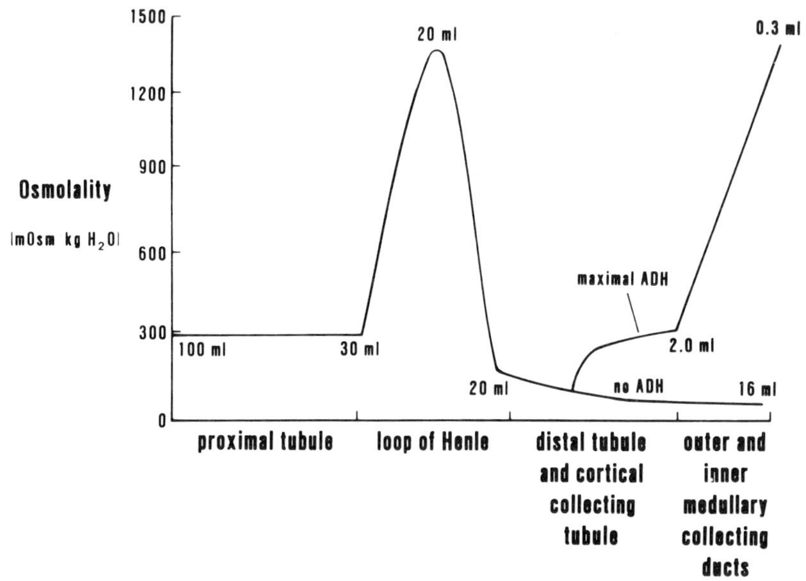

formed. If we assume plasma osmolality to be 285 mosm/liter, then

$$\frac{1.4 \text{ mosm/ml} \times 0.3 \text{ ml/min}}{0.285 \text{ mosm/ml}} = \frac{0.420}{0.285}$$

$$= 1.5 \text{ ml/min} = \text{Cosm}$$

$$V - \text{Cosm} = -\text{CH}_2\text{O or } T^c\text{H}_2\text{O}$$

$$0.3 - 1.5 = -1.2 \text{ ml/min}$$

The magnitude of the negative free-water clearance, or the rate of solute-free water resorption in the overall concentrating process, equals 1.2 ml/min.

Conversely, if 20 ml of hypotonic fluid were delivered into the distal tubule in the absence of AVP and 90 percent of the solute were resorbed without water, approximately 20 ml of a dilute fluid (osmolality of 28.5 mosm/liter) would be delivered into the final segment or medullary collecting duct. In the absence of AVP a minimal amount of fluid (4 ml/min) would be removed, leaving 16 ml of urine with a final concentration of 30 mosm/liter.

$$\text{CH}_2\text{O} = V - \text{Cosm}$$

$$\text{Cosm} = \frac{0.030 \text{ mosm/ml} \times 16 \text{ ml/min}}{0.285 \text{ mosm/ml}} = 1.7 \text{ ml/min}$$

$$\text{CH}_2\text{O} = 16 - 1.7 = 14.3 \text{ ml/min}$$

The changes in fluid absorption along the nephron during diuresis and antidiuresis are depicted in Fig. 5-6.

A distinction should be drawn between *standard free water clearance* (CH_2O) and *electrolyte free water clearance* [$CH_2O(E)$].[165a] Standard clearance formulas use terms that include the *total* serum and the *total* urine osmolality, not the more physiologically relevant terms that use only the electrolyte contribution to total osmolalities. Measurements of total serum and urine osmolality incorporate values for all the solute present in solution; thus both *effective* and *ineffective* osmoles are included in these assays. Urea accounts for the vast bulk of the ineffective urinary osmoles. Since urea freely crosses cell membranes it cannot establish transcellular osmotic gradients and therefore does not influence water movement between body fluid compartments. Since the retention or excretion of urea does not influence the serum sodium concentration or the release of vasopressin, its inclusion in the terms used for serum and urine osmolality is not physiologically relevant. It should be replaced with the calculated terms for electrolyte osmolality. Serum electrolyte osmolality can be approximated by doubling the serum sodium concentration, whereas urinary electrolyte osmolality can be approximated by doubling the sum of sodium and potassium concentrations. When nonrenal metabolic acidosis is present, the contribution of $NH_4^+Cl^-$ should be included in the calculation.

These points are vividly illustrated by the common clinical setting of volume contraction and dehydration. Renal conservation of electrolytes and water in this circumstance spawns a concentrated urine of low volume containing minimal amounts of sodium and potassium. The hyperosmolality of this urine is accounted for by the presence of urea at high concentration. Excretion of 500 ml of this (relatively) electrolyte-free urea solution depletes body water by 500 ml and so raises the serum sodium concentration by an amount dictated by the loss of this amount of electrolyte-free water.

Formulas for calculating electrolyte-free water clearance are:

$$\text{CH}_2\text{O(E)} = V - \text{Cosm(E)}$$

and

$$\text{Cosm(E)} = \frac{U\text{osm(E)}V}{P\text{osm(E)}} = \frac{2(U\text{Na} + U\text{K})V}{2(P\text{Na})}$$

In recent years, the generation of a positive CH_2O during a maximal sustained water diuresis in dogs and humans has been used as an index of sodium chloride resorption in the diluting segment of the nephron, and maximal urine volume (V) under these conditions has been used as an index of sodium chloride delivery to this site(s). The anatomic location of this segment is not precisely known. In the state of physiologic diabetes insipidus (no apparent circulating AVP), it includes at least the thick ascending limb, and distal convoluted tubule, and the cortical collecting duct, and some have even included the medullary collecting duct. To use CH_2O and V in this manner as an approximation of distal nephron sodium chloride resorption, one must assume little or no back-diffusion of water in the nephron beginning with the ascending limb. If this were true, urinary flow rate (V) would equal the rate at which fluid is delivered to the ascending limb. In recent years, to enhance the reliability and correctness of these calculations, the renal clearance of lithium has been utilized as a measure of maximal tubular sodium and water resorption. The lithium ion is almost totally resorbed in the proximal tubule, and thus, its clearance closely approximates the volume of sodium and water delivery to the descending limb of Henle's loop. If relatively early in the ascending limb the fluid becomes isosmotic and the sodium concentration is near that of glomerular filtrate, then V can be used to estimate the rate of sodium delivery to the subsequent diluting site $(V \times P\text{Na})/\text{GFR} \times P\text{Na} = V/\text{GFR}$ = percentage of filtered water or sodium delivered to the "diluting site." If we further assume that sodium resorption at this site accounts for the dilution of the urine, then $CH_2O \times P\text{Na}$ = the amount of sodium resorbed in the diluting segment(s), and

$$\frac{CH_2O \times P\text{Na}}{\text{GFR} \times P\text{Na}} = \frac{CH_2O}{\text{GFR}}$$

and therefore the fraction of filtered sodium resorbed at the diluting site. Also,

$$\frac{CH_2O/\text{GFR}}{V/\text{GFR}} = \frac{CH_2O}{V}$$

or the fraction of filtered sodium delivered to the diluting site that is resorbed.

As mentioned earlier, these calculations and the assumptions upon which they are based have been widely utilized in humans and animals because of their simplicity and analytic reliability. Unfortunately, the assumptions are incorrect, and Jamison and Kriz, in their most comprehensive monograph,[113] have described why this is so. Their analysis deserves to be quoted in its entirety:

> It has become increasingly clear, however, that of the foregoing assumptions at least two are not even good approximations. At the end of the thick ascending limb, the point where obligatory water reabsorption ends and facultative water reabsorption begins, the percentage of filtered water has been found to be 30 percent in the dog and 25 percent in the monkey, rather than the 8 to 15 percent estimated from V/GFR. Furthermore, in studies of the Brattleboro rat, a strain with hereditary hypothalamic diabetes insipidus in a state of perpetual water diuresis, the fraction of filtered water remaining at the beginning of the collecting tubule system was 20 percent, which declined to 10 percent at the end, indicating that the reabsorption of water along the collecting tubule system amounted to 10 percent of the GFR. This finding could not be accounted for by a disproportionately lower delivery of water to the collecting tubule system from the juxtamedullary nephron than from the superficial nephron since in another study of rats, approximately 1.5 percent of filtered water was reabsorbed in the terminal millimeter of the collecting duct system alone. These findings indicate that even in maximum water diuresis (absence of ADH), substantial water reabsorption occurs beyond the supposed diluting site.
>
> The assumption that dilution by NaCl reabsorption occurs exclusively in the thick ascending limb was also shown to be incorrect. The Brattleboro rat experiments cited above disclosed that the average osmolality of fluid entering the beginning of the collecting duct, 94 mosm/kg H_2O, was reduced to 65 mosm/kg H_2O in the final urine and was entirely accounted for by the reabsorption of sodium and an accompanying anion equivalent to 5 percent of the filtered load, indicating that the collecting tubule also participates in the process of urinary dilution. Similar findings were reported by Sonnenberg[214] in the rat in vivo and by Hanley and Kokko in the isolated cortical collecting duct of rabbit perfused in vitro.[94]
>
> How important to the interpretation of CH_2O is the disclosure that at least two assumptions are incorrect? It was estimated, for example, that CH_2O underestimates sodium reabsorption by the thick ascending limb by as much as 40 percent.[118] Of greater significance, however, is the fact that fractional sodium reabsorption by the thick ascending limb and distal tubule is higher and that by the collecting duct system lower in antidiuresis than in water diuresis.[114] Malnic et al.[149] found, for example, that in the collecting duct approximately 1.5 percent of the filtered sodium is reabsorbed in antidiuresis, while, as noted above,[114] in water diuresis three times as much sodium was reabsorbed by the same segment. *Thus the induction of water diuresis alters segmental sodium reabsorption—* reducing it in the distal tubule and increasing it in the collecting tubule. A reasonable explanation for this phenomenon is that the sodium concentration in the distal tubule fluid cannot be lowered below a certain minimum value.[149,232] When the volume of fluid remaining in the distal tubule is increased in water diuresis, less sodium is reabsorbed by that segment and more is delivered to the collecting duct, which reabsorbs the extra sodium to maintain sodium balance.
>
> In summary, while the use of CH_2O probably is a reliable estimate of directional change in overall sodium reabsorption by the thick ascending limb-distal tubule-collecting duct system, it cannot be used as a quantitative measure of sodium reabsorption by the thick ascending limb. In man, of course, a more precise index is unavailable.

The negative free-water clearance, or T^cH_2O, that is,

$$T^cH_2O = -CH_2O = \text{Cosm} - V$$
$$= V \times U\text{osm}/P\text{osm} - 1$$

is a reasonable estimate of one component of the concentrating process, the magnitude of the abstraction of free water from the isosmotic luminal fluids in the process of forming a urine hypertonic to the simultaneously measured plasma. From all the available in vivo micropuncture studies, the sites in the mammalian nephron where ADH-induced water resorption changes the luminal fluid from hypotonic to isotonic and then to hypertonic are the cortical and medullary collecting ducts, respectively. This process will now be examined in detail.

VASOPRESSIN: STRUCTURE AND CELLULAR ACTION

The ADH vasopressin (see Chap. 4) is depicted in Fig. 5-7. In most mammalian species, including humans, position 8 is occupied by arginine; in the pig and several nonmammalian species lysine is substituted. AVP is composed of a cyclic hexapeptide, the ring of which is closed by a disulfide bond, and a linear tripeptide tail. The conformation of the molecule includes two beta turns, each composed of four amino acids.[228,229] All peptide bonds display the *trans* configuration;[79] significant intramolecular hydrogen bonding occurs within the ring structure.[230]

The sequence of events culminating in increased water permeability of the luminal membrane is initiated by the binding of AVP to a specific receptor on the basolateral cell membrane. The conformational factors responsible for the binding process and the subsequent initiation of biological activity have been partially elucidated. The side chains of each of the four amino acids located in the corner positions of the beta turns appear critical for binding of the molecule to its receptor; of these, asparagine is the most important.[233] Conversely, the basic moiety in position 8 (either arginine or lysine) and the carboxamide group of asparagine in position 5 are critical to the intrinsic activity of the hormone.[67] A few other generalizations regarding structure-activity relationships may be made. No single amino acid is absolutely essential for biological activity; however, any modification of the asparagine residue leads to a diminution of activity.[190,195] If the length of the side chain is altered (either increased or decreased), biological activity is decreased but not completely lost.[15] While a ring configuration in some form is essential for biological activity, neither the size of the ring nor the presence of a disulfide bond is an absolute requirement.[191] Deamination of cysteine in position 1 and lipophilic substitution of the side chain in position 4 both increase the antidiuretic-to-pressor activity ratio of the molecule.[235] Finally, replacement of L-arginine in position 8 with D-arginine (DAVP) further increases the antidiuretic-pressor activity ratio.[194] Thus, in comparison to AVP, 1-deamino-8-D-AVP (dDAVP) has a longer duration of action, three times the antidiuretic effect, and reduced pressor activity; and 1-deamino-4-valine (8-D-AVP), abbreviated dVDAVP, has a more prolonged duration of action, four times the antidiuretic potency, and undetectable pressor effects, making it the most specific antidiuretic peptide reported.[194]

Arginine-vasopressin

Cys-Tyr-Phe-Glu(NH_2)-Asp(NH_2)-Cys-Pro-Arg-Gly-NH_2

FIGURE 5-7 • Amino acid sequence of arginine vasopressin.

MECHANISM OF VASOPRESSIN ACTION

The first step in the action of vasopressin (Fig. 5-8) on its target tissues in the kidney requires binding to its receptor. Studies directed at characterizing the ADH receptor have been performed with membrane preparations of porcine, bovine, and rat kidneys utilizing tritiated lysine and AVP.[117] Unfortunately, these membrane preparations are heterogeneous with respect to their cellular origin. Furthermore, they lack the intracellular machinery that is potentially important in the regulation of surface receptors. Cells of porcine origin have been studied both in monolayer and in suspension.[187] The K_d value of 5 to 20 nM is in excellent agreement with those reported earlier.[117] A dimeric ADH receptor has been postulated, with receptor transition from high affinity to low affinity occurring upon hormone binding to the first dimer.[187] This transition could serve to increase the likelihood of uniform adenylyl cyclase activation along the collecting tubule by limiting receptor occupancy within a certain radius of the already occupied receptor and allowing binding elsewhere in preferential fashion.[188] While these studies are intriguing, they too were performed in cells of undefined origin. Further studies in other, more physiological systems would be of great interest.

Binding of AVP to its receptor results in increased adenylyl cyclase activity, which, provided sufficient magnesium is present,[78] catalyzes the formation of adenosine cyclic 3′,5′-monophosphate (cAMP) from adenosine triphosphate (ATP). The AVP receptor is coupled to the catalytic unit of adenylyl cyclase by the stimulatory guanine nucleotide-binding regulatory protein, G_s.[78,156] This is a heterotrimeric protein whose α subunit binds and hydrolyzes GTP. In the absence of AVP the α chain is bound to GDP and does not stimulate the catalytic unit. Receptor occupancy catalyzes the exchange of GDP for GTP; this results in a conformational change in the α subunit that allows it to stimulate the catalytic unit to form cAMP. Hydrolysis of the bound nucleotide then returns the system to the inactive state. In similar fashion, the activity of the catalytic unit is subject to modulation by G_i, a family of proteins that mediate inhibition of

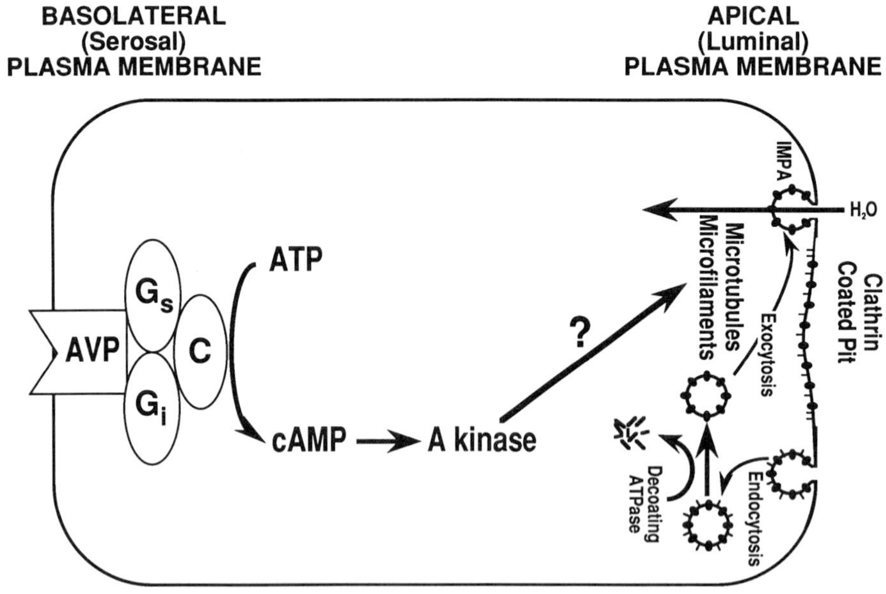

FIGURE 5-8 • Schematic representation of the cellular action of vasopressin. AVP, arginine vasopressin; G_s,G_i, stimulatory and inhibitory guanine nucleotide-binding regulatory proteins; C, catalytic unit of adenylyl cyclase; ATP, adenosine triphosphate; cAMP, cyclic adenosine monophosphate; A kinase, cyclic nucleotide-dependent protein kinase; IMPA, intramembrane particle aggregates. See text for details. (Modified from Brown D: *Am J Physiol* 256:F1–F12, 1989.)

adenylyl cyclase.[78,156] The exotoxin of *Bordetella pertussis* catalyzes ADP-ribosylation of a cysteine residue near the carboxyl terminus of the G protein ∝ chain.[78,156] This prevents receptor stimulation of G_i and results in the elimination of G_i-mediated inhibition of cyclase. In addition to G proteins, the activity of vasopressin-sensitive adenylyl cyclase is apparently modulated by calmodulin.[6]

The AVP-induced increase in adenylyl cyclase activity results in heightened cAMP formation, which ultimately causes the apical (luminal) cell membrane to become more permeable to water.[52] Administration of exogenous cAMP or its analogues mimics the effect of ADH on the collecting tubule,[56,85] as does inhibition of cAMP phosphodiesterase with either theophylline[86] or the synthetic analogue 1-methyl-3-isobutyl-xanthine (MIX).[51] Whereas the pivotal role played by cAMP has been clearly demonstrated, details of the mechanism beyond this point are uncertain. cAMP activates protein kinase(s) in a dose-dependent fashion;[54,63] protein kinase activity correlates well with the observed increase in apical permeability.[196] While preliminary data do support a functional role for activation of protein kinase A in the hydroosmotic response to AVP,[213] it has yet to be determined whether the increase in protein kinase activity is directly responsible for the increase in permeability or is merely an epiphenomenon reflecting the metabolic status of the cell.

The role of the cytoskeleton in the hydro-osmotic response to vasopressin is under investigation. The two most important components of the cytoskeletal system are microfilaments (actin filaments) and microtubules. Microfilaments consist of two strands of globular molecules about 4 nm in diameter twisted into a helix; microtubules are much larger structures formed by the organization of 13 tubulin protofilaments into a cylinder. Both microfilaments and microtubules appear to be necessary for the proper expression of vasopressin action. Toad bladders exposed to inhibitors of either microtubules (e.g., colchicine, vinblastine, or podophyllotoxin) or microfilaments (e.g., cytochalasin B) exhibit marked attenuation of osmotic water flow in response to vasopressin or exogenous cAMP.[223] It must be pointed out, however, that the effect of colchicine may in part be due to stimulation of prostaglandin synthesis. Pretreatment of toad bladders with cyclo-oxygenase inhibitors completely reversed the inhibitory effects of colchicine on vasopressin-stimulated water flow.[33] Cyclo-oxygenase inhibition failed to reverse inhibition of cAMP-stimulated water flow, suggesting a dual mode of action for colchicine. Intraperitoneal administration of colchicine or vinblastine prevents urinary concentration in the rat despite normal levels of adenylyl cyclase, cAMP phosphodiesterase, and protein kinase activity.[53] These observations permit one to speculate on the role of protein kinase, namely, that protein phoshorylation by protein kinase is necessary for the aggregation and action of microtubules and microfilaments.[221]

Freeze fracture electron microscopy has demonstrated the formation of characteristic intramembranous particle aggregates (IMPAs) in the protoplasmic surface of toad bladder or collecting duct apical membranes in response to ADH[26,40,95,123] or exogenous cAMP.[58,119] These IMPAs obey a dose-response relationship to vasopressin and dissipate upon withdrawal of the hormone.[96] They correlate numerically with, and are specific for, vasopressin-induced osmotic water flow.[58,119,124] IMPA formation and ADH-induced osmotic water flow exhibit similar temperature dependence;[122] likewise, the time course of intramembranous particle aggregation most likely parallels that of water flow.[62,121,123] The previously described decrease in ADH-induced osmotic water flow in the presence of microtubule or microfilament inhibitors is accompanied by a decrease in the number and surface density of IMPAs.[120] Once the response to vasopressin is established, however, subsequent administration of microtubule inhibitors is without effect, while microfilament inhibitors do diminish the response. This suggests that both microtubules and microfilaments are required for the initiation of intramembrane particle aggregation but that only microfilaments are needed for their maintenance.[120] As depicted in Fig. 5-8, IMPAs exist as preformed structures in the membranes of subapical intracytoplasmic organelles. They are inserted into the apical cell membrane in response to ADH[101,163] via a process akin to exocytosis. When ADH is withdrawn, they are retrieved from the membrane in clathrin-coated pits via a process akin to endocytosis.[5,29,230] The fusion of these organelles with the apical membrane requires microtubules;[163] it has been suggested that microtubules may act as "tracks" guiding the movement of cytoplasmic organelles.[164] This could perhaps explain the need for microtubules in the fusion process but not for the maintenance of the aggregates.

ADH causes an increase in the number of small (0.1- to 0.2-nm) aqueous channels, or pores, in the apical membrane rather than increasing the size of such channels or diffusely altering membrane fluidity.[92,98] Evidence in support of this concept is derived from studies of proton conductance[80] and examination of the relative changes in permeability to lipophilic solutes and water in response to ADH (i.e., molecular sieving[68]). Protons in aqueous solution travel by "jumping" from one water molecule to another. If ADH induces aqueous pores, it should also increase proton conductance, since protons will be able to "jump" from a water molecule in the bulk solution to another in the pore. On the other hand, if ADH increases water permeability by virtue of a generalized increase in membrane fluidity, there would be no increase in proton conductance, since the dielectric constant* of even very fluid lipids is low. In the toad bladder, vasopressin induces a threefold increase in proton conductance.[80] In artificial lipid bilayer membranes, the ratio of the diffusional water permeability coefficient (Pd_w) to the permeability coefficient of a small lipophilic solute (Pd_s) remains constant over a wide range of conditions. The finding that the Pd_w/Pd_s ratio in toad urinary bladder increases approximately 25-fold in the presence of ADH is most consistent with an increased number of small aqueous channels.[68] It has been determined over a range of temperatures that 6 to 20 molecules of water in single file occupy each channel.[98,143]

As previously mentioned, IMPA formation and osmotic water flow are similarly temperature-dependent,[122] exhibit a similar time course,[119] and are both decreased in the presence of microtubule or microfilament inhibitors.[120] These observations suggest that the IMPAs are the actual sites of water flow. (At 45 to 60 nm in diameter, the aggregates are clearly too large to be the actual pore; they may, however, house smaller channels within them.) The recent observation that toad bladders treated with a mild nonionic surfactant display a reversible decrease in ADH-induced osmotic water flow, correlating with a decrease in the number of IMPAs, lends support to this hypothesis.[181] Recent studies utilizing fluorescent fluid-phase markers have confirmed the presence of water channels in IMPAs.[5,230] Studies aimed at identifying the protein contents of IMPAs and elucidating the factors that control their membrane cycling are currently in progress.

* The dielectric constant of a medium is the ratio of the flux density of electric lines of force through a medium to that through a vacuum.

MODULATION OF AVP ACTION

An increasing number of factors have been recognized as capable of modulating the hydro-osmotic effect of AVP. They include a number of hormones, drugs, and metabolic abnormalities. Some of these factors are discussed below.

Hormonal factors

Catecholamines

Given systemically to the dog, rat, or humans, alpha-adrenergic agonists cause a diuresis,[70,146,197] while beta-adrenergic agonists cause an anti-diuresis.[19,141,198] Given intrarenally[197,198] or to a hypophysectomized subject,[19,197] they are without effect, suggesting that the effect of systemically administered catecholamines on water excretion is exerted via changes in vasopressin release. However, studies in the amphibian bladder demonstrated that while adrenergic agents alone do not alter apical membrane water permeability, they do change the membrane's response to vasopressin. Alpha-adrenergic stimulation decreases the hydro-osmotic response to ADH or theophylline but not to exogenous cAMP, indicating that it interferes with adenylyl cyclase stimulation.[12,91] Likewise, studies in the isolated cortical collecting tubule have shown that alpha agonists decrease AVP-induced cAMP accumulation,[39] resulting in diminished water resorption.[134] This appears to occur more specifically by an alpha$_2$-adrenergic effect.[135,226] Alpha$_2$-adrenergic inhibition of AVP-stimulated adenylyl cyclase activity in cultured inner medullary collecting duct cells does not occur in cells pretreated with pertussis toxin, indicating that inhibition is transduced by a member of the G_i family of guanine nucleotide-binding regulatory proteins.[226] Similarly, pertussis toxin significantly attenuates alpha$_2$-adrenergic inhibition of AVP-stimulated water flux in isolated perfused rabbit cortical collecting ducts.[180] The role played by beta agonists is not as well defined; while toad bladder and collecting duct studies have demonstrated an increase in cAMP accumulation,[12,220] no hydro-osmotic effect has been observed in the isolated perfused tubule.[134] It appears, therefore, that an intrarenal effect of beta-adrenergic stimulation to enhance water resorption is not operant in vivo.

Prostaglandins

While the cell or cells responsible for prostaglandin (see Chap. 15) production have not been fully identified, the renal papilla and, to a somewhat lesser degree, the renal medulla are clearly sites of prostaglandin (primarily PGE_2) synthesis.[60] A number of in vivo and in vitro studies have addressed the question of whether AVP stimulates renal prostaglandin synthesis.[13] In vivo studies in the rat clearly demonstrated an increase in PGE_2 and $PGF_{2\alpha}$ excretion following ADH administration. This effect is not due to the vasoconstrictor action of ADH, since it is observed with dDAVP as well.[59] Results in other species, including the dog, are less consistent. Thus, while some have noted an effect in humans,[61] others have not.[13] The effects of ADH on prostaglandin synthesis in in vitro systems, including the toad bladder,[22,240] isolated collecting duct,[109] and cell culture[88] are likewise inconsistent, but the majority of studies seem to suggest a stimulatory effect.

While there is little controversy that prostaglandins antagonize ADH action,[1,170,231] a number of mechanisms could account for this observation. A mechanism involving an effect on the adenylyl cyclase system has received considerable experimental support from in vitro experiments.[86] In cultured canine cortical collecting duct cells, low concentration of PGE_2 antagonizes vasopressin-mediated cAMP production.[76] This appears to be due to coupling of the PGE_2 receptor to the inhibitory guanine nucleotide-binding protein, G_i.[165,215] Recent evidence suggests a possible role for PGE_2-mediated activation of protein kinase C as well.[97] A mechanism involving a decrease in interstitial tonicity by (1) decreased urea reabsorption from the inner medullary collection duct,[239] (2) decreased sodium chloride reabsorption in the medullary thick ascending limb,[219] or (3) increased medullary blood flow[126] could also be operant in vivo (Fig. 5-9).

Thromboxanes

Thromboxanes (see Chap. 15) are a class of compounds derived from arachidonic acid that are closely related to the prostaglandins. Like prostaglandin production, thromboxane production increases upon administration of AVP.[31,32] Thromboxane B_2 increases AVP-induced water flow sevenfold.[30] Furthermore, inhibition of thromboxane synthesis by imidazole results in a significant decrease in AVP-stimulated water flow.[34] It should

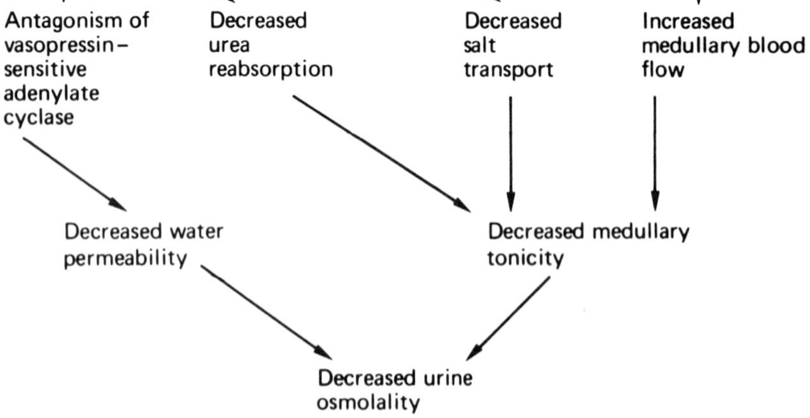

FIGURE 5-9 • Possible mechanisms whereby prostaglandins may impair the urinary concentrating ability. (From Beck TR, Dunn NJ: *Miner Electrolyte Metab* 6:46, 1981. Used by permission.)

be emphasized, however, that at present these findings are confined to toad bladder studies; thus, relevance to the hydro-osmotic effect of AVP on the mammalian collecting duct remains to be determined.

Kinins

Both exogenously administered and endogenously released kinins (see Chap. 15) possess significant diuretic activity.[166] The mechanism responsible for this diuretic effect is uncertain. In vivo, bradykinin has been reported to stimulate secretion of AVP,[183] whereas administration of AVP has been reported to have either no effect upon[23] or to increase[65] urinary kallikrein excretion. It is clear, however, that in the amphibian bladder either administration of bradykinin or kinase inhibition decreases vasopressin-stimulated water flow,[38,74] while kallikrein inhibition by aprotinin significantly increases the hydro-osmotic effect of AVP.[37] This antagonistic relationship between AVP and the kinin system may be due to the ability of bradykinin to stimulate phospholipase A_2[76,204] or C.[48,203] Studies in the perfused cortical collecting tubule of the rabbit suggest a prostaglandin-mediated effect.[199] As with thromboxanes, the relevance of these findings to the mammalian collecting duct remains to be elucidated.

Adrenal steroids

Though not recognized as often as the defect in urinary diluting capacity, adrenal insufficiency is also associated with a diminution in urinary concentrating ability in both humans and experimental animals.[45,201,205,237] Initially thought to be due to decreased medullary tonicity,[45,205] it now appears that the major defect is a reduction in tubular responsivity to vasopressin. Toad bladder studies have demonstrated an increase in vasopressin-stimulated water flow in the presence of adrenal steroids (see Chap. 14),[93,218] and a recent study examining the water permeability characteristics of isolated perfused cortical collecting tubules removed from adrenalectomized rabbits revealed a marked decrease in vasopressin-stimulated water flow, which corrected upon addition of either a mineralocorticoid (deoxycorticosterone) or a glucocorticoid (dexamethasone) to the tubular perfusate.[201] Coupled with the observations that the defect in vasopressin-stimulated water flow is corrected by inhibition of phosphodiesterase activity and that the response to exogenous cAMP is unaltered,[201] these findings strongly suggest a decrease in cAMP accumulation, most likely due to enhanced phosphodiesterase activity in the absence of adrenal steroids. This has been confirmed[108] by the direct measurement of cAMP phosphodiesterase activity in the papillary collecting duct of adrenalectomized rats.

Adrenal insufficiency may interfere with vasopressin-stimulated water flow by two other mechanisms as well: (1) some investigators have reported diminished vasopressin-sensitive adenylyl cyclase activity in the absence of adrenal steroids, although this is not a uniform finding;[108,138,177] and (2) in the toad bladder, glucocorticoid deficiency is associated with increased prostaglandin synthesis, which may, as noted above, attenuate the hydro-osmotic response to vasopressin.[242]

Electrolyte changes

Hypokalemia

Hypokalemia (see Chap. 22) has long been known to cause polyuria and diminished renal concentrating ability.[179] Polyuria appears prior to any detectable defect in urinary concentration and is due to a primary effect of potassium depletion to stimulate water intake.[20] It is clear, however, from a number of observations that a renal concentrating defect that is independent of the high rate of water turnover eventually supervenes. These observations include the demonstration of normal vasopressin levels in hypokalemic subjects,[16] the occurrence of the concentrating defect in hypokalemic rats whose water intake has been restricted to match that of normokalemic controls,[20] and the observation that exogenous vasopressin fails to correct the concentrating defect.[100a] Much speculation as to the nature of this defect has centered on the known decrease in medullary interstitial tonicity in hypokalemia.[16,84] The mechanism underlying the decreased tonicity remains to be elucidated, but is most likely a consequence of a decrease in sodium chloride reabsorption in the thick ascending limb.[89] However, the elaboration of hypotonic urine by hypokalemic dogs[77] and humans[189] irrefutably implicates a defect in the collecting duct's response to vasopressin, independent of the decreased but still hypertonic medullary tonicity. This effect is not mediated by prostaglandins, since inhibition of their synthesis with indomethacin does not improve urinary concentrating ability in the hypokalemic rat.[18] Thus, a direct effect of hypokalemia on the collecting tubule is likely. Indeed, studies in the toad bladder have shown decreased vasopressin-stimulated water flow when potassium is removed from the bathing solution.[69] Similarly, papillary collecting ducts of hypokalemic rats exhibit diminished diffusional water permeability in response to vasopressin as compared to normokalemic controls.[36] This is associated with decreased cAMP accumulation, apparently due to decreased adenylyl cyclase activity.[125] The observation in the toad bladder that the hydro-osmotic response to exogenous cAMP is inhibited in the absense of potassium[69] raises the possibility of a "postcyclic" defect as well; the nature of such defect, if present, is unknown.

Hypercalcemia

Hypercalcemia (see Chap. 32) is another well-recognized cause of impaired urinary concentrating ability.[225] Although polydipsia may contribute,[142] the defect is primarily intrarenal. A decrement in medullary tonicity is undoubtedly present[7,142] and is most likely related to a decrement in solute reabsorption in the thick ascending limb.[174] This defect is also associated with an impairment in AVP-stimulated adenylyl cyclase in this segment.[17] The elaboration of urine hypotonic to plasma in the presence of vasopressin[64] implies a defect intrinsic to the collecting tubule. Toad bladder studies have demonstrated a direct effect of increased serosal calcium on adenylyl cyclase activity, resulting in a decreased hydro-osmotic response to vasopressin with no effect on the response to exogenous cAMP. The vasopressin-dependent osmotic permeability coefficient (Pf) was found to be decreased in the papillary collecting duct of hypercalcemic rats;[36] no change in cAMP accumulation was observed, however, implying a postcyclic defect. Studies in the isolated perfused cortical collecting duct have yielded conflicting results, with increases in the bath calcium concentration reported both to increase[81] and decrease[73] osmotic water flow.

An increase in cellular calcium appears to decrease the hydroosmotic[2] and cAMP stimulating effect of vasopressin.[225] Administration of verapamil (calcium channel blocker) decreases cellular calcium uptake and decreases vasopressin-stimulated water flow in the toad bladder while increasing cAMP-stimulated water flow.[102] The latter effect is presumably due to phosphodiesterase inhibition by verapamil. Three structurally dissimilar calcium channel blockers were shown to inhibit vasopressin-stimulated water flow.[145] This effect is at least in part independent of calcium fluxes, since the drugs were shown to decrease cAMP generation in cellular homogenates and membrane-free supernates as well.

The ubiquitous calcium-binding protein calmodulin has recently been suggested to be of importance in vasopressin-stimulated water flow. In the toad bladder, trifluoperazine (TFP, a phenothiazine with known calmodulin-inhibiting properties has been shown to decrease osmotic water flow in response to vasopressin, cAMP, or MIX.[9,144] Diminished flow with MIX implies a postcyclic defect, an assumption that is corroborated by the finding that IMPA frequency is decreased 50 percent in TFP-treated bladders.[144] Evidence has also been proffered for a precyclic role for calmodulin based upon studies performed on renal cells of porcine origin (LLC-PK_1) grown in culture in which calmodulin enhanced adenylate cyclase activity.[6]

In summary, the precise cellular mechanisms responsible for the effects of calcium on vasopressin-stimulated water flow have not been fully elucidated.

TABLE 5-6 • Pharmacologic agents that alter vasopressin action

Agents that inhibit the peripheral action of vasopressin	Agents that potentiate the peripheral action of vasopressin
Lithium[207]	Nonsteroidal anti-inflammatory agents (short-term)[1]
Demeclocycline[205]	Acetaminophen[168]
Colchicine[223]	Chlorpropamide[4]
Vinblastine[223]	Tolbutamide[66]
Methoxyflurane[43]	
Glyburide, acetohexamide, and tolazamide[161]	
Amphotericin B[49]	
Gentamicin[82]	
Propoxyphene[27]	
Furosemide and ethacrynic acid[222]	
Radiocontrast agents[131]	

Pharmacologic agents

A number of pharmacologic agents are known to either enhance or impair the renal action of vasopressin (Table 5-6). This section briefly dicusses four drugs that are employed therapeutically because of their ability to alter water excretion.

Chlorpropamide

Chlorpropamide (see Chaps. 20 and 21) is known to increase urinary concentrating ability and decrease urine volume in patients with central, but not nephrogenic, diabetes insipidus.[4,153] Studies in both humans and rats with central diabetes insipidus have suggested that low levels of endogenous vasopressin are required for chlorpropamide to function.[21,155] Chlorpropamide was therefore felt to increase either secretion of or tubular responsiveness to the remaining vasopressin. However, no change in plasma vasopressin was demonstrable in a group of subjects receiving intravenous chlorpropamide.[103] Toad bladder studies have demonstrated an effect of chlorpropamide to enhance vasopressin or theophylline-stimulated water flow with no response to chlorpropamide alone.[107,154] Yet, cAMP levels were elevated in medullary tissue of rats fed chlorpropamide in vivo but were decreased in medullae exposed to chlorpropamide in vitro only.[11] In similar fashion, chlorpropamide caused a decrease in cAMP-stimulated water flow in the toad bladder,[147,154] although it has no effect on cAMP phosphodiesterase.[11,162] The possibility that the effects of chlorpropamide are mediated by an effect on prostaglandin inhibition has been proposed from studies in the toad bladder,[241] but has not been confirmed.

The results of a more recent study suggest that the enhanced response to vasopressin in chlorpropamide-treated animals is due to an effect of the drug to enhance solute resorption in the medullary ascending limb, thereby increasing interstitial tonicity and the osmotic drive for water resorption rather than to a cAMP-mediated alteration in collecting duct water permeability.[137]

Carbamazepine

The anticonvulsant drug carbamazepine (see Chaps. 20 and 21) is known to possess antidiuretic properties and has in fact been used in the treatment of diabetes insipidus.[99] Its mechanism of action is even less well understood than that of chlorpropamide. Plasma vasopressin levels were reported to be elevated in two patients with carbamazepine-induced water intoxication,[212] suggesting increased vasopressin secretion as the drug's mode of action. This concept is supported by the demonstration that carbamazepine alone had no effect on water flow in either the toad bladder or the rat with hereditary hypothalamic diabetes insipidus, whereas it did increase urinary osmolality and decrease the magnitude of diuresis in the normal water-diuresing rat.[227] However, other studies in humans[152,216] employing sensitive radioimmunoassay techniques have demonstrated low levels of AVP in patients taking carbamazepine; in one study, in fact, AVP levels fell during antidiuresis. Further investigation into this drug's mechanism is clearly needed.

Demeclocycline

Since it was first recognized as a cause of nephrogenic diabetes insipidus,[206] demeclocycline (see Chaps. 20 and 21) has become the drug of choice for the treatment of the syndrome of inappropriate ADH secretion.[72] It has yet to be determined if demeclocycline reduces AVP secretion. It is, however, clear that demeclocycline induces dose-dependent decreases in human renal medullary adenylyl cyclase activity[57] and in vasopressin-stimulated water flow in the toad bladder.[206] Demeclocycline also decreases cAMP-stimulated water flow,[206] implying the existence of a "postcyclic" defect. Indeed, in addition to its effects on cAMP generation, demeclocycline has been shown to decrease protein kinase activity; phosphodiesterase activity is mildly diminished as well.[57] The multiple sites of action suggest a mechanism mediated by the cation-chelating properties of the drug.[38] The role of prostaglandins in the action of demeclocycline is unclear; one study showed a modest decrease in polyuria when urinary prostaglandin E_2 excretion was decreased 60 percent by indomethacin.[202]

Lithium

By virtue of its widespread use in the treatment of affective disorders, lithium (see Chaps. 20 and 21) has emerged as perhaps the most common cause of nephrogenic diabetes insipidus.[178] Animal studies have demonstrated an effect of lithium to stimulate thirst very early in the course of its administration,[157,209] which is not evident later on.[8,71] The suggestion that lithium impairs vasopressin secretion from the pituitary[207] is not supported by the observation that in response to an infusion of hypertonic saline solution animals receiving lithium exhibit a similar degree of depletion of vasopressin from the hypophysis as control animals do.[100] Furthermore, plasma vasopressin levels in subjects on lithium are normal or increased,[8,71] implying a primary renal defect; indeed, both the rat[100]and humans[148] with lithium-induced diabetes insipidus are unresponsive to exogenous vasopressin. The mechanism underlying this defect is unclear. Despite its effect on sodium transport,[208] lithium apparently does not interfere with the accumulation of medullary solutes.[41] Thus, an intrinsic tubular defect is postulated. Lithium has been reported to decrease vasopressin-stimulated water flow in the toad bladder with no effect on cAMP-stimulated water flow, suggesting a defect in cAMP generation;[208] in fact, vasopressin-sensitive adenylyl cyclase activity was reported to be decreased in rat,[110] rabbit,[55] and human[50] medullary tissue in the presence of lithium. In another toad bladder study, however, lithium caused no change in vasopressin-stimulated water flow in the presence of theophylline,[14] suggesting that lithium may increase phosphodiesterase activity. Phosphodiesterase activity has been demonstrated to be increased in rat medullary tissue exposed to lithium.[10,110] Evidence exists also for a "postcyclic" defect, since rats with central diabetes insipidus, but not those treated with lithium, increased their urinary osmolality above that of plasma in response to dibutyryl cAMP.[71]

REFERENCES

1. Anderson RJ et al: Evidence for an in vivo antagonism between vasopressin and prostaglandin in the mammalian kidney. *J Clin Invest* 56:420, 1975.
2. Ando Y et al: Phorbol ester and A23187 have additive but mechanistically separate effects on vasopressin action in rabbit collecting tubule. *J Clin invest* 81:1578, 1988.
3. Andreoli TE et al: Questions and replies: Renal mechanisms for urinary concentrating and diluting processes. *Am J Physiol* 235:F1, 1978.
4. Arduino F et al: Antidiuretic action of chlorpropamide in idiopathic diabetes insipidus. *J Clin Endocrinol Metab* 26:1325, 1966.
5. Ausiello DA: Cellular biology of the water channel. *Kidney Int* 36:497, 1989.
6. Ausiello DA, Hall D: Regulation of vasopressin-sensitive adenylate cyclase by calmodulin. *J Biol Chem* 256:9796, 1981.

6a. Babiker MM, Rankin JE: Neurohypophyseal control of kidney function in the European (Anguilla-Anguilla L.) Adapted to sea water or fresh water. *Endocrinol* 76:347, 1958.

7. Bank N, Aynedjian HS: On the mechanism of hyposthenuria in hypercalcemia, *J Clin Invest* 44:681, 1965.

8. Baylis PH, Heath DA: Water disturbances in patients treated with oral lithium carbonate. *Ann Intern Med* 88:607, 1978.
9. Beauwens R, Rentmeesters M: Role of calmodulin in antidiuretic hormone mediated water transport. *Biochem Biophys Res Commun* 99:491, 1981.
10. Beck N, Davis BB: Effects of lithium on vasopressin-dependent cyclic AMP in rat renal medulla. *Endocrinology* 97:202, 1975.
11. Beck N et al: Effect of chlorpropamide on cyclic AMP in rat renal medulla. *Endocrinology* 95:771, 1974.
12. Beck N et al: Effects of catecholamines and their interaction with other hormones on cyclic 3′,5′-adenosine monophosphate of the kidney. *J Clin Invest* 51:939, 1972.
13. Beck TR, Dunn MJ: The relationship of antidiuretic hormone and renal prostaglandins. *Miner Electrolyte Metab* 6:46, 1981.
14. Bentley PJ, Wasserman A: The effects of lithium on the permeability of an epithelial membrane, the toad urinary bladder. *Biochim Biophys Acta* 226:285, 1972.
15. Berde B, Boissonnas RA: *Berde Handbook of Experimental Pharmacology,* in Berde B (ed): Berlin, Springer-Verlag, 1968.
16. Berl T: Water metabolism in potassium depletion. *Miner Electrolyte Metab* 4:209, 1980.
17. Berl T: The cAMP system in vasopressin sensitive nephron segments of the vitamin D treated rat. *Kidney Int* 31:1065, 1987.
18. Berl T et al: Renal concentrating defect in the hypokalemic rat is prostaglandin independent. *Am J Physiol* 238:F37, 1980.
19. Berl T et al: Effect of alpha and beta adrenergic stimulation on renal water excretion in normal subjects and patients with diabetes insipidus. *Kidney Int* 6:247, 1974.
20. Berl T et al: On the mechanism of polyuria in potassium depletion: The role of polydipsia. *J Clin Invest* 60:620, 1977.
21. Berndt WO et al: Potentiation of the antidiuretic effect of vasopressin by chlorpropamide. *Endocrinology* 86:1028, 1970.
22. Bisordi JE et al: Interaction of vasopressin and prostaglandins in the toad urinary bladder. *J Clin Invest* 66:1200, 1980.
23. Bonner G et al: The renal kallikrein-kinin system in Brattleboro rats with hereditary hypothalamic diabetes insipidus. *Acta Endocrinol* 98:36, 1981.
24. Bonventre JV, Lechene CP: Renal medullary concentrating process: an integrative hypothesis. *Am J Physiol* 239:F578, 1980.
25. Bonventre JV et al: Effect of urea concentration of pelvic fluid on renal concentrating ability. *Am J Physiol* 239:F609, 1980.
26. Bourguet J et al: Alterations in membrane-associated particle distribution during antidiuretic challenge in frog urinary bladder epithelium. *Biophys J* 16:627, 1976.
27. Bower BF et al: In vitro studies of the mechanism of polyuria induced by dextro propoxyphene (Darvon). *Proc Soc Exp Biol Med* 120:155, 1965.
28. Braun EJ: Glomerular filtration in birds: Its control. *Fed Proc* 41:2377, 1982.
29. Brown D: Membrane recycling and epithelial cell function. *Am J Physiol* 256:F1, 1989.
30. Burch RM, Halushka PV: Thromboxane and stable prostaglandin endoperoxide analogs stimulate water permeability in the toad urinary bladder. *J Clin Invest* 66:1251, 1980.
31. Burch RM, Halushka PV: Vasopressin stimulates prostaglandin and thromboxane synthesis in toad bladder epithelial cells. *Am J Physiol* 243:F593, 1982.
32. Burch RM et al: Vasopressin stimulates thromboxane synthesis in the toad urinary bladder: Effects of imidazole. *J Pharmacol Exp Ther* 210:344, 1979.
33. Burch RM, Halushka PV: Inhibition of prostaglandin synthesis antagonizes the colchicine-induced reduction of vasopressin-stimulated water flow in the toad urinary bladder. *Mol Pharmacol* 21:142, 1982.
34. Burch RM et al: Vasopressin-stimulated water flow is decreased by thromboxane synthesis inhibition or antagonism. *Am J Physiol* 239:F388, 1980.
35. Burg MB, Green N: Function of the thick ascending limb of Henle's loop. *Am J Physiol* 224:659, 1973.
36. Carney S et al: A study in vitro of the concentrating defect associated with hypokalemia and hypercalcemia. *Pfluegers Arch* 366:11, 1976.
37. Carvounis CP et al: Role of the endogenous kallikrein-kinin system in modulating vasopressin-stimulated water flow and urea permeability in the toad urinary bladder. *J Clin Invest* 67:1792, 1981.
38. Casell AH, Hutchison JD: Selectivity of cation chelation to tetracyclines: Evidence for special conformation of calcium chelate. *Biochem Biophys Res Commun* 43:625, 1971.
39. Chabardes D et al: Inhibition of alpha$_2$-adrenergic agonists on AVP-induced cAMP accumulation in isolated collecting tubule of the rat kidney. *Mol Cell Endocrinol* 37:263, 1984.
40. Chevalier J et al: Membrane associated particles: Distribution in frog urinary bladder epithelium at rest and after oxytocin treatment. *Cell Tissue Res* 152:129, 1974.
41. Christensen S: Acute and chronic effects of vasopressin in rats with lithium-polyuria. *Acta Pharmacol Toxicol* 38:241, 1976.
42. Chuang EL et al: Studies on the mechanism of reduced urinary osmolality after exposure of the renal papilla. *J Clin Invest* 61:633, 1978.
43. Churchill D et al: Persisting renal insufficiency after methoxyflurane anesthesia: A report of two cases and review of literature. *Am J Med* 56:575, 1974.
44. Clapp WL et al: Morphologic heterogeneity along the rat inner medullary collecting duct. *Lab Invest* 60:219, 1989.
45. Cooke CR, Steenburg RW: Effects of aldosterone and cortisol on the renal concentrating mechanism. *J Lab Clin Med* 82:784, 1973.
46. Culpepper RM, Andreoli TE: Interactions among prostaglandin E$_2$, antidiuretic hormone, and cyclic adenosine monophosphate in modulating Cl-absorption in single mouse medullary thick ascending limbs of Henle. *J Clin Invest* 71:1588, 1983.
47. Dantzler WH: Reptilian glomerular and tubular function and their control. *Fed Proc* 41:2371, 1982.

48. Dixon BS et al: Bradykinin activates protein kinase C in cultured collecting tubular cells. *Am J Physiol* 257:F808, 1989.
49. Douglas JB, Healy JK: Nephrotoxic effects of amphotericin B, including renal tubular acidosis. *Am J Med* 46:154, 1969.
50. Dousa TP: Interaction of lithium with vasopressin-sensitive cyclic AMP system of human renal medulla. *Endocrinology* 95:1359, 1974.
51. Dousa TP, in Martinez-Maldonado (ed): *Methods in Pharmacology, Renal Pharmacology*. New York, Plenum, 1976, vol 4.
52. Dousa TP: Cellular action of antidiuretic hormone. *Miner Electrolyte Metab* 5:144, 1981.
53. Dousa TP, Barnes LD: Effects of colchicine and vinblastine on the cellular action of vasopressin in mammalian kidney: A possible role of microtubules. *J Clin Invest* 54:252, 1974.
54. Dousa TP, Barnes LD: Regulation of protein kinase by vasopressin in renal medulla in situ. *Am J Physiol* 232:F50, 1977.
55. Dousa TP, Hechter O: The effect of sodium chloride and lithium chloride on vasopressin-sensitive adenylate cyclase: 1. *Life Sci* 9:765, 1970.
56. Dousa TP, Valtin H: Cellular actions of vasopressin in the mammalian kidney. *Kidney Int* 10:46, 1976.
57. Dousa TP, Wilson DM: Effects of demethylchlortetracycline on cellular action of antidiuretic hormone in vitro. *Kidney Int* 5:279, 1974.
58. Dratwa M et al: Intramembranous particle aggregation in toad urinary bladder after vasopressin stimulation. *Lab Invest* 40:46, 1979.
59. Dunn MJ et al: Renal excretion of prostaglandin E_2 and F_2 in diabetes insipidus rats. *Am J Physiol* 235:E624, 1978.
60. Dunn MJ, Zambraski FJ: The effects on the kidney of drugs which inhibit prostaglandin synthesis. *Kidney Int* 18:609, 1980.
61. Dusing R et al, in Samuelsson B et al (eds): *Advances in PG and Thromboxane Research*. New York, Raven Press, 1980, vol 7, pp 1111.
62. Edwards BR et al: Intramembranous particle clusters in collecting duct cells of rats. Influence of water balance. *Renal Physiol* 6:25, 1983.
63. Edwards et al: Protein kinase activity in isolated tubules of rat renal medulla. *Am J Physiol* 238:F269, 1980.
64. Epstein FH et al: Changes in renal concentrating ability produced by parathyroid extract. *J Clin Invest* 38:1214, 1959.
65. Fejes-Toth G et al: Effect of vasopressin on renal kallikrein excretion. *Am J Physiol* 239:F388, 1980.
66. Fichman MP, Brooker G: Deficient renal cyclic adenosine 3′-5′ monophosphate production in nephrogenic diabetes insipidus. *J Clin Endocrinol Metab* 35:35, 1972.
67. Fink ML, Bodansiszky Z: Synthesis and hormonal activities of 8-L-homonorleucine vasopressin. *J Med Chem* 16:1324, 1973.
68. Finkelstein A: Nature of the water permeability increase induced by antidiuretic hormone (ADH) in toad urinary bladder and related tissues. *J Gen Physiol* 68:137, 1976.
69. Finn AL et al: Relation between toad bladder potassium content and permeability response to vasopressin. *Am J Physiol* 210:1279, 1966.
70. Fisher DA: Norepinephrine inhibition of vasopressin antidiuresis. *J Clin Invest* 47:540, 1968.
71. Forrest JN Jr et al: On the mechanism of lithium-induced diabetes insipidus in man and the rat. *J Clin Invest* 53:1115, 1974.
72. Forrest JN Jr et al: Superiority of demeclocycline over lithium in the treatment of chronic syndrome of inappropriate secretion of antidiuretic hormone. *N Engl J Med* 298:173, 1978.
73. Frindt G et al: Hydroosmotic response of collecting tubules to ADH or cAMP at reduced peritubular sodium. *Am J Physiol* 243:F503, 1982.
74. Furtado MRF: Inhibition of the permeability response to vasopressin and oxytocin in the toad bladder: Effect of bradykinin, kallidin, eledoisin, and physalaemin. *J Membr Biol* 4:165, 1971.
75. Gamble JL et al: An economy of water in renal function referable to urea. *Am J Physiol* 109:139, 1934.
76. Garcia-Perez A, Smith WL: Apical-basolateral membrane asymmetry in canine cortical collecting tubule cells: Bradykinin, arginine vasopressin, prostaglandin E_2 interrelationships. *J Clin Invest* 74:63, 1984.
77. Giebisch G, Lozano R: The effects of adrenal steroids and potassium depletion on the elaboration of an osmotically concentrated urine. *J Clin Invest* 38:843, 1959.
78. Gilman AG: G proteins: Transducers of receptor-generated signals. *Ann Rev Biochem* 56:615, 1987.
79. Glickson JD et al: Method for correlation of proton magnetic resonance assignments in different solvents: Conformational transition of oxytocin and lysine vasopressin from dimethylsulfoxide to water. *Proc Natl Acad Sci U S A* 69:2566, 1972.
80. Gluck S, Al-Awqati Q: Vasopressin increases water permeability by inducing pores. *Nature* 284:631, 1980.
81. Goldfarb S: Effects of calcium on ADH action in the cortical collecting tubule perfused in vitro. *Am J Physiol* 243:F481, 1982.
82. Gordon JA et al: The renal concentrating defect after gentamicin administration in the rat. *J Lab Clin Med* 101:903, 1983.
83. Gottschalk CW, Mylle M: Micropuncture study of the mammalian urinary concentrating mechanism: Evidence for the countercurrent hypothesis. *Am J Physiol* 196:927, 1959.
84. Gottschalk CW et al: Osmolality of renal tubular fluids in potassium-depleted rodents. *Clin Sci* 29:249, 1965.
85. Grantham JJ, Burg MB: Effect of vasopressin and cyclic AMP on permeability of isolated collecting tubules. *Am J Physiol* 211:255, 1966.
86. Grantham JJ, Orloff J: Effect of prostaglandin E_1 on the permeability response of the isolated collecting tubule to vasopressin, adenosine 3′,5′-monophosphate and theophylline. *J Clin Invest* 47:1154, 1968.
87. Greger RF, Schlatter E: Coupled transport of $2Cl^-/Na^+/K^+$ of the luminal membrane of the rabbit thick ascending limb of Henle. *Kidney Int* 21:274, 1982.
88. Grenier FC et al: Kinin-induced prostaglandin synthesis

by renal papillary collecting tubule cells in culture. *Am J Physiol* 241:F94, 1981.
89. Gutsche HU et al: In vivo evidence of impaired solute transport by the thick ascending limb of potassium depleted rats. *J Clin Invest* 73:908, 1984.
90. Hall DA, Varney DM: Effect of vasopressin on electrical potential difference and chloride transport in mouse medullary thick ascending limb of Henle's loop. *J Clin Invest* 66:792, 1980.
91. Handler JS et al: Effect of adrenergic agents on toad bladder response to ADH, 3′,5′-cyclic AMP and theophylline. *Am J Physiol* 215:1024, 1968.
92. Handler JS, Orloff J: *Antiduretic hormone,* in Edelman IS, Schultz SG (eds): *Annual Reviews of Physiology.* Palo Alto: Annual Reviews, 1981, vol 43, p 611.
93. Handler JS et al: Effect of adrenal steroid hormones on the response of the toad's urinary bladder to vasopressin. *J Clin Invest* 48:823, 1969.
94. Hanley MJ, Kokko JP: A study of chloride transport across the rabbit collecting tubule. *J Clin Invest* 62:399, 1978.
95. Harmanci MC et al: Antidiuretic hormone-induced intramembranous alterations in mammalian collecting ducts. *Am J Physiol* 235:F440, 1978.
96. Harmanci MC et al: Vasopressin and collecting duct intramembranous particle clusters: a dose-response relationship. *Am J Physiol* 239:F560, 1980.
96a. Hays RM: Water transport in epithelia in urinary concentrating mechanisms, in Kinne RKH (ed): *Comp Physiology Ed.* Basel, Karger, 1990, vol 2, p 1.
97. Hebert RL et al: PGE_2 inhibits AVP induced water flow in cortical collecting ducts by protein kinase C activation. *Am J Physiol* 259:F318, 1990.
98. Hebert SC et al: The effects of antidiuretic hormone (ADH) on solute and water transport in the mammalian nephron. *J Membr Biol* 58:1, 1981.
99. Henry DA et al: Hyponatremia during carbamazepine treatment. *Br Med J* 1:83, 1977.
100. Hochman S, Gutman Y: Lithium: ADH antagonism and ADH independent action in rats with diabetes insipidus. *Eur J Pharmacol* 28:100, 1974.
100a. Hollander W Jr et al: Defect in the renal tubular reabsorption of water associated with potassium depletion in rats. *Am J Physiol* 189:557, 1957.
101. Humbert F et al: Particle aggregates in plasma and intracellular membranes of toad bladder (granular cell). *Experientia* 33:1364, 1977.
102. Humes HD et al: Effect of verapamil on the hydroosmotic response to antidiuretic hormone in toad urinary bladder. *Am J Physiol* 239:F250, 1980.
103. Huupponen R et al: Plasma AVP after intravenous chlorpropamide. *Int J Clin Pharmacol Ther Toxicol* 19:6, 1981.
104. Imai M, Kokko JP: Sodium chloride, urea, and water transport in the thin ascending limb of Henle: Generation of osmotic gradients by passive diffusion of solutes. *J Clin Invest* 53:393, 1974.
105. Imai M, Kokko JP: Mechanism of sodium and chloride transport in the thin ascending limb of Henle. *J Clin Invest* 58:1054, 1976.
106. Imai M et al: Transition of permeability properties along the descending limb of long-loop nephrons. *Am J Physiol* 254:F323, 1988.
107. Inglefinger JR, Hays RM: Evidence that chlorpropamide and vasopressin share a common site of action. *J Clin Endocrinol Metab* 29:738, 1969.
108. Jackson BA et al: Concentrating defect in the adrenalectomized rat: Abnormal vasopressin-sensitive cyclic adenosine monophosphate metabolism in the papillary collecting duct. *J Clin Invest* 72:997, 1983.
109. Jackson BA et al: Vasopressin-prostaglandin interactions in isolated tubules from rat outer medulla. *J Lab Clin Med* 96:119, 1980.
110. Jackson BA et al: Lithium-induced polyuria: Effect of lithium on adenylate cyclase and adenosine 3′,5′-monophosphate phosphodiesterase in medullary ascending limb of Henle's loop and in medullary collecting tubules. *Endocrinology* 107:1693, 1980.
111. Jacobson HR: Functional segmentation of the mammalian nephron. *Am J Physiol* 241:F203, 1981.
112. Jamison RL: Micropuncture study of segments of thin loops of Henle in the rat. *Am J Physiol* 215:236, 1968.
113. Jamison RL, Kriz W: *Urinary Concentrating Mechanism, Structure and Function.* New York, Oxford University Press, 1982.
114. Jamison RL, Lacy FB: Evidence for urinary dilution by the collecting tubule. *Am J Physiol* 223:898, 1972.
115. Jamison RL, Maffly RH: The urinary concentrating mechanism. *N Engl J Med* 295:1059, 1976.
116. Jamison RL, Oliver RE: Disorders of urinary concentration and dilution. *Am J Med* 72:308, 1982.
117. Jard S et al: Comparative studies with the ADH receptors from pig and rat kidney: Structure activity relationships and receptor-adenylate cyclase coupling. *Proceedings of the Seventh International Congress on Nephrology.* Basel, Karger, 1978, p 307.
118. Johnston PA et al: Evidence for a concentration gradient favoring outward movement of sodium from the thin loop of Henle. *J Clin Invest* 59:234, 1977.
119. Kachadorian WA et al: Time course of ADH-induced intramembranous particle aggregation in toad urinary bladder. *Am J Physiol* 234:F461, 1978.
120. Kachadorian WA et al: Possible roles for microtubules and microfilaments in ADH action on toad urinary bladder. *Am J Physiol* 236:F14, 1979.
121. Kachadorian WA et al: Relationship of aggregated intramembranous particles to water permeability in vasopressin-treated toad urinary bladders. *J Clin Invest* 59:576, 1977.
122. Kachadorian WA et al: Temperature dependence of ADH-induced water flow and intramembranous particle aggregates in toad bladder. *Science* 205:910, 1979.
123. Kachadorian WA et al: Vasopressin-induced structural change in toad bladder luminal membrane. *Science* 190:67, 1975.
124. Kachadorian WA et al: Membrane structural and functional responses to vasopressin in toad bladder. *J Membr Biol* 30:381, 1977.
125. Kim J, Berl T: The cyclic AMP system in the inner medullary collecting duct of the potassium depleted rat. *Kidney Int* 26:384, 1984.
126. Kirschenbaum MA et al: Redistribution of renal cortical

blood flow during inhibition of prostaglandin synthesis. *Am J Physiol* 227:801, 1974.

127. Knepper MA: Urea transport in isolated thick ascending limb and collecting ducts from rats. *Am J Physiol* 245:F634, 1983.
128. Knepper MA, Star R: The vasopressin regulated urea transporter in renal inner medullary collecting duct. *Am J Physiol* 259:F393, 1990.
129. Kokko JP, Rector FC Jr: Countercurrent multiplication system without active transport in inner medulla. *Kidney Int* 2:214, 1972.
130. Kondo Y, Imai M: Effect of glutaraldehyde on renal tubular function. II. Selective inhibition of Cl^- transport in the hamster thin ascending limb of Henle's loop. *Pflugers Arch* 408:484, 1987.
131. Kovnat PJ et al: Azotemia and nephrogenic diabetes insipidus after arteriography. *Radiology* 108:541, 1973.
132. Kriz W: Structural organization of the renal medulla: Comparative and functional aspects. *Am J Physiol* 241:R3, 1981.
133. Kriz W: Structural organization of the renal medullary counterflow system. *Fed Proc* 42:2379, 1983.
134. Krothapalli RK et al: Modulation of the hydro-osmotic effect of vasopressin on the rabbit cortical collecting tubule by adrenergic agents. *J Clin Invest* 72:287, 1983.
135. Krothapalli RK, Suki WN: Functional characterization of the alpha-adrenergic receptor modulating the hydro-osmotic effect of vasopressin on the rabbit cortical collecting tubule. *J Clin Invest* 73:740, 1984.
136. Kuhn W, Ryffel K: Herstellung Konzentrierter Losungen aus Verdunnten durch Blosse Membranwirkung: Ein Modellversuch zur Funktion der Niere. *Z Physiol Chem* 276:145, 1942.
137. Kusano E et al: Chlorpropamide action on renal concentrating mechanism in rats with hypothalamic diabetes insipidus. *J Clin Invest* 72:1298, 1983.
138. Lang MA, Edelman IS: Effects of aldosterone and vasopressin on adenyl cyclase activity of rat kidney. *Am J Physiol* 222:21, 1972.
139. Layton HE: Urea transport in a distributed model of the urinary concentrating mechanism. *Am J Physiol* 258: F1110, 1990.
140. Lenley KV, Kriz W: Cycles and separations. The histotopography of the urinary concentrating process. *Kidney Int* 31:538, 1987.
141. Levi J et al: Effect of isoproterenol on water diuresis in the rats with congenital diabetes insipidus. *Am J Physiol* 221:1728, 1971.
142. Levi M et al: Mechanism of concentrating defect in hypercalcemia: Role of polydipsia and prostaglandins. *Kidney Int* 23:489, 1983.
143. Levine SD et al: The water permeability of toad urinary bladder. *J Gen Physiol* 83:543, 1984.
144. Levine SD et al: Effects of trifluoperazine on function and structure of toad urinary bladder: Role of calmodulin in vasopressin-stimulation of water permeability. *J Clin Invest* 67:662, 1981.
145. Levine SD et al: Calcium flow-independent actions of calcium channel blockers in toad urinary bladder. *Am J Physiol* 244:C243, 1983.
146. Lieberman B et al: Effect of adrenergic blocking agents on the vasopressin inhibiting action of norepinephrine. *Proc Soc Exp Biol Med* 133:131, 1970.
147. Lozada ES et al: Studies of the mode of action of the sulfonylureas and phenylacetamides in enhancing the effect of vasopressin. *J Clin Endocrinol Metab* 34:704, 1972.
148. MacNeil S et al: Lithium and the antidiuretic hormone. *Br J Clin Pharmacol* 3:304, 1976.
149. Malnic G et al: Micropuncture study of distal tubular potassium and sodium transport in the rat nephron. *Am J Physiol* 211:529, 1966.
150. Marsh DJ: Solute and water flows in thin limbs of Henle's loop in the hamster kidney. *Am J Physiol* 218:824, 1970.
151. Marsh DJ, Azen SP: Mechanism of NaCl reabsorption by hamster thin ascending limbs of Henle's loops. *Am J Physiol* 228:71, 1975.
152. Meinders AE et al: Antidiuretic action of carbamazepine. *Clin Sci* 47:289, 1974.
153. Meinders AE et al: Chlorpropamide treatment in diabetes insipidus. *Lancet* 2:544, 1967.
154. Mendoza SA: Effect of chlorpropamide on the permeability of the urinary bladder of the toad and the response to vasopressin, adenosine-3′,5′-monophosphate and theophylline. *Endocrinology* 84:411, 1969.
155. Miller M, Moses AM: Mechanism of chlorpropamide action in diabetes insipidus. *J Clin Endocrinol Metab* 30:488, 1970.
156. Miller TR: Transmembrane signalling through G proteins. *Kidney Int* 39:421, 1991.
157. Mishkind MH et al: Studies of lithium induced polyuria (abstract). *Clin Res* 25:596A, 1977.
158. Molony DA et al: Na^+:K^+:$2Cl^-$ cotransport and the thick ascending limb. *Kidney Int* 36:418, 1989.
159. Morel F: Sites of hormone action in the mammalian nephron. *Am J Physiol* 240:F159, 1981.
160. Morgan T, Berliner RW: Permeability of the loop of Henle, vasa recta, and collecting duct to water, urea, and sodium. *Am J Physiol* 215:108, 1968.
161. Moses AM et al: Diuretic action of three sulfonylureas. *Ann Intern Med* 78:541, 1973.
162. Moses AM, Coulson R: Augmentation by chlorpropamide of 1-deamino-8-D-arginine vasopressin-induced antidiuresis and stimulation of renal medullary adenylate cyclase and accumulation of adenosine 3′,5′-monophosphate. *Endocrinology* 106:967, 1980.
163. Muller J et al: Evidence that ADH-stimulated intramembrane particle aggregates are transferred from cytoplasmic to luminal membranes in toad bladder epithelial cells. *J Cell Biol* 85:83, 1980.
164. Murphy DB, Tilney LG: The role of microtubules in the movement of pigment granules in teleost melanophores. *J Cell Biol* 61:757, 1974.
165. Nadler SP et al: PGE_2, forskolin, and cholera toxin interactions in rabbit cortical collecting tubule. *Am J Physiol* 250;F127, 1986.

165*a*. Narins RG et al: Polyuria: Simple and mixed disorders. *Am J Kidney Dis* 17:237, 1991.

166. Nasjletti A et al: Disappearance of bradykinin in the renal circulation of dogs: Effects of kininase inhibition. *Circ Res* 37:59, 1975.

167. Nishimura H, Masashi I: Control of renal function in fresh water and marine teleosts. *Fed Proc* 41:2355, 1982.
168. Nusynowitz ML, Forsham PH: The antidiuretic action of acetoaminophen. *Am J Med Sci* 252:429, 1966.
169. Oliver RE et al: Urinary concentration in the papillary collecting duct of the rat: Role of the ureter. *J Clin Invest* 59:157, 1982.
170. Orloff J, Zusman R: Role of prostaglandin E (PGE) in the modulation of the action of vasopressin on water flow in the urinary bladder of the toad and mammalian kidney. *J Membr Biol* 40:297, 1978.
171. Osgood RW et al: Further studies on segmental sodium transport in the rat kidney during expansion of the extracellular fluid volume. *J Clin Invest* 62:311, 1978.
172. Pang PKP et al: Endocrine and neural control of amphibian renal functions. *Fed Proc* 41:2365, 1982.
173. Pennell JP et al: An in vivo study of the concentrating process in the descending limb of Henle's loop. *Kidney Int* 5:337, 1974.
173a. Perks AM: The neurohypophysis: The place of comparative studies in biology and medicine, in Pang PKT et al (eds): *Vertebrate Endocrinology: Fundamentals and Biomedical Implications.* New York, Academic Press, 1989, vol 2, p 9.
174. Peterson LN: Vitamin D induced hypercalcemia inhibits thick ascending limb NaCl reabsorption in vivo. *Am J Physiol* 259:F122, 1990.
175. Philips JE: Hormonal control of renal function in insects. *Fed Proc* 41:2348, 1982.
176. Rabinowitz L et al: Effect of acute urea administration on urinary nonurea solute concentration. *Am J Physiol* 221:242, 1971.
177. Rajerison R et al: The vasopressin-sensitive andenylate cyclase of the rat kidney: Effect of adrenalectomy and corticosteroids on hormonal receptor-enzyme coupling. *J Biol Chem* 249:6390, 1974.
178. Ramsey TA, Cox M: Lithium and the kidney: A Review. *Am J Psychiatry* 139:443, 1982.
179. Relman AS, Schwartz WB: The kidney in potassium depletion. *Am J Med* 24:764, 1958.
180. Ribeiro CP et al: Prevention of α_2-adrenergic inhibition of ADH action by pertussis toxin in rabbit CCT. *Am J Physiol* 253:C105, 1987.
181. Ripoche P et al: Detergent extraction of membrane proteins related to the action of antidiuretic hormone. *Biochim Biophys Acta* 693:497, 1982.
182. Rocha AS, Kokko JP: Sodium chloride and water transport in the medullary thick ascending limb of Henle: Evidence for active chloride transport. *J Clin Invest* 52:612, 1973.
183. Rocha E et al: Release of antidiuretic hormone by bradykinin. *J Pharmacol Exp Ther* 146:24, 1964.
184. Roman RJ, Lechene C: Meclofenamate and urine concentration with and without exposure of the renal papilla. *Am J Physiol* 240:F423, 1981.
185. Rouffignac C de: Physiological role of the loop of Henle in urinary concentration. *Kidney Int* 2:297, 1972.
186. Rouffignac C de, Morel F: Micropuncture study of water, electrolytes, and urea movements along the loops of Henle in *Psammomys*. *J Clin Invest* 48:474, 1969.
187. Roy C, Ausiello DA: Characterization of (8-lysine)-vasopressin binding sites on a pig kidney cell line (LLC-PK_1): Evidence for hormone-induced receptor transition. *J Biol Chem* 256:3415, 1981.
188. Roy C et al: Relationship of (8-lysine)-vasopressin receptor transition to receptor functional properties in a pig kidney cell line (LLC-PK_1). *J Biol Chem* 256:3423, 1981.
189. Rubini ME: Water excretion in potassium deficient man. *J Clin Invest* 40:2215, 1961.
190. Rudinger J: The design of peptide hormone analogs, in Ariens EJ (ed): *Drug Design.* New York, Academic Press, 1971, vol 2, p 319.
191. Rudinger J, Jost K: A biologically active analog of oxytocin not containing a disulfide group. *Experientia* 20:570, 1964.
192. Sands JH, Knepper MA: Urea permeability of mammalian inner medullary collecting duct system and papillary surface epithelia. *J Clin Invest* 79:138, 1987.
193. Sands JM, Kokko JP: Countercurrent system. *Kidney Int* 38:695, 1990.
194. Sawyer WH et al: Structural changes in the arginine vasopressin molecule that enhance antidiuretic activity and specificity. *Endocrinology* 94:1106, 1974.
195. Sawyer WH, Manning M: Synthetic analogs of oxytocin and the vasopressins. *Annu Rev Pharmacol* 13:5, 1973.
196. Schlondorff D, Franki N: Effect of vasopressin on cyclic AMP-dependent protein kinase in toad urinary bladder. *Biochim Biophys Acta* 628:1, 1980.
196a. Schmidt-Nielsen B, Forster RP: Comparative physiology of electrolyte and water regulation with emphasis on sodium, potassium, chloride, urea, and osmotic pressure, in Maxwell MH, Kleeman CR (eds): *Clinical Disorders of Water and Electrolyte Metabolism,* 3d ed. New York, McGraw-Hill, 1980, p 37.
197. Schrier RW, Berl T: Mechanism of effect of alpha adrenergic stimulation with norepinephrine on renal water excretion. *J Clin Invest* 52:502, 1973.
198. Schrier RW et al: Mechanism of antidiuretic effect of beta adrenergic stimulation. *J Clin Invest* 51:97, 1972.
199. Schuster VL et al: Interactions of lysyl-bradykinin and antidiuretic hormone in the rabbit cortical collecting tubule. *J Clin Invest* 73:1659, 1984.
200. Schutz W, Schnermann J: Pelvic urine composition as a determinant of inner medullary solute concentration and urine osmolality. *Pfluegers Arch* 334:154, 1972.
201. Schwartz MJ, Kokko JP: Urinary concentrating defect of adrenal insufficiency: Permissive role of adrenal steroids on the hydroosmotic response across the rabbit cortical collecting tubule. *J Clin Invest* 66:234, 1980.
202. Serros ER et al: Effect of prostaglandin inhibition on demeclocycline administration in conscious rats. *Prostaglandins Med* 5:175, 1980.
203. Shayman JA, Morrison AR: Bradykinin-induced changes in phosphatidylinositol turnover in cultured rabbit papillary collecting tubule cells. *J Clin Invest* 76:987, 1985.
204. Shayman JA et al: Islet activating protein inhibits kinin-stimulated inositol phosphate production, calcium mobi-

lization, and prostaglandin E_2 synthesis in renal papillary collecting tubule cells independent of cyclic AMP. *J Biol Chem* 262:17083, 1987.
205. Sigler MH et al: Renal concentrating ability in the adrenalectomized rat. *Clin Sci* 28:29, 1965.
206. Singer I, Rotenberg D: Demeclocycline-induced nephrogenic diabetes insipidus: In vivo and in vitro studies. *Ann Intern Med* 79:679, 1973.
207. Singer I, Rotenberg D: Mechanisms of lithium action. *N Engl J Med* 289:254, 1973.
208. Singer I et al: Lithium-induced nephrogenic diabetes insipidus: In vivo and in vitro studies. *J Clin Invest* 51:1081, 1972.
209. Smith DF, Balagura S: Sodium appetite in rats given lithium. *Life Sci* 11:1021, 1972.
210. Smith HW: *Principles of Renal Physiology*. New York: Oxford University Press, 1956.
211. Smith HW: *The Kidney: Structure and Function in Health and Disease.* New York: Oxford University Press, 1951.
212. Smith NJ et al: Raised plasma AVP concentration in carbamazepine-induced water intoxication. *Br Med J* 2:804, 1977.
213. Snyder HM, Breyer MD: Synergy between site-selective cyclic AMP analogues supports a role for cAMP-dependent protein kinase in mediating vasopressin stimulated water flow in rabbit cortical collecting duct (abstract). *J Am Soc Nephrol* 1:678, 1990.
214. Sonnenberg H: Medullary collecting duct function in antidiuretic and in salt and water diuretic rats. *Am J Physiol* 226:501, 1974.
215. Sonnenburg WK, Smith WL: Regulation of cyclic AMP metabolism in rabbit cortical collecting tubule cells by prostaglandins. *J Biol Chem* 263:6155, 1988.
216. Stephens WP: Plasma AVP concentration and antidiuretic action of carbamazepine. *Br Med J* 1:1445, 1978.
217. Stephenson JL: Concentration of urine in a central core model of the renal counterflow system. *Kidney Int* 2:85, 1972.
218. Stoff JS et al: The effect of aldosterone on the accumulation of adenosine 3′,5′-cyclic monophosphate in toad bladder epithelial cells in response to vasopressin and theophylline. *Proc Natl Acad Sci U S A* 69:805, 1972.
219. Stokes JB: Effect of prostaglandin E_2 on chloride transport across the rabbit thick ascending limb of Henle. *J Clin Invest* 64:495, 1979.
220. Strauch BS, Langton RG: Tyramine, catecholamines and the action of vasopressin on stimulation of water efflux in toad bladder. *Arch Biochem Biophys* 129:277, 1969.
221. Strewler GJ, Orloff J: Roll of cyclic nucleotides in the transport of water and electrolytes. *Adv Cyclic Nucleotide Res* 8:311, 1977.
222. Szatalowicz VL et al: Comparative effect of diuretics on renal water excretion in hyponatremic oedematous disorders. *Clin Sci* 62:235, 1982.
223. Taylor A et al: Vasopressin: Possible role of microtubules and microfilaments in its action. *Science* 181:347, 1973.
224. Teitelbaum I, Berl T: Water metabolism in electrolyte disorders. *Semin Nephrol* 4:354, 1984.
225. Teitelbaum I, Berl T: effect of calcium on vasopressin-mediated cAMP formation in cultured rat inner medullary collecting tubule cells. *J Clin Invest* 77:1574, 1986.
226. Teitelbaum I et al: Adrenergic control of cAMP generation in rat inner medullary collecting tubule cells. *Kidney Int* 35:647, 1989.
227. Uhlich E et al: Zur Antidiuretischen Wirkung von Carbamazepin bei Diabetes Insipidus. *Klin Wochenschr* 50:1127, 1972.
228. Urry DW, Ohnishi M, in Urry DW (ed): *Spectroscopic Approaches to Biomolecular Conformation.* Chicago, American Medical Association, 1969, p 263.
229. Venkatachalam CM: Stereochemical criteria for polypeptides and proteins: 5. Conformation of a system of three linked peptide units. *Biopolymers* 6:1425, 1968.
230. Verkman AS: Mechanisms and regulation of water permeability in renal epithelia. *Am J Physiol* 257:C839, 1989.
231. Walker LA et al: Antidiuretic hormone increases renal prostaglandin synthesis in vivo. *Am J Physiol* 235:F180, 1978.
232. Walser M: Sodium excretion, in Rouiller C, Muller A (eds): *The Kidney: Morphology Biochemistry Physiology.* New York, Academic Press, 1971, p 135.
233. Walter R et al: Relation of the conformation of oxytocin to the biology of neurohypophyseal hormones. *Proc Natl Acad Sci U S A* 68:1355, 1971.
234. Walter R et al: Conformational considerations of vasopressin as a guide to development of biological probes and therapeutic agents, in Andreoli TE et al (eds): *Disturbances in Body Fluid Osmolality.* Bethesda, American Physiological Society, 1977, p 1.
235. Walter R, du Vigneaud V: 1-deamino-1,6-L-selenocystine oxytocin, a highly potent analog of 1-deamino oxytocin. *J Am Chem Soc* 77:1331, 1966.
236. Wesson LG, Anslow WP: Effect of osmotic diuresis and mercurial diuresis in simultaneous water diuresis. *Am J Physiol* 170:255, 1952.
237. Willson DM, Sunderman FW: Studies in serum electrolytes: 12. The effect of water restriction in a patient with Addison's disease receiving sodium chloride. *J Clin Invest* 18:35, 1939.
238. Wirz H et al: Lokalisation des Konzentrierungsprozesses in der Niere durch Direkte Kryoskopie. *Helv Physiol Acta* 9:196, 1951.
239. Zook TE, Strandhoy JW: Inhibition of ADH-enhanced urea and water movement by prostaglandins. *Prostaglandins* 20:1, 1980.
240. Zusman RM et al: Vasopressin stimulated prostaglandin E biosynthesis in the toad urinary bladder effect on water flow. *J Clin Invest* 60:1339, 1977.
241. Zusman RM et al: Inhibition of vasopressin-stimulated prostaglandin E biosynthesis by chlorpropamide in the toad urinary bladder. *J Clin Invest* 60:1348, 1977.
242. Zusman RM et al: Effect of adrenal steroids on vasopressin-stimulated PGE synthesis and water flow. *AM J Physiol* 234:F532, 1978.

CHAPTER • 6

Regulation of extrarenal potassium metabolism

Ronald D. Perrone • Edward A. Alexander

The purpose of this chapter is to review those nonrenal mechanisms which influence the distribution of potassium within the body. While renal excretion is the major determinant of potassium regulation, nonrenal mechanisms assume greater importance as renal function diminishes.

The total body potassium content of a normal human is approximately 50 meq per kilogram of body weight, with a volume of distribution of about 1.1 liters per kilogram of body weight.[61,201] Exchangeable potassium is estimated to be 90 to 99 percent of total body potassium.[61] Roughly 98 percent of body potassium is intracellular, and muscle cells house most of this fraction. Total body potassium is a function of body size and decreases significantly with increasing age.[48,70,130] A concentration gradient of approximately 30:1 is maintained between intracellular and extracellular compartments by an energy-consuming process. It should be appreciated that the cellular concentration of potassium is not uniform within cells or among various cell types and the concentration gradient varies with physiologic and pathophysiologic perturbations. This gradient is the major determinant of the transmembrane potential, a critical factor in the functioning of muscle, nerve, and transporting epithelia.

The dynamic interrelationship of total body potassium content, potassium excretion, and the distribution of potassium between intracellular and extracellular fluid compartments determines the concentration of plasma potassium. After an acute oral or intravenous potassium load, about 50 percent of administered potassium appears in the urine within 4 to 6 h.[52,96] Of the retained cation, 80 to 90 percent is rapidly transported from the extracellular to the intracellular space, thus preventing potentially lethal hyperkalemia.

Total body potassium is a critical determinant of its own internal distribution. As total body potassium decreases, the fraction of a given exogenous load taken up by cells is increased. Conversely, when total body potassium is increased, the cellular uptake diminishes. The relationship between total body potassium and cellular uptake is linear but not proportional. As total body potassium decreases, the percentage remaining within cells increases.[201] Sterns and coworkers[201] studied the disposition of an intravenous potassium infusion in five hemodialysis patients who were virtually anuric. Changes in plasma potassium were best described by a two-compartment kinetic model that accounted for bidirectional flux between intra- and extracellular compartments.

EFFECTS OF HORMONES

INSULIN

The well-established clinical use of insulin in the acute treatment of hyperkalemia is based upon the ability of this hormone to increase directly the cellular uptake of potassium by hepatic and muscle cells. The cellular mechanism by which insulin stimulates potassium uptake has not been resolved definitively. Although most[41,82,151,231,232,236] but not all[195,196] investigators have demonstrated that insulin hyperpolarizes muscle and adipose cells in the presence or absence of glucose, there is disagreement regarding the mechanism by which this is achieved. Some suggest that primary stimulation of Na^+-K^+ ATPase mediates the insulin effect;[41,42,82,151] others suggest that the hormone decreases permeability of the cell membrane to sodium relative to potassium while secondarily enhancing potassium influx.[232,235]

The increase in muscle Na^+-K^+ pumping is independent of an increase in the number of sodium pumps.[38] In adipocytes, insulin increases the affinity of the alpha-+ (probably alpha-2) subunit of Na^+-K^+ ATPase for sodium.[131] The mechanism whereby insulin increases the sodium affinity of Na^+-K^+ ATPase is unknown.

The physiologic role of insulin in maintaining a normal plasma potassium concentration is not as well established. Controversy exists as to whether insulin participates in a physiologic feedback control loop responsive to changes in plasma potassium or whether it has a permissive effect, in which its mere presence is sufficient for optimal potassium entry into cells.

Infusions of potassium that substantially elevate the plasma concentration (>1.5 meq/liter) in dogs[109,166,177] are associated with significant increases in plasma insulin. Conversely, pancreatectomy[110] or alloxan-induced diabetes[177] causes animals to tolerate potassium chloride infusions poorly. This effect can be reversed with administration of insulin. Similar findings were noted in diabetic humans.[200,201] Lesser degrees of elevation of the plasma potassium concentration (<1.0 meq/liter) are associated with little or no measurable increment in peripheral insulin levels.[49]

The use of somatostatin, an inhibitor of insulin release, indicates an important role for basal insulin secretion in extrarenal potassium homeostasis in humans and animals.[216] Infusion of somatostatin into maturity-onset diabetics or into nondiabetic subjects elevated plasma potassium levels approximately 0.6 meq/liter, whereas no change was noted after infusion into juvenile-onset diabetics lacking endogenous insulin[53] (Fig. 6-1). Infusion of potassium chloride into dogs at a rate that raises plasma potassium by 0.5 to 0.6 meq/liter does not result in increased peripheral insulin levels.[53] Simultaneous administration of somatostatin with potassium chloride results in decreased insulin levels and a threefold increase in plasma potassium concentration; the addition of insulin to the somatostatin infusion restores potassium levels to normal. In human and animal studies[53] somatostatin had no effect on urinary potassium excretion; thus, the effects noted in the above-mentioned studies appear to be entirely extrarenal.

Failure of induced increments in plasma potassium concentration to increase peripheral insulin levels has suggested that the hormone has a permissive but not active role in extrarenal potassium homeostasis. It is important to recognize, however, that portal insulin levels are substantially higher than peripheral levels and that increments in insulin secretion would initially be perceived by the liver, an important site of potassium uptake (see below). In fact, Hiatt and associates[109] demonstrated increased pancreaticoduodenal vein insulin concentrations with small increments in plasma potassium. Using the insulin clamp technique, DeFronzo and colleagues[55] demonstrated a dose-related increment in splanchnic (primarily hepatic) uptake of potassium with increases in plasma insulin as low as 37 μU/ml. Net splanchnic glucose uptake was reduced during the period of increased potassium uptake, indicating a dissociation of the action of insulin on potassium uptake from its effect on glucose uptake. Others have shown that potassium up-

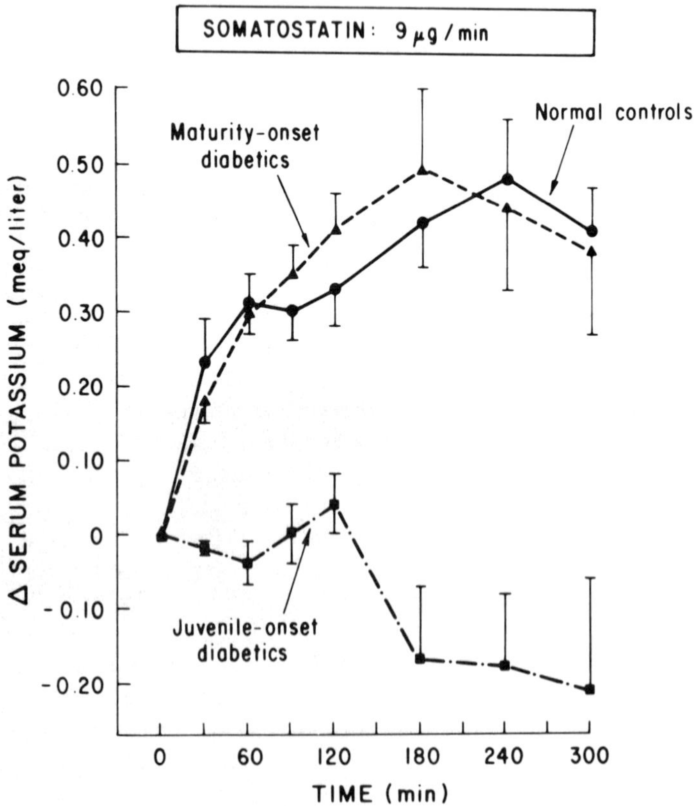

FIGURE 6-1 • The effect of infusion of somatostatin (an inhibitor of insulin secretion) on the change in serum potassium concentration in healthy volunteers (●, n = 9); maturity-onset diabetics (▲, n = 6); and juvenile-onset diabetics (■, n = 3). Values are mean ± standard error. (From DeFronzo RA et al: *J Clin Invest* 61:472, 1978.)

take in forearm tissues (muscle and adipose) was also stimulated in a dose-dependent fashion[10,236] by an intra-arterial infusion of insulin. The intermediate dose of insulin used (estimated to increase insulin levels by 40 μU/ml) caused no increase in net glucose uptake while increasing potassium uptake. In vitro studies using muscle[234,235] or isolated perfused liver[33] have also demonstrated a dissociation between potassium and glucose uptake.

The available evidence suggests but does not establish that a physiologic negative feedback control loop exists between insulin and potassium. Total insulin deficiency is clearly associated with abnormal potassium homeostasis, indicating that basal insulin levels are required. Insulin is an important component of the extrarenal defense against hyperkalemia and acts in both physiologic and pharmacologic concentrations.

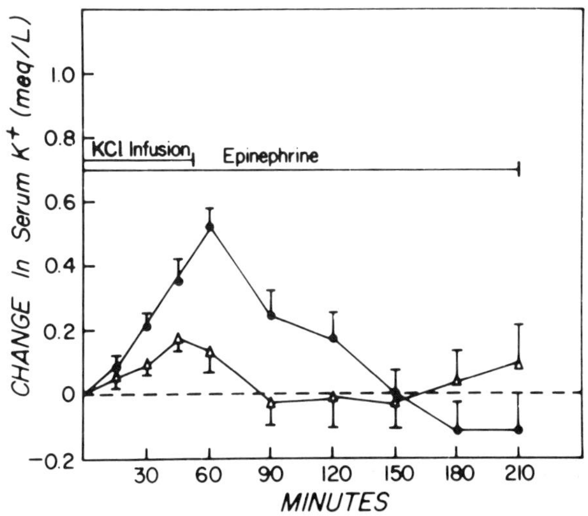

FIGURE 6-2 • Effect of epinephrine on the increment in serum potassium induced by an intravenous potassium infusion in the same five healthy subjects, with (△) and without (●) epinephrine infusion. Values are mean ± standard error. (From Rosa RM et al: *N Engl J Med* 302:431, 1980.)

CATECHOLAMINES

Catecholamines have been demonstrated to play an important role in extrarenal potassium homeostasis. Administration of epinephrine to animals produces a biphasic response of the plasma potassium, consisting of transient hyperkalemia followed by a prolonged period of hypokalemia.[59,60,212,213,219] Hyperkalemia is thought to result from hepatic potassium release[60,189] and is blocked by alpha-[69,212] and beta-adrenergic blockers, the latter in high doses.[34,212] Administration of a pure alpha-adrenergic agonist such as phenylephrine elevates the plasma potassium; this effect is prevented by alpha-adrenergic blockade.[225]

Combined administration of alpha and beta agonists surprisingly results in more profound initial hyperkalemia than that seen with pure alpha agonists alone.[212] The hypokalemic action of epinephrine and other catecholamines is unaffected by peripheral alpha-adrenergic blockade but is blocked by beta or beta 2 blockers and enhanced by mixed beta or selective beta 2 agonists. Recent studies have demonstrated conclusively that the hypokalemic action of the catecholamines is mediated solely by beta 2 receptors.[25,30]

It is thought that transient hepatic potassium release accounts for the initial hyperkalemic action of catecholamines,[60] whereas both liver and muscle participate in subsequent uptake of potassium and resultant hypokalemia.[219] These actions are independent of, and do not require changes in, plasma insulin, aldosterone, glucagon, glucose, or urinary potassium excretion. Catecholamine-induced potassium uptake has been demonstrated in vitro in skeletal muscle and is inhibited by propranolol but not by alpha-adrenergic blockade.[40] Exposure to catecholamines enhances potassium uptake and sodium extrusion, which occur in association with hyperpolarization of the muscle cell. This can be inhibited by ouabain, indicating that Na^+-K^+ ATPase participates in this action. The intracellular events leading to activation of Na^+-K^+ ATPase and potassium uptake are thought to result from beta 2 receptor-mediated stimulation of adenylate cyclase, which catalyzes the production of cAMP.[40] Propranolol enhances and epinephrine diminishes urinary potassium excretion;[56] however, propranolol and other mixed beta or beta 2 antagonists elevate the plasma potassium, whereas epinephrine and mixed beta and beta 2 agonists lower the plasma potassium. Furthermore, this effect may persist chronically,[162] as demonstrated by mild degrees of elevation of the plasma potassium concentration in hypertensive patients treated for several months with beta blockers alone. No changes were noted in exchangeable potassium and sodium, suggesting that total body potassium balance did not change.

Participation of catecholamines in the physiologic regulation of the plasma potassium concentration is suggested by the studies of Rosa and coworkers[175] (Fig. 6-2) and DeFronzo and associates.[56] These workers observed significant effects on plasma potassium levels during infusions of physiologic amounts of epinephrine, which raised the plasma catechole's concentrations into the stimulated physiologic range. Significant changes in plasma catecholamines were not noted during potassium chloride infusions that elevated the plasma potassium by 0.7 to 0.8 meq/liter, which may be due to rapid reuptake by sympathetic neurons. Alterations in the basal plasma potassium level in many clinical situations attest to the quantitatively important effect that catecholamines exert on potassium homeostasis. Increased endogenous catecholamine levels from anxiety,[141] cardiac arrest,[176] myocardial infarction,[154] induction of anesthesia,[118] or stroke[154] decrease plasma potassium. Administration of beta 2 agonists for treatment of bronchospasm,[43] as a local dental anesthetic,[146] or for tocolysis[152,210] results in clinically important hypokalemia. Prior treatment with a diuretic augments the hypokalemic effect of albuterol (salbutamol), presumably by depletion of total body potassium stores.[127] The hypokalemic effect of beta 2 agonists has even been used to therapeutic advantage for the acute treatment of hyperkalemia in dialysis patients.[5,150] Administration of beta blockers usually increases plasma potassium concentration by less than 0.5 meq/liter in the absence of potassium loads or impaired ability to excrete the cation. In the presence of renal failure, cardiac bypass, diabetes, or hypoaldosteronism, substantially greater elevations of the plasma potassium may occur.[12,24,129]

Catecholamines appear to have an important physiologic role in regulation of potassium distribution. Furthermore, decreased and increased plasma potassium levels, respectively, are associated with therapeutic administration of beta agonists and antagonists. (For a further discussion of catecholamines see Chap. 49.)

ALDOSTERONE

Although a role for aldosterone (see Chap. 14) in extrarenal potassium homeostasis has been suggested by several in vivo and in vitro studies, the issue remains controversial. The role of aldosterone in promoting potassium excretion by the colon is well established and will be discussed separately.

Both increased and decreased intracellular potassium content have been demonstrated following in vitro incubation of rat muscle or kidney with aldosterone.[1,126,159] Similarly conflicting results have been noted in intracellular potassium following adrenalectomy.[86,199] Studies in humans and animals in which administration of aldosterone lowered the plasma potassium concentration in the absence of negative potassium balance have been viewed as evidence for an extrarenal action of the hormone[15,51,52,92,114,128,157,202] While these data are suggestive of such an action, it is important to recognize that balance studies lack sufficient sensitivity to detect the very small changes in total body potassium that may result in a lowered plasma potassium concentration. In addition, gastrointestinal potassium loss was not accounted for in some of these studies.[15,92]

A large dose of aldosterone acutely administered to glucocorticoid-replaced adrenalectomized-nephrectomized rats infused with potassium chloride partially normalizes extrarenal potassium tolerance.[26] One may calculate from these results that an additional 5 percent of the infused potassium load is transferred out of the extracellular compartment by the acute administration of aldosterone. The site of potassium removal in the study cited above was not fully defined and might well be accounted for by acute enhancement of potassium excretion by the colon.[63]

Little dispute exists regarding the ability of an increased plasma potassium concentration to stimulate aldosterone secretion. Small increases in plasma potassium result in increased plasma aldosterone.[49] This may also be demonstrated in vitro and in anephric humans and dogs. Potassium is thought to be a direct-acting aldosterone secretagogue; however, blockage of angiotensin II formation with the converting enzyme inhibitor captopril inhibits potassium-induced but not adrenocorticotropic hormone-induced (ACTH-induced) aldosterone secretion in normal dogs.[171] This suggests that there is some in vivo dependence of potassium-induced aldosterone secretion on angiotensin II. Recent studies have shown that both potassium and angiotensin II stimulate aldosterone secretion via an increase in cytosolic free calcium.[172]

The role of aldosterone in modulating potassium movement into liver or muscle cells is still uncertain despite many attempts to directly or indirectly demonstrate such an effect. The magnitude of this possible effect is small, particularly when compared to the renal excretory action.[163]

GLUCOCORTICOIDS

In addition to the effect on intestinal epithelia, glucocorticoids (see Chap. 14) have been shown in some studies to have an effect on plasma potassium that is independent of the effect on urinary potassium excretion. Glucocorticoid administration produces significant kaluresis[16,50,120] that is not usually associated with sodium retention and only lasts for 24 h. Despite this kaliuresis, several studies,[16,120] although not all,[125,147] have demonstrated transient increases in plasma potassium levels following acute administration of glucocorticoids. Longer periods of follow-up show that the plasma potassium concentration returns to normal within 12 to 24 h. There is little information concerning the mechanism of this effect.

GLUCAGON

The physiological role of glucagon in potassium homeostasis is probably not of great significance except for its interaction with other hormones. Glucagon levels increase following infusion of potassium.[177] The defect in extrarenal potassium tolerance caused by pancreatectomy,[110] alloxan-induced diabetes,[177] or somatostatin infusion[53] is completely corrected by insulin replacement, suggesting there is no contribution of glucagon to this response in the intact animal. Furthermore, tolerance to infused potassium is unimpaired when glucagon secretion is suppressed by simultaneous glucose infusion.[177] Thus, the role of glucagon in response to administered potassium loads appears to be limited to maintenance of normal glucose levels in the presence of increased insulin secretion.

Administration of glucagon in pharmacologic doses to intact or nephrectomized animals is associated with a biphasic response similar to that with epinephrine.[167,228] Initial hyperkalemia and hyperglycemia are followed by hypokalemia and return of glucose levels toward normal. The initial hyperkalemic effect is due to hepatic potassium release[33,94,189] and is blocked by the alpha-adrenergic blocker dibenamine.[69] Subsequent hypokalemia requires an intact pancreas for full expression.[167] That this effect is dependent on insulin is further suggested by studies of humans infused with somatostatin and glucagon.[137] Absence of insulin ameliorates the hypokalemic phase of glucagon administration. Physiologic levels of glucagon were achieved in this study, indicating that under conditions of insulin deficiency increases in plasma glucagon may increase plasma potassium.

Glucagon-mediated hepatic potassium release is usually associated with glucose release[189,228] but may be dissociated from it. Hepatic glycogen depletion induced by fasting or repetitive glucagon injection results in a diminished hyperglycemic response, whereas the hyperkalemic response persists.[69] Further evidence for dissociation is provided by the use of dibenamine,[69] which blocks the hyperkalemic but not the hyperglycemic action of glucagon. Therefore, hepatic glucose and potassium efflux mediated by glucagon appear to be independent actions that occur over approximately the same time period.

Glucagon produces kaliuresis when given in pharmacologic but not in physiologic doses.[71,173,185,197] Elevation of plasma glucagon in the physiologic range appears to have no important role in extrarenal potassium homeostasis, except possibly in insulin-deficient states, where slight elevations of plasma potassium are produced.

PARATHYROID HORMONE

An effect of the intracellular calcium concentration on potassium movement across cell membranes has been recognized for over 30 years; increasing cell calcium increases potassium efflux,[90,145,222] whereas decreasing cell calcium has the opposite effect.[174] The mechanism whereby changes in the cytosolic calcium concentration alter transcellular potassium movement has not been firmly established but is likely to be mediated via potassium channels.[145] Since parathyroid hormone (PTH) increases the calcium content of many tissues,[138] it is not surprising that administration of the hormone interferes with extrarenal potassium uptake. Studies in acutely nephrectomized rats demonstrate clearly that disposal of an intravenous potassium load is impaired when PTH is simultaneously infused and that this effect is independent of plasma pH and the levels of insulin, aldosterone, catecholamines, calcium, and bicarbonate.[204] It is unlikely that hyperparathyroidism significantly affects the plasma potassium concentration when renal excretory capacity for the cation is maintained. The importance of PTH to extrarenal potassium homeostasis in chronic renal failure is discussed below.

THYROID HORMONE

A physiologic role for thyroid hormone in the regulation of potassium distribution has not been delineated. Clinical disturbances of thyroid function, however, are associated with altered potassium homeostasis, despite normal plasma potassium concentrations. Severely thyrotoxic patients with muscle weakness have been demonstrated to have reduced total exchangeable potassium[66] and normal[180] or reduced[179] intracellular potassium concentration in skeletal muscle. Treatment of hypothyroid children with thyroxine, however, significantly increased the intracellular potassium concentration in skeletal muscle in one study.[68] Animal studies revealed normal[28] or increased[112,113] muscle potassium and increased total exchangeable potassium[67] following administration of thyroid hormone. A simple explanation for these differences is not apparent, but the possibilities include species variation, alterations in intracellular water content, and differences in duration and amount of thyroid hormone administration.

A recent study examined the complex interactions of thyroid hormone and the sympathetic nervous system as related to extrarenal potassium disposal. Cellular uptake of an intravenous potassium load in acutely nephrectomized rats was impaired in hypothyroid animals and enhanced in thyrotoxic animals.[124] Complex interactions with the sympathetic nervous system were evident. In the hypothyroid state, increased alpha-adrenergic tone, or responsiveness, contributed to the impaired extrarenal potassium uptake, whereas in the thyrotoxic state, increased beta-adrenergic and decreased alpha-adrenergic tone, or responsiveness, contributed to the increased extrarenal potassium uptake. Because tissue potassium levels were not determined, the role of prior depletion of tissue potassium stores could not be assessed.

Thyroid hormone increases the activity of Na^+-K^+ ATPase by direct and indirect mechanisms.[13,28,100,112] Ouabain-sensitive oxygen consumption, potassium uptake, and sodium efflux are all increased by the hormone. This increased Na^+-K^+ ATPase activity is due to both the enhanced action of individual pumps and the increased number of pumps, as reflected by an increase in ouabain binding sites. Conversely, absence of thyroid hormone decreases the number of sodium pumps.[75]

Combined potassium deficiency and triiodothyronine (T_3) administration enhances $Na^+ - K^+$ ATPase activity to an even greater degree.[188]

GROWTH HORMONE

Participation of growth hormone in the regulation of potassium homeostasis has been suggested by numerous studies. Administration of growth hormone to growth hormone–deficient humans or animals results in diminished urinary potassium excretion without changes in plasma potassium.[31,108] Chronic administration of growth hormone to hypophysectomized rats results in increased muscle potassium concentrations.[20] Zierler and colleagues[236] have demonstrated increased forearm muscle potassium uptake, comparable to that produced by large doses of insulin, in human subjects given pharmacologic amounts of growth hormone. Similar changes were noted in fasting and acromegaly,[236] states associated with elevated growth hormone levels.

Recombinant human growth hormone has also been used to promote anabolism or growth in patients without growth hormone deficiency. In surgical patients, short-term administration of recombinant human growth hormone results in nitrogen and potassium retention and a reduction in the serum potassium level.[136,230] By contrast, chronic administration of growth hormone to children or adults with long-standing renal insufficiency has not been reported to affect the serum potassium level.[214]

Potassium infusion results in increased plasma growth hormone levels in normal[57] and hypertensive[217] human subjects. These changes appear to be independent of alterations in insulin and glucose levels. An interrelationship between growth hormone and potassium homeostasis is also supported by the finding of reduced hormone levels in potassium deficiency, which return to normal following potassium administration.[168,169] The physiologic role of growth hormone on in vivo extrarenal potassium homeostasis remains to be established.

SUMMARY OF HORMONAL EFFECTS

Much of our knowledge regarding the extrarenal effects of hormones on potassium homeostasis is derived from experiments designed to isolate the effect of one or more of these agents. The quantitative importance of each factor is difficult to determine precisely. Furthermore, the relative importance of one hormone may be greatly modified by the presence or absence of another. Hormones not only may affect potassium distribution but may directly or indirectly stimulate the secretion or release of other hormones; for example, catecholamines stimulate hyperglycemia and hyperinsulinemia.[56] Despite these limitations, it is possible to estimate the relative importance of several hormones. Catecholamines and insulin clearly have the best-defined and quantitatively most important effects on potassium distribution. Glucagon and aldosterone have small effects, and considerable doubt exists as to their importance in physiologic regulation of potassium distribution. In the presence of diabetes mellitus, renal failure, or beta-adrenergic blockade, glucagon and aldosterone may become more important. Possible roles for glucocorticoids, parathyroid hormone, thyroid hormone, or growth hormone remain speculative at this time.

ACID-BASE EFFECTS

It had been generally accepted that acute acid-base changes produce concurrent alterations in the distribution of potassium between body fluid compartments, with acidemia raising and alkalemia lowering plasma potassium concentration.[32,158,183,206] Recent studies, however, indicate clearly that this simple relationship is incomplete. Oster and associates[160,161] showed conclusively that the relationship between acidemia and plasma potassium in the dog is markedly influenced by the nature of the acid infused. Infusion of mineral acids (HCl, NH_4Cl) raised plasma potassium concentration significantly more than equally acidifying infusions of such organic acids as lactic, β-hydroxybutyric, or methylmalonic. Three hours of organic acidemia did not cause significant hyperkalemia, although blood pH was reduced to 7.15.[160] Changes in potassium excretion or insulin or glucose levels could not account for the differences noted. However, Adrogué and coworkers[2] explained these findings by showing that ketoacid infusion stimulates portal hyperinsulinemia with hepatic uptake of potassium. Mineral acid infusion, on the other hand, increases glucagon levels without an increase in insulin secretion, thus accounting for the hyperkalemia. Fulop[89] reviewed the findings in patients with lactic and ketoacidoses of varying causes and could find no direct correlation between the level of acidemia and the plasma potassium concentration. Adrogué and Madias carefully reviewed the available literature relating changes in blood pH to potassium concentration. They concluded, as did Oster and associates[160] and others[133] that there was a significant inverse correlation between the change in blood pH and plasma potassium during mineral acidemia but not during organic acidemia.[3] During respiratory acidosis the increment in plasma potassium concentration for any change in pH was less than during mineral acidemia but greater than during organic acidemia. Alkalosis, whether metabolic or respiratory, is accompanied by a small decrement in plasma potassium levels, which is apparently unrelated to changes in hormonal factors.[205] The mechanism whereby acid-base changes elicit an alteration in plasma potassium concentration is unclear, but simple $H^+ - K^+$ exchange cannot explain all the available data. A recent study in nephrectomized rats demonstrated that the acidosis induced by a potassium load could be prevented by amiloride.[7] Thus, hyperkalemia appears to activate the $Na^+ - H^+$ exchanger leading to extracellular acidosis. The multiple influences on potassium flux discussed in this chapter certainly modify the response to the acid-base change, but the specific influences are not yet precisely defined. This is particularly pertinent in attempting to predict the plasma potassium level on the basis of blood pH in patients, where total body potassium and internal environment vary so widely. From the available data no clear stoichiometric relationship exists between changes in blood pH and changes in plasma potassium concentration.

OSMOLALITY

When effective plasma osmolality (i.e., tonicity) is raised, hyperkalemia often is noted. This is thought to occur because diffusion of water out of cells and the resulting increased intracellular concentration of potassium favor its outward diffusion. This hyperkalemic effect is especially important in patients with diabetes mellitus, who develop hypertonicity secondary to hyperglycemia. Diabetics are particularly at risk for hyperkalemia, since they are more likely also to have hypoaldosteronism.[128,135,156] The hyperkalemic effect of hypertonicity has also been demonstrated in patients with chronic renal failure after infusion with hypertonic saline.[46]

EXERCISE

Release of intracellular potassium with transient hyperkalemia (0.3 to 0.6 meq/liter) is regularly found after exercise but may be particularly severe after exhaustive physical activity, where a doubling has been observed.[144] The mechanism for this increase in cellular potassium efflux appears to be fully explained by the electrical excitatory events occurring in exercising muscles.[44,106,111,144] The increment in potassium released from cells for a given amount of work is less in subjects tested after physical training. In addition, baseline plasma potassium concentration in conditioned subjects is often lowered, although total body potassium is not decreased.[121] This response is similar to that described below for potassium adaptation. The mechanism for the decrease in muscle potassium efflux was evaluated in dogs by Knochel. He found that inhibition of aldosterone, insulin, and epinephrine had no effect on the reduction of exercise-induced hyperkalemia after training.[122]

DRUGS

DIGITALIS

Digitalis is a well-known inhibitor of $Na^+ - K^+$ ATPase. In view of this enzyme's importance in membrane transport of potassium into cells, it is not surprising that hyperkalemia may result from serious digitalis overdoses and release of intracellular potassium. In fact, 11 of 23 patients with severe digitalis toxicity experienced significant hyperkalemia.[190] In patients chronically digitalized, total body and muscle potassium were reduced.[73]

SUCCINYLCHOLINE

Succinylcholine, a muscle relaxant used in anesthesia, induces the release of a small amount of potassium from normal muscles[99] by increasing permeability of the muscle membrane. This effect occurs as part of the normal depolarization induced by the drug, but the effect may be markedly exaggerated in damaged or denervated muscle, from which potentially lethal amounts of potassium may be released. This abnormal response may be elicitable for weeks to months after muscle injury[99] and presents a risk for such patients who require surgery.

CALCIUM CHANNEL BLOCKING AGENTS

Calcium channel blockers (CCBs) increase the disposal of an intravenous potassium load in acutely nephrectomized rats; this effect is independent of adrenal function and peripheral sympathetic activity.[203] In humans, administration of the CCB nitrendipine for 4 to 7 days enhances epinephrine's hypokalemic effects; there is no effect on basal plasma potassium levels prior to epinephrine administration.[149]

Alterations in the cytosolic calcium concentration are known to alter transcellular potassium movements, as discussed above (see "Parathyroid Hormone"). The mechanism whereby increased intracellular calcium increases potassium efflux and decreased intracellular calcium decreases potassium efflux has not been established. Recently, it has been determined that elevation of the intracellular calcium concentration within the physiologic range inhibits the $alpha_2$ subunit of $Na^+ - K^+$ ATPase.[142] Increased activity of $Na^+ - K^+$ ATPase from decreased intracellular calcium concentration could possibly account for the enhancement of net potassium uptake by CCBs.

THIAZIDE DIURETICS

Plasma potassium concentration was shown to decrease in anephric patients after they received thiazides. The authors postulated an extrarenal effect of the drug on transcellular potassium movement.[76]

GENERALIZED INHIBITION OF $Na^+ - K^+$ ATPase

A patient with hyperkalemia due to defects in both extrarenal uptake and renal excretion of potassium has been described.[207] The finding of blunted extrarenal uptake of potassium in response to insulin and albuterol, exaggerated hyperkalemia after administration of propranolol, unexplained defective tubular secretion (excretion) of potassium, and the association with high circulating levels of digoxin-like factors suggest generalized inhibition of $Na^+ - K^+$ ATPase activity.[207]

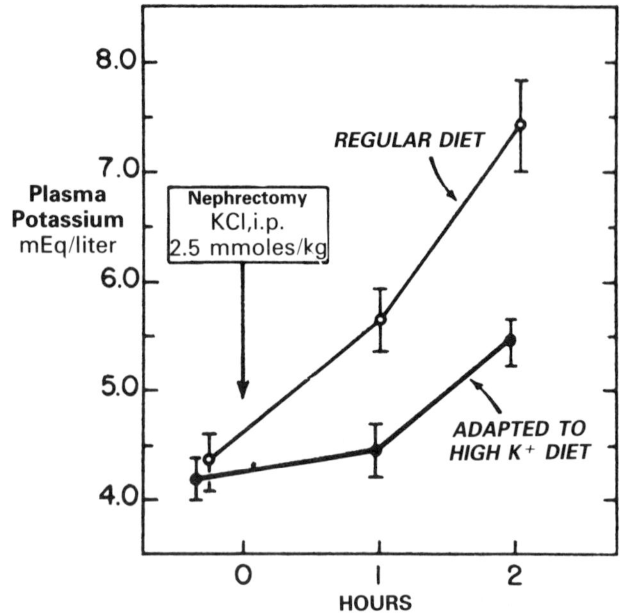

FIGURE 6-3 • Extrarenal potassium adaptation in rats; the response of acutely nephrectomized rats to an acute potassium load after five days of either a regular or high-potassium diet. (From Alexander EA, Levinsky NG: *J Clin Invest* 47:740, 1968.)

POTASSIUM ADAPTATION

Chronic potassium loading protects against hyperkalemia from acute potassium infusions. This phenomenon, termed potassium adaptation, is a function of both renal and extrarenal changes in potassium handling. Adaptation has been utilized as an experimental model to help clarify the mechanisms of potassium transport. Renal adaptation is discussed in Chap. 7. Conclusive evidence for extrarenal potassium adaptation (EKA) was provided by Alexander and Levinsky[4] and subsequently confirmed by others.[81,117,163,166,167,181,193,194] They noted that rats fed a high-potassium diet for several days maintained a lower plasma potassium after acute bilateral nephrectomy and potassium challenge (Fig. 6-3). Since prior adrenalectomy prevented this adaptation, it was concluded that chronic mineralocorticoid stimulation was necessary for EKA. The sites and mechanism(s) of this extrarenal removal of potassium have not been precisely defined, but increased muscle, liver, and colon uptake are highly likely.

The role in the potassium adaptation response of the other hormones that affect potassium transport has not been evaluated. Hayslett, Binder, and associates[104,117,119] have demonstrated that increased potassium ingestion is reflected in increased potassium secretion by the rat colon. They found an increase in the basolateral cell membrane area, an increase in $Na^+ - K^+$ ATPase density, and an increase in transepithelial potential difference, results similar to those noted in the kidney.[181] These changes probably reflect an increase in cell potassium uptake at the basolateral border, with secondary potassium efflux across the luminal membrane.

While definitive evidence for increased potassium uptake by muscle is limited,[4] this probably reflects the methodologic difficulty of finding a small increment in muscle potassium within the vast muscle potassium pool. It is possible that enhanced cellular uptake after acute loading might occur because chronic potassium feeding stimulates chronic hyperaldosteronism, which leads to renal and gastrointestinal potassium loss and eventually cellular potassium depletion. The reduction in intracellular potassium thus provides a storage site more avid for the acute potassium load than is present in rats eating a regular diet.[4,21,193,194] It is of interest that normal aging impairs extrarenal and renal potassium adaptation in the rat.[21] The response to acute potassium loading when ingesting a regular diet, however, is not different from that found in young rats. The latter finding is consistent with that observed in aging humans where insulin- and beta-adrenergic-mediated potassium uptake were normal.

CHRONIC RENAL FAILURE

Extrarenal potassium uptake is impaired in end-stage renal failure (see Chap. 39),[9,79,96,115] but the mechanism underlying this impairment is undefined. The levels of total exchangeable potassium and intracellular potassium in patients with chronic renal failure are consistently reduced or normal but are never elevated.[74] Thus, there should be an adequate "cell sink" for potassium, but acute uptake is impaired. Any of the mechanisms influencing the distribution of potassium discussed in this chapter might be contributory, but no clear experimental evidence implicating a particular mechanism is available. Gastrointestinal potassium secretion is increased in renal failure and thus is excluded as a cause.[17,103] The hormones important in extrarenal potassium uptake—insulin, epinephrine, and aldosterone (except in patients with hypoaldosteronism)—are normal or elevated in patients with renal failure; these hormones would contribute to impaired extrarenal uptake only if there was tissue insensitivity to them.

Impaired hypokalemic responses to infused epinephrine and inhaled albuterol (specific beta 2 agonist) have been demonstrated in uremic patients.[93,198,218] It is thought that this tissue insensitivity to catecholamines is due to abnormal responsivity of the $beta_2$ adrenoceptor.[198] This resistance may be due to greater receptor occupancy caused by higher endogenous epinephrine levels.[218] This defect is specific for catecholamine-mediated potassium uptake, whereas insulin-mediated uptake across splanchnic and femoral vascular beds is normal in uremic human subjects[8] and normal or increased in skeletal muscle from uremic rats.[58,95] Simultaneous administration of intravenous insulin and glucose with nebulized albuterol reduces plasma potassium more effectively than administration of either modality alone.[6] Of interest, the presence of glucose in dialysate increases plasma insulin levels and decreases the total removal of potassium compared to glucose-free dialysate.[220] This effect is achieved without any differences between dialysate formulations or in pre- or postdialysis plasma potassium levels. Thus, there is decreased removal of intracellular potassium due to insulin-mediated potassium uptake.[220] Increased glucagon levels in uremia[72,184] may be important also, but this possibility has not been tested. Since Na^+-K^+ ATPase plays a major role in the cellular influx of potassium, it is possible that the uremic milieu adversely affects the functioning of transport by the ATPase.

There are, in fact, two known abnormalities of Na^+-K^+ pumping in uremia: decreased catalytic turnover of Na^+-K^+ ATPase, possibly due to circulating toxins, and decreased numbers of Na^+-K^+ ATPase pump sites. Both findings can increase intracellular sodium concentrations. Welt and associates[221] reported that erythrocytic concentrations of sodium were increased in approximately 25 percent of uremic subjects. Although such defects in Na^+-K^+ pumping have been reasonably well characterized in erythrocytes from uremic patients,[45,116] there is only limited proof for the existence of such defects in skeletal muscle and liver, the major sites of extrarenal potassium disposal. Marked abnormalities in the uremic muscle cell, including decreased intracellular water content[22] and sodium concentration,[47] and the tendency to normal or reduced total body potassium[74] are findings suggestive of decreased Na^+-K^+ pump activity. Hypopolarization of human skeletal muscle membrane potential is found in uremic subjects and is corrected after two to three weeks of regular hemodialysis.[47] Decreased Na^+-K^+ pump activity has also been found in isolated muscle obtained from uremic rats[58,95] without an alteration in the number of skeletal muscle pump sites, as determined by ouabain binding.[58] More recent evidence indicates that steady-state levels of messenger RNA coding for the $alpha_2$ isoform of Na^+-K^+ ATPase are decreased in uremic rat tissues;[209] whether this decrease in message translates into decreased numbers of pump sites remains to be determined.

PTH increases intracellular calcium and increases potassium efflux in acutely nephrectomized rats, as described earlier in this chapter. In rats with chronic renal failure, both parathyroidectory and the CCB verapamil enhance extrarenal potassium disposal. Administration of PTH impairs extrarenal potassium uptake whether or not the parathyroid glands are intact.[191] The effect of PTH on potassium uptake in human subjects with chronic renal failure has not yet been examined; nor has it been determined whether the effect of PTH is mediated by an increase in intracellular calcium, which inhibits the $alpha_2$ subunit of Na^+-K^+ ATPase.[142]

In summary, several possible mechanisms may account for the impaired extrarenal potassium disposal that is characteristic of end-stage renal failure. These possibilities include decreased transport by Na^+-K^+ ATPase, tissue insensitivity to catecholamines, and elevation of intracellular calcium by PTH. When insulin is secreted or administered, potassium is rapidly taken up by extrarenal tissues; however, decreased insulin secretion secondary to fasting or starvation leaves the organism particularly vulnerable to hyperkalemia as renal excretory function and catecholamine-mediated potassium uptake are diminished.

GASTROINTESTINAL TRACT

Intestinal transport of potassium, like transport in the kidney, is altered by various physiologic and pathologic perturbations. States of acute or chronic potassium loading are associated with increased fecal potassium excretion.[17,18,81,119] Similarly, potassium deficiency is associated with increased potassium absorption.[18,105] The portion of potassium excretion accounted for by the gut is normally less than 10 to 20 percent of total potassium excretion[192] even in states of potassium excess.[81] Clearly the kidney has the major excretory role when renal function is well preserved.

MECHANISMS OF POTASSIUM TRANSPORT

A detailed discussion of gastrointestinal potassium transport is beyond the scope of this chapter; the topic is treated further in Chap. 7. Potassium transport in human small bowel is thought to be entirely passive,[215] but colonic potassium transport is mediated by active processes that are modifiable under various conditions. Excretion of potassium by the colon may play a significant role in extrarenal potassium homeostasis in certain situations.

Unlike nonepithelial tissues, in which potassium entry and egress take place across a simple cell membrane, colonic potassium excretion necessitates net movement across the entire intestinal wall. Both paracellular and transcellular pathways are known to operate in this tissue.[104] Since most studies have examined rat and rabbit intestinal epithelium and since species differences exist, great caution must be exercised in applying these data to human intestinal potassium transport.

With these limitations in mind, a simplified scheme for colonic potassium secretion follows.

Potassium secretion by the colon, as in other transporting epithelia, is closely linked to sodium absorption. Sodium entry across the luminal membrane is a passive process facilitated by a favorable electrochemical gradient. Exit of sodium across the serosal membrane is mediated by Na^+-K^+ ATPase and is coupled asymmetrically to potassium entry. After entering the cell, potassium may exit across the luminal surface, destined for potential excretion, or may exit across the serosal surface and thereby return to the bloodstream. The lumen-negative electrical potential difference favors potassium secretion. However, most available evidence,[11,62,64,101,117,139,226] but not all,[18,87] suggests that net potassium secretion exceeds that which the potential difference alone could cause. Other factors that enhance potassium secretion include increased plasma potassium concentration,[17] increased Na^+-K^+ ATPase,[81] cAMP,[83,153] cholinergic agents,[153] metabolic acidosis,[77] and the laxative bisacodyl.[153] Respiratory acid-base disturbances have no effect on colonic potassium transport,[36,78] whereas metabolic alkalosis decreases its secretion.[77] Luminal factors also are important with regard to secretion or absorption of potassium. A high luminal sodium concentration (140 meq/liter) causes potassium secretion, whereas absence of luminal sodium markedly stimulates potassium absorption.[164] Changes in luminal flow rate have no effect on colonic potassium secretion,[18] in contrast to the situation in the kidney.[97] Paracellular pathways may provide a mode of potassium secretion entirely dependent on the transepithelial potential difference. There is increasing evidence supporting the existence in rat distal colon of a luminal potassium absorptive pump, possibly a proton-potassium ATPase.[85,143,164,165] The activity of this pump is increased by dietary potassium restriction,[85,208] hyperaldosteronism,[164] and decreasing pH.[164]

RENAL FAILURE

A significant role for intestinal potassium excretion evolves in severe renal insufficiency, when as much as 30 to 80 percent of total potassium intake may be excreted in the feces (Fig. 6-4).[102,103,123,182] The underlying mechanism for this substantial increase in secretion is probably similar to that occurring in potassium adaptation (see below). Increased activity of Na^+-K^+ ATPase occurs in rats with increased dietary potassium intake and 70 percent renal ablation.[17] Although aldosterone levels are elevated in renal failure,[107] its role in stimulating colonic potassium excretion is unclear. Dietary sodium restriction[102,103,182] and deoxycorticosterone[202] or spironolactone administration[103,202] had no effect on fecal potassium excretion in balance studies performed in human subjects. Wilson and colleagues,[227] however, demonstrated a reversal of low sodium/potassium ratios in fecal water in two uremic subjects after spironolactone administration.

HORMONES IN THE GASTROINTESTINAL TRACT

Aldosterone is known to modify potassium transport in various segments of the gastrointestinal tract in parallel

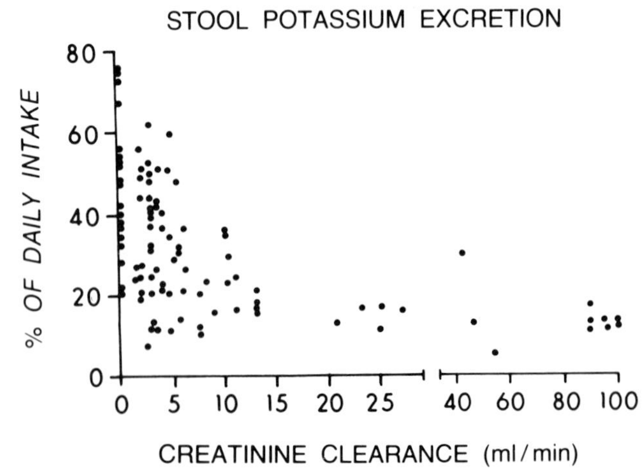

FIGURE 6-4 • Relationship between the degree of renal insufficiency and fecal potassium excretion. Data points are compiled from three studies[103,227,229] comprising 98 balance periods in 40 patients. Variation in dietary protein or sodium intake did not produce consistent changes in fecal potassium excretion; thus data points from these balance periods were included without special designation.

with its effects on the kidney. Both saliva and gastric juice have increased concentrations of potassium following mineralocorticoid stimulation.[140] Distal small bowel (ileum) has been demonstrated to respond to aldosterone administration in animal studies.[223] The jejunum, however, does not respond to mineralocorticoid stimulation.[35] Elevation of endogenous aldosterone levels[80,155] or administration of fludrocortisone[98] to patients with ileostomies results in increased potassium excretion. Changes in net potassium excretion are usually less than 10 meq/day.[80,98,155] Thus, in most situations, there is little quantitative contribution from these changes to external potassium balance.

The large intestine of humans and animals also responds to mineralocorticoid stimulation with increased fecal potassium excretion.[14,65,186,211,229] This may be demonstrated during acute[64,88] or chronic[65,211] administration of mineralocorticoid and, like the renal response,[91] is associated with increased $Na^+ - K^+$ ATPase activity.[35,211,223] Some, but by no means all, patients with primary hyperaldosteronism have inappropriately high fecal potassium excretion for their plasma potassium concentration. In one patient, fecal potassium excretion was 47 to 61 meq/day with varying potassium intakes.[29] Increases in fecal potassium excretion in primary hyperaldosteronism are usually less than 30 meq/day when renal function is normal and contribute substantially less than the kidney to total potassium excretion.[37,132,148,187] As indicated above, in vitro studies performed using sodium-free solutions demonstrate that hyperaldosteronism stimulates the activity of a potassium absorptive pump.[164]

Effects similar to those of aldosterone on ileum and colon have been demonstrated with dexamethasone or methylprednisolone in animal studies.[19,27,35,223] Furthermore, glucocorticoids have been shown to act on the jejunum.[35] Increased $Na^+ - K^+$, ATPase, sodium absorption, and potassium excretion were also documented to occur in these stuudies. Administration of hydrocortisone to humans also results in enhancement of fecal potassium excretion and sodium absorption.[37] Until recently, it has been unclear whether these glucocorticoid effects resulted from binding to mineralocorticoid receptors or from a distinct effect mediated via binding to a specific glucocorticoid receptor. Studies by Bastl and coworkers have persuasively defined the specificity of the glucocorticoid effect (see Chap. 14). The role of other hormones in regulating colonic potassium excretion has not been evaluated. Further consideration of hormone action in the gastrointestinal system is given in Chap 7.

POTASSIUM ADAPTATION

Acute or chronic potassium loading enhances colonic potassium excretion.[17,18,81,117] The jejunum does not participate in this adaptive response;[17] other segments of the gastrointestinal tract have not been studied in this regard. The mechanism responsible for the increased colonic potassium secretion is not completely understood. Both in vivo[117] and in vitro[83] studies suggest that potassium excretion is mediated by an active transport process. Chronic potassium loading increases both the activity and number of $Na^+ - K^+$ ATPase pump sites.[81,104] These increases correlate well with increases in basolateral membrane surface area noted in histologic studies.[117] Although transepithelial potential difference is increased under these conditions,[17,81] little[117] or no[17,81] change is noted in sodium, chloride, and water movement. Increased $Na^+ - K^+$ ATPase and potassium secretion are also seen in adrenalectomized animals maintained on replacement doses of mineralocorticoid,[81] suggesting that increased aldosterone secretion is not the sole stimulus for colonic potassium adaptation. In fact, the full expression of colonic potassium adaptation results from two distinct mechanisms: increased aldosterone secretion and an aldosterone-independent mechanism induced by dietary potassium loading.[84]

POTASSIUM DEFICIENCY

Chronic potassium depletion produced by feeding a potassium-deficient diet to rats greatly diminishes potassium secretion[18] and may result in net absorption.[85,105,208]

REFERENCES

1. Adler S: An extrarenal action of aldosterone on mammalian skeletal muscle. *Am J Physiol* 218:616, 1970.
2. Adrogué HJ et al: Role of the endocrine pancreas in the kalemic response to acute metabolic acidosis in conscious dogs. *J Clin Invest* 75:798, 1985.
3. Androgué HJ, Madias NE: Changes in plasma potassium concentration during acute acid base disturbances. *Am J Med* 71:456, 1981.
4. Alexander EA, Levinsky NG: An extrarenal mechanism of potassium adaptation. *J Clin Invest* 47:740, 1968.
5. Allon M et al: Nebulized albuterol for acute hyperkalemia in patients on hemodialysis. *Ann Intern Med* 11:426, 1989.
6. Allon M, Copkney C: Albuterol and insulin for treatment of hyperkalemia in hemodialysis patients. *Kidney Int* 38:869, 1990.
7. Altenberg GA et al: Amiloride prevents the metabolic acidosis of a KCl load in nephrectomized rats. *Clin Sci* 76:649, 1989.
8. Alvestrand A et al: Insulin-mediated potassium uptake is normal in uremic and healthy subjects. *Am J Physiol* 246:E174, 1984.
9. Alvo M et al: Effect of a simultaneous potassium and carbohydrate load on extrarenal K homeostasis in end-stage renal failure. *Nephron* 53:133, 1989.

10. Andres R et al: Effect of insulin on carbohydrate metabolism and on potassium in the forearm of man. *J Clin Invest* 41:108, 1962.
11. Archampong EQ et al: The absorption and secretion of water and electrolytes across the healthy and the diseased human colonic mucosa measured in vitro. *Gut* 13:880, 1972.
12. Arthur S, Greenberg A: Hyperkalemia associated with intravenous labetalol therapy for acute hypertension in renal transplant recipients. *Clin Nephrol* 33:269, 1990.
13. Asano Y: Increased cell membrane permeability to Na^+ and K^+ induced by thyroid hormone in rat skeletal muscle. *Experientia* 32(suppl):199, 1978.
14. August JT et al: Response of normal subjects to large amounts of aldosterone. *J Clin Invest* 37:1549, 1958.
15. Barbour GL, Keller AW: Distal renal tubular acidosis in selective hypoaldosteronism. *South Med J* 71:1397, 1956.
16. Bartter FC, Fourman P: The different effects of aldosterone-like steroids on urinary excretion of potassium and acid. *Metabolism* 11:6, 1962.
17. Bastl CP et al: Increased large intestinal secretion of potassium in renal insufficiency. *Kidney Int* 12:9, 1977.
18. Bastl CP et al: Characteristics of potassium secretion in the mammalian colon. *Am J Physiol* 234:F48, 1978.
19. Bastl CP et al: Role of glucocorticoids and aldosterone in maintenance of colonic cation transport. *Am J Physiol* 238:F181, 1980.
20. Batts AA et al: The effect of growth hormone on muscle potassium and on extracellular fluid. *Endrocrinology* 55:456, 1954.
21. Bengele HH et al: Impaired renal and extrarenal potassium adaptation in old rats. *Kidney Int* 23:684, 1983.
22. Bergstrom J et al: Muscle intracellular electrolytes in patients with chronic uremia. *Kidney Int* 24:S153, 1983.
23. Berlyne GM et al: Exchangeable potassium and renal potassium handling in advanced chronic renal failure in man. *Nephron* 8:264, 1971.
24. Bethune DW, McKay R: Paradoxical changes in serum-potassium during cardiopulmonary bypass in association with non-cardioselective beta-blockade. *Lancet* 2:381, 1978.
25. Bia MJ, DeFronzo RA: Extrarenal potassium homeostasis. *Am J Physiol* 240:F257, 1981.
26. Bia MJ et al: Regulation of extrarenal potassium homeostasis by adrenal hormones in rats. *Am J Physiol* 242:F641, 1982.
27. Binder HJ: Effect of dexamethasone on electrolyte transport in the large intestine of the rat. *Gastroenterology* 75:212, 1978.
28. Biron R et al: Thyroid hormones and the energetics of active sodium-potassium transport in mammalian skeletal muscles. *J Physiol* (*Lond*) 297:47, 1979.
29. Brooks RV et al: Potassium deficiency of renal and adrenal origin. *Am J Med* 23:391, 1957.
30. Brown RS: Extrarenal potassium homeostasis. *Kidney Int* 30:116, 1986.
31. Bunner DL et al: Comparative potency of subtilisin-cleaved and intact human growth hormone measured in growth hormone-deficient human subjects. *J Clin Endocrinol Metab* 48:293, 1979.
32. Burnell JM et al: Effect in humans of extracellular pH change in relationship between serum potassium concentration and intracellular potassium. *J Clin Invest* 35:935, 1956.
33. Burton SD et al: Dissociation of potassium and glucose efflux in isolated perfused rat liver. *Am J Physiol* 212:261, 1967.
34. Castro-Tavares J: A comparison between the influence of pindolol and propranolol on the response of plasma potassium to catecholamines. *Arzneim Forsch* 26:238, 1976.
35. Charney AN et al: Na-K-activated adenosine triphosphatase and intestinal electrolyte transport. *J Clin Invest* 56:653, 1975.
36. Charney AN et al: Acute respiratory alkalosis and acidosis and rabbit intestinal ion transport in vivo. *Am J Physiol* 244:G145, 1983.
37. Charron RC et al: The effect of adrenal steroids on stool composition, as revealed by in vivo dialysis of faeces. *Clin Sci* 37:151, 1969.
38. Clausen T: Regulation of active Na^+-K^+ transport in skeletal muscle. *Physiol Rev* 66:542, 1986.
39. Clausen T, Everts ME: Regulation of the Na,K-pump in skeletal muscle. *Kidney Int* 35:1, 1989.
40. Clausen T, Flatman JA: The effect of catecholamines on Na-K transport and membrane potential in rat soleus muscle. *J Physiol (Lond)* 270:383, 1977.
41. Clausen T, Hansen O: Active Na-K transport and the rate of ouabain binding: The effect of insulin and other stimuli on skeletal muscle and adipocytes. *J Physiol (Lond)* 270:415, 1977.
42. Clausen T, Kohn PG: The effect of insulin on the transport of sodium and potassium in rat soleus muscle. *J Physiol (Lond)* 265:19, 1977.
43. Clifton GD et al: Effects of sequential doses of parenteral terbutaline on plasma levels of potassium and related cardiopulmonary responses. *Am Rev Respir Dis* 141:575, 1990.
44. Coester N et al: Plasma electrolytes, pH and ECG during and after exhaustive exercise. *J Appl Physiol* 34:677, 1973.
45. Cole CH: Decreased ouabain-sensitive adenosine triphosphatase activity in the erythrocyte membrane of patients with chronic renal disease. *Clin Sci* 45:775, 1973.
46. Conte G et al: Acute increase in plasma osmolality as a cause of hyperkalemia in patients with renal failure. *Kidney Int* 38:301, 1990.
47. Cotton JR et al: Resting skeletal muscle membrane potential as an index of uremic toxicity. *J Clin Invest* 63:501, 1979.
48. Cox JR, Shalaby WA: Potassium changes with age. *Gerontology* 27:340, 1981.
49. Cox M et al: The defense against hyperkalemia: The roles of insulin and aldosterone. *N Engl J Med* 299:525, 1978.
50. Davis JO, Howell DW: Comparative effect of ACTH, cortisone and DCA on renal function, electrolyte excretion and water exchange in normal dogs. *Endocrinology* 52:245.
51. Dawborn JK, Watson L: Effect of prolonged administration of aldosterone on potassium and magnesium metabolism in the rabbit. *Med J Aust* 2:304, 1968.
52. DeFronzo RA: Hyperkalemia and hyporeninemic hypoaldosteronism. *Kidney Int* 17:118, 1980.

53. DeFronzo RA et al: Influence of basal insulin and glucagon secretion on potassium and sodium metabolism: Studies with somatostatin in normal dogs and in normal diabetic human beings. *J Clin Invest* 61:472, 1978.
54. DeFronzo RA et al: Impaired renal tubular potassium secretion in sickle cell disease. *Ann Intern Med* 90:310, 1979.
55. DeFronzo RA et al: Effect of graded doses of insulin on splanchnic and peripheral potassium metabolism in man. *Am J Physiol* 238:E421, 1980.
56. DeFronzo RA et al: The effect of epinephrine on potassium homeostasis. *Kidney Int* 20:83, 1981.
57. Dluhy RG et al: Serum immunoreactive insulin and growth hormone response to potassium in normal man. *J Appl Physiol* 33:22, 1972.
58. Druml W et al: Abnormal cation transport in uremia. *J Clin Invest* 81:1197, 1988.
59. D'Silva JL: The action of adrenaline on serum potassium. *J Physiol (Lond)* 82:393, 1934.
60. D'Silva JL: The action of adrenaline on serum potassium. *J Physiol (Lond)* 86:219, 1936.
61. Edelman IS, Leibman J: Anatomy of body water and electrolytes. *Am J Med* 27:256, 1959.
62. Edmonds CJ: The gradient of electrical potential difference and of sodium and potassium of the gut contents along the caecum and colon of normal and sodium-depleted rats. *J Physiol (Lond)* 193:571, 1967.
63. Edmonds CJ: Amiloride sensitivity of the transepithelial electrical potential and of sodium and potassium transport in rat distal colon in vivo. *J Physiol (Lond)* 313:547, 1981.
64. Edmonds CJ, Godfrey RC: Measurement of electrical potentials of the human rectum and pelvic colon in normal and aldosterone-treated patients. *Gut* 11:330, 1970.
65. Edmonds CJ, Marriott J: Factors influencing the electrical potential across the mucosa of rat colon. *J Physiol (Lond))* 194:457, 1968.
66. Edmonds CJ, Smith T: Total body potassium in relation to thyroid hormones and hyperthyroidism. *Clin Sci* 60:311, 1981.
67. El Shahawy M et al: Hyperthyroidism and potassium. *JAMA* 217:969, 1971.
68. Elliott DA, Cheek DB: Muscle electrolyte patterns during growth, in Cheek DB (ed): *Human Growth*. Philadelphia, Lea & Febiger, 1968, p 260.
69. Ellis S, Beckett SB: Mechanism of the potassium mobilizing action of epinephrine and glucagon. *J Pharmacol Exp Ther* 142:318, 1963.
70. Ellis KJ et al: A predictor for total body potassium in man based on height, weight, sex, and age: application in metabolic disorders. *J Lab Clin Med* 83:716, 1974.
71. Elrick H et al: Effects of glucagon on renal function in man. *J Clin Endocrinol Metab* 18:813, 1958.
72. Emmanouel DS et al: Pathogenesis and characterization of hyperglucogonemia in the uremic rat. *J Clin Invest* 58:1266, 1976.
73. Ericsson F et al: Effect of digoxin upon intracellular potassium in man. *Scand J Clin Lab Invest* 41:457, 1981.
74. Ericsson F: Intracellular potassium in man. *Scand J Clin Lab Invest* 42 (Suppl) 163:36, 1982.
75. Everts ME et al: $Na^+ - K^+$ pump in rat muscle: Effects of hypophysectomy, growth hormone, and thyroid hormone. *Am J Physiol* 259:E278, 1990.
76. Ezra D et al: Evidence for an extrarenal action of chlorothiazide on serum potassium. *Miner Electrolyte Metab* 7:285, 1982.
77. Feldman GM, Charney AN: Effect of acute metabolic alkalosis and acidosis on intestinal electrolyte transport in vivo. *Am J Physiol* 239:G427, 1980.
78. Feldman GM, Charney AN: Effect of acute respiratory alkalosis and acidosis on intestinal ion transport in vivo. *Am J Physiol* 242:G486, 1982.
79. Fernandez J et al: Impaired extrarenal disposal of an acute oral potassium load in patients with endstage renal disease on chronic hemodialysis. *Miner Electrolyte Metab* 12:125, 1986.
80. Field H et al: Electrolyte changes in ileal contents and in feces during restriction of dietary sodium with and without the administration of cation-exchange resin. *Circulation* 12:625, 1955.
81. Fisher KA et al: Potassium secretion by colonic mucosal cells after potassium adaptation. *Am J Physiol* 251:987, 1976.
82. Flatman JA, Clausen T: Combined effects of adrenaline and insulin on active electrogenic $Na^+ - K^+$ transport in rat soleus muscle. *Nature* 281:580, 1979.
83. Foster ES et al: Cyclic adenosine monophosphate stimulates active potassium secretion in the rat colon. *Gastroenterology* 84:324, 1983.
84. Foster ES et al: Role of aldosterone and dietary potassium in potassium adaptation in the distal colon of the rat. *Gastroenterology* 88:41, 1985.
85. Foster ES et al: Dietary potassium modulates active potassium absorption and secretion in rat distal colon. *Am J Physiol* 251:G619, 1986.
86. French W, Manery JF: The effect of aldosterone on electrolytes in muscle, kidney cortex and serum. *Can J Biochem* 42:1459, 1964.
87. Frizzell RA et al: Ion transport by rabbit colon: 1. Active and passive components. *J Membr Biol* 27:297, 1976.
88. Fromm M, Hegel U: Segmental heterogeneity of epithelial transport in rat large intestine. *Pfluegers Arch* 378:71, 1978.
89. Fulop M: Serum potassium in lactic acidosis and ketoacidosis. *N Engl J Med* 300:1087, 1979.
90. Gardos G: The function of calcium in the potassium permeability of human erythrocytes. *Biochim Biophys Acta* 30:653, 1958.
91. Garg LC et al: Mineralocorticoid effects on Na-K-ATPase in individual nephron segments. *Am J Physiol* 240:F536, 1981.
92. Gerstein A et al: Aldosterone deficiency in chronic renal failure. *Nephron* 5:90, 1968.
93. Gifford JD et al: Control of serum potassium during fasting in patients with end-stage renal disease. *Kidney Int* 35:90, 1989.
94. Glinsmann WH, Mortimore GE: Influence of glucagon and 3′, 5′-AMP on insulin responsiveness of the perfused rat liver. *Am J Physiol* 215:553, 1968.
95. Goecke IA et al: Enhanced insulin sensitivity in extrarenal potassium handling in uremic rats. *Kidney Int* 39:39, 1991.

96. Gonick HD et al: Functional impairment in chronic renal disease. Studies of potassium excretion. *Am J Med Sci* 216:281, 1971.
97. Good DW, Wright FS: Luminal influences on potassium secretion: Sodium concentration and fluid flow rate. *Am J Physiol* 236:F192, 1979.
98. Goulston D et al: Effect of mineralocorticoids on the sodium/potassium ratio of human ileostomy fluid. *Lancet* 2:541, 1963.
99. Gronert GR, Theye RA: Pathophysiology of hyperkalemia induced by succinylcholine. *Anesthesiology* 43:89, 1975.
100. Haber RS, Loeb JN: Effect of 3, 5, 3′-triiodothyronine treatment on potassium efflux from isolated rat diaphragm: role of increased permeability in the thermogenic response. *Endocrinology* 11:1217, 1982.
101. Hawker PC et al: Mechanisms of transport of Na, Cl, and K in the human colon. *Gastroenterology* 74:1241, 1978.
102. Hayes CP, Robinson RR: Fecal potassium excretion in patients on chronic intermittent hemodialysis. *Trans Am Soc Artif Intern Organs* 11:242, 1965.
103. Hayes CP et al: An extrarenal mechanism for the maintenance of potassium balance in severe chronic renal failure. *Trans Assoc Am Physicians* 80:207, 1964.
104. Hayslett JP et al: Mechanism of increased potassium secretion in potassium loading and sodium deprivation. *Am J Physiol* 239:F378, 1980.
105. Hayslett JP et al: Demonstration of net potassium absorption in mammalian colon. *Am J Physiol* 242:G209, 1982.
106. Hazeyama Y, Sparks HV: A model of potassium efflux during exercise of skeletal muscle. *Am J Physiol* 236:R83, 1979.
107. Hene RJ et al: Plasma aldosterone concentrations in chronic renal disease. *Kidney Int* 21:98, 1982.
108. Henneman PH et al: Effects of human growth hormone in man. *J Clin Invest* 39:1223, 1960.
109. Hiatt N et al: The effect of potassium chloride on insulin secretion in vivo. *Horm Metab Res* 4:64, 1972.
110. Hiatt N et al: Necessity for insulin in transfer of excess infused K to intracellular fluid. Metabolism 23:43, 1974.
111. Hirche HE et al: Extracellular K^+ concentration and K^+ balance of the gastrocnemius muscle of the dog during exercise. *Pfluegers Arch* 387:231, 1980.
112. Ismail-Beigi F, Edelman IS: Mechanism of thyroid calorigenesis: role of active sodium transport. *Proc Natl Acad Sci USA* 67:1071, 1970.
113. Ismail-Beigi F, Edelman IS: Effects of thyroid status on electrolyte distribution in rat tissues. *Am J Physiol* 225:1172, 1973.
114. Jacobs DR, Posner JB: Isolated analdosteronism: 2. The nature of the adrenal cortical enzymatic defect, and the influence of diet and various agents on electrolyte balance. *Metabolism* 13:522, 1964.
115. Kahn T et al: Factors related to potassium transport in stable chronic renal disease. *Clin Sci* 54:661, 1978.
116. Kaji DM, Kahn T: Na^+–K^+ pump in chronic renal failure. *Am J Physiol* 252:F785, 1987.
117. Kashgarian M et al: Amplification of cell membrane surface in potassium adaptation. *Lab Invest* 42:581, 1980.
118. Kharasch ED, Bowdle TA: Hypokalemia before induction of anesthesia and prevention by β_2 adrenoceptor antagonism. *Anesth Analg* 72:216, 1991.
119. Kliger AS et al: Demonstration of active potassium transport in the mammalian colon. *J Clin Invest* 67:1189, 1981.
120. Knight RP et al: Effects of intravenous hydrocortisone on electrolytes of serum and urine in man. *J Clin Endocrinol* 15:176, 1955.
121. Knochel JP: Personal communication.
122. Knochel JP et al: Muscle cell hyperpolarization and potassium tolerance induced by exercise training. *Clin Res* 25:445A, 1977.
123. Kopple JD, Coburn JW: Metabolic studies of low protein diets in uremia: 1. Nitrogen and potassium. *Medicine* 52:583, 1973.
124. Kubota K, Ingbar SH: Influences of thyroid status and sympathoadrenal system on extrarenal potassium disposal. *Am J Physiol* 258:E428, 1990.
125. Levitt MF, Bader ME: Effect of cortisone and ACTH on fluid and electrolyte distribution in man. *Am J Med* 11:715, 1951.
126. Lim VS, Webster GD: The effect of aldosterone on water and electrolyte composition of incubated rat diaphragms. *Clin Sci* 33:261, 1967.
127. Lipworth BJ et al: Prior treatment with diuretic augments the hypokalemic electrocardiographic effects of inhaled albuterol. *Am J Med* 86:653, 1989.
128. Loeb RD et al: Electrolyte balance studies in adrenalectomized dogs with particular reference to the excretion of sodium. *J Exp Med* 57:775, 1933.
129. Lundborg P: The effect of adrenergic blockade on potassium concentrations in different conditions. *Acta Med Scand Suppl* 672:121, 1983.
130. Lye M: Distribution of body potassium in healthy elderly subjects. *Gerontology* 27:286, 1981.
131. Lytton J: Insulin affects the sodium affinity of the rat adipocyte (Na^+,K^+)-ATPase. *J Biol Chem* 260:10075, 1985.
132. Mader IJ, Iseri LT: Spontaneous hypopotassemia, hypomagnesemia, alkalosis and tetany due to hypersecretion of corticosterone-like mineralocorticoid. *Am J Med* 19:976, 1955.
133. Magner PO et al: The plasma potassium concentration in metabolic acidosis: A re-evaluation. *Am J Kidney Dis* 3:220, 1988.
134. Makoff DL et al: Hypertonic expansion: acid-base and electrolyte changes. *Am J Physiol* 218:1207, 1970.
135. Makoff DI et al: On the mechanism of hyperkalemia due to hyperosmotic expansion with saline or mannitol. *Clin Sci* 41:383, 1971.
136. Manson JM, Wilmore DW: Positive nitrogen balance with human growth hormone and hypocaloric intravenous feeding. *Surgery* 100:188, 1986.
137. Massara F et al: Influence of glucagon on plasma levels of potassium in man. *Diabetologia* 19:414, 1980.
138. Massry SG: The toxic effects of parathyroid hormone in uremia. *Semin Nephrol* 3:306, 1983.
139. McCabe R et al: Potassium transport by rabbit descending colon. *Am J Physiol* 242:C81, 1982.
140. McCance RA: The effect of salt deficiency in man on the volume of the extracellular fluids, and on the composition of sweat, saliva, gastric juice and cerebrospinal fluid. *J Physiol* 92:208, 1938.
141. McCleane GJ, Watters CH: Pre-operative anxiety and serum potassium. *Anesthesia* 45:583, 1990.

142. McGeoch JE: The alpha-2 isomer of the sodium pump is inhibited by calcium at physiological levels. *Biochem Biophys Res Commun* 173:99, 1990.
143. McLaughlin ML et al: Secondary hyperaldosteronism stimulates acidification in rat distal colon. *Pfluegers Arch* 416:639, 1990.
144. Medbo JI, Sejersted OM: Plasma potassium changes with high intensity exercise. *J Physiol* 421:105, 1990.
145. Meech RW: Calcium-dependent potassium activation in nervous tissues. *Annu Rev Biophys Bioeng* 7:1, 1978.
146. Meechan JG, Rawlins MD: The effect of adrenaline in lignocaine anaesthetic solutions on plasma potassium in healthy volunteers. *Eur J Clin Pharmacol* 32:81, 1987.
147. Mills JN et al: The acute effect of hydrocortisone, deoxycorticosterone and aldosterone upon the excretion of sodium, potassium and acid by the human kidney. *J Physiol* 151:312, 1960.
148. Milne MD et al: Primary aldosteronism. *Q J Med* 26:317, 1957.
149. Mimran A et al: Nitrendipine enhances the effect of epinephrine on serum potassium in normal man. *J Hyperten* 4(suppl 5):S213, 1986.
150. Montoliu J et al: Potassium-lowering effect of albuterol for hyperkalemia in renal failure. *Arch Intern Med* 147:713, 1987.
151. Moore RD, Rabovsky JL: Mechanism of insulin action on resting membrane potential of frog skeletal muscle. *Am J Physiol* 236:C249, 1979.
152. Moravec MA, Hurlbert BJ: Hypokalemia associated with terbutaline administration in obstetrical patients. *Anesth Analg* 59:917, 1980.
153. Moreto M et al: Effects of secretagogues on the K^+ permeability of mucosal and serosal borders of rabbit colonic mucosa. *Biochim Biophys Acta* 648:215, 1981.
154. Morgan DB, Young RM: Acute transient hypokalaemia: New interpretation of a common event. *Lancet* 2:751, 1982.
155. Moss S et al: Water and electrolyte composition of urine and ileal fluid and its relationship to renin and aldosterone during dietery sodium deprivation in patients with ileostomies. *Clin Sci* 61:407, 1981.
156. Nicolis GL et al: Glucose-induced hyperkalemia in diabetic subjects. *Arch Intern Med* 141:49, 1981.
157. Norby LH et al: Possible role for impaired renal prostaglandin production in pathogenesis of hyporeninaemic hypoaldosteronism. *Lancet* 2:1118, 1978.
158. Nuttall FQ: Serum electrolytes and their relation to acid-base balance. *Arch Intern Med* 116:670, 1965.
159. Osore H: Effects of D-aldosterone on sodium and potassium concentrations of incubated renal slices: A dual mechanism of action. *East Afr Med J* 58:912, 1981.
160. Oster JR et al: Relationship between blood pH and potassium and phosphorus during acute metabolic acidosis. *Am J Physiol* 235:F345, 1978.
161. Oster JR et al: Plasma potassium response to acute metabolic acidosis induced by mineral and nonmineral acids. *Miner Electrolyte Metab* 4:28, 1980.
162. Pedersen G, Pedersen EB: Effect of propranolol on total exchangeable body potassium and total exchangeable body sodium in essential hypertension. *Scand J Clin Lab Invest* 39:167, 1979.
163. Perrone RD et al: Mineralocorticoid activity of 19-nor-DOC and 19-OH-DOC in adrenalectomized rat. *Am J Physiol* 242:E305, 1982.
164. Perrone RD, McBride DE: Aldosterone and P_{CO_2} enhance rubidium absorption in rat distal colon. *Am J Physiol* 254:G898, 1988.
165. Perrone RD et al: Aldosterone induces apical vesicles in rat distal colon. *Am J Physiol* 259:F65, 1990.
166. Pettit G et al: Plasma K^+ and insulin: Changes during KCl infusion in normal and nephrectomized dogs. *Am J Physiol* 228:107, 1975.
167. Pettit GW et al: The contribution of renal and extrarenal mechanisms to hypokalemia induced by glucagon. *Eur J Pharmacol* 41:437, 1977.
168. Podolsky S, Melby JC: Improvement of growth hormone response to stimulation in primary aldosteronism with correction of potassium deficiency. *Metabolism* 25:1027, 1976.
169. Podolsky S et al: Potassium depletion in hepatic cirrhosis: A reversible cause of impaired growth-hormone and insulin response to stimulation. *N Engl J Med* 288:644, 1973.
170. Ponce SP et al: Drug-induced hyperkalemia. *Medicine* 64:357, 1985.
171. Pratt JH: Role of Angiotensin II in potassium-mediated stimulation of aldosterone secretion in the dog. *J Clin Invest* 70:567, 1982.
172. Pratt JH et al: Evidence that angiotensin-II and potassium collaborate to increase cytosolic calcium and stimulate the secretion of aldosterone. *Endocrinology* 125:2463, 1989.
173. Pullman TN et al: Direct effects of glucagon on renal hemodynamics and excretion of inorganic ions. *Metabolism* 16:358, 1967.
174. Putney JW Jr: Stimulus permeability coupling: Role of calcium in the receptor regulation of membrane permeability. *Pharmacol Rev* 30:209, 1979.
175. Rosa RM et al: Adrenergic modulation of extrarenal potassium disposal. *N Engl J Med* 302:431, 1980.
176. Salerno DM: Postresuscitation hypokalemia in a patient with a normal prearrest serum potassium level. *Ann Intern Med* 108:836, 1988.
177. Santeusanio F et al: Evidence for a role of endogenous insulin and glucagon in the regulation of potassium homeostasis. *J Lab Clin Med* 81:809, 1973.
178. Saris S et al: Lack of effect of nonsteroidal anti-inflammatory drugs on exercise-induced hyperkalemia. *N Engl J Med* 307:559, 1982.
179. Satoyoshi E et al: Myopathy in thyrotoxicosis. *Neurology* 13:645, 1963.
180. Savoie JC, Jungers P: Intracellular potassium in hyperthyroidism, in Cassano C, Andreoli M (eds): *Current Topics in Thyroid Research*. New York, Academic Press, 1965, p 1065.
181. Schon DA et al: Mechanism of potassium excretion in renal insufficiency. *Am J Physiol* 227:1323, 1974.
182. Schrier RW, Regal EM: Influence of aldosterone on sodium, water and potassium metabolism in chronic renal disease. *Kidney Int* 1:156, 1972.
183. Scribner BH, Burnell JM: Interpretation of the serum potassium concentration. *Metabolism* 5:468, 1956.
184. Sherwin RS et al: Influence of uremia and hemodialysis on the turnover and metabolic effects of glucagon. *J Clin Invest* 57:722, 1976.

185. Sherwin RS et al: Influence of physiologic hyperglucagonemia on urinary glucose, nitrogen and electrolyte excretion in diabetes. *Metabolism* 26:53, 1977.
186. Shields R et al: Action of aldosterone upon the intestinal transport of potassium, sodium, and water. *Gut* 7:686, 1966.
187. Shields R et al: Absorption and secretion of water and electrolytes by the intact colon in a patient with primary aldosteronism. *Br Med J* 1:93, 1968.
188. Shishiba Y et al: Potassium deficiency enhances the effect of thyroid hormone on NaK-ATPase in liver and kidney. *Endocrinol Jpn* 27:329, 1980.
189. Shoemaker WC, Finder AG: Relation of potassium and glucose release from the liver in the unanesthetized dog. *Proc Soc Exp Biol Med* 108:248, 1961.
190. Smith TW et al: Treatment of life-threatening digitalis intoxication with digoxin-specific Fab antibody fragments: Experience in 26 cases. *N Engl J Med* 307:1357, 1982.
191. Soliman AR et al: Parathyroid hormone interferes with extrarenal disposition of potassium in chronic renal failure. *Nephron* 52:262, 1989.
192. Spencer RP: Potassium metabolism and gastrointestinal function: A review. *Am J Dig Dis* 4:145, 1959.
193. Spital A, Sterns RH: Paradoxical potassium depletion: A renal mechanism for extrarenal potassium adaptation. *Kidney Int* 30:532, 1986.
194. Spital A, Sterns RH: Extrarenal potassium adaptation: The role of aldosterone. *Clin Sci* 76:213, 1989.
195. Stark RJ, O'Doherty J: Intracellular Na^+ and K^+ activities during insulin stimulation of rat soleus muscle. *Am J Physiol* 242:E193, 1982.
196. Stark RJ et al: Continuous measurements of intracellular sodium and potassium activities during insulin stimulation of adipocytes. *Diabetes* 29:1040, 1980.
197. Staub A et al: A renal action of glucagon. *Proc Soc Exp Biol Med* 94:57, 1957.
198. Stemmer CL et al: Impairment of beta 2-adrenoceptor-stimulated potassium uptake in end-stage renal disease. *J Clin Pharmacol* 27:628, 1987.
199. Stern TN et al: Dynamic aspects of sodium metabolism in experimental adrenal insufficiency using radioactive sodium. *Am J Physiol* 164:437, 1951.
200. Sterns RH et al: Role of insulin in human K^+ homeostasis. *Kidney Int* 12:475, 1977.
201. Sterns RH et al: Disposition of intravenous potassium in anuric man: A kinetic analysis *Kidney Int* 15:651, 1979.
202. Sugarman A, Brown RS: The role of aldosterone in potassium tolerance: Studies in anephric humans. *Kidney Int* 34:397, 1988.
203. Sugarman A, Kahn T: Calcium channel blockers enhance extrarenal potassium disposal in the rat. *Am J Physiol* 250:F695, 1986.
204. Sugarman A, Kahn T: Parathyroid hormone impairs extrarenal potassium tolerance in the rat. *Am J Physiol* 254:F385, 1988.
205. Suzuki H et al: Role of hormonal factors in plasma K alterations in acute respiratory and metabolic alkalosis in dogs. *Am J Physiol* 258:F305, 1990.
206. Swan RC, Pitts RF: Neutralization of infused acid by nephrectomized dogs. *J Clin Invest* 34:205, 1955.
207. Szylman P et al: Nonazotemic hyperkalemia with renal and extrarenal defects in potassium transport: Association with high levels of digoxin-like immunoreactive factor. *J Lab Clin Med* 116:315, 1990.
208. Tannen RL et al: K^+ transport by rat colon: Adaptation to a low potassium diet. *Am J Physiol* 250:F483, 1984.
209. Teixeira da Silva JC Jr et al: Na,K-ATPase mRNA isoform expression in uremia (abstract). *J Am Soc Nephrol* 1:643, 1990.
210. Thomas DJB, Dove AF: Metabolic effects of salbutamol infusion during premature labor. *Br J Obstet Gynecol* 84:497, 1977.
211. Thompson BD, Edmonds CJ: Comparison of effects of prolonged aldosterone administration on rat colon and renal electrolyte excretion. *J Endocrinol* 50:163, 1971.
212. Todd EP, Vick RL: Kaleotropic effect of epinephrine: Analysis with adrenergic agonists and antagonists. *Am J Physiol* 220:1963, 1971.
213. Todd EP et al: The influence of the rate of infusion on the kaleotropic effect of epinephrine. *Arch Intern Physiol Biochim* 77:33, 1969.
214. Tonshoff B et al: Disturbance of growth hormone-insulin-like growth factor axis in uraemia. *Pediatr Nephrol* 4:654, 1990.
215. Turnberg LA: Potassium transport in the human small bowel. *Gut* 12:811, 1971.
216. Unger RH, Dobbs RE: Insulin, glucagon, and somatostatin secretion in the regulation of metabolism. *Annu Rev Physiol* 40:307, 1978.
217. Useda Y et al: Response of plasma ACTH and adrenocortical hormones to potassium loading in essential hypertension. *Jpn Circ J* 46:317, 1982.
218. Vea AM et al: Beta adrenergic modulation of extrarenal potassium disposal in terminal uraemia. *Proc Eur Dialysis Transplant Assoc* 19:756, 1982.
219. Vick RL et al: Epinephrine-induced hypokalemia: Relation to liver and skeletal muscle. *J Pharmacol Exp Ther* 181:139, 1972.
220. Ward RA et al: Hemodialysate composition and intradialytic metabolic, acid-base and potassium changes. *Kidney Int* 32:129, 1987.
221. Welt LG et al: An ion transport defect in erythrocytes from uremic patients. *Trans Assoc Am Physicians* 77:169, 1986.
222. Whittam R: The control of membrane permeability to potassium in red blood cells. *Nature* 219:610, 1968.
223. Will PC et al: Induction of amiloride-sensitive sodium transport in the rat colon by mineralocorticoids. *Am J Physiol* 238:F261, 1980.
224. Will PC et al: Induction of amiloride-sensitive sodium transport in the intestines by adrenal steroids. *Ann NY Acad Sci* 372:64, 1981.
225. Williams ME et al: Impairment of extrarenal potassium disposal by α-adrenergic stimulation. *N Engl J Med* 311:145, 1984.
226. Wills NK, Biagi B: Active potassium transport by rabbit descending colon epithelium. *J Membr Biol* 64:195, 1982.
227. Wilson DR et al: The chemical composition of faeces in uraemia as revealed by in-vivo faecal dialysis. *Clin Sci* 35:197, 1968.

228. Wolfson SK, Ellis S: Effects of glucagon on plasma potassium. *Proc Soc Exp Biol Med* 91:226, 1958.
229. Wrong O, Metcalfe-Gibson A: The electrolyte content of faeces. *Proc R Soc Med* 58:1007, 1965.
230. Ziegler TR et al: Metabolic effects of recombinant human growth hormone in patients receiving parenteral nutrition. *Ann Surg* 208:6, 1988.
231. Zierler KL, Rogus EM: Rapid hyperpolarization of rat muscle induced by insulin. *Biochim Biophys Acta* 640:687, 1981.
232. Zierler KL, Rogus E: Insulin does not hyperpolarize rat muscle by means of a ouabain-inhibitable process. *Am J Physiol* 241:C145, 1981.
233. Zierler KL: Effect of insulin on membrane potential and potassium content of rat muscle. *Am J Physiol* 197:515, 1959.
234. Zierler KL: Effect of insulin on potassium efflux from rat muscle in the presence and absence of glucose. *Am J Physiol* 198:1066, 1960.
235. Zierler KL: Insulin, ions, and membrane potentials, in Greep RO, Astwood EB (eds): *Handbook of Physiology, Endocrinology*. Washington DC, American Physiolog Society, 1973, section 7, vol 1, p. 347.
236. Zierler KL, Rabinowitz D: Roles of insulin and growth hormone, based on studies of forearm metabolism in man. *Medicine* 42:385, 1963.
237. Zierler KL, Rabinowitz D: Effect of very small concentrations of insulin on forearm metabolism: Persistence of its action on potassium and free fatty acids without its effect on glucose. *J Clin Invest* 43:950, 1964.

CHAPTER • 7

Regulation of renal potassium metabolism

Michael J. Field • Robert W. Berliner • Gerhard H. Giebisch

POTASSIUM HOMEOSTASIS

IMPORTANCE

Potassium ions occupy an important place in the body's electrolyte composition despite their relatively low concentration in the extracellular fluid. This is principally because potassium is the most abundant cation present in intracellular fluid and, as such, it subserves several functions crucial to the normal workings of the cell, and hence of the whole organism. Furthermore, the steep concentration gradient resulting from this differential pattern of distribution across cell membranes is responsible for many of the electrical properties of body cells in both nonexcitable tissues, such as the transporting epithelia of the kidney and gut, and in excitable tissues, including nerve and muscle fibers.

The principal physiologic roles of potassium are listed in Table 7-1. Cell potassium contributes the majority of intracellular solute and thus has a critical role in maintaining normal cell volume.[140,243] An important relationship also exists between intracellular potassium and hydrogen ion concentrations, such that relatively small changes in the former can greatly perturb intracellular pH,[2,250] which, in turn, regulates many metabolic processes. Less well defined roles of cell potassium include an influence on many cell enzyme systems,[231] including those affecting nucleic acid synthesis and hence protein synthesis and cell growth.[28,139] The precise maintenance of the potassium concentration gradient across cell membranes contributes significantly to the resting membrane potential of all cells.[250] It has a crucial role in nerve and muscle excitation. This process involves electrical impulse propagation that is based on rapidly altering the contributions of sodium and potassium electrochemical potential gradients to the cell membrane potential.[102] The important clinical consequences of even quite small variations in extracellular potassium concentration for the normal function of striated, smooth, and cardiac muscle will be considered further in Chap. 22, "Hypokalemic States."

TABLE 7-1 • Physiologic roles of potassium

	References
ROLES OF INTRACELLULAR POTASSIUM	
Cell volume maintenance	140,243
Intracellular pH regulation	2,250
Cell enzyme function	231
DNA/protein synthesis	28
Cell growth	139
ROLES OF TRANSCELLULAR POTASSIUM CONCENTRATION RATIO	
Resting cell-membrane potential	231,250
Neuromuscular excitability	102,231
Cardiac pacemaker rhythmicity	102

Two processes together determine the steady-state relationship between potassium concentrations inside and outside body cells: (1) ATPase-driven sodium-potassium exchange is responsible for active potassium uptake into cells against an electrochemical potential gradient, and (2) the potassium permeability of the cell membrane determines the rate at which potassium ions passively leak out of cells. These two processes are also important in transepithelial potassium transport, by which certain specialized cells, principally in the tubules of the kidney, are able to achieve vectorial potassium transport. In these tissues, active potassium pumping and passive potassium leaks are asymmetrically localized in the basolateral and luminal membranes of the cells. In addition, these two processes are sensitive to a variety of modulating factors. Thus, the same potassium-translocating elements that maintain the high potassium concentration in body cells in general are also responsible for vectorial net potassium transport at the sites in the nephron that control potassium excretion.

COMPONENTS

It is clear from the foregoing that effective mechanisms must exist to maintain both the total body potassium content and the precise partitioning of potassium between the intracellular and extracellular fluid compartments.

Estimates of total body potassium content in humans, based on chemical and isotopic measurements, yield an average of 53 to 55 meq per kilogram of body weight.[151,171] Most of this amount, totaling some 3700 meq in an average male, is located inside cells, primarily within skeletal muscle (3000 meq), liver (200 meq), and erythrocytes (235 meq). Even under conditions of widely varying potassium intake, it has been shown that the surplus or deficit in total body potassium is rarely greater than 5 percent,[171,224] implying a remarkable capacity for the excretory mechanisms to maintain overall potassium balance. Thus, on a typical western diet, providing approximately 1 meq of potassium per kilogram per day, balance is achieved through daily excretion of the same amount, largely via the kidney (>90 percent), although a smaller and less finely regulated loss also occurs via the colon. Fluctuations in the level of intake are matched, within 3 to 5 days, by appropriate adjustments in renal potassium excretion. It has been noted, however, that renal adaptation to potassium depletion is less efficient than to potassium loading,[73,194,224] reflecting perhaps the evolution of a mammalian kidney poised for effective excretion of the relatively high potassium content of a mixed diet. The bulk of this chapter will be devoted to an analysis of the mechanisms by which the kidney effects this regulation.

Although only 2 percent of body potassium is located in the extracellular fluid, its concentration there is held relatively constant, between 3.5 and 5.0 meq/liter, over a wide range of dietary potassium intake. In contrast to the paramount role of the kidney in adjusting to chronic changes in steady-state potassium balance, a variety of extrarenal mechanisms are largely responsible for acute regulation of the extracellular potassium concentration. Chief among these factors are acid-base status[2,59] and the hormones epinephrine, aldosterone, and insulin,[17,18,33,36,37,126,145] all of which influence the distribution of potassium across cell membranes. These mechanisms, which are particularly important in determining the organism's tolerance of an acute load of potassium, are discussed in greater detail in Chap. 6.

In summary, three processes interact in the establishment and maintenance of potassium homeostasis (Fig. 7-1): gastrointestinal intake, internal distribution between intracellular and extracellular fluid compartments, and excretion, very largely a function of the kidney under normal physiologic conditions.

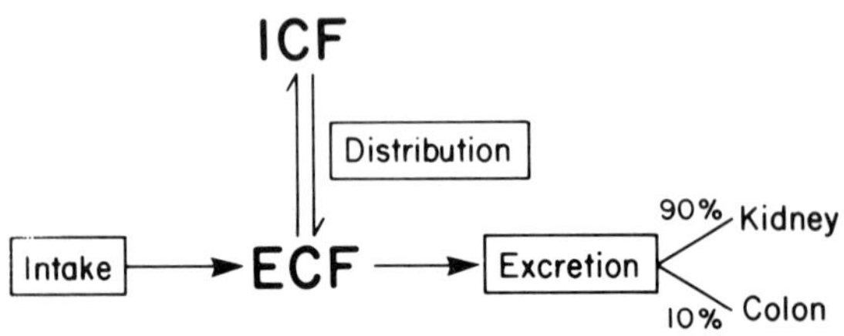

FIGURE 7-1 • Components of potassium homeostasis.

NEPHRON SITES OF POTASSIUM TRANSPORT

GLOMERULAR FILTRATION

Potassium is freely filtered across the glomerular membranes, resulting in concentrations in glomerular ultrafiltrate similar to those in plasma. Small corrections for the effect of the transmembrane Donnan equilibrium, which tends to lower ultrafiltrate potassium concentration, and for plasma water, which tends to elevate it, approximately cancel each other. The rate of glomerular filtration does not in general act as an important physiologic regulator of final urinary potassium excretion rates.[16,137]

PATTERN OF POTASSIUM TRANSPORT ALONG THE TUBULE SYSTEM

Micropuncture profile of superficial nephrons

Since conventional cortical micropuncture techniques provide access only to superficially situated nephrons, it is in these structures that we have the most information concerning the sequential pattern of potassium transport along the tubule system. Dividing the tubule fluid-to-plasma ratio for potassium. $(TF/P)_{K^+}$, by that for inulin, $(TF/P)_{In}$, yields an estimate of the fraction of the filtered potassium that reaches the point from which the micropuncture sample is collected.[72] Data obtained in this way from several studies are summarized in Fig. 7-2.

Proximal tubule

The accessible portion of the proximal convoluted tubule absorbs some 50 to 70 percent of the filtered potassium.[20,142,143,147,177,258] This process has been shown to commence in the very earliest parts of the proximal convolution in Munich-Wistar rats, in which superficial glomeruli are found,[136] it continues, moreover, in late proximal segments accessible for study at the kidney surface. In general, potassium reabsorption appears to be closely tied to reabsorption of sodium and water, since the potassium concentration in tubule fluid shows no great deviation from that in plasma. However,

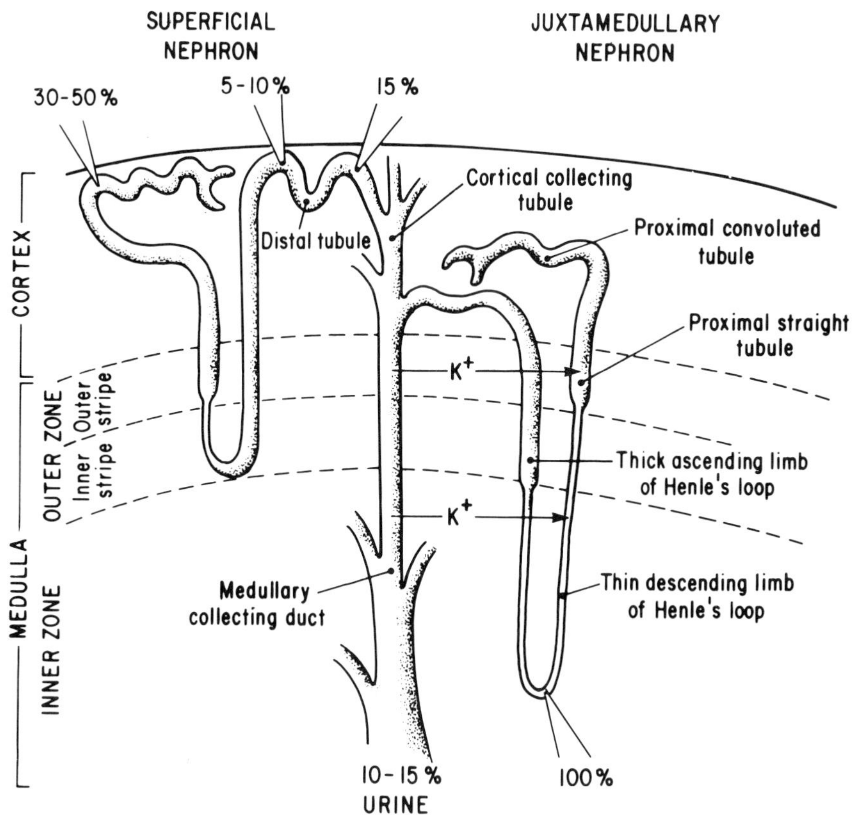

FIGURE 7-2 • Sites of potassium handling by the nephron. Representative superficial and juxtamedullary (deep) portions of nephron are shown, together with typical values, in an animal on a normal potassium diet, for fractional delivery of potassium (percent of filtered load) at sites accessible by micropuncture. Arrows on the juxtamedullary nephron indicate the proposed route for recycling of potassium within the medulla. (Adapted from Tannen RL, in Massry SG, Glassock RJ, eds: *Textbook of Nephrology,* Baltimore, Williams & Wilkins, 1983.)

at least two circumstances have been described in which proximal potassium reabsorption behaves independently of that of sodium and water. First, after acetazolamide administration, potassium reabsorption has been shown to continue normally despite inhibition of proximal bicarbonate, sodium, and fluid transport.[14] Second, the reduction in proximal sodium and fluid reabsorption in the remaining kidney following contralateral nephrectomy is not associated with impaired potassium reabsorption.[42] Whether this dissociation is of importance under more physiologic conditions is not certain.

Despite the extensive potassium reabsorption in the proximal tubule, this process is not generally important in determining rates of final urinary potassium excretion, since small variations in the degree of reabsorption may be compensated for in the loop of Henle.

Loop of Henle

The micropuncturist studies the loop of Henle indirectly by comparing tubular aspirates from the last accessible portion of the proximal convolution and the earliest available segment of the distal tubule. The filtrate is thus altered by the diverse intervening epithelial structures: the pars recta of the proximal tubule, the thin descending limb and thick ascending limb of the loop itself, and the earliest segment of the distal tubule, situated beyond the macula densa. Hence, deductions as to overall loop function gained from micropuncture studies cannot be used to infer the transport characteristics of any particular well-defined segment. Moreover, data obtained by puncturing the hairpin bend of the loop via an approach on the exposed papilla reflect the function only of nephrons originating deeper in the cortex; since these nephrons do not contribute convolutions to the cortical surface, it is not possible to describe confidently in full the segmental transport properties of either superficial or juxtamedullary loops from currently available data.

Setting aside these limitations for the moment, it is possible to deduce for superficial nephrons (which constitute the majority of nephrons in most mammalian species) that the loop segment, as defined above, reabsorbs a further 20 to 40 percent of the filtered potassium load under a wide variety of conditions (Fig. 7-2). As a result, fractional delivery to the earliest accessible distal tubule site usually approximates 10 percent. Although small changes in early distal potassium delivery have been reported following acute potassium infusions,[222] in general, transport of potassium up to this nephron site is little altered.[142,143]

However, acute potassium loading, by stimulating medullary potassium recycling (see "Pattern of Potassium Transport in Juxtamedullary Nephrons," below), enhances the delivery of potassium to the early distal tubule.[109] Potassium depletion stimulates potassium reabsorption,[29] as does the administration of aldosterone, whereas adrenalectomy reduces potassium retrieval and increases the delivery of potassium into the early distal tubule.[204] Ammonium ions compete with potassium ions for reabsorption. The competition of potassium and ammonium ions on the Na-2Cl-K cotransporter explains the fact that hyperkalemia diminishes ammonium deposition in the renal medulla and impedes ammonium excretion into the urine.[78] It is now known from in vitro microperfusion experiments that the greater part of the reabsorptive flux in the loop occurs across the thick ascending limb epithelium[25,218] in parallel with significant reabsorption of sodium and chloride. Agents that interfere with the reabsorptive function of this loop segment, such as the powerful loop diuretics furosemide and ethacrynic acid, result in delivery of increased amounts of potassium to the early distal tubule.[46,154,174] The cellular mechanism responsible for these effects will be discussed below.

Distal tubule

Early clearance and stop-flow studies suggested that the distal tubule represented a potential site of potassium secretion. This prediction was confirmed by micropuncture experiments in which fluid was sampled along the accessible segments of the superficial distal tubule.[122,123] Moreover, the extent of potassium secretion in this segment was highly variable, responding appropriately to a wide range of metabolic challenges (Fig. 7-3). Thus, during potassium loading, appreciable net entry of potassium was evident by the end of the distal tubule, accounting in fact for the greater part of potassium appearing in the final urine under these conditions.[142] Conversely, during potassium depletion, a tendency toward reabsorption was evident along the accessible distal segment, thus contributing to optimum potassium conservation. When urinary excretion rates were 10 to 15 percent of the amount filtered, as seen in animals on a normal diet, a moderate degree of secretion was observed along the distal tubule. Subsequent studies confirmed the importance, at least in the rat, of the "late" portion of the distal tubule as a key regulatory site of potassium excretion. Potassium entry into the late distal tubule was shown to be affected by changes in acid-base status,[145] mineralocorticoid hormones,[32,98,100] plasma potassium concentration,[123,206,260] and many diuretic agents.[71] The details of these and other influences on distal potassium secretion will be treated more fully later in this chapter.

It is important at this stage to emphasize the anatomical basis of the functional studies described above. It is convenient for the micropuncturist to define the "distal tubule" as that nephron segment extending from the macula densa to the first junction with another distal tubule.[72,76] However, it is now clear that this somewhat arbitrary definition takes no account of the well-documented heterogeneity of this portion of the nephron in the rat and hence obscures potentially important differences in the transport characteristics of the component segments.[10,118,209,251] Moreover, since important species differences exist in this regard, extrapolation of classical micropuncture findings, derived chiefly from studies in the rat, to the situation in humans or other animals should be made with caution.

Current nomenclature for the accessible part of the distal tubule in the rat[130] divides this structure into three segments, in which electron microscopic criteria have been used to define at least four cell types,[205] as shown in Fig. 7-4. The first segment, the distal convoluted tubule proper, is composed entirely of a *distal cell* type, characterized by short apical microvilli and deep basolateral membrane infoldings stuffed with mitochondria. This segment, about 1 mm long, constitutes the *early distal tubule,* as identified during micropuncture. It changes gradually, below the kidney surface, to a shorter connecting tubule (also called the mid-distal tubule or transition region) comprising two cell types: *connecting tubule cells,* with smooth luminal membranes and less prominent basolateral infoldings and mitochondria than distal cells, and *intercalated cells,* which are flatter cells with luminal

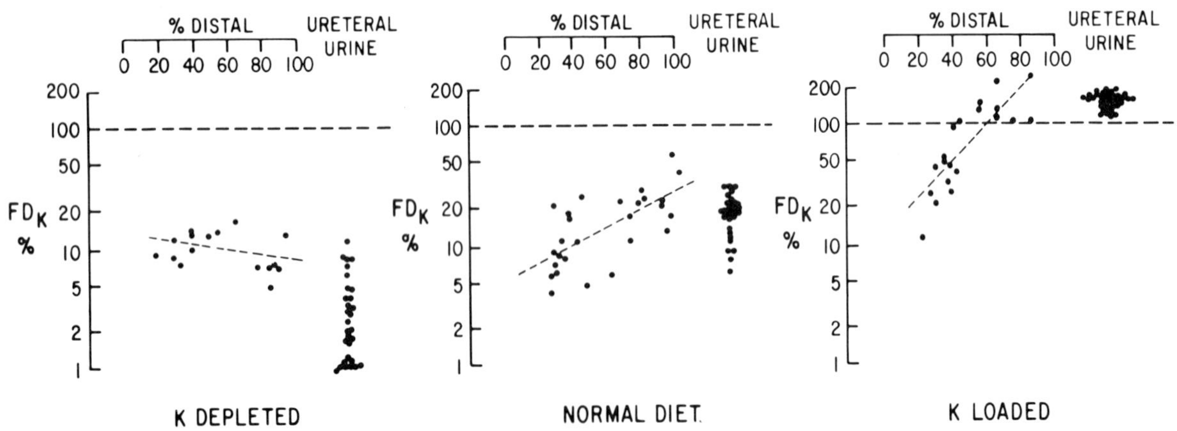

FIGURE 7-3 • Pattern of fractional delivery of potassium (FD$_K$; percent of filtered load) along the distal tubule in rats on low-, normal-, and high-potassium diets. (Adapted from Malnic G et al: *Am J Physiol* 206:674, 1964.)

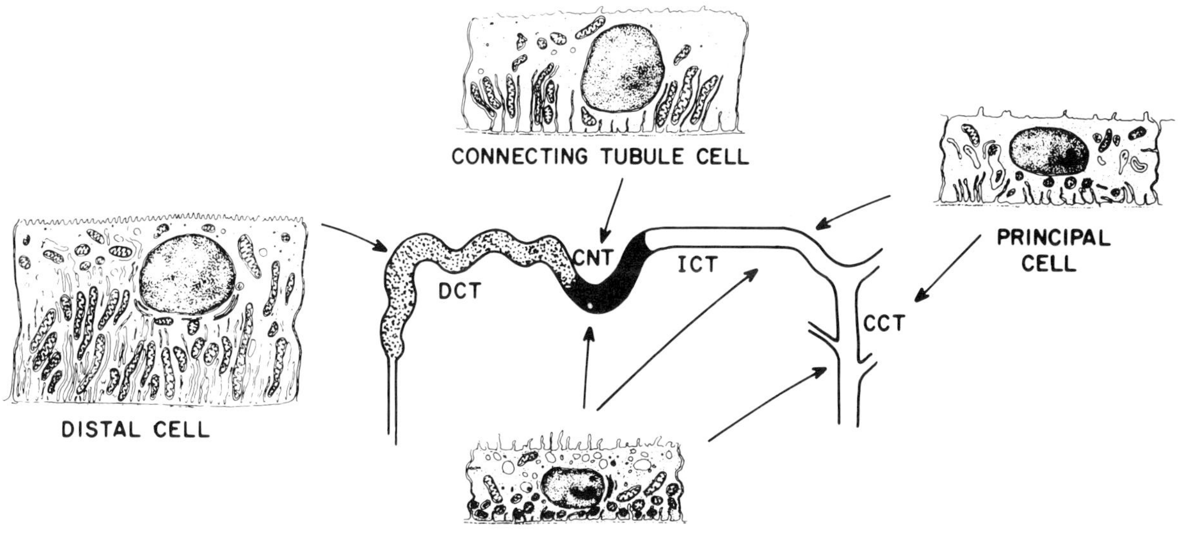

FIGURE 7-4 • Schematic representation of the superficial distal nephron of the rat. Principal morphological features of the four distinct cell types found within the regions indicated are shown in the sketches, based on electron microscope observation. DCT, distal convoluted tubule; CNT, connecting tubule; ICT, initial collecting tubule; CCT, cortical collecting tubule. (From Stanton BA et al: *Kidney Int* 19:36, 1981. Used by permission.)

microplicae, abundant apical vesicles, and basal mitochondria.

The third segment returns to the kidney surface (the *late distal* site of the micropuncturist) as the *initial collecting tubule,* and consists of principal cells (with smooth luminal membranes, shallow basolateral infoldings, and no cytoplasmic vesicles) and intercalated cells, as already described. A broadly similar description applies to the rabbit, where the terms "bright," "granular," and "light" have been used for the three successive segments.[118] Important differences have also been noted, however:[34,255] the junctions between the three zones are more sharply defined in the rabbit than the rat, and the middle ("granular") segment is relatively longer, extending in inner cortical nephrons beyond the confluence of two distal tubules.

This morphological heterogeneity has important functional correlates. Both $Na^+ - K^+$ ATPase activity[119] and hormone-sensitive adenylate cyclase activity[153] have been shown to be distributed in a segmental pattern paralleling the divisions described above. Most important, potassium secretion appears to be chiefly a property of the connecting and initial collecting tubules; the "true" distal convoluted tubule (early distal segment) expresses this capacity to a relatively minor extent under normal circumstances. This has been clearly demonstrated by selective and separate microperfusion, in vivo, of the early and late accessible portions of the distal tubule in the rat.[49,206,209] Supportive evidence also comes from morphological studies during adaptation to a high potassium intake. Dramatic changes in cell ultrastructure are confined to the principal and connecting cell types during adaptation,[209] making it reasonable to suggest that these cells mediate potassium secretion.

A complementary suggestion has been advanced as to the function of the intercalated ("dark") cells, at least in the medullary collecting duct.[215] In this segment potassium depletion causes a specific and sharply localized increase only in the length of the luminal membrane of the intercalated cell. This finding is consistent with the idea that a potassium-uptake mechanism mediating potassium reabsorption is located in the apical membrane of these cells (see below).

Collecting duct system

Individual divisions of the collecting duct system—the cortical collecting tubule and the outer and inner medullary collecting duct—are not directly accessible to superficial micropuncture. However, an overall assessment of the contribution of these structures to renal potassium handling can be made by comparing the delivery of potassium at the latest accessible distal tubule site on the renal surface to the final excretion of potassium into the urine.[73] This approach, though, does not allow for detection of oppositely directed net transport across successive portions of this duct system. It also assumes that nephrons lying deeper within the cortex behave the same way as those located closer to the surface.

Considerable interest has been focused on the latter objection in recent years, largely on the basis of accumulating evidence that significant differences may exist between these two nephron populations with respect to potassium handling.[113] This subject is discussed further below. Specifically, it has been proposed that under some circumstances, the deeper nephrons may contribute more potassium into the collecting ducts than do superficial ones. Thus, under experimental conditions in which net addition of potassium to the urine has been demonstrated to occur between the superficial late distal tubule and the beginning of the papillary collecting ducts,[142,143,260] it has not been possible to determine whether this is the result of potassium secretion into more proximal segments of the collecting duct tree or of disproportionately greater potassium delivery out of juxtamedullary nephrons. Two indirect lines of evidence suggest that the former explanation is more likely. Using a chemical agent to induce selective destruction of the renal papilla, Reineck and coworkers[179] showed that this procedure did not diminish the previously observed addition of potassium between the superficial late distal tubule and the early papillary collecting duct. Had the deep nephron population contributed proportionately more potassium than the superficial nephrons, this result would not be expected. Second, a variety of approaches to sampling fluid moving down the distal reaches of the collecting duct system[112] have not in general demonstrated successive increases in potassium entry, as would be expected if juxtamedullary nephrons added large amounts of potassium to the collecting duct urine. The more direct technique of in vitro perfusion of isolated cortical collecting tubules from rabbit kidney[84,169,221] has clearly demonstrated that this segment *can* secrete potassium, and it is reasonable to assume that this process accounts in vivo for the portion of potassium added to the urine beyond the distal tubule in micropuncture experiments. This segment is morphologically similar to the initial collecting duct (late distal tubule) in the rat[251,255] and has a similar embryological origin,[255] being derived from the ureteric bud outgrowth. It also shares with the initial collecting duct a sensitivity to amiloride,[169,221] mineralocorticoids,[127,155,166,183,194,220] and antidiuretic hormone (ADH).[83,186,188,189]

In contrast, the medullary portions of the collecting duct appear in general to reabsorb potassium.[112,113,219] This can be directly demonstrated by micropuncture of the terminal few millimeters of the papillary collecting duct[41] or by retrograde catheterization of individual collecting ducts via the exposed papilla.[97,203] Although potassium reabsorption in this segment is most marked during hydropenia[178] and in animals on a low-sodium or low-potassium diet,[41] it can also be detected in animals on a normal potassium diet and during water diuresis.[203]

Pattern of potassium transport in juxtamedullary nephrons

Although there is no clear evidence from free-flow micropuncture studies that potassium enters the lumen of superficial nephrons earlier than the middistal tubule, it has been clearly demonstrated that there is net potassium entry into the descending limb of Henle's loop in nephrons originating deeper in the cortex.[113] By sampling fluid from the hairpin bend of the loop in the exposed papilla, Jamison and colleagues,[111] confirming an earlier observation by DeRouffignac and associates,[39] showed that in rats on a normal diet the amount of potassium delivered to the end of the descending limb exceeded the amount filtered by some 13 percent. Assuming that the proximal convoluted tubule of these nephrons reabsorbed potassium, it was clear that appreciable entry must have occurred into the pars recta and/or the thin descending limb of the loop of Henle. It was also shown that this potassium addition to loop fluid was suppressed by treatment with furosemide[111] or amiloride,[11] or by short-term dietary potassium deprivation,[44] administration of calcitonin,[48] and adrenalectomy.[101] On the other hand, under conditions of dietary potassium loading, the amount of potassium reaching the tip of Henle's loop increased to 180 percent of the filtered load.[11] Vasopressin also increases the recycling of potassium.[155]

A schematic summary of the main transport events underlying potassium recycling is given in Fig. 7-5. It is thought that the potassium added to the thin descending limb originates in the medullary collecting duct rather than the thick ascending limb, since the potassium increment was markedly suppressed by amiloride treatment, which is known to inhibit potassium secretion into initial

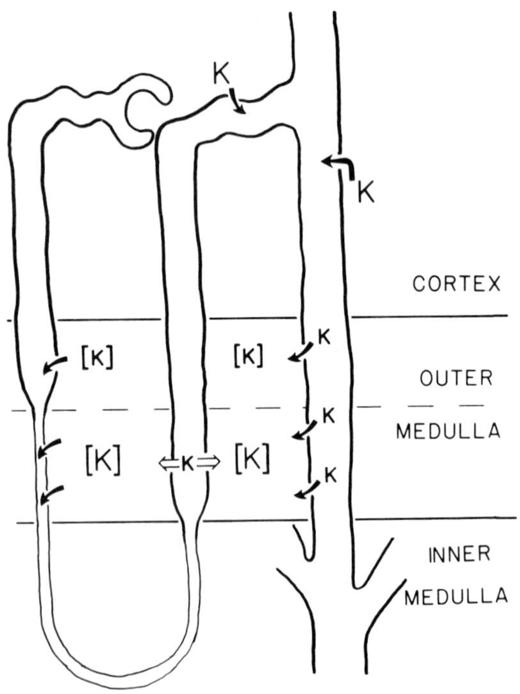

FIGURE 7-5 • Schematic summary of transport events in medullary potassium recycling. See text for details. (From Stokes JB: *J Clin Invest* 70:219, 1982. Used by permission.)

and cortical collecting tubules.[11] By raising the potassium concentration in the medullary interstitium, reabsorption of potassium from the medullary collecting duct would provide a favorable concentration gradient for passive potassium entry into the pars recta and thin descending limb,[113] although the former segment has also been shown in vitro to be capable of active potassium secretion.[252] However, the resulting "recycling" of potassium within the renal medulla would not be expected to contribute to the net transfer of potassium from the blood into the urine. One possible function of this process has been suggested by the finding that an elevated ambient potassium concentration inhibits sodium chloride reabsorption by the medullary thick ascending limb of Henle's loop.[217,218] If this effect were to occur in the medulla, an increase in sodium chloride delivery from the loop into the distal tubule of deep nephrons would be expected, which in turn could accentuate distal potassium secretion in this nephron population. Although such a sequence of events could not influence the efficiency of potassium excretion under steady-state conditions, it may play such a role in response to acute changes in potassium intake.[222]

Many of the features of the hypothesis of medullary potassium recycling have been documented experimentally, and appropriate transport characteristics have been demonstrated for most of the participating tubule segments. However, it must be emphasized that direct verification of all the details of potassium recycling in vivo is limited by the inaccessibility to study of distal tubules of deep nephrons and the tip of Henle's loop of superficial nephrons. Thus it remains uncertain whether there is a fundamental difference between superficial and deep nephrons in the delivery of potassium from the distal tubule into the collecting duct system. The possible involvement of recycling in pathological states remains to be fully explored.

CELL MECHANISMS OF POTASSIUM TRANSPORT

Since an adequate description of the factors regulating renal potassium excretion is dependent on knowledge of the underlying mechanisms, the following sections will outline the basic characteristics of transepithelial potassium transport at successive points along the nephron.

PROXIMAL TUBULE

The mechanisms involved in reabsorption of potassium in the proximal tubule are not fully understood. It is likely that different mechanisms are involved in early compared to later segments of the proximal convolution, and different processes again may operate in the proximal straight tubule.

Evidence for active transfer of potassium from glomerular filtrate to blood is strongest in the early portions of the proximal tubule. Here the transepithelial electrical potential is most often lumen-negative by some 2 to 5 mV relative to the interstitium, and the luminal-fluid potassium activity falls slightly, implying that movement occurs against its electrochemical gradient.[23,73] Confirmatory data come from experiments in which acetazolamide is given to inhibit bicarbonate reabsorption.[14] Under these conditions, proximal sodium and fluid reabsorption are markedly reduced, and yet potassium reabsorption is unimpaired, proceeding against an even more pronounced concentration gradient. Direct measurements of intracellular potassium activity, together with values for the electrical potential profile across the epithelium, indicate that potassium must be accumulated actively across the basolateral membranes.[61,131] Transcellular potassium reabsorption must by implication involve both paracellular and transcellular pathways (Fig. 7-6*a*), but Weinstein has recently suggested that active potassium reabsorption could also occur by its movement into the proximal tubule cell via the intercellular pathway.[241a] Paradoxically, recent electrophysiological studies[120,135] have demonstrated the presence of potassium channels in this membrane, through which the ions may move passively in a secretory direction (cell to lumen). While the physiological function of these channels is presently uncertain, they may have a role in cell volume regulation or in stabilizing the apical membrane voltage.[88] Movement from the cell into the interstitium may proceed by electrodiffusion, since a potassium conductive pathway has also been demonstrated in the basolateral membrane.[30,74,182] However, it is clear that potassium exit may also occur via KCl cotransport,[6,52] although the relative contribution of these two mechanisms has not been well defined.

It seems likely that at least some component of potassium reabsorption in later portions of the proximal convoluted tubule may proceed passively. This follows from the fact that the transepithelial electrical potential becomes slightly lumen-positive with respect to the interstitium.[74] Passively reabsorbed potassium most likely moves by diffusion across the significant intercellular shunt pathway in this epithelium (Fig. 7-6*a*). A second passive force acting on potassium in the proximal tubule is bulk fluid movement, secondary to active sodium reabsorption. This mechanism, transporting potassium through cellular junctions by solvent drag, has been highlighted by microperfusion experiments, in which the direction of net potassium transport across rat proximal tubules could be reversed by changing the direction of net fluid volume movement when the tubule lumen is perfused with hypertonic mannitol solutions.[21] That such a mechanism is of physiologic importance is suggested by

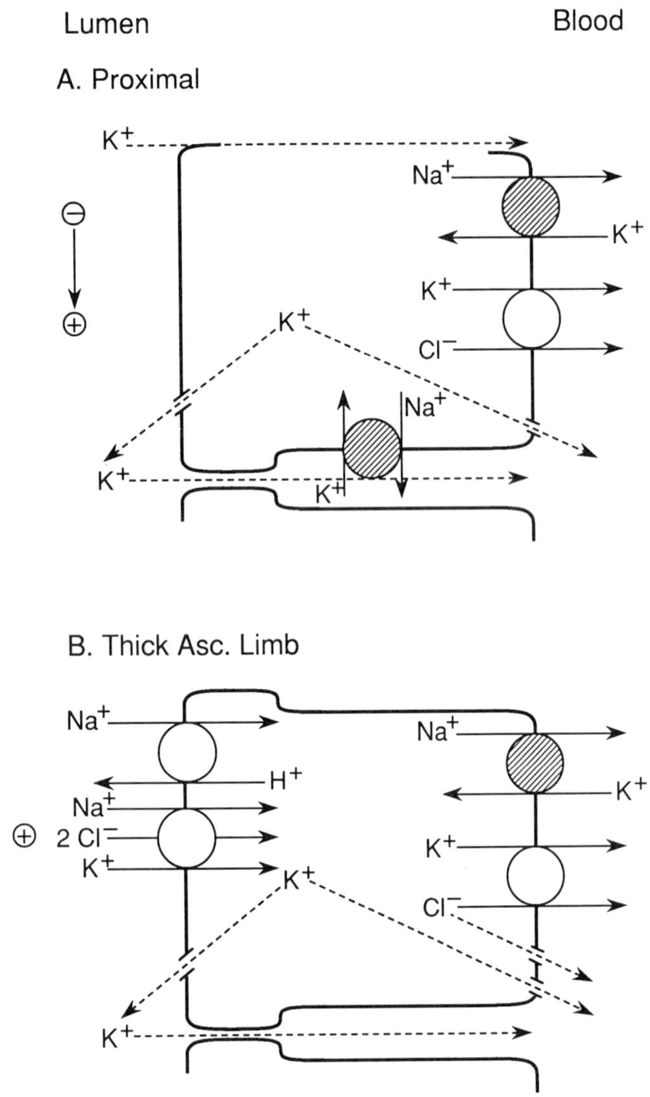

FIGURE 7-6 • Schematic cell models depicting possible mechanisms involved in transepithelial potassium transport. (*a*) Proximal tubule; (*b*) thick ascending limb of Henle's loop. Broken arrows are passive electrodiffusive pathways; solid arrows are active or facilitated transport mechanisms. Plus and minus signs in the lumen signify the electrical polarity of the lumen relative to the interstitium under free-flow conditions.

the observation that maneuvers such as extracellular volume expansion, which depress proximal sodium and fluid absorption, also inhibit potassium reabsorption in this segment.[14,73]

Potassium transport in the pars recta of the proximal tubule (proximal straight tubule) appears to involve processes different from those described above. When this segment is isolated and studied in vitro, appreciable net secretion of sodium and fluid can be induced by including a high concentration of *p*-aminohippurate in the bathing medium. Under these conditions net entry of potassium also occurs, the luminal concentration rising significantly above that in the bath.[85] Potassium secretion into the proximal straight tubule has also been shown to occur when media of more physiologic composition are used, and volume reabsorption rather than secretion is present.[241,252] These studies have been taken to imply that this segment has a relatively high potassium permeability.[113] However, it should be noted that, since proximal straight tubules are inaccessible to direct study in vivo, the exact extent and significance of potassium entry into the proximal straight tubule in superficial and deep nephrons cannot be established with certainty and will be highly dependent upon the potassium concentration in the surrounding interstitial medium.

LOOP OF HENLE

The thin descending limb of the loop of Henle is probably a site of net potassium entry into the lumen (see above). It has been demonstrated[111] that, given the measured potassium permeability for this segment obtained by in vitro perfusion,[180] potassium entry into the lumen would be expected along the entire length of the descending thin limb, assuming a uniformly rising gradient of interstitial potassium concentration between the corticomedullary junction and the tip of the papilla. This could account, at least in the deep population of nephrons, for the observed high mass flow of potassium at the bend of the loop of Henle.[113] Both morphological[110] and biochemical[119] considerations make it likely that transepithelial ion movements in thin Henle's loop segments are driven by passive rather than active forces.

The thick ascending limb of Henle's loop has been studied extensively in vitro, and much of what is known of potassium movement across this nephron segment is derived from electrophysiological and ion-flux data obtained with the in vitro preparation.[25] Potassium reabsorption is usually observed in the isolated thick ascending limb, especially when the sodium concentration of the perfusion fluid is relatively low and the lumen-positive transepithelial potential is high.[26] This observation, together with a high potassium permeability in the thick limb,[113] suggests that a component of potassium reabsorption could be driven passively through the intercellular pathway.[195] However, an important transcellular route is indicated, at least in the cortical segment, by studies on the isolated cortical thick ascending limb in the rabbit[89] showing that luminal potassium is a prerequisite for active sodium chloride transport. This has given rise to the concept of a cotransport mechanism for sodium, potassium, and chloride in the luminal membrane, operating in an electroneutral manner with the stoichiometry $1Na^+:2Cl^-:1K^+$[87,156] The luminal membrane also possesses an appreciable potassium conductance, resulting in extensive recirculation of potassium back from the cell into the lumen[90] (Fig. 7-6*b*). However, potassium can also leave the cell across the basolateral membrane, either conductively or as electrically neutral KCl cotransport.[91] This exit process offsets the active uptake of potassium in exchange for sodium at the basolateral surface.

Findings essentially identical to those described above have been reported for the medullary portion of the mouse thick ascending limb[95] and for the diluting segment (early distal tubule) of the amphibian *Amphiuma*.[157] It has been possible with the latter preparation to explore the operation of the transport process in the luminal membrane in more detail, by the use of cellular impalements with ion-sensitive microelectrodes. Thus it has been shown that intracellular sodium activity is sharply reduced by lowering the concentration of either chloride *or* potassium in the lumen[159,160] and also by luminal application of furosemide, which interferes with the cotransport process in the apical membrane.[158,160] These maneuvers, which inhibit potassium uptake from the lumen while leaving cell-to-lumen diffusion of potassium unopposed, may even result in reversal of the direction of net potassium transfer from reabsorption to secretion. Indeed, net entry of potassium into superficial loops of Henle perfused with furosemide-containing fluids had been noted previously in several micropuncture studies.[154,174,259]

Finally, several factors that modulate the potassium conductance of the luminal membrane in this segment have been identified. Adaptation to a high potassium intake has been shown to be associated with an increase in the conductance of the apical membrane in amphibian diluting segment,[160] a change that facilitates net potassium secretion under these conditions. Application of ADH to the basolateral surface has also been shown to increase the potassium conductance of the luminal membrane in mouse medullary thick ascending limb, leading in this case to stimulation of net sodium chloride reabsorption.[95] Similar responses have recently been demonstrated in this segment following treatment with aldosterone.[40,93] Interstitial acid-base changes may also influence this apical conductance. Acidification of the solution bathing isolated *Amphiuma* diluting segments causes a reduction in the potassium conductance of the luminal membrane,[210] presumably acting to minimize potassium loss during acidosis.

INITIAL AND CORTICAL COLLECTING TUBULES

As pointed out earlier in this chapter, potassium secretion is an important property of the epithelium lining the late portions of the distal tubule accessible to micropuncture in the rat ("initial collecting tubule") and of the cortical collecting tubule, studied most extensively by perfusion in vitro after isolation from rabbit kidney.[84,169,216,221] Since net potassium transport does not appear to be a major feature of the true "distal convoluted tubule" (a term now reserved for the early part of the accessible distal tubule),[205,208,255] the following paragraphs contain no further reference to that segment of the nephron.

Principal cells of the initial and cortical collecting tubules are thought to effect potassium secretion as the result of sequential transport across the basolateral and luminal membranes (Fig. 7-7*a*). The basolateral membrane is the site of an active mechanism for the uptake of potassium from the extracellular fluid in exchange for sodium, mediated by a typical membrane-bound ATPase enzyme system. Supportive evidence for such a mechanism comes from three approaches: (1) cytochemical localization of ATPase along the basolateral border of cortical collecting tubules;[51] (2) abolition of both sodium reabsorption and potassium secretion by this segment after basolateral exposure to cyanide,[163] implying ATP-

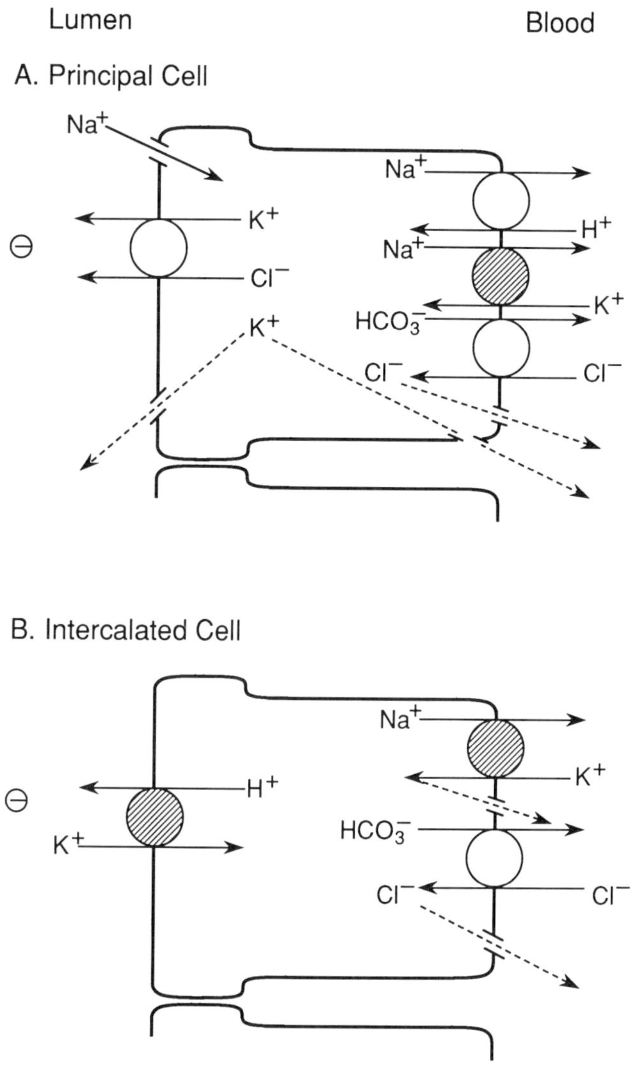

FIGURE 7-7 • Schematic models of cells from the initial and cortical collecting tubules of the rat. (*a*) Principal cell; (*b*) intercalated cell. The apical $K^+ - H^+$ countertransport mechanism depicted in the luminal membrane of the intercalated cell is based on indirect evidence. Symbol conventions are as in Fig. 7-6.

dependence; and (3) similar abolition of cation fluxes by basolateral ouabain,[84] a specific inhibitor of the $Na^+ - K^+$ pump. The operation of this exchange pump is ultimately responsible for the interdependence of the processes of distal sodium reabsorption and potassium secretion, although, as has frequently been pointed out,[73] the degree of "coupling" of these two fluxes is highly variable and clearly subject to other influences.

Although it has not been demonstrated in mammalian tubules that potassium uptake across the basolateral membrane is an active process, the intracellular potassium activities in amphibian distal tubules are higher than can be accounted for by the electrical potential across the basolateral membrane.[131] It also appears likely that, as in other tissues, the pump operates electrogenically, removing three sodium ions from the cell in exchange for the uptake of two potassium ions, since rapid alterations in the rate of transepithelial sodium transport lead to prompt parallel changes in basolateral membrane potential.[73] A more direct piece of evidence has been provided by Koeppen and coworkers,[128] who found that addition of ouabain to the medium bathing the basolateral surface of the isolated cortical collecting tubule of the rabbit caused an initial rapid depolarization followed by a more gradual and sustained depolarization of the basolateral membrane. This response is consistent with inhibition of an electrogenic sodium-potassium pump in the first phase and a progressive dissipation of the potassium gradient from cell to bath in the second. The latter conclusion is based on the evidence that the basolateral membrane has an appreciable potassium conductance, such that under normal circumstances a portion of potassium accumulated in the cell leaks back into the interstitium. This process generates an outwardly directed potassium diffusion potential, which, together with the potential generated by electrogenic operation of the pump, is thought to account for the electrical potential across the basolateral cell face. This potential has been measured at values between 65 and 90 mV (cell interior negative) in initial collecting duct cells[129] and approximately 84 mV in isolated collecting ducts.[128]

The relative importance of basal potassium uptake in the regulation of the final rate of potassium secretion has been emphasized in tracer kinetic studies of potassium transfer across the distal tubule.[150] The uptake process is stimulated during chronic high dietary intake of potassium, acute increases in plasma potassium concentration, and alkalosis, all of which lead to an increase in the intracellular potassium pool. In general, these stimuli bring about augmented rates of potassium secretion without altering the rate constants for transfer across the luminal membrane. Other lines of evidence, elaborated below, suggest that the activity of the basolateral pump is also regulated by adrenal steroids. Stimulation of the pump by increases in extracellular potassium concentration may be limited by saturation behavior.[206]

The second step involved in potassium secretion is movement of the ion across the apical membrane of the cell into the tubule lumen. Most evidence suggests that this occurs passively, since the electrochemical gradient is favorable for diffusion into the lumen and the potassium conductance of the apical membrane is high.[73] Preferential transfer of potassium into the lumen, rather than back into the interstitium, is favored because the electrical potential difference is lower across the luminal membrane than across the basolateral membrane.[128] It is this asymmetrical electrical polarization of the two cell membranes that gives rise to the overall lumen-negative transepithelial potential difference in both initial[10,94,143,253] and cortical[92,128,169,216,221] collecting tubules. The potential of about 70 mV (cell interior negative) across the apical membrane of cortical collecting tubules[128] results largely from the outwardly directed potassium diffusion potential, partly opposed by an inward diffusion potential for sodium. Sodium entry from the lumen into both initial and cortical collecting tubule cells occurs down its electrochemical gradient through specific membrane channels, which can be blocked by amiloride. Since adding this agent (or lowering the sodium concentration in luminal fluid) results in hyperpolarization of the potential across the apical membrane,[128] net potassium secretion in both initial[46] and cortical[221] collecting tubules is inhibited (for further discussion see "Factors Influencing Renal Potassium Transport").

The properties of the potassium channel that is responsible for the apical potassium permeability have been defined.[249] The channel has a high open probability that allows potassium ions to recycle effectively between cell and lumen. Interestingly, the apical potassium channel is inhibited by millimolar concentrations of ATP. The functional role of the sensitivity of apical potassium channels to ATP remains to be further explored but could be involved in the coupling between basolateral $Na^+ - K^+$ pump activity and apical potassium conductance. With enhanced basolateral Na^+ and K^+ transport, ATP concentration may decrease and unblock apical potassium channels. Stimulation of apical potassium recycling would follow and accelerate cotransport turnover. The observations that the concentration of ATP rises in cells of the thick ascending limb after ouabain or furosemide supports the view that cell ATP levels may change with modulation of the activity of the basolateral $Na^+ - K^+$ pump.[116]

Although previous studies in the cortical collecting duct[84] were interpreted to imply the existence of an active secretory mechanism located in the luminal membrane of this segment,[73,254] it is now generally not considered necessary to postulate such a mechanism (distinct from active basolateral uptake) to account for the data.[164] However, evidence is available to support the presence of an electroneutral KCl cotransporter in the apical membrane of principal cells,[49,238,248] and it has been proposed that this mechanism may contribute to potassium secretion, particularly when chloride concentration in tubule fluid falls to very low levels.

Intercalated cells located within the initial and cortical collecting duct epithelium are not thought to take part in the process of potassium secretion but are now considered to play a role in the reabsorption of potassium and the secretion of hydrogen ions under appropriate metabolic conditions. Evidence for active potassium reabsorption by the distal tubule is largely indirect, being based on the observation that during potassium depletion, distal potassium secretion is abolished despite persistence of a lumen-negative transepithelial potential.[46,142] Furthermore, steady-state potassium concentrations in the lumens of normal rats were generally found to be below those predicted from passive distribution, according to the simultaneously measured electrical potential difference.[144] The suggestion that the potassium uptake mechanism resides in the apical membrane of the intercalated cells is based chiefly on morphological evidence, namely, that potassium depletion induces a selective hypertrophy of this membrane in intercalated cells in the cortical and medullary collecting ducts (Fig. 7-7).[209,215] Several pieces of data suggest that the mechanism for this potassium uptake process may involve a $K^+ - H^+$ ATPase resembling that found in gastric parietal cells. The following observations are most pertinent: (1) inhibitors of this pump reduce hydrogen ion secretion and potassium absorption in the distal tubule of potassium-depleted rats, and (2) morphological alterations in apical membranes of intercalated cells occur in metabolic acidosis as they do in potassium depletion.[141,238] It remains possible, however, that other forms of K^+ ATPase, and indeed of H^+ ATPase, may exist in this membrane and that these structures may in fact reside in different types of intercalated cells.[238] It should also be noted that the mechanism of potassium exit across the basolateral membrane of intercalated cells performing potassium absorption is unknown.

FACTORS INFLUENCING RENAL POTASSIUM TRANSPORT

As previously discussed, the rate of urinary potassium excretion under physiologic conditions is largely determined by the level of activity of the potassium secretory mechanism located in the distal portions of the cortical nephron. The factors modulating this mechanism are therefore responsible for control of renal potassium excretion in response to a wide variety of metabolic challenges. Since all of these influences are known to act, at least in part, on the superficial distal tubule and since this segment is readily accessible at the kidney surface and has been extensively studied, the following account will focus

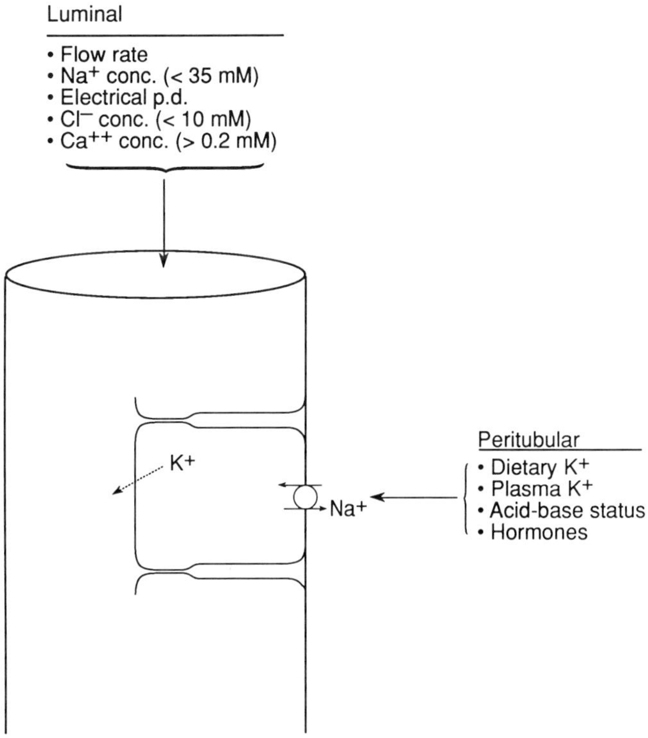

FIGURE 7-8 • Factors influencing potassium secretion by the distal tubule.

on information obtained from investigations of potassium transport at this nephron site in the rat.

The factors to be discussed can be conveniently considered in two groups, illustrated schematically in Fig. 7-8: (1) those acting primarily from the luminal side of the epithelium and (2) those acting from the peritubular (blood) side.

LUMINAL FACTORS

Flow rate

The rate of fluid flow through the distal tubule has been shown to be a potent factor influencing potassium secretion at this site. Under a wide variety of circumstances, an increase in luminal flow rate results in an increase of potassium secretion.[71,123,133,174,178] A corresponding relationship is generally also observed between final urinary flow rate and potassium excretion when changes in urine flow reflect changes in solute excretion. Thus, increased potassium excretion is seen after volume expansion due to saline infusion,[43,143] in mannitol-induced osmotic diuresis,[198] following release of ureteric obstruction[149] or removal of the opposite kidney,[172] and as a result of diuretic therapy (discussed further below).

Studies on single nephrons have confirmed the role of both sodium delivery and flow rate in potassium secretion.[257] Figure 7-9 shows the results of a microperfusion

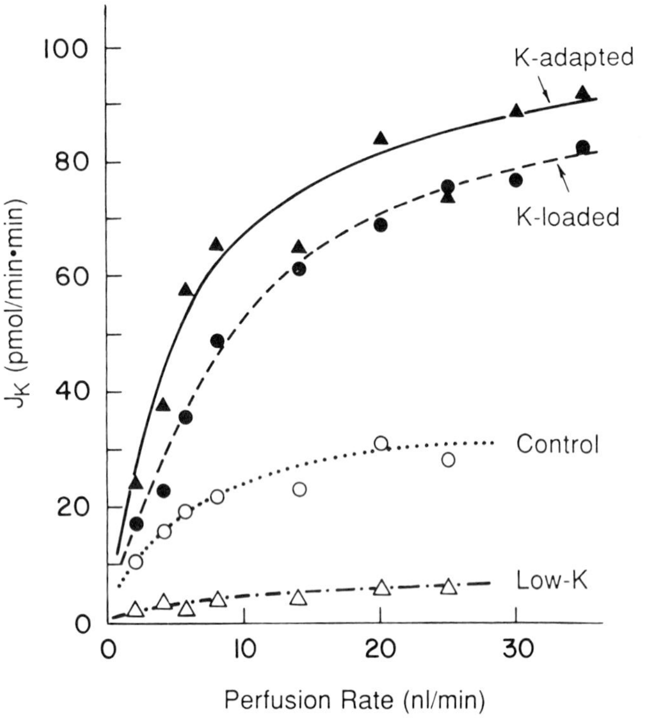

FIGURE 7-9 • Relationship between rate of potassium secretion and tubule perfusion rate in control, low-potassium, acutely potassium-loaded, and potassium-adapted animals. (From Malnic G et al: *Am J Physiol* 256:F932, 1989. Used by permission.)

study in which flow rate was altered from the physiologic range of a few nanoliters per minute to high values.[146] It is clear that potassium secretion rises sharply, particularly over the lower range of flow rates. Similar results have been obtained in isolated cortical collecting tubules.[50] It is also apparent from inspection of Fig. 7-9 that, for a given flow rate, potassium secretion is relatively diminished in potassium depletion and enhanced by a high-potassium diet. In perfused cortical collecting tubules, mineralocorticoids also have a stimulating effect on potassium secretion over a wide range of flow rates.[50]

Two mechanisms have been invoked to explain the flow-dependent increase of potassium excretion. The first places emphasis on increased sodium reabsorption with delivery of larger amounts of fluid and sodium ions into the distal nephron.[123,162] Increasing sodium delivery is thought to enhance sodium entry into principal tubule cells, stimulating basolateral potassium uptake and enhancing potassium secretion into the lumen. Potassium concentrations in the lumen would thus be well maintained over a wide range of luminal flow rates, provided the basolateral pump is normally unsaturated and responds to increased sodium delivery with enhanced turnover.

A second mechanism to explain flow-dependent stimulation of potassium secretion is based on microperfusion experiments in which increased flow rate led to stimulation of potassium secretion without enhanced sodium transport.[79] Significantly, potassium concentrations fell with increased flow rate, thus increasing the concentration gradient of potassium across the apical membrane. This mechanism of stimulation of potassium secretion plays a more important role in conditions in which basolateral pump activity may be compromised or lumen flow rate has increased to such an extent that pumping cannot rise in proportion to sodium delivery.

As mentioned before, several lines of evidence indicate that the epithelium of the late distal tubule has a high overall potassium permeability, probably reflecting high potassium conductances of both the apical and basolateral membranes (the extent of potassium permeation through the intercellular shunt pathway is not known). Phenomenologically, this is manifested by rapid attainment (< 1 s) of steady-state potassium concentrations in the lumen,[70] resulting in no reduction[123] or only modest reductions[133,178] in concentrations of potassium in the lumen as distal flow rate increases over a wide range. Thus, the result of a proportionately smaller fall in concentration for a given increase in flow rate is a rise in net secretion into the lumen.[255-257] This model also requires that cell potassium concentration be maintained during flow stimulation of its secretion, and this is probably achieved under physiologic conditions by increased Na^+ reabsorption associated with enhanced activity of the basolateral Na^+-K^+ ATPase, bringing increased amounts of potassium into the cell.[146,199]

As will be discussed further, changes in flow rate frequently accompany other factors that influence the distal potassium secretory apparatus. The net effect of such combined disturbances, then, depends upon which influence has the predominant effect.

Sodium concentration in the lumen

The concentration of sodium in the late distal tubule has been shown to increase under many circumstances in which there is increased flow rate and potassium secretion.[123,124] However, as noted above, microperfusion studies demonstrate that if flow rate is held constant, changing sodium concentration in the lumen over the physiologic range observed in free flow (between 40 and 100 m*M*) does not affect the rate of potassium secretion.[79] Sodium concentration appears to be limiting for potassium secretion only when reduced below 35 m*M*.[81,82] A possible mechanism for this effect was suggested by measurements of transepithelial electrical potential under similar conditions. Although the sensitivity of this potential to the sodium concentration in the lumen had been previously demonstrated when the concentration was varied in large steps,[75] reexamination of this relationship over a narrower range revealed that the potential is relatively insensitive to increases in sodium concentration above 40 m*M* but that there is a sharp reduction as the concentration is reduced below this level.[81,82] Since this relationship parallels that between potassium secretion and sodium concentration,[81,82] it may be surmised that the reduced electrical potential (presumably the result of hyperpolarization of the luminal membrane due to attenuation of the inward sodium diffusion potential) at very low luminal sodium concentrations acts to impede potassium movement into the lumen. A very similar relationship between luminal sodium concentration and transepithelial potential on the one hand and net potassium secretion on the other has been demonstrated in the isolated cortical collecting tubule.[216]

Since luminal sodium concentration rarely falls below 40 m*M* in the distal tubule under physiologic conditions, it is unlikely that this variable normally acts to regulate potassium secretion at this site. Very low sodium concentrations may, however, develop in cortical collecting tubules during water diuresis, when this segment normally contains fluid with a sodium concentration in the range 20 to 25 m*M*[57] potassium secretion may be limited under these conditions and so contribute to the failure of potassium excretion to increase during water diuresis[4,230] (an additional influence of ADH levels has also been proposed to explain this phenomenon; see below). Similar considerations may apply during marked sodium depletion or mineralocorticoid excess.[173]

Electrical potential difference

It is evident that at least one step in the process of potassium secretion, the passive movement of potassium from cell to lumen across the apical membrane, would be expected to be sensitive to the prevailing transmembrane electrical potential. Data from several experimental situations appear to confirm a relationship between potassium secretion and the potential difference measured across the epithelium as a whole.[255] Furthermore, it has been shown by direct voltage clamping of late segments of the distal tubule that potassium secretion is enhanced in proportion to the degree of lumen negativity imposed.[63] However, it should be stressed that in many situations, most notably in acute potassium loading,[260] transepithelial potential and luminal potassium concentrations vary independently,[255] underscoring the importance of alterations in other components of the secretory mechanism (particularly uptake at the basolateral surface) in determining the final rate of secretion.

The above considerations indicate that the transepithelial electrical potential, while frequently correlating with changes in potassium secretion, is not the sole determinant of this process. Indeed, as noted previously, one of the most frequently activated stimuli for secretion, an increase in flow rate of tubule fluid, operates independently of (and often in the direction opposite to) changes in potential difference.[80] On the other hand, electrical effects may sometimes play a secondary role as partial mediators of the action of certain of the primary factors discussed elsewhere in this section (e.g., mineralocorticoid treatment).

Although the transepithelial potential itself cannot generally be considered to act as a primary regulator of potassium secretion under physiologic conditions, it may play such a role in a number of situations of clinical interest. Thus, the diuretic amiloride, which acts in the late distal[9,46] and cortical collecting tubules[128,167,221] by blocking entry of sodium into the cell through luminal membrane channels, causes a dramatic inhibition of potassium secretion at these sites.[46,221] Since this agent abolishes the inward sodium diffusion potential, which normally partially depolarizes the apical transmembrane potential, it leads to hyperpolarization of the apical membrane and hence reduces the transepithelial potential.[128] In this way, the change it induces in potential difference may be considered the proximate (if not the primary) cause of the observed fall in potassium secretion. Conversely, recent evidence suggests that the antitumor agent *cis*-dichlorodiamineplatinum (cisplatinum) may increase the sodium conductance of the apical membrane,[232] an effect that depolarizes this membrane, making the lumen-negative transepithelial potential larger. This effect can be blocked by amiloride.[5] Since cisplatinum therapy is known to be associated with renal potassium (and magnesium) wasting, it is likely that the increased transtubular electrical gradient enhances distal potassium secretion. This suggestion has led to a successful preliminary trial of amiloride therapy to prevent potassium loss during cisplatinum administration.[117] Finally, potassium disturbances in some forms of distal renal tubular acidosis (RTA) may have a basis in electrical changes in the distal tubule.[12] For example, it has been proposed that "chloride shunt" RTA, which is associated with potassium retention and hyperkalemia,[187] may be caused by a primary defect in which chloride permeability of the distal tubule is increased, resulting in a reduced transepithelial potential and a drop in the electrical driving force for secretion of both hydrogen ion and potassium.

Chloride concentration in the lumen

In early studies of renal potassium handling it was frequently observed that the administration of salts of sodium in which the anion was relatively poorly reabsorbed resulted in increased rates of potassium excretion.[7,229] Since it was at that time also found that the presence in the lumen of relatively impermeant anions, such as sulfate, was associated with increased luminal negativity in the distal tubule,[31,143] it was proposed that potassium secretion was stimulated by the increase in the transepithelial electrical gradient.[7,31]

A reexamination of this question has introduced another possible explanation of the effect of the infusion of nonchloride salts.[237] During microperfusion of superficial distal tubules with sulfate solutions, it was found that although a small increase in transepithelial potential occurred, it was inadequate to account for the simultaneously measured stimulation of potassium secretion. Indeed, addition of amiloride to the sulfate-containing perfusate revealed a dissociation between net potassium secretion and electrical potential, the latter falling somewhat while secretion still increased. After measuring net potassium secretory rates over a wide range of luminal chloride concentrations, it was found that chloride concentrations below about 10 m*M* were always associated with an increase in net potassium secretion.[237] These results would appear to justify considering low lumen chloride concentration an independent factor influencing potassium secretion, especially since such low chloride concentrations in the distal tubule may well be achieved in vivo under various conditions involving high distal delivery of nonchloride anions, such as bicarbonate in metabolic alkalosis, or after treatment with carbonic anhydrase inhibitors. The cellular mechanism of this effect most likely relates to the operation of the potassium chloride cotransporter located on the apical membrane of cells in the potassium-secreting distal nephron segments.[49b,238,248] Finally, in interpreting clearance studies it should also be remembered that systemic infusions of nonchloride salts provoke a marked diuresis; thus, increased distal tubule flow must be considered another factor acting to increase potassium secretion under these circumstances.

Calcium concentration in the lumen

Microperfusion studies of superficial distal tubules in the rat indicate that the calcium concentration in the tubule lumen also controls potassium secretion.[162] Elevating calcium from 0.2 to 0.8 m*M* depressed both potassium secretion and the lumen-negative transepithelial potential difference. It is likely that the primary effect of increasing lumen calcium concentration is to depress the apical sodium permeability. The hyperpolarization of the apical membrane would reduce the driving force for potassium entry into the lumen. The modulation of distal potassium secretion by calcium is of interest because both loop and thiazide diuretics alter distal calcium delivery. Loop diuretics tend to increase calcium by blocking its reabsorption in the thick ascending limb of Henle's loop; on the other hand, thiazide diuretics decrease distal calcium concentration by enhancing reabsorption.[162]

PERITUBULAR FACTORS

Several important influences on potassium secretion can be grouped for convenience under this heading, in that their action on distal potassium transport is exerted primarily from the blood-facing side of the tubule epithelium.

Dietary potassium intake

Since an *increase in dietary intake of potassium* is associated with a parallel increase in urinary potassium excretion, external balance is quickly reestablished, usually at a normal level of extracellular potassium concentration.[209,260] The sites at which such adaptive increases in renal potassium transport occur have been shown by micropuncture studies to include the distal tubule,[142,260] but microcatheterization of medullary collecting ducts shows that these structures may also contribute.[193] Kinetic studies in the late distal tubule using[42] K-tracer flux analysis suggest that the mechanism underlying the enhancement of potassium secretion in this segment is an increase in uptake of potassium at the basolateral membrane,[150] leading to an increase in the cell potassium pool and hence providing an increased chemical gradient for diffusion into the lumen. Consistent with this model is the direct demonstration of elevated intracellular potassium activity in distal tubule cells during chronic potassium loading.[122]

Both biochemical and morphological observations support the concept that adaptation to a high dietary potassium intake involves stimulation of active basolateral potassium uptake in initial and cortical collecting tubules. Thus, an increase in Na^+-K^+ ATPase,[202] localized especially to cortical collecting tubules,[45] has been demonstrated during adaptation to a high potassium intake. On the basis of kinetic analysis, this change has been attributed to an increase in the number of ATPase sites rather than a change in the binding properties of the enzyme.[201,202] A correlate of this biochemical analysis is the demonstration by morphometric techniques of an amplification of the surface area of basolateral membrane in principal cells in the initial collecting tubule[209] and outer medullary collecting tubule[76] after continued ingestion of a high-potassium diet. These observations thus are also consistent with an increase in the number of ATPase pump units per cell in potassium-secreting epithelial segments.

Although the stimulus for this adaptive change is not precisely understood, two factors may be considered. First, the elevated levels of circulating aldosterone that are found in this situation may contribute to the increase in ATPase activity, since mineralocorticoids have been shown to activate ATPase in other settings.[64,191] Evidence against this possibility is the observation that potassium loading increases renal Na^+-K^+ ATPase activity in adrenalectomized rats that are given only small maintenance doses of mineralocorticoid replacement,[201] implying that high concentrations of aldosterone are not necessary for increased ATPase activity but may play a permissive role. A second factor that may be involved is the rise in plasma potassium concentration that occurs during potassium loading. Recent physiologic studies designed to evaluate the independent contributions of aldosterone and hyperkalaemia confirmed the importance of potassium per se in inducing adaptive changes in its tubular secretion, although maximum rates of potassium excretion were achieved in animals given *both* high aldosterone and potassium.[212]

One aspect of adaptation to dietary potassium-loading is potassium *tolerance*, defined as the ability to survive an otherwise lethal, acute potassium challenge. Thus, rats receiving a diet high in potassium for some weeks are able to excrete a higher proportion of an acutely infused load of potassium, and to do so at a lower plasma potassium concentration, than nonadapted rats.[1,227,260] The nephron segments involved in this response include both the late distal tubule[260] and the medullary collecting duct.[193] At the former site, the increased potassium secretory capacity has been shown to be independent of the increase in the flow rate of tubule fluid that accompanies both acute and chronic potassium loading.[206] It should be pointed out, however, that an important component of potassium tolerance is the increase in uptake of potassium by extrarenal tissues that occurs in this situation,[3] thereby limiting the rise in plasma potassium in adapted animals. Finally, potassium adaptation similar to that described above can also be demonstrated after experimental subtotal nephrectomy,[132,192] serving as a model for chronic renal failure in which renal potassium secretion per functioning nephron is also enhanced.[233]

Dietary deprivation of potassium results in a state of renal potassium retention, in which urinary potassium excretion may fall to levels below 2 percent of the filtered load.[46,138,142] Micropuncture studies indicate that this state is associated with complete suppression of potassium secretion along the length of the distal tubule,[142] with appreciable net potassium reabsorption in the initial and medullary collecting ducts.[41,178] In the established phase of potassium depletion, kinetic studies suggest that the cell potassium transport pool is reduced in the late distal epithelium due to suppression of uptake at the basolateral membrane,[150] and intracellular potassium activity has been shown to be depressed.[122] This change would be expected to result in a reduction of the potassium flux from cell into lumen in this segment and may leave unopposed an active uptake mechanism.[73] Although administration of the mineralocorticoid hormone deoxycorticosterone acetate (DOCA) cannot restore potassium excretion to normal in this phase,[138] DOCA can increase potassium excretion during the first 24 h of depletion. This suggests a role for falling endogenous aldosterone levels in curtailing potassium losses during the early phase of renal potassium conservation.[138] It should be mentioned that a role for other, as yet undefined, factors mediating short-term potassium conservation has been proposed from studies in the isolated perfused kidney.[170]

It is of interest that potassium depletion enhances the content of K^+-H^+ ATPase in the initial and medullary collecting ducts[47,65] and accounts for the fact that active net potassium reabsorption replaces net potassium secretion in the initial collecting duct. Passive potassium permeability in the outer medullary collecting ducts is also increased by potassium depletion,[247] possibly favoring passive potassium reabsorption in the renal medulla.

Although physiologic studies on individual cell types in the distal tubule epithelium have not yet been possible, the results of morphologic studies have strongly suggested that the intercalated cell may have specific responsibility for potassium reabsorption. Thus, during potassium depletion, marked amplification of the luminal membrane surface area,[215] with increased apical microplicae, has been demonstrated in the intercalated cells of the medullary collecting duct, while the morphology of principal cells is essentially unchanged.

Plasma potassium concentration

Although some studies on potassium excretion, measured over a range of plasma potassium levels, had demonstrated an approximately linear increase in excretion as potassium concentration rose,[229] interpretation of this result was complicated by simultaneous changes in other relevant variables produced by potassium infusion. In particular, since hyperkalemia is known to inhibit proximal sodium and fluid reabsorption,[24] the resulting increase in the delivery of sodium and fluid into the distal nephron may contribute to stimulating potassium secretion as a purely secondary effect. Furthermore, in intact animals, potassium infusion is also associated with increased aldosterone secretion, which may also contribute to enhanced potassium excretion.

Experiments involving continuous microperfusion, in vivo, of distal tubule segments in the rat have helped to clarify these issues. Tubules were perfused at a constant rate with fluid of constant composition while the animals were given a range of acute and chronic potassium loads. Potassium secretion increased linearly as the plasma concentration rose to approximately 6 m*M*; above that level no further increase in transport was observed,[207] as seen in Fig. 7-10. Thus, an apparent saturation of the secretory mechanism could be demonstrated when the additional effect of increased flow was controlled. This behavior suggests that the limitation on secretory rate may be due to saturation of the uptake mechanism at the basolateral surface of the cell, leading to a maximal value of intracellular potassium activity, which limits the rate of secretion.[207] Since, however, these experiments did not control the systemic level of aldosterone, which was higher in the more hyperkalemic animals, a subsequent series of microperfusion studies in adrenalectomized rats was designed to "clamp" the plasma aldosterone concentration at a fixed level during acute potassium infusion. These experiments clearly demonstrate a marked direct effect of hyperkalemia, independent of flow and

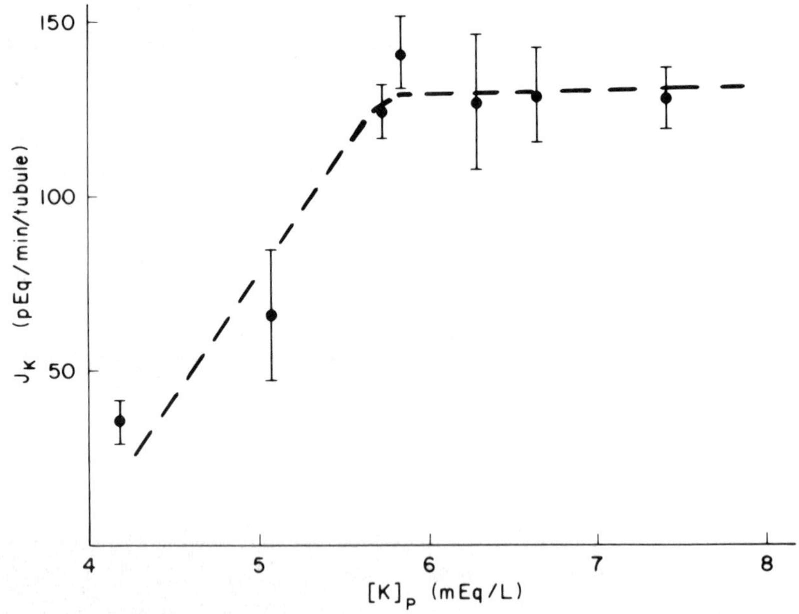

FIGURE 7-10 • Potassium secretion (J_K) by distal tubules microperfused in vivo at a fixed rate with a constant perfusion fluid. Plasma potassium concentration $[K]_P$ was changed by a variety of acute and chronic potassium loads. Line of best fit drawn by hand. (Adapted from Stanton BA, Giebisch GH: *Am J Physiol* 243:F487, 1982.)

aldosterone, on distal potassium secretion (Fig. 7-11). Similar conclusions have been reached in relation to whole-kidney potassium excretion in longer-term studies in adrenalectomized dogs.[261]

Acid-base status

Observations over many years have indicated that disturbances in systemic acid-base balance have significant effects upon renal potassium handling. In general, it has been found that metabolic and respiratory alkalosis are associated with increased urinary potassium excretion, whereas acidosis usually reduces potassium excretion. A somewhat variable response has been noted, however, with metabolic acidosis, particularly when chronic,[68] the reasons for this will be explored below. Free-flow micropuncture experiments have demonstrated that these alterations in potassium excretion are brought about, at least in part, in the distal tubule, where potassium secretion is altered dramatically by disturbances in acid-base status. These effects on potassium secretion were evident despite simultaneous changes in plasma potassium concentration that would tend in themselves to have the opposite effects on secretion.

The mechanisms underlying the stimulation of potassium secretion by alkalosis and depression of potassium secretion by acidosis involve changes of both apical and basolateral transport. Alkalosis stimulates both basolateral $Na^+ - K^+$ turnover and potassium permeability and thus augments both basolateral potassium uptake and apical transfer into the lumen.[184,242] Extracellular acidosis has the opposite effect. Once a new steady state has been reached, potassium concentrations, measured in principal cells by electron probe analysis,[13] are within the normal range in alkalosis and acidosis. Apparently, potassium movement across both basolateral and apical membranes has increased in proportion to the altered rate of potassium secretion.

Although the foregoing account is consistent with most of the available data concerning changes at the cell level during alterations of systemic pH, some questions regarding overall renal potassium handling are not fully

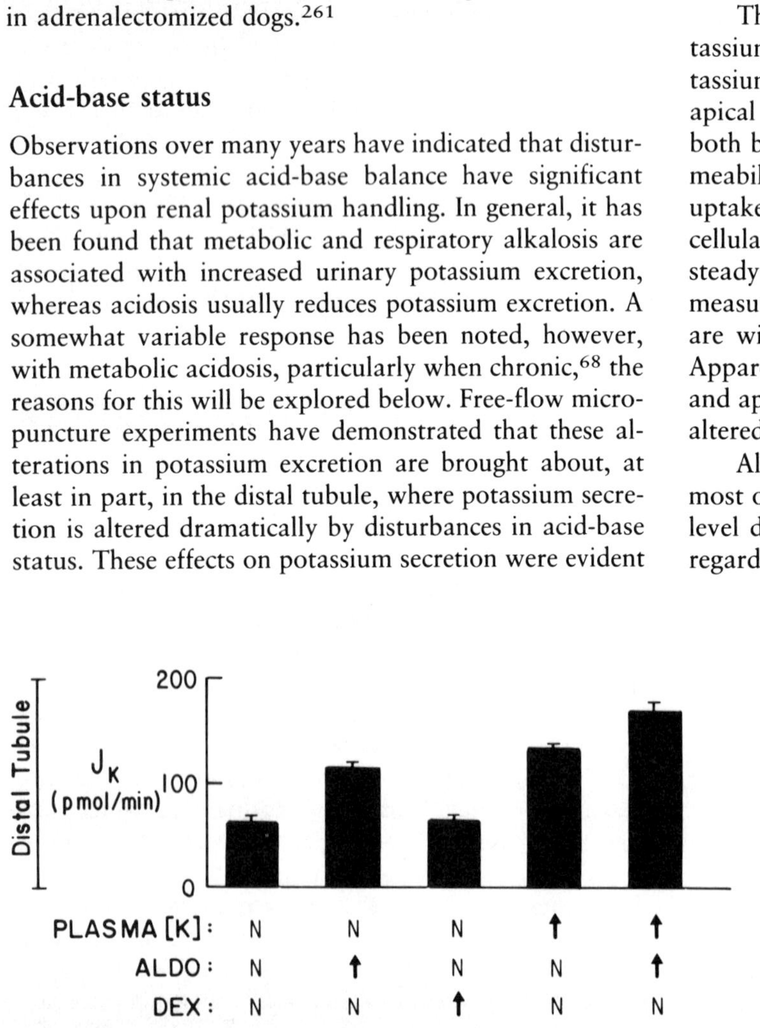

FIGURE 7-11 • Potassium secretion (J_K) by distal tubules microperfused in vivo at a fixed rate with a constant perfusion fluid. Rats were adrenalectomized and given basal replacement doses of both aldosterone and dexamethasone, resulting in "normal" (N) levels of these hormones. In addition, aldosterone, dexamethasone, or neither was infused acutely during the transport study, resulting in elevated (↑) levels of the appropriate hormone. Plasma potassium was either "normal" (N), or elevated (↑) by acute infusion of KCl. (Compiled from data in Field et al.[56,58])

answered by the studies cited. It is possible that secondary effects of acid-base disturbances may also influence urinary potassium excretion. For example, during alkalosis, the presence of unreabsorbed bicarbonate in the distal tubule might itself lead to stimulation of potassium secretion, both by increasing the flow rate of fluid past the secretory site and by depressing chloride concentration in the initial collecting tubule.[237] Conversely, during acidosis, an intrinsic inhibitory effect on potassium secretion might be masked or overwhelmed by an opposing stimulatory effect of increased distal flow, secondary in this case to depression of proximal sodium and fluid reabsorption by low bicarbonate levels.[86] To examine these questions, Stanton and Giebisch[207] perfused distal tubules in vivo at a constant rate while inducing systemic metabolic acidosis and alkalosis. Under these conditions, potassium secretion was shown to be directly stimulated during alkalosis and depressed during acidosis. However, data obtained by free-flow collection during acidosis in this study demonstrated an increase in potassium secretion at the late distal tubule and in the final urine, consequent upon elevated distal flow rates. This observation may provide a basis for the lack of consistency in published accounts of the effect of acidosis on potassium excretion,[68] since the magnitude of the diuretic response is highly variable from study to study.

The effect of changes in the pH of the luminal fluid on potassium secretion by the distal tubule appears much less important than that of the changes in the peritubular environment discussed above;[145,207] the same may not apply, however, in the cortical collecting ducts.[22]

Closely related to the influence of acid-base disturbances on renal potassium handling is the role of ammonia metabolism. In general, a reciprocal relationship exists between renal ammonium and potassium excretion.[223] Thus, administration of glutamine to stimulate ammonia production and excretion of ammonium results in a reduction in potassium excretion[226] due to depression of potassium secretion at sites beyond the late distal tubule.[108] Conversely, potassium loading inhibits ammonia production and excretion, while potassium depletion is a powerful stimulus to ammonia production and excretion.[108] These relationships have suggested the possibility of a feedback control loop between potassium and ammonia metabolism,[223,224] and quantitative considerations suggest that ammonium is a physiologically significant determinant of potassium excretion.[225]

Hormones

Adrenal corticosteroids

It is well known that the native mineralocorticoid hormone *aldosterone* has an influence on renal potassium excretion. This effect is most easily recognized under conditions of chronic exposure to excessive or inadequate amounts of the hormone. In human primary hyperaldosteronism (Conn's syndrome), for example, potassium depletion and hypokalemia are classical hallmarks of the disease,[69,181] while potassium retention and hyperkalemia are characteristically found in adrenocortical insufficiency.[98] In both conditions, an important effect of dietary sodium intake on potassium balance is recognized: high sodium availability exaggerates the urinary potassium losses in the presence of excess aldosterone, while low sodium intake exacerbates potassium retention in adrenal failure.[73,98] These observations underscore the importance of the previously discussed factors of flow and/or luminal sodium concentration in modulating potassium transport at secretory sites in the distal nephron.

Recent experiments in adrenalectomized dogs have clarified the steady-state relationships between the circulating aldosterone level and plasma potassium concentration.[263] By fixing the aldosterone dose at discrete levels over a wide physiologic range, it was shown that for a given level of potassium intake, external balance was achieved at a lower plasma potassium concentration when aldosterone was high than when it was low. Two factors probably contribute to this relationship: on one hand, increased aldosterone levels lead to increased urinary potassium excretion before steady-state conditions are reestablished, but on the other, aldosterone causes movement of potassium from the extracellular to the intracellular fluid compartment.[17,18,262]

It is not clear that *acute* changes in aldosterone concentration are important in the physiologic regulation of renal potassium excretion.[175] Although a kaliuretic response to mineralocorticoid injection was reported in several early studies,[8,62] many investigators subsequently have been unable to demonstrate this effect using lower, more physiologic doses of hormone.[175] Furthermore, in studies in which potassium excretion is found to be stimulated, it is often only with sodium loading or potassium deficiency,[59,103,105,244] conditions that are not in the physiologic context of increased aldosterone secretion. The basis for these discrepancies has been clarified by microperfusion experiments in adrenalectomized rats.[56] When electrolyte transport was studied in individual distal tubules perfused at a constant rate and with a fluid of constant composition, an acute infusion of aldosterone significantly stimulated net potassium secretion (Fig. 7-11). However, final urinary potassium excretion, measured at the same time, was unchanged. It seems likely that the explanation for this disparity lies in the marked reduction in urinary sodium concentration and excretion, and hence in luminal flow rates, which develop during acute aldosterone administration. The changes secondarily limit the extent of distal potassium secretion during free-flow conditions. In contrast, during more chronic exposure to elevated aldosterone levels, urinary potassium excretion can increase, since the initially depressed flow rates are restored to normal as a result of plasma volume expansion (the phenomenon of mineralocorticoid "escape," Fig. 7-12).[152]

The mechanism of the direct effect of aldosterone on epithelial potassium secretion has been investigated with electrophysiological techniques. A series of experiments on the rat kidney in vivo[244-246] suggested that the response of the late distal tubule to aldosterone could be interpreted in terms of two components: a stimulatory action on uptake of potassium, at the basolateral surface, and an effect on the apparent potassium permeability of the luminal membrane.[99] Sodium reabsorption is also known to be stimulated by aldosterone in this nephron segment, and the resulting increase in the electrical negativity of the lumen would also favor potassium secretion. Although the data in regard to potassium are conflicting,[104,244] most evidence supports the hypothesis that induction of new protein synthesis plays a role in mediating the effects of aldosterone on both sodium and potassium transport in the kidney.[104,148] Furthermore, there is morphological evidence that amplification of the basolateral membrane area, presumably reflecting an increase in pump sites, follows mineralocorticoid treatment in both initial and cortical collecting tubules.[211,240] A model of the actions of mineralocorticoids on Na^+ and K^+ transport in principal cells of the cortical collecting tubule is shown in Fig. 7-13.[15]

More recently, transepithelial ion-flux and electrical data obtained with rabbit cortical collecting tubules perfused in vitro[169,194,216] have provided further evidence consistent with stimulation of potassium secretion in this nephron segment by mineralocorticoids. The relative contributions of changes at the apical and basolateral membranes to this process have been revealed by the application of intracellular microelectrode techniques.[127,128] As shown in Fig. 7-13, chronic pretreatment of rabbits with the mineralocorticoid DOCA results in an increase in the transepithelial potential difference, due to both depolarization of the apical membrane and hyperpolarization of the basolateral membrane, the latter presumably the result of stimulation of ATPase pump activity. Ion-substitution and ion-blocker experiments indicate that the apical membrane conductances to both sodium and potassium are increased after DOCA administration.[127] Thus, enhanced potassium secretion results from the combined effects of (1) increased basolateral uptake by both active and electroconductive pathways, (2) an increased electrochemical gradient favoring movement across the apical membrane from the cell into the lumen, and (3) increased potassium conductance of the luminal membrane.

Subsequent work has further clarified the time course of the component cellular responses following sustained mineralocorticoid treatment in rabbit cortical collecting tubules.[165] As shown in Fig. 7-14, the earliest effect is increased apical membrane sodium conductance, with increases in apical potassium conductance and basolateral Na^+-K^+ ATPase activity following in parallel 1 to 2 days later. Indeed, it appears that basal pump stimulation is dependent on increased apical sodium entry,

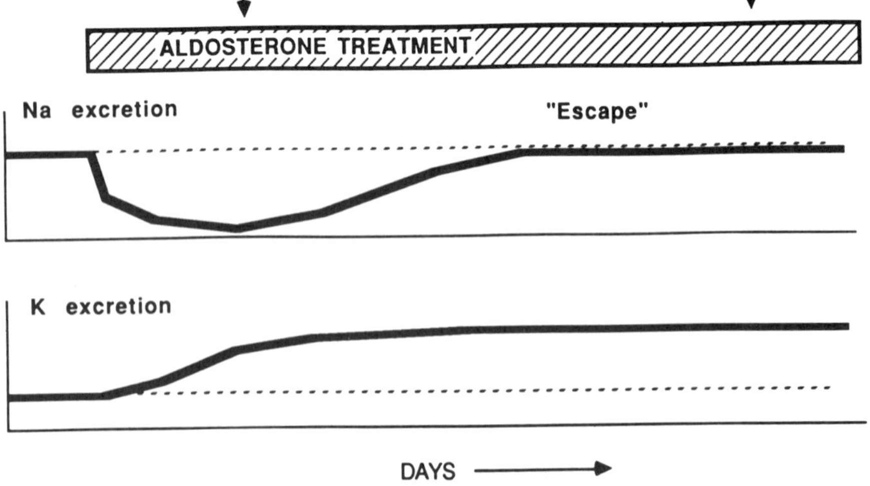

FIGURE 7-12 • Diagram of events during development of aldosterone escape. In phase 1, distal sodium reabsorption is stimulated and curtails urine sodium excretion. In phase 2, extracellular volume expansion develops during sodium retention and leads to secondary inhibition of proximal sodium transport and increased distal sodium and fluid delivery. With attainment of a new state of sodium balance, potassium excretion remains elevated as distal potassium secretion is stimulated by an enhanced flow rate past the distal nephron sites of potassium secretion. (From Field M, Giebisch G in Laragh JH, Brenner BM, eds: *Hypertension: Pathophysiology, Diagnosis and Management,* New York, Raven Press, 1990. Used by permission.)

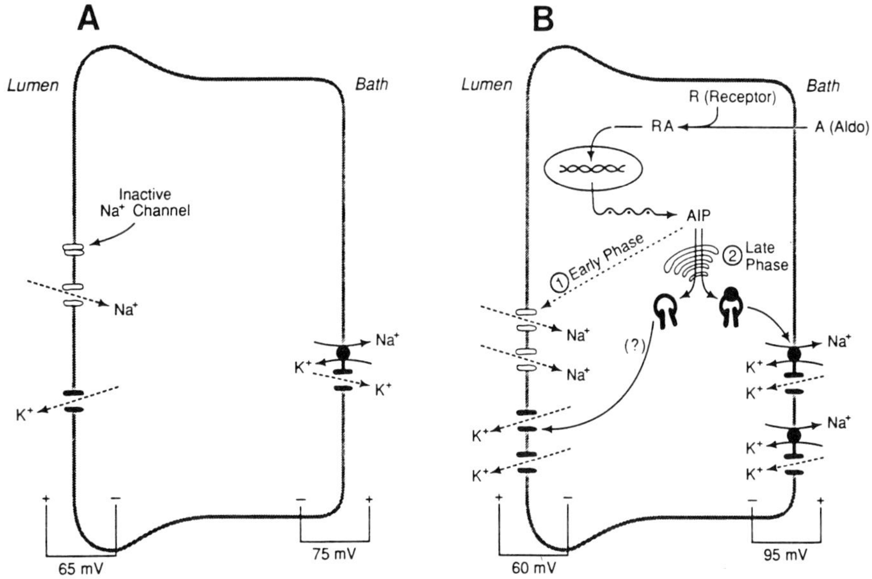

FIGURE 7-13 • Cell model of the actions of aldosterone on sodium and potassium transport in principal cells of the cortical collecting tubule. (*a*) Model of transport in the absence of aldosterone; (*b*) model of transport in the presence of aldosterone. Shown are binding of aldosterone to a cytoplasmic receptor (R), synthesis of aldosterone-induced proteins (AIPs), early activation of apical sodium-channels, and increased turnover and up-regulation of basolateral $Na^+ - K^+$ ATPase. Note also the activation of apical and basolateral potassium-channels. (From O'Neil RG in Giebisch G, ed: *Current Topics in Membranes and Transport,* Orlando, Academic Press, vol 28, 1987. Used by permission.)

since it can be abolished by pretreatment with the sodium channel blocker amiloride.[168]

Less information is available on the effects of *glucocorticoids* on potassium transport. Although it has been recognized for some time that infusion of potent glucocorticoids such as dexamethasone can stimulate renal potassium excretion,[19,66,96] it has been uncertain from clearance experiments whether this effect represents a direct action of the steroid on the potassium secretory mechanism or results secondarily from the increases in glomerular filtration, sodium excretion, and tubule flow rate that accompany dexamethasone infusion. The latter appears to be the correct explanation,[58] since, when distal tubules of adrenalectomized rats were perfused in vivo at a constant rate, acute systemic infusion of dexamethasone did not affect the rate of net potassium secretion in the perfused tubules (Fig. 7-11), while final urinary potassium excretion was enhanced, along with excretion of sodium and fluid.[58]

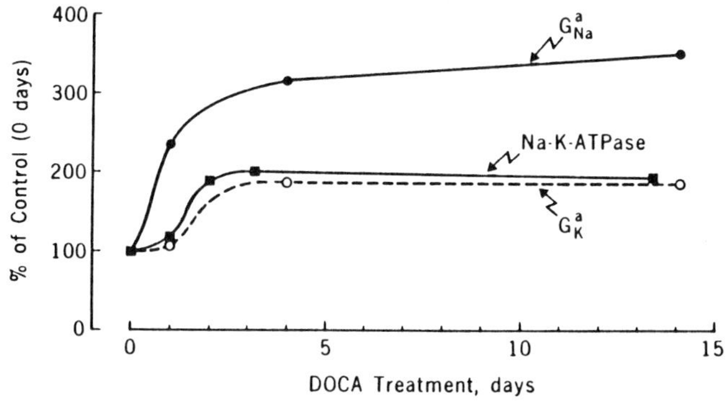

FIGURE 7-14 • Time course of apical and basolateral changes of membrane function in principal cells of cortical collecting tubule. Shown are alterations of apical sodium (G^a_{Na}) and potassium (G^a_K) conductance and of basolateral $Na^+ - K^+$ ATPase. (From O'Neil RG: *Sem Nephrol* 10:365, 1990. Used by permission.)

Antidiuretic hormone

In many experiments, infusion of ADH has been noted to increase potassium excretion despite variable effects on sodium excretion and a marked slowing of urinary flow rate that would otherwise be expected to decrease potassium secretion.[35,115,200] Conversely, the induction of water diuresis, during which ADH levels are suppressed, does not stimulate potassium excretion[4,230] despite high fluid flow rates through the distal nephron.

To explore the possibility of a direct effect of ADH on potassium secretion by the tubules, distal tubules of ADH-deficient rats were microperfused with an isotonic fluid.[57] Infusion of ADH into the peripheral circulation was associated with a marked stimulation of potassium secretion in perfused tubules in the absence of significant changes in luminal sodium delivery or flow rate. A similar response has been obtained following the addition of ADH to the solution bathing isolated perfused rat cortical collecting tubules.[185,228] In this preparation, increased apical sodium conductance secondarily enhances the driving force for potassium secretion into the lumen.[189] It is of interest that adrenal corticosteroids greatly enhance this response of the cortical collecting duct to ADH.[186]

When considered together, the acute effects on renal potassium transport described above for aldosterone and ADH suggest a possible homeostatic role for these hormones in protecting body potassium balance against acute changes in extracellular fluid volume or hydration status.[197] Thus, as shown in Fig. 7-15, an abrupt fall in extracellular volume leads to marked antinatriuresis and antidiuresis, but these effects do not result in depression

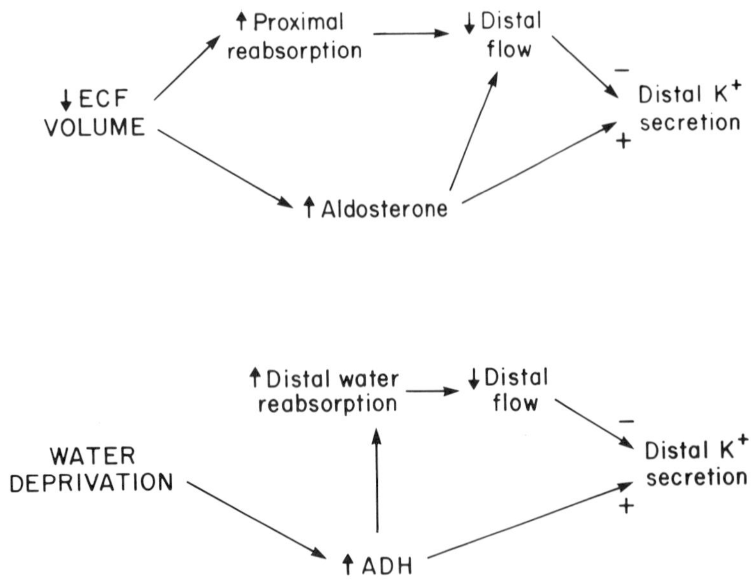

FIGURE 7-15 • Homeostatic interaction among factors influencing potassium secretion by the distal tubule during acute reduction of extracellular fluid volume (top) and water deprivation (bottom).

of potassium excretion because of the simultaneous direct effect of aldosterone to stimulate potassium secretion by the tubules. Similarly, pure water deprivation does not lead to significant potassium retention because of the direct effect of increased ADH levels in augmenting potassium secretion. It should be noted, as pointed out previously, that changes in sodium concentration of luminal fluid may also influence potassium secretion under these conditions.

Other hormones

An inhibitory effect of *epinephrine* on renal potassium excretion has recently been described.[37,114] This agent is known to enhance uptake of potassium by extrarenal tissues. Therefore, the observed fall in urinary potassium excretion might be mediated indirectly, since a reduction in plasma potassium concentration would be expected to inhibit potassium secretion by the distal tubule. However, when plasma potassium levels of epinephrine-infused and control-group rats were matched by giving different acute potassium infusions, the epinephrine group still excreted less potassium.[38] This effect was shown to be mediated at sites beyond the superficial late distal tubule and would be consistent with the demonstration that catecholamines can inhibit potassium secretion by the isolated cortical collecting tubule,[125] possibly by decreasing the transepithelial potential difference.[107] This action of epinephrine in the kidney appears to be mediated by betaadrenoreceptors.[38,125]

Of potential therapeutic interest is the observation that alpha-2 adrenoreceptor agonists indirectly inhibit potassium secretion by opposing the action of ADH at the level of the collecting duct. Thus, infusion of such agents increases urinary sodium and water excretion without increasing potassium excretion.[67,213]

Insulin is also known to exert a stimulatory effect upon potassium uptake by cells and, like epinephrine, plays an important role in the regulation of "internal" potassium balance.[17,36,126,214] Less is known, however, about its direct or indirect influence on renal potassium transport. (See also Chap. 14 for a comprehensive discussion of adrenal hormones.)

INTERACTIONS AMONG FACTORS

It is evident from the foregoing analysis of the factors that influence potassium secretion by the distal tubule that the net effect of a given systemic disturbance on final potassium excretion frequently represents the result of two or more interacting forces. In particular, the powerful effect of changes in the flow rate of tubular fluid often augments or opposes the "intrinsic" response of the tubules to several primary influences. As shown in Table 7-2, the final effect of these interactions in some cases

TABLE 7-2 • Interactions between flow and other factors influencing distal tubular potassium secretion

	Direct	Flow	Net
Hyperkalemia	↑	↑	↑↑
Acidosis	↑	↓	—
Alkalosis	↑	↑	↑↑
Aldosterone			
Acute	↑	↓	—
Chronic	↑	—	↑
Dexamethasone	—	↑	↑
ADH	↑	↓	—

(e.g., prolonged acidosis and acute aldosterone and ADH release) is to minimize the "direct" effect of the initial disturbance on potassium excretion, although the exact balance point reached depends on the relative magnitudes of the primary influence on one hand and the alteration in flow on the other. In other disturbances (e.g., acute hyperkalemia and systemic alkalosis), the direct and flow-mediated influences are additive. Although this results in maximally efficient potassium excretion in the case of acute potassium loading, it is clearly detrimental to overall potassium balance in prolonged metabolic alkalosis.

EFFECT OF DIURETICS

Although clearly not part of the normal physiology of renal potassium metabolism, the influence of diuretic drugs on potassium excretion is of some interest in the context of the mechanisms for renal potassium transport discussed in this chapter and in relation to interactions among the control factors involved. Details of the pharmacology and primary mechanisms of action of diuretics are given more fully elsewhere in this book (see Chap. 19), and the present discussion is limited solely to their effects on potassium transport.[106,236]

From the point of view of renal potassium handling, diuretic agents can be broadly divided into two groups: those that tend to depress potassium excretion (kaliopenic diuretics) and those that enhance it (kaliuretic diuretics).

Kaliopenic diuretics include amiloride, triamterene, and the spironolactones. While the potassium-sparing action of the first two of these is largely independent of mineralocorticoid activity, that of the spironolactone group is directly related to circulating aldosterone levels.[77] This is in accord with the concept that these steroidlike compounds antagonize the actions of mineralocorticoids at or near the receptor sites in the target tissue. Although micropuncture studies with this group of drugs have not been reported, stop-flow experiments are consistent with a distal site of action,[234] in accord with a similar distribution of mineralocorticoid receptors within the kidney.[53,54] Therapeutic usefulness of this group is greatest in states of primary or secondary aldosterone overproduction.

Amiloride and triamterene also act at a distal site within the nephron. In the case of amiloride, for which the most information is available, a clear inhibition of potassium secretion in the distal tubule[46] and cortical collecting duct[221] has been demonstrated directly. As described earlier in this chapter, this action is thought to be mediated by a hyperpolarization of the electrical potential across the apical membrane in the potassium-secreting cells of these nephron segments, due in turn to specific blockade by the drug of conductance channels for sodium in this membrane.[128,167] Since sodium reabsorption at these distal sites normally accounts for only some 2 to 5 percent of the filtered load, these drugs are weak natriuretic agents but are useful when used in combination with most other classes of diuretics (see below) to antagonize the potassium loss induced by the latter.

Kaliuretic diuretics include all the other drugs in clinical use as natriuretic agents. While the effects of carbonic anhydrase inhibitors, cardiac glycosides, and mercurials are of some theoretical and historical interest,[71,77] the following discussion will be confined to the three classes of diuretics commonly used in current therapeutics: osmotic agents, "loop" diuretics, and thiazide-like diuretics.

Osmotic agents such as mannitol and urea act primarily by reducing sodium and water reabsorption in the proximal tubule.[71] The resulting increase in delivery of fluid into the distal tubule results in a stimulation of potassium secretion, as previously discussed. It has also been mentioned earlier that infusions of sodium salts of poorly reabsorbed anions (e.g., sulfate and bicarbonate) have both a flow-dependent effect on potassium secretion and an effect due to depression of chloride concentration in the distal tubule.

Loop diuretics such as furosemide, ethacrynic acid, and bumetanide inhibit sodium chloride reabsorption by the thick ascending limb of Henle's loop.[77,87,154,156,158,190] Since the mechanism for this process is now known to involve electrically neutral cotransport of one Na^+ with one K^+ and two Cl^- ions (see above), it is clear that one potential site of potassium loss is the loop itself, especially since the abolition of the normal lumen-positive electrical potential would further minimize any passive (intercellular) potassium reabsorption in this segment. The major cause of potassium loss with these agents, however, is undoubtedly the sharp increase in delivery of sodium and fluid into the distal tubule.[71] Although an additional effect of furosemide[236] and related agents[55] on sodium chloride reabsorption by the microperfused distal tubule itself has been described, this action is unlikely to be of major quantitative importance in accounting for the natriuresis or kaliuresis. However, at least two additional factors may compound the potassium loss during therapy with these drugs. First, increased levels of aldosterone associated both with the underlying condition (cardiac failure, nephrotic syndrome, etc.) and with the extracellular volume reduction produced by the diuretic are likely to play a role, especially when dietary salt is restricted at the same time (see Chap. 19).[77,121,197] Second, it is possible that ADH, also released by the stimulus of volume reduction, may aggravate potassium loss, because such losses are reduced if furosemide is given during water diuresis.[121]

Thiazide diuretics include a wide range of chemically related agents that are thought to act in the early distal tubule.[49,77,134] The specific membrane mechanism influenced by thiazide appears to be a coupled sodium chloride cotransport process located in the luminal membrane of the cells of the early distal tubule.[49,235,236] Potassium losses are consequent upon flow increases into the late distal site of potassium secretion, compounded by hormonal responses to volume depletion.

REFERENCES

1. Adam WR, Dawborn JK: Potassium tolerance in rats. *Aust J Exp Biol Med Sci* 50:757, 1972.
2. Adler S, Fraley D: Potassium and intracellular pH. *Kidney Int* 11:433, 1977.
3. Alexander EA, Levinsky NG: An extrarenal mechanism for potassium adaptation. *J Clin Invest* 47:740, 1968.
4. Ali MN et al: Electrolyte excretion in diuretic and nondiuretic dogs. *J Physiol* 141:177, 1958.
5. Allen GG, Barratt LJ: Effect of cis-platinum on the transepithelial potential difference of the rat distal tubule. *Kidney Int* 27:842, 1985.
6. Avison MJ et al: Na^+ and K^+ fluxes stimulated by Na^+-coupled glucose transport: Evidence for a Ba^{2+}-insensitive K^+ efflux pathway in rabbit proximal tubules. *J Membr Biol* 105:197, 1988.
7. Bank N, Schwartz WB: The influence of anion penetrating ability on urinary acidification and the excretion of titratable acid. *J Clin Invest* 39:1516, 1960.
8. Barger AC et al: Infusion of aldosterone, 9α-fluorohydrocortisone and antidiuretic hormone into the renal artery of normal and adrenalectomized, unanesthetized dogs: Effect on electrolyte and water excretion. *Endocrinology* 62:804, 1958.
9. Barratt LJ: The effect of amiloride on the transepithelial potential difference of the distal tubule of the rat kidney. *Pfluegers Arch* 361:251, 1976.
10. Barratt LJ et al: Transepithelial potential difference profile of the distal tubule of the rat kidney. *Kidney Int* 8:368, 1975.
11. Battilana CA et al: Effect of chronic potassium loading on potassium secretion by the pars recta or descending limb of the juxtamedullary nephron in the rat. *J Clin Invest* 62:1093, 1978.
12. Battle D, Kurtzman NA: Acid-base physiology and pathophysiology, in Klahr S, Massry SG (eds): *Contemporary Nephrology*. New York, Plenum, 1983, vol 2, p 193.
13. Beck FX et al: The distribution of potassium, sodium and chloride across the apical membrane of renal tubular cells: Effect of acute metabolic alkalosis. *Pfluegers Arch* 411:259, 1988.
14. Beck FX et al: Effect of acute metabolic acidosis on transmembrane electrolyte gradients in individual renal tubule cells. *Pfluegers Arch* 412:427, 1988.
15. Beck LH et al: Sodium-independent active potassium reabsorption in proximal tubule of the dog. *J Clin Invest* 52:2641, 1973.
16. Berliner RW: Renal Mechanisms for Potassium Excretion, Harvey Lecture Series 55. New York, Academic Press, 1961, p 141.
17. Bia MJ, DeFronzo RA: Extrarenal potassium homeostasis. *Am J Physiol* 240:F257, 1981.
18. Bias MJ et al: Regulation of extrarenal potassium homeostasis by adrenal hormones in rats. *Am J Physiol* 242:F641, 1982.
19. Bia MJ et al: The effect of dexamethasone on renal electrolyte excretion in the adrenalectomized rat. *Endocrinology* 111:882, 1982.
20. Bloomer HA et al: The mechanism of potassium reabsorption in the proximal tubule of the rat. *J Clin Invest* 42:277, 1963.
21. Bomsztyk K, Wright FS: Effects of transepithelial fluid flux on transepithelial voltage and transport of calcium, sodium, chloride and potassium by renal proximal tubule. *Kidney Int* 21:269, 1982.
22. Boudry J et al: The effect of lumen pH on potassium transport in renal cortical collecting tubules. *Am J Physiol* 230:239, 1976.
23. Boulpaep EL: Recent advances in electrophysiology of the nephron. *Annu Rev Physiol* 38:20, 1976.
24. Brandis M et al: Potassium-induced inhibition of proximal tubular fluid reabsorption in rats. *Am J Physiol* 222:421, 1972.
25. Burg MB: Thick ascending limb of Henle's loop. *Kidney Int* 22:454, 1982.
26. Burg MB, Green N: Effect of ethacrynic acid on the thick ascending limb of Henle's loop. *Kidney Int* 4:301, 1973.
27. Burg MB, Orloff J: Perfusion of isolated renal tubules, in Orloff J, Berliner RW (eds): *Handbook of Physiology*. Washington, DC, American Physiological Society, sec 8, 1973, p 145.
28. Bygrave, FL: The ionic environment and metabolic control. *Nature* 214:667, 1967.
29. Capasso G et al: Water and electrolyte transport along the rat loop of Henle: Effect of chronic dietary potassium adaptation and restriction. Proc 11th Int Congress of Nephrol. Tokyo, 1990, p 493A.
30. Cardinal J et al: Luminal and peritubular ionic substitutions and intracellular potential of the rabbit proximal convoluted tubule. *Am J Physiol* 247:F352, 1984.
31. Clapp JR et al: Effect of unreabsorbed anions on proximal and distal transtubular potentials in rats. *Am J Physiol* 202:781, 1962.
32. Cortney MA: Renal tubular transfer of water and electrolytes in adrenalectomized rats. *Am J Physiol* 216:589, 1969.
33. Cox M et al: The defense against hyperkalemia: The roles of insulin and aldosterone. *N Engl J Med* 299:525, 1978.
34. Crayen M, Thoenes W: Architektur und cytologische Charakterisierung des distalen Tubulus der Rattenniere. *Fortschr Zool* 23:279, 1975.
35. Cross RB et al: The effect of vasopressin on water and electrolyte excretion by the sheep. *Aust J Exp Biol* 41:629, 1963.
36. DeFronzo RA et al: The effect of insulinopenia and adrenal hormone deficiency on acute potassium tolerance. *Kidney Int* 17:586, 1980.
37. DeFronzo RA et al: Epinephrine and potassium homeostasis. *Kidney Int* 20:83, 1981.
38. DeFronzo RA et al: Inhibitory effect of epinephrine on

renal potassium secretion: A micropuncture study. *Am J Physiol* 245:F303, 1983.

39. DeRouffignac C et al: Micropuncture study of water, electrolyte and urea movements along the loop of Henle in *Psammomys. J Clin Invest* 48:474, 1969.
40. Dietl P et al: Adrenal corticosteroid action on the thick ascending limb. *Sem Nephrol* 10:350, 1990.
41. Diezi J et al: Micropuncture study of electrolyte transport across papillary collecting duct of the rat. *Am J Physiol* 224:623, 1973.
42. Diezi J et al: Effects of nephrectomy on renal salt and water transport in the remaining kidney. *Kidney Int* 10:450, 1976.
43. Dirks JH, Seeley JF: Effect of saline infusions and furosemide on the dog distal nephron. *Am J Physiol* 219:114, 1970.
44. Dobyan DC et al: Suppression of potassium recycling in the renal medulla by short-term potassium deprivation. *Kidney Int* 16:704, 1979.
45. Doucet A, Katz AI: Renal potassium adaptation: Na,K-ATPase activity along the nephron after chronic potassium loading. *Am J Physiol* 238:F380, 1980.
46. Duarte CG et al: Effect of amiloride, ouabain, and furosemide on distal tubular function in the rat. *Am J Physiol* 221:632, 1971.
47. Doucet A et al: Characterization of K-ATPase activity in distal nephron: Stimulation by potassium depletion. *Am J Physiol* 253:F418, 1987.
48. Elalouf J-M et al: Effects of human calcitonin on water and electrolyte movements in rat juxtamedullary nephrons: Inhibition of medullary K recycling. *Pfluegers Arch* 406:502, 1986.
49. Elalouf J-M et al: Stimulation by human calcitonin of electrolyte transport in distal tubules of rat kidney. *Pfluegers Arch* 399:111, 1983.

49*a*. Elalouf J-M et al: Effects of dDAVP on rat juxtamedullary nephrons: stimulation of medullary K recycling. *Am J Physiol* 249:F291, 1985.

49*b*. Ellison DH et al: Thiazide-sensitive sodium chloride cotransport in early distal tubule. *Am J Physiol* 253:F546, 1987.

50. Engbretson BG et al: Flow-dependence potassium secretion by rabbit cortical collecting tubule in vitro. *Am J Physiol* 253:F896, 1987.
51. Ernst SA: Transport ATPase cytochemistry: Ultrastructural localization of potassium-dependent and potassium-independent phosphatase activities in rat kidney cortex. *J Cell Biol* 66:586, 1975.
52. Eveloff J, Warnock DG: K-Cl transport systems in rabbit renal basolateral membrane vesicles. *Am J Physiol* 252:F883, 1987.
53. Farman N, Bonvalet JP: Aldosterone binding in isolated tubules: 3. Autoradiography along the rat nephron. *Am J Physiol* 245:F606, 1983.
54. Farman N et al: Binding sites of mineralo and glucocorticoids along the mammalian nephron (rat and rabbit), in Morel F (ed): *Biochemistry of Kidney Functions*, INSERM Symposium no. 21. New York, Elsevier, 1982, p. 285.
55. Field MJ et al: Effects of enantiomers of indacrinone (MK-196) on cation transport by the loop of Henle and distal tubule studied by microperfusion in vivo. *J Pharm Exp Ther* 230:62, 1984.
56. Field MJ et al: Independent effects of aldosterone (*A*) and plasma K concentration on distal tubular K secretion. *Kidney Int* 25:300, 1984.
57. Field MJ et al: Influence of ADH on renal potassium handling: A micropuncture and microperfusion study in Brattleboro rats. *Kidney Int* 25:502, 1984.
58. Field MJ et al: Differential acute effects of aldosterone and dexamethasone and hyperkalemia on distal tubular potassium secretion in the rat kidney. *J Clin Invest* 74:1792, 1984.

58*a*. Field M, Giebisch G: Physiologic actions of aldosterone on the kidney, in Laragh JH, Brenner BM (eds): *Hypertension: Pathophysiology, Diagnosis and Management*. New York, Raven Press, 1990, pp 1273–1285.

59. Fimognari GM et al: Induction of RNA and protein synthesis in the action of aldosterone in the rat. *Am J Physiol* 213:954, 1967.
60. Fraley D, Adler S: Isohydric regulation of plasma potassium by bicarbonate in the rat. *Kidney Int* 9:333, 1976.
61. Fujimoto M et al: Electrochemical profile of K and Cl ions across the proximal tubule of bullfrog kidneys, in Kobayashi K et al (eds): *Renal Research*. Basel, Karger, 1977, vol 6, p 114.
62. Ganong WF, Mulrow PJ: Rate of change in sodium and potassium excretion after injection of aldosterone into the aorta and renal artery of the dog. *Am J Physiol* 195:337, 1958.
63. Garcia-Filho E et al: Effects of changes in electrical potential difference on tubular potassium transport. *Am J Physiol* 238:F235, 1982.
64. Garg LC et al: Mineralocorticoid effects on NaK-ATPase in individual nephron segments. *Am J Physiol* 240:F536, 1981.
65. Garp LC et al: Ouabain-insensitive K-adenosine triphosphate in distal nephron segments of the rabbit. *J Clin Invest* 81:1204, 1988.
66. Garrod O et al: The action of cortisone and desoxycorticosterone acetate on glomerular filtration rate and sodium and water in the adrenalectomized dog. *J Clin Invest* 34:761, 1955.
67. Gellai M, Edwards RM: Mechanism of alpha 2-adrenoceptor agonist-induced diuresis. *Am J Physiol* 255: F317, 1988.
68. Gennari FJ, Cohen JJ: Role of the kidney in potassium homeostasis: Lessons from acid-base disturbances. *Kidney Int* 8:1, 1975.
69. George JM et al: The syndrome of primary aldosteronism. *Am J Med* 48:343, 1970.
70. Giebisch GH: Some reflections on the mechanism of renal tubular potassium transport. *Yale J Biol Med* 8:315, 1975.
71. Giebisch GH: Effects of diuretics on renal transport of potassium, in Martinez-Maldonado M (ed): *Methods in Pharmacology*. New York, Plenum, 1976, vol 4A.
72. Giebisch GH: micropuncture techniques, in Gupta BL, Moreton RB (eds): *Transport of Ions and Water in Animals*. New York, Academic Press, 1977.

73. Giebisch GH: Renal potassium transport, in Giebisch GH et al (eds): *Membrane Transport in Biology*. New York, Springer-Verlag, 1978, vol 4A, p 215.
74. Giebisch GH, Windhager EE: Electrolyte transport across renal tubular membranes, in Orloff J, Berliner RW (eds): *Handbook of Physiology*. Washington, DC, American Physiological Society, sec 8, 1973, p. 315.
75. Giebisch GH et al: Effect of ionic substitutions on distal potential differences in rat kidney. *Am J Physiol* 211:560, 1966.
76. Giebisch GH et al: Renal transport and control of potassium excretion, in Rector FC Jr, Brenner BM (eds): *The Kidney*, 2d ed. Philadelphia, Saunders, 1981, p 408.
77. Goldberg M: The renal physiology of diuretics, in Orloff J, Berliner RW (eds): *Handbook of Physiology*. Washington, DC, American Physiological Society, 1973, sec 8, p 1003.
78. Good DW: Active absorption of NH_4 by rat medullary thick ascending limb: Inhibition by potassium. *Am J Physiol* 255:F78, 1988.
79. Good DW, Wright FS: Luminal influences on potassium secretion: Sodium concentration and fluid flow rate. *Am J Physiol* 236:F192, 1979.
80. Good DW, Wright FS: Luminal influences on potassium secretion: Transepithelial voltage. *Am J Physiol* 239: F289, 1980.
81. Good DW et al: Effects of low lumen sodium concentrations on potassium secretion and transepithelial voltage in renal distal tubule. *Fed Proc* 40:395, 1981.
82. Good DW et al: Luminal influences on potassium secretion: Low sodium concentration. *Am J Physiol* 246:F609, 1984.
83. Grantham JJ, Burg MB: Effect of vasopressin and cyclic AMP on permeability of isolated collecting tubules. *Am J Physiol* 211:255, 1966.
84. Grantham JJ et al: The nature of transtubular Na and K transport in isolated rabbit collecting tubules. *J Clin Invest* 49:1815, 1970.
85. Grantham JJ et al: Net fluid secretion in proximal straight renal tubules in vitro: Role of PAH. *Am J Physiol* 226:191, 1974.
86. Green R, Giebisch GH: Ion requirements of proximal tubular sodium transport: 1. Bicarbonate and chloride. *Am J Physiol* 229:1205, 1975.
87. Greger R: Ion transport mechanisms in thick ascending limb of Henle's loop of mammalian nephrons. *Physiol Rev* 65:760, 1985.
88. Greger R, Gögelein H: Role of K^+ conductive pathways in the nephron. *Kidney Int* 31:1055, 1987.
89. Greger R, Schlatter E: Presence of luminal K^+, a prerequisite for active NaCl transport in the cortical thick ascending limb of Henle's loop of rabbit kidney. *Pfluegers Arch* 392:92, 1981.
90. Greger R, Schlatter E: Properties of the lumen membrane of the cortical thick ascending limb of Henle's loop of rabbit kidney. *Pfluegers Arch* 396:315, 1983.
91. Greger R, Schlatter E: Properties of the basolateral membrane of the cortical thick ascending limb of Henle's loop of rabbit kidney: A model for secondary active chloride transport. *Pfluegers Arch* 396:325, 1983.
92. Gross JB et al: A functional comparison of the cortical collecting tubule and the distal convoluted tubule. *J Clin Invest* 55:1284, 1975.
93. Guggino WB et al: The amphibian diluting segment. *Am J Physiol* 254:F615, 1988.
94. Hayslett JP et al: Electrical characteristics of the mammalian distal tubule: Comparison of Ling-Gerard and macroelectrodes. *Kidney Int* 12:324, 1977.
95. Hebert SC et al: The effects of antidiuretic hormone on cellular conductive pathways in mouse medullary thick ascending limbs of Henle: 1. ADH increases transcellular conductance pathways. *J Membr Biol*, 80:201, 1984.
96. Hiatt N et al: Adrenal hormones and the regulation of serum potassium in potassium-loaded adrenalectomized dog. *Endocrinology* 105:215, 1979.
97. Hierholzer K: Secretion of potassium and acidification in collecting ducts of mammalian kidney. *Am J Physiol* 201:318, 1961.
98. Hierholzer K, Lange S: The effects of adrenal steroids on renal function, in Thurau K (ed): *Kidney and Urinary Tract Physiology*, MTP International Review of Science, Physiology Series 1. London, Butterworth, 1974, p 273.
99. Hierholzer K, Wiederholt M: Some aspects of distal tubular solute and water transport. *Kidney Int* 9:198, 1976.
100. Hierholzer K et al: Micropuncture study of renal transtubular concentration gradients of sodium and potassium in adrenalectomized rats. *Pfluegers Arch* 285:193, 1965.
101. Higashihara E et al: Effects of aldosterone on potassium recycling in the kidney of adrenalectomized rats. *Am J Physiol* 248:F219, 1985.
102. Hodgkin AL: *The Conduction of the Nervous Impulse*. Springfield, IL, Thomas, 1964.
103. Horisberger J-D, Diezi J: Effects of mineralocorticoids on Na^+ and K^+ excretion in the adrenalectomized rat. *Am J Physiol* 245:F89, 1983.
104. Horisberger J-D, Diezi J: Inhibition of aldosterone-induced antinatriuresis and kaliuresis by actinomycin-D. *Am J Physiol* 246:F201, 1984.
105. Howell DS, Davis JO: Relationship of sodium retention to potassium excretion by the kidney during administration of desoxycorticosterone acetate to dogs. *Am J Physiol* 179:359, 1954.
106. Hropot M et al: Tubular action of diuretics: Distal effects on electrolyte transport and acidification. *Kidney Int* 28:477, 1985.
107. Iino Y et al: Effects of catecholamines on electrolyte transport in cortical collecting tubule. *J Membr Biol* 61:67, 1981.
108. Jaeger P et al: Ammonium transport in rat cortical tubule: Relationship to potassium metabolism. *Am J Physiol* 245:F593, 1983.
109. Jamison RL: Potassium recycling. *Kidney Int* 31:695, 1987.
110. Jamison RL, Kriz W: *Urinary Concentrating Mechanism: Structure and Function*. New York, Oxford University Press, 1982.
111. Jamison RL et al: Potassium secretion by the descending limb of pars recta of the juxtamedullary nephron in vivo. *Kidney Int* 9:323, 1976.
112. Jamison RL et al: Questions and replies: Role of the collecting tubule in fluid, sodium, and potassium balance. *Am J Physiol* 237:F247, 1979.

113. Jamison RL et al: New pathways for potassium transport in the kidney, *Am J Physiol* 242:F297, 1982.
114. Johnson MD, Barger C: Circulating catecholamines in control of renal electrolyte and water excretion. *Am J Physiol* 240:F192, 1981.
115. Johnson MD et al: Effects of AVP and DDAVP on plasma renin activity and electrolyte excretion in conscious dogs. *Am J Physiol* 236:F66, 1979.
116. Jung KY et al: Cellular adenosine triphosphate production and consumption in the descending thin limb of Henle's loop in the rat. *Renal Physiol Biochem* 13:248, 1990.
117. Jureidini KF et al: Prevention of cis-platinum nephrotoxicity with amiloride hydrochloride. Abstracted in *Second Asian Pacific Congress of Nephrology*. 1983, p 41.
118. Kaissling B, Kriz W: *Structural Analysis of Rabbit Kidney*. Berlin, Springer, 1979.
119. Katz AI et al: Na-K-ATPase activity along the rabbit, rat and mouse nephron. *Am J Physiol* 237:F114, 1979.
120. Kawahara et al: Potassium channels in *Necturus* proximal tubule. *Am J Physiol* 253:F488, 1987.
121. Kelly RA et al: Effects of aldosterone and ADH on potassium excretion with furosemide (abstract). *Kidney Int* 25:169, 1984.
122. Khuri RN et al: Intracellular potassium in cells of the distal tubule. *Pfluegers Arch* 335:297, 1972.
123. Khuri RN et al: Effects of flow rate and potassium intake on distal tubular potassium transfer. *Am J Physiol* 228:1249, 1975.
123a. Weinstein AM: Modeling the proximal tubule: Complications of the paracellular pathway. *Am J Physiol* 254:F297, 1988.
124. Khuri RN et al: Effects of graded solute diuresis on renal tubular sodium transport in the rat. *Am J Physiol* 228:1262, 1975.
125. Kimmel P, Goldfarb S: Effect of isoproterenol, cyclic AMP and antidiuretic hormone on potassium transport in cortical collecting tubule, abstracted. *Clin Res* 30:453A, 1982.
126. Knochel JP: Role of glucoregulatory hormones in potassium homeostasis. *Kidney Int* 11:443, 1977.
127. Koeppen BM, Giebisch GH: Mineralocorticoid regulation of sodium and potassium transport by the cortical collecting duct, in Graves JS (ed): *Regulation and Development of Membrane Transport Processes*. New York, Wiley, 1985, p 90.
128. Koeppen BM et al: Intracellular microelectrode characterization of the rabbit cortical collecting duct. *Am J Physiol* 244:F35, 1983.
129. Koeppen BM et al: Electrophysiology of mammalian renal tubules: Inferences from intracellular microelectrode studies. *Annu Rev Physiol* 45:497, 1983.
130. Kriz W, Bankir L: A standard nomenclature for structures of the kidney. *Am J Physiol* 254:F1, 1988.
131. Kubota T et al: Intracellular potassium activity measurements in single proximal tubules of *Necturus* kidney. *J Membr Biol* 73:51, 1983.
132. Kunau RT, Whinnery MA: Potassium transfer in distal tubule of normal and remnant kidneys. *Am J Physiol* 235:F186, 1978.
133. Kunau RT et al: Characteristics of the relationship between the flow rate of tubular fluid and potassium transport in the distal tubule of the rat. *J Clin Invest* 54:1488, 1974.
134. Kunau RT Jr et al: Clarification of the site of action of chlorothiazide in the rat nephron. *J Clin Invest* 56:401, 1975.
135. Lapointe JY et al: Characterization of the apical membrane ionic permeability of the rabbit proximal convoluted tubule. *Am J Physiol* 250:F339, 1986.
136. LeGrimellec C: Micropuncture study along the proximal convoluted tubule. *Pfluegers Arch* 354:133, 1975.
137. LeGrimellec C et al: ^{3}H-inulin and electrolyte concentrations in Bowman's capsule in rat kidney. *Pfluegers Arch* 354:117, 1975.
138. Linas SL et al: Mechanism of renal potassium conservation in the rat. *Kidney Int* 15:601, 1979.
139. Lubin M: Cell potassium and the regulation of protein synthesis, in Hoffman JF (ed): *The Cellular Functions of Membrane Transport*. Englewood Cliffs, NJ, Prentice-Hall, 1964, p 193.
140. Macknight ADC, Leaf A: Regulation of cellular volume, in Andreoli TA et al (eds): *Physiology of Membrane Disorders*. New York, Plenum, 1978, p 315.
141. Madsen KM, Tisher CC: Structural-functional relationships along the distal nephron. *Am J Physiol* 250:F1, 1986.
142. Malnic G et al: Micropuncture study of renal potassium excretion in the rat. *Am J Physiol* 206:674, 1964.
143. Malnic G et al: Micropuncture study of distal tubular potassium and sodium transport in rat nephron. *Am J Physiol* 211:529, 1966.
144. Malnic G et al: Microperfusion study of distal tubular potassium and sodium transfer in rat kidney. *Am J Physiol* 211:548, 1966.
145. Malnic G et al: Potassium transport across renal distal tubules during acid-base disturbances. *Am J Physiol* 221:1192, 1971.
146. Malnic G et al: Flow dependence of K secretion in cortical distal tubules of the rat. *Am J Physiol* 256:F932, 1989.
147. Marsh DJ et al: Micropuncture analysis of the behaviour of potassium ions in rat cortical tubules. *Pfluegers Arch* 277:107, 1963.
148. Marver D, Kokko JP: Renal target sites and the mechanism of action of aldosterone. *Miner Electrolyte Metab* 9:1, 1983.
149. McDougal WS, Wright FS: Defect in proximal and distal sodium transport in post-obstructive diuresis. *Kidney Int* 2:304, 1972.
150. Mello-Aires M et al: Kinetics of potassium transport across single distal tubules of rat kidney. *J Physiol* 232:47, 1973.
151. Miller CE, Remenchik AP: Problems involved in accurately measuring the K content of the human body. *Ann NY Acad Sci* 110:175, 1963.
152. Möhring J, Möhring B: Reevaluation of DOCA escape phenomenon. *Am J Physiol* 223:1237, 1972.
153. Morel F: Sites of hormone action in the mammalian nephron. *Am J Physiol* 240:F159, 1981.
154. Morgan T et al: Effect of furosemide on Na and K transport studied by microperfusion of the rat nephron. *Am J Physiol* 218:292, 1970.
155. Muto S et al: An acute increase of peritubular K stimulates

K transport through cell pathways of CCT. *Am J Physiol* 255:F108, 1988.
156. Murer H, Greger R: Membrane transport in the proximal tubule and thick ascending limb of Henle's loop: Mechanisms and their alterations. *Klin Wochenschr* 60:1103, 1982.
157. Oberleithner H, Giebisch GH: Mechanism of potassium transport across distal tubular epithelium of *Amphiuma*, in Macknight ADC, Leader JP (eds): *Epithelial Ion and Water Transport*. New York, Raven Press, 1981.
158. Oberleithner H et al: Cellular mechanism of the furosemide sensitive transport system in the kidney. *Klin Wochenschr* 60:1173, 1982.
159. Oberleithner H et al: Effects of inhibition of chloride transport on intracellular sodium activity in distal amphibian nephron. *Pfluegers Arch* 394:55, 1982.
160. Oberleithner H et al: The effect of furosemide on luminal sodium, chloride and potassium transport in the early distal tubule of *Amphiuma* kidney: Effects of potassium adaptation. *Pfluegers Arch* 396:27, 1983.
161. Oberleithner H et al: Effect of luminal potassium on cellular sodium activity in the early distal tubule of Amphiuma kidney. *Pfluegers Arch* 396:34, 1983.
162. Okusa MD et al: Luminal calcium regulates potassium transport by the renal distal tubule. *Am J Physiol* 258:F423, 1990.
163. O'Neil RG: Effects of DOCA and amiloride on sodium and potassium transport by the isolated cortical collecting tubule of the rabbit, PhD dissertation. Urbana, University of Illinois 1976 (cited in *Fed Proc* 40:2403, 1981).
164. O'Neil RG: Potassium secretion by the cortical collecting tubule. *Fed Proc* 40:2403, 1981.
165. O'Neil RG: Adrenal steroid regulation of potassium transport, in Giebisch G (ed): *Current Topics in Membranes and Transport*. Orlando, Academic Press, 1987, vol 28, p 185.
166. O'Neil RG: Aldosterone regulation of sodium and potassium transport in the cortical collecting tubule. *Sem Nephrol* 10:365, 1990.
167. O'Neil RG, Boulpaep E: Effect of amiloride on the apical cell membrane cation channels of a sodium-absorbing, potassium-secreting renal epithelium. *J Membr Biol* 50:365, 1979.
168. O'Neil RG, Hayhurst RA: Sodium-dependent modulation of the renal Na-K-ATPase: Influence of mineralocorticoids on the cortical collecting duct. *J Memb Biol* 85:169, 1985.
169. O'Neil RG, Helman SI: Transport characteristics of renal collecting tubules: Influences of DOCA and diet. *Am J Physiol* 233:F544, 1977.
170. Ornt DB, Tannen RL: Demonstration of an intrinsic renal adaptation for K^+ conservation in short-term K^+ depletion. *Am J Physiol* 245:F329, 1983.
171. Patrick J: Assessment of body potassium stores. *Kidney Int* 11:476, 1977.
172. Peters G: Compensatory adaptation of renal functions in the unanesthetized rat. *Am J Physiol* 205:1042, 1963.
173. Peterson LN, Wright FS: Effect of sodium intake on renal potassium excretion. *Am J Physiol* 233:F225, 1977.
174. Quamme GA: Effect of furosemide on calcium and magnesium transport in the rat nephron. *Am J Physiol* 241:F340, 1981.
175. Rabinowitz L: Aldosterone and renal potassium excretion. *Renal Physiol* 2:229, 1979–80.
176. Rastegar A: Changes in membrane surfaces of collecting duct cells in potassium adaptation. *Kidney Int* 18:293, 1980.
177. Rector FC Jr et al: Proximal tubular reabsorption of potassium during mannitol diuresis in rats. *J Lab Clin Med* 63:100, 1964.
178. Reineck HJ et al: Potassium transport in the distal tubule and collecting duct of the rat. *Am J Physiol* 229:1403, 1975.
179. Reineck HJ et al: Studies on the role of nephron heterogeneity in the rat. *Am J Physiol* 239:F187, 1980.
180. Rocha AS, Kokko JP: Membrane characteristics regulating potassium transport out of the isolated perfused descending limb of Henle. *Kidney Int* 4:326, 1973.
181. Ross EJ: *Aldosterone and Aldosteronism*. London, Lloyd-Luke, 1975.
182. Sackin H, Palmer LG: Basolateral potassium channels in renal proximal tubule. *Am J Physiol* 253:F476, 1987.
183. Sansom SC et al: Na-dependent effects of DOCA on cellular transport properties of CCD's from ADX rabbits. *Am J Physiol* 253:F753, 1987.
184. Schäfer Ch et al: Antagonistic action of H^+ and Ca^{++} on K^+-transport in diluting segment of frog kidney. *J Cell Physiol Biochem* in press.
185. Schafer JA, Troutman SL: Effect of ADH on rubidium transport in isolated perfused rat cortical collecting tubule. *Am J Physiol* 250:F1063, F1072, 1986.
186. Schafer JA, Troutman SL: Potassium transport in cortical collecting tubules from mineralocorticoid-treated rat. *Am J Physiol* 253:F76, 1987.
187. Schambelan M et al: Mineralocorticoid resistant renal hyperkalemia without salt wasting (type II pseudohypoaldosteronism): Role of increased renal chloride reabsorption. *Kidney Int* 19:716, 1981.
188. Schlatter E: Antidiuretic hormone regulation of electrolyte transport in the distal nephron. *Renal Physiol Biochem* 12:65, 1989.
189. Schlatter E, Schafer JA: Electrophysiological studies in principal cells of rat cortical collecting tubules: ADH increases the apical membrane Na^+-conductance. *Pfluegers Arch* 409:81, 1987.
190. Schlatter E et al: Effect of "high ceiling" diuretics on active salt transport in the cortical thick ascending limb of Henle's loop of rabbit kidney: Correlation of chemical structure and inhibitory potency. *Pfluegers Arch* 396:210, 1983.
191. Schmidt U et al: Sodium and potassium-activated ATPase: A possible target of aldosterone. *J Clin Invest* 55:655, 1975.
192. Schon DA et al: Mechanism of potassium excretion in renal insufficiency. *Am J Physiol* 227:1323, 1974.
193. Schon DA et al: Role of the medullary collecting duct in potassium excretion in potassium-adapted animals. *Kidney Int* 20:655, 1981.
194. Schultze RG, Nissenson AR: Potassium: Physiology and pathophysiology, in Maxwell MH, Kleeman CR (eds):

Clinical Disorders of Fluid and Electrolyte Metabolism, 3d ed. New York, McGraw-Hill, 1980, p 113.
195. Schwab A, Oberleithner H: Trans- and paracellular K^+ transport in diluting segment of frog kidney. *Pfluegers Arch* 411:268, 1988.
196. Schwartz GJ, Burg MB: Mineralocorticoid effects on cation transport by cortical collecting tubules in vitro. *Am J Physiol* 235:F576, 1978.
197. Sealey JE, Laragh JH: A proposed cybernetic system for sodium and potassium homeostasis: coordination of aldosterone and intrarenal physical factors. *Kidney Int* 6:281, 1974.
198. Seely JF, Dirks JH: Micropuncture study of hypertonic mannitol diuresis in the proximal and distal tubule of the dog kidney. *J Clin Invest* 48:2330, 1969.
199. Sejersted OM et al: Dependency of renal potassium excretion on Na, K-ATPase transport rate. *Acta Physiol Scand* 123:9, 1985.
200. Shade RE: Changes in sodium and potassium excretion, PRA and heart rate with vasopressin infusion in the acutely hypophysectomized dog. *Physiologist* 25:289, 1982.
201. Silva P et al: The role of Na-K-activated adenosine triphosphatase in potassium adaptation: Stimulation of enzymatic activity by potassium loading. *J Clin Invest* 52:2665, 1973.
202. Silva P et al: Adaptation to potassium. *Kidney Int* 11:466, 1977.
203. Sonnenberg H: Medullary collecting duct function in antidiuretic and in salt- or water-diuretic rats. *Am J Physiol* 226:501, 1974.
204. Stanton B: Regulation by adrenal corticosteroids of sodium and potassium transport in loop of Henle and distal tubule of rat kidney. *J Clin Invest* 78:1612, 1986.
205. Stanton BA, Giebisch GH: Mechanism of urinary potassium excretion. *Miner Electrolyte Metab* 5:100, 1981.
206. Stanton BA, Giebisch GH: Potassium transport by the renal distal tubule and effects of potassium loading. *Am J Physiol* 243:F487, 1982.
207. Stanton BA, Giebisch GH: Effects of pH on potassium transport by renal distal tubule. *Am J Physiol* 242:F544, 1982.
208. Stanton BA, Giebisch GH: Regulation of potassium homeostasis, in Corradino RA (ed): *Functional Regulation at the Cellular and Molecular Levels*. Amsterdam, Elsevier/North-Holland, 1982, p 259.
209. Stanton BA et al: Structural and functional study of the rat distal nephron: Effects of potassium adaptation and depletion. *Kidney Int* 19:36, 1981.
210. Stanton BA et al: Acidification of the basolateral solution reduces potassium conductance of the apical membrane. *Fed Proc* 41:1006, 1982.
211. Stanton BA et al: Role of physiological levels of aldosterone in regulation of distal tubule morphology and potassium transport, abstracted. *Kidney Int* 23:267, 1983.
212. Stanton B et al: Independent effects of aldosterone and potassium on induction of potassium adaptation in rat kidney. *J Clin Invest* 79:198, 1987.
213. Stanton B et al: Localization of alpha 2-adrenoreceptor-mediated increase in renal Na^+, K^+ and water excretion. *Am J Physiol* 252:F1016, 1987.
214. Sterns RH et al: Internal potassium balance and the control of the plasma potassium concentration. *Medicine* 60:339, 1981.
215. Stetson D et al: Morphological alterations in the rat medullary collecting duct following K^+ depletion. *Kidney Int* 17:45, 1980.
216. Stokes JB: Potassium secretion by cortical collecting tubule: Relation to sodium absorption, luminal sodium concentration, and transepithelial voltage. *Am J Physiol* 241:F395, 1981.
217. Stokes JB: Effect of elevated [K] on ion transport in the medullary thick ascending limb of Henle's loop (mTALH), abstracted. *Kidney Int* 21:289, 1982.
218. Stokes JB: Consequences of potassium recycling in the renal medulla: Effects on ion transport by the medullary thick ascending limb of Henle's loop. *J Clin Invest* 70:219, 1982.
219. Stokes JB: Ion transport by the cortical and outer medullary collecting tubule. *Kidney Int* 22:473, 1982.
220. Stokes JB et al: Heterogeneity of the rabbit collecting tubule: Localization of mineralocorticoid hormone action to the cortical portion. *Kidney Int* 20:340, 1981.
221. Stoner LC et al: Ion transport in cortical collecting tubule: Effect of amiloride. *Am J Physiol* 227:453, 1974.
222. Sufit CR, Jamison RL: Effect of acute potassium load on reabsorption in Henle's loop in the rat. *Am J Physiol* 245:F569, 1983.
223. Tannen RL: Relationship of renal ammonia production and potassium homeostasis. *Kidney Int* 11:453, 1977.
224. Tannen RL: Control of potassium excretion, in Massry SG, Glassock RJ (eds): *Textbook of Nephrology*. Baltimore, Williams & Wilkins, 1983, p 3.31.
225. Tannen RL: Effect of potassium on renal acidification and acid-base homeostasis. *Sem Nephrol* 7:263, 1987.
226. Tannen RL, Terrien T: Potassium-sparing effect of enhanced renal ammonia production. *Am J Physiol* 228:699, 1975.
227. Thatcher JS, Radike AW: Tolerance to potassium intoxication in the albino rat. *Am J Physiol* 151:138, 1947.
228. Tomita K et al: Control of sodium and potassium transport in the cortical collecting duct of the rat: Effects of bradykinin, vasopressin, and deoxycorticosterone. *J Clin Invest* 76:132, 1985.
229. Toussaint C, Vereerstraeten P: Effects of blood pH changes on potassium excretion in the dog. *Am J Physiol* 202:768, 1962.
230. Urbach JR et al: Effect of water diuresis on renal excretion of certain urinary solutes in normal man. *J Appl Physiol* 6:243, 1953.
231. Ussing HH: The alkali metal ions in isolated systems and tissues, in *Handbuch der Experimentellen Pharmacologie*. Heidelberg, Springer-Verlag, 1960, p 1.
232. Van Den Berg EK et al: Cisplatin-induced changes in sodium, chloride and urea transport by the frog skin. *Kidney Int* 19:8, 1981.
233. van Ypersele de Strihou C: Potassium homeostasis in renal failure. *Kidney Int* 11:491, 1977.
234. Vander AJ et al: Stop-flow analysis of aldosterone and

steroidal antagonist, SC8109, on renal tubular transport kinetics. *Proc Soc Exp Biol Med* 103:525, 1960.
235. Velazquez H: Thiazide diuretics. *Renal Physiol* 10:184, 1987.
236. Velazquez H, Wright FS: Renal distal tubule pathways for sodium, chloride and potassium transport assessed by diuretics, abstracted. *Kidney Int* 23:269, 1983.
237. Velazquez H et al: Luminal influences on potassium secretion: Chloride replacement with sulfate. *Am J Physiol* 242:F46, 1982.
238. Velazquez H et al: Chloride-dependent potassium secretion in early and late renal distal tubules. *Am J Physiol* 253:F555, 1987.
239. Verlander JW et al: Effect of acute respiratory acidosis on two populations of intercalated cells in rat cortical collecting duct. *Am J Physiol* 253:F1142, 1987.
240. Wade JB et al: Modulation of cell membrane area in renal collecting tubules by corticosteroid hormones. *J Cell Biol* 81:439, 1979.
241. Wasserstein AG, Agus ZS: Potassium secretion in the rabbit proximal straight tubule. *Am J Physiol* 245:F167, 1983.
241a. Weinstein AM: Modelling the proximal tubule: Complications of the paracellular pathway. *Am J Physiol* 254:F297, 1988.
242. Westphale H-J et al: Aldosterone stimulates cellular K^+ uptake and K release in the diluting segment of the frog kidney. *J Cell Physiol Biochem*, 1:89, 1991.
243. Whittembury G, Grantham JJ: Cellular aspects of renal sodium transport and cell volume regulation. *Kidney Int* 9:103, 1976.
244. Wiederholt M et al: Effect of aldosterone on sodium and potassium transport in the kidney. *J Steroid Biochem* 3:151, 1972.
245. Wiederholt M et al: Mechanism of action of aldosterone on potassium transfer in the rat kidney. *Pfluegers Arch* 345:159, 1973.
246. Wiederholt M et al: Intracellular potassium in the distal tubule of the adrenalectomized and aldosterone-treated rat. *Pfluegers Arch* 347:117, 1974.
247. Wingo CS: Potassium transport by the medullary collecting tubule of the rabbit: Effects of variation in K intake. *Am J Physiol* 253:F1136, 1987.
248. Wingo CS: Potassium secretion by the cortical collecting tubule: Effect of Cl gradients and ouabain. *Am J Physiol* 256:F306, 1989.
249. Wang W et al: Regulation of the small conductance channel in the apical membrane of rat cortical collecting tubule. *Am J Physiol* 259:F494, 1990.
250. Woodbury DM: Physiology of body fluids, in Ruch TC et al (eds): *Physiology and Biophysics*. Philadelphia, Saunders, 1974, vol 2, p 450.
251. Woodhall PB, Tisher CC: Response of the distal tubule and cortical collecting duct to vasopressin in the rat. *J Clin Invest* 52:3095, 1973.
252. Work J et al: Transport of potassium in the rabbit pars recta. *Am J Physiol* 242:F226, 1982.
253. Wright FS: Increasing magnitude of electrical potential along the renal distal tubule. *Am J Physiol* 220:624, 1971.
254. Wright FS: Potassium transport by the renal tubule, in Thurau K (ed): *Kidney and Urinary Tract Physiology*, MTP International Review of Science, Physiology Series 1. Baltimore, University Park Press, 1974, vol 6, p 79.
255. Wright FS: Sites and mechanisms of potassium transport along the renal tubule. *Kidney Int* 11:415, 1977.
256. Wright FS: Potassium transport by successive segments of the mammalian nephron. *Fed Proc* 40:2398, 1981.
257. Wright FS: Flow-dependent transport processes: Filtration, absorption, secretion. *Am J Physiol* 243:F1, 1982.
258. Wright FS, Giebisch GH: Renal potassium transport: Contributions of individual nephron segments and populations. *Am J Physiol* 235:F515, 1978.
259. Wright FS, Schnermann J: Interference with feedback control of glomerular filtration rate by furosemide, triflocin, and cyanide. *J Clin Invest* 53:1695, 1974.
260. Wright FS et al: Potassium secretion by distal tubule after potassium adaptation. *Am J Physiol* 221:437, 1971.
261. Young DB: Relationship between plasma potassium concentration and renal potassium excretion. *Am J Physiol* 242:F599, 1982.
262. Young DB, Jackson TE: Effects of aldosterone on potassium distribution. *Am J Physiol* 243:R526, 1982.
263. Young DB, Paulsen AW: Interrelated effects of aldosterone and plasma potassium on potassium excretion. *Am J Physiol* 244:F28, 1983.

CHAPTER • 8

Control of ventilation: central chemical drive

Homayoun Kazemi • Bernard Hitzig

PHYSIOLOGICAL SIGNIFICANCE OF AND BASIC CONCEPTS RELATED TO RESPIRATORY CONTROL

Respiratory control mechanisms regulate ventilation, matching the metabolic needs of the organism with the gas content of its respiratory environment. This system must function efficiently over a diverse range of activities and external conditions, necessitating highly accurate sensors or receptors and rapidly responding controller and effector mechanisms. Additionally, alterations in ventilation must simultaneously be integrated with appropriate changes in cardiac output so as to ensure normalcy of the gaseous environment of the tissues. The integration of these responses serves to provide the oxygen necessary for cellular metabolic processes and to regulate total body acid-base homeostasis. In order to accomplish this remarkable task, a wide diversity of receptors monitoring the gas content of the lungs and the chemical environment of several body fluids must feed information to an integrative center (controller) that stimulates the effector system to produce the proper changes in ventilation.

The respiratory receptors must initiate rapid responses to transient changes in both the internal and external environments of the organism, and maintain ventilatory adaptations to such sustained perturbations as living at high altitudes, various illnesses, sleep, and exercise. Receptors vary as to structure and function and include mechanical and irritant receptors in the lung, chemoreceptors in the carotid body and aortic arch, and brain stem (*central*) chemoreceptors. The receptor neurons function via feedback mechanisms that relay to the brain respiratory centers error signals caused by changes in their metabolism or in their immediate external chemical environment. The centers in the brain respond by producing appropriate alterations in ventilation. There is great variation in receptor type, in the kinds of stimuli perceived, and in the ventilatory responses elicited. The system contains considerable redundancy, which creates a large ventilatory reserve. The great diversity in the types of receptors and the stimuli affecting them as well as the multiplicity of interrelated ventilatory responses and voluntary control optimize the plasticity of the organism. This chapter will focus upon chemical control of ventilation and the interaction between acid-base homeostasis of body fluids and chemoreception. Before embarking on these considerations, however, it is important to realize that by concentrating on the chemical control of ventilation we are emphasizing only one aspect of respiratory control. The level of ventilation, that is, the volume of air moved in and out of the lungs per unit time, is ultimately decided by several factors, only one of which is the chemical drive of ventilation. For the respiratory apparatus to function properly one needs: (1) the respiratory centers within the brain, including the integrative loci, and intact and responsive inspiratory and expiratory neurons in the midbrain; (2) transmission of impulses from the brain to the respiratory muscles (diaphragm and intercostals); (3) properly functioning respiratory muscles; and (4) a lung and thoracic cage mechanically capable of responding to the action of respiratory muscles. Abnormalities in respiratory control can become clinically apparent if there is dysfunction anywhere along the complex pathway. Since this book deals with electrolyte and fluid imbalance, the subsequent discussion will be confined to chemoreception and chemical drive to ventilation.

Aerobic metabolism involves the utilization of O_2 and the release of CO_2. Anaerobic productions of ATP by glycolysis produces lactic acid, which is released into the blood. Other metabolically produced fixed acids appear in extracellular fluids during certain disease states, such as diabetes mellitus. Excess volatile (CO_2) and fixed acids stimulate both peripheral and central chemoreceptors to produce increases in ventilation. Hypoxemia also causes the carotid and aortic arch chemoreceptors to increase ventilation.

PERIPHERAL ARTERIAL CHEMORECEPTORS

The carotid and aortic bodies contain the peripheral arterial chemoreceptors. The carotid body receptors are located at the bifurcation of the common carotid arteries; the aortic body chemoreceptors are found between the arch of the aorta and the pulmonary artery and on the dorsal surface of the pulmonary artery. Although both chemoreceptors are associated with baroreceptors, they remain anatomically separate entities. Afferent fibers from the aortic receptors ascend to the medulla via the vagus nerve, while those of the carotid body reach the brain by passing through Hering's nerves to the glossopharyngeal nerves. Blood flow through the carotid body is very high relative to the oxygen extraction and utilization by carotid body cells. The oxygen and CO_2 tensions in the immediate environment of the chemosensitive cells, therefore, remain close to that of arterial blood. Presumably, this facilitates accurate monitoring of arterial acid-base status and oxygen tension by the receptor cells.

The carotid receptors have been much more thoroughly studied than the aortic bodies, because of accessibility, and are thought to be the more important in humans. Carotid chemoreceptor stimulation produces approximately a sevenfold greater increase in ventilation than similar stimulation of the aortic bodies.[10] Decreases in arterial P_{O_2} and/or increases in arterial P_{CO_2} produce an increase in the firing rate of both chemoreceptors. Increased arterial hydrogen ion concentration also increases chemoreceptor discharges and therefore increases ventilation. This has been established by experiments in which inactivation of the nerves connecting these receptors to the medulla eliminated the ventilatory increases.[10] Additionally, perfusion of isolated peripheral chemoreceptors has shown that they respond to chemical changes in the arterial blood they monitor.

Five histologically distinguishable cell types are found in the carotid body. The carotid afferent nerve cells and/or the glomus cells (type I cells) are thought to possess the chemoreceptor function. Microelectrode recordings of the responses of single chemoreceptor afferent nerve fibers demonstrate increased activity with decreased arterial P_{O_2}, increased arterial P_{CO_2}, or increased arterial hydrogen ion concentration, indicating that the same chemoreceptor cell may be responding to all three stimuli; however, more recent experiments indicate that the mechanism of action of hypoxemia and hypercapnia may be different.[18] Currently, it is thought that the firing rate of afferent fibers is particularly sensitive to changes in Pa_{O_2} when these values are between 30 and 60 torr. Several investigators have demonstrated a synergistic action of decreased arterial P_{O_2} and increased arterial P_{CO_2} on carotid chemoreceptor discharge.[24,59] For example, a greater increase in ventilation can be elicited for a given decrease in arterial P_{O_2} at normal arterial P_{CO_2} than during hypocapnia. The converse is also true; increases in ventilation mediated by carotid chemoreceptors during hypercapnia are much greater at normal (or slightly below normal) arterial P_{O_2} than during hyperoxia. The combination of hypercapnia and hypoxia produces a much greater increase in ventilation than the total ventilatory change calculated by adding the responses seen when each stimulus is applied alone.

The relationship between stimulus and receptor is not very well understood. The mechanisms involved in the interaction of chemical stimuli with the chemoreceptive cells, which result in increased ventilation, remain undefined. The possibility exists that the known chemical stimuli exert an indirect effect on receptor function through an intermediary mechanism that has yet to be elucidated. New ideas have recently been advanced concerning the nature of stimulus-receptor interaction and its relationship to the maintenance of total body acid-base homeostasis. Current data suggest that impulses transmitted through the cranial nerves from the peripheral chemoreceptors cause release of the excitatory amino acid glutamate, probably at the nucleus tractus solitarius, which in turn increases ventilation. Data in support of this concept are persuasive for hypoxia and just beginning to appear for metabolic acidosis.[33,34]

The role of the peripheral chemoreceptors in the normal regulation of ventilation is a question of considerable interest. Initially, it was believed that peripheral chemoreceptors were not involved in regulating respiration during steady-state breathing. More recent studies, however, estimate that denervation of these receptors, in an unanesthetized preparation, results in a 12 to 20 percent reduction in resting ventilation coupled with a 5- to 10-torr increase in arterial P_{CO_2}.[4,55,64] Several studies that dealt with central chemical control of ventilation have provided indirect evidence concerning the hierarchy of receptor control of ventilation during central nervous system (CNS) acid-base stress.[11,28,71] Perfusion of the brain extracellular fluid (ECF) spaces of unanesthetized animals with a markedly acidic mock cerebrospinal fluid (CSF) consistently drove ventilation at a greatly elevated rate despite marked alkalosis in the arterial blood. These results indicate that the central chemosensors exert the dominant influence over chemical control of ventilation during acid-base stress.

Under physiological conditions, arterial acidosis coincides with CNS acidosis. In many instances, however, the normal acid-base status of arterial blood is restored by ventilatory change before that of the CNS. This is particularly true for acid-base stress induced by increases in fixed acid (e.g., lactic acidosis), since fixed acid is cleared relatively slowly from the CNS. Under these conditions, ventilation remains increased, and a systemic respiratory alkalosis coexists with a slowly improving metabolic acidosis in the CNS. Javaheri and coworkers,[39] using the technique of peripheral chemoreceptor denervation, have shown that ventilatory increases seen during acute metabolic acidosis are not dependent upon peripheral chemoreceptors.

CHEMICAL STIMULI AFFECTING THE CONTROL OF VENTILATION

One of the basic physiological questions concerning the control of ventilation is the nature of the chemical stimuli producing alterations in respiration. The difficulty in resolving this involves integrating total body responses with cellular processes occurring within the receptors. The most widely used research techniques extrapolate chemical changes in various fluid compartments of the body to alterations in receptor function by measuring ventilatory change. Clearly, ascribing effector function directly to alterations in receptor mediation ignores the role of the integrative system and other modulating effects on the receptors themselves. Additionally, several receptors may respond to the same chemical stimulus, making correlation of the overall ventilatory response with the function of any specific receptor difficult. These are specific problems involved in understanding chemical control of ventilation. Since many of the current concepts concerning the nature of the stimuli affecting respiratory chemosensors have developed from central chemoreceptor research,[12] we will concentrate on this system.

In 1954, Leusen published his classic studies noting that changes in the acid-base status of mock CSF perfusing the brain ventriculocisternal system of anesthetized dogs resulted in predictable alterations in ventilation.[56,57] Similar ventilatory increases were produced by increases in fixed or volatile acid in the perfusate. These studies established that there were areas of chemosensitivity within the CNS that were sensitive to the acid-base status of brain ECF. Additionally, they provided a factual basis for the concept that the chemosensitive areas were being stimulated by increases in the hydrogen ion concentration of the perfusate. Previously, it had been thought that molecular CO_2 had a direct effect on ventilation that was independent of increases in proton concentration. The evidence for this idea came from the fact that ventilatory changes produced by a given decrease in arterial pH are much greater with increases in P_{CO_2} than those seen with increases in arterial fixed acid. However, it has subsequently been shown that arterial fixed acid does not as readily cross the blood-brain barrier as does CO_2 and therefore is not as effective a stimulant to the central chemoreceptors. Many lines of evidence have since shown that the CO_2 ventilatory drive is mediated by changes in acidity at the receptor sites.

Pappenheimer and associates[71] subsequently demonstrated that increases in alveolar ventilation produced by ventriculocisternal perfusion in unanesthetized goats were much greater than those seen in anesthetized animals for a given change in CNS $[H^+]$ and did not correlate well with acid-base changes in large-cavity CSF. The increases could be described as a single function of the acid concentration of brain interstital fluid (ISF) measured three-quarters of the distance along the bicarbonate concentration gradient between the large-cavity CSF and brain capillary blood. This hypothesis makes the assumption that the ionic composition of brain ISF can be predicted from that of the mock CSF perfusate. Implicit in this view is the concept that the ependyma present no barrier to simple diffusion between CSF and brain ISF. Fencl and colleagues[14] demonstrated that this is true during steady-state conditions and certain chronic metabolic acid-base disturbances.[16] However, recent work has shown that there is a dichotomy in the acid-base status, and possibly the ionic composition, of brain ISF and CSF, and that ventilation may be tracking brain ISF.[12,51]

The proton concentration of ISF in a particular area of the brain is a function of metabolic production of CO_2 and fixed acid, localized brain blood flow, temperature, and the ionic composition of the local ISF. This can be modified by alterations in ventilation, physiochemical buffering, and/or acidic processes (i.e., ion pumping). Studies utilizing pH or P_{CO_2} brain surface microelectrodes have shown that transient localized pH changes do not correlate well with changes in large-cavity CSF.[12] Ventilatory changes observed during acute CO_2 inhalation temporally match alterations in the acidity of localized ECF in the area of the fourth cerebral ventricle.[54] Fencl and coworkers[17] were able to show disparities between estimates of brain ISF hydrogen ion concentration and bicarbonate concentration and those of large-cavity CSF in goats acclimatized to high altitude for 5 days. The brain ISF acidosis was caused by increased production of lactic acid by brain cells, presumably due to increased glycolysis brought about by chronic hypoxia. These data show that certain chronic acid-base disturbances are capable of producing an acid-base disequilibrium between brain ISF and CSF, and lend credence to the concept that acid concentration within ISF is the stimulus affecting central chemoreceptors. Since brain ISF is physically closer than CSF to the blood-brain interface, it is possible that plasma acid-base disturbances (particularly those involving CO_2) may have much more of an effect on central chemical control of ventilation than previously supposed.[39]

Even though the exact location of the central chemosensitive areas is in dispute, much of the evidence for an acid-concentration stimulus comes from studies aimed at locating the central sites of chemoreception. Applications of fixed acid to the ventrolateral surface of the medulla in the region of the seventh through twelfth cranial nerves resulted in large increases in ventilation that could be blocked with localized application of procaine.[60] These studies led to the hypothesis that the receptors responsible for central chemical control of ventilation are separate from the medullary respiratory control centers. Localized application of fixed acid, coupled with the results of the ventricular perfusion studies, lent credence to the hypothesis that the proton concentration is the regulating variable concerned with chemical control of ventilation. Subsequent investigations have provided evidence that the location of the chemosensitive areas is not on the medullary surface in contact with cisternal CSF, but is concentrated in two distinct regions several hundred microns deep in the tissue overlying the lateral medullary surface, in close proximity to brain ISF.[3,61,62,72] Clearly, separate chemoreceptors must involve neurotransmission, and recent in vitro and in vivo work has suggested the involvement of acetylcholine in chemoreception in the central ventilatory response to H^+.[6,20,22]

Other studies challenge the concept of the existence of chemoreceptors as separate entities independent of the respiratory control center.[8,9,52,58] These investigators contend that a rich vascular network on the surface of the medulla conducts H^+ to the medullary respiratory control centers, which respond with appropriate alterations in ventilation. Anatomical evidence supporting the existence of such a vascular network has recently been obtained.[13,52] Adherents of both models, however, accept the concept that increases in ventilation are tied to localized increases in acidity despite the lack of a defined mechanism for acid mediation of receptor or neuronal excitation.

ACID-BASE REGULATION OF THE CHEMORECEPTOR ENVIRONMENT

To our knowledge, all of the pertinent research on receptive structures involved in control of ventilation has, at least in part, involved the acid-base status of their immediate fluid environment. Appropriate ventilatory adjustments are dependent upon, among other things, acid-base parameters of plasma and brain ECF.[69]

Plasma has a relatively high concentration of protein, which is essentially absent from tissue ISF. The concentrations of several ions in brain ISF and CSF differ from those in plasma and peripheral tissue ISF (an ultrafiltrate of plasma). Potassium, calcium, and bicarbonate ion concentrations are significantly lower in brain ECF, and the concentrations of magnesium and chloride ions are higher. These ionic concentration differences have led to the concept that active processes are involved in the formation of brain ECF.

REGULATION OF CSF ACID-BASE STATUS

The regulation of CSF acidity during acid-base stress has been a major area of active research. It is generally recognized that CSF acidity changes less than that of blood during acute metabolic acid-base derangements, while it more closely resembles that of arterial blood during respiratory acid-base disturbances. Regulation of the CSF bicarbonate concentration during acid-base disturbances has also been extensively investigated. A large body of research (which has produced equivocal results) has been devoted to determining whether the regulation of brain ISF $[HCO_3^-]$ and/or $[H^+]$ is active or passive.

Another major focus of many investigators has involved the relationship between plasma $[HCO_3^-]$, $[H^+]$, and P_{CO_2} on one hand and CSF acid-base regulation on the other. Usually these experiments are accomplished by experimentally varying two of the plasma variables while holding the third constant. Measurements of the same variables in large-cavity CSF are then made after a predetermined period of time. Increases in arterial P_{CO_2} under these experimental conditions result in rapid and stable increases in CSF $[HCO_3^-]$ and concomitant decreases in CSF $[H^+]$.[67,73] In experiments in which the arterial P_{CO_2} is increased without holding plasma $[HCO_3^-]$ constant, there is a larger and more rapid increase in CSF $[HCO_3^-]$ than in plasma.[47,65] A stepwise increase in plasma $[HCO_3^-]$ under isocapnic conditions results in a slow but significant rise in CSF $[HCO_3^-]$; a decrease in plasma $[HCO_3^-]$ produces a slow decrease in CSF $[HCO_3^-]$. This decrease in CSF $[HCO_3^-]$ is significantly less, however, than the experimental decrease produced in arterial blood. These results have been interpreted as demonstrating that the acid-base status of the brain's ECF compartment is more closely regulated than that of arterial blood.

The underlying mechanisms involved in regulating CSF acid-base homeostasis are very complicated, and their elucidation has only recently been approached. Much of the difficulty can be ascribed to confusion concerning the dependent and independent variables affecting the acid-base status of dilute salt solutions. An independent variable is defined as one that can be changed only from outside of the system. Dependent variables cannot be changed directly from outside of the system; they can be altered only when one (or more) of the independent variables determining the dependent variables' behavior changes. Recently, investigators have begun to appreciate the effects of the completely dissociated ions on traditional acid-base variables. The strong ions in brain ISF are Na^+, K^+, Mg^{2+}, Ca^{2+}, Cl^-, and lactate. The *strong ion difference* (SID) has been defined by Stewart[79] as the sum of the completely dissociated cations of a solution minus the sum of the completely dissociated anions, all expressed in meq/liter. This concept reflects the electroneutrality constraints present in any dilute salt solution.

According to this model, changes in $[H^+]$, $[OH^-]$, and $[HCO_3^-]$ must be effected by changes in one of the independent variables of the solution. The independent variables in ISF that determine the concentration of the products of weakly dissociating electrolytes (i.e., $[H^+]$, $[OH^-]$, and $[HCO_3^-]$) are the ISF SID and P_{CO_2}. Plasma contains a significant concentration of protein, a weak-acid buffer, which is an additional independent variable affecting plasma acid-base behavior. Bradbury[5] has advanced a similar interpretation, calling the SID "buffer base." Implicit in this view of the system is the requirement that there can be no net change in the activity of a dependent variable without a concomitant change in one or more of the independent variables within the compartment in question. This means that there would have to have been an increase in the CSF SID in order for $[HCO_3^-]$ in the CSF to increase. A good approximation for ISF, in general, is that the SID is equal to the $[HCO_3^-]$, since P_{CO_2} in ISF has very little effect on $[HCO_3^-]$ at CO_2 pressures above 4 torr. ISF $[HCO_3^-]$ is therefore a good measure of changes in ISF SID. This is not, however, true for plasma, due to the presence of weak-acid buffer in the form of plasma proteins.

This approach has important implications for understanding the regulation of brain ISF $[H^+]$. Infusions of fixed acid, such as HCl, into plasma (while arterial P_{CO_2} is held constant) are known to produce very small changes in CSF $[H^+]$. Traditionally, this has been taken to mean that the blood-brain barrier is not very permeable to H^+; however, application of the SID model reveals that the impermeability of the blood-brain barrier is to excess plasma strong anions, in this case, Cl^-. This interpretation fits the evidence, since it is well known that brain ISF ion concentrations involved in the determination of SID (Na^+, K^+, Ca^{2+}, Mg^{2+}, Cl^-, and lactate) are well regulated and are maintained at significantly different concentrations from their concentrations in plasma. A similar analysis can be applied to experiments in which there are no plasma infusions of fixed base. This does not mean that a dependent variable, in a particular compartment, cannot be the regulating variable of an unrelated process, for example, brain ISF $[H^+]$ as a stimulus for ventilation.

Recent work has emphasized the importance of measuring strong ions in CSF during acid-base stress. In turtles, a variety of acid-base stresses, such as anoxia, hypercapnia, and anoxia plus hypercapnia, produced large changes in CSF strong ions that coud be directly equated with equimolar increases in CSF $[HCO_3^-]$.[29] The major change involved a large increase in CSF sodium ion concentration ~15 meq/liter, relative to an increase in plasma $[Na^+]$ of only a few milliequivalents per liter. In rats exposed to hypercapnia the initial change in the CSF SID was a result of an increase in CSF sodium ion concentration, usually in the first 30 min after the increase in P_{CO_2}. After 3 h of exposure, however, $[Na^+]$ in CSF had returned to normal, and the increase in $[HCO_3^-]$ was a result of decreases in chloride ion concentration.[68] Kazemi and Choma[50] have demonstrated that during hypercapnia brain ECF $[H^+]$ is dependent upon $Na^+ - K^+$ ATPase-mediated Na^+ movement from the blood into the ECF by the choroid plexus and glia. Javaheri and Kazemi[41] have shown that 4 h of acid-base stress (respiratory and/or metabolic acidosis) in dogs resulted in reciprocal equimolar changes in concentrations of chloride and bicarbonate in cisternal CSF. They concluded that, for CSF, $[HCO_3^-]$ in acid-base disorders is determined by the difference between $[Na^+]$ and $[Cl^-]$. Other evidence supports the concept that in acid-base disturbances Cl^- is the key regulated ion in the central nervous system. Blocking chloride regulation by intrathecal injection of chloride-transport inhibitors such as DIDS (4,4′-diisothiocyano-2,2′-disulfonate stilbene) and pyridoxal-5′-phosphate prevents Cl^- entry into the CSF. For any given increase in P_{CO_2}, there is a greater increase in bicarbonate concentration in CSF.[21]

In an effort to integrate acid-base homeostasis and receptor function with basic cellular function, Rahn[74] and Reeves[75–77] have advanced the hypothesis that animals and humans are not regulating arterial and intracellular pH per se, but are regulating the constancy of the fractional dissociation of the imidazole moiety of histidine (α-imidazole) contained in proteins throughout the body. α-Imidazole is defined as the ratio of unprotonated imidazole to total imidazole:

$$\alpha\text{-imidazole} = \frac{\text{Im}}{\text{HIm}^+ + \text{Im}} \qquad (1)$$

α-Imidazole regulation would have the effect of maintaining cellular protein charge states and enzymatic functions constant. In addition, the regulation of protein charge states would keep Donnan ratios constant and therefore maintain constancy in the ionic composition of various body fluids. Much of the evidence for this concept has been developed in extensive studies of air-breathing, ecotothermic (body temperature varies with ambient temperature) vertebrates. It is well known that, in many of these animals, arterial hydrogen ion concentration and P_{CO_2} increase with increasing body temperature, while CO_2 stores remain constant. At any given body temperature, however, arterial pH and P_{CO_2} are well protected. Jackson and coworkers[36–38] demonstrated that CO_2 production and O_2 consumption in turtles increase dramatically with increasing body temperature, while arterial [HCO_3^-] and ventilation remain relatively constant. Jackson explained that increases in CO_2 production that are not matched by increased ventilation are responsible for the temperature-produced elevations in arterial P_{CO_2} and, therefore, arterial acidity.

Reeves and his coworkers[75–77] provided evidence that the imidazole ring structure, because of its ubiquity and relatively high concentration (~40 m*M*), pK in the physiological range (7.00), and enthalpy of ionization of (7 kcal/mol), is responsible for the pH-temperature relationship seen in the blood and tissue of many animals. They also demonstrated the constancy of α-imidazole with alterations in body temperature in dilute salt solutions, arterial blood plasma, red blood cells, and in the cells of various tissues of several animals. Clearly, for the hypothesis of Rahn and Reeves to be correct, chemical control of ventilation would have to follow the α-imidazole model. Reeves hypothesized[75] that the protein charge state of receptor membranes controlling ventilation depended on α-imidazole regulation. Changes in the acid-base status of the immediate environment of the receptors would alter the protein charge state of the membranes and, therefore, alter ion channels and fluxes. As a result, firing rates and ventilation would change. This hypothesis permits the prediction that even when body temperature varies, α-imidazole, unlike pH and P_{CO_2}, should remain constant. Under these conditions ventilation should be independent of metabolism.

This concept has been applied to central chemical control of ventilation in turtles, where pH and P_{CO_2} in CSF vary significantly over a wide excursion of body temperature while ventilation remains constant.[30] At a given body temperature, however, small changes in CSF pH resulted in large increases in ventilation. CNS α-imidazole for turtles at three different body temperatures and for goats at 39°C[71] is the same (~0.80). In addition, alterations in relative ventilation, for turtles at different body temperatures and for goats at 39°C plot as a single function of the changes in CNS α-imidazole (Fig. 8-1). These results strongly imply that regulation of ventilation utilizes the same mechanisms in air-breathing ectothermic vertebrates and mammals, and that the ectothermic model was incorporated into the mammalian scheme of acid-base regulation. Application of an imidazole blocker to the chemosensitive area of the medulla in cats blocked increases in ventilation caused by local application of acid[70] and provides further evidence for this hypothesis.

These results also suggest that the basic mechanism involved in the regulation of ventilation and, therefore, acid-base homeostasis is essentially a passive physicochemical one. Much of the previous work has concentrated on active regulation, involving negative feedback loops, using control system theory as a model. This type of regulation would, of necessity, require greater expenditure of energy on the part of the organism than passive

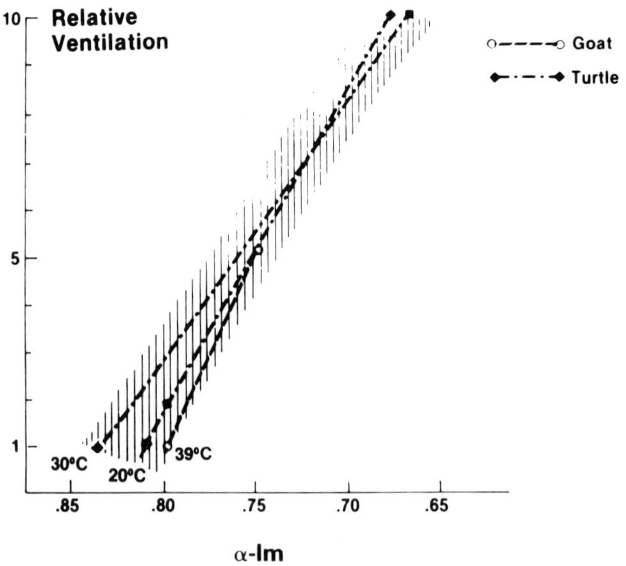

FIGURE 8-1 • The relationship between changes in relative ventilation and the fractional dissociation of α-imidazole (α-Im) is illustrated for the turtle and goat at different body temperatures.

physicochemical processes. α-Imidazole regulation is, therefore, thermodynamically more conservative, requiring minimal energy expenditure and then only during severe acid-base stress. In addition, the α-imidazole hypothesis unifies cellular processes, receptor function, acid-base homeostasis, and the control of ventilation into one coherent theory that applies to all vertebrates, including humans.

So far in this discussion, we have reviewed the mechanisms and concepts of central regulation of ventilation, particularly in relation to electrolyte and acid-base homeostasis. Central ventilatory drive, by altering alveolar ventilation, changes the arterial P_{CO_2}. The relationship between alveolar ventilation ($\dot{V}_A$), P_{CO_2} and CO_2 output ($\dot{V}_{CO_2}$) is given by equation 2:

$$P_{CO_2} = \frac{\dot{V}_{CO_2}}{\dot{V}_A} \tag{2}$$

Thus, for any given CO_2 output, whether in the steady state or otherwise, arterial P_{CO_2} is inversely related to alveolar ventilation. In humans, at 37°C, P_{CO_2} is extremely well regulated, remaining within the narrow range of 38 to 42 mmHg. This implies that alveolar ventilation is exquisitely regulated. It is adjusted when CO_2 output changes, in order to maintain P_{CO_2} constant. In terms of central mechanisms of respiratory drive, this suggests that the environment of chemoreceptors must be sensitive to changes brought about by changes in P_{CO_2}. Thus, ventilation is either increased or decreased to keep P_{CO_2} constant. In addition to changes in central drive specifically ascribed to the hydrogen ion or α-imidazole hypotheses, other phenomena also operate within the

CNS in response to changes in P_{CO_2}. These events concern alterations in brain and CSF content of organic acids, ammonia, and aminoacids, some of which are either excitatory or inhibitory neurotransmitters.

These alterations and adaptations will be described for respiratory acid-base disorders. As an extension of this basic concept, respiratory compensation for metabolic acid-base disorders will be briefly reviewed.

The key to the entire scheme resides in the fact that the brain's ionic composition and hydrogen ion concentration must remain relatively constant for neurons to function properly. With this central theme, the issue of central chemical drive in respiratory acidosis and alkalosis can be addressed.

RESPIRATORY CONTROL IN SYSTEMIC ACID-BASE DISORDERS

RESPIRATORY ACID-BASE DISORDERS

The primary event in respiratory acid-base disorders is an alteration in arterial P_{CO_2}. Implicit in this is the fact that *elevation in* P_{CO_2} indicates *alveolar hypoventilation;* too little alveolar ventilation ($\dot{V}_A$) occurs in relation to CO_2 output ($\dot{V}_{CO_2}$). A *lowered* P_{CO_2} indicates *alveolar hyperventilation;* too much alveolar ventilation occurs in relation to CO_2 output. The earlier discussion in this section emphasized the fact that in central chemical control of ventilation the key factor is H^+ homeostasis and α-imidazole regulation ("alpha stat") in the CNS. This phenomenon accounts for the precise regulation of alveolar ventilation and its matching to CO_2 output. Thus, elevation or reduction of P_{CO_2} signifies failure of this stimulus-response feedback loop. The factors responsible for this failure are varied and, obviously, are different in respiratory acidosis as compared to respiratory alkalosis. However, once the P_{CO_2} remains elevated or reduced for any length of time, adaptive biochemical mechanisms within the CNS are activated that tend to restore the hydrogen ion concentration toward normal. How quickly these biochemical mechanisms become operative is not known, but they are probably active within minutes of a change in P_{CO_2} and reach full compensation within hours—varying from 1 to 6 h, depending on the magnitude of change in P_{CO_2}.

It can be shown that when P_{CO_2} in humans has been elevated or reduced for several days, the sensitivity of the respiratory centers to CO_2 is altered. In normal subjects the ventilatory response to CO_2 is quite brisk. The mean increase in ventilation is 2.5 liters for each 1-mmHg increase in P_{CO_2}; that is, the CO_2-ventilatory response curve has a slope of 2.5. In patients with chronic CO_2 retention, it has been known for over 40 years that the ventilatory response to CO_2 is diminished.[81] Conversely, subjects with sustained low P_{CO_2} (e.g., after adaptation to high altitude) have a heightened ventilatory response to CO_2.[78] The task at hand has been to define the central mechanisms responsible for this change in ventilatory response to CO_2 in chronic hyper- and hypocapnia. If the central drive is critically dependent on the acidity of the environment of the chemoreceptors, then the buffering capacity of the brain must increase with chronic hypercapnia and diminish with chronic hypocapnia. Various factors that go into regulating CNS ionic homeostasis have already been reviewed. Specific mechanisms in respiratory acidosis and alkalosis will not be discussed here. (See Chap. 30.)

Respiratory acidosis

The sustained elevation of P_{CO_2} is associated with increased bicarbonate concentration in the CSF and an equimolar reduction in CSF chloride concentration.[21,41] As brain cells increase their bicarbonate content the brain becomes a better buffer (brain CO_2 dissociation curve shifts to the left).[46] Studies show that brain intracellular $[H^+]$ is indeed restored toward normal.[2] These increases in central bicarbonate concentration and buffering capacity can explain the diminished ventilatory response to CO_2 seen in chronic CO_2 retainers. With the increased brain $[HCO_3^-]$, a given change in P_{CO_2} causes a lesser increase in $[H^+]$ and thus becomes a lesser stimulus to respiration. As outlined earlier, a number of mechanisms have been advanced to explain the increased CNS $[HCO_3^-]$ and brain buffering capacity. The major group of cells within the CNS responsible for acid-base regulation are the glial cells and cells of the choroid plexus, which can generate bicarbonate and allow for exit of protons formed in the CO_2 hydration reaction.

$$CO_2 + H_2O \rightleftharpoons H_2CO_3 \rightleftharpoons H^+ + HCO_3^- \qquad (3)$$

These cells contain carbonic anhydrase,[23,84] which catalyzes the reaction in equation 3. They also have an abundance of $Na^+ - K^+$ ATPase, which allows for exchange of H^+ for Na^+ from blood.[50] A number of experiments injecting acetazolamide, an inhibitor of carbonic anhydrase, into the cerebral ventricles have shown that the expected increase in CSF bicarbonate concentration does not occur in response to hypercapnia.[84] Hypercapnia also fails to alter CSF bicarbonate when an inhibitor of $Na^+ - K^+$ ATPase pump activity, ouabain, is injected into the cerebral ventricles.[50] Further studies have also demonstrated that bicarbonate enters the CNS from plasma during hypercapnia as a consequence of its increased plasma concentration. Thus the increase in CNS bicarbonate has two potential sources, one within the CNS, generated by carbonic anhydrase-containing glial and choroid plexus cells, and a second one from the blood. This has been termed the "dual contribution theory" of CNS bicarbonate regulation in hypercapnia.[25]

In addition to changes in [HCO_3^-] in the CNS in response to hypercapnia, there are changes in levels of amino acids and ammonia that have implications both for proton regulation and for neuronal discharge. There are alterations in brain organic buffers and ammonia in hypercapnia.[48,49,83] Brain and CSF ammonia concentrations are increased independently of changes in blood ammonia. The increase in brain ammonia helps in H^+ buffering and increases the CSF [HCO_3^-] by buffering the hydrogen ions produced in the CO_2 hydration reaction.

$$\begin{array}{c} CO_2 + H_2O \rightleftharpoons H_2CO_3 \rightleftharpoons H^+ + HCO_3^- \\ \downarrow \\ NH_3 + H^+ \rightarrow NH_4^+ \end{array} \qquad (4)$$

The source of CNS ammonia is unknown but probably derives from certain of the amino acids in the brain.[19] The absolute magnitude of buffering by the increased ammonia content, however, is relatively small.[84]

More important, the increase in ammonia in the brain is associated with reduction in α-ketoglutarate and glutamic acid content but an increase in glutamine. Thus, one can look at this reaction as the "detoxification" pathway for the increased ammonia:

$$\begin{array}{l} \alpha\text{-ketoglutarate} + NH_3 \rightleftharpoons \text{glutamic acid} \\ \quad + NH_3 \xrightleftharpoons[]{\text{GLUTAMINE SYNTHETASE}} \text{glutamine} \end{array} \qquad (5)$$

It is of interest that the enzyme glutamine synthetase, which is necessary for glutamine formation from glutamic acid, is found only in the glial cells,[63] the same cells so critical in H^+ and HCO_3^- regulation.

Increases in P_{CO_2} are also associated with changes in other amino acids.[83] They include reduced levels of aspartate in the brain and increases in brain γ-amino aminobutyric acid (GABA). These changes are related to CO_2 fixation in the brain. Their relationship to CO_2 and ammonia metabolism is depicted in Fig. 8-2.

The changes in amino acid content of the brain are important in several ways. First, the reductions in aspartate and glutamate reduce the overall hydrogen ion load in the brain and thus reduce the degree of "local acidosis" in response to hypercapnia. Probably more significant are the alterations in GABA and glutamate content in terms of neuronal discharge. Glutamate is an excitatory neurotransmitter; GABA is an inhibitory one. These two amino acids have opposing effects on the membrane potential difference of individual medullary respiratory neurons,[80] and when administered by ventriculocisternal perfusion (VCP) in the animal, glutamate increases ventilation and GABA depresses ventilation.[7,53] Other studies have also shown that increases in endogenous brain content of GABA and glutamate also cause the same changes in ventilation as their exogenous administration,[26,32] indicating their importance in the central control of ventilation. Thus, the fall in CNS glutamate and increase in GABA during hypercapnia has the effect of depressing neuronal excitation and can account not only for the diminished central respiratory drive, but also for some of the neurological manifestations of hypercapnia. Recent data show that infusion of GABA into the cisternal CSF is associated with significant depression of tidal volume and frequency in the cat; with higher concentrations total cessation of respiration, as well as hypotension

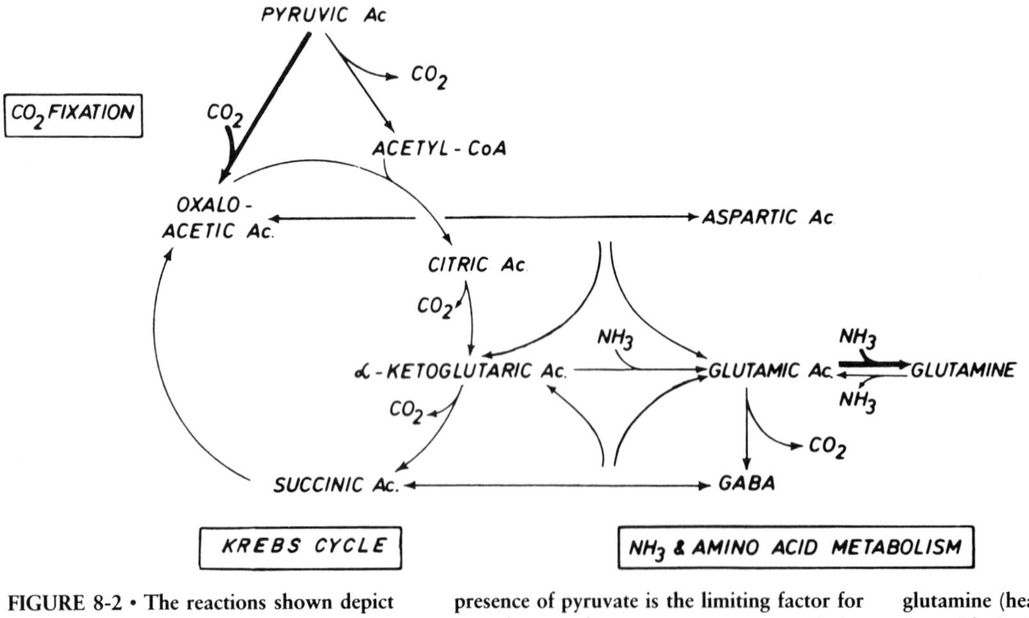

FIGURE 8-2 • The reactions shown depict the fixation of CO_2 within the CNS and its relationship to Krebs cycle intermediates and amino acid and ammonia metabolism. The presence of pyruvate is the limiting factor for CO_2 fixation (heavy arrow). Hypercapnia is associated with increased NH_3 availability and enhanced incorporation of the latter into glutamine (heavy arrow). See text for details. Ac, acid; CoA, coenzyme A; GABA, α-aminobutyric acid.

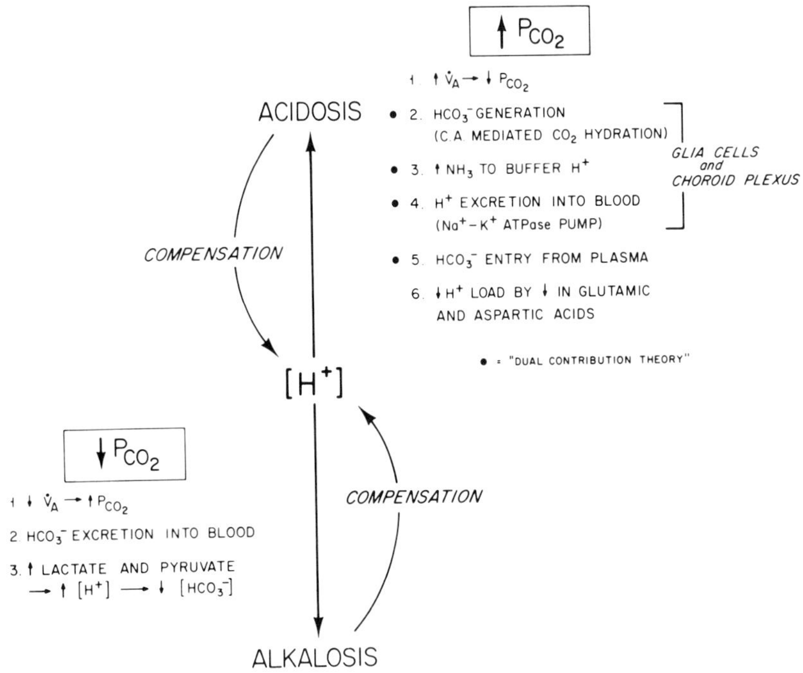

FIGURE 8-3 • Mechanisms of CNS proton homeostasis in respiratory acid-base disturbances. The primary aim is to return central [H^+] toward normal.

and bradycardia may occur.[85] These changes in neurotransmitters may be responsible for the observed depressed hypoxic ventilatory drive in patients with CO_2 retention.[27,66]

The relationship between central [H^+] regulation and amino acid metabolism is a complex one, and many of the steps need to be elucidated, but clearly H^+ regulation and amino acid metabolism in hypercapnia occur in parallel and in many instances are closely linked.[31]

Figure 8-3 summarizes the foregoing discussion on respiratory acidosis, making H^+ homeostasis the central theme in CNS respiratory drive. The primary aim is to keep [H^+] constant. The central drive's major regulator is the level of alveolar ventilation, which adjusts the P_{CO_2} and restores the milieu of the brain and respiratory chemoreceptors within it. If alveolar ventilation cannot be adequately adjusted, because, for example, of mechanical impairment of the chest, neuromuscular disease, primary disease of the respiratory tract, or CNS depressant drugs, then mechanisms within the CNS involving HCO_3^- formation and other ionic changes in the brain are activated to restore [H^+]. In this process there are also changes in ammonia and amino acids that help with H^+ regulation but also have direct effects of their own on respiratory neuronal transmission and central respiratory drive.

Respiratory alkalosis

The theme of central [H^+] regulation can also be invoked to explain the central chemical drive in respiratory alkalosis (see also Chap. 30). Numerous studies have shown that in chronic hypocapnia the CSF bicarbonate concentration is reduced, brain [HCO_3^-] diminishes, and the brain CO_2 dissociation curve is shifted to the right.[2,46] All of these observations confirm the fact that the central [H^+] has been returned toward normal. The actual stimulus to sustained increased ventilation in chronic hypocapnia, once [H^+] compensation has occurred, is not completely clear; the extensive literature on the subject has recently been reviewed by Dempsey and Forster.[12] The major conclusion of their review is that CSF acidity is not responsible for the increased respiratory drive, although some site within brain ISF sensitive to H^+ could be. In terms of mechanisms available to the CNS in reducing [HCO_3^-] in CSF, the best evidence suggests that HCO_3^- moves into blood as a function of reduction in P_{CO_2}.[40] This movement is almost independent of plasma [HCO_3^-]. What role Cl^- regulation plays in this adjustment in [HCO_3^-] of CSF is not known. In terms of the strong ion difference, however, [Cl^-] would have to increase when hypocapnia induces a reduction in CSF [HCO_3^-]. The other mechanism that augments the lowering of CNS bicarbonate content in hypocapnia is the increased accumulation of brain organic acids, specifically, lactic acid and to a lesser extent pyruvic acid.[47] Three mechanisms are involved in the increased availability of CNS lactate in this setting. They include (1) an increase in anaerobic glycolysis secondary to the reduction in brain blood flow caused by the reduced P_{CO_2} and local CNS alkalosis;[15] (2) a reduction in P_{CO_2} directly affecting the intermediates in the Krebs cycle by reducing conversion of fumarate to succinate and thus limiting the source of energy to brain cells;[40] and (3) (less important) an alkalosis-induced shift of the oxyhemoglobin dissociation curve to the left, which reduces tissue oxygen extraction for any given P_{O_2} and thus leads to brain hypoxia.

The role of neurotransmitters in sustaining the respiratory drive in chronic hypocapnia is not known but may be very significant, particularly in the ventilatory adaptation to high altitude.[12]

Figure 8-3 shows that, in hypocapnia, the first response of central chemical drive to lowered P_{CO_2} is to reduce alveolar ventilation, thus tending to increase P_{CO_2} and restore CNS [H^+] toward normal. If this cannot be accomplished, bicarbonate moves into blood; this transport is directly related to the prevailing level of P_{CO_2}. Brain acidity is further increased by the accumulation of lactic and pyruvic acids. The end result is the restoration of the CNS [H^+] to or toward normal.

METABOLIC ACID-BASE DISORDERS

In this presentation of respiratory control, it is relevant to indicate that there is hyperventilation in metabolic acidosis and hypoventilation in metabolic alkalosis.[35] (Chapter 25 reviews metabolic acid-base disturbances in greater detail.) The mechanisms by which compensatory changes in ventilation are elicited by metabolic acid-base disorders have been the subject of much controversy. There is ample evidence to support the thesis that peripheral chemoreceptors—carotid and aortic bodies—are sensitive to changes in blood pH and that metabolic acidosis causes increased peripheral chemoreceptor discharge and metabolic alkalosis diminishes chemoreceptor discharge. Data from animal experiments, however, indicate that the same degree of respiratory compensation occurs with and without peripheral chemoreceptors.[39,45] This implies that changes in [H^+] in the blood are appreciated by the central chemoreceptors and that the blood-brain barrier *is not* completely impermeable to H^+ from blood. Electrodes sensitive to brain surface pH and Cl^- show that cerebral-surface ECF pH, HCO_3^-, and Cl^- change in the same direction as they do in blood following an acute intraarterial injection of acid or alkali.[1] More recent work shows that there is direct and significant exchange of bicarbonate between blood and brain.[44]

Thus, in terms of respiratory compensation for metabolic acid-base disorders, one can state that peripheral chemoreceptors are responsible for some of the adaptation but are not entirely essential and that changes in blood pH are appreciated by the central receptors.

Normal subjects in steady-state metabolic acidosis and alkalosis demonstrated a predictable and consistent respiratory compensation for both acidosis and alkalosis,[42] and a linear relationship was shown between P_{CO_2} and plasma [HCO_3^-]. This linearity was the same in both acidosis and alkalosis. The slope of 0.7 (Fig. 8-4) is close to the slope of 0.75 reported in patients whose plasma bicarbonate was changed while undergoing hemodialysis.[82] This slope of 0.7 also holds for a whole host of subjects whose serum bicarbonate level was elevated up to 40 meq/liter or more.[43]

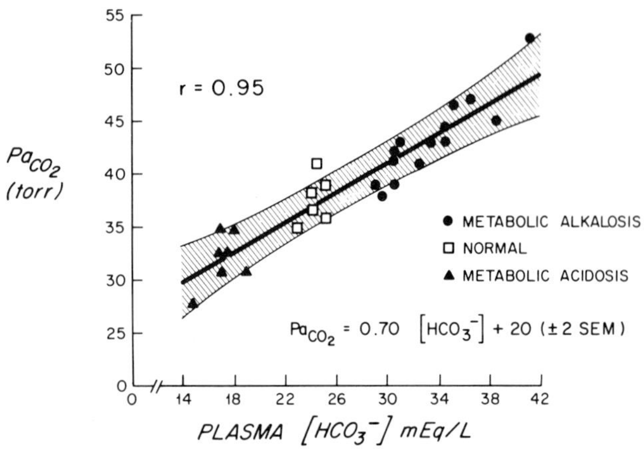

FIGURE 8-4 • Respiratory compensation in metabolic acid-base disorders. The changes in P_{CO_2} were measured in six healthy subjects during steady-state episodes of metabolic acidosis and alkalosis. Note the linear relationship between P_{CO_2} and bicarbonate concentration in both acidosis and alkalosis (slope of 0.7). The solid black line is the mean regression line; the shaded area represents 95 percent confidence limits. (From Javaheri S et al: *Chest* 81:296, 1982. Used by permission.)

The respiratory compensation in metabolic acidosis and alkalosis can be viewed from the standpoint of hydrogen ion homeostasis in the area of the chemoreceptors. In these terms the response minimizes the change in acidity in the immediate environment of the chemoreceptors. Reduced [H^+] occurring in metabolic alkalosis depresses ventilation by diminishing the integrated neural output of the receptors. Compensatory hypocapnia in metabolic acidosis and hypercapnia in metabolic alkalosis tend to restore [H^+] in the receptor areas toward normal. Whether the central or peripheral receptors are more important in this compensation is not entirely relevant, but the available animal data show that the respiratory compensation can occur without the peripheral chemoreceptors.

REFERENCES

1. Ahmad HR, Loeschke HH: Fast bicarbonate-chloride exchange between plasma and brain extracellular fluid at maintained PCO_2. *Pfluegers Arch* 295:300, 1982.
2. Arieff AI et al: Intracellular pH of brain: Alterations in acute respiratory acidosis and alkalosis. *Am J Physiol* 230:804, 1976.
3. Berndt J et al: Untersuchungen zum zentralen chemosensiblen Mechanismus der Atmung: 2. Die Steuerung der Atmung durch das extracellulare pH im Gewebe der Medulla oblongata. *Pfluegers Arch* 332:146, 1972.
4. Bouverot P et al: Etude du role des chemorecepteurs arteriels dans la regulation de la respiration pulmonaire chez le chien eveille. *Arch Int Pharmacodyn Ther* 157:253, 1965.

5. Bradbury M: *The Concept of a Blood-Brain Barrier*. New York, Wiley, 1979.
6. Burton MD et al: CSF acidosis augments ventilation through cholinergic mechanisms. *J Appl Physiol* 66:2562, 1989.
7. Chiang C-H et al: Central cardiorespiratory effects of glutamate in dogs. *J Appl Physiol* 60:2056, 1986.
8. Cozine RA, Nagai SH: Medullary surface chemoreceptors and regulation of respiration in the cat. *J Appl Physiol* 22:117, 1967.
9. Cragg P et al: The pH of brain extracellular fluid in the cat. *J Physiol* 272:137, 1977.
10. deBurgh Daly M, Ungar A: Comparison of the reflex responses elicited by stimulation of the separately perfused carotid and aortic body chemoreceptors in the dog. *J Physiol* 182:379, 1966.
11. Dempsey JA et al: The brain's role in exercise hyperpnea. *Med Sci Sports Exerc* 11:213, 1979.
12. Dempsey JA, Forester HV: Mediation of ventilatory adaptation. *Physiol Rev* 62:262, 1982.
13. Dermietzel R: Central chemosensitivity, morphological studies in acid-base homeostasis, in Loeschke HH (ed): *Acid-Base Homeostasis of the Brain Extracellular Fluid and Respiratory Control System*. Stuttgart, Thieme, 1976, p 52.
14. Fencl V et al: Studies on the respiratory response to disturbances of acid-base balance, with deductions concerning ionic composition of cerebral interstitial fluid. *Am J Physiol* 210:459, 1966.
15. Fencl V et al: Respiration and cerebral blood flow in metabolic acidosis and alkalosis in humans. *J Appl Physiol* 27:67, 1969.
16. Fencl V: Distribution of H^+ and HCO_3^- in cerebral fluids, in Siesjo BK, Sorensen SC (eds): *Homeostasis of the Brain*. Copenhagen, Munksgaard, 1971, p 175.
17. Fencl V et al: Composition of cerebral fluids in goats adapted to high altitude. *J Appl Physiol* 47:508, 1979.
18. Fitzgerald RS et al: Testing of ionic pumps in the carotid body, in Lahiri S et al (eds): *Chemoreceptors and Reflexes in Breathing: Cellular and Molecular Aspects*. New York, Oxford University Press, 1989, p 74–84.
19. Folbergrova J et al: Carbohydrate and amino acid metabolism in rat cerebral cortex in moderate and extreme hypercapnia. *J Neurochem* 25:457, 1975.
20. Folgering H et al: Stimulation of phrenic nerve activity by an acetylcholine releasing drug: 4-aminopyridine. *Pfluegers Arch* 379:181, 1979.
21. Frankel H, Kazemi H: Regulation of CSF composition-blocking chloride bicarbonate exchange. *J Appl Physiol* 55:177, 1983.
22. Fukuda Y, Loeschke HH: A cholinergic mechanism involved in the neuronal excitation by H^+ in the respiratory chemosensitive structures of the ventral medulla oblongata of rats *in vivo*. *Pfluegers Arch* 376:229, 1978.
23. Giacobini E: Cytochemical study of the localization of carbonic anhydrase in the nervous system. *J Neurochem* 9:169, 1962.
24. Greco EC Jr et al: Respiratory responses to intravenous and intrapulmonary CO_2 in awake dogs. *J Appl Physiol* 45:109, 1978.
25. Hasan FM, Kazemi H: Dual contribution theory of regulation of CSF HCO_3^- in respiratory acidosis. *J Appl Physiol* 40:559, 1976.
26. Hedner J et al: An analysis of the mechanism by which gamma-aminobutyric acid depresses ventilation in the rat. *J Appl Physiol* 56:849, 1984.
27. Herrera L, Kazemi H: Modification of phrenic nerve output to hypoxia after two hours of hypercapnia and increased cerebrospinal fluid [HCO_3^-]. *Am Rev Respir Dis* 126:70, 1982.
28. Hitzig BM, Jackson DC: Central chemical control of ventilation in the unanesthetized turtle. *Am J Physiol* 235:R257, 1978.
29. Hitzig BM, Nattie EE: Cerebrospinal fluid acid-base homeostasis during asphyxic diving, hypercapnia, and anoxia in turtles (abstract). *Physiologist* 22:56, 1979.
30. Hitzig BM: Temperature-induced changes in turtle CSF pH and central control of ventilation. *Respir Physiol* 49:205, 1982.
31. Hoop B et al: Relationship between CNS H^+ regulation and amino acid metabolism in hypercapnia. *Am Rev Respir Dis* 128:45, 1983.
32. Hoop B et al: Central respiratory effects of glutamine synthesis inhibition in dogs. *J Appl Physiol* 65:1099, 1988.
33. Hoop B et al: Brain glutamate metabolism during hypoxia and peripheral chemodenervation. *J Appl Physiol* 69:147, 1990.
34. Housley GD, Sinclair JD: Localization by kainic acid lesions of neurons transmitting the carotid chemoreceptor stimulus for respiration in rat. *J Physiol* (London), 406:99, 1988.
35. Irsigler GB et al: Relationship of CSF pH, O_2 and CO_2 responses in metabolic acidosis and alkalosis in humans. *J Appl Physiol* 48:355, 1980.
36. Jackson DC: The effect of temperature on ventilation in the turtle, *Pseudeymys scripta elegans*. *Respir Physiol* 12:131, 1971.
37. Jackson DC et al: The effects of temperature and carbon dioxide breathing on ventilation and acid-base status of turtles. *Respir Physiol* 20:131, 1974.
38. Jackson DC: Respiratory control and CO_2 conductance: Temperature effects in a turtle and a frog. *Respir Physiol* 33:103, 1978.
39. Javaheri S et al: Ventilatory drive in acute metabolic acidosis. *J Appl Physiol* 46:913, 1979.
40. Javaheri S et al: Role of PCO_2 as determinant of CSF [HCO_3^-] in metabolic acidosis. *Respir Physiol* 36:155, 1979.
41. Javaheri S, Kazemi H: Electrolyte composition of cerebrospinal fluid in acute acid-base disorders. *Respir Physiol* 45:141, 1981.
42. Javaheri S et al: Compensatory hypoventilation in metabolic alkalosis. *Chest* 81:296, 1982.
43. Javaheri S, Kazemi H: Metabolic alkalosis and hypoventilation in humans. *Am Rev Respir Dis* 136:1011, 1987.
44. Johnson DC et al: Movement of CO_2 and HCO_3^- from blood to brain in dogs. *J Appl Physiol* 54:989, 1983.
45. Kaehny WD, Jackson JT: Respiratory response to HCl acidosis in dogs after carotid body denervation. *J Appl Physiol* 46:1138, 1979.
46. Kazemi H et al: CO_2 buffering capacity of brain in respiratory acidosis and alkalosis. *J Appl Physiol* 22:241, 1967.
47. Kazemi H et al: Brain and cerebrospinal fluid lactate concentration in respiratory acidosis and alkalosis. *Respir Physiol* 6:178, 1969.

48. Kazemi H et al: Brain organic buffers in respiratory acidosis and alkalosis. *J Appl Physiol* 34:478, 1973.
49. Kazemi H et al: The CSF HCO_3^- increase in hypercapnia; relationship to HCO_3^- glutamate, glutamine and NH_3 in brain. *Respir Physiol* 28:387, 1976.
50. Kazemi H, Choma L: H^+ transport from CNS in hypercapnia and regulation of CSF [HCO_3^-]. *J Appl Physiol* 43:667, 1977.
51. Kazemi H, Johnson DC: Regulation of cerebrospinal fluid acid-base balance. *Physiol Rev* 66:953, 1986.
52. King GW: Brain stem blood vessels and the organization at the lateral reticular formation in the medulla oblongata of the cat. *Brain Res* 191:253, 1980.
53. Kneussl M et al: Reversible depression of ventilation and cardiovascular function by ventriculocisternal perfusion with gamma-aminobutyric acid in dogs. *Am Rev Respir Dis* 133:1024, 1986.
54. Lambertsen CJ: Carbon dioxide and respiration in acid-base homeostasis. *Anesthesiology* 21:642, 1960.
55. Lambertsen CJ: Chemical control of respiration at rest, in Mountcastle VB (ed): *Medical Physiology,* 14th ed. St. Louis, Mosby, 1980, p 1774.
56. Leusen IR: Chemosensitivity of the respiratory center: Influence of CO_2 in the cerebral ventricles on respiration. *Am J Physiol* 176:39, 1954.
57. Leusen IR: Chemosensitivity of the respiratory center: Influence of changes in the H^+ and total buffer concentrations in the cerebral ventricles on respiration. *Am J Physiol* 176:45, 1954.
58. Lipscomb WT, Boyarsky LL: Neurophysiological investigations of medullary chemosensitivity areas of respiration. *Respir Physiol* 16:362, 1972.
59. Loeschke HH, Gertz KH: Einfluss des O_2-Druckes in der Einatmungsluft auf die inter Konstanthaltung des alveolaren CO_2^- Druckes. *Pfluegers Arch* 267:460, 1958.
60. Loeschke HH: Central nervous chemoreceptors, in Widdicombe JE (ed): *MTP International Review of Science: Respiratory Physiology.* London, Butterworth, 1974, p 167.
61. Loeschke HH: Functional aspects of central chemosensitivity, in von Euler C. Lagercrantz H (eds): *Central Nervous Control Mechanisms in Breathing.* New York, Pergamon, 1979, p 13.
62. Loeschke HH et al: Does CO_2 act on the respiratory centers? *Pfluegers Arch* 381:249, 1979.
63. Martinez-Hernandez A et al: Glutamine synthetase: Glial localization in brain. *Science* 195:1356, 1977.
64. Mitchell RA et al: Respiratory response and CSF pH during disturbances in blood acid-base balance in awake dogs with denervated aortic and carotid bodies (abstract). *Physiologist* 7:208, 1964.
65. Monroe CB, Kazemi H: Effect of changes in plasma bicarbonate level on CSF bicarbonate in respiratory acidosis. *Respir Physiol* 17:386, 1973.
66. Mountain R et al: Hypoventilation in obstructive lung disease. *N Engl J Med* 298:521, 1978.
67. Nattie EE, Romer L: CSF HCO_3^- regulation in isosmotic conditions: The role of brain PCO_2 and plasma HCO_3^-. *Respir Physiol* 33:177, 1978.
68. Nattie EE: Brain and cerebrospinal fluid ionic composition and ventilation in acute hypercapnia. *Respir Physiol* 40:309, 1980.
69. Nattie EE: Ionic mechanisms of cerebrospinal fluid acid-base regulation. *J Appl Physiol* 54:3, 1983.
70. Nattie EE: Intracisternal diethylpyrocarbonate inhibits central chemosensitivity in conscious rabbits. *Respir Physiol* 64:161, 1986.
71. Pappenheimer JR et al: Role of cerebral fluids in control of respiration as studied in unanesthetized goats. *Am J Physiol* 208:436, 1965.
72. Pappenheimer JR: The ionic composition of cerebral extracellular fluid and its relation to the control of breathing. *Harvey Lect* 6:73, 1967.
73. Pavlin EG, Hornbein TF: Distribution of H^+ and HCO_3^- between CSF and blood during respiratory acidosis in dogs. *Am J Physiol* 228:1145, 1975.
74. Rahn H: Gas transport from the external environment to the cells, in deReuck AVS, Porter R (eds): *Development of the Lung.* Boston, Little, Brown, 1967, p 3.
75. Reeves RB: An imidazole alphastat hypothesis for vertebrate acid-base regulation: Tissue carbon dioxide content and body temperature in bullfrogs. *Respir Physiol* 14:219, 1972.
76. Reeves RB: The interaction of body temperature and acid-base balance in ectothermic vertebrates. *Annu Rev Physiol* 40:752, 1977.
77. Reeves RB, Rahn H: Patterns in vertebrate acid-base regulation, in Wood S, Lenfant C (eds): *Evolution of the Respiratory Process: A Comparative Approach.* New York, Marcel Dekker, 1979, p 225.
78. Severinghaus JW et al: Respiratory control at high altitude suggesting active transport regulation of CSF pH. *J Appl Physiol* 18:1155, 1963.
79. Stewart PA: *How to Understand Acid-Base.* New York, Elsevier/North-Holland, 1981, pp 32–33.
80. Tapia R: Glutamine metabolism in brain, in Mora J, Palacios R (eds): *Glutamine: Metabolism, Enzymology and Regulation.* New York, Academic Press, 1980, p 285.
81. Tenney SM: Ventilatory response to carbon dioxide in pulmonary emphysema. *J Appl Physiol* 6:477, 1954.
82. van Ypersele de Stirhou C, Frans A: The respiratory response to metabolic alkalosis and acidosis in disease. *Clin Sci* 45:439, 1973.
83. Weyne J et al: Selected brain amino acid and ammonium during chronic hypercapnia in conscious rats. *J Appl Physiol* 44:333, 1978.
84. Wichser J, Kazemi H: CSF bicarbonate regulation in respiratory acidosis and alkalosis. *J Appl Physiol* 38:504, 1975.
85. Yamada KA et al: Medullary ventral surface GABA receptors affect respiratory and cardiovascular function. *Brain Res* 248:71, 1982.

CHAPTER • 9

Acid production

Jack G. Kleinman • Jacob Lemann, Jr.

INTRODUCTORY CONCEPTS

The multiple biochemical reactions of metabolism result in both the production and consumption, or removal, of both acids and bases from body fluids. Nevertheless, in the healthy steady state the acidity of body fluids, reflected by pH and the state of titration of body buffers that determine pH, is closely regulated and very stable. In the extracellular fluid (ECF), the concentrations of bicarbonate and carbonic acid (which is proportional to and reflected by the P_{CO_2}), which constitute the most important buffer system determining extracellular pH, are similarly stable. In population studies *arterial* or *arterialized capillary* serum or plasma bicarbonate concentration averages 24 ± 1 SD meq/liter, and arterial P_{CO_2} averages 39 ± 2 mmHg (5.2 ± 0.3 kPa). Thus, arterial pH averages 7.42 ± 0.02.[7] Similarly, mean *venous* serum or plasma bicarbonate concentration values (which are higher than arterial levels because bicarbonate shifts from red blood cells to plasma as hemoglobin buffers incoming CO_2) average 27 ± 2 meq/liter, and venous P_{CO_2} (which is also higher than arterial P_{CO_2} because of CO_2 production by tissues) averages 47 ± 4 mmHg. Since the increment in P_{CO_2} of venous blood relative to arterial blood is greater than the relative increment in bicarbonate concentration, venous pH is slightly lower than arterial pH, averaging 7.38 ± 0.02.[1,48,52,53,109] When venous bicarbonate concentration, P_{CO_2}, and pH were repetitively measured over 4 to 10 days in the same 32 subjects eating constant diets of normal composition, the average coefficients of variation (average of individual standard deviations divided by individual means × 100) were bicarbonate concentration, 3.3 percent; P_{CO_2}, 6.9 percent; and pH (calculated as $[H^+]$, neq/liter), 5.2 percent. All of these observations emphasize the closely controlled regulation of the titration of body buffers and the acidity of the ECF in health.

The stability of these values involves the integrated regulation of acid and base production, consumption, distribution, buffering, and excretion. Ultimately, all acid-base disturbances must reflect alterations in rates of production and/or excretion of acid or base. This chapter focuses primarily on the sources of H^+ production and, to a lesser extent, on organic acid distribution among different organs in health and disease, together with a consideration of the metabolic consumption of H^+. Renal net acid excretion will also be considered in the context of the quantification of fixed acid production (see also Chaps. 10 and 27).

Body composition in healthy adults is essentially constant from day to day. The body stores and concentrations in body fluids of nitrogen (urea), sodium, potassium, calcium, and other minerals are stable. The daily intakes of calories, nitrogen, and minerals are equaled by their expenditure or excretion. Similarly the acidity and buffering capacity of body fluids in health are stable from day to day so that daily production and excretion of hydrogen ions must also be equal.

In health, the rate of production of the volatile acid, carbonic acid, from neutral foods such as carbohydrate, fat, and protein is equaled by the simultaneous rate of pulmonary carbon dioxide excretion; thus, the arterial as well as venous carbon dioxide tension, the respiratory component of the acid-base equilibrium in ECF, is held nearly constant at about 40 mmHg. Clearly, variations in the gradient for pulmonary carbon dioxide excretion will alter P_{CO_2}. A discussion of primary respiratory acid-base disorders is considered in Chap. 30.

Similarly, in health there is production each day of so-called nonvolatile or fixed acids. As soon as an acid with a pK' that is lower than ambient pH is produced in cells by the metabolism either of ingested food or of tissue constituents, the hydrogen ions released by the dissociation of the acid react with body buffers (see Chap. 24 for a review of acid pK'). The bicarbonate ion is one such body buffer. Buffering of the hydrogen ion by bicarbonate results in the formation of carbonic acid, which is transported to the lungs, where it is dehydrated and excreted as CO_2:

$$HA \rightarrow H^+ + A^- + Na^+ + HCO_3^- \rightarrow Na^+ + A^- + H_2CO_3 \rightarrow Na^+ + A^- + CO_2 + H_2O \quad (1)$$

Obviously, such a process could not continue for long without the regeneration of the bicarbonate ions that are consumed in these buffering reactions. This regeneration process is accomplished by the renal excretion of hydrogen ions as urinary titratable acid (titration of buffer filtered through the glomeruli, principally phosphate) and ammonium (buffer generated and secreted by the kidney) less any bicarbonate that, having escaped renal tubular reabsorption, appears in the urine. Thus, each hydrogen ion secreted into the urine as net acid excretion [titratable acid + ammonium − (HCO_3^-)] identifies a bicarbonate ion that has been synthesized and returned to renal venous blood, thus restoring the bicarbonate ion consumed as fixed acid was produced and buffered (see also Chap. 10).

Historically, healthy subjects eating normal diets and having normal and stable serum bicarbonate concentrations, P_{CO_2}, and blood pH levels were assumed to be in acid balance; that is to say, rates of fixed acid production and renal net acid excretion were assumed to have been equal or acid balance was approximately zero (i.e., net fixed acid production − renal net acid excretion = zero). The rate of net acid excretion could readily be quantitated as the sum of urinary titratable acid and ammonium minus excreted bicarbonate. However, all of the reactions leading to the production of fixed acid or the net production of bicarbonate had not been identified. Techniques have now been devised to identify and quantitate the sources of net fixed acid production in human beings. These methods are, of necessity, indirect, identifying products of metabolism which, by biochemical reasoning, must have been associated with hydrogen ion production or consumption. In healthy subjects eating normal diets the major sources of fixed acid production, base production, or base loss include

1. The *oxidation of dietary organic sulfur* in the sulfur-containing amino acids to inorganic sulfate, quantitated by the measurement of urinary sulfate excretion:

$$R\text{—}SH + 2O_2 \rightarrow R + SO_4^{2-} + 2H^+ \quad (2)$$

2. The *production of organic acids* that are not oxidized to CO_2 and H_2O and that are quantified by the urinary excretion of organic anion. This measurement identifies hydrogen ions added to body fluid as neutral precursors are metabolized to acids:

$$\text{Glucose} \rightarrow 2\ \text{lactate}^- + 2H^+ \quad (3)$$

$$\text{Triglycerides} \rightarrow \text{acetate}^- + H^+ \quad (4)$$

$$\text{Nucleoproteins} \rightarrow \text{urate}^- + H^+ \quad (5)$$

3. *Dietary intake of potential base*, principally as potassium salts of metabolizable organic bases, such as citrate in fruits and vegetables:

$$R\text{—}COO^-K^+ + O_2 \rightarrow \text{urea} + CO_2 + K^+ + HCO_3^- \quad (6)$$

This reaction is quantitated by measurement of the dietary content of unmeasured anion:

$$(\Sigma Na^+ + K^+ + Ca^{2+} + Mg^{2+}, \text{meq/day}) - (\Sigma Cl^-, \text{meq/day} + 1.8\ PO_4, \text{mmol/day}) \quad (7)$$

(See "Phosphorus: Phosphoproteins and Phosphate Esters" for an explanation of the use of 1.8 for PO_4.) Average diets contain approximately 40 to 90 meq of unmeasured anion per day. When the diet contains relatively more protein and purified carbohydrate, the unmeasured anion content of the diet may actually have a negative value, indicating that the diet contains unmeasured cation (presumably amino groups) metabolizable to H^+.[53] On the other hand, diets containing mostly fruits and vegetables may provide as much as 150 meq/day or more of unmeasured anion. As shown in Fig. 9-1, daily urinary organic anion excretion ranges from about 30 to 65 meq/day and is primarily related to the dietary intake of unmeasured anion.[1,48,53,109] A relationship to body weight is not evident.

4. The *excretion of actual or potential base in the feces*, which normally contains both bicarbonate as well as inorganic salts of short-chain fatty acids such as potassium acetate, potassium proprionate, and so on.[111] This source of base loss (which may also be thought of as H^+ gain to body fluids) can be quantitated by measurement of the fecal unmeasured anion in a manner identical to that applied to the diet. As shown in Fig. 9-2, the fecal unmeasured anion excretion among healthy adults eating a variety of diets may vary from about 5 to 60 meq/day. Fecal unmeasured anion is related primarily to dietary unmeasured anion and to fecal weight and less closely to body weight.[1,48,53,109]

When net fixed acid production is estimated in this manner and compared to the simultaneously measured rate of renal net acid excretion, net external acid balance can be evaluated. A representative example of the acid balance in a healthy adult eating a constant normal diet is shown in Fig. 9-3. This man weighed 77.2 kg and his serum bicarbonate concentration, P_{CO_2} and blood pH were stable, averaging 24.6 meq/liter, 40 mmHg, and

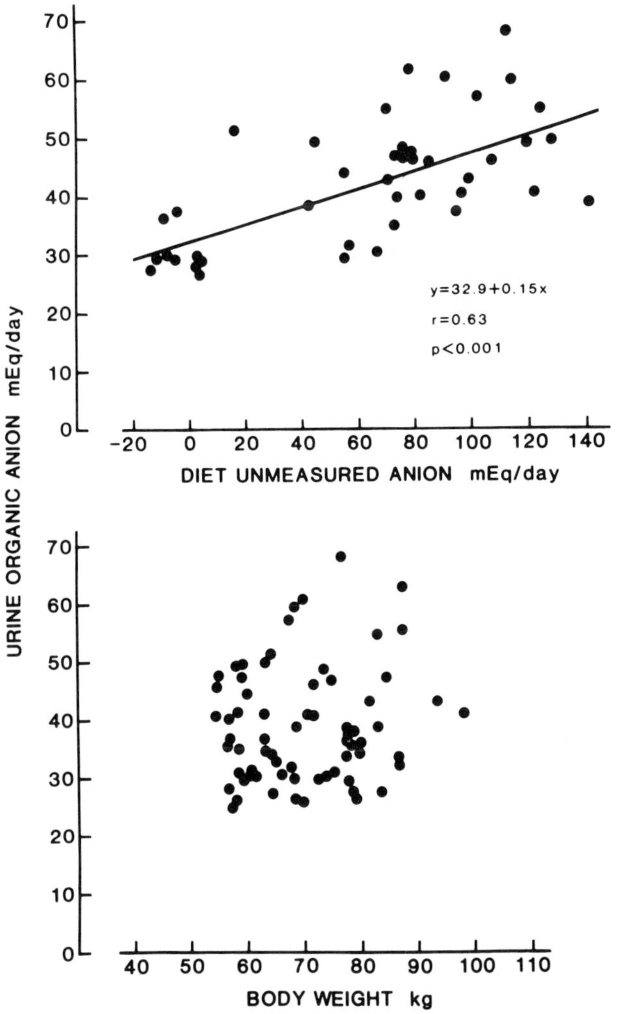

FIGURE 9-1 • Daily urinary organic anion excretion in healthy adults in relation to daily dietary unmeasured anion intake (upper panel) and body weight (lower panel).[1,48,53,109]

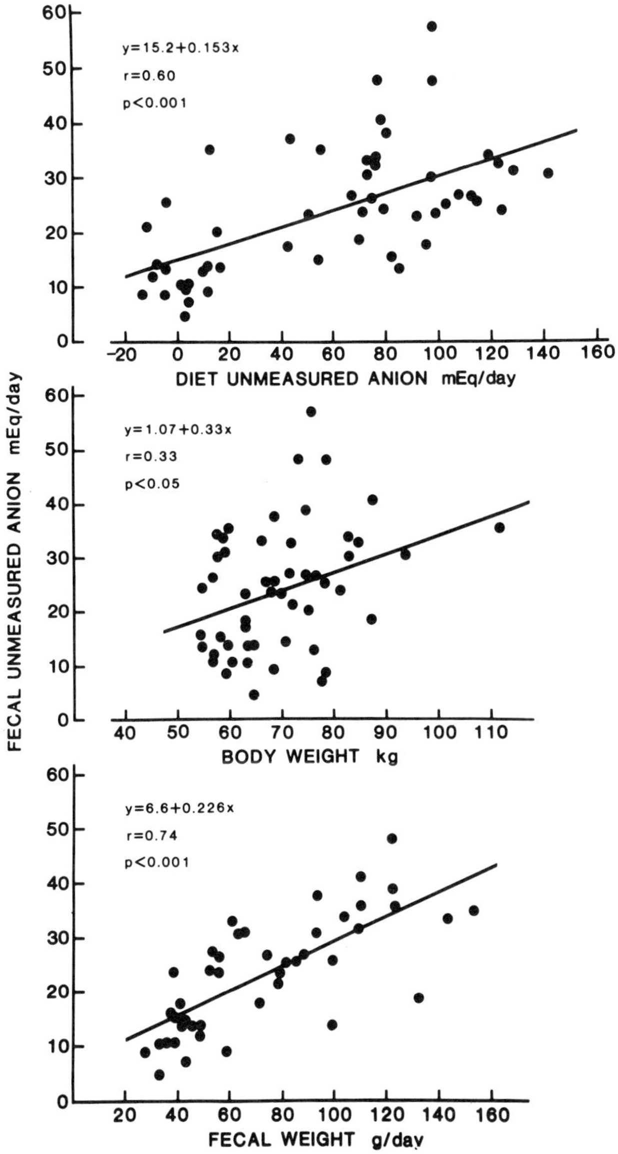

FIGURE 9-2 • Daily unmeasured anion content of the feces in healthy adults in relation to daily dietary unmeasured anion intake (upper panel), body weight (middle panel), and daily fecal wet weight (lower panel).[1,48,53,109]

7.41 units, respectively. His normal whole food diet provided 110 meq Na^+, 63 meq K^+, 22 meq Ca^{2+}, and 19 meq Mg^{2+} per day as well as 158 meq Cl^- and 26 mmol PO_4 (mean valence = 1.8; see "Phosphorus: Phosphoproteins and Phosphate Esters") per day. Thus, the unmeasured anion of his diet was 10 meq/day. His average daily fecal content of unmeasured anion was calculated in a similar manner and averaged 17 meq/day. Mean daily urinary sulfate excretion averaged 30 meq/day and organic anion 46 meq/day. Thus, net fixed acid production averaged [sulfate (30 meq/day) plus organic anion (46 meq/day)] minus [dietary unmeasured anion (10 meq/day) minus fecal unmeasured anion (17 meq/day)] = 83 meq/day. The simultaneous rate of renal net acid excretion averaged 83 meq/day. Thus, average daily acid balance, calculated as the difference between fixed acid production and net renal acid excretion, was zero meq/day. For a group of 16 healthy adults in which individual rates of net acid production calculated in this manner ranged from 21 to 120 meq/day, net acid excretion similarly ranged from 29 to 112 meq/day, and daily acid balance averaged -1 ± 12 meq/day, a value not significantly different from zero ($p > .70$).[53] Rather than actually measure the dietary and fecal content of unmeasured anion in order to assess net intestinal absorption of potential base, it has been proposed that in the acute steady state, estimation of the daily rate of urinary excretion of unmeasured anion (estimated as for the diet or the feces) will provide equivalent data.[67]

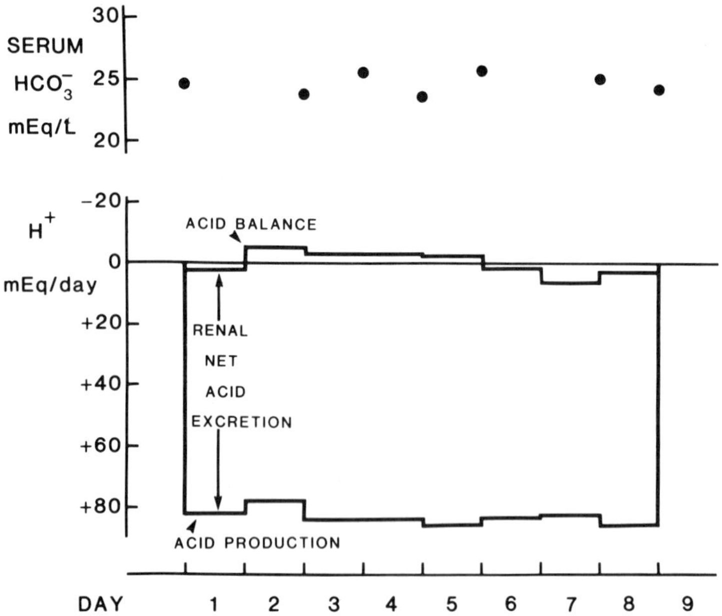

FIGURE 9-3 • Serum bicarbonate and acid balance in a healthy man. Daily fixed acid production is plotted downward from the zero line, and daily renal net acid excretion is plotted upward from acid production. Thus, open areas below the zero line indicate positive acid balance, and extensions above zero indicate negative acid balance (see text).[53]

ACID PRODUCTION

SULFURIC ACID: THE OXIDATION OF THE SULFUR-CONTAINING AMINO ACIDS, METHIONINE AND CYSTEINE

More than 75 years ago, Sherman and Gettler recognized that the urinary excretion of inorganic sulfate reflected the oxidation of organic sulfur contained in amino acids either ingested in the diet or derived from the catabolism of tissue proteins.[93] More recent studies have clearly documented the quantitative relationships between the oxidation of amino acid sulfur and acid production in men.[38,50] Following a control period, five subjects were given 13.0 g of supplementary methionine daily representing 93 mmol of sulfur (or 186 meq of potential sulfate, SO_4^{2-}). Observations were continued after the methionine loads were discontinued. Methionine loading augmented urinary sulfate excretion and was accompanied by acidification of the urine and augmentation of net acid excretion. During the period of methionine loading and the recovery period that followed, the cumulative increment in urinary inorganic sulfate excretion, which averaged 730 meq, was matched by a nearly equivalent cumulative increment in net acid excretion, which averaged 684 meq, or 93 percent of the sulfate.[50] These observations indicated that the administration of methionine resulted in the production of 2 meq H^+/mmol of sulfur oxidized or 1 meq H^+/meq of sulfate produced. The known biochemical pathways involved in the oxidation of methionine and cysteine are

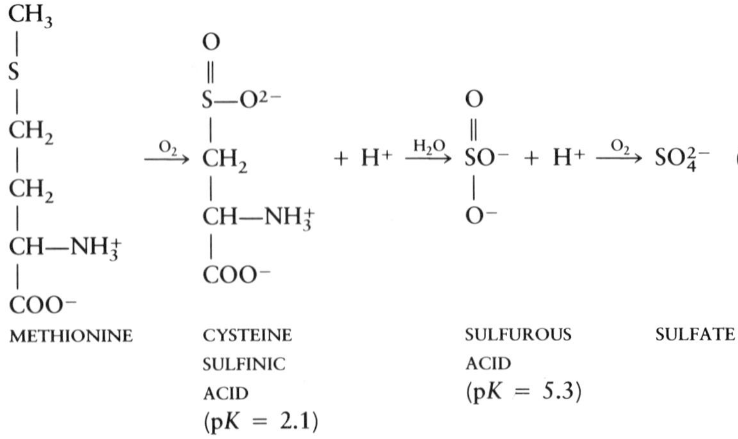

(8)

Although hydrogen ions are released in two intermediate steps, the overall reaction can be summarized as

$$R{-}SH \rightarrow R + SO_4^{2-} + 2H^+ \qquad (9)$$

Serum bicarbonate concentration fell by approximately 5 meq/liter during methionine loading, providing further evidence for acidification of body fluids as acid production was increased by this process.[49] The decline in serum bicarbonate concentration was accompanied by a comparable rise in serum chloride concentration, presumably because sulfate is poorly reabsorbed by the renal tubule relative to chloride. Thus, there was no significant rise in the serum unmeasured anion concentration during methionine loading.

During methionine loading, only about 72 percent of the administered sulfur could be accounted for by an increase in urinary sulfate excretion. Sulfate was not detected in the feces. Presumably, the remaining portion of the methionine administered was either incorporated into tissue proteins such as hair, skin, and nails or converted to thiols (neutral sulfur-containing molecules) such as taurine, which would have no net effect on acid production. Figure 9-4 reemphasizes this point by showing the relationship between urinary sulfate excretion and estimated dietary intake of sulfur in subjects eating various constant diets, including diets on which subjects were placed in order to study methionine loading. Approximately 0.71 meq of sulfate appears in the urine per 1 meq of sulfur (potential SO_4^{2-}) fed over this wide range of sulfur intakes, indicating that approximately 70 percent of dietary sulfur results in acid production by augmentation of urinary sulfate excretion.

Under normal conditions, dietary protein constitutes the sole source of organic sulfur intake. The quantitative importance of dietary protein, and of the sulfur content of the protein to the urinary excretion of inorganic sulfate and, thus, to acid production, is illustrated in Fig. 9-5. Urinary sulfate excretion rises progressively as dietary protein intake increases. The rise is greater when the protein is provided as egg white, which contains 1.25 meq potential SO_4^{2-} per gram of protein, than when the diet protein is provided as mixed proteins (meat, milk, and cereals), which contain about 0.56 meq potential SO_4^{2-} per gram of protein, or soy protein, which contains 0.4 meq potential SO_4^{2-} per gram of protein. Thus, high protein diets, or starvation and the catabolism of tissue protein, will augment sulfur oxidation, acid production, and urinary sulfate excretion, while low protein diets with adequate total calories will minimize acid production from these sources.[38]

PHOSPHORUS: THE ROLE OF PHOSPHOPROTEINS AND PHOSPHATE ESTERS

Although phosphorus is the commonly applied term, all phosphorus in biological systems exists as phosphate ($H_2PO_4^-$, HPO_4^{2-}, and PO_4^{3-}; see Chap. 12). In the blood, at pH 7.4, the pK_2 of approximately 6.8 for the dissociation $H_2PO_4^- \rightarrow HPO_4^{2-} + H^+$ dictates that the molar concentration ratio of $HPO_4^{2-}/H_2PO_4^-$ be 4:1. Thus, the apparent valence of phosphate per millimole of phosphorus is $(0.8 \times 2) + (0.2 \times 1) = 1.8$.

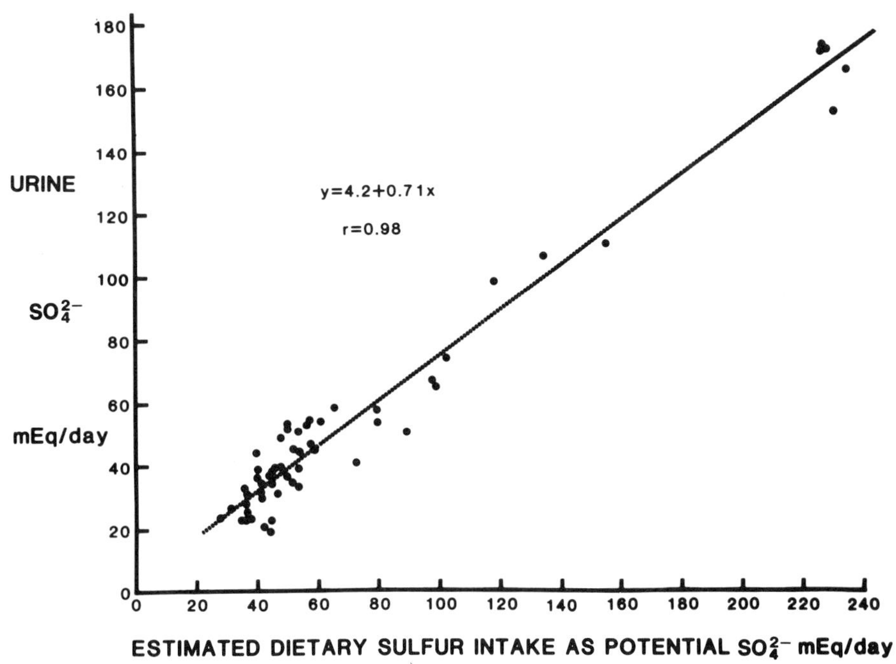

FIGURE 9-4 • Daily urinary SO_4^{2-} excretion as a function of estimated dietary sulfur intake, as potential SO_2^{2-}, in meq/day (1 mmol sulfur = 2 meq = 32 mg).[1,48,50,54,78,109]

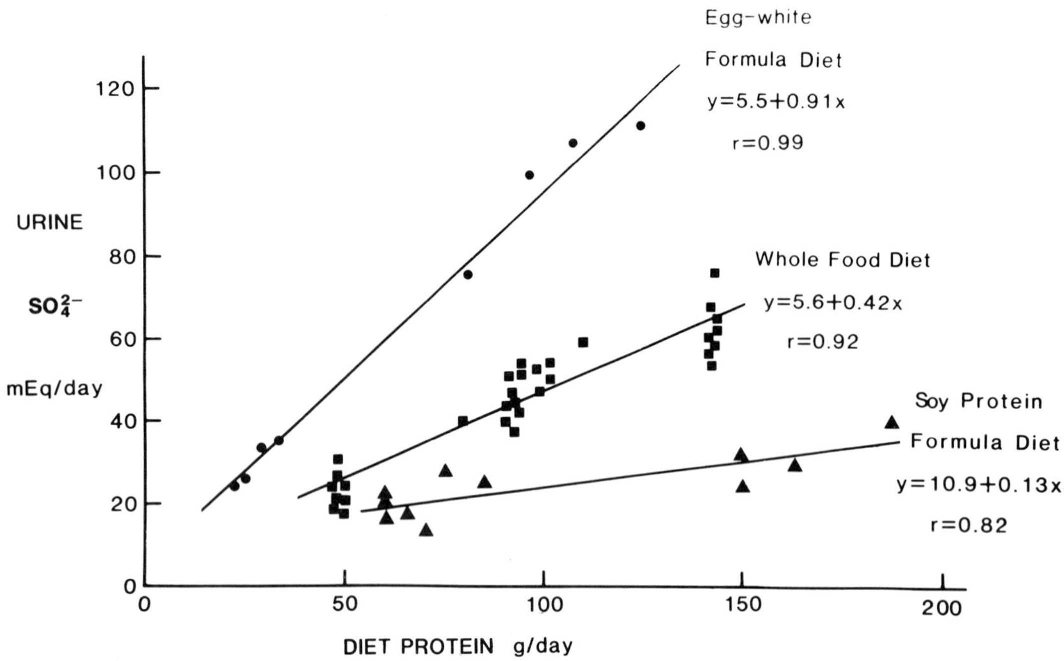

FIGURE 9-5 • Daily urinary SO_4^{2-} excretion in subjects fed varying amounts of protein either as egg white (1.25 meq potential sulfate per gram), mixed protein (average of 0.6 meq potential sulfate per gram), or soy protein (0.4 meq potential sulfate per gram).[1,48,52,53,109]

If the dietary phosphate were present as all orthophosphate diesters, neutralized by metabolizable cations (amino groups) such as serine or threonine esters in proteins, the hydrolysis and metabolism of such a substance with conversion of the phosphate to its state in plasma would be a source of acid production:

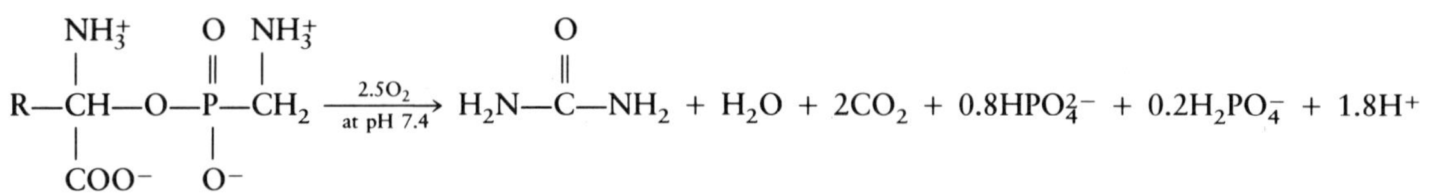 (9)

In fact, when a purified phosphoprotein, free of inorganic cations, was fed to healthy volunteers, acid production from this source could be identified and was quantitated as approximately 1.8 meq H^+ generated per millimole phosphorus ingested.[54]

However, most foods contain phosphate esters of compounds involved in carbohydrate metabolism, such as glucose-6-phosphate, as well as phosphoproteins, phospholipids, and ribose-phosphate in nucleic acids. Many, if not most, of these intracellular compounds are neutralized by intracellular inorganic cations such as K^+ and Mg^{2+}. The hydrolysis and metabolism of such compounds to the state of phosphate in plasma would in fact consume hydrogen ions through net bicarbonate production:

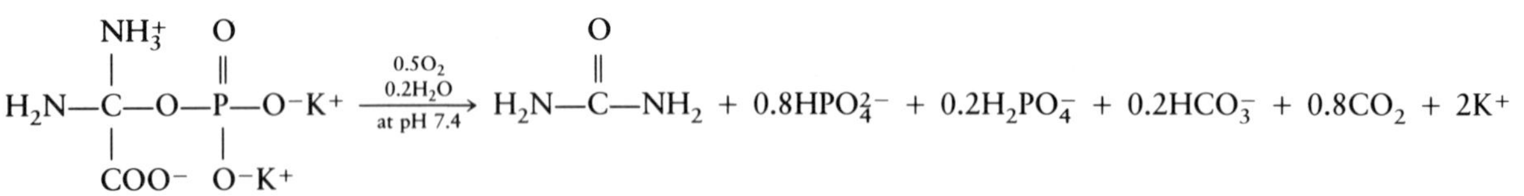 (10)

When a pure phosphorprotein in the diet was neutralized by the addition of $Ca(OH)_2$ and $Mg(OH)_2$ in quantities that titrated the phosphate to its state in plasma (0.8 HPO_4^{2-}/0.2 $H_2PO_4^-$), it was shown that no net fixed acid production from the phosphoprotein could be detected.[78]

Since the precise states of phosphates in food are not known, the development of techniques to estimate acid balance has involved the arbitrary assignment of a mean valence of 1.8 for phosphate in the diet (see below). The actual valence of phosphate in feces is also not precisely known. Feces are composed of a mixture of cells (bacterial, intestinal, and undigested diet), fiber, various precipitates, and a fluid phase. It has been shown that only about 5 percent of fecal phosphorus is dialyzable, suggesting it is either confined within cells or present as precipitated calcium and magnesium phosphates.[111] It would appear, therefore, that the true valence of phosphorus in the feces is greater than 1.8 but less than the maximum value of 3. However, as shown in Table 9-1, the effect on the calculation of acid balance of the arbitrary assignment of the valence of phosphate as 1.8 in the diet takes into account the fact that if the true valence were higher or lower, phosphate would, respectively, bind or liberate H^+ upon digestion and entry into extracellular fluid at pH 7.4.[49] Similarly, in the calculation of the acid balance, assigning phosphate a valence of 1.8 in feces (the same value as assigned in the diet) automatically takes into account any quantities of H^+ that would have been bound or liberated if the valence of phosphate changed during passage through the intestine. Thus, healthy adults eating diets that result in rates of acid production ranging from about 20 to 120 meq/day appear to be in approximate acid balance when phosphate is assigned a valence of 1.8 in both diet and stool.

Subjects in steady-state phosphorus balance quantitatively excrete ingested phosphate, and the proportionality between urinary HPO_4^{2-} and $H_2PO_4^-$ is largely determined by the daily acid load. Conversion of filtered HPO_4^{2-} to excreted $H_2PO_4^-$ by the tubular secretion of protons creates titratable acid, which helps to rid the body of excess acid. Analysis of dietary phosphate reveals that half is present as HPO_4^{2-} and the remainder as $H_2PO_4^-$ or its equivalent.[31a] Since urinary pH is usually 1 log unit below the pK of $H_2PO_4^-$ (6.8), 90 percent of excreted phosphate appears as $H_2PO_4^-$. It can be shown that excreted phosphate accounts for the net removal of roughly 15 meq of acid. Thus, gastrointestinal absorption of "acid phosphate" ($H_2PO_4^-$) frees up protons but also generates its own buffer (HPO_4^{2-}), which eventually carries the protons into the urine. Absorption of dietary "alkaline phosphate" (HPO_4^{2-}) generates bicarbonate by absorbing body protons and via the renal generation of titratable acid. With normal diets the impact of ingested phosphate on acid-base homeostasis is generally rather small.

To summarize, net fixed acid production will increase principally as a result of increased dietary intake of protein and, thus, sulfur-containing amino acids, leading to the generation of H^+ as sulfur is metabolized to SO_4^{2-}. Acid production will be reduced as the diet contains greater amounts of unmeasured anion relative to protein.

TABLE 9-1 • Theoretical effects of alterations in the valence of phosphorus (P) in diet and stool on the estimation of net fixed acid production (meq)*

Valence of P	Calculated diet OA†	Calculated fecal OA	Net OA absorbed (reduction in net acid production)	H^+ added to body fluid from absorbed P	H^+ added to body fluid from unabsorbed (fecal) P	Sum of changes in H^+ added (increase in net acid production)	Total true change in calculated net acid production
1.8 in diet and stool	68	40	28	0	0	0	−28
1.0 in diet and stool	100	48	52	24	0	24	−28
3.0 in diet and stool	20	28	−8	−36	0	−36	−28
1.0 in diet and 1.8 in stool	100	40	60	24	8	32	−28
1.0 in diet and 3.0 in stool	100	28	72	24	20	44	−28
1.8 in diet and 3.0 in stool	68	28	40	0	12	12	−28
3.0 in diet and 1.0 in stool	20	48	−28	−36	−20	−56	−28

* Calculated on the basis of the following: a daily diet composition of Σ cations, 300 meq; Cl, 160 meq; and P, 40 mM; and a mean daily stool composition of Σ cations, 60 meq; Cl, 2 meq; and P, 10 mmol.

† OA, organic anions (actual or potential bicarbonate).

SOURCE: From Lemann J Jr, Lennon EJ: Role of diet, gastrointestinal tract and bone in acid-base homeostasis. *Kidney Int* 1:275, 1972. Used by permission.

THE RELATIONSHIP AMONG FIXED ACID PRODUCTION, RENAL NET ACID EXCRETION, ACID BALANCE, AND THE SERUM BICARBONATE CONCENTRATION

Daily renal net acid excretion varies directly with the rate of fixed acid production. This relationship is shown in Fig. 9-6 for subjects eating normal diets or diets supplemented with either NH_4Cl to increase acid production or $NaHCO_3$ to decrease acid production. As acid production is increased, net renal acid excretion does not rise to levels that would serve to completely dispose of the increased acid load. In other words, the slope of renal net acid excretion as a function of fixed acid production (Fig. 9-6) is significantly less than unity: $p < .001$. Consequently, as acid production increases, acid is retained in the body. A portion of the retained acid is buffered by bicarbonate in the ECF and readily available tissue buffers, while another portion is buffered by bone.[52] Figure 9-7 shows the relationships among serum bicarbonate concentrations and rates of fixed acid production, renal net acid excretion, and acid balance in normal subjects when rates of fixed acid production were experimentally varied over a wide range. Serum bicarbonate concentration falls by 1.8 meq/liter for each 1-meq/kg-per-day increment in acid production, and serum bicarbonate concentration falls similarly with increments in renal net acid excretion and as acid balance becomes more positive. Other studies have shown that serum bicarbonate concentration also declines as daily net acid excretion varies over the range of 14 to 154 meq/day or 0.2 to 2.0 meq/kg per day in subjects eating a range of normal diets.[46] In individuals with impaired renal function and, thus, limitations in renal net acid excretion, any increment in fixed acid production would result in a greater reduction in serum bicarbonate concentration than in individuals with normal renal function.[28]

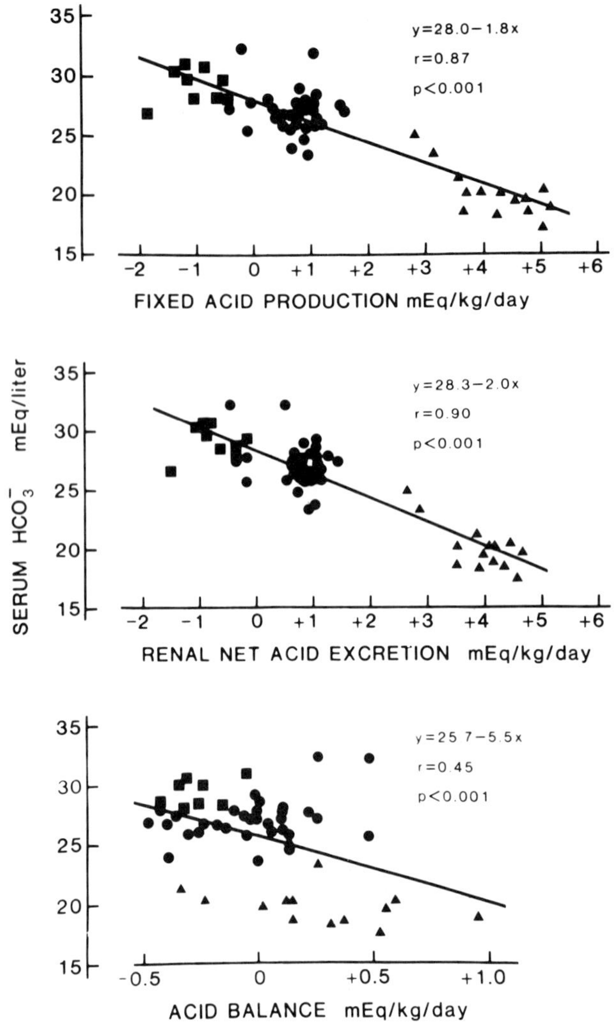

FIGURE 9-7 • Serum bicarbonate concentrations in healthy adults eating normal diets (circle), diets supplemented with NH_4Cl (triangle), or diets supplemented with $NaHCO_3$ (square) in relation to daily fixed acid production per kilogram of body weight (upper panel), daily renal net acid excretion (same units; middle panel), and daily acid balance (same units; lower panel).[1,48,51,52,107]

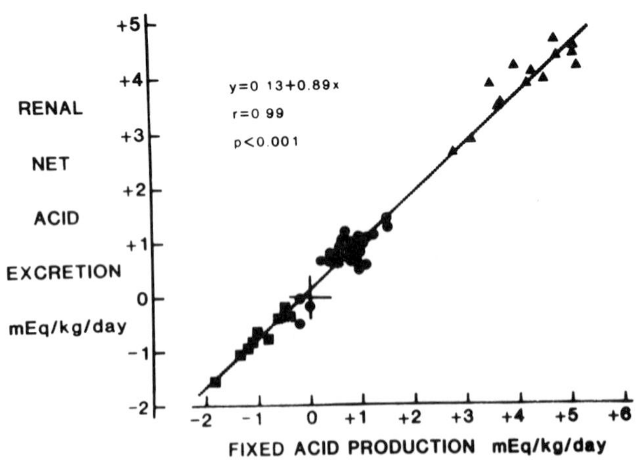

FIGURE 9-6 • Daily renal net acid excretion per kilogram of body weight in healthy adults in relation to daily fixed acid production per kilogram. Circle, normal diets; triangle, NH_4Cl; square, $NaHCO_3$.[1,48,51,52,53,109]

ORGANIC ACID PRODUCTION

Disorders of organic acid production and disposal are the most common clinical causes of increased acid production and acidosis. Consideration of the contribution of organic acids to acid production requires review of the turnover of endogenous organic acids in health.

The quantitatively important acid-producing metabolic reactions are those involving the hydrolysis of ATP to yield ADP, HPO_4^{2-}, and H^+, and the reduction of ferrichrome respiratory enzymes and pyridine nucleotides.[4] At an average cellular pH of 7.2, these reactions can be summarized by the following equations:

$$MgATP^{2-} + H_2O \rightarrow MgADP^{2-} + 0.72HPO_4^{2-} + 0.28H_2PO_4^- + 0.72H^+ \quad (11)$$

$$NADH + H^+ + FADH_2 + 4 \text{ cytochrome } c^+ \rightarrow NAD^+ + FAD + 4 \text{ cytochrome } c + 4H^+ \quad (12)$$

Under normal conditions ATP synthesis has been estimated at 120 mol/day.[42] Assuming the steady state, ATP hydrolysis would also equal this figure, leading to 86.4 mol of H^+ per day produced by the first of these reactions. Comparable figures derived from the NADH and $FADH_2$ production attendant upon glucose and triglyceride turnovers are 24 mol H^+ and 58 mol H^+, respectively.[42] In health, however, there is no net gain of H^+ from these reactions, since the pyridine nucleotides, flavoproteins, and cytochromes are reoxidized and ATP hydrolysis is balanced by ATP synthesis.[103]

Studies of carbohydrate metabolism have traditionally focused attention on glycolysis as a net acid-producing pathway. The conversion of glucose to lactate can be summarized as follows:

$$C_6H_{12}O_6 \rightarrow 2CH_3CHOHCOO^- + 2H^+ + 2ATP \quad (13)$$

Since this pathway is linked to ATP synthesis under normal circumstances, there is no net gain of H^+. As many reactions consume H^+ as produce it.

In the anaerobic state, which occurs in exercising skeletal muscle at a threshold that depends on the exercise training of the individual,[108] the pathway is unable to replenish ATP at a rate fast enough to consume the H^+ generated by rapid ATP hydrolysis. The net effect, therefore, is production of H^+ as lactic acid. Organs or tissues that can engage in gluconeogenesis from lactate or that can oxidize this substrate will either consume H^+, as in the reverse of the above reaction, or will produce bicarbonate (which amounts to the same thing), as follows:

$$2CH_3CHOHCOO^- + 6O_2 \rightarrow 4CO_2 + 2HCO_3^- + 4H_2O \quad (14)$$

Cycling of glucose to glycogen and back and of fatty acid to triglyceride and back also produces H^+, but in health this acid is also consumed in the final and complete metabolism of these substrates to CO_2 and H_2O.[4] Incomplete metabolism, however, results in H^+ accumulation. In the case of carbohydrate, as previously indicated, this will be associated with rapid ATP hydrolysis as well as the accumulation of H^+ and lactate.

In the case of fatty acid oxidation the situation is more complex. In addition to the H^+ produced during triglyceride hydrolysis, acid is also formed during the production of acylcoenzyme A (acyl-CoA), the beta oxidation of fatty acids, and the formation of 3-hydroxy-3-methylglutaryl-CoA.[4]

$$C_{51}H_{98}O_6 + 3H_2O \rightarrow C_3H_8O_3 + 3C_{16}H_{31}O_2^- + 3H^+ \quad (15)$$

$$3CH_3(CH_2)_{14}COO^- + 3MgATP^{2-} + 3CoA^{4-} \rightarrow 3CH_3(CH_2)_{14}COSCoA^{4-} + 3AMP^{2-} + 6P_i^{2-} + 3Mg^{2+} + 3H^+ \quad (16)$$

$$CH_3(CH_2)_{12}CH_2CH_2COSCoA + FAD + NAD^+ + HSCoA + H_2O \rightarrow CH_3(CH_2)_{12}COSCoA + CH_3COSCoA + FADH_2 + NADH + H^+ \quad (17)$$

$$CH_3COSCoA + CH_3COCH_2COSCoA + H_2O \rightarrow CH_3COH(CH_2COO^-)CH_2COSCoA + HSCoA + H^+ \quad (18)$$

The cleavage of this compound to form acetoacetate and acetyl-CoA is not accompanied by additional H^+ production, and the reactions resulting in the formation of β-hydroxybutyrate and acetone result in net consumption of H^+. As in the case of other acid-producing reactions, no net H^+ production will ensue if the H^+ is reutilized. Under normal circumstances, brain, muscle, and kidney oxidize acetoacetate and β-hydroxybutyrate, thus consuming H^+.

Other than the reaction of CO_2 with water, the only metabolic reactions that result in significant net H^+ production under ordinary conditions are those that produce acids with incompletely metabolized or nonmetabolizable anions. As indicated earlier, these reactions include organic acids produced by the incomplete metabolism of carbohydrate, fat, or protein; the oxidation of the sulfur-containing amino acids, methionine and cysteine;[38,50] and, under certain circumstances, the metabolism of phosphoproteins.[54] The most important factors involved in the acute regulation of H^+ in body fluids are the competence of respiratory function and the presence of various buffer systems. Discussion of how these factors affect acid-base balance is beyond the purview of this chapter. A number of other factors, however, can affect reactions resulting in H^+ production, H^+ removal, or both so as to produce net H^+ accumulation or dissipation. These factors include the state of tissue oxygenation, exercise, circulatory competence between H^+-producing and H^+-consuming organs, acid-base balance itself, hormones, toxins, enzyme deficiencies, and diet composition, as well as gastrointestinal and renal function.

As indicated earlier, *anaerobiasis* or ischemia is associated with an imbalance between the hydrolysis of ATP and its resynthesis and the reduction and oxidation of respiratory enzymes and pyridine nucleotides.[4,34] These processes are accomplished, for all practical purposes, by the electron transport chain of mitochondria. This system is sensitive to the availability of O_2, anoxia leading to cessation of function, and accumulation of reduced enzyme forms and substrates. NADH can be reoxidized to NAD to some extent by conversion of pyruvate to lactate in cytosol. This reaction accounts for the accumulation of lactate in anoxic states. A buildup of H^+ in cells or a fall in cell pH in a variety of tissues and organs has been demonstrated to occur within minutes of the onset of anoxia using such techniques as phosphorus nuclear magnetic resonance and indicator compounds.[44,75] The mechanism responsible for the extracellular acidosis associated with tissue anoxia appears to primarily involve cation exchange ($Na^+ - H^+$) and operates as long as a favorable gradient remains for Na^+ transport into cells.[82]

Although the body as a whole operates in the aerobic state under normal conditions, some organs or tissues are often called upon to function in a relatively anaerobic state. Thus, the blood flowing from exercising muscles has a lower pH than systemic venous blood, and muscle lactate production increases so as to produce metabolic acidosis, increased muscle lactate content, and lactic acidemia.[33,107,108] Lactic acid production in short-term, intense exercise can reach 300 to 500 meq/min.[69] The initial rise in serum lactate levels under these circumstances, about 10 to 12 meq/liter, will be mirrored by an equivalent fall in serum bicarbonate concentration.[15] Even though ATP levels are well maintained in exercising muscle, the decreases in creatine phosphate observed indicate an increase in ATP turnover leading to a decline in muscle cell pH.[84] Thus it is clear that increased organic anion production by exercising skeletal muscle is accompanied by net H^+ production.

Even in the basal state in healthy humans a number of organs and tissues are capable of net lactate and, presumably, H^+ production. This organic acid production is quantitatively summarized in Table 9-2.[73] These net acid-producing tissues must be balanced by organs that consume H^+ by metabolizing lactate or utilizing it to resynthesize glucose. As indicated in Table 9-2, the liver and kidney are largely responsible for lactate utilization under normal circumstances. In addition, these organs have a large capacity for augmenting their lactate utilization.[13] That such utilization results in consumption of H^+ is demonstrated by the direct relationship between lactate uptake and cell pH in the isolated perfused liver.[17] The maximal rate of elimination of lactate by metabolism in otherwise normal individuals has been estimated to be between 5 and 10 mmol/min, the liver being responsible for at least half this total.[91] At normal hepatic blood flow rates, hepatic lactate uptake increases linearly until a blood concentration of 5 mmol/liter is reached.[92]

Since H^+ is consumed stoichiometrically when lactate is utilized by gluconeogenesis or oxidation, five to ten times the normal rate of H^+ production by reactions associated with glycolysis could be eliminated in this manner. However, whether lactate and H^+ production ever exceeds these levels in situations other than exhausting exercise has been questioned.[73] Thus, while it is conceptually possible to envision an increase in net lactate and, therefore, H^+ production solely as the result of an increase in the activity of glycolytic pathways in tissues having this capability, actual clinical situations are more likely to result from a decrease in activity of lactate- and H^+-consuming pathways in the liver and kidneys or from a combination of increased production and decreased utilization.

When the balance of lactate and H^+ production and utilization is upset, lactic acidosis results. A list of some of the major clinical conditions associated with lactic acidosis is given in Table 9-3. This list is not meant to be comprehensive but includes the important situations arranged according to current thinking as to whether increased lactate and H^+ production, reduced removal of lactate and H^+, or a combination of these two mechanisms is the important factor in their pathogenesis (see Chap. 25).

The other major organic acids produced in pathologic states are those that result from the incomplete *oxidation of fatty acids*. The reactions involved have been presented earlier (equations 15 through 18). As indicated, H^+ is produced at several points in the pathway from triglycerides to *ketone bodies*, but only acetoacetic and β-hydroxybutyric acids unequivocally identify net H^+ addition to body fluids (see Chap. 26). Each mole of fatty acid, if metabolized solely to ketoacids, can be associated with the production of 11 mol of free H^+ and 12 mol of H^+ linked to flavoproteins and pyridine nucleotides.[4]

In health, significant quantities of ketoacids are produced in the liver at a rate of approximately 2 μmol/min per kilogram of body weight, or about 200 mmol/day in a

TABLE 9-2 • Basal lactate production and utilization by various tissues

Tissue	Basal lactate production, mmol/day/70 kg	Tissue	Basal lactate utilization, mmol/day/70 kg
Skin	353	Liver	722
Red blood cells	302	Kidney	386
Brain	235	Heart	80
Muscle	218	Other	102
Intestinal mucosa	112		
Leukocytes, platelets	70		
Total	1290	Total	1290

SOURCE: From Park R, Arieff AI: Lactic acidosis, in Stollerman GH et al (eds): *Advances in Internal Medicine*, Chicago, Year Book Medical, 1980, vol 25. Used by permission.

TABLE 9-3 • Causes of lactic acidosis

INCREASED LACTATE AND H^+ PRODUCTION
Pyruvate dehydrogenase deficiency
Defects in oxidative phosphorylation
REDUCED LACTATE AND H^+ REMOVAL
Type I glycogen storage disease; glucose-6-phosphatase deficiency
Fructose-1,6-diphosphatase deficiency
Liver disease
Hepatotoxins (ethanol, methanol, salicylates, ethylene glycol, phenformin, isoniazide)
INCREASED LACTATE AND H^+ PRODUCTION COMBINED WITH DECREASED UTILIZATION
Reduced perfusion of large tissue mass
Shock
Severe anemia
Carbon monoxide poisoning
Hematologic malignancies and tumors

SOURCE: Adapted from Relman AS, Lactic acidosis, in Brenner BM, Stein JH (eds): *Acid-Base and Potassium Homeostasis, Contemporary Issues in Nephrology,* New York, Churchill Livingstone, 1978, vol 2, p 65.

70-kg individual.[62] In health, as in the case of lactic acid, these ketoacids are almost completely oxidized in all peripheral tissues, especially in the kidney and brain.[4] This rate of oxidation increases with elevations of blood ketones up to 7 meq/liter and may be somewhat dependent on insulin.[12]

Ketone production, primarily related to the delivery of free fatty acids to the liver, can increase above normal in a number of circumstances.[91] Fasting and insulin deficiency are the most common examples of situations associated with increases in ketoacid synthesis. Other less common conditions associated with accumulation of ketones and acidosis include certain inborn errors of metabolism, such as glycogen storage diseases, glycogen synthetase deficiency, carbamyl phosphate synthetase deficiency, and tyrosinosis.[10,18,23,104] In addition, poisoning with ethanol or overdose of beta-adrenergic agonists can also increase serum ketoacids.[41,55,100]

Data on rates of ketone body production in humans are available mainly from studies of starvation and diabetes. An overnight fast is enough to increase hepatic ketone production to 5 to 6 μmol/min per kilogram of body weight.[92] After about 3 days this value may be as high as 24 μmol/min per kilogram of body weight in obese subjects.[11] Values available in the literature, however, vary widely between these two levels.[24,72,76,110] These reports generally utilized hepatic vein catheterizations and isotope dilution determinations to estimate production values. Studies utilizing methodology for estimating net endogenous acid production presented earlier in this chapter were applied to a number of volunteers who fasted for 14 days in an environmental chamber at 16°C.[39] Acid production increased by about 0.7 to 0.8 μmol/min per kilogram of body weight above the mean of control days due to an increase in urinary organic anion excretion. Presumably the increment represented ketoacids. Further supporting this view was the observation that urinary net acid excretion increased by similar amounts so that cumulative acid balances were unchanged during the period of the fast.

These data indicate that after the first few days of starvation, the rate of ketoacid production appears to stabilize and is matched by an increased rate of ketone utilization and renal excretion. This leads to steady-state blood ketone concentrations (acetoacetic and β-hydroxybutyric acids) of between 5 and 8 meq/liter.[11] Assuming a space of distribution for ketoacids of 300 ml per kilogram of body weight, a plasma level of 8 meq/liter identifies an accumulation of 168 meq of H^+ in a 70-kg individual. Were this to be completely buffered by extracellular mechanisms, it would be associated with a fall in serum bicarbonate concentration of approximately 6 meq/liter. The data available in the literature appear to confirm that in starvation serum bicarbonate values decline to this degree.[24,72]

In contrast to starvation, diabetic ketosis is often progressive (see Chap. 20). It may result in severe metabolic acidosis, with blood pH values below 7.2 and bicarbonate concentrations below 10 meq/liter, and a fatal outcome may ensue. This situation may be brought about by large increases in ketoacid production, decreases in ketone utilization, or a combination of both mechanisms. Clinically, other factors, such as the patient's state of nutrition, perfusion status of ketone-producing and -consuming organs, the level of renal function, and hormonal or pharmacologic status, may alter the relative contributions of ketone production and utilization to the pathophysiology of diabetic ketoacidosis.[63]

Cessation of insulin therapy in diabetics is associated with a progressive increase in ketone production to rates of almost 20 μeq/min per kilogram of body weight after 10 h.[64] Net utilization also increased in these studies, but always lagged behind production so that plasma ketones rose progressively. This is equivalent to the addition to body fluids of about 125 meq of H^+ over 10 h, or about 300 meq of H^+ per day. This considerable acid load would very rapidly deplete the extracellular buffers and produce severe acidosis. Thus, it may be that ketone overproduction alone can initiate ketoacidosis. However, a number of factors can reduce ketone utilization so as to contribute to the intensity of acidosis. A number of other factors modulate ketone production during the course of diabetic ketoacidosis. In addition to the presence or absence of insulin, hepatic blood flow affects the rate of ketone production through variations in the rate of free fatty acid uptake.[92] Catecholamines (including therapeutic beta agonists) also increase this rate by making free fatty acids more available.[62] Other hormones, including glucagon, growth hormone, and glucocorticoids, also intensify the ketogenesis of insulin deficiency.[62,63,87,88] Vasopressin, on the other hand, decreases hepatic ketone production, and plasma free fatty acids also exert a suppressive effect on ketone production by inhibiting lipolysis.[16,32,81] It is of some interest with regard to the treatment of diabetic ketoacidosis that the antilipolytic effect of insulin appears to require higher blood levels than are needed to suppress glucose production, perhaps because of antagonism by other hormones.[101]

In contrast to starvation ketosis, patients with diabetic ketoacidosis are not in a steady state. Thus their urinary excretion rates of organic acid and net acid are not accurate reflections of the net acid production. Furthermore, due to uncertainties regarding the space of distribution of ketoacids and bicarbonate in the face of the alterations in body fluid volumes that occur in these patients, neither the level of serum ketones nor the fall in serum bicarbonate concentration appears to precisely estimate the amount of acid added to body fluids. In addition, it is clear that the increase in plasma unmeasured anions may correspond poorly to the fall in serum bicarbonate concentration, further complicating attempts to estimate the amount of acid added during the development of ketoacidosis[3] (see Chaps. 26 and 30). Net renal acid excretion will, however, play a significant role in H^+ elimination during diabetic ketoacidosis even though it does not serve to identify the magnitude of H^+ addition. Values of 4 to 5 μeq/min per kilogram of body weight early in the hospital course of patients with ketoacidosis have been reported.[3,71] It is of interest that these values appear to somewhat exceed the ketone accumulation rate of about 3 μmol/min per kilogram of body weight estimated from production and utilization measurements for the first 10 h after insulin withdrawal.[64] Even during the years before the availability of insulin, when experiments under controlled conditions were not possible, it was reported that early in the course of diabetic acidosis the renal acid excretory rate rises promptly and is little different from the excretion rate of ketones.[105] Thus, it seems likely that other factors serve to depress ketone utilization so that net H^+ production significantly exceeds maximal rates of renal H^+ excretion. It also seems likely that the associated volume depletion leads to impairment in hepatic, renal, and peripheral blood flow and, thus, to depressed ketone oxidation. Acute or chronic depressions of the glomerular filtration rate will also act to decrease renal net acid excretion, thus rendering acid balance more positive. Finally, because of the acidosis, the liver may switch from being a net lactate utilizer to a lactate producer, resulting in lactic acidemia, which would contribute to the severity of the metabolic acidosis.[54,58]

Another aspect of acid balance that has been indicated by these studies of acid excretion is the loss of potential base represented by the urinary excretion of ketones that are not in the form of free acid or NH_4^+ salts. When ketone excretion is not hampered by severe volume contraction, the loss of the Na^+ and K^+ salts of the ketoacids may exceed the rate of net acid excretion.[70] This is directly analogous to the fecal loss of potential base in the form of organic anions discussed earlier. When acid overproduction is curtailed by insulin administration, serum ketoacids can be metabolized to bicarbonate. The prior urinary loss of ketoacid salts (unaccompanied by H^+) may delay the recovery from acidosis.[68] This anion loss is also thought to be responsible for the hyperchloremic acidosis observed in approximately 10 to 50 percent of patients admitted with diabetic ketosis.[3]

Organic acid accumulation may also suppress organic acid production. This concept has been specifically applied to alterations in either lactic or ketoacid production secondary to either experimental manipulations of acid-base balance or alkali therapy in pathophysiological states of acid overproduction. In vitro studies utilizing a variety of tissues appear to support the idea that low pH inhibits and high pH stimulates lactic and ketoacid production.[5,25,31,43,65,79,89] In the latter case, however, this effect may be mediated by increasing pH or HCO_3^- concentration, which make free fatty acids more available through the activation of fat lipolysis.[106] Similar in vitro studies of lactic and ketoacid utilization are less clear, with alterations in pH causing gluconeogenesis and oxidation to increase, decrease, or remain unchanged, depending on the organ or tissue studied.[35] In vivo studies, however, have been more uniform regarding the effects of maneuvers that alter acid-base status. Administration of acid or alkali to fasted animals or humans blunts or stimulates, respectively, the fasting ketonemia.[36,60,86,97] Balance studies are consistent with acid administration inhibiting net ketone production and alkali administration stimulating net ketone production.[37] Acid has rarely been given intentionally in pathologic acidotic states. However, there is evidence that bicarbonate administration to diabetics with ketoacidosis and both patients and experimental animals with lactic acidosis increases the production of organic acids.[2,8,21,22,56,96] There are, however, major difficulties with these studies. While it seems clear that alkali or acid administration may affect organic acid production, it is by no means certain that it is some component of systemic acid-base status that controls this phenomenon. The changes in systemic pH, bicarbonate, and P_{CO_2} induced by alkali administration are much smaller than the alterations that have been reported to affect organic acid production in vitro as well as the activity of even the most exquisitely sensitive enzyme systems.[61,49,102] Although dogs with experimental lactic acidosis treated with sodium bicarbonate had a decrease in liver cell pH, this parameter was not correlated with decreases in hepatic lactate extraction.[8] In fact, the difference in blood lactate between animals treated with sodium bicarbonate and those treated with sodium chloride appears to be largely related to a major increase in splanchnic lactate production in the former in the face of essentially comparable acid-base parameters. In sum, although acid-base maneuvers appear to affect organic acid production in pathologic states, there is very little evidence for true "feedback" control in the sense of acid-base parameters acting to signal a change that limits their own excursions. The administration of $NaHCO_3$ as part of the treatment of organic acidosis has been reported to have an adverse effect on recovery, perhaps because of the accompanying increase in P_{CO_2} that accentuates intracellular acidosis, especially in the presence of hypoxia.[94] A mixture of $NaHCO_3$ and Na_2CO_3 that prevents the rise in P_{CO_2}[45] or dichloroacetate, a stimulator of pyruvate dehydrogenase,[59,95] are currently being evaluated as therapeutic agents for the treatment of severe organic acidosis.

Enzyme deficiencies, by preventing the normally complete oxidation of metabolic intermediates, can result in the accumulation of H^+. Those that can cause accumulation of H^+ as lactic acid are shown in Table 9-3.[77] Other enzyme deficiencies are associated with the accumulation of other acids and involve abnormalities in the metabolism of carbohydrates and the amino acids, especially leucine, isoleucine, and lysine. These defects, which are usually manifest at birth or during early infancy, are listed in Table 9-4. A review of this literature, however, reveals little in the way of quantitative data. In particular, few investigations of total organic acid production or net acid excretion have been performed, so that, in fact, there are no reliable estimates available of acid balance in these conditions.

To recapitulate, in health, large quantities of organic acids are produced and consumed in the body in nearly equivalent quantities each day. This endogenous acid turnover has little or no net affect on serum bicarbonate concentration, P_{CO_2}, or pH levels. Similarly, the relatively small quantities of acid that are produced in relation to the oxidation of dietary sulfur and fecal and urinary organic anion excretion are matched by the excretion of an equivalent quantity of acid in the urine, thus maintaining acid-base homeostasis. In disease, metabolic acidosis is the consequence of either augmented rates of acid production or impaired renal net acid excretion, or both.

TABLE 9-4 • Defects in carbohydrate, peptide or amino acid metabolism causing metabolic acidosis

Pathway	Enzyme defect	Organic acid accumulated	References
Tricarboxylic acid cycle	NADH-cytochrome c reductase	Succinic acid, ketoacids, lactic acid	9
Glycogen	Glycogen synthetase	Ketoacids	10
	Hepatic phosphorylase	Ketoacids	104
Glutathione	Glutathione synthetase	Pyroglutamic	30,40,47
Urea cycle	Carbamyl phosphate synthetase	Ketoacids	23
Lysine	Glutaconyl CoA decarboxylase	Glutaric, glutaconic and 3-hydroxyglutaric	29
	Multiple (glutaric aciduria type II)	Glutaric, lactic, α-hydroxybutyric, etc.	74
Leucine	Branched-chain ketoacid dehydrogenase (maple syrup urine disease)	2-Ketoisocaproic, 2-keto-3-methylvaleric, 2-keto-isovaleric	98
	Isovalerate CoA dehydrogenase	Isovaleric	14
	β-methylcrotonyl CoA carboxylase	β-methylcrotonic β-hydroxyisovaleric	27,85
	3-hydroxy-3-methylglutaryl CoA lyase	Hydroxymethylglutaric, 3-methylglutaconic, 3-hydroxyisovaleric 3-methylglutaric	20,90
Isoleucine	β-ketothiolase	α-methyl-β-hydroxybutyric 3-hydroxybutyric, lactic, acetoacetic, 2-methylacetoacetic, 3-hydroxyisovaleric	19,80
	Propionyl CoA carboxylase	Propionic	26
	Methylmalonyl CoA mutase	Methylmalonic, ketoacids	66,83
Tyrosine	*p*-Hydroxyphenylpyruvate oxidase	*p*-Hydroxyphenyllactic, *p*-hydroxyphenylacetic, *p*-hydroxyphenylpyruvic, and ketoacids	18
Glutamate-aspartate	Unknown (transport defect)	Ketoacids	99

REFERENCES

1. Adams ND et al: The calciuria of increased fixed acid production in humans: Evidence against the role for parathyroid hormone and 1,25-$(OH)_2$-vitamin D. *Calcif Tissue Int* 27:233, 1979.
2. Adlersberg D: Acetonurie und Acidose. *Biochem Z* 143:527, 1923.
3. Adrogué HJ et al: Plasma acid-base patterns in diabetic ketoacidosis. *N Engl J Med* 307:1603, 1982.
4. Alberti KGMM, Cuthbert C: The hydrogen ion in normal metabolism: A review, in Porter R, Lawrenson G (eds): *Metabolic Acidosis,* Ciba Foundation Symposium 87. London, Pitman, 1982, p 1.
5. Albrecht V et al: The influence of pH and methyline blue on the pathways of glucose utilization and lactate formation in erythrocytes of man. *Eur J Biochem* 20:44, 1971.
6. Allen LH et al: Protein-induced hypercalciuria: A longer term study. *Am J Clin Nutr* 32:741, 1979.
7. Altman PL, Katz DD (eds): *Human Health and Disease.* Bethesda: Federation of American Societies for Experimental Biology, 1977, p 194.
8. Arieff AI et al: Systemic effects of $NaHCO_3$ in experimental lactic acidosis in dogs. *Am J Physiol* 242:F586, 1982.
9. Asano K et al: Succinic acidemia: A new syndrome of organic acidemia associated with congenital lactic acidosis and decreased NADH-cytochrome c reductase activity. *Clin Chim Acta* 173:305, 1988.
10. Aynsley-Green A et al: Hepatic glycogen synthetase deficiency: Definition of syndrome from metabolic and enzyme studies on a 9-year-old girl. *Arch Dis Child* 52:573, 1977.
11. Balasse EO: Kinetics of ketone body metabolism in fasting humans. *Metabolism* 28:41, 1979.
12. Balasse EO, Havel RJ: Evidence for an effect of insulin on the peripheral utilization of ketone bodies in dogs. *J Clin Invest* 50:801, 1971.
13. Berry MN: The liver and lactic acidosis. *Proc R Soc Lond* 60:1260, 1967.
14. Budd MD et al: Isovaleric acidemia: Clinical features of a new genetic defect of leucine metabolism. *N Engl J Med* 277:321, 1967.
15. Buono MJ, Roby FB: Acid-base, metabolic, and ventilatory responses to repeated bouts of exercise. *J Appl Physiol* 53:436, 1982.
16. Burns TW et al: Site of free-fatty-acid inhibition of lipolysis by human adipocytes. *Metabolism* 24:265, 1975.
17. Cohen RD et al: The effect of changes in lactate uptake on the intracellular pH of the perfused rat liver. *Clin Sci* 41:159, 1971.
18. Danks DM et al: A new form of prolonged transient tyrosinemia presenting with severe metabolic acidosis. *Acta Paediatr Scand* 64:209, 1975.
19. Daum RS et al: An inherited disorder of isoleucine catabolism causing accumulation of α-methylacetoacetate and α-methyl-β-hydroxybutyrate, and intermittent acidosis. *Pediatr Res* 7:149, 1973.
20. Faull K et al: Patient with defect in leucine metabolism. *N Engl J Med* 294:1013, 1976.
21. Fields ALA et al: Chronic lactic acidosis in a patient with cancer: Therapy and metabolic consequences. *Cancer* 47:2026, 1981.
22. Fraley DS et al: Stimulation of lactate production by administration of bicarbonate in a patient with a solid neoplasm and lactic acidosis. *N Engl J Med* 303:1100, 1980.
23. Freeman JM et al: Congenital hyperammonemia. *Arch Neurol* 23:430, 1970.
24. Garber AJ et al: Hepatic ketogenesis and gluconeogenesis in humans. *J Clin Invest* 54:981, 1974.
25. Gevers W, Dowdle E: The effect of pH on glycolysis in vitro. *Clin Sci* 25:343, 1963.
26. Gompertz D et al: Localization of enzymatic defect in propionicacidemia. *Lancet* 1:1140, 1970.
27. Gompertz D et al: Biotin-responsive β-methylcrotonylglycinuria. *Lancet* 2:22, 1971.
28. Goodman AD et al: Production, excretion and net balance of fixed acid in patients with renal acidosis. *J Clin Invest* 44:495, 1965.
29. Goodman SI et al: Glutaric aciduria: Biochemical and morphological considerations. *J Pediatr* 90:746, 1977.
30. Hagenfeldt L et al: Pyroglutamic aciduria. *Acta Paediatr Scand* 63:1, 1974.
31. Halperin M et al: Factors that control the effect of pH on glycolysis in leukocytes. *J Biol Chem* 244:384, 1969.

31a. Halperin ML, Jungas RL: Metabolic production and renal disposal of hydrogen ions. *Kidney Int* 24:709, 1983.

32. Hems DA: Rapid hormonal control of hepatic catabolism in health and disease. *Clin Sci* 56:197, 1979.
33. Hermansen L, Vaage O: Lactate disappearance and glycogen synthesis in human muscle after maximal exercise. *Am J Physiol* 233:E422, 1977.
34. Hochachka PW, Mommsen TP: Protons and anaerobiasis. *Science* 219:1391, 1983.
35. Hood VL, Tannen RL: pH control of lactic acid and keto acid production: A mechanism of acid-base regulation. *Miner Electrolyte Metab* 9:317, 1983.
36. Hood VL et al: Impact of hydrogen ion on fasting ketogenesis: Feedback regulation of acid production. *Am J Physiol* 242:F238, 1982.
37. Hood VL et al: Systemic pH modifies ketone body production rates and lipolysis in humans. *Am J Physiol* 259:E327, 1990.
38. Hunt JN: The influence of dietary sulfur on the urinary output of acid in man. *Clin Sci* 15:119, 1956.
39. Iampietro PF et al: Composition and caloric density of weight loss during caloric restriction in cold. *J Appl Physiol* 16:624, 1961.
40. Jellum E et al: Pyroglutamic aciduria: A new inborn error of metabolism. *Scand J Clin Lab Invest* 26:327, 1970.
41. Jenkins DW et al: Alcoholic ketoacidosis. *JAMA* 217:177, 1971.
42. Johnston DG, Alberti KGMM: Acid-base balance in metabolic acidosis. *Clin Endocrinol Metab* 12:267, 1983.
43. Katzman R et al: Effect of increased carbon dioxide concentrations on fixed acid production in vitro. *Am J Physiol* 172:317, 1953.
44. Kleinman JG et al: Cell pH and acid transport in renal cortical tissue. *Am J Physiol* 239:F440, 1980.
45. Kucera RR et al: Brain pH effects of $NaHCO_3$ and Carbicarb® in lactic acidosis. *Crit Care Med* 17:1320, 1989.

46. Kurtz I et al: Effect of diet on plasma acid-base composition in normal humans. *Kidney Int* 24:670, 1983.
47. Larsson A et al: Pyroglutamic aciduria (5-oxoprolinuria), an inborn error in glutathione metabolism. *Pediatr Res* 8:852, 1974.
48. Lemann J Jr: Unpublished observations.
49. Lemann J Jr, Lennon EJ: Role of diet, gastrointestinal tract and bone in acid-base homeostasis. *Kidney Int* 1:275, 1972.
50. Lemann J Jr, Relman AS: The relation of sulfur metabolism to acid-base balance and electrolyte excretion: The effects of DL-methionine in normal man. *J Clin Invest* 38:2215, 1959.
51. Lemann J Jr et al: The net balance of acid in subjects given large loads of acid or alkali. *J Clin Invest* 44:507, 1965.
52. Lemann J Jr et al: The effects of chronic acid loads in normal man: Further evidence for the participation of bone in the defense against chronic metabolic acidosis. *J Clin Invest* 45:1608, 1966.
53. Lennon EJ et al: The effects of diet and stool composition on the net external acid balance of normal subjects. *J Clin Invest* 45:1601, 1966.
54. Lennon EJ et al: The effects of phosphoproteins on acid balance in normal subjects. *J Clin Invest* 41:637, 1962.
55. Levy LJ et al: Ketoacidosis associated with alcoholism in nondiabetic subjects. *Ann Intern Med* 78:213, 1973.
56. Lipsky SR et al: The effects of alkalosis upon ketone body production and carbohydrate metabolism in man. *J Clin Invest* 33:1269, 1954.
57. Lloyd MH et al: Effect of phenformin on gluconeogenesis from lactate and intracellular pH in the isolated perfused guinea pig liver. *Diabetes* 24:618, 1975.
58. Lloyd MH et al: The effect of simulated metabolic acidosis in intracellular pH and lactate metabolism in the isolated perfused rat liver. *Clin Sci* 45:543, 1973.
59. Ludvik B et al: Effects of dichloroacetate and bicarbonate on haemodynamic parameters in healthy volunteers. *Clin Sci* 80:47, 1991.
60. Mackay EM et al: The influence of alkalosis and acidosis upon fasting ketosis. *J Biol Chem* 138:63, 1941.
61. Mansour TE: Studies on heart phosphofructokinase: Purification, inhibition and activation. *J Biol Chem* 238:2285, 1963.
62. Miles JM et al: Effects of free fatty acids, insulin, glucagon and adrenalin on ketone body production in humans, in Porter R, Lawrenson G (eds): *Metabolic Acidosis,* Ciba Foundation Symposium 87. London, Pitman, 1982, p 192.
63. Miles JM, Gerich JE: Glucose and ketone body kinetics in diabetic ketoacidosis. *Clin Endocrinol Metab* 12:303, 1983.
64. Miles JM et al: Effects of acute insulin deficiency on glucose and ketone body turnover in man: Evidence for the primary of overproduction of glucose and ketone bodies in the genesis of diabetic ketoacidosis. *Diabetes* 29:926, 1980.
65. Minakami S et al: Hydrogen ion concentrations and erythrocyte glycolysis. *Biochem Biophys Res Commun* 17:748, 1964.
66. Oberholzer VG et al: Methylmalonic aciduria: An inborn error of metabolism leading to chronic metabolic acidosis. *Arch Dis Child* 42:492, 1967.
67. Oh MS: A new method for estimating G-I absorption of alkali. *Kidney Int* 36:915, 1989.
68. Oh MS et al: The mechanism of hyperchloremic acidosis during the recovery phase of diabetic ketoacidosis. *Diabetes* 30:310, 1981.
69. Osnes J-B, Hermansen L: Acid-base balance after maximal exercise of short duration. *J Appl Physiol* 32:59, 1972.
70. Oster JR, Epstein M: Acid-base aspects of ketoacidosis. *Am J Nephrol* 4:137, 1984.
71. Owen OE et al: Renal function and effects of partial rehydration during diabetic ketoacidosis. *Diabetes* 30:510, 1981.
72. Owen OE et al: Liver and kidney metabolism during prolonged starvation. *J Clin Invest* 48:574, 1969.
73. Park R, Arieff AI: Lactic acidosis. *Adv Intern Med* 25:33, 1980.
74. Przyrembel H et al: Glutaric aciduria type II: Report of a previously undescribed metabolic disorder. *Clin Chim Acta* 66:227, 1976.
75. Radda GK et al: Energy metabolism and cellular pH, in Porter R, Lawrenson G (eds): *Metabolic Acidosis,* Ciba Foundation Symposium 87. London, Pitman, 1982, p 36.
76. Reichard GA Jr et al: Ketone body production and oxidation in fasting obese humans. *J Clin Invest* 53:508, 1974.
77. Relman AS: Lactic acidosis, in Brenner BM, Stein JH (eds): *Acid-Base and Potassium Homeostasis, Contemporary Issues in Nephrology.* New York, Churchill Livingstone, 1978, vol 2, p 65.
78. Relman AS et al: Endogenous production of fixed acid and the measurement of the net balance of acid in normal subjects. *J Clin Invest* 40:1621, 1961.
79. Relman AS: Metabolic consequences of acid-base disorders. *Kidney Int* 1:347, 1972.
80. Robinson BH et al: Acetoacetyl CoA thiolase deficiency: A cause of severe ketoacidosis in infancy simulating salicylism. *J Pediatr* 95:228, 1979.
81. Rodbell M: Modulation of lipolysis in adipose tissue by fatty acid concentration in fat cell. *Ann N Y Acad Sci* 131:302, 1965.
82. Roos A, Boron WF: Intracellular pH. *Physiol Rev* 61:296, 1981.
83. Rosenberg LE et al: Methylmalonic aciduria: An inborn error of metabolism leading to chronic metabolic acidosis, long-chain ketonuria and intermittent hyperglycinemia. *N Engl J Med* 278:1319, 1968.
84. Ross BD et al: Preliminary observations on the metabolic response to exercise in humans using ^{31}phosphorus nuclear magnetic resonance, in Porter R, Lawrenson G (eds): *Metabolic Acidosis,* Ciba Foundation Symposium 87. London, Pitman, 1982, p 145.
85. Roth K et al: Beta-methylcrotonic aciduria associated with lactic acidosis. *J Pediatr* 88:229, 1976.
86. Sapir DG et al: The role of potassium in the control of ammonium excretion during starvation. *Metabolism* 25:211, 1976.
87. Schade D et al: The regulation of plasma ketone body concentrations by counter-regulatory hormones in man:

2. Effects of growth hormone in diabetic man. *Diabetes* 27:916, 1978.
88. Schade D et al: Glucocorticoid regulation of plasma ketone body concentration in insulin deficient man. *J Clin Endocrinol Metab* 44:1069, 1977.
89. Scheuer J, Berry MN: Effect of alkalosis on glycolysis in the isolated rat heart. *Am J Physiol* 213:1143, 1967.
90. Schutgens RBH et al: Lethal hypoglycemia in a child with a deficiency of 3-hydroxy-3-methylglutarylcoenzyme A lyase. *J Pediatr* 94:89, 1979.
91. Sestoft L, Bartels PD: Biochemistry and differential diagnosis of metabolic acidosis. *Clin Endocrinol Metab* 12:287, 1983.
92. Sestoft L et al: Regulation of gluconeogenesis and ketogenesis during rest and exercise in diabetic subjects and normal men. *Clin Sci* 53:411, 1977.
93. Sherman HC, Gettler AO: The balance of acid-forming and base-forming elements in food, and its relation to ammonia metabolism. *J Biol Chem* 11:323, 1912.
94. Stacpoole PW: Lactic acidosis: The case against bicarbonate therapy. *Ann Intern Med* 105:276, 1986.
95. Stacpoole PW et al: Dichloroacetate in the treatment of lactic acidosis. *Ann Intern Med* 108:58, 1988.
96. Staubli C: Beiträge sur Patholgic and Therapie des Diabetes Mellitus. *Deutsch Arch Klin Med* 93:107, 1908.
97. Stinebaugh BJ et al: Mechanism for the paradoxical aciduria following alkali administration to prolonged-fasted patients. *Metabolism* 24:915, 1975.
98. Sweetman L: Branched chain organic aciduria, in Scriver CR et al (eds): *The Metabolic Basis of Inherited Disease,* 6th ed. New York, McGraw-Hill, 1989, p 791.
99. Teijema HL et al: Dicarboxylic aciduria: An inborn error of glutamate and asparatate transport with metabolic implications, in combination with a hyperprolinemia. *Metabolism* 23:115, 1974.
100. Thomas DJB et al: Salbutamol-induced diabetic ketoacidosis. *Br Med J* 2:438, 1977.
101. Thomas S et al: Insulin action on adipocytes. *Biochem J* 184:355, 1979.
102. Trivedi B, Danforth WH: Effect of pH on the kinetics of frog muscle phosphofructokinase. *J Biol Chem* 241:4110, 1966.
103. Vaghy PL: Role of mitochondrial oxidative phosphorylation in the maintenance of intracellular pH. *J Mol Cell Cardiol* 11:933, 1979.
104. Van Creveld S, Huiying F: Glycogen storage disease. Biochemical and clinical data in sixteen cases. *Am J Med* 38:554, 1965.
105. Van Slyke DD, Palmer WW: Studies of acidosis: 16. The titration of organic acids in urine. *J Biol Chem* 41:567, 1920.
106. Vega FU, de Cingolani GEC: Effect of pH on epinephrine induced lipolysis in isolated fat cells. *Am J Physiol* 227:168, 1974.
107. Wasserman K et al: Interaction of physiological mechanisms during exercise. *J Appl Physiol* 22:71, 1967.
108. Wasserman K et al: Gas exchange theory and the lactic acidosis (anaerobic) threshold. *Circulation* 81:II-14, 1990.
109. Weber HP et al: The lack of effect of chronic metabolic acidosis on 25-OH-vitamin D metabolism and serum parathyroid hormone in humans. *J Clin Endocrinol Metab* 43:1047, 1976.
110. Wolfe BM et al: Effect of a 3-day fast and of ethanol on splanchnic metabolism of FFA, amino acids and carbohydrates in healthy young men. *J Clin Invest* 57:329, 1976.
111. Wrong OD et al: *The Large Intestine: Its Role in Mammalian Nutrition and Homeostasis.* New York, Wiley, 1981, p 15.

CHAPTER • 10

Renal regulation of acid-base metabolism

Orson W. Moe • Floyd C. Rector, Jr. • Robert J. Alpern

Extracellular pH must be precisely regulated because the function of almost all physiologic processes is impaired when pH is not maintained within the normal physiologic range. Extracellular pH is a determinant of the fraction of extracellular calcium that is ionized. It directly affects the solubility of bone salts and may influence the affinity of plasma transport proteins for their substrates. The most important role of extracellular pH, however, is in the regulation of cell pH. Almost all cellular functions are mediated by enzymes whose structure and function is dependent on the pH of the intracellular milieu. Thus, pathologic changes in cell pH have marked effects on cell function. In addition, small changes in cell pH are often involved in the regulation of key cell functions such as metabolism and cell division.

A number of mechanisms help to regulate extracellular and intracellular pH. First are the extracellular and intracellular buffer systems, which serve to minimize the pH change that occurs in response to addition of acid or base. Second, the lungs protect pH by altering systemic P_{CO_2}. Finally, the kidneys excrete acid or base so as to return the pH of extracellular fluid to normal.

Cells, in addition, possess independent mechanisms that protect intracellular pH in the presence of changes in extracellular pH. These include the ability to alter the rate of acid generation from metabolism, and active hydrogen ion extruding mechanisms. This chapter will briefly discuss the importance of buffers in pH regulation, the mechanisms that regulate cellular pH, and some of the nonrenal mechanisms that contribute to the regulation of the extracellular pH. It will then concentrate on the renal mechanisms by which extracellular pH is regulated.

BUFFER CHEMISTRY

GENERAL

Both intracellular and extracellular fluid contain buffers that help prevent large changes in pH. All buffer systems include an acidic and a basic moiety, which participate in the following reaction:

$$\text{Acid} \rightleftharpoons H^+ + \text{base}$$

Addition of H^+ to a solution of buffer permits base molecules to accept the H^+ and form the conjugate acid. This tends to decrease the magnitude of the change in free hydrogen ion concentration and thus to reduce the change in pH.

Buffers are characterized by a dissociation constant, K_d, which defines the concentrations of the different moieties at equilibrium:

$$K_d = \frac{[\text{base}]\,[H^+]}{[\text{acid}]} \quad (1)$$

Because acid-base reactions are extremely rapid, acid-base components are essentially always at equilibrium, and their concentrations therefore are always described by equation 1. If one defines pX as the negative logarithm of X, equation 1 can be rearranged to yield the Henderson-Hasselbalch equation:

$$\text{pH} = \text{p}K + \log\frac{[\text{base}]}{[\text{acid}]} \quad (2)$$

Buffer capacity is the number of moles of strong acid or base needed to lower or raise the pH of one liter of buffer solution by one pH unit.

Buffer systems can be "closed" or "open." The more typical system is closed, the total concentration of the acidic and basic moieties (total buffer content) being constant. In a closed system, if one acidic molecule is removed, a basic molecule must be formed. Closed buffers exert their greatest effect when pH is equal to pK and essentially lose all buffer capacity when pH is more than 2 units away from pK. In an open buffer system, one of the components of the acid-base pair can enter or leave the system. The concentration of this component is usually held constant while the concentration of the other component varies with pH. Open buffers are unusual in that they can function as good buffers many pH units away from their pK. When an open buffer's acid can enter or leave the system, it exerts a greater buffer capacity at higher pH values (e.g., the bicarbonate–carbonic acid buffer system). Conversely, when an open buffer's base can enter or leave the system, it exerts a greater buffer capacity at lower pH (e.g., the ammonia-ammonium buffer system). Phosphate, hemoglobin, and albumin are physiologically important closed buffer systems; bicarbonate-CO_2 and ammonia-ammonium are important open buffer systems.

BICARBONATE–CARBONIC ACID–CO_2 BUFFER SYSTEM

Bicarbonate, carbonic acid, and carbon dioxide form the major buffer system in extracellular fluid. This buffer system provides the first line of defense in protecting extracellular fluid pH. Like all other buffer systems, it includes an acid (carbonic acid), which is capable of donating a proton, and a base (bicarbonate), which is capable of accepting a proton:

$$\underset{\text{Carbonic acid}}{H_2CO_3} \rightleftharpoons \underset{\text{Proton}}{H^+} + \underset{\text{Bicarbonate}}{HCO_3^-}$$

The dissociation constant for the reaction is given by equation 3:

$$K_{d_{H_2CO_3}} = \frac{[H^+]\,[HCO_3^-]}{[H_2CO_3]} = 2.7 \times 10^{-4}M \qquad (3)$$

The bicarbonate buffer system is an open buffer system due to the dissociation reaction:

$$\underset{\text{Carbonic acid}}{H_2CO_3} \rightleftharpoons \underset{\text{Water}}{H_2O} + \underset{\text{Carbon dioxide}}{CO_2}$$

Carbon dioxide can enter or leave this system, thus effectively allowing carbonic acid to enter or leave. The complete equilibrium reactions, therefore, are

$$H^+ + HCO_3^- \rightleftharpoons H_2CO_3 \rightleftharpoons H_2O + CO_2$$

In extracellular fluid, the concentration of CO_2 is held constant by ventilation (see below), and the concentration of water is constant. Thus, if the buffer system is at equilibrium, the concentration of carbonic acid is maintained constant by the lungs. Addition of 1 meq of protons to a liter of extracellular fluid causes 1 meq of bicarbonate to form carbonic acid. The transient increase in carbonic acid and carbon dioxide concentration stimulates ventilation so that these values are returned to baseline. Thus, the concentration of bicarbonate drops by 1 meq/liter, but the concentration of carbonic acid remains constant.

If the CO_2 reactions are included in the acid-base equilibrium reactions, the relevant equation is

$$K = \frac{[H^+]\,[HCO_3^-]}{\alpha P_{CO_2}} = 8.1 \times 10^{-7}M \qquad (4)$$

where α is the CO_2 solubility coefficient. In most physiologic solutions, α is approximately 0.03 mM/mmHg. Equation 4 can be rewritten in the Henderson-Hasselbalch form as shown in equation 5:

$$\text{pH} = \text{p}K' + \log\frac{[HCO_3^-]}{\alpha P_{CO_2}} \qquad (5)$$

where the pK' equals 6.1. This form has the advantage that it clearly shows that regulation of pH is performed by two separate mechanisms: (1) the bicarbonate concentration is maintained by the kidney, and (2) the P_{CO_2} is regulated by the lungs. It must be emphasized, however, that these equations, which include CO_2, are only valid if carbonic acid and CO_2 are in equilibrium. As will be discussed below, this is a valid assumption in blood and in many other compartments of the body.

CARBONIC ANHYDRASE

The dissociation of carbonic acid to form protons and bicarbonate occurs instantaneously and is thus essentially always at equilibrium. The hydration of CO_2 to form carbonic acid and the dehydration of carbonic acid to form CO_2, however, do not occur as quickly and thus are often not at equilibrium. In certain key locations, such as red blood cells, lungs, and kidneys, this reaction must be accelerated for normal function. For this purpose, there is an enzyme, carbonic anhydrase, that accelerates both the hydration and the dehydration reaction equally and thus does not change the equilibrium constant. In the presence of carbonic anhydrase, the hydration and dehydration reactions occur extremely rapidly such that the system is essentially always at equilibrium and equation 5 is valid. Because carbonic anhydrase is present in red blood cells, the Henderson-Hasselbalch equation (equation 5) is valid for blood. The physiologic importance of this enzyme will be discussed repeatedly throughout this chapter.

REGULATION OF INTRACELLULAR pH

Maintenance of cell pH is important for optimal functioning of the complex metabolic machinery of the cell. In addition, certain cellular functions, such as glycolysis and cell division, appear to be regulated by small changes in cell pH.

Cell membranes are permeable to some extent to protons (H^+) and/or hydroxyl ions (OH^-). Consequently, the membrane potential difference of 60 to 90 mV, interior negative, will tend to cause hydrogen ions to enter the cell and hydroxyl (or bicarbonate) ions to leave the cell. If there were no energy input into cell pH regulation, the cell would be more acidic than its exterior by 1.0 to 1.5 pH units. Nontransporting cells are more acidic inside than outside, but they are not as acidic internally as the potential difference would dictate.[226]

Cell pH is kept constant by a balance of processes that add or remove protons from the cell. Because cells are more alkaline than would be predicted for electrochemical equilibrium, a driving force is always present, causing hydrogen ions to enter the cell and bicarbonate (and hydroxyl) ions to diffuse out of the cell. In addition, metabolic processes generate intracellular acid. Cell pH is maintained by processes that actively remove hydrogen ions from the cell at the same rate at which acid is generated within the cell from metabolism and from passive leak pathways.

The active removal of acid from cells occurs by different mechanisms in different cell types.[226] These mechanisms are shown in Fig. 10-1. All of these mechanisms are classified as secondary-active, in that active transport processes establish electrochemical gradients for sodium (Na^+) or chloride (Cl^-), and these gradients are then able secondarily to transport hydrogen and bicarbonate against their respective electrochemical gradients. The inward coupled movement of sodium and bicarbonate in exchange for the coupled outward movement of a proton and chloride (Fig. 10-1, mechanism 2) appears to be the predominant mechanism in lower animal forms; in *Necturus* and mammalian cells sodium-proton exchange (Fig. 10-1, mechanism 1) is the predominant mechanism of cellular proton extrusion. These secondary-active transport mechanisms are capable of achieving a greater degree of cellular alkalinity than actually exists. If the cell sodium concentration is 10 times less than that of plasma, one can calculate that a neutral sodium-proton antiporter would be capable of raising the cell's pH 1.0 unit above extracellular pH. Cells also can defend against an alkaline cell pH. For this purpose, most cells utilize a Cl/HCO_3 exchange (Fig. 10-1, mechanism 3).

Thus, maintenance of cell pH involves a steady state in which multiple processes proceed simultaneously. Acid is continuously leaking into the cell and is being generated by metabolism. Acid is also being removed from the cell by active transport mechanisms at the same rate at which it is being formed. Regulatory changes in the rate of acid extrusion, accomplished by altering the activity of the sodium-proton exchanger, can lead to changes in cell pH that are used to regulate certain processes, such as glycolysis or cell division.[134]

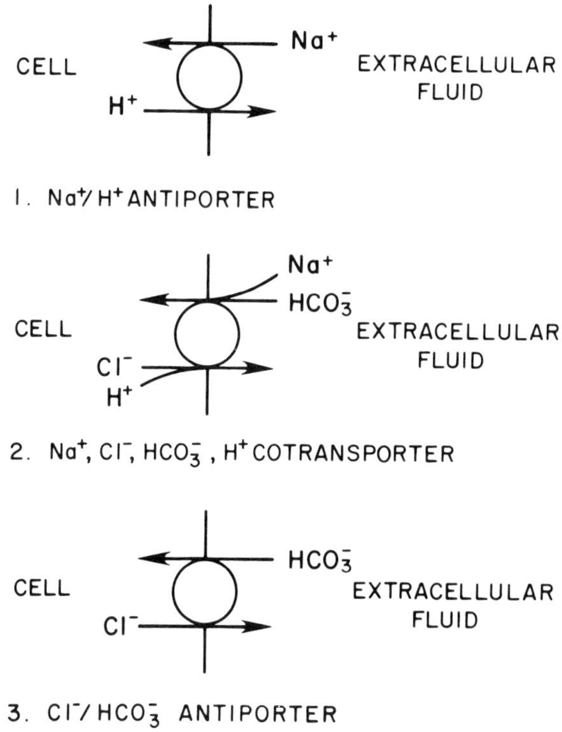

FIGURE 10-1 • Mechanisms of cellular pH regulation.

Sudden addition of acid or base to the cell (as would occur with changes in extracellular pH) lead to only small changes in cell pH because of the large buffer capacity of the cells. In addition, these small changes in cell pH lead to changes in the rate of metabolism and of active acid extrusion that tend to return cell pH toward normal. Of particular importance is the finding that the activity of the sodium-proton exchanger increases in a nonlinear fashion as internal hydrogen ion concentration increases.[16] Changes in extracellular fluid pH do lead to changes in cell pH, but the mechanisms described above make these changes small.

EXTRARENAL ACID-BASE BALANCE

CO_2 PRODUCTION AND EXCRETION

The cells of the body normally produce approximately 13 mol of CO_2 per day. Since tissue CO_2 tensions are greater than the CO_2 tension of arterial plasma, CO_2 diffuses into the plasma. In plasma, CO_2 is carried in one of three ways:

1. The process of *simple solution* is limited by the solubility coefficient of CO_2 (0.03 m*M*/mmHg).
2. *Bicarbonate formation* occurs as follows:

$$CO_2 + H_2O \rightarrow H_2CO_3 \rightarrow H^+ + HCO_3^-$$

This process is limited by two factors. The first is that there is *no* carbonic anhydrase in plasma, which makes carbonic acid formation slow. Second, hydrogen ions formed must be buffered, and the buffering capacity of plasma is small.
3. Reaction of CO_2 with amino groups of proteins forms *carbamino* compounds:

$$R{-}NH_2 + CO_2 \rightarrow R{-}NH{-}COO^- + H^+$$

Once again, a hydrogen ion is formed, and it must be buffered.

Thus, because of the low buffering capacity of plasma and the absence of carbonic anhydrase, the CO_2-carrying capacity of plasma is small. CO_2 can, however, enter red blood cells, which contain carbonic anhydrase and hemoglobin (which has a large buffering capacity in the physiologic pH range). CO_2 that enters red blood cells can remain dissolved. It can also rapidly form hydrogen ion and bicarbonate; the hydrogen ion is buffered by hemoglobin, and the bicarbonate leaves the cell in exchange for chloride. In this manner, increases in P_{CO_2} cause chloride to enter red blood cells; the process is referred to as the *chloride shift*. Finally, the CO_2 can form carbamino compounds with hemoglobin; the hydrogen ion formed will be buffered by the hemoglobin. Thus, the majority of CO_2 is carried effectively by red blood cells.

Pulmonary interstitial CO_2 tension is very low, causing CO_2 to leave the blood and consequently reverse all of the abovementioned processes. The kidney takes no part in the excretion of CO_2. If cellular CO_2 generation exceeds pulmonary CO_2 excretion, blood CO_2 tension rises, leading to an increase in hydrogen ion and bicarbonate concentrations. Conversely, if pulmonary CO_2 excretion exceeds cellular CO_2 generation, blood CO_2 tension decreases, leading to a decrease in hydrogen ion and bicarbonate concentrations. In general, however, the balance between metabolic production of CO_2 by tissues and excretion of CO_2 by the lungs is very precise, maintaining arterial P_{CO_2} at approximately 40 mmHg.

EXTRARENAL NONVOLATILE ACID PRODUCTION

In addition to producing the volatile acid CO_2 as described above, the body generates nonvolatile acids. An average person generates approximately 1 meq of nonvolatile acid per kilogram of body weight per day. This leads to a small increase in the hydrogen ion concentration of the extracellular fluid and subsequent titration of bicarbonate and nonbicarbonate buffers. The nonbicarbonate buffers titrated include cellular and bone buffers. Thus, for every 1 meq of net acid generated, 1 meq of bicarbonate is consumed or nonbicarbonate buffer is acidified. In the absence of kidneys, this acidification would gradually lead to a progressive metabolic acidosis.

The kidneys prevent this acidosis by excreting hydrogen ions each day in an amount equivalent to the quantity of hydrogen ions generated by extrarenal mechanisms. This is one of the two major functions of the kidney in acid-base balance. It is referred to as *bicarbonate regeneration* but actually represents the regeneration of both bicarbonate and basic nonbicarbonate buffer. Exactly how the renal tubules regenerate base is discussed below.

ROLE OF THE KIDNEY IN ACID-BASE BALANCE

As stated earlier, one of the major roles of the kidney in acid-base regulation is to regenerate base consumed by extrarenal acid production. The kidney performs this role by the excretion of acid. Net acid excretion (NAE) is defined by the equation:

$$\text{NAE} = (r_{NH_4} + r_{TA}) - r_{HCO_3^-} \qquad (6)$$

where r_{NH_4} = rate of ammonium excretion
r_{TA} = rate of titratable acid excretion
$r_{HCO_3^-}$ = rate of bicarbonate excretion

Ammonium and titratable acids are the two types of urinary buffers that help to excrete acid. These buffers are described in depth in the following section.

Any bicarbonate that appears in the urine is equivalent to net base excretion and thus must be subtracted from the NAE. Under normal conditions, approximately 4300 meq of bicarbonate is filtered by the glomerulus each day. It is obvious that if even small fractions of this filtered bicarbonate were excreted, NAE would become negative and acidosis would quickly develop. The second major function of the kidney in acid-base balance is therefore to reabsorb or reclaim most of this filtered bicarbonate. This process is referred to as *bicarbonate reclamation*.

Certain organic anions, such as citrate, ketoanions, and lactate, are metabolized to bicarbonate and can be viewed as bicarbonate equivalents. Strictly speaking, these anions should be represented in equation 6 because their loss in the urine amounts to loss of bicarbonate. Normally, 24-h citrate excretion is between 5 and 10 meq, and that of lactate and ketoanions is virtually zero. In metabolic alkalosis, urinary citrate can increase up to 17 meq/day and will contribute significantly to net base excretion. Similarly, in keto- and lactic acidosis, urinary loss of these organic anions can amount to substantial loss of potential bicarbonate. Therefore, in appropriate clinical situations, the bicarbonate term in equation 6 should be modified to "bicarbonate equivalent" to include organic anions.

In summary, the kidney serves two major functions in acid-base balance. First, it reclaims most of the filtered bicarbonate. Second, it regenerates base by excreting ammonium and titratable acid. In order for the body to remain in acid-base balance, the rate of renal NAE must equal the rate of extrarenal nonvolatile acid production.

FILTRATION OF BICARBONATE

From the foregoing discussion, it is clear that the glomerulus does not participate in renal acidification but actually contributes to the load placed on the kidney. Decreases in glomerular filtration rate (GFR) do not impaír renal acidification except as they correlate with loss of renal mass and consequent reduction of ammonia production. GFR can, however, be an important regulator of the plasma bicarbonate concentration by affecting the load placed on the kidney. At normal plasma bicarbonate concentrations, GFR is not very important because increases in it are accompanied by concomitant increases in tubular bicarbonate absorption; acid excretion is thus unaffected (Fig. 10-2*a*).[56,210] This glomerulotubular balance is due to increases in tubular flow rate, secondary to the increased GFR, that markedly stimulate proximal tubular bicarbonate absorption (a thorough discussion of the mechanism of this phenomenon is presented below).[14,47] In the presence of high plasma bicarbonate concentrations (metabolic alkalosis), however, GFR becomes very important. In this situation, bicarbonate absorption is no longer flow-dependent and remains constant as GFR increases (Fig. 10-2*b*).[55] Increases in GFR in this condition lead to marked bicarbonaturia; decreases in GFR can prevent bicarbonaturia. Cogan and Liu have emphasized that this is an important mechanism by which alkalosis is maintained in volume depletion and potassium deficiency.[55]

URINARY BUFFERS

As described earlier, the kidney must excrete about 70 meq/day of hydrogen ions that have been generated extrarenally. If this quantity of H^+ were excreted in 2 liters of water, the pH of the solution would be 1.5. This would force the kidney to secrete hydrogen ions against a large chemical gradient and would markedly increase the energy requirements of acid-base balance. This problem is prevented by the excretion of large amounts of buffer in the urine. Thus, 70 meq of hydrogen ions can be excreted by merely lowering the urine pH to appproximately 6.0 and titrating 70 meq of buffer with the H^+. There are two major buffer systems in the urine: titratable acid and ammonia.

TITRATABLE ACID EXCRETION

Titratable buffers include a group of "closed system" buffers that are filtered by the glomerulus and are capable of being titrated within the pH range achieved in the kidney. A good example, and certainly the most important, of the titratable buffers is phosphate. The phosphate buffer system includes four components: phosphoric acid and mono-, di-, and tribasic phosphates:

$$\underset{\text{Phosphoric acid}}{H_3PO_4} \rightleftharpoons H^+ + \underset{\text{Monobasic phosphate}}{H_2PO_4^-} \rightleftharpoons 2H^+ + \underset{\text{Dibasic phosphate}}{HPO_4^{2-}}$$
$$\rightleftharpoons 3H^+ + \underset{\text{Tribasic phosphate}}{PO_4^{3-}}$$

Phosporic acid exists only in solutions of pH far below those achieved in the plasma or urine. Conversely, tribasic phosphate exists only in solutions of pH far above those achieved in plasma or urine. Thus, the only relevant moieties in this buffer system are the monobasic and dibasic buffer pair:

$$H_2PO_4^- \rightleftharpoons H^+ + HPO_4^{2-}$$

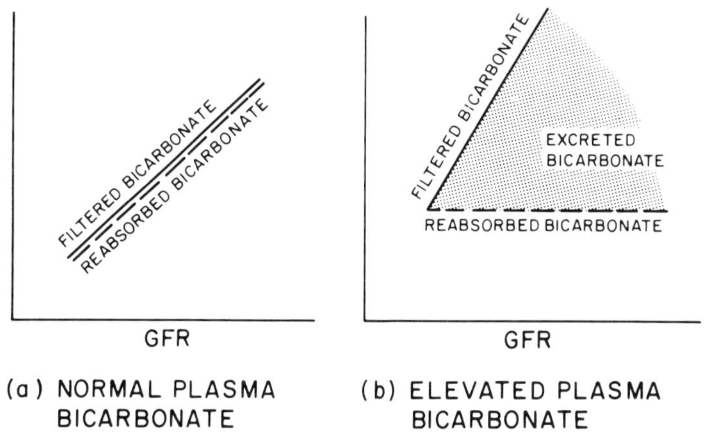

FIGURE 10-2 • Effect of glomerular filtration rate (GFR) on bicarbonate reabsorption and excretion. In the presence of a normal plasma bicarbonate concentration, bicarbonate reabsorption increases with GFR; the rate of bicarbonate excretion is unaffected. In the presence of an elevated plasma bicarbonate concentration, bicarbonate reabsorption is relatively fixed; bicarbonate excretion increases as GFR increases.

This buffer system has a pK of 6.9. The relative concentrations of the two forms of phosphate are determined by

$$pH = 6.9 + \log\frac{[HPO_4^{2-}]}{[H_2PO_4^-]} \quad (7)$$

or

$$[HPO_4^{2-}] = [H_2PO_4^-] \times 10^{(pH - 6.9)} \quad (8)$$

Because the phosphate buffer system is a closed buffer system, the total concentration of phosphate is not affected by urinary acidification. At pH 6.9, half of the total phosphate buffer is in the acid form and half in the basic form. In plasma at pH 7.4, one-fourth of the phosphate is in the acid form. When this phosphate appears in urine at pH 6.0, 90 percent of the phosphate is in the acid form. The number of protons secreted by the kidney and buffered by phosphate (TA_{PHOS}) in this situaton can be calculated as

$$TA_{PHOS} = (0.90 - 0.25)\ (r_{t,PO_4}) \quad (9)$$

where r_{t,PO_4} is equal to the total rate of phosphate excretion. Since 90 percent of phosphate is already in the acid form at pH 6.0, further acidification would add little more acid phosphate to the urine. There are, however, other titratable acids in the urine.

Because there are many closed, titratable buffer systems in the urine, it is impractical to calculate the amount of titratable acid in the urine from urinary and plasma pH and total buffer excretion as in equation 9. A more practical way is to titrate the urine from its pH back to 7.4 using NaOH. The number of milliequivalents of hydroxyl ions required to titrate back to pH 7.4 is equal to the number of milliequivalents of hydrogen ions which were added by the kidney to titrate these buffers down to the pH of the urine.

Ammonia synthesis and excretion

Ammonia synthesis

Several complete reviews of ammonia metabolism have been published.[15,212,273] In this section we will briefly review the synthesis and renal handling of ammonia and then emphasize its importance in acid-base regulation.

The majority of ammonia is synthesized in the kidney from glutamine.[212] Glutamine is actively taken up by the apical and basolateral membranes of the proximal tubule and is then transported into the mitochondria.[15] Present evidence suggests that the mitochondria constitute the major site of ammonia synthesis.

In the mitochondria, glutamine is deamidated by phosphate-dependent glutaminase. This reaction forms ammonia and glutamate. Glutamate is then converted to α-ketoglutarate, either by transamination (donating its amino group to another ketoacid) or by deamination (releasing another ammonia). Mitochondrial and cellular accumulation of tricarboxylic acid cycle intermediates is prevented by transporting malate or oxaloacetate out of the mitochondria and converting them to phosphoenolpyruvate. This compound can either be converted to glucose (by gluconeogenesis) or can reenter the mitochondria and form CO_2 and H_2O.

Ammonia synthesis is stimulated by chronic acidosis and chronic K deficiency. In both of these states, phosphate-dependent glutaminase and phosphoenolpyruvate carboxykinase activities are increased.[15,273] Pitts has estimated that in chronic metabolic acidosis, approximately one-third of the ammonia that leaves the kidney in the urine or the renal vein is derived from the renal artery.[212] Of the remaining two-thirds, 66 percent is formed by the kidney from the amide nitrogen of glutamine, 28 percent from the amino nitrogen of glutamine, and the rest from the amino nitrogens of alanine and glycine (by transamination to form glutamate from α-ketoglutarate) or from glutamate.[212]

Tubular handling of ammonia

The proximal tubule is the major site of ammonia synthesis. Rector and Orloff found that glutaminase was present in far greater amounts in cortical slices than in medullary slices.[219] Curthoys and Lowry found that glutaminase was present primarily in the proximal tubule.[64] Good and Burg found that all segments of the nephron were able to synthesize ammonia, but only in the proximal tubule did the rate increase in response to acidosis.[98] In addition, Good and Burg found that the rates of ammonia synthesis were greatest in the proximal and distal convoluted tubule.[98]

This leads to an obvious problem. The majority of excreted ammonia is trapped in the tubular fluid in the medullary collecting tubules; yet most ammonia synthesis occurs in the proximal tubule. The kidney therefore must possess a mechanism to transport ammonia to the medullary collecting tubule, where it can be trapped.

Transport of total ammonia can occur by NH_3 movement (nonionic diffusion)[211] or NH_4^+ movement (ionic transport). The relative importance of these two modes of transport depends upon the relative concentrations of the two substrates and their relative permeabilities. The pK of ammonia at 37°C is approximately 9.0. Thus, in fluids of pH 7.0, the concentration of NH_4^+ is 100-fold greater than the concentration of NH_3. If a membrane has a 100-fold greater permeability to NH_3 than to NH_4^+, transport will occur 50 percent by nonionic diffusion and 50 percent by ionic transport. Thus, the relative amounts of nonionic and ionic transport will depend on the relative permeabilities. Whereas lipid-soluble compounds may have extremely large permeabilities across cell membranes, NH_3 is not very lipid-soluble; its partition coefficient between chloroform and water is only 0.04.[25]

PROXIMAL TUBULE Micropuncture studies have shown that 75 to 125 percent of excreted ammonia enters the tubular fluid in the proximal tubule.[39,232] The first step in ammonia transport is the movement of ammonia synthesized in the proximal tubule cell into the lumen of the proximal tubule. Nagami and coworkers have demonstrated that ammonia synthesized in the in vitro perfused mouse proximal tubule is preferentially transported into the luminal fluid.[199-201] This preferential transport of ammonia into the luminal fluid could occur by one of three mechanisms. First, NH_3 could diffuse preferentially into the luminal fluid because apical membrane NH_3 permeability is higher than basolateral membrane NH_3 permeability. Second, NH_3 could diffuse preferentially into the luminal fluid due to trapping by the low luminal pH. Finally, NH_4^+ could move preferentially into the luminal fluid because of the polarized location of an NH_4^+ transporter on the apical membrane.

Preisig and Alpern examined the apical and basolateral membrane pathways for NH_3-NH_4^+ transport by measuring the effect of luminal or peritubular addition of NH_3-NH_4^+ on proximal tubule cell pH.[215] These investigators found that apical membrane NH_3 permeability was 6.2×10^{-2} cm/s and basolateral membrane NH_3 permeability was 7×10^{-2} cm/s. Thus permeability to NH_3 was equal on both membranes and was large. In addition, these investigators found that NH_4^+ was transported on the apical membrane Na^+-H^+ antiporter, an effect that was blocked by luminal amiloride. Kinsella and Aronson have also found that NH_4^+ could serve as a substrate for the Na^+-H^+ antiporter.[145] Based on these studies, it appears that selective ammonia transport into the luminal fluid could be accounted for by ammonium transport on the apical membrane Na^+-H^+ antiporter or by nonionic diffusion of NH_3 into the luminal fluid driven by the low luminal pH.

The relative importance of these two mechanisms has been addressed by studying the effect of amiloride and amiloride analogues on ammonia secretion into the proximal tubule. Nagami found that luminal amiloride blocked ammonia transport into the proximal tubule,[201] while Simon and associates found only a small effect.[253] Thus, it is not clear which of these two mechanisms is quantitatively most important. Most likely, both mechanisms contribute to the selective transport of ammonia into the luminal fluid. It is interesting that nonionic diffusion of NH_3 into the luminal fluid is enhanced by the presence of an acid disequilibrium pH. This may provide a teleologic reason for the absence of luminal carbonic anhydrase in the S3 segment of the proximal tubule (see below).[157]

LOOP OF HENLE Once secreted into the lumen of the proximal tubule, ammonium must be delivered to the medullary interstitium. Approximately 40 percent of ammonia delivered to the end proximal tubule is no longer present in the early distal tubule.[39] Good and coworkers found that the rat thick ascending limb perfused in vitro absorbed NH_3-NH_4^+. Because luminal fluid was acidified this transport could not be accounted for by nonionic diffusion, driven by a pH gradient.[99] To further investigate the mechanisms by which NH_4^+ was absorbed from the thick ascending limb, Garvin and associates varied transepithelial voltage in the rabbit thick ascending limb by varying the NaCl concentration gradient.[84] When tubules were voltage-clamped to a transepithelial voltage of 0, 35 percent of NH_4^+ absorption was inhibited. This component presumably represents voltage-driven paracellular NH_4^+ transport. At a transepithelial voltage of 0 mV, furosemide inhibited another 35 to 40 percent of NH_4^+ absorption, suggesting that this component is transported on the Na^+-K^+-$2Cl^-$ cotransporter. Presumably, the remaining 25 to 30 percent of NH_4^+ absorption occurs on another transporter. In parallel studies, Good addressed this question in the rat medullary thick ascending limb perfused in vitro.[95] NH_4^+ permeability was measured and accounted for approximately 35 percent of ammonia absorption. The remaining NH_4^+ absorption was inhibited by raising luminal K^+ concentration from 4 to 24 meq/liter, suggesting that NH_4^+ was able to be transported at the K^+ site of apical membrane transporters in this segment.

Combining the results of Garvin and associates and Good,[84,95] the best explanation appears to be that there are three components of NH_4^+ absorption: (1) NH_4^+ diffusion driven by the lumen-positive voltage, (2) the Na^+-K^+-$2Cl^-$ cotransporter, and (3) apical membrane K^+ conductance. In vesicles generated from the thick ascending limb, Kinne and colleagues found that NH_4^+ competed with K^+ on the Na^+-K^+-$2Cl^-$ cotransporter and that NH_4^+ could be transported as a substrate in place of K^+ on this transporter.[142] The mechanism of basolateral membrane NH_3-NH_4^+ transport has not been addressed.

In addition to active NH_4^+ transport in the thick ascending limb, nonionic diffusion may also contribute to ammonia absorption in the loop of Henle. As tubular fluid passes down into the loop of Henle, it is alkalinized.[40,73,100] This alkalinization of fluid in the descending limb of the loop of Henle is due to water abstraction, which concentrates the dissolved CO_2 and the bicarbonate. The CO_2 can diffuse out, but the bicarbonate is trapped. DuBose and associates and Buerkert and colleagues have found tubular fluid at the tip of the loop of Henle to have a pH of 7.4 and a bicarbonate concentration of 21 m*M*.[40,73] Alkalinization causes an increase in luminal NH_3 concentration, which can then leave the loop of Henle by nonionic diffusion.

The mechanisms described above allow for the transport of NH_4^+ from the loop of Henle into the medullary interstitium. The countercurrent system in the vasa recta helps keep the NH_3-NH_4^+ in the medullary interstitium. In addition, ammonia in the outer medullary interstitium can enter the S3 proximal tubule, aided by the acid disequilibrium pH (see below), and reenter the medulla.

COLLECTING DUCT Studies in in vitro perfused tubules suggest that entry of ammonia into the lumen of the collecting tubule occurs by nonionic diffusion. Knepper and coworkers and Star and associates have found that an acid disequilibrium pH increases ammonia transport into the lumen of the cortical collecting duct and outer medullary collecting duct, respectively.[148,261] Hamm and colleagues found that total ammonia flux in the cortical collecting duct correlated better with NH_3 than NH_4^+ concentration gradients.[109] They estimated an NH_3 permeability of 5×10^{-3} cm/s in this segment.

In summary, ammonia is synthesized in the proximal tubule but requires transport to the lumen of the collecting duct in order to be excreted (Fig. 10-3). Ammonia moves from the proximal tubule cell into the lumen both by nonionic diffusion, being trapped by the luminal acid pH, and by NH_4^+ transport on the Na^+-H^+ antiporter. Ammonia is then reabsorbed from the loop of Henle by NH_4^+ transport in the thick ascending limb and by nonionic diffusion. Ammonia accumulates in the medullary interstitium, helped by the countercurrent system, and is then trapped in the lumen of the cortical collecting duct by nonionic diffusion of NH_3.

Regulation of ammonia excretion

It is obvious from the preceding discussion that ammonia excretion can be regulated by two means. First, the rate of ammonia synthesis can be changed. Increases in ammonia synthesis increase the amount of ammonia appearing in the urine and in the renal vein. Second, the quantity of ammonia trapped in the urine can be affected. Lowering the pH of the collecting duct tubular fluid traps ammonia in the urine. In this situation, total ammonia production is unaffected; the increment in urinary ammonia excretion is balanced by a decrement in renal vein ammonia.

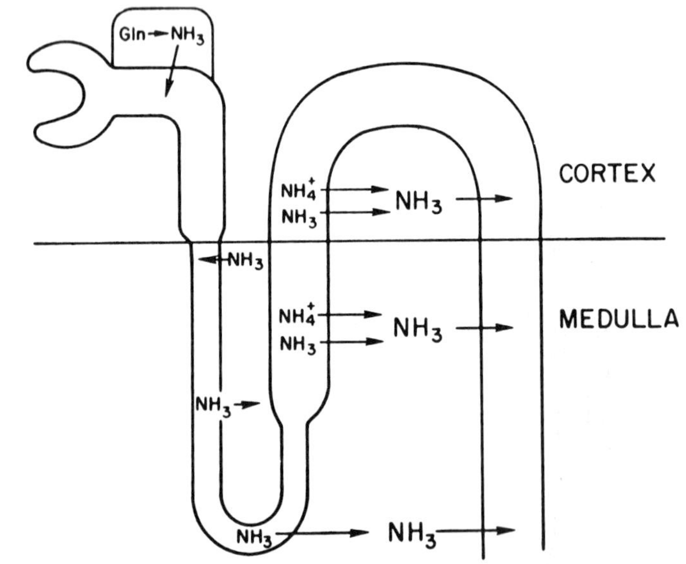

FIGURE 10-3 • Delivery of ammonia synthesized by the proximal tubule in the cortex to the collecting tubule in the medulla. See text for explanation. (From Alpern RJ et al, in Brenner BM, Rector FC (eds): *The Kidney,* 4th ed, Philadelphia, Saunders, 1990. Used by permission.)

Pitts emphasized the dual regulation of ammonia excretion (Fig. 10-4).[211] In control dogs, urinary ammonia excretion increased as urine pH fell, presumably due to trapping. In chronic acidosis, urinary ammonia excretion also increased as urine pH decreased (again due to trapping). However, for any urine pH, urinary ammonia excretion in dogs with chronic acidosis was higher than in controls. This was due to stimulation of ammonia synthesis during chronic metabolic acidosis.

In addition to chronic metabolic acidosis, other factors have been shown to affect the rate of ammonia synthesis. Tannen and colleagues found that potassium deficiency increases ammonia synthesis and that hyperkalemia suppresses ammonia synthesis.[272,274,275] This effect is very important in type IV renal tubular acidosis (RTA; see Chap. 27). In addition, respiratory acidosis affects the rate of ammonia synthesis. This effect differs from the effect of metabolic acidosis with respect to its time course. Acute respiratory acidosis stimulates ammonia synthesis;[203] the stimulation disappears as respiratory acidosis becomes chronic.[225]

MECHANISMS AND REGULATION OF RENAL ACIDIFICATION

PROXIMAL TUBULE

Role in acidification

After it is formed in the glomerulus, the tubular fluid first comes in contact with the proximal convoluted tubule (PCT). The fluid entering the PCT has an approximate pH of 7.26, a P_{CO_2} of 60 mmHg, and a bicarbonate concentration of 24 meq/liter.[70] This high P_{CO_2} is present throughout the renal cortex[69,86] and is currently thought to be due to CO_2 generated from metabolism in combination with CO_2 acquired by vascular-vascular exchange (i.e., through a modified countercurrent system.)[33,175]

Acidification occurs along the length of the PCT such that the pH and bicarbonate concentration decrease to approximately 6.70 and 8 meq/liter, respectively.[56,70] Because of the removal of 50 percent of the filtered water in the PCT, this decrease in bicarbonate concentration reflects reabsorption of approximately 75 percent of filtered bicarbonate. Thus, the PCT reclaims the majority of filtered bicarbonate. Further bicarbonate reabsorption occurs in the proximal straight tubule. The proton secretory capacity is, however, far less in this segment than in the PCT.[42,181,287]

In addition, by acidifying its lumen, the proximal tubule converts titratable buffer to its acid form; am-

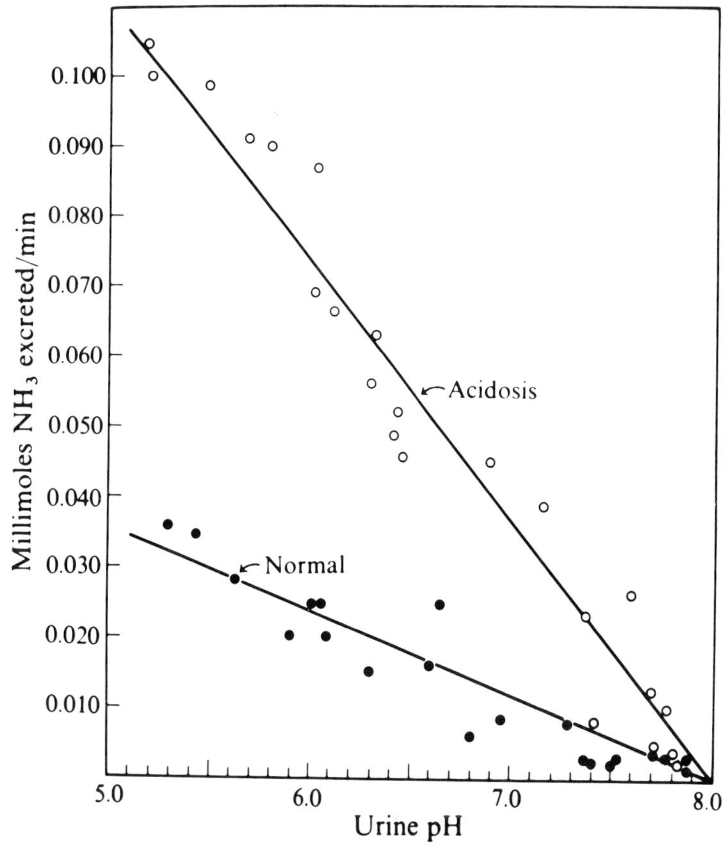

FIGURE 10-4 • Ammonia excretion as a function of urine pH. Decreases in urine pH increase ammonia excretion, presumably through trapping. In addition, for any given urine pH, animals with chronic acidosis excrete more ammonia than controls, presumably because of increased synthesis. (From RF Pitts: *Fed Proc* 7:418, 1948. Used by permission.)

monia is trapped in the tubular fluid. As discussed above, ammonia trapping in the proximal tubule is important for the transport of synthesized ammonia to the collecting duct.

Cellular mechanism of acidification

Site of active transport

Because acidification raises the hydrogen ion concentration of luminal fluid, hydrogen ions are secreted against a chemical gradient. This therefore is an active process that requires the input of energy. Acidification in the proximal tubule requires the net movement of acid from the blood into the cell across the basolateral membrane and then from the cell to the luminal fluid across the apical membrane.

Proximal tubular cell pH is between 7.2 and 7.3.[7,18] If the cell voltage of approximately −60 mV (which will attract hydrogen ions) is considered, it is clear that hydrogen ions can passively cross the basolateral membrane from blood to cell. The secretion of hydrogen ions from the cell into the lumen, however, requires energy input. This relationship is depicted in Fig. 10-5, which shows the voltage, pH, and electrochemical potential for hydrogen ions in the three compartments. Hydrogen ions are able to move from a higher to a lower electrochemical potential (blood to cell) spontaneously but require energy

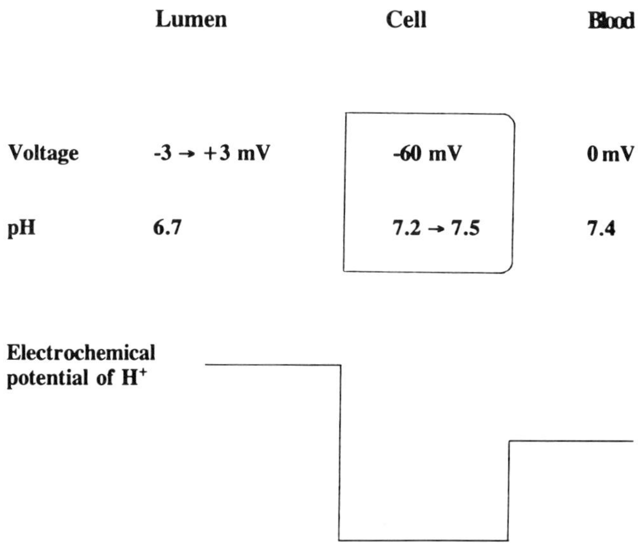

FIGURE 10-5 • Site of the active step in proton secretion. The negative cell potential leads to a low electrochemical potential in the cell, which allows protons to enter the cell from the blood passively. Ejecting protons across the luminal membrane to the higher electrochemical potential in the lumen, however, requires active transport.

input to move from a lower to a higher electrochemical potential (cell to lumen). In general, similar results have been found for all acidifying epithelia: the site of hydrogen ion extrusion is the site of the active step.

Proton secretion versus bicarbonate absorption

The reabsorption of bicarbonate could occur by one of the two mechanisms shown in Fig. 10-6. First, as shown in Fig. 10-6*a*, there could be secretion of a hydrogen ion or proton across the apical membrane. This proton is generated from carbonic acid in the cell; upon addition to the lumen it reacts with any basic buffer there to form the conjugate acid of the buffer. Since the most prevalent buffer in the lumen is bicarbonate, most of the secreted protons react with bicarbonate, forming carbonic acid. Carbonic acid then dehydrates to CO_2, which can diffuse out of the lumen. Generation of a proton from carbonic acid in the cell leaves a bicarbonate ion, which then exits across the basolateral membrane. The net result is the translocation of bicarbonate from the lumen to the peritubular capillary.

A second possible mechanism, shown in Fig. 10-6*b*, entails direct absorption of bicarbonate. As bicarbonate concentration is lowered, carbonic acid dissociates to form bicarbonate and hydrogen, thus acidifying the lumen. Carbonic acid concentration is maintained by carbon dioxide diffusing into the lumen and being hydrated to carbonic acid. Thus, proton secretion generates carbonic acid (Fig. 10-6*a*), while direct bicarbonate absorption consumes carbonic acid (Fig. 10-6*b*).

The determination as to which of these mechanisms was present came about through manipulation of the bicarbonate–carbonic acid–CO_2 buffer system. As stated earlier in this chapter, the bicarbonate–carbonic acid reactions are instantaneous; this system is always at equilibrium. The carbonic acid–carbon dioxide hydration-dehydration reactions, however, are slow, and thus these components are not in equilibrium. When carbonic anhydrase is present, these reactions are markedly accelerated and the entire system is in equilibrium. The *equilibrium pH* is defined as the pH that is calculated from the bicarbonate concentration and P_{CO_2} using the Henderson-Hasselbalch equation. The *in situ pH* is the actual pH present in the proximal tubule. The *disequilibrium pH* is defined as the difference between the in situ pH and the equilibrium pH.

If carbonic anhydrase is present, or if carbonic acid is neither being generated nor consumed, in situ pH equals equilibrium pH and disequilibrium pH is zero. This is found in the proximal tubule.[71,221,282] When inhibitors of carbonic anhydrase are infused, carbonic acid is not maintained in equilibrium with CO_2. If carbonic acid is being formed from proton secretion as in Fig. 10-6*a*, carbonic acid and hydrogen ion concentrations will be higher than those calculated from the bicarbonate concentration and P_{CO_2} (i.e., disequilibrium pH is acid). If there is direct bicarbonate absorption with consumption of carbonic acid as in Fig. 10-6*b*, the concentrations of carbonic acid and hydrogen ion will be lower than calculated (i.e., alkaline disequilibrium pH). If there is no acidification, with no addition or removal of carbonic acid, there should be no disequilibrium pH. These values have now been measured by three groups in the proximal tubule, and all have found an acid disequilibrium pH after inhibition of carbonic anhydrase.[71,221,282]

The results of these experiments therefore provided two important findings. First, they demonstrated that acidification in the proximal tubule occurs by proton secretion with generation of carbonic acid (Fig. 10-6*a*). Second, they showed that carbonic anhydrase is normally present in the luminal membrane of the proximal tubule (and has functional contact with the luminal fluid), such that a disequilibrium pH only exists when carbonic

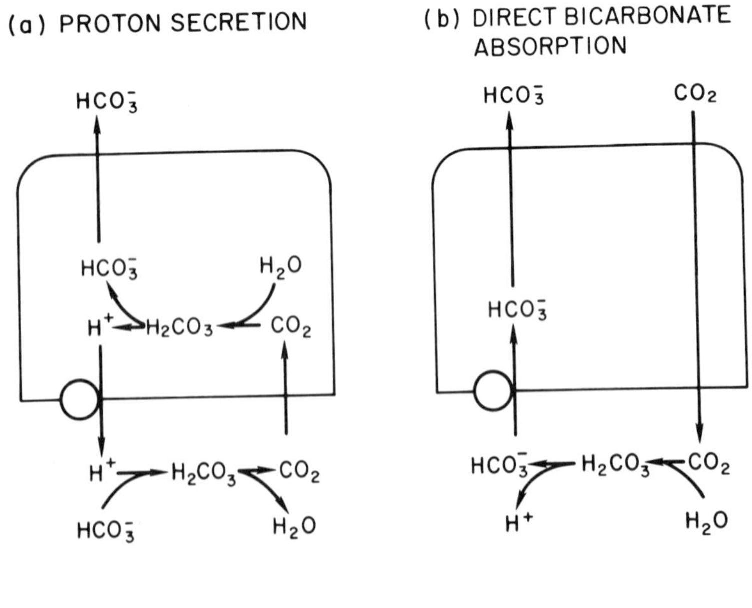

FIGURE 10-6 • Proton secretion versus direct bicarbonate absorption.

anhydrase inhibitors are administered. The significance of this second finding will be discussed below.

Transcellular pathway

Apical membrane H secretion

Apical membrane H^+ secretion is an active process. Active H secretion has been divided into primary active, secondary active, and tertiary active mechanisms. *Primary active H^+ secretion* involves direct coupling of H^+ secretion to metabolism. *Secondary active H^+ secretion* involves coupling of H^+ secretion to the transport of another solute, for which a concentration gradient has been generated by coupling to metabolism. Finally, *tertiary active transport* involves a system where metabolism generates a concentration gradient for solute X; a coupled transport mechanism then allows solute X to generate a favorable gradient for solute Y; a second coupled transporter allows solute Y to actively transport H^+ ions. At present, most of the evidence suggests an important role for primary and secondary active transport, and these mechanisms will be discussed further below. The interested reader is referred to other references that describe the mechanisms of H^+-HCO_3^- transport in more depth.[8,15]

PRIMARY ACTIVE TRANSPORT: H^+-ATPASE Five lines of evidence support the presence of an apical membrane H^+-translocating ATPase in the proximal tubule. First, an H^+-translocating ATPase has been found in apical membrane vesicle preparations.[143] Unfortunately, because these membrane preparations are frequently contaminated by other cell membranes and because many intracellular vesicles contain H^+ ATPases, these results were not definitive. The second line of evidence in support of an H^+ ATPase is the finding of Na^+-independent cell alkalinization in perfused proximal tubules.[156,202] The third line of evidence is the demonstration of an acidification-dependent, lumen-positive voltage in the proximal tubule.[80,81] In these studies, proximal tubules were perfused with synthetic solutions in the absence of any organic solutes that might generate a lumen-negative voltage. A lumen-positive voltage was found that was inhibited by acetazolamide and unaffected by ouabain. The fourth line of evidence is the staining of proximal tubular apical membrane with antibodies generated against a purified H^+ ATPase.[38]

Finally, it has been found that inhibition of the Na^+-H^+ antiporter with amiloride is unable to completely inhibit HCO_3^- absorption.[46,121,217] When all appropriate corrections were made, it was calculated that approximately 65 percent of proximal tubular HCO_3^- absorption could be accounted for by an amiloride-sensitive mechanism (see below), but that 35 percent of HCO_3^- absorption was mediated by a Na^+-independent amiloride-insensitive apical membrane transport mechanism.[217]

SECONDARY ACTIVE TRANSPORT: Na^+-H^+ ANTIPORTER The majority of proximal tubule $NaHCO_3$ absorption is mediated by an apical membrane Na^+-H^+ antiporter. There are three major lines of evidence supporting this. First, studies in apical membrane vesicles have demonstrated that Na^+ gradients lead to the countertransport of H^+ and pH gradients lead to countertransport of Na^+ ions.[144,197,289]

The second line of studies have demonstrated effects of luminal Na^+ on cell pH in the proximal tubule. In these studies, it was demonstrated that luminal Na^+ removal causes a cell acidification, luminal Na^+ addition causes a cell alkalinization, and these pH changes are blocked by amiloride and amiloride analogues.[9,217] Amiloride and its analogues are inhibitors of Na^+-H^+ exchange. The last line of evidence supporting an important role is the inhibition of $NaHCO_3$ absorption in the proximal tubule by amiloride and amiloride analogues.[46,121,217]

The molecular nature of this Na^+-H^+ antiporter is presently under investigation. Na^+-H^+ antiporter activity is ubiquitously found in mammalian cells. At present, this transporter protein is believed to exist in two pharmacological forms: a form that is relatively resistant to inhibition by amiloride present in apical membranes of epithelia, where it mediates transepithelial transport, and an amiloride-sensitive form present in all cells, where it regulates cell volume, growth, and intracellular pH. Sardet and coworkers recently cloned a cDNA for human Na^+-H^+ antiporter that predicts a protein of 815 amino acids with an N-terminal hydrophobic domain that spans the lipid membrane 10 to 12 times, followed by a C-terminal cytoplasmic hydrophilic domain.[234] Expression studies have shown this cDNA to be a functional Na^+-H^+ antiporter that exhibits characteristics of the growth factor-activatable amiloride-sensitive transporter.[235] This Na^+-H^+ antiporter is highly conserved in the animal kingdom, and cDNAs cloned from numerous mammalian species all exhibit high degrees of homology (>90 percent) to the human protein.[118,209,222,269] Recently, the genomic organization and 5′-regulatory region of the human Na^+-H^+ antiporter gene has been characterized, and the gene has been localized to human chromosome 1p.[163,192]

The mRNA of this Na^+-H^+ antiporter is present in kidney cortex and renal tubules, but since the cloned Na^+-H^+ antiporter exhibits characteristics of the amiloride-sensitive isoform present in nonepithelial cells, it is not clear whether these renal transcripts represent the apical membrane Na^+-H^+ antiporter that effects transepithelial transport. Recently, a second distinct molecular isoform was cloned from intestinal epithelia that might code for the isoform involved in epithelial transport.[235]

At present, it is not known whether the same Na^+-H^+ antiporter resides on the intestinal and renal apical membranes. It is possible that Na^+-H^+ antiporters exist as multiple isoforms in a multigene family.

Basolateral membrane HCO_3^- exit

Because cell pH is above electrochemical equilibrium, basolateral membrane base efflux can occur passively. The passive mechanism appears to be an electrogenic Na^+-$3HCO_3^-$ cotransport mechanism. Three lines of evidence support this conclusion. First, studies have investigated the effect of peritubular composition on cell pH, cell Na^+ concentration, and cell voltage. These studies have found that decreases in peritubular pH or Na^+ concentration lead to a cell depolarization that is inhibited by disulfonic stilbenes.[29,30,34,41,297,298] While the effect of a decrease in peritubular pH on cell voltage is consistent with a basolateral membrane HCO_3^- conductance, the effect of peritubular Na^+ concentration on cell voltage is in the wrong direction for a simple basolateral membrane Na^+ conductance and in fact is more consistent with a Na^+-coupled transport mechanism carrying a net negative charge. Using microelectrodes and pH-sensitive fluorescent dyes to measure cell pH, it has been found that decreasing peritubular pH or Na^+ concentration leads to cell acidification.[7,34,298] In addition, these effects on cell pH are inhibited by disulfonic stilbenes (inhibitors of anion transport). Using Na^+-selective microelectrodes to measure cell Na^+ activity, it has been found that decreases in peritubular pH or Na^+ concentration cause a decrease in cell Na^+ activity that is inhibited by disulfonic stilbenes.[34,298] These studies also have demonstrated that complete Na^+ removal from luminal and peritubular solutions leads to inhibition of 90 to 100 percent of basolateral membrane H^+-HCO_3^- permeability.[7,298] Finally, these studies have found that the transporter is not dependent on the presence of Cl.[10,34] All of these studies together demonstrate the presence of an electrogenic Na^+-coupled HCO_3^- transport mechanism that carries a net negative charge and is inhibited by disulfonic stilbenes.

The second set of studies demonstrating the presence of this transporter has been generated from isolated basolateral membrane vesicles.[1,106] These studies have demonstrated that in the presence of HCO_3^-, $^{22}Na^+$ uptake is enhanced. Addition of SITS (a compound that inhibits bicarbonate exit from the cell) blocks the $^{22}Na^+$ uptake in the presence of HCO_3^- but has no effect in the absence of HCO_3^-. Finally, when an inside positive voltage is established in the vesicles, $^{22}Na^+$ uptake is enhanced in the presence of HCO_3^- but unaffected in the absence of HCO_3^-. This latter voltage effect is in the wrong direction for a Na^+ conductance but is in the correct direction for a Na^+ flux occurring on a transporter that carries a net negative charge. All of these vesicle studies have been performed in the absence of Cl^-. All of these studies are consistent with $^{22}Na^+$ uptake on an electrogenic Na^+-HCO_3^- cotransporter.

In subsequent studies, the stoichiometry of the transporter has been found to be 1 Na^+:3 HCO_3^-:2 negative charges.[255,298] In further studies, it has been found that the actual substrates carried on the transporter are 1 Na^+, 1 HCO_3^-, and 1 CO_3^{2-}.[254]

The last set of studies examining this issue have examined the effect of a number of maneuvers on transepithelial HCO_3^- absorption and have generated a number of findings suggesting that the Na^+-$3HCO_3^-$ cotransporter is responsible for almost all of HCO_3^- absorption. First, HCO_3^- absorption in the proximal tubule is almost completely inhibited by luminal and peritubular Na^+ removal but is unaffected by luminal and peritubular Cl^- removal.[42,46,49,181,236] Second, SITS, an inhibitor of the Na^+-$3HCO_3^-$ cotransporter, inhibits HCO_3^- absorption.[47] Finally, maneuvers that depolarize the cell, such as the addition of barium, inhibit HCO_3^- absorption.[236] Based on all of these studies, it appears that the basolateral membrane Na^+-$3HCO_3^-$ cotransporter mediates most of basolateral membrane HCO_3^- movement effecting transcellular acid secretion.

Paracellular pathway

All of the previous discussion has referred to how protons are actively secreted into the lumen from the peritubular capillary. This results in a high luminal proton concentration (low pH) and a low luminal bicarbonate concentration. This provides a driving force for diffusion of protons and bicarbonate around the cell through the paracellular pathway. The permeability of the paracellular pathway is thought to be determined by the size of the pores in the tight junction.

Protons have an extremely high mobility in free solution because they are small and because they are able to "jump" from one water molecule to another. The amount of diffusion, however, is linearly related to the mobility and the concentration gradient. In physiologic solutions, protons exist in extremely low concentrations (at pH 7.0, the proton concentration is 10^{-7} *M*, which is approximately 10^5 times smaller than the bicarbonate concentration); thus, proton diffusion in these solutions is extremely slow and not physiologically important. Measurements of proton permeability in the rabbit PCT have confirmed this. Although proton permeability is higher than bicarbonate permeability, it is not sufficiently high to compensate for the low proton concentrations present in vivo.[108,244]

Bicarbonate permeability has been measured in the rat and the rabbit PCT by numerous investigators, who find that it is small compared to sodium or chloride permeability (values range from 0.9 to 3.5×10^{-5} cm/s).[12,48,119,238,288] However, it is large enough to be an important determinant of acidification. At the beginning of the PCT, luminal bicarbonate concentration is similar to that of plasma; thus, paracellular bicarbonate diffusion is extremely slow. As the filtrate proceeds along the tubule, luminal bicarbonate concentration decreases, which accelerates the rate of bicarbonate diffusion back into the lumen. When rat PCTs are perfused with a solution containing 5m*M* bicarbonate, the net rate of bicarbonate absorption is 12 pmol/mm·min.[12] This includes an active transcellular proton secretory flux of 42 pmol/mm·min in parallel with a paracellular bicarbonate backleak flux of −30 pmol/mm·min.[12] Thus, with low luminal bicarbonate concentrations, the rate of bicarbonate diffusion into the lumen can approach 75 percent of the rate of active proton secretion.

Carbonic anhydrase

The importance of carbonic anhydrase in acidification has been alluded to multiple times in this chapter. When carbonic anhydrase inhibitors are infused intravenously or perfused into the proximal tubule, proximal tubular bicarbonate absorption is inhibited by 80 to 100 percent.[47,57,171,172] Histologic studies have found that carbonic anhydrase is present on the apical membrane, in the cytoplasm, and on the basolateral membrane.[168] However, the relative importance of these sites of carbonic anhydrase activity is incompletely understood.

As discussed above, carbonic anhydrase on the apical membrane appears to have functional contact with the luminal fluid and is very important in acidification.[71,221,282] Normally, when protons are secreted into the proximal tubular lumen, they react with bicarbonate to form carbonic acid, which is then dehydrated to form CO_2, which diffuses out of the lumen (Fig. 10-6*a*). In the absence of carbonic anhydrase, carbonic acid concentration increases, as do the proton and bicarbonate concentrations. The increased proton concentration (disequilibrium pH) slows the rate of proton secretion by creating a more unfavorable chemical proton gradient (see below). Indeed, when a dextran-bound carbonic anhydrase inhibitor (which does not enter the cell) is perfused into the lumen of the proximal tubule, a very large disequilibrium pH develops, and 80 percent of bicarbonate absorption is inhibited.[174] This is a clear demonstration of the importance of apical membrane-bound carbonic anhydrase.

In contrast, when acetazolamide, a carbonic anhydrase inhibitor that *does* enter the cell, is perfused into the proximal tubule, bicarbonate absorption is inhibited by 90 to 100 percent, but there is only a small disequilibrium pH.[172] This strongly suggests that carbonic anhydrase at sites other than the apical membrane plays a key role. Cytoplasmic and basolateral membrane carbonic anhydrase catalyze the conversion of CO_2 to carbonic acid, which supplies protons to the apical membrane Na^+-H^+ antiporter and H^+ pump, and HCO_3^- to the basolateral membrane Na^+-$3HCO_3^-$ transporter. Inhibition of carbonic anhydrase at either of these two sites can alkalinize the cell and secondarily inhibit acidification.[147]

Summary

In summary, proximal tubule acidification is mediated by apical membrane H^+ ATPase and apical membrane Na^+-H^+ antiporters working in parallel (Fig. 10-7). These transporters eject protons into the luminal fluid and generate base within the cell; base efflux then occurs by a Na^+-$3HCO_3^-$ cotransport mechanism. A number of other H^+-HCO_3^- transporters have been demonstrated to be present in proximal tubule cells but appear to play no role in transepithelial acidification.[8]

Regulation of proximal acidification

Luminal bicarbonate concentration and pH

As described earlier, proximal tubular acidification involves secretion of protons from cell to lumen. Acidification would therefore be expected to be sensitive to the proton concentration or pH of the luminal fluid. The first study to examine the question measured the pH as a function of time in luminal split droplets containing bicarbonate. The rate of acidification was found to be proportional to the luminal concentration of bicarbonate.[180] Similar results have been found in tubular microperfusion studies.[12,238] Fig. 10-8 (solid line) shows the measured rate of bicarbonate absorption as a function of luminal bicarbonate concentration.

In these studies, when luminal bicarbonate concentration was altered, a gradient was created for paracellular bicarbonate diffusion. In order to assess the magnitude of this passive bicarbonate diffusion, bicar-

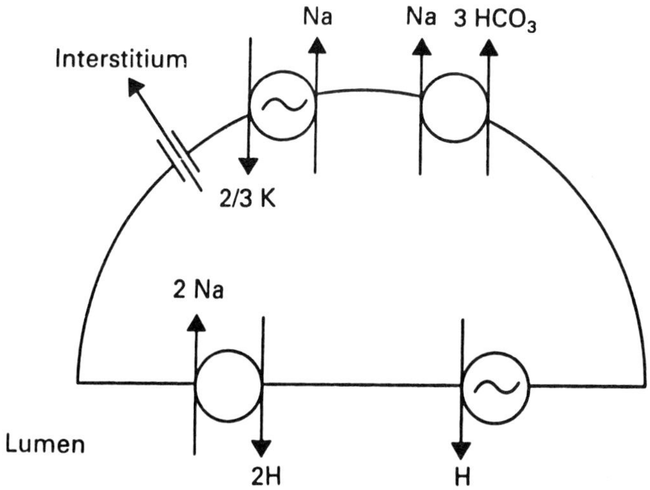

FIGURE 10-7 • Mechanism for acidification of the proximal tubule.

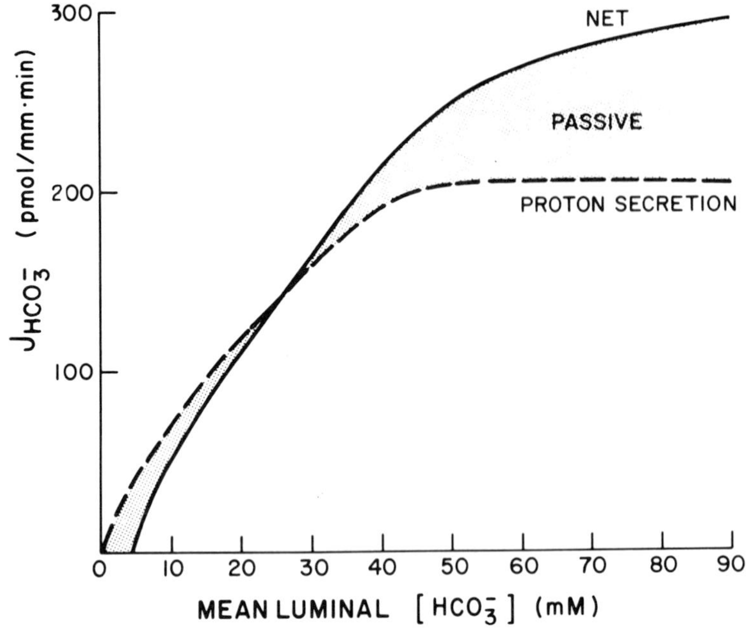

FIGURE 10-8 • Effect of luminal bicarbonate concentration on net bicarbonate absorption, passive bicarbonate diffusion, and active transcellular proton secretion in the PCT. (From Alpern RJ et al: *Am J Physiol* 243:F53, 1982. Used by permission.)

bonate permeability was measured and multiplied by the concentration gradients measured in the abovementioned studies. The shaded area in Fig. 10-8 represents the calculated rates of passive bicarbonate diffusion expressed as a function of luminal bicarbonate concentration.[12] When luminal bicarbonate concentration is less than 25 meq/liter (the bicarbonate concentration of plasma), bicarbonate diffuses from blood to lumen. When luminal bicarbonate concentration is greater than 25 meq/liter, bicarbonate diffuses from lumen to blood. At a luminal concentration of 25 meq/liter there is no diffusion.

When the measured rates of net bicarbonate absorption are corrected for the calculated rates of passive bicarbonate diffusion, the remaining portion represents the rate of transcellular proton secretion (Fig. 10-8, dashed line). This transcellular component varies as a function of luminal bicarbonate concentration and pH. Thus, both the rates of transcellular proton secretion and of paracellular bicarbonate diffusion vary as luminal bicarbonate concentration and pH vary. Sasaki and coworkers found similar results in the microperfused rabbit PCT.[238] Vesicle studies have found that the rate of Na^+-H^+ exchange across brush border membranes varies with extravesicular (luminal) pH.[17]

Figure 10-8 shows that proton secretion reaches its maximal rate at a luminal HCO_3^- concentration of 45 meq/liter. This decreased sensitivity to high luminal concentrations of HCO_3^- is most likely due to the fact that apical membrane transporters are in fact H^+ transporters and are thus sensitive to luminal H^+ concentration. At high HCO_3^- concentrations, even large changes in the concentration of the anion have only small effects on H^+ concentration.

The finding that the rate of bicarbonate absorption varies as luminal pH varies has important physiologic implications. First, the highest rate of bicarbonate absorption occurs in the early proximal tubule, where luminal bicarbonate concentration and pH are high. Toward the end of the PCT, where luminal bicarbonate concentration and pH are low, proton secretion slows, and the rate of bicarbonate diffusion into the lumen increases. Both of these effects tend to slow the net rate of acidification. These findings also explain the effect of dextran-bound carbonic anhydrase inhibitors on acidification.[174] These agents block luminal carbonic acid conversion to CO_2, elevating proton concentration (disequilibrium pH). This decrease in luminal pH then slows the rate of transcellular proton secretion.

An additional result of this concentration dependence is to moderate any effects on proximal tubular acidification.[11] Inhibition of acidification due to any factor prevents luminal bicarbonate concentration from falling as rapidly as normal. The higher luminal bicarbonate concentrations then stimulate acidification, thus moderating the inhibitory effect. The reverse occurs in response to a stimulatory effect.

Luminal flow rate

When the GFR increases, the filtered load of bicarbonate increases. If the rate of tubular bicarbonate absorption does not increase in proportion, massive bicarbonaturia results, leading to severe acidosis. In studies where dogs were fed protein to increase their GFR, bicarbonate reabsorption was found to increase proportionately with GFR.[210] Micropuncture studies have demonstrated that stimulation of bicarbonate absorption by increases in GFR occurs at least in part in the proximal tubule.[56]

One possible mechanism for the "flow dependence" of bicarbonate absorption is that flow alters the luminal concentration profile of bicarbonate.[22,296] Increases in luminal flow rate cause luminal bicarbonate concentration to drop at a reduced rate. This leads to higher luminal bicarbonate concentrations and higher pH, which stimulates the rate of acidification. Microperfusion studies from two laboratories have, however, found that this mechanism explains only 15 percent of the observed flow dependence of bicarbonate absorption.[14,47]

When the rate of proton secretion was examined as a function of luminal bicarbonate concentration, it was found that increases in luminal flow rate stimulated proton secretion at low luminal bicarbonate concentrations but had little effect at luminal concentrations sufficient to achieve the maximal rate of proton secretion (Fig. 10-9). These findings are most consistent with the presence of a flow-dependent diffusion barrier in the proximal tubule. When protons are secreted by the cell, a thin layer is created with a high proton concentration and a low bicarbonate concentration. As described earlier, proton diffusion at physiologic concentrations is extremely slow. Thus, the pH in this layer will be determined by the relative rates of proton secretion by the cell and bicarbonate diffusion from the lumen. In order for such a layer to exist, a barrier to bicarbonate diffusion must exist. This diffusion barrier would presumably be adjacent to the microvilli of the brush border membrane. If increases in flow rate decreased the magnitude of this diffusion barrier, pH would rise in the layer adjacent to the cell, and proton secretion would be stimulated. If, however, luminal bicarbonate concentrations were high so that the rate of proton secretion was maximal and thus independent of luminal pH, increases in the pH of this thin layer would not stimulate proton secretion.[295] Thus, at the maximal rate, proton secretion would not be expected to be flow-dependent. This is exactly the kinetic behavior that was found (Fig. 10-9).[14]

In summary, increases in luminal flow rate markedly stimulate bicarbonate absorption by altering the luminal bicarbonate concentration and pH in the vicinity of the apical membrane. This concentration is affected by flow rate in two ways (Fig. 10-10). First, increases in flow rate increase the bicarbonate concentration in the center of the lumen (bulk phase) by altering the axial luminal concentration profile. This effect accounts for only 15 percent of flow-dependent stimulation of bicarbonate absorption. Second, increases in flow rate decrease the magnitude of a luminal diffusion barrier, which produces decreases in the magnitude of radial concentration gradients. This appears to represent the major effect of flow rate on the bicarbonate concentration in the vicinity of the luminal membrane and thus on bicarbonate absorption. Flow dependence of bicarbonate absorption is an important homeostatic mechanism that prevents increases in GFR from leading to massive bicarbonaturia and acidosis. In certain conditions, however, the maximal rate of proton secretion is markedly reduced, and flow dependence is therefore attenuated (see below).

In addition to the acute effects of flow rate on the rate of HCO_3^- absorption, there are also chronic adaptive effects of changes in GFR. If single-nephron GFR is increased chronically, either by decreases in renal mass, protein feeding, or hyperglycemia, a number of changes in proximal tubular H^+ transport are provoked. In tubules perfused at identical flow rates, rates of HCO_3^- absorption are greater in tubules from hyperfiltering animals.[216] In addition, apical membrane Na^+-H^+ antiporter activity and basolateral membrane Na^+-$3HCO_3^-$ cotransporter activity are increased in proximal tubules

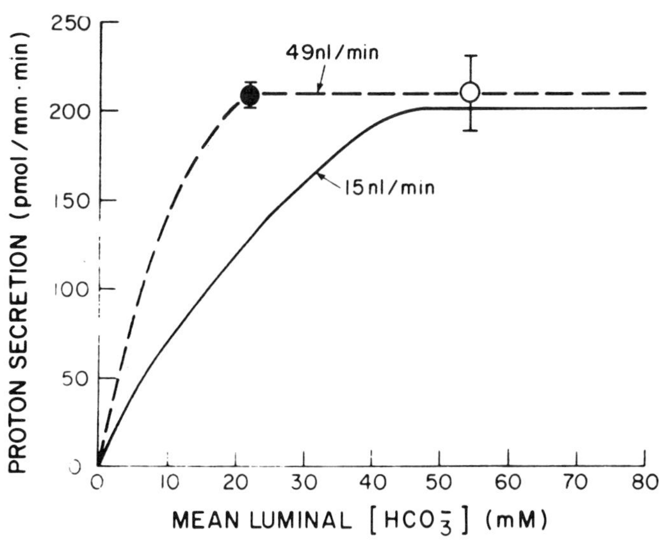

FIGURE 10-9 • Effect of luminal flow rate on transcellular proton secretion in the PCT expressed as a function of luminal bicarbonate concentration . The solid line represents tubules perfused at a low rate (15 nl/min); the dashed line, tubules perfused at a high rate (49 nl/min). The closed circle represents tubules perfused with 25 m*M* bicarbonate; the open circle, tubules perfused with 60 m*M* bicarbonate. (From Alpern RJ et al: *Am J Physiol* 245:F478, 1983. Used by permission.)

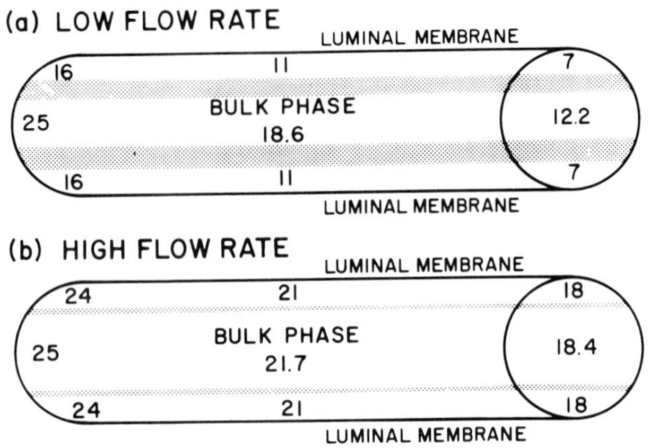

FIGURE 10-10 • Effect of luminal flow rate on concentration profiles in the proximal tubule. Tubules are perfused from left to right. Bicarbonate concentrations in the bulk phase are shown in the center of the tubule, and bicarbonate concentrations in the vicinity of the luminal membrane are shown at the top and bottom of the tubule. The shaded area represents the luminal barrier to bicarbonate diffusion. (From Alpern RJ et al: *Am J Physiol* 245:F478, 1983. Used by permission.)

from hyperfiltering animals.[111,112,216,233] These effects can be demonstrated after the transporters have been removed from the hyperfiltering environment, either by vesicle preparation or by luminal and peritubular perfusion. These effects thus represent an adaptation in proximal tubular function. In addition, increases in the Na^+-H^+ antiporter and the Na^+-$3HCO_3^-$ cotransporter activities occur in parallel.[216]

Peritubular pH, bicarbonate concentration, and P_{CO_2}

Peritubular pH can be varied by altering peritubular bicarbonate concentration or P_{CO_2}. When luminal determinants of acidification (luminal pH and flow rate) remain constant, increases in peritubular bicarbonate concentration inhibit bicarbonate absorption,[13,47,90,189,238] and decreases in peritubular bicarbonate concentration stimulate bicarbonate absorption.[13,155] This effect could be due to an effect on passive bicarbonate diffusion or on transcellular proton secretion. However, proximal tubular bicarbonate permeability is low and is not affected by peritubular pH.[13] Thus, peritubular alkalemia inhibits, and peritubular acidemia stimulates, transcellular proton secretion.[13,238] When the rate of transcellular proton secretion is examined as a function of luminal bicarbonate concentration in the presence of normal and increased concentrations of peritubular bicarbonate, increases in peritubular bicarbonate concentration are found to reduce the maximal rate of proton secretion (Fig. 10-11).[13]

These observations can be explained as follows. Decreases in peritubular pH and HCO_3^- concentration will accelerate the rate of base efflux on the Na^+-$3HCO_3^-$ cotransporter. This leads to cell acidification, which can increase apical membrane H^+ secretion by three mechanisms. First, a decrease in cell pH will increase the driving force across apical membrane transporters. Second, the Na^+-H^+ antiporter is regulated allosterically by cell pH.[16] Third, decreases in cell pH may lead to exocytotic insertion of membranes containing H^+ transporters.[245]

In addition to these acute mechanisms, the proximal tubule also adapts to chronic changes in blood pH. Ullrich and coworkers perfused the lumen and pertitubular capillary of a proximal tubule with solutions of similar pH and examined the rates of acidification using the split-droplet technique. Rats pretreated with $NaHCO_3$ had a lower rate of acidification than control rats.[278] In addition, Kunau and associates found that acidification rates were increased in acid-fed rats compared to control rats when all determinants of H^+ secretion were corrected for.[155]

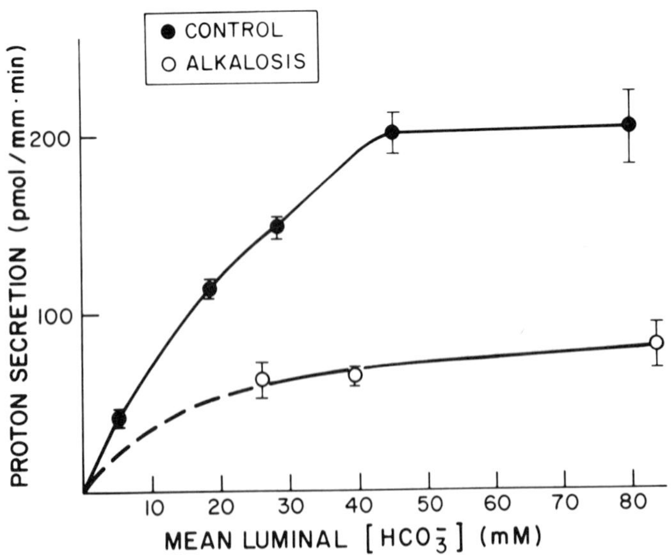

FIGURE 10-11 • Effect of alkalosis on transcellular proton secretion in the PCT expressed as a function of luminal bicarbonate concentration. (From Alpern RJ et al: *J Clin Invest* 71:736, 1983. Used by permission.)

The mechanisms responsible for these chronic adaptations to acidosis have been further elucidated. Na^+-H^+ antiporter activity, as assayed in vesicles or in perfused tubules, is increased.[2,63,144,214,276] This effect involves an increase in the V_{max} of the Na^+-H^+ antiporter.[2,276] In addition, the activity of the basolateral membrane Na^+-$3HCO_3^-$ cotransporter is increased.[2,214] In that all of these transporter assays are done after the transporter has been removed from the inducing environment, these effects represent memory effects.

The signals responsible for eliciting these adaptations have been difficult to determine precisely in vivo because of the inability to rule out possible changes in hormone levels, renal hemodynamics, or renal nerve activity. Horie and colleagues have recently studied this phenomenon in cultured proximal tubule cells.[120] Confluent primary cultures of rabbit proximal tubule cells were rendered quiescent and then exposed to either control or acid media for 2 days. Following this preincubation, cells were removed from the preincubation media, and Na^+-H^+ antiporter activity was assayed 1 h later. Preincubation in acidified, low-HCO_3^- media elicited an increase in Na^+-H^+ antiporter activity, demonstrating that a decrease in extracellular pH was sufficient to elicit this adaptation. It is interesting to note that when cultured fibroblasts were incubated under the same acidic conditions, Na^+-H^+ antiporter activity was inhibited, suggesting that the stimulatory effect is tissue specific. A similar increase in Na^+-H^+ antiporter activity has also been demonstrated in a number of renal cell lines, including MCT, OKP, and LLC-PK1.[131,194] In the primary cultures, the increase in Na^+-H^+ antiporter activity was inhibited by cycloheximide, suggesting a dependence on protein synthesis.[120] In addition, in MCT cells and LLC-PK1 cells, incubation in acid media increases the abundance of messenger RNA for the Na^+-H^+ antiporter.[131,194] In fibroblasts, incubation in acid media decreases the abundance of Na^+-H^+ antiporter mRNA.[194] In summary, these studies suggest that chronic acidosis leads to an increase in synthesis of Na^+-H^+ antiporters, associated with increased mRNA abundance and possibly transcriptional activation of the gene. Similar mechanisms may underlie the effects of chronic acidosis on the Na^+-$3HCO_3^-$ cotransporter and on the ammoniagenic enzymes phosphate-dependent glutaminase and PEPCK.

These results have a number of important physiologic implications. When subjects are fed large amounts of $NaHCO_3$ they excrete it in their urine and do not develop a chronic metabolic alkalosis. This is because the induction of a mild metabolic alkalosis leads to a marked inhibition of proton secretion in the proximal tubule. In addition, Cogan and Liu have found that the ability to maintain an alkalosis is markedly dependent on GFR.[55] When GFR is increased in alkalotic animals, proximal bicarbonate absorption does not increase, as it does in nonalkalotic animals.[55,56] This implies that increases in luminal flow rate do not stimulate bicarbonate absorption in alkalotic animals (Fig. 10-2). These observations are exactly what would be predicted from the results of microperfusion studies. In alkalosis the maximal rate of proton secretion is reduced, and thus the rate of proton secretion is close to maximal at low flow rates (Fig. 10-11).[13] Since increases in flow rate cannot cause the rate of proton secretion to exceed the maximal rate (Fig. 10-9),[14] flow dependence is limited in this situation. Thus, in the presence of metabolic alkalosis, increases in GFR are *not* associated with large increases in proximal bicarbonate absorption and therefore are associated with bicarbonaturia (Fig. 10-2). This makes GFR an important determinant of bicarbonate excretion in the presence of metabolic alkalosis.

Peritubular pH can also be altered by changing peritubular P_{CO_2}. Micropuncture studies have demonstrated that increases in P_{CO_2} stimulate proximal bicarbonate absorption and that decreases in P_{CO_2} inhibit it.[54,160] Stationary microperfusion studies in vivo and continuous microperfusion studies in vitro have also found that the rate of bicarbonate absorption increases as the ambient P_{CO_2} increases.[137,189,238] The cellular mechanisms are probably similar to those discussed above for changes in peritubular bicarbonate concentration.

Chronic changes in P_{CO_2} also elicit chronic adaptations in proximal tubule transporters. Cogan showed that proximal tubules from animals with chronic respiratory acidosis demonstrate increased H^+ secretion compared to tubules in animals with acute respiratory acidosis.[58] In addition, apical membrane Na^+-H^+ antiporter activity and basolateral membrane Na^+-$3HCO_3^-$ transporter activity are increased in chronic respiratory acidosis.[153,228] These transporter effects involve a V_{max} effect.[228] In addition, cultured proximal tubule cells incubated in high P_{CO_2} media demonstrate increased Na^+-H^+ antiporter activity[120] and increased Na^+-H^+ antiporter mRNA abundance.[194] Thus, the adaptations to chronic changes in P_{CO_2} resemble in many respects the adaptations to chronic changes in the serum HCO_3^-. In summary, peritubular pH is a potent regulator of proximal tubule H^+ secretion. This involves acute and chronic effects on H^+-HCO_3^- transport mechanisms.

Extracellular fluid volume

Extracellular fluid volume is extremely important in acid-base regulation. Most forms of chronic metabolic alkalosis are associated with extracellular fluid volume depletion. This volume depletion counterbalances the effect of peritubular alkalemia in causing bicarbonaturia and leads to maintenance of metabolic alkalosis (reabsorption of all of the filtered bicarbonate).[59]

It has long been thought that the proximal tubule is the major site where extracellular fluid volume regulates acidification.[59] Micropuncture studies have demonstrated that if GFR is maintained constant, extracellular fluid volume expansion inhibits proximal bicarbonate absorption. This effect is, however, much smaller than the effect of volume status on chloride absorption.[53,208] Microperfusion studies have further characterized this effect. These studies have confirmed that the effect on bicarbonate absorption is smaller than the effect on chloride absorption.[13,48] In addition, Alpern and coworkers have found that volume status does not directly affect the rate of transcellular proton secretion. Rather, volume expansion increases bicarbonate permeability and thus increases the rate of bicarbonate backleak.[13]

Recently, the effect of chronic changes in dietary NaCl on Na^+-H^+ antiporter activity was examined in apical membrane vesicles. Na^+-H^+ antiporter V_{max} was found to be higher in rats given a low-salt diet than in those rats ingesting a high-salt diet.[195] This suggests that small but chronic changes in extracellular fluid volume can lead to an adaptation in the Na^+-H^+ antiporter. An increase in Na^+-H^+ antiporter activity would increase both proximal tubular $NaHCO_3$ and NaCl absorption in chronic volume contraction.

Potassium

Potassium depletion frequently accompanies alkalosis and stimulates acidification. Chan and coworkers have used luminal and capillary microperfusion to examine whether such an effect occurs in the proximal tubule. When the potassium concentration of the peritubular capillary was lowered from 4 to 2 meq/liter, proximal acidification was unaffected.[47] However, when rats were placed on a diet containing no potassium and allowed to become potassium-deficient, acidification was stimulated by 23 percent.[47] This effect of a low-potassium diet has been demonstrated to be due to parallel increases in apical membrane Na^+-H^+ antiporter and basolateral membrane Na^+-$3HCO_3^-$ cotransporter activities.[256] Once again, this transporter effect is demonstrable in vesicles removed from the inducing environment.

Calcium, phosphate, and PTH

The role of calcium, phosphate, and parathyroid hormone (PTH) in the regulation of acidification is extremely complex due to the interactions of these determinants with each other. PTH infusion into rats or dogs inhibits volume and bicarbonate absorption in the proximal tubule, as assessed by in vivo micropuncture.[20,218] In these studies, the inhibition of acidification could be due to PTH or hypercalcemia. In vitro microperfusion of rabbit proximal tubules has shown that PTH directly inhibits proximal tubular fluid and bicarbonate absorption in the absence of changes in calcium concentration.[132,186,187] This inhibition of proximal bicarbonate absorption could be due to a decrease in the rate of active bicarbonate absorption (active proton secretion) or an increase in the rate of bicarbonate backleak (increased bicarbonate permeability). Indeed, studies in the rat and rabbit PCT have found that PTH and cAMP increase permeability to sucrose and mannitol.[136,169,170] McKinney and Myers addressed this question by examining the effect of PTH on the rate of bicarbonate backleak during inhibition of active transport.[186,187] In this setting, they found no effect of PTH. They therefore suggested that the major effect of PTH on acidification was to inhibit active proton secretion.

The direct effect of PTH on acidification has now been studied at the cellular level. PTH increases adenyl cyclase activity, increasing cell cAMP levels and secondarily stimulating cAMP-dependent protein kinase. Through this mechanism, PTH has been demonstrated to inhibit the apical membrane Na^+-H^+ antiporter.[139,213] Cyclic AMP-dependent protein kinase has been demonstrated to directly inhibit Na^+-H^+ antiporter activity in brush border membrane vesicles.[291,292] Recently, Sasaki and colleagues have demonstrated that PTH does not affect basolateral membrane Na^+-$3HCO_3^-$ cotransporter activity.[237] However, studies in basolateral membrane vesicles have found that cAMP-dependent protein kinase inhibits Na^+-$3HCO_3^-$ cotransporter activity.[229] PTH is also known to activate phospholipase C, with secondary increases in cell calcium and activation of protein kinase C.[122] However, no role of this effect in acidification has been demonstrated.

Whether there is a direct effect of calcium on proximal acidification has also been studied successfully in the in vitro perfused rabbit PCT. Increases in bath calcium concentration had a small but significant stimulatory effect on the rate of bicarbonate absorption.[188]

Although PTH is a potent inhibitor of proximal acidification, it appears that its net effect along the entire nephron is to stimulate acidification. Indeed, Bank and Aynedjian found that while PTH inhibited proximal bicarbonate absorption, total kidney titratable acid, ammonia, and net acid excretion rose and urine pH decreased.[20] Puschett and Zurbach found bicarbonate excretion and urinary pH unaffected in spite of inhibition of proximal acidification.[218] These results suggest that PTH stimulates distal acidification.

Clearance studies have examined the effect of chronic PTH administration in the rat and dog. These studies found that increased levels of PTH led to a primary metabolic alkalosis.[128,129,193] The metabolic alkalosis occurred whether increased levels of PTH were associated with hypercalcemia or hypocalcemia,[129] and was due to extrarenal and renal factors. The extrarenal effect is related to PTH-induced mobilization of bone bicarbonate;[128,129] the renal effect is most likely a stimulation of distal acidification. This stimulation of distal acidification may be due to increases in distal delivery of phosphate.[31]

Clearance studies have also found that administration of 1α,25-dihydroxycholecalciferol (1,25-DHCC) leads to hypercalcemia and metabolic alkalosis.[128,193] Here, the metabolic alkalosis occurs in the absence of increased PTH and is related to extrarenal vitamin D-induced mobilization of bone bicarbonate and renal hypercalcemia-induced stimulation of acidification.[129] This stimulation of acidification may be what is observed in the proximal tubule when bath calcium is raised.[188]

Phosphate depletion is also an important determinant of renal acidification. Gold and colleagues first reported that phosphate depletion in dogs caused a metabolic acidosis. Because of marked bicarbonaturia at abnormally low plasma bicarbonate concentrations, this defect was attributed to the proximal tubule.[93] Emmett and associates found similar results in rats but also found that phosphate depletion led to mobilization of bone bicarbonate. This initially prevented metabolic acidosis in spite of a similar acidification defect.[75]

In summary, PTH inhibits proximal bicarbonate absorption but stimulates distal acidification. The result is an increased rate of renal acidification. Hypercalcemia stimulates proximal and possibly distal acidification. Phosphate depletion inhibits proximal acidification. In addition to these renal effects, any maneuver that leads to bone calcium mobilization also leads to bone bicarbonate mobilization.

Hormones

In addition to PTH, discussed above, a number of other hormones regulate rates of H^+ secretion in the proximal tubule. In addition to hemodynamic effects, *angiotensin II* (AII) has been demonstrated to directly stimulate Na^+ and volume absorption in the proximal tubule.[110,241] This effect is dose-dependent in that stimulation is seen at low concentrations of 10^{-12} to 10^{-10} *M*, with inhibition seen at high concentrations around 10^{-7} to 10^{-6} *M*. As might be expected, this increase in Na^+ absorption is accompanied by an increase in H^+ secretion.[164,165] The effect of AII on H^+ secretion is greatest in the S_1 proximal tubule, where AII receptors are most dense.[165] Angiotensin II has been demonstrated to increase Na^+-H^+ antiporter and Na^+-$3HCO_3^-$ cotransporter activity.[85,231] The mechanism of action by which AII stimulates this transporter is still under investigation, but one mechanism appears to be inhibition of adenyl cyclase by an inhibitory G-protein (G_i)-coupled process with subsequent decreases in cell cAMP levels.[68,166]

The effect of *catecholamines* on proximal tubule function is more complex. A number of investigators have found that various catecholamine receptors mediate effects on proximal tubule function. The only clear demonstration of regulation of an H^+ transporter has been by alpha 2 receptors, which have been demonstrated to increase Na^+-H^+ antiporter activity.[204] The stimulation of Na^+-H^+ antiporter is consistent with the previous finding of stimulation of proximal tubule bicarbonate absorption by alpha-adrenergic agonists.[44] This has been shown to be due to inhibition of adenyl cyclase.[52] *Dopamine* has also been demonstrated in proximal tubule cells to activate adenyl cyclase and to inhibit the Na^+-H^+ antiporter.[76]

LOOP OF HENLE

The loop of Henle includes the thin descending limb, the thin ascending limb, and the thick ascending limb. Micropuncture studies have evaluated the importance of the loop of Henle by comparing the compositions of tubular fluid at the end of the PCT and at the early distal tubule. These studies have found that the pH and bicarbonate concentrations are similar in these locations.[40,73,100] However, because water is abstracted in the loop, maintenance of constant pH involves absorption of 50 to 70 percent of the bicarbonate delivered out of the PCT.[40,73] Since pH is not altered in this segment, titratable acid content is not altered. As discussed previously, ammonium is absorbed in the loop of Henle such that the quantity arriving in the distal convoluted tubule is less than the quantity leaving the PCT.[39,40]

In these micropuncture studies, the segment examined included the proximal straight tubule and the loop of Henle. Since the proximal straight tubule has been shown to absorb bicarbonate,[181,287] these studies do not provide information concerning the contribution of the loop segments. That question has been studied effectively using the in vitro perfused thick ascending limb of the loop of Henle.

Iino and Burg perfused the rabbit cortical thick ascending limb of the loop of Henle at 1.1 nl/mm·min and found no significant bicarbonate absorption.[133] These results agree with studies that have demonstrated that carbonic anhydrase is absent from the rabbit thick ascending limb.[66] Good and coworkers found that rat cortical and medullary thick ascending limbs perfused at 1 nl/mm·min absorb bicarbonate at a rate of approximately 5 pmol/mm·min.[99] These results agree with histologic studies that have demonstrated carbonic anhydrase in the rat thick ascending limb.[66] Friedman and Andreoli found no significant bicarbonate absorption in the mouse thick ascending limb,[79] which possesses carbonic anhydrase.[66] These authors, however, perfused at a rapid rate (10.9 nl/min) and may have been unable to detect the small rates of bicarbonate absorption measured by Good and coworkers.

The mechanism of HCO_3^- absorption in the thick ascending limb of the loop of Henle of the rat has been investigated by Good.[94] HCO_3^- absorption was inhibited by acetazolamide, implying a dependence on carbonic anhydrase. In addition, HCO_3^- absorption was dependent on Na^+ absorption in that it was inhibited by Na^+ removal, luminal amiloride, or inhibition of the basolateral membrane Na^+-K^+ ATPase. All of these studies point to an apical membrane Na^+-H^+ antiporter. Finally, these studies found that furosemide stimulated Na^+-H^+ exchange, possibly by inhibiting NaCl entry into the cell, lowering cell Na^+, and secondarily stimulating the Na^+-H^+ antiporter.

Krapf measured cell pH in the in vitro perfused rat cortical thick ascending limb and studied the transport mechanisms present.[152] Decreases in peritubular pH or in peritubular Na^+ concentration caused a cell acidification that was partially blocked by SITS and independent of Cl. This effect was dependent on the presence of CO_2-HCO_3^-. In addition, depolarization of cells caused them to alkalinize. All of these results are similar to those present in the proximal tubule and suggest the presence of a basolateral membrane Na^+-$3HCO_3^-$ cotransporter. Similar results have been found in the salamander diluting segment.[286] Thus, based on the abovementioned results, it appears that HCO_3^- absorption is mediated by an apical membrane Na^+-H^+ antiporter working in series with a basolateral membrane Na^+-$3HCO_3^-$ cotransporter. This mechanism is very similar to that present in the proximal tubule.

More recent studies have addressed the regulation of HCO_3^- absorption in the rat thick ascending limb. Tubules dissected from rats with chronic metabolic acidosis were found to have increased rates of HCO_3^- absorption, whereas tubules dissected from rats with chronic metabolic alkalosis were found to have decreased rates.[96] In addition, adrenalectomy decreased HCO_3^- absorption, and application of aldosterone in vitro reversed this decrease.[96] Finally, conditions that increased Na^+ delivery to the thick ascending limb in vivo increased HCO_3^- absorption in the in vitro perfused tubule.[96]

A number of hormones known to activate adenyl cyclase in the thick ascending limb also regulate HCO_3^- absorption. *Arginine vasopressin* (AVP), *glucagon*, and *PTH* all inhibit HCO_3^- absorption.[97] Application of 8-bromocyclic AMP was also found to inhibit HCO_3^- absorption. This effect was not due to stimulation of NaCl absorption in that AVP still inhibited HCO_3^- absorption in the presence of 10^{-4} *M* furosemide.

Micropuncture studies have evaluated the role of these effects by comparing the quantity of HCO_3^- at the end proximal tubule and the early distal tubule. AVP and glucagon inhibited HCO_3^- absorption in the loop of Henle.[32,191] PTH, however, stimulated HCO_3^- absorption in thyroparathyroidectomized rats.[190] The reason for the discrepancy between this result and that in the in vitro perfused tubule is currently unexplained.

DISTAL NEPHRON

Role in acidification

Fluid delivered to the distal nephron is normally low in both bicarbonate (5 to 7 meq/liter) and pH (6.5 to 6.7).[70] It is the role of the distal nephron to reabsorb most of the remaining bicarbonate and to further lower the pH of the tubular fluid so as to trap ammonium and titrate filtered buffers to form titratable acid. The distal nephron is composed of multiple segments. Each segment poses different technical problems for the investigator, and thus the techniques used to examine each segment have been different. We will first describe the role of each segment in acidification and then examine the cellular mechanism and regulation of acidification.

"Surface distal tubule"

This segment is defined as the portion of a superficial distal tubule that comes to the surface of the kidney and thus is accessible to micropuncture. The surface distal tubule includes four discrete segments: the *thick ascending limb of the loop of Henle,* the *distal convoluted tubule,* the *connecting tubule,* and the *initial cortical collecting tubule.*[196] The connecting tubule and the initial cortical collecting tubule contain intercalated cells, which have been found in other segments of the nephron to mediate H^+-HCO_3^- transport (see below). Studies have demonstrated that the surface distal tubule is capable of either net H^+ secretion or net HCO_3^- secretion, depending on the dietary history of the animal.[173]

Cortical collecting duct

This segment has been studied by in vitro perfusion of tubular segments that have been dissected out from the kidney. McKinney and Burg found that this segment is capable of absorbing bicarbonate (acidification) or secreting bicarbonate (alkalinization). If animals are pretreated with acid, the cortical collecting tubule absorbs bicarbonate; if animals are pretreated with alkali, the cortical collecting tubule secretes bicarbonate. Both processes are relatively slow compared to the rates of proton secretion observed in the proximal tubule and the medullary collecting tubule. When tubules are perfused in the absence of pH gradients, the rates of bicarbonate absorption are approximately 6 pmol/mm·min in the cortical collecting tubule,[182-184] 11 pmol/mm·min in the medullary collecting tubule,[167] and 80 pmol/mm·min in the PCT.[42]

Outer medullary collecting duct

This segment has been studied extensively by in vitro microperfusion. Thus far it has been demonstrated to acidify its luminal contents at a higher rate than does the cortical collecting tubule.[167] No bicarbonate secretion has been identified. The medullary collecting tubule differs from other segments in that it has been found to acidify its luminal contents but not to perform any active sodium or potassium transport.[266]

Papillary (inner medullary) collecting duct

The papillary collecting duct has been studied in vivo with micropuncture and in vivo microcatheterization. The papillary collecting duct does acidify its luminal contents[72,104,277] and is capable of absorbing bicarbonate.[105,223,277] No net bicarbonate secretion has been observed, but the possibility of a bicarbonate secretory pathway has been raised (see below).[277]

Cell types mediating H^+-HCO_3^- transport

H^+-HCO_3^- transport in the connecting tubule, cortical collecting duct, and portions of the outer medullary collecting duct is mediated by the *intercalated cell.* This cell stains intensely for carbonic anhydrase and is found immunocytochemically to contain the type II isoenzyme of carbonic anhydrase. This cell has a darker cytoplasm and numerous mitochondria. Recent data suggest that other cells in the distal nephron may mediate H^+ secretion. In the rat inner medullary collecting duct, there are few intercalated cells;[51] yet these segments secrete H^+. In the inner stripe of the rabbit outer medullary collecting duct, intercalated cells are also scarce. However, in this segment the predominant cell type is one that is functionally very similar to the intercalated cell. Ridderstrale and colleagues have found that this segment ultrastructurally contains one cell type with apical membrane rod-shaped particles, subapical vesicles, and weak carbonic anhydrase staining.[224] Electrophysiologically, these cells have a voltage of approximately 30 mV with a very high apical membrane resistance and a basolateral Cl selective membrane, characteristics similar to those of a typical intercalated cell.[151,198] Functionally, these cells have an apical membrane *N*-ethylmaleimide (NEM)-sensitive H^+ pump and a basolateral membrane stilbene-sensitive Cl^--HCO_3^- exchanger, also typical of acid-secreting intercalated cells.[36,113,114] In spite of these similarities, these cells do not stain with antibodies against carbonic anhydrase isoenzyme II.[179]

Intercalated cells have also been further subdivided into two types: *type A* and *type B intercalated cells.* Type A intercalated cells are believed to mediate H^+ secretion. As noted above, these cells are similar to the H^+-secreting cells of the outer medullary collecting duct. The type A intercalated cell stains with antibodies against a vacuolar H^+ ATPase on the apical membrane and stains with antibodies against the band 3 Cl^--HCO_3^- exchanger on the basolateral membrane.[38,243] These cells demonstrate luminal endocytosis.[245] In addition, these cells have an extensive microplicated apical membrane.[178]

A second cell type, the type B intercalated cell, is believed to mediate HCO_3^- secretion in the connecting tubule, initial cortical collecting tubule, and cortical collecting duct. This cell has a more well-developed basolateral membrane with a less well-developed microvillus apical membrane.[178] It has basolateral membrane staining with antibodies against a vacuolar H^+ pump but no staining with antibodies against band 3.[38,243] In the rabbit, these cells stain apically with peanut lectin. Functionally, these cells have been demonstrated to possess an apical membrane Cl^--HCO_3^- exchanger, confirming their role in HCO_3^- secretion (see below).

Cellular mechanism of acidification

Proton secretion versus bicarbonate absorption

As in the proximal tubule, bicarbonate absorption in the distal nephron could occur by proton secretion (Fig. 10-6*a*) or direct bicarbonate absorption (Fig. 10-6*b*). The approach to this problem has been similar to that used with the proximal tubule.

Disequilibrium pH has been measured in the surface distal convoluted tubule, the outer medullary collecting duct, and the papillary collecting duct. DuBose and associates found that if distal acidification was stimulated by a combined respiratory acidosis-metabolic alkalosis, an acid disequilibrium pH was observed in the surface distal tubule.[71] DuBose and colleagues also found that this acid disequilibrium pH occurred in the absence of carbonic anhydrase inhibition and was prevented by carbonic anhydrase infusion. These results suggest that luminal fluid does not have functional contact with carbonic anhydrase in the distal convoluted tubule.

Graber and coworkers measured disequilibrium pH along the length of the medullary collecting tubule using microcatheterization.[104] DuBose measured disequilibrium pH in the papillary collecting duct using micropuncture.[72] Both groups found that control rats possessed an acid disequilibrium pH that was abolished by infusion of carbonic anhydrase.[72,104] These results once again suggest that acidification in the collecting tubule occurs by proton secretion and that fluid in the collecting tubule lumen is not in functional contact with carbonic anhydrase.

Star and coworkers measured the disequilibrium pH in segments from the rabbit collecting duct perfused in vitro. In these studies, an acid disequilibrium pH was present in the cortical collecting duct and in the outer stripe of the outer medullary collecting duct.[260,261] The disequilibrium pH was eliminated by addition of carbonic anhydrase to the lumen. By contrast, the inner stripe of the outer medullary collecting tubule did not possess an acid disequilibrium pH but developed one upon inhibition of luminal carbonic anhydrase. The latter finding suggested that this segment is unique in that the luminal fluid is exposed to carbonic anhydrase. Recently, Wall and associates have found a similar presence of luminal carbonic anhydrase in the rat inner medullary collecting duct.[284]

Apical membrane H^+ secretion

Initial studies examined whether H^+ secretion was mediated by Na^+-H^+ exchange or electrogenic proton secretion. Koeppen and Hellman perfused the cortical collecting tubule in vitro at very low rates and measured transepithelial potential difference (PD) and the pH of collected fluid.[150] When tubules were perfused with sodium-free solutions or exposed to ouabain (maneuvers that should eliminate the sodium transport-dependent negative potential) luminal PD became positive. This positive PD was reduced by carbonic anhydrase inhibition and peritubular SITS and was unaffected by chloride removal from the perfusates. These data suggest that the lumen-positive PD is due to acidification and represents electrogenic proton secretion. In addition, these studies show that this process does not require sodium transport.

Ullrich and Papavassiliou also found that bicarbonate absorption in the papillary collecting duct is unaffected by sodium removal from luminal and peritubular perfusates.[277] Data in the medullary collecting tubule have also suggested an electrogenic, sodium-independent process. Lombard, Stone, and coworkers have demonstrated bicarbonate absorption in this segment.[167,267,268] Stokes, however, found that his segment does not actively transport sodium.[266] Stone and associates found that the medullary collecting tubule possessed a lumen-positive PD that was dependent on the magnitude of acidification.[267] In these studies both the lumen-positive PD and the rate of acidification were unaffected by sodium removal.

Further evidence in favor of an apical membrane H^+ ATPase has been provided by measuring cell pH in the inner stripe of the outer medullary collecting tubule using fluorescent techniques.[113] In these studies, Hays and Alpern examined the recovery of cell pH from an acid load. Addition of luminal Na^+ had no effect on the rate of cell alkalinization. Luminal NEM, an inhibitor of vaculolar H^+ ATPases, inhibited cell pH recovery. Addition of NEM to the basolateral solution had no effect. These studies thus suggested that the apical membrane has an NEM-sensitive H^+ pump. Gluck and coworkers have purified an H^+ ATPase of the vaculolar type from renal medullary membranes.[91] Using antibodies against a number of the subunits of the purified H^+ ATPase, apical membranes of H^+-secreting intercalated cells were labeled.[38] In summary, these results suggest that acidification in the distal nephron is due to electrogenic, sodium-independent proton secretion.

Basolateral membrane bicarbonate exit

Stone and coworkers found that the rate of chloride secretion in the medullary collecting tubule was equal to the rate of proton secretion.[268] They also found that chloride gradients affected the rate of proton secretion (a bath Cl > lumen Cl gradient-stimulated proton secretion; a lumen Cl > bath Cl gradient-inhibited proton secretion). This effect was not mediated by chloride gradient-induced changes in transepithelial PD. In addition, total chloride removal from luminal and bath fluids abolished proton secretion. Stone and colleagues also found that SITS inhibits proton secretion when applied from the bath side but has no effect when applied from the lumen.[268] SITS is a known inhibitor of the red blood cell chloride-bicarbonate exchanger;[43,149] thus, these results suggest the presence of a chloride-bicarbonate exchanger on the basolateral membrane. However, SITS may affect other anion transporters and thus may not be very specific.

Once again, studies have utilized the measurement of cell pH to examine basolateral membrane H^+-HCO_3^- transport mechanisms. These studies have found that H^+-secreting intercalated cells and cells of the outer medullary collecting duct inner stripe have a Cl^--HCO_3^- exchanger.[36,114,247] Chloride addition to the peritubular fluid causes cell acidification, and Cl^- removal causes cell alkalinization. This effect is partially inhibited by removal of exogenous CO_2-HCO_3^- and is unaffected by Na^+ removal or voltage-clamping the tubule.[114] Studies have also examined whether antibodies generated against the red blood cell band 3 Cl^--HCO_3^- exchanger stain kidney membranes. These studies have demonstrated that most antibodies will stain the basolateral membrane of H^+-secreting cells.[242,243,283] However, monoclonal antibodies generated against the amino terminal portion of the red blood cell band 3 Cl^--HCO_3^- exchanger do not stain the kidney sections.[283] A renal Cl^--HCO_3^- exchanger has now been cloned from renal cDNA libraries by two groups.[37,154] Both groups have found that the renal Cl^--HCO_3^- exchanger is identical to the red blood cell Cl^--HCO_3^- exchanger with the exception that the N-terminal portion of the protein is deficient. This has been demonstrated to be due to transcription from the same gene but utilizing an alternative start site.

In addition to the Cl^--HCO_3^- exchanger, a number of groups have found basolateral membrane Na^+-H^+ antiporters in the collecting tubule. This was first demonstrated by Chaillet and Boron[45] and has subsequently been found in both H^+-secreting and HCO_3^--secreting intercalated cells as well as in the inner stripe of the outer medullary collecting duct.[36,113,290] It is currently not clear what the role of a basolateral membrane Na^+-H^+ antiporter is in these cells. Presumably, it is related to "housekeeping functions" and is not relevant to transepithelial H^+ secretion.

In summary, base efflux across the basolateral membrane of H^+-secreting cells occurs by Cl^--HCO_3^- exchange. Although these cells possess a Na^+-H^+ antiporter, it would function in the wrong direction to mediate base efflux. Chloride that enters the cell on the Cl^--HCO_3^- exchanger could exit across the apical or basolateral membrane. Koeppen has demonstrated that the basolateral membrane has a high conductance to Cl^-, while the apical membrane has an extremely low ionic conductance.[151] Thus, most likely Cl^- that enters the cell

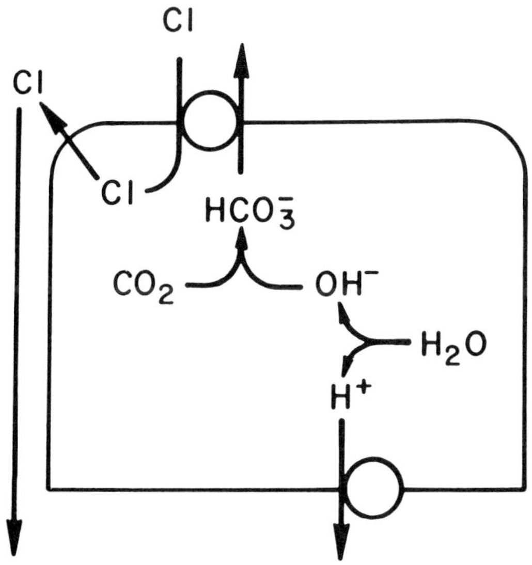

FIGURE 10-12 • Mechanism of proton secretion in the distal nephron. (From Alpern RJ in Brenner BM, Rector FC (eds): *The Kidney,* 4th ed, Philadelphia, Saunders, 1990. Used by permission.)

on the Cl^--HCO_3^- exchanger exits the basolateral membrane. The lumen positive voltage generated by electrogenic H^+ secretion will then drive Cl^- across the tight junction into the lumen. Figure 10-12 shows the mechanism of H^+ secretion in the distal nephron.

Leak pathways

Leak pathways are extremely small in the collecting tubule. Although bicarbonate permeability has not been measured, it is assumed to be low because of the high electrical resistance of this epithelium.[117] Hydrogen ion permeability measured in the cortical collecting tubule was 1.3×10^{-3} cm/s (two orders of magnitude less than in the proximal tubule).[108]

Cellular mechanism of bicarbonate secretion

When cortical collecting tubules are perfused in vitro with solutions containing 25 meq/liter bicarbonate on their luminal and peritubular sides, some tubules actively absorb bicarbonate, while some tubules actively secrete bicarbonate. McKinney and Burg found that if rabbits were pretreated with NH_4Cl, their cortical collecting tubules absorbed bicarbonate,[182,183] whereas if they were pretreated with $NaHCO_3$, their cortical collecting tubules secreted bicarbonate.[182,184] It appears that both secretion and absorption of bicarbonate proceed simultaneously, although pretreatment of the animals determines which process proceeds at the faster rate.

The cellular mechanism of HCO_3^- secretion has been best studied in tubules perfused from animals with DOCA-induced metabolic alkalosis.[258] In these tubules, rates of HCO_3^- secretion were equal to rates of Cl^- absorption. In addition, HCO_3^- secretion was dependent on the presence of Cl^- and was independent of the presence of Na^+. These results suggest that active basolateral membrane H^+ extrusion is mediated by a Na^+-independent mechanism, namely a H^+ ATPase. The Cl^- dependence may be related to apical membrane base efflux. Indeed, basolateral membrane Cl^--HCO_3^- exchange has been demonstrated in beta intercalated cells using the fluorescent measurement of cell pH.[247,290] This Cl^--HCO_3^- exchanger is different from the red blood cell Cl^--HCO_3^- exchanger in that antibodies generated against the red blood cell transporter do not stain the apical membrane of the HCO_3^--secreting cells. In addition, luminal disulfonic stilbenes do not inhibit HCO_3^- secretion in the mammalian cortical collecting tubule.[240]

The presence of a basolateral membrane H^+ ATPase in beta intercalated cells has been confired by immunocytochemical studies. Antibodies generated against the H^+ ATPase of Gluck and associates stain the basolateral membrane in HCO_3^--secreting cells.[38] Fluorescent pH measurements have demonstrated a basolateral membrane Na^+-H^+ antiporter in these cells,[290] but as stated above, the lack of Na^+ dependence of HCO_3^- secretion implies that this mechanism is not related to HCO_3^- secretion. In addition, peritubular amiloride, an inhibitor of the Na^+-H^+ antiporter, does not affect the rate of HCO_3^- secretion.[240]

Based on these results, the best model for HCO_3^- secretion appears to be basolateral membrane H^+ extrusion by a vacuolar H^+ ATPase. Base generated within the cell exits across the apical membrane in exchange for chloride. Once again, the results of electrophysiologic studies suggest that the basolateral membrane of these cells contains a high Cl^- conductance, while the apical membrane is poorly conductive to all ions.[198] Therefore, Cl^- that enters the cell in exchange for HCO_3^- most likely exits the basolateral membrane. This mechanism would be electroneutral in that apical and basolateral membrane net charge movement is zero. Figure 10-13 shows the cellular model for bicarbonate secretion in type B intercalated cells.

Carbonic anhydrase

Histologic studies show that carbonic anhydrase is present in large amounts in intercalated cells.[66,168] Intercalated cells are absent from the outer medulla, but carbonic anhydrase is present in the remaining cells. Carbonic anhydrase is, however, totally absent from the papilla.[66,168]

Microperfusion studies have found that both proton secretion and bicarbonate secretion in the cortical collecting tubule and proton secretion in the outer medullary collecting tubule are inhibited by inhibitors of carbonic anhydrase.[167,183,184] Similarly, micropuncture and stationary microperfusion studies have found that these in-

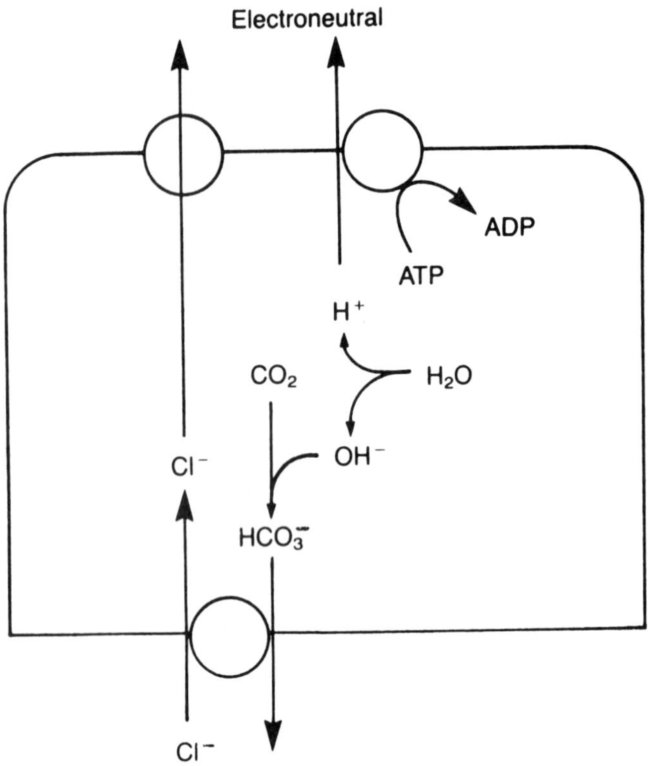

FIGURE 10-13 • Mechanism of bicarbonate secretion in the cortical collecting tubule. (From Alpern RJ in Brenner BM, Rector FC (eds): *The Kidney,* 4th ed, Philadelphia, Saunders, 1990. Used by permission.)

hibitors reduce the rate of bicarbonate absorption in the papillary collecting duct.[223,277] The latter finding is somewhat surprising in that histologic studies have been unable to find carbonic anhydrase in the papillary collecting duct.[66,168] The most likely explanation for this is that small amounts of carbonic anhydrase, in concentrations too low for detection, are present and are required for normal rates of acidification.

As discussed above, most segments of the distal nephron have an acid disequilibrium pH under control conditions. This implies that under control conditions the luminal fluid is not at equilibrium and thus is not exposed to carbonic anhydrase. Addition of luminal carbonic anhydrase causes the disequilibrium pH to disappear.[72,104,260,261] In addition, Lönnerholm and Ridderstrale found no carbonic anhydrase on the luminal membrane of the collecting tubule.[168] The lack of exposure of luminal fluid to carbonic anhydrase is very important in the genesis of the high CO_2 tension of alkaline urine, as will be discussed below. As noted above, in the outer medullary collecting tubule inner stripe of the rabbit and the inner medullary collecting duct of the rat, luminal fluid is exposed to carbonic anhydrase.

Other models for studying distal acidification

As discussed above, recent developments in tubular microperfusion technology have greatly increased our understanding of distal nephron acidification mechanisms. Other techniques have also been used to approach this problem and have added greatly to our knowledge.

Turtle urinary bladder

One experimental model that has been particularly useful has been the turtle urinary bladder. The turtle bladder is an epithelium with a high electrical resisitance. The epithelium absorbs sodium from and acidifies its luminal fluid. It offers the technical advantage that it can be studied in a chamber as a sheet separating two bathing solutions: mucosal (luminal) and serosal (peritubular). In this chamber, transepithelial voltage can be measured and can be maintained at set values (voltage clamp).

Acidification in the turtle bladder involves proton secretion rather than direct bicarbonate absorption.[263] Proton secretion occurs by a sodium-independent process and is electrogenic.[263] Acidification is inhibited by serosal SITS[62] or by removal of chloride from the serosal fluid.[77] Therefore, the base exit step on the serosal membrane appears to involve chloride-hydroxyl exchange. The epithelium is electrically tight (has high resistance); thus, leak pathways are unimportant.[24,263] Measurements of cell pH have demonstrated that proton secretion across the mucosal membrane is active, whereas hydroxyl exit across the serosal membrane is passive.[262] Acidification appears to be performed by only one of the cell types. These cells, referred to as mitochondrial rich cells, contain many mitochondria and large amounts of carbonic anhydrase.[250,263]

The proton secretory flux exists in the absence of CO_2 or bicarbonate. This flux therefore involves hydrogen or hydroxyl ion movement. If CO_2 and bicarbonate are added to the serosal solution so as to maintain serosal pH steady, a bicarbonate secretory flux is observed.[159] This flux is electroneutral and involves 1:1 exchange with chloride.[159] Thus, addition of bicarbonate to the serosal solution causes a serosal-to-mucosal bicarbonate flux and a mucosal-to-serosal chloride flux. Although the bicarbonate concentration gradient is sufficient to drive the bicarbonate and chloride fluxes, these fluxes are coupled to aerobic metabolism and are inhibited by deoxygenation, dinitrophenol, cyanide, and deoxyglucose.[206] Chloride-bicarbonate exchange is also a unidirectional process; addition of bicarbonate to the mucosal solution does *not* lead to chloride secretion.[159]

It is clear from the foregoing discussion that the turtle bladder provides an ideal opportunity for the examination of cellular mechanisms of acidification in the distal nephron. Recent perfusion studies have found a remarkable degree of similarity between the mechanisms of acidification in the turtle bladder and in the mammalian cortical collecting tubule. This is not surprising, since both segments are electrically tight epithelia (electrical resistance is high) that provide the final acidification of the luminal fluid. Both epithelia possess electrogenic proton secretion and can actively secrete bicarbonate. The turtle bladder offers the opportunity to inhibit proton secretion or bicarbonate secretion independently, allowing the study of the remaining flux. This presents a significant experimental advantage over the cortical collecting tubule.

Urine-minus-blood P_{CO_2}

Another technique that has proved useful for the examination of distal acidification has been the urine-minus-blood P_{CO_2} (U-B P_{CO_2}). In the presence of an acid urine, urinary P_{CO_2} is slightly less than or similar to blood P_{CO_2}. In the presence of bicarbonaturia (alkaline urine), the urinary P_{CO_2} rises and becomes greater than the P_{CO_2} of blood. The mechanism leading to a positive U-B P_{CO_2} in alkaline urine was first addressed by Ochwadt and Pitts. They found that intravenous infusions of carbonic anhydrase lowered the U-B P_{CO_2} from about 40 mmHg to zero.[205] Such an infusion leads to carbonic anhydrase in the urine and presumably in the tubular fluid.

These results imply that the high urinary P_{CO_2} is due to delayed dehydration of carbonic acid. Carbonic acid is formed in a compartment of the kidney by the combining of a proton and a bicarbonate ion (compartment 1, Fig. 10-14). This compartment has a high CO_2 permeability. If carbonic anhydrase is present in the luminal fluid, the carbonic acid will dehydrate to form CO_2, which then diffuses into the blood, and the urinary P_{CO_2} becomes equal to that of blood (Fig. 10-14*a*). However, if carbonic anhydrase is absent from the luminal fluid of this compartment, the dehydration of carbonic acid is delayed, and tubular fluid passes into a second compartment (Fig. 10-14*b*) with higher concentrations of carbonic acid, bicarbonate, and acidified nonbicarbonate buffer. In this second compartment, acidified nonbicarbonate buffer can react with bicarbonate to form carbonic acid, which then slowly dehydrates to form CO_2. The rate of CO_2 diffusion in this compartment is limited (compartment 2, Fig. 10-14), and the majority of CO_2 formed appears in the urine. Thus, carbonic anhydrase infusion causes the U-B P_{CO_2} to become zero by allowing all of the carbonic acid to be converted to CO_2 in compartment 1, where the CO_2 can easily diffuse into the blood.

The compartment in which CO_2 diffusion is limited (compartment 2) was initially felt to be the urinary pelvis, ureters, and bladder. CO_2 diffusion out of the urine is limited in these locations because of the limited surface area. Graber and colleagues, however, found that the P_{CO_2} of medullary collecting duct fluid was elevated above that of blood and that the level rose along the length of the medullary collecting tubule.[103] DuBose found similarly that the P_{CO_2} in the papillary collecting duct was elevated above that in blood and that the P_{CO_2} rose along the length of the papillary collecting duct. DuBose also found that the P_{CO_2} in the vasa recta was elevated and equal to the P_{CO_2} in the neighboring collecting tubule.[72] From these results, it appears that the medullary collecting tubule is also part of compartment 2 in that outward CO_2 diffusion is limited. This limitation of CO_2 diffusion is due to the countercurrent system, not

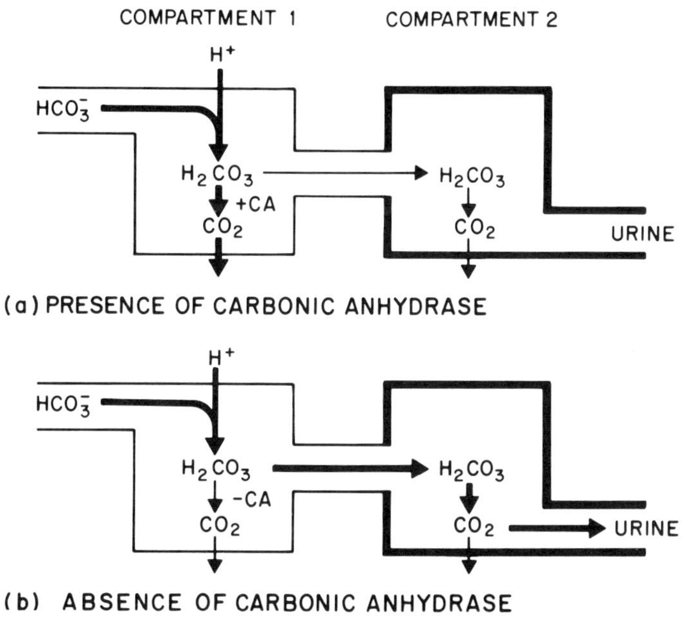

FIGURE 10-14 • Generation of the urine-minus-blood P_{CO_2} in alkaline urine. Protons are added to the luminal contents in compartment 1, which is very permeable to CO_2. Compartment 2 is impermeable to CO_2. (*a*) If carbonic anhydrase is present in the luminal fluid, the bulk of CO_2 is formed in compartment 1, from which it can diffuse out; urine P_{CO_2} will be equal to that of blood. (*b*) If carbonic anhydrase is absent from the luminal fluid, the bulk of CO_2 is formed in compartment 2, where it is unable to leave; it thus appears in the urine as a high P_{CO_2}.

to low CO_2 permeability of the medullary collecting tubule. The countercurrent system, designed to prevent sodium chloride and urea from diffusing out of the inner medulla, also prevents CO_2 from diffusing out of the inner medulla. Thus, the inner medulla, pelvis, ureters, and bladder all represent structures where CO_2 diffusion is limited. Sabatini and coworkers have found that papillary necrosis does not affect the U-B P_{CO_2} in rats, suggesting that the inner medulla, among these structures, is not required for generation of U-B P_{CO_2}.[230] As noted above, the rabbit outer medullary collecting duct inner stripe and the rat inner medullary collecting duct have apical membrane carbonic anhydrase to which the luminal fluid is exposed. While this will allow rapid formation of CO_2, the limitations on CO_2 diffusion from these structures prevent collapse of the U-B P_{CO_2}.

The process by which protons are released to react with bicarbonate (compartment 1) has been very controversial. Arruda and coworkers examined the U-B P_{CO_2} in a number of different experimental situations and found that the U-B P_{CO_2} correlated with the ability of the animal to concentrate its urine.[18] These authors postulated that urinary concentration (water abstraction) increased the concentration of bicarbonate, which gave rise to the following reaction:

$$2HCO_3^- \rightarrow H^+ + CO_3^{2-} + HCO_3^- \rightarrow H_2CO_3 + CO_3^{2-}$$

This reaction, referred to as the *ampholyte reaction*, involves the net conversion of two bicarbonate ions to form a carbonate ion and a carbonic acid molecule. The carbonic acid then dissociates to form CO_2.

In support of the ampholyte hypothesis is the observation that the U-B P_{CO_2} is directly related to urinary bicarbonate concentration, increasing as urinary bicarbonate concentration increases. However, Giammarco and coworkers have found in rabbits that the U-B P_{CO_2} is approximately zero at any urinary bicarbonate concentration.[89] This finding rules out the possibility that the U-B P_{CO_2} is due to a simple chemical reaction such as the ampholyte reaction, which should occur in all species.

A second hypothesis for the generation of protons to react with bicarbonate is the *mixing hypothesis*. This theory states that tubular fluid from one set of nephrons contains large amounts of bicarbonate, while tubular fluid from another set of nephrons contains no bicarbonate and a large quantity of titratable acid. When these fluids mix in the collecting tubule, carbonic acid is generated. There is very little basis for this theory. No nephron segment has been found that contains a large quantity of titratable acid in animals undergoing a bicarbonate diuresis. In addition, this theory predicts that the U-B P_{CO_2} would decrease if titratable buffer excretion markedly decreased. Rector and associates found that a large U-B P_{CO_2} could be generated in the presence of very low titratable buffer excretion.[220]

Thus, neither of the above theories can explain the source of protons added to the tubular fluid. The best theory appears to be that it is proton secretion by the collecting tubule that provides the source of luminal hydrogen ions. On the basis of this thesis, the U-B P_{CO_2} has been very useful for the study of the regulation of distal acidification.

In summary, it appears that the U-B P_{CO_2} is an index of proton secretion in the cortical and medullary portions of the collecting tubule. Protons secreted in these structures combine with luminal bicarbonate to form carbonic acid. Because carbonic anhydrase is not present in the lumen of the collecting tubule, dehydration to CO_2 is delayed. Thus, very little CO_2 is formed in the cortex, where diffusion into the blood would be rapid. Rather, CO_2 is formed in the deep medulla, where it is trapped by the countercurrent system, and in the urinary pelvis, where limited surface area prevents its outward diffusion.

Regulation of distal acidification

Luminal pH

As discussed above, acidification in the distal nephron involves proton secretion across the luminal membrane. The rate of such a process may or may not vary in response to changes in luminal pH. This question has been best examined using the turtle bladder.[24,264]

Steinmetz and Lawson found that the rate of net proton secretion in the turtle bladder decreased as mucosal pH decreased (solid line, Fig. 10-15).[264] In order to define which components of this net flux were active and which were passive, proton fluxes were examined at various values of mucosal pH in the presence of deoxygenation and acetazolamide. Passive fluxes did not exist when mucosal pH was greater than 4.5; thus, the rate of active proton secretion was equal to the rate of net proton secretion (Fig. 10-15). With mucosal pH less than 4.5, where active proton secretion stops, a significant passive backleak flux developed.[264]

Beauwens and Al-Awqati examined the simultaneous effects of mucosal pH on proton secretion and on glucose metabolism.[24] They found that changes in mucosal pH affected proton secretion and metabolism in a similar manner, such that the ratio of the change in proton secretion to the change in metabolism remained constant. Such results show that proton secretion is tightly coupled to metabolism and confirm that leak pathways are insignificant.

The effect of luminal pH in the mammalian nephron has not been addressed in perfusion studies. However, the fact that U-B P_{CO_2} increases with increases in urinary bicarbonate concentration is probably due to an effect of increased luminal buffer to increase luminal pH, which secondarily stimulates proton secretion.

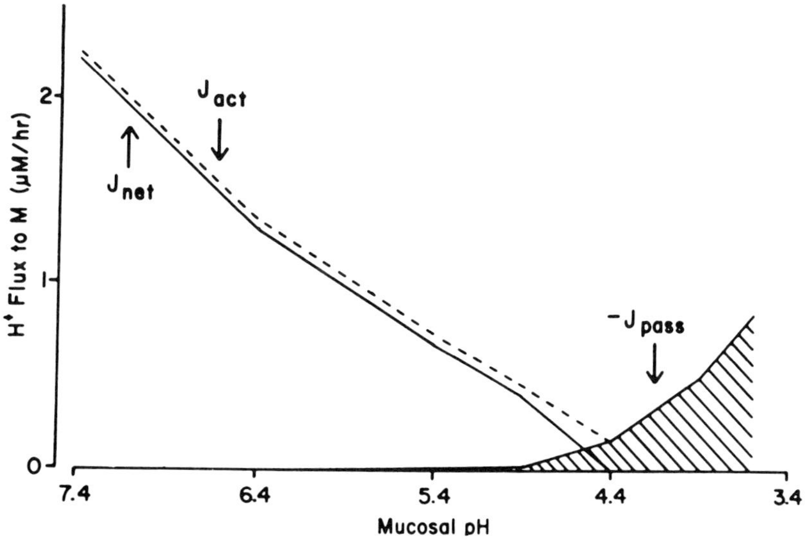

FIGURE 10-15 • Effect of mucosal pH on net proton secretion, active proton secretion, and passive proton diffusion in the turtle urinary bladder. (From Steinmetz PR, Lawson LR: *Am J Physiol* 220:1573, 1971. Used by permission.)

In summary, proton secretion in the distal nephron is stimulated by increases in luminal pH. This causes distal nephron proton secretion to modulate any effects occurring in a more proximal segment. Inhibition of proximal bicarbonate absorption leads to distal delivery of a more alkaline tubular fluid, which stimulates distal proton secretion.

Sodium delivery, nonreabsorbable anions, and potential difference

The type of anion delivered distally is an important determinant of acidification. Schwartz and colleagues examined the effect of sodium sulfate infusion on urine pH, acid, and electrolyte excretion in human subjects.[251] In subjects on an unrestricted-salt diet, the infusion led to increased sodium and potassium excretion but did not affect urinary pH or net acid excretion. However, in subjects maintained on a low-salt diet or given mineralocorticoids, sodium sulfate infusion markedly decreased urinary pH, decreased bicarbonate excretion, and increased ammonia excretion. This, if distal acidification is stimulated by mineralocorticoids or volume depletion, sodium sulfate further stimulates it.

Sodium sulfate is thought to stimulate distal acidification by two mechanisms. First, sulfate is not well absorbed in the proximal tubule. This causes large amounts of sodium sulfate to be delivered distally and thus increases distal sodium delivery. If distal avidity is high (as it is in volume depletion or with exogenous mineralocorticoids), increased distal sodium delivery leads to increased distal sodium absorption and a more electronegative lumen. In addition, chloride, to which the tubule is relatively permeable, normally diffuses out of the distal tubular lumen in response to the negative PD and thus shunts the PD. If a large amount of sodium is delivered distally with a nonreabsorbable anion that cannot follow sodium (e.g., sulfate), the luminal PD becomes more negative.

In these studies, it is possible that the anion is directly regulating bicarbonate secretion. The importance of PD in this effect was confirmed by studies that compared the effects of various anions on urinary pH and acid excretion.[21] Whereas sodium phosphate, sodium sulfate, and sodium ferrocyanide infusions were all associated with low urinary pH and increased acidification, sodium chloride and sodium thiocyanate infusions were not. Thiocyanate is a very lipophilic anion; biological membranes are thus very permeable to it. Thiocyanate is therefore even more capable than chloride of shunting the lumen-negative PD.

The importance of anions in chronic acid-base balance has been demonstrated in studies comparing the effects of chronic hydrochloric acid (HCl), sulfuric acid (H_2SO_4), and nitric acid (HNO_3) feeding in dogs on a low-salt diet.[65] After 2 to 3 weeks of acid administration, the dogs were in balance, with plasma bicarbonate concentration down 8.6 meq/liter in dogs fed HCl, down 3.7 meq/liter in dogs fed H_2SO_4, and unchanged in dogs fed HNO_3. In all three groups net acid excretion was increased. In the HCl-fed dogs, the increase in net acid excretion was due to the severe acidosis. However, in the sulfate and nitrate-fed groups, net acid excretion was equally increased in the presence of only mild or no acidosis. Thus, sulfate and nitrate are able to stimulate acidification and secondarily to modify the degree of acidosis produced.

There is also evidence that increased distal sodium delivery in the *absence* of nonreabsorbable anions can regulate distal acidification. Tam and associates examined the effect of sodium excretion rate on the U-B P_{CO_2} in dogs.[271] Dogs were divided into two groups: normal and increased extracellular fluid volume. Volume-expanded dogs had a low U-B P_{CO_2} that did not correlate with changes in sodium excretion rate. In dogs with normal extracellular fluid volume, U-B P_{CO_2} increased as sodium excretion increased. Administration of amiloride, which inhibits distal sodium absorption, lowered the U-B P_{CO_2} in the dogs with normal extracellular fluid volume but had no effect in the volume-expanded dogs. These results suggest that in the presence of sodium avidity, distal delivery of sodium and the rate of distal sodium absorption are important determinants of distal acidification.

Increased distal delivery of sodium is most likely responsible for the alkalosis-producing effect of loop diuretics. Loop diuretics lead to a decrease in urinary pH, an increase in net acid excretion, an increase in plasma bicarbonate concentration,[35,107] and an increase in the U-B P_{CO_2}.[87] Prevention of volume contraction does not prevent the alkalosis but does reduce its magnitude; previous adrenalectomy has a similar effect.[35] In addition, amiloride abolishes the decrease in urine pH seen with loop diuretics.[107] These data suggest that loop diuretics increase delivery of sodium to the distal nephron, increasing distal sodium absorption and PD. This effect is enhanced by diuretic-induced volume contraction, which increases distal sodium avidity, at least partially by increasing mineralocorticoids. Amiloride inhibits distal sodium absorption and thus prevents this effect.

Thus, increases in distal delivery of sodium and of nonreabsorbable anions stimulate distal nephron acidification, partly at least, by making the luminal PD more negative. Clapp and coworkers examined the effect of an intravenous sodium sulfate infusion on PD in the distal tubule.[50] Sodium sulfate infusion caused the PD to become 17 mV more negative in sodium-fed rats and 31 mV more negative in sodium-deprived rats. Velasquez and colleagues have recently confirmed these results: they found that distal tubules perfused with chloride-free perfusates containing sulfate had a more negative PD than that seen with chloride-containing perfusates.[280] The effect on PD was, however, only 2 mV, far smaller than that seen by Clapp and associates.

Al-Awqati and coworkers examined the effect of potential difference on the rate of proton secretion in the turtle bladder.[4,6] These authors found that imposing a lumen-positive difference slowed the rate of proton secretion (Fig. 10-16). In addition, they found that a 60-mV gradient was equivalent to a one-unit pH change, or a tenfold difference in hydrogen ion concentration. This implies that the proton pump is equally sensitive to electrical and chemical gradients. Ziegler and associates have also found that proton secretion in the toad bladder is sensitive to transepithelial PD.[299]

As mentioned earlier, Koeppen and Helman found that proton secretion in the cortical collecting tubule was electrogenic and thus might be expected to be PD-

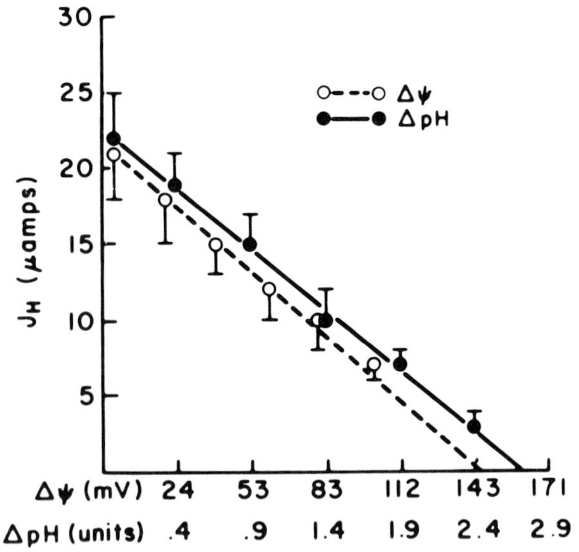

FIGURE 10-16 • Effect of transepithelial pH and PD (Δ Ψ) gradients on proton secretion in the turtle urinary bladder. (From Al-Awqati Q et al: *Am J Physiol* 233:F502, 1977. Used by permission.)

sensitive.[150] Laski and coworkers found that ouabain applied to the peritubular membrane or lithium applied to the luminal surface decreased the lumen-negative PD of the cortical collecting tubule and resulted in inhibition of acidification.[158] These data suggest that proton secretion in the cortical collecting tubule is voltage-dependent and that changes in distal sodium delivery and in the anion delivered distally may affect acidification through changes in the PD.

The medullary collecting tubule appears to be somewhat different from the cortical collecting tubule. Although acidification is also electrogenic in this segment[267] and may be PD-sensitive, active sodium transport does not occur.[266] Thus, changes in sodium delivery are not expected to alter the PD. Indeed, Laski and colleagues found no effect of ouabain on PD or on the rate of bicarbonate absorption in the medullary collecting duct.[158]

Stone and associates, however, found an additional mechanism for an anion effect in this segment.[268] These authors have found that replacement of luminal chloride with gluconate stimulates bicarbonate absorption. This stimulation was not due to an effect on PD; the authors thought it to be due to a chloride-bicarbonate exchanger on the basolateral membrane. These results provide another explanation for the effect of nonchloride anions on acidification. In addition, luminal anions can affect the rate of bicarbonate secretion in the cortical collecting duct. The previously discussed thiocyanate data, however, suggest that the major renal effect is electrical.[21]

In summary, conditions that lead to increased distal sodium reabsorption (increased distal delivery of sodium) or decreased distal chloride reabsorption lead to a more lumen-negative PD. By altering the electrochemical gradient across the epithelium, the change in PD can stimulate distal acidification. In addition, luminal anion composition may affect the rate of acidification by mechanisms not related to PD.

Mineralocorticoids

Clearance studies have demonstrated that mineralocorticoids stimulate tubular acidification in the absence of effects on volume status, serum potassium, or ammonia excretion rate.[123,125,252] This effect occurs in the mineralocorticoid-sensitive segment of the nephron: the collecting tubule. One mechanism for this effect is stimulation of sodium absorption in the cortical collecting tubule by mineralocorticoids, which causes the luminal voltage to become more negative.[207,246]

There also appears, however, to be a direct effect of mineralocorticoids of transepithelial proton secretion that is independent of its effect on sodium absorption. This effect has been studied using the turtle bladder. Al-Awqati and coworkers found that aldosterone applied in vitro stimulated proton secretion in the turtle bladder within 2 h.[5] The stimulation of proton secretion was direct; it occurred before sodium transport was stimulated, it was observed in the presence of total inhibition of sodium transport by ouabain, and it was observed in the short-circuited state in which changes in transepithelial PD are prevented.[5] Actinomycin D, an inhibitor of transcription, blocked the effect of aldosterone, suggesting that the effect is dependent on protein synthesis.[5] Al-Awqati also found that the metabolic coupling ratio is altered by aldosterone. Thus, bladders treated with aldosterone transport more protons per glucose molecule metabolized than do untreated bladders.[3]

Figure 10-17*a* shows the effect of mucosal pH on the rate of proton secretion in turtle bladders in the absence (open circles) and presence (closed circles) of aldosterone.[3,5] When mucosal pH is elevated, aldosterone increases the rate of proton secretion. However, the mucosal pH at which proton secretion stops is not affected by aldosterone. Thus, the capacity of the system to secrete protons is limited in aldosterone-deficient bladders, but the minimum urinary pH that can be obtained is not affected.

These results agree with the results of clearance studies in dogs (Fig. 10-17*b*).[123] When large amounts of ammonia are excreted in the urine, the capacity to secrete protons is limited in mineralocorticoid-deficient dogs; thus, urine pH is elevated. However, when ammonia synthesis is impaired and ammonia excretion is low, mineralocorticoid-deficient dogs are able to lower their urine pH to the same level as mineralocorticoid-replete dogs. This explains the observation in patients with hypoaldosteronism that urine pH is appropriately low in spite of

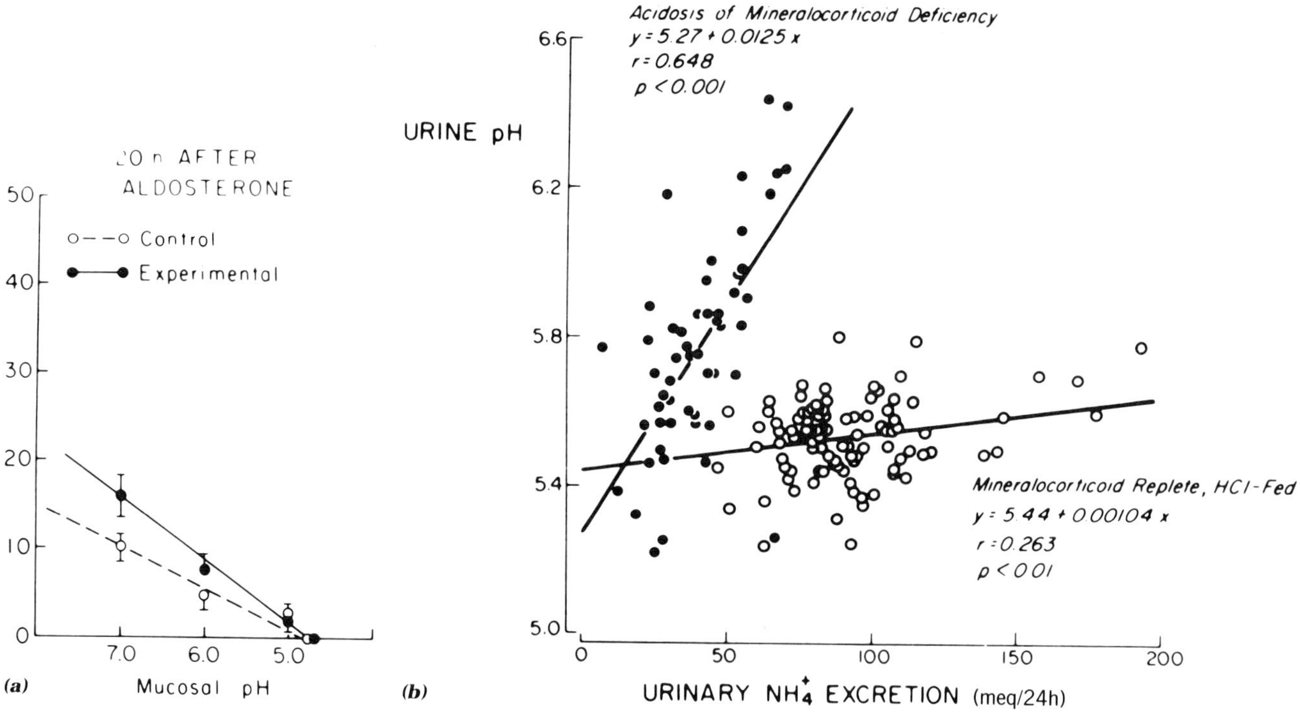

FIGURE 10-17 • (*a*) Effect of aldosterone on proton secretion in the turtle urinary bladder expressed as a function of mucosal pH. (From Al-Awqati Q et al: *J Clin Invest* 58:351, 1976. Used by permission.) (*b*) Urine pH expressed as a function of urinary ammonium excretion in dogs with similar degrees of acidosis; dogs are mineralocorticoid-deficient (●) or replete (○). (From Hulter HN et al: *Am J Physiol* 232:F136, 1977. Used by permission.)

low net acid excretion.[252] Hyperkalemia in these patients suppresses ammonia synthesis,[274] and in the presence of limited distal ammonia delivery, these patients are able to excrete an appropriately acid urine.[252]

A direct effect of aldosterone on proton secretion has also been demonstrated in the mammalian collecting tubule. Koeppen and Hellman found that removal of sodium from lumen and bath led to a lumen-positive PD, which was due to electrogenic proton secretion (see above). This lumen-positive PD was increased significantly in tubules from rabbits pretreatd with mineralocorticoids.[150] Stone and colleagues found that medullary collecting tubules from previously adrenalectomized rabbits did not secrete protons and that this defect was reversed by addition of aldosterone to the bath.[267] Since the medullary collecting tubule does not actively transport sodium,[266] the aldosterone-modulated proton secretion must represent a direct effect on the acidification process.

In summary, mineralocorticoids affect acidification in three ways. First, mineralocorticoids stimulate sodium absorption and create a more lumen-negative PD, which stimulates proton secretion. Second, mineralocorticoids directly stimulate collecting tubule proton secretion. Third, mineralocorticoids lower serum potassium, stimulating ammonia synthesis and increasing buffer delivery to the collecting tubule.

Potassium

Potassium has several effects on acid-base balance. Some of those discussed previously are (1) hypokalemia-induced stimulation and hyperkalemia-induced inhibition of ammonia synthesis, (2) stimulation of proximal tubular acidification by potassium deficiency, and (3) reduction in glomerular filtration rate secondary to potassium deficiency. There are, however, a number of additional effects on distal acidification.

Jones and coworkers found that simple potassium depletion in normal human subjects caused the serum bicarbonate concentration to increase only slightly.[138] Hulter and associates examined the effect of potassium depletion in dogs.[127] These authors found that potassium deficiency caused a metabolic acidosis. The metabolic acidosis was due to decreased aldosterone levels, which resulted from suppressed secretion and accelerated metabolic clearance of aldosterone during potassium deficiency. Jones and colleagues also found that potassium-depleted human subjects suppressed their aldosterone levels.[138]

When dogs receive exogenous mineralocorticoid, however, they develop a metabolic alkalosis. The magnitude of the alkalosis is greater if they were previously on a potassium-restricted diet.[124,227] Hulter and coworkers found that the more severe alkalosis was due to a greater increase in net acid excretion in potassium-deficient dogs than in controls.[124] For any urine pH, potassium-deficient dogs had a greater rate of ammonia excretion. The increased ammonia excretion rate suggests that synthesis of ammonia had increased; increased ammonia synthesis had been demonstrated previously in potassium deficiency.[272,274]

If increased excretion of ammonia were the only effect of potassium deficiency, these dogs would be expected to have a higher urine pH. Increases in distal buffer delivery would increase net acid excretion but would also increase urine pH. In fact, potassium-deficient dogs had a lower urinary pH.[124] Thus, in addition to increasing ammonia synthesis, potassium deficiency causes enhanced mineralocorticoid-induced proton secretion. The increase in H^+ secretion was blocked by amiloride, suggesting that it occurred in the distal nephron.[126]

Further studies have examined the effect of a K-deficient diet using the in vitro perfused tubule. McKinney and Davidson found that K-deficient rabbits developed a metabolic acidosis, which was associated with inhibition of H^+ secretion in the outer medullary collecting duct.[185] This inhibition was associated with a decrease in aldosterone levels, which most likely was responsible for the decreased rates of H^+ transport and the metabolic acidosis. In the studies of Hays and colleagues, K deficiency caused a metabolic alkalosis in rabbits.[115] Cortical collecting ducts demonstrated no net acid transport, in spite of the presence of a metabolic alkalosis. Rates of H^+ secretion in the inner stripe of the outer medullary collecting duct were not different than control, despite expected low aldosterone levels. These results were interpreted as indicating an increase in H^+ secretion in the cortical and outer medullary collecting tubule in K deficiency. The difference between the results of McKinney and Davidson and Hays and coworkers most likely relates to different dietary protocols.

Morphologic examination of intercalated cells has indicated a number of effects of K deficiency. Stetson and colleagues found that K depletion caused a decrease in the number of subapical vesicles associated with a 3.3-fold increase in the amount of apical membrane. These results suggested exocytotic membrane insertion in response to K depletion.[265] Wingo has found that outer medullary collecting ducts dissected from K-deficient animals absorb K^+, and in this setting, both K^+ absorption and H^+ secretion are blocked by omeprazole, a sulfhydryl reacting agent.[293] Doucet and Marsay found increased K-dependent ATPase activity in the collecting tubule of K-deficient animals, raising the question of the presence of a gastric H^+-K^+ ATPase.[67] More recently, Wingo and associates have demonstrated staining of intercalated cells with antibodies directed against the gastric H^+-K^+ ATPase.[294]

Based on all these results, it is tempting to speculate that intercalated cells have an H^+-K^+ ATPase similar to that present in the stomach. This is distinct from the vacuolar H^+ ATPase. Hays and Alpern did not find any evidence for an apical membrane H^+-K^+ ATPase in outer medullary collecting ducts dissected from control animals.[113] It is thus possible that K deficiency induces exocytotic insertion of membranes containing H^+-K^+ ATPase, leading to increased rates of H^+ secretion and K^+ absorption in the collecting duct.

In summary, potassium deficiency affects renal acidification in many ways. It decreases GFR, which can lower the filtered load of bicarbonate. It stimulates proton secretion and ammonia synthesis in the proximal tubule. In the distal nephron, potassium deficiency directly stimulates proton secretion but inhibits proton secretion by suppressing aldosterone levels. In a normal patient, the suppression of aldosterone is able to counterbalance the other effects, and acid-base balance is not markedly altered. However, if mineralocorticoid levels are high and cannot be suppressed, potassium deficiency markedly enhances the tendency toward alkalosis. This explains the observation of Kassirer and coworkers that the severity of alkalosis in patients with unsuppressed mineralocorticoid activity correlates with the degree of potassium depletion.[140]

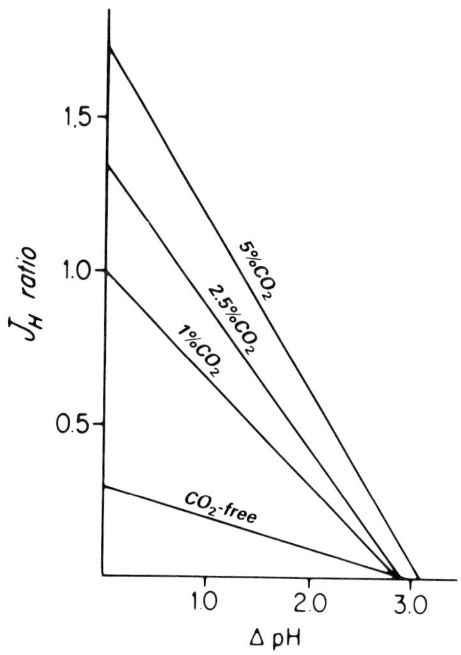

FIGURE 10-18 • Effect of serosal CO_2 tension on proton secretion in the turtle urinary bladder, expressed as a function of the transepithelial pH gradient. (From Al-Awqati Q et al: *Am J Physiol* 233:F502, 1977. Used by permission.)

Peritubular pH

Alterations in peritubular pH lead to changes in renal acidification that tend to return peritubular pH toward normal. As discussed previously, a major part of this response occurs in the proximal tubule; the distal nephron also appears to play an important part. Gougoux and coworkers found that when all other determinants are controlled, U-B P_{CO_2} increases during metabolic acidosis and decreases during metabolic alkalosis.[101,102] Graber and coworkers have confirmed these findings in microcatheterization studies of the medullary collecting duct. Medullary collecting duct acidification increased markedly in metabolic acidosis.[105] In contrast, Bengele and associates, who also used microcatheterization of the medullary collecting duct, observed no net acid addition along the medullary collecting duct in acute respiratory acidosis.[26] A possible explanation for their finding is offered below.

Once again, turtle bladder studies have contributed greatly to an understanding of the mechanisms involved in pH regulation. Schwartz and Steinmetz first found that acidification is very sensitive to CO_2 in the absence of bicarbonate.[249] Schwartz found that in the presence of bicarbonate, proton secretion was also stimulated by increasing P_{CO_2}; proton secretion reached a maximal rate at approximately 4 percent CO_2.[248] Al-Awqati and colleagues found that increases in CO_2 tension stimulated proton secretion but did not affect the minimum mucosal pH that the epithelium could establish (Fig. 10-18).[4,6]

Bengele and associates found that in respiratory acidosis acidification proximal to the medullary collecting duct was markedly stimulated such that the fluid delivered to the medullary collecting duct had a low pH.[26] The studies of Al-Awqati (Fig. 10-18) suggest that the effect of P_{CO_2} becomes smaller as luminal pH decreases and disappears when the limiting pH is reached.[6] This, together with the suppressive effect of low luminal pH may explain the failure to observe acidification in this setting.

Cohen and Steinmetz[61] examined the role of cell pH in the regulation of proton secretion by varying serosal bicarbonate concentration and/or P_{CO_2} and measuring cell pH (DMO) and the rate of proton secretion. Decreasing serosal bicarbonate concentration increased serosal and cellular hydrogen ion concentrations, and the rate of proton secretion increased. The rate of proton secretion, examined as a function of cellular hydrogen ion concentration, demonstrated saturation kinetics (Fig. 10-19). Although the mechanistic significance of these kinetics is not known, it is clear that the rate of proton secretion is more sensitive to cellular hydrogen ion concentrations in the alkaline range. In the studies in which serosal P_{CO_2} was altered, cell pH was not measured; the authors estimated it. When the rate of proton secretion was examined as a function of cell pH in these studies, the relationship was the same as when serosal bicarbonate concentration was varied.[61] It therefore appears that both serosal bicarbonate concentration and P_{CO_2} regulate the rate of proton secretion through changes in cell pH.

Cell pH can affect the rate of proton secretion in a number of ways. First, it can alter the electrochemical

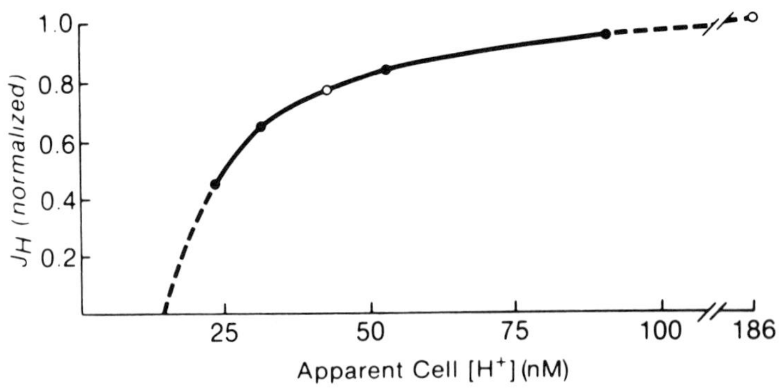

FIGURE 10-19 • Effect of cellular hydrogen ion concentration on the rate of proton secretion in the turtle urinary bladder. (From Cohen LH, Steinmetz PR: *J Gen Physiol* 76:381, 1980. Used by permission.)

gradient for protons across the luminal membrane. Second, it can cause insertion into the luminal membrane of membrane that contains proton pumps. In this regard, Arruda, Dykto, and their respective coworkers found that microtubular and microfilament function are required for CO_2-induced stimulation of proton secretion in the turtle bladder.[19,74] Gluck and colleagues found that increasing CO_2 led to exocytosis, which caused insertion of new membrane into the luminal membrane.[92] Colchicine inhibited the CO_2-induced exocytosis and the CO_2-induced stimulation of proton secretion.[92] Ultrastructural studies by Madsen and Tisher have shown that respiratory and metabolic acidosis lead to exocytosis and luminal membrane insertion in the mammalian outer medullary collecting tubule.[176,177]

In addition to effects of cell pH, previous acid-base status causes a chronic adaptation in the turtle bladder. Cohen examined the effect of acid-base treatment on the subsequent rate of turtle bladder acidification.[60] Turtles received either sodium bicarbonate, ammonium chloride, or tap water for 4 days. Bladders were then removed, and the rates of proton secretion and chloride-bicarbonate exchange were measured. Bladders from alkalotic turtles had an increased rate of chloride-bicarbonate exchange, but proton secretion was unaffected. Since chloride-bicarbonate exchange functions only in the direction of bicarbonate secretion,[159] stimulated exchange provides a mechanism for increasing elimination of bicarbonate in alkalotic turtles. Bladders from acidotic turtles had an increased rate of proton secretion, but chloride-bicarbonate exchange was unaffected.[60]

Chronic adaptation to previous acid-base status is also important in mammalian tubules. McKinney and Burg found that rabbit cortical collecting tubules perfused in vitro sometimes absorbed bicarbonate and sometimes secreted bicarbonate.[182] However, tubules from rabbits treated with ammonium chloride absorbed bicarbonate, while tubules from rabbits treated with sodium bicarbonate secreted bicarbonate.[182-184] Lucci and associates found similarly that in vivo microperfused superficial distal convoluted tubules did not exhibit net bicarbonate transport.[173] However, if rats were made chronically acidotic, there was net bicarbonate absorption. Levine and coworkers found that surface distal tubules of rats fed acid showed net H^+ secretion, while those of rats fed alkali had secreted alkali.[130,161]

Ullrich and Papavassiliou found that microperfused papillary collecting ducts from acidotic rats reabsorbed bicarbonate at an accelerated rate. Collecting ducts from alkalotic rats reabsorbed bicarbonate at a slower rate.[277] These authors also found that the rate of glycodiazine absorption was unaffected by acid-base status.*[277] Taken together, the results of Ullrich and Papavassiliou imply that net acidification in the papillary collecting tubule includes two fluxes. One occurs in the absence of bicarbonate and is not regulated by previous acid-base status; it is presumably proton secretion. A second flux only occurs in the presence of bicarbonate and is modulated by the animal's previous acid-base status. Further studies need to be performed to examine whether this second flux is similar to the chloride-bicarbonate exchange identified in the turtle bladder.

A number of studies have addressed the possible cellular mechanisms responsible for this apparent memory effect. Schwartz and associates examined the number of type A and type B intercalated cells in cortical collecting tubules from acid- and alkali-loaded rabbits.[247] Type A intercalated cells were defined by luminal endocytosis, and type B intercalated cells were defined by peanut lectin binding. These investigators found that dietary changes had no effect on the total number of intercalated cells but that acid-fed animals had a greater number of type A intercalated cells and alkali-fed animals had a greater number of type B intercalated cells. Because no mitotic spindles were found, it was concluded that this transition did not involve cell death or cell proliferation but, rather, involved interconversion between type A and type B intercalated cells.

As noted above, type A intercalated cells have an apical membrane H^+ ATPase, while type B intercalated cells have a basolateral membrane H^+ ATPase. This raises the possibility that interconversion between type A

* Glycodiazine is a weak acid which is neutral and lipid-soluble in its acid form. It is therefore very similar to bicarbonate; glycodiazine absorption can be used as an index of proton secretion.

and type B intercalated cells could merely involve a "reversal of polarity."[247] In addition, type A intercalated cells have a basolateral membrane Cl^--HCO_3^- exchange, while type B intercalated cells have apical Cl^--HCO_3^- exchange. However, as noted above, these Cl^--HCO_3^- exchangers are molecularly distinct.

Recent studies by Kim and colleagues have suggested an alternative explanation. These investigators examined the effect of dietary acid on the ultrastructural characteristics of the rat cortical collecting duct.[141] In addition, cells were stained for band 3 protein immunocytochemically. In tubules from acid-fed animals, type A intercalated cells had more extensive apical microprojections and increased staining for basolateral Cl^--HCO_3^- exchanger in the basal region and for carbonic anhydrase in the apical region. Type B cells were small and difficult to identify with certainty. The relative numbers of type A and type B cells were not altered. These investigators thus concluded that chronic changes in acid-base status do not alter the relative numbers of type A and type B intercalated cells but, rather, affect the relative activities of the two cell types.

In summary, distal acidification is regulated by peritubular bicarbonate concentration and P_{CO_2} in three ways: (1) acute alterations affect the electrochemical gradient for hydrogen ions; (2) acute alterations lead to exocytotic addition and endocytotic removal of proton secretory sites from the luminal membrane; (3) chronic alterations lead to adaptive changes in the epithelium. The acute effects of peritubular bicarbonate concentration and P_{CO_2} are mediated by changes in cell pH.

Extracellular fluid volume

Extracellular fluid volume is an important determinant of renal acidification.[59] We have already discussed its important effects on GFR and proximal acidification. The question of an effect in the distal nephron has received surprisingly little attention. Tam and coworkers found that extracellular volume contraction increased U-B P_{CO_2}.[270] These authors also found that volume expansion eliminated the correlation between distal delivery of sodium (estimated by sodium excretion) and the U-B P_{CO_2}.[271]

These results suggest that volume status affects distal acidification. This effect is probably at least partially secondary to changes in sodium transport. These changes in sodium transport could be due to changes in aldosterone, natriuretic factors, or other factors. In addition, as discussed earlier, extracellular fluid volume–induced changes in aldosterone can directly affect acidification.

Hormones

As discussed earlier, PTH inhibits proximal acidification[20,132,186,187,218] but stimulates whole kidney acidification.[20,128,129,193] These results suggest that PTH stimulates distal acidification. Studies using the toad bladder have found such a stimulation,[78] but similar studies in the turtle bladder have not.[162] As the turtle does not possess parathyroid glands, these results are not surprising. In support of an effect on distal acidification, Bengele and associates have found that thyroparathyroidectomy inhibits acidification in the medullary collecting duct.[27] Measuring U-B P_{CO_2}, Mercier and colleagues found that PTH increased distal acidification in thyroparathyroidectomized rats. This effect, however, was attributable to increases in distal phosphate delivery rather than to a direct effect of PTH.[190]

Bichara and coworkers found that DDAVP, a V_2 agonist, stimulated H^+ secretion in the distal nephron.[32] Mercier and associates found that glucagon inhibited distal acidification.[191] The physiologic significance of the effects of PTH, AVP, and glucagon has not been determined.

Hays and colleagues examined the regulation of H^+ secretion in the inner stripe of the outer medullary collecting duct of the rabbit perfused in vitro.[116] In these studies, 8-bromo cAMP and forskolin, a direct activator of adenyl cyclase, stimulated H^+ secretion. Prostaglandin E_2 inhibited H^+ secretion. Cyclic AMP may mediate the AVP effect described above.

REFERENCES

1. Akiba T et al: Electrogenic sodium/bicarbonate cotransport in rabbit renal cortical basolateral membrane vesicles. *J Clin Invest* 78:1472, 1986.
2. Akiba T et al: Parallel adaptation of the rabbit renal cortical sodium/proton antiporter and sodium bicarbonate cotransporter in metabolic acidosis and alkalosis. *J Clin Invest* 80:308, 1987.
3. Al-Awqati Q: Effect of aldosterone on the coupling between H^+ transport and glucose oxidation. *J Clin Invest* 60:1240, 1977.
4. Al-Awqati Q: H^+ transport in urinary epithelia. *Am J Physiol* 235:F77, 1978
5. Al-Awqati Q et al: Characteristics of stimulation of H^+ transport by aldosterone in turtle urinary bladder. *J Clin Invest* 58:351, 1976.
6. Al-Awqati Q et al: Transport of H^+ against electrochemical gradients in turtle urinary bladder. *Am J Physiol* 233:F502, 1977.
7. Alpern RJ: Mechanism of basolateral membrane H/OH/HCO_3 transport in the rat proximal convoluted tubule: A sodium-coupled electrogenic process. *J Gen Physiol* 86:613, 1985.
8. Alpern RJ: Cell mechanisms of proximal tubule acidification. *Physiol Rev* 70:79, 1990
9. Alpern RJ, Chambers M: Cell pH in the rat proximal convoluted tubule: Regulation by luminal and peritubular pH and sodium concentration. *J Clin Invest* 78:502, 1986.
10. Alpern RJ, Chambers M: Basolateral membrane Cl/HCO_3 exchange in the rat proximal convoluted tubule: Na de-

pendent and independent modes. *J Gen Physiol* 89:581, 1987.
11. Alpern RJ, Rector FC Jr: A model of proximal tubular bicarbonate absorption. *Am J Physiol* 17:F272, 1985.
12. Alpern RJ et al: Effect of luminal bicarbonate concentration on proximal acidification in the rat. *Am J Physiol* 243:F53, 1982.
13. Alpern RJ et al: Effects of extracellular fluid volume and plasma bicarbonate concentration on proximal acidification in the rat. *J Clin Invest* 71:736, 1983.
14. Alpern RJ et al: Flow dependence of proximal tubular bicarbonate absorption. *Am J Physiol* 245:F478, 1983.
15. Alpern RJ et al: Renal acidification mechanisms, in Brenner BM, Rector FC Jr (eds): *The Kidney*, 4th ed. Philadelphia, Saunders, 1990, p 318.
16. Aronson PS et al: Modifier role of internal H^+ in activating the Na^+-H^+ exchanger in renal microvillus membrane vesicles. *Nature* 299:161, 1982.
17. Aronson PS et al: Interaction of external H^+ with the Na^+-H^+ exchanger in renal microvillus membrane vesicles. *J Biol Chem* 258:6767, 1983.
18. Arruda JAL et al: The critical importance of urinary concentrating ability in the generation of urinary carbon dioxide tension. *J Clin Invest* 60:922, 1977.
19. Arruda JAL et al: Inhibition of H^+ secretion in the turtle bladder by colchicine and vinblastine. *J Lab Clin Med* 96:450, 1980.
20. Bank N, Aynedjian HS: A micropuncture study of the effect of parathyroid hormone on renal bicarbonate reabsorption. *J Clin Invest* 58:336, 1976.
21. Bank N, Schwartz WB: The influence of anion penetrating ability on urinary acidification and the excretion of titratable acid. *J Clin Invest* 39:1516, 1960.
22. Barfuss DW, Schafer JA: Flow dependence of nonelectrolyte absorption in the nephron. *Am J Physiol* 236:F163, 1982.
23. Baum M, Berry CA: Evidence for neutral transcellular NaCl transport and neutral basolateral chloride exit in the rabbit proximal convoluted tubule. *J Clin Invest* 74:205, 1984.
24. Beauwens R, Al-Awqati Q: Active H^+ transport in the turtle urinary bladder: Coupling of transport to glucose oxidation. *J Gen Physiol* 68:421, 1976.
25. Bell JM, Field AL: The distribution of ammonia between water and chloroform. *J Am Chem Soc* 33:940, 1911.
26. Bengele HH et al: Effect of respiratory acidosis on acidification by the medullary collecting duct. *Am J Physiol* 244:F89, 1983.
27. Bengele HH et al: Effect of acute thyroparathyroidectomy on nephron acidification. *Am J Physiol* 246:F569, 1984.
28. Berry CA: Electrical effects of acidification in the rabbit proximal convoluted tubule. *Am J Physiol* 240:F459, 1981.
29. Biagi BA, Sohtell M: pH sensitivity of the basolateral membrane of the rabbit proximal tubule. *Am J Physiol* 250:F261, 1986.
30. Biagi BA, Sohtell M: Electrophysiology of basolateral bicarbonate transport in the rabbit proximal tubule. *Am J Physiol* 250:F267, 1986.
31. Bichara M et al: Effects of parathyroid hormone on urinary acidification. *Am J Physiol* 251:F444, 1986.
32. Bichara M et al: Effects of antidiuretic hormone on urinary acidification and on tubular handling of bicarbonate in the rat. *J Clin Invest* 80:621, 1987.
33. Bidani A et al: Analysis of the determinants of renal cortical P_{CO_2}. *Am J Physiol* 247:F466, 1984.
34. Boron WF, Boulpaep EL: Intracellular pH regulation in the renal proximal tubule of the salamander: Basolateral HCO_3^- transport. *J Gen Physiol* 81:53, 1983.
35. Bosch JP et al: Effect of chronic furosemide administration on hydrogen and sodium excretion in the dog. *Am J Physiol* 232:F397, 1977.
36. Breyer MD, Jacobson HR: Regulation of rabbit medullary collecting duct cell pH by basolateral Na/H and Cl/base exchange. *J Clin Invest* 84:996, 1989.
37. Brosius FC et al: The major kidney band 3 gene transcript predicts an amino-terminal truncated band 3 polypeptide. *J Biol Chem* 264:7784, 1989.
38. Brown D et al: Localization of a proton-pumping ATPase in rat kidney. *J Clin Invest* 82:2114, 1988.
39. Buerkert J et al: Ammonium handling by superficial and juxtamedullary nephrons in the rat: Evidence for an ammonia shunt between the loop of Henle and the collecting duct. *J Clin Invest* 70:1, 1978.
40. Buerkert J et al: Segmental analysis of the renal tubule in buffer production and net acid formation. *Am J Physiol* 244:F442, 1983.
41. Burckhardt BC et al: Electrophysiological analysis of bicarbonate permeation across the peritubular cell membrane of rat kidney proximal tubule. Basic observations. *Pfluegers Arch* 401:34, 1984.
42. Burg MB, Green N: Bicarbonate transport by isolated perfused rabbit proximal convoluted tubules. *Am J Physiol* 233:F307, 1977.
43. Cabantchik ZI et al: The anion transport system of the red blood cell: The role of membrane protein evaluated by the use of probes. *Biochim Biophys Acta* 515:239, 1978.
44. Chan YL: Adrenergic control of bicarbonate absorption in the proximal convoluted tubule of the rat kidney. *Pfluegers Arch* 388:159, 1980.
45. Chaillet JR et al: Basolateral Na/H exchange in the rabbit cortical collecting tubule. *J Gen Physiol* 86:795, 1985.
46. Chan YL, Giebisch G: Relationship between sodium and bicarbonate transport in the rat proximal convoluted tubule. *Am J Physiol* 240:F222, 1981.
47. Chan YL et al: Control mechanisms of bicarbonate transport across the rat proximal convoluted tubule. *Am J Physiol* 242:F532, 1982.
48. Chan YL et al: Passive driving forces of proximal tubular fluid and bicarbonate transport: Gradient dependence of H^+ secretion. *Am J Physiol* 245:F622, 1983.
49. Chantrelle B et al: Evidence for coupled sodium/hydrogen exchange in the rat superficial proximal convoluted tubule. *Pfluegers Arch* 395:186, 1982.
50. Clapp JR et al: Effect of unreabsorbable anions on proximal and distal transtubular potentials in rats. *Am J Physiol* 202:781, 1962.
51. Clapp WL et al: Intercalated cells of the rat inner medullary collecting duct. *Kidney Int* 31:1080, 1987.
52. Clark JD et al: α_2-adrenergic receptors regulate Na-H exchange via a cAMP-dependent mechanism. *Am J Physiol* 259:F977, 1990.

53. Cogan MG: Extracellular volume expansion predominantly inhibits NaCl rather than $NaHCO_3$ reabsorption in the rat proximal convoluted tubule. *Am J Physiol* 245:F272, 1983.
54. Cogan MG: Effects of acute alterations in P_{CO_2} on proximal bicarbonate, chloride and water reabsorption. *Am J Physiol* 246:F21, 1984.
55. Cogan MG, Liu F-Y: Metabolic alkalosis in the rat. *J Clin Invest* 71:1141, 1983.
56. Cogan MG et al: Control of proximal bicarbonate reabsorption in normal and acidotic rats. *J Clin Invest* 64:1168, 1979.
57. Cogan MG et al: Effect of acetazolamide on bicarbonate reabsorption in the proximal tubule of the rat. *Am J Physiol* 237:F447, 1979.
58. Cogan MG et al: Chronic hypercapnia stimulates proximal bicarbonate reabsorption in the rat. *J Clin Invest* 74:1942, 1984.
59. Cohen JJ: Selective Cl retention in repair of metabolic alkalosis without increasing filtered load. *Am J Physiol* 218:165, 1970.
60. Cohen LH: HCO_3-Cl exchange transport in the adaptive response to alkalosis by turtle bladder. *Am J Physiol* 239:F167, 1980.
61. Cohen LH, Steinmetz PR: Control of active proton transport in turtle urinary bladder by cell pH. *J Gen Physiol* 76:381, 1980.
62. Cohen LH et al: Inhibition of the bicarbonate exit step in urinary acidification by a disulfonic stilbene. *J Clin Invest* 61:981, 1978.
63. Cohn D et al: Metabolic acidosis and parathyroidectomy increase Na^+-H^+ exchange in brush border vesicles. *Am J Physiol* 245:F217, 1983.
64. Curthoys NP, Lowry OH: The distribution of glutaminase isoenzymes in the various structures of the nephron in normal, acidotic, and alkalotic rat kidney. *J Biol Chem* 248:162, 1973.
65. DeSousa RC et al: Renal regulation of acid-base equilibrium during chronic administration of mineral acid. *J Clin Invest* 53:465, 1974.
66. Dobyan DC, Bulger RE: Renal carbonic anhydrase. *Am J Physiol* 243:F311, 1982.
67. Doucet A, Marsy S: Characterization of K-ATPase activity in distal nephron: Stimulation by potassium depletion. *Am J Physiol* 253:F418, 1987.
68. Douglas JG: Angiotensin receptor subtypes of the kidney cortex. *Am J Physiol* 253:F1, 1987.
69. DuBose TD Jr et al: Direct determination of P_{CO_2} in the rat renal cortex. *J Clin Invest* 62:338, 1978.
70. DuBose TD Jr et al: Micropuncture determination of pH, P_{CO_2}, and total CO_2 concentration in accessible structures of the rat renal cortex. *J Clin Invest* 64:476, 1979.
71. DuBose TD Jr et al: Determination of disequilibrium pH in the rat kidney in vivo: Evidence for hydrogen secretion. *Am J Physiol* 240:F138, 1981.
72. DuBose TD Jr: Hydrogen ion secretion by the collecting duct as a determinant of the urine to blood P_{CO_2} gradient in alkalotic urine. *J Clin Invest* 69:145, 1982.
73. DuBose TD Jr et al: Comparison of acidification parameters in superficial and deep nephrons of the rat. *Am J Physiol* 244:F497, 1983.
74. Dykto G et al: Stimulation of urinary acidification by CO_2 in the turtle bladder: Possible role of calcium, microfilaments and microtubules (abstract). *Clin Res* 31:427A, 1983.
75. Emmett M et al: The pathophysiology of acid-base changes in chronically phosphate-depleted rats: Bone-kidney interactions. *J Clin Invest* 59:291, 1977.
76. Felder et al: Dopamine inhibits Na-H exchanger activity in renal brush border membrane vesicles by stimulation of adenylate cyclase activity. *Am J Physiol* 259:F297, 1990.
77. Fischer JL et al: Chloride dependence of the HCO_3 exit step in urinary acidification by the turtle bladder. *Am J Physiol* 245:F564, 1983.
78. Frazier LW: Effects of parathyroid hormone on H^+ and NH_4^+ excretion in toad urinary bladder. *J Membr Biol* 30:187, 1976.
79. Friedman PA, Andreoli TA: CO_2-stimulated NaCl absorption in the mouse renal cortical thick ascending limb of Henle: Evidence for synchronous Na^+/H^+ and Cl^-/HCO_3^- exchange in apical plasma membranes. *J Gen Physiol* 80:683, 1982.
80. Frömter E, Gessner K: Active transport potentials, membrane diffusion potentials and streaming potentials across rat kidney proximal tubule. *Pfluegers Arch* 351:85, 1974.
81. Frömter E, Gessner K: Effect of inhibitors and diuretics on electrical potential differences in rat kidney proximal tubule. *Pfluegers Arch* 357:209, 1975.
82. Frömter E, Sato K: Electrical events in active H^+/HCO_3^- transport across rat proximal tubular epithelium, in Kasbeker D et al (eds): *Gastric Hydrogen Ion Secretion*. New York, Marcel Dekker, 1976, p 382.
83. Frömter E et al: Permeability properties of the proximal tubular epithelium of the rat kidney studied with electrophysiological methods, in Giebisch G (ed): *Electrophysiology of Epithelial Cells*. Stuttgart, Schattaur Verlag, 1970, p 119.
84. Garvin JL et al: Active NH_4 absorption by the thick ascending limb. *Am J Physiol* 255:F57, 1988.
85. Geibel J et al: Angiotensin II stimulates both Na/H and Na/HCO_3 cotransport in the rabbit proximal tubule. *Proc Natl Acad Sci U S A* 87:7917, 1990.
86. Gennari FJ et al: P_{CO_2} measurements in the surface proximal tubules and peritubular capillaries of the rat kidney. *Am J Physiol* 242:F78, 1982.
87. Giammarco RA: Effect of furosemide on collecting duct hydrogen ion secretion in the rabbit. *J Lab Clin Med* 97:390, 1981.
88. Giammarco RA et al: The effect of hyperventilation on distal nephron hydrogen ion secretion. *J Clin Invest* 58:77, 1976.
89. Giammarco RA et al: Collecting duct hydrogen ion secretion in the rabbit: Role of potassium. *J Lab Clin Med* 91:948, 1978.
90. Giebisch G et al: Kinetics of luminal acidification in cortical tubules of the rat kidney. *J Physiol* 267:571, 1977.
91. Gluck S, Caldwell J: Immunoaffinity purification and characterization of vacuolar H-ATPase from bovine kidney. *J Biol Chem* 262:15780, 1987.
92. Gluck S et al: Exocytosis regulates urinary acidification in turtle bladder by rapid insertion of H^+ pumps into the luminal membrane. *Proc Natl Acad Sci U S A* 79:4327, 1982.

93. Gold LW et al: Renal bicarbonate wasting during phosphate depletion: A possible cause of altered acid-base homeostasis in hyperparathyroidism. *J Clin Invest* 52:2556, 1973.
94. Good DW: Sodium-dependent bicarbonate absorption by cortical thick ascending limb of rat kidney. *Am J Physiol* 248:F821, 1985.
95. Good DW: Active absorption of NH_4 by rat medullary thick ascending limb: Inhibition by potassium. *Am J Physiol* 255:F78, 1988.
96. Good DW: Adaptation of HCO_3 and NH_4 transport in rat MTAL: Effects of chronic metabolic acidosis and Na intake. *Am J Physiol* 27:F1345, 1990.
97. Good DW: Inhibition of bicarbonate absorption by peptide hormones and cyclic AMP in rat medullary thick ascending limb. *J Clin Invest* 85:1006, 1990.
98. Good DW, Burg MB: Ammonia production by individual segments of the rat nephron. *J Clin Invest* 73:602, 1984.
99. Good DW et al: Ammonia and bicarbonate transport by thick ascending limb of rat kidney. *Am J Physiol* 247:F35, 1984.
100. Gottschalk CW et al: Localization of urine acidification in the mammalian kidney. *Am J Physiol* 198:581, 1960.
101. Gougoux A et al: Effect of blood pH on distal nephron hydrogen ion secretion. *Kidney Int* 17:615, 1980.
102. Gougoux A et al: Studies on the mechanism whereby acidemia stimulates collecting duct hydrogen ion secretion in vivo. *Kidney Int* 20:643, 1981.
103. Graber ML et al: Elevated urinary P_{CO_2} in the rat: An intrarenal event. *Kidney Int* 21:795, 1982.
104. Graber ML et al: pH and P_{CO_2} profiles of the rat inner medullary collecting duct. *Am J Physiol* 241:F659, 1981.
105. Graber ML et al: Acute metabolic acidosis augments collecting duct acidification rate in the rat. *Am J Physiol* 241:F669, 1981.
106. Grassl SM, Aronson PS: Na/HCO_3 cotransport in basolateral membrane vesicles isolated from rabbit renal cortex. *J Biol Chem* 261:8778, 1986.
107. Györy AZ, Lessner D: Independence of ethacrynic acid-induced renal hydrogen ion excretion of sodium-volume depletion in man. *Clin Sci* 53:125, 1977.
108. Hamm LL et al: Hydrogen ion (H^+) permeability of the rabbit proximal convoluted tubule. *Am J Physiol* 246:F3, 1984.
109. Hamm LL et al: Transport of ammonia in the rabbit cortical collecting tubule. *J Clin Invest* 75:478, 1985.
110. Harris PJ, Young JA: Dose-dependent stimulation and inhibition of proximal tubule sodium reabsorption by angiotensin II in the rat kidney. *Pfluegers Arch* 367:295, 1977.
111. Harris RC et al: Adaptation of Na-H exchange in renal microvillus membrane vesicles: Role of dietary protein and uninephrectomy. *J Clin Invest* 74:1979, 1984.
112. Harris RC et al: Sodium-hydrogen exchange and glucose transport in renal microvillus membrane vesicles from rats with diabetes mellitus. *J Clin Invest* 77:724, 1986.
113. Hays SR, Alpern RJ: Apical and basolateral membrane H extrusion mechanisms in inner stripe of rabbit outer medullary collecting duct. *Am J Physiol* 28:F628, 1990.
114. Hays SR, Alpern RJ: Basolateral membrane Na-independent Cl/HCO_3 exchange in the inner stripe of the rabbit outer medullary collecting duct. *J Gen Physiol* 95:347, 1990.
115. Hays SR et al: Effect of K depletion on HCO_3 transport across rabbit collecting duct segments. *Kidney Int* 29:386, 1986.
116. Hays SR et al: Hormonal regulation of proton secretion in rabbit medullary collecting duct. *J Clin Invest* 78:1279, 1986.
117. Helman SI et al: Effect of vasopressin on electrical resistance of renal cortical collecting tubules. *Am J Physiol* 220:1825, 1971.
118. Hildebrandt F et al: Cloning of a cDNA encoding a rabbit renal Na/H antiporter. *Kidney Int* 37:204, 1990.
119. Holmberg C et al: Determination of chloride and bicarbonate permeabilities in proximal convoluted tubules. *Am J Physiol* 241:F386, 1981.
120. Horie S et al: Preincubation in acid medium increases Na/H antiporter activity in cultured renal proximal tubule cells. *Proc Natl Acad Sci U S A* 87:4742, 1990.
121. Howlin K et al: Amiloride inhibition of proximal tubular acidification. *Am J Physiol* 17:F773, 1985.
122. Hruska et al: Stimulation of inositol triphosphate and diacylglycerol production in renal tubular cells by parathyroid hormone. *J Clin Invest* 70:230, 1987.
123. Hulter HN et al: Impaired renal H^+ secretion and NH_3 production in mineralocorticoid-deficient glucocorticoid-replete dogs. *Am J Physiol* 232:F136, 1977.
124. Hulter HN et al: K^+ deprivation potentiates the renal alkalosis-producing effect of mineralocorticoid. *Am J Physiol* 235:F298, 1978.
125. Hulter HN et al: Renal acidosis in mineralocorticoid deficiency is not dependent on NaCl depletion or hyperkalemia. *Am J Physiol* 236:F283, 1979.
126. Hulter HN et al: K^+ deprivation potentiates the renal acid excretory effect of mineralocorticoid: Obliteration by amiloride. *Am J Physiol* 236:F48, 1979.
127. Hulter HN et al: Pathogenesis of renal hyperchloremic acidosis resulting from dietary potassium restriction in the dog: Role of aldosterone. *Am J Physiol* 238:F79, 1980.
128. Hulter HN et al: Renal and systemic acid-base effects of the chronic administration of hypercalcemia-producing agents: Calcitriol, PTH, and intravenous calcium. *Kidney Int* 21:445, 1982.
129. Hulter HN et al: Metabolic alkalosis in models of primary and secondary hyperparathyroid states. *Am J Physiol* 245:F450, 1983.
130. Iacovitti M et al: Distal tubule bicarbonate accumulation in vivo. *J Clin Invest* 78:1658, 1986.
131. Igarashi P et al: Metabolic acidosis stimulates transport activity and transcript levels of the basolateral Na/H exchanger in LLC-PK1 cells. *J Am Soc Nephrol* 1:21, 1990.
132. Iino Y, Burg MB: Effect of parathyroid hormone on bicarbonate absorption by proximal tubules in vitro. *Am J Physiol* 236:F387, 1979.
133. Iino Y, Burg MB: Effect of acid-base status in vivo on bicarbonate transport by rabbit renal tubules in vitro. *Jpn J Physiol* 31:99, 1981.
134. Ives HE, Rector FC Jr: Proton transport and cell function. *J Clin Invest* 73:285, 1984.
135. Ives HE et al: Mixed-type inhibition of the renal Na^+/H^+ antiporter by Li^+ and amiloride: Evidence for a modifier site. *J Biol Chem* 258:9710, 1983.

136. Jacobson HR: Altered permeability in the proximal tubule response to cyclic AMP. *Am J Physiol* 236:F71, 1979.
137. Jacobson HR: Effects of CO_2 and acetazolamide on bicarbonate and fluid transport in rabbit proximal tubules. *Am J Physiol* 240:F54, 1981.
138. Jones JW et al: Systemic and renal acid-base effects of chronic dietary potassium depletion in humans. *Kidney Int* 21:402, 1982.
139. Kahn AM et al: Parathyroid hormone and dibutyryl cAMP inhibit Na/H exchange in renal brush border vesicles. *Am J Physiol* 248:F212, 1985.
140. Kassirer JP et al: On the pathogenesis of metabolic alkalosis in hyperaldosteronism. *Am J Med* 49:306, 1970.
141. Kim J et al: Structural-functional adaptation of intercalated cells in rat collecting duct. *J Am Soc Nephrol* 1:651, 1990.
142. Kinne R et al: Ammonium transport in medullary thick ascending limb of rabbit kidney: Involvement of the Na/K/Cl cotransporter. *J Membr Biol* 94:279, 1986.
143. Kinne-Saffran E et al: An ATP-driven proton pump in brush-border membranes from rat renal cortex. *J Membr Biol* 64:67, 1982.
144. Kinsella JL, Aronson PS: Properties of the Na^+-H^+ exchanger in renal microvillus membrane vesicles. *Am J Physiol* 238:F461, 1980.
145. Kinsella JL, Aronson PS: Interaction of NH_4 and Li with the renal microvillus membrane Na-H exchanger. *Am J Physiol* 241:C220, 1981.
146. Kinsella JL et al: Na/H exchange activity in renal brush border membrane vesicles in response to metabolic acidosis: The role of glucocorticoids. *Proc Natl Acad Sci U S A* 81:630, 1984.
147. Kleinman JG et al: Cell pH and acid transport in renal cortical tissue. *Am J Physiol* 239:F440, 1980.
148. Knepper M et al: Mechanism of ammonia secretion by cortical collecting ducts of rabbits. *Am J Physiol* 16:F729, 1984.
149. Knauf PA, Rothstein A: Chemical modification of membranes: 1. Effects of sulfhydryl and amino reactive reagents on anion and cation permeability of the human red blood cell. *J Gen Physiol* 58:190, 1971.
150. Koeppen BM, Helman SI: Acidification of luminal fluid by the rabbit cortical collecting tubule perfused in vitro. *Am J Physiol* 242:F521, 1982.
151. Koeppen BM: Conductive properties of the rabbit outer medullary collecting duct: Inner stripe. *Am J Physiol* 248:F500, 1985.
152. Krapf R: Basolateral $H/OH/HCO_3$ transport in the rat cortical thick ascending limb. *J Clin Invest* 82:234, 1988.
153. Krapf R: Mechanisms of adaptation to chronic respiratory acidosis in the rabbit proximal tubule. *J Clin Invest* 83:890, 1989.
154. Kudrycki K, Shull GE: Primary structure of the rat kidney band 3 anion exchange protein deduced from a cDNA. *J Biol Chem* 14:8185, 1989.
155. Kunau RT et al: Effect of metabolic acidosis on proximal tubule tCO_2 absorption. *Am J Physiol* 249:F62, 1985.
156. Kurtz I: Apical Na/H antiporter and glycolysis-dependent H-ATPase regulate intracellular pH in the rabbit S3 proximal tubule. *J Clin Invest* 80:928, 1987.
157. Kurtz I et al: Spontaneous luminal dysequilibrium pH in S3 proximal tubules. *J Clin Invest* 78:989, 1986.
158. Laski ME, Kurtzman NA: Characterization of acidification in the cortical and medullary collecting tubule of the rabbit. *J Clin Invest* 72:2050, 1983.
159. Leslie BR et al: Coupling between Cl^- absorption and HCO_3^- secretion in turtle urinary bladder. *Am J Physiol* 225:610, 1973.
160. Levine DZ: Effect of acute hypercapnia on proximal tubular water and bicarbonate absorption. *Am J Physiol* 221:1164, 1971.
161. Levine DZ et al: An in vivo microperfusion study of distal tubule bicarbonate reabsorption in normal and ammonium chloride rats. *J Clin Invest* 78:1658, 1986.
162. Lief PD et al: Effect of cyclic AMP on hydrogen ion secretion by turtle urinary bladder. *Kidney Int* 16:103, 1979.
163. Lifton RP et al: Cloning of the human genomic amiloride-sensitive Na/H antiporter gene, identification of genetic polymorphisms, and localization on the genetic map of chromosome 1p. *Genomics* 7:131, 1990.
164. Liu F-Y, Cogan MG: Angiotensin II: A potent regulator of acidification in the rat early proximal convoluted tubule. *J Clin Invest* 80:272, 1987.
165. Liu F-Y, Cogan MG: Angiotensin II stimulation of hydrogen ion secretion in the rat early proximal tubule. *J Clin Invest* 82:601, 1988.
166. Liu F-Y, Cogan MG: Angiotensin II stimulates early proximal bicarbonate absorption in the rat by decreasing cyclic adenosine monophosphate. *J Clin Invest* 84:83, 1989.
167. Lombard WE et al: Bicarbonate transport in cortical and outer medullary collecting tubules. *Am J Physiol* 244:F289, 1983.
168. Lönnerholm G, Ridderstrale Y: Intracellular distribution of carbonic anhydrase in the rat kidney. *Kidney Int* 17:162, 1980.
169. Lorentz WB Jr: The effect of cyclic AMP and dibutyryl cyclic AMP on the permeability characteristics of the renal tubule. *J Clin Invest* 53:1250, 1974.
170. Lorentz WB Jr: Effect of parathyroid hormone on renal tubular permeability. *Am J Physiol* 231:1401, 1976.
171. Lucci, MS et al: Carbonic anhydrase-dependent bicarbonate reabsorption in the rat proximal tubule. *Am J Physiol* 236:F58, 1979.
172. Lucci MS et al: Direct evaluation of acidification by rat proximal tubule: Role of carbonic anhydrase. *Am J Physiol* 238:F372, 1980.
173. Lucci MS et al: Evaluation of bicarbonate transport in rat distal tubule: Effects of acid-base status. *Am J Physiol* 243:F335, 1982.
174. Lucci MS et al: Function of proximal tubule carbonic anhydrase defined by selective inhibition. *Am J Physiol* 245:F443, 1983.
175. Maddox D et al: Proximal bicarbonate reabsorption and the determinants of tubular and capillary P_{CO_2} in the rat. *Am J Physiol* 247:F73, 1984.
176. Madsen KM, Tisher CC: Cellular response to acute respiratory acidosis in rat medullary collecting duct. *Am J Physiol* 245:F670, 1983.
177. Madsen KM, Tisher CC: Response of intercalated cells (IC) in the outer medullary collecting duct to chronic metabolic acidosis. *Lab Invest* 51:268, 1984.

178. Madsen KM et al: Structural-functional relationships along the distal nephron. *Am J Physiol* 250:F1, 1986.
179. Madsen KM et al: Identification of intercalated cells in rabbit medullary collecting duct. *Kidney Int* 35:458A, 1989.
180. Malnic G, de Mello-Aires M: Kinetic study of bicarbonate reabsorption in proximal tubule of the rat. *Am J Physiol* 220:1759, 1971.
181. McKinney TD, Burg MB: Bicarbonate and fluid absorption by renal proximal straight tubules. *Kidney Int* 12:1, 1977.
182. McKinney TD, Burg MB: Bicarbonate transport by rabbit cortical collecting tubules: Effect of acid and alkali loads in vivo on transport in vitro. *J Clin Invest* 60:766, 1977.
183. McKinney TD, Burg MB: Bicarbonate absorption by rabbit cortical collecting tubules in vitro. *Am J Physiol* 234:F141, 1978.
184. McKinney TD, Burg MB: Bicarbonate secretion by rabbit cortical collecting tubules in vitro. *J Clin Invest* 61:1421, 1978.
185. McKinney TD, Davidson KK: Effect of potassium depletion and protein intake in vivo on renal tubular bicarbonate transport in vitro. *Am J Physiol* 252:F509, 1987.
186. McKinney TD, Myers P: Bicarbonate transport by proximal tubules: Effect of parathyroid hormone and dibutyryl cyclic AMP. *Am J Physiol* 238:F166, 1980.
187. McKinney TD, Myers P: PTH inhibition of bicarbonate transport by proximal convoluted tubules. *Am J Physiol* 239:F127, 1980.
188. McKinney TD, Myers P: Effect of calcium and phosphate on bicarbonate and fluid transport by proximal tubules in vitro. *Kidney Int* 21:433, 1982.
189. de Mello-Aires M, Malnic G: Peritubular pH and P_{CO_2} in renal tubular acidification. *Am J Physiol* 228:1766, 1975.
190. Mercier O et al: Effects of parathyroid hormone and urinary phosphate on collecting duct hydrogen ion secretion. *Am J Physiol* 251:F802, 1986.
191. Mercier O et al: Effects of glucagon on H/HCO_3 transport in Henle's loop, distal tubule and collecting ducts in the rat. *Am J Physiol* 257:F1003, 1989.
192. Miller RT et al: Structure of the human Na/H exchanger gene and 5′-flanking region. *J Biol Chem* 266:10813, 1991.
193. Mitnick P et al: Effects of two models of hypercalcemia on renal acid-base metabolism. *Kidney Int* 21:613, 1982.
194. Moe OW et al: Differential regulation of Na/H antiporter by acid in renal epithelial cells and fibroblasts. *J Clin Invest* 88:1703, 1991.
195. Moe OW et al: Dietary NaCl modulates Na/H antiporter activity in renal cortical apical membrane vesicles. *Am J Physiol* 260:F130. 1991.
196. Morel F et al: Functional segmentation of the rabbit distal tubule by microdetermination of hormone-dependent adenylate cyclase activity. *Kidney Int* 9:264, 1976.
197. Murer H et al: Sodium/proton antiport in brush-border membrane vesicles isolated from rat small intestine and kidney. *Biochem J* 154:597, 1976.
198. Muto S et al: Electrophysiological identification of α and β intercalated cells and their distribution along the distal nephron segments. *J Clin Invest* 86:1829, 1990.
199. Nagami G et al: Regulation of ammonia production by mouse proximal tubules perfused in vitro. *J Clin Invest* 75:844, 1985.
200. Nagami G et al: Ammonia production by isolated mouse proximal tubules perfused in vitro. *J Clin Invest* 78:124, 1986.
201. Nagami G et al: Luminal secretion of ammonia in the mouse proximal tubule in vitro. *J Clin Invest* 81:159, 1988.
202. Nakhoul NL et al: Intracellular pH regulation in the S3 segment of the rabbit proximal tubule in HCO_3-free solutions. *J Gen Physiol* 92:369, 1988.
203. Narins RG et al: Effects of acute acid-base changes on in vivo total ammonia synthesis in the rat. *Contrib Nephrol* 31:47, 1982.
204. Nord E et al: α_2-adrenergic agonists stimulate Na-H antiporter activity in the rabbit renal proximal tubule. *J Clin Invest* 80:1755, 1987.
205. Ochwadt BK, Pitts RF: Effects of intravenous infusion of carbonic anhydrase on carbon dioxide tension of alkaline urine. *Am J Physiol* 185:426, 1956.
206. Oliver JA et al: Energy dependence of urinary bicarbonate secretion in turtle bladder. *J Clin Invest* 55:1003, 1975.
207. O'Neil RG, Helman SI: Transport characteristics of renal collecting tubules: Influences of DOCA and diet. *Am J Physiol* 233:F544, 1977.
208. Paillard M et al: Proximal reabsorption of HCO_3, Cl, and water during isohydric extracellular fluid volume expansion (VE) in Sprague Dawley rats (abstract). *Kidney Int* 23:237A, 1983.
209. Pearce D et al: Cloning of a partial length rat kidney cDNA homologous to the human Na/H antiporter. *Kidney Int* 37:233, 1990.
210. Pitts RF, Lotspeich WD: Bicarbonate and the renal regulation of acid-base balance. *Am J Physiol* 147:138, 1946.
211. Pitts RF: Renal excretion of acid. *Fed Proc* 7:418, 1948.
212. Pitts RF: Production and excretion of ammonia in relation to acid-base regulation, in Orloff J, Berliner RW (eds): *Handbook of Physiology*. Washington DC, American Physiological Society, 1973, Section 8, p 455.
213. Pollock AS et al: Parathyroid hormone inhibition of Na-H antiporter activity in a cultured renal cell line. *Am J Physiol* 250:F217, 1986.
214. Preisig PA, Alpern RJ: Chronic metabolic acidosis causes an adaptation in the apical membrane Na/H antiporter and basolateral membrane Na/3HCO_3 symporter in the rat proximal convoluted tubule. *J Clin Invest* 82:1445, 1988.
215. Preisig PA, Alpern RJ: Pathways for apical and basolateral membrane NH_3 and NH_4 movement in rat proximal tubule. *Am J Physiol* 28:F587, 1990.
216. Preisig PA, Alpern RJ: Increased Na/H antiporter and Na/3HCO_3 symporter activities in chronic hyperfiltration. *J Gen Physiol* 97:195, 1991.
217. Preisig PA et al: Role of Na/H antiporter in rat proximal tubule bicarbonate absorption. *J Clin Invest* 80:970, 1987.
218. Puschett JB, Zurbach P: Acute effects of parathyroid hormone on proximal bicarbonate transport in the dog. *Kidney Int* 9:501, 1976.
219. Rector FC Jr, Orloff J: The effect of the administration of sodium bicarbonate and ammonium chloride on the ex-

cretion and production of ammonia. The absence of alterations in the activity of renal ammonia-producing enzymes in the dog. *J Clin Invest* 38:366, 1959.
220. Rector FC Jr et al: Examination of the mixing hypothesis as an explanation for elevated urinary CO_2 tensions. *Am J Physiol* 197:861, 1959.
221. Rector FC Jr et al: The mechanism of bicarbonate reabsorption in the proximal and distal tubules of the kidney. *J Clin Invest* 44:278, 1965.
222. Reilly RF et al: Cloning and immunolocalization of an Na/H exchanger in LLC-PK_1 cells. *J Am Soc Nephrol* 1:745, 1990.
223. Richardson RMA, Kunau RT Jr: Bicarbonate reabsorption in the papillary collecting duct: Effect of acetazolamide. *Am J Physiol* 243:F74, 1982.
224. Ridderstale Y et al: Morphological heterogeneity of the rabbit collecting duct. *Kidney Int* 34:655, 1988.
225. Rodriguez-Nichols F et al: Response of renal NH_3 production to chronic respiratory acidosis. *Am J Physiol* 247:F896, 1984.
226. Roos A, Boron WF: Intracellular pH. *Physiol Rev* 61:296, 1981.
227. Roth DG, Gamble JR Jr: Deoxycorticosterone-induced alkalosis in dogs. *Am J Physiol* 208:90, 1965.
228. Ruiz OS et al: Na/HCO_3 and Na/H antiporter in chronic respiratory acidosis and alkalosis. *Am J Physiol* 256:F414, 1989.
229. Ruiz O, Arruda JAL et al: Modulation of renal Na/HCO_3 cotransporter by protein kinases A and C. *Kidney Int* 37:544, 1990.
230. Sabatini S et al: The effects of chronic papillary necrosis on acid excretion. *Pfluegers Arch* 393:262, 1982.
231. Saccomani G et al: Angiotensin II stimulation of Na-H exchange in proximal tubule cells. *Am J Physiol* 258:F1188, 1990.
232. Sajo IM et al: Sites of ammonia addition to tubular fluid in rats with chronic metabolic acidosis. *Kidney Int* 20:353, 1981.
233. Salihagic AM et al: Short-term and long-term stimulation of Na/H exchange in cortical brush-border membranes during compensatory growth of the rat kidney. *Pfluegers Arch* 413:190, 1988.
234. Sardet C et al: Molecular cloning, primary structure and expression of the human growth factor activatable Na/H antiporter. *Cell* 56:271, 1989.
235. Sardet C et al: Molecular properties of Na/H exchangers, in De Santo NG, Capasso G (eds): *Acid-Base Balance: Molecular, Cellular and Clinical Aspects*. Italy, Editoriale Bios, 1990, p 13.
236. Sasaki S, Berry CA: Mechanism of HCO_3^- exit across the basolateral membrane of rabbit proximal convoluted tubules. *Am J Physiol* 246:F889, 1984.
237. Sasaki S, Marumo F et al: Cellular mechanisms of inhibition of proximal acidification by PTH. *J Am Soc Nephrol* 1:658, 1990.
238. Sasaki S et al: Effect of luminal and peritubular HCO_3^- concentrations and PCO_2 on HCO_3^- reabsorption in rabbit proximal convoluted tubules perfused in vitro. *J Clin Invest* 70:639, 1982.
239. Sasaki S et al: Effect of potassium concentration on bicarbonate reabsorption in the rabbit proximal convoluted tubule. *Am J Physiol* 224:F122, 1983.
240. Schuster VL: Cyclic adenosine monophosphate-stimulated bicarbonate secretion in rabbit cortical collecting tubules. *J Clin Invest* 75:2056, 1985.
241. Schuster VL et al: Angiotensin II directly stimulates sodium transport in rabbit proximal convoluted tubules. *J Clin Invest* 73:507, 1984.
242. Schuster VL et al: Two types of collecting duct mitochondria-rich (intercalated) cells: Lectin and band 3 cytochemistry. *Am J Physiol* 251:C347, 1986.
243. Schuster VL et al: Co-localization of H-ATPase and band 3 Cl-HCO_3 exchanger in rabbit collecting duct intercalated cells. *Am J Physiol* 260:F506, 1991.
244. Schwartz GJ: Na^+-dependent H^+ efflux from proximal tubule: Evidence for reversible Na^+-H^+ exchange. *Am J Physiol* 224:F380, 1981.
245. Schwartz GJ, Al-Awqati Q: Carbon dioxide causes exocytosis of vesicles containing H pumps in isolated perfused proximal and collecting tubules. *J Clin Invest* 75:1638, 1985.
246. Schwartz GJ, Burg MB: Mineralocorticoid effects on cation transport by cortical collecting tubules in vitro. *Am J Physiol* 235:F576, 1978.
247. Schwartz GJ et al: Plasticity of functional epithelial polarity. *Nature (London)* 318:368, 1985.
248. Schwartz JH: H^+ current response to CO_2 and carbonic anhydrase inhibition in turtle bladder. *Am J Physiol* 231:565, 1976.
249. Schwartz JH, Steinmetz PR: CO_2 requirements for H^+ secretion by the isolated turtle bladder. *Am J Physiol* 220:2051, 1971.
250. Schwartz JH et al: Specialized function of carbonic anhydrase-rich and granular cells of turtle bladder. *Am J Physiol* 242:F627, 1982.
251. Schwartz WB et al: Acidification of the urine and increased ammonium excretion without change in acid-base equilibrium: Sodium reabsorption as a stimulus to the acidifying process. *J Clin Invest* 34:673, 1955.
252. Sebastian A et al: Amelioration of metabolic acidosis with fludrocortisone therapy in hyporeninemic hypoaldosteronism. *N Engl J Med* 297:576, 1977.
253. Simon EE et al: Determinants of ammonia entry along the rat proximal tubule during chronic metabolic acidosis. *Am J Physiol* 256:F1104, 1989.
254. Soleimani M, Aronson PS: Ionic mechanism of $NaHCO_3$ cotransport in rabbit renal basolateral membrane vesicles. *J Biol Chem* 264:18302, 1989.
255. Soleimani M et al: Stoichiometry of Na-HCO_3 cotransport in basolateral membrane vesicles isolated from rabbit renal cortex. *J Clin Invest* 79:1276, 1987.
256. Soleimani M et al: Potassium depletion increases luminal Na/H exchange and basolateral Na:CO_3:HCO_3 cotransport in rat renal cortex. *J Clin Invest* 86:1076, 1990.
257. Sonnenberg H et al: Ammonia addition into the medullary collecting duct of the rat. *Kidney Int* 19:281, 1981.
258. Star RA: Basolateral membrane sodium-independent Cl/HCO_3 exchanger in rat inner medullary collecting duct cell. *J Clin Invest* 85:1959, 1990.
259. Star RA et al: Bicarbonate secretion and chloride absorption by rabbit collecting ducts: Role of chloride bicarbonate exchange. *J Clin Invest* 76:1123, 1985.
260. Star RA et al: Dysequilibrium pH and ammonia transport

in isolated perfused cortical collecting ducts. *Am J Physiol* 253:F1232, 1987.
261. Star RA et al: Luminal dysequilibrium pH and ammonia transport in outer medullary collecting duct. *Am J Physiol* 252:F1148, 1987.
262. Steinmetz PR: Acid-base relations in epithelium of turtle bladder: Site of active step in acidification and role of metabolic CO_2. *J Clin Invest* 48:1258, 1969.
263. Steinmetz PR: Cellular mechanisms of urinary acidification. *Physiol Rev* 54:890, 1974.
264. Steinmetz PR, Lawson LR: Effect of luminal pH on ion permeability and flows of Na^+ and H^+ in turtle bladder. *Am J Physiol* 220:1573, 1971.
265. Stetson DL et al: Morphological alteration in the rat medullary collecting duct following potassium depletion. *Kidney Int* 17:45, 1980.
266. Stokes JB: Na and K transport across the cortical and outer medullary collecting tubule of the rabbit: Evidence of diffusion across the outer medullary portion. *Am J Physiol* 242:F514, 1982.
267. Stone DK et al: Mineralocorticoid modulation of rabbit medullary collecting duct acidification: A sodium-independent effect. *J Clin Invest* 72:77, 1983.
268. Stone DK et al: Anion dependence of rabbit medullary collecting duct acidification. *J Clin Invest* 71:1505, 1983.
269. Takaichi K et al: Sequence analysis of Na/H antiporter cDNAs from human tissues. *J Am Soc Nephrol* 1:745, 1990.
270. Tam SC et al: Effect of extracellular fluid volume contraction on distal-nephron hydrogen ion secretion in vivo. *J Lab Clin Med* 96:442, 1980.
271. Tam SC et al: Studies on the regulation of hydrogen ion secretion in the collecting duct in vivo: Evaluation of factors that influence the urine minus blood PCO_2 difference. *Kidney Int* 20:636, 1981.
272. Tannen RL: The effect of uncomplicated potassium depletion on urine acidification. *J Clin Invest* 49:813, 1970.
273. Tannen RL: Ammonia metabolism. *Am J Physiol* 235:F265, 1978.
274. Tannen RL, McGill J: Influence of potassium on renal ammonia production. *Am J Physiol* 231:1178, 1976.
275. Tannen RL et al: Renal adaptation to a high potassium intake: The role of hydrogen ion. *J Clin Invest* 52:2089, 1973.
276. Tsai CJ et al: Increased Vmax for Na/H antiporter in proximal tubule brush border vesicles from rabbits with metabolic acidosis. *Am J Physiol* 247:F339, 1984.
277. Ullrich KJ, Papavassiliou F: Bicarbonate reabsorption in the papillary collecting duct of rats. *Pflügers Arch* 389:271, 1981.
278. Ullrich KJ et al: Renal proximal tubular buffer-(glycodiazine) transport. *Pflügers Arch* 357:149, 1975.
279. Ullrich KJ et al: Coupling between proximal tubular transport processes: Studies with ouabain, SITS and HCO_3^- free solutions. *Pflügers Arch* 368:245, 1977.
280. Velazquez H et al: Luminal influences on potassium secretion: Chloride replacement with sulfate. *Am J Physiol* 242:F46, 1982.
281. Verkman AS, Alpern RJ: Kinetic transport model for cellular regulation of pH and solute concentration in the renal proximal tubule. *Biophys J* 51:533, 1987.
282. Vieira FL, Malnic G: Hydrogen ion secretion by rat renal cortical tubules as studied by an antimony microelectrode. *Am J Physiol* 214:710, 1968.
283. Wagner S et al: Immunochemical characterization of a band 3-like anion exchanger in collecting duct of human kidney. *Am J Physiol* 253:F213, 1987.
284. Wall SM et al: Net acid transport by isolated perfused inner medullary collecting ducts. *Am J Physiol* 258:F75, 1990.
285. Wallin JD et al: Effect of increased distal bicarbonate delivery on free water reabsorption in the dog. *Am J Physiol* 224:209, 1973.
286. Wang W: Evidence for Na-dependent rheogenic HCO_3 in fused cells of frog distal tubules. *Pfluegers Arch* 408:291, 1987.
287. Warnock DG, Burg MB: Urinary acidification: CO_2 transport by the rabbit proximal straight tubule. *Am J Physiol* 232:F20, 1977.
288. Warnock DG, Yee VJ: Anion permeabilities of the isolated perfused rabbit proximal tubule. *Am J Physiol* 242:F395, 1982.
289. Warnock DG et al: Na^+/H^+ antiporter of brush border vesicles: Studies with acridine orange uptake. *Am J Physiol* 242:F733, 1982.
290. Weiner ID, Hamm LL: Regulation of intracellular pH in the rabbit cortical collecting tubule. *J Clin Invest* 85:274, 1990.
291. Weinman EJ et al: cAMP-associated inhibition of Na-H exchanger in rabbit kidney brush-border membranes. *Am J Physiol* 252:F19, 1987.
292. Weinman EJ et al: Reconstitution of cAMP-dependent protein kinase regulated renal Na-H exchanger. *J Membr Biol* 101:11, 1988.
293. Wingo CS: Active proton secretion and potassium absorption in the rabbit outer medullary collecting duct. *J Clin Invest* 84:361, 1989.
294. Wingo CS et al: H-K-ATPase immunoreactivity in cortical and outer medullary collecting duct. *Kidney Int* 38:985, 1990.
295. Winne D: Unstirred layer, source of biased Michaelis constant in membrane transport. *Biochim Biophys Acta* 298:27, 1973.
296. Wright FS: Flow-dependent transport processes: Filtration, absorption, secretion. *Am J Physiol* 243:F1, 1982.
297. Yoshitomi K, Fromter E: Cell pH of rat proximal tubule in vivo and the conductive nature of peritubular HCO_3/OH exit. *Pfluegers Arch* 402:300, 1984.
298. Yoshitomi K et al: Rheogenic $NaHCO_3$ cotransport in the peritubular membrane of rat renal proximal tubule. *Pluegers Arch* 405:360, 1985.
299. Ziegler TW et al: Influence of transepithelial potential difference on acidification in the toad urinary bladder. *Kidney Int* 10:279, 1976.

CHAPTER • 11

Calcium Metabolism

James E. Bourdeau • Maurice F. Attie

The physiologic roles played by calcium vary from that of a rapidly fluctuating intracellular messenger[119,194,475,476] to that of a stable component of crystals providing structural support.[417,465] Plasma calcium stabilizes the membranes of excitable cells, such as muscle and nerve, and binds to macromolecules, such as the proteins of the blood clotting cascade.

The low calcium concentrations in cytoplasm and the high calcium content in bone necessitate energy-requiring transport mechanisms to maintain the steep gradients for this ion at interfaces with plasma. Cytosolic calcium expresses much of its messenger role by binding with high affinity to a homologous class of proteins that include calmodulin, troponin C, and vitamin D-dependent calcium-binding protein (calbindin-D). Through these interactions, cytoplasmic calcium regulates muscle and microtubule contraction, initiation of mitosis, and a host of enzymes, including adenylate cyclase and cyclic adenosine monophosphate (cAMP) phosphodiesterase. Much of the information from cytoplasmic calcium is transmitted through protein kinases (mediators of protein phosphorylation), both dependent on and independent of calmodulin.

Of the ionic components of plasma, only sodium is regulated more strictly than calcium (when expressed as the ratio between the mean and one standard deviation of the normal plasma concentration). The parathyroid glands regulate plasma calcium concentration by secreting parathyroid hormone (PTH) in response to hypocalcemia. PTH raises the level of circulating calcium by enhancing resorption of bone, by increasing reabsorption of calcium by the renal tubules, and by augmenting intestinal absorption of calcium. The latter effect is indirect; that is, PTH increases synthesis of 1α,25-dihydroxyvitamin D_3 [1α,25-$(OH)_2D_3$, or calcitriol], a steroid hormone, synthesized in the proximal tubules of the kidney, that acts on the intestine. Large amounts of calcium must cross both renal tubular and intestinal epithelia without perturbing the messenger function of calcium in the cytosol. This chapter discusses the state of calcium in body compartments; calcium fluxes across organellar, plasma, and epithelial membranes; and the factors regulating these calcium fluxes.

CALCIUM DISTRIBUTION AND CONTENT

Calcium is the most abundant electrolyte in the human body, a 70-kg male containing approximately 1300 g (or 1.9 percent of total body mass),[427] primarily as a result of its considerable storage in the skeleton (Table 11-1). Greater than 99 percent of skeletal calcium is unavailable for day-to-day regulation of plasma calcium concentration.

CELLULAR AND CYTOSOLIC CALCIUM

The calcium content of soft tissues varies from 1 to 10 mmol per kilogram of body weight.[445] This variability reflects differences in calcium adsorbed to cell membranes and in the content of calcium within organelles.

TABLE 11-1 • Distribution of calcium in the body of a 70-kg adult

Organ	Calcium, g
Bone	1300(99)*
Teeth	7(0.6)
Soft tissues	7(0.6)
Extravascular fluid	0.70(0.06)
Plasma	0.35(0.03)

* Numbers in parentheses indicate percent of total.

SOURCE: From Nordin BEC: Nutritional considerations, in Nordin BEC (ed): *Calcium, Phosphate, and Magnesium Metabolism,* New York, Churchill Livingstone, 1976, p 3. Used by permission.

The density of calcium within organelles such as sarcoplasmic reticulum, endoplasmic reticulum, and mitochondria can be high and may be stabilized therein in noncrystalline forms by ligands such as magnesium-ATP and phosphocitrate.[31,335] The free calcium concentration in the cytosol is only 10^{-8} to 10^{-6} *M*. This very low level is maintained by extrusion mechanisms that transport calcium against steep gradients across the cell membrane and into the mitochondria and endoplasmic and sarcoplasmic reticula. Less than 1 percent of total body calcium is in solution in extracellular and intracellular fluid compartments.

PHYSICOCHEMICAL STATE OF CALCIUM IN BIOLOGICAL SOLUTIONS

Plasma

Because of its accessibility, blood plasma (or serum; Fig. 11-1) is the biological solution most frequently analyzed for calcium. Inasmuch as the ionic calcium (Ca^{2+}) concentration of the extracellular fluid (ECF), of which the plasma is a part, is the focal point for the endocrine regulation of calcium homeostasis, the choice of this solution for analysis is logical and useful. Nonetheless, the correct description of the physicochemical states of calcium in the plasma and their accurate measurement remain difficult problems in physiologic chemistry because plasma is a complex aqueous solution.

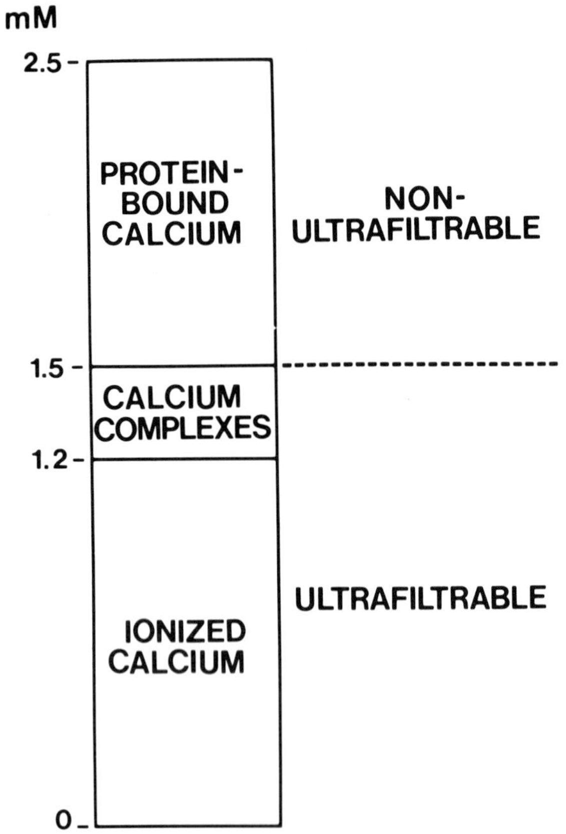

FIGURE 11-1 • Typical distribution of the components of plasma total calcium concentration in normal adult humans. Values may be converted from millimoles (m*M*) per liter to milligrams per deciliter by multiplying by 4 (the atomic weight of calcium is 40.08 g/mol).

The *plasma total calcium concentration* of adult humans is 2.10 to 2.60 m*M* (8.4 to 10.4 mg/dl).[181,324,539] It may be measured by isotope dilution mass spectrometry, the definitive method;[392] by atomic absorption spectrometry, the reference method;[99] by fluorescence-quenching titration of a calcium-sensitive fluorescent dye, such as calcein;[49] or by colorimetric methods.[177,324,628] These methods are accurate and precise, and although clinical laboratory reference ranges for plasma total calcium concentration vary slightly,[628] there is no controversy about the meaning of this measurement (in contrast to the measurement of ionized calcium).

In the plasma, approximately 40 percent of the total calcium is *bound to proteins*, as assessed by ultrafiltration[391,455,592,616] or gel filtration.[590,591] Most of this protein-bound calcium is in chemical equilibrium with the *ultrafilterable calcium*, but the former does not participate in reactions that involve Ca^{2+}, such as myocardial contractility, neuromuscular activity, or blood coagulation. Between 75 and 90 percent of the protein-bound calcium is associated with albumin,[391, 455, 591] which—although a zwitterion—has a net ionic charge of −19 per molecule at pH 7.4.[456] Electrostatic interactions between albumin and divalent calcium cations would be expected to play a role in calcium binding,[246,293,312,456] and most evidence indicates that anionic carboxylate groups of glutamate and aspartate residues in albumin are ligands that interact electrostatically with calcium ions.[178,179,340,341,638] Irons and Perkins[293] and Pedersen[455] have proposed that albumin contains specific calcium-binding sites. The molecular nature of these hypothetical binding sites is unknown, but if they do exist, they may contain neutral oxygen donor atoms from uncharged peptide carbonyl or hydroxyl groups that, in conjunction with anionic carboxylate groups, form multi-oxygen atom coordination sites for stereospecific Ca^{2+} binding.[179,340,341,638] Alternatively, the neutral atom donors for the calcium-binding sites may be provided by nitrogen atoms within imidazole groups, the latter being uncharged at pH 7.4.[453,454] Calcium binding to albumin is strongly pH-dependent between pH values of 7 and 8: binding decreases or increases as the pH decreases or increases, respectively.[246,293,312,453,592] Because most carboxyl groups in albumin are negatively charged even at pH 5, Katz and Klotz concluded that the increase in calcium binding as the pH increases in the physiologic range is due to increased electrostatic attraction as the net negative charge of the protein increases,[312] presumably resulting from the loss of protons from imidazole nitrogens. Eastman and associates[178] suggested that the swelling of the albumin molecule that occurs as the pH is increased above 7 unmasks anionic carboxylate groups that bind calcium. This hypothesis is consistent with the experimental findings of Fogh-Andersen.[211] Conversely, Pedersen has proposed that removal of hydrogen ions from cationic imidazole groups of the albumin molecule allows calcium ions to bind as the pH increases.[452,455] According to Pedersen, calcium ions are individually bound to albumin as at least a bidentate chelate* that contains two anionic carboxylate groups.[454] He has hypothesized that the imidazole group at or near the calcium-binding site may be either a neutral nitrogen donor that forms a tridentate chelate of calcium in conjunction with the anionic carboxylate groups or a cationic protonated nitrogen donor that forms a salt linkage with one of the anionic carboxylate groups, thereby preventing calcium binding.[453] Regardless of the exact sites and mechanisms, in normal plasma only a small fraction of the calcium-binding sites within albumin are occupied.[452,455] Long-chain fatty acids—such as palmitic, stearic, and oleic—enhance calcium binding to albumin.[325,642] The remaining protein-bound calcium, approximately 10 to 25 percent of the total, is associated with α2-macroglobulin, haptoglobins, and the major immunoglobulins: IgG, IgA, and IgM.[591] The total protein-bound calcium concentration has been measured directly by gel filtration[590,591] or has been calculated as the difference between the plasma (or serum) total calcium concentration and the calcium concentration of plasma ultrafiltrates.[389,455,592,616,642] The distribution of protein-bound calcium among serum proteins has been examined with gel filtration chromatography.[591]

Approximately 60 percent of the total plasma calcium is ultrafilterable because it is not protein-bound, consisting of low-molecular weight calcium complexes and ionized calcium.[389,455,590,592,616,642] In descending order of concentration, the former include calcium bicarbonate, calcium citrate, calcium phosphate, calcium lactate, and calcium sulfate.[590,615,616] Calcium bicarbonate and calcium lactate are monovalent positively charged ion pairs, calcium phosphate and calcium sulfate are uncharged ion pairs, and calcium citrate is a monovalent anionic chelate at pH 7.4.[615] Changes in serum bicarbonate concentration in vitro are inversely related to changes in ionized calcium concentration independent of changes in pH.[282] This relationship reflects the formation or dissolution of calcium bicarbonate complexes under physiologic conditions.[512] Likewise, increases in plasma lactate or citrate concentrations promote the formation of their respective calcium complexes. The latter are derived not only from interactions of these anions with ionic calcium but also from their removal of calcium that is bound to plasma proteins.[588,589] In serum, the total concentration of low-molecular weight calcium complexes, which have been isolated from serum by gel-filtration column chromatography, is 0.26 to 0.31 m*M*.[587,590]

The majority of the plasma ultrafilterable calcium is ionized. The *plasma ionized calcium* concentration in normal humans, 1.12 to 1.23 m*M*,[181] is 44 to 59 percent of the plasma total calcium concentration, as measured either by the murexide method[455,616] or by Ca^{2+}-selective electrodes.[389,397] As the biologically active component of the ECF calcium with respect to myocardial contractility, neuromuscular activity, and blood coagulation—and perhaps with respect to mineralization of bone as well—and as the reference variable for the endocrine regulation of calcium homeostasis, the ECF ionized calcium has been the plasma calcium component of greatest interest, despite the substantial theoretical and practical difficulties associated with its measurement.[89]

Calcium salts studied by x-ray crystallography demonstrate a calcium ionic radius of between 0.094 and 0.099 nm, values that approximate those of sodium ions.[341,357,449] In aqueous solutions, the divalent calcium cation is surrounded locally by a small number of "bound" water molecules. This hydration sheath, or shell, results primarily from the electrostatic interactions between the positively charged calcium ion and the electrical dipoles of the adjacent water molecules.[91,257,485] Because the electrostatic charge of the calcium ion is twice that of the sodum ion, despite nearly identical ionic radii, the surface charge density of the former is higher, resulting in a greater surrounding electrical field. The larger electrical field around the calcium ion explains why the hydration number* of calcium chloride is three to four times greater than that of sodium chloride.[485] On the other hand, because the magnesium ion is smaller than the calcium ion (the ionic radius of magnesium is 0.065 nm),[341,357,449] despite identical electrostatic charge, the hydration number of magnesium is larger than that of calcium. Consequently, the hydrated magnesium ion is larger than the hydrated calcium ion, which in part is responsible for the smaller ionic mobility of magnesium in comparison to calcium in aqueous solutions.

In addition to the specific interactions with certain anions and with protein discussed above, calcium ions interact nonspecifically with all other ions that are present in plasma.[417] The extent of these interactions, which are also primarily electrostatic, is determined by the dielectric constant of water and by the ionic strength of plasma, which in turn determine the electrochemical ac-

* *Chelate:* a binding configuration in which a central ion is joined by ordinary or coordinate bonds to two or more nonmetallic atoms of the same binding site. *Bidentate:* characterized by having two ligands (i.e., bonds) per binding site. *Tridentate:* characterized by having three ligands per binding site.

* The hydration number should be thought of as an index of the degree of ion hydration and not as the specific number of water molecules in a rigid shell surrounding the naked ion.

tivity of the calcium ion.[91,417] It is the activity of the calcium ions that is measured in blood plasma by Ca^{2+}-selective electrodes.[389,532] Values of Ca^{2+} activity, which are electrochemical potentials that are measured in millivolts, are converted to "concentrations of free ions" by dividing the Ca^{2+} activity by the activity coefficient for calcium ions in plasma.[183,391] A fundamental theoretical and practical problem is that the latter value is unknown and cannot be easily determined because the chemical composition of plasma is incompletely defined and varies from individual to individual.[532,615] Therefore, the calibration methods for Ca^{2+}-selective electrodes—that is, the methods of choosing the Ca^{2+} activity coefficient for plasma—are somewhat arbitrary, with the consequence that values of free calcium ion concentrations determined by such methods must be considered estimations.[183,532,615]

Other extracellular fluids

Despite its physiologic importance, the physicochemical state of calcium in the microscopic extracellular environment of bone is poorly understood, because of the technical difficulties of directly sampling fluid from this site.[416] Calcification of growth plate cartilage has been studied by analysis of fluid obtained by direct micropuncture of surgically exposed cartilage, which reveals ultrafilterable calcium concentrations that deviate only slightly from those of the serum.[276] Microelectrode studies of fluid sequestered between osteoclasts and crypt walls of osteoporotic bone fragments in rabbit ear chambers revealed pH values as low as 4.7 and Ca^{2+} concentrations as high as 40 m*M*.[534] Consistent with these latter observations, it has been hypothesized that the ionic composition of bone ECF, including calcium concentration, must differ from that of an ultrafiltrate of plasma.[416,445] In addition, it seems likely that the former might vary with the physiologic state of the organism, such as blood PTH concentration.

Total calcium concentrations in macroscopic samples of cerebrospinal fluid derived from normal humans vary between 1.05 and 1.35 m*M*.[181] By means of a Ca^{2+}-selective micropipette, the tip of which was inserted just beneath the pial surface of exposed cerebellum in the anesthetized rat, the calcium ion concentrations in the microscopic ECF of the brain were shown to change significantly with neuronal activity.[423] This finding supports Neuman's speculation that "nearly every organ system may, in fact, regulate the composition of its own [extracellular] fluid medium"[416] and indicates that analysis of bulk-phase cerebrospinal fluid[136] is inadequate to describe the physicochemical state of calcium in the microenvironment of the ECF surrounding functional central nervous system tissue.

The physicochemical state of calcium in the luminal fluid of the kidney tubules differs from that of calcium in the plasma for several reasons.[53] First, ultrafiltration of plasma at the renal corpuscle excludes protein from the tubule lumen, allowing only ionic calcium and ultrafilterable calcium complexes to enter. Second, tubular transport processes—such as absorption of bicarbonate and secretion of hydrogen ions; tubular transport of phosphate, oxalate, sulfate, and citrate; and tubular secretion of organic anions—alter the chemical composition of tubular luminal fluid in ways that may be expected to alter the physicochemical state of calcium. Finally, active and passive transport of calcium by the epithelia of the various nephron segments, processes that are influenced by the physicochemical state of calcium, cause changes in the concentration of ionized calcium along the kidney tubule. Likewise, the physicochemical state of calcium in the final urine is different than that in plasma. In normal humans, approximately 28 percent of urinary calcium is bound to citrate, 12 percent to sulfate, and 9 percent to phosphate.[615] On a 10-mmol calcium diet, normal humans excrete urine in which the total calcium concentration is 2.29 ± 0.27 m*M* (SE, $n = 34$), and the ionic calcium concentration is estimated to be 0.90 ± 0.09 m*M* (SE, $n = 34$).[295] Supersaturation of the urine with calcium oxalate or phosphate salts and the role of urinary inhibitors of crystal growth and nucleation in preventing calcium urolithiasis are discussed in several monographs.[141–143,545]

CALCIUM FLUXES

ACROSS EPITHELIA

Calcium exchange between nonlactating mammalian organisms and their environment occurs via the intestinal tract, the kidneys, and the sweat glands. When calcium losses in sweat are small,* urinary calcium excretion should closely approximate net calcium absorption from the intestinal tract of adults that are in external calcium balance. Both the intestinal tract and the nephrons are composed sequentially of several different types of specialized epithelia (Table 11-2), across each of which there may be calcium movement. As depicted in Fig. 11-2, these epithelia consist of a single cell layer. The luminal borders of the cells are contiguous and are joined together by tight junctions. The lateral intercellular spaces, which together with the apical tight junctions form the *paracellular pathway*, extend to the bases of the cells, which lie upon a porous basement membrane (not shown in the figure).

Calcium ion movement may proceed either between the cells via the paracellular pathway or through the cells via a pathway that involves Ca^{2+} interaction with both

* In the discussion that follows, the role of the sweat glands in calcium excretion has been neglected. In normal adults, the average excretion of calcium in sweat is 0.25 to 0.37 mmol/day.[154,438] These rates may increase significantly with high rates of perspiration.[610]

cellular metabolism. In most instances, active calcium transport occurs against a transepithelial electrochemical potential difference for Ca^{2+} movement and occurs in the absorptive (i.e., lumen-to-blood) direction.[53,342]

The first step in this process is the entry of calcium ions from the lumen into the cell across the luminal plasmalemma (Fig. 11-2). Because the luminal Ca^{2+} concentration greatly exceeds that in the cytosol and the interior of the epithelial cell is highly electronegative with respect to the lumen, a large electrochemical potential difference favors Ca^{2+} diffusion into the cell. However, because pure lipid bilayers have a very low ionic permeability, specific transport mechanisms must exist for Ca^{2+} to cross the apical plasmalemma.[271,353] At present, little is known about the molecular nature of these entry mechanisms, but the available information (which will be discussed subsequently) suggests that they differ, depending upon epithelial cell type.

Inside the cell, calcium ions must be translocated from the luminal to the basolateral plasmalemma, where they are extruded. One possibility is that they diffuse through the cytosol down a favorable, albeit small, concentration gradient. In segments of the intestine or the nephron where active transcellular calcium absorption occurs—the duodenum[70,624] and the distal convoluted and connecting tubules,[53,150,152] respectively—the cells contain a vitamin D-dependent, cytosolic, calcium-binding protein, calbindin-D.[12,70,342,497,573,622] Both experimental[203,204,206] and theoretical[321] evidence suggests that this protein, which was discovered by Wasserman and Taylor in the intestine of chicks,[625] facilitates Ca^{2+} diffusion through aqueous solutions. Accordingly, calbindin-D may play an important role in intracellular Ca^{2+} movement between the luminal cell membrane entry sites and the Ca^{2+} extrusion mechanisms located in the basolateral plasmalemma.

The final step in transcellular calcium absorption is the extrusion of calcium ions from the cell interior across the basolateral plasmalemma into the serosal interstitial space. Because this process occurs against a large electrochemical potential difference, it is active. Two possible mechanisms in intestinal[398] and renal[572,639] epithelial cells have been identified (Fig. 11-2). One is a high-affinity, Ca^{2+}-dependent, calmodulin-stimulated adenosine triphosphatase (Ca^{2+}-ATPase),[109–112,114–116,158,167,175,227,228,232,233] which couples the extrusion of one Ca^{2+} to the hydrolysis of one molecule of adenosine triphosphate. It is a single polypeptide with a M_r of about 135 kilodaltons and a K_m for Ca^{2+} of about 0.16 μM.[109,114–116,232] The K_m for Ca^{2+} is decreased, and the V_{max} of ATP hydrolysis is increased by a cAMP-dependent, protein kinase–mediated phosphorylation of this plasma membrane calcium pump.[298] In the small intestine of the rat, the Ca^{2+}-ATPase is vitamin D-dependent[227] and is regulated by calmodulin.[410] A second potentially important mechanism for active Ca^{2+} extrusion from the cell is a calcium-sodium antiporter.[114–116,232,233,330,398,460,600,640] This process obligatorily couples the efflux of one Ca^{2+} to the influx of three Na^+,[111,114,116] the latter driven by a favorable electrochemical potential difference established by the Na^+-K^+-dependent ATPase (Na^+-K^+ ATPase) located in the basolateral cell membranes. In heart sarcolemma this electrogenic exchange is activated by a calcium- and calmodulin-dependent protein kinase–mediated phosphorylation step and inactivated by a phosphatase-mediated dephosphorylation.[123] The energy for Ca^{2+} extrusion is derived from the Na^+ electrochemical potential difference, and therefore Ca^{2+} efflux by this mechanism is an example of secondary active transport.[13] The relative importance of these two active Ca^{2+} extrusion mechanisms in either intestinal or renal epithelial cells through which calcium transport occurs is at present unclear. The calculated electrochemical potential differences for calcium and sodium across the basolateral plasmalemma predict that the exchanger, when functioning with a stoichiometry of $3Na^+:1Ca^{2+}$, is inactive under steady-state physiologic conditions.[58,232] Accordingly, it would not effect net calcium transport. Alternatively, it has been suggested that the antiporter is a major calcium influx pathway in kidney cells.[547] Under such circumstances, calcium ions would cycle across the basolateral cell membrane: Ca^{2+} influx would be coupled to Na^+ extrusion, and Ca^{2+} efflux would occur via the Ca^{2+}-pumping ATPase. Such a process could play an important role in the regulation of cytosolic free Ca^{2+} concentration but would not participate directly in effecting net calcium transport. Finally, the Ca^{2+}-Na^+ exchanger could serve as a limited Ca^{2+} influx mechanism that would raise cytosolic Ca^{2+} concentration in response to an increase in cell Na^+, thereby coupling luminal entry and basolateral exit of Na^+.[232,572,639] In those epithelia across which calcium fluxes are primarily paracellular, these active Ca^{2+} extrusion mechanisms in concert probably serve to regulate intracellular Ca^{2+} concentrations at their low steady-state values.

The sites, mechanisms, and regulation of calcium transport across the intestine and the renal tubule are discussed later (see "Kidneys" and "Intestines").

ACROSS THE MEMBRANES OF INTRACELLULAR ORGANELLES

Cytosolic Ca^{2+} concentrations in nonexcitable cells are maintained in the steady state at values of about 0.1 μM despite the approximately $1-mM$ concentration of calcium ions in the extracellular fluids. As pointed out by Carafoli,[117] the continuous influx of calcium across the plasma membranes requires that calcium be extruded continuously from the cytoplasm by mechanisms that also reside in the plasma membranes, namely, the Ca^{2+}

ATPase and/or the Ca^{2+}-Na^+ antiporter. In their absence, the cells could not maintain their low steady-state cytosolic calcium concentrations and would accumulate calcium. However, except for the erythrocyte, which lacks intracellular organelles, it is unlikely that the plasma membrane Ca^{2+} pump-leak system alone either establishes the set-point concentration around which cytosolic Ca^{2+} concentration is controlled or is involved in the rapid regulation of transient changes in cytosolic Ca^{2+} concentrations. The latter are important in intracellular signaling and the regulation of epithelial cell functions.[117,119] One example is the PTH-stimulated, inositol 1,4,5-trisphosphate–mediated, spikelike rise in cytosolic Ca^{2+} concentration that increases gluconeogenesis and shortens apical microvilli in renal proximal tubular cells.[236,237,277,279] Other examples are the regulation of intestinal and renal tubular sodium transport.[170,172,272] In cells of excitable tissues, such as nerve synapses and cardiac muscle, rapid alterations in Ca^{2+} concentrations in the micromolar range are critical to normal function. In general, under normal circumstances, the rapid control of transient changes in cytosolic Ca^{2+} concentration is achieved by Ca^{2+} transport across the membranes of subcellular organelles, including the endoplasmic reticulum and, in muscle, the sarcoplasmic reticulum. Although their capacity to remove calcium from or to add calcium to the cytoplasm is finite, and therefore incapable of maintaining calcium homeostasis in the presence of long-term alterations in calcium transport across the plasma membranes, they are able to respond rapidly to acute changes in cytoplasmic Ca^{2+} concentration and to buffer the latter around a set point in the submicromolar range.[111,117]

Reticula

Under physiologic conditions, most cell calcium is stored in the endoplasmic reticulum,[134] and this organelle is responsible for the fine regulation of cytosolic Ca^{2+} concentration at its resting level.[111,114] Calcium is transported into both endoplasmic [114] and sarcoplasmic[291] reticula by a high-affinity Ca^{2+} ATPase (K_m for $Ca^{2+} < 0.5\ \mu M$).[114] Unlike the plasmalemmal enzyme, which transports one Ca^{2+} per hydrolyzed ATP, the Ca^{2+}-pumping ATPase of endoplasmic reticulum has a stoichiometry of $2Ca^{2+}$:1ATP.[114] Inositol-trisphosphate rapidly releases the calcium stores of the endoplasmic reticulum into the cytoplasm,[111,114,134] resulting in a transient spikelike increase in cytosolic Ca^{2+}. The latter is an important intracellular signal of the occupation of plasmalemmal receptors by extracellular peptide hormones, including PTH in proximal tubular cells.[236,237,279] The mechanism mediating Ca^{2+} efflux from the endoplasmic reticulum is not well understood but may involve calcium-induced release via a "channel."[114]

Mitochondria

Mitochondria previously were believed to be important in the regulation of cytosolic Ca^{2+} concentration.[369] However, as pointed out by Carafoli,[114] the low affinity of the Ca^{2+} uptake mechanism compared to known values of the cytosolic Ca^{2+} concentration and the low total calcium content of mitochondria in situ have led to the opposite conclusion.[163,245,256] Mitochondrial calcium transport has been studied extensively.[5,97,98,113,118,210,336,421,422] Calcium cycling across the mitochondrial inner membrane occurs as follows.* Electrogenic hydrogen ion extrusion from the mitochondrion to the cytoplasm, driven by the energy of electron transport through the respiratory chain (i.e., mitochondrial respiration), creates a large electrical potential difference across the inner mitochondrial membrane, the mitochondrial matrix (or inside) being negative with respect to the cytoplasm. This voltage drives Ca^{2+} into the mitochondrion electrophoretically via a Ca^{2+} uniport. Ca^{2+} movement from the inside of the mitochondrion to the cytoplasm occurs via a separate pathway that, depending on the cell type, includes either a Ca^{2+}-$2Na^+$ antiporter or a sodium- and ATP-independent calcium efflux mechanism (the mitochondrial inner membranes are devoid of Ca^{2+}-ATPase). A calcium-hydrogen antiporter has been proposed[210] for the latter but is not universally accepted.[5] Under normal conditions an important role of the calcium transport processes across the mitochondrial inner membrane is the regulation of matrix calcium.[163,245,256] By transmitting changes in cytosolic Ca^{2+} concentration into the mitochondrial matrix, this system regulates the activity of three Ca^{2+}-sensitive dehydrogenases that are important in intramitochondrial oxidative metabolism: pyruvate dehydrogenase, NAD^+-isocitrate dehydrogenase, and oxoglutarate dehydrogenase.[163,245,256] Accordingly, hormones that raise cytosolic Ca^{2+} concentrations while stimulating energy-requiring processes within cells stimulate the production of ATP.

A descriptive summary of Ca^{2+} transport mechanisms in plasma membranes and the membranes of subcellular organelles is shown in Fig. 11-3.

BONE

ORGANIZATION OF THE SKELETON

Approximately 80 percent of the skeleton is *compact* or *cortical bone* that forms the dense outer surface of all bones and is the major type of bone in the appendicular

* The mitochondrial outer membrane is believed to be freely permeable to calcium ions.[97] Therefore, it is assumed that the Ca^{2+} concentration in the space between the inner and outer membranes is equal to—and in diffusion equilibrium with—the cytoplasm.

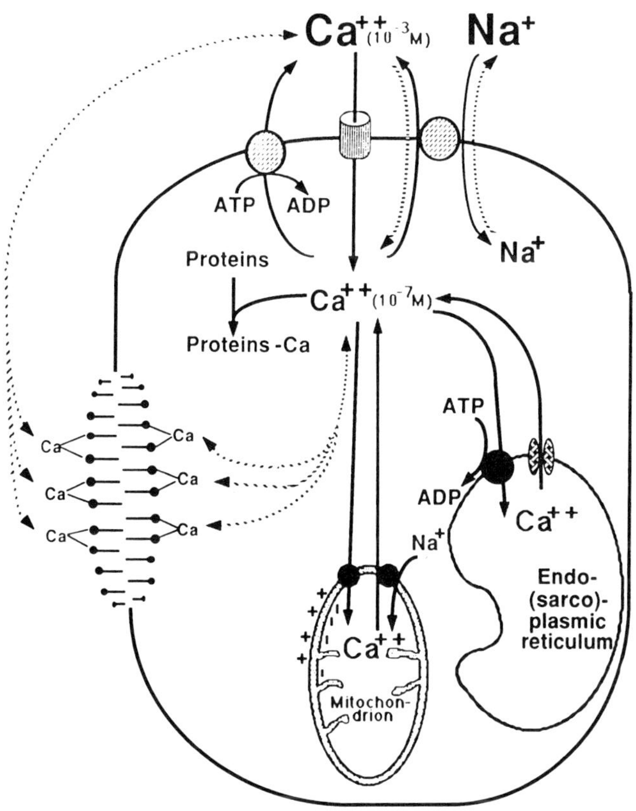

FIGURE 11-3 • Summary of the Ca^{2+}-transporting systems in eucaryotic cells. The figure shows seven transporting systems: three in the plasma membrane (a Ca^{2+}-ATPase, a Na^{+}-Ca^{2+} exchanger, and a Ca^{2+} channel), two in the endosarcoplasmic reticulum (a Ca^{2+}-ATPase and a release channel) and two in the inner membrane of mitochondria (an electrophoretic uptake uniporter and a Ca^{2+}-releasing Na^{+}-Ca^{2+} exchanger). The systems in the Golgi membranes and in the lysosomes have not been inserted in the figure because they are still insufficiently characterized. The soluble Ca^{2+}-binding proteins of the cytosol and the acidic phospholipids of the plasma membrane have been included in the figure as participants in the Ca^{2+}-buffering function. (From Carafoli E, *J Cardiovasc Pharmacol* 12:S77, 1988. Used by permission.)

skeleton. Its principal role is physical support. The overall structure of cortical bone is one of concentric lamellae of mineral penetrated by a fine network of cellular processes originating from osteocytes (Fig. 11-4). The other 20 percent of the skeleton is *trabecular* or *cancellous bone*, a complex network of interconnecting plates and bars found predominantly in the central core of bones in the axial skeleton (pelvis and spine) and flat bones and in the metaphyses of long bones (Fig. 11-4). The surface area–to–volume ratio in trabecular bone is much greater than that in cortical bone, and two-thirds of the total surface of the skeleton is trabecular.[444] All bone surfaces are covered by a layer of flat cells that separate bone from ECF and mediate the exchange of mineral between ECF and bone. The surfaces of cortical bone are also active; the endosteal, or inner, surface is usually more metabolically active than the periosteal, or outer, surface.

MINERAL AND ORGANIC COMPOSITION

Bone is a mineralized connective tissue, a framework of proteins with mineral crystals embedded in the protein, and a surface covered by cells. Hydrated bone is approximately 40 percent mineral, 30 percent organic material, and 30 percent water in cells, vascular spaces, and ground substance. The mineral in bone is mainly calcium, phosphate, and carbonate in a molar ratio of approximately 10:6:1. Most of the mineral is in the form of spindle-shaped crystals of *hydroxyapatite* with a unit cell content of $Ca_{10}(PO_4)_6(OH)_2$. During mineralization of bone, it is likely that mineral is initially deposited as amorphous *brushite* ($CaHPO_4 \cdot H_2O$) before organizing into hydroxyapatite crystals.[465] A small fraction of the apatite in bone has substitution of fluoride or chloride for OH. *Fluoride*-substituted apatite, fluorapatite, is less soluble than hydroxyapatite; in supersaturated solutions, fluoride induces a faster growth of crystals. Some hydroxyapatite on bone surfaces contains *carbonate* (CO_3) in the PO_4 position, disrupting the crystal and making it more soluble.[465] The carbonate in bone is mostly on surfaces and probably plays a role in buffering the pH of extracellular fluids.

Approximately 90 percent of the protein in bone is *type I collagen*, which is also the most abundant collagen in the body and is also found in skin, tendon, and most other connective tissues except cartilage. It is also the major secretory product of the osteoblast. The collagen molecule has a molecular weight of 300 kD and is composed of two identical α_1(I) chains and a structurally similar but genetically different α_1(I) chain. The chains are wound around each other in a tight triple-helix configuration. The primary amino acid sequence of collagen consists of a Gly-X-Y repeating triplet, where X is often proline and Y hydroxyproline. The triple-helix configuration gives the molecule its semirigid and stable structure. The three-dimensional fiber structure of collagen is made up of collagen molecules stacked and staggered side by side. Posttranslational cross-linking between collagen molecules strengthens this configuration.

Approximately 10 to 15 percent of the protein in bone consists of noncollagenous proteins (Table 11-3). Around 25 percent of these proteins are from ECFs and are trapped or adsorbed to bone. The noncollagenous proteins in bone can be divided into the following four general groups:

1. *Cell attachment proteins* provide sites and receptors for cell attachment. They include fibronectin, thrombospondin, osteopontin, and bone sialoprotein.
2. *Proteoglycans* contain a protein core and covalently attached side chains consisting of acidic polysaccharides or glycosaminoglycans (GAGs). The two main GAGs in bone are chondroitin sulfate and heparin sulfate, and they are found attached to two proteins, decorin and biglycan.[484] These pro-

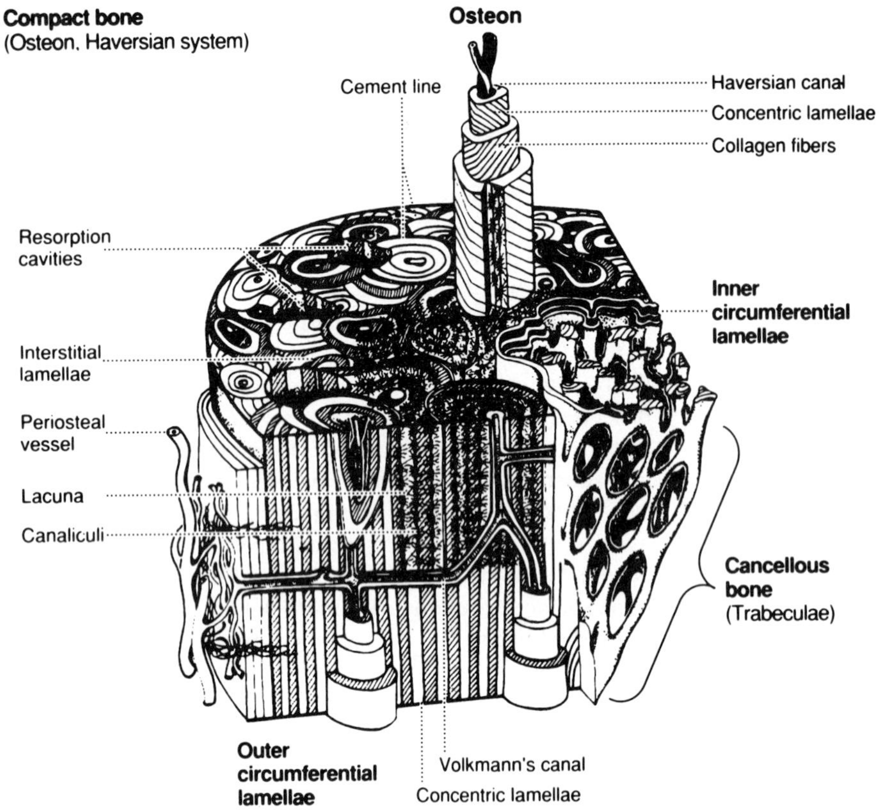

FIGURE 11-4 • Schematic view of a section of the proximal shaft of a long bone with cortical (left) and trabecular (right) bone. Cortical bone is made up of osteons (Haversion systems) and circumferential lamellae at the endosteal (inner) and periosteal (outer) surfaces. The osteons have a central Haversian canal surrounded by concentric lamellae with a common orientation of collagen fibers. A cement line marks the edge of the osteon. Osteocytes are embedded in the lacunae and interconnected by canaliculi. The osteons are connected by Volkmann's canals. Three resorption cavities are shown. (From Weiss L (ed): *Cell and Tissue Biology: A Textbook of Histology,* Baltimore, Urban and Schwarzenberg, 1989. Used by permission.)

TABLE 11-3 • Principal noncollagen bone matrix proteins

	Molecular mass $\times 10^{-3}$	Possible role in bone
OSTEOBLAST-DERIVED PROTEINS		
Thrombospondin	450	Cell attachment, spreading
Fibronectin	440	Cell attachment, spreading
Biglycan (proteoglycan I)	170	Unknown
Decorin (proteoglycan II)	120	Unknown
Bone sialoprotein	75	Cell attachment
Osteopontin	50	Cell attachment, spreading
Osteonectin	35	Ca^{2+} binding, hydroxyapatite binding
Matrix gla protein	9	Unknown
Osteocalcin	6	Ca^{2+} binding
Platelet-derived growth factor	30	Increase bone resorption, induce formation of new cartilage and bone
BONE MORPHOGENETIC PROTEINS		
Transforming growth factor-β	25	Increase bone formation, decrease bone resorption
PLASMA-DERIVED PROTEINS		
α_2HS-glycoprotein	50	Recruitment of osteoclast precursors

SOURCE: Modified from Termine JD, Bone matrix proteins and the mineralization process, in Favus MJ (ed): *Primer on the Metabolic Bone Diseases and Disorders of Mineral Metabolism*, Kelseyville, Calif, American Society for Bone and Mineral Research, 1990, p 17. Used by permission.

teoglycans are not unique to bone and are found in other connective tissues. Their role is currently a subject of speculation. Highly negatively charged proteoglycans containing chondroitin sulfate swell to a large volume with hydration and probably function as scaffolding for collagen assembly. The heparin sulfate proteoglycans are membrane-associated and may facilitate interaction of the osteoblast with extracellular matrix proteins.[27]

3. *Hydroxyapatite- and calcium-binding proteins* also occur in bone. Osteonectin, the most abundant noncollagen binding protein, is a phosphorylated glycoprotein that binds hydroxyapatite, calcium, collagen, and thrombospondin.[40,577] Binding of collagen and hydroxyapatite suggests that osteonectin plays a role in nucleation and organization of hydroxyapatite. Osteocalcin is a small calcium-binding protein that constitutes as much as 10 to 20 percent of the noncollagenous protein of bone.[209,484] It binds calcium by means of three negatively charged γ-carboxyglutamic acid (GLA) residues.[344] The γ-carboxylation of these residues is a vitamin K-dependent process, as it is for other GLA proteins, such as the clotting factors in blood. Osteocalcin binds to hydroxyapatite and is incorporated into the bone matrix, but some also leaks out into the circulation. Levels of osteocalcin in serum correlate with the rate of bone formation and turnover measured by quantitative bone histomorphometry. Osteocalcin levels are used as an index of osteoblast activity and bone turnover in patients with metabolic bone diseases.[86,125,131,176,186] The synthesis of osteocalcin by osteoblasts and its release into plasma is stimulated by $1\alpha,25\text{-(OH)}_2D$ and inhibited by glucocorticoids,[180,345,425,655] most likely by effects of these steroid hormones on transcription of the osteocalcin gene.[394] Matrix GLA protein (MGP) is another calcium-binding protein with GLA residues with partial structural homology to osteocalcin. It is found in cartilage and bone, and its function is not known.[484]
4. Several *growth factors* have been purified from mineralized bone matrix. These factors are manufactured by osteoblasts, although some may also be adsorbed from plasma. Large amounts of *transforming growth factor* β are found in bone and released by bone resorption. As described below, this protein inhibits osteoclasts and stimulates bone formation, and thus its release from matrix may modulate resorption and couple bone resorption and formation. The bone morphogenetic proteins are a family of proteins that induce endochondral bone formation when implanted into soft tissues and may have a role in fracture repair and embryonic bone development.[644] α_2HS-glycoprotein is derived from liver but is avidly concentrated in bone.[225] It is known to be a chemoattractant for monocytes and is speculated to have a role in recruiting osteoclast precursors.

Although tissues such as skin and tendon have a protein composition that is similar to that of bone, only bone becomes mineralized. Moreover, ECFs are supersaturated with respect to calcium and phosphate. Mineralization is not ubiquitous, because of the presence of crystal inhibitors such as pyrophosphate and calcium-binding proteins. Mineralization of the bone matrix deposited by osteoblasts does not occur for 3 to 10 days after it has been synthesized. The osteoblast regulates the deposition of mineral in matrix through its protein products and by reducing the concentration inhibitors of mineralization, such as pyrophosphatase with the enzyme *alkaline phosphatase*. A high-alkaline phosphatase activity on the cell surface appears to be critical for mineralization. Cell lines of osteosarcoma cells without alkaline phosphatase do not form mineral in culture, but after transfecting with a full-length cDNA of alkaline phosphatase, they do mineralize.[651] The expression of this enzyme by a cell is not the only requisite for bone mineralization, since alkaline phosphatase-producing cells, like hepatocytes, do not mineralize. It has been speculated that the noncollagenous bone matrix proteins are responsible for the mineralization of bone matrix; however, studies using immunohistochemistry and in situ hybridization have shown that these proteins are not unique to bone.[484] Mineral is deposited in bone matrix by a process regulated by cells and cell products in the microenvironment of bone-forming regions.

The mechanism of nucleation of bone mineral crystals and deposition in bone is unknown. In calcified cartilage and woven bone, mineralization is initiated by matrix vesicles containing mineral crystals.[10] The vesicles are small membrane-bound particles that arise from "pinched-off" regions of the plasma membrane. These vesicles are rich in alkaline phosphatase and have a lipid-rich inner membrane that becomes the nidus for hydroxyapatite crystal formation. The crystal grows until it destroys the vesicle. In mature bone matrix, vesicles have not been shown to initiate mineralization. Instead, it is likely that nucleation is mediated by some of the proteins decorating collagen, since collagen does not mineralize without these proteins.

MODELING AND REMODELING

Modeling is a term used for the process by which bone alters its shape through resorption and formation at different sites. For example, the shafts of most long bones continue to increase in diameter throughout adult life by a process of net resorption of bone at the endosteal surface and formation of bone at the periosteal surface.

Remodeling refers to the process in which resorption of a quantum of bone is followed by formation at the same site. The entire skeleton undergoes a slow but inexorable turnover by this process. Remodeling serves to repair skeletal microdamage and to release calcium into the circulation to satisfy homeostatic demands. The effects of systemic hormones and local factors such as mechanical stress on bone are mediated by way of remodeling. Normally, the close coordination between bone resorption and formation during remodeling preserves skeletal mass and structure. Trabecular bone, because of its large surface area, turns over most rapidly and is subject to the greatest changes with metabolic demands. In humans, approximately 5 percent of cortical bone is replaced per year, while 20 to 40 percent of trabecular bone is replaced.[445] An extreme example is seen in the egg-laying chicken. A typical egg may contain 2 g of calcium, equivalent to 10 percent of the skeletal calcium content; to turn over this large quantity of calcium, a uniquely vascular trabecular bone appears during periods of egg-laying under the stimulus of estrogen.[286]

Remodeling occurs in discreet units on bone surfaces at foci called bone remodeling units (BRUs), which lead to the formation of a unit structure of bone called a bone structural unit (BSU). BSUs can be seen in bone sections because they are separated by a highly mineralized, collagen-poor cement line marking the farthest extent of BRU bone resorption. In compact bone, the BSU is the secondary osteon, or *Haversian system*, a cylinder of about 200 to 250 μm in diameter that is usually parallel to the long axis of the bone (Fig. 11-5).[444] In trabecular bone the BSU is a flatter, bowl-shaped structure (Fig. 11-6). Resorption and formation occur sequentially or in a coupled manner, with osteoclasts excavating a cavity that is then filled in by osteoblasts (Fig. 11-6). Bone surfaces that are not undergoing remodeling are covered by a layer of lining cells that are probably of osteoblast lineage.

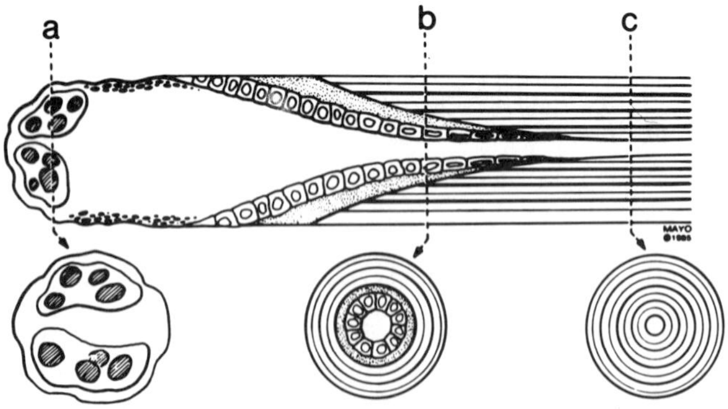

FIGURE 11-5 • A bone multicellular unit in cortical bone. The osteoclasts excavate a cone-shaped structure known as the "cutting cone." Osteoclastic resorption is followed by osteoblasts, which form new bone and refill the cavity. (From Eriksen EF et al: *Endocrinol Metab Clin North Am* 18:919, 1989. Used by permission.)

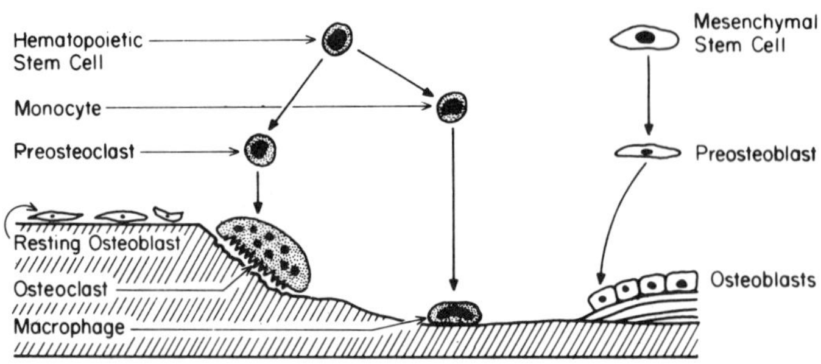

FIGURE 11-6 • Bone remodeling in a single bone remodeling unit (BRU). A quiescent surface at left is covered with flat lining cells of osteoblast lineage. Activation appears to involve an interaction of these resting osteoblasts and osteoclasts. The osteoclasts derive from a hematopoietic stem cell that may also be the precursor of the macrophage. During the reversal phase, macrophages migrate to the bone surface. After the reversal phase, osteoblasts fill in the resorption cavity with a layer of lamellar bone. The osteoblasts derive from mesenchymal stem cells in marrow. (From Raisz LG: *N Engl J Med* 318:818, 1988. Used by permission.)

The remodeling process begins with the recruitment of osteoclasts to a site on a surface of bone, perhaps by lining cells that are themselves responding to hormonal or mechanical stimuli, a process termed *activation* (Fig. 11-6). The recruiting message from lining cell to osteoclast is not known; one possibility is that lining cells retract to expose the naked surface of bone that is chemoattractive to osteoclasts. It is likely that the initial message for activation is received by osteoblastic cells, since activators of bone resorption such as PTH cannot activate osteoclasts directly (see below). Once in contact with bone, osteoclasts excavate a cavity referred to as a *Howship's lacuna*, of about 50 μm in depth in trabecular bone or 100 μm in depth in cortical bone over a period of one to three weeks.[444] Osteoclasts then disappear from the cavity and are replaced by mononuclear cells of uncertain origin that deposit a thin layer of cement substance. These cells are then followed by osteoblasts that fill the cavity with new bone over a period of three months. The duration of the cycle of bone formation in cortical and trabecular bone is around three to four months, but an additional three to six months is needed for the bone to become fully mature.[440] Some osteoblasts remain embedded in the new bone and become osteocytes. Osteocytes maintain contact with each other and with surface osteoblasts through the network of microcanals.

Osteoblasts synthesize bone by initially depositing a protein matrix that mineralizes after 5 to 10 days. The biochemical events that explain the lag in mineralization of osteoid are not known; the lag may be related to further cross-linking of collagen or removal of inhibitors of mineralization. As a result of this lag in mineralization, osteoblasts forming bone are seen in histologic sections overlying a thin layer of unmineralized matrix. The rate of mineralization can be measured with a technique known as *double tetracycline labeling*. Tetracycline accumulates on mineralizing surfaces, and the tetracycline can be seen in bone sections because of its fluorescence (Fig. 11-7). Typically, a pulse of tetracycline is given over 1 to 2 days, followed by a second pulse 14 days later. A bone biopsy is performed after the second pulse. The rate of bone mineralization can be calculated by dividing the mean distance between the two bands by the interdose duration. This technique allows direct assessment of the rate of osteoid formation and the rate of osteoid mineralization; it thus can define high or low turnover states and states of impaired mineralization (osteomalacia).

Estimates of the amount of bone turned over by the remodeling process account for far less calcium turnover than is predicted from total body analyses based on the kinetics of calcium isotopes. For example, 10 percent skeletal turnover predicts calcium turnover of 6 to 8 mmol/day. However, kinetic analyses using injected isotopes give estimates of 50 to 100 mmol/day.[131,370] This discrepancy suggests that the remodeling process contributes little to hour-to-hour calcium homeostasis; instead, remodeling may have more of a structural role and a role in the long-term regulation of mineral exchange with the skeleton. On a morphologic basis, the mineral homeostatic function has been attributed to all bone surfaces. Most of these surfaces are lined with so-called quiescent cells or with the fine processes from osteocytes that occupy a delicate network of canaliculi throughout cortical and trabecular bone.[445] The full network of microcanaliculi may increase the mineral surface by 3000 times. This network is intimately related to bone of all degrees of maturity such that in young adults no mineral is more than 5 mm from a canaliculus.

CELLS

Three morphologically distinct cell types have been identified in bone: *osteoclasts*, *osteoblasts*, and *osteocytes*. In addition, flat, surface-lining cells and marrow cells are believed to play important but less well-known roles.

Osteoclasts are specialized, usually multinucleated cells that resorb bone.[262,281,426] Osteoclasts attach to bone, forming a sealed space and a characteristic ruffled border consisting of projections of plasma membrane similar to the brush borders of intestinal and kidney cells. In this sealed space, the osteoclast creates an acidic environment (pH 4.5 to 5) that dissolves bone mineral and activates proteases secreted by the osteoclasts that degrade the matrix.[19,605] Protons are pumped into this

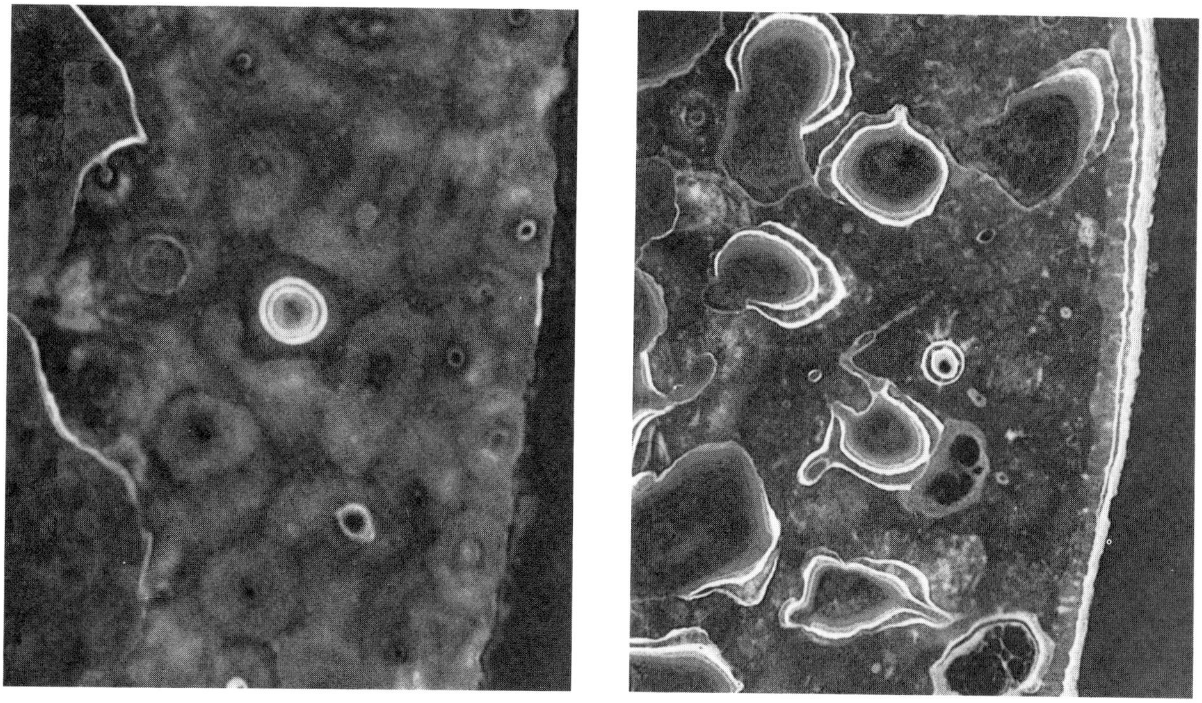

FIGURE 11-7 • Fluorescent micrographs of tetracycline-labeled section of rib from dogs treated (right) and untreated (left) with human parathyroid hormone. The tetracycline appears as bright fluorescence. The section from the untreated dog shows only one tetracycline-labeled osteon and one resorption cavity, whereas most of the surfaces exhibit formation in the treated dog. (From Inoue K, Takahashi H in Weiss L (ed): *Cell and Tissue Biology: A Textbook of Histology* Used by permission.)

space with a H^+-K^+-ATPase similar to that of kidney tubule acidifying cells. *Carbonic anhydrase*, the enzyme that catalyzes the conversion of CO_2 to carbonic acid, provides protons for this pump. The carbonic anhydrase is critical, since inhibitors of this enzyme inhibit bone resorption. Moreover, a rare autosomal recessive form of osteopetrosis (a disease characterized by dense bones as a result of impaired osteoclastic resportion) is associated with a deficiency of the carbonic anhydrase type II.[542] The osteoclast does not produce collagenase but instead degrades collagen and other bone matrix proteins with proteases such as cathepsin B. Urinary measurements of small peptides containing hydroxyproline residues, which result from the breakdown of collagen, are used clinically as an index of the rate of bone resorption.

Osteoclasts are formed by the fusion of mononuclear cells that are most likely derived from pluripotent hematopoietic stem cells.[516,605] The precursor of the osteoclast may be delivered to bone from the circulation; the evidence for this derives from studies with humans and animals with osteopetrosis. Mice with osteopetrosis can be cured by parabiosis with a normal litter mate or by infusion of spleen cells from normal litter mates.[515] Humans with osteopetrosis have been effectively treated by marrow cell transplantation.[140] The osteoclast does not derive from the macrophage itself, since its immunologic, histochemical, and functional properties are entirely different.[275] It is likely that these cells have a common precursor (but diverge at an early stage of differentiation), since in some forms of osteopetrosis both osteoclasts and macrophages have functional defects.[480] Multinucleated cells with features of osteoclasts—such as the capacity to form a ruffled border, to resorb bone, and to retract their cytoplasm in response to calcitonin—can be induced from cells in bone marrow.[352,564]

Osteoblasts are the cells that are responsible for synthesizing bone matrix. They also play a role in the mineralization process. The osteoblast has the typical appearance of a protein-synthesizing cell;[473] it is cuboidal and has a large Golgi apparatus and abundant endoplasmic reticula. Cytoplasmic processes from the osteoblast extend deep into the osteoid matrix and are also in contact with the osteocyte processes in their canaliculi. The osteoblast surface contains alkaline phosphatase. This enzyme might serve to hydrolyze organic phosphates and pyrophosphate, an inhibitor of calcium-phosphate crystal growth. This function is supported by the mineralization defect (rickets and osteomalacia) that occurs with hereditary deficiency of the enzyme (hypophosphatasia).[636]

After completion of a synthetic cycle, the osteoblast is thought to become either an *osteocyte* or a flat, surface-lining cell. While osteocyte function has been impossible to measure directly, it seems likely that this cell can modulate calcium flux in both directions between ECF and bone.

The osteoblast derives from a local marrow stem cell and may be a cousin of the fibroblast, with which it shares many synthetic functions, including collagen synthesis.[489] Bone matrix is made up of 90 percent type I collagen and a long list of other proteins that participate in the mineralization of matrix, since type I collagen in other tissues, such as skin, does not mineralize (see below). They may also have a role in the structure of bone, and some appear to modulate the activity of osteoclasts during bone resorption.[225,593] The bone remodeling cycle is initiated by osteoclasts and most humoral modulators of remodeling primarily affect resorption. However, the osteoblast is the cell that receives these signals and in turn modulates the activity of the osteoclast.[488] Activators of bone resorption, such as PTH, prostaglandins, and growth factors (interleukin I; platelet-derived, epidermal, and transforming growth factors) act through osteoblasts. Isolated osteoclasts require the presence of osteoblasts to respond to hormonal enhancement of bone resorption.

Mineralization of bone matrix requires a supersaturated solution of calcium and phosphate. A marked reduction in the concentrations of these ions is associated with impaired mineralization and accumulation of large amounts of unmineralized matrix (rickets or osteomalacia). Part of the process involves the hydrolysis of certain organic phosphate esters and pyrophosphate, which are inhibitors of mineralization by alkaline phosphatase on the surface of osteoblasts.[384] The initiator of mineralization is not collagen and may be one of the noncollagenous proteins in bone.

SIGNALS

Bone cells are regulated by a complex hierarchy of local and systemic factors. At one level, bone participates in the regulation of ECF calcium concentration and therefore responds to systemic hormones such as PTH and $1\alpha,25\text{-}(OH)_2D$. At another level, bone cells respond to physical deformation, which leads to changes in the shape of bone (modeling). During bone remodeling, resorption and formation are tightly coordinated or coupled by signals between bone cells.

Investigators in the past decade have found several local factors that modulate bone cell activity.[126,472] These factors include prostaglandins and a wide range of peptide growth factors synthesized by bone cells or adjacent marrow cells. These factors can have effects on the same cell that makes the factor (autocrine factors) or on other nearby cells (paracrine factors). The effects include replication and differentiation of bone cell precursors and modification of the activity of bone cells. To complicate matters further, some of the effects of systemic factors such as PTH on bone cells may be mediated by local factors produced in response to PTH. The list of potential paracrine and autocrine factors that modulate bone cells is long. However, since these are produced within the microenvironment of the bone cells, sorting out their contribution is a complex effort. Extrapolating the results of in vitro studies to explain in vivo physiologic or pathophysiologic phenomena is perilous, since differing culture conditions and varying hormone concentrations have led, on occasion, to contradictory findings. Although isolation of specialized bone cells has led to a better understanding of their phenotype, isolated cell cultures cannot provide information about the intricate cell-to-cell relationships that exist in bone in vivo. With the exciting new tools of histochemistry and in situ hybridization, however, further information should be forthcoming from bone sections.

Calcium-regulating hormones

Parathyroid hormone

Acute increases in the level of PTH stimulate bone resorption by osteocytes and osteoclasts and inhibit osteoblastic bone formation, thereby releasing calcium into the circulation. The response to increases in PTH occurs within minutes. Chronic and severe hyperparathyroidism is associated with enhanced bone turnover; in this circumstance, increased resorption is coupled with an increase in bone formation, but the net effect is progressive bone loss, particularly in regions of cortical bone. The increased bone formation with chronically high levels of PTH may be an indirect effect of the enhanced remodeling or a direct stimulatory effect of PTH on osteoblasts. Although one of the principal target cells of PTH is the osteoclast, this cell does not have receptors for PTH.[533] The action of PTH on osteoclasts is indirect and most likely mediated by factors released by PTH-stimulated osteoblasts. McSheedy and Chambers have shown that PTH does not increase bone resorption by isolated osteoclasts unless they are cocultured with osteoblasts.[383] It appears, therefore, that the stimulatory effect of PTH on differentiated osteoclasts is mediated by factors produced by osteoblastic cells. In addition, on stimulation, lining cells (quiescent osteoblasts) become smaller and flat, possibly providing access to bone surfaces that are normally covered with a layer of cells by osteoclasts. There is evidence that some of the effects of PTH are mediated by insulin-like growth factor I (IGF-I), transforming growth factor β (TGF-β), and possibly other local growth factors.[107,472] In contrast to the effect of PTH on differentiated osteoclasts, Takahashi has shown that PTH promotes the formation of multinucleated osteoclast-like cells in long-term human bone marrow cultures.[564]

Although the classical effect of PTH on bone is catabolic, intermittent injections of low doses of PTH can increase bone mass, particularly in trabecular bone. In 1970, Kalu and associates observed that injections of parathyroid extract increased the density of the femoral metaphysis in rats.[307] In dogs, Tam and coworkers found that intermittent injections of human $PTH_{1\text{-}34}$ at doses that did not cause hypercalcemia increased bone formation surfaces and bone appositional rate but had no effect on bone resorption.[568] In contrast, continuous infusion of the same doses caused less stimulation of bone formation and markedly increased resorption. This anabolic effect of intermittent PTH has been seen by exposing cultured rat calvariae transiently, rather than continuously, to PTH. The cultures that were transiently exposed to PTH (24 h, followed by 48 h without PTH) had markedly increased levels of IGF-I; incubation with antibodies to IGF-I blocked the anabolic effects of PTH.[107] These studies suggest that the anabolic effect of PTH on bone depends on intermittent stimulation of bone cells and may be mediated by IGF-I. The increase in trabecular bone induced by PTH in the animal models suggests that the response of bone cells to PTH is modulated not only by the concentration of PTH but also by the pattern of its daily concentration, or pulsatility.[266] PTH is known to be secreted in a pulsatile manner, and recently Silverberg and colleagues showed that the rise in PTH in response to hypocalcemia is less in women with osteoporosis than in age- and sex-matched controls.[537] Perhaps the lack of PTH pulsatility causes bone loss in the women with osteoporosis.

Vitamin D

The earliest recognized effect of vitamin D was in preventing rickets. In the absence of vitamin D, bone mineralization is impaired, and in children, vitamin D deficiency causes rickets, which is characterized by painful bone deformities and growth retardation. Vitamin D deficiency in adults also causes impaired mineralization and weak bones but does not produce deformities; this syndrome is known as *osteomalacia*. The effects of $1\alpha,25\text{-}(OH)_2D$ on bone development and mineralization appear to be a result of providing adequate levels of calcium and phosphorus for mineralization of bone as a result of the effects of $1\alpha,25\text{-}(OH)_2D$ on intestinal absorption, rather than a direct effect on bone cells. In the absence of $1\alpha,25\text{-}(OH)_2D$, circulating levels of calcium and phosphate are too low for adequate mineralization of bone. Underwood and DeLuca have shown that provision of normal levels of calcium and phosphate by intravenous infusion to rats that are vitamin D deficient leads to normal growth and mineralization.[602] Moreover, in a child with severe rickets lacking $1\alpha,25\text{-}(OH)_2D$ receptors (vitamin D-dependent rickets type II), infusion of calcium over a period of several months led to healing of rachitic lesions.[17]

Although these studies suggest that the effects of $1\alpha,25\text{-}(OH)_2D$ on bone growth and mineralization are entirely indirect, osteoblasts have $1\alpha,25\text{-}(OH)_2D$ receptors, and 1α,25-$(OH)_2$D directly influences the expression of several osteoblastic proteins. In cultured osteoblast-like cells[365,432,440] and in vivo,[655] 1α,25-$(OH)_2$D induces the synthesis of noncollagenous matrix proteins such as osteocalcin and also down-regulates the production of type I collagen by fetal rat calvariae.[500] In addition, 1α,25$(OH)_2$D increases epidermal growth factor receptors and transforming growth factor β-like activity in osteoblast-like cell lines.[457] These studies suggest that 1α,25-$(OH)_2$D directly modulates bone metabolism, but the physiologic relevance of these direct effects remains to be determined.

As part of its calcemic effect, 1α,25-$(OH)_2$D also enhances bone resorption. The increased bone resorption mediated by 1α,25-$(OH)_2$D is a result of an increase in the number and activity of osteoclasts.[481] However, osteoclasts apparently do not contain receptors for vitamin D. The increase in the number of osteoclasts may be a result of effects of 1α,25-$(OH)_2$D on osteoclast precursors to differentiate into mature osteoclasts.[492] In long-term cultures of human bone marrow, 1α,25-$(OH)_2$D markedly increases the number of multinucleated osteoclast-like cells.[564] Osteoclast stem cells, like several other hematopoietic cells, could have 1α,25-$(OH)_2$D receptors. Similarly to its effect on other cell lines, 1α,25-$(OH)_2$D may promote the maturation of these stem cells. In addition, 1α,25-$(OH)_2$D enhances osteoclast activity by stimulating osteoblasts to produce a soluble factor that influences osteoclasts to increase bone resorption.[382]

Calcitonin

The principal effect of an acute infusion of calcitonin (CT) on calcium metabolism is a prompt inhibition of bone resorption. The reduced flux of calcium from bone can mildly reduce the level of circulating calcium. The effect of CT on bone is a result of a rapid and direct inhibitory effect on bone resorption by osteoclasts and perhaps also by osteocytes. Isolated osteoclasts in vitro undergo dramatic reductions in migration and morphological changes when exposed to CT.[127,128] The ruffled border of the osteoclast decreases within minutes of exposure to CT, and the cell begins to withdraw from bone-resorbing surfaces. Receptors for CT have been shown on rat osteoclasts,[424] where CT appears to act by stimulating cAMP. CT receptors have not been found on osteoblasts. During chronic administration, CT causes a reduction in bone turnover rather than hypocalcemia; presumably the inhibitory effect on osteoclasts slows the activation of bone remodeling units and, in parallel, reduces bone formation. In addition, osteoclasts appear to "escape" from the action of CT within days of administration, so that the hypocalcemic action is markedly blunted. This phenomenon may be the result of down-regulation of CT receptors in bone.[571]

Sex steroids

Sex steroids have an important role in skeletal development and the maintenance of the integrity of bone. The rise in the level of sex steroids—androgens in men and estrogens in women—is associated with a large increase in bone mass and closure of the epiphyses. Loss of estrogens at the time of menopause or after removal of the ovaries leads to a transient acceleration of bone loss over a four- to seven-year period. During this period, histomorphometric analysis of bone shows that bone remodeling is markedly increased. Administration of estrogens prevents this bone loss[21,348] and reduces the rate of bone remodeling. The bone changes after menopause are mostly a result of the large drop in the circulating concentration of estradiol, the principal premenopausal estrogen. Menopause is also associated with a reduction in the concentration of testosterone,[611] which may also play a role in maintaining bone mass. Men do not undergo a major loss of sex steroids in middle age, but testosterone appears to have a similar role in maintaining their bone mass. When men fail to produce testosterone as a result of loss of testicular or pituitary function, they lose significant amounts of bone, particularly in the spine,[208,553] and their rate of bone remodeling transiently accelerates.[294]

Early attempts to demonstrate estrogen receptors in bone were negative, and the effects of estrogens were felt to be an indirect effect of estrogen on the levels of osteotropic hormones. Recent studies suggest that the levels of PTH, CT, and 1α,25-$(OH)_2$D do not significantly change after menopause compared to premenopausal levels.[195] Administration of estrogens to postmenopausal women increases both total and free 1α,25-$(OH)_2$D levels; however, this may be a pharmacologic effect.[131a] Moreover, estrogens may modulate the secretion and effects of PTH on bone. Estrogens partly block PTH stimulation of bone resorption. In postmenopausal women with primary hyperparathyroidism, estrogen administration commonly reduces the level of serum calcium.[363a]

It now appears that a major component of the effect of both estrogens and androgens on bone is a result of a direct action of these hormones on the osteoblast.[191] Recent studies have shown specific, high-affinity binding of estradiol and the presence of estrogen receptor mRNA in osteosarcoma cell lines with osteoblast-like features[317] and in osteoblast cells derived from human trabecular bone explants.[187] In addition, androgen receptors have been demonstrated in several osteoblast-like cell strains.[147] Moreover, estrogens appear to have direct anabolic actions on bone. 17β-estradiol stimulates the proliferation of cell lines with osteoblastic features[190] and rat calvarial cells[189] and also enhances transcription of α_1(I) procollagen mRNA in rat calvarial osteoblasts.[190] Testosterone also stimulates the proliferation of calvarial cells. The mechanism by which estrogens block the PTH stimulation of bone resorption is probably direct as well, since exposure to 17β-estradiol inhibits PTH stimulation of cAMP accumulation.[191] The most conclusive demonstration of a direct effect of estrogen on bone is an experiment by Takano-Yamamoto and Rodan in which they infused physiologic concentrations of 17β-estradiol locally and continuously into femoral trabecular bone of ovariectomized rats through a hole in the distal metaphysis. After 8 days, 17β-estradiol infusion markedly increased trabecular bone volume and reduced the number of osteoclasts and increased the number of osteoblasts.[565]

In addition to stimulating the expression of bone proteins, estrogens enhance the production of growth factors that may mediate the effect on the cell itself in an autocrine manner or on other cells, such as osteoclasts, that do not have receptors for estrogens. 17β-estradiol enhances the production of IGF-I from rat calvarial osteoblasts, and incubation of 17β-estradiol–exposed cells with antibodies to IGF-I blocks the stimulation of cell proliferation by 17β-estradiol.[190] 17β-estradiol also reduces the level of PGE_2 released from rat calvarial explants;[207] PGE_2 is a potent stimulator of bone resorption.

Local signals

In addition to systemic factors, bone cell activity is governed by a large number of factors (peptides and prostaglandins) produced or released in the vicinity of the target bone cells (Table 11-4). These local factors may modulate the effects of systemic hormones like PTH; PTH stimulates release of growth factors from osteoblasts that modulate the activity of osteoclasts and the osteoblasts themselves. Local factors also modulate the local coupling of bone formation and resorption and may mediate the response of bone to strain, injury, and inflammation. These factors derive from the bone cells themselves or from nearby marrow cells and function in an autocrine or paracrine fashion. In addition, factors that modulate bone cell activity are embedded in bone matrix and released with bone resorption or injury. The local factors, unlike systemic hormones, have little cell specificity; they are produced in many tissues and their activity is a function of highly localized concentration. Thus, the common endocrine paradigm of assessing the role of a hormone by systemic infusion is not valid in assessing the role of these factors. Instead, their activity must be surmised by localizing their production and by determining their effects on organ or cell cultures or in in vivo models in which expression has been altered. Understanding the physiologic and pathologic role of these factors remains one of the major challenges of bone biology.

TABLE 11-4 • Local regulators of bone remodeling

FACTORS SYNTHESIZED BY BONE CELLS
Insulin-like growth factor I (IGF-I)
Transforming growth factor-β (TGF-β)
$β_2$ microglobulin ($β_2$m)
Platelet-derived growth factor (PDGF)
Fibroblast growth factors (FGFs)
Prostaglandins
Bone morphogenetic proteins (BMPs)
FACTORS MADE BY CELLS IN THE VICINITY OF BONE
Tumor necrosis factor-α (TNF-α)
Fibroblast growth factors (FGFs)
Lymphotoxin
Interferon-γ (IFN-γ)
Platelet-derived growth factor (PDGF)
Interleukin 1 (IL-1)

Transforming growth factors

The transforming growth factors (TGFs) are a multifunctional family of peptide growth factors that can induce growth and neoplastic changes in normal cells. TGF-β is secreted by bone cells and present in large amounts in bone matrix.[106] Bone and platelets are the major sources of this factor, but most cells in the body have receptors for TGF-β. It is likely that TGF-β plays an important role in the coupling of bone formation and resorption. TGF-β causes proliferation of cells of osteoblastic lineage and enhances collagen production by cultured osteoblastic cells. It also inhibits osteoclastic bone resorption and differentiation of osteoclast precursors in long-term cultured human bone marrow.[133,459] Although synthesis of TGF-β is not known to be enhanced by hormones such as PTH that enhance bone resorption, enhanced bone resorption would release TGF-β from stores in bone matrix.[458] TGF-β fits the role of a factor that couples bone formation to bone resorption, since its release from bone during resorption would enhance the number and activity of osteoblasts in the vicinity of resorption and depress the activity of the osteoclasts. TGF-β plays an important role in wound healing. It is released from platelets and acts as a chemoattractant for wound fibroblasts and a stimulator of type I collagen synthesis. It probably also has a role in fracture healing, since it would be released by platelets and disrupted matrix. Injection of TGF-β into the periosteum of an uninjured rat bone stimulates the local accumulation of osteoblasts and chondrocytes that form a typical callus.[304]

Insulin-like growth factors

IGF-I (also called somatomedin C) and IGF-II are two similar growth-promoting peptides. IGF-I is made in several tissues, including bone, in response to growth hormone and functions as both a local autocrine-paracrine factor and a systemic hormone.[654] Circulating levels of IGF-I are derived from growth hormone-stimulated secretion from the liver. IGF-I is also secreted by osteoblasts, and both synthesis and secretion are stimulated by PTH, estradiol, and to a lesser extent growth hormone.[378] IGF-I enhances collagen and matrix synthesis by osteoblasts (to a lesser extent, IGF-II has the same effect) and enhances proliferation of osteoblastic cells.[106,379] It also stimulates the expression of osteoblastic proteins such as alkaline phosphatase and osteocalcin.[103] As discussed above, it appears likely that the anabolic effect of PTH on bone is mediated by IGF-I released from osteoblasts. It is likely that IGF-I has several roles in bone. It modulates the anabolic effects of hormones such as estrogens and PTH. In addition, it probably plays a role in growth hormone-stimulated bone growth.

Prostaglandins

The prostaglandins alter the activity of both bone osteoblasts and osteoclasts, but their net effect on any of these cells depends on the type and concentration of the prostaglandin and perhaps the stage of differentiation of the cell.[472] PGE_2 is produced in large amounts in bone and has been shown to stimulate bone resorption in vitro (but not in vivo), and at high concentrations it stimulates bone formation. When PGE_2 is infused into newborn humans to maintain the patency of the ductus arteriosus, it increases periosteal bone formation.[597] In rats, PGE_1 infusion causes an increase in new-woven trabecular bone and cortical endosteal bone formation.[300] The prostaglandins may also function as local modulators of bone remodeling. Their production in bone is stimulated by PTH and inhibited by glucocorticoids.[471] Prostaglandin production in bone is also stimulated by growth factors such as EGF and platelet-derived growth factor (PDGF), by mechanical stress, and by mediators of inflammation and injury such as IL-1.[472]

Platelet-derived growth factor

Although PDGF was originally named because of its presence in platelets, bone matrix and cultured osteosarcoma cells (as well as other nonosteoid tissues) are a rich source.[106] PDGF stimulates bone resorption and bone cell replication, suggesting that it has a role in bone remodeling. Its release from matrix and platelets also suggests that it has a role in fracture repair.

Bone morphogenetic proteins

Injection of demineralized bone matrix into soft tissues in rodents leads to a cascade of events, including cartilage formation and eventual formation of ectopic bone; this process mirrors the normal in vivo process of cartilage and bone formation.[603,604] The partially purified protein(s) in bone matrix leading to this process were called bone morphogenetic protein by Urist.[604] Four peptides from highly purified preparations of bone morphogenetic proteins (BMPs) from bovine bone have been sequenced and their human cDNAs cloned: BMP 1, BMP 2A, BMP 2B, and BMP 3.[619,644] These peptides are similar in sequence to the TGF-β family of growth and differentiation factors. Each induces cartilage formation.[619,644] In a recent study, subcutaneous implantation of BMP 2A in rats led to a local sequence of development including cartilage growth; mineralization of cartilage; osteoblast induction and growth of vessels into the developing ectopic bone; and development of marrow precursors, then marrow, and finally mature bone.[620] TGF-β does not stimulate cartilage formation.[644] The similarity of this progression to the repair of fractures and to embryonic long bone development suggests that BMPs have a role in these processes. Using in situ hybridization, BMP 2A mRNA has been shown to be expressed in developing limbs and tooth buds as well as in nonskeletal tissues like heart and hair follicle, indicating a role for BMPs in morphogenesis.[351]

β_2-microglobulin

β_2 microglobulin (β_2M) is a protein present on the surface of most cells and enhances the stimulatory effect of IGF-I, perhaps by modulating its binding to receptors.[104,106] β_2M is also found embedded in bone matrix.

Fibroblast growth factors

Acidic and basic fibroblast growth factors (FGFs) are made by a variety of tissues, where they participate in angiogenesis. In addition, both α-FGF and β-FGF stimulate bone cell replication but do not directly affect bone resorption or bone matrix synthesis.[105,106] These factors are released by cell injury or death and therefore may contribute to bone repair.

Several cytokines affect bone cells and generally stimulate bone resorption. These include interleukin-1 (IL-1), tumor necrosis factor-α (TNF-α), and lymphotoxin (TNF-β). An exception among these immune response products is interferon-γ, which inhibits bone resorption. IL-1 is a monocyte product that stimulates T lymphocytes. In bone, it stimulates bone resorption and has biphasic effects on collagen synthesis; at low doses it increases synthesis, and at high doses synthesis is inhibited.[102] It is probably the major component of the bone resorption–stimulating activity present in stimulated peripheral leukocytes and previously was known as osteoclast-activating factor.[168] It also may be the mediator of the bone resorption and hypercalcemia in some hematologic malignancies with bone invasion and rheumatoid arthritis. Lymphotoxin and TNF-α are released by activated T lymphocytes and activated macrophages, respectively. They both stimulate the proliferation of osteoclast progenitors and stimulate bone resorption.[582] They also cause hypercalcemia when injected in vivo and may play a role in the local bone resorption and hypercalcemia associated with multiple myeloma and leukocyte malignancies.[224,472] An increase of osteoclast-like cells has been observed in marrow cultures after treatment with granulocyte and macrophage colony-stimulating factor.

Physical stress

Within a range of genetically determined shape, a bone can adapt its architecture in response to mechanical stresses. This notion dates back to 1892, when the German anatomist Julian Wolff stated that "every change in the function of bone is followed by certain changes in internal architecture and external conformation in accordance with mathematical laws."[641] Bone size and thickness reflect the size and weight of an individual as well as the history of stresses on that bone. In general, larger and more muscular individuals who are physically active have wider and more dense bones than individuals who are physically inactive. One illustration of these phenomena is the finding that professional tennis players have a cortical thickness of the humerus in their tennis playing arm that is 20 to 30 percent greater than that in the nonplaying arm,[303] while in nonathletes there is little or no discrepancy between the two arms. On the other hand, immobilization and loss of gravity are known to lead to brisk bone loss.

An interesting insight into the nature of the mechanical stimulus comes from experiments performed with disarticulated ulnae of roosters subjected to mechanical stress.[501] In the absence of any mechanical load, the limbs lost 15 to 20 percent of their bone mass over an eight-week period. When the ulnae were subjected to only four precisely measured daily deformations (of a magnitude similar to wing flapping), bone loss was prevented.[501] The amount of bone mass stimulated by these stresses was most dependent on the amount of strain or deformation of the bone.[326,451,501] Thus, it appears that bone deformation itself is an osteogenic stimulus. The critical question is how this deformation of the extracellular calcified matrix by mechanical stress is translated into a stimulus for bone cells.

The mechanism by which the mechanical deformation of bone is transduced into a signal for bone cells is not known. One proposal is that tissue strains cause interstitial fluid flow and that these strain-induced flows generate electrical signals.[302,461] These electrical signals, known as zeta or streaming potentials, may be messengers for bone cells.

NATURAL HISTORY OF BONE MASS

Skeletal mineralization occurs rapidly during the third trimester of fetal gestation. The fetal skeletal calcium content is 28 g; thus, approximately 320 mg of calcium per day is accumulated over 90 days. Over the next 20 years, another 700 to 1000 g of calcium is accumulated; accumulation rates vary from a low of 60 to 80 mg/day between ages 3 and 6 years up to 400 mg/day during the peak of adolescent growth.

Cortical bone thickness reaches a maximum in the third and perhaps early part of the fourth decade of life, although modeling at the periosteal (outer) surface and endosteal (inner) surface continues throughout life.[222,444] With age, endosteal resorption outstrips periosteal apposition, and therefore the shafts of most long bones in the elderly are wider but have a thinner cortex.[222] At the mid-femur, one radiographic study showed that the diameter increased by approximately 20 percent between the ages of 45 and 49 years and after age 75.[546] A more centripetal distribution of bone mass provides more resistance to bending, which is the mechanism of fracture of the shafts of most long bones. Lifetime skeletal losses (estimated in population-based surveys by neutron activation analysis) range from 30 percent in women to 20 percent in men. Women lose 3.8 g of calcium per year (10 mg/day) between the ages of 30 and 54 and 7.6 g/year (21 mg/day) after age 55 years.[144,145] Men lose a constant 2.6 g/year (7 mg/day). Elderly men have a greater bone mass than elderly women because they achieve a higher peak bone mass and lose bone more gradually, in large part because levels of sex hormones do not drop as drastically as in women.

Lifetime trabecular bone losses are greater than cortical bone loss; women lose approximately 50 percent of vertebral trabecular bone[108] compared to a 40 percent loss of cortical bone in the mid-forearm[377] and a 30 percent loss in the second metacarpal.[222] Vertebral trabecular bone loss accelerates in the perimenopausal period for 5 to 10 years after menopause. After the abrupt loss of hormones with oophorectomy, bone mass in the trabecular region of vertebral bodies fell by 9 percent per year,[226] more than double the rate of change after natural menopause.[192] Loss of bone in the midshaft of the radius was only 2 percent.

It should be noted that, with few exceptions, estimates of bone loss are based on cross-sectional data that are influenced by secular trends. For example, the improved nutrition and increased height in the population of the United States over the past several decades may have increased bone mass in young adults (since bone mass is proportional to body size); this would exaggerate estimates of bone loss in cross-sectional studies.

Determinants of bone mass

Individuals at age 65 years may have a low bone mass because they have been briskly losing bone or because they acquired a low peak bone mass. Peak skeletal mass is 25 to 30 percent higher in males than in females and about 10 percent higher in African-Americans than in whites.[144,145] Even within demographic groups the variance of peak bone mass is large; one standard deviation is as much as 15 percent of the average peak bone mass.[444] The lower 2.5 percent of the population would have a bone mass 30 percent below the mean, the same as the bone mass of an elderly person. Thus, the variance in peak bone mass accounts for much of the variance of bone mass in later age. Factors that could affect the variance of peak bone mass or involutional bone loss are described below.

Genetic factors

Evidence from several types of studies suggests that a large component of bone mass, particularly peak bone mass, is genetically determined. One example of genetic influence is the difference in bone mass between Caucasians and Africans or African-Americans (see below). Studies have found strong evidence for genetic transmission of bone mass by showing a greater degree of resemblance of bone mass between monozygotic than between dizygotic twins.[165,390,543] These studies assume that environmental factors influencing bone mass affect both types of twins equally, but since monozygotic twins are genetically identical, their intrapair differences arise only from environmental factors. The hereditary effects were large; most of the variance in bone mass was accounted for by hereditary influences. In addition, Seeman and coworkers recently showed that daughters of women with osteoporosis had a lower bone mass at all sites (corrected for height, weight, and age) than daughters of nonosteoporotic women.[520] The strength of this familial influence was as great as that for height. Taken together, these studies suggest that a large component of the variance in bone mass in the population is genetic.

Ethnic group

African-Americans of both sexes have more bone mass than whites.[462] These racial differences were first quantitated in the 1950s by showing that dry defatted skeletons of African-American males were 7 percent more dense than those of white males and bones of African-Americans females were 13 percent more dense than their white counterparts.[65,594] Racial differences in bone mass are apparent even in infancy. These differences are due in part to the fact that in early childhood and throughout adult life African-Americans are larger and have a greater lean body mass.[220,435] Even after adjusting for height, weight, and lean body weight, African-American women and men have a greater total body calcium and bone mass in the spine, radius, and hip.[145,166]

Calcium intake

Clearly, some level of calcium intake is critical to achieve and maintain a proper bone mass, but the level of intake needed is a subject of controversy. A typical woman must absorb an average of 110 mg more calcium per day than she loses in stool, sweat, or urine (two to three times this amount is needed during the adolescent growth spurt) to accumulate a normal peak bone mass. The calcium intake required for children and adolescents to achieve positive balance is not known. Young adult women in some studies are in negative calcium balance when their intakes are below 800 to 1000 mg/day.[261] This is an alarming value, since the mean calcium intake of young adults is approximately 600 mg/day. In part as a result of these studies, the National Research Council has set the recommended daily allowance (RDA) at 1200 mg/day for people between the ages of 10 and 18 years of age.[154]

A population study of bone mineral density in two rural districts of Yugoslavia with an almost twofold difference in calcium intake (500 versus 1100 mg/day) found that the major difference between the two districts was in peak bone mass rather than rate of bone loss after maturity.[373] Studies in the United States have shown a small but significant relationship between dietary calcium and forearm bone mass.[36,308,549] Although these studies suggest that calcium intake has a small influence on peak bone mass, the effect of calcium may be underestimated because of the inaccuracy of the methods used to assess past dietary history. On the other hand, calcium intake within the range of normal human consumption may not be critical. It is likely that adaptive mechanisms maintain skeletal homeostasis over a wide range of calcium intakes. Stores of calcium in bone are not tapped to maintain homostasis in this range. At the upper end of intake, there is no evidence that a high calcium intake pushes calcium into bone. On the lower end of intake there is a "threshold" below which calcium absorption cannot keep up with insensible losses of calcium and intake becomes rate limiting for skeletal mass.[260] The level of this threshold depends on the capacity to absorb calcium efficiently and reduce urinary calcium losses, which varies with age (see below) as well as ethnic and genetic makeup. An example of adaptation to a low calcium intake is the Bantu population in South Africa, who consume approximately 200 to 400 mg/day of calcium and yet have an incidence of hip fractures that is much lower than that of their white South African neighbors, who consume more calcium.[548] African-Americans also may be particularly well adapted to a low calcium intake. There may be a hormonal explanation for this adaptation. African-Americans have higher PTH levels[24] and lower bone turnover than whites, suggesting that their skeletons are less sensitive to PTH.[631] The higher levels of PTH enhance calcium absorption by increasing $1\alpha,25\text{-}(OH)_2D$ levels (which increases the efficiency of calcium absorption) and lowering urinary calcium losses. This skeletal resistance to PTH could explain how a population preserves its bone mass in the presence of a low dietary calcium.

In summary, calcium plays a permissive role in determining bone mass; above a certain level of calcium intake, bone mass is not influenced by calcium.[260] Below a critical level or threshold, the supply of calcium is rate limiting. This is similar to the role of nutrients such as essential amino acids. Low intake of essential amino acids leads to a negative protein balance, with depletion of protein from tissues such as muscle. However, high intake of amino acids is not anabolic itself but allows protein accumulation in response to stimuli such as exercise.

With advancing age the efficiency of calcium absorption in the intestine falls,[221,292] in part as a result of an age-related decline in circulating $1\alpha, 25\text{-}(OH)_2D$, a critical modulator of intestinal calcium absorption.[220,221,541,595] Two age-related changes in vitamin D metabolism contribute to the low levels of $1\alpha,25\text{-}(OH)_2D$: older individuals synthesize less $1\alpha,25\text{-}(OH)_2D$, even after PTH infusions,[541] and there is a decline in the body stores of vitamin D. In a recent survey, healthy elderly women living in the sunny American Southwest had levels of 25-hydroxyvitamin D 25-(OH)D, the precursor of $1\alpha,25\text{-}(OH)_2D$, that were half those of young adults living in the same area.[433] Levels of 25-(OH)D are even lower in institutionalized or home-bound elderly persons. The mechanism appears to be an age-related decline in the capacity of skin to manufacture vitamin D under the influence of ultraviolet light.[354] The net result is that the elderly need more calcium to remain in balance; they have a higher threshold.

Anthropomorphic dimensions and muscle mass

The known tendency of small persons with a thin habitus to have bones that are smaller and less dense than large individuals[144,182,222,540] fits with anthropologic data showing that the cross-sectional area of long bones is proportional to the square of its length.[504] This relationship is not surprising, since a longer bone needs a wider shaft to resist bending. In a study of 86 normal women between the ages of 20 and 35 years, the relationship between height and bone mineral content of the radius was highly significant ($r = 0.6$, $p < .01$), indicating that height accounts for 35 percent of the variance in bone mass.[549] Independently of height, body weight appears to influence weight-bearing bones such as the spine and femoral neck, but not the radius.[346]

Physical activity

At one extreme, paralysis, weightlessness, and immobilization cause profound bone loss. For example, within weeks of immobilizing a fractured arm in a cast, there is a 20 to 25 percent loss of density,[635] and after three months the tibia loses almost 50 percent of its mass.[598] In several studies, individuals who are physically active have been shown to have a greater bone mass than sedentary individuals, although the difference between the most active individuals and the least active individuals is usually less than 10 percent,[308,323,364] a modest effect compared to the influence of immobilization. This suggests that the response of bones to physical activity is near maximal at a level of loading that is within the range of our sedentary population. Thus, increasing the activity level of a sedentary person causes a small increase in bone mass, but the response to pathologic decreases in activity or stress—for example, bedrest or immobilization—is a profound reduction in bone mass. Perhaps it should not be a surprise that bone does not atrophy or hypertrophy to a major extent in response to the changes in activity that humans are likely to be engaged in.

The role of physical inactivity in age-related bone loss is supported (circumstantially) by the studies showing that bone and lean body mass atrophy in parallel with age. In cross-sectional studies, physical activity measured by questionnaire has been shown to correlate with bone mass.[323,556] In one intriguing study, the grip strength of postmenopausal women over a three-year period predicted the increase in cross-sectional area of the radius rather than the change in density.[510] Thus, it is possible that the periosteal expansion of long bones described above is the parameter that is influenced by physical stress.

Sex hormones

Sex hormones have a critical role in the development and maintenance of bone mass in both sexes. Puberty is associated with a large increase in bone mass in males and females; individuals with impaired sex hormone production at puberty end up with a subnormal peak bone mass. In addition, the higher levels of androgens in men could account for their greater bone mass. It is likely that some of the variance in bone mass in women is a result of differences in sex hormone levels. In one study of young women, estradiol levels and androgen levels (androstenedione or testosterone) each independently accounted for a small though significant portion of the variance in vertebral trabecular bone density.[87] High levels of androgens are bone anabolic in women, since women with hirsutism and abnormally high serum testosterone levels have been shown to have a higher spine bone mass than nonhirsute women.[88] From these data it appears that in the vast majority of women differences in sex steriods explain only a small component of bone mass. Only in the unusual cases of hyperandrogenism or ovarian deficiency do they appear to affect bone mass.

The effect of estrogen deficiency on bone mass is most dramatic after oophorectomy when bone loss transiently accelerates over a four- to six-year period.[347] The greatest amount of bone loss occurs in trabecular bone in the axial skeleton, where as much as 9 percent per year is lost, versus 2 percent in the mid-shaft of the radius.[226] The hormonal changes of natural menopause are less abrupt, and, not surprisingly, the rate of bone loss is more gradual than after oophorectomy.[195,283] Bone loss is spread out over more years after natural menopause, since estrogen levels begin to fall before cessation of menses, and longitudinal studies indicate that bone loss accelerates even before menopause (cessation of menses) begins.[483]

In summary, loss of estrogens accounts for a transient but large component of age-related bone loss. The mechanism appears to be a direct effect of estrogens on bone. It is not clear why bone loss resulting from estrogen withdrawal decelerates. Sex hormone levels also decline in men, although the reduction is relatively less and not as abrupt as in women. Hypogonadism in men is associated with large losses of bone. At present the role of senescent decline in testosterone levels in involutional bone loss in men is not known.

Bone loss and changes in bone cells

Bone loss implies an imbalance between the amount of bone formed and the amount resorbed in each BRU as a result of an increase in bone resorbed by osteoclasts, a decrease in bone synthesized by osteoblasts, or both. The *rate* of bone loss is a function of the discrepancy between the activity of the osteoclasts and the osteoblasts in each BRU (each unit's deficit) and the rate of remodeling, or the number of units (Fig. 11-6).

Is involutional bone loss caused by a change in the activity in bone of these cell types? With age there is a decline in the mean wall thickness of old remodeling units or trabecular packets.[349] This parameter measures the amount of bone formed during the entire osteoblastic phase of bone remodeling. Since mineral and osteoid appositional rates measured with tetracycline labeling are normal, this implies that the active life span of osteoblasts is reduced; that is, the rate of matrix synthesis is normal over a shorter time span. The cause of this change in osteoblast function is not known. It may be a general phenomenon associated with aging since other cells, such as fibroblasts, also have a reduced activity with age. The defect in bone formation is not evident in early postmenopausal women, where bone turnover and osteoclastic activity are increased. The evidence for increased osteoclastic activity comes from the finding that the depth of resorption cavities is increased.[444] Thus, bone loss is accelerated because more bone is resorbed than formed in each remodeling unit and because the increased activation of remodeling units magnifies the impact of this deficit on bone mass.

KIDNEYS

OVERVIEW

In mammals, urinary calcium excretion is the difference between its glomerular filtration and net tubular reabsorption. Net tubular secretion of calcium has never been demonstrated in vivo.[562] Normal adults consuming a typical North American diet (600 to 1200 mg of calcium per day)[339] filter approximately 270 mmol (10,800 mg) daily:

$$\underset{\text{Glomerular filtration rate}}{180 \text{ liter/day}} \times \underset{\text{Plasma total [calcium]}}{2.5 \text{ mmol/liter}} \times \underset{\text{Ultrafilterable fraction of plasma calcium}}{0.6} = 270 \text{ mmol}$$

In this setting, urinary calcium excretion typically ranges from 1.25 to 7.5 mmol/day (50 to 300 mg/day).[337,339] Therefore, the renal tubules normally reabsorb between 97 and 99.5 percent of the filtered calcium. In humans urinary calcium excretion varies directly with dietary intake, but large changes in dietary calcium are associated with only modest changes in urinary excretion (Fig. 11-8).[184,337,339] Additional dietary factors influence normal urinary calcium excretion: *sodium chloride* or *protein* ingestion promote hypercalciuria, whereas increased

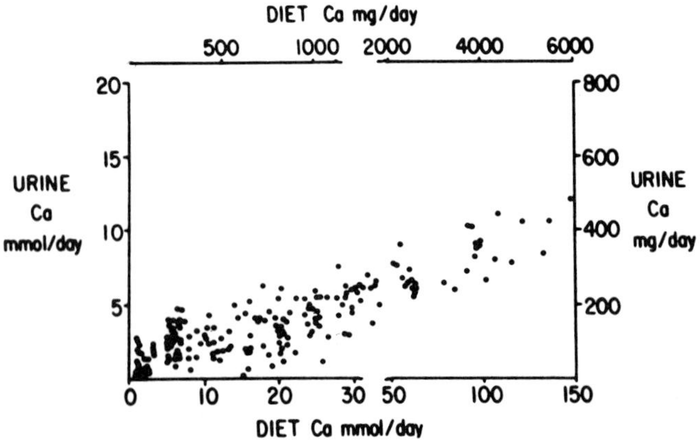

FIGURE 11-8 • Urinary calcium excretion as a function of dietary calcium intake in healthy adults. (From Lemann J Jr et al: *N Engl J Med* 301:535, 1979. Used by permission.)

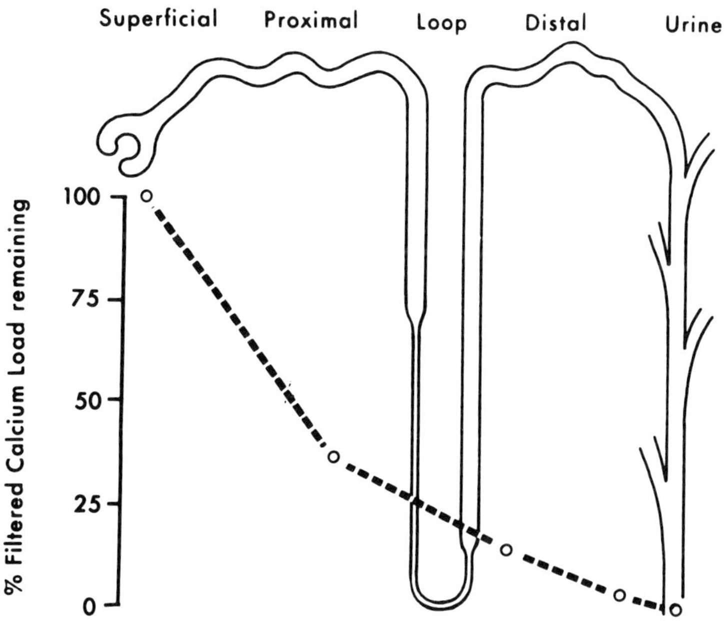

FIGURE 11-9 • Profile of calcium reabsorption along the nephron derived from micropuncture data obtained from superficial proximal and distal tubules in the rat and the dog. (From Sutton RAL, Dirks JH in Brenner BM, Rector FC (eds): *The Kidney,* 2d ed, Philadelphia, Saunders, 1981, p 551. Used by permission.)

dietary *phosphate* causes hypocalciuria.[184,337,339] Consumption of a diet that causes fixed *acid production* and thus renal net acid excretion causes hypercalciuria, reflecting increased bone resorption.[338]

Physiologically, *PTH,* which increases renal tubular calcium reabsorption, is the most important hormone regulating urinary calcium excretion.[3,53,314,498,560] Although potentially important in the chronic regulation of urinary calcium excretion, the role of *calcitriol* remains uncertain.[53,139,258,259,648] Pharmacologically, several diuretics cause hypercalciuria—the most prominent being *furosemide*—whereas others, including the *thiazides* and *amiloride,* cause hypocalciuria.[4,53,314,498,560]

The general sites of calcium reabsorption along the nephron are shown in Fig. 11-9. Of the calcium filtered at the renal corpuscles, approximately 65 percent is reabsorbed in the proximal tubule, 20 percent in the loop of Henle, and the majority of the remainder in the distal tubule.[558] Five percent or less is reabsorbed by the collecting ducts.*

In the mammalian nephron, there are at least 12 discrete tubular segments beyond the renal corpuscle (Table 11-2).[92,305] The mechanisms and the regulation of calcium transport in each of these segments differ.[53] In addition, the "nephron segments are arranged in series so that the function of each depends in part on changes in the tubule fluid composition caused by transport that occurred earlier."[92]

* This description ignores possible differences in the reabsorption of calcium between superficial and juxtamedullary nephrons, an issue that remains to be investigated.

Renal corpuscle

Calcium is filtered at the glomerulus by solvent drag during the ultrafiltration of blood plasma in the renal corpuscle. Under normal circumstances the movement of Ca^{2+} and low molecular-weight calcium complexes from the glomerular capillary lumen into Bowman's space is not restrained by the filtration membrane, the concentrations of calcium in the glomerular filtrate and ultrafiltrates of plasma being equal.[562] Protein-bound calcium is not filtered. In hypercalcemia, both the GFR and the ultrafilterable fraction of plasma calcium are reduced.[562]

Proximal tubule

The proximal tubules of superficial or juxtamedullary nephrons consist of at least three different segments (Table 11-2). Each has a distinct structure and function.[296,514] Therefore, although the different segments may have common mechanisms of calcium transport, it also is possible that differences exist.

Net fluid reabsorption occurs in each proximal tubule segment under normal circumstances, driven by osmotic forces that ultimately are generated by or linked to active sodium transport.[30,92,296,513,514] Where measured, the epithelial hydraulic conductivity is high,[30,513] and a significant fraction of osmotically driven fluid reabsorption may occur via the paracellular pathway.[30,239] If the *reflection coefficient* for calcium (σ_{Ca}) at the apical tight junctions is less than unity, it is theoretically possible that a portion of calcium reabsorption in proximal tubule segments occurs by *solvent drag* via the paracellular pathway. Supporting this hypothesis, a micropuncture study showed that artificially induced changes in net volume flux can affect calcium transport in the rat proximal convoluted tubule in vivo.[42] Under normal conditions the absorption of fluid was related directly to that of calcium. Reduction or reversal of the volume flux by addition of mannitol to the perfusate reduced or reversed the calcium flux, respectively.[42] The σ_{Ca} was estimated to be 0.28.[42] In contrast, in the rabbit proximal convoluted tubule studied in vitro, σ_{Ca} was estimated to be only 0.89, a value that would preclude significant absorption by solvent drag.[419] In summary, a portion of calcium absorption by the proximal tubules may occur by solvent drag, but the importance of this mechanism compared to diffusional or active transport is unknown.

The total calcium concentration in proximal tubular luminal fluid may exceed the ultrafilterable plasma calcium concentration by 20 percent but does not vary with axial length, at least through the mid-portion of segment 2.[562] The causes of the increased luminal fluid calcium concentration and the question of whether the difference in total calcium concentrations between luminal fluid and an ultrafiltrate of plasma reflects a difference in Ca^{2+} concentrations are not certain.[53, 562] Possibilities for the former include molecular sieving of calcium at the apical tight junctions, secretory calcium diffusion occurring via the paracellular pathway (driven by the lumen-negative voltage in segment 1), and the formation of nonabsorbable calcium complexes in the tubule lumen.[53,562] The permeability of the paracellular pathway to calcium is high in segment 1,[43,600] so that a favorable electrochemical potential difference (lumen > peritubular space) would result in net calcium efflux by diffusion.[43,600] Since the voltage is lumen-negative, however, this would have to be the result of a higher luminal than peritubular fluid Ca^{2+} concentration.

Changes in the composition of the glomerular filtrate between the renal corpuscle and the cortical segment-2 proximal tubules establish a lumen-positive voltage and a higher luminal ionized calcium concentration than the peritubular space.[52,508,514] The former results from a chloride-bicarbonate bi-ionic electrical potential difference, the ionic gradients for which are established by transport processes in the segment 1 proximal tubule.[92] The latter results from the lower pH and bicarbonate concentration of the tubular fluid compared to plasma in this segment of the nephron.[52] Because of its low electrical resistance and high calcium permeability, the lumen-positive voltage and higher luminal Ca^{2+} concentration drive net Ca^{2+} efflux by diffusion in this segment.[52,411,508]

Calcium reabsorption in both segment 1[41,43,600] and segment 2[499] may in part be active.[53] In segment 1 there is evidence for both a high-affinity, Ca^{2+}-Mg^{2+}-dependent ATPase[175] and a basolateral cell membrane Ca^{2+}-Na^{+} antiporter.[233] Basolateral plasma membrane vesicles derived from the renal cortex of rats, which are predominantly from proximal tubular cells, demonstrate a high-affinity, calmodulin-dependent Ca^{2+}-pump.[233,234,474,607] Of interest, these Ca^{2+} pumps are not detected by monoclonal antibodies that recognize epitopes on the distal tubular Ca^{2+} pump,[45] thus suggesting the existence of isoforms of this enzyme. Similarly, Ca^{2+}-Na^{+} exchange activity has been detected in basolateral plasmalemmal vesicles derived from bovine,[567] canine,[518,519] porcine,[447] and rat[254,299,474,607] renal cortices. In intact proximal tubular cells derived from the kidneys of both rats[171,254,474] and rabbits,[474] there is functional evidence for a Ca^{2+}-Na^{+} antiporter. Thus, several studies suggest that the transporters necessary for active calcium absorption in the proximal tubule exist. Functional evidence also exists for an active component of proximal tubular Ca^{2+} absorption.[562] The latter process is stimulated by luminal bicarbonate, suggesting that it is linked to proton secretion.[41] Recently, the Ca^{2+}-pumping function of the Ca^{2+}-Mg^{2+}-dependent ATPase and the existence of the Ca^{2+}-Na^{+} antiporter in proximal tubular cells have been disputed, thus questioning whether either could subserve active calcium transport.[44,389,474]

In conclusion, calcium absorption in the proximal tubules appears to have both passive and active components. The former derives from both solvent drag and diffusion, whereas the latter is linked to luminal fluid acidification. The relative importance of the two components to net calcium efflux is presently unknown. Correspondingly, the roles of the Ca^{2+}-pumping ATPase and the Ca^{2+}-Na^{+} exchanger vis-à-vis effecting transcellular calcium absorption versus maintaining the normally low cytosolic free Ca^{2+} concentration in these cells is unclear.

Conditions that inhibit fluid reabsorption in the proximal tubules also inhibit calcium reabsorption, in some instances resulting in increased urinary calcium excretion. Extracellular fluid volume expansion, whether induced by sodium chloride ingestion or mineralocorticoid excess, is an important example. In conjunction with the inhibitory effects of NaCl-induced volume expansion[4] and mineralocorticoid excess[57] on calcium reabsorption by the collecting ducts, this proximal tubular inhibition of calcium reabsorption results in increased urinary calcium excretion. In contrast, although acetazolamide, which inhibits proximal tubular sodium bicarbonate and fluid reabsorption, inhibits calcium reabsorption in proximal tubules, it does not increase urinary calcium excretion because of increased calcium reabsorption in subsequent nephron segments.[562]

Thin limbs of Henle's loop

The thin limbs of Henle's loop play a minor role in calcium transport by the renal tubule.[53] The descending thin limb essentially is a conduit for luminal calcium flow between the end of the proximal tubule and the beginning of the thin ascending limb, because net calcium transport is absent.[486,499] Calcium concentration increases along the descending limb as water is reabsorbed.[486] The thin ascending limb may serve as a passive calcium exchanger between tubule lumen and medullary interstitium but does not transport calcium actively.[486]

Thick ascending limb of Henle's loop

A lumen-positive transepithelial voltage that is associated with active sodium chloride reabsorption is present in the medullary and cortical thick ascending limbs of Henle's loop.[93,94] Its magnitude increases substantially along the length of these segments, and it drives Ca^{2+} diffusion out of the lumen via the paracellular pathway, resulting in net calcium reabsorption.[55,523,561] Active calcium reabsorption also is present in the cortical portion of the thick ascending limb.[216,289,486,561] The luminal plasma membrane entry step may be a dihydropyridine-sensitive Ca^{2+} channel,[17] and the extrusion mechanism probably is a Ca^{2+}-pumping ATPase, because the Ca^{2+}-Na^{+} antiporter is not present in these cells.[255] Of note, calbindin-D_{28k}, which is present in most epithelia that actively absorb calcium, is absent.[497,573] Calcium reabsorption in the medullary portion of the thick ascending limb is increased by *calcitonin* and in the cortical portion by *PTH*.[53,412] These hormones, via their individual receptors, stimulate basolateral cell membrane adenylate cyclase to produce intracellular cAMP.[53,412] In the cortical thick ascending limb, cAMP—through stimulation of a cAMP-dependent protein kinase—may increase the Ca^{2+} conductance of the apical tight junctions, thereby augmenting paracellular diffusional calcium absorption.[51] Alternatively, or in addition, cAMP may activate dihydropyridine-sensitive Ca^{2+} channels in the luminal plasmalemma, thus increasing Ca^{2+} uptake into the cytosol. This action would increase cytosolic Ca^{2+} concentration, which in turn would drive increased basolateral cell membrane Ca^{2+} extrusion via the Ca^{2+}-pumping ATPase. Together, these effects would accelerate transcellular active calcium absorption.[16] Furosemide reduces sodium chloride reabsorption and consequently diminishes the associated lumen-positive transepithelial voltage in both portions of the thick ascending limb.[93,94,412] By reducing the electrical driving force, it inhibits diffusional calcium reabsorption at these sites.[53,60] This action explains the potent, clinically useful, calciuric effect of furosemide when it is administered to humans.[562]

Distal convoluted and connecting tubules

In the distal convoluted and connecting tubule segments, calcium ions are actively reabsorbed against both chemical concentration and electrical potential differences.[150,290,523] This absorption is transcellular, because the transepithelial electrochemical potential difference for Ca^{2+} favors net secretion via the paracellular pathway. The molecular mechanisms of Ca^{2+} entry into the cells of these two segments are unknown. Ca^{2+} diffusion through the cytosol may be facilitated by calbindin-D_{28k},[72,74] which is absent from cells in preceding portions of the nephron.[497,573] Calcium ions are extruded actively across basolateral cell membranes against a large electrochemical potential difference. Specifically, the voltages across this membrane in rabbit distal convoluted and connecting tubule cells are −78 and −77 mV, respectively.[400,652] Since the plasma Ca^{2+} concentrations in this species average 1.75 m*M*,[164] but the cytosolic values are only 100 to 150 n*M*,[56,58,59,328] a substantial chemical concentration difference also exists. Active extrusion is effected by a high-affinity Ca^{2+}-Mg^{2+} ATPase.[45–48] In the rabbit, distal convoluted and connecting tubules contain the highest activity of this enzyme.[175] Since calbindin-D_{28k} has many of the physicochemical properties of calmodulin, including calcium binding, and since calmodulin stimulates the Ca^{2+}-pumping ATPases in other cells,[617] the coexistence of these two proteins has led to the speculation that calbindin-D_{28k} may stimulate the calcium pump.[47] Definitive evidence for such a role, however, remains to be established.

A high-activity Ca^{2+}-Na^{+} antiporter also exists in the basolateral plasmalemmae of distal convoluted and connecting tubule cells.[58,474] This exchanger, the stoichiometry of which is estimated to be $3Na^{+}:1Ca^{2+}$,[567] also could extrude cytosolic Ca^{2+} if operating in a calcium efflux mode. Calculations of the electrochemical potential differences for Ca^{2+} and Na^{+} movements across the basolateral cell membrane, however, predict that the exchanger does not effect net ion fluxes under physiologic conditions.[58] Rather, the antiporter probably participates in the regulation of cytosolic Ca^{2+} concentration in response to changes in luminal sodium entry, a process that may be important in regulating transcellular Na^{+} absorption.[58,232,572,639]

PTH increases calcium absorption in the distal nephron. In the rat, this occurs in both the distal convoluted and connecting tubules,[151] consistent with the presence of PTH-sensitive adenylate cyclase in cells of both segments.[393] In the rabbit, PTH increases calcium reabsorption in connecting tubules,[290,523,528] which also possess PTH-sensitive adenylate cyclase.[393] In both species, the action of the hormone is mediated via cAMP.[290,523,528] At the cellular level PTH, acting through cAMP, increases Ca^{2+} influx (from the lumen into the cytosol) across the apical plasmalemma of connecting tubules.[56,59] This action, mediated by a cAMP-dependent protein kinase, is an important step in accelerating transcellular Ca^{2+} absorption.[327] Concomitantly, PTH stimulates peritubular influx of Ca^{2+}, the physiologic role of which is uncertain.[56,59] These actions raise cytosolic Ca^{2+} concentration.[56,58,59,327] The molecular nature of these phosphorylation-stimulated Ca^{2+} entry pathways is unknown. The distal convoluted and connecting tubules are the last nephron segments that contain PTH-sensitive adenylate cyclase and PTH-sensitive calcium transport. The rabbit distal convoluted tubule contains a CT-sensitive adenylate cyclase[393] and is the site of CT-stimulated, cAMP-mediated acceleration of calcium absorption.[528]

Thiazides or amiloride, acting at the luminal plasmalemma, increase calcium reabsorption in the distal nephron.[149,153,562] Both diuretics—thiazides by inhibiting electroneutral Na^+-Cl^- cotransport and amiloride by inhibiting conductive Na^+ entry—lower cytosolic Na^+ concentration.[530] By increasing the electrochemical potential for Na^+ entry across the basolateral plasmalemma, the reduced intracellular Na^+ activity may allow the Ca^{2+}-Na^+ antiporter to operate in a Ca^{2+} extrusion mode, thereby increasing transcellular Ca^{2+} absorption.[529] These actions contribute to the hypocalciuric effect of these diuretics, which are used clinically to treat hypercalciuria.[7,337,437]

In summary, the distal convoluted and connecting tubules actively reabsorb calcium. Calcium transport is increased by CT and thiazide diuretics in the former and by PTH and amiloride in the latter. Although only 9 to 10 percent of the calcium filtered at the glomeruli is reabsorbed in these nephron segments, it is here that urinary calcium excretion is finely regulated, primarily by PTH.

Collecting ducts

During antidiuresis, tubular fluid entering the cortical collecting duct is hypoosmotic compared to interstitial fluid. The transepithelial voltage is lumen-negative,[92] and the luminal fluid Ca^{2+} concentration is below that of the peritubular fluid. Therefore, a large electrochemical potential difference favors net Ca^{2+} secretion via the paracellular pathway. However, because of the low calcium permeability of this tubular segment, this calcium "leak" is very small under normal circumstances.[57] Indeed, under conditions of antidiuresis, reabsorption of hypocalciuric fluid raises the luminal fluid Ca^{2+} concentration, thereby reducing the driving force for net calcium secretion. When the lumen-negative voltage is large in the cortical collecting duct, as occurs with chronic mineralocorticoid excess, this secretory calcium "leak" may become significant and contribute to hypercalciuria.[53,57] Ca^{2+}-Na^+ antiporters, which may regulate cytosolic Ca^{2+} concentration and thereby apical cell membrane Na^+ entry,[218,439,639] are present in the basolateral plasmalemmae of rat cortical collecting duct cells.[570]

In the rat, calcium is reabsorbed in the outer and inner medullary collecting ducts by a mechanism that is in part Na^+-dependent.[25,356]

In summary, cortical collecting ducts transport only small amounts of calcium under normal circumstances and therefore play only a minor role in determining urinary calcium excretion. In contrast, inner medullary collecting ducts absorb an important fraction of the calcium delivered to them. The increase in tubular fluid calcium concentration that occurs between the end of the connecting tubule and the urine results primarily from osmotic reabsorption of water across the collecting duct.

PARATHYROID HORMONE

PTH increases calcium reabsorption in both the cortical thick ascending limb of Henle's loop and the connecting tubule. In the kidney in vivo, these actions determine the relationship between serum ultrafilterable calcium concentration and urinary calcium excretion (Fig. 11-10). Notably, for any serum calcium concentration, hypoparathyroid and hyperparathyroid individuals excrete more or less calcium in the urine, respectively, than euparathyroid individuals. In addition, at low serum calcium concentrations hypoparathyroid individuals may be hypocalciuric, whereas at high serum calcium concentrations hyperparathyroid individuals may be hypercalciuric, due in large part to the differences in the filtered loads of calcium between these two conditions and not to the tubular effects of PTH.[450]

CALCITONIN

CT increases calcium reabsorption in both the medullary thick ascending limb of Henle's loop and the distal con-

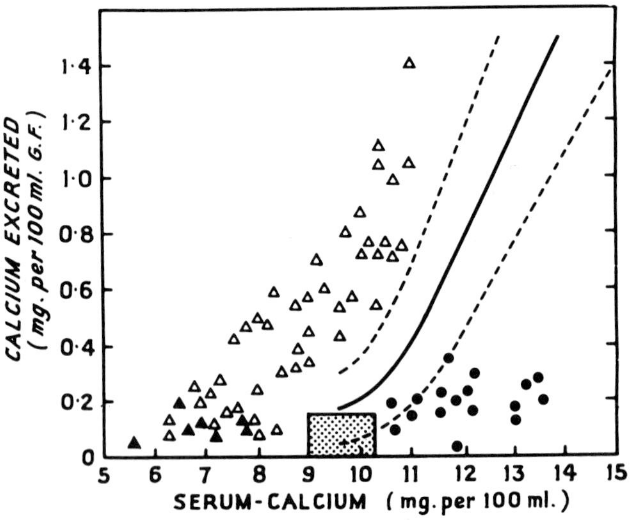

FIGURE 11-10 • Relationship between serum calcium concentration and urinary calcium excretion (expressed as calcium excreted = $[Ca]_{urine} \times [creatinine]_{serum}$ $[creatinine]_{urine}$) during calcium-loading experiments in humans. The stippled rectangle represents the normal ranges in euparathyroid individuals. The solid line surrounded by dotted lines indicates the mean ± 2 SD for normal subjects. The triangles indicate values for hypoparathyroid individuals, and the closed circles represent values for hyperparathyroid individuals. (From Nordin BEC, Peacock M: *Lancet* 2:1280, 1969. Used by permission.)

voluted tubule,[528,559] thereby decreasing urinary calcium excretion.[29,121,468,478] CT also reduces the physiologic hypercalcemia and increased glomerular filtration of calcium that accompany postprandial intestinal calcium absorption. These concurrent actions, decreased glomerular filtration and increased tubular reabsorption, minimize urinary loss of dietary calcium.[15,566]

CT stimulates adenylate cyclase activity in the medullary thick ascending limbs and distal convoluted tubules,[393] thereby increasing calcium reabsorption via a cAMP-dependent process.[468,528,559] The molecular mechanisms by which CT increases calcium transport are unknown.

CALCITRIOL

The effects of calcitriol on renal tubular calcium reabsorption are controversial. Increased, decreased, or unchanged values have been observed in response to this hormone, depending upon the experimental conditions.[53,61,95,314,560,608,648] Analogously to its stimulatory effects on active Ca^{2+} absorption by duodenal enterocytes (vide infra), calcitriol has been hypothesized to increase active Ca^{2+} reabsorption across cells of the distal convoluted and connecting tubules. Direct evidence for such an action, however, is lacking. In healthy men with normal renal function consuming a modestly calcium-restricted diet, oral administration of calcitriol increased urinary calcium excretion in excess of dietary intake.[2] The dose of calcitriol administered in these studies did not raise serum calcium concentration and probably did not demineralize bone.[2] These observations suggest that the most important effect of calcitriol is to stimulate intestinal calcium absorption and provide no evidence that tubular calcium reabsorption is increased substantially.[2]

IONIC FACTORS

Magnesium

Hypermagnesemia, whether from a high dietary intake or parenteral infusion, causes hypercalciuria.[562,615] Conversely, low magnesium intake in growing rats causes hypocalciuria in spite of normal or increased plasma calcium concentrations.[615] A calcium-magnesium interaction at the basolateral cell membranes of the thick ascending limb has been proposed to control calcium transport.[122,469,470] It is hypothesized that increases in magnesium concentration in the peritubular interstitium inhibit transcellular calcium absorption by an unknown mechanism. This hypothesis has been disputed because no evidence for such a mechanism could be found in the cortical thick ascending limb of Henle's loop in the rabbit.[522] In addition to a possible direct inhibitory effect, hypermagnesemia also suppresses PTH secretion, resulting in decreased renal tubular calcium reabsorption.[235,372]

Hydrogen ions

Chronic metabolic acidosis increases the renal clearance of calcium by inhibiting its tubular reabsorption.[498,560,562] Sodium bicarbonate therapy for the acidosis reestablishes normal calcium reabsorption, perhaps by stimulating a luminal cell membrane Ca^{2+}-H^+ antiporter in both proximal[41] and connecting[328] tubules.

Anions

Approximately 20 percent of the calcium in the glomerular filtrate is complexed by anions such as bicarbonate, citrate, phosphate, lactate, and sulfate, among others. Their concentrations, as well as those of urate and oxalate, in luminal fluid are continuously changing due to their reabsorption and secretion by proximal tubules. In addition, they are concentrated in the lumen as water is reabsorbed in the later portions of the nephron. These anions affect calcium transport across the tubular epithelia by their effects on Ca^{2+} concentrations. Higher concentrations of anionic ligands reduce the luminal Ca^{2+} concentration and vice versa. Lower concentrations of Ca^{2+} in the tubular lumen decrease both active and passive calcium reabsorption. Given the large number of potentially important anions, both endogenous and exogenous, that may form complexes with calcium and given the variety of transport processes for each anion in the various segments of the nephron, their integrated effects on urinary calcium excretion are complicated and a clear understanding of their roles in determining urinary calcium excretion awaits further investigation.[53,615] From a therapeutic viewpoint, it is noteworthy that phosphate administration, either orally or parenterally, lowers urinary calcium excretion.[372,562,615] The mechanism by which phosphate administration reduces urinary calcium excretion is uncertain but may be due to stimulation of PTH release by a reduction in plasma Ca^{2+} concentration.[498] Conversely, chronic phosphate depletion increases urinary calcium excretion.[53,164,372,562]

INTESTINES

OVERVIEW

In normal individuals, dietary intake is the sole source of external calcium. A fraction of dietary calcium is absorbed by the intestines; the remainder appears in the feces. When calcium losses in sweat are small, urinary calcium excretion closely approximates net intestinal calcium absorption in adults in external calcium balance. When calcium is eliminated from the diet, it is lost in the feces and urine, resulting in negative external balance.

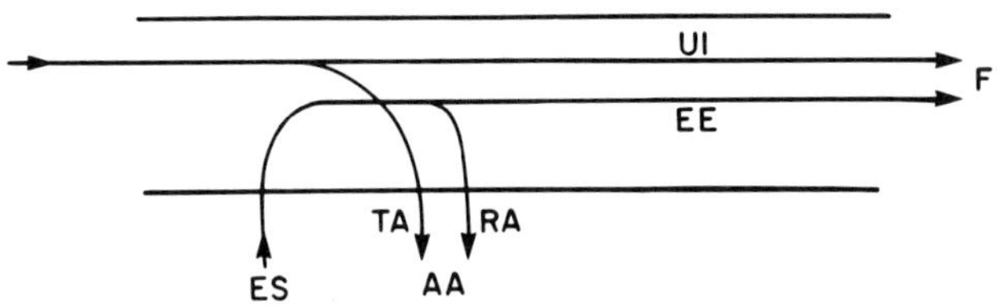

FIGURE 11-11 • Transfers of calcium in the gastrointestinal tract. I, dietary calcium intake; ES, endogenous calcium secretion; TA, true absorption of dietary calcium; RA, reabsorption of endogenous calcium that was secreted; AA, absolute absorption of calcium (AA = TA + RA); UI, unabsorbed dietary calcium (UI = I − TA); EE, excretion of endogenous calcium that was secreted (EE = ES − RA); F, fecal excretion of calcium (F = UI + EE). Net calcium absorption is defined as I − F. (From Parfitt AM, Kleerekoper M in Maxwell MH, Kleeman CR (eds): *Clinical Disorders of Fluid and Electrolyte Metabolism,* 3d ed, New York, McGraw-Hill, 1980, p 269. Used by permission.)

Fecal calcium in the absence of dietary calcium indicates that endogenous calcium is secreted into the gastrointestinal tract and that a fraction of it is not reabsorbed. In fact, endogenous calcium is added to the alimentary canal from salivary, gastric, biliary, pancreatic, and intestinal secretions. These net calcium transfers are summarized in Fig. 11-11.

In healthy men, external calcium balance can be maintained with dietary intakes as low as 5 to 10 mmol/day, with a negative balance ensuing below these values.[8,154] For adults, the recommended dietary allowance for calcium is 20 mmol/day.[154] During gestation or lactation, it increases to 30 mmol/day because mineralization of the fetal skeleton and milk production each draw from calcium stores in the maternal skeleton, which can be maintained by increasing dietary intake.[154]

Approximately 25 to 27 mmol of calcium enter the gastrointestinal tract daily, 20 mmol from the diet and 5 to 7 mmol by endogenous secretion.[8,306,438,445] Normal individuals in calcium balance absorb 8 to 10 mmol; 15 to 19 mmol is eliminated in the stool (Fig. 11-12). Accordingly, although 33 percent of the total calcium load presented to the intestinal tract is absorbed, only 20 percent of dietary intake is retained, as measured by oral intake minus fecal output, because of endogenous calcium secretion. Intestinal calcium absorption varies with age. It is high during the skeletal growth of childhood and adolescence[306,342] but decreases steadily with advancing age, particularly after the seventieth year.[12,221] Calcium absorption increases both with pregnancy and with lactation.[38,66–68,306,342,624] When dietary calcium is reduced, its fractional absorption is increased, a phenomenon that is referred to as *adaptation*.[20,342,624] The changes in intestinal calcium absorption that occur with old age, reproduction and lactation, and decreased dietary intake are, at least in considerable part, mediated by changes in the plasma concentration of 1α,25-$(OH)_2$D.[12,62,221,624]

Physiologically, 1α,25-$(OH)_2$D (calcitriol) is the primary regulator of intestinal calcium absorption.[8,70,160,306,342,409,429,438,445,621,622,624] This hormone begins to augment active calcium absorption late in the suckling period[251] and remains the dominant influence on this process throughout life. Luminal *lactose* increases intestinal calcium absorption in adult humans by an unknown mechanism whose action is independent of and additive to that of calcitriol.[11] Similarly, luminal *glucose* and *galactose* increase epithelial calcium absorp-

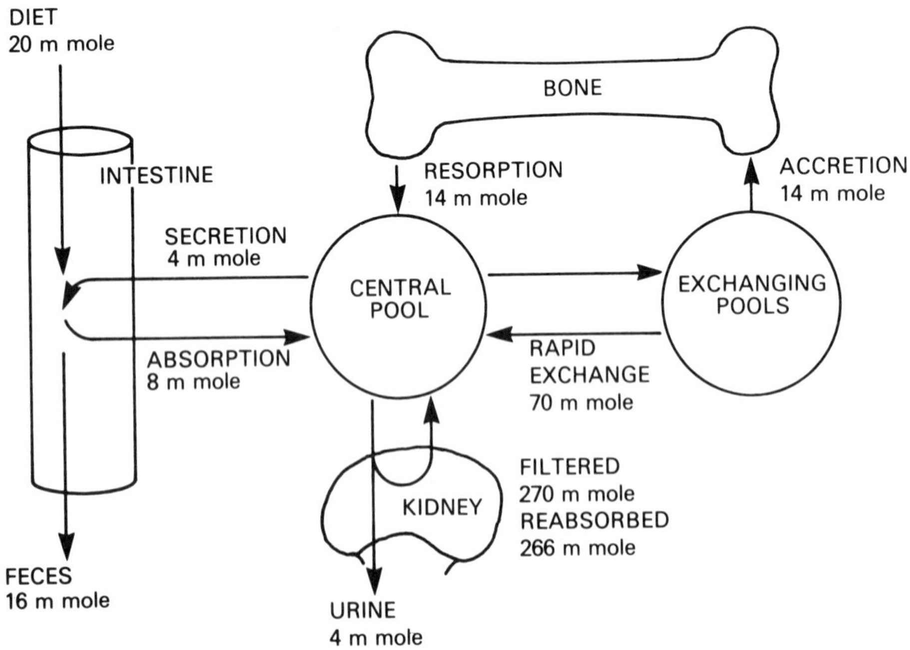

FIGURE 11-12 • Calcium fluxes between body pools for a 70-kg adult with unchanging total body calcium (i.e., in external balance for calcium). All fluxes are in millimoles per day.

tion in the intestine.[124,242] Pharmacologic inhibitors of calcium absorption include *cellulose phosphate*,[337] *glucocorticoids*,[306,342,438,624] and *phenytoin*.[342,624] The first complexes Ca^{2+} in the intestinal lumen and thereby increases fecal calcium excretion.[337] The second inhibits active calcium absorption in the duodenum[331,517] but may stimulate absorption in the distal colon.[331] The mechanism by which the third acts is unclear but may be multifactorial, involving inhibition of both $1\alpha,25\text{-(OH)}_2D$ synthesis and Ca^{2+} movement through the intestinal epithelial cells.[342]

With adequate luminal concentrations, calcium may be absorbed in all segments of the intestine beyond the stomach.[75,196,320] Normally, the highest rates occur in the *duodenum* and *early jejunum*.[445,624] Although the rate of calcium absorption per unit length is lower in the *ileum*, it accounts for as much as 70 percent of the net efflux from the intestinal lumen because of its substantial length.[320,405] The *colon* also may absorb calcium but generally at lower rates and only when dietary intake is low. Colonic absorption becomes important during adaptation to a low calcium diet.[199] In humans calcium absorption is nil when dietary intake falls to about 5 mmol/day and changes to net secretion at values below these.[359,429] Similarly to the renal tubule, intestinal segments are arranged in series. Likewise, the function of each depends in part on the changes in luminal fluid composition caused by more proximal digestive and transport processes. In this regard, one important factor is intraluminal pH.[438] In the proximal duodenum, the pH is low because of gastric hydrochloric acid secretion. The low pH favors ionization of calcium, which favors absorption. An important clinical correlate is that calcium absorption from its carbonate salt is impaired by achlorhydria under fasting conditions.[479] Conversely, the alkaline pH of the ileum favors the formation of calcium complexes, which may limit absorption, despite a total calcium concentration that is greater than that in either the duodenum or jejunum (see reference 33 in reference 624 herein).

When the segments of the small intestine are viewed as a whole, calcium absorption during normal dietary calcium intake may be separated kinetically into two components. The first is a saturable *transcellular flux* occurring primarily through enterocytes of the duodenum and proximal jejunum that is regulated by calcitriol. The second is a nonsaturable *paracellular flux* occurring primarily between enterocytes of the distal jejunum and the ileum that is independent of nutritional or hormonal regulation. In the cecum and colon the paracellular pathway plays a minor, if any, role in calcium absorption during normal conditions. However, the transcellular pathway in these segments becomes important in calcium reclamation from the luminal contents when dietary calcium is restricted. Of the two pathways, paracellular absorption occurring in the distal small intestine predominates when dietary calcium intake is normal and luminal ionized calcium concentrations exceed those of plasma, whereas the calcitriol-regulated transcellular absorptive pathway becomes essential for calcium conservation during adaptation to a low calcium intake.[69,71,75,405]

Although such kinetic analyses are helpful in understanding calcium absorption by the gut as a whole, to understand the details of these processes, it is necessary to study the mechanisms and regulation of calcium transport in each of its segments (Table 11-2). In general, such studies have been performed in intestinal segments from the chick or the rat.

DUODENUM

Calcium absorption in the duodenum occurs via two parallel processes.[70,624] *Diffusional absorption* occurs when the concentration of Ca^{2+} in the luminal contents is high (e.g., following a calcium-rich meal). Under these conditions, the electrochemical potential difference across the duodenum favors calcium movement from lumen to blood by diffusion, apparently via the *paracellular pathway*.[342,624]

In addition to this passive absorption, *active calcium transport* occurs in the duodenum.[8,70,306,342,398,409,438,445,487,621,622,624] Active Ca^{2+} absorption occurs *transcellularly* and is regulated by $1\alpha,25\text{-(OH)}_2D$.[71,160,429,623] In this process calcium enters the duodenal mucosal cells across their luminal membranes and diffuses through the cytosol to the basolateral cell membranes, where extrusion is effected by energy-requiring mechanisms (Fig. 11-2). When the concentration of Ca^{2+} in the duodenal lumen is high, this mechanism operates in parallel with paracellular diffusion to achieve net calcium absorption. When the concentration of Ca^{2+} in the lumen is low, the active calcium transport mechanism alone effects calcium absorption. Whereas the passive diffusional component of calcium transport is linearly related to the electrochemical driving forces for Ca^{2+} movement and is nonsaturable, the active calcium transport process demonstrates saturation kinetics.[70,342,624]

The first step in transcellular Ca^{2+} movement is its entry into the cell across the luminal membrane. It has been hypothesized that *IMCal*, a membrane-associated vitamin D-induced calcium-binding protein of approximately 200 kilodaltons, effects Ca^{2+} entry into rat duodenal cells from the intestinal lumen—perhaps by serving as a specific Ca^{2+} channel for passive diffusion into the cytosol.[318,511] (As of this writing the presence or absence of Ca^{2+} channels in the apical plasmalemmae of these cells remains to be established, either by patch-clamp or other related electrophysiologic experiments.) Alternatively, it has been proposed that $1\alpha,25\text{-(OH)}_2D$ regulates calcium entry across the luminal membrane of chick duodenal mucosal cells by altering apical membrane phosphatidylcholine content and thereby membrane structure.[212,322,477] The altered lipids might serve as calcium ionophores,[622] or, as has been suggested for dog kidney proximal tubule brush-border membranes, they might be involved in a dynamic calcium-binding process that translocates calcium ions from the luminal to the cytoplasmic aspect of the cell membrane.[278] Such "liponomic" control of calcium movement across the luminal plasmalemma, although vitamin D-dependent, does not require the synthesis of new protein. The molecular mechanisms by which 1α,25-$(OH)_2D$ alters lipid turnover and structure and how these effects increase Ca^{2+} entry across this membrane are unclear.[622] Similarly, alterations, predominantly involving lipids, have been found in the topography of duodenal luminal cell membranes from the chick intestine in response to 1α,25-$(OH)_2D$.[430] Attempts to elucidate the Ca^{2+} entry step at the mucosal cell membrane by measuring uptake into brush-border vesicles isolated from rat duodena[387] were inconclusive because of extensive calcium binding to the vesicle interiors, which was not related to calcium transport. Calcitriol stimulated initial calcium uptake rates when injected intraperitoneally to vitamin D-deficient rats 16 h prior to membrane isolation.[387] Calcium-binding studies of isolated duodenal brush-border membranes demonstrated both high- and low-affinity sites.[388] The former were protein or phosphoprotein, whereas the latter were primarily phospholipids. It was speculated that the high-affinity binding sites might regulate Ca^{2+} movement through a selective Ca^{2+} channel. In summary, although 1α,25-$(OH)_2D$ affects the apical plasmalemma of duodenal enterocytes, the mechanism by which it increases Ca^{2+} entry into these cells is unresolved.

The second step in transcellular Ca^{2+} movement is diffusion from the apical cell membrane entry site to the basolateral cell membrane extrusion site. Since the cytosolic free Ca^{2+} concentration in duodenal enterocytes is about 100 n*M*,[33] the concentration gradient for Ca^{2+} diffusion between these two sites, which is the driving force for this movement, must be quite small. Based upon the diffusion coefficient of calcium ions in water at 37° C and a presumed Ca^{2+} concentration difference of 200 n*M*, it has been estimated that simple intracellular diffusion can account for only about $\frac{1}{70}$ of the observed calcium flux through these cells.[75] Accordingly, this process is facilitated by a vitamin D-dependent, high-affinity, calcium-binding protein (*calbindin*).[203,204,206,321] In the chick this protein is about 30 kilodaltons (calbindin-D_{28k}), whereas in the rat it is about 9 kilodaltons (calbindin-D_{9k}).[244,622] Calbindin-D_{28k} and -D_{9k} bind four or two calcium ions per molecule, respectively; the affinity constant of each protein for Ca^{2+} is about $2 \times 10^6\ M^{-1}$.[244,622] In vitamin D-deficient animals, the protein is absent from the duodenal mucosal cells and appears within 2.5 h after injection of calcitriol.[622] This pathway of calcium absorption recently has been visualized by ion microscopic imaging of ^{44}Ca in chicken duodenal enterocytes,[129] and the notion has been espoused that calbindin-facilitated intracellular Ca^{2+} diffusion is the rate-limiting step in calcitriol-stimulated active calcium absorption.[71,73,75,442,443,487] However, an examination of the quantitative relationship between calcium absorption and calbindin-D_{28k} in the chick duodenum, although suggesting that this protein is one part of the calcium absorptive process, demonstrated dissociations between the calbindin-D_{28k} content of the cells and calcium absorption rates under certain circumstances, implying that 1α,25-$(OH)_2D$ affects other steps in this process as well.[205]

The final step in transcellular Ca^{2+} movement is active extrusion from the cytosol across the basolateral plasmalemma into the interstitial fluid, which occurs against a large electrochemical potential difference. The nature and regulation of this step are not fully agreed upon. One mechanism of Ca^{2+} extrusion is a high-affinity *Ca^{2+}-pumping ATPase*.[158,228] In vitamin D-deficient rats, this enzyme is regulated by 1α,25-$(OH)_2D$, which increases its activity by augmenting V_{max}.[227] In contrast, in vitamin D-replete rats, calcitriol increases the epithelial mucosal-to-serosal unidirectional calcium flux by mechanisms that apparently do not involve ATP-dependent basolateral cell membrane calcium extrusion.[199] The latter observations question whether, under physiologic conditions, transcellular calcium absorption is driven by a Ca^{2+}-pumping ATPase, the synthesis of which is regulated by 1α,25-$(OH)_2D$. Independently of calcitriol, calmodulin increases the activity of the Ca^{2+}-pumping ATPase by increasing its affinity for Ca^{2+}.[230] Although early studies failed to show it,[230] calbindin-D_{9k} stimulated Ca^{2+} transport by the basolateral cell membrane calcium pump in duodenal enterocytes when the experimental methods were modified.[617] As with calmodulin, this effect was independent of calcitriol. A second potential, but minor, mechanism for Ca^{2+} extrusion is a *Ca^{2+}-Na^+ exchanger*.[229,606] The direction in which this process translocates calcium ions—either into or out of the cell—under physiologic conditions is unknown. Even assuming it effects Ca^{2+} extrusion, its activity is only 10 percent of that of the Ca^{2+}-ATPase and is not regulated by 1α,25-$(OH)_2D$.[229] These biochemical findings are consistent with calcium transport studies that failed to demonstrate a significant role for Ca^{2+}-Na^+ exchange in duodenal calcium absorption.[200] Within the duodenum, vitamin D-dependent calcium absorption takes place primarily in the mid- to upper villus—and not in the crypt—region.[606,618]

An unsettled issue is whether 1α,25-$(OH)_2D$ stimulates duodenal calcium transport solely via mechanisms that require interaction of the hormone with the epithelial cell nucleus, resulting in DNA-directed protein synthesis.

The work of Rasmussen and associates[212,322,477] showing rapid changes in the lipid composition of the plasma membrane would dispute this hypothesis. Conversely, the work of DeLuca and coworkers[35,160,161,215] examining the temporal relationship between the action of $1\alpha,25\text{-}(OH)_2D$ on duodenal mucosal cell calcium transport and the induction of calbindin-D synthesis may be interpreted as supporting a strictly genomic mechanism. Wasserman and colleagues[621,626] have proposed that $1\alpha,25\text{-}(OH)_2D$ has a biphasic action on duodenal cellular calcium transport. First, the hormone induces changes in luminal cell membrane phospholipid metabolism that correlate with increased calcium permeation—an effect independent of protein synthesis. Second, the hormone induces the synthesis of calbindin-D, and possibly Ca^{2+}-ATPase, resulting in increased transfer of calcium through and out of the cell. This formulation is consistent with previous speculation by Norman and coworkers[430] and Bronner and coworkers[76] that both genomic and nongenomic effects of $1\alpha,25\text{-}(OH)_2D$ play roles in the stimulation of duodenal calcium absorption.

Recently, Norman and colleagues showed that physiologic concentrations of serosal—but not mucosal—calcitriol promptly (within 2 min) stimulate intestinal calcium absorption, presumably by nongenomic mechanisms.[156,157,411,429] This very rapid increase in transport, which is observed only in duodena harvested from vitamin D-replete—and not vitamin D-deficient—chicks, has been termed *transcaltachia*. From the results of studies with stimulators or inhibitors of mucosal-to-serosal ^{45}Ca fluxes across perfused intestinal segments, they have proposed that calcitriol activates basolateral plasmalemmal Ca^{2+} channels, allowing an influx of serosal calcium that initiates this response.[157] Protein kinase C and cAMP-dependent protein kinase have been suggested as mediators of this action.[156] Finally, they have speculated that calcium is transported through these cells in vesicles that are attached to microtubules by calbindin-D_{28k}.[411] Though speculative, this hypothesis is provocative. An important test of its physiologic relevance will be to assess whether variations in serosal calcitriol concentrations, as might be expected acutely in vivo, are related to concurrent changes in calcium absorption.

Less conventional pathways and mechanisms for intracellular calcium transport, which have been reviewed by Wasserman,[621,622] have been proposed by Weringer and associates,[634] Reith,[482] and Terepka and associates.[575]

JEJUNUM

Calcium may be absorbed or secreted by the jejunum, depending upon the conditions of the studies.[196,333,613] Under normal circumstances, *passive calcium movement* plays a more important role than in the duodenum, because the electrical conductance of the jejunum is twice as high.[369] Conversely, *active calcium transport* is much lower, or even absent, in the jejunum.[70,196,333,613] When the jejunum is exposed to high concentrations of $1\alpha,25\text{-}(OH)_2D$, active calcium absorption is detectable,[333,438] but the magnitude is lower than in the duodenum.[196,333] In healthy humans calcium is absorbed in the jejunum when luminal calcium concentration is adequate, and this absorption is stimulated by calcitriol.[320] Likewise, *IMCal* content[318] and *Ca^{2+} ATPase* activity[227] are lower in jejunal than duodenal cells. A *Ca^{2+}-Na^+* antiporter is present in the basolateral cell membranes. Its activity is equal to that in the duodenum and likewise is not regulated by $1\alpha,25\text{-}(OH)_2D$.[229]

ILEUM

Calcium may be *secreted* or *absorbed* by the ileum.[196,614] In rats ingesting a high-calcium diet throughout life, there is net calcium secretion.[614] Conversely, in rats placed on a low-calcium diet, a maneuver that increases the plasma concentration of $1\alpha,25\text{-}(OH)_2D$, calcium is absorbed during the growth period.[614] Calcium secretion by the ileum initially was thought to be an active process,[614] but subsequently it has been proposed to result from solvent drag of calcium from the lateral intercellular spaces, across the tight junctions, and into the gut lumen.[407,409,608]

Active calcium absorption,[196,408] calcium entry across the ileal cell luminal membrane,[333] and the activity of the Ca^{2+} ATPase[230] are all increased by $1\alpha,25\text{-}(OH)_2D$. Under appropriate conditions—for example, low luminal Ca^{2+} concentration and high plasma concentrations of $1\alpha,25\text{-}(OH)_2D$—$Ca^{2+}$ is absorbed actively via the transcellular pathway. In addition, calcium absorption may occur by solvent drag via the paracellular pathway in the ileum.[22]

COLON

The *cecum actively absorbs calcium* at a high rate.[406] Apparently, the luminal cell membranes have the highest density of calcium entry sites in the rat intestine. These cells possess parallel mechanisms for extrusion of calcium ions that move transcellularly to the basolateral plasmalemmae. Both the Ca^{2+}-Na^+ exchanger and the Ca^{2+}-ATPase may extrude calcium from cecal cells into the lamina propria. In young rats, a low-calcium diet did not stimulate calcium absorption, but it was decreased in response to either a high-calcium[406] or vitamin D-deficient diet.[196]

Under normal circumstances, the colon plays a small—but important—role in overall calcium absorption.[287] However, when rats are fed a low-calcium diet, active absorption is induced in the ascending[196,198,331] and descending,[196,198] but not the transverse,[196] portions. Likewise, when normal rats were treated with supraphysiologic doses of 1α,25-$(OH)_2D$, calcium absorption occurred in the ascending[196,310] and descending,[196,201,202,331] but not the transverse,[196] portions of the colon. Similar results have been reported in healthy humans.[243] Favus and coworkers[198] suggested that the Ca^{2+} ATPase located in the basolateral membranes of descending colon cells is the primary mechanism for active calcium transport. In addition to a calcium pump, Lee[331] found a parallel sodium-dependent calcium extrusion process. Recently, Wiener and coworkers[637] confirmed the existence of a high-affinity (K_m = 90 n*M*) Ca^{2+},Mg^{2+}-dependent ATPase in basolateral cell membranes of rabbit distal colon. Despite using three different approaches to detect it, these investigators could not find a Ca^{2+}-Na^{+} exchanger. Since the affinity of the calcium pump is appropriate for the resting cytosolic free Ca^{2+} concentration in these cells (about 140 n*M*),[612] it is likely that it serves as the extrusion mechanism.

1α,25-$(OH)_2$D

Calcitriol increases calcium absorption in most segments of the intestines. Normally, the predominant effect is on the duodenum, but as plasma concentrations of this hormone increase, the jejunum, ileum, and ascending and descending colon are recruited to absorb calcium as well. In normal humans (with plasma calcitriol concentrations between 35 and 48 pg/ml) consuming a 900-mg calcium diet, vitamin D-dependent (transcellular) calcium absorption accounts for approximately three times more calcium absorption than the vitamin-D independent (paracellular) pathway.[524] However, since the vitamin D-dependent mechanism is nearly saturated, even at lower calcium intakes, all of the increment in calcium absorption that occurs when normal calcium meals are supplemented with extra calcium is mediated by the vitamin D-independent mechanism. In vitamin D deficiency, calcium absorption by the intestines is reduced, because without adequate plasma concentrations of this hormone, active transport of calcium is minimal or absent and hypocalcemia ensues. During periods of calcium need, such as pregnancy, lactation, and growth, plasma 1α,25-$(OH)_2$D concentrations are elevated, and they promote increased intestinal calcium absorption. When dietary calcium intake is low, 1α,25-$(OH)_2$D concentrations are elevated, and they stimulate active intestinal calcium transport to maximize the fractional absorption of calcium. Administration of excessive amounts of vitamin D_3 (or its analogues) causes hypercalcemia and hypercalciuria from the hormone's action on the gastrointestinal tract and bone.

REGULATION OF CALCIUM METABOLISM

PARATHYROID HORMONE

Synthesis and secretion

The parathyroid gland is the principal regulator of ionized calcium concentration in plasma. Within it are the sensors for recognizing the concentration of ionized calcium and the components for synthesizing and secreting PTH. The release of PTH from the parathyroid gland is stimulated by a small decrease in extracellular ionized calcium concentration and inhibited by small increases. PTH enhances the flux of calcium into the circulation from bone, kidney, and—indirectly, via calcitriol—intestine. This feedback system maintains the level of calcium in ECF at a remarkably constant level.

PTH is a single-chain polypeptide with 84 amino acids and a molecular weight of approximately 9300 daltons. The predominant species secreted by the parathyroid gland is the full 84–amino acid peptide, but biological activity of PTH only requires the amino-terminal one-third of the molecule.[495] The function of the remainder of the peptide is unknown. Deletion of the middle and carboxyl-terminal region of the peptide does not eliminate its biological activity. Studies using chemically synthesized fragments of bovine and human PTH have shown that the amino acid sequence 7 to 34 can bind to PTH receptors without activating them. The first three to seven amino acids of the NH_2 terminal are critical for activating the receptor.[494]

Like other peptide hormones, PTH is synthesized as a large–molecular weight (115 amino acids) precursor, *preproPTH* (Fig. 11-13).[264,265] The amino terminus of this precursor, termed the signal or leader sequence, directs the nascent peptide into the cisternae of the rough endoplasmic reticulum as it is being assembled on membrane-bound ribosomes. The leader sequence of the nascent peptide binds to the so-called signal-recognition particle, which then binds to a receptor on the rough endoplasmic reticulum, thereby bringing the molecule to the endoplasmic reticulum as it is assembled.[495] The "pre," or leader, sequence is removed by a signal peptidase as the protein traverses the membrane of the rough endoplasmic reticulum.[496] Therefore, preproPTH does not exist as a full-length protein. The resulting peptide, *proPTH,* is not secreted from the parathyroid cell and has no hormonal bioactivity;[238] its role may be to direct hormone transport within intracellular organelles. ProPTH is transported to the Golgi apparatus, where the six–amino acid "pro" sequence is removed within minutes of synthesis. PTH is then packaged in secretory granules, from which it leaves the cell after fusion of the secretory granules with the plasma membrane. A small proportion of PTH molecules are cleaved to smaller frag-

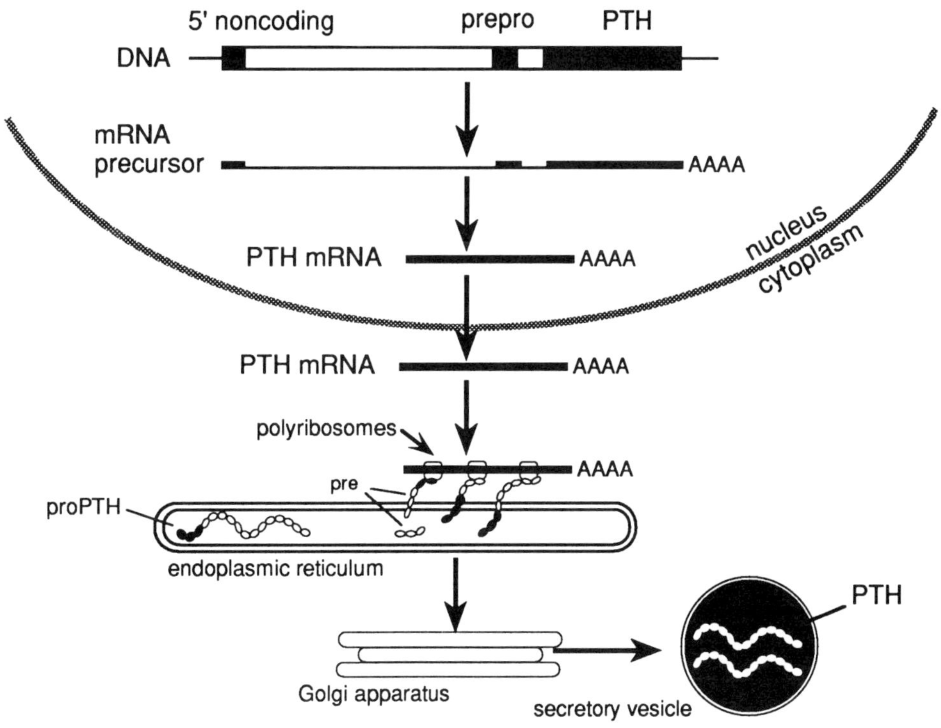

FIGURE 11-13 • Schematic representation of the biosynthesis and secretion of precursor and secretory forms of PTH. Transcription of the gene encoding preproPTH in the nucleus is followed by removal of intervening sequences. The mature mRNA migrates to the cytoplasm and binds to polyribosomes. The pre, or signal, portion of the nascent peptide binds to the signal-recognition particle, and this complex in turn binds to a docking protein on the endoplasmic reticulum, facilitating entry of the peptide into the endoplasmic reticulum. During this entry and before the synthesis of the peptide is completed, the pre sequence is removed. The remaining proPTH is transported to the Golgi apparatus, where the pro sequence is removed. The remaining 84-amino acid mature hormone, PTH, is packaged into secretory vesicles for secretion. A variable fraction of hormone is transported to lysosomes and degraded into bioinactive fragments (not shown).

ments in lysosomes; some of these fragments, which are most likely bioinactive, are secreted.

The structure of both the PTH gene and mRNA have been determined using recombinant DNA technology.[264,609,629] The human PTH gene exists as only one copy per haploid cell and is located on the short arm of chromosome 11.[404] The gene has two introns, or intervening sequences, that are transcribed but then removed and not found in the mature PTH mRNA; there is no evidence for alternative splicing of this gene. Important information on the regulation of PTH synthesis will derive from ongoing efforts to identify DNA sequences outside the promoter region of the PTH gene that function as either enhancers stimulating transcription or silencers inhibiting transcription. It is likely that cellular receptors and second messengers that are in turn influenced by calcium, vitamin D, and other modulators of parathyroid function bind to these regions of the gene. For example, $1\alpha,25\text{-(OH)}_2D$ appears to inhibit PTH gene transcription[536] by binding with its receptor to a region flanking the PTH gene.[432]

Regulation of synthesis and secretion

Parathyroid gland secretion of PTH is principally regulated by extracellular ionized calcium.[14] Secretion of PTH is maximally inhibited by as little as a 10 percent increase in calcium concentration and near maximally stimulated by a 10 percent drop in calcium.[374] This demonstrates that control of hormone secretion is exerted within the physiologic range of calcium concentrations. The secretory response curve to variation in extracellular calcium can be characterized by four independent parameters: *maximal secretory rate*, *basal secretory rate* (minimum output), *set point* (calcium level required to give half of maximal suppression), and *sensitivity* (slope of the response curve; Fig. 11-14). These parameters can be altered in various physiologic and pathologic states. The maximal secretory capacity is increased by prolonged hypocalcemia because it leads to cellular proliferation and gland enlargement. The basal secretory rate may be abnormally high in some cases of primary hyperparathyroidism and may be the cause of excess PTH secretion.[81] In other cases of hyperparathyroidism, the set point is shifted so that the level of calcium required to inhibit PTH secretion is raised.[81] The set point is also increased in the neonatal period (in cows and perhaps in humans),[79] and this may account for the transient hypercalcemia of human and bovine neonates.

The normal parathyroid gland turns over its supply of PTH once every 6 h. Compared to glands that secrete hormone in a mostly episodic manner (such as insulin-secreting islet cells), relatively little hormone is stored in parathyroid cells. To coordinate secretion and glandular stores of PTH, calcium regulates not only secretion but also the synthesis and catabolism of the hormone in the gland. Recent studies suggest that hypocalcemia enhances transcription of the PTH gene while hypercalcemia has

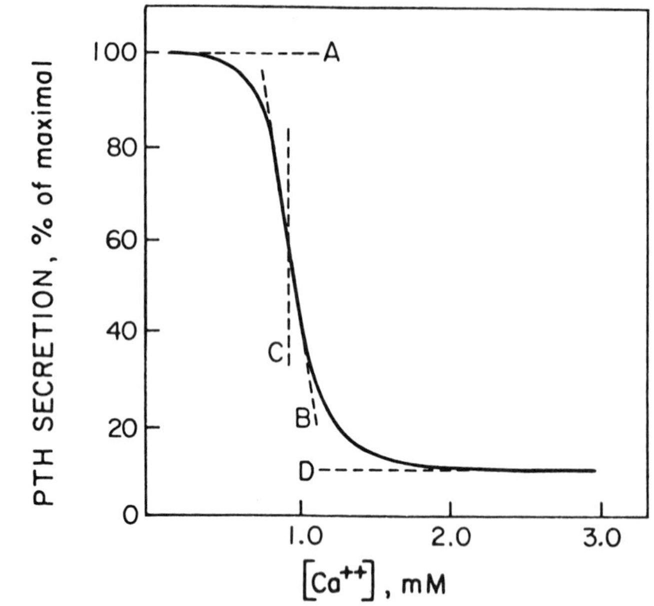

FIGURE 11-14 • Sigmoidal relationship between extracellular calcium and PTH secretion determined with bovine parathyroid cells in vitro. The secretory response of parathyroid cells can be characterized by four parameters: maximal secretory rate (A); minimum secretory rate (D); sensitivity or slope of the response curve (B); and set point or calcium level required to give half of maximal suppression (C). (From Brown EM: *J Clin Endocrinol Metab* 56:572, 1983. Used by permission.)

little effect on transcription.[535] Rats made hypocalcemic by three weeks of a low calcium diet had a threefold increase in the level of PTH mRNA in their parathyroid glands compared to normocalcemic rats on a normal diet (an increase in the number of parathyroid cells may have also contributed to the higher levels of PTH mRNA).[403] Hypercalcemia, on the other hand, did not reduce the level of PTH mRNA in rats fed a high-calcium diet.[403] Compared to controls, there was no detectable change in the level of PTH mRNA in such rats. It is surprising that studies in vitro with cultured parathyroid cells have shown that low ionized calcium concentration has little effect on PTH mRNA levels while high levels of calcium markedly reduce transcription.[505] This discrepancy may be a result of effects of calcium in vitro on cellular proliferation that are unique to culture situations.[535] Although hypercalcemia does not inhibit PTH synthesis, it reduces stores of hormone by catabolizing PTH within lysosomal enzymes.[376] Some of the resulting fragments (which are bioinactive) are secreted.

These studies of parathyroid hormone synthesis and secretion suggest that when serum calcium is increased above the normal range, the parathyroid gland continues to produce basal levels of PTH; suppressing secretion with hypercalcemia does not lead to accumulation of PTH, because hormone degradation is enhanced. Enhanced output of PTH during hypocalcemia is a result of increased synthesis of hormone. To some degree the increase in hormone output after chronic hypocalcemia is a result of an increase in the number of parathyroid gland cells, since chronic hypocalcemia stimulates parathyroid cell proliferation and an increase in parathyroid cell mass (hyperplasia). The mechanism by which low levels of calcium stimulate parathyroid cell proliferation is not known.

Regulation of PTH secretion by calcium

The modulation of hormone secretion by changes in ionized calcium within the physiologic range is a unique property of three cell types: parathyroid cells, renin-secreting cells of the juxtaglomerular apparatus, and perifollicular (calcitonin-secreting) C cells. Only in parathyroid and renin-secreting cells is hormone secretion inversely related to the calcium level. The mechanism of this unusual response to extracellular calcium has not been entirely worked out, but evidence now points to a parathyroid cell surface receptor that binds calcium and modulates the levels of at least two second messengers in the cell: cAMP and the phosphoinositides. These second messengers in turn modulate PTH secretion.[82,412,413] The putative calcium receptor on the external surface of the plasma membrane of the parathyroid cell is linked to these second messenger systems by guanine-nucleotide regulatory (G) proteins.

Agents that affect cAMP levels in the parathyroid cell cause parallel changes in PTH secretion.[85] The parathyroid cell plasma membrane contains receptors that can either activate adenylyl cyclase (dopamine type 1, histamine type 2, β-adrenergic, secretin, and prostaglandin E_2) or inhibit adenylyl cyclase (alpha 1 and prostaglandin $F_{2\alpha}$). At present there is no evidence that agents acting through these receptors are important in parathyroid physiology, since administration of β-adrenergic catecholamines and their blockers in vivo do not affect PTH secretion. However, they may underlie the rapid pulsatile release[214,266,316,366] or stress-associated release[37] of PTH. High levels of calcium in vitro decrease cAMP levels in the parathyroid cells, but not sufficiently to account for its suppressive effects on PTH secretion.[85] Moreover, incubation of parathyroid cells with high levels of calcium diminishes the secretory effects of agents that release PTH by way of a cAMP mechanism without having large effects on cellular cAMP.[85] The calcium-mediated changes in cAMP levels most likely account for a component of the parathyroid's response to changes in calcium but do not account for the entire effect. Current evidence suggests that calcium inhibits cAMP formation through an inhibitory G protein–coupled receptor (G_i); uncoupling of the receptor from the inhibitory actions on adenylyl cyclase by ADP-ribosylation of G_i with pertussis toxin eliminates the calcium-induced inhibition of cAMP production.[132]

Increases in extracellular calcium provoke a brisk increase in cytosolic calcium that can be detected in vitro using intracellular calcium-sensitive fluorescent dyes such as fura-2.[329,413,414] The calcium is mobilized from cellular stores and from outside the cell through voltage-insensitive calcium channels. Mobilization of cellular calcium results from activation of phospholipase C, which leads to increased formation of inositol 1,4,5-trisphosphate (IP_3) and diacylglycerol from phosphatidylinositol bisphosphate.[83,531] The increased level of calcium in the cell is most likely not the inhibitor of secretion, since raising the calcium concentration of cells that have been rendered partially permeable by electroshock does not inhibit secretion.[431] IP_3 releases calcium from cellular stores[185] and thereby increases cytosolic calcium levels. Diacylglycerol activates protein kinase C; the role of protein kinase C in PTH secretion, if any, is controversial.[82]

There are at least three lines of evidence for a calcium receptor on the plasma membrane of parathyroid cells. One is that the trivalent cation lanthanum which does not penetrate cell membranes mimics the effect of calcium on mobilizing cell pools of calcium[415] and inhibiting PTH secretion.[83] Another is that inhibition of adenylyl cyclase and most likely activation of phospholipase C is mediated by G proteins that interact with cell surface receptors. Finally, Gylfe and colleagues have found a monoclonal antibody that binds to parathyroid cell surfaces that prevents the high calcium mediated mobilization of cellular calcium stores.[247] If this antibody truly binds to the calcium receptor, it may be a key to identifying and sequencing this protein.

Regulation of PTH secretion by vitamin D

1α,25-$(OH)_2$D provides a second negative feedback loop that modulates parathyroid gland function and reinforces the feedback effect of calcium. A wide range of in vivo and in vitro experiments suggest that 1α,25-$(OH)_2$D inhibits PTH synthesis and secretion. Parathyroid cells have been shown to contain receptors for 1α,25-$(OH)_2$D.[630] The addition of 1α,25-$(OH)_2$D to primary cultures of parathyroid cells reduces the level of PTH mRNA and the secretion of PTH.[536] Injection of 1α,25-$(OH)_2$D into rats reduces the PTH mRNA levels by more than 95 percent.[403] The action of 1α,25-$(OH)_2$D appears to be a direct effect on transcription[536] of the PTH gene and may be mediated by a hormone response element flanking the PTH gene. Okazaki and colleagues transfected constructs of the 5′ flanking region of the human PTH gene linked to a reporter gene into a rat pituitary cell line containing a 1α,25-$(OH)_2$D receptor.[432] Addition of 1α,25-$(OH)_2$D reduced reporter gene transcription; the response was not blocked by cycloheximide, suggesting that 1α,25-$(OH)_2$D and its receptor were acting directly on a hormone response element in the 5′ flanking region of the gene.

These studies indicate that 1α,25-$(OH)_2$D modulates hormone synthesis in the parathyroid but do not answer the physiologically more important question of whether secretion is modulated by 1α,25-$(OH)_2$D. The in vivo effect of 1α,25-$(OH)_2$D on PTH secretion has been difficult to discern because administration of 1α,25-$(OH)_2$D raises the level of calcium, which also feeds back on the parathyroid gland. In one interesting study, Madsen showed that 1α,25-$(OH)_2$D markedly reduced the level of PTH in patients with acute oliguric renal failure in whom the serum calcium was maintained by peritoneal dialysis.[355] The in vivo role of 1α,25-$(OH)_2$D in modulating the function of the parathyroid gland has been mostly studied in the setting of chronic renal failure because 1α,25-$(OH)_2$D deficiency in renal failure has been hypothesized to be a cause of secondary hyperparathyroidism in these patients. Delmez and colleagues found that after patients with chronic renal failure were treated with 1α,25-$(OH)_2$D intravenously for two weeks, PTH levels fell during a calcium infusion at a lower level of ionized plasma calcium than before treatment.[159] These data suggest that 1α,25-$(OH)_2$D modulates sensitivity to calcium of the parathyroid gland.

The possibility that 1α,25-$(OH)_2$D, in addition to calcium, feeds back on the parathyroid gland raises the question of whether there is any teleologic advantage to such a system. One advantage is that it may protect the skeleton when calcium intake is low. The increase in PTH in response to a decrease in calcium intake would increase bone resorption and 1α,25-$(OH)_2$D; the increase in 1α,25-$(OH)_2$D would not only correct the hypocalcemia but also suppress PTH directly and direct more of the adaptive response to diminished calcium intake to the intestine and away from PTH-mediated bone resorption.

Regulation of PTH secretion by magnesium

Magnesium levels also modulate PTH secretion (see Chaps. 13 and 34). The best known and most clinically important relationship is the hypocalcemia and relative hypoparathyroidism associated with chronic severe hypomagnesemia. The hypocalcemia and hypoparathyroidism are in large part a result of impaired secretion of PTH, and both are promptly restored after repletion of magnesium.[9,502,503,649] Chronic hypomagnesemia associated with impaired PTH secretion and hypocalcemia may occur in malnourished alcoholics and in the magnesium-wasting renal tubular disease associated with cisplatinum therapy. In contrast to the effect of chronic hypomagnesemia, acute reductions of magnesium concentration in vitro stimulate PTH secretion, and hypermagnesemia inhibits PTH in vivo and in vitro and potentiates the effect of hypercalcemia.[84,135,249,375] On a molar basis, magnesium is a less potent modulator of secretion than calcium, and the concentrations that influence PTH secretion are far beyond the normal range.[80] Acute hypomagnesemia is unlikely in vivo, but severe hypermagnesemia may occur in renal failure or during therapy of eclampsia.

Periodic secretion

PTH levels are generally constant, but careful inspection reveals a circadian variation with two main secretory peaks and smaller increases in PTH levels approximately every hour.[101,214,316,366] These variations in circulating levels of PTH have been shown most conclusively by recent studies using immunoassays specific for the intact PTH molecule.[101,316,366] The fluctuation of PTH levels is less than that of hormones such as luteinizing hormone or adrenocortical stimulating hormone; peak levels are approximately 30 percent greater than nadir concentrations. In some studies there is an inverse relationship between the increases in PTH and slight declines in serum calcium concentrations but no relationship to meals.[101,316,366] The stimulus for the periodicity of PTH or calcium is not known. One could speculate that secretion of PTH may be mediated by the nervous system through catecholamine-containing nerve endings in the gland. These periodic fluctuations of PTH levels may have a physiologic role in altering the action of the hormone on its target tissues. Intermittent administration of PTH to several animal species leads to stimulation of osteoblastic bone formation and an increase in bone mass; continuous administration of the same amount of hormone does not increase bone mass and even causes bone loss.[107,307,568]

Structure-function relationships and mechanism of action

The amino terminal end of the PTH molecule binds to cell surface receptors with hormone specificity, high affinity, and low capacity in classic target tissues such as bone and kidney as well as nonclassic target tissues such as smooth muscle, liver, and lymphocytes. The mechanism of action of the hormone is consistent with the emerging model of signal transduction across cell membranes of other peptide hormones and amines. The internal cell-signaling domain of the PTH receptor activates two second messenger systems by stimulating the enzymes adenylyl cyclase and phospholipase C (Fig. 11-15).[137,647] Each of these enzymes activates a cascade of second messengers that mediate the effects of the hormone. Adenylate cyclase generates cAMP, which activates cAMP-dependent protein kinase A and leads to the phosphorylation of cellular proteins. These phosphorylated proteins modulate a wide range of cellular processes, including secretion, membrane transport, intermediary metabolism, and gene transcription. The effects of cAMP on gene transcription are mediated by a family of newly discovered cAMP response element (CRE) binding proteins that, upon phosphorylation, bind to specific sequences in non-

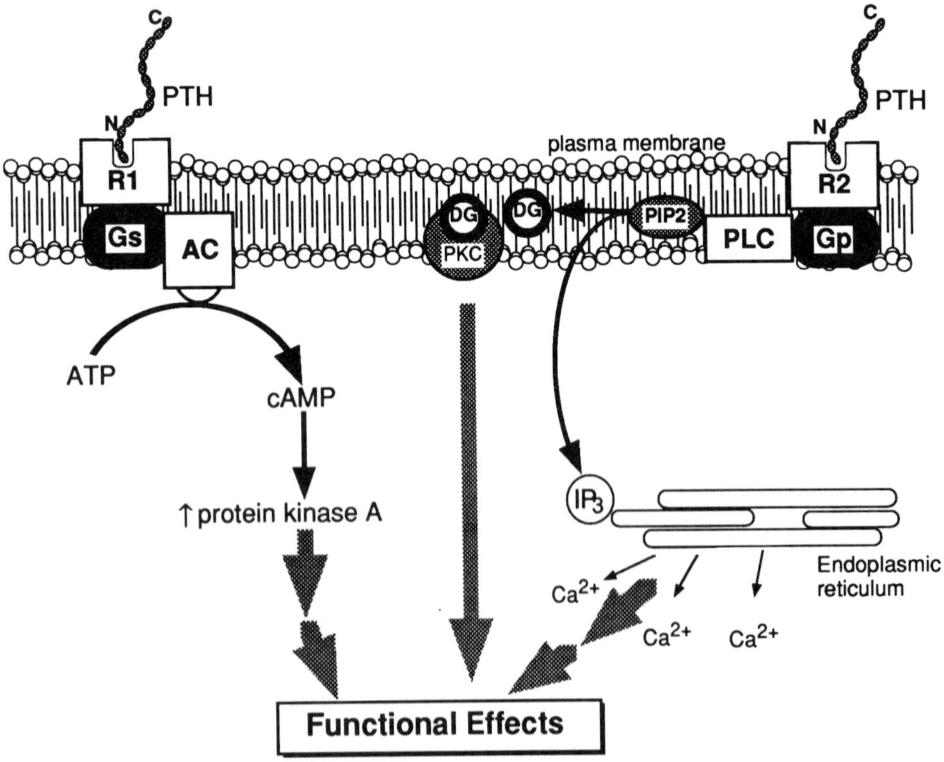

FIGURE 11-15 • Cellular mechanism of action of PTH. The N terminal of PTH binds to receptors (R1 and R2) activating two second messenger systems. The receptors are coupled to their second messenger pathways by G proteins, G_S and G_P. The first leads adenylyl cyclase (AC), stimulating formation of cAMP. cAMP activates protein kinase A, which phosphorylates proteins that modulate a wide range of cellular activities. The other receptor system activates phospholipase C (PLC), which increases the levels of inositol 1,4,5-trisphosphate (IP_3) and diacylglycerol (DAG). IP_3 raises intracellular calcium by releasing stores in the endoplasmic reticulum and by opening channels in the plasma membrane (not shown), modifying the activity of calcium-binding proteins. DAG activates protein kinase C (PKC) in the plasma membrane. The combined effects of increased cAMP, intracellular calcium, DAG, and IP_3 lead to the effects of PTH on its target cells.

transcribed regions flanking regions of genes and modulate their transcription.[248] The portions of the genome that are regulated by PTH have not yet been identified but will probably provide important insight into the mechanism of action of this hormone.

Activation of phospholipase C cleaves the membrane-bound lipid phosphatidylinositol 4,5 bisphosphate (PIP_2) to form IP_3 and diacylglycerol (DAG). IP_3 diffuses into the cell, causing release of calcium stored in the endoplasmic reticulum and a rapid rise in intracellular calcium.[137,647] IP_3 may also stimulate entry of calcium through calcium channels in the plasma membrane.[137,279,518] Rapid shift of calcium into cells probably accounts for the fact that the earliest effect of a large pulse of PTH on serum calcium in vivo is a decrease of 0.2 meq/liter with a nadir at 10 min.[446] A rise in intracellular calcium can initiate a cascade of intracellular events by activating calcium-binding proteins such as calmodulin, which in turn stimulate the activity of another protein kinase, calcium-calmodulin kinase II. DAG, the other product of PIP_2, remains membrane bound and activates yet another protein kinase, protein kinase C.

Receptor-mediated activation of both enzymes is mediated by guanine nucleotide-binding proteins, or G proteins.[301,557] In the case of adenylyl cyclase, PTH binding to the receptor causes G_s, one of the G proteins, to bind GTP, which converts it to the activated state. Activated G_s then stimulates the catalytic subunit of adenylyl cyclase to convert ATP to cAMP. The G protein then hydrolyzes GTP to GDP and is inactivated. The G proteins consist of an α subunit, which binds and hydrolyzes GTP, as well as β and γ subunits. Activation of phospholipase C is also dependent on a G protein called G_p. It is not known whether the PTH receptors coupled to these second messenger systems are the same molecule.

In the rare disorder known as *pseudohypoparathyroidism*, we can see the consequences of an abnormal G_s. Patients with pseudohypoparathyroidism have hypocalcemia and hyperphosphatemia as a result of resistance to the action of PTH; their circulating levels of PTH are elevated.[343] These patients may also have resistance to the effects of other hormones as well as abnormal physical features. In many of these patients, the genetic basis of the abnormality is known to be one of several mutations of the α subunit of G_s.[448]

As of the time of this writing, the full sequence of the PTH receptor has not been determined, but partial purification suggests that it is a glycoprotein, similar to other transmembrane receptors, with a molecular mass of 58 kilodaltons.[311] It is not known whether there are several forms of receptor in different tissues or whether separate types of receptors are linked to the different second messenger systems, similar to the case of receptors for glucagon and vasopressin. Prolonged exposure to high levels of PTH has been shown to *down-regulate* the number of receptors and blunts the response to PTH.[358] The number of receptors on bone cells is increased by high levels of *glucocorticoids*.[526] The physiologic role of this modulation is not known, but patients taking high doses of glucocorticoids lose bone in part as a result of enhanced osteoclastic bone resorption, an effect that may be mediated by enhanced response to PTH.[385]

Nephrogenous urinary cAMP

Urinary cAMP is derived from cAMP filtered at the glomerulus and cAMP produced in the kidney and spilled over into the urine (nephrogenous urinary cAMP).[63] Most of the cAMP produced in renal cells is metabolized intracellularly. Under normal circumstances half of urinary cAMP is derived from plasma and half is nephrogenous.[63,64] Although hormones such as vasopressin and CT stimulate cAMP production by renal cells, their contribution to basal levels of urinary cAMP, even when these hormones are at high levels, is insignificant. Basal nephrogenous urinary cAMP is almost entirely PTH-dependent; in hypoparathyroidism it is less than 20 percent of normal.

Measurement of nephrogenous cAMP can be employed as an in vivo bioassay of circulating PTH. Total urinary cAMP is often measured instead of nephrogenous cAMP because the latter requires measuring cAMP in plasma, which is technically demanding. Total urinary cAMP is an accurate index of PTH activity because the background of nonnephrogenous cAMP is relatively constant.

"Classical" actions

The principal actions of PTH on mineral metabolism, the "classical" actions of PTH, are confined to the *kidney* and *bone*. PTH acts on the kidney to increase the clearances of phosphorus and possibly bicarbonate and to decrease the clearances of calcium (see the section on "Kidneys") and magnesium. PTH also acts on the kidney to stimulate the production of $1\alpha,25\text{-}(OH)_2D$ (see "Synthesis and Metabolism of Vitamin D"). In bone, PTH inhibits osteoblast function and increases osteoclast and osteocyte function (see section on "Bone").

"Nonclassical" actions

Receptors for PTH have been identified in several cell types and organs (macrophages, lymphocytes, dermal fibroblasts, vascular and nonvascular smooth muscle, placenta, and brain) without a known role in mineral homeostasis. For example, PTH relaxes vascular and non-vascular smooth muscle in vitro, and injections of PTH in vivo cause hypotension.[389] In brain, PTH increases calcium transport of synaptosomal membranes, and high levels of PTH such as those seen in renal failure are thought to mediate the CNS dysfunction of uremia.[371] The physiologic role of these receptors has been an enigma for many years. The recent discovery of PTH-related proteins (PTHrPs) suggests that the responses to PTH in these tissues are mediated by receptors intended for PTHrPs that are generated locally and act in a paracrine manner.

PTH-RELATED PROTEINS

Certain malignancies cause hypercalcemia by producing a humoral factor that has long been suspected as being either PTH itself[6] or a protein resembling PTH in activity.[555] The search for a factor responsible for the so-called humoral hypercalcemia of malignancy led to the recent discovery of PTHrP, a protein expressed in many tissues, which resembles PTH and has PTH-like bioactivity. PTHrP was purified from cell lines derived from tumors causing the syndrome and the cDNAs cloned from libraries derived from these cells.[563]

PTHrP is approximately twice the size of PTH. In the amino terminal, 8 of the first 13 amino acids are identical to those of PTH (Fig. 11-16). Thereafter the peptides diverge in sequence, but the primary structure of the first 34 amino acids gives PTHrp a conformation that binds to and activates PTH receptors. Synthetic peptides with the first 34 amino acids of PTHrp produce hypercalcemia after injection in rats, increase bone resorption in vivo and in vitro, increase renal calcium reabsorption, and produce phosphaturia.[273,490,650] The function of the remainder of the molecule is not known. The domain between amino acids 34 and 111 is highly conserved between species, suggesting that it has an important—although unknown—function. This region also contains potential amidation sites, suggesting that the peptide undergoes posttranslational processing. The carboxyl terminal domain can contain one of three segments that arise as a result of alternative splicing of the 3′ exon of the PTHrP gene.[362,580]

The PTHrP gene contains nine exons that predict protein species of 139, 141, and 173 amino acids in length. The middle portion of the PTHrP gene containing exons 2 to 4 has an intron-exon organization identical to that of the three exons of the PTH gene.[367] The PTHrP gene has been located on chromosome 12, while the gene for PTH is on chromosome 11.[361] It is likely that the PTH and PTHrP genes have arisen from duplication of a common ancestral gene. Several other related genes are on both chromosome 12 and 11, and the short arms of both chromosomes are thought to have arisen from a duplication event. The 3′ untranslated region of PTHrP mRNA contains multiple copies of an AU motif that is associated with mRNA instability and rapid turnover.[288] Several cytokines and proto-oncogenes with short mRNAs carry this motif, which may provide a mechanism for rapid dissipation of a paracrine or autocrine signal.[554]

PTHrP levels in plasma are elevated in a high percentage of patients with hypercalcemia associated with solid tumors, including squamous cell carcinoma of the lung, head and neck, and esophagus; genitourinary cancers; and breast cancers.[96,263,309] In addition, a small percentage of patients with hypercalcemia associated with hematologic neoplasms (lymphoma and multiple myeloma) also have increased levels of PTHrP.[94,261,307] In contrast, PTHrP levels are not elevated in most normocalcemic patients with malignancy or in patients with primary hyperparathyroidism.

PTHrP is also produced by several normal tissues, where it may have a role that is not related to its effects on classic target tissues of PTH. Using Northern analysis, mRNA transcripts of PTHrP have been found in lactating breast; brain; placenta; keratinocytes; parathyroid gland; thyroid gland; fetal, but not adult, liver; and gravid rat

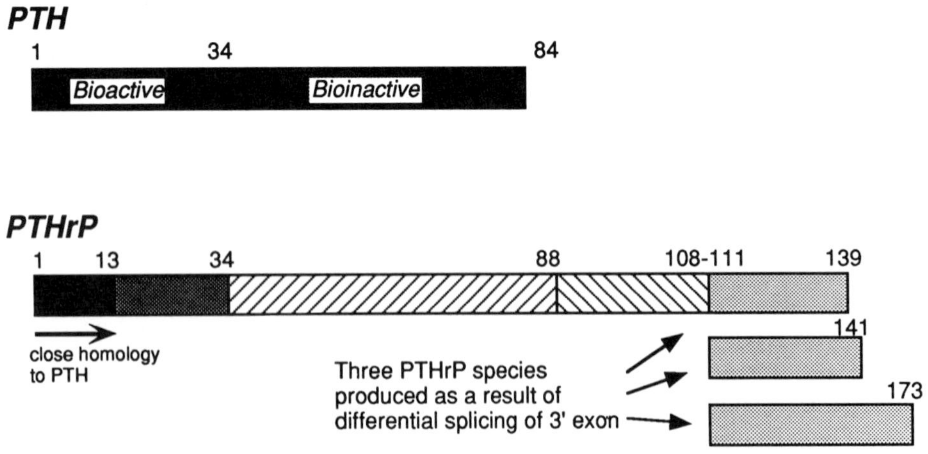

FIGURE 11-16 • Protein structure of PTH and PTH-related proteins (PTHrPs). There is a high degree of homology between the two peptides in the first 13 amino acids of the N terminal. The remainder of the first 34 amino acids are dissimilar, but synthetic fragments of PTHrP containing the first 25 residues bind to PTH receptors and have full PTH bioactivity. The region of PTHrP between 34 and 88 is highly conserved across several species, but its function is not known. The region between residues 88 and 111 contains several amidation sites. The carboxyl terminal region can contain one of three sequences of different lengths as a result of alternate splicing of mRNA.

myometrium.[554] In most of these tissues PTHrP appears to have a paracrine or autocrine role. To date there is no evidence that there is a distinct PTHrP receptor that is different from the receptor for PTH. One interesting role of PTHrP is in the rat breast, where PTHrP is produced transiently after suckling.[579] Suckling is known to stimulate pituitary secretion of prolactin, which augments milk production, and injection of prolactin into rats enhances production of PTHrP mRNA.[578] PTHrP is also transported into the milk, where levels are nearly 1000-fold those in plasma.[90,315] The role of PTHrP in milk production is currently unknown but likely to be a local one. There is no evidence that lactation increases circulating PTHrP, although PTHrP (perhaps produced locally in other tissues) may have a role in mobilizing calcium for breast milk; it is known that women with hypoparathyroidism paradoxically need less calcium and vitamin D supplements when they are lactating.[155] The capacity of breast to make PTHrP is not surprising, since hypercalcemia associated with breast cancer is likely mediated by PTHrP.

PTHrP is produced in large quantities by human epidermal keratinocytes, and it appears to stimulate differentiation of keratinocytes into cornified epithelium.[434] PTHrP from the placenta or the parathyroid gland may modulate the placental calcium pump, which maintains the plasma calcium in the mammalian fetus at a higher level than maternal plasma level.[367,491] Thyroparathyroidectomy of fetal calves results in hypocalcemia that is not ameliorated by infusion of PTH,[120] but infusion of partially purified preparations of PTHrP in isolated placentae enhances placental calcium transport.[491] PTHrP is also expressed in the last 48 h of gestation in rat uterine myometrium.[582] Since PTHrP is known to relax smooth muscle[389] and uterine contractions,[441] it may have a role in relaxing the uterus during the phases of contraction and relaxation that occur in the last few days of pregnancy.[582]

The cloning and sequencing of the PTHrP gene confirmed that a PTH-like peptide was responsible for the humoral hypercalcemia associated with malignancy. The discovery of the diverse roles of this peptide and its receptor in a growing range of tissues has been an unexpected and fascinating insight. The story that has emerged from the first three years of investigation is that several tissues use PTHrP and the PTH receptor to transmit a wide range of local messages, which in most cases are not related to classic actions of PTH or effects on calcium metabolism.

CALCITONIN

CT is a 32-amino acid peptide that is secreted by *C cells in the thyroid* as well as several other tissues. At high concentrations, CT inhibits osteoclastic bone resorption. The *role of calcitonin in normal human physiology, if any, is unknown.*

Origin and biosynthesis

The main sources of circulating CT in mammals are the C cells, or parafollicular cells, that are dispersed within the upper and lateral portions of the thyroid gland. These cells derive from the neural crest and become the ultimobranchial body in lower vertebrates. In mammals, the ultimobranchial body fuses with the thyroid gland. CT is also present in tissues such as lung, brain, gastrointestinal tract, and pituitary gland, where it is usually made by cells of neuroendocrine origin. Although these tissues contribute to circulating CT, only secretion from the C cell is responsive to hypercalcemia.

The sequencing of the CT gene has led to the elucidation of a pathway of biosynthesis of unusual complexity. CT derives from a large gene with six exons on chromosome 11. Two of the exons encode two other secreted peptides, katacalcin and CT gene–related peptide (CGRP; Fig. 11-17). The physiologic role of katacalcin, if any, is not known. CGRP is a neurotransmitter and a potent vasodilator. The single primary mRNA transcript from the CT gene is spliced in C cells to yield either a precursor mRNA that encodes a 141-amino acid peptide with CT and katacalcin. In other tissues the same precursor is spliced to yield a 128-amino acid CGRP precursor (Fig. 11-17). Most tissues with an active CT gene express CGRP. The C cells mostly express CT but also synthesize and secrete CGRP. A second CT gene, the β-CGRP gene, has been found also on chromosome 11.[334,551] It contains a sequence that codes for a CT-like peptide, but this sequence is preceded by a termination codon that prevents expression.[334,506,551]

CT is a single-chain peptide with a disulfide bridge between amino acids 1 and 7. The sequence of CT from several species is known. The CTs from different species differ mostly in the mid-portion of the molecule. Analysis of the structure of these CTs as well as modifications of the human CT have shown that the amino-terminal disulfide bridge and the carboxy-terminal proline amide residue are critical for biological activity, although the disulfide bridge can be replaced with a $-CH_2-CH_2-$ bridge. Surprisingly, fish CTs are more potent in humans than the native human peptide. The unusual potency of these molecules results both from resistance to degradation and from an exceptionally high receptor affinity.

The presence of CGRP in nerve and brain suggests that it functions as a neurotransmitter. CGRP is a potent vasodilator, and high concentrations of the peptide have been found in perivascular nerves,[396] where it may modulate regional blood flow. It also has a hypocalcemic effect similar to that of CT but is two to three orders of magnitude less potent than CT.[586]

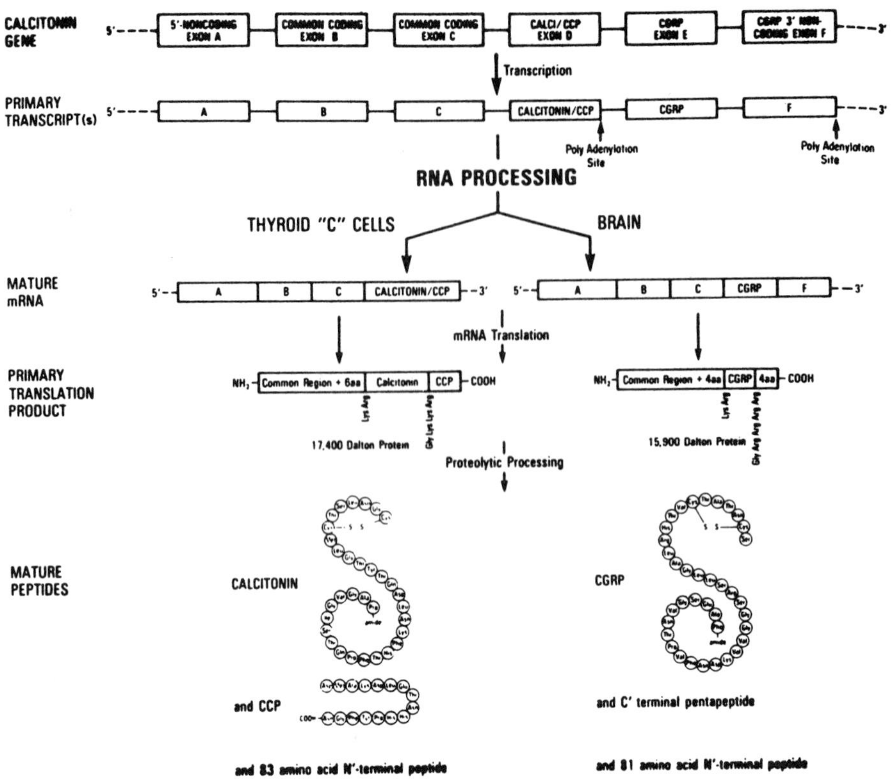

FIGURE 11-17 • Structural organization and processing of the α-calcitonin/CGRP gene. The primary transcript has two polyadenylation sites and, by differential tissue-specific processing, can yield two different mRNAs, one coding for the CGRP precursor and one coding for the calcitonin precursor.

Secretion

Extracellular calcium appears to be the most important factor that enhances CT secretion from C cells. An acute rise in the level of calcium provokes a brisk increase in CT secretion. Since high levels of CT have a hypocalcemic effect, CT is presumed to have a role in protecting against acute hypercalcemia. Chronic hypercalcemia does not increase circulating levels of CT.[584] Histopathologic studies show that hypercalcemia causes only modest hyperplasia of C cells; depletion of granule storage is a more prominent finding.[653] Several gastrointestinal peptides, including gastrin, cholecystokinin, secretin, and cerulein, stimulate CT secretion when infused at pharmacologic concentrations. The effect of calcium and the gastrointestinal peptides on CT secretion suggests that CT responds to meals, especially those that are high in calcium, but attempts to demonstrate such a response have been negative.[436] Similarly, 1α,25-$(OH)_2D$ has been shown to inhibit synthesis of CT,[401,402] but there is no evidence that changes in the blood levels of 1α,25-$(OH)_2D$ in normal or in pathologic states influence CT levels.

Circulating CT exists as several immunochemical species.[15,39] In patients with medullary carcinoma of the thyroid and in patients with lung cancers, a substantial proportion of their circulating hormone exists as higher-molecular weight moieties of CT.[39] The heterogeneity may be a result of dimerization of CT by means of disulfide linkages as well as monomers bound to plasma proteins and high-molecular weight forms that are incompletely processed. This heterogeneity of CT in plasma has complicated the interpretation of many studies. More recent assays performed with plasma extracts have increased the sensitivity and specificity of measuring monomeric CT and allowed measurement in the physiologic range.[39] One area of controversy that has been resolved with assays for monomeric CT is whether the level of CT and its responsiveness to calcium decline with age or are lower in women. This issue has received considerable attention because it has been hypothesized that low levels of CT have a pathogenetic role in osteoporosis.[380] Assays for monomeric CT show that there is no aging-associated decline in the level of CT or secretory reserve, but levels of CT are lower in women than in men.[39,585]

Actions

The principal effect of an acute infusion of CT on calcium metabolism is a prompt inhibition of bone resorption. The reduced flux of calcium from bone can cause a mild reduction in the level of circulating calcium. The effect of CT on bone is a result of a rapid and direct inhibitory effect on bone resorption by osteoclasts and perhaps also by osteocytes. Isolated osteoclasts in vitro undergo dramatic reductions in migration and morphological changes when exposed to CT.[127,128] The ruffled border of the osteoclast decreases within minutes of exposure to CT, and the cell begins to withdraw from bone-resorbing surfaces. Receptors for CT have been shown on rat osteoclasts,[424] where CT appears to act by stimulating cAMP formation. CT receptors have not been found on osteoblasts. During chronic administration, CT reduces bone turnover rather than causing hypocalcemia; presumably the inhibitory effect on osteoclasts leads to reduced activation of bone remodeling units and a parallel reduction in bone formation. In addition, osteoclasts appear to "escape" from other actions of CT within days of administration, so that the hypocalcemic action is markedly blunted. This phenomenon may be the result of down-regulation of CT receptors in bone.[571]

Acute infusion of pharmacologic doses of CT increases urinary excretion of sodium, calcium, and phosphate[32] and enhances renal synthesis of $1\alpha,25\text{-}(OH)_2D$.[297] These actions, while important in pharmacology, may not contribute to normal physiology of kidney or bone, since the levels required for these effects may be above those achieved during normal CT secretion.

Although CT was discovered and named because of its capacity to lower serum calcium, it is possible that this peptide has other functions. In submammalian vertebrates without a bony skeleton, such as the shark, CT produces hypercalcemia via effects on calcium-transporting organs such as the kidney, intestine, or gills.[231] CT acts upon the salmon gill to increase efflux of calcium and phosphorus and to decrease perfusate flow rate.[386] High levels of CT in utero (a stage wherein circulating calcium is controlled by mother and not fetus) suggest that it has a trophic effect on bone development.[509] Indeed, CT directly stimulates proliferation of immature, but not of mineralizing, fetal cartilage.[633]

Actions in CNS and other tissues

CT is found in several tissues, including lung, parathyroid gland, gastrointestinal tract, hypothalamus, and pituitary gland. The distribution of CT is similar to that of other peptides made in neuroendocrine cells, such as somatostatin, cholecystokinin, and bombesin. In these tissues CT may play a role as a neurotransmitter. Pharmacologic doses of CT decrease the secretion of pancreatic enzymes, gastrin, and gastric acid as well as secretion of potassium, chloride, sodium, and water by the small intestine. Administration of CT intracerebrally induces analgesia and enhances glucose-stimulated insulin release from the pancreas.[241]

Physiologic role in humans

CT has been proposed to have two effects in normal human physiology. One is to blunt abrupt increases in serum calcium during sudden calcium entry into the circulation after a calcium-rich meal. Although this effect of CT is evident during acute calcium infusions, there is no evidence that under normal circumstances humans are challenged with acute increases of calcium that would stimulate CT secretion. Chronic increases in the level of serum calcium do not enhance CT secretion.

CT has also been proposed to have an anabolic effect on the skeleton, but this remains an unproven hypothesis. According to this hypothesis, the rise in CT in response to calcium from a meal or in response to gastrointestinal hormones would inhibit bone resorption and blunt the rise in the level of serum calcium, keeping calcium in bone and preventing its loss in urine. However, there is no demonstrable rise in the level of CT in response to meals.[436] The notion of an anabolic skeletal effect of CT is supported by some studies showing that patients who have had their thyroids removed have less bone mass than controls with intact thyroid glands,[381] but bone loss in these patients may have been a result of administration of supraphysiologic doses of thyroid hormones or other factors besides CT. Hurley and coworkers recently found that bone mineral density in patients who had had total thyroidectomy was not lower than in patients with intact thyroid glands.[285] There is also no evidence that CT plays a major role in the genesis of osteoporosis, since recent studies have not shown a decrease in plasma levels of CT or secretory reserve in patients with osteoporosis.[28,467,583] Finally, the markedly elevated levels of CT associated with C-cell tumors and medullary carcinoma of the thyroid are not associated with increased bone mineral density,[285] although bone turnover in these patients is markedly reduced.

CALCIFEROLS

The calciferols are a class of fat-soluble secosteroids (i.e., a steroid with an open ring; the B-ring of calciferols is open) that are more properly considered a steroid hormone than a vitamin. The parent compounds are cholecalciferol, vitamin D_3, which is made in the skin upon exposure to ultraviolet (UV) light and ergocalciferol, vitamin D_2, which is produced by irradiating the plant sterol ergosterol. Vitamin D (the term D refers to D_3 and/or D_2) is a prohormone that is metabolized in the liver and kidney to form $1\alpha,25\text{-}(OH)_2D$, which activates receptors in target tissues and plays a critical role in maintaining calcium homeostasis. The discovery of vitamin D followed observations in the nineteenth century that a high percentage of children raised in crowded, polluted, industrial cities had a deforming bone disease called rickets. In 1919, Mellanby[384] and Huldschinsky[284] showed that addition of cod liver oil to the diet or skin exposure to sunlight could cure rickets. In 1924, Steenbock[552] and Hess[267] discovered independently that foods exposed to a mercury vapor lamp had antirachitic activity. This led to fortification of foods with irradiated provitamin D and eventually vitamin D and to the elucidation of the structure of vitamin D and its derivatives.

Synthesis and metabolism of vitamin D

Sources of vitamin D

Vitamin D_3 is synthesized from 7-dehydrocholesterol in skin nonenzymatically under the influence of UV light (Fig. 11-18). In the first step of the reaction, UV light with a wavelength between 280 and 310 nm penetrates into the basal layer of the epidermis and produces previtamin D_3. Previtamin D_3 undergoes thermal isomerization to vitamin D_3 over a 3-day period. Once formed, vitamin D_3 diffuses into the capillary bed.

The amount of vitamin D produced in skin is primarily a function of the amount of exposure to UV light, but other factors also influence this process. Large amounts of the skin pigment melanin compete for absorption of UV light, and persons with dark skin require several times the sunlight exposure of lightly pigmented individuals to make the same amount of vitamin D.[269,270] Therefore, dark skin pigment is an advantage in regions of the world where sun exposure is intense. Holick and colleagues have found a second mechanism that may be more important in protecting against vitamin D intoxication from sun exposure.[270] Previtamin D in skin also absorbs UV light and isomerizes to lumisterol or tachysterol, which remain in the skin and are shed with the epidermis.[270] Holick and associates have shown that, regardless of the extent of skin pigmentation, only 10 to 20 percent of 7-dehydrocholesterol is converted to vitamin D.[270] These two mechanisms can prevent excess production of vitamin D with long exposure to sunlight. Vitamin D_3 production in skin is also known to decline with age. The mechanism appears to be an age-related decline in the amount of 7-dehydrocholesterol in the skin.[354]

Most of the vitamin D in residents of the United States derives from sun exposure. Only a few foods naturally contain vitamin D. These include fish and mammalian livers and egg yolks. In much of the world, foods are fortified with vitamin D. In the United States, milk is fortified with 10 μg (400 IU) of either vitamin D_2 or D_3 per quart; the recommended daily allowance for adults is 5 mg. Dietary vitamin D is absorbed in the small bowel with the aid of bile salts, incorporated into chylomicrons in the intestinal wall, and transported to the circulation and liver via the thoracic duct.[250]

Vitamin D is very fat soluble and is mostly stored in fat tissue. The half-life of tissue stores of vitamin D is several months, which allows vitamin D stores to be maintained in normal individuals living at high latitudes who only get sun exposure during a small part of the year. Krall and associates have shown that postmenopausal women (mean age 58 years) in Massachusetts who consumed less than 220 IU of vitamin D daily had mild though significant increases of PTH levels, presumably to compensate for inadequate vitamin D supplies, during the late winter months, while PTH levels did not increase in women consuming more than 220 IU.[319] In older individuals, not only is the synthesis of vitamin D reduced in

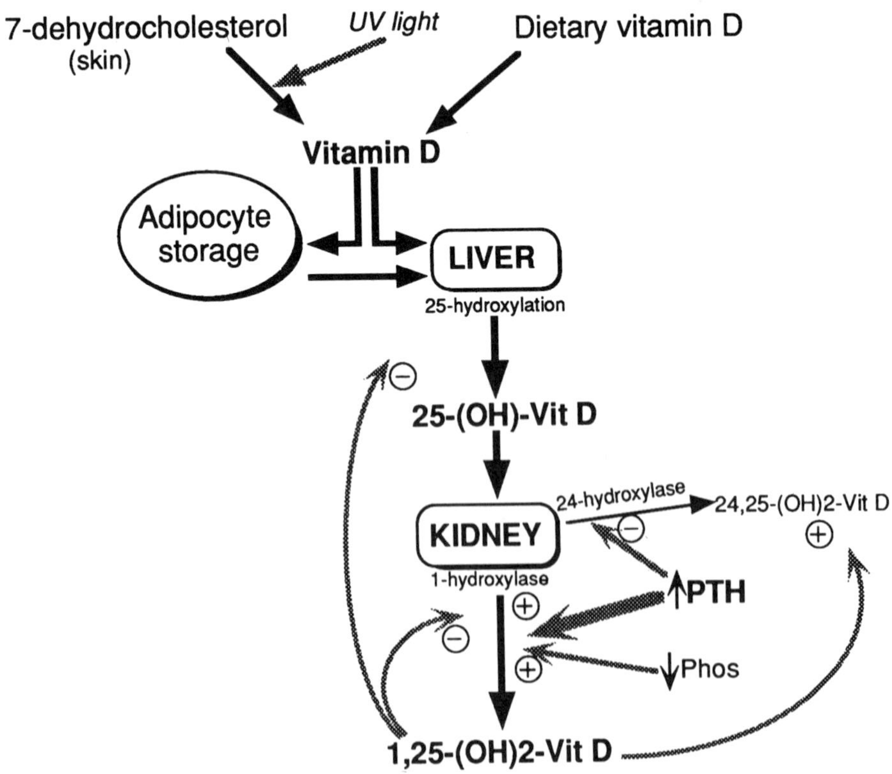

FIGURE 11-18 • Schematic depiction of sequence of activation of vitamin D to form 1α,25-$(OH)_2$D.

skin, but intake of foods fortified with vitamin D is often reduced. The other implication of the long half-life of vitamin D is that hypervitaminosis D (usually a result of chronic administration of daily doses in excess of 1 mg or 40,000 IU) may persist for several months.

Synthesis of 25-(OH)D

The first step in the synthesis of the metabolically active vitamin D, 1α,25-$(OH)_2D$, is 25-hydroxylation in the liver by a cytochrome P_{450} monooxygenase (Fig. 11-18).[507] This step is loosely regulated. The rate of synthesis of 25-(OH)D is primarily determined by the concentration of substrate, vitamin D. Since there is a close relationship between stores of vitamin D and levels of 25-(OH)D, the serum level of 25-(OH)D is an index of the cumulative exposure to sunlight and dietary intake of vitamin D and is a useful clinical tool. Circulating 25-(OH)D is tightly bound to vitamin D–binding protein (DBP). Although 25-(OH)D does not have biologic activity at physiologic concentrations, at supraphysiologic levels it may have the same actions as high levels of 1α,25-$(OH)_2D$, producing hypercalcemia.

The half-life of 25-(OH)D in the circulation is around 15 days. Studies in rats have shown that the clearance of 25-(OH)D is enhanced by high levels of 1α,25-$(OH)_2D$ produced either by administration of 1α,25-$(OH)_2D$ or by a low-calcium diet.[138,252] The increased clearance of 25-(OH)D is primarily in the liver, since a substantial amount of the 25-(OH)D is excreted in the bile.[138] Feedback lowering of 25-(OH)D levels by high levels of 1α,25-$(OH)_2D$ may explain the low levels of 25-(OH)D in gastrointestinal or hepatic disorders characterized by intestinal malabsorption of calcium and secondary hyperparathyroidism.

Renal synthesis of 1α,25-$(OH)_2D$

The final step in the activation of vitamin D is 1α-hydroxylation of 25-(OH)D to form 1α,25-$(OH)_2D$, which has 500 to 1000 times greater biologic activity than its precursor, 25-(OH)D (Fig. 11-18). 1α,25-$(OH)_2D$ is the biologically active form of vitamin D and appears to be responsible for all of the known effects of vitamin D on calcium metabolism. It is also the most potent sterol in promoting calcium transport and bone calcium mobilization. Circulating levels of 1α,25-$(OH)_2D$ in humans are 500-fold to 1000-fold lower than those of 25-(OH)D. 1α,25-$(OH)_2D$ is transported in the circulation bound to DBP but less avidly so than 25-(OH)D. It has a circulating half-life of 4 to 6 h.[240]

The principal site for 1α-hydroxylation is in the renal proximal tubule.[313] The enzyme is a mixed-function cytochrome P_{450} hydroxylase. Although several other tissues have been shown to be capable of metabolizing 25-(OH)D to 1α,25-$(OH)_2D$ (see below), the kidney is the only one that significantly contributes to circulating levels of 1α,25-$(OH)_2D$. The best evidence for this is that in patients who have had bilateral nephrectomy, circulating concentrations of 1α,25-$(OH)_2D$ are low or undetectable.[525] The exception to this generalization is the placenta; during pregnancy the placenta produces 1α,25-$(OH)_2D$, and levels of both total and free 1α,25-$(OH)_2D$ are elevated.

Renal synthesis of 1α,25-$(OH)_2D$ is tightly regulated, in contrast to synthesis of 25-(OH)D, and closely related to the body economy of calcium. The principal regulator of 1α,25-$(OH)_2D$ synthesis is PTH. A drop in serum calcium provokes a corrective rise in the level of PTH, which enhances renal calcium conservation and bone resorption. The rise in 1α,25-$(OH)_2D$ in response to PTH enhances the PTH effect on bone and stimulates intestinal absorption of calcium. The increase in 1α,25-$(OH)_2D$ in response to PTH may lag as much as 12 h behind the rise in PTH and the calcemic effect several hours more, since it requires induction of protein synthesis in intestine and bone. Synthesis of 1α,25-$(OH)_2D$ is also directly inhibited by 1α,25-$(OH)_2D$ in cultured kidney cells.[569]

The rate of synthesis of 1α,25-$(OH)_2D$ in the kidney is inversely related to the level of circulating inorganic phosphate, but the level of phosphate itself may not be the modulator. One possibility is that it is related in some way to transport across the renal tubule. A low phosphorus intake enhances renal tubular reabsorption of phosphate and increases production of 1α,25-$(OH)_2D$, while diseases of the renal tubule with impaired tubular reabsorption of phosphate (such as hypophosphatemic rickets) are associated with low levels of 1α,25-$(OH)_2D$.[23] Extreme changes in dietary phosphorus intake (625 to 2300 mg/day) can provoke almost twofold changes in the level of 1α,25-$(OH)_2D$ (Fig. 11-19).[464] However, variations in dietary phosphorus within the range of a typical diet most likely have little influence on the level of 1α,25-$(OH)_2D$. Calvo and colleagues showed that when normal adults were switched from a typical normal diet containing 930 mg/day of phosphorus and

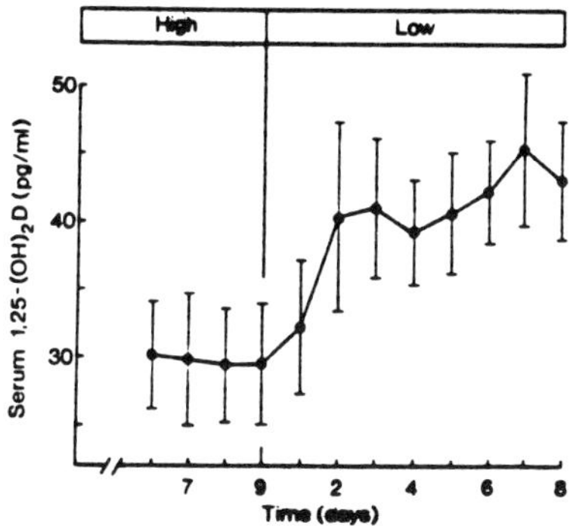

FIGURE 11-19 • Effect of a reduction of dietary intake of phosphorus from 2300 mg/day to 625 mg/day 1α,25-$(OH)_2D$.

820 mg/day calcium to a diet more typical of an adolescent ingesting large quantities of soda pop with 1660 mg/day phosphorus and 420 mg/day calcium, the serum concentration of 1α,25-$(OH)_2D$ increased.[101] This study suggests that the suppressive effect of phosphorus on 1,25-$(OH)_2D$ synthesis is overridden by the increase in PTH caused by the hypocalcemic effect of both high phosphorus and low calcium intake. The suppressive effects of phosphate on 1α,25-$(OH)_2D$ synthesis are probably more important in patients with renal insufficiency.[463] In normal individuals, phosphorus intake most likely plays a minor role in modulating serum levels of 1α,25-$(OH)_2D$, since phosphorus is a constitutive component of most diets, and (unlike calcium) extremes of dietary intake are unusual.

24-hydroxylation of vitamin D

The most abundant dihydroxyvitamin D metabolite in the circulation is 24,25-$(OH)_2D$. In general, 24-hydroxylation of 25-(OH)D is regulated in a direction opposite that for 1-hydroxylation.[368] 1α,25-$(OH)_2D$ stimulates 24-hydroxylation, and PTH inhibits this enzyme.[146] In the vitamin D–deficient state, the activity of the 24-hydroxylase is low, and 1-hydroxylation in increased. When vitamin D is replete, 24-hydroxylase activity is increased, and 1-hydroxylation is inhibited.

Both hydroxylase enzymes have a similar distribution in the kidney, but 24-hydroxylase activity has been found in nearly all tissues known to have 1α,25-$(OH)_2D$ receptors.[481] The distribution of the principal calciferol metabolites in the body is quantitated in Table 11-5. The physiologic role of 24,25-$(OH)_2D$ has long been a subject of investigation and debate. At present the best evidence is that 24,25-$(OH)_2D$ has no biologic activity and merely represents a degradation product of 1α,25-$(OH)_2D$.[269,274] 1α,25-$(OH)_2D$ is also a substrate for the 24-hydroxylase enzyme; 1α,24,25-$(OH)_3D$ appears to be minor but active metabolite of 1α,25-$(OH)_2D$.

Extrarenal synthesis of 1α,25-$(OH)_2D$

In vitro studies have shown that a wide range of tissues can metabolize 25-(OH)D to 1α,25-$(OH)_2D$. These include normal human bone cells, chick intestinal cells, human neonatal keratinocytes, and cultured human melanoma cells.[23,269] 1α,25-$(OH)_2D$ production by cultured macrophages is enhanced when these cells are stimulated by lipopolysaccharides from cell walls of gram-negative bacteria or γ-interferon.[269] This finding may explain the enhanced 1α,25-$(OH)_2D$ production and hypercalcemia in some patients with granulomatous diseases such as *sarcoidosis* and *tuberculosis*. In sarcoidosis, high levels of 1α,25-$(OH)_2D$ are not produced in the kidney, since they persist after nephrectomy.[18] The best evidence is that the 1α,25-$(OH)_2D$ is made by inflammatory cells in the granuloma; cultured pulmonary alveolar macrophages from patients with sarcoidosis produce 1α,25-$(OH)_2D$[1] and lymph node homogenates from these patients can 1α-hydroxylate ^3H-25-(OH)D. Occasional patients with Hodgkin's or non-Hodgkin's lymphomas, which are tumors of the lymphocyte line, have hypercalcemia as a result of enhanced production of 1α,25-$(OH)_2D$.

Aside from late stages of pregnancy, the contribution of extrarenal production of 1α,25-$(OH)_2D$ to circulating levels is minor. As discussed below, under "Biological Actions of 1α,25-$(OH)_2D$," this sterol may have a local or paracrine role in extrarenal tissues, particularly immune cells.

Transport of vitamin D and its metabolites

Vitamin D and all its metabolites are bound in the circulation to DBP. This protein has been sequenced and shown to consist of 458 amino acids with a high degree of homology to albumin and α-fetoprotein.[148] It has been hypothesized that all three proteins arose from a common progenitor.[148] DBP has only one sterol-binding site per molecule, and this binding site has a higher affinity for

TABLE 11-5 • Metabolic parameters of the major calciferols in humans

Metabolite	Serum concentration, ng/ml	Serum half-life, days	Body pool, μg	Turnover, μg/day
Vitamin D*	10	30	1000	15
25-(OH)D	30	15	200	7
1α, 25-$(OH)_2D$	0.03	0.2	0.5	1

NOTE: These are estimates of average values; the normal ranges vary approximately from one-third to three times the mean.
* D refers to D_2 plus D_3.

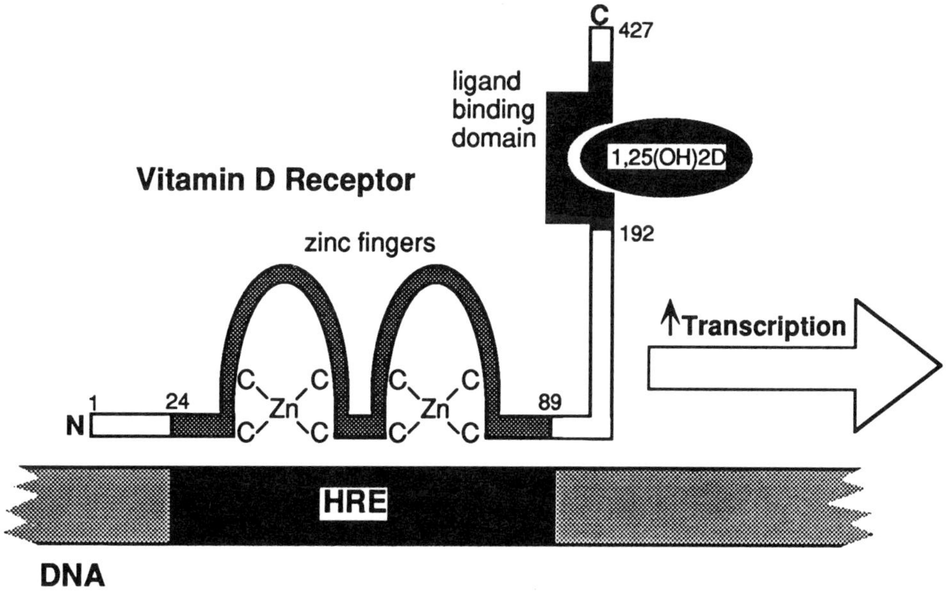

FIGURE 11-20 • Interaction of vitamin D receptor protein containing 1α,25-$(OH)_2D$ with the hormone response element (HRE) of a target gene.

25-(OH)D than for 1α,25-$(OH)_2D$ or vitamin D. Since the concentration of the plasma binding sites is far in excess of the concentrations of vitamin D, less than 5 percent of available binding sites are generally occupied. Levels of DBP are not known to be modified in disorders of calcium metabolism. In pregnancy and during estrogen therapy, DBP synthesis in the liver is increased. This increases the total concentration of vitamin D metabolites in serum, although an increased synthesis of 1α,25-$(OH)_2D$ leads to an increase in the levels of free 1α,25-$(OH)_2D$ as well.

There is no evidence that DBP has any role in facilitating access of 1α,25-$(OH)_2D$ to its target tissues. Its most likely function is to facilitate the solubility of vitamin D and its metabolites in serum and provide a reservoir of vitamin D and its metabolites.

Biological actions of 1α,25-$(OH)_2D$

Modes of action

With regard to mineral metabolism, 1α,25-$(OH)_2D$ should be viewed as a hormone produced by the kidney under feedback regulation and acting on distant target tissues. The target organs for the hormonal effects of 1α,25-$(OH)_2D$ are *bone, intestine, kidney,* and *parathyroid gland.* In addition, 1α,25-$(OH)_2D$ has effects on cells such as lymphocytes, monocytes, and keratinocytes, where it may function as a paracrine or autocrine factor.

1α,25-$(OH)_2D$ acts on its target cells by binding to the nuclear vitamin D receptor (VDR). The VDR then binds to selective regions of target genes, the hormone response elements (HREs), to up-regulate or down-regulate transcription of these genes. The VDR is a 48-kilodalton protein that has been cloned and shown to be structurally related to the nuclear receptors for other steroid hormones. These receptors are also known as the superfamily of intracellular receptors and include receptors for estrogen, thyroid hormone, glucocorticoids, retinoic acid, and androgens as well as the v-erbA oncogene.[193] The receptor proteins share a highly conserved DNA binding domain with two "zinc fingers" and a hormone binding domain that is less highly conserved. The zinc fingers are loops of amino acids with basic amino acids at the base of the loops that bind zinc (Fig. 11-20). The positively charged amino acids interact with the negatively charged DNA. Specific amino acids in the region of the zinc finger closest to the N terminal determine whether the receptor binds to the HRE for 1α,25-$(OH)_2D$ or another steroid hormone.[213] The carboxyl terminal of the steroid receptor proteins contains a region with high-affinity, steroid-specific recognition sites that are less well conserved, reflecting the specificity for their different ligands.

The sequence of the vitamin D response element (VDRE) has been determined by deletion and reconstruction of DNA sequences within the promoter region of the osteocalcin gene.[162,394] The sequence of the VDRE is similar to the sequence of HRE of other steroid hormones.

The VDRE of the osteocalcin gene has been extensively studied and is located about 500 base pairs upstream from the site of initiation of transcription.[162,280,365] It contains a complex palindromic sequence that has similarity to the estrogen response element as well as the thyroid hormone response element.[394] It is known that glucocorticoids inhibit the effects of 1α,25-$(OH)_2D$ on calcium absorption in the intestine and inhibit 1α,25-$(OH)_2D$ induction of osteocalcin synthesis in bone. Using promoter expression constructs of the human osteocalcin gene transfected into stable cell lines, Morrison and coworkers showed that the glucocorticoid repression of osteocalcin transcription acted through a response element proximal to and distinct from the VDRE.[394]

Absence of the VDR produces target hormone resistance to the action of 1α,25-$(OH)_2D$. Patients with *hereditary 1α,25-(OH)₂D-resistant rickets (HVDRR)*, have severe rickets, hypocalcemia, secondary hyperparathyroidism, and increased levels of 1α,25-$(OH)_2D$.[77,493] They also frequently have total scalp and body *alopecia*, the mechanism of which is not known. In a recent study of seven family branches of an extended kindred with this disorder, DNA sequence revealed a nonsense mutation in the steroid-binding domain of the VDR, causing premature termination of the protein.[360] Little of this protein is produced, perhaps because the mRNA is unstable.

Although there is consensus that the major effects of 1α,25-$(OH)_2D$ are exerted via the nuclear vitamin D receptor, 1α,25-$(OH)_2D$ may have other modes of action on its target cells that are too rapid to be a result of modification of protein synthesis. 1α,25-$(OH)_2D$ has been shown to increase rat duodenal alkaline phosphatase activity within 10 min of incubation.[26] These effects are not blocked by inhibitors of transcription or translation.[477] 1α,25-$(OH)_2D$ has been postulated to have a "liponomic" action, since it alters the plasma membrane lipid composition and fluidity in various cell types.[477] Recent studies using rat colonic epithelium in vitro have shown that 1α,25-$(OH)_2D$ stimulates membrane phosphoinositide turnover within 15 s and leads to a brisk rise in cytosolic calcium.[612]

Bone

Vitamin D has two main effects on bone. One is to provide, via effects on intestinal absorption, the necessary concentrations of calcium and inorganic phosphate for normal bone mineralization. The second is a calcemic effect; 1α,25-$(OH)_2D$ stimulates osteoclastic resorption of bone. The increased bone resorption mediated by 1α,25-$(OH)_2D$ is a result of an increase in the number and activity of osteoclasts.[481] The mechanisms of the effects of vitamin D on bone are described in more detail under the earlier main section on "Bone."

Intestine

The principal means by which 1α,25-$(OH)_2D$ maintains calcium and phosphorus homeostasis is to enhance the intestinal absorption of calcium and phosphorus. The mechanism by which 1α,25-$(OH)_2D$ enhances the efficiency of intestinal absorption of calcium and phosphorus is not known. Intestinal mucosa cells have 1α,25-$(OH)_2D$ receptors, and 1α,25-$(OH)_2D$ increases the synthesis and the level of a calcium-binding protein known as calbindin-D or calcium-binding protein (CaBP),[550,627] as well as calmodulin and several brush-border–associated proteins. The level of calbindin-D correlates with the level of intestinal absorption of calcium.[205] However, 1α,25-$(OH)_2D$ can enhance calcium absorption from perfused rat duodena during exposure to 1α,25-$(OH)_2D$ before significant changes in the levels of proteins such as calbindin-D would occur.[411] These studies suggest that part of the effect of 1α,25-$(OH)_2D$ on calcium absorption is mediated by nongenomic effects. As discussed above, 1α,25-$(OH)_2D$ may mediate these effects by stimulating membrane phosphoinositide turnover.

Other target tissues

1α,25-$(OH)_2D$ has been shown to bind to 1α,25-$(OH)_2D$ receptors and modulate growth and differentiation of hematopoietic cells, cancer cells, and skin cells. In vitro studies with myeloid leukemic cell lines have shown that 1α,25-$(OH)_2D$, at concentrations that may be supraphysiologic, reduces proliferation and promotes differentiation toward cells that express macrophage-related antigens and enzymes including phagocytic activity.[481] In the human promyelocytic leukemia cell line (HL-60), reduced cellular proliferation was accompanied by a rapid decline in the level of c-myc oncogene mRNA.[538] Proliferating, but not quiescent, T and B lymphocytes express 1α,25-$(OH)_2D$ receptors, and 1α,25-$(OH)_2D$ has been shown to inhibit proliferation, lymphokine production, and immunoglobulin production.[596] 1α,25-$(OH)_2D$ inhibits the in vitro proliferation of cells from several nonleukemia cancers, including melanoma and lung and colon cancer. 1α,25-$(OH)_2D$ also promotes the differentiation of immature, cultured basal-layer skin cells into mature squamous cells.[544]

These studies in a wide range of tissues have a common theme: the presence of 1α,25-$(OH)_2D$ receptors in immature proliferating cells and an effect of 1α,25-$(OH)_2D$ in promoting differentiation and inhibiting proliferation. Together they suggest that these cells possess a system modulating these functions and that a hormone response element is conserved as part of this system. 1α,25-$(OH)_2D$ may function in these tissues as a paracrine or autocrine hormone, since many have the capacity to 1α-hydroxylate 25-(OH)D. Their relevance to human physiology is unclear, since clear-cut abnormalities are not well described in vitamin D deficiency, with the exception of anemia and a tendency toward increased infection in vitamin D deficiency. Patients with absent receptors for 1α,25-$(OH)_2D$ are not known to have hematopoietic abnormalities, although they commonly have total alopecia.

INTEGRATED REGULATION OF SERUM CALCIUM CONCENTRATION

PTH regulates the serum calcium concentration through its direct actions on mineral transport in bone and kidney and through its secondary actions [mediated directly by 1α,25-$(OH)_2D$] on mineral transport in intestine and bone (Fig. 11-12). The parathyroid gland is the principal sensor and regulator of circulating calcium levels; 1α,25-$(OH)_2D$, by its actions on intestinal calcium transport, is the principal determinant of long-term mineral balance. The coordinated effects of PTH and 1α,25-$(OH)_2D$ determine net fluxes of calcium between the principal calcium pools. Although only small amounts of calcium enter and leave the body each day, the unidirectional fluxes between internal pools are relatively large (Fig. 11-12), providing opportunity for large hormonal effects. In the absence of PTH, the level of calcium in plasma is maintained in the range of 1.25 to 1.5 m*M* (5 to 6 mg/dl) by the combination of nearly complete renal tubular reabsorption plus equilibrium with large pools in bone.

A decrease in the plasma ionized calcium concentration immediately stimulates secretion of PTH; the level of PTH increases by several times in response to acute hypocalcemia and increases further if secondary hyperparathyroidism lasts long enough to stimulate parathyroid hyperplasia. Figure 11-21 illustrates the homeostatic response to acute hypocalcemia in patients with Paget's disease of bone treated with plicamycin (mithramycin), an inhibitor of osteoclasts.[34] The level of PTH and urinary cAMP (which reflects PTH bioactivity) in these patients increased promptly in response to hypocalcemia. The urinary calcium fell as a result of a reduction in the filtered load of calcium and increased tubular reabsorption. The time course of the increase in PTH was coincident with the fall in calcium, but the peak 1α,25-$(OH)_2D$ levels occurred 12 to 24 h after the lowest calcium level. The lag between the increase in PTH and the increase in 1α,25-$(OH)_2D$ most likely is a result of the fact that stimulation of 1α,25-$(OH)_2D$ synthesis requires induction of 1α-hydroxylase in the kidney.

If a calcipenic challenge persists for longer than one to two days, the skeletal response becomes progressively greater as more osteoclasts are recruited by the coordinate action of PTH and 1α,25-$(OH)_2D$. A sustained calcipenic challenge usually occurs as a result of reduced calcium intake, which also stimulates PTH and 1α,25-$(OH)_2D$. The latter increases the fractional absorption of calcium in the gut, which in turn feeds back on PTH. The high 1α,25-$(OH)_2D$ also feeds back on the parathyroid gland, blunting the parathyroid response to hypocalcemia; the consequence is to shift the burden of maintaining the circulating level of calcium from bone to the intestine. Another consequence of prolonged secondary hyperparathyroidism is that renal clearance of phosphate increases. Although PTH mobilizes phosphate from bone into plasma, this is more than compensated for by the phosphaturic action of PTH; the consequence is that serum calcium concentration is maintained, while serum phosphorus falls.

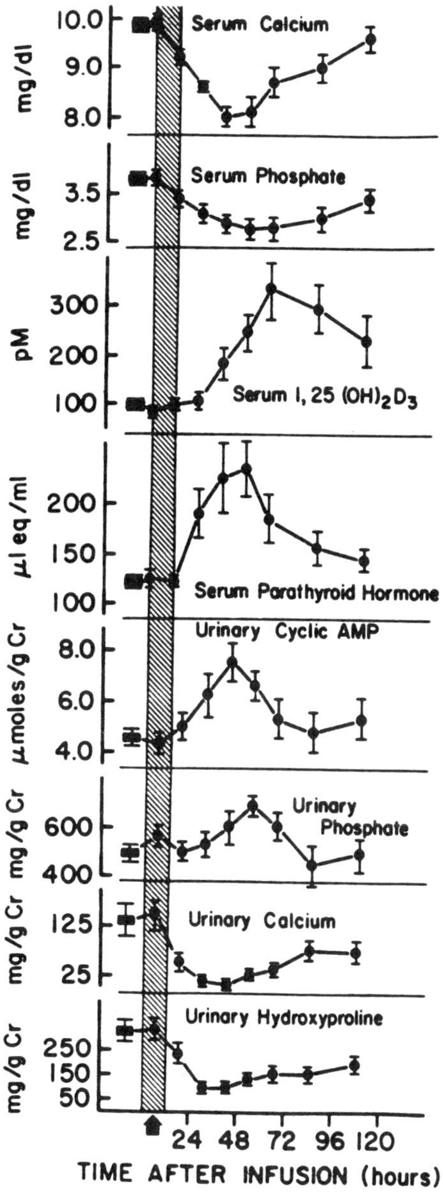

FIGURE 11-21 • Response of serum 1α,25-$(OH)_2D$, PTH, and other indexes of mineral metabolism to hypocalcemia induced by infusion of Plicamycin (mithramycin). Plicamycin was infused over the 12-h period shown by the vertical band. (From Bilezikian JP et al: *N Engl J Med* 299:437, 1978. Used by permission.)

The response to a rise in serum calcium is largely the converse of the response to a fall. Increased urinary calcium excretion unloads a relatively large portion of a hypercalcemic challenge. The kidneys can excrete substantial calcium despite only a modest increase in the filtered load because the fall in the level of PTH, which occurs within minutes of a rise in calcium, reduces renal tubular reabsorption. With suppression of PTH, renal clearance of phosphate decreases, raising the serum phosphate concentration. Lower PTH and higher serum phosphate levels inhibit $1\alpha,25\text{-}(OH)_2D$ production, causing intestinal absorption and skeletal release of calcium to decrease.

REFERENCES

1. Adams JS et al: Isolation and structural identification of 1,25-dihydroxyvitamin D_3 produced by cultured alveolar macrophages in sarcoidosis. *J Clin Endocrinol Metab* 60:960, 1985.
2. Adams ND et al: Effects of calcitriol administration on calcium metabolism in healthy men. *Kidney Int* 21:90, 1982.
3. Agus ZS, Goldfarb S: Renal regulation of calcium balance, in Seldin DW, Giebisch G (eds): *The Kidney: Physiology and Pathophysiology*. New York, Raven Press, 1985, vol. 2, p 1323.
4. Agus ZS et al: Regulation of urinary calcium excretion in the rat. *Am J Physiol* 232:F545, 1977.
5. Akerman KEO, Nicholls DG: Physiological and bioenergetic aspects of mitochondrial calcium transport. *Rev Physiol Biochem Pharmacol* 95:149, 1983.
6. Albright F: Case 27461, Case records of the Massachusetts General Hospital. *N Engl J Med.* 225:789, 1941.
7. Alon U et al: Additive hypocalciuric effects of amiloride and hydrochlorothiazide in patients treated with calcitriol. *Miner Electrolyte Metab* 10:379, 1984.
8. Alpers DH: Absorption of water-soluble vitamins, folate, minerals and vitamin D, in Sleisenger MH, Fordtran JS (eds): *Gastrointestional Disease*, 3d ed. Philadelphia, Saunders, 1983, p 830.
9. Anast CS et al: Impaired release of parathyroid hormone in magnesium deficiency. *J Clin Endocrinol Metab* 42:707, 1976.
10. Anderson HC: Mechanism of mineral formation in bone. *Lab Invest* 60:320, 1989.
11. Armbrecht HJ: Effect of age and the milk sugar lactose on calcium absorption by the small intestine. *Adv Exp Med Biol* 249:185, 1989.
12. Armbrecht HJ et al: Effects of vitamin D metabolites on intestinal calcium absorption and calcium-binding protein in young and adult rats. *Endocrinology* 106:469, 1980.
13. Aronson PJ: Identifying secondary active solute transport in epithelia. *Am J Physiol* 240:F1, 1981.
14. Aurbach GD: Regulation of secretion of parathyroid hormone. *Adv Nephrol* 11:131, 1982.
15. Austin LA, Heath H: Calcitonin: Physiology and pathophysiology. *N Engl J Med* 304:269, 1981.
16. Bacskai BJ, Friedman PA: Activation of latent Ca^{2+} channels in renal epithelial cells by parathyroid hormone. *Nature* 347:388, 1990.
17. Balsan S et al: Long-term calcium infusions can cure osteomalacia and promote normal mineralization in hereditary resistance to 1,25-dihydroxyvitamin D. *J Clin Invest* 77:1661, 1986.
18. Barbour GL et al: Hypercalcemia in an anephric patient with sarcoidosis: Evidence for extrarenal generation of 1,25-dihydroxyvitamin D. *N Engl J Med* 305:440, 1981.
19. Baron R et al: Cell-mediated extracellular acidification and bone resorption: Evidence for a low pH in resorbing lacunae and localization of a 100 kD lysosomal membrane protein at the osteoclast ruffled border. *J Cell Biol* 101:2210, 1985.
20. Barr DR et al: Characterization of the renal and intestinal adaptations to dietary calcium deprivation in growing female rabbits. *Miner Electrolyte Metab* 17:32, 1991.
21. Barzel US: Estrogens in the prevention and treatment of postmenopausal osteoporosis: A review. *Am J Med* 85:847, 1988.
22. Behar J, Kerstein MD: Intestinal calcium absorption: Differences in transport between duodenum and ileum. *Am J Physiol* 230:1255, 1976.
23. Bell NH: The vitamin D-endocrine system. *J Clin Invest* 76:1, 1985.
24. Bell NH et al: Evidence for alteration of the vitamin D-endocrine system in obese subjects. *J Clin Invest* 76:370, 1985.
25. Bengele HH et al: Calcium and magnesium transport along the inner medullary collecting duct of the rat. *Am J Physiol* 239:F24, 1980.
26. Ben-Nasr L et al: Rapid (10 minute) stimulation of rat duodenal alkaline phosphatase activity by 1,25-dihydroxyvitamin D_3. *Endocrinology* 123:1778, 1988.
27. Beresford JN et al: Analysis of the proteoglycans synthesized by human bone cells *in vitro*. *J Biol Chem* 262:13120, 1987.
28. Beringer TRO et al: Absence of evidence for a role of calcitonin in the etiology of femoral neck fracture. *Calcif Tissue Int* 39:300, 1986.
29. Berndt TJ, Knox FG: Effect of parathyroid hormone and calcitonin on electrolyte excretion in the rabbit. *Kidney Int* 17:473, 1980.
30. Berry CA, Rector FC Jr: Renal transport of glucose, amino acids, sodium, chloride, and water, in Brenner BM, Rector FC Jr (eds): *The Kidney*, 4th ed. Philadelphia, Saunders, 1991, vol 1, p 245.
31. Betts F et al: Atomic structure of intracellular amorphous calcium phosphate deposits. *Proc Natl Acad Sci U S A* 72:2088, 1975.
32. Bijvoet OLM et al: Natriuretic effect of calcitonin in man. *N Engl J Med* 284:681, 1971.
33. Bikle D et al: 1,25-dihydroxyvitamin D increases the intracellular free calcium concentration of duodenal epithelial cells, in Norman AW et al (eds): *Vitamin D: Chemical, Biochemical and Clinical Update*. Berlin, DeGruyter, 1985, p 416.

34. Bilezikian JP et al: Response of 1α,25-dihydroxyvitamin D_3 to hypocalcemia in human subjects. *N Engl J Med* 299:437, 1978.
35. Bishop CW et al: Induction of calcium-binding protein before 1,25-dihydroxyvitamin D_3 stimulation of duodenal calcium uptake. *J Biol Chem* 258:1305, 1983.
36. Black-Sandler R et al: Postmenopausal bone density and milk consumption in childhood and adolescence. *Am J Clin Nutr* 42:270, 1985.
37. Blum JW et al: Plasma catecholamine and parathyroid hormone responses in cattle during treadmill exercise at simulated high altitude. *Horm Metab Res* 11:246, 1979.
38. Boass A et al: Calcium metabolism during lactation: Enhanced intestinal calcium absorption in vitamin D-deprived hypocalcemic rats. *Endocrinology* 109:900, 1981.
39. Body J, Heath H: Estimates of circulating monomeric calcitonin: Physiologic studies in normal and thyroidectomized man. *J Clin Endocrinol Metab* 57:897, 1983.
40. Bolander ME et al: Osteonectin cDNA sequence reveals potential binding regions for calcium and hydroxyapatite and shows homologies with both a basement membrane protein (SPARC) and a serine proteinase inhibitor (ovomucoid). *Proc Natl Acad Sci U S A* 85:2919, 1988.
41. Bomsztyk K, Calalb MB: Bicarbonate absorption stimulates active calcium absorption in the rat proximal tubule. *J Clin Invest* 81:1455, 1988.
42. Bomsztyk K, Wright FS: Dependence of ion fluxes on fluid transport by rat proximal tubule. *Am J Physiol* 250:F680, 1986.
43. Bomsztyk K et al: Effects of luminal fluid anions on calcium transport by proximal tubule. *Am J Physiol* 246:F600, 1984.
44. Bonventre JV, Cheung JY: Cytosolic free calcium concentration in cultured renal epithelial cells. *Am J Physiol* 250:F329, 1986.
45. Borke JL et al:Co-localization of erythrocyte Ca^{++}-Mg^{++} ATPase and vitamin D-dependent 28-kDa-calcium binding protein. *Kidney Int* 34:262, 1988.
46. Borke JL et al: Monoclonal antibodies to human erythrocyte membrane Ca^{++}-Mg^{++} adenosine triphosphatase pump recognize an epitope in the basolateral membrane of human kidney distal tubule cells. *J Clin Invest* 80:1225, 1987.
47. Borke JL et al: Plasma membrane calcium pump and 28-kDA calcium binding protein in cells of rat kidney distal tubules. *Am J Physiol* F842:257, 1989.
48. Borke JL et al: Recent advances in calcium transport by the kidney. *Semin Nephrol* 10:15, 1990.
49. Borle AB, Briggs FN: Microdetermination of calcium in biological material by fluorometric titration. *Anal Chem* 40:339, 1968.
50. Boskey AL et al: Formation of hydroxyapatite at low supersaturation. *J Phys Chem* 80:40, 1976.
51. Bourdeau JE: Calcium transport across the cortical thick ascending limb of Henle's loop, in Bronner F, Peterlik M (eds): *Calcium and Phosphate Transport across Biomembranes*. New York, Academic Press, 1981, p. 199.
52. Bourdeau JE: Calcium transport across the pars recta of cortical segment 2 proximal tubules. *Am J Physiol* 251:F718, 1986.
53. Bourdeau JE: Renal handling of calcium, in Brenner BM, Stein JH (eds): *Divalent Ion Homeostasis, Contemporary Issues in Nephrology*. New York, Churchill Livingstone, 1983, vol 11, p 1.
54. Bourdeau JE, Burg MB: Effect of PTH on calcium transport across the cortical thick ascending limb of Henle's loop. *Am J Physiol* 239:F121, 1980.
55. Bourdeau JE, Burg MB: Voltage dependence of calcium transport in the thick ascending limb of Henle's loop. *Am J Physiol* 236:F357, 1979.
56. Bourdeau JE, Eby BK: Cyclic AMP-stimulated rise of $[Ca^{2+}]_i$ in rabbit connecting tubules: Role of peritubular Ca. *Am J Physiol* 258:F751, 1990.
57. Bourdeau JE, Hellstrom-Stein RJ: Voltage-dependent calcium movement across the cortical collecting duct. *Am J Physiol* 242:F285, 1982.
58. Bourdeau JE, Lau K: Basolateral cell membrane Ca-Na exchange in single rabbit connecting tubules. *Am J Physiol* 258:F1492, 1990.
59. Bourdeau JE, Lau K: Effects of parathyroid hormone on cytosolic free calcium concentration in individual rabbit connecting tubules. *J Clin Invest* 83:373, 1989.
60. Bourdeau JE et al: Inhibition of calcium absorption in the cortical thick ascending limb of Henle's loop by furosemide. *J Pharmacol Exp Ther* 211:815, 1982.
61. Bourdeau JE et al: Parathyroid hormone-stimulated calcium absorption in cTAL from vitamin D-deficient rabbits. *Kidney Int* 31:913, 1987.
62. Bourdeau JE et al: Renal responses to calcium deprivation in young rabbits. *Miner Electrolyte Metab* 14:150, 1988.
63. Broadus AE: Nephrogenous cyclic AMP. *Recent Prog Horm Res* 37:667, 1981.
64. Broadus AE: Nephrogenous cyclic AMP as a parathyroid function test. *Nephron* 23:136, 1979.
65. Broman GE et al: The density of selected bones of the human skeleton. *Am J Phys Anthropol* 16:197, 1958.
66. Brommage R: Measurement of calcium and phosphorus fluxes during lactation in the rat. *J Nutr* 119:428, 1989.
67. Brommage R, Baxter DC: Elevated calcium, phosphorus and magnesium retention in pregnant rats prior to the onset of fetal skeletal mineralization. *J Bone Miner Res* 3:667, 1988.
68. Brommage R et al: Vitamin D-independent intestinal calcium and phosphorus absorption during reproduction. *Am J Physiol* 259:G631, 1990.
69. Bronner F: Intestinal calcium absorption: Mechanisms and applications. *J Nutr* 117:1347, 1987.
70. Bronner F: Intestinal calcium absorption and transport, in Carafoli E (ed): *Membrane Transport of Calcium*. New York, Academic Press, 1982, p 237.
71. Bronner F: Intestinal calcium transport: The cellular pathway. *Miner Electrolyte Metab* 16:94, 1990.
72. Bronner F: Renal calcium transport: Mechanisms and regulation: An overview. *Am J Physiol* 257:F707, 1989.
73. Bronner F: Vitamin D-dependent active calcium transport: The role of CaBP. *Calcif Tissue Int* 43:133, 1988.
74. Bronner F, Stein WD: $CaBP_r$ facilitates intracellular diffusion for Ca pumping in distal convoluted tubule. *Am J Physiol* 255:F558, 1988.

75. Bronner F et al: An analysis of intestinal calcium transport across the rat intestine. *Am J Physiol* 13:G561, 1986.
76. Bronner F et al: Molecular and transport effects of 1,25-dihydroxyvitamin D_3 in rat duodenum. *Fed Proc* 41:61, 1982.
77. Brooks MH et al: Vitamin D-dependent rickets type II: Resistance of target organs to 1,25-dihydroxyvitamin D. *N Engl J Med* 298:996, 1978.
78. Brown EM: Four-parameter model of the sigmoidal relationship between parathyroid hormone release and extracellular calcium concentration in normal and abnormal parathyroid tissue. *J Clin Endocrinol Metab* 56:572, 1983.
79. Brown EM: Set-point for calcium: Its role in normal and abnormal parathyroid secretion, in Cohn DV et al (eds): *Hormonal Control of Calcium Metabolism*. Princeton, Excerpta Medica, 1981, p 35.
80. Brown EM, Chen CJ: Calcium, magnesium and the control of PTH secretion. *Bone Miner* 5:249, 1989.
81. Brown EM et al: Calcium-regulated parathyroid hormone release in primary hyperparathyroidism. *Am J Med* 66:923, 1979.
82. Brown EM et al: Ca^{2+}-sensing, second messengers, and the control of parathyroid hormone secretion. *Cell Calcium* 11:333, 1990.
83. Brown EM et al: A comparison of the effects of divalent and trivalent cations on parathyroid hormone release, 3′,5′-cyclic-adenosine monophosphate accumulation, and the levels of inositol phosphates in bovine parathyroid cells. *Endocrinology* 127:1064, 1990.
84. Brown EM et al: Extracellular calcium potentiates the inhibitory effects of magnesium on parathyroid function in dispersed bovine parathyroid cells. *Metabolism* 33:171, 1984.
85. Brown EM et al: Relationship of intracellular 3′,5′-adenosine monophosphate accumulation to parathyroid hormone release from dispersed bovine parathyroid cells. *Endocrinology* 103:2323, 1978.
86. Brown JP et al: Serum bone Gla protein, a specific marker for bone formation in postmenopausal osteoporosis. *Lancet* 1:1091, 1984.
87. Buchanan JR et al: Determinants of peak trabecular bone density in women: The role of androgens, estrogen and exercise. *J Bone Miner Res* 3:673, 1989.
88. Buchanan JR et al: Effect of excess endogenous androgens on bone density in young women. *J Clin Endocrinol Metab* 67:937, 1988.
89. Buckley BM, Russell LJ: The measurement of ionized calcium in blood plasma. *Ann Clin Biochem* 25:447, 1988.
90. Budayr AA et al: High levels of parathyroid hormone-like protein in milk. *Proc Natl Acad Sci U S A* 86:7183, 1989.
91. Bull HW: *An Introduction to Physical Biochemistry*. Philadelphia, Davis, 1964, pp 64–65, 75–79.
92. Burg MB: Renal handling of sodium, chloride, water, amino acids, and glucose, in Brenner BM, Rector FC Jr (eds): *The Kidney*, 2d ed. Philadelphia, Saunders, 1981, vol 1, p 328.
93. Burg MB: Thick ascending limb of Henle's loop. *Kidney Int* 22:454, 1982.
94. Burg MB, Green N: Function of the thick ascending limb of Henle's loop. *Am J Physiol* 224:659, 1973.
95. Burnatowska MA et al: Effects of vitamin D on renal handling of calcium, magnesium and phosphate in the hamster. *Kidney Int* 27:864, 1985.
96. Burtis WJ et al: Immunochemical characterization of circulating parathyroid hormone-related protein in patients with humoral hypercalcemia of cancer. *N Engl J Med* 322:1106, 1990.
97. Bygrave FL: Calcium transport in mitochondria isolated from normal and injured tissue, in Anghileri LJ, Tuffet-Anghileri AM (eds): *The Role of Calcium in Biological Systems*. Boca Raton, Fl, CRC Press, 1982, vol 1, p 121.
98. Bygrave FL: Mitochondria and the control of intracellular calcium. *Biol Rev* 53:43, 1978.
99. Cali JP et al: A referee method for the determination of total calcium in serum. *Clin Chem* 19:1208, 1973.
100. Calvo MS et al: Circadian variation in ionized calcium and intact parathyroid hormone: Evidence for sex differences in calcium homeostasis. *J Clin Endocrinol Metab* 72:69, 1991.
101. Calvo MS et al: Elevated secretion and action of parathyroid hormone in young adults consuming high phosphorus, low calcium diets assembled from common foods. *J Clin Endocrinol Metab* 66:823, 1988.
102. Canalis E: Interleukin-1 has independent effects on DNA and collagen synthesis in cultures of rat calvariae. *Endocrinology* 118:74, 1986.
103. Canalis E, Lian JB: Effects of bone associated growth factors on DNA, collagen and osteocalcin synthesis in cultured fetal rat calvariae. *Bone* 9:243, 1988.
104. Canalis E et al: A bone-derived growth factor isolated from rat calvariae is $beta_2$-microglobulin. *Endocrinology* 121:1198, 1987.
105. Canalis E et al: Effects of basic fibroblast growth factor on bone formation *in vitro*. *J Clin Invest* 81:1572, 1988.
106. Canalis E et al: Growth factors and the regulation of bone remodeling. *J Clin Invest* 81:277, 1988.
107. Canalis E et al: Insulin-like growth factor I mediates selective anabolic effects of parathyroid hormone in bone cultures. *J Clin Invest* 83:60, 1989.
108. Cann CE, Genant HK: Cross-sectional studies of vertebral mineral using quantitative computed tomography. *J Comput Assist Tomogr* 6:216, 1983.
109. Carafoli E: Calcium pump of the plasma membrane. *Physiol Rev* 71:129, 1991.
110. Carafoli E: Calmodulin in the membrane transport of Ca^{++}. *Cell Calcium* 2:353, 1981.
111. Carafoli E: Intracellular calcium homeostasis. *Ann Rev Biochem* 56:395, 1987.
112. Carafoli E: Intracellular calcium regulation, with special attention to the role of the plasma membrane calcium pump. *J Cardiovasc Pharmacol* 12:S77, 1988.
113. Carafoli E: Mitochondrial calcium transport: An overview, in Siegel FL et al (eds): *Calcium-Binding Proteins: Structure and Function*. New York, Elsevier/North-Holland, 1980, p 121.
114. Carafoli E: The intracellular homeostasis of calcium: An overview. *Ann N Y Acad Sci* 551:147, 1988.
115. Carafoli E: The plasma membrane calcium pump: Struc-

ture, function, and regulation. *Biochem Soc Trans* 17:808, 1989.
116. Carafoli E: The plasma membrane calcium transporting systems in the regulation of cell calcium, in Adelstein R et al (eds): *Advances in Second Messenger and Phosphoprotein Research.* New York, Raven Press, 1988, p 147.
117. Carafoli E: The regulation of the cellular functions of Ca^{2+}, in Bronner F, Coburn JW (eds): *Disorders of Mineral Metabolism, Calcium Physiology.* New York, Academic Press, 1982, vol 2, p 1.
118. Carafoli E: The transport of calcium across the inner membrane of mitochondria, in Carafoli E (ed): *Membrane Transport of Calcium.* New York, Academic Press, 1982, p 109.
119. Carafoli E, Penniston JT: The calcium signal. *Sci Am* 253:70, 1985.
120. Care AD et al: The effect of fetal thyroparathyroidectomy on the transport of calcium across the bovine placenta to the fetus. *Placenta* 7:417, 1986.
121. Carney SL, Thompson L: Acute effect of calcitonin on rat renal electrolyte transport. *Am J Physiol* 240:F12, 1981.
122. Carney SL et al: Effect of magnesium deficiency on renal magnesium and calcium transport in the rat. *J Clin Invest* 65:180, 1980.
123. Caroni P, Carafoli E: The regulation of the Na^{+}-Ca^{2+} exchanger of heart sarcolemma. *Eur J Biochem* 132:451, 1983.
124. Carroll KM et al: Glucose enhancement of transcellular calcium transport in the intestine. *Am J Physiol* 255:G339, 1988.
125. Catherwood BD et al: Determinants of bone gamma-carboxyglutamic acid-containing protein in plasma of healthy aging subjects. *Bone* 6:9, 1985.
126. Centrella M, Canalis E: Local regulators of skeletal growth: A perspective. *Endocr Rev* 6:544, 1985.
127. Chambers TJ, Magnus CJ: Calcitonin alters behaviour of isolated osteoclasts. *J Pathol* 136:27, 1982.
128. Chambers TJ et al: The effect of human calcitonin on the cytoplasmic spreading of rat osteoclasts. *J Clin Endocrinol Metab* 63:1080, 1986.
129. Chandra S et al: Ion microscopic imaging of calcium transport in the intestinal tissue of vitamin D-deficient and vitamin D-replete chickens: A ^{44}Ca stable isotope study. *Proc Natl Acad Sci U S A* 87:5715, 1990.
130. Chang EB et al: Secretagogue-induced changes in membrane calcium permeability in chicken and chinchilla ileal mucosa: Selective inhibition by loperamide. *J Clin Invest* 78:281, 1986.
131. Charles P et al: Estimation of bone turnover evaluated by ^{47}Ca-kinetics: Efficiency of serum bone gamma-carboxyglutamic acid-containing protein, serum alkaline phosphatase, and urinary hydroxyproline excretion. *J Clin Invest* 76:2254, 1985.
131a. Cheema C et al: Effects of estrogen on circulating "free" and total 1,25-dihydroxyvitamin D and on the parathyroid–vitamin D axis of postmenopausal women. *J Clin Invest* 83:537–542, 1989.
132. Chen CJ et al: Divalent cations suppress 3′,5′-adenosine monophosphate accumulation by stimulating a pertussis toxin-sensitive guanine nucleotide-binding protein in cultured bovine parathyroid cells. *Endocrinology* 124:233, 1989.
133. Chenu C et al: Transforming growth-factor-β inhibits formation of osteoclast-like cells in long-term human marrow cultures. *Proc Natl Acad Sci U S A* 85:5683, 1988.
134. Cheung JY et al: Regulation of cytosolic free calcium concentration in cultured renal epithelial cells. *Am J Physiol* 251:F690, 1986.
135. Cholst IN et al: The influence of hypermagnesemia on serum calcium and parathyroid hormone levels. *N Engl J Med* 301:1221, 1984.
136. Chutkow JG: Magnesium and calcium in the cerebrospinal fluid of the rat. *Proc Soc Exp Biol Med* 128:555, 1968.
137. Civitelli R et al: PTH elevates inositol polyphosphates and diacylglycerol in a rat osteoblast-like cell line. *Am J Physiol* 255:E660, 1988.
138. Clements MR et al: A new mechanism for induced vitamin D deficiency in calcium deprivation. *Nature* 325:62, 1987.
139. Coburn JW et al: Interactions between vitamin D and the kidney, in Martinez-Maldonado M (ed): *Methods in Pharmacology, Renal Pharmacology.* New York: Plenum Press, 1976, vol 4a, p 227.
140. Coccia PF et al: Successful bone-marrow transplantation for infantile malignant osteopetrosis. *N Engl J Med* 302:701, 1980.
141. Coe FL (ed): *Hypercalciuric States.* Orlando, Grune & Stratton, 1984.
142. Coe FL (ed): *Nephrolithiasis,* in Brenner BM, Stein JH (eds): *Contemporary Issues in Nephrology.* New York, Churchill Livingstone, 1980, vol 5.
143. Coe FL, Parks JH: *Nephrolithiasis: Pathogenesis and Treatment,* 2d ed. Chicago, Year Book Medical, 1988.
144. Cohn SH et al: Changes in body chemical composition with age measured by total-body neutron activation. *Metabolism* 25:85, 1976.
145. Cohn SH et al: Comparative skeletal mass and radial bone mineral content in black and white women. *Metabolism* 26:171, 1977.
146. Colston K, Feldman D: 1,25-dihydroxyvitamin D_3 receptors and functions in cultured pig kidney cells (LLCPK1): Regulation of 24,25-dihydroxyvitamin D_3 production. *J Biol Chem* 257:2504, 1982.
147. Colvard DS et al: Identification of androgen receptors in normal human osteoblast-like cells. *Proc Natl Acad Sci U S A* 86:854, 1989.
148. Cooke NE, Haddad JG: Vitamin D binding protein (Gc-globulin). *Endocr Rev* 10:294, 1989.
149. Costanzo LS: Localization of diuretic action in microperfused rat distal tubules: Ca and Na transport. *Am J Physiol* 248:F527, 1985.
150. Costanzo LS, Windhager EE: Calcium and sodium transport by the distal convoluted tubule of the rat. *Am J Physiol* 235:F492, 1978.
151. Costanzo LS, Windhager EE: Effects of PTH, ADH and cyclic AMP on distal tubular Ca and Na reabsorption. *Am J Physiol* 239:F478, 1980.

152. Costanzo LS, Windhager EE: Sodium-calcium interaction in the distal tubule, in Vogel HG, Ullrich KJ (eds): *New Aspects of Renal Function.* Amsterdam, Excerpta Medica, 1978, p 147.
153. Costanzo LS et al: Comparison of calcium and sodium transport in early and late rat distal tubules: Effect of amiloride. *Am J Physiol* 246:F937, 1984
154. Council, National Research: *Recommended Dietary Allowances: Report of the Committee on Dietary Allowances, Food and Nutrition Board, Division of Biological Sciences, Assembly of Life Sciences.* Washington, DC, National Academy Press, 1980.
155. Cundy T et al: Remission of hypoparathyroidism during lactation: Evidence for a physiological role for prolactin in the regulation of vitamin D metabolism. *Clin Endocrinol (Oxford)* 26:667, 1987.
156. de Boland AR, Norman A: Evidence for involvement of protein kinase C and cyclic adenosine 3′,5′ monophosphate-dependent protein kinase in the 1,25-dihydroxyvitamin D_3-mediated rapid stimulation of intestinal calcium transport (transcaltachia). *Endocrinology* 127:39, 1990.
157. de Boland AR et al: Ca^{2+}-channel agonist BAY K8644 mimics 1,25$(OH)_2$-vitamin D_3 rapid enhancement of Ca^{2+} transport in chick perfused duodenum. *Biochem Biophys Res Commun* 166:217, 1990.
158. De Jonge HR et al: Phosphorylated intermediates of Ca^{2+}-ATPase and alkaline phosphatase in plasma membranes from rat duodenal epithelium. *Biochim Biophys Acta* 647:140, 1981.
159. Delmez JA et al: Parathyroid hormone suppression by intravenous 1,25-dihydroxyvitamin D: A role for increased sensitivity to calcium. *J Clin Invest* 83:1349, 1989.
160. DeLuca HF: Vitamin D-dependent calcium transport. *Soc Gen Physiol Ser* 39:160, 1985.
161. DeLuca HF et al: Molecular events involved in 1,25-dihydroxyvitamin D_3 stimulation of intestinal calcium transport. *Fed Proc* 41:66, 1982.
162. Demay MB et al: DNA sequences in the rat osteocalcin gene that bind the 1,25-dihydroxyvitamin D_3 receptor and confer responsiveness to 1,25-dihydroxyvitamin D_3. *Proc Natl Acad Sci U S A* 87:369, 1990.
163. Denton RM, McCormack JG: Ca^{2+} transport by mammalian mitochondria and its role in hormone action. *Am J Physiol* 249:E543, 1985.
164. DePalo D et al: Renal responses to phosphorus deprivation in young rabbits. *Miner Electrolyte Metab* 14:313, 1988.
165. Dequeker J et al: Genetic determinants of bone mineral content at the spine and radius: A twin study. *Bone* 8:207, 1987.
166. DeSimone DP et al: Influence of body habitus and race on bone mineral density of the midradius, hip, and spine in aging women. *J Bone Miner Res* 4:828, 1989.
167. De Smedt H et al: Phosphorylated intermediates of (Ca^{2+} + Mg^{2+})-ATPase and alkaline phosphatase in renal plasma membranes. *Biochim Biophys Acta* 728:409, 1983.
168. Dewhirst FE et al: Purification and partial sequence of human osteoclast activating factor: Identity with interleukin-1. *J Immunol* 135:2562, 1985.
169. Dillingham MA et al: Calcium modulates vasopressin effect in rabbit cortical collecting tubule. *Am J Physiol* 252:F115, 1987.
170. Dominguez JH et al: Intracellular messenger for action of angiotensin II on fluid transport in rabbit proximal tubule. *Am J Physiol* 252:F423, 1987.
171. Dominguez JH et al: Na^+ electrochemical gradient and Na^+-Ca^{2+} exchange in rat proximal tubule. *Am J Physiol* 257:F531, 1989.
172. Donowitz M: Ca^{2+} and cyclic AMP in regulation of intestinal Na, K, and Cl transport. *Ann Rev Physiol* 48:135, 1986.
173. Donowitz M, Asarkof N: Calcium dependence of basal electrolyte transport in rabbit ileum. *Am J Physiol* 243:G28, 1982.
174. Donowitz M et al: Calcium dependence of serotonin-induced changes in rabbit ileal electrolyte transport. *J Clin Invest* 66:341, 1980.
175. Doucet A, Katz AI: High-affinity Ca-Mg-ATPase along the rabbit nephron. *Am J Physiol* 242:F346, 1982.
176. Duda RJ et al: Concurrent assays of circulating bone-gla protein and bone alkaline phosphatase: Effects of sex, age and metabolic bone disease. *J Clin Endocrinol Metab* 66:951, 1988.
177. Durham ACH, Walton JM: A survey of the available colorimetric indicators for Ca^{2+} and Mg^{2+} ions in biological experiments. *Cell Calcium* 4:47, 1983.
178. Eastman JW et al: Ultrafiltrable calcium and the conformation of albumin. *Clin Chim Acta* 58:233, 1975.
179. Einspahr H, Bugg CE: Crystal structures of calcium complexes of amino acids, peptides and related model systems, in Wasserman RH et al (eds): *Calcium-Binding Proteins and Calcium Function.* New York, Elsevier/North-Holland Press, 1977, p 13.
180. Ekenstam E et al: The acute effect of high dose corticosteroid treatment on serum osteocalcin. *Metabolism* 37:141, 1988.
181. Elin RJ: Reference intervals and laboratory values of clinical importance, in Wyngaarden JB, Smith LH (eds): *Cecil Textbook of Medicine,* 18th ed. Philadelphia, Saunders, 1988, vol 2, p 2395.
182. Ellis KJ, Cohn SH: Correlation between skeletal calcium and muscle mass in man. *J Appl Physiol* 230:143, 1975.
183. Engel K et al (eds): Ionized Calcium Workshop No. 1. *Scand J Clin Lab Invest* 43(suppl 165):1, 1983.
184. Epstein FH: Calcium and the kidney. *Am J Med* 45:700, 1968.
185. Epstein PA et al: Modulation of intracellular Ca^{2+} in the parathyroid cell: Release of Ca^{2+} from the non-mitochondrial pools by inositol trisphosphate. *FEBS Lett* 188:141, 1985.
186. Epstein S: Serum and urinary markers of bone remodeling: Assessment of bone turnover. *Endocr Rev* 9:437, 1988.
187. Eriksen EF et al: Evidence of estrogen receptors in normal human osteoblast-like cells. *Science* 241:84, 1988.
188. Eriksen EF et al: Histomorphometric analysis of bone in metabolic bone disease. *Endocrinol Metabol Clin North Am* 18:919, 1989.
189. Ernst M et al: Enhanced osteoblast proliferation and collagen gene expression by estradiol. *Proc Natl Acad Sci U S A* 85:2307, 1988.

190. Ernst M et al: Estradiol effects on proliferation, messenger ribonucleic acid for collagen and insulin-like growth factor-I, and parathyroid hormone-stimulated adenylate cyclase activity in osteoblastic cells from calvariae and long bones. *Endocrinology* 125:825, 1989.
191. Ernst M et al: Evidence for a direct effect of estrogen on bone cells *in vitro*. *J Steroid Biochem Mol Biol* 34:279, 1989.
192. Ettinger B et al: Long-term estrogen replacement therapy prevents bone loss and fractures. *Ann Intern Med* 102:319, 1985.
193. Evans RM: The steroid and thyroid hormone receptor superfamily. *Science* 240:889, 1988.
194. Exton JH: Mechanisms of action of calcium-mobilizing agonists: Some variations on a young theme. *FASEB J* 2:2670, 1988.
195. Falch JA et al: Early postmenopausal bone loss is not associated with a decrease in circulating levels of 25-hydroxyvitamin D, 1,25-dihydroxyvitamin D, or vitamin D-binding protein. *J Clin Endocrinol Metab* 64:836, 1987.
196. Favus MJ: Factors that influence absorption and secretion of calcium in the small intestine and colon. *Am J Physiol* 248:G147, 1985.
197. Favus MJ, Langman CB: Effects of 1,25-dihydroxyvitamin D_3 on colonic calcium transport in vitamin D-deficient and normal rats. *Am J Physiol* 246:G268, 1984.
198. Favus MJ et al: Effects of diet calcium and 1,25-dihydroxyvitamin D_3 on colon calcium active transport. *Am J Physiol* 238:G75, 1980.
199. Favus MJ et al: Effects of $1,25(OH)_2D_3$ on enterocyte basolateral membrane Ca transport. *Am J Physiol* 256:G613, 1989.
200. Favus MJ et al: Effects of trifluoperazine, ouabain, and ethacrynic acid on intestinal calcium transport. *Am J Physiol* 244:G111, 1983.
201. Favus MJ et al: Evidence for *in vivo* upregulation of the intestinal vitamin D receptor during dietary calcium restriction in the rat. *J Clin Invest* 82:218, 1988.
202. Favus MJ et al: Kinetic characteristics of calcium absorption and secretion by rat colon. *Am J Physiol* 240:G350, 1981.
203. Feher JJ: Facilitated calcium diffusion by intestinal calcium-binding protein. *Am J Physiol* 244:C303, 1983.
204. Feher JJ: Measurement of facilitated calcium diffusion by a soluble calcium binding protein. *Biochim Biophys Acta* 773:91, 1984.
205. Feher JJ, Wasserman RH: Calcium absorption and intestinal calcium-binding protein: Quantitative relationship. *Am J Physiol* 236:E556, 1979.
206. Feher JJ et al: Comparison of the enhanced steady-state diffusion of calcium by calbindin-D_{9k} and calmodulin: Possible importance in intestinal calcium absorption. *Cell Calcium* 10:189, 1989.
207. Feyen JHM, Raisz LG: Prostaglandin production by calvariae from sham-operated and ovariectomized rats: Effects of 17β-estradiol *in vivo*. *Endocrinology*, 121:819, 1987.
208. Finkelstein JS et al: Osteoporosis in men with idiopathic hypogonadotropic hypogonadism. *Ann Intern Med* 106:354, 1987.
209. Fisher LW, Termine JD: Noncollagenous proteins influencing the local mechanisms of calcification. *Clin Orthop Relat Res* 200:362, 1985.
210. Fiskum G, Lehninger AL: Mitochondrial regulation of intracellular calcium, in Cheung WY (ed): *Calcium and Cell Function*. New York, Academic Press, 1982, vol 2, p 39.
211. Fogh-Andersen N: Albumin/calcium association at different pH, as determined by potentiometry. *Clin Chem* 23:2122, 1977.
212. Fontaine O et al: Liponomic control of Ca^{2+} transport: Relationship to mechanism of action of 1,25-dihydroxyvitamin D_3. *Proc Natl Acad Sci U S A* 78:1751, 1981.
213. Forman BM, Samuels HH: Interactions among a subfamily of nuclear hormone receptors: The regulatory zipper model. *Mol Endocrinol* 4:1293, 1990.
214. Fox J et al: Episodic secretion of parathyroid hormone in the dog. *Am J Physiol* 241:E171, 1981.
215. Franceschi RT, DeLuca HF: The effect of inhibitors of protein and RNA synthesis on 1α,25-dihydroxyvitamin D_3-dependent calcium uptake in cultured embryonic chick duodenum. *J Biol Chem* 256:3848, 1981.
216. Friedman PA: Basal and hormone-activated calcium absorption in mouse renal thick ascending limbs. *Am J Physiol* 254:F62, 1988.
217. Friedman PA et al: Sodium-calcium interactions in the renal proximal convoluted tubule of the rabbit. *Am J Physiol* 240:F558, 1981.
218. Frindt G, Windhager EE: Ca^{2+}-dependent inhibition of sodium transport in rabbit cortical collecting tubules. *Am J Physiol* 258:F568, 1990.
219. Frindt G et al: Hydroosmotic response of collecting tubules to ADH or cAMP at reduced peritubular sodium. *Am J Physiol* 243:F503, 1982.
220. Gallagher JC et al: Effect of estrogen on calcium absorption and serum vitamin D metabolites in postmenopausal osteoporosis. *J Clin Endocrinol Metab* 51:1359, 1980.
221. Gallagher JC et al: Intestinal calcium absorption and serum vitamin D metabolites in normal subjects and osteoporotic patients: Effect of age and dietary calcium. *J Clin Invest* 64:729, 1979.
222. Garn SM: *The Earlier Gain and the Later Loss of Cortical Bone*, Springfield, Ill, Thomas, 1970.
223. Garn SM, Clark DC: Nutrition, growth, development and maturation: Findings from the Ten-State Survey 1968–1970. *Pediatrics* 56:306, 1975.
224. Garrett IR et al: Production of the bone resorbing cytokine lymphotoxin by cultured human myeloma cells. *N Engl J Med* 317:526, 1987.
225. Gehron-Robey P et al: The biochemistry of bone, in Riggs BL, Melton LJ (eds): *Osteoporosis: Etiology, Diagnosis, and Management*, New York, Raven Press, 1988.
226. Genant HK et al: Quantitative computed tomography of vertebral spongiosa: A sensitive method for detecting early bone loss after oophorectomy. *Ann Intern Med* 97:699, 1982.
227. Ghijsen WEJM, van Os CH: 1α,25-dihydroxyvitamin D_3 regulates ATP-dependent calcium transport in basolateral plasma membranes of rat enterocytes. *Biochim Biophys Acta* 689:170, 1982.
228. Ghijsen WEJM et al: ATP-dependent calcium transport and its correlation with Ca^{2+}-ATPase activity in baso-

lateral plasma membranes of rat duodenum. *Biochim Biophys Acta* 689:327, 1982.

229. Ghijsen WEJM et al: Kinetic properties of Na^+/Ca^{2+} exchange in basolateral plasma membranes of rat small intestine. *Biochim Biophys Acta* 730:85, 1983.
230. Ghijsen WEJM et al: Regulation of duodenal Ca^{2+} pump by calmodulin and vitamin D-dependent Ca^{2+} binding protein. *Am J Physiol* 251:G223, 1986.
231. Glowacki J et al: Calcitonin produces hypercalcemia in leopard sharks. *Endocrinology* 116:827, 1985.
232. Gmaj P, Murer H: Calcium transport mechanisms in epithelial cell membranes. *Miner Electrolyte Metab* 14:22, 1988.
233. Gmaj P et al: Calcium ion transport across plasma membranes isolated from rat kidney cortex. *Biochem J* 178:549, 1979.
234. Gmaj P et al: A high-affinity, calmodulin-dependent Ca^{2+} pump in the basal-lateral plasma membranes of kidney cortex. *Eur J Biochem* 136:71, 1983.
235. Goldberg M et al: Renal handling of phosphate, calcium, and magnesium, in Brenner BM, Rector FC Jr (eds): *The Kidney*. Philadelphia, Saunders, 1976, vol 1, p 344.
236. Goligorsky MS et al: Cytoplasmic calcium in individual proximal tubular cells in culture. *Am J Physiol* 251:F938, 1986.
237. Goligorsky MS et al: Hormonal regulation of gluconeogenesis in cultured proximal tubular cells: Role of cytosolic calcium. *Am J Physiol* 253:F802, 1987.
238. Goltzman D et al: Studies of the multiple forms of bioactive parathyroid hormone and parathyroid hormone-like substances. *Recent Prog Horm Res* 42:665, 1986.
239. Gonzalez E et al: Cell osmotic water permeability of isolated rabbit proximal straight tubules. *Am J Physiol* 242:F321, 1982.
240. Gray RW et al: Metabolism and excretion of ^3H-1,25-$(OH)_2$-D_3 in healthy adults. *J Clin Endocrinol Metab* 46:756, 1978.
241. Greeley GH et al: Intracerebroventricular administration of calcitonin enhances glucose-stimulated release of insulin. *Regul Pept* 24:259, 1989.
242. Griessen M et al: Effect of absorbable and nonabsorbable sugars on intestinal calcium absorption in humans. *Gastroenterology* 96:769, 1989.
243. Grinstead WC et al: Effect of 1,25-dihydroxyvitamin D_3 on calcium absorption in the colon of healthy humans. *Am J Physiol* 247:G189, 1984.
244. Gross M, Kumar R: Physiology and biochemistry of vitamin D-dependent calcium binding proteins. *Am J Physiol* 259:F195, 1990.
245. Gunter TE et al: Mechanisms of mitochondrial calcium transport. *Adv Exp Med Biol* 232:1, 1988.
246. Gurd FRN, Wilcox PE: Complex formation between metallic cations and proteins, peptides, and amino acids. *Adv Protein Chem* 11:311, 1956.
247. Gylfe E et al: Monoclonal antiparathyroid antibodies: Tools for studies of the regulation of cytoplasmic calcium and function of parathyroid and other antibody-reactive cells. *Cell Calcium* 11:329, 1990.
248. Habener JF: Cyclic AMP response element binding proteins: A cornucopia of transcription factors. *Mol Endocrinol* 4:1087, 1990.
249. Habener JF, Potts JT: Relative effectiveness of magnesium and calcium on the secretion and biosynthesis of parathyroid hormone *in vitro*. *Endocrinology* 98:197, 1976.
250. Haddad JG et al: Vitamin D uptake and metabolism by perfused rat liver: Influences of carrier proteins. *Endocrinology* 123:498, 1988.
251. Halloran BP, DeLuca HF: Calcium transport in small intestine during early development: Role of vitamin D. *Am J Physiol* 239:G473, 1980.
252. Halloran BP et al: Chronic 1,25-dihydroxyvitamin D_3 administration in the rat reduces the serum concentration of 25-hydroxyvitamin D by increasing metabolic clearance rate. *J Clin Invest* 78:622, 1986.
253. Hammerman MR, Hruska KA: Cyclic AMP-dependent protein phosphorylation in canine renal brush border membrane vesicles is associated with decreased phosphate transport. *J Biol Chem* 257:992, 1982.
254. Hanai H et al: Parathyroid hormone increases sodium/calcium exchange activity in renal cells and the blunting of the response in aging. *J Biol Chem* 261:5419, 1986.
255. Hanaoka K et al: Evidence for pH-dependent active Ca^{2+} transport in the basolateral membrane of rabbit cortical thick ascending limb. *J Am Soc Nephrol* 1:576, 1990.
256. Hansford RG: Relation between mitochondrial calcium transport and control of energy metabolism. *Rev Physiol Biochem Pharmacol* 102:1, 1985.
257. Harned HS, Owen BB: *The Physical Chemistry of Electrolytic Solutions,* 3d ed. New York, Reinhold, 1958, pp 383, 514.
258. Haussler MR, Brickman AS: Vitamin D: Metabolism, actions, and disease states, in Bronner F, Coburn JW (eds): *Disorders of Mineral Metabolism, Calcium Physiology.* New York, Academic Press, 1982, vol 2, p 359.
259. Haussler MR, McCain TA: Basic and clinical concepts related to vitamin D metabolism and action. *N Engl J Med* 297:974 and 1040, 1977.
260. Heaney RP: Nutritional factors in bone health, in Riggs BL, Melton LJ (eds): *Osteoporosis: Etiology, Diagnosis, and Management.* New York, Raven Press, 1988, p 359.
261. Heaney RP et al: Calcium balance and calcium requirements in middle-aged women. *Am J Clin Nutr* 30:1603, 1977.
262. Heersche JNM: Bone cells and bone turnover: The basis for pathogenesis in metabolic bone disease: Cellular and tissue mechanisms, in Tam C et al (eds): *Metabolic Bone Disease: Cellular and Tissue Mechanisms.* Boca Raton, Fla, CRC Press, 1989.
263. Henderson JE et al: Circulating concentrations of parathyroid hormone-like peptide in malignancy and hyperparathyroidism. *J Bone Miner Res* 5:105, 1990.
264. Hendy GN et al: Cloning and nucleotide sequence of DNA coding for bovine pre-proparathyroid hormone. *Proc Natl Acad Sci U S A* 78:7365, 1979.
265. Hendy GN et al: Nucleotide sequence of cloned cDNAs encoding human preproparathyroid hormone. *Proc Natl Acad Sci U S A* 78:7365, 1981.
266. Hesch RD et al: Pulsatile secretion of parathyroid hormone and its action on a type I and type II PTH receptor: A hypothesis for understanding osteoporosis. *Calcif Tissue Int* 42:341, 1988.
267. Hess AF, Weinstock M: Antirachitic properties imparted

to inert fluids and green vegetables by ultraviolet irradiation. *J Biol Chem* 62:301, 1924.
268. Hirose RP, Chang EB: Effects of serotonin on Na^+-H^+ exchange and intracellular calcium in isolated chicken enterocytes. *Am J Physiol* 254:G891, 1988.
269. Holick MF: Vitamin D: Biosynthesis, metabolism and mode of action, in DeGroot LJ (ed): *Endocrinology*. Philadelphia, Saunders, 1989, p 902.
270. Holick MF et al: Factors that influence the cutaneous photosynthesis of previtamin D_3. *Science* 211:590, 1981.
271. Holmes RP et al: The effect of membrane lipid composition on the permeability of membranes to Ca^{2+}. *Ann N Y Acad Sci* 414:44, 1983.
272. Homaidan FR et al: Two calcium channels in basolateral membranes of rabbit ileal epithelial cells. *Am J Physiol* 257:G86, 1989.
273. Horiuchi N et al: Similarity of synthetic peptide from human tumor to parathyroid hormone *in vivo* and *in vitro*. *Science* 238:1566, 1987.
274. Horst RL et al: 24-hydroxylation of 1,25-dihydroxyergocalciferol: An unambiguous deactivation process. *J Biol Chem* 261:9250, 1986.
275. Horton MA et al: Identification of human osteoclasts with monoclonal antibodies. *N Engl J Med* 312:923, 1985.
276. Howell DS, Pita JC: Calcification of growth plate cartilage with special reference to studies on micropuncture fluids. *Clin Orthop* 118:208, 1976.
277. Hruska KA et al: Effects of parathyroid hormone on cytosolic calcium in renal proximal tubular primary cultures. *Am J Physiol* 251:F188, 1986.
278. Hruska KA et al: Phosphorylation of renal brush-border membrane vesicles: Effect on calcium uptake and membrane content of polyphosphoinositides. *J Biol Chem* 258:2501, 1983.
279. Hruska KA et al: Stimulation of inositol trisphosphate and diacylglycerol production in renal tubular cells by parathyroid hormone. *J Clin Invest* 79:230, 1987.
280. Huang YC et al: Effect of hormones and development on the expression of the rat 1,25-dihydroxyvitamin D_3 receptor gene: Comparison with calbindin gene expression. *J Biol Chem* 264:17454, 1989.
281. Huffer WE: Morphology and biochemistry of bone remodeling: Possible control by vitamin D, parathyroid hormone and other substances. *Lab Invest* 59:418, 1988.
282. Hughes WS et al: The effect of the bicarbonate anion on serum ionized calcium concentration *in vitro*. *J Lab Clin Med* 103:93, 1984.
283. Hui SL, Wiske PS: A prospective study of change in bone mass with age in post-menopausal women. *J Chron Dis* 35:715, 1982.
284. Huldschinsky K: Heilung von Rachitis durch Kunstliche Hohensonne. *Dtsch Med Wochenschr* 14:712, 1919.
285. Hurley D et al: Axial and appendicular bone mineral density in patients with long-term deficiency or excess of calcitonin. *N Engl J Med* 317:537, 1987.
286. Hurwitz SL: Calcium metabolism in birds, in Florkin M, Scheer BJ (eds): *Chemical Zoology*. New York, Academic Press, 1978, vol 10, p 273.
287. Hylander E et al: Calcium absorption after intestinal resection: The importance of a preserved colon. *Scand J Gastroenterol* 25:705, 1990.
288. Ikeda K, Broadus AE: Regulation of parathyroid hormone–related peptide gene expression by cycloheximide. *J Biol Chem* 265:5398, 1990.
289. Imai M: Calcium transport across the rabbit thick ascending limb of Henle's loop perfused *in vitro*. *Pfluegers Arch* 374:255, 1978.
290. Imai M: Effects of parathyroid hormone and N^6, $O^{2'}$-dibutyryl cyclic AMP on Ca^{2+} transport across the rabbit distal nephron segments perfused *in vitro*. *Pfluegers Arch* 390:145, 1981.
291. Inesi G: Mechanism of calcium transport. *Ann Rev Physiol* 47:573, 1985.
292. Ireland P, Fordtran JS: Effect of dietary calcium and age on jejunal calcium absorption in humans studied by intestinal perfusion. *J Clin Invest* 52:2672, 1973.
293. Irons LI, Perkins DJ: Studies on the interaction of magnesium, calcium and strontium ions with native and chemically modified human serum albumin. *Biochem J* 84:152, 1962.
294. Jackson JA et al: Bone histomorphometry in hypogonadal and eugonadal men with spinal osteoporosis. *J Clin Endocrinol Metab* 65:53, 1987.
295. Jacobson AL et al: Urinary ionic calcium and binding sites in normocalciuric idiopathic calcium urolithiasis. *Invest Urol* 17:218, 1979.
296. Jacobson HR: Transport characteristics of *in vitro* perfused proximal convoluted tubules. *Kidney Int* 22:425, 1982.
297. Jaegar P et al: Evidence that calcitonin stimulates 1,25-dihydroxyvitamin D production and intestinal absorption of calcium *in vivo*. *J Clin Invest* 78:456, 1986.
298. James PH et al: Primary structure of the cAMP-dependent phosphorylation site of the plasma membrane calcium pump. *Biochem* 28:4253, 1989.
299. Jayakumar A et al: Sodium gradient-dependent calcium uptake in renal basolateral membrane vesicles: Effect of parathyroid hormone. *J Biol Chem* 259:10827, 1984.
300. Jee WSS et al: The effects of prostaglandin E_2 in growing rats: Increased metaphyseal hard tissue and cortico-endosteal bone formation. *Calcif Tissue Int* 37:148, 1985.
301. Johnson GL, Dhanasekaren N: The G-protein family and their interaction with receptors. *Endocr Rev* 10:317, 1989.
302. Johnson MW: Behavior of fluid in stressed bone and cellular stimulation. *Calicif Tissue Int* 34:(suppl)S72, 1984.
303. Jones HH et al: Humeral hypertrophy in response to exercise. *J Bone Joint Surg* 59-A:204, 1977.
304. Joyce ME et al: Transforming growth factor-β initiates cartilage and bone formation *in vivo*, in Cohn DV et al (eds): *Calcium Regulation and Bone Metabolism: Basic and Clinical Aspects*. Amsterdam, Excerpta Medica, 1990.
305. Kaissling B, Kriz W: Structural analysis of the rabbit kidney, in Brodal A et al (eds): *Advances in Anatomy, Embryology, and Cell Biology*, Berlin, Springer-Verlag, vol 56, 1979.
306. Kalser MH: Water and mineral transport, in Bockus HLB et al (eds): *Gastroenterology*, 3d ed. Philadelphia, Saunders, 1976, vol 2, p 79.

307. Kalu DN et al: Parathyroid hormone and experimental osteoporosis. *Lancet* 1:1363, 1970.
308. Kanders B et al: Interaction of calcium nutrition and physical activity on bone mass in young women. *J Bone Miner Res* 3:145, 1988.
309. Kao PC et al: Parathyroid hormone-related peptide in plasma of patients with hypercalcemia and malignant lesions. *Mayo Clin Proc* 65:1399, 1990.
310. Karbach U, Rummel W: Calcium transport across the colon ascendens and the influence of 1,25-dihydroxyvitamin D_3 and dexamethasone. *Eur J Clin Invest* 17:368, 1987.
311. Karpf DB et al: Molecular determinants of parathyroid hormone function, in Cohn DV et al (eds): *Calcium Regulation and Bone Metabolism: Basic and Clinical Aspects.* Amsterdam, Exerpta Medica, 1990, p 15.
312. Katz S, Klotz IM: Interactions of calcium with serum albumin. *Arch Biochem Biophys* 44:351, 1953.
313. Kawashima H et al: Localization of 25-hydroxyvitamin D_3-1,α-hydroxylase and 24-hydroxylase along the rat nephron. *Proc Natl Acad Sci U S A* 76:1199, 1981.
314. Kelepouris E: Renal handling of calcium. *Am J Nephrol* 8:226, 1988.
315. Khosla S et al: Parathyroid hormone related peptide in lactation and in umbilical cord blood. *Mayo Clin Proc* 65:1408, 1990.
316. Kitamura N et al: Episodic fluctuation in serum intact parathyroid hormone concentration in men. *J Clin Endocrinol Metab* 70:252, 1990.
317. Komm BS et al: Estrogen binding receptor mRNA and biological response in osteoblast-like cells. *Science* 241:84, 1988.
318. Kowarski S, Schachter D: Intestinal membrane calcium-binding protein: Vitamin D-dependent membrane component of the intestinal calcium transport mechanism. *J Biol Chem* 255:10834, 1980.
319. Krall EA et al: Effect of vitamin D intake on seasonal variations in parathyroid hormone secretion in postmenopausal women. *N Engl J Med* 321:1777, 1989.
320. Krejs GJ et al: Effect of 1,25-dihydroxyvitamin D_3 on calcium and magnesium absorption in the healthy human jejunum and ileum. *Am J Med* 75:973, 1983.
321. Kretsinger RH et al: Model of facilitated diffusion of calcium by the intestinal calcium binding protein, in Norman AW et al (eds): *Vitamin D: Chemical, Biochemical and Clinical Endocrinology of Calcium Metabolism.* Berlin, de Gruyter, 1982, p 233.
322. Kreutter D et al: The effect of essential fatty acid deficiency on the stimulation of intestinal calcium transport by 1,25-dihydroxyvitamin D_3. *J Biol Chem* 258:4977, 1983.
323. Kriska AM et al: The assessment of historical physical activity and its relation to adult bone parameters. *Am J Epidemiol* 127:1053, 1988.
324. Ladenson JH: Clinical chemistry of disorders of mineral homeostasis, in Sonnenwirth AC, Jarrett L (eds): *Gradwohl's Clinical Laboratory Methods and Diagnosis,* 8th ed. St. Louis, Mosby, 1980, vol 1, p 324.
325. Ladenson JH, Shyong JC: Influence of fatty acids on the binding of calcium to human serum albumin. *Clin Chim Acta* 75:293, 1977.
326. Lanyon LE: Functional strain in bone tissue as an objective and controlling stimulus for adaptive bone remodelling. *J Biomech* 20:1083, 1987.
327. Lau K, Bourdeau JE: Evidence for cAMP-dependent protein kinase in mediating the parathyroid hormone-stimulated rise in cysotolic free calcium in rabbit connecting tubules. *J Biol Chem* 264:4028, 1989.
328. Lau K, Bourdeau JE: Evidence for luminal Ca:H exchange in rabbit connecting tubules. *J Am Soc Nephrol* 1:724, 1990.
329. LeBoff MS et al: Role of cytosolic calcium in the control of cAMP content by calcium in bovine parathyroid cells. *Mol Cell Endocrinol* 45:127, 1986.
330. Lee CO et al: Cytosolic calcium ion activity in epithelial cells of *Necturus* kidney. *Nature* 287:859, 1980.
331. Lee DBN: Unanticipated stimulatory action of glucocorticoids on epithelial calcium absorption: Effect of dexamethasone on rat distal colon. *J Clin Invest* 71:322, 1983.
332. Lee DBN et al: Calcium and inorganic phosphate transport in rat colon: Dissociated response to 1,25-dihydroxyvitamin D_3. *J Clin Invest* 65:1326, 1980.
333. Lee DBN et al: Intestinal and metabolic effect of 1,25-dihydroxyvitamin D_3 in normal adult rat. *Am J Physiol* 240:G90, 1981.
334. Leff SG et al: Production of a novel neuropeptide encoded by the calcitonin gene via tissue-specific RNA processing. *Nature* 304:129, 1983.
335. Lehninger AL: Mitochondria and the physiology of Ca^{++}. *Trans Am Clin Climatol Assoc* 83:83, 1973.
336. Lehninger AL et al: Transport and accumulation of calcium in mitochondria. *N Y Acad Sci* 307:160, 1978.
337. Lemann J Jr: Idiopathic hypercalciuria, in Coe FL et al (eds): *Nephrolithiasis, Contemporary Issues in Nephrology.* New York, Churchill Livingstone, 1980, vol 5, p 86.
338. Lemann J Jr et al: The importance of renal net acid excretion as a determinant of fasting urinary calcium excretion. *Kidney Int* 29:743, 1986.
339. Lemann J Jr et al: Urinary calcium excretion in human beings. *N Engl J Med* 301:535, 1979.
340. Levine BA, Williams RJP: Calcium binding to proteins and other large biological anion centers, in Cheung WY (ed): *Calcium and Cell Function.* New York, Academic Press, 1982, vol 2, p 1.
341. Levine BA, Williams RJP: The chemistry of calcium ion and its biological relevance, in Anghileri LJ, Tuffet-Anghileri AM (eds): *The Role of Calcium in Biological Systems.* Boca Raton, Fla, CRC Press, 1982, vol 1, p 3.
342. Levine BS et al: Intestinal absorption of calcium: Its assessment, normal physiology, and alterations in various disease states, in Bronner F, Coburn JW (eds): *Disorders of Mineral Metabolism, Calcium Physiology.* New York, Academic Press, 1982, vol 2, p 103.
343. Levine MA, Aurbach GD: Pseudohypoparathyroidism, in DeGroot LJ (ed): *Endocrinology.* Philadelphia, Saunders, 1989, vol 2, p 1065.
344. Lian JB, Gundberg CM: Osteocalcin: Biochemical considerations and clinical applications. *Clin Orthop* 226:267, 1988.
345. Lian JB et al: Studies of hormonal regulation of osteocalcin synthesis in cultured fetal rat calvariae. *J Biol Chem* 260:931, 1985.

346. Liel Y et al: Effects of race and body habitus on bone mineral density of the radius, hip, and spine in premenopausal women. *J Clin Endocrinol Metab* 66:1247, 1988.
347. Lindsay R et al: Bone response to termination of oestrogen treatment. *Lancet* 1:1325, 1978.
348. Lindsay R et al: Long-term prevention of spinal osteoporosis by estrogens. *Lancet* 1:1038, 1976.
349. Lips P et al: Mean wall thickness of trabecular bone packets in the human iliac crest: Changes with age. *Calcif Tissue Res* 26:13, 1978.
350. Lorenzen M et al: Quinidine effect on hydroosmotic response of collecting tubules to vasopressin and cAMP. *Am J Physiol* 252:F1103, 1987.
351. Lyons KM et al: Organogenesis and pattern formation in the mouse: RNA distribution patterns suggest a role for bone morphogenetic protein-2A (BMO-2A). *Development* 109:833, 1990.
352. MacDonald BR et al: Formation of multinucleated cells which respond to osteotropic hormones in long-term human bone marrow cultures. *Endocrinology* 120:2326, 1987.
353. MacDonald RC: Energetics of permeation of thin lipid membranes by ions. *Biochim Biophys Acta* 448:193, 1976.
354. MacLaughlin J, Holick MF: Aging decreases the capacity of human skin to produce vitamin D_3. *J Clin Invest* 76:1536, 1985.
355. Madsen S et al: Suppressive effect of 1,25-dihydroxyvitamin D_3 on circulating parathyroid hormone in acute renal failure. *J Clin Endocrinol Metab* 53:823, 1981.
356. Magaldi AJ et al: Calcium transport across rat inner medullary collecting duct perfused *in vitro*. *Am J Physiol* 257:F738, 1989.
357. Mahan BH: *University Chemistry*. Reading, Mass, Addison-Wesley, 1965, pp 470, 477.
358. Mahoney CA, Nissenson RA: Canine renal receptors for parathyroid hormone: Down regulation *in vivo* by exogenous parathyroid hormone. *J Clin Invest* 72:411, 1983.
359. Maierhofer WJ et al: Phosphate deprivation increases serum 1,25-$(OH)_2$-vitamin D concentrations in healthy men. *Kidney Int* 25:571, 1984.
360. Malloy PJ et al: The molecular basis of hereditary 1,25-dihydroxyvitamin D_3 resistant rickets in seven related families. *J Clin Invest* 86:2071, 1990.
361. Mangin M et al: Identification of a cDNA encoding a parathyroid hormone-like peptide from a human tumor associated with humoral hypercalcemia of malignancy. *Proc Natl Acad Sci U S A* 85:597, 1988.
362. Mangin M et al: Two distinct tumor-derived parathyroid hormone-like peptides result from alternative ribonucleic acid splicing. *Mol Endocrinol* 2:1049, 1988.
363. Mann S. Molecular recognition in biomineralization. *Nature* 1:119, 1988.
363a. Marcus R et al: Conjugated estrogens in the treatment of postmenopausal women with hyperparathyroidism. *Ann Intern Med* 100:633–640, 1984.
364. Marcus R et al: Menstrual function and bone mass in elite women distance runners. *Ann Intern Med* 102:158, 1985.
365. Markose E et al: Vitamin D-mediated modifications in protein-DNA interactions at two promoter elements of the osteocalcin gene. *Proc Natl Acad Sci U S A* 87:1701, 1990.
366. Markowitz ME et al: Temporal interrelationships between the circadian rhythms of serum parathyroid hormone and calcium concentrations. *J Clin Endocrinol Metab* 67:1068, 1988.
367. Martin TJ, Suva LJ: Parathyroid hormone-related protein in hypercalcemia of malignancy. *Clin Endocrinol* 31:631, 1989.
368. Marx SJ et al: Calciferols: Actions and deficiencies in action. *Vitam Horm* 40:235, 1983.
369. Marx SJ, Bourdeau JE: Calcium metabolism, in Maxwell MH et al (eds): *Clinical Disorders of Fluid and Electrolyte Metabolism,* 4th ed. New York, McGraw-Hill, 1987, p 214.
370. Massin JP et al: Compartmental analysis of calcium kinetics in man: Application of a four-compartmental model. *Metabolism* 23:399, 1974.
371. Massry SG.: The toxic effects of parathyroid hormone in uremia. *Semin Nephrol* 3:306, 1983.
372. Massry SG, Coburn JW: Divalent ions and the kidney, in Kurtzman NA, Martinez-Maldonado M (eds): *Pathophysiology of the Kidney*. Springfield, Ill, Thomas, 1977, p 596.
373. Matkovic V et al: Bone status and fracture rates in two regions of Yugoslavia. *Am J Clin Nutr* 32:540, 1979.
374. Mayer GP: Effect of calcium and magnesium on parathyroid hormone secretory rate in calves, in Owen, M. et al (eds): *Calcium Regulating Hormones*. Amsterdam, Exerpta Medica, 1975.
375. Mayer GP, Hurst JG: Comparison of the effects of calcium and magnesium on parathyroid hormone secretion rate in calves. *Endocrinology* 102:1803, 1978.
376. Mayer GP et al: Effects of plasma calcium concentration on the relative proportion of hormone and carboxyl fragments in parathyroid venous blood. *Endocrinology* 105:1778, 1979.
377. Mazess RB: On aging bone loss. *Clin Orthop* 165:239, 1982.
378. McCarthy TL et al: Parathyroid hormone enhances the transcript and polypeptide levels of insulin-like growth factor I in osteoblast-enriched cultures from fetal rat bone. *Endocrinology* 124:1247, 1989.
379. McCarthy TL et al: Regulatory effects of insulin-like growth factor I and II on bone collagen synthesis in rat calvarial cells. *Endocrinology* 124:301, 1989.
380. McDermott MT, Kidd GS: The role of calcitonin in the development and treatment of osteoporosis. *Endocr Rev* 8:377, 1987.
381. McDermott MT et al: Reduced bone mineral content in totally thyroidectomized patients: Possible effect of calcitonin deficiency. *J Clin Endocrinol Metab* 56:936, 1983.
382. McSheehy PMJ, Chambers TJ: 1,25-dihydroxyvitamin D_3 stimulates rat osteoblastic cells to release a soluble factor that increases osteoclastic bone resorption. *J Clin Invest* 80:425, 1987.
383. McSheehy PMJ, Chambers TJ: Osteoblastic cells mediate osteoclastic responsiveness to parathyroid hormone. *Endocrinology* 118:824, 1986.

384. Mellanby E. An experimental investigation of rickets. *Lancet* 1:407, 1919.
385. Meunier PJ et al: Bone histomorphometry in corticosteroid-induced osteoporosis and Cushing's syndrome. *Adv Exp Med Biol* 171:191, 1984.
386. Milhaud G et al: Calcitonin, a major gill hormone. *Proc Natl Acad Sci U S A* 77:6935, 1980.
387. Miller A, Bronner F: Calcium uptake in isolated brush-border vesicles from rat small intestine. *Biochem J* 196:391, 1981.
388. Miller A et al: Characterization of calcium binding to brush-border membranes from rat duodenum. *Biochem J* 208:773, 1982.
389. Mok LL et al: Parathyroid hormone as a smooth muscle relaxant. *Endocr Rev* 10:420, 1989.
390. Moller M et al: Metacarpal morphometry in monozygotic and dizygotic elderly twins. *Calcif Tissue Res* 25:197, 1978.
391. Moore EW: Ionized calcium in normal serum, ultrafiltrates, and whole blood determined by ion-exchange electrodes. *J Clin Invest* 49:318, 1970.
392. Moore LJ, Machlan LA: High accuracy determination of calcium in blood serum by isotope dilution mass spectrometry. *Anal Chem* 44:2291, 1972.
393. Morel F: Sites of hormone action in the mammalian nephron. *Am J Physiol* 240:F159, 1981.
394. Morrison N et al: 1,25-dihydroxyvitamin D-responsive element and glucocorticoid repression in the osteocalcin gene. *Science* 246:1158, 1989.
395. Moy TC et al: Intestinal basolateral membrane Ca-ATPase activity with properties distinct from those of the Ca-pump. *Biochem Biophys Res Commun* 141:979, 1986.
396. Mulderry PK et al: Calcitonin gene-related peptide in cardiovascular tissues of the rat. *Neuroscience* 14:947, 1985.
397. Müller-Plathe O, Lindmann K: Ionized calcium versus total calcium. *Scand J Clin Lab Invest* 43(suppl 165):71, 1983.
398. Murer H, Hildmann B: Transcellular transport of calcium and inorganic phosphate in the small intestinal epithelium. *Am J Physiol* 240:G409, 1981.
399. Murphy E et al: Effects of calcitonin on cytosolic Ca in a suspension of rabbit medullary thick ascending limb tubules. *Am J Physiol* 251:C491, 1986.
400. Muto S et al: Electrophysiological identification of α- and β-intercalated cells and their distribution along the rabbit distal nephron segments. *J Clin Invest* 86:1829, 1990.
401. Naveh-Many T et al: Calcium regulates parathyroid hormone messenger ribonucleic acid (mRNA), but not calcitonin mRNA *in vivo* in the rat: Dominant role of 1,25-dihydroxyvitamin D. *Endocrinology* 125:275, 1989.
402. Naveh-Many T, Silver J: Regulation of calcitonin gene transcription by vitamin D metabolites *in vivo* in the rat. *J Clin Invest* 81:270, 1988.
403. Naveh-Many T, Silver J: Regulation of parathyroid hormone gene expression by hypocalcemia, hypercalcemia, and vitamin D in the rat. *J Clin Invest* 86:1313, 1990.
404. Naylor SL et al: Human parathyroid hormone gene (PTH) is on short arm of chromosome 11. *Somatic Cell Genet* 9:609, 1983.
405. Nellans HN: Intestinal calcium absorption: Interplay of paracellular and cellular pathways. *Miner Electrolyte Metab* 16:101, 1990.
406. Nellans HN, Goldsmith RS: Transepithelial calcium transport by rat cecum: High efficiency absorptive site. *Am J Physiol* 240:G424, 1981.
407. Nellans HN, Kimberg DV: Anomalous calcium secretion in rat ileum: Role of paracellular pathway. *Am J Physiol* 236:E473, 1979.
408. Nellans HN, Kimberg DV: Cellular and paracellular calcium transport in rat ileum: Effects of dietary calcium. *Am J Physiol* 235:E726, 1978.
409. Nellans HN, Kimberg DV: Intestinal calcium transport: Absorption, secretion, and vitamin D, in Crane RK (ed): *Gastrointestinal Physiology III, International Review of Physiology.* Baltimore, University Park Press, 1979, vol 19, p 227.
410. Nellans HN, Popovitch JE: Calmodulin-regulated, ATP-driven calcium transport by basolateral membranes of rat small intestine. *J Biol Chem* 256:9932, 1981.
411. Nemere I, Norman AW: Transcaltachia, vesicular calcium transport, and microtubule-associated calbindin-D_{28k}: Emerging views of 1,25-dihydroxyvitamin D_3-mediated intestinal calcium absorption. *Miner Electrolyte Metab* 16:109, 1990.
412. Nemeth EF: Regulation of cytosolic calcium by extracellular divalent cations in C-cells and parathyroid cells. *Cell Calcium* 11:323, 1990.
413. Nemeth EF, Carafoli E: The role of extracellular calcium in the regulation of intracellular calcium and cell function. *Cell Calcium* 11:319, 1990.
414. Nemeth EF, Scarpa A: Cytosolic Ca^{2+} and the regulation of secretion in parathyroid cells. *FEBS Lett* 203:15, 1986.
415. Nemeth EF, Scarpa A: Rapid mobilization of cellular Ca^{2+} in bovine parathyroid cells evoked by extracellular divalent cations: Evidence for a cell surface calcium receptor. *J Biol Chem* 262:5188, 1987.
416. Neuman WF: The *milieu interieur* of bone: Claude Bernard revisited. *Fed Proc* 28:1846, 1969.
417. Neuman WF, Neuman MW: *The Chemical Dynamics of Bone Mineral.* Chicago, University of Chicago Press, 1958, pp 1–19.
418. Neuman WF, Neuman MW: Studies of diffusion in calvaria. *Calcif Tissue Int* 33:441, 1981.
419. Ng RCK et al: Calcium transport in the rabbit superficial proximal convoluted tubule. *J Clin Invest* 74:834, 1984.
420. Ng RCK et al: Divalent cation transport in isolated tubules. *Kidney Int* 22:492, 1982.
421. Nicholls DG, Åkerman K: Mitochondrial calcium transport. *Biochim Biophys Acta* 683:57, 1982.
422. Nicholls DG, Crompton M: Mitochondrial calcium transport. *FEBS Lett* 111:261, 1980.
423. Nicholson C et al: Calcium modulation in brain extracellular microenvironment demonstrated with ion-selective micropipette. *Proc Natl Acad Sci U S A* 74:1287, 1977.
424. Nicholson GC et al: Abundant calcitonin receptors in isolated rat osteoclasts: Biochemical and autoradiographic characterization. *J Clin Invest* 78:355, 1986.
425. Nielsen HK et al: The effects of high dose glucocorticoid administration on serum bone gamma-carboxyglutamic

acid-containing protein, serum alkaline phosphatase, and vitamin D metabolites in normal subjects. *Bone Miner* 4:105, 1988.

426. Nijweide PJ et al: Cells of bone: Proliferation, differentiation and hormonal regulation. *Physiol Rev* 66:855, 1986.
427. Nordin BEC: Nutritional considerations, in Nordin BEC (ed): *Calcium, Phosphate, and Magnesium Metabolism.* New York, Churchill Livingstone, 1976, p 3.
428. Nordin BEC, Peacock M: Role of the kidney in regulation of plasma calcium. *Lancet* 2:1280, 1969.
429. Norman AW: Intestinal calcium absorption: A vitamin D-hormone-mediated adaptive response. *Am J Clin Nutr* 51:290, 1990.
430. Norman AW et al: Intestinal calcium transport: Pleiotropic effects mediated by vitamin D. *Fed Proc* 41:78, 1982.
431. Oetting M et al: Permeabilization reveals classical stimulus-secretion coupling in bovine parathyroid cells. *Endocrinology* 121:1571, 1987.
432. Okazaki T et al: 5′-flanking region of the parathyroid hormone gene mediates negative regulation by 1,25-dihydroxyvitamin D_3. *J Biol Chem* 263:2203, 1988.
433. Omdahl JL et al: Nutritional status in a healthy elderly population: Vitamin D. *Am J Clin Nutr* 36:1225, 1982.
434. Orloff JJ et al: Parathyroid hormone-like proteins: Biochemical responses and receptor interactions. *Endocr Rev* 10:476, 1989.
435. Owen GM, Lubin LH: Anthropometric differences between black and white preschool children. *Am J Dis Child* 126:168, 1973.
436. Owyang C et al: Comparison of the effects of pentagastrin and meal-stimulated gastrin on plasma calcitonin in normal man. *Am J Dig Dis* 23:1084, 1978.
437. Pak CYC: Physiological basis for absorptive and renal hypercalciurias. *Am J Physiol* 237:F415, 1979.
438. Pak CYC, Fordtran JS: Disorders of mineral metabolism, in Sleisenger MH, Fordtran JS (eds): *Gastrointestinal Disease,* 2d ed. Philadelphia, Saunders, 1978, p 251.
439. Palmer LG, Frindt G: Effects of cell Ca and pH on Na channels from rat cortical collecting tubule. *Am J Physiol* 253:F333, 1987.
440. Pan LC, Price PA: The effect of transcriptional inhibitors on the bone gamma-carboxyglutamic acid protein response to 1,25-dihydroxyvitamin D_3 in osteosarcoma cells. *J Biol Chem* 259:5844, 1984.
441. Pang PKT et al: Inhibition of uterine contraction by synthetic parathyroid hormone fragment. *Life Sci* 28:1317, 1981.
442. Pansu D et al: Duodenal and ileal calcium absorption in the rat and effects of vitamin D. *Am J Physiol* 244:G695, 1983.
443. Pansu D et al: Theophylline inhibits transcellular Ca transport in intestine and Ca binding by CaBP. *Am J Physiol* 257:G935, 1989.
444. Parfitt AM: Bone remodeling: Relationship to the amount and structure of bone and the pathogenesis and prevention of fractures, in Riggs BL, Melton LJ (eds): *Osteoporosis: Etiology, Diagnosis, and Management.* New York, Raven Press, 1988.
445. Parfitt AM, Kleerekoper M: The divalent ion homeostatic system: Physiology and metabolism of calcium, phosphorus, magnesium, and bone, in Maxwell MH, Kleeman CR (eds): *Clinical Disorders of Fluid and Electrolyte Metabolism,* 3d ed. New York, McGraw-Hill, 1980, p 269.
446. Parsons JA, Robinson CJ: Calcium shift into bone causing transient hypocalcemia after injection of parathyroid hormone. *Nature* 230:581, 1971.
447. Parys JB et al: Characterization of ATP-driven calcium uptake in renal basal-lateral and renal endoplasmic reticulum membrane vesicles. *Cell Calcium* 6:413, 1985.
448. Patten JL et al: Mutation in the gene encoding the stimulatory G protein of adenylate cyclase in Albright's hereditary osteodystrophy. *N Engl J Med* 322:1412, 1990.
449. Pauling L: *The Nature of the Chemical Bond and the Structure of Molecules and Crystals: An Introduction to Modern Structural Chemistry,* 3d ed. Ithaca, NY, Cornell University Press, 1960, p 514.
450. Peacock M et al: Relation between serum and urinary calcium with particular reference to parathyroid activity. *Lancet* 1:384, 1969.
451. Pead MJ et al: Direct transformation from quiescence to bone formation in the adult periosteum following a single brief period of bone loading. *J Bone Miner Res* 3:647, 1988.
452. Pedersen KO: Binding of calcium to serum albumin: 1. Stoichiometry and intrinsic association constant at physiological pH, ionic strength, and temperature. *Scand J Clin Lab Invest* 28:459, 1971.
453. Pedersen KO: Binding of calcium to serum albumin: 2. Effect of pH via competitive hydrogen and calcium ion binding to the imidazole groups of albumin. *Scand J Clin Lab Invest* 29:75, 1972.
454. Pedersen KO: Binding of calcium to serum albumin: 4. Effect of temperature and thermodynamics of calcium-albumin interaction. *Scand J Clin Lab Invest* 30:89, 1972.
455. Pedersen KO: Protein-bound calcium in human serum: Quantitative examination of binding and its variables by a molecular binding model and clinical implications for measurement of ionized calcium. *Scand J Clin Lab Invest* 30:321, 1972.
456. Peters T: Serum albumin. *Adv Clin Chem* 13:37, 1970.
457. Petkovich PM et al: 1,25-dihydroxyvitamin D_3 increases epidermal growth factor receptors and transforming growth factor β-like activity in a bone-derived cell line. *J Biol Chem* 262:13424, 1987.
458. Pfeilschifter J, Mundy GR: Modulation of type β transforming growth factor activity in bone cultures by osteotropic hormones. *Proc Natl Acad Sci U S A* 84:2024, 1987.
459. Pfeilschifter J et al: Transforming growth factor β inhibits bone resorption in fetal rat long bone cultures. *J Clin Invest* 82:680, 1988.
460. Philipson KD: Sodium-calcium exchange in plasma membrane vesicles. *Annu Rev Physiol* 47:561, 1985.
461. Pollack SR et al: The electrical double layer in bone and its influence on stress-generated potentials. *Calcif Tissue Int* 35:577, 1984.
462. Pollitzer WS, Anderson JJB: Ethnic and genetic differences in bone mass: A review with a hereditary vs environmental perspective. *Am J Clin Nutr* 50:1244, 1989.
463. Portale AA et al: Effect of dietary phosphorus on circulating concentrations of 1,25-dihydroxyvitamin D and im-

munoreactive parathyroid hormone in children with moderate renal insufficiency. *J Clin Invest* 73:1580, 1984.

464. Portale AA et al: Physiologic regulation of the serum concentration of 1,25-dihydroxyvitamin D by phosphorus in normal men. *J Clin Invest* 83:1494, 1989.
465. Posner AS: The mineral of bone. *Clin Orthop Relat Res* 200:87, 1985.
466. Powell DW: Barrier function of epithelia. *Am J Physiol* 241:G275, 1981.
467. Prince RL et al: Plasma calcitonin levels are not lower than normal in osteoporotic women. *J Clin Endocrinol Metab* 68:684, 1989.
468. Quamme GA: Effect of calcitonin on calcium and magnesium transport in rat nephron. *Am J Physiol* 238:E573, 1980.
469. Quamme GA, Dirks JH: Intraluminal and contraluminal magnesium on magnesium and calcium transfer in the rat nephron. *Am J Physiol* 238:F187, 1980.
470. Quamme GA, Dirks JH: Magnesium transport in the nephron. *Am J Physiol* 239:F393, 1980.
471. Raisz LG: Effects of parathyroid hormone and cortisol on prostaglandin production by neonatal rat calvaria *in vitro*. *Endocr Res* 6:311, 1985.
472. Raisz LG: Local and systemic factors in the pathogenesis of osteoporosis. *N Engl J Med* 318:818, 1988.
473. Raisz LG, Kream BE: Regulation of bone formation: 1. *N Engl J Med* 309:29, 1983; 2. *N Engl J Med* 309:83, 1983.
474. Ramachandran C, Brunette MG: The renal Na^+/Ca^{2+} exchange system is located exclusively in the distal tubule. *Biochem J* 257:259, 1989.
475. Rasmussen H: The calcium messenger system: 1. *N Engl J Med* 314:1094, 1986; 2. *N Engl J Med* 314:1164, 1986.
476. Rasmussen H et al: Information flow in the calcium messenger system, in Poste G, Crooke, ST (eds): *New Insights into Cell and Membrane Transport Processes*. New York, Plenum Press, 1986, p 145.
477. Rasmussen H et al: Role of changes in membrane lipid structure in the action of 1,25-dihydroxyvitamin D_3. *Fed Proc* 41:72, 1982.
478. Rasmussen H et al: Thyrocalcitonin, EGTA, and urinary electrolyte excretion. *J Clin Invest* 46:746, 1967.
479. Recker RR: Calcium absorption and achlorhydria. *N Engl J Med* 313:70, 1985.
480. Reeves JD et al: Host defense in infantile osteopetrosis. *Pediatrics* 64:202, 1979.
481. Reichel H et al: The role of the vitamin D endocrine system in health and disease. *N Engl J Med* 320:980, 1989.
482. Reith EJ: A model for transcellular transport of calcium based on membrane fluidity and movement of calcium carriers within the more fluid microdomains of the plasma membrane. *Calcif Tissue Int* 35:129, 1983.
483. Riggs BL et al: Rates of bone loss in the appendicular and axial skeletons of women: Evidence of substantial vertebral bone loss before menopause. *J Clin Invest* 77:1487, 1986.
484. Robey PG et al: The biochemistry of bone, in Riggs BL, Melton LJ (eds): *Osteoporosis: Etiology, Diagnosis, and Management*. New York, Raven Press, 1988.
485. Robinson RA, Stokes RH: *Electrolyte Solutions: The Measurement and Interpretation of Conductance, Chemical Potential and Diffusion in Solutions of Simple Electrolytes*. London, Butterworth, 1955, pp 239–253.
486. Rocha AS et al: Calcium and phosphate transport in isolated segments of rabbit Henle's loop. *J Clin Invest* 59:975, 1977.
487. Roche C et al: Localization of vitamin D-dependent active Ca^{2+} transport in rat duodenum and relation to CaBP. *Am J Physiol* 251:G314, 1986.
488. Rodan GA, Martin TJ: Role of osteoblasts in hormonal control of bone resorption: A hypothesis. *Calcif Tissue Int* 33:349, 1981.
489. Rodan GA, Rodan SB: Expression of the osteoblastic phenotype, in Peck W (ed): *Bone and Mineral Research*. Amsterdam, Elsevier, 1983.
490. Rodan SB et al: Comparison of postreceptor effects of 1-34 human hypercalcemia factor and 1-34 human parathyroid hormone in rat osteosarcoma cells. *J Clin Invest* 81:924, 1988.
491. Rodda CP et al: Evidence for a novel parathyroid hormone-related protein in fetal lamb parathyroid glands and sheep placenta: Comparisons with a similar protein implicated in humoral hypercalcemia of malignancy. *J Endocrinol* 117:261, 1988.
492. Roodman GD et al: 1,25-dihydroxyvitamin D_3 causes formation of multinucleated cells with several osteoclast characteristics in cultures of primate marrow. *Proc Natl Acad Sci U S A* 82:8213, 1985.
493. Rosen JF et al: Rickets with alopecia: An inborn error of vitamin D metabolism. *J Pediatr* 94:729, 1979.
494. Rosenblatt M: Peptide hormone antagonists that are effective *in vivo:* Lessons from parathyroid hormone. *N Engl J Med* 315:1004, 1986.
495. Rosenblatt M et al: Parathyroid hormone: Physiology, chemistry, biosynthesis, secretion, metabolism, and mode of action, in DeGroot LJ (ed): *Endocrinology*. Philadelphia, Saunders, 1989.
496. Rosenblatt MR et al: Synthesis of a fragment of parathyroid hormone, bPTH-(28-48): An inhibitor of hormone cleavage *in vivo*. *Biochemistry* 16:2811, 1977.
497. Roth J et al: Localization of the vitamin D-dependent calcium-binding protein in mammalian kidney. *Am J Physiol* 243:F243, 1982.
498. Rouse D, Suki WN: Renal control of extracellular calcium. *Kidney Int* 38:700, 1990.
499. Rouse D et al: Calcium transport in the pars recta and thin descending limb of Henle of the rabbit, perfused *in vitro*. *J Clin Invest* 65:37, 1980.
500. Rowe DW, Kream BE: Regulation of collagen synthesis in fetal rat calvaria by 1,25-dihydroxyvitamin D_3. *J Biol Chem* 257:8009, 1982.
501. Rubin CT, Lanyon LE: Regulation of bone formation by applied dynamic loads. *J Bone Joint Surg* 66A:397, 1984.
502. Rude RK et al: Functional hypoparathyroidism and PTH end organ resistance in human magnesium deficiency. *Clin Endocrinol* 5:209, 1976.
503. Rude RK et al: Parathyroid hormone secretion in magnesium deficiency. *J Clin Endocrinol Metab* 60:800, 1978.
504. Ruff CB, Hayes WC: Sex differences in age-related remodeling of the femur and tibia. *J Orthop Res* 6:886, 1988.

505. Russell J et al: Direct regulation by calcium of cytoplasmic messenger ribonucleic acid coding for pre-proparathyroid hormone in isolated bovine parathyroid cells. *J Clin Invest* 72:1851, 1983.
506. Russo A et al: Differential regulation of the coexpressed calcitonin/α-CGRP and β-CGRP neuroendocrine genes. *J Biol Chem* 263:5, 1988.
507. Saarem K et al: Subcellular localization of vitamin D_3 25-hydroxylase in human liver. *J Biol Chem* 259:10936, 1984.
508. Sacks P, Bourdeau JE: Ca^{2+} absorption in the pars recta of cortical segment 2 rabbit proximal tubules: Role of diffusion. *Am J Physiol* 257:F262, 1989.
509. Samaan NA et al: Immunoreactive calcitonin in the mother, neonate, child, and adult. *Am J Obstet Gynecol* 121:622, 1975.
510. Sandler RB et al: The effect of grip strength on radial bone in postmenopausal women. *J Orthop Res* 7:440, 1989.
511. Schachter D, Kowarski S: Isolation of the protein IMCal, a vitamin D-dependent membrane component of the intestinal transport mechanism for calcium. *Fed Proc* 41:84, 1982.
512. Schaer H: Decrease in ionized calcium by bicarbonate in physiological solutions. *Pfluegers Arch* 347:249, 1974.
513. Schafer JA: Salt and water absorption in the proximal tubule. *Physiologist* 25:95, 1982.
514. Schafer JA, Barfuss DW: The study of pars recta function by the perfusion of isolated tubule segments. *Kidney Int* 22:434, 1982.
515. Schneider GB. Cellular specificity of the cure for osteopetrosis: Isolation of and treatment with pluripotent hemopoietic stem cells. *Bone* 6:241, 1985.
516. Schneider GB et al: Pluripotent hemopoietic stem cells give rise to osteoclasts. *Am J Anat* 177:505, 1986.
517. Schultz TD et al: Decreased intestinal calcium absorption *in vivo* and normal brush border membrane vesicle calcium uptake in cortisol-treated chickens: Evidence for dissociation of calcium absorption from brush border vesicle uptake. *Proc Natl Acad Sci U S A* 79:3542, 1982.
518. Scoble JE et al: Calcium transport in canine renal basolateral membrane vesicles: Effects of parathyroid hormone. *J Clin Invest* 75:1096, 1985.
519. Scoble JE et al: Na^{+}-Ca^{2+} exchange and calcium permeability in canine basolateral membrane vesicles: The effects of dibutyryl cAMP and specific inhibitors. *Biochim Biophys Acta* 944:233, 1988.
520. Seeman E et al: Reduced bone mass in daughters of women with osteoporosis. *N Engl J Med* 320:554, 1989.
521. Semrad CE, Chang EB: Calcium-mediated inhibition of Na-H exchange in small intestine. *Am J Physiol* 252:C315, 1987.
522. Shareghi GR, Agus ZS: Magnesium transport in the cortical thick ascending limb of Henle's loop of the rabbit. *J Clin Invest* 69:759, 1982.
523. Shareghi GR, Stoner LC: Calcium transport across segments of the rabbit distal nephron *in vitro*. *Am J Physiol* 235:F367, 1978.
524. Sheikh MS et al: Role of vitamin D-dependent and vitamin D-independent mechanisms in absorption of food calcium. *J Clin Invest* 81:126, 1988.
525. Shephard RM et al: Determination of vitamin D and its metabolites in plasma from normal and anephric man. *Biochem J* 182:55, 1979.
526. Shigeno C et al: Photoaffinity labeling of parathyroid hormone receptors in clonal rat osteosarcoma cells. *J Biol Chem* 263:2864, 1988.
527. Shimizu T et al: Effect of parathyroid hormone on the connecting tubule from the rabbit kidney: Biphasic response of transmural voltage. *Pfluegers Arch* 416:254, 1990.
528. Shimizu T et al: Effects of PTH, calcitonin, and cAMP on calcium transport in rabbit distal nephron segments. *Am J Physiol* 259:F408, 1990.
529. Shimizu T et al: Interaction of trichlormethiazide or amiloride with PTH in stimulating calcium absorption in the rabbit connecting tubule. *Am J Physiol* 261:F36, 1991.
530. Shimizu T et al: Site and mechanism of action of trichlormethiazide in rabbit distal nephron segments perfused *in vitro*. *J Clin Invest* 82:721, 1988.
531. Shoback DM et al: High calcium and other divalent cations increase inositol trisphosphate in bovine parathyroid cells. *Endocrinology* 124:838, 1988.
532. Siggaard-Andersen O et al: What is "ionized calcium?" *Scand J Clin Lab Invest* 43(suppl 165):11, 1983.
533. Silve CM et al: Parathyroid hormone receptor in intact embryonic chicken bones: Characterization and cellular localization. *J Cell Biol* 93:379, 1982.
534. Silver IA: Microelectrode studies on the acid microenvironment beneath adherent macrophages and osteoclasts. *Exp Cell Res* 175:266, 1988.
535. Silver J et al: Regulation of parathyroid hormone and calcitonin gene expression by 1,25-dihydroxyvitamin D_3 and calcium, in Cohn DV et al (eds): *Calcium Regulation and Bone Metabolism: Basic and Clinical Aspects.* Amsterdam, Exerpta Medica, 1990, p 140.
536. Silver J et al: Regulation by vitamin D metabolites of parathyroid hormone gene transcription *in vivo* in the rat. *J Clin Invest* 78:1296, 1986.
537. Silverberg SJ et al: Abnormalities in parathyroid hormone secretion and 1,25-dihydroxyvitamin D_3 formation in women with osteoporosis. *N Engl J Med* 320:277, 1989.
538. Simpson RU et al: Transcriptional regulation of the c-myc proto-oncogene by 1,25-dihydroxyvitamin D_3 in HL-60 promyelocytic leukemia cells. *J Biol Chem* 262:4104, 1987.
539. Sinton TJ et al: Reference intervals for calcium, phosphate, and alkaline phosphatase as derived on the basis of multichannel analyzer profiles. *Clin Chem* 32:76, 1986.
540. Slemenda CW et al: Predictors of bone mass in perimenopausal women: A prospective study of clinical data using photon absorptiometry. *Ann Intern Med* 112:96, 1990.
541. Slovik DM et al: Deficient production of 1,25-dihydroxyvitamin D in elderly osteoporotic patients. *N Engl J Med* 305:372, 1981.
542. Sly WS et al: Carbonic anhydrase II deficiency identified as the primary defect in the autosomal recessive syndrome of osteopetrosis with renal tubular acidosis and cerebral calcification. *Proc Natl Acad Sci U S A* 80:2752, 1983.
543. Smith DM et al: Genetic factors in determining bone mass. *J Clin Invest* 52:2800, 1973.

544. Smith EL et al: Effect of 1,25-dihydroxyvitamin D_3 on the morphologic and biochemical differentiation of cultured human epidermal keratinocytes grown in serum-free conditions. *J Invest Dermatol* 86:709, 1986.
545. Smith LH et al (eds): *Urolithiasis: Clinical and Basic Research.* New York, Plenum Press, 1981.
546. Smith RW, Walker RR: Femoral expansion in aging women: Implications for osteoporosis and fractures. *Science* 145:156, 1964.
547. Snowdowne KW, Borle AB: Effects of low extracellular sodium on cytosolic ionized calcium: Na^+-Ca^{2+} exchange as a major calcium influx pathway in kidney cells. *J Biol Chem* 260:14998, 1985.
548. Solomon L: Osteoporosis and fracture of the femoral neck in the South African Bantu. *J Bone Joint Surg* 50B:2, 1968.
549. Sowers M et al: Correlates of forearm bone mass among women during maximal bone mineralization. *Prev Med* 14:585, 1985.
550. Spencer R et al: Stimulation of intestinal calcium-binding protein mRNA synthesis in the nucleus of vitamin D-deficient chicks by 1,25-dihydroxyvitamin D. *Biochem J* 175:1089, 1978.
551. Steenbergh PH et al: The second human calcitonin/CGRP gene is located on chromosome 11. *Hum Genet* 70:259, 1985.
552. Steenbock H: The induction of growth-promoting and calcifying properties in a ration exposed to light. *Science* 60:224, 1924.
553. Stepan JJ et al: Castrated men exhibit bone loss: Effect of treatment on biochemical indices of bone remodeling. *J Clin Endocrinol Metab* 69:523, 1989.
554. Stewart AF, Broadus AE: Parathyroid hormone-related proteins: Coming of age in the 1990s. *J Clin Endocrinol Metab* 71:1410, 1990.
555. Stewart AF et al: Biochemical evaluation of patients with malignancy-associated hypercalcemia: Evidence for humoral and non-humoral groups. *N Engl J Med* 303:1377, 1980.
556. Stillman RJ et al: Physical activity and bone mineral content in women aged 30 to 85 years. *Med Sci Sports Exercise* 18:576, 1986.
557. Stryer L, Bourne HR: G proteins: A family of signal transducers. *Annu Rev Cell Biol* 2:391, 1986.
558. Suki WN: Calcium transport in the nephron. *Am J Physiol* 237:F1, 1979.
559. Suki WN, Rouse D: Hormonal regulation of calcium transport in thick ascending limb renal tubules. *Am J Physiol* 241:F171, 1981.
560. Suki WN, Rouse D: Renal transport of calcium, magnesium, and phosphorus, in Brenner BM, Rector FC Jr (eds): *The Kidney,* 4th ed. Philadelphia, Saunders, 1991, vol 1, p 380.
561. Suki WN et al: Calcium transport in the thick ascending limb of Henle: Heterogeneity of function in the medullary and cortical segments. *J Clin Invest* 66:1004, 1980.
562. Sutton RAL, Dirks JH: Calcium and magnesium: Renal handling and disorders of metabolism, in Brenner BM, Rector FC Jr (eds): *The Kidney,* 3d ed. Philadelphia, Saunders, 1986, vol 1, p 551.
563. Suva LJ et al: A parathyroid hormone-related protein implicated in malignant hypercalcemia: Cloning and expression. *Science* 242:893, 1987.
564. Takahashi N et al: Osteoclast-like cells form in long-term human bone marrow but not in peripheral blood cultures. *J Clin Invest* 83:543, 1989.
565. Takano-Yamamoto T, Rodan GA: Direct effects of 17 β-estradiol on trabecular bone in ovariectomized rats. *Proc Natl Acad Sci U S A* 87:2172, 1990.
566. Talmage RV et al: Evidence for an important physiological role for calcitonin. *Proc Natl Acad Sci U S A* 77:609, 1980.
567. Talor Z, Arruda JAL: Partial purification and reconstitution of renal basolateral Na^+-Ca^{2+} exchanger into liposomes. *J Biol Chem* 260:15473, 1985.
568. Tam CS et al: Parathyroid hormone stimulates the bone apposition rate independently of its resorptive action: Differential effects of intermittent and continuous administration. *Endocrinology* 110:506, 1982.
569. Tanaka Y et al: The role of 1,25-dihydroxyvitamin D_3 and parathyroid hormone in the regulation of renal 25-hydroxyvitamin D_3-24-hydroxylase. *Arch Biochem Biophys* 171:521, 1975.
570. Taniguchi et al: Na/Ca exchangers in collecting cells of rat kidney: A single tubule fura-2 study. *Pfluegers Arch* 415:191, 1989.
571. Tashjian AH et al: Calcitonin binding sites in bone: Relationships to biological response and escape. *Recent Prog Horm Res* 34:285, 1978.
572. Taylor A, Windhager EE: Possible role of cytosolic calcium and Na-Ca exchange in regulation of transepithelial sodium transport. *Am J Physiol* 236:F505, 1979.
573. Taylor AN et al: Immunocytochemical localization of vitamin D-dependent calcium-binding protein in renal tubules of rabbit, rat, and chick. *Kidney Int* 21:765, 1982.
574. Teitelbaum I, Berl T: Effects of calcium on vasopressin-mediated cyclic adenosine monophosphate formation in cultured rat inner medullary collecting tubule cells: Evidence for the role of intracellular calcium. *J Clin Invest* 77:1574, 1986.
575. Terepka AR et al: Transcellular transport of calcium. *Symp Soc Exp Biol* 30:117, 1976.
576. Termine JD: Bone matrix proteins and the mineralization process, in Favus MJ (ed): *Primer on the Metabolic Bone Disorders and Diseases of Mineral Metabolism.* Kelseyville, Calif, American Society for Bone and Mineral Research, 1990, p 16.
577. Termine JD et al: Osteonectin, a bone-specific protein linking mineral to collagen. Cell 26:99, 1981.
578. Thiede MA: The mRNA encoding a parathyroid hormone-like peptide is produced in mammary tissue in response to elevations in serum prolactin. *Mol Endocrinol* 3:1443, 1989.
579. Thiede MA, Rodan GA: Expression of a calcium-mobilizing parathyroid hormone-like peptide in lactating mammary tissue. *Science* 242:278, 1988.
580. Thiede MA et al: Human renal carcinoma expresses two messages encoding a parathyroid hormone-like peptide: Evidence for the alternative splicing of a single-copy gene. *Proc Natl Acad Sci U S A* 85:4605, 1988.
581. Thiede MA et al: Intrauterine occupancy controls expression of the parathyroid hormone-related peptide gene

in preterm rat myometrium. *Proc Natl Acad Sci U S A* 87:6969, 1990.

582. Thomson BM et al: Tumor necrosis factors α and β induce osteoblastic cells to stimulate osteoclastic bone resorption. *J Immunol* 138:775, 1987.
583. Tiegs RD et al: Calcitonin secretion in postmenopausal osteoporosis. *N Engl J Med* 312:1097, 1985.
584. Tiegs RD et al: Plasma calcitonin in primary hyperparathyroidism: Failure of C-cell response to sustained hypercalcemia. *J Clin Endocrinol Metab* 63:785, 1986.
585. Tiegs RD et al: Secretion and metabolism of monomeric human calcitonin: Effects of age, sex and thyroid damage. *J Bone Miner Res* 1:339, 1986.
586. Tippins JR et al: The myotropic and calcium modulating effects of calcitonin gene-related peptide (CGRP). *Neuropeptides* 4:425, 1984.
587. Toffaletti J: Physiological importance of calcium complexes, in Anghileri LJ, Tuffet-Anghileri AM (eds): *The Role of Calcium in Biological Systems.* Boca Raton, Fla, CRC Press, 1982, vol 2, p 69.
588. Toffaletti J, Abrams B: Effects of *in vivo* and *in vitro* production of lactic acid on ionized, protein-bound, and complex-bound calcium in blood. *Clin Chem* 35:935, 1989.
589. Toffaletti J et al: Influence of continuous infusion of citrate on responses of immunoreactive parathyroid hormone, calcium and magnesium components and other electrolytes in normal adults during plateletapheresis. *J Clin Endocrinol Metab* 60:874, 1985.
590. Toffaletti J et al: Separation and quantitation of serum constituents associated with calcium by gel filtration. *Clin Chem* 22:1968, 1976.
591. Toffaletti J et al: Use of gel filtration to examine the distribution of calcium among serum proteins. *Clin Chem* 23:2306, 1977.
592. Toribara TY et al: The ultrafiltrable calcium of human serum: 1. Ultrafiltration methods and normal values. *J Clin Invest* 36:738, 1957.
593. Triffitt JT. The special proteins of bone tissue. *Clin Sci* 72:399, 1987.
594. Trotter M et al: Densities of bones of white and negro skeletons. *J Bone Joint Surg* 42A:104, 1960.
595. Tsai KS et al: Impaired vitamin D metabolism with aging in women: Possible role in pathogenesis of senile osteoporosis. *J Clin Invest* 73:1668, 1984.
596. Tsoukas CD et al: 1,25-dihydroxyvitamin D_3, a novel immunoregulatory hormone. *Science* 221:1181, 1984.
597. Ueda K et al: Cortical hyperostosis following long-term administration of prostaglandin E_1 in patients with cyanotic congenital heart disease. *J Pediatr* 97:834, 1980.
598. Ulivieri FM et al: Quantification by dual photon absorptiometry of local bone loss after fracture. *Clin Orthop Rel Res* 250:291, 1990.
599. Ullrich KJ: Permeability characteristics of the mammalian nephron, in Orloff J, Berliner RW (eds): *Handbook of Physiology,* sec 8, *Renal Physiology.* Washington, DC, American Physiological Society, 1973, p 377.
600. Ullrich KJ et al: Active Ca^{2+} reabsorption in the proximal tubule of the rat kidney. *Pfluegers Arch* 364:223, 1976.
601. Ullrich KJ et al: Prinzipien des epithelialen Transportes in Niere und Darm. *Klin Wochenschr* 57:977, 1979.
602. Underwood J, DeLuca HF: Vitamin D is not directly necessary for bone growth and mineralization. *Am J Physiol* 246:E493, 1984.
603. Urist MR: Bone formation by auto-induction. *Science* 81:680, 1983.
604. Urist MR et al: Solubilized and insolubilized bone morphogenetic protein. *Proc Natl Acad Sci U S A* 76:1828, 1979.
605. Vaes G: Cellular biology and biochemical mechanism of bone resorption: A review of recent developments on the formation, activation, and mode of action of osteoclasts. *Clin Orthop* 231:239, 1988.
606. van Corven EJJM et al: Distribution of Ca^{2+}-ATPase, ATP-dependent Ca^{2+}-transport, calmodulin and vitamin D-dependent Ca^{2+}-binding protein along the villus-crypt axis in rat duodenum. *Biochim Biophys Acta* 820:274, 1985.
607. van Heeswijk MPEM et al: Kinetic properties of the ATP-dependent Ca^{2+} pump and the Na^+/Ca^{2+} exchange system in basolateral membranes from rat kidney cortex. *J Membr Biol* 79:19, 1984.
608. van Os CH: Transcellular calcium transport in intestinal and renal epithelial cells. *Biochim Biophys Acta* 906:195, 1987.
609. Vasicek T et al: Nucleotide sequence of the human parathyroid hormone gene. *Proc Natl Acad Sci U S A* 80:2127, 1983.
610. Verde T et al: Sweat composition in exercise and in heat. *J Appl Physiol* 53:1540, 1982.
611. Vermeulen A: The hormonal activity of the postmenopausal ovary. *J Clin Endocrinol Metab* 42:247, 1976.
612. Wali RK et al: $1,25(OH)_2$-vitamin-D_3 stimulates membrane phosphoinositide turnover, activates protein kinase C, and increases cytosolic calcium in rat colonic epithelium. *J Clin Invest* 85:1296, 1990.
613. Walling MW: Intestinal Ca and phosphate transport: Differential responses to vitamin D_3 metabolites. *Am J Physiol* 233:E488, 1977.
614. Walling MW, Kimberg DV: Calcium absorption or secretion by rat ileum *in vitro*: Effects of dietary calcium intake. *Am J Physiol* 226:1124, 1974.
615. Walser M: Divalent cations: Physicochemical state in glomerular filtrate and urine and renal excretion, in Orloff J, Berliner RW (eds): *Handbook of Physiology,* sec 8, *Renal Physiology.* Washington, DC, American Physiological Society, 1973, p 555.
616. Walser M: Ion association: 6. Interactions between calcium, magnesium, inorganic phosphate, citrate and protein in normal human plasma. *J Clin Invest* 40:723, 1961.
617. Walters JRF: Calbindin-D_{9k} stimulates the calcium pump in the rat enterocyte basolateral membranes. *Am J Physiol* 256:G124, 1989.
618. Walters JRF, Weiser MM: Calcium transport by rat duodenal villus and crypt basolateral membranes. *Am J Physiol* 252:G170, 1987.
619. Wang EA et al: Purification and characterization of other distinct bone-inducing factors. *Proc Natl Acad Sci U S A* 84:7109, 1988.
620. Wang EA et al: Recombinant human bone morphogenetic protein induces bone formation. *Proc Natl Acad Sci U S A* 87:2220, 1990.

621. Wasserman RH: Intestinal absorption of calcium and phosphorus. *Fed Proc* 40:68, 1981.
622. Wasserman RH, Fulmer CS: Calcium transport proteins, calcium absorption, and vitamin D. *Annu Rev Physiol* 45:375, 1983.
623. Wasserman RH, Fulmer CS: On the molecular mechanism of intestinal calcium transport. *Adv Exp Biol Med* 249:45, 1989.
624. Wasserman RH, Taylor AN: Gastrointestinal absorption of calcium and phosphorus, in Aurbach GD (ed): *Handbook of Physiology,* sec 7, *Endocrinology, Parathyroid Gland.* Washington, DC, American Physiological Society, 1976, vol 7, p 137.
625. Wasserman RH, Taylor AN: Vitamin D_3-induced calcium-binding protein in chick intestinal mucosa. *Science* 152:791, 1966.
626. Wasserman RH et al: Evidence for multiple effects of vitamin D_3 on calcium absorption: Response of rachitic chicks, with or without partial vitamin D_3 repletion, to 1,25-dihydroxyvitamin D_3. *Proc Natl Acad Sci U S A* 79:7939, 1982.
627. Wasserman RH et al: Vitamin D-dependent calcium-binding protein: Purification and some properties. *J Biol Chem* 243:3978, 1968.
628. Weatherburn MW et al: Serum calcium methodology: A Canadian assessment based on the application of the reference method. *Clin Biochem* 15:222, 1982.
629. Weaver CA et al: Isolation and complete nucleotide sequence of the gene for bovine parathyroid hormone. *Gene* 28:319, 1984.
630. Wecksler WR et al: Studies on the mode of action of calciferol: Subcellular localization of 1,25-dihydroxyvitamin D in chicken parathyroid gland. *Arch Biochem Biophys* 183:168, 1977.
631. Weinstein RS, Bell NH: Diminished rates of bone formation in normal black adults. *N Engl J Med* 319:1698, 1988.
632. Weiss L: *Cell and Tissue Biology: A Textbook of Histology.* Baltimore, Urban and Schwarzenberg, 1989.
633. Weiss RE et al: Calcitonin stimulates bone formation when administered prior to initiation of osteogenesis. *J Clin Invest* 68:815, 1981.
634. Weringer EJ et al: A proposed cellular mechanism for calcium transport in the intestinal epithelial cell. *Calcif Tissue Res* 26:71, 1978.
635. Westlin NE: Loss of bone mineral after Colles' fracture. *Clin Orthop Relat Res* 102:194, 1974.
636. Whyte MP: Hypophosphatasia, in Scriver CR et al (eds): *The Metabolic Basis of Inherited Disease,* 3d ed. New York, McGraw-Hill, 1989, vol 2, p 2843.
637. Wiener H: Active Ca^{2+} transport systems in basolateral membranes from rabbit distal colon. *J Intern Med* 228 (suppl 1):119, 1990.
638. Williams RJP: Calcium chemistry and its relation to protein binding, in Wasserman RH et al (eds): *Calcium Binding Proteins and Calcium Function.* New York, Elsevier/North-Holland Press, 1977, p 3.
639. Windhager EE, Taylor A: Regulatory role of intracellular calcium ions in epithelial Na transport. *Annu Rev Physiol* 45:519, 1983.
640. Windhager EE et al: Sodium-calcium interaction in renal tubular epithelium, in Bronner F, Peterlik M (eds): *Calcium and Phosphate Transport across Biomembranes.* New York, Academic Press, 1981, p 203.
641. Wolff J: *Das Gesetz der Transformation der Knochen.* Berlin, Hirschwald, 1892.
642. Wortsman J, Traycoff RB: Biological activity of protein-bound calcium in serum. *Am J Physiol* 238:E104, 1980.
643. Wortsman J et al: A rapid method for the determination of ultrafilterable calcium in serum. *J Lab Clin Med* 98:691, 1981.
644. Wozney JM et al: Novel regulators of bone formation: Molecular clones and activities. *Science* 242:1528, 1988.
645. Wuthier RE: Electrolytes of isolated epiphyseal chondrocytes, matrix vesicles, and extracellular fluid. *Calcif Tissue Res* 23:125, 1977.
646. Yada T et al: Intestinal secretagogues increase cytosolic free Ca^{2+} concentration and K^+ conductance in a human intestinal epithelial cell line. *J Membr Biol* 112:159, 1989.
647. Yamaguchi DT et al: Parathyroid hormone-activated calcium channels in an osteoblast-like clonal osteosarcoma cell line: cAMP-dependent and cAMP-independent calcium channels. *J Biol Chem* 262:7711, 1987.
648. Yamamoto M et al: Vitamin D deficiency and renal calcium transport in the rat. *J Clin Invest* 74:507, 1984.
649. Yamamoto T et al: Primary hypomagnesemia with secondary hypocalcemia: Report of a case and review of the world literature. *Magnesium* 4:153, 1985.
650. Yates AJP et al: Effects of a synthetic peptide of a parathyroid hormone-related protein on calcium homeostasis, renal tubular calcium reabsorption and bone metabolism *in vivo. J Clin Invest* 81:932, 1988.
651. Yoon K et al: Alkaline phosphatase cDNA transfected cells promote calcium and phosphate deposition. *Connect Tissue Res* 22:17, 1989.
652. Yoshitomi K et al: Electrophysiological characterization of rabbit distal convoluted tubule cell. *Pfluegers Arch* 414:457, 1989.
653. Young DM, Capen CC: Thyrocalcitonin content of thyroid glands from cows with vitamin D-induced hypercalcemia. *Endocrinology* 86:1463, 1970.
654. Zapf J, Froesch ER: Insulin-like growth factors/somatomedins: Structure, secretion, biological actions and physiological role. *Horm Res* 24:1528, 1986.
655. Zerwekh JE et al: Short-term 1,25-dihydroxyvitamin D_3 administration raises serum osteocalcin in patients with postmenopausal osteoporosis. *J Clin Endocrinol Metab* 60:615, 1985.

CHAPTER • 12

Physiology of phosphorus metabolism

Norimoto Yanagawa • Farid Nakhoul

Kiyoshi Kurokawa • David B. N. Lee

PLASMA PHOSPHORUS

COMPOSITION AND UNITS

The composition of total plasma phosphorus is listed in Fig. 12-1. The discussion in this chapter will revolve around the homeostasis of the inorganic orthophosphate fraction, which may be taken to represent the total plasma inorganic phosphate, since the quantity represented by the pyrophosphate fraction is relatively small. Orthophosphates are derived from sequential dissociation of orthophosphoric acid:

$$\begin{array}{l} H_3PO_4 \rightleftharpoons H^+ + H_2PO_4^- \\ \qquad\qquad\qquad\quad \upharpoonleft\downharpoonright \\ \qquad\qquad\qquad H^+ + HPO_4^{2-} \\ \qquad\qquad\qquad\quad \upharpoonleft\downharpoonright \\ \qquad\qquad\qquad H^+ + PO_4^{3-} \end{array} \qquad (1)$$

Within the range of pH compatible with life, the quantities of undissociated orthophosphoric acid and of the completely dissociated trivalent phosphate found in body fluids are extremely small and need not be considered further for our present discussion. Therefore, for practical purposes the term plasma (inorganic) phosphate embraces two orthophosphate components: $H_2PO_4^-$ and HPO_4^{2-}. The relative proportion of the two ionic species in the circulation may be derived as follows:

$$H_2PO_4^- \rightleftharpoons H^+ + HPO_4^{2-} \qquad (2)$$

From the law of mass action and where K_a represents the ionization or dissociation constant, it follows that

$$[H^+] = K_a \times [H_2PO_4^-]/[HPO_4^{2-}] \qquad (3)$$

The expression can be further transformed using the Henderson-Hasselbalch equation:

$$-\log[H^+] = -\log K_a + -\log[H_2PO_4^-]/[HPO_4^{2-}] \qquad (4)$$

Substituting pH for $-\log[H^+]$, pK_a for $-\log K_a$ and log $[HPO_4^{2-}]/[H_2PO_4^-]$ for $-\log[H_2PO_4^-]/[HPO_4^{2-}]$,

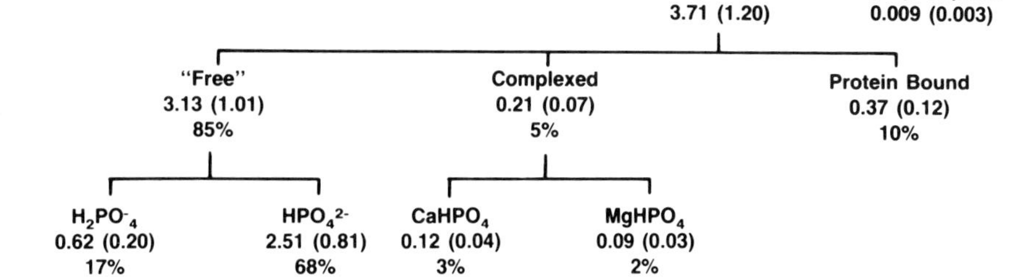

FIGURE 12-1 • Distribution of phosphorus in various phosphate fractions of human plasma. Representative values are in milligrams per 100 milliliters, with the equivalent millimoles per liter indicated in parentheses. (From Lee DBN et al, in Bronner F, Coburn JW, eds: *Disorders of Mineral Metabolism,* New York, Academic Press, 1981, vol 3, pp 283–421. Used by permission.)

$$pH = pK_a + \log[HPO_4^{2-}]/[H_2PO_4^-] \quad (5)$$

For equation 5, the proportion of the two inorganic phosphate species in the circulation at normal pH 7.40 can be calculated from the Henderson-Hasselbalch equation ($pK_a = 6.80$):

$$7.40 = 6.80 + \log [HPO_4^{2-}]/[H_2PO_4^-]$$

$$\log[HPO_4^{2-}]/[H_2PO_4^-] = 0.60$$

Since the antilog of 0.60 is 4, it follows that

$$[HPO_4^{2-}]/[H_2PO_4^-] = 4$$

The same proportion can be derived from the law of mass action (equation 3), substituting the known value of 160 nmol/liter for K_a and the normal $[H^+]$ of 40 nmol/liter:

$$40 = 160 \times [H_2PO_4^-]/[HPO_4^{2-}]$$

Therefore,

$$[HPO_4^{2-}]/[H_2PO_4^-] = 160/40 = 4$$

Thus, at normal plasma pH there are 4 mm (8 meq) of the divalent HPO_4^{2-} phosphate to every 1 mm (1 meq) of the monovalent $H_2PO_4^-$. Stating this another way, a solution containing the two phosphate molecules in the above proportion would have a "neutral" pH of 7.40. Such solutions are indeed prepared for clinical use and are commonly labeled as "neutral phosphate" solutions.

Since plasma phosphate contains a mixture of monovalent and divalent ionic species, it has an intermediate valence (charge per millimole), which can be calculated as follows: at pH 7.40, for every 5 mmol of plasma phosphate, 4 mmol will be the divalent HPO_4^{2-}, containing a total of eight negative charges, and 1 mmol will be the monovalent $H_2PO_4^-$, containing one negative charge. This would give rise to a total of nine negative charges per 5 mmol of phosphate and thus a composite valence of 1.8 ($9/5 = 1.8$). The interconversion of plasma phosphate from millimole to milliequivalent can thus be calculated from the formula mmol × 1.8 = meq.

Plasma phosphate concentration is measured in terms of the elemental phosphorus contained in the phosphate molecules. A normal plasma phosphorus concentration of 3.1 mg/100 ml (31 mg/liter) is equivalent to 1 mmol of phosphorus per liter (since the atomic weight of phosphorus is 30.98), which is the same as 1 mmol of phosphate per liter or 1.7 meq of phosphate per liter. Although the term plasma phosphate concentration is often used interchangeably with the term plasma phosphorus concentration, it should be apparent that the practice is not strictly correct when the unit milligram per 100 milliliters is used. A plasma phosphorus concentration of 3.1 mg/100 ml is quite different from a plasma phosphate concentration of 3.1 mg/100 ml. The former represents 1 mmol of phosphorus (or 1 mmol of phosphate), while the latter represents 31/96.3 or 0.32 mmol of phosphorus or phosphate. The number 96.3 represents the composite molecular weight of the two phosphate species at pH 7.40. The molecular weights of HPO_4^{2-} and $H_2PO_4^-$ are 96 and 97, respectively, and therefore 1 mmol of plasma phosphate at pH 7.40 would weigh

$$\tfrac{2}{3}(96) + \tfrac{1}{3}(97) = 96.3 \text{ mg}$$

USE OF TERMS PHOSPHORUS AND PHOSPHATE

The phosphate content in various biological materials, such as food, plasma, tubular fluid, urine, tissue, and feces, is measured and expressed in terms of total elemental phosphorus in the sample and generally uses units such as milligrams per 100 milliliters (mg/100 ml). On the other hand, phosphorus participates in physiologic and biochemical events in the body as phosphate molecules; for example, the glomerulus filters and the tubule transports phosphate, not phosphorus. For such purposes it is more convenient to use units such as milliequivalents per liter or millimoles per liter. With this in mind we will now use the abbreviation P interchangeably for either phosphorus or phosphate for the rest of the chapter. As discussed, normal plasma P concentration can be expressed as 3.1 mg/100 ml, 1 mmol/liter (1 m*M*), or 1.7 meq/liter.

RENAL HANDLING OF PHOSPHATE

GLOMERULAR ULTRAFILTERABILITY

Under normal conditions, about 6 to 20 percent of plasma P is protein-bound (Table 12-1). A small fraction of plasma P that complexes with calcium and magnesium is also nondiffusible. Although a significant amount of plasma P is protein-bound, when measured directly, the ratio of ultrafilterable P to total plasma P concentration is close to unity.[307,427] This apparent discrepancy is explained by two factors. The first is that in measuring plasma P concentration, the volume occupied by plasma proteins (7 percent) is not taken into account. The second is that the presence of impermeant, anionic proteins on only one side (blood side) of the glomerular filtration membrane would result in a Gibbs-Donnan distribution such that on the protein side there would be a lesser concentration of diffusible negative ions such as P. The Gibbs-Donnan correction factor for P is 0.915.[667] If all plasma P were freely ultrafilterable, the glomerular filtrate P concentration would have been 1/(0.93 × 0.915), or 1.175, times that of plasma P concentration. Since the actual filterable plasma P is approximately 85 percent of the total plasma P concentration, the ultrafilterable P concentration would then be 0.85/(0.93 × 0.915), or 1.0, times that of the total plasma P concentration, thus confirming the accuracy of the actual measurements.[307,427]

It is important to point out that the ultrafilterability of P may be influenced by factors other than protein binding. For example, it has been observed that raising

TABLE 12-1 • Ultrafilterable phosphate in normal subjects

Reference	Ultrafilterable phosphate, mg/100 ml	Corrected value, mg/100 ml	Total phosphate, mg/100 ml	Protein binding, %
Benjamin and Hess[66]				
Adults	4.45	3.8	4.2	10
Infants	7.0	6.0	6.9	13
Hopkins et al.[333]	3.9	3.3	3.5	6
Walser[676]	3.64	3.10	3.56	13
Robertson and Peacock[581]	3.10	2.64	3.28	20
Weeke and Friis[681]	4.00	3.40	3.93	13

NOTE: All values are mean values. Corrected value = ultrafilterable phosphate/1.175.

SOURCE: From Robertson WG, in Nordin EC, ed: *Calcium, Phosphate and Magnesium Metabolism*, Edinburgh, Churchill Livingstone, 1976, pp 217–219. Used by permission.

the serum calcium (Ca) concentration in vitro would result in a fall in the ultrafilterable fraction of P. This has been attributed to the formation of a nondiffusible calcium-phosphate-protein colloid complex.[332,465] The influence of Ca in reducing the ultrafilterability of P appears to occur in vivo as well as in vitro. Thus, Cuche and associates[186] demonstrated an inverse linear relationship between the percentage of ultrafilterability of serum inorganic phosphate and the serum calcium-phosphate product during calcium infusion into thyroparathyroidectomized (TPTX) dogs receiving an infusion of parathyroid hormone (PTH). Peraino and Suki[531] also demonstrated a consistent trend of reduction in ultrafilterability of serum P in TPTX dogs receiving a Ca infusion. The effect was observed whether simultaneous PTH infusion was given or not. In addition to its effect on the filtrability of P, Ca infusion also causes an increase in serum P concentration.[186,531] The mechanism is not clear but may result, at least in part, from the exodus of organic P from red blood cells.[142] This phosphatemic effect does not appear to depend on the presence of PTH or calcitonin.[24,134,279,317,328,336] It appears that the phosphatemic effect of Ca is generally greater than its influence on lowering the ultrafilterability of P, so that the filtered load of P is generally increased during Ca infusion.[531] In the presence of a normal Ca concentration, elevating P concentration to 8 mmol/liter (24.8 mg/100 ml) does not affect the diffusibility of either P or Ca.[333]

SITES OF PHOSPHATE TRANSPORT ALONG THE NEPHRON

In his classical whole-kidney clearance studies, Pitts concluded that the renal handling of P in the mammalian species could be accounted for by ultrafiltration at the glomerulus followed by regulated tubular reabsorption.[538,539] He observed that the maximum P clearance, measured at plasma P concentrations ([P]) up to above 20 mmol/liter, could be accounted for by filtration alone and therefore suggested that renal tubules did not secrete phosphate. Although several subsequent studies have produced contrary conclusions, the bulk of the current evidence continues to uphold Pitt's original conclusion and fails to document net P secretion in mammalian kidneys.[598] Therefore, currently it is generally accepted that any factor that alters renal P excretion in the mammalian kidney must do so by changing either the filtered load (glomerular filtration rate [GFR] × plasma [P]) or the tubular reabsorption rate.

Attempts at defining segmental P reabsorption characteristics along the nephron began with stop-flow studies that indicated that P reabsorption in mammalian nephron occurred predominantly in the proximal tubule (PT).[538,688] Subsequent free-flow micropuncture studies of the proximal convoluted tubule (PCT) in dog and rat with normal plasma [P] suggested that between 60 and 70 percent of the filtered load of P was reabsorbed by the last segment of the cortical superficial nephron.[5,623,638] In the first 10 to 20 percent of PT length, where 15 percent of the filtered sodium (Na) and fluid has been reabsorbed, the tubular fluid–to–ultrafiltrate concentration ratio of P ($[TF/UF]_P$) has already fallen significantly from 1.0 in Bowman's capsule to approximately 0.6 to 0.7, suggesting a proportionately greater reabsorption of P than of Na and fluid.[5,19,427,638,684] Simple calculation would indicate that 40 percent of the filtered P (or 50 percent of the P reabsorbed by the whole nephron, assuming an overall fractional P reabsorption of 80 percent) is reabsorbed in the first few convolutions of the PCT. In the remainder of the accessible PT, $[TF/UF]_P$ remained roughly constant, while Na and fluid reabsorption increased to approximately 65 percent of the filtered load. Thus, P reabsorption continued in the more distal portion of PCT, but now at a rate proportional to Na and fluid reabsorption. In TPTX animals, the $[TF/UF]_P$ continued to fall in this more distal portion of the PCT,[52,250,443] although even in these experimental models the early convolutions still demonstrated relatively greater activity for P reabsorption.[48] This relative decline in tubular reabsorptive rate as a function of distance from the glomerulus has also been observed in studies of the isolated perfused rabbit tubule and is currently termed axial or intranephron heterogeneity of P transport.[48,201,386,463] The question whether deeper nephrons reabsorb greater, equal, or lesser fractions of filtered P than superficial nephrons (internephron heterogeneity) remains unresolved. McKeown and associates[463] using an in vitro microperfusion technique, found no difference in net P reabsorption by representative PCTs from these two nephron populations. On the other hand, micropuncture data from the laboratory of Knox and associates suggest greater deep nephron P reabsorption under conditions of dietary P deprivation or absence of PTH and greater deep nephron P rejection under the condition of P loading or PTH infusion.[386,406]

Reabsorption of P in nephron segments between the late proximal and early distal tubule has been measured in a number of micropuncture studies performed under a variety of different experimental conditions, such as in intact, acute, or chronic TPTX animal models and with or without P and/or saline loading. In some studies P reabsorption in this intermediate site is derived from micropuncture of the proximal and distal tubule of the same nephron, while in other studies it is derived from micropuncture of the proximal and distal tubules of different nephrons. It is not surprising that the overall data demonstrated P reabsorption in this intermediate portion of the nephron in some reports and not in others. Amiel, Kuntziger and their respective associates demonstrated P reabsorption in this portion of the nephron in acutely TPTX but not in intact or chronically TPTX rats.[17,19,394] Pastoriza and associates also found P reabsorption between the late proximal and early distal segments of TPTX rats, and this was reduced by infusion of PTH.[529] The tubular segment(s) in which this reabsorption occurs is not certain. Lang and associates[407] attempted to evaluate P transport in segments beyond the proximal micropuncture site by injecting and positioning isolated droplets of perfusion fluid in various nephron segments between late proximal and early distal tubules and subsequent reaspiration of the fluid for analysis. They found P reabsorption in the descending, but not in the ascending, segments. The P transport in the descending segments probably represents reabsorption by the terminal convoluted and straight portions of the PT. This conclusion gains credence from the observation of Dennis and associates,[201] who, using in vitro microperfusion, have also demonstrated P reabsorption in rabbit PT segments beyond the point of in vivo micropuncture. However, no net P transport was noted in either the thin ascending limb or thick ascending limb of Henle's loop.[583] These data taken together suggest that P is reabsorbed between the late proximal and the early distal tubule and that this reabsorption probably occurs in the remainder of PCT beyond the point accessible to micropuncture, as well as in the straight portion of the PT: the pars recta.

The question of whether there is P reabsorption in the distal convoluted tubule remains open. In free-flow micropuncture experiments, the finding of a reduction in tubular fluid P delivery between early and late distal puncture sites has led to the conclusions that up to 10 percent of the filtered load is reabsorbed in the superficial distal tubules[411,413,529] and that this transport system may be inhibited by PTH. However, using other techniques, including split droplet, microinjection, and microinfusion, radioactive P recovery was complete in Munich-Wistar strain rats, suggesting the absence of net P reabsorption.[108,202,286,623] On the other hand, P tracer recovery was incomplete (80 to 90 percent) in two other Wistar strains, the Saclay and Bordeaux strains,[545] suggesting the presence of a P reabsorptive mechanism.

Various studies, usually employing different techniques, have also provided dissimilar data and conclusions concerning P handling in the terminal nephron. A difference in P recovery between the late superficial distal tubules and urine has often been taken as a measure of P transport by the terminal nephron. Thus, a lower urinary P recovery is used as evidence for P reabsorption, and a higher urinary P recovery is used as evidence for P secretion by this segment of the nephron. Such interpretation is of course not strictly correct, since the urine P delivery may be modified by tubular fluid from deep nephrons (Fig. 12-2). The data in the figure suggest that under the conditions of both acute and chronic TPTX, P reabsorption is more avid in deep than in superficial nephrons, since the P recovery (in percent of the filtered load) at the tip of the Henle's loop of the deep nephron is already lower than that in the distal tubule of the superficial nephron. This fluid with a lower P content could then dilute the P concentration of fluid draining into the collecting duct from the distal tubule of the superficial nephron. The final urine would therefore have a lower P concentration than the tubular fluid collected from the superficial distal tubule. Thus, it should be quite clear that a urinary P delivery lower than that found in the tubular fluid collected from superficial distal tubule does not necessarily prove P reabsorption in the intervening tubular segments. Parenthetically, Fig. 12-2 also provides data suggesting that under condition of P loading, deep nephrons reject more P than the superficial nephrons. Further scrutiny of Fig. 12-2, however, reveals that the urinary P is not only lower than the tubular fluid P collected from the distal tubule of the superficial nephron but is also lower than the tubular fluid P collected from the ascending limb of the deep nephron. This would suggest that some P reabsorption occurred beyond either or both of these micropuncture sites. Possible distal sites where P transport may take place are the granular, confluent segments of the distal convoluted tubule and the early branched segment of the collecting duct. These are

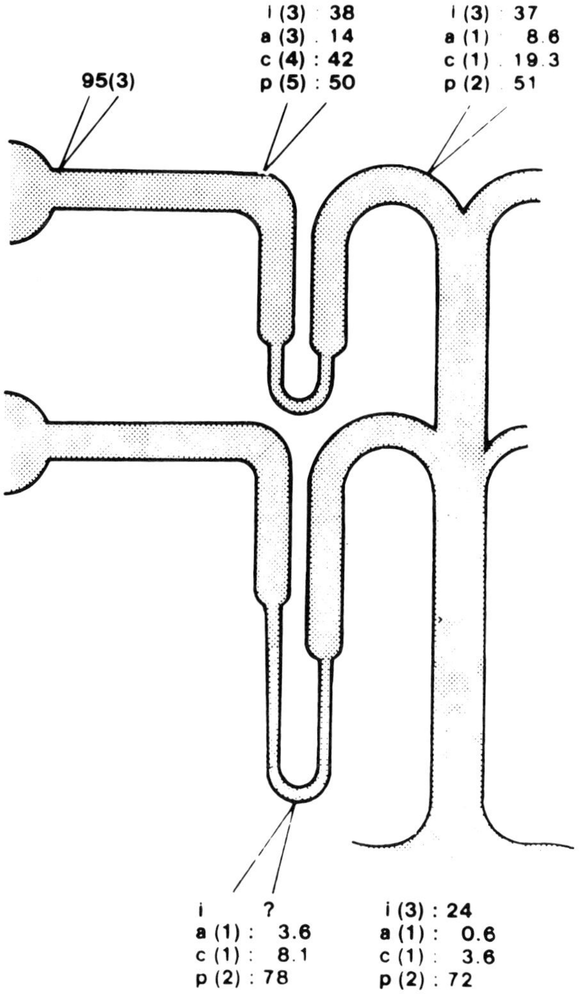

FIGURE 12-2 • Segmental reabsorption of phosphate in superficial and deep nephrons. Summary of free-flow micropuncture data. The phosphate recovery rate in percentage of filtered load is shown for the various nephron segments. The superscript numbers indicate one source in the literature: (1) Hass et al;[316] (2) Knox et al;[387] (3) Greger et al;[286] (4) Amiel et al;[18] and (5) Boudry et al.[87] i, intact; a, acute parathyroidectomy; c, chronic parathyroidectomy; p, phosphate loading following acute parathyroidectomy. In general, similar recoveries at the equivalent puncture sites have been reported in different studies, and thus data from several references are combined. (From Lang F et al: *Renal Physiol Basel* 4:1, 1981. Used by permission.)

the only distal segments sensitive to PTH in terms of cAMP response.[132] They form arcades that are especially well developed in deep nephrons. The observation that there is no PTH-sensitive adenylate cyclase system in the collecting duct appears to fit well with the finding of a lack of PTH effect on P reabsorption in the cortical collecting duct of the rabbit using in vitro microperfusion techniques.[202] Bengele and associates,[63] employing a collecting duct microcatheterization technique, were also unable to demonstrate a PTH effect on P transport along the inner medullary collecting duct of rat. These workers, however, found P reabsorption in this terminal segment of nephron in the acute TPTX state, when the delivery of P to this portion of the nephron is markedly reduced. In the in vitro perfused collecting duct, Shareghi and associates also found a small, PTH-insensitive, P outflux.[606] However, measurements obtained from micropuncture studies have failed to demonstrate net P reabsorption in this tubule segment.[315]

Thus, the weight of current evidence suggests that most, and perhaps all, of the filtered P is reabsorbed in the PT. The reabsorptive capacity is greatest in the early convolutions but continues in convolutions and pars recta distal to segments accessible to micropuncture. The P reabsorption in the late PT probably accounts for the bulk of the "distal" P reabsorption observed in a large number of studies. There is little evidence to suggest net P transport in the thin and thick ascending loops of Henle. While the question whether the distal convoluted tubule reabsorbs P remains open, increasing, but not conclusive, evidence supports the existence of a P reabsorptive mechanism in the PTH-responsive, adenylate cyclase-containing distal "arcades." A P reabsorptive mechanism in the collecting ducts has been proposed but requires further experimental validation.

MECHANISMS OF PHOSPHATE TRANSPORT

The cellular events involved in P movement from the luminal fluid to the peritubular capillary blood have been studied in the PTs, where the principal portion of the filtered P is reabsorbed. In the PT, P reabsorption occurs principally by a unidirectional process that proceeds transcellularly with minimal intercellular backflux from the plasma to the lumen. As previously discussed, the [P] in the luminal fluid when it enters the PT is similar to that in the plasma (i.e., 2.0 to 2.5 m*M*) and is normally reduced to 1.0 to 1.5 m*M* when it leaves the PT. In contrast, since the P content in freeze-clamped kidney tissue is approximately 5 m*M*/kg of tissue water[324,334] and about 27 percent of the total cellular P is free in solution, as was determined by ^{31}P nuclear magnetic resonance (NMR) in the isolated perfused kidney,[246] the concentration of cytosolic free P in the PT cells can be estimated to be approximately 1 m*M*. On the other hand, with a 60- to 65-mV potential difference (intracellularly negative) across the PT cell membrane, the free cellular [P] at equilibrium is expected to be 10 times lower than that in the ECF. The estimated free [P] in the PT cells thus seems to be higher than the predicted equilibrium value. This would imply that P enters the cell from the lumen against its electrochemical gradient by an energy-requiring mechanism and leaves the cell on the contraluminal membrane down the electrochemical gradient (Fig. 12-3). Thus, P absorption by PT cells is not determined passively by thermodynamic driving forces but, rather, by the spe-

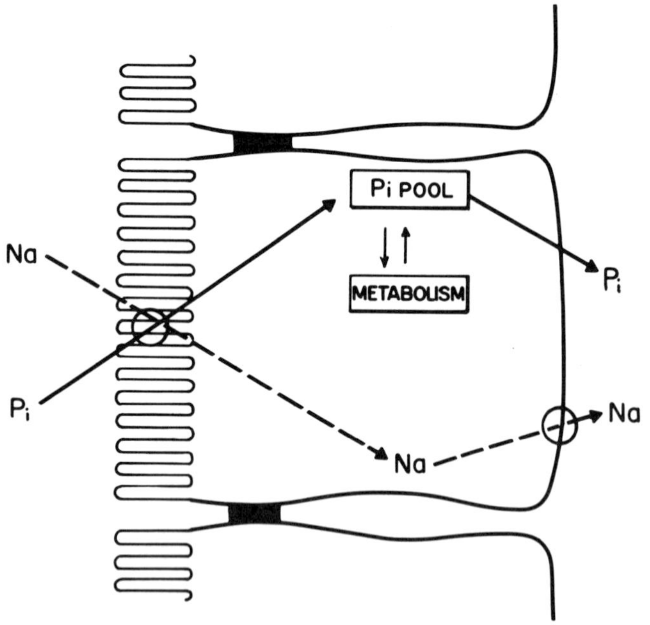

FIGURE 12-3 • Schematics of transcellular P transport across the proximal tubule cell. For details see the text.

cific transport systems located on the brush border and the basolateral membranes.

BRUSH BORDER MEMBRANE

Na^+-P cotransporter

The lipid bilayer structure of the brush border membrane consists of a hydrophobic inner core of hydrocarbons. This forms a barrier for hydrophilic molecules such as P to traverse the membrane and provides a framework for protein anchoring. Thus, P can cross the membrane more rapidly via a specific transport system associated with one or more membrane proteins. Current evidence indicates that most of the proteins involved in transmembrane transport processes are "intrinsic" membrane proteins that span the lipid bilayer in a fixed and asymmetric orientation. The process of movement of P is thought to involve subtle conformational changes in the transport protein assembly. Thus, P may have access to a polar pocket in a protein that traverses the membrane and releases P on the other side. Alternatively, the tertiary structure of the protein may form a channel that spans the membrane and opens upon P binding to a site exterior to the bilayer.

Until recently, attempts to identify the brush border membrane P transporter have met with limited success. Alkaline phosphatase, a known brush border membrane enzyme, was once thought to be involved in P transport. This proposal was based essentially on the observations of parallel changes of alkaline phosphatase and P transport activity under various experimental conditions.[211,212] However, further in vitro studies demonstrated that inhibition of alkaline phosphatase by levamisole or proteases did not affect the brush border membrane P transport and rendered the role of alkaline phosphatase highly unlikely.[110,585,636,653] Covalent labeling of brush border membrane P transport proteins by reagents reacting with various amino acids has also been attempted. For example, brush border membrane P transport is inhibited by reagents that react with carboxyl (carbodiimides), tyrosine (fluorodinitrobenzene), arginine (phenylglyoxal), and lysine (pyridoxal phosphate) residues, indicating the functional importance of these residues.[177,433,637,696] A P-binding proteolipid, "phosphorin," has also been extracted and purified from the brush border membranes.[366,367] While some common properties of P binding to this proteolipid and of P transport in brush border membrane suggest its involvement in P transport, it lacks other important features of the P transporter, such as sodium dependency of P binding. Recently, by using molecular biology techniques, a single clone mRNA isolated from rabbit renal cortex was found to express P transport activity similar to that of the brush border membrane when injected into *Xenopus laevis* oocytes.[685] It is clear that the success in the isolation of this P transporter will provide a useful tool for future studies in this field.

Brush border membrane P transport is active and sodium-dependent. Figure 12-4 shows a typical experiment demonstrating Na^+-P cotransport by the isolated brush border membrane vesicles. In the presence of an inward Na^+ gradient, P is rapidly accumulated in the vesicles to concentrations that transiently exceed the equilibrium values and is released back to the medium when the sodium gradient is dissipated. The sodium dependency has also been found for the transport systems for other solutes, such as glucose and amino acids. In PT cells, the energy required to maintain the favorable electrochemical gradient for sodium is generated by Na^+-K^+ ATPase at the basolateral membrane. It thus appears that the sodium gradient across the brush border membrane that favors sodium transport provides a common force for these transport activities. However, the exact mechanism coupling sodium to P transport remains unknown. It is possible that the structure of the P transporter is such that binding of sodium to an adjacent site enhances the binding of P to the transporter. At pH 7.4, Na^+-P cotransport in the brush border membrane is not sensitive to membrane potential, whereas at more acidic extravesicular pH values, an electrogenic component of P transport becomes apparent; it transfers positive charges from the luminal to the cytoplasmic membrane surface.[114] These findings thus suggest an electroneutral cotransport of two Na^+ ions and one divalent P ion at physiologic pH and an electrogenic cotransport of two Na^+ ions and one monovalent P ion at acid pH.

It is not known whether the electroneutral and the electrogenic components of Na^+-P cotransport are mediated by one transporter molecule or by two different transporter molecules. The observation of different kinetic characteristics of P uptake by brush border membrane vesicles derived from either the same region or different regions of the kidney indicates the existence of heterogeneity in the Na^+-P cotransport system. Na^+-P cotransport in brush border membranes isolated from superficial kidney cortex was found to be resolved into two kinetic components having similar V_{max} but significantly different K_m for P.[111] In contrast, in vesicles isolated from deep kidney cortex, only one system with high P affinity was found. The P transport system in vesicles isolated from deep cortex was also found to be more susceptible to the regulation by P content in the diet.[111]

Regulation of the Na^+-P cotransporter

ALLOSTERIC REGULATION BY NA+ AND H+ In general, the rate of P reabsorption in the PT increases with increasing pH of the tubular fluid.[494] With isolated brush border membrane vesicles, the rate of P uptake also increases when the extravesicular (or luminal) pH increases.[139,590] Since pH changes alter the composition of P between monovalent form, $H_2PO_4^-$, and divalent form, HPO_4^{2-}, the apparent inhibitory effect of luminal H^+ on P transport was first considered to indicate that the divalent form is the preferred species for renal brush border membrane P transport.[139,140,330,590] However, later studies showed that the effect of pH was sodium-dependent in such a way that the effect of pH was greatest at low, while diminished at high, sodium concentrations.[20] Kinetic analysis also revealed that pH affects the affinity of the brush border membrane P transport system for sodium but not for P. The K_m for sodium was 70 m*M* at pH 7.4 and 190 m*M* at pH 6.4, while the K_m for P was the same at both high and low pH. Irrespective of pH value, the affinity of the transporter for P was strongly increased by sodium, while the affinity for sodium was not affected by P. The Hill coefficient for sodium interaction was 2 and for P interaction was 1 under conditions of different pH, suggesting that the 2Na:1P stoichiometry of Na^+-P cotransport was not changed by pH. Collectively, these results indicate that sodium and H^+ are powerful allosteric modulators of brush border membrane P transport that interact with the transporter at sites different from the P-binding site and, by mutual interaction, control the affinity for P (Fig. 12-5). Since the estimated K_m for P in the PT in vivo (0.7 to 1.7 m*M*) is close to the physiologic P concentration in the PT luminal fluid, it is conceivable that changes in luminal fluid pH can effectively modulate the P reabsorption rate.

The interactions of sodium and protons with the cytosolic side of the P transporter are less well characterized. In isolated brush border membrane vesicles, P transport is stimulated when the pH of the intravesicular space (or cytosolic side of the membrane) is lowered.[20,590] These results suggest that H^+ has similar effects on the internal and external membrane surface: a decrease of the intravesicular pH could reduce the affinity for Na^+ and facilitate its discharge, followed by the discharge of P at the cytosolic side of the membrane, and thereby accelerate the transport cycle.[20] Alternatively, these results may provide evidence for a preferential transport of divalent P, because at low intravesicular pH,

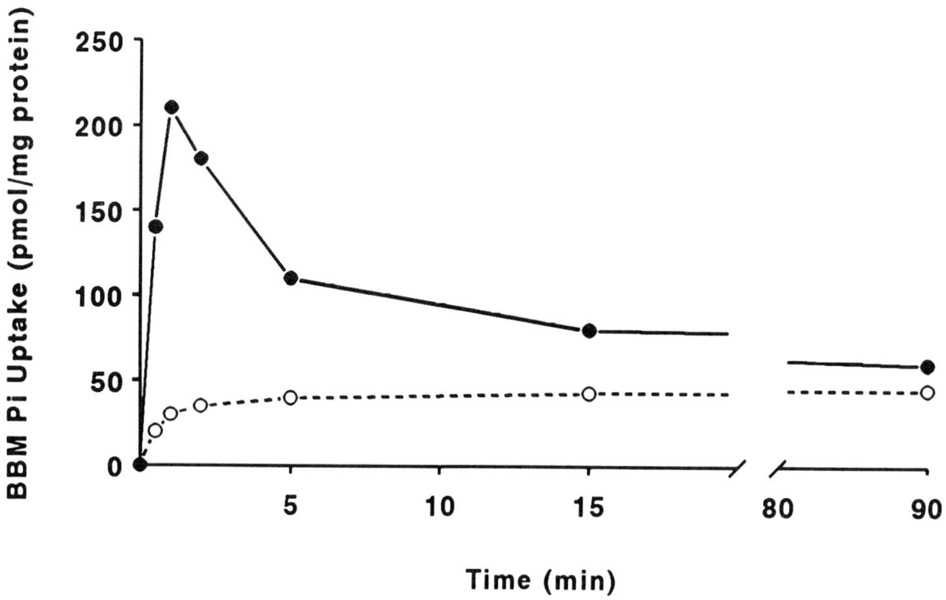

FIGURE 12-4 • Uptake of P by renal brush border membrane vesicles in the presence of an inward-directed Na^+ gradient (●—●) or in the absence of Na^+ (○—○). For details see the text.

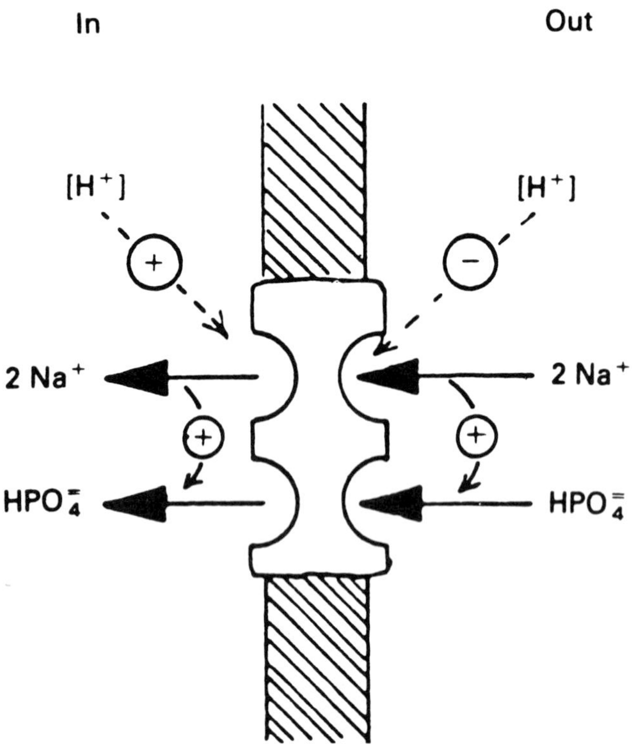

FIGURE 12-5 • Schematic representation of interaction of P, Na^+, and H^+ with the Na^+–P cotransport system of the renal brush border membrane. Broken lines and minus and plus signs denote inhibition and stimulation, respectively, of reactions indicated by solid arrows. (From Gmaj P, Murer H: *Physiol Rev* 66:36, 1986. Used by permission.)

P may be trapped inside the vesicles as $H_2PO_4^-$ and facilitate the uptake of HPO_4^{2-}.[590]

Regardless of the underlying mechanism, these results suggest that H^+ acts on both sides of the brush border membrane and influences P transport (Fig. 12-5). Fluctuations of cytosolic pH may be expected to have more pronounced effects on P transport than changes of luminal pH, because the sensitivity of P transporter to pH is higher at the low [Na^+] that prevails inside the cell. However, in contrast to the direct effect of luminal pH, the effect of intracellular pH on P transport across PT cells is probably more complex, because in addition to its direct interaction with the P transporter from the cytosolic side of the brush border membrane, intracellular pH may interact with P transport through changes in other parameters, such as cellular metabolism and membrane composition. Indeed, as will be discussed later, conflicting evidence has been reported regarding the effect of intracellular pH on P transport.[381]

COVALENT MODIFICATION BY PHOSPHORYLATION, ADP-RIBOSYLATION, AND THIOL REDOX Studies on the inhibition of PT P transport by PTH and cAMP led to the proposition that cAMP-dependent protein phosphorylation may correlate with decreased Na^+-P cotransport in brush border membrane. PTH-sensitive adenylate cyclase is present on the basolateral membrane of the PT,[137,607] and cAMP-dependent protein kinase exists in both the cytosol and the brush border membrane.[263,371] Na^+-P cotransport was decreased in brush border membranes isolated from kidneys of animals treated with PTH,[111,337] and the cAMP-dependent phosphorylation of several protein bands was demonstrated in brush border membrane vesicles in vitro.[72,297,298,300,448] Furthermore, correlation was demonstrated between cAMP-dependent phosphorylation and decreased Na^+-P cotransport in brush border membrane vesicles in vitro. In some studies, a modest inhibition (up to 15 percent) of the Na^+-dependent P uptake was observed when brush border membranes were phosphorylated by cAMP in the presence of ATP.[297,299] However, in other studies, when the kinetics of Na^+-P cotransport were measured, no effect of cAMP on either the K_m or V_{Max} of the Na^+-P cotransport system could be demonstrated.[72,448] The interpretation of these results is complicated by the methodological difficulties involved in the measurements of the effects of nucleotides on P transport in the isolated brush border membrane vesicles, where the added nucleotides are rapidly hydrolyzed by alkaline phosphatase, 5′-nucleotidase, and nucleotide pyrophosphatase.[92,99,408,652] The hydrolysis of nucleotides results not only in rapid depletion of the added nucleotides but also in isotope dilution during the subsequent ^{32}P uptake measurements. The other difficulty involves the need to open the sealed vesicles to let the added nucleotides into the intravesicular space, since their effects are relevant only when they locate at the cytosolic side of the membrane. This maneuver may adversely affect the regulatory systems of the Na^+-P cotransport system. It is also possible that protein phosphorylation may occur in leaky vesicles while the ^{32}P uptake is measured in sealed vesicles. Furthermore, it is not certain if the phosphorylated proteins represent the intrinsic membrane proteins or other nonmembrane cytoskeletal elements contained in the vesicles. With these pitfalls and the inconsistent results reported so far, the involvement of protein phosphorylation in the regulation of Na^+-P cotransport remains to be verified.

Another covalent modification proposed to be involved in the regulation of Na^+-P cotransport is the ADP ribosylation related to the NAD hypothesis.[92,98,211,299] According to this concept, brush border membrane proteins are ADP-ribosylated by intracellular NAD catalyzed by membrane-bound ADP ribosyltransferase, which results in an inhibition of Na^+-P cotransport.[299,302,361] This hypothesis arose from the observed inverse correlation between gluconeogenesis and P transport in renal PTs. Stimulation of renal gluconeogenesis was associated with reduced P reabsorption under various conditions, such as administration of PTH or glucocorticoid, starvation, and chronic metabolic acidosis.[211,361] Since gluconeogenesis occurs in the direction of utilizing the reducing equivalents of NADH in the cytosol, stimulation of gluconeogensis is expected to be associated with an increased NAD/NADH ratio or increased free NAD in the cytosol of the PT cells.[211,361,564] In an in vitro study, brush border membrane ^{32}P uptake was inhibited when NAD was added to the suspension of the brush border membrane vesicles.[298] The ^{32}P from ^{32}P-NAD was further demonstrated to be incorporated into brush border membrane proteins, suggesting that ADP ribosylation occurs in association with a decrease of brush border membrane P uptake.[299,361] The inhibition of P uptake by ADP ribosylation was also suggested to be involved in the effect of cholera toxin.[15] However, the methodological pitfalls that complicated the studies of protein phosphorylation also apply to these studies with NAD: NAD was rapidly hydrolyzed by the brush border membrane vesicles in vitro. The subsequent release of P from NAD could result in isotope dilution of ^{32}P during the uptake measurements. Indeed, NAD did not inhibit ^{32}P uptake when hydrolysis of the nucleotide had been prevented.[652] When NAD was introduced into the intravesicular space and removed from the extravesicular space, no inhibition of P uptake was observed.[274] Moreover, in the isolated perfused kidney[38] and in isolated perfused PTs[700,701] the oxidation and reduction of intracellular NAD with pyruvate and lactate resulted in no appreciable changes in P reabsorption. In isolated perfused PTs[701] it was also demonstrated that gluconeogenesis activity can be dissociated from P transport, therefore negating a direct cause-effect correlation between gluconeogenesis and P transport in PT.

Results from these studies have rendered the proposed scheme that PT gluconeogenesis activity directly regulates brush border membrane P transport through changes in cellular NAD content highly unlikely. The widely observed inverse correlation between brush border membrane P transport and cellular gluconeogenesis and NAD content thus remains unexplained. As an alternative mechanism, recent studies showed that modification of brush border membrane thiol redox by reducing or oxidizing thiol reagents caused a respective increase or decrease in Na^+-dependent P uptake.[641] Since the cellular NAD content is intimately linked to that of NADP and oxidized glutathione (GSSG), which in turn governs the thiol redox of various cellular proteins, it is possible that changes in cellular NAD content may indirectly alter the brush border membrane thiol redox and affect its P uptake. In support of this possibility, it was further found that preincubation of PTs with nicotinamide, an agent that raises the cellular NAD content, caused an oxidation of the thiol redox as well as an inhibition of Na^+-dependent P uptake in the subsequently isolated brush border membrane vesicles.[641]

In summary, although cAMP-dependent protein phosphorylation, NAD-dependent ADP ribosylation, and thiol redox have been demonstrated to modulate brush border membrane P uptake, their definitive regulatory roles remain uncertain. The mechanisms underlying the reciprocal correlation of gluconeogenesis and cellular NAD content with P reabsorption in renal proximal tubules remain to be elucidated.

OTHER REGULATORY FACTORS The lipid microenvironment in which the Na^+-P cotransporters are immersed may play an important role in the regulation of their transport rate.[481] Fluorescence polarization and electron spin resonance experiments indicated a higher order of membrane lipid orientation in the brush border membrane than in the basolateral membrane. Lipid analyses demonstrated that the cholesterol-to-phospholipid molar ratios are significantly higher in the brush border membrane than in the basolateral membrane, which may explain the higher order of lipid orientation, or the lower fluidity, of the brush border membrane.[423,483] Changes in membrane lipid composition may therefore alter its fluidity state, which in turn may affect the rate of movement of the transport proteins. Indeed, changes in brush border membrane lipid composition and fluidity state have been shown to be associated with changes in its P transport rate under conditions such as dietary P deprivation[482] or direct addition of $1\alpha,25\text{-}(OH)_2D_3$ to the brush border membrane.[397] However, contradictory conclusions have also been reported recently.[426]

The membrane recycling by endocytosis and exocytosis can be a rapid process affecting membrane protein insertion and removal. In renal PTs, reabsorption of the filtered proteins occurs through endocytosis at the brush border membrane,[176,441] and it has been demonstrated that exocytosis accounts for the insertion of proton pumps into the brush border membrane.[602] Recent studies in an established renal cell line derived from opossum kidney (OK cells), which retain PT transport characteristics, have demonstrated a reciprocal relationship between the changes in endocytosis and that in Na^+-dependent P uptake and suggested that membrane recycling may play a role in the regulation of Na^+-P cotransport.[359] Evidence has also been provided to suggest the role of membrane transport in the PTH action and the early adaptation to P deprivation. Exposure of OK cells to PTH was found to alter apical membrane protein content,[573] and inhibition of endocytosis by exposing these cells to hyperosmolar medium was found to attenuate the inhibitory effect of PTH on Na^+-dependent P uptake.[360] On the other hand, exposure of renal epithelial cells to P-free medium has been found to induce a rapid increase in Na^+-dependent P uptake independent of new protein synthesis.[70,129] Recent studies showed that this adaptive response was abolished when intracellular protein transport was inhibited by brefeldin, suggesting the participation of membrane protein transport in the early response of P uptake to P deprivation.[702]

BASOLATERAL MEMBRANE

P transport across the basolateral membrane is less well characterized. This is mainly because of the technical difficulties involved in the studies on ion transport by the isolated basolateral membrane. In contrast to the brush border membranes, which form a mostly uniform population of tightly sealed, right-side-out-oriented vesicles, the basolateral membrane preparations consist of a mixture of open sheets, inside-out, and right-side-out vesicles and only a small fraction of tightly sealed, transport-competent vesicles.[273] In addition, the preparations are usually contaminated with a small but significant amount of brush border membranes. These and other methodological considerations preclude the exact interpretation of the results obtained so far in the isolated basolateral membranes. Nevertheless, the available data suggest the existence in the basolateral membranes of both Na^+-independent[330] and -dependent[601] P transport pathways. The Na^+-independent uptake of P by basolateral membrane vesicles isolated from rat kidney cortex was found to be inhibited by 4,4¹-diisothiocyanatostilbene-2,2¹-disulfonic acid (DIDS), suggesting the involvement of an anion exchange mechanism.[287] However, contradictory reports exist with regard to whether P and other anions are transported through a common anion transport pathway or through separate transport pathways. In dog kidney basolateral membrane preparation, a Na^+-dependent P transport pathway was described.[601] Compared to brush border membrane, this transport system was electrogenic and insensitive to pH changes. Kinetic parameters showed that the Na^+-dependent P transport system represents a high-affinity, low-capacity transport system, whereas the Na^+-independent P transport system is one of low affinity and high capacity. Since the driving forces of Na^+ gradient and cell potential are always directed toward the cell interior, the Na^+-dependent P transport system in the basolateral membrane probably functions, not for P exit from the cell, but rather for P entry from the contraluminal side when the P entry from the lumen becomes restricted.[601] On the other hand, the Na^+-independent P transport system probably is involved mainly for P exit from the cell. The kinetic characteristics found for the Na^+-independent and -dependent P transport systems thus seem to be appropriate for their respective functions.

TRANSCELLULAR PHOSPHATE TRANSPORT

Since intracellular P plays a major role in governing various aspects of cell metabolism and function, it is expected that the net P transport across the PT cell will take place without large fluctuations of free [P] in the cytosol. This implies that P entry into the cell across the brush border membrane must be tightly coupled with its exit across the basolateral membrane (Fig. 12-3). The mechanisms involved in the maintenance of constant free [P] in the cytosol are not clear. Although it is likely that most of the P absorbed across the brush border membrane is rapidly discharged into the blood across the basolateral membrane, the small portion of the P that may be esterified into organic P compounds probably plays a critical role in the cell function. Information on the respective importance of P entry from the brush border membrane versus that from the basolateral membrane can be derived from studies in isolated perfused kidneys and in isolated perfused PT.[97,98,248] When isolated rat kidneys were perfused with P-free medium, the total tissue P and the cytosolic free P concentration, as determined by ^{31}P NMR, decreased initially and then remained constant for hours.[248] The kidney remained viable under these conditions, as indicated by the normal Na^+ reabsorption and O_2 uptake. Thus, it appears that the net P efflux from the cell was completely inhibited after P supply was stopped and a certain amount of P had been lost. In the isolated perfused rabbit PT, omission of P from the luminal fluid resulted in an inhibition of net fluid absorption, whereas omission of P from the peritubular fluid had no effect on fluid absorption rate.[98] The inhibition of fluid absorption and respiration was dependent on the presence of glucose in the luminal fluid and did not occur when glucose transport was inhibited with phlorizin or when glycolysis was inhibited by 2-deoxyglucose. This suggests the occurrence of the so-called crabtree effect: hexose-induced inhibition of respiration that occurs when intracellular P is incorporated into glycolytic intermediates and becomes a limiting factor for oxidative phosphorylation. Results from these studies also indicate that P transport across the brush border membrane is necessary for the maintenance of normal P concentration in the cell and that P entry across the basolateral membrane cannot fully compensate for the reduced P transport across the brush border membrane.

REGULATION OF RENAL PHOSPHATE EXCRETION

HORMONAL FACTORS

Parathyroid hormone

Since the early work of Greenwald and Gross,[285] it has been repeatedly demonstrated that PTH administration leads to phosphaturia by reducing the maximal transport rate of P reabsorption: *T*mP/GFR.[275,457] The influence of normal or basal circulating concentrations of PTH on renal P handling is clearly demonstrated in a number of studies. For example, in intact dogs, extracellular fluid (ECF) volume expansion with saline solution inhibits both Na and P reabsorption in the PCT, with a rise in $[TF/UF]_P$ in the late PT (Fig. 12-6). In the presence of PTH (intact dogs), most of the increase in the fraction of

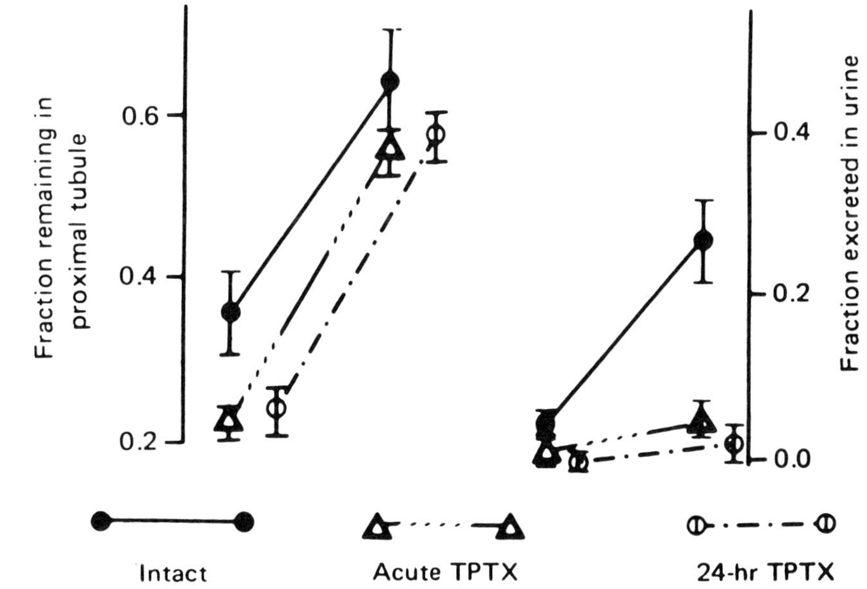

FIGURE 12-6 • Effect of saline expansion on the fraction of filtered phosphate remaining in the late proximal tubule (left) and on urinary fractional phosphate excretion (right) in intact and thyroiparathyroidectomized (TPTX) dogs. Lines connect mean values before and after saline expansion. (From Beck LH, Goldberg M: *Kidney Int* 6:18, 1974. Used by permission.)

filtered P load delivered to this point (0.6 − 0.4 = 0.2) is excreted in the urine. In TPTX animals, the basal, preexpansion $[TF/UF]_P$ in the late PT is lower (0.2 versus 0.4 in intact animal). This suggests the presence of a P reabsorptive mechanism in the early portions of PCT, which is normally inhibited by the presence of "physiologic" concentrations of PTH. This reabsorptive mechanism, however, appears to be inhibitable also by volume expansion, since the postsaline phosphaturia in the late PT of TPTX dogs was not different from that measured in intact dogs. However, in marked contrast to intact dogs, this large increase in distal delivery was not translated into a similar increase in urinary P in the TPTX dogs. This observation strongly suggests that TPTX has unmasked an important P reabsorptive mechanism distal to the last accessible puncture sites of the PCT and that this mechanism is not inhibited by systemic saline administration, thus blunting the volume expansion-induced phosphaturia in these TPTX dogs. Similar data and conclusions have been provided by Knox and Lechene in rats.[380]

Goldfarb and associates,[277] using a micropuncture recollection technique, measured proximal nephron and whole-kidney *T*mP in dogs and calculated the distal nephron *T*mP. They suggested that there was a proximal, as well as a distal (i.e., distal to the proximal micropuncture site) *T*mP: a concept entirely consistent with the conclusion of two P reabsorptive mechanisms just discussed. Knox attributed the distal *T*mP to P transport in the terminal segments of PT. Using microperfusion technique, he estimated a maximal P transport rate of 14 pmol/(mm·min) with a K_m of 1 mmol/liter in the PCT. The corresponding figures for the "descending portion of the tubule including the terminal PT and pars recta" were 6 pmol/mm·min and 0.2 mmol/liter, respectively.[379] The study of Beck and Goldberg[52] suggests that basal or "physiologic" levels of circulating PTH appeared to put a "brake" on both proximal and distal P reabsorptive systems, whereas saline loading inhibited proximal P reabsorptive system only. The proximal system is also sensitive to inhibition by a variety of other factors, including carbonic anhydrase inhibition,[51,383] mild hypercalcemia,[278] hyperglycemia,[198] and metolazone administration.[234] The common denominator for inhibition of P reabsorption in this portion of the PCT appears to revolve around the inhibition of Na transport, which is known to be closely linked to PT P reabsorption (see "Plasma Phosphate Homeostasis"). On the other hand, in segments inaccessible to micropuncture, the P reabsorptive mechanism appears to be uniquely responsive to PTH and apparently is not influenced by maneuvers that are known to inhibit Na reabsorption.

Although it is generally accepted that PTH is the most important physiologic influence on renal P excretion[275] and is the major determinant of plasma P concentrations[74,525] through its effect on *T*mP/GFR, it should be pointed out that there is no compelling evidence supporting the importance of this hormone in overall P balance. Repeated observations have confirmed that the balance between urinary excretion and dietary input of P is maintained not only in normal humans but also in patients with hyper- and hypoparathyroidism.[134,524] Furthermore, in experimental studies, Foulks and Perry have demonstrated that parathyroidectomy in dogs did not consistently modify the renal P transport regulation in response to fasting or to exogenous P administration.[242] Moreover, parathyroidectomized (PTX) rats given constant doses of PTH were able to regulate P excretion in response to changes in P load as efficiently as normal rats and with as little fluctuation in plasma P concentration.[668] Similarly, the adaptive changes in P threshold or *T*mP/GFR to changes in P load can also occur in the absence of PTH activity. Thus, P loading reduces *T*mP both in patients with untreated hypoparathyroidism[656] and in PTX dogs.[242] It is important to note that the bulk of available information on PTH regulation of renal P excretion has been obtained under conditions of either abnormally high (hyperparathyroid patients or subjects and animals given pharmacologic doses of PTH) or abnormally low (hypoparathyroid patients or post-TPTX or post-PTX subjects and animals) PTH levels. The study of Parsons and Reit first highlighted the fundamentally different physiologic response to sustained administration of a near-physiologic dose of PTH.[526] Continuous infusion of 0.2 units (100 ng) of PTH per kilogram per hour to dogs for up to three weeks resulted in a prompt and sustained hypercalemia of 13 to 14 mg/100 ml. However, the examination of bone biopsy materials revealed no signs of osteocytic osteolysis and no increase in the number of osteoclasts. Alcohol-soluble hydroxyproline in plasma (an index of collagen breakdown and bone resorption) was found to be unchanged during hypercalcemia. Furthermore, intestinal Ca absorption rose, urinary Ca clearance fell, and the animals were in fact in positive Ca balance. Clearly, when administered at such "physiologic" doses, PTH did not exhibit its more well-known bone-destructive and overall Ca catabolic properties. Unfortunately, the only information on P was limited to the comment that no change in urine or plasma P concentration was observed during the study. It is clear that the action of PTH under more physiologic settings (rather than under conditions of excessively high levels or complete absence of circulating PTH) and its exact role in overall P metabolism require additional studies.

A large body of evidence supports the thesis that the phosphaturic effect of PTH is mediated through its stimulatory effect on adenylate cyclase. PTH-sensitive adenylate cyclase has been identified in the following sites along the rabbit nephron: PCT; pars recta; the cortical portion of the thick ascending limb; the granular, confluent segments of the distal convoluted tubule, including the connecting tubule; and the early branched segment of the collecting duct.[485,486] The PTH-responsive segments of the terminal nephrons form arcades, which are especially well developed in deep nephrons. However, the presence of PTH-sensitive adenylate cyclase does not necessarily imply the simultaneous existence of a PTH-sensitive P transport system. Whether or not the stimulation of adenylate cyclase in distal tubules correlates with changes in P transport or is primarily associated with the known changes in calcium transport is not known. In TPTX animals, the discrepancy between PT P excretion and urinary P excretion can also be explained by the heterogeneous PTH effect between nephron populations. Indeed, in TPTX rats, P reabsorption is greater in deep than in superficial PTs.[276,316] Following an acute infusion of a high dose of PTH, fractional P reabsorption decreased to similar levels in both superficial and deep nephrons, suggesting a possibly greater PTH effect in deep nephrons.

In renal PT, PTH inhibits P, bicarbonate, Na^+, and fluid reabsorption[200,342,351,464] and stimulates glucose[400,497,699] and ammonia production.[144,145,535] The sequence of biochemical steps involved with PTH action begins with receptor binding and activation of adenylate cyclase on the basolateral membrane. The PTH-sensitive adenylate cyclase complex in the basolateral membrane consists of a membrane receptor, a nucleotide regulatory component (G protein), and a catalytic subunit.[61,62] Guanine nucleotides interact with G protein and promote the coupling between PTH receptor and the catalytic subunit. Activation of adenylate cyclase catalyzes the conversion of adenosine triphosphate to cAMP. Since many of the biological effects of peptide hormones are mediated through cAMP-dependent protein phosphorylation, it has been postulated that PTH-stimulated cAMP may lead to phosphorylation of renal brush border membranes and mediate the hormonal effect of P transport.[297,298,299] In support of this thesis, the P uptake was found to be decreased in brush border membranes isolated from kidneys of animals treated with PTH,[111,337,371] and cAMP-dependent protein kinase was found to be present in the brush border membrane;[263,371] the latter phosphorylates several protein bands in brush border membrane in vitro.[72,297,299,300,448] Furthermore, phosphorylation of brush border membranes by cAMP in the presence of ATP was found to reduce P uptake, and the effect of cAMP was reversed when brush border membranes were dephosphorylated by phosphoprotein phosphatase.[297,298]

In contrast to these observations, an increasing body of evidence has accumulated to indicate that cAMP-dependent protein phosphorylation alone cannot fully account for the PTH effect on P transport. For example, in rabbit kidneys, PTH-sensitive adenylate cyclase has been identified in both proximal convoluted and straight tubules.[485] However, the in vitro perfusion of these segments showed that PTH and cAMP, although inhibiting the Na^+-H^+ exchange system in both segments, affect P transport only in the straight, but not in the convoluted, portion of the PT.[202,699] In isolated brush border membrane, despite the phosphorylation of several protein bands by cAMP in the presence of ATP, no effect of cAMP on either the K_m or V_{max} of the Na^+-P cotransport system could be demonstrated.[72,448] Resistance to the phosphaturic effect of PTH and cAMP has been observed in starvation,[334,384] in P depletion,[271,528,629] in respiratory alkalosis,[334] after lithium administration, and in type II pseudohypoparathyroidism.[26] The responsiveness to PTH under these conditions can be restored by various means without affecting the PTH-cAMP axis.[25,26,631,632]

Besides activation of adenylate cyclase, alternative pathways of PTH-stimulated signal generation in the PT have been reported. In particular, intracellular calcium-dependent mechanisms have received increasing attention. It has been well demonstrated that an increase in intracellular calcium is important in mediating the effect of PTH to stimulate PT glucose production.[400,497,699] The involvement of intracellular calcium-dependent mechanisms in mediating the effect of PTH on PT P transport has also been suggested recently. Thus, in isolated perfused rabbit PCT, PTH inhibits bicarbonate reabsorption but fails to stimulate glucose production or inhibit P reabsorption.[202,699] It was found that these PTH responses could be restored by raising the extracellular calcium concentration.[202] Furthermore, addition of intracellular calcium antagonists was found to abolish these PTH actions in PTs and in brush border membranes.[202,698] The involvement of a calcium-dependent mechanism has been further supported by the discovery of a calcium, phospholipid-dependent protein kinase: protein kinase C.[504] Thus, in renal PT cells, PTH activates phospholipase C and stimulates inositol 1,4,5-triphosphate (IP_3) and diacylglycerol production.[339] The IP_3 thus produced releases calcium from intracellular storage and raises cytosolic calcium levels.[283,338] The increase in cytosolic calcium and the formation of diacylglycerol together lead to the activation of protein kinase C.[504] Similarly to cAMP-dependent protein kinase, protein kinase C is present in the brush border membrane[81] and may inhibit P transport through protein phosphorylation. The possibility that activation of protein kinase C leads to inhibition of P transport has been examined in an established renal cell line from opossum kidneys: OK cells. These cells contain PTH-sensitive adenylate cyclase, and both PTH and cAMP inhibit P uptake by these cells.[131,360,446,557,573] However, the concentration of PTH required for adenylate cyclase activation was found to be higher than that required for P uptake inhibition by a threefold magnitude.[161,162] On the other hand, in OK cells, it was found that PTH activates phospholipase C and increases IP_3 and diacylglycerol formation,[339] and that activation of protein kinase C by phorbol esters inhibited P uptake by these cells.[447,483] Recently, it was also found that, although PTH increases cAMP production in all clones of OK cells, there exist certain clonal sublines that show resistance to PTH inhibition of P uptake.[160] By monitoring changes in intracellular calcium in response to PTH, a close correlation has been observed between the stimulation of transient elevations in cytosolic calcium and the inhibition of P uptake by PTH.[478] These studies therefore strongly suggest that PTH regulates P transport in PT cells through dual mechanisms; one involves activation of adenylate cyclse and cAMP-dependent protein kinase A, and the other involves activation of phospholipase C and protein kinase C.

The inhibition of PT P transport by PTH is associated with a decrease in the apparent maximal rate of P transport (V_{max}). Protein phosphorylation, through either protein kinase A or protein kinase C, can conceivably phosphorylate and modify the activity of P transport proteins already present in the brush border membrane. An alternative possibility, which is also consistent with a V_{max} change, is that PTH may influence membrane recycling. There is good evidence that active membrane recycling, including both endocytosis and exocytosis, occurs in renal PTs.[176,441,602] The recycling of membrane transport proteins could allow for rapid up- or down-regulation of the capacity of the brush border membrane for solute transport. Indirect support for the involvement of membrane recycling in the PT response to PTH has been provided by the observations that pretreatment of rats with colchicine, a microtubule-disrupting agent, blocked the normal inhibitory action of PTH on renal P transport.[213] In OK cells, stimulation of endocytosis caused an inhibition of P uptake[359] and abrogated the inhibitory effect of PTH.[360]

Vitamin D metabolites

Many early studies have demonstrated that vitamin D increased renal tubular P reabsorption in rachitic dogs[309] and patients.[149,376] However, since these conditions are associated with secondary hyperparathyroidism, the antiphosphaturic effect of vitamin D may be attributed to its primary effect on inhibiting PTH secretion, either as a result of an increase in serum calcium concentration or as a consequence of a direct suppressive action of vitamin D on the parathyroid glands.[515] The reduction in urine P excretion can also be explained by an increased deposition of P into the skeleton as a result of vitamin D administration in these states. Other investigators attempted to demonstrate a direct tubular P conserving effect of vitamin D in the absence of PTH. Constanzo and associates studied the effect of 100 units of vitamin D_3 on renal P handling in vitamin D-deficient rats fed a low-P diet.[165] Vitamin D repletion was carried out 48 h and TPTX was performed 2 h prior to clearance studies. Vitamin D-repleted rats demonstrated higher P reabsorption measured over a wide range of filtered loads. It should be pointed out that the TPTX rats in this study were hypophosphatemic rather than hyperphosphatemic, as anticipated in the parathyroid-deprived state. The hypophosphatemia in these TPTX rats may be the result of the low P content in the diet. The acuteness of the parathyroid ablation would also allow little time for the development of the anticipated elevation in plasma P concentration. However, an antiphosphaturic effect of vitamin D_3, 25-hydroxyvitamin D_3 [25-$(OH)D_3$], or 1α,25-dihydroxyvitamin D_3 [1α,25-$(OH)_2D_3$] has also been demonstrated in more chronic TPTX animal models. These include vitamin D-replete TPTX dogs[510,549,551] and vitamin D-replete PTX rats.[541,543] It should be pointed out that in these studies, a vitamin D-induced increase in renal P reabsorption was demonstrated under conditions in which urinary P excretion was first increased by the administration of a variety of phosphaturic agents, such as vasopressin, saline solution, PTH, or calcitonin (CT) alone or in combination. When the effect of vitamin D and its metabolites on plasma and urinary P is examined in the hypoparathyroid state, unmodified by maneuvers that caused, or would cause, hypophosphatemia and/or phosphaturia, quite different results were obtained. The administration of vitamin D to hypoparathyroid patients resulted in a reduction in tubular P reabsorption, with a consequent fall in plasma P levels.[12] Similar results have been observed in TPTX or PTX rats.[82,182,257,502] Bonjour and associates[82] demonstrated that the administration of $1\alpha,25\text{-}(OH)_2D_3$ decreased serum P level and increased urinary P excretion in hyperphosphatemic TPTX rats. It is interesting that, in similar TPTX rats rendered hypophosphatemic by low-P diet feeding, the same metabolite increased P concentration and did not change urine P excretion, which remained low at 0.6 nmol/ml glomerular filtrate. Recent studies suggest that vitamin D may increase brush border membrane P transport by directly altering membrane lipid composition.[222,397]

It appears, therefore, that vitamin D and its metabolites have an antiphosphaturic and plasma P-elevating effect in hypophosphatemic (e.g., vitamin D deficiency or P deprivation) states or in situations in which basal urinary P excretion is first augmented by maneuvers such as volume expansion or the administration of vasopressin, PTH, or CT. On the other hand, the administration of vitamin D and its metabolites has a phosphaturic and plasma P-lowering effect in hyperphosphatemic or P-repleted states. In this context, it is interesting to note that Gekle and associates,[260] using a micropuncture technique, found that in normal and rachitic (hypophosphatemic) rats, vitamin D_3, 20 to 1800 IU/min per 100 g body weight, led to a decrease in $[TF/UF]_P$ (increased tubular P reabsorption) in the PT, while in TPTX (hyperphosphatemic) rats vitamin D_3 caused an increase in this ratio (reduced tubular P reabsorption). Garabedian and associates[257] and Lee and associates[280] also noted that $1\alpha,25\text{-}(OH)_2D_3$ has a plasma P-lowering effect in hyperphosphatemic rats and a plasma P-elevating effect in hypophosphatemic rats. One possible explanation for the apparent "paradoxical" effects of vitamin D is to postulate that this hormone may participate in the maintenance of normal plasma P by sustaining renal P reabsorptive capacity at its normal (optimal or maximal) rate. Its administration under conditions characterized by a submaximal reabsorptive rate (e.g., vitamin D deficiency or the various phosphaturic maneuvers mentioned above) would restore reabsorption of P to or toward normal; that is, it would increase renal P reabsorption and correction of hypophosphatemia. In situations in which renal P reabsorption is already at its optimal or maximal rate (e.g., normal, P-repleted state, or hypoparathyroid state), the administration of vitamin D would have little or no further effect on renal handling of P. The observation of phosphaturia under such conditions would simply be the result of an increase in P entry into the ECF from an increase in intestinal P absorption and/or an increase in bone P mobilization. Since the body is in P balance, this increased P load would simply be excreted in the urine, and thus "phosphaturia" would ensue.

Thus, in addition to a direct action on renal tubular P handling, vitamin D also causes changes in a number of other systems, many of which may independently cause additional changes in renal P reabsorption or excretion. The overall action of vitamin D on renal P handling represents the summation of a multiplicity of other vitamin D effects, among which are its action on PTH secretion and its action on P handling by the nonrenal organs such as the intestine and the skeleton. In addition, the effect of vitamin D on renal P handling would also be modified by the underlying metabolic status and the doses (physiologic or pharmacologic) of the hormone used. Thus, the induction of active bone formation in the treatment of rickets would be expected to cause antiphosphaturia, while the administration of toxic quantities of vitamin D could cause unbridled bone resorption and consequent increases in renal P excretion. In view of these considerations, it is hardly surprising to find that, while a number of studies have reported vitamin D or its metabolites to cause "antiphosphaturia," other studies have observed that these vitamin D sterols act to cause "phosphaturia."

Growth hormone

Growth hormone (GH) administration is followed by acute reduction in urinary P excretion in humans,[175] dogs,[173] and rats.[216] Long-term administration of either human GH to normal subjects and patients with hypopituitarism or bovine GH to dogs is associated with consistent increases in *T*mP/GFR.[74,175] Although acute GH administration caused no change or only a slight increase in plasma [P],[175,325] long-term administration of the hormone is associated with significant elevation in plasma [P].[175] Clinically, both plasma [P] and *T*mP/GFR are higher in active acromegalics than in adult control patients and patients in whom acromegaly is successfully treated.[59,174] Higher serum [P] has also been observed in postmenopausal women, in whom a direct correlation between this parameter and plasma GH levels has been observed.[7] Higher serum [P] in babies and children[112,659] and its "normalization" after puberty[654] have also been taken as evidence of a GH-related effect on serum and renal P homeostasis. However, the observation that serum [P] and *T*mP/GFR in pituitary dwarfs were also higher than those found in normal adults[174] suggests that age-dependent variations in P regulation cannot be solely attributed to changes in GH metabolism. In fact, Boucher has failed to demonstrate any striking difference in plasma GH concentrations between children and adults.[86] It may be appropriate to point out that reduced tetra-*S*-carbamidomethyl-GH has been found to duplicate the effect of GH on serum and urinary P, suggesting that the biological effect of GH is not dependent on the presence of disulfide bridges, which, on the other hand, are critical for the immunoreactivity of GH.[164]

The mechanism of action of GH on renal P reabsorption is not clear. GH receptors have not been described in renal tissue, and the hormone does not appear to influence cAMP generation or gluconeogenesis in isolated PTs.[288] Since the effect of GH on growth is mediated by somatomedin,[666] it is possible that the action of GH on P homeostasis is also effected through the same agent. The report that the age-adjusted serum [P] may be low in patients with hereditary somatomedin deficiency (Loron dwarfs)[410] appears to lend some credence to such a postulate.[501]

Altenahr and Kampf[16] have reported ultrastructural evidence for suppressed parathyroid gland activity in GH treated rats. This finding dovetails well with the observation that GH stimulates intestinal Ca absorption[173] and that it increases $1\alpha,25\text{-}(OH)_2D_3$ synthesis,[620] which may directly suppress parathyroid gland activity.[515] Hypercalcemia has also been reported in some acromegalic patients.[496] However, other observations suggest that the antiphosphaturic effect of GH is not mediated through the PTH axis. Thus, GH is found to increase *T*mP/GFR in TPTX dogs.[173] Moreover, the effect of PTH in lowering the *T*mP/GFR is observed in dogs both before and after GH treatment, suggesting that GH does not modify the action of PTH on renal P handling.

In addition to raising renal P reabsorptive capacity, GH has a number of other renal effects. The hormone is known to increase GFR in both normal subjects and in patients with hypopituitarism.[264] in dogs, GH raises GFR, renal plasma flow, tubular maximal secretion of para-aminohippurate,[21,194] and tubular maximal reabsorption of sulfate.[265] Its action on renal hemodynamics is particularly relevant to our discussion because the effect of GH on tubular P reabsorption may simply reflect an adjustment in glomerular-tubular balance resulting from an increase in filtered load for P. Indeed, Cattaneo and associates[126] demonstrated in five acromegalic patients a parallel increase in GFR and *T*mP, suggesting that *T*mP/GFR is unchanged in patients with excessive GH secretion. However, the bulk of evidence, including that reviewed above, indicates that GH raises *T*mP/GFR and therefore would suggest that it raises the intrinsic tubular reabsorptive capacity for P. Such a notion was further supported by the finding that administration of GH increased P uptake by renal brush border membrane.[303] An alternative antiphosphaturic mechanism for GH is suggested by the micropuncture observation in rats, indicating that the hormone increased proximal Na reabsorption.[612] Other studies have also demonstrated a GH-associated retention of Na in humans[192] and rats.[46] Since Na and P transport is coupled, at least in part, in the PT, the action of GH on Na may cause secondary effects on P reabsorption. However, the antinatriuretic action of GH is not consistently demonstrated in all studies.[559]

Since renal P excretion is dependent on the net flux of P from the intestine and the tissue-bone P pool into the ECF compartment (see "Plasma Phosphate Homeostasis"), any extrarenal effect of GH on P metabolism will have important effects on renal P excretion. In both humans and animals, GH administration causes positive P balance.[50,343] The P retention is a result of tissue anabolism and is accompanied by increases in intestinal P absorption.[216] The net effect of GH on bone is variable,[562] ranging from stimulation of bone growth and bone remodeling to net bone resorption. Intracellular shift of P for GH-induced anabolism would be expected to reduce the P load for renal excretion and, thus, antiphosphaturia.

In summary, the bulk of clinical and experimental evidence suggests that GH increases plasma [P], renal *T*mP/GFR, intestinal P reabsorption, and net P retention. The renal effect on P handling is not secondary to other GH-induced changes in kidney functions and is not dependent on the presence or absence of PTH. It is more likely to be related to the extrarenal effect of GH on general anabolism and therefore a greater tissue need for P. The site of action of GH on renal P handling is still not clearly defined.

Vasopressin (antidiuretic hormone)

Supraphysiologic doses of antiduretic hormone (ADH) paradoxically cause diuresis characterized by an increase in Na, K, Cl, and P excretion (see Chap. 4). The diuresis is observed in both diuretic and antidiuretic animals[106,135,341,453] and is not directly attributable to ADH-induced hemodynamic changes. Thus, the diuretic action of ADH is observed in the absence of changes in GFR and RPF and under conditions in which the rise in systemic blood pressure is prevented by the use of nitroprusside.[18,401] The phosphaturic action of ADH can also be induced by direct injection of the hormone into the renal artery of dogs undergoing hypotonic saline diuresis,[453] further suggesting that the phosphaturic effect of ADH is mediated directly through the kidney rather than through an indirect effect secondary to some systemic effects. As one might anticipate, direct renal artery infusion of cAMP elicited a similar phosphaturic response.[453] In addition, acute supraphysiologic doses of ADH also cause a consistent increase in serum [P] that is not dependent on the presence or absence of PTH, since it occurs in both intact and PTX animals.[31,32] Since this increase in serum [P] after ADH administration occurs in the presence of an increased urinary P excretion, the possibility that this hormone mobilizes P from tissue-skeletal pools into the ECF compartment must be entertained. Heidenreich and associates[322] have demonstrated that ADH increases hepatic glycogenolysis, with a concomitant decrease in hepatic glycogen content and an increase in serum glucose and lactate levels. This would lead to increased delivery of P from the tissue pool into the extracellular space.

Wen attempted to define the site of action of ADH on P reabsorption and carried out PT micropuncture studies in TPTX dogs given pressor doses of ADH.[683] A consistent increase in the TF/plasma ratio for P was observed, suggesting an inhibitory effect of ADH on proximal P reabsorption. Interestingly, the TF/plasma ratio for inulin was unchanged in face of a clear natriuresis exhibited by the whole kidney, suggesting that the effect of ADH on Na is dissociated from that on P in the PT and that its natriuretic effect is mediated through nephron segments distal to the proximal puncture site. The study of Kurtzman and associates[401] suggests that the ADH action on P reabsorption appears to be quite specific, since no effect was observed on the maximal rate of bicarbonate and glucose reabsorption. The demonstration that the effect of ADH on renal P reabsorption may be duplicated by cAMP[453] suggests that the inhibitory effect may be mediated through the ADH-cAMP axis. This would raise a conceptual difficulty, since no ADH-sensitive adenylate cyclase has been demonstrated in the pars convoluta and the pars recta of PTs.[486]

In conclusion, ADH in supraphysiologic doses inhibits its renal P excretion by a mechanism that is independent of changes in systemic blood pressure, renal hemodynamics, or the presence or absence of PTH. The phosphaturic effect can be mimicked by cAMP and appears to be expressed, at least in part, through inhibition of PT P reabsorption. The fact that high doses of ADH also elevate plasma [P] suggests that the augmented renal P excretion may reflect an extrarenal effect of ADH in mobilizing P from tissue pool into the ECF compartment. The question of whether supraphysiologic doses of ADH affect intestinal P absorption has not been answered.

Calcitonin

The association between CT administration and phosphaturia has been demonstrated in humans[76,519,618] and in most of the animal species studied.[45,589,591,618,691] In dogs, the phosphaturic effect of CT is less consistently demonstrated and appears to require the presence of parathyroid glands.[154,520,552,589] Puschett and coworkers[552] propose that CT aborts the antiphosphaturic effect of 25-(OH)D_3 in ECF-volume expanded dogs. In pigs, phosphaturia appears to be induced by large doses of CT used in the presence of intact parathyroid glands.[154,589] In other animal species, including humans, the contribution of CT-induced hypocalcemia in the production of phosphaturia, either directly or through its stimulation of PTH, is considered less likely. Thus, the phosphaturic effect of CT was observed in studies in which hypocalcemia is corrected by simultaneous Ca infusion.[519] The CT-mediated phosphaturia is also not PTH-dependent, since the action is also observed in hypoparathyroid humans[76,519] and in TPTX animals.[452,582]

Since the increase in renal P excretion occurs in face of steady or falling plasma [P] and in the absence of changes in GFR,[28,519] it has been concluded that CT causes phosphaturia through inhibition of tubular P reabsorption rather than increases in filtered load. The nephron site or sites at which CT acts to reduce P reabsorption are uncertain. PT micropuncture data demonstrated increases in P reabsorption in one study[425] and decreased P reabsorption in another study.[258]

There is now convincing evidence for the presence of CT receptors, as demonstrated by high-affinity binding of radiolabeled salmon CT and CT-sensitive adenylate cyclase in renal tissue.[454,558] A close association between the presence of CT receptors and CT-activated adenylate cyclase has been demonstrated. Thus, there is a link between the distribution of high-affinity CT-binding sites and the presence of hormone-sensitive adenylate cyclase; CT binding and activation of adenylate cyclase occurs at similar hormone concentrations; and the relative potencies of CT analogues were similar whether measured by competition for high-affinity binding sites or by their effects on adenylate cyclase. In addition, in maneuvers in which the CT-binding sites were reduced,[438,454] a parallel reduction in the CT-sensitive adenylate cyclase activity was also observed.

Based on in vitro assays, CT-dependent adenylate cyclase has been located in three nephron segments: the medullary and cortical portions of the thick ascending limb of the loop of Henle and the bright portion of the distal convoluted tubule.[136] It therefore appears that the PTH-sensitive and the CT-sensitive adenylate cyclase systems have quite different sites of distribution in nephron segments and there is no overlap of both systems in any segment, except for the cortical portion of the thick ascending limb. The effect of PTH and CT on cAMP generation was found to be additive by some workers[321] and not by others.[399]

Although the close association between CT-receptors and CT-activated adenylate cyclase appears well established, the question whether the CT-induced phosphaturia is mediated through this system has not been convincingly answered. Kurokawa and associates demonstrated that CT caused increases in renal generation of cAMP in rats under both in vivo and in vitro conditions and that this cAMP response preceded the observed phosphaturia.[399] In humans, Ardaillou also observed a CT-induced increase in urinary cAMP excretion, but this increase is secondary to a rise in serum cAMP and thus filtered cAMP.[28] The extrarenal cAMP is thought to be of osseous origin. The nephrogenous cAMP was unchanged, although a clear natriuresis was observed. Of greater interest is the finding that phosphaturia and natriuresis have been shown in dogs and cows in which CT receptors and CT-activated adenylate cyclase could not be demonstrated.[210,454] It is possible that the failure to demonstrate these entities may be related to the insensitivity of the existing methods, but the possibility that the renal action of CT on P is mediated by mechanisms other than adenylate cyclase is also a viable alternative. The latter possibility is highlighted by the observation that CT induces definite changes in P transport in rat PT,[258] although the rat does not possess a CT-sensitive adenylate cyclase system in the proximal nephron. A recent report that CT treatment causes a reduction in P uptake by isolated brush border membrane vesicles would implicate the PT as one of the nephron segments where CT may modulate P transport.[708]

CT exerts important extrarenal effects on P homeostasis. In rats, CT administration lowers serum [P]. This hypophosphatemic effect is also observed in nephrectomized or PTX animals,[645] suggesting that the underlying mechanism is not a result of increased renal P loss and is PTH-independent. CT also lowers serum [Ca], and this has been attributed to the known inhibitory effect of the hormone on bone resorption.[558] CT may also increase the flux of Ca from the ECF compartment into soft tissue.[697] Borle has concluded that CT stimulates cellular uptake of Ca and inhibits Ca efflux.[83] It has been suggested that CT causes hypophosphatemia through similar mechanisms: inhibition of the movement of P from bone to ECF; stimulation of P movement from the ECF compartment into soft tissues; and, in addition, an increase in urinary P excretion.[646] Evidence of soft tissue sequestration of P is, however, not strong. Kenny and Heiskell[365] failed to find consistent changes in P content of kidney, small intestine, submaxillary salivary glands, and lens in rats given subcutaneous, crude CT preparations. However, Meyer and Meyer[472] observed an increase in liver P in CT-treated rats.

The physiologic role of CT in humans is less well defined. No consistent alterations of serum P levels are known in patients with CT oversecretion secondary to medullary thyroid carcinoma[467] or in patients with no endogenous CT, that is, thyroidectomized patients.[459] Administration of pharmacologic doses of porcine or salmon CT to patients with Paget's disease[291,295] or those with hypercalcemia[712] is also not invariably followed by hypophosphatemia. However, in normal subjects and in patients with hypoparathyroidism, net intestinal absorption of P was significantly diminished upon administration of high doses of synthetic salmon CT.[350] The phosphaturic effect of porcine, bovine, human, and salmon CT in humans has also been documented in a larger number of studies.[76,158,314,451,519]

Glucocorticoids

In humans the acute administration of ACTH or high doses of hydrocortisone or dexamethasone is associated with a reduction in serum [P] and an increase in urinary P excretion.[22,345,669] Similar observations have been documented in rats.[262,409,692] The hypophosphatemic and phosphaturic responses were observed in both intact and PTX rats, suggesting that the action of glucocorticoids (GCs; see Chap. 14) is not PTH-dependent.[409] More recently GCs have also been reported to abolish the hypophosphaturic response to P deprivation.[661] However, starvation abolishes the GC-induced increment in P excretion, and this is attributed to the preexisting high basal endogenous secretion of adrenal GCs in the fasting state.[409] Thompson and associates[658] demonstrated that the hypophosphatemic effects of CT and GCs were additive. Goldsmith and associates,[281] on the other hand, failed to observe a hypophosphatemic effect of acute, high-dose hydrocortisone administration in normal individuals and in subjects with a variety of endocrine disorders. Of further interest is the observation that urinary P, rather than increasing, actually decreased. The antiphosphaturic effect of GCs was also reported by Laidlaw and coworkers.[405] Goldsmith and associates further demonstrated an ipsilateral decrement in fractional P excretion (FEP) during direct infusion of hydrocortisone into the renal artery in amounts too small to produce systemic effects. Goldsmith and associates documented an inverse correlation between plasma hydrocortisone concentration and renal FEP and proposed that the diurnal rhythm of P excretion (forenoon troughs and afternoon-evening peaks) is a reflection of circadian changes in plasma hydrocortisone concentrations.

The reason for the divergent observations on the effect of GCs on renal P handling is not immediately apparent. At least two additional factors must be considered in the determination of the overall effect of GCs on renal P excretion. These are the extrarenal effects of GCs and the influence of GCs on other renal functions, which may secondarily influence P excretion in the urine.

The general catabolic effect of GCs is well known. This tissue-wasting effect would provide an endogenous P load that would end up in urine for excretion. Less expected is the possibility that GCs may cause an opposite, tissue P-sequestrating effect. Thompson and associates made the interesting observation that the GC-induced fall in serum [P] occurred even in bilaterally nephrectomized rats, suggesting that the extracellular P may be disposed through nonrenal routes.[658] This possibility gains additional credence from the observation that in normal subjects treated with hydrocortisone, urinary P fell below the control levels after an acute initial rise, while serum [P] continued to fall.[475,533] In individuals who had been given intravenous P infusions, the loss of P from the ECF space under the influence of cortisol could not be entirely accounted for by the increase in urinary excretion of P.[475] All these observations suggest the possibility of increased intracellular sequestration of P under the influence of GC. Support for such a hypothesis may be derived from the findings that ACTH increases P turnover in tissues of hypophysectomized rats and that adrenalectomy diminishes significantly the uptake of radiophosphate in muscle.[262] After treatment with ACTH, increased uptake of radiophosphate into various P-containing fractions of the brain of normal and hypophysectomized rats was observed.[389] Other extrarenal effects of GCs that may influence renal P excretion include its stimulatory effects on the parathyroid gland,[253,692] renal 25-(OH)D-1α-hydroxylase activity,[619] and growth hormone synthesis.[102] The effect of GCs on intestinal absorption of P is not well delineated. Loron observed an increase in intestinal absorption of P after short-term administration of cortisone in rats,[437] while Clark and Smith[153] failed to observe any change in P absorption after short-term treatment with hydrocortisone in the same animal model. Caniggia and Gennari[119] reported reduction in intestinal P absorption in patients on long-term steroid therapy.

GCs exert several important effects on the kidney that may influence the urinary excretion of P, including increasing GFR and renal plasma flow (RPF),[289] and stimulation of renal sodium reabsorption and consequent expansion of the ECF space.[289,345] The latter effect may not be a simple consequence of renal Na retention, since acute ECF expansion is also observed in rats in negative external Na balance.[289] Such observations would suggest a GC-induced internal redistribution of Na. Relman and Schwartz showed that rigid Na restriction modified the effect of compound F acetate on the excretion of P.[572] The GCs also have important effects on net tubular hydrogen ion excretion and the acid-base status of the final urine.[567] Systemic acidosis has been demonstrated to abolish the hypophosphaturic response to P deprivation.[429] Long-term administration of GCs leads to a fall in serum K levels and K depletion. Renal wasting of P has been demonstrated in individuals with K-losing renal disease.[444] The P uptake is reduced in brush border membranes isolated from GC-treated animals.[246,661] On the other hand, the simultaneous increase in brush border membrane Na^+-H^+ exchange and the resultant luminal acidification could also contribute to the phosphaturic effect of GCs.[246] GCs have also been implicated in mediating the phosphaturic effect of metabolic acidosis.[85]

In contrast to GCs, deoxycorticosterone acetate (DOCA) administration in humans is not associated with either a reduction in serum [P] or an increase in urinary P excretion.[475] DOCA also has no clear effect on P excretion in dogs.[577] Rastegar and associates[565] observed that fractional excretion of P in humans is not increased during mineralocorticoid "escape" and concluded that the natriuretic response to volume expansion occurs in nephron segments other than the PT, the predominant site of P reabsorption.

Thus, it is quite clear that GCs can substantially modify renal P handling. These steroidal effects are mediated through alterations in extrarenal P metabolism; through GC-induced changes in PTH, vitamin D, and growth hormone availability; and through changes in Na and K metabolism. Altered cation balance can, in turn, modify renal P handling. The phosphaturic response to GCs is vitally dependent upon the dose administered. Large amounts elicit a catabolic response, and the ensuing phosphaturia reflects the appropriate renal clearance of P released from dying cells. Low doses of GCs administered to subjects with adrenal insufficiency elicits an anabolic response, characterized by incorporation of P into growing cells. The ensuing hypophosphaturia reflects the beneficial renal conservation.

The many extrarenal effects of GCs—often left uncontrolled in many studies—have beclouded the question of whether these steroids exert a direct effect on renal P handling.

Estrogens

Experimental studies have demonstrated renal receptors with high affinity for estrogens in various species.[205,432] The estradiol receptor complexes are different from those formed with aldosterone and are found in both cytosol and nuclei. Estrogen is also known to induce renal ultrastructural changes, mainly in the PTs.[353] In clinical practice, mostly in subjects with osteoporosis, the administration of estrogens is associated with a lowering of serum [P].[566,707] Urinary P excretion has been reported to decrease by some[707] and to remain unchanged or to increase by others.[499,574] The former observation may be attributed, at least in part, to the lower plasma [P], which in turn may be the result of the anabolic influence of estrogen, while the latter observation may be explained by the estrogen-induced increase in PTH and mobilization of bone minerals (see below). Riggs and associates[574] did not observe any change in tubular reabsorption of P (TRP) in osteoporotic patients treated with long-term estrogen therapy, although serum [P] consistently fell in all subjects studied. In experimental studies Forland[239] reported a phosphaturic effect of estrogens in rats but did not explore the mechanism in detail. No measurements were made of serum [P], GFR, or indexes of PTH activity. Other studies, however, have revealed little influence of estrogens on renal hemodynamics[353] and Na or K excretion[236] in rodents.

Observations on physiologic states characterized by various circulating concentrations of estrogen have also yielded different conclusions. The daily urinary P excretion rate progressively increases in males for the first three decades and in females for the first two decades in life (Fig. 12-7a); thereafter, the excretion rate steadily falls in both sexes with increasing age. Men also excrete more P than women through most of the adult life span. When P excretion is expressed in relation to creatinine excretion, an index of lean body mass, both the age- and sex-dependency of the P excretion rate disappeared (Fig. 12-7b). The variation in daily urinary P output

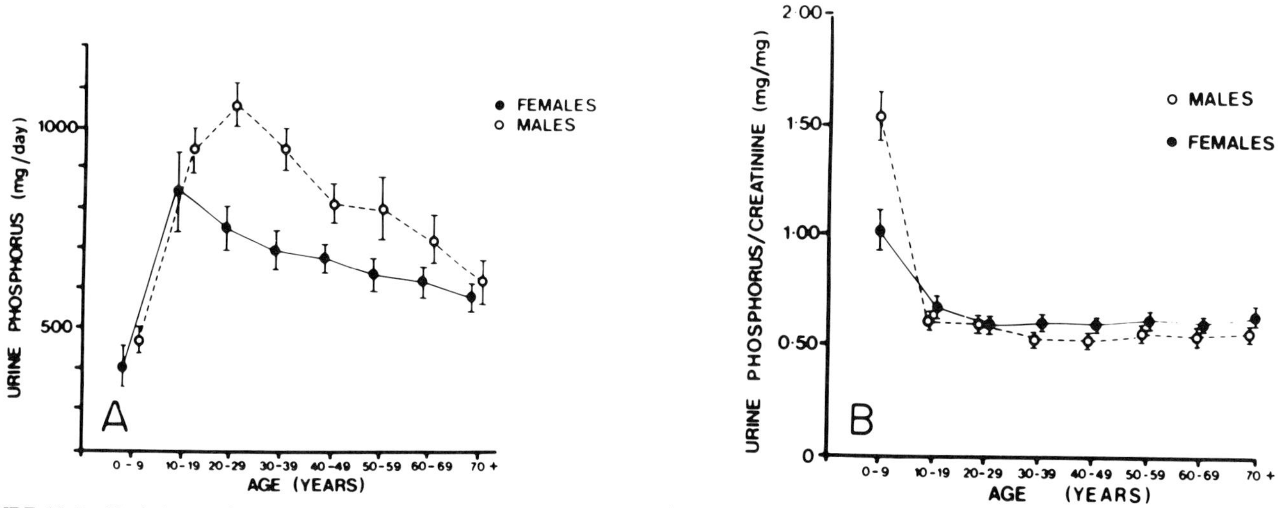

FIGURE 12-7 • Variation with age in the mean (± SEM) daily (*a*) urine phosphorus and (*b*) urinary phosphorus/creatinine ratio in healthy men and women. (From Robertson WG, in Nordin BEC, ed: *Calcium, Phosphate and Magnesium Metabolism,* Edinburgh, Churchill Livingstone, 1976, pp 113–161. Used by permission.)

probably results from differences in P intake, which, like the lean body mass, is lower in females and decreases with age. During pregnancy, serum P does not change during the first two trimesters but falls significantly during the third trimester;[647] this has been attributed to the increased production of estrogens, but unequivocal validation of the hypothesis is still lacking. Information on renal handling of P during pregnancy has not been well documented. Plasma [P] has been reported to rise in postovariectomized and postmenopausal women by some investigators[488,706] but not by others.[355,644] In studies in which a rise in plasma [P] was observed, the possible role of estrogen withdrawal has been postulated, since Aitken and associates[8] have reported an inverse relationship between *T*mP/GFR and circulating estradiol levels. Moreover, the elevated *T*mP/GFR[499] and plasma [P][8] in these estrogen-deprived states could be reversed by estrogen replacement therapy. On the other hand, Young and associates[707] have reported an increase in urinary P/creatinine ratio (suggestive of decreased TRP) in fasting postmenopausal women, and this was attributed to increased bone resorption and elevation in plasma [P] found in these subjects.

Estrogens also interact with other hormones that may in turn influence P homeostasis. Beginning with PTH, Heany theorized that estrogens regulate bone sensitivity to PTH and that estrogen deprivation causes increased bone sensitivity to PTH.[318] The theory would predict a rise in bone remodeling after menopause and that estrogen replacement and/or Ca supplementation should reduce the remodeling. The study of Recker and associates[566] appears to validate these predictions and thus lends credence to the hypothesis. The observation that estrogen administration reduces urinary excretion of Ca and hydroxyproline is also consistent with the postulate that the hormone reduces net bone resorption.[574] This may also be the basis for the observed fall in both fasting levels of plasma and urine Ca and 24-h urine excretion of Ca and hydroxyproline in postmenopausal, hyperparathyroid patients treated with estrogen preparations.[255] Finally, Orimo[516] and coworkers observed that estrogens decreased bone tissue response to PTH under tissue culture conditions. A possible complication of this effect on reducing bone resorption is a net reduction in delivery of Ca into ECF with consequent fall in serum [Ca] and stimulation of PTH. Indeed, Riggs and associates[575] observed an elevated PTH in estrogen-treated osteoporotic women, which was inversely proportional to the fall in serum [Ca]. This elevation in PTH may theoretically reverse the estrogen effect and cause a "paradoxical" increase in bone resorption. The lack of a consistent single effect on bone dynamics may explain the findings of both "phosphaturic" and "antiphosphaturic" effect of estrogens by different investigators.

An estrogen-1α,25-$(OH)_2$D interaction has also been observed. Estrogen injection in birds is associated with an increase in renal 25-(OH)/D-1α-hydroxylase.[364] Conversely, ovariectomy or antiestrogen agents decrease the synthesis of 1α,25-$(OH)_2D_3$.[39,40] In physiologic states characterized by an increase of endogenous estrogen, such as egg laying in the hen[537] and pregnancy in women,[393,537] circulating 1α,25-$(OH)_2D_3$ concentration is also elevated. In male animals, the 1α,25-$(OH)_2D_3$-stimulating effect of estrogen appears to depend on the simultaneous presence of testosterone. Thus, a single injection of estradiol-17β-OH into a normal male bird results in a marked increase in renal 25-(OH)D-1α-hydroxylase activities, while in castrated male chicks, such a response is only observed in animals pretreated with testosterone.[364,649] However, as we have discussed, the effect of $1\alpha,25\text{-}(OH)_2D_3$ on renal P handling is, by itself, not fully understood. The effect of estrogen on plasma and renal P homeostasis may also be influenced by the interaction between this hormone and the growth hormone. Thus, it has been observed that females usually have higher plasma GH levels during fasting, exercise, and stress than males.[244] This difference in response to stress is eliminated by a few days of estrogen treatment in men.[470] Postmenopausal women, like men, showed blunted GH response to stress. Since GH is an "antiphosphaturic" hormone, these observations would support those studies which suggest that estrogens are antiphosphaturic agents. Along this line of argument, Aitken reported increased GH levels in postmenopausal-women and suggested that elevation in serum [P] in estrogen-deprived individuals could be attributed to increases in GH.[7] The increase in intestinal absorption of Ca in pregnant women has also been attributed to an interaction between estrogens and placental lactogen, which is chemically related to GH.[319] It has been postulated that the placental lactogen may mimic the effect of GH in stimulating renal 1α-hydroxylase and increase circulating $1\alpha,25\text{-}(OH)_2D_3$.[620]

In summary, there is no convincing evidence either for or against a direct action of estrogens on renal reabsorption of P. Most of the studies documenting changes in renal P excretion associated with changes in estrogen status could be explained by the influence of the hormone on systemic P metabolism or on the action of other hormones, which in turn may affect the metabolism and renal excretion of P.

Thyroid hormones

Several reports have attested to the observation that serum [P] is higher in patients with hyperthyroidism than in euthyroid subjects.[489] The elevation in serum [P] is correlated with serum T_4 levels[576] and falls after successful treatment.[527] Conversely, hypothyroid patients have lower serum [P] than do normal individuals,[445] and the low [P] is reversed after therapy with thyroid extract.[9] In experimental studies, administration of T_3 to dogs[58] and T_4 to rats[80] is associated with increases in serum [P]. A number of investigators have reported decreased FEP[2] and a normal[511] or low[306] P excretion index (PEI) in patients with hyperthyroidism, while other investigators observed that T_3 administration results in a reduction in TRP, that is, an increase in FEP.[58] The divergent results are not totally unexpected, since the indexes used for accessing TRP do not reliably reflect the intrinsic capacity of the tubule to reabsorb P and are in fact markedly influenced by exogenous and endogenous P load as well as changes in renal hemodynamics. The validity of the various indexes used for measuring the intrinsic renal P reabsorptive capacity will be discussed in greater detail in a later section. More rigorous measurements tend to suggest that thyroid hormones increase intrinsic TRP. Thus, Bijvoet and Majoor[77] demonstrated a positive correlation between *T*mP/GFR and the level of protein-bound iodine, while Gellissen and Brodehl[261] observed reduced *T*mP in infants with congenital absence of thyroid glands and an increase in this parameter with appropriate replacement therapy. In experimental studies, the rate of TRP P (measured at several different serum [P]s) is increased in thyrotoxic rats[80] and decreased in hypothyroid rats[79] when compared with controls. In primary cultured renal cells, addition of triiodothyronine or thyroxine was found to stimulate P uptake.[512] On the other hand, pretreatment with thyroid hormone also enhances P uptake by the renal brush border membrane.[229,372,710] The increase in cellular and brush border membrane P uptake in response to thyroid hormone is sensitive to RNA and protein synthesis inhibitors, suggesting an involvement of protein synthesis in its effect.[512]

The observation that urinary P excretion is higher in hyperthyroid patients,[445] in subjects given T_3[58] or T_4,[9] and in thyrotoxic rats than in pair-fed controls[80] may be explained by the extrarenal effect of thyroid hormones on dietary intake, intestinal absorption, and bone and soft tissue metabolism. It is well known that thyrotoxicosis may be manifested by an increase in appetite and food consumption. Net intestinal P absorption, as measured by balance studies, is either increased[9] or unchanged[349] in thyrotoxic patients. Increased intestinal P absorption has also been reported in rats treated with T_4.[80] It is interesting that thyroid hormone appears to inhibit intestinal Ca absorption in humans[614] and experimental animals.[80,507] Thyroid hormones are known to cause a PTH-independent reduction in bone mass and an increase in bone resorption in thyrotoxic humans[471] and experimental animals.[78] The effect on bone is reflected by elevation in fasting urinary Ca[508] and hydroxyproline[373] excretion. The effect of thyroid hormones on soft tissue metabolism is complex, but weight loss and tissue catabolism per se may increase urinary P excretion by releasing endogenous tissue P.

The effect of thyroid hormones on renal P transport is further complicated by their interaction with various other hormones that are also known to influence renal P handling. Thus, thyrotoxicosis may affect vitamin D metabolism, as reflected by an elevated 24,25-dihydroxyvitamin D [$24,25\text{-}(OH)_2D_3$] and a lower $1\alpha,25\text{-}(OH)_2D_3$ in the circulation of hyperthyroid patients.[346,461] GH is found to be elevated in thyrotoxic patients[91] and to increase in hypothyroid rats following T_4 administration.[369,689] The possibility that the hyperphosphatemia in thyrotoxic patients may be a reflection of parathyroid supression has also been entertained. However, serum immunoreactive PTH levels in these patients have been found to be elevated[115] and normal or reduced.[88] In animal studies, the effect of T_4 on serum [P] and renal tubular P reabsorptive capacity can be demonstrated even in PTX rats.[80] Experimental studies have also demonstrated that T_4 stimulates Na^+-K^+ ATPase in various tissues, including the kidney,[354] raising the possibility of a primary effect of T_4 on Na^+-K^+ ATPase and thereby enhancing Na-P cotransport across the apical membranes.

In summary, thyroid hormones probably directly stimulate renal P reabsorptive capacity. This effect may be masked by their extensive extrarenal actions on P metabolism as well as their complex interacations with other hormone systems, which by themselves have important influence on renal P handling.

Neoplastic "phosphaturic" factors

The syndrome of tumoral or oncogenic osteomalacia is characterized by hypophosphatemia, normocalcemia, decreased renal P reabsorptive capacity, elevated alkaline phosphatase, and rickets or osteomalacia refractory to "physiologic" doses of vitamin D. Resection of the tumor tissue is generally followed by clinical, biochemical, and skeletal remission, with restoration of plasma [P] and renal P reabsorptive capacity to normal.[4,214] Although most reported cases were found in patients with bone and soft tissue tumors of mesenchymal origin, the syndrome has also been observed in association with fibrous dysplasia of bone,[203] malignant neurinoma,[592] and neurofibromatosis.[594] Based on a detailed study of one patient, Drezner and Feinglos[214] proposed that the primary lesion may elaborate a factor that inhibits $1\alpha,25\text{-}(OH)_2D_3$ synthesis. Complete resolution of the biochemical abnormalities and healing of bone pathology was observed after oral administration of physiologic amounts of $1\alpha,25\text{-}(OH)_2D_3$. However, $1\alpha,25\text{-}(OH)_2D_3$ deficiency is unlikely to be the only cause of the syndrome, or one would expect close similarities between the biochemical features of this syndrome and those of vitamin D-deficient or -dependent rickets. Yet, in the patient studied, both serum Ca and PTH levels were normal. Of great interest is the report of a patient with epidermal nevus syndrome with nonfamilial hypophosphatemic rickets, in whom excision of the fibrous tumors was followed by healing of bone lesion. An extract of the tumor, which contained no immunoassayable PTH or CT, caused phosphaturia in a puppy.[34]

Insulin

Insulin decreases plasma P concentration because of shifts from the extracellular space into the intracellular space.[576] Despite this profound extrarenal effect, insulin exerts only a modest antiphosphaturic effect.[576] Pretreatment of PTs with insulin leads to an increase in P uptake by the subsequently isolated brush border membrane vesicles,[296,301] providing evidence of a direct tubular effect. This has been substantiated further by the observation that insulin stimulates P transport in OK cells.[1] As discussed earlier, insulin may play an important role in mediating the antiphosphaturic effect of P deprivation.[14]

Atrial natriuretic factor

In addition to its natriuretic effect, infused atrial natriuretic factor (ANF) increases urinary excretion of many other solutes, including P.[116,305] The phosphaturic effect of ANF occurs through its inhibition of P transport in PT brush border membranes.[304,709] The underlying cellular mechanisms of this effect are not clear, but recent studies suggest a potential role of ANF in the higher fractional excretion of P in rats with reduced renal mass.[517]

Catecholamines

Epinephrine decreases plasma P, presumably by shifting P into the intracellular space.[576] The hypophosphatemic response was also observed after isoproterenol[368] and was blocked by propranolol,[455] suggesting the involvement of a beta-adrenergic receptor mechanism. Epinephrine, norepinephrine, and isoproterenol are all hypophosphaturic.[487] Although the decrease in P excretion occurs in the absence of changes in renal hemodynamics, it is difficult to separate these effects from changes in the filtered load of P due to the concomitant hypophosphatemia. On the other hand, dopamine increases P excretion without changing plasma [P].[188] The role of the renal nerves in P handling has been examined.[643] Renal denervation causes phosphaturia. This effect is believed to be part of a general effect of denervation on proximal transport processes and thus a consequence of decreased sodium reabsorption.

Concluding remarks

It is apparent that a large number of hormones are known to influence renal P excretion. However, the effects of many of these hormones on the magnitude and direction of changes in renal P transport, as well as the mechanisms through which and the location (within the nephron) at which these changes are mediated, are not entirely clarified. Each of these hormones is also known to have important actions on extrarenal metabolism of P and other related substances, which may in turn cause additional changes in renal P excretion. All these hormones also significantly influence various aspects of renal function and transport processes of other solutes, which in turn may further modify the direct effect of a given hormone on renal P reabsorption. It is important to point out that major P regulation and overall P balance can occur in the absence of any of the hormones discussed.

OTHER FACTORS INFLUENCING RENAL PHOSPHATE EXCRETION

Variation in phosphorus intake

The renal tubule has an intrinsic ability to adjust the reabsorption rate of P according to the need and the availability of P to the body. P reabsorption is increased under the conditions of greater P need, such as rapid growth, pregnancy, lactation, and dietary restriction. Conversely, in times of surfeit, such as slow growth, chronic renal failure, or dietary excess, the renal P reabsorption is curtailed. Micropuncture and microperfusion studies have shown that these adaptive responses occur in, although are not limited to, the PT.[96,385,492,528,665] Once these changes were induced in vivo, they persisted in vitro. Segments of PTs from rabbits fed a low-P diet showed an enhanced P (but not Na^+ or glucose) transport rate, whereas PTs from rabbits fed a high-P diet exhibited a low P transport rate.[96] The degree of adaptation may be greater in the deep than in the superficial nephrons.[386,406] The adaptation to P deprivation is independent of PTH, and the phosphaturic response to PTH and cAMP is severely blunted in P-depleted animals.[271,528,629] In rats fed low-P diets, the response to PTH disappears in the early PT but is retained in the late PT.[665] In fasted hamsters, the response to PTH can be restored by metabolic acidosis and by acetazolamide administration.[334,384] The adaptation to a low-P diet is fast; enhanced P transport can be detected after 2 to 4 h of P deprivation.[128,426] The reaction to P overload also occurs with similar promptness.[141]

The adaptive response to dietary P intake can clearly be demonstrated in the brush border membrane. The Na^+-dependent P uptake across the brush border membrane is markedly increased within hours of dietary P restriction or, conversely, decreased with short-term elevation of dietary P.[140,141,212,361,605,634,635] The triggering mechanism and the intracellular response to dietary P restriction are not known. Characteristically, the adaptation is expressed as an increase of V_{max} of Na^+-P cotransport, while K_m is not changed,[111,140,426,495] which suggests that the number of P transport systems in the membrane is increased. A similar adaptive response to P restriction has also been demonstrated in renal epithelial cells grown in culture.[70,71,73,107,129] These studies showed that the Na^+-dependent P uptake by these cells was increased when they were maintained in media low in P. These studies also suggested that the adaptive response consisted of an immediate response involving activation of P transporters on the apical membrane and a second, long-term response involving new protein synthesis.[70,129] It is not clear whether the activation of P transporters on the apical membrane is due to the uncovering of latent carriers within the membrane; an exocytic insertion of transport assemblies, either from a readily available intracellular reservoir or from de novo synthesis; or a combination of all three processes. Further evidence has also been provided suggesting a role for an increase in brush border membrane fluidity resulting from alterations in its lipid composition.[482] Such a notion, however, has been challenged by the observation that, during the early phase of P deprivation, isolated renal brush border membranes showed an increase in P uptake without detectable changes in fluidity or cholesterol content, and that in vitro alteration in brush border membrane fluidity did not correlate with P uptake.[426] Recently, a role of insulin has been proposed in the acute response to dietary P restriction.[14] Thus, in rats fed a low-P diet, suppression of endogenous insulin secretion by infusion of somatostatin was found to prevent the adaptive increase in P reabsorption despite a lower plasma [P]. The addition of exogenous insulin to these rats restored the antiphosphaturic effect of the low-P diet.[14]

It is of interest that P deprivation by fasting does not result in similar P handling by the kidney. P excretion is higher in fasted rats than in rats fed either a normal or a low-P diet.[202,204] Moreover, the fasted rats retain partial responsiveness to PTH, in contrast to the resistance present in rats on a low-P diet.[57] The higher excretion rate of P in fasting is likely to be due to effects at the PT cell, because fasting does not increase the P uptake into brush border membrane vesicles.[362] Furthermore, when rats adapted to a low-P diet are subsequently starved, fasting reverses the increased uptake of P by the brush border membrane vesicles.[362] How the kidneys differentiate between selective and total dietary intake is not known.

Effective circulating volume

Clearance studies in rats,[250] dogs,[458,550,639] and humans[626] have shown that acute expansion of the ECF with saline solution leads to an increase in P excretion associated with natriuresis. A direct correlation can be demonstrated between the fraction of filtered P excreted and that of Na. An exaggerated phosphaturic response to ECF expansion has also been observed in subjects with essential hypertension, a finding that is compatible with the general mechanisms of Na reabsorption in these subjects.[133] Since acute reduction in GFR does not abort the increase in P excretion, it was concluded that saline expansion inhibits tubular P reabsorption independent of the filtered load. In whole animal studies, the effect of saline expansion on P excretion occurs both in the presence and in the absence of parathyroid glands, although the magnitude of phosphaturia is greater in intact than in PTX animals.[312,313] This suggests that the full expression of saline-induced phosphaturia requires not only the presence of a natriuresis but also the presence of intact parathyroid glands. When ECF expansion is induced with hyperoncotic albumin, the increase in P excretion can be completely abolished by preventing the fall in the plasma-ionized [Ca].[388]

Micropuncture studies[5,52,250,380] indicate that saline-induced volume expansion leads to a decrease in proximal reabsorption of both Na and P. The magnitude of inhibition is not significantly influenced by the removal of parathyroid glands. The reduction in proximal P reabsorption is paralleled by an increase in urinary P excretion in intact animals[52,380] and in animals several days after thyroparathyroidectomy (chronic TPTX).[250,326] In the latter instance, the magnitude of phosphaturia was reduced compared to that observed in intact animals. However, saline expansion in animals several hours to a day after thyroparathyroidectomy (acute TPTX) is not accompanied by any increases in urinary P excretion, although proximal P reabsorption is reduced to the same extent as in intact animals.[52,380] The abolition of ECF expansion-induced phosphaturia by acute TPTX, PTX, or Ca infusion (acute PTH suppression) has also been demonstrated in a number of other studies.[249,284,600] The acute withdrawal of circulating PTH probably unmasked a powerful distal P reabsorptive mechanism, clearing the increased, volume-induced P delivery from upstream, which otherwise would have been excreted in the urine. The partial restoration of the saline-induced phosphaturia in chronic TPTX animals may be related to the rise in plasma [P] in these animals, leading to an increase in filtered load and presumably the saturation of this distal P reabsorptive mechanism. In this context it is interesting to note that Herbert and associates[326] have demonstrated that the difference in the phosphaturic response to saline infusion between acute and chronic TPTX animals can be abolished when serum P levels are the same in both conditions. Recent clearance studies by Frick and Durasin[251] have also shown that extracellular volume expansion reduced TRP in intact as well as acutely TPTX rats, provided P infusions were given during the study.

The combination of micropuncture and clearance data suggests that the inhibition of proximal P reabsorption by saline infusion is largely PTH-independent and is most likely the result of the generalized increase in passive backflux induced by ECF volume expansion. The translation of this reduced proximal P reabsorption into whole-kidney phosphaturia requires the presence of parathyroid glands, which appear to exercise a "braking" effect on a potent distal P reabsorptive mechanism. The acute withdrawal of this parathyroid influence would result in the elimination of this saline-induced phosphaturia. Chronically, the influence of PTH withdrawal is minimized and saline-induced phosphaturia is restored, at least partially. This may be the result of an increased filtered load of P, secondary to the increment in plasma [P], or may be the result of other, PTH-independent tubular adaptive mechanisms for P reabsorption.

Thus, Na and P transport appear to parallel each other in the PT but are dissociated more distally. This distal dissociation has been used to explain the lack of phosphaturic response during the natriuresis associated with chronic ECF expansion in patients with hyperaldosteronism and in normal subjects given a chronic Na load.[565] Under these conditions the natriuresis is attributed to changes in distal segments where Na and P transport may be completely dissociated.

The role of PTH in the production of ECF expansion-induced phosphaturia has already been discussed. The possibility that the dilutional hypocalcemia per se may directly mediate the ECF expansion-induced phosphaturia is considered less likely, since a 25 percent reduction of this ion by the infusions of edetic acid (EDTA) into the renal artery did not have a significant effect on the renal handling of P.[187] The finding that renal vasodilatation also increases P excretion in dogs[6,188,599] raises a further possible mechanism for phosphaturia of ECF expansion. Renal vasodilatation, with its consequent diminished filtration fraction, lowers peritubular protein concentration and increases peritubular hydrostatic pressure, which may account for the phosphaturia. However, pharmacologic vasodilatation does not always lead to phosphaturia. Dopamine, for example, is phosphaturic, whereas isoproterenol is not.[188] Again, acetylcholine and prostaglandin E_1 (PGE_1) are phosphaturic, whereas low doses of bradykinin or prostaglandin E_2 (PGE_2) are nonphosphaturic.[599] Thus, it appears that mechanisms other than vasodilatation per se may be important in the induction of phosphaturia by these agents. For example, one possible explanation as to why low doses of bradykinin and PGE_2 do not cause phosphaturia is the finding that these agents also do not interfere with proximal tubular reabsorption which, as we have already discussed, may play an important role in the mediation of whole-kidney phosphaturia in the intact animal. By contrast, dopamine inhibits fluid (J_v) reabsorption in isolated perfused PTs.[60] It is possible that properties other than vasodilatation may be operative in vasodilator-induced phosphaturia.

Epstein and coworkers studied the effect of neck-out water immersion on renal P handling.[227] This model allows central blood volume expansion without saline infusion, and ionized Ca and PTH concentrations were unaltered. Despite a natriuresis (maximal fractional Na excretion was 1.4 percent) equivalent to acute administration of 2 liters of saline solution, phosphaturia was not observed. Since there was also a simultaneous bicarbonaturia, the authors proposed that the site of action for natriuresis was in the PT. If that is the case, then the dissociation between natriuresis and phosphaturia would suggest a distal site for P reabsorption, compensating for the presumed reduction in proximal P reabsorption.

Diuretics

Acetazolamide

Many diuretics increase urinary P excretion. Carbonic anhydrase inhibitors are probably the most potent phosphaturic diuretics and have an effect that is equal to that of PTH. Acetazolamide administration markedly increases the fraction of filtered P excreted in relation to that for Na in dogs[35,51,221,254,383] and in humans.[548] The effect of acetazolamide does not appear to be mediated by PTH, since it also induces phosphaturia in chronically PTX animals.[221] In acutely TPTX animals, the phosphaturia is less than that seen in chronically TPTX or intact dogs.[51] Knox and coworkers[383] noted that the action of PTH was additive to the effect of maximal inhibition of carbonic anhydrase by acetazolamide, suggesting that the two agents may have different mechanisms and sites of action on P reabsorption. In addition, P reabsorption was inhibited to a greater degree by PTH than by acetazolamide beyond the point of micropuncture.

Because acetazolamide and PTH have similar actions on P, bicarbonate, and Na excretion and manifest an interaction on bone PTH-activated adenylate cyclase,[476] a number of studies have examined the effect of acetazolamide on the adenylate cyclase system in the kidney. Rodriguez and coworkers[584] found that in both normal and PTX rats, acetazolamide duplicated the action of PTH by increasing urinary excretion of cAMP. A similar effect was demonstrated with cAMP generation by renal cortical slices in vitro. Alkalinization of the urine with bicarbonate infusions, on the other hand, failed to result in a change in the excretion of either P or cAMP. Indirect evidence for a role of the adenylate cyclase system in the phosphaturic effect of acetazolamide has been generated by clearance studies in normal dogs and in dogs treated with lithium, an inhibitor of adenylate cyclase.[33] Acetazolamide administration led to natriuresis and bicarbonaturia in both normal and lithium-treated dogs. On the other hand, phosphaturia was observed only in the normal dogs, but not in the lithium-treated dogs. These data suggest that acetazolamide causes natriuresis and bicarbonaturia through inhibition of carbonic anhydrase and causes phosphaturia through activation of the adenylate cyclase system. On the other hand, in humans, the infusion of acetazolamide in patients with hypoparathyroidism or pseudohypoparathyroidism has been shown to result in augmented excretion of P without an increase in urinary cAMP.[615]

The question of whether the acetazolamide-induced phosphaturia is secondary to its effect on bicarbonaturia is also not clearly settled. It has been suggested that alkalinization of luminal fluid increases the intratubular concentration of the more polar and less transportable divalent P ion HPO_4^{2-} over that of the more easily reabsorbed monovalent ion $H_2PO_4^-$.[254,548] On the other hand, isolated brush border membrane vesicle studies would suggest that the divalent P ion is the preferred molecule for reabsorption, since increased P uptake was observed in an alkaline medium.[330] However, although carbonic anhydrase inhibition causes bicarbonaturia in the "bulk" luminal fluid, its effect on the "microenvironment" of the brush border is uncertain. Indeed, acetazolamide may cause a fall in luminal pH because of the development of "disequilibrium" pH.[568] There are, however, other data supporting the importance of the presence of bicarbonate in the expression of the phosphaturic effect of acetazolamide. In studies of the isolated perfused kidney, the presence or absence of bicarbonate in the perfusion medium did not alter the basal FEP (7 percent). The FEP remained unaltered when acetazolamide was added in the absence of bicarbonate but increased sixfold (to 43 percent) following acetazolamide in the presence of bicarbonate.[68]

Thiazides

Thiazides cause significant phosphaturia with fractional excretions approaching those attained with acetazolamide.[101,221,630] These diuretics also augment the urinary excretion of sodium chloride, bicarbonate, and potassium. The carbonic anhydrase inhibitory activity of these agents, although less than that of acetazolamide (Table 12-2), is nevertheless significant and may account for the reduced bicarbonate reabsorption in the PT. Simultaneous micropuncture and clearance studies demonstrated a marked decline in the proximal fractional reabsorption of P following the administration of chlorothiazide or metolazone.[234] As in the case of acetazolamide, it is uncertain whether the phosphaturic effect of thiazides is a direct result of carbonic anhydrase inhibition or is mediated through separate mechanisms. The possibility that the thiazides may cause phosphaturia through the adenylate cyclase–cAMP axis needs to be entertained, since this group of diuretics has been shown to inhibit phosphodiesterase, which inhibits cAMP conversion to 5′-monophosphate.[604] A number of studies, however, suggest that the phosphaturic action of the thiazides and the carbonic anhydrase inhibitors may be fundamentally different. Thus, whereas acetazolamide causes a significant phosphaturia in acutely PTX rats, chlorothiazide fails to do so except during P infusion.[540] In chronically PTX animals, the filtered load of P is higher than in acutely PTX animals and the phosphaturic response can again be elicited.[221,540]

Furosemide and ethacrynic acid

Both furosemide and ethacrynic acid have their major action on the medullary portion of the ascending limb of the loop of Henle. Both agents also detectably inhibit proximal tubular reabsorption, especially when studied under conditions in which the urinary losses are replaced to prevent volume depletion.[150,382] When studied under such conditions, both diuretics also clearly increase urinary P excretion.[215,221,290,625] Bumetanide, a new diuretic with a site of action similar to that of furosemide and ethacrynic acid, is also phosphaturic in humans.[89]

TABLE 12-2 • Effect of diuretics on renal phosphate excretion

Diuretics	CA inhibition activity*	Inhibition of Na reabsorption: sites and potency				Peak fractional excretion, %		Reference/species
			Ascending limb					
		Proximal	Medullary	Cortical	Distal	Na	P	
PROXIMAL								
Acetazolamide	1.0	+ + +			+	5	30–60	Knox et al., 1976/dog;[383] Beck and Goldberg, 1973/ dog;[51] Eknoyan et al., 1970/ dog;[221] Fulop and Brazeau, 1968/dog[254]
LOOP								
Furosemide	0.02	+	+ + +	+		25	20–45	Puschett and Goldberg, 1968/ humans;[547] Steele, 1971/ humans;[625] Hass et al., 1977/dog;[290] Duarte, 1974/ dog[215]
Ethacrynic acid	0.000003	+	+ + +	+ +		25	25–30	Steele, 1971/humans;[625] Duarte, 1974/dog[215]
DISTAL								
Thiazides	0.15	+			+ + +	8	30	Steinmuller and Puschett, 1972/humans;[630] Brickman et al., 1972/humans;[101] Weinmann and Eknoyan, 1975/rat;[682] Fernandez and Puschett, 1973/rat[234]
Triamterene Amiloride Spironolactone					+ + +	2	†	Ben Ishay et al., 1972;[65] Walker et al., 1972/ humans;[670] Johny et al., 1969[348]
OSMOTIC								
Mannitol		+	+ + +			8	23	Maesaka et al., 1976/rat[442]

KEY: +, minor action; + + +, major action.
* Relative to the concentration of acetazolamide required for 50% inhibition of carbonic anhydrase (CA), considered as unity.
† No effect on P reabsorption.
SOURCE: Based on data from Martinez-Maldonado and Eknoyan.[452]

The modest carbonic anhydrase inhibitory activity of furosemide (Table 12-2) has been proposed as a possible mechanism for its phosphaturic action. In this context, it is interesting to note that in dogs given acetazolamide, the subsequent administration of furousemide caused no further phosphaturia or bicarbonaturia.[290] Furosemide, however, differs from acetazolamide in that it has no effect on urinary excretion of cAMP or on the activity of adenylate cyclase in the renal cortex.[584] On the other hand, furosemide, like the thiazides, has inhibitory action on phosphodiesterase activity in rat renal cortical tissue.[604] Whether this increases intracellular cAMP concentration and inhibits P reabsorption remains to be established. A further difference from acetazolamide is the observation of Haas and coworkers that the phosphaturic action of furosemide is dependent on the presence of PTH.[290] These workers noted that in acutely PTX dogs, furosemide did not increase FEP except when given during the constant infusion of bovine PTH. However, it should be pointed out that the reduction in GFR was more marked in dogs given furosemide alone (−40 to −50 percent) than in dogs given both PTH and furosemide (−20 to −26 percent). Since furosemide is secreted by the PT[569] and acts on the luminal side of the distal nephron,[207] a reduction in GFR could also result in a decreased distal delivery of the proximally secreted furosemide to act on more distal luminal sites. The dependency of furosemide on PTH in mediating its phosphaturic action has also been challenged by the observation that this agent inhibits P reabsorption in isolated perfused kidney, obviously in the total absence of PTH.[505]

Amiloride, spironolactone, and triamterene

None of the distal potassium-sparing diuretics has been shown to inhibit renal TRP.[65,348,670]

Osmotic diuretics

Mannitol, the most commonly utilized osmotic diuretic, exerts its major inhibition on Na reabsorption on the loop of Henle.[603] A lesser degree of inhibition of Na reabsorption is also observed in the PT. Although a number of studies have demonstrated that neither urea nor mannitol increases P excretion, Maesaka and coworkers more recently provided evidence for a phosphaturic effect of mannitol.[442] A possible explanation for the discrepant observation may be attributed to the fact that, in the earlier studies, the occurrence of phosphaturia may have been missed because mannitol interferes with the Fisk and Subbarrow method used for determination of P.[166] The mechanism underlying mannitol-induced phosphaturia has not been clearly established. The study of Maesaka and coworkers suggests that the phosphaturic effect of mannitol is mediated through PTH stimulation. Thus, when calcium and magnesium were given to counteract the dilutional effect of mannitol administration, the phosphaturic effect was blunted. Moreover, a phosphaturic effect was not observed in TPTX animals, except when a constant infusion of PTH was simultaneously administered.

Acid-base status

It has been well demonstrated that changes in acid-base balance result in changes in urinary P excretion. However, the relationships are complex, and the results obtained by various experimental techniques are divergent or even contradictory. Considering the fact that systemic acid-base balance is likely to affect the pH of different compartments in and around the PT, such as luminal fluid, cytosol, and peritubular fluid, and that these pH changes may have diverse effects on P reabsorption, the inconsistent results reported in these studies can probably be attributed to the complex interactions among these various components.

Effect of luminal pH

In microperfusion experiments in rat PTs, Bank and coworkers[43] found that the reabsorption of 2 m*M* P was greater at acid than at alkaline pH of the perfusion solution. In another microperfusion study in rat PT but with much higher [P] concentration (100 m*M*) in the perfusion solution, Cassola and Malnic[125] also found that the rate of P reabsorption was greater with acid than with alkaline perfusion solutions. Similar results were also reported in isolated perfused rabbit PTs by Ham and associates.[294] In these studies, the reabsorption of 10 m*M* P was found to be higher at acid than at alkaline pH in the lumen.

In contrast to these reports, other studies showed an opposite effect of luminal pH on P reabsorption. In microperfusion experiments in rat PTs, Baumann and colleagues[47] found the reabsorption of 2 m*M* P was twice as high at pH 7.4 as at pH 6.8 in the lumen. In double microperfusion experiments of rat PTs and peritubular capillaries, Ullrich and coworkers[665] found that the reabsorption of 4 m*M* P was higher at alkaline than at acid luminal pH. In another microperfusion study in rat PTs, Quamme and Wong[556] also showed that P reabsorption was twice as high as pH 7.6 than at pH 6.5 in the lumen.

The apparent discrepancies among these results were in part resolved by the studies reported by Lang and associates.[406] These studies showed that P reabsorption in rat PT was stimulated by alkaline luminal pH when [P] in the lumen was low, but it was inhibited by high pH at high luminal [P]. In the studies reported by Quamme and Wong,[556] it was also found that systemic infusion of P or administration of a high-P diet diminished the dependency of P reabsorption on luminal pH. It thus appears that the luminal pH dependence of P reabsorption is under the influence of P availability to the PT cells. Alkaline pH in the lumen enhances P reabsorption only when P is not in excess to the PT cells. These observations are in good agreement with the properties of the Na^+-P cotransporter described in the isolated brush border membrane. In isolated brush border membrane vesicles, alkaline pH at the outer (or luminal) solution stimulates the Na^+-dependent P uptake by increasing the affinity of the Na^+-P cotransporter for Na^+ and, consequently, for P. Thus, at [P] in the lumen above saturation, the luminal pH will no longer have direct effect on P reabsorption.

Effect of intracellular pH

Changes in intracellular pH may play a key role in regulating PT P reabsorption. Unfortunately, no direct evidence exists to evaluate this possibility or its mechanism. In isolated brush border membrane vesicles, acidic pH in the intravesicular space (or cytosolic side of the membrane) enhances P uptake.[20,590] As discussed earlier, this is considered to be due to either an increased rate of P dissociation from the carrier or the trapping of the monovalent P. However, the effect of intracellular pH may be more complex than its direct effect on brush border membrane because changes in intracellular pH can produce profound metabolic changes, which in turn may exert additional effects on P reabsorption.

Ullrich and colleagues[665] observed that P reabsorption was decreased after acetazolamide infusion and concluded that intracellular alkalosis reduces P reabsorption. On the contrary, by using citrate reabsorption and cellular citrate content as an intracellular pH indicator, Knox and coworkers[381] suggested that intracellular alkalosis enhances, while intracellular acidosis suppresses, PT P reabsorption. On the other hand, results from the systemic acid-base effects have frequently been used to infer the effects of intracellular pH on P reabsorption. Such practice, however, could also be misleading because changes in systemic bicarbonate concentration and pH do not necessarily reflect changes in intracellular pH. For example, the systemic metabolic alkalosis in potassium-depleted subjects may in fact be associated with an intracellular acidosis. Reciprocally, the systemic metabolic acidosis after acute lithium administration could actually accompany intracellular alkalosis. It is clear that studies that allow simultaneous measurements of intracellular pH and P transport are needed to clarify these issues.

Effect of systemic acid-base balance

Changes in respiratory acid-base balance have direct effects on renal P handling. Respiratory acidosis leads to a consistent depression in renal P reabsorption.[680] This occurs independently of other factors, such as PTH, filtered P load, bicarbonate reabsorption, and extracellular pH.[680] Respiratory alkalosis, on the other hand, results in an increased renal P reabsorption.[334] This again appears to be dependent on P_{CO_2} tension rather than on extracellular alkalosis, because HCl infusion did not affect the respiratory effect. Furthermore, respiratory alkalosis blunts the phosphaturic effect of PTH and cAMP, suggesting an effect independent of PTH. These observations may suggest a yet unknown, but potentially important, role of intracellular P_{CO_2} in controlling P reabsorption.

Acute metabolic acidosis induced by acute acid infusion does not alter basal P excretion but does attenuate the phosphaturic effect of PTH.[541] In contrast, chronic metabolic acidosis causes a significant decrease in P reabsorption.[55] Studies in isolated brush border membrane vesicles showed that chronic metabolic acidosis leads to a lower Na^+-dependent P uptake, with a decrease in V_{max}.[356] This is quite different from the direct stimulatory effect of intravesicular H^+ on brush border membrane P uptake. The mechanisms leading to this change in the brush border membrane are not known, but an increase in GC hormone levels has been implicated to be involved in this down-regulation of P transport.[85] In addition, the simultaneous increase in Na^+-H^+ exchange activity induced by metabolic acidosis and the resultant changes in luminal as well as intracellular pH could also contribute to the inhibition of P reabsorption. Acute metabolic alkalosis by sodium bicarbonate infusion also reduces P reabsorption by a mechanism independent of PTH, ECF volume expansion, or plasma calcium.[395,711] This effect, however, is critically dependent on the antecedent dietary P intake,[553,624] so that bicarbonate infusion in animals on normal dietary P intake leads to an enhanced P reabsorption but causes a decrease in P reabsorption in animals on high P dietary intake. This is similar to the effect of luminal alkalinization, as discussed earlier, and suggests a possible role of luminal pH in mediating the effect of acute metabolic alkalosis. Chronic alkalosis, on the other hand, increases P reabsorption, presumably by mechanisms similar to those in chronic acidosis but working in the opposite direction.[479]

Calcium

The effect of Ca on renal P handling is generally studied by measuring changes in renal P reabsorption and excretion associated with changes in serum [Ca] induced by intravenous infusion or by the administration of chelators.

The infusion of Ca may influence renal P handling by a number of different mechanisms,[531] including its effect on PTH secretion, and renal hemodynamics and a possible direct effect on renal TRP. As discussed earlier (see "Plasma Phosphorus"), Ca infusion may also affect renal P excretion by its influence on the physicochemical states of circulating P.

Acute infusions of Ca in normal subjects result in an increase in both renal P reabsorption and plasma [P]. Since the absolute urinary P excretion was also increased during infusion, the possibility of net P mobilization from bone and soft tissue was suggested.[328,335,510] The change in renal P reabsorption has been attributed to secondary inhibition of PTH secretion, since the antiphosphaturic effect was reversed when exogenous PTH was given simultaneously.[328,403] Moreover in some hypoparathyroid patients, Ca infusions and increases in serum [Ca] (from baseline hypocalcemic levels) did not reduce renal P excretion.[218,279,328,336,510] These studies therefore suggest that in humans, Ca infusion increases renal P reabsorption and that this action is mediated through suppression of PTH secretion. Glorieux and Scriver,[272] in their studies on *x*-linked hypophosphatemia, proposed that renal

TRP is mediated through two mechanisms: a larger, PTH-responsive component and a smaller, PTH-insensitive, but Ca-responsive component. In patients with *x*-linked hypophosphatemia, the Ca-responsive component remains intact, thus giving rise to the observation that Ca infusion in these patients was associated with an increase in renal P reabsorption. The existence of a PTH-independent, P reabsorptive mechanism that is sensitive to Ca infusions has also been sought in patients with postsurgical or idiopathic hypoparathyroidism. Unfortunately, the results have been quite variable, with reduction in urine P excretion observed only in some of the patients studied.[134,404] In fact, in a number of studies, sustained correction of hypocalcemia in hypoparathyroid patients has quite the opposite effect and has been found to result in an increase in both absolute and FEP.[218,279,328,336] In some patients this increase in P excretion may be attributed to a Ca infusion–associated increase in serum [P] (discussed earlier), but in others this increase in P excretion occurred in the absence of overt changes in serum [P].[218] Thus, observations in humans suggest that Ca infusion could cause an increase in renal P reabsorption by the suppression of PTH secretion. In addition, it appears that Ca also has a direct, PTH-independent effect on renal tubular handling of P. In conditions such as *x*-linked hypophosphatemia and in some cases of hypoparathyroidism, Ca infusion is associated with an increase in renal P reabsorption, while in other cases of hypoparathyroidism the same maneuver is associated with a decrease in renal P reabsorption as reflected by an increase in renal P excretion. The reasons for these variable responses remain to be defined.

A number of animal studies appear to lend support to the thesis that Ca enhances renal P reabsorption. Lavender and Pullman[415] demonstrated an ipsilateral decrease in urinary P excretion during acute infusion of Ca into one renal artery. However, these changes could have resulted from the effect of hypercalcemia on renal hemodynamics rather than from its direct effect on tubular P transport, since both renal plasma flow and GFR were also reduced. Acute hypercalcemia-associated vasoconstriction could decrease renal P excretion by reducing the GFR, thus decreasing the filtered load of P,[146,411,438,671] or by inducing a disproportionate reduction in RPF, thus increasing the filtration fraction and consequently increasing proximal solute and P reabsorption.[146,411,671] In addition, acute Ca infusions have been shown to decrease the glomerular ultrafiltration coefficient, K_f,[340] thus providing an additional factor for reducing GFR. However, a number of other studies also appear to support the contention that Ca infusions cause a PTH-independent increase in renal P reabsorption. Thus, Popovtzer and associates[542] observed that the induction of hypercalcemia clearly reduced the phosphaturia induced by volume expansion in PTX rats. Employing micropuncture techniques, Amiel and associates[19] noted that elevating Ca concentration from the basal hypocalcemic level increased P reabsorption by the PT, loop of Henle, and distal nephron of PTX rats. In both studies, plasma [P] was not altered significantly. Rouse and Suki,[588] using an in vitro microperfusion technique, further demonstrated that in rabbit PCT (both superficial and deep), elevating the [Ca] in both the perfusate and the bathing medium led to an increase in the lumen-to-bath (reabsorptive) flux of P. This Ca-associated action on P reabsorption was not observed in the proximal straight tubule.

Unfortunately, other experimental studies led to contrary conclusions.[186,531] Cuche and associates[186] demonstrated that Ca infusion caused a clear increase in both absolute and fractional P excretion in TPTX dogs, and this phosphaturic effect was seen whether the dogs were given PTH infusions or not. Measurement of PT P reabsorption also demonstrated that acute hypercalcemia decreased this parameter in both rats[206] and dogs.[217]

As with the data in humans, the reasons for these divergent findings in animal studies is not clear. It is clear, however, that changes in proximal P handling may not be paralleled by similar changes in the final urine. Indeed, Goldfarb and associates[278] demonstrated that the acute hypercalcemia-induced reduction in proximal P reabsorption was not translated into an increase in P excretion by the whole kidney. This observation suggested that hypercalcemia unmasked or stimulated important distal tubular reabsorptive mechanisms for P. Peraino and Suki infused Ca into TPTX dogs and found significant increases in serum [P] (4.6 ± 0.2 increasing to 6.1 ± 0.2 mg/100 ml), filtered P load, and tubular P reabsorption.[391] Similar studies were carried out in dogs in which serum [P] was first raised with appropriate infusions. The infusion of Ca caused further increases in the already elevated serum P levels (7.4 ± 0.3 to 8.6 ± 0.2 mg/100 ml) and filtered P load.[531] However, the preinfusion, already elevated tubular P reabsorptive rate was not further increased by Ca infusion. This study suggests that the enhancing effect of Ca on P reabsorption can only be demonstrated in dogs reabsorbing P at rates below maximum. This study also emphasizes that because Ca infusion may also change the filtered load of P, a change in urinary P excretion cannot be used to extrapolate a reciprocal change in P reabsorption. Thus, in response to Ca infusions, dogs that received prior P infusions manifested an increase in the filtered load of P in the absence of any further change in the P reabsorption rate. One would thus observe a rise in urinary P excretion even though the renal P reabsorption was not decreased. In dogs not receiving prior P administration, Ca infusions caused an increase in the calculated urinary P excretion (rising from 0.08 to 0.16 mg/min) even though the tubular P reabsorption was clearly increased.

In dogs, the induction of acute hypocalcemia was associated with increased urinary P excretion.[586] Although this has been attributed to stimulation of PTH secretion because the phosphaturic effect was abolished immediately after TPTX, a direct effect of hypocalcemia on TRP has not been excluded.[249,284] Cuche and coworkers[187] provided additional evidence supporting the participation of changes in PTH secretion in the mediation of hypocalcemia-induced increases in renal P excretion. They noted that EDTA infusions failed to cause a phosphaturia when PTH levels were held constant by infusion of exogenous hormone in TPTX dogs. However, when the chelator is given to parathyroid-intact animals, increases in the FEP were noted. Other studies, however, support a direct effect of hypocalcemia on renal P reabsorption. Thus, Rasmussen and associates,[561] using ethyleneglycol-bis(β-aminothyl ether)-N,N,N^1,N^1-tetraacetic acid (EGTA) in TPTX rats, have demonstrated a clear phosphaturic effect of hypocalcemia. Peraino and Suki[531] also demonstrated in TPTX dogs that EGTA-induced hypocalcemia augments FEP. Estep and associates[231] reported that acute hypocalcemia induced by EDTA infusion increased P clearance in normal human subjects but decreased it in nine of eleven hyperparathyroid and five hypoparathyroid patients. They proposed that Ca and PTH have opposing effects on the renal handling of P and that the net result of a change in serum [Ca] depends on the relative predominance of either of these factors in a given set of clinical or experimental conditions. However, in contrast to these studies, in recent studies with cultured renal epithelial cells, lowering the extracellular calcium from 2 to 0.02 m*M* was actually found to increase the cellular P uptake.[127]

In summary, the circulating [Ca] may modify renal P reabsorption through mechanisms other than those dependent on PTH secretion. Examples of such mechanisms include the effect of Ca on plasma P concentration, on the glomerular ultrafiltration coefficient, on renal hemodynamics, and possibly also directly on renal tubular cell function. These PTH-independent effects may either increase or decrease P reabsorption. The directional change in P reabsorption appears to be dictated by factors such as the basal [Ca] and whether the renal tubule is already at or well below its maximal reabsorptive capacity for P.

Magnesium

Short-term magnesium (Mg) infusions were associated with suppression of PTH and decreased urinary P excretion.[456] Increased dietary Mg was shown to reduce urinary P excretion.[152] On the other hand, Mg depletion in rats caused phosphaturia, which was not abolished by parathyroidectomy.[268,270] Knochel[378] summarized experimental and clinical evidence supporting the notion that hypomagnesemia or Mg depletion may cause hypophosphatemia and an inappropriate degree of phosphaturia. However, hyperphosphatemia may also occur with selective Mg deficiency in humans.[466] Muldowney and associates[493] found that P clearance was reduced in Mg depletion. This abnormality was corrected by Mg repletion or following the infusion of parathyroid extract. On the other hand, Estep and associates[230] found no phosphaturic response to infusion of parathyroid extract in Mg-depleted patients. Levi and associates[425] found a reduced phosphaturic response to parathyroid extract in Mg-depleted dogs compared to the same dogs repleted with Mg. Medalle and Waterhouse[466] found no phosphaturic response to parathyroid extract in a patient both during Mg depletion and after Mg repletion.

Lithium

Arruda and associates[33] demonstrated that the intraperitoneal administration of lithium (Li) chloride (3 meq/kg) for 3 days not only blocked the renal cortical adenylate cyclase–cAMP system but also interfered with reactions distal to the formation of cAMP because the phosphaturic effect of both PTH and cAMP was clearly inhibited in the Li-treated dogs. It is of interest to note that, in humans, Li ingestion is associated with an increased incidence of hyperparathyroidism[148] as well as several other metabolic abnormalities, such as nephrogenic diabetes insipidus and thyroid hypofunction.[225,240]

Diurnal rhythm

The diurnal variation in P excretion is well known in humans[686] and also has been observed in dogs, even during prolonged anesthesia.[456] The circadian rhythm of P excretion is depicted in Fig. 12-8. Generally, P excretion is lowest between 8 A.M. and 12 noon, increasing progressively during the afternoon and evening and reaching its peak at approximately midnight. This rhythm in P excretion is paralleled by a similar pattern of change in plasma [P] and [PTH]. However, the diurnal changes in P excretion cannot be attributed to changes in PTH secretion because a similar circadian rhythm has also been observed in patients with hypoparathyroidism.[293] Furthermore, in normal subjects cAMP excretion (an indicator of circulating PTH activity) does not display a similar diurnal pattern.[138] The rhythm also appears intact in vitamin D-resistant rickets[44] and in hyperparathyroidism.[281] In one patient with a parathyroid adenoma, however, variation in diurnal P excretion was not observed until the adenoma was removed.[705]

The circadian rhythm of P excretion cannot be attributed to changes in GFR.[621,686] It follows a pattern different from those for Na, K, Cl, and Ca.[491,660] The excretory rhythm is not changed by progesterone[344] or aldosterone[660] administration. Schaaf and Kyle[595] docu-

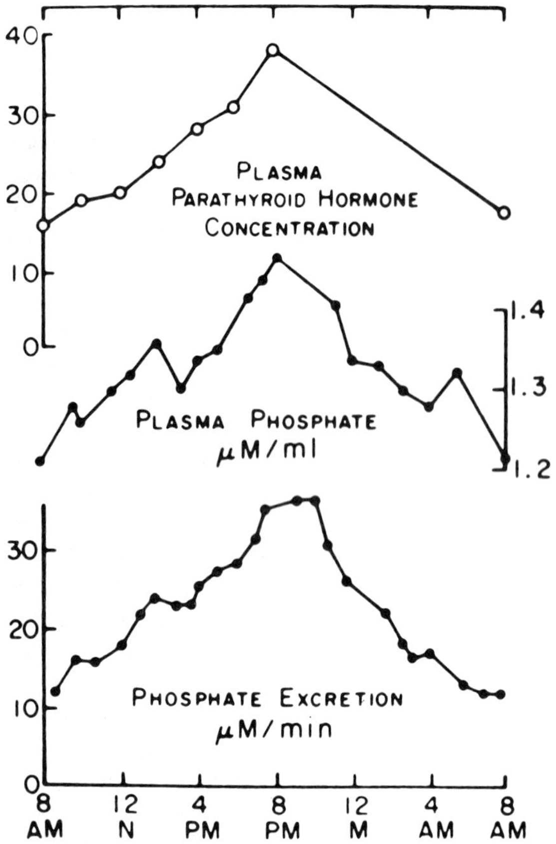

FIGURE 12-8 • Schematic summary of circadian rhythm of phosphate excretion. Data are from Stanbury[621] and Arnaud and coworkers[29] on normal human subjects under similar, but not identical, conditions. (From Mudge GH et al, in Orloff J et al, eds: *Handbook of Physiology,* Baltimore, Williams & Wilkins, 1973, sec 8, pp 587–652. Used by permission.)

mented that the diurnal rhythm of P excretion was not affected by feedings every 4 h but could be altered by either night feeding or 48-h fasting. Others, however, reported that diurnal P excretion was insensitive to food intake.[320] Goldsmith and associates,[281] in studies limited to the forenoon, found a progressive reduction in circulating hydrocortisone levels associated with a rising renal P clearance. With cortisone administration, P clearance decreased. They also demonstrated that the P excretory rhythm was absent or abnormal in patients with abnormal adrenocortical or pituitary dysfunction. The circadian rhythm of P excretion can also be blunted by metapyrone, a known inhibitor of adrenocortical function.[344] Alteration in sleep patterns also alters the P excretion pattern such that a minimal excretion rate tends to coincide with the period of awakening.[474]

Although the mechanism underlying the diurnal variation in the P excretion rate is still not precisely known, awareness of its existence is important in the design and interpretation of acute studies involving changes in the P excretory rate.

Miscellaneous factors influencing phosphorus excretion

Purkerson and coworkers[546] observed reduction in urinary P and Na excretion in unilateral postobstructed kidneys. In contrast, Beck[56] reported increased phosphaturia and natriuresis following release of bilateral ureteral obstruction in rats. The presence or absence of PTH and variations in ECF volume did not significantly influence the phosphaturia, but the prevention of hyperphosphatemia associated with bilateral ureteral obstruction abolished the anticipated postobstructive phosphaturia.

The variation in urinary P excretion (in milligrams per day) in various parts of the world in all likelihood can be accounted for by differences in P intake.[580] The apparent influence of sex and aging on the urinary P excretion rate has been discussed.

INTESTINAL PHOSPHATE TRANSPORT

GENERAL REMARKS

Dietary phosphorus exists in both inorganic and organic forms. Most of the P in milk is inorganic, and most of the P in vegetables, meat, and other nondairy sources is found inside the cells and is complexed as phosphoproteins, phosphosugars, and phospholipids. Organic P is usually hydrolyzed in the gut, liberating the inorganic P for absorption,[484,663] although certain phospholipids may be absorbed in organic forms.[193] After administration of [^{32}P]phosphate, plasma radioactivity peaked at about 60 min.[118,123] The maximum increase in stable plasma P after an oral load occurred after 90 min.[163] Based on deconvolutional analysis, after sequential administration of two doses of [^{32}P]phosphate (with 50 mg carrier P as Na_2HPO_4), the peak absorptive rate was rapidly attained at 30 min.[450]

Phosphate absorption in humans has been traditionally measured by balance techniques. The difference between dietary and fecal P is termed "net P absorption" and is expressed either as the absolute amount or as a percentage of the intake. In normal subjects net P absorption is a linear function of dietary P intake.[690] For a dietary P range of 4 to 30 mg/kg per day, the percentage of net P absorption is between 60 and 65 percent of intake. Thus, net P absorption differs from net Ca absorption in a number of aspects (Fig. 12-9). First, over the customary range of P intake, net P absorption is a linear function of P intake, whereas net Ca absorption is related to Ca intake in a curvilinear manner, rising steeply initially as Ca intake rises and thereafter less steeply when Ca intake exceeds 10 mg/kg per day. Second, net fractional absorption of P (60 to 65 percent) is about two times higher than that for Ca (20 to 30 percent). Finally, when dietary P supply is low, fecal P decreases proportionately, whereas fecal Ca exceeds dietary Ca at the lower range of Ca intake. Endogenous fecal P in four normal subjects was estimated to be approximately 100 mg/day.[374] In six subjects with osteoporosis, hypoparathyroidism, or Paget's disease, Wilkinson[690] found an average value for P of 0.86 mg/kg of body weight per day, which is a close approximation of the earlier estimate. Dominguez and associates[208] measured an average of 4.6 mg fecal P per kilogram of body weight per day in normal volunteers whose stools were collected from days 7 to 24 of dietary P restriction.

MECHANISM OF PHOSPHATE ABSORPTION

Extensive data summarized elsewhere[185,415] are consistent with a model requiring intestinal P absorption to occur via two "routes": a cellularly mediated active transport and a diffusional flux, largely through the paracellular shunt pathway.

Transcellular absorption

Transcellular transport of P across an intestinal cell would involve at least three steps: entry across the luminal membrane, ferry through the cytoplasm, and exit across the basolateral membrane.

Luminal P entry

Energetic considerations would predict an energy-dependent luminal entry for the anionic P, since the cell interior is highly electronegative.[513] Definitive cytosolic P activity remains to be determined, although available evidence suggests that it is higher than that of the ECF.[391,396] There is now convincing evidence indicating that the active entry of P across the luminal membrane is mediated by a vitamin D- and Na-dependent mechanism.[185,192,419] The K_m for this luminal P entry is estimated at 0.2 mM, thus exhibiting about a tenfold higher affinity than the K_m for active, *transepithelial* P absorption (2 mM), discussed below in the section on "Diffusional Absorption." Active vitamin D sterols enhance this Na-dependent P transport system through stimulation of maximal velocity (V_{max}), leaving K_m unchanged. Of interest, and less expected from energetic considerations, is the finding of a Na- and vitamin D-independent, nonsaturable component of P influx across the apical border of enterocytes. The regulation and the physiologic significance of this P transport process are not well characterized.

As one might anticipate, much interest has centered on the molecular characterization of the Na^+-P cotransporter. Debiec and Lorenc have identified a 155-kilodalton Na^+-P–binding protein in rabbit intestinal brush border membrane.[196] The protein has a high affinity for P binding (K_m = 10μM) and also binds Na^+ with a K_m of 7.5 mM. Substrates that inhibited vesicular Na^+-P transport also inhibited P binding by the protein. Peerce labeled the Na^+-P cotransporter in rabbit intestinal brush border membrane using arginine group-specific inhibitors and has also identified a polypeptide (molecular weight = 130) that most likely contained the Na^+ and P binding sites.[530] While Na^+-P cotransport is clearly the major mechanism for P entry into the enterocytes, Shirazy-Beechey and associates have observed that in the proximal intestine of the lamb the driving force for apical membrane P uptake is dependent on a hydrogen, rather than a sodium, gradient.[608]

Much better characterized is the highly specific P-binding protein (PBP) in bacterial cells. It consists of a single polypeptide chain with a relative molecular mass of 34,400, estimated from the sequence of 321 residues, and contains one tight P-binding site with a K_d of 1 μM at

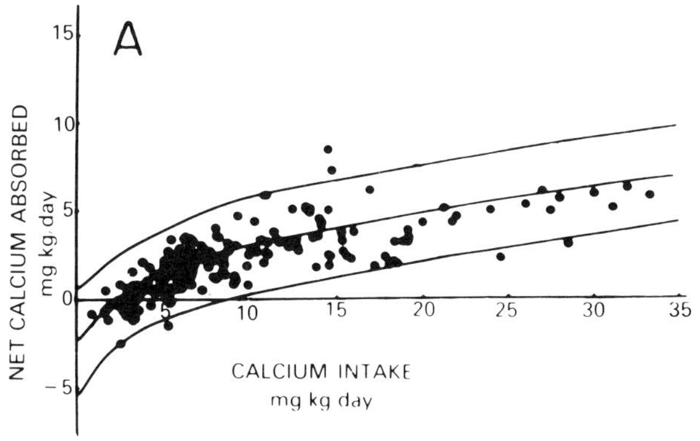

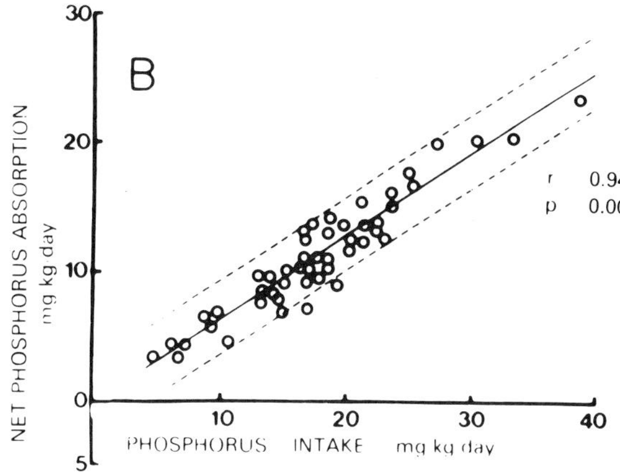

FIGURE 12-9 • The relationship between (*a*) net Ca absorbed and dietary Ca intake and (*b*) net P absorbed and dietary P intake in normal subjects. (From Wilkinson R, in Nordin BEC, ed: *Calcium, Phosphate and Magnesium Metabolism,* Edinburgh, Churchill Livingstone, 1976, pp 36–112. Used by permission.)

pH 8.3. Recently, Luecke and Quiocho have described the x-ray structure of the liganded form of this protein.[440] It consists of two separate, similarly folded globular domains. The bound P is situated in the deep cleft between the domains and is totally buried below the protein surface. The submerged P is anchored by 12 strong hydrogen bonds, all formed with protein groups. PBP binds both monobasic and dibasic P, although the latter may be slightly preferred. The researchers pointed out that the hydrogen bonds, involving primarily main-chain peptide and hydroxyl groups, not only confer specificity and affinity for charged ligands, but are also important for efficient active transport and rapid ion movement.

In addition to the protein transporter, the membrane lipid environment and its associated protein kinase systems[555] and the cytoskeleton[252] may also influence P uptake across the apical membrane. PTH, cAMP, and vitamin D metabolites have all been described to cause changes in membrane phospholipid turnover and composition and the incorporation of P into membrane phospholipids.[245,555,563]

Transcytoplasmic P ferrying

Relatively little is known about the movement of P from the apical pole to the basolateral pole. Sampson and Matthews, based on electron microscopic autoradiography, demonstrated the distribution of orally administered [^{32}P] phosphate in practically every subcellular organelle within the enteroctye of rat duodenum.[593] However, absorbed [^{32}P] phosphate mixed with only a small fraction of the total intracellular P pool, suggesting passage through restricted channels such as the microtubules. A similar conclusion has been proposed in the earlier study of Kowarski and Schachter.[391] The work of Brazy and colleagues suggested that essential metabolic P utilized by rabbit PT cells originated through apical, not basolateral, membrane.[98]

Basolateral P exit

Thermodynamic considerations discussed in relation to apical P entry would predict that P exit across the basolateral membrane could occur passively down its electrochemical gradients. This may be facilitated by carriers. Danisi and coworkers[191] have reported a carrier-mediated, Na^+-independent P transport mechanism in basolateral membrane vesicles from rat small intestine. Others, however, have found a Na^+-dependent P transport mechanism in basolateral membrane vesicles from rat[267] and human small intestine.[368] The role of these basolateral Na^+-dependent processes in overall transcellular P transport is not clear.

Diffusional absorption

Studies of P carrier kinetics in rat jejunum have revealed an estimated K_m (the concentration of ambient P at which active transport is one-half the maximal rate) of 2 m*M* for the absorptive mucosal-to-serosal flux.[675] The relatively low K_m is a likely explanation for the failure to demonstrate active P absorption in a number of earlier studies. For example, McHardy and Parsons[462] perfused rat jejunum in vivo and found that P absorption is mediated by a diffusional process; that is, the rate of P absorption was linearly correlated to the perfusate [P] with no tendency toward saturation. However, the [P] in the perfusion solution used ranged between 12.5 and 100 m*M*, which was clearly above the saturation concentration for the active mechanism, and therefore the finding of only a diffusional process for P movement is not unexpected. In vivo measurements of jejunal P absorption in humans also yielded data consistent with the presence of an active, saturable process with an estimated K_m of about 2 m*M*.[677,690] Thus, measurements made at luminal [P] greater than 2 to 3 m*M* would be expected to produce data consistent with absorption by a diffusional process with no tendency toward saturation. When measurements were made under fasting conditions, intraluminal [P] at all levels of the small intestine in humans is about 2 m*M*.[352] With feeding, one would clearly expect higher luminal [P]. Indeed, the [P] in human fecal fluid as determined by in vivo dialysis was 5 m*M*.[695] Thus, the observation that net P absorption in humans is a linear function of dietary P intake (Fig. 12-9*b*) becomes entirely explicable. Equally explicable would be the observation that the fraction of P absorbed from the diet is about 0.6, and no adaptive changes have been demonstrated over a wide range of P intake (4 to 30 mg/kg of body weight per day). Thus, although there is convincing evidence for the existence of an active P absorptive process that is sensitive to $1\alpha,25\text{-}(OH)_2D_3$, under normal circumstances intestinal P absorption is probably accomplished almost entirely through a diffusional process. The active component probably becomes important only under unusual conditions, such as when dietary P is extremely low,[416,675] a condition that is also associated with increased synthesis and intestinal localization of $1\alpha,25\text{-}(OH)_2D_3$.[648]

PHOSPHATE ABSORPTION IN UREMIA

In advanced renal failure, the reduction in $1\alpha,25\text{-}(OH)_2D_3$ synthesis would be expected to affect the active component of P absorption and thus could cause reduction in net P absorption. Lower intestinal P absorption in uremic patients has indeed been demonstrated using balance studies[390,622] and radiophosphate markers.[120] However, since under normal dietary conditions (i.e., with adequate P intake), the bulk of intestinal P absorption is accomplished through diffusion, the loss of the active P absorptive component may cause relatively little disruption in overall P absorption by the intestine. The lack of a perceptible effect of uremia on P absorption may indeed be deduced from a number of studies. The external balance data of Brickman and associates[100] may serve as a representative example. Recalculation of the data [excluding the three patients who received $Al(OH)_3$ gel throughout the study] indicates that the uremic patients absorbed 15.8 of the 26.2 mmol of P eaten in the diet, representing a fractional absorption of 0.60. This compares favorably with the normal controls, who retained 32.5 of the 51.2 mmol of P consumed, a fractional P absorption of 0.63. Following $1\alpha,25\text{-}(OH)_2D_3$ or $1\alpha\text{-}(OH)D_3$ therapy, the fractional absorption rose to 0.72 and 0.70 for uremic patients and controls, respectively. Farrington and associates[232] measured the fraction of an orally administered ^{32}P dose in plasma (αPO_4) at various time intervals for 3 h. They noted that at 60 min, chronic renal failure (CRF) patients had a marginally lower αPO_4 than did the normals. However, at 3 h the αPO_4 was not different for normal controls, CRF patients, or patients on hemodialysis. These data lend further credence to the thesis that neither uremia nor its anticipated $1\alpha,25\text{-}(OH)_2D_3$ deficiency affects intestinal P absorption in any important fashion. A reduction in net P absorption in uremic patients, if demonstrated, was usually accounted for by other factors, such as decreased availability of dietary P for absorption (e.g., reduced intake and/or the use of P binders) or as part of a generalized malabsorptive process associated with uremia. The universal practice of giving P binders (to cause "iatrogenic P malabsorption") to uremic patients attests to the fact that, relative to the body's need, the intestine is not underabsorbing P.

In summary, the bulk of intestinal P absorption appears to be mediated by a diffusional process, presumably through the paracellular space, and therefore is primarily a function of P intake. Because most diets contain an abundance of P, the quantity of P absorbed always exceeds the need both under normal circumstances and in uremia. Active, transcellular P absorption becomes predominant under conditions of low luminal P availability, such as dietary P deprivation and/or excessive luminal P binding.

FACTORS AFFECTING INTESTINAL PHOSPHATE ABSORPTION

Dietary and luminal P availability

Figure 12-7*b* clearly indicates that net P absorption increases in proportion to dietary P intake. As discussed earlier, this intake-dependent P absorption is most likely mediated through a diffusional process across the intercellular pathway. Based on available data on the electrochemical gradients across the intestinal epithelium, it can be predicted that net diffusional absorption of P would occur whenever luminal [P] exceeds 1.8 m*M*, a concentration that is attained even under fasting conditions (see above). Thus, under normal dietary conditions, P intake is probably the most important factor in the determination of net P absorption. This diffusional process would clearly cease when luminal P becomes extremely low under conditions such as dietary P deprivation or excessive administration of P binders. Under such conditions the active, transcellular P transport would be expected to become the predominant mode for P absorption. It is interesting that the K_m (the luminal [P] at which active transport is one-half the maximal rate) for this process is around 2m*M* (see above), a level close to the predicted concentration (1.8 m*M*) at which the chemical gradient-driven diffusional absorption would cease. Portale and associates have demonstrated in healthy humans that low P and high P intake induced rapid, large, inverse, and sustained changes in circulating concentrations of $1\alpha,25\text{-}(OH)_2D_3$, a major regulator of active P absorption (see below). This change in circulating $1\alpha,25(OH)_2D_3$ was the result of changes in production rate and was not associated with changes in the metabolic clearance rate of $1\alpha,25\text{-}(OH)_2D_3$.[544]

Vitamin D

Extensive clinical and experimental studies have generated compelling evidence for the existence of an active P transport mechanism in intestine and the regulation of this mechanism by the active metabolite of vitamin D: $1\alpha,25\text{-}(OH)_2D_3$.[185,415,555] As discussed earlier, this regulatory step is mediated through P entry across the apical membrane via the Na^+-P cotransport mechanism. It is of interest to note that the Harrisons have observed that vitamin D not only stimulated active Ca absorption but also augmented diffusional Ca absorption in all segments of the small intestine.[311] Thus, the possibility exists that vitamin D can also increase P absorption through the diffusional pathway. It should also be pointed out that vitamin D is important in maximizing the intestinal absorptive surface and in maintaining its integrity,[282] and thereby influences P absorption.

Physiologic need for P

It is well known that under conditions of increased P demand, such as active growth and pregnancy, $1\alpha,25\text{-}(OH)_2D_3$ synthesis is increased and P absorption stimulated. However, experimental studies suggest that physiologic mechanisms other than those dependent on vitamin D may also participate in the regulation of intestinal P absorption under the stress of heightened physiologic needs for P.[105,179,417] For example, in face of severe vitamin D depletion, continued active P absorption can still be demonstrated in jejunum from young rats. On the other hand, in mature rats, despite normal vitamin D nutritional status, active P secretion (rather than active P absorption) is demonstrated in the same intestinal segment. These observations suggest that factors such as the demand for P to satisfy the stress of growth (as in younger, vitamin D-deficient rats) or the lack of such demand for P when growth plateaus (as in older rats in normal vitamin D balance) may modulate net jejunal P absorption and that such factors operate independently from the prevailing status of vitamin D nutrition.[417]

Parathyroid hormone

Although PTH is a major regulator of renal P reabsorption, there is no convincing evidence that PTH has a direct influence on intestinal P absorption. PTH administration to normal subjects did not alter radiophosphorus absorption.[121] In rat balance studies, PTH also failed to cause any changes in P absorption,[151] a finding consistent with the observation that parathyroidectomy did not influence absorption of labeled P from the perfused loops of rat duodenum and ileum in vivo.[678] Direct application of PTH to intestinal preparations of adult and growing rats also failed to elicit either an intestinal adenylate cyclase or a mucosal cAMP response.[673] In studies on rat jejunum using the Ussing technique, direct application of dibutyryl-cAMP to the serosal compartment markedly increased (212 percent) short-circuit current (primarily the result of active chloride secretion) without causing any discernible changes in active P absorption.[418,673] These data suggest that neither PTH nor its second messenger has a direct influence on intestinal P absorption. Several other studies, however, have produced a contrary conclusion,[21,84,436] and therefore the question should still be considered open.

The demonstration of a direct PTH effect on intestinal P absorption must be carefully distinguished from an indirect effect of the hormone on 1α,25-$(OH)_2D$ synthesis. The clear influence of the latter hormone on P absorption has already been discussed. It has been shown that 1α,25-$(OH)_2D_3$ stimulates intestinal cAMP levels and adenylate cyclase in rats.[673,674]

Alkaline phosphatase

Wasserman and Taylor[679] have attempted to isolate a P carrier molecule (a counterpart to Ca-binding protein) in the supernatant fraction obtained from intestinal mucosal homogenates. After equilibration dialysis, they detected only minimal binding of labeled P by this soluble fraction and observed no difference between rachitic and vitamin D-repleted chicks. Their study, however, did not rule out the possibility that binders or carrier molecules might be present in particulate fractions that were not examined; for example, brush borders or basolateral membrane fractions may well have vitamin D-inducible changes in P-binding capacity. One of the possible candidates involved in active P absorption is alkaline phosphatase. Since phosphorylated compounds are not readily absorbed,[587,693] it has been suggested that intestinal alkaline phosphatase may serve a hydrolytic function to free inorganic P for absorption. This enzyme is clearly increased by vitamin D repletion of vitamin D-deficient animals. The orthophosphoric monoester phosphohydrolase has its highest activity in duodenum[402] and has been localized to both the brush border membrane[67] and the basolateral membrane[477] of the intestine. A correlation between [^{32}P]-phosphate uptake and the activity of alkaline phosphatase has been demonstrated in mouse intestine.[484] The finding that 1-phenylalanine and disodium ethane-1-hydroxy-1,1-diphosphonate (EHDP) both reduced P absorption in the chick intestinal loop preparation[679] has been used as further evidence of the participation of alkaline phosphatase in intestinal P absorption. However, these two agents might also affect P transport through other mechanisms, such as via altered metabolism of vitamin D. Studies of binding affinity of alkaline phosphatase for P in *Escherichia coli* yielded values sufficiently high to suggest a possible carrier-mediated mechanism.[27]

An apparent paradox is the finding that alkaline phosphatase, with a high optimal pH, is predominantly located in the duodenum, where the pH is usually low. If this enzyme were important in P absorption, one also would expect it to concentrate in the jejunum, where P absorption is greatest.[308,391] Such difficulty clearly reflects the complexity of this enzyme, which not only exists in several isoenzymes in the small intestine but also has an affinity for a large number of substrates, ranging from paranitrophenol phosphate to ATP. It can also function as a phosphotransferase.[693]

Recent progress toward the identification of the Na^+-P cotransporter (see above) clearly excludes alkaline phosphatase as the possible carrier. Loghman-Adham and colleagues have also demonstrated that phosphonocarboxylic acids that specifically inhibited Na^+-P cotransporter in rat small intestinal brush border membrane vesicle preparations did not affect the activity of alkaline phosphatase.[434]

Sodium

The role of sodium in P absorption has been known for a long time. In vitro studies of McHardy and Parsons[462] in the rat demonstrated that P absorption increased in parallel with an increase in [Na] in the perfusate. Harrison and Harrison[310] also documented a direct correlation between concentrative P transport by everted sacs of rat intestine and [Na] in the incubation media. Taylor[651] examined the relationship of Na to P transport by everted sacs of chick ileum and found that replacement of Na with choline (in both mucosal and serosal media) decreased the accumulation of [^{32}P] in the mucosa and reduced the transfer of this marker into the serosal compartment of the sac. Inhibition of Na^+-K^+ ATPase with 1 m*M* ouabain did not affect the mucosal accumulation but decreased the transfer of the tracer into the serosal compartment. It was concluded that Na^+-K^+ ATPase activity was important for P transport out of the cell.

The stimulatory effect of Na^+ on P absorption is most likely a reflection of the activities of the 1α,25-$(OH)_2$D-sensitive apical Na^+-P cotransporter discussed earlier. Figure 12-10*A* demonstrates the effect of ambient [Na^+] on mucosal P influx in intact jejunal epithelium from 1α,25-$(OH)_2$D-replete rats. The anticipated increases in P influx with increasing incubation [Na^+] was observed up to a [Na^+] of about 100 m*M*.[419,673] Thereafter, further increase in [Na^+] caused a decrease rather than an increase in P influx. It should be pointed out that, although in *renal* brush border membrane vesicle studies a direct correlation between P uptake and inwardly directed Na^+ gradient was observed up to a [Na^+] of 300 m*M*,[20] in rat *intestinal* brush border membrane vesicle preparations the Na^+-dependent P uptake (measured at pH 7.4) reached a plateau at [Na^+] of 60 to 80 m*M*, with no further increase in P uptake as [Na^+] increased to 140 m*M*.[67] The data of Danisi and coworkers[190] on rabbit duodenal brush border membrane vesicle studies also revealed that the Na^+-dependent P influx (measured at both pH 6.8 and 7.6) reached a maximum at an extravesicular [Na^+] of 50 to 75 m*M* and that further increases in [Na^+] to 300 m*M* caused no further increase in P influx. While the observation that the Na^+-P cotransport appears to "saturate" at [Na^+] of 100 m*M* (Fig. 12-10*b*) is consistent with these brush border membrane vesicle studies, the finding that, at higher [Na^+], P influx in fact decreased does not parallel the findings in these resealed vesicles. This drop in P influx is not likely the result of changes in tissue viability or changes in general tissue transport functions, since the short circuit current (SCC) increased predictably throughout the range of [Na^+] studied (Fig. 12-10*b*). It is possible that the exhibition of the biphasic response in P influx across the mucosal membrane is a characteristic of intact enterocytes locked into an intact epithelium by tight junction complexes and that the second phase of the response can no longer occur when the brush border is separated and resealed in isolation. It is interesting to note that virtually all reported P uptake studies in renal or intestinal brush border membrane vesicle preparations have used an extravesicular [Na^+] of 100 m*M*. It is possible that this is because at this [Na^+], P influx can be most predictably measured.

In contrast to P influx, transepithelial P transport, both in the absorptive, mucosal-to-serosal (J_{ms}) direction and in the secretory, serosal-to-mucosal (J_{sm}) direction, increased in parallel with increases in buffer [Na] up to

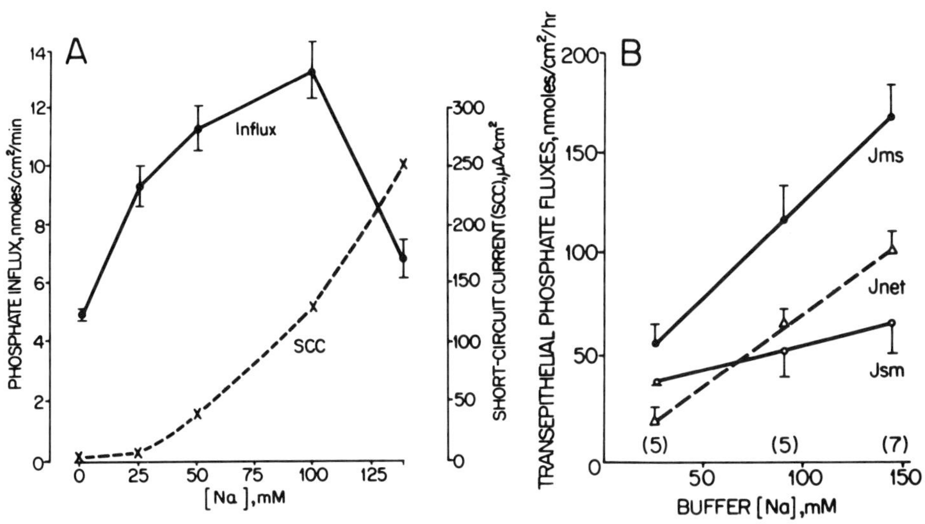

FIGURE 12-10 • Effect of varying extracellular [Na] on 1,25$(OH)_2D_3$-stimulated P transport in rat jejunal epithelium, measured in vitro under short-circuited conditions. Buffer pH = 7.4 and [P] = 2.4 mM. (*a*) Mucosal P influx and transepithelial short-circuit current (I_{SC}; n = 8 for each pH studied). (*b*) Transepithelial P fluxes: mucosal to serosal (J_{ms}), serosal to mucosal (J_{sm}), and net (J_{net}, i.e., J_{ms} − J_{sm}) fluxes. Figures in parentheses indicate the number of studies at each [Na]. (From Lee DBN et al: *Am J Physiol* 251:G90, 1986. Used by permission.)

TABLE 12-3 • Additional factors that may modify intestinal phosphate absorption

Agents	Animals	Findings and/or conclusions	References
HORMONES			
Thyroid	Humans	P malabsorption in hypothyroid subjects (balance technique)	578
	Humans	Decreased radioactive P absorption in hypothyroid subjects; reversed by TSH	118
	Humans	Normal P absorption in hypothyroid subjects, and T_3 treatment did not produce any change (balance technique)	468
	Humans	Thyroxine treatment increased radioactive P influx into intestine	536
	Humans	P malabsorption in hyperthyroidism by balance technique	168
	Humans	Normal P absorption in hyperthyroid cases	349
	Humans	Normal radioactive P absorption in hyperthyroidism	118
	Humans	Increased net P absorption in thyrotoxic patients	9,597
	Rats	P transfer decreased in duodenum, but no effect on distal segments with thyroxine pretreatment	
	Rats	T_4 increased P absorption	80
	Chicks	Thyroxine and T_3 increased Na^+-dependent P accumulation by cultured embryonic jejunum	184
	Chicks	T_3 increased Na^+-P cotransport by brush border membrane vesicle from cultured embryonic jejunum	185
	Chicks	T_3 further enhances the stimulatory action of $1\alpha,25\text{-}(OH)_2D_3$ on Na^+-P uptake by cultured embryonic jejunum	185
Calcitonin (CT)	Humans	20 MRC units/day for 3 days increased radioactive P absorption in normal subjects	122
	Humans	Salmon CT decreased P absorption	350
	Dogs	P transport in perfused jejunal loops was not affected by CT administration	180
	Rats	CT inhibited intestinal P absorption	650
Corticosteroids (C)	Humans	Dexamethasone increased fecal P	113
	Humans	Chronic C therapy decreased radioactive P absorption	118
	Rats	Hydrocortisone pretreatment did not affect in vivo P absorption	153
	Rats	Hydrocortisone inhibits intestinal phosphate absorption	235
	Rats	C stimulated vitamin D-independent active P uptake; effect of two hormones additive	704
	Rats	C may stimulate passive P absorption through effect on passive fluid movement	703
	Chicks	C stimulated vitamin D-independent active P uptake by embryonic duodenum; effect of two hormones synergistic	172
Insulin (I)	Rats	Brush border membrane vesicle from streptozotocin diabetic rats exhibited greater Na^+-dependent P accumulation than those from controls	266
	Chicks	Sustained exposure of cultured small intestine to I depressed vitamin D-independent Na^+-P uptake	183
	Chicks	I enchanced vitamin D-dependent P uptake in cultured embryonic jejunum	530

150 m*M* (Fig. 12-10*b*). Because the rise in J_{ms} was proportionately greater than that in J_{sm}, the net P absorption ($J_{net} = J_{ms} - J_{sm}$) also increased with increasing buffer [Na^+].

The dissociation between mucosal P influx and transepithelial P absorption at buffer [Na^+] above 100 m*M* suggests that a mechanism other than the Na^+-dependent P influx (Na^+-P cotransporter) may participate in P absorption. Convective and diffusive absorption through the paracellular pathway may constitute additional modes for P absorption that is responsive to Na^+. In terms of convective absorption, Pappenheimer and colleagues have recently proposed the general principle that the bulk of luminal nutrients are absorbed through the paracellular route.[522,523] They proposed that the primary function of active transcellular solute transport is to set up conditions that will facilitate solute traffic through the intercellular space in the absorptive direction. Thus, active solute transport from the lumen leads to high solute concentration in the lateral spaces on the antiluminal side of the occluding junction, providing the osmotic force for absorption of fluid. The activation of the Na^+-coupled solute transport mechanism also triggers contraction of circumferential actomyosin fibers in the terminal web of

TABLE 12-3 • (*Continued*)

Agents	Animals	Findings and/or conclusions	References
DIETARY FACTORS			
Carbohydrates	Rats	Presence of luminal glucose did not affect P absorption (in vivo gut loop)	462
	Rats	Glucose required on concentrative P transport (in vivo gut sacs)	308
Lysine	Chicks	Inhibited radioactive P absorption from ligated intestinal loops	147
L-Phenylalanine	Chicks	Decreased radioactive P absorption in in vivo loops	679
	Chicks	No effect on radioactive P transport in in vivo loops	651
	Mice	Decreased P uptake by intestine in vitro	484
CATIONS			
Magnesium (Mg)	Humans	Increased Mg intake led to decreased P absorption	103
	Rats	Increased P absorption in in vitro gut loops from Mg-deficient rats or in normal rats but with Mg removed from ambient medium	437
	Rats	Increased dietary Mg led to decreased P absorption in vivo	151
Potassium (K)	Rats	Increased K in bathing medium led to increased concentrative transport of P (everted sacs)	308
	Sheep	Increased K intake led to decreased fecal P in balance studies	640
Ammonium	Chicks	Ammonium chloride inhibited radioactive P absorption in ligated duodenal loops	147
DRUGS			
Antacids	Humans	Nonabsorbable aluminum and magnesium compounds increased fecal P	156,439
Diphosphonates	Chicks	Decreased radioactive P transport across in vivo ileal loops	679
Cyclophosphamide	Humans	Decreased radioactive P absorption in patients with leukemias and cancers	118
Anaerobiosis and cyanide	Rats	Decreased concentrative transport of P in everted gut loops	308
Iodoacetate, arsenite, 2,4-dinitrophenol	Rats	Decreased P influx and tissue uptake in everted duodenal loops	84
Ouabain	Chicks	Decreased in vitro ileal P transport	651
Arsenate	Chicks	Decreased [^{32}P] phosphate transfer	679
Cyanide	Humans	Decreased P uptake by small intestinal mucosa in vitro	609
TONICITY			
Mannitol, urea	Rats	Mannitol- or urea-induced changes in perfusing fluid tonicity did not affect P absorption	462
Urea	Chicks	Urea-induced changes in tonicity had no effect on P absorption	147

the microvillar cytoskeletal complex, thereby increasing occluding junction permeability and further facilitating the osmotically driven bulk absorption of luminal nutrients.

In addition to absorption by solvent drag, a Na^+-dependent diffusive driving force may also participate in P absorption through the paracellular route. Thus, in the same study that is depicted in Fig. 12-8*b*, the transepithelial potential difference (PD) was found to increase from −0.3 mV to +4.8 mV (serosal positive) as the extracellular [Na^+] increased from 25 to 144 m*M*. Since the phosphate ion is negatively charged, this Na^+-dependent change in PD would constitute an increasing driving force for diffusive P flux in the absorptive direction.

Hydrogen ion concentration

At physiologic pH, P exists in two anionic forms: HPO_4^{2-} and $H_2PO_4^-$. In experimental studies, P absorption was found to rise with increases in perfusion fluid pH, suggesting that the transport of the divalent molecule was favored.[178,462] The effect of pH on transcellular P absorption has been examined by studying the effect of varying external pH on P influx across the apical membrane in intact rat jejunal epithelium,[419] and brush border membrane vesicles of rat small intestine[67] and rabbit duodenum.[190] In all these studies an increase in P influx was observed with reduction in medium pH. This is in marked contrast to P uptake across the apical membrane of renal tubular cells which exhibited an increase with increases in external pH (refer to earlier discussion on renal P transport). On the other hand, in brush border membrane vesicles from chicken duodenum[554] and in colon-derived CaCo^2 cell lines,[480] no preference for either P molecules was observed.

The observation on the preferred acidic environment for P transport in rat jejunum appears consistent with the measurement of pH in the intestinal microenvironment.

An unequilibrated region (about 700 μm thick) has been demonstrated in the immediate vicinity of the mucosal surface of the rat jejunum with pH one to two orders of magnitude lower than the bulk solution pH.[607] Thus, the effective pH (approximately 5.4) at the transporting surface would dictate that all P in the immediate ambience would be in the monobasic form. Danisi et al proposed that the pH-dependence of P-uptake is not the result of a differential preference for monovalent or divalent phosphate ions, but rather is secondary to the effect of pH on the transporter, in part related to changes in affinity of the transporter for Na.[190] Theoretically, in addition to its effect on the dissociation of the P molecule and the conformation of the cell membrane or carrier-molecules in the membrane, changes in transmembrane pH gradients can change Na^+ fluxes through the Na^+/H^+ exchanger. This change in Na^+ flux may, in turn, affect P influx through the cotransport mechanism already discussed. H^+ ions may also influence membrane and/or epithelial permeability[419] and thereby changes in P transport.

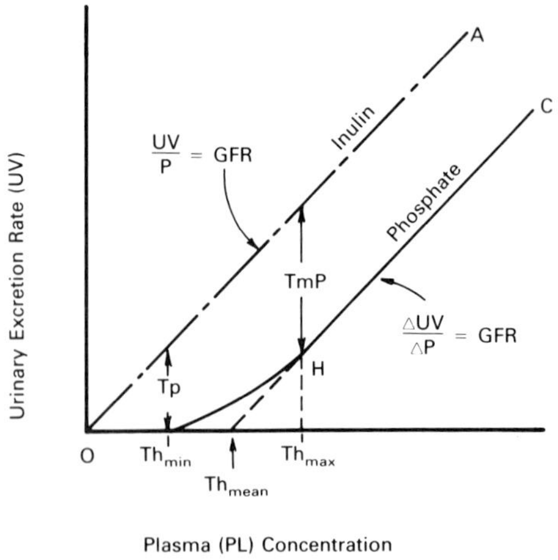

FIGURE 12-11 • Schematic relationship between urinary excretion rate (UV) and plasma concentrations (PL). Th_{min} minimal threshold; Th_{mean}, theoretical mean threshold, and Th_{max} maximal threshold. For details see the text. (Modified from Mudge GH et al, in Orloff J et al, eds: *Handbook of Physiology,* Baltimore, Williams & Wilkins, sec 8, 1973, pp 587–652. Used by permission.)

Other factors

Other factors that may affect intestinal P absorption are listed in Table 12-3.

PLASMA PHOSPHATE HOMEOSTASIS

*Tm*P/GFR AND ITS RELATIONSHIP TO PLASMA PHOSPHORUS CONCENTRATION

Under normal circumstances, the intestine is the only organ through which exogenous P is added to the ECF, while the kidney is the only organ from which excess P is removed from the ECF and excreted. Although intermediary mechanisms, including P exchange between the ECF and the skeleton or the soft tissues, play important roles in the overall metabolism of P, the fundamental process of P homeostasis integrates intestinal P absorption and renal P excretion. While the gut intermittently floods the ECF with P through absorption, it is the kidney that continuously regulates the plasma [P] and overall P homeostasis by excreting precisely the amount that is absorbed in excess of the body's need.

The amount of urinary P (U_PV, or urine [P] × urine volume), which in a steady state reflects the amount of P absorbed by the intestine, represents the difference between the filtered P load (PL_P × GFR, or plasma [P] × GFR) and the rate of tubular P reabsorption (T_P) (Fig. 12-11). The dynamics of renal P handling is best described by comparing it to the renal handling of inulin. As plasma inulin (PL_{in}) is progressively increased by inulin infusion, $U_{in}V$ rises proportionately. Since inulin is filtered entirely at the glomerulus and is not reabsorbed or secreted by the tubules, the rate at which it is excreted ($U_{in}V$) is the same as the rate at which it is filtered at the glomerulus. Thus,

$$PL_{in} \times GFR = U_{in}V$$
$$GFR = U_{in}V/PL_{in}$$

That is, the slope of the inulin line OA (Fig. 12-11) is equal to the GFR. If all the filtered P were also excreted without reabsorption, the same (inulin) line would describe the relation between U_pV and PL_p. However, in measurements when PL_p is progressively increased by P infusion, the urinary excretion of P (represented by the curve O-Th_{min}-H-C in (Fig. 12-11) is always less than the rate filtered (represented by the line OA) by an amount indicated by the vertical line depicted as T_p or *Tm*P. The magnitude of this line reflects the difference between the filtration rate and the excretion rate for P and is thus equal to the T_p. As plasma P is raised from O to Th_{min}, the T_p increases in step with the filtration rate so that no P is excreted. As PL_p is progressively increased above Th_{min}, T_p continues to increase, although now no longer at the same rate, so that P begins to appear in urine in increasing quantities. Finally, as PL_p reaches Th_{max} or above, T_p reaches a maximum rate and ceases to increase with further increases in PL_p. This maximum rate is generally known as the maximum tubular reabsorptive rate for P or *Tm*P. When the plasma P is raised above Th_{max}, the increased filtered load is not reabsorbed and will therefore be excreted as would a glomerular filtration marker such as inulin. Therefore, the slope of this portion of the P titration curve (HC) is identical to that for inulin (OA). GFR derived from the relationship of PL_p and U_pV at sufficiently high P-filtered loads is indeed identical with inulin clearance over a wide range of GFRs.[30] Downward extrapolation of CH intersects the abscissa at Th_{mean}, which is called the mean P threshold. This is the plasma [P] below which virtually all the filtered P is reabsorbed and above which virtually all the filtered P is excreted. Figure 12-11 also depicts two other thresholds: the minimal threshold (Th_{min}), representing the lowest plasma [P] above which P first appears in the urine, and the maximal threshold (Th_{max}), representing the plasma [P] at which the tubular reabsorptive capacity for P is saturated. In common practice, and for convenience, the P threshold refers to the mean threshold (Th_{mean}), which is in fact derived rather than directly measured and is also known as the theoretical renal P threshold.[491] The curvilinear portion of the relationship (Th_{min}-H) represents the "phosphate splay" in standard titration studies. If this splay is temporarily dropped from consideration, the P titration curve can be reduced into O-Th_{mean}-H-C, giving a single threshold, Th_{mean}. At this plasma [P], the P reabsorption rate would just attain its maximum (*T*mP). By definition,

$$T_p = (PL_p \times GFR) - U_pV$$

at the point when PL_p just attains Th_{mean}, U_pV would still momentarily be at zero, and T_p would have just reached *T*mP, and thus

$$TmP = Th_{mean} \times GFR$$

or

$$Th_{mean} = TmP/GFR$$

Thus, the P threshold representing a plasma [P] (mass/volume) is equal to the maximum tubular reabsorptive rate per unit volume of GFR, *T*mP/GFR, which also is described in terms of mass/volume (mass/time ÷ volume/time = mass/volume). The reason for the equality of plasma P threshold and *T*mP/GFR is not difficult to comprehend. Under normal conditions the kidney rejects about 10 to 20 percent of the filtered P, suggesting that the *T*mP is either approached or exceeded. Thus, the amount of P reabsorbed per minute would be expected to approximate *T*mP, and this amount of P will be diluted in the volume of fluid reabsorbed over the same period of time. Since under normal circumstances only 1 percent of the filtered fluid reaches the urine, the rate of fluid reabsorbed would approach GFR. Thus, the P in the reabsorbate (*T*mP) will be diluted in a fluid volume equal to GFR, or the [P] of the reabsorbate would be *T*mP/GFR. If *T*mP is 3.2 mg/min and GFR is 100 ml/min, then the reabsorbate will have a [P] of 3.2 mg/100 ml. Since the reabsorbate is continuously returned to the blood, plasma [P] will move toward the value represented by *T*mP/GFR.

The argument for the existence of a P threshold in humans was advanced over half a century ago.[3,90] Albright and associates[10] and Ellsworth[223] proposed that alterations in the P threshold were the basis for the hyper- and hypophosphatemia observed in hypo- and hyperparathyroid states, respectively. It was not until much later that the existence of *T*mP was demonstrated in dogs by Harrison and Harrison[309] and in humans by Schiess and associates.[596] Initially, *T*mP was proposed as a bio-

TABLE 12-4 • Variables that influence the tubular reabsorption of phosphate in normal subjects

Variable	Symbol	Calculation	Dimensions	Average	Range
Plasma phosphate	[P]		Mass/vol (mg/100 ml)	3.2	2.3–4.4
Glomerular filtration rate	GFR		Vol/time (ml/min)	100	80–120
Filtered load	L	[P] × GFR	Mass/time (mg/min)	3.2	
Urinary excretion rate	UV		Mass/time (mg/min)	0.36	0.14–0.57
Tubular reabsorption rate	*T*	L − UV	Mass/time (mg/min)	2.84	
Maximum tubular reabsorption rate	*T*m	See Fig. 12-11	Mass/time (mg/min)	3.2	
Limit, or threshold phosphate concentration	*T*mP/GFR	See Fig. 12-11 and related text	Mass/vol (mg/100 ml)	3.2	2.5–4.2
Phosphate clearance	C_{PO_4}	UV/P	Vol/time (ml/min)	12	
Phosphate/creatinine clearance	C_{PO_4}/C_{creat}	UV/L	No dimensions	0.12	
Fractional reabsorption of filtered load	%TRP	T/L = 1 − UV/L	No dimensions	0.88	
Phosphate excretion index	PEI	*			±0.09
Index of phosphate excretion	IPE	†	Mass/vol (mg/100 ml)		±0.50

NOTE: Also included are the various indexes for measurement of tubular phosphate reabsorption activity.

* $PEI = C_{PO_4}/C_{creat} - 0.055[P] + 0.07$; [P] in mg/100 ml.[511]

† $IPE = UV/GFR - \frac{[P] - 2.5}{2}$; [P] in mg/100 ml.[509]

SOURCE: From Bijvoet OLM, in Avioli L et al, eds: *Phosphate Metabolism: Kidney and Bone*, Paris, Armour Montagu, 1976, pp 421–474. Used by permission.

logic constant, independent of GFR.[37] The substantiation of this concept became problematic when considerable variations in *Tm*P were observed among various individuals and under various experimental conditions.[657] Subsequent studies clearly demonstrated a direct correlation between *Tm*P and GFR, and when measurements were expressed as *Tm*P/GFR, much of the variation could be eliminated.[23,75]

INDEXES FOR ACCESSING RENAL PHOSPHATE REABSORPTIVE ACTIVITY

The maximum tubular reabsorption of P per unit volume of GFR, *Tm*P/GFR, most likely reflects the quantity of transporting carrier available per unit of kidney mass. Physiologically, *Tm*P/GFR is probably the most meaningful measurement of renal TPR, providing more precise information than most of the other available indexes listed in Table 12-4. Figure 12-12 depicts the relationship between urinary P excretion (P_E, expressed in milligrams per 100 ml of glomerular filtrate) and plasma [P] in two groups of subjects: normal volunteers and patients with primary hyperparathyroidism. In both groups, urinary P_E reflects appropriately the changes in dietary P load: lower P_E with lower dietary P and higher P_E with higher dietary P. The excretory response to changes in P load appears to parallel the relationship described by the two curves representing *Tm*P/GFR of 2.5 and 4.2 mg/100 ml, respectively. These two curves would delineate 95 percent of the titration curves found in normal volunteers.[75] While the adaptive response in normal volunteers (light and dark dots) moves up and down the normal range of *Tm*P/GFR curves, patients with primary hyperparathyroidism (light and dark triangles) appear to move along similar curves but displaced to the left of the normals; that is, hyperparathyroid patients excrete similar amounts of P at lower plasma [P] when compared to normal volunteers. Stating it differently, hyperparathyroid patients have lower *Tm*P/GFR. Hypoparathyroid patients (not shown in Fig. 12-12) were also able to regulate urinary P_E in response to changes in dietary P load; however, the adjustment moved along *Tm*P/GFR curves displaced to the right of the normal range; that is, hypoparathyroid patients have higher *Tm*P/GFR.[74,524] In Fig. 12-13, the same normal limits of *Tm*P/GFR are represented by the two thick lines (with splays eliminated). In addition, a family of lines are plotted radiating from the origin, each representing a given fractional P reabsorption (% TRP). Thus, the 90 percent line, for example, would represent a urinary excretion rate of 10 percent of the filtered load. If one were to superimpose on this figure data points similar to those in Fig. 12-12, it would be immediately apparent that the measured values in normal subjects and hyperparathyroid patients conform more closely to the *Tm*P/GFR model than the percent TRP model. The geometric relationship between *Tm*P/GFR and percent TRP shown in Figs. 12-12 and 12-13 clearly illustrates that an increase or decrease in dietary P load (therefore a parallel increase or decrease in P_E) would inevitably lead to a reduction or augmentation in percent TRP, even in the absence of any change in tubular reabsorptive capacity (i.e., with *Tm*P/GFR remaining unchanged). The problem with using common indexes of P reabsorption such as percent TRP or FEP becomes clear when one considers that by simple manipulation of dietary P one may obtain TRP values characteristic of hyperparathyroidism in patients who actually have hypoparathyroidism and vice versa.

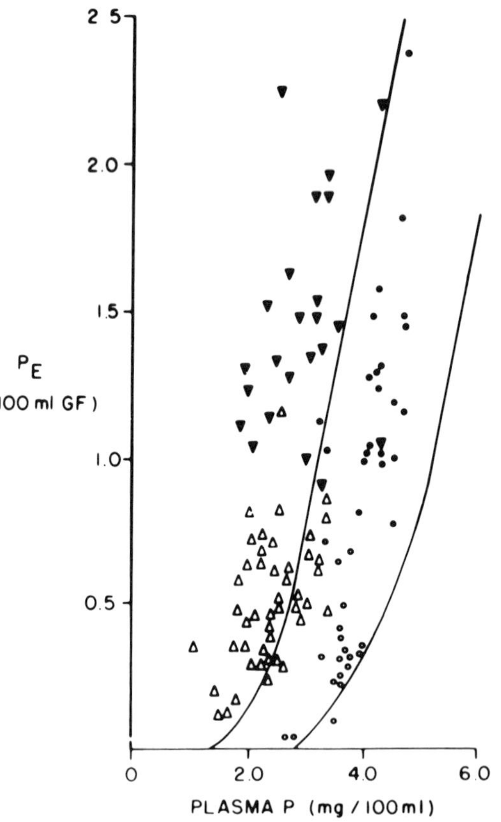

FIGURE 12-12 • Relationship between urinary phosphate excretion (P_E) and plasma P concentration. Dark and light triangles represent hyperparathyroid patients on high-P and normal or low-P diets, respectively, and dark and light dots represent normal volunteers on high-P and normal or low-P diets, respectively. See the text for discussion. (From Parfitt AM, Frame B, in Avioli L et al, eds: *Phosphate Metabolism: Kidney and Bone,* Paris, Armour Montagu, 1976, pp 179–196. Used by permission.)

HOMEOSTASIS UNDER CONDITIONS OF NORMAL RENAL FUNCTION

Under normal conditions the rate of P input into the plasma pool balances its rate of removal. The sources of P input include intestinal absorption, bone mineral resorp-

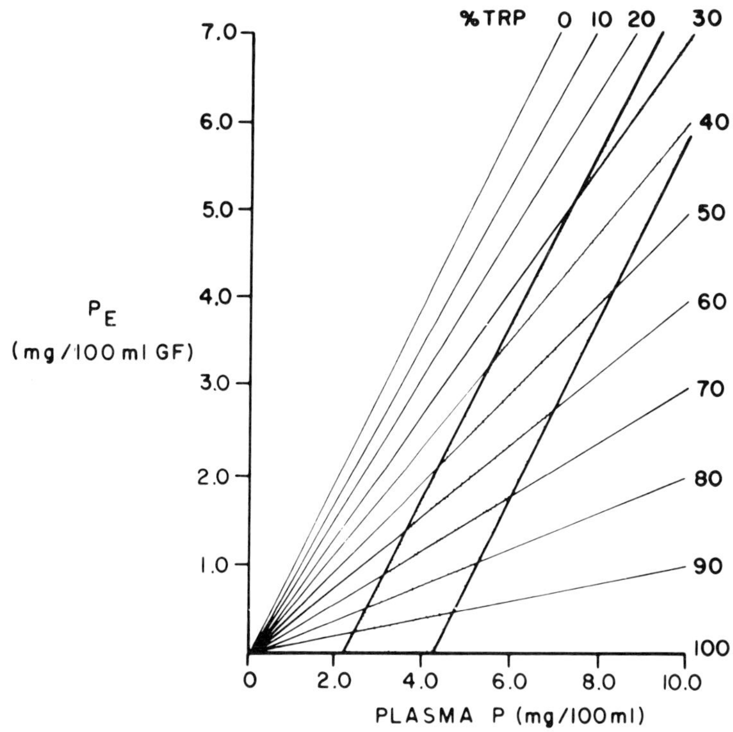

FIGURE 12-13 • Comparison of *Tm*P/GFR and percent TRP as two models of P reabsorption. Values of equal percent TRP are represented by a family of lines radiating from the origin. See the text for discussion. (From Parfitt AM, Frame B, in Avioli L et al, eds: *Phosphate Metabolism, Kidney and Bone,* Paris, Armour Montagu, 1976, pp 179–196. Used by permission.)

tion, renal tubular reabsorption, and transfer from skeletal and nonskeletal tissue. Routes for P exit from plasma would include intestinal secretion, transfer into skeletal and nonskeletal tissue, and glomerular filtration. A convenient model[579] for conceptualizing plasma P homeostasis is illustrated in Fig. 12-14. A steady-state plasma [P] is attained when the rate of renal P output exactly balances the sum of net rates of input from all extrarenal sources:

$$dF/dt - dR/dt = dA/dt + dB/dt + dS/dt$$

where dF/dt and dR/dt are rates of glomerular filtration and tubular reabsorption of P and dA/dt, dB/dt, and dS/dt are net rates of P input from intestine, bone, and soft tissue. Since the GFR of P, dF/dt, is equal to the product of PL_p (plasma [P]) and GFR, the equation may be written as

$$PL_P \times GFR = dA/dt + dB/dt + dS/dt + dR/dt$$

or

$$PL_P = (dA/dt + dB/dt + dS/dt)/GFR + P_R$$

where P_R is the rate of tubular P reabsorption factored by GFR [(dR/dt)/GFR], generally expressed in milligrams per 100 ml of glomerular filtration. As disussed earlier, under normal conditions the kidney rejects about 10 to 20 percent of the filtered P. This would suggest that P_R is close to or equal to *Tm*P/GFR. The term (dA/dt + dB/dt + dS/dt) represents the total load of P added to the plasma pool and will therefore be equal to the rate of urinary P excretion (dU/dt); thus,

$$PL_P = P_U + P_R$$

where P_U is the rate of urinary P excretion factored by GFR [(dU/dt)/GFR]. Therefore, the steady-state plasma [P] is determined by the extrarenal P load, reflected by P_U, and the renal tubular P reabsorption, P_R.

The relative contribution of each of the parameters has been estimated in a number of metabolic states, and the results are summarized in Table 12-5. It is clear that in the presence of normal GFR (100 ml/min), the renal P reabsorptive activity, P_R, is by far the most important determinant of plasma [P] (79 to 92 percent) in all conditions studied. With progressive reduction in GFR, the contribution of P_R to plasma P homeostasis diminishes. This will be discussed in more detail in the following section. In the fasting state (i.e., $dA/dt = 0$), the transfer rate of P from bone or soft tissue into the plasma varies with different metabolic states but contributes significantly to plasma P homeostasis. The contribution of the soft tissue is always greater than that from bone. In the normal, nonfasting state, intestinal absorption constitutes the only source of net P load added to the plasma P pool. A number of factors, including carbohydrate feeding and acid-base changes, can cause rapid and sometimes profound changes in plasma [P] by translocating P into or out of cells. These factors may account, at least in part, for the observed fluctuations in plasma [P] when this

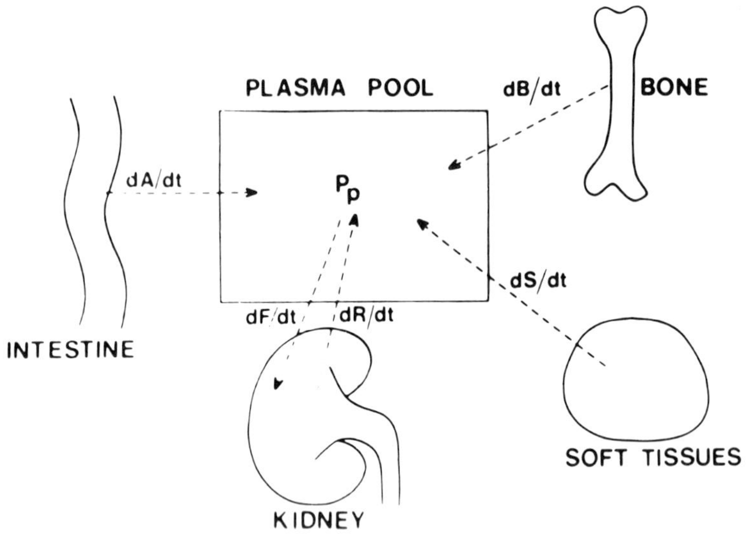

FIGURE 12-14 • A schematic representation of the main sources of P transfer to and from the plasma pool. See text and the legend for Table 12-5 for a key to the abbreviations used. (From Robertson WG, in Nordin BEC, ed: *Calcium, Phosphate and Magnesium Metabolism,* Edinburgh, Churchill Livingstone, 1976, pp 217–219. Used by permission.)

TABLE 12-5 • Relative transfer of phosphate into and out of the plasma pool in various metabolic states

Metabolic state	GFR, ml/min	PL_p, mg/100 ml	P_R mg/100 ml GF	P_R %	*dA/dt*(1/GFR) mg/100 ml GF	*dA/dt*(1/GFR) %	*dB/dt*(1/GFR) mg/100 ml GF	*dB/dt*(1/GFR) %	*dS/dt*(1/GFR) mg/100 ml GF	*dS/dt*(1/GFR) %	T_mP/GFR, mg/100 ml GF
Normal, fasting	100	3.3	2.9	88	~0	0	~0.05	1	~0.35	11	3.1
Normal, nonfasting	100	3.6	3.0	83	~0.6	17	~0	0	~0	0	3.0
Hyper-para-thyroid, fasting	100	2.4	1.9	79	~0	0	~0.15	6	~0.35*	15	1.9
Hypo-para-thyroid, fasting	100	5.3	4.9	92	~0	0	~0.05	1	~0.35*	7	5.5
Mild renal failure, fasting	25	4.2	2.2	53	~0	0	~0.6	14	~1.4*	33	2.2
Severe renal failure, fasting	10	6.5	1.5	23	~0	0	~1.5	23	~3.5*	54	1.5

KEY: GFR, glomerular filtration rate; PL_p, plasma phosphate concentration; P_R, renal tubular phosphate reabsorptive rate; *dA/dt, dB/dt,* and *dS/dt,* net rates of input of phosphate from intestinal absorption, bone, and soft tissue, respectively; *T*mP, maximum tubular reabsorptive rate for phosphate.

* Assuming that the rate of release of P (in mg/min) from soft tissues and the labile pool of bone does not vary from that in the normal fasting state.

SOURCE: From Robertson WG, in Nordin BEC, ed: *Calcium, Phosphate and Magnesium Metabolism*, Edinburgh, Churchill Livingstone, 1976, pp 217–219. Used by permission.

parameter is sequentially measured over short intervals. However, in contrast to the kidney, the operation of these factors is not sustained and therefore probably contributes little toward overall, long-term regulation of normal plasma [P]. In various pathologic conditions, net bone resorption, net loss from cells, or dissolution of ectopic "calcification" may also contribute P load into the plasma pool and therefore urinary P output.

HOMEOSTASIS UNDER CONDITIONS OF RENAL FAILURE

As just discussed, P_R or *T*mP/GFR is the major regulator of normal plasma [P]. Regulation is achieved by the excretion of appropriate amounts of filtered P. Thus,

$$U_PV = (PL_P \times GFR) - TmP$$

or

$$PL_P = TmP/GFR + U_PV/GFR$$

From this equation a theoretical relationship between plasma [P] and GFR can be calculated for a given U_PV and *T*mP/GFR. In the upper panel of Fig. 12-15 the relationship between PL_P and GFR is calculated using a constant, normal *T*mP/GFR of 3.2 mg/100 ml, with the two interrupted curves representing the lower and upper limits of normal U_PV of 0.14 and 0.57 mg/min. U_PV, in steady state, would of course represent the amount of P absorbed from the intestine. Thus, assuming a fractional P absorption of 0.6, the limits of U_PV selected would represent a dietary P intake of 336 to 1368 mg/day, respectively. The derived relationships predicted very well the data obtained by direct measurement of plasma [P] and GFR in a group of healthy subjects and patients with various degrees of CRF (see Chaps. 42 and 43) taken from the work of Kleeman and associates.[375] The preceding equation can be further transformed by dividing each term by PL_P:

$$1 = (TmP/GFR)/PL_P + U_PV/(GFR \times PL_P)$$

since P clearance, C_P, = U_PV/PL_P,

$$1 - C_P/GFR = (TmP/GFR)PL_P$$

or

$$TRP = (TmP/GFR)/PL_P$$

The calculated relationship between TRP (in percent) and GFR (in milliliters per minute) is illustrated in the lower panel of Fig. 12-15, using the same given conditions as those used in the upper panel. Again the calculated relationship conforms well with direct measurements reported by Slatopolsky and colleagues[616] in healthy individuals and in patients with varying degrees of CRF.

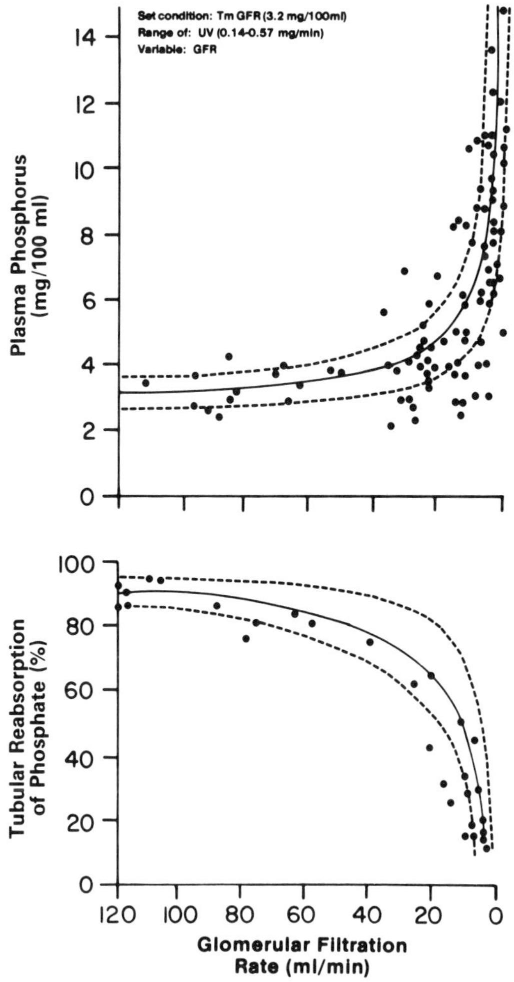

FIGURE 12-15 • The relationship between plasma phosphate concentrations and GFR (upper panel) and percent tubular reabsorption of phosphate and glomerular filtration rate (lower panel). The solid dots represent data from normal individuals and patients with chronic renal disease taken from Kleeman et al[375] for upper panel and from Slatopolsky et al [616] for lower panel. They can be seen to conform to the curve derived from calculations based on a constant TmP/GFR (From Bijvoet OLM, in Avioli L et al (eds): *Phosphate Metabolism. Kidney and Bone,* Paris, Armour Montagu, 1976, pp 421–442. Used by permission.)

A number of important observations are contained in Fig. 12-15. First, when GFR is 30 ml/min or higher, variations in dietary P, as reflected by U_PV, have relatively small effect on plasma [P]. When the GFR falls below 30 ml/min, plasma [P] becomes increasingly more sensitive to changes in U_PV or further reduction in GFR. For example, at a GFR of 20 ml/min, increasing U_PV from 0.14 to 0.57 mg/min raises plasma [P] from 3.8 to 6.0 mg/100 ml (58 percent), and at a GFR of 10 ml/min, the same maneuver increases plasma [P] from 4.8 to 8.6 mg/100 ml (80 percent). The steep slope of the portion of the curve at GFRs below 30 ml/min clearly indicates a relationship characterized by large changes in plasma [P] for very small changes in GFR. Inspection of the equation

$$PL_P = U_PV/GFR + TmP/GFR$$

further illustrates the point that a variation in dietary P load would have little influence on PL_P when GFR is normal. This is because the magnitude of the term U_PV/GFR is relatively insignificant when the denominator (GFR) is much larger than the numerator (U_PV). Under such conditions, PL_P would be mainly a function of the remaining term, *T*mP/GFR. Thus, assuming a daily dietary P intake of 1000 mg and a fractional intestinal P absorption of 0.6, the amount absorbed, therefore, the amount excreted (U_PV) would be 600 mg/24 h or 0.42 mg/min. At a normal GFR of 100 ml/min, the term U_PV/GFR would have a value of 0.42 mg/100 ml. This would account for only 11 percent [0.42/(3.2 + 0.42) = 0.11] of the total plasma [P], assuming *T*mP/GFR = 3.2 mg/100 ml. On the other hand, if the GFR is reduced to 5 ml/min, the same dietary load would result in a U_PV/GFR value of 8.4 mg/100 ml GF. Thus, the intestinal P absorption would account for 72 percent of the total plasma [P] [8.4/(3.2 + 8.4)]. This illustration again emphasizes the point that, in subjects with normal GFRs, plasma [P] is mainly a function of *T*mP/GFR, while in subjects with low GFRs, diet or other forms of P input into the ECF becomes a major factor in determining plasma [P]. The exaggerated fluctuation in PL_P observed in uremic patients or patients on intermittent dialysis therapy should therefore occasion no surprise. Sudden P influx into the ECF occurs with each meal, and sudden P efflux occurs with each dialysis. In the interim, the P load varies with the amount of intestinal P binders ingested, the rate of catabolism and destruction of soft tissue, and the net rate of bone resorption or lysis. The "paradoxical" fall in PL_P following parathyroidectomy in some uremic patients (in contrast to the expected rise in PL_P following the extirpation of hyperfunctioning parathyroid tissue in subjects with normal renal function) may be accounted for by the reduction in PTH-induced transfer of bone P into ECF.

The lower panel of Fig. 12-15 illustrates the requirement of the mathematical relationship between the TRP and the GFR for the former to decrease curvilinearly with a reduction in the latter even when the TRP, *T*mP/GFR, remains constant at its normal value of 3.2 mg/100 ml. Changes in TRP do not distinguish the effect of altered GFR from the effect of altered TRP. Like plasma [P], at low GFR, the TRP can change markedly with small changes in either U_PV or GFR. Even in the face of very low GFR, the theoretical curves for either PL_P versus GFR or TRP versus GFR would predict that a simple reduction of U_PV could restore highly abnormal PL_P or TRP to normal without the necessity of invoking changes in *T*mP/GFR. It bears repeating that the mathematically derived curves, which predicted closely the actual measurements in human subjects, were based on a fixed value of *T*mP/GFR of 3.2 mg/100 ml. This implies that the observed changes in PL_P and TRP associated with progressive reduction in GFR could in fact occur without the necessity of inducing adaptive changes in *T*mP/GFR by factors such as PTH. Indeed, several groups of investigators have provided evidence in favor of the argument that the normalization of the TRP and the maintenance of plasma P homeostasis in CRF may not necessarily require, or reflect, the participation of PTH.[130,241,642]

THE REGULATION OF TOTAL BODY PHOSPHORUS

Although the mechanism of plasma P homeostasis has been studied extensively, direct information on the regulation of total body P is relatively unexplored. There is a lack of systematic understanding of the sensing mechanism, the afferent limb, the integrating center, the efferent limb, and the effector mechanism in the homeostasis of total body P.

As discussed earlier, intake of a P load leads to an increase in renal P excretion. This regulatory response can occur in the absence of PTH, but whether other hormonal or nonhormonal factors are involved is not clear. As mentioned earlier, Brazy and associates[96] have suggested that the renal P adaptation to P loading may be mediated through extrarenal signals.

Interest in the syndrome of experimental P depletion has provided some insight into the fundamental adaptative processes that conserve and maintain total body, and particularly vital soft tissue, P stores. This syndrome is discussed in detail in Chap. 33, but several aspects of possible relevance to total body P regulation will be dealt with here.

The response to dietary P deprivation involves several components: virtual elimination of external P loss, metabolic adaptations that reduce the need for P, and a mobilization of bone P to meet soft tissue needs. The efficiency of the P-conserving mechanism in face of P deprivation is depicted in Fig. 12-16. Rapidly growing rats fed a normal P (0.3 percent) diet, either ad lib (NP) or pair-fed (NP-PF) with rats on a very low P (0.03 percent) diet, were clearly in positive P balance and excreted significant amounts of P in both urine and stool throughout the three weeks of balance studies. In rats fed a low-P diet (LP), the negative balance (mainly through stool loss) observed during the first week was corrected during the second week as a consequence of a reduction in fecal P loss and complete renal conservation of P. Stool P fell even further in the third week, and there was, in fact, a small but measurable amount of P in the urine. Duodenal segments from rats fed a low-P diet demonstrated a clear increase in P uptake during the second and third weeks of P deprivation when

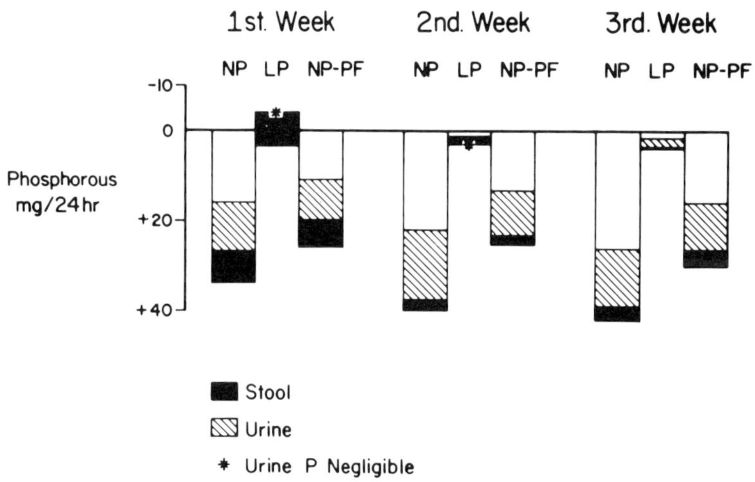

FIGURE 12-16 • Effect of dietary P deprivation on P balance in normal rats. P intake is plotted from the "0" line (neutral balance) downward, and the stool and urine output are plotted successively from the intake line upward. A positive balance is indicated by an open column below the "0" line and a negative balance by the dark column above the "0" line. See text for further details. (From Lee DBN et al: *Am J Physiol* 236(4):E451–E457, 1979. Used by permission.)

compared to their pair-fed mates on a normal P diet.[414] Growth in the P-deprived rats in terms of weight gain was markedly reduced or completely arrested. Thus, growing rats under conditions of severe P deprivation were able to achieve P balance by avid renal and intestinal conservation of P coupled with cessation of growth, which would reduce the anabolic need for P not vital for survival. A minimal but continued fecal P loss (1 to 2 mg/day) in rats placed on a low-P diet probably represents the obligatory shedding of epithelial cells and P secretion as well as other unregulated losses rather than indicating defective P absorption.

There are convincing data supporting the presence of skeletal breakdown and/or demineralization in the syndrome of P deprivation.[49,64,93,155,157,169,189,195,226,233,247,392,439,460,610,655] A number of observations lend support to the thesis that under such circumstances the P removed from bone is utilized in soft tissue. Several studies[93,169,233] have demonstrated that, with the exception of blood and its components, the total P in nonskeletal tissues is normal in "P-depleted" rats. The analysis of total tissue P, however, does not answer the more critical question of the possible changes in the inorganic and various organic P components and their distribution in the subcellular fractions. In this context, it is interesting that Kreusser and associates[392] observed that the renal content of inorganic P did not decrease until two weeks after dietary P deprivation, while the ATP level remained normal for six weeks. Emmett and associates[226] also found a normal renal cortical ATP level in rats deprived of dietary P for 18 days.

Rickets and osteomalacia, the lesion that has received the most attention from early investigators of the P-depletion syndrome, may indeed be only a consequence of the body's attempt to sustain the survival of other, more vital nonskeletal tissues in the face of critical P deficiency. This concept gains support from the study of Day and McCollum in rats[195] reported over five decades ago. Figure 12-17, constructed from their data, indicates that P deficiency resulted initially in a marked inhibition of growth, as reflected by a failure to gain weight. This may, however, be attributed to poor appetite and decreased food intake, since the pair-fed mates that received equal quantities of food with normal P content had similar reduction in weight gain, especially during the first four weeks. One of the most striking effects of P deprivation was the negative Ca balance, in large measure attributable to a marked increase in urinary Ca throughout the experimental period. However, the rate of Ca excretion decreased progressively after the second week so that the P-deprived animals were soon able to achieve zero or neutral Ca balance. The urinary excretion of P immediately became negligible in the P-deprived rats, but the small, constant P losses in stool accounted for the progressively more negative P balance. A positive nitrogen balance was observed during the first four weeks, when the rate of urinary Ca loss was greatest and weight gain in the P-deficient rats was not different from that in the pair-fed mates. In later periods, when the Ca balance approached "zero," weight gain ceased and nitrogen balance became negative in the low-P rats.

While the reduction in urinary Ca may be attributable in part to a decrease in intake, the major cause was probably the exhaustion of the exchangeable or metabolically active component of bone minerals. This assumption was supported by x-ray evidence of extreme osteopenia and the autopsy finding of markedly subnormal mineralization of the skeleton. These observations suggest that sustained P deprivation in growing rats led to a prompt, marked, and continuous release of bone minerals. The P released was used for P turnover in, and maintenance and growth of, soft tissue, while the Ca released was excreted in the urine. The degree of Ca excretion thus provides an indication of both the rate of bone demineralization and the extent of soft tissue demand for P. As bone minerals became depleted, growth ceased and the

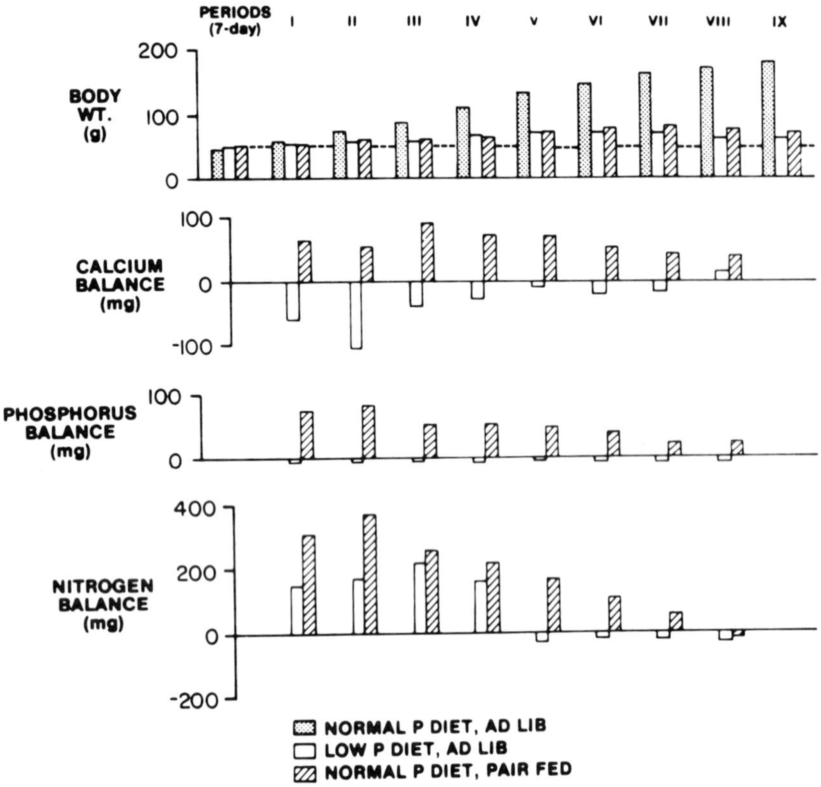

FIGURE 12-17 • Effect of P depletion on body weight and Ca, P, and N balance in young rats. (From Lee DBN et al, in Bronner F, Coburn JW (eds): *Disorders of Mineral Metabolism,* New York, Academic Press, 1981, vol III, pp 283–421. Used by permission.)

animal became catabolic. This is reflected by weight loss and negative nitrogen balance. It is likely that death in these rats reflected an exhaustion of P reserves so that the various P-dependent life-sustaining processes were no longer able to function. The inference that in P deprivation bone P is sacrificed to meet the critical soft tissue need for P would lead to the prediction that pathophysiologic states or maneuvers that reduce the anabolic need for P would spare the skeleton and ameliorate the severity of the P-depletion syndrome.

It is therefore of great interest to note that McCollum and Simmonds[460] in 1922 observed that simple starvation, and therefore cessation of growth, led to improvement in rickets in P-depleted rats. As a corollary, Copp and Suiker[169] observed that fasting in young P-deficient rats resulted in rapid correction of hypophosphatemia and hypercalcemia. Within 48 h the rats in fact developed frank hyperphosphatemia and hypocalcemia. Clarkson and associates[155] studied a leukemic patient with clinical and laboratory evidence of P depletion in whom hyperphosphatemia and hypocalcemia developed rapidly with the administration of GC, a known tumor-lytic as well as catabolic agent. Moreover, dietary P deprivation in young growing animals rapidly leads to overt manifestations of P deficiency, whereas it takes longer and is more difficult to induce the deficiency syndrome in grown animals. In grown animals, P-binding compounds such as $Al(OH)_3$ may be required in addition to produce P-deficiency syndrome.[64,157] Copp and Suiker[169] were able to produce experimental P deficiency in young rats in 5 weeks, but it took 26 weeks in adult rats.

Although reduction in growth and a consequent decrease in anabolic need for P may ameliorate the adverse effect of P deprivation, the acceleration of growth or an increase in anabolic need for P will induce P deficiency or exacerbate the effect of a relatively inadequate P supply. The unique syndrome of fatal hyperalimentation mimics P depletion with remarkable exactitude.[610,611] The catastrophe is most likely the result of a sudden induction in anabolic activities, creating a precipitous and often fatal imbalance between P demand and P supply. As one would anticipate, the malignancy of the syndrome is exacerbated when hyperalimentation is instituted in hosts that are rapidly losing weight (breakdown of lean tissue). Of further interest is the demonstration that certain biochemical features of P depletion may develop in rats fed a diet considered adequate in P for normal growth but that exhibited spontaneously accelerated growth.[95,416] In this connection it is interesting to recall that x-ray signs of rickets have been seen in infants that grow rapidly but exhibit no other disturbance in mineral metabolism.[237]

Thus, selective P deprivation (to be distinguished from starvation or total caloric deprivation) leads to changes directed toward restoring external P balance and maintaining soft tissue P needs by P mobilization from bone. These adaptive changes are manifested by a constellation of measurable abnormalities, the severity of which is modified by the difference between metabolic P need and exogenous P supply. Adaptive responses of P deprivation appear to have evolved whenever the body "sees" a relative excess of P demand over P supply; they become resolved when demand balances supply. However, the sensor, the messenger, and the mechanisms by which these responses are initiated and sustained are not known.

It is probable that these changes do not depend critically on hormones considered important in mineral homeostasis, such as PTH and CT,[49,157,189] vitamin D,[94] or GH.[420] Many changes characteristic of P depletion can also be observed in face of normal or even elevated plasma [P].[53,95,271,416,628,629] Of the four major laboratory indexes of dietary P deprivation (i.e., hypophosphatemia, hypercalcemia, hypophosphaturia, and hypercalciuria), all of which may occur within 4 to 24 h after placing animals on a low-P diet,[428,560] hypophosphaturia is probably the most reliable, since it can develop and persist even if plasma [P] tends toward normal.[53,95,628,629] The promptness with which hypophosphaturia develops suggests a possible sensing mechanism in the proximal gastrointestinal tract. The message would then be transmitted to the kidney and bone in some manner that may not always involve changes in plasma [P]. The sensor may be a "ratio" sensor, responding to the ratio of calories to P rather than to the absolute level of P in the diet. This is because complete starvation does not elicit a similar sequence of events. Beck and associates[57] have demonstrated in rats that fasting was associated with increased rather than decreased urinary P excretion. Also, increase in P uptake by renal cortical brush border membrane vesicles was observed only in rats fed a low-P diet, but not in rats totally starved.[362,426] The promptness with which the various characteristic features of P deprivation develop also suggests that a change in body P stores is not an important signal, since it is unlikely that a significant reduction in body P content can occur within several hours. Measurements of total P,[93,169,233] inorganic P,[392] and ATP content[226,392] of cells are not consistent with a distinct reduction in intracellular P, at least in the early stages. Moreover, acute respiratory alkalosis[490] and glucose hyperalimentation[69,610,611] both shift P into cells and do not cause external P loss but lead promptly to biochemical changes characteristic of P deprivation. All these observations suggest that the basic signal that leads to the various changes associated with P deprivation may be precipitated by a change in the ratio of P to glucose (calories) entering the cell or a metabolic pool, rather than by an alteration in gross parameters such as the total P, inorganic P, or ATP content. The messenger that transmits the postulated proximal gastrointestinal tract recognition of low dietary intake to the target organs is completely unknown. Two studies have postulated the existence of hormone(s) responsible for inducing hypercalciuria[64] and hypophosphaturia[627] as observed in experimental P depletion.

REFERENCES

1. Abraham MI et al: Insulin stimulates phosphate transport in opossum kidney eithelial cells. *Am J Physiol* 258: F1592, 1990.
2. Adams PH et al: Effects of hyperthyroidism on bone and mineral metabolism in man. *Q J Med* 36:1, 1967.
3. Adolph EF: The chemical sensitiveness of the kidneys. *Am J Physiol* 74:93, 1925.
4. Agus ZS: Oncogenic hypophosphatemic osteomalacia. *Kidney Int* 24:113, 1983.
5. Agus ZS et al: Mode of action of parathyroid hormone and cyclic adenosine 3′,5′-monophosphate on renal tubular phosphate reabsorption in the dog. *J Clin Invest* 50:617, 1971.
6. Ahumada JJ, Massry SG: Renal vasodilatation: Effect on renal handling of phosphate. *Clin Sci* 41:109, 1971.
7. Aitken JM et al: Plasma growth hormone and serum phosphorous concentrations in relation to the menopause and to estrogen therapy. *J Endocrinol* 59:593, 1973.
8. Aitken JM et al: The effect of long-term mestranol administration on calcium and phosphorous homeostasis in oophrectomized women. *Clin Sci* 41:233, 1971.
9. Albright F et al: Studies of calcium and phosphorous metabolism: 8. The influence of the thyroid gland and parathyroid hormone upon the total acid-base metabolism. *J Clin Invest* 10:187, 1931.
10. Albright F et al: Studies on parathyroid physiology: 3. The effect of phosphate ingestion and clinical hyperparathyroidism. *J Clin Invest* 2:411, 1932.
11. Albright F, Ellsworth R: Studies on the physiology of the parathyroid glands: 1. Calcium and phosphorus studies on a case of idiopathic hypoparathyroidism. *J Clin Invest* 7:183, 1929.
12. Albright F, Reifenstein EC: Mode of action of vitamin D and dihydrotachysterol, in *The Parathyroid Glands and Metabolic Bone Disease.* Baltimore, Williams & Wilkins, 1948, p 122.
13. Allen FN et al: The relationship of phosphate and carbohydrate metabolism. *Am J Physiol* 70:333, 1925.
14. Allon M et al: Insulin in the acute renal adaptation to dietary phosphate restriction in the rat. *Kidney Int* 37:14, 1990.
15. Al-Mahrouq HA et al: Cholera toxin action on rabbit renal brush border membranes inhibits phosphate transport. *Biochim Biophys Acta* 981:200, 1988.
16. Altenahr E, Kampf E: Parathyroid function in rats treated with growth hormone. *Virchows Arch Pathol Anat Physiol* 371:363, 1976.
17. Amiel C: Sites of renal tubular reabsorption of phosphate, in Fliesch H, Massry SG (eds): *Renal Handling of Phosphate.* New York, Plenum, 1980, p 39.
18. Amiel C et al: Evidence for a parathyroid hormone-

independent calcium modulation of phosphate transport along the nephron. *J Clin Invest* 57:256, 1976.
19. Amiel C et al: Micropuncture study of handling of phosphate by proximal and distal nephron in normal and parathyroidectomized rat: Evidence for distal reabsorption. *Pfluegers Arch* 317:93, 1970.
20. Amstutz M et al: Effect of pH on phosphate transport in rat renal brush border membrane vesicles. *Am J Physiol* 248:F705, 1985.
21. Anderson GH, Draper HH: Effect of dietary phosphorus on calcium metabolism in intact and parathyroidectomized adult rats. *J Nutr* 102:1123, 1972.
22. Anderson J, Foster JB: Effect of cortisone on urinary phosphate excretion in man. *Clin Sci* 18:437, 1959.
23. Anderson J, Parsons V: The tubular maximal resorptive rate for inorganic phosphate in normal subjects. *Clin Sci* 25:431, 1963.
24. Anderson JBB, Talmage RV: The effect of calcium infusion and calcitonin on plasma phosphate in sham-operated and thyroparathyroidectomized dogs. *Endocrinology* 93:1222, 1973.
25. Angielski S et al: Reversible resistance to the phosphaturic effect of cAMP in lithium treated rats. *Acta Physiol* 33:463, 1982.
26. Angielski S et al: The effect of maleate and lithium on renal function and metabolism, in Schmidt V, Dubach VC (eds): *Renal Metabolism in Relation to Renal Function.* Bern, Huber, 1976, p 142.
27. Applebury ML et al: Phosphate binding to alkaline phosphatase. *J Biol Chem* 245:4968, 1970.
28. Ardaillou R: Kidney and calcitonin. *Nephron* 15:250, 1975.
29. Arnaud CD et al: Radioimmunoassay of human parathyroid hormone in serum. *J Clin Invest* 50:21, 1971.
30. Arner B: Phosphate disappearance from plasma and the renal handling of phosphate after intravenous loading in man. *Acta Med Scand* 415(suppl):1, 1964.
31. Arruda JAL et al: Effects of vasopressin administration on sodium excretion and plasma phosphate concentration. *Proc Soc Exp Biol Med* 155:308, 1977.
32. Arruda JAL et al: Interaction of arginine vasopressin and parathyroid hormone on renal bicarbonate handling. *Miner Electrolyte Metab* 1:139, 1978.
33. Arruda JAL et al: Lithium administration and phosphate excretion. *Am J Physiol* 231:1140, 1976.
34. Aschinberg LC et al: Vitamin D-resistant rickets associated with epidermal nevus syndrome: Demonstration of a phosphaturic substance in the dermal lesions. *J Pediatr* 91:56, 1977.
35. Aurbach GD, Heath DA: Parathyroid and calcitonin regulation of renal function. *Kidney Int* 6:331, 1974.
36. Aurbach GD et al: Structure, synthesis and mechanism of action of parathyroid hormone. *Recent Prog Horm Res* 28:353, 1972.
37. Ayer JL et al: Independence of phosphate reabsorption and glomerular filtration in dog. *Am J Physiol* 151:168, 1947.
38. Baines AD, Ross BD: Gluconeogenesis and phosphate reabsorption in isolated lactate or pyruvate-perfused rat kidneys. *Miner Electrolyte Metab* 10:286, 1984.
39. Baksi SN, Kenny AD: Effects of administration of antiestrogen tomoxifen in vivo on the metabolism of 25-hydroxyvitamin D3 in vitro in the Japanese quail. *Biochem Pharmacol* 26:2439, 1977.
40. Baksi SN, Kenny AD: Ovarian influence on 25-hydroxyvitamin D3 metabolism in Japanese quail (abstract). *Fed Proc* 35:665, 1976.
41. Banerjee RK et al: Purification and reconstitution of the phosphate transporter from bovine heart mitochondria. *Biochem Biophys Res Commun* 75:772, 1977.
42. Bank N, Malnic G: Effect of urinary alkalinization on renal phosphate reabsorption, in Massry SG, Fleisch H (eds): *Renal Handling of Phosphate.* New York: Plenum, 1980, p 209.
43. Bank N et al: A micropuncture study of phosphate reabsorption by the rat proximal renal tubule. *J Clin Invest* 54:1040, 1974.
44. Barbour BH et al: Studies on the mechanism of phosphorus excretion in vitamin D resistant rickets. *Nephron* 3:40, 1966.
45. Barlet JP et al: Effect of porcine, salmon and human calcitonin in cows and sheep. *Horm Metab Res* 3:363, 1971.
46. Batts, AA et al: The effect of growth hormone on muscle potassium and on extracellular fluid. *Endocrinology* 55:456, 1955.
47. Baumann K et al: pH dependence of phosphate reabsorption in the proximal tubule of rat kidney. *Pfluegers Arch* 360:183, 1975.
48. Baumann K et al: Renal phosphate transport: Inhomogeneity of local-proximal transport rates and sodium dependence. *Pfluegers Arch* 356:287, 1985.
49. Baylink D et al: Formation, mineralization and resorption of bone hypophosphatemic rats. *J Clin Invest* 50:2519, 1971.
50. Beck JC et al: Metabolic effects of human and monkey growth hormone in man. *Science* 125:884, 1957.
51. Beck LH, Goldberg M: Effects of acetazolamide and parathyroidectomy on renal transport of sodium, calcium and phosphate. *Am J Physiol* 224:1136, 1973.
52. Beck LH, Goldberg M: Mechanism of the blunted phosphaturia in saline-loaded thyroparathyroidectomized dogs. *Kidney Int* 6:18, 1974.
53. Beck N: Effect of dietary phosphorus (P) intake on renal actions of parathyroid hormone (PTH) and cyclic AMP (cAMP). *Kidney Int* 10:487, 1976.
54. Beck N: Effect of metabolic acidosis on renal action of parathyroid hormone. *Am J Physiol* 228:1483, 1975.
55. Beck N: Effect of metabolic acidosis on renal response to parathyroid hormone in phosphorus deprived rats. *Am J Physiol* 241:F23, 1981.
56. Beck N: Phosphaturia after release of bilateral ureteral obstruction in rats. *Am J Physiol* 237:F14, 1979.
57. Beck N et al: Effect of fasting on tubular phosphorus reabsorption. *Am J Physiol* 237:F241, 1979.
58. Beisel WR et al: Phosphaturesis: A direct renal effect of triiodothyronine. *Am J Physiol* 195:357, 1958.
59. Belforte L et al: Long-term treatment with 2-Br-alpha-ergocryptine in acromegaly. *Acta Endocrinol* 85:235, 1977.

60. Bello-Reuss E et al: Dopamine decreases fluid reabsorption in straight portions of rabbit proximal tubule. *Am J Physiol* 242:F634, 1982.
61. Bellorin-Font E, Martin KJ: Regulation of the PTH receptor cyclase system of canine kidney: Effects of calcium, magnesium and guanine nucleotides. *Am J Physiol* 241:F364, 1981.
62. Bellorin-Font E et al: Regulation of PTH receptor adenylate cyclase system of canine kidney: Influence of Mn^{2+} on effects of Ca^{2+}, PTH and GTP. *Am J Physiol* 242:F457, 1982.
63. Bengele HH et al: Phosphate transport along the inner medullary collecting duct of the rat. *Am J Physiol* 237:F48, 1979.
64. Ben-Isaac C et al: Evidence for humoral factor responsible for the hypercalciuria of phosphate depletion. *Clin Res* 23:134, 1975.
65. Ben Ishay D et al: Effect of spironolactone on urinary calcium excretion. *Isr J Med Sci* 8:495, 1972.
66. Benjamin HR, Hess AF: The forms of inorganic phosphorus in human and animal sera: 1. Normal, rachitic, hypercalcemic and other conditions. *J Biol Chem* 70:35, 1933.
67. Berner W et al: Phosphate transport into brush border membrane vesicles isolated from rat small intestine. *Bio chem J* 160:467, 1976.
68. Besarb A et al: Bicarbonate and sodium reabsorption by the isolated perfused kidney. *Am J Physiol* 228:1525, 1975.
69. Betro MG, Pain RW: Hypophosphatemia in a hospital population. *Br Med J* 1:273, 1972.
70. Biber J, Murer H: Na-Pi cotransport in LLC-PK_1 cells: Fast adaptive response to Pi deprivation. *Am J Physiol* 249:C430, 1985.
71. Biber J et al: Modulation of Na^+-Pi cotransport in opossum kidney cells by extracellular phosphate. *Am J Physiol* 255:C155, 1988.
72. Biber J et al: Phosphorylation of rat kidney proximal tubular brush border membranes: Role of cAMP-dependent protein phosphorylation in the regulation of phosphate transport. *Pfluegers Arch* 398:221, 1983.
73. Biber J et al: Sodium-dependent transport of phosphate in LLC-PK_1 cells. *Biochim Biophys Acta* 735:325, 1983.
74. Bijvoet OLM: The importance of the kidneys in phosphate homeostasis, in Avioli L et al (eds): *Phosphate Metabolism: Kidney and Bone.* Paris, Armour Montagu, 1976, p 421.
75. Bijvoet OLM: Relation of plasma phosphorus concentration to renal tubular reabsorption of phosphate. *Clin Sci* 37:23, 1969.
76. Bijvoet OLM, Froeling PCAM: Calcitonin, parathyroid hormone, and the kidney, in Frame B, Parfitt AM (eds): *Clinical Aspects of Metabolic Bone Disease.* Amsterdam, Excerpta Medica, 1973, p 184.
77. Bijvoet OLM, Majoor CLH: The renal tubular reabsorption of phosphate in thyrotoxicosis. *Clin Chim Acta* 11:181, 1965.
78. Bommer J et al: Bone cell metabolism in experimental hyper- and hypothyroidism. *Eur J Clin Invest* 3:215, 1973.
79. Bommer J et al: Parathyroid activity in hyperthyroidism. *Calcif Tissue Res* 21(suppl):288, 1976.
80. Bommer J et al: Parathyroid-independent change in the renal handling of phosphate in hyperthyroid rats. *Kidney Int* 15:325, 1979.
81. Boneh A, Tenenhouse HS: Protein kinase C in mouse kidney: Subcellular distribution and endogenous substrates. *Biochem Cell Biol* 66:262, 1988.
82. Bonjour J-P et al: Effect of 1,25-dihydroxy-vitamin-D3 on the renal handling of Pi in thyroparathyroidectomized rats. *J Clin Invest* 60:1419, 1977.
83. Borle AB: Regulation of cellular calcium metabolism and calcium transport by calcitonin. *J Membr Biol* 21:125, 1975.
84. Borle AB et al: Role of parathyroid hormone in phosphate transport across rat duodenum. *Am J Physiol* 204:705, 1963.
85. Borowitz SM, Ghishan FK: Maturation of jejunal phosphate transport by rat brush border membrane vesicles. *Pediatr Res* 19:1308, 1985.
86. Boucher BJ: The assay of human growth hormone and its clinical application, in Mason AS (ed): *Human Growth Hormone.* London, Heinemann, 1972, p 94.
87. Boudry J-F et al: Secretion of inorganic phosphate in the rat nephron. *Clin Sci* 48:475, 1975.
88. Bouillon R, de Moor P: Parathyroid function in patients with hyper or hypothyroidism. *J Clin Endocrinol Metab* 38:999, 1974.
89. Bourke E et al: The site of action of bumetamide in man. *Eur J Pharmacol* 23:283, 1973.
90. Brain RT et al: Observations on phosphates in blood and on the urinary excretion of phosphates. *Biochem J* 22:628, 1928.
91. Braumann H et al: Comparative study of growth hormone response to hypoglycemia in normal subjects and in patients with primary myxedema or hyperthyroidism before and after treatment. *J Clin Endocrinol Metab* 36:1162, 1973.
92. Braun-Werness JL et al: Binding of nicotinamide adenine dinucleotide by the renal brush border membrane fraction from rat kidney cortex. *Biochim Biophys Acta* 732:553, 1983.
93. Brautbar N et al: Influence of dietary magnesium in experimental phosphate depletion: Bone and soft tissue mineral changes. *Am J Physiol* 237:E152, 1979.
94. Brautbar N et al: Interactions between vitamin D deficiency and phosphorus depletion in the rat. *J Clin Invest* 63:335, 1979.
95. Brautbar N et al: Normophosphatemic phosphate depletion in the growing rat. *Am J Physiol* 236:E283, 1979.
96. Brazy PC et al: Comparative effect of dietary phosphate, unilateral nephrectomy, and parathyroid hormone on phosphate transport by the rabbit proximal tubule. *Kidney Int* 17:788, 1980.
97. Brazy PC et al: Inhibition of renal metabolism: Relative effects of arsenate on sodium, phosphate and glucose transport by the rabbit proximal tubule. *J Clin Invest* 66:1211, 1980.
98. Brazy PC et al: Metabolic requirement for inorganic phos-

phate by the rabbit proximal tubule: Evidence for a crabtree effect. *J Clin Invest* 70:53, 1982.

99. Brendt TJ et al: Nicotinamide adenine dinucleotide and renal response to parathyroid hormone. *Endocrinology* 108:2005, 1981.
100. Brickman AS et al: Actions of 1α-hydroxyvitamin D3 and 1α,25-dihydroxyvitamin D3 on mineral metabolism in man: 1. Effects of net absorption of phosphorus. *Am J Clin Nutr* 30:1064, 1977.
101. Brickman AS et al: Changes in serum and urinary calcium during treatment with hydrochlorothiazide: Studies on mechanism. *J Clin Invest* 51:945, 1972.
102. Bridson WE, Kohler PO: Cortisol stimulation of growth hormone production by human pituitary tissue in culture. *J Clin Endocrinol* 30:538, 1970.
103. Briscoe AM, Ragan C: Effect of magnesium on calcium metabolism in man. *Am J Clin Nutr* 19:296, 1966.
104. Brodehl J, Gellissen K: Der Einfluss des Angiotensins II auf die tubulare Phosphatruckresorption beim Menschen. *Klin Wochenschr* 44:1171, 1966.
105. Brommage R et al: Vitamin D-independent intestinal calcium and phosphorus absorption during reproduction. *Am J Physiol* 259:G631, 1990.
106. Brooks FP, Pickfore M: The effect of posterior pituitary hormones on the excretion of electrolytes in dogs. *J Physiol* 142:486, 1958.
107. Brown CD et al: Sodium-dependent phosphate transport by apical membrane vesicles from a cultured renal epithelial cell line (LLC-PK_1). *Biochim Biophys Acta* 769:471, 1984.
108. Brunette MG et al: Effect of parathyroid hormone on phosphate reabsorption along the nephron of the rat. *Am J Physiol* 225:1076, 1973.
109. Brunette MG et al: Effect of temperature and pH on phosphate transport through brush border membrane vesicles in rats. *Can J Physiol Pharmacol* 62:229, 1984.
110. Brunette MG, Dennis VW: Effects of L-bromotetramisole on phosphate transport by the proximal renal tubule: Failure to demonstrate a direct involvement of alkaline phosphatase. *Can J Physiol Pharmacol* 62:229, 1982.
111. Brunette MG et al: Phosphate uptake by superficial and deep nephron brush border membranes: Effect of dietary phosphate and parathyroid hormone. *Pfluegers Arch* 400:356, 1984.
112. Bullock JK: Physiologic variations in inorganic blood phosphorus content at different age periods: Attempt to explain these in growing child. *Am J Dis Child* 40:725, 1930.
113. Bunim JJ et al: Studies on dexamethasone, a new synthetic steroid in rheumatoid arthritis: A preliminary report. *Arthritis Rheum* 1:313, 1958.
114. Burckhardt G et al: The influence of pH on phosphate transport into rat renal brush border membrane vesicles. *Pfleugers Arch* 390:191, 1981.
115. Burman KD et al: Ionized and total serum calcium and parathyroid hormone in hyperthyroidism. *Ann Intern Med* 84:668, 1976.
116. Burnett JC et al: Effects of synthetic atrial natriuretic factor on renal function and renin release. *Am J Physiol* 247:F863, 1984.
117. Butturini U, Bonomini V: Uber die Wirkung von Blukagon und Insulin auf Nierenfunktion, Harnausscheidung der Phosphat-, Bicarbonat- und Ammoniakionen und titrierbare Aciditat beim Menschen. *Helv Chir Acta* 5:617, 1958.
118. Caniggia A, Gennari C: Absorption du phosphate radioactif chez l'homme et sa regulation, in Hioco DJ (ed): *Phosphate et metabolisme phosphocalcique*. Paris, Editions Sandoz, 1971, p 209.
119. Caniggia A, Gennari C: Effect of 25-hydroxycholecalciferol (25-HCC) on intestinal absorption of 47-Ca in four cases of iatrogenic Cushing's syndrome. *Helv Chir Acta* 37:221, 1974.
120. Caniggia A, Gennari C: Intestinal absorption of radiophosphate after physiologic doses of 25(OH)D3 in normals, liver cirrhosis and chronic renal failure patients, in Normal AW et al (eds): *Vitamin D: Biochemical, Chemical and Clinical Aspects Related to Calcium Metabolism*. Berlin, de Gruyter, 1977, p 755.
121. Caniggia A et al: Early effects of synthetic bovine parathyroid hormone and synthetic salmon calcitonin on urinary excretion of cyclic AMP, phosphate and calcium in man. *Calcif Tissue Res* 20:209, 1976.
122. Caniggia A et al: Influenze della tirocalcitonia sull'assorbimento intestinale del radiocalcio (Ca-47) nell'nono. *Boll Soc Ital Biol Sper* 44:458, 1968.
123. Caniggia A et al: Intestinal absorption of radiophosphate in osteomalacia before and after vitamin D treatment. *Calcif Tissue Res* 2:299, 1968.
124. Case records of the Massachusetts General Hospital, Case 20. *N Engl J Med* 292:1117, 1975.
125. Cassola AC, Malnic G: Phosphate transfer and tubular pH during renal stopped-flow microperfusion experiments in the rat. *Pfluegers Arch* 367:249, 1977.
126. Cattaneo C et al: The maximum tubular reabsorption of phosphate in acromegaly. *Acta Endocrinol* 45:203, 1964.
127. Caverzasio J, Bonjour JP: Influence of calcium on phosphate transport in cultured kidney epithelium. *Am J Physiol* 254:F217, 1988.
128. Caverzasio J, Bonjour JP: Mechanism of rapid phosphate transport adaptation to a single low Pi meal in rat renal brush border membrane. *Pfluegers Arch* 409:333, 1987.
129. Caverzasio J et al: Adaptation of phosphate transport in phosphate-deprived LLC-PK_1 cells. *Am J Physiol* 248:F122, 1985.
130. Caverzasio J et al: Parathyroid hormone independent adaptation of tubular phosphate transport to renal mass reduction. *Kidney Int* 17:856, 1980.
131. Caverzasio J et al: Sodium dependent phosphate transport inhibited by parathyroid hormone and cyclic AMP stimulation in an opossum kidney cell line. *J Biol Chem* 261:3233, 1986.
132. Chabardes D et al: PTH sensitive adenyl cyclase activity: Different segments of the rabbit nephron. *Pfluegers Arch* 354:229, 1975.
133. Chaimovitz C et al: Exaggerated phosphaturic response to volume expansion in patients with essential hypertension. *Clin Sci* 49:207, 1975.
134. Chambers EL Jr et al: Tests for hyperparathyroidism: Tubular reabsorption of phosphate, phosphate deprivation and calcium infusion. *J Clin Endocrinol Metab* 16:1507, 1956.

135. Chan WY, Sawyer WH: Natriuresis in conscious dogs during arginine vasopressin infusion and after oxytocic injection. *Proc Soc Exp Biol Med* 110:697, 1962.
136. Charbardes D et al: Distribution of calcitonin-sensitive adenylate cyclase activity along the rabbit kidney tubule. *Proc Natl Acad Sci U S A* 73:3608, 1976.
137. Charbardes D et al: PTH sensitive adenyl cyclase activity in different segments of the rabbit nephron. *Pfluegers Arch* 354:229, 1975.
138. Chase LR et al: Pseudohypoparathyroidism: Defective excretion of 3′5′-AMP in response to parathyroid hormone. *J Clin Invest* 48:1832, 1969.
139. Chen L, Sacktor B: Sodium gradient-dependent phosphate transport in renal brush border membrane vesicles. *J Biol Chem* 256:1556, 1981.
140. Chen L et al: Phosphate uptake by renal membrane vesicles of rabbits adapted to high and low phosphorus diets. *Am J Physiol* 245:F175, 1983.
141. Chen L et al: Renal adaptation to phosphate load in the acutely thyroparathyroidectomized rat: Rapid alteration in brush border membrane phosphate transport. *Am J Physiol* 246:F488, 1984.
142. Chen PS Jr, Neuman WF: Renal excretion of calcium by the dog. *Am J Physiol* 180:623, 1955.
143. Chen TC et al: Role of vitamin D metabolites in phosphate transport of rat intestine. *J Nutr* 104:1056, 1974.
144. Chen WYC et al: Role of parathyroid hormone in rat remnant kidney ammonium metabolism. *Miner Electrolyte Metab* 17:46, 1991.
145. Chobanian MC, Hammerman MR: Parathyroid hormone stimulates ammoniagenesis in canine renal proximal tubular segments. *Am J Physiol* 255:F847, 1988.
146. Chomdej B et al: Renal hemodynamics and autoregulatory responses to acute hypercalcemia. *Am J Physiol* 232:490, 1977.
147. Chow K et al: Effects of ammonia on the absorption and accumulation of glucose, 45Ca and 32P from the ligated intestinal loop in the chick. *J Nutr* 102:1513, 1972.
148. Christiansen C et al: Lithium-induced "primary" hyperparathyroidism. *Calcif Tissue Res* 22(suppl):341, 1977.
149. Chu HI et al: Calcium and phosphorus in osteomalacia: Further studies on vitamin D action—early signs of depletion and effects of minimal doses. *J Clin Invest* 19:349, 1940.
150. Clapp JR et al: Proximal site of action of ethacrynic acid: Importance of filtration rate. *Am J Physiol* 220:1335, 1971.
151. Clark I: The effects of dietary and hormone factors on phosphate metabolism in the rat, in Hioco DJ (ed): *Phosphate et metabolisme phosphocalcique*. Paris, Editions Sandoz, 1971, p. 89.
152. Clark I: Effects of magnesium ions on calcium and phosphorus metabolism. *Am J Physiol* 214:348, 1968.
153. Clark I, Smith MR: Effects of parathyroidectomy and hydrocortisone on the intestinal absorption of calcium and phosphate. *Endocrinology* 74:421, 1964.
154. Clark JD, Kenny AD: Hog thyrocalcitonin in the dog: Urinary calcium phosphorus, magnesium and sodium responses. *Endocrinology* 84:1199, 1969.
155. Clarkson DR et al: Phosphate depletion and glucocorticoid-induced hyperphosphatemia in lymphoblastic leukemia. *Metabolism* 22:611, 1973.
156. Clarkson EM et al: The effect of aluminium hydroxide on calcium, phosphorus and aluminium balances, the serum parathyroid hormone concentration and the aluminium content of bone in patients with chronic renal failure. *Clin Sci* 43:519, 1972.
157. Coburn JW, Massry SG: Changes in serum and urinary calcium during phosphate depletion: Studies on mechanisms. *J Clin Invest* 49:1073, 1970.
158. Cochran M et al: Renal effects of calcitonin. *Br Med J* 1:135, 1970.
159. Cohen JJ et al: Renal tubular reabsorption of acetoacetate, inorganic sulfate and inorganic phosphate in the dog as affected by glucose and phlorhizin. *Am J Physiol* 184:91, 1956.
160. Cole JA et al: Clonal sublines that are morphologically and functionally distinct from parental OK cells. *Am J Physiol* 256:F672, 1989.
161. Cole JA et al: A dual mechanism for regulation of kidney phosphate transport by parathyroid hormone. *Am J Physiol* 253:E221, 1987.
162. Cole JA et al: Regulation of sodium dependent phosphate transport by parathyroid hormone in opossum kidney cells: Adenosine 3′5′-monophosphate dependent and independent mechanisms. *Endocrinology* 122:2981, 1988.
163. Condon JR et al: Defective intestinal phosphate absorption in familial and non-familial hypophosphatemia. *Br Med J* 3:138, 1970.
164. Connors MH et al: Retention of biologic activity of human growth hormone in man after reduction and alkylation. *J Clin Endocrinol Metab* 37:499, 1973.
165. Constanzo LS et al: Renal actions of vitamin D in D-deficient rats. *Am J Physiol* 226:1490, 1974.
166. Cook BS, Simmons DH: Mannitol interference in phosphate determination: Method of correction. *J Lab Clin Med* 60:160, 1962.
167. Cook GMW, Stoddart RW: *Surface Carbohydrates of the Eukaryotic Cell.* New York, Academic Press, 1973.
168. Cook PB et al: The effect of thyrotoxicosis upon the metabolism of calcium, phosphorus and nitrogen. *Q J Med* 28:505, 1959.
169. Copp DH, Suiker AP: Study of calcium kinetics in calcium and phosphorus-deficient rats with the aid of radiocalcium, in Mclean FC et al (eds): *Radioisotopes and Bone*. Oxford, Blackwell, 1962.
170. Corman B et al: Glucose-mediated inhibition of phosphate reabsorption in rat kidney. *Am J Physiol* 235:F430, 1978.
171. Corradino RA: Hydrocortisone and vitamin D_3 stimulation of ^{32}Pi-phosphate accumulation by organ-culture chick embryo duodenum. *Hor Metab Res* 11:519, 1979.
172. Corry BC et al: Intestinal absorption of phosphate, in Massry SG, Glassock RJ (eds): *Textbook of Nephrology*, 2d ed. Baltimore, Williams & Wilkins, 1989, p 328.
173. Corvilain J, Abramow M: Effect of growth hormone on tubular transport of phosphate in normal and parathyroidectomized dogs. *J Clin Invest* 43:1608, 1964.
174. Corvilain J, Abramow M: Growth and renal control of plasma phosphate. *J Clin Endocrinol* 34:452, 1972.
175. Corvilain J, Abramow M: Some effects of human growth

hormone on renal hemodynamics and on tubular phosphate transport in man. *J Clin Invest* 41:1230, 1963.

176. Coudrier E et al: Cytoskeleton organization and submembranous interactions in intestinal and renal brush borders. *Kidney Int* 34:309, 1988.
177. Craik JD, Reithmeier RAF: Inhibition of phosphate transport in human enthrocytes by water-soluble carbodiimides. *Biochim Biophys Acta* 778:429, 1984.
178. Cramer CF: Effect of Ca/P ratio and pH on calcium and phosphorus absorption from dog gut loop in vivo. *Can J Physiol Pharmacol* 461:171, 1968.
179. Cramer CF, McMillan J: Phosphorus adaptation in rats in absence of vitamin D or parathyroid glands. *Am J Physiol* 239:G261, 1980.
180. Cramer CF et al: The effect of chicken and hog calcitonin on some parameters of Ca, P and Mg metabolism in dogs. *Can J Physiol Pharmacol* 47:181, 1969.
181. Crawford AL et al: The effect of glucagon on blood sugar and inorganic phosphorus levels in normothermic and hypothermic rats. *Can J Physiol Pharmacol* 43:601, 1965.
182. Crawford JD et al: Mechanisms of renal tubular phosphate reabsorption and the influence thereon of vitamin D in completely parathyroidectomized rats. *Am J Physiol* 180:156, 1955.
183. Cross HS, Peterlik M: Effects of vitamin D and insulin on phosphate transport in the differentiating chick small intestine, in Bronner F, Peterlik M (eds): *Calcium and Phosphate Transport across Biomembranes.* New York, Academic Press, 1981, p 293.
184. Cross HS et al: Intestinal phosphate and calcium absorption: Joint regulation by thyroid hormones and 1,25-dihydroxyvitamin D_3. *Acta Endocrinol (Copenhagen)* 113:96, 1986.
185. Cross HS et al: Mechanism and regulation of intestinal phosphate absorption. *Miner Electrolyte Metab* 16:115, 1990.
186. Cuche JL et al: Intrarenal calcium in phosphate handling. *Am J Physiol* 230:790, 1976a.
187. Cuche JL et al: Lack of effect of hypocalcemia on renal phosphate handling. *J Lab Clin Med* 88:271, 1976.
188. Cuche JL et al: Phosphaturic effect of dopamine in dogs. *J Clin Invest* 58:71, 1976.
189. Cuisinier-Gleizes P et al: Phosphorus deficiency, parathyroid hormone and bone resorption in the growing rats. *Calcif Tissue Int Res* 20:235, 1976.
190. Danisi G et al: Effect of pH on phosphate transport into intestinal brush-border membrane vesicles. *Am J Physiol* 246:G180, 1984.
191. Danisi G et al: Phosphate transport across brush border and basolateral membrane vesicles of small intestine, in Bronner F, Peterlik H (eds): *Epithelial Calcium and Phosphate Transport: Molecular and Cellular Aspects.* New York, Liss, 1984, p 229.
192. Danisi G et al: Regulation of Na-dependent phosphate influx across the mucosal border of duodenum by 1,25-dihydroxycholecalciferol. *Pfluegers Arch* 388:227, 1980.
193. Davenport HW (ed): *Physiology of the Digestive Tract.* Chicago, Year Book Medical, 1966.
194. Davis JO et al: II. Renal hemodynamic function, electrolyte metabolism and water exchange in adrenalectomized hypophysectomized dogs. *Am J Physiol* 176:411, 1954.
195. Day HG, McCollum EV: Mineral metabolism, growth, symptomatology of rats on diet extremely deficient in phosphorus. *J Biol Chem* 130:269, 1939.
196. Debiec H, Lorenc R: Identification of Na^+-Pi-binding protein in kidney and intestinal brush-border membranes. *Biochem J* 225:185, 1988.
197. DeFronzo RA et al: The effect of insulin on renal handling of sodium, potassium, calcium and phosphate in man. *J Clin Invest* 55:845, 1975.
198. DeFronzo RA et al: The effects of glucose and insulin on renal electrolyte transport. *J Clin Invest* 58:83, 1976.
199. Dennis VW: Influence of bicarbonate on parathyroid hormone-induced changes in fluid absorption by the proximal tubule. *Kidney Int* 10:373, 1976.
200. Dennis VW, Brazy PC: Divalent anion transport in isolated renal tubules. *Kidney Int* 22:498, 1982.
201. Dennis VW et al: Characteristics of phosphate transport in isolated proximal tubule. *Am J Physiol* 231:979, 1976.
202. Dennis VW et al: Response of phosphate transport to parathyroid hormone in segments of rabbit nephron. *Am J Physiol* 233:F29, 1977.
203. Dent CE, Gartner JM: Hypophosphatemia osteomalacia in fibrous dysplasia. *Q J Med* 45:411, 1976.
204. deRouffignac C et al: Micropuncture study of water and electrolyte movement along the loop of Henle in *Psammomys* with special reference to magnesium, calcium and phosphorus. *Pfluegers Arch* 344:309, 1973.
205. DeVries JR et al: Estradiol renal receptor molecules and estradiol-dependent antinatriuresis. *Kidney Int* 2:95, 1972.
206. DiBona GF: Effect of hypercalcemia on renal tubular sodium handling in the rat. *Am J Physiol* 220:49, 1971.
207. Dirks JH, Seely JF: Effect of saline infusions and furosemide on the dog distal nephron. *Am J Physiol* 219:114, 1970.
208. Dominguez JH et al: Dietary phosphate deprivation in women and men: Effects of mineral and acid balances, parathyroid hormone and the metabolism of 25-OH-vitamin D. *J Clin Endocrinol Metab* 43:1056, 1976.
209. Donker AJM et al: Indomethancin in Bartter's syndrome. *Nephron* 19:200, 1977.
210. Dousa TP: Effects of hormone on cyclic AMP formation in kidneys of nonmammalian vertebrates. *Am J Physiol* 226:1193, 1974.
211. Dousa TP, Kempson SA: Regulation of renal brush border membrane transport of phosphate. *Miner Electrolyte Metab* 7:113, 1982.
212. Dousa TP et al: Adaptive changes in renal cortical brush border membrane. *Adv Exp Med Biol* 128:69, 1980.
213. Dousa TP et al: Effect of colchicine on urinary phosphate and regulation by parathyroid hormone. *Am J Physiol* 231:61, 1976.
214. Drezner MK, Feinglos MN: Osteomalacia due to 1α,25-dihydroxycholecalciferol deficiency. *J Clin Invest* 60:1046, 1977.
215. Duarte CG: Effects of ethacrynic acid and furosemide on urinary phosphate in the dog. *Clin Sci* 46:671, 1974.
216. Durand D et al: Effets precoces de l'hormone de crois-

sance sur les phosphates seriques et urinaires du rat. *Experientia* 32:120, 1976.
217. Edwards BR et al: Effect of calcium infusion on renal tubular reabsorption in the dog. *Am J Physiol* 227:13, 1974.
218. Eisenberg E: Effects of serum calcium level and parathyroid extracts on phosphate and calcium excretion in hypoparathyroid patients. *J Clin Invest* 44:942, 1965.
219. Eisenberg E: Effects of varying phosphate intake in primary hyperparathyroidism. *J Clin Endocrinol Metab* 28:651, 1968.
220. Eisenberg E: Renal effects of parathyroid hormone, in Talmage RV, Belanger LF (eds): *Parathyroid Hormone and Thyrocalcitonin (Calcitonin)*. Amsterdam, Excerpta Medica, 1968, p 465.
221. Eknoyan G et al: Effect of diuretics on urinary excretion of phosphate, calcium and magnesium in thyroparathyroidectomized dogs. *J Lab Clin Med* 76:257, 1970.
222. Elganish A et al: In vitro effects of vitamin D3 on the phospholipids of isolated renal brush border membranes. *J Membr Biol* 72:85, 1983.
223. Ellsworth R: Studies on the physiology of the parathyroid glands: 5. Action of parathyroid extract on the renal threshold of phosphorus. *J Clin Invest* 11:1011, 1932.
224. Elrick H et al: Effects of glucagon on renal function in man. *J Clin Endocrinol Metab* 18:813, 1958.
225. Emmerson GH et al: Serum thyrotropin and thyroxine concentration in patients receiving lithium carbonate. *J Clin Endocrinol Metab* 36:338, 1973.
226. Emmett M et al: The pathophysiology of acid-base changes in chronically phosphate-depleted rats: Bone-kidney interaction. *J Clin Invest* 59:291, 1977.
227. Epstein M et al: Failure of water immersion to influence parathyroid hormone secretion and renal phosphate handling in normal man. *J Lab Clin Med* 87:218, 1976.
228. Escoubet B et al: Adaptation to P_i deprivation of cell Na-dependent P_i uptake: A widespread process. *AM J Physiol* 256:C322, 1989.
229. Espinosa RE et al: Effects of thyroxine administration on phosphate transport across renal brush border membrane. *Am J Physiol* 246:F133, 1984.
230. Estep HL et al: Hypocalcemia due to hypomagnesemia and reversible parathyroid hormone unresponsiveness. *J Clin Endocrinol Metab* 29:842, 1969.
231. Estep HL et al: Phosphate excretion patterns following intravenous injection of ethylenediaminetetraacetate (EDTA). *J Clin Endocrinol Metab* 25:1385, 1965.
232. Farrington K et al: Dissociation of absorption of calcium and phosphate after successful cadavaric renal transplantation. *Br Med J* 1:712, 1979.
233. Feaster JP et al: P32 distribution and excretion in rats fed vitamin D-free and low phosphorus diets. *J Nutr* 51:381, 1953.
234. Fernandez PD, Puschett JB: Proximal tubular actions of metolazone and chlorothiazide. *Am J Physiol* 225:954, 1973.
235. Ferraro C et al: Intestinal absorption of phosphate: Action of protein synthesis inhibitors and glucocorticoids in the rat. *J Nutr* 106:1752, 1976.
236. Fimognari GM et al: Induction of RNA and protein synthesis in the action of aldosterone in the rat. *Am J Physiol* 213:954, 1967.
237. Follis HR Jr: Diseases, particularly of bone, associated with derangements of calcium and phosphorus metabolism, in Reifenstein EC Jr (ed): *Metabolic Interactions*. New York, Josiah Macy Jr Foundation, 1953, p 210.
238. Fordtran JS, Locklear TW: Ionic constituents and osmolarity of gastric and small-intestinal fluids after eating. *Am J Dig Dis* 11:503, 1966.
239. Forland M: Effect of estradiol on phosphorus excretion in intact and hypophysectomized rats. *Endocrinology* 83:516, 1968.
240. Forrest JN et al: On the mechanism of lithium induced diabetes insipidus in man and the rat. *J Clin Invest* 53:1115, 1974.
241. Fotino S: Phosphate excretion in chronic renal failure: Evidence for a mechanism other than circulating parathyroid hormone. *Clin Nephrol* 8:499, 1977.
242. Foulks JG, Perry FA: Renal excretion of phosphate following parathyroidectomy in dog. *Am J Physiol* 196:554, 1959.
243. Fox MS et al: Impaired renal tubular function induced by sugar infusion in man. *J Clin Endocrinol Metab* 24:1318, 1964.
244. Frantz AG, Rabkin MT: Effects of estrogen and sex difference on secretion of human growth hormone. *J Clin Endocrinol Metab* 25:1470, 1965.
245. Frarese RV et al: The phosphatidate-polyphosphoinositide cycle: Activation by parathyroid hormone and dibutyryl-cAMP in rabbit kidney cortex, in Scott WN, Goodman DB (eds): Hormonal regulation of epithelial transport of ions and water. *Ann N Y Acad Science* 372:539, 1981.
246. Freeman D et al: Energetics of sodium transport in the kidney: Saturation transfer ^{31}P-NMR. *Biochim Biophys Acta* 762:325, 1983.
247. Freeman S, McLean FC: Experimental rickets: Blood and tissue changes in puppies receiving a diet very low in phosphorus with and without vitamin D. *Arch Pathol Lab Med* 32:387, 1941.
248. Freiberg JM et al: Glucocorticoids increase the Na^+-H^+ exchange and decrease the Na^+-gradient dependent phosphate uptake system in renal brush border membrane vesicles. *Proc Natl Acad Sci U S A* 79:4932, 1982.
249. Frick A: Mechanism of inorganic phosphate diuresis secondary to saline infusions in the rat. *Pfluegers Arch* 313:106, 1969.
250. Frick A: Proximal tubule reabsorption of inorganic phosphate during saline infusion in the rat. *Am J Physiol* 223:1034, 1972.
251. Frick A, Durasin I: Effect of expansion of extracellular fluid volume on the maximal reabsorptive capacity for inorganic phosphate in parathyroidectomized and intact rats. *Pfluegers Arch* 370:115, 1977.
252. Fuchs R, Peterlik M: Intestinal phosphate transport, in Massry SG et al (eds): *Phosphate and Minerals in Health and Disease*. New York, Plenum, 1980, p 381.
253. Fuick RF et al: Effect of glucocorticoids on function of the parathyroid glands in man. *J Clin Endocrinol Metab* 40:152, 1975.

254. Fulop M, Brazeau P: The phosphaturic effect of sodium bicarbonate and acetazolamide in dogs. *J Clin Invest* 47:983, 1968.
255. Gallagher JC, Nordin BEC: Treatment with estrogens of primary hyperparathyroidism in post-menopausal women. *Lancet* 1:503, 1972.
256. Gantt CL, Carter WJ: Acute effects of angiotensin on calcium, phosphorus, magnesium and potassium excretion. *Can Med Assoc J* 90:287, 1964.
257. Garabedian M et al: 1,25-dihydroxycholecalciterol effect on serum phosphorus homeostasis in rats. *Endocrinology* 98:794, 1976.
258. Gekle D: Der Einfluss von synthetischem Calcitonin auf die proximal-tubulare Phosphatresorption. *Klin Wochenschr* 50:527, 1972.
259. Gekle D, von Carlowitz B: Micropuncture investigations on the effect of angiotensin on the inorganic phosphate reabsorption in the proximal tubule of the rat. *Pfluegers Arch* 342:73, 1973.
260. Gekle D et al: The effect of vitamin D on renal inorganic phosphate reabsorption of normal rats, parathyroidectomized rats, and rats with rickets. *Pediatr Res* 5:40, 1971.
261. Gellissen K, Brodehl J: Clearance-Untersuchungen bei Sauglingen mit angeborene Athyreosen. *Klin Wochenschr* 43:1063, 1965.
262. Gemzell CA, Samuels LT: The effect of hypophysectomy, adrenalectomy and of ACTH administration on the phosphorus metabolism of rats. *Endocrinology* 47:48, 1950.
263. George ER et al: Cyclic adenosine monophosphate dependent and independent protein kinase activity of renal brush border membranes. *Arch Biochem Biophys* 180:429, 1977.
264. Gershberg H: Metabolic and renotropic effects of human growth hormone in disease. *J Clin Endocrinol Metab* 20:1107, 1960.
265. Gershberg H, Gash J: Effect of growth hormone on sulfate Tm, urea clearance and fasting blood glucose. *Proc Soc Exp Biol Med* 91:46, 1956.
266. Ghishan FK et al: Phosphate transport by jejunal brush border membrane vesicles of the streptozo tocin-diabetic rat. *Diabetes* 34:7323, 1985.
267. Ghishan FK et al: Phosphate transport by rat intestinal basolateral-membrane vesicles. *Biochem J* 243:641, 1987.
268. Ginn HE, Shanbour LL: Phosphaturia in magnesium deficient rats. *Am J Physiol* 212:1347, 1967.
269. Ginsburg JM: Effect of glucose and free fatty acid oı phosphate transport in dog kidney. *Am J Physiol* 222:1153, 1972.
270. Gitleman HJ et al: The influence of parathyroid glands on the hypercalcemia of experimental magnesium depletion in the rat. *J Clin Invest* 47:118, 1968.
271. Gloor HJ et al: Resistance to the phosphaturic and calcemic actions of parathyroid hormone during phosphate depletion: Prevention by 1,25-dihydroxyvitamin D3. *J Clin Invest* 63:371, 1979.
272. Glorieux F, Scriver CR: Loss of a parathyroid hormone-sensitive component of phosphate transport in X-linked hypophosphatemia. *Science* 175:997, 1972.
273. Gmaj P et al: Calcium transport in isolated and reconstituted basolateral plasma membranes of rat kidney cortex, in Bronner F, Peterlik M (eds): *Epithelial Calcium and Phosphate Transport: Molecular and Cellular Aspects.* New York, Liss, 1984, p 337.
274. Gmaj P et al: Intravesicular NAD has no effect on sodium-dependent phosphate transport in isolated renal brush border membrane vesicles. *Pfluegers Arch* 400:60, 1984.
275. Goldberg M et al: Renal handling of phosphate, calcium and magnesium, in Brenner BM, Rector FC Jr (eds): *The Kidney.* Philadelphia, Saunders, 1976, vol 1, p 344.
276. Goldfarb S: Juxtamedullary and superficial nephron phosphate reabsorption in the cat. *Am J Physiol* 239:F336, 1980.
277. Goldfarb S et al: Dissociation between the sites of action of PTH and saline on renal phosphate reabsorption. *Clin Res* 22:528A, 1974.
278. Goldfarb S et al: Effects of calcium on renal tubular phosphate reabsorption. *Am J Physiol* 234:F22, 1978.
279. Goldman R, Bassett SH: Effect of intravenous calcium gluconate upon the excretion of calcium and phosphorus in patients with idiopathic hypoparathyroidism. *J Clin Endocrinol Metab* 14:278, 1954.
280. Goldman R, Bassett SH: Renal regulation of phosphorus excretion. *J Clin Endocrinol Metab* 18:981, 1958.
281. Goldsmith RS et al: Primary role of plasma hydrocortisone concentration in the regulation of normal forenoon pattern of urinary phosphate excretion. *J Clin Endocrinol Metab* 25:1649, 1965.
282. Goldstein DA et al: The duodenal mucosa in patients with renal failure: Response to $1{,}25(OH)_2D_3$. *Kidney Int* 19:324, 1981.
283. Goligorsky MS et al: Cytoplasmic Ca^{2+} in individual proximal tubular cells in culture: Effects of parathyroid hormone. *Am J Physiol* 251:F938, 1986.
284. Gradowska L et al: On the mechanism of the phosphaturia of extracellular fluid volume expansion in the dog. *Kidney Int* 3:230, 1973.
285. Greenwald I, Gross J: The effect of the administration of a potent parathyroid extract upon the excretion of nitrogen, phosphorus, calcium and magnesium, with some remarks on the solubility of calcium phosphate in serum and on the pathogenesis of tetany. *J Biol Chem* 66:217, 1925.
286. Greger RF et al: Site of renal phosphate reabsorption: Micropuncture and microinfusion study. *Pfluegers Arch* 369:111, 1977.
287. Grinstein S et al: Inorganic anion transport in kidney and intestinal brush border and basolateral membranes. *Am J Physiol* 238:F452, 1980.
288. Guder WG: Hormonal regulation of renal gluconeogenesis in isolated tubule fragments, in Schmidt U, Dubach UC (eds): *Current Problems in Clinical Biochemistry*, vol 6, *Renal Metabolism in Relation to Renal Function.* Bern, Hans Huber 1976, p 202.
289. Haack D et al: Comparative study on development of corticosterone and DOCA hypertension in rats. *Am J Physiol* 233:F403, 1977.
290. Haas JA et al: Phosphaturic effect of furosemide: Role of PTH and carbonic anhydrase. *Am J Physiol* 232:F105, 1977.
291. Haddad JG Jr et al: Effects of prolonged thyrocalcitonin administration on Paget's disease of bone. *N Engl J Med* 283:549, 1970.

292. Hadvarg P, Kadenbach B: Identification of a membrane protein involved in mitochondrial phosphate transport. *Eur J Biochem* 67:573, 1976.
293. Halden A et al: Parathyroid hormone and phosphate homeostasis in man. *Acta Endocrinol* 46:285, 1964.
294. Ham LL et al: Effect of luminal pH and HCO_3^- on phosphate reabsorption in the rabbit proximal convoluted tubule. *Am J Physiol* 247:F25, 1984.
295. Hamilton CR: Effects of synthetic salmon calcitonin in patients with Paget's disease of bone. *Am J Med* 56:315, 1970.
296. Hammerman MR: Interaction of insulin with renal proximal tubular cell. *Am J Physiol* 249:F1, 1985.
297. Hammerman MR, Hruska KA: Cyclic AMP-dependent protein phosphorylation in canine renal brush border membrane vesicles is associated with decreased phosphate transport. *J Biol Chem* 257:992, 1982.
298. Hammerman MR, Schwab SJ: Phosphate transport in the kidney. Studies with isolated membrane vesicles, in Bronner F, Peterlik M (eds): *Epithelial Calcium and Phosphate Transport: Molecular and Cellular Aspects.* New York, Liss, 1984, p 325.
299. Hammerman MR et al: ADP ribosylation of canine renal brush border membrane vesicle proteins is associated with decreased phosphate transport. *J Biol Chem* 257:12380, 1982.
300. Hammerman MR et al: Effect of parathyroid hormone on Na^+-dependent phosphate transport and cAMP-dependent ^{32}P phosphorylation in brush border vesicles from isolated perfused canine kidneys. *Arch Biochem Biophys* 227:91, 1983.
301. Hammerman MR et al: Insulin stimulates Pi transport in brush border vesicles from proximal tubular segments. *Am J Physiol* 247:E616, 1984.
302. Hammerman MR et al: NAD^+-induced inhibition of phosphate transport in canine renal brush border membranes: Mediation through a process other than or in addition to NAD^+ hydrolysis. *Biochim Biophys Acta* 732:110, 1983.
303. Hammerman MR et al: Regulation of canine renal vesicle Pi transport by growth hormone and parathyroid hormone. *Biochim Biophys Acta* 603:322, 1980.
304. Hammond TG et al: Administration of atrial natriuretic factor inhibits sodium-coupled transport in proximal tubules. *J Clin Invest* 75:1983, 1985.
305. Hammond TG et al: Synthetic atrial natriuretic factor decreases renal tubular phosphate reabsorption in rats. *Am J Physiol* 249:F315, 1985.
306. Harden R McG et al: Phosphate excretion and parathyroid function in thyrotoxicosis. *J Endocrinol* 28:281, 1964.
307. Harris CA et al: Composition of mammalian glomerular filtrate. *Am J Physiol* 227:972, 1974.
308. Harrison HE, Harrison HC: Intestinal transport of phosphate: Action of vitamin D, calcium and potassium. *Am J Physiol* 201:1007, 1961.
309. Harrison HE, Harrison HC: The renal excretion of inorganic phosphate in relation to the action of vitamin D and parathyroid hormone. *J Clin Invest* 20:47, 1941.
310. Harrison HE, Harrison HC: Sodium, potassium and intestinal transport of glucose, L-tyrosine, phosphate and calcium. *Am J Physiol* 295: 107, 1963.
311. Harrison HE, Harrison HC: Vitamin D and permeability of intestinal mucosa to calcium. *Am J Physiol* 208:370, 1965.
312. Harrop GA Jr, Benedict EM: The participation of inorganic substances in carbohydrate metabolism. *J Biol Chem* 59:683, 1924.
313. Harrop GA Jr, Benedict EM: The role of phosphate and potassium in carbohydrate metabolism following insulin administration. *Proc Soc Exp Biol Med* 20:430, 1923.
314. Hass HG, Dambacher M: Thyrocalcitonin effects in man. *Helv Chir Acta* 34:327, 1968.
315. Hass JA et al: Failure to detect papillary collecting duct phosphate reabsorption in thyroparathyroidectomized rats. *Miner Electrolyte Metab* 3:146, 1980.
316. Hass JA et al: Nephron heterogeneity of phosphate reabsorption. *Am J Physiol* 234:F287, 1978.
317. Hausmann E: Change in plasma phosphate concentration on infusion of calcium gluconate or Na2EDTA. *Proc Soc Exp Biol Med* 134:182, 1970.
318. Heany RP: Evaluation and interpretation of calcium-kinetics data in man. *Clin Orthop* 31:153, 1963.
319. Heany RP, Skillman TG: Calcium metabolism in normal human pregnancy. *J Clin Endocrinol Metab* 33:661, 1971.
320. Heaton FW, Hodgkinson A: External factors affecting diurnal variation in electrolyte excretion with particular reference to calcium and magnesium. *Clin Chim Acta* 8:246, 1963.
321. Heersche JNM et al: Calcitonin and the formation of 3′,5′-AMP in bone and kidney. *Endocrinology* 94:241, 1974.
322. Heidenreich O et al: Stoffwechselwirkungen von synthetischem Angiotensin II. *Arch Int Pharmacodyn Ther* 148:309, 1964.
323. Heidland A et al: Untersuchungen zur Pathophysiologie der renalen Phosphatexkretion bei essentieller und renovascularer Hypertonie, Pyelonephritis und Blomerulonephritis. *Klin Wochenschr* 49:1121, 1971.
324. Hems DA, Gaja G: Carbohydrate metabolism in the isolated perfused rat kidney. *Biochem J* 128:412, 1972.
325. Henneman PH et al: Effects of human growth hormone in man. *J Clin Invest* 39:1223, 1960.
326. Herbert CS et al: Decreased phosphate reabsorption by volume expansion in the dog. *Kidney Int* 7:247, 1972.
327. Hevesy G, DalSanto G: Effect of adrenalin on the interaction between plasma and tissue constituents. *Acta Physiol Scand* 32:339, 1954.
328. Hiatt HH, Thompson DD: Some effects of intravenously administered calcium on inorganic phosphate metabolism. *J Clin Invest* 36:573, 1957.
329. Ho MK, Guidotti G: A membrane protein from human erythrocytes involved in anion exchange. *J Biol Chem* 250:675, 1975.
330. Hoffman N et al: Phosphate transport by isolated renal brush border vesicles. *Pfluegers Arch* 362:147, 1976.
331. Hopfer UK et al: Differences in neutral amino acid and glucose transport between brush border and basolateral membrane of intestinal epithelial cells. *J Cell Physiol* 89:805, 1976.

332. Hopkins TR et al: Ultrafiltration studies on calcium and phosphorus in human serum. *Bull Johns Hopkins Med J* 93:249, 1952.
333. Hopkins TR et al: Ultrafiltration studies on calcium and phosphorus in pathological human serum. *Bull Johns Hopkins Med J* 93:249, 1953.
334. Hoppe A et al: Effect of respiratory alkalosis on renal phosphate excretion. *Am J Physiol* 243:F471, 1982.
335. Howard JE: Normal calcium and phosphorus transport in body fluid homeostasis, in Reifenstein EC Jr (ed): *Metabolic Interactions*. New York, Josiah Macy Jr Foundation, 1953, p 11.
336. Howard JE et al: On certain physiologic responses to intravenous injection of calcium salts into normal, hyperparathyroid and hypoparathyroid persons. *J Clin Endocrinol Metab* 13:1, 1953.
337. Hruska KA, Hammerman MR: Parathyroid hormone inhibition of phosphate transport in renal brush border vesicles from phosphate-depleted dogs. *Biochim Biophys Acta* 645:351, 1981.
338. Hruska KA et al: Effects of parathyroid hormone on cytosolic calcium in renal proximal tubular primary cultures. *Am J Physiol* 251:F188, 1986.
339. Hruska KA et al: Stimulation of inositol triphosphate and diacylglycerol production in renal tubular cells by parathyroid hormone. *J Clin Invest* 79:230, 1987.
340. Humes HD et al: Evidence for a parathyroid hormone dependent influence of calcium on the glomerular ultrafiltration coefficient. *J Clin Invest* 61:32, 1978.
341. Humphreys MH et al: Natriuresis produced by vasopressin or hemorrhage during water diuresis in the dog. *Am J Physiol* 219:658, 1970.
342. Iino Y, Burg MB: Effect of parathyroid hormone on bicarbonate absorption by proximal tubules in vitro. *Am J Physiol* 236:F387, 1979.
343. Ikkos D et al: The effect of human growth hormone in man. *Acta Endocrinol* 32:341, 1959.
344. Imrie MJ et al: Circadian variations in renal and adrenal-function: Are they connected? in Williams PC (ed): *Hormone and the Kidney*. New York, Academic Press, 1973, p 3.
345. Ingbar SH et al: The effects of ACTH and cortisone on the renal tubular transport of uric acid, phosphorus, and electrolytes in patients with normal renal and adrenal function. *J Lab Clin Med* 38:533, 1951.
346. Jastrup B et al: Serum levels of vitamin D metabolites and bone remodeling in hyperthyroidism. *Metabolism* 31:126, 1982.
347. Jobin J et al: Effect of acetazolamide on renal bicarbonate reabsorption in volume-expanded dogs. *Am J Physiol* 232:F484, 1977.
348. Johny KV et al: Amiloride hydrochloride, a hypercalciuric diuretic. *Aust N Z J Med* 18:267, 1969.
349. Jones JE et al: Magnesium metabolism in hyperthyroidism and hypothyroidism. *J Clin Invest* 45:891, 1966.
350. Juan D et al: Absorption of inorganic phosphate in the human jejunum and its inhibition by salmon calcitonin. *J Clin Endocrinol Metab* 43:517, 1976.
351. Karlinsky ML et al: Effect of parathormone and cyclic AMP on renal bicarbonate reabsorption. *Am J Physiol* 227:1226, 1974.
352. Karr WC, Abbott WO: Intubation studies of the human small intestine: 4. Chemical characteristics of the intestinal contents in the fasting state and as influenced by the administration of acids, of alkalines and of water. *J Clin Invest* 14:893, 1935.
353. Katz AI, Lindheimer MD: Actions of hormones on the kidney. *Annu Rev Physiol* 39:97, 1977.
354. Katz AI, Lindheimer MD: Renal sodium- and potassium-activated adenosine triphosphatase and sodium reabsorption in the hypothyroid rat. *J Clin Invest* 52:796, 1973.
355. Kelly P et al: Relationship between serum phosphate concentration and bone resorption in osteoporosis. *J Lab Clin Med* 69:110, 1967.
356. Kempson SA: Effect of metabolic acidosis on renal brush border membrane adaptation to low phosphate diet. *Kidney Int* 22:225, 1982.
357. Kempson SA, Dousa TP: Phosphate transport across renal cortical brush border membrane vesicles from rats stabilized on a normal, high or low phosphate diet. *Life Sci* 24:881, 1979.
358. Kempson SA, Curthoys NP: NAD^+-dependent ADP-ribosyltransferase in renal brush border membranes. *Am J Physiol* 245:C449, 1983.
359. Kempson SA et al: Endocytosis and Na^+/solute cotransport in renal epithelial cells. *J Biol Chem* 264:18451, 1989.
360. Kempson SA et al: Parathyroid hormone action on phosphate transport is inhibited by high osmolality. *Am J Physiol* 258:F1336, 1990.
361. Kempson SA et al: Possible role of nicotinamide adenine dinucleotide as an intracellular regulator of renal transport of phosphate in the rat. *J Clin Invest* 67:1347, 1981.
362. Kempson SA et al: Renal brush border membrane adaptation to phosphorus deprivation: Effects of fasting versus low-phosphorus diet. *Kidney Int* 18:36, 1980.
363. Kenny AD: Effect of catecholamines on serum calcium and phosphorus levels in intact and parathyroidectomized rats. *Naunyn-Schmiedeberg's Arch Exp Pathol Pharmakol* 248:144, 1964.
364. Kenny AD: Vitamin D metabolism: Physiological regulation in egg-laying Japanese quail. *Am J Physiol* 230:1609, 1976.
365. Kenny AD, Heiskell CA: Effect of crude thyrocalcitonin on calcium and phosphorus metabolism in rats. *Proc Soc Exp Biol Med* 120:269, 1965.
366. Kessler RJ, Vaughn DA: Divalent metal is required for both phosphate transport and phosphate binding to phosphorin, a proteolipid isolated from brush border membrane vesicles. *J Biol Chem* 259:9059, 1984.
367. Kessler RJ et al: Phosphate-binding proteolipid from brush border. *J Biol Chem* 257:14311, 1982.
368. Kikuchi K, Ghishan FK: Phosphate transport by basolateral plasma membranes of human small intestine. *Gastroenterology* 93:106, 1987.
369. Kikuyama S et al: Effect of perinatal hypothyroidism on pituitary secretion of growth hormone and prolactin in rats. *J Endocrinol* 62:213, 1974.
370. Kimmich GA: Energetics of Na^+-dependent sugar transport by isolated intestinal cells: Evidence for a major role for membrane potential. *Am J Physiol* 233:E357, 1977.
371. Kinne R et al: Distribution of membrane bound cyclic

AMP-dependent protein kinase in the plasma membrane of cells of the kidney cortex. *J Membr Biol* 24:145, 1975.
372. Kinsella J, Sacktor B: Thyroid hormones increase Na^+-H^+ exchange activity in renal brush border membranes. *Proc Natl Acad Sci U S A* 82:3606, 1985.
373. Kivirikko KI et al: Value of urine and serum hydroxyproline in the diagnosis of thyroid disease. *J Clin Endocrinol* 25:1347, 1965.
374. Kjerult-Jenson K: Excretion of phosphorus by the bowel. *Acta Physiol Scand* 3:1, 1941.
375. Kleeman CR et al: Calcium and phosphorus metabolism and bone disease in uremia. *Clin Orthop* 68:210, 1970.
376. Klein R, Gow RC: Interactions of parathyroid hormone and vitamin D on the renal excretion of phosphate. *J Clin Endocrinol Metab* 13:271, 1953.
377. Klisiechi A, Pytasz M: Uber die Rolle einiger Neurohormone auf die renale Phosphatausscheidung. *Helv Physiol Pharmacol Acta* 58:81, 1961.
378. Knochel JP: The pathophysiology and clinical characteristics of severe hypophosphatemia. *Arch Intern Med* 127:203, 1977.
379. Knox FG: The intrarenal metabolism of phosphate. *Physiologist* 20:25, 1977.
380. Knox FG, Lechenen C: Distal site of action of parathyroid hormone on phosphate reabsorption. *Am J Physiol* 229:1556, 1975.
381. Knox FG et al: Cellular mechanisms of phosphate transport, in Massry SG, Fleisch H (eds): *Renal Phosphate Handling of Phosphate*. New York, Plenum, 1980, p 79.
382. Knox FG et al: Effect of furosemide on sodium reabsorption by the proximal tubule in the dog. *Am J Physiol* 217:192, 1969.
383. Knox FG et al: Effect on parathyroid hormone on phosphate reabsorption in the presence of acetazolamide. *Kidney Int* 10:216, 1976.
384. Knox FG et al: Mechanisms of resistance to the phosphaturic effect of the parathyroid hormone in the hamster. *J Clin Invest* 59:675, 1977.
385. Knox FG et al: Nephron sites of adaptation to changes in dietary phosphate. *Adv Exp Med Biol* 151:13, 1982.
386. Knox FG et al: Phosphate transport along the nephron. *Am J Physiol* 233:F261, 1977.
387. Knox FG et al: Phosphate transport in superficial and deep nephrons in phosphate-loaded rats. *Am J Physiol* 233:F150, 1977.
388. Knox FG et al: Proximal tubule reabsorption after hyperoncotic albumin infusion. *J Clin Invest* 53:501, 1974.
389. Kocsis JJ: Uptake of P-32 into various phosphorus-containing fractions in the brain of normal, hypophysectomized and ACTH-treated hypophysectomized rats. *Endocrinology* 59:591, 1956.
390. Kopple JD, Coburn JW: Metabolic studies of low protein diets in uremia: 2. Calcium, phosphorus and magnesium. *Medicine* 52:597, 1973.
391. Kowarski S, Schachter D: Effects of vitamin D on phosphate transport and incorporation into mucosal constituents of rat intestinal mucosa. *J Biol Chem* 244:211, 1969.
392. Kreusser WJ et al: Phosphate depletion: Effect on renal inorganic phosphate and adenine nucleotides, urinary phosphate and calcium, and calcium balance. *Miner Electrolyte Metab* 1:30, 1978.
393. Kumar R et al: Elevated 1,25-dihydroxyvitamin D plasma levels in normal pregnancy and lactation. *J Clin Invest* 63:342, 1979.
394. Kuntziger HE et al: Effects of parathyroidectomy and cyclic AMP on renal transport of phosphate, calcium and magnesium. *Am J Physiol* 227:905, 1974.
395. Kuntziger HE et al: Localization of parathyroid hormone-independent sodium bicarbonate inhibition of tubular phosphate reabsorption. *Kidney Int* 17:749, 1980.
396. Kupfer S, Kosovsky JD: Renal intracellular phosphate and phosphate excretion. *Mt Sinai J Med* 37:359, 1970.
397. Kurnik BRC et al: 1,25-Dihydroxycholexcalciferol stimulates renal phosphate transport by directly altering membrane phosphatidylcholine composition. *Biochim Biophys Acta* 917:81, 1987.
398. Kuroda S et al: Relationship between proximal tubule total CO_2 and phosphate reabsorption in acute and chronic PTX rats. *Renal Physiol* 3:171, 1979.
399. Kurokawa K et al: Effects of calcitonin on the concentration of cyclic adenosine 3′,5′-monophosphate in rat kidney in vivo and in vitro. *Endocrinology* 94:1514, 1974.
400. Kurokawa K et al: Ionic control of renal gluconeogenesis: 2. The effects of Ca^{++} and H^+ upon the response to parathyroid hormone and cyclic AMP. *Biochim Biophys Acta* 313:32, 1973.
401. Kurtzman NA et al: The effect of infusion of pharmacologic amounts of vasopressin on renal electrolyte excretion. *Am J Physiol* 228:890, 1975.
402. Kwawitt EL et al: Calcium absorption and brush border phosphatases following dietary calcium restriction. *Am J Physiol* 224:548, 1973.
403. Kyle LH et al: Inhibitory effects of induced hypercalcemia on secretion of parathyroid hormone. *J Clin Endocrinol Metab* 22:52, 1962.
404. Kyle LH et al: The metabolic effects of intravenous administration of calcium. *J Lab Clin Med* 43:123, 1954.
405. Laidlaw JC et al: Comparison of metabolic effects of cortisone and hydrocortisone in man. *Ann N Y Acad Sci* 61:315, 1955.
406. Lang F et al: Factors modulating the renal handling of phosphate. *Renal Physiol* 4:1, 1981.
407. Lang F et al: Stationary microperfusion study of phosphate reabsorption in proximal and distal nephron segments. *Pfluegers Arch* 368:45, 1977.
408. Lang RP et al: Nucleotide inhibition of phosphate transport in the renal proximal tubule. *Am J Physiol* 245:F263, 1983.
409. Lau K et al: Chronic phosphate depletion: Changes in segmental calcium and phosphate reabsorption, in *Abstracts of the 10th Annual Meeting of the American Society of Nephrology*. Washington, DC, American Society of Nephrology, 1977, p 6.
410. Lau K et al: The effects of parathyroid hormone on renal phosphate handling, in Massry SG, Fleisch H (eds): *Renal Handling of Phosphate*. New York, Plenum, 1980, p 115.
411. Lavender AR, Pullman TN: Changes in inorganic phosphate excretion induced by renal arterial infusion of calcium. *Am J Physiol* 205:1025, 1963.
412. Lechene C et al: Electron probe microanalysis of the renal effect of parathyroid hormone, in Copp DH, Talmage PV

(eds): *Endocrinology of Calcium Metabolism.* Amsterdam, Excerpta Medica, 1978, p 230.

413. Lee DBN et al: The biochemical indices of experimental phosphorus depletion: A re-examination of their physiological significance, in Massry SG et al (eds): *Homeostasis of Phosphate and Other Minerals.* New York, Plenum, 1978, p 382.
414. Lee DBN et al: Calcium and inorganic phosphate transport in rat colon: Dissociated response to 1,25-dihydroxyvitamin D3. *J Clin Invest* 65:1326, 1980.
415. Lee DBN et al: Disorders of phosphorus metabolism, in Bronner F, Coburn JW (eds): *Disorders of Mineral Metabolism.* New York, Academic Press, 1981, vol 3, p 283.
416. Lee DBN et al: Effect of phosphorus depletion on intestinal calcium and phosphorus absorption. *Am J Physiol* 236:E451, 1979.
417. Lee DBN et al: Intestinal phosphate absorption: Influence of vitamin D and non-vitamin D factors. *Am J Physiol* 250: G369, 1986.
418. Lee DBN et al: Jejunal phosphate transport is not mediated by the PTH-adenylate cyclase system: Further evidence on the contrasting features between intestinal and renal phosphate transport mechanisms. *Miner Electrolyte Metab* 12:293, 1986.
419. Lee DBN et al: Phosphate transport across rat jejunum: Influence of sodium, pH and 1,25-dihydroxyvitamin D_3. *Am J Physiol* 251:G90, 1986.
420. Lee DBN et al: Regulation of serum phosphorus by $1,25(OH)_2D_3$, in Norman AW et al (eds): *Vitamin D: Basic Research and Its Clinical Applications.* Berlin, de Gruyter, 1979, p 939.
421. Lee DBN et al: The role of growth hormone in experimental phosphorus depletion. *Calcif Tissue Int* 32:105, 1980.
422. LeGrimellec C, Lechene C: Renal effects of thyroid calcium infusion in parathyroidectomized rats: Electron probe analysis, in *Abstracts of the 4th Annual Meeting of the American Society of Nephrology.* Washington, DC, American Society of Nephrology, 1970, p 45.
423. LeGrimellec C et al: Fluidity of brush border and basolateral membranes from human kidney cortex. *Am J Physiol* 245:F227, 1983.
424. LeGrimellec C et al: 3-H insulin and elecrolyte concentrations in Bowman's capsule in rat kidney. *Pfluegers Arch* 354:117, 1975.
425. Levi J et al: Effect of magnesium (Mg) depletion on serum calcium (SCa) and on the response of bone and kidney to parathyroid hormone. *Clin Res* 20:192, 1972.
426. Levine BS et al: Early renal brush border membrane adaptation to dietary phosphorus. *Miner Electrolyte Metab* 10:222, 1984.
427. Levine BS et al: Effect of metabolic acidosis on phosphate transport by the renal brush border membrane. *Biochim Biophys Acta* 727:7, 1983.
428. Levine BS et al: Renal adaptation to dietary phosphate deprivation: Role of proximal tubule brush-border membrane fluidity. *Am J Physiol* 260:F613, 1991.
429. Levitan BA: Effect in normal man of hyperglycemia and glycosuria on excretion and reabsorption of phosphate. *J Appl Physiol* 4:224, 1951.
430. Li JJ et al: An estrogen binding protein in the renal cytosol of intact, castrated and estrogenized golden hamsters. *Endocrinology* 95:1134, 1974.
431. Lifshitz F et al: Influence of parathyroid function upon the in vitro transport of calcium and phosphate by the rat intestine. *Endocrinology* 84:912, 1969.
432. Lifshitz F et al: Intestinal transport of calcium and phosphate in experimental magnesium deficiency. *Proc Soc Exp Biol Med* 125:19, 1967.
433. Lin JT et al: Structural state of the Na^+/D-glucose cotransporter in calf kidney brush-border membranes. *Biochim Biophys Acta* 819:66, 1985.
434. Loghman-Adham M et al: Inhibition of Na-Pi cotransport in small gut brush border by phosphonocarboxilic acids. *Am J Physiol* 252:G244, 1987.
435. Loreau N et al: Calcitonin-sensitive adenylate cyclase in rat renal tubular membranes. *Biochem J* 150:305, 1975.
436. Loreau N et al: Renal calcitonin receptors and adenylate cyclase in rats immunized against tubular basement membrane. *Kidney Int* 12:184, 1977.
437. Loron Z et al: Phosphaturic effect of cortisone in normal and parathyroidectomized rats. *Proc Soc Exp Biol Med* 96:649, 1957.
438. Loron Z et al: Pituitary dwarfism with high serum levels of growth hormone. *Isr J Med Sci* 4:883, 1968.
439. Lotz M et al: Evidence for phosphorus depletion syndrome in man. *N Engl J Med* 278:409, 1968.
440. Luecke H, Quiocho FA: High specificity of a phosphate transport protein determined by hydrogen bonds. *Nature* 347:402, 1990.
441. Maack T et al: Renal filtration, transport and metabolism of proteins, in Seldin DW, Giebisch G (eds): *The Kidney: Physiology and Pathophysiology.* New York, Raven Press, 1985, p 1773.
442. Maesaka JK et al: Effect of mannitol on phosphate transport in intact and acutely thyroparathyroidectomized rats. *J Lab Clin Med* 87:680, 1976.
443. Maesaka JK et al: Effect of saline infusion on phosphate transport in intact and thyroparathyroidectomized rats. *Am J Physiol* 225:1421, 1973.
444. Mahler RF, Stanbury SW: Potassium losing renal disease. Renal and metabolic observations on a patient sustaining renal wastage of potassium. *Q J Med* 25:21, 1956.
445. Malamos B et al: The renal handling of phosphate in thyroid disease. *J Endocrinol* 45:269, 1969.
446. Malmstrom K, Murer H: Parathyroid hormone inhibits phosphate transport in OK cells but not in LLC-PK_1 and JTC-12.P3 cells. *Am J Physiol* 251:C23, 1986.
447. Malmstrom K et al: Intracellular cascades in the parathyroid hormone dependent regulation of Na^+/phosphate cotransport in OK cells. *Biochem J* 251:207, 1988.
448. Malmstrom K et al: Possible mechanisms for the regulation of the Pi transport in brush border membrane vesicles, in Bronner F, Peterlik M (eds): *Epithelial Calcium and Phosphate Transport: Molecular and Cellular Aspects.* New York, Liss, 1984, p 325.
449. Malvin RL, Lotspeich WD: Relation between tubular transport of inorganic phosphate and bicarbonate in the dog. *Am J Physiol* 187:51, 1956.
450. Marshall DH: Calcium and phosphate kinetics, in Nordin BEC (ed): *Calcium, Phosphate and Magnesium Metabolism.* Edinburgh, Churchill Livingstone, 1976, p 259.
451. Martin TJ, Melick RA: The acute effects of porcine calcitonin in man. *Aust N Z J Med* 18:258, 1969.
452. Martinez-Maldonado M, Eknoyan G: Role of extra-

cellular fluid volume expansion and diuretics in renal handling of phosphate, in Massry SG, Fleisch H (eds): *Renal Handling of Phosphate*. New York: Plenum, 1980, p 265.
453. Martinez-Maldonado M et al: Natriuretic effects of vasopressin and cyclic AMP: Possible site of action in the nephron. *Am J Physiol* 220:2013, 1971.
454. Marx SJ, Aurbach GD: Renal receptors for calcitonin: Coordinate occurrence with calcitonin-activated adenylate cyclase. *Endocrinology* 97:448, 1975.
455. Massara F, Camanni F: Propranolol block of adrenalin-induced hypophosphatemia in man. *Clin Sci* 38:245, 1970.
456. Massry SG et al: Evidence for suppression of parathyroid gland by hypermagnesemia. *J Clin Invest* 49:1619, 1970.
457. Massry SG et al: Excretion of phosphate and calcium. Physiology of their renal handling and relation to clinical medicine. *Arch Intern Med* 131:878,1983.
458. Massry SG et al: The influence of extracelluar volume expansion on renal phosphate reabsorption in the dog. *J Clin Invest* 48:1237, 1969.
459. Mazzuoli GF et al: Long-term observation of the effect of thyroidectomy in patients with elevated thyroid thyrocalcitonin content, in Taylor S (ed): *Calcitonin: Proceedings of the Symposium on Thyrolcacitonin and the C Cells*. London, Heinemann, 1967, p 364.
460. McCollum EV, Simmonds N: Studies on experimental rickets: 15. The effect of starvation on the healing of rickets. *Bull Johns Hopkins Med J* 33:31, 1922.
461. McFarland IA et al: Vitamin D metabolism in hyperthyroidism. *Clin Endocrinol* 17:51, 1982.
462. McHardy GJR, Parsons DS: The absorption of inorganic phosphate from the small intestine of the rat. *Q J Exp Physiol* 41:398, 1956.
463. McKeown JS et al: Intrarenal heterogeneity for fluid, phosphate and glucose absorption in the rabbit. *Am J Physiol* 6:F312, 1979.
464. McKinney TD, Myers P: PTH inhibition of bicarbonate transport by proximal convoluted tubules. *Am J Physiol* 239:F127, 1980.
465. McLean FC, Hinrichs MA: The formation and behavior of colloidal calcium phosphate in the blood. *Am J Physiol* 121:580, 1938.
466. Medalle R, Waterhouse C: A magnesium-deficient patient presenting with hypocalcemia and hypophosphatemia. *Ann Intern Med* 79:76, 1973.
467. Melvin KEM, Tashjian AH Jr: The syndrome of excessive thyrocalcitonin produced by medullary carcinoma of the thyroid. *Proc Natl Acad Sci U S A* 59:1216, 1968.
468. Menczel J et al: Effect of triiodothyronine on calcium and phosphorus metabolism in hypothyroidism. *Isr J Med Sci* 3:761, 1967.
469. Mercado A et al: On the mechanisms responsible for the phosphaturia of bicarbonate administration. *J Clin Invest* 56:1386, 1975.
470. Merimee TJ et al: Sex determined hormone responses to amino acid stimulation. *J Clin Endocrinol Metab* 26:79, 1966.
471. Meunier PJ et al: Bone manifestations of thyrotoxicosis. *Orthop Clin North Am* 3:745, 1972.
472. Meyer RA Jr, Meyer MH: Thyrocalacitonin infection to rats increases the liver inorganic phosphate. *Endocrinology* 96:1048, 1975.
473. Milhaud G, Mouhktar MS: Antagonistic and synergistic actions of thyrocalcitonin and parathyroid hormone on the levels of calcium and phosphate in the rat. *Nature* 211:1186, 1966.
474. Mills JN: Circadian rhythms during and after three months in solitude underground. *J Physiol* 174:217, 1964.
475. Mills JN, Thomas S: The acute effect of adrenal hormones and carbohydrate metabolism upon plasma phosphate and potassium concentration in man. *J Endocrinol* 16:164, 1957.
476. Minkin C, Jennings JM: Carbonic anhydrase and bone remodeling: Sulfonamide inhibition of bone reabsorption in organ culture. *Science* 176:1931, 1972.
477. Mircheff AK, Wright EM: Analytical isolation of plasma membranes of intestinal epithelial cells: Identification of Na, K-ATPase rich membranes and the distribution of enzyme activities. *J Membr Biol* 28:309, 1976.
478. Miyauchi A et al: Stimulation of transient elevations in cytosolic Ca^{2+} is related to inhibition of Pi transport in OK cells. *Am J Physiol* 259:F485, 1990.
479. Mizgala CL, Quamme GA: Renal handling of phosphate. *Physiol Rev* 65:431, 1985.
480. Mohrmann I et al: Sodium-dependent transport of Pi by an established intestinal epithelial cell line ($CaCo^2$). *Am J Physiol* 250:G323, 1986.
481. Molitoris BA: Membrane fluidity: Measurement and relationship to solute transport. *Semin Nephrol* 7:61, 1987.
482. Molitoris BA et al: Renal apical membrane cholesterol and fluidity in regulation of phosphate transport. *Am J Physiol* 249:F12, 1985.
483. Molitoris BA, Simon FR: Renal cortical brush border and basolateral membranes: Cholesterol and phospholipid composition and relative turnover. *J Membr Biol* 83:207, 1985.
484. Moog F, Glazier HS: Phosphate absorption and alkaline phosphatase activity in the small intestine of the adult mouse and of the chick embryo and hatched chick. *Comp Biochem Physiol* 42A:321, 1972.
485. Morel F: Sites of hormone action in the mammalian nephron. *Am J Physiol* 240:159, 1981.
486. Morel F et al: Measurement of hormone dependent adenylate cyclase activity in single pieces of rabbit kidney tubules, in Schmidt U, Dubach UC (eds): *Current Problems in Clinical Biochemistry*, vol 6, *Renal Metabolism in Relation to Renal Function*. Bern, Hans Huber, 1976, p 214.
487. Morey ER, Kenny AD: Effects of catecholamines on urinary calcium and phosphorus in intact and parathyroidectomized rats. *Endocrinology* 75:18, 1964.
488. Morgan DB: *Osteomalacia, Renal Osteodystrophy and Osteoporosis*. Springfield, Ill, Thomas, 1973.
489. Mosekilde L et al: Bone changes in hyperthyroidism: Interrelationship between bone morphometry, thyroid function and calcium-phosphorus metabolism. *Acta Endocrinol* 85:515, 1977.
490. Mostellar ME, Tuttle EP Jr: The effects of alkalosis on plasma concentration and urinary excretion of phosphate in man. *J Clin Invest* 43:138, 1964.
491. Mudge GH et al: Tubular transport of urea, glucose, phosphate, uric acid, sulfate and thiosulfate, in Orloff RW

et al (eds): *Handbook of Physiology*. Baltimore, Williams & Wilkins, 1973, sec 8, p 587.

492. Muhlbauer RC et al: Tubular localization of adaptation to dietary phosphate in rats. *Am J Physiol* 233:F342, 1977.
493. Muldowney FB et al: Parathormone-like effect on magnesium replenishment in steatorrhea. *N Engl J Med* 282:61, 1970.
494. Murer H, Burckhardt G: Membrane transport of anions across epithelia of mammalian small intestine and kidney proximal tubule. *Rev Physiol Biochem Pharmacol* 96:1, 1983.
495. Murer H et al: Sodium-dependent transport of inorganic phosphate across the renal brush border membrane. *Adv Exp Med Biol* 128:11, 1980.
496. Nadarajah A et al: Calcium metabolism in acromegaly. *Br Med J* 4:797, 1968.
497. Nagata N, Rasmussen H: Parathyroid hormone, cAMP, Ca^{++} and gluconeogenesis. *Proc Natl Acad Sci U S A* 64:368, 1970.
498. Nakai M et al: Phorbol esters inhibit phosphate uptake in opossum kidney cells: A model of proximal tubular cells. *Biochem Biophys Res Commun* 145:303, 1987.
499. Nassim Jr et al: The effect of stilbestrol on urinary phosphate excretion. *Clin Sci* 15:367, 1956.
500. Neville DM, Glossmann H: Plasma membrane protein subunit composition: A comparative study by discontinuous electrophoresis in sodium dodecyl sulfate. *J Biol Chem* 246:6335, 1971.
501. New MI et al: Pseudo hypopituitary dwarfism with normal plasma growth hormone and low serum sulfation factor. *J Pediatr* 20:620, 1972.
502. Ney RL et al: Actions of vitamin D independent of parathyroid glands. *Endocrinology* 82:760, 1968.
503. Nishimoto H: On relation between carbohydrate metabolism and inorganic phosphate. *Jpn J Exp Med* 7:207, 1929.
504. Nishizuka Y: Studies and perspectives of protein kinase C. *Science* 225:1365, 1984.
505. Nizet A: Excretion and tubular reabsorption of sodium, glucose and phosphate by isolated dog kidneys: Influence of blood dilution. *Pfluegers Arch* 332:248, 1972.
506. Nizet A et al: Hormone and non-specific humoral factors in the interferences between sodium, glucose and phosphate handling by the dog kidney, in Schmidt U, Dubach UC (eds): *Current Problems in Clinical Biochemistry*, vol 6, *Renal Metabolism in Relation to Renal Function*. Bern, Hans Huber, 1976, p 262.
507. Noble HM, Matty AJ: The effect of thyroxine on the movement of calcium and inorganic phosphate through the small intestine of the rat. *J Endocrinol* 37:111, 1967.
508. Nordin BEC (ed): *Calcium, Phosphate and Magnesium Metabolism*. Edinburgh, Churchill Livingstone, 1976.
509. Nordin BEC, Bulusu L: A modified index of phosphate excretion. *Postgrad Med J* 44:93, 1968.
510. Nordin BEC, Fraser R: Assessment of urinary phosphate excretion. *Lancet* 1:947, 1960.
511. Nordin BEC, Fraser R: The effect of intravenous calcium on phosphate excretion. *Clin Sci* 12:477, 1954.
512. Noronha-Blob L et al: Stimulation by thyroid hormone of phosphate transport in primary cultured renal cells. *J Cell Physiol* 137:95, 1988.
513. Nseir NZ et al: Mechanism of the renal tubular effects of 25-hydroxy and 1,25-dihydroxyvitamin D3 in the absence of parathyroid hormone. *Miner Electrolyte Metab* 1:48, 1978.
514. Okada Y et al: Effects of potassium ions and sodium ions on membrane potential of epithelial cells in rat duodenum. *Biochim Biophys Acta* 413:104, 1975.
515. Oldham SB et al: The acute effect of 1,25-dihydroxycholecalciferol on serum immunoreactive parathyroid hormone (iPTH) in the dog. *Endocrinology* 104:248, 1979.
516. Orimo H et al: Increased sensitivity of bone to parathyroid hormone in ovariectomized rats. *Endocrinology* 90:760, 1972.
517. Ortola FV et al: Endogenous ANP augments fractional excretion of Pi, Ca and Na in rats with reduced renal mass. *Am J Physiol* 255:F1091, 1988.
518. Oxender DL, Quay SC: Isolation and characterization of membrane binding proteins, in Korn ED (ed): *Methods in Membrane Biology*. New York, Plenum, 1976, vol. 6, p 183.
519. Paillard F et al: Renal effects of salmon calcitonin in man. *J Lab Clin Med* 80:200, 1972.
520. Pak CYC et al: Renal effects of porcine thyrocalcitonin in the dog. *Endocrinology* 87:262, 1970.
521. Paloyan E et al: Glucagon-induced hypocalcemia. *Metabolism* 16:35, 1967.
522. Pappenheimer JR: Physiological regulation of transepithelial impedance in the intestinal mucosa of rat and hamsters. *J Membr Biol* 100:137, 1987.
523. Pappenheimer JR, Reiss KZ: Contribution of solvent drag through intercellular junctions to absorption of nutrients by the small intestine of the rat. *J Membr Biol* 100:123, 1987.
524. Parfitt AM, Frame B: Phosphate loading and depletion in vitamin D treated hypoparathyroidism, in Avioli L et al (eds): *Phosphate Metabolism: Kidney and Bone*. Paris, Armour Montagu, 1976, p 179.
525. Parfitt AM, Kleerekoper M: The divalent ion homeostatic system: Physiology and metabolism of calcium, phosphorus, magnesium, and bone, in Maxwell MH, Kleeman CR (eds): *Clinical Disorders of Fluid and Electrolyte Metabolism*, 3d ed. New York, McGraw-Hill, 1980, p 269.
526. Parsons JA, Reit B: Chronic response of dogs to parathyroid infusion. *Nature* 250:254, 1974.
527. Parsons V, Anderson J: The maximum renal tubular reabsorptive rate for inorganic phosphate in thyrotoxicosis. *Clin Sci* 27:313, 1964.
528. Pastoriza-Munoz E et al: Effect of phosphate deprivation on phosphate reabsorption in rat nephron: Role of PTH. *Am J Physiol* 244:F140, 1983.
529. Pastoriza-Munoz E et al: Effects of purified parathyroid hormone (PTH) on phosphate (P) reabsorption along the nephron in acutely parathyroidectomized (TPTX) rats. *Physiologist* 19:325, 1976.
530. Peerce BE: Identification of the intestinal Na-phosphate cotransporter. *Am J Physiol* 256:G645, 1989.
531. Peraino RA, Suki WN: Influence of calcium on renal handling of phosphate, in Massry SG, Fleisch H (eds): *Renal Handling of Phosphate*. New York, Plenum, 1980, p 287.
532. Perlzweig WA et al: The behavior of inorganic phosphate

in the blood and urine of normal and diabetic subjects during carbohydrate metabolism. *Proc Soc Exp Biol Med* 21:33, 1923.

533. Persky M et al: Acute effects of intravenous hydrocortisone on glucose and insulin tolerances, and levels of serum and urinary inorganic phosphorus. *J Clin Endocrinol Metab* 15:1247, 1955.
534. Peterlik M et al: Intestinal phosphate transport: Mechanistic and regulatory aspects, in Hurwitz S, Sela J (eds): *Current Advances in Skeletogenesis.* Jerusalem, Heiliger, vol 3, 1987, p 287.
535. Pfeifer U, Guder WG: Stimulation of cellular autophagy by parathyroid hormone and cAMP in isolated tubular fragments from the rat's kidney cortex. *Virchows Arch B Cell Pathol* 19:51, 1975.
536. Pfleger K et al: Phosphat Durchtritt am isolierten darm unter Dinitrophenol und Thyoxin. *Biochem J* 330:303, 1958.
537. Pike JW et al: Circulating 1α,25-$(OH)_2D3$ during physiological states of calcium stress, in Norman AW et al (eds): *Vitamin D: Biochemical, Chemical and Clinical Aspects Related to Calcium Metabolism.* Berlin, de Gruyter, 1977, p 187.
538. Pitts RF: The excretion of urine in the dog. *Am J Physiol* 106:1, 1933.
539. Pitts RF, Alexander RS: The renal reabsorptive mechanism for inorganic phosphate in normal and acidotic dogs. *Am J Physiol* 142:648, 1944.
540. Popovtzer MM: Renal response to phosphaturic agents in acutely and chronically parathyroidectomized rats. *Proc Soc Exp Biol Med* 154:522, 1977.
541. Popovtzer MM et al: The acute effect of 25-hydroxycholecalciferol on renal handling of phosphorus: Evidence for a parathyroid hormone-dependent mechanism. *J Clin Invest* 53:913, 1974.
542. Popovtzer MM et al: Effect of Ca^{++} on renal handling of PO_4^{3-}: Evidence for two reabsorptive mechanisms. *Am J Physiol* 229:901, 1975.
543. Popovtzer MM et al: Evidence for interference of 25(OH) vitamin D3 with phosphate effect of calcitonin. *Am J Physiol* 232:E515, 1977.
544. Portale AA et al: Oral intake of phosphorus can determine the serum concentration of 1,25-dihydroxyvitamin D by determining its production rate in humans. *J Clin Invest* 77:7, 1986.
545. Poujeol P et al: Phosphate reabsorption in rat nephron terminal segments: Intrarenal heterogeneity and strain differences. *Pfluegers Arch* 371:39, 1977.
546. Purkerson ML et al: Tubular reabsorption of phosphate after release of complete ureteral obstruction in the rat. *Kidney Int* 5:326, 1974.
547. Puschett JB, Goldberg M: The acute effects of furosemide on acid and electrolyte excretion in man. *J Lab Clin Med* 71:666, 1968.
548. Puschett JB, Goldberg M: The relationship between the renal handling of phosphate and bicarbonate in man. *J Lab Clin Med* 73:956, 1969.
549. Puschett JB et al: The acute renal effects of 1,25-dihydroxycholecalciferol. *Proc Soc Exp Biol Med* 141:379, 1972.
550. Puschett JB et al: Effects of saline loading and aortic obstruction on proximal phosphate transport. *Am J Physiol* 223:851, 1972.
551. Puschett JB et al: Evidence for a direct action of cholecalciferol and 25-hydroxycholecalciferol on the renal transport of phosphate, sodium, and calcium. *J Clin Invest* 51:373, 1972.
552. Puschett JB et al: Study of the renal tubular interactions of thyrocalcitonin, cyclic adenosine 3′,5′-monophosphate, 25-hydroxycholecalciferol, and calcium ion. *J Clin Invest* 53:756, 1974.
553. Quamme GA: Effects of metabolic acidosis, alkalosis and dietary hydrogen ion intake on phosphate transport in the convoluted tubule. *Am J Physiol* 249:F769, 1985.
554. Quamme GA: Phosphate transport in intestinal brush-border membrane vesicles: Effect of pH and dietary phosphate. *Am J Physiol* 249:G168, 1985.
555. Quame GA, Shapiro RJ: Membrane controls of epithelial phosphate transport. *Can J Physiol Pharmacol* 65:275, 1987.
556. Quamme GA, Wong NLM: Phosphate transport in the proximal convoluted tubule: Effect of intraluminal pH. *Am J Physiol* 246:F323, 1984.
557. Quamme G et al: Sodium phosphate cotransport in OK cells: Inhibition by PTH and adaptation to low phosphate. *Am J Physiol* 257:F967, 1989.
558. Queener SF, Bell NH: Calcitonin: A general survey. *Metabolism* 24:555, 1975.
559. Rabkin R et al: Effect of growth hormone on renal sodium and water excretion. *Horm Metab Res* 7:139, 1975.
560. Rader JJ et al: Calcium and phosphorus deficiency in rats: Effect on PTH and 1,25-dihydroxyvitamin D3. *Am J Physiol* 236:E118, 1979.
561. Rasmussen H et al: Thyrocalcitonin, EGTA, and urinary electrolyte excretion. *J Clin Invest* 46:746, 1967.
562. Rasmussen H, Bordier P: *The Physiological Basis of Metabolic Bone Disease.* Baltimore, Williams & Wilkins, 1974.
563. Rasmussen H et al: Liponomic regulation of calcium transport by $1,25(OH)_2D3$, in Scott WN, Goodman DB (eds): *Hormonal Regulation of Epithelial Transport of Ions and Water. Ann N Y Acad Sci* 372:518, 1981.
564. Rasmussen HD et al: Ionic control of metabolism, in Greep RO, Astwood EB (eds): *Handbook of Physiology: Endocrinology.* Washington, DC, American Physiological Society, 1976, vol 7, p 225.
565. Rastegar A et al: Renal handling of calcium and phosphate during mineralocorticoid "escape" in man. *Kidney Int* 2:279, 1972.
566. Recker RR et al: Effect of estrogens and calcium carbonate on bone loss in postmenopausal women. *Ann Intern Med* 87:649, 1977.
567. Rector FC Jr: Acidification of the urine, in Orloff J, Berliner RW (eds): *Handbook of Physiology,* sec 8, *Renal Physiology.* Baltimore, Williams & Wilkins, 1973, p 431.
568. Rector FC Jr et al: The mechanism of bicarbonate reabsorption in the proximal and distal tubule of the kidney. *J Clin Invest* 44:278, 1965.
569. Rector FC Jr et al: The mechanism of suppression of proximal tubular reabsorption by saline infusions. *J Clin Invest* 46:47, 1967.
570. Reifenstein EC et al: Observations on the use of the serum phosphorus level as an index of pituitary growth hormone

activity: The effect of estrogen therapy in acromegaly. *Endocrinology* 39:71, 1946.
571. Reiss E et al: The role of phosphate in the secretion of parathyroid hormone in man. *J Clin Invest* 49:2146, 1970.
572. Relman AS, Schwartz WB: The metabolic effects of compound F acetate in man. *J Clin Invest* 31:656, 1952.
573. Reshkin SJ et al: Parathyroid hormone-induced alterations of protein content and phosphorylation in enriched apical membranes of opossum kidney cells. *J Biol Chem* 265:15261, 1990.
574. Riggs BL et al: Effect of sex hormones on bone in primary osteoporosis. *J Clin Invest* 48:1065, 1969.
575. Riggs BL et al: Short- and long-term effects of estrogen and synthetic anabolic hormone in postmenopausal osteoporosis. *J Clin Invest* 51:1959, 1972.
576. Ritz E et al: Effects of hormones other than parathyroid hormones on renal handling of phosphate, in Massry SG, Fleisch H (eds): *Renal Handling of Phosphate.* New York, Plenum, 1980, p 137.
577. Roberts KE, Pitts RF: The effects of cortisone and desoxycorticosterone on the renal tubular reabsorption of phosphate and the excretion of titratable acid and potassium in dogs. *Endocrinology* 52:324, 1953.
578. Robertson JD: Calcium and phosphorus studies in myxedema. *Lancet* 2:216, 1941.
579. Robertson WG: Plasma phosphate homeostasis, in Nordin BED (ed): *Calcium, Phosphorus and Magnesium Metabolism.* Edinburgh, Churchill Livingstone, 1976, p 217.
580. Robertson WG: Urinary excretion, in Nordin BED (ed): *Calcium, Phosphorus and Magnesium Metabolism.* Edinburgh, Churchill Livingstone, 1976, p 113.
581. Robertson WG, Peacock M: New techniques for the separation and measurement of the calcium fractions of normal human serum. *Clin Chim Acta* 20:315, 1968.
582. Robinson CJ et al: Phosphaturic effect of thyrocalcitonin. *Lancet* 1:83, 1966.
583. Rocha AS et al: Calcium and phosphate transport in isolated segments of rabbit Henle's loop. *J Clin Invest* 59:975, 1977.
584. Rodriguez HJ et al: Effect of acetazolamide on the urinary excretion of cyclic AMP and on the activity of renal adenyl cyclase. *J Clin Invest* 53:122, 1974.
585. Rohn R et al: Effect of protease treatment on enzyme content, protein content and transport function of brush border membrane isolated from rat small intestine and kidney cortex. *Mol Physiol* 3:3, 1983.
586. Rosenbaum JL et al: Effect of sudden blood calcium depletion on phosphorus excretion. *Endocrinology* 74:266, 1964.
587. Rothstein A et al: Relationship of cell surface to metabolism: 9. Digestion of phosphorylated compounds by enzymes located on surface of intestinal cell. *Am J Physiol* 173:41, 1953.
588. Rouse D, Suki WN: Calcium (Ca)-mediated phosphate (PO_4) transport in proximal convoluted tubule (PCT) of the rabbit. *Miner Electrolyte Metab* 9:178, 1983.
589. Russell RGG, Fleisch W: The renal effects of thyrocalcitonin in the pig and dog, in Taylor S (ed): *Calcitonin: Proceedings of the Symposium on Thyrocalcitonin and the C Cells.* London, Heinemann, 1968, p 297.
590. Sacktor B, Cheng L: Sodium gradient-dependent phosphate transport in renal brush border membrane vesicles: Effect of an intravesicular greater than extravesicular proton gradient. *J Biol Chem* 256:8080, 1981.
591. Salako LA et al: The effects of porcine calcitonin on renal function in the rabbit. *Endocrinology* 50:485, 1971.
592. Salveson H, Boe J: Osteomalacia: Report on two cases with the Milkman's syndrome. *Acta Med Scand* 266(suppl):863, 1952.
593. Sampson HW, Matthews JL: Electron microscope autoradiographic investigation of ^{32}P in the intestinal epithelium of rachitic, normal and vitamin D-treated rats. *Calcif Tissue Res* 10:58, 1972.
594. Saville PD et al: Osteomalacia in von Recklinghausen's neurofibromatosis: Metabolic study of a case. *Br Med J* 1:1311, 1955.
595. Schaat M, Kyle LH: Diurnal variations of calcium and phosphorus in blood and urine. *Clin Res* 6:139, 1958.
596. Schiess WA et al: The renal regulation of acid-base balance in man: 2. Factors affecting the excretion of titratable acid by the normal human subject. *J Clin Invest* 29:57, 1948.
597. Schittenhelm A, Eisler B: Untersuchungen uber die Wirkung des Thyroxins auf den Eiwieb-Wasser-und Mineralstoffwechsel. *Z Gesamte Exp Med* 61:239, 1928.
598. Schneider EG et al: Is phosphate secreted by the kidney? in Massry SG, Fliesch H (eds): *Renal Handling of Phosphate.* New York, Plenum, 1980, p 59.
599. Schneider EG et al: Relationship between proximal sodium reabsorption and excretion of calcium, magnesium and phosphate. *Kidney Int* 4:369, 1973.
600. Schneider EG et al: Role of parathyroid hormone in the phosphaturia or extracellular fluid volume expansion. *Kidney Int* 7:317, 1975.
601. Schwab SJ et al: Na^+ gradient-dependent Pi uptake in bsolateral membrane vesicles from dog kidney. *Am J Physiol* 246:F663, 1984.
602. Schwartz GJ, Al-Awqati Q: Carbon dioxide causes exocytosis of vesicles containing H^+ pumps in isolated perfused proximal and collecting tubules. *J Clin Invest* 75:1638, 1985.
603. Seely JF, Dirks JH: Micropuncture study of hypertonic mannitol diuresis in the proximal and distal tubule of the dog kidney. *J Clin Invest* 48:2330, 1969.
604. Senft G et al: Der Einfluss von Hydrochlorothiazide und anderen sulfonamidierten Diuretica auf die 3′,5′ AMP phosphodiesterase: Activitat in der Rattenniere. *Arch Exp Pathol Pharmakol* 259:344, 1968.
605. Shah SV et al: Renal adaptation to low phosphate diet in rats: Blockade by actinomycin D. *J Clin Invest* 64:955, 1979.
606. Shareghi GR, Agus ZS: Phosphate transport in the light segment of the rabbit cortical collecting tubule (CCT1), in Massry SG et al (eds): *Phosphate and Minerals in Health and Disease.* New York, Plenum, 1980.
607. Shiau Y-F et al: Mechanism maintaining a low-pH microclimate in the intestine. *Am J Physiol* 248:G608, 1985.
608. Shirazy-Beechey SP et al: Changes in the functions of the intestinal brush border membranes during the development of the ruminant habit in lambs. *Compar Biochem Physiol* 94B:801, 1989.

609. Short EM et al: Familial hypophosphatemic rickets: Defective transport of inorganic phosphate by intestinal mucosa. *Science* 179:700, 1973.
610. Silvis SE, Paragus PD Jr: Fatal hyperalimentation syndrome: Animal studies. *J Lab Clin Med* 78:918, 1971.
611. Silvis SE, Paragus PD Jr: Parasthesias, weakness, seizures and hypophosphatemia in patients receiving hyperalimentation. *Gastroenterology* 62:513, 1972.
612. Simone PG, Solomon S: Aldosterone: Effect on incorporation of leucine into the trichloroacetic acid precipitable fraction of rabbit renal cortical tissue. *Experientia* 26:656, 1970.
613. Simoni RD: Macromolecular characterization of bacterial transport systems, in Fos CF, Keith AD (eds): *Membrane Molecular Biology*. Stamford, Conn: Sinauer Associates, 1972, p 289.
614. Singhelakis P et al: Intestinal calcium absorption in hyperthyroidism. *Metabolism* 23:311, 1974.
615. Sinha PK et al: Effect of acetazolamide on the renal excretion in hypoparathyroidism and pseudohypoparathyroidism. *J Lab Clin Med* 89:1188, 1977.
616. Slatopolsky E et al: Control of phosphate excretion in uremic man. *J Clin Invest* 47:1865, 1968.
617. Snyder JA, McIntosh JR: Biochemistry and physiology of microtubules. *Annu Rev Biochem* 45:699, 1976.
618. Sorensen OH, Hindberg I: The acute and prolonged effect of porcine calcitonin on urine electrolyte excretion in intact and parathyroidectomized rats. *Acta Endocrinol* 70:295, 1972.
619. Spanos E, McIntyre I: Effect of glucocorticoids on vitamin D metabolism, in Norman AW et al (eds): *Vitamin D: Biochemical, Chemical and Clinical Aspects Related to Calcium Metabolism*. Berlin, de Gruyter, 1977, p 191.
620. Spanos E et al: Effect of growth hormone on vitamin D metabolism. *Nature* 273:246, 1978.
621. Stanbury SW: Some aspects of disordered renal tubular function. *Adv Intern Med* 9:231, 1958.
622. Stanbury SW, Lumb GA: Metabolic studies of renal osteodystrophy: 1. Calcium, phosophorus and nitrogen metabolism in rickets, osteomalacia and hyperparathyroidism complicating chronic uremia and in the adult Fanconi syndrome. *Medicine* 41:1, 1962.
623. Staum BB et al: Tracer microinjection study of renal tubular phosphate reabsorption in the rat. *J Clin Invest* 51:2271, 1972.
624. Steele TH: Bicarbonate-induced phosphaturia *Pfluegers Arch* 370:291, 1977.
625. Steele TH: Dual effect of potent diuretics on renal handling of phosphate in man. *Metabolism* 20:749, 1971.
626. Steele TH: Increased urinary phosphate excretion following volume expansion in normal man. *Metabolism* 19:129, 1970.
627. Steele TH, Underwood JL: Renal response to phosphorus deprivation in the isolated rat kidney. *Kidney Int* 13:124, 1978.
628. Steele TH et al: Phosphatremic actions of 1,25-dihydroxyvitamin D3. *Am J Physiol* 229:489, 1975.
629. Steele TH et al: Renal resistance to parathyroid hormone during phosphorus deprivation. *J Clin Invest* 58:1461, 1976.
630. Steinmuller SR, Puschett JB: Effects of metolazone in man: Comparison with chlorothiazide. *Kidney Int* 1:169, 1972.
631. Stepinski J et al: Effect of lithium on renal gluconeogenesis. *Acta Biochim Pol* 31:229, 1984.
632. Stepinski J et al: Inhibition of 2-oxoglutarate metabolism by lithium in the isolated rat kidney cortex tubules. *Acta Biochim Pol* 31:241, 1984.
633. Stern PH, Bell NH: Effect of glucagon on serum calcium in the rat and on bone resorption in tissue culture. *Endocrinology* 87:111, 1970.
634. Stoll R et al: Effect of dietary phosphate intake on phosphate transport by isolated rat renal brush border vesicles. *Biochem J* 180:465, 1979.
635. Stoll R et al: Phosphate transport by rat renal brush border membrane vesicles: Influence of dietary phosphate, parathyroidectomy, and 1,25-dihydroxy D_3. *Pfluegers Arch* 380:47, 1979.
636. Storelli C, Murer H: On the correlation between alkaline phosphatase and phosphate transport in rat renal brush border membrane vesicles. *Pfluegers Arch* 384:149, 1980.
637. Strevey J et al: Effect of arginine modification on kidney brush border membrane transport activity. *Biochem J* 223:793, 1984.
638. Strickler JC et al: Micropuncture study of inorganic phosphate excretion in the rat. *J Clin Invest* 43:1596, 1964.
639. Suki WN et al: Effect of expansion of extracellular fluid volume on renal phosphate handling. *J Clin Invest* 48:1888, 1969.
640. Suttle NF, Field AC: Studies on magnesium on ruminant nutrition: 8. Effect of increased intakes of potassium and water on the metabolism of magnesium, phosphorus, sodium, potassium and calcium in sheep. *Br J Nutr* 21:819, 1967.
641. Suzuki M et al: Thiol redox and phosphate transport in renal brush-border membrane: Effect of nicotinamide. *Biochim Biophys Acta* 1021:85, 1990.
642. Swenson RS et al: Evidence that parathyroid hormone is not required for phosphate homeostasis in renal failure. *Metabolism* 24:199, 1975.
643. Szenasi G et al: Tubular transport and urinary excretion of phosphate after renal denervation in the anesthetized rat. *Am J Physiol* 240:F481, 1981.
644. Szymendera J, Mandajewicz S: Calcium metabolism after castration. *Lancet* 2:1091, 1967.
645. Talmage RV, Anderson JJB: The effect of calcitonin on 32-P disappearance from plasma in parathyroidectomized and nephrectomized rats. *Proc Soc Exp Biol Med* 141:982, 1974.
646. Talmage RV et al: The influence of calcitonin on the disappearance of radiocalcium and radiophosphorus from plasma. *Endocrinology* 90:1185, 1972.
647. Tan CM et al: Serum ionic calcium levels during pregnancy. *Br J Obstet Gynaecol* 79:694, 1972.
648. Tanaka Y, DeLuca HF: Intestinal calcium transport: Stimulation by low phosphorus diets. *Science* 181:564, 1973.
649. Tanaka Y et al: Control of renal vitamin D hydroxylases in birds by sex hormones. *Proc Natl Acad Sci U S A* 73:2701, 1976.
650. Tanzer FS, Navia JM: Calcitonin inhibition of intestinal phosphate absorption. *Nature* 242:221, 1963.
651. Taylor AN: In vitro phosphate transport in chick ileum:

Effect of cholecalciferol, calcium, sodium and metabolic inhibitors. *J Nutr* 104:489, 1974.
652. Tenenhouse HS, Chu YL: Hydrolysis of nicotinamide adenine dinucleotide by purified renal brush border membranes. *Biochem J* 204:635, 1982.
653. Tenenhouse HS et al: Alkaline phosphatase activity does not mediate phosphate transport in the renal-cortical brush border membrane. *Biochem J* 190:473, 1980.
654. Thalassinos NC et al: Urinary excretion of phosphate in normal children. *Arch Dis Child* 45:269, 1970.
655. Theiler A, Green HH: Aphosphorosis in ruminants. *Nutr Rev* 1:359, 1932.
656. Thompson DD, Hiatt HH: Effect of phosphate loading and depletion on the renal excretion and reabsorption of inorganic phosphate. *J Clin Invest* 36:566, 1956.
657. Thompson DD, Hiatt HH: Renal absorption of phosphate in normal human subjects and in patients with parathyroid disease. *J Clin Invest* 36:550, 1957.
658. Thompson JS et al: Dissociation of the lowering effect of calcitonin on plasma Ca and P in cortisone-treated nephrectomized rats. *Endocrinology* 94:799, 1974.
659. Todd WR et al: Blood calcium and phosphorus in newborn. *Am J Dis Child* 57:1278, 1939.
660. Toor M et al: Diurnal variations in the composition of blood and urine in man living in hot climate. *Nephron* 2:334, 1965.
661. Turner ST et al: Mechanism of glucocorticoid effect on renal transport of phosphate. *Am J Physiol* 243:C227, 1982.
662. Tyson GF, Bulger RE: Effect of vinblastine sulfate on the fine structure of proximal tubule cell of rat kidney. *J Biol Chem* 59:349, 1973.
663. Ugolev AM: *Physiology of Membrane Digestion*. New York, Plenum, 1968.
664. Ullrich KJ et al: Coupling between proximal tubular transport processes: Studies with ouabain, SITS and HCO_3^--free solutions. *Pfluegers Arch* 368:245, 1977.
665. Ullrich KJ et al: Phosphate transport in the proximal convolution of the rat kidney: 1. Tubular heterogeneity, effect of parathyroid hormone in acute and chronic parathyroidectomized animals and effect of phosphate diet. *Pfluegers Arch* 372:269, 1977.
666. Van den Brande JL: Plasma somatomedin, in Pacile A, Muller E (eds): *Growth Hormone and Related Peptides: Proceedings of the 3rd International Symposium*. Amsterdam, Excerpta Medica, 1975, p 271.
667. Van Slyke DD et al: Studies of gas and electrolyte equilibria in the blood: 5. Factors controlling electrolyte and water distribution in the blood. *J Biol Chem* 56:765, 1923.
668. Van Stone JC, Perry FA: Phosphate excretion in the parathyroidectomized rat receiving parathyroid hormone. *Metabolism* 21:849, 1972.
669. Wajchenberg BL et al: Antagonism between adrenal steroids and parathyroid hormone. *J Clin Endocrinol Metab* 25:1677, 1965.
670. Walker BR et al: Effect of triamterene on the renal clearance of calcium, magnesium, phosphate and uric acid in man. *Clin Pharmacol Ther* 13:145, 1972.
671. Wallach S, Carter AC: Metabolic and renal effects of acute hypercalcemia in dogs. *Am J Physiol* 200:359, 1961.
672. Walling MW: Effects of 1α,25-dihydroxyvitamin D3 on active intestine inorganic phosphate absorption, in Norman W et al (eds): *Vitamin D: Biochemical, Chemical and Clinical Aspects Related to Calcium Metabolism*. Berlin, de Gruyter, 1977, p 321.
673. Walling MW: Intestinal inorganic phosphate transport, in Massry SG et al (eds): *Homeostasis of Phosphate and Other Minerals*. New York, Plenum, 1978, p 131.
674. Walling MW et al: Elevation of cyclic AMP levels and adenylate cyclase activity in duodenal mucosa from vitamin D-deficient rats by 1α,25-dihydroxycholecalciferol. *Endocr Res Commun* 3:83, 1976.
675. Walling MW et al: Jejunal phosphate (Pi) active transport: Effects of phosphorus depletion and vitamin D. *Fed Proc* 36:1097, 1977.
676. Walser M: Ion association: 6. Associations between calcium, magnesium, inorganic phosphate, citrate and protein in normal human plasma. *J Clin Invest* 40:723, 1961.
677. Walton J, Gray TK: Absorption of intestinal phosphate in the human small intestine. *Clin Sci* 56:407, 1979.
678. Wasserman RH, Comar CL: The parathyroids and the intestinal absorption of Ca, Sr and phosphate ions in the rat. *Endocrinology* 69:1074, 1961.
679. Wasserman RH, Taylor AN: Intestinal absorption of phosphate in the chick: Effect of vitamin D3 and other parameters. *J Nutr* 103:586, 1973.
680. Webb RK et al: Relationship between phosphaturia and acute hypercapnia in the rat. *J Clin Invest* 60:829, 1977.
681. Weeke E, Friis T: Serum fractions of calcium and phosphorus in uremia. *Acta Med Scand* 189:79, 1971.
682. Weinman EJ, Eknoyan G: Chronic effects of chlorothiazide on reabsorption by the proximal tubule of the rat. *Clin Sci* 49:107, 1975.
683. Wen SF: The effect of vasopressin on phosphate transport in the proximal tubule of the dog. *J Clin Invest* 53:660, 1974.
684. Wen SF: Micropuncture studies of phosphate transport in the proximal tubule of the dog. *J Clin Invest* 53:143, 1974.
685. Werner A et al: Cloning of the renal Na^+/Pi cotransporter system. *J Am Soc Nephrol* 1:746A, 1990.
686. Wesson LG Jr: Electrolyte excretion in relation to diurnal cycles of renal function: Plasma electrolyte concentrations and aldosterone secretion before and during salt and water balance changes in normotensive subjects. *Medicine* 43:547, 1964.
687. White HL et al: Enhancing effects of growth hormone on renal function. *Am J Physiol* 157:47, 1949.
688. Wilde WS, Malvin RL: Graphical placement of transport segment along the nephron from urine concentration pattern developed with stop flow technique. *Am J Physiol* 195:153, 1958.
689. Wilkins, JN et al: The effect of hyperthyroidism and 2,4-dinitrophenol on growth hormone synthesis. *Endocrinology* 95:1259, 1974.
690. Wilkinson R: Absorption of calcium, phosphorus and magnesium, in Nordin BEC (ed): *Calcium, Phosphate and Magnesium Metabolism*. Edinburgh, Churchill Livingstone, 1976, p 36.
691. Williams CC et al: The effects of synthetic human and salmon calcitonins on electrolyte excretion in the rat. *Clin Sci* 42:129, 1972.
692. Williams GA et al: Interrelationship of parathyroid and

adrenocortical function in calcium homeostasis in the rat. *Endocrinology* 95:707, 1974.
693. Wilson TH, Wilson DW: Studies in vitro of digestion and absorption of pyrimidine nucleotides by the intestine. *J Biol Chem* 233:1544, 1958.
694. Wolosin JM et al: Functional characterization of anion transport system isolated from human erythrocyte membranes. *J Biol Chem* 252:2419, 1977.
695. Wrong O et al: In vivo dialysis of faeces as a method of stool analysis: 1. Technique and results in normal subjects. *Clin Sci* 28:357, 1965.
696. Wuarin F et al: The Na^+/Pi-cotransporter of OK cells: Reaction and tentative identification with N-acetylimidazole. *Biochim Biophys Acta* 981:185, 1989.
697. Yamaguchi M et al: Effect of thyrocalcitonin on calcium concentration in liver and intact and thyroparathyroidectomized rats. *Endocrinology* 96:1004, 1975.
698. Yanagawa N, Jo OD: Possible role of calcium in parathyroid hormone action on phosphate transport by rabbit renal brush border membrane. *Biochem Biophys Res Commun* 128:278, 1985.
699. Yanagawa N, Jo OD: Possible role of calcium in parathyroid hormone actions in rabbit renal proximal tubules. *Am J Physiol* 250:F942, 1986.
700. Yanagawa N et al: Cytosolic redox potential and phosphate transport in the proximal tubule of the rabbit: A study in the isolated perfused tubules. *Miner Electrolyte Metab* 11:57, 1985.
701. Yanagawa N et al: Dissociation of gluconeogenesis from fluid and phosphate reabsorption in isolated rabbit proximal tubules. *Kidney Int* 25:869, 1984.
702. Yanagawa N et al: Intracellular protein transport and the adaptation to phosphate deprivation in OK cells. *J Am Soc Nephrol* 1:736A, 1990.
703. Yeh JK, Aloia JF: Effect of glucocorticoids on the passive transport of phosphate on different segments of the intestine in the rat. *Bone Miner* 2:11, 1987.
704. Yeh JK et al: Interrelation of cortisone and 1,25-dihydroxycholecalciferol on intestinal calcium and phosphate absorption. *Calcif Tissue Int* 36:608, 1984.
705. Yendt ER, Jaworski ZF: The relationship of urinary phosphate changes to parathyroid activity, in Greep RO, Talmage RV (eds): *The Parathyroids.* Springfield, Ill, Thomas, 1961, p 439.
706. Young MM, Nordin BEC: Effects of natural and artificial menopause on plasma and urinary calcium and phosphorus. *Lancet* 2:118, 1967.
707. Young MM et al: Some effects of ethinyl oestradiol on calcium and phosphorus metabolism in osteoporosis. *Clin Sci* 34:411, 1968.
708. Yusufi ANK et al: Calcitonin inhibits Na^+ gradient dependent phosphate uptake across renal brush border membranes *Am J Physiol* 252:F598, 1987.
709. Yusufi ANK et al: Effect of atrial natriuretic factor on brush border membrane transport of phosphate in phosphate deprived rats. *Biochem Pharmacol* 37:4027, 1988.
710. Yusufi ANK et al: Modulatory effect of thyroid hormones on uptake of phosphate and other solutes across luminal brush border membrane of kidney cortex. *Endocrinology* 116:2438, 1985.
711. Zilenovski Am et al: Effect of sodium bicarbonate on phosphate excretion in acute and chronic PTX rats. *Am J Physiol* 236:F184, 1979.
712. Zilva JF, Nicholson JP: Plasma phosphate and potassium levels in the hypercalcemia of malignant disease. *J Clin Endocrinol Metab* 36:1091, 1973.

CHAPTER • 13

Magnesium metabolism

Gary A. Quamme • John H. Dirks

OVERVIEW OF MAGNESIUM METABOLISM

Magnesium is the fourth most abundant cation in the human body and the second most common cation in the intracellular fluid (ICF). The abundance and distribution of the Mg^{2+} ion implies that it plays an essential role in intracellular metabolism. Although no single homeostatic control has been demonstrated for Mg^{2+}, the ion's cellular availability is closely regulated by the gastrointestinal tract, kidney, and bone.

Intracellular magnesium plays a critical role in many metabolic processes, including production and utilization of energy. Hydrolysis of adenosine triphosphate (ATP) via the various magnesium-dependent ATPases is involved in maintenance of intracellular electrolyte composition. In addition, magnesium is necessary for a large number of enzymatic reactions, including those involving DNA transcription, RNA aggregation, and protein synthesis. Extracellular magnesium is broadly implicated in neuronal control, neuromuscular transmission, and cardiovascular tone. It is not surprising that disturbances in the metabolism of magnesium result in a wide spectrum of clinical signs and symptoms.

Intracellular magnesium concentration, $[Mg^{2+}]_i$, and, more important, its availability to essential metabolic processes appear to be the determining factors in magnesium homeostasis. Recent evidence indicates that only 1 to 2 percent of the total cell magnesium is in the free form, Mg^{2+}, the levels of which are carefully controlled within the cell. Cellular magnesium content is maintained at the expense of extracellular fluid (ECF) and bone magnesium levels. Bone reservoirs are more important over the long term, since they contain about two-thirds of total body magnesium. Bone turnover rates are slow, and the hourly or daily requirements are met by a balance between intestinal absorption and renal excretion.

Approximately 30 to 40 percent of dietary magnesium is absorbed by the gastrointestinal tract, principally from the small bowel. The absolute absorption appears to be dependent on the magnesium content of the diet and on total body magnesium. Relatively higher magnesium absorption occurs in patients who have previously ingested low-magnesium diets or subjects who are in overall negative magnesium balance. The factors controlling intestinal magnesium absorption are not well delineated but appear to involve the vitamin D metabolites and parathyroid hormone (PTH). Absorption may also be affected by intraluminal complexing agents such as phytates, found in cereal grains.

The excretory side of magnesium balance involves appropriate changes in renal magnesium handling. Present evidence suggests that the renal handling of magnesium is normally a filtration-reabsorption process; experimental support for secretion remains unconvincing. Renal magnesium reabsorption has distinctive features when compared with reabsorption of sodium and calcium. The concentration of magnesium in the proximal tubule rises to 1.5 to 2.0 times that of glomerular filtrate. Some 20 to 30 percent of filtered magnesium is reabsorbed in the proximal tubule, compared to 50 or 60 percent absorption of sodium or calcium. Although the fractional reabsorption of magnesium is only half that of sodium, magnesium reabsorption changes in parallel with that of sodium in response to alterations in ECF volume. Approximately two-thirds of filtered magnesium is reabsorbed in the loop of Henle, mainly in the thick ascending limb. Recent evidence suggests that magnesium reabsorption in the ascending limb may be voltage-dependent and secondary to active sodium chloride reabsorption. Evidence also suggests an important competition between magnesium and calcium for transport at the basolateral surface of ascending limb cells. The loop of Henle appears to be the major nephron site where magnesium reabsorption is controlled. The principal factors that alter magnesium reabsorption in the loop include hormones such as PTH, glucagon, calcitonin, changes in plasma magnesium and calcium concentrations, and the loop diuretics. About 5 percent of filtered magnesium is delivered into the distal nephron, where only a small fraction is reabsorbed. The transport capacity of the distal segments is readily exceeded with increased magnesium delivery. Urinary magnesium excretion is principally determined within the thick ascending limb of Henle's loop.

BIOCHEMICAL AND PHYSIOLOGICAL EFFECTS

CHEMICAL PROPERTIES OF MAGNESIUM

Magnesium is the eighth most abundant element in the earth's crust. It does not occur free but is found in large deposits in the composite form as magnesite, dolomite, and other minerals. Although magnesium and calcium share the property of being the major divalent cations in the biological systems, they have very different chemical and physiological characteristics in the dilute aqueous salt solutions that are normally present in the body. The coordination number of magnesium is six, whereas that of calcium is eight. Accordingly, affinities for specific binding sites may be distinctive. In addition, the hydrated Mg^{2+} ion is relatively larger than calcium, and the hydrated forms of magnesium salts are relatively more soluble and able to participate in many metabolic processes. It is believed that Mg^{2+} differs from Ca^{2+} because of its interaction with water, the rate of exchange of water molecules on its inner shell of hydration being three or four orders of magnitude slower than for the other ions.[49,99] These properties are presumably the basis of the markedly different roles of magnesium and calcium within the respective intracellular and extracellular compartments. Moreover, this chemical property of magnesium enhances the solubility of calcium when the latter is complexed with anions such as phosphate and oxalate.[184] This may be beneficial in some patients with recurrent calcium oxalate or calcium phosphate stones.[122]

DISTRIBUTION OF TOTAL BODY MAGNESIUM

The adult human body contains 21 to 28 g (3400 to 4500 mmol) of magnesium.[191] Less than 2 percent of the total body magnesium store is located in the ECF compartment (Tables 13-1, 13-2). The principal stores of magnesium are bone (67 percent), muscle (20 percent), and nonmuscle soft tissues (11 percent, Fig. 13-1). The normal ratio of calcium to magnesium in bone is 50:1; trabecular bone contains more magnesium than cortical bone.[5,6] The major portion of magnesium is complexed to the apatite crystal rather than to bone matrix. Normal magnesium concentration in muscle is 3.8 mmol/kg of fat-free solids; much of this is complexed to intracellular organophosphates and proteins.[184] The normal magnesium level in red blood cells (RBCs) is about 2.3 m*M*, of which 84 percent is thought to be complexed to ATP.[46] Magnesium content of the erythrocyte appears to be inversely related to the age: reticulocytes contain about twice as much magnesium as do older RBCs. Recent studies suggest that magnesium enters these cells only during erythropoiesis and then is progressively lost as circulating RBCs age.[185] Accordingly, erythrocyte magnesium levels may not adequately reflect intracellular or total body magnesium content.

EXCHANGEABLE MAGNESIUM

The earliest change observed in experimental magnesium depletion in man or animals is a fall in extracellular magnesium concentration.[6,7,166,180] Intracellular magne-

TABLE 13-1 • Distribution of magnesium in the adult human body

Tissue	Total Mg concentration, mmol/liter	Free Mg^{2+}, m*M*	% of total body Mg
ECF	0.75–1.05	0.25–0.5	1.3
ICF			
Erythrocyte	2.3–3.1	0.5–1.0	0.7
Muscle	3.8	0.5–1.0	20
Other cells	8	0.5–1.0	10
Bone			
Cortical	107*		67
Trabecular	126*		
CSF	1.25		
Sweat	0.3		
Total body magnesium	**12***		**100**

ABBREVIATIONS: ECF, extracellular fluid; ICF, intracellular fluid; CSF, cerebrospinal fluid.
* In mmol/kg.

TABLE 13-2 • Magnesium in normal plasma

	Concentration, m*M*	% of total
Free Mg^{2+}	0.53	55
Protein-bound Mg	0.30	32
$MgHPO_4$	0.03	3
Mg citrate	0.04	4
Other Mg complexes	0.06	6
Total	**0.96**	100

SOURCE: Abstracted from Walser.[184]

sium concentrations have been reported to be either normal or low when serum magnesium levels are low (see below). However, controversy exists as to the relative magnitude of changes in magnesium content of ECF, muscle, and bone. Alfrey and colleagues determined magnesium levels in muscle, erythrocyte, and bone of patients with low, normal, and elevated levels of plasma and total body magnesium.[6] They showed a better correlation between serum and bone magnesium levels than between serum and muscle concentrations.[6,7] These data suggest that bone and ECF magnesium are the major pools that respond to deficits or surfeits of magnesium. Under normal physiological conditions about one-third of the bone magnesium is absorbed to the surface of the apatite crystal and is thought to be exchangeable with the bone ECF.[7] However, bone ECF and circulating ECF may not be in equilibrium. Throughout life there is a continuous process of bone formation and bone removal; under normal conditions magnesium is released in association with calcium phosphates. Such continuous bone remodeling probably contributes little to mineral homeostasis. In addition, the availability of the bone magnesium reservoir is dependent on age.[27] Thirty percent of the magnesium content of bone is thought to be exchangeable in young individuals, whereas only a small fraction of this may be exchangeable in the elderly.[5,27] The available magnesium may also increase in circumstances of increased bone turnover or bone dissolution, such as with rapid skeletal growth or in Pagets' disease.

The intracellular-to-extracellular distribution of magnesium is similar to that of potassium. Potassium is the most abundant cation within cells, found mostly within muscle. Minute changes in intracellular potassium may rapidly result in dramatic changes in the extracellular potassium concentration. However, these rapid intracellular-to-extracellular cation shifts observed for potassium do not occur with magnesium. Magnesium, unlike potassium, is bound to intracellular ligands and is not readily available for exchange; less than a third of muscle and erythrocyte magnesium is thought to be exchangeable.[5] Bone studies using the short-half-life ^{28}Mg for compartmental analysis of the plasma and the nonplasma whole body compartments suggest that exchangeable magnesium is less than 15 percent of total body magnesium; turnover half-times are at least 60 days.[185] Long-term balance studies and compartmental analysis of magnesium turnover have been plagued with technical difficulties, due principally to the absence of a stable isotope with an appropriate half-life. ^{28}Mg has a half-life of 21.3 h, which is short compared to the turnover rates of magnesium. The use of a more stable isotope of magnesium, such as ^{26}Mg, and analysis with neutron activation techniques have not been rewarding.[158] In summary, bone and muscle cells are the major intracellular magnesium storage pools in humans, of which only a small fraction is exchangeable with the ECF.

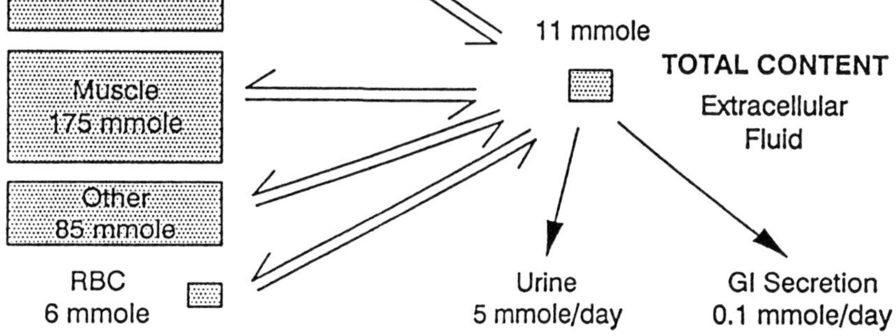

FIGURE 13-1 • Distribution of magnesium in the body, including dietary intake, gastrointestinal absorption, and urinary excretion.

INTRACELLULAR FREE Mg^{2+} ACTIVITY

Although magnesium is abundant within the cell, most is chelated to various organic substrates and not available for biochemical processes or transport.[64] The important fraction of intracellular magnesium is the free form Mg^{2+}. A number of studies have indicated that intracellular Mg^{2+} levels may be on the order of 0.5 to 1.0 m*M*,[23,79,125,140,149] although other studies have reported somewhat higher values.[1,25,29,40,66,86,116] In 1989, a fluorescent dye was developed to measure intracellular free Mg^{2+} concentrations, $[Mg^{2+}]_i$, within single living cells.[125,144,145,149] The use of this fluorescent probe has clarified some of the controversies concerning Mg^{2+} concentrations within the cytosol (Fig. 13-2). $[Mg^{2+}]_i$ appears to be about 0.5 m*M* and as such makes up only 1 to 2 percent of the total cellular magnesium. The small fraction of total magnesium that is in the free Mg^{2+} form should be considered when reviewing the older literature concerning magnesium exchanges based on total cell magnesium.

The transmembrane electrical potential of most cells is in the order of −65 mV, inside with respect to outside; accordingly, it has been speculated for some time that Mg^{2+} may move passively into the cell down the transmembrane electrical gradient. As $[Mg^{2+}]_i$ was not known, it was unsure what role the transmembrane chemical gradient played in this influx. The fluorescent studies indicate that $[Mg^{2+}]_i$ is 0.5 m*M*, which is about 1 percent of total cellular magnesium.[9,41] Thus, the principal driving force for Mg^{2+} movement into the cell is the transmembrane electrical gradient at extracellular magnesium concentration, $[Mg^{2+}]_o$, of 0.5 to 0.75 m*M*.

Recently, we have performed a number of experiments to define the entry of Mg^{2+} into the cell. This was done by depleting cells of Mg^{2+} for a prolonged period of time and subsequently observing the change in $[Mg^{2+}]_i$ when the cells were placed in a buffer containing high $[Mg^{2+}]_o$ (Fig. 13-2). The refill rate, a measure of concentration change per time, was sufficiently rapid to be detected with changes in fluorescence of mag-fura-2. Two aspects of this refill were of interest. First, the pattern of refill did not asymptote but was linear with time, which suggests that the principal driving force for entry is the transmembrane electrical potential rather than the transmembrane chemical gradient. Second, the entry of Mg^{2+} appears to be highly regulated. We consistently observed that the change in $[Mg^{2+}]_i$ of Mg^{2+}-depleted cells after refill abruptly stopped at or near the normal cell $[Mg^{2+}]_i$. This is in contrast to cells cultured in normal Mg^{2+} media where $[Mg^{2+}]_i$ was not altered over the same time frame of study. $[Ca^{2+}]_i$ was not altered throughout these manipulations. These observations suggest that Mg^{2+} entry is regulated and specific to Mg^{2+}. At the present time, we do know whether this entry pathway is a channel or some other transporter. Magnesium channels have previously been identified through electrophysiological approaches,[8,126,127,133] and evidence has been provided for transporters such as Na^+-Mg^{2+} exchange.[61,62,65,76,105] It is not known whether the Mg^{2+} entry we have demonstrated in Fig. 13-2 is involved in transepithelial transport or simply with housekeeping duties, thereby providing appropriate Mg^{2+} levels for intracellular metabolism.

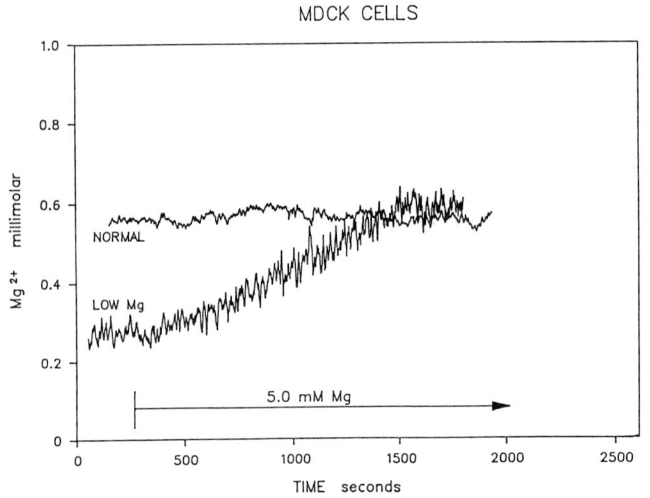

FIGURE 13-2 • Intracellular free Mg^{2+} concentration in normal Mg^{2+}-depleted Madin-Darby canine kidney (MDCK) cells. Confluent MDCK cells were cultured in either normal (0.5 m*M* magnesium) or Mg^{2+}-free media (less than 0.01 m*M*) for 16 to 20 h. Isolated cells were loaded with 5 μ*M* mag-fura-2 AM, and the fluorescence signal was monitored at 505 nm with excitation wavelengths alternating between 340 and 385 nm using a Deltascan (Photon Technologies, Inc.) spectrofluorometer. The $[Mg^{2+}]_i$ was calculated with a K_D of 1.45 m*M*, for the fluorescent dye–cation complex corrected for fluorescence from extracellular dye and autofluorescence. The basal $[Mg^{2+}]_i$ was determined, and the cells were subsequently placed in buffer solution containing high $MgCl_2$ (5.0 m*M*). The rate of Mg^{2+} refill, $d([Mg^{2+}]_i)/dt$, was determined by using linear regression on the increase in $[Mg^{2+}]_i$ versus time following placement into solutions containing 5 m*M* $MgCl_2$. Note that Mg^{2+} increased only in magnesium-depleted cells and that the $[Mg^{2+}]_i$ abruptly leveled off near normal basal Mg^{2+} levels, indicating that the entry pathway is regulated. (From *Am J Physiol* 259:C521, 1990. Used by permission.)

Other factors may also alter intracellular Mg^{2+} concentration. As most (more than 90 percent) of the intracellular ATP is tightly complexed to Mg^{2+}, any changes in ATP levels may alter $[Mg^{2+}]_i$.[60,62] Indeed, this is the basis for ^{31}P nuclear magnetic resonance (NMR) determination of intracellular Mg^{2+}.[77] We have shown that the application of a mitochondrial uncoupler and glycolytic inhibitor depresses ATP levels and increases free Mg^{2+}, presumably from the dissociation of an ATP-Mg^{2+} complex.[60] However, intracellular Mg^{2+} does not go much above 1.0 m*M* with diminished ATP levels of about 5.0 m*M*. Accordingly, other intracellular complexes or compartmentalization may limit the rise in intracellular free Mg^{2+} under these conditions. These "buffering" processes remain to be determined. In addition, we have shown that intracellular Mg^{2+} may be controlled by intracellular compartmentalization, possibly by specific processes of the endoplasmic or sarcoplasmic reticulum. Free Mg^{2+} concentration is not uniform throughout the cell, being higher in the cytosol near the plasma membrane and lower within the nucleus.[60] This heterogenous distribution of Mg^{2+} may have important ramifications in cell metabolism. These and other controls[147] will be elucidated within the present decade due in major part to the availability of sensitive and specific fluorescent probes for intracellular Mg^{2+}.

In summary, a typical cell contains between 12 and 15 m*M* magnesium, of which about 1 to 2 percent is ionized. Because the ECF contains about 0.53 m*M* free Mg^{2+} (Table 13-2) and the transmembrane electrical potential is normally −65 mV, magnesium appears to be actively extruded from the cell into the ECF. The details of such a process are unknown, but it may be accomplished through ATP-requiring magnesium pumps[170] or by a sodium-magnesium antiport exchange system. The driving force for sodium-magnesium exchange resides in the low intracellular sodium concentration and the high transmembrane potential difference, which are largely determined by the sodium pump, Na^+-K^+ ATPase. The backleak of sodium into the cell may be coupled to active magnesium efflux.[15,129] The precise description of cellular magnesium transport and its controls are fruitful areas for research.

BIOCHEMICAL AND PHYSIOLOGICAL FUNCTIONS OF MAGNESIUM

Magnesium plays a critical and necessary role in intracellular metabolism. One of its essential roles is to activate a wide spectrum of enzymatic reactions. These incude the various phosphokinases and phosphateses that are involved in energy storage and utilization. The most commonly recognized is the activation of ATPases involved in establishing and controlling intracellular electrolyte content. Magnesium may function primarily to form Mg^{2+}-ATP^{2-}, which is a substrate for these enzymes. Accordingly, activation of these ATPases by specific ions results in hydrolysis of ATP and the net transport of the ions from one compartment to another. The ion-sensitive ATPases are situated in the intracellular compartments and membranes and regulate the flow of potential energy from the mitochondria and cytoplasm. Recognized Mg^{2+}-ATPases include ouabain-sensitive Mg^{2+} + (Na^+-K^+) ATPase, ouabain-insensitive Mg^{2+} + H^+ ATPase, and the Ca^{2+}-Mg^{2+} ATPase, which are associated with sodium pumps, proton pumps, and calcium pumps, respectively. The sodium pump maintains cell distribution of Na^+ and K^+; the proton pumps are essential in mitochondrial ATP generation and pH balance; and the calcium pump is most notable in preserving low intracellular calcium concentrations. Specific magnesium pumps have not yet been demonstrated but may well present in some, if not all, cells. The Mg^{2+}-dependent ATPases are distributed in all cell compartments and may have several functions other than ion transport, particularly in the many endergonic processes requiring ATP hydrolysis. ATP is also utilized in substrate interconversions and for such biosynthetic processes as gluconeogenesis and the formation of phospholipids and proteins. Magnesium is indirectly involved in protein synthesis through its action on nucleic acid polymerization, its role in binding of ribosomes to RNA, and the synthesis and degradation of DNA.[92]

There is abundant evidence to indicate that Mg^{2+} may have regulatory functions in the matrix of mitochondria controlling fatty acid metabolism, volume homeostasis, and energy generation.[19,67,90,171] In addition to its direct involvement in phosphorylation of glucose along the anaerobic pathway, magnesium may indirectly control mitochondrial oxidative metabolism. Mitochondria contain large amounts of magnesium, which may be involved with the alteration of Na^+ and K^+ permeability and the pH-regulated anion uniporter across the inner mitochondrial membrane.[97,171] Permeability to these ions is normally low; an increase in permeability may lead to the dissipation of the hydrogen ion concentration gradient across the inner mitochondrial membrane. Since this gradient is thought to be involved in forming ATP from ADP and inorganic phosphate (by a reaction involving the mitochondrial proton ATPase), its dissipation would result in a decrease in electron transport and an uncoupling of oxidative phosphorylation. Competitors of magnesium control of permeability at the inner mitochondrial membrane, such as mercury, gentamicin, cisplatin (cis-dichlorodiammineplatinum), cyclosporine and other cytotoxins, may lead to mitochondrial swelling, increased mitochondrial respiration, and uncoupled oxidative phosphorylation.[18,186] This may provide a common biochemical pathway in the pathogenesis of cytotoxicity.

It is not likely that intracellular Mg^{2+} plays a direct role in signal transduction mechanisms analogous to that of intracellular Ca^{2+}.[22] However, it is apparent that Mg^{2+} may indirectly affect cell regulation through its actions on essential enzyme reactions involved in signal transduction. For example, adenylate cyclase, which is critical in the generation of the intracellular second messenger, cAMP, has also been shown to require magnesium. The substrate for this enzyme reaction is Mg^{2+}-ATP, which is converted to cAMP in the presence of adenylate cyclase.[30] Mg^{2+} has also been shown to regulate phosphatidylinositol-specific phospholipase C at appropriate intracellular concentrations, 0.3 to 1.0 m*M*.[36] Accordingly, intracellular Mg^{2+} may modulate levels of the second messenger, diacylglycerol. Magnesium may also be involved in the modulation of specific peptide hormones through interaction with their respective cell surface receptors.[93,109] The other product of phospholipase C activity, inositol 1,4,5-tris phosphate (IP_3) may also be influenced by Mg^{2+}, leading to diminished IP_3-induced Ca^{2+} release.[177]

Over the last decade, it has become increasingly clear that Mg^{2+} plays an important role in altering the activity of a number of ion channels. Nowak and coworkers first demonstrated Mg^{2+} blockage of *N*-methyl-D-aspartate (NMDA) receptors.[128] This is one of the glutamate receptors involved in fast excitatory neurotransmission.[106] Mg^{2+} apparently blocks these channels from both extracellular and intracellular sides by different binding sites.[81,82] Mg^{2+} is also partly responsible for inward rectification of a number of potassium channels, including the muscarinic receptor–operated K^+ channel,[87,88] the Na^{2+}-activated K^+ channel,[114] the Ca^{2+}-activated K^+ channel,[34] and the inwardly rectifying K^+ channel,[113,172,176] and for blocking the outward currents of the ATP-regulated K^+ channel.[89] Unidirectional and voltage-dependent blockage by internal Mg^{2+} seems to be a common mechanism causing inward rectification of K^+ channels. However, the sensitivity to Mg^{2+} differs among the kinds of channels.[114] Cytosolic Mg^{2+} also modulates Ca^{2+} channel activity in various cell types.[2,190] Voltage-gated Ca^{2+} channels are present in most, if not all, excitable cells and play a key role in the initiation and maintenance of excitation and contraction of neural and cardiac cells.[81] Evidence shows that Mg^{2+} ions enter the Ca^{2+} channel and bind to one or more specific sites, interfering with Ca^{2+} transport. Outward Na^+ currents through tetrodotoxin (TTX)-sensitive Na^+ channels are blocked in a voltage- and time-dependent fashion by intracellular Mg^{2+}.[134] The effects of Mg^{2+} on ionic channels may be more complicated than simple obstruction of the permeation pathway.[82,173] Further electrophysiological studies will clarify our understanding of these effects; nevertheless, it is evident that intracellular Mg^{2+} plays an important role in modulating channel activity.

In addition to magnesium's role in intracellular metabolism, it has a number of specific functions in different organ systems. Magnesium plays an essential role in the central nervous and peripheral neuromuscular systems. Most of the available knowledge has been gained from clinical observation of magnesium deficiency or subsequent to administration of pharmacological amounts of magnesium salts.

Table 13-3 summarizes some of the common manifestations of hypomagnesemia and hypermagnesemia (see Chap. 34). The mechanisms of these alterations are not understood. Magnesium depletion leads to an increase in central neuronal excitability and enhanced neuromuscular transmission, whereas hypermagnesemia results in neuromuscular blockade. Magnesium excess is thought to displace membrane-bound Ca^{2+}, leading to an inhibition of the prejunctional release of acetylcholine and a decrease in the sensitivity of the motor end plate to the depolarizing action of acetylcholine.[68] This may result in increased muscle fasciculations, tetany when magnesium is deficient, and flaccid muscular paralysis when magnesium is in excess. In addition, hypomagnesemia may lead to more central disturbances such as disorientation, convulsions, and psychotic behavior.[167] Anorexia, nausea, and apathy frequently occur prior to peripheral neurological manifestations.[167] Brain or spinal cord trauma leads to a decline in free Mg^{2+} levels as measured by ^{31}P NMR techniques,[178,179] and subsequent magnesium infusions have been reported to mitigate cell damage and hasten recovery.[117]

Magnesium has a number of effects on the cardiovascular system. Magnesium excess causes increased atrioventricular and intraventricular conduction time, with lengthened PR and QRS intervals of the ECG.[160] Severe hypomagnesemia leads to a prolongation of the Q-T interval, which may predispose the heart to ventricular arrhythmias.[91] The underlying mechanism of these cardiac effects is not well understood but probably involves an interaction of magnesium with calcium channels. Intracellular Mg^{2+} has been implicated in energy disturbances resulting from damage and recovery from myocardial ischemia.[10,67] Peripheral vascular tone is also influenced by the ambient magnesium concentration;[146] for instance, hypomagnesemia commonly results in increased arteriolar tone.[175] When extracellular magnesium is lowered, there is increased uptake of calcium and an enhanced intracellular calcium concentration, which may lead to increased tension of vascular smooth muscle.[174] This suggests a physiological role for magnesium in the control of cellular arteriolar calcium extrusion and peripheral tone.[10] Intracellular Mg^{2+} has been claimed by many investigators to be a biological antagonist of Ca^{2+}, in effect buffering the overzealous actions of Ca^{2+} within the cell. Many of these general interpretations are based on pharmacological experiments using very large Mg^{2+} concentrations.[44] As intracellular Mg^{2+} is normally within the range of 0.5 to 1.0 m*M*, it is likely that the protective effects are specific.

Magnesium appears to be interrelated with potassium, the other major intracellular cation. Changes in the intracellular concentration of one tend to lead to similar changes in the other. This is particularly evident in muscle cells, where the magnesum concentration was shown to vary directly with the potassium level.[6] In magnesium-deficient humans or animals, total body potassium is often reduced; conversely, intracellular magnesium may be low in animals with potassium deficiency.[16,95] This association is further strengthened by several clinical observations that suggest that correction of the intracellular potassium and magnesium deficits is facilitated if both are included in the replacement ther-

TABLE 13-3 • Some common manifestations of altered magnesium metabolism

	Manifestation	Mechanism
MAGNESIUM DEFICIENCY		
Biochemical	Hypocalcemia	Impaired PTH secretion PTH resistance to end organs Resistance to vitamin D
	Hypokalemia	Renal K^+ wasting
Neuromuscular	Neuromuscular irritability (muscle tremors, weakness, fasciculations, tetany)	Hypocalcemia Hypomagnesemia
	Central nervous system (nystagmus, ataxia, vertigo psychiatric abnormalities)	
Cardiovascular	Cardiac arrhythmia (tachycardia, prolonged P-R and Q-T intervals, abnormal T wave)	Hypokalemia Hypomagnesemia
Gastrointestinal	Dysphagia	Neuromuscular irritability
Hematologic	Anemia (reticulocytosis, spherocytosis, microcytosis, erythroid hyperplasia)	
MAGNESIUM EXCESS		
Biochemical	Hypocalcemia	Renal calcium wasting Impaired PTH secretion
Neuromuscular	Neuromuscular depression (decrease in deep tendon reflexes, paralysis)	Impaired nerve transmission Decrease in postsynaptic response
	Central nervous system (depression, somnolence)	Hypermagnesemia
Cardiovascular	Cardiac arrhythmia (bradycardia, increased QRS duration)	Hypermagnesemia Hypocalcemia

apy. Accordingly, it is difficult to replace potassium during magnesium depletion without also repairing the magnesium deficit. Cronin and colleagues examined the effect of pure magnesium deficiency on muscle composition in the dog.[43] Magnesium deficiency led to severe hypomagnesemia over a 10-week period, with only modest changes in muscle magnesium content. However, skeletal muscle phosphorus decreased significantly with increases in calcium, sodium, and chloride, and no change in potassium. These data led the authors to conclude that intracellular phosphorus deficiency may be the critical change in magnesium depletion. The basis for the coexistence of intracellular phosphorus depletion in the face of a normal serum phosphate concentration is not known. However, it would appear that intracellular magnesium is directly or indirectly important in the maintenance of normal electrolyte distribution. Perhaps magnesium depletion retards ATP generation so that the cell is no longer able to maintain the normal transmembrane electrolyte gradients.[189]

BONE MAGNESIUM

Bone magnesium is localized in the bone cells; in the bone surface pool, either in the hydrated form or absorbed to the crystal surface; and in the mineralized matrix, replacing calcium in the apatite crystal.[183] As in other cells, magnesium is involved in enzyme activation and mitochondrial energy transfer in bone cells. Osteoblasts, osteoclasts, and associated cells have an abundance of enzymes, such as the acid and alkaline phosphatases and the pyrophosphatases, that are involved in the calcification process. These enzymes are important in the normal functioning of matrix vesicles. Osteoblasts and chondrocytes form matrix vesicles, which may provide nucleation sites for calcification of the osteoid and cartilage matrix. These vesicles are rich in calcium, phosphate, alkaline phosphatase, pyrophosphatase, ATP, and magnesium. Mg^{2+}-ATP may stabilize and perhaps regulate the amorphous calcium phosphate granules prior to apatite formation.[132] In addition to metabolic functions within the bone cells, magnesium is involved with structural aspects of bone, replacing calcium in the apatite crystal. This appears to be a nonspecific event, because the incorporation and release of magnesium is associated with calcium. The significance of this is unknown because bone mineralization, bone remodeling, and marrow differentiation continue even in the presence of severe magnesium depletion, but at an impaired rate.[151,157] These events are under the control of PTH, vitamin D metabolites, and possibly calcitonin.

DIETARY INTAKE AND GASTROINTESTINAL ABSORPTION

INTESTINAL MAGNESIUM HANDLING

Dietary magnesium

The average daily diet in North America contains approximately 10 to 15 mmol (240 to 370 mg) of elemental magnesium.[94,159] The daily dietary requirement for magnesium is about 9 to 16 mmol for young adult males and 7.5 to 14 mmol for females (Table 13-4). Although this requirement is not sharply defined, it suggests that the average North American diet is only adequate for maintenance of body magnesium levels. Moreover, magnesium requirements increase with rapid growth in infancy and adolescence and during pregnancy and lactation. Despite the suggestive borderline dietary insufficiency, overt magnesium deficiency from dietary causes alone is uncommon. This is probably because of the ubiquity of magnesium in the North American diet, especially if the diet is high in seafood, nuts, grains, and vegetables rich in chlorophyll, a magnesium chelator.[159] In addition, under normal circumstances, the gastrointestinal tract and kidney absorb and conserve appropriate quantities of magnesium.

TABLE 13-4 • Dietary requirements and gastrointestinal absorption

Daily requirements	9–18 mmol (220–400 mg)
Normal daily dietary content	10–15 mmol (250–370 mg)
Intestinal dietary absorption	30–40%
Flux rate at luminal Mg = 5 m*M*	
Jejunum	0.12 mmol/30 $cm \cdot h^{-1}$
Ileum	0.12 mmol/30 $cm \cdot h^{-1}$

SOURCE: Abstracted from Brannan et al,[26] Levine et al,[103] and Walser.[184]

Gastrointestinal absorption

About 30 to 40 percent of ingested magnesium is absorbed when dietary intake of magnesium is normal. Fractional magnesium absorption may increase to as high as 80 percent when dietary intake is restricted to about 1 mmol and decrease to 25 percent of intake on magnesium intakes as high as 25 mmol/day.[4] Accordingly, intestinal absorption is controlled by a factor or factors that respond appropriately to dietary magnesium content.

Magnesium absorption in humans and animals occurs primarily in the distal portion of the small intestine.[4,20,26,72,107,121,148] Normally, the flux rates for magnesium are greater in the ileum than in the duodenum or jejunum, but this may be related to the length of the individual segments and transit time through each.[26] Brannan and colleagues demonstrated similar fluxes for magnesium from perfused human jejunal and ileal segments when the intraluminal magnesium concentration was above 5 m*M*. Somewhat higher rates were observed in the ileum than in the jejunum at concentrations below this value (Fig. 13-3*a*). These observations help explain the high incidence of magnesium deficiency following surgical resection or bypass of the ileum for either obesity or diseases of the distal small bowel. The colon absorbs small amounts of magnesium, which may be significant under certain circumstances.[4,96,119] For instance, hypermagnesemia has been reported following enemas with epsom salts (magnesium sulfate).[59]

Intestinal magnesium absorption may occur through transcellular or paracellular pathways.[78] In the transcellular pathway, magnesium may cross the brush border membrane of the intestinal epithelial cell down an electrochemical gradient. Evidence has been presented that this may be facilitated by a carrier that demonstrates a limiting transport rate of about 10 m*M* (Fig. 13-3*a*). Movement across the basolateral membrane is active, since transport occurs against an electrochemical gradient. Details of these steps have not yet been described. In the paracellular pathway, magnesium is transported between the enterocytes. The driving force for paracellular magnesium absorption is probably a chemical, rather than an electrical, gradient, since magnesium concentration in the intestinal lumen may be higher than that in plasma but the electrical potential is normally about 5 mV, lumen-negative with respect to plasma.[26,96] Magnesium absorption may also be affected by paracellular water absorption and solvent drag of magnesium through the paracellular pathway. Moreover, water movement can increase or decrease the luminal volume, which tends to affect magnesium concentration. As both transcellular

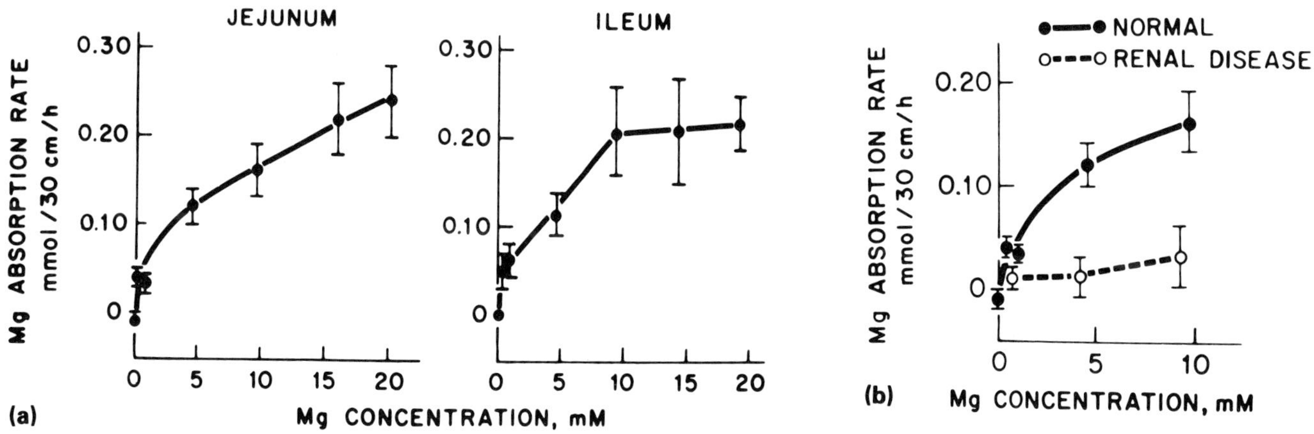

FIGURE 13-3 • (*a*) Magnesium absorption rate in the normal human jejunum and ileum at various luminal magnesium concentrations. (*b*) Comparison of jejunal magnesium absorption in normal subjects and patients with chronic renal failure at various luminal magnesium concentrations. (From *Clin Invest* 57:1412, 1976. Used by permission of the American Society for Clinical Investigations.)

and paracellular magnesium fluxes are dependent on luminal magnesium concentration, magnesium absorption is deeply influenced by water movement. For instance, prolonged diarrhea results in intestinal malabsorption of magnesium.

Factors that alter intestinal magnesium handling

VITAMIN D AND PTH Little is known about the control of intestinal magnesium absorption. Balance studies suggest that vitamin D may augment magnesium absorption in the small intestine, as it does calcium absorption.[26,103] Other studies have failed to demonstrate an enhanced uptake of magnesium following administration of vitamin D. Serum magnesium concentrations are not high in patients with vitamin D intoxication.[24,118,121] Brannan and colleagues[26] found decreased magnesium and calcium absorption in uremic patients and suggested that the impaired absorption of both was the result of a 1α,25-dihydroxyvitamin D_3 [1α,25-$(OH)_2D_3$] deficiency (Fig. 13-3*a*). On balance, evidence indicates vitamin D acts on intestinal magnesium absorption. Accordingly, magnesium absorption may decrease with age which is associated with a progressive decrease in the ability to generate 1α25-$(OH)_2D_3$.

PTH has also been implicated in the control of intestinal magnesium absorption. MacIntyre and Robinson reported that administration of PTH augments magnesium absorption from duodenal, jejunal, and ileal loops of parathyroidectomized (PTX) rats.[107] They concluded that absorption of magnesium by the gut is largely controlled by PTH. Accordingly, intestinal magnesium absorption may well be under regulatory influences similar to those observed for calcium. Development of hypomagnesemia or hypocalcemia due to a low-magnesium diet or a low-calcium diet results in stimulation of PTH secretion. PTH may act directly on the gut or, more likely, activate renal 25-hydroxyvitamin D [25-(OH)D], 1α hydroxylase, and increase 1α,25-$(OH)_2D_3$ synthesis, which in turn acts on the gut to increase magnesium and calcium absorption. One notable exception in this common control of magnesium and calcium is that, unlike the stimulation of intestinal calcium absorption by low dietary calcium that persists after thyroparathyroidectomy (TPTX), the low dietary magnesium effect on calcium transport is abolished by removal of the parathyroid glands.[181] Further studies are needed to clarify the specific roles of PTH and vitamin D in intestinal magnesium absorption.

The effects on magnesium transport of such hormones as growth hormone, estrogens, androgens, adrenal glucocorticoids, thyroid hormone, and somatostatin remain to be studied. These hormones may exert their effects on magnesium transport in part by altering vitamin D metabolism. It is thought that growth hormone, prolactin, and estrogens increase generation of 1α,25-$(OH)_2D_3$, whereas the others may decrease vitamin D generation.

A number of early studies concluded that luminal calcium may influence magnesium absorption.[3,28,37,84,169] These reports have allowed others to suggest a common absorptive pathway for magnesium and calcium. Recent intestinal perfusion studies of Brannan and associates have not supported these postulations.[26] High luminal concentrations of either calcium (20 m*M*) or magnesium (10m*M*) failed to influence the absorption of the other divalent cation. This suggests that the absorptive mechanisms are independent. As indicated above, chronic administration of either calcium or magnesium may alter PTH and vitamin D balance and thereby indirectly affect intestinal absorption of calcium, magnesium, or both. Present evidence indicates that there are separate mechanisms for calcium and magnesium at similar luminal concentrations.

AVAILABILITY OF DIETARY MAGNESIUM The amount of available intraluminal magnesium also affects intestinal absorption. Presumably only the ionized magnesium, Mg^{2+}, is transported by the intestinal epithelium. Precipitation of magnesium as insoluble phosphates, carbonates, and soaps begins in the ileum, progresses further in the colon, and is very extensive in the stool. This may influence the amount of magnesium that is not absorbed; for instance, total fecal phosphate is correlated closely with the sum of total fecal calcium and magnesium.[45] Any alteration in the luminal concentration of calcium or phosphate may also indirectly affect magnesium absorption. Accordingly, elevation of intraluminal magnesium may precipitate phosphate and allow for greater calcium absorption.[83] Fats may also make magnesium unavailable for absorption. Steatorrhea may cause or potentiate magnesium malabsorption through formation of nonabsorbable magnesium-lipid salts.[24] Formation of magnesium salts with lipids that are normally absorbed in the small bowel may predispose patients with ileal bypass surgery to further magnesium deficiency.

The major portion of the magnesium found in the stool is derived from the diet. Magnesium concentrations in saliva, gastric secretions, bile, and pancreatic and intestinal secretions range from 0.3 to 0.7 m*M* and amount to only 1.2 percent of the daily fecal output.

PRIMARY MALABSORPTION OF MAGNESIUM A small number of patients have been reported with primary hypomagnesemia due to an isolated defect in the gastrointestinal absorption of magnesium (see Chap. 34).[120,130,168] Severe magnesium deficiency occurs when these patients are on normal dietary intakes of magnesium, but plasma magnesium concentration may be normalized by greatly increasing the oral intake of magnesium. This finding suggests that the problem lies with regulation of magnesium absorption rather than with an absence of membrane carriers. There appears to be no common link between primary gastrointestinal hypomagnesemia and the rare condition of primary renal magnesium wasting.[69] Although of interest, these diseases are uncommon, and no experimental animal models are presently available for study.

RENAL HANDLING OF MAGNESIUM

SEGMENTAL MAGNESIUM HANDLING

Glomerular filtration

Unfilterable magnesium constitutes 70 to 80 percent of total plasma Mg^{2+} as determined by direct sampling of surface glomeruli of Munich-Wistar rats and by the use of artificial membranes, while the ultrafilterable part of plasma calcium is 60 to 65 percent of total Ca^{2+} concentration in plasma. Only 70 to 80 percent of the filterable magnesium is thought to be in the ionic form Mg^{2+}; the remainder is predominantly complexed to anions, particularly phosphate, citrate, and oxalate.[184] The ultrafilterability of plasma magnesium is not affected by magnesium deficiency, magnesium excess, or elevation of plasma calcium concentration.[35] Other factors that may affect glomerular ultrafilterability, such as acidosis, alkalosis, and alterations of plasma anion and protein constituents, remain to be evaluated. Since 20 to 30 percent of plasma magnesium is bound to plasma proteins, it may be assumed that the free Mg^{2+}, or ultrafilterable, portion changes with alteration in plasma concentration, which should be borne in mind when interpreting plasma magnesium levels.

Proximal convoluted tubule

The proximal convoluted tubule reabsorbs less than 25 percent of the magnesium filtered at the glomerulus (Fig. 13-4). Luminal magnesium concentration rises with respect to ultrafilterable magnesium along the length of the proximal convoluted tubule (Fig. 13-5). Morel and colleagues[123] were the first investigators to demonstrate this occurrence in the rat. The mean tubule fluid to ultrafilterable (TF/UF) magnesium ratio was 1.7 at a point in the nephron where 50 to 55 percent of sodium and water had been reabsorbed.[123] This appears to be a common phenomenon in all species studied to date.[142] The overall fractional magnesium reabsorption in the proximal tubule is some 20 to 30 percent of the filtered load; this is about 50 to 70 percent of the fractional reabsorption rate of sodium and calcium. Overall magnesium reabsorption in the proximal tubule closely follows changes in salt and water reabsorption, but at a lower fractional rate. The profile for the TF/UF magnesium ratio relative to the inulin concentration ratio remains largely unchanged in a variety of experimental circumstances, including volume expansion, diuretic administration, metabolic acidosis and alkalosis, and changes in plasma levels of calcium and phosphate.[142]

The observation that the tubule fluid magnesium concentration may be about 1.5 times greater than the plasma concentration suggests that the proximal tubule epithelium possess a low permeability for magnesium relative to sodium or calcium. A detailed analysis of magnesium transport in the proximal tubule was made using in vivo microperfusion.[135] Tubules were perfused with Ringer's solutions containing various amounts of magnesium chloride. Magnesium was measured by electron microprobe analysis in the samples collected downstream from the perfusion site. Absolute magnesium concentration increased along the perfused tubule in a linear manner, with net water reabsorption similar to that

FIGURE 13-4 • Summary of magnesium handling in renal tubules.

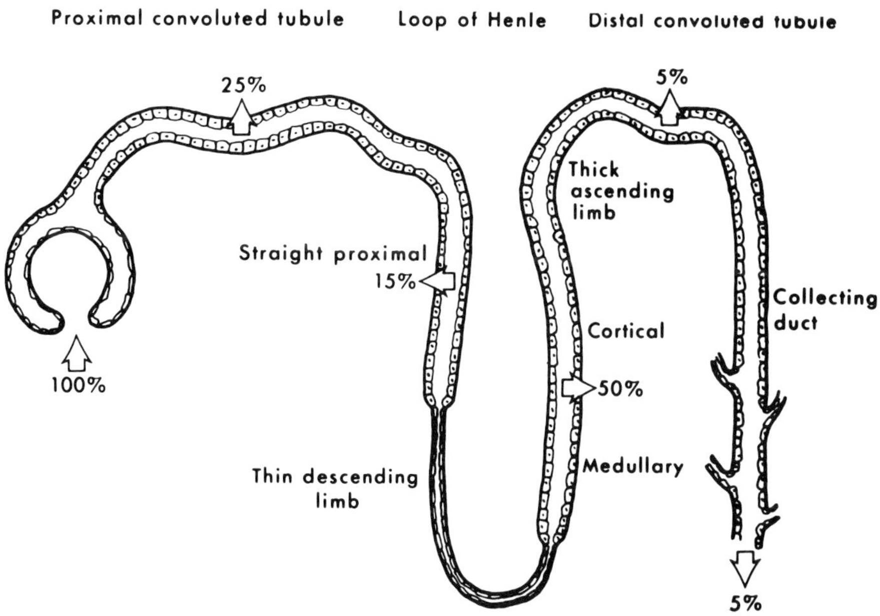

observed in free-flow micropuncture studies. The collected-to-perfusate concentration ratio of magnesium rose whether luminal magnesium concentrations were markedly below or even very significantly (tenfold) above the ultrafilterable plasma magnesium level, indicating a relatively low permeability of the superficial proximal tubule to magnesium relative to sodium and calcium.

In the above mentioned in vivo perfusion studies it was demonstrated that magnesium reabsorption is dependent on intraluminal magnesium concentration. Perfusion of rat proximal tubules with solutions containing magnesium in excess of 5 to 7 m*M* failed to saturate the transport system. Further studies in dogs given magnesium chloride infusions support these observations.[194] Graded elevations of plasma magnesium resulted in enhanced absolute magnesium reabsorption (Fig. 13-5).

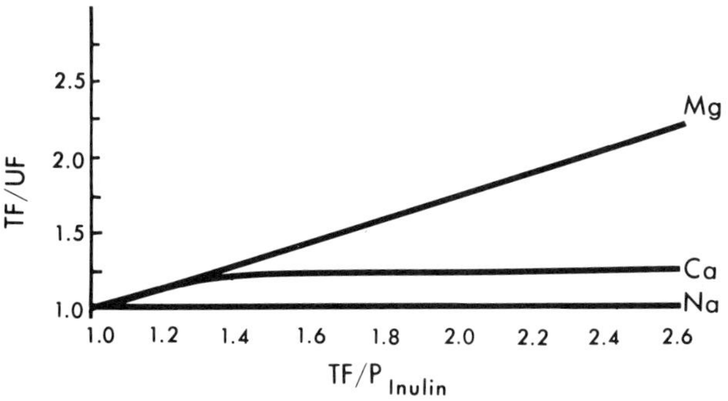

FIGURE 13-5 • Concentration profile of magnesium, calcium, and sodium along the proximal convoluted tubule. TF/UF, tubule fluid–to–ultrafilterable cation concentration ratio; TF/P inulin, tubule fluid–to–plasma inulin concentration ratio (an index of water absorption).

The last observation is possibly the basis of the glomerulotubular balance observed for magnesium. The reabsorptive rate is dependent on the luminal magnesium concentration, which in turn is determined by the concurrent sodium and water transport. In summary, magnesium transport by the superficial proximal tubule is mainly a unidirectional process and is dependent on luminal or filtered magnesium concentration; magnesium is reabsorbed proportionally to sodium and water transport but at a lower rate.

Proximal straight tubule and thin descending limb of Henle's loop

Present knowledge of magnesium transport by the proximal straight tubule has been gained indirectly by evaluating the fluid collected by micropuncture from the bend of the loop of the surgically exposed papilla of the young rat or desert rodent. As such, these data describe the function of the proximal convoluted and proximal straight segments of the deep nephrons, which may function quite differently from the superficial tubules described above. De Rouffignac and colleagues examined fluid collected from the late superficial proximal tubule and the tip of the long loops in the desert rat.[46] They determined that there was greater fractional magnesium concentration present at the end of the deep descending limb than at the end of the superficial proximal tubule. Because the rise in intraluminal magnesium correlated with osmolality of the tubule fluid rather than with water reabsorption, they postulated a net entry of magnesium in some segment prior to the hairpin turn of the loop. Furthermore, the concentration of sodium, potassium, chloride, and, to a lesser extent, calcium also rose toward the bend of the loop and correlated better with the rise in osmolality than with water absorption. It was proposed that the rise in electrolyte concentrations, including that of magnesium, could be explained by entry into the pars recta or thin descending limb of the loop with subsequent removal by the thick ascending limb and possibly the distal tubule, that is, by a process of medullary recycling.[46] Brunette and coworkers[31] observed little addition of magnesium up to the bend of papillary loops of normal rats. However, in rats given large infusions of $MgCl_2$, magnesium was present in amounts greater than could be accounted for by filtration and water absorption, suggesting that there is net secretion of magnesium from the vasa recta or interstitium into the lumen of the straight proximal tubule or the thin descending limb of the juxtamedullary nephrons.[32,33]

The existence of magnesium secretion has not been supported by other studies of the loop. Superficial loops from the late proximal convoluted tubule were perfused in vivo with magnesium-free solutions.[135] Little magnesium was detected in the fluid collected from the early distal tubule, suggesting that the epithelium of short cortical loops of the rat nephron is relatively impermeable to magnesium. More recently, we have investigated magnesium transport in isolated straight proximal segments from the rabbit kidney.[143] In vitro perfusion of superficial or juxtamedullary tubule segments with magnesium-free solutions resulted in little influx of magnesium from the bath to the lumen. Moreover, secretion was not detected when the bath magnesium concentration was elevated to 3.0 m*M*. The isolated straight proximal segments from the rabbit absorbed magnesium when they were perfused with artificial solutions resembling late proximal fluid. The collected-to-perfusate magnesium concentration ratio rose with water abstraction, not unlike the rise in concentration ratio observed for fluid from the proximal convoluted tubule. Thus, the reabsorptive rate for magnesium is fractionally lower compared with the transport rates of water and sodium in both the cortical and the juxtamedullary straight proximal tubules of the rabbit.

In summary, the straight proximal tubule has a low permeability to magnesium and has a low reabsorption rate, which depends on the luminal magnesium concentration. The luminal magnesium level is influenced in turn by the magnesium delivery rate and the concurrent rate of sodium transport.

Magnesium transport in the thin descending limb has not been directly investigated with in vivo perfusion techniques. If the thin limb is permeable to magnesium, it should diffuse from the interstitium into the lumen and account for the observations mentioned above in the rat.[46] The magnitude of this predicted backflux would depend on the transepithelial concentration gradient and electrical potential. Confirmation of this hypothesis, particularly with in vitro perfusion, would explain many reports suggesting that the long, deep loop nephrons contribute more magnesium to the final urine than do the short, superficial loops.[100]

Ascending limb of Henle's loop

The early micropuncture studies of Morel and colleagues indicated that the loop of Henle was the major site of magnesium reabsorption.[123] Magnesium concentration in the early distal tubule fluid was distinctly lower than the ultrafilterable magnesium concentration, with a TF/UF ratio of 0.5 to 0.6. Hence, some 50 to 60 percent of the filtered magnesium was reabsorbed between the last accessible proximal tubule on the surface of the kidney and the early distal tubule (Fig 13-4). This represents a fractional reabsorption rate greater than that of sodium and calcium, based on the amount filtered at the glomerulus. The more recent micropuncture studies of Brunette and coworkers[31] in the rat and De Rouffignac and coworkers in *Psammomys* showed an increase in the mean TF/UF magnesium concentration ratio at the bend of the descending limb of the loop, which indicated that the major site of the marked magnesium reabsorption must be located in the ascending limb of Henle's loop, most likely in the thick segment of the ascending limb. Magnesium transport in the thin ascending limb has not been investigated, but a number of studies have been directed at the thick ascending limb.[52,53,165,192,193]

We have used in vivo perfusion techniques to examine magnesium reabsorption within the loop of Henle. Although the loop is composed of straight portions of the proximal tubule and segments of the thin ascending limb as well as the thick ascending limb, it seems likely that the major changes in transport occurred within the thick ascending limb.[48] Experiments in which the loop was perfused at constant flow rates with elevated magnesium concentrations and in the presence of normal plasma magnesium provided evidence that the loop of Henle has a remarkable capacity to increase its absolute reabsorption with increased delivery.[135] There was no indication of a saturation of magnesium transport, or a *Tm*, when the luminal magnesium concentrations were increased from 0 to 5 m*M*. Reabsorption approximated 80 percent of the delivery load at any level of luminal magnesium concentration; this was not unlike the fractional reabsorptive rates of sodium and calcium. In contrast to the effects of changing luminal magnesium concentration, elevation of plasma magnesium concentration (i.e., at the basolateral membrane) resulted in a marked depression of magnesium absorption. As plasma magnesium concentration was progressively raised, absolute and fractional magnesium reabsorption fell sharply and independently of luminal magnesium concentration. This suggests that hypermagnesemia retards magnesium reabsorption in the loop of Henle by inhibition of magnesium transport at the basolateral membrane. No change in

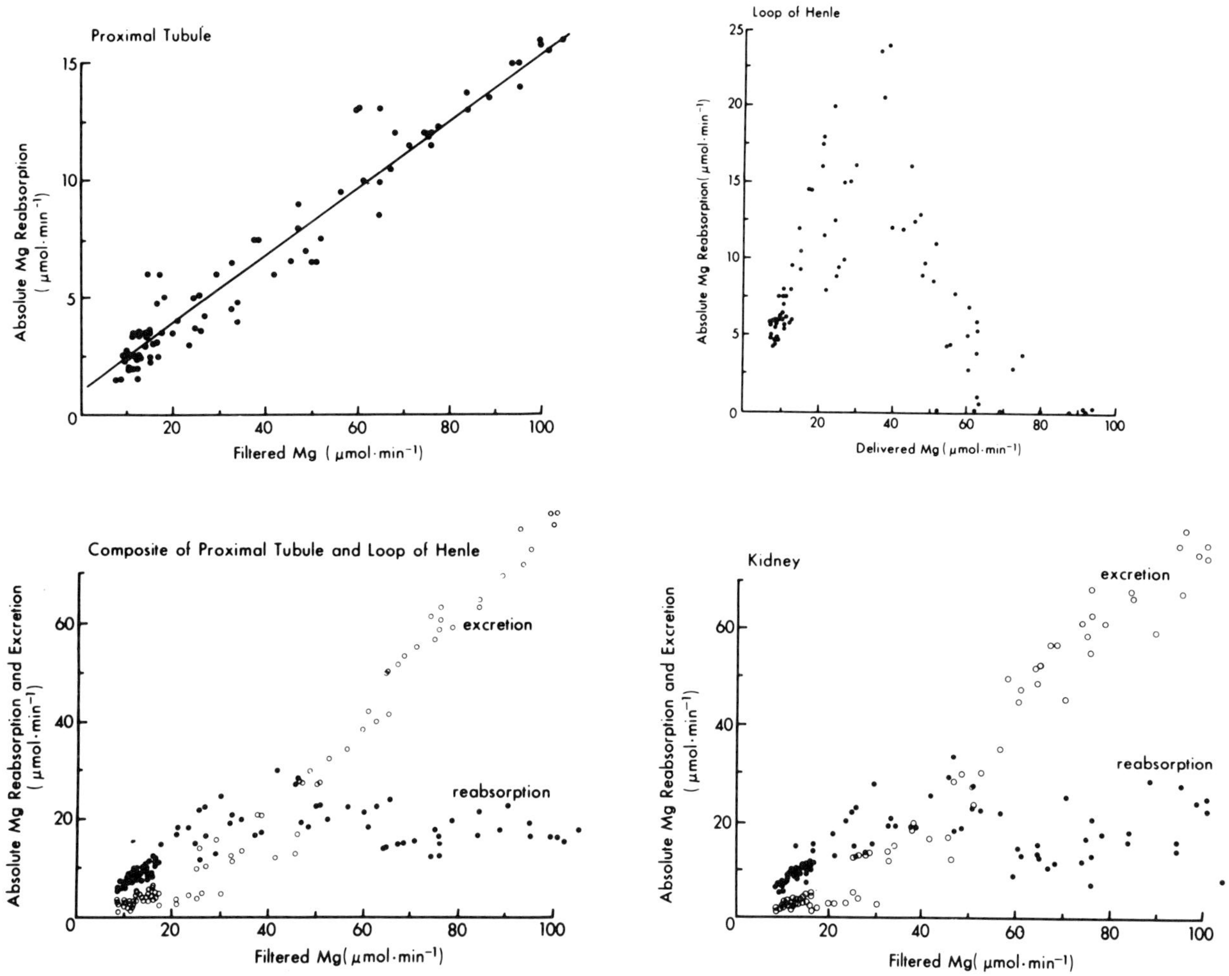

FIGURE 13-6 • Evaluation of the tubular reabsorptive capacity for magnesium in the TPTX dog. Dogs were given an acute $MgCl_2$ load, and reabsorptive capacity in the proximal tubule, loop of Henle, and distal tubule was assessed by micropuncture studies. Apparent *Tm* for magnesium absorption is a composite of transport effects occuring in the proximal tubule and loop of Henle.

sodium chloride absorption occurred during these studies, suggesting a direct effect on magnesium transport.

These observations provided the basis for the *Tm* of magnesium that has previously been reported (Fig. 13-6). Massry and colleagues[111] progressively elevated the plasma magnesium concentration in dogs and performed standard clearances. Overall kidney reabsorption of magnesium initially increased, reached an apparent saturation point, and at extreme levels appeared to fall. This phenomenon suggested there was a tubular maximum transport process (*Tm*) for magnesium. However, free-flow micropuncture studies in dogs subjected to progressive hypermagnesemia indicated that the apparent *Tm* of magnesium transport may reflect a fortuitous composite of increasing proximal tubular magnesium reabsorption and simultaneously declining magnesium reabsorption in the loop, due to an action of magnesium on the basolateral side of the tubule (Fig. 13-7). Shareghi and Agus[165] have supported this concept using the technique of in vitro perfusion of isolated rabbit tubules. They

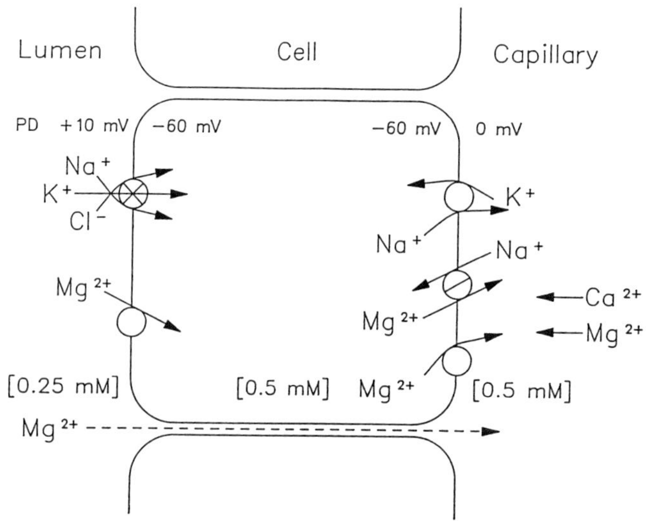

FIGURE 13-7 • Schematic illustration of cellular magnesium transport within the cortical thick ascending limb of the loop of Henle.

reported that elevation of bath magnesium significantly decreased magnesium transport in the cortical thick ascending limb segment, whereas elevation of luminal magnesium concentration increased magnesium absorption. These studies confirmed the earlier observations obtained by in vivo techniques in the rat. It is now clear that the many cell-types that make up the nephron handle magnesium in very different ways; this should be noted when interpreting overall renal magnesium handling and the meaning of changes in *Tm* for magnesium.[111,151,152]

Clearance studies have indicated that hypercalcemia also inhibits magnesium reabsorption.[38,112,184] In vivo microperfusion studies have shown that hypercalcemia inhibits both magnesium and calcium reabsorption in the loop of Henle with no change in sodium chloride absorption.[101,137] Thus, there is suggestive evidence of calcium-magnesium interaction on the basolateral side of the ascending limb cell that is not directly related to sodium chloride reabsorption.[135] Generally, high plasma calcium and high plasma magnesium retard magnesium reabsorption relatively more than that of calcium. Normally, hypercalcemia and hypermagnesemia inhibit both calcium and magnesium absorption.

In addition to the effect of alteration in basolateral magnesium and calcium concentrations, magnesium reabsorption within the loop in influenced by the existing sodium chloride transport.[142] Normally, changes in sodium chloride transport in the loop of Henle are reflected in proportional changes in magnesium reabsorption. Furthermore, sodium chloride reabsorption in the loop of Henle and presumably in the thick ascending limb may be altered by changes in the luminal flow rate as well as by direct changes in active sodium chloride transport. These observations are readily explained if magnesium transport is passive and depends on the sodium chloride-generated transmembrane potential. Evidence for this has recently come from studies on isolated cortical and medullary segments.[165] The transmembrane voltage has been demonstrated to be positive in the cortical and medullary segments of the thick ascending limb. The positive luminal voltage may be the basis for passive calcium and magnesium movement from the lumen to the blood.

Recent microperfusion studies have clarified our understanding of NaCl absorption within the thick ascending limb.[73,85] It is now known that Na^+-$2Cl^-$-K^+ transport is coupled at the luminal membrane of both medullary and cortical segments. Movement of these ions across the luminal membrane occurs due to sodium moving down its electrochemical gradient from the tubule fluid into the cell. The ATP-dependent sodium pump (Na^+-K^+ ATPase) located at the basolateral or peritubular side of the cell maintains the favorable sodium electrochemical gradient across the luminal membrane. Sodium exits across the basolateral membrane via the Na^+-K^+ pump, whereas chloride is thought to move passively from the cell into the peritubular interstitium, perhaps coupled in part with potassium. Greger has reasoned that the presence of a large potassium conductance across the luminal membrane may provide the basis for the lumen-positive transepithelial electrical potential observed in the thick ascending limb.[73] In addition to transcellular absorption, ions may move around the cell through the paracellular pathways according to the latter's permselective properties. With respect to this model, it is thought that about half of the sodium is transported through the cell and the remainder moves passively through the paracellular pathway, facilitated by the lumen-positive electrical potential.[73] According to this view, the intercellular spaces may be in virtual diffusion equilibrium with the peritubule,[85] and the electromotive force for the transepithelial voltage is dependent on active cellular Na^+-K^+ transport.

A positive luminal voltage has been postulated to be important in the passive reabsorption of cations such as sodium, potassium, and possibly magnesium and calcium.[73] This passive movement has the beneficial effect of reducing the expenditure of metabolic energy for electrolyte reabsorption, but as a consequence of this tenet, factors that influence NaCl transport would be expected to affect the transepithelial voltage and thus the passive transport of magnesium and calcium.

Two interesting observations pertain to these speculations. First, furosemide inhibits absorption of calcium and magnesium as well as of sodium chloride in the loop of Henle.[138] This suggests some dependence of calcium and magnesium transport on sodium chloride absorption. Furthermore, the reabsorption of calcium and magnesium, particularly the latter, is inhibited to a greater degree than is that of sodium chloride. This may indicate that the permeability coefficient for magnesium is lower than that for sodium and that magnesium transport is less for any given level of sodium chloride absorption. Second, increased flow rates into the thick ascending segment, such as with extracellular volume expansion, leads to a greater fractional excretion of magnesium than sodium; for example, a 1 to 2 percent increase in fractional sodium excretion is usually accompanied by 10 to 15 percent increment in magnesium excretion. These observations are readily explained if magnesium transport is entirely passive in nature, but an active mechanism may also exist within the cells.

Some recent evidence has also been published that indicates that a portion of magnesium absorption may be active in nature, possibly through a transcellular route.[139] The thick ascending limb is composed of two distinct portions based on morphological and functional characteristics: the medullary and cortical segments. Greger and De Rouffignac and colleagues perfused cortical segments at low perfusion rates and measured net electrolyte movement as well as simultaneously determining the transepithelial electrical potential difference (PD) and resistance values.[192,193] Basal transport of magnesium was appreciable and was increased by about 50 percent with the application of either antidiuretic hormone (ADH) or glucagon. Both hormones increased magnesium transport with little, if any, alteration in PD, transepithelial resistance, or NaCl absorption. Based on the comparatively large changes in net magnesium transport relative to the PD values, these studies suggest that there may be an active component of magnesium transport in the cortical thick ascending limb. These workers have consistently observed little or no magnesium transport in the medullary segment of the thick ascending limb.[52,53,192,193]

In summary, there is good evidence for both active and passive magnesium transport in the cortical thick ascending limb. The evidence for passive transport is based on the observation of the dependence of magnesium movement on transepithelial voltage and the inhibition of magnesium absorption by furosemide.[138] Support for active magnesium transport has come from recent studies demonstrating a stimulation of magnesium movement by ADH and glucagon in the absence of changes in transepithelial PD or resistance.[192,193] It should be mentioned that the early studies of Shareghi and Agus that provided evidence for only passive movement were performed in the absence of hormones.[165] Accordingly, active transport may have been small and undetectable in this preparation.

We can speculate on some of the mechanisms involved in paracellular absorption and transcellular magnesium movement across the luminal and basolateral membranes (Fig. 13-7). As mentioned above, magnesium may move passively across the epithelium or between the cells (paracellular pathway), driven by a transepithelial positive voltage.[165] It is not evident at the present time how hypermagnesemia and hypercalcemia affects these pathways.[73,139] Magnesium may cross the luminal membrane in a mediated manner, down the electrical gradient established by the active Na^+-K^+ ATPase system on the basolateral membrane. It is not known whether magnesium moves in the divalent form or the monovalent form (e.g., with chloride). Transfer of magnesium across the basolateral membrane occurs against its electrochemical gradient and must therefore involve an active or secondary active transport process. Both these situations are schematically illustrated in Fig. 13-7. Either of these processes may exist, since a Mg^{2+} ATPase has been identified in prokaryote cells[170] and Na^+-Mg^{2+} exchange has been identified in RBCs.[61,62,65,74,75,76,105] and squid axons.[15,50,71] This may also apply to magnesium transport in the loop, although at present there is no a priori evidence that this may occur. Factors that influence transcellular magnesium flux may affect any one of these steps, such as the effects of furosemide at the luminal membrane, alterations of Na^+-K^+ ATPase activity and changes in the intracellular magnesium pool, and the direct effects of hypermagnesemia and hypercalcemia on the active or secondary active transport process at the basolateral membrane.

Distal convoluted tubule and collecting duct

Information about magnesium reabsorption in the distal convoluted tubule has come from free-flow micropuncture studies of the superficial nephron. The TF/UF magnesium concentration ratio has been observed to rise along the accessible distal tubule, although this rise is usually less than that of the inulin ratio, indicating the presence of magnesium absorption within this segment. Under normal conditions the distal convoluted tubule has the capability of reabsorbing a small but significant portion of delivered magnesium, accounting for approximately 2 to 5 percent of the filtered magnesium. Fractional reabsorption is approximately one-third of either fractional sodium or calcium reabsorption in the distal tubule. Distal magnesium reabsorption is normally close to capacity, whereas the calcium and sodium transport is ordinarily unsaturated.[135,138] Micropuncture and microperfusion studies of the distal tubule[42] have demonstrated that calcium reabsorption is independent of sodium transport and is not affected by the existing potential difference, suggesting that unique transport mechanisms exist for these two cations. Moreover, the lumen-negative potential difference may be large in this segment, implying that calcium is actively transported. Distal magnesium reabsorption may also involve active transport. It appears that the distal convoluted tubule is another site where magnesium may be dissociated from sodium and calcium; details remain to be elucidated.

All studies reported to date suggest that the collecting tubules and collecting ducts play a very limited role in renal magnesium transport[33,35,46] and may account for the reabsorption of less than 1 to 3 percent of the filtered magnesium. Most of our information concerning magnesium transport in the terminal segments is indirect and involves comparison of the magnesium remaining in late distal fluid with that appearing in the excreted urine. Inferences drawn from differences between delivery rates at the distal tubule and final urine may lead to interpretative errors due to the cellular heterogeneity of tubule segments and also because the collecting ducts receive distal tubules from both superficial and deep nephrons, which may have very different functional properties. Only recently has the collecting tubule been investigated by direct means. Brunette and coworkers[33] found little magnesium transport when they compared samples collected from early and late sites of the same collecting duct of exposed papillae of young rats. This was confirmed by Bengele and colleagues,[21] who determined magnesium transport by microcatheterization methods along the inner medullary collecting duct of rats. They were unable to demonstrate magnesium transport in these segments.

Shareghi and Agus,[165] using in vitro perfusion techniques, were not able to detect net transport of either magnesium or calcium in the late segment of the rabbit cortical collecting tubule. These results suggest that little or no reabsorption takes place in either the cortical or the medullary collecting ducts.

FACTORS THAT ALTER RENAL MAGNESIUM HANDLING

Table 13-5 summarizes some of the factors that have been reported to influence magnesium excretion. The more important of these influences are elaborated in this section.

Renal plasma flow and glomerular filtration

Magnesium absorption appears to be in balance with the filtration rate, that is, there exists a glomerular tubule balance. Coburn and associates studied the effects of increased glomerular filtration rate (GFR) on magnesium excretion in the dog.[39] They observed relatively little changes in fractional magnesium excretion with alterations in filtration rates. Similar studies using acetylcholine, bradykinin, and other agents evaluated the effects exerted by the resulting renal vasodilation on magnesium excretion. Only small increases were found, which were proportional to the increases in sodium excretion.[112] The tubule segments responsible for these changes have not been systematically studied but are probably within the proximal tubule and the thick ascending limb.[194]

Chronic renal failure, with its attendant reduction in GFR, results in a rise in fractional magnesium excretion similar in magnitude to that observed for urinary calcium and sodium excretion[197] (see Chaps. 34 and 39). Studies were performed on dogs with experimentally induced uremia. Like patients with chronic renal failure, these animals have a reduced number of nephrons and demonstrate marked hyperfiltration per nephron. Observations from micropuncture studies demonstrate that the fractional magnesium reabsorption was reduced in proportion to sodium and calcium transport within the loop of Henle. Thus, a decrease in the single nephron GFR and the filtration fraction increases the peritubular capillary hydrostatic pressure and decreases colloid osmotic pressure, which in turn diminishes proximal salt and water reabsorption and enhances delivery into the loop of Henle. Enhanced distal salt delivery, and perhaps natriuretic hormones and factors, may affect magnesium transport in a manner similar to sodium reabsorption in chronic renal failure. Accordingly, as the nephron population diminishes, each individual nephron adapts by excreting more of the filtered salt, including magnesium, to maintain the fine balance between dietary intake and renal excretion. These adaptive mechanisms fail only in end stage renal failure, when there is not a sufficient number of nephrons to excrete the dietary magnesium, leading to retention of magnesium and hypermagnesemia.[112]

TABLE 13-5 • Factors in altered renal magnesium excretion

Increased excretion	Decreased excretion
Extracellular fluid volume expansion	Extracellular fluid volume depletion
Hypermagnesemia	Magnesium depletion
Hypercalcemia	Hypocalcemia
Loop diuretics (e.g., furosemide, ethacrynic acid)	Peptide hormones (PTH, calcitonin, glucagon, antidiuretic hormone)
Osmotic diuretics (e.g., urea, mannitol)	Metabolic alkalosis
Phosphate depletion	Hyperthyroidism
Metabolic acidosis	
Carbohydrate, protein, alcohol intake	

Sodium balance and ECF volume

Extracellular volume expansion with saline or Ringer's solution produces an immediate increase in magnesium excretion. The response of magnesium excretion parallels that of sodium and calcium, but the fractional magnesium excretion rate is approximately twice that of these other two cations. The high fractional magnesium excretion rate secondary to volume expansion persists despite reduction in renal artery perfusion pressure. The reduction in salt and water reabsorption occurs principally in the proximal tubule, so that fractional reabsorption falls from 30 to 15 percent when the extracellular volume is expanded by 5 percent of body weight.[194] The increased amount of magnesium delivered to the loop is largely excreted unchanged in the urine, due to the concomitant increase in distal salt delivery from the proximal tubule.

Hypermagnesemia

The most striking changes in magnesium excretion occur in response to alterations in plasma magnesium concentration. With marked hypermagnesemia, due to high dietary intake or intravenous infusion, the rate of magnesium excretion can approximate the rate of filtration. Conversely, severe hypomagnesemia results in almost complete renal conservation of this cation. Thus, the plasma Mg^{2+} concentration appears to be a major determinant of renal magnesium excretion.

The magnesuria caused by hypermagnesemia is due to the combined effects of increased filtered load, reduced fractional reabsorption in the proximal tubule, and a reduction in reabsorption in the ascending limb of Henle's loop. In the presence of hypermagnesemia, the fractional sodium and water reabsorption is modestly reduced in the proximal tubule due to inhibition of unidirectional and net sodium efflux. This leads to a proportional reduction in fractional magnesium reabsorption. Evidence indicates that magnesium reabsorption in the loop of Henle is markedly reduced during hypermagnesemia due to the direct action of magnesium from the basolateral membrane of the thick ascending limb. Magnesium concentration rises sharply in the distal tubule, exceeding this segment's limited reabsorptive capacity and thereby resulting in excretion of most of the magnesium rejected by the loop of Henle. As mentioned earlier, the inhibitory effects of hypermagnesemia on the proximal tubule and the loop of Henle result in an apparent *Tm* of magnesium. The concept of a *Tm* of maximal reabsorptive capacity has been valuable in assessing body magnesium stores.[151,152,161,182] The threshold value for magnesium, above which magnesuria occurs, is close to the normal plasma magnesium concentration. The reabsorptive capacity is appropriately elevated in states of magnesium deficiency and lowered in states of magnesium surfeit. These changes reflect processes occurring principally in the loop of Henle.

Some evidence of magnesium secretion has been obtained in the presence of marked hypermagnesemia. Averill and Heaton reported a fractional magnesium excretion exceeding 164 percent in rats chronically given magnesium salts, thus demonstrating magnesium secretion.[11] Wen and coworkers demonstrated that the fraction of filtered magnesium remaining in the distal tubule was 15 to 20 percent less than that excreted in the urine, suggesting that magnesium addition occurred beyond the distal tubule.[188] However, others were unable to demonstrate secretion either by clearance techniques or by micropuncture studies of the distal tubule and collecting ducts.[32,35] Present evidence indicates that magnesium is not secreted to any great extent by the nephron.

Hypomagnesemia and magnesium depletion

Primary magnesium depletion by dietary means in humans is extremely uncommon because the kidney has the remarkable ability to conserve magnesium. When depletion does occur, it is usually due to gross absorptive abnormalities, such as bowel resection, or due to a compromise of rental function, such as occurs with overzealous use of diuretics, longstanding hypercalcemia, or chronic administration of drugs such as cisplatin, cyclosporine, and so on.[51]

It has been clinically recognized for a long time that diminished magnesium intake or intestinal malabsorption leads to appropriate renal magnesium conservation in an effort to maintain magnesium balance. The basis for this alteration in magnesium transport is not fully understood. Evidence has been given that renal magnesium conservation resulting from low intake may be related to a fall in plasma magnesium and therefore decreased filtered load.[35,70,150,166,167,187] This conclusion is based on the close association of changes in urinary magnesium excretion with alterations of plasma magnesium concentration. Recent studies in the rat clearly indicate that a fall in plasma magnesium is not necessary for appropriate conservation.[162] In these studies, changes in tubular magnesium reabsorption and urinary magnesium excretion occur 15 to 20 h prior to a fall in filtered load. Accordingly, the rat kidney adapts to magnesium availability independently of an alteration in filtered load. This adaptation occurs in the loop of Henle, most probably in the thick ascending limb. Moreover, the cellular adaptation is (1) rapid, occurring within 5 h of dietary restriction; (2) specific, not affecting sodium or calcium transport; and (3) independent of circulating PTH and calcitonin levels.[162] The conclusions from these data are consonant with clinical reports that showed that urinary magnesium excretion may be significantly decreased without an alteration in plasma magnesium concentration.[54,63]

It is interesting to speculate on the cellular basis by which acute dietary magnesium restriction alters the transport rate within the thick ascending limb. Our studies with isolated cortical thick ascending limb cells showed that magnesium uptake was greater when the cells were cultured in low-magnesium media compared to normal. This indicates that the adaptation of transport function is intrinsic to the cell.[141] Thick ascending limb cells adapt appropriately independently of hormonal factors. The mechanism for this adjustment in transport rates is unknown at the present time.

Hypercalcemia and hypocalcemia

Hypercalciuria of any etiology, such as hyperparathyroidism, malignancy, or vitamin D excess, markedly increases magnesium excretion.[112,142] Moreover, the fractional excretion of magnesium usually rises more markedly than the excretion of calcium. Conversely, as mentioned above, hypermagnesemia results in a greater magnesuria than it does in calciuria. A common pathway for calcium-magnesium reabsorption, presumably more sensitive to magnesium transport than to calcium reabsorption, has been suggested. Coburn and colleagues[39] demonstrated, in a number of clearance studies in the dog, that the elevation of plasma calcium concentration progressively reduced the maximum ability of the kidney to reabsorb magnesium. This has been extensively reviewed by Massry and associates.[112] Subsequent micropuncture and microperfusion studies have provided additional understanding of magnesium transport during hypercalcemia. Le Grimellec and coworkers[101] demonstrated that calcium and magnesium absorption were depressed principally in the distal tubular segments. These studies were performed on rats with intact parathyroid glands. Suppression of PTH release may have contributed to the increase in urinary calcium and magnesium excretion. Microperfusion studies performed on TPTX rats have demonstrated that elevation of plasma calcium per se reduces calcium and magnesium reabsorption in the loop of Henle.[142] Moreover, magnesium reabsorption is inhibited to a greater degree than is that of calcium, while sodium reabsorption remains near control values. Absolute reabsorption of magnesium in the distal tubule is modestly increased because of its augmented delivery from the loop, but because the distal reabsorptive capacity is low, most of this magnesium is excreted. That increases in plasma calcium and magnesium mutually inhibit the reabsorption of each other in the loop of Henle strongly supports the existence of calcium-magnesium membrane interaction. This competition appears to occur at the basolateral membrane, since elevations of the luminal calcium concentration have little effect on the reabsorption rate of magnesium and vice versa.[139] Hypocalcemia may lead to enhanced magnesium reabsorption.[136] Hypocalcemia may permit more complete calcium and magnesium reabsorption in the loop as the result of reduced competition for the transport system at the basolateral membrane.

Phosphate depletion

Dietary phosphate restriction affects appropriate renal conservation by enhancing phosphate reabsorption and impairing the phosphaturic action of PTH. It is interesting that the syndrome of phosphate depletion also results in marked hypercalciuria and hypermagnesuria. In fact, the renal magnesium wasting may be sufficient to lead to overt hypomagnesemia.[38,98] Micropuncture experiments in phosphate-depleted dogs indicated that this defect occurs in the thick ascending limb and distal tubule and may be corrected by the acute administration of PTH (see below) or neutral phosphate infusions.[198] The cellular mechanisms responsible for the inability of the kidney to normally conserve magnesium in phosphate deficiency are unclear. However, this syndrome has been receiving more attention recently as phosphate depletion is becoming more frequently recognized in such common disorders as dietary malabsorption and chronic alcoholism.

Hormonal control of magnesium absorption in the thick ascending limb

It has been known for some time that PTH enhances the tubular reabsorption of magnesium and diminishes urinary Mg excretion.[112,142,184] Many of the early micropuncture studies were performed on TPTX animals and the data compared with subsequent collections following hormone replacement. The hormonal effects were marginal or often not detected,[139] and many required special circumstances to demonstrate segmental action.[80,111,138,194] However, the studies of De Rouffignac and colleagues have clearly shown that PTH increases magnesium absorption in the cortical thick ascending limb.[48] PTH, acting in concert with other hormonal factors mentioned below, is sufficient for adequate control of renal magnesium balance.

A large number of hormones act within the thick ascending limb; many of which have been demonstrated to alter magnesium absorption.[12-14,55-58] De Rouffignac's studies have added greatly to our understanding of hormonal controls for magnesium handling within the thick ascending limb.[48] Morel and associates[124] showed that PTH, calcitonin, and glucagon stimulate the generation of cAMP in the cortical thick ascending limb, whereas ADH, calcitonin, and glucagon release the same second messenger in the medullary thick ascending limb. Moreover, these hormones appear to act on the same adenylyl cyclase pool within the target cells. Accordingly, each one of these hormones should lead to similar functional responses predicated on receptor distribution within each segment.[124] De Rouffignac and colleagues developed a novel approach to test this theory.[47,48] They used Brattleboro rats with hereditary diabetes insipidus, which lack endogenous ADH, and they infused either glucose or somatostatin to inhibit glucagon secretion. Furthermore, they thyroparathyroidectomized the animals to eliminate circulating PTH and calcitonin. Thus, a "hormone-deprived" animal model was created to serve as a basis for evaluating the respective actions of each hormone. Micropuncture studies were then performed to determine the single and combined effects of hormone administration; it is important to note that these studies were all performed with physiological hormone concentrations. They determined that the hormonal responses were in the loop of Henle, probably the thick ascending limb. Moreover, the changes in fractional urinary excretion were associated with those observed within the thick ascending limb for each hormone. All four hormones—PTH, glucagon, calcitonin, and the ADH analogue 1-desamino-8-arginine vasopressin—reduced the concentration of magnesium and calcium in distally collected tubular fluid as a consequence of enhanced reabsorption in the loop and Henle.[12,13,55-57] Calcitonin, ADH, and glucagon, but not PTH, stimulated NaCl transport in the thick ascending limb. These authors also showed that many of the actions of these hormones were additive.[58] Thus, one hormone may stimulate magnesium transport in the presence of the others. For example, the infusion of supramaximal doses of glucagon and ADH to hormone-deprived animals resulted in greater reabsorption than in animals receiving either hormone alone. Accordingly, the concerted actions of two or more hormones may be important in controlling thick ascending limb functions.

A number of in vitro studies have been performed to isolate the site and mechanism of action. These studies have necessarily been performed on species other than the rat because of the ease of obtaining isolated tubule segments. Shareghi and Agus[165] observed a 1.5- to 2.0-fold increase in magnesium and calcium absorption in rabbit cortical thick ascending limb without a change in the transepithelial PD or alteration of NaCl transport following the addition of PTH to the bathing solution. De Rouffignac and colleagues reported that ADH increased net magnesium and calcium absorption in mouse cortical thick ascending limb in the absence of alterations in transepithelial voltage or resistance measurements. In parallel experiments, glucagon increased magnesium, calcium, and NaCl flux with no effect on concurrently measured transepithelial PD or resistance parameters. There was no observable stimulation of magnesium transport in the medullary thick ascending limb in the latter studies;[52,53,192,193] absorption remained essentially zero despite the presence of appreciable NaCl flux. These data are entirely harmonious with the findings obtained in the hormone-deprived rat model.[48]

Adrenocortical steroids

It has not yet been demonstrated that glucocorticoids or mineralocorticoids exert any regulatory effect on Mg^{2+} excretion. Chronic administration of glucocorticoids usually leads to an increase in urinary excretion of both magnesium and calcium in animals and humans.[112] This may be related to the catabolic effect of glucocorticoids on bone, with release of magnesium; or it may be due to the rise in GFR that is often observed in this situation. The acute administration of methylprednisolone to adrenalectomized dogs did not change the excretion of magnesium.[110] Short-term administration of mineralocorticoids, such as aldosterone, to dogs decreased sodium excretion but did not influence excretion of calcium or magnesium. The transport of these three cations can therefore probably be dissociated at the level of the distal tubule. Long-term administration of aldosterone increased calcium and magnesium excretion; this effect was reversed by spironolactone administration or adrenal insufficiency.[112] The modest increase in magnesium excretion with chronic mineralocorticoid administration probably reflects the associated volume expansion, which increases the delivery of sodium, calcium, and magnesium to the distal tubule. There, mineralocorticoids may enhance sodium reabsorption without affecting calcium and magnesium transport.

Thyroid hormone

Magnesium metabolism is altered in hyperthyroidism and in hypothyroidism. Thyrotoxic patients often have a decreased serum magnesium concentration with increased fractional magnesium excretion. This may be explained by the associated increase in plasma calcium concentration and hypercalciuria in such patients.[142] Hypothyroidism, on the other hand, is consistently associated with an increase in mean plasma magnesium concentration, possibly due to renal magnesium retention. Moreover, intracellular magnesium has been reported to be low in thyroid hormone deficiency.[180] The mechanisms responsible for these changes are unknown. Overall, the changes observed in renal magnesium reabsorption in hypothyroidism and hyperthyroidism are small compared to the more marked metabolic changes intrinsic to these disorders.

Other hormones

A variety of other hormones are thought to influence renal magnesium handling, although their specific roles are not well understood. Isoproterenol increases magnesium and calcium absorption in the thick ascending limb.[14] A few studies have been directed at the role of vitamin D metabolites on magnesium homeostasis.[142] Growth hormone has been reported to increase urinary magnesium as well as calcium. In addition, infusion of angiotensin II or catecholamines increases the urinary excretion of magnesium in proportion to calcium and sodium excretion.[112] Estrogens and androgens have been reported either to increase or to have little effect on magnesium excretion.[112] The mechanisms of the changes appear to involve extrarenal events of hemodynamic alterations induced by the hormones rather than direct action on the tubule.

Acidosis and alkalosis

Metabolic acidosis has long been known to be associated with increased urinary excretion of calcium; however, the effects of acidosis on magnesium excretion have been less clear.[184] Increases in urinary magnesium excretion have been found in some, but not all,[102] studies of experimental metabolic acidosis in humans. The explanation for these disparate results is not apparent. Acute metabolic acidosis in experimental animals uniformly results in increases in urinary magnesium excretion; the site of action appears to be the loop of Henle.[163] The changes observed in metabolic alkalosis are more consistent. Acute and chronic bicarbonate infusion leads to a fall in urinary magnesium excretion.[131,196] The mechanisms responsible, however, are unclear. The data are hard to interpret because many of the earlier reports failed to determine and control the plasma concentrations of ionized calcium and magnesium.

Diuretics

A number of drugs may increase renal magnesium excretion. The most important of these are the loop diuretics, such as furosemide, ethacrynic acid, and bumetanide, which cause massive magnesuria along with marked natriuresis and calciuresis. The loop diuretics increase magnesium excretion relatively more than they increase excretion of calcium and sodium.[138] As previously mentioned, furosemide inhibits sodium chloride transport in the loop of Henle and produces an associated inhibition of magnesium transport. It is not known whether furosemide has any additional effects on magnesium transport within this segment. Ethacrynic acid and mercurial diuretics exert effects similar to those of furosemide.

The acute and chronic administration of thiazide diuretics may produce a mild magnesuria, but this response is variable. It is probably related to the magnitude of the inhibition of proximal salt and water reabsorption and their subsequent delivery to the loop. Depending on the loop flow rate, modest amounts of magnesium may escape reabsorption, accounting for the variable magnesuric response that is seen in clinical studies. Thiazide diuretics inhibit sodium reabsorption in the distal convoluted tubule and increase calcium transport. Data obtained from micropuncture studies of the hamster demonstrate little or no change in magnesium reabsorption in the distal tubule following the administration of thiazides, whereas the reabsorption of sodium was inhibited and that of calcium increased.[195] These observations support previous findings that hydrochlorothiazide may alter calcium absorption with little effect on magnesium transport.[28,104] However, thiazides are useful alternatives to the loop diuretics since they do not compromise the renal conservation of magnesium because they act within the distal convoluted tubule, not the loop of Henle.[154]

The osmotic diuretics mannitol and urea increase magnesium excretion in proportion to the magnitude of the osmotic load.[199] Magnesium excretion may rise to 40 to 50 percent of filtered magnesium following administration of mannitol or urea. Micropuncture studies have demonstrated that both these agents reduce magnesium reabsorption in the loop of Henle.[199] Hyperglycemia similarly causes pronounced increases in magnesium excretion; these effects have not been specifically studied. In summary, osmotic diuretics appear to reduce reabsorption of magnesium, principally within the loop of Henle, by increasing the flow rate and by decreasing NaCl transport in the loop.

Other factors

A host of other factors have been examined for their effects on magnesium excretion. By and large, the results are often equivocal and usually of little apparent significance. The ingestion of a variety of metabolizable substrates, such as glucose, galactose, fructose, and protein, produces a magnesuria without an accompanying natriuresis.[112,184] Alcohol administered acutely or chronically increases fractional magnesium excretion by 5 to 10 percent.[95,180] The mechanisms underlying these effects are unclear; indirect effects of rapidly metabolizable products on the tubule may be involved. A number of pharmacological agents, such as cyclosporine, gentamicin, and cisplatin,[51,155,156] may selectively reduce magnesium reabsorption. Most likely these agents always alter magnesium reabsorption in the loop of Henle.[108,115,119] The acquired renal magnesium leak persists for a number of years following cessation of treatment.[156] A primary inherited defect in renal reabsorption of magnesium has been reported in humans.[17,69,153] It is unknown whether this defect is related to other abnormalities for the hypercalciuria, hypokalemia, and hypophosphaturia also observed in these patients.

The interrelationship between potassium and magnesium homeostasis is not well understood. Many patients who present with hypomagnesemia of various etiologies also have an associated hypokalemia.[183] Since renal potassium handling differs markedly from that of magnesium, it is not obvious that the basis of the association is a renal defect.[142] A number of studies have demonstrated that a cellular potassium deficit cannot be corrected with potassium supplements alone, but the prior correction of magnesium depletion is necessary. This suggests that intracellular potassium exchange may require magnesium.[167] Others have suggested that magnesium depletion may lead to hypokalemia because it increases renin secretion, which markedly elevates aldosterone secretion.[142]

Summary of factors

The present concept of renal tubular magnesium reabsorption suggests that it is largely a unidirectional process throughout the whole nephron. Magnesium reabsorption proceeds at a slower rate in the proximal tubule than does reabsorption of sodium and calcium. The primary site of modifications of magnesium reabsorption is in the ascending limb of Henle's loop. Magnesium reabsorption in the loop is affected by a number of drugs, such as diuretics and osmotic agents, as well as plasma calcium and magnesium levels. No specific hormonal controls have yet been identified as regulators of magnesium transport. Rather, a number of factors, such as plasma magnesium and calcium concentrations; ECF volume balance; and peptide hormones, such as PTH, glucagon, and calcitonin, may act in concert to control day-to-day renal magnesium homeostasis.

REFERENCES

1. Adam et al: Problems in the assessment of magnesium depletion in the rat by in vivo ^{31}P-NMR. *Magn Reson Med* 7:300, 1988.
2. Agus ZS et al: Cytosolic magnesium modulates calcium channel activity in mammalian ventricular cells. *Am J Physiol* 256:C456, 1989.
3. Alcock N, MacIntyre I: Interrelation of calcium and magnesium absorption. *Clin Sci* 22:185, 1962.

4. Aldor TAM, Moore EW: Magnesium absorption by everted sacs of rat intestine and colon. *Gastroenterology* 59:3019, 1973.
5. Alfrey AC, Miller N: Bone magnesium pools in uremia. *J Clin Invest* 52:3019, 1973.
6. Alfrey AC et al: Evaluation of body magnesium stores. *J Lab Clin Med* 84:158, 1974.
7. Alfrey AC et al: Effect of age and magnesium depletion on bone magnesium pools in rats. *J Clin Invest* 54:1074, 1974.
8. Almers W, Palade PT: Slow calcium and potassium currents across frog muscle membrane: Measurements with a vaseline-gap technique. *J Physiol (Lond)* 312:159, 1981.
9. Altshuld RA, Brierley GP: Cation homeostasis in isolated cardiac myocytes, in Piper HM, Isenberg G (eds): *Isolated Adult Cardiomyocytes.* Boca Raton, Fla, CRC, 1989, p 83.
10. Altura BM, Altura BT: Role of magnesium in the pathogenesis of hypertension: Relationship to its actions on cardiac and muscular smooth muscle, in Laragh JH, Brenner BM (eds): *Hypertension: Pathophysiology, Diagnosis, and Management.* New York, Raven Press, 1990, p 1003.
11. Averill CM, Heaton FW: The renal magnesium reabsorption in the rat. *Clin Sci* 31:353, 1966.
12. Bailly C, Amiel C: Effect of glucagon on renal magnesium reabsorption in the rat. *Pfluegers Arch* 392:360, 1982.
13. Bailly C et al: PTH-like glucagon stimulation of Ca and Mg reabsorption in Henle's loop of the rat. *Am J Physiol* 246:F205, 1984.
14. Bailly C et al: Isoproterenol increases Ca, Mg and NaCl reabsorption in the mouse thick ascending limb. *Am J Physiol* 258:F1221, 1990.
15. Baker PF, Crawford AC: Mobility and transport of magnesium in squid axons. *J Physiol (Lond)* 337:351, 1972.
16. Baldwin D et al: Interrelations of magnesium, potassium, phosphorus, and creatinine in skeletal muscle of man. *J Clin Invest* 31:850, 1952.
17. Bar SR et al: Hypomagnesemic hypocalcemia secondary to renal magnesium wasting. *Ann Intern Med* 82:646, 1975.
18. Beavis AD: *N*-ethylmaleimide and mercurials modulate inhibition of the mitochondrial inner membrane anion channel by H^+, Mg^{2+} and cationic amphiphiles. *Biochim Biophys Acta* 1063:111, 1991.
19. Beavis AD, Powers MF: On the regulation of the mitochondrial inner membrane anion channel by magnesium and protons. *J Biol Chem* 164:17148, 1989.
20. Behar J: Magnesium absorption by the rat ileum and colon. *Am J Physiol* 227:334, 1974.
21. Bengele HH et al: Calcium and magnesium transport along the inner medullary collecting duct of the rat. *Am J Physiol* 239:F24, 1981.
22. Berridge MJ: Inositol trisphosphate and diacylglycerol: Two interacting second messengers. *Ann Rev Biochem* 56:159, 1987.
23. Blatter LA, McGuigan JAS: Free intracellular magnesium concentration in ferret ventricular muscle measured with ion selective microelectrode. *J Exp Physiol* 71:451, 1986.
24. Booth CC et al: Incidence of hypomagnesemia in intestinal malabsorption. *Br Med J* 2:141, 1963.
25. Borchgrevink PC et al: Magnesium and reperfusion of ischemic rat heart as assessed by ^{31}P-NMR. *Am J Physiol* 256:H195, 1989.
26. Brannan PG et al: Magnesium absorption in human small intestine: Results in normal subjects, patients with chronic renal disease and patients with absorptive hypercalciuria. *J Clin Invest* 52:1412, 1976.
27. Breibart S et al: Relation of age to radiomagnesium exchange in bone. *Proc Soc Exp Biol Med* 105:361, 1960.
28. Brickman AS et al: Changes in serum and urinary calcium during treatment with hydrochlorothiazide: Studies on mechanisms. *J Clin Invest* 51:945, 1972.
29. Brinley FJ Jr et al: The concentration of ionized magnesium in barnacle muscle fibers. *J Physiol (Lond)* 266:545, 1977.
30. Brown EM, Thatcher JG: Adenosine 3′,5′-monophosphate (cAMP)-dependent protein kinase and the regulation of parathyroid hormone release by divalent cations and agents elevating cellular cAMP in dispersed bovine parathyroid cells. *Endocrinology* 110:1374, 1982.
31. Brunette MG et al: Micropuncture study of renal magnesium transport along the nephron in the young rat. *Am J Physiol* 227:891, 1974.
32. Brunette MG et al: Micropuncture study of renal magnesium transport in renal magnesium-loaded rats. *Am J Physiol* 229:1695, 1975.
33. Brunette MG et al: Magnesium handling by the papilla of the young rat. *Pfluegers Arch* 373:29, 1978.
34. Callewaert et al: Existence of a calcium-dependent potasium channel in the membrane of cow cardiac Purkinje cells. *Pfluegers Arch* 406:424, 1986.
35. Carney SL et al: Effect of magnesium deficiency on renal magnesium and calcium transport in the rat. *J Clin Invest* 65:180, 1980.
36. Chien MM, Cambier JC: Divalent cation regulation of phosphoinositide metabolism: Naturally occurring B lymphoblasts contain a Mg^{2+}-regulated phosphatidylinositol-specific phospholipase C. *J Biol Chem* 265:920, 1990.
37. Clarkson EM et al: The effect of high intake of calcium on magnesium metabolism in normal subjects and patients with chronic renal failure. *Clin Sci* 32:11, 1967.
38. Coburn JW, Massry SG: Changes in serum and urinary calcium during phosphate depletion: Studies on mechanism. *J Clin Invest* 49:1073, 1970.
39. Coburn JW et al: The effect of calcium infusion on renal handling of magnesium with normal and reduced glomerular filtration rate. *Nephron* 7:108, 1970.
40. Cohen SM, Burt CT: ^{31}P nuclear magnetic relaxation studies of phosphocreatine in intact muscle: Determination of intracellular free magnesium. *Proc Natl Acad Sci U S A* 74:4271, 1977.
41. Corkey BE et al: Regulation of free and bound magnesium in rat hepatocytes and isolated mitochondria. *J Biol Chem* 261:2567, 1986.
42. Costanzo LS, Windhager EE: Calcium and sodium transport by the distal convoluted tubule of the rat. *Am J Physiol* 235:492, 1978.
43. Cronin RE et al: Skeletal muscle injury after magnesium depletion in the dog. *Am J Physiol* 243:113, 1982.
44. Crosby G, Szabo MD: Excess Mg^{2+} and central nervous system metabolism, in Strata P, Carbone E (eds): *Mg^{2+} and Excitable Membranes.* Heidelberg, Springer-Verlag, 1990, p 119.

45. Dempsey EF et al: A study of factors determining fecal electrolyte excretion. *Metabolism* 7:108, 1950.
46. De Rouffignac C et al: Micropuncture study of water and electrolyte movements along the loop of Henle in *Psammomys* with special reference to magnesium, calcium and phosphate. *Pfluegers Arch* 344:309, 1973.
47. De Rouffignac C et al: Stimulation by antidiuretic hormone of electrolyte tubular reabsorption in rat kidney. *Am J Physiol* 244:F309, 1983.
48. De Rouffignac C et al: Physiological control of the urinary concentrating mechanism by peptide hormones. *Kidney Int* 31:611, 1987.
49. Diebler H et al: Kinetics and mechanisms of reactions of main group metal ions with biological carriers. *Pure Appl Chem* 20:93, 1969.
50. Dipolo, Beaugé L: An ATP-dependent Na^+/Mg^{2+} counter transport is the only mechanism of Mg^{2+} extrusion in squid axons. *Biochim Biophys Acta* 946:424, 1988.
51. Dirks JH: The kidney and magnesium regulation. *Kidney Int* 23:771, 1983.
52. Di Stefano A et al: Effects of glucagon on Na^+, Cl^-, K^+, Mg^{2+} and Ca^{2+} transport in cortical and medullary thick ascending limbs of mouse kidney. *Pfluegers Arch* 414:640, 1989.
53. Di Stefano A et al: Effects of parathyroid hormone and calcitonin on Na^+, Cl^-, K^+, Mg^{2+} and Ca^{2+} transport in coritical and medullary thick ascending limbs of mouse kidney. *Pfluegers Arch* 417:161, 1990.
54. Dunn MJ, Walser MR: Magnesium depletion in normal man. *Metabolism* 15:844, 1964.
55. Elalouf JM et al: Stimulation by human calcitonin of electrolyte transport in distal tubules of rat kidney. *Pfluegers Arch* 399:111, 1983.
56. Elalouf JM et al: Effects of antidiuretic hormone on electrolyte reabsorption and secretion in distal tubules of rat kidney. *Pfluegers Arch* 401:167, 1984.
57. Elalouf JM et al: ADH-like effects of calcitonin on electrolyte transport by Henle's loop of rat kidney. *Am J Physiol* 246:F213, 1984.
58. Elalouf JM et al: Additivity of the effects of glucagon and vasopressin on renal Mg reabsorption and urine concentration ability in the rat. *Pfluegers Arch* 407:566, 1986.
59. Fawcett DW, Gens JP: Magnesium poisoning following an enema of epsom salt solution. *JAMA* 123:1028, 1943.
60. Feng A et al: Intracellular Mg^{2+} concentration following inhibition of ATP generation in isolated cardiomyocytes. *Clin Res* 39:257A, 1991.
61. Féray J-C, Garay R: A Na^+-stimulated Mg^{2+}-transport system in human red blood cells. *Biochim Biophys Acta* 856:26, 1986.
62. Féray J-C, Garay R: A one-to-one Mg^{2+}:Mn^{2+} exchange in rat erythrocytes. *J Biol Chem* 262:5763, 1987.
63. Fitzgerald MG, Fourman P: An experimental study of magnesium deficiency in man. *Clin Sci* 15:635, 1956.
64. Flatman PW: Magnesium transport across cell membranes. *J Membr Biol* 80:1, 1984.
65. Frenkel EJ et al: ATP requirement of the sodium-dependent magnesium extrusion from human red blood cells. *J Physiol (Lond)* 414:385, 1989.
66. Fry CH: Measurements and control of intracellular magnesium ion concentration in guinea pig and ferret ventricular myocardium. *Magnesium* 5:306, 1986.
67. Garfinkel et al: Magnesium in cardiac energy metabolism. *J Mol Cell Cardiol* 18:1003, 1986.
68. Ghoneim MM, Long JP: The interaction between magnesium and other neuromuscular blocking agents. *Anesthesiology* 32:23, 1970.
69. Gitelman HJ et al: A new familial disorder characterized by hypokalemia and hypomagnesemia. *Trans Assoc Am Physicians* 79:221, 1966.
70. Gitelman HJ et al: Influence of parathyroid glands on hypercalcemic of experimental magnesium depletion in rat. *J Clin Invest* 47:118, 1968.
71. Gonzalaz-Serratos H, Rasgado-Flores H: Extracellular magnesium-dependent sodium influx in squid giant axons. *Am J Physiol* 259:C541, 1990.
72. Graham LA et al: Gastrointestinal absorption and excretion of ^{28}Mg in man. *Metabolism* 9:646, 1960.
73. Greger R: Ion transport mechanism in thick ascending limb of Henle's loop of mammalian nephron. *Physiol Rev* 65:760, 1985.
74. Günther T: Functional compartmentalization of intracellular magnesium. *Magnesium* 5:53, 1986.
75. Günther T, Vorman J: Characterization of Na^+/Mg^{2+} antiport by simultaneous $^{28}Mg^{2+}$ influx. *Biochem Biophys Res Commun* 148:1069, 1987.
76. Günther T et al: Characterization of Na^+-depleted Mg^{2+} efflux from Mg^{2+}-loaded rat erythrocytes. *Biochim Biophys Acta* 1023:455, 1990.
77. Gupta RK, Moore RD: ^{31}P NMR studies of intracellular free Mg^{2+} in intact frog skeletal muscles. *J Biol Chem* 255:3987, 1980.
78. Hardwick LL et al: Site and mechanism of intestinal magnesium absorption. *Miner Electrolyte Metab* 16:174, 1990.
79. Harman AW et al: Cytosolic free magnesium, ATP, and blebbing during chemical hypoxia in cultured rat hepatocytes. *Biochem Biophys Res Comm* 170:477, 1990.
80. Harris CA et al: Effects of parathyroid hormone on electrolyte transport in the hamster nephron. *Am J Physiol* 236:346, 1978.
81. Hartzell HC, White RE: Effects of magnesium on inactivation of the voltage-gated calcium current in cardiac myocytes. *J Gen Physiol* 94:745, 1989.
82. Hartzell HC, White RE: Regulation of the voltage-gated Ca^{2+} current by intracellular free Mg^{2+} studied by internal perfusion of single cardiac myocytes, in Strata P, Carbone E (eds): *Mg^{2+} and Excitable Membranes*. Heidelberg, Springer-Verlag, 1990, p 71.
83. Heaton FW, Parsons FM: The metabolic effect of high magnesium intake. *Clin Sci* 21:273, 1961.
84. Heaton FW et al: Observations on the relationship between calcium and magnesium metabolism in man. *Clin Sci* 27:1, 1964.
85. Hebert SC, Andreoli TE: Control of NaCl transport in the thick ascending limb. *Am J Physiol* 246:F745, 1984.
86. Hess P, Weingart R: Intracellular magnesium concentration determination with ion-selective microelectrodes. *J Physiol (Lond)* 318:14, 1981.
87. Horie M, Irisawa H: Rectification of muscarinic K^+ current by magnesium ion in guinea pig atrial cells. *Am J Physiol* 253:H210, 1987.
88. Horie M, Irisawa H: Dual effects of intracellular magnesium on muscarinic potassium channel current in single

guinea-pig ventricular cells. *J Physiol (Lond)* 408:313, 1989.
89. Horie M et al: Voltage-dependent magnesium block of adenosine-triphosphate-sensitive potassium channel in guinea-pig atrial cells. *J Physiol (Lond)* 387:251, 1987.
90. Igbavboa U, Pfeiffer DR: Regulation of reverse uniport activity in extramitochondrial divalent cations: Dependence on a soluble intermembrane space component. *J Biol Chem* 266:4283, 1991.
91. Iseri LT et al: Magnesium deficiency and cardiac disorders. *Am J Med* 58:837, 1975.
92. Ishijima et al: External magnesium-dependent early stimulation of nucleotide synthesis in Swiss 3T3 cells. *Am J Physiol* 257:C1113, 1989.
93. Jackowski MM et al: Regulation of adrenergic stimulation of hepatic adenylate cyclase by divalent cations. *Biochim Biophys Acta* 714:74, 1982.
94. Jones JE et al: Magnesium requirements in adults. *Am J Clin Nutr* 20:632, 1967.
95. Jones JE et al: Magnesium balance studies in chronic alcoholism. *Ann N Y Acad Sci* 162:935, 1969.
96. Karbach U: Cellular-mediated and diffusive magnesium transport across the descending colon of the rat. *Gastroenterology* 96:1282, 1989.
97. Jung et al: Matrix free Mg^{2+} changes with metabolic state in isolated heart mitochondria. *Biochemistry* 29:4121, 1990.
98. Kreusser W et al: Effect of PO_4 depletion on magnesium metabolism in rats. *J Clin Invest* 61:573, 1978.
99. Lansman JB et al: Blockade of current through single channels by Cd^{2+}, Mg^{2+} and Ca^{2+}: Voltage and concentration dependence of calcium entry into the pore. *J Gen Physiol* 88:321, 1986.
100. LeGrimellec C et al: Simultaneous Mg, Ca, P, K, Na and Cl analysis in rat tubular fluid: 2. During acute Mg plasma loading. *Pfluegers Arch* 340:197, 1973.
101. LeGrimellec C et al: Simultaneous Mg, Ca, P, K, Na and Cl analysis in rat tubular fluid: 3. During acute Ca plasma loading. *Pfluegers Arch* 346:171, 1974.
102. Lennon EJ, Piering WF: A comparison of the effects of glucose ingestion and NH_4Cl acidosis on urinary calcium and magnesium excretion in man. *J Clin Invest* 49:1458, 1970.
103. Levine BS et al: Effects of vitamin D and diet magnesium on magnesium metabolism. *Am J Physiol* 239:G515, 1980.
104. Ljunghall S et al: Calcium and magnesium metabolism during long-term treatment with thiazides. *Scand J Urol Nephrol* 15:257, 1981.
105. Lüdi H, Schatzmann HJ: Some properties of a system for sodium-dependent outward movement of magnesium from metabolizing human red blood cells. *J Physiol (Lond)* 390:367, 1987.
106. MacDermott AB, Dale N: Receptors, ion channels and synaptic potentials underlying the integrative actions of excitatory amino acids. *Trends Neurosci* 10:280, 1987.
107. MacIntyre I, Robinson CJ: Magnesium and the gut: Experimental and clinical observation. *Ann N Y Acad Sci* 162:865, 1969.
108. Magil AB et al: Long-term morphological and biochemical observation in cisplatin-induced hypomagnesemia in rats. *Nephron* 43:223, 1986.
109. Maquire ME: Magnesium regulation of the beta-receptor adenylate cyclase complex: 2. Sc^{3+} as a Mg^{2+} antagonist. *Mol Pharmacol* 22:274, 1982.
110. Massry SG et al: The acute effect of adrenal steroids on the interrelationship between the renal excretion of sodium, calcium and magnesium. *J Lab Clin Med* 70:563, 1967.
111. Massry SG et al: Renal handling of magnesium in the dog. *Am J Physiol* 216:1460, 1969.
112. Massry SG, Coburn JW: The hormonal and non-hormonal control of renal excretion of calcium and magnesium. *Nephron* 10:66, 1973.
113. Matsuda et al: Ohmic conductance through the inwardly rectifying K channel and blocking by internal Mg^{2+}. *Nature* 325:156, 1987.
114. Matsuda H: Voltage-dependent blockage of cardiac inwardly rectifying K^+ channels by internal Mg^{2+}, in Strata P, Carbone E (eds): *Mg^{2+} and Excitable Membranes.* Heidelberg, Springer-Verlag, 1990, p 51.
115. Mavichack V et al: Studies on the pathogenesis of cisplatin-induced hypomagnesemia in rats. *Kidney Int* 28:914, 1985.
116. McGuigan JAS et al: Use of ion selective microelectrodes to measure intracellular free Mg^{2+}, in Strata P, Carbone E (eds): *Mg^{2+} and Excitable Membranes.* Heidelberg, Springer-Verlag, 1990, p 1.
117. McIntosh TK et al: Magnesium protects against neurological deficit after brain injury. *Brain Res* 482:252, 1989.
118. Meintzer RB, Steenbock H: Vitamin D and magnesium absorption. *J Nutr* 56:285, 1955.
119. Meneely R et al: Intestinal maturation: In vivo magnesium transport. *Pediatr Res* 16:295, 1982.
120. Milla P et al: Studies in primary hypomagnesemia: Evidence for defective carrier-mediated small intestine transport of magnesium. *Gut* 20:1028, 1979.
121. Miller ER et al: Mineral balance studies with the baby pig: Effect of dietary vitamin D_2 level upon calcium, phosphorus and magnesium balance. *J Nutr* 85:255, 1965.
122. Moore CA, Bunce GI: Reduction in frequency of renal calculus formation by oral magnesium administration: a report. *Invest Urol* 2:7, 1964.
123. Morel F et al: Electron probe analysis of tubular fluid composition. *Nephron* 6:350, 1969.
124. Morel F: Sites of hormone action in the mammalian nephron. *Am J Physiol* 240:159, 1981.
125. Murphy E et al: Cytosolic free magnesium levels in ischemic rat heart. *J Biol Chem* 264:5622, 1989.
126. Nakatani K, Yua K: Calcium and magnesium fluxes across the plasma membrane of the toad rod outer segment. *J Physiol* 395:695, 1988.
127. Narita K et al: Mn and Mg influxes through Ca channels of motor nerve terminals are prevented by verapamil in frogs. *Brain Res* 510:289, 1990.
128. Nowak L et al: Magnesium gates glutamate-activated channels in mouse central neurons. *Nature* 307:462, 1984.
129. Palaty V: Regulation of the cell magnesium in vascular smooth muscle. *J Physiol* 242:555, 1974.
130. Paunier L et al: Primary hypomagnesemia with secondary hypocalcemia in an infant. *Pediatrics* 41:385, 1968.
131. Periano RA et al: Renal excretion of calcium and magne-

sium during correction of metabolic acidosis by bicarbonate infusion in the dog. *Miner Electrolyte Metab* 3:87, 1980.
132. Posner AS: Intramitochondrial storage of stable amorphous calcium phosphate. *Ann N Y Acad Sci* 307:248, 1978.
133. Preston RP: A magensium current in *Paramecium*. *Science* 250:258, 1991.
134. Pusch et al: Intracellular magnesium blocks sodium outward currents in a voltage- and dose-dependent manner. *Biophys J* 55:1267, 1989.
135. Quamme GA, Dirks JH: Effect of intraluminal and contraluminal magnesium on magnesium and calcium transfer in the rat nephron. *Am J Physiol* 238:F187, 1980.
136. Quamme GA: Effect of calcitonin on calcium and magnesium transport in the rat nephron. *Am J Physiol* 238:573, 1980.
137. Quamme GA: Effect of hypercalcemia on renal tubular handling of calcium and magnesium. *Can J Physiol Pharmacol* 60:1275, 1980.
138. Quamme GA: Effect of furosemide on calcium and magnesium transport in the rat nephron. *Am J Physiol* 241:F340, 1981.
139. Quamme GA: Control of magnesium transport in the thick ascending limb. *Am J Physiol* 256:F197, 1989.
140. Quamme GA, Rabkin SW: Cytosolic free magnesium in cardiac myocytes: Identification of a Mg^{2+} influx pathway. *Biochem Biophys Res Comm* 167:1406, 1990.
141. Quamme GA, Dai L-J: Presence of a novel influx pathway for Mg^{2+} in MDCK cells. *Am J Physiol* 259:C521, 1990.
142. Quamme GA, Dirks JH: Renal magnesium transport. *Rev Physiol Biochem Pharmacol* 97:69, 1983.
143. Quamme GA, Smith C: Magnesium transport in isolated proximal straight tubule of the rabbit. *Am J Physiol* 246:F483, 1984.
144. Quamme GA, Dai L-J: Determination of intracellular Mg^{2+} activity in isolated cortical thick ascending limb cells. *Kidney Int* 37:461, 1990.
145. Raju BE et al: A fluorescent indicator for measuring cytosolic free magnesium. *Am J Physiol* 256:C540, 1989.
146. Resnick LM et al: Divalent cations in essential hypertension: Relations between serum ionized calcium, magnesium, and plasma renin activity. *N Engl J Med* 309:888, 1983.
147. Romani A, Scarpi A: Hormonal control of Mg^{2+} transport in the heart. *Nature* 346:841, 1990.
148. Ross DB: In vitro studies on the transport of magnesium across the intestinal wall of the rat. *J Physiol* 16:C417, 1962.
149. Rotevatn et al: Cytosolic free magnesium concentration in cultured chick heart cells. *Am J Physiol* 257:C141, 1989.
150. Roy DR: Magnesium absorption in the juxtamedullary loop of Henle: Effect of magnesium deprivation. *Can J Physiol Pharmacol* 65: 1918, 1987.
151. Rude RK et al: Renal tubular maximum for magnesium in normal, hypoparathyroid, and hyperparathyroid man. *J Clin Endocrinol Metab* 51:70, 1980.
152. Rude RK, Ryzen E: *Tm* Mg and renal Mg threshold in normal man and in certain pathophysiologic conditions. *Magnesium* 5:273, 1986.
153. Runeber L et al: Hypomagnesemia due to renal disease of unknown etiology. *Am J Med* 59:873, 1975.
154. Ryan MP: Magnesium and potassium-sparing diuretics. *Magnesium* 5:282, 1986.
155. Schilsky RL, Anderson T: Hypomagnesemia and renal magnesium wasting in patients receiving cisplatin. *Ann Intern Med* 90:929, 1979.
156. Schilsky RL et al: Persistent hypomagnesemia following cisplatin chemotherapy for testicular cancer. *Cancer Treat Rep* 66:15, 1979.
157. Schwartz R, Reddi AH: Influence of magnesium depletion on matrix induced endochondrial bone formation. *Calcif Tissue Int* 26:18, 1979.
158. Schwartz R: ^{26}Mg as a probe in research on the role of magnesium in nutrition and metabolism. *Fed Proc* 41:2709, 1982.
159. Seelig MS: The requirement of magnesium by the normal adult: Summary and analysis of published data. *Am J Clin Nutr* 13:212, 1964.
160. Seelig MS: Electrocardiographic patterns of magnesium depletion appearing in alcoholic heart disease. *Ann N Y Acad Sci* 162:906, 1969.
161. Seelig MS: Magnesium deficiency in the pathogenesis of disease: Early roots of cardiovascular skeletal and renal abnormalities, in Avioli LV (ed): *Topics in Bone and Renal Disorders*. New York, Plenum, 1980, p 1.
162. Shafik IM, Quamme GA: Early adaptation of renal magnesium reabsorption in response to magnesium restriction. *Am J Physiol* 257:F974, 1989.
163. Shapiro RJ et al: Influence of chronic dietary acid on renal tubular handling of magnesium. *Pfluegers Arch* 409:492, 1987.
164. Shareghi GR, Agus ZS: Phosphate transport in the late segment of the rabbit cortical collecting tubule. *Clin Res* 27:430A, 1979.
165. Shareghi GR, Agus ZS: Magnesium transport in the cortical thick ascending limb of Henle's loop of the rabbit. *J Clin Invest* 69:759, 1982.
166. Shils ME: Experimental human magnesium depletion: 1. Clinical observations and blood chemistry alterations. *Am J Clin Nutr* 15:133, 1964.
167. Shils ME: Experimental human magnesium depletion. *Medicine* 48:61, 1969.
168. Skyberg D et al: Neonatal hypomagnesemia with selective malabsorption of magnesium-clinical entity. *Scand J Clin Lab Invest* 21:355, 1968.
169. Smith RH: Net exchange of certain inorganic ions and water in the alimentary tract of the milk-fed calf. *Biochem J* 83:151, 1962.
170. Snavely MD et al: The Mg + B Mg^{2+} transport locus of *Salmonella typhimurium* encodes a P-type ATPase. *J Biol Chem* 266:815, 1991.
171. Somlyo AV et al: Electron probe x-ray microanalysis of Ca^{2+}, Mg^{2+}, and other ions in rapidly frozen cells. *Methods Enzymol* 172:203, 1989.
172. Tarr et al: Intracellular magnesium affects I_k in single frog atrial cells. *Am J Physiol* 257:H1663, 1989.
173. Tsien RW et al: Calcium channels: Mechanisms of selectivity, permeation, and blockage. *Ann Rev Biophys Chem* 16:265, 1987.
174. Turlapaty PD, Altura BM: Extracellular magnesium ions control calcium exchange and content of vascular smooth muscle. *Eur J Pharmacol* 52:421, 1978.
175. Turlapaty PD, Altura BM: Magnesium deficiency pro-

duces spasms of coronary arteries: Relationship to etiology of sudden death ischemic heart disease. *Science* 208:198, 1980.
176. Vandenberg C: Inward rectification of a potassium channel in cardiac ventricular cells depends on internal magnesium ions. *Proc Nat Acad Sci U S A* 84:2560, 1987.
177. Volpe et al: Regulation of inositol 1,4,5-trisphosphate induced Ca^{2+} release: 1. Effect of Mg^{2+}. *Am J Physiol* 258:C1077, 1990.
178. Vink R et al: Decline in intracellular free magnesium concentration is associated with irreversible tissue injury following brain trauma. *J Biol Chem* 263:757, 1988.
179. Vink R et al: Traumatic spinal cord injury in rabbits decreases intracellular free magnesium concentration as measured by ^{31}P MRS. *Brain Res* 490:144, 1989.
180. Wacker WEC, Parisi AE: Magnesium metabolism. *N Engl J Med* 278:658, 1968.
181. Waling MW et al: Effects of magnesium deficiency and thyroparathyroidectomy on active calcium transport by rat duodenum. *Proc Soc Exp Biol Med* 148:1038, 1975.
182. Wallach S: Availability of body magnesium during magnesium deficiency. *Magnesium* 7:692, 1988.
183. Wallach S: Effects of magnesium on skeletal metabolism. *Magnesium Trace Elem* 9:1, 1990.
184. Walser M: Magnesium metabolism. *Ergeb Physiol* 59:185, 1967.
185. Watson WS, Hildi TE: Magnesium metabolism in blood and the whole body in man using ^{28}magnesium. *Metabolism* 28:90, 1979.
186. Weinberg JM: The cell biology of ischemic renal injury. *Kidney Int* 39:477, 1991.
187. Welt LG: Experimental magnesium depletion. *Yale J Biol Med* 36:325, 1969.
188. Wen SF et al: Evidence for a renal magnesium secretion during magnesium infusion in the dog. *Am J Physiol* 220:33, 1971.
189. Whang R, Welt IG: Observations in experimental magnesium depletion. *J Clin Invest* 42:305, 1963.
190. White RE, Hartzell HC: Effects of intracellular free magnesium on calcium current in isolated cardiac myocytes. *Science* 239:778, 1988.
191. Widdowson EM et al: Chemical composition of human body. *Clin Sci* 10:113, 1951.
192. Wittner M et al: Differential effects of ADH on sodium, chloride, potassium, calcium and magnesium transport in cortical and medullary thick ascending limbs of mouse nephron. *Pfluegers Arch* 412:516, 1988.
193. Wittner M, Di Stefano A: Effects of ADH, PTH and glucagon on the cortical and medullary thick ascending limb of Henle's loop of the mouse nephron. *Pfluegers Arch* 415:707, 1990.
194. Wong NLM et al: Tubular maximum reabsorptive capacity for magnesium in the dog. *Am J Physiol* 13:F78, 1983.
195. Wong NLM et al: Effect of chlorothiazide on renal calcium and magnesium handling in the hamster. *Can J Physiol Pharmacol* 60:1160, 1982.
196. Wong NLM et al: The effect of acidosis and alkalosis on renal handling of magnesium. *Kidney Int* 22:113, 1983.
197. Wong NLM et al: Divalent ion transport in dogs with experimental chronic renal failure. *Can J Physiol Pharmacol* 60:1296, 1982.
198. Wong NLM et al: Renal and tubular transport in phosphate depletion: A micropuncture study. *Can J Physiol Pharmacol* 58:1063, 1980.
199. Wong NLM et al: Effects of mannitol on water and electrolyte transport in the dog kidney. *J Lab Clin Med* 68:3, 1979.

SECTION I-3

PHYSIOLOGIC EFFECTS OF THE ENDOCRINE SYSTEM AND GASTROINTESTINAL TRACT ON FLUID AND ELECTROLYTE METABOLISM

CHAPTER • 14

Adrenal steroid hormones

Henry N. Hulter

ADRENAL STEROID BIOCHEMISTRY

BIOCHEMISTRY AND PHYSIOLOGIC REGULATION OF ADRENAL STEROID SECRETION

The mammalian adrenal cortex comprises two functionally and anatomically distinct subdivisions. The human inner fasciculata-reticularis zone secretes 15 to 20 mg/24 h of cortisol, a steroid hormone with predominantly glucocorticoid activity. The more superficial glomerulosa zone of the adrenal cortex produces aldosterone, the major mammalian mineralocorticoid hormone. When measured under conditions of normal North American dietary intake, aldosterone secretion varies between 50 and 150 μg/24 h.[69,196]

The adrenal steroid structure is composed of three six-carbon rings and a single five-carbon ring (Fig. 14-1). Cholesterol, derived from dietary sources or from endogenous synthesis, is the precursor for adrenal steroidogenesis. Each of the adrenal steroids contains 21 carbons, including a two-carbon side chain. The addition of an hydroxyl group at position 17 converts progesterone to a family of 17-hydroxylated steroids and ultimately to cortisol. As an alternative to 17-hydroxylation, metabolism of progesterone through additional pathways results in the production of the mineralocorticoid steroids desoxycorticosterone (DOC), 18-hydroxycorticosterone, and aldosterone.

Once secreted, approximately 90 percent of plasma cortisol is bound to plasma proteins. About 75 percent of the plasma cortisol is bound tightly to the plasma protein corticosteroid-binding globulin (CBG), and the remainder is bound loosely to albumin.[30,196] The bound fraction of circulating aldosterone has been reported at approximately 65 percent[44,165,370] and is accounted for by both albumin and nonalbumin proteins. The extent to which CBG accounts for nonalbumin binding of aldosterone has not been resolved.[165,370]

Cortisol synthesis and secretion are controlled chiefly by the acute and chronic actions of the peptide adrenocorticotropic hormone (ACTH), which is stored in and released from the anterior pituitary gland. ACTH is normally released in a diurnal pattern by the anterior pituitary gland and is controlled by corticotropin-releasing factor (CRF). The normal diurnal pattern of cortisol secretion yields to rapid increases in secretion rates in response to stressful stimuli such as trauma, exercise, hypoglycemia, pyrogens, and surgery. ACTH-regulated adrenal cortisol synthesis results from the binding of ACTH to its receptors, leading to an activation of the intracellular enzyme adenylyl cyclase, resulting in an increase in cellular levels of adenosine 3′, 5′, monophosphate (cAMP). Substantial evidence supports the notion that all of the actions of ACTH are mediated by an increase in cytosolic cAMP concentration, which leads to an activation of cAMP-dependent protein kinase. A wide variety of evidence supports the conclusion that both acute and chronic effects of ACTH result from regulation of steroidogenesis at an early step: the removal of a six-carbon fragment from the side chain of cholesterol to form pregnenolone. The initial event in ACTH action is thought to be an intramitochondrial step that depends on the integrity of mitochondrial membranes.[310]

The control of aldosterone synthesis appears to be much more complex than the control of cortisol synthesis.[29,87,258] The renin-angiotensin system is the most potent regulatory influence on aldosterone secretion (see Chap. 16). The activity of the renin-angiotensin system is modulated by a variety of factors, the most important of which are the effective extracellular fluid volume (ECFV),

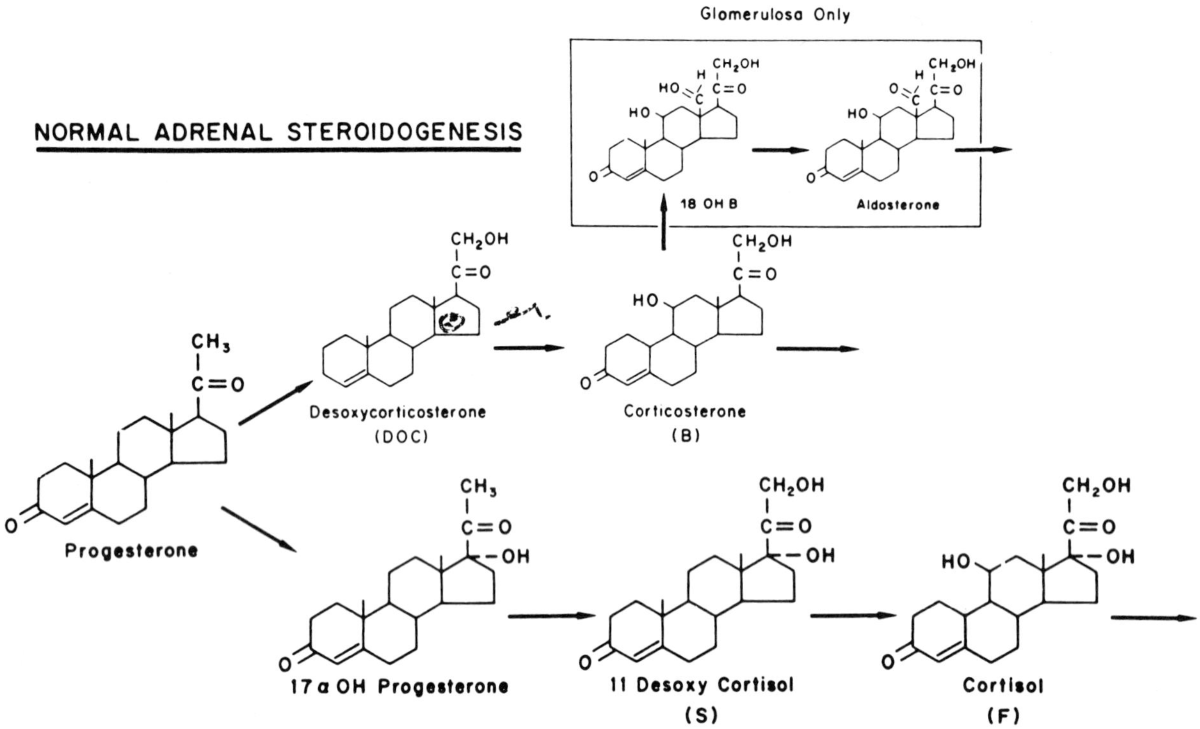

FIGURE 14-1 • Final pathways of aldosterone and cortisol biosynthesis. (From Ehrlich EN in DeGroot LJ, ed: *Endocrinology*, Philadelphia, Saunders, 1989. Used by permission.)

the adrenergic nervous system, distal tubular Cl^- concentration, potassium, and prostaglandin synthesis. Angiotensin II (AII) is an octapeptide degradation product of the sequential enzymatic actions of renin and converting enzyme on circulating renin substrate (angiotensinogen). The source of secreted plasma renin activity is accounted for nearly exclusively by the juxtaglomerular apparatus of the kidney. Therefore, most of the effects of the renin-angiotensin system on adrenal zona glomerulosa function have been attributed to modulation of AII levels in systemic plasma rather than to local tissue concentrations. However, renin has also been localized recently to the outer zona glomerulosa[58,232] and, more specifically, to an intracellular location in zona glomerulosa cells by in situ hybridization assay of renin messenger RNA.[54] Regulation of adrenal renin concentration may be important physiologically, since a low-sodium diet markedly stimulates both adrenal renin content and systemic plasma renin activity. A recent report suggests that adrenal renin is necessary for an intact aldosterone response to hyperkalemia in rats.[231]

The stimulatory action of AII on aldosterone synthesis is signaled through binding to specific receptors in the plasma membrane (Fig. 14-2). Incomplete evidence suggests that the AII receptor may be coupled to one or more G regulatory proteins within the plasma membrane. The G protein, activated by its ability to reversibly bind to cytosolic guanosine triphosphate (GTP), regulates the activity of phospholipase C in the plasma membrane. Thus, AII receptor occupancy results in the hydrolysis of phosphatidylinositol 4,5-bisphosphate (PIP_2) by phospholipase C, resulting in the formation of inositol trisphosphate (IP_3) and 1,2-diacylglycerol (1,2-DG).[76,78] Increased cytosolic levels of IP_3 result in rapid elevation of cytosolic calcium concentration from two sources: release of intracellular calcium stores and entry of extracellular calcium. The increase in cytosolic calcium is dependent on the dose of AII and correlates well with aldosterone synthesis.[28] Not all studies have confirmed an effect of AII on cellular calcium influx.[71] The positive studies have found that the enhanced influx of calcium was blocked by the dihydropyridine class of calcium channel blockers, which indicates a role for voltage-dependent calcium channels.[174,176] AII's effects on aldosterone secretion are not mediated via the cAMP system. In fact, AII has been shown to slightly decrease cAMP generation.[129] Thus, depletion of effective arterial blood volume by physiologic and pathophysiologic perturbations enhances renal production and subsequent release of renin and thereby increases the AII synthetic rate. The elevated plasma AII concentration increases aldosterone production, which thereby promotes renal tubular sodium reabsorption and so reestablishes a normal effective arterial blood volume. According to current concepts, this feedback control system is judged to be the most sensitive final regulator of effective arterial blood volume in humans. Physiologic increments in AII levels have also been shown to have direct stimulatory effects on proximal tubule Na^+ and HCO_3^- reabsorption in rats.[198-200]

Potassium is also a potent secretagogue of aldosterone, which, in turn, is a potent stimulus for potassium secretion by the distal nephron (vide infra). The acute infusion of potassium in normal subjects increases plasma aldosterone concentration.[57,134,289] Chronic increases in dietary potassium intake enhance the aldosterone secretion rate, while low potassium intake has a suppressive effect.[57,147] Chronic changes in dietary potassium intake either complement or oppose concomitant volume/sodium-induced AII-mediated changes in aldosterone secretion. Thus, under most physiologic conditions, the control of aldosterone secretion is codetermined by variation in intake of these two major dietary cations. Whereas effective control of aldosterone secretion by potassium is demonstrable in circumstances in which endogenous renin and AII levels are quite low (e.g., in nephrectomized humans[12,41]), it has been shown that during an acute potassium infusion in vivo, the aldosterone secretory response is completely inhibited by systemic administration of captopril, a potent inhibitor of converting enzyme responsible for AII production.[254] Thus, low levels of AII in plasma and possibly in adrenal tissue may be sufficient for operation of the potassium secretagogue mechanism, but a more effective degree of elimination of AII reveals its important permissive effect on potassium-induced aldosterone secretion. In addition to this permissive effect, acute and chronic increments in plasma potassium and AII concentrations have more than additive effects on aldosterone secretion when both secretagogues are varied simultaneously (Fig. 14-3).[254,367] Potassium enhances the aldosterone-stimulating action of AII either through an increase in intracellular potassium concentration or by increasing the number of AII receptors on glomerulosa cells.[62,63]

The cellular transduction mechanism whereby potassium stimulates aldosterone secretion is quite dissimilar to that of other aldosterone secretagogues. An elevation in extracellular potassium concentration acts at the plasma membrane by diminishing the outwardly directed diffusion gradient for intracellular potassium.[257]

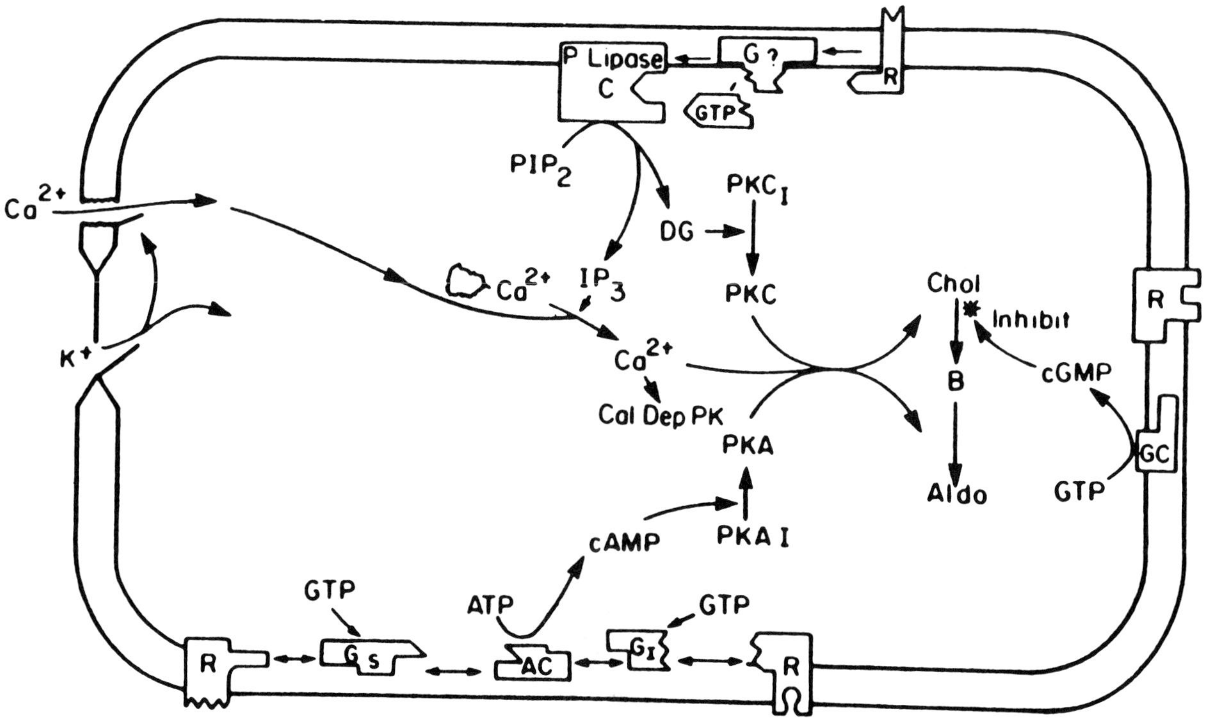

FIGURE 14-2 • Diagram of the relationship among the factors regulating aldosterone secretion. Angiotensin II and vasopressin both activate phospholipase C, as shown at the top of the cell. ACTH at low concentrations may also have this effect. ACTH, melanocyte-stimulating hormone (MSH), and serotonin all utilize the G_s-cAMP system as shown at the bottom of the cell. Angiotensin II, dopamine, ANP, and somatostatin may use G_I to inhibit adenylyl cyclase. ANP may increase cGMP production, but whether this is the mechanism by which ANP inhibits aldosterone secretion is unclear. AC, adenylyl cyclase; Aldo, aldosterone; cAMP, cyclic adenosine monophosphate; ATP, adenosine triphosphate; B, corticosterone; Cal Dep PK, calmodulin-dependent protein kinase; Chol, cholesterol; DG, 1,2-diacylglycerol; G?, unidentified other G protein; GC, guanylyl cyclase; cGMP, cyclic guanosine monophosphate; G_s, stimulatory G protein; GTP, guanosine triphosphate; IP_3, inositol triphosphate; PIP_2, phosphatidylinositol 4,5-biphosphate; PKA, protein kinase A; PKA_I, inactive PKA; PKC, protein kinase C; PKC_I, inactive PKC; P Lipase C, phospholipase C; R, receptor. (From Quinn SJ, Williams GH: *Annu Rev Physiol* 50:409, 1988. Used by permission.)

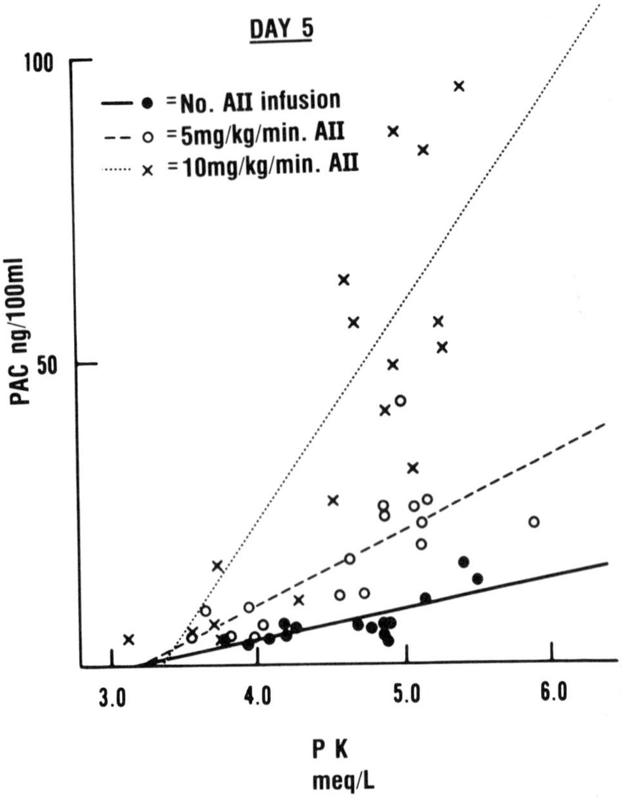

FIGURE 14-3 • Plasma aldosterone concentration (PAC) plotted as a function of plasma potassium concentration during the sustained infusion of angiotensin II in dogs. Values plotted represent data from the fifth day of infusion. (From Young DB et al: *Am J Physiol* 247:E328, 1984. Used by permission.)

The diminished rate of potassium efflux due to increased extracellular potassium concentration causes electrical depolarization of the plasma membrane, which is thought to activate voltage-dependent calcium channels present in the plasma membrane.[175] Activation of voltage-dependent calcium channels increases the cytosolic calcium concentration due to passive calcium influx from the extracellular fluid (ECF), which appears to be well correlated with the aldosterone production rate.[32] The specific role of calcium-induced activation of calmodulin-dependent protein kinase in this process remains to be elucidated.

ACTH, an aldosterone secretagogue, appears to operate only acutely. The response to intravenous ACTH is maximal after 15 min of infusion, but in contrast to the effects of AII or potassium, the adrenal response to a sustained stimulus diminishes rapidly, and by 24 h aldosterone output in humans is actually lower than control values.[264] Although multiple transduction mechanisms have been suggested for ACTH-induced stimulation of aldosterone secretion, most studies have suggested that the dominant mechanism is the binding of ACTH to a specific receptor that couples the signal via a G regulatory protein (G_s) to activation of adenylyl cyclase (Fig. 14-2).[90]

Accumulating evidence indicates that plasma osmolality is a potent mediator of aldosterone secretion. In studies in dogs, acute and chronic hyponatremia substantially increases aldosterone secretion,[36,39] whereas acute and chronic hypernatremia suppresses aldosterone secretion.[36,293,330] Studies in the isolated perfused canine adrenal gland indicate that the effect is specific for changes in osmolality rather than in sodium concentration.[293,330] The cellular transduction pathways for the effect of osmolality on aldosterone secretion have not been elucidated.

Numerous studies in vivo have demonstrated a role for the adrenergic system in modulating aldosterone secretion. Aldosterone secretion in humans is significantly enhanced by administration of the dopaminergic antagonist metoclopramide, indicating that its production is ordinarily tonically suppressed by dopamine.[33] Characterization of adrenal dopamine receptors indicates the existence of D_2 and possibly D_1 classes.[222] Details of the dopaminergic cellular transduction mechanism are conflicting. Controversy has emerged as to the physiologic importance of dopamine as a regulator of aldosterone secretion.[97]

Chronic metabolic acidosis induced by NH_4Cl feeding to normal human subjects has been reported to increase the aldosterone secretion rate.[181,290] Since mineral acid feeding induces negative sodium balance and hyperreninemia, these studies do not necessarily suggest a direct effect of acidosis on aldosterone secretion.[290] However, direct acid-base effects on glomerulosa cells are possible, inasmuch as studies in the isolated canine adrenal gland have shown that a hypobicarbonatemic, acidemic perfusate potentiates ACTH-stimulated aldosterone secretion.[260] Whether acidosis can stimulate aldosterone secretion in the absence of exogenous ACTH stimulation remains to be established. A recent report of measurements of intracellular pH in bovine glomerulosa cells demonstrated a correlation between AII-stimulated aldosterone production and amiloride-inhibitable cell alkalinization.[140] Whether the observed changes in cell pH directly determine the aldosterone synthetic rate or whether altered cell pH is a nonspecific effect of cell stimulation remains to be determined.

Atrial natriuretic peptide (ANP) appears to decrease aldosterone secretion by at least two mechanisms: ANP decreases renin secretion[204] and also may have a direct action on glomerulosa cells.[116] Whether the direct effect of synthetic ANP on isolated glomerulosa cells is dependent on modulation by the renin-angiotensin system within those cells remains to be determined.

Parathyroid hormone (PTH) has been reported recently to bind specifically to bovine adrenal glomerulosa and outer fasiculata.[152a] Moreover, PTH was shown to stimulate aldosterone secretion in a dose-dependent manner and to potentiate the secretory response to AII in isolated glomerulosa cells. Addition of PTH alone elicited a small increase in cytosolic Ca^{++} concentration, but in cells pretreated with AII or K^+, the intracellular Ca^{++} response to PTH was potentiated markedly.[152a] These results are consistent with the results of studies using long-term PTH infusion to normal human subjects in which experimental hyperparathyroidism was associated with evidence of increased aldosterone secretion.[151a]

In most physiologic and pathophysiologic circumstances, plasma aldosterone concentration is modulated predominantly by changes in secretion rate. However, changes in the aldosterone metabolic clearance rate can also have a large impact on circulating aldosterone levels. High aldosterone extraction rates by the splanchnic and hepatic circulations have been demonstrated in both dogs and humans. Thus, changes in hepatic blood flow and hepatic extraction can account for the impaired metabolic clearance rate seen with acute postural changes and in chronic liver disease.[45,221] In chronically potassium-depleted dogs, a significant increase in the aldosterone metabolic clearance rate, as well as a decreased aldosterone secretion rate, has been documented to participate in hypoaldosteronism.[147] The mechanism by which potassium depletion increases the aldosterone metabolic clearance rate has not been defined.

ADRENAL STEROID RECEPTOR BIOCHEMISTRY AND PHYSIOLOGY

In the past several years, the primary structures of each of the known steroid hormone receptors have been characterized following cloning and sequencing of their cDNAs. These advances, facilitated by modern molecular biology techniques, have dramatically, although still incompletely, clarified how steroid hormones control gene expression. The high lipid solubility of steroid hormones enables diffusion through the target cell membranes, where they interact with cytosolic receptors. Binding of steroid hormones to their receptors induces a change in the structure of the receptor such that the receptor-hormone complex is thereby permitted to bind to specific DNA sequences in nuclear chromatin. These critically important regulatory DNA sequences are generally termed *hormone response elements* and function to modulate the transcription of the nearby hormone target genes. Historically, adrenal steroid hormones have been subdivided into those with primarily mineralocorticoid activity and those with glucocorticoid activity, based on the relative potency of the particular steroid to influence sodium and potassium transport versus the steroid's ability to influence carbohydrate metabolism. The mineralocorticoid and glucocorticoid potency of a particular steroid hormone correlates with its relative affinity for the so-called mineralocorticoid (type I) and glucocorticoid (type II) receptors.[277] Based on studies of $[^3H]$-labeled steroid binding in vitro, the high-affinity (type I) aldosterone binding sites were shown to have an equivalently high affinity for aldosterone and for DOC but a much lower affinity for corticosterone and dexamethasone (a potent synthetic glucocorticoid).[92,93] Based on this steroidal specificity profile, type I sites were designated as the structural counterpart of mineralocorticoid receptor activity. Similarly, dexamethasone's greater binding to the lower affinity (type II) site defined the glucocorticoid receptor.

Both the mineralocorticoid and glucocorticoid receptors have been cloned and expressed in a variety of cell systems.[7,135,215,348] However, despite these powerful advances, studies have not been reported in which definitive quantitative localization of receptors has been assessed by monoclonal antibody binding to type I and II receptors in the target epithelial cells of interest. An initial report of qualitative immunostaining of rabbit nephron segments using monoclonal antibodies directed against at least one isoform of type I and type II receptors has found extensive antibody localization of both receptor types in all postproximal segments. The absence of staining by anti-type II antibody in the proximal tubule suggests that the documented proximal effects of type II agonists are derived from an alternative isotype of the type II receptor or that proximal effects of glucocorticoids are mediated by a nonreceptor mechanism of action.[81a]

Localization of adrenal steroid binding sites along the nephron has been performed by autoradiography and also by segmental binding of ^3H steroid to isolated tubular segments or whole kidney preparations. Both techniques can be influenced by postbinding dissociation of the steroid. The autoradiographic technique has the advantage of discriminating cytosolic binding from nuclear binding and permits the observation of temperature-dependent transitions from cytosolic labeling at low temperatures to nuclear translocation of label at physiologic temperatures. Both techniques have been employed to define type I sites of action, and both techniques suggest that the cortical collecting tubule (CCT), connecting tubule (CNT), and medullary collecting tubule (MCT) are specific targets for aldosterone in the rabbit (Table 14-1).[60,79,80,188,208] Similar autoradiographic findings have been reported for aldosterone binding in isolated rat nephron segments.[81] When CCT was used as the source of receptor, aldosterone had a higher affinity for binding sites than did DOC or dexamethasone. Renal aldosterone binding by autoradiography is saturable, and the equilibrium dissociation constants have been found to average between 0.5 and 2.2 n*M*.[60,79] Since the plasma concentration of aldosterone is less than 1 n*M*,[69,196,295] the values depicted in Table 14-1 are consistent with the conclusion that roughly half of the receptors are occupied at normal plasma aldosterone concentrations.

TABLE 14-1 • Localization of corticosteroid binding sites

Species	^{3}H-steroid	Temperature, °C	K_d nM	Concentration used, nM	Relative binding								Units	Characteristics	Reference
					PCT	PR	mTALH	cTALH	DCT	CNT	CCT	MCT			
Rabbit	Aldosterone	25	2.2	6	0.07	0.01	0.03	0.04	0.04	0.92	1.00	0.96	mol/cm	A > DOCA > DEX	60
Rabbit	Aldosterone	30	0.5	0.3	0.04	0.17	0.26	0.45	0.13	1.47	1.00	0.39	nuclear	A > DEX	79
				1.5	< 0.01	0.04	0.14	0.23	0.82	0.91	1.00	0.45	grains/100		79
				20	0	0.43	0.35	0.82	1.09	0.96	1.00	1.09	μm^2		79
Rabbit	Dexamethasone	30	30	53	1.14	1.77	0.06	0.14	0.34	0.63	1.00	0.11	nuclear grains/100 μm^2	DEX ≥ B >> A*	80
Rat	Corticosterone	25	25	80	0.11	0.06	0.03	0.03	0.28		1.00	0.27	mol/cm	B > DOCA > A >> DEX,F	188

* Competition on whole kidney, not isolated tubules.

ABBREVIATIONS: PCT, proximal convoluted tubule; PR, pars recta; mTALH, medullary thick ascending limb of Henle; cTALH, cortical TALH; DCT, distal convoluted tubule; CNT, connecting tubule; CCT, cortical collecting tubule; MCT, medullary collecting tubule.

SOURCE: Adapted from Marver D: *Am J Physiol* 246:F111, 1984. Used by permission.

Whether type I receptors found in the distal convoluted tubule (DCT), the medullary thick ascending limb of Henle (mTALH), the cortical thick ascending limb of Henle (cTALH), and the inner MCT represent true aldosterone receptors or illicit occupancy of type II receptors is unclear.[59,79] In the most detailed studies, substantial aldosterone binding was observed only at high concentrations, and competition with dexamethasone was as effective as that with aldosterone in these segments.[79] Outer MCT has not been studied extensively in this regard.

The autoradiographic nuclear labeling pattern for the type II glucocorticoid receptor differs substantially from that for the type I receptor inasmuch as type II receptors are much more abundant in the proximal tubule than in distal segments; type II sites have only a modest presence in the distal nephron (Table 14-1).[188] The type II receptor binding hierarchy is dexamethasone > corticosterone > aldosterone. The presence of glucocorticoid type II receptors in both proximal and distal nephron segments is consistent with widespread presence of type II receptors in all segments of the intestine in which they have been sought.[34,131,207,209,255] In contrast, intestinal type I receptors have been localized only in distal colon.[20] Firm conclusions regarding the nature and physiologic significance of both proximal nephronal and intestinal type II receptors (demonstrable by autoradiography but not by monoclonal antibody) will await future investigation.[81a,188]

Recent detailed studies of interorgan variation in the characteristics of type I binding sites have revealed a pattern of inherent nonselectivity. The hippocampus has, in addition to classical type II receptors, a type I class of binding site with a higher affinity for corticosterone and aldosterone than for dexamethasone.[49,50,51,52,53,234] The hippocampal type I receptor was thought initially to be quite different from the renal type I receptor inasmuch as renal cytosolic fractions from adrenalectomized rats incubated with [^{3}H] steroids demonstrated a steroid specificity pattern different from that seen in the hippocampus.[182] In these studies, corticosterone was a substantially less potent competitor for aldosterone binding in the renal cytosolic fraction, whereas in the hippocampus, corticosterone binding potency was equivalent to that of aldosterone. Subsequent studies established that these differences were due, not to variation in the intrinsic characteristics of these receptors, but to corticosterone binding to extravascular CBG (transcortin) present in kidney cytosol but not in brain.[306,307]

A number of studies have attempted to explain the heretofore occult renal mechanisms that underlie the aldosterone selectivity of type I receptors. An explanation was required for how the renal type I receptor could function physiologically to receive information from nanomolar concentrations of circulating aldosterone when circulating concentrations of cortisol (human) or corticosterone (rat and rabbit) were much higher and should therefore have dominated type I receptor binding despite the presence of cytosolic CBG. To simplify the system, studies were carried out in adrenalectomized 10-day-old rats with very low levels of CBG. Under these conditions, renal cytosolic in vitro binding of aldosterone and that of corticosterone were equivalent, yet when these steroids were injected into the animal in vivo, very much higher binding of aldosterone relative to corticosterone was found in the kidney, parotid, and colon but not the hippocampus.[307,308] These findings fostered the hypothesis that aldosterone target tissues in vivo can exclude corticosterone and cortisol from epithelial but not hippocampal mineralocorticoid receptors. Such an exclusion mechanism would cause aldosterone activity to be greater than that of corticosterone in vivo, but the differences would disappear with cytosolic preparations.

Evidence derived from several laboratories has given strong support to the thesis that the enzyme 11-β-hydroxysteroid dehydrogenase (11-HSD) is responsible for providing aldosterone-specificity to mineralcorticoid receptors. The enzyme, which converts cortisol to cortisone, is found in the kidney, parotid gland, and colon but not in the hippocampus or heart. By converting cortisol, with its substantial mineralocorticoid activity, to the inactive cortisone, this enzyme limits competition for type I receptors. Moreover, 11-HSD activity in homogenates of epithelial tissues could be blocked by prior in vivo administration of carbenoxolone, a hemisuccinate salt of the active component of licorice (glycyrrhetinic acid) and a known potent inhibitor of 11-HSD.[94] These observations help to clarify the pathophysiologic basis of the syndrome of apparent mineralocorticoid excess[318] and the apparent mineralocorticoid activity of glycrrhetinic and glycrrhizic acids, the active compounds in licorice.[318] In the former syndrome, patients are deficient in 11-HSD activity and manifest severe hypertension, hypokalemia, and suppression of the renin-aldosterone system. These clinical and chemical findings undoubtedly result from the excess cortisol that accumulates near renal type I receptors in the absence of the 11-HSD.[235,318] Metabolic balance studies in normal human subjects have demonstrated that licorice-induced sodium retention is associated with alterations in cortisol metabolism indicating inhibition of 11-HSD. Moreover, the reaction products of 11-HSD activity, the 11-keto analogues of cortisol and corticosterone, do not bind to type I receptors.[94] Conversion of the hydroxyl at C-11 in a certain steroid structure to a keto group clearly renders this particular steroid incapable of interacting with its receptor. The question is therefore raised as to how the prototypical mineralocorticoid, aldosterone, eludes in vivo metabolism to its less active 11-keto analogue. Although crystalline aldosterone possesses a hydroxyl group at C-11, the molecule does not exist in this form in aqueous solution but cyclizes to hemiketal/hemiacetal forms which protect the C-11 hydroxyl group from acting as a substrate for 11-HSD. It is notable that neither progesterone nor DOC possesses a hydroxyl group at C-11, and therefore neither steroid is metabolized by 11-HSD, a characteristic that permits their unmitigated action as mineralocorticoids at the type I receptor.

If 11-HSD exerts a key influence on mineralocorticoid activity, it is important to demonstrate its presence in the same distal nephron segments that respond to aldosterone. Recent studies have addressed this point and examined the conversion of corticosterone to its 11-keto analogue in discrete isolated segments of rabbit tubules and have shown that 11-HSD activity is very high in aldosterone-sensitive tubular segments in comparison with proximal nephron segments (Fig. 14-4).[24]. Although 11-HSD bioactivity and aldosterone binding sites co-localize to distal nephron segments, 11-HSD immunostaining does not localize to these segments. This observation has been explained by the demonstration of several isoforms of 11-HSD (some not necessarily immunoreactive) despite the finding of a unique 11-HSD mRNA. Using in situ hybridization, this mRNA was found to be highly expressed in all nephron segments in the rat.[363b]

Recent studies using an in vivo rat model and an in vitro collecting duct tissue culture model have raised the surprising possibility that not all classic mineralocorticoid effects on sodium, potassium, and hydrogen ion transport are mediated by activation of type I receptors. It was suggested that, under certain conditions, perhaps some of these epithelial transport effects might be mediated by occupancy of type II glucocorticoid receptors. In vivo studies in adrenalectomized rats have demonstrated that systemic administration of RU-28362, a pure glucocorticoid agonist with unmeasureable type I affinity, results in kaliuresis and antinatriuresis. Moreover, after pretreatment with carbenoxolone, the effect of RU-28362 on urinary electrolytes was comparable in magnitude to a maximal aldosterone response.[95] Recent studies utilizing primary cultures of rabbit CCT cells grown as an epithelium show that not only aldosterone, but also Ru-28362, can cause nearly identical increments in transepithelial voltage, short-circuit current, Na^+ absorption, and K^+ secretion in tight epithelia. It is most interesting to note that the effect of RU-28362 was completely prevented by cotreatment with the glucocorticoid receptor antagonist RU-38486, whereas the specific mineralocorticoid receptor antagonist ZK-91587 did not block its effect.[82] It seems possible that certain steroid hormone response elements within nuclear chromatin may be activated indiscriminately by steroid agonists bound to either type I or type II receptors (see below). Additional possibilities have been raised to explain the effects of predominantly glucocorticoid steroids (e.g., corticosterone) in stimulating sodium transport. Using

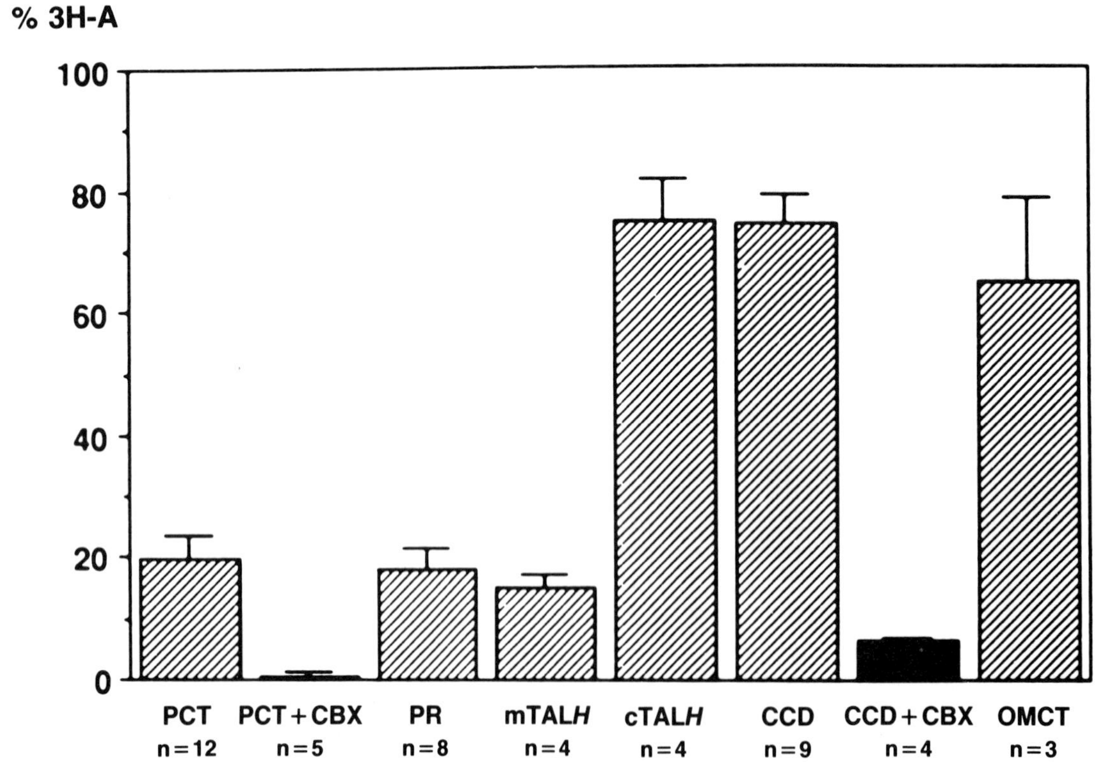

FIGURE 14-4 • Percent conversion of [^{3}H]-corticosterone to [^{3}H]-11-dehydrocorticosterone by various rabbit tubular segments in vitro. Mean values are given ± SEM. The number of tubular segments is indicated under each column. Black columns correspond to results in the presence of carbenoxolone (CBX). PCT, proximal convoluted tubule; mTAL, medullary thick ascending limb; cTAL, cortical thick ascending limb; CCD, cortical collecting duct; OMCT, outer medullary collecting tubule. (From Bonvalet J-P et al: *J Clin Invest* 86:832, 1990. Used by permission.)

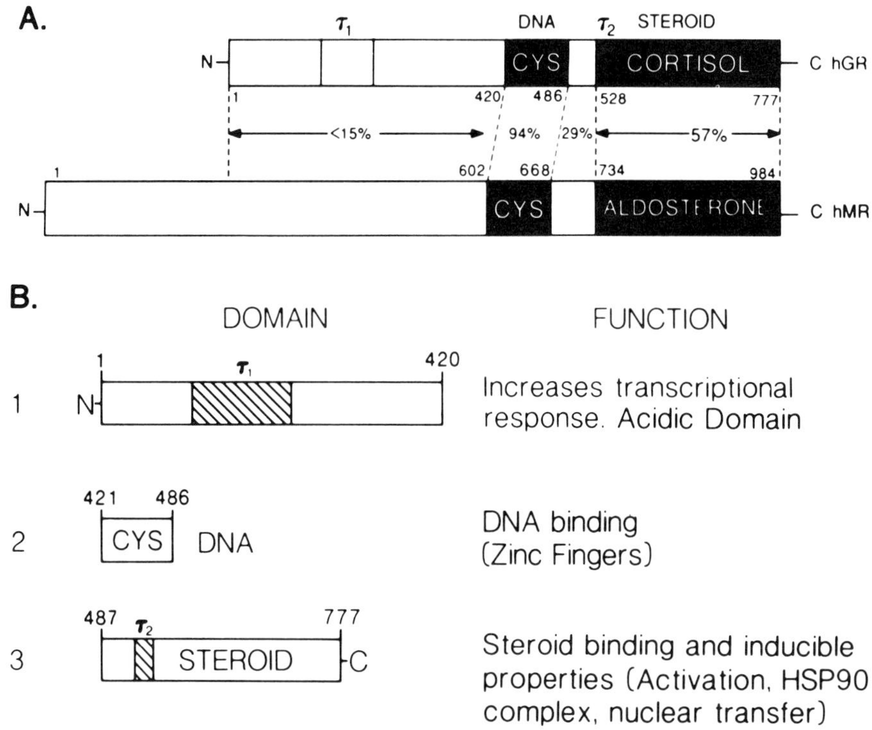

FIGURE 14-5 • Structural homologies and functional domains of the human glucocorticoid receptor. (*a*) Schematic comparison of the primary amino acid sequences of the human glucocorticoid receptor (hGR) and human mineralocorticoid receptor (hMR). Regions of structural homologies and their percent amino acid sequence identity are indicated between the dashed lines. The degree of sequence identity between hGR and hMR is most significant in regions associated with the DNA-binding (CYS) and ligand-binding (steroid) functions. Cortisol and aldosterone are glucocorticoid and mineralocorticoid hormones, respectively, and τ_1 and τ_2 refer to sequences that stimulate gene transcription. N and C represent the amino and carboxyl termini. (*b*) For conceptual simplicity, the hGR can be subdivided into three functional domains. The amino terminus (N) is variable in size and sequence among the steroid receptors. In the hGR it contains a region (τ_1), somewhat acidic in nature, that is important for stimulating gene transcription. The DNA-binding region, characterized by invariant cysteine residues (CYS), appropriately positions the receptor on target DNA sequences. The carboxyl terminal region (C) contains the hormone-binding function, and the interactions of hormone with this region are postulated to induce a number of additional activities determined by this region. These activities may include dissociation from a receptor-heat shock protein (HSP90) complex, nuclear translocation, and stimulation of transcription by the region indicated as τ_2. (From Evans RM, Arriza JL: *Neuron* 2:1105, 1989. Used by permission.)

A6 cells from a continuous cell line derived from the kidney of *Xenopus laevis* (a typical tight epithelium when grown on permeable supports), sodium transport has been stimulated by endogenous conversion of corticosterone to 6β-OH-corticosterone. These studies have shown that 6β-OH-corticosterone binds preferentially to a third (putative type IV) receptor, which, when activated, accounts for 90 percent of the maximum short-circuit current in epithelia exposed to corticosterone for 24 h.[66] This receptor has been designated type IV to avoid confusion with the type III "CBG-like" renal cytosolic binding site for corticosterone, which is not a true receptor.[208] Whether mammalian epithelia utilize a type IV receptor for sodium transport remains to be determined. Moreover, it is not yet clear whether 6β-hydroxylation occurs in the mammalian kidney. However, preliminary evidence suggests a significant antinatriuretic response to 6β-OH-corticosterone following systemic administration in adrenalectomized rats.[66,157]

The metabolism of aldosterone may also affect its cellular action. An accumulating body of evidence suggests that, at least in rat kidney and toad bladder, mineralocorticoid target cells may regulate their sensitivity to extracellular aldosterone levels. This change is effected by the metabolic reduction of aldosterone at its C-4 and C-5 positions, creating more potent metabolites.[225] These metabolites appear to be produced in the nucleus and may represent a postreceptor regulatory event. The renal metabolites are produced to a greater extent in male than in female rats[224] and have been shown to be potent mineralocorticoid agonists.[225] This postreceptor regulatory step might explain the greater antinatriuretic and kaliuretic effects of aldosterone in male rats.[223] Whether these reduced aldosterone metabolites play important roles in the target cells of additional mammalian species remains to be explored.

Considerable information is available on the properties and structure of the glucocorticoid and mineralocorticoid receptors, as well as the hormone response elements (HRE). Several functional domains of the glucocorticoid and mineralocorticoid receptors are depicted in Fig. 14-5. As shown, the receptor molecules can be divided into domains that determine DNA binding, hormone binding, and transcriptional activation properties. The central region of the receptor is responsible for DNA recognition and is highly conserved among steroid receptors. Point mutations within this region can eradicate the ability of the glucocorticoid receptor to bind DNA.[137,305] It appears that this domain specifically positions the receptor onto target gene promoters within the nuclear chromatin. The carboxyl terminal region determines the hormone binding specificity, as well as a number of hormone-inducible functions, including nuclear translocation[253] and stimulation of transcription.[137,347] The amino terminal portions of these receptors provide an important activation function in an acidic segment, termed τ_1, which has been shown to be necessary for efficient stimulation of gene transcription.[110,136]

The structure of the centrally located DNA binding domain of both steroid receptors permits two receptor molecules to dimerize in a fashion whereby both molecules contact the specific HRE in the DNA double helix. Only after steroid ligand-receptor binding has occurred does dimer formation of this higher affinity DNA binding species occur.[30a] However, the apparent identity of the HREs for the glucocorticoid, mineralocorticoid, androgen, and progesterone receptors represents a dilemma for the physiologist, considering the great differences in observed hormone responses to these various agonists.[91a] Each cell's diversity of response may depend on a variety of unexplored factors:

1. Subtle variations from consensus HRE DNA sequences that might affect the affinity of the HRE for each species of ligand receptor complex.
2. Each cell type may possess specific additional transcription factors that compete for or interact with the receptor dimer.[54a]
3. Additional potential diversity of the cell's response is accounted for by the presence of DNA binding sites for various factors that modify or contribute to the response.[54a]
4. Multiple copies of the same HRE permit increased transcriptional efficiency dependent on HRE number.
5. Negative response elements exist that depress transcription in some tissues but enhance transcription in other tissues as modulated by various transcription factors.[54a] An example is the composite or negative glucocorticoid HRE (nGRE) in the mouse proliferin gene that overlaps with a binding site for AP-1, a phorbol ester-activated transcription factor.[54a] The nGRE is bound selectively in vitro by both the glucocorticoid receptor and by c-Jun and c-Fos, components of the AP-1 transcription factor. c-Jun and c-Fos serve as selectors of hormone responsiveness: The nGRE is inactive in the absence of c-Jun, whereas it confers a positive glucocorticoid effect in the presence of c-Jun and a negative glucocorticoid effect in the presence of c-Jun plus high levels of c-Fos (c-Jun/c-Fos heterodimers). Thus, the net response in a given cell depends on the ratio of c-Fos to c-Jun in that cell.

   Several groups have reported repression by the glucocorticoid receptor and the AP-1 complex of their respective response elements.[157a,202a,293a,363a] Repression by the glucocorticoid receptor has been reported to occur via a direct protein-protein interaction between the DNA binding domain of the receptor and the DNA binding region of the c-Jun monomer.[363a]

EFFECTS OF ADRENAL STEROIDS TO INCREASE ENZYME ACTIVITY

Localization of aldosterone action has also been investigated by determining whether the hormone could increase RNA synthesis (transcription products) or the activity of such putatively aldosterone-induced proteins (translation products) as Na^+-K^+ ATPase, citrate synthase and flavokinase in specific tubular segments.[166,219] Chronic systemic mineralocorticoid administration significantly increases RNA synthesis in rabbit CCT, MCT, and DCT. No significant alterations in RNA synthesis were observed in segments proximal to the DCT, a finding that is generally consistent with the receptor localization studies noted above.

It has been demonstrated that following mineralocorticoid administration, the activity of citrate synthase, a mitochondrial Krebs cycle enzyme, is greatly increased in mammalian kidney, toad bladder, and cultured collecting duct cells.[210,211,220] Microassay of citrate synthase activity in isolated segments of rabbit kidney has shown that aldosterone administration increases enzyme activity acutely in the CCT, $OMCT_{is}$, and mTALH.[211] No significant aldosterone-stimulated citrate synthase activity was observed in other nephron segments. Thus, with the exception of stimulation in the mTALH, citrate synthase activation studies agree with the specific aldosterone receptor studies noted above.

Activity of the important transport enzyme renal Na^+-K^+ ATPase is in part under the control of adrenal steroids. Enzyme activity is reduced by adrenalectomy and elevated to normal levels by the administration of adrenal steroids.[74,166,219] Acute or chronic mineralocorticoid excess increases Na^+-K^+ ATPase activity most consistently in the CCT, but increases have also been noted in the CNT and the OMCT.[59,121,152,208,210,237,295] Chronic enzyme stimulation has been achieved both by exogenous mineralocorticoid (DOC) and by increasing endogenous aldosterone levels secondary to a low-sodium diet.[100,189] These changes were limited to the CNT and the CCT and were associated with a corresponding increase in basolateral cell membrane (the cellular site of this transport protein) area.[160,189] The mineralocorticoid-induced effects on enzyme activity appear to be specific, since the changes in collecting duct enzyme activity can be prevented by administration of spironolactone, a specific mineralocorticoid antagonist.[73,189,251]

Mineralocorticoid hormones have similar effects in the distal colon. Stimulated Na^+-K^+ ATPase activity, citrate synthase activity, and aldosterone receptors have been found uniquely in this intestinal segment.[5,34,162,209]

Glucocorticoids are potent stimulators of Na^+-K^+ ATPase activity within specific nephron segments. Despite the high numbers of specific type II receptors in the CCT, there is no evidence that glucocorticoids can stimulate Na^+-K^+ ATPase activity in this segment.[229,251] Supraphysiologic doses of dexamethasone have been shown to increase enzyme activity in the CCT, but this effect was abolished by spironolactone, indicating its probable operation via type I receptors.[73] Glucocorticoids have a large effect on Na^+-K^+ ATPase activity following either acute or chronic dexamethasone administration in DCT, mTALH, and proximal convoluted tubule (PCT).[73,75,101] In PCT, dexamethasone effects were not inhibitable by spironolactone, indicating the likelihood of a specific type II receptor effect.[73] Neither mineralocorticoid nor glucocorticoid hormones appear to regulate Na^+-K^+ ATPase activity in proximal straight tubule (PST) or cTALH.[72]

It has been suggested recently that adrenal steroids may provide tonic stimulation of the renal adenylyl cyclase system.[61] Although a number of studies have demonstrated that adrenal steroids can modulate the degradation rate of cAMP, there has been little evidence that they influence the production rate of cAMP. In chronically adrenalectomized rats, adenylyl cyclase stimulation by arginine vasopressin (AVP), glucagon, and calcitonin was reduced in the mTALH, whereas only the response to AVP was decreased in CCT and MCT. Chronic administration of a physiologic dose of dexamethasone reversed the impaired stimulation of adenylyl cyclase in mTALH, but the adenylyl cyclase defect in the collecting duct was prevented only by mineralocorticoid hormone. Detailed investigations of the mechanism(s) underlying these effects suggested that the total adenylyl cyclase was probably unaltered but that steroid hormones affect the activation state of the regulatory G_s protein.[61]

In the intestinal tract, glucocorticoids diffusely stimulate Na^+-K^+ ATPase activity. Enzyme activity is increased in the jejunum, the ileum, and throughout the colon.[34,360] This distribution pattern of enzyme stimulation is similar to that for the specific glucocorticoid receptors.[209,255]

PHYSIOLOGIC EFFECTS OF ADRENAL STEROIDS

EFFECT OF ADRENAL STEROIDS ON RENAL AND SYSTEMIC HEMODYNAMICS

Mineralocorticoids

The major hemodynamic effects of mineralocorticoid steroids are secondary to the induction of salt retention and ECF volume (ECFV) expansion.[124,163,365] Plasma renin activity is suppressed in response to mineralocorticoid-induced ECFV expansion and is increased in response to contraction of the ECFV (see Chap. 16).[259,319,365] Peripheral and renal vascular resistance increase in parallel with an increase in plasma renin and AII activity.[155] Whereas cardiac output increases in mineralocorticoid excess states in response to increments in ECFV, there is substantial evidence that mineralocorticoids can cause hemodynamic changes even in the absence of sodium retention and ECFV expansion.[8,178,226,256,340] Rabbit arterial and venous tissue has been found to possess high-affinity binding sites for mineralocorticoid steroids, including aldosterone.[178] Aldosterone stimulates arterial contraction and delays relaxation in rabbit tissue studied in vitro.[256] Aldosterone can also greatly augment cardiac contractile force in the isolated rat heart,[8] but this result has not been obtained by all investigators.[340] Aldosterone exerts the following effects on vascular smooth muscle in vitro: stimulation of Na^+-K^+ ATPase-mediated Na^+ efflux, stimulation of Na^+ efflux independent of the Na^+ pump, and increased K^+ permeability.[206,227] A recent preliminary report demonstrates that, in vitro, aldosterone can also increase the number of AII surface receptors in vascular smooth muscle cells and can prevent down-regulation of the receptor number by AII. Moreover, aldosterone increased the production of IP_3 in proportion to the hormone-induced increment in the AII receptor number.[339] In rat models, mineralocorticoid-induced hypertension has been prevented with a low-NaCl diet.[191,298,368] Since hypertension does not occur in NaCl-restricted, mineralocorticoid-treated subjects or animals, it seems likely that ECFV expansion is a prerequisite (and perhaps even sufficient) for the increase in blood pressure by type I agonists. The impact of direct vascular action of type I agonists may, therefore, be quite small. One intensively studied model of spontaneous hypertension in the SHR rat is characterized by an abnormal pattern of aldosterone metabolism relative to that found in normotensive strains of this rat.[226] The possibility is thereby raised that an alteration in aldosterone metabolism might be related to the pathogenesis of hypertension in this model.

Glucocorticoids

Glucocorticoids appear to have more complex interrelationships with systemic hemodynamics than do mineralocorticoids. In glucocorticoid deficiency, cardiac stroke volume and blood pressure decrease, while peripheral vascular resistance is either unchanged or increases and renal vascular resistance increases.[26,354] A number of interactions have been described between glucocorticoids and the renin-angiotensin system. Plasma renin activity is inappropriately low in glucocorticoid deficiency, despite hypotension and low cardiac output.[179,180,319] Renin substrate production is under glucocorticoid control,[268,319] with low levels increasing after glucocorticoid administration.[179,180,319] It therefore appears that the low circulating renin activity complicating glucocorticoid deficiency is caused, in large part, by the limitation in renin substrate levels. States of glucocorticoid excess cause chronic hypertension even in animals ingesting a low-salt diet.[191,298,368] Renin activity has been elevated[180] in some models of glucocorticoid hypertension, while in others levels have remained normal despite increased concentration of substrate.[236] A role for the renin-angiotensin system in glucocorticoid-induced hypertension remains unclear, since captopril administration does not prevent its development.[70,173] Although plasma catecholamines are not altered by glucocorticoid-induced hypertension in the rat,[263] the steroids potentiate the pressor effects of epinephrine,[17,187] a phenomenon that is abolished by indomethacin administration.[127] This finding raises the possibility that altered prostaglandin metabolism might play a role in the hypertension induced by glucocorticoids. A role for vasopressin in glucocorticoid-induced hypertension seems unlikely, since the antidiuretic hormone (ADH)-deficient Brattleboro rat is as sensitive as the normal Wistar rat.[262] Dexamethasone increases Na^+-K^+ ATPase activity in rat arteries.[244] Whether secondary alterations in cytosolic Na^+ or K^+ activity within vascular tissues play a role in glucocorticoid-induced hypertension remains to be determined. Although it is now clear that the acute and chronic administration of certain glucocorticoids expands the ECFV by their weak mineralocorticoid activity, there is also strong evidence in several species to show that this volume expansion is mediated by extrarenal mechanisms.[55,117,124,193,278,327,346] Numerous reports in humans, rats, and dogs have documented large increases in ECFV, plasma volume, and cardiac output following administration of glucocorticoid steroids.[55,117,193,278,327,346,354] Prolonged administration of cortisone to humans resulted in a 30 percent increase in ECFV, despite a lack of weight gain and a near-zero

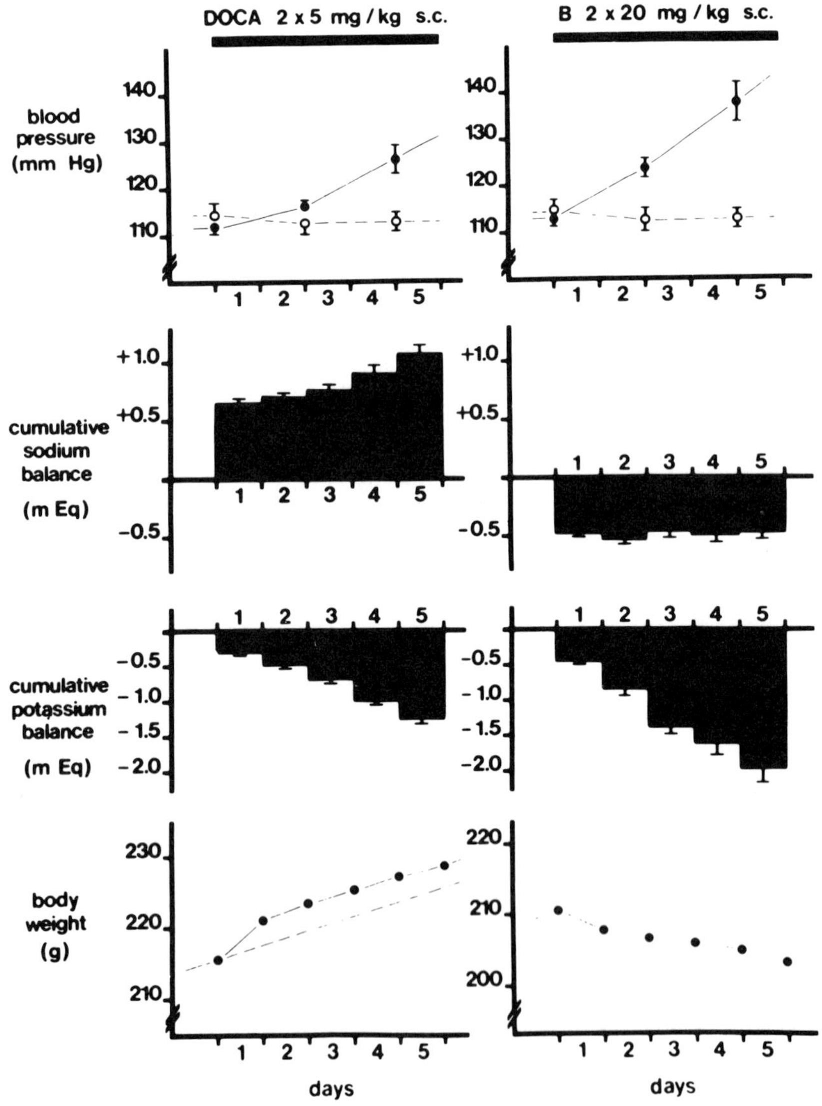

FIGURE 14-6 • Effect of DOCA and corticosterone (B) on blood pressure, cumulative change in sodium and potassium balances, and body weight in normal rats. For blood pressure and body weight, solid circles indicate steroid-treated rats and open circles untreated control animals. Cumulative balance data were calculated using a presteroid 5-day control period as baseline. Values are means ± SEM. (From Haack D et al: *Am J Physiol* 233:F403, 1977. Used by permission.)

sodium intake.[193] The proximate cause of such large shifts in sodium, chloride, and water from the intracellular to the extracellular space has not been elucidated, but these observations are consistent with the observed widespread activation of Na^+-K^+ ATPase by glucocorticoid hormones.[345] Whether a generalized cellular extrusion of sodium could result in sufficient expansion of ECFV remains to be determined.

Figure 14-6 highlights the results of balance studies that have emphasized the major pathophysiologic differences between the administration of excess mineralocorticoid hormones (e.g., DOC) and that of excess glucocorticoid hormones (e.g., corticosterone and compound B) in rats. The prolonged administration of either steroid resulted in ECFV and plasma volume expansion and hypertension.[124] Plasma renin activity and AII levels declined in both circumstances. Since ECFV expansion is sustained, the kidney is responsible for retention of at least a portion of Na^+ and Cl^- shifted from the intracellular fluid (ICF) to the ECF (see below). The pathogenesis of this expansion and hypertension appears quite different during DOC administration. Positive sodium balance from renal retention accounts for the volume expansion, whereas corticosterone administration causes negative sodium balance, suggesting that the documented ECFV expansion occurred by an extrarenal mechanism and that the kidney was responding, in part, to an overexpanded state with natriuresis. Thus, glucocorticoid-induced ECFV expansion is accompanied by weight loss, whereas mineralocorticoid-induced expansion is accompanied by weight gain. Negative potassium balance induced by glucocorticoids is due at least in part to tissue catabolism and in part to ECFV expansion, resulting in enhanced distal nephron sodium delivery and/or luminal flow rate at potassium secretory sites (see below).

Administration of large doses of glucocorticoid hormones to both human beings[40,193,247] and animals[47,125] causes large increases in the glomerular filtration rate (GFR). The hormone-induced increment in GFR may not be due solely to increased ECFV. However, the observation that the effect is still observed during concurrent rigid sodium restriction does not eliminate extrarenal ECFV expansion (noted above) as a mediator or prerequisite.[47,125] Increased GFR is accompanied by an increase in renal plasma flow.[40,47,125] Studies in animals have shown either no change or decreases in filtration fraction, whereas in humans this parameter increases,[40] suggesting a preferential increase in vasomotor tone at the efferent arteriole. Studies in rats have documented that increased renal blood flow is accompanied by decreases in afferent and efferent arteriolar resistance.[13,98] The changes in single-nephron GFR appear to be relatively independent of changes in net ultrafiltration pressure, plasma oncotic pressure, and glomerular ultrafiltration coefficient (a permeability and surface area parameter). The mechanism of glucocorticoid-induced renal vasodilatation remains to be determined. Although possible roles for AII, ANP, and prostaglandins have been invoked to explain these effects, no consensus has emerged in support of any of these mediators.[14] It is interesting to note that the glomerular hemodynamic changes caused by glucocorticoids are nearly identical to those observed following an acute infusion of amino acids.[125,214] Since glucocorticoid administration produces a large increase in plasma concentration of various amino acids,[125] it is tempting to speculate that amino acids and/or ECFV expansion might modulate the alterations in GFR associated with glucocorticoid administration.

EFFECTS OF ADRENAL STEROIDS ON SODIUM TRANSPORT

Mineralocorticoids

Renal effects of mineralocorticoids

The major mammalian mineralocorticoid hormones, aldosterone and DOC, decrease urinary sodium excretion.[31,42,124,128,144,151,163,190,216,217,269] Aldosterone's antinatriuresis occurs as early as 30 min after administration and is the most reproducible effect of mineralocorticoids, regardless of variations in physiologic conditions. Sustained renal retention of sodium and water maintains the ECFV expansion as long as the mineralocorticoid excess persists. After several days, the expanded ECFV fails to increase further despite continued mineralocorticoid administration. This characteristic of the normal kidney to restore daily sodium balance after creating a large positive balance is called mineralocorticoid escape (see below). Mineralocorticoid-induced sodium transport is observed to the greatest extent in the mammalian CCT.[240,295] The CCT consists of at least three cell types. *Principal cells* are responsible for sodium and potassium transport and constitute two-thirds of the cell population (see Chap. 7). The remaining cells comprise two populations of *intercalated cells*, one responsible for H^+ secretion (α intercalated cell) and another responsible for HCO_3^- secretion (β intercalated cell). Sodium reabsorption by principal cells of the CCT occurs in a multistep sequence. Filtered sodium ions are transported passively down their electrochemical gradient from the luminal fluid into the cytosol through amiloride-inhibitable plasma membrane channels.[240,326] At the basolateral plasma membrane, sodium ions are actively transported into the ECF by Na^+-K^+ ATPase, the enzymatic equivalent of the sodium pump. Aldosterone stimulates this pathway, simultaneously decreasing overall transepithelial electrical resistance. Based largely on investigations in the amphibian urinary bladder, it has been suggested that the physiologic action of aldosterone can be divided into three phases: (1) a latent period of about 1 h; (2) the "early response," during the second and third hours; and (3) the "late response," from the fourth hour and beyond.[77,103,219,275]

The cellular components of principal cell sodium transport stimulated by mineralocorticoid hormones are shown in Fig. 14-7. Apical membrane sodium and potassium channels increase their conductance in response to aldosterone, facilitating sodium uptake and potassium secretion. Na^+-K^+ ATPase activity is augmented greatly, thereby providing a route for cellular sodium exit at the basolateral membrane as well as a tendency for intracellular potassium concentration to rise. Large increases in cytosolic potassium concentration are prevented because aldosterone increases basolateral potassium conductance. The magnitude of increased cytosolic potassium concentration-induced basolateral membrane hyperpolarization is minimized by mineralocorticoid-induced increments in basolateral potassium and chloride conductances.[172,230,282] Although the outwardly directed potassium diffusion gradient at the basolateral membrane augments the cell-negative voltage present at the basolateral membrane in control conditions, the potassium concentration gradient alone cannot account for the observed mineralocorticoid-induced increase in basolateral potential to −100 mV. The major mechanism accounting for the hyperpolarization is thought to be the augmented activity of the Na^+-K^+ ATPase pump, which exports three sodium ions for each two potassium ions that it imports, rendering the interior of the cell negatively charged. This basolateral hyperpolarization is sufficient to reverse the direction of net potassium flux from cellular exit to cellular entry. That is, the more favorable electrical gradient for potassium entry across the basolateral membrane effectively counterbalances the relatively unchanged chemical gradient favoring potassium exit and thereby results in a mineralocorticoid-induced enhancement in the supply of cellular potassium for luminal secretion. The cellular potassium secretory flux can thus exceed that predicted by the stoichiometry of the Na^+-K^+ pump. The primacy of hormonal stimulation of the Na^+-K^+ ATPase pump in hyperpolarizing the basolateral membrane is evidenced by the effect of luminal amiloride. By inhibiting sodium entry through its luminal channel, amiloride limits the availability of substrate to the cation pump and so depolarizes the membrane despite the continuing presence of mineralocorticoids.[282] As depicted in Fig. 14-7, transepithelial hyperpolarization results primarily from the hyperpolarization of the basolateral membrane. Mineralocorticoid-induced changes in apical voltage tend to be much less pronounced than changes at the basolateral membrane.

Minor species differences between rats and rabbits exist in the chloride conductance of the principal cell basolateral membrane of the CCT. The normally high basolateral chloride conductance of the rabbit (Fig. 14-7)[281,282] further increases with chronic administration of large doses of mineralocorticoid hormone despite increasing values of transepithelial lumen-nega-

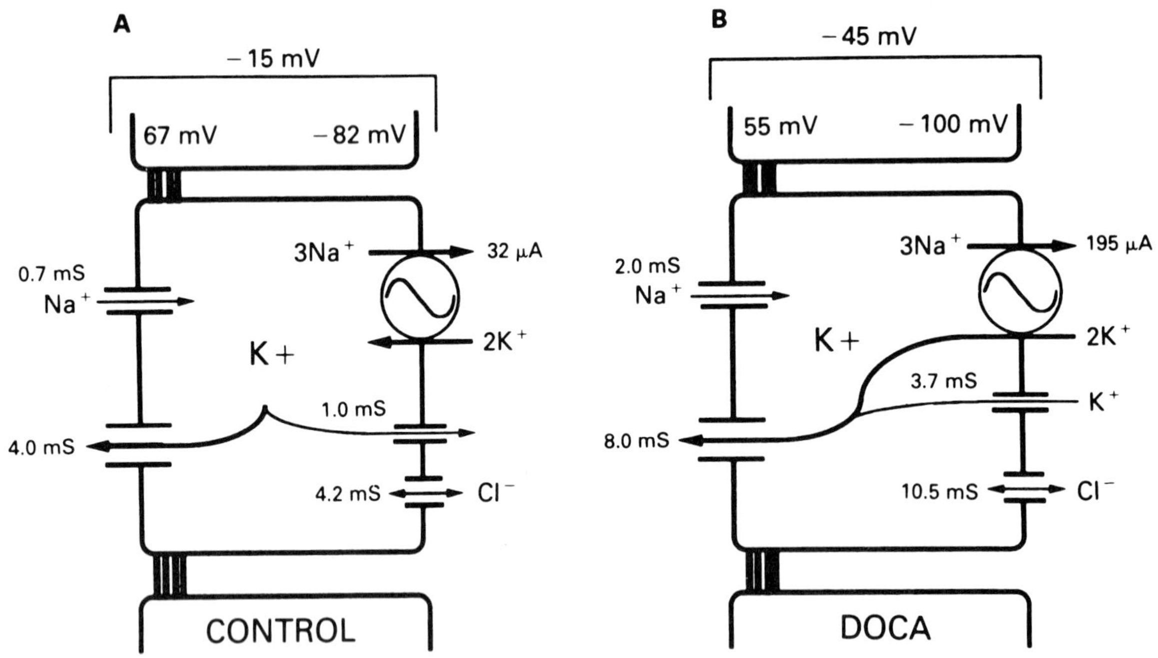

FIGURE 14-7 • Pathways of Na^+ and K^+ transport in control and mineralocorticoid-treated (DOCA) rabbit CCT principal cells. The apical (luminal) membrane is on the left. Electrical values are representative of those reported by several investigators. Increased apical Na^+ conductance stimulates Na^+ transport, which, because of the electrogenicity of the Na^+-K^+ pump, hyperpolarizes the basolateral membrane, thereby enhancing K^+ entry into the cell through the basolateral K^+ channel. Thus, the cell's K^+ supply is increased, thereby enhancing apical K^+ secretion through a more conductive channel. (From Stokes JB: *Kidney Int* 38:679, 1990. Used by permission.)

tive voltage.[282] In the basolateral membrane of the principal cells of rat CCT the chloride conductance is very small, particularly compared to the large potassium conductance.[282,291] The functional consequence of this difference remains to be investigated.

In contrast to the CCT, isolated perfused rabbit OMCT demonstrates no detectable active transport of Na^+, K^+, or Cl^-, even with chronic mineralocorticoid stimulation.[321] In the isolated perfused rat papillary collecting duct ($IMCD_{2+3}$), significant sodium transport has not been demonstrated by all investigators,[183,280,316] but when observed, it was significantly inhibited by ouabain.[183] Transepithelial voltage in this segment, however, was not significantly altered by DOC administration.[270] Micropuncture studies have demonstrated that acute aldosterone administration increased net sodium reabsorption in IMCD.[337,338] That chronic DOC administration increased Na^+-K^+ ATPase activity throughout the rat IMCD suggests that mineralocorticoids can enhance sodium and potassium transport in this segment.[331] The quantitative importance of this segment in the renal response to mineralocorticoids is undetermined but appears to be small.

The cell biology of the response to aldosterone has become increasingly complex and is still poorly understood (Table 14-2 and Fig. 14-8). The biochemical features of the response are as follows: (1) an increase in Na^+-K^+ ATPase activity (see above); (2) an increase in the activity of mitochondrial citric acid cycle enzymes (see above); (3) synthesis of additional Na^+-K^+ ATPase molecules;[104,105,106,241,273,274,342] (4) synthesis of aldosterone-induced proteins;[15,23,107,108,186,267,299,300,301,334,328] (5) protein glycosylation;[22] and (6) methylation of phospholipids and proteins.[218,285,333,357] Most theories of aldosterone action postulate that the induced proteins may be (1) mitochondrial enzymes such as citrate synthase and flavokinase (see above), which could provide additional ATP for energizing active transport; (2) Na^+-K^+ ATPase located at the basolateral membrane (see above); and (3) other aldosterone-induced proteins of unknown function.

Stimulation of Na^+-K^+ ATPase activity has been demonstrated as early as 1 h[292] or as late as 7 h after hormone administration.[228] With respect to the late re-

TABLE 14-2 • Biochemistry of mineralocorticoid response

1. Activation of preformed subunits of Na^+-K^+ ATPase
2. Increased activity of citric acid cycle enzymes
3. Increased net synthesis of Na^+-K^+ ATPase subunits
4. Synthesis of aldosterone-induced proteins with unknown function
5. Protein glycosylation
6. Methylation of phospholipids and proteins
7. Increased cystolic Ca^+ activation of calmodulin

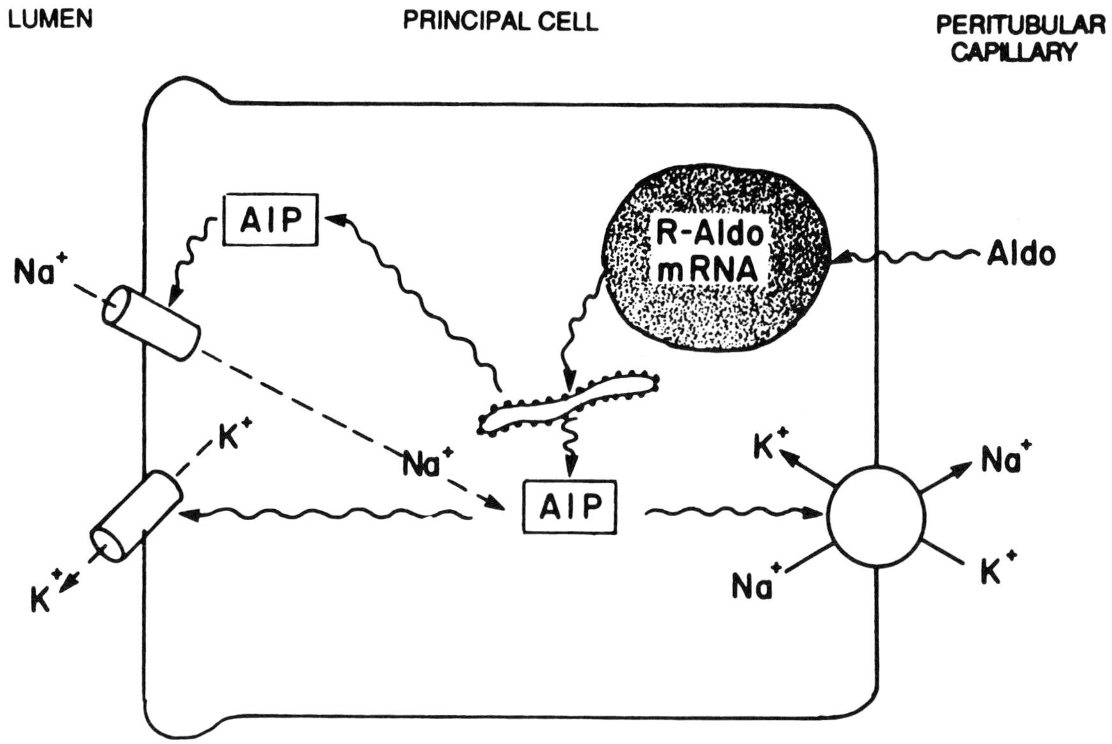

FIGURE 14-8 • Cell model for the proposed mechanism of action of mineralocorticoids on principal cells of the rabbit CCT. AIP is aldosterone-induced protein. The straight broken line represents rapid movement of ions through chanels. The wavy solid line represents slower cell processes. (From Sansome S et al: *Am J Physiol* 253:F753, 1987. Used by permission).

sponse to aldosterone, there has been a correlation between the synthesis of new Na^+-K^+ ATPase subunits and the late increase in sodium transport.[104,158,274,342] This correlation was even better when sodium butyrate, an inhibitor of steroid-induced transcription from DNA, blocked aldosterone-induced synthesis of Na^+-K^+ ATPase molecules and simultaneously inhibited the late increase in sodium transport.[333,334] These results are consistent with the thesis that de novo synthesis of Na^+-K^+ ATPase molecules plays no major role in the early response to aldosterone. However, numerous investigators have shown that the enzymatic activity of the sodium pump can increase during the first 3 h after exposure to aldosterone.[72,141,251,266,292] A role for the intracellular sodium concentration of principal cells in modulating the activity of preexisting Na^+-K^+ ATPase units was first raised by the observation that amiloride (an inhibitor of luminal sodium channels in principal cells) could abolish the aldosterone-induced increase in enzymatic activity of the sodium pump.[251] Subsequent studies in rabbits showed that animals maintained on a low-NaCl diet (with secondary hyperaldosteronism) exhibited a large increase in enzymatic Na^+-K^+ ATPase activity after 3 to 4 days on the low-sodium regimen. Enzymatic activity subsequently declined, returning to control levels after 2 weeks of dietary NaCl restriction. The decline in sodium pump enzymatic activity was preceded by a decrease in urinary sodium concentration (and presumably excretion) suggestive of a limiting decrease in sodium delivery to the CCT. A combination of high distal delivery of sodium to the CCT concomitant with chronic administration of DOC resulted in similar elevations in enzymatic Na^+-K^+ ATPase activity after 3 to 4 days, but in this case activity remained stable thereafter for 2 weeks. In rabbits simultaneously treated with DOC and the sodium channel blocker, amiloride, the effect of mineralocorticoid on the enzymatic activity of the Na^+-K^+ ATPase was reduced markedly. Since it is well known that chronic mineralocorticoid administration induces de novo synthesis of Na^+-K^+ ATPase subunits (see above), the presence of sodium is most likely exerting its influence on the sodium pump by virtue of its modulation of a posttranslational process.[239] Posttranslational modification of enzyme activity is consistent with data that have demonstrated large increases in Na^+-K^+ ATPase subunits even in the presence of effective blockade of apical sodium entry with amiloride.[104] Thus, during the early response to mineralocorticoid hormone, the steroid enhances sodium entry through the apical sodium channel which activates preformed Na^+-K^+ ATPase subunits. This increase in enzymatic activity translates to greater rates of sodium efflux at the basolateral membrane and may thus be secondary to enhanced sodium influx through apical sodium channels. During the late response, an increased rate of synthesis of Na^+-K^+ ATPase subunits appears to sustain the increase in sodium transport at the basolateral membrane. During both early and late phases, the ATP energy pool available to the sodium pump is under the control of mineralocorticoid hormone as modulated by increased enzymatic activity of mitochondrial enzymes (see above).

Recent studies of Na^+-K^+ ATPase heterodimer gene expression in A_6 kidney cells from *Xenopus laevis* indicate that aldosterone increases the transcription of both alpha and beta subunit genes as early as 15 min after administration. This suggests that there is a direct effect of the hormone-receptor complex on steroid response elements within nuclear chromatin.[343] However, inhibition of protein synthesis by cycloheximide completely abolished the mineralocorticoid-induced rapid increase in the Na^+-K^+ ATPase gene transcription rate. This finding is consistent with the notion that aldosterone acts indirectly on gene expression or that a direct effect of the activated hormone receptor complex on the gene promoter requires the presence of a short-lived protein.[343]

In addition to aldosterone-induced proteins of known identity (e.g., citrate synthase and Na^+-K^+ ATPase), numerous others with unknown function are also found in cytosol following mineralocorticoid administration.[77,103,219] Most of those investigated to date are associated with the early response to mineralocorticoid administration. However, some of these proteins appear only after 6 h of hormone incubation.[334] In addition to stimulating the synthesis of proteins, aldosterone has been shown to repress the synthesis of at least five proteins in toad bladder epithelia.[334] It is currently unknown whether down-regulation of cytosolic proteins is caused by direct transcriptional effects or by posttranscriptional regulation. The mechanism whereby aldosterone increases the transport of sodium through luminal sodium channels has not yet been determined. The channels appear to have the biochemical characteristics of proteins.[16,286] The number of conducting sodium channels increases within the first 3 h following administration of mineralocorticoid.[43,102,103,242,243] Whether the increase in functional channels results from an integration of newly synthesized channels into apical membrane or whether preexisting sodium channels are activated by modification of the channels (phosphorylation, methylation, and glycosylation) requires further investigation. Most studies to date support the hypothesis that aldosterone-induced events at the luminal membrane are caused by activation of preformed sodium channels (Fig. 14-8).[283] Numerous studies have investigated the possibility that methylation of preexisting channels increases their number.[218,285,357] Administration of the methyl group donator *S*-adenosylmethionine instead of aldosterone has been shown to enhance Na^+ transport as well as to increase the number of methylations of cellular phospholipids and proteins in A_6 cells.[285] Additional evi-

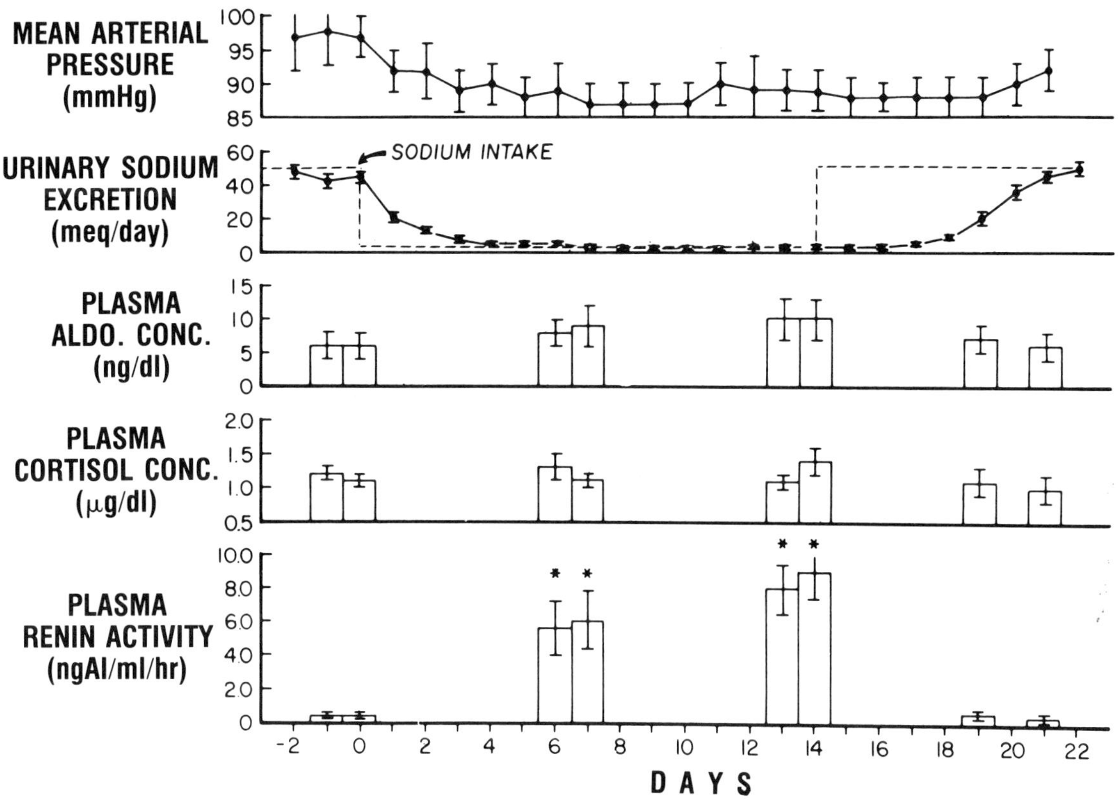

FIGURE 14-9 • Changes in mean arterial pressure, urinary sodium excretion, plasma aldosterone concentration, plasma cortisol concentration, and plasma renin activity during two weeks of sodium restriction in ADX dogs (n = 5) infused continuously with maintenance ("sodium-replate") amounts of aldosterone and cortisol (* indicates $p < 0.05$ compared with control). (From Lohmeier TE et al: *Hypertension* 2:497, 1980. Used by permission.)

dence supports a role for aldosterone-induced modification of carboxyl groups of the sodium channel in stimulating sodium transport.[170,245,246]

A role for the cytosolic calcium concentration in regulating aldosterone-induced renal sodium reabsorption is also possible. Studies of apical membrane vesicles from toad bladder and studies of frog skin have suggested that increases in cytosolic calcium might decrease apical membrane permeability to sodium.[35] Recent studies with A_6 cells, however, have demonstrated that exposure of the cells to aldosterone transiently increased cytosolic calcium, which correlated with the onset of amiloride-sensitive increases in electrogenic sodium absorption. Prevention of the rise in cytosolic calcium concentration by pretreatment with the intracellular calcium chelator BAPTA inhibited the aldosterone-induced increase in sodium absorption.[252] Additional studies have demonstrated that calmodulin antagonists are capable of inhibiting the aldosterone-induced increments in sodium transport. These studies raise the intriguing possibility that a calcium signal-induced activation of calmodulin might modulate mineralocorticoid-induced increases in apical sodium conductance.[252]

Whereas it is well established that complete aldosterone deficiency causes renal sodium wasting, hypotension, and ECF volume depletion, there have been few studies critically examining the putative requirement for an increase in aldosterone secretion in response to reduction in sodium intake for preventing renal sodium wasting and hypotension.[132,133] Chronic balance studies in dogs have compared the response to sodium restriction in adrenalectomized (ADX) animals receiving fixed normal amounts of aldosterone and cortisol with those of intact animals.[201] As shown in Fig. 14-9, reduction in NaCl intake in the fixed-steroid ADX animals did not result in greater negative sodium balance than that observed in intact animals, despite unchanged plasma steroid concentrations. Changes in GFR and renal plasma flow were also not different in intact and ADX groups. Mean arterial pressure fell by only 8 mmHg in dogs with fixed levels of aldosterone. These results, from a prolonged period of experimental sodium restriction, indicate that maintenance of sodium balance and arterial pressure during sodium depletion is not critically dependent on enhanced aldosterone secretion.[201]

MINERALOCORTICOID ESCAPE When large doses of exogenous mineralocorticoid hormones are administered or when endogenous secretion of mineralocorticoid hormones is stimulated in normal subjects or experimental animals, an initial period of sodium retention occurs, leading to a large increase in ECFV. In the chronic steady-state of mineralocorticoid excess, the persistent action of the hormone results in renal potassium wasting, metabolic alkalosis, polyuria, hypercalciuria, and hypertension. However, after several days of sodium retention, daily sodium balance is restored; that is, no further positive sodium balance occurs, and no further weight gain is documented. This phenomenon has been designated mineralocorticoid escape because, contrary to what might be expected from the mechanism of action of mineralocorticoid hormones, renal mechanisms are induced that overcome the deleterious effects of persistent and relentless positive sodium balance.[112] The kidney escapes only from the sodium transport effects; potassium and hydrogen ion hypersecretion continues.

Mineralocorticoid escape has been attributed to a variety of factors, including increases in plasma ANF,[118,369] increases in renal arterial pressure,[126] decreases in plasma renin activity,[21] and decreases in renal sympathetic nerve activity.[271] Micropuncture studies have suggested a role for the proximal tubule and the loop of Henle in mediating the escape.[112,113,194] Indicators of suppressed proximal sodium reabsorption, such as increased lithium clearance, appear by the second day of aldosterone infusion in dogs.[113] Mean arterial pressure increases during the first day of exposure to the hormone.[113,126] Utilizing an elegant protocol in which renal arterial pressure was prevented from increasing with an electronically servo-controlled aortic occluder, investigators have found that sustained aldosterone infusion in dogs dramatically decreases urinary sodium excretion on the first day and that sodium excretion remains similarly depressed on each of the six subsequent days of continued infusion.[126] As depicted in Fig. 14-10, when renal arterial pressure was permitted to subsequently increase during a more prolonged period of aldosterone infusion, urinary sodium excretion increased dramatically and the animals

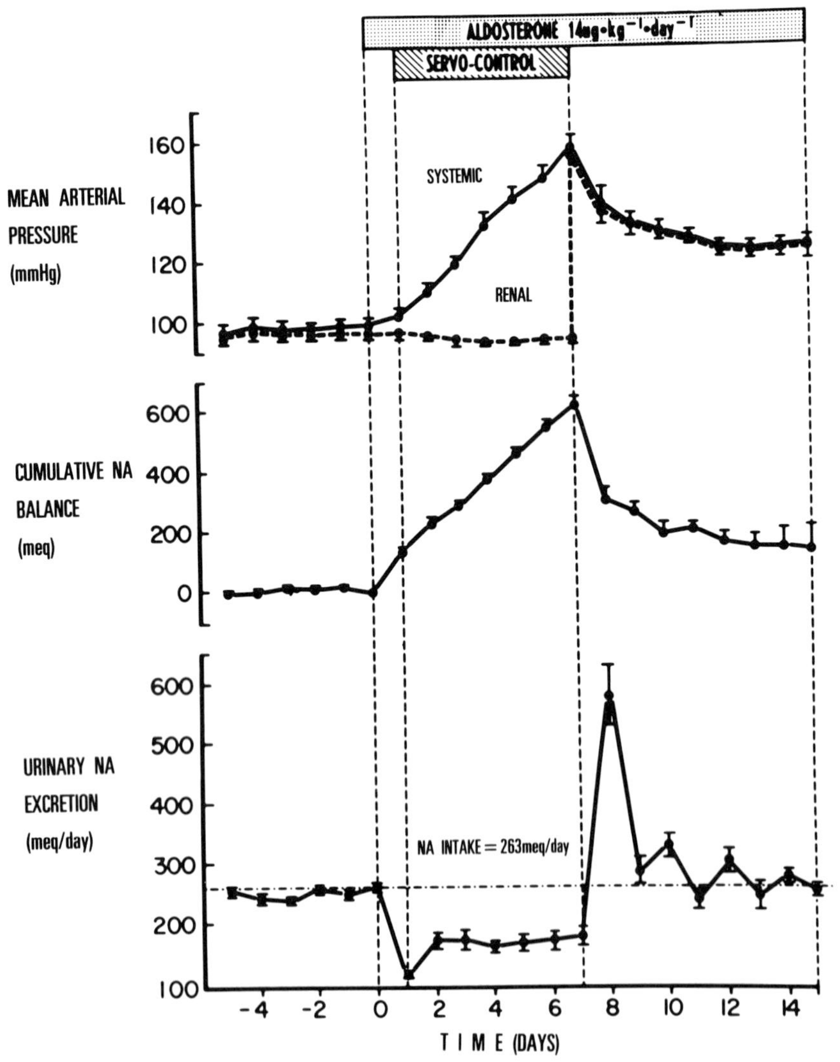

FIGURE 14-10 • Effects of an aldosterone infusion on mean arterial pressure, cumulative change in sodium balance, and urinary sodium excretion when renal perfusion pressure was servo-controlled at the normal level. Values represent means ± SEM in seven dogs (From Hall JE et al: *Hypertension* 2:139, 1980. Used by permission.)

returned promptly to daily neutral sodium balance. The GFR increased significantly as renal arterial pressure was permitted to rise. In the animals in which mineralocorticoid escape was prevented by controlling renal arterial pressure, relentless sodium retention occurred and was accompanied by massive abdominal swelling and ascites formation. Thus, it appears that increased renal perfusion pressure plays a critical role in modulating the extent of sodium retention during states of mineralocorticoid excess.

Clearance studies in rats have suggested that the hypercalciuria of mineralocorticoid excess is independent of parathyroid hormone (PTH) and perhaps independent of suppressed proximal tubule sodium reabsorption.[109] Whether the hypercalciuria complicating mineralocorticoid excess occurs in the absence of suppressed proximal sodium reabsorption remains to be determined.

Intestinal effects of mineralocorticoids

The colon is analogous to the distal nephron, since it absorbs sodium and secretes potassium under the influence of adrenal steroids (see Chap. 17). The intestinal effects of aldosterone are probably limited to the distal colon,[10,34,355,359] since specific mineralocorticoid receptors are present at least at this site.[5] Elevated plasma levels of aldosterone increase active, amiloride-sensitive sodium transport and active potassium secretion.[86,279] However, administration of glucocorticoids (e.g., dexmethasone and methylprednisolone) cause similar changes in distal colon transport.[86,279] This confusion has been resolved recently in studies comparing the effects of aldosterone and the specific glucocorticoid agonist RU28,362. These studies have demonstrated that occupation of the type II receptor with a pure glucocorticoid stimulates only electroneutral NaCl absorption and not electrogenic amiloride-inhibitable sodium absorption.[10] It seems likely (although unproven) that whenever glucocorticoids appear to stimulate electrogenic sodium reabsorption, it is due to excess binding to the type I receptor.[335] The cellular mechanism of type II receptor-mediated NaCl reabsorption remains to be determined. The observation that aldosterone can stimulate electroneutral NaCl absorption to a small extent, in addition to its major effect on electrogenic sodium reabsorption, is probably explained by its affinity for the type II receptor. As in the collecting duct, aldosterone increases Na^+-K^+ ATPase and citrate synthase activity in the distal colon.[34,209]

Replacement of aldosterone to ADX rats fails to fully restore sodium transport in the distal colon, whereas replacement of glucocorticoids (e.g., dexamethasone) completely normalizes sodium flux.[9] This observation has not been explained but may be related to glucocorticoid-mediated increments in intestinal blood flow. Whether a full expression of aldosterone action might require permissive preexisting elevations in blood flow in an ADX rat has not been investigated.

Recent studies of cation transport in rat distal colon have provided evidence for a large dissociation between the effects of replacement doses of aldosterone on Na^+ and their effects on K^+ transport.[9] Aldosterone restored potassium secretion to control levels but was without detectable effect on Na^+ transport. This finding has also been observed in human and dog colon in vivo[192,309] after acute aldosterone administration. The mechanism for this interesting dissociation is not known.

Glucocorticoids

Effect of glucocorticoids on renal sodium reabsorption

Acute administration of glucocorticoids increases renal sodium excretion (Fig. 14-6; see above).[124] In part, this effect is due to glucocorticoid-induced ECFV expansion and increased GFR, as discussed above. However, since the filtered load of sodium is increased, the net renal reabsorptive rate for sodium is also increased by glucocorticoid hormones. Whether glucocorticoids have a specific stimulatory effect on tubular sodium transport or whether it is a nonspecific effect of an increased filtered sodium load remains to be elucidated. As described above, glucocorticoids are potent stimulators of both renal cortical and medullary Na^+-K^+ ATPase. These effects appear to be specific for the type II receptors. Increases in Na^+-K^+ ATPase activity appear to be independent of GFR, since they are observed even when the GFR is held constant by concomitant renal arterial or ureteral clamping.[85]

Directly applied dexamethasone does not increase sodium absorption in the cortical collecting duct,[295] but its effects on other segments have not been reported. In the proximal tubule, glucocorticoid administration has been shown to increase the activity (V_{max}, maximal rate) of the Na^+-H^+ exchanger (antiporter) located in the luminal brush border membrane. Since this transporter is responsible for a large fraction of proximal sodium reabsorption, these findings raise the possibility that glucocorticoids might mediate proximal sodium transport. The time course for inducing the Na^+-H^+ antiporter activity in isolated cells is nearly identical to that for the induction of the Na^+-K^+ ATPase by glucocorticoids.[311] This observation raises the possibility that a primary increase in Na^+-H^+ antiporter activity might increase the cytosolic sodium concentration and thereby stimulate basolateral Na^+-K^+ ATPase activity.[91,296] On the other hand, a primary stimulation of Na^+-K^+ ATPase activity might secondarily activate the Na^+-H^+ antiporter by virtue of a decrement in cellular sodium concentration. Thus, whether glucocorticoids can directly or indirectly increase Na^+-H^+ exchange activity remains to be determined.

Intestinal effects of glucocorticoids on sodium transport

The intestine has to date provided the most extensive evidence for glucocorticoid-stimulated sodium absorption.[9,11,19,159] Increased Na^+ absorption and increased Na^+-K^+ ATPase have been demonstrated in every segment of both the large and the small intestine.[9,34,360,361] In the ileum, glucocorticoid deficiency inhibits electrogenic Na^+ absorption and simultaneously stimulates Cl^- secretion. This novel observation is consistent with reports of secretory-type diarrhea in patients with Addison's disease.[349]

EFFECTS OF ADRENAL STEROIDS ON POTASSIUM HOMEOSTASIS

Mineralocorticoids

Effects of mineralocorticoids on renal potassium transport

The acute effect of aldosterone on the renal excretion of potassium is more variable than its effect on sodium (see Chap. 7). The acute kaliuretic response to aldosterone administration depends on both preexisting sodium[128,139,269] and potassium[84,138] balance. In animals and humans ingesting a low NaCl diet, mineralocorticoid hormone administration does not cause a kaliuresis.[128,269] Moreover, the kaliuretic effect is greatly enhanced in both animals and humans in direct relation to NaCl intake.[128,138,269] Two reports of acute aldosterone administration in rats have raised the possibility that a mild degree of preexisting potassium depletion might potentitiate the magnitude of mineralocorticoid-induced kaliuresis.[84,138] However, this observation has not been evident in dogs[144,151] and has not been evaluated in humans.

Chronic mineralocorticoid administration to NaCl-replete animals and humans uniformly increases the renal clearance of potassium (i.e., there is a greater excretion rate at any plasma concentration), regardless of the state of potassium balance.[128,144,269,366] The increased ECFV from sustained mineralocorticoid-induced sodium retention eventually increases the delivery of sodium and water to the CCT, where these factors modulate renal potassium excretion and secretion (see below). In glucocorticoid-replete humans and dogs, renal hyperkalemia is a predictable consequence of aldosterone deficiency.[143,146,302,366] Since potassium is a potent secretagogue for aldosterone and aldosterone, in turn, is a

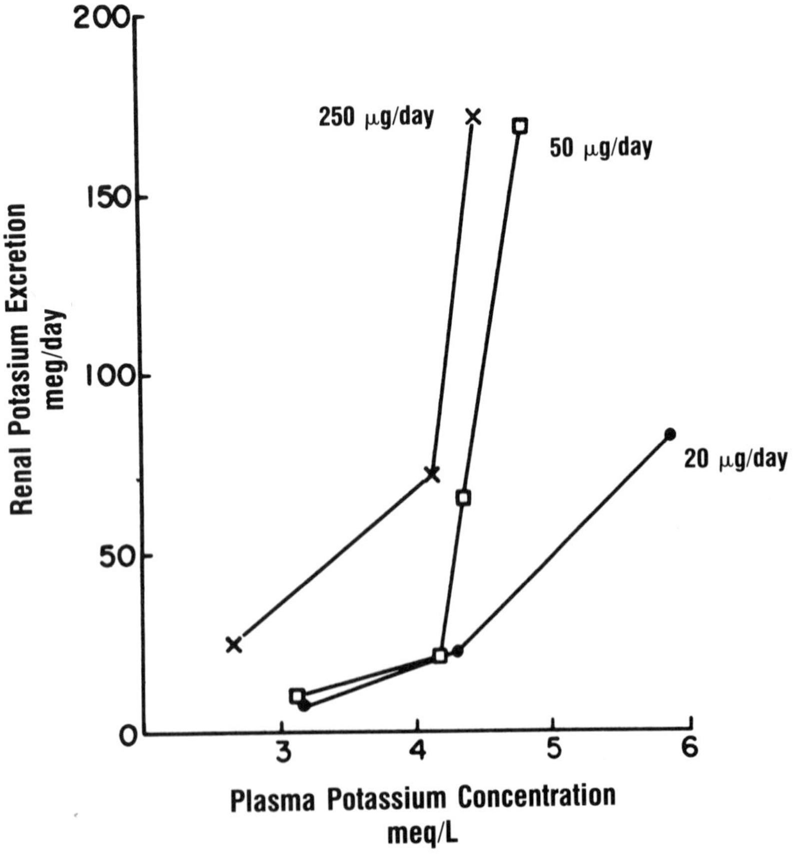

FIGURE 14-11 • Mean values for plasma potassium concentration and urinary potassium excretion in dogs receiving continuous infusions of aldosterone at rates of 20, 50, and 250 μg/24h. (From Young DB, Paulsen AW: *Am J Physiol* 244:F28, 1983. Used by permission.)

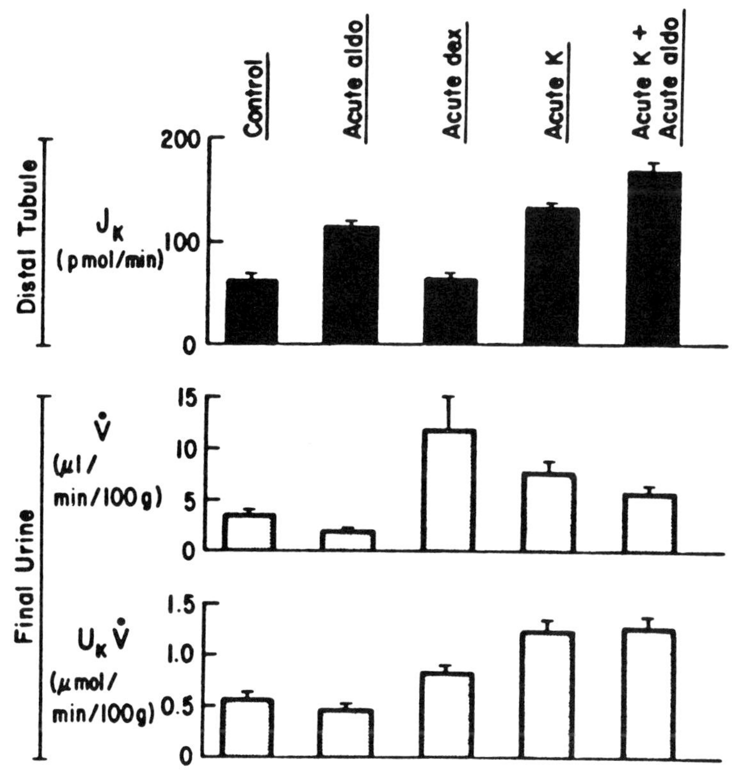

FIGURE 14-12 • Distal tubule and urinary potassium excretion in ADX rats in which aldosterone and dexamethasone were maintained at constant levels by chronic infusion. The animals received superimposed acute infusions of steroids and/or potassium as indicated. J_K, potassium secretory flux; $\dot{V}$, urine flow; $U_K\dot{V}$, urinary potassium excretion. (From Field MJ et al: *J Clin Invest* 74:1792, 1984. Used by permission.)

potent stimulus for increased renal potassium clearance, elucidation of the quantitative interrelationships has been difficult. The best quantitative assessment of this dual feedback regulatory system was obtained from ADX, glucocorticoid-replaced dogs randomized into several groups, each receiving a different amount of dietary potassium.[366] The varied potassium diet provided each group with a different but stable level of plasma and urinary potassium. Each group then received graded amounts of aldosterone, and measurements were made in the steady state.[366] The potent effect of the chronically imposed aldosterone level on the renal clearance of potassium is indicated by the shift in the relationship between renal potassium excretion and plasma potassium concentration (Fig. 14-11). The increased aldosterone infusion rate increased the renal clearance of potassium. The sustained hypokalemia with "normal" daily rates of potassium excretion (reflecting normal dietary potassium intake) indicates that supranormal (250 µg/24 h) infusions of aldosterone cause renal potassium wasting. Chronic renal potassium wasting is characteristic of states of mineralocorticoid excess in which dietary NaCl intake and excretion rates reflect those of a typical North American diet (80-150 mmol/24 h).[163,269]

Distal tubule micropuncture studies in rats[132,250,355,356] and studies utilizing the isolated perfused rabbit CCT[114,320] indicate that aldosterone stimulates transepithelial potassium secretion at these sites. Identification of specific segments responsible for changes in ion flux in most of the reported "distal tubule" micropuncture studies is difficult. As previously noted, the "distal tubule" includes the cTALH, DCT, CNT, and CCT. Since increased luminal flow rates stimulate distal nephron potassium secretion, a flow-independent effect of aldosterone could only be demonstrated in vivo under conditions of constant luminal flow rate in the microperfused rat distal tubule.[83] The results of these distal tubule potassium flux studies in ADX rats receiving fixed steroid doses are shown in Fig. 14-12. Net potassium secretory flux is significantly stimulated by the acute administration of aldosterone and/or potassium but not by the acute administration of dexamethasone. Urinary potassium excretion in these studies, however, did not reflect the increase in distal nephron potassium secretion in response to aldosterone. The failure to observe an increase in urinary potassium excretion was presumably due to aldosterone-induced diminution in distal nephron flow rate owing to stimulation of sodium and water reabsorption at upstream locations. In addition to tubular flow rate, decreased luminal fluid sodium concentration, at levels below 35 mmol/liter, has been demonstrated to inhibit potassium secretion in both distal tubule[115] and isolated perfused CCT.[320] It is difficult to separate the effects of distal luminal flow rate and distal sodium concentration under most in vivo circumstances, since decreased distal sodium delivery is ordinarily accompanied by a decrease in fluid delivery rate. Thus, acute or chronic sodium loading presumably enhances expression of aldosterone-induced kaliuresis by minimizing any upstream effect of aldosterone to limit CCT fluid and sodium delivery. The dependence of potassium secretion on distal flow is lost, at least in rats, after a brief period of dietary potassium restriction.[167] This finding may explain why acute aldosterone administration is more kaliuretic in potassium-depleted rats than in potassium-repleted rats.

The rate of potassium secretion in the mineralocorticoid-stimulated CCT is directly related to the simultaneous rate of sodium absorption and to the magnitude of the lumen-negative voltage created by sodium transport.[320] Eliminating sodium from luminal fluid abolishes potassium secretion. Ultimately, then, distal nephron potassium secretion is regulated by the activity of the Na^+-K^+ pump located at the basolateral membrane. The finding that inhibition of Na^+-K^+ ATPase with ouabain eliminates net potassium secretion in the mineralocorticoid-stimulated rabbit CCT gives credibility to the aforementioned hypothesis.[363] Further evidence supporting this relationship is provided by the finding that amiloride-induced inhibition of luminal sodium conductance markedly inhibits mineralocorticoid-stimulated potassium secretion in rabbit CCT.[130,238,240] Mineralocorticoid hormones exert potent effects on both apical and basolateral membrane conductances in the principal cell of rabbit CCD (Fig. 14-7). It is therefore difficult to be certain whether an increase in apical membrane potassium conductance is required for mineralocorticoids to stimulate potassium secretory flux. Apical membrane depolarization is induced by chronic mineralocorticoid administration, thereby increasing the apical electrical driving force for potassium exit. A recent electrophysiologic study using the isolated perfused rat CCT has shown that the hormone-induced apical membrane depolarization in principal cells is sufficient to explain the observed increment in apical potassium secretory flux.[288]

Effects of aldosterone on intestinal potassium transport

In addition to its renal effects, aldosterone also increases net potassium secretion in the distal colon (see Chap. 17).[9,67,86,89] Enhanced potassium transport is accompanied by increased activity of Na^+-K^+ ATPase and increased basolateral membrane surface area.[162,344]

Glucocorticoids

Effects of glucocorticoids on renal potassium transport

Acute administration of glucocorticoids causes a kaliuresis in rats (Fig. 14-6). Glucocorticoid-induced renal potassium secretion is attributable to enhanced distal nephron potassium secretory flux,[83] which can be prevented if the flow rate is held constant during luminal microperfusion.[83] As noted above, glucocorticoid-induced acute ECFV expansion and increased GFR appear to be responsible for the increased distal delivery rate. Chronic dexamethasone administration also causes a kaliuresis in ADX rats during acute potassium loading, although extrarenal potassium tolerance remains impaired.[18,48] Chronic administration of large doses of triamcinolone to dogs causes a sustained increase in urinary potassium excretion, partly due to the persistent catabolic effect of glucocorticoids.[148] Thus, sustained urinary losses of potassium during glucocorticoid excess are associated with enhanced urinary nitrogen excretion and a negative nitrogen balance.

Effects of glucocorticoids on intestinal potassium transport

Glucocorticoids also stimulate potassium secretion in the distal colon.[9,19] In distal colon of ADX rats, replacement doses of dexamethasone increase potassium secretion to normal levels while simultaneously increasing to normal the transmural lumen-negative voltage.[9] Whether large increases in lumen-negative voltage alone can restore normal levels of potassium secretion remains to be determined.

Effect of adrenal steroids on internal potassium balance

Controversy has arisen regarding the role of aldosterone on internal potassium balance in general and its specific role in the extrarenal adaptation to sustained potassium loading.[6,313,314] This subject is reviewed in Chap. 6.

Glucocorticoids may affect internal potassium balance.[96,161] Humans receiving large doses of prednisone or dexamethasone demonstrated significant decreases in erythrocyte sodium concentration and significant increases in intracellular potassium concentration.[161] Maximum ouabain binding was markedly higher in erythrocytes from glucocorticoid-treated subjects. These findings suggest that glucocorticoids can increase the number of Na^+-K^+ pump sites in nonepithelial tissues and that a larger number of pump sites might cause the acute and/or chronic sequestration of potassium in nonepithelial tissues. This observation is also consistent with the finding that glucocorticoids effect acute shifts in sodium from intracellular to ECF compartments (see above).

EFFECTS OF ADRENAL STEROIDS ON ACID-BASE METABOLISM

The metabolic acidosis complicating adrenal insufficiency has been attributed, at least in part, to a reduction in the rate of renal hydrogen ion secretion, since the rate of net acid excretion is subnormal.[156,287,364] Adrenal regulation of renal acid excretion is a complex process involving modulation of renal H^+ secretion, renal ammoniagenesis, and systemic endogenous acid production. Additional indirect actions of adrenal steroids on net acid excretion are mediated through changes in sodium, potassium, and chloride transport.[56,143,144,145,146,151,358]

Mineralocorticoids

The role of aldosterone in the renal regulation of the plasma HCO_3^- concentration

Administration of mineralocorticoids to normal human subjects increases net acid excretion.[42,46,190,195,205,216,217,269] Within hours of aldosterone administration, urine pH decreases[42,216,217,312] and net acid excretion increases.[42,190,216,217] The administration of large amounts of aldosterone to normal subjects for many weeks increases plasma bicarbonate concentration, causing a metabolic alkalosis.[163]

In each of the three mammalian species investigated to date (human, dog, and rat), experimental induction of mineralocorticoid deficiency, unaccompanied by glucocorticoid deficiency, diminishes net acid excretion, causing a hyperchloremic metabolic acidosis.[64,143,146,177,302] The latter is accounted for by reduced distal nephron proton secretion. Although the hyperkalemia and aldosterone deficiency per se can reduce renal ammonia production,[143,146,329,352] the putative role of the latter in the impairment of renal net acid excretion has not been established. In fact, no experimental protocol has yet been reported in any species that indicates that a primary increase or decrease in renal ammoniagenesis can result in an increase or decrease, respectively, in net acid excretion.

In mineralocorticoid-deficient dogs and humans, NH_4^+ excretion rates vary inversely with the magnitude of the hyperkalemia.[143,302] However, an inverse relationship between net acid excretion and plasma potassium concentration does not obtain. The two key components of net acid excretion are NH_4^+ and titratable acid ($H_2PO_4^-$). By diminishing entry of NH_3 (in states of decreased renal NH_3 production) to the tubular lumen, free H^+ concentration rises, since protons are no longer titrated by NH_3. The falling pH now titrates HPO_4^{2-}, forming $H_2PO_4^-$, which can substitute for the reduced NH_4^+ excretion. The inability of the hyperkalemia complicating hypoaldosteronism to alter the renal regulation of plasma bicarbonate concentration is illustrated in Figs. 14-13 and 14-14. Figure 14-13 depicts the development of hypobicarbonatemia following withdrawal of mineralocorticoid hormones in ADX dogs given fixed steroid doses and ingesting a normal potassium diet.[143] The

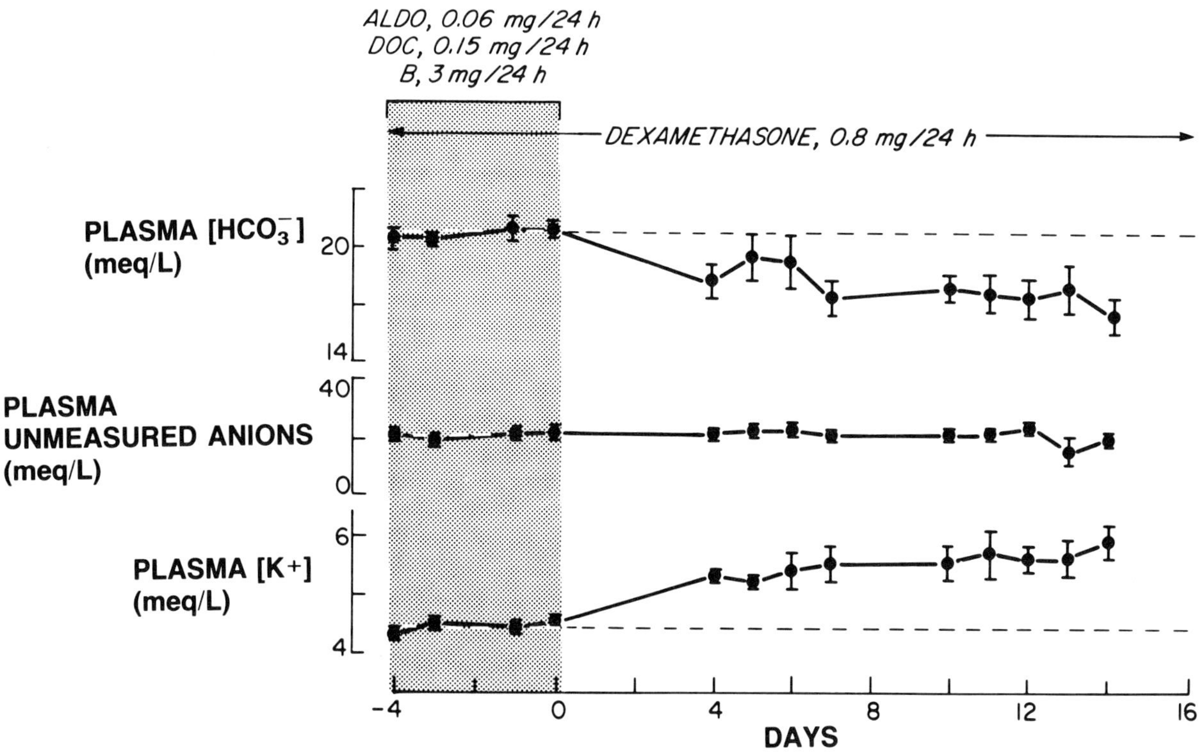

FIGURE 14-13 • Mean plasma bicarbonate, unmeasured anion, and potassium concentrations before and after discontinuation of mineralocorticoid hormones in dogs (n = 10) fed a normal potassium diet. Values are means ± SEM. (From Hulter HN et al: *Am J Physiol* 232:F136, 1977. Used by permission.)

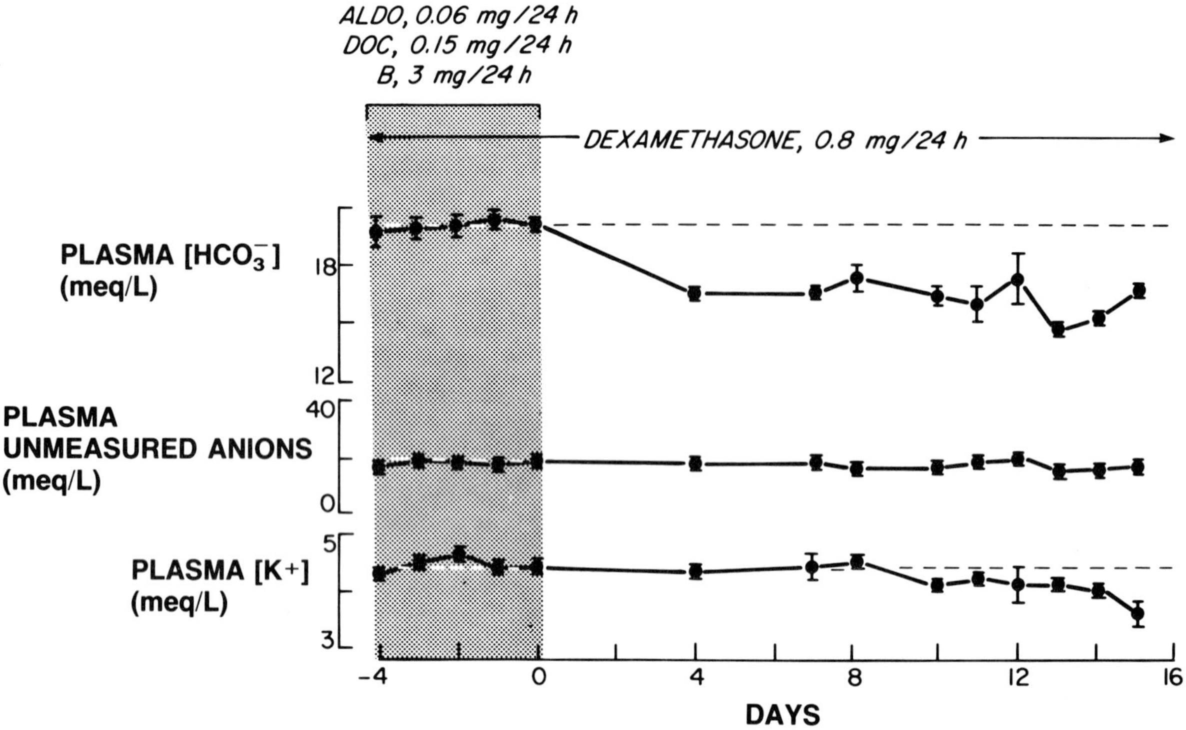

FIGURE 14-14 • Mean plasma bicarbonate, unmeasured anion, and potassium concentrations before and after discontinuation of mineralocorticoid hormones in dogs (*n* = 11). Dietary sodium phosphate was substituted for potassium phosphate at the time of mineralocorticoid discontinuation to maintain plasma potassium concentration constant. Values are means ± SEM. (From Hulter HN et al: *Am J Physiol* 232:F136, 1977. Used by permission.)

onset of mineralocorticoid deficiency is accompanied by both hyperkalemia and hypobicarbonatemia. This circumstance is contrasted in Fig. 14-14, in which an identical protocol was undertaken to induce mineralocorticoid deficiency except that hyperkalemia was prevented by substituting sodium phosphate for potassium phosphate in the diet when mineralocorticoids were discontinued. This modification of the protocol did not significantly alter the magnitude of the hyperchloremic acidosis and caused no significant difference in the accumulated deficit of net acid excretion. Dogs developing mineralocorticoid-deficiency acidosis under conditions of hyperkalemia decreased net acid excretion by virtue of a decrease in NH_4^+ excretion, whereas normokalemic dogs demonstrated a decrease in net acid excretion due to decreased titratable acid excretion. That is, since both NH_3 and HPO_4^{2-} are major urinary buffers under ordinary metabolic circumstances, it is difficult to demonstrate impaired acid excretion based on the diminution of only one of these two buffers. To date, an experimental model of hypophosphaturia in dogs has provided the only evidence to show that deficiency of any urinary buffer can impair renal net acid excretion.[149]

Since aldosterone deficiency causes both renal sodium wasting and renal acidosis,[143,302] it is possible that the ECFV depletion could impair distal nephron acidification by decreasing renal hemodynamics and/or distal nephron sodium delivery. Figure 14-15 depicts the results of chronic balance studies in dogs in which negative sodium balance was prevented during mineralocorticoid deficiency by increasing the rate of NaCl administration in a chronic continuous intravenous infusion. Careful and continuous prevention of negative sodium balance had no appreciable acid-base effect and did not ameliorate diminished net acid excretion or metabolic acidosis.[146]

Studies in the mineralocorticoid-deficient dog indicate that the renal H^+ secretion-rate capacity is reduced, while the ability to establish transepithelial H^+ concentration gradients is unimpaired.[143,146] When luminal buffer concentration (NH_4^+) is low, as when renal production and urinary excretion of ammonia are reduced by hyperkalemia, urine pH is highly acidic and does not differ from that in normal dogs with similar degrees of metabolic acidosis (Fig. 14-16). However, at higher values of luminal NH_4^+ concentration, urine pH increases to a greater degree in mineralocorticoid-deficient than in mineralocorticoid-repleted animals. Thus, mineralocorticoid deficiency decreases the rate capacity for H^+ secretion in response to increasing availability of luminal buffer content (luminal entry of basic NH_3).

Cellular mechanism of mineralocorticoid-dependent renal H^+ secretion

The cellular mechanism of acidification in the mammalian collecting duct has not been defined (see

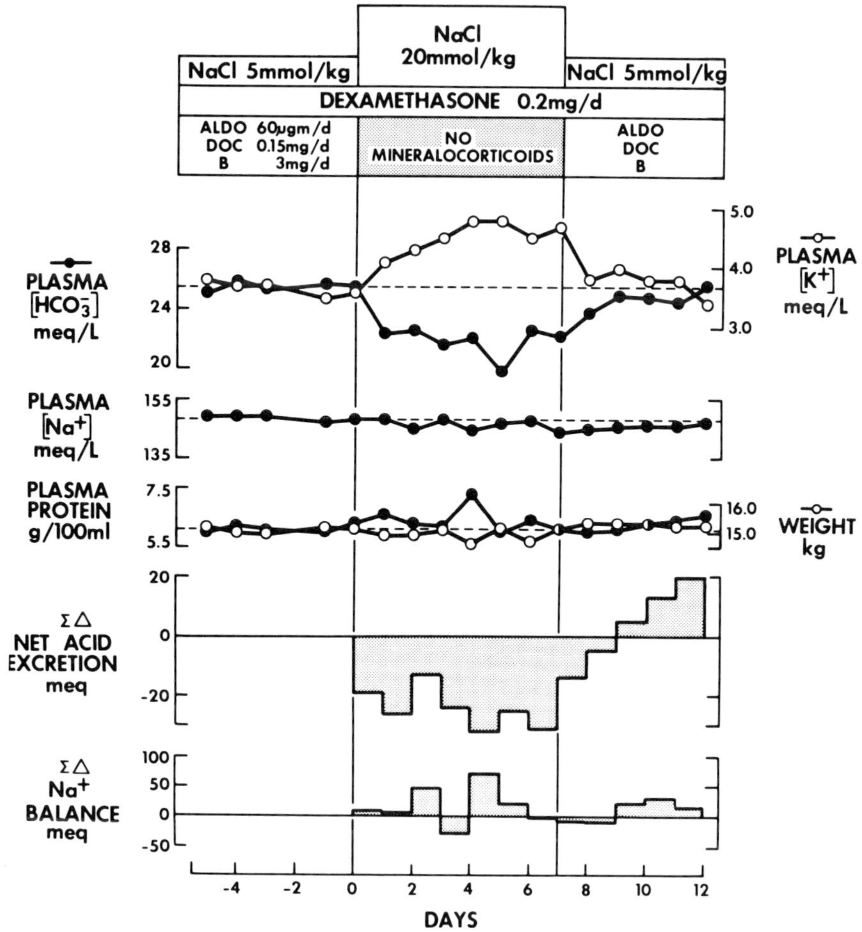

FIGURE 14-15 • Effect of mineralocorticoid discontinuation on plasma and urinary acid-base and electrolyte composition in a representative dexamethasone-replaced ADX dog maintained in normal NaCl balance by chronic continuous intravenous infusion of NaCl. The period of recovery from mineralocorticoid deficiency is also depicted. (From Hulter HN et al: *Am J Physiol* 236:F283, 1979. Used by permission.)

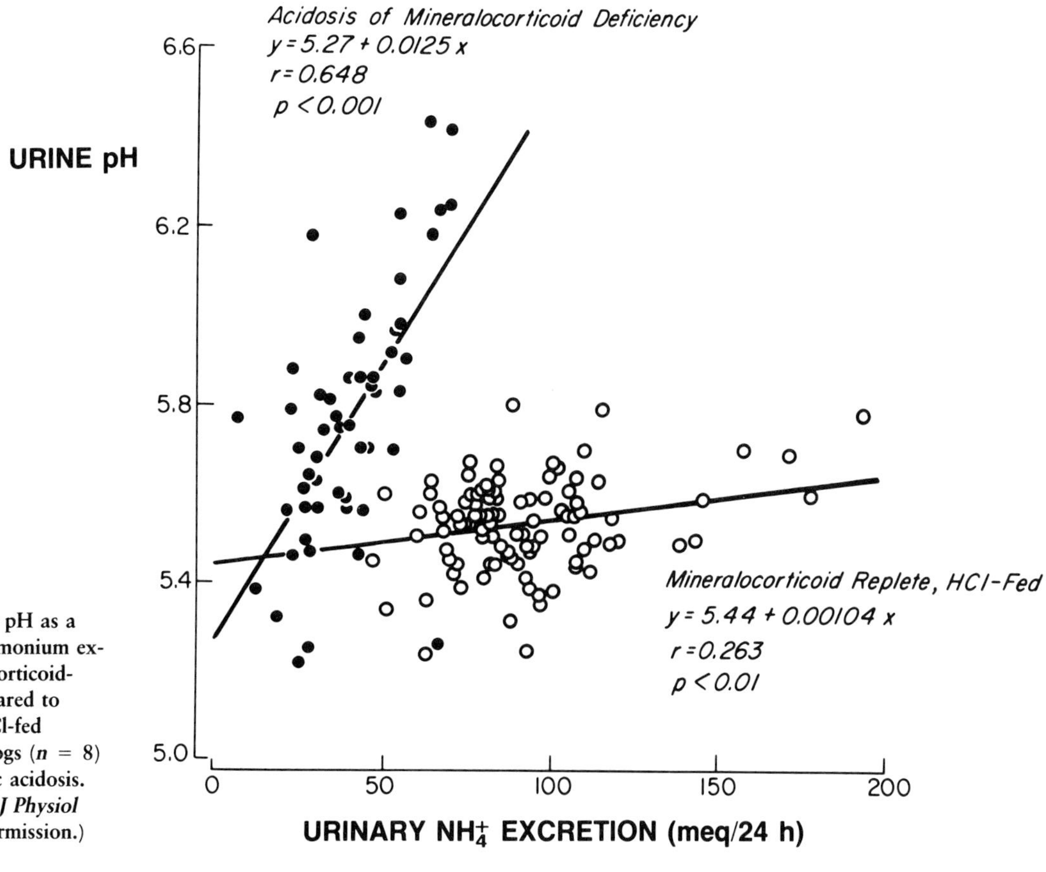

FIGURE 14-16 • Daily urine pH as a function of daily urinary ammonium excretion in acidotic mineralocorticoid-deficient dogs ($n = 5$) compared to similar values in acidotic HCl-fed mineralocorticoid-repleted dogs ($n = 8$) during steady-state metabolic acidosis. (From Hulter HN et al: *Am J Physiol* 232:F136, 1977. Used by permission.)

Chap. 10). A widely employed model for its study utilizes the urinary bladder of the Colombian toad and the freshwater turtle. These H^+-secreting epithelia are embryologically and physiologically analogous to collecting duct epithelia.[3,203,317] In these epithelia, the H^+ secretory mechanism is electrogenic (capable of transporting net positive charge into the apical solution) and is not dependent directly on Na^+ absorption.[317] The H^+ secretory rate may, however, be influenced by the transepithelial voltage, which is dependent on the rate of active sodium reabsorption.[3,4] As in the collecting duct principal cells discussed above, bladder epithelia contain sodium-transporting cells that render the apical solution voltage-negative. Protons are secreted in bladder epithelia by mitochondria-rich cells analogous to the intercalated cells of the collecting duct. The rate of H^+ secretion decreases in response to an unfavorable increase in the transepithelial H^+ gradient and also decreases in response to an imposed unfavorable electrical gradient. The magnitude of the transepithelial H^+ concentration gradient required to nullify continued net H^+ secretion is an index of the driving force, or "proton-motive" force, of the H^+ secretory pump.[2-4] The rate of H^+ secretion at nonlimiting H^+ gradients is an index of the conductance of H^+ through the active transport pathway (or an index of the number of functional pumps). As demonstrated in Fig. 14-17, aldosterone increases the rate of H^+ secretion at nonlimiting pH gradients but does not influence the proton-motive force of the H^+ secretory pump.[2-4] This finding is consistent with studies of mammalian mineralocorticoid deficiency that indicate that mineralocorticoids increase the rate capacity for acidification without altering the maximal pH gradient achieved (Fig. 14-16).

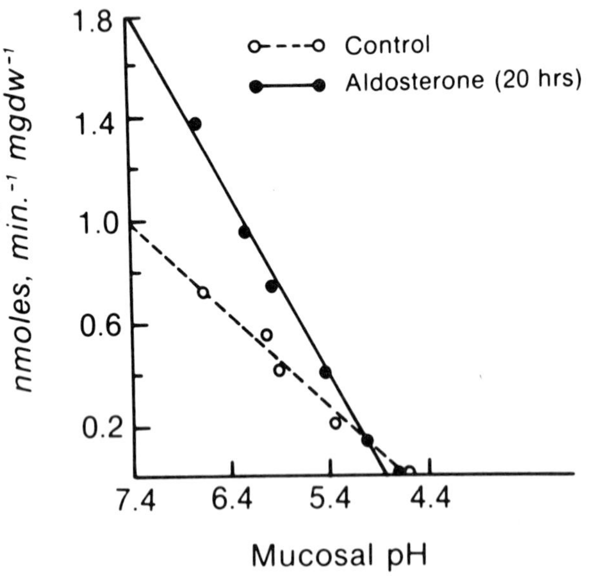

FIGURE 14-17 • The relationship of H^+ secretion (J_H) to the applied pH gradient (against which H^+ is secreted) in ouabain-treated freshwater turtle bladders studied under short-circuit conditions in both control and aldosterone-treated hemibladders. Aldosterone increased the rate of H^+ secretion at nonlimiting H^+ concentration gradients (increased slope) but did not alter the applied H^+ gradient at which net H^+ secretion ceases (the "proton motive force" of the pump). (From Al-Awqati Q: *J Clin Invest* 58:351, 1976. Used by permission.)

Recent studies of rabbit CCT acidification indicate that its characteristics are similar to those in the urinary bladders of the toad and the turtle.[171,185] Electrogenic H^+ secretion is stimulated by treatment of the animal with large doses of mineralocorticoid hormone.[171] These studies have also demonstrated that mineralocorticoid-dependent acidification in the CCT is due in part to active sodium reabsorption, which increases the electronegativity of the lumen and thus stimulates the H^+ secretion rate. Inhibition of active sodium transport converts the lumen-negative potential to lumen-positive potential, the latter being attributed to the electrogenic proton secretion.[171] The sodium-dependent component of CCT acidification has been demonstrated in rabbit tubules utilizing various inhibitors of transepithelial sodium transport.[185] It is interesting to note that the CCT does not always appear to reabsorb bicarbonate during mineralocorticoid stimulation.[99] When chronic mineralocorticoid administration caused an in vivo metabolic alkalosis, in vitro studies of the CCT demonstrated HCO_3^- secretion. If sufficient NH_4Cl was administered to decrease plasma HCO_3^- concentration by 5 mmol/liter, CCT bicarbonate secretion was eliminated. Whether this apparent reversal of direction of bicarbonate secretion was due to alterations in systemic acid-base equilibrium or to other factors (e.g., sodium depletion, more severe renal potassium wasting, alterations in anion delivery, and alterations in calcium balance and/or delivery) remains to be determined. The possibility that mineralocorticoid hormone, under certain conditions, stimulates HCO_3^- secretion directly has not been excluded.

Figure 14-18 depicts a simplified version of our current concepts of proton- and HCO_3^--secreting cells within the collecting duct.[294] Proton secretion is thought to occur primarily in the alpha cell, more heavily represented in the OMCD. This cell possesses an apical H^+ ATPase and a basolateral chloride-bicarbonate exchanger that stains immunocytochemically positive for the erythrocyte band 3 anion exchange protein. The beta cell appears to be responsible for HCO_3^- secretion and is located only in the CCT. This cell is band 3-negative and disposes of protons into ECF using a basolateral H^+ ATPase.

The OMCT contrasts with the CCT in that active sodium and potassium transport does not occur in the former segment. Moreover, mineralocorticoids do not alter transepithelial voltage, which is lumen-positive.[321-323] The lumen-positive potential results from electrogenic H^+ secretion accompanied by Cl^- secretion at nearly identical rates.[202,322,323] The chronic administration of DOC or acutely applied aldosterone significantly increases the H^+ secretory rate. Chronic dexa-

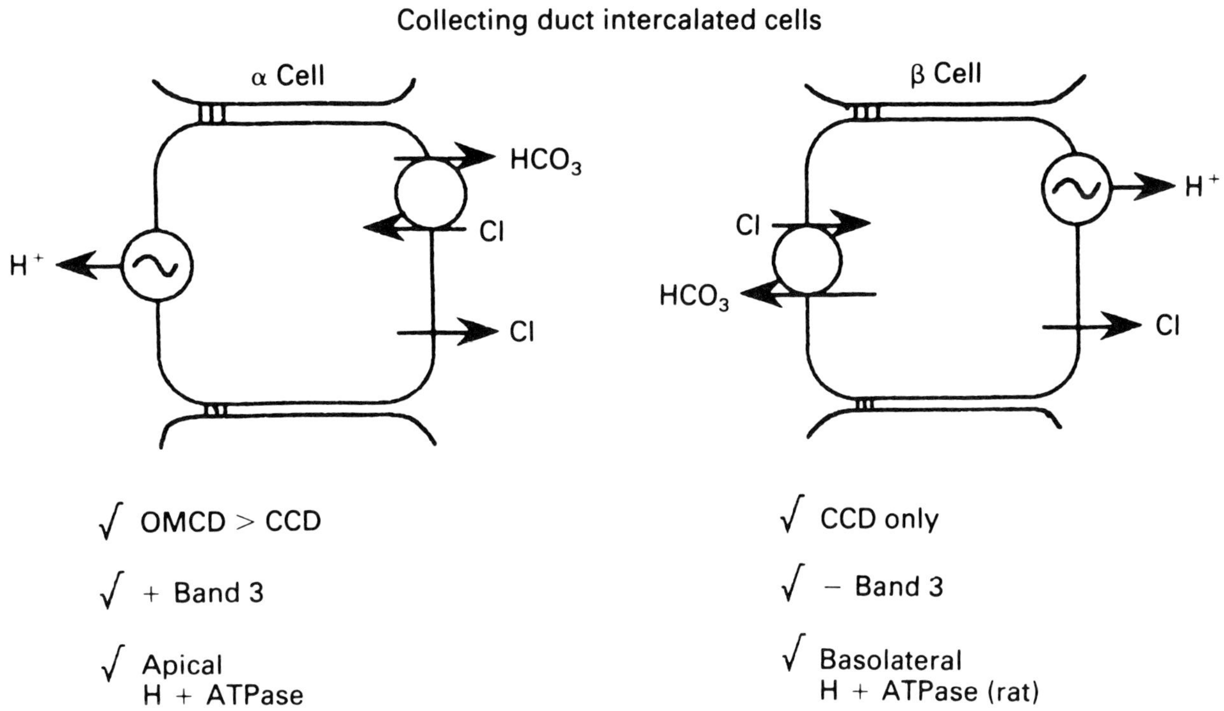

FIGURE 14-18 • Model of transporters and transport proteins in the alpha and beta cells of the collecting duct. (From Schuster VL: *Kidney Int* 38:668, 1990. Used by permission.)

methasone administration and in vitro dexamethasone application have no effect.[323]

Recent micropuncture studies have thoroughly investigated aldosterone-stimulated acidification in the accessible portion of the rat IMCD. These in vivo studies assessed the role of this segment in generating a pH gradient and in the formation of NH_4^+, titratable acid, and net acid. Rats with metabolic acidosis induced by acid loading secreted significant amounts of net acid [(NH_4^+ + titratable acid) − HCO_3^-] between the base and tip of the IMCD (Fig. 14-19). Rats with a similar degree of metabolic acidosis from mineralocorticoid deficiency did not exhibit an increment in net acid secretion in this segment.[64] These studies indicate that aldosterone-dependent acidification takes place in the IMCD. Whether the impairment in acid secretion is due to the observed diminution in the NH_3 concentration gradient between the loop of Henle and collecting duct lumen or whether it is due to the loss of a primary effect of aldosterone on proton secretion remains to be determined.

Considerable information is available regarding the structure and biochemistry of the proton-translocating ATPase located at the apical membrane of alpha cells and the basolateral membrane of beta cells in the collecting duct.[324,325] This proton pump has been classified as a vacuolar proton pump. Characterization of its physiologic role has been hampered by the lack of a highly specific inhibitor. Recently, however, a potentially specific inhibitor, bifilomycin A-1, has been identified, and this tool may facilitate our future understanding of pump function.[25] It is not yet clear whether aldosterone administration increases the synthesis of additional copies of the H^+ ATPase, increases the efficiency of glucose utilization,[4] or enhances the net insertion rate of preformed proton pumps in subapical vesicles into apical membranes. Recent studies in rat distal colon may provide a clue to the mechanism by which aldosterone facilitates acidification.[213,248,249] In this tissue, secondary hyperaldosteronism results in enhanced in vitro acidification in a manner consistent with enhanced operation of an H^+-K^+ ATPase.[213] Additional studies in the distal colon from aldosterone-infused rats demonstrated significant increases in the number, surface density, and total volume of subapical vessels.[249] It is possible that these aldosterone-induced morphologic changes represent an increase in the number of proton pumps available for subsequent shuttling into the apical membrane, whereby transepithelial hydrogen ion secretion could be augmented. Although previous studies of apical membrane morphology in CCT intercalated cells have not discerned mineralocorticoid-stimulated subapical morphologic changes, the findings in the colon suggest that this question should be reexamined and perhaps examined in medullary intercalated cells as well.

Whereas numerous questions remain concerning the cellular mechanism whereby aldosterone stimulates renal acidification, it has been firmly established that potassium depletion is a necessary cofactor in the pathogenesis

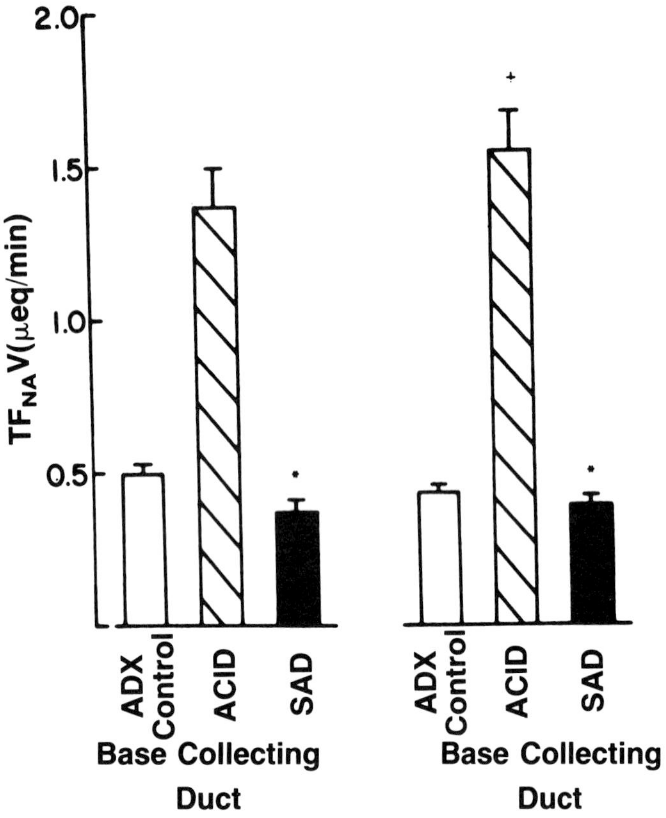

FIGURE 14-19 • Absolute delivery of net acid (NA) in tubular fluid from ADX control animals receiving fixed steroid replacement, acid-fed acidotic animals (acid), and acidotic rats with selective aldosterone deficiency (SAD). Paired micropuncture-derived delivery values are depicted for both the base and the tip of papillary collecting duct sites. (*, $p < 0.01$ for SAD versus CMA; +, $p < 0.05$ for tip values versus base values in CMA). (From DuBose TD Jr, Caflisch CR: *J Clin Invest* 82:1624, 1988. Used by permission.)

of metabolic alkalosis induced by excess mineralocorticoid hormones.[120,144,151,184,276] Chronic administration of mineralocorticoids with minimal glucocorticoid activity results in little or no increase in plasma bicarbonate concentration in human beings or dogs when dietary intake of potassium is not reduced.[120,144,184,276] Even four-times daily administration of ten-times normal amounts of aldosterone for 90 days fails to increase plasma bicarbonate concentration by more than 15 percent in normal subjects.[163] Preexisting or coexisting restriction of potassium intake, however, permits the prompt development of frank metabolic alkalosis that persists until potassium is resupplied or hormone administration is discontinued (Fig. 14-20).[120,144,164,184,276] The cellular mechanisms whereby potassium depletion potentiates the alkalosis-producing effect of mineralocorticoids have not been elucidated. However, observations in dogs have raised the possibility that potassium depletion enhances distal nephron lumen-negative voltage. This is borne out by the finding that amiloride obliterates the enhancement of the mineralocorticoid effect on renal acidification and alkalosis by potassium depletion.[145] Observations in dogs receiving normal, fixed amounts of mineralocorticoids are consistent with the hypothesis of enhanced lumen-negative voltage. In this model, dietary potassium depletion accelerates renal chloride conservation in response to dietary chloride restriction but impairs maximal renal chloride conservation in response to mineralocorticoid excess.[151] Figure 14-21 depicts the relationships of additional factors that modulate the severity of metabolic alkalosis induced by mineralocorticoid excess.[342] These factors include ECFV expansion, which diminishes renal bicarbonate reabsorption and the proximal effect of potassium depletion and/or hypokalemia to enhance bicarbonate reabsorption prior to its delivery to mineralocorticoid-responsive sites in the CCT and the OMCT. The direct effect of hypokalemia and/or potassium depletion on renal net acid excretion, as modulated by accentuated lumen-negative voltage, would be predicted to occur in the CCT.

Role of glucocorticoids in acid-base homeostasis

The combined deficiency of both mineralocorticoid and glucocorticoid hormones (Addison's disease) is associated with metabolic acidosis. Since the rate of net acid excretion is reduced, the acidosis is at least partly attributable to a reduction in the rate of renal H^+ secretion.[156,287,364] It has not yet been established whether glucocorticoids are essential for acid excretion when renal hemodynamics are maintained at normal levels.[65,358] Although systematic studies of the acid-base effects of glucocorticoids have not been reported in human subjects, studies in both rats and dogs suggest that renal ammonia production varies directly with glucocorticoid availability.[148,350] This effect of glucocorticoids on ammoniagenesis in vivo is depicted in Fig. 14-22.[148] This finding is consistent with the observation that ADX animals have decreased plasma levels of the ammoniagenic precursor glutamine and cannot normally increase these levels during acidosis.[142,284] Renal extraction of glutamine is also decreased.[142] Administration of replacement doses of glucocorticoids increases plasma glutamine concentration.[284] Although acute administration of glucocorticoids to ADX rats increases titratable acid and NH_4^+ excretion,[358] it is unclear whether this is due to a change in renal hemodynamics and/or in the distal sodium delivery or to a specific effect on renal acidification. The effects of glucocorticoid replacement or discontinuation on chronic renal and systemic acid-base equilibrium have not been evaluated.

Controversy has arisen as to whether the normal renal response to acute or chronic acid loading requires an increase in adrenal secretion of glucocorticoids.[350,353] Although significant increases in plasma corticosterone and urinary corticosterone have been reported in response to both acute and chronic acid loading in rats,[212,350] a similar glucocorticoid response has not been documented in other species.[150,181,290] Although it has been argued that an acidosis-induced increment in glucocorticoid secretion might require severe acidosis, no increase in urinary cortisol excretion has been reported in normal human subjects, even when sufficient NH_4Cl has been administered (4.2 mmol/kg per 24 h) to result in a steady-state mean plasma HCO_3^- concentration of 11 mmol/liter.[181] Additional studies in normal subjects given smaller doses of NH_4Cl also found no significant change in the plasma concentration of ACTH-dependent steroids, including cortisol. Moreover, no increase in 17-hydroxysteroid excretion (an index of cortisol secretion rate) was observed during acid feeding.[290] These studies indicate that, at least in human beings, persistent metabolic acidosis of either moderate or severe magnitude is not associated with an increased secretion rate or plasma concentration of cortisol.

Metabolic alkalosis occurs in states of hyperglucocorticoidism.[37,120,123,148,303,315] Administration of large doses of hydrocortisone to humans has been shown to increase net acid excretion[190,351] and plasma bicarbonate concentration,[123,303,315] but the specificity of this effect for type II receptor activation is uncertain, since hydrocortisone is known to possess substantial mineralocorticoid activity.[11,31] In rats, large doses of triamcinolone, a pure glucocorticoid, increase renal ammonia production and excretion and increase plasma HCO_3^- concentration. Studies in the rat have not evaluated all the components of net acid excretion or the potential alterations in endogenous acid production.[351]

The renal and systemic acid-base effects of prolonged administration of the specific glucocorticoid triamcinolone have provided information relative to the occur-

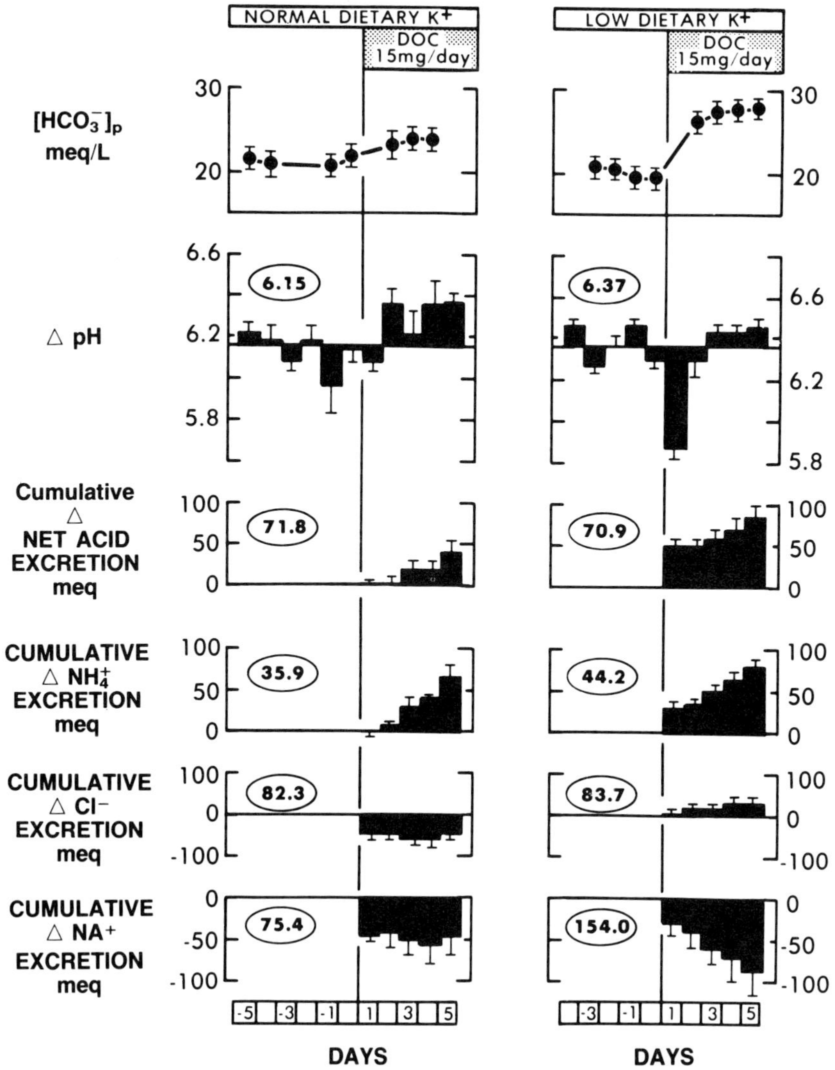

FIGURE 14-20 • Changes in mean plasma bicarbonate concentration, urine pH, and net acid, NH_4^+, Cl^-, and Na^+ excretion in potassium-replete and potassium-restricted dogs (left panel, $n = 5$, normal dietary K^+; right panel, $n = 9$, low dietary K^+) prior to and during DOC administration. Cumulative Δ excretion represents the accumulated sum of daily differences from the mean control daily excretion value (encircled). (From Hulter HN et al: *Am J Physiol* 235:F298, 1978. Used by permission.)

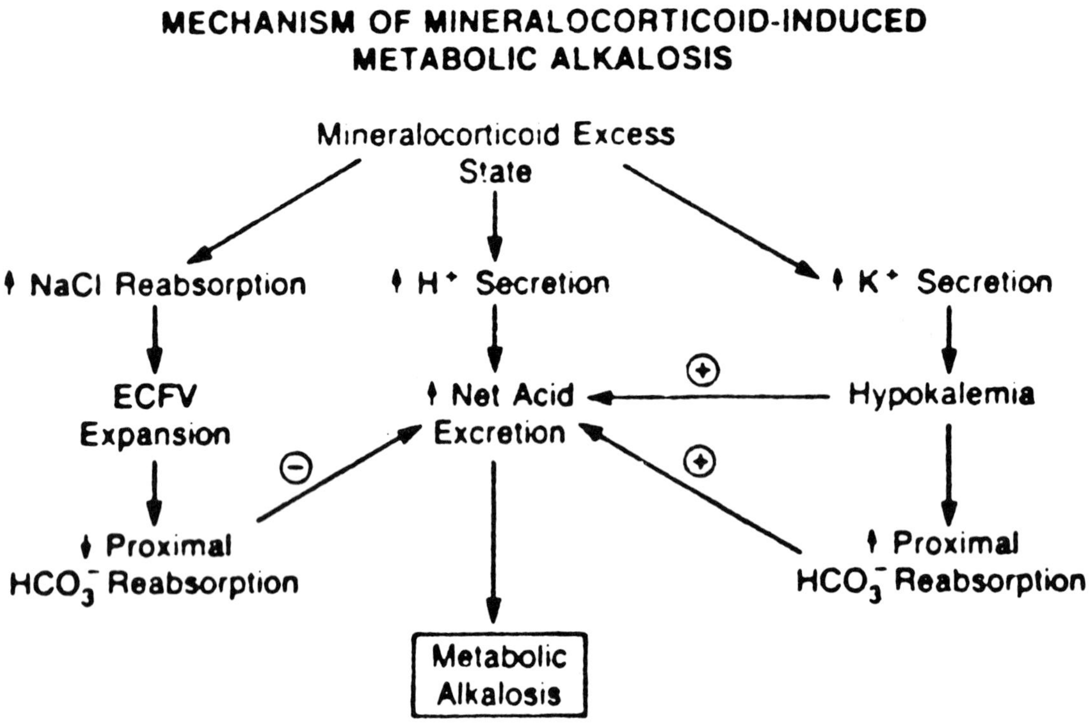

FIGURE 14-21 • Schematic representation of the generation and maintenance of metabolic alkalosis associated with primary mineralocorticoid excess. Accelerated renal H^+ secretion is associated with increased renal sodium reabsorption and renal K^+ wasting. (From Toto RD in Kokko JP, Tannen RL, eds: *Fluids and Electrolytes*, 2d ed, Philadelphia, Saunders, 1990. Used by permission.)

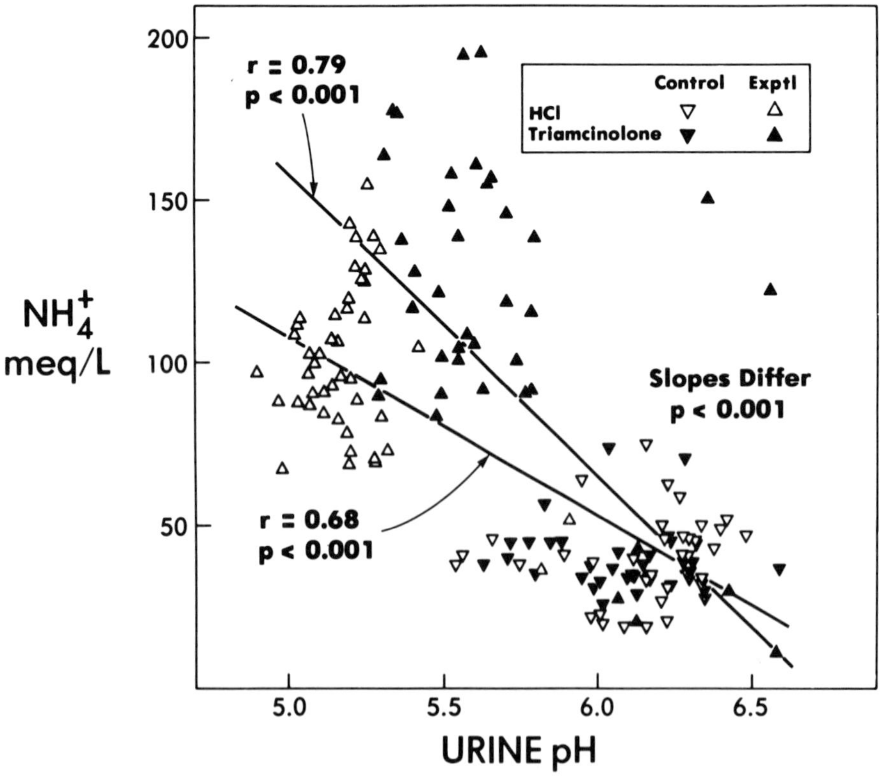

FIGURE 14-22 • Relationship between urine ammonium concentration and urine pH in dogs during chronic triamcinolone administration in comparison with animals receiving chronic HCl feeding. (From Hulter HN et al: *Am J Physiol* 239:F30, 1980. Used by permission.)

rence of metabolic alkalosis in naturally occurring hyperglucocorticoid states as well as insight into the mechanism of glucocorticoid-induced stimulation of renal acidification.[148] Administration of a very large dose of triamcimolone (1.0 mg/kg per 24 h) persistently reduces urine pH and increases net acid excretion (Fig. 14-23). The glucocorticoid also increases the urinary unmeasured anion excretion, which reflects the excretion rate of organic anions and sulfate (derived from organic acids and H_2SO_4). Initially, triamcinolone's catabolic effect increased endogenous acid production, causing a metabolic acidosis on the first day of its administration. However, with sustained triamcinolone administration, net acid excretion cumulatively increased to values that exceeded urinary unmeasured anion excretion (an index of endogenous acid production), thereby returning plasma bicarbonate concentration to stable control values. In the steady state, triamcinolone administration did not alter plasma potassium concentration or renal potassium clearance, in contrast to the hypokalemia and enhanced renal potassium clearance that complicate chronic administration of the mineralocorticoid DOC. Triamcinolone did not significantly change sodium or chloride excretion. Thus, at the highest dose of triamcinolone, endogenous acid production was stimulated along with renal H^+ secretion. The latter reflects an increased sum of net acid excretion and HCO_3^- reabsorption. The increase in renal hydrogen ion secretion was related partly to an increase in filtered bicarbonate load and partly to increased net acid excretion. Chronic administration of one-tenth the dose of triamcinolone to dogs also persistently reduced the urine pH and increased net acid excretion. Because the latter exceeded the unmeasured anion excretion, plasma bicarbonate concentration increased significantly, and a stable metabolic alkalosis of modest magnitude ensued. This finding suggested that the lower dose of triamcinolone was a lesser stimulus to organic and sulfuric acid production while still independently enhancing the renal H^+ secretory capacity. This effect of glucocorticoid is similar to that of dexamethasone, which stimulates acidification when applied directly to toad bladder epithelia.[203] These glucocorticoid effects are not likely to be mediated via type I receptors, since alterations in chloride excretion and potassium clearance were not observed.[148] Whether naturally occurring alkalosis in states of cortisol excess is due to the mineralocorticoid activity of cortisol or to specific type II receptor-mediated action, as demonstrable in the dog, remains to be determined.

The tubular site mediating the effects of glucocorticoids on renal acidification has not been determined. Since these steroids stimulate acid secretion by the toad bladder epithelia, it is likely that the collecting duct is the target site in the mammalian kidney.[203] As noted above, glucocorticoids increased the level of the Na^+-H^+ antiporter in proximal tubule brush border membranes, and

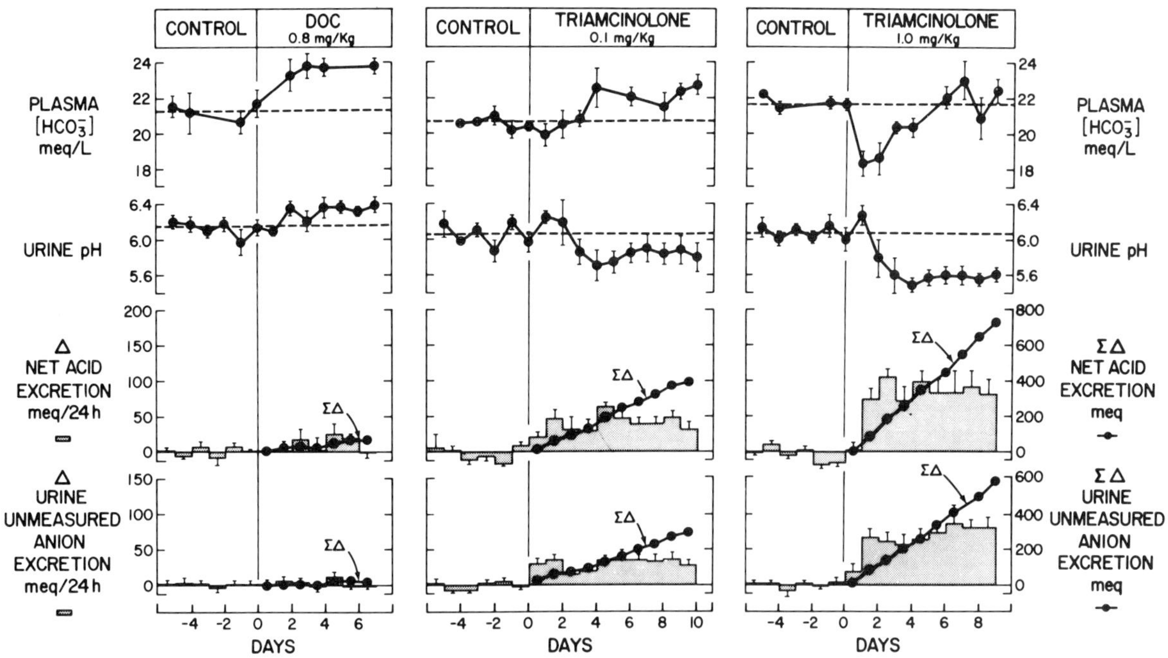

FIGURE 14-23 • Effect of chronic administration of triamcinolone compared with chronic DOC administration on plasma bicarbonate concentration, urine pH, and urinary excretion of net acid and unmeasured anions. Unmeasured anions were calculated as (NH_4^+ + Na^+ + K^+) − (Cl^- + HCO_3^- + HPO_4^{2-} + $H_2PO_4^-$ in milliequivalents per 24 h. Values are means ± SEM. (From Hulter HN et al: *Am J Physiol* 239:F30, 1980. Used by permission.)

it has been suggested that this effect might increase NH_4^+ excretion inasmuch as this antiporter can also function to exchange Na^+ for NH_4^+.[168,169] It is also possible that inhibition of proximal luminal membrane phosphate uptake by glucocorticoids might serve to enhance titratable acid excretion.[88] The latter possibility will await studies of chronic glucocorticoid deficiency to test the hypothesis that variation in phosphate excretion might modulate net acid excretion under these conditions.[149] A recent preliminary report suggests that dexamethasone (but not aldosterone) can stimulate bicarbonate reabsorption in rat loop of Henle.[341] The relative role of this segment in the renal alkalosis-producing effect of glucocorticoids remains to be determined.

ROLE OF ADRENAL STEROIDS IN WATER METABOLISM

Diluting ability

Role of mineralocorticoid hormones in renal diluting ability

Adrenal steroids are necessary for maximal dilution of the urine and thereby for maintenance of normal body tonicity (see Chap. 5).[1,26,111,259] Thus, in human beings and experimental animals with adrenal insufficiency, ingested free water cannot be normally excreted, and the host is thereby sensitized to hyponatremia and/or hypo-osmolality. The mechanisms proposed to explain the impaired diluting ability in adrenal insufficiency include ECFV depletion as well as the selective deficiency of either glucocorticoid or mineralocorticoid hormones.[26,111] Careful studies in patients with Addison's disease have suggested that both minimal urinary osmolality and free water clearance could be normalized with prior ECFV expansion in the absence of hormonal therapy.[111] This study has not been repeated, but the results underscore the possibility that in humans ECFV depletion is the sole defect responsible for impaired urinary diluting ability in adrenal insufficiency.

A major role for ECFV status in mineralocorticoid deficiency was also documented in studies in dogs that examined the effect of ECFV depletion on diluting ability in ADX animals given glucocorticoid replacement.[336] In these studies a severe renal diluting defect was corrected either by repair of ECFV depletion with saline solution or by sustained physiologic doses of mineralocorticoid hormones. Subsequently, a role for elevated ADH levels in similarly treated mineralocorticoid-deficient dogs was postulated, based on the finding of elevated plasma ADH levels in animals with impaired diluting capacity.[27] Evidence that nonosmotic ADH release was not fully responsible for impaired diluting ability in mineralocorticoid-deficient rats was provided in studies utilizing an ADH antagonist.[153] In these studies, the ADH antagonist could not fully correct diluting ability in mineralocorticoid-deficient rats, providing evidence supporting the role of a large ADH-independent mechanism for impaired diluting ability. These results were consistent with studies in Brattleboro rats with congenital central diabetes insipidus that, when rendered mineralocorticoid-deficient, continued to have a severe renal diluting defect.[119] The ADH-independent renal diluting ability of mineralocorticoid deficiency might thereby be postulated to result from decreased delivery of filtrate to the renal diluting segment (TAL).

Role of glucocorticoids in maintenance of renal diluting ability

Several lines of evidence point to a specific role for glucocorticoid deficiency in the impaired diluting ability of adrenal insufficiency. Studies in glucocorticoid-deficient, mineralocorticoid-repleted, ADX dogs demonstrated impaired cardiac function and elevated plasma ADH levels following, but nor prior to, receiving a large water load.[26] The failure of these glucocorticoid-deficient dogs to excrete a water load in the presence of a significant decrease in stroke volume led to the conclusion that baroreceptor-mediated release of ADH was responsible for the renal diluting defect. The relative importance of elevated ADH levels and hemodynamic impairment in the distal delivery of filtrate remains to be determined. Studies in glucocorticoid-deficient rats are consistent with the hypothesis that two potent mechanisms are operative, involving both ADH-dependent and ADH-independent defects in renal diluting capacity. Studies in Brattleboro rats devoid of ADH have been utilized to assess the ADH-independent defect.[197] These studies indicate that a significant renal diluting defect persists after two weeks of glucocorticoid deficiency despite the absence of ADH. Glucocorticoid-deficient, mineralocorticoid-repleted rats with diabetes insipidus demonstrated large and significant reductions in cardiac output, arterial pressure, and renal blood flow in association with significant increases in systemic and renal vascular resistance. Thus, it appears that hemodynamic derangements consequent to glucocorticoid deficiency are responsible for an ADH-independent component of the renal diluting defect. This interpretation is consistent with the results of additional studies from the same laboratory in which glucocorticoid-deficient rats without diabetes insipidus underwent acute water loads in the presence and absence of an ADH-antagonist.[153] Administration of the ADH antagonist improved but did not normalize free water excretion or maximal lowering of urinary osmolality.

Glucocorticoid deficiency might impair renal dilution by enhancing collecting duct permeability to water under either basal or ADH-stimulated conditions. This hypothesis has been tested in both rat papillary collecting duct and in isolated perfused CCT.[265,297] These studies provide no evidence that glucocorticoid deficiency can enhance either basal or ADH-stimulated diffusional water permeability. Although it seems most likely that the ADH-independent impairment in renal diluting ability is caused by hemodynamically mediated decrements in delivery of sodium and water to the diluting segment (TAL), it is also possible that glucocorticoid deficiency impairs solute efflux from either the TAL, DCT, CNT, or collecting duct.

Role of adrenal steroids in renal concentrating ability

In addition to maintaining normal renal and systemic hemodynamics and GFR, adrenal steroids are also necessary for free water reabsorption.[362] Studies in both rat papillary collecting duct and rabbit CCT indicate that adrenal steroids are necessary for a normal accumulation of cAMP in response to ADH.[154,297] As discussed in detail in Chap. 5, elevated cAMP concentration in collecting duct cytosol is thought to mediate the ADH-induced increase in transepithelial water permeability required to maximally concentrate the urine. Although studies in the isolated collecting duct have suggested that adrenal steroids control the degradation of cAMP through activation of phosphodiesterase, studies of isolated rat medullary membrane preparations suggested that adrenalectomy might also reduce ADH-stimulated adenylyl cyclase activity.[261] Recent studies in isolated tubular segments from mineralocorticoid- and glucocorticoid-deficient rats have confirmed the finding that adrenalectomy decreases ADH-stimulated adenylyl cyclase activity in both mTALH and MCT.[61] Dexamethasone restored adenylyl cyclase activity in the mTALH, whereas aldosterone restored it in the MCT. The results of additional studies evaluating the mechanism of steroid-induced stimulation of adenylyl cyclase activity were consistent with the hypothesis that glucocorticoid and mineralocorticoid deficiency in mTALH and MCT, respectively, impair adenylyl cyclase activity at the level of the regulatory protein G_s.

A role for prostaglandins (PGs) in modulating steroid-induced alterations in free water reabsorption is also possible. Studies in toad bladder epithelia have suggested that the stimulatory effects of aldosterone and dexamethasone in increasing hydraulic water permeability were due in part to inhibition of ADH-stimulated PG synthesis.[371] The relevance of the in vitro toad bladder data to in vivo mammalian physiology, however, is open to question. Rather than the decrease predicted from in vitro data, urinary excretion of PGE_2 and $PGF_2\alpha$ excretion increase significantly after glucocorticoid treatment in both humans and rats.[38,233,262,272] These observations are consistent with the finding that renal papillary PGE_2 production was increased after prolonged administration of dexamethasone to rats.[122] These results suggest that in vivo effects of glucocorticoids on renal water metabolism are probably not mediated by effects on PG production.

REFERENCES

1. Ackerman GL, Miller CL: Role of hypovolemia in the impaired water diuresis of adrenal insufficiency. *J Clin Endocrinol Metab* 30:252, 1970.
2. Al-Awqati Q et al: Characteristics of stimulation of H^+ transport by aldosterone in turtle urinary bladder. *J Clin Invest* 58:351, 1976.
3. Al-Awqati Q et al: Transport of H^+ against electochemical gradients and glucose oxidation. *Am J Physiol* 233:F502, 1977.
4. Al-Awqati Q: Effect of aldosterone on the coupling between H^+ transport and glucose oxidation. *J Clin Invest* 60:1240, 1977.
5. Alberti KG, Sharp GW: The isolation of bound aldosterone from the nuclei of human toad and rat colon. *Ann Endocrinol* 31(suppl 4):777, 1970.
6. Alexander EA, Levinsky NG: An extrarenal mechanism of potassium adaptation. *J Clin Invest* 47:740, 1968.
7. Arriza JL et al: Cloning of human mineralocorticoid receptor complementary DNA: Structural and functional kinship with the glucocorticoid receptor. *Science* 237:268, 1987.
8. Ballard K et al: Effect of aldosterone and of plasma extracts on a rat heart-lung preparation. *Am J Physiol* 199:221, 1960.
9. Bastl CP et al: Role of glucocorticoids and aldosterone in maintenance of colonic cation transport. *Am J Physiol* 238:F181, 1980.
10. Bastl CP: Regulation of cation transport by low doses of glucocorticoids in in vivo adrenalectomized rat colon. *J Clin Invest* 80:348, 1987.
11. Bastl CP, Marver D: The mechanism of action of aldosterone and glucocorticoids and their effects on fluid-electrolyte metabolism: Review of ongoing and emerging controversies, in Narins RG (ed): *Controversies in Nephrology and Hypertension*. New York, Churchill Livingstone, 1984, p 579.
12. Bayard F et al: The regulation of aldosterone secretion in anephric man. *J Clin Invest* 50:1585, 1971.
13. Baylis C, Brenner BM: Mechanism of the glucocorticoid-induced increase in glomerular filtration rate. *Am J Physiol* 234:F166, 1978.
14. Baylis C et al: Glucocorticoids and control of glomerular filtration rate. *Semin Nephrol* 10:320, 1990.
15. Benjamin WB, Singer, J: Aldosterone-induced protein in toad urinary bladder. *Science* 186:269, 1974.
16. Benos DJ et al: Purification and characterization of the amiloride-sensitive sodium channel from A_6 cultured cells and bovine renal papilla. *Proc Natl Acad Sci U S A* 83:8252, 1986.
17. Besse JC, Bass AD: Potentiation by hydrocortisone of responses to catecholamines in vascular smooth muscle. *J Pharmacol Exp Ther* 154:224, 1966.

18. Bia MJ et al: Regulation of extrarenal potassium homeostasis by adrenal hormones in rats. *Am J Physiol* 242:F641, 1982.
19. Binder HJ: Effect of dexamethasone on electrolyte transport in the large intestine of the rat. *Gastroenterology* 75:212, 1978.
20. Binder HJ et al: Demonstration of specific high affinity receptors for aldosterone in cytosol of rat colon. *Endocrinology* 118:628, 1986.
21. Biollaz J et al: Escape from mineralocorticoid excess: The role of angiotensin II. *J Clin Endocrinol Metab* 54:1187, 1982.
22. Blazer-Yost B, Cox M: Aldosterone-induced proteins: Characterization using lectin-affinity chromatography. *Am J Physiol* 249:C215, 1985.
23. Blazer-Yost B et al: Aldosterone-induced proteins in renal epithelia. *Biochim Biophys Acta* 719:158, 1982.
24. Bonvalet JP et al: Distribution of 11β-hydroxysteroid dehydrogenase along the rabbit nephron. *J Clin Invest* 86:832, 1990.
25. Bowman EJ et al: Bafilomycins: A class of inhibitors of membrane ATPases from microorganisms, animal cells and plant cells. *Proc Natl Acad Sci U S A* 85:7972, 1988.
26. Boykin J et al: Role of plasma vasopressin in impaired water excretion of glucocorticoid deficiency. *J Clin Invest* 62:738, 1978.
27. Boykin J et al: Mechanisms of impaired water excretion in mineralocorticoid deficient dogs. *Miner Electrolyte Metab* 2:310, 1979.
28. Braley LM et al: Comparative effect of angiotensin II, potassium, adrenocorticotropin, and cyclic adenosine 3′, 5′-monophosphate on cytosolic calcium in rat adrenal cells. *Endocrinology* 119:1010, 1986.
29. Bravo EL: Regulation of aldosterone secretion: Current concepts and newer aspects. *Adv Nephrol* 1:105, 1977.
30. Brien TG: Human corticosteroid binding globulin. *Clin Endocrinol* 14:193, 1981.
30a. Cairns W et al: Assembly of a glucocorticoid receptor complex prior to DNA binding enhances its specific interaction with a glucocorticoid response element. *J Biol Chem* 266:11221, 1991.
31. Campen TJ et al: Mineralo- and glucocorticoid effects on renal excretion of electrolytes. *Pfluegers Arch* 399:93, 1983.
32. Capponi AM et al: Correlation between cytosolic free Ca^{++} and aldosterone production in bovine adrenal glomerulosa cells. *J Biol Chem* 259:8863, 1984.
33. Carey RM et al: Effects of metoclopramide and bromocriptine on the renin-angiotensin-aldosterone system in man: Dopaminergic control of aldosterone. *J Clin Invest* 63:727, 1979.
34. Charney AN et al: Na^+-K^+ activated, adenosine triphosphatase and intestinal electrolyte transport: Effect of adrenal steroids. *J Clin Invest* 56:653, 1975.
35. Chase HS Jr: Does calcium couple the apical and basolateral membrane permeabilities in epithelia? (editorial review). *Am J Physiol* 247:F869, 1984.
36. Childers JW, Schneider EG: The effects of hypertonic and hypotonic sodium chloride infusions on urinary sodium excretion in conscious dogs. *Clin Sci (London)* 61:191, 1981.
37. Christy NP, Laragh JH: Pathogenesis of hypokalemic alkalosis in Cushing's syndrome. *N Engl J Med* 265:1083, 1961.
38. Codde JP, Beilin LJ: Dietary fish oil prevents dexamethasone-induced hypertension in the rat. *Clin Sci* 69:691, 1985.
39. Cohen JJ, Hulter HN et al: The critical role of the adrenal gland in the renal regulation of acid-base equilibrium during chronic hyptonic expansion: Evidence that chronic hyponatremia is a potent stimulus to aldosterone secretion. *J Clin Invest* 48:1201, 1976.
40. Connell JMC et al: Effects of ACTH and cortisol administration on blood pressure, electrolyte metabolism, atrial natriuretic peptide and renal function in normal man. *J Hypertens* 5:425, 1987.
41. Cooke CR et al: Modulation of plasma aldosterone concentration by plasma potassium in anephric man in the absence of a change in potassium balance. *J Clin Invest* 52:3028, 1973.
42. Crabbe J, Thorn GW: Effects de l'aldosterone sur la fonction renale de l'homme normal. *Rev Fr Etud Clin Biol* 9:729, 1964.
43. Cuthbert AW, Shum NK: Effects of ADH and aldosterone on amiloride binding in toad bladder epithelial cells. *Proc R Soc Lond [Biol]* 189B:543, 1975.
44. Daughaday WH et al: Binding of corticosteroids by plasma proteins: 6. The binding of cortisol and aldosterone by corticosteroid-binding globulin and by the estrogen-induced binding system of plasma. *J Clin Endocrinol Metab* 21:53, 1960.
45. Davis JO et al: Metabolism of aldosterone in several experimental situations with altered aldosterone secretion. *J Clin Invest* 44:1433, 1965.
46. Dawborn JK: The effect of prolonged intravenous infusion of aldosterone in a normal human subject. *Med J Aust* 1:1079, 1969.
47. DeBermudez L, Hayslett JP: Effect of methylprednisolone on renal function and the zonal distribution of blood flow in the rat. *Circ Res* 31:44, 1972.
48. DeFronzo RA et al: Effect of insulinopenia and adrenal hormone deficiency on acute potassium tolerance. *Kidney Int* 17:586, 1980.
49. de Kloet ER et al: Differences in corticosterone and dexamethasone binding to rat brain and pituitary. *Endocrinology* 96:598, 1975.
50. de Kloet ER et al: Interaction in vivo and in vitro of corticoids and progesterone with cell nuclei and soluble macromolecules from rat brain regions and pituitary. *Brain Res* 105:129, 1976.
51. de Kloet ER et al: Decreased serotonin turnover in the dorsal hippocampus of rat brain shortly after adrenalectomy: Selective normalization after corticosterone substitution. *Brain Res* 239:659, 1982.
52. de Kloet ER et al: Aldosterone blocks the response to corticosterone in the raphe-hippocampal serotonin system. *Brain Res* 264:323, 1983.
53. de Kloet ER et al: Selective control by corticosterone of $serotinin_1$ receptor capacity in the raphe-hippocampal system. *Neuroendocrinology* 42:513, 1986.
54. Deschepper CF et al: Analysis by immunocytochemistry and in situ hybridization of renin and its mRNA in

kidney, testis, adrenal and pituitary of the rat. *Proc Natl Acad Sci U S A* 83:7552, 1986.
54a. Diamond MI et al: Transcription factor interactions: Selectors of positive or negative regulation from a single DNA element. *Science* 249:1266, 1990.
55. Dingman JF et al: Influence of intravenously administered adrenal steroids on sodium and water excretion in normal and addisonian subjects. *Metabolism* 7:608, 1958.
56. DiTella PJ et al: Mechanism of the metabolic acidosis of selective mineralocorticoid deficiency. *Kidney Int* 14:466, 1978.
57. Dluhy, RG et al: Studies of the control of plasma aldosterone concentration in normal man:2. Effect of dietary potassium and acute potassium infusion. *J Clin Invest* 51:1950, 1972.
58. Doi Y et al: Effects of changes in sodium or potassium balance and nephrectomy, on adrenal renin and aldosterone concentrations. *Hypertension* 6(suppl):I-124, 1983.
59. Doucet A, Katz AI: Determination of Na-K-ATPase activity in single segments of the mammalian nephron. *Am J Physiol* 7:F105, 1979.
60. Doucet A, Katz AI: Mineralocorticoid receptors along the nephron: [^{3}H] aldosterone binding in rabbit tubules. *Am J Physiol* 241:F605, 1981.
61. Doucet A et al: Gluco- and mineralocorticoid control adenylate cyclase in specific nephron segments. *Am J Physiol* 258:F812, 1990.
62. Douglas JC: Potassium ion as a regulator of adrenal angiotensin II receptors. *Am J Physiol* 239:E317, 1980.
63. Douglas JC: Mechanism of adrenal angiotensin II receptor changes after nephrectomy in rats. *J Clin Invest* 67:1171, 1981.
64. Dubose TD Jr, Caflisch CR: Effect of selective aldosterone deficiency on acidification in nephron segments of the rat inner medulla. *J Clin Invest* 82:1624, 1988.
65. Dubrovsky AHE et al: Renal net acid excretion in the adrenalectomized rat. *Kidney Int* 19:516, 1981.
66. Duncan RL et al: Corticosterone's metabolite is an agonist for Na^+ transport stimulation in A6 cells. *Am J Physiol* 255:F736, 1988.
67. Edmonds CJ, Marriott JC: The effect of aldosterone and adrenalectomy on the electrical potential difference of rat colon and in the transport of sodium, potassium, chloride and bicarbonate. *J Endocrinol* 39:517, 1967.
68. Edwards CRW et al: Localization of 11β-hydroxysteroid dehydrogenase: Tissue specific protector of the mineralocorticoid receptor. *Lancet* 2:986, 1988.
69. Ehrlich EN: Adrenocortical regulation of electrolyte and water metabolism, in DeGroot LJ (ed): *Endocrinology*, 2d ed. Philadelphia, Saunders, 1989, vol 2, p 1582.
70. Elijovich F, Krakoff LR: Mechanism of the response to captopril in glucocorticoid hypertension. *Clin Exp Hypertens [A]* 4:1795, 1982.
71. Elliott ME et al: Angiotensin effects on calcium and steroidogenesis in adrenal glomerulosa cells. *Endocrinology* 116:1051, 1985.
72. El Mernissi G, Doucet A: Short-term effect of aldosterone on renal sodium transport and tubular Na-K-ATPase in the rat. *Pfluegers Arch* 399:139, 1983.
73. El Mernissi G, Doucet A: Short-term effects of aldosterone and dexamethasone on Na-K-ATPase along the rabbit nephron. *Pfluegers Arch* 399:147, 1983.
74. El Mernissi G et al: Changes in tubular basolateral membrane markers after chronic DOCA treatment. *Am J Physiol* 245:F100, 1983.
75. El Mernissi G, Doucet A: Specific activity of Na-K-ATPase after adrenalectomy and hormone replacement along the rabbit nephron. *Pfluegers Arch* 402:258, 1984.
76. Enyedi P et al: Polyphosphoinositide metabolism in adrenal glomerulosa cells. *Mol Cell Endocrinol* 41:105, 1985.
77. Fanestil DD, Park CS: Steroid hormones and the kidney. *Annu Rev Physiol* 43:637, 1981.
78. Farese RV: Phospholipids as intermediates in hormone action. *Mol Cell Endocrinol* 35:1, 1984.
79. Farman NA et al: Aldosterone binding in isolated tubules: 2. An autoradiographic study of concentration dependency in the rabbit nephron. *Am J Physiol* 242:F69, 1982.
80. Farman N et al: Autoradiographic determination of dexamethasone binding sites along the rabbit nephron. *Am J Physiol* 244:F325, 1983.
81. Farman N, Bonvalet JP: Aldosterone binding in isolated tubules: 3. Autoradiography along the rat nephron. *Am J Physiol* 245:F606, 1983.
81a. Farman N et al: Immunolocalization of gluco- and mineralocorticoid receptors in rabbit kidney. *Am J Physiol* 260:C226, 1991.
82. Fejes-Toth A, Fejes-Toth G: Glucocorticoid receptors mediate mineralocorticoid-like effects in cultured collecting duct cells. *Am J Physiol* 259:F672, 1990.
83. Field MJ et al: Differential acute effects of aldosterone, dexamethasone and hyperkalemia on distal tubular potassium secretion in the rat kidney. *J Clin Invest* 74:1792, 1984.
84. Fimognari GM et al: Induction of RNA and protein synthesis in the action of aldosterone in the rat. *Am J Physiol* 213:954, 1967.
85. Fisher KW et al: Dissociation of Na-K-ATPase specific activity and net reabsorption of Na. *Am J Physiol* 228:1745, 1975.
86. Foster ES et al: Corticosteroid alteration of active electrolyte transport in rat distal colon. *Am J Physiol* 245:G668, 1983.
87. Fraser R et al: Control of aldosterone secretion. *Clin Sci* 56:389, 1979.
88. Freiberg JM et al: Glucocorticoids increase the Na:H exchange and decrease the Na gradient-dependent phosphate-uptake systems in renal brush border membrane vesicles. *Proc Natl Acad Sci U S A* 79:4932, 1982.
89. Frizzell RA et al: Effect of aldosterone on ion transport by rabbit colon in vitro. *J Membr Biol* 39:1, 1978.
90. Fujita K et al: The role of cyclic AMP in aldosterone production by isolated zona glomerulosa cells. *J Biol Chem* 254:8567, 1979.
91. Fukuda Y, Aperia A: Differentiation of Na^+-K^+ pump in rat proximal tubule is modulated by Na^+-H^+ exchanger. *Am J Physiol* 255:F552, 1988.
91a. Fuller P J: The steroid receptor superfamily: Mechanisms of diversity. *FASEB J* 5:3092, 1991.

92. Funder JW et al: The roles of plasma binding and receptor specificity in the mineralocorticoid action of aldosterone. *Endocrinology* 92:994, 1973.
93. Funder JW et al: Glucocorticoid receptors in the rat kidney: The binding of tritiated dexamethasone. *Endocrinology* 92:1005, 1973.
94. Funder JW et al: Mineralocorticoid action: Target-tissue specificity is enzyme, not receptor, mediated. *Science* 242:583, 1988.
95. Funder JW et al: Apparent mineralocorticoid excess, pseudohypo-aldosteronism, and urinary electrolyte excretion: Toward a redefinition of mineralocorticoid action. *FASEB J* 4:3234, 1990.
96. Gall G et al: Effects of aldosterone and cortisol on human erythrocyte Na^+ efflux. *J Clin Endocrinol Metab* 32:555, 1971.
97. Ganguly A: Dopaminergic regulation of aldosterone secretion: How credible? *Clin Sci* 66:631, 1984.
98. Garcia DL et al: Chronic glucocorticoid therapy amplifies glomerular injury in rats with renal ablation. *J Clin Invest* 80:867, 1987.
99. Garcia-Austt J et al: Deoxycorticosterone-stimulated bicarbonate secretion in rabbit cortical collecting ducts: Effects of luminal chloride removal and in vivo acid loading. *Am J Physiol* 249:F205, 1985.
100. Garg LC et al: Mineralocorticoid effects on Na-K-ATPase in individual nephron segments. *Am J Physiol* 240:F536, 1981.
101. Garg LC et al: Glucocorticoid effects on Na-K-ATPase in rabbit nephron segments. *Am J Physiol* 248:F487, 1985.
102. Garty H et al: Metabolic regulation of apical sodium permeability in toad urinary bladder in the presence and absence of aldosterone. *J Membr Biol* 74:15, 1983.
103. Garty H: Mechanism of aldosterone action in tight epithelia. *J Membr Biol* 90:193, 1986.
104. Geering K et al: Hormonal regulation of (Na, K)-ATPase biosynthesis in the toad bladder. *J Biol Chem* 257:10338, 1982.
105. Geering K et al: Effects of thyromimetic drugs on aldosterone-dependent sodium transport in the toad bladder. *J Membr Biol* 77:15, 1984.
106. Geering K et al: Receptor occupancy vs. induction of Na-K-ATPase and Na transport by aldosterone. *Am J Physiol* 248:C102, 1985.
107. Geheb M et al: Aldosterone-induced proteins in toad urinary bladders. *J Biol Chem* 256:11716, 1981.
108. Geheb M et al: Mineralocorticoid-specificity of aldosterone-induced protein synthesis in giant toad (*Bufo marinus*) urinary bladders. *Biochem J* 214:29, 1983.
109. Gehr MK, Goldberg M: Hypercalciuria of mineralocorticoid escape: Clearance and micropuncture studies in the rat. *Am J Physiol* 251:F879, 1986.
110. Giguere V et al: Functional domains of the human glucocorticoid receptor. *Cell* 46:645, 1986.
111. Gill JR et al: Restoration of water diuresis in addisonian patients by expansion of volume of extracellular fluid. *J Clin Invest* 41:1078, 1962.
112. Gonzalez-Campoy JM et al: Escape from the sodium-retaining effects of mineralocorticoids: Role of ANF and intrarenal hormone systems. *Kidney Int* 35:767, 1989.
113. Gonzalez-Campoy JM et al: Proximal tubule response in aldosterone escape. *Am J Physiol* 256:R86, 1989.
114. Good DW, Wright FS: Luminal influences on potassium secretion: Sodium concentration and fluid flow rate. *Am J Physiol* 236:F192, 1979.
115. Good DW et al: Luminal influences on potassium secretion: Low sodium concentration. *Am J Physiol* 246:F609, 1984.
116. Goodfriend TJ et al: Actions of synthetic atrial natriuretic factor on bovine adrenal glomerulosa. *Life Sci* 35:1675, 1984.
117. Gotshall RW, LeBrie SJ: Water and electrolyte distribution in adrenalectomized-nephrectomized rats. *Am J Physiol* 223:198, 1972.
118. Granger JP et al: Elevated levels of atrial natriuretic peptide during aldosterone escape. *Am J Physiol* 252:R878, 1987.
119. Green HH et al: On the role of antidiuretic hormone in the inhibition of acute water diuresis in adrenal insufficiency and the effects of gluco- and mineralocorticoids in reversing the inhibition. *J Clin Invest* 49:1724, 1970.
120. Grollman AP, Gamble JL Jr: Metabolic alkalosis, a specific effect of adrenocortical hormones. *Am J Physiol* 196:135, 1959.
121. Gross JB et al: A functional comparison of the cortical collecting tubule and the distal convoluted tubule. *J Clin Invest* 55:1284, 1975.
122. Grunfeld JP et al: Effects of glucocorticoids and antiglucocorticoids on renal and aortic prostaglandin synthesis. *Am J Physiol* 251:F810, 1986.
123. Gwinup G et al: The production of hypokalemic alkalosis with hydrocortisone in subjects with adrenal insufficiency. *Metabolism* 9:831, 1964.
124. Haack D et al: Comparative study on development of corticosterone and DOCA hypertension in rats. *Am J Physiol* 233:F403, 1977.
125. Hall JE et al: Control of arterial pressure and renal function during glucocorticoid excess in dogs. *Hypertension* 2:139, 1980.
126. Hall JE et al: Role of renal hemodynamics and arterial pressure in aldosterone "escape." *Hypertension* 6(suppl I): I183, 1984.
127. Handa M et al: Dexamethasone hypertension in rats: Role of prostaglandins and pressor sensitivity to norepinephrine. *Hypertension* 6:236, 1984.
128. Harrington JT, Hulter HN et al: Mineralocorticoid-stimulated renal acidification in the dog: The critical role of dietary sodium. *Kidney Int* 30:43, 1986.
129. Hausdorff WP et al: Control of aldosterone production by angiotensin II is mediated by two guanine nucleotide regulatory proteins. *Endocrinology* 120:1668, 1987.
130. Helman SI, O'Neil RG: Model of active transepithelial Na and K transport of renal collecting tubules. *Am J Physiol* 233:F559, 1977.
131. Henning SJ et al: A study of the cytoplasmic receptors for glucocorticoids in intestine of pre and post weanling rats. *J Biol Chem* 220:2073, 1975.
132. Hierholzer K et al: Micropuncture study of renal transtubular concentration gradients of sodium and potassium in adrenalectomized rats. *Pfluegers Arch* 285:193, 1965.
133. Hierholzer K. Wiederholt, M: Some aspects of distal tubular solute and water transport. *Kidney Int* 9:198, 1976.

134. Himathongkam T et al: Potassium-aldosterone-renin interrelationships. *J Clin Endocrinol Metab* 41:153, 1975.
135. Hollenberg SM et al: Primary structure and expression of a functional human glucocorticoid receptor cDNA. *Nature* 318:635, 1985.
136. Hollenberg SM et al: Colocalization of DNA-binding and transcriptional activation functions in the human glucocorticoid receptor. *Cell* 49:39, 1987.
137. Hollenberg SM, Evans RM: Multiple and cooperative transactivation domains of the human glucocorticoid receptor. *Cell* 55:899, 1988.
138. Horisberger JD, Diezi J: Effect of mineralocorticoids on Na^+ and K^+ excretion in the adrenalectomized rat. *Am J Physiol* 245:F89, 1983.
139. Horisberger JD, Diezi J: Inhibition of aldosterone-induced antinatriuresis and kaliuresis by actomycin D. *Am J Physiol* 246:F201, 1984.
140. Horiuchi T et al: Regulation of aldosterone biosynthesis by Na^+/H^+ antiport: Relationships between intracellular pH and angiotensin II. *Endocrinology* 124:1925, 1989.
141. Horster M et al: Aldosterone in vitro restores nephron Na-K-ATPase of distal segments from adrenalectomized rabbits. *Pfluegers Arch* 384:203, 1980.
142. Hughey RA et al: Acute acidosis and renal arteriovenous differences of glutamine in normal and adrenalectomized rats. *Am J Physiol* 238:F199, 1980.
143. Hulter HN et al: Impaired renal H^+ secretion and NH_3 production in mineralocorticoid-deficient glucocorticoid-replete dogs. *Am J Physiol* 232:F136, 1977.
144. Hulter HN et al: K^+ deprivation potentiates the renal alkalosis-producing effect of mineralocorticoid. *Am J Physiol* 235:F298, 1978.
145. Hulter HN et al: K^+ deprivation potentiates the renal acid excretory effect of mineralocorticoid: Obliteration by amiloride. *Am J Physiol* 236:F48, 1979.
146. Hulter HN et al: Renal acidosis in mineralocorticoid deficiency is not dependent on NaCl depletion or hyperkalemia. *Am J Physiol* 236:F283, 1979.
147. Hulter HN et al: Pathogenesis of renal hyperchloremic acidosis resulting from dietary potassium restriction in the dog: Role of aldosterone. *Am J Physiol* 238:F79, 1980.
148. Hulter HN et al: Effects of glucocorticoid steroids on renal and systemic acid-base metabolism. *Am J Physiol* 239:F30, 1980.
149. Hulter HN: Hypophosphaturia impairs the renal defense against metabolic acidosis. *Kidney Int* 26:302, 1984.
150. Hulter HN et al: Effects of ECF volume depletion on renal regulation of acid-base and potassium equilibrium during chronic mineral acid administration. *J Lab Clin Med* 103:854, 1984.
151. Hulter HN et al: Effects of dietary potassium depletion and mineralocorticoid excess on renal Cl^- conservation in the dog. *Am J Physiol* 248:F104, 1985.
151a. Hulter HN et al: Chronic continuous PTH infusion results in hypertension in normal subjects. *J Clin Hypertens* 4:360, 1986.
152. Imai M: The connecting tubule: A functional subdivision of the rabbit distal nephron segments. *Kidney Int* 15:346, 1979.
152a. Isales CM et al: Parathyroid hormone modulates angiotensin II: Induced aldosterone secretion from the adrenal glomerulosa cell. *Endocrinology* 129:489, 1991.
153. Ishikawa S, Schrier RW: Effect of arginine vasopressin antagonists in glucocorticoid and mineralocorticoid deficient rats. *Kidney Int* 22:587, 1982.
154. Jackson BA et al: Concentrating defect in the adrenalectomized rat: Abnormal vasopressin-sensitive cyclic adenosine monophosphate metabolism in the papillary collecting duct. *J Clin Invest* 72:997, 1983.
155. Jackson EK et al: Physiological functions of the renal prostaglandin, renin and kallekrein systems, in Seldin DW, Giebisch G (eds): *The Kidney: Physiology and Pathophysiology*. New York, Raven Press, 1985, vol 1, p 613.
156. Jiminez-Diaz, C: Death in Addison's disease. *Lancet* 2:1135, 1936.
157. Johnson, JP et al: A metabolite of corticosterone is antinatriuretic but not kaliuretic in rats (abstract). *Kidney Int* 27:258, 1985.
157a. Jonat C et al: Antitumor promotion and anti-inflamation: Down modulation of AP-1 (fos/jun) activity by glucocorticoid hormone. *Cell* 62:1189, 1990.
158. Jorgensen PL: Structure, function and regulation of Na-K-ATPase in the kidney. *Kidney Int* 29:10, 1986.
159. Jorkasky D et al: Differential effects of corticosteroids on Na^+ transport in rat distal colon in vitro. *Am J Physiol* 248:G424, 1985.
160. Kaissling B, Le Hir M: Distal tubular segments of the rabbit kidney after adaptation to altered Na- and K-intake: 1. Structural changes. *Cell Tissue Res* 224:469, 1982.
161. Kaji DM et al: Glucocorticoid-induced alterations in the sodium potassium pump of the human erythrocyte. *J Clin Invest* 68:422, 1981.
162. Kashgarian M: Changes in cell membrane surfaces associated with alterations of transepithelial ion movement, in Boulpaep EL (ed): *Current Topics in Membranes and Transport*. New York, Academic Press, 1980, vol 13, p 149.
163. Kassirer JP et al: On the pathogenesis of metabolic alkalosis in hyperaldosteronism. *Am J Med* 49:306, 1970.
164. Kassirer, JP et al: Aldosterone-induced metabolic alkalosis in man (abstract). Proc Annu Meet Am Soc Nephrol, 5th, Washington, DC, 1971, p 36.
165. Katayama S, Yamaji T: A binding protein for aldosterone in human plasma. *J Steroid Biochem* 16:185, 1982.
166. Katz AI: Corticosteroid regulation of Na-K-ATPase along the mammalian nephron. *Semin Nephrol* 10:388, 1990.
167. Khuri RN et al: Effects of flow rate and potassium intake on distal tubular potassium transfer. *Am J Physiol* 228:1249, 1975.
168. Kinsella JL et al: Na^+-H^+ exchange activity in renal brush border membrane vesicles in response to metabolic acidosis: The role of glucocorticoids. *Proc Natl Acad Sci U S A* 81:630, 1984.
169. Kinsella JL et al: Glucocorticoid activation of Na^+/H^+ exchange in renal brush border vesicles: Kinetic effects. *Am J Physiol* 248:F233, 1985.

170. Kipnowski J et al: Modification of carboxyl of Na-channels inhibits aldosterone action on Na transport. *Am J Physiol* 245:F726, 1983.
171. Koeppen BM, Helman SI: Acidification of luminal fluid by the rabbit cortical collecting tubule perfused in vitro. *Am J Physiol* 242:F521, 1982.
172. Koeppen BM et al: Intracellular microelectrode characterization of the rabbit cortical collecting duct. *Am J Physiol* 244:F35, 1983.
173. Kohlmann O et al: Effect of captopril on glucocorticoid excess hypertension (abstract). *Clin Res* 28:333A, 1980.
174. Kojima I et al: Characteristics of angiotensin II-, K^+- and ACTH-induced calcium influx in adrenal glomerulosa cells: Evidence that angiotensin II, K^+, and ACTH may open a common calcium channel. *J Biol Chem* 260:9171, 1985.
175. Kojima I et al: Intracellular calcium and adenosine 3′, 5′-cyclic monophosphate as mediator of potassium-induced aldosterone secretion. *Biochem J* 228:69, 1985.
176. Kojima K et al: Dihydropyridine calcium agonist and antagonist effects on aldosterone secretion. *Am J Physiol* 247:E645, 1984.
177. Kornandakieti C, Tannen RL: H^+ transport by the aldosterone deficient rat distal nephron. *Kidney Int* 25:629, 1984.
178. Kornel L et al: Evidence for the presence in arterial walls of an intracellular-molecular mechanism for action of mineralocorticoids. *Clin Exp Hypertens [A]*4:1561, 1982.
179. Krakoff LR et al: Pathogenesis of hypertension in Cushing's syndrome. *Am J Med* 58:216, 1975.
180. Krakoff LR et al: Effect of methlprednisolone upon arterial pressure and the renin angiotensin system in the rat. *Am J Physiol* 288:613, 1975.
181. Krapf R et al: Chronic respiratory alkalosis: The effect of sustained hyperventilation on renal regulation of acid-base equilibrium. *N Engl J Med* 324:1394, 1991.
182. Krozowski ZS, Funder JW: Renal mineralocorticoid receptors and hippocampal corticosterone binding species have identical intrinsic steroid specificity. *Proc Natl Acad Sci U S A* 80:6056, 1983.
183. Kudo LH et al: Effect of vasopressin on sodium transport across inner medullary collecting duct. *Am J Physiol* 258:F1438, 1990.
184. Kurtzman NA et al: Pathophysiology of metabolic alkalosis. *Arch Intern Med* 131:702, 1973.
185. Laski ME, Kurtzman NA: Characterization of acidification in the cortical and medullary collecting tubule of the rabbit. *J Clin Invest* 72:2050, 1983.
186. Law PY, Edelman IS: Effect of aldosterone on incorporation of amino acids into renal medullary proteins. *J Membr Biol* 41:15, 1978.
187. Lecomte J et al: Potentiation per l'hydrocortisone des effects moteurs del l'adrenaline. *Arch Int Pharmacodyn Ther* 119:133, 1959.
188. Lee SM et al: Corticosteroid binding sites along the rat nephron. *Am J Physiol* 244:F504, 1983.
189. Le Hir M et al: Distal tubular segments of the rabbit kidney after adaptation to altered Na- and K-intake: 2. Changes in Na-K-ATPase activity. *Cell Tissue Res* 224:493, 1982.
190. Lemann J Jr et al: Studies of the acute effects of aldosterone and cortisol on the interrelationship between renal sodium, calcium and magnesium excretion in normal man. *Nephron* 7:117, 1970.
191. Lesnik H et al: The release of antidiuretic hormone from the pituitary stalk after intravenous calcium chloride or magnesium chloride infusions in rats. *J Endocrinol* 45:83, 1969.
192. Levitan R, Ingelfinger FJ: Effect of D-aldosterone on salt and water absorption from the intact human colon. *J Clin Invest* 44:801, 1965.
193. Levitt MF, Bader ME: Effect of cortisone and ACTH on fluid and electrolyte distribution in man. *Am J Med* 11:715, 1951.
194. Leyssac PP, Holstein-Rathlou NH: Comments on the lithium clearance method for estimating renal tubular function. *News Physiol Sci* 3:77, 1988.
195. Liddle GW: Aldosterone antagonists. *Arch Intern Med* 102:998, 1958.
196. Liddle GW: The adrenal cortex, in Williams RH (ed): *Textbook of Endocrinology*, 5th ed. Philadelphia, Saunders, 1974, p 233.
197. Linas SL et al: Role of vasopressin in the impaired water excretion of glucocorticoid deficiency. *Kidney Int* 18:58, 1980.
198. Liu F-Y, Cogan MG: Angiotensin II: A potent regulator of acidification in the rat early proximal convoluted tubule. *J Clin Invest* 80:272, 1987.
199. Liu F-Y, Cogan MG: Role of protein kinase C in proximal bicarbonate absorption and angiotensin signaling. *Am J Physiol* 258:F927, 1990.
200. Liu F-Y, Cogan MG: Roles of protein kinase C and calcium in S_1 proximal bicarbonate absorption and angiotensin II signaling (abstract). *Kidney Int* 37:541, 1990.
201. Lohmeier TE et al: Is aldosteronism important in the maintenance of arterial blood pressure and electrolyte balance during sodium depletion? *Hypertension* 2:497, 1980.
202. Lombard WE et al: Collecting duct bicarbonate transport: Comparison of cortical and medullary segments. *Kidney Int* 16:827, 1979.
202a. Lucibello FC et al: Mutual transrepression of Fos and the glucocorticoid receptor: Involvement of a functional domain in Fos which is absent in FosB. *EMBO J* 9:2827, 1990.
203. Ludens JH, Fanestil DD: Aldosterone stimulation of acidification of urine by isolated urinary bladder of the Colombian toad. *Am J Physiol* 226:1321, 1974.
204. Maack T et al: Effects of auriculin (atrial natriuretic factor) on blood pressure, renal function, and the renin-aldosterone system in dogs. *Am J Med* 77:1069, 1984.
205. Mach RS et al: Action clinique et metabolique de l'aldosterone (electrocortine). *Schweiz Med Wochenschr* 84:407, 1954.
206. Magliola L et al: Alterations in active Na^+-K^+ transport during mineralocorticoid-salt hypertension in the rat. *Am J Physiol* 250:C540, 1986.
207. Marusic ET et al: Corticosteroid binding studies in cytosol of colonic mucosa of the rat. *Am J Physiol* 240:G417, 1981.
208. Marver D: Evidence of corticosteroid action along the

nephron. *Am J Physiol* 246:F111, 1984.
209. Marver D: Assessment of mineralocorticoid activity in the rabbit colon. *Am J Physiol* 246:F437, 1984.
210. Marver D, Kokko JP: Renal target sites and the mechanism of action of aldosterone. *Miner Electrolyte Metab* 9:1, 1983.
211. Marver D, Schwartz MJ: Identification of mineralocorticoid target sites in the isolated rabbit cortical nephron. *Proc Natl Acad Sci U S A* 77:3672, 1980.
212. May RC et al: Metabolic acidosis stimulates protein degradation in rat muscle by a glucocorticoid-dependent mechanism. *J Clin Invest* 77:614, 1986.
213. McLaughlin ML et al: Secondary hyperaldosteronism stimulates acidification in rat distal colon. *Pfluegers Arch* 416:639, 1990.
214. Meyer TW et al: The renal hemodynamic response to amino acid infusion in the rat. *Trans Assoc Am Physicians* 96:76, 1983.
215. Miesfeld R et al: Genetic complementation of a glucocorticoid receptor deficiency by expression of cloned receptor cDNA. *Cell* 46:389, 1986.
216. Mills JN et al: The acute effect of hydrocortisone, deoxycorticosterone and aldosterone upon the excretion of sodium, potassium and acid by the human kidney. *J Physiol* 151:312, 1960.
217. Mills JN et al: The effects of intravenous aldosterone and hydrocortisone on the urinary electrolytes of the recumbent human subject. *J Physiol* 156:415, 1961.
218. Minuth WW et al: Methylation of cytosolic proteins may be a possible biochemical pathway of early aldosterone action in cultured renal collecting duct cells. *Differentiation* 36:23, 1987.
219. Minuth WW et al: Complex physiological and biochemical action of aldosterone in toad urinary bladder and mammalian renal collecting duct cells. *Renal Physiol* 10:297, 1987.
220. Minuth WW et al: Action of aldosterone on citrate synthase in cultured renal collecting duct cells. *Renal Physiol* 12:85, 1989.
221. Mitch WE et al: Plasma levels and hepatic extraction of renin and aldosterone in alcoholic liver disease. *Am J Med* 66:804, 1979.
222. Missale C et al: Characterization of dopamine receptors associated with aldosterone secretion in rat adrenal glomerulosa. *Endocrinology* 119:2227, 1986.
223. Morris DJ et al: The physiological response to aldosterone in adrenalectomized and intact rats and its sex dependence. *Endocrinology* 92:989, 1973.
224. Morris DJ: The metabolism and mechanisms of action of aldosterone. *Endocr Rev* 2:234, 1981.
225. Morris DJ, Brem AS: Metabolic derivatives of aldosterone. *Am J Physiol* 252:F365, 1987.
226. Morris DJ, Kenyon CJ: Aldosterone and its metabolism in spontaneously hypertensive rats (SHR) *Clin Exp Hypertens [A]*4:1613, 1982.
227. Moura AM et al: Extrarenal effects of aldosterone and antimineralocorticoid compounds. *Kidney Int* 34(suppl 26):S8, 1988.
228. Mujais SK et al: Regulation of renal Na-K-ATPase in the rat: Role of the natural mineralo- and glucocorticoid hormones. *J Clin Invest* 73:13, 1984.
229. Mujais SK et al: Relationship between adrenal steroids and renal Na-K-ATPase: Effect of short-term hormone administration on the rat cortical collecting tubule. *Pfluegers Arch* 402:48, 1984.
230. Muto S et al: An acute increase of peritubular K stimulates K transport through cell pathways of CCT. *Am J Physiol* 225:F108, 1988.
231. Nakamura M et al: A role for the adrenal renin-angiotensin system in the regulation of potassium-stimulated aldosterone production. *Endocrinology* 117:1772, 1985.
232. Naruse M et al: Renin exists in human adrenal tissue. *J Clin Endocrinol Metab* 57:482, 1983.
233. Nasjletti A et al: Plasma concentration, renal excretion and tissue release of prostaglandins in the rat with dexamethasone-induced hypertension. *Endocrinology* 114: 1033, 1984.
234. Nestler EJ et al: Corticosterone increases the amount of protein I, neuron specific phosphoprotein, in rat hippocampus. *Science* 212:1162, 1981.
235. Oberfield SE et al: Metabolic and blood pressure responses to hydrocortisone in the syndrome of apparent mineralocorticoid excess. *J Clin Endocrinol Metab* 56:332, 1983.
236. Okuno T et al: Dexamethasone hypertension in rats. *Clin Exp Hypertens [A]*3:1075, 1981.
237. O'Neil RG: Modulation of Na^+K^+-ATPase expression in renal collecting duct. *Curr Top Membr Transp* 34:209, 1989.
238. O'Neil RG, Boulpaep EL: Effect of amiloride on the apical cell membrane cation channels of a sodium-absorbing, potassium-secreting renal epithelium. *J Membr Biol* 50:365, 1979.
239. O'Neil RG, Hayhurst RA: Sodium dependent modulation of the renal Na/K-ATPase: Influence of mineralocorticoids on the cortical collecting duct. *J Membr Biol* 85:169, 1985.
240. O'Neil RG, Helman SI: Transport characteristics of renal collecting tubules: Influences of DOCA and diet. *Am J Physiol* 233:F544, 1977.
241. Paccolat MP et al: Aldosterone regulation of Na^+- transport and Na-K-ATPase in A6 cells: Role of growth conditions. *Am J Physiol* 252:C468, 1987.
242. Palmer LG et al: Current-voltage analysis of apical sodium transport in toad urinary bladder: Effects of inhibitors of transport and metabolism. *J Membr Biol* 57:59, 1980.
243. Palmer LG et al: Aldosterone control of the density of Na channels in the toad urinary bladder. *J Membr Biol* 64:91, 1982.
244. Pamnani MB et al: Altered activity of the sodium-potassium pump in arteries of rats with steroid hypertension. *Clin Sci Mol Med* 55:41s, 1978.
245. Park CS et al: Role of carboxyl group in Na-entry step at apical membrane of toad urinary bladder. *Am J Physiol* 245:F707, 1983.
246. Park CS, Fanestil DD: Functional groups of the Na-channel: Role of carboxyl and histidyl groups. *Am J Physiol* 245:F716, 1983.
247. Pechet MM et al: Metabolic studies with a new series of 1,4-dienesteroids: 2. Effects of normal subjects of prednisone, prednisolone, and 9α-fluoroprednisolone. *J Clin Invest* 38:691, 1959.

248. Perrone RD et al: Aldosterone induces apical vesicles in rat distal colon. *Am J Physiol* 259:F65, 1990.
249. Perrone RD, McBride DE: Aldosterone and P_{CO_2} enhance K^+-dependent chloride absorption in rat distal colon. *Pfluegers Arch* 416:632, 1990.
250. Peterson LN, Wright FS: Effect of sodium intake on renal potassium excretion. *Am J Physiol* 233:F225, 1977.
251. Petty KJ et al: Secondary effect of aldosterone on Na-K-ATPase activity in the rabbit cortical collecting tubule. *J Clin Invest* 68:1514, 1981.
252. Petzel D et al: Correlates of aldosterone-induced increases in Ca_i^{++} and I_{sc} suggest that Ca_i^{++} is the second messenger for stimulation of apical membrane conductance. *J Clin Invest* 89:150, 1992.
253. Picard D, Yamamoto KR: Two signals mediate hormone-dependent nuclear localization of the glucocorticoid receptor. *EMBO J* 6:3333, 1987.
254. Pratt JH: Role of angiotensin II in potassium mediated stimulation of aldosterone secretion in the dog. *J Clin Invest* 70:667, 1982.
255. Pressley L, Funder JW: Glucocorticoid and mineralocorticoid receptors in gut mucosa. *Endocrinology* 97:588, 1975.
256. Purdy RE et al: Vasconstrictor effects of aldosterone in isolated vascular tissue. *Clin Exp Hypertens[A]*4:1583, 1982.
257. Quinn SJ et al: Electrical properties of isolated rat adrenal glomerulosa and fasciculata. *Endocrinology* 120:903, 1987.
258. Quinn SJ, Williams GH: Regulation of aldosterone secretion. *Annu Rev Physiol* 50:409, 1988.
259. Quintanilla AP et al: Renal hemodynamics and water excretion in Addison's disease. *Metabolism* 25:419, 1976.
260. Radke KJ et al: Effect of hydrogen ion concentration on corticosteroid secretion. *Am J Physiol* 250:E259, 1986.
261. Rajerison RM et al: The vasopressin-sensitive adenylate cyclase of the rat kidney: Effect of adrenalectomy and corticosteroids on hormonal receptor-enzyme coupling. *J Biol Chem* 249:6390, 1974.
262. Ramos-Frendo B et al: Methyl-prednisonolone-induced hypertension in the rat: Evidence against the role of plasma volume changes, vasopressin and renal prostaglandin E_2. *J Hypertens* 3:461, 1985.
263. Rascher W et al: Plasma catecholamines: Noradrenaline metabolism and vascular response in deoxycorticosterone acetate hypertension of rats. *Eur J Pharmacol* 75:255, 1981.
264. Rayfield EJ et al: Aldosterone secretory and glucocorticoid excretory responses to alpha 1-24 (Cortrosyn) in sodium-depleted normal man. *J Clin Endocrinol Metab* 36:30, 1973.
265. Rayson BMR et al: The effect of adrenal cortical hormones on water permeability of the collecting duct of the rat. *Pfluegers Arch* 373:105, 1978.
266. Rayson BM, Lowther SO: Steroid regulation of Na-K-ATPase: Differential sensitivities along the nephron. *Am J Physiol* 246:F656, 1984.
267. Reich JM et al: Mechanism of hormonal modulation of ion transport in the toad's urinary bladder: Subcellular localization of aldosterone-induced proteins. *Biochim Biophys Acta* 676:379, 1981.
268. Reid IA et al: Studies concerning the regulation and importance of plasma angiotensinogen concentration in the dog. *Endocrinology* 93:107, 1973.
269. Relman AS, Schwartz WB: The effect of DOCA on electrolyte balance and its relation to sodium chloride intake. *Yale J Biol Med* 24:540, 1952.
270. Rocha AS, Kudo LH: Water, urea, sodium, chloride and potassium transport in the in vitro isolated perfused papillary collecting duct. *Kidney Int* 22:485, 1982.
271. Romero JC et al: Contribution of sympathetic neural reflexes to mineralocorticoid escape. *Fed Proc* 44:2382, 1985.
272. Rosenkrantz B et al: Dexamethasone effect on prostanoid formation in healthy man. *Clin Sci* 68:681, 1985.
273. Rossier BC et al: Kinetics of RNA labeling in toad bladder epithelium: Effects of aldosterone and related steroids. *Proc Natl Acad Sci U S A* 71:3101, 1974.
274. Rossier BC: Biosynthesis of Na-K-ATPase in amphibian epithelial cells. *Curr Top Membr Trans* 20:25, 1984.
275. Rossier BC: Mechanisms of action of mineralocorticoid hormones. *Endocr Res* 15:203, 1989.
276. Roth DG, Gamble JL Jr: Deoxycorticosterone-induced alkalosis in dogs. *Am J Physiol* 208:90, 1965.
277. Rousseau G et al: Glucocorticoid and mineralocorticoid receptors for aldosterone. *J Steroid Biochem* 3:219, 1972.
278. Sambhi M et al: Acute pharmacodynamic effects of glucocorticoids. *Circulation* 31:523, 1965.
279. Sandle GI, Binder HJ: Corticosteroids and intestinal ion transport. *Gastroenterology* 93:188, 1987.
280. Sands JM et al: Hormone effects on NaCl permeability of rat inner medullary collecting duct. *Am J Physiol* 255:F421, 1988.
281. Sansom SC et al: Microelectrode assessment of chloride conductive properties of cortical collecting duct. *Am J Physiol* 247:F291, 1984.
282. Sansome SC, O'Neil RG: Effects of mineralocorticoids on transport properties of cortical collecting duct basolateral membrane. *Am J Physiol* 251:F743, 1986.
283. Sansome S et al: Na-dependent effects of DOCA on cellular transport properties of CCDs from ADX rabbits. *Am J Physiol* 253:F753, 1987.
284. Sapir DG et al: The role of alanine and glutamine in steroid-induced nitrogen wasting in man. *Clin Sci* 53:215, 1977.
285. Sariban-Sohraby S et al: Methylation increases Na-transport into A6 apical membrane vesicles: Possible mode of aldosterone action. *Science* 225:745, 1984.
286. Sariban-Sohraby S, Benos DJ: The amiloride-sensitive sodium channel. *Am J Physiol* 250:C175, 1986.
287. Sartorius OW et al: Studies on the interrelationships of the adrenal cortex and renal ammonia excretion by the rat. *Endocrinology* 52:256, 1953.
288. Schafer JA et al: Vasopressin and mineralocorticoid increase apical membrane driving force for K^+ secretion in rat CCD. *Am J Physiol* 258:F199, 1990.
289. Schambelan M et al: Prevalence, pathogenesis, and functional significance of aldosterone deficiency in hyperkalemic patients with chronic renal insufficiency. *Kidney Int* 17:89, 1980.
290. Schambelan M et al: Adrenocortical hormone secretory

response to chronic NH_4Cl-induced metabolic acidosis. *Am J Physiol* 252:E454, 1987.

291. Schlatter E, Schafer JA: Electrophysiological studies in principal cells of rat cortical collecting tubules: ADH increases the apical membrane Na^+-conductance. *Pfluegers Arch* 409:81, 1987.
292. Schmidt U et al: Sodium- and potassium-activated ATPase. *J Clin Invest* 55:655, 1975.
293. Schneider EG et al: Effect of sodium concentration on aldosterone secretion by isolated perfused canine adrenal glands. *Endocrinology* 115:2195, 1984.
293a. Schule R et al: Functional antagonism between oncoprotein c-jun and the glucocorticoid receptor. *Cell* 62:1217, 1990.
294. Schuster VL: Organization of collecting duct intercalated cells. *Kidney Int* 38:668, 1990.
295. Schwartz GJ, Burg MB: Mineralocorticoid effects on cation transport by cortical collecting tubules in vitro. *Am J Physiol* 235:F576, 1978.
296. Schwartz GJ, Evan AP: Development of solute transport in rabbit proximal tubule: 3. Na-K-ATPase activity. *Am J Physiol* 246:F845, 1984.
297. Schwartz MJ, Kokko JP: Urinary concentrating defect of adrenal insufficiency: Permissive role of adrenal steroids on the hydroosmotic response across the rabbit collecting tubule. *J Clin Invest* 66:234, 1980.
298. Scoggins BA et al: Adrenocorticotropic hormone-induced hypertension in sheep. *Circ Res* 43(suppl I):176, 1978.
299. Scott WN, Sapirstein US: Identification of aldosterone induced proteins in the toad's urinary bladder. *Proc Natl Acad Sci U S A* 72:4056, 1975.
300. Scott WN et al: Comparison of toad bladder aldosterone-induced proteins and proteins synthesized in vitro using aldosterone-induced messenger RNA as template. *J Membr Biol* 213, 1978.
301. Scott WN et al: Inhibition of fatty acid synthesis prevents the incorporation of aldosterone-induced proteins into membranes. *J Biol Chem* 254:4957, 1979.
302. Sebastian A et al: Effect of mineralocorticoid replacement therapy on renal acid-base homeostasis in adrenalectomized patients. *Kidney Int* 18:762, 1980.
303. Seldin DW, Rector FC Jr: The generation and maintenance of metabolic alkalosis. *Kidney Int* 1:306, 1972.
304. Spelling JH, Field M: Physiologic and pharmacologic effects of glucocorticoids on ion transport across rabbit ileal mucosa in vitro. *J Clin Invest* 67:770, 1981.
305. Severne Y et al: Metal finding 'finger' structures in the glucocorticoid receptor defined by site-directed mutagenesis. *EMBO J* 7:2053, 1988.
306. Sheppard KE, Funder JW: Cortisol 17β acid, transcortin, and the heterogeneity of rat brain glucocorticoid receptors. *J Steroid Biochem* 25:285, 1986.
307. Sheppard K, Funder JW: Mineralocorticoid specificity of renal type I receptors: In vivo binding studies. *Am J Physiol* 252:E224, 1987.
308. Sheppard K, Funder JW: Type I receptors in parotid, colon and pituitary are aldosterone-selective in vivo. *Am J Physiol* 253:E467, 1987.
309. Shields R et al: Action of aldosterone upon the intestinal-transport of potassium, sodium and water. *Gut* 7:686, 1966.
310. Simpson ER, Waterman MR: Steroid hormone biosynthesis in the adrenal cortex and its regulation by adrenocorticotropin, in De Groot LJ (ed): *Endocrinology*, 2d ed. Philadelphia, Saunders, 1989, vol 2, p 1543.
311. Sinha SK et al: Mechanism of activation of renal $(Na^+ + K^+)$-ATPase in the rat: Effect of acute and chronic administration of dexamethasone. *Biochim Biophys Acta* 641:20, 1981.
312. Sonnenblick EH et al: The nature of the action of intravenous aldosterone: Evidence for a role of the hormone in urinary dilution. *J Clin Invest* 40:903, 1961.
313. Spital A, Sterns RH: Paradoxical potassium depletion: A renal mechanism for extrarenal potassium adaptation. *Kidney Int* 30:532, 1986.
314. Spital A, Sterns RH: Extrarenal potassium adaptation: The role of aldosterone. *Clin Sci* 76:213, 1989.
315. Sprague RG et al: Observations on the physiologic effects of cortisone and ACTH in man. *Arch Intern Med* 85:199, 1950.
316. Stanton BA: Characterization of apical and basolateral membrane conductances of rat inner medullary collecting duct. *Am J Physiol* 256:F862, 1989.
317. Steinmetz PR: Characteristics of hydrogen ion transport in urinary bladder of fresh water turtle. *J Clin Invest* 46:1531, 1967.
318. Stewart PM et al: The syndrome of apparent mineralocorticoid excess: A defect in the cortisol-cortisone shuttle. *J Clin Invest* 82:340, 1988.
319. Stockigt JR et al: Renin and renin substrate in primary adrenal insufficiency: Contrasting effects of glucocorticoids and mineralocorticoid deficiency. *Am J Med* 66:915, 1979.
320. Stokes JB: Potassium secretion by cortical collecting tubule: Relation to sodium absorption, luminal sodium concentration and transepithelial voltage. *Am J Physiol* 10:F395, 1981.
321. Stokes JB et al: Heterogeneity of the rabbit collecting tubule: Localization of mineralocorticoid hormone action to the cortical portion. *Kidney Int* 20:340, 1981.
322. Stone DK et al: Anion dependence of rabbit medullary collecting duct acidification. *J Clin Invest* 71:1505, 1983.
323. Stone DK et al: Mineralocorticoid modulation of rabbit medullary collecting duct acidification: A sodium-independent effect. *J Clin Invest* 72:77, 1983.
324. Stone DK, Xie XS: Proton translocating ATPases. *Kidney Int* 33:767, 1988.
325. Stone DK et al: Structure of vacuolar proton pumps. *Semin Nephrol* 10:159, 1990.
326. Stoner LC et al: Ion transport in cortical collecting tubule: Effect of amiloride. *Am J Physiol* 227:453, 1974.
327. Swingle WW, Swingle AJ: Effect of adrenal steroids upon plasma volume of intact and adrenalectomized dogs. *Proc Soc Exp Biol Med* 119:452, 1965.
328. Szerlip HM et al: Aldosterone-induced proteins: Purification and localization of GP65,70. *Am J Physiol* 256:C865, 1989.
329. Tannen RL:Relationship of renal ammonia production and potassium homeostasis. *Kidney Int* 11:453, 1977.

330. Taylor RE Jr et al: Specificity of the effects of osmolality on aldosterone secretion. *Am J Physiol* 252:E118, 1987.
331. Terada Y, Knepper MA: Na-K-ATPase activities in renal tubule segments of rat inner medulla. *Am J Physiol* 256:F218, 1989.
332. Toto RD: Metabolic acid-base disorders, in Kokko JP, Tannen RL (eds): *Fluids and Electrolytes*, 2d ed. Philadelphia, Saunders, 1990, p 301.
333. Truscello A et al: Effects of butyrate on histone deacetylation and aldosterone-dependent Na-transport in the toad bladder. *J Biol Chem* 258:3388, 1983.
334. Truscello A et al: Thyroid hormone antagonizes an aldosterone-induced protein: A candidate mediator for the late mineral corticoid response. *J Membr Biol* 89:173, 1986.
335. Turnamian SG, Binder HJ: Regulation of active sodium and potassium transport in the distal colon of the rat: Role of aldosterone and glucocorticoid receptors. *J Clin Invest* 84:1924, 1989.
336. Ufferman R, Schrier RW: Importance of sodium intake and mineralocorticoid hormone in the impaired water excretion of adrenal insufficiency. *J Clin Invest* 51:1639, 1972.
337. Uhlich E et al: Einfluss von Aldosteron auf den Natriumtransport in den Sammelrohren der Saugetierniere. *Pfluegers Arch* 308:111, 1969.
338. Uhlich E et al: Einfluss von Aldosteron auf den Ausstrom markierten Natriums aus den Sammelrohren der Ratte. *Pfluegers Arch* 320:261, 1970.
339. Ullian ME, Linas SL: Effect of aldosterone on angiotensin II receptor function in rat cultured vascular smooth muscle cells (abstract). *Kidney Int* 37:359, 1990.
340. Ullrick WC, Hazlewood RL: Influence of aldosterone on isometric tension development in the rat heart. *Am J Physiol* 204:1001, 1963.
341. Unwin R et al: Effect of adrenal steroids on loop of Henle bicarbonate transport (abstract). *Kidney Int* 37:548, 1990.
342. Verrey F et al: Regulation by aldosterone of Na-K-ATPase in RNAs, protein synthesis and sodium transport in cultured kidney cells. *J Cell Biol* 104:1231, 1987.
343. Verrey F et al: Aldosterone induces a rapid increase in the rate of Na, K-ATPase gene transcription in cultured kidney cells. *Mol Endocrinol* 3:1369, 1989.
344. Wade JB: Hormonal modulation of epithelial structure, in Boulpaep E (ed): *Current Topics in Membranes and Transport.* New York, Academic Press, 1980, vol 13, p 123.
345. Wambach G et al: Na-K pump activity in erythrocytes of patients with endogenous and exogenous glucocorticoid excess. *Cardiology* 72(suppl 1):95, 1985.
346. Webel ML: Effects of a large dose of methylprednisone on renal function. *J Lab Clin Med* 80:765, 1972.
347. Webster NJG et al: The hormone-binding domains of the estrogen and glucocorticoid receptors contain an inducible transcription activation function. *Cell* 54:199, 1988.
348. Weinberger C et al: Domain structure of human glucocorticoid receptor and its relationship to the V-erbA oncogene product. *Nature (London)* 318:670, 1985.
349. Welbourn RB: Endocrine causes of diarrhea. *Proc Soc Med* 56:1080, 1963.
350. Welbourne TC: Acidosis activation of the pituitary adrenal renal glutaminase I axis. *Endocrinology* 99:1071, 1976.
351. Welbourne TC et al: Trimacinolone activation of renal ammonia production. *Proc Soc Exp Biol Med* 153:539, 1976.
352. Welbourne TC, Francoeur D: Influence of aldosterone on renal ammonia production. *Am J Physiol* 233:E56, 1977.
353. Welbourne TC: Glucocorticoid control of ammoniagenesis in the proximal tubule. *Semin Nephrol* 10:339, 1990.
354. Whitworth JA: Mechanisms of glucocorticoid-induced hypertension. *Kidney Int* 31:1213, 1987.
355. Weiderholt M et al: Effect of aldosterone on sodium and potassium transport in the kidney. *J Steroid Biochem* 3:151, 1972.
356. Weiderholt M et al: Mechanism of action of aldosterone on potassium transfer in the rat kidney. *Pfluegers Arch* 345:159, 1973.
357. Weismann WP: Aldosterone-stimulated transmethylations are linked to sodium transport. *Am J Physiol* 248:F43, 1985.
358. Wilcox CS et al: Differential effects of acute mineralo- and glucocorticoid administration on renal acid elimination. *Kidney Int* 21:546, 1982.
359. Will PC et al: Induction of amiloride sensitive sodium transport in rat colon by mineralocorticoids. *Am J Physiol* 238:F261, 1980.
360. Will PC et al: Induction of amiloride-sensitive sodium transport in the intestines by adrenal steroids. *Proc N Y Acad Sci* 372:64, 1981.
361. Will PC et al: Regulation of amiloride-sensitive electrogenic sodium transport in the rat colon by steroid hormones. *Am J Physiol* 248:G124, 1985.
362. Willson PM, Sunderman FW: Studies in serum electrolytes: 12. The effect of water restriction in a patient with Addison's disease receiving sodium chloride. *J Clin Invest* 18:35, 1939.
363. Wingo CS: Effect of ouabain on K secretion in cortical collecting tubules from adrenalectromized rabbits. *Am J Physiol* 247:F588, 1984.
363a. Yang-Yen H-F et al: Transcriptional interference between c-jun and the glucocorticoid receptor: Mutual inhibition of DNA binding due to direct protein-protein interaction. *Cell* 62:1205, 1990.
363b. Yau JLW et al: 11β-hydroxysteroid dehydrogenase mRNA expression in rat kidney. *Am J Physiol* 260:F764, 1991.
364. Yoshimura H et al: Study on the mechanism of acid and ammonia excretion by the kidney after acid load. *Jpn J Physiol* 21:143, 1962.
365. Young DB, Guyton AC: Steady-state aldosterone dose-response relationships. *Circ Res* 40:138, 1977.
366. Young DB, Paulsen AW: Interrelated effects of aldosterone and plasma potassium on potassium excretion. *Am J Physiol* 244:F28, 1983.

367. Young DB et al: Multiplicative interaction between angiotensin II and K^+ concentration in stimulation of aldosterone. *Am J Physiol* 247:E328, 1984.
368. Zimmerman G, Fleischer N: Role of calcium ions in the release of ACTH from rat pituitary tissue in vitro. *Endocrinology* 87:426, 1970.
369. Zimmerman RS et al: Atrial natriuretic peptide during mineralocorticoid escape in the human. *J Clin Endocrinol Metab* 64:624, 1987.
370. Zipser RD et al: Characteristics of aldosterone binding in human plasma. *J Clin Endocrinol Metab* 50:158, 1980.
371. Zusman RM et al: Effect of adrenal steroids on ADH-stimulated PGE synthesis and water flow. *Am J Physiol* 234:F532, 1978.

CHAPTER • 15

Renal prostaglandins and kinins

Kamal F. Badr • Barry M. Brenner

RENAL PROSTAGLANDINS

Prostaglandins (PGs) influence a variety of physiologic processes in the mammalian kidney. By their direct action and by modulation of the action of other hormones, PGs participate in the regulation of renal blood flow; glomerular filtration rate (GFR); and the urinary excretion of acid, electrolytes, and water. Knowledge of these regulatory functions has led to a broadened understanding of the biochemical effects of hormones on the kidney. From a pathophysiologic point of view, the potentially detrimental effects on renal function of the many drugs commonly used to inhibit PG synthesis are now better comprehended. In addition, derangements in PG metabolism have been implicated in an increasing number of disease states.

This chapter summarizes current knowledge of the biochemistry, physiology, and pathophysiology of the renal PGs.

BIOSYNTHESIS AND METABOLISM

Overview of renal PG synthesis

Since PGs are not stored in tissues, their biologic action must be immediately preceded by de novo synthesis. Furthermore, ambient tissue concentrations of PGs are determined not only by the rate of synthesis but also by the rate and routes of catabolism. Since virtually all experimental work has demonstrated that PGs are locally active, not circulating, hormones, it is the PGs synthesized within the kidney that are believed to affect renal function. Therefore, the actions of PGs in the kidney are regulated by changes in intrarenal production and degradation.

PGs are derived from unsaturated 20-carbon fatty acids, the most abundant of which is arachidonic acid (AA; 5,8,11,14-eicosatetraenoic acid; C20:4; Fig. 15-1). AA is a polyunsaturated fatty acid with 20 carbon atoms and 4 double bonds (C20:4) that is formed in the liver via elongation and desaturation of its precursor, linoleic acid (C18:2). The latter is an essential fatty acid (EFA) ingested at the rate of approximately 10 g/day in adults, of which only about 1 mg/day is eliminated as an end product of AA metabolism.[208,379,380] The latter gives rise to PGs of the dienoic series, indicated by the subscript 2 in the abbreviation (e.g. PGE_2). The triene (C20:3) and pentaene (C20:5) analogues of AA (which yield PGE_1 and PGE_3, respectively) do not exist in significant quantities within the kidney.

Following stimuli that lead to the activation of cellular phospholipases (PLs), principally phospholipase A_2 (PLA_2) and phospholipase C (PLC), membrane-bound AA undergoes esterolytic cleavage, yielding free AA, a rate-limiting step in its subsequent metabolism into biologically relevant end products.[34,86,89,135,143,244,470] In the case of PLA_2 activation, a reaction probably involving activation of guanine nucleotide-binding (G) proteins, AA is released directly from membrane phospholipids.[132] Activation of PLC, on the other hand, probably involves release of AA from diacylglycerol (DAG) via the sequential activation of DAG lipase. DAG is itself formed as a result of PLC-mediated breakdown of membrane-bound phosphatidylinositol-bisphosphate (PIP_2).[39,41,85,141,343,413] In cells of glomerular mesangial origin[276,392] and early passage proximal tubule cells in culture,[470] PLA_2-mediated AA release appears to be the preferred mechanism. Following deesterification, free AA becomes a possible substrate for one of three major enzymatic transformations the common result of which is the incorporation of oxygen atoms at various sites of the fatty acid backbone, with accompanying changes in its molecular structure (such as ring formation). This process results in the formation of biologically active molecules, often referred to as eicosanoids. The specific nature of the products generated is a function of the initial stimuli for AA release as well as the cell types involved.[86,201,206,303,386,390,393,394,470] These products will, in turn, either *mediate* or *modulate* the biological actions of the agonist in question. All three enzymatic pathways of AA metabo-

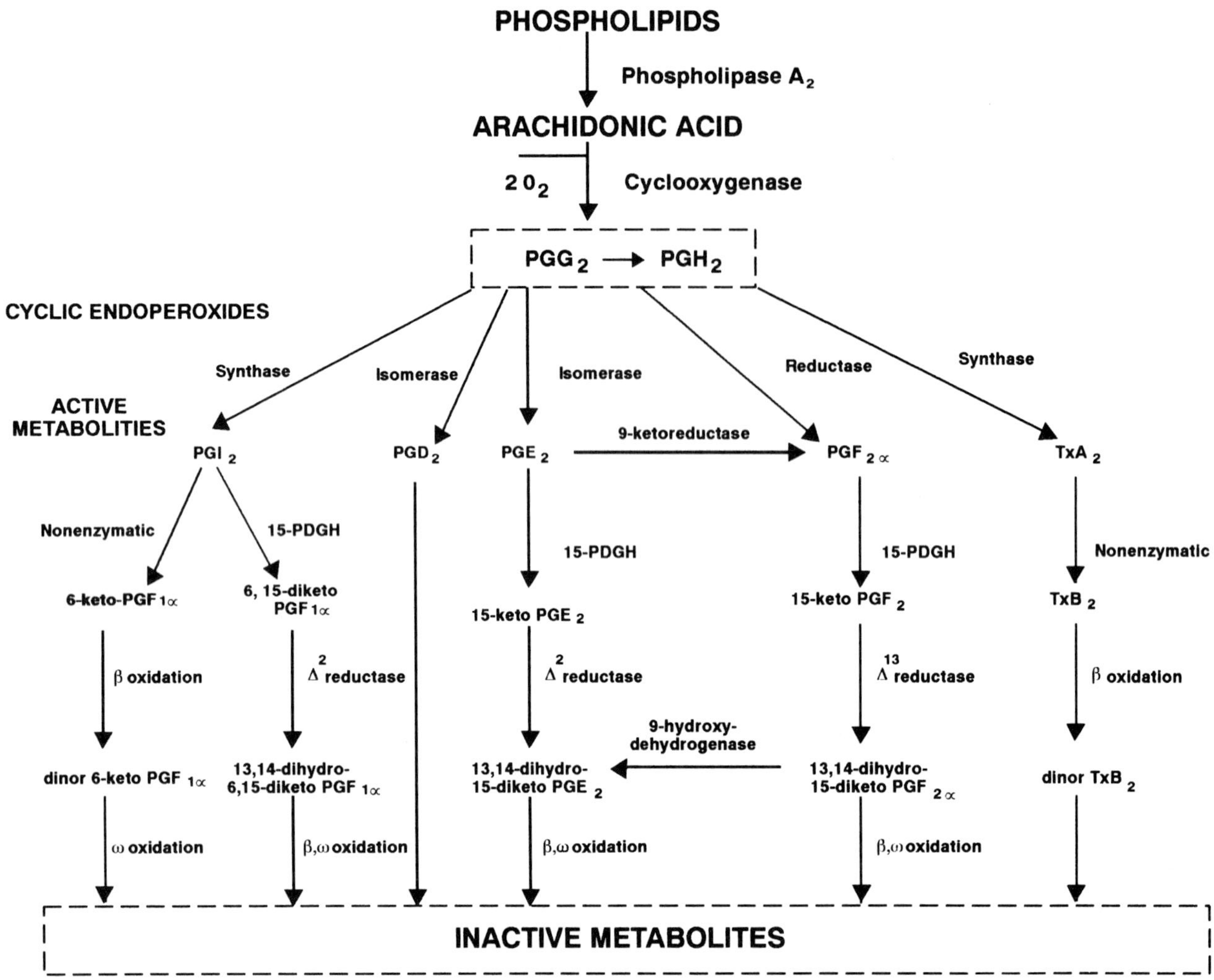

FIGURE 15-1 • Cyclooxygenase pathway reactions.

lism are present in the kidney: the cyclooxygenase pathway, leading to the formation of PGs and thromboxanes; the lipoxygenase pathway, leading to the formation of mono-, di-, and trihydroxy eicosatetraenoic acids (HETEs) and leukotrienes (LTs); and the cytochrome P-450-mediated oxygenation of AA, leading to the formation of epoxyeicosatrienoic acids (EETs), their corresponding diols, HETEs, and monooxygenated AA derivatives.

Molecular oxygen is added to free AA by the action of the enzyme cyclooxygenase, yielding the first of the unstable endoperoxide intermediates, PGG_2 (Fig. 15-1). The enzyme is a 72-kilodalton protein present in endoplasmic, nuclear, and possibly mitochondrial membranes;[377] in arterial and arteriolar endothelial cells,[383,390] mesangial cells,[11,133,161,386,392,395,414,452] glomerular epithelial cells,[414] and renal interstitial cells;[50,498,500] and along most segments of the tubule, although in markedly varying concentrations.[3,47,95,213,330,391,396,398,424,455,487] The second enzyme of the cyclooxygenase complex is a peroxidase that converts PGG_2 to PGH_2.[181] These short-lived compounds can exert constrictor effects on the renal vasculature,[334,450] but whether these transient metabolic species exist in sufficient concentrations to influence the intact kidney is controversial. At physiologic pH, PGH_2 undergoes spontaneous hydrolysis to a mixture of PGE_2, $PGE_{2\alpha}$, and PGD_2.[437] More important, however, are specific enzymes that convert PGH_2 to PGE_2, PGI_2 (prostacyclin), and the closely related thromboxane A_2 (TXA_2). A specific PGD_2 isomerase has been described in some tissues, although not in kidney; renal PGD_2 synthesis appears to be nominal compared to that of the other PGs. Thromboxane synthetase is active in normal renal tissue at low levels. Renal thromboxane generation increases dramatically, however, under certain pathologic conditions (see below).

Regulation of renal PG synthesis

PL-mediated release of AA appears to be the rate-limiting step in PG biosynthesis. Not all arachidonate associated with membrane phospholipids is equivalent. Rather, there appear to be at least two distinct pools of AA; they have been referred to as the *hormone-specific pool* and the *nonspecific pool.*[119,402] Those hormones that can sharply increase renal PG synthesis, of which the best studied are bradykinin, arginine vasopressin (AVP), and angiotensin II (AII), stimulate PL activity and thereby the release of AA.[34,110,193,194,289,290,321,401,499] The fatty acid released from the hormone-specific pool is tightly coupled to cyclooxygenase, such that a large percentage is ultimately converted to PGs.[194] Release of arachidonate from the nonspecific pool can be triggered in vivo by ischemia and in vitro by the calcium ionophore A23187. This pool of arachidonate is less tightly coupled to cyclooxygenase, so that even though these stimuli increase PG synthesis, a much larger fraction of the released arachidonate is reincorporated into the membrane or perhaps metabolized by the lipoxygenase system.[119,193] Furthermore, this nonspecific pool is less specific for AA release and can lead to the liberation of fatty acids that are not PG precursors.[194]

Although AA release is the most important and best-studied determinant of transient changes of PG synthesis in response to discrete manipulations, more distal components of the synthetic pathway are also subject to regulation. Certain persistent (i.e., lasting for several hours or days) stimuli, such as ureteral occlusion[415] or the hormones bradykinin[321] and AVP[24] increase renal cyclooxygenase activity. It is interesting to note that the latter two hormones also can abruptly stimulate PL activity. The vasoconstrictor conformation of the AVP molecule has been shown to be related to stimulation of the PL activity,[32,494,495] whereas prolonged administration of a pure antidiuretic analogue enhances cyclooxygenase activity.[33] Similarly, ureteral obstruction not only increases cyclooxygenase activity but also selectively enhances TXA_2 generation, suggesting that specific stimulation of the enzyme thromboxane synthetase occurs.[305] Although the regulation of both PGE_2 insomerase and PGI_2 synthetase has not been studied in any detail in vivo, certain in vitro regulatory factors have been identified. For example, reduced glutathione strongly stimulates PGE_2 synthesis,[320,409] whereas hydroperoxy fatty acids (products of the lipoxygenase pathway) inhibit prostacyclin generation.[175] The physiologic role of these various factors is unclear.

Effects of dietary manipulations

EFA deficiency, which selectively depletes the hormone-responsive phosphatidylinositol pool of AA, markedly blunts its intracellular availability in response to hormonal stimulation and thereby abrogates hormone-induced eicosanoid release.[247,248,250] Fish oil diets, rich in ω-3 polyunsaturated fatty acids (in which the double bond farthest from the carboxyl group is three carbons away from the terminal, or ω carbon atom; AA is thus an ω-6 fatty acid) will result in competition by these substrates for AA oxygenation pathways, resulting in the formation of biologically inactive end products.[217] Steroid administration, on the other hand, exerts an opposing effect in the kidney,[120-122] which may explain the increased urinary excretion and glomerular synthesis of AA metabolites following dexamethasone treatment despite the known inhibitory effects of corticosteroids on phospholipase activity.

Sources and nephronal distribution of cycloxygenase products

AA metabolites exert biological actions on renal cells due to their local release in discrete anatomical microenvironments along the nephron (e.g., glomerulus, proximal tubule, collecting tubule, etc.). Such release may occur either from cells indigenous to that nephron segment (autocrine/paracrine actions) or from infiltrating cells of nonrenal origin, such as leukocytes or platelets during inflammatory reactions. To assess cyclooxygenase activity in the kidney, investigators have utilized bioanalytic techniques such as radioimmunoassay (RIA), enzyme-linked RIA, high-pressure liquid chromatography (HPLC), and gas chromatography/mass spectrometry (GC/MS), as applied either to whole kidney effluents, tissue slice incubates from various anatomic sections, microdissected or isolated glomeruli and tubule segments, and freshly isolated or cultured renal cells.[3,47,95,213,330,391,396,398,424,455,487] In addition, histochemical, immunohistochemical, and immunofluorescence techniques have been employed to define the distribution of cyclooxygenase pathway enzymes such as cyclooxygenase,[303] endoperoxide synthase,[161,487] and PGI_2 synthase.[161] In general, these approaches have yielded consistent results, although differences in relative generation rates among the various metabolites in the same nephron segments have been reported.[47] These differences are probably due to interspecies variations and to the lack of sensitivity of some of the earlier methodologies. Herein follows a general description of the cyclooxygenase products generated along the various segments of the nephron.

GLOMERULUS Glomeruli can be isolated either by differential sieving or by microdissection. The differential sieving method may subject glomeruli to hypoxic injury, but recent modifications have improved cell viability in this preparation.[250] Cyclooxygenase activity is present in arterial and arteriolar endothelial cells, including glomerular afferent and efferent arterioles.[447] The predominant metabolite from these vascular endothelial cells is PGI_2.[447] Whole glomeruli generate PGE_2, PGI_2, $PGF_{2\alpha}$ and TXA_2.[26,125,178,391,424,455] The predominant product in the rat and in the rabbit is PGE_2, followed by PGI_2 and $PGF_2\alpha$ and finally TXA_2.[26,125,178,391,424,455] Quan-

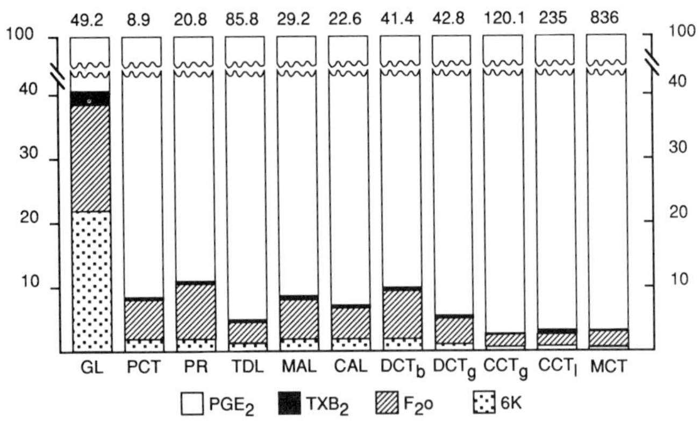

FIGURE 15-2 • Percent contribution of PGE_2, TXB_2, $PGF_{2}\alpha$, and 6-keto $PGF_{1}\alpha$ (6K) to prostanoid synthesis in rabbit nephron. Total synthesis in picograms per half-hour per millimeter of tubule length is given above each bar. GL, glomerulus; PCT, proximal convoluted tubule; PR, pars recta; TDL, thin descending limb; MAL, medullary ascending limb; CAL, cortical ascending limb; DCTb, bright portion of distal tubule; DCT, granular portion of distal tubule; CCTg, granular cortical collecting tubule; CCTl, light CCT; MCT, medullary collecting tubule. (From Farman N et al: *Am J Physiol* 252:F53, 1987. Used by permission.)

titative analysis of these eicosanoids in the glomerulus has been controversial, but the results of a recent study by Farman and coworkers utilizing microdissected rabbit nephrons and a highly sensitive enzyme-linked RIA are depicted in Fig. 15-2 and are, in general, consistent with previously published data in the rat.[125] In human[424] and pig[264] glomeruli, the predominant metabolite appears to be PGI_2, rather than PGE_2, as seen in the rat and rabbit. In the pig, glomerular $PGF_{2\alpha}$ synthesis exceeds that of PGE_2 and TXA_2.[264] In dog cortical slices, PGI_2 production also appears to exceed that of PGE_2 and $PGF_{2\alpha}$,[330] and in isolated dog glomerular preparations, PGI_2 release in response to exogenous AA is dose-dependent and correlates more closely with physiologically relevant responses, such as renin release, than does that of PGE_2.[398]

Analysis of individual glomerular cell subpopulations has provided insight into the intraglomerular localization of prostanoid synthesis. Cultured *mesangial cells* of the smooth muscle-containing variety from rat and human sources are capable of generating PGE_2.[2,232,270,275,378,386,392,394,395,412,452] Human mesangial cells are also capable of producing $PGF_{2\alpha}$ and PGI_2[11] and, when stained by immunofluorescence techniques in biopsy, nephrectomy, and necropsy specimens, are positive for PG endoperoxide synthase and prostacyclin synthase.[161] The latter also stains intensely in peritubular capillaries and their adjacent interstitial cells.[161] Recent attention has focused on the eicosanoid-generating capacity of glomerular tissue macrophages, initially described by Schreiner and colleagues,[397] also localized in the mesangium but derived from the bone marrow and bearing Ia determinants on their surface. These glomerular macrophages, which normally constitute less than 5 percent of the glomerular cell population, increase markedly in response to such specific stimuli as circulating macromolecules, immune complexes, and endotoxin. These cells have been repeatedly proposed as a potential source for the intraglomerular release of eicosanoids, particularly in the absence of an overt inflammatory lesion.[16,249,397] That such release is indeed relevant has been confirmed recently by depleting normal rat glomeruli of macrophages consequent to the induction of fatty acid deficiency.[249,250] In these animals, severe blunting of hormone-stimulated glomerular eicosanoid-generating potential was documented in vitro.

Glomerular *epithelial cells* also appear to participate in PG synthesis, but the profile of cyclooxygenase products generated in these cells remains controversial. While some authors find a pattern of PG production in rat glomerular epithelial cells that is similar to that of mesangial cells ($PGE_2 > PGF_{2\alpha} > PGI_2 = TXA_2$), others have found a predominance of PGI_2 in the same cells.[390] Glomerular capillary *endothelial cell* PG generation profiles remain undefined.

TUBULE Figure 15-2 depicts the synthesis of PG metabolites along the rabbit tubule. Clearly, the predominant synthetic site is in the collecting tubule (CT), particularly its medullary portion (MCT). This pattern has also been observed by other investigators, utilizing a host of analytic techniques, in a variety of species.[11,47,161,303,330,390,398,487] As seen in Fig. 15-2, PGE_2 is the predominant PG formed in the tubule, the variations among the other products being insignificant.[125] Within the microdissected CT, Schlondorff and associates[396] have observed regional heterogeneity, with the MCT and nonbranched cortical CTs producing significantly greater amounts of PGE_2 than branched cortical CTs. PGE_2 is also the major cyclooxygenase metabolite generated in *medullary interstitial cells*.[280]

Renal PG catabolism

The ambient concentration of a substance within a given organ is determined not only by its rate of synthesis but also by its rate of degradation. Certain prostanoids are intrinsically unstable. The vasodilator PGI_2 undergoes spontaneous hydrolysis to 6-keto-$PGF_{1\alpha}$, with a half-life at 37° C of 2 to 4 min, whereas the vasoconstrictor TXA_2 degrades spontaneously to TXB_2, with a half-life of 30 s.[379] Neither of these hydrolysis products possesses biological activity, but the assays for 6-keto-$PGF_{1\alpha}$ and TXB_2 are useful determinants of the synthetic rates of their respective parent compounds.

The initial step in the enzymatic degradation of PGE_2 and $PGE_{2\alpha}$ is catalyzed by PG dehydrogenase (PGDH).[177,303,390,418,453] Two forms of this enzyme exist in kidney. Type I PGDH is confined to the renal cortex. It is highly specific for the 15-hydroxy group common to all PGs and requires NAD^+ as a cofactor.[240,241,481] The enzyme catalyzes the formation of the inactive 15-keto PGs. Type II PGDH is found in both renal cortex and medulla and uses $NADP^+/NADPH$ as a cofactor. This relatively nonspecific enzyme catalyzes the reversible interconversion of hydroxyl and keto groups at the C-9 and C-15 positions.[65,236] The most abundant product of the isomerism is also the appropriate 15-keto PG. It now appears that two enzymes previously described as separate, 9-ketoreductase and $NADP^+$-dependent 15-hydroxy PGDH, are associated with a single protein. In association with the type I PGDH, the enzyme Δ^{13}-reductase reduces the Δ^{13} double bond of a 15-keto PG irreversibly, giving rise to the 13,14-dihydro-15-keto PG. The cofactor can be either NADH or NADPH.

Beyond these relatively specific steps in the catabolism of PGs, the products undergo beta oxidation, the sequential removal of two or four carbon atoms from the carboxyl terminus, giving rise to the dinor and tetranor products.[247] In addition, kidney cortex contains an ω and ω-1 hydroxylation system, which adds OH groups to the aliphatic terminus of the molecule.[356] Both beta oxidation and omega hydroxylation are nonspecific processes in the catabolism of fatty acids. Another PG-specific enzyme is a separate 9-hydroxy PGDH. This enzyme oxidizes the biologically inactive hydrolysis product of PGI_2, 6-keto $PGF_{1\alpha}$, to 6-keto PGE_1.[180,478] The latter compound has been shown to possess vasodilatory activity comparable to that of authentic PGI_2.[362]

Physiologically relevant transformations of cyclooxygenase products in the kidney include the NADPH-dependent 9-ketoreductase reaction, which converts PGE_2 into $PGF_{2\alpha}$, a biologically active compound.[296] This enzymatic activity is detectable in homogenates from cortex, medulla, or papilla but is particularly enriched in suspensions from the thick ascending limb of Henle (TALH).[296] This reaction and the documented conversion of PGD_2 into an apparently biologically active metabolite (9α, 11b-PGF2α)[263] may significantly contribute to the measurements of urinary $PGF_{2\alpha}$ in response to exogenously administered agonists or to other experimental manipulations. One could therefore erroneously conclude that the renal responses observed under these conditions were due to $PGF_{2\alpha}$.

Other key aspects of renal PG metabolism include the occurrence of an epoxidation pathway for the metabolism of PGI_2, leading to the formation of 5-hydroxy-6-keto $PGF_{1\alpha}$,[479] and the occurrence of an unusual PGF_2 metabolite (9,15-dioxo,11-hydroxyprost-5,13-dienoic acid) under conditions of low enzyme-to-substrate ratio.[304] A high-salt diet augments 9α-reductase activity,[469] while hyperthyroidism inhibits the activity of PGDH.[302]

Renal receptors and intracellular signals for cyclooxygenase metabolites

Of the cyclooxygenase metabolites known to exert biological effects in the kidney, only the PGE_2 receptor has been sufficiently characterized to warrant consideration. Limas and Limas reported the presence of receptors for PGE_2 in 1984 using radioligand binding and microdissection techniques.[259] They found the greatest concentration of PGE_2 receptors in the outer medulla, with lesser degrees of binding in the inner medulla and cortex. Receptor density for PGE_2 was calculated at 2.12 pmol/mg, compared to 0.44 for $PGF_{2\alpha}$ and 1.12 for PGE_1. In subsequent studies, the same investigators demonstrated down-regulation of the PGE_2 receptor by endogenously generated or exogenously added homoligand, likely mediated through a reversible cycling mechanism.[261] Despite predominance of the PGE_2 receptor density in the outer medulla, inhibition of endogenous synthesis by indomethacin reveals binding in virtually all nephron segments, as demonstrated by Eriksen and coworkers using radiohistochemical techniques.[118] In these studies, the authors, using nonlinear direct binding plots and linear regression data as applied to binding of 3H-PGE_2 to rat kidney cryostate sections, estimated a binding density (B_{max}) of 2.1 to 3.2 fmol/cm^2, a Hill coefficient of 1.0, and a dissociation constant (K_d) ranging from 1.4 to 3.3 n*M*.[118]

Attempts at biochemical characterization of the PGE_2 receptor have yielded important information regarding the mechanism of action of this eicosanoid in the kidney. Using membranes from canine renal outer medulla, Watanabe and colleagues detected specific, reversible, high-affinity (K_d = 20 n*M*) and protein-dependent binding of PGE_2 to a single class of receptors.[467] Solubilization and biochemical characterization of the binding activity revealed association of the PGE_2 receptor to a pertussis toxin-sensitive guanine nucleotide regulatory protein (N_i; see "Water Transport," below).

In addition to the renal medulla, PGE_2 binding has also been characterized in isolated rat glomeruli, where radioligand binding revealed the presence of specific binding sites with a K_d of 14.3 n*M* and a B_{max} of 81.4 fmol/mg protein.[70] The rank order of other eicosanoids by potency of specific binding inhibition was $PGE_1 = PGE_2 >> TXB_2 = PGD_2 >> PGF_{2\alpha} >$ 6-keto $PGF_{1\alpha}$.[70] Rat mesangial cell responses to PGE_2, as well as to $PGF_{2\alpha}$ and the TXA_2 endoperoxide analogue U-46619, were described by Mene and associates.[293] All three agonists were found to induce rapid and dose-dependent increases in intracellular free Ca^{2+} concentrations, which, in the case of U-46619, were abolished by a TXA_2 receptor antagonist. In addition, these eicosanoids all effected an increase in cellular accumulation of total inositol phosphates, suggesting the involvement of PLC in the mediation of their biological effects in mesangial cells.

Stimuli for renal generation of cyclooxygenase products

The generation and local release of AA cyclooxygenase products in various segments of the nephron can result from a variety of hormonal, chemical, or physical stimuli. AII-mediated PG release is best characterized with respect to cellular mechanisms and physiologic importance. In mesangial cells and whole glomeruli, activation of AII receptors is coupled to a PLC-dependent increase in intracellular Ca^{2+} concentration, which in turn results in PLA_2 activation and AA release from membrane phosphoinositol lipids.[250,386,391-393,395,402,424,455] A similar mechanism occurs in AVP-mediated PG generation in these tissues.[275,386]

Biological actions of cyclooxygenase products in the kidney

A principal role of cyclooxygenase products of AA metabolism in renal physiology is their mediation and/or modulation of the actions of other hormones or autacoids, in particular with regard to the physiologic actions of these hormones or autacoids on renal vascular tone, mesangial and glomerular functions, and the handling of salt and water. Inhibition of cyclooxygenase activity in the absence of exogenous administration or endogenous release of hormones such as AII or AVP has little effect on renal functional parameters.[310,492] Once their local release is stimulated by exogenous or endogenous hormones or autacoids, cyclooxygenase products may themselves stimulate the local generation of other hormones. PG-stimulated renin release is an example of this mode of action.[133] It is important to note that under *pathophysiologic* conditions such as inflammatory injury, *excessive* local release of cyclooxygenase products, whether by resident renal cells or by infiltrating cellular elements, may mediate the functional derangements that characterize such conditions (see below). TXA_2-mediated renal vasoconstriction during obstructive injury is a case in point.[5,267]

Effects on vascular smooth muscle and mesangial cell function

A large body of experimental evidence clearly divides cyclooxygenase products into smooth muscle relaxants (PGE_2 and PGI_2) and smooth muscle constrictors (TXA_2 and $PGF_{2\alpha}$). The renal vasculature is no exception, although these responses there do appear to have some species-specific characteristics. For example, PGE_2 relaxes rat and rabbit afferent arterioles.[114] PGI_2, a potent vasodilator in humans, appears to have little intrinsic vasoactive effect in the rat kidney[488] but is a highly potent relaxant of rabbit afferent, efferent, and interlobular arteriolar smooth muscle[114] and is a vasodilator in the dog.[46,153,179] $PGF_{2\alpha}$ is without effect on any arterial segment in the rabbit kidney[114] but is a mild vasoconstrictor in the dog.[153,179] TXA_2 analogues exert constrictor effects on rat arteriolar smooth muscle, but no micropuncture measurements are available to exactly define the effector locus of these effects. However, administration of a TXA_2-like stable PGH_2 analogue, U-44069, to the isolated perfused rat kidney results in renal vasoconstriction accompanied by a severe reduction in filtration fraction, suggesting a predominantly preglomerular action.[268]

The contribution of these vasoactive properties of cyclooxygenase products to the regulation of renal vascular tone under normal conditions is probably minimal.[310,492] Inhibition of cyclooxygenase activity[492] or selective antagonism of TXA_2 synthesis[310] or actions[29] does not result in any change in renal vascular resistance in the conscious or anesthetized euvolemic male rat[310] or in humans.[492] However, inhibition of cyclooxygenase in the anesthetized female rat leads to augmentation of the GFR and relaxation of afferent and efferent arterioles.[310] This response is not observed in conscious female rats; ovariectomized, anesthetized female rats; or male rats. The involvement of cyclooxygenase products in the regulation of renal vascular tone is thus a peculiarity of the anesthetized female rat, and its mechanism remains undefined.

Mesangial cell synthesis and release of PGE_2 and PGI_2 clearly modulate the constrictor actions of AII, norepinephrine, and AVP[239,288,349,385,386,390,392,458] in these cells. In the presence of cyclooxygenase inhibitors, the mesangial cell and glomerular constrictor actions of these hormones are markedly enhanced.[385,386,390,392] These in vitro studies have been confirmed by in vivo experiments demonstrating that the reductions in renal blood flow and in the glomerular capillary ultrafiltration coefficient (K_f) in response to the exogenous administration of these hormones is also accentuated in the presence of cyclooxygenase inhibitors.[31,160,464,486] The PG endoperoxide analogue U-44069 is a potent mesangial cell constrictor, and its addition to cultured mesangial cells is also associated with dose-dependent stimulation of PGE_2 release from these cells,[294] thereby extending the counter-regulatory role of mesangial cell PGE_2 release to the modulation of eicosanoid-induced contractions. In addition to their effects on mesangial cells smooth muscle tone and adherence properties, PGs exert other effects on mesangial cell function, including inhibition of their proliferation in response to mitogenic stimuli.[192]

The release of vasodilator PGs (PGE_2 and PGI_2) in response to renal vasoconstrictors such as AII, AVP, norepinephrine, platelet-activating factor (PAF), and serotonin is a highly relevant biological response with important consequences with regard to the preservation of renal perfusion under conditions in which the local or systemic relese of these agents is enhanced.[31,133,160,161,464,484] Numerous experimental and clinical studies have established that the vasodilatory action of PGs on the afferent arteriole serves to maintain renal vascular resistance at a relatively low value compared to that of the systemic vasculature in the face of elevated levels of AII and/or enhanced sympathoadrenal activity. This results in the preservation of renal blood flow and GFR during congestive heart failure and intravascular volume depletion[17] or during exogenous administration of AII[31,160] and AVP.[464,484] Inhibition of PG generation in these and other conditions may result in acute renal insufficiency.[17] Vasodilator PGs, particularly PGI_2, may also counteract the vasoconstrictor responses to calcium in humans.[315]

In addition to modulating the actions of vasoconstrictors, endogenous PGs also mediate the actions of some vasodilator agents. For example, PGI_2 mediates the vasorelaxant actions of dopamine[274] and magnesium[313] in humans and of hydralazine[340] and epidermal growth factor (EGF)[146] in dogs. In addition, PGs may mediate the renal vasodilatory response to a protein meal in humans.[457] Atrial natriuretic peptide, a known renal vasodilator, does not appear to invoke PG release in rat glomeruli.[181,375]

Effects on renin release

Extensive evidence in the whole animal, in isolated perfused kidney, and in isolated glomeruli, as well as in mesangial cells in culture, supports the capacity of PGs, particularly PGE_2 and PGI_2, to release renin.[21,37,68,100,138-140,142,154,182,234,262,408,438,473] PG-mediated renin release is independent of stretch receptors or beta-adrenergic mechanisms.[37,100,138,438] Renin release in response to renal nerve stimulation, however, is not enhanced by PG generation.[37,154,234,438] PG-mediated renin release may also mediate the canine vasodilator response to exogenously administered glucagon.[460]

Effects on salt and water transport

It is now well established that arachidonate metabolites of the cyclooxygenase pathway have important effects on salt and water transport in the kidney through direct actions on the epithelial cells that line the nephron. Thus, functional effects can be observed that are thought to be independent of any hemodynamic changes produced by these compounds.

Proximal tubule

Neither the proximal convoluted tubule nor the proximal straight tubule is a significant source of biologically active cyclooxygenase metabolites of AA.[51,63] When factored per millimeter of tubule length, the proximal convoluted tubule and pars recta of rabbit nephron produce 1/20 to 1/100 of the cyclooxygenase products produced by collecting duct segments.[47,125] Since oxygenated metabolites of AA function predominantly as autacoids, it is not surprising that very little evidence has accumulated to show that these metabolites exert functional effects on the tubule. Early whole animal studies suggested that infusion of PGE_2 in thyroparathyroidectomized rats blocks the phosphaturic action of parathyroid hormone (PTH).[136] More recently, PGE_2 has been shown to block the activation of adenyl cyclase by PTH, and, furthermore, this activation was attenuated by pretreatment with pertussis toxin.[107] Subsequent studies utilizing in vitro perfused proximal tubules showed that PGE_2 had no effect on sodium chloride or phosphate transport in the proximal convoluted tubule, whereas in the proximal straight tubule, high concentrations of PGE_2 had a mild effect on sodium chloride absorption and phosphate absorption, decreasing them by 33 and 12 percent respectively.[106] In vitro microperfusion studies with $PGF_{2\alpha}$ failed to show an effect on sodium chloride or phosphate transport.[106]

Loop of Henle

The nephron segments making up the loop of Henle also display limited metabolism of AA through the cyclooxygenase pathway.[47,125] No direct effects of cyclooxygenase metabolites on function of the thin limbs of Henle have been demonstrated. However, the thick ascending limb has recently been shown to exhibit PGE_2 receptors in high density.[118,259] In normal rat kidney, the greatest density of PGE_2 receptors was found in the medullary thick ascending limb, while some receptors were found in cortical thick ascending limbs.[118] However, after indomethacin pretreatment, there was a significant increase in receptor density in the inner medulla, probably representing the inner medullary collecting duct.[118] This is probably due to inhibition of endogenous PGE_2 production and thus a decrease in competition for receptor binding between exogenous and endogenous ligand. The possibility of up-regulation of inner medullary PG receptors also exists.

The observation of specific binding of PGE_2 on the medullary thick ascending limb is consistent with prior studies suggesting that PGE_2 inhibits sodium chloride absorption in this nephron segment.[434] In the medullary thick ascending limb of certain species, antidiuretic hormone (ADH) and cAMP stimulate sodium chloride absorption.[172,186,381] Indeed, the stimulatory effect of ADH is mediated through cAMP generation.[198] Subsequent to the demonstration that PGE_2 inhibits sodium chloride absorption in the medullary thick ascending limb of the rabbit perfused in vitro, it was shown that PGE_2 blocks ADH- but not cAMP-stimulated sodium chloride absorption in the medullary thick ascending limb of the mouse.[92] It is likely that the mechanism involves activation of G_i and inhibition of adenyl cyclase by PGE_2.[93] Such a mechanism is in keeping with the previously mentioned inhibition of cAMP generation in response to parathyroid hormone PTH in proximal tubules and the inhibition of ADH-induced cAMP generation in the collecting duct, which will be discussed later. The source of the PGE_2 that inhibits medullary thick ascending limb cell transport is unclear, if such an event occurs in vivo. This nephron segment has finite but limited PGE_2 production,[47,125] and its regulation by AVP is unexplored.

In contrast to the medullary portion of the thick ascending limb of Henle, there is much less evidence that cyclooxygenase products exert functional effects in the cortical thick ascending limb of Henle. This nephron segment exhibits the same low rates of synthesis of cyclooxygenase products[47,125] but in addition demonstrates small numbers of receptors.

Collecting duct system

In almost all mammalian species studied thus far, the collecting ducts are the major nephron segments responsible for PG synthesis.[47,125,199,205,225,396] Recent careful microdissection studies with segmental analysis of eicosanoid generation[47,125] have demonstrated that medullary collecting ducts produce greater amounts of cyclooxygenase products than do cortical collecting ducts. As with all other nephron segments, the predominant cyclooxygenase metabolite produced by collecting ducts is PGE_2, which accounts for more than 95 percent of the cyclooxygenase products, followed by $PGF_{2\alpha}$, which accounts for less than 5 percent.[47,125] In keeping with the concept that these metabolites behave predominantly as autacoids, the majority of receptors for PGE_2 in the kidney are found on collecting ducts (also thick ascending limbs, as mentioned above).[118] In addition, this distribution of PGE_2 production is predominantly localized to the collecting duct in the outer and inner medulla.[118]

Solute transport

Infusion of AA or the cyclooxygenase products PGE_2 or PGI_2 directly into the renal artery results in natriuresis.[45,166,199,205,209,225,227,344,431,442,463] While hemodynamic changes probably contribute to this effect, studies confirm that the proximal tubule is not the locus of action.[145,190,425] Similarly, sodium delivery to the early distal tubule was not increased,[145] suggesting that the natriuresis originates either from the deep nephrons or distal to the surface distal tubule (i.e., the collecting ducts).[147,228,229] That PGE_2 can inhibit sodium transport in the collecting ducts was confirmed by in vitro perfusion studies of rabbit cortical collecting tubule.[197,434] Effects of PGE_2 on outer and inner collecting duct segments have also been described, with the lack of an effect on the former[129] and possibly an effect on the latter, since inhibition of cyclooxygenase appears to enhance salt reabsorption in the papillary collecting duct.[474] It should be noted that in studies on the in vitro perfused rat cortical collecting tubule, PGE_2 had no effect on sodium transport.[187]

This discrepancy in the observed effect of PGE_2 on the isolated cortical collecting duct of the rat versus that of the rabbit leaves some uncertainty regarding the effect of PGE_2 on sodium transport in the human cortical collecting duct. In spite of this, it is relevant to ask what mechanism PGE_2 exerts its inhibitory effect on sodium transport. In the rabbit cortical collecting duct, inhibition of sodium transport is paralleled by a major reduction in lumen negative transepithelial voltage.[197,434] Sodium transport in the cortical collecting duct is electrogenic and proceeds through the principal cell. Sodium enters the cell through the apical membrane via a conductive sodium channel and exits across the basolateral membrane through the electrogenic Na^+-K^+ ATPase.[187,233,338,389,432] Inhibition of either sodium entry across the apical membrane or its exit via the Na^+-K^+ ATPase across the basolateral membrane could be the site of action of PGE_2. Recent preliminary studies utilizing indirect methods suggest that the primary effect of PGE_2 may be at the apical cell membrane.[285] Further direct studies utilizing electrophysiologic techniques that can identify apical sodium conductance changes or patch clamp studies of the apical membrane will be necessary to confirm this.

The identified signal transduction pathways utilized by PGE_2 in the cortical collecting duct modulate intracellular cAMP levels. PGE_2 can stimulate[416] or suppress cAMP accumulation.[64,416,451] The latter may also involve stimulation of phosphodiesterase.[451] Although modulation of cAMP levels may play an important role in PGE_2 effects on water transport in the cortical collecting duct (see "Water Transport," below), it is less clear that PGE_2 affects sodium transport via modulation of cAMP levels.[384,399] Recently, PGE_2 has been shown to increase cell calcium and activate protein kinase C in in vitro perfused cortical collecting ducts.[185] Either the elevated cell calcium[444] or the activation of protein kinase C[184] may be responsible for the inhibition of sodium transport. Further studies are required to identify which processes are involved.

Much less is known about direct epithelial actions of PGs on outer and inner medullary collecting ducts. In vitro studies have shown that PGE_2 inhibits net bicarbonate absorption in the outer medullary collecting duct.[183] With respect to the inner medullary collecting duct, in vivo studies suggest that cyclooxygenase products may inhibit sodium absorption in the papillary collecting duct. Inhibition of cyclooxygenase with ibuprofen produces antinatriuresis and increased accumulation of sodium in the renal papillae.[344] This accumulation of sodium in the papillae was disproportionately greater than the accumulation of urea and potassium, suggesting that decreased papillary blood flow was not solely responsible.

Water transport

Hormonally regulated water transport (see Chap. 5) across the collecting duct appears to be a major process under the influence of cyclooxygenase products, especially PGs. The early classical studies of Grantham and Orloff demonstrated that PGE_1 stimulated basal hydraulic conductivity of the isolated pefused cortical collecting tubule but that PGE_2 also blunted the subsequent hydraulic conductivity response to AVP.[162] In these early studies, the action of PGE_1 appeared to be at a pre-cAMP step. These early studies were confirmed with respect to PGE_2.[316] PGE_2 also stimulates basal hydraulic conductivity and suppresses the hydraulic conductivity response to AVP in rabbit cortical collecting duct.[316] Since the effect of AVP to increase the hydraulic conductivity of the cortical collecting duct is known to be mediated via increased accumulation of cAMP, a number of studies have determined the effect of PGE_2 on cAMP metabolism in this nephron segment.[64,115,202,416,451] These studies clearly demonstrate that PGE_2 can stimulate cAMP generation and also suppress cAMP generation in response to AVP (Fig. 15-3). Although there is some discrepancy, generally, inhibition of cAMP generation is seen at lower concentrations of PGE_2, while stimulation is observed at higher concentrations. In studies on immunodissected rabbit cortical collecting duct cells,[416] nanomolar quantities of PGE_2 suppressed AVP-stimulated cAMP generation, and higher concentrations stimulated cAMP generation. In contrast, in microdissected rabbit cortical collecting ducts, there appeared to be a dose-dependent effect of PGE_2 to suppress cAMP generation in response to AVP, although high concentrations of PGE_2 did modestly stimulate cAMP accumulation.[64] The reason for this discrepancy in results with two different preparations is at present unclear. A component of the suppression by PGE_2 of cAMP accumulation may be secondary to the activation of phosphodiesterase.[451] In immunodissected rabbit cortical collecting duct cells, the inhibitory effect of PGE_2 on AVP-stimulated cAMP generation could be reversed by pertussis toxin pretreatment, suggesting that the effect of PGE_2 is mediated through the pertussis toxin-sensitive inhibitory guanine nucleotide-binding protein, G_i.[416]

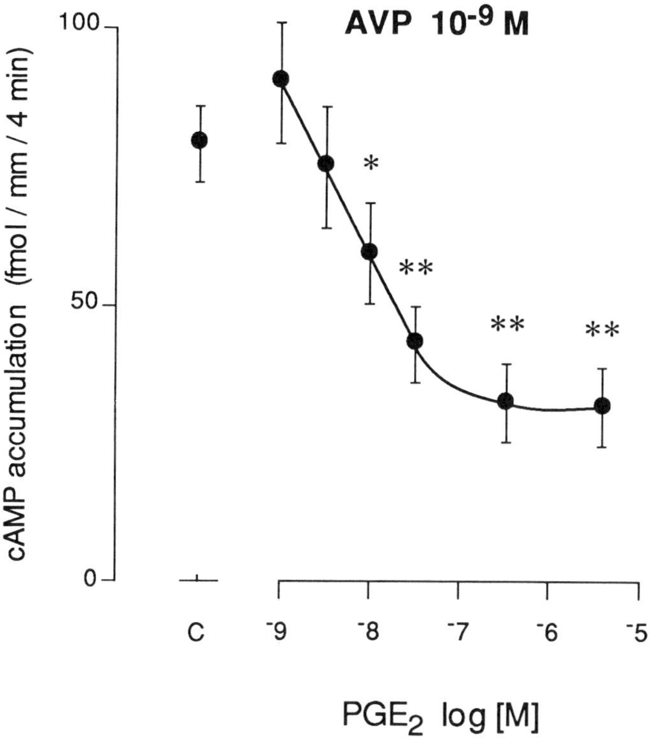

FIGURE 15-3 • PGE_2 inhibition of AVP-induced cAMP accumulation in rabbit CCT. All media contained 5 μM indomethacin. CCTs were incubated in presence of 1 mM IBMX and either 1 nM AVP only (C) or 1 nM AVP plus various concentrations of PGE_2. *,$P < .005$; **,$P < .001$ versus AVP.

In addition to affecting the water flow response through modulation of cAMP levels, PGE_2 has recently been shown to inhibit AVP-induced osmotic water flow through stimulation of protein kinase C activity.[185] Furthermore, PGE_2 raises intracellular calcium activity in cortical collecting ducts.[185] Both activation of protein kinase C and elevation of cell calcium inhibit AVP-induced osmotic water flow in the cortical collecting duct.[9,10] The action of protein kinase C to inhibit AVP-induced osmotic water flow is effected at both a pre- and a post-cAMP step.[10,185] It is also possible that activation of protein kinase C affects the cAMP response to AVP, not only through an action on adenyl cyclase,[105] but also through stimulation of cAMP phosphodiesterase.[104] It should be noted that more recent preliminary studies on the toad bladder also confirm a protein kinase C-dependent mechanism for the inhibition of water flow in response to PGE_2.[254] The three possible signaling pathways that PGE_2 can utilize in the cortical collecting duct are depicted in Fig. 15-4.

Physiologic relevance of PGE_2-AVP interactions

In vitro functional studies clearly show that PGE_2 interferes with AVP-induced hydraulic conductivity in the collecting duct and analogous tissues, as summarized above. To characterize the functional significance of these observations, a number of questions must be answered: (1) Is there strong evidence from in vivo studies for this PGE_2-AVP interaction?, (2) What is the source of the PGE_2?, and (3) Is there evidence of the self-regulation of AVP action through AVP-mediated PGE_2 production and action? Both AVP and 1-desamino-8-D-arginine vasopressin (dDAVP) acutely increase urinary PG excretion in conscious Brattleboro rats and water diuresing Long-Evans rats.[111,128] While some discrepancies exist among

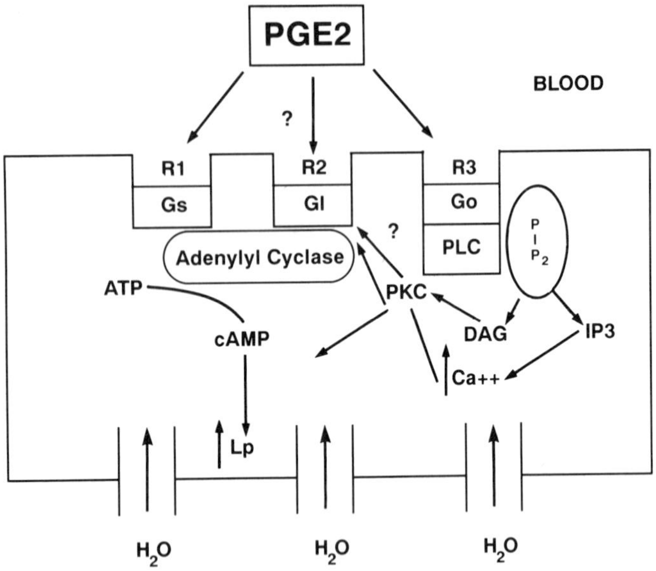

FIGURE 15-4 • Summary of three signaling pathways utilized by PGE_2 in the rabbit CCD. PGE_2 binding to receptor 1 (R1) increases the hydraulic conductivity (*Lp*) by increasing cAMP generation through G_s (stimulatory guanine nucleotide-binding protein). PGE_2 binding to receptor 2 decreases AVP-stimulated *Lp* through G_i (inhibitory guanine nucleotide-binding protein). PGE_2 binding to receptor 3 acts through phospholipase C (PLC; presumably through a pertussis toxin-insensitive G protein, G_O), generating inositol triphosphate (IP3), which causes release of intracellular calcium. Diacylglycerol (DAG) is generated and activates protein kinase C (PKC). PKC inhibits AVP action through both precyclic AMP and post-cAMP mechanisms. The precyclic AMP mechanism is likely to involve activation of G_i. The question marks refer to the fact that we currently do not know to what extent G_i is activated directly through R2 or indirectly through R3. Also shown is the possibility that elevated intracellular calcium can also suppress cAMP accumulation through a mechanism involving G_i.

studies in humans, the general consensus is that urinary PGE_2 excretion also increases in response to AVP and dDAVP.[113,309,465,494,495] In agreement with the functional role for the increased urinary PGE_2 excretion seen with AVP infusion are numerous observations of enhanced renal concentrating ability in animals or humans pretreated with inhibitors of PG production.[7,103,127,237,431] These functional studies, along with observations of urinary PGE_2 excretion, are certainly compatible with the in vitro studies reporting an inhibitory role of PGE_2 on the action of AVP in the collecting duct and are also compatible with the hypothesis that AVP action is autoregulated by AVP-induced PGE_2 synthesis. How good is the evidence that AVP stimulates PGE_2 production at the level of the collecting duct?

Numerous studies have explored the ability of AVP to increase PGE_2 synthesis by collecting tubules or collecting tubule cells.[148,149,207,226,396,482] However, in virtually all of these studies, the concentration of AVP required to produce even barely detectable PG synthesis was at least 1 to 2 log orders of magnitude greater than the AVP concentration providing a maximal water flow response in the isolated collecting tubule. In addition, exogenous AA is required for observing the AVP stimulation of PGE_2 production. The dose of AVP required raises some question about the physiologic significance of these studies. In addition, the requirement for exogenous AA suggests that in many of the in vitro systems the experimental conditions are associated with depletion of AA from the hormonally responsive pool.

Studies performed on isolated perfused tubules suggest that normal concentrations of AVP are not associated with functionally significant PGE_2 production, since indomethacin has no effect on the water flow response observed with 2 to 230 p*M* AVP (Fig. 15-5).[8,400,433] Indeed, in a recent study,[8] the counterregulatory and inhibitory role of PGE_2 on AVP-induced water flow could only be demonstrated when AVP concentrations 3 log units above maximal physiologic levels were utilized. At this concentration, AVP has been shown in a number of systems (the perfused collecting duct[8] and isolated principal cells from the rabbit cortical collecting duct[53]) to acutely increase intracellular calcium and activate protein kinase C. The latter events are probably mediated by activation of phospholipase C and subsequent hydrolysis of phosphotidylinositol bis-phosphate. Similar effects of AVP have recently been described in inner medullary collecting tubule cells and in medullary interstitial cells.[24,445] Indeed, studies on the inner medullary collecting duct cells suggest that this action of AVP is not mediated by an AVP receptor but, rather, by the oxytocin receptor.[445] Thus, at least with respect to isolated collecting duct segments or cells or cultured cells from cortical and medullary collecting ducts, the data proving a physiologic role for AVP-stimulated PG production is unconvincing. This uncertainty exists in spite of the fact that one can demonstrate clear-cut biochemical actions of high concentrations of AVP that may be mediated by the V_1 receptor subtype or possibly the oxytocin receptor.

Cyclooxygenase metabolites and potassium homeostasis

The inhibition of PG synthesis is at times associated with the development of hyperkalemia that is out of proportion to accompanying reductions in renal function.[128a] The mechanisms underlying this phenomenon probably involve inhibition of potassium secretion in aldosterone-sensitive segments of the distal tubule,[326a] thereby creating a state similar to hyporeninemic hypoaldosteronism. Since PGs are a significant stimulus for renin release in the kidney, this has been hypothesized as a probable principal cause of the resulting hyperkalemia, although direct impairment of potassium secretion may also be involved. The hyperkalemia associated with the administration of NSAIDs may be particularly severe in the presence of accompanying interstitial nephritis, such as in gouty nephropathy.[128a] Conversely, hypokalemia has been associated with increased renal PG synthesis, but the data in human beings and rats are somewhat conflicting.[441a]

Other effects of cyclooxygenase products on renal function

Conflicting evidence exists regarding involvement of cyclooxygenase products, particularly TXA_2, in the mediation of tubuloglomerular feedback responses.[137] Tubuloglomerular feedback is the term applied to the preglomerular vasoconstrictor stimulus that appears to be evoked in response to increased solute (probably chloride) delivery to the cells of the macula densa. The inhibition of TXA_2 synthesis has been associated with some amelioration of renal vasoconstriction, which accompanies the activation of tubuloglomerular feedback. In addition, PGs may modulate the autoregulation of renal blood flow (RBF) in young rats[71] and participate in the maintenance of renal perfusion in the fetal kidney.[287]

INVOLVEMENT OF CYCLOOXYGENASE METABOLITES IN RENAL PATHOPHYSIOLOGY

Cyclooxygenase products of AA have been implicated in the mediation of renal functional changes in a number of disorders, including glomerular injury, various forms of acute renal failure (ARF), chronic renal failure, allograft rejection and cyclosporine nephrotoxicity, hepatorenal syndrome, diabetic nephropathy, essential hypertension, and Bartter's syndrome. These areas will be reviewed here, as will be the proposed roles for these eicosanoids in the renal adaptations to pregnancy.

Experimental and human glomerular injury

In view of their synthesis by glomerular mesangial and epithelial cells, their possible local generation and release by infiltrating leukocytes and platelets, and their potent effects on renal vascular tone and mesangial cell function, the involvement of AA cyclooxygenase products in the mediation of glomerular injury has been the subject of much vigorous research. For the sake of clarity, we shall divide the available evidence into two main areas: glomerular inflammatory injury and glomerular noninflammatory immune injury (usually proteinuric).

Glomerular inflammatory injury

In examining the role of AA cyclooxygenase products in the mediation of inflammatory glomerular injury, investigators have focused on two models: experimentally induced antiglomerular basement membrane antibody (anti-GBM Ab)-induced glomerulonephritis (often referred to as nephrotoxic serum, or NTS, nephritis) and the naturally occurring model of lupus-like disease in the F_1 hybrid of NZBxNZW mice.

NTS-induced glomerulonephritis, produced in the rat by the administration of antibody directed against glomerular basement membrane antigens (anti-GBM), has proven to be a highly useful tool for evaluating the pathogenesis of glomerulonephritic injury. Induction of

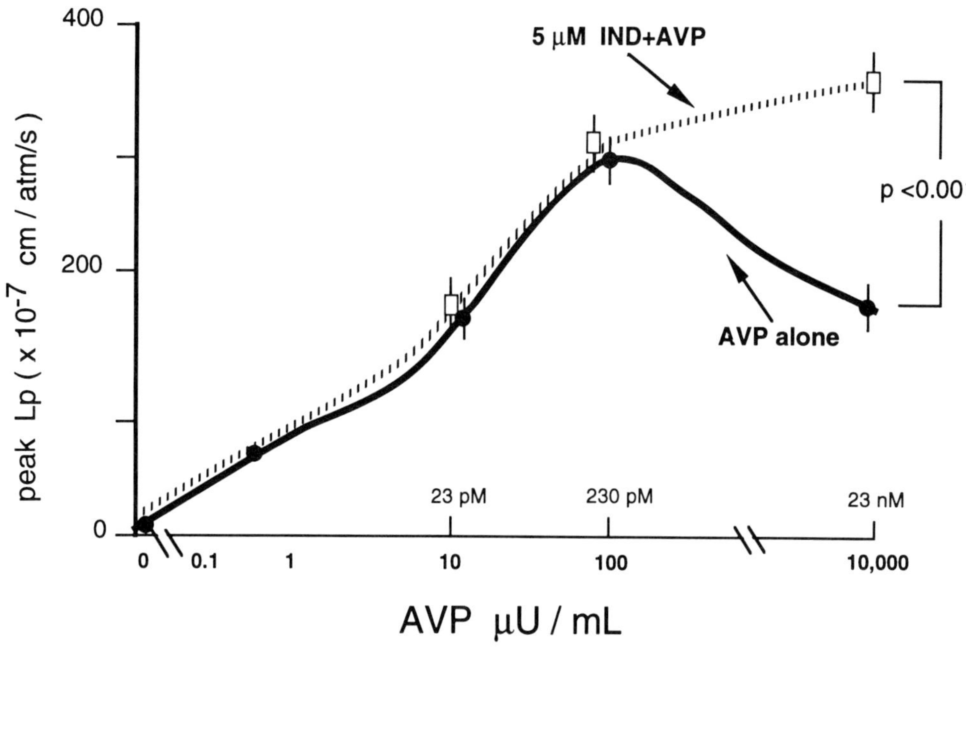

FIGURE 15-5 • Concentration dependence of collecting duct hydraulic conductivity (peak *Lp*) response to AVP. The solid line represents data from tubules exposed to AVP alone, while the interrupted line refers to data from tubules exposed to 5 μM indomethacin (IND) and AVP. Indomethacin does not augment the response to AVP at concentrations of AVP up to 230 p*M*. Only when pharmacologic concentrations of AVP are used (23 n*M*) is there evidence for an enhancing effect of indomethacin. Note that *Lp* actually declines with 23 n*M* AVP and is "restored" by pretreatment with indomethacin.

this form of injury in the Munich-Wistar rat, uniquely endowed with surface glomeruli accessible to direct measurement of glomerular dynamics, has allowed investigators to describe the pattern of glomerular microcirculatory derangements underlying the depressed filtration rates observed during the acute (heterologous) as well as the delayed (autologous) phases of this experimental model. Consensus has emerged from numerous studies performed during both the heterologous and autologous phases that the principal factor accounting for the fall in filtration rates in this model of injury was a marked reduction in the glomerular capillary ultrafiltration coefficient (K_f).[19,42,43,272,441] While K_f is low throughout both phases of the disease process, renal vascular resistence (RVR) is initially elevated during the heterologous phase[19,42] but eventually falls as the lesion transforms into the autologous phase, and, at 10 to 14 days after initiation of injury, RVR may be equal to or even less than that observed in control animals.[19] It is interesting that micropuncture measurements reveal that, in the heterologous phase, both pre (R_a) and post (R_e) glomerular resistances are elevated, but since R_e is proportionately greater, intraglomerular capillary pressure (P_{GC}) and transcapillary hydraulic pressure (ΔP) are higher than normal.[19,42,43,272,441] In the late phase, however, RVR is low due to a dramatic reduction in R_a with relative maintenance of R_e, resulting in persistently elevated P_{GC} and ΔP.[19] Evidence from a number of laboratories strongly suggests that the evolving changes in arteriolar tone during the course of this inflammatory lesion are mediated principally by locally released cyclooxygenase and lipoxygenase metabolites of AA.[19,42,43,441]

The studies of Lianos and coworkers[257] and of Stork and Dunn[435] have established an important role for TXA_2 release in mediating the increased RVR observed during the early phase of this disease. Their studies also suggest that by day 1, the increasing rate of PGE_2 generation may account for the progressive dilatation of renal arterioles, leading to progressive increases in RBF at this and later stages.[257,435] In these studies, TXA_2 antagonism appeared to ameliorate the falls in RBF and GFR 2 h post-NTS but not at 1 day.[435] As will be discussed later, it is likely that lipoxygenase products play a more significant role with regard to the falls in K_f and GFR during this early phase than do cyclooxygenase metabolites.[19] During the heterologous phase, the weight of current evidence favors a predominant role for cyclooxygenase products in mediating both the renal vasodilation[441] and the reduction in K_f[441] that characterize this phase. The net functional result of cyclooxygenase inhibition during this phase of experimental glomerulonephritis, therefore, would depend on the relative importance of renal perfusion versus the preservation of K_f to the maintenance of GFR.[211,435] It is interesting that evidence from a number of investigators also assigns a role for cyclooxygenase products in modifying the nature of the pathologic lesion[245,246] and the extent of accompanying proteinuria.[224,441] It should be emphasized, however, that the potency and dose of the antibody used, the time at which measurements are performed, and the nature of the histopathologic lesion present are all major determinants of the prevailing functional parameters, and presumably of their modification by cyclooxygenase inhibitors.[19,42,43,211,257,272,435,441] Early studies by Kelley and colleagues[217] and others[373] reported a beneficial effect of fish oil diets (enriched in eicosapentaenoic acid) on the course of genetic murine lupus (MRL-lpr) mice and an accompanying reduction in the generation of cyclooxygenase products. In subsequent studies, enhanced renal TXA_2 and PGE_2 generation was demonstrated in this model, as well as that arising in the F_1 offspring of NZBxNZW mice.[218] These animal studies were supported further by the studies of Patrono and associates in humans, in which they demonstrated an inverse relationship between TXA_2 biosynthesis and GFR.[346] More recently, these authors have presented evidence demonstrating improvement of renal function in patients with lupus nephritis following short-term therapy with a thromboxane receptor antagonist but not with aspirin.[352] Taken together, these data, as well as others from animal and human studies,[40,74,96,176,220,428,439] support a major role for the intrarenal generation of TXA_2 in mediating renal vasoconstriction during inflammatory and lupus-associated glomerular injury.

The demonstration of a functionally significant role for cyclooxygenase metabolites in experimental and possibly human inflammatory glomerular injury has raised the question of the cellular sources of these eicosanoids in the glomerulus. In addition to infiltrating inflammatory cells, resident glomerular macrophages, glomerular mesangial cells, and glomerular epithelial cells represent likely sources for eicosanoid generation (see above). It is interesting that macrophage/monocyte-mediated interleukin-1 (IL-1) release stimulates mesangial cell PGE_2 synthesis,[269] a phenomenon that may be of relevance in the chronic phase of NTS-induced injury. Furthermore, complement components, particularly C5b6, C7, C8, and C9, which are known to be involved in the inflammatory models described above, have been implicated in the stimulation of PGE_2 synthesis in glomerular epithelial cells.[176] Finally, Sraer and associates[419] have demonstrated that glomerular synthesis of long-chain saturated or monoenoic fatty acids is associated with stimulation of TXA_2 from coincubated platelets.

Glomerular noninflammatory injury

A number of primary human glomerulopathies, such as minimal change disease, focal sclerosing glomerulopathy, and membranous glomerulopathy, are characterized by heavy proteinuria in the absence of an overt glomerular inflammatory reaction. In these disorders, some clinical studies have shown an amelioration of proteinuria upon treatment of patients with cyclooxygenase inhibitors.[4,325,390] This observation has prompted investigation into the possible role of intrarenal eicosanoid generation in the pathogenesis of proteinuria in these disorders. A number of experimental models have been developed in which the glomerular histologic picture mimics that of minimal change disease, such as puromycin- and adriamycin-induced nephroses, or that of membranous nephropathy, such as passive Heyman (PHN) or cationic bovine gamma globulin (CABG)-induced nephroses. Common to all of these models is a paucity of inflammatory cells in the glomerulus, coupled with fusion of foot processes in the epithelial cells and heavy proteinuria. Experiments in the isolated perfused kidney, as well as in vivo, have established an absolute requirement for complement activation in the development of these lesions and in the accompanying enhancement of glomerular prostanoid synthesis.[176] It is especially interesting that neutralization of the negative charge on glomerular epithelial cells in culture by polycationic molecules, which is the probable mechanism leading to foot process fusion and proteinuria in vivo, is associated with marked stimulation of PGE_2 and PGI_2 generation by these cells.[359] The mechanism whereby changes in membrane charge stimulate prostanoid synthesis remains undefined but is probably related to increased availability of AA secondary to changes in membrane structure.[359] Similarly, enhanced glomerular synthesis and/or urinary excretion of both PGE_2 and TXA_2 has been demonstrated in PHN[96,224,420] and in CABG-[84,365] and adriamycin-[36,369,497] induced glomerulopathies in rats. Controversy exists, however, with respect to the pathogenetic significance of TXA_2 generation and the development of proteinuria. Whereas TXA_2 inhibition was associated with a reduction in proteinuria in adriamycin-induced nephrosis[369] and in some studies of PHN,[96,224] other studies in this same model[420] and in CABG-induced glomerulopathy[84,365] failed to confirm these observations. It does appear, however, that enhanced PGE_2 generation may mediate renal vasodilatation in CABG-induced disease.[365]

Acute renal failure

The pathophysiologic significance of cyclooxygenase metabolites has been investigated in various models of prerenal, intrinsic, and postrenal (obstructive) ARF. Of the major causes of ARF, an important homeostatic and/or pathophysiologic role for PGs and TXA_2 has been established during hemodynamic (pre-) renal failure,[17,126,312,355] endotoxin-induced ARF,[18,54,446] and obstructive injury.[5,15,22,98,144,196,230,267,331,367,448,480]

When cardiac output is compromised, as in extracellular fluid volume depletion or congestive heart failure, systemic blood pressure is preserved by the action of high circulating levels systemic vasoconstrictors (norepinephrine, AII, and AVP). Diminution of their effects within the renal vasculature serves to blunt the marked depression of RBF that would otherwise develop. As noted above, the intrarenal generation of vasodilator products of AA, including PGE_2 and PGI_2, is a central part of this protective adaptation. Studies in rats have shown that the increase in RVR induced by exogenously administered AII or renal nerve stimulation (increased beta-adrenergic tone) is exaggerated during concomitant inhibition of PG synthesis.[31,349] Experiments in animals with volume depletion have demonstrated the existence of intrarenal AVP-PG interactions similar to those described above for AII.[104] Although a direct demonstration of vasoconstrictor activity of AVP in humans is still lacking, the demonstration of high circulating levels of PGs in patients with congestive heart failure suggest important interactions between vasoconstrictors and PGs in humans as well. In fact, studies in patients with congestive heart failure have confirmed that enhanced PG synthesis is crucial in protecting kidneys from various vasoconstrictor influences present in this condition.[17,126,312] Figure 15-6 schematizes the role of vasoconstrictor-PG interactions in the preservation of renal perfusion when systemic hemodynamics are compromised. Should renal hypoperfusion be sufficiently severe, intrinsic (structural) hypoxemic ARF develops. Evidence from animal studies suggests that augmented synthesis of TXA_2 may exacerbate postischemic renal failure[251] and that elevated levels of PGI_2 may exert a cytoprotective effect, limiting renal structural and functional deterioration.[130,251] The clinical relevance of these findings remains uncertain.

ARF accompanying the acute administration of endotoxin in rats is characterized by progressive reductions

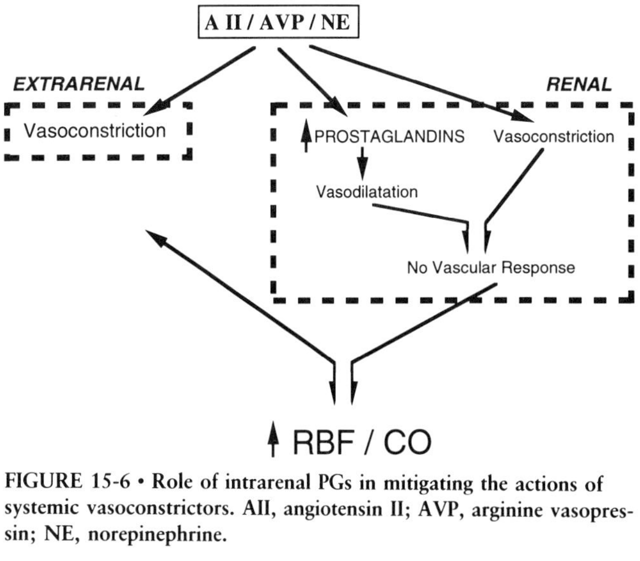

FIGURE 15-6 • Role of intrarenal PGs in mitigating the actions of systemic vasoconstrictors. AII, angiotensin II; AVP, arginine vasopressin; NE, norepinephrine.

TABLE 15-1 • Documented renal effects of nonsteroidal anti-inflmmatory drugs (NSAID)

Drug class	Generic name	Brand name/ manufacturer	Renal effects				
			Edema	ARF	NS	PN	↑K
Salicylates							
Acetylated	acetylsalicylic acid	Many	X	X		?	
Nonacetylated	sodium salicylate	Pabalate/Robins					
	choline salicylate	Arthropan/Purdue Frederick					
	choline magnesium trisalicylate	Trilisate/Purdue Frederick					
	salsalate	Disalcid/Riker					
Propionic acid derivatives	ibuprofen	Many	X	X			
	naproxen	Naprosyn/Syntex	X	X	X		
	fenoprofen calcium	Nalfon/Dista	X	X	X	?	
Indoleacetic acid derivatives	indomethacin	Indocin/MSD	X	X	X		X
	sulindac	Clinoril/MSD					
	tolmetin	Tolectin/McNeil	X	X	X		
Anthranilic acid derivatives	meclofenamate sodium	Meclomen/ Parke-Davis	X			?	
Pyrazolone derivatives	phenylbutazone	Butazolidin/Geigy	X	X		X	

ABBREVIATIONS: ARF, acute renal failure; NS, nephrotic syndrome; PN, papillary necrosis; ↑K, hyperkalemia.

SOURCE: Stoff JS, Clive DM: Role of arachidonic acid metabolites in acute renal failure, in Brenner BM, Lazarus JM (eds), *Acute Renal Failure*, 2d ed. New York, Churchill Livingstone, 1988, p 155. Used by permission.

in RBF and GFR in the absence of hypotension.[18,54,446] Results of renal histologic studies in such animals are normal, but cortical generation rates of AA cyclooxygenase metabolites are markedly elevated.[18] A number of reports have provided evidence of a role for TXA_2-induced renal vasoconstriction in this model of renal dysfunction.[18,54,446] In addition, the literature abounds with isolated reports regarding the roles of PGs and TXA_2 in modulating or modifying renal injury in a number of models of toxin-mediated acute tubular injury, including those induced by uranyl nitrate,[69] aminoglycosides,[12,189] glycerol,[342,468] oxygen radicals,[28] and analgesics.[49] Similar roles have been proposed in other inflammatory reactions, such as those associated with anaphylactic injury[13,14] and interstitial nephritis,[219] but these observations await further confirmation and a more rigorous definition of the underlying mechanisms.

Following induction of chronic (more than 24 h) ureteral obstruction in the rabbit,[5,305,331,367,448] cat,[367] rat,[134,144,196,230] dog,[22,267,480] and human,[15] renal PG and TXA_2 synthesis is markedly enhanced, particularly in response to stimuli such as endotoxin or bradykinin.[5,6,55,150,306,307,337,448] This phenomenon can be demonstrated in the in vivo preparation.[15,22,94,144,196,267,331,367,448,480] as well as in the isolated perfused kidney subjected to obstruction in vivo.[5] Enhanced prostanoid synthesis probably arises from infiltrating mononuclear cells,[5] proliferating fibroblast-like cells,[331] interstitial macrophages,[5] and interstitial medullary cells.[98] The enhancement of TXA_2 synthesis can be modified by dietary protein intake.[196] Considerable evidence suggests a causal relationship between increased renal generation of this eicosanoid and the intense vasoconstriction that characterizes the hydronephrotic or postobstructed kidney.[5,15,22,144,195,196,267,331,367,448,480,485] Hydronephrotic injury can thus be regarded as a form of subacute inflammatory insult in which intrarenal eicosanoid generation from infiltrating leukocytes contributes to the pathophysiologic process.[5,230,331] Finally, TXA_2 has been implicated in the resetting of the tubuloglomerular feedback mechanism observed in hydronephrotic kidneys.[308]

Allograft rejection and cyclosporine nephrotoxicity

Allograft rejection

Coffman and colleagues demonstrated that acute administration of a TXA_2 synthesis inhibitor was associated with significant improvement in rat renal allograft function.[79] These studies, in which GFR, RBF, and eicosanoid measurements were performed in the renal venous effluent of ex vivo perfused kidneys, provided a strong impetus to further assess the role of this eicosanoid in the altered glomerular function of renal allografts during acute rejection. A number of other experimental and clinical studies have also demonstrated increased TXA_2 synthesis during allograft rejection,[80,159,221,252,443] suggesting that increased urinary TXA_2 excretion may be an early indicator in renal and cardiac allograft rejection.[221] More recently, Coffman and colleagues demonstrated little effect of dietary fish oil supplementation on the rejection process or renal functional parameters 6 days after transplantation in the rat, despite generalized reduction in PG and TXA_2 generation, a finding inconsistent with their earlier studies utilizing a TXA_2 synthesis inhibitor,[80] indicating a possible necessary role for vasodilator PGs in the preservation of renal function.

Cyclosporine-A nephrotoxicity

Repeated observations in clinical and experimental models of cyclosporine-A (CY-A) nephrotoxicity have established the presence of a significant component of intrarenal vasoconstriction in its pathogenesis.[368] In a number of cell systems, addition of CY-A has been shown to increase intracellular calcium concentrations[81] and to augment receptor-mediated cellular calcium fluxes,[322] a condition that may lead to stimulation of cyclooxygenase activity. Whisler and coworkers[475] demonstrated that addition of CY-A to human peripheral blood monocytes resulted in increased PGE_2 synthesis due to increased availability of free intracellular AA. This finding raises the possibility that, in activated cells in which AA release is already stimulated, the addition of CY-A may further augment the availability of this substrate to the cyclooxygenase. Furthermore, CY-A administration has been associated with activation of the renin-angiotensin system intrarenally as well as systemically,[368] constituting a potential intermediary signal for intrarenal PG production. Numerous investigators have demonstrated effects for CY-A on renal PG and/or TXA_2 synthesis and provided evidence of a major role for renal and leukocyte TXA_2 synthesis in mediating acute as well as chronic CY-A nephrotoxicity in rats.[78,311,350,351,376,476] Fish oil-rich diets,[80,376] TXA_2 antagonists,[368] or administration of CY-A in fish oil as a vehicle[116] have all been shown to reduce renal TXA_2 synthesis and afford protection against nephrotoxicity. The clinical applicability of these observations has not been tested yet. (See also Chap. 42.)

Hepatorenal syndrome

A number of clinical studies have documented diminished renal synthesis of vasodilator PGs, in particular PGI_2, in patients with liver cirrhosis complicated by functional (vasoconstrictive) renal failure.[167,169,242,243,370] In addition to diminished renal synthesis, systemic PGI_2 generation may actually be increased in these patients, leading to a reduction in systemic arterial pressure and hence further compromising renal perfusion.[168] Diminished renal PG synthesis has also been implicated in the pathogenesis of the severe sodium retention in these patients, as well as in their resistance to diuretic therapy.[117,292] The sodium-retaining properties of nonsteroidal anti-inflammatory drugs (NSAIDs) are particularly exaggerated in patients with cirrhosis of the liver, attesting to the dependence of renal salt excretion on vasodilatory PGs.[99,364] It is unlikely that the severe degree of renal vasoconstriction seen in these patients is due solely to the absence of the renal synthesis of a vasodilator in the absence of an active vasoconstrictor stimulus. Such a mediator, however, remains elusive; TXA_2 appears not to be involved.[496]

Chronic renal insufficiency

Following experimental reduction in renal mass, glomerular[423] and urinary excretion of PGs and TXA_2 increases several fold, particularly when factored for the number of remaining nephrons.[20,319,360] This increase in prostanoid synthesis has been postulated as being necessary for the compensatory hypertrophy that follows renal ablation.[222,253,265,266,299,422] In studies employing acute inhibition of cyclooxygenase activity, Nath and associates have demonstrated reductions in nephron perfusion rate and K_f in remnant kidneys but not in intact controls,[319] and similar hemodynamic consequences have been documented by others.[265,266,299] Selective inhibition of TXA_2 synthesis, however, is associated with an increase in GFR[483] and, in chronic studies, with improvement in GFR, lessening of proteinuria, and preservation of renal histologic conditions.[360,483] Other investigators have documented increases in vasodilator PG synthesis in response to ingestion of high-protein diets in rats with reduced renal mass[253,422] and prevention of dietary protein-induced renal vasodilatation in these animals in the presence of cyclooxygenase inhibition. Dietary manipulations aimed at decreasing cyclooxygenase product synthesis (fish oil diets),[387] however, have been associated with worsening of proteinuria and glomerular sclerosis.[387] Linoleic acid-rich diets, on the other hand, seem to preserve GFR following nephrectomy, although this phenomenon could not be correlated with enhanced prostanoid synthesis as compared to low linoleic acid diet-fed nephrectomized controls.[204] It thus appears that generalized induction of cyclooxygenase activity may be a feature of the remnant kidney, at least in the rat, and that AA cyclooxygenase products may contribute to the regulation of glomerular perfusion and filtration rates in this model, with a predominantly salutary role for vasodilator PGs.

In patients with chronic renal insufficiency secondary to glomerular inflammatory injury or chronic immune complex-mediated glomerulonephritis,[75,326,348] a beneficial role for renal vasodilator PGs (PGI_2) and detrimental effects for renal TXA_2 have been demonstrated. For these reasons, selective inhibition of renal TXA_2 synthesis with low-dose aspirin or TXA_2 synthetase inhibitors or receptor antagonists has been advocated in these patients, but more controlled clinical trials are needed.[75,326,348,352]

Diabetes mellitus

A number of studies in patients with insulin-dependent diabetes have demonstrated elevated urinary excretion rates of vasodilatory PGs and TXA_2[123,124,212,286] and reductions in abnormally elevated values of GFR and renal plasma flow rate (RPF) in these patients upon treatment with cyclooxygenase inhibitors.[124] Similarly, glomerular PG and TXA_2 generation in rats with streptozotocin-induced diabetes was found to be elevated,[52,88,223,301,363] and treatment with indomethacin[88] and aspirin[301] was associated with reversal of the hyperfiltration characteristic of this disease as well as prevention of progressive functional detorioration.[301] These findings in both patients and rats, however, were challenged by similar studies yielding opposing results.[23,25,72,97,223] Barnett and associates[25] found that the alterations in glomerular eicosanoid biosynthesis were limited to streptozotocin-treated animals but were absent in genetically diabetic BB-D rats. Similarly, studies involving selective antagonism of TXA_2 synthesis have yielded contradictory data with respect to its role in the pathogenesis of diabetic nephropathy.[97] In patients with hyporeninemic hypoaldosteronism, deficient basal, as well as stimulated, PGI_2 production has been proposed as an underlying mechanism for the low active renin concentration and the altered vasomotor tone.[314]

In summary, the roles played by cyclooxygenase products in mediating diabetic nephropathy remain controversial. Beneficial clinical responses to platelet inhibitory therapy (aspirin and/or dipyridamol)[108] raise the possibility that the effects of cyclooxygenase inhibition may be related to inhibition of platelet, rather than renal, thromboxane generation.

Pregnancy

Studies in pregnant rats and humans have documented increased glomerular synthesis[163,164] and urinary excretion[486] of PGE_2, $PGF_{2\alpha}$, and PGI_2 without significant changes in TXA_2 generation. The increased renal levels of these cyclooxygenase products may be related to the documented decrease in the activity of 15-PGDH, the principal enzyme involved in the metabolism of PGs,[56,66,67] in pregnant animals, probably due to the elevated levels of estrogen.[66] The latter has been shown to selectively decrease the V_{max} for this enzyme in the kidney (but not the lung) while not affecting the K_m.[56,66,67] Augmented PG synthesis in gravid animals and humans has therefore been postulated as the basis for the increased levels of GFR and RPF normally seen during pregnancy. PG inhibition, however, is without effect on these parameters in anesthetized or conscious[30,82,83] rats. While stimulated vasodilator PG synthesis does not appear to contribute to the regulation of GFR and RPF in normal pregnancy, diminished synthesis of PGI_2 has been demonstrated in human[298] and animal[216] models of pregnancy-induced hypertension. In the latter, inhibition of TXA_2 synthetase has been associated with resolution of the hypertension, suggesting a possible pathophysiologic role.[216] A beneficial effect of reducing TXA_2 generation, while preserving PGI_2 synthesis, by low-dose (60 to 100 mg/day) aspirin therapy has been demonstrated convincingly in two recent studies in patients at risk for pregnancy-induced hypertension.[35,388]

Hypertension

Several lines of evidence suggest the involvement of cyclooxygenase products in accentuating the salt-retaining stimuli that characterize patients with some forms of essential hypertension. This evidence is derived mainly from studies of salt balance and blood pressure measurements in hypertensive individuals receiving NSAIDs. These agents lead to increased salt retention in hypertensive patients but not in normal persons.[347,430,449] In particular, cyclooxygenase inhibition is associated with resistance to the diuretic actions of thiazides[112,235,477] and furosemide.[347] They also decrease responsiveness to the blood pressure-lowering effects of beta-adrenergic blockers.[477] This effect is probably due to the counterregulatory role of endogenous renal PGs in antagonizing the vasoconstrictive effects of alpha-adrenergic nerve activity.[200] For this reason, those NSAIDs not associated with inhibition of renal cyclooxygenase, such as sulindac, are better tolerated in the hypertensive patient.[358] The extent to which sulindac spares renal cyclooxygenase remains controversial,[48,73,102,188,332,345,347,358,372,404,417] however, and any effect is likely to be dose-dependent.

In patients with renal artery stenosis, increased renal venous PG secretion is observed from the stenotic side, probably reflecting renin-stimulated PG synthesis.[440] This local release of PGs in such patients maintains a relatively low RVR, thereby mitigating the effects of decreased perfusion pressure on ipsilateral renal perfusion.

Finally, attempts at treating hypertension with PG analogues have generally been disappointing,[371] while those involving dietary manipulations have achieved only modest results.[231]

At the experimental level, two models of hypertension in the rat appear to involve derangements in cyclooxygenase product generation: the salt-sensitive Dahl rat model (Dahl-S) and the spontaneously hypertensive rat (SHR). Papillary collecting tubule cell synthesis and urinary excretion of PGE_2 from Dahl-S rats are markedly depressed compared to salt-resistant controls.[366] This observation is true under baseline as well as A23187-stimulated conditions both before and after the development of hypertension.[366] This effect may be due to decreased availability of substrate (AA), since PLA_2 activity in renomedullary tissue from these rats is reduced.[260] In the SHR, on the other hand, the opposite appears to be true: PLA_2 activity is enhanced[214] leading to increased synthesis of PGs and TXA_2. However, these effects are accompanied by an apparent resistance to the actions of vasodilatory PGs, such as PGE_2, probably due to a postreceptor intracellular defect.[456] The result is unopposed action of the vasoconstrictor TXA_2, leading to elevations in renal and systemic vascular resistances, a fall in GFR, and salt retention.[341] In fact, therapy with thromboxane antagonists affords protection against the development of hypertension in these rats, particularly if initiated at an early age.[165,361,410,454]

In two-kidney one-clip (Goldblatt) hypertension, increased PG synthesis is observed from the clipped side and, as in humans, cyclooxygenase inhibition leads to detorioration of renal function on that side.[421] In additon, increases in sensitivity to the constrictor effects of TXA_2 analogues have been documented two weeks after clipping.[490] DOCA salt-induced hypertension does not appear to be influenced by cyclooxygenase pathway products,[77] while that associated with glucocorticoid excess may be exacerbated by a relative deficiency of vasodilator PGs.[76]

Bartter's syndrome

Bartter's syndrome is a rare disorder characterized by normotensive hypokalemia, urinary potassium and chloride wasting, renal concentrating defect, metabolic alkalosis, and increased levels of renin, angiotensin II, and aldosterone. Also found are hypomagnesemia, elevated plasma concentrations of catecholamines and bradykinins, and reduced urinary kinin excretion.[156,411] The renal juxtaglomerular apparatus and prostaglandin-producing medullary interstitial cells are hyperplastic and hypertrophied.[26,459] Symptoms of weakness, muscle cramps, polyuria, and malaise are common; they may generally be attributed to severe chronic potassium depletion.

Excessive PG production has been recognized as a feature of Bartter's syndrome. Serum PG concentrations and urinary excretion of PGE_2 and PGI_2 metabolites are generally elevated compared to normal individuals.[156,170,369] In view of the recognized capacity of PGs to promote renin secretion and induce natriuresis, it has been proposed that primary overproduction of PGs could account for both activation of the renin-angiotensin system, with secondary urinary potassium wasting, and urinary sodium loss, which would explain the absence of hypertension. However, elevated PG production and excretion are not uniform features of Bartter's syndrome.[156] Furthermore, urinary potassium wasting is not attributable to activation of the renin-angiotensin-aldosterone system, since bilateral adrenalectomy or pharmacologic inhibition of aldosterone action does not correct it.[382] In addition, inhibition of PG synthesis with NSAIDs does not fully correct the hypokalemia[382,493] despite lowering PGE_2 and PGI_2 excretion; reducing elevated plasma renin, aldosterone, and bradykinin levels; and restoring normal vascular reactivity to AII and norepinephrine.[109,171,174,411,459,461] Other evidence suggests that activation of PG production is a secondary abnormality and that the primary defect is diminished chloride reabsorption in the thick ascending limb of Henle's loop.[157] The beneficial ability of cyclooxygenase inhibitors to normalize sensitivity of vessels to pressor agents may be the result of removal of competing vasodilator compounds.

THE RENAL KALLIKREIN-KININ SYSTEM

Of the various hormones that regulate renal function, the renal kallikrein-kinin system is the least understood. It is clear that kinins generated within the kidney can exert profound effects on RBF and salt excretion. However, it has been more difficult to define the precise role played by the kinins in specific physiologic and pathophysiologic situations. Part of the difficulty in assigning a precise activity to the kinins is due to methodological difficulties in measuring the activity of the integrated system. An additional problem confounding specific understanding of renal kinin action is the involvement of many other hormone systems, particularly the PGs, in mediating kinin activity. Despite these problems, it has become clear in recent years that the renal kallikrein-kinin system is a potentially powerful mediator of renal function.[89,255]

BIOSYNTHESIS AND METABOLISM

Kallikreins are serine proteases that act on a class of protein substrates, the *kininogens*, to liberate biologically active peptides, referred to collectively as *kinins*. There are two main classes of kallikreins: plasma and glandular. The two systems differ in several ways, including molecular size, substrate specificity, and primary product (bradykinin or lysyl-bradykinin). *Plasma kallikrein*, also known as *Fletcher factor*, is an important mediator of inflammation and blood coagulation. *Glandular kallikreins* are found in the kidney as well as in the sweat glands, pancreas, salivary glands, and intestine.

Renal kallikrein can release kinins from both high- and low-molecular-weight kininogen. However, the preferred substrate in vivo appears to be the low-molecular-weight type. There is no evidence for renal synthesis of kininogen; it is generally concluded that the substrate is derived from plasma. Renal kallikrein releases *kallidin* (lysyl-bradykinin), a decapeptide, which is then partially converted by an aminopeptidase to the nonapeptide *bradykinin*. Kinins are rapidly converted by enzymes, referred to as *kininases*, to inactive peptide fragments. The two main kininases are *kininase I* and *kinase II*. Kininase II is also known as *angiotensin-converting enzyme* and is, in fact, a relatively nonspecific dicarboxypeptidase.

The difficulty in precisely defining the physiologic role of the renal kallikrein-kinin system is due to the limitations in currently available experimental methods. As with any other hormone system, there are basically two experimental approaches for evaluating the function and regulation of renal kinins. Some studies aim to identify the factors that regulate the activity of the system by measuring increases or decreases in end products in response to various manipulations. This approach assumes the existence of an accurate assay of the system, something analogous to plasma renin activity in the case of the renin-angiotensin system or urinary PG excretion in the case of renal PGs. Other studies seek to evaluate the functional consequences of altering active kinin concentration within the kidney. Such changes can be effected by direct infusion of peptide into the renal artery or by the administration of drugs that specifically alter intrarenal kinin generation.

The primary means of assessing the activity of the renal kallikrein-kinin system has been the assay of urinary kallikrein activity. The assumptions underlying this approach are that kallikrein activity is the rate-limiting step in renal kinin accumulation and that urinary excretion of the enzyme parallels intrarenal activity. Until recently, the assay of urinary kallikrein employed synthetic substrates (e.g., tosyl *l*-arginine methyl ester, or TAME, esterase assay) to measure urinary protease activity.[277] Recently, non-kallikrein proteases hve been found in urine, motivating researchers to develop far more specific assays that use authentic kininogens as substrates.[152,333] An alternative approach has been the direct determination of the mass of urinary kallikrein by radioimmunoassay.[61,333] The disadvantage of this approach is that it measures both active and inactive forms of the enzyme, a significant problem, since inactive kallikrein can account for as much as half of the total found in urine.[63,258] Although measurement of the biologically active product of the system would seem to be more relevant than measurement of the enzyme mass, there are severe methodological problems in measuring the quantity of urinary kinins, including their instability and the presence of renal, bladder, and urinary kininases. Recently, Scicli and coworkers[403] assayed kinins in urine obtained from ureteral catheters in rats and found that various maneuvers (e.g., urinary acidification and diuretic administration) changed urinary kallikrein and kinins in opposite directions.[403] At this point, it is difficult to know which available method, if any, most accurately assesses the activity of the renal kallikrein-kinin system.

Direct infusion of kinins has been employed in order to assess their effect on renal function. A basic problem with this approach is that infused kinins are not known to achieve, necessarily, the same distribution as do kinins generated within the kidney, particularly since it appears that most kinin synthesis occurs within the distal nephron.[318] Changes in renal function after administration of aprotinin (a protease inhibitor that reduces kallikrein activity) have been attributed to changes in renal kinin concentration.[303] However, aprotinin is a relatively nonspecific inhibitor; studies employing aprotinin should be interpreted with some caution.[191] Similarly, studies that have used kininase II (i.e., converting enzyme) inhibitors to modulate kinin levels also have changed other determinants of renal function and should likewise be regarded with caution.

The state of the art is therefore hard to define. The kinins are clearly chemically and physiologically potent substances. Yet there is no universally agreed upon assay for them, nor are there known specific inhibitors of their synthesis or action. Clearly, a more accurate picture of the role played by kinins in renal physiology awaits future methodological advances.

COMPONENTS OF THE RENAL KALLIKREIN-KININ SYSTEM

Renal kallikrein, like other glandular kallikreins, is a glycoprotein with a molecular weight in the range of 25,000 to 45,000. It is enzymatically and immunologically identical to the kallikrein obtained from glandular sources such as the pancreas and the salivary gland.[353] Some researchers have suggested that renal kallikrein exists as a proenzyme (prekallikrein) requiring activation; this would explain why approximately half the urinary kallikrein is inactive.[354] However, to date, only active kallikrein has been found within the kidney. It is reasonably certain that renal kallikrein is synthesized by the kidney.[327,374] Elegant immunological and enzymatic studies by Proud and colleagues have mapped the distribution of kallikrein along the nephron.[357] There is virtually no activity in the early proximal tubule. Activity becomes detectable in the later portion of the proximal tubule and peaks in the connecting tubule, but activity is still found in appreciable amounts in the cortical collecting tubule. Immunofluorescence experiments have demonstrated that kallikrein is concentrated in a rim of cytoplasm immediately below the luminal plasma membrane.[339] Glandular kallikrein in several organs is regulated by a series of inhibitors, most of which are small peptides (molecular weight, 5 to 20,000) capable of inhibiting a variety of proteases in addition to kallikrein (e.g., aprotinin). Two nonspecific protease inhibitors have been identified in urine, and a single specific kallikrein inhibitor has been isolated from kidney.[151] The relationship of these inhibitors to the regulation of kallikrein activity in vivo is uncertain.

Renal kininogen, the substrate for renal kallikrein, is probably not synthesized within the kidney; it originates in the liver and gains access to the kidney by glomerular filtration.[51] Peptidase activity is high in the proximal tubule, but it has been estimated that enough kininogen gains access to the distal tubule and presents itself to kallikrein to account for renal kinin synthesis. There are two circulating forms of kininogen: low molecular weight (LMWK) and high molecular weight (HMWK). Renal kallikrein can cleave active products from either substrate. However, the preferred substrate in vivo is LMWK, since patients with congenital deficiency of HMWK (Fitzgerald trait) excrete normal amounts of urinary kinins.[60]

Renal kallikrein, like other glandular kallikreins, releases kallidin (lysyl-bradykinin) from kininogen.[51] A renal aminopeptidase converts a portion of kallidin to the nonapeptide bradykinin. However, most of the kallidin remains uncleaved; kallidin is the predominant kinin excreted in the urine.[472] Kallidin and bradykinin are of equal physiologic potency. One hundred-fold increases of plasma bradykinin concentration have only trivial effects on urinary bradykinin excretion, demonstrating that urinary kinins are generated within the kidney.[317]

The kidney possesses high levels of kininase activity, most of which is attributable to kininase II (angiotensin-converting enzyme). The major portion of the enzyme is located in the proximal tubule brush border.[173,466] This localization ensures that any filtered kinins are catabolized immediately. However, kinins delivered by microinjection into the distal tubule are excreted into the urine, revealing the relative lack of kininase activity in this nephron segment.[58] It is generally agreed that kinins synthesized within the kidney are not added to the plasma but are either excreted in the urine or catabolized within the kidney.

PHYSIOLOGIC AND PATHOPHYSIOLOGIC ROLE OF THE RENAL KALLIKREIN-KININ SYSTEM

Despite the methodological difficulties in studying their synthesis and activity, there is general agreement that the renal kinins are vasodilatory, natriuretic, and diuretic. The conclusions regarding the action of bradykinin on the renal vasculature are based largely on infusion studies[158,291,471] that have shown that, like other renal vasodilators, bradykinin preferentially increases deep cortical flow without affecting GFR.[203,426] Although the suggestion has never been verified experimentally, kinin-mediated increases in deep cortical flow may be accompanied by increases in medullary blood flow, which is relevant to understanding kinin action on salt and water excretion.

Bradykinin does not directly affect sodium transport, at least in those nephrons of the outer cortex accessible to micropuncture.[427] Therefore, the brisk natriuresis induced by bradykinin must be due either to a direct effect on sodium transport selectively acting on heterogeneous inner cortical nephrons or to changes in intrarenal hemodynamics. Similarly, the water diuresis and concentrating defect observed with infused bradykinin may be attributable to dissipation of the medullary osmotic gradient, which is in turn caused by increased medullary blood flow.

Bradykinin and the renal PGs (specifically, PGE_2 and PGI_2) have identical effects on renal blood flow and salt and water excretion. Bradykinin is known to be a potent stimulator of renal PG synthesis, inviting speculation about the extent to which the actions of renal kinins are mediated by PG intermediates. The question, while apparently straightforward, has led to a long and at times contentious debate in the literature.[44,131,238,273,291,295,436,489]

Despite general agreement about the actions of the renal kallikrein-kinin system, definition of the role played by the system in regulating renal function has proved elusive. The most thoroughly explored possibility has been the kinin response to brief saline loading. Many investigators argue that the renal kinins mediate the natriuresis of fluid space expansion, since kallikrein excretion is enhanced under these conditions.[281] Marin-Grez demonstrated that administration of an anti-bradykinin antibody attenuated the natriuretic response to an exogenous saline load by 50 percent.[283] Some workers have reported observing a direct relationship between dietary sodium and urinary kallikrein.[1,90,91,101] Studies by Levy and associates and by Margolius and associates failed to demonstrate an increase in urinary kallikrein in response to acute saline loading in human subjects.[256,277] There are no apparent explanations for these discrepancies.

A potentially confounding variable in the interpretation of the role of renal kinins in the physiologic regulation of natriuresis is the effect of mineralocorticoids. Most workers agree that administration of a mineralocorticoid to salt-loaded animals increases urinary kallikrein excretion.[1,277] This effect is not observed during the first few days of hormone administration, leading to the suggestion that kinins mediate the phenomenon of mineralocorticoid escape.[282] Investigators who subscribe to the belief that kinin production increases with volume increase attribute the mineralocorticoid effect to progressive sodium retention. Margolius and coworkers have argued, on the other hand, that steroids have a direct effect on renal kallikrein activity.[277] This group has reported an increase in urinary kallikrein level after salt restriction; the increase was found to be blocked by spironolactone.[279] They have also reported that aldosterone exerts a direct stimulatory influence on kallikrein activity in kidney cell suspensions.[210] Thus, data exist suggesting that salt loading and mineralocorticoids may both stimualte the renal kallikrein system. Since under physiologic conditions these two factors are inversely related, it remains difficult to define the role played by the kallikrein system in renal salt handling.

All classes of diuretics apparently enhance urinary kallikrein excretion.[59,62,87,271,278,297,323,324,335,336,405,406,491] Enhanced kallikrein excretion has also been consistently seen as the response to a variety of renal vasodilators.[271,297] Since thiazides and acetazolamide, which do not increase RBF, also stimulate urinary kallikrein output, the diuretic effect cannot simply be due to renal vasodilatation. The response is also not attenuated by pretreatment with beat-adrenergic blockers, implying that it is independent of renin release. Since all diuretics and renal vasodilators increase delivery of filtrate to distal nephron segments, the site of renal kallikrein synthesis, a unifying hypothesis would be that enhanced distal tubular flow rates nonspecifically increase urinary kallikrein activity.

Renal kinins and hypertension

Since renal kinins are natriuretic and vasodilatory, the possibility that a deficiency in the system might be involved in the pathogenesis of hypertension has excited much active research.[59] Early epidemiologic studies did detect a decrease in urinary kallikrein activity in patients with essential hypertension.[278,405,406,491] Subsequent studies made the observation that blacks excreted less kallikrein than did whites and that the urinary kallikrein level was further reduced in black family members of hypertensive patients.[491] These deficiencies in urinary kallikrein excretion parallel the decreased natriuresis observed following abrupt volume loading in black hypertensive patients and their first-degree relatives. It is tempting to speculate that a genetically determined deficiency in renal kallikrein activity is somehow causally related to the increased frequency and severity of essential hypertension in the black population. However, since salt excretion itself can alter urinary kallikrein excretion, the fundamental defect could be increased tubular sodium reabsorption, to which changes in kallikrein are secondary.

Many studies have demonstrated a decrease in urinary kallikrein activity in various experimental models of hypertension. For example, the Dahl salt-sensitive rat has markedly decreased urinary kallikrein activity. Similar results have been obtained in genetically hypertensive rats as well as in surgically created models, such as Goldblatt one-kidney hypertension.[62,63] The possibility still exists that changes in kallikrein excretion are secondary to the hypertensive state. However, these data, coupled with the clinical observations, argue that deficiencies in the system may well exacerbate hypertensive tendencies. The one experimental model of hypertension associated with increased urinary kallikrein output is mineralocorticoid-salt hypertension.[62] This result is not surprising in view of the recognized stimulatory effect of both mineralocorticoids and salt on renal kallikrein. Increases in renal kallikrein activity may therefore not serve to completly protect against hypertension. The renal kallikrein-kinin system can reasonably be considered to represent one of many components involved in the regulation of blood pressure under physiologic and pathologic conditions.

Kinins and renal disease

Urinary excretion of kallikrein has been assessed in several forms of experimental renal injury. In rats with acute renal failure induced by injection of methemoglobin, urinary kallikrein concentration is markedly decreased.[284] Salt loading protects against the development of renal failure and simultaneously raises kallikrein excretion to normal. Urinary kallikrein decreases in response to acute ureteral ligation.[329] The role played by decreases in kallikrein activity in the pathogenesis of these forms of disease is unknown.

Patients with chronic renal insufficiency have been reported to excrete normal[57] or increased[1] amounts of kallikrein. Both of these studies noted an increase in excretion of kallikrein when adjusted for GFR. The adaptation to progressive nephron loss may involve an increase in kallikrein synthesis per remaining nephron. Alternatively, other factors acting to increase single-nephron GFR might, by increasing distal tubular flow rates in the remnant nephrons, raise kallikrein excretion. Kallikrein concentration is markedly decreased in the urine of patients with renal insufficiency and hypertension.[300] In such patients, blood pressure and urinary kallikrein concentration are inversely correlated; another possible cause-and-effect relationship may be involved.

REFERENCES

1. Adetuyibi A, Mills IH: Relation between urinary kallikrein and renal function, hypertension, and excretion of sodium and water in man. *Lancet* 2:203, 1972.
2. Adler S et al: Biphasic effect of oxygen radicals on prostaglandin production by rat mesangial cells. *Am J Physiol* 252:F743, 1987.
3. Alavi N et al: Prostaglandin and thromboxane synthesis by highly enriched rabbit proximal tubular cells in culture. *J Lab Clin Med* 110:338, 1987.
4. Alavi N et al: Reduction of proteinuria by indomethacin

in patients with nephrotic syndrome. *Am J Kidney Dis* 8:397, 1986.
5. Albrightson CR et al: Effect of endogenously produced leukotrienes and thromboxane on renal vascular resistance in rabbit hydronephrosis. *Circ Res* 61:514, 1987.
6. Allen JT et al: The effect of indomethacin on renal blood flow and ureteral pressure in unilateral ureteral obstruction in awake dogs. *Invest Urol* 15:324, 1978.
7. Anderson R et al: Evidence for in vivo antagonism between vasopressin and prostaglandin in the mammalian kidney. *J Clin Invest* 56:420, 1975.
8. Ando Y et al: Dose-dependent heterogenous actions of vasopressin in rabbit cortical collecting ducts. *Am J Physiol* 25:F556, 1989.
9. Ando Y et al: Phorbol myristate acetate, dioctanoylglycerol, and phosphatidic acid inhibit the hydrooxmotic effect of vasopressin on the rabbit collecting tubule. *J Clin Invest* 80:590, 1987.
10. Ando Y et al: Phorbol ester and A23187 have additive but mechanistically separate effects on vasopressin action in rabbit collecting tubule. *J Clin Invest* 81:1578, 1988.
11. Ardaillou N et al: Prostaglandin synthesis by human glomerular cells in culture. *Prostaglandins* 26:773, 1983.
12. Assael BM et al: Prostaglandins and aminoglycoside nephrotoxicity. *Toxicol Appl Pharmacol* 78:386, 1985.
13. Assem ES et al: Mast cells and IgE-mediated release of histamine and arachidonate metabolites from human kidney. *Agents Actions* 23:177, 1988.
14. Assem ES, Abdullah NA: Release of thromboxane B_2 and leukotriene C_4 and reduction in renal perfusion in experimental anaphylactic reaction of isolated guinea pig kidney. *Int Arch Allergy Appl Immunol* 82:212, 1987.
15. Badr KF, Brenner BM: Renal circulatory and nephron function in experimental obstruction of the urinary tract, in Brenner BM, Lazarus JM (eds): *Acute Renal Failure*, 2d ed. Philadelphia, Saunders, 1988, p. 91.
16. Badr KF et al: Glomerular responses to platelet activating factor in the rat: Role of thromboxane A_2. *Am J Physiol* 256:F35, 1989.
17. Badr KF, Ichikawa I: Prerenal failure: A deleterious shift from renal compensation to decompensation. *N Engl J Med* 319:623, 1988.
18. Badr KF et al: Roles for thromboxane A_2 and leukotrienes in endotoxin-induced acute renal failure. *Kidney Int* 30:474, 1986.
19. Badr KF et al: Preservation of the glomerular capillary ultrafiltration coefficient during rat nephrotoxic serum nephritis by a specific leukotriene D_4 receptor antagonist. *J Clin Invest* 81:1702, 1988.
20. Baer PG, Nasjletti A: Effect of uninephrectomy on urinary prostaglandin E_2, F_{2alpha}, and 6-ketoprostaglandin F_{1alpha} excretion in rats. *Clin Sci* 66:407, 1984.
21. Balckshear JL et al: Dissociation of renin release and renal vasodilation by prostaglandin synthesis inhibitors. *Am J Physiol* 237:F20, 1979.
22. Balint P, Laszlo K: Effect of imidazole and indomethacin on hemodynamics of the obstructed canine kidney. *Kidney Int* 27:892, 1985.
23. Bank N et al: Vasoregulatory hormones and the hyperfiltration of diabetes. *Am J Physiol* 254:F202, 1988.
24. Barnett R et al: Vasopressin (AVP) stimulation of phosphatidylinositol (PI) hydrolysis and calcium channel activation in rat medullary interstitial cells (RMIC). *Kidney Int* 37:205, 1990. (Abst.)
25. Barnett R et al: Comparison of glomerular and mesangial prostaglandin synthesis and glomerular contraction in two rat models of diabetes mellitus. *Diabetes* 36:1468, 1987.
26. Bartter FC et al: Hyperplasia of the juxtaglomerular complex with hyperaldosteronism and hypokalemic alkalosis. *Am J Med* 33:821, 1962.
27. Basci A et al: Effect of stimulated neutrophils on cyclic nucleotide content in isolated rat glomeruli. *Am J Physiol* 252:F429, 1987.
28. Baud L, Ardaillou R: Reactive oxygen species: Production and role in the kidney. *Am J Physiol* 251:F765, 1986.
29. Baylis C: Effects of administered thromboxanes on the intact normal rat kidney. *Renal Physiol* 10:110, 1987.
30. Baylis C: Renal effects of cyclooxygenase inhibition in the pregnant rat. *Am J Physiol* 253:F158, 1987.
31. Baylis C, Brenner BM: Modulation by prostaglandin synthesis inhibitors of the action of exogenous angiotensin II on glomerular ultrafiltration in the rat. *Circ Res* 43:899, 1978.
32. Beck TR et al: Effect of arginine vasopressin and its analogues on the synthesis of PGE_2 by rat renal medullary interstitial cells in culture. *J Pharmacol Exp Ther* 215:15, 1980.
33. Beck TR et al: Desamino-D-arginine vasopressin induces fatty acid cyclo-oxygenase activity in the renal medulla of diabetes insipidus rats. *J Pharmacol Exp Ther* 221:269, 1982.
34. Benabe JE et al: Effects of angiotensin II on phosphatidylinositol and polyphosphoinositide turnover in rat kidney. *J Biol Chem* 257:7430, 1982.
35. Benigni A et al: Effect of low-dose aspirin on fetal and maternal generation of thromboxane by platelets in women at risk for pregnancy-induced hypertension. *N Engl J Med* 321:357, 1989.
36. Benigni A et al: Role of renal prostaglandins in normal and nephrotic rats with diet-induced hyperfiltration. *J Lab Clin Med* 108:230, 1986.
37. Berl T et al: Prostaglandins in the betaadrenergic and baroreceptor-mediated secretion of renin. *Am J Physiol* 236:F472, 1979.
38. Berl T et al: Prostaglandin synthesis inhibition in the action of vasopressin: Studies in man and rat. *Am J Physiol* 232:F529, 1977.
39. Berridge MJ: Inositol trisphosphate and diacylglycerol: Two interacting second messengers. *Annu Rev Biochem* 56:159, 1987.
40. Bertani T et al: Effect of aspirin and sulindac in rabbit nephrotoxic nephritis. *J Lab Clin Med* 107:261, 1986.
41. Blackshear PJ et al. Protein kinases 1988: A current perspective. *FASEB J* 2:2957, 1988.
42. Blantz RC et al: Glomerular immune injury in the rat: The influence of angiotensin II rat nephrotoxic serum nephritis, effects on renal hemodynamics. *J Clin Invest* 72:1439, 1981.
43. Blantz RC et al: The acute effect of antiglomerular basement membrane antibody upon glomerular filtration in the rat: The influence of dose and complement depletion. *J Clin Invest* 59:910, 1977.

44. Blasingham MC, Nasjletti A: Contribution of renal prostaglandins to the natriuretic action of bradykinin in the dog. *Am J Physiol* 237:F182, 1979.
45. Bolger PM et al: Effects of PGD_2 on canine renal function. *Nature* (London) 267:628, 1977.
46. Bolger PM et al: Renal action of prostacyclin. *Nature* (*London*) 271:467, 1978.
47. Bonvalet JP et al: Segmental synthesis and actions of prostaglandins (PGs) along the nephron. *Am J Physiol* 253:F377, 1987.
48. Brater DC et al: Effects of ibuprofen, naproxen, and sulindac on prostaglandins in men. *Kidney Int* 27:66, 1985.
49. Brezis M et al: Inhibition of prostaglandin synthesis in rat kidney perfused with and without erythrocytes: Implication for analgesic nephropathy. *Miner Electrolyte Metab* 12:326, 1986.
50. Brown CA et al: Identification of an angiotensin receptor in rabbit renomedullary interstitial cells in culture: Correlation with prostaglandin biosynthesis. *Circ Res* 46:802, 1980.
51. Bryan FT et al: Bradykininogen synthesis by liver, in Back N et al (eds): *Vasopeptides: Chemistry, Pharmacology and Pathophysiology*. New York, Plenum Press, 1972, p 43.
52. Bunke M, Itskovitz H: Urinary excretion and renal production of prostaglandins E_2, F_{2alpha}, and thromboxane B_2 in experimental diabetes mellitus. *J Lab Clin Med* 108:332, 1986.
53. Burnatowska-Hledin MA, Spielman WS: Vasopressin V_1 receptors on the principal cells on the rabbit cortical collecting tubule. *J Clin Invest* 83:84, 1989.
54. Burnier M et al: Effects of nonhypotensive endotoxemia in conscious rats: Role of prostaglandins. *Am J Physiol* 254:H509, 1988.
55. Cadnapaphornchai P et al: Prostaglandin-mediated hyperemia and renin-mediated hypertension during acute ureteral obstruction. *Prostaglandins* 16:965, 1978.
56. Cagen L et al: Estradiol is responsible for reduced renal prostaglandin dehydrogenase activity in female rats. *Biochim Biophys Acta* 833:372, 1985.
57. Cannella G et al: l'escrezione urinaria di callicreina nella glomerulonefrite. *Boll Soc Ital Biol Sper* 49:580, 1973.
58. Carone FA et al: Micropuncture evidence of rapid hydrolysis of bradykinin by rat proximal tubule. *Am J Physiol* 230:1420, 1976.
59. Carretero OA, Scicli AG: The renal kallikrein-kinin system in human and experimental hypertension. *Klin Wochenschr* 56(suppl 1):113, 1978.
60. Carretero OA, Scicli AG: The renal kallikrein-kinin system. *Am J Physiol* 238:F247, 1980.
61. Carretero OA et al: Measurement of urinary kallikrein activity by kinin radioimmunoassay. *Biochem Pharmacol* 25:2265, 1976.
62. Carretero OA et al: Urinary kallikrein, plasma renin and aldosterone in New Zealand genetically hypertensive (GH) rats. *Clin Exp Pharmacol Physiol* 3(suppl):55, 1976.
63. Carretero OA et al: Urinary kallikrein in rats bred for their susceptibility and resistance to the hypertensive effect of salt: A new radioimmunoassay for its direct determination. *Circ Res* 42:727, 1978.
64. Chabardes D et al: Effect of PGE_2 and alpha-adrenergic agonists on AVP-dependent cAMP levels in rabbit and rat CCT. *Am J Physiol* 255:F43, 1988.
65. Chang DG, Tai HH: Characterization of two enzyme proteins catalyzing $NADP^+$/NADPH-dependent oxidoreduction of prostaglandin at C-9 and C-15 from swine kidney. *Arch Biochem Biophys* 214:464, 1982.
66. Chang WC: Effects of steroids on renal NAD^+-dependent 15-hydroxyprostaglandin dehydrogenase activity in ovariectomized rats. *Prostaglandins Leukotrienes Med* 29:25, 1987.
67. Chang WC, Tai HH: Induction of a decrease in renal NAD^+-dependent 15-hydroxyprostaglandin dehydrogenase activity by estradiol in rats. *Biochem Pharmacol* 34:2073, 1985.
68. Chansel D et al: Identification and regulation of renin in human cultured mesangial cells. *Am J Physiol* 252:F32, 1987.
69. Chaudhari A, Kirschenbaum MA: Altered glomerular eicosanoid biosynthesis in uranyl nitrate-induced acute renal failure. *Biochim Biophys Acta* 792:135, 1984.
70. Chaudhari A, Kirschenbaum MA: Specific prostaglandin E_2 binding sites in isolated rat glomeruli: Evidence for glomerular PGE receptors. *Prostaglandins Leukotrienes Med* 20:55, 1985.
71. Chevalier RL et al: Endogenous prostaglandins modulate autoregulation of renal blood flow in young rats. *Am J Physiol* 253:F66, 1987.
72. Christiansen JS et al: Short-term inhibition of prostaglandin synthesis has no effect on the elevated glomerular filtration rate of early insulin-dependent diabetes. *Diabetic Med* 2:17, 1985.
73. Cibattoni G et al: Effects of sulindac on renal and extrarenal eicosanoid synthesis. *Clin Pharmacol Ther* 41:380, 1987.
74. Ciabattoni G et al: Effects of sulindac and ibuprofen in patients with chronic glomerular disease: Evidence for the dependence of renal function on prostacyclin. *N Engl J Med* 310:279, 1984.
75. Ciabattoni G et al: Effects of sulindac and ibuprofen in patients with chronic glomerular disease: Evidence for the dependence of renal function on prostacyclin. *N Engl J Med* 310:279, 1984.
76. Codde JP, Beilin LJ: Dietary fish oil prevents dexamethasone induced hypertension in the rat. *Clin Sci* 69:691, 1985.
77. Codde JP et al: Dietary suppression of prostaglandin synthesis does not accelerate DOCA/salt hypertension in rats. *Clin Exp Pharmacol Physiol* 14:513, 1987.
78. Coffman TM et al: Evidence that renal prostaglandin and thromboxane production is stimulated in chronic cyclosporine nephrotoxicity. *Transplantation* 43:282, 1987.
79. Coffman TM et al: Functional role of thromboxane production by acutely rejecting renal allografts in rats. *J Clin Invest* 75:1242, 1985.
80. Coffman TM et al: Effect of dietary fish oil supplementation on eicosanoid production by rat renal allografts. *Transplantation* 45:470, 1988.
81. Colombani P et al: Cyclosporine A binding to calmodulin: A possible site of action on T lymphocytes. *Science* 228:337, 1985.
82. Conrad KP, Colpoys MC: Evidence against the hypothesis

that prostaglandins are the vasodepressor agents of pregnancy: Serial studies in chronically instrumented, conscious rats. *J Clin Invest* 77:236, 1986.
83. Conrad KP, Dunn MJ: Renal synthesis and urinary excretion of eicosanoids during pregnancy in rats. *Am J Physiol* 253:F1197, 1987.
84. Cook HT et al: Effect of a thromboxane synthesis inhibitor on eicosanoid synthesis and glomerular injury during acute unilateral glomerulonephritis in the rat. *Clin Nephrol* 26:195, 1986.
85. Cooper CL, Malik KU: Evidence that bradykinin stimulates renal prostaglandin synthesis by a mechanism distinct from that of other vasoactive substances. *Circ Res* 60:914, 1987.
86. Cooper CL et al: Mechanism of action of angiotensin II and bradykinin on prostaglandin synthesis and vascular tone in the isolated rat kidney: Effect of Ca^{++} antagonists and calmodulin inhibitors. *Circ Res* 56:97, 1985.
87. Croxatto HR et al: Effect of furosemide upon urinary kallikrein excretion. *Agents Actions* 3:267, 1973.
88. Craven PA et al: Sequential alterations in glomerular prostaglandin and thromboxane synthesis in diabetic rats: Relationship to the hyperfiltration of early diabetes. *Metabolism* 36:95, 1987.
89. Craven PA, DeRobertis FR: Ca-calmodulin-dependent release of arachidonic acid for renal medullary prostaglandin synthesis; Evidence for involvement of phospholipases A_2 and C. *J Biol Chem* 258:4814, 1983.
90. Croxatto HR et al: The effect of water, sodium overloading and diuretics upon urinary kallikrein. *Adv Exp Med Biol* 70:361, 1975.
91. Croxatto HR et al: Renal urinary kallikrein in normotensive and hypertensive rats during enhanced excretion of water and electrolytes. *Clin Sci* 51:259S, 1976.
92. Culpepper RM, Andreoli TE: Interactions among prostaglandin E_2, antidiuretic hormone and cyclic adenosine monophosphate in modulating Cl absorption in single mouse medullary thick ascending limbs of Henle. *J Clin Invest* 71:1588, 1983.
93. Culpepper RM, Andreoli TE: PGE_2, forskolin, and cholera toxin interactions in modulating NaCl transport in mouse mTALH. *Am J Physiol* 247:F784, 1984.
94. Currie M et al: The mechanism and site of the enhanced arachidonate metabolism in ureter obstruction, in Dunn MJ et al (eds): *Prostaglandins and the Kidney*. New York, Plenum Press, 1983, p 299.
95. Currie MG et al: Cell culture of renal epithelium derived from rabbit microdissected cortical collecting tubules. *Am J Physiol* 244:F724, 1983.
96. Cybulsky AV et al: A role for thromboxane in complement-mediated glomerular injury. *Am J Pathol* 128:45, 1987.
97. Dallinger KJ et al: Specific thromboxane synthetase inhibition and haemostasis in insulin-dependent diabetics. *Diabetes Res* 3:377, 1986.
98. Danon A et al: Eicosanoid synthesis by rabbit hydronephrotic cortical interstitial cells in culture. *J Pharmacol Exp Ther* 238:95, 1986.
99. Daskalopoulos G et al: Sulindac and indomethacin suppress the diuretic action of furosemide in patients with cirrhosis and ascites: Evidence that sulindac affects renal prostaglandins. *Am J Kidney Dis* 6:217, 1985.
100. Data JL et al: The prostaglandin system: A role in baroreceptor control of renin release. *Circ Res* 42:454, 1978.
101. Debono E, Mills IH: Simultaneous increases in kallikrein in renal lymph and urine during saline infusion. *J Physiol* 241:127P, 1974.
102. Deermann B et al: A double blind comparison of naproxen and sulindac in female patients with heart failure. *Scand J Rheumatol* 62(suppl):32, 1986.
103. Dixey JJ et al: The effect of indomethacin on the renal response to arginine vasopressin in man. *Clin Sci* 70:409, 1986.
104. Dixon BS et al: Protein kinase C (PKC) regulates cAMP phosphodiesterase activity in LLC-PK: cells. *Kidney Int* 37:207, 1990. (Abstr.)
105. Dixon BS et al: Phorbol esters inhibit adenylate cyclase activity in cultured collecting tubular cells. *Am J Physiol* 254:C183, 1988.
106. Dominguez JH et al: Prostaglandin E_2 and parathyroid hormone: Comparisons of their actions on the rabbit proximal tubule. *Kidney Int* 26:404, 1984.
107. Dominguez JH et al: Prostaglandin E_2 is an inhibitor of adenylate cyclase in rabbit proximal tubule. *Am J Physiol* 254:C304, 1988.
108. Donadio JV et al: Platelet-inhibitor treatment of diabetic nephropathy: A 10-year prospective study. *Mayo Clin Proc* 63:3, 1988.
109. Donher AJ: Indomethacin in Bartter's syndrome. *Nephron* 19:200, 1977.
110. Dunn MJ et al: Renal excretion of prostaglandins E_2 and $F_{2\alpha}$ in diabetes insipidus rat. *Am J Physiol* 235:E624, 1978.
111. Dunn MJ et al: Renal excretion of prostaglandin E_2 and $F_{2\alpha}$ in diabetes insipidus rat. *Am J Physiol* 255:E629, 1978.
112. Dunn MJ, Grone HJ: The relevance of prostaglandins in human hypertension. *Adv Prostaglandin Thromboxane Leukotriene Res* 13:179, 1985.
113. Dusing R et al: Renal prostaglandin and water balance: Studies in normal volunteer subjects and in patients with central diabetes insipidus. *Clin Sci* 61:61, 1981.
114. Edwards RM: Effects of prostaglandins on vasoconstrictor action in isolated renal arterioles. *Am J Physiol* 248:F779, 1985.
115. Edwards RM et al: ADH-sensitive cAMP system in papillary collecting duct: Effect of osmolality and PGE_2. *Am J Physiol* 240:F311: 1981.
116. Elzinga L et al: modification of experimental nephrotoxicity with fish oil as the vehicle for cyclosporine. *Transplantation* 43:271, 1987.
117. Epstein M, Lifschitz M: Renal eicosanoids as determinants of renal function in liver disease. *Hepatology* 7:1359, 1987.
118. Eriksen EF et al: Prostagladin-E_2 receptors in the rat kidney: Biochemical characterization and localization. *Kidney Int* 32:181, 1987.
119. Erman A et al: Different pools of esterified arachidonic acid in rabbit kidney medulla: Relationship to Ca^{2+}-stimulated prostaglandin biosynthesis. *Lipids* 17:119, 1982.
120. Erman A et al: Augmentation of unesterified arachidonic acid in the renal inner medulla of dexamethasone-treated rats: Relationship to altered triglyceride metabolism. *J Biol Chem* 260:4679, 1985.

121. Erman A et al: Treatment with dexamethasone increases glomerular prostaglandin synthesis in rats. *J Pharmacol Exp Ther* 239:296, 1986.
122. Erman A, Nasjletti A: Enhancement of renal medulla prostaglandin synthetase following dexamethasone treatment in the rat. *Biochem Biophys Res Commun* 121:255, 1984.
123. Esmatjes E et al: Renal hemodynamic abnormalities in patients with short term insulin-dependent diabetes mellitus: Role of renal prostaglandins. *J Clin Endocrinol Metab* 60:1231, 1985.
124. Esmatjes E et al: Renal excretion of prostaglandin E_2 and plasma renin activity in type I diabetes mellitus: Relationship to normoglycemia achieved with artificial pancreas. *Diabetes Care* 10:428, 1987.
125. Farman N et al: PGE_2, $PGF_{2\alpha}$, 6-keto-$PGF_{1\alpha}$, and TXB_2 synthesis along the rabbit nephron. *Am J Physiol* 252:F53, 1987.
126. Favre L et al: Reversible acute renal failure from combined triemterene and indomethacin: A study in healthy subjects. *Ann Int Med* 96:317, 1982.
127. Fejes-Toth G et al: Renal response to vasopressin after inhibition of prostaglandin synthesis. *Am J Physiol* 232:F416, 1977.
128. Fejes-Toth G et al: Acute effects of antidiuretic hormone on urinary prostaglandin excretion. *J Pharmacol Exp Ther* 227:215, 1983.
128a. Findling JW et al: Indomethacin-induced acute renal failure in three patients with gouty arthritis. *JAMA* 244:1127, 1980.
129. Fine LG, Trizna WP: Influence of prostaglandins on sodium transport of isolated medullary nephron segments. *Am J Physiol* 232:F383, 1977.
130. Finn WF et al: Protective effect of prosyacycline on postischemic acute renal failure in the rat. *Kidney Int* 32:479, 1987.
131. Flamenbaum W et al: Bradykinin-induced renal hemodynamic alterations: Renin and prostaglandin relationships. *Am J Physiol* 237:F433, 1979.
132. Flower RJ, Blackwell GJ: The importance of phospholipase A_2 in prostaglandin synthesis. *Biochem Pharmacol* 25:286, 1976.
133. Foidart JB, Mahieu P: Glomerular mesangial cell contractility in vitro is controlled by an angiotensin-prostaglandin balance. *Mol Cell Endocrinol* 47:163, 1986.
134. Folkert VW, Schlondorff D: Altered prostaglandin synthesis by glomeruli from rats with unilateral ureteral ligation. *Am J Physiol* 241:F289, 1981.
135. Folkert VW, Schlondorff D: Prostaglandin synthesis linked to phosphatidyl inositol turnover in isolated rat glomeruli. *Biochem Biophys Acta* 794:206, 1984.
136. Fragola J et al: Inhibition of the renal tubular effects of PTH on phosphate transport by PGE_2. *Endocrinology* 109:2267, 1981.
137. Franco M et al: Evaluation of prostaglandins as mediators of tubuloglomerular feedback. *Am J Physiol* 254:F642, 1988.
138. Franco-Saenz R et al: Prostaglandin stimulation of renin release: Independence of β-adrenergic receptor activity and mechanism of action. *Endocrinology* 106:1400, 1980.
139. Fransisco LL et al: Prostaglandins in renin release during sodium deprivation. *Am J Physiol* 243:F537, 1982.
140. Freeman RH et al: Role of renal prostaglandins in the control of renin release. *Circ Res* 54:1, 1984.
141. Friedlander G et al: Benzyl alcohol increases membrane fluidity and modulates cyclic AMP synthesis in intact renal epithelial cells. *Biochim Biophys Acta* 903:341, 1987.
142. Frohlich JC et al: Reduction of plasma renin activity by inhibition of the fatty acid cyclooxygenase in human subjects. *Circ Res* 44:781, 1979.
143. Fujimoto Y et al: Triacylglycerol lipase-mediated release of arachidonic acid for renal medullary prostaglandin synthesis. *Arch Biochem Biophys* 261:368, 1988.
144. Fukuda S et al: Increase in enzyme activities of prostaglandin biosynthesis and catabolism by acute ureteral ligaton in rat kidney. *Life Sci* 37:1249, 1985.
145. Fulgraff G, Meiforth A: Effects of prostaglandin E_2 on excretion and reabsorption of sodium and fluid in rat kidneys (micropuncture studies). *Pfluegers Arch* 330:243, 1971.
146. Gan BS et al: Epidermal growth factor-urogastrone causes vasodilatation in the anesthetized dog. *J Clin Invest* 80:199, 1987.
147. Ganguli M et al: Evidence that prostaglandin synthesis inhibitors increase the concentration of sodium and chloride in rat medulla. *Circ Res* 40:135, 1977.
148. Garcia-Perez A, Smith WL: Apical-basolateral membrane asymmetry in canine cortical collecting tubule cells. *J Clin Invest* 74:63, 1984.
149. Garcia-Perez A, Smith WL: Use of monoclonal antibodies to isolate cortical collecting tubule cells: AVP induces PGE release. *Am J Physiol* 244:C211, 1983.
150. Gaudio KM et al: Renal perfusion and intratubular pressure during utereral occlusion in the rat. *Am J Physiol* 238:F205, 1980.
151. Geiger R, Mann K: A kallikrein-specific inhibitor in rat kidney tubules. *Hoppe Seylers Z Physiol Chem* 357:553, 1976.
152. Geiger R et al: Isolation of human urinary kallikrein by affinity chromatography. Determination of human urinary kallikrein. *J Clin Chem Clin Biochem* 12:479, 1977.
153. Gerber JG et al: Prostaglandins and renin release: 2. Assessment of renin secretion following infusion of PGI_2, E_2, and D_2 into the renal artery of anesthetized dogs. *Prostaglandins* 15:81, 1978.
154. Gerber JG et al: Control of canine renin release: Macula densa requires prostaglandin synthesis. *J Physiol* 319:419, 1981.
155. Gibbons CP et al: Cortical and vascular prostaglandin synthesis during renal allograft rejection in the rat. *Transplantation* 43:472, 1987.
156. Gill JR: Bartter's syndrome. *Annu Rev Med* 30:405, 1980.
157. Gill JR, Bartter FC: Evidence for a prostaglandin-independent defect in chloride reabsorption in the loop of Henle as a proximal cause of Bartter's syndrome. *Am J Med* 65:766, 1978.
158. Gill JR et al: Bradykinin and renal function in normal man: Effects of adrenergic blockade. *Am J Physiol* 209:844, 1965.
159. Gill JR et al: Bartter's syndrome: A disorder characterized

by high urinary prostaglandins and a dependence of hyperreninemia on prostaglandin synthesis. *Am J Med* 61:43, 1976.
160. Goto F et al: Effect of cyclooxygenase and thromboxane synthase inhibition on the response to angiotensin II in the hypoperfused canine kidney. *J Pharmacol Exp. Ther* 243:799, 1987.
161. Govindarajan S et al: Immunohistochemical distribution of renal prostaglandin endoperoxide synthase and prostacyclin synthase: Diminished endoperoxide synthase in the hepatorenal syndrome. *Hepatology* 7:654, 1987.
162. Grantham JJ, Orloff J: Effect of prostaglandin E_1 on the permeability response of the isolated collecting tubule to vasopressin, adenosine 3′,5′-monophosphate, and theophylline. *J Clin Invest* 47:1154, 1968.
163. Gregoire I et al: Effect of pregnancy on plasma renin activity and glomerular synthesis of prostaglandins and thromboxane in rats. *Agents Actions* 22(suppl):147, 1987.
164. Gregiore I et al: Prostanoid synthesis by isolated rat glomeruli: Effect of oestrous cycle and pregnancy. *Clin Sci* 73:641, 1987.
165. Grone HJ et al: Role of thromboxane in control of arterial pressure and renal function in young spontaneously hypertensive rats. *Am J Physiol* 250:F488, 1986.
166. Gross JB, Bartter FC: Effects of prostaglandins E_1, A_1, and F_2 on renal handling of salt and water. *Am J Physiol* 225:218, 1973.
167. Guarner C et al: Renal prostaglandins in cirrhosis of the liver. *Clin Sci* 70:477, 1986.
168. Guarner F et al: Increased synthesis of systemic prostacyclin ion cirrhotic patients. *Gastroenterology* 90:687, 1986.
169. Guarner F et al: Renal function in fulminant hepatic failure: Hemodynamics and renal prostaglandins. *Gut* 28:1643, 1987.
170. Güllner H-G: Prostacyclin overproduction in Bartter's syndrome. *Lancet* 2:767, 1979.
171. Güllner H-G: Correction of increased prostacyclin synthesis in Bartter's syndrome by indomethacin treatment. *Prostaglandins Med* 4:65, 1980.
172. Hall DA, Varney DM: Effect of vasopressin on electrical potential difference and chloride transport in mouse medullary thick ascending limb of Henle. *J Clin Invest* 66:792, 1980.
173. Hall ER et al: Angiotensin I-converting enzyme in the nephron. *Life Sci* 18:1299, 1976.
174. Halushka PV et al: Bartter's syndrome: Urinary prostaglandin E-like material and kallikrein, indomethacin effects. *Ann Intern Med* 87:281, 1977.
175. Ham EA et al: Peroxidase dependent deactivation of prostacylcin synthetase. *J Biol Chem* 254:2191. 1979.
176. Hansch GM et al: The complement membrane attack complex stimulates the prostanoid production of cultured glomerular epithelial cells. *Int Arch Allergy Appl Immunol* 85:87, 1988.
177. Hansen HS: 15-hydroxyprostaglandin dehydrogenase: A review. *Prostaglandins* 12:647, 1976.
178. Harris RC et al: Involvement of cyclooxygenase and cytochrome P450 metabolites of arachidonic acid in rat renal responses to epidermal growth factor. *Kidney Int* 35:312, 1989.
179. Hashimoto T: Effects of prostaglandin E_2, I_2, and $F_{2\alpha}$ on systemic and renal hemodynamics, renal function, and renin secretion in anesthetized dogs. *Jpn J Pharmacol* 30: 173, 1980.
180. Hassid A et al: Metabolism of prostaglandin by human renal enzymes: Presence of 9,15-hydroxyprostaglandin dehydrogenase activity in human kidney. *Adv Prostaglandin Thromboxane Res* 11:49, 1983.
181. Haylor J: Prostaglandin synthesis and renal function in man. *J Physiol* 298:383, 1980.
182. Hayashi Y et al: Role of prostaglandins in norepinephrine and renin release in canine kidney. *Am J Physiol* 253:F929, 1987.
183. Hays S et al: Hormonal regulation of proton secretion in rabbit medullary collecting duct. *J Clin Invest* 78:1279, 1986.
184. Hays SR et al: Effects of protein kinase C activation on sodium, poyassium, chloride and total CO_2 transport in the rabbit cortical collecting tubule. *J Clin Invest* 80:1561, 1987.
185. Hebert RL et al: Prostaglandin E_2 raises cell calcium in rabbit cortical collecting duct (CCD): An action distinct from its effects on AVP-stimulated water flow. *Am J Physiol* 259:F318, 1990.
186. Hebert SC et al: NaCl transport in mouse medullary thick ascending limbs: 1. Functional nephron heterogeneity and ADH-stimulated NaCl cotransport. *Am J Physiol* 241:F412, 1981.
187. Helman SI, O'Neil RG: Model of active transepithelial Na and K transport of renal collecting tubules. *Am J Physiol* 233:F55, 1977.
188. Henrich WL et al: Renal hemodynamic effects of therapeutic plasma levels of sulindac sulfide during hemorrhage. *Kidney Int* 29:484, 1986.
189. Higa EM et al: Role of the prostaglandin and kallikrein-kinin systems in aminoglycoside-induced acute renal failure. *Braz J Med Biol Res* 18:355, 1985.
190. Higashihara E et al: Cortical and papillary micropuncture examination of chloride transport in segments of the rat kidney during inhibition of prostaglandin production: Possible role for prostaglandins in the chloriuresis of acute volume expansion. *J Clin Invest* 64:1277, 1979.
191. Hochstrasser K et al: Proteinase inhibitors of the respiratory tract: Studies on the structural relationship between acid-stable inhibitors present in the respiratory tract, plasma and urine, in Bayer-Symposium V, *Proteinase Inhibitors*. Berlin, Springer-Verlag, 1974, p 11.
192. Homma T et al: Prostaglandins of mesangium origin inhibit mesangial cell proliferation and matrix synthesis. *Kidney Int* 33:268, 1988.
193. Hseuh W, Needleman P: Sites of lipase activation and prostaglandin synthesis in isolated, perfused rabbit hearts and hydronephrotic kidneys. *Prostaglandins* 16:661, 1978.
194. Hseuh W et al: Hormone selective lipase activation. *Prostaglandins* 13:1073, 1977.
195. Ichikawa I, Brenner BM: Local intrarenal vasoconstrictor-vasodilator interactions in mild partial ureteral obstruction. *Am J Physiol* 236:F131, 1979.

196. Ichikawa I et al: Dietary protein intake conditions the degree of renal vasoconstriction in acute renal failure caused by ureteral obstruction. *Am J Physiol* 249:F54, 1985.
197. Ino Y, Imai M: Effects of prostaglandins on sodium transport in isolated collecting tubules. *Pfluegers Arch* 373:125, 1978.
198. Imbert-Teboul M et al: Vasopressin-dependent adenylate cyclase activities in the rat kidney medulla: Evidence for two separate sites of action. *Endocrinology* 102:1254, 1978.
199. Imbert-Teboul M et al: Sites of prostaglandin E_2 synthesis along the rabbit nephron. *Mol Cell Endocrinol* 45:1, 1986.
200. Inokuchi K, Malik KU: Attenuation by prostaglandins of adrenergically induced renal vasoconstriction in anesthetized rats. *Am J Physiol* 246:R228, 1984.
201. Isakson PC et al: Hormonal stimulation of arachidonate release from isolated perfused organs: Relationship to prostaglandin biosynthesis. *Prostaglandins* 14:853, 1977.
202. Ishikawa S et al: Calmodulin regulation of cellular cyclic AMP production in response to arginine vasopressin, prostaglandin E_2 and forskolin in rat renal papillary collecting tubule cells in culture. *J Endocrinol* 107:15, 1985.
203. Itskovitz HD, Campbell WB: Vasodilators, intrarenal distribution of blood flow and renal function in isolated perfused canine kidneys. *Proc Soc Exp Biol Med* 153:161, 1976.
204. Izumi Y et al: Effects of dietary linoleic acid on blood pressure and renal function in subtotally nephrectomized rats. *Proc Soc Exp Biol Med* 183:193, 1986.
205. Jackson BA et al: Vasopressin-prostaglandin interactions in isolated tubules from rat outer medulla. *J Lab Clin Med* 96:119, 1980.
206. Jackson RM et al: Production of arachidonic acid metabolites by endothelial cells in hyperoxia. *J Appl Physiol* 61:584, 1986.
207. Jaisser F et al: Effects of AVP and dDAVP on PGE_2 synthesis in superfused cortical collecting tubules. *Am J Physiol* 256:F1044, 1989.
208. Johnson M et al: Alternate pathways of arachidonate metabolism: Prostaglandins, thromboxane, and leukotrienes, in Cambell PN, Marshall RD (eds): *Essays in Biochemistry*. New York, Academic Press, 1983.
209. Johnston HH et al: Effect of prostaglandin E: On renal hemodynamics, sodium, and water excretion. *Am J Physiol* 213:939, 1967.
210. Kaizu T, Margolius HS: Studies on rat renal cortical cell kallikrein: 1. Separation and measurement. *Biochim Biophys Acta* 411:305, 1975.
211. Kaizu K et al: Role of prostaglandins and angiotensin II in experimental glomerulonephritis. *Kidney Int* 28:629, 1985.
212. Katayama S et al: Increased thromboxane B_2 excretion in diabetes mellitus. *J Lab Clin Med* 109:711, 1987.
213. Katayama S et al: Estradiol stimulates rat renopapillary prostaglandin E_2 (PGE_2), but not PGF_2 alpha biosynthesis. *Endocrinology* 117:656, 1985.
214. Kawaguchi H et al: Renal prostaglandins and phospholipase A_2 in spontaneously hypertensive rats. *J Hypertens* 5:299, 1987.
215. Hayashi K et al: Atrial natriuretic factor does not stimulate prostaglandin synthesis in isolated rat glomeruli. *Endocrinol Jpn* 33:369, 1986.
216. Keith JC Jr et al: Beneficial effects of U-63,557A, a thromboxane synthetase inhibitor, in an ovine model of pregnancy-induced hypertension. *Am J Obstet Gynecol* 157:199, 1987.
217. Kelley VE et al: A fish oil diet rich in eicosapentaenoic acid reduces cyclooxygenase metabolites, and suppresses lupus in MRL-lpr mice. *J Immunol* 134:1914, 1985.
218. Kelley VE et al: Increased renal thromboxane production in murine lupus nephritis. *J Clin Invest* 77:252, 1986.
219. Kelly CJ et al: Prostaglandin E_1 inhibits effector T cell induction and tissue damage in experimental murine interstitial nephritis. *J Clin Invest* 79:782, 1987.
220. Kher V et al: Protective effect of polyunsaturated fatty acid supplementation in apoferritin induced murine glomerulonephritis. *Prostaglandins Leukotrienes Med* 22:323, 1986.
221. Khirabadi BS et al: Urine immunoreactive thromboxane B_2 in rat cardiac allograft rejection. *Transplantation* 39:6, 1985.
222. Kirschenbaum MA: Prostanoids and renal failure: A hypothetical role for prostanoids in progressive renal disease. *Contrib Nephrol* 50:36, 1986.
223. Kirschenbaum MA, Chaudhari A: Effect of experimental diabetes on glomerular filtration rate and glomerular prostanoid production in the rat. *Miner Electrolyte Metab* 12:352, 1986.
224. Kirschenbaum MA et al: Effect of indomethacin on proteinuria in rats with autologous immune complex nephropathy. *Prostaglandins* 30:295, 1985.
225. Kirschenbaum MA et al: Regulation of vasopressin action by prostaglandins. *J Clin Invest* 70:1193, 1982.
226. Kirschenbaum MA et al: Regulation of vasopressin action by prostaglandins: Evidence for prostaglandin synthesis in the rabbit cortical collecting tubule. *J Clin Invest* 70:1193, 1982.
227. Kirschner KA: Indomethacin antagonizes furosemide's intratubular effects during loop segment microperfusion. *J Pharmacol Exp Ther* 243:881, 1987.
228. Kirschner KA: Prostaglandin inhibitors alter loop segment chloride uptake during furosemide diuresis. *Am J Physiol* 248:F698, 1985.
229. Kirschner KA et al: Prostaglandin E_2 but not I_2 restores furosemide response in indomethacin-treated rats. *Am J Physiol* 250:F980, 1986.
230. Klotman PE et al: Thromboxane synthesis inhibition improves function of hydronephrotic rat kidneys. *Am J Physiol* 250:F282, 1986.
231. Knapp HR, Fitzgerald G: The antihypertensive effects of fish oil: A controlled study of polyunsaturated fatty acid supplementation in essential hypertension. *N Engl J Med* 320:1037, 1989.
232. Knauss T, Abboud HE: Effect of serotonin on prostaglandin synthesis in rat cultured mesangial cells. *Am J Physiol* 251:F844, 1986.
233. Koeppen BM et al: Intracellular microelectrode characterization of the rabbit cortical collecting duct. *Am J Physiol* 244:F35, 1983.
234. Kopp U et al: The role of prostaglandin in alpha and beta

adrenoceptor mediated renin release response to graded renal nerve stimulation. *Pfluegers Arch* 391:1, 1981.
235. Koopmans PP et al: The effects of sulindac and indomethacin on the antihypertensive and diuretic action of hydrochlorothiazide in patients with mild to moderate essential hypertension. *Br J Clin Pharmacol* 21:417, 1986.
236. Korff JM, Jarabak J: An NADP-linked prostacyclin dehydrogenase in rabbit kidney. *Prostaglandins* 21:719, 1981.
237. Kramer H: Effects of inhibition of prostaglandin synthesis on renal electrolyte excretion and concentrating ability. *Prostaglandins Med* 1:341, 1978.
238. Kramer HJ et al: Effects of aprotinin on renal function and urinary prostaglandin excretion in conscious rats after acute salt loading. *Clin Sci* 56:547, 1979.
239. Kreisberg JI, Venkatachalam MA: Vasoactive agents affect mesangial cell adhesion. *Am J Physiol* 251:C505, 1986.
240. Kung-Chao DTY, Tai HH: NAD^+ dependent 15-hydroxyprostaglandin dehydrogenase from porcine kidney: 1. Purification and partial characterization. *Biochim Biophys Acta* 614:1, 1980.
241. Kung-Chao DTY, Tai HH: NAD^+dependent 15-hydroxyprostaglandin dehydrogenase from porcine kidney: 2. Kinetic studies. *Biochim Biophys Acta* 614:14, 1980.
242. Laffi G et al: Effects on sulindac and ibuprofen in patients with cirrhosis and ascites: An explanation for the renal-sparing effect of sulindac. *Gastroenterology* 90:182, 1986.
243. Laffi G et al: Altered renal and platelet arachidonic acid metabolism in cirrhosis. *Gastroenterology* 90:274, 1986.
244. Lands WEM: The biosynthesis and metabolism of prostaglandins. *Annu Rev Physiol* 41:633, 1979.
245. Lavelle KJ: Effect of indomethacin and benoxaprofen on immune complex interaction with cultured glomerular cells. *Immunol Invest* 14:211, 1985.
246. Lavelle KJ et al: Effect of prostaglandins on immune complex interaction with glomerular cells in vitro. *Immunol Invest* 14:57, 1985.
247. Lefkowith JB et al: Paradoxical conservation of cardiac and renal arachidonate content in essential fatty acid deficiency. *J Biol Chem* 260:15736, 1985.
248. Lefkowith JB et al: Metabolic and functional alterations in macrophages induced by essential fatty acid deficiency. *J Biol Chem* 262:6668, 1987.
249. Lefkowith JB et al: Murine glomerular leukotriene B_4 synthesis. Manipulation by (ω-6) fatty acid deprivation and cellular origin. *J Clin Invest* 82:1655, 1988.
250. Lefkowith JB, Schreiner G: Essential fatty acid deficiency depletes rat glomeruli of resident macrophages and inhibits angiotensin II-induced eicosanoid synthesis. *J Clin Invest* 80:947, 1987.
251. Lelcuk S et al: Prostacyclin and thromboxane A_2 moderate postischemic renal failure. *Surgery* 98:207, 1985.
252. Lenhard V et al: Transfusion-induced enhancement of prostaglandin and thromboxane release in prospective kidney graft recipients. *Proc Eur Dial Transplant Assoc Eur Ren Assoc* 21:923, 1985.
253. Levine MM et al: Effect of protein on glomerular filtration rate and prostanoid synthesis in normal and uremic rats. *Am J Physiol* 251:F635, 1986.
254. Levine SD, Jacoby M: High concentrations of prostaglandin E_2 (PGE_2) inhibit water flow across toad bladder via a kinase-C dependent mechanism. *Kidney Int* 37:209, 1990. (Abstr.)
255. Levinsky NG: The renal kallikrein-kinin system. *Circ Res* 44:441, 1979.
256. Levy SB et al: The relationship of urinary kallikrein activity to renal salt and water excretion. *Clin Sci* 54:39, 1978.
257. Lianos EA et al: Glomerular prostaglandin and thromboxane synthesis in rat nephrotoxic serum nephritis: Effects on renal hemodynamics. *J Clin Invest* 72:1439, 1983.
258. Lieberthal W et al: Reduced ratio of active-to-total urinary kallikrein in essential hypertension. *Hypertension* 4:603, 1983.
259. Limas C, Limas CJ: Prostaglandin receptors in rat kidney. *Arch Biochem Biophys* 233:32, 1984.
260. Limas C, Limas CJ: Renomedullary phospholipases in salt-sensitive and salt-resistant Dahl rats. *Am J Med Sci* 290:185, 1985.
261. Limas C, Limas CJ: Homologous regulation of prostaglandin E_2 receptors in rat renal medulla. *Arch Biochem Biophys* 259:89, 1987.
262. Lin CS et al: Prostaglandins and renin release in vitro. *Am J Physiol* 240:E609, 1981.
263. Liston TE, Roberts LJ: Metabolic fate of radiolabeled prostaglandin D_2 in a normal human male volunteer. *J Biol Chem* 260:13172, 1985.
264. Livio M et al: Metabolism of arachidonic acid in isolated glomeruli from pig kidney. *Biochem Biophys Acta* 961:110, 1988.
265. Logan JL, Benson B: Further studies on the effects of cyclooxygenase inhibitors on compensatory renal growth. *Prostaglandins Leukotrienes Med* 30:9, 1987.
266. Logan JL et al: Inhibition of compensatory renal growth by indomethacin. *Prostaglandins* 31:253, 1986.
267. Loo M et al: Effect of thromboxane inhibition on renal blood flow in dogs with complete unilateral ureteral obstruction. *J Urol* 136:1343, 1986.
268. Loutzenhiser R et al: Reversal of renal and smooth muscle actions of the thromboxane mimetic U-44069 by diltiazem. *Am J Physiol* 250:F619, 1986.
269. Lovett DH et al: Interleukin I and the glomerular mesangium: 1. Punification and characterization of a mesangial-derived outgrowth factor. *J Immunol* 136:3700, 1986.
270. Lovett D: Interleukin I and the glomerular mesangium: 2. Monokine stimulation of mesangial cell prostanoid secretion. *Am J Pathol* 129:543, 1987.
271. MacFarlane NAA et al: Changes in kallikrein excretion during arterial infusion of angiotensin, abstracted. *J Endocrinol* 61:72P, 1974.
272. Maddox DA et al: Determinants of glomerular filtration in experimental glomerulonephritis in the rat. *J Clin Invest* 55:305, 1975.
273. Malik KU, Nasjletti A: Attenuation by bradykinin of adrenergically-induced vasoconstriction in the isolated perfused kidneys of the rabbit: Relationship to prostaglandin synthesis. *Br J Pharmacol* 67:269, 1979.
274. Manoogian C et al: The renal vasodilating effect of

dopamine is mediated by calcium flux and prostacyclin release in man. *J Clin Endocrinol Metab* 66:678, 1988.

275. Margolis BL et al: Epidermal growth factor is synergistic with phorbol esters and vasopressin in stimulating arachidonate release and prostaglandin production in renal glomerular mesangial cells. *Biochem J* 249:587, 1988.
276. Margolis BL et al: Epidermal growth factor stimulates phospholipase A_2 in vasopressin treated rat glomerular mesangial cells. *Biochem J* 256:469, 1988.
277. Margolius HS et al: Urinary kallikrein excretion in normal man: Relationships to sodium intake and sodium-retaining steroids. *Circ Res* 35:812, 1974.
278. Margolius HS et al: Urinary kallikrein excretion in hypertensive man: Relationships to sodium, intake and sodium-retaining steroids. *Circ Res* 35:820, 1974.
279. Margolius HS et al: The effects of aldosterone and spironolactone on renal kallikrein in the rat. *Clin Sci* 51:279S, 1976.
280. Maridonneau-Parini I et al: Effect of intracellular oxygen-free radicals on the formation of lipid derived mediators in rat renomedullary interstitial cells. *Biochem Pharmacol* 34:4137, 1985.
281. Marin-Grez M et al: Evidence for an involvement of kinins in regulation of sodium excretion. *Am J Physiol* 223:794, 1972.
282. Marin-Grez M et al: The involvement of urinary kallikrein in the renal escape from the sodium retaining effect of mineralocorticoids. *Henry Ford Hosp Med J* 21:85, 1973.
283. Marin-Grez M: The influence of antibodies against bradykinin on isotonic saline diuresis in the rat. Evidence for kinin involvement in renal function. *Pfluegers Arch* 350:231, 1974.
284. Martin RA et al: Urinary kallikrein and pathophysiology of acute renal failure in the rat. *Medicine* 36:223, 1976.
285. Marver D: PGE_2 and PMA secondarily inhibit rabbit CCT Na-K-ATPase activity by a primary effect on luminal membrane Na permeability. *Kidney Int* 37, 1990.
286. Mathiesen ER et al: Elevated urinary prostaglandin excretion and the effect of indomethacin on renal function in incipient diabetic nephropathy. *Diabetic Med* 5:145, 1988.
287. Mathson JR et al: Effect of inhibition of prostaglandin synthesis on fetal renal function. *Kidney Int* 20:621, 1981.
288. Matsumura Y et al: Synergistic action of angiotensin II on norepinephrine-induced prostaglandin release from rat glomeruli. *Am J Physiol* 250:F811, 1986.
289. McGiff JC et al: Release of prostaglandin-like substance into renal venous blood in response to angiotensin II. *Circ Res* 26/27(suppl I):1121, 1970.
290. McGiff JC et al: Release of a prostaglandin E-like substance from canine kidney by bradykinin. *Circ Res* 31:36, 1972.
291. McGiff JC et al: The actions of bradykinin and eledoisin in the canine isolated kidney: Relationships to prostaglandins. *Clin Sci* 49:125, 1975.
292. Medina JF et al: Effect of spironolactone on renal prostaglandin excretion in patients with liver cirrhosis and ascites. *J Hepatol* 3:206, 1986.
293. Mene P et al: Stimulation of cytosolic free calcium and inositol phosphates by prostaglandins in cultured rat mesangial cells. *Biochem Biophys Res Commun* 142:579, 1987.
294. Mene P, Dunn MJ: Contractile effects of TXA_2 and endoperoxide analogues on cultured rat glomerular mesangial cells. *Am J Physiol* 251:F1029, 1986.
295. Messina EJ et al: Inhibition of bradykinin vasodilation and potentiation of norepinephrine and angiotensin vasoconstriction by inhibitors of prostaglandin synthesis in skeletal muscle of the rat. *Circ Res* 37:430, 1975.
296. Miller MJ et al: Enriched prostaglandin E-9 ketoreductase activity in outer medullary cells of the rabbit kidney. *Prostaglandins* 30:867, 1985.
297. Mills IH et al: The renal kallikrein-kinin system and the regulation of salt and water excretion. *Fed Proc* 35:181, 1976.
298. Minuz P et al: Reduced excretion of vasodilator prostaglandins in preeclampsia. *Agents Actions* 22(suppl):175, 1987.
299. Mistry CD et al: Effects of sulindac on renal function and prostaglandin synthesis in patients with moderate chronic renal insufficiency. *Clin Sci* 70:501, 1986.
300. Mitas JA et al: Urinary kallikrein (UKa): Relationship to hypertension in renal parenchymal disease (RPD). *Clin Res* 26:366A, 1978.
301. Moel DI et al: Effect of aspirin on experimental diabetic nephropathy. *J Lab Clin Med* 110:300, 1987.
302. Moore PK, Hoult JRS: Experimental hyperthyroidism in rats suppresses in vitro prostaglandin metabolism in lung and kidney. *Prostaglandins* 16:355, 1978.
303. Morrison AR: Biochemistry and pharmacology of renal arachidonic acid metabolism. *Am J Med* 80(suppl 1A):3, 1986.
304. Morrison AR, Crowley JR: Identification of an unusual cyclooxygenase metabolite of arachidonic acid in rabbit renal medulla. *Arch Biochem Biophys* 234:413, 1984.
305. Morrison AR et al: Unmasking of thromboxane A_2 synthesis by ureter obstruction in the rabbit kidney. *Nature (London)* 267:259, 1977.
306. Morrison AR et al: Thromboxane A_2 biosynthesis in the ureter obstructed isolated perfused kidney of the rabbit. *J Pharmacol Exp Ther* 205:1, 1978.
307. Morrison AR et al: Mechanism of enhanced renal prostaglandin biosynthesis in ureter obstruction: Role of de novo protein synthesis. *J Biol Chem* 253:8210, 1978.
308. Morsing P et al: Effect of thromboxane inhibition on tubuloglomerular feedback in hydronephrotic kidneys. *Kidney Int* 36:447, 1989.
309. Moses AM et al: Antidiuretic and PGE_2 responses to AVP in subjects with central and nephrogenic diabetes insipidus. *Am J Physiol* 248:F354, 1985.
310. Munger K, Baylis, C: Sex differences in renal hemodynamics in rats. *Am J Physiol* 254:F223, 1988.
311. Murray BM et al: Effect of cyclosporine administration on renal hemodynamics in conscious rats. *Kidney Int* 28:767, 1985.
312. Muther RS et al: Aspirin-induced depression of glomerular filtration rate in normal humans: Role of sodium balance. *Ann Intern Med* 94:317, 1981.
313. Nadler JL et al: Evidence that prostacyclin mediates the vascular action of magnesium in humans. *Hypertension* 9:379, 1987.
314. Nadler JL et al: Evidence of prostacyclin deficiency in the syndrome of hyporeninemic hypoaldosteronism. *N Engl J Med* 314:1015, 1986.

315. Nadler JL et al: Evidence that prostacyclin modulates the vascular actions of calcium in man. *J Clin Invest* 77:1278, 1986.
316. Nadler SP et al: PGE_2, forskolin, and cholera toxin interactions in rabbit cortical collecting tubule. *Am J Physiol* 19:F127, 1986.
317. Nasjletti A et al: Disappearance of bradykinin in the renal circulation of dogs: Effects of kininase inhibition. *Circ Res* 37:59, 1975.
318. Nasjletti A, Colina-Chourio J: Interaction of mineralocorticoids, renal prostaglandins, and the renal kallikrein-kinin system. *Fed Proc* 35:189, 1976.
319. Nath KA et al: Regulatory role of prostanoids in glomerular microcirculation of remnant nephrons. *Am J Physiol* 252:F829, 1987.
320. Navarro J et al: Hydroxylation of prostaglandin E_1 by kidney cortex microsomal monoxygenase in the guinea pig. *Arch Biochem Biophys* 191:125, 1976.
321. Needleman P et al: Specific regulation of peptide-induced renal prostaglandin synthesis. *J Biol Chem* 254:9772, 1979.
322. Nicchitta CV et al: Cyclosporine augments receptor-mediated cellular Ca fluxes in isolated hepatocytes *J Biol Chem* 260:13613, 1985.
323. Nielson CK, Arrigoni-Martelli E: Effects on rat urinary kallikrein excretion of bumetanide, bendroflumethiazide and hydralazine. *Acta Pharmacol Toxicol* 40:267, 1977.
324. Nielson CK et al: Investigations on the antihypertensive activity of timolol and bendroflumethiazide and the combination in dogs and rats. *Acta Pharmacol Toxicol* 39:500, 1976.
325. Niwa T et al: Prostaglandin E_1 infusion therapy in chronic glomerulonephritis: A double-blind, crossover trial. *Prostaglandins Leukotrienes Med* 19:227, 1985.
326. Niwa T et al: Urinary prostaglandins and thromboxane in patients with chronic glomerulonephritis. *Nephron* 46:281, 1987.
326a. Norby LH et al: Possible role of impaired renal prostaglandin production in pathogenesis of hyporeninemic hypoaldosteronism. *Lancet* 2:1118, 1978.
327. Nustad K et al: The relationship between kidney and urinary kininogenase. *Br J Pharmacol* 39:73, 1970.
328. Oates JA et al: Metabolism of prostaglandins and thromboxane. *Adv Prostaglandin Thromboxane Res* 6:35, 1980.
329. O'Connor GJ et al: Urinary kallikrein (UKAL) and postobstructive nephropathy. *Kidney Int* 12:532, 1977.
330. Okahara T et al: Zonal heterogeneity of prostaglandin and thromboxane release in the dog kidney. *Prostaglandins* 25:373, 1983.
331. Okegawa T et al: Metabolic and cellular alterations underlying the exaggerated renal prostaglandin and thromboxane synthesis in ureter obstruction in rabbits: Inflammatory response involving fibroblasts and mononuclear cells. *J Clin Invest* 71:81, 1983.
332. Olanoff LS et al: Sulindac does not preserve renal prostacyclin synthesis during endotoxemia. *Prostaglandins* 29:1031, 1985.
333. Ole-MoiYoi O et al: Immunologic reactivity of purified human urinary kallikrein (urokallikrein) with antiserum directed against human pancreas. *J Immunol* 118:667, 1977b.
334. Oliver JA et al: Renal vascular and excretory responses to prostaglandin endoperoxides in the dog. *Am J Physiol* 236:H427, 1979.
335. Olsen UB: Prostaglandin/kinin activity related to changed renal compliance after bumetanide in dogs. *Acta Pharmacol Toxicol* 40:430, 1977.
336. Olsen UB, Ahnfelt-Ronne I: Bumetanide induced increase of renal blood flow in conscious dogs and its relation to local renal hormones (PGE, kallikrein and renin). *Acta Pharmacol Toxicol* 38:219, 1976.
337. Olsen UB et al: Prostaglandins, a link between renal hydro- and hemodynamics in dogs. *Acta Physiol Scand* 97:369, 1976.
338. O'Neil RG, Sansom SC: Characterization of apical cell membrane Na^+ and K^+ conductances of cortical collecting duct using microelectrode techniques. *Am J Physiol* 247:F14, 1984.
339. Orstavik T et al: Cellular origin of urinary kallikrein. *J Histochem Cytochem* 24:1037, 1976.
340. Panzenbeck M et al: Prostaglandins participate in the renal vasodilation due to hydralazine in dogs. *J Pharmacol Exp Ther* 237:525, 1986.
341. Papanicolaou N et al: Selective inhibition of renal thromboxane biosynthesis increased sodium excretion rate in normal and saline-loaded rats. *Clin Sci* 68:79, 1985.
342. Papanicolaou N et al: Selective inhibition of thromboxane synthesis partially protected while inhibition of angiotensin II formation did not protect rats against acute renal failure induced with glycerol. *Prostaglandins Leukotrienes Med* 21:29, 1986.
343. Parker J et al: Evidence of protein kinase C involvement in phorbol diester-stimulated arachidonic acid release and prostaglandin synthesis. *J Biol Chem* 262:5385, 1987.
344. Passmore JC et al: Urinary and renal papillary solutes during cyclooxygenase inhibition with ibuprofen. *J Lab Clin Med* 110:807, 1987.
345. Patrono C: Inhibition of renal prostaglandin synthesis in man: Methodological and clinical implications. *Scand J Rheumatol* 62(suppl):14, 1986.
346. Patrono C et al: Functional significance of renal prostacyclin and thromboxane A_2 production in patients with systemic lupus erythematosus. *J Clin Invest* 76:1011, 1985.
347. Patrono C, Dunn MJ: The clinical significance of inhibition of renal prostaglandin synthesis. *Kidney Int* 32:1, 1987.
348. Patrono C, Pierucci A: Renal effects on nonsteroidal anti-inflammatory drugs in chronic glomerular disease. *Am J Med* 81:71, 1986.
349. Pelayo JC: Renal adrenergic effector mechanisms: Glomerular sites for prostaglandin interaction. *Am J Physiol* 254:F184, 1988.
350. Perico N et al: Functional significance of exaggerated renal thromboxane A_2 synthesis induced by cyclosporine A. *Am J Physiol* 251:F581, 1986.
351. Perico N et al: Effect of short-term cyclosporine administration in rats on renin-angiotensin and thromboxane A2: Possible relevance to the reduction in glomerular filtration rate. *J Pharmacol Exp Ther* 239:229, 1986.
352. Pierucci A et al: Improvement of renal function with selec-

tive thromboxane antagonism in lupis nephritis. *N Engl J Med* 320:421, 1989.

353. Pisano JJ: Chemistry and biology of the kallikrein-kinin system, in Proteases and biological control. *Cold Spring Harbor Conf Cell Prolif* 2:199, 1975.
354. Pisano JJ et al: The kallikrein-kinin system in the kidney. *Contrib Nephrol* 12:116, 1978.
355. Podjarny E et al: Prostanoids in renal failure induced by converting enzyme inhibition in sodium-depleted rats. *Am J Physiol* 254:F358, 1988.
356. Powell WS; Distribution of prostaglandin omega-hydroxylases in different tissues. *Prostaglandins* 19:701, 1980.
357. Proud D et al: Distribution of immunoreactive kallikrein along the rat nephron. *Am J Physiol* 244:F510, 1983.
358. Puddey IB et al: Differential effects of sulindac and indomethacin on blood pressure in treated essential hypertensive subjects. *Clin Sci* 69:327, 1985.
359. Pugliese F et al: Glomerular epithelial cell, polyanion neutralization is associated with enhanced prostanoid production. *Kidney Int* 32:57, 1987.
360. Purkerson ML et al: Inhibition of thromboxane synthesis ameliorates the progressive kidney disease of rats with subtotal renal ablation. *Proc Natl Acad Sci U S A* 82:193, 1985.
361. Purkerson ML et al: Thromboxane synthesis and blood pressure in spontaneously hypertensive rats. *Hypertension* 8:1113, 1986.
362. Quilley CP et al: 6-Keto-PGE$_1$: A possible metabolite of prostacyclin having platelet antiaggregatory effects. *Hypertension* 2:524, 1980.
363. Quilley J, McGiff JC: Influence of insulin on urinary eicosanoid excretion in rats with experimental diabetes mellitus. *J Pharmacol Exp Ther* 238:606, 1986.
364. Quintero E et al: Sulindac reduces the urinary excretion of prostaglandins and impairs renal function in cirrhosis with ascites. *Nephron* 42:298, 1986.
365. Rahman MA et al: Immune complex effects on glomerular eicosanoid production and renal hemodynamics. *Kidney Int* 31:1317, 1987.
366. Reid GM et al: Papillary collecting tubule synthesis of prostaglandin E$_2$ in Dahl rats. *Hypertension* 11:179, 1988.
367. Reingold DF et al: Differential biosynthesis of prostaglandins by hydronephrotic rabbit and cat kidneys. *J Pharmacol Exp Ther* 216:510, 1981.
368. Remuzzi G, Bertani T: Renal vascular and thrombotic effects of cyclosporine. *Am J Kidney Dis* 13:261, 1989.
369. Remuzzi G et al: Increased glomerular thromboxane synthesis as a possible cause of proteinuria in experimental nephrosis. *J Clin invest* 75:94, 1985.
370. Rimola A et al: Urinary excretion of 6-keto-prostaglandin F$_{1\alpha}$, thromboxane B$_2$ and prostaglandin E$_2$ in cirrhosis with ascites: Relationship to functional renal failure (hepatorenal syndrome). *J Hepatol* 3:111, 1986.
371. Ritter JM et al: Effects of a stable prostaglandin analogue, L-644,122, in healthy and hypertensive men. *Eur J Clin Pharmacol* 28:685, 1985.
372. Roberts DG et al: Sulindac is not renal sparing in man. *Clin Pharmacol Ther* 38:258, 1985.
373. Robinson DR et al: The protective effect of dietary fish oil on murine lupus. *Prostaglandins* 30:51, 1985.
374. Roblero J et al: Kallikrein-like activity in perfusates and urine of isolated rat kidneys. *Am J Physiol* 231:1383, 1976.
375. Rodriguez-Puyol D et al: Lack of a direct regulatory effect of atrial natriuretic factor on prostaglandins and renin release by isolated rat glomeruli. *Biochem Biophys Res Commun* 138:496, 1986.
376. Rogers TS et al: Selective enhancement of thromboxane in macrophages and kidneys in cyclosporine-induced nephrotoxicity. Dietary protection by fish oil. *Transplantation* 45:153, 1988.
377. Rollins TE, Smith WL: Subcellular localization of prostaglandin forming cyclooxygenase in swiss mouse 3T3 fibroblasts by electron microscopic immunocytochemistry. *J Biol Chem* 255:4872, 1980.
378. Roszinski S, Jelkmann W: Effect of P_{O_2} on prostaglandin E$_2$ production in renal cell cultures. *Respir Physiol* 70:131, 1987.
379. Samuelsson B: An elucidation of the arachidonic acid cascade: Discovery of prostaglandins, thromboxane, and leukotrienes. *Drugs* 33(suppl 1):2, 1987.
380. Samuelsson B: Prostaglandins and thromboxanes, in Greep RO (ed): *Recent Progress in Hormone Research*. New York, Academic Press, 1978, vol 34, p 239.
381. Sasaki S, Imai M: Effects of vasopressin on water and NaCl transport across the in vitro perfused medullary thin ascending limb of Henle's loop of mouse. *Pfluegers Arch* 383:215, 1980.
382. Sato M: Bartter's syndrome with normal urinary excretion of prostaglandin E: Therapeutic effects of propranolol, spironolactone, indomethacin and potassium chloride. *Tohoku J Exp Med* 131:151, 1980.
383. Satoh H, Satoh S: Prostaglandin E$_2$ and I$_2$ production in isolated dog renal arteries in the absence or presence of vascular endothelial cells. *Biochem Biophys Res Commun* 118:873, 1984.
384. Schafer JA, Troutman SL: Cyclic AMP mediated the stimulation of Na^+ transport by arginine vasopressin in isolated perfused rat cortical collecting tubules. *J Physiol* 394:13P, 1987.
385. Scharschmidt LA et al: Angiotensin II and eicosanoids in the control of glomerular size in the rat and human. *Am J Physiol* 250:F348, 1986.
386. Scharschmidt LA, Dunn MJ: Prostaglandin synthesis by rat glomerular mesangial cells in culture: Effects of angiotensin II and arginine vasopressin. *J Clin Invest* 71:1756, 1983.
387. Scharschmidt LA et al: Effects of dietary fish oil on renal insufficiency in rats with subtotal nephrectomy. *Kidney Int* 32:700, 1987.
388. Schiff E et al: The use of aspirin to prevent pregnancy-induced hypertension and lower the ratio of thromboxane A$_2$ to prostacyclin in relatively high risk pregnancies. *N Engl J Med* 321:351, 1989.
389. Schlatter E, Schafer JA. Electrophysiological studies in principal cells of rat cortical collecting tubules. *Pfluegers Arch* 409:81, 1987.
390. Schlondorff D, Ardaillou R: Prostaglandins and other arachidonic acid metabolites in the kidney. *Kidney Int* 29:108, 1986.
391. Schlondorff D et al: In vivo demonstration of glomerular

PGE_2 responses to physiological manipulations and experimental agents. *Am J Physiol* 252:F717, 1987.

392. Schlondorff D et al: Angiotensin II stimulates phospholipases C and A_2 in cultured rat mesangial cells. *Am J Physiol* 253:C113, 1987.
393. Schlondorff D et al: Differential stimulation of PGE_2 synthesis in mesangial cells by angiotensin and A23187. *Am J Physiol* 248:C119, 1985.
394. Schlondorff D et al: Differential stimulation of PGE_2 synthesis in mesangial cells by angiotensin and A23187. *Am J Physiol* 248:C119, 1985.
395. Schlondorff D et al: Different concentrations of pertussis toxin have opposite effects on agonist-induced PGE_2 formation in mesangial cells. *Biochem Biophys Res Commun* 141:39, 1986.
396. Schlondorff D et al: Synthesis of prostaglandin E_2 in different segments of isolated collecting tubules from adult and neonatal rabbits. *Am J Physiol* 248:F134, 1985.
397. Schriener GF et al: Characterization of resident glomerular cells expressing Ia determinants and manifesting restricted interactions with lymphocytes. *J Clin Invest* 68:920, 1981.
398. Schryver S et al: Cortical distribution of prostaglandin and renin in isolated dog glomeruli. *Kidney Int* 25:512, 1984.
399. Schuster VL: Mechanism of bradykinin, ADH, and cAMP interaction in rabbit cortical collecting duct. *Am J Physiol* 249:F645, 1985.
400. Schuster VL et al: Interactions of lysyl-bradykinin and antidiuretic hormone in the rabbit cortical collecting tubule. *J Clin Invest* 73:1659, 1984.
401. Schwartzman M, Rax A: Biochemical actions of vasoactive peptide hormones. *Biochem J* 192:127, 1980.
402. Schwartzman M et al: Bradykinin and angiotensin II activation of arachidonic acid deacylation and prostaglandin E_2 formation in rabbit kidney: Hormone-sensitive versus hormone-insensitive lipid pools of arachidonic acid. *J Biol Chem* 256:2329, 1981.
403. Scicli AG et al: Effect of pH and amiloride in the intrarenal formation of kinins. *Am J Physiol* 245:F198, 1983.
404. Sedor JR et al: Effects of sulindac and indomethacin on renal prostaglandin synthesis. *Clin Pharmacol Ther* 36:85, 1984.
405. Seino M et al: Urinary kallikrein excretion and sodium metabolism in hypertensive patients. *Tohoku J Exp Med* 116:359, 1975.
406. Seino M et al: Effect of spironolactone on urinary kallikrein excretion in patients with essential hypertension and in primary aldosteronism. *Tohoku J Exp Med* 121:111, 1977.
407. Seto S et al: The effect of aprotinin (a serine protease inhibitor) on renal function and renin release. *Hypertension* 5:893, 1983.
408. Seymour AA, Zehr JE: Influence of renal prostaglandin synthesis on renin control mechanisms in the dog. *Circ Res* 45:13, 1979.
409. Sheng WY et al: Kinetic comparison and regulation of the cascade of microsomal enzymes involved in renal arachidonate and endoperoxide metabolism. *J Biol Chem* 258:2188, 1983.
410. Shibouta Y et al: Delay of the initiation of hypertension in spontaneously hypertensive rats by CV-4151, a specific thromboxane A_2 synthetase inhibitor. *Eur J Pharmacol* 109:135, 1985.
411. Silverberg AB et al: Resistance to endogenous norepinephrine in Bartter's syndrome. Reversion during indomethacin administration. *Am J Med* 64:231, 1978.
412. Singhal PC et al: Endocytosis by cultured mesangial cells and associated changes in prostaglandin E_2 synthesis. *Am J Physiol* 252:F627, 1987.
413. Slivka SR, Insel PA: Alpha 1-adrenergic receptor-mediated phosphoinositide hydrolysis and prostaglandin E_2 formation in Madin-Darby canine kidney cells: Possible parallel activation of phospholipase C and phospholipase A_2. *J Biol Chem* 262:4200, 1987.
414. Smith WL, Bell TG: Immunohistochemical localization of the prostaglandin-forming cyclooxygenase in renal cortex. *Am J Physiol* 235:F451, 1978.
415. Smith WL, Bell TG: Increased renal tubular synthesis of prostaglandins in the rabbit kidney in response to ureteral obstruction. *Prostaglandins* 18:269, 1979.
416. Sonnenburg WK, Smith WL: Regulation of cyclic AMP metabolism in rabbit cortical collecting tubule cells by prostaglandins. *J Biol Chem* 263:6155, 1988.
417. Spence JD: The arthritic patient with hypertension: Selection of an NSAID. *Scand J Rheumatol* 62(suppl):36, 1986.
418. Speziale E et al: Rat renal medulla possess high capacity to catabolize prostaglandins. *Biochem Biophys Res Commun* 124:69, 1984.
419. Sraer J et al: Human glomeruli release fatty acids which stimulate thromboxane synthesis in platelets. *Kidney Int* 32:62, 1987.
420. Stahl RA et al: Enhanced glomerular prostaglandin formation in experimental membranous nephropathy. *Kidney Int* 31:1126, 1987.
421. Stahl RA et al: Glomerular prostaglandin formation in two-kidney, one-clip hypertensive rats. *Am J Physiol* 247:F975, 1984.
422. Stahl RA et al: High protein intake stimulates glomerular prostaglandin formation in remnant kidneys. *Am J Physiol* 252:F1088, 1987.
423. Stahl RA et al: Prostaglandin and thromboxane formation in glomeruli from rats with reduced renal mass. *Nephron* 42:252, 1986.
424. Stahl RA et al: Angiotensin II stimulation of prostaglandin E_2 and 6-keto-F_{1alpha} formation by isolated human glomeruli. *Kidney Int* 26:30, 1984.
425. Standhoy JW et al: Effects of prostaglandins E_1 and E_2 on renal sodium reabsorption and Starling force. *Am J Physiol* 226:1015, 1974.
426. Stein JH et al: Effect of renal vasodilation on the distribution of cortical blood flow in the kidney of the dog. *J Clin Invest* 50:1429, 1971.
427. Stein JH et al: The effect of bradykinin on proximal tubular sodium reabsorption in the dog: Evidence for functional nephron heterogeneity. *J Clin Invest* 51:1709, 1972.
428. Steinhauer HB et al: Studies on thromboxane B_2 and prostaglandin E_2 production in the course of murine autoimmune disease: Inhibition by oral histidine and zinc supplementation. *Clin Nephrol* 24:63, 1985.
429. Steinhauer HB et al: Thromboxane B_2 and beta 2-micro-

globulin as early indicators of renal allograft rejection. *Proc Eur Dial Transplant Assoc Eur Ren Assoc* 21:1032, 1985.

430. Stoff JS: Prostaglandins and hypertension. *Am J Med* 80:56, 1986.
431. Stoff JS et al: Indomethacin impairs water diuresis in the DI rat: Role of prostaglandins independent of ADH. *Am J Physiol* 241:F231, 1981.
432. Stokes JB: Ion transport by the cortical and outer medullary collecting tubule. *Kidney Int* 22:473, 1982.
433. Stokes JB: Modulation of vasopressin-induced water permeability of the cortical collecting tubule by endogenous and exogenous prostaglandins. *Miner Electrolyte Metab* 11:240, 1985.
434. Stokes JB, Kokko JF: Inhibition of sodium transport by prostaglandin E_2 across isolated perfused rabbit collecting tubule. *J Clin Invest* 59:1099, 1977.
435. Stork JE, Dunn MJ: Hemodynamic roles of thromboxane A_2 and prostaglandin E_2 in glomerulonephritis. *J Pharmacol Exp Ther* 233:672, 1985.
436. Strand JC, Gilmore JP: Prostaglandins do not mediate the renal effects of bradykinin. *Renal Physiol* 5:286, 1982.
437. Sun FF et al: Metabolism of prostaglandins in the kidney. *Kidney Int* 19:760, 1981.
438. Suzuki S et al: The role of renal prostaglandins in the renin response to isoproterenol in the rat in vitro. *Endocrinology* 108:1654, 1981.
439. Suzuki Y et al: Antinephritic effect of Y-19018, a thromboxane A synthetase inhibitor, on crescentic-type anti-GBM nephritis in rats. *Jpn J Pharmacol* 45:177, 1987.
440. Tabuchi Y et al: Renal vein prostaglandins in renovascular hypertensive patients. *Prostaglandins Leukotrienes Med* 19:219, 1985.
441. Takahashi K et al: Predominant functional roles for thromboxane A_2 and prostaglandin E_2 during late nephrotoxic serum glomerulonephritis in the rat. *J Clin Invest* 85:1974, 1990.

441a. Tannen RL: Disorders of potassium balance, in Brenner BM, Rector FC Jr (eds): *The Kidney*, 4th ed. Philadelphia, Saunders, 1991, p 805.

442. Tannenbaum J et al: Enhanced renal prostaglandin production in the dog: 1. Effects on renal function. *Circ Res* 36:197, 1975.
443. Tannenbaum JS et al: Prostaglandin synthesis associated with renal allograft rejection in the dog. *Transplantation* 37:438, 1984.
444. Taylor A, Windhager EE: Possible role of cytosolic calcium and Na-Ca exchange in regulation of transepithelial sodium transport. *Am J Physiol* 236:F505, 1979.
445. Teitelbaum I, Strasheim A: Vasopressin (AVP)-stimulated phospholipase C (PLC) activity in the rat inner medullary collecting tubule (RIMCT) is mediated by the oxytocin receptor. *Kidney Int* 37:203, 1990. (Abst.)
446. Tempel GE et al: Improvement in organ blood flow by inhibition of thromboxane synthetase during experimental endotoxic shock in the rat. *J Cardiovasc Pharmacol* 8:514, 1986.
447. Terragno NA et al: Endogenous prostaglandin synthesis inhibitor in the renal cortex: Effects on production of prostacycline by renal blood vessels. *Clin Sci* 55(suppl):199, 1978.
448. Thomasson DL et al: Cortical interstitial cell interactions induce sensitivity of hydronephrotic kidney to bradykinin. *Kidney Int* 33:71, 1988.
449. Timarco B et al: Role of prostaglandins in the renal handling of a salt load in essential hypertension. *Am J Cardiol* 55:116, 1985.
450. Toda N: Responses to prostaglandin H_2 and I_2 of isolated dog cerebral and peripheral arteries. *Am J Physiol* 238:H111, 1980.
451. Torikai S, Kurokawa K: Distribution of prostaglandin E_2 sensitive adenylate cyclase along the rat nephron. *Prostaglandins* 21:427, 1981.
452. Troyer DA et al: Effects of vasopressin on phosphoinositides and prostaglandin production in cultured mesangial cells. *Am J Physiol* 249:F139, 1985.
453. Uchida S et al: Localization and properties of NAD^+-dependent 15-hydroxyprostaglandin dehydrogenase activity in the rat kidney. *Pfluegers Arch* 404:278, 1985.
454. Uderman HD et al: Thromboxane synthetase inhibitor UK38,485 lowers blood pressure in the adult spontaneously hypertensive rat. *J Cardiovasc Pharmacol* 6:969, 1984.
455. Uemasu J et al: Prostaglandin E_2 production by glomeruli and collecting tubules isolated from rat kidney. *Jpn J Physiol* 37:631, 1987.
456. Umemura S et al: Defective renal adenylate cyclase response to prostaglandin E_2 in spontaneously hypertensive rats. *J Hypertens* 3:159, 1985.
457. Vanrenterghem YF et al: Role of prostaglandins in protein-induced glomerular hyperfiltraton in normal humans. *Am J Physiol* 254:F463, 1988.
458. Venkatachalam MA, Kreisberg JI: Agonist-induced isotonic contraction of cultured mesangial cells after multiple passage. *Am J Physiol* 249:C48, 1985.
459. Verberkmoes R et al: Bartter's syndrome with hyperplasia of renomedullary cells: Successful treatment with indomethacin. *Kidney Int* 9:302, 1976.
460. Vikse A et al: Dissociation between renal prostaglandin E_2 and renin release: Effects of glucagon, dopamine and cyclic AMP in dogs. *Acta Physiol Scand* 125:619, 1985.
461. Vinci JM et al: The kallikrein-kinin system in Bartter's syndrome and its response to prostaglandin synthetase inhibition. *J Clin Invest* 61:1671, 1978.
462. Wahl MI et al: Antiphosphotyrosine recovery of phospholipase C activity after EGF treatment of A-431 cells. *Science* 241:968, 1988.
463. Walker BR: Antidiuresis and decreased sodium excretion during cyclooxygenase inhibition in the conscious dog. *Renal Physiol* 6:53, 1983.
464. Walker BR et al: Potentiated vasoconstrictor response to vasopressin following meclofenamate in conscious rats. *Proc Soc Exp Biol Med* 187:157, 1988.
465. Walker RM et al: Role of renal prostaglandin during antidiuresis and water diuresis in man. *Kidney Int* 21:365, 1981.
466. Ward PE et al: Isolation of membrane-bound renal enzymes that metabolize kinins and angiotensins. *Biochem J* 157:642, 1976.
467. Watanabe T et al: Association of a solubilized prostaglandin E_2 receptor from renal medulla with a pertussis toxin-reactive guanine nucleotide regulatory protein. *J Biol Chem* 261:13430, 1986.

468. Watson AJ et al: Selective inhibition of thromboxane synthesis in glycerol-induced acute renal failure. *Am J Kidney Dis* 8:26, 1986.
469. Weber PC et al: Prostaglandin E_2 9-keto-reductase is a mediator of salt intake-related prostaglandin-renin interactions. *Nature (London)* 266:65, 1977.
470. Welsh C et al: Relationship between phospholipase C activation and prostaglandin E_2 and cyclic adenosine monophosphate production in rabbit tubular epithelial cells: Effects of angiotensin, bradykinin, and arginine vasopressin. *J Clin Invest* 81:710, 1988.
471. Webster ME, Gilmore JP: Influcence of kallidin-10 on renal function. *Am J Physiol* 206:714, 1964.
472. Webster ME, Pierce JV: The nature of kallidins released from human plasma by kallikreins and other enzymes. *Ann N Y Acad Sci* 104:91, 1963.
473. Wilcox CS et al: Intrarenal prostaglandin release: Effects of arachidonic acid and hyperchloremia. *Kidney Int* 28:43, 1985.
474. Wilson D et al: Prostaglandin synthesis inhibition during volume expansion: Collecting duct function. *Kidney Int* 22:1, 1982.
475. Whisler R et al: Characteristics of cyclosporine induction of increased prostaglandin levels from human peipheral blood monocytes. *Transplantation* 38:377, 1984.
476. Whiting PH et al: Interactions between cyclosporin A, indomethacin and 16,16-dimethyl prostaglandin E_2: Effects on renal, hepatic and gastrointestinal toxicity in the rat. *Br J Exp Pathol* 68:777, 1987.
477. Wong DG et al: Effect of non-steroidal anti-inflammatory drugs on control of hypertension by beta-blockers and diuretics. *Lancet* 1:997, 1986.
478. Wong P et al: Hepatic metabolism of prostacyclin in rabbit: Formation of a potent new inhibitor of platelet aggregation. *Biochem Biophys Res Commun* 93:486, 1980.
479. Wong PY et al: Epoxidation of prostacyclin in the rabbit kidney. *J Biol Chem* 260:9150, 1985.
480. Wong PY et al: Deficiency in 15-hydroxyprostaglandin dehydrogenase activity after unilateral ureteral obstruction of the dog kidney. *J Pharmacol Exp Ther* 232:470, 1985.
481. Wright JT, Corder CN: NAD^+15-hydroxyprostaglandin dehydrogenase distribution in rat kidney. *J Histochem Cytochem* 27:657, 1979.
482. Wuthrich RP, Vallotton MB: Prostaglandin E_2 and cyclic AMP response to vasopressin in renal medullary tubular cells. *Am J Physiol* 251:F499, 1986.
483. Yamashita W et al: A thromboxane synthetase antagonist ameliorates progressive renal disease of Dahl-S rats. *Kidney Int* 33:77, 1988.
484. Yared A et al: Mechanism of preservation of glomerular perfusion and filtration during acute extracellular volume depletion: Importance of intrarenal vasopressin-prostaglandin interaction for protecting kidneys from constrictor action of vasopressin. *J Clin Invest* 75:1477, 1985.
485. Yarger WE et al: Obstructive nephropathy in the rat: Possible roles for the renin-angiotensin system, prostaglandins and thromboxanes in post-obstructive renal function. *J Clin Invest* 65:400, 1980.
486. Ylikorkala O et al: Renal prostacyclin and thromboxane in normotensive and preeclamptic pregnant women and their infants. *J Clin Endocrinol Metab* 63:1307, 1986.
487. Yoshimoto T et al: Regional distribution of prostaglandin endoperoxide synthase studied by enzyme-linked immunoassay using monoclonal antibodies. *Biochim Biophys Acta* 877:141, 1986.
488. Yoshioka T et al: In vivo influence of prostaglandin I_2 on systemic and renal circulation in the rat. *Hypertension* 7:867, 1985.
489. Yun J et al: Effect of bradykinin on renal function in dogs treated with indomethacin or propranolol. *Renal Physiol* 5:31, 1982.
490. Zimmerman BG: Renal vascular reactivity to U46619 and adrenergic agonists in Goldblatt hypertension. *Am J Physiol* 253:H1523, 1987.
491. Zinner SH et al: Stability of blood pressure rank and urinary kallikrein concentratoin in childhood: An eight-year follow-up. *Circulation* 58:908, 1978.
492. Zipser RD: Effects of selective inhibition of thromboxane synthesis on renal function in humans. *Am J Physiol* 248:F753, 1985.
493. Zipser RD: Regulation of urinary prostaglandins in Bartter's syndrome. *Am J Med* 67:263, 1979.
494. Zipser RD et al: Stimulation of renal prostaglandin synthesis by the pressor activity of vasopressin. *Endocrinology* 108:495, 1981.
495. Zipser RD et al: Dual effects of antidiuretic hormone on urinary prostaglandin E_2 in man. *J Clin Endocrinol Metab* 53:522, 1981.
496. Zipser RD et al: Therapeutic trial of thromboxane synthesis inhibition in the hepatorenal syndrome. *Gastroenterology* 87:1228, 1984.
497. Zoja et al: Indomethacin reduces proteinuria in passive Heymann nephritis in rats. *Kidney Int* 31:1335, 1987.
498. Zusman RL, Keiser HR: Prostaglandin biosynthesis by rabbit renomedullary interstitial cells in tissue culture: Stimulation by angiotensin II, bradykinin, and arginine vasopressin. *J Clin Invest* 60:215, 1977.
499. Zusman RL, Keiser HR: Prostaglandin E_2 biosynthesis by rabbit renomedullary interstitial cells in tissue cultures. *J Biol Chem* 252:2069, 1977.
500. Zusman RM, Keiser HR: Regulation of PGE_2 synthesis by angiotensin II, potassium, osmolality, and dexamethasone. *Kidney Int* 17:277, 1980.

CHAPTER • 16

The renin-angiotensin system

Norman K. Hollenberg • Julie R. Ingelfinger • Victor J. Dzau

RENIN-ANGIOTENSIN CASCADE

RENIN: CHARACTERISTICS AND CHEMISTRY

Renin is the first enzyme in the biochemical cascade of the renin-angiotensin system. It is synthesized and stored in the juxtaglomerular cells of the afferent arteriole of the kidney and is released into circulation in response to a variety of stimuli. Renin is an aspartyl proteinase. It cleaves its substrate, angiotensinogen, to generate the decapeptide angiotensin I. By definition, aspartyl proteinases belong to the acid proteinase family. Like other acid proteinases, the active site of renin contains two carboxyl groups, contributed by aspartic acid residues at positions 32 and 215, which are essential for catalytic function.[120] The amino acid sequence of the primary renin resembles, to a large extent, those of other acid proteinases, such as pepsin and chymosin. Comparison of the amino acid sequence of renin with that of porcine pepsin indicated a 40 percent sequence homology.[121] Renin, however, is distinct from other acid proteinases in several respects. It is active at neutral pH, has free sulfhydryl groups, and is highly selective for its substrate.[121] Acid proteinases, in general, are nonspecific enzymes capable of degrading a large number of proteins. The substrate specificity of renin is stringently limited to one particular peptide bond of angiotensinogen.

Mouse, rat, and human renin genes (as well as cDNAs) have been cloned and sequenced.[21,63,83,93,126] While in the human and the rat a single renin locus has been identified, in the mouse certain strains possess two renin genes that are closely linked. (These loci are termed *Ren-1^c*, from the one-gene C57BL/10 mouse, and *Ren-1^d* and *Ren-2^d*, from the two-gene DBA/2 mouse.) Mouse strains with two renin genes have higher extrarenal renin levels (especially in the submandibular gland) than do strains with only one gene. The renin gene from these three species (mouse, rat, and human) has a high degree of homology and similarity to genes that encode other acid proteases. Analysis of the regulatory region of the renin gene reveals a number of *cis*-acting elements in the 5′-flanking region for cAMP-responsive elements; activator protein 1 (AP1) binding sites; and glucocorticoid-, estrogen-, and progesterone-responsive elements.

Studies of mRNA regulation show that sodium depletion, angiotensin-converting enzyme (ACE) inhibition, beta-adrenergic receptor activation, and renal ischemia all increase renal renin mRNA expression.[52,96,123,130] Depletion of sodium also stimulates cardiac and adrenal renin mRNA expression but does not affect submandibular gland or testis renin mRNA expression. While androgen and estrogen both stimulate extrarenal renin mRNA expression, these hormones do not affect renal renin mRNA levels.[54] The number of cells in the kidney expressing renin decrease after birth, and the intrarenal distribution is more widespread early in development.[74]

Structure and synthesis

Renin has been completely purified from various species.[31,43,70,94,186] There appears to be a high degree of structural conservation between renins of different species.[32,47] Renal renin is a glycoprotein with a molecular weight of 37,000 to 40,000. Its isoelectric point is between 5.2 and 5.8, and the pH optimum for reaction with angiotensinogen is 5.5 to 5.6. Studies of the structure of mouse submandibular gland renin indicate that renin is composed of a heavy chain (molecular weight 31,000) and a light chain (molecular weight 5500) linked by a single disulfide bond.[121] The active site is located in the heavy chain; the function of the light chain has not yet been exactly elucidated. Based on the known amino acid sequence of mouse submandibular gland renin, a three-dimensional structural model has been proposed using high-performance computer graphics.[11] The catalytic site of renin is formed as a cleft between two lobes of the enzyme molecule. Despite the large extent of sequence conservation between the active sites of renin and other aspartyl proteinases, there are some remarkable differences at the edges of the active site cleft. Some of the variability involves surface loops and a "flap" containing basic residues.

Renin is synthesized from its mRNA as a preproenzyme[46,102] and is rapidly translocated into the lumen of the endoplasmic reticulum. In the lumen of the rough endoplasmic reticulum and Golgi apparatus, prorenin is processed into the mature, active enzyme, which is finally packaged and stored in secretory granules. Two proteolytic cleavages are necessary in the processing and maturation of prorenin to renin. The first cleavage occurs at arginine-63–serine–64 and converts prorenin to a single-chain polypeptide. The second cleavage removes the dipeptide arginine-352–arginine–353, resulting in two chains.[121,149] The biosynthetic sequence of human renin has recently been characterized.[91,106,137,143] Biosynthesis and secretion of human renin has been studied in both renal and extrarenal tumor tissue, in normal kidney, and in cultured cells transfected with and thus expressing the human renin gene.[106,137,143] Translation of human renin mRNA results in preprorenin, which then undergoes cotranslational removal of the signal peptide, followed by glycosylation during transfer into the cisternae of the rough endoplasmic reticulum. Within the juxtaglomerular cells of the kidney, prorenin appears to be sorted by one of two pathways: a regulated pathway mediated by secretory granules, where a thiol protease cleaves the amino terminal of the 43-amino acid prosegment, or a constitutive pathway.[143] Studies using site-directed mutagenesis suggest that neither the prosegment nor glycosylation is necessary for sorting, although they may influence or participate in it.[89] In the human, markedly increased levels of circulating prorenin (also called inactive renin) occur both as a normal physiologic response and as a response to disease. Prorenin level may participate in the regulation of renal renin production.

Some insight into the genetic regulation of renin has been provided by studies of mouse submandibular gland renin. As mentioned above, inbred strains of mice with low levels of submandibular gland renin have a single renin gene (*Ren-1*^{c}), while strains that have high submandibular gland renin levels carry duplicated renin genes (*Ren-1*^{d}, *Ren- 2*^{d}).[135,141] Both genes have been mapped to the same region of mouse chromosome 1. The available data suggest that *Ren-1* is primarily expressed in the kidney and therefore determines the structure of the physiologically important isoenzyme. The regulation of the renin synthesis appears to occur at the level of translatable renin.

In addition to the active enzyme, heavier forms of renin, ranging in molecular weight from 50,000 to 140,000, have been reported.[95,154] The high-molecular weight forms of renin can be broadly divided into two groups based on the presence or absence of enzymatic activity. The first group includes inactive enzyme, which may be activated by limited proteolysis using trypsin, pepsin, or kallikrein or by acidification or prolonged cold exposure. These "inactive renins" have been demonstrated in plasma and kidneys of humans, hogs, and possibly dogs and cats, as well as in human amniotic fluid.[95,154] Plasma inactive renin appears to originate primarily from the kidney.[90] Recent purification of hog renal inactive renin indicates that it has a molecular weight of 50,000 and is probably a single-chain polypeptide.[167] In addition, antibodies to the prosegment of prorenin have provided strong data showing that inactive renin and prorenin are immunlogical homologues and are likely to be the same molecule.[13,103] Based on these observations, inactive renin appears to be the zymogen (biological precursor) of the active, mature enzyme. For this reason, inactive renin has also been named prorenin by many investigators,[70,154] although definitive evidence of its precursor nature is lacking.

The second group of high-molecular weight forms do have intrinsic enzymatic activity. They tend to be larger than inactive renin (molecular weight approximately 60,000) and can be isolated from renal extracts in the presence of sulfhydryl-oxidizing agents such as sodium tetrathionate or *N*- ethylmaleimide.[68] Available evidence suggests that these forms represent renin complexed with protein; that is, postsynthetic modification of the enzyme has occurred.[100] Although it has been postulated that these forms are renin-inhibitor complexes, in vitro artifacts of the extraction process cannot be ruled out.

Extrarenal renin-angiotensin system

Several investigators have demonstrated that reninlike enzymes exist in many tissues besides the kidney. While some of the enzymes may be cathepsin D, immunoreactive renin has clearly been identified in brain, arterior pituitary, uterus, arterial tissue, and adrenal cortex.[26,44,48,71,131,145] Renin mRNA has also been identified in these tissues.[54,106] In most of these tissues, other components of the renin-angiotensin system have also been identified, suggesting that the entire system exists locally in these sites. The brain renin-angiotensin system may play a role in control of blood pressure, release of antidiuretic hormone and catecholamines, and regulation of thirst.[144] The role of the other local renin-angiotensin system in unclear, although the vascular enzyme may contribute to the local regulation of flow and vascular resistance.

ANGIOTENSINOGEN: CHARACTERISTICS AND BIOCHEMISTRY

The renin substrate angiotensinogen is an alpha 2 globulin synthesized and released by the liver. It has been purified from plasma of several species.[12,172] Angiotensinogen is a glycoprotein that exists in two forms: molecular weight 62,000 and molecular weight 65,000. The

14 NH_2-terminal amino acid residues of angiotensinogen, the tetradecapeptide, contains the angiotensin I sequence and is functional as renin substrate in vitro. Renin cleaves angiotensinogen specifically at the leucine-leucine bond present at positions 10 and 11 in all species[12] except human, to release the physiologically inactive peptide angiotensin I. The human NH_2-terminal sequence differs from those in equine and rat angiotensinogen: the cleavage site is a leucine-valine bond.[172] Human angiotensinogen is not hydrolyzed by nonprimate renins. However, human renin is capable of hydrolyzing nonprimate angiotensinogen. This species specificity may be due to structural differences in renins and angiotensinogens of different species. Indeed, monoclonal antibodies directed at the active site of human renin do not inhibit renin activities of rat, dog, mouse, and rabbit.[51]

The angiotensinogen genes for rat, mouse, and human have been cloned and sequenced and are all present as a single copy.[29,69,107,114,133,168] cDNA and genomic clone analyses show that the angiotensinogen gene encodes a single protein product. The mRNA for rat angiotensinogen is approximately 1800 nucleotides in length, with 61 in the 5′ untranslated region, 1431 in the coding region, and 200 to 400 in the 3′ untranslated sequence. The mRNA is heterogeneous in size because it has at least four polyadenylation sites.[133] The rat angiotensinogen gene, 12 kilobase (kb) pairs long, has been studied the most thoroughly and has five exons separated by four introns.[168] It is interesting to note that the first exon is separated from the others by a 5-kb intron and encodes solely a portion of the 5′ untranslated region of the mRNA. The region of the gene immediately flanking the structural portion has several identifiable promoter elements, such as a TATA box at position −30 base pair (bp; relative to the transcription start site) as well as two putative glucocorticoid-responsive elements, at −586 and −477 bp. There are several transcriptionally active elements[29,30,147,148] in the 5′-flanking region, including ones for glucocorticoid, estrogen, and bacterial endotoxin inducibility; there is also a cytokine-responsive element.

Angiotensinogen secretion

Angiotensinogen is stored in low quantities in the liver, but in response to an appropriate stimulus it is rapidly synthesized and released. Somewhat paradoxically, hepatic angiotensinogen production is stimulated by angiotensisn II and inhibited by renin or des(angiotensin II)-angiotensinogen, a product of the reaction of renin and angiotensinogen.[82] This observation may explain, in part, the decrease in plasma angiotensinogen concentration observed with captopril therapy. Hepatic angiotensinogen production is also stimulated by several hormones, including glucocorticoids, estrogens (including the oral contraceptives), and thyroxine.[49] Hypophysectomy results in a marked decrease in the rate of angiotensinogen production and plasma substrate concentration, which can be normalized with replacement of these hormones.[50] Although plasma angiotensinogen concentration usually reflects the rate of hepatic angiotensinogen production, changes in degradation due to alterations in plasma renin concentration can also affect plasma substrate levels. The influence of these hormones on hepatic angiotensinogen release may explain the elevated plasma substrate levels observed in patients with Cushing's disease or hyperthyroidism and in women on oral contraceptives and during pregnancy.[49] Other clinical conditions that affect plasma angiotensinogen levels include bilateral nephrectomy, which increases the plasma concentration, and hepatic cirrhosis, which decreases it.

Plasma angiotensinogen may be rate-limiting in the generation of angiotensin I and thus important in the regulation of blood pressure. Under normal conditions, plasma angiotensinogen concentration is significantly lower than the K_m of renin and angiotensinogen reaction.[49] In conditions where plasma angiotensinogen concentration is primarily increased, the rate of angiotensin II production also increases. The importance of plasma angiotensinogen in blood pressure control has been demonstrated by in vivo experiments in which antiangiotensinogen antibody was administered to rats. Substrate excess may contribute to the hypertension in Cushing's syndrome and with the use of oral contraceptives.

Assays of renin activity

The standard renin assay assesses enzymatic activity by measuring the rate of generation of angiotensin I, the product of renin and angiotensinogen, by radioimmunoassay. Plasma renin *activity* (PRA) is assessed by measuring the rate of angiotensin I generation in vitro from the reaction of endogenous renin and endogenous substrate. The measurement is made by incubating the plasma sample at 37°C in the presence of angiotensinase inhibitors (8-hydroxyquinolone-dimercaptopropranolol and EDTA) at pH 5.7 or 7.4.[78] On the other hand, plasma renin *concentration* (PRC) measures the in vitro generation of angiotensin I by endogenous renin in the presence of excess substrate. Here, excess substrate is added to the sample, and the incubation is carried out as described. Hence, the rate of angiotensin I generation in this assay is not potentially limited by substrate concentration. If plasma angiotensinogen concentration is rate-limiting under physiologic conditions, changes in plasma concentration within a certain range would affect PRA but not PRC. Under normal circumstances, a close correlation exists between PRA and concentration of circulating renin. However, under certain conditions, such as hyperthyroidism and pregnancy, in which plasma substrate concentration increases out of proportion to the rise in PRC, the relationship between PRA and PRC is altered.[49] Similarly, in conditions associated with a primary fall in plasma substrate concentration, such as in thyroidectomized rats, decreases in PRA as well as in the PRA/PRC ratio are observed.

ANGIOTENSIN-CONVERTING ENZYME

Angiotensin-converting enzyme (ACE) is a dipeptidyl peptidase that cleaves the carboxyl-terminal dipeptide of angiotensin I, releasing angiotensin II. It is present in high concentration on the luminal membrane surface of endothelial cells of pulmonary capillaries. Although it is also found in the plasma, the plasma concentration is only a small fraction of that in the lung. Thus, the majority of plasma angiotensin I is converted to angiotensin II in a single pass through the pulmonary circulation.[150] ACE and its isoenzyme(s) are also found in the kidney, brain, liver, epididymis, and most vascular beds.[23] Based on current information, it appears that the conversion of angiotensin I to angiotensin II takes place at local tissue sites as well, accounting for much of local tissue angiotensin II.

ACE is a glycoprotein with a molecular weight of 150,000, including an anchor peptide with a molecular weight of approximately 4000, which is submerged in the lipid bilayer of the plasma membrane; the anchor peptide is clipped after solubilization with trypsin.[178] ACE is a metalloprotease that is inhibited by EDTA and other chelating agents. The enzyme is activated by chloride and other monovalent anions. The active site of ACE contains three stereospecific groups (resembling carboxypeptidase A in this respect). A catalytically essential zinc atom in the active site appears to be directly involved in the hydrolysis of the sessile bond. Further components of the active site are the carboxyl group of an aspartyl or glutamyl residue and tyrosyl, arginyl, and lysyl residues. The last two are probably involved in mediating the anion activition. ACE is also capable of cleaving COOH-terminal dipeptides of bradykinin ("kinase II") and enkephalins, as well as a variety of protected tripeptides.[60]

The study of ACE cDNA in mouse, human, and rabbit has shown that the protein is highly conserved among mammalian species.[9,56,57,156,160] The genomic DNA 5′ to the mouse and human ACE also has two distinct regions of conserved sequence.[156] ACE mRNA (about 4000 bp) encodes 1306 amino acids containing a presequence of 29 amino acids. The protein has much internal homology, with a section at the amino terminal that is 67 percent homologous to a region in the carboxyl half; this pattern suggests gene duplication. Residues 1231 to 1247 exhibit hydrophobicity, suggesting a membrane-spanning domain (membrane anchor). This structure would be consistent with the cell surface location of the enzyme, and the protein would enter the circulation after the removal of the anchor. Many tissues show evidence of this 4.3-kb mRNA. However, the testis expresses a 3-kb mRNA, which appears by sequence analysis to be identical to the 3′ end of endothelial ACE. Testicular ACE has unique residues at the 5′ end (222 residues). It appears that alternative promotor use accounts for the differences in endothelial and testicular mRNAs. With cDNA available, a number of investigators have begun to study regulation of the gene expression of ACE.

The plasma ACE appears to originate from the endothelial enzyme. The factors that control its release are not known. Endothelial ACE synthesis is stimulated by dexamethasone and captopril and inhibited by low oxygen tension.[67,118] In active sarcoidosis or other granulomatous diseases involving the lung, plasma ACE concentration is elevated; changes in plasma ACE levels may be useful as an index of the activity of these diseases.[38] Plasma ACE concentration has been shown to be decreased in patients with a variety of diseases of pulmonary parenchyma, including chronic obstructive lung disease, carcinoma, and cystic fibrosis.[79,109] It is also elevated, for unknown reasons, in Gaucher's disease, hyperthyroidism, and diabetes mellitus.[110,111,187]

ANGIOTENSINS

Angiotensin II, the physiologically active octapeptide, has multiple sites of action. It is one of the most potent vasoconstrictors formed in the mammalian body. The renal and splanchnic circulations are particularly sensitive to the vasoconstrictor action of angiotensin II. Angiotensin II can cause contraction of isolated glomeruli and may alter glomerular dynamics and filtration coefficient.[9,22] In vitro experiments have suggested that angiotensin II can modify tubular sodium handling.[108] Large amounts of angiotensin II appear to be produced within the glomerulus and proximal tubule.[155] The octapeptide is a potent stimulus for aldosterone release from the adrenal cortex. It has also been shown to stimulate release of catecholamines from the adrenal medulla and from peripheral sympathetic nerve endings.[102,117] Injection of angiotensin II into the central nervous system can stimulate thirst, increase systemic blood pressure, and evoke secretion of antidiuretic hormone and catecholamines.[44]

Angiotensin I is probably physiologically inactive, although some observations suggest that it is capable of stimulating catecholamine release from the adrenal medulla and inducing thirst when injected into the central nervous system.[64,139] Angiotensin II can be cleaved by aminopeptidases to yield des-(aspartyl^1)-angiotensin II, or "angiotensin III." This heptapeptide is a potent stimulator of aldosterone release in situ and in vitro; it induces renal vasoconstriction, stimulates prostaglandin release from perfused vessels in vitro, and is a potent inhibitor of renin release.[10,75] The physiologic importance of angiotensin III, however, remains unclear. Angiotensin III appears to interact with the product of an oncogene, termed *mas*, which has many characteristics of an angiotensin receptor. The *mas* gene product reacts with angiotensin III in preference to angiotensin II, which binds less strongly.[188]

ANGIOTENSIN RECEPTORS

The actions of angiotensin II are mediated by specific receptors located on a variety of target organs, including the kidney, adrenal cortex, vascular smooth muscle cells, uterus, bladder, several regions of the brain, and sympathetic nerve endings.[5,25,41,119,125] These receptors have been characterized pharmacologically and biochemically. The binding of angiotensin to these receptors is stereospecific and saturable. Angiotensin is displaceable from its receptors by structurally related agonists and antagonists. The dissociation constant, K_d, is approximately $10^{-9}M$. On the basis of much experimental data, it appears that there are multiple isoforms of angiotensin receptors that display distinct tissue and organ distributions and are affected by the normal progression of development and by physiologic and pathophysiologic changes. The coupling of these various receptor forms to intracellular signals may differ. The pharmacologic inhibition of such receptors started with saralasin, but this substance is a competitive partial agonist.[179] Recently, a series of nonpeptide antagonists to the angiotensin II receptors have been discovered.[27,173,183,184] These are selective and have facilitated the characterization of at least two types of receptors, AT_1 and AT_2, which are being further classified into subtypes. The AT_1 receptor, the cDNA for which has been cloned,[127,152] has multiple functions in mediating the role of angiotensin II. The AT_1 receptor appears to be G protein-linked. The AT_2 receptor appears to be expressed during development yet is of uncertain significance.[76] High levels of angiotensin II have tissue-specific effects on its receptor. For example, angiotensin II upregulates angiotensin II receptors in the adrenal cortex, while in the vasculature, angiotensin II downregulates receptors.

Smooth muscle receptors are regulated by sodium intake; the influence of sodium intake on adrenal receptors is more complex, as reviewed in detail below. In vivo studies have shown that the sensitivity of the adrenals to angiotensin II increases during sodium depletion, whereas the vascular sensitivity decreases.[1,85] The converse occurs during sodium loading. The effects of a low-sodium diet on vascular receptors can be reproduced by infusion of angiotensin II and blocked by captopril, indicating that changes in circulating angiotensin II are responsible for the regulation of angiotensin II receptors.[77] Recent studies indicate that changes in glomerular angiotensin II receptors resemble those of vascular smooth muscle receptors with respect to sodium intake. The change in the number of glomerular angiotensin II receptors parallels the changes in glomerular contractility and dynamics and thus may be important in the regulation of glomerular filtration.[65] Regulatory influences on brain and pituitary angiotensin II receptors have not yet been characterized.

Knowledge of how angiotensin regulates gene expression is only just emerging. Angiotensin II appears to act, at least in part, through stimulation of proto-oncogenes, such as c-fos and c-myc.[129,166] Some evidence indicates that some of the gene effects of angiotensin II may be associated with activation (via protein kinase C) of an enhancer element called AP-1, which is key to the transcriptional control of several genes.

RENIN RELEASE

FACTORS CONTROLLING RENIN RELEASE

Renin is the first and the rate-limiting enzyme of the biochemical renin-angiotensin system cascade. Its concentration in plasma appears to depend primarily on the rate of secretion from the kidney. Little is known about control of or variations in its degradation.

The release of renin is influenced by a number of factors.[101] The major signals controlling renin secretion are (1) renal perfusion pressure, monitored by an intrarenal baroreceptor; (2) the adrenergic nervous system, via renal sympathetic nerves or circulating catecholamines that act on a beta receptor; (3) distal tubular sodium concentration at the macula densa; and (4) other humoral signals (potassium, angiotensin II, prostaglandins, and possibly kinins).

Tobian originally proposed the existence of an intrarenal baroreceptor that regulates renin release in response to change in the stretch of the arteriolar wall.[174] Although there is much debate as to the nature and site of this baroreceptor, the weight of evidence indicates that changes in renal perfusion pressure, per se, influence renin release. Conversely, elevated renal perfusion pressure suppresses renin secretion. The stimulus-response curve of pressure and renin secretion has recently been defined in the conscious dog.[62] Renin release is relatively unresponsive to the initial 10 to 20-mmHg reduction from a normal basal blood pressure. The threshold pressure is 80 to 90 mmHg; below the threshold, renin secretion is a steep and linear function of renal perfusion pressure.

Sodium also exerts a major influence on renin release. Both intrarenal infusion of sodium chloride and an increase in dietary sodium intake are capable of inhibiting renin release. Dietary sodium restriction is associated witih increased renin secretion. There are at least two possible mechanisms by which sodium may influence renin release. Sodium may have an indirect effect by changing extracellular sodium content and fluid volume (leading to an altered volume or neural signal); or there may be, potentially, a direct effect of sodium on the juxtaglomerular apparatus (either on the juxtaglomerular cells or on macula densa sensors). There is probably little or no direct effect on renin release by juxtaglomerular cells or changes in plasma sodium concentration within the physiologic range. The effect of sodium concentration in the distal nephron on renin release is unresolved. Kotchen and coworkers have suggested that chloride rather than sodium is responsible for the control of renin release via the macula densa.[105]

Effects of adrenergic receptor stimulation

The activity of two intrarenal adrenergic receptors (beta and dopaminergic) influence renin release. The contribution of alpha receptors is unclear. The beta and dopaminergic receptors on the juxtaglomerular cells are responsive to both neurally released and circulating catecholamines.[101] Electrical stimulation of renal sympathetic nerves or selective areas of the vasomotor center or hypothalamus results in renin release, which is blocked by propranolol. Epinephrine and isoproterenol stimulate renin release both in vivo and in vitro. Specific dopaminergic nerve endings and receptors have been demonstrated in the kidney. Stimulation of dopaminergic receptors also results in renin release.[122]

The role of the alpha-adrenergic receptor in regulation of renin secretion is less clear. Since presynaptic and postsynaptic alpha receptors are present in the intact innervated kidney, the responses to nonsubtype-selective adrenergic agonists or antagonists may vary, depending on the dose of the agent and the physiologic condition of the study. To date, the data appear to favor an inhibitory effect of the alpha-adrenergic receptor on renin release.[101]

Other influences on renin release

Several other humoral factors also influence the secretion of renin.[101] Hypokalemia stimulates renin release. Vasopressin inhibits renin secretion, but its effect of renin release is probably mediated by systemic or renal hemodynamic changes. Vasodilator prostaglandins (PGs), PGE_2 and PGI_2, appear to stimulate renin release, as does arachidonic acid. The contribution of endogenous PGs to the control of renin release in the intact subject is less clear. It appears that in the basal state in the sodium-replete dog, the PG synthetase inhibitor indomethacin has no effect on renin release.[36] On the other hand, indomethacin reduces basal renin release in the sodium-depleted dog. Similarly, decreased cardiac output by vena caval constriction and hemorrhage evokes secretion of renin, which can be attenuated by indomethacin.[55] In addition, endogenous PGs may mediate many stimulatory signals, such as the renal baroreceptor signals.[6]

Studies on the effect of calcium on the secretion of renin have yielded conflicting results. Several investigators have demonstrated that intrarenal infusion of calcium chloride reduces renin secretion. A few others have reported an increase in renin release.[177,185] Moreover, removal of calcium from cell-free perfusate of isolated kidneys increases basal renin release;[66,139] but Viskoper and coworkers reported no effect of calcium chelation with EGTA in the blood-perfused isolated kidney.[176] The addition of lanthanum, a cation that "locks" calcium channels and blocks calcium efflux, to isolated perfused kidneys[112] or glomeruli[4] decreased renin release.[112]

These experiments using intact preparations have several limitations. Calcium infusion may lead to changes in sodium excretion and/or alterations in renal hemodynamics that may indirectly influence renin release. Removal of calcium from the perfusate or use of chelating agents can produce nonspecific effects on cell volume or membrane permeability. Furthermore, increasing calcium concentration may lead to increased calcium influx into nerve terminals or endothelial cell membranes, evoking catecholamine release in the first instance or resulting in PG release from the endothelial cells; both catecholamine and PG secretions can secondarily stimulate renin secretion from juxtaglomerular cells. Overall, the data favor the existence of an inhibitory effect of calcium on renin secretion; such an inhibition is in contrast to the effect of calcium on the secretion of most other hormones.

FEEDBACK REGULATION OF RENIN RELEASE

Renin release is subject to feedback regulation. For example, within minutes after renal artery constriction in the experimental animal, pressure distal to constriction begins to rise toward baseline pressure as systemic pressure rises. This rise in distal pressure is also associated with rising intrarenal resistance, after the initial autoregulatory vasodilation, partly due to angiotensin-mediated renal vasoconstriction.[2,45] This increase in distal pressure is at least in part responsible for the subsequent inhibition of renin release.

Angiotensin II also has a direct inhibitory effect on renin release by the juxtaglomerular cells, known as the short feedback loop. A third mechanism of feedback inhibition involves sodium retention and extracellular fluid (ECF) volume expansion induced by elevated plasma aldosterone or by other factors; it is known as the long feedback loop.

CELLULAR MECHANISMS OF RENIN RELEASE

Despite extensive studies identifying the factors that influence renin release, the cellular messengers of these signals are poorly understood. The best candidates for second messengers are calcium, endogenous PGs, and cAMP.

Manipulations that increase intracellular calcium concentration, such as increasing extracellular calcium, lanthanum, and calcium ionophores, tend to depress renin secretion. An increase in intracellular calcium concenetration may be the mechanism by which angiotensin II, norepinephrine, vasopressin, and other vasoconstrictors inhibit renin secretion. Conversely, when calcium influx is reduced by the addition of verapamil, the inhibitory effect of these agents on renin release is attenuated.[128,136] Increased extracellular potassium and increased intraluminal pressure in renal arterioles may exert inhibitory effects by a similar mechanism. Harada and Rubin have shown that renin release mediated by the beta-adrenergic receptor is associated with a dose- and time-related calcium efflux, providing indirect evidence that a decrease in intracellular calcium may be the stimulatory signal to renin release.[81]

Since many cellular events controlled by intracellular calcium are mediated by calmodulin, the cellular calcium-binding protein, Churchill and Churchill studied the effect of trifluoperazine, a putative calmodulin inhibitor, on renin release. Trifluoperazine produced a dose-dependent increase in renin release and blocked the inhibitory effect of a high extracellular potassium concentration.[28] These investigators postulate that changes in calmodulin-calcium complex mediate the influence of calcium on renin release.

Endogenous PGs may also act as second messengers, mediating the response to several stimuli that promote renin release, including sodium depletion, beta-adrenergic stimulation, and reduction of renal perfusion pressure in the autoregulatory range. However, the role of PGs in renin release in response to reduction of pressure below the autoregulatory range (60 mmHg) is less clear.

Other cellular mechanisms, such as adenylate cyclase activity, may also be second messengers in response to certain stimuli of renin release.[34]

In summary, the dominant factor leading to renin release appears to be a threat to ECF volume. When such a threat occurs, the various factors that stimulate release—fall in renal perfusion pressure, increased sympathetic activity to the kidney, decreased distal tubule sodium concentration—would all act in concert to promote renin release. Indeed, this represents a good example of a biological amplification system for homeostasis.

PHARMACOLOGIC INTERRUPTION OF THE RENIN-ANGIOTENSIN SYSTEM

Since the late 1960s, our understanding of the role of the renin-angiotensin system in physiology and pathophysiology has advanced greatly in major part due to the sequential development of agents for blocking the system at one of several sites. Why did these agents find such a rapid and wide use? Haber has pointed out the central role played by ablation of endocrine organs in proving that a given biological response is mediated by a specific hormone.[80] In the special case of the renin-angiotensin, where the kidney is both the source of the hormone and a major responding organ, ablation has not been possible. The pharmacologic agents have therefore come to play a special role as a replacement for ablation. However (as is frequently forgotten), no agent has a single action, and no agent provides data that are of unquestioned validity. Researchers are eager to draw physiologic conclusions from pharmacologic data.

TYPES OF ANTAGONISTS

The renin-angiotensin cascade offers a series of sites that have been exploited for more or less selected inhibition (Table 16-1). Renin release from the kidney is mediated in part by a neural action that is blocked by beta-adrenergic blocking agents.[34,101] Clonidine, acting as a post-synaptic alpha-receptor agonist, also blunts renin release.[140]

The action of renin on its substrate is antagonized by nonspecific proteases (e.g., pepstatin), by antibody to renin, and more specifically by structural analogues of the substrate itself.[19,80,116,140,146] This approach offers great promise of specificity for dissecting pathophysiologic data. Because of the species specificity of renin, renin inhibitors generated for one species often lack efficacy on others. Emphasis has been given to the development of renin inhibitors specific for primates, although a renin inhibitor specific for rats has been developed.[92] A variety of effective renin inhibitors have been devel-

TABLE 16-1 • Pharmacologic Interruption of the Renin-Angiotensin System

Disrupted mechanism	Product	Pharmacologic blocker
Renin release	Renin	Beta-adrenergic blocking agents* Alpha-adrenergic agonists*
Renin's action on substrate	AI	Substrate analogues Pepstatin
AI conversion to AII	AII	Peptide inhibitors of peptidyl-dipeptide hydrolase* Nonpeptide inhibitors QL of peptidyl-dipeptide hydrolase*
AII and AIII action on receptor	Response	Peptide analogues of AII Peptide analogues of AIII

* Applied clinically.

Abbreviations: AI, Angiotension I; AII, Angiotensin II; AIII, Angiotensin III.

oped[37,98,158] and are now being used in humans. In general, the agents available to date have shown limited bioavailability when taken by mouth, which has limited their initial use to short-term studies. Their availability should clarify some of the issues concerning the contribution of the renin-angiotensin system to the physiology and pathophysiology of hypertension.

Angiotensin I, as reviewed above, is hydrolyzed by an enzyme in lung and peripheral tissue that cleaves the carboxyl-terminal histidine-leucine dipeptide bond, thereby generating the active octapeptide angiotensin II. The same enzyme is also responsible for the degradation of bradykinin and for the hydrolysis of other peptides, such as the beta chain of insulin. Thus, the same enzyme is variously known as *converting enzyme, kininase II*, and *dipeptidyl-peptide hydrolase*.[59] These names imply a functional specificity that does not exist. This enzyme can be blocked by a number of agents, including a series of peptides first isolated from snake venom.[134] Because the first biological activity demonstrated was inhibition of the degradation of bradykinin, these agents were termed bradykinin-potentiating factors (BPF). The most widely studied peptide in this series is a nonapeptide distributed under the name SQ 20881. Decapeptide analogues have also been shown to compete with angiotensin I for converting enzyme.[116]

A series of novel nonpeptide blockers of converting enzyme have been synthesized, all based on proline, the carboxyl-terminal amino acid in angiotensin I. These agents have been designed on the basis of a working model of the receptor site on the enzyme.[33,165] This class of agent has played an important role in defining normal mechanisms, exacting pathophysiologic data, and treating hypertension and congestive heart failure.

Octapeptide analogues of angiotensin II act as antagonists by competing with angiotensin at its receptor site in vascular smooth muscle, the adrenal cortex, cardiac muscle, and the nervous system.[116,146]

The major limitation of the angiotensin antagonists developed in the 1970s was that they were partial agonists. Thus, these analogues elicited an angiotensin-like response in systems especially sensitive to angiotensin II, especially when endogenous angiotensin II levels were reduced. The original structure of these compounds prevented the separation of their agonist and antagonist properties.[19,115,146] The agonist properties in some cases proved useful, for example, in examining affinity of receptors and characterizing excitation-contraction coupling,[116] but limited the usefulness of these compounds in exploring the physiology of the system. When appropriate doses were employed, the direction, but not the magnitude, of the response provided useful information.[87,171] The recent development of a series of nonpeptide competitive antagonists based on an imidazole structure appears very promising.[27,183,184] These agents are effective angiotensin antagonists with great specificity, lack the partial agonist action, and have been shown to be effective in a number of models. As in the case of the renin inhibitors, their availability should clarify the contribution of the renin-angiotensin system to the pathogenesis of disease.

Until 1971 it was believed that aminopeptidase-mediated removal of the NH_2-terminal aspartyl residue was the first step in degradation, because the heptapeptide was inactive as a pressor agent and had no effect on one smooth muscle preparation, the uterus. As reviewed above, it has become clear that in some systems—especially those involving the renal blood supply, aldosterone release by the adrenal cortex, and renin release—the heptapeptide has substantial biological activity, approaching or matching that of angiotensin II; indeed, some have described the heptapeptide as "angiotensin III." Analogues of angiotensin III have shown preferential blockade of aldosterone release and effects on the renal blood supply, with much lesser effects on systemic blood pressure.[16,171]

SPECIFICITY AND SENSITIVITY

The angiotensin analogues and converting enzyme inhibitors have found wide application in the assessment of a variety of systems, and the converting enzyme inhibitors are playing an ever-increasing clinical role. The difference in their structure, mechanism of action, and potential lack of specificity often have resulted in uncertainty in interpreting experimental data. Application of the angiotensin analogues and enzyme inhibitors in parallel has been especially powerful for distinguishing angiotensin's specific contribution. In those mechanisms in which they have induced an identical response, little doubt was left that angiotensin was the responsible mediator. Problems, of course, have arisen when responses to the two classes of agent were disparate.

The major problem with the use of converting enzyme inhibitors has been the lack of specificity of peptidyl-dipeptide hydrolase, an enzyme that hydrolyzes a wide variety of dipeptides, including angiotensin II and bradykinin. The hypotensive or vasodilatory effect of the inhibitor could reflect either a reduction in angiotensin II or an increase in bradykinin concentration, since the latter is an active vasodilator.[59] Moreover, evidence has been presented indicating that inhibition of converting enzyme with captopril results in PGE_2 release.[163] Moreover, the depressor response to captopril is blunted by PG synthetase inhibitors.[124] Whether the PG release occurs as a direct response to captopril or indirectly through bradykinin accumulation has not been established.

A powerful approach to enhancing the specificity of converting enzyme inhibition, as indicated above, has involved a comparison of the response to an angiotensin analogue and a converting enzyme inhibitor. Kimbrough and coworkers, for example, demonstrated an identical degree of renal vasodilatation in response to the two classes of agent in dogs ingesting a restricted-sodium diet.[104] Few would doubt, therefore, that this response must reflect reversal of the local action of angiotensin II. A potentially even more powerful approach involves superimposition of converting enzyme inhibition on an angiotensin analogue administered in sufficient dosage that the local actions of angiotensin II would be vitiated.[89,189] The new renin inhibitors and angiotensin antagonists will prove useful in clarifying many of the remaining issues in the pathogenesis of disease.

THE PHYSIOLOGY OF THE RENIN-ANGIOTENSIN SYSTEM

Renin was identified as a potent pressor agent late in the nineteenth century and ranks among the earliest hormones identified. Workers have been able to measure plasma renin and angiotensin II for over two decades. During the same period, the factors that determined renin release and its plasma concentration have come into sharp focus. The structure of angiotensin was identified over 30 years ago; synthetic angiotensin has been available for administration for almost as long. Despite these advances, the physiologic and pathophysiologic roles played by the system have remained obscure, but the forces obscuring our understanding have become increasingly apparent.

Reasons for the difficulty in elucidating specific actions of the renin-angiotensin system seem to be several. First, as reviewed above, the sensitivity of the kidney, the adrenal gland, and the blood pressure to angiotensin II is more variable than is the concentration of angiotensin II itself. For this reason it has been difficult to predict the biological response from the measurement of a plasma concentration of angiotensin II. Second, in the case of the renin-angiotensin system, where the kidney is both the source of the hormone and the major responding organ, the experimental approach of gland ablation has not been feasible. This tool, so useful in endocrinology, is not available. Pharmacologic interruption of the system, as emphasized above, makes use of the data derived from studies of angiotensin II analogues and converting enzyme inhibitors to compensate for the deficiency. (Pharmacologic methods are discussed further in the forthcoming sections.)

EXTRACELLULAR FLUID VOLUME CONTROL: PHYLOGENY

Recent investigation of the physiologic role of the renin-angiotensin-aldosterone sytem has focused primarily on its contribution to blood pressure homeostasis, ignoring its primary involvement in regulating ECF volume. Examination of the evolutionary development of the system highlights the primacy of volume regulation rather than the control of blood pressure.

In its evolution, the kidney and the control systems that converge on the kidney have adapted to progressively more difficult challenges in the regulation of body sodium and water as our predecessors shifted from life in salt water to fresh water and finally to air. The most primitive vertebrates, the cyclostomes and elasmobranchs, appear not to have renin activity or juxtaglomerular granules in their kidneys. The enzyme and its secretory granules appear early, however; they became evident in teleosts and tetrapods.[159] What was the function of this system early in phylogeny?

Little is known concerning blood pressure control in primitive organisms, but the lungfish, as a representative example, has an arterial blood pressure of about 15 mmHg. At this level it would appear that blood pressure is effectively unregulated.[153]

What evolutionary data are available regarding the response of aldosterone to activation of the renin-angiotensin system? Phylogenetically, the amphibian was the first vertebrate to venture from the protective environment of water to air, where the defense of ECF volume became substantially more difficult. Capelli and coworkers pointed out that the appearance of the recurrent nephron and the macula densa in the amphibian represents the "beginnings of a structural element within the nephron to aid electrolyte and volume homeostasis, by sampling fluids reaching the distal segments of the nephron."[24] Bern concluded that aldosterone was an "invention of land-living vertebrates,"[7] appearing late in phylogeny. Vinson and colleagues expressed a contrary view: none of the studies they cited of earlier aldosterone synthesis documented significant plasma concentrations of aldosterone, an important role of aldosterone in sodium handling, or responsiveness of the adrenal gland to angiotensin.[175] What had been documented was a capacity to synthesize aldosterone; however, even in reptiles and amphibia, angiotensin II may have little influence on the adrenal gland.

The simplest interpretation of this overview is that the renin-angiotensin system initially evolved as a primitive ECF volume control system. It acted primarily on the glomerular circulation by controlling renal plasma flow and pressure in the glomerulus and thus affected glomerular filtration rate. The role of this system broadened with increasingly ambitious ventures into new and more hostile environments. The primary role of this system was to control the ECF volume via sodium homeostasis; its influence on blood pressure is best seen as incidental to volume control.

Maneuvers that lead to increased renin secretion generally involve a challenge to ECF volume.[34] The primary determinant of the enzyme's secretion is total body sodium. Certainly, an excellent association has been widely documented among sodium intake, sodium excretion, and the state of this system. A reduction in venous return to the human heart, by quiet standing, for example, results in a rapid burst of renin release. Conversely, a translocation of blood from the lower portion of the body to the thorax by immersion in water to the neck suppresses the system.[58] Clearly, the receptors responsible for volume control and serving as the afferent limb for renin release lie, at least in part, in the thorax and are sensitive to thoracic blood volume. Both neural and metabolic factors can also influence the renin-angiotensin system. Thus, potassium homeostasis, on one hand, and neural influences acting via beta receptors in the juxtaglomerular apparatus, on the other, also influence renin release.[34] These influences are best seen, however, as playing a modulating, rather than a central, role in control of the system.

THE ROLE OF RENIN AND ANGIOTENSIN IN ALDOSTERONE SECRETION

The important contribution of aldosterone to sodium handling by the kidney and thus to sodium homeostasis has been unequivocally proven (Chap. 3). There is also no doubt that angiotensin administration increases aldosterone secretion. What once was disputed is the primacy of the renin system in mediating the adrenal response to reduced sodium intake. One major objection had been the failure of angiotensin, when administered to normal subjects with a high sodium intake, to reproduce the increase in aldosterone secretion evinced by restriction of sodium intake.[14] Two studies answered this objection by documenting an enhanced adrenal response to angiotensin in normal subjects ingesting a restricted-sodium diet.[85,132] Both studies demonstrated a virtually identical increase in the slope of the relationship between plasma angiotensin II and plasma aldosterone concentration. At any given plasma angiotensin II concentration, whether endogenously or exogenously derived, individuals on a low sodium intake showed a striking enhancement of adrenal aldosterone release. Because vascular smooth muscle responsiveness to angiotensin II was already known to be depressed during reduced sodium intake, it became apparent that there was a reciprocal control of the sensitivity of the adrenal gland and vascular smooth muscle with changes in sodium intake.

A second objection to the dominance of the renin-angiotensin system in mediating aldosterone release was the inconsistent change in secretion of aldosterone upon blockade of angiotensin action. Steele and Lowenstein reported that saralasin, the angiotensin antagonist, failed to reduce plasma aldosterone levels in sodium-depleted rabbits.[161] As pointed out above, saralasin is not a pure competitive antagonist; it is a partial agonist, exerting an angiotensin-like action in settings in which endogenous angiotensin is reduced.[86] Indeed, even when the renin-angiotensin system is activated, the use of excessive amounts of saralasin leads to an agonist response.

As converting enzyme inhibitors have become more potent and long-acting, it has become clear that angiotensin represents the dominant mediator of adrenal responses to changes in sodium intake in healthy humans.[164,183]

THE INFLUENCE OF RENIN AND ANGIOTENSIN II ON THE RENAL BLOOD SUPPLY

The major local intrarenal action of angiotensin II early in phylogeny has continued in higher vertebrates and in human beings. In normal dogs and humans ingesting a high-salt diet, neither saralasin nor teprotide, the first available converting enzyme inhibitor, increased renal blood flow.[87,104] When the renin-angiotensin system was activated and renal blood flow was reduced by restriction of sodium intake, both inhibitors induced a dose-related increase in renal blood flow. A brisk natriuresis followed blockade of the renal actions of angiotensin II when sodium intake was restricted; this result suggested that the local action of angiotensin had contributed to renal sodium handling.[104] A contribution of angiotensin II, independent of aldosterone, to renal sodium handling in humans was evident when natriuresis appeared within 20 min of administration of a converting enzyme inhibitor. The response occurred far too soon to reflect the natriuretic effect of a fall in plasma aldosterone; the response more closely paralleled the rise in renal blood flow.

Administration of angiotensin II reduces renal blood flow but exerts a smaller influence on glomerular filtration rate (GFR), so that filtration fraction increases. Because of the remarkable sensitivity of the renal blood supply to angiotensin II, the quantity required to induce a renal vascular response is less than 10 percent of that required to increase blood pressure.[85] In subjects on a high-salt diet, sodium excretion decreases with these very small amounts, perhaps reflecting the increase in filtration fraction and thus the physical forces within the kidney. On the other hand, there is substantial interest in the tubular actions of angiotensin II.[96] There are important species differences in the intraglomerular actions of angiotensin II. Although earlier studies had shown that subpressor quantities of angiotensin II increased proteinuria in the rat, due to a change in the characteristics of the filtration barrier, in humans even pressor concentrations of angiotensin II had no influence on barrier size selectivity.[113] Indeed, a reduction in proteinuria occurred, which probably reflected the decrease in the GFR.

THE INFLUENCE OF RENIN AND ANGIOTENSIN ON BLOOD PRESSURE

When the renin-angiotensin system in normal humans is suppressed by the liberal intake of sodium and potassium, angiotensin II antagonists and converting enzyme inhibition both reduce recumbent arterial blood pressure minimally.[151] Indeed, the modest activation of the renin-angiotensin system induced by quiet standing does not potentiate markedly the depressor response to either class of agent. When the system is activated further by restriction of sodium intake, however, both classes of agent induce a reproducible reduction in arterial blood pressure despite recumbency. The response to interruption of the system is modest. Diastolic blood pressure, for example, fell by only 5 ± 2.5 (±SD) mmHg when 50 normal subjects in salt balance, ingesting 10 meq/day of sodium, were treated with a converting enzyme inhibitor.[88] Thus, a fall in diastolic blood pressure exceeding 10 mmHg is abnormal.[88] Increasing degrees of negative sodium balance increase the importance of angiotensin II in maintaining arterial pressure. Indeed, aggressive depletion of sodium makes even the "low-renin hypertensive" dependent on angiotensin II for blood pressure maintenance.[72]

Although the vasoconstriction caused by the direct vascular action of angiotensin II can account for the hormone's pressor effect, there has been continuing interest in the details of the vascular response. Renin substrate, for example, can induce vascular smooth muscle contraction through pathways not specific to the renin-angiotensin cascade.[20] Adrenergic mechanisms might contribute to the local endothelial renin-angiotensin system,[169] but subpressor angiotensin II infusions did not stimulate sympathetic activity in humans.[73] In some systems, such as the canine cerebral artery, angiotensin II produced endothelium-dependent contraction through an indirect pathway that probably involved stimulation of thromboxane A2 formation.[115] Aldosterone release and sodium retention provide additional indirect mechanisms by which angiotensin II can induce a pressor response.

Interpretation of the responses to converting enzyme inhibition has been complicated by the likelihood that these agents have other actions in addition to suppressing angiotensin II formation. Associated reactions include the release of vasodilator PGs[163] and raising the plasma concentration of bradykinin by depressing its degradation.[181]

RESPONSIVENESS TO ANGIOTENSIN II: VASCULAR SMOOTH MUSCLE AND THE ADRENAL GLAND

The importance of responsiveness to angiotensin II as a variable has been discussed in several of the preceding sections. The past decade has seen important advances in our understanding of the determinants of responsiveness to angiotensin II, but important areas of controversy still exist.

That pressor responses to angiotensin II varied with the state of sodium balance was long recognized,[99] but it was not until 1972 that evidence first appeared to indicate that the variation in the pressor response reflected a change in vascular smooth muscle, a change that was still evident when isolated arterial muscle strips were placed in tissue bath.[162] Localization of the information in the smooth muscle strip and specificity of the influence of sodium intake made it likely that the angiotensin II receptor was involved. The blunted response to restriction of sodium intake and the enhanced response to a high sodium intake in animals and in humans was specific for angiotensin II; norepinephrine showed no such shift in vascular responsiveness.[84,162]

Blood pressure and the vascular bed of the limb changed in sensitivity to angiotensin II as sodium intake changed. In a consistent but substantially greater way, renal blood supply responsiveness changed with sodium intake.[84] A tenfold reduction in responsiveness of the renal blood supply occurred on a low-salt diet. Since the shift in responsiveness was substantially larger than the change in plasma angiotensin II concentration, the interesting possibility arose that free angiotensin II concentration in the kidney increased more than that in plasma during the restriction of sodium intake.

The development of techniques for assessing tissue binding of radioactively labeled ligands and their application to the assessment of receptors have provided a clear indication that the shifts in responsiveness to angiotensin II reflect a reciprocal relationship between plasma angiotensin II concentration and the number of receptors in a wide variety of smooth muscle preparations.[39,77] The radioligand studies, furthermore, are supported by pharmacologic evidence favoring a receptor locus for alterations in sensitivity.[180] The interpretation of the shifts in sensitivity in vivo, therefore, was straightforward.

Changes in the responsiveness of the adrenal gland to angiotensin II are related to a more complex underlying mechanism. In healthy humans, as indicated above, restriction of sodium intake substantially enhances the adrenal response to angiotensin II.[85,132] The application of radioligand binding techniques to studying the adrenal angiotensin II receptor and alternative pharmacologic approaches have not led to a clear understanding of why adrenal sensitivity changes. Some radioligand studies have suggested a receptor mechanism;[1,17,42] others have not.[40,180] The complexity of the regulatory mechanisms is evident from the fact that restriction of calcium intake produced a directionally opposite effect on adrenal and smooth muscle binding of labeled angiotensin II.[3]

What of humans? Such direct inquiries, of course, are not possible. An alternative approach to assessing whether the modification in responsiveness of these target tissues reflects changes in circulating angiotensin II or is linked to other factors dependent on dietary sodium intake is possible, based on the ability of converting enzyme inhibitors to reduce circulating angiotensin II concentration. This approach reversed the reduction in both the pressor response and the renal vascular response to angiotensin in normal subjects with a low sodium intake, returning the response toward that anticipated on a high-salt diet.[35,157] This response to converting enzyme inhibition is, therefore, precisely that anticipated from the in vitro studies.

In the case of the adrenal gland and aldosterone release in normal human subjects, however, converting enzyme inhibition did nothing to responsiveness to angiotensin; this finding favors a different mechanism in determining adrenal responsiveness.[35,157] The most likely candidate as a regulatory mechanism in adrenal sensitivity to angiotensin is the late pathway in aldosterone biosynthesis.[182]

The recent emphasis on shifts in sensitivity reflects not only growing insight into the role of sensitivity modulation as a determinant of normal physiologic processes but also the belief that changes in sensitivity may make a substantial contribution to the pathogenesis of disease.

REFERENCES

1. Aquilera G et al: Angiotensin II receptors: Properties and regulation in adrenal glomerulosa cells. *Circ Res* 46 (suppl 1):1–118, 1980.
2. Ayers CR et al: Effect of 1-sarcosine-8-alanine angiotensin II and converting enzyme inhibitor on renin release in dog acute renovascular hypertension. *Circ Res* 34/35(suppl 1):1–27, 1974.
3. Baksi SN et al: Low-calcium diet increases blood pressure and alters peripheral but not central angiotensin II binding sites in rats. *J Hypertens* 7:423, 1989.
4. Baumbach L, Leyssac PP: Studies on the mechanism of renin release from isolated superfused rat glomeruli: Effects of calcium, calcium ionophore and lanthanum. *J Physiol* 273:745, 1977.
5. Bennett JP, Snyder SH: Angiotensin II binding to mammalian brain membranes. *J Biol Chem* 251:7423, 1976.
6. Berl T et al: Prostaglandins in the beta-adrenergic and baroreceptor-mediated secretion of renin. *Am J Physiol* 236:F472, 1979.
7. Bern HA: Hormones and endocrine glands of fishes. *Science* 158:455, 1967.
8. Bernstein KE et al: The isolation of angiotensin-converting enzyme cDNA. *J Biol Chem* 263:11021, 1988.
9. Blantz RC et al: Angiotensin II effects upon the glomerular microcirculation and ultrafiltration coefficient of the rat. *J Clin Invest* 57:419, 1976.
10. Blumberg AS et al: Angiotensin III induced prostaglandin release. *Prostaglandins* 11:195, 1976.
11. Blundell T et al: Three-dimensional structure, specificity and catalytic mechanism of renin. *Nature (London)* 304:273, 1983.
12. Bouhnik J et al: Rat angiotensinogen and des (angiotensin I) angiotensinogen: Purification, characterization and partial sequencing. *Biochemistry* 20:7010, 1981.
13. Bouhnik J et al: Immunologic identification of both plasma and human renal inactive renin as prorenin. *J Clin Endocrinol Metab* 60:399m, 1985.
14. Boyd GW et al: The role of angiotensin II in the control of aldosterone in man. *Clin Sci* 42:91, 1972.
15. Brasier AR et al: Multiple cis-acting DNA regulatory elements mediate hepatic angiotensinogen gene expression. *Mol Endocrinol* 3:1022, 1989.
16. Bravo EL et al: Action of [1-des (aspartic acid), 8-isoleucine] angiotensin II upon the pressor and steroidogenic activity of angiotensin II. *J Clin Endocrinol Metab* 40:530, 1974.
17. Bravo EL: Regulation of aldosterone secretion: Current concepts and newer aspects. *Adv Nephrol* 7:105, 1977.
18. Budisavljevic M et al: Antagonist effect of a receptor-mimicking peptide encoded by human angiotensin II complementary RNA. *Hypertension* 19:345, 1992.
19. Bumpus FM: Recognition and management of renal vascular hypertension, in Davis JO et al (eds): *Hypertension: Mechanisms, Diagnosis and Management*. New York, HP Publishing, 1977, p 254.
20. Bund SJ et al: The contractile effects of porcine tetradecapeptide renin substrate in human resistance vessels: Evidence of activation by vascular wall renin and serine proteases. *J Hypertens* 7:741, 1989.
21. Burnham CE et al: Molecular cloning of rat renin cDNA and its gene. *Proc Natl Acad Sci U S A* 84:5605, 1987.
22. Caldicott WJH et al: Angiotensin receptors in glomeruli differ from those in renal arterioles. *Kidney Int* 19:687, 1981.
23. Caldwell PRB et al: Angiotensin converting enzyme: Vascular endothelial localization. *Science* 191:1050, 1976.
24. Capelli JP et al: A phylogenetic study of the renin-angiotensin system. *Am J Physiol* 218:1171, 1970.
25. Capponi AM, Catt KJ: Angiotensin II receptors in adrenal cortex and uterus. *J Biol Chem* 254:5120, 1979.
26. Celio MR et al: Renin in anterior pituitary, pineal and neural cells of mouse brain. *J Biomed Mater Res* 1:427, 1980.
27. Chiu AT et al: Nonpeptide angiotensin II receptor antagonists: 7.1. Cellular and biochemical pharmacology of PuP 753, an orally active antihypertensive agent. *J Pharmacol Exp Ther* 252:711, 1989.
28. Churchill PC, Churchill MC: Effects of trifluoperazine on renin secretion of rat kidney slices. *J Pharmacol Exp Ther* 224:68, 1983.
29. Clouston WM et al: Molecular cloning of the mouse angiotensinogen gene. *Genomics* 2:240, 1988.
30. Clouston WM et al: The angiotensinogen gene is located on mouse chromosome 8. *FEBS Lett* 255:419, 1989.
31. Cohen S et al: Isolation and characterization of renin-like enzymes from mouse submaxillary glands. *Biochemistry* 11:4286, 1972.
32. Corvol P et al: Structure of the mouse submaxillary gland renin precursor and a model for renin processing. *Hypertension* 5(suppl 1):1–3, 1983.
33. Cushman DW et al: Design of potent competitive inhibitors of angiotensin-converting enzyme: Carboxylalkanoyl and mercaptoalkanoyl amino acids. *Biochemistry* 16:5484, 1977.
34. Davis JO, Freeman RH: Mechanisms regulating renin release. *Physiol Rev* 56:1, 1976.
35. Dawson-Hughes BF et al: Plasma angiotensin concentration regulates vascular but not adrenal responsiveness to restriction of sodium intake in normal man. *Clin Sci* 61:527, 1981.

36. Defforrest JM et al: Effects of indomethacin and meclofenamate on renin release and renal hemodynamic function during chronic sodium depletion in conscious dogs. *Circ Res* 47:99, 1980.
37. Delabays A et al: Hemodynamic and humoral effects of the new renin inhibitor enalkiren in normal humans. *Hypertension* 13:941, 1989.
38. De Remee RA, Rohrbach J: Serum angiotensin converting enzyme activity in evaluating the clinical course of sarcoidosis. *Ann Intern Med* 92:361, 1980.
39. Devynck MA, Meyer P: Angiotensin receptors in vascular tissue. *Am J Med* 61:758, 1976.
40. Douglas JG: Effects of high potassium diet on angiotensin-induced aldosterone production in rat adrenal glomerulosa cells. *Endocrinology* 106:983, 1980.
41. Douglas JG: Angiotensin receptor subtypes of the kidney cortex. *Am J Physiol* 253:F1, 1987.
42. Doulgas JG, Catt KJ: Regulation of angiotensin II receptors in the rat adrenal cortex by dietary electrolytes. *J Clin Invest* 58:834, 1976.
43. Dzau VJ et al: Complete purification of dog renal renin. *Biochemistry* 18:5224, 1979.
44. Dzau VJ et al: Characterization of renin-like enzymes in the rabbit uterus by renin specific antibody. *Circulation* 62(suppl III): III-238, 1980.
45. Dzau VJ et al: Sequential renal hemodynamics in experimental benign and malignant hypertension. *Hypertension* 3(suppl 1): I-63, 1981.
46. Dzau VJ et al: Studies of the biosynthesis of renin using a cell-free translation system. *Clin Sci* 61:241S, 1981.
47. Dzau VJ et al: Characterization of antibody to canine renal renin: Studies of interspecies homology of renin using antibody as probe. *Hypertension* 4:341, 1982.
48. Dzau VJ et al: Evidence for renin in rat brain: Differentiation from other renin-like enzymes. *Am J Physiol* 242:E292, 1982.
49. Dzau VJ, Hermann HC: Hormonal regulation of angiotensinogen synthesis. *Life Sci* 30:577, 1982.
50. Dzau VJ, Sands K: Role of the pituitary gland in regulation of angiotensinogen production. *Fed Proc* 41:6265, 1982.
51. Dzau VJ et al: Antibodies as specific renin inhibitors: Studies with polyclonal and monoclonal antibodies and Fab fragments. *Clin Exp Hypertens* A5(suppl 7, 8):1207, 1983.
52. Dzau VJ et al: Sequential changes in renin secretion-synthesis coupling in response to acute beta adrenergic stimulation (abstract). *Clin Res* 35:604A, 1987.
53. Dzau VJ et al: Tissue specific regulation of renin expression in the mouse. *Hypertension* 9(supppl 3):3-36, 1987.
54. Dzau VJ et al: Molecular biology of the renin-angiotensin system. *Am J Physiol* 255:F563, 1988.
55. Echtenkamp SF et al: Effects of indomethacin, renal denervation and propranolol on plasma renin activity in conscious dogs with chronic thoracic caval constriction. *Circ Res* 49:492, 1981.
56. Ehlers MR et al: Molecular cloning of human testicular angiotensin-converting enzyme. *Proc Natl Acad Sci U S A* 86:7741, 1989.
57. Ehlers MRW, Riordan JF: Angiotensin-converting enzyme: New concepts concerning its biological role. *Biochemistry* 28:5311, 1989.
58. Epstein M: Studies of volume homeostasis in man utilizing the model of head out water immersion. *Nephron* 22:9, 1978.
59. Erdos EG: Angiotensin I converting enzyme. *Circ Res* 36:247, 1975.
60. Erdos EG et al: Hydrolysis of enkephalin by cultured endothelial cells and purified dipeptidyl peptidase. *Biochem Pharmacol* 27:843, 1978.
61. Erdos EG, Gaford JT: Human angiotensin-converting enzyme. *Clin Exp Hypertens* A5(suppl 7, 8):1251, 1983.
62. Farhi ER et al: Interactions between intrarenal epinephrine receptors and the renal baroreceptor in the control of PRA in conscious dogs. *Circ Res* 50:477, 1982.
63. Field LF et al: Tissue and gene specificity of mouse renin expression. *Hyptertension* 6:597, 1984.
64. Fitzsimons JT: The effect on drinking of peptide precursors and of short chain peptide fragments of angiotensin II injected into the rat's diencephalon. *J Physiol* 214:295, 1971.
65. Foidart J et al: Evidence for mesangial glomerular recepetors for angiotensin II linked to mesangial cell contractility. *FEBS Lett* 121:333, 1980.
66. Fray JCS et al: Stimulation of renin release in perfused kidney by low calcium and high magnesium. *Am J Physiol* 232:F377, 1977.
67. Friedland JC et al: Angiotensin converting enzyme: Induction by steroids in rabbit alveolar macrophages in culture. *Science* 197:64, 1977.
68. Funakawa S et al: Conversion between renin and high molecular weight renin in the dog. *Biochem J* 176:977, 1978.
69. Gaillard I et al: Structure of human angiotensinogen gene. *DNA* 8:87, 1989.
70. Galen FX et al: Multiple forms of human renin: Purification and characterization. *J Biol Chem* 254:4848, 1979.
71. Ganten D et al: Iso-renin of extrarenal origin: The tissue angiotensinogenase systems. *Am J Med* 60:760, 1976.
72. Gavras H et al: Reciprocal relation between renin dependency and sodium dependency in essential hypertension. *N Engl J Med* 295:1278, 1976.
73. Goldsmith SR et al: Subpressor angiotensin II infusions do not stimulate sympathetic activity in humans. *Am J Physiol* 258:H179, 1990.
74. Gomez RA et al: Distribution of renin mRNA and its protein in the developing kidney. *Am J Physiol* 257:F850, 1988.
75. Goodfriend TL, Peach MJ: Angiotensin III: Evidence and speculation for its role as an important agonist in the renin-angiotensin system. *Circ Res* 36/37(suppl 1):38, 1975.
76. Grady EF et al: Expression of AT2 receptors in the developing rat fetus. *J Clin Invest* 88:921, 1991.
77. Gunther S et al: Regulation by angiotensin II of its receptors in resistance blood vessels. *Nature (London)* 287:230, 1980.
78. Haber E et al: Application of a radioimmunoassay for angiotensin I to the physiologic measurements of plasma renin activity in normal human subjects. *J Clin Endocrinol Metab* 29:1349, 1969.

79. Haber E et al: Sites and mechanisms of the conversion of angiotensin I to II, in Genest J, Koiw E (eds): *Hypptertension '72*. Berlin, Springer-Verlag, 1972, p 563.
80. Haber E: The role of renin in normal and pathological cardiovascular homeostasis. *Circulation* 54:849, 1976.
81. Harada E, Rubin RP: Stimulation of renin secretion and calcium efflux from the isolated perfused cat kidney by noradrenaline after prolonged calcium deprivation. *J Physiol* 274:367, 1978.
82. Hermann HC, Dzau VJ: Feedback regulation of angiotensinogen production by components of the renin-angiotensin system. *Circ Res* 328, 1983.
83. Hobart PM et al: Human renin gene: Structure and sequence analysis. *Proc Natl Acad Sci U S A* 81:5026, 1984.
84. Hollenberg NK et al: Renal vascular response to angiotensin and norepinephrine in normal man: Effect of salt intake. *Circ Res* 31:750, 1972.
85. Hollenberg NK et al: Reciprocal influence of salt intake on adrenal glomerulosa and renal vascular responses to angiotensin II in normal man. *J Clin Invest* 54:34, 1974.
86. Hollenberg NK et al: Blockade and stimulation of renal, adrenal and vascular angiotensin II receptors with 1-sar 8-ala angiotensin II in normal man. *J Clin Invest* 57:39, 1976.
87. Hollenberg NK et al: Renal vascular response to interruption of the renin-angiotensin system in normal man. *Kidney Int* 12:285, 1977.
88. Hollenberg NK et al: Response to saralasin and angiotensin's role in essential and renal hypertension. *Medicine* 58:115, 1979.
89. Hollenberg NK, Passan DR: Specificity of renal vasodilation with captopril: Saralasin prevents the response in the DOCA-treated, salt-loaded rabbit. *Life Sci* 31:329, 1982.
90. Hsueh W et al: Characterization of inactive renin from human kidney and plasma: Evidence of a renal source of circulating inactive renin. *J Clin Invest* 71:506, 1983.
91. Hsueh WA, Baxter JE: Human prorenin: Brief review. *Hypertension* 17:469, 1991.
92. Hui KY et al: Design of rat renin inhibitory peptides. *J Med Chem* 31:1679, 1988.
93. Imai T et al: Cloning and sequence of cDNA for human renin precursor. *Proc Natl Acad Sci U S A* 80:7405, 1983.
94. Inagami T, Murakami K: Pure renin isolation from hog kidney and characterization. *J Biol Chem* 252:2978, 1977.
95. Inagami T, Murakami K: Prorenin. *J Biomed Mater Res* 1:456, 1980.
96. Ingelfinger JR et al: Sodium regulation of kidney angiotensinogen messenger RNA expression in rat kidney cortex and medulla. *J Clin Invest* 78:1311, 1986.
97. Ingelfinger JR et al: In situ hybridization evidence for angiotensinogen messenger RNA in the rat proximal tubule. *J Clin Invest* 85:417, 1990.
98. Jeunemaitre X et al: Plasma angiotensins, renin, and blood pressure during acute renin inhibition by CGP 38 560A in hypertensive patients. *Am J Hypertens* 2:819, 1989.
99. Kaplan NM, Silah JG: The effect of angiotensin II on the blood pressure in humans with hypertensive disease. *J Clin Invest* 43:659 1964.
100. Kawamura M et al: Characteristics of a renin-binding substance for the conversion of renin into a higher molecular-weight form in the dog. *Clin Sci* 57:345, 1979.
101. Keeton TK, Campbell WB: The pharmacologic alteration of renin release. *Pharmacol Rev* 32:81, 1980.
102. Khairallah PA: Action of angiotensin on adrenergic nerve endings: Inhibition of norepinephrine uptake. *Fed Proc* 31:1351, 1972.
103. Kim SJ et al: Identification of plasma inactive renin as prorenin with a site-directed antibody. *Biochem Biophys Res Commun* 126:641, 1985.
104. Kimbrough HM Jr et al: Effect of intrarenal AII blockade on renal function in conscious dogs. *Circ Res* 40:174, 1977.
105. Kirchner KA et al: Importance of chloride for acute inhibition of renin by sodium chloride. *Am J Physiol* 235:F444, 1978.
106. Krieger JE, Dzau VJ: Molecular biology of hypertension. *Hypertension* 18(suppl 1):1–3, 1991.
107. Kunapuli SP, Kumar A: Molecular cloning of human angiotensinogen cDNA and evidence for the presence of its mRNA in rat heart. *Circ Res* 60:786, 1987.
108. Leyssac PP: Intrarenal function of angiotensin. *Fed Proc* 26:55, 1967.
109. Lieberman J: A new confirmatory test for sarcoidosis—serum angiotensin converting enzyme: Effect of steroids and chronic lung disease. *Annu Rev Resp Dis* 109:743, 1974.
110. Lieberman J, Buetler E: Elevation of serum angiotensin-converting enzyme in Gaucher's disease. *N Engl J Med* 294:1442, 1976.
111. Lieberman J, Sastre A: Serum angiotensin converting enzyme: Elevation in diabetes mellitus. *Ann Intern Med* 93:825, 1980.
112. Logan AG et al: The effect of lanthanum on renin secretion and renal vasoconstriction. *Proc R Soc London* 195:327, 1977.
113. Loon N et al: Effect of angiotensin II infusion on the human glomerular filtration barrier. *Am J Physiol* 26:F608, 1989.
114. Lynch KR et al: Localization of angiotensinogen mRNA sequences in rat brain. *Hypertension* 8:540, 1986.
115. Manabe K et al: Endothelium-dependent contractions induced by angiotensin I and angiotensin II in canine cerebral artery. *J Pharmacol Exp Ther* 251:317, 1989.
116. Marshall GR: Structure-activity relations of antagonists of the renin-angiotensin system. *Fed Proc* 35:2494, 1976.
117. McCubbin JW: Peripheral effects of angiotensin on the autonomic nervous system, in Page IH, Bumpus FM (eds): *Angiotensin*. New York, Springer-Verlag, 1974, p 417.
118. Mellins RB: Metallic functions of the lung and their clinical relevance. *Am J Roentgenol* 138:999, 1982.
119. Mendelsohn FAO et al: Angiotensin II receptors in the kidney. *Fed Proc* 45:1420, 1986.
120. Misono KS, Inagami TT: Characterization of the active site of mouse submandibular gland renin. *Biochemistry* 19:2616, 1980.
121. Misono KS et al: Amino acid sequence of mouse submaxillary gland. *Proc Natl Acad Sci U S A* 79:4858, 1982.
122. Mizoguchi H et al: Effect of intrarenal administration of dopamine on renin release in conscious dogs. *Am J Physiol* 224:H39, 1983.
123. Moffat RB et al: Modulation of kidney renin messenger RNA levels during experimentally induced hypertension. *Hypertension* 9(suppl 3):3–36, 1987.

124. Moore TJ et al: Contribution of prostaglandins to the antihypertensive action of captopril in essential hypertensin. *Hypertension* 3:168, 1981.
125. Moore TJ, Williams GH: Angiotensin II receptors in human platelets. *Circ Res* 51:314, 1981.
126. Morris BJ et al: Human renin gene sequence, gene regulation and prorenin processing. *J Hypertens* 2(suppl 3):231, 1984.
127. Murphy TJ: Isolation of a cDNA encoding the vascular type-1 angiotensin II receptor. *Nature (London)*:351:233, 1991.
128. Naftilan A, Oparil S: The role of calcium in the control of renin release. *Hypertension* 4:670, 1982.
129. Naftilan AJ et al: Induction of the proto-oncogene c-jun by angiotensin II. *Mol Cell Biol* 10:5536, 1990.
130. Nakamura N et al: Nonproportional changes in plasma renin concentration, renal renin content, and rat renin messenger RNA. *Hypertension* 7:855, 1985.
131. Naruse M, Inagani T: Markedly elevated specific renin levels in the adrenal gland of genetically hypertensive rats. *Proc Natl Acad Sci U S A* 79:3295, 1982.
132. Oelkers W et al: Sensitization of the adrenal cortex to angiotensin II in sodium-deplete man. *Circ Res* 34:69, 1974.
133. Ohkubo H et al: Cloning and sequence analysis of cDNA for angiotensinogen. *Proc Natl Sci U S A* 80:2196, 1983.
134. Ondetti MA et al: Angiotensin-converting enzyme inhibitors from the venom of *Bothrops jararaca*: Isolation, elucidation of structure, and synthesis. *Biochemistry* 10:4033, 1971.
135. Panthier JJ et al: The mouse RN locus: S allele of the renin regulator gene results from a single structural gene duplication. *EMBO J* 1:1417, 1982.
136. Park CS et al: Calcium in the control of renin secretion: Ca^{2+} influx as an inhibitory signal. *Am J Physiol* 240:F70, 1980.
137. Paul M et al: Glycosylation influences intracellular transit time and secretion rate of human prorenin in transfected cells. *J Hyptertens Suppl* 6:S487, 1988.
138. Peach MJ: Adrenal medulla, in Page IH, Bumpus FM (eds): *Angiotensin*. New York, Springer-Verlag, 1974, p 17.
139. Peart WS et al: The effects of EDTA and EGTA on renin secretion. *Br J Pharmacol* 59:247, 1977.
140. Pettinger WA: Evidence for a renal alpha-adrenergic receptor inhibiting renin release in rats. *Circ Res* 38:1, 1976.
141. Piccini N et al: A DNA polymorphism consistent with gene duplication correlates with high renin levels in mouse submaxillary gland. *Cell* 30:205, 1982.
142. Poulsen K et al: Renin is synthesized as a 50,000 dalton single-chain polypeptide in cell-free translation systems. *FEBS Lett* 93:135, 1979.
143. Pratt RE et al: Human renin biosynthesis and secretion in normal and ischemic kidneys. *Proc Natl Acad Sci U S A* 84:7837, 1987.
144. Printz D et al: The brain renin angiotensin system (minireview), in Gaunter D et al (eds): *The Renin Angiotensin System in the Brain*. Heidelberg, Springer-Verlag, 1982, p 3.
145. Re R et al: Renin synthesis by canine aortic smooth muscle cells in culture. *Life Sci* 30:99, 1982.
146. Regoli D et al: Pharmacology of angiotensin. *Pharmacol Rev* 26:69, 1974.
147. Ron D et al: An inducible 50-kilodalton NFkB-like protein and a constitutive protein both bind the acute-phase element of the angiotensinogen gene. *Mol Cell Biol* 10:1023, 1990.
148. Ron D et al: The permissive role of glucocorticoids on interleukin-1 stimulation of angiotensinogen gene transcription is mediated by an interaction between inducible enhancers. *Mol Cell Biol* 10:4389, 1990.
149. Rouger F et al: Molecular cloning of a mouse submaxillary gland renin with DNA. *Proc Natl Acad Sci U S A* 78:6367, 1981.
150. Ryan JW et al: Metabolism of angiotensin I in the pulmonary circulation. *Biochem J* 120:221, 1970.
151. Sancho J et al: The role of the renin-angiotensin-aldosterone system in cardiovascular homeostasis in normal human subjects. *Circulation* 53:400, 1976.
152. Sasaki K et al: Cloning and expression of a complementary DNA encoding a bovine adrenal angiotensin II type-1 receptor. *Nature (London)*: 351:230, 1991.
153. Sawyer WH et al: Renal responses of Australian lungfish to vasotocin, angiotensin II, and NaCl infusion. *Am J Physiol* 231:593, 1976.
154. Sealey J et al: Prorenin and other large molecular weight forms of renin. *Endocr Rev* 1:365, 1980.
155. Seikaly M et al: Endogenous angiotensin concentrations in specific intrarenal fluid compartments of the rat. *J Clin Invest* 86:1352, 1989.
156. Shai S-Y et al: Genomic DNA 5′ to the mouse and human angiotensin converting enzyme gene contains two distinct regions of conserved sequence. *Biochem Biophys Res Commun* 167:1128, 1990.
157. Shoback D et al: Endogenous angiotensin II as a determinant of sodium modulated changes in tissue responsiveness to angiotensin II in normal man. *J Clin Endocrinol Metab* 57:764, 1983.
158. Siragy HM et al: Intrarenal renin inhibition increases renal function by an angiotensin II-dependent mechanism. *Am J Physiol* 255:F749, 1988.
159. Sokabe H: Phylogeny of the renal effects of angiotensin. *Kidney Int* 6:263, 1974.
160. Soubrier FF et al: Two putative active centers in human angiotensin I-converting enzyme revealed by molecular cloning. *Proc Natl Acad Sci U S A* 35:9386, 1988.
161. Steele JM, Lownestein J: Differential effects of an angiotensin II analogue on pressor and adrenal receptors in the rabbit. *Circ Res* 35:592, 1974.
162. Strewler GJ et al: Sodium intake and vascular smooth muscle responsiveness to norepinephrine and angiotensin in the rabbit. *Circ Res* 31:758, 1972.
163. Swartz SL et al: Increase in prostaglandins during converting enzyme inhibition. *Clin Sci* 59:133S, 1980.
164. Swartz SL et al: Primacy of the renin-angiotensin system in mediating the aldosterone response to sodium restriction. *J Clin Endocrinol Metab* 50:1071, 1980.
165. Sweet CTR: Antihypertensive activity of *N*(*S*)-1-(ethoxycarbonyl)-3-phenylpropyl-L-Ala-L-Pro (MK-421), an orally active converting enzyme inhibitor. *J Pharmacol Exp Ther* 216:558, 1981.
166. Takeuchi K et al: Angiotensin II can regulate gene expression by the AP-1 binding sequence via a protein kinase

C-dependent pathway. *Biochem Biophys Res Commun* 172:1189, 1990.

167. Takii Y, Inagami T: Purification of a completely inactive renin from hog kidney and identification of renin zymogen. *Biochem Biophys Res Commun* 104:133, 1982.
168. Tanaka T et al: Common structural organization of the angiotensinogen and the a1-antitrypsin genes. *J Biol Chem* 259:8063, 1984.
169. Tang S-S et al: Endothelial renin-angiotensin pathway: Adrenergic regulation of angiotensin secretion. *Circ Res* 66:103, 1990.
170. Tang S-S et al: Characterization of nuclear angiotensin-II binding sites in rat liver and comparison with plasma membrane receptors. *Endocrinology* 131:374, 1992.
171. Taub KJ: Angiotensin antagonists with increased specificity for the renal vasculature. *J Clin Invest* 59:528, 1977.
172. Tewksbury DA et al: The amino terminal amino acid sequence of human angiotensinogen. *Biochem Biophys Res Commun* 99:1311, 1981.
173. Timmermans PBMWM et al: Angiotensin II receptor antagonists: From discovery to antihypertensive drugs. *Hypertension* 18(suppl 3):3–136, 1991.
174. Tobian L: Interrelationship of electrolytes, juxtaglomerular cells, and hypertension. *Physiol Rev* 40:280, 1960.
175. Vinson GP et al: Comparative and evolutionary aspects of aldosterone secretion and zona glomerulosa function. *J Endocrinol* 81:5P, 1979.
176. Viskoper RJ et al: Effect of Ca^{2+} binding by EGTA on renin release in the isolated perfused rabbit kidney. *Proc Soc Exp Biol Med* 152:415, 1976.
177. Watkins BE et al: Intrarenal site of action of calcium on renin secretion in dogs. *Circ Res* 39:847, 1976.
178. Weare J et al: Purification of human angiotensin converting enzyme using reverse immunoadsorption chromatography. *Anal Biochem* 123:310, 1982.
179. Whitebread S et al: Preliminary biochemical characterization of two angiotensin II receptor subtypes. *Biochem Biophys Res Commun* 163:284, 1989.
180. Williams GH et al: Influence of sodium intake on vascular and adrenal angiotensin II receptors. *Endocrinology* 98:1343, 1976.
181. Williams GH, Hollenberg NK: Accentuated vascular and endocrine response to SQ 20881 in hypertension. *N Engl J Med* 297:184, 1977.
182. Williams GH et al: Adrenal responses to pharmacological interruption of the renin-angiotensin system in sodium restricted normal man. *J Clin Endocrinol Metab* 47:725, 1978.
183. Wong PC et al: Nonpeptide angiotensin II receptor antagonists: 8.1. Characterization of functional antagonism displayed by DuP 753, an orally active antihypertensive agent. *J Pharmacol Exp Ther* 252:719, 1989.
184. Wong PC et al: Nonpeptide angiotensin II receptor antagonists: 9.1. Antihypertensive activity in rats of DuP 753, an orally active antihypertensive agent. *J Pharmacol Exp Ther* 252:726, 1989.
185. Yamamoto K et al: Effect of Ca^{2+} on renin release in vitro and in vivo. *Jpn Circ J* 38:1127, 1974.
186. Yokosawa H et al: Human renal renin: Complete purification and characterization. *J Biol Chem* 255:3498, 1980.
187. Yotsumoto H et al: Increased levels of serum angiotensin converting enzyme activity in hyperthyroidism. *Ann Intern Med* 96:326, 1982.
188. Young D et al: Isolation and characterization of a new cellular oncogene encoding a protein with multiple transmembrane domains. *Cell* 45:711, 1986.
189. Zimmerman BG, Wong PC: Alterations in renal function produced by angiotensin converting enzyme inhibitors, in Horovitz ZP (ed): *Angiotensin Converting Enzyme Inhibitors: Mechanism of Action and Clinical Implications*. Baltimore, Urban and Schwarzenberg, 1981, p 239.

CHAPTER • 17

Transport of water and electrolytes in the gastrointestinal tract: physiological mechanisms, regulation, and methods of study

Kim E. Barrett • Kiertisin Dharmsathaphorn

The primary function of the gastrointestinal tract is to digest and absorb nutrients. In support of this function, the amount of water in the intestinal lumen must be closely regulated to control the physical passage of intestinal contents, to permit the access of digestive enzymes to food particles, and to allow the diffusion of digested nutrients to the epithelial cells, where they are absorbed. Despite the importance of intestinal water balance, it is not directly regulated. Water moves passively into and out of the intestinal lumen in response to the active transport of electrolytes and other solutes. Thus, it is the control of epithelial electrolyte transport that makes possible the control of the fluidity of intestinal contents. In addition, some areas of the gastrointestinal tract and organs that drain into it have developed specialized electrolyte transport functions related to digestion, such as acid secretion in the stomach and bicarbonate secretion in the duodenum. The stomach has an important secretory function; a large quantity of hydrochloric acid is secreted by its parietal cells. This function, which is very well preserved in the animal kingdom, probably has a role in host defense against microorganisms. Bicarbonate (HCO_3^-) is secreted by cells that line the surface of the stomach and duodenum and may play an important role in protecting the upper gastrointestinal tract from acid injury. Large amounts of bicarbonate are also secreted via the biliary and pancreatic ducts to neutralize the gastric acid in the small intestine.

Studies from the authors' laboratories have been supported by grants from the National Institutes of Health (AM 28305, AM 01146, AI 24992) and the National Foundation for Ileitis and Colitis.

This chapter describes the physiology of intestinal electrolyte transport and how it is regulated at the intracellular, epithelial, and organ levels. It also briefly reviews some of the experimental methods that have yielded our present state of knowledge or may be expected to provide important information in this area in the future. Disease correlations will be mentioned only in passing; for more specific information on clinical aspects of intestinal electrolyte transport, see Chap. 36.

GENERAL AND ANATOMICAL FEATURES OF INTESTINAL WATER BALANCE

The gastrointestinal tract displays considerable ability to both secrete and conserve fluid. While the average daily oral fluid intake is usually about 2000 ml (depending on the type and number of meals taken), the gastrointestinal tract and the organs that drain into it supply at least another 7000 ml (Fig. 17-1). In health, most of the fluid load presented to the small intestine is absorbed to osmotically balance the absorption of nutrients and electrolytes; the 1500 to 2000 ml that remains to be presented to the colon is also largely absorbed, leaving approximately 100 ml to be excreted in the stool. Both the small and large intestines have considerable reserve capacity for absorption and can readily accommodate increases in the fluid load without a concomitant increase in fecal water. Conversely, the intestines have a substantial reserve of ability to secrete fluid and electrolytes. The

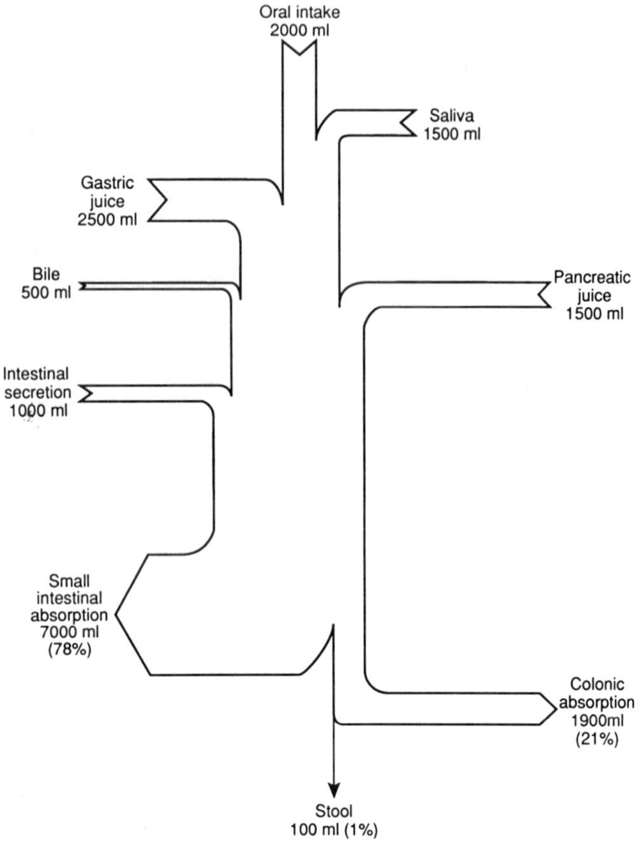

FIGURE 17-1 • Daily water balance in the healthy human gastrointestinal tract. The small intestine is responsible for absorbing approximately 78 percent of the daily fluid load, largely in association with nutrient uptake. The colon absorbs the majority of the remaining fluid, with an efficiency of approximately 95 percent, leaving only about 1 percent of the fluid load to be excreted in the stool.

1000 ml secreted each day under normal circumstances can be augmented many times in the presence of toxins or endogenous secretagogues. The most dramatic examples are patients with cholera, who can secrete more than 30 liters of stool water a day. Despite this vast capacity, the intestine has a relatively minor role in the physiological regulation of water and electrolyte balance; its importance becomes more apparent in pathological conditions wherein alarming and life-threatening amounts of fluid and electrolytes can be lost.

The discussion of anatomical features contributing to water transport focuses on the intestine because of its importance in fluid and electrolyte balance. The stomach, liver and biliary tract, and pancreas are discussed only briefly. The reserve capacity of the intestine for fluid absorption and secretion is a functional correlate of intestinal anatomy; the gastrointestinal tract has a massive amplification in surface area afforded by folds, villi, and microvilli.[157,204,205] The overall surface area of the gastrointestinal tract (Fig. 17-2) in human beings is larger than a doubles tennis court (>200 m^2). The capacity of the intestine afforded by surface area is further supplemented by the ability to control gastrointestinal motility. Coordinated contractions of intestinal smooth muscle regulate the flow of the luminal contents to ensure adequate contact time for absorption to take place. There-

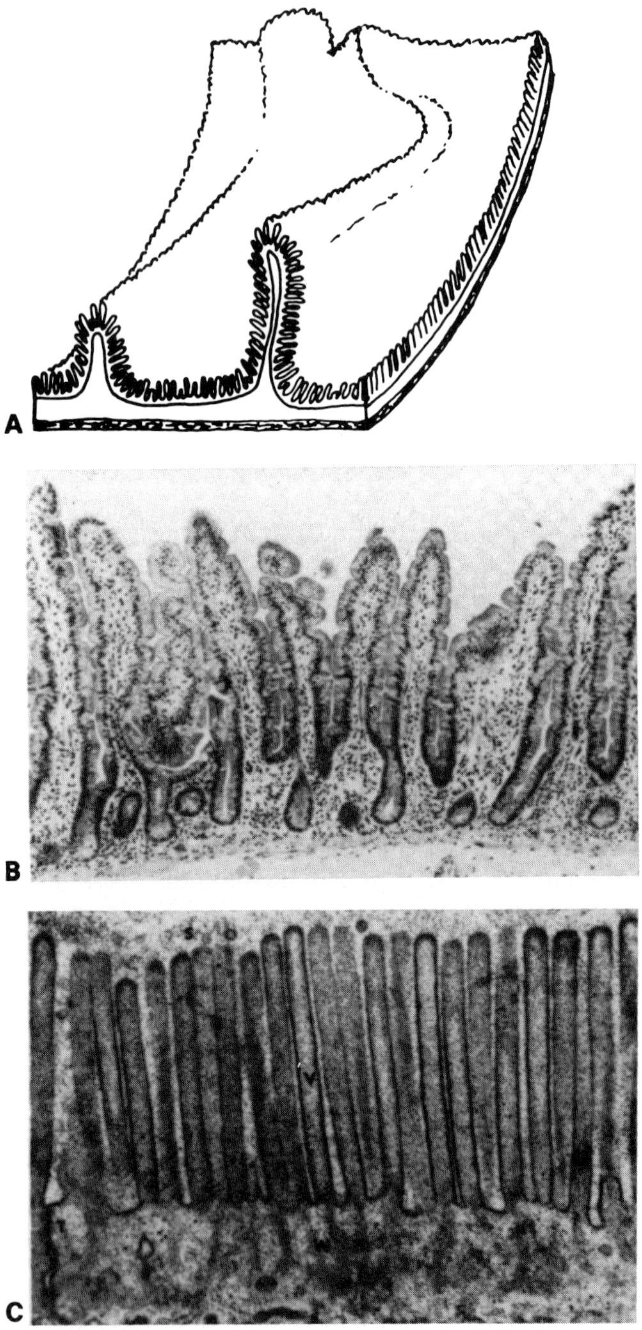

FIGURE 17-2 • Amplification of intestinal surface area by (*a*) intestinal folds (plicae conniventes), (*b*) villi, and (*c*) microvilli. Compared with a flat surface, intestinal folds increase the surface area by a factor of 3, villi by a factor of 10, and microvilli by a factor of 20. Together, these features increase the surface area approximately 600 times. (Micrographs from Trier JS et al, in Sleisenger MH, Fordtran JS, eds: *Gastrointestinal Disease: Pathophysiology, Diagnosis, Management, 3d ed,* Philadelphia, Saunders, 1983. Used by permission.)

fore, under normal circumstances, deficiency of mucosal absorptive function is rarely observed except in (1) patients with massive intestinal resections, (2) patients with diseases that destroy the absorptive cells, or (3) patients with diseases that form a submucosal barrier to the absorptive process. Pathological fluid and electrolyte losses arise more often from excessive stimulation of intestinal secretion than from failure of absorption. If the secretory process alone is activated, the patient loses large amounts of fluid and electrolytes in the stool.

It should be noted that the absorptive and secretory functions of the intestine are at least partially unrelated, and they may have different regulatory mechanisms. Therefore, the absorptive function may remain intact while the secretory function is abnormally affected by toxins or other secretagogues. A potential anatomical

TABLE 17-1 • Gastrointestinal secretory stimuli

Stimulus	Intracellular mediator	References
ENDOGENOUS INTESTINAL AGENTS		
Prostaglandins	cAMP	5,26,122,152,143
VIP	cAMP	38,130,187,210
Secretin	cAMP	103,159
PHI	cAMP	8
Glucagon	cAMP	87,103
GIP	Unknown	102
Gastrin	Unknown	
Calcitonin	Ca^{2+} ?	11,89,125,211
Substance P	Ca^{2+}	116,211
Neurotensin	Ca^{2+}	116
Bombesin	Unknown	11,115
Vasopressin	cAMP	100
Cholecystokinin	Ca^{2+} ?	159
Cholinergic agonists	Ca^{2+}	111,203,227,228
Serotonin	Ca^{2+}	51
Adenosine	Unknown	13,49
Prolactin	Unknown	147
Histamine	Ca^{2+}	214–216
Bradykinin	cAMP	80
Hydrogen peroxide	Unknown	118
INTESTINAL LUMEN-ACTIVE AGENTS		
Bacterial enterotoxins		
V. cholerae	cAMP	4,10,62,83,122
E. coli (heat-labile)	cAMP	
E. coli (heat-stable)	cGMP	65
Other bacterial endotoxins		
Shigella	Unknown	121
Salmonella	Unknown	82
Clostridium	Unknown	158
Viruses	Unknown	
Parasites	Unknown	
Bile salts and other fatty acids	Ca^{2+}	7,20,25,154
EXOGENOUS PHARMACEUTICAL AGENTS		
Laxatives	Mostly unknown	
ENDOGENOUS GASTRIC STIMULI		
Histamine	cAMP	196
Gastrin	Ca^{2+}	197,198,206
Acetylcholine	Ca^{2+}	197,198

ABBREVIATIONS: VIP, vasoactive intestinal peptide; PHI, peptide histidine, isoleucine amide; GIP, glucose-dependent insulinotropic peptide

TABLE 17-2 • Intestinal absorptive stimuli

Stimulus	Intracellular mediator	References
ENDOGENOUS INTESTINAL AGENTS		
Glucocorticoids	Unknown	63,138
Enkephalins and other opioids	Ca^{2+} ?	48,114,144
Alpha-adrenergic agonists	Ca^{2+} ?	56,66,108
Somatostatin	Ca^{2+} ?	28,43,92
Angiotensin	Unknown	137
INTESTINAL LUMEN-ACTIVE AGENTS		
Nutrients	None	72
EXOGENOUS PHARMACEUTICAL AGENTS		
Prostaglandin synthesis inhibitors (e.g., indomethacin, aspirin)	cAMP	67
Phenothiazines	Ca^{2+}-calmodulin	111,172,193
Propranolol	Unknown	67
Nicotinic acid	Unknown	67
Local anesthetics	Unknown	67
Chloroquine	Unknown	67
Lithium	Unknown	67

basis for these distinct functions is provided by the belief that the crypt cells are responsible for secretion while the villous and surface cells are responsible for absorption.[52,96,175,219] The absorptive and secretory functions of the epithelial cells are regulated by a large array of peptide hormones and neurotransmitters released from the endocrine cells, immunologic effector cells, and nerve endings, as well as a number of lumenally active agents (see Tables 17-1 and 17-2).[188,195,212,213] The endocrine cells are located in the crypt region (Fig. 17-3). The messengers (peptides or other substances) contained in these cells are released in response to the luminal environment and provide *paracrine* regulation of the adjacent epithelial cells.[133] Many of these compounds stimulate electrolyte secretion; others stimulate electrolyte absorption or inhibit secretion. As in the skin, the nerve cells and nerve endings in the gut are in close proximity to the epithelial cells and provide another modality of control, *neurocrine* regulation (see Fig. 17-4 and 17-5).[33,109,225] The neurons also innervate the intestinal smooth muscles and provide local coordination for the epithelial transport functions and gut motility.[85,225] For example, the endogenous opiates locally constrict circular smooth muscle, which delays transit time and increases mucosal absorption.[21,48]

In addition to paracrine and neurocrine regulation, *endocrine* regulation provides distant coordination among various portions of the gastrointestinal tract or between the gut and other organs (Fig. 17-5). This endocrine effect results from the release of peptides or neurotransmitters from the endocrine cells, and possibly the nerve cells, into the bloodstream. As stated above, lumi-

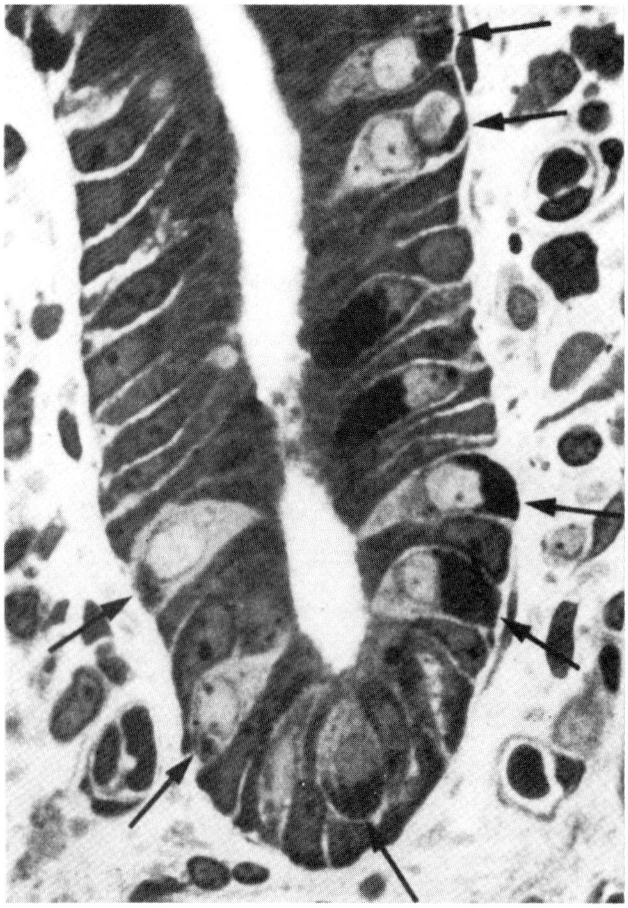

FIGURE 17-3 • A crypt region from human duodenum. Endocrine cells (arrows) are situated between epithelial cells. (From Fujita T, in Suda T, Matsuo Y, eds: *Structure and Function of the Digestive System,* Tokyo, Nakayam Shoten, 1976. Used by permission.)

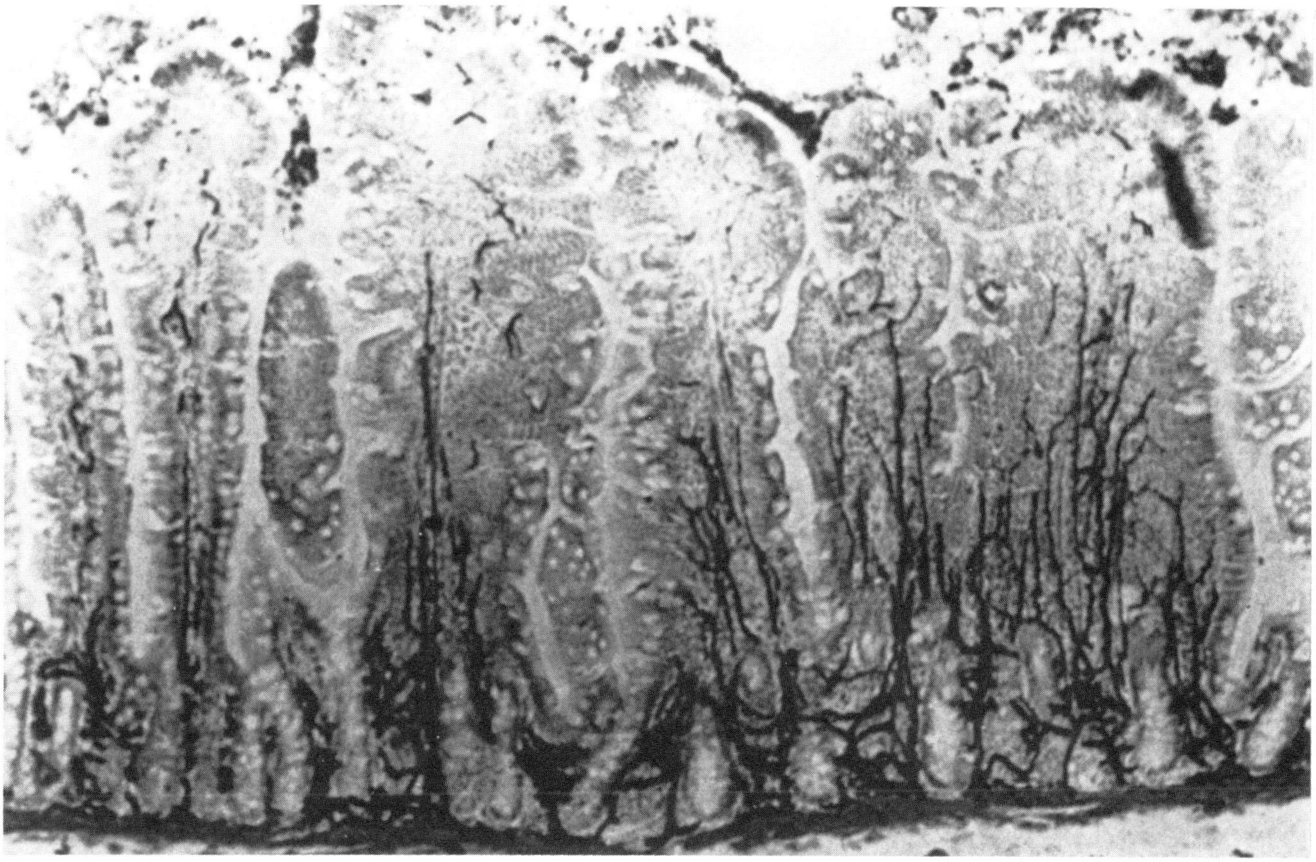

FIGURE 17-4 • Section of human jejunal mucosa stained for nerve fibers. Nerve fibers are abundant in the submucosal region around the crypts and extending up to the villi. (From Isaacs et al: *J Clin Invest* 58:540, 1976. Used by permission.)

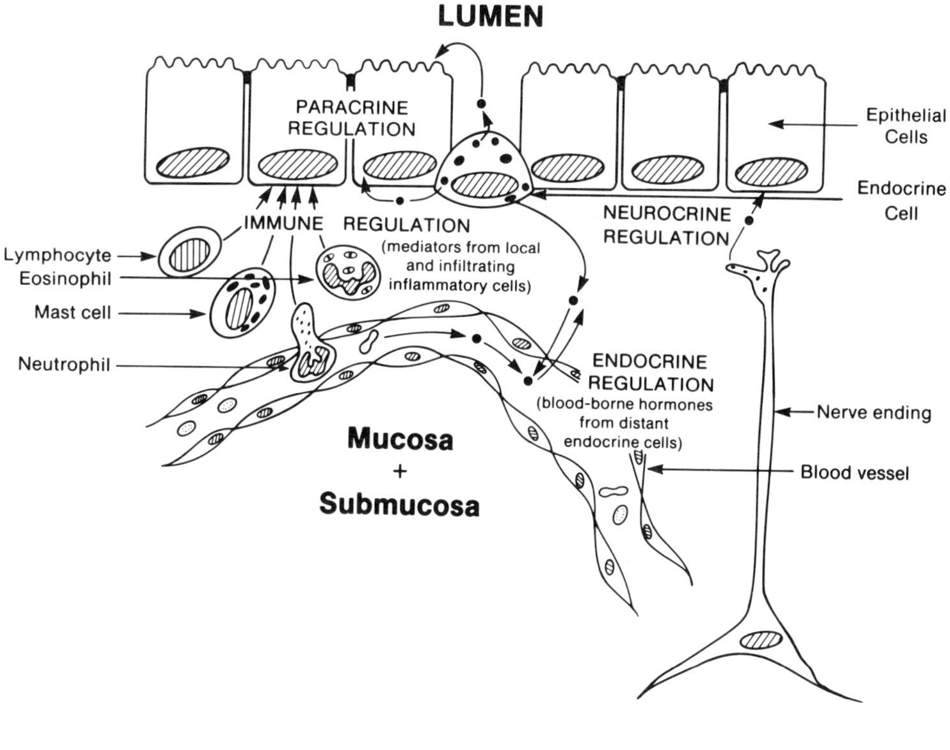

FIGURE 17-5 • Neurohormonal and immune regulation of the intestinal epithelium. Endocrine cells in the crypt region release across their basolateral membranes peptides or other substances that regulate electrolyte-transporting cells nearby (paracrine regulation). These substances or others from distant organs can also enter the bloodstream to regulate distant parts of the epithelium (endocrine regulation). Nerve cells can release peptides or neurotransmitters from the nerve endings to regulate the epithelial cells or muscle cells (neurocrine regulation). Immunologic effector cells (mast cells, eosinophils, neutrophils, and lymphocytes) in the lamina propria respond to antigenic and cytokine stimuli with release of mediators that also regulate the epithelium (immune regulation). There is evidence of substantial interaction among these various modes of regulation. (From Barrett KE, Dharmsathaphorn K, in Yamada T ed: *Textbook of Gastroenterology,* New York, Lippincott, 1991, p 265. Used by permission.)

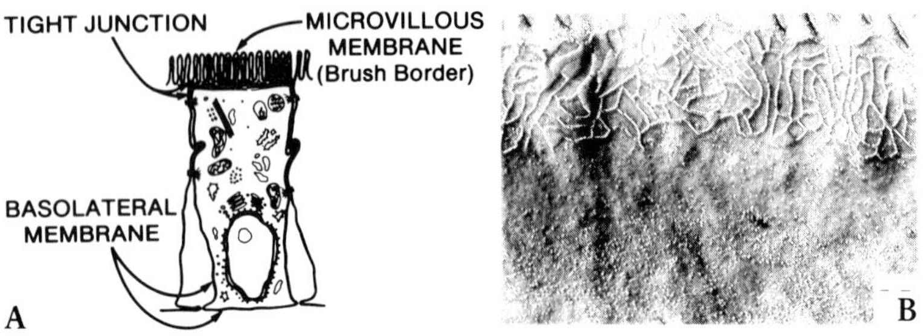

FIGURE 17-6 • Tight junctions (occluding junctions). These structures tightly seal adjacent epithelial cells, making them into a relatively impermeable epithelial sheet. (*a*) The tight junction serves to separate the apical (microvillous) and basolateral membranes. (*b*) Freeze fracture replicas of tight junctions on lateral surface of villous cell, demonstrating a network of tight junction strands. (From Madera et al: *Gastroenterology* 78:970, 1980. Used by permission.)

nal contents, including bile salts, may also participate directly and indirectly in regulating gastrointestinal function.

Recently, a fourth control mechanism for epithelial function has been increasingly recognized:[171] *immunologic* regulation (Fig. 17-5). Mediators and cytokines released from immunocytes such as mast cells, neutrophils, eosinophils, and lymphocytes resident in the lamina propria can directly stimulate epithelial cells or can act in concert with hormones or neurotransmitters. Such immunologic regulation is presumably of importance in disorders of electrolyte and fluid transport associated with intestinal inflammation.

The epithelium itself is anatomically highly specialized, in keeping with its role as the major intestinal barrier to fluid and electrolyte flow. Its makeup allows for two major pathways of solute movement. The plasma membrane of the epithelial cell, being a lipid bilayer, is impermeable to water, but the epithelial cells can actively transport certain electrolytes transcellularly via specialized transport pathways. Water and oppositely charged ions follow passively and paracellularly through an intercellular structure called the tight junction. These junctions, which seal the luminal side of the epithelial cells,[58,78,185] are analogous to the plastic holder that holds together a six-pack of beer (Fig. 17-6). Thus, the gastrointestinal tract can be considered a semipermeable membrane with the tight junctions serving as pores to allow passive paracellular movement of smaller molecules, according to the direction of the osmotic gradient. At an ultrastructural level, the tight junctions are comprised of a number of approximately parallel strands. In general, the permeability of the tight junction varies directly with the number of tight junction strands.[31,151] The number of strands is small in the upper intestine but gradually increases distally. The upper gut is therefore significantly more permeable than the colon to passive movement of fluids and electrolytes.[40,71] Variations of tight junction permeability also exist locally in the same segment of intestine. The villous region is much "tighter" than the crypt; most of the passive paracellular movement of water and electrolytes probably occurs in the crypt region.[151] Recent studies have demonstrated that the cytoskeleton of the cells inserts itself directly into the tight junction strand; the number of strands increases with hypertonicity and decreases with agents that disrupt the cytoskeleton. It is likely that tight junction permeability can be regulated, but the regulatory factors involved are currently unknown.[15]

The stomach is a highly specialized organ. It is lined with surface mucous cells, which secrete mucus and bicarbonate.[112] Numerous glandular structures develop in the thick wall of the stomach. These *oxyntic glands* contain both the parietal cells, which secrete hydrochloric acid and intrinsic factor, and the chief cells, which secrete pepsin (Fig. 17-7). The parietal cells are very active cells,

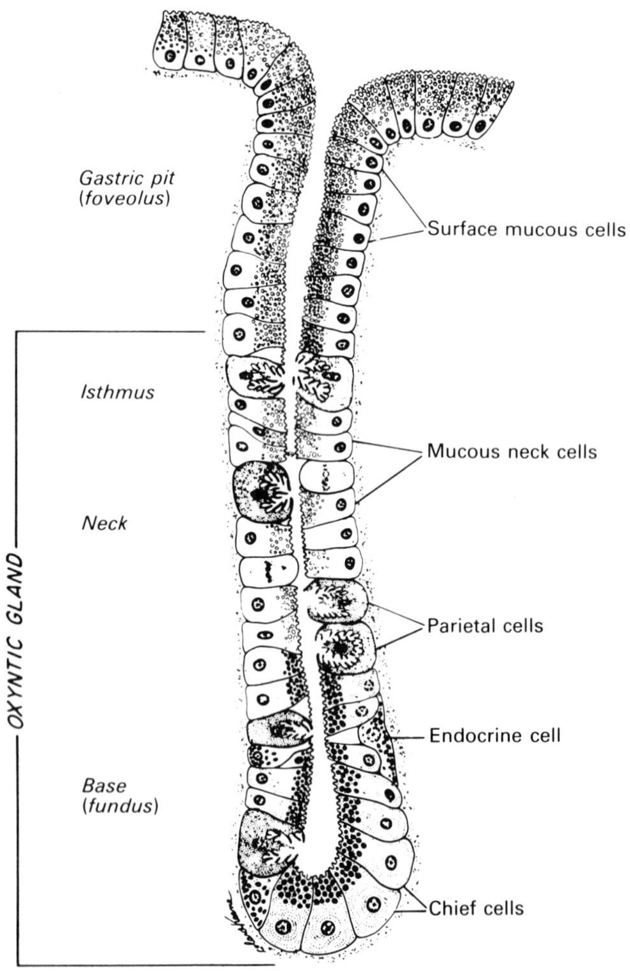

FIGURE 17-7 • Simplified diagram of a tubular oxyntic gland of the stomach. (From Ito S, in Johnson LR, ed: *Physiology of the Gastrointestinal Tract*, New York, Raven, 1981. Used by permission.)

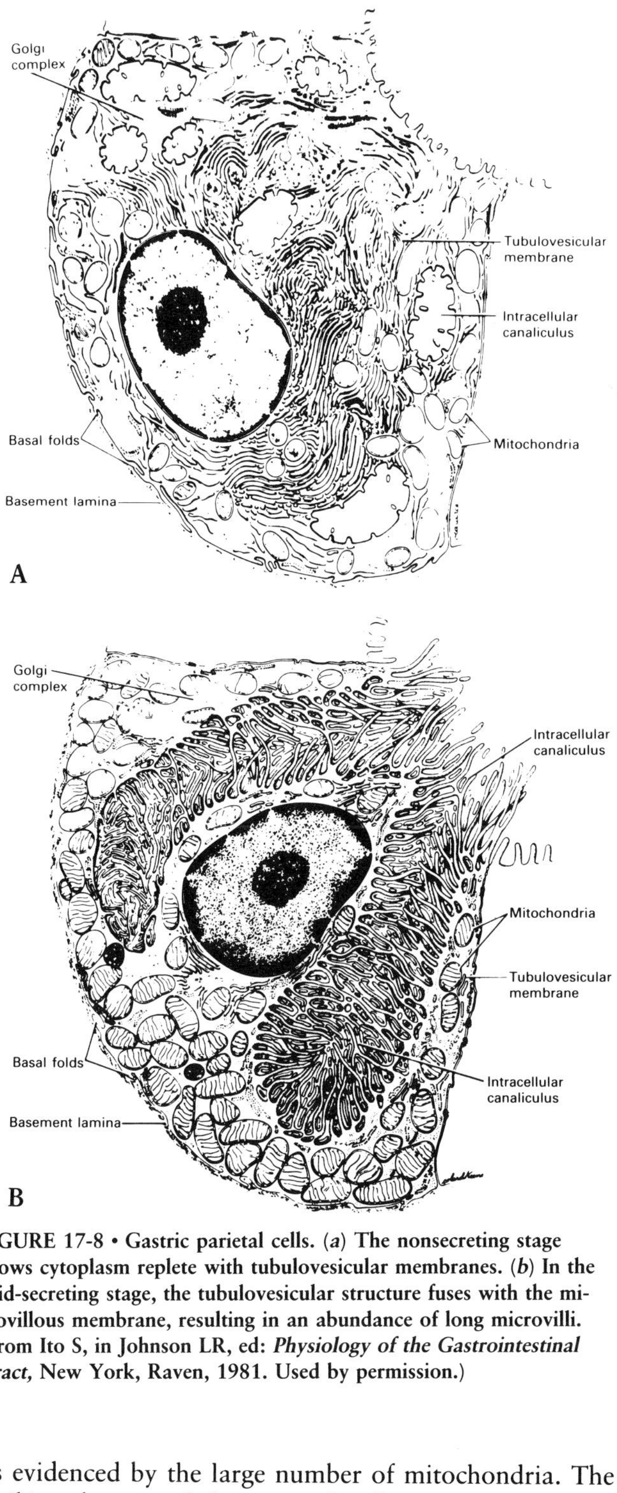

FIGURE 17-8 • Gastric parietal cells. (*a*) The nonsecreting stage shows cytoplasm replete with tubulovesicular membranes. (*b*) In the acid-secreting stage, the tubulovesicular structure fuses with the microvillous membrane, resulting in an abundance of long microvilli. (From Ito S, in Johnson LR, ed: *Physiology of the Gastrointestinal Tract,* New York, Raven, 1981. Used by permission.)

as evidenced by the large number of mitochondria. The striking feature of the parietal cell is its extensive tubulovesicular membrane, which can fuse with the microvillous membrane when stimulated to secrete acid (Fig. 17-8). These tubulovesicular structures, like the microvillous membrane, contain K^+-H^+ATPase, which is crucial for the acid secretory process.[73,112] They connect oxyntic glands with the more superficial gastric pits lined by surface mucous cells.

Less is known about water and electrolyte transport in the liver and biliary tract because of their relatively poor accessibility. The hepatocytes secrete bile salts, which are "followed," osmotically, by water, into the canaliculi. In the literature, this portion of the secretion is called *bile salt-dependent bile flow*. It is distinct from the other portion of hepatic canalicular secretion: *bile salt-independent bile flow*. The latter secretion is electrolyte-dependent, much as is water and electrolyte transport in other organs. The bile ducts and gallbladder, like other epithelia, are lined with epithelial cells that can secrete or absorb electrolytes. In the gallbladder, where bile is stored, abosrption of Na^+, Cl^-, and water predominates;[176] in the rest of the biliary tract, secretion of HCO_3^- predominates.[113] The epithelium of the pancreas and pancreatic duct also secrete primarily bicarbonate.[155]

ELECTROLYTE TRANSPORT PATHWAYS

Transport mechanism is the term used here to express a net transcellular movement of an ion across an epithelium in either the absorptive or the secretory direction. The term *transport pathway* is used for a carrier, a channel, or a pump in the cell membrane. The absorptive or secretory mechanism in each organ may be considered a specialized function of the epithelial cells the organ possesses. Each epithelial cell type that carries out a specialized function itself possesses a number of electrolyte transport pathways, that is, carriers, channels, or pumps in the plasma membrane. In general, each active transport mechanism requires the participation of usually three transport pathways: an uptake step across one plasma membrane, an exit step across another plasma membrane, and a pump, which provides the energy. The pump may also serve as an uptake or exit step; thus, a minimum of two different transport pathways is required for each absorptive or secretory mechanism (see Figs. 17-9 to 17-14, below). It is worth noting that each transport pathway usually drives the absorption or secretion of only one electrolyte.

Technological advances in experimental techniques, particularly the use of membrane vesicles, cultured cell lines, and patch-clamp and molecular biological techniques, have recently enhanced our ability to define the pathways involved in a variety of transport mechanisms. An increasing number of pumps, carriers, and channels have been identified at both the physiological and the biochemical level.[209] Evidence that these transport pathways are regulated by peptides or neurotransmitters is accumulating rapidly and is providing insight into the overall regulation of each transport mechanism. Cells may adjust for longer-term regulation by increasing or decreasing the number of pumps or carriers, while regulation of the channels, due to their large capacity (discussed below), may better serve short-term regulation. The electrolyte transport pathways known to exist in the gastrointestinal epithelia are summarized in Table 17-3,

TABLE 17-3 • Electrolyte transport pathways

Transport pathway	Transport mechanism	Endogenous regulation	Specific inhibitors	References
TRANSCELLULAR PATHWAYS				
Pumps				
Na^+-K^+ ATPase	Most active transport process involving Na^+,K^+, or Cl^-	Aldosterone or corticosteroid	Ouabain	63,117
K^+-H^+ ATPase	H^+ secretion by gastric parietal cells; possibly colonic absorption of K^+	Unknown	Omeprazole	73,141
Ca^{2+} and Mg^{2+} ATPases	Cellular handling of Ca^{2+} and Mg^{2+}	cAMP or calmodulin	Lanthanum or vanadate	99
Carriers				
Na^+-H^+ exchange	Electroneutral NaCl absorption in the intestine and gallbladder	Calmodulin ?	Amiloride	14,127
Cl^--HCO_3^- exchange	Electroneutral NaCl absorption in the intestine and gallbladder; HCO_3^- secretion in the gastrointestinal tract	Calmodulin ?	Disulfonic stilbenes	140,142
Na^+-K^+-Cl^- cotransport	Cl^- secretory processes in the intestine and probably in other organs, possibly involved in HCl secretion in the stomach or HCO_3^- secretion in the pancreas, biliary tree, and intestinal tract	Unknown	Bumetanide or furosemide	45,97,165
Na^+-glucose cotransport	Glucose absorption	Unknown	Phlorizin	84,105,123,162
Other Na^+ contransport pathways	Absorption of other nutrients	Unknown	Unknown	1–3,35,161,177
Channels				
Na^+ channel	Electrogenic Na^+ absorption in the colon	Aldosterone	Amiloride	221
Cl^- channel	Cl^- secretion in the gastrointestinal tract	cAMP and Ca^{2+}	Anthracene-9-COOH or picrotoxin	170,218
K^+ channel	Cl^- secretion in the gastrointestinal tract; possibly involved in K^+ absorptive and secretory mechanisms	cAMP and Ca^{2+}	Barium, quinidine, or tetraethylammonium	134,146,150
PARACELLULAR PATHWAYS				
Tight junction	Allowing oppositely charged ion and water to follow actively transported ion	Cytoskeleton	Unknown	15

together with the specific ion-absorptive or -secretory mechanism in which they are thought to participate. At present, the individual electrolyte transport pathways involved in each transport mechanism are not as well understood as is the overall transport phenomenon itself.

Subsequent portions of this chapter review properties of various types of transport pathways and how different arrangements of these transport pathways enable each portion of the gastrointestinal tract to carry out its specialized functions.

PROPERITIES OF PUMPS, CARRIERS, AND CHANNELS

ATPase PUMPS

Active transport of an ion implies that it is moved by the cell against an energy barrier. This movement requires an input of energy from the cell via the activity of a so-called pump. In mammalian cells, ATPases serve this energy-providing function. Among the ATPases, the Na^+-K^+ ATPase is the best understood, but other ATPases (e.g., K^+-H^+, Ca^{2+}, and Mg^{2+} ATPases) have also been described.[73,99,117]

Na^+-K^+ ATPase pumps are localized basolaterally.[46,200] The role of these pumps in active transport of nutrients and electrolytes has been well characterized. Most, if not all, active transport processes are related to this pump, as evidenced by the fact that the cardiac glycosides (e.g., ouabain), which inactivate this pump, inhibit all of the active transport mechanisms currently known to exist. The Na^+-K^+ ATPase pump catalyzes outward movement of three Na^+ ions and inward movement of two K^+ ions per cycle across the basolateral membrane; one ATP molecule is used each time.[124] Since more cations are pumped out than are replaced, a negative intracellular electrical potential is created. The action of this ATPase pump keeps the intracellular Na^+ concentration relatively low. Thus, the pump creates electrochemical gradients favoring passive Na^+ influx across the plasma membrane via either Na^+ channels or Na^+-requiring cotransport and exchange carriers (Figs. 17-11, 17-12, and 17-14 below). The Na^+ cotransport and exchange carriers allow the energy provided by the Na^+-K^+ ATPase to be used effectively for the absorption of many nutrients and electrolytes. The Na^+-K^+ ATPase pump also provides energy for secretory mechanisms, such as Cl^- secretion (discussed below and illustrated in Fig. 17-9).

Biochemical characterization of the two subunits of the Na^+-K^+ ATPase, α and β, has been made. Monoclonal antibodies have been developed that may provide useful insight into the synthesis of this important pump and its insertion into the basolateral membrane.[181,209]

Another ATPase pump that has received substantial attention is the K^+-H^+ ATPase pump.[73] It is present on parietal cells of the gastric mucosa and has been found in other acid-secreting epithelia as well. For HCl secretion, an apically localized K^+-H^+ ATPase pump on the parietal cell exchanges K^+ for H^+; the H^+ taken up is secreted along with Cl^-, providing for the unique acid-secretory function of the gastric cells (Fig. 17-10). Other ATPases, including various Ca^{2+} and Mg^{2+} ATPases, are distributed on the membranes of cellular organelles as well as on the plasma membrane.[99] These ATPases are important in the regulation of cellular Ca^{2+} and Mg^{2+} distribution.

CARRIERS

Even with a limited number of ATPases serving as pumps, a wide diversity of active transport mechanisms is possible because of the availability of various carriers that serve to convert the energy provided by the pump into specialized functions. Although carriers do not actively move ions against energy barriers themselves, they serve as secondary active transport pathways because they are integral parts of a number of active transport mechanisms. They are best described as facilitated transport pathways that may catalyze ion movement either into or

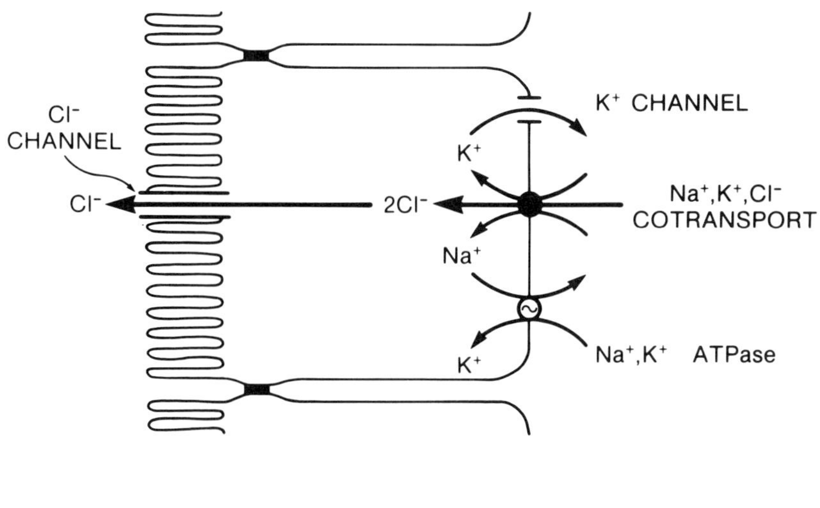

FIGURE 17-9 • Chloride secretory mechanism. The Na^+-K^+-Cl^- cotransport mechanism on the basolateral membrane serves as the uptake step, with the Na^+-K^+ ATPase pump providing the driving force and recycling Na^+. The excess K^+ is recycled via K^+ channels on the basolateral membrane. The Cl^- exists via a Cl^- channel on the apical membrane. Regulatory sites for the Cl^- secretory process are at the Cl^- channels and/or K^+ channels.

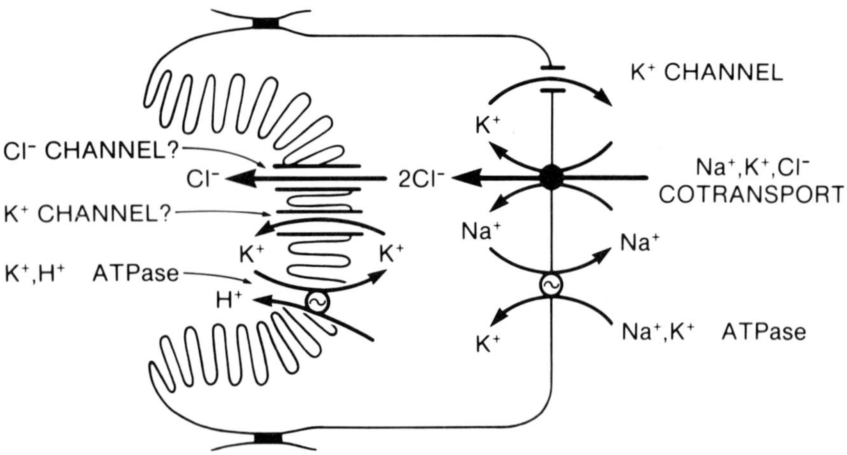

FIGURE 17-10 • Gastric acid secretions. Although the exact mechanism remains to be elucidated, H^+ ions are believed to be made available through the action of carbonic anhydrase, which catalyzes the reversible hydration of carbon dioxide ($CO_2 + H_2O \rightleftharpoons H^+ + HCO_3^-$); HCO_3^- produced is transported back to the bloodstream (not shown). The key component is the K^+-H^+ ATPase (which exchanges K^+ for H^+). Secretion of K^+ and Cl^- across the apical membrane may occur via K^+ and Cl^- channels or by a K^+-Cl^- cotransport pathway. The Cl^- uptake mechanisms on the basolateral membrane probably are similar to those described for intestinal Cl^- secretion (Fig. 17-9).

out of the cell, in sharp contrast to the pumps, which drive movement of a given ion in only one direction. A carrier may be either a cotransport carrier, also called a *symport*, or an exchange carrier, an *antiport*. In the case of a contransport carrier, the carrier protein binds to specific ions or other molecules on one side of the plasma membrane and shuttles them across to the other, according to the existing net electrochemical gradient. In the case of an exchange carrier, one molecule is transported in exchange for another molecule that has a favorable chemical gradient. Carriers are saturable transport pathways that allow certain ions to move across the plasma membrane faster than could be expected by diffusion along the existing electrochemical gradient. Many carriers catalyze a cotransport process that includes Na^+, taking advantage of the Na^+ gradient set up by the Na^+-K^+ ATPase pump. In a cotransport mechanism, the net chemical gradient is a function of the product of the concentrations of the molecules involved on each side of the membrane. For example, in the case of Na^+-glucose cotransport, the effective gradient can be calculated as the difference between $[Na^+]$[glucose] on one side of the membrane and $[Na^+]$[glucose] on the other side. By coupling the transport of important molecules with Na^+, it is possible for the cell to take advantage of the favorable Na^+ electrochemical gradient and to move such molecules "uphill," against their own chemical gradients.

The cotransport carriers are major transport pathways for absorption of a wide variety of nutrients and electrolytes by the intestine. Of the nutrient-related carriers, the Na^+-glucose cotransport carrier has been studied most (Fig. 17- 11).[84,105,123,162] Besides glucose, many other food-derived products (e.g, amino acids, di- and tripeptides, vitamins, bile salts, etc.) are taken up by similar mechanisms, each involving a different carrier protein.[1-3,35,161,177] The primary role of the Na^+-glucose cotransporter is nutrient absorption, but the process also brings in Na^+ and water. This phenomenon has been exploited clinically with the use of glucose-saline oral rehydration solutions for the treatment of dehydration associated with severe diarrhea.[70,72] The Na^+ that is absorbed along with glucose promotes positive electrolyte and water balance and has been widely applied in the treatment of diarrhea. Intestinal cotransport carriers

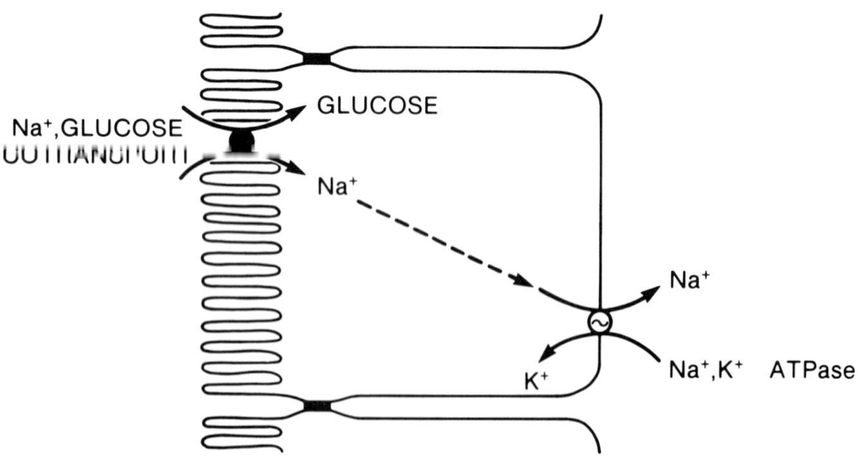

FIGURE 17-11 • Na^+-glucose absorption. A Na^+-glucose cotransport carrier on the apical membrane serves to bring glucose and Na^+ into the cell. Sodium is then pumped out via the Na^+-K^+ ATPase; glucose proceeds across the basolateral membrane via another facilitated transport carrier for glucose. Similar Na^+ cotransport mechanisms also exist for amino acids, dipeptides, tripeptides, many B vitamins, and bile salts.

that deal only with electrolytes also exist. Among these is the Na^+-K^+-Cl^- cotransport carrier, which is required for the Cl^- secretory mechanism (Fig. 17-9).[45,220] Many other cotransport pathways, such as a K^+-Cl^- cotransport, have been proposed. At present, it is unclear whether these pathways truly exist and what role they may have in the gut; they are not discussed here.

The *exchange* carriers or antiports carry a needed ion into the cell in exchange for a readily available intracellular ion. There are two major intestinal ion exchange carriers: the Na^+-H^+ exchange[127,163] and Cl^--HCO_3^- exchange pathways.[140,142] They are both involved in the so-called electroneutral NaCl absorptive process. The exchanges make good sense, since these pathways effectively exchange the waste product CO_2, which in the presence of carbonic anhydrase forms H^+ and HCO_3^-, for Na^+ and Cl^- (Fig. 17-12). An exchange carrier that may be important for cellular Ca^{2+} homeostasis is the Na^+-Ca^{2+} exchanger.[57] This carrier moves Ca^{2+} out of the cells and keeps the intracellular Ca^{2+} concentration one or two orders of magnitude lower than that in the extracellular fluid.

CHANNELS

The ionic channel serves a function similar to that of a carrier but distinct from it. While both systems are constituents of transport mechanisms, the channel is a high-flow system capable of moving a large number of ions rapidly; it also catalyzes the movement of only one kind of electrolyte.[199] The carrier system, on the other hand, moves smaller numbers of molecules but can do so against a chemical gradient for at least one of the species being transported because of its more complicated cotransport or exchange mechanism. The channel may be compared to a gate: when the gate is open, it allows a large amount of a selected ion to flow downstream according to the existing electrochemical gradient. Each channel on the plasma membrane, when open, may allow a large number of ions—10^6 to 10^8—to move across each second. Because of its large capacity, the physiological capability of a channel approaches that of passive diffusion, which is not saturable. Also because of their capacity, ionic channels are probably the most important transport pathways for electrolytes. Regulation of channel activity is likely to have a very dramatic response. It is possible that the immediate actions of many peptides or neurotransmitters are the result of the opening or closing of ionic channels.

The body of knowledge regarding ionic channels in the gastrointestinal tract is still relatively small. However, the patch-clamp technique (see the Appendix of this chapter) is expanding information in this area rapidly. Specific ionic channels for Na^+, Cl^-, K^+, and Ca^{2+} have been described. The Na^+ channel is a classic example; its role in colonic Na^+ absorption and its regulation by aldosterone are well recognized.[221] Na^+ channels can be blocked by amiloride; many studies of the Na^+ channel before the availability of the patch-clamp technique were indirect, using amiloride sensitivity as an indicator. The biochemical nature of the channel is beginning to be understood.[98,128,202,209]

Chloride channels have not been studied as thoroughly as Na^+ channels. Their existence has been suggested by the observation that Cl^- ions can be secreted alone in response to many peptides or neurotransmitters. Recent microelectrode and patch-clamp studies confirmed their presence on the apical membrane and suggest that there is more than one Cl^- channel. The lack of a known specific chemical blocker for these Cl^- channels has slowed progress in this area. However, studies of the defective gene in cystic fibrosis, a disease where cellular Cl^- transport is disregulated, have identified a protein called CFTR (cystic fibrosis transmembrane conductance regulator) the predicted structure of which makes it likely that it is an ion channel or an ion channel accessory protein.[173] The observation that this protein is made by

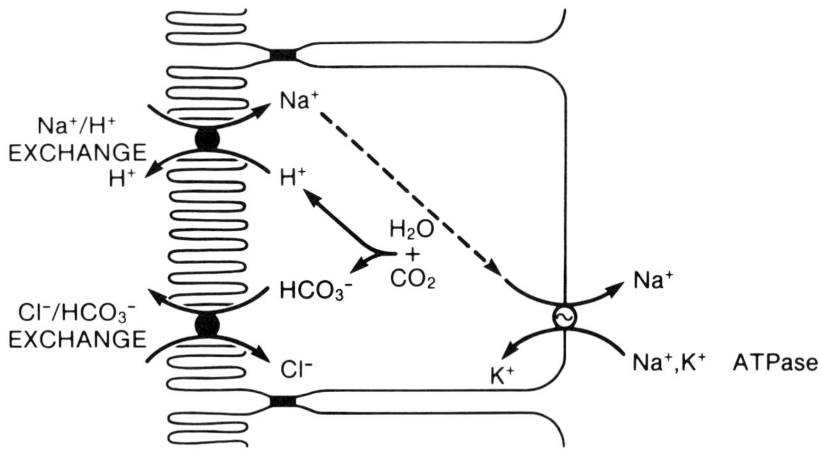

FIGURE 17-12 • Electroneutral NaCl absorption. It is currently believed that the electroneutral NaCl cotransport mechanism in the intestine results from a dual exchange system composed of a Na^+-H^+ exchange and a Cl^--HCO_3^- exchange working in concert. These exchange carriers serve to bring Na^+ and Cl^- across the apical membrane into the cell. Sodium is then pumped out by the Na^+-K^+ ATPase; Cl^- follows the Na^+.

T_{84} colonic epithelial cells, which secrete chloride, suggests that the cystic fibrosis gene product could be the chloride channel. Besides the obvious implications that these recent studies have for the diagnosis and treatment of cystic fibrosis, where Cl^- transport is deficient, they will improve our understanding of Cl^- transport in the gut in health and in conditions such as secretory diarrhea, where it is excessive. Other authors have recently reported the successful purification and reconstitution into lipid bilayers of chloride channels from the kidney and the trachea.[131] These channels may be similar, if not identical, to those present in intestinal epithelial cells.

Enough evidence is available to postulate the existence of multiple K^+ channels in the gastrointestinal tract and to link them to the Cl^- secretory process (Fig. 17-9).[146] These postulated K^+ channels are thought to be localized in the basolateral membrane of mucosal epithelial cells. Direct verification of their existence and regulation on intestinal epithelial cells, using the patch-clamp technique, is awaited. This procedure may prove technically difficult due to the presumed basolateral location of the majority of these channels, as opposed to the apical location of Na^+ and Cl^- channels. It is not known whether K^+ channels are involved in active K^+ absorption or secretion.

The ability of Ca^{2+} channel blockers to inhibit certain secretory mechanisms of the epithelium of the gut has convinced many of the existence of Ca^{2+} channels in this site. Ca^{2+} transport in the intestine is relatively complex; certain mechanisms that have been attributed to Ca^{2+} channels may actually involve the Na^+-Ca^{2+} exchange carrier. As is true for other ionic channels, the role of Ca^{2+} channels in the intestine awaits further investigation with the patch-clamp technique.

OTHER TRANSPORT PATHWAYS

Transport pathways for other ions (e.g., bicarbonate, sulfate, phosphate, organic ions, and divalent cations) are much less well defined, although they undoubtedly exist. There may exist a bicarbonate channel in addition to the Cl^--HCO_3^- exchange carrier; special transport mechanisms for sulfate and phosphate may exist. Discussion of these pathways is beyond the scope of this chapter. Additional information on pumps, carriers, and channels can be found in Chap. 2.

ELECTROLYTE TRANSPORT MECHANISMS IN THE GASTROINTESTINAL TRACT

The diversity of transport functions exhibited by the intestinal tract and other organ systems is shown in Table 17-4. This diversity results from various combinations of the basic transport pathways. The same transport pathway can be called upon to work in concert with others to serve a variety of different functions (e.g., the Na^+- K^+ ATPase provides energy for most transport mechanisms). It should be pointed out that similar physiological and

TABLE 17-4 • Diversity of transport properties along the gastrointestinal tract

Organ	Major transport mechanisms	Pathological conditions	Diseases
Salivary glands	Cl^- and HCO_3^- secretion	Decreased secretion	Sjögren's syndrome
Esophagus	None known		
Stomach	HCl secretion	Excessive HCl secretion	Gastric and duodenal ulcers
	HCO_3^- secretion	Decreased HCO_3^- secretion	? Gastric ulcer
Duodenum	HCO_3^- secretion	Decreased HCO_3^- secretion	Duodenal ulcer
Liver and biliary tract	Bile acid secretion	Decreased bile salt level	Gallstones
	HCO_3^- secretion	Unknown	
Pancreas	HCO_3^- secretion	Decreased HCO_3^- secretion	? Pancreatitis
Small intestine	Electroneutral NaCl absorption	Decreased NaCl absorption	Secretory diarrhea
	Absorption of glucose and other nutrients	Decreased nutrient digestion and absorption	Osmotic diarrhea
	Cl^- and HCO_3^- secretion	Excessive Cl^- secretion	Secretory diarrhea
Large intestine	Electrogenic Na^+ absorption	Decreased Na^+ absorption	Secretory diarrhea
	Electroneutral NaCl absorption	Decreased NaCl absorption	Secretory diarrhea
	Cl^- and HCO_3^- secretion	Excessive Cl^- secretion	Secretory diarrhea

regulatory mechanisms are shared by epithelial cells in many different organs. This fact is particularly true for the gastrointestinal tract, kidney, respiratory tract, choroid plexus, sweat glands, and the cornea and ciliary body of the eye. Clearly, knowledge acquired from one cell system may be applicable to others.

The diversity of transport mechanisms in the gut serves one specific purpose: to facilitate absorption of useful substances and to excrete waste or harmful substances. Under normal circumstances, the small intestine absorbs the bulk of nutrients and water. The absorption of carbohydrates, amino acids, dipeptides, tripeptides, fat, minerals, vitamins, and bile salts is the key function of the small intestine. Many of these substances are absorbed by a cotransport pathway together with Na^+.

Another key function is the absorption of water, which passively follows via a paracellular mechanism along the osmotic gradient created by the absorption of nutrients and Na^+. In addition, the intestine can be stimulated to absorb more water by increasing its absorptive capacity for Na^+ and Cl^-. Only 1500 to 2000 ml of the 9000 ml entering the small intestine daily escapes absorption there. (Fig. 17-1).

In contrast to the small intestine, the human large intestine does not absorb nutrients but serves as a reservoir for unabsorbable carbohydrates, protein, and other substances, which together probably account for 10 percent of ingested calories. Colonic bacteria can absorb short-chain fatty acids produced by their own catabolism of unabsorbed carbohydrates.[22,180] The major role played by the colon is to conserve the fluid and electrolytes presented to it (Fig. 17-1). Only approximately 100 ml of water is lost to the stool each day.[41] Of course, the colon also has a large secretory capacity, which can be stimulated by luminal toxins or endogenous hormones.

SECRETORY MECHANISMS

Except in the liver, where bile salts are secreted, the secretory mechanisms throughout the gastrointestinal tract center on the Cl^- ion. Hydrochloric acid is the major secretory product of the stomach;[148] in other parts of the tract, the predominant ion secreted is either Cl^- or HCO_3^-,[47,189,207] the latter probably a result of Cl^--HCO_3^- exchange.[39,107]

Gastrointestinal Cl^- secretion (electrogenic Cl^- secretion)

The Cl^- secretory mechanism has been reasonably well defined (Fig. 17-9).[37] It is called *electrogenic* Cl^- secretion because Cl^- is the only ion actively secreted by the epithelium, and its movement can thus be detected by monitoring electrical potentials. In the Cl^- secretory process, cells take up Cl^- from the blood across the basolateral membrane via the Na^+-K^+-Cl^- cotransport pathway.[45,220] An appropriate gradient for this uptake is set up by the energy-requiring Na^+-K^+ ATPase pathway, while K^+ channels on the basolateral membrane allow for K^+ recycling.[150,220] Chloride accumulates intracellularly above its electrochemical equilibrium and exits through the apical membrane via Cl^- channels. The sites of regulation by intracellular messengers such as cAMP and Ca^{2+} are at the Cl^- and/or K^+ channels.[29,220] Once the Cl^- ion is secreted transcellularly, Na^+ and K^+ passively follow.

Gastrointestinal HCO_3^- secretion

HCO_3^- is the predominant ion in biliary and pancreatic secretions.[113,155,176,186] The recent emphasis on gastric and duodenal HCO_3^- secretory mechanisms is due to their possible role in mucosal defense against ulcer formation.[68,69] Bicarbonate secretion is also important in the small intestine, where it gradually becomes the predominant luminal anion, probably as a means of conserving Cl^-.[39,47,189,207] Although the HCO_3^- secretory mechanisms have not been fully elucidated, involvement of the Cl^--HCO_3^- exchanger on the apical membrane appears important.[39,107] Disulfonic stilbenes, which inhibit Cl^--HCO_3^- exchange, block HCO_3^- secretion. It is possible that Cl^- secretion acts as an integral component of the HCO_3^- secretory process by providing Cl^- for exchange with the HCO_3^- (Fig. 17-13). Bicarbonate can either be produced intracellularly by the action of carbonic anhydrase or, possibly, be transported from the blood. Other mechanisms of HCO_3^- secretion by the gastrointestinal epithelium that do not involve Cl^--HCO_3^- exchange may exist but have yet to be explored.

Gastric acid secretion

Hydrochloric acid is secreted in the stomach by the parietal cells, which have special morphological features (Fig. 17-8).[60,90,196-198] These cells contain numerous tubulovesicular structures, which fuse with the apical membrane upon stimulation by histamine, gastrin, or acetylcholine.[73,112,179] Similar structures are also present in acid-secreting cells of the renal tubule. These tubulovesicular organelles, as well as the apical membrane, contain K^+-H^+ ATPase. Fusion of the tubulovesicular structure to the apical membrane effectively increases the apical membrane surface area as well as the number of K^+-H^+ ATPase pumps on the membrane, and thus increases H^+ secretion. The mechanism involved in hydrochloric acid secretion remains to be fully elucidated. A tentative mechanism is proposed in Fig. 17-10. Chloride is required for acid secretion.[149] The Cl^- secretory component may be very similar to that which occurs in the intestine. It appears to involve a bumetanide-sensitive mechanism, which is likely to be the Na^+-K^+-Cl^-

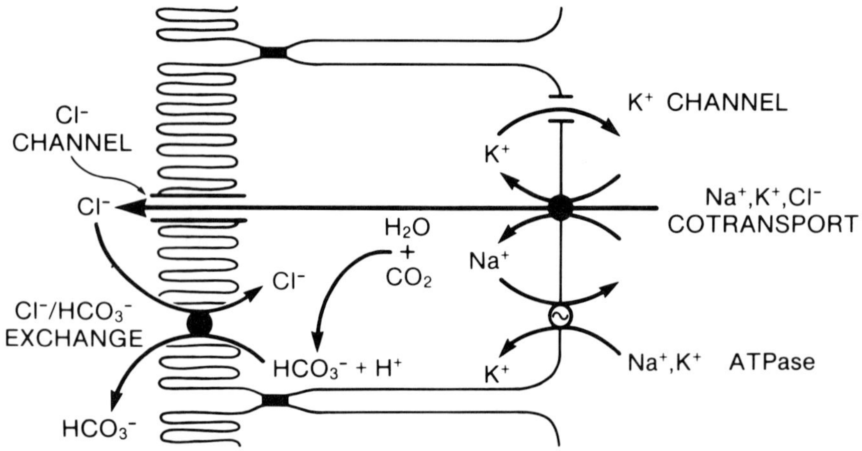

FIGURE 17-13 • Bicarbonate secretory mechanism. Bicarbonate ions are products of the reaction catalyzed by carbonic anhydrase ($H_2O + CO_2 \rightleftharpoons H^+ + HCO_3^-$). The HCO_3^- secretory mechanism appears to involve a Cl^--HCO_3^- exchange on the apical membrane, as depicted. Chloride secretion similar to that described in Fig. 17-9 may be a prerequisite for HCO_3^- secretion. Each milliequivalent of HCO_3^- secreted results in the return of 1 meq of H^+ to the body. The mechanism by which protons are returned is not well defined.

cotransport pathway, as well as a barium-sensitive K^+ channel.[145] The Na^+-K^+ ATPase pump, which provides energy for this uptake step, recycles the Na^+, leaving K^+ and Cl^- to accumulate intracellularly. How K^+ and Cl^- exit through the apical membrane is not known with certainty but is presumed to occur via specific channels or a K^+-Cl^- cotransport mechanism.[224] The unique feature of this acid secretory mechanism is that the secreted K^+ is taken back by the cell in exchange for H^+ through the action of the K^+-H^+ ATPase pump on the apical membrane. The net result is HCl secretion. This process can be inhibited by omeprazole, which inactivates the K^+-H^+ ATPase pump.[61,132,141]

ABSORPTIVE MECHANISMS

Sodium is the primary ion that drives intestinal water absorption. In the small intestine, cotransport of Na^+ with nonelectrolyte food-derived products and electroneutral NaCl aborption are together responsible for most, if not all, of the water and electrolyte absorption.[17-19,67,174,184,192] In addition, cotransport of Na^+ with bile salts provides for the bile salt uptake step in the terminal ileum. The large intestine absorbs Na^+ avidly via both the Na^+ channel and the electroneutral NaCl absorptive mechanism shared by the small intestine.[17-19,86,174,183,192]

Na^+-glucose cotransport and similar mechanisms in the small intestine

Glucose is absorbed via a Na^+-glucose cotransport carrier on the apical membrane of the small intestinal epithelium[84,105,123,162] (Fig.17-11). Na^+ and glucose bind to the carrier, which shuttles them from the outer surface of the apical membrane to the inner surface. There, both are released before the carrier returns to the outer surface. Because transport carriers function in both directions, an appropriate electrochemical gradient must exist to direct vectorial transport. The Na^+ gradient created by the Na^+-K^+ ATPase pump provides the needed energy for the absorptive direction. Absorbed glucose diffuses across the basolateral membrane by another facilitated transport pathway,[106] and the Na^+ is pumped out basolaterally by the Na^+-K^+ ATPase. The charge of the absorbed Na^+ promotes absorption of an anion, primarily Cl^-, via the paracellular pathway. Water follows passively to maintain osmolality. Therefore, the intestinal glucose transport mechanism also serves to drive water and electrolyte absorption.[72]

Many cotransport mechanisms for other nutrients depend on sodium ion gradients across the apical membrane created by the Na^+-K^+ ATPase pump. Of the large number of cotransport mechanisms that involve Na^+, most exist only in the small intestine, and not in the large intestine. Cotransport of Na^+ with amino acids, dipeptides, or tripeptides provides for the absorption of protein constituents.[1-3,88,161] Cotransport of Na^+ and many B vitamins has been recognized.[6,177] Finally, ileal uptake of bile acids also occurs via a Na^+ cotransport mechanism.

Electroneutral Na^+ and Cl^- absorption in the intestine

A Na^+-Cl^- cotransport mechanism has been proposed because in the isolated intestine a significant portion of Na^+ uptake requires the presence of Cl^-, and vice versa.[54,76,77,166] This mechanism is called electroneutral Na^+-Cl^- cotransport, to distinguish it from an electrogenic Na^+ absorptive mechanism (discussed below). However, the interdependence of Na^+ and Cl^- transport could not be demonstrated easily when apical membrane vesicles were studied, which raised questions about the nature of this cotransport phenomenon.[139] The debate about the nature of this mechanism is likely to continue. Many investigators now believe that the electroneutral

Na^+-Cl^- cotransport is actually composed of a Na^+-H^+ exchange working in concert with a Cl^--HCO_3^- exchange mechanism.[16,127,140,142,163] This mechanism allows both Na^+ and Cl^- to enter the cell, in exchange for H^+ and HCO_3^- (Fig. 17-12). Protons and HCO_3^- are produced intracellularly by the action of carbonic anhydrase on CO_2. Sodium, which enters the cell, is then pumped out by the Na^+-K^+ ATPase, with Cl^- following. This Na^+-Cl^- cotransport mechanism appears to be widely distributed in the epithelium of the gastrointestinal tract, including the gallbladder, the small intestine, and the proximal part of the large intestine.[54,76,77,166, 176]

Electrogenic Na^+ absorption in the colon

Electrogenic Na^+ absorption predominates in the colon.[86] It is so called because the absorbed Na^+ ion is the only ion moving transcellularly, permitting its transport to be detected with electrical equipment. The Na^+ ion enters the cell via a Na^+ channel on the apical membrane. It is pumped out across the basolateral membrane by the Na^+-K^+ ATPase pump (Fig. 17-14). The absorbed Na^+ is followed paracellularly by water and anions, resulting in net water and electrolyte movement from the luminal side to the bloodstream side of the colon.

K^+ absorption and secretion

Only recently have active intestinal transport mechanisms for K^+ been recognized and investigated.[101,126,194] In the past, it was felt that K^+ simply leaked through the epithelial tight junction according to the existing gradient or by a solvent drag mechanism. However, active participation of the colonic mucosa in K^+ homeostasis has now been verified.[74,101,194] Many investigators believe that a transcellular mechanism for K^+ transport is in fact the predominant one. However, the transport pathways involved in the K^+ absorptive or secretory mechanisms have only been postulated.[194] For K^+ absorption, it is possible that K^+-H^+ ATPase serves to exchange intracellular H^+ for K^+. The accumulated K^+ then diffuses across the basolateral membrane via a K^+ channel or other K^+ carriers. For K^+ secretion, it is postulated that transcellular movement of K^+ is achieved by an increase in the activity of either the basolateral Na^+- K^+ ATPase, an apical K^+ conductance, or both.

Absorption and secretion of other ions

In general, the body does not permit the absorption of important substances to occur by passive routes. Rather, mechanisms exist to regulate their absorption or secretion, allowing for adaptation to environmental changes. It is probably reasonable to assume that active intestinal transport processes exist for all of the important ions, including divalent cations, sulfate, phosphate, and organic anions. Unfortunately, the transport mechanisms of many of these ions are at present poorly understood. Luminal absorption of calcium is regulated by vitamin D and its metabolites, specifically 1α,25-dihydroxyvitamin D_3 (see Chap. 11).[24,59,164] Parathyroid hormone (PTH) and calcitonin also influence calcium homeostasis.[89,125] Calcium in different intracellular pools serves different functions, made possible through its segregation by different calcium-binding proteins. Some of the binding proteins bind absorbed calcium, regulating its absorption, while others bind free cytosolic calcium, thereby modifying various cellular functions.[53] These two pools of calcium do not appear to interact. Therefore, transport of absorbed calcium across the epithelial cell need not affect any calcium-mediated cellular functions. The transport pathways involved are thought to be a Na^+-Ca^{2+} exchange and various Ca^{2+} ATPases, which may

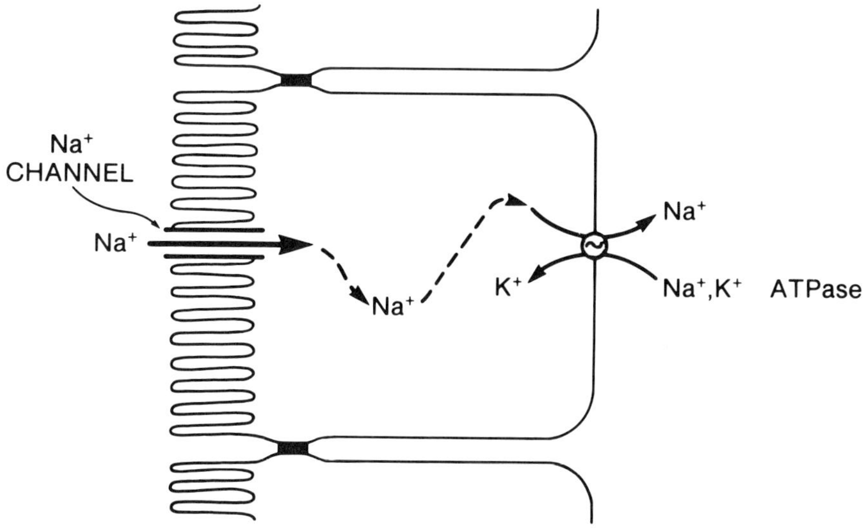

FIGURE 17-14 • Electrogenic Na^+ absorption. Na^+ enters the apical membrane via a Na^+ channel. The basolateral Na^+-K^+ ATPase pump extrudes cellular Na^+, thereby driving luminal absorption.

be important in keeping calcium in different intracellular compartments.[57,99]

REGULATION OF ELECTROLYTE TRANSPORT

BIOCHEMICAL REGULATION

Our understanding of the regulation of electrolyte transport mechanisms could be very useful clinically. Drugs that structurally resemble hormones or neurotransmitters with known actions have been designed and used clinically. Those with antisecretory properties have been used successfully in the treatment of diarrhea. Others with secretory properties have been used for constipation. Some of the drugs were widely used before their mechanisms of action were well understood. A classic example is the use of synthetic opiates to treat diarrhea.

For the purpose of discussing peptide or neurotransmitter regulation, the intestine may be considered a self-modulated organ. The endocrine cells, nerve cells, and immune cells serve as sensors responding to various stimuli, and the hormones, neurotransmitters, and mediators released serve as messengers.[195] These messengers then modulate and coordinate the functions of the intestine and other digestive organs. The regulation can be paracrine, neurocrine, endocrine, or immunologic in nature.[188,212,213]

The mechanism by which a given peptide or neurotransmitter causes secretion has gradually become clearer with the advent of new methods of investigation. In the past only cAMP and cGMP could be measured; now, free cytosolic calcium, phospholipids, inositol phosphates, free fatty acids, and other intracellular messengers can be measured directly. The role of protein kinases, calmodulin, and G proteins can also be examined experimentally. These technological advancements, in conjunction with the growth of knowledge regarding the participation of basic transport pathways in a given transport mechanism, should allow better mapping of cellular regulatory mechanisms from the receptor site to the transport pathway level. Clearly, knowledge in this regard is still quite limited.

Theoretically, sites for intervention in electrolyte transport mechanisms include any step in the cascade of biochemical events following receptor binding and activation. For practical purposes, the receptor-mediated regulation can be divided into three steps: (1) receptor binding and activation, (2) activation of intracellular mediators (secondary messengers), and (3) activation of the transport pathway.

Receptor binding and activation usually occurs on the basolateral membrane for endogenous stimuli.[44] The receptor recognizes the signal (hormone or neurotransmitter) released by sensor cells (endocrine, immunologic, or nerve cells) and initiates the biological event. A large number of hormones and neurotransmitters may affect or modulate the transport function of the epithelial cells. The assortment of hormones and neurotransmitters that increase fluid and electrolyte secretion or absorption and the intracellular mediators involved in their action are summarized in Tables 17-1 and 17-2, respectively. The physiological role of each peptide or neurotransmitter cannot yet be clearly delineated because pharmacological doses are needed for most of the biological studies, and relatively few specific receptor antagonists are available.

The ability of cells and products (mediators and cytokines) of the immune system to influence intestinal electrolyte transport is becoming increasingly recognized.[171] Immunocytes can be considered specialized sensors of the intestinal environment that utilize highly specific mechanisms (antibodies) to respond to local stimuli. Mast cells and neutrophils have been examined most extensively for their ability to induce intestinal secretion; both cell types release substances that can directly stimulate epithelial cells to secrete chloride ions. It is also apparent that immune regulation can occur through indirect pathways, via interactions with nerves, through the stimulation of prostaglandin production by mesenchymal elements, or by alteration of epithelial sensitivity to the normal neurohormonal "tone."[12]

After binding to the receptor, the hormones or neurotransmitters activate a cascade of intracellular mediators (secondary messengers), which stimulate or inhibit certain epithelial electrolyte transport mechanisms. In contrast to the large number of receptors, the intracellular mediators are relatively few. Many hormones and neurotransmitters activate the same intracellular event. A number of secondary messengers have been recognized (Fig. 17-15). Activation of these secondary messengers and interactions between them regulate various absorptive or secretory processes in the intestine. Substances causing intestinal secretion can at present be divided into two groups: those with effects mediated by cyclic nucleotides and those with effects transduced by levels of free cytosolic calcium.[29,53,64,143] Prostaglandins and vasoactive intestinal peptide (VIP), for example, cause secretion via a cAMP-mediated mechanism. They activate adenylate cyclase and increase cellular cAMP production.[122,187,210] Cholera toxin also increases cAMP levels, by retarding the degradation of adenylate cyclase.[83] In both cases, increased cAMP levels lead to the activation of a cAMP-dependent protein kinase and electrolyte secretion.[27,190,191] cGMP appears to regulate the secretory process activated by the heat-stable toxin of *Escherichia coli*. The mechanism in this case may involve a cGMP-dependent protein kinase.[23,65]

There are at least two mechanisms for calcium-dependent control of intestinal ion transport; one involves calmodulin and the other phosphoinositide metabo-

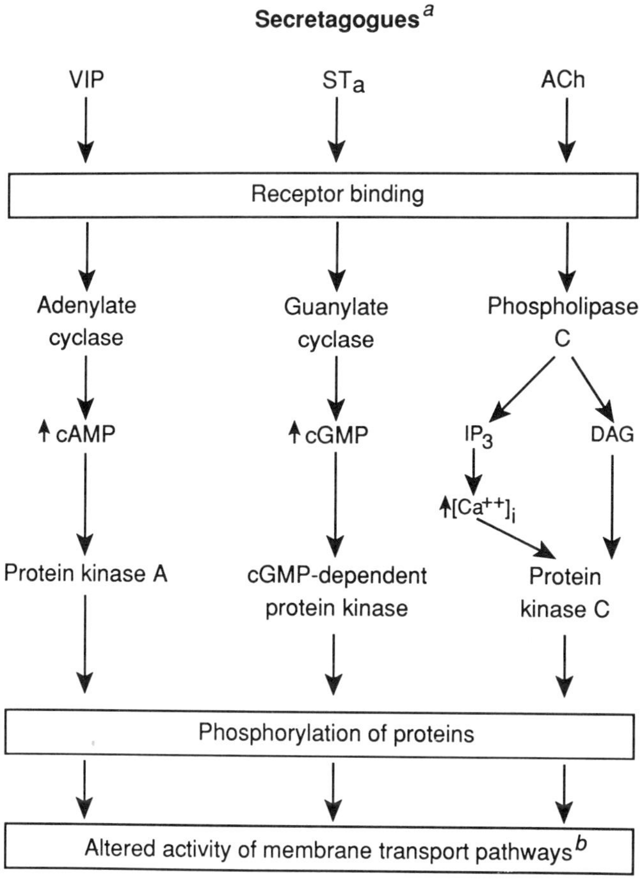

FIGURE 17-15 • Second messenger systems hypothetically involved in epithelial electrolyte transport. Secretagogues bind receptors on either the basolateral (endogenous stimuli) or apical (exogenous stimuli) aspect of epithelial cells. Depending on the nature of the stimulus, a second messenger or messengers are produced. This activates a specific protein kinase to phosphorylate proteins, which may be transport pathways or accessory proteins. a, secretagogues given are examples of cAMP-, cGMP-, and Ca^{2+}-dependent agents; VIP, vasoactive intestinal polypeptide; ST_a, heat stable toxin of *Escherichia coli;* ACh, acetylcholine; b, protein phosphorylation may result in both up- and downregulation of transport pathway activity; $[Ca^{2+}]i$, free cytosolic calcium concentration; DAG, diacylglycerol; IP_3, inositol trisphosphate.

lites.[167,168,222] This information is relatively new; thus, it is not clear which calcium-mediated responses listed in Tables 17-1 and 17-2 involve calmodulin and which involve phosphoinositide metabolites. Acetylcholine probably mobilizes calcium from intracellular pools[160] by a phosphoinositide-related mechanism and subsequently activates protein kinase C.[32,50] The calmodulin-dependent mechanisms are known to be important because trifluoperazine and chlorpromazine, which inactivate the calcium-calmodulin complex, have antisecretory properties.[110] However, calcium-calmodulin may be more involved in the regulation of basal absorption than in the control of stimulated secretion.[50] It is likely that the calmodulin-related mechanism and the phosphoinositide-related mechanism activate distinct protein kinases. The calmodulin-related mechanism may activate a protein kinase that regulates an apical membrane transport pathway to inhibit electrolyte absorption. The phosphoinositide-related mechanism, on the other hand, apparently activates protein kinase C.

The final event regulated by intracellular mediators is at the transport pathway level, either at the basolateral or apical membrane. All the peptide hormones and neurotransmitters that regulate electrolyte transport function apparently do so in the short term by activating or inactivating a transport pathway. For example, aldosterone or corticosteroids increase flow through the Na^+ channel on the colonic apical membrane to increase Na^+ absorption.[221] VIP and prostaglandin $E_1(PGE_1)$ open a cAMP-dependent Cl^- channel on the apical membrane, permitting Cl^- secretion.[220] Acetylcholine opens a calcium-dependent K^+ channel on the basolateral membrane, indirectly creating a favorable gradient for Cl^- secretion across the apical membrane.

OTHER FACTORS THAT INFLUENCE INTESTINAL WATER AND ELECTROLYTE TRANSPORT

Several other factors may influence water and electrolyte transport by intestinal epithelial cells. These factors include intestinal motility,[30,120,217] intestinal permeability,[75] plasma oncotic pressure, and arterial, venous, and luminal hydrostatic pressures.[95,169,201,226] Of these, in clinical practice, only intestinal motility appears to play an important role in water and electrolyte transport,[30,120,217] although this may simply reflect our lack of knowledge of the complex interactions and contributions of these physiological control mechanisms. Coordinated gastrointestinal transit allows more contact time for absorption, which may decrease stool volume significantly.[30,119,120,182,217] Many antidiarrheal drugs, such as the synthetic opiates, are effective mainly because of their inhibitory effect on gut motility.[21,182] Other factors, such as any alteration of intestinal permeability, may affect the balance between absorption and secretion. Intestinal permeability may increase a great deal in diseases that cause mucosal injury; bile salts and fatty acids also increase the permeabilty of colonic mucosa.[75] An increased permeability may allow many smaller molecules, which normally are not absorbed, to diffuse across the intestinal mucosa more easily and may allow the oncotic pressure and venous hydrostatic pressure to have a more prominent effect on electrolyte secretion or absorption.

Finally, there has been a recent increase in the amount of information available regarding control of electrolyte transport by the central nervous system. While this is clearly a controlling system of substantial clinical relevance, it has been difficult to design studies to assess its contribution. Central control has been shown to be important for gastric acid secretion, duodenal bicarbonate secretion, and intestinal chloride secretion.[33,136] It is likely that our improved ability to understand central control of transport phenomena will enhance our ability to treat conditions such as stress-induced duodenal ulceration.

IMPLICATION IN DISEASES

In clinical gastroenterology, the area of electrolyte transport physiology is applied mainly to the management of hypersecretory states (e.g., peptic ulcer disease and diarrhea). Pharmacological bypass of the secretory defect in cystic fibrosis is another topic of investigation.

Treatment of acid-peptic disease currently centers around the inhibition of acid secretion, although in the future stimulation of bicarbonate secretion may gain more acceptance. Inhibition of gastric acid secretion can be achieved by the use of histamine H_2 blockers or vagotomy, which interfere with receptor-mediated stimulation. On the other hand, inhibition of H^+ exit by an inhibition of H^+-K^+ ATPase has recently become a possible alternative.[141]

When discussing the treatment of diarrhea, two basic approaches should be considered: stimulation of the existing absorptive mechanism, which typically remains functional, and interruption of the excessive secretory function.[129] For the former, glucose-salt solution has been successfully applied clinically. The latter approach may be applied by manipulating the receptor-mediated process, or in theory by blocking Cl^- exit. At present, only pharmacological manipulation of the receptor sites is used clinically. Opiates, alpha 2-adrenergic agents, and somatostatin are all useful in the treatment of diarrhea. Approaches to the therapy for diarrhea that could be considered experimental include the administration of fluid-phase toxin receptors and interruption of the secretory process at the intracellular mediator stage (e.g., by the use of trifluoperazine). In the future, inhibition of the transport pathway directly, similar to the use of omeprazole to inhibit gastric acid secretion, may be possible. If a suitable Cl^- channel blocker that is active luminally could be developed, Cl^- exit at the apical membrane could be inhibited.

APPENDIX: METHODOLOGIES FOR INTESTINAL ELECTROLYTE TRANSPORT STUDIES

IN VIVO PERFUSION

In vivo perfusion techniques are used to study water and electrolyte transport in healthy humans. The techniques are also widely implemented in whole animals. The two variations of this method are double-lumen perfusion and triple-lumen perfusion. Both techniques use a nonabsorbable marker, such as polyethylene glycol or polymeric dyes, to calculate the amount of water absorbed or secreted between two points of an intestinal segment.[34,55] These in vivo perfusion techniques allow measurement of the rate of disappearance or appearance of material in the intestinal lumen. With these techniques, it is assumed that what disappears has been absorbed and what appears has been secreted. In general, this assumption is valid, and the technique is useful for identification and study of absorptive or secretory phenomena. These techniques allow for the influence of most contributing factors, including gut motility and blood flow; therefore, the results are representative of what happens normally. These perfusion studies have significant limitations when employed in hopes of elucidating the mechanisms and transport pathways involved in absorptive or secretory processes. Mechanistic studies can be better carried out with the in vitro techniques described below.

Double-lumen perfusion

A number of early studies in humans used double-lumen perfusion (Fig. 17-16). In human studies, a double-lumen tube is inserted into the intestine via the mouth. The intestinal segment of interest may be occluded proximally with a balloon built into the tube (to prevent interference from the normal flow of intestinal contents); in animal studies, a segment of the intestine is usually isolated surgically. The infusate is instilled at the proximal port and effusate is collected from the distal port. The use of nonabsorbable markers avoids problems of incomplete collection. The amount of water absorbed or secreted can be calculated from the relative concentration of the nonabsorbable marker at the two ports. If water is absorbed, the concentration of the nonabsorbable marker in the effusate is increased compared to the infused concentration; if water is secreted, the marker is diluted. The amount of any electrolyte or other substance absorbed or secreted can also be calculated from the differences between the concentration entering the segment and concentration collected distally, once the amount of water absorption or secretion is known.

Triple-lumen perfusion

Double-lumen perfusion is not ideal for human studies where it is impossible to isolate the test segment completely from the normal flow of intestinal contents from the upper tract. To compensate for this problem, a third lumen is introduced to sample the intestinal content after the infusate is mixed with the existing luminal contents (Fig. 17-17).[34] This allows sampling of well-mixed contents between two points of an intestinal segment. Calculation of the amount of water and electrolyte absorbed

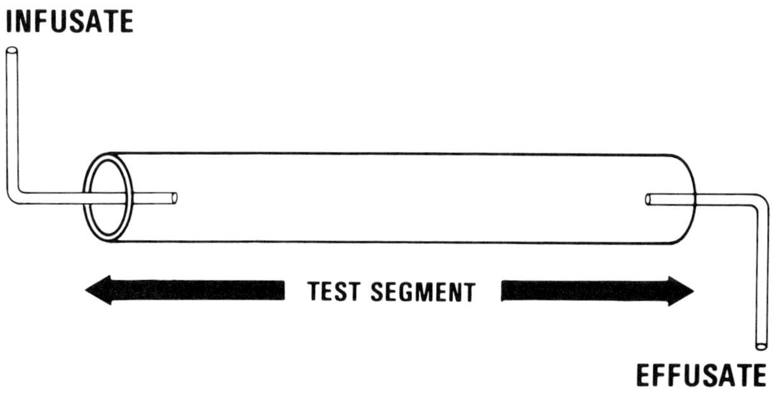

FIGURE 17-16 • Double-lumen perfusion. A segment of the intestine can be isolated surgically or by occlusion with a balloon at the infusion site. An infusate containing a known concentration of the substance of interest and a nonabsorbable marker is infused at the proximal end of the test segment while effusate is collected at the distal end. Measurement of the concentrations of the nonabsorbable marker and a substance of interest in the effusate allows calculation of the amounts of water and other substances absorbed or secreted in the test segment. (Adapted from Moore EW: *Gastroenterology: Liver Disease, Teaching Material,* American Gastroenterological Association, 1976. Used by permission.)

between the points follows the same principle as the double-lumen perfusion technique.

IN VITRO TECHNIQUES

In vitro techniques use either isolated segments of the intestine, isolated enterocytes, cells grown in tissue culture, or plasma membranes isolated from enterocytes. The advantages of each method arise mainly from its ability to exclude certain confounding factors. Isolated intestine stripped of the muscular layers excludes the effects of blood flow and motility. Isolated enterocytes or cell cultures exclude the influence of preexisting peptides or neurotransmitters and the effects of resident lamina proprial cells. Isolated apical or basolateral membranes allow precise identification and localization of transport pathways. Conversely, with the progressive simplification of each experimental model, the preparation is increasingly isolated from normal regulatory factors. The phenomena observed may therefore not be pertinent to whole organs. It is likely that a full appreciation of the regulation of intestinal transport will be derived from the combined use of a number of techniques.

Everted gut sac

This simple technique permits gross estimation of absorptive or secretory functions (Fig. 17-18): a segment of the intestine is everted, tied at both ends, and suspended in the same solution that fills the sac.[223] Potential stimuli of absorption or secretion can then be added to the bathing medium. The everted sac enlarges upon absorption and shrinks with secretion. The preparation retains most intestinal structures and regulatory mechanisms. Except for blood flow and central nervous system control, the phenomena observed should be pertinent to the whole intestine. One of the potential problems is that only those absorbed substances that also penetrate the muscular layers and the serosa can be detected by this technique.

Ussing chamber

The Ussing chamber is designed to detect active transort mechanisms. Electrochemical driving forces for passive ion movement are eliminated by the design of the equipment. In essence, it consists of two fluid-filled reservoirs with a piece of the isolated intestine separating them (Fig.

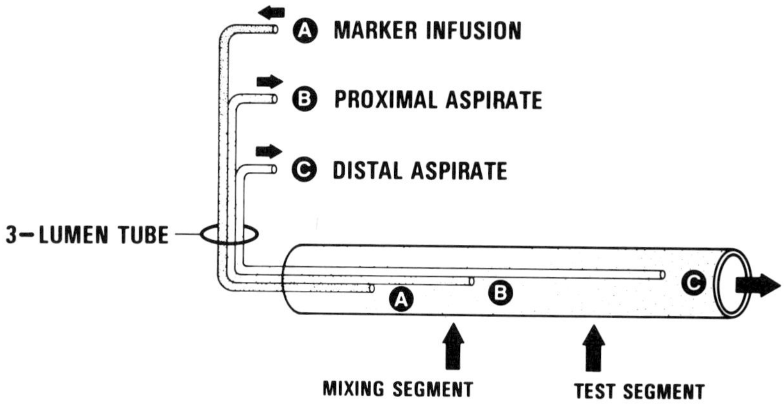

FIGURE 17-17 • Triple-lumen perfusion. The technique is based on the same principle as double-lumen perfusion (described in Fig. 17-16). Rather than using the infusate at the starting point, the infusate (marker infusion) is allowed to mix with the intestinal contents in the mixing segment, between points A and B. Point B, where proximal aspirate is collected, corresponds to the infusion point in the double-lumen perfusion; the test segment is therefore between points B and C. The amount of water or other substances absorbed from the segments can be calculated from the difference between B and C, using proximal aspirate and distal aspirate samples. (Adapted from Moore EW: *Gastroenterology: Liver Disease, Teaching Material,* American Gastroenterological Association, 1976. Used by permission.)

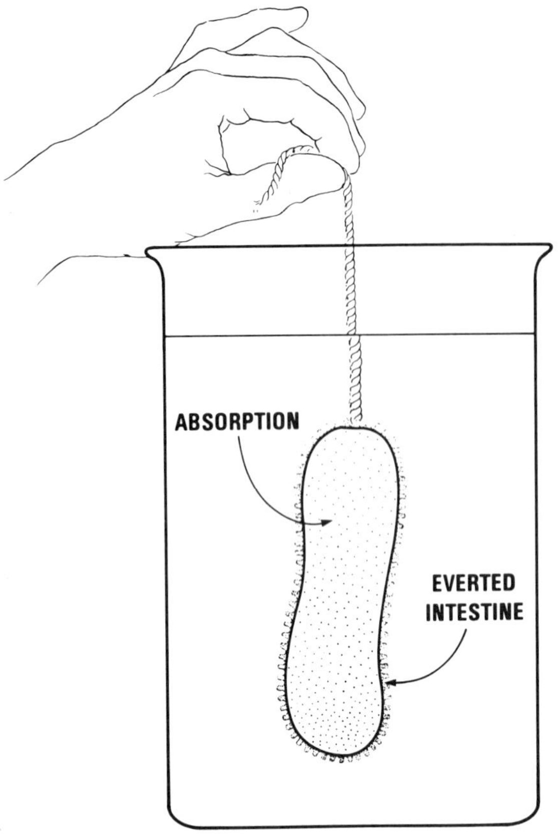

FIGURE 17-18 • Everted gut sac. A segment of intestine is everted and tied at both ends. Absorption of water enlarges the sac; secretion shrinks it.

17-19).[36,208] The mucosa or the luminal surface is bathed by one reservoir, while the serosal or basolateral surface is bathed by the other. To eliminate the chemical gradient, both surfaces are exposed to similar bathing solutions; to eliminate the electrical gradient, a voltage-clamp apparatus generates an electrical current sufficient to nullify the spontaneous electrical potential difference existing across the tissue. The current needed is called the short-circuit current. It reflects the net transport of charged species and can be used to monitor electrolyte transport activity. Movement of a specific ion from one side of the intestine to the other can also be directly measured by the use of radioisotope tracers. The Ussing chamber allows active transport phenomena across an epithelial sheet to be identified without the confounding effects of gut motility and blood flow. It is an excellent method of studying the absorptive or secretory mechanisms for a specific molecule. The involvement of a given transport pathway (on the apical or basolateral membrane) in a transport mechanism can be identified, provided that a specific inhibitor for the pathway exists (see Table 17-3). Similarly, the involvement of an intracellular mediator can be inferred if a specific inhibitor of that secondary messenger is found to inhibit the transport phenomenon.

Microelectrodes

The principle of the ion-selective electrode is similar to that of the pH electrode. An ion-selective substance at the tip of the electrode allows a specific ion to pass through

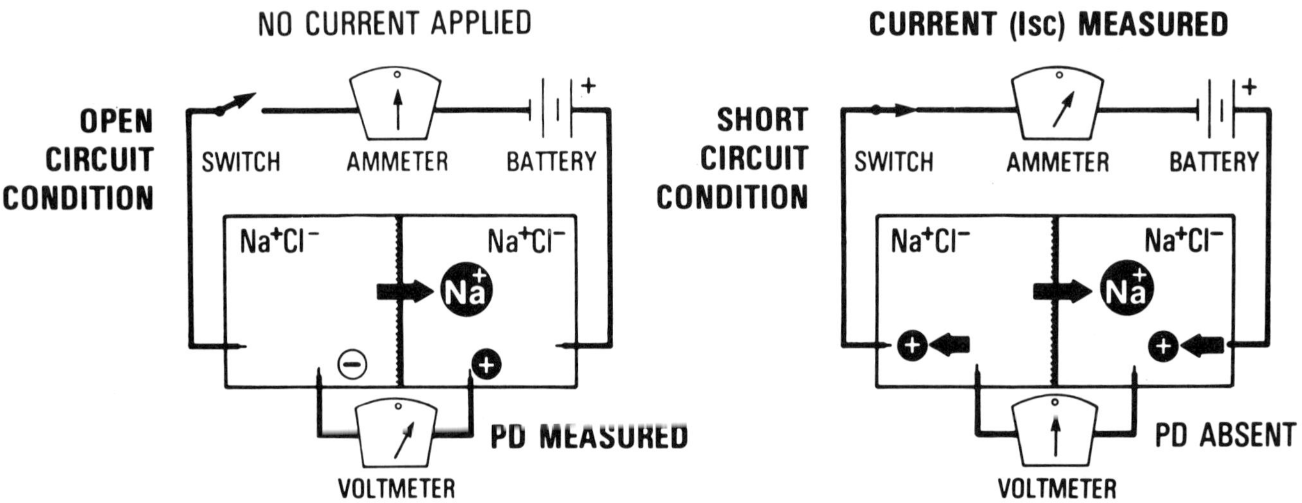

FIGURE 17-19 • Ussing chamber. A piece of intestine or an epithelial sheet is clamped between baths containing warm, oxygenated physiological saline solution. Chemical gradients across the tissue are eliminated by the use of similar bathing solutions on each side; the electrochemical gradient that may result from active transport is nullified by an electrical current supplied by a voltage clamp apparatus. (*a*) Open-circuit condition: the voltmeter measures the potential difference (PD) resulting from the active transport. (*b*) Short-circuited condition: the battery with ammeter adjusts the potential difference to zero; under this condition, there is no electrochemical gradient across the isolated intestine or epithelial sheet. The amount of current needed to nullify the potential difference quantifies the net active transport of charged ions. Radioactive tracers can be used to identify the ionic species being actively transported. (Adapted from Moore EW: *Gastroenterology: Liver Disease, Teaching Material,* American Gastroenterological Association, 1976. Used by permission.)

and results in a detectable electrical current.[79,81,93] Use of an ion-selective microelectrode permits measurement of the electrical potential across the plasma membrane (apical or basolateral) in an intact cell, and determination of the conductance across the membrane for the ion of interest. The latter quantity reflects the activity of a channel or carrier and can be used to detect changes induced by peptides or other compounds. The concentration of a specific ion in the epithelial cell can also be estimated. The advantage of the technique is that it allows studies to be carried out in a single cell, avoiding many confounding factors resulting from the multiple cell types in an intact tissue. The principal disadvantage is the limitation inherent in interpreting the results; as they are based on an electrical profile, which may be similar for a number of ions, the results are somewhat indirect.

Another method, electron probe microanalysis, also provides information about the intracellular content of ions, but the technique requires specialized equipment that is not readily available.[135]

Patch-clamp techniques

The principle of the patch-clamp technique is similar to that of the ion-selective microelectrode. In this case, the tip of the electrode is sealed with a tiny patch of plasma membrane from the epithelial cell.[178] The tip of the electrode therefore contains one or several ionic channels of interest rather than an ion-selective substance. When exposed to proper ion gradients, a small burst of electrical current can be detected if an ionic channel is present and open. Patch-clamping provides a direct method of verifying and studying ionic channels. It has accordingly become an important and widely used technique.

Radionuclide uptake and efflux studies in isolated cells

Uptake of radionuclide into whole cells or efflux of radionuclide out of cells can be studied using isolated enterocytes. Recently, the ability to apply these techniques to intact cultured monolayers has allowed verification that various transport pathways are localized at the apical or basolateral membrane.[146] Employing ion substitution or pH gradients in conjunction with the use of a radionuclide can verify whether a cotransport (symport) or ion exchange (antiport) mechanism is present. An ionic channel can also be readily detected, but the method cannot directly differentiate a channel from a carrier. Activation or inhibition of these pathways by peptides or other compounds can also be tested.

Membrane vesicles

The apical and basolateral membranes of intestinal epithelial cells can be isolated, separated, and purified on the basis of their different densities.[9,94,104,156] The apical membrane, with its attached cytoskeleton, is somewhat denser. The enzyme markers, which are integral to the membrane, allow one to detect and estimate the extent of purification of the membrane preparations. The broken plasma membrane fragments, which contain carriers, channels, and/or pumps, tend to seal as round vesicles. Radionuclide uptake and efflux studies can be carried out on vesicles in a manner similar to the whole cell studies. The concentration of ions inside and outside the vesicle can be better controlled than in whole cells. Shorter time courses can be studied more easily, and a better estimation of the stoichiometry of a given transport pathway can be obtained. Fluorescent dyes have also been widely applied for ion transport studies.[91] The membrane vesicles are also expected to present a better preparation for biochemical studies of the transporter protein.

Cell culture

Cultured epithelial cells, especially continuous cell lines, exclude confounding factors introduced by the endocrine cells, nerve endings, and immunocytes normally present in isolated tissue.[42] A culture line containing only one cell type can serve as a model for the study of transport mechanisms. Recently, a number of colonic cell lines have been successfully used to study the Cl^- secretory mechanism. Many techniques mentioned above can be easily applied to cultured cells, including the Ussing chamber, radionuclide uptake and efflux, microelectrode, and patch-clamp techniques. Application of these techniques to cultured cells should provide results quite complementary to the studies of whole or isolated intestine.

REFERENCES

1. Adibi SA et al: Evidence for two different modes of tripeptide disappearance in human intestine. *J Clin Invest* 56:1355, 1975.
2. Adibi SA: Intestinal transport of dipeptides in man: Relative importance of hydrolysis and intact absorption. *J Clin Invest* 50:2266, 1971.
3. Adibi SA, Kim YS: Peptide absorption and hydrolysis, in Johnson LR et al (eds): *Physiology of the Gastrointestinal Tract.* New York, Raven Press, 1981, p 1073.
4. Al-Awqati Q et al: Electrolyte transport in human ileum: Effect of purified cholera exotoxin. *Am J Physiol* 224:818, 1973.
5. Al-Awqati Q, Greenough WB III: Prostaglandins inhibit intestinal sodium transport. *Nature (London)* 238:26, 1972.
6. Alpers DH: Absorption of water-soluble vitamins, folate, minerals and vitamin D, in Sleisenger MH, Fordtran JS (eds): *Gastrointestinal Disease: Pathophysiology, Diagnosis, Management*, 3d ed. Philadelphia, Saunders, 1983, p 830.

7. Ammon HV, Phillips SF: Inhibition of ileal water absorption by intraluminal fatty acids: Influence of chain length, hydroxylation and conjugation of fatty acids. *J Clin Invest* 53:205, 1974.
8. Anagnostides AA et al: Peptide histidine isoleucine (PHI): A secretagogue in porcine intestine. *Dig Dis Sci* 28:893, 1983.
9. Aronson PS: Identifying secondary active solute transport in epithelia. *Am J Physiol* 240:F1, 1981.
10. Banwell JG et al: Intestinal fluid and electrolyte transport in human cholera. *J Clin Invest* 49:183, 1970.
11. Barbezat GO et al: Effects of bombesin, calcitonin, and enkephalin on canine jejunal water and electrolyte transport. *Dig Dis Sci* 28:273, 1983.
12. Barrett KE, Dharmsathaphorn K: Secretion and absorption: Small intestine and colon, in Yamada T (ed): *Textbook of Gastroenterology*. New York, Lippincott, 1991, p 265.
13. Barrett KE et al: Immune-related intestinal chloride secretion: II. Effect of adenosine on T_{84} cell line. *Am J Physiol* 258:C902, 1990.
14. Benos DJ: Amiloride: A molecular probe of sodium transport in tissues and cells. *Am J Physiol* 242:C131, 1982.
15. Bentzel CJ et al: Cytoplasmic regulation of tight-junction permeability: Effect of plant cytokinins. *Am J Physiol* 239:C75, 1980.
16. Binder HJ et al: Mechanism of electroneutral sodium chloride absorption in distal colon of the rat. *Gastroenterology* 93:449, 1987.
17. Binder HJ: Absorption and secretion of water and electrolytes by small and large intestine, in Sleisenger MH, Fordtran JS (eds): *Gastrointestinal Disease: Pathophysiology, Diagnosis, Management*, 3d ed. Philadelphia, Saunders, 1983, p 811.
18. Binder HJ, Sandle GI: Electrolyte absorption and secretion in the mammalian colon, in Johnson LR et al (eds): *Physiology of the Gastrointestinal Tract*, 2d ed. New York, Raven Press, 1987, p 1389.
19. Binder HJ (ed): *Mechanisms of Intestinal Secretion*. New York, Alan R. Liss, 1979.
20. Binder HJ, Rawlins CL: The effect of conjugated dihydroxy bile salts on electrolyte transport in rat colon. *J Clin Invest* 52:1460, 1973.
21. Bitar KN, Makhlouf GM: Opiate receptors are present on circular and selectively absent from longitudinal muscle cells of the intestine (abstract). *Gastroenterology* 84:1107, 1983.
22. Bond JH et al: Colonic conservation of malabsorbed carbohydrate. *Gastroenterology* 78:444, 1980.
23. Brasitus TA et al: Intestinal mucosal cyclic GMP: Regulation and possible role in ion transport. *Am J Physiol* 231:275, 1976.
24. Brautbar N et al: Intestinal absorption of calcium: Role of dietary phosphate and vitamin D. *Am J Physiol* 241:G49, 1981.
25. Bright-Asare P, Binder HJ: Stimulation of colonic secretion of water and electrolytes by hydroxy fatty acids. *Gastroenterology* 64:81, 1973.
26. Bukhave K. Rask-Madsen J: Saturation kinetics applied to in vitro effects of low prostaglandins E_2 and $F_{2\alpha}$ concentrations on ion transport across human jejunal mucosa. *Gastroenterology* 78:32, 1980.
27. Burnham DB, Fondacaro JD: Secretagogue-induced protein phosphorylation and chloride transport in Caco-2 cells. *Am J Physiol* 256:G808, 1989.
28. Carter RF et al: Inhibition of VIP-stimulated intestinal secretion and cyclic AMP production by somatostatin in the rat. *Gastroenterology* 74:726, 1978.
29. Cartwright CA et al: Synergistic action of cyclic AMP and calcium mediated chloride secretion in a colonic epithelial cell line. *J Clin Invest* 76:1837, 1985.
30. Christensen J: Motility of the colon, in Johnson LR et al (eds): *Physiology of the Gastrointestinal Tract*, 2d ed. New York, Raven Press, 1987, p 665.
31. Claude P. Goodenough DA: Fracture faces of zonulae occludentes from "tight" and "leaky" epithelia. *J Cell Biol* 58:390, 1973.
32. Cohn JA: Protein kinase C mediates cholinergically regulated protein phosphorylation in a Cl-secreting epithelium. *Am J Physiol* 258:C227, 1990.
33. Cooke HJ: Role of the "little brain" in the gut in water and electrolyte homeostasis. *FASEB J* 3:127, 1989.
34. Cooper HR et al: A method for studying absorption of water and solute from the human small intestine. *Gastroenterology* 50:1, 1966.
35. Curran PF et al: Kinetic relations of the Na-amino acid interaction at the mucosal border of intestine. *J Gen Physiol* 50:1261, 1967.
36. Curran PF, Schultz SG: Transport across membranes: General principles, in Code CF (ed): *Handbook of Physiology: Alimentary Canal.* Washington DC, American Physiological Society, 1968, p 1217.
37. Davis GR et al: Active chloride secretion in the normal human jejunum. *J Clin Invest* 66:1326, 1980.
38. Davis GR et al: Effect of vasoactive intestinal polypeptide on active and passive transport in the human jejunum. *J Clin Invest* 67:1687, 1981.
39. Davis GR et al: Evaluation of chloride/bicarbonate exchange in the human colon in vivo. *J Clin Invest* 71:201, 1983.
40. Davis GR et al: Permeability characteristics of human jejunum, ileum, proximal colon and distal colon: Results of potential difference measurements and unidirectional fluxes. *Gastroenterology* 83:844, 1982.
41. Devroede GJ, Phillips SF: Conservation of sodium, chloride and water by the human colon. *Gastroenterology* 56:421, 1969.
42. Dharmsathaphorn K et al: A human colonic tumor cell line that maintains vectorial electrolyte transport. *Am J Physiol* 246:G204, 1984.
43. Dharmsathaphorn K et al: Effect of somatostatin on ion transport in rat colon. *J Clin Invest* 66:813, 1990.
44. Dharmsathaphorn K et al: Preferential binding of vasoactive intestinal polypeptide to basolateral membrane of rat and rabbit enterocytes. *J Clin Invest* 71:27, 1983.
45. Dharmsathaphorn K et al: VIP- induced chloride secretion by a colonic epithelial cell line: Direct participation of a basolaterally localized Na^+,K^+,Cl^- cotransport system. *J Clin Invest* 75:462, 1985.
46. DiBona DR, Mills JW: Distribution of Na-pump sites in transporting epithelia. *Fed Proc* 38:134, 1979.
47. Dietz J, Field M: Ion transport in rabbit ileal mucosa: IV. Bicarbonate secretion. *Am J Physiol* 225:858, 1973.
48. Dobbins JW et al: Effect of D-Ala, met-enkephalin amide

on ion transport in rabbit ileum. *J Clin Invest* 66:19, 1980.
49. Dobbins JW et al: Adenosine and adenosine analogues stimulate adenosine cyclic 3′,5′-monophosphate-dependent chloride secretion in the mammalian ileum. *J Clin Invest* 74:929, 1984.
50. Donowitz M et al: Elevated intracellular Ca^{2+} acts through protein kinase C to regulate rabbit ileal NaCl absorption: Evidence for sequential control by Ca^{2+}/calmodulin and protein kinase C. *J Clin Invest* 83:1953, 1989.
51. Donowitz M et al: Calcium dependence of serotonin-induced changes in rabbit ileal electrolyte transport. *J Clin Invest* 66:341, 1980.
52. Donowitz M, Madara JL: Effect of extracellular calcium depletion on epithelial structure and function in rabbit ileum: A model for selective crypt or villus epithelial cell damage and suggestion of secretion by villus epithelial cells. *Gastroenterology* 83:1231, 1982.
53. Donowitz M, Sharp GWG (eds): *Mechanisms of Intestinal Electrolyte Transport and Regulation by Calcium.* New York, Alan R. Liss, 1984.
54. Duffey ME et al: Intracellular chloride activities in rabbit gallbladder: Direct evidence for the role of the sodium-gradient in energizing "uphill" chloride transport. *J Membr Biol* 42:229, 1978.
55. Dupas J-L et al: Polymeric dyes: Useful nonabsorbable reference markers for intestinal perfusion studies in animals. *J Pharm Sci* 74:328, 1985.
56. Durbin T et al: Clonidine and lidamidine (WHR-1142) stimulate sodium and chloride absorption in the rabbit ileum. *Gastroenterology* 82:1352, 1982.
57. Eisner DA, Lederer WJ: Na-Ca exchange: Stoichiometry and electrogenicity. *Am J Physiol* 248:C189, 1985.
58. Farquhar MG, Palade GE: Junctional complexes in various epithelia. *J Cell Biol* 17:375, 1963.
59. Favus MJ: Factors that influence absorption and secretion of calcium in the small intestine and colon. *Am J Physiol* 248:G147, 1985.
60. Feldman M, Richardson CT: Gastric acid secretion in humans, in Johnson LR et al (eds): *Physiology of the Gastrointestinal Tract.* New York, Raven Press, 1981, p 693.
61. Fellenius E et al: Substituted benzimidazoles inhibit gastric acid secretion by blocking (H^+ + K^+)ATPase. *Nature (London)* 290:159, 1981.
62. Field M et al: Effect of cholera enterotoxin on ion transport across isolated ileal mucosa. *J Clin Invest* 51:796, 1972.
63. Field M: Corticosteroids, Na, K-ATPase and intestinal water and electrolyte transport. *Gastroenterology* 75:317, 1978.
64. Field M et al: Ion transport in rabbit ileal mucosa: II. Effects of cyclic 3′,5′-AMP. *Am J Physiol* 221:992, 1971.
65. Field M et al: Heat stable enterotoxin of *Escherichia coli:* In vitro effects on guanylate cyclase activity, cyclic GMP concentration, and ion transport in small intestine. *Proc Natl Acad Sci U S A* 75:2800, 1978.
66. Field M, McColl I: Ion transport in rabbit ileal mucosa: III. Effects of catecholamines. *Am J Physiol* 225:852, 1973.
67. Field M: Secretion by the small intestine, in Johnson LR et al (eds): *Physiology of the Gastrointestinal Tract.* New York, Raven Press, 1981, p 963.
68. Flemstrom G, Garner G: Gastroduodenal HCO_3^- transport: Characteristics and proposed role in acidity regulation and mucosal protection. *Am J Physiol* 242:G183, 1982.
69. Flemstrom G: Gastric and duodenal mucosal bicarbonate secretion, in Johnson LR et al (eds): *Physiology of the Gastrointestinal Tract*, 2d ed. New York, Raven Press, 1987, p 1011.
70. Fordtran JS, Ingelfinger FJ: Absorption of water, electrolytes, and sugars from the human gut, in Code CF (ed): *Handbook of Physiology: Alimentary Canal*, Washington DC, American Physiological Society, 1968, p 1457.
71. Fordtran JS et al: Permeability characteristics of the human small intestine. *J Clin Invest* 44:1935, 1965.
72. Fordtran JS: Stimulation of active and passive sodium absorption by sugars in the human jejunum. *J Clin Invest* 55:728, 1975.
73. Forte JG et al: Mechanisms of gastric H^+ and Cl^- transport. *Annu Rev Physiol* 42:111, 1980.
74. Foster ES et al: Role of aldosterone and dietary potassium in potassium adaptation in the distal colon of the rat. *Gastroenterology* 88:41, 1985.
75. Freel RW et al: Role of tight-junctional pathways in bile salt-induced increases in colonic permeability. *Am J Physiol* 245:G816, 1983.
76. Frizzell RA et al: Sodium chloride transport by rabbit gallbladder: Direct evidence for a coupled NaCl influx process. *J Gen Physiol* 65:769, 1975.
77. Frizzell RA et al: Sodium-coupled chloride transport by epithelial tissues *Am J Physiol* 236:F1, 1979.
78. Fromter E, Diamond J: Route of passive ion permeation in epithelia. *Nature (London)* 235:9, 1972.
79. Fromter E: Viewing the kidney through microelectrodes. *Am J Physiol* 247:F695, 1984.
80. Gaginella T, Kachur JF: Kinins as mediators of intestinal secretion. *Am J Physiol* 256:G1, 1989.
81. Garcia-Diaz JF et al: Electronic device for micro-electrode recordings in epithelial cells. *Am J Physiol* 246:C339, 1984.
82. Giannella RA et al: Pathogenesis of salmonella-mediated intestinal fluid secretion. *Gastroenterology* 69:1238, 1975.
83. Gill DM: Mechanism of action of cholera toxin. *Adv Cyclic Nucleotide Res* 8:85, 1977.
84. Goldner AM et al: Sodium and sugar fluxes across the mucosal border of rabbit ileum. *J Gen Physiol* 53:362, 1969.
85. Goyal RK: Neurology of the gut, in Sleisenger MH, Fordtran JH (eds): *Gastrointestinal Disease: Pathophysiology, Diagnosis, Management*, 3d ed. Philadelphia, Saunders, 1983, p 97.
86. Grady GF et al: Active transport of sodium by human colon in vitro. *Gastroenterology* 59:583, 1970.
87. Granger DN et al: Mechanism of glucagon-induced intestinal secretion. *Am J Physiol* 239:G30, 1980.
88. Gray GM: Mechanisms of digestion and absorption of food, in Sleisenger MH, Fordtran JH (eds): *Gastrointestinal Disease: Pathophysiology, Diagnosis, Management*, 3d ed. Philadelphia, Saunders, 1983, p 844.
89. Gray TK et al: Thyrocalcitonin and the jejunal absorption

of calcium, water and electrolytes in normal subjects. *J Clin Invest* 52:3084, 1973.

90. Grossman MI: Regulation of gastric acid secretion, in Johnson LR et al (eds): *Physiology of the Gastrointestinal Tract*. New York, Raven Press, 1981, p 659.
91. Grover AK et al: Ion movements in membrane vesicles: A new fluorescence method and application to smooth muscle. *Am J Physiol* 248:C372, 1985.
92. Guandalini S et al: In vitro effects of somatostatin on ion transport in rabbit intestine. *Am J Physiol* 238:G67, 1980.
93. Gupta BL et al: Microprobe measurement of Na, K and Cl concentration profiles in epithelial cells and intercellular spaces of rabbit ileum. *Nature (London)* 272:70, 1978.
94. Gustin MC, DBP Goodman: Isolation of brush-border membrane from the rabbit descending colon epithelium. *J Biol Chem* 256:10651, 1981.
95. Hakim AA et al: Mechanism of production of intestinal secretion by negative luminal pressure. *Am J Physiol* 2:E416, 1977.
96. Hallback D-A et al: Evidence for cholera secretion emanating from the crypts: A study of villus tissue osmolarity and fluid and electrolyte transport in the small intestine of the cat. *Gastroenterology* 83:1051, 1982.
97. Hannafin J et al: Presence of a sodium-potassium chloride cotransport system in the rectal gland of squalus acanthias. *J Membr Biol* 75:73, 1983.
98. Hartshorne RP, Catterall WA: The sodium channel from rat brain. *J Biol Chem* 259:1667, 1984.
99. Haynes DH: Mechanism of Ca^{2+} transport by Ca^{2+}-Mg^{2+}-ATPase pump: Analysis of major states and pathways. *Am J Physiol* 244:G3, 1983.
100. Hays RM: Alteration of luminal membrane structure by antidiuretic hormone. *Am J Physiol* 245:C289, 1983.
101. Hayslett JP, Binder HJ: Mechanism of potassium adaption. *Am J Physiol* 243:F103, 1982.
102. Helman CA, Barbezat GO: The effect of gastric inhibitory polypeptide on human jejunal water and electrolyte transport. *Gastroenterology* 72:376, 1977.
103. Hicks T, Turnberg LA: The effect of glucagon and secretin on salt and water transport in the human jejunum. *Gut* 13:854, 1972.
104. Hopfer U: Isolated membrane vesicles as tools for analysis of epithelial transport. *Am J Physiol* 233:E445, 1977.
105. Hopfer U et al: Glucose transport in isolated brush border membrane from rat small intestine. *J Biol Chem* 248:25, 1973.
106. Hopfer U et al: Differences in neutral amino acid and glucose transport between brush border and basolateral plasma membrane of intestinal epithelial cells. *J Cell Physiol* 89:805, 1976.
107. Hubel KA: Bicarbonate secretion in rat ileum and its dependence on intraluminal chloride. *Am J Physiol* 231:1409, 1967.
108. Hubel KA: Intestinal ion transport: Effect of epinephrine, pilocarpine, and atropine. *Am J. Physiol* 231:252, 1976.
109. Hubel KA: Intestinal nerves and ion transport: Stimuli, reflexes, and responses. *Am J Physiol* 248:G261, 1985.
110. Ilundain A, Naftalin RJ: Role of Ca^{2+} dependent regulator protein in intestinal secretion. *Nature (London)* 279:446, 1979.
111. Isaacs PET et al: In vitro behavior of human intestinal mucosa: The influence of acetylcholine on ion transport. *J Clin Invest* 58:535, 1976.
112. Ito S: Functional gastric morphology, in Johnson LR et al (eds): *Physiology of the Gastrointestinal Tract*, 2d ed. New York, Raven Press, 1987, p 817.
113. Jones RS, Myers WC: Regulation of hepatic biliary secretion. *Annu Rev Physiol* 41:67, 1979.
114. Kachur J et al: Control of guinea pig intestinal electrolyte secretin by a δ-opiate receptor. *Proc Natl Acad Sci U S A* 77:2753, 1980.
115. Kachur JF et al: Neurohumoral control of ileal electrolyte transport: I. Bombesin and related peptides. *J Pharmacol Exp Ther* 220:449, 1982.
116. Kachur JF et al: Neurohumoral control of ileal electrolyte transport: II. Neurotensin and substance P. *J Pharmacol Exp Ther* 220:456, 1982.
117. Kaplan HJ: Sodium ions and the sodium pump: Transport and enzymatic activity. *Am J Physiol* 245:G327, 1983.
118. Karayalcin SS et al: Hydrogen peroxide stimulates rat colonic prostaglandin production and alters electrolyte transport. *J Clin Invest* 86:60, 1990.
119. Kelly KA: Motility of the stomach and gastroduodenal junction, in Johnson LR et al (eds): *Physiology of the Gastrointestinal Tract*, 2d ed. New York, Raven Press, 1987, 613.
120. Kerlin P et al: Relationship of motility to flow of contents in the human small intestine. *Gastroenterology* 82:701, 1982.
121. Keusch GT et al: The pathogenesis of *Shigella* diarrhea: I. Enterotoxin production by *Shigella dysenteriae*. *J Clin Invest* 51:1212, 1972.
122. Kimberg DV et al: Stimulation of intestinal mucosal adenyl cyclase by cholera enterotoxin and prostaglandins. *J Clin Invest* 50:1218, 1971.
123. Kimmich GA: Intestinal absorption of sugar, in Johnson LR et al (eds): *Physiology of the Gastrointestinal Tract*. New York, Raven Press, 1981, p 1035.
124. Kirk KL et al: Active sodium transport by turtle colon via an electrogenic Na-K exchange pump. *Nature (London)* 287:237, 1980.
125. Kisloff B, Moore EW: Effects of intravenous calcitonin on water, electrolyte, and calcium movement across in vivo rabbit jejunum and ileum. *Gastroenterology* 72:462, 1977.
126. Kliger AS et al: Demonstration of active potassium transport in the mammalian colon. *J Clin Invest* 67:1189, 1981.
127. Knickelbein R et al: Sodium and chloride transport across rabbit ileal brush border. I. Evidence for Na-H Exchange. *Am J Physiol* 245:G504, 1983.
128. Kosower EM: A structural and dynamic molecular model for the sodium channel of *Electrophorus electricus*. *FEBS Lett* 182:234, 1985.
129. Krejs GJ, Fordtran JS: Diarrhea, in Sleisenger MH, Fordtran JS (eds): *Gastrointestinal Disease: Pathophysiology, Diagnosis, Management*, 3d ed. Philadelphia, Saunders, 1983, p. 257.
130. Krejs GJ, Fordtran JS: Effect on VIP infusion on water and ion transport in the human jejunum. *Gastroenterology* 78:722, 1980.
131. Landry DW et al: Purification and reconstitution of chlo-

ride channels from kidney and trachea. *Science* 244:1469, 1989.
132. Larsson H et al: Inhibition of gastric acid secretion by omeprazole in the dog and rat. *Gastroenterology* 85:900, 1983.
133. Larsson LI et al: Somatostatin cell processes as pathways for paracrine secretion. *Science* 205:1393, 1980.
134. Latorre R, Miller C: Conduction and selectivity in potassium channels. *J Membr Biol* 71:11, 1983.
135. Lechene C: Electron probe microanalysis of biological soft tissues: Principle and technique. *Fed Proc* 39:2871, 1980.
136. Lenz HJ, Brown MR: Cerebroventricular calcitonin gene-related peptide inhibits rat duodenal bicarbonate secretion by release of norepinephrine and vasopressin. *J Clin Invest* 85:25, 1990.
137. Levens NR: Modulation of jejunal ion and water absorption by endogenous angiotensin after dehydration. *Am J Physiol* 246:G700, 1984.
138. Levitan R, Ingelfinger FJ: Effect of D-aldosterone on salt and water absorption from the intact human colon. *J Clin Invest* 44:801, 1965.
139. Liedtke CM, Hopfer U: Mechanism of Cl^- translocation across small intestinal brush border membrane: II. Absence of Na^+-Cl^- cotransport *Am J Physiol* 242:G263, 1982.
140. Liedtke CM, Hopfer U: Mechanism of Cl^- translocation across small intestinal brush border membrane: II. Demonstration of Cl^--OH^- exchange and Cl^- conductance. *Am J Physiol* 242:G272, 1982.
141. Lind T et al: Effect of omeprazole—a gastric proton pump inhibitor—on pentagastrin stimulated acid secretion in man. *Gut* 24:270, 1983.
142. Lowe AG, Lambert A: Chloride-bicarbonate exchange and related transport processes. *Biochim Biophys Acta* 694:353, 1983.
143. McCabe RD, Smith PL: Colonic potassium and chloride secretion: Role of cAMP and calcium. *Am J Physiol* 248:G103, 1985.
144. McKay JS et al: The influence of opiates on ion transport across rabbit ileal mucosa. *Gastroenterology* 80:279, 1981.
145. McLennan WL et al: Ba^{2+}-inhibition of electrogenic Cl^- secretion in vitro frog and piglet gastric mucosa. *Am J Physiol* 239:G151, 1980.
146. McRoberts JA et al: Cyclic AMP and Ca^{++}-activated K^+ transport in a human colonic epithelial cell line. *J Biol Chem* 260:14163, 1985.
147. Mainoya JR: Effect of prolactin on fluid and NaCl absorption by the rat proximal and distal colon. *Experientia* 35:1060, 1979.
148. Makhlouf GM: Electrolyte composition of gastric secretion, in Johnson LR et al (eds): *Physiology of the Gastrointestinal Tract.* New York, Raven Press, 1981, p 551.
149. Malinowska DH et al: Cl^- requirement of acid secretion in isolated gastric glands. *Am J Physiol* 245:G573, 1983.
150. Mandel KG et al: Ba^{2+} inhibition of VIP- and A23187-stimulated Cl^- secretion by T_{84} cell monolayers. *Am J Physiol* 250:C486, 1986.
151. Marcial MA et al: Partitioning of paracellular conductance along the ileal crypt-villus axis: A hypothesis based on structural analysis with detailed consideration of tight junction structure-function relationships. *J Membr Biol* 80:59, 1984.
152. Matuchansky C, Bernier JJ: Effect of prostaglandin F_1 on glucose, water and electrolyte absorption in the human jejunum. *Gastroenterology* 64:1111, 1973.
153. Matuchansky C et al: Further studies on prostaglandin E-induced jejunal secretion of water and electrolytes in man. *Gastroenterology* 71:274, 1976.
154. Mekhjian HS et al: Colonic secretion of water and electrolytes induced by bile acids: Perfusion studies in man. *J Clin Invest* 50:1569, 1971.
155. Meyer JH: Control of pancreatic exocrine secretion, in Johnson LR et al (eds): *Physiology of the Gastrointestinal Tract.* New York, Raven Press, 1981, p 821.
156. Mircheff AK et al: Preparative scale isolation of basal-lateral plasma membranes from rat intestinal epithelial cells. *Membr Biochem* 1:177, 1978.
157. Moog F: The lining of the small intestine. *Sci Am* 245:154, 1981.
158. Moore R et al: *C. difficile* toxin A increases intestinal permeability and induces Cl^- secretion. *Am J Physiol* 259:G165, 1990.
159. Moritz M et al: Effect of secretin and cholecystokinin on the transport of electrolytes and water in human jejunum. *Gastroenterology* 64:76, 1973.
160. Muallem S, Sachs G: Ca^{2+} metabolism during cholinergic stimulation of acid secretion. *Am J Physiol* 248:G216, 1985.
161. Munck BG: Intestinal absorption of amino acids, in Johnson LR et al (eds): *Physiology of the Gastrointestinal Tract.* New York, Raven Press, 1981, p 1097.
162. Murer H, Hopfer U: Demonstration of electrogenic Na^+-dependent D-glucose transport in intestinal brush border membranes. *Proc Natl Acad Sci U S A* 71:484, 1974.
163. Murer H et al: Sodium proton antiport in brush border membrane vesicles isolated from rat small intestine. *Biochem J* 154:597, 1976.
164. Murer H, Hildmann B: Transcellular transport of calcium and inorganic phosphate in the small intestinal epithelium. *Am J Physiol* 240:G409, 1981.
165. Musch MW et al: Na^+-K^+-Cl^- co-transport in the intestine of a marine teleost. *Nature (London)* 300:331, 1982.
166. Nellans HN et al: Coupled sodium-chloride influx across the brush border of rabbit ileum. *Am J Physiol* 225:467, 1973.
167. Nellans HN, Popovitch JE: Calmodulin-regulated, ATP-driven calcium transport by basolateral membranes of rat small intestine. *J Biol Chem* 256:9932, 1981.
168. Nishizuka Y: Turnover of inositol phospholipids and signal transduction. *Science* 225:1365, 1984.
169. Norman DA et al: Water and electrolyte movement and mucosal morphology in the jejunum of patients with portal hypertension. *Gastroenterology* 79:707, 1980.
170. Peterson K-U, Reuss L: Cyclic AMP-induced chloride permeability in the apical membrane of *Necturus* gallbladder epithelium. *J Gen Physiol* 81:705, 1983.
171. Powell DW: The immunophysiology of intestinal electrolyte transport, in Frizzell RA, Field M (eds): *Handbook of Physiology: Absorptive and Secretory Processes of the Intestine.* Bethesda MD, American Physiological Society, 1991, p 591.

172. Rabbini GH et al: Chlorpromazine reduces fluid-loss in cholera. *Lancet* 1:410, 1979.
173. Riordan JR et al: Identification of the cystic fibrosis gene: Cloning and characterization of complementary DNA. *Science* 245:1066, 1989.
174. Robinson JWL (ed): *Intestinal Ion Transport*. Lancaster, UK, MTP Press, 1976.
175. Roggin GM et al: Unimpaired response of rabbit jejunum to cholera toxin after selective damage to villus epithelium. *Gastroenterology* 63:981, 1972.
176. Rose RC: Absorptive functions of the gallbladder, in Johnson LR et al (eds): *Physiology of the Gastrointestinal Tract*, 2d ed. New York, Raven Press, 1987, p 1455.
177. Rose RC: Intestinal absorption of water-soluble vitamins, in Johnson LR et al (eds): *Physiology of the Gastrointestinal Tract*, 2d ed. New York, Raven Press, 1987, p 1581.
178. Sakmann B, Neher E (eds): *Single Channel Recording*. New York, Plenum Press, 1983.
179. Sachs G, Berglindh T: Physiology of the parietal cell, in Johnson LR et al (eds): *Physiology of the Gastrointestinal Tract*. New York, Raven Press, 1981, p 567.
180. Saunders DR, Wiggins HS: Conservation of mannitol, lactulose and raffinose by the human colon. *Am J Physiol* 241:G397, 1981.
181. Schenk DB et al: Use of a monoclonal antibody to quantify (Na^+,K^+)-ATPase activity and sites in normal and regenerating rat liver. *J Biol Chem* 259:14941, 1984.
182. Schiller LR et al: Mechanism of the antidiarrheal action of codeine. *Gastroenterology* 80:1275, 1981.
183. Schultz SG: Ion transport by mammalian large intestine, in Johnson LR et al (eds): *Physiology of the Gastrointestinal Tract*. New York, Raven Press, 1981, p 991.
184. Schultz SG: Salt and water absorption by mammalian small intestine, in Johnson LR et al (eds): *Physiology of the Gastrointestinal Tract*. New York, Raven Press, 1981, p 983.
185. Schultz SG: The role of paracellular pathways in isotonic fluid transport. *Yale J Biol Med* 50:99, 1977.
186. Schulz I: Electrolyte and fluid secretion in the exocrine pancreas, in Johnson LR et al (eds): *Physiology of the Gastrointestinal Tract*, 2d ed. New York, Raven Press, 1987, p 1147.
187. Schwartz CJ et al: Vasoactive intestinal peptide stimulation of adenylate cyclase and active electrolyte secretion in intestinal mucosa. *J Clin Invest* 54:536, 1974.
188. Scott WN, Goodman DBP (eds): Hormonal regulation of epithelial transport of ions and water. *Ann N Y Acad Sci* 372:1, 1981.
189. Sheerin HF, Field M: Ileal HCO_3 secretion: Relationship to Na and Cl transport and effect of theophylline. *Am J Physiol* 228:1065, 1975.
190. Shlatz LJ et al: Cyclic nucleotide-dependent phosphorylation of rat intestinal microvillus and basal lateral membrane proteins by an endogenous protein kinase. *Gastroenterology* 75:838, 1978.
191. Shlatz LJ et al: Phosphorylation of specific rat intestinal microvillus and basal-lateral membrane proteins by cyclic nucleotides. *Gastroenterology* 76:293, 1979.
192. Skadhauge E (ed): *Intestinal Absorption and Secretion*. Lancaster, UK, MTP Press, 1984.
193. Smith PL, Field M: In vitro antisecretory effects of trifluoperazine and other neuroleptics in rabbit and human small intestine. *Gastroenterology* 78:1545, 1980.
194. Smith PL, McCabe RD: Mechanism and regulation of transcellular potassium transport by the colon. *Am J Physiol* 247:G445, 1984.
195. Solcia E et al: Endocrine cells of the digestive system, in Johnson LR et al (eds): *Physiology of the Gastrointestinal Tract*, 2d ed. New York, Raven Press, 1987, p 111.
196. Soll AH, Wollin A: Histamine and cyclic AMP in isolated canine parietal cells. *Am J Physiol* 237:E444, 1979.
197. Soll AH, Berglindh T: Physiology of isolated gastric glands and parietal cells: Receptors and effectors regulating function, in Johnson LR et al: (eds): *Physiology of the Gastrointestinal Tract*, 2d ed. New York, Raven Press, 1987, p 883.
198. Soll AH, Walsh JH: Regulation of gastric acid secretion. *Annu Rev Physiol* 41:35, 1979.
199. Steven CF: Biophysical studies of ion channels. *Science* 225:1346, 1984.
200. Stirling CE: Radioautographic localization of sodium pump sites in rabbit intestine. *J Cell Biol* 53:704, 1972.
201. Swabb EA et al: Acute elevation of intraluminal hydrostatic pressure alters small intestinal but not rat colonic water transport and permeability. *Gastroenterology* 76:1257, 1979.
202. Tamkun MM et al: The sodium channel from rat brain: Reconstitution of neurotoxin- activated ion flux and scorpion toxin binding from purified components. *J Biol Chem* 259:1676, 1984.
203. Tapper EJ et al: Cholinergic-adrenergic interaction of intestinal ion transport *Am J Physiol* 235:E402, 1978.
204. Trier JS et al: Anatomy, embryology, and developmental abnormalities of the small intestine and colon, in Sleisenger MH, Fordtran JS (eds): *Gastrointestinal Disease: Pathophysiology, Diagnosis, Management*, 3d ed. Philadelphia, Saunders, 1983, p 780.
205. Trier JS, Madara JL: Functional morphology of the mucosa of the small intestine, in Johnson LR et al (eds): *Physiology of the Gastrointestinal Tract*. New York, Raven Press, 1981, p 925.
206. Trudeau WL, McGuigan JE: Relations between serum gastrin levels and rates of gastric hydrochloric acid secretion. *N Engl J Med* 284:408, 1971.
207. Turnburg DA et al: Interrelationships of chloride, bicarbonate, sodium and hydrogen transport in the human ileum. *J Clin Invest* 49:557, 1970.
208. Ussing HH, Zerahn K: Active transport of sodium as the source of electric current in the short circuited frog skin. *Acta Physiol Scand* 214:110, 1951.
209. Wade JB, Lewis SA (eds): *Molecular Approaches to Epithelial Transport: Current Topics in Membranes and Transport*. London, Academic Press, vol 20, 1984.
210. Waldman DB et al: Effects of vasoactive intestinal peptide on rat colonic transport and adenylate cyclase activity. *Gastroenterology* 73:518, 1977.
211. Walling MV et al: Effects of calcitonin and substance P on the transport of Ca, Na and Cl across rat ileum in vitro, *Gastroenterology* 73:89, 1977.
212. Walsh JH: Gastrointestinal hormones, in Johnson LR et al (eds): *Physiology of the Gastrointestinal Tract*, 2d ed. New York, Raven Press, 1987, p 181.
213. Walsh JH: Gastrointestinal peptide hormones, in

Sleisenger MH, Fordtran JS (eds): *Gastrointestinal Disease: Pathophysiology, Diagnosis, Management*, 3d ed. Philadelphia, Saunders, 1983, p 54.
214. Wang YZ et al: Histamine augments colonic secretion in guinea pig distal colon. *Am J Physiol* 258:G432, 1990.
215. Wang YZ, Cooke HJ: H_2 receptors mediate cyclical chloride secretion in guinea pig distal colon. *Am J Physiol* 258:G887, 1990.
216. Wasserman SI et al: Immune-related intestinal Cl^- secretion: I. Effect of histamine on the T_{84} cell line. *Am J Physiol* 254:C53, 1988.
217. Weisbrodt NW: Motility of the small intestine, in Johnson LR et al (eds): *Physiology of the Gastrointestinal Tract*, 2d ed. New York, Raven Press, 1987, p 631.
218. Welsh MJ: Anthracene-9-carboxylic acid inhibits an apical membrane chloride conductance in canine tracheal epithelium. *J Membr Biol* 78:61, 1984.
219. Welsh MJ et al: Crypts are the site of intestinal fluid and electrolyte secretion. *Science* 218:1219, 1982.
220. Weymer A et al: Chloride secretory mechanisms induced by prostaglandin E_1 in a colonic epithelial cell line. *J Clin Invest* 76:1828, 1985.
221. Will PC et al: Introduction of amiloride-sensitive sodium transport in the rat colon by mineralocorticoids. *Am J Physiol* 238:F261, 1980.
222. Williamson JR et al: Inositol trisphosphate and diacylglycerol as intracellular second messengers in liver. *Am J Physiol* 248:C203, 1985.
223. Wilson TH, Wiseman G: The use of sacs of everted small intestine for the study of transference of substances from the mucosal to the serosal surface. *J Physiol* 123:116, 1954.
224. Wolosin JM, Forte JG: Stimulation of oxyntic cell triggers K^+ and Cl^- conductances in apical H^+-K^+-ATPase membrane. *Am J Physiol* 246:C537, 1984.
225. Wood JD: Enteric neurophysiology. *Am J Physiol* 247:G585, 1984.
226. Yablonski ME, Lifson N: Mechanism of production of intestinal secretion by elevated venous pressure. *J Clin Invest* 57:904, 1976.
227. Zimmerman TW et al: Mechanism of cholinergic regulation of electrolyte transport in rat colon in vitro. *Am J Physiol* 242:G116, 1982.
228. Zimmerman TW et al: Role of calcium in the regulation of colonic secretion in the rat. *Am J Physiol* 244:G552, 1983.

PART II

CLINICAL SYNDROMES OF DISORDERED FLUID AND ELECTROLYTE METABOLISM

CHAPTER • 18

Pathophysiology of the edema-forming states

Murray Epstein • Guido O. Perez

Edema is one of the most vexing problems to afflict patients. By definition, edema is an excessive accumulation of fluid within the interstitial space, that is, within the nonvascular portion of the extracellular fluid (ECF) space. Edema may be localized or generalized. Localized edema is restricted to a discrete vascular territory, such as the edema that accompanies inflammation and the localized edema that follows mastectomy. Generalized edema exists when the potential for fluid to leave the vascular space exists for all vascular beds within the body.

Generalized edema (Table 18-1) is important in the clinical practice of medicine, since it signals the presence of a number of important disease states. Edema may not be detectable until several liters of fluid are retained. The following sections consider the pathophysiologic events responsible for edema formation and some of the major clinical disorders associated with generalized edema. Later parts of this chapter develop the pathophysiologic principles that form the basis of edema therapy (see Chap. 19 for further consideration of this topic).

According to the traditional concept, generalized edema requires two conditions for its development.[98] First, there must be an imbalance of the forces that regulate the movement of fluid between intravascular and interstitial compartments, referred to as *Starling forces*, so that an outward movement of fluid across the capillary wall into the interstitial space is favored. Second, this perturbation of the Starling forces must be accompanied by the renal retention of sodium. In the absence of renal sodium retention, edema formation would be largely self-limited because the imbalance of Starling forces tends to correct itself as fluid accumulation progresses.

In general, the hydrostatic pressure in the vascular tree, the tissue fluid oncotic pressure, and the negative hydrostatic pressure in the interstitial compartment favor the movement of fluid out of the vascular space.[68] Only

TABLE 18-1 • Causes of Generalized Edema

COMMON CAUSES
Congestive heart failure
Cirrhosis
Nephrotic syndrome
Acute nephritic syndrome
Pregnancy
Normal
Toxemic
Idiopathic edema
Premenstrual tension syndrome
Nutritional or "hunger," edema
UNUSUAL CAUSES
Arteriovenous fistulas
Hypothyroidism
Diabetes mellitus ("insulin edema")
Associated with microangiopathy (rare)
Associated with insulin treatment of ketoacidosis
Entry into tropical environment
Capillary leak syndrome
Hereditary angioneurotic edema
Drugs
Estrogens, oral contraceptives
Vasodilator antihypertensive drugs
Nonsteroidal anti-inflammatory drugs
Lithium

plasma oncotic pressure promotes movement of fluid into the vascular compartment. Excess fluid filtered into the interstitial space is returned to the circulation by way of the lymphatics. If capillary permeability (to protein) increases or the aforementioned mechanisms are altered, a net movement of fluid into the interstitial compartment takes place.

Although the major edematous states differ with regard to both anatomic and functional abnormalities, they share a common deranged regulatory mechanism for maintaining sodium homeostasis. Thus, in cirrhosis of the liver, the volume receptors appear to be intact and functioning normally, but circulating blood volume is maldistributed such that the kidney behaves as if it were underperfused. In congestive heart failure (CHF), it has been proposed that sodium retention occurs because altered volume receptors are incapable of adequately signaling the kidney to excrete sodium.

All of the major edematous disease states are characterized by the unrelenting accumulation of salt and water. Even when fluid retention has become massive, the kidney often continues to retain salt and water, behaving as though it were responding to a volume deficit. It has been proposed that the stimulus for sodium retention is a reduction of the "effective" blood volume (EBV), a feature common to all major edematous states ("underfill theory"). Effective blood volume represents the part of the total circulating volume that is capable of stimulating volume receptors. The concept is somewhat elusive because the actual volume receptors remain incompletely defined. A diminished EBV may reflect subtle alterations in systemic hemodynamic factors such as decreased filling of the arterial tree, diminished central blood volume, or both. In normal circumstances, but not in the major edema states, EBV correlates with total ECF volume. Despite massive retention of salt and water, EBV remains functionally contracted because of a disturbance in the factors governing the distribution of fluid within the ECF compartment.

It is possible to understand why, according to this theory, the retained fluid in major edematous states fails to determine or modify the stimulus for continuing sodium and water retention. Despite a progressive increase in total ECF volume, fluid is sequestered in one or more of the other fluid compartments (i.e., the venous circulation or interstitial space) without normalizing EBV. Only a normalization of the disturbance in the forces governing fluid distribution can permit reexpansion of EBV to its original level. Recently, however, an alternative formulation, the *overflow theory*, has held that renal sodium retention is the *primary* event (see "Afferent Events").

In summary, in two of the major edematous disorders (i.e., CHF and cirrhosis), the kidney is not the culprit; rather, it is best seen as an innocent victim: the kidney's response is appropriate to the information it receives. What are inappropriate in these settings are the signals being transmitted to the kidney.

No attempt is made in this chapter to examine in detail the entire spectrum of the edematous disorders. Emphasis is instead given to the five major disorders frequently encountered in clinical practice; the minor disorders receive only brief consideration.

CONGESTIVE HEART FAILURE

It has been known for many years that the kidney plays a prominent role in the pathogenesis of CHF. Initially, the circulatory congestion characterizing CHF was thought to be merely a mechanical phenomenon, but subsequently workers realized that a more complex series of events is involved and that renal mechanisms play a key role in this process.[143,155] It is apparent that, regardless of the initial changes in cardiac or systemic hemodynamics that occur in CHF, the resultant expansion of the ECF volume requires that renal salt retention participate. That is, an inability to excrete ingested sodium is a fundamental component of this disease process.

It has been clearly demonstrated that the ability of the kidney to excrete sodium and water diminishes as the pumping ability of the heart declines, and that this derangement occurs early in CHF.[72] Thus, even though patients with *mild* heart failure may not be edematous, a reduced ability to excrete a sodium load can still be demonstrated.[98] In advanced heart failure, marked renal sodium retention is present, and only a small fraction of an infused or ingested salt load can be excreted.[11,72]

AFFERENT EVENTS

Two major theories have been offered to explain the initial events leading to sodium retention in CHF. Neither adequately encompasses all types of heart failure. The *backward failure* theory advocated by Starling[142] postulates that, as the heart failure worsens, venous pressure on the right side of the heart increases progressively. This rise is associated with increased hydrostatic pressure in the peripheral capillary beds, which promotes net transudation of fluid from the intravascular to the interstitial space. Intravascular hypovolemia results, which signals the kidney to conserve salt and water.

The *forward failure* theory promulgated by Starr and coworkers[143] and Warren and Stead[155] holds that decreasing cardiac output initiates the CHF process. This results in a reduction in renal perfusion, requiring the kidney to restore circulatory adequacy; the kidney attempts to do so by retaining salt and water. The retention of fluid causes expansion of the plasma volume, which, in the face of diminishing cardiac output, causes venous pressure to rise and excess fluid to accumulate in the interstitial space.

These two theories are not necessarily mutually exclusive. As pointed out by Homer Smith,[140] Starling originally incorporated elements of a forward failure theory into his formulation of the pathogenesis of edema formation in CHF.

The pathways signaling the kidney to retain sodium and water probably involve an afferent receptor system, the nature of which has not been definitively established. Considerable evidence exists of the presence of such receptors in both the low-pressure (central venous or pulmonary) circulation as well as in the high-pressure arterial side of the circulation.

Low-pressure receptors

Although considerable uncertainty exists as to the location of the critical receptors in the low-pressure circulation, it appears that the atria are likely sites.[61,125] Both atria have dense populations of nerve fibers that could respond to changes in central volume or pressure. Furthermore, numerous studies have shown that distension of either the left or the right atrium leads to enhanced sodium and water excretion.

High-pressure receptors

Considerable evidence suggests that volume or pressure receptors found in the high-pressure arterial circulation also modulate renal sodium excretion.[34,98] Although the responsible sensors have not yet been adequately defined, available data support the importance of baroreceptors of the aortic arch and carotid sinus in modifying renal sodium handling.

The nature of the afferent signals has not been precisely established. On one hand, it has been proposed that a reduction in cardiac output is itself the afferent stimulus.[103,129,130] Migdal and associates have suggested, as an alternative, that changes in intracardiac hemodynamics may be more important than arterial receptors in mediating the antinatriuresis of experimental CHF.[108] In their study, three separate maneuvers each lowered cardiac output by 25 to 30 percent in dogs; these procedures were pulmonary artery banding, thoracic inferior vena cava (TIVC) ligation, and left ventricular infarction. Sodium excretion, however, declined significantly only in the TIVC group.[108] Measurements of central pressure changes showed the only difference to be in the right ventricular end-diastolic pressure, which was reduced in the TIVC dogs and increased in the pulmonary artery-banded dogs. Similar findings in studies on conscious non-hydrated dogs have supported these conclusions.[162]

EFFERENT MECHANISMS

A cascade of events occurs in CHF that eventuates in renal sodium retention. Impaired cardiac emptying results in a rise in ventricular end-diastolic pressure. As depicted in Fig. 18-1, the increased venous pressure promotes transudation of fluid out of the vascular channel through several mechanisms. First, the mean capillary hydrostatic pressure is increased. Edema forms because the resulting rate of fluid transfer from peripheral capillaries to the interstitial space exceeds the rate of return of interstitial fluid to the intravascular compartment. Second, increased peripheral venous pressure may, in addition, cause a neurogenic resetting of pre- and postcapillary resistances, leading to increased capillary hydrostatic pressure and transudation of fluid from the intravascular to the interstitial space. Third, an increase in systemic venous pressure often leads to hepatic congestion, which may depress both plasma renin clearance and the hepatic metabolism of aldosterone. Fourth, there is reason to believe that an increase in systemic venous pressure per se may contribute to sodium retention via afferent pathways. Evidence exists supporting the presence of volume receptors in the venous portion of the central circulation (referred to as *low-pressure volume receptors*). It is thus possible that an increased venous pressure activates such receptors, leading to sodium retention by the kidneys. Furthermore, salt and water retention in CHF leads to a slight decrease in systemic plasma protein concentration, reducing the oncotic pressure gradient and thereby favoring edema formation. Finally, several lines of evidence

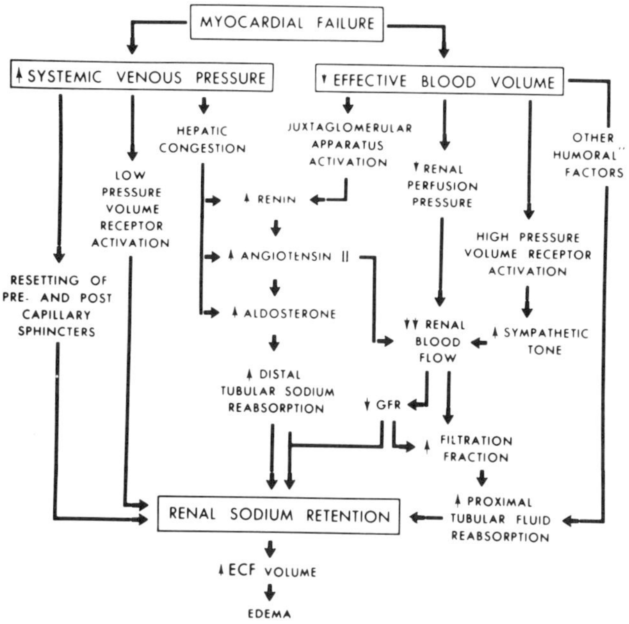

FIGURE 18-1 • The major pathophysiologic mechanisms leading to renal sodium retention in CHF. The increased systemic venous pressure promotes transudation of fluid out of the vascular channel by several mechanisms. A concomitant diminution in effective blood volume promotes renal sodium retention through several hormonal, hemodynamic, and neural mechanisms. (Modified from Humes HD et al in Brenner BM, Stein JH (eds): *Contemporary Issues in Nephrology: Sodium and Water Homeostasis*, New York, Churchill Livingstone, 1978. Used by permission.)

suggest that the increase in central venous pressure in CHF retards lymph flow in the thoracic duct, thereby decreasing lymphatic drainage of peripheral interstitial spaces.[73]

The kidneys respond to the diminished EBV by retaining salt. Several mechanisms participate. The reduced EBV activates the renin-angiotensin-aldosterone system, promoting sodium reabsorption in the distal segments of the nephron. Similarly, an increase in sympathetic tone appears to contribute to the observed elevations in peripheral and renal vascular resistance in CHF.

The decrease in renal plasma flow (RPF) is attributable to several mechanisms acting in concert (Fig. 18-1). The decline in renal perfusion is usually associated with little or no concurrent decline in the glomerular filtration rate (GFR), thereby resulting in a rise in the GFR/RPF ratio, or *filtration fraction*; the elevated filtration fraction is thought to play a fundamental role in promoting sodium retention (see Chap. 3).

Creager and colleagues[23] assessed the effects of angiotensin II in mediating the alterations in renal function in CHF in humans. These workers determined the effects of a converting-enzyme inhibitor (CEI) on renal hemodynamics and sodium handling. It was observed that CEI increased RPF by 60 percent in the absence of significant changes in GFR. As a consequence, the filtration fraction decreased from 0.41 to 0.33. Urinary sodium excretion doubled, and plasma aldosterone concentration decreased by two-thirds. These findings suggest that the renin-angiotensin system contributes to the impaired renal perfusion and sodium retention in CHF. However, the multiple effects of CEI, including lowering systemic vascular resistance and enhancing myocardial function, obscure the interpretation of the data.

As discussed earlier, enhanced sodium reabsorption mediated by these various mechanisms reexpands the *total* blood volume to values usually far in excess of normal. Despite such increases in ECF, EBV remains decreased; because the cardiac output remains low and central venous pressure remains elevated, the stimulus for salt retention persists.

Successful therapy for CHF consists of interrupting this vicious self-perpetuating cycle. Improvement of the pumping action of the heart increases EBV and lowers systemic venous pressure. Consequently, the two major afferent mechanisms that lead to salt and water retention in CHF are vitiated. Diuretic agents promote salt and water excretion; they are used in an attempt to control excessive fluid retention. Traditional teaching has been that diuretic-induced improvement in CHF derives from altering left ventricular function so as to displace its presumed position on the plot of Starling's law away from the descending limb of the curve (Fig. 18-2). Recent evidence, however, suggests that improved left ventricular performance results from reduced afterload, not from decreased preload.[157] Nevertheless, excessive diuresis might lead to marked intravascular volume depletion and decreases in cardiac output and renal perfusion.

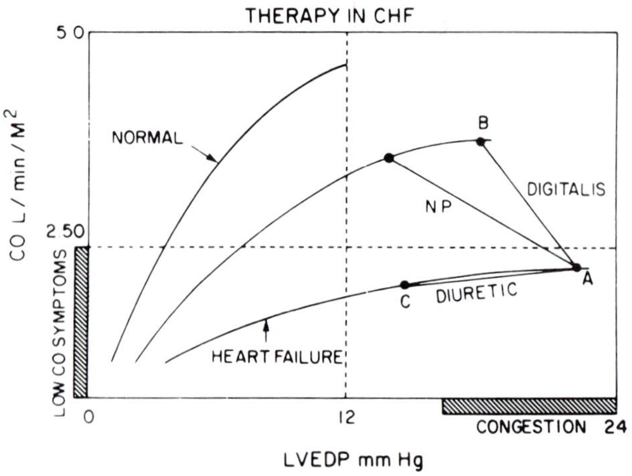

FIGURE 18-2 • An illustration of Starling's law of the heart. There is normally a dependence of cardiac output on left ventricular end diastolic pressure (LVEDP). The normal relationship is shown at the top of the figure; the relationship in severe congestive heart failure is at the bottom. Digitalis (point B) shifts the curve toward the normal relationship by virtue of its inotropic action on the myocardium. Diuretics (point C) do not shift the curve but, rather, decrease congestive symptoms owing to a decrease in plasma volume and LVEDP. Peripheral vasodilators such as nitroprusside (NP) reduce the afterload on the myocardium to simultaneously increase cardiac output and decrease congestion in the pulmonary circuit. (From Grantham JJ, Chonko AM in Brenner BM, Stein JH (eds): *Contemporary Issues in Nephrology: Sodium and Water Homeostasis*, New York, Churchill Livingstone, 1978. Used by permission.)

CIRRHOSIS

The clinical course of patients with decompensated Laennec's cirrhosis is complicated frequently by progressive renal sodium retention, leading to the formation of ascites and peripheral edema.[35,36,38,50,59,79,115] It should be underscored that cirrhotic patients who are unable to excrete sodium continue to gain weight and accumulate ascites and edema as long as dietary sodium content exceeds maximal urinary sodium excretion. If access to sodium is not curtailed, the relentless retention of salt may lead to the accumulation of vast amounts of ascites (on occasion 20 liters or more). Weight gain and ascites formation promptly cease when sodium intake is sufficiently limited. It should further be noted that the impairment of renal sodium handling in such patients is not an unalterable condition. Cirrhotic patients may undergo a spontaneous diuresis followed by a return to avid salt retention.[35,36,152]

A consideration of the pathogenetic events leading to the deranged sodium homeostasis of cirrhosis is simplified by consideration of the afferent and efferent mechanisms.

AFFERENT EVENTS

Traditionally, it has been thought that ascites formation in cirrhotic patients begins when a critical imbalance of Starling forces (portal hypertension and hypoalbuminemia) in the hepatic sinusoids and splanchnic capillaries causes an excessive amount of lymph to form, overwhelming the capacity of the thoracic duct to return the lymph to the circulation.[158] Consequently, lymph accumulates in the peritoneal space as ascites; circulating plasma volume then contracts. Thus, as ascites develops, there is a progressive redistribution of plasma volume. Even though *total* plasma volume may be increased in this setting, the physiologic circumstance may mimic a reduction in plasma volume (reduced EBV).[36,38,118,132] The diminished effective volume constitutes an afferent signal to the renal tubule to augment salt and water reabsorption. Although an imbalance of Starling forces in the hepatosplanchnic microcirculation is thought to make an important contribution to the relative decrease in EBV, this is not the sole mechanism. An additional determinant is total peripheral resistance, which is diminished

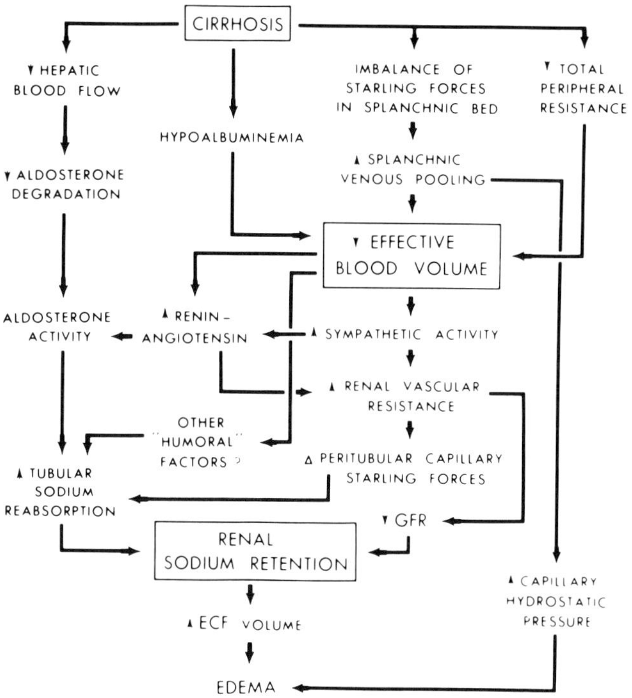

FIGURE 18-3 • Schematic drawing of the factors operative in the traditional, underfiling theory of sodium retention in cirrhosis. The figure shows that an imbalance of Starling forces in the hepatosplanchnic microcirculation is not the sole mechanism of sodium retention. Acting in concert, these factors promote a reduction in effective plasma volume.

significantly in most patients with cirrhosis who are retaining sodium and water (see below). This decrease in peripheral vascular resistance is related in part to the presence of arteriovenous shunts, but a role for some putative vasodilator (not yet defined, but either produced by or at least not inactivated by the diseased liver) has been proposed. Thus, despite an increase in *total* plasma volume, the relative "fullness" of the vascular tree is diminished. As shown in Fig. 18-3, several hemodynamic events act in concert to diminish effective volume, thereby activating the mechanisms promoting sodium retention.

In summary, the traditional formulation suggests that the renal retention of sodium in cirrhosis is a secondary rather than a primary event.

Peripheral arterial vasodilation hypothesis

Recently, an alternative hypothesis, termed the *peripheral arterial vasodilation hypothesis*, has been proposed to account for the initiation of sodium and water retention in cirrhosis.[133] One may regard this theory as a revision of the underfill theory. The principal distinguishing feature of this newly proposed theory is that the decrease in effective blood volume is attributable primarily to an early increase in vascular capacitance. Thus, peripheral vasodilatation is the initial determinant of intravascular underfilling, and an imbalance between the expanded capacitance and the available volume constitutes a diminished effective volume. This formulation recognizes that total peripheral resistance is diminished significantly in most edematous cirrhotic patients and in animals with toxic cirrhosis[95,96] or with bile duct ligation.[136] Furthermore, this concept brings the hypothesis into accord with some experimental observations that were not consistent with the original postulate. For example, careful balanced studies in animals with experimental cirrhosis have clearly shown that sodium retention precedes ascites formation.[95,96]

Both underfill theories provide a possible explanation of why fluid retention may fail to attenuate the stimulus for continuing sodium and water retention. Despite a progressive increase in total ECF volume, fluid is sequestered into one or more of the other fluid compartments without normalizing EBV. Only correction of the disturbance in the forces governing fluid distribution will permit a reexpansion of EBV.

Overflow theory

During the past two decades, an alternative hypothesis has been proposed. Lieberman and associates proposed the *overflow theory* of ascites formation.[100,101] In contrast to the traditional model, the overflow theory proposes that the primary event in ascites formation is the inappropriate retention of sodium by the kidneys, with resulting expansion of plasma volume. The mechanisms underlying primary renal sodium retention have not been defined, although Levy[95] has suggested that elevated intrahepatic pressure causes reflex stimulation of efferent renal sympathetic nerve activity. In the setting of abnormal Starling forces (venous hypertension and reduced plasma colloid osmotic pressure, or COP) in the portal venous bed and hepatic sinusoids, the increased plasma volume is sequestered preferentially in the peritoneal space as ascites. Thus, according to this scheme, renal sodium retention and plasma volume expansion precede rather, than follow, the formation of ascites.

The overflow theory of ascites formation has provoked much controversy. In support of the theory, one can cite the demonstration of increased plasma volume in cirrhosis with ascites and the finding that increases in measured plasma volume have not been observed in ascitic cirrhotic patients undergoing a spontaneous diuresis. Additional support has come from a series of elegant investigations carried out by Levy and coworkers on dogs.[95,96,97] The animals were fed dimethylnitrosamine to produce experimental portal cirrhosis. Levy's group demonstrated in sequential studies that renal sodium retention precedes ascites formation.

Although the abovementioned observations collectively support the overflow theory of ascites formation, a number of clinical observations in humans are inconsistent with such a formulation. Thus, rapid volume expansion by exogenous solutions, including saline solution, frequently results in a transient improvement in renal sodium and water handling.[128,148,154] However, the volume of *all* ECF compartments is increased by these maneuvers; concomitant alterations in plasma composition are presumed to occur. This lack of specificity has precluded definitive statements regarding the etiologic role of a diminished EBV. Thus, the results of many earlier studies must be questioned because of uncertainties inherent in the experimental designs and the confounding of plasma volume effects by changes in plasma composition.

Studies from our laboratory over the past 20 years have circumvented many of these problems by applying a unique investigative tool, the water immersion model, to the assessment of the relationships of renal function to volume changes and hormonal alterations.[34,42,45,94] Before these findings are enumerated, the differences between water immersion and more traditional attempts at achieving expansion of ECF volume should be emphasized.

In contrast to saline administration, water immersion is associated with a decrease in body weight. The volume stimulus of immersion is promptly reversible after cessation of immersion: hypervolemia from saline administration, in contrast, is relatively sustained.[94] The reversibility of immersion-induced ECF volume expansion constitutes an important attribute in minimizing any risk to the patient. Also unlike saline administration, immersion stimulates volume change in the absence of changes in plasma composition.[34] Immersion may be thought of as a potent "central volume stimulus" that does not entail infusing exogenous volume expanders. Its potency suggested that it might be used to assess the role of changes in *effective* plasma volume in modifying renal sodium homeostasis in cirrhosis.

Studies in 32 patients with decompensated cirrhosis demonstrated that water immersion strikingly normalized renal sodium handling.[36] As shown in Fig. 18-4,

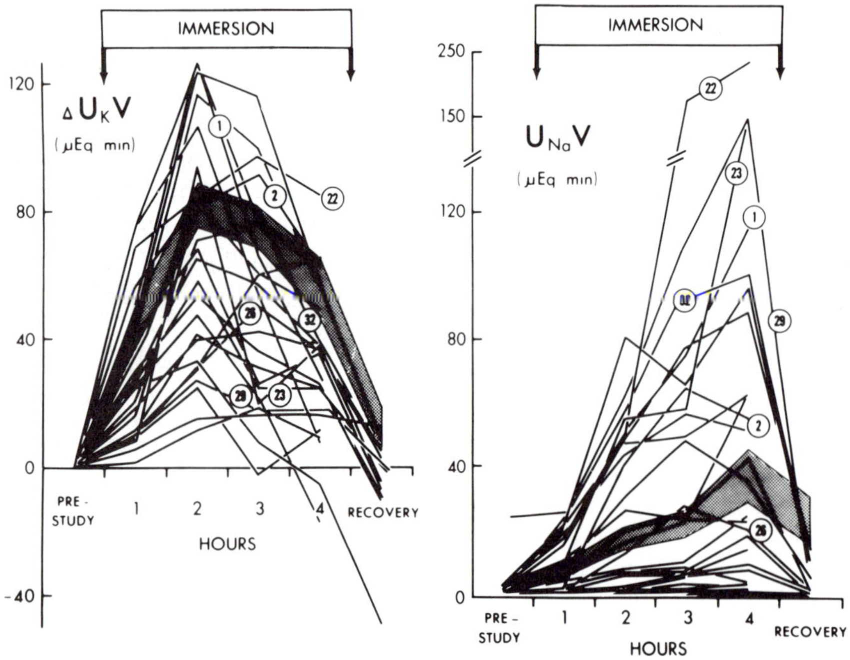

FIGURE 18-4 • Effects of water immersion, following 1 h of quiet sitting (prestudy), on the sodium excretion rate ($U_{Na}V$) and potassium excretion rate ($U_K V$) in a large group of alcoholic liver disease patients. Circled numbers represent individual patients. Data for $U_K V$ are expressed in terms of absolute changes from the rate during the preimmersion period, $\Delta U_K V$. The shaded area represents the mean plus or minus of 14 normal control subjects undergoing an identical immersion study while ingesting an identical 10 meq sodium/100 meq potassium diet. Over half of the cirrhosis patients manifested an appropriate or "exaggerated" natriuretic response. In general, the increase in $U_{Na}V$ was associated with a concomitant increase in $\Delta U_K V$. (From Epstein M in Epstein M, (ed): *The Kidney in Liver Disease*, 3d ed, New York, Elsevier/North Holland, 1983. Used by permission.)

immersion resulted in marked natriuresis and kaliuresis in the majority of these patients. During the final 1 h of immersion, the rate of sodium secretion ($U_{Na}V$) was 20 times greater than it was during the 1 h before the study. Thus, the marked antinatriuresis of cirrhosis was promptly reversed by a manipulation that altered the distribution of plasma volume without increasing total plasma volume; indeed, plasma volume often decreased. These studies lend strong support to the concept that a diminished EBV is a major determinant of the enhanced tubular reabsorption of sodium in cirrhosis.

We believe that the available evidence favors a prominent role for diminished EBV in mediating the avid sodium retention of many cirrhotic patients. It should be emphasized, though, that the two models described above may not be mutually exclusive. As already noted, cirrhosis is a dynamic clinical disorder.[36,59] Yet, virtually all the available clinical studies of deranged sodium homeostasis were carried out at a single *stage* of the disease, at a time when decompensation was well established, with little information available during the incipient stage of sodium retention. In contrast, the studies with the canine cirrhosis model deal with the relatively early stage of sodium retention. Any formulation that suggests that the same antinatriuretic forces are operative throughout the evolution of sodium retention in human cirrhosis is probably a marked oversimplification. The pathogenesis of abnormal sodium retention in cirrhosis may be viewed as involving differing forces that participate in varying degrees.

EFFERENT EVENTS

The decreased GFR that commonly accompanies advanced liver disease was initially thought to be the sole cause of salt retention. It is now clear that the same abnormalities of renal sodium handling can occur despite preserved or, at times, supranormal GFRs.[16,84] These observations emphasize that the renal sodium retention accompanying cirrhosis is attributable primarily to enhanced tubular reabsorption rather than to alterations in the filtered load of sodium.[16,44]

The mediators of the enhanced tubular reabsorption of sodium in cirrhosis and their relative importance have not been completely elucidated. Nevertheless, several hormonal, neural, and hemodynamic mechanisms have been implicated or suggested. Those mechanisms for which there is some evidence, and their interrelationships, are summarized schematically in Fig. 18-5.

Hyperaldosteronism

The diminution of effective plasma volume results in activation of the renin-angiotensin system. As a consequence, aldosterone secretion is augmented, which in

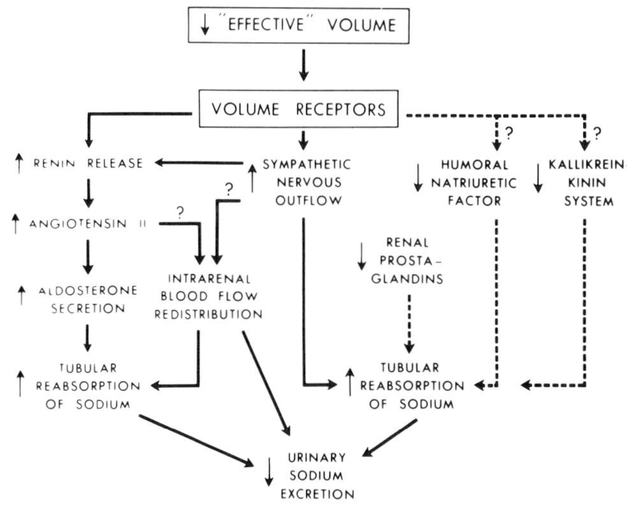

FIGURE 18-5 • Schematic drawing of possible mechanisms whereby a diminished *effective* volume results in sodium retention in cirrhosis. The heavy arrows indicate pathways for which corroboratory evidence is available. The dashed lines represent proposed pathways, the existence of which remains to be established. (From Epstein M et al: *Gastroenterology* 76:622, 1979. Used by permission.)

turn stimulates sodium reabsorption in the distal segments of the nephron. The increased urinary[22] and plasma[49,127] aldosterone levels in many patients with decompensated cirrhosis has led many observers to propose that this hormone is the major determinant of sodium retention.

A number of recent studies have questioned the validity of this formulation, suggesting that the increased plasma aldosterone levels and the sodium retention of cirrhosis may not be causally related. As discussed in several recent reviews,[36,50] investigators have demonstrated a dissociation of sodium excretion and plasma aldosterone concentration in cirrhotic patients. Renal sodium excretion has been demonstrated to vary independently of plasma aldosterone in patients undergoing a spontaneous diuresis following aminoglutethimide administration[127] and following long-term oral sodium loading.[18] The application of the immersion model to an assessment of the relationship of plasma aldosterone levels to renal sodium handling has amplified such earlier observations.[36,40,43]

Immersion of patients with decompensated cirrhosis promptly and profoundly (66 percent) reduced plasma aldosterone concentration in 15 of 16 patients.[40] Despite suppression of plasma aldosterone to similar low levels in all patients, 8 patients manifested markedly blunted or no natriuretic response during immersion. This demonstration that the suppression of circulating aldosterone is dissociated from the absence of natriuresis lends strong support to the interpretation that aldosterone is not the primary determinant of the impaired sodium excretion in cirrhosis. Additional studies with spironolactone administration during immersion have supported this interpretation.[40]

Taken together, all the evidence currently available therefore favors the postulate that the hyperaldosteronism of cirrhosis is a permissive factor only and that the predominant component of the abnormal renal sodium handling is a diminished distal delivery of filtrate. Only when distal filtrate delivery is enhanced by an experimental or pharmacological maneuver does the effect of aldosterone on renal sodium handling in cirrhosis become evident.

The demonstration that hyperaldosteronism cannot completely account for sodium retention in cirrhosis has prompted a search for other hormonal mediators that participate in this derangement.

Role of the renin-angiotensin system

One attractive explanation for the sodium retention of cirrhosis is derived from the recent observation that the intrarenal renin-angiotensin system influences renal sodium handling independently of changes in plasma aldosterone concentration. Studies in conscious, uninephrectomized dogs have demonstrated that the intrarenal infusion of the angiotensin II antagonist, 1-sar-8-ala angiotensin II, or a converting enzyme inhibitor, SQ 20881, resulted in significant increases in urinary sodium excretion.[83] Such observations suggest that endogenous angiotensin II may exert intrarenal effects leading to salt retention. Perhaps the most compelling evidence of the role of intrarenal angiotensin in mediating enhanced sodium reabsorption is derived from studies utilizing an inhibitor of angiotensin-converting enzyme in humans. Hollenberg and associates[74] have demonstrated that the administration of teprotide (an inhibitor of angiotensin-converting enzyme) to patients with essential hypertension induced a significant natriuresis in every patient. Since the natriuresis occurred within as little as 20 min of teprotide administration and since the offset in aldosterone's renal action is measured in hours, the natriuresis was clearly independent of a suppression of aldosterone. If such a mechanism applies to cirrhotic humans, it is conceivable that the stimulated renin-angiotensin system observed in many patients with cirrhosis may contribute directly to impaired renal sodium handling.

Renal prostaglandins

Within the past two decades, increasing evidence has accumulated suggesting that alterations in renal prostaglandins (PGs) may be important in mediating sodium retention (see Chap. 15).[10] Administration of inhibitors of synthetase (both indomethacin and ibuprofen) significantly decreases both GFR and effective renal plasma flow (ERPF) in patients with alcoholic liver disease.[9,48a,164] The decrements in renal hemodynamics varied directly with the degree of sodium retention: the patients with the most avid sodium retention manifested the largest decrements in GFR.[20,164]

We believe that the abovementioned findings are not isolated observations. As noted in a recent review,[48,48a] renal PGs may be thought of as critical modulators of renal function during conditions or disease states involving volume reduction. The demonstration that PG synthetase inhibition affects renal function only in decompensated but not in compensated cirrhotic patients, (i.e., in the presence of ascites and/or edema) and that the effects of synthetase inhibition vary as a function of the degree of renal sodium avidity, is consistent with this formulation.[164]

Since the studies cited above examined the effect of inhibiting endogenous production of renal PGs, it was important to assess the effect of an increased level of *endogenous* PGs on changes in renal function. Our recent demonstration that water immersion up to the neck constitutes a unique means of augmenting urinary PG excretion, and presumably renal PG synthesis,[47] prompted an examination of the relationship of immersion-induced changes in PGs and renal sodium handling. Immersion of cirrhotic patients promptly increased mean PGE excretion three times more than that observed in normal subjects studied under identical conditions.[41] That the GFR increased in most of these patients in response to immersion, and that all manifested a marked natriuresis, is consistent with the importance of renal PG synthesis as a determinant of renal hemodynamics and renal sodium handling in decompensated cirrhosis. When interpreted in concert with the earlier studies using PG synthetase inhibitors, these findings suggest that perturbations of renal PGE production contributes to the renal dysfunction in cirrhosis. Specifically, it is tempting to postulate that, in the setting of cirrhosis of the liver (and presumably other disorders characterized by diminished EBV), enhanced PG synthesis acts as a compensatory or adaptive response to incipient renal ischemia. The corollary of this proposition is that the administration of agents that impair or attenuate such an adaptation might result in a clinically important deterioration of renal function. Additional studies are necessary to characterize further the role of PG alterations in determining renal sodium retention in cirrhosis.

If this formulation is valid, one may inquire how it can be reconciled with discrepant reports of both elevated and depressed PGE levels in patients with advanced cirrhosis and sodium retention.[41,164] Previous proposals suggesting that urinary PGE levels are increased in cirrhotic patients with ascites are not totally consistent with the literature. As we have noted elsewhere, others have found either normal or depressed levels in patients with advanced cirrhosis.[41] In our view, the enhanced PGE excretory levels in some patients with decompensated cirrhosis should be viewed as an insufficient (and thus failing) attempt at natriuresis. Patients with "normal" or modestly elevated levels are considered to be unable to mount a sufficient compensatory response; they may be at an even higher risk of renal failure and sodium retention. The finding of elevated PG levels in some patients with decompensated cirrhosis does not militate against the theory that an impairment of a compensatory response of renal PGs contributes to the sodium retention.

Sympathetic nervous system

An increase in sympathetic nervous system activity may contribute to the sodium retention of cirrhosis. It is now well established that alterations in the input from cardiopulmonary receptors induce changes in renal sympathetic activity.[145,163] Thus, a decrease in blood volume can modify the afferent input from these receptors, thereby increasing sympathetic nerve activity.[34,163] Alterations in adrenergic nervous activity can modify urinary sodium excretion by several mechanisms: (1) by influencing Starling forces in the peripheral capillary bed, (2) by affecting the central blood volume and thus the distribution of the ECF, or (3) by influencing renal sympathetic nerve activity.

The mechanisms whereby renal sympathetic nerves modulate renal sodium reabsorption are multiple. Increases in efferent renal sympathetic nerve activity (ERSNA) produce renal vasoconstriction with decreases in renal blood flow and GFR. In addition, increased ERSNA favors sodium retention by possibly altering intrarenal hemodynamics with a preferential redistribution toward the outer cortical nephrons.[144] Recently, much attention has been directed to the ability of increased sympathetic tone to promote an antinatriuresis without eliciting changes in GFR, renal blood flow, or intrarenal distribution of blood flow.[26-28] It should be noted that this direct renal tubular effect of increased ERSNA acts at several loci in the nephron. Recent evidence suggests that increased ERSNA enhances reabsorption in the proximal convoluted tubule, Henle's loop, and the distal convoluted tubule.

Despite such theoretical considerations, there are relatively few data bearing on the importance of alterations in the sympathetic nervous system in cirrhotic individuals. Studies by Epstein and coworkers[39] have raised the possibility that adrenergic activity may be enhanced in cirrhosis. In the course of assessing intrarenal hemodynamics in cirrhotic patients, these investigators observed that the intrarenal infusion of the alpha-adrenergic blocker phentolamine failed to increase renal blood flow significantly in cirrhotic patients. Although the failure of phentolamine to enhance renal perfusion was interpreted initially as indicating the absence of increased renal adrenergic tone, caution is required in reaching such a conclusion. It should be underscored that a majority of patients who received an intrarenal infusion of phentolamine manifested transient hypotension with significant reductions in arterial blood pressure. It is conceivable that such concomitant alterations in systemic hemodynamics would have masked any phentolamine-induced enhancement of renal perfusion.

The important question of whether renal sympathetic nerve activity is increased in cirrhosis has been assessed by measuring norepinephrine levels in peripheral plasma and renal venous blood, measuring renal veno-arterial norepinephrine concentration differences, assessing kidney norepinephrine secretion and extraction, and looking for increased rates of norepinephrine spillover to plasma for the body as a whole.[58,71,110,163] Metabolism of norepinephrine has also been studied in individual organs and in specific vascular territories, such as the kidneys.[70,71]

Bichet and coworkers[6] have reported that patients with advanced cirrhosis manifest elevated concentrations of plasma catecholamines. These investigators proposed that the encountered catecholamine changes accounted for the impaired sodium handling in their patients.

Although most observers agree that mean peripheral norepinephrine levels are elevated in cirrhotic patients, it is an oversimplification to suggest that such alterations in catecholamine metabolism affect all cirrhotic patients with deranged sodium and water homeostasis.[131] Recently, we examined the relationship between plasma norepinephrine levels and renal sodium and water handling during immersion-induced central blood volume expansion.[46] Although mean norepinephrine levels were elevated for the group as a whole, more than half of the patients with decompensated cirrhosis manifested appropriate (i.e., not elevated) norepinephrine levels. Furthermore, norepinephrine levels did not correlate with alterations in renal sodium or water excretion (Fig. 18-6).

In summary, despite an incomplete data base, the available evidence suggests that the sympathetic nervous system is of prime importance in mediating sodium retention in cirrhosis. In studies in experimental models of cirrhosis, including bile duct-ligated animals the sympathetic nervous system has been implicated in mediating sodium retention. Studies in cirrhotics have begun to show correlations between increased peripheral and/or renal sympathetic nervous system activity and renal sodium retention.

Kallikrein-kinin system

Preliminary evidence has suggested that diminished kinin formation may contribute to sodium retention in liver disease.[112] Wong and colleagues observed that "functional plasma prekallikrein" (i.e., esterase) was reduced in patients with severe cirrhosis and patients with the hepatorenal syndrome, and plasma bradykinin was also decreased.[160] As would be expected, plasma renin ac-

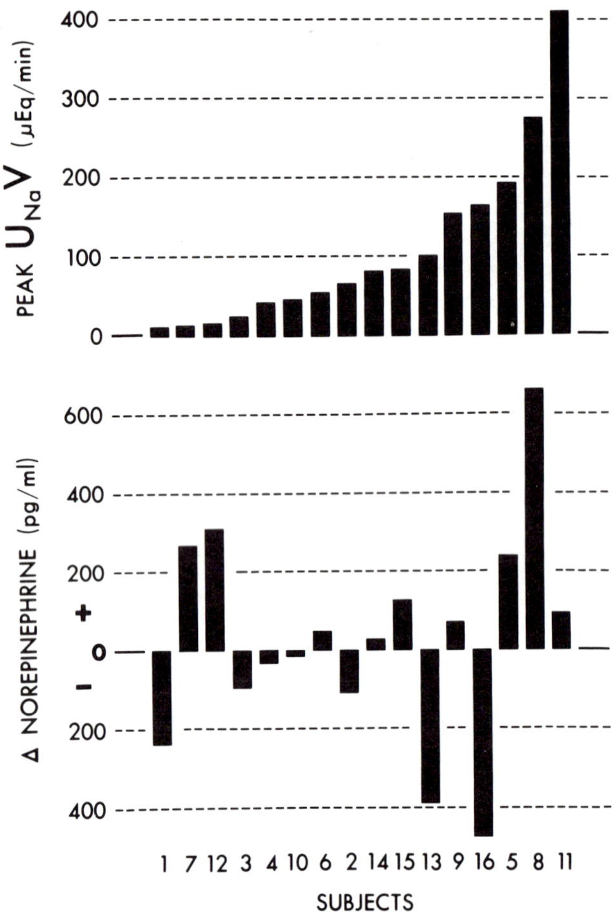

FIGURE 18-6 • Relationship of renal sodium excretion *(upper panel)* to alterations in plasma norepinephrine *(lower panel)* during immersion in 16 cirrhotic patients. The numbers along the horizontal axis designate the individual patients. As can be seen, the magnitude of the natriuresis, as assessed by peak $U_{Na}V$, varied independently of Δ norepinephrine (nadir minus prestudy norepinephrine) during immersion (r = 0.256; NS). (From Epstein M et al: *Miner Electrolyte Metab*, 11:25, 1985. Used by permission.)

tivity (PRA) was greatly increased in both groups. The authors speculated that the vasodilator (kinin) deficiency (perhaps in conjunction with vasoconstrictor excess) may contribute to the pathogenetic mechanisms mediating both sodium retention and renal failure.

More recently, Zipser and associates studied a series of patients with alcoholic cirrhosis. Urinary kallikrein excretion was diminished in cirrhotic patients, with or without ascites, despite elevated plasma aldosterone concentrations and increased urinary PGE excretion in the patients with ascites.[165] PG synthetase inhibition reduced creatinine clearance in the group, but neither PG synthetase inhibition nor spironolactone appreciably altered kallikrein excretion in the individuals with cirrhosis.[165] These findings were interpreted by the authors as suggesting not only that activity of the renal kallikrein-kinin system is diminished in cirrhosis, but also that kallikrein excretion in dissociated in cirrhotic patients from its usual modulating influences.

The preliminary studies cited above are of interest, but additional studies encompassing evaluations of the *renal* kallikrein-kinin system are necessary to characterize further the role of the kallikrein-kinin system as a determinant of the abnormal sodium retention of cirrhosis.

Role of humoral natriuretic factors

Within the past several years, increasing evidence has accumulated pointing to the existence of a circulating natriuretic factor that normally depresses renal tubular reabsorption in response to ECF volume expansion.[15,24] Buckalew and Gruber have recently published a scholarly review summarizing the evidence of the existence of a natriuretic hormone and the recent developments in its characterization.[15] Preliminary indications suggest that this hormone is a low-molecular weight peptide, which is formed by enzymatic degradation of a larger precursor. Its release is controlled, at least in part, by mechanoreceptors in the low-pressure circulation,[15,34,61] and it appears to function as an endogenous digitalis-like substance. Biologic effects that have been ascribed to the putative natriuretic hormone include (1) the ability to induce natriuresis, (2) inhibition of sodium transport (antinatriferic activity), (3) inhibition of Na^+-K^+ ATPase, and (4) increased vascular reactivity.

The possible existence of such a natriuretic factor is relevant to considerations of the mechanisms of sodium retention and edema formation in cirrhosis.[57,109] A hypothesis that is implicit in this concept is that sodium retention results from a failure to elaborate natriuretic hormone when renal sodium retention causes ECF volume to increase. In cirrhosis, release of such a natriuretic hormone might be suppressed because the splanchnic sequestration of ECF prevents restoration of "effective" arterial filling, despite surpluses of salt and water in the vascular and interstitial spaces.

Role of atrial natriuretic factor

It recently has been shown that mammalian atria contain potent natriuretic and vasoactive peptide(s), which have been referred to as atrial natriuretic factor (ANF; see Chap. 3).[105] Several laboratories have purified, sequenced, and synthesized atrial peptides that have the natriuretic and vasoactive properties of crude atrial extract. Maack and associates[105] characterized the renal hemodynamic and hormonal effects of ANF by investigating the effects of a continuous infusion of the synthetic hormone on blood pressure, renal hemodynamics, GFR, and renal excretory functions in intact dogs. The results demonstrate that this peptide of atrial origin decreases blood pressure and increases GFR and sodium excretion without a sustained increase in RPF. In addition, synthetic ANF decreased the renin secretory rate, plasma renin levels, and plasma aldosterone levels. Taken together, these observations suggest an important potential role for ANF in the regulation of blood pressure, renal function, and sodium-volume homeostasis.

It is tempting to attribute a cardinal role to this peptide in modulating renal sodium handling under normal and edematous conditions in light of several lines of evidence suggesting that stretch receptors residing in the atria may participate in regulating volume homeostasis.[36,38,61] Specifically, the sodium retention and activation of the renin-angiotensin-aldosterone system in patients with cirrhosis may result from a failure to elaborate ANF when ECF volume increases in response to renal sodium retention.

Despite such theoretical considerations, recent evidence indicates that a deficiency of circulating ANF levels per se does not account for the sodium retention.[1,37,52,53] Determinations of plasma ANF levels have disclosed that they are not suppressed in such patients; indeed, they tend to be elevated, exceeding those of normal subjects studied under similar conditions. Studies of ANF responsiveness utilizing stimulatory maneuvers, including water immersion and portal-systemic venous shunting, disclosed that ANF is released appropriately (Fig. 18-7).[1,37,51,52,139] Collectively, these findings indicate that a deficiency of ANF synthesis and release does not contribute substantively to the sodium and water retention that afflicts many patients with advanced liver disease.

In summary, it is apparent that the renal sodium retention of advanced liver disease is a complex pathophysiologic constellation with numerous and diverse causes. Increasing evidence demonstrates that the attribution of deranged sodium handling to abnormalities of aldosterone is an oversimplification and that, more likely, this disordered physiology is due to the combined effects of perturbations of several regulatory systems. Several lines of evidence point strongly to the importance of the renal PG system in contributing to sodium retention. Provocative suggestions regarding the participation of the sympathetic nervous system have been advanced, but the contribution of that system remains to be established.

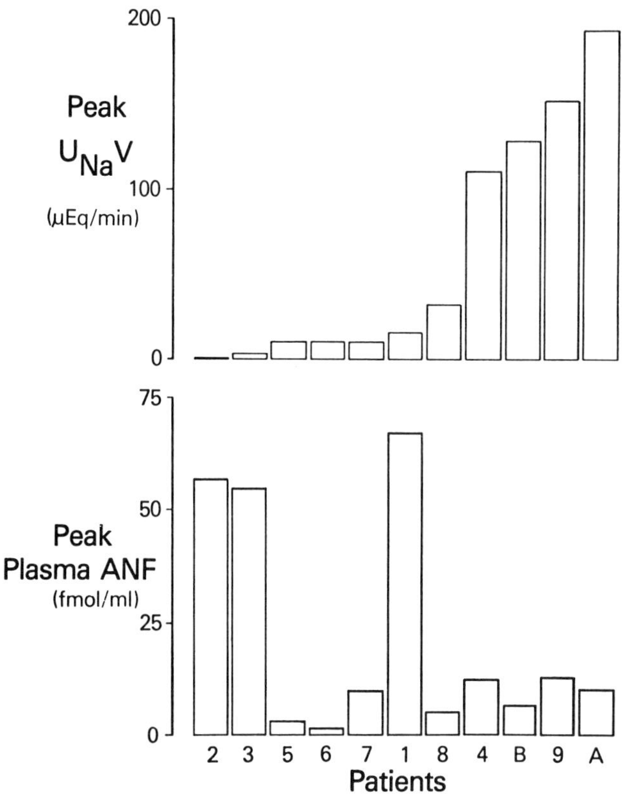

FIGURE 18-7 • Relationship of renal sodium excretion *(upper panel)* to peak plasma ANF *(lower panel)* during immersion in 11 cirrhotic patients. As can be seen, the magnitude of the natriuresis, as assessed by peak $U_{Na}V$, varied independently of peak plasma ANF during immersion ($r = 0.36$; $p > 0.2$). (Modified from Epstein M et al: *Am J Nephrol* 133, 1989. Used by permission.)

RENAL DISEASE

Sodium retention in glomerular disease is mediated by two major mechanisms. The first mechanism is associated with heavy proteinuria and hypoalbuminemia, leading to an alteration of the Starling forces across capillaries and translocation of fluid into the interstitial space (nephrotic edema). The resultant contraction of plasma volume activates several humoral, neural, and hemodynamic mechanisms that signal the kidney to retain sodium. The other mechanism is intrarenal in nature; it involves decreases in GFR and other incompletely understood events that lead to stimulation of sodium reabsorption (nephritic edema; Table 18-2).

TABLE 18-2 • Comparison Between Nephritic and Nephrotic Edema

	Nephritic edema	Nephrotic edema
Glomerular filtration rate	↓	→ ↓
Plasma volume	↑	→ ↓
Blood pressure	↑	→ ↓
Plasma renin activity	↓	→ ↑
Plasma aldosterone concentration	↓	→ ↑
Plasma oncotic pressure	→	↓
Extracellular fluid volume	↑	↑
Urinary sodium excretion	↓	↓
Filtration fraction	↓	↓

NOTE: ↓ is decreased, ↑ is increased, → is unchanged.

NEPHROTIC SYNDROME

Adult humans normally excrete up to 150 mg/day of protein in the urine. In the setting of renal disease with involvement of the glomerulus, proteinuria (>150 mg/day) often ensues. When the magnitude of protein losses and catabolism exceed that of hepatic albumin production, the concentration of plasma albumin declines, and the signs and symptoms of the nephrotic syndrome develop. The nephrotic syndrome may be defined as heavy proteinuria (≥3.5 g/day), predominantly albuminuria, with concomitant hypoalbuminemia, edema, and hyperlipidemia. Edema is the most prominent manifestation of the nephrotic syndrome and often provides the first evidence of disease noted by patients.

Afferent events

The pathogenesis of sodium retention in the nephrotic syndrome remains incompletely understood.[5,31] The traditional formulation holds that the reduction of the plasma colloid osmotic pressure (COP) associated with heavy and sustained proteinuria alters the Starling forces in the systemic capillaries; a translocation of fluid from the intravascular compartment to the interstitial space is therefore induced (Fig. 18-8).[12,64,75,161] The resultant contraction of the intravascular compartment is thought to activate a variety of mechanisms that signal the kidney to retain sodium and water. The retained fluid may not correct the diminished vascular volume. In fact, fluid retention may lead to a further decrease in the plasma COP, which then results in additional movement of fluid to the interstitial space. Eventually, a steady state is achieved due to the progressive increase in tissue hydrostatic pressure and to other factors that slow down the redistribution of fluid between the two extracellular fluid compartments.

The albumin concentration in lymph is decreased in the nephrotic syndrome;[111] hence, there is no evidence of a capillary permeability defect. Likewise, there are no reported abnormalities in lymphatic drainage in nephrotic patients.[75,92]

The traditional concept that reduced intravascular volume activates renal sodium-retaining mechanisms has not always stood up to scrutiny.[33,60,78] Meltzer and associates[107] used measurements of plasma renin activity (PRA) as an index of EBV in 16 patients with nephrotic syndrome. They found that only 25 percent of their patients had elevated PRA levels, suggesting that intravascular volume depletion was not the most important mechanism of sodium retention in their patients. Patients with high PRA had minimal-change disease and less hypertension and azotemia than did those with low PRA. These observations suggest that additional factors, such as superimposed decreases in GFR, may participate in the pathogenesis of edema formation.

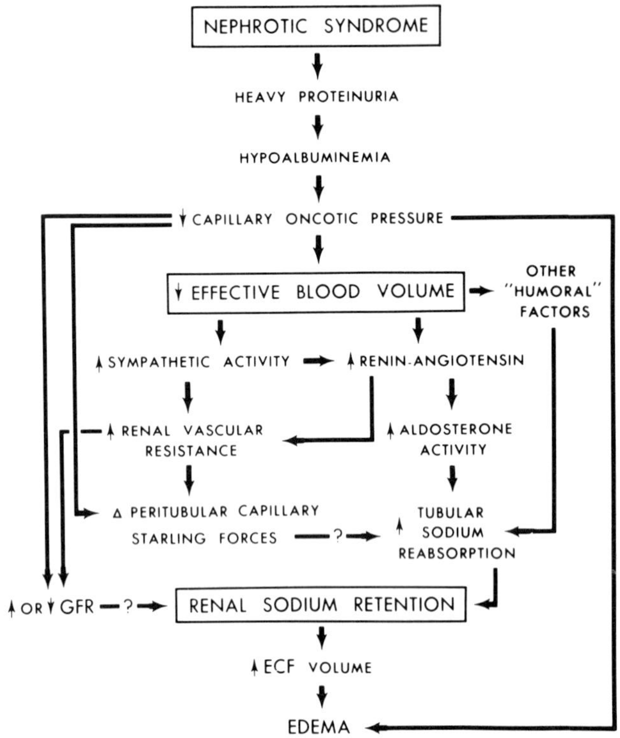

FIGURE 18-8 • The major pathophysiologic mechanisms leading to renal sodium retention in the nephrotic syndrome according to the traditional theory. Massive proteinuria leads to hypoalbuminemia and decreased plasma oncotic pressure, with resultant diminution in total blood volume and effective blood volume. The figure shows the sequence of potential hormonal, hemodynamic, and neural events that may be activated as a consequence and the manner in which they may interact to promote sodium retention.

Plasma aldosterone concentrations and PRA are increased in fewer than 50 percent of patients with the nephrotic syndrome,[13,31,134] and plasma norepinephrine and vasopressin levels are normal.[134] In contrast, Rascher and Tulassay[124] and Tulassay and coworkers[149] reported that edematous nephrotic children with minimal-change disease had higher plasma levels of PRA, aldosterone, vasopressin, and norepinephrine than did healthy controls. The results of their studies and those of Usberti and associates[151] and Trachtman and associates[147] suggest that nonosmotic stimuli may be responsible for the elevated vasopressin levels and water retention in the nephrotic syndrome. Of interest, ANF levels were found to be normal or decreased in several studies.[120,122,124] Nevertheless, end-organ resistance to ANF has been postulated to play a role in the pathogenesis of nephrotic edema.[119,120]

Several investigators have recently reported that blood volume was reduced in only one-third or fewer of their patients, the rest exhibiting normal or high values.[13,55,87,88,137] Dorhout Mees and colleagues evaluated adult patients with minimal-change disease before and after corticosteroid-induced remissions.[31] Prior to treatment, all subjects exhibited moderately expanded plasma volumes. Remission was associated with a decrease in blood pressure and plasma volume. More recently, these investigators confirmed that plasma volume is usually normal or increased in nephrotic patients.[62] In contrast, a group of 16 adults, 8 of whom had minimal-change disease, exhibited blood volumes that were less than those in control subjects and were inversely and significantly related to PRA.[151]

Several studies have examined the effect of acute volume expansion on urinary sodium excretion in nephrotic subjects. Koomans and coworkers[85] showed that, although plasma volume increased substantially with hyperoncotic albumin, urinary sodium excretion increased only slightly, suggesting that plasma volume contraction was not the important sodium-retaining stimulus. Likewise, Brown and coworkers[113] gave 40 g of salt-poor albumin for three days to nephrotic patients and failed to induce a negative sodium balance.

Expansion of central blood volume induced by water immersion resulted in moderate increases in sodium and water excretion in two studies.[3,89] However, preimmersion plasma volume was normal or increased in many of the patients. Nevertheless, water immersion and albumin infusions resulted in a reduction of PRA, aldosterone, vasopressin, and norepinephrine levels and a rise in sodium and water excretion in nephrotic children.[123,124] Plasma ANP increased fivefold during albumin infusions.[123]

Methodological differences could account for some of the reported discrepancies in blood volume in nephrotic patients. The overestimation of plasma volume using radiolabeled albumin, however, could not account for the observed discrepancies.[5,62,114] Nonetheless, blood volume measurements were not corrected for body weight in some studies and were expressed per kilogram of dry weight or wet weight in others.

Other important variables that might account for the discrepancies in blood volume estimation in nephrotic patients include (1) the phase of nephrotic syndrome during which the study was done (edema-forming, stable, and edema-mobilizing periods); (2) differences in GFR, renal histopathology, heart, and liver functions; and (3) uncontrolled posture, sodium intake, and the use of medications that may influence sodium balance.

It is difficult to envisage how plasma volume could be normal in hypoalbuminemic states. However, many patients with hypoalbuminemia, including those with congenital analbuminemia, are edema-free. Compensatory mechanisms seem to exist, therefore, that guard against contraction of plasma volume and the development of edema when plasma COP is decreased. One of the factors that possibly aids in preventing edema in this setting is the compliance characteristics of the interstitial fluid compartment.[68,69] The relatively noncompliant nature of the interstitial compartment at normal or slightly increased volumes results in marked increases in interstitial fluid pressure, which could prevent the translocation of fluid. Another factor that prevents the formation of edema in hypoalbuminemic states is a decrease in the COP of the interstitial tissues, probably caused by an increased lymph flow.[166] Human subcutaneous tissue has a protein concentration 30 to 60 percent of that in plasma, corresponding to a COP of 10 to 15 mmHg. In hypoalbuminemic states, the osmotic pressure of the interstitial fluid may be reduced to less than 5 mmHg.[86,88] Finally, studies of hypoalbuminemic edema induced by plasmapheresis suggest that capillary permeability to albumin varies directly with changes in plasma albumin concentration and inversely with changes in plasma volume.[159] Thus, if interstitial fluid protein concentration decreases, the osmotic gradient across the capillary bed can be maintained or could even increase in spite of hypoalbuminemia.

An additional explanation for why the plasma volume may be normal or increased in some hypoalbuminemic patients with the nephrotic syndrome is the observation that sodium retention in these patients may be mediated not only by extrarenal mechanisms but also by intrinsic renal mechanisms. For example, the nephrotic patients with expanded plasma volume and low PRA evaluated by Meltzer and associates appeared to have greater reductions in GFR than did those with high PRA and hypovolemia.[107] Important observations were reported in a recent study in which rats were rendered nephrotic by injection of sheep anti-FX-IA antibody.[81] The rats showed no changes in plasma volume, ^{22}Na space, or PRA despite marked hypoalbuminemia (serum albumin, 0.67 g/100 ml). When the antibody was given to rats with chronic renal failure, plasma volume and ^{22}Na space increased and PRA decreased. Thus, it appears that concomitant decreases in GFR or a "nephritic" component with subsequent renal sodium retention and expansion of plasma volume may be a necessary factor for the clinical expression of edema in the nephrotic syndrome. Two additional studies of puromycin aminonucleoside (PAN)-induced nephrotic syndrome have also produced direct evidence of renal sodium retention as a consequence of one or more intrarenal abnormalities.[17,76]

Efferent events

As mentioned above, sodium retention in the nephrotic syndrome appears to be mediated, at least in part, by intrarenal mechanisms. Based on Starling forces, glomerular filtration in the presence of hypoalbuminemia would be expected to increase and proximal tubular reabsorption to decrease. In contrast to the anticipated increase in GFR, however, most studies in humans and experimental animals indicate that GFR is normal or decreased. The scarcity of reports showing an increased GFR in nephrotic patients suggests that other factors, presumably a decrease in ultrafiltration coefficient (K_f), dampen the favorable osmotic pressure gradient for filtration. On the other hand, the expected decrease in proximal tubular sodium reabsorption as a result of the low peritubular protein concentration has been suggested by several studies in humans[66] and in experimental animals.[4,76]

Bernard and colleagues[4] evaluated sodium handling in rats with autologous immune complex nephritis, a model of nephrotic syndrome in which the GFR after volume expansion is not different from that found in adjuvant-injected controls. They found that sodium delivery into the loop of Henle was equal in nephrotic and control rats, since the slightly lower filtered load of sodium in nephrotic rats offset the depression in proximal reabsorption. The authors concluded that the inability to excrete sodium in this model was due either to enhanced reabsorption by the collecting duct or to abnormal function of deep nephrons. In contrast to most reported observations, results of the micropuncture studies by Kurodo and associates, performed during the period of active accumulation of sodium and water, showed that fractional reabsorption of fluid in the proximal tubule was increased.[91]

Ichikawa and associates investigated a model of unilateral albuminuria induced by PAN to ascertain whether the avid sodium retention in the nephrotic syndrome is due to an intrinsic inability of the proteinuric kidney to excrete salt and water or whether salt retention merely represents a normal renal response to an extrarenal stimulus.[76] They excluded the latter possibility by observing that reductions of GRF and salt excretion occurred only in the PAN-treated kidneys, even though systemic plasma protein concentration was not reduced. Acute hypoalbuminemia reduces K_f,[2] a noteworthy finding in that it could help explain why GFR is often reduced in patients with glomerulopathy, even in the absence of severe structural damage. Of the intrinsic renal mechanisms evaluated, a reduction in GFR did not appear to be required for salt retention, since, despite a rise in GFR induced by saralasin, sodium excretion did not increase in the PAN-treated kidneys. The authors confirmed previous observations that proximal tubular sodium and water reabsorption is decreased in experimental glomerulopathies. They showed that the mechanism responsible for this reduction was the lower K_f and filtration fraction in the PAN-perfused golmeruli, which resulted in lower peritubular capillary plasma protein concentration. Peritubular capillary hydrostatic pressure did not differ between the control and experimental kidneys. As with proximal tubules, superficial loop segments also failed to account for the observed salt retention by proteinuric kidneys. The authors concluded that neither a fall in the filtered load of sodium nor changes in the various superficial nephron segments proximal to the end of the distal tubule account for the antinatriuretic response of PAN-treated nephrons. It is interesting that the results of studies in rats with aminonucleoside nephrosis suggest that an intact inner renal medulla is not necessary for sodium retention to occur.[82]

Relatively few studies have been conducted in humans to determine the nephron sites of excessive tubular sodium reabsorption in patients with the nephrotic syndrome. Grausz and coworkers used the technique of distal tubular blockade.[66] They concluded that sodium retention in the nephrotic syndrome is due to excessive distal reabsorption rather than abnormalities of proximal tubular function. Although the demonstration by Usberti and colleagues that glucose reabsorption is decreased in these patients[150] is consistent with a reduction in proximal tubular reabsorption, such an approach is inferential and open to challenge. In contrast, the impaired renal handling of water found in children with lipoid nephrosis was cited as supporting decreased delivery of sodium to the ascending limb because of *increased* proximal reabsorption.[67] In that study, however, the roles of other mechanisms that might have contributed to abnormal renal water excretion were not directly examined.

It is unlikely that the increased distal sodium reabsorption in the nephrotic syndrome is mediated primarily by increased aldosterone levels. Elevated levels of aldosterone have been reported in many, but not all, patients with the nephrotic syndrome.[18,93] Many studies have demonstrated a dissociation of renal salt retention from aldosterone levels in nephrotic patients.[13,14] In addition, suppression of aldosterone levels in these patients did not reverse the sodium-retaining state.[14,32] Furthermore, administration of saralasin resulted in an increased GFR in the PAN-perfused kidney, but it did not affect sodium handling.[76] This observation was thought to suggest that the renin-angiotensin system did not play an important role in mediating the overall salt retention of the proteinuric kidney. On the other hand, a recent study[135] in which an aldosterone antagonist reversed the positive sodium balance in nephrotic patients supports the existence of an important role for aldosterone.

Evidence consistent with renal nerve stimulation of increased renal tubular sodium reabsorption has been presented. Plasma norepinephrine is increased in patients with the nephrotic syndrome,[123] as is urinary catecholamine excretion,[113] possibly reflecting heightened renal nerve activity. Moreover, using the rat model of adriamycin nephrosis, DiBona and colleagues[29] have shown that the inability of these animals to excrete a saline load was corrected by renal denervation. Nevertheless, the contribution of this factor to renal salt retention in the nephrotic syndrome remains undefined; the expected increase in proximal reabsorption induced by renal nerve stimulation[26,28] has not been found in most studies.

Increased PG production has been reported in the nephrotic syndrome.[77,137] Nevertheless, findings in human beings[117] and experimental animals[99] suggest that PG excretion is suppressed during relapse and is increased in the recovery phase. Finally, a role for other hormonal factors, including ANF (see above) in the sodium retention in the nephrotic syndrome has not been established with certainty.

Summary

No single mechanism can be invoked to explain sodium retention in patients with the nephrotic syndrome. Discrepancies in the estimation of ECF volume among some of the studies could be explained by methodological differences. It appears, however, that plasma volume is not reduced in many patients with the nephrotic syndrome. This finding implies that sodium retention is mediated by intrarenal mechanisms, related perhaps to the underlying glomerular disease; the effects of such processes is expansion of plasma volume despite low plasma COP. The intrarenal mechanisms may include decreases in GFR and in the filtered load of sodium, increased distal sodium reabsorption, or sodium retention by deep nephrons. In the presence of an expanded plasma volume and therefore increased capillary hydrostatic pressure, the aforementioned compensatory mechanisms, which usually act to prevent translocation of fluid to the interstitial compartment in the presence of hypoalbuminemia, may fail, leading to the development of edema.

NEPHRITIC SYNDROME

Acute glomerulonephritis results in variable reductions in GFR and a fall in sodium excretion, which may lead to expanded plasma volume, hypertension, and CHF.[64] For unknown reasons, the expanded plasma volume does not induce the anticipated adjustment in sodium handling that normally leads to an accelerated natriuresis and restoration of sodium balance.

Most studies of experimental glomerulonephritis[104,106,126,153,156] have shown that the absolute rate of sodium reabsorption in the proximal tubule is decreased, due primarily to a fall in filtration fraction and in peritubular blood oncotic pressure. Therefore, the avid sodium retention in the nephritic syndrome must be due either to decreases in K_f and (consequently) GFR or to enhanced reabsorption of sodium in the distal or deep nephrons.

There is no direct evidence to show that sodium retention in acute glomerulonephritis is related to humoral factors. The PRA is usually low, reflecting the expanded ECF volume.[8,121] Aldosterone secretion does not increase in this setting, although it could be argued that aldosterone levels are inappropriately high, considering the extent of intravascular volume expansion. The role of nonaldosterone humoral factors has been examined by Godon and associates.[65] They suggested that sodium retention in the nephritic syndrome is the consequence of the lack of a natriuretic factor. On the other hand, in animals with acute unilateral nephrotoxic nephritis, avid sodium reabsorption was found only in the experimental kidney, suggesting that a systemic humoral mechanism was not operative. The studies of experimental glomerular disease mentioned above also support the idea that intrarenal mechanisms have a role in the pathogenesis of sodium retention in glomerulonephritis.

There is no evidence to show that either impaired myocardial function or altered capillary permeability plays a role in the pathogenesis of nephritic edema. CHF, when it occurs in acute nephritis, is largely the consequence of renal sodium retention and expanded plasma volume and is thought not to be a primary event.[7]

Sodium retention in acute glomerulonephritis thus appears to be due to a decline in GFR and/or to changes in the distal tubule or juxtamedullary nephrons that prevent or blunt the adaptive natriuresis per nephron associated with progressive expansion of ECF volume. Edema in this setting is probably secondary to an elevation of capillary pressure, which disturbs the steady-state Starling forces across capillary walls.

In summary, two important factors contribute to renal sodium retention in glomerular diseases. The first factor is an extrarenal mechanism that is primarily related to hypoproteinemia and the consequent reduction in plasma COP. The resultant alteration of the Starling forces leads to translocation of fluid from the intravascular compartment to the interstitial space. The reduced plasma volume then activates several humoral and hemodynamic mechanisms, which signal the kidney to retain sodium. The second factor consists of intrarenal mechanisms, including a decrease in K_f, with consequent decreases in GFR and filtered load, and/or factors that stimulate sodium reabsorption in the distal tubule or in deep nephrons. There is insufficient evidence to establish that activation of the renin-angiotensin-aldosterone system plays an important role in the pathogenesis of sodium retention associated with glomerulopathies.

The interplay between these two pathogenetic factors determines the pathophysiologic characteristics of the disease in a given patient. These factors may operate in sequence or simultaneously. As shown in Fig. 18-9, it is likely that both factors eventually become operative in many patients. In cases of pure nephrotic edema associated with severe hypoproteinemia, only the extrarenal mechanisms are activated. In these patients, one might expect normal or low blood pressure, contracted plasma volume, and high PRA levels. On the other hand, in

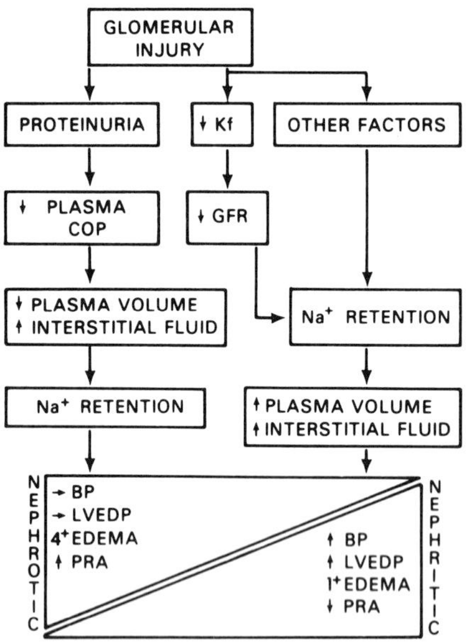

FIGURE 18-9 • Schematic diagram of the two proposed pathogenic pathways responsible for sodium retention in glomerular diseases. In *nephrotic edema*, sodium retention is presumed to be mediated by tubular mechanisms, since it may occur without any appreciable reduction in GFR. The reduced plasma colloid osmotic pressure (COP) results in movement of fluid into the interstitial space. The reduced plasma volume causes activation of various mechanisms that signal the kidney to retain sodium. Patients with nephrotic edema would theoretically be expected to have normal blood pressure, *severe* edema, and decreased plasma renin activity (PRA). In *nephritic edema*, sodium retention seems to be due to reduced distal delivery of filtrate, which results from impaired GFR coupled with constant or enhanced distal sodium reabsorption. Patients with nephritic edema may manifest hypertension, congestive heart failure (LVEDP), and suppressed PRA. The lower part of the figure highlights the considerable overlap that may exist between the nephrotic and nephritic mechanisms of edema formation.

patients with predominantly nephritic-type edema, sodium retention is the primary event, and plasma COP is normal. It is characterized by hypertension, expanded plasma volume, congested circulation, and suppressed PRA (Table 18-2).

This formulation does not include other pathogenetic factors, such as chronic renal insufficiency, accelerated hypertension, or administration of drugs that may affect renal sodium handling. It is important to emphasize that these considerations have great clinical relevance and may dictate the urgency and risks of aggressive diuretic or antihypertensive therapy.

IDIOPATHIC EDEMA

Idiopathic edema is a common disorder that occurs almost exclusively in women. It is characterized by salt retention in the absence of known causes of edema. This is a diagnosis of exclusion; common conditions, such as subtle CHF, renal disease, hepatic disease with hypoproteinemia, and other less common etiologies must be considered and excluded before this diagnosis can be established.[25,90,146]

Several unique features of idiopathic edema suggest that it is different from edema of a known etiology. Idiopathic edema rarely occurs in males and occurs in females only after puberty. Although the edema may be episodic (the disorder has been called cyclical edema), it can be persistent. It often increases prior to the onset of menses, due perhaps to the sodium-retaining effects of estrogen. In women afflicted with this disorder, edema of the face, hands, and feet develop rapidly; edema is frequently accompanied by symptoms of headache, irritability, and depression. Some women gain as much as 10 to 12 pounds during a 24-h period; a decrease in urine output occurs concomitantly.

There is an important postural component to the occurrence of edema. Although upright posture is associated with hyperaldosteronism and sodium retention in normal subjects, edema rarely occurs. In contrast, patients with idiopathic cyclical edema seem to have an exaggerated response to upright posture; the antinatriuresis of upright posture results in significant pitting edema of their lower extremities.

Many observers have emphasized that prominent psychological problems afflict these women. Indeed, one author has referred to the condition as "psyclical edema."[146] Whether such psychological problems are overemphasized, however, must be considered. The disorder is common, and those women who are ultimately referred to university hospitals for evaluation probably represent a small percentage of those with the problem. As with any chronic disease, the emotional response to the condition varies. If edema is associated in the patient's mind with cardiac or renal disease, there may be a great deal of anxiety about sodium retention. In addition, many of these women are obese; there frequently is great anxiety about their appearance and weight.

The altered self-image of these patients compels many of them to take diuretics constantly and surreptitiously. The salient clinical features with which the patients present include unexplained hypokalemia, urinary potassium wasting, and elevated PRA. Mistaken diagnoses, including that of Bartter's syndrome, are possible. In any patient being evaluated for unexplained hypokalemia with urinary potassium wasting, the urine should be tested for the presence of diuretics; the procedure can be readily performed by chromatography in many toxicology laboratories.[141]

PATHOGENESIS

Despite much study, the mechanisms responsible for the salt retention in idiopathic edema have not been established. Occasionally, cyclic edema may occur as a result of occult hepatic, renal, or cardiac disease or in response to subtle changes in capillary permeability. Possible mechanisms leading to idiopathic edema include a reduction in arterial blood pressure when standing; intermittent alteration in capillary permeability; increased aldosterone secretion; alteration in estrogen, progesterone, or catecholamine metabolism; and hypoproteinemia.[25,63,90,138]

It should be emphasized that, in some instances, treatment of idiopathic edema may exacerbate the symptoms. DeWardener has proposed that the edema in most patients with this syndrome is caused by the use of a diuretic.[25] According to his hypothesis, the continued use of a diuretic, regardless of the reason for initiating its use, causes a persistent rise in plasma renin activity and secondary aldosteronism. Eventually the juxtaglomerular apparatus of such patients becomes enlarged;[25] it is probable, therefore, that there is an associated increase in the size of the adrenal glands. The resultant hyperaldosteronism may induce sustained antinatriuresis for as long as two weeks following cessation of diuretic treatment. A vicious cycle ensues: irregularity in the dose of diuretics may cause a sharp fall in urinary sodium excretion, a gain in weight, and rapid onset of the characteristically uncomfortable edema. The edema prompts a quick return to the use of diuretics, which in turn aggravates the secondary aldosteronism. Edema rarely is present while the patient is regularly taking diuretics.

Many of the patients have been paramedical workers who have easy access to diuretics. Long-term diuretic therapy is associated with potassium depletion, which can potentiate the problem by producing symptoms of weakness, malaise, and irritability. Possibly the most convincing evidence that idiopathic edema is due to the continuous use of diuretics is the response of most patients when the diuretics are stopped. Body weight and edema increase transiently, but within the next two to three weeks the weight returns to baseline and the edema clears (Fig. 18-10).

Several anecdotal reports suggest that captopril, an inhibitor of angiotensin-converting enzyme, decreases the sodium retention associated with idiopathic edema. The salutary effects of the drug suggest an important role of angiotensin II and/or aldosterone in the pathogenesis of idiopathic edema. These preliminary results have been confirmed in one recent study.[30] Another investigation, however, suggests that captopril may have an additional effect on vascular permeability.[56] Although captopril is known to increase PGE_2 synthesis, the inhibitory effects of captopril on edema were not prevented by indomethacin, suggesting that captopril's salutary effect is mediated independently of PGs.

Deficient catecholamine levels, especially of dopamine, have been reported in some patients with idiopathic edema; this finding awaits confirmation. The use of agents with dopaminergic activity has not been universally successful to date.

THE IATROGENIC EDEMA STATES

With the increasing complexity and sophistication of medical practice, physician-induced sodium retention looms more important as a cause of sodium retention and

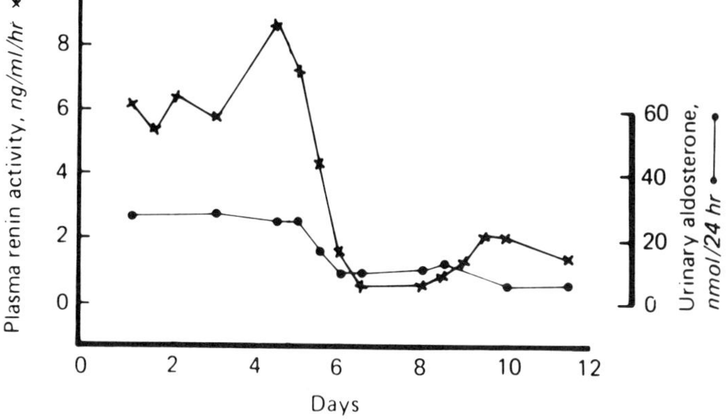

FIGURE 18-10 • Changes in body weight in relation to diuretic administration in a patient with idiopathic edema. ***(Upper panel)*** **body weight in kilograms;** ***(lower panel)*** **PRA and urinary aldosterone excretion. The area to the left of the vertical line represents the period of diuretic (bendroflumethiazide) administration. (From deWardener HE:** ***Kidney Int*** **19:881, 1981. Used by permission.)**

edema. Two settings in which iatrogenic edema appears are following the administration of certain drugs and the excessive, rapid intravenous infusion of sodium-containing solutions. On occasion, excessive oral salt-loading may also permit iatrogenic edema to develop.

A variety of drugs have been shown to promote sodium retention. These include estrogens, vasodilator drugs used in treatment of hypertension, and, more recently, nonsteroidal anti-inflammatory drugs (NSAIDs).

ESTROGENS

Estrogens, either by themselves or as oral contraceptives, promote sodium retention.[80] The mechanism of action has not been completely elucidated but is thought to have both intra- and extrarenal components. Since estrogens do not influence GFR or RPF in human beings in any significant manner, the observed renal effects must occur at the level of the tubule. The indirect actions are not well defined; they may be mediated in part through mineralocorticoids and possibly through alterations in prolactin.

VASODILATOR-INDUCED EDEMA

The pathogenesis of sodium retention induced by antihypertensive agents is not completely understood. One contributing factor appears to be a decrease in renal perfusion pressure with alteration of proximal tubular sodium reabsorption. Potent vasodilators such as minoxidil or diazoxide have a more marked antinatriuretic effect because of the marked stimulation of the activity of the renin-aldosterone and sympathetic nervous systems. In addition, it has been suggested that relaxation of precapillary sphincters may expose systemic capillaries to a higher hydrostatic pressure. The resultant disruption of Starling forces would favor the translocation of fluid into the interstitial compartment. The increase of blood flow to the skin and other organs with high capillary flow is consistent with this formulation.

NONSTEROIDAL ANTI-INFLAMMATORY DRUGS

Numerous studies have been performed to address the possible role of the renal PGs in regulating renal sodium handling.[47,102] Studies in animals have demonstrated that the intrarenal infusion of vasodilating PGs leads to increases in sodium excretion. Whether these results are a direct result of PGs acting at the level of the nephron or are a consequence of changes in hemodynamic factors is difficult to ascertain. An alternative approach to this question has employed inhibitors of PG synthesis; such as NSAIDs. Under most circumstances, when normal animals were studied there was either a transient decrease or no change in sodium excretion. When NSAIDs were administered, however, under conditions in which the kidney is avidly retaining sodium, a further increase in tubular sodium reabsorption was observed.[102]

Recent studies have suggested that NSAIDs may induce sodium retention in humans. In the course of examining the frequency and severity of side effects of NSAIDs during community use, Coles and colleagues noted that peripheral edema was associated with NSAID administration with a frequency ranging from 2 to 23 percent.[21]

Recently, it has been suggested that sulindac differs from other NSAIDs by sparing *renal* but inhibiting *systemic* PG synthesis. This possibility is reflected by the lack of an effect on urinary PGE_2 excretion and on other putative endpoints of renal PG synthesis, such as renin release and response to furosemide, whereas inhibition of systemic PGs is reflected by the decreased production of thromboxane by platelets.[19] Ciabattoni and associates[19] compared one week of treatment with 1.2 g/day of ibuprofen to 400 mg/day sulindac in a large group of women with chronic glomerular diseases. Sulindac did not affect urinary excretion of PGE_2 or keto $PGF_{1\alpha}$ or cause renal function to deteriorate, whereas serum thromboxane B_2 decreased 85 percent. In contrast, ibuprofen caused approximately 80 percent decreases in both urinary PGs, a 30 percent decrease in creatinine clearance, and a 35 percent decrease in PAH clearance. If such findings are extrapolated to normal subjects, one might anticipate that sulindac would be associated with the lowest incidence of peripheral edema. Despite these impressive preliminary results, it is unsettled whether sulindac is indeed renal sparing after long-term use in patients with other edematous disorders or in normal human beings.

An additional mechanism whereby NSAIDs promote edema formation occurs in sodium-retaining patients who are receiving diuretics. It is well established that NSAIDs impair the natriuretic action of diuretic agents.[116] Thus, when taken concurrently with diuretic agents, NSAIDs may interfere with the action of diuretics, thus promoting salt and water retention.

REFERENCES

1. Atlas SA, Epstein M: Atrial natriuretic factor: Implications in cirrhosis and other edematous disorders, in Epstein M (ed): *The Kidney in Liver Disease*, 3d ed. Baltimore, Williams & Wilkins, 1988, p 429.
2. Baylis C et al: Dynamics of glomerular ultrafiltration: 9. Effects of plasma protein concentration. *Am J Physiol* 232:F58, 1977.
3. Berlyne GM et al: Water immersion in nephrotic syndrome. *Arch Intern Med* 141:1275, 1981.

4. Bernard D et al: Renal sodium retention during volume expansion in experimental nephrotic syndrome. *Kidney Int* 14:478, 1978.
5. Bernard DB: Extrarenal complications of the nephrotic syndrome. *Kidney Int* 33:1184, 1988.
6. Bichet DG et al: Potential role of increased sympathetic activity in impaired sodium and water excretion in cirrhosis. *N Engl J Med* 307:1552, 1982.
7. Binak K et al: Circulatory changes in acute glomerulonephritis at rest and exercise. *Br Heart J* 37:833, 1975.
8. Birkenhager WH et al: Interrelations between arterial pressure fluid volume and plasma renin concentration in the course of acute glomerulonephritis. *Lancet* 1:1086, 1970.
9. Boyer TD et al: Effect of indomethacin and prostaglandin A_1 on renal function and plasma renin activity in alcoholic liver disease. *Gastroenterology* 77:215, 1979.
10. Brater DC et al: Effects of ibuprofen, naproxen, and sulindac on prostaglandins in men. *Kidney Int* 27:66, 1985.
11. Braunwald E et al: A method for the detection and quantification of impaired sodium excretion: Results of an oral sodium tolerance test in normal subjects and in patients with heart disease. *Circulation* 32:223, 1965.
12. Brown EA et al: Blood volume and its regulation. *Annu Rev Physiol* 19:231, 1957.
13. Brown EA et al: Evidence that some mechanism other than the renin system causes sodium retention in nephrotic syndrome. *Lancet* 2:1237, 1982.
14. Brown EA et al: Lack of effect of captopril on the sodium retention of nephrotic syndrome. *Nephron* 37:43, 1984.
15. Buckalew VM: Natriuretic hormone, in Epstein M (ed): *The Kidney in Liver Disease*, 3d ed. Baltimore, Williams & Wilkins, 1988, p 417.
16. Chaimovitz C et al: Mechanism of increased renal tubular sodium reabsorption in cirrhosis. *Am J Med* 52:198, 1972.
17. Chandra M et al: Renal function in rats with unilateral proteinuria produced by renal perfusion with aminonucleoside. *Pediatr Res* 15:340, 1981.
18. Chonko AM et al: The role of renin and aldosterone in the salt retention of edema. *Am J Med* 63:881, 1977.
19. Ciabottoni G et al: Effects of sulindac and ibuprofen in patients with chronic glomerular disease: Evidence for the dependence of renal function on prostacyclin. *N Engl J Med* 310:279, 1984.
20. Clive DM, Stoff JS: Renal syndromes associated with nonsteroidal anti-inflammatory drugs. *N Engl J Med* 310:563, 1984.
21. Coles LS et al: From experiment to experience: Side effects of nonsteroidal anti-inflammatory drugs. *Am J Med* 74:820, 1983.
22. Coppage WS et al: The metabolism of aldosterone in normal subjects and in patients with hepatic cirrhosis. *J Clin Invest* 41:1672, 1962.
23. Creager MA et al: Acute regional circulatory and renal hemodynamic effects of converting-enzyme inhibition in patients with congestive heart failure. *Circulation* 64:483, 1981.
24. deWardener HE: Natriuretic hormone. *Clin Sci* 53:1, 1977.
25. deWardener HE: Idiopathic edema: Role of diuretic abuse. *Kidney Int* 19:881, 1981.
26. DiBona GD: Neurogenic regulation of renal tubular sodium reabsorption. *Am J Physiol* 233:F73, 1977.
27. DiBona GD: The functions of the renal nerves. *Rev Physiol Biochem Pharmacol* 94:75, 1982.
28. DiBona GD et al: Neurogenic control of renal tubular sodium reabsorption in the dog. *Circ Res* 40:51, 1977.
29. DiBona et al: Neural control of renal function in edema forming states. *Am J Physiol* 254:R1017, 1988.
30. Docci D et al: Therapeutic response of idiopathic edema to captopril. *Nephron* 34:198, 1983.
31. Dorhout Mees EJ et al: Observations on edema formation in the nephrotic syndrome in adults with minimal lesions. *Am J Med* 67:378, 1979.
32. Dussing R et al: The renin-angiotensin-aldosterone system in patients with nephrotic syndrome: Effect of 1-sar-8-ala-angiotensin II. *Nephron* 25:187, 1980.
33. Eisenberg G: Blood volume in persons with the nephrotic syndrome. *Am J Med Sci* 255:320, 1968.
34. Epstein M: Renal effects of head-out water immersion in man: Implications for an understanding of volume homeostasis. *Physiol Rev* 58:529, 1978.
35. Epstein M: Deranged sodium homeostasis in cirrhosis. *Gastroenterology* 76:622, 1979.
36. Epstein M: Renal sodium handling in liver disease, in Epstein M (ed): *The Kidney in Liver Disease*, 3d ed. Baltimore, Williams & Wilkins, 1988, p 3.
37. Epstein M: Atrial natriuretic factor in patients with liver disease. *Am J Nephrol* 9:89, 1989.
38. Epstein M: Treatment of refractory ascites. *N Engl J Med* 321:1675, 1989.
39. Epstein M et al: Renal failure in the patient with cirrhosis: The role of active vasoconstriction. *Am J Med* 49:175, 1970.
40. Epstein M et al: Characterization of the renin-aldosterone system in decompensated cirrhosis. *Circ Res* 41:818, 1977.
41. Epstein M et al: Characterization of renal PGE responsiveness in decompensated cirrhosis: Implications for renal sodium handling. *Clin Sci* 63:555, 1982.
42. Epstein M et al: Comparison of water immersion and saline infusion as a means of inducing volume expansion in man. *J Appl Physiol* 39:66, 1975.
43. Epstein M et al: Determinants of deranged sodium and water homeostasis in decompensated cirrhosis. *J Lab Clin Med* 87:822, 1976.
44. Epstein M et al: Interrelationship of renal sodium and phosphate handling in cirrhosis. *Miner Electrolyte Metab* 7:305, 1982.
45. Epstein M et al: Comparison of the suppressive effects of water immersion and saline administration on renin-aldosterone in normal man. *J Clin Endocrinol Metab* 49:358, 1979.
46. Epstein M et al: Effect of water immersion on plasma catecholamines in decompensated cirrhosis. *Miner Electrolyte Metab* 11:25, 1985.
47. Epstein M et al: Relationship between renal prostaglandin E and renal sodium handling during water immersion in normal man. *Circ Res* 45:71, 1979.
48. Epstein M, Lifschitz MD: Volume status as a determinant of the influence of renal PGE on renal function. *Nephron* 25:157, 1980.
48a. Epstein M, Lifschitz M: Renal eicosanoids as determin-

ants of renal function in liver disease. *Hepatology* 7:1359, 1987.

49. Epstein M, Norsk P: Aldosterone in liver disease, in Epstein M (ed): *The Kidney in Liver Disease*, 3d ed. Baltimore, Williams & Wilkins. 1988, p 356.
50. Epstein M: The sodium retention of cirrhosis: A reappraisal. *Hepatology* 6:312, 1986.
51. Epstein M et al: Effects of water immersion on ANP release in humans. *Am J Nephrol* 9:1, 1989.
52. Epstein M et al: Relationship of increased plasma ANF and renal sodium handling during immersion-induced central hypervolemia in normal humans. *J Clin Invest* 79:738, 1987.
53. Epstein M et al: Relationship between plasma ANF responsiveness and renal sodium handling in cirrhotic humans. *Am J Nephrol* 133, 1989.
54. Erdmann AJ et al: Effect of increased vascular pressure on lung fluid balance in unanesthetized sheep. *Circ Res* 37:271, 1975.
55. Fadnes et al: A study on oedema mechanism in nephrotic syndrome. *Scand J Clin Invest* 46:533, 1986.
56. Fantone JC et al: Inhibition of vascular permeability changes in rats by captopril. *J Clin Invest* 69:1207, 1982.
57. Favre H: Role of the natriuretic factor in the disorders of sodium balance., in Hamburger J et al (eds): *Advances in Nephrology*. Chicago, Year Book Medical, 1981, vol 2, p 3.
58. Folkow B et al: Measurements of plasma norepinephrine concentrations in human primary hypertension. *Hypertension* 5:399, 1983.
59. Gabuzda GJ: Cirrhosis, ascites and edema: Clinical course related to management. *Gastroenterology* 58:546, 1970.
60. Garnett ES, Webber CE: Changes in blood-volume produced by treatment in the nephrotic syndrome. *Lancet* 2:798, 1967.
61. Gauer OH: Mechanoreceptors in the intrathoracic circulation and plasma volume control, in Epstein M (ed): *The Kidney in Liver Disease*. New York, Elsevier, 1978, p 3.
62. Geers AB et al: Plasma volume (PV) measurements in patients with nephrotic syndrome (NS): A methodological study on the labelled albumin method. *Kidney Int* 23:123, 1983.
63. Gill JR Jr et al: Idiopathic edema. 2. Pathogenesis of edema in patients with hypoalbuminemia. *Am J Med* 52:452, 1972.
64. Glassock RJ: Sodium homeostasis in acute glomerulonephritis and the nephrotic syndrome. *Contrib Nephrol* 23:181, 1980.
65. Godon JP: Evidence of increased proximal sodium and water in experimental glomerulonephritis: Role of natriuretic factor of renal origin. *Nephron* 21:145, 1978.
66. Grausz H et al: Effect of plasma albumin on sodium reabsorption in patients with nephrotic syndrome. *Kidney Int* 1:47, 1972.
67. Gur A et al: A study of the renal handling of water in lipoid nephrosis. *Pediatr Res* 10:197, 1976.
68. Guyton AC: Interstitial fluid pressure: 2. Pressure-volume curves of the interstitial space. *Circ Res* 16:452, 1976.
69. Guyton AC et al: Dynamics of edema and the safety factor against edema. In *Circulatory Physiology*. Philadelphia, Saunders, 1975, vol 2, p 149.
70. Henriksen J et al: Splanchnic and renal elimination and release of catecholamines in cirrhosis: Evidence of enhanced sympathetic nervous activity in patients with decompensated cirrhosis. *Gut* 25:1034, 1984.
71. Henriksen J et al: Sympathetic nervous activity in cirrhosis: A survey of plasma catecholamine studies. *J Hepatol* 1:55, 1985.
72. Hollander W, Judson WE: The relationship of cardiovascular and renal hemodynamic function to sodium excretion in patients with severe heart disease but without edema. *J Clin Invest* 35:970, 1956.
73. Hollander W et al: Lymphatic flow in human subjects as indicated by the disappearance of I^{131}-labelled albumin from the subcutaneous tissue. *J Clin Invest* 40:223, 1961.
74. Hollenberg NK et al: Increased glomerular filtration rate after converting-enzyme inhibition in essential hypertension. *N Engl J Med* 301:9, 1979.
75. Hopper J et al: Lipoid nephrosis in 31 adult patients: Renal biopsy study by light, electron and fluorescence microscopy with experience in treatment. *Medicine* 49:321, 1970.
76. Ichikawa I et al: Role of intrarenal mechanisms in the impaired salt excretion of experimental nephrotic syndrome. *J Clin Invest* 71:91, 1983.
77. Januszewicz P et al: Abnormal prostaglandin excretion in children with minimal change nephrotic syndrome. *Prostagland Med* 7:149, 1981.
78. Jensen H et al: Albumin metabolism in the nephrotic syndrome in adults. *Clin Sci* 33:445, 1967.
79. Jones RA et al: Reversal of diurnal variation in renal function in cases of cirrhosis with ascites. *J Clin Invest* 31:326, 1952.
80. Katz AI, Lindheimer MD: Actions of hormones on the kidney. *Annu Rev Physiol* 39:97, 1977.
81. Kaysen GA et al: Plasma volume expansion necessary for edema formation in the rat with Heymann nephritis. *Am J Physiol* 248:F247, 1985.
82. Keeler R: Chemical medullectomy does not prevent sodium retention in nephrotic rats. *Miner Electrolyte Metab* 15:241, 1989.
83. Kimbrough HM et al: Effect of intrarenal angiotensin II blockade on renal function in conscious dogs. *Circ Res* 40:174, 1977.
84. Klingler EL et al: Renal function changes in cirrhosis of the liver. *Arch Intern Med* 125:1010, 1970.
85. Koomans HA et al: Effects of plasma volume expansion on renal salt handling in patients with the nephrotic syndrome. *Am J Nephrol* 4:227, 1984.
86. Koomans HA et al: Lowered protein content of tissue fluid in patients with nephrotic syndrome: Observations during disease and recovery. *Nephron* 40:391, 1985.
87. Koomans HA et al: The importance of plasma protein for blood volume and blood pressure homeostasis. *Kidney Int* 30:730, 1986.
88. Koomans HA et al: Lowered tissue-fluid oncotic pressure protects the blood volume in the nephrotic syndrome. *Nephron* 42:317, 1986.
89. Krishna GG, Danovitch GM: The effects of water immersion on renal function in the nephrotic syndrome. *Kidney Int* 21:395, 1982.
90. Kuchel O et al: Inappropriate response to upright posture:

A precipitating factor in the pathogenesis of idiopathic edema. *Ann Intern Med* 73:245, 1970.
91. Kuroda S et al: A micropuncture study of renal sodium retention in nephrotic syndrome rats: Evidence for increased resistance to tubular fluid flow. *Kidney Int* 16:561, 1979.
92. Langgard H: Den subkutane absorption af albumin ved odemtilstande. *Ugeskr Laeger* 126:69, 1964.
93. Laragh JH: Hormones and the pathogenesis of congestive heart failure: Vasopressin, aldosterone and angiotensin II. *Circulation* 253:1015, 1962.
94. Levinson R et al: Comparison of the effects of water immersion and saline infusion on central hemodynamics in man. *Clin Sci* 52:343, 1977.
95. Levy M: Pathophysiology of ascites formation, in Epstein M (ed): *The Kidney in Liver Disease*, 3d ed. Baltimore, Williams & Wilkins, 1988, p 209.
96. Levy M: Sodium retention in dogs with cirrhosis and ascites: Efferent mechanisms. *Am J Physiol* 233:F586, 1977.
97. Levy M et al: Sodium retention in dogs with experimental cirrhosis following removal of ascites by continuous peritoneovenous shunting. *J Lab Clin Med* 94:933, 1979.
98. Levy M, Seely JF: Pathophysiology of edema formation, in Brenner BM, Rector FC Jr (eds): *The Kidney*, 2d ed. Philadelphia, Saunders, 1981, p 723.
99. Lianos EA et al: Glomerular prostaglandin and nephrotoxic serum nephritis. *J Clin Invest* 72:1439, 1983.
100. Lieberman FL et al: Effective plasma volume in cirrhosis with ascites: Evidence that a decreased value does not account for renal sodium retention, a spontaneous reduction in glomerular filtration rate (GFR) and a fall in GFR during drug-induced diuresis. *J Clin Invest* 48:975, 1969.
101. Lieberman FL et al: The relationship of plasma volume, portal hypertension, ascites and renal sodium retention in cirrhosis: The overflow theory of ascites formation. *Ann N Y Acad Sci* 170:202, 1970.
102. Lifschitz MD: Renal effects of nonsteroidal anti-inflammatory agents. *J Lab Clin Med* 102:313, 1983.
103. Lifschitz MD, Schrier RW: Alterations in cardiac output with chronic constriction or thoracic inferior vena cava. *Am J Physiol* 225:1364, 1973.
104. Lubowitz H et al: Experimental glomerulonephritis in the rat. *Kidney Int* 5:356, 1975.
105. Maack T et al: Atrial natriuretic factor: Structure and functional properties (editorial review). *Kidney Int* 27:607, 1985.
106. Maddox DA et al: Control of proximal tubule fluid reabsorption in experimental glomerulonephritis. *J Clin Invest* 55:1315, 1975.
107. Meltzer JI et al: Nephrotic syndrome: Vasoconstriction and hypervolemic types indicated by sodium-renin profiling. *Ann Intern Med* 91:688, 1979.
108. Migdal S et al: Evidence that decreased cardiac output is not the stimulus to sodium retention during acute constriction of the vena cava. *J Lab Clin Med* 89:809, 1977.
109. Naccarato R et al: Renal handling of sodium and water in early chronic liver disease. *Gastroenterology* 81:205, 1981.
110. Nicholls K et al: Elevated plasma norepinephrine concentrations in decompensated cirrhosis: Association with increased secretion rates, normal clearance rates, and suppressibility by central blood volume expansion. *Circ Res* 56:457, 1985.
111. Noddeland H et al: Interstitial fluid colloid osmotic and hydrostatic pressures in subcutaneous tissue of patients with nephrotic syndrome. *Scand J Clin Lab Invest* 42:139, 1982.
112. O'Connor DT, Stone RA: The renal kallikrein-kinin system: Description and relationship to liver disease, in Epstein M (ed): *The Kidney in Liver Disease*, 2d ed. New York, Elsevier/North Holland, 1983, p 469.
113. Oliver NJ et al: Demonstration of increased catecholamine excretion in the nephrotic syndrome. *Proc Soc Exp Biol Med* 125:1176, 1967.
114. Olmer M et al: Determination of blood volume in nephrotic patients. *Am J Nephrol* 9:211, 1989.
115. Papper S, Saxon L: The diuretic response to administered water in patients with liver disease: 2. Laennec's cirrhosis of the liver. *Arch Intern Med* 103:750, 1959.
116. Patak RV et al: Antagonism of furosemide by indomethacin in normal and hypertensive man. *Prostaglandins* 10:649, 1975.
117. Pedersen EB et al: Urinary prostaglandin E_2 aned F_2 excretion in nephrotic syndrome during basal conditions, after water loading, and after remission of the syndrome. *Acta Med Scand* 69:224, 1988.
118. Perez GO et al: Role of dialysis and ultrafiltration in the treatment of the renal complications of liver disease, in Epstein M (ed): *The Kidney in Liver Disease*, 3d ed. Baltimore, Williams & Wilkins, 1988, p 613.
119. Perico N et al: Renal response to atrial peptides is reduced in experimental nephrosis. *Am J Physiol* 252:F654, 1987.
120. Peterson C et al: Atrial natriuretic peptide and the renal response to hypervolemia in nephrotic humans. *Kidney Int* 34:825, 1988.
121. Powell HR et al: Plasma renin activity in acute poststreptococcal glomerulonephritis and the hemolytic-uremic syndrome. *Arch Dis Child* 49:802, 1974.
122. Rabelink AJ et al: Renal response to atrial natriuretic peptide in nephrotic syndrome. *Nephrol Dial Transplant* 2:510, 1987.
123. Rascher W et al: Diuretic and hormonal responses to head-out water immersion in nephrotic syndrome. *J Pediatr* 109:609, 1986.
124. Rascher W, Tulassay T: Hormonal regulation of water metabolism in children with nephrotic syndrome. *Kidney Int* 32:583, 1987.
125. Reinhardt HW et al: Left atrial pressure and sodium balance in conscious dogs on a low sodium intake. *Pfluegers Arch* 370:59, 1977.
126. Rocha A et al: Micropuncture studies in rats with experimental glomerulonephritis. *Kidney Int* 3:356, 1974.
127. Rosoff L Jr et al: Studies of renin and aldosterone in cirrhotic patients with ascites. *Gastroenterology* 69:698, 1975.
128. Schedl HP, Bartter FC: An explanation for and experimental correction of the abnormal water diuresis in cirrhosis. *J Clin Invest* 39:248, 1960.
129. Schrier RW, Humphreys MH: Factors involved in the antinatriuretic effects of acute constriction of the thoracic and abdominal inferior vena cava. *Circ Res* 29:479, 1971.
130. Schrier RW et al: Role of cardiac output and the autonomic nervous system in the antinatriuretic response to acute

constriction of the thoracic superior vena cava. *Circ Res* 29:490, 1971.
131. Schrier RW: Pathogenesis of sodium and water retention in high-output and low-output cardiac failure, nephrotic syndrome, cirrhosis and pregnancy: 1. *N Engl J Med* 319:1065, 1988.
132. Schrier RW: Pathogenesis of sodium and water retention in high-output and low-output cardiac failure, nephrotic syndrome, cirrhosis and pregnancy: 1. *N Engl J Med* 319:1065, 1988; 2. *N Engl J Med* 319: 1127, 1988.
133. Schrier RW et al: Peripheral arterial vasodilation hypothesis: A proposal for the initiation of renal and water retention in cirrhosis. *Hepatology* 8:1151, 1988.
134. Shapiro MD et al: Role of glomerular filtration rate in the impaired sodium and water excretion in patients with the nephrotic syndrome. *Am J Kidney Dis* 8:81, 1986.
135. Shapiro M et al: Role of aldosterone in the Na retention of patients with nephrotic syndrome (abstract). *Kidney Int* 29:203, 1986.
136. Shasha SM et al: Haemodynamic studies in dogs with chronic bile duct ligation. *Clin Sci* 50:533, 1976.
137. Shehadeh et al: Indomethacin and the nephrotic syndrome. *JAMA* 141:1264, 1979.
138. Sims E et al: The relation of capillary angiopathy and diabetes mellitus to idiopathic edema. *Ann Intern Med* 63:972, 1965.
139. Skorecki KL et al: Role of atrial natriuretic peptide in the natriuretic response to central volume expansion induced by head-out water immersion in sodium-retaining cirrhotic subjects. *Am J Med* 85:375, 1988.
140. Smith HW: *The Kidney: Structure and Function in Health and Disease*. New York, Oxford University Press, 1951.
141. Sohn D et al: Detection of diuretics in the urine. *J Chromatogr* 87:570, 1973.
142. Starling EH: Physiological factors involved in the causation of dropsy. *Lancet* 2:1405, 1896.
143. Starr J Jr et al: The absence of conspicuous increments of venous pressure after severe damage to the right ventricle of the dog, with a discussion of the relation between clinical congestive heart failure and heart disease. *Am Heart J* 26:291, 1943.
144. Stein JH et al: Alterations in intrarenal blood flow distribution: Methods of measurement and relationship to sodium balance. *Circ Res* 32(suppl 1):61, 1973.
145. Thames MD: Neural control of renal function: Contribution of cardiopulmonary baroreceptors to the control of the kidney. *Fed Proc* 37:1209, 1977.
146. Thorn GW: Approach to the patient with "idiopathic edema" or "periodic swelling." *JAMA* 206:333, 1968.
147. Trachtman H et al: Platelet vasopressin levels in childhood idiopathic nephrotic syndrome. *Am J Dis Child* 142:1313, 1988.
148. Tristani FE, Cohn JN: Systemic and renal hemodynamics in oliguric hepatic failure: Effect of volume expansion. *J Clin Invest* 46:1894, 1967.
149. Tulassay T et al: Atrial natriuretic peptide and other vasoactive hormones in nephrotic syndrome. *Kidney Int* 31:1391, 1987.
150. Usberti M et al: Relationship between serum albumin concentration and tubular reabsorption of glucose in renal disease. *Kidney Int* 16:546, 1979.
151. Usberti M et al: Role of plasma vasopressin in the impairment of water excretion in nephrotic syndrome. *Kidney Int* 25:422, 1984.
152. Vaamonde CA: Renal water handling in liver disease, in Epstein M (ed): *The Kidney in Liver Disease*, 3d ed. Baltimore, Williams & Wilkins, 1988, p 31.
153. Van Liew JB, Von Baeyer HR: Proximal tubule volume reabsorption in anti-GBM nephritic rats. *Physiologist* 17:348, 1974.
154. Vlahcevic ZR et al: Renal effects of acute expansion of plasma volume in cirrhosis. *N Engl J Med* 272:387, 1965.
155. Warren JV, Stead EA: Fluid dynamics in chronic congestive heart failure: An interpretation of the mechanisms producing edema, increased plasma volume and elevated venous pressure in certain patients with prolonged congestive failure. *Arch Intern Med* 73:138, 1944.
156. Wen SF, Wagnild JP: Acute effect of nephrotoxic serum on renal sodium transport in the dog. *Kidney Int* 9:243, 1976.
157. Wilson JR et al: Effect of diuresis on the performance of the failing left ventricle in man. *Am J Med* 70:234, 1981.
158. Witte MH et al: Progress in liver disease: Physiological factors involved in the causation of cirrhotic ascites. *Gastroenterology* 61:742, 1971.
159. Wraight EP: Capillary permeability of protein as a factor in the control of plasma volume. *J Physiol* 277:39, 1974.
160. Wong PY et al: Kallikrein-kinin and renin-angiotensin systems in functional renal failure of cirrhosis of the liver. *Gastroenterology* 73:1114, 1977.
161. Yamauchi H, Hopper J Jr: Hypovolemic shock as a complication in the nephrotic syndrome: Report of ten cases. *Ann Intern Med* 60:242, 1964.
162. Yaron M, Bennet CM: Renal sodium handling in acute right-sided heart failure in dogs. *Miner Electrolyte Metab* 1:303, 1978.
163. Zambraski EJ, DiBona GF: Sympathetic nervous system in hepatic cirrhosis, in Epstein M (ed): *The Kidney in Liver Disease*, 3d ed. Baltimore, Williams & Wilkins, 1988, p 469.
164. Zipser RD et al: Prostaglandins: Modulators of renal function and pressor resistance in chronic liver disease. *J Clin Endocrinol Metab* 48:895, 1971.
165. Zipser RD et al: Renal kallikrein excretion in alcoholic cirrhosis: Relation to other vasoactive systems. *Am J Gastroenterol* 75:183, 1980.
166. Zweifach BW: Capillary filtration and mechanisms of edema formation. *Pfluegers Arch* 336(suppl 81):S81, 1972.

CHAPTER 19

Treatment of edema states

Arnold M. Chonko • Jared J. Grantham

Edema is defined as an abnormal collection of body fluid. In most instances the edema accumulates in intercellular (interstitial) tissue spaces because of an alteration in the forces that control the transcapillary transfer of fluid. Edema may be generalized when these forces are abnormal in all capillary beds, as may be seen in cardiac failure, cirrhosis, and the nephrotic syndrome. By contrast, edema may develop within a circumscribed area of the body owing to localized venous, lymphatic, or inflammatory disease. Common to all edematous conditions is the accumulation of excess total body sodium chloride and water.

EDEMA FORMATION

STARLING FORMULATION OF TISSUE FLUID BALANCE

All edema is due to alterations of the forces, described by Starling in 1896, that govern the transcapillary movement of fluid between the intracellular and interstitial fluid compartments of the extracellular fluid space.[319] These forces include (1) hydrostatic pressure within the capillary (P_c), which provides the major force favoring outward fluid movement; (2) tissue, hydrostatic pressure (P_t), which limits the outward movement of capillary fluid; (3) oncotic pressure of plasma proteins, which favors movement of fluid into the vascular space; and (4) the permeability or filtration coefficient (K_f) of the capillary membrane, characterizing physical properties of the membrane that determine how fast fluid moves through it in response to a pressure gradient.[338] These forces are illustrated in Fig. 19-1 and summarized in equation 1 in simplified algebraic form.

$$J_V = K_f (P_c - P_t) - \sigma (\pi_c - \pi_i) \qquad (1)$$

where
J_V = net volume flow between intravascular and interstitial spaces
K_f = permeability or ultrafiltration coefficient of capillary membrane
P_c = intracapillary hydrostatic pressure
P_t = interstitial hydrostatic pressure
σ = reflection coefficient for plasma protein
$\pi_c - \pi_i$ = colloid osmotic pressures of plasma and interstitial fluid

Under normal circumstances the net hydrostatic pressure gradient ($P_c - P_t = \Delta P$) slightly exceeds the net colloid osmotic pressure gradient ($\pi_c - \pi_i = \Delta\pi$), so that fluid is primarily filtered out of the capillary into the

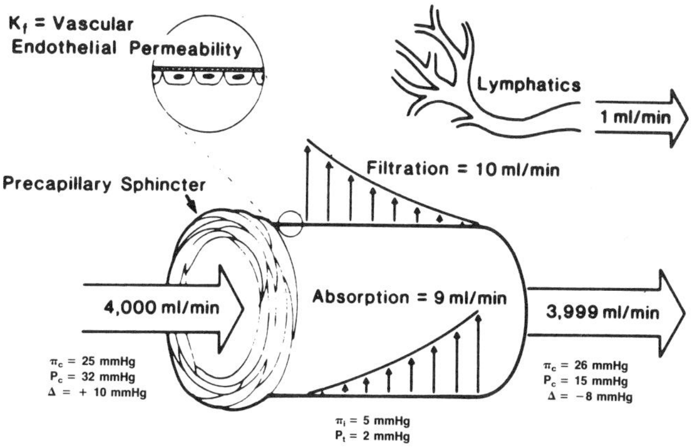

FIGURE 19-1 • Diagrammatic representation of fluid exchange across the capillaries. Plasma flow through the capillaries is about 4000 ml/min. K_f, hydraulic permeability coefficient of the capillaries; π_c and π_i, oncotic pressures of plasma and interstitial fluid; P_c and P_t, hydrostatic pressures within capillaries and interstitial tissues; ΔmmHg, algebraic sum of forces favoring filtration of fluid out of (or into) the capillaries. The precapillary sphincter can constrict, decreasing plasma flow and the hydrostatic pressure delivered to a capillary bed. P_t is assumed to be 2 mmHg, although in some investigations this pressure has been found to be lower.[165] Net forces favor filtration at the proximal end (+ 10 mmHg, leading to 10 ml/min filtration) and reabsorption at the distal end (−8 mmHg, leading to 9 ml/min reabsorption into capillaries). The lymphatics return to the systemic circulation fluid that is filtered but not reabsorbed. (Adapted from Earley LE, Forland M: Nephrotic syndrome, in Earley LE, Gottschalk CW (eds): *Strauss and Welt's Diseases of the Kidney*, 3d ed. Boston, Little, Brown, 1979.)

interstitial space. A smaller volume of fluid than was originally filtered at the arteriolar end of the capillary bed is reabsorbed into the venules. Under steady-state conditions $J_V = J_L$, where J_L is the net return of fluid from the lymphatic circulation into the vascular compartment. Thus, the normal relationship between the intravascular volume and the interstitial volume of the extracellular fluid (ECF) space remains constant at a ratio of 3:1, and the volume of the ECF space remains constant at approximately 20 percent of that individual's lean body weight.

ALTERATIONS OF STARLING FORCES

The following abnormalities can lead to a translocation of fluid from the intravascular to the interstitial fluid compartment (refer to Fig. 19-1): (1) increase in capillary hydrostatic pressure (as seen in cerebral edema formation due to malignant hypertension); (2) decrease in plasma colloid osmotic pressure (as in nephrotic syndrome); (3) impaired venous outflow (venous thrombosis of an extremity); (4) impaired lymphatic flow (carcinomatous obstruction of lymphatics); or (5) increase in capillary permeability with a change in K_f ("leaky" pulmonary capillaries in acute respiratory distress syndrome with pancreatitis).

Edema formation is ultimately opposed by hydrostatic pressure generated within the interstitial fluid space, which is normally a very low pressure system; the hydrostatic pressure favors return of fluid and solutes to the vascular fluid space. Thus, in the case of acute lymphatic obstruction, interstitial fluid accumulates in the area drained by the obstructed system until P_t increases, owing to local tissue swelling, sufficient to stop the usual small net ultrafiltration. In burn injury with tissue necrosis K_f is increased such that capillaries become highly permeable to plasma albumin, thereby decreasing the plasma colloid osmotic pressure (and increasing the tissue colloid osmotic pressure). In this example, interstitial fluid accumulates until the tissue hydrostatic pressure P_t increases to match the capillary hydrostatic pressure P_c. In congestive heart failure, particularly in so-called right-sided heart disease, increased venous pressure is transmitted to the capillaries, causing an increase in P_c. Edema accumulates in dependent portions of the body until tissue pressure P_t offsets the elevated venous pressure. Even in individuals with severe nephrotic syndrome, edema accumulation, which is thought to result primarily from the fall in normal plasma oncotic pressure, diminishes with time as the interstitial space becomes engorged with fluid. In this case P_t slowly rises to the point that a new steady state is reached. Movement of fluid from the vascular space (J_v) then equals the return of fluid from the lymphatics (J_L) to the veins. A price is paid in the stabilization process, however: enlargement of the somatic part to the point that tissue pressure is increased.

ROLE OF KIDNEY IN EDEMA FORMATION AND MAINTENANCE

All edema, whether circumscribed or generalized, is ultimately dependent upon the kidney for maintenance. As pointed out in Chap. 18, there are multiple tubular mechanisms that lead to enhanced absorption of filtered salt and water within the nephron, particularly when the plasma volume is contracted. Thus, in conditions of localized edema accumulation, such as lymphatic or venous obstruction of an extremity, or in an area of circumscribed burn injury, the kidney increases tubular absorption of glomerular filtrate in response to a transient decrease in the intravascular volume. As illustrated in Fig. 19-2, a fall in the effective intravascular volume leads to a transient fall in cardiac output. This causes the kidney tubules to hyperabsorb glomerular filtrate, reexpand intravascular volume, and return the cardiac output to a normal value. However, as illustrated in Fig. 19-2, the patient's body weight is increased as the volume of the ECF compartment (in particular, the interstitial volume) is increased. There is a trade-off of sorts, in which renal tubules reabsorb extra salt and water to expand an inadequate circulatory volume. One "trades" edema for improved cardiac output. Thus, the kidney participates in a *secondary* fashion in the maintenance of localized edema accumulation. In such situations it is clearly appropriate for the kidney to hyperabsorb glomerular filtrate in order to refill the shrunken intravascular volume. If the injury to the local area persists, as illustrated in Fig. 19-2, each wave of edema accumulation causes a decrease in cardiac output and renal retention of additional salt and water. This is perceived clinically as a progressive increase in body weight.

In acute glomerulonephritis the kidney plays a *primary* pathogenetic role in the genesis and maintenance of generalized edema. In this instance the glomerular filtration rate (GFR) is decreased; continued oral intake of salt and water may not be accompanied by an appropriately balanced rate of salt and water excretion. Plasma volume is expanded as an initial response to the impairment in glomerular filtration. The total ECF volume is expanded as fluid "overflows" into the interstitium in consequence of "dilution" of the normal colloid osmotic force within the vascular tree. In this clinical situation, measurements of blood volume or cardiac output reveal normal or elevated values. Thus, the decline of salt and water excretion by the kidney in this circumstance cannot be viewed as an appropriate renal response. The kidney is clearly damaged and unable to perform its normal excretory and regulatory functions, and thereby contributes to the *primary* genesis and the *secondary* maintenance of edema.

Congestive heart failure illustrates another example of a "trade-off phenomenon" in which the renal response (hyperabsorption of glomerular filtrate) initially produces a beneficial effect (expansion of the effective intravascular volume to increase cardiac preload and return

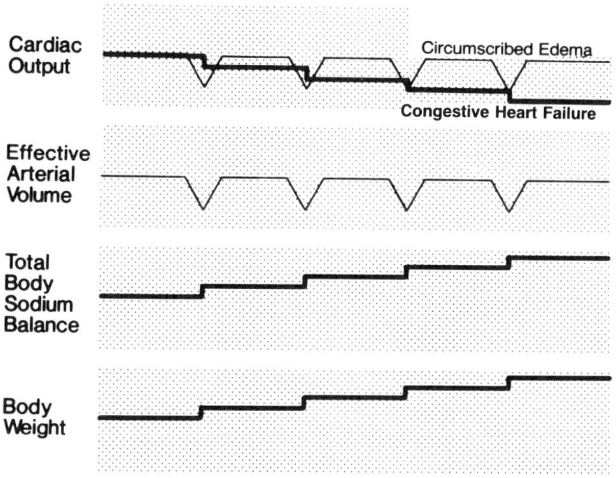

FIGURE 19-2 • Trade-off hypothesis for edema formation and maintenance in conditions of circumscribed edema and congestive heart failure. In congestive heart failure (heavy line, top) a decrease in cardiac output decreases effective arterial volume; in circumscribed edema (light line, top) effective arterial volume is decreased because fluid is translocated into tissues as a result of venous or lymphatic obstruction, increased K_f, or increased capillary hydrostatic pressure. In both cases renal response of increased sodium (and water) retention restores effective arterial volume at the expense of net increases in total body sodium and body weight. Further episodes of impairment of cardiac output or local fluid accumulation result in additional increments in sodium and weight.

cardiac output toward normal levels), albeit at the expense of an expanded ECF volume and edema. However, as illustrated in Fig. 19-2, many cardiac disease states are progressive. A transient stabilization of cardiac output or a transient return to normal cardiac output occurs, owing to the enhanced cardiac "preload" of plasma volume expansion that results from tubular hyperabsorption of glomerular filtrate. However, the effective arterial volume and cardiac output eventually decline and trigger another round of enhanced renal tubular reabsorption of sodium chloride and water. The ultimate consequence of this trade-off of enhanced renal retention of salt and water for effective arterial volume is the gradual expansion of total body salt and water content, reflected by weight gain and edema accumulation. The benefits of the trade-off (augmented cardiac output, increased cardiac preload) reach a limit when the Starling forces within the pulmonary capillary tree are tipped in the direction of filtration into the interstitium and alveolar spaces. Peripheral edema is not life-threatening; pulmonary edema is.

CONCEPT OF "EFFECTIVE" ARTERIAL VOLUME

In generalized edematous conditions, most evidence supports the notion that the plasma volume is the portion of the ECF volume that is primarily adjusted by renal mechanisms. The interstitial fluid volume is regulated secondarily by the balance of transcapillary Starling forces. It is important to note that renal salt and water balance is not controlled to hold intravascular volume constant; rather, plasma volume is regulated so as to achieve an "effective" blood volume adequate to meet the metabolic requirements of the peripheral tissues. Unfortunately, the "effective" arterial volume cannot now be quantified, and it probably bears no precise relationship to plasma volume measured using dilution principles. In other words, measurements of blood volume, erythrocyte mass, or plasma volume are probably not sufficiently accurate to determine whether or not the arterial blood volume matches the capacity of the arterial circulation.

The notion of an "ineffective" circulating blood volume is difficult to conceptualize. Consider, however, that at the instant of death from an arrhythmia the victim has a normal blood volume; it could even be measurably normal. Nevertheless, in the corpse the blood volume is not "effective." There are clinical conditions, such as severe congestive heart failure or hepatorenal syndrome, in which the patient is technically alive and the measured blood volume (assessed by isotopic techniques) is within the acceptable range for the individual's age and body weight or surface area. However, the blood volume is not much more effective in providing perfusion to the peripheral tissues and organs of these individuals than in our absurd analogy.

This is not to suggest that with congestive heart failure syndrome, severe changes in left ventricular dysfunction are necessary to induce abnormal salt and water retention by the kidney. Seminal studies by Barger and colleagues pointed out that alterations in sodium excretion can be detected even with the mildest forms of experimental heart failure before venous pressure is changed.[28] More recently, studies conducted in rats with acute myocardial infarction indicated that sodium excretion is reduced in animals with little or no change in maximal ventricular pumping capacity.[181]

SMALL ERRORS IN RENAL EXCRETION COMPOUNDED WITH TIME

In circumstances leading to an arterial volume that is inadequate for tissue perfusion, the kidneys are signaled to increase the tubular reabsorption of glomerular filtrate. Although the nature of the signal is not yet clear, increased tubular absorption is apparently the primary renal mechanism that accounts for the development of positive salt and water balance, since the GFR is often normal in many patients in the early stages of edema formation. The increase in renal salt and water excretion that is triggered inappropriately, because of an "ineffective" arterial volume, does not have to be very large to cause severe fluid retention and edema. Normally, the

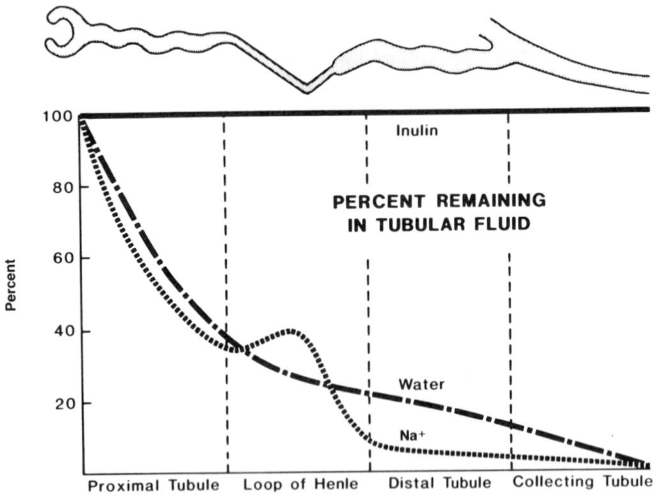

FIGURE 19-3 • Quantitative view of tubule salt and water reabsorption. Most filtered salt and water is reabsorbed in the proximal tubule without developing appreciable transtubule osmotic gradients. Sodium (Na^+) is actually added to tubule fluid in the descending limb of Henle's loop, but there is absorption of sodium without water in the ascending portion (the diluting segment). Only a small fraction of filtered sodium is reabsorbed in the distal and collecting tubules. Inulin, a marker of glomerular filtration, is neither reabsorbed nor secreted.

human body filters about 150 to 180 liters of ECF per day, of which all but 1 percent (1.5 liters) is reabsorbed by the renal tubules (see Fig. 19-3). If the kidneys make only a 0.5 percent error in reabsorption, so that 99.5 percent of the filtered salt and water is reabsorbed in the face of a constant fluid intake and constant GRF, then the individual will retain about 0.75 liter of water each day. In one week, 5.25 liters of extra water will be retained, which is a weight gain of about 11.5 pounds (5.25 kg). Thus, small errors in the reabsorption of filtered salt and water can build up to large excesses of body water and cause profound edema formation.

PRINCIPLES OF EDEMA MANAGEMENT

The best way to remove edema is to reverse whatever disease process initiated the sequence of events that led to the excessive renal retention of salt and water. For example, cardiac failure due to hypothyroidism can be reversed with thyroid hormone replacement; cardiac failure due to hyperthyroidism can be improved with ablation of thyroid tissue. Cardiac failure due to valvular insufficiency may be benefited by surgical prosthetic replacement. The nephrotic syndrome that occurs secondary to systemic vasculitis or minimal change glomerulopathy often responds to treatment with corticosteroids or a combination of cyclophosphamide and corticosteroids. Drugs such as nonsteroidal anti-inflammatory agents can induce the nephrotic syndrome; discontinuing such drugs can reverse edema formation.[123,245] One should attempt to uncover factors contributing to the pathogenesis of the sodium and water retention and treat appropriately those factors that can be reversed.

Several other supportive measures can be used to improve edema mobilization. These include bedrest, elevation of the lower extremities, elastic stockings and other pneumatic devices applied to edematous extremities, water immersion, and dietary restriction of salt and water intake. In the nephrotic syndrome, dietary supplementation of protein and calories will maximize the hepatic production of albumin; most foods that contain protein, however, also contain NaCl. Sodium intake must be monitored and restricted.

Bedrest decreases the hydrostatic pressure within the lower leg capillaries by eliminating a portion of the gravitational component. Thus, the sum of Starling forces is tipped to favor return of fluid from interstitium to capillaries. The metabolic requirements of the peripheral tissues are often decreased with bedrest, so that, in congestive heart failure, less demand is placed on a compromised myocardium. With this simple maneuver as much as 400 to 500 ml of tissue fluid can be transferred in a few days into the central venous circulation.[194,278] Other beneficial effects of bedrest include decreased circulating levels of catecholamines, aldosterone and antidiuretic hormone (ADH). Natriuresis and diuresis are thus facilitated.[281]

Diuretics are chemical substances that promote increased urine flow. With the exception of life-threatening pulmonary edema, diuretic drugs should not be used first in the treatment of edematous states. Diuretics should not be used for the treatment of *localized* edema (with the possible exception of pulmonary edema secondary to acute respiratory distress syndrome); these drugs should be used with caution in states of *generalized* edema accumulation. Diuretics inhibit salt and water reabsorption by the kidney tubules; as a result, they decrease plasma volume. As plasma volume transiently diminishes because of the loss of salt and water into the urine, plasma oncotic pressure rises and capillary hydrostatic pressure falls. In most instances forces favoring translocation of fluid from the interstitial to the intravascular compartment are enhanced and edema fluid "refills" the vascular volume. Since, in general, edema results from an ineffective arterial blood volume, diuretic therapy may lead to *further diminution* of the effective arterial blood volume. The rapid decrase of plasma volume may cause severe hypoperfusion of vital organs. For this reason other therapeutic measures should be considered prior to the use of diuretic drugs.

Despite the foregoing admonitions, diuretics can be used safely and judiciously to the comfort of the edematous patient. In fact, the use of diuretics may be the only means to mobilize edema in certain patients.

DIURETIC DRUGS

RENAL HANDLING OF DIURETIC DRUGS

Most diuretic drugs, except spironolactone and the osmotic agents such as mannitol, are organic anions at physiologic pH. They bind tightly to serum proteins and are not freely filtered into the urine (Table 19-1). Following gastrointestinal absorption or parenteral administration, these agents appear in the urine at much higher concentrations than in the plasma. They are actively transported (secreted) into the urine by the proximal tubules.[151,152] Certain endogenous organic anions, such as urate, lactate, and b-hydroxybutyrate, and certain common drugs such as penicillin, probenecid, and the cephalosporin antibiotics, are also secreted into the urine in the proximal tubule.[152,185] This rather indiscriminate secretory transport mechanism in the basolateral membrane of proximal tubules may be responsible for some of the drug interactions and side effects that occur with the use of diuretics.

Amiloride and triamterene are organic cations at physiologic pH, are extensively protein-bound, and appear in the urine in very high concentrations (Table 19-1).[24,164] They are secreted by the organic cation transport system also located within the basolateral membrane of proximal tubule cells. Thus, it appears that most diuretic drugs (with the possible exception of spironolactone) enter the urine via a transport step that moves the drug from the basolateral portion of the proximal epithelium through the cell into the urine. There, the drug exerts it inhibitory effect on salt and water transport in nephron segments farther downstream.

The affinity of diuretic drugs for the proximal tubule secretory transporter may determine to some extent the duration of action of these drugs. For instance, furosemide, ethacrynic acid, bumetanide, and chlorothiazide are highly protein-bound in plasma; yet these drugs are transported into the urine within minutes after appearing in the plasma. Urinary levels of these drugs build rapidly and disappear within several hours. In contrast, chlorthalidone and metolazone do not appear in the urine as rapidly. Instead, these drugs enter the urine in low concentrations and over a longer time; the drugs are found in the urine 20 to 24 h following administration. Hepatic excretion of some diuretic drugs may also determine the speed of onset and duration of their action.

It appears that the potent, rapidly acting diuretic drugs are organic anions that must enter the urine to effect a solute diuresis.[74] Hook and Williamson were the first to show that probenecid blocked the *acute* natriuresis and chloruresis usually caused by furosemide.[180] Probenecid evidently competes for the same basolateral secretory sites as furosemide and diminishes the entry of the diuretic into the urine. Brater and colleagues[71] have shown that probenecid delays entry of the diuretic into the urine (Fig. 19-4). In the presence of probenecid, furosemide enters the urine primarily by filtration rather than tubular secretion. Since furosemide is highly protein-bound, glomerular filtration is a rather inefficient way to excrete the drug. Consequently, low levels of furosemide are excreted in the urine for longer periods in the presence of probenecid than in the absence of probenecid. Figure 19-4 emphasizes how furosemide recirculates in the renal plasma when tubular secretion of the drug is blocked by probenecid. Probenecid also blocks the hepatic excretion of furosemide, thereby prolonging the life span of the diuretic in plasma and urine.[71,216,344]

Furosemide's brisk natriuresis and chloruresis of relatively short duration, when prlonged by probenecid, is shown in Fig. 19-5. The time course of drug activity is shifted to the right. Similar findings have been obtained with probenecid plus chlorothiazide in humans.[48] Interestingly, the overall natriuretic effects of standard doses of both furosemide and chlorothiazide (40 and 500 mg, respectively) were greater when probenecid was administered with the diuretic than when the drug was given without probenecid. Thus, it appears that the amount of diuretic-related inhibition of solute transport depends on the duration of drug action at the nephron, as well as on the concentration of the drug in the urine. The thiazide diuretics and those agents that work within the medullary portion of the loop of Henle (furosemide, ethacrynic acid, and bumetanide) seem to be such potent inhibitors of sodium chloride movement across the cells of the nephron that a *small* amount of drug present in the urine for a *long* period of time can elicit natriuretic and chloruretic responses that are as large as or greater than those seen with a *higher* concentration of drug given over a *shorter* time. In other words, in patients with normal rates of glomerular filtration, maximal inhibition of tubular salt reabsorption can be reached with modest doses of potent diuretics. Higher doses of potent diuretics given over short intervals are not as effective in removing excess body salt and water as smaller doses given more frequently, if GFR is normal. However, when the GFR is decreased, doses of diuretics must be increased significantly to reach a "threshold" for effect.[282,344] Often this requires progressive doubling of the dose of diuretic until diuresis occurs.

The work of Rose and colleagues gives some insight into the relative resistance to diuretics of individuals with azotemia.[283] Even though less furosemide is bound to plasma proteins in azotemic patients, and a larger fraction of plasma furosemide is filtered into the urine, furosemide given to azotemic subjects does not elicit the sharp rise in urine levels of the diuretic drug usually obtained following administration to normal subjects. Grantham and colleagues showed that certain aryl acids accumulate in the plasma of individuals with chronic renal insufficiency.[148,153,274] Furthermore, these aryl anions are transported into the urine by proximal tubules and they may interfere with the secretion of furosemide

TABLE 19-1 • Characteristics of drugs used for diuretic therapy

Drug	pk	Protein binding (%)	Major excretory routes	Normal dosing interval (h)	Dose adjustment with GFR decrease*			Comments and extrarenal effects
					>50	10–50	<10	
Acetazolamide	7.2	90–95	Renal	6	6	12	av	Decreases aqueous humor formation in the eye; diuresis ceases with development of metabolic acidosis
Amiloride	8.7	65–75	Renal	24	?	?	?	Blocks potassium excretion; tends to induce hyperkalemia
Bumetanide	3.6	95–97	Renal/ hepatic	6	6	nc	nc	Similar to furosemide but more potent; can be substituted for furosemide in allergic patients
Chlorthalidone	9.4	76	Renal/ hepatic	24	24	24	48	Tends to produce exaggerated urine potassium loss if patient fails to restrict sodium intake
Ethacrynic acid	3.5	90	Renal/ hepatic	6	6	6	av	Potentially ototoxic due to effects of cochlear endolymph solute transport Increases renal blood flow and increases venous capacitance Can be substituted for furosemide in allergic patients
Furosemide	3.8	91–99	Renal	6	6	6	6	Potentially ototoxic due to effects on cochlear solute transport
Indapamide	—	71–79	Renal	24	24	24	av	Has direct vasodilatory action
Mannitol	—	0	Renal	6	6	av	av	Avoid in renal failure
Mercurials	—	—	Renal	24	24	av	av	Relatively potassium-sparing; replaced by newer drugs
Metolazone	9.7	95	Renal/ hepatic	24	24	nc	nc	Appears to be useful when GFR < 30 ml/min
Spironolactone	—	98	Hepatic	6	6–12	12–24	av	Blocks potassium excretion; tends to induce hyperkalemia
Thiazides	6.3–6.8	65–95	Renal	12	12	12	av	Usually not useful when GFR < 30 ml/min
Triamterene	6.2	70–80	Renal/ hapatic	12	12	12	av	Blocks potassium excretion; produces hyperkalemia; can cause nephrolithiasis; acts as folic acid antagonist

* In ml/min.

Abbreviations: GFR, glomerular filtration rate; av, avoid; nc, no change.

SOURCE: Adapted from Bennett WM et al: *Ann Intern Med* 93:62, 1980; and Heel KC, Avery GS, in Avery GS (ed): *Principles and Practice of Clinical Pharmacology Therapeutics*, 2d ed. Australia, ADIS Press, 1980.

and other diuretics. Rose and colleagues found that the amount of furosemide entering the urine was decreased in azotemic patients; the natriuretic and chloruretic response to furosemide was also diminished.[283] Conceivably, some of the aryl anions in the urine of azotemic patients block the luminal action of furosemide in the loop of Henle.[152,153]

Inhibitors of prostaglandin (PG) synthesis may diminish the response to diuretics.[47,72] Although PG synthesis inhibitors are organic acids that can, potentially, block transport of the organic acid diuretics to their sites of action,[185] Brater and coworkers found that indomethacin decreased the diuretic response to furosemide in human volunteers without affecting the total amount and

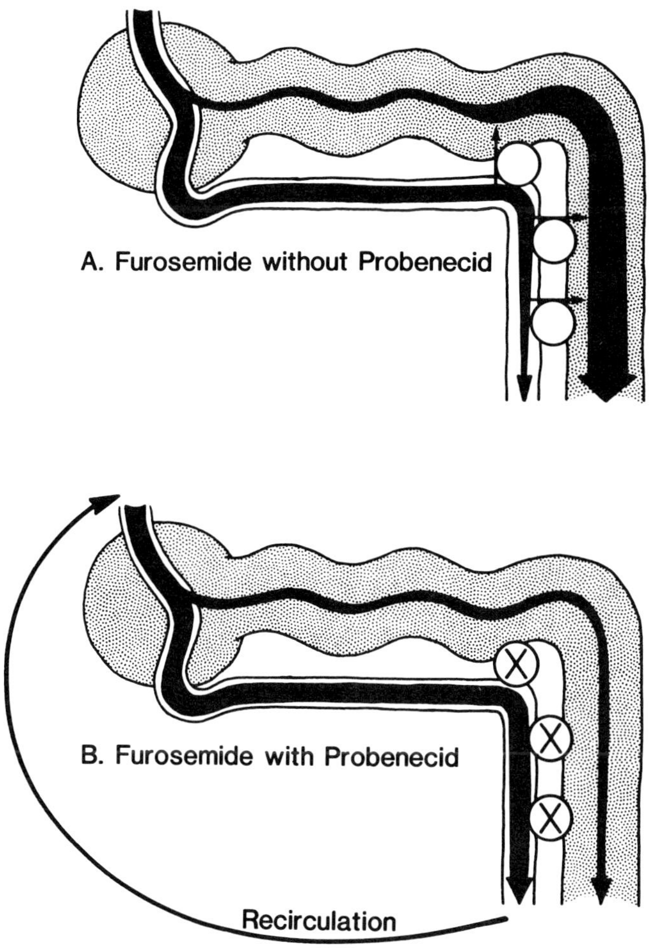

FIGURE 19-4 • Schematic representation of the renal clearance of furosemide. Furosemide is significantly bound to plasma proteins. Only a small portion enters the urine by filtration. A. The drug is primarily secreted into the urine under normal conditions. B. With probenecid administration furosemide secretion is blocked: furosemide recirculates in the plasma and enters the urine more slowly via glomerular filtration.

time course of delivery of the diuretic into the urine.[47] This effect was also associated with a decrease in furosemide-stimulated PG appearance in the urine.[24,25] Thus, it remains unclear whether indomethacin interferes with the inhibitory effects of urinary furosemide on the tubule or whether indomethacin blunts the diuretic effects of furosemide by means of hemodynamic alterations (see below).

EXTRARENAL EFFECTS OF DIURETIC DRUGS

Diuretic drugs have extrarenal as well as renal effects. For example, acetazolamide decreases aqueous humor formation in the eye,[238] and ethacrynic acid and furosemide decrease cochlear endolymph solute transport[58,204] (they are also potentially ototoxic in high doses); both drugs increase peripheral venous capacity,[96] which may prove beneficial in lowering pulmonary hydrostatic capillary pressure in individuals with pulmonary edema in the setting of acute myocardial infarction[96] (see below). Most of the important extrarenal effects of diuretic drugs are listed in Table 19-1. The table also highlights several pharmacologic characteristics of these drugs.

GENERAL NATURE OF DIURETIC ACTION

Most drugs used clinically to cause diuresis inhibit solute reabsorption in the renal tubule. Agents that increase GFR primarily through a direct action on renal plasma flow (e.g., dopamine) or by expanding plasma volume (e.g., albumin) may be regarded as diuretics. Many other drugs increase cardiac output, for instance, by reducing the pressure opposing the muscle contraction of the left ventricle. These *cardiac afterload reducers*, hydralazine,

FIGURE 19-5 • The natriuretic response to intravenous furosemide in human volunteers with and without probenecid pretreatment. *Left panel*, relationship between concentrations of furosemide in serum and sodium excretion rate. *Right panel*, relationship between urinary excretion rate of furosemide and sodium excretion rate. Note that probenecid delays the entry of furosemide into the urine; probenecid does not interfere with the natriuretic effect of furosemide once the drug reaches the urine. (From Chennavasin et al: Reprinted from *Kidney Int* 16:193, 1979.)

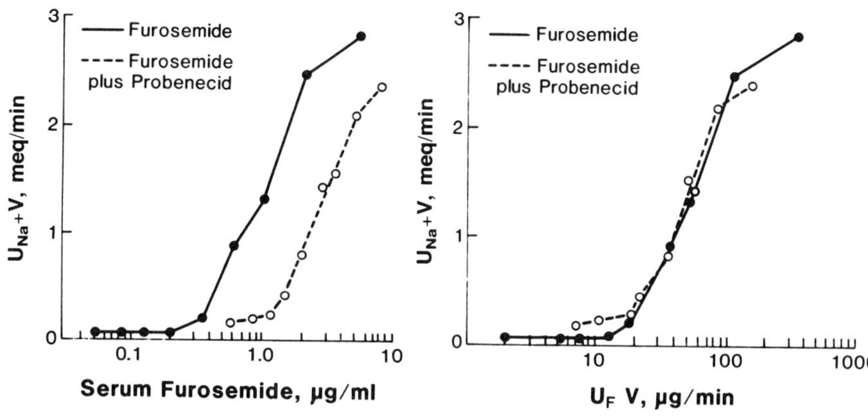

prazosin, angiotensin converting enzyme inhibitors (captopril, enalapril, lisinopril) nitroprusside and minoxidil, can at times increase renal blood flow and serve to increase both GFR and urine flow rate. (These drugs will be discussed later in this chapter.)

There are two general types of diuresis, solute and water diuresis (Fig. 19-6). Solute diuresis develops when the transtubular reabsorption of solute is impaired and the solute entering the tubule lumen by glomerular filtration is not reabsorbed to a normal extent. Since water reabsorption is tied to solute transport in the renal tubule, the inhibition of salt transport diminishes osmotic water reabsorption; *solute diuresis* ensues.

Salt reabsorption can be inhibited in two ways. First, a substance such as mannitol may be filtered into the urine freely; however, unlike glucose, mannitol is not reabsorbed by tubules and thereby the impermeant solute constrains the osmotic reabsorption of water.[137,259] Agents that act principally as nonreabsorbable filtered solutes are known collectively as *osmotic diuretics* (a rather poor name: *all* diuretics interfere with osmotic water reabsorption). The second type of solute diuresis derives from inhibition of active salt reabsorption in the tubule cell (Fig. 19-6). In this context, pharmacologic agents interfere with the machinery of active transport to slow the reabsorption of solute and, secondarily, the osmotic reabsorption of fluid. There are several steps in the sequence of salt reabsorption in which drugs might interfere:

1. The entry of solute into the cell at the urinary plasma membrane
2. The energizing step at which intracellular ATP fuels the solute pump
3. The exit of solute from the cell across the peritubular plasma membrane

Most potent diuretic drugs interfere with solute entry at the urinary plasma membrane.

Water diuresis without a corresponding increase in solute loss may be induced by pharmacologic means (Fig. 19-6). Antidiuretic hormone normally modulates the reabsorption of water along the distal nephron and collecting system.[149,154,172] Agents that block the cellular action of vasopressin (i.e., ADH) may cause water loss to a remarkable degree, without a concurrent increase in solute excretion. Some of these drugs, however, do increase sodium chloride excretion to a mild degree.[310]

CELLULAR MECHANISMS OF DIURETIC ACTION

The principal pharmacologic diuretics increase urinary salt excretion by decreasing the transepithelial reabsorption of sodium chloride.The cellular loci for inhibition of salt transport have been evaluated extensively for decades, and recently, a unitary view has begun to emerge.

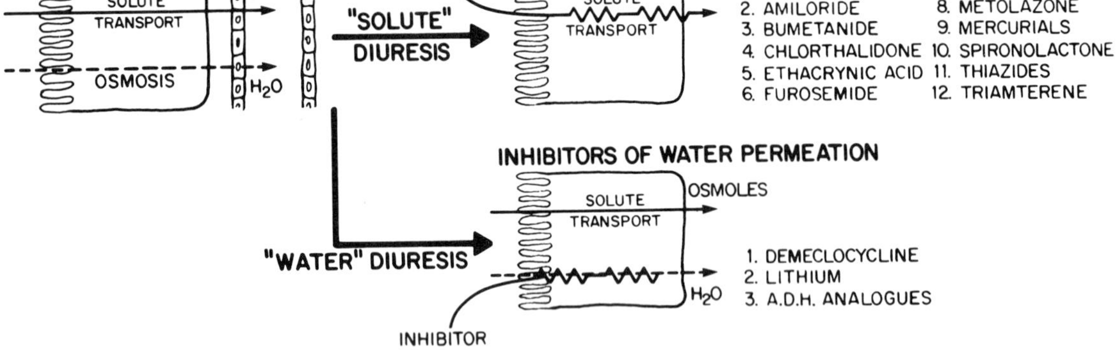

FIGURE 19-6 • General mechanisms of diuresis. Glomerular filtrate is absorbed in renal tubules due to the active transport of solute and the passive transport of water (osmosis). Interference with tubular absorption can result in two types of diuresis: (1) solute diuresis follows the glomerular filtration of nonreabsorbable solute or in consequence of the inhibition of solute pumps; (2) water diuresis follows the selective decrease in osmotic permeability to water. (Adapted from Grantham JJ, Chonko AM: The physiological basis and clinical use of diuretics, in Brenner BM, Stein JH (eds): *Sodium and Water Homeostasis.* New York, Churchill Livingstone, 1978.)

Energy derived from metabolism within renal cells is imparted to a solute pump on the blood or basolateral side of tubule cells. This pump is driven by energy stored as ATP. It effects the movement of three Na^+ ions from cytoplasm to interstitium in exchange for two K^+ ions that move from interstitium to cytoplasm. This imbalance between Na^+ and K^+ movement gives rise to a potential difference that is instrumental in the movement of anions in the absorptive direction.[14] The sodium pump (Na^+-K^+ ATPase) also establishes gradients for Na^+ and K^+ between cytoplasm and the urine and interstitial fluids. Thus, there is a tendency for Na^+ to diffuse into the cytoplasm from the urine and from the interstitium.

All along the renal tubule processes may be found that take advantage of the transmembrane Na^+ gradients. Specialized membrane proteins (transporters) permit absorption of certain solutes with Na^+ into the cell. We know the most about the coupling of Na^+ and Cl^- in the ascending limb of Henle's loop (Fig. 19-7). Here Na^+ and Cl^- are absorbed as the two ions enter the cytoplasm on a common carrier protein. The Na^+ ion is then pumped out of the cytoplasm by the Na^+ pump: Cl^- exits down a favorable electrochemical gradient. In this example, the energy for Na^+ and Cl^- transport is derived from metabolism, and transduced through the ion gradients generated by the Na^+-K^+ ATPase in the basolateral membrane. Urinary potassium appears to be essential for sodium chloride absorption.[159,160]

Recent studies have revealed many other interesting ways that Na^+ movement from urine to cell can be coupled to the movement of other ions. Na^+: H^+; Na^+: K^+; Na^+: HCO_3^-; Na^+: phosphate; Na^+: glucose; Na^+: amino acid; and Na^+: K^+: 2 Cl^- cotransport mechanisms have been postulated.[14,38,61,173,186] Experiments in rats indicate that the terminal Na^+: H^+ exchanger plays a major role in bulk transport in the proximal tubule since inhibition of this antiport system inhibits a major portion of transcellular chloride transport.[274a]

Recently, a novel chloride-anion (formate, hydroxyl, oxalate) luminal exchanger has been described in the proximal tubule.[293] The quantitative significance of this transport system remains to be elucidated.

Diuretics act primarily from the urine side to interfere with the coupling of movement of Na^+ to movement of other solutes from urine to cytoplasm. It is clear that the loop diuretics act to block NaCl cotransport. In the cortical distal tubule and collecting tubules, amiloride and triamterene inhibit Na^+: H^+ cotransport.[164,325]

Acetazolamide does not interact with Na^+ directly in the luminal membrane. This carbonic anhydrase inhibitor effectively acts from the urinary side by diminishing the reabsorption of HCO_3^- from the urine; Na^+ reabsorption is inhibited as a consequence.[211,239]

Only one diuretic, spironolactone, may act on the basolateral side of the tubule cells. Spironolactone competes with aldosterone for cellular receptors, and in this way the effect of the hormone is diminished.[85,232] Aldosterone potentiates Na^+ reabsorption by increasing the activity of the Na^+ pump and by increasing the movement of Na^+ from urine to cytoplasm. Recent work

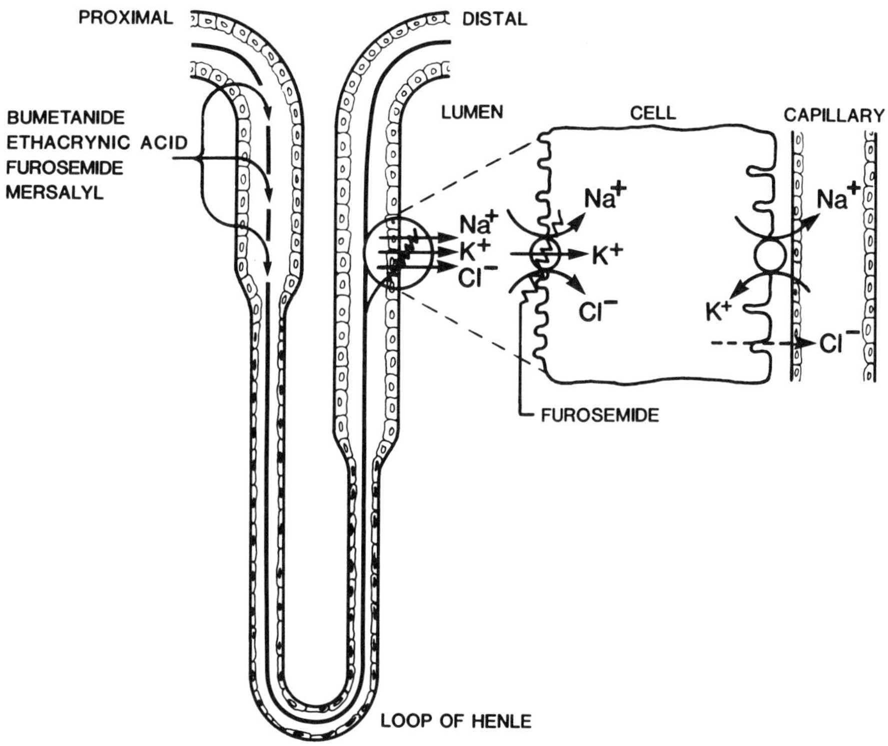

FIGURE 19-7 • Mechanism of action of furosemide in the loop of Henle. Furosemide is actively secreted into the urine in the proximal tubule and interferes with sodium and potassium chloride transport at the luminal membrane of the ascending limb to decrease net solute absorption. Note that the driving force for sodium and potassium chloride cotransport across the luminal membrane is created by the basolateral sodium-potassium pump fueled by ATP. Bumetanide, ethacrynic acid (cysteine adduct of the drug), and mersalyl probably have similar actions in this nephron segment.

suggests that the luminal effect of aldosterone may be primary.[241]

There are several interesting consequences of the site and mechanism of action of diuretics. Since they act primarily from the urine side, they must be either filtered or secreted into the urine to be effective. Many of the drugs that are tightly protein-bound are therefore not filtered appreciably (Table 19-1). The concentration of the diuretics in the urine by the combined processes of water reabsorption and tubular diuretic secretion leads to extraordinarily high levels of diuretic in the tubule fluid. This feature gives a measure of selective action within the kidney and spares other organs from the effects of the agents. Finally, by inhibiting the movement of salt and water from urine to cytoplasm diuretics, cellular swelling is avoided. Were their effect primarily to block the Na^+-K^+ ATPase, diuretics would cause the cells to swell as transepithelial transport of NaCl was blocked; this could lead to altered hydrodynamic performance in tubules and blood vessels.

ORGANIZATION OF THE RENAL TUBULE

To guide the discussion of diuretic mechanisms it is useful to divide the nephron into its respective axial components (see Fig. 19-8). In the proximal segment large amounts of salt and water are absorbed without the development of major differences in solute concentrations between urine and blood. By contrast, the distal nephron, which arbitrarily begins at the bend of Henle's loop, absorbs salt and water at a lower rate than proximally and generates great differences in concentration across the tubule wall.

It is clear that the nephron is much more heterogeneous than conveyed by the postwar concept of the bipartite tubule. The proximal tubule is composed of at least three distinct portions, ending in the descending limb of Henle's loop.[186,291,309] The ascending limb of Henle's loop has papillary and medullary thin segments;[206] medullary and cortical segments are somewhat different types of cells.[5,60] The distal convoluted tubule comprises four contiguous segments, all of which appear to function differently in respect to solute and water transport.[190,214] The collecting system begins in the cortex, where several connecting tubules unite to form the cortical collecting tubule.[6,184] The cortical collecting tubule descends unbranched into the medulla where several collecting tubules unit to form the medullary and thence the papillary collecting ducts.[280] Obviously, diuretics may interfere with solute and water reabsorption at several morphologically distinct sites along the renal tubule.[136] Figure 19-9 shows the nephron loci in which these drugs exert their major inhibitory actions on salt and water transport.

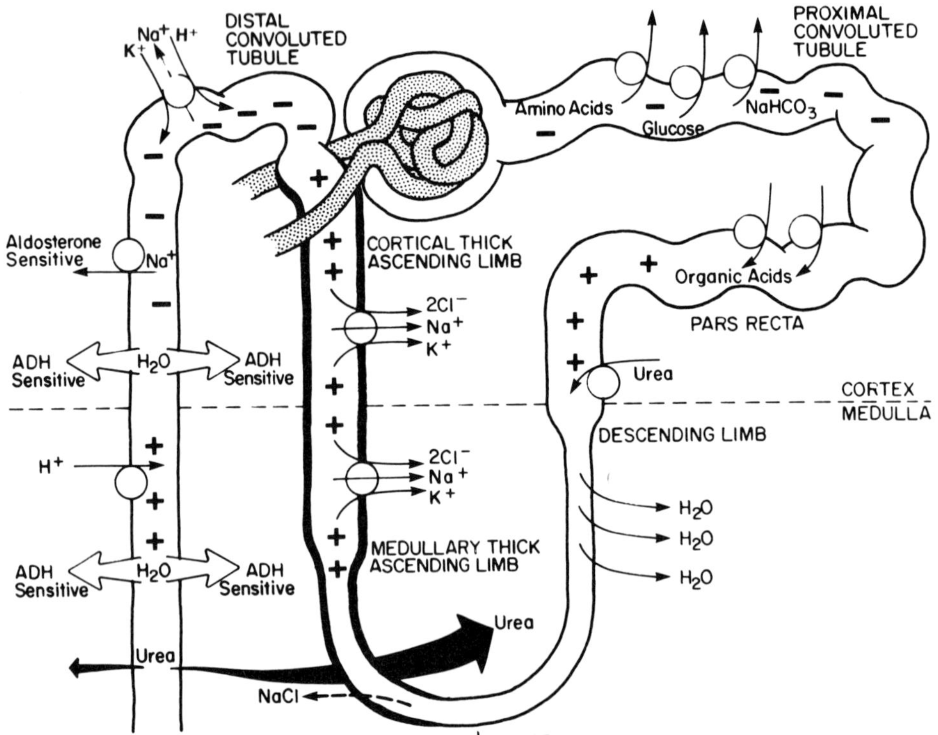

FIGURE 19-8 • Sites of tubule salt and water absorption. Sodium is reabsorbed with inorganic anions, amino acids, and glucose in the proximal tubule against an electrical gradient that is lumen negative. In the late part of the proximal tubule (pars recta), sodium and water are reabsorbed to a lesser extent and organic acids (hippurate, urate) and urea are secreted into the urine. The electrical potential is lumen positive in the pars recta. Water, but not salt, is removed from tubule fluid in the thin descending limb of Henle's loop, but in the ascending portion salt is reabsorbed without water, rendering the tubule fluid hyposmotic with respect to the interstitium Sodium, chloride, and potassium are reabsorbed by the medullary and cortical portions of the ascending limb; the lumen potential is positive. Sodium is reabsorbed and potassium and hydrogen ions are secreted in the distal tubule and collecting ducts. Water absorption in these segments is regulated by antidiuretic hormone (ADH). The electrical potential is lumen negative in the cortical sections and positive in the medullary segments. Urea is concentrated in the interstitium of the medulla and assists in the generation of maximally concentrated urine.

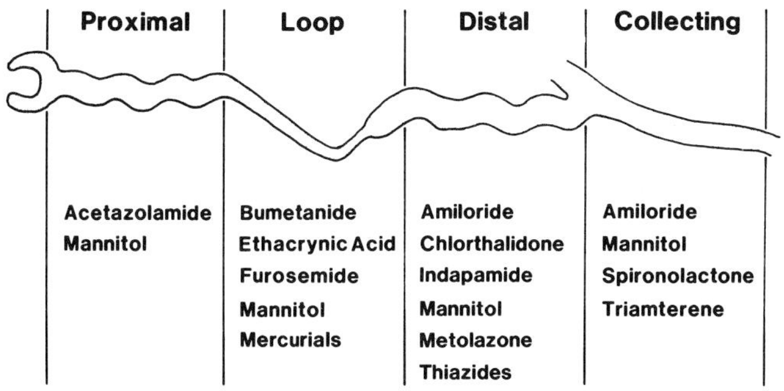

FIGURE 19-9 • Nephron loci in which diuretic drugs exert their major inhibitory actions on salt and water transport.

ACTION OF DIURETICS ON NEPHRON SEGMENTS

Glomerulus

It has been exceedingly difficult to determine if diuretics have a direct glomerular action, since most agents may alter tubular salt transport as they modify GFR. For example, thiazide diuretics decrease GFR; but these agents also inhibit distal salt reabsorption; the latter effect could alter GFR indirectly through either the renin-angiotensin or PG systems. By contrast, furosemide inhibits salt reabsorption in the loop of Henle and causes the GFR to increase in the early phase of drug action.[22,23,103] Heretofore, it had been impossible to separate the glomerular from the tubular effects of diuretic drugs; however, Brenner and associates[53,93] and Savin and colleagues[288] have devised experimental techniques that allow for a direct examination of glomerular effects. From these studies, it appears that physiologic and pharmacologic substances may alter GFR directly by changing either the rate of renal plasma flow, by means of afferent and efferent arteriolar constriction or dilation, or the K_f of the filtration barrier. Diuretic drugs set into motion a cascade of secondary events such as renin release and consequent generation of angiotensin, aldosterone, ADH, and intrarenal PGs. These substances may exert significant influences upon the glomerular filtration barrier. There are currently no reports to indicate that diuretics have direct effects on the hydraulic permeability of the glomerular filtration barrier.

PROXIMAL TUBULE

Approximately 70 percent of the glomerular filtrate is reabsorbed isosmotically in the proximal tubule. In this segment sodium is reabsorbed actively as well as coupled to reabsorption of glucose and amino acids (see Fig. 19-8).[61,205,208,290] This portion of the nephron reabsorbs the majority of the filtered bicarbonate by means of hydrogen ion secretion that is catalyzed by carbonic anhydrase.[37,239] These transport events in the early proximal tubule establish several passive forces that favor continued salt and water reabsorption in the later portions of the proximal nephron. These forces include a chloride diffusion gradient that results from the removal of bicarbonate from the filtrate; the osmotic effects of higher peritubular capillary concentrations of glucose, acetate, bicarbonate, and amino acids; and a lumen-positive diffusion potential created by the passive movement of chloride out of the tubule lumen.[61,205,207,208] Obviously, the proximal tubule is a segment in which even weakly active diuretics could exert profound effects on urinary salt excretion. The operation of the osmotic diuretic, mannitol, described above (see "general nature of diuretic action") is an example.[137,151] When the proximal tubules are modestly inhibited from transporting the usual amounts of filtrate out of the tubule lumen, proportionately more of the glomerular filtrate is delivered to the loop of Henle and tubule segments beyond. Because these later segments are able to compensate somewhat better than the proximal tubule for the presence of non-reabsorbed solutes, the overall effect of osmotic diuretics is relatively mild.

There is good evidence to show that many other diuretics have the ability to inhibit proximal salt and water reabsorption. The inhibition of absorptive capacity has been demonstrated in well-controlled laboratory studies in which high doses of the drugs were used;[64,74,97,203] in the usual clinical setting it appears that in sustained states of reduced plasma volume, the proximal tubules reabsorb proportionally more salt and water than normal. The increased reabsorption occurs even after administration of diuretics that can inhibit solute transport in proximal tubules. This paradoxical feature of many diuretics is a reflection of the so-called *braking phenomenon* observed with the chronic use of diuretics. The braking phenomenon is treated more fully in a later section.

Although acetazolamide is filtered somewhat, it enters the tubule cell and urine principally by active secretion through the aryl acid transport mechanism.[211,238,239] This drug causes diuresis by inhibiting carbonic anhydrase, which catalyzes the reaction between carbon dioxide and water shown in equation 2 or its equivalent in alkaline solution, equation 3.

$$CO_2 + H_2O \rightleftharpoons H_2CO_3 \qquad (2)$$

or

$$CO_2 + OH^- \rightleftharpoons HCO_3^- \qquad (3)$$

Inhibitors of this enzyme severely retard the formation of bicarbonate ion from carbon dioxide and water. In the context of renal solute reabsorption, a significant amount of solute is reabsorbed in the proximal tubule (a lesser amount in the distal tubule) as sodium bicarbonate. With its reabsorption impaired, bicarbonate behaves as an impermeant anion in the urine.

Bicarbonate reabsorption may occur by two principal mechanisms. One mechanism involves the luminal secretion of hydrogen ion that is inextricably tied to the catalytic action of carbonic anhydrase; the other mechanism involves reabsorption of bicarbonate as an anion much in the same way that chloride is transported. It is the catalytic reabsorption, the former, that is inhibited by acetazolamide in modest doses. Maren projected that approximately 25 percent of bicarbonate reabsorption is dependent on catalysis of carbon dioxide hydrolysis.[239] In a series of studies, Maren's group has shown that 99.99 percent of carbonic anhydrase can be inhibited by a dose of acetazolamide (10 mg per kilogram of body weight) sufficient to achieve a blood level of $10^{-4}M$. The increase in bicarbonate clearance resulting from such a moderate dose of the drug reflects the "catalyzed" component of bicarbonate reabsorption. It is also clear from Maren's work that additional bicarbonate excreted in response to higher blood concentrations of carbonic anhydrase inhibitor probably represents the component that is normally reabsorbed by the "noncatalytic" anion transport mechanism.[238,239] Thus, it appears that acetazolamide may increase urinary loss of solute and water in two ways: (1) by the specific inhibition of carbonic anhydrase in renal tubule cells; (2) (at high dose) by the nonspecific inhibition of anion reabsorption.

Many diuretics possess some carbonic anhydrase inhibitory activity; by virtue of their chemical properties as organic acids, many diuretics are accumulated and secreted by the proximal tubules. Thus, the action of furosemide, chlorothiazide, and chlorthalidone in the proximal tubule may all reflect the weak carbonic anhydrase inhibitory effect of each drug, amplified by cellular accumulation.

To summarize, in the proximal tubule sodium is actively reabsorbed, bicarbonate is reabsorbed in consequence of the secretion of hydrogen ion, and chloride is reabsorbed passively. Diuretics with carbonic anhydrase inhibitor activity interfere with hydrogen secretion and, in consequence, a bicarbonate-rich fluid enters the descending limb of Henle's loop. The reabsorption of sodium and chloride can be interfered with by several diuretics in the proximal tubule, but by mechanisms that are not understood. The clinical effectiveness of any agent acting in the proximal tubule depends heavily on the relative volume of the plasma compartment. With plasma volume expansion, acetazolamide, thiazides, furosemide, ethacrynic acid, and metolazone provoke solute and water loss from the proximal tubule; with plasma volume contraction they probably do not. Mannitol and other substances that are freely filtered into the urine and not actively transported by the tubules inhibit salt and water reabsorption from the proximal tubule lumen;[137,259] to a smaller extent they also operate in more distal tubule segments (Fig. 19-9). However, with plasma volume contraction the diuretic effect of mannitol also wanes.

Loop of Henle

The descending branch of the loop of Henle principally exchanges water from lumen to interstitium; no active solute transport is discernible in this segment. In the thin ascending segment sodium chloride is reabsorbed passively, owing to a steep gradient for urea from interstitium to tubule fluid.[206] No diuretics are known to be effective in this initial portion of the ascending limb of Henle's loop. In the medulla and cortex, however, solute reabsorption occurs in consequence of the active transport of solutes from lumen to blood.[62,63,279] Several studies indicate that sodium, potassium, and chloride may be reabsorbed by a cotransport process that operates in the luminal membranes of cells in the ascending loop of Henle (Fig. 19-7).[159,160]

In these segments salt is reabsorbed and dilute urine is formed due to the tubule wall's relatively low permeability to water. The ascending limb is the major source of free-water formation in the kidney.[59-63] Vasopressin (antidiuretic hormone, or ADH) does not change water permeability in this segment, but it does, apparently, stimulate salt reabsorption.[167,168,173]

The ascending limb is the site of action of several potent diuretics: bumetanide, furosemide, ethacrynic acid, and the mercurials;[63,74,204,344] thiazides, it appears, do not act in this segment from either side of the tubule. Each agent causes a diuresis typified by chloruresis. Each drug is more active from the urinary than from the peritubular side of the tubule.[74,151] The mechanism by which sodium, potassium, and chloride reabsorption across this segment is forestalled has not been completely resolved; currently available evidence favors the view that the diuretics block the entry of these solutes into the cell at a common cotransport carrier located at the urinary plasma membrane (Fig. 19-7).

Distal convoluted tubule

Sodium chloride and water are reabsorbed in the distal convoluted tubule, a segment that generates salt gradients. Kunau and associates[212] showed that thiazides unequivocally inhibit salt transport in this segment of the rat; Costanzo and Windhager[87] have shown that thiazides act primarily from the urinary side of the distal tubule. Inhibitors of carbonic anhydrase may act in this segment as well, but the inhibition of salt reabsorption is difficult to detect by micropuncture. Amiloride, a diuretic related to the more widely used triamterene, inhibits salt and water transport in the distal convoluted tubule by blocking sodium channels in the cell's luminal membrane.[23,100,327] Probably, sodium chloride reabsorption is modulated by aldosterone in this segment, although micropuncture studies have not yielded convincing results in this regard.[241,344]

Collecting system

Sodium, chloride, and water are normally reabsorbed to a varying extent along the entire course of the collecting system. This terminal segment is probably a key locus for the fine regulation of salt and water balance.[150,322] The collecting system is crucial in the context of all diuretic action, for any inhibitory action of diuretics proximal to the collecting segments can be outweighed by enhanced salt and water reabsorption in the terminal segments.

Several diuretics act directly in the collecting tubule (see Fig. 19-10). Amiloride rapidly inhibits sodium reabsorption in isolated cortical collecting tubules by interfering with the transport of sodium across the urinary membrane.[324,325] The blockade of sodium reabsorption interferes in turn with net potassium secretion.[262,263,337] In intact animals an amiloride (or triamterene) effect is evinced by incrased sodium and decreased potassium excretion.[163,164,351] Amiloride, triamterene, and spironolactone have only weak or moderate natriuretic effects because at the sites of their activity only small amounts of sodium chloride are reabsorbed.

Aldosterone has the important function in the collecting system of increasing sodium chloride reabsorption and potassium secretion. Salt reabsorption that is dependent on aldosterone can be inhibited with spironolactone, a competitive inhibitor of a variety of mineralocorticoids.[85] The effectiveness of spironolactone as a diuretic depends upon the influence of aldosterone in the distal nephron in a clinical setting of hyperaldosteronism (primary or secondary).

The collecting system is the principal segment where ADH mediates increased water reabsorption. Inhibition of the hormone leads to a water diuresis. Several drugs have been found to block the renal action of ADH, probably in the collecting system. Lithium, a cation used in the treatment of manic-depressive psychosis, caused nephrogenic diabetes insipidus. The cellular basis for the inhibitory effect on the ADH response is not clear, but lithium more than likely interferes with the intracellular production and action of cAMP.[310] Demeclocycline, a tetracycline derivative, also blocks the action of ADH on the kidney.[73,310] This drug has been used successfully in the treatment of patients with the syndrome of inappropriate ADH secretion.[73] It appears that newer synthetic analogues of ADH, which bind to the collecting tubule ADH receptor sites but do not elicit hydroosmotic effects, may be useful in the treatment of this syndrome.[237]

Abramow[3] reported that ethacrynic acid and furosemide inhibit the action of ADH in isolated perfused collecting tubules. Such an inhibitory action, if exercised in vivo, could explain the observation that slightly dilute urine may be excreted transiently when these potent loop diuretics are infused into patients with the syndrome of inappropriate ADH secretion.[169]

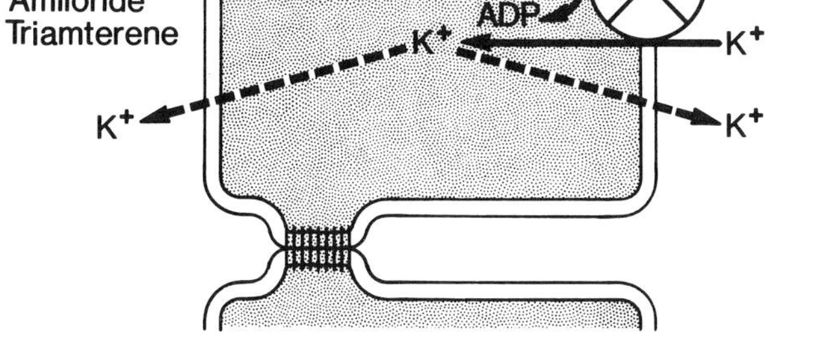

FIGURE 19-10 • Mechanism of action of distal and collecting tubule diuretics. Spironolactone interferes with the effect of aldosterone to increase the rate of sodium-potassium exchange at the basolateral surface. Amiloride and triamterene interact with lumen membrane transporters to prevent the entry of urinary sodium into the cytoplasm. The net effect of all these drugs is to decrease sodium absorption and potassium secretion.

HEMODYNAMIC EFFECTS OF DIURETICS

Several diuretics have hemodynamic effects in the kidney. Intravenous furosemide and ethacrynic acid cause a significant decrease in renal vascular resistance and an increase in renal blood flow.[22,27,103,292] The mechanism of this renal response remains controversial. It may be due to enhanced intrarenal genesis or release of vasodilatory (and natriuretic) PG derivatives; these PG derivatives are found in increased amounts in the urine and renal venous effluent following administration of furosemide (see Fig. 19-11).[1,2,354,355] Moreover, PG synthetase inhibitors have been found to block the furosemide-induced renal vasodilatation in most,[23,25,103,228] although not all,[26] investigations. It is of interest that furosemide and ethacrynic acid do not significantly increase GFR when renal blood flow is increased.[187] By contrast, acetazolamide, benzolamide, and chlorothiazide administered intravenously decrease both renal blood flow and GFR.[23,103,243] The mediation of this response remains uncertain. However, there is evidence that stimulation of the renin-angiotensin system may be responsible, since the fall in both renal blood flow and GFR is vitiated by concurrent blockade of angiotensin.[341]

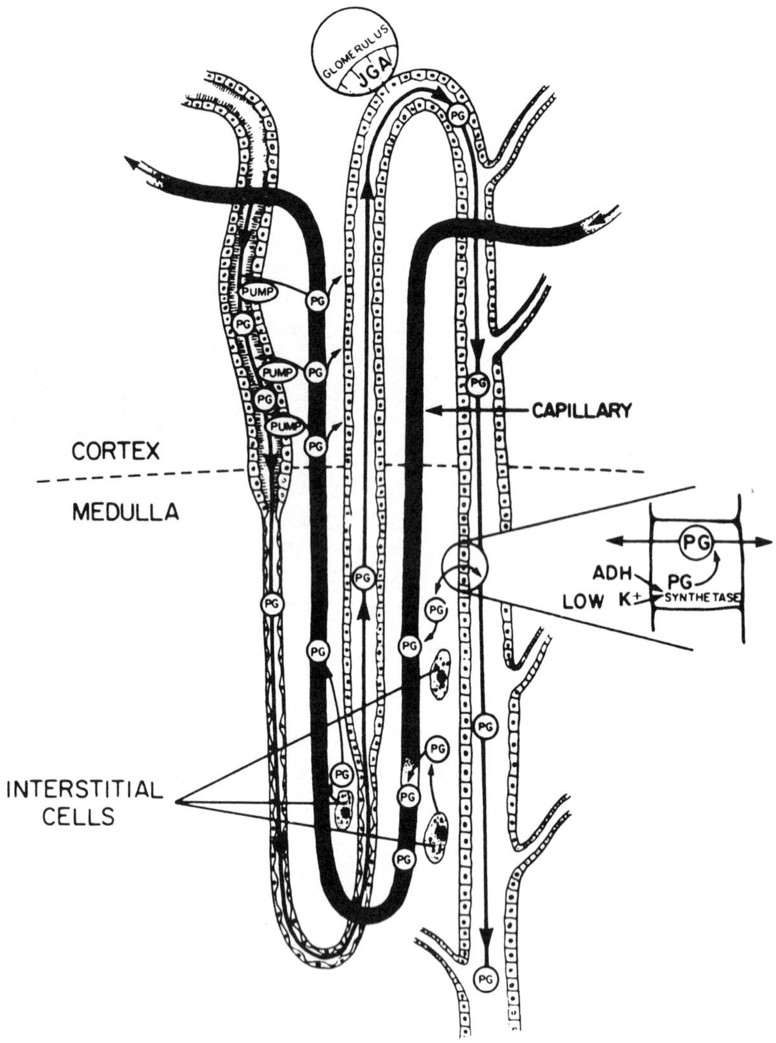

FIGURE 19-11 • Hypothetical scheme for the intrarenal delivery and tubule transport of endogenous prostaglandins. Vasopressin (ADH) and hypokalemia stimulate the synthesis of prostaglandins in the interstitial and collecting tubule (duct) cells. The prostaglandins may enter the peritubular capillaries and vasa recta to be transported to cortical structures. The prostaglandins are extracted from the cortical capillaries and secreted into the urine by the proximal tubules. [From Grantham JJ, Chonko AM, in Brenner BM, Stein JH (eds): *Sodium and Water Homeostasis.* New York, Churchill Livingstone, 1978, p. 178. Used with permission.]

In the past decade, specific dopaminergic receptors have been located within the renal cortical vasculature.[144,166,294] Dopamine infusions in low dose (approximately 2 to 3 μg/kg per min) produce significant increases in renal blood flow and, at times, increased GFR in experimental animals[103,249] and in clinical studies.[143] In most situations augmented urine flow is elicited with intravenous administration of this alpha-adrenergic agonist regardless of the rate of glomerular filtration. Bello-Reuss and colleagues[31] have shown that dopamine blocks net salt and water reabsorption in proximal rabbit tubules perfused in vitro. Thus, although the primary effect of low-dose dopamine may be related to augmentation of renal blood flow to the glomeruli, and perhaps to increased K_f, the drug also inhibits tubular reabsorption of glomerular filtrate.[31,229] Increasing urine flow in the face of a falling GFR is beneficial in certain clinical situations (e.g., oliguric acute renal failure). However, reports of occult plasma volume contraction and "polyuric" prerenal failure (i.e., prerenal azotemia due to plasma volume contraction) in patients treated with dopamine (either alone or in combination with nephrotoxic antibiotics such as the aminoglycoside derivatives) have appeared.[252] Since dopamine causes the kidney to produce urine even in the setting of reduced plasma volume, an adequate plasma volume is essential in any individual who receives the drug.

INTEGRATED RENAL MECHANISMS AND DIURETIC EFFECTS

Diuretic effects of the renin-angiotensin, renal kallikrein-kinin, and renal prostaglandin systems

There are multiple and complex interactions among the three major vasoactive hormone systems (renin-angiotensin, kallikrein-kinin, and PG systems) that have been demonstrated to exist within the mammalian kidney. Renal PGs appear to play a pivotal role in the relationships among the three systems (see Fig. 19-11).[22,24,138] For instance, PGs enhance renin production both in vitro[350] and in vivo.[22,343] Prostaglandins also appear to mediate both baroreceptor-initiated[22] and sympathetically stimulated release of renin by the kidney.[65] Moreover, products of the renin-angiotensin and kallikrein-kinin systems serve as positive feedback to stimulate PG production.[246,364] In addition, the renin-angiotensin-aldosterone system stimulates release of kallikrein, probably through an effect of aldosterone.[240] Since the renin-angiotensin system primarily constricts the renal cortex vessels, whereas the kinin and PG systems primarily dilate them, a complex vascular "tug of war" is going on within the kidney at most times. Prostaglandin synthetase inhibitors, such as the nonsteroidal anti-inflammatory drugs, can tip the balance of forces in the direction of vasoconstriction, and thus reduce renal blood flow significantly. Glomerular filtration rate is usually steady under normal circumstances, despite the use of these drugs; it is kept constant by means of compensating mechanisms that provide for GFR autoregulation.[102,138] However, if the renal parenchyma has previously been injured (for instance, by obstruction, ischemia, or inflammation), inhibition of PGs with pharmacologic agents can produce declines in both renal blood flow and GFR.[102,256,346]

Diuretic drugs, in particular bumetanide, furosemide, ethacrynic acid, and the thiazide derivatives, have a complicated impact on the three renal vasoactive hormone systems. These diuretic agents cause an increased release of renin, PGs, and kinin from the mammalian kidney. The most consistent reaction pattern seen following administration of diuretic drugs is one of augmented renin release from the juxtaglomerular apparatus, which may[24,25,130] or may not[1,2] be related primarily to PG release. Renin release eventuates in generation of angiotensins I and II within the kidney (and the lung). Angiotensin II is a potent pressor substance owing to its ability to induce peripheral arteriolar constriction. However, the renal vasoconstrictive effects of angiotensin II are opposed under normal circumstances: angiotensin II simultaneously stimulates the intrarenal synthesis of vasodilating PGs (and perhaps kinin release).[295,364] Edwards[108] found that angiotensin II, when applied in vitro to isolated afferent and efferent arterioles dissected from the rabbit cortex, preferentially constricts the efferent, but not the afferent arteriole. It appears that under conditions of decreased renal perfusion and relative cortex ischemia, activation of the renin-angiotensin system might provide a protective mechanism for maintaining filtration pressure across the glomerular capillary by means of selective postglomerular efferent arteriolar constriction.[88,182]

A complete discussion of the interactions among the vasoactive hormone systems of the kidney is beyond the scope of this review. This topic is more completely covered in Chap. 14 to 16; in addition, several excellent reviews have appeared in the literature recently.[12,22,27,102,295]

Renal compensatory responses to diuretics: "The braking phenomenon"

It is intuitively obvious that the diuresis induced by any drug is inherently self-limited. Extracellular fluid volume depletion sufficient to cause marked arterial hypotension could theoretically stop the formation of glomerular filtrate; the example is extreme, akin to the surgical aphorism that "all bleeding stops." Long before frank arterial hypotension develops owing to severe depletion of the ECF compartment, intrarenal adjustments occur that curtail the loss of salt and water into the urine. In general, the administration of any diuretic sufficient to decrease the plasma volume causes the compensatory increase of solute and water reabsorption in portions of the nephron not inhibited by the drug. In other words, when a diuretic blocks solute and water transport across one particular nephron segment, the fractional reabsorption of glomerular filtrate can increase across other segments of the nephron located proximal and/or distal to the inhibited segment.

The compensatory increases in reabsorption that occur in segments of the nephron not directly inhibited by diuretic drugs have been detailed in studies of acetazolamide, which exerts its primary effect in the proximal tubule.[37,211] As increased amounts of glomerular filtrate rich in sodium bicarbonate leave the proximal tubule, the more distal segments, particularly the loop of Henle, increase the reabsorption of sodium chloride. Consequently, the natriuretic and diuretic effect of the drug is much less than would be predicted from its selective action on the proximal tubule alone. Indeed, the loop of Henle responds so proficiently to increases in sodium chloride delivery that it has been suggested that changes in proximal tubule reabsorption may be of little consequence to the overall regulation of sodium excretion.[137,203]

In addition to the rapid renal adjustment to the loss of salt from the proximal tubule, other conserving mechanisms come into play when a proximally acting diuretic is given. Depletion of the extracellular fluid volume causes the release of renin from the kidney.[77] Elevated levels of plasma renin increase the generation of angiotensin, which in turn stimulates adrenal secretion of aldosterone. Elevated levels of plasma aldosterone increase sodium reabsorption and potassium secretion across the distal nephron. Thus, the proximal diuretic action of acetazolamide increases salt reabsorption in the loop of Henle and the more distal portions of the nephron to counteract the primary action of the drug. Overall, however, there is an increased rate of urinary salt excretion in response to acetazolamide, although the effect of the drug on the proximal tubule is not fairly represented by what appears in the final urine.

The intrarenal adjustments in response to diuretics tend to slow down or brake the urinary excretion of salt. This is the *braking phenomenon*[74,352,353] Conceptually, the braking phenomenon appears to be the mirror image of the so-called escape phenomenon seen in patients on a high salt intake and exogenous mineralocorticoid (see Chap. 3). The braking phenomenon is not limited to diuretics with primary actions in the proximal segments of the nephron. As illustrated in Fig. 19-12, normal subjects on a fixed daily salt intake, when given a potent loop diuretic, quickly develop negative salt balance. There is weight loss during the first few days of diuretic administration as the ECF volume decreases. After the initial phase of diuretic action the amount of salt appearing in the urine progressively diminishes; within a week the urinary salt losses fall to a level equal to the oral salt intake: the point of *salt balance*. At this point fractional reabsorption of salt in the proximal tubules and distal nephron is increased sufficiently to offset the saliuretic action of the diuretic in the loop of Henle. Here, the braking phenomenon diminishes the net excretion of salt. The phenomenon in this case is due to multiple factors operating in the proximal tubule (perhaps including suppression of a "third factor"), and increased salt absorption in the distal nephron; the distal effect is mediated through stimulation of aldosterone upon volume reduction.

Recent experiments in animal models and in human volunteers are consistent with the notion that diuretic-induced stimulation of the renin-angiotensin-aldosterone axis and sympathetic nervous system is central to the blunting of diuretic effect (braking phenomenon). It has been shown that angiotensin II and norepinephrine directly stimulate Na^+-H^+ antiporter transport activity and increase the proximal reabsorption of sodium, chloride, and water.[230] These hormones can enhance proximal tubule reabsorption by their effects on peritubular capillary hemodynamics.[74,282]

In the distal nephron, aldosterone increases the size of responsive cells in the collecting tubule, particularly when distal tubule sodium delivery is high.[112,191,192,316-318] Thus, compensatory distal tubule cell growth as well as augmented transport rate serve to decrease the natriuresis obtained with chronic diuretic administration. Wilcox and associates were the first to confirm the braking phenomenon hypothesis in normal volunteers.[352,353] Loon and colleagues have recently extended these observations and identified increased distal convoluted tubule transport as an adaptation to chronic diuretic treatment in humans.[231]

CLINICAL COMPLICATIONS OF DIURETIC DRUGS (TABLE 19-2)

A clear understanding of the tubular adjustments that account for the development of the braking phenomenon is important when the clinical complications commonly induced by diuretic drugs are considered. Many of these complications derive from the increased reabsorption of glomerular filtrate mediated by plasma volume contraction in portions of the nephron not affected directly by the diuretic. The reabsorption of most filtered solutes, not just the sodium ion, is affected by the state of expansion or contraction of the ECF compartment. Therefore, most

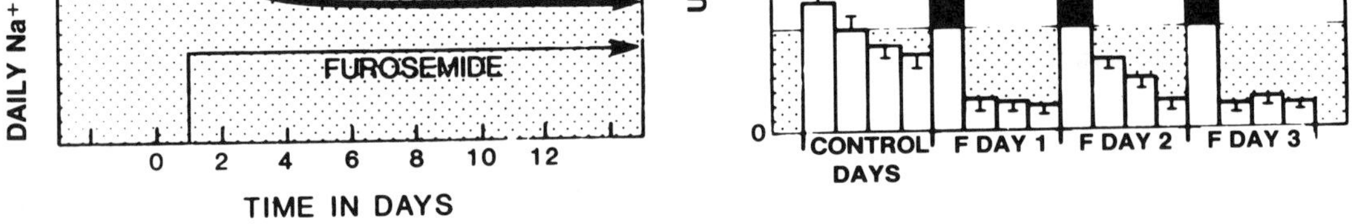

FIGURE 19-12 • Illustration of the "braking phenomenon" that accounts for how salt (and fluid) balance is established during the administration of furosemide. (*Left*) Relationship between sodium intake and excretion, before and after daily furosemide administration. Note that the urinary excretion of sodium exceeds dietary intake for several days, during which time the person loses 1 to 2 kg of weight. After 7 to 8 days, the urinary excretion of sodium once again equals the daily intake of sodium as "hyperabsorption" of filtered sodium occurs across tubule segments not blocked by furosemide. (*Right*) Relationship between sodium intake and excretion in human volunteers taking furosemide and adhering to a constant intake of sodium. Note that the urine excretion of sodium exceeds intake only for several hours each day when furosemide is being excreted in the urine; the remainder of each day the urine sodium excretion is diminished to levels below the control excretory values (stippled area) as tubule segments hyperabsorb glomerular filtrate in response to mild plasma volume contraction. The net effect of the pulse use of furosemide is to defeat the goal of producing a persistent decrease in ECF volume. [Adapted from Grantham JJ, Chonko AM: Diuretics, in Brenner BM, Stein JH (eds): *Topics in Nephrology*. New York, Churchill Livingstone, 1978, p. 178; and Wilcox CS et al: Response of the kidney to furosemide. 1. Effects of salt intake and renal compensation. *J Lab Clin Med* 102:450, 1983.]

TABLE 19-2 • **Complications of diuretic therapy**

FLUID, ELECTROLYTE, AND ACID-BASE DISORDERS
Extracellular fluid volume depletion
Potassium depletion
Magnesium depletion
Metabolic alkalosis
Metabolic acidosis
Hyponatremia
Hypercalcemia
METABOLIC DISORDERS
Hyperuricemia
Hyperglycemia
Hyperlipidemia
Gynecomastia/sexual dysfunction
Osteomalacia
TOXIC DISORDERS
Ototoxicity
Hypersensitivity

of the important complications of diuretics can be explained within the framework of our understanding of segmental nephron reabsorptive characteristics. Most fluid and electrolyte complications occur within the first several weeks of therapy provided that dose, dietary intake, and renal function remain stable.[33,282,331,337]

Fluid, electrolyte, and acid-base complications

Depletion of the extracellular fluid volume

Extracellular fluid volume depletion is a common complication of diuretic use, particularly when the potent loop-acting diuretics are employed.[112,204,282] As discussed above, patients are protected against ECF depletion to some degree by the braking phenomenon. The patients most prone to develop ECF depletion are those individuals with gastrointestinal tract complications such as nausea, vomiting, or diarrhea who are unable to ingest appropriate amounts of salt and water to replace the major portion of the ongoing daily urinary losses. In patients with underlying renal insufficiency, ECF depletion can lead to the development of overt uremia, although in many individuals prerenal azotemia develops with a ratio of blood urea nitrogen (BUN) to creatinine of 15:1 to 20:1; orthostatic hypotension and a tendency toward oliguria result. Increased tubule absorption of filtered urea and increased urea appearance due to release of amino acids from peripheral tissues and increased hepatic degradation contribute to the prerenal azotemia.[193] This complication underlies another complication of diuretic treatment, the genesis and maintenance of metabolic alkalosis. Both ECF depletion and metabolic alkalosis respond to replenishment of the ECF fluid with isotonic saline and/or discontinuation or dose reduction of the diuretic drugs.

Potassium depletion

Potassium depletion is another complication of diuretic use. This subject has received extensive attention in the recent medical literature.[101,178,179,260,313] Some investigators think that concern about this complication is exaggerated.[171,222,255] That does not mean that potassium depletion is not a serious problem, since it can lead to defects in renal concentration[32,59] and eventually to the development of interstitial fibrosis.[276,277,337] Severe potassium depletion may cause malfunction of other organ systems: cardiac muscle irritability, particularly in conjunction with digitalis therapy;[323] decreased striated-muscle blood flow and predisposition to rhabdomyolysis;[202] and sluggish pancreatic insulin release with attendant carbohydrate intolerance.[118] Patients taking diuretics who suffer a myocardial infarction may experience significant shifts of potassium into cells in consequence of catecholamine release; this may provoke increased ventricular ectopy.[284]

Inhibition of potassium reabsorption in the proximal tubule may contribute to urinary potassium loss. Acetazolamide, bumetanide, furosemide, and ethacrynic acid may increase the amount of potassium reaching the bend of Henle's loop. How much of the unreabsorbed potassium escapes into the final urine is not known, because potassium reabsorption in the collecting system may modify substantially the composition of the terminal urine.

Acetazolamide, bumetanide, furosemide, ethacrynic acid, the thiazides, and osmotic diuretics also may promote urinary potassium loss by an indirect action on the distal convoluted and cortical collecting tubules. Urinary potassium secretion is strongly dependent on the rate of volume flow past these distal sites.[316,317,337] Other factors that favor potassium loss into the urine include enhanced delivery of sodium chloride to the distal nephron, enhanced delivery of relatively impermeant anions to the distal nephron, and the presence of elevated plasma levels of aldosterone.[316,317,337] Even a slight decrease in the ECF volume activates the renin-angiotensin-aldosterone system; aldosterone increases potassium secretion in the distal nephron. Thus, increased urine flow together with increased levels of aldosterone promote high rates of potassium secretion into the urine.

With the development of hypokalemia, the secretion of aldosterone by the adrenal gland drops.[44,45,77,337] It is also important to note that with sustained contraction of the ECF compartment, enhanced proximal reabsorption of glomerular filtrate diminishes the flow of urine into the distal nephron. Consequently, with sustained volume contraction and potassium depletion, excretion of the cation may be sharply curtailed. Other factors responsible for increased distal tubule potassium secretion include metabolic alkalosis[316] and increased ADH levels.[122]

In patients taking diuretics, exaggerated kaliuresis usually does not occur if an appropriate decrease in the volume of the ECF compartment is achieved. Davidson and associates[90] studied 83 patients with organic heart disease who were taking either furosemide or a thiazide derivative over a long period. Only 15 percent of these patients developed mild hypokalemia (serum potassium levels < 3.5 meq/liter); none developed severe hypokalemia (serum potassium levels ≤ 3.0 meq/liter). The deficit in total-body potassium was only 3 to 5 percent (100 to 150 meq/liter) in the mildly hypokalemic individuals. Similar findings have been reported in patients with hypertension who were given long-term thiazide treatment.[222] Urinary potassium loss and potassium depletion are most pronounced in those patients who take diuretics and ingest large loads of solute and water. In these patients supplemental intake of potassium chloride may be necessary. However, restriction of dietary sodium intake (to about 87 meq/day) is the most appropriate way to abolish excessive urinary potassium wasting.

All diuretics do not increase losses of potassium into the urine. Spironolactone, a competitive antagonist of aldosterone, and amiloride and triamterene, which are not structurally related to aldosterone, act on the distal nephron to block potassium secretion. These agents are most effective when used in combination with the more potent loop inhibitors to reduce the urinary potassium loss of intense diuresis.

Angiotensin converting enzyme inhibitors also decrease kaliuresis induced by thiazide and loop diuretics. A portion of this decrease can be attributed to diminished aldosterone levels.[106,337] Physicians are cautioned not to use antikaliuretic drugs routinely in patients with renal insufficiency since life-threatening hyperkalemia and metabolic acidosis may develop.[106,132,157] The metabolic acidosis that results may be due in part to decreased ammonia generation by the renal epithelium in the face of hyperkalemia.[335,336]

Metabolic alkalosis

Metabolic alkalosis is often seen together with total body potassium depletion upon the use of diuretics. Seldin and Rector[300] and Kurtzman and coworkers[215] have extensively reviewed the mechanisms by which alkalosis may occur. It is generally held that potassium depletion causes increased secretion of hydrogen ion by renal tubules together with an increased excretion of ammonia into the urine. Ammonium is excreted as a chloride salt. Consequently, for each equivalent of ammonium excreted one equivalent of bicarbonate appears in the plasma compartment in place of chloride. Owing to contraction of the ECF compartment the metabolic alkalosis is maintained by increased reabsorption of sodium bicarbonate. Metabolic alkalosis can also result from the intense renal loss of sodium chloride. *Contraction alkalosis* was first reported with the clinical use of ethacrynic acid, a potent chloruretic agent.[67] In most cases of diuretic- induced metabolic alkalosis, reduction of the dose of diuretic results in correction of the alkalosis.[195] Potassium supplementation to a level exceeding normal dietary potassium intake is sometimes required.[135]

Metabolic acidosis

Metabolic acidosis may occur as a complication of acetazolamide, amiloride, spironolactone, or triamterene therapy. Acetazolamide induces renal sodium bicarbonate wasting which halts when the plasma bicarbonate level falls to about 18 to 19 meq/liter. The effect of the drug is due to carbonic anhydrase inhibition; the diuretic effect of the drug ceases when the mild metabolic acidosis develops.

Spironolactone may also produce hyperchloremic metabolic acidosis.[132] The blockade of aldosterone diminishes urinary potassium excretion such that a surfeit of potassium builds within the renal tubular epithelium. The excess potassium reduces ammonia extraction by the tubules and decreases net ammonium chloride excretion into the urine. Amiloride and triamterene can produce a similar syndrome of hyperkalemic metabolic acidosis. Reducing the body potassium stores (with polystyrene sulfonate resin, Kayexalate) often diminishes the acidosis.[333]

Hyponatremia

Hyponatremia is seen relatively frequently in patients taking diuretics. Fichman and coworkers[121] reported on 10 patients with severe, symptomatic hyponatremia due to thiazides. All of the patients were depleted of potassium. Their plasma ADH activity levels were paradoxically elevated. Since the subsequent correction of hyponatremia could not be attributed to the retention of exogenous sodium, it was suggested that potassium depletion may have facilitated the entry of sodium into cells during the loss of potassium chloride in the urine. The resultant volume contraction due to the loss of extracellular solute may have provoked the release of ADH to promote the development of hyponatremia.

Diuretics active in the ascending loop of Henle impair the generation of dilute urine by blocking salt reabsorption.[74,94] Thus a limit is set on the amount of solute-free water the kidney can excrete. If the patient ingests free water faster than the ascending limb can generate dilute urine, hyponatremia is certain to follow.[94] Potent loop diuretics also cause contraction of the ECF compartment, whereupon ADH may be released into the blood. The increased reabsorption of free water in the distal nephron caused by ADH contributes further to the development of hyponatremia.[172] Ashraf and colleagues[17] reported on a series of hyponatremic patients who displayed extraordinary depression of free water clearance while taking routine doses of thiazide diuretics. Friedman and associates recently demonstrated that the response to a single dose of hydrochlorothiazide (50 mg) predicted the development of hyponatremia in patients at risk for this abnormality.[129] Increased weight gain due to polydypsia was implicated as the cause. Thus, patients taking potent diuretics that work in the loop of Henle or distal convolution should be cautioned against excessive water intake.

Effects on calcium, phosphorus, and magnesium

A comprehensive discussion of the effects of diuretics on the renal excretion of calcium, phosphorus, and magnesium is beyond the scope of this review (see Chaps. 12, 32, and 34). Several excellent reviews have been published which emphasize the interdependency of these solutes in the tubular reabsorbate and the roles of sodium, parathyroid hormone, and vitamin D in the renal handling of divalent ions.[303,329,331] Several points merit emphasis here. First, most diuretics acutely increase the renal excretion of calcium, phosphorus, and magnesium. In general, the increased rate of elimination reflects the natriuretic or chloruretic potency of the particular diuretic. Second, the chronic administration of diuretics causes the calciuria and phosphaturia to return to (or fall below) the control values. Third, there have been no reports of sustained diuretic-induced phosphaturia or calciuria that have resulted in overt phosphate or calcium depletion syndromes. On the contrary, long-term thiazide administration may lead to overt hypercalcemia.[177] Thus, it seems that compensatory mechanisms, perhaps related to increased proximal tubular reabsorption due to extracellular volume contraction, counteract the acute phosphaturic and calciuric effects of certain diuretics.

There are a few important exceptions to these general rules. Thiazide diuretics decrease calcium excretion with both short- and long-term use.[54] Amiloride also has this effect[86] Evidence obtained from micropuncture experiments is compatible with the notion that the thiazides have a direct effect on the distal tubule to augment calcium reabsorption and inhibit sodium reabsorption.[87,107] This property of the thiazides is central to their use in the treatment of calcium renal lithiasis.[360] By contrast, furosemide and ethacrynic acid increase calcium excretion regardless of schedule of drug administration. Bourdeau has demonstrated that furosemide interferes with the reabsorption of calcium across the thick medullary portion of the loop of Henle.[43] Bumetanide, furosemide, and ethacrynic acid are useful in the treatment of acute hypercalcemic conditions. Since overt calcium depletion has not resulted from long-term therapy with these drugs, it is likely that extrarenal mechanisms such as increased gastrointestinal calcium reabsorption occur to compensate for the increased calcium losses into the urine. When using furosemide (or bumetanide or ethacrynic acid) to induce calciuresis in the treatment of hypercalcemia it is important to recall that isotonic saline should be given in generous amounts in order to match or somewhat slightly exceed the loss of sodium chloride into the urine.[328] At times this requires massive amounts of isotonic saline in order to keep pace.[175]

Magnesium depletion

Thiazide and loop diuretics, such as furosemide, can produce magnesium depletion when administered chronically.[18,99,105,287,303,307,312] The resulting cellular magnesium depletion may contribute to the genesis of cardiac arrhythmias.[104,334] Magnesium depletion can produce hypocalcemia by reducing parathormone secretion.[286,329] Thiazide and furosemide induced magnesium excretion is probably diminished by amiloride, triamterene, and spironolactone.[287,303]

Metabolic complications

Hyperuricemia

Urate is freely filtered into the urine. Bidirectional transport of urate takes place along the course of the proximal tubule with net reabsorption occurring early in the proximal convolution (S_1 segment), net secretion occurring in the middle portion (S_2 segment) of the proximal tubule, and net reabsorption again occurring in the last portion of the proximal tubule (S_3 segment, probably the locus of "postsecretory" reabsorptive transport).[151,320] Beyond the proximal tubule a small amount of urate absorption occurs along favorable concentration gradients between lumen and bloodstream, established by salt and water removal from the tubule fluid. Urate secretion does not occur appreciably beyond the S_2 portion of the proximal tubule.[75,309] Since many of the potent diuretics are organic acids, and are secreted into the urine by the proximal straight tubule, interference with the secretion of uric acid may account in part for the hyperuricemia observed with theses drugs.[78] On the other hand, there is evidence to indicate that enhanced tubular reabsorption of uric acid, secondary to plasma volume contraction, is also involved in the elevation of plasma urate concentration during the chronic use of diuretics. Urate is reabsorbed in the proximal tubule to a greater extent than normal in response to diuretic-induced volume contraction.[345] However, inhibition of secretion of urate into the urine may occur with plasma volume contraction. Steele and Oppenheimer[321] showed that simultaneous replacement of urinary salt losses induced with a diuretic agent prevented the fall in uric acid clearance obtained with the same drug if volume contraction developed.

Reduction in dose of the offending diuretic often corrects the hyperuricemia. However, such a reduction in dose may not be feasible in certain patients with avid salt retention. The addition of a uricosuric drug, such as probenecid, has proved beneficial in our hands since the diuretic effect is only delayed, not vitiated, when probenecid blocks the rapid excretion of the diuretic into the urine (Fig. 19-4). Both the natriuretic effect of the diuretic and the uricosuric effect of the probenecid are preserved when they are administered together.

An alternative strategy is to use the xanthine oxidase inhibitor allopurinol to reduce the plasma urate level. However, this drug may cause hepatitis and exfoliative dermatitis and may be involved in cataract formation.[4,128,188,223] Therefore, it seems prudent to use allopurinol only in those patients with recurrent gouty arthritis or acute uric acid nephropathy, who have GFRs below 40 ml/min in whom probenecid is ineffective.[66,151] It appears that sustained plasma urate elevations up to 10 to 12 ng/dl have no deleterious effects on renal function.[34,66]

Hyperglycemia

Glucose intolerance induced by chlorothiazide therapy was first reported by Wolff in 1963.[357] Impaired carbohydrate metabolism has also been reported with the use of furosemide[156,349] and ethacrynic acid.[11,357] The mechanism(s) by which the thiazide derivatives and the loop of Henle agents induce glucose intolerance remains controversial. Decreased insulin secretion by the pancreas,[176] peripheral tissue resistance to insulin,[273,332,348] and increased insulin output accelerating the development of insulin depletion in the prediabetic state[302] have all been suggested. Since it is now well established that potassium and insulin homeostasis are closely linked,[147] investigators have focused upon the relationships among diuretic therapy, net potassium balance, and the state of glucose tolerance in an individual. Helderman and associates,[174] in a series of carefully controlled experiments which made use of a glucose-clamp technique, found that individuals taking hydrochlorothiazide for 10 days did not develop alterations in glucose tolerance, beta-cell sensitivity to glucose or gastric inhibitory polypeptide, or tissue sensitivity to insulin, as long as hypokalemia was prevented. Thus, it appears (in the short term) that potassium loss may be the most important factor relating the development of overt glucose intolerance to the use of potent diuretic drugs. Long-term studies of nondiabetic hypertensive patients taking diuretics indicate that less than 5 percent of this population are overtly glucose-intolerant.[35] There may be considerably more risk of decreasing glucose control, however, in insulin-dependent diabetics who require potent diuretics to control hypertension or edema formation.[146,258] Hyperglycemia has not been seen with isolated use of potassium-sparing diuretics such as triamterene, amiloride, or spironolactone.

Recently, several investigators have found that glucose intolerance and hyperinsulinemia are commonly present in persons with high blood pressure.[119,273,332] It has also been demonstrated that resistance to insulin-stimulated glucose uptake is present in nonobese patients with hypertension. Moreover, hypertensive patients treated with hydrochlorothiazide, in contrast to those treated with the angiotensin converting enzyme inhibitor captopril, had increased basal insulin concentration and an enhanced late insulin response to a glucose challenge.[273] These findings have led to a reassessment of the use of diuretics as first-line therapy for hypertension.

Hyperlipidemia

In 1964 Schoenfield and Goldberger reported that serum cholesterol increased in five of six cardiac patients treated with a thiazide diuretic; the cholesterol levels returned to normal when the diuretic was withdrawn.[296] Ames and Hill extended these observations to a group of 39 hypertensive patients treated with chlorthalidone or hydrochlorothiazide and found increases in both serum cholesterol and triglyceride concentrations (11 mg/dl and 34 mg/dl, respectively).[7] Grimm and associates reported that hydrochlorothiazide or chlorthalidone increased plasma total cholesterol, very-low density and low-density lipoprotein cholesterol, and plasma triglyceride concentrations, with triglyceride concentrations showing the largest increase. High-density lipoprotein cholesterol remained stable during thiazide diuretic treatment.[162] Although the magnitude of the increase in plasma lipid content appears to be related to the dose of the thiazide diuretic drugs, the mechanism responsible for the increased lipid levels remains unclear. Furosemide and spironolactone administered under similar conditions increased serum cholesterol and triglyceride levels.[8,9] Several investigators have advanced the notion that the lipid-elevating properties of the thiazide diuretics may offset some of the beneficial antihypertensive effects of these drugs, particularly in regard to the pathogenesis of atherosclerosis.[8,9,189] Indapamide does not alter lipids in an unfavorable manner.[250]

Gynecomastia and sexual dysfunction

Spironolactone use has been reported to cause gynecomastia, irregular menses, and impotence.[157,232] These effects may relate to the drug's ability to compete for cytosolic protein receptors for androgenic hormones.[232]

Impotence has also been strongly associated with chronic thiazide use. A study by the Medical Research Council in Great Britain found a 19 percent incidence of impotence in hypertensive patients taking thiazide diuretics.[155]

Osteomalacia

Osteomalacia related to chronic anticonvulsant therapy has been reported to worsen when acetazolamide therapy is given concurrently.[236] The mechanism of this effect is unclear; it may be related to the diuretic-induced mild metabolic acidosis.

Toxic reactions

Ototoxicity

Ototoxicity has been reported following use of furosemide and ethacrynic acid;[89] reversible hearing loss associated with high-dose therapy has been reported in patients with renal insufficiency.[299]

Hypersensitivity reactions

Hypersensitivity reactions also have been reported with diuretic drug use, particularly use of the thiazides and furosemide. These reactions include skin rash,[170] leukopenia,[270,363] thrombocytopenia,[26,363] necrotizing vasculitis,[42] and acute hypersensitivity pneumonitis.[29,30,275] The common ground for these reactions may be the presence of sulfur within the ring structure of the thiazides, bumetanide, and furosemide. Amiloride, triamterene, and ethacrynic acid do not contain sulfur; they can be substituted for the former drugs when an idiosyncratic reaction develops.

DIURETICS IN THE TREATMENT OF EDEMATOUS CONDITIONS

CONGESTIVE HEART FAILURE

Heart failure is a pathophysiologic state in which an abnormality of cardiac function is responsible for the inability of the heart to pump at a rate commensurate with the requirements of metabolizing tissues.[197,221,347,356,361] In congestive heart failure (see Chap. 18) it is the heart that fails, not the kidney.[55,248,315,347,361] As shown in Fig. 19-13, a failing heart has a higher left ventricular end-diastolic volume for a given ventricular performance; furthermore, with exercise, end-diastolic pressure may increase with little increase in stroke volume. The failure of cardiac output to increase with effort results in underperfusion of tissues, which is translated into symptoms of increased fatigue and dyspnea on exertion. The initial response of the cardiovascular system to an added hemodynamic burden or insult to myocardial contractility is to recruit several compensatory mechanisms: an increase in catecholamine release, activation of the renin angiotensin-aldosterone axis, and an increase in renal tubular sodium and water retention (capable of enhancing the cardiac output via the Frank-Starling phenomenon), or development of myocardial hypertrophy.[347,356,361] When these compensatory mechanisms are insufficient to return cardiac output to normal the clinical manifestations of congestive heart failure become evident. Thus, the response of the kidney can be viewed as a protective mechanism in the course of pump failure (Figs. 19-2 and 19-13). As the cardiac output decreases, the kidney responds with increased retention of fluid. In consequence, the venous return to the heart is increased and the myocardium is stretched further (i.e., preload increases) to permit an increased stroke volume and cardiac output (Fig. 19-13). This mechanism eventually becomes less effective as the heart fails progressively and actin:myosin sarcomere units are stretched beyond optimum contraction length.[315] Ultimately plasma volume expansion leads to pulmonary vascular congestion and translocation of fluid from the pulmonary capillaries into the alveoli (pulmonary edema). Diuretics are beneficial in this condition by virtue of their ability to reduce both the plasma volume and the venous return to the heart, so that the symptoms of dyspnea caused by pulmonary congestion are ameliorated.

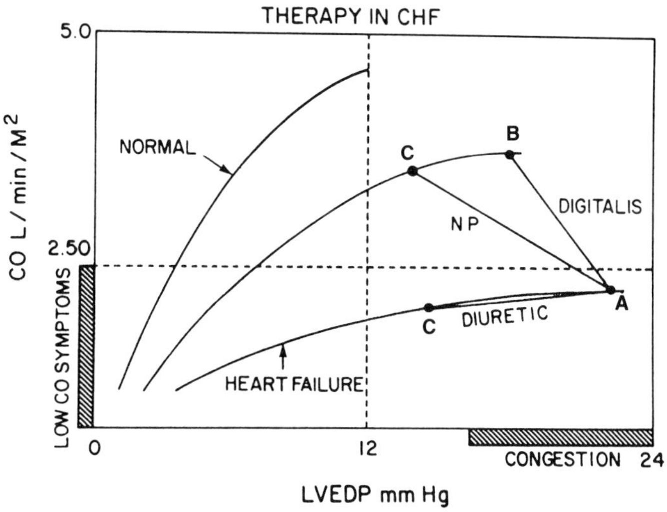

FIGURE 19-13 • An illustration of the Frank-Starling law of the heart, relating left ventricular "preload" (left ventricular end-diastolic pressure, LVEDP) to cardiac index (CI). The normal relationship is shown at the top of the figure; the relationship in severe congestive heart failure is at the bottom (A). Digitalis (B) shifts the curve toward the normal relationship by virtue of its inotropic action on the myocardium. Peripheral vasodilator drugs (nitroprusside, NP) that reduce both the myocardial "afterload" and the "preload" simultaneously increase cardiac output and decrease pulmonary vascular congestion (C). Diuretic drugs do not usually shift the curve upward; they reduce pulmonary vascular congestion owing to a decrease in plasma volume and LVEDP.

Diuretics do not necessarily improve myocardial performance by a direct mechanism (Fig. 19-13); nevertheless, diuretics may improve myocardial performance indirectly by relieving pulmonary vascular congestion and increasing oxygenation of the blood. Diuretics may also lower arterial blood pressure and improve cardiac hemodynamics by lessening the afterload of resistance against which the left ventricle must contract.[356]

Bumetanide, furosemide, and ethacrynic acid may be particularly useful in the treatment of acute pulmonary edema *in the setting of acute myocardial infarction* since these drugs may provide a beneficial extrarenal hemodynamic effect, namely, augmented peripheral venous capacitance, within minutes of intravenous administration (Fig. 19-14). The augmentation occurs independently of the diuretic effects of these agents.[41,52,96] This phenomenon may not take place in conditions of acute pulmonary edema associated with *chronic cardiomyopathic disease*. In fact, transient hemodynamic deterioration has been reported following intravenous administration of furosemide in patients with chronic heart failure.[127] An increase in mean arterial pressure, systemic vascular resistance, and left ventricular filling pressure, along with decreased cardiac output, were observed. The precise mechanism for this transient increase in left ventricular outflow resistance which causes worsening of left ventricular pump function remains unclear; however, there was evidence for activation of the neurohumoral axis since plasma renin activity, plasma norepinephrine, and arginine vasopressin levels increased concomitantly. The clinical relevance of these transient effects remains to be elucidated.

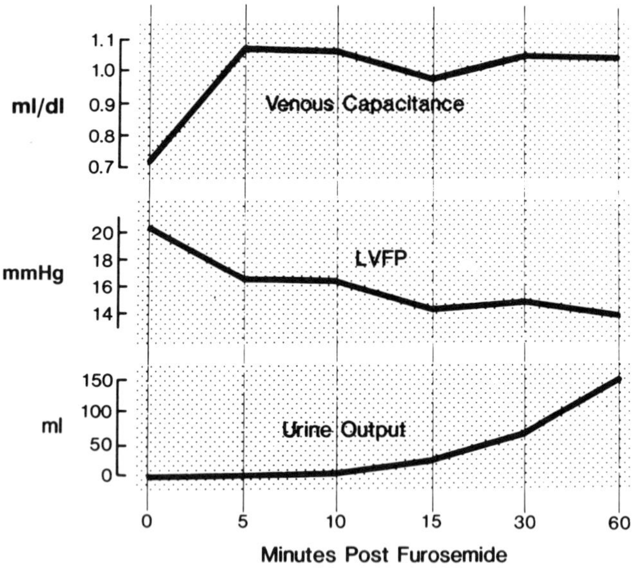

FIGURE 19-14 • The beneficial hemodynamic effects of intravenous furosemide administration in a patient with acute myocardial infarction and pulmonary edema. Temporal changes in calf venous capacitance (*top*), mean left ventricular filling pressure (*middle*), and urine output (*bottom*) are illustrated. Note that the decrease in left ventricular filling pressure and the simultaneous increase in calf venous capacitance preceded significantly increased urine output during the initial 15-min interval after furosemide was administered. (From Dikshit K et al: *N Engl J Med* 288:1087, 1971.)

In the treatment of chronic congestive heart failure diuretic drugs should be used as adjunctive therapeutic agents. Therapeutic measures that *directly* improve myocardial performance should be employed prior to diuretic use. Three classes of drugs are useful to improve myocardial performance: cardiac glycosides, vasodilator drugs, and inotropic catecholamine derivatives.

Digitalis, by virtue of its inotropic effect on the failing left ventricular myocardium, improves the Frank-Starling relationship between pressure and cardiac output (Fig. 19-13). Digitalis partially inhibits myocardial Na^+-K^+ ATPase, causing an increase in intracellular calcium that augments myocardial contractility and cardiac output. The improved hemodynamic state that follows the use of digitalis reduces efferent sympathetic nerve impulse traffic; this can lead to enhanced renal perfusion.[339] The decreased sympathetic input to the kidney may result from a direct effect of digitalis on afferent nerve fiber endings in the heart, since it has been demonstrated in dogs that cardiac glycosides injected into the coronary circulation or applied to the epicardium of the animal cause a rapid decrease in sympathetic nerve activity in the kidneys.[339] Thus, enhanced renal perfusion may occur before the positive inotropic effects of digitalis. Considerable controversy has developed in recent years regarding the efficacy of digitalis use in heart failure patients with a normal sinus rhythm. Two recent studies with digoxin and placebo have proved the efficacy of glycoside use. In both studies symptoms of congestive failure were improved and were paralleled by increased ejection fraction determinations[68] and improved exercise tolerance.[69]

Unfortunately, digitalis possesses significant cardiac and extracardiac toxic side effects, particularly when used in older individuals with damaged myocardial tissue; injured heart muscle may become an arrhythmogenic focus.[50,301,323] Moreover, although most patients respond favorably to conventional treatment with cautious use of digitalis and diuretics, relatively refractory heart failure that is not amenable to operative intervention may develop in advanced myocardial heart disease. An important advance in the medical therapy for such patients with acute and chronic pump dysfunction has been the use of systemic vasodilator drugs (exclusive of diuretic agents) to reduce excessive left ventricular afterload. Their effects are to raise the lowered cardiac output and reduce elevated pulmonary venous pressure.[19,20,56,70,79,124] Several excellent reviews are available as a guide to proper use of these drugs.[82,125,196,197,242,265,266]

A few principles bear emphasis. First, as illustrated in Table 19-3, most *vasodilator drugs* have simultaneous effects on both the venous and arterial beds. Thus, afterload reduction in consequence of arterial dilatation and preload reduction in consequence of venous dilatation take place concomitantly with application of most of these drugs;[125,196,197,242,265,266] the exceptions are the nitrates, which work predominantly on the venous bed,

TABLE 19-3 • Spectrum of actions of systemic vasodilator drugs

Venous bed	Arterial tree	
SL nitroglycerine	Nitroprusside	Hydralazine
T nitroglycerine	Phentolamine	Minoxidil
IV nitroglycerine	Trimethaphan	
Long-acting nitrates	Prazosin	
	Trimazosin	
	Phenoxybensamine	
	Hydralazine-nitrate	
	Hydralazine-prazosin	
	Captopril	
	Enalapril	
	Lisinopril	
↓ LVEDV ↓ MVO_2	↑ CO(EDP > 12) ↓ LVEDV ↓ MVO_2	↑ CO ↓ MVO_2

Spectrum of actions of systemic vasodilator drugs on peripheral venous and arterial vascular beds. LVEDV, left ventricular end-diastolic volume; MVO_2, myocardial oxygen consumption; CO, cardiac output; EDP, left ventricular end-diastolic pressure; SL, sublingual; T, topical; IV, intravenous. Note that many vasodilators have simultaneous effects on both the venous and arterial beds. The net effects of these drugs often include increased cardiac output, reduction in LVEDV, and reduction in MVO_2. (Adapted from Mason DT et al: *Arch Intern Med* 140:1577, 1980.)

and hydralazine and minoxidil, which work primarily on the arterial bed.[82,125,196,197,242,265,266] Fortunately, relatively noninvasive techniques, such as isotopic cardiac scans and sonographic measurements of left ventricular contractility, are available as an aid in determining the efficacy of these drug regiments. A maintained or improved GFR points to improved cardiac function.

Second, it used to be taught that a decreased preload (i.e., *pure venous dilatation*) usually did not produce an increased cardiac output. Franciosa and associates have reported, however, that reduction of left ventricular filling pressure to within the low normal range by nitroprusside infusion, in patients with *chronic* left ventricular failure, can raise cardiac output.[126] The elevated output may exceed the levels observed at the so-called optimum left ventricular filling pressure, 14 to 18 mmHg, in patients with *acute* myocardial dysfunction due to ischemia.[82,126,127] This study is supported by the reports that oral long-acting isosorbide dinitrate improves myocardial function and response to diuretic administration over the long term.[81,125,220] Moreover, recent trials have demonstrated a life-prolonging effect of the combination of oral hydralazine and nitrate.[80-82]

Third, inhibition of *angiotensin-converting enzyme (ACE)* has been shown in several well-controlled trials to improve the disordered hemodynamics, alleviate the symptoms, and improve survival in patients suffering from congestive heart failure.[84,91,106,209,221,264,304] ACE inhibitors reduce both preload and afterload and can increase cardiac output while simultaneously lowering pulmonary vascular congestion. When administered with a diuretic, the ACE inhibitor minimizes the loss of serum potassium and blunts the reflex renin-angiotensin stimulating effect of diuretic therapy.[106,221,264,304,330] ACE inhibitors have significant side effects: hypotension, angioedema, chronic cough, hyperkalemia in patients with renal insufficiency,[257] and a tendency to produce worsening azotemia in individuals with renal underperfusion states such as bilateral renal artery stenosis, or renal artery stenosis in a solitary kidney.[88,182] The most limiting feature of these drugs is their tendency to produce hypotension in patients with low cardiac output. However, this untoward effect can be minimized by starting with low doses (6.25 mg of captopril twice daily or 2.5 mg of enalapril once daily) and titrating upward. It is best to withhold diuretics, if possible, for 48 h prior to the start of ACE inhibition therapy for treatment of left ventricular dysfunction. Since Edwards' original demonstration that angiotensin II preferentially constricts the efferent arterioles of the renal microvasculature,[108] it has become clear that individuals with a stimulated renin-angiotensin axis with poor renal perfusion, due to congestive heart failure, can experience sudden declines in GFR with the start of ACE inhibition.[257] Fortunately, the azotemia usually reverses with discontinuation of the ACE inhibitor therapy in these situations.[88,182,257] Conversion from ACE inhibitors to other vasodilator drugs is indicated if renal dysfunction does not reverse with lessened diuretic therapy in patients with congestive heart failure.

Fourth, individuals with severe left ventricular dysfunction not responsive to combined vasodilator therapy and cardiac glycoside therapy may benefit from intermittent, intravenous infusions of catecholamine derivatives such as dopamine or dobutamine.[21,197,265,266] Leier and associates were the first to demonstrate that 48- to 72-h infusions of intravenous dobutamine (approximately 10 μg/kg/min) to hospitalized patients could significantly improve left ventricular performance and relieve symptoms of congestive heart failure.[218,219] Dobutamine acts on both beta- and alpha-adrenergic receptors to produce a strong positive inotropic action while reducing pulmonary and systemic vascular resistance. In most patients dobutamine increases stroke output and decreases systemic vascular resistance while maintaining renal perfusion. Dobutamine can produce lowering of serum potassium by causing a shift of potassium into cells via modulation of the sodium:potassium-ATPase responsible for maintaining intracellular-extracellular potassium gradients.[145,284] This tendency to move potassium intracellularly with dobutamine infusions (as well as other catecholamines) may produce hypokalemia in patients taking diuretic drugs for pulmonary congestive symptoms. Recently, Miller reported relief of symptoms of congestive heart failure in patients with severe cardiomyopathies given intravenous dobutamine at home.[251]

Last, occasional patients with congestive heart failure appear to be refractory to the effects of furosemide or other potent loop diuretics even when the drug is administered intravenously. Studies by Brater and coworkers point out this unresponsiveness is not due to lack of entry of furosemide into the urine (Fig. 19-15).[49,51] The lack of diuretic response in this clinical circumstance is more likely related to avid reabsorption of glomerular filtrate at nephron sites not blocked by furosemide (probably the proximal tubule and the late portions of the nephron). An inappropriate or unbridled braking phenomenon probably operates in this state. Although combined therapy with multiple diuretic drugs that work at several loci within the nephron (for instance, combining furosemide with thiazide derivates simultaneously blocks the loop of Henle and distal convoluted tubule) at times proves useful,[113,358] often it is more beneficial to use vasodilator drugs—hydralazine or ACE inhibitors, for example—to effect enhancement of cardiac output and renal blood flow.[82,84,106,124,221,235,304]

CIRRHOSIS WITH ASCITES (SEE CHAP. 18)

Two theories have been proposed to account for the excessive sodium retention that is seen in individuals who have cirrhosis with ascites formation: *underfill* theory and *overflow* theory.[114,226,254,359] The classic explanation argues that an altered Starling equilibrium in the portal circulation causes peritoneal transudation of fluid such that the effective circulating blood volume is reduced; the kidney responds to the ECF contraction by increasing the tubular reabsorption of glomerular filtrate.[224,226] Ascites formation occurs as a primary event in this scenario; it results from the translocation of fluid from the plasma into the peritoneal cavity due to the development of a high portal venous pressure. Thus, the kidney is signaled that the circulating arterial volume is "underfilled"; it responds in a protective manner, by hyperabsorbing glomerular filtrate in order to prevent collapse of the plasma volume.

The alternative hypothesis suggests that the initiating event is increased renal sodium retention. The increase in retention is presumed to be set off primarily by the development of hepatic parenchymal disease; how the damaged liver signals to the healthy kidney to alter sodium transport remains a mystery but may relate to increased nitric oxide synthesis by peripheral blood vessels.[342] The excessive renal sodium and water retention results secondarily in ascites formation because of the alteration in Starling forces within the hepatic-portal circulation (i.e., because of portal hypertension). Lieberman and associates first proposed this overflow theory for ascites formation in 1969 when they found that plasma volume determinations were normal or increased, not decreased or underfilled, in patients who had cirrhosis with ascites.[227] Moreover, these individuals did not experience drops in plasma volume or hepatic wedge pressure (an index of portal venous pressure) when spontaneous diuresis occurred with bedrest. Experiments by

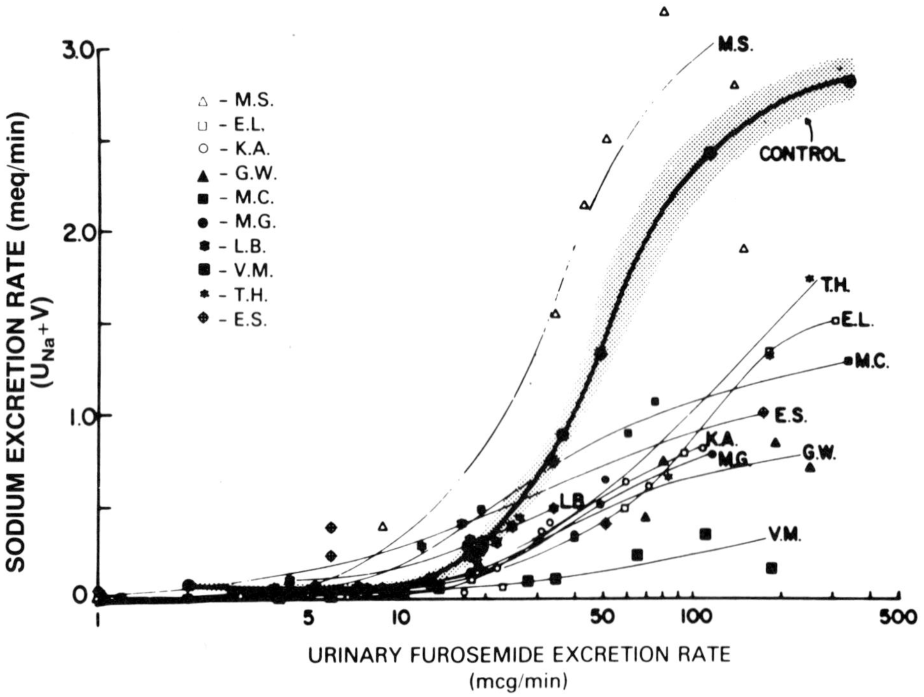

FIGURE 19-15 • Relationship between urinary furosemide delivery and natriuretic response in 10 patients with congestive heart failure (individual curves labeled with initials) and 8 normal controls (heavy line connecting large solid circles). Note that patients with heart failure, in general, experienced less natriuresis per amount of furosemide excretion. (From Brater DC et al: *Clin Pharmacol Ther* 28:182, 1980.)

Levy, in a model of cirrhosis in dogs, also support the overflow theory. The dogs showed urinary retention of sodium and water in advance of either ascites formation or a measurable change in total peripheral resistance or cardiac output.[225,226,359]

Regardless of the exact mechanism responsible for the genesis of excessive sodium and water retention by the kidney, the patient with cirrhosis and ascites has an "ineffective" circulating volume.[226,359] The ineffectiveness of the circulation is often reflected in persistently elevated plasma renin activity (PRA) and plasma aldosterone concentration.[285,297] However, when challenged with an oral salt load, PRA and plasma aldosterone levels fell into the normal range in some cirrhotic subjects (Fig. 19-16); the fall in PRA occurred with a price: excessive weight gain and sodium retention compared to normal volunteers.[76] Perhaps the former patients reflect individuals in a phase of underfilling of the vascular tree, while the latter patients reflect individuals in a phase of overfilling. Furthermore, measures of PRA may be predictive of long-term survival in individuals with cirrhosis and ascites who are fed a diet containing 40 meq of sodium and no diuretics.[15] The individuals with high PRA ($>$ 7.5 $\pm$ 3.8 ng/ml per h) survived approximately 6 months; individuals with relatively normal PRA (1.1 $\pm$ 0.7 ng/ml per h) survived 28 months on the average. There was also a close correlation between the degree of renal sodium retention and the degree of elevation of the PRA. This association may reflect renal ischemia in patients who succumbed early. In support of this concept, Bichet and coworkers reported that both plasma ADH and plasma norepinephrine levels are increased in patients with hepatic ascites.[39,40] The increased tendency for these patients to develop hyponatremia when given excessive water loads and prerenal azotemia at the time of gastrointestinal hemorrhage

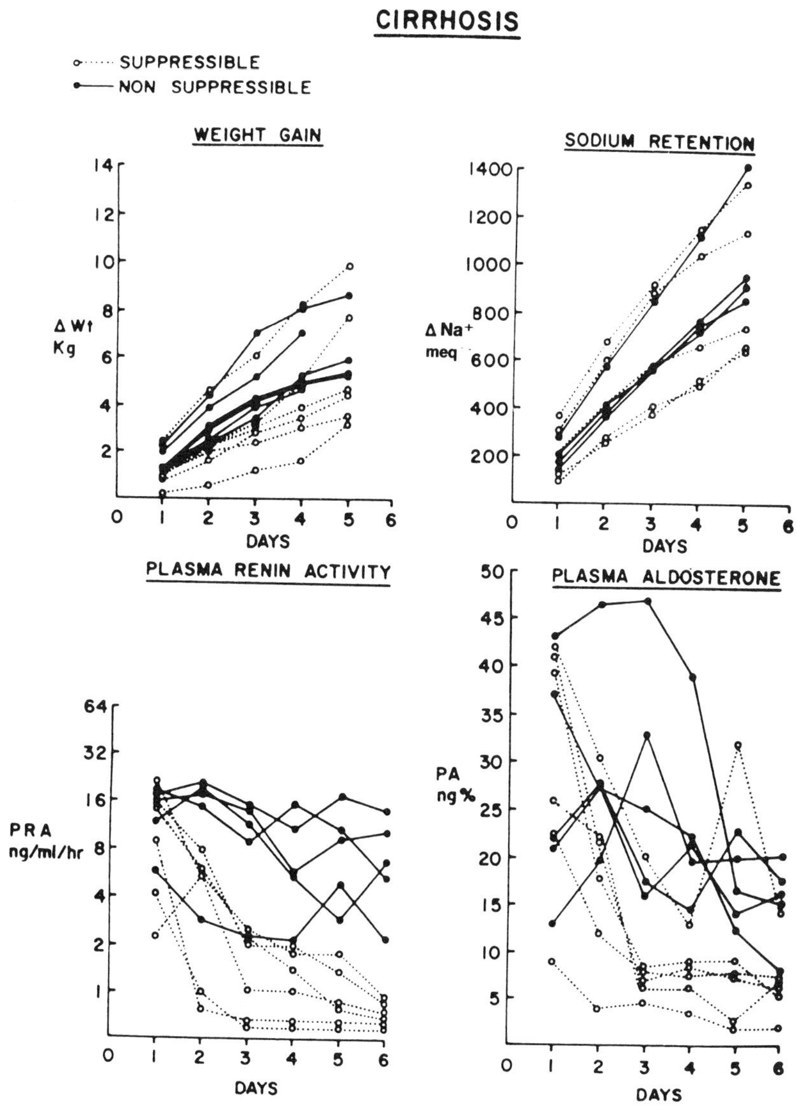

FIGURE 19-16 • Weight gain, cumulative sodium retention, plasma renin activity, and plasma aldosterone over 5 days of high sodium intake in 11 patients with cirrhosis and ascites. Note that plasma renin and aldosterone concentrations were suppressed into the normal range during salt retention in 5 patients; in 6 patients these plasma hormones remained elevated during salt retention. (From Chonko AM et al: *Am J Med* 63:881, 1977.)

is a clinical correlate of the experiments reported by Bichet and associates.

Diuretics must be used cautiously to treat edema and ascites in cirrhotic patients because such individuals are susceptible to vascular collapse. The cornerstone of therapy is sodium restriction. Since most patients lose about 22 meq of sodium per day by extrarenal means, a diet including 40 to 45 meq (1000 mg) of sodium will minimize weight gain and effect weight loss if reasonable amounts of sodium are excreted in the urine. Approximately 28 percent of patients hospitalized with cirrhosis and ascites experience spontaneous diuresis with bedrest and sodium restriction alone.[117,161]

All nephrotoxic drugs, in particular aminoglycoside antibiotics, should be avoided in cirrhotic patients. Nonsteroidal anti-inflammatory drugs and other drugs that interfere with the synthesis of intrarenal PGs should also be strictly avoided. It is clear from several studies that cirrhotic individuals have elevated levevls of PGE_2 in the urine; the PG elevation probably reflects an increased intrarenal genesis of these fatty acids as a protective response to maintain renal blood flow and GFR.[226,362] Inhibition of PG synthesis in cirrhotic individuals by administration of indomethacin,[46] ibuprofen,[362] and acetylsalicylic acid[271] results in sharp declines in GFR and blunts the diuretic response to furosemide.

Previously, it has been suspected that patients treated with diuretics had an increased frequency of complications compared to those treated with salt and fluid restriction alone.[133,306] A controlled trial discounts this idea; it showed that a modest diuresis can be accomplished without complications attributable to fluid and electrolyte shifts in seriously ill patients with abdominal discomfort due to tense ascites.[161] It is prudent to recall that although patients with hepatic ascites may experience a profound pharmacologic diuresis, the urine is derived principally from the plasma and peripheral interstitial fluid rather than from the ascitic pool. Shear and associates demonstrated that the maximum rate at which ascites fluid can be reabsorbed is about 900 ml/day.[305] This finding has been recently confirmed by Pockros and Reynolds.[272] Therefore, in patients with ascites and no peripheral edema, a forced diuresis that exceeds a net fluid loss of 900 ml/day may lead to rapid depletion of the plasma volume, vascular collapse, and renal hypoperfusion. Functional acute renal failure, the so-called hepatorenal syndrome, has resulted from the overly aggressive use of diuretic agents to cirrhotic individuals.[308]

Spironolactone is the diuretic favored by most experts as initial therapy in the cirrhotic patient who continues to accumulate ascites and edema while he or she adheres to a sodium-restricted diet.[117] Up to 75 percent of patients respond to spironolactone without other diuretic intervention.[110] Daily doses of 100 to 200 mg are usually successful; an upper limit of 400 mg daily is recommended, since hyperchloremic metabolic acidosis ("type IV" distal renal tubular acidosis) can result with higher doses.[132] Since spironolactone takes several days to achieve maximum benefit, the dose should not be increased unless there is still no evidence of weight loss or diuresis after 4 to 5 days.[110,117]

If diuresis does not occur with spironolactone alone, 40 mg of furosemide with stepwise increases every 2 to 3 days can be added; a dose of 120 mg per day should be the maximum administered. Furosemide kinetics have been found to be normal[289] and abnormal[131,269] in studies of cirrhotic patients. Some individuals apparently are resistant to furosemide, owing to poor transport of the drug to the loop of Henle in the tubular fluid. A trial with bumetanide or ethacrynic acid can prove beneficial in a small percentage of these patients. Potassium depletion must be avoided when furosemide or other potent loop diuretics are used, since increased ammonia generation by the renal epithelium is triggered by the exaggerated kaliuresis that attends cellular potassium depletion.[335,336] Hepatic encephalopathy has been precipitated in the setting of potassium depletion.[134]

Eknoyan and colleagues[111] demonstrated that the combination of ascites "reinfusion" and furosemide in patients with massive ascites results in reduced natriuresis. Experience with warm water immersion is in agreement with Eknoyan's observation and is consonant with the notion that return of ascitic fluid to the central venous circulation improves renal blood flow, GFR, and responsiveness to diuretic drugs.[114] In this regard, a series of studies have reported beneficial effects of a peritoneovenous (LeVeen) shunt.[116,200] Schroeder and colleagues found that LeVeen shunt placement resulted in significant reductions in ascites accumulation, enhanced diuresis, and improvement in GFR in five individuals with tense hepatic ascites.[298] Unfortunately, peritoneovenous shunt therapy is associated with a long list of medical complications, including sepsis, intravascular coagulopathy, hepatic encephalopathy, and pulmonary vascular congestion.[115,116] Several authorities do not recommend LeVeen shunt placement if the prothrombin time in a cirrhotic individual is prolonged six seconds beyond control.[116,158]

Recently, high-volume paracentesis with removal of 3 to 5 liters of ascitic fluid over several hours followed with intravenous infusion of albumin concentrates (averaging 60 to 80 g) has proved beneficial in patients with intense ascites refractory to diuretic therapy.[16,141,142,199] Surprisingly, this procedure did not produce vascular collapse, electrolyte imbalance, or progressive azotemia if plasma volume was adequately replaced. Whether the risk of infection and inconvenience of the paracentesis procedure will limit the effectiveness of such therapy remains to be elucidated. Follow-up treatment with spironolactone may help delay reaccumulation of ascites.[268,269]

NEPHROTIC SYNDROME

Generalized edema is a cardinal feature of the nephrotic syndrome (see Chap. 18). The classic explanation for the abnormal renal salt and water retention suggests that this process is a normal renal response to plasma volume reduction induced by decreases in plasma colloid concentration; plasma colloid levels may drop owing to albumin loss into the urine and increased albumin catabolism by the renal epithelium.[254,359] A significant portion of the plasma proteins that leak into the urine because of glomerular injury are reabsorbed by the proximal tubule cells;[359] the albumin is broken down into amino acids in the course of transport through the tubule cells.[359] Recently, Ichikawa and associates have obtained evidence that intrarenal factors unrelated to the systemic development of hypoalbuminemia may contribute to enhanced salt and water retention by the kidney.[183] The tubular hyperabsorption of glomerular filtrate appears to take place beyond the distal convolution. Thus, there may be several mechanisms operative in the pathogenesis of avid renal salt and water retention in the nephrotic syndrome. In this condition the arterial circulation is perceived by the kidney as "ineffective"; enhanced tubular reabsorption of glomerular filtrate occurs, then, even when the GFR is normal.

Plasma renin and aldosterone variations

As found in patients with cirrhosis and ascites, plasma renin and aldosterone levels (markers that are presumed to reflect the adequacy of the arterial circulation) have been found to vary considerably in individuals with nephrotic edema. Initial studies reported persistent elevations of both of these substances in the plasma of nephrotic patients; increased amounts of aldosterone were also found in the urine.[10,233] However, Chonko and colleagues found that both plasma renin and aldosterone levels in several nephrotic individuals were suppressed to the normal range when the patient was challenged with a salt load (Fig. 19-17).[76] Brown and associates have confirmed this finding in 6 of 12 edematous nephrotic patients previously unexposed to

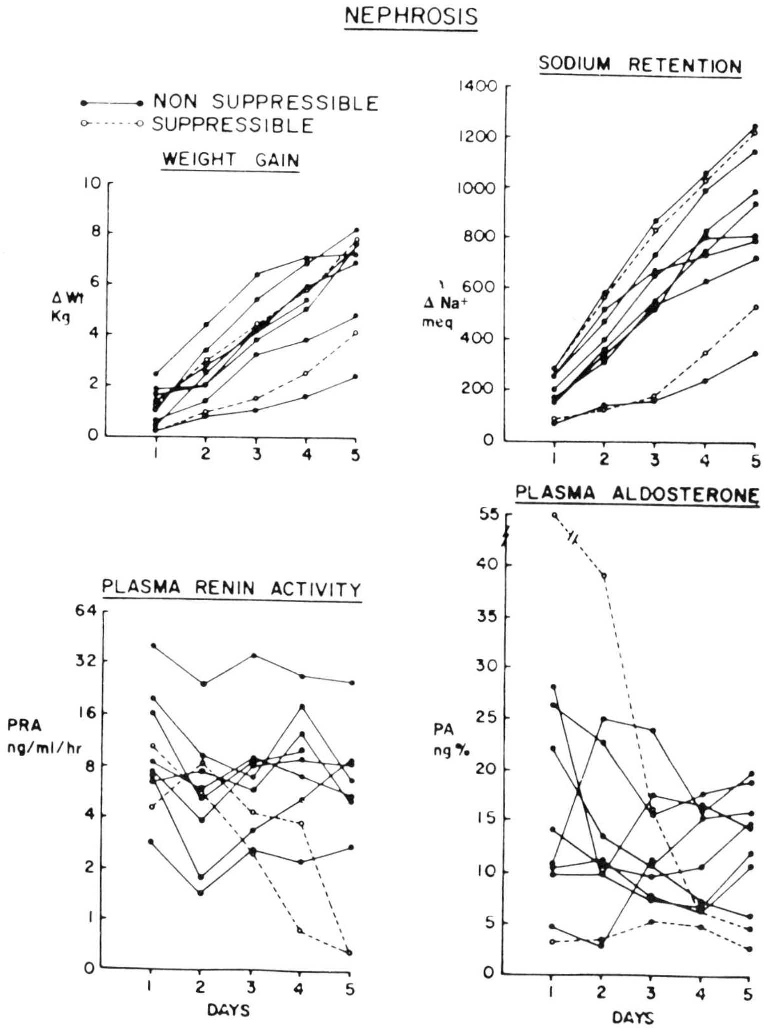

FIGURE 19-17 • Weight gain, cumulative sodium retention, plasma renin activity, and plasma aldosterone over 5 days of high sodium intake in 10 patients with nephrotic syndrome. Note that 2 of 10 patients showed suppressed plasma renin and aldosterone concentrations, into the normal range, during salt retention. (From Chonko AM et al: *Am J Med* 63:881, 1977.)

diuretic drugs. Blood volume was increased in the individuals with normal plasma renin and aldosterone levels.[57] It appears that patients with edema formation due to nephrotic proteinuria represent a heterogeneous population in regard to the adequacy of filling of their plasma volumes. Meltzer and coworkers found that determination of the relationship between PRA and urine sodium excretion in a nephrotic population revealed a spectrum of disease the extremes of which suggested two different pathophysiologic forms.[247] One group had persistently elevated plasma renin and aldosterone levels and appeared to be "vasoconstrictive." These individuals had normal GFRs, were normotensive, and often achieved complete remission with steroid therapy. A second group had decreased plasma renin and aldosterone levels; they were termed "hypervolemic." These individuals had decreased GFRs, were hypertensive, and did not respond to steroids. Of the two groups, the former would probably be more prone to vascular collapse if aggressive pharmacologic diuresis were instituted.

Although the classic theory of salt retention in the nephrotic syndrome may not apply in all nephrotic patients, it is clear that proteinuria is ultimately involved in the pathogenesis of edema formation.[359] The most satisfactory approach to treating the nephrotic syndrome is eradication of the underlying glomerular disease; both drug-induced and spontaneous remissions of proteinuria are associated with the clearing of edema and restoring of normal sodium balance. Unfortunately, only a portion of the nephrotic population responds to treatment with corticosteroids or immunosuppressive drugs. Nonsteroidal anti-inflammatory agents have been reported to diminish proteinuria in nephrotic patients with a variety of glomerulopathies.[13] However, these agents inhibit renal PG generation and have been reported to cause reversible and irreversible renal failure in nephrotic individuals.[244,245] Paradoxically, these drugs can cause nephrotic proteinuria; this may be a result of hypersensitivity.[123] Nonsteroidal anti-inflammatory agents should probably be avoided in all individuals with nephrotic proteinuria unless these drugs are given by a nephrologist who will closely monitor the renal effects.

Edema-mobilizing treatment

Dietary manipulations are important in the management of the nephrotic syndrome. Sodium restriction, preferably to 40 to 60 meq per day (1000 to 1500 mg), is effective in arresting or slowing the rate of edema formation in most individuals; in conjuction with cautious use of diuretics, dietary limitation can often lead to resolution of edema. Protein supplementation to intakes of 2 to 3 g per kilogram of body weight per day, particularly using proteins of high biologic quality (i.e., rich in essential amino acids), can induce positive nitrogen balance and increase hepatic albumin synthesis.[359] A positive nitrogen balance is associated with a decreased incidence of infectious complications, which constitute a major risk to nephrotic individuals.[359]

Other maneuvers can be used to help mobilize peripheral edema accumulation. Rest periods scattered throughout the day, during which time the feet are elevated to the level of the heart, can mobilize edema fluid, particularly if small doses of a rapidly acting diuretic drug are used in conjunction with these periods of rest.[194] Swimming is also useful since redistribution of peripheral edema fluid to the central venous circulation can occur as the limbs are immersed. Berlyne and colleagues reported that four hours of immersion to the neck in warm water led to the loss of about 2 kg of fluid in each of 5 adult nephrotic patients.[36]

Drug-induced diuresis

The decision to use diuretics to mobilize nephrotic edema should not be taken lightly, particularly since the plasma volume may be chronically contracted. Consequently, these individuals may develop vascular collapse when treated too aggressively with diuretics.

For initial diuretic use a thiazide is a safe choice. If the edema is massive and resistant to therapy, and the patient does not have a symptomatic reduction in plasma volume, bumetanide, furosemide, or ethacrynic acid may be substituted or added to the thiazide. If serious hypokalemia results, the addition of amiloride, triamterene, or spironolactone to the diuretic regimen may prove useful in effecting both reduction of urinary potassium wasting and enhanced natriuresis. Results of several micropuncture investigations are compatible with the notion that early in the course of the nephrotic syndrome the distal, and not the proximal, portions of the nephron make up the site of avid sodium absorption.[183,213]

Some nephrotic individuals are resistant to the effects of potent diuretic drugs. Keller and associates found that furosemide kinetics were not severely compromised in nephrotic patients with normal GFRs but the natriuretic responses to appropriate urinary levels of furosemide were reduced in comparison to normal individuals.[198] There was no correlation between the lack of response and urine protein content in this study. However, other investigators have found that intratubule albumin blunts the response to furosemide.[201,311] The magnitude of the latter effect remains to be clarified. Overall, it appears that an exaggerated braking phenomenon probably accounts for the hyperabsorption of glomerular filtrate across noninhibited portions of the nephron.

In diuretic-resistant individuals combination therapy with metolazone and spironolactone[217] has been useful. Infusion of colloid, or "salt poor" albumin, in combination with diuretic agents is useful in mobilizing huge collections of edema.[92] Unfortunately, such measures provide only temporary benefit since the infused protein is rapidly lost into the urine.

IDIOPATHIC EDEMA

Idiopathic edema is a common disorder of women characterized by cyclical episodes of sodium retention and edema formation in the absence of cardiac, endocrine, hepatic, or renal disease.[267] The etiology of this disorder remains unclear. Exaggerated orthostatic pooling of blood, exaggerated renal response to estrogen or to sympathetic nerve discharge, hypoalbuminemia, and alteration in peripheral capillary premeability have each been proposed to explain the tendency to retain salt.[83,109,139,140,210,267,326,340] None of these mechanisms is unequivocally supported by data from clinical studies of affected women. Plasma renin activity and plasma aldosterone levels have been found to fall to the normal range in several of these women when each was challenged with a high-salt diet.[120] Moreover, MacGregor and associates described several patients with idiopathic edema who were persuaded to stop diuretic therapy (see Fig. 19-18). These women gained several kilograms and noticed increased edema formation during the initial five-day period after discontinuing diuretics. However, they then experienced a spontaneous diuresis and were free of edema within four weeks.[234] Further observations by this group of investigators led to the suggestion that the major cause of idiopathic edema is prolonged use of diuretics; extended laxative use may also be involved.[95] The intermittent use of potent loop-acting diuretics in the setting of wide variations in daily sodium, water, and carbohydrate intake may be particularly responsible.

Many women with idiopathic edema appear to be extraordinarily conscious of their appearance and exhibit a dietary pattern of intermittent starvation followed by salt and carbohydrate refeeding; this sequence of events is known to precipitate the renal retention of sodium and water.[95] The initial edema formation in this syndrome may occur upon refeeding; the edema then is exacerbated by diuretic intake. In patients who have intermittent reductions in potassium intake and continue to take diuretic drugs chronically, potassium and magnesium depletion may develop. Depletion of these cations can potentiate the common clinical symptoms of this syndrome: weakness, malaise, irritability, abdominal bloating, and increased thirst.[331,337] Idiopathic edema may be treated most effectively by withdrawing all diuretics and instituting a moderate dietary sodium and water restriction (87 meq sodium and 1500 ml water per day). Dietary counseling to avoid a pattern of intermittent starvation and gluttony and the institution of an exercise program (daily swimming or bicycling) are also important therapeutic measures. Patients who stop using diuretics and follow the dietary restrictions but do not become edema-free within four weeks should be reexamined for the presence of occult thyroid or cardiac disease.[95,261] Recently, several patients with idiopathic edema have benefited from captopril therapy following discontinuation of diuretics.[98,253] Moreover, Sowers and associates described several women who benefited from the oral administration of the dopamine agonist, bromocriptine.[314] It appears that idiopathic edema is truly a syndrome with variable causes and responses to therapy.

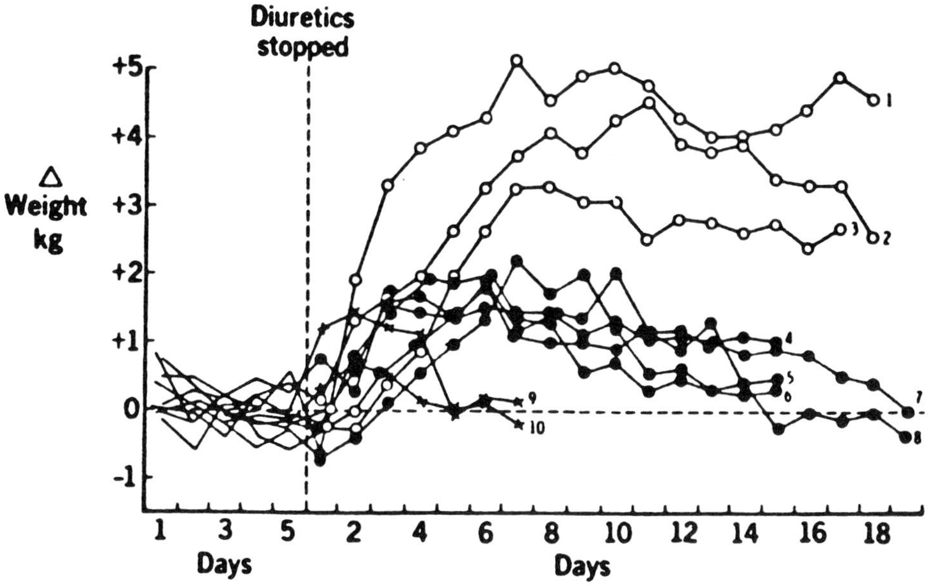

FIGURE 19-18 • The effect of stopping diuretics in women with idiopathic edema. Note that more than half of the patients eventually lost weight and became edema-free. (From MacGregor GA et al: Is "idiopathic" edema idiopathic? *Lancet* 1:397, 1979, with permission.)

REFERENCES

1. Abe K et al: Effect of furosemide on urinary excretion of prostaglandin E in normal volunteers and patients with essential hypertension. *Prostaglandins* 14:513, 1977.
2. Abe K et al: The kallikrein-kinin system and prostaglandins in the kidney. *Circ Res* 43:254, 1978.
3. Abramow M: Effects of ethacrynic acid on the isolated collecting tubule. *J Clin Invest* 53:796, 1974.
4. Al-Kawas FH et al: Allopurinol hepatotoxicity. Report of two cases and review of the literature. *Ann Intern Med* 95:588, 1981.
5. Allen F, Tisher CC: Morphology of the ascending thick limb of Henle. *Kidney Int* 9:8, 1976.
6. Almeida AJ, Burg MB: Sodium transport in the rabbit connecting tubule. *Am J Physiol* 243:F330, 1982.
7. Ames RP, Hill P: Elevation of serum lipid levels during diuretic therapy of hypertension. *Am J Med* 61:748, 1976.
8. Ames RP: The influence of non-beta-blocking drugs on the lipid profile: Are diuretics outclassed as initial therapy for hypertension? *Am Heart J* 114:998, 1987.
9. Ames RP, Hill P: Improvement of glucose tolerance and lowering of glycohemoglobin and seruum lipid concentrations after discontinuation of antihypertensive drug therapy. *Circulation* 65:899, 1982.
10. Ammenti A et al: Mineralocorticoids in the nephrotic syndrome of children. *Clin Nephrol* 14:238, 1980.
11. Andersen OO, Persson I: Carbohydrate metabolism during treatment with chlorthalidone and ethacrynic acid. *Br Med J* 2:798, 1968.
12. Anggard E, Oliw E: Formation and metabolism of prostaglandins in the kidney. *Kidney Int* 19:771, 1981.
13. Arisz L et al: The effect of indomethacin on proteinuria and kidney function in the nephrotic syndrome. *Acta Med Scand* 199:121, 1976.
14. Aronson P: Identifying secondary active solute transport in epithelia. *Am J Physiol* 240:F1, 1981.
15. Arroyo V et al: Plasma renin activity and urinary sodium excretion as prognostic indicators in nonazotemic cirrhosis with ascites. *Ann Intern Med* 94:198, 1981.
16. Arroyo V et al: Paracentesis in the management of cirrhotics with ascites, in Epstein M (ed): *The Kidney in Liver Disease*, 3d ed. Baltimore, Williams & Wilkins, 1988.
17. Ashraf N et al: Thiazide-induced hyponatremia associated with death or neurologic damage in outpatients. *Am J Med* 70:1163, 1981.
18. Auamme GA: Effect of furosemide on calcium and magnesium transport in the rat nephron. *Am J Physiol* 241:F340, 1981.
19. Awan NA et al: Efficacy of oral angiotensin-converting enzyme inhibition with captopril therapy in severe chronic normotensive congestive heart failure. *Am Heart J* 101:22, 1981.
20. Awan NA et al: Clinical pharmacology and therapeutic application of prazosin in acute and chronic refractory congestive heart failure. Balanced systemic venous and arterial dilation improving pulmonary congestion and cardiac output. *Am J Med* 65:146, 1978.
21. Ayres SM: Using inotropes effectively to manage ventricular failure: Which agents are most effective and safe? *J Crit Illness* 1:59, 1986.
22. Badr KF, Jacobson HR: Arachidonic acid metabolites and the kidney, in Brenner BM, Rector FC Jr (eds): *The Kidney*, 4th ed. Philadelphia, Saunders, 1991, p 584.
23. Baer JE et al: The potassium-sparing and natriuretic activity of *N*-amidino-3,5-diamino-6-chloropyrazine-carboxamide hydrochloride dihydrate (amiloride hydrochloride). *J Pharmacol* 157:472, 1967.
24. Bailie MD et al: Effects of indomethacin on furosemide-induced changes in renal blood flow (38711). *Proc Soc Exp Biol Med* 148:1173, 1975.
25. Bailie MD et al: Natriuretic effect of furosemide after inhibition of prostaglandin synthetase[1]. *J Pharmacol Exp Ther* 199:469, 1976.
26. Ball P: Thrombocytopenia and purpura in patients receiving chlorothiazide and hydrochlorothiazide. *JAMA* 173:663, 1960.
27. Ballermann BJ et al: Vasoactive peptides and the kidney, in Brenner BM, Rector FC Jr (eds): *The Kidney*, 4th ed. Philadelphia, Saunders, 1991, p 510.
28. Barger AC et al: Reduced sodium excretion in dogs with mild valvular lesions of the heart, and in dogs with congestive heart failure. *Am J Physiol* 180:249, 1955.
29. Beaudry C, LaPlante L: Severe allergic pneumonitis from hydrochlorothiazide. *Ann Intern Med* 78:251, 1973.
30. Bell RT, Lippmann M: Hydrochlorothiazide-induced pulmonary edema. *Arch Intern Med* 319:817, 1979.
31. Bello-Reuss E et al: Dopamine decreases fluid reabsorption in straight portions of rabbit proximal tubule. *Am J Physiol* 242:F634, 1982.
32. Bennett CM: Urine concentration and dilution in hypokalemic and hypercalcemic dogs. *J Clin Invest* 49:1447, 1970.
33. Bennett WM et al: Drug therapy in renal failure: Dosing guidelines for adults. *Ann Intern Med* 93:62, 1980.
34. Berger L, Yü T: Renal function in gout: 4. An analysis of 524 gouty subjects including long-term followup studies. *Am J Med* 59:605, 1975.
35. Berglund G, Andersson O: Beta blockers or diuretics in hypertension? A six year follow-up of blood pressure and metabolic side-effects. *Lancet* i:744, 1971.
36. Berlyne GM et al: Water immersion in nephrotic syndrome. *Arch Intern Med* 131:1275, 1981.
37. Bernstein BA, Clapp JR: Micropuncture study of bicarbonate reabsorption by the dog nephron. *Am J Physiol* 214:251, 1968.
38. Berry CA, Warnock DG: Acidification in the in vitro perfused tubule. *Kidney Int* 22:507, 1982.
39. Bichet DG et al: Potential role of increased sympathetic activity in impaired sodium and water excretion in cirrhotic patients. *N Engl J Med* 307:1552, 1982.
40. Bichet DG et al: Role of vasopressin in abnormal water excretion in cirrhotic patients. *Ann Intern Med* 96:413, 1982.
41. Biddle TL, Yu PN: Effect of furosemide on hemodynamics and lung water in acute pulmonary edema secondary to myocardial infarction. *Am J Cardiol* 43:86, 1979.
42. Bjornberg A, Gisslen H: Thiazides: A cause of necrotising vasculitis? *Lancet* 2:982, 1965.

43. Bourdeau JE et al: Inhibition of calcium absorption in the cortical thick ascending limb of Henle's loop by furosemide. *J Pharmacol Exp Ther* 221:815, 1982.
44. Boyd JE et al: Role of potassium in the control of aldosterone secretion in the rat. *Endocrinology* 88:556, 1971.
45. Boyd JE et al: Importance of potassium in the regulation of aldosterone production. *Circ Res* 32/33(suppl 1):39, 1973.
46. Boyer TD et al: Effect of indomethacin and prostaglandin A, on renal function and plasma renin activity in alcoholic liver disease. *Gastroenterology* 77:215, 1979.
47. Brater DC: Analysis of the effect of indomethacin on the response to furosemide in man: Effect of dose of furosemide. *J Pharmacol Exp Ther* 210:386, 1978.
48. Brater DC: Increase in diuretic effect of chlorothiazide by probenecid. *Clin Pharmacol Ther* 28:259, 1978.
49. Brater DC et al: Furosemide in patients with heart failure: Shift in dose-response curves. *Clin Pharmacol Ther* 28:182, 1980.
50. Brater DC, Morrelli HF: Systemic alkalosis and digitalis related arrhythmias. *Acta Med Scand* 79:S647, 1981.
51. Brater DC et al: Absorption and disposition of furosemide in congestive heart failure. *Kidney Int* 22:171, 1982.
52. Brater DC et al: Bumetanide and furosemide in heart failure. *Kidney Int* 26:183, 1984.
53. Brenner BM et al: The dynamics of glomerular ultrafiltration in the rat. *J Clin Invest* 50:1776, 1971.
54. Breslau N et al: The role of volume contraction in the hypocalciuric action of chlorothiazide. *Kidney Int* 10:164, 1976.
55. Bristow MR et al: Decreased catecholamine sensitivity and β-adrenergic-receptor density in failing human hearts. *N Eng J Med* 307:205, 1982.
56. Brodie BR et al: Effects of sodium nitroprusside on left ventricular diastolic pressure-volume relations. *J Clin Invest* 59:59, 1977.
57. Brown EA et al: Is the renin-angiotensin-aldosterone system involved in the sodium retention in the nephrotic syndrome? *Nephron* 32:102, 1982.
58. Brusilow SW, Gordes E: The mutual independence of the endolymphatic potential and the concentrations of sodium and potassium in endolymph. *J Clin Invest* 52:2517, 1973.
59. Buckalew V et al: Free water reabsorption during solute diuresis in normal and potassium-depleted rats. *Am J Physiol* 212:381, 1967.
60. Burg MB: Thick ascending limb of Henle's loop. *Kidney Int* 22:454, 1982.
61. Burg MB, Good D: Sodium chloride coupled transport in mammalian nephrons. *Annu Rev Physiol* 45:533, 1983.
62. Burg MB, Green N: Function of the thick ascending limb of Henle's loop. *Am J Physiol* 224:659, 1973.
63. Burg MB et al: Furosemide effect on isolated perfused tubules. *Am J Physiol* 225:119, 1973.
64. Burke TJ et al: Determinants of the effect of furosemide on the proximal tubule. *Kidney Int* 1:12, 1972.
65. Campbell WB et al: Role of renal prostaglandins in sympathetically mediated renin release in the rat. *J Clin Invest* 64:448, 1979.
66. Campion EW et al: Asymptomatic hyperuricemia: Risks and consequences in the normative aging study. *Am J Med* 82:421, 1987.
67. Cannon PJ et al: "Contraction" alkalosis after diuresis of edematous patients with ethacrynic acid. *Ann Intern Med* 62:979, 1965.
68. Captopril Multicenter Research Group: A placebo controlled trial of captopril in refractory chronic congestive heart failure. *J Am Coll Cardiol* 2:755, 1983.
69. Captopril-Digoxin Multicenter Research Group: Comparative effects of therapy with captopril and digoxin in patients with mild to moderate heart failure. *JAMA* 259:539, 1988.
70. Chatterjee K et al: Long-term outpatient vasodilator therapy of congestive heart failure. *Am J Med* 65:134, 1978.
71. Chennavasin P et al: Pharamcodynamic analysis of the furosemide-probenecid interaction in man. *Kidney Int* 16:187, 1979.
72. Chennavasin P et al: Pharmacokinetic-dynamic analysis of the indomethacin-furosemide interaction in man. *J Pharmacol Exp Ther* 215:77, 1980.
73. Cherrill DA et al: Demeclocycline treatment in the syndrome of inappropriate antidiuretic hormone secretion. *Ann Intern Med* 83:654, 1975.
74. Chonko AM, Grantham JJ: The use of the isolated tubule preparation for the investigation of diuretics, in Martinez-Maldonado M (ed): *Methods in Pharmacology*. New York, Plenum Press, 1976, vol 4A, p 43.
75. Chonko AM: Urate secretion in isolated rabbit renal tubules. *Am J Physiol* 239:F545, 1980.
76. Chonko AM et al: The role of renin and aldosterone in the sale retention of edema. *Am J Med* 63:881, 1977.
77. Chonko AM et al: Renin and the kidney. *Nephron* 15:279, 1975.
78. Chonko AM, Stewart RJ: Pharmacologic inhibition of urate transport across perfused and nonperfused rabbit proximal straight tubules. *Clin Res* 28:748A, 1980.
79. Cohn JN, Franciosa JA: Vasodilator therapy of cardiac failure *N Engl J Med* 297:27, 1977.
80. Cohn JN et al: Effect of vasodilator therapy on mortality in chronic congestive heart failure: Results of a Veterans Administration Cooperative Study (V-HeFT). *N Engl J Med* 314:1547, 1986.
81. Cohen JN et al: Veterans Administration Cooperative Study on vasodilator therapy of heart failure: Influence of prerandomization variables on the reduction of mortality by treatment with hydralazine and isosorbide dinitrate. *Circulation* 75:IV49, 1987.
82. Cohn JN: Current therapy of the failing heart. *Circulation* 78:1099, 1988.
83. Coleman M et al: Idiopathic edema—Studies demonstrating protein-leaking angiopathy. *Am J Med* 49:106, 1969.
84. The CONSENSUS Trial Study Group: Effects of enalapril on mortality in severe congestive heart failure: Results of the cooperative North Scandinavian enalapril survival study (CONSENSUS). *N Engl J Med* 315:1429, 1987.
85. Corvol P et al: Mechanism of the antimineralocorticoid effects of spironolactones. *Kidney Int* 20:1, 1981.
86. Costanzo LS: Comparison of calcium and sodium trans-

port in early and late rat distal tubules: Effect of amiloride. *Am J Physiol* 246:F937, 1984.
87. Costanzo LS, Windhager EE: Calcium and sodium transport by the distal convoluted tubule of the rat. *Am J Physiol* 235:F492, 1978.
88. Curtiss JJ et al: Inhibition of angiotensin-converting enzyme in renal-transplant recipients with hypertension. *N Engl J Med* 308:377, 1982.
89. David DS, Hitzig P: Diuretics and ototoxicity. *N Eng J Med* 284:1328, 1971.
90. Davidson C et al: Effect of long-term diuretic treatment on body-potassium in heart disease. *Lancet* 2:1044, 1976.
91. Davis R et al: Treatment of chronic congestive heart failure with captopril, an oral inhibitor of angiotensin-converting enzyme. *N Engl J Med* 301:117,1979.
92. Davison AM et al: Salt-poor human albumin in management of nephrotic syndrome. *Br Med J* 1:481, 1974.
93. Deen WM et al: Dynamics of glomerular ultrafiltration in the rat: 4. Determination of the ultrafiltration coefficient. *J Clin Invest* 52:1500, 1973.
94. DeFronzo RA, Thier SO: Pathophysiologic approach to hyponatremia. *Arch Intern Med* 140:897, 1980.
95. DeWardener HE: Idiopathic edema: Role of diuretic abuse. *Kidney Int* 19:881, 1981.
96. Dikshit K et al: Renal and extrarenal hemodynamic effects of furosemide in congestive heart failrue after acute myocardial infarction. *N Engl J Med* 288:1087, 1971.
97. Dirks JH et al: Micropuncture study of the effect of various diuretics on sodium reabsorption by the proximal tubules of the dog. *J Clin Invest* 45:1875, 1966.
98. Docci D et al: Therapeutic response of idiopathic edema to Captopril. *Nephron* 34:198, 1983.
99. Duarte CF: Effects of ethacrynic acid and furosemide on urinary calcium, phosphate and magnesium. *Metabolism* 17:876, 1968.
100. Duarte CF et al: Effect of amiloride, ouabain, and furosemide on distal tubular function in the rat. *Am J Physiol* 221:632, 1971.
101. Duke M: Thiazide-induced hypokalemia association with acute myocardial infarction and ventricular fibrillation. *JAMA* 239:43, 1978.
102. Dunn M, Hood VL: Prostaglandins and the kidney, editorial. *Am J Physiol* 233:F169, 1977.
103. Dworkin LD, Brenner BM: The renal circulations, in Brenner BM, Rector FC Jr (eds): *The Kidney*, 4th ed. Philadelphia, Saunders, 1991.
104. Dyckner T, Wester PO: Ventricular extrasystoles and intracellular electrolytes before and after potassium and magnesium infusions in patients on diuretic treatment. *Am Heart J* 97:12, 1979.
105. Dyckner T, Wester PO: Effects of magnesium infusions in diuretic induced hyponatraemia. *Lancet* 1:585, 1981.
106. Dzau VJ et al: Sustained effectiveness of converting enzyme inhibition in patients with severe congestive heart failure. *N Engl J Med* 302:1373, 1980.
107. Edwards BR et al: Micropuncture study of diuretic effects on sodium and calcium reabsorption in the dog nephron. *J Clin Invest* 52:2418, 1973.
108. Edwards RM: Segmental effects of norepinephrine and angiotensin II on isolated renal microvessels *Am J Physiol* 244:F526, 1983.
109. Edwards OM, Bayliss RIS: Idiopathic edema of women. *Q J Med* 177:125, 1976.
110. Eggert RC: Spironolactone diuresis in patients with cirrhosis and ascites. *Br Med J* 4:401, 1970.
111. Eknoyan G et al: Combined ascitic fluid and furosemide infusion in the management of ascites. *N Engl J Med* 282:713, 1970.
112. Ellison DH et al: Adaptation of the distal convoluted tubule of the rat. Structural and functional effects of dietary salt intake and chronic diuretic infusion. *J Clin Invest* 83:113, 1989.
113. Ellison DH: The physiologic basis of diuretic synergism: Its role in treating diuretic resistance. *Ann Intern Med* 114:886, 1991.
114. Epstein M et al: Determinants of deranged sodium and water homeostasis in decompensated cirrhosis. *J Lab Clin Med* 87:822, 1976.
115. Epstein M: Peritoneovenous shunt in the management of ascites and the hepatorenal syndrome. *Gastroenterology* 82:790, 1982.
116. Epstein M: Role of the peritoneovenous shunt in the management of ascites and the hepatorenal syndrome, in Epstein M (ed): *The Kidney in Liver Disease*, 3d ed. Baltimore, Williams & Wilkins, 1988, p 146.
117. Epstein M: Diuretic therapy in liver disease, in Epstien M (ed): *The Kidney in Liver Disease*, 3d ed. Baltimore, Williams & Wilkins, 1988, p 121.
118. Fajans S et al: Benzothiadiazine suppression of insulin release from normal and abnormal islet cell tissue in man. *J Clin Invest* 45:481, 1966.
119. Ferannini E et al: Insulin resistance in essential hypertension. *N Eng J Med* 317:350, 1987.
120. Ferris TF et al: Studies of the mechanism of sodium retention in idiopathic edema. *Trans Assoc Am Physicians* 86:310, 1973.
121. Fichman MP et al: Diuretic-induced hyponatremia. *Ann Intern Med* 75:83, 1971.
122. Field MJ et al: Influence of ADH on renal potassium handling: A micropuncture and microperfusion study. *Kidney Int* 25:502, 1984.
123. Finkelstein A et al: Fenoprofen nephropathy: Lipoid nephrosis and interstitial nephritis. *Am J Med* 72:81, 1982.
124. Franciosa JA et al: Hemodynamic improvement after oral hydralazine in left ventricular failure. *Ann Intern Med* 86:388, 1977.
125. Franciosa JA, Cohn JN: Hemodynamic responsiveness to short- and long-acting vasodilators in left ventricular failure. *Am J Med* 65:126, 1978.
126. Franciosa JA et al: "Optimal" left ventricular filling pressure during nitroprusside infusion for congestive heart failure. *Am J Med* 74:457, 1983.
127. Francis GS et al: Acute vasoconstrictor response to intravenous furosemide in patients with chronic congestive heart failure. *Ann Intern Med* 103:1, 1985.
128. Fraunfelder FT et al: Cataracts associated with allopurinol therapy. *Am J Ophthalmol* 94:137, 1982.

129. Friedman E et al: Thiazide-induced hyponatremia. *Ann Intern Med* 110:24, 1989.
130. Frolich J et al: Effect of indomethacin on furosemide stimulated renin and sodium excretion. *Circ Res* 52:II, 99, 1975.
131. Fuller R et al: Furosemide kinetics in patients with hepatic cirrhosis with ascites. *Clin Pharmacol Ther* 30:461, 1981.
132. Gabow PA et al: Spironolactone-induced hyperchloremic acidosis in cirrhosis. *Ann Intern Med* 90:338, 1979.
133. Gabuzda GJ: Cirrhosis, ascites and edema, clinical course related to management. *Gastroenterology* 48:546, 1970.
134. Gabuzda GJ, Hall PW: Relation of potassium depletion to renal ammonium metabolism and hepatic coma. *Medicine* 45:481, 1966.
135. Garella S: Saline-resistant metabolic alkalosis or "chloride-wasting nephropathy." *Ann Inern Med* 73:31, 1970.
136. Garg LC, Narang N: Effects of hydrochlorothiazide on Na-K-ATPase activity along the rat nephron. *Kidney Int* 31:918, 1987.
137. Gennari FJ, Kassirer JP: Osmotic diuresis. *N Engl J Med* 291:714, 1974.
138. Gerber JG, Nies AS: The role of prostaglandins in the control of renal hemodynamics. *Miner Electrolyte Metab* 6:27, 1981.
139. Gill JR et al: Idiopathic edema: 1. The occurrence of hypoalbuminemia and abnormal albumin metabolism in women with unexplained edema. *Am J Med* 52:444, 1972.
140. Gill JR et al: Idiopathic edema: 2. Pathogenesis of edema in patients with hypoalbuminemia. *Am J Med* 52:452, 1972.
141. Gines P et al: Comparison of paracentesis and diuretics in the treatment of cirrhotics with tense ascites: Results of a randomized study. *Gastroenterology* 93:234, 1987.
142. Gines P et al: Randomized comparative study of therapeutic paracentesis with and without intravenous albumin in cirrhosis. *Gastroenterology* 94:1493, 1988.
143. Goldberg LI: Cardiovascular and renal actions of dopamine: Potential clinical applications. *Pharmacol Rev* 24:1, 1972.
144. Goldberg LI et al: A comparison of the vascular dopamine receptor with other dopamine receptors. *Annu Rev Pharmacol Toxicol* 18:57, 1978.
145. Goldenberg IF et al: Effect of dobutamine on plasma potassium in congestive heart failure secondary to idiopathic or ischemic cardiomyopathy. *J Am Coll Cardiol* 63:843, 1989.
146. Goldner MG et al: Hyperglycaemia and glycosuria due to thiazide derivatives administered in diabetes mellitus. *N Engl J Med* 262:403, 1960.
147. Gordon P: Glucose intolerance with hypokalemia. Failure of short-term potassium depletion in normal subjects to reproduce the glucose and insulin abnormalities of clinical hypokalemia. *Diabetes* 22:544, 1973.
148. Grantham JJ: Studies of organic anion and cation transport in isolated segments of proximal tubules. *Kidney Int* 22:519, 1982.
149. Grantham JJ, Burg MB: Effect of vasopressin and cyclic AMP on permeability of isolated collecting tubules. *Am J Physiol* 211:255, 1966.
150. Grantham JJ et al: The nature of transtubular Na and K transport in isolated rabbit renal collecting tubules. *J Clin Invest* 49:1815, 1970.
151. Grantham JJ, Chonko AM: Renal handling of organic anions and cations; excretion of uric acid, in Brenner BM, Rector FC Jr (eds): *The Kidney*, 4th ed. Philadelphia, Saunders, 1991, p 483.
152. Grantham JJ, Irish JM: Organic acid transport and fluid secretion in the pars reca (PST) of the proximal tubule. *Excerpta Medica Int Congress Series* 422:83, 1977.
153. Grantham JJ et al: Fluid secretion in isolated proximal straight renal tubules. Effect of human uremic serum. *J Clin Invest* 52:2441, 1973.
154. Grantham JJ, Orloff J: Effect of prostaglandin E_1 on the permeability response of the isolated collecting tubule to vasopressin, adenosine 3′, 5′-monophosphate, and theophylline. *J Clin Invest* 47:1154, 1968.
155. Greenberg G et al: Adverse reactions to bendrofluazide and propranolol for the treatment of mild hypertension. *Lancet* 2:539, 1981.
156. Greenblatt DJ et al: Clinical toxicity of furosemide in hospitalized patients. *Am Heart J* 94:6, 1977.
157. Greenblatt DJ, Koch-Weser J: Adverse reactions to spironolactone. *JAMA* 225:40, 1973.
158. Greenlee HB et al: Intractable ascites treated with peritoneovenous shunts (LeVeen). *Arch Surg* 116:518, 1981.
159. Greger R: Cation selectivity of the isolated perfused cortical thick ascending limb of Henle's loop of rabbit kidney. *Pflugers Arch* 390:30, 1981.
160. Greger R, Schlatter E: Presence of luminal K^+, a prerequisite for active NaCl transport in the cortical thick ascending limb of Henle's loop of rabbit kidney. *Pflugers Arch* 392:92, 1981.
161. Gregory PB et al: Complications of diuresis in the alcoholic patient with ascites: A controlled trial. *Gastroenterology* 73:534, 1977.
162. Grimm RH et al: Effects of thiazide diuretics on plasma lipids and lipoproteins in mildly hypertensive patients. *Ann Intern Med* 94:7, 1981.
163. Guignard JP, Peters G: Effects of triamterene and amiloride on urinary acidification and potassium excretion in the rat. *Eur J Pharmacol* 10:255, 1970.
164. Gussin RZ: Potassium-sparing diuretics. *J Clin Pharmacol* 17:651, 1977.
165. Guyton AC: A concept of negative interstitial pressure based on pressures in implanted perforated capsules. *Circ Res* 12:399, 1963.
166. Hahn RA, Wardell JR: Renal vascular activity of SK&F 38393 and dopamine in anesthetized dogs. *J Cardiovasc Pharmacol* 2:583, 1980.
167. Hall DA, Varney DM: Effect of vasopressin on electrical potential difference and chloride transport in mouse medullary thick ascending limb of Henle's loop. *J Clin Invest* 66:792, 1980.
168. Hall DA, Varney DM: Effect of vasopressin on chloride transport by mouse medullary thick ascending limb of Henle's loop perfused in vitro. *Kidney Int* 16:751, 1979.

169. Hantman D et al: Rapid correction of hyponatremia in the syndrome of inappropriate secretion of antidiuretic hormone. *Ann Intern Med* 78:870, 1973.
170. Harber LC et al: Photosensitivity due to chlorothiazide and hydrochlorothiazide. *N Engl J Med* 261:1378, 1959.
171. Harrington JT et al: Our national obsession with potassium. *Am J Med* 73:155, 1982.
172. Hebert SC, Andreoli TE: Water movement across the mammalian cortical collecting duct. *Kidney Int* 22:526, 1982.
173. Hebert SC et al: Salt absorption in the thick ascending limb of Henle's loop: NaCl cotransport mechanisms. *Semin Nephrology* 2:316, 1982.
174. Helderman JH et al: Prevention of the glucose intolerance of thiazide diuretics by maintenance of body potassium. *Diabetes* 32:106, 1983.
175. Helzberg J et al: Refractory hypercalcemia. *J Kans Med Soc* 84:16, 1983.
176. Hicks BH et al: A controlled study of clopamine, clorexolone, and hydrochlorothiazide in diabetes. *Metabolism* 22:101, 1973.
177. Higgins BA et al: The effect of bendrofluazide on urine calcium excretion. *Clin Sci* 27:457, 1964.
178. Holland OB et al: Diuretic-induced ventricular ectopic activity. *Am J Med* 70:762, 1981.
179. Hollifield JW, Slaton PE: Thiazide diuretics, hypokalemia and cardiac arrhythmias. *Acta Med Scand* 647:67, 1981.
180. Hook JB, Williamson HE: Influence of probenecid and alterations in acid-base balance of the saluretic activity of furosemide. *J Phamarcol Exp Ther* 149:404, 1965.
181. Hostetter TH et al: Cardiorenal hemodynamics and sodium excretion in rats with myocardial infarction. *Am J Physiol* 245:H98, 1983.
182. Hricik DE et al: Captopril-induced functional renal insufficiency in patients with bilateral renal-artery stenoses or renal-artery stenosis in a solitary kidney. *N Engl J Med* 308:373, 1983.
183. Ichikawa I et al: Role for intrarenal mechanisms in the impaired salt excretion of experimental nephrotic syndrome. *J Clin Invest* 71:91, 1983.
184. Imai M, Nakamura R: Function of distal convoluted and connecting tubules studied by isolated nephron fragments. *Kidney Int* 22:465, 1982.
185. Irish JM: Secretion of prostaglandin E_2 by rabbit proximal tubules. *Am J Physiol* 237:F268, 1979.
186. Jacobson HR: Transport characteristics of in vitro perfused proximal convoluted tubules. *Kidney Int* 22:425, 1982.
187. Jarnberg PO et al: Acute effects of furosemide and mannitol on renal function in the early postoperative period. *Acta Anaesthesiol Scand* 22:173, 1978.
188. Jick H et al: Potentiation of ampicillin skin reactions by allopurinol or hyperuricemia. *J Clin Pharmacol* 21:456, 1981.
189. Johnson BF: The emerging problem of plasma lipid changes during antihypertensive therapy. *J Cardiovasc Pharmacol* 4:S213, 1982.
190. Kaissling B, Wilhelm K: Axial heterogeneity of the "Distal Tubule." *Contrib Nephrol* 33:29, 1982.
191. Kaissling B: Structural aspects of adaptive changes in renal electrolyte excretion. *Am J Physiol* 243:F211, 1982.
192. Kaissling B, Stanton BA: Adaptation of distal tubule and collecting duct to increased sodium delivery: 1. Ultrastructure. *Am J Physiol* 255:F1256, 1988.
193. Kamm DE et al: Contribution of the urea appearance rate to diuretic-induced azotemia in the rat. *Kidney Int* 32:47, 1987.
194. Karnard DR et al: Head-down tilt as a physiological diuretic in normal controls and in patients with fluid-retaining states. *Lancet* 2:525, 1987.
195. Kassirer JP, Schwartz WB: Correction of metabolic alkalosis in man without repair of potassium deficiency. *Am J Med* 40:19, 1966.
196. Katz AM: Potential deleterious effects of inotropic agents in the therapy of chronic heart failure. *Circulation* 73:III-184, 1986.
197. Katz AM: Changing strategies in the management of heart failure. *J Am Coll Cardiol* 13:513, 1989.
198. Keller E et al: Disposition and diuretic effect of furosemide in the nephrotic syndrome. *Clin Pharmacol Ther* 32:442, 1982.
199. Kellerman PS, Linas SL: Large-volume paracentesis in treatment of ascites. *Ann Intern Med* 112:899, 1990.
200. Kinney MJ et al: The "hepatorenal" syndrome and refractory ascites. *Nephron* 23:228, 1979.
201. Kirchner KA et al: Intratubular albumin blunts the response to furosemide—a mechanism for diuretic resistance in the nephrotic syndrome. *J Pharmacol Exp Ther* 252:1097, 1990.
202. Knochel JP, Schlein EM: On the mechanism of rhabdomyolysis in potassium depletion. *J Clin Invest* 51:1750, 1972.
203. Knox FG: Role of the proximal tubule in the regulation of urinary sodium excretion. *Mayo Clin Proc* 48:565, 1973.
204. Koechel DA: Ethacrynic acid and related diuretics: Relationship of structure to beneficial and detrimental actions. *Annu Rev Pharmacol Toxicol* 21:265, 1981.
205. Kokko JP: Proximal tubule potential difference—Dependence on glucose, HCO_3, and amino acids. *J Clin Invest* 52:1362, 1973.
206. Kokko JP: Transport characteristics of the thin limbs of Henle. *Kidney Int* 22:449, 1982.
207. Kokko JP, Rector FC Jr: Flow dependence of transtubular potential difference in isolated perfused segments of rabbit proximal convoluted tubule. *J Clin Invest* 50:2745, 1971.
208. Kokko JP et al: Characteristics of NaCl and water transport in the renal proximal tubule. *J Clin Invest* 50:69, 1971.
209. Kramer BL et al: Controlled trial of captopril in chronic heart failure: A rest and exercise hemodynamic study. *Circulation* 67:807, 1983.
210. Kuchel O et al: Inappropriate response to upright posture. A precipitating factor in the pathogenesis of idiopathic edema. *Ann Intern Med* 73:245, 1970.
211. Kunau RT Jr: The influence of the carbonic anhydrase inhibitor, benzolamide (CL-11,366), on the reabsorption of chloride, sodium, and bicarbonate in the proximal tubule of the rat. *J Clin Invest* 51:294, 1972.
212. Kunau RT Jr et al: Clarification of the site of action of chlorothiazide in the rat nephron. *J Clin Invest* 56:401, 1975.
213. Kuroda S et al: A micropuncture study of renal sodium

retention in nephrotic syndrome in rats: Evidence for increased resistance to tubular fluid flow. *Kidney Int* 16:561, 1979.
214. Kurokawa K et al: Metabolic heterogeneity of the nephron. *Miner Electrolyte Metab* 7:225, 1982.
215. Kurtzman NA et al: Pathophysiology of metabolic alkalosis. *Arch Intern Med* 131:702, 1973.
216. Lambert C et al: Nonrenal clearance of furosemide as a cause of diuretic response variability in the rat. *J Pharmacol Exp Ther* 222:232, 1982.
217. Lang GR et al: Metolazone and spironolactone in cirrhosis and the nephrotic syndrome. *Clin Pharmacol Ther* 21:234, 1976.
218. Leier CV et al: The cardiovascular effects of the continuous infusion of dobutamine in patients with severe cardiac failure. *Circulation* 56:468, 1977.
219. Leier CV et al: Drug-induced conditioning in congestive heart failure. *Circulation* 65:1382, 1982.
220. Leier CV et al: Improved exercise capacity and differing arterial and venous tolerance during chronic isosorbide dinitrate therapy for congestive heart failure. *Circulation* 67:817, 1983.
221. Le Jemtel TH et al: Effects of acute angiotensin converting enzyme inhibition on renal blood flow in patients with stable congestive heart failure. *Am J Med Sci* 292:123, 1986.
222. Lemieux G et al: Hypokalemia during the treatment of arterial hypertension with diuretics. *CMA Journal* 122:905, 1980.
223. Lerman S et al: Allopurinol therapy and cataractogenesis in humans. *Am J Ophthalmol* 94:141, 1982.
224. Levinsky NG: Refractory ascites in cirrhosis. *Kidney Int* 14:93, 1978.
225. Levy M: Sodium retention and ascites formation in dogs with experimental portal cirrhosis. *Am J Physiol* 233:F572, 1977.
226. Levy M: Pathophysiology of ascites formation, in Epstein M (ed): *The Kidney in Liver Disease*, 3d ed. Baltimore, Williams & Wilkins, 1988, p 88.
227. Lieberman FL et al: Effective plasma volume in cirrhosis with ascites. Evidence that a decreased value does not account for renal sodium retention, a spontaneous reduction in glomerular filtration rate (GFR), and a fall in GFR during drug-induced diuresis. *J Clin Invest* 48:975, 1969.
228. Lifschitz MD: Prostaglandins and renal blood flow: In vivo studies. *Kidney Int* 19:781, 1981.
229. Lindner A et al: Synergism of dopamine plus furosemide in preventing acute renal failure in the dog. *Kidney Int* 16:158, 1979.
230. Liu F-Y, Cogan MG: Angiotensin II stimulates early proximal bicarbonate absorption in the rat by decreasing cyclic adenosine monophosphate. *J Clin Invest* 84:83, 1989.
231. Loon NR et al: Mechanism of impaired natriuretic response to furosemide during prolonged therapy. *Kidney Int* 36:682, 1989.
232. Loriaux DL et al: Spironolactone and endocrine dysfunction. *Ann Intern Med* 85:630, 1976.
233. Luetscher JA Jr et al: Observations on the sodium-retaining corticoid (aldosterone) in the urine of children and adults in relation to sodium balance and edema. *J Clin Invest* 33:1441, 1954.
234. MacGregor GA et al: Is "idiopathic" edema idiopathic? *Lancet* 1:397, 1979.
235. Magorien RD et al: Prazosin and hydralazine in congestive heart failure. *Ann Intern Med* 95:5, 1981.
236. Mallette LE: Acetazolamide-accelerated anticonvulsant osteomalacia. *Arch Intern Med* 137:1013, 1977.
237. Manning M, Sawyer W: Antagonists of vasopressor and antidiuretic responses to arginine vasopressin. *Ann Intern Med* 96:520, 1982.
238. Maren TH: Relations between structure and biological activity of sulfonamides. *Annu Rev Pharmacol Toxicol* 16:309, 1976.
239. Maren TH: Use of inhibitors in physiological studies of carbonic anhydrase. *Am J Physiol* 232:F291, 1977.
240. Margolius HS et al: The effects of aldosterone and spironolactone on renal kallikrein in the rat. *Clin Sci* 51:279S, 1976.
241. Marver D, Kokko JP: Renal target sites and the mechanism of action of aldosterone. *Miner Electrolyte Metab* 9:1, 1983.
242. Mason DT et al: Treatment of acute and chronic congestive heart failure by vasodilator-afterload reduction. *Arch Intern Med* 140:1577, 1980.
243. Mathisen O et al: Effect of acetazolamide on glomerulotubular balance and renal metabolic rate. *Scand J Clin Lab Invest* 36:617, 1976.
244. McCarthy JT et al: Acute intrinsic renal failure induced by indomethacin. *Mayo Clin Proc* 57:289, 1982.
245. McCarthy JT et al: Reversible nonoliguric acute renal failure associated with zomepirac therapy. *Mayo Clin Proc* 57:351, 1982.
246. McGiff JC et al: Release of a prostaglandin E-like substance from canine kidney by bradykinin. *Circ Res* 31:36, 1972.
247. Meltzer J et al: Nephrotic syndrome: Vasoconstriction and hypervolemic types indicated by renin-sodium profiling. *Ann Intern Med* 91:688, 1979.
248. Mettauer B et al: Sodium and water excretion abnormalities in congestive heart failure. *Ann Intern Med* 105:161, 1986.
249. Meyer MG et al: Effects of dopamine on renal function and hemodynamics in the dog. *J Pharmacol Exp Ther* 156:186, 1967.
250. Meyer-Sabellek W et al: Serum lipoprotein levels during long-term treatment of hypertension with indapamide. *Hypertension* 7:170, 1985.
251. Miller LW: Outpatient dobutamine for refractory congestive heart failure: Advantages, techniques, and results. *J Heart Lung Transplant* 10:482, 1991.
252. Miller PD et al: Polyuric prerenal failure. *Arch Intern Med* 140:907, 1980.
253. Mimran A, Targhetta R: Captopril treatment of idiopathic edema. *N Engl J Med* 301:1289, 1979.
254. Moe GW et al: Control of extracellular fulid volume and pathophysiology of edema formation, in Brenner BM, Rector FC Jr (eds): *The Kidney*, 4th ed. Philadelphia, Saunders, 1991, p 623.
255. Morgan DB et al: The relation between plasma, erythrocyte and total body potassium in patients with hypokalaemia. *Miner Electrolyte Metab* 5:233, 1981.
256. Morrison AR, Benabe JE: Prostaglandins and vascular

tone in experimental obstructive nephropathy. *Kidney Int* 19:786, 1981.

257. Murphy BF et al: Renal insufficiency with combinations of angiotensin converting enzyme inhibitors and diuretics. *B Med J* 288:844, 1984.
258. Murphy MG et al: Glucose intolerance in hypertensive patients treated with diuretics: A fourteen-year follow-up. *Lancet* Dec:1293, 1982.
259. Nissenson AR et al: Mannitol. *West J Med* 131:277, 1979.
260. Nordrehaug JE: Malignant arrhythmias in relation to serum potassium values in patients with an acute myocardial infarction. *Acta Med Scand* 101:S647, 1981.
261. Obeid AI et al: Cardiac function in idiopathic edema. *Arch Intern Med* 134:253, 1974.
262. O'Neil RG, Boulpaep EL: Ionic conductive properties and electrophysiology of the rabbit cortical collecting tubule. *Am J Physiol* 243:F81, 1982.
263. O'Neil RG, Boulpaep EL: Effect of amiloride on the apical cell membrane cation channels of a sodium-absorbing, potassium-secreting renal epithelium. *J Membr Biol* 50:365, 1979.
264. Packer M et al: Comparison of captopril and enalapril in patients with severe chronic heart failure. *N Engl J Med* 315:847, 1986.
265. Packer M: Vasodilator and inotropic drugs for the treatment of chronic heart failure: Distinguishing hype from hope. *J Am Coll Cardiol* 12:1299, 1988.
266. Packer M: Therapeutic options in the management of chronic heart failure: Is there a drug of first choice? *Circulation* 79:198, 1989.
267. Paller MS, Ferris TF: Idiopathic edema, in Dirks JH, Sutton RA (eds): *Diuretics Physiology, Pharmacology and Clinical Use*. Philadelphia, Saunders, 1986, p 193.
268. Perez-Ayuso RM et al: Randomized comparative study of efficacy of furosemide versus spironolactone in nonazotemic cirrhosis with ascites: Relationship between the diuretic response and the activity of the renin-aldosterone system. *Gastroenterology* 84:961, 1983.
269. Pinzani M et al: Altered furosemide pharmacokinetics in chronic alcoholic liver disease with ascites contributes to diuretic resistance. *Gastroenterology* 92:294, 1987.
270. Pisciotta V: Drug-induced agranulocytosis. *Drugs* 15:132, 1978.
271. Planas R et al: Acetylsalicylic acid suppresses the renal hemodynamic effect and reduces the diuretic action of furosemide in cirrhosis with ascites. *Gastroenterology*, 84:247, 1983.
272. Pockros PJ, Reynolds TB: Rapid diuresis in patients with ascites from chronic liver disease: The importance of peripheral edema. *Gastroenterology* 90:1827, 1986.
273. Pollare T et al: A comparison of the effects of hydrochlorothiazide and captopril on glucose and lipid metabolism in patients with hypertension. *N Engl J Med* 321:868, 1989.
274. Porter RD et al: Secretory activity and aryl acid content of serum, urine, and cerebrospinal fluid in normal and uremic man. *J Lab Clin Med* 85:723, 1975.

274a. Preisig PA, Rector FC Jr: Role of Na^+-H^+ antiport in rat proximal tubule NaCl absorption. *Am J Physiol* 255:F461, 1988.

275. Prupas HM, Brown D: Acute idiosyncratic reaction to hydrochlorothiazide ingestion. *West J Med* 138:101, 1983.
276. Relman AS, Schwartz WB: The nephropathy of potassium depletion. *N Engl J Med* 255:195, 1956.
277. Relman AS, Schwartz WB: The kidney in potassium depletion. *Am J Med* 24:764, 1958.
278. Ring-Larsen H et al: Diuretic treatment in decompensated cirrhosis and congestive heart failure: Effect of posture. *Br Med J* 292:1351, 1986.
279. Rocha AS, Kokko JP: Sodium chloride and water transport in the medullary thick ascending limb of Henle. *J Clin Invest* 52:612, 1973.
280. Rocha AS, Kudo LH: Water, urea, sodium, chloride, and potassium transport in the in vitro isolated perfused papillary collecting duct. *Kidney Int* 22:485, 1982.
281. Rondeau E et al: High plasma antidiuretic hormone in patients with cardiac failure: Influence of age. *Miner Electrolyte Metab* 8:267, 1982.
282. Rose BD: Diuretics: Nephrology forum. *Kidney Int* 39:336, 1991.
283. Rose HJ et al: Depression of renal clearance of furosemide in man by azotemia. *Clin Pharmacol Ther* 21:141, 1976.
284. Rose RM et al: Adrenergic modulation of extrarenal potassium disposal. *N Engl J Med* 302:431, 1980.
285. Rosoff L et al: Studies of renin and aldosterone in cirrhotic patients with ascites. *Gastroenterology* 69:698, 1975.
286. Rude RK et al: PTH secretion in magnesium deficiency. *J Clin Endocrinol Metab* 47:800, 1978.
287. Ryan MP et al: Effects of diuretics on the renal handling of magnesium. *Drugs* 28(suppl 1):167, 1984.
288. Savin VJ, Terreros DA: Filtration in single isolated mammalian glomeruli. *Kidney Int* 20:188, 1981.
289. Sawhney VK et al: Furosemide disposition in cirrhotic patients. *Gastroenterology* 81:1012, 1981.
290. Schafer JA: Salt and water absorption in the proximal tubule. *Physiologist* 25:95, 1982.
291. Schafer JA, Barfuss DW: The study of pars recta function by the perfusion of isolated tubule segments. *Kidney Int* 22:434, 1982.
292. Scheinman M et al: Hemodynamic effects of ethacrynic acid in patients with refractory acute left ventricular failure. *Am J Med* 50:291, 1971.
293. Schild L et al: Effect of formate on volume reabsorption in the rabbit proximal tubule. *J Clin Invest* 79:32, 1987.
294. Schmidt M, Imbs JL: Pharmacological characterization of renal vascular dopamine receptors. *J Cardiovasc Pharmacol* 2:595, 1980.
295. Schnermann J, Briggs JP: Participation of renal cortical prostaglandins in the regulation of glomerular filtration rate. *Kidney Int* 19:802, 1981.
296. Schoenfield MR, Goldberger E: Hypercholesterolemia induced by thiazides: A pilot study. *Curr Ther Res* 6:180, 1964.
297. Schroeder ET et al: Effect of blockade of angiotensin II on blood pressure, renin and aldosterone in cirrhosis. *Kidney Int* 9:511, 1976.

298. Schroeder ET et al: Effects of a portocaval or peritoneovenous shunt on renin in the hepatorenal syndrome. *Kidney Int* 15:54, 1979.
299. Schwartz GH et al: Ototoxicity induced by furosemide. *N Engl J Med* 282:1413, 1970.
300. Seldin DW, Rector FC Jr: The generation and maintenance of metabolic alkalosis. *Kidney Int* 1:306, 1972.
301. Selzer A: Digitalis in cardiac failure—Do benefits justify risks? *Arch Intern Med* 141:18, 1981.
302. Shapiro AP et al: Effect of thiazides on carbohydrate metabolism in patients with hypertension. *N Engl M Med* 265:1028, 1961.
303. Shareghi GT, Agus ZS: Magnesium transport in the cortical thick ascending limb of Henle's loop of the rabbit. *J Clin Invest* 69:759, 1982.
304. Sharpe DN et al: Enalapril in patients with chronic heart failure: A placebo-controlled, randomized, double-blind study. *Circulation* 70:271, 1984.
305. Shear L et al: Compartmentalization of ascites and edema in patients with hepatic cirrhosis. *N Engl J Med* 282:1391, 1970.
306. Shear L et al: Renal failure in patients with cirrhosis of the liver: 1. Clinical and pathologic characteristics. *Am J Med* 39:184, 1965.
307. Sheehan J, White A: Diuretic-associated hypomagnesaemia. *Br Med J* 285:11576, 1982.
308. Sherlock S et al: Complications of diuretic therapy in hepatic cirrhosis. *Lancet* 1:1049, 1986.
309. Shimomura A et al: The nature of urate transport in isolated rabbit proximal tubules. *Am J Physiol* 241:F565, 1981.
310. Singer I, Forrest JN Jr: Drug-induced states of nephrogenic diabetes insipidus. *Kidney Int* 10:82, 1976.
311. Smith DE et al: Urinary protein binding, kinetics and dynamics of furosemide in nephrotic patients. *J Pharm Sci* 74:603, 1985.
312. Smith WO et al: Magnesium depletion induced by various diuretics. *Okla State Med Assoc* 55:248, 1962.
313. Solomon HJ, Cole AG: Importance of potassium in patients with acute myocardial infarction. *Acta Med Scand* 87:S647, 1981.
314. Sowers J, Catania R et al: Effects of bromocriptine on renin, aldosterone and prolactin responses to posture and metoclopramide in idiopathic edema: Possible therapeutic approach. *J Clin Endocrinol Metab* 54:510, 1982.
315. Spotnitz HM et al: Relation of ultrastructure to function in the intact heart: Sarcomere structure relative to pressure volume curves of intact left ventricles of dog and cat. *Circ Res* 18:49, 1966.
316. Stanton BA, Giebisch G: Effects of pH on potassium transport by renal distal tubule. *Am J Physiol* 242 (*Renal Fluid Electrolyte Physiol* 11):F544, 1982.
317. Stanton BA, Kaissling B: Adaptation of distal tubule and collecting duct to increased sodium delivery: 2. Na^+ and K^+ transport. *Am J Physiol* 255:F1269, 1988.
318. Stanton BA, Kaissling B: Regulation of renal ion transport and cell growth by sodium. *Am J Physiol* 257:F1, 1989.
319. Starling EH: On the absorption of fluid from the connective tissue space. *J Physiol* 19:312, 1896.
320. Steele TH, Boner G: Origins of the uricosuric response. *J Clin Invest* 52:1368, 1973.
321. Steele TH, Oppenheimer S: Factors affecting urate excretion following diuretic administration in man. *Am J Med* 47:564, 1969.
322. Stein JH, Reineck HJ: The role of the collecting duct in the regulation of excretion of sodium and other electrolytes. *Kidney Int* 6:1, 1974.
323. Steiness E: Diuretics, digitalis and arrhythmias. *Acta Med Scand* 75:S647, 1981.
324. Stokes JB: Ion transport by the cortical and outer medullary collecting tubule. *Kidney Int* 22:473, 1982.
325. Stoner LC et al: Ion transport in cortical collecting tubules: Effect of amiloride. *Am J Physiol* 227:453, 1974.
326. Streeten DHP et al: Studies of the pathogenesis of idiopathic oedema: The roles of postural changes in plasma volume, plasma renin activity, aldosterone secretion rate and glomerular filtration rate in the retention of sodium and water. *Clin Sci* 45:347, 1973.
327. Sudou K, Hoshi T: Mode of action of amiloride in toad urinary bladder. *J Membr Biol* 32:115, 1977.
328. Suki WN et al: Acute treatment of hypercalcemia with furosemide. *N Engl J Med* 283:836, 1970.
329. Suki WN, Rouse D: Renal transport of calcium, magnesium and phosphorus, in Brenner BM, Rector FC Jr (eds): *The Kidney*, 4th ed. Philadelphia, Saunders, 1991, p 380.
330. Sullivan JM: Drug suppression of the angiotensin system in congestive heart failure. *Annu Rev Med* 344:169, 1983.
331. Sutton RAL, Dirks JH: Disturbances of calcium and magnesium metabolism, in Brenner BM, Rector FC Jr (eds): *The Kidney*, 4th ed. Philadelphia, Saunders, 1991, p 841.
332. Swislocki ALM et al: Insulin resistance, glucose intolerance and hyperinsulinemia in patients with hypertension. *AJH* 2:419, 1989.
333. Szylman P et al: Role of hyperkalemia in the metabolic acidosis in isolated hypoaldosteronism. *N Engl J Med* 294:351, 1976.
334. Tackett RL, Holl JE: Increased automaticity and decreased inotropism of ouabain in dogs with furosemide induced hypomagnesemia. *J Cardiovasc Pharmacol* 3:1269, 1981.
335. Tannen RL: Relationship of renal ammonia production and potassium homeostasis. *Kidney Int* 11:453, 1977.
336. Tannen RL, McGill J: Influence of potassium on renal ammonia production. *Am J Physiol* 231:1178, 1976.
337. Tannen RL: Disorders of potassium balance, in Brenner BM, Rector FC Jr (eds): *The Kidney*, 4th ed. Philadelphia, Saunders, 1991, p 805.
338. Taylor AE: Capillary fluid filtration—Starling forces and lymph flow. *Circ Res* 49:557, 1981.
339. Thames MD: Acetylstrophanthidin-induced reflex inhibition of canine renal sympathetic nerve activity mediated by cardiac receptors with vagal afferents. *Circ Res* 44:8, 1979.
340. Thibonnier M et al: Abnormal regulation of antidiuretic hormone in idiopathic edema. *Am J Med* 67:67, 1979.
341. Tucker BJ, Blantz RC: Inhibition of tubulo-glomerular feedback (TGF) induced reduction in nephron filtration rate (SNGFR) with saralasin (S). *Kidney Int* 14:784, 1978.

342. Vallance P, Moncada S: Hyperdynamic circulation in cirrhosis: A role for nitric oxide? *Lancet* 337:776, 1991.
343. Weber PC et al: Effect of stimulation and inhibition of the renal prostaglandin synthetase system on renin release in vivo and in vitro. *Clin Sci* 51:271S, 1976.
344. Weiner IM: General pharmacological aspects of diuretics, in Dirks JH, Sutton RA (eds): *Diuretics Physiology, Pharmacology and Clinical Use.* Philadelphia, Saunders, 1986, p 12.
345. Weinman EJ et al: The influence of the extracellular fluid volume on the tubular reabsorption of uric acid. *J Clin Invest* 55:283, 1975.
346. Weismann DN: Altered renal hemodynamic and urinary prostaglandin response to acute hypoxemia after inhibition of prostaglandin synthesis in the anesthetized dog. *Circ Res* 48:632, 1981.
347. Weissler AM. The heart in heart failure *Ann Intern Med* 69:929, 1968.
348. Weller JN, Borondy PE: Effects of benzothiadiazine drugs on carbohydrate metabolism. *Metabolism* 14:708, 1965.
349. Weller JM, Borondy M: Effect of furosemide on glucose metabolism. *Metabolism* 16:532, 1967.
350. Whorton AR et al: Prostaglandins and renin release: 1. Stimulation of renin release from rabbit renal cortical slices by PGI_2. *Prostaglandins* 14:1095, 1977.
351. Wiebelhaus VD et al: The natriuretic and diuretic characteristics of triamterene in the dog. *Arch Int Pharmacodyn Ther* 169:429, 1967.
352. Wilcox CS et al: Response of the kidney to furosemide: 1. Effects of salt intake and renal compensation. *J Lab Clin Med* 102:450, 1983.
353. Wilcox CS et al: Factors affecting potassium balance during furosemide administration. *Clin Sci* 67:195, 1984.
354. Williamson HE et al: Furosemide induced release of prostaglandin E to increase renal blood flow. *Proc Soc Exp Biol Med* 150:104, 1975.
355. Williamson HE et al: Ethacrynic acid induced release of prostaglandin E to increase renal blood flow. *Prostaglandins* 11:519, 1976.
356. Wilson JR et al: Effects of diuresis on the performance of the failing left ventricle in man. *Am J Med* 70:234, 1981.
357. Wolff FW et al: Drug induced diabetes. *JAMA* 185:568, 1963.
358. Wollam GL et al: Diuretic potency of combined hydrochlorothiazide and furosemide therapy in patients with azotemia. *Am J Med* 72:929, 1982.
359. Yanover MJ et al: Cirrhosis and ascites and the nephrotic syndrome, in Dirks JH, Sutton RA (eds): *Diuretics Physiology, Pharmacology and Clinical Use.* Philadelphia, Saunders, 1986, p 168.
360. Yendt ER et al: The use of thiazides in the prevention of renal calculi. *Can Med Assoc J* 102:614, 1970.
361. Young JB, Roberts R: Heart failure, in Dirks JH, Sutton RA (eds): *Diuretics Physiology, Pharmacology and Clinical Use.* Philadelphia, Saunders, 1986, p 85.
362. Zipser RD et al: Prostaglandins: Modulators of renal function and pressor resistance in chronic liver disease. *J Clin Endocrinol Metab* 48:895, 1979.
363. Zuckerman AJ, Chazan AA: Agranulocytosis with thrombocytopenia following chlorothiazide therapy. *Br Med J* 29:1, 1960.
364. Zusman RM, Keiser HR: Prostaglandin biosynthesis by rabbit renomedullary interstitial cells in tissue culture. *J Clin Invest* 60:215, 1977.

CHAPTER • 20

Hyponatremia: pathophysiology, diagnosis, and therapy

Richard H. Sterns • Helen Ocdol • Robert W. Schrier • Robert G. Narins

PHYSIOLOGIC PRINCIPLES

Seizures, coma, and brain death are potential consequences of untreated hyponatremia. Unquestionably, this serious electrolyte abnormality demands prompt diagnosis and effective therapy. On the other hand, if hyponatremia is corrected too rapidly, equally devastating neurologic sequelae can develop.

Only by clearly appreciating the physiologic principles underlying normal water and electrolyte homeostasis can one construct rational therapeutic regimens to effectively reverse this potentially dangerous disorder while avoiding iatrogenic complications. This chapter reviews these key concepts and develops a diagnostic and therapeutic approach derived from these guiding fundamental principles. The physiologic and biochemical concepts outlined below are discussed in greater depth in Chaps. 1 through 5. The following sections highlight those practical aspects that provide a basis for understanding and treating hyponatremia.

OSMOLALITY, TONICITY, AND SOLUTE DISTRIBUTION

Although the qualitative distribution of solute between the intracellular fluid (ICF) and the extracellular fluid (ECF) differs strikingly (Fig. 20-1), a key physiological principle prevails: *The concentration of solute particles must always be the same in the ICF as it is in the ECF.*[91,107,303] Water movement across semipermeable membranes rapidly dissipates any pathologic attempt to create a transcellular concentration gradient. Thus, when a solute such as sodium selectively accumulates in the ECF, solute-free water will move from the ICF to the ECF, down its concentration gradient. Net water movement continues until equality of transmembrane solute concentration is again achieved. Shrinkage of the intracellular space and expansion of the extracellular space are necessary consequences of this asymmetrical solute accumulation. Conversely, when the concentration of sodium and other extracellular solutes is reduced, preservation of osmotic equilibrium requires cell swelling.

The osmotic pressure that attracts water is solely dependent upon the number of solute particles per unit volume of solvent. The molecular weight, size, and shape of the particles are virtually irrelevant. Biologically, this pressure is defined by the number of milliosmoles of solute (mosmol) per kilogram of water. A milliosmole is simply the number of millimoles (i.e., milligrams divided by atomic or molecular weight of a given substance) of solute per liter of water. Solutes such as NaCl exist in biological solutions as admixtures of the un-ionized molecule and as its dissociated components, Na^+ and Cl^-. Thus, the addition of 5800 mg (100 mmol) of NaCl (molecular weight 58) to 1 liter of ECF adds 100 mmol/liter. Since approximately 80 percent of the NaCl ionizes, 20 mmol (mosmol) remains as the undissociated NaCl, 80 mmol (mosmol) as Na^+, and a like amount as Cl^-. The number of particles added to the solution (20 + 80 + 80) is 180 mmol (mosmol). By contrast, the nondissociable solute, urea (molecular weight 60), contributes a total of only 100 mmol when 6000 mg is added to the same 1 liter. Thus, the dissociability of the solute is important to its osmotic contribution. The following general formulas may be used to determine the osmotic distribution of a substance:

$$\text{mmol} = \text{mg/mol wt (at wt)} \qquad (1)$$

$$\text{mosmol} = n \times \text{mmol} \qquad (2)$$

The authors acknowledge support from the University Medical Research Foundation.

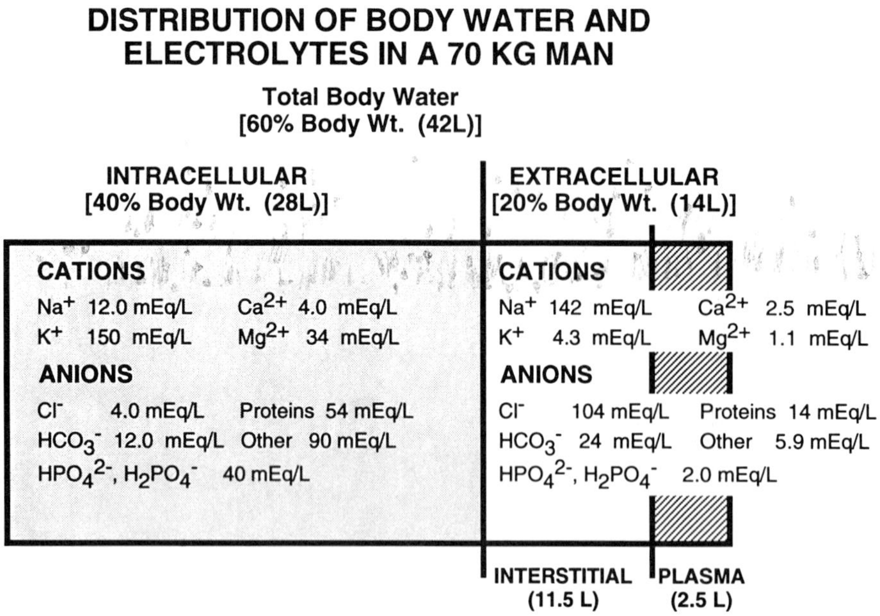

FIGURE 20-1 • Distribution of body water electrolytes in a young 70-kg man.

where *n* is the number of particles into which the parent compound dissociates. Tables defining the dissociability of chemicals should be consulted for values for *n*.

Total osmolality is composed of both *effective* and *ineffective* components (Fig. 20-2).[107,303,377] Effective osmoles cannot freely permeate cell membranes and are restricted to either the ICF or the ECF. The asymmetrical accumulation of effective osmoles in either the ECF (e.g., Na^+, glucose, mannitol, and glycine) or the ICF (e.g., K^+, amino acids, and organic acids) causes transcompartmental movement of water (see above). The effective osmolality of a solution is synonymous with its *tonicity*. Ineffective osmoles freely cross cell membranes and therefore are unable to effect shifts in water between fluid compartments. Such ineffective solutes (e.g., urea, ethanol, and methanol) contribute to total osmolality but not to tonicity. It follows that the plasma of patients with renal failure and increased blood urea concentrations may be hyperosmolar but not hypertonic because the concentration of urea in the ICF is equal to that in the ECF. Similarly, azotemic, hyponatremic patients may have normal serum osmolalities (e.g., 280 mosm/liter) due to unrelated but offsetting increases in urea and decreases in sodium concentrations, but have expanded ICF volumes due to their hypotonicity. Tonicity, not osmolality, is the physiologic parameter that the body strives to regulate. It also follows that excreted urea does not change the tonicity of urine or that of the body fluid from which it is removed.

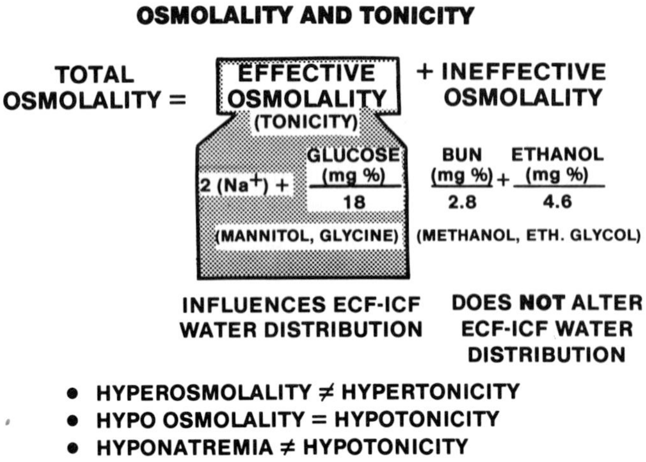

FIGURE 20-2 • Osmolality versus tonicity.

Calculation of plasma osmolality (and therefore of intracellular osmolality, because they are equal) is easily accomplished and is clinically useful (Fig. 20-2). Unlike plasma osmolality, plasma tonicity cannot routinely be measured by a single assay. Rather, tonicity requires separate measurements for each of the contributing solutes (sodium, glucose, mannitol, etc.).

Comparison of the calculated plasma osmolality with the value measured by an osmometer (the osmolal gap; Fig. 20-2) is a useful screening technique for identifying circulating toxins (see Chap. 25) and for identifying pseudohyponatremia (see below).[107,145] The two components of the calculated osmolality include the electrolytes (essentially sodium and its balancing anions) and the normally appearing nonelectrolytes (urea and glucose). When the measured osmolality exceeds the calculated value by more than 10 mosmol/liter, some solute, not accounted for by sodium and its anions or by glucose or urea, must be present in the ECF. Various low–molecular weight toxins can account for this solute.

The particles contributing to ICF and ECF osmolality are qualitatively quite different but equivalent in concentration (Fig. 20-1). Particle size, diffusibility, and membrane transport processes create this asymmetrical distribution of solute. Large-molecular weight proteins and phosphorylated metabolic intermediates remain imprisoned within cells, whereas glucose and albumin are largely restricted to the ECF. Although both cations are permeable to cell membranes, ICF and ECF concentrations of sodium and potassium differ markedly. The Na^+-K^+ ATPase electrolyte pump, inserted into cell membranes, utilizes high-energy phosphate stores to create and maintain this altered electrolyte distribution, which subserves several key functions. The osmotic pressure of the ICF tends to exceed that of the ECF because of cellular synthesis, accrual, and retention of phosphorylated and high-molecular weight osmotically active particles. Cells would burst were water movement allowed to follow the dictates of the unmodified osmotic pressure of the ICF. Sodium export, mediated by the Na^+-K^+ ATPase, reduces cell solute content, thereby removing the risk of potentially lethal ICF expansion. Normal pump activity ensures that K^+ will account for the vast bulk of cellular osmoles, whereas Na^+ serves a similar function in the ECF. Thus, by doubling the exchangeable total body sodium (Na^+_E) and doubling the exchangeable potassium (K^+_E) content, thereby accounting for counterbalancing anions, one can account for almost all extracellular, intracellular and therefore, total body solute. Division of this total body solute by total body water approximates the prevailing osmolality of all body fluids:

$$\text{Osmolality (ECF, ICF)} = 2(Na^+_E + K^+_E)/\text{total body water} \quad (3)$$

It follows logically from equation 3 that hypoosmolality may result from any one or a combination of three pathogenic mechanisms: loss of body sodium and/or potassium and gain of body water with or without loss of one or both electrolytes.[91,270,303,307,308]

OSMOREGULATION

The solute concentration of body fluids is held virtually constant by tightly regulating the ebb and flow of body water. Examination of equation 3 suggests that gain of either Na^+ or K^+ ought to increase osmolality, but this increase is transient, since water-retaining forces (see below) are stimulated, which returns solute concentration to normal. The price paid for sustaining isotonicity by the accrual of water is weight gain and volume expansion. Conversely, selective loss of either Na^+ or K^+ transiently decreases osmolality, which suppresses these water-retaining forces, allowing renal water excretion to reestablish isotonicity; weight loss and volume contraction result.

The control of water balance regulates solute concentration, whereas separate forces (see Chap. 3) regulating sodium and (to a lesser extent) potassium balance maintain body fluid volume. Because Na^+ is restricted to the ECF, where it accounts for the vast majority of solute, control of sodium balance by secondarily influencing water balance regulates ECF volume. Shrinkage of cell volume occurs when loss of cell solute (largely K^+) or gain of ECF solute causes water to exit cells. Conversely, expansion of cell volume results when ECF water moves intracellularly in response to accumulation of cell solute or (more commonly) secondary to selective loss of ECF solute (i.e., Na^+).

Water balance determines the concentration of solute in all body fluid compartments, whereas sodium balance determines the volume of the ECF. It is not surprising that such vital parameters are closely guarded by sensitive and multifaceted control systems. Indeed, each of these vigilant regulatory systems is characterized by afferent sensors that continuously monitor effective osmolality (i.e., tonicity) and ECF volume and transmit signals to efferent systems that enhance retention or excretion of water or salt.[22,23,263-265,278,303] "Cross-talk" must occur between these regulatory systems, because pathologic gain or loss of water not only alters solute concentration but eventually effects significant change in ECF volume. Thus, complicated clinical conditions often spawn complex and coexisting changes in solute concentration and ECF volume.

The constancy of serum sodium concentration despite minute-to-minute challenges from our capricious appetites for salt and water underscores the vital importance of the osmoregulatory system. Water retention, hypotonicity, and lethal degrees of cellular swelling are avoided by a system that integrates thirst, tonicity of body fluids, and renal water excretion. Voluntary ingestion of 20 liters of water over a 20-h period can increase urine volume by a similar amount, while serum sodium concentration remains within the normal range. The proper functioning of this osmoregulatory system obviously affords great protection from hypotonicity. The interplay of these forces is outlined below.

Osmoreception

Hypothalamic receptors, exquisitely sensitive to changes in tonicity (effective osmolality), thirst, and antidiuretic hormone (i.e., arginine vasopressin, or AVP) release ensure that regulated water intake and excretion maintain serum tonicity normal (Fig. 20-3).[379] Although its sensitivity is much less, this system also responds to the dictates of extreme changes in ECF volume, blood pressure, and several other nonosmotic stimuli (Fig. 20-4).[181,217,229,279]

Long before the advent of highly sensitive and specific immunoassays, Verney deduced that brain cells, sensitive to changes in effective ECF osmolality, released a principal that caused renal water retention and the elaboration of highly concentrated urine.[343] Rapid intracarotid infusions of effective—but not ineffective—osmoles reduced urine volume while increasing its os-

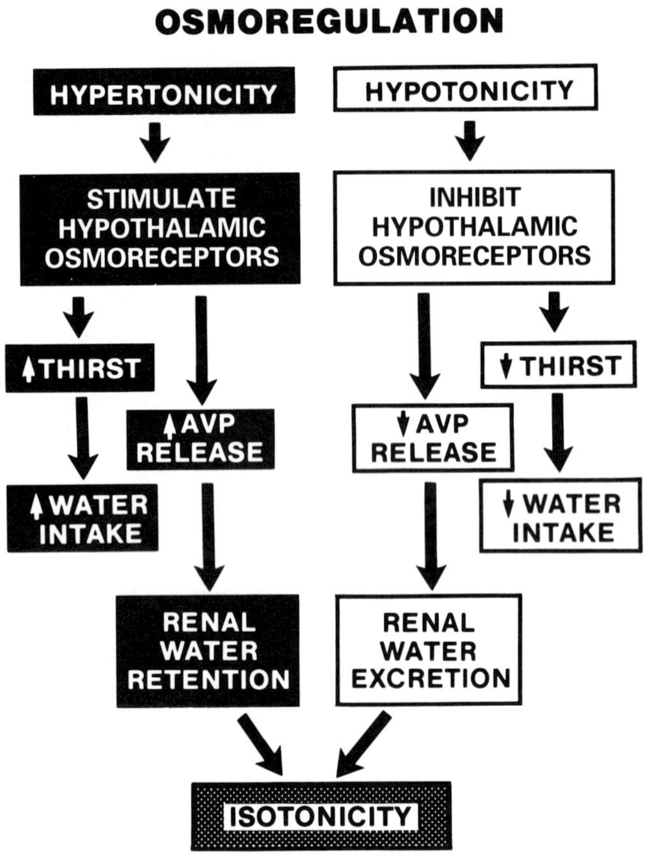

FIGURE 20-3 • Overview of water balance.

molality. We now know that when tonicity changes by as little as 1 percent, osmoreceptors that alter the synthesis and release of AVP are triggered in the hypothalamus.[22,23,263,264] This hormone, synthesized by neurons located in the supraoptic and paraventricular nuclei, is complexed to neurophysin, its carrier protein, and then delivered via axonal flow to storage sites in the posterior pituitary.[379] Under steady-state conditions of isotonicity (serum osmolality 285 mosm/liter), plasma AVP levels average 2.5 pg/ml but vary directly with induced changes in serum tonicity (Fig. 20-5). Indeed, serum AVP levels are unmeasurable when serum osmolality falls below 280 mosm/liter, and consequently torrential volumes of maximally dilute urine (osmolality 40 to 50 mosm/liter) are excreted (Fig. 20-5). Conversely, as rising serum osmolality approximates 295 mosm/liter, plasma AVP levels approximate 5.0 pg/ml, and urine volume contracts to well less than 1 liter of maximally concentrated fluid (1200 mosm/liter). Further increases in serum osmolality elicit further increments in plasma AVP concentrations, but no further change in urinary volume or concentration is realized. However, the vasoconstrictive effect of these high circulating levels of hormone may help to sustain normotension.

Hypotensive or volume-contracted subjects continue to retain proffered water despite worsening hypotonicity. In teleological terms, tonicity in this setting is sacrificed for maintenance of plasma volume, hemodynamic stability being the more vital function. Neural impulses from baroreceptors in the great vessels and atria, stimulated by an 8 to 10 percent reduction in ECF volume or by hypotension, are carried via cranial nerves IX and X to the hypothalamus.[229,278] A large hemodynamic stimulus elicits higher AVP levels than does an osmotic stimulus. Thus, although AVP release is more sensitive to changes in tonicity, the AVP release stimulated by volume contraction can override the less potent inhibitory effects of hypotonicity.

A variety of noxious stimuli, acting through higher centers, also stimulate AVP release (Fig. 20-4). These secretagogues include pain, emotional stress, nausea, hy-

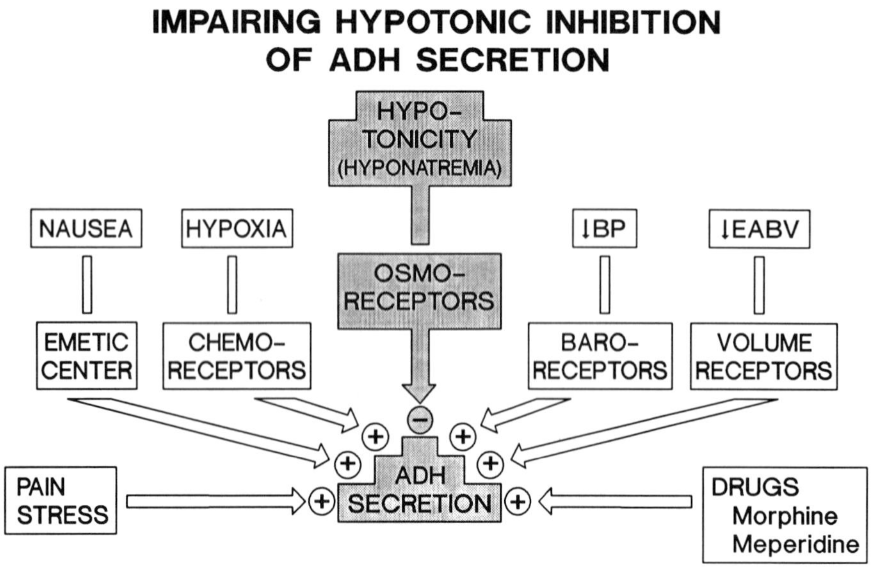

FIGURE 20-4 • Nonosmotic stimuli of AVP secretion.

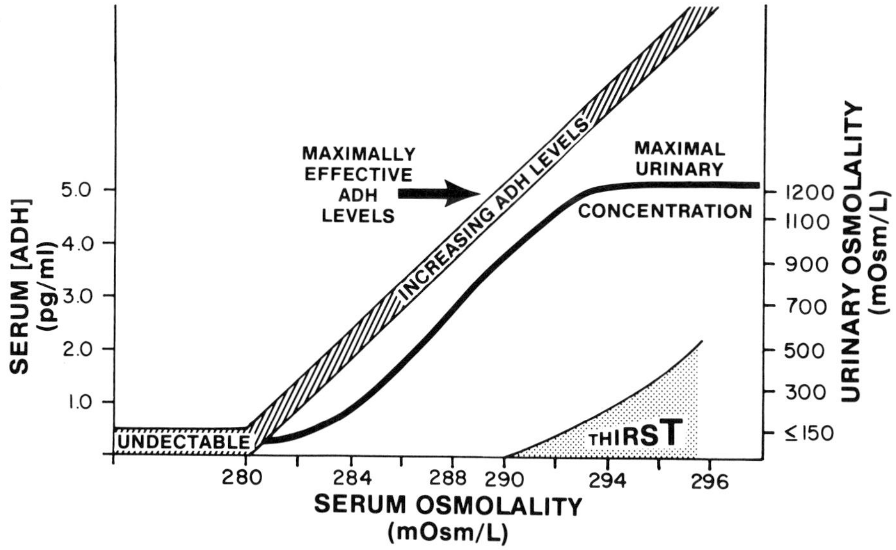

FIGURE 20-5 • Plasma tonicity, thirst, and AVP secretion.

poxia, hypoglycemia, and various drugs.[119,217,264,265,266,274,303] Hypotonicity results from excessive exposure to water when volume contraction or one of these other stimuli is present.

Renal water handling

Guided by varying plasma AVP concentrations, the kidney excretes or retains precisely the right amount of water to prevent more than a 1 to 2 percent variation in serum sodium concentration. If sodium and potassium are excreted at a concentration equal to the cation concentration of plasma water (150 m*M*), the level of serum sodium remains unchanged; reduced ECF volume is the only result of this proportionate excretion of sodium and water. If, however, sodium and potassium are excreted with proportionately more water (i.e., excreted urine is dilute), the serum sodium concentration will increase. Finally, serum sodium levels decrease if cations are excreted with proportionately less water (i.e., concentrated urine is excreted).[270,303]

For the kidney to excrete the water we ingest, *adequate volumes of glomerular filtrate must be delivered to the distal nephron, where sodium chloride is selectively removed* from the filtrate, leaving ("electrolyte-free") water in the tubule. In the absence of AVP, the distal nephron remains relatively "waterproof," allowing this dilute fluid to be excreted. The medullary interstitium, through which course the collecting ducts with their dilute filtrate, is always hypertonic to plasma. AVP increases the water channels in the walls of the collecting duct, which allows for osmotic equilibration between the dilute luminal and the hypertonic interstitial fluids.[303] Thus, in the presence of AVP water is conserved as it moves into the medulla and eventually back to the systemic circulation. Failure to suppress AVP secretion during periods of excess water exposure limits its excretion by the kidney and thereby predisposes one to hyponatremia. The numerous conditions that sustain inappropriately high levels of circulating AVP are outlined in Table 20-1. Disorders that severely limit glomerular filtration or increase its proximal reabsorption (hypovolemic and hypoalbuminemic states) may also predispose one to water retention and hyponatremia by limiting delivery of filtrate to the diluting sites of the distal nephron. Impaired sodium reabsorption in the diluting sites will also limit the amount of dilute (electrolyte-free) urine that can be excreted. Loop-active diuretics (furosemide, bumetanide, and ethacrynic acid) and thiazide diuretics impair dilution by inhibiting sodium reabsorption in the thick ascending limb and early distal tubule, respectively.

Thirst

The forces that stimulate and suppress thirst are remarkably similar to those affecting AVP release.[11,22,247,265,268,303,321,377] Thus, hypertonicity and hypovolemia both provoke release of the hormone and elicit the sensation of thirst. The physiologic benefit derived from both ingesting and retaining water needed for the repair of hypernatremia or hypovolemia is obvious. The osmoreceptors for thirst are located in the anterior portion of the hypothalamus, overlapping but at least partially separate from those mediating vasopressin release.[379] They respond to an increase in tonicity (e.g., from sodium or mannitol) but not to an increased concentration of an ineffective osmole such as urea.[377] While some studies suggest that the osmotic threshold for thirst is higher than that for AVP release,[263,265] other data show remarkably similar thresholds.[22,23,247,321] In any case, thirst is experienced at plasma osmolalities within the physiologic

TABLE 20-1 • Causes of SIADH

CNS disorders
- Psychosis
- Trauma
- Neoplasms: primary and metastatic
- Vascular: hemorrhage, infarction, and vasculitits
- Infection: meningitis, brain abscess, and encephalitis
- Miscellaneous: Guillain-Barré syndrome, multiple sclerosis, hydrocephalus, and Shy-Drager syndrome

Pulmonary disorders
- Infectious: pneumonia (viral, bacterial, and fungal) and tuberculosis
- Functional: asthma, acute respiratory failure, and mechanical ventilation

Tumors
- Bronchogenic (small-cell), pancreas, duodenum, ureter, nasopharynx, leukemia, Hodgkin's disease, and thymoma

Drugs
- Antidiuretic hormones: AVP, dDAVP, and oxytocin
- Psychotropic agents: amitriptyline, desipramine, protriptyline, haloperidol, trifluoperazine, thioridazine, fluphenazine, tranylcypromine, thiothixene, monoamine oxidase inhibitors, and carbamazepine
- Antineoplastic agents: cyclophosphamide, vincristine, and vinblastine
- Diabetic agents: chlorpropamide and tolbutamide
- Miscellaneous: bromocriptine and nicotine

Trauma (surgery)

Other
- Nausea, alcohol withdrawal, and AIDS

range. The drinking response to hypovolemia appears to be mediated through the renin-angiotensin system. Angiotensin II, a potent dipsogen, activates receptors located in the subfornical organ.[11,379]

ADAPTATIONS TO HYPOTONICITY

When osmoregulatory systems fail to maintain tonicity within the normal range, cells must adapt to the disturbance in order to preserve their volume.[173,190,374] On exposure to a hypotonic environment, all cells initially swell as water diffuses into the cytoplasm until the osmolality of intracellular and extracellular fluids equalizes. Within seconds, however, many cells begin to adjust their volume back toward its original size. This response, known as a *volume regulatory decrease*, occurs at widely varying rates, depending on cell type, and is explained in part by a loss of potassium, chloride, and, in some cells, sodium ions. Volume regulatory losses of intracellular potassium are mediated by the opening of stretch-activated potassium channels.[190]

Most cells also maintain relatively high cytoplasmic concentrations of small, osmotically active organic molecules known as *organic osmolytes* (Table 20-2).[177,374] The major organic osmolytes are limited to a few classes of compounds—polyols, methylamines, and free amino acids—which are shared by species from widely diverse phyla. The few organic osmolytes found in nature are *nonperturbing solutes*; unlike sodium and potassium, their intracellular concentrations may vary widely without affecting tertiary protein structure.[374]

Variation in the cellular content of organic osmolytes explains the ability of osmoconforming marine animals to survive without major alterations in cell volume or intracellular electrolyte concentrations when they travel from the sea (salt water) to fresh water (as in an estuary). The same adaptation explains why the cells of the inner renal medulla can maintain their volume and electrolyte

TABLE 20-2 • Major cellular organic osmolytes

Amino acids
- Glutamate
- Glutamine
- Aspartate
- Taurine (β-amino acid)

Methylamines
- Betaine
- Glycerophosphorylcholine
- Creatine/creatine phosphate

Polyhydric alcohols
- Myoinositol

concentrations despite wide variations in the osmolality of interstitial fluid under conditions of water diuresis and antidiuresis. Other mammalian cells, particularly those of the brain and heart, accumulate organic osmolytes under hypertonic conditions and lose them when confronted with hypotonicity.[177,183,190,322,329,331,341]

BRAIN ADAPTATIONS TO HYPOTONICITY

The need for a volume-regulatory adaptation to hyponatremia is most imperative in the brain, where the rigid calvarium places sharp limits on the degree of tissue expansion; an increase in brain water content of more than approximately 10 percent is incompatible with life (Fig. 20-6).[308] While the blood-brain barrier resists the permeation of most osmotically active solutes, it is permeable to water. Thus, when the serum sodium concentration falls, a transient osmotic gradient forms between the systemic capillary blood and the brain, causing water to flow rapidly across the barrier into brain cells, thereby restoring osmotic equilibrium. If the brain were to behave as a perfect osmometer, swelling in proportion to the change in tonicity, a reduction in sodium concentration from 140 to 127 mmol/liter (a 10 percent change) would be all that could be tolerated. The fact that humans may survive unharmed with serum sodium concentrations below 100 mmol/liter (low enough to cause a 40 percent increase in brain volume) is living testimony to the resistance of the brain to osmotic swelling.[308]

Total cerebral volume is, of course, largely determined by the volume of each of its two major fluid compartments: the interstitial fluid (ISF) space and the ICF space. Adaptive changes in the size of both compartments limit the degree of cerebral edema in hypotonicity.[303,308] When water is drawn osmotically across the blood-brain barrier, the hydrostatic pressure of the interstitial space rises, forcing fluid out of the brain through extracellular channels interconnecting the interstitial space with the cerebrospinal fluid (CSF).[199,221,303,308] Transfer of ISF into the CSF (and hence to the general circulation via the arachnoid villae) limits brain swelling to about one-half of what would be predicted by ideal osmotic behavior.

Reduction of the brain sodium content (caused primarily by the exit of ISF) begins within minutes of the onset of hyponatremia.[199] Volume regulatory responses by brain cells require more time. Cellular potassium loss begins after a few hours of sustained hypotonicity, and within 24 h this adaptive response becomes maximal.[138,199,275,310] Because the amount of potassium that can be extruded is limited, other intracellular solutes must also be exported to allow for the realization of the full adaptive response to severe hyponatremia.[3,85,138,190,275,310]

The brain cell cytoplasm normally contains high con-

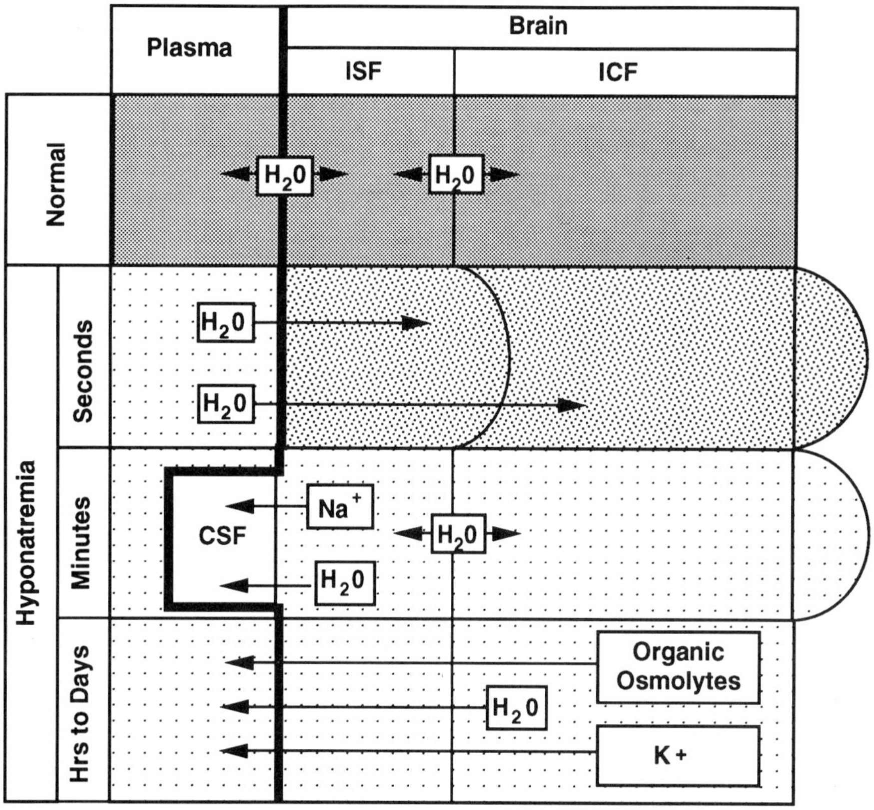

FIGURE 20-6 • Brain adaptation to hyponatremia. The consequences of an acute reduction in plasma sodium concentration are illustrated by time course. *Seconds:* Water (but no solute) flows across the blood-brain barrier to reestablish osmotic equilibrium; expansion of the brain's ISF and ICF spaces results. *Minutes:* bulk flow of Na^+, Cl^-, and water through extracellular channels linking the brain's ISF and the CSF restores ISF volume to normal. *Hours to days:* ICF volume returns to normal as cell K^+ and organic osmolytes are lost, allowing excess cell water to return to the plasma.

centrations of several amino acids (most notably taurine, glutamine, and glutamate), methylamines (phosphocreatine and betaine), and the polyhidric alcohol myoinositol.[177,183,190,322,323,329,331,341] The concentration of these organic osmolytes (once known as *idiogenic osmoles*) rises in hypernatremia and falls in response to hypotonic hyponatremia.[183,189,322,323,329,330,331,341] The time required for this adaptation is uncertain, but in experimental animals, it appears to require at least 1 to 2 days.[310,341] Similarly, during correction of hyponatremia, the reuptake of organic osmolytes is slower than the reuptake of electrolytes by the brain.[183,310,341] In rodents, replenishment of myoinositol and taurine requires several days.

Because adjustments in cell solute content take time to fully develop, the brain is imperiled by rapid osmotic changes.[3,138,190,303,310] Thus, acute hyponatremia may be fatal at serum sodium concentrations that are well tolerated chronically.[12,13,100,132,184,255,259,345] Moreover, while the extrusion of organic osmolytes from brain cells ultimately protects against lethal cerebral edema, an accumulation of these compounds in the brain's interstitial space during the initial stages of the adaptation may cause neurologic symptoms because many of these organic osmolytes are neurotransmitters.[177,183,189,190,322,329,341] The adaptations that defend against cerebral edema in chronic hyponatremia also predispose to brain injury when the electrolyte disturbance is corrected too rapidly (Fig. 20-7). As the serum sodium concentration returns to normal, cellular solutes lost in the adaptive phase must be recovered. Unless this process keeps pace with the rising serum sodium concentration, brain dehydration may result.[183,190,303,310,329] As will be discussed later, this phenomenon appears to underlie most of the neurologic complications of chronic hyponatremia.

CAUSES OF HYPONATREMIA (Table 20-3)

NONHYPOTONIC HYPONATREMIA

Pseudohyponatremia

Approximately 92 to 94 percent of normal serum is accounted for by water. The remaining 6 to 8 percent is mainly composed of lipids and protein. Because sodium ions dissolve only in the water phase, the content of sodium in a liter of serum is defined by the product of its

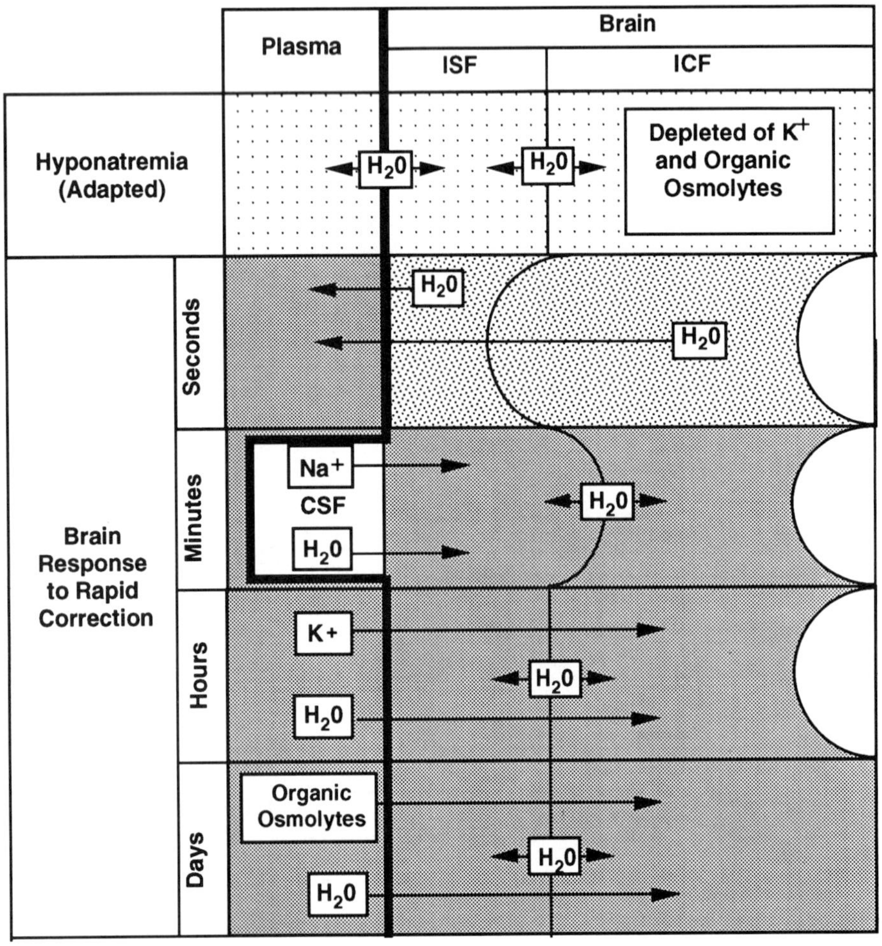

FIGURE 20-7 • Rapid correction of chronic hyponatremia. Before correction, the brain and plasma are in osmotic equilibrium, and ICF volume is normal because of an adaptive loss of cellular solute (K^+ and organic osmolytes). The effects of rapid correction on the brain are illustrated by time course. *Seconds:* Osmotic equilibrium between brain and plasma osmolalities is reestablished as water (but no solute) flows across the blood-brain barrier, dehydrating the brain's ICF and ISF spaces. *Minutes:* Bulk flow of CSF restores ISF volume and brain Na^+ content to supernormal levels. *Hours:* Recovery of cellular K^+ partially restores ICF volume. *Days:* Full repair of ICF volume does not occur until cellular organic solute content returns to normal.

TABLE 20-3 • Physiologic classification of hyponatremia

- **Nonhypotonic hyponatremia**
  - **Pseudohyponatremia**
    - Hyperlipidemia
    - Hyperproteinemia (multiple myeloma and macroglobulinemia)
  - **Hyperglycemia**
  - **Exogenous solutes**
    - Hypertonic mannitol
    - Postprostatectomy syndrome (isotonic)
      - Mannitol
      - Sorbitol
      - Glycine
- **Hypotonic hyponatremia**
  - **Intact (minimally impaired) diluting ability**
    - Psychotic polydipsia
    - Beer potomania
    - Infants
  - **Impaired diluting ability independent of AVP**
    - Renal failure
    - Diuretics
  - **Impaired diluting ability from hemodynamic stimulus to AVP**
    - **Volume depletion**
      - Extrarenal losses
      - Renal losses
        - Addison's disease
        - Cerebral salt wasting
        - Renal salt-wasting disorders
      - Renal and extrarenal losses
        - Vomiting or nasogastric suction
    - **Edematous conditions**
      - Congestive heart failure
      - Cirrhosis
      - Nephrotic syndrome
  - **Inappropriate secretion of AVP (SIADH; see Table 20-1)**

concentration in water and the percentage of water in each liter of serum. The actual concentration of sodium in serum water averages 154 meq/liter, and because the average percentage of water in serum is 93 percent, 143 meq of sodium resides in each *total liter of serum* (0.93 × 154 meq/liter). Thus, because the sodium concentration is reported by clinical laboratories in terms of milliequivalents per liter of *total serum*, normal values average 143 meq/liter. Hypertriglyceridemia severe enough to cause serum to become lactescent and hyperproteinemia from advanced multiple myeloma or macroglobulinemia, artifactually lower the serum sodium concentration.[16,102,104,116,139,141,303,318,361] As lipid or protein accumulates and is homogeneously dispersed throughout the serum, more nonsodium solid and less water will be present in each liter. Water is displaced from each unit volume of serum to accommodate the additional solid (Fig. 20-8). Reported values for serum sodium concentration are low because each unit volume of serum assayed in these instances has more solid and less water and sodium (Fig. 20-8). A clinical corollary of this observation is that 1 liter of the normal saline solution used for intravenous therapy contains sodium at a concentration of 154 meq/liter. No solids are present to "dilute" the saline solution and lower the sodium concentration.

Measurement of the serum sodium concentration with direct ion-selective electrodes can *theoretically* avoid the problem of "pseudohyponatremia."[62,171,361] The electrodes "recognize" the sodium concentration only in the aqueous phase, and their calibration allows values to be reported in the usual range of 143 meq/liter. Such instruments are most commonly found in intensive care and surgical areas. However, clinical laboratories using an ion-selective electrode dilute the serum prior to the analysis, and this dilution step introduces an artifact that allows hyperlipidemia and hyperproteinemia to effect the

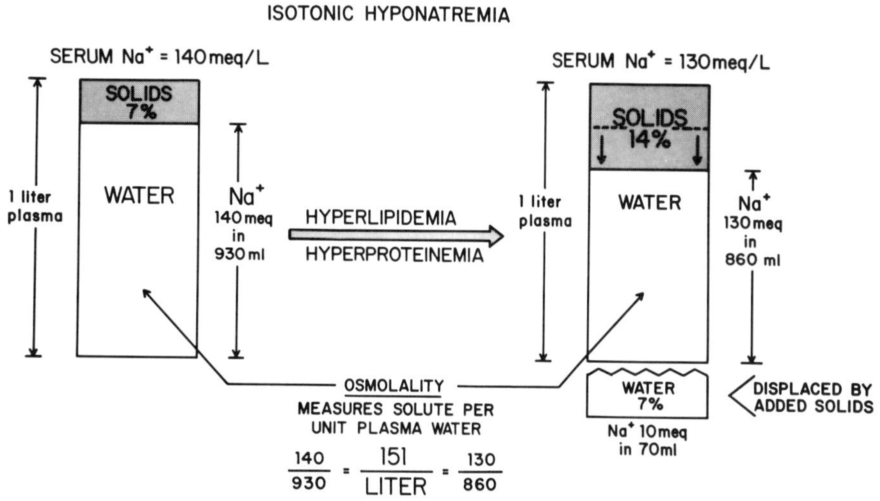

FIGURE 20-8 • Pseudohyponatremia. High concentrations of lipid and protein artifactually lower the serum sodium concentration. (From Narins RG, Lazarus JM, in Vandam LD, ed: *To Make the Patient Ready for Anesthesia: Medical Care of the Surgical Patient*, Menlo Park, CA, Addison-Wesley, 1980. Used by permission.)

same errors as seen with flame photometry. The basis of the artifact is that, even though the electrode always reads the sodium concentration in the aqueous phase, when diluting a fat- or protein-laden sample, the technician unknowingly delivers less sodium for dilution. Adding 1 ml of either of the abnormal samples to 9 ml of water creates a dilution that is greater than 1:10 because less water and salt are delivered in the 1 ml of hyperlipidemic or hyperproteinemic samples. Thus, even though the electrode correctly "reads" the sodium concentration of the aqueous phase, the artifact introduced by fat and lipid remains. Automatic dilution devices inject another possible error: true volumes of highly viscous hyperproteinemic serum may not be delivered by diluting pumps to the assay electrode. If the hyperviscosity causes less than 1 ml to be delivered, for example, the dilution will unknowingly be greater than the technician thinks, causing the final calculation to erroneously further reduce the serum concentration.

Neither fat nor protein alters the freezing point depression of plasma, as measured by an osmometer. Thus, suspected pseudohyponatremia may be documented by comparing the measured serum osmolality with the plasma osmolality calculated from the concentrations of sodium, blood urea nitrogen (BUN), and glucose, as discussed earlier in this chapter. The normal measured osmolality and the artifactually low calculated value cause the osmolal gap to increase. Thus, pseudohyponatremia or the circulation of low-molecular weight compounds can increase the osmolal gap.[107,145] While conceptually fascinating, pseudohyponatremia is rarely an important clinical problem. Only extremely severe hyperlipidemia and hyperproteinemia introduce major errors in the measured serum sodium concentration. For example, if the serum triglyceride level reached the extreme value of 10,000 mg/dl, the serum sodium concentration would decrease from 140 meq/liter to 120 meq/liter. Because such levels of hypertriglyceridemia are so uncommon, it follows that profound hyponatremia (values below 125 meq/liter) are almost never due to lipid accumulation alone. Multiplication of the plasma lipid level (expressed in milligrams per dl) by 0.002 yields the artifactual reduction in serum sodium level (meq/liter).[219] This factor is derived as follows. The density of serum lipid (i.e., the number of milliliters occupied by each g/liter) is 0.7. Dividing the measured serum triglyceride level in mg/liter by its density yields the number of ml of serum water that have been displaced. If, for example, the serum triglyceride level was 1000 mg/dl (i.e., 10,000 mg/liter), 14.3 ml of water would be displaced, diluting the serum by 14.3:1000; thus, the serum sodium concentration will decrease by 140 × 0.0143, or approximately 2 meq/liter, or each mg/dl of lipid reduces the concentration by 0.002 meq/liter (this derivation was pointed out by Dr. Robert Kreisberg). Multiplication of the increment in serum proteins (g/dl) above 8 g/dl by 0.25 approximates the number of meq/liter that the serum sodium concentration is reduced.

Hyperglycemia

Hyponatremia may be associated with hypertonicity (*hypertonic hyponatremia*).[156,212,250,269,355] This form of hyponatremia occurs most commonly in uncontrolled diabetes mellitus. In diabetic hyperglycemia, sodium-free water shifts out of the cells into the ECF, diluting the serum sodium concentration because, without adequate insulin, glucose is an impermeant (and therefore "effective") osmole. Thus, in hyperglycemia, the serum sodium concentration is commonly reduced, giving the false impression of hypotonicity. With insulin therapy, glucose becomes an ineffective osmole as it enters cells and is metabolized. Water then reenters cells, and the serum sodium concentration rises. Thus, it is useful to adjust the serum sodium concentration for the effect of hyperglycemia by calculating what the serum sodium concentration would be if the glucose concentration were returned to normal. For every 100 mg/100 ml increase in plasma glucose, the osmotic water shift causes the serum sodium concentration to fall by approximately 1.3 to 1.6 mmol/liter.[156,269]

Exogenous solutes

Like hyperglycemia, hypertonic infusions of impermeant solutes, such as mannitol and glycerol, decrease the serum sodium concentration by drawing water into the extracellular space to reestablish osmotic equilibrium. Under such conditions, the low serum sodium concentration accurately portrays the sodium concentration in plasma water and in the ISF. However, the measured plasma osmolality (and tonicity) will be high due to the presence of the low-molecular weight solutes in the ECF.[30]

Absorption of large volumes of isotonic mannitol from irrigants used during prostate surgery causes marked hyponatremia with a normal plasma osmolality.[123,209] Though the absorbed solute is confined to the extracellular space, no shift of water from the ICF occurs because plasma osmolality is unaltered. In other words, this is an example of *isotonic hyponatremia*. Isotonic sorbitol and isotonic (2.2 percent) or slightly hypotonic (1.5 percent) glycine solutions are also used in modern urologic surgery. Like mannitol, sorbitol and 2.2 percent glycine are initially confined to the extracellular space, causing marked hyponatremia without altering osmolality.[42,123,228,273,303,380] (The 1.5 percent glycine solution has an osmolality of 200 mosm/kg and thus reduces plasma osmolality moderately.) However, unlike mannitol, sorbitol and glycine are ultimately metabolized (leaving water behind), causing hypotonicity as a late complication. When large amounts of glycine are absorbed during surgery, hypotonicity, direct neurotoxic effects of the amino acid, and increased blood ammonia levels generated in its metabolism conspire to create severe neurologic symptoms.[123,157,228,273,303,380]

HYPOTONIC HYPONATREMIA

We classify hypotonic hyponatremia in terms of the kidney's ability to dilute the urine and excrete electrolyte-free water. Further subclassification is based on the various forces that modify renal dilution.

Normal or minimally impaired diluting ability

Psychotic polydipsia

Extreme polydipsia is relatively common in psychiatric patients, and in some cases it can be complicated by severe symptomatic hyponatremia.[19,62,112,128,140,149,261,286,293,296,315] The mechanism for hyponatremia in this condition is unclear. Approximately one-half of the reported cases have had maximally dilute urine (urine osmolalities below 100 mosm/kg) at the time of presentation. In such cases, a massive water diuresis rapidly returns the serum sodium concentration to nearly normal levels.[128,303,306] It is surprising that severe hyponatremia can develop in patients with maximally dilute urine. Assuming daily solute excretion of 900 mosm, it should be possible to excrete 9 to 18 liters of urine daily (375 to 750 ml/h) if the urine is diluted to 50 to 100 mosm/kg. However, daily intakes of 10 to 15 liters have been recorded in psychotic patients, and much of this water may be ingested over a few hours (from garden hoses, shower heads, etc.).[19,303,347] During periods of frantic water ingestion, intake can easily overwhelm the maximal excretory rate of 750 ml/h.

Transient release of AVP may also contribute to hyponatremia in polydipsic patients.[76,140,303] There is evidence indicating that nicotine-induced AVP secretion caused by smoking often plays a role.[7,150,303] AVP release caused by psychosis itself, by nausea associated with massive water intake (see below), or even by cerebral edema induced by hypotonicity may all conspire to impair urinary dilution. Drugs used to treat psychosis have often been suspected as a cause of the syndrome, but none of the major tranquilizers, with the exception of carbamazepine (see below), has been clearly shown to have an antidiuretic effect.[92,276,303,375] Thiazide diuretics (which impair the ability to generate a maximally dilute urine) have been responsible for episodes of severe acute hyponatremia in polydipsic patients.[92,182,255,287,293,303]

During recovery from self-induced water intoxication, some patients initially excrete a maximally dilute urine and then concentrate their urine inappropriately when the plasma osmolality rises above 250 mosm/kg.[128] Such resetting of the osmostat does not explain why the plasma osmolality fell far below the apparent setpoint for AVP release during episodes of extreme polydipsia. This finding does, however, establish a lower starting point for the serum sodium concentration. Indeed, in subjects who have recovered from water intoxication, the osmotic threshold for AVP secretion is slightly reduced, and baseline plasma sodium concentrations have averaged 133 mmol/liter.[115] These patients also have enhanced sensitivity to the antidiuretic effect of very low levels of AVP, a finding that could be explained by up-regulation of AVP receptors in response to hormone levels that have been chronically suppressed by a persistently large water intake.

Beer potomania

Beer contains very little protein or electrolyte. Subjects who subsist on large volumes of beer without other dietary intake (a practice known as beer potomania)[77,129,135,151] excrete much less urea, sodium, and potassium in their urine than do patients with a more adventurous palate. Even with a maximally dilute urine, water excretion is limited by the small amount of urinary solute. For example, if the total solute available for urinary excretion were reduced to 300 mosm/day from the usual 900 mosm and the urine could still be diluted to 50 mosm/kg, each liter of urine would contain 50 mosm of solute, and the daily solute load of 300 mosm would be excreted in only 6 liters. Enthusiastic beer drinkers can thus imbibe a larger volume of fluid than they can eliminate. As in psychotic water drinkers, hyponatremia is especially likely to develop in beer drinkers when the urine is less than maximally dilute (e.g., when thiazide diuretics are prescribed or when gastrointestinal fluid losses result in a hemodynamic stimulus for AVP release).

Hyponatremia in infants

Acute hyponatremia may develop in infants after they ingest large amounts of water.[113,158,277,333] Water intoxication caused by feeding excessively dilute formula (or substituting plain water for formula in a baby's bottle) is becoming increasingly common among the urban poor. Although infants can excrete a maximally dilute urine, their ability to excrete free water is limited by a low glomerular filtration rate. Once water intake is restricted, the serum sodium concentration is normalized as large volumes of urine are excreted.

Imparied diluting ability independent of AVP secretion

Renal failure

The smaller volume of fluid filtered each day by the failing kidney limits the range of water excretion.[97] If, for example, the glomerular filtration rate is 5 ml/min, only 7 liters of filtrate are formed daily, of which only approximately 30 percent reaches the diluting segments of the nephron. Even with complete suppression of AVP and absolute impermeability of the collecting duct, a maximum of only 2 liters of electrolyte-free water can be generated. If daily water intake exceeds this amount, positive water balance and hyponatremia will ensue.

Diuretics

In two recent series, diuretics were the sole etiologic agent or a major contributing factor in over half the patients admitted to the hospital for severe hyponatremia.[1,96,306] Diuretic-induced hyponatremia is primarily a complication of thiazide diuretics and metolazone.[1,14,15,21,96,147,196,356] By blocking the reabsorption of sodium and chloride in the cortical diluting segment, these agents prevent the generation of a maximally dilute urine. Because they do not affect salt reabsorption in the ascending limb of the loop of Henle, thiazides allow excretion of a maximally concentrated urine. Consequently, thiazide diuretics permit simultaneous retention of water and depletion of sodium, potassium, and chloride.[15] When a patient is taking thiazides, the cation concentration of the urine may exceed that of plasma, resulting in a positive electrolyte-free water balance.[270] Since loop diuretics (furosemide, bumetanide, and ethacrynic acid) impair both the renal concentrating and diluting mechanisms, they are less often associated with hyponatremia.

Impaired renal diluting ability by itself causes hyponatremia only when a large water intake requires a dilute urine to achieve water balance. Thus, as previously discussed, thiazides are particularly likely to cause severe hyponatremia in polydipsic subjects.[182,287] However, severe hyponatremia may also develop in patients with only moderate fluid intake.[103] Nonosmotic release of AVP caused by diuretic-induced volume depletion may explain this complication. However, while some patients with diuretic-induced hyponatremia are clinically volume-depleted, the majority appear isovolemic.[1,96,306] Intercurrent illnesses that decrease dietary protein and salt intake and transiently increase AVP secretion often precede episodes of hyponatremia in patients taking diuretics. Indeed, when measured, AVP levels have been increased in most, but not all, patients.[110]

Primarily a disease of the elderly,[1,14,21,33,41,161,208,312] severe diuretic-induced hyponatremia affects women much more often than it affects men (in four recent series, over 80 percent with the disorder were female).[1,96,306] Small, elderly women are particularly susceptible to diuretic-induced hyponatremia because relatively small gains in water and losses of salt are required. Patients typically present with hyponatremia, hypokalemia, and a metabolic alkalosis. As previously mentioned, potassium depletion contributes to the lowering of the serum sodium concentration. However, hypokalemia is not universal, and hyponatremia may occur in patients receiving combinations of thiazides and potassium-sparing diuretics.[21,147,196]

Impaired diluting ability: hemodynamic release of AVP

Volume depletion

Hypotension and/or hypovolemia are perhaps the most common nonosmotic stimuli for AVP secretion. The relationship between plasma AVP levels and arterial blood pressure is exponential; thus, AVP secretion is less sensitive to small hemodynamic stimuli than to small changes in osmolality, but a large change in intravascular volume or blood pressure elicits higher levels of AVP than are achieved through osmotic stimuli. Volume depletion changes the setpoint, or threshold, of AVP secretion such that, at any given level of plasma osmolality, AVP levels are higher than in normovolemia.[22,23,181,263-265,278]

Hypovolemia caused by extrarenal fluid losses

Hypovolemic hyponatremia is most often associated with gastrointestinal fluid loss, as in vomiting, diarrhea, or laxative abuse. "Third space" losses of ECF into the abdominal cavity in pancreatitis or peritonitis, into the bowel lumen in intestinal ileus, or into peripheral tissues in patients with burns or muscle damage may also produce this syndrome.

Extrarenal fluid losses cannot cause hyponatremia by themselves. Indeed, the fluid lost is sometimes hypotonic to plasma and therefore should raise the serum sodium concentration. Hyponatremia occurs when isotonic or hypotonic fluid losses result in a hemodynamic stimulus for thirst and AVP secretion. Increased water intake (either by the patient or from ill-conceived intravenous fluid management) coupled with hormonally mediated renal water retention causes the hyponatremia. A rather spectacular example of this phenomenon is seen in long-distance runners who have collapsed with severe hyponatremia at the end of a race after replacing large hypotonic sweat losses (up to 20 liters) with sugar water.[105,137,142,166,224,225,242] Because splanchnic blood flow is reduced during strenuous exercise, absorption of much of the ingested water is delayed; symptomatic hyponatremia may then emerge explosively after the race is over.

Hypovolemia caused by renal salt wasting

Diseases associated with impaired renal sodium conservation may cause hyponatremia, particularly if the renal concentrating mechanism is preserved. Inappropriate natriuresis triggers physiologic antidiuresis via hemodynamic stimuli for AVP secretion. Disordered secretion of the hormones that control sodium excretion most commonly causes this syndome.

In Addison's disease, combined mineralocorticoid deficiency (which causes renal sodium wasting and volume depletion as well as hyperkalemia) and glucocorticoid deficiency (which independently enhances AVP secretion) conspire to increase AVP levels.[170,279,281,301,341] It is important to recognize that hyponatremia without hypovolemia may complicate isolated glucocorticoid deficiency in patients with anterior pituitary insufficiency in whom mineralocorticoid secretion is intact (see below).[43,185,188,230] Hyponatremia may also complicate isolated mineralocorticoid deficiency when glucocorticoid secretion is normal (as in patients with hyporeninemic hypoaldosteronism), although this is less common.

Excessive secretion of atrial natriuretic peptide or other natriuretic hormones may occasionally cause renal salt wasting and hyponatremia.[86,348,353,367] Release of these hormones from injured brain tissue appears to be the mechanism for some cases of "cerebral salt wasting."[152,290,359,365] As inappropriate AVP secretion is commonly seen in neurologic disorders, the distinction between inappropriate natriuresis and inappropriate antidiuresis may be difficult.[86,218,222,223,237,249,291,292,348,353,373] In either case, urinary sodium excretion may be high, and increased levels of atrial natriuretic peptide may be found.[54,90,118,178,193,284] Documentation of renal sodium wasting prior to water retention, clinical evidence of hypovolemia,[86,223,367,368] and a fall in AVP levels in response to volume repletion are required to make this diagnosis; in most published cases of alleged cerebral salt wasting, these details have been lacking. The distinction is more than academic, however. Hypovolemia may impair cerebral blood flow in patients with subarachnoid hemorrhage when vasospasm develops.[130,223,366] Consequently, many authors have advocated volume expansion, rather than water restriction, when hyponatremia complicates subarachnoid hemorrhage.[87,222,366]

A variety of salt-losing renal diseases, such as chronic interstitial nephritis, medullary cystic disease, polycystic disease, and partial urinary tract obstruction may exhibit hypovolemic hyponatremia.[303] As renal concentrating ability is typically lost in these disorders, hyponatremia will occur only when water intake is large and dietary sodium intake is low. Hyponatremia is more likely to occur when proximal tubular sodium reabsorption is impaired, with relative preservation of distal concentrating mechanisms, as in platinum toxicity.[335]

Hypovolemia caused by combined renal and extrarenal losses

Surprisingly, patients who continue to drink while vomiting repeatedly (a feat most often accomplished by alcoholics) can still absorb enough ingested water to become hyponatremic. Electrolyte losses in the vomitus, coupled with urinary sodium and potassium losses induced by metabolic alkalosis, contribute to hypovolemia, which provides a hemodynamic stimulus for AVP secretion. Because nausea is a potent primary stimulus for AVP secretion,[274] some vomiting patients may become hyponatremic without clinically apparent volume depletion.[60]

Edematous disorders

Any disease that can cause edema can cause hyponatremia. The same hemodynamic stimuli that promote sodium retention also stimulate nonosmotic release of AVP.[282,283] Elevated AVP levels have been documented in edematous patients with congestive heart failure, hepatic cirrhosis, and nephrotic syndrome. These conditions are all characterized by relative "underfilling" of the arterial circulation.[283]

CONGESTIVE HEART FAILURE In congestive heart failure, baroreceptors and ventricular receptors that sense pulse pressure (i.e., stroke volume) and cardiac output appear to provide the afferent stimulus for AVP release.[32,125,167,202,260,332] Improvement of these variables (despite a decrease in mean arterial blood pressure) with afterload reduction using captopril or prazosin reduces AVP levels and increases water excretion.[89,210,235,236] Theoretically, the stimulus for AVP secretion provided by a decreased effective arterial blood volume should be offset by inhibition of AVP release due to left atrial distension. However, chronic atrial distension is associated with blunted left atrial receptor sensitivity. Thus, the effect of high-pressure baroreceptor stimulation appears to override any inhibitory input from the atria.[282]

Most patients with hyponatremia associated with congestive heart failure have detectable plasma immunoreactive AVP levels (30 of 37 cases in one series).[314] Because hyponatremia is usually associated with prerenal azotemia, an intrarenal mechanism (independent of AVP) may also play a role in the impaired water excretion of this disease. Evidence supporting an intrarenal mechanism is provided by the improvement in urinary dilution afforded by furosemide and mannitol, agents that increase fluid delivery to more distal diluting sites.[280] However, other explanations can be invoked to account for these results. Mannitol infusion may produce ECF volume expansion, thereby suppressing baroreceptor-mediated AVP release, while furosemide may antagonize the action of AVP on the collecting duct.

HEPATIC CIRRHOSIS A substantial number of patients with advanced hepatic cirrhosis complicated by ascites and edema are unable to excrete a water load. Cirrhotic patients with hyponatremia have been shown to have a faster heart rate, lower plasma albumin, and higher plasma concentrations of AVP, renin, aldosterone, and norepinephrine than those who excrete a water load normally.[31,44,94,238,282] Head-out water immersion partially reverses these abnormalities, and water immersion combined with norepinephrine infusion (to prevent peripheral vasodilatation) completely normalizes water excretion. Suppression of plasma AVP during water immersion alone is comparable to that achieved when immersion is combined with norepinephrine, but the combined maneuver results in a higher blood pressure, potentially decreasing proximal tubular fluid reabsorption and increasing sodium and water delivery to the distal nephron.[282]

As with cardiac failure, the hyponatremic cirrhotic patient may excrete a hypotonic urine during other maneuvers that increase distal fluid delivery (infusion of mannitol, saline solution, saline solution with albumin, or ascitic fluid).[198,282] Experimental models of altered liver function also show that impaired excretion of water in the disease is caused by nonosmotic release of AVP and diminished distal delivery of fluid to the diluting segments of the nephron.[282] In some experimental models, sodium retention can be shown to occur prior to the onset of ascites and without evidence of underfilling of the circulation, suggesting that at least in early cirrhosis, ascites develops because of primary sodium retention and overflow edema.

Taken together, these results suggest that cirrhotic patients who are susceptible to hyponatremia have a decreased effective arterial blood volume.[282,283] Hemodynamic abnormalities associated with the disease (peripheral vasodilatation, splanchnic venous pooling, and decreased plasma oncotic pressure due to hypoalbuminemia) cause nonosmotic release of AVP.[67,94,202,282,283] Either these same hemodynamic abnormalities or, alternatively, a primary abnormality in renal sodium handling reduces delivery of fluid to the diluting segments of the nephron, compounding the defect in water excretion.

NEPHROTIC SYNDROME In some patients with the nephrotic syndrome, particularly children with minimal-change disease and a normal glomerular filtration rate, a decreased effective arterial blood volume (caused by decreased plasma oncotic pressure) initiates AVP release and water retention.[29,122,240,282] In such patients, administration of hyperoncotic albumin and head-out water immersion reduce plasma AVP, renin, aldosterone, and norepinephrine and increase levels of atrial natriuretic factor, causing natriuresis and diuresis. However, in most adults with the nephrotic syndrome, blood volume is increased and blood pressure is often elevated. Consequently, hyponatremia is less common in the nephrotic syndrome than in other edematous disorders.

Impaired diluting ability: "inappropriate" AVP secretion

Secretion of AVP is considered inappropriate when it persists in the absence of appropriate osmotic and hemodynamic stimuli. Inappropriate secretion of antidiuretic hormone impairs the excretion of water, but the controls of sodium balance are unaffected, and there is no tendency to retain sodium. In fact, when hyponatremia occurs from retention of ingested or infused water, the expanded ECF volume triggers a natriuresis. Thus, urinary sodium excretion may transiently exceed sodium intake, giving the false impression of salt wasting. Negative sodium balance may exacerbate the hyponatremia.

The consequences of relentless AVP secretion are illustrated by Leaf's classic experiment in which water intake was varied while continuously infusing AVP (Fig. 20-9).[178] When the rate of water intake approximated that of urinary water excretion, no change in body weight, serum sodium concentration, or urinary sodium excretion occurred. However, at higher rates of water intake, the AVP infusion caused net water retention, an increase in weight, natriuresis, and a fall in serum sodium concentration. Restriction of water intake restored all parameters to baseline levels despite the continued infusion of AVP.

Leaf's experiment mimics the clinical findings of the syndrome of inappropriate antidiuretic hormone secretion (SIADH).[58,284] The clinical syndrome caused by this abnormality was first described by Schwartz and Bartter in two patients with bronchogenic carcinoma who were found to have concentrated urine despite hyponatremia and hypoosmolality.[284] Since this report, SIADH has been recognized in a wide variety of pathologic states (see below).[10,79,120,134,168,303,357]

Patients with this syndrome become hyponatremic if they are given enough electrolyte-free water, but unlike patients with a hemodynamic cause for AVP secretion, they have no tendency to retain sodium and do not develop edema.[58,117,340] Because the controls of sodium excretion are intact (and independent of the level of the

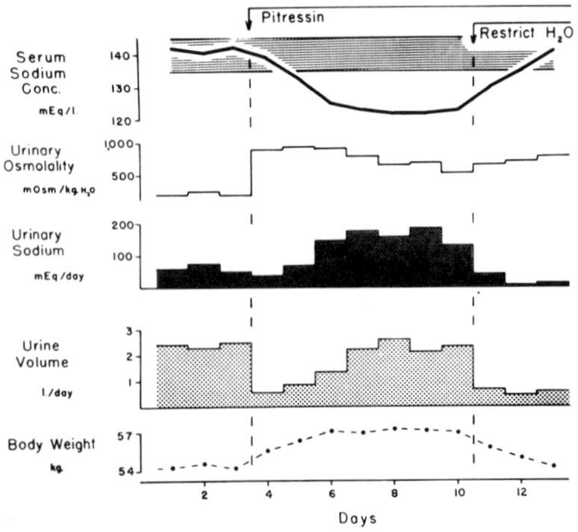

FIGURE 20-9 • Experimental SIADH. During a constant infusion of AVP, increasing water intake causes weight gain, hyponatremia, and natriuresis. Restriction of water intake restores all parameters to baseline despite continued infusion of AVP. (From Goldberg M, *Med Clin North Am* 47:915, 1963. Used by permission.)

serum sodium concentration), urinary sodium excretion eventually matches intake. Extreme dietary sodium restriction can lead to a urine that is nearly sodium-free, while a large sodium load is followed by a rapid increase in sodium excretion.[226]

Several patterns of inappropriate AVP secretion have been recognized.[376] These various patterns reflect the many different diseases that can be responsible for the syndrome (see below). Abnormal AVP secretion may be caused by ectopic production of the hormone by tumors[339] (classically, but not limited to, small-cell carcinoma of the lung) or by disordered secretion by the neurohypophysis.

While AVP secretion is sometimes erratic and totally independent of osmotic stimuli, some responsiveness to changes in plasma tonicity has been found in the majority of patients with SIADH who have been studied.[376] In some cases, AVP secretion is qualitatively normal, but the osmoreceptor threshold is "reset" at a lower than normal value.[75,204,376] Below the reset osmotic threshold, plasma AVP levels become undetectable, allowing excretion of a maximally dilute urine. Thus, while such patients are hyponatremic, they are not in danger of progressive hypotonicity if they are given additional water. It is surprising, however, that this pattern of abnormal AVP secretion (often called a "reset osmostat") can be found in patients with SIADH associated with tumors as well as in patients with more benign causes of the syndrome. Thus, while a reset osmostat is usually not a cause of severe symptomatic hyponatremia, it may be a sign of severe underlying disease. In another pattern of release, known as "vasopressin leak," the basal level of AVP is elevated and unresponsive to osmotic stimuli, but plasma AVP levels increase appropriately as plasma osmolality is elevated into the normal range. Unlike patients with the reset osmostat variant, patients with a vasopressin leak are unable to dilute their urine no matter how low the serum sodium falls, and they will retain water and become severely hyponatremic if water intake is not restricted.

In about 10 percent of patients with SIADH, AVP levels remain at a low basal level that fails to increase even as the plasma osmolality is elevated.[311,376] This finding would be expected if an antidiuretic substance not measured by the AVP radioimmunoassay were produced or if there were an increased sensitivity of the tubules to the normally secreted hormone. The reason for this pattern of secretion has not yet been established.

Endocrine abnormalities

Glucocorticoid deficiency caused by anterior pituitary insufficiency or isolated ACTH deficiency is often complicated by hyponatremia.[43,185,188,230,252] There is no evidence of hypovolemia, which occurs in Addison's disease, and the disorder presents with all the clinical features of SIADH. Plasma AVP levels are elevated and respond promptly to glucocorticoid replacement. Impaired water excretion is also found in humans and animals with *hypothyroidism*.[8,143,279,294] AVP levels are also increased, possibly because of diminished cardiac output; reduced renal blood flow and glomerular filtration rate may also contribute to the defect.[8,279,362] Though abnormal hemodynamics may be responsible for the abnormal water metabolism of hypothyroidism, hyponatremic patients with the disease may be free of edema, responding in all respects as do other patients with SIADH.

Drug-induced SIADH

Several drugs that impair the renal diluting capacity and cause hyponatremia are listed in Table 20-1. Some of these agents mimic the effect of AVP on the collecting duct, while others stimulate the release of AVP or potentiate its action.[179,206] Several of the more important offending agents are reviewed here.

Desamino-8-D-AVP (dDAVP) is an analogue of AVP that selectively stimulates V2 receptors.[267] Used in the treatment of diabetes insipidus, dDAVP in excessive doses can cause hyponatremia, particularly in patients with coexisting thirst disorders. Because dDAVP improves platelet function in patients with von Willebrand's disease, the drug has also been used perioperatively to decrease bleeding. When given intravenously in multiple doses along with hypotonic fluids, the dDAVP has been associated with severe symptomatic hyponatremia.[288,295,360]

Oxytocin, used to induce labor or abortion, has a direct antidiuretic effect at high doses similar to that of AVP. When administered with excess electrolyte-free water, hyponatremia will result.[184,213,215] In some cases, severe hyponatremia has developed after the infusion of less than 3 liters of fluid. Because oxytocin has a short half-life, its discontinuation is typically followed by a water diuresis, which returns the serum sodium concentration to normal.

Chlorpropamide, an oral hypoglycemic agent used in the treatment of diabetes mellitus, is second only to thiazides as a cause of hyponatremia.[153,215,256,344] Approximately 4 percent of chlorpropamide-treated patients develop hyponatremia with the clinical characteristics of SIADH. Since the introduction of newer hypoglycemic agents, the chlorpropamide syndrome is seen much less frequently. These newer agents do not cause hyponatremia. Sulfonylurea drugs increase AVP release from the neurohypophysis and also augment the action of AVP on the kidney.[215] The latter effect appears to be caused by sulfonylurea-induced inhibition of AVP-stimulated prostaglandin E (PGE) synthesis. The net water-retaining effect of AVP reflects the algebraic sum of its two mutually offsetting effects on the kidney. The direct water-retaining tubular effect is partially inhibited by the simultaneous stimulation of PGE synthesis by AVP.[121] By eliminating the inhibitory effect of PGE, chlorpropamide increases the net effect of a given amount of hormone.

Nonsteroidal anti-inflammatory drugs decrease water excretion by potentiating the end-organ action of AVP via decreased synthesis of the AVP inhibitor PGE (see above). Hyponatremia attributable solely to nonsteroidal anti-inflammatory drugs has been reported only rarely, possibly because prostaglandin inhibition may also directly suppress AVP secretion centrally.[51,245] However, these commonly used drugs may exacerbate other causes of SIADH.[358]

Carbamazepine, used as an anticonvulsant and for treatment of tic douloureux, also causes hyponatremia by inducing AVP release.[155,159,172,375] The defect in water excretion caused by carbamazepine is dose-related, and a negative correlation between serum sodium concentrations and drug levels has been demonstrated. Carbamazepine-induced hyponatremia is particularly common in psychiatric institutions among patients with polydipsia. One report suggests that hyponatremia associated with carbamazepine therapy can be reversed with phenytoin.[298]

Vincristine, an antineoplastic agent, has a neurotoxic effect on the hypothalamic microtubular assembly, altering the normal osmoreceptor control of AVP secretion.[262] Hyponatremia caused by the drug tends to be accompanied by clinical evidence of peripheral neuropathy.

Cyclophosphamide, when administered intravenously, can impair water excretion, causing acute hyponatremia.[36,74,358] The antidiuretic effect of the drug begins 4 to 12 h after injection and lasts as long as 12 h. The defect in water metabolism is temporally related to urinary excretion of active alkylating metabolites. Patients receiving cyclophosphamide are particularly susceptible to hyponatremia because they are encouraged to drink large volumes of water to prevent chemical cystitis.

Nicotine decreases renal water excretion by stimulating AVP release despite elevation of systemic arterial blood pressure.[134] Central cholinergic pathways for AVP release possess nicotinic properties. Smoking appears to play an important role in the hyponatremia of psychotic water drinkers.[7]

Psychotropic agents have often been implicated in the etiology of hyponatremia, including the monoamine oxidase inhibitor tranylcypramine; the phenothiazines thioridazine, trifluoperazine, and fluphenazine; the butyrophenone haloperidol; the thithixenes; and the tricyclic antidepressants amitryptyline, protriptyline, and desipramine.[5,25,55,78,83,186,239,244,248,254] Nevertheless, it must be emphasized that hyponatremia in emotionally disturbed or psychotic patients may not be a direct consequence of these medications.[179,206,276] Causality has been more convincingly demonstrated with the tricyclic antidepressants.[25,83,186,248,276]

Similarly, *morphine and other opiates* have frequently been cited as causes of inappropriate secretion of AVP. However, there is no convincing evidence showing a direct effect of the agents on AVP release (see Chap. 4). Indirect stimulation of AVP caused by opiate-induced nausea or hypotension may occur.

Tumor-induced SIADH

Since the first report of SIADH in association with bronchogenic carcinoma, a long list of other tumors have been reported to cause hyponatremia (see below).[35,216,339] Small-cell carcinoma of the lung is the most common neoplasm associated with SIADH.[187]

Some tumors have been found to synthesize and secrete AVP.[9,108,180] Tumor extracts have been shown to contain antidiuretic activity by bio- and immunoassay. Many tumors contain typical secretory granules of the hormone, and in vitro synthesis of AVP has been demonstrated in cultured neoplastic tissue. However, AVP has been found in only about half of the tumors taken from patients with hyponatremia, suggesting that other factors may be responsible for the syndrome in many patients. Some tumors may stimulate AVP secretion from the neurohypophysis; in other cases, hyponatremia has occurred without elevated AVP levels, implying that another antidiuretic substance may be responsible.

Usually, tumors are clinically evident when hyponatremia is discovered. However, the electrolyte disturbance may precede the diagnosis of malignancy by months or even years. Thus, unexplained, persistent hyponatremia meeting the criteria for SIADH should be considered a marker for an underlying malignancy.

Pulmonary disorders

Hyponatremia is a frequent complication of pneumonia.[88,169,271,272] AVP levels are elevated but fall within a few days during treatment, so that with water restriction hyponatremia corrects about twice as rapidly as it does in SIADH associated with tumors. SIADH is also common in tuberculosis, and bioassays have demonstrated antidiuretic activity in tuberculous lung tissue.[13,350] Acute respiratory failure may also be associated with hyponatremia.[314] Hypoxemia and hypercapneic acidosis alone or in combination stimulate nonosmotic release of AVP.[95,258] Plasma AVP levels are best correlated with P_{CO_2}, which decreases as hypercapneia diminishes. Severe asthma without hypercarbia has also been associated with hyponatremia. Elevated AVP concentrations correlate with increased airway obstruction as measured by a decrease in FEV1.[271] Chronic obstructive airway disease severe enough to cause cor pulmonale causes both sodium and water retention, but in stable chronic obstructive pulmonary disease (COPD), water balance is usually normal.[95,271] Mechanical ventilation, particularly when combined with positive expiratory pressure, provides a nonosmotic stimulus for AVP release by impeding venous return, thus decreasing cardiac output.

Central nervous system disorders

SIADH complicates a wide range of disorders in which there is damage to or inflammation of the central nervous system (CNS; Table 20-1).[218,237,249,291,292,359] The possibility of CNS pathology should always be considered in hyponatremic patients who present with neurologic symptoms, particularly when the symptoms fail to improve during correction of the electrolyte disturbance.

As previously discussed, hyponatremia in at least some CNS conditions, most notably subarachnoid hemorrhage, may not always be caused by inappropriate AVP release.[86,152,222,290,348,365,373] Sodium wasting induced by release of natriuretic substances from the brain may provide a hemodynamic stimulus for AVP secretion.

Surgery

AVP levels amost invariably rise in response to anesthesia and surgery and may remain elevated for up to 5 days.[49,53,131,148,200,299,320] These patients are subject to the full range of nonosmotic stimuli that sustain AVP secretion: hypoxia, pain, nausea, hypotension, narcotics, and hypoglycemia. The tendency of the postoperative patient to retain water has long been recognized, prompting warnings against excessive use of electrolyte-free water after surgery.[20,132,133,284,372,378] Unfortunately, even today, this advice is not always heeded.[13,82,100] In a recent prospective study, 4.4 percent of surgical patients developed a plasma sodium concentration below 130 mmol/liter within 1 week of their operation.[49]

Nausea

Nausea is one of the most potent stimuli to AVP secretion known in humans, resulting in as much as a 1000-fold increase in plasma AVP levels. The nausea need not be associated with vomiting to stimulate AVP release.[60,274]

Alcohol withdrawal

Alcoholics in withdrawal fail to excrete a water load normally and have higher AVP levels than do normal volunteers despite lower levels of serum sodium concentration.[93,328] This situation occurs in the absence of hypovolemia as measured by blood pressure, BUN, and plasma renin levels. The pattern of AVP hypersecretion in patients with alcohol withdrawal contrasts with the inhibition of AVP that follows the acute ingestion of alcohol.

Acquired immunodeficiency syndrome

Surveys of admitted patients with the acquired immunodeficiency syndrome (AIDS) have found a 35 to 56 percent incidence of hyponatremia.[4,64,317,349] Many of these patients have features of SIADH associated with opportunistic infections causing pneumonia and meningitis. Others have clinical signs of volume depletion without low urine sodium values, a finding that may indicate coexistent renal disease or adrenal insufficiency. Hyponatremia often occurs after the administration of antibiotics in hypotonic intravenous solutions, a practice that should be avoided in this population.

CLINICAL CONSEQUENCES OF HYPONATREMIA

ACUTE HYPONATREMIA

When hyponatremia develops faster than the brain can adapt to the disturbance, cerebral edema accompanied by a syndrome known as *water intoxication* results.[20,132,133,234] The neurologic manifestations of this disorder, first recognized in the early 1920s, include headache, nausea, vomiting, weakness, incoordination, tremors, delirium, and ultimately seizures and decerebrate posturing.[12,20,144,165,247,316,372] Computed tomography of the brain may show narrowing of the third and lateral ventricles, representing diffuse brain edema that resolves after treatment.[26] Occasionally, however, brain edema may be severe enough to cause transtentorial herniation, a complication that is typically heralded by respiratory arrest and ultimately death.[12,13,28,100,132,184,254,259,345]

The few published cases of fatal cerebral edema have involved patients whose serum sodium concentration was still falling at the time of herniation and in whom severe hyponatremia had developed in less than 48 h. A recent review of the literature found that deaths and severe sequelae most commonly occur when the serum sodium concentration falls below 120 mmol/liter and falls by more than 0.5 mmol/liter per hour (Fig. 20-10).[52] Indeed, these complications become increasingly more common when sodium's rate of fall exceeds 1 mmol/liter per hour. Based on this experience and what is known of the rate of adaptation to hyponatremia in animals, it is reasonable to call hyponatremia acute when the serum sodium level has fallen by more than 12 mmol/liter per day and has been low for less than 48 h.

Young women account for most of the reported fatalities from acute hyponatremia.[13,100] This observation

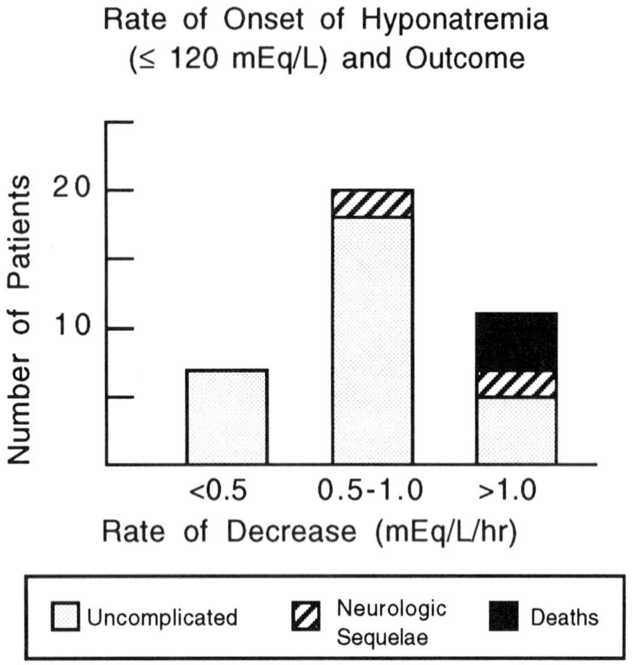

FIGURE 20-10 • Complications of acute hyponatremia: effect of rate of onset.[51]

has led some investigators to conclude that women in their reproductive years are less tolerant of hyponatremia than are men.[101] The most striking evidence of a female susceptibility to brain injury is provided by two recent papers that reported 26 previously healthy young women who became severely hyponatremic after routine elective procedures and subsequently suffered permanent neurologic complications, including 14 deaths from documented brain herniation.[13,100] These frightening reports underscore the potential dangers of severe acute hyponatremia, but they may not be representative of the usual course of the disorder. Cases were identified over many years from 26 different medical centers and were referred to the authors for review by families, physicians, and lawyers. Reports of acute hyponatremia without this selection bias suggest that the majority of young women survive without sequelae.[303,308] Nevertheless, the potential lethality of the chemical abnormality should not be minimized.

Among published reports of patients with seizures and coma caused by psychotic polydipsia, oxytocin infusion, or inappropriate postoperative fluid management, the mortality rate is less than 5 percent.[308] The widespread belief that survival is only 50 percent is based on individual case reports of fatalities and series devoted solely to patients with adverse outcomes. The relatively low mortality rate, however, should not diminish respect for the potential dangers of this condition.

In addition to the neurologic findings that dominate the clinical presentation of acute hyponatremia, the electrolyte disturbance may also be complicated by rhabdomyolysis that can be severe enough to precipitate acute renal failure.[211,326]

CHRONIC HYPONATREMIA

In general, the symptoms of chronic hyponatremia are more subtle, vague, and nonspecific than those of acute water intoxication, and they tend to occur at lower serum sodium levels.[12,65,79,303,306,308] Typically, the symptoms include anorexia, nausea, emesis, muscular weakness, and cramps. The patients may also become irritable and may show striking personality changes, becoming uncooperative, confused, or hostile.[106,191] With extremely low serum sodium concentrations, gait disturbances, stupor, and, more rarely, seizures may occur.[65,79] Chronic hyponatremia has not been known to cause herniation, even when the serum sodium concentration falls below 105 mmol/liter; indeed, computed tomography shows no evidence of brain swelling in patients with sustained hyponatremia at this level, including those who present with seizures or other severe neurologic symptoms.[34,109,308,352] However, patients with prolonged hyponatremia are susceptible to iatrogenic complications when their electrolyte disturbance is corrected too rapidly (Fig. 20-11).

RAPID CORRECTION OF HYPONATREMIA AND OSMOTIC DEMYELINATION

When the serum sodium concentration is returned to normal, solutes lost in the adaptation to hyponatremia must be recovered by the brain. Unless this process keeps pace with the rising serum sodium concentration, brain dehydration and injury may result (Fig. 20-7).[183,310,322] For reasons that remain unclear, the clinical manifesta-

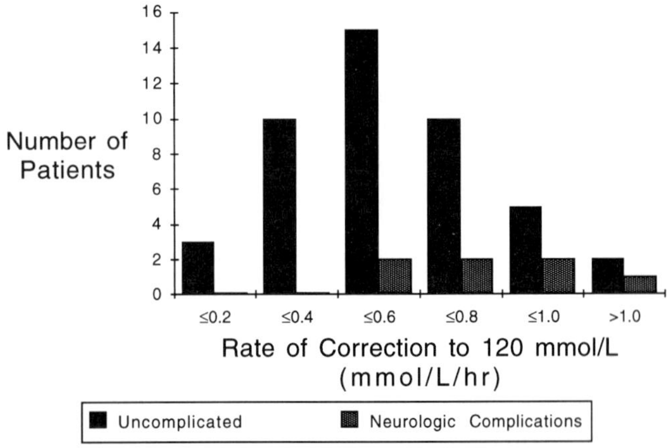

FIGURE 20-11 • Complications of chronic hyponatremia: effect of rate of correction. Data are from a survey of patients at a single medical center with serum sodium values 110 mmol/liter.[302]

tions of this injury are delayed, evolving 1 to several days after treatment in a characteristic fashion that has been dubbed the *osmotic demyelination syndrome*.[28,50,109,302]

A spectrum of neurologic findings distinct from the original hyponatremic symptoms can occur. Mild cases may be manifested by transient behavioral disturbances,[197,246,251] seizures,[302,306,363] movement disorders,[84,194,324,325] or akinetic mutism.[304,306] More severe cases develop clinical features of a pontine disorder (pseudobulbar palsy, quadriparesis, and unresponsiveness).[28,37,40,45,57,59,111,201,302,327,352,369] In its most dramatic form, patients may be awake but unable to move or communicate and may require ventilator support. Marked improvement can occur even after several weeks of severe disability, but some patients are left with significant permanent sequelae.[253,302,351] In fatal cases of the clinical syndrome, demyelination with relative sparing of neurons and axons is found in the center of the basal pons (a pathologic finding known as central pontine myelinolysis, or CPM[2] and in a symmetrical distribution in other areas of the brain in which there is a close admixture of gray and white matter.[34,154,176,371] Evidence of demyelination can often be documented with magnetic resonance images obtained 3 to 4 weeks after the clinical onset (Fig. 20-8).[38,39,98,205,214]

The osmotic demyelination syndrome has been reproduced in animal models of hyponatremia. The experiments have shown that the disorder is caused by a large, rapid increase in serum sodium concentration rather than hyponatremia itself.[162-164,174,183,203,233,300,310,334,342] The susceptibility to injury is much greater after 3 or more days of hyponatremia than it is after 1 day. In the rat and the dog, the minimum increase capable of producing lesions is approximately 15 to 17 mmol/liter per day, and both the frequency and the severity of lesions increase with more rapid rates of correction (Fig. 20-12).

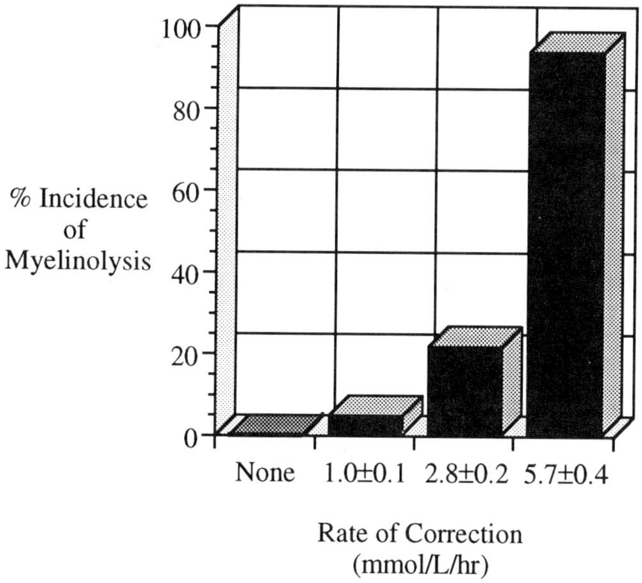

FIGURE 20-12 • Experimental myelinolysis in chronically hyponatremic rats.[338]

Similar observations have been made in humans.[28,38,52,175,176,227,232,302,303,305-310,337] Patients at greatest risk for osmotic demyelination have been hyponatremic for more than 2 days, usually with very low serum sodium concentrations (≤ 105 mmol/liter).[39,52,302,306,308] Almost invariably, correction has exceeded 12 mmol/liter during any 24-h period, and most patients with fatal disease have undergone correction by more than 20 mmol/liter within 1 to 2 days.[18,28,227,302] Alcoholism, severe liver disease, and other debilitating illnesses appear to increase the susceptibility to osmotic demyelination, but they are not prerequisites for it.[2,40,46,56,201] Many cases have been reported in patients with no illness other than severe chronic hyponatremia (and its subsequent rapid correction) to explain their neurologic sequelae.[34,38,39,50,57,59,109,303,305-310] Acute hyponatremia can usually be corrected rapidly without sequelae, but even in this setting there have been occasional reports of CPM.[310]

DIAGNOSTIC APPROACH TO HYPONATREMIA

Hyponatremia is, of course, merely a laboratory finding. Its evaluation demands a logical stepwise approach.

HYPOTONIC VERSUS NONHYPOTONIC HYPONATREMIA

The first step in the evaluation of hyponatremia is to verify that the low serum sodium concentration represents hypotonicity. If the patient is hyperglycemic, the serum sodium must be corrected for the osmotic effect of the elevated blood glucose (see above). Measurement of plasma osmolality is indicated when pseudohyponatremia is suspected because of lactescent serum or multiple myeloma or when the patient has received exogenous solutes (see above).

Differential diagnosis of hypotonic hyponatremia

Once it has been established that hypotonicity is in fact present, the differential diagnosis can proceed in a logical fashion. The cause of acute hyponatremia is usually evident from the clinical setting. The major diagnostic challenge comes in distinguishing among various causes of chronic hyponatremia. Since almost all patients with sustained hyponatremia have a defect in water excretion (and therefore a less than maximally dilute urine), the question to be answered is, "Why is water excretion impaired?" Except for patients with advanced renal failure and some patients treated with thiazide-type diuretics, persistent nonosmotic secretion of AVP is usually responsible for water retention. The diagnostic goal is to identify the reason that AVP is being secreted despite a low serum sodium concentration.

To facilitate the differential diagnosis, it is useful to divide patients into three general hypotonic syndromes: (1) hypovolemic hyponatremia, (2) edematous hyponatremia, and (3) isovolemic hyponatremia (Fig. 20-13). In some cases, the distinctions among these syndromes are obvious from the history and physical examination. For example, in a massively edematous patient with a low cardiac output, the diagnostic evaluation of hyponatremia need proceed no further. Blood pressure, pulse (response to postural changes), and skin turgor are other obvious clues to the sufficiency of vascular volume. In more subtle cases, laboratory findings may be helpful in making this diagnostic division.

Prerenal azotemia in the absence of edema suggests a diagnosis of hypovolemia, but the increase in BUN may be blunted in patients with a poor dietary protein intake. The serum uric acid may provide a helpful supplementary clue.[24,68,71,192,289,297] Uric acid clearance is reduced in volume-depleted and increased in volume-expanded conditions. Because clinically "isovolemic" patients with water retention and hyponatremia actually have slight (and clinically inapparent) volume expansion, serum uric acid levels are usually low, often extremely so. Conversely, serum uric acid concentration tends to be elevated in hypovolemia. Subtle, clinically inapparent volume depletion may also be identified by a low urinary sodium concentration (or chloride concentration in alkalotic subjects).[27,48,219] Urine chemistries in patients with prerenal azotemia from vomiting often demostrate generous amounts of sodium, while chloride is virtually absent.[219] The volume contraction from vomiting stimulates renal reabsorption of filtered sodium chloride, but

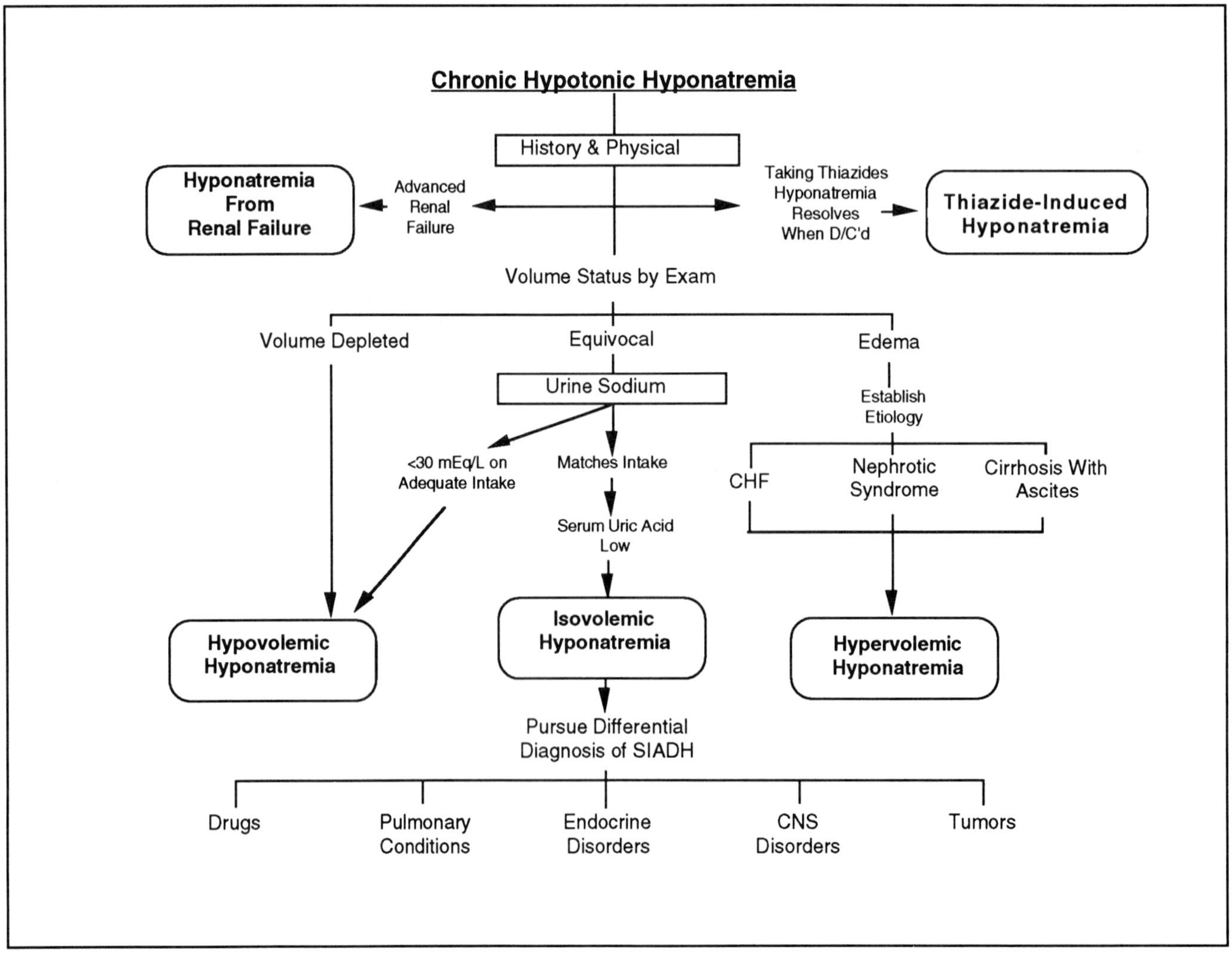

FIGURE 20-13 • Differential diagnosis of chronic hypotonic hyponatremia.

the gastric production of sodium bicarbonate overwhelms renal reabsorption of the alkali. The relative resistance of the HCO_3^- anion to reabsorption obligates excretion of neutralizing cation (Na^+ and K^+). In this setting, the low urinary chloride concentration is a better reflection of the ECF volume contraction.

In isovolemic patients, urinary sodium excretion matches or exceeds intake such that the urine sodium concentration typically exceeds 30 mmol/liter.[178,226,284] This finding must, however, be interpreted with caution. The "isovolemic" patient with SIADH may have a low urinary sodium concentration if dietary salt intake is very low or if there are ongoing extrarenal losses. Conversely, patients who are hypovolemic because of a primary renal salt-wasting disorder of Addison's disease have high urinary sodium concentrations. It must also be emphasized that edematous patients with decreased effective arterial blood volumes, as well as hypovolemic patients, have a low urine sodium concentration. Thus, laboratory findings must be correlated with physical findings. A diagnosis of absolute volume depletion is rarely correct in a patient with edema.

In some cases, it may be difficult to distinguish between subtle volume depletion and isovolemic hyponatremia. In such cases, it may be useful to monitor the changes in serum and urine sodium concentration and urine osmolality during a brief infusion of isotonic saline solution. In volume depletion, much of the infused saline solution is retained (and the urine sodium concentration remains low); as the volume deficit is repaired and plasma AVP levels fall, the urine becomes more dilute and the serum sodium level rises as free water excretion increases. In isovolemic hyponatremia, the infused sodium is promptly excreted in the urine and urine sodium concentration increases; the urine remains inappropriately concentrated and the serum sodium concentration fails to rise or may even fall. A saline trial should be used with extreme caution in patients with severe hyponatremia: volume-depleted patients may respond with a large, rapid rise in serum sodium concentration that may lead to severe neurologic complications (see below).

Differential diagnosis of SIADH

In isovolemic hyponatremia, AVP secretion is independent of any obvious hemodynamic stimulus and is thus termed "inappropriate." This, however, is not a complete diagnosis. In all patients with SIADH, a specific etiology for inappropriate AVP secretion must be sought. In some cases, particularly when a previously normonatremic patient becomes hyponatremic in the hospital, the cause for SIADH is obvious (e.g., drugs, pneumonia, acute respiratory failure, cerebrovascular accident, etc.) and further diagnostic testing is unnecessary.

When there is no obvious cause for SIADH, a more extensive evaluation is indicated. Malignancy must be excluded, and because small-cell carcinoma of the lung is one of the more common causes of SIADH, computed tomography of the chest should be strongly considered. Diseases of the CNS should also be excluded, and an endocrine evaluation to exclude hypothyroidism and cortisol deficiency is also indicated. Occasionally, in psychotic, mentally retarded, alcoholic, or elderly patients, no cause for SIADH will be found. Careful follow-up is essential because malignancies may become clinically apparent years after a diagnosis of "idiopathic" SIADH.[194]

EVALUATION OF THIAZIDE-ASSOCIATED HYPONATREMIA

Patients who become hyponatremic while taking thiazide diuretics do not fit well into the diagnostic grouping described above. By physical examination, they usually appear isovolemic, and this clinical impression is often bolstered by low BUN and serum uric acid levels and a high urine sodium concentration (because of the natriuretic effect of the diuretic).[1,96] The diagnosis of thiazide-induced hyponatremia is based on a history of diuretic use and the finding that hyponatremia is resolved when the offending agent is discontinued. Most patients become normonatremic and are able to dilute their urine maximally when diuretics are discontinued, but full resolution of hyponatremia and full recovery of diluting ability may be delayed for 1 to 2 weeks, during which the patient commonly exhibits evidence of a "reset osmostat."[110,124,354] Unless there is clinical evidence to suggest an underlying cause for SIADH, an extensive diagnostic evaluation should be postponed for 2 to 3 weeks. However, because thiazides may exacerbate the hyyponatremia caused by SIADH, an evaluation is indicated if even mild hyponatremia persists after this diagnostic waiting period.

THERAPEUTIC APPROACH TO HYPONATREMIA

Because the treatment of hyponatremia can be at least as dangerous as the disorder itself, care must be taken to avoid correction that is more aggressive than it needs to be. A balance must be struck between the need to elevate the serum sodium concentration urgently and the risks of raising it by too much in too short a time.[17,28,52,302,303,305-309,313,337,338]

Complications of therapy can be seen when hyponatremia is corrected by more than 12 mmol/liter within 24 h or by more than 18 mmol/liter within 48 h.[52,302,308] In asymptomatic patients with long-standing hyponatremia, the dangers of the electrolyte disturbance are so minimal that the rate of correction can be maintained far below this limit.[52,81,302,306,308,313] At the other extreme, severely symptomatic patients with acute hyponatremia may require correction by as much as 6 to 12 mmol/liter within a few hours to avoid injury from seizures or cerebral edema.[28,52,277] While such treatment risks an inadvertent increase of more than 12 mmol/liter per day the relatively low incidence of iatrogenic injury in this setting justifies a more aggressive therapeutic approach.[28,306,337,370] However, even when emergency measures are clearly indicated, there is never any need to deliberately raise the serum sodium concentration by more than 12 mmol/liter within 24 h.[308]

ACUTE HYPONATREMIA

The benefits of therapy are clearest in the severely symptomatic patient who has been hyponatremic for a short time (≤ 36 h). Because acute symptomatic hyponatremia is potentially lethal, the serum sodium concentration must be rapidly increased to reduce the degree of cerebral edema.[133] Emergency therapy is obviously indicated for seizures and coma, but even relatively minor symptoms (headache, vomiting, or confusion) should be considered ominous in a patient receiving hypotonic fluids intravenously. Because the serum sodium concentration is still decreasing, cerebral edema may be worsening when the diagnosis of hyponatremia is first made. Seizures, respiratory arrest, and even herniation may emerge explosively, sometimes without warning.[12,13,28,100,132,184,254,259,345]

Reversible defects in water excretion

For many patients with acute hyponatremia, therapeutic interventions (beyond restricting water intake) may be largely superfluous because the provoked water diuresis soon corrects the electrolyte disturbance. For example, many psychotic patients with self-induced water intoxication have a nearly maximally dilute urine at presentation. By the time that hyponatremia is recognized, it has already begun to improve, and active therapeutic interventions may not be necessary.[128,303,306] Similarly, hyponatremia associated with oxytocin infusion usually improves rapidly when the drug is discontinued.[184,213,215] Patients with psychotic polydipsia usually tolerate extremely large and rapid increases in the serum sodium concentration (presumably because severe hyponatremia is not sustained long enough to permit the brain to adapt to it),[310] and it is often difficult to prevent such increases from occurring.[46,306]

Fixed defects in water excretion

Acutely hyponatremic patients who are unable to excrete dilute urine should be treated promptly with intravenously administered hypertonic saline solution.[17,18,28,52,133,277,303,305,307-309,337] To avoid excessive volume expansion, the infusion can be combined with furosemide. The diuretic promotes a hypotonic diuresis, and resultant urinary sodium losses are replaced with 3% saline solution (0.5 mmol/ml).[127] Thus, the excreted salt is returned, millimole for millimole, in a smaller volume (i.e., more concentrated), which keeps body sodium content constant while allowing for electrolyte-free water loss. Since in a furosemide-induced diuresis the urine approximates a one-half normal saline solution, the sodium and chloride lost in a liter of such urine can generally be replaced with 150 ml of 3 percent saline solution. The net effect is a negative free water balance of 850 ml.

Consider the following example. A 75-year-old woman weighing 50 kg is given an excessive amount of fluid postoperatively, lowering her serum sodium concentration from 140 to 116 mmol/liter over 36 h. She now has neurologic symptoms. The objectives of treatment are (1) to increase the serum sodium by 4 mmol/liter, to 120 mmol/liter, within the next 4 h and (2) using furosemide and saline solution, to remove the appropriate amount of water, leaving total body sodium content unchanged. The following are the necessary calculations:

1. Calculate the total body water content. Since muscle mass and body water content decrease with age (see Chap. 1), assume the preoperative total body water content to have been 40 percent of the body weight, or 20 liters.
2. Calculate the amount of total body cation. Total body cation content is defined by the product of the total body water content and the serum sodium concentration (140 mmol/liter × 20 liters = 2800 mmol).
3. Calculate the new body water content. The amount of total body cation (2800 mmol) is distributed in an increased volume of total body water, lowering the serum sodium concentration to 116 mmol/liter. Thus, 2800 mmol/X liters = 116 mmol/liter. The new body water content (X) is 24.1 liters, indicating that the patient has gained 4.1 liters of water.
4. Calculate the amount of water to be removed. To determine how much water must be removed to achieve the desired sodium level of 120 mmol/liter, ask "In what volume of water must 2800 mmol of cation be distributed to yield a serum sodium concentration of 120 mmol/liter?" Thus, 2800 mmol/X liters = 120 mmol/liter. The amount of water to be removed (X) is 23.3 liters, indicating that 0.8 liters must be removed within 4 h, or approximately 200 ml of electrolyte-free water should be lost hourly to raise the serum sodium concentration by 1 mmol/liter per hour.
5. Achieve net water removal with a furosemide-induced diuresis. Initiate a diuresis with 10 to 20 mg

of diuretic, repeating the dose as needed to sustain a diuresis of 250 ml/h. Begin replacement of cation losses by assuming the sum of urine sodium and potassium concentrations to be 75 mmol/liter; at a urine output of 250 ml/h, 19 mmol of cation will be lost each hour. Replacing these losses with 3 percent saline solution requires an infusion of approximately 35 ml/h. Since 250 ml of urine is lost each hour and 40 ml of fluid is infused, the net water loss is 210 ml/h, slightly more than is needed.

As serum and urinary electrolyte data return, adjustments in the rate of saline solution administration can be made to achieve the desired increase in serum sodium concentration. Intensive therapy can be stopped after 3 to 4 h (or earlier if symptoms subside completely), and a more conservative regimen appropriate for chronic hyponatremia should be substituted (see below). The patient must be continuously monitored to ensure that serum sodium levels do not increase by more than 10 to 12 mmol/liter in the first 24 h or by more than 16 to 18 mmol/liter in the first 48 h. Larger changes are of no added benefit and increase the risk of iatrogenic injury.

CHRONIC HYPONATREMIA

In practice, the duration of hyponatremia is seldom precisely known because most patients develop the disturbance outside the hospital. However, when a patient who is not a psychotic water drinker becomes hyponatremic at home, it is reasonable to presume that the electrolyte disturbance is chronic.[306] With a normal water intake, it usually takes at least 2 days to lower the serum sodium concentration enough to cause symptoms. Even when hyponatremia develops in the hospital, the precise duration of the disturbance may be unclear if chemistry determinations have been infrequent.[120,220,306,357] Still, it is usually possible to approximate the rate of onset by examining fluid orders and by considering the duration of symptoms. In most cases of uncertainty, it is best to assume that the disorder has been present long enough to make excessive correction potentially dangerous.

Predicting the rate of correction

As noted earlier, the serum sodium concentration is determined by the total cation content of body fluids and by the total body water content, as described in the following equation (Na_E: exchangable sodium; K_E: exchangable potassium):[91]

$$\text{Serum [Na]} = \frac{\text{total body } Na_E + \text{total body } K_E}{\text{total body water}}$$

Thus, the serum sodium concentration will increase when either a potassium or a sodium deficit is replaced at a given body water content. In predicting how much correction is likely to occur with a given therapeutic maneuver, urinary water losses as well as sodium and potassium administration must be considered. It must also be remembered that the total body water content varies with age and sex as well as weight, ranging from about 0.6 liter/kg in a young man to 0.4 liter/kg in an elderly woman (see Chap. 1).

Reversible defects in water excretion

The risks of rapid correction are greatest in chronically hyponatremic patients with reversible defects in water excretion. If a water diuresis develops during treatment, the serum sodium concentration will increase extremely rapidly.[231,306] For example, in a 50-kg woman, free water excretion of 500 ml/h will increase the serum sodium concentration by about 2 mmol/liter per hour. A water diuresis may emerge when extracellular volume repletion abolishes a hemodynamic stimulus to AVP release or when some other factor impairing diluting ability is removed (e.g., after thiazide diuretics, oral hypoglycemic agents, oxytocin, or AVP are discontinued; after cortisol deficiency or hypothyroidism are treated; or after acute respiratory failure is resolved).

Hyponatremia caused by thiazide diuretics is particularly susceptible to rapid correction.[302,306] The typical patient is a small elderly woman with a correspondingly small body water content. Severe potassium depletion is often present, and, as noted earlier, its repair contributes to the increase in serum sodium concentration. Finally, as the diuretic is withdrawn and volume deficits are replaced, diluting ability is restored, allowing a water diuresis to develop. Because most patients with thiazide-induced hyponatremia are not clinically volume-depleted, sodium replacement should be limited to that of a regular diet (about 150 to 200 mmol/day).

Volume-depleted patients with chronic hyponatremia can be treated with isotonic saline solution. However, careful monitoring of the urine output is mandatory during therapy, and volume replacement should be limited to the amount required to effect hemodynamic stability. If a water diuresis develops despite this cautious approach, electrolyte-free net water losses may have to be slowed by administering hypotonic fluids, or the diuresis may have to be temporarily interrupted with AVP or dDAVP to prevent excessive rates of correction.

Fixed defects in water excretion

Hyponatremia associated with edema and with SIADH tends to be relatively resistant to rapid correction.[306] In both cases, water restriction is the cornerstone of therapy. The lower the serum sodium concentration and the more severe the symptoms, the more stringent water restriction must be. In nonedematous patients who are alert enough to eat and drink, a high salt intake (which can be attained with salt tablets if necessary), combined with a modest fluid restriction, limits the intake of electrolyte-free water. If the patient is less than fully alert, all oral intake of fluids should be discontinued, completely eliminating the intake of electrolyte-free water. Tube feedings and intravenously administered fluids required for nutrition or medications should contain sodium and potassium in a combined concentration of at least 15 mmol/liter.

Restriction of free water intake will increase the serum sodium concentration regardless of the cause of hyponatremia. However, in patients who excrete a very concentrated urine, this approach alone may result in an unacceptably slow resolution of the electrolyte disturbance and an unhappy patient. Isotonic saline solution will not be helpful in speeding the process, and it may be hazardous. In congestive heart failure and cirrhosis, it will, of course, worsen edema. In SIADH, the serum sodium concentration may actually fall as administered salt is excreted in a concentrated urine, causing net accumulation of free water.

There are several approaches for facilitating gradual correction of hyponatremia. By impairing urinary concentrating ability, furosemide and other "loop" diuretics increase electrolyte-free water excretion. It is a common error to assume that "overdiuresis" is responsible for hyponatremia in patients with severe biventricular heart failure; in fact, the electrolyte disturbance usually reflects oliguria due to diuretic resistance. Although thiazides are contraindicated, adequate doses of a loop diuretic will actually increase free water excretion and improve hyponatremia, particularly if dietary salt intake is liberalized once a larger urine output has been achieved. Angiotensin-converting enzyme inhibitors enhance the effectiveness of furosemide in treating the hyponatremia of heart failure. There are several explanations for the beneficial effect: (1) angiotension II-mediated thirst may be reduced; (2) nonosmotic release of AVP may be prevented because of improved cardiac output and/or diminished angiotensin II-mediated AVP secretion; (3) delivery of glomerular filtrate to diluting sites may be increased because of a fall in filtration fraction; and (4) these agents may directly impair the hydroosmotic effect of AVP on the renal collecting duct.

In SIADH, loop diuretics may be combined with orally administered salt or a slow infusion (10 to 20 ml/h) of 3% saline solution to gradually return the serum sodium concentration to normal.[66,73] Salt tablets and diuretics are also effective as maintenance therapy. Some investigators have advocated urea therapy for SIADH.[69,70,72,257] Urea given orally or by infusion induces an osmotic diuresis that obligates water excretion in excess of sodium. It has been used for emergency treatment of hyponatremia and for its long-term management. In one study, five patients required 30 g of urea daily to maintain a serum sodium concentration greater than 120 mmol/liter. However, in two patients who drank 2 to 3 liters of water each day, 60 g of urea was needed, a dose that may be quite unpalatable.

Lithium carbonate and demeclochlortetracycline (demeclocycline), drugs that block the effect of AVP on the collecting duct, causing nephrogenic diabetes insipidus, have been used in the long-term management of SIADH. (More specific agents that directly block the effect of AVP on V2 receptors are still in the developmental stage.)[146,160] The side effects of lithium limit its usefulness, but demeclocycline in a dose of 600 to 1200 mg/day is usually effective and well tolerated.[47,99] However, this drug also has several disadvantages: (1) its effect on water excretion is delayed for several days, and its effect persists for a similar period after treatment has been discontinued; (2) it is nephrotoxic when hepatic function is impaired;[80,207] and (3) by causing nephrogenic diabetes insipidus, it predisposes to dehydration those patients who are unable to seek water. In the authors' experience, demeclocycline is seldom necessary because most patients can be managed with fluid restriction, salt, and diuretics (or urea). However, the drug may be useful in polydipsic, psychotic patients with SIADH who will not restrict their water intake;[6,345] in such patients, even loop diuretics should be avoided because a maximally dilute urine is necessary to eliminate the large daily water load.

Chronic hyponatremia with severe symptoms

Chronic hyponatremia should not be equated with asymptomatic hyponatremia. Very low serum sodium concentrations usually cause some neurologic symptoms.[65,79,306,319] If there is an underlying neurologic problem or if there has been a recent abrupt decrease in sodium concentration, patients with long-standing hyponatremia may present with seizures and coma. Clearly, patients who present with severe neurologic symptoms must be treated more aggressively than would be appropriate for patients with more moderate symptoms. In such cases, treatment should be initiated in a similar fashion as for patients with known acute hyponatremia. However, since the risks of iatrogenic injury are much higher in chronic hyponatremia, extreme care is necessary to limit the first day's correction to 12 mmol/liter or less, and the rate of correction should be even slower in the days that follow.

REFERENCES

1. Abramow M, Cogan E: Clinical aspects and pathophysiology of diuretic-induced hyponatremia. *Adv Nephrol Necker Hosp* 13:1, 1984.
2. Adams RD et al: Central pontine myelinolysis. *Arch Neurol Psychiatry* 81:154, 1959.
3. Adler S, Simplaceanu V: Effect of acute hyponatremia

on rat brain pH and rat brain buffering. *Am J Physiol* 256:F113, 1989.

4. Agarwal A et al: Hyponatremia in patients with the acquired immunodeficiency syndrome. *Nephron* 53:317, 1989.
5. Ajlouni K et al: Thiothixene-induced hyponatremia. *Arch Intern Med* 134:1103, 1974.
6. Alexander RC et al: A double blind, placebo-controlled trial of demeclocycline treatment of polydipsia-hyponatremia in chronically psychotic patients. *Biol Psychiatry* 15:417, 1991.
7. Allon M et al: Role of cigarette use in hyponatremia in schizophrenic patients. *Am J Psychiatry* 35:268, 1990.
8. Allon M et al: Renal sodium and water handling in hypothyroid patients: The role of renal insufficiency. *J Am Soc Nephrol* 1:205, 1990.
9. Amatruda TT et al: Carcinoma of the lung with inappropriate antidiuresis: Demonstration of antidiuretic hormone-like activity in tumor tissue. *N Engl J Med* 269:544, 1963.
10. Anderson RJ et al: Hyponatremia: A prospective analysis of its epidemiology and the pathogenetic role of vasopressin. *Ann Intern Med* 102:164, 1985.
11. Andersson B, Rundgren M: Thirst and its disorders. *Annu Rev Med* 33:231, 1982.
12. Arieff AI et al: Neurologic manifestations and morbidity of hyponatremia: Correlation of brain water and electrolytes. *Medicine (Baltimore)* 55:121, 1976.
13. Arieff AI: Hyponatremia, convulsions, respiratory arrest, and permanent brain damage after elective surgery in young healthy women. *N Engl J Med* 314:1529, 1986.
14. Ashouri OS: Severe diuretic hyponatremia in the elderly: A series of eight patients. *Arch Intern Med* 146:1355, 1986.
15. Ashraf N et al: Thiazide-induced hyponatremia associated with death or neurologic damage in outpatients. *Am J Med* 70:1163, 1981.
16. Aw TC, Kiechle FL: Pseudohyponatremia. *Am J Emerg Med* 3:236, 1985.
17. Ayus JC et al: Changing concepts in treatment of severe symptomatic hyponatremia: Rapid correction and possible relation to central pontine myelinolysis. *Am J Med* 78:897, 1985.
18. Ayus JC et al: Treatment of symptomatic hyponatremia and its relation to brain damage: A prospective study. *N Engl J Med* 317:1190, 1987.
19. Barlow ED, DeWardener HE: Compulsive water drinking. *Q J Med* 28:235, 1959.
20. Bartholomew LG, Scholz DA: Reversible post-operative neurological symptoms: Report of five cases secondary to water intoxication and sodium depletion. *JAMA* 162:22, 1956.
21. Bayer AJ et al: Plasma electrolytes in elderly patients taking fixed combination diuretics. *Postgrad Med J* 62:159, 1986.
22. Baylis PH, Thompson CJ: Osmoregulation of vasopressin secretion and thirst in health and disease. *Clin Endocrinol* 29:549, 1988.
23. Baylis PH: Osmoregulation and control of vasopressin secretion in healthy humans. *Am J Physiol* 253:R671, 1987.
24. Beck LH: Hyporuricemia in the syndrome of inappropriate secretion of antidiuretic hormone. *N Engl J Med* 301:528, 1979.
25. Beckstrom D et al: Syndrome of inappropriate antidiuretic hormone secretion associated with amytryptiline administration. *JAMA* 241:133, 1979.
26. Berginer VM et al: CT brain scan in acute water intoxication. *J Neurol Neurosurg Psychiatry* 48:841, 1985.
27. Berl T et al: Clinical disorders of water metabolism. *Kidney Int* 10:117, 1976.
28. Berl T: Treating hyponatremia: Damned if we do and damned if we don't. *Kidney Int* 37:1006, 1990.
29. Berlyne GM et al: Renal salt and water handling in water immersion in the nephrotic syndrome. *Arch Intern Med* 141:1275, 1981.
30. Berry AJ, Peterson ML: Hyponatremia after mannitol administration in the presence of renal failure. *Anesth Analg* 60:165, 1981.
31. Bichet D et al: Role of vasopressin in abnormal water excretion in cirrhotic patients. *Ann Intern Med* 96:413, 1982.
32. Bichet DG: Water disturbances in cardiac failure. *Baillieres Clin Endocrinol Metab* 3:559, 1989.
33. Booker JA: Severe symptomatic hyponatremia in elderly outpatients. *J Am Geriatr Soc* 32:108, 1984.
34. Boon AP, Potter AE: Extensive extrapontine and central pontine myelinolysis associated with correction of profound anoxic hyponatremia. *Neuropathol Appl Neurobiol* 13:1, 1987.
35. Bower BF et al: Bronchogenic carcinoma with inappropriate antidiuretic activity in plasma and tumor. *N Engl J Med* 217:934, 1964.
36. Bressler RB, Huston DP: Water intoxication following moderate-dose intravenous cyclophosphamide. *Arch Intern Med* 145:548, 1985.
37. Brunner JE: Central pontine myelinolysis in a patient with adrenal insufficiency. *Henry Ford Hosp Med J* 33:45, 1985.
38. Brunner JE et al: Central pontine myelinolysis after rapid correction of hyponatremia: A magnetic resonance imaging study. *Ann Neurol* 23:389, 1988.
39. Brunner JE et al: Central pontine myelinolysis and pontine lesions after rapid correction of hyponatremia: A prospective magnetic resonance imaging study. *Ann Neurol* 27:61, 1990.
40. Burcar PJ et al: Hyponatremia and central pontine myelinolysis. *Neurology* 27:223, 1977.
41. Byatt CM et al: Diuretics and electrolyte disturbances in 1000 consecutive geriatric admissions. *J R Soc Med* 83:704, 1990.
42. Campbell HT et al: Severe hyponatremia without severe hypoosmolality following transurethral resection of the prostate (TURP) in end-stage renal disease. *Am J Kidney Dis* 12:152, 1988.
43. Carroll PB et al: Isolated adrenocorticotrophic hormone deficiency presenting as chronic hyponatremia. *N Y State J Med* 90:210, 1990.
44. Castellano G et al: Antidiuretic hormone and renal function after water loading in patients with cirrhosis of the liver. *Scand J Gastroenterol* 26:49, 1991.
45. Castillo RA et al: Central pontine myelinolysis and pregnancy. *Obstet Gynecol* 73:459, 1989.
46. Cheng JC et al: Long-term neurologic outcome in psycho-

genic water drinkers with severe symptomatic hyponatremia: The effect of rapid correction *Am J Med* 88:561, 1990.
47. Cherill DA et al: Demeclocyline treatment in the syndrome of inappropriate antidiuretic hormone secretion. *Ann Intern Med* 83:654, 1975.
48. Chung HM et al: Clinical assessment of extracellular fluid volume in hyponatremia. *Am J Med* 83:905, 1987.
49. Chung HM et al. Post-operative hyponatremia. *Arch Intern Med* 314:1529, 1986.
50. Clifford DB et al: Osmotic demyelination syndrome: Lack of pathologic and radiologic imaging correlation. *Arch Neurol* 46:343, 1989.
51. Clive DM, Stoff JS: Renal syndromes associated with nonsteroidal antiinflamatory drugs. *N Engl J Med* 310:563, 1984.
52. Cluitmans FH, Meinders AE: Management of severe hyponatremia: Rapid or slow correction? *Am J Med* 88:161, 1990.
53. Cochrane JPS et al: Arginine vasopressin release following surgical operations. *Br J Surg* 68:209, 1981.
54. Cogan E et al: Natriuresis and atrial natriuretic factor secretion during inappropriate antidiuresis. *Am J Med* 84:409, 1988.
55. Cohen BJ et al: More cases of SIADH with fluxetine. *Am J Psychiatry* 147:948, 1990.
56. Cohen BJ et al: Pontine myelinolysis after correction of hyponatremia during burn resuscitation. *J Burn Care Rehabil* 12:153, 1991.
57. Conger JD et al: Central pontine myelinolysis associated with inappropriate antidiuretic secretion. *Am J Med* 47:813, 1969.
58. Cooke RC et al: The syndrome of inappropriate antidiuretic hormone secretion (SIADH): Pathophysiologic mechanisms in solute and volume regulation. *Medicine* 58:240, 1979.
59. Copeland PM: Diuretic abuse and central pontine myelinolysis. *Psychother Psychosom* 52:101, 1989.
60. Coslovsky R et al: Hypo-osmolar syndrome due to prolonged nausea. *Arch Intern Med* 144:191, 1984.
61. Cowell DC, McGrady PM: Direct-measurement ion-selective electrodes: Analytical error in hyponatremia. *Clin Chem* 31:2009, 1985.
62. Crammer JL: Drinking, thirst and water intoxication *Br J Psychiatry* 159:83, 1991.
63. Cronin RE: Psychogenic polydipsia with hyponatremia: Report of eleven cases. *Am J Kidney Dis* 9:410, 1987.
64. Cusano AJ et al: Hyponatremia in patients with acquired immune deficiency syndrome. *J Acquir Immune Defic Syndr* 3:949, 1990.
65. Daggett P et al: Neurological aspects of hyponatraemia. *Postgrad Med J* 58:737, 1982.
66. Decaux G et al: Treatment of the syndrome of inappropriate secretion of antidiuretic hormone with furosemide. *N Engl J Med* 304:329, 1981.
67. Decaux G et al: Role of vagal neuropathy in the hyponatraemia of alcoholic cirrhosis. *Br Med J Clin Res* 293:1534, 1986.
68. Decaux G et al: Mechanisms of hypouricemia in the syndrome of inappropriate secretion of antidiuretic hormone. *Nephron* 39:164, 1985.
69. Decaux G, Genette F: Urea for long-term treatment of syndrome of inappropriate secretion of antidiuretic hormone. *Br Med J Clin Res* 283:1081, 1981.
70. Decaux G et al: Use of urea for treatment of water retention in hyponatraemic cirrhosis with ascites resistant to diuretics. *Br Med J Clin Res* 290:1782, 1985.
71. Decaux G et al: Dissociation between uric acid and urea clearances in the syndrome of inappropriate secretion of antidiuretic hormone related to salt excretion. *Clin Sci* 78:451, 1990.
72. Decaux G et al: Hyponatremia in the syndrome of inappropriate secretion of antidiuretic hormone: Rapid correction with urea, sodium chloride, and water restriction therapy. *JAMA* 247:471, 1982.
73. Decaux G et al: Inappropriate secretion of antidiuretic hormone treated with frusemide. *Br Med J Clin Res* 285:89, 1982.
74. DeFronzo RA et al: Water intoxication in man after cyclophosphamide therapy: Time course and relation to drug activation. *Ann Intern Med* 78:861, 1973.
75. DeFronzo RA et al: Normal diluting capacity in hyponatremic patients: Reset osmostat or varient of SIADH. *Ann Intern Med* 84:538, 1976.
76. Delva NJ et al: Vasopressin in chronic psychiatric patients with primary polydipsia. *Br J Psychiatry* 157:703, 1990.
77. Demanet JC et al: Coma due to water intoxication in beer drinkers. *Lancet* 2:1115, 1971.
78. DeRiviera JLG: Inappropriate secretion of antidiuretic hormone from fluphenazine therapy. *Ann Intern Med* 82:811, 1975.
79. DeTroyer A, Demanet JC: Clinical, biological and pathogenic features of the syndrome of inappropriate secretion of antidiuretic hormone. *Q J Med* 45:521, 1976.
80. DeTroyer A et al: Demeclocycline treatment of water retention in cirrhosis. *Ann Intern Med* 87:195, 1976.
81. DeTroyer A: Treatment of syndrome of inappropriate antidiuretic hormone secretion. *JAMA* 237:2723, 1977.
82. DeVita MV et al: Incidence and etiology of hyponatremia in an intensive care unit. *Clin Nephrol* 34:163, 1990.
83. Dhar SK, Ramos RR: Inappropriate antidiuresis during desipramine therapy. *Arch Intern Med* 138:1750, 1978.
84. Dickoff DJ et al: Striatal syndrome following hyponatremia and its rapid correction: A manifestation of extrapontine myelinolysis confirmed by magnetic resonance imaging. *Arch Neurol* 45:112, 1988.
85. Dila CJ, Pappius HM: Cerebral water and electrolytes. *Arch Neurol* 26:85, 1972.
86. Diringer M et al: Sodium and water regulation in a patient with cerebral salt wasting. *Arch Neurol* 46:928, 1989.
87. Diringer MN et al: Hypervolemic therapy prevents volume contraction but not hyponatremia following subarachnoid hemorrhage. *Ann Neurol* 31:543, 1992.
88. Dixon BS, Anderson RJ: Pneumonia and the syndrome of inappropriate antidiuretic hormone secretion: Don't pour water on the fire. *Am Rev Respir Dis* 138:512, 1988.
89. Dzau VJ, Hollenberg NK: Renal response to captopril in severe heart failure: Role of furosemide in natriuresis and reversal of hyponatremia. *Ann Intern Med* 100:777, 1984.
90. Eadington DW, Cowan FM: Dissociation between the secretion and renal action of endogenous atrial natriuretic

peptide in the syndrome of inappropriate antidiuresis. *Postgrad Med J* 66:20, 1990.
91. Edelman IS et al: Interrelations between serum sodium concentration, serum osmolality and total exchangeable sodium, total exchangeable potassium and total body water. *J Clin Invest* 37:1236, 1958.
92. Emsley RA et al: Inappropriate antidiuretic state in long-term psychiatric inpatients. *S Afr Med J* 77:307, 1990.
93. Emsley RA et al: Impaired water excretion and elevated plasma vasopressin in patients with alcohol-withdrawal symptoms. *Q J Med* 244:671, 1987.
94. Epstein M: Derangements of renal water handling in liver disease. *Gastroenterology* 89:1415, 1985.
95. Farber MO et al: Abnormalities of sodium and H_2O handling in chronic obstructive lung disease. *Arch Intern Med* 142:1326, 1982.
96. Fichman MP et al: Diuretic-induced hyponatremia. *Ann Intern Med* 75:853, 1971.
97. Fine LG, Salehmoghaddam S: Water homeostasis in acute and chronic renal failure. *Semin Nephrol* 4:289, 1984.
98. Fong VH et al: Antemortem diagnosis of central pontine myelinolysis: Report of a case. *Chang Keng I Hsueh* 13:336, 1990.
99. Forest JM Jr et al: Superiority of demeclocyline over lithium in the treatment of chronic syndrome of inappropriate antidiuretic hormone. *N Engl J Med* 298:173, 1978.
100. Fraser CL, Arieff AL: Fatal central diabetes mellitus and insipidus resulting from untreated hyponatremia: A new syndrome. *Ann Intern Med* 112:113, 1990.
101. Fraser CL et al: Sex differences result in increased morbidity from hyponatremia in female rats. *Am J Physiol* 256:R880, 1989.
102. Frick PG et al: Hyponatremia associated with hyperproteinemia in multiple myeloma. *Helv Med Acta* 33:317, 1967.
103. Friedman E et al: Thiazide-induced hyponatremia: Reproducibility by single dose rechallenge and an analysis of pathogenesis. *Ann Intern Med* 110:24, 1989.
104. Frier BM et al: Misleading plasma electrolytes in diabetic children with severe hyperlipidemia. *Arch Dis Child* 55:771, 1980.
105. Frizzell RT et al: Hyponatremia and ultramarathon running. *JAMA* 255:772, 1986.
106. Gehi MM et al: Psychiatric manifestations of hyponatremia. *Psychosomatics* 22:739, 1981.
107. Gennari FJ: Current concepts. Serum osmolality: Uses and limitations. *N Engl J Med* 310:102, 1984.
108. George JM et al: Biosynthesis of vasopressin in vitro and ultrastructure of a bronchogenic carcinoma: Patient with the syndrome of inappropriate secretion of antidiuretic hormone. *J Clin Invest* 51:141, 1972.
109. Gerard E et al: MR demonstration of mesencephalic lesions in osmotic demyelination syndrome (central pontine myelinolysis). *Neuroradiology* 29:582, 1987.
110. Ghose RR: Plasma arginine vasopressin in hyponatraemic patients receiving diuretics. *Postgrad Med J* 61:1043, 1985.
111. Gledhill RF, Thompson PD: Central pontine myelinolysis and the correction of hyponatraemia. *S Afr Med J* 72:328, 1987.
112. Godleski LS et al: Prevalence of polyuria among chronically psychotic men. *Psychiatr Med* 6:114, 1988.
113. Goldberg GN et al: Infantile water intoxication after a swimming lesson. *Pediatrics* 70:599, 1982.
114. Goldman MB: A rational approach to disorders of water balance in psychiatric patients. *Hosp Community Psychiatry* 42:488, 1991.
115. Goldman MB et al: Mechanisms of altered water metabolism in psychotic patients with polydipsia and hyponatremia. *N Engl J Med* 318:397, 1988.
116. Goldman MH, Kashani M: Spurious hyponatremia in diabetic ketoacidosis with massive lipid elevations. *J Med Soc N J* 79:591, 1982.
117. Graber M, Corish D: The electrolytes in hyponatremia. *Am J Kidney Dis* 18:527, 1991.
118. Gross P et al: Natriuretic factors and lithium clearance in patients with the syndrome of inappropriate antidiuretic hormone (SIADH). *Eur J Clin Invest* 19:11, 1989.
119. Gross P et al: Vasopressin in hyponatremia: What stimuli? *J Cardiovasc Pharmacol* 8(suppl 7):S92, 1986.
120. Gross PA et al: Pathogenesis of clinical hyponatremia: Observations of vasopressin and fluid intake in 100 hyponatremic medical patients. *Eur J Clin Invest* 17:123, 1987.
121. Gross PA et al: Prostaglandins and water metabolism: A review with emphasis on in vivo studies. *Kidney Int* 19:839, 1981.
122. Gur A et al: A study of the renal handling of water in lipid nephrosis. *Pediatr Res* 20:197, 1976.
123. Hahn RG: The transurethral resection syndrome. *Acta Anaesthesiol Scand* 35:557, 1991.
124. Hamburger S et al: Thiazide-induced syndrome of inappropriate secretion of antidiuretic hormone: Time course of resolution. *JAMA* 246:1235, 1981.
125. Hamilton RW, Buckalew VM Jr: Sodium, water, and congestive heart failure. *Ann Intern Med* 100:902, 1984.
126. Hammerman C et al: Severe hyponatremia with indomethacin: A more serious toxicity than previously realized? *Dev Pharmacol Ther* 8:260, 1985.
127. Hantman D et al: Rapid correction of hyponatremia in the syndrome of inappropriate secretion of antidiuretic hormone: An alternative treatment to hypertonic saline. *Ann Intern Med* 78:870, 1973.
128. Hariprasad MK et al: Hyponatremia in psychogenic polydipsia. *Arch Intern Med* 140:1639, 1980.
129. Harrow AS: Beer potomania syndrome in an alcoholic. *Va Med Q* 116:270, 1989.
130. Hasan D et al: Hyponatremia is associated with cerebral ischemia in patients with aneurysmal subarachnoid hemorrhage. *Ann Neurol* 27:106, 1990.
131. Hass M, Glick SM: Radioimmunoassayable plasma vasopressin associated with surgery. *Arch Surg* 113:597, 1978.
132. Helwig FC et al: Water intoxication: Report of a fatal human case, with clinical, pathologic and experimental studies. *JAMA* 104:1569, 1935.
133. Helwig FC et al: Water intoxication: Moribund patient cured by administration of hypertonic salt solution. *JAMA* 110:644, 1938.
134. Heslop H et al: Hyponatraemic-hypertensive syndrome due to unilateral renal ischaemia in women who smoke heavily. *N Z Med J* 98:739, 1985.

135. Hilden T, Svendsen TL: Electrolyte disturbances in beer drinkers. *Lancet* 2:245, 1975.
136. Hill AR et al: Altered water metabolism in tuberculosis: Role of vasopressin. *Am J Med* 88:357, 1990.
137. Hiller WD: Dehydration and hyponatremia during triathlons. *Med Sci Sports Exerc* 21(suppl 5):S219, 1989.
138. Holliday MA et al: Factors that limit brain volume changes in response to acute and sustained hyper- and hyponatremia. *J Clin Invest* 47:1916, 1968.
139. Howard JM, Reed J: Pseudohyponatremia in acute hyperlipemic pancreatitis: A potential pitfall in therapy. *Arch Surg* 120:1053, 1985.
140. Illlowsky BP, Kirch DG: Polydipsia and hyponatraemia in psychiatric patients. *Am J Psychiatry* 145:675, 1988.
141. Ionescu-Tirgosviste C, Cheta D: Misleading hyponatraemia in hyperlipidaemic states. *Lancet* 1:212, 1980.
142. Irving RA et al: Evaluation of renal function and fluid homeostasis during recovery from exercise-induced hyponatremia. *J Appl Physiol* 70:342, 1991.
143. Iwasaki Y et al: Osmoregulation of plasma vasopressin in myxedema. *J Clin Endocrinol Metab* 1:205, 1990.
144. Jabre A et al: Decerebrate posturing with the syndrome of inappropriate secretion of antidiuretic hormone. *Surg Neurol* 23:56, 1985.
145. Jacobsen D et al: Anion and osmolal gaps in the diagnosis of methanol and ethylene glycol poisoning. *Acta Med Scand* 212:17, 1982.
146. Jard S: Vasopressin antagonists. *Adv Nephrol* 16:1, 1987.
147. Johnston C et al: Hyponatraemia and Moduretic-grand mal seizures: A review. *J R Soc Med* 82:479, 1989.
148. Jones DG: The Schwartz-Bartter syndrome in patients admitted to a general surgical unit following trauma. *Injury* 16:413, 1985.
149. Jose CJ, Perez-Cruet J: Incidence and morbidity of self-induced water intoxication in state mental hospital patients. *Am J Psychiatry* 136:221, 1979.
150. Jose CJ, Perez-Cruet J: Self-induced water intoxication: A comparison of 34 cases with matched controls. *J Clin Psychiatry* 47:368, 1986.
151. Joyce SM, Potter R: Beer potomania: An unusual cause of symptomatic hyponatremia. *Ann Emerg Med* 15:745, 1986.
152. Juul R et al: Atrial natriuretic peptide following subarachnoid haemorrhage in man. *Acta Neurochir (Wien)* 106:18, 1990.
153. Kadowaki T et al: Chlorpropamide-induced hyponatremia: Incidence and risk factors. *Diabetes Care* 6:468, 1983.
154. Kalnins RM et al: Central pontine myelinolysis with widespread extrapontine lesions: A report of two cases. *Clin Exp Neurol* 20:189, 1984.
155. Kastner T et al: Carbamazepine-induced hyponatremia in patients with mental retardation. *Am J Ment Retard* 96:536, 1992.
156. Katz MA: Hyperglycemia-induced hyponatremia: Calculation of expected serum sodium depression. *N Engl J Med* 289:843, 1973.
157. Kay MC et al: Vision loss following transurethral resection of the prostate. *J Clin Neuro Ophthalmol* 5:273, 1985.
158. Keating JP et al: Oral water intoxication in infants: An American epidemic. *Am J Dis Child* 145:985, 1991.
159. Kimura T et al: Mechanism of carbamazepine (Tegretol)-induced antidiuresis: Evidence for release of antidiuretic hormone and impaired excretion of a water load. *J Clin Endocrinol Metab* 38:356, 1974.
160. Kinter LB et al: Antagonists of the antidiuretic activity of vasopressin. *Am J Physiol* 254:F165, 1988.
161. Kleinfeld M et al: Hyponatremia as observed in a chronic disease facility. *J Am Geriatr Soc* 27:156, 1979.
162. Kleinschmidt-DeMasters BK, Norenberg MD: Rapid correction of hyponatremia causes demyelination: Relation to central pontine myelinolysis. *Science* 211:1068, 1981.
163. Kleinschmidt-DeMasters BK, Norenberg MD: Cerebellar degeneration in the rat following rapid correction of hyponatremia. *Ann Neurol* 10:561, 1981.
164. Kleinschmidt-DeMasters BK, Norenberg MD: Neuropathologic observations in electrolyte-induced myelinolysis in the rat. *J Neuropathol Exp Neurol* 41:67, 1982.
165. Knochel JP: Neuromuscular manifestations of electrolyte disorders. *Am J Med* 72:521, 1982.
166. Knochel JP: Catastrophic medical events with exhaustive exercise: "White collar rhabdomyolysis." *Kidney Int* 38:209, 1990.
167. Kortas C et al: Vasopressin in congestive heart failure. *J Cardiovasc Pharmacol* 8:S107, 1986.
168. Kovacs L, Robertson GL: Disorders of water balance: Hyponatraemia and hypernatraemia. *Baillieres Clin Endocrinol Metab* 6:107, 1992.
169. Kudva BT et al: Syndrome of inappropriate ADH secretion: Prevalence in respiratory disorders. *J Postgrad Med* 28:92, 1982.
170. Laczi F et al: Osmoregulation of arginine-8-vasopressin secretion in primary hypothyroidism and in Addison's disease. *Acta Endocrinol (Copenh)* 114:389, 1987.
171. Ladenson JH et al: Misleading hyponatremia due to hyperlilpidemia: A method-dependent error. *Ann Intern Med* 95:707, 1981.
172. Lahr MB: Hyponatremia during carbamazepine therapy. *Clin Pharmacol Ther* 37:693, 1985.
173. Lang MA: Correlation between osmoregulation and cell volume regulation. *Am J Physiol* 252:R768, 1987.
174. Laureno R: Experimental pontine and extrapontine myelinolysis. *Trans Am Neurol Assoc* 105:354, 1980.
175. Laureno R: Rapid correction of hyponatremia: Cause of pontine myelinolysis? *Am J Med* 71:846, 1981.
176. Laureno R, Karp BI: Pontine and extrapontine myelinolysis following rapid correction of hyponatraemia. *Lancet* 1:1439, 1988.
177. Law RO: Amino acids as volume-regulatory osmolytes in mammalian cells. *Comp Biochem Physiol* 99:263, 1991.
178. Leaf A et al: Evidence in man that urinary electrolyte loss induced by pitressin is a function of water retention. *J Clin Invest* 32:868, 1953.
179. Lee MR: Effects of drugs on water metabolism. *Br J Clin Pharmacol* 12:289, 1981.
180. Legros JJ et al: Neurophysins as markers of vasopressin and oxytocin release: A study in carcinoma of the lung. *Horm Res* 34:151, 1990.
181. Leimbach WN Jr et al: Baroreflex control of plasma arginine vasopressin in humans. *Am J Physiol* 247:H638, 1984.
182. Levine S et al: Fatal water intoxication, schizophrenia and

diuretic therapy for systemic hypertension. *Am J Med* 82:153, 1987.
183. Lien YH et al: Study of brain electrolytes and organic osmolytes during correction of chronic hyponatremia: Implications for the pathogenesis of central pontine myelinolysis. *J Clin Invest* 88:303, 1991.
184. Lillien A: Oxytocin-induced water intoxication: A report of a maternal death. *Obstet Gynecol* 32:171, 1968.
185. Linas SL et al: Role of vasopressin in the impaired water excretion of glucocorticoid deficiency. *Kidney Int* 18:58, 1980.
186. Liskin B et al: Imipramine-induced inappropriate ADH secretion. *J Clin Psychopharmacol* 4:146, 1984.
187. Lokich JJ: The frequency and clinical biology of the ectopic hormone syndromes of small cell carcinoma. *Cancer* 50:2111, 1982.
188. Luboshitzky R et al: Hypopituitarism with water intoxication and coma: Favorable outcome following early treatment. *J Endocrinol Invest* 2:423, 1979.
189. Lundbaek JA et al: Brain interstitial composition during acute hyponatremia. *Acta Neurochir Suppl (Wien)* 51:17, 1990.
190. Macknight ADC et al: Physiologic and pathophysiologic responses to changes in extracellular osmolality, in Seldin DW, Giebisch G (eds): *The Kidney: Physiology and Pathophysiology*, 2d ed. Raven Press, 1992.
191. MacMillan HL et al: Hyponatremia and depression. *J Nerv Ment Dis* 178:720, 1990.
192. Maesaka JK et al: Hyponatremia and hypouricemia: Differentiation from SIADH. *Clin Nephrol* 33:174, 1990.
193. Manoogian C et al: Plasma atrial natriuretic hormone levels in patients with the syndrome of inappropriate antidiuretic hormone secretion. *J Clin Endocrinol Metab* 67:571, 1988.
194. Maraganore DM et al: Movement disorders as sequelae of central pontine myelinolysis: Report of three cases. *Mov Disord* 7:142, 1992.
195. Martinez-Maldonado M: Inappropriate antidiuretic hormone secretion of unknown origin. *Kidney Int* 17:554, 1980.
196. Mathew TH et al: Hyponatraemia due to the combination of hydrochlorothiazide and amiloride (Moduretic): Australian spontaneous reports 1977–1988. *Med J Aust* 152:308, 1990.
197. McColl P, Kelly C: A misleading case of central pontine myelinolysis: Risk factors for psychiatric patients. *Br J Psychiatry* 160:550, 1992.
198. McCormick PA et al: Intravenous albumin infusion is an effective therapy for hyponatraemia in cirrhotic patients with ascites. *Gut* 31:204, 1990.
199. Melton JE et al: Volume regulatory loss of Na, Cl, and K from rat brain during acute hyponatremia. *Am J Physiol* 252:F661, 1987.
200. Melville RJ et al: Stimulus for vasopressin release during elective intraabdominal operations. *Br J Surg* 72:979, 1985.
201. Messert B et al: Central pontine myelinolysis: Considerations on etiology, diagnosis and treatment. *Neurology* 29:147, 1979.
202. Mettauer B et al: Sodium and water excretion abnormalities in congestive heart failure: Determinant factors and clinical implications. *Ann Intern Med* 105:161, 1986.
203. Mickel HS et al: Protein oxidation and myelinolysis occur in brain following rapid correction of hyponatremia. *Biochem Biophys Res Commun* 172:92, 1990.
204. Miles AI, Needle MA: Fixed hyponatremia with normal responses to varying salt and water intakes. *N Engl J Med* 284:26, 1971.
205. Miller GM et al: Central pontine myelinolysis and its imitators: MR findings. *Radiology* 168:795, 1988.
206. Miller M, Moses AM: Drug-induced states of impaired water excretion. *Kidney Int* 10:96, 1976.
207. Miller PD et al: Plasma demeclocycline levels and nephrotoxicity: Correlation in hyponatremic cirrhotic patients. *JAMA* 243:2513, 1980.
208. Misra SC, Mansharamani GG: Hyponatremia in elderly hospital in-patients. *Br J Clin Pract* 43:295, 1989.
209. Mitnick PD, Bell S: Rhabdomyolysis associated with severe hyponatremia after prostatic surgery. *Am J Kidney Dis* 16:73, 1990.
210. Montgomery AJ et al: Severe hyponatraemia and cardiac failure successfully treated with captopril. *Br Med J Clin Res* 284:1085, 1982.
211. Mor F et al: Rhabdomyolysis in self-induced water intoxication. *J Nerv Ment Dis* 175:742, 1987.
212. Moran SM, Jamison RL: The variable hyponatremic response to hyperglycemia. *West J Med* 142:49, 1985.
213. Morgan DB et al: Water intoxication and oxytocin infusion. *Br J Obstet Gynecol* 84:6, 1977.
214. Morlan L et al: Central pontine myelinolysis following correction of hyponatremia: MRI diagnosis. *Eur Neurol* 30:149, 1990.
215. Moses AM et al: Mechanism of chlorpropamide-induced antidiuresis in man: Evidence for release of ADH and enhancement of peripheral action. *Metabolism* 22:59, 1973.
216. Moses AM, Scheinman SJ: Ectopic secretion of neurohypophyseal peptides in patients with malignancy. *Endocrinol Metab Clin North Am* 20:489, 1991.
217. Moses AM et al: Pathophysiologic and pharmacologic alterations in the release and action of ADH. *Metabolism* 25:697, 1976.
218. Murty GE et al: Early inappropriate secretion of antidiuretic hormone after transsphenoidal pituitary adenomectomy. *J Laryngol Otol* 104:894, 1990.
219. Narins RG et al: Diagnostic strategies in disorders of fluid, electrolyte and acidbase homeostasis. *Am J Med* 72:496, 1982.
220. Natkunam A et al: Hyponatremia in a hospital population. *J Med* 22:83, 1991.
221. Nattie EE, Edward WH: Brain and CSF water and ions in newborn puppies during acute hypo- and hypernatremia. *J Appl Physiol* 51:1086, 1981.
222. Nelson PB et al: Hyponatremia in intracranial disease: Perhaps not the syndrome of inappropriate secretion of antidiuretic hormone (SIADH). *J Neurosurg* 55:938, 1981.
223. Nelson RJ: Blood volume measurement following subarachnoid haemorrhage. *Acta Neurochir Suppl (Wien)* 47:114, 1990.
224. Noakes TD: Hyponatremia during endurance running: A physiological and clinical interpretation. *Med Sci Sports Exerc* 24:403, 1992.
225. Noakes TD et al: The incidence of hyponatremia during

prolonged ultraendurance exercise. *Med Sci Sports Exerc* 2:165, 1990.
226. Nolph KD, Schrier RW: Sodium, potassium and water metabolism in the syndrome of inappropriate antidiuretic hormone secretion. *Am J Med* 49:534, 1970.
227. Norenberg MD et al: Association between rise in serum sodium and central pontine myelinolysis. *Ann Neurol* 11:128, 1982.
228. Norlen H et al: Glycine solution as an irrigating agent during transurethral prostatic resection. *Scand J Urol Nephrol* 20:19, 1986.
229. Norsk P: Influence of low- and high-pressure baroreflexes on vasopressin release in humans. *Acta Endocrinol* 121 (suppl 1):1, 1989.
230. Oelkers W: Hyponatremia and inappropriate secretion of vasopressin (antidiuretic hormone) in patients with hypopituitarism. *N Engl J Med* 321:492, 1989.
231. Oh MS et al: Central pontine myelinolysis following isotonic saline. *Am J Med Sci* 298:40, 1989.
232. Oh MS, Carroll HJ: Disorders of sodium metabolism: Hypernatremia and hyponatremia. *Crit Care Med* 20:94, 1992.
233. Oh MS et al: Prevention of myelinolysis in rats by dexamethasone or colchicine. *Am J Nephrol* 10:158, 1990.
234. Okura M et al: Electroencephalographic changes during and after water intoxication. *Jpn J Psychiatry Neurol* 44:729, 1990.
235. Packer M et al: Identification of hyponatremia as a risk factor for the development of functional renal insufficiency during converting enzyme inhibition in severe chronic heart failure. *J Am Coll Cardiol* 10:837, 1987.
236. Packer M et al: Correction of dilutional hyponatremia in severe chronic heart failure by converting-enzyme inhibition. *Ann Intern Med* 100:782, 1984.
237. Padilla G et al: Vasopressin levels in infants during the course of aseptic and bacterial meningitis. *Am J Dis Child* 145:991, 1991.
238. Papadakis MA et al: Hyponatraemia in patients with cirrhosis. *Q J Med* 76:675, 1990.
239. Peck V, Shenkman L: Haloperidol-induced syndrome of inappropriate secretion of antidiuretic hormone. *Clin Pharmacol Ther* 26:442, 1979.
240. Pedersen ED et al: Defective renal water excretion in nephrotic syndrome. The relationship between renal water excretion and kidney function, arginine-vasopressin, angiotensin II and aldosterone in plasma before and after water loading. *Eur J Clin Invest* 15:24, 1985.
241. Perucca E et al: Water intoxication in epileptic patients receiving carbamazepine. *J Neurol Neurosurg Psychiatry* 41:713, 1978.
242. Pestell RG et al: Biochemical and hormonal changes during a 1000 km ultramarathon. *Clin Exp Pharmacol Physiol* 16:353, 1989.
243. Peters KR et al: Intraocular pressure after transurethral prostatic surgery. *Anesthesiology* 55:327, 1981.
244. Petersen JC et al: Inappropriate antidiuretic hormone secondary to monoamine oxidase inhibitor. *JAMA* 239:1422, 1978.
245. Petersson I et al: Water intoxication associated with nonsteroidal anti-inflammatory drug therapy. *Acta Med Scand* 221:221, 1987.
246. Pfister HW et al: Mild central pontine myelinolysis: A frequently undetected syndrome. *Eur Arch Psychiatry Neurol Sci* 235:134, 1985.
247. Phillips PA et al: Osmotic thirst and vasopressin release in humans: A double blind crossover study. *Am J Physiol* 248:R745, 1985.
248. Pledger DR, Mathew H: Hyponatremia and clomipramine therapy. *Br J Psychiatry* 154:263, 1989.
249. Poon WS et al: Secretion of antidiuretic hormone in neurosurgical patients: Appropriate or inappropriate? *Aust N Z J Surg* 59:173, 1989.
250. Popli S et al: Asymptomatic, nonketotic, severe hyperglycemia with hyponatremia. *Arch Intern Med* 150:1962, 1990.
251. Price BH, Mesulam MM: Behavioral manifestations of central pontine myelinolysis. *Arch Neurol* 44:671, 1987.
252. Raff H: Glucocorticoid inhibition of neurohypophysial vasopressin secretion. *Am J Physiol* 252:R635, 1987.
253. Ragland RL et al: Central pontine myelinolysis with clinical recovery: MR documentation. *J Comput Assist Tomogr* 13:316, 1989.
254. Rao K et al: Water intoxication and thioridazine (Mellaril). *Ann Intern Med* 82:61, 1975.
255. Raskind M: Psychosis, polydipsia, and water intoxication: Report of a fatal case. *Arch Gen Psychiatry* 30:112, 1974.
256. Ravat HK, Joshi VR: Chlorpropamide induced syndrome of inappropriate secretion of antidiuretic hormone. *J. Assoc Physicians India* 39:645, 1991.
257. Reeder RF, Harbaugh RE: Administration of intravenous urea and normal saline for the treatment of hyponatremia in neurosurgical patients. *J Neurosurg* 70:201, 1989.
258. Reihman DH et al: Effect of hypoxemia on sodium and water excretion in chronic obstructive lung disease. *Am J Med* 78:87, 1985.
259. Rendell M et al: Fatal compulsive water drinking. *JAMA* 240:2557, 1978.
260. Riegger GA et al: Antidiuretic hormone in congestive heart failure. *Am J Med* 72:49, 1982.
261. Riggs AT et al: A review of disorders of water homeostasis in psychiatric patients: Department of Medicine, University of Minnesota. *Psychosomatics* 32:133, 1991.
262. Robertson GL et al: Vincristine neurotoxicity and abnormal secretion of antidiuretc hormone. *Arch Intern Med* 132:717, 1973.
263. Robertson GL et al: The osmoregulation of vasopressin. *Kidney Int* 10:25, 1976.
264. Robertson GL: Physiology of ADH secretion. *Kidney Int* 32 (suppl 21):520, 1987.
265. Robertson GL: Thirst and vasopressin function in normal and disordered states of water balance. *J Lab Clin Med* 101:351, 1983.
266. Robertson GL et al: Neurogenic disorders of osmoregulation. *Am J Med* 72:339, 1982.
267. Robinson AG: dDAVP in the treatment of central diabetes insipidus. *N Engl J Med* 294:507, 1976.
268. Rolls BJ et al: Thirst following water deprivation in humans. *Am J Physiol* R476, 1980.
269. Roscoe JM et al: Hyperglycemia-induced hyponatremia: Metabolic considerations in calculation of serum sodium depression. *Can Med Assoc J* 112:452, 1975.

270. Rose BD: New approach to disturbances in the plasma sodium concentration. *Am J Med* 81:1033, 1986.
271. Rose CE et al: Water metabolism in respiratory disorders. *Semin Nephrol* 4:295, 1984.
272. Rosenow EC III et al: Inappropriate antidiuretic hormone secretion in pneumonia. *Mayo Clin Proc* 47:169, 1972.
273. Rothenberg DM et al: Isotonic hyponatremia following transurethral prostate resection. *J Clin Anesth* 2:48, 1990.
274. Rowe JW et al: Influence of the emetic reflex on vasopressin release in man. *Kidney Int* 16:729, 1979.
275. Rymer MM, Fishman RA: Protective adaptation of brain to water intoxication. *Arch Neurol* 28:49, 1973.
276. Sandifer MG: Hyponatremia due to psychotropic drugs. *J Clin Psychiatry* 44:301, 1983.
277. Sarnaik AP et al: Management of hyponatremic seizures in children with hypertonic saline: A safe and effective strategy. *Crit Care Med* 19:758, 1991.
278. Schrier RW et al: Osmotic and nonosmotic control of vasopressin release. *Am J Physiol* 236:F321, 1979.
279. Schrier RW, Goldberg JP: The physiology of vasopressin release and the pathogenesis of impaired water excretion in adrenal, thyroid and edematous disorders. *Yale J Biol Med* 53:525, 1980.
280. Schrier RW et al: Effect of furosemide on free water excretion in edematous patients with hyponatremia. *Kidney Int* 3:30, 1973.
281. Schrier RW, Linas SL: Mechanisms of the defect in water excretion in adrenal insufficiency. *Miner Electrolyte Metab* 4:1, 1980.
282. Schrier RW: Pathogenesis of sodium and water retention in high output and low output cardiac failure, nephrotic syndrome, cirrhosis and pregnancy. *N Engl J Med* 319:1065, 1988.
283. Schrier RW: Body fluid volume regulation in health and disease: A unifying hypothesis. *Ann Intern Med* 113:155, 1990.
284. Schwartz WB et al: Syndrome of renal sodium loss and hyponatremia probably resulting from inappropriate secretion of antidiuretic hormone. *Am J Med* 23:529, 1957.
285. Scott JC Jr et al: Water intoxication and sodium depletion in surgical patients. *Obstet Gynecol* 26:168, 1965.
286. Shah PJ, Greenberg WM: Polydipsia with hyponatremia in a state hospital population. *Hosp Community Psychiatry* 43:509, 1992.
287. Shah PJ, Greenberg WM: Water intoxication precipitated by thiazide diuretics in polydipsic psychiatric patients. *Am J Psychiatry* 148:1424, 1991.
288. Shepherd LL et al: Hyponatremia and seizures after intravenous administration of desmopressin acetate for surgical hemostasis. *J Pediatr* 114:470, 1989.
289. Shichiri M et al: Renal handling of urate in the syndrome of inappropriate secretion of antidiuretic hormone. *Arch Intern Med* 145:2045, 1985.
290. Shimoda M et al: Atrial natriuretic polypeptide in patients with subarachnoid haemorrhage due to aneurysmal rupture: Correlation to hyponatremia. *Acta Neurochir (Wien)* 97:53, 1989.
291. Shucart W: Hyponatremia in neurosurgical patients. *Clin Neurosurg* 35:93, 1989.
292. Sica DA, Culpepper RM: Severe hyponatremia in spinal cord injury. *Am J Med Sci* 298:331, 1989.
293. Singh S et al: Water intoxication in psychiatric patients. *Br J Psychiatry* 146:127, 1985.
294. Skowsky WR, Kikuchi TA: The role of vasopressin in the impaired water excretion of myxedema. *Am J Med* 64:613, 1978.
295. Smith TJ et al: Hyponatremia and seizures in young children given dDAVP. *Am J Hematol* 31:199, 1989.
296. Smith WO, Clark ML: Self-induced water intoxication in schizophrenic patients. *Am J Psychiatry* 137:1055, 1980.
297. Sonnenblick M, Rosin A: Increased uric acid clearance in the syndrome of inappropriate secretion of antidiuretic hormone. *Isr J Med Sci* 24:20, 1988.
298. Sordillo P et al: Carbamazapine-induced syndrome of inappropriate antidiuretic hormone secretion. *Arch Intern Med* 138:299, 1978.
299. Soroker D et al: Symptomatic hyponatraemia due to inappropriate antidiuretic hormone secretion following minor surgery. *Can J Anaesth* 38:225, 1991.
300. Soupart A et al: Limits of brain tolerance to daily increments in serum sodium in chronically hyponatraemic rats treated with hypertonic saline or urea: Advantages of urea. *Clin Sci* 80:77, 1991.
301. Spital A: Hyponatremia in adrenal insufficiency: Review of pathogenetic mechanisms. *South Med J* 75:581, 1982.
302. Sterns RH et al: Osmotic demyelination syndrome following correction of hyponatremia. *N Engl J Med* 314:1535, 1986.
303. Sterns RH, Spital A: Disorders of water balance, in Kokko JP, Tannen RL (eds): *Fluids and Electrolytes*. Philadelphia, Saunders, 1990, p 280.
304. Sterns RH: Neurological deterioration following treatment for hyponatremia. *Am J Kidney Dis* 13:434, 1989.
305. Sterns RH: Severe hyponatremia: The case of conservative management. *Crit Care Med* 20:534, 1992.
306. Sterns RH: Severe symptomatic hyponatremia: Treatment and outcome, a study of 64 cases. *Ann Intern Med* 107:656, 1987.
307. Sterns RH: The management of hyponatremic emergencies. *Crit Care Clin* 7:127, 1991.
308. Sterns RH: The management of symptomatic hyponatremia. *Semin Nephrol* 10:503, 1990.
309. Sterns RH: The treatment of hyponatremia: First, do no harm. *Am J Med* 88:557, 1990.
310. Sterns RH et al: Brain dehydration and neurologic deterioration after rapid correction of hyponatremia. *Kidney Int* 35:69, 1989.
311. Sugama T et al: A case of syndrome of inappropriate secretion of antidiuretic hormone (SIADH) with low plasma concentrations of antiduretic hormone. *Intern Med* 31:246, 1992.
312. Sunderam SG, Mankikar GD: Hyponatremia in the elderly. *Age Ageing* 12:77, 1983.
313. Swales JD: Management of hyponatremia. *Br J Anaesth* 67:146, 1991.
314. Szatalowicz VL et al: Plasma antidiuretic hormone in acute respiratory failure. *Am J Med* 72:583, 1982.
315. Tallis GA: Hyponatraemia in psychiatric patients. *Med J Aust* 150:151, 1989.
316. Tang WY et al: Chorea, a manifestation of hyponatraemia? *Singapore Med J* 22:92, 1981.
317. Tanneau RS et al: The finding among AIDS patients of

paradoxical hypouricemia in the presence of volume depletion combined with hyponatremia and high fractional excretion of sodium. *Am J Kidney Dis* 17:724, 1991.

318. Tarail R et al: Misleading reductions of serum sodium and chloride associated with hyperproteinemia in patients with multiple myeloma. *Proc Soc Exp Biol Med* 110:145, 1962.
319. Thomas TH et al: Severe hyponatremia: A study of 17 patients. *Lancet* 1:621, 1978.
320. Thomas TH, Morgan DB: Post-surgical hyponatremia: The role of intravenous fluids and arginine vasopressin. *Br J Surg* 66:540, 1979.
321. Thompson CF et al: The osmotic thresholds for thirst and vasopressin release are similar in healthy man. *Clin Sci* 71:651, 1986.
322. Thurston JH et al: Adaptive decreases in amino acids (taurine in particular), creatine, and electrolytes prevent cerebral edema in chronically hyponatremic mice: Rapid correction (experimental model of central pontine myelinolysis) causes dehydration and shrinkage of the brain. *Metab Brain Dis* 2:223, 1987.
323. Thurston JH et al: Myo-inositol: A newly identified nonnitrogenous osmoregulatory molecule in mammalian brain. *Pediatr Res* 26:482, 1989.
324. Tinker R et al: Pontine myelinolysis presenting with acute parkinsonism as a sequel of corrected hyponatraemia. *J Neurol Neurosurg Psychiatry* 53:87, 1990.
325. Tison FX et al: Delayed onset movement disorders as a complication of central pontine myelinolysis. *Mov Disord* 6:171, 1991.
326. Tomiyama J et al: Water intoxication and rhabdomyolysis. *Jpn J Med* 29:52, 1990.
327. Tomlinson BE et al: Central pontine myelinolysis: Two cases with associated electrolyte disturbance. *Q J Med* 179:373, 1976.
328. Trabert W et al: Inappropriate vasopressin secretion in severe alcohol withdrawal. *Acta Psychiatr Scand* 85:376, 1992.
329. Trachtman H: Cell volume regulation: A review of cerebral adaptive mechanisms and implications for clinical treatment of osmolal disturbances: II. *Pediatr Nephrol* 6:104, 1992.
330. Trachtman H et al: Taurine and osmoregulation: 3. Taurine deficiency protects against cerebral edema during acute hyponatremia. *Pediatr Res* 27:85, 1990.
331. Trachtman H et al: The role of polyols in cerebral cell volume regulation in hypernatremic and hyponatremic states. *Life Sci* 49:677, 1991.
332. Uretsky BF et al: Plasma vasopressin response to osmotic and hemodynamic stimuli in heart failure. *Am J Physiol* 248:H396, 1985.
333. Vanapruks V, Prapaitrakul K: Water intoxication and hyponatraemic convulsions in neonates. *Arch Dis Child* 64:734, 1989.
334. Van Reeth O, Decaux G: Rapid correction of hyponatraemia with urea protect against brain damage in rats. *Clin Sci* 77:351, 1989.
335. Vassal G et al: Hyponatremia and renal sodium wasting in patients receiving cisplatinum. *Pediatr Hematol Oncol* 4:337, 1987.
336. Verbalis JG, Drutarosky MD: Adaptation to chronic hypoosmolality in rats. *Kidney Int* 34:351, 1988.
337. Verbalis JG: Hyponatraemia. *Baillieres Clin Endocrinol Metab* 3:499, 1989.
338. Verbalis JG: Hyponatremia: Answered and unanswered questions. *Am J Kidney Dis* 18:546, 1991.
339. Verbalis JG: Tumoral hyponatremia. *Arch Intern Med* 146:1686, 1986.
340. Verbalis JG et al: Adaptive responses to sustained volume expansion in hyponatraemic rats. *J Endocrinol* 122:421, 1989.
341. Verbalis JG, Gullans SR: Hyponatremia causes large sustained reductions in brain content of multiple organic osmolytes in rats. *Brain Res* 567:274, 1991.
342. Verbalis JG, Martinez AJ: Neurological and neuropathological sequelae of correction of chronic hyponatremia. *Kidney Int* 39:1274, 1991.
343. Verney EB: Absorption and excretion of water: Antidiuretic hormone. *Lancet* 2:739, 1946.
344. Vieweg WV et al: Hypocalcemia: An additional complication of the syndrome of selfinduced water intoxication and psychosis (SIWIP). *Psychiatr Med* 4:291, 1986.
345. Vieweg WV et al: Death from self-induced water intoxication among patients with schizophrenic disorders. *J Nerv Ment Dis* 173:161, 1985.
346. Vieweg WV et al: The use of demeclocycline in the treatment of patients with psychosis, intermittent hyponatremia, and polydipsia (PIP syndrome). *Psychiatr Q* 59:62, 1988.
347. Vieweg WVR et al: Correlation of parameters of urinary excretion with serum osmolality among patients with psychosis, intermittent hyponatremia, and poydipsia (PIP syndrome). *Psychiatric Med* 6:81, 1988.
348. Vingerhoets F, de Tribolet N: Hyponatremia hypoosmolarity in neurosurgical patients: "Appropriate secretion of ADH" and cerebral salt wasting syndrome. *Acta Neurochir (Wien)* 91:50, 1988.
349. Vitting KE et al: Frequency of hyponatremia and nonosmolar vasopressin release in the acquired immunodeficiency syndrome. *JAMA* 263:973, 1990.
350. Vorherr H et al: Antidiuretic principle in tuberculous lung tissue of a patient with pulmonary tuberculosis and hyponatremia. *Ann Intern Med* 72:383, 1970.
351. Wakui H et al: Dramatic recovery from neurological deficits in a patient with central pontine myelinolysis following severe hyponatremia. *Jpn J Med* 30:281, 1991.
352. Walker JV, Englander RN: Central pontine myelinolysis following rapid correction of hyponatremia in an alcoholic. *Am J Kidney Dis* 12:531, 1988.
353. Walker V: Fluid balance disturbances in neurosurgical patients: Physiological basis and definitions. *Acta Neurochir Suppl (Wien)* 47:95, 1990.
354. Wall BM et al: Reversible changes in osmoregulation of vasopressin release due to impaired water excretion. *Am J Kidney Dis* 18:269, 1991.
355. Walters E, Hallam L: Association of hyperglycaemia with hyponatraemia. *Br Med J Clin Res* 288:1146, 1984.
356. Walters EG et al: Hyponatraemia associated with diuretics. *Br J Clin Pract* 41:841, 1987.
357. Wattad A et al: Hyponatremia in hospitalized children. *Clin Pediatr (Phila)* 31:153, 1992.
358. Webberley MJ, Murray JA: Life-threatening acute hyponatraemia induced by low dose cyclophosphamide and indomethacin. *Postgrad Med J* 65:950, 1989.

359. Weinand ME et al: A study of serum antidiuretic hormone and atrial natriuretic peptide levels in a series of patients with intracranial disease and hyponatremia. *Neurosurgery* 25:781, 1989.
360. Weinstein RE et al: Severe hyponatremia after repeated intravenous administration of desmopressin. *Am J Hematol* 32:258, 1989.
361. Weisberg LS: Pseudohyponatremia: A reappraisal. *Am J Med* 86:315, 1989.
362. Weiss NW, Robertson GL: Water metabolism in endocrine disorders. *Semin Nephrol* 4:303, 1984.
363. Weissman JD, Weissman BM: Pontine myelinolysis and delayed encephalopathy following the rapid correction of acute hyponatremia. *Arch Neurol* 46:926, 1989.
364. Weissman PW: Chlorpropamide hyponatremia. *N Engl J Med* 284:65, 1971.
365. Wijdicks EF et al: Atrial natriuretic factor and salt wasting after aneurysmal subarachnoid hemorrhage. *Stroke* 22:1519, 1991.
366. Wijdicks EF et al: Hyponatremia and cerebral infarction in patients with ruptured intracranial aneurysms: Is fluid restriction harmful? *Ann Neurol* 17:137, 1985.
367. Wijdicks EF et al: Volume depletion and natriuresis in patients with a ruptured intracranial aneurysm. *Ann Neurol* 18:211, 1985.
368. Wijdicks EF et al: Hyponatraemia and volume status in aneurysmal subarachnoid haemorrhage. *Acta Neurochir Suppl (Wien)* 47:111, 1990.
369. Woods C: Central pontine myelinolysis: A case study. *Axone* 12:77, 1991.
370. Worthley LI, Thomas PD: Treatment of hyponatraemic seizures with intravenous 29.2 percent saline. *Br Med J* 292:168, 1986.
371. Wright DG et al: Pontine and extrapontine myelinolysis. *Brain* 102:361, 1979.
372. Wynn V, Robb CG: Water intoxication: Differential diagnosis of the hypotonic syndromes. *Lancet* 1:587, 1954.
373. Yamaki T et al: Cerebral salt wasting syndrome distinct from the syndrome of inappropriate secretion of antidiuretic hormone (SIADH). *Acta Neurochir (Wien)* 115:156, 1992.
374. Yancey PH et al: Living with water stress: Evolution of osmolyte systems. *Science* 217:1214, 1982.
375. Yassa R et al: Carbamazepine and hyponatremia in patients with affective disorder. *Am J Psychiatry* 145:339, 1988.
376. Zerbe R et al: Vasopressin function in the syndrome of inappropriate antidiuresis. *Annu Rev Med* 31:315, 1980.
377. Zerbe RL, Robertson GL: Osmoregulation of thirst and vasopressin secretion in human subjects: Effect of various solutes. *Am J Physiol* 244:E538, 1983.
378. Zimmermann B, Wagensteen OH: Observations on water intoxication in surgical patients. *Surgery* 34:654, 1952.
379. Zimmerman EA et al: Anatomical basis of thirst and vasopressin secretion. *Kidney Int* 32:S14, 1987.
380. Zucker JR, Bull AP: Independent plasma levels of sodium and glycine during transurethral resection of the prostate. *Can Anaesth Soc J* 31:307, 1984.

CHAPTER • 21

Hyperosmolal states

Gail Morrison • Irwin Singer

An elaborate network of regulatory systems maintains the quantity of total body water, and both the quantity and composition of total body solute within narrow ranges. Under normal circumstances, therefore, the solute concentration or osmolality of body fluids, that is, the ratio of solute content to water content in any body fluid compartment, is fairly constant, and varies only slightly from day to day. However, many clinical conditions can disrupt the normal homeostatic mechanisms, resulting in the retention or loss of water and/or solute; the body fluids may then be too concentrated (hyperosmolal) or too dilute (hyposmolal). Both hyperosmolality and hyposmolality can significantly impair neurological function. This chapter will focus on those conditions associated with hyperosmolal states, that is, states associated with abnormally concentrated body fluids.[11,90,202]

The first sections of this chapter review the salient features of normal water metabolism and its servoregulatory systems. (See Chap. 5 for more detail.) Next, the distribution of solute and water between different body fluid compartments is addressed, with the mechanisms governing that distribution under normal and abnormal conditions.[196] (See Chap. 1 for more detail.) The last part discusses in detail those clinical conditions associated with hyperosmolality.[106]

NORMAL OSMOREGULATORY SERVOMECHANISMS

Most clinical conditions associated with hyperosmolality result from net loss of total body water (TBW). This net loss implies a significant defect in the regulation of water balance because under normal circumstances the average quantity of water accrued daily, that is, by direct ingestion and by catabolic production, equals the average quantity of water excreted daily by renal, cutaneous, gastrointestinal, and pulmonary routes.[2] As long as water and solute balance are achieved on a daily basis, body fluid osmolality is maintained within a narrow range. Two osmoregulatory systems control water balance, and therefore control body fluid osmolality: thirst[3,84] and antidiuretic hormone (ADH).[30,192] There is little or no osmoregulatory control over the other aspects of water accrual and excretion. The two osmoregulatory systems are coordinated by the "osmostat," a group of closely interconnected hypothalamic neurons, with cortical connections that mediate thirst and hypophyseal connections that mediate ADH release. The overall functioning of the osmoregulatory servomechanism is shown in Fig. 21-1. With ideal regulation, either system (thirst or ADH) should suffice to maintain water balance; in practice, defects are usually present in both systems when water balance is not maintained near normal.[2,3]

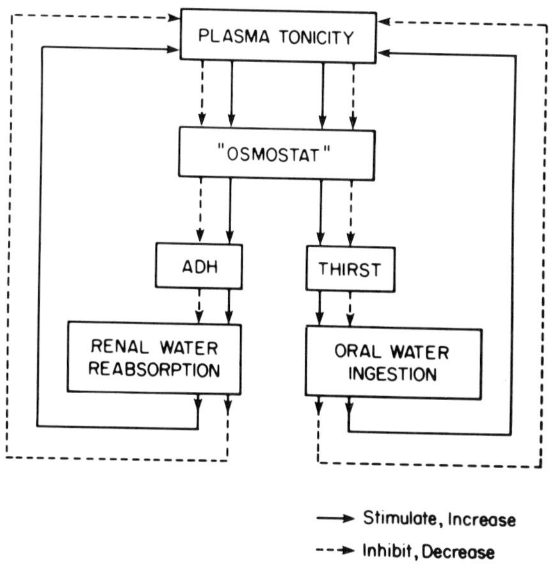

FIGURE 21-1 • Control of body fluid tonicity (normal osmolal servoregulation).

NORMAL ANTIDIURETIC HORMONE REGULATION

ADH and the central nervous system

The regulation of renal water excretion depends on the release of ADH and the ability of the kidneys to respond to it.[192,193,195] (These aspects of normal water physiology are discussed in more detail in Chaps. 4 and 5.)

ADH is synthesized in the hypothalamus (principally in the supraoptic and paraventricular nuclei) along with the ADH carrier protein, neurophysin.[36] The hormone-carrier complex is transported intraaxonally to the neurohypophysis for storage. The complex is normally released from the neurohypophysis, and in some cases from the hypothalamus, in response to an increase in intracellular "effective" osmolality or tonicity (discussed in Hyperosmolality, effective osmolality, and tonicity, below), and/or to a decrease in effective arterial blood volume (EABV). However, all solutes are not equally effective in stimulating ADH release, and the rate of solute administration may also be important.[210] For example, when sodium chloride or mannitol induces a given increment in plasma osmolality, a similar release of ADH is elicited.[10] However, urea and glucose are less effective stimuli for ADH release.[10] Urea stimulates ADH release only slightly, if at all; glucose may actually decrease ADH release. If urea (or glucose) is administered very rapidly, there may be a transient increase in ADH release, but in the steady state there is little or no stimulation because the urea or glucose enters the cells and is no longer an effective osmole. Glucose may have additional actions to suppress ADH release after cellular entry.[243]

The relationships between the plasma osmolality (P_{osm}), the level of plasma ADH concentration (P_{ADH}), and urine osmolality (U_{osm}) are shown in Fig. 21-2. When P_{osm} is less than 280 mosm/kg circulating levels of ADH are undetectable (less than about 0.5 pg/ml), and U_{osm} is generally less than 150 mosm/kg. On the other hand, when P_{osm} is greater than 295 mosm/kg, circulating levels of ADH exceed 5.0 pg/ml, and U_{osm} is generally greater than 850 mosm/kg. Note that the P_{ADH} becomes undetectable at the same time that the urine osmolality reaches a minimum (U_{min} or min U_{osm}) and that ADH levels greater than 5.0 pg/ml do not produce greater increases in U_{osm} (i.e., the max U_{osm} or U_{max} has already been reached). Since the threshold for the perception of thirst is about 295 mosm/kg, the thirst mechanism generally does not become active until P_{ADH} is already sufficient to produce the max U_{osm}. In other words, oral water intake does not increase in response to hyperosmolality until renal water conservation is already maximal.[195]

The relationships of P_{ADH}, P_{osm}, and U_{osm} show a remarkable regulatory responsiveness with respect to maintaining P_{osm} and water balance in a narrow normal range.[195] A change of only 5 percent in P_{osm} can produce a fivefold increase in P_{ADH}, which spans the full range of renal water conservation from U_{min} to U_{max}. This change in U_{osm} can represent a tenfold reduction in urine volume, with most of the water conservation occurring at low levels of P_{ADH}. When the P_{osm} rises by only 1 to 2 percent, P_{ADH} rises from 1.0 to 2.0 pg/ml, U_{osm} doubles, and the urine volume is halved; each successive rise in P_{osm} and P_{ADH} results in successively smaller amounts of additional water reabsorption.

Changes in EABV also have important effects on ADH release and thirst.[193,195,210] These effects of EABV are mediated by stretch or volume receptors in the left atrium and by baroreceptors (pressure) in the aortic arch

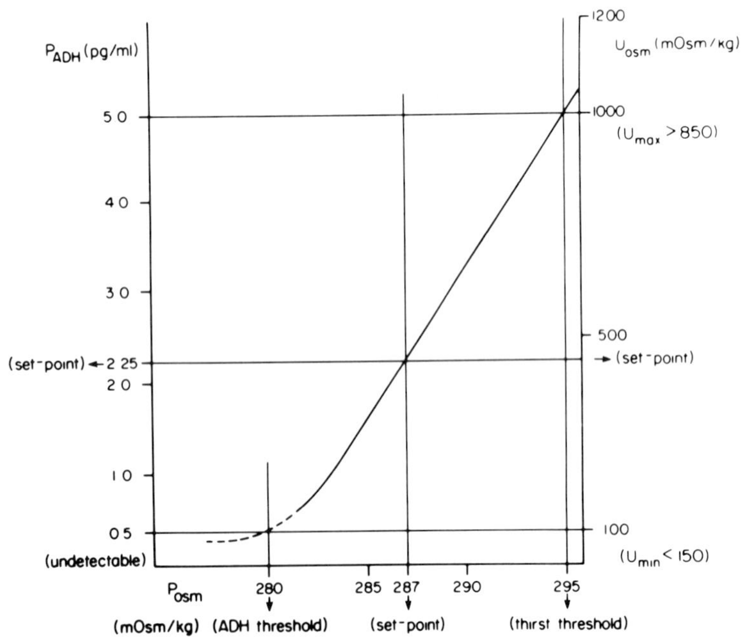

FIGURE 21-2 • Relationship between plasma osmolality (P_{osm}), plasma level of antidiuretic hormone (P_{ADH}), and urine osmolality (U_{osm}).

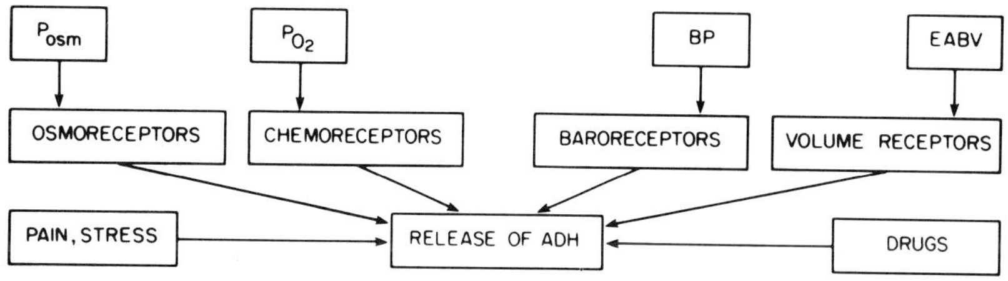

FIGURE 21-3 • Control of ADH release.

and carotid sinus. ADH release is very sensitive to changes in EABV: a 10 percent decrease in blood pressure can increase P_{ADH} to levels sufficient to achieve U_{max}. Although further decreases in blood pressure elevate P_{ADH} still more, renal water conservation is already at its limit. When acting in concert, a decrease in EABV increases the sensitivity of the ADH response to a given rise in P_{osm}; an increase in EABV has the opposite effect. Effective osmolality has a similar influence on the ADH response to a given change in EABV. When conflicting stimuli (e.g., a decrease in EABV and a decrease in P_{osm}) are received by the osmostat, the response to changes in EABV takes precedence over the response to changes in P_{osm}; in other words, the servomechanisms protect EABV even if a normal P_{osm} must be sacrificed.[210] For example, a decrease in EABV caused by hemorrhage will result in an increase in P_{ADH}; if water is available, the increased intake will be conserved by the kidney, resulting in a decreased P_{osm}, but without a decrease in P_{ADH} to the level expected by the lower P_{osm} alone. The result is hyponatremia, a common finding in states associated with EABV depletion.

In a sense, osmolality and EABV may be considered "physiological," or normal, stimuli for ADH release and thirst because the responses to these stimuli serve a recognizable homeostatic function. However, there are many other stimuli which influence ADH release and thirst which have no obvious homeostatic roles, and which can actually take precedence over the usual physiological stimuli.[194] For example, much of our water intake is conditioned by social and cultural influences that are not well related to physiological (osmotic or volumetric) needs. Such nonphysiological stimuli may also cause ADH release and excessive water retention (Fig. 21-3); both volume expansion and hyponatremia may result. (Chapter 4 provides more discussion of ADH regulation.)

ADH and the kidney

A detailed discussion of the mechanism of ADH action and the role of the kidney in water conservation is outside the scope of this chapter, and will only be outlined below (Chaps. 3 and 5 present extensive discussions).[69,91,113,195] ADH is thought to work by activating adenylate cyclase in the serosal (basolateral) membranes of the epithelial cells of the renal collecting tubules.[203,224] Through a series of intermediate biochemical steps, probably including protein phosphatases and phosphorylases, eventually the mucosal (luminal) membranes are made more permeable to water (see Fig. 21-4). The water flow occurs in response to the osmotic gradient from the lumen of the collecting duct to the interstitium of the renal medulla, and therefore strongly depends on the ability of the kidney to generate and maintain the osmotic gradient. Several anatomical elements of the epithelial cells, including intramembranous particle aggregates, cytoplasmic microfilaments, and intracellular microtubules, may be important in the transepithelial pathway.[195] Many other regulatory systems (e.g., calmodulin, prostaglandins, other cyclic nucleotides and hormones) are thought to be involved in modulating ADH-induced transepithelial water flow.[43,107,112,126,130]

Recent evidence suggests that as renal prostaglandin synthesis increases (e.g., as seen after an acute water load), the hydroosmotic actions of ADH are inhibited, possibly hastening the excretion of a water load and preventing over-hydration.[212]

With the development of new antagonists the physiological function of vasopressin may be further defined.[205]

Although an understanding of the fine mechanism of ADH action is of some importance in understanding de-

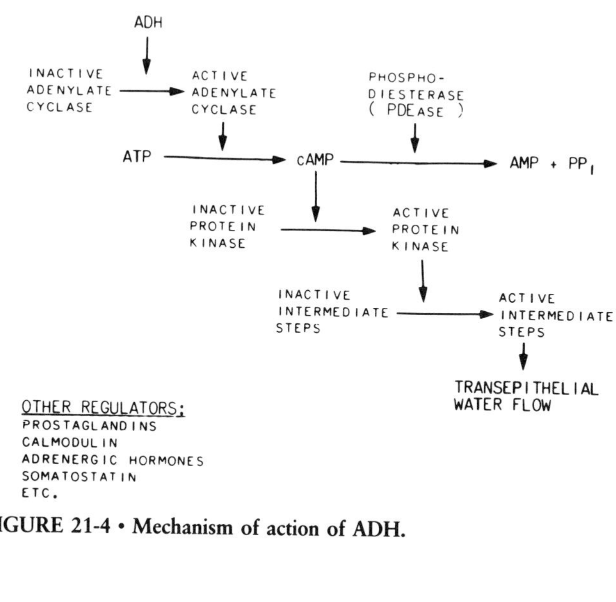

FIGURE 21-4 • Mechanism of action of ADH.

fects in renal water metabolism (particularly nephrogenic diabetes insipidus), a broad view is often more useful as a clinical starting point. In brief, when P_{ADH} levels are low (usually in response to a low P_{osm}), the distal portions of the nephron, particularly the collecting duct, are relatively impermeable to water. The result is the excretion of a relatively large volume of urine with a low U_{osm}, which would tend to raise the P_{osm} toward normal. In contrast, when P_{ADH} levels are high, the distal nephron is relatively permeable to water. Water may then be reabsorbed into the hyperosmolar interstitium of the renal medulla, allowing the U_{osm} to rise and the urinary volume to fall. The result is the excretion of a small volume of urine with a high U_{osm}, which would increase water conservation and lower P_{osm}. Thus, a normal end-organ (renal) response to the appropriate level of ADH is required for proper water balance.

NORMAL THIRST REGULATION

Although the perception of thirst and its regulation are the least well characterized aspects of human water metabolism,[2,76,84,85,88,108,194] there is little doubt that the afferent stimuli for the sensation of thirst include both osmolal and volumetric signals, both in animals and in humans. However, it is not clear how these signals are transmitted to the thirst center. For example, increases in either plasma or cerebrospinal fluid (CSF) sodium concentration can stimulate thirst (and ADH release), but it is not clear if changes in osmolality or in sodium concentration per se are the primary stimuli. Similar controversy surrounds the mediation of volumetric stimuli, which arrive at least from cardiac (left atrial) and from arterial (carotid, and probably renal) baroreceptors. The renin-angiotensin system plays a major role, but not the exclusive one, in mediating volumetric (but probably not osmolal) stimuli for thirst and ADH release. The relative importance of both centrally produced angiotensin II and peripherally produced, centrally acting angiotensin II,[88,139,195] enkephalins and other opiate mediators,[195] prostaglandins,[195] tachykinins,[15] and other neuroactive substances is still under investigation.[195]

Although it has traditionally been believed that the thirst center lies specifically in the hypothalamus and overlaps with the ADH-regulating center, the thirst system is at least partially separable from the ADH system; specific thirst-regulating neurons reside in the anterior wall of the third ventricle. Furthermore, the neuronal pathways mediating the osmolal and volumetric stimuli from their respective receptors to the higher (cortical) thirst centers probably have different neurotransmitters: the pathways mediating osmolal stimuli are probably cholinergic; at least some of the pathways mediating volumetric stimuli (via angiotensin II) are probably dopaminergic.

The study of thirst in humans is far more complicated than in animals.[85] The two normal physiological stimuli for thirst, increasing osmolality and decreasing EABV, are often obscured by cultural and social determinants of drinking behavior that have little or no relationship to physiological processes concerned with maintaining water balance. This situation is somewhat analogous to the inappropriate release of ADH in response to various stresses unrelated to either osmolal or volumetric stimuli. In contrast to studies of ADH release, there are no strictly quantitative, clinically well-accepted, standardized tests to evaluate the sensation of thirst in humans (see "Thirst testing," below).

Furthermore, many studies suggest that the state of EABV conditions the thirst response for a given osmolal stimulus, in a manner similar to that described for ADH release;[133] thus, the administration of hypertonic saline increases the osmolal but decreases the volumetric stimulus for thirst and ADH release, whereas the use of dehydration increases both stimuli (for the two responses). Consequently, the "threshold" at which the sensation of thirst appears, and the "sensitivity" ("gain") of thirst as a function of changes in either stimulus, are not rigorously defined with respect to either stimulus alone, or by a standardized procedure. Although some of the same problems exist in characterizing ADH release with respect to osmolal and volumetric stimuli in humans, standardized testing and measurements of ADH levels have permitted a greater understanding of ADH regulation than of thirst regulation under clinical conditions.

The detailed mechanism of regulating water intake is less well understood; Chap. 4 provides additional details. There does not seem to be any facultative control over the gastrointestinal absorption of water, and most of the regulation seems to depend on varying intake, that is, the sensation of thirst. It is clear that if thirst were solely dependent on the normal physiological stimuli, alterations in water intake alone might achieve water balance; this is an important consideration if the ADH-renal mechanism is not functioning properly. Unfortunately, many nonphysiological influences affect water intake, and many CNS disorders simultaneously disturb the ADH and thirst mechanisms.[85,137,189,195]

INTEGRATION OF ADH AND THIRST

The relationships between ADH and thirst in normal individuals have been characterized to a limited degree.[192,194] At a normal P_{osm} of 287 mosm/kg, the P_{ADH} level is set at about 2.25 pg/ml, which is just about the level needed to produce nearly half-maximal urine osmolality (about 500 mosm/kg; see Fig. 21-2). However, a normal individual does not usually experience thirst at this level of P_{osm}, which is the normal set point. If a standard overnight dehydration test is performed (see

"Dehydration tests," below), thirst is usually first expressed when the P_{osm} reaches about 295 mosm/kg, about a 2 percent increase in P_{osm}, and this is often considered a normal "osmolal threshold" for thirst, although the stimulus is complex (see "Thirst testing," below). At this P_{osm}, the level of P_{ADH} has risen to over 5.0 pg/ml, more than sufficient to achieve the max U_{osm} of about 1200 mosm/kg. Thus, the thirst mechanism for increased water intake in response to "osmolal" stimuli does not seem to become active in humans until after the ADH mechanism for renal water retention is already at its highest activity.

Animal data suggest that ADH release is also more sensitive than thirst to volumetric stimuli; about a 10 percent decrease in EABV (produced by hemorrhage) will increase P_{ADH}, but a 20 percent decrease in EABV may be needed to elicit thirst.[2,3] If these conclusions are applicable to humans, the steady state for water metabolism must be maintained primarily by variations in ADH release (renal water retention). Thirst only becomes important when renal water conservation is inadequate to maintain acceptable values for EABV and osmolality.

On the other side of the normal set point, water loading sufficient to reduce P_{osm} by about 3 percent reduces P_{ADH} to undetectable levels (less than about 0.5 pg/ml) and achieves a min U_{osm} (usually less than 75 mosm/kg); the sensation of thirst is absent over this entire range of P_{osm} (from about 287 to 291 mosm/kg). After the apparent threshold for thirst is reached by dehydration, water ingestion usually proceeds until a P_{osm} well below the threshold is attained; thus the sensation of thirst does not reappear immediately after water intake ceases.[2,3,85,195] There is also preabsorptive suppression of thirst following water ingestion, but the mechanism is not well understood.

SUMMARY OF NORMAL OSMOREGULATORY SERVOMECHANISMS: ADH AND THIRST

Thirst regulation is similar in many ways to ADH regulation. The two regulatory functions reside in partially overlapping areas in the CNS, respond to similar osmolal and volumetric stimuli, and act in the same direction with respect to TBW and osmolality. However, there are important differences in the two regulatory systems. Thirst regulation is much less well studied in humans, at least partly owing to a lack of standardized clinical tests. In general, thirst seems more sensitive to nonosmolal, nonvolumetric influences than is ADH release, although both systems can be governed by such influences. Finally, ADH release seems critical for regulation around euvolemia and the normal osmolal set point in humans; thirst and increased water intake only become important after substantial increases in P_{osm} or decreases in EABV, when the P_{ADH} has already reached levels sufficient for max U_{osm}.[195]

PHYSIOLOGY AND PATHOPHYSIOLOGY OF HYPEROSMOLAR STATES

The following sections describe the regulation of water and solute transfer between the extracellular fluid (ECF) and intracellular fluid (ICF) compartments, emphasizing pathophysiological mechanisms.[78] A more detailed discussion of the regulation of cell volume and the compartmentation of body water may be found in Chap. 1.

ISOSMOLALITY AND HYPEROSMOLALITY

Normal distribution of water and solute

Water accounts for approximately 60 percent of body weight in males, but closer to 50 percent in females (reflecting the slightly greater adipose tissue content of women).[28] Two-thirds of the TBW is located inside cells (ICF compartment); the remaining one-third is extracellular. The intravascular fluid accounts for one-quarter of the ECF; the remaining three-quarters is contained in the interstitial fluid compartment. (See Fig. 21-5.)

The ECF and ICF differ in size and solute composition.[28,162] Sodium salts (principally chloride and bicarbonate) are the major ECF solutes, whereas potassium and magnesium salts (principally phosphates, proteinates, and sulfates) are the major intracellular solutes. The cell membranes which separate the ICF and ECF are relatively permeable to water, but are not freely permeable to these osmotically active solutes.[28,196] Since two-thirds of the total quantity of solutes is located in the ICF and one-third in the ECF, and since water distributes

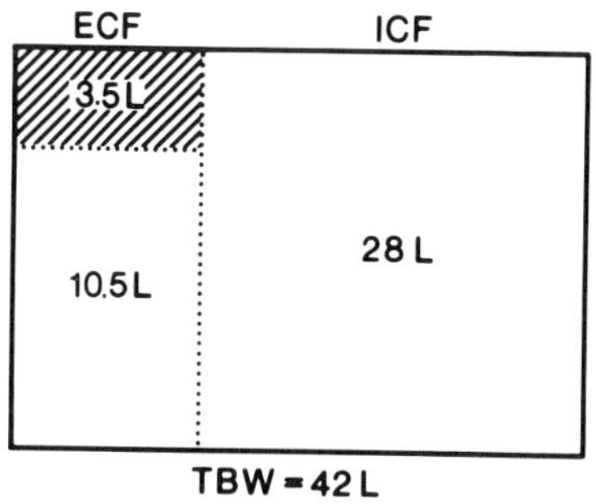

FIGURE 21-5 • Body fluid compartments. Total body water (TBW) accounts for 60 percent of lean body mass in a 70-kg man (42 liters). Two-thirds of TBW (28 liters) is located in the intracellular fluid compartment (ICF) and one-third (14 liters) is located in the extracellular fluid compartment (ECF). One-quarter of the ECF (3.5 liters) is intravascular (shaded area); three-quarters (10.5 liters) of ECF is interstitial.

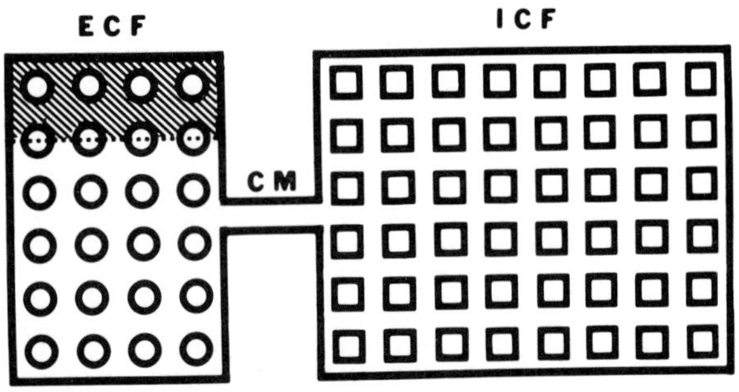

FIGURE 21-6 • Distribution of water and solute. The larger square (right) represents the intracellular fluid (ICF) compartment and the smaller square (left) represents the extracellular fluid (ECF) compartment. The bridge connecting the two compartments represents the cell membranes. The volumes of the two compartments are represented by the areas of the outer squares. The small symbols (open squares, open circles) represent intracellular solutes (largely potassium salts) and extracellular solutes (largely sodium salts), respectively. The number of small symbols represents the solute content of each compartment, and the density of symbols represents the solute concentration (osmolality) of the compartment. Under normal circumstances, the ICF contains two-thirds and the ECF contains one-third of the total body solute (TBS). Since all membranes are completely permeable to water, the osmolalities of the two compartments are equal in the steady state. Consequently, two-thirds of the total body water (TBW) is located in the ICF and one-third is located in the ECF. The volumes of the two compartments then reflect their respective "effective" solute contents. (From Feig PU, McCurdy DK: *N Engl J Med* 297:1444, 1977, with permission.)

according to the amount of osmotically active solute contained in each compartment, the ICF in the steady state contains two-thirds of TBW and the ECF contains one-third (Fig. 21-6). The compartmental distribution of water reflects the more restricted compartmental distribution of solutes; except in the renal medulla, water moves to dissipate any osmotic gradients (see Chap. 5).

Sodium salts (chloride and bicarbonate) and glucose (in the absence of insulin) are considered *impermeant* solutes because they are relatively restricted to the ECF, and "effective osmoles" because they exert an osmotic force for water movement across cell membranes. Glucose is most effective as an osmole when given very rapidly in the absence of insulin; glucose is least effective as an osmole when given very slowly in the presence of insulin.[79,80] In contrast, solutes which distribute evenly between ECF and ICF are called *permeant*; they are not effective osmoles because they do not generate an osmotic force across the cell membranes and do not promote water transfer between the ECF and the ICF. Urea, methanol, and ethanol are examples of permeant solutes.[7,79,80,123,143,157]

Under normal circumstances, the plasma osmolality is the measurement used in clinical medicine to determine the concentration of ECF solutes. Since the osmolalities of almost all body fluids (both ICF and ECF) are the same in the steady state, the measured P_{osm} represents the osmolality of all body fluid compartments. Note that the measured ECF osmolality is the sum of both impermeant solutes (e.g., sodium salts, glucose) and permeant solutes (e.g., urea). The freezing-point-depression method of determining P_{osm} used by most clinical laboratories depends on the total number of osmotically active particles, not on their permeability.

If direct measurement of P_{osm} is not available, it can be estimated from the following relationship:

$$P_{osm} = 2[Na^+] + \frac{[glucose]}{18} + \frac{[BUN]}{2.8} \qquad (1)$$

Here, $[Na^+]$ is given in meq/liter, [glucose] and [BUN] (blood urea nitrogen) in mg/100 dl.* For example, with $[Na^+]$ = 140 meq/liter, [glucose]L = 100 mg/dl, and [BUN] = 20 mg/dl, the calculation for estimating P_{osm} is

$$P_{osm} = 2(140) + \frac{100}{18} + \frac{20}{2.8} = 293 \text{ mosm/kg} \qquad (2)$$

The normal range of P_{osm} is 280 to 295 mosm/kg. Under certain conditions the equation for calculating P_{osm} must be expanded to include other solutes (permeant and impermeant) which could be present in substantial quantities (i.e., solutes other than sodium salts, glucose, and urea). For example, the presence of ethanol, methanol, mannitol, sorbitol, or glycerol in the ECF elevates the measured P_{osm} and must be considered in calculating an estimate of P_{osm}. If any of these substances is present, Equation 1 must be modified as follows:

$$P_{osm} = 2[Na^+] + \frac{[glucose]}{18} + \frac{[BUN]}{2.8} + [X] \qquad (3)$$

where [X] is given (in mg/dl) by

$$\frac{[ethanol]}{4.6} \text{ or } \frac{[methanol]}{3.2} \text{ or } \frac{[mannitol]}{18} \text{ or } \frac{[sorbitol]}{18}$$

$$\text{or } \frac{[glycerol]}{9}$$

In Equation 3, [X] = the concentration of the substance in mg/dl divided by 1/10 of its molecular weight in grams. If more than one such substance is present, each should be added as a separate term. By definition, if P_{osm} exceeds 295 mosm/kg, then body fluids are *hyperosmolal* (too concentrated); if P_{osm} is

* The concentration of glucose (mg/dl) is converted to osmolality (mosm/kg) by assuming that the molecular weight of glucose is 180 g/mole and the density of water is 1 kg/liter. Therefore, the blood glucose concentration is divided by 180 (to convert to mmol/dl) and multiplied by 10 (to convert to mmol/liter). These two corrections are usually combined (180/10), so blood glucose is divided by 18 to convert to mmol/liter. Since for a nondissociable species such as glucose, 1 mole = 1 osmole, the same correction converts to mosm/kg (1 liter = 1 kg, for water under standard conditions). The contribution of urea to the osmolality is derived in a similar fashion; however, BUN refers only to the two nitrogen atoms in urea, whose molecular weight = 14 g/atom, and not to the whole urea molecule (molecular weight = 60 g/atom). Therefore, the BUN in mg/dl is divided by 2.8, that is, by 14 × (2/10) to arrive at mmol/liter (= mosm/kg).

below 280 mosm/kg, body fluids are *hyposmolal* (too dilute).[79,80]

Hyperosmolality, effective osmolality, and tonicity

A clinical determination more useful than plasma osmolality is "effective" osmolality; whereas P_{osm} includes the concentrations of all ECF solutes, both permeant and impermeant, "effective" osmolality is determined only by the concentrations of impermeant solutes, that is, those solutes that cause water to transfer between the ICF and the ECF. "Effective" osmolality is more conveniently termed *tonicity*. The tonicity of the ECF is not measured; it is estimated from an equation that includes only those substances which remain restricted outside cell membranes. Under normal clinical conditions the following equation is used to estimate the effective osmolality or tonicity of ECF:

$$\text{Effective } P_{osm} \text{ or tonicity} = 2[\text{Na}^+] + \frac{[\text{glucose}]}{18} \qquad (4)$$

where $[\text{Na}^+]$ is given in meq/liter and [glucose] is given in mg/dl. For example, if the Na^+ concentration is 140 meq/liter and the glucose concentration is 100 mg/dl, then the effective P_{osm} or tonicity would be estimated by the equation:

$$\text{Effective } P_{osm} \text{ or tonicity} = 2(140) + \frac{100}{18} \qquad (5)$$

$$= 286 \text{ mosm/kg}$$

The normal range for effective P_{osm} is 275 to 290 mosm/kg. Both ethanol and methanol are similar to urea in that they contribute to the P_{osm} but not to the effective P_{osm} or tonicity. In contrast, mannitol, sorbitol, and glycerol are relatively restricted to the ECF; they therefore contribute to both P_{osm} and effective P_{osm} (tonicity) (see Fig. 21-7).[79,80]

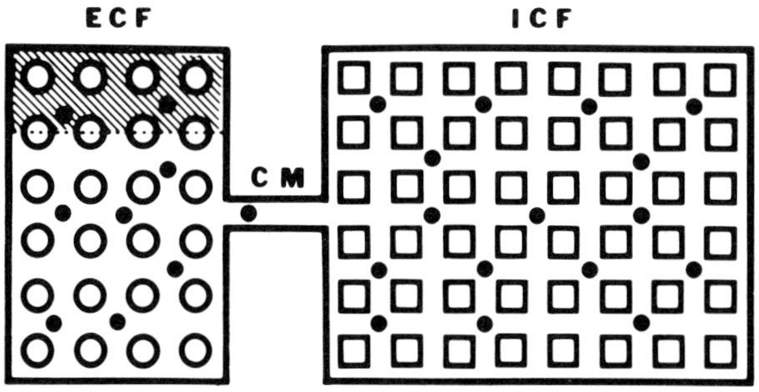

FIGURE 21-7 • Hyperosmolality without hypertonicity (permeant solute gain). An "ineffective" (permeant) solute, such as urea or ethanol (small solid circles), diffuses across all cell membranes; it therefore distributes throughout TBW. Thus, permeant solutes do not exert an osmotic force for water movement from one compartment to another, and there is no change in the volumes of the ECF or ICF. Hyperosmolality, but not hypertonicity, is the result of addition of a permeant solute. See Fig. 21-6 for explanation of symbols. (From Feig PU, McCurdy DK: *N Engl J Med* 297:1444, 1977, with permission.)

In the steady state, the tonicities of the ECF and ICF are (like the osmolalities) equal, because water moves freely across the separating cell membranes. In most normal individuals, a value two times the ECF sodium concentration corresponds well to the effective P_{osm} or tonicity. Furthermore, conditions that initially elevate the ECF sodium content eventually increase the osmolality and tonicity of both ECF and ICF. Because sodium is restricted to the ECF, the rise in ECF sodium content results in increases in ECF sodium concentration, osmolality, and tonicity. In response to the osmotic gradient water moves from the ICF to the ECF until the gradient is dissipated and the osmolalities of the ECF and ICF are equal. Therefore, in the steady state, conditions associated with hypernatremia, with hyperglycemia, or with the presence of other effective osmoles, cause similar increases in tonicity and water movement; the effective P_{osm} is therefore a reasonable estimate of the steady-state tonicity of both ECF and ICF.

Since those clinical conditions associated with hypertonicity often have neurological sequelae, whereas those associated with hyperosmolality in the absence of hypertonicity are not usually associated with such neurological sequelae, the distinction between hyperosmolal and hypertonic states is important. While the presence of hypertonicity always implies hyperosmolality, hyperosmolality does not always mean hypertonicity. Readers are warned that (unfortunately) many textbooks of clinical medicine use these terms interchangeably.[10]

PATHOPHYSIOLOGY OF HYPEROSMOLALITY

Hyperosmolality without hypertonicity

Pathophysiological conditions that increase the BUN (e.g., uremia), and some other clinical conditions (e.g., ethanol or methanol ingestion) raise the plasma osmolality but do not result in ECF expansion because these permeant solutes distribute evenly between ECF and ICF (Fig. 21-7). For ineffective osmoles like urea there are increased but equal solute concentrations in the two compartments. Azotemia, for example, does not produce an alteration in relative compartment volumes because the absence of an osmotic gradient precludes an intercompartmental shift of water. A patient with uremia who has a [BUN] = 210 mg/dl, serum $[\text{Na}^+]$ = 125 meq/liter, and [glucose] = 90 mg/dl is hyperosmolal, as shown by applying Equation 1,

$$P_{osm} = 2(125) + \frac{90}{18} + \frac{210}{2.8} = 330 \text{ mosm/kg} \qquad (6)$$

Such a patient is also hypotonic, as Equation 4 shows,

$$\text{Effective } P_{osm} = 2[125] + \frac{[90]}{18} = 255 \text{ mosm/kg} \qquad (7)$$

The distribution of urea in this hyperosmolal but not hypertonic patient is shown in Fig. 21-7. Any condition that affects the concentrations of solutes in all body compartments, but that does not alter the effective osmolality or tonicity of any body compartment, does not create a primary problem with water regulation.

Hyperosmolality with hypertonicity

There are three forms of hyperosmolality with hypertonicity: pure water loss, hypotonic fluid loss, and impermeant solute gain. Each of these forms has some unique characteristics, but they also have several features in common.

Pure water loss

Body fluid tonicity was defined above as the ratio of the molar quantity of impermeant solute (or effective osmole) in a compartment to its water content (by mass). Consequently, hypertonicity can occur as a result of either net loss of water or net gain of impermeant solute.[79,80] Net water loss can occur when the body loses excessive quantities either of electrolyte-free fluids (pure water) or of relatively more water than electrolyte (hypotonic fluid). Loss of electrolyte-free water results in the contraction of both ECF and ICF compartments in the same proportion as the original distribution of TBW; thus two-thirds of the water loss comes from the ICF and one-third comes from the ECF (Fig. 21-8). Since there is no change in the solute content of either compartment, the water loss concentrates all solutes and raises both the osmolality and the tonicity of the two compartments. The loss from the intravascular compartment (which represents one-fourth of the ECF) is thus only one-twelfth of the total body water loss (Table 21-1). Most of the water loss comes from the ICF, rather than the ECF; most of the ECF loss comes from the interstitial compartment. For these reasons conditions associated with loss of electrolyte-free fluids rarely present with clinical hypotension or shock until the losses are extreme.

TABLE 21-1 • Physiological changes due to pure water loss

Loss of 1 liter of electrolyte-free water	
PARAMETER	NET CHANGE
P_{osm}	+ 7.5 mosm/liter
Sodium content	0
TBW	− 1000 ml
ECF volume	− 333 ml
Plasma volume	− 83 ml

Hypotonic fluid loss

When hypotonic fluids (water in excess of electrolyte) are lost, both the ICF and the ECF compartments contract appreciably (Fig. 21-9). The hypotonic losses may be considered as consisting of two components: a volume of pure water (i.e., with no electrolyte content) and a volume of solution that has an electrolyte content equal to that of TBW. For example (Table 21-2), the loss of 2 liters of half-isotonic saline (with a total electrolyte content equal to that of 1 liter of normal ECF)) can be thought of as the loss of 1 liter of pure water and 1 liter of isotonic saline. The loss of pure water results in contraction of both ICF and ECF compartments in proportion to their original distribution.[79,80] However, the loss of iso-

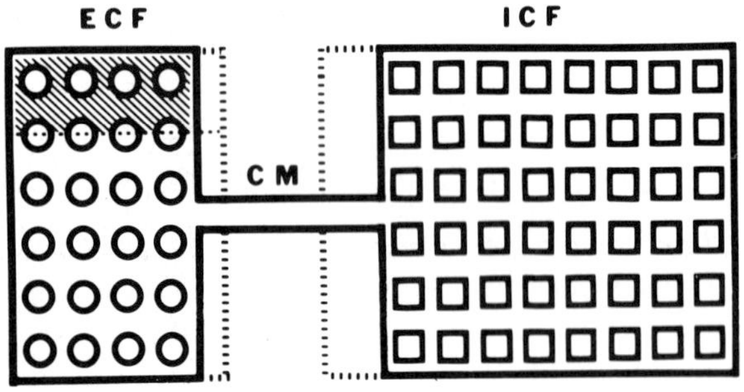

FIGURE 21-8 • Hypertonicity due to pure water loss. A pure water deficit is shared proportionally by all body fluid compartments, according to the "effective" solute content of each compartment. Therefore, both the ECF and the ICF will contract; ⅔ of the deficit will be derived from the ICF and ⅓ from the ECF. Only $\frac{1}{12}$ of the total water loss will be derived from the intravascular compartment. (The dotted lines indicate the normal volumes of the body fluid compartments, as shown in Fig. 21-6.) The total amount of solute in each compartment remains constant, but the solute concentration (osmolality) increases. See Fig. 21-6 for explanation of symbols. (From Feig PU, McCurdy DK: *N Engl J Med* 297:1444, 1977, with permission.)

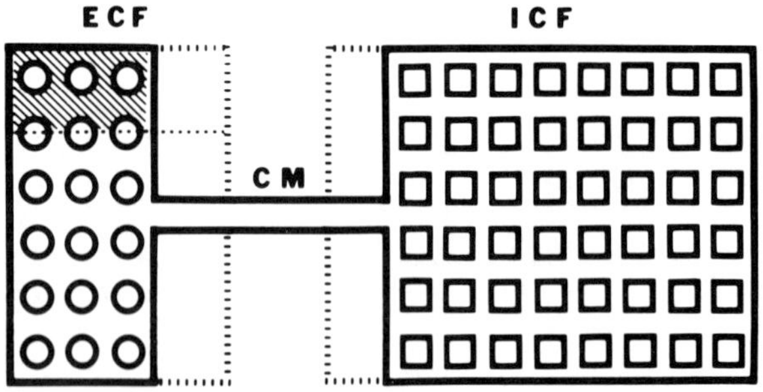

FIGURE 21-9 • Hypertonicity due to hypotonic fluid loss. Loss of hypotonic fluid from the ECF causes ECF and intravascular volume to contract to a greater degree than does the loss of pure water. In this figure, it is assumed that the hypotonic fluid loss has an electrolyte content of about ⅓ of normal ECF. Although the total volume loss is only 50 percent more than with pure water loss (compare Figure 21-8), the contraction of the intravascular volume exceeds that of a pure water loss by 150 percent. The degree of ICF contraction and the degree of hypertonicity are the same in the two cases. See Fig. 21-6 for explanation of symbols. (From Feig PU, McCurdy DK: *N Engl J Med* 297:1444, 1977, with permission.)

TABLE 21-2 • **Physiological changes due to hypotonic fluid loss**

	Loss of 2 liters of half-isotonic NaCl solution			
PARAMETER	LOSS OF 1 LITER ISOTONIC SALINE	+	LOSS OF 1 LITER H_2O	NET CHANGE
P_{osm}	0		+ 7.5 mosm/liter	+ 7.5 mosm/liter
Sodium content	− 150 meq		0	− 150 meq
TBW	− 1000 ml		− 1000 ml	− 2000 ml
ECF volume	− 1000 ml		− 333 ml	− 1333 ml
Plasma volume	− 250 ml		− 83 ml	− 333 ml

tonic saline results in a selective contraction of the ECF because sodium salts are essentially restricted to the ECF. Since the volume of the intravascular compartment is one-quarter of the ECF volume, a substantial decrease in the intravascular volume occurs, and in contrast to loss of pure water, the loss of even moderate quantities of sodium-containing hypotonic fluids can result in hypotension. In other words, the loss of electrolyte-containing fluids results in disproportionate contraction of that compartment to which that electrolyte is normally restricted. Hence, the loss of fluids containing only potassium salts would result in the disproportionate contraction of the ICF. Loss of fluids containing both sodium and potassium salts would result in contractions of the ECF and ICF compartments, respectively, in proportion to the relative content of the two electrolytes in the fluids lost.

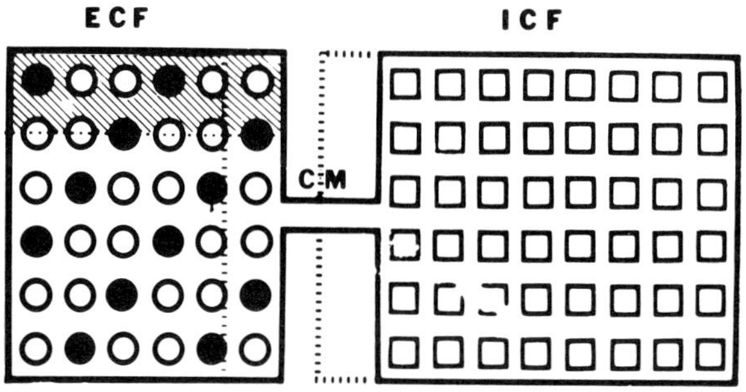

FIGURE 21-10 • Hypertonicity due to impermeant solute gain. The addition of an "effective" solute to the ECF expands the ECF compartment and contracts the ICF compartment as water moves from the ICF to the ECF in response to the osmotic gradient. The relative volumes of the two compartments change to reflect their present relative solute contents. Therefore, when the steady state (osmolal equilibrium) is reached, all body fluids are equally hypertonic. See Fig. 21-6 for explanation of symbols. (From Feig PU, McCurdy DK: *N Engl J Med* 297:1444, 1977, with permission.)

Impermeant solute gain

As previously discussed, only the addition of an impermeant solute can increase the tonicity of TBW. The addition of such a solute (e.g., a sodium salt) to the ECF immediately increases ECF osmolality (and tonicity). Since the solute in this case is restricted to the ECF, the osmotic gradient promotes water movement from the ICF to the ECF, increasing the osmolality (and tonicity) of the ICF. The result is an increase in the volume of the ECF and a decrease in the volume of the ICF. When the steady state is reached, the osmolality (and tonicity) of the two compartments will be the same and there will be no further net water transfer between ICF and ECF (Fig. 21-10). Note that the selective addition of a *potassium* salt would result in an *increase* in the volume of the ICF since potassium is restricted thereto; water would then move from the ECF to the ICF, resulting in contraction of the ECF until the osmolalities of ECF and ICF are equal. Both osmolalities, of course, would be elevated: since total body salt (TBS) has increased, with no change in TBW, the osmolality (TBS/TBW) must increase. The selective increase in ICF volume, occasioned by a shift in water from the ECF, has an important clinical correlate: when insulin is used in the treatment of hyperglycemia, the shift of glucose from the ECF to the ICF may be faster than glucose metabolism to CO_2 and H_2O inside the cells; this transient increase in ICF solute results in a corresponding shift of water from the ECF, including the intravascular compartment, and can cause hypotension.

In summary, the presence of hyperosmolality does not always mean hypertonicity is present; but the presence of hypertonicity always means that hyperosmolality is present. Hypertonicity is always associated with an increase in total body impermeant solute content, a decrease in TBW content, or both.

Consequences of hypertonicity

The effects of hypertonicity are discussed in detail in Chap. 4 and will be treated only briefly here. The response of cells to ECF hypertonicity depends on the cell type, the specific impermeant solute, and the rapidity with which hypertonicity develops.[9,10] Rapid development of hypertonicity dehydrates all cells, but when hypertonicity develops slowly or has been present for some time (hours to days) some cells (e.g., red blood cells) gain intracellular solute and partially correct their dehydration.

The brain is particularly vulnerable to water loss because rapid cerebral dehydration can rupture the blood

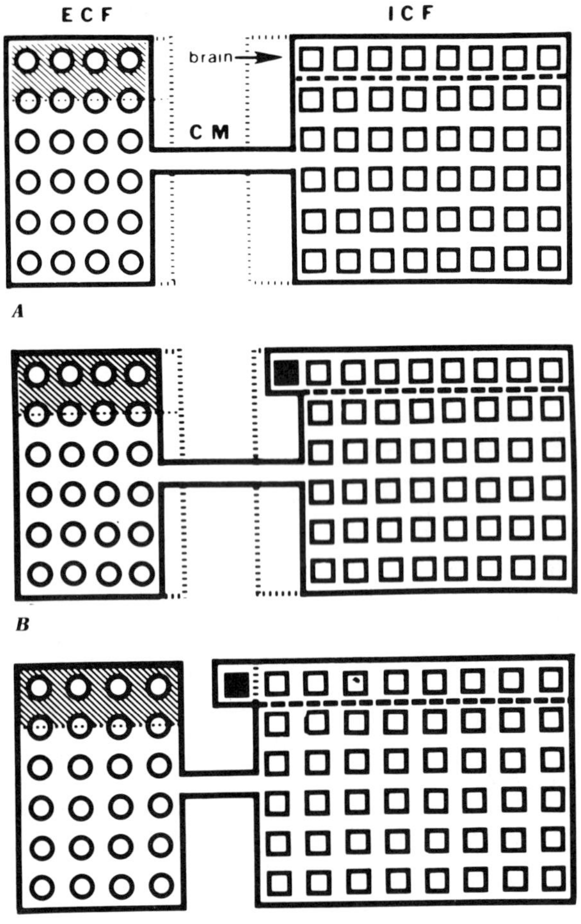

FIGURE 21-11 • The brain in hypertonic states. (A) The dashed line in the upper portion of the larger square (ICF, right) separates the brain from the rest of the ICF (the size of the brain is exaggerated relative to the whole ICF). In the early phase of hypertonicity the brain shares the water loss incurred by the rest of the ICF, in proportion to its solute content. (B) Later in the course of hypertonicity, the appearance of idiogenic osmoles (solid square) allows the brain to expand somewhat back toward its volume. (C) Correction of hypertonicity by rapid replacement of water deficits results in overexpansion of the brain due to the presence of the extra osmoles. The hypertonicity must be corrected slowly enough to allow the idiogenic osmoles to disappear if cerebral edema is to be avoided. See Fig. 21-6 for explanation of symbols. (From Feig PU, McCurdy DK: *N Engl J Med* 297:1444, 1977, with permission.)

vessels that connect the brain to the rigid calvarium.[219] To protect itself from cellular dehydration, the brain appears to generate new intracellular solute (sometimes called "idiogenic osmoles") (Fig. 21-11). Intracellular osmolality is thus increased, reducing the loss of intracellular water associated with hypertonicity.[79,80] The identities of many idiogenic osmoles are still uncertain, although evidence seems to implicate three major groups of organic molecules that serve as biological osmoles: polyols (e.g., myoinositol, sorbitol), trimethylamines (e.g., betaine, glycerophosphorylcholine), and amino acids and their derivatives (e.g., glutamate, glutamine, taurine) in addition to sodium, potassium, and urea.[141] The speed of formation and the composition of the idiogenic osmoles depend on the cause and time course of the hypertonicity. Idiogenic osmoles normally are produced slowly. During hypertonicity they can maintain brain cell volume close to normal.[9] However, if there is insufficient time to form these idiogenic osmoles, brain cell dehydration occurs and neurological disturbances follow.[166]

Thus, brain cells (and perhaps some other cell types) may have special adaptive mechanisms for maintaining cell volume. Although the production of idiogenic osmoles could be an accidental effect of brain cell injury, most investigators believe it represents a true homeostatic mechanism. This unique brain adaptation has important clinical implications. If hyperosmolality were to be rapidly corrected by intake of electrolyte-free water, the increased amount of intracellular water associated with idiogenic osmoles could lead to cerebral edema and the syndrome of *isotonic water intoxication*. This clinical hazard would persist until the idiogenic osmoles were removed or inactivated; the kinetics of their disposition is unknown.[10]

CLINICAL DISORDERS ASSOCIATED WITH HYPEROSMOLALITY

HYPEROSMOLALITY WITHOUT HYPERTONICITY

Although many disorders of body fluid osmolality are associated with corresponding changes in tonicity, this is not the case when an "ineffective" (permeant) solute like urea or ethanol accounts for the hyperosmolar state.[10] The distinction is clinically important because the presence of hyperosmolality without hypertonicity does not necessarily indicate a need to increase TBW, whereas hyperosmolality associated with hypertonicity almost always indicates a need to increase TBW.

Hyperosmolality due to urea content

In normal individuals, urea, the major nitrogenous end product of protein catabolism, is primarily eliminated from the body by urinary excretion. With constant urea production the amount of urea excreted in a given time period represents the difference between the load of urea filtered [i.e., the product of the blood urea concentration (mol/liter) and the GFR (liters/min)] and the flow-dependent reabsorption of urea in the distal portions of the nephron. Patients with steady-state renal failure have a diminished GFR and an increased flow rate per nephron. However, the decrease in urea reabsorption cannot compensate for the decrease in GFR, and the concentration of urea in the blood rises as a result, until the filtered load is nearly normal. After three to four days of acute renal failure[8,178] or after two weeks of chronic renal failure,[17] the steady state both in humans and in experimental animals is characterized by reduced GFR, elevated concentration of urea in all body fluids, and normal urinary urea excretion. Assuming a constant rate of production, urea excretion is nearly equal to urea production.

An elevation in ECF urea concentration causes hyperosmolality (Equation 1) but not hypertonicity (Equation 4), because the urea concentration has risen to the same degree in the intracellular water. In fact, individuals with renal failure often have a low serum sodium concentration, which might indicate an increased TBW (see Chaps. 41 and 43). In such a circumstance the plasma tonicity might be reduced while the plasma osmolality is elevated. For example, consider an individual with plasma $[Na^+]$ = 125 meq/liter, blood [glucose] = 100 mg/dl, and [BUN] = 150 mg/dl. The (measured or calculated) $P_{osm} = (2)(125) + (100/18) + (150/2.8) = 308.5$ mosm per kilogram of water, which is clearly greater than normal (hyperosmolal); however, the calculated plasma tonicity would be $P_{tonicity} = (2)(125) + (100/18) = 255.5$ mosm per kilogram of water, which is clearly below normal (hypotonic). In fact, water restriction might be clinically indicated to deal with hypotonicity, although the patient is hyperosmolal (see Chap. 20).

In addition to patients with renal failure, patients with normal renal function but markedly increased protein catabolism (as, for example, in postoperative states or corticosteroid administration), or who receive large quantities of protein- or amino acid-containing solutions (as are used for hyperalimentation) may have elevated BUN levels. In these circumstances urea production from endogenous or exogenous protein catabolism exceeds urea excretion by the kidney (and to a lesser extent, by the liver and gastrointestinal tract); the blood urea concentration rises until the elimination rate equals the production rate. Some hyperalimentation solutions (e.g., Fre-Amine E) have been designed to provide only eight essential amino acids with glucose and water, to minimize the symptomatic elevation in BUN in patients with renal failure. The amino acids are metabolized by pathways that do not lead to urea production; adequate calories are provided to minimize endogenous protein catabolism. However, both hyperalimentation and hypercatabolic states can be associated with hyperosmolality, which may or may not be associated with hypertonicity.

Direct infusion of urea presents a special problem because the rate of infusion is an important consideration. Although rarely used today, rapid urea infusion was formerly used as osmotic diuretic therapy to treat cerebral edema.[216] Rapid urea infusions can cause water to shift from the ICF to the ECF and produce an osmotic diuresis, because the rate of water movement from ICF to ECF exceeds the rate of urea movement in the opposite direction, at least transiently. The resultant water shifts in the CNS are probably responsible for the clinical findings (headaches, seizures, muscular twitching, coma, EEG abnormalities),[216] since slower infusions of urea do not produce these neurological effects although the same BUN may be achieved. This hypothesis is supported by animal studies that show that urea equilibration between plasma and muscle water occurs in 1 h after urea infusion,[127] but may not be complete between plasma and CSF water even after 4 to 10 h.[127] Thus, rapid urea infusions produce a transient increase in effective osmolality, although urea is a relatively permeant solute. Slower urea infusions, or longer equilibration times, confirm that urea is a permeant solute, with no effect on tonicity when the steady state is reached.

Hyperosmolality due to alcohol content

Alcohols such as methanol and ethanol are very permeant and increase P_{osm} without a change in plasma tonicity even at rapid rates of infusion (Equation 3). Clinical alcohol intoxication can usually be recognized (by euphoria or impaired coordination) at blood ethanol levels of 30 to 50 mg/dl; ataxia may be evident at about 100 mg/dl, and stupor or coma may develop at concentrations above 300 to 400 mg/dl. Over this range of plasma ethanol concentrations (30 to 400 mg/dl), ethanol raises the P_{osm} from 6.5 to 86.9 mosm/kg water above normal. The P_{osm} returns to normal as the ethanol (mol wt = 46 g) is eliminated and plasma levels fall to zero.

Methanol intoxication has a less predictable clinical course, but death has been observed after an ingestion of as little as 20 ml. In contrast to ethanol intoxication, methanol poisoning is usually manifested by severe metabolic acidosis and damage to the retina and the optic nerve, often leading to blindness (see Chap. 25). As long as methanol is present in the plasma the P_{osm} will be elevated, but there will be no increase in plasma tonicity because methanol distributes rapidly throughout TBW. Management of methanol intoxication includes treatment of the metabolic acidosis, removal of methanol by peritoneal dialysis or hemodialysis, and administration of ethanol to compete with methanol and inhibit the metabolism of methanol to toxic metabolites. The elevation in plasma osmolality is not indicative of hypertonicity or cellular dehydration in either methanol or ethanol intoxication.

HYPEROSMOLALITY WITH HYPERTONICITY

Pure water loss: Diabetes insipidus, insensible loss, hypodipsia

Clinical disorders that cause essentially "pure" water loss are important but relatively uncommon causes of hypertonicity. Such disorders result from (1) inadequate water intake alone (e.g., primary hypodipsia), (2) excessive urinary loss of relatively electrolyte-free water (e.g., diabetes insipidus), or (3) increased insensible (cutaneous and pulmonary) losses (e.g., hyperthermia). Conditions that cause pure water loss concentrate the solutes of all body fluids; the water is lost in the same proportion as it is normally distributed in the body (two-thirds from the ICF and one-third from ECF). Since sodium is a primary ECF solute, pure water loss produces hypernatremia. As Equation 4 indicates, the effective plasma osmolality (tonicity) increases. The pathophysiological consequences of pure water loss are shown in Fig. 21-8.

General characteristics and types of diabetes insipidus

Diabetes insipidus (DI) is the term used for all clinical disorders that impair renal water conservation.[196] The clinical presentation is usually independent of etiology: polydipsia and polyuria are characteristic, with the excretion of large quantities of relatively electrolyte-free urine. The urine is inappropriately dilute relative to plasma tonicity and the patient's needs. There is also a tendency toward rapid and severe volume depletion if water intake is restricted. These disorders result from either an ADH deficiency originating in the CNS (central diabetes insipidus) or a lack of renal responsiveness to normal P_{ADH} levels (nephrogenic diabetes insipidus, NDI).[28]

A transient DI, either arginine vasopressin (AVP)-responsive (central) or AVP-resistant (nephrogenic) occurs infrequently during pregnancy (2 to 4 cases/100,000 pregnancies). A high incidence of such AVP-sensitive DI occurs in families with asymptomatic carriers for central DI. In such women, the increase in the metabolic clearance of AVP,[61] especially near term, probably exceeds the pituitary's capacity for AVP production. Following delivery, the DI generally resolves, but it has a tendency to recur and occasionally be more severe in subsequent pregnancies.

A different transient DI, unresponsive to exogenous AVP, has occurred in some pregnant women who have abnormal liver and renal function and a high incidence of hypertension. The etiology for the resistance to AVP is unknown. In other women who develop AVP-resistant DI, treatment with dDAVP is effective, suggesting inactivation of circulating endogenous AVP is etiologic. Because the placenta produces large quantities of the cystine aminopeptidase, vasopressinase, which inactivates AVP and oxytocin in vitro, it is possible the production of this enzyme during pregnancy causes rapid inactivation of AVP and results in the development of DI. Within 2 to 4 months of delivery, both of these forms of AVP-resistant DI resolve spontaneously.[73]

Central diabetes insipidus

Central diabetes insipidus (CDI) results from either absolute (complete CDI) or relative (partial CDI) lack of circulating ADH.[28,195,196] Defects at any of the following anatomical sites in the pathway of ADH production and release can cause CDI: (1) the osmoreceptor or "osmostat," (2) the hypothalamic nuclei responsible for ADH synthesis, (3) the axons of these nuclei, which transport ADH to the neurohypophysis, and (4) the neurohypophysis itself. Disorders that affect the osmostat often affect the nuclei, and disorders that affect one or both of these sites are often associated with disorders of thirst regulation as well.

ETIOLOGY OF CENTRAL DIABETES INSIPIDUS Table 21-3 details a variety of clinical disorders that can cause complete or partial CDI. Damage to the neurohypophysis, either accidental or secondary to surgical hypophysectomy, is the most common cause of CDI today. Destruction by invasive tumors, either primary or metastatic, is the next most common cause; the third most prevalent etiology is idiopathic and familial.

TABLE 21-3 • Etiology of central diabetes insipidus (CDI)

ACQUIRED
Posthypophysectomy
Posttrauma
Tumors (intracranial):
Primary
Craniopharyngioma
Pinealoma
Pituitary adenoma
Secondary (metastatic):
Breast
Leukemia
Infections:
Encephalitis
Meningitis
Guillain-Barré syndrome
Vascular disorders:
Hypoxia
Aneurysms
Sheehan's syndrome
Granulomas:
Histiocytosis X
Eosinophilic granuloma
Schüller-Christian disease
Sarcoidosis
Drugs:
Clonidine
Phencyclidine
Idiopathic syndromes:
Autoimmune diseases
HEREDITARY
X-linked
Congenital anomalies

CDI following hypophysectomy, tumors, and trauma In selected cases, hypophysectomy is performed for hypophyseal and hypothalamic tumors.[48] Either transient or permanent CDI occurs in at least 50 percent of these cases. The transient CDI may last for a few hours or for much longer; reversal is still possible after many years. Such surgery interrupts the hypothalamohypophyseal tract at the level of the sella turcica or above the median eminence, often resulting in retrograde degeneration of the hypothalamic nuclei. The extent (complete or partial) and the duration (transient or permanent) of postsurgical CDI depends on the degree of degeneration. Persistent and/or complete CDI do not result unless degeneration of the hypothalamic nuclei is extensive.[195] This suggests that ADH can be released directly into the systemic circulation in response to normal physiological stimuli, without being stored or released by the neurohypophysis.

A triphasic pattern often characterizes the disturbed osmoregulation following hypothalamohypophyseal surgery: (1) transient polyuria and polydipsia (CDI) usually appear immediately following surgery due to the traumatic, functional suppression of ADH release; (2) inappropriate antidiuresis (transient SI-ADH) appears after four or five days as ADH is released from the damaged or necrotic hypothalamohypophyseal neurons; and, finally, (3) polyuria and polydipsia return, usually reflecting permanent CDI.[6,28,213,214] On occasion (particularly with limited hypophyseal resections), there is a fourth phase, where normal osmoregulation resumes at the hypothalamic level.[195] In this case, the "third phase" would also have been a transient CDI.

Head trauma is now a very frequent cause of CDI, and may show a pattern of disturbed osmoregulation quite similar to that following hypophysectomy. More commonly, head trauma results in a transient edema and swelling of the brain (including the hypothalamus), which temporarily prevents the release of ADH, thereby causing transient CDI. Resolution of the cerebral edema usually results in complete restoration of neurohypophyseal function.[231]

Destruction and/or degeneration of the hypothalamic neurons (either nuclei or axons) are the probable mechanisms by which tumors cause CDI. The most common tumors associated with CDI are craniopharyngiomas, pinealomas, gliomas, chromophobe and other pituitary adenomas,[217] and metastatic tumors;[4,244] other space-occupying lesions, such as sarcoid granulomas,[165] behave in a similar fashion.[48] Central DI has frequently been found in children with Langerhans cell histiocytosis (histiocytosis X).[71] Within four years of the diagnosis 42 percent of children in one study developed CDI.[71] Rarely, a tumor may be associated with NDI, rather than CDI.[78]

As indicated previously, AVP-sensitive and AVP-resistant DI have developed in association with pregnancy.[38,72,73,117,132,142,215] Transient CDI has also been reported in association with hypoxic states,[19] hemorrhagic states,[237] or fevers of unknown origin (FUO).[187] When severe, untreated hyponatremia causes brain damage, both CDI and diabetes mellitus have developed and proved fatal.[87]

A newly recognized, rare congenital disorder, Wolfram's syndrome (WS), is also associated with DI. In its complete form, it is characterized by insulin-dependent diabetes mellitus (IDDM), optic atrophy (OA), DI, deafness, and dilatation of the urinary tract; the acronym for these characteristics is DIDMOAD. DI responds to the administration of vasopressin. At least 75 percent of these individuals have HLA-DRZ haplotype.[32,179]

Idiopathic and familial CDI Sporadic cases of CDI present in childhood with polyuria and polydipsia.[28,105,195] It is a result of selective and virtually complete destruction of the hypothalamic ADH-producing neurons. The etiology of the lesion is unknown. A familial form of this disorder is transmitted as an autosomal dominant trait; an X-linked recessive form has also been described.[28,195,200] Familial CDI appears early in life; its pathology and pathophysiology are indistinguishable from the sporadic variety.[180] Recent studies[206,207] have revealed that approximately one-third of patients with presumed idiopathic DI have autoantibodies to the vasopressin-secreting cells of the human hypothalamus, suggesting a variant of this disorder has an autoimmune component. A significant number of individuals with antivasopressin antibodies have hypothalamic invasion by histiocytosis X.[207,208,209] Furthermore, in individuals with CDI of childhood observed for up to 26 years, anterior pituitary dysfunction was a frequent association.[58] Confirmation of this provocative new finding is awaited.

CLINICAL PRESENTATION OF CDI Complete CDI is characterized by massive polyuria and polydipsia, in conjunction with an inability to concentrate the urine. Under most circumstances in adults, CDI has such an abrupt onset that the patient can often pinpoint the day it began.[48] The U_{osm} is always low (usually less than 100 mosm/kg) relative to P_{osm}. With adequate access to water and an intact thirst mechanism, which is frequently found in individuals with CDI,[229] the P_{osm} will be normal or only slightly elevated, despite the production of large volumes of hypotonic urine. With continued loss of such large volumes of relatively electrolyte-free urine, hypodipsia, or even modest water restriction results in severe dehydration, hypernatremia, and increased plasma osmolality and tonicity. If net loss exceeds 7 liters of electrolyte-free water, the ECF compartment is sufficiently contracted to produce clinical evidence of volume depletion.

One consequence of diminishing volume is increased proximal tubular reabsorption of sodium and water.[196] This adjustment decreases the delivery of sodium and water to the distal nephron, and therefore decreases urine output. Urine osmolalities as high as 200 to 400 mosm/kg can be found under these conditions of slow urinary flow, even if ADH levels are undetectable. However, when volume depletion is corrected, severe polyuria recurs. Coexisting anterior pituitary insufficiency (due, for example, to a pinealoma) causes a similar reduction in the degree of polyuria. In this condition, the decrease in cortisol resulting from ACTH deficiency increases the permeability of the collecting duct to water, even without detectable levels of ADH. Following cortisol replacement, the CDI defect is unmasked, and the polyuria becomes apparent.[165]

In partial CDI, impairment of renal concentrating ability is less severe; consequently, only moderate degrees of polyuria and polydipsia develop.[161] When stressed by prolonged water deprivation, the inability to elaborate maximally concentrated urine can still result in severe dehydration and hypertonicity.

DIAGNOSIS AND TREATMENT OF DI AND CDI Diabetes insipidus should be suspected in any polyuric patient whose urine is dilute and essentially electrolyte-free.[48,161,185,199] Clinical features relate to dehydration, including dry mucous membranes, increased thirst, decreased tissue turgor, decreased sweat, and, in severe cases, shock and neurological complications. The patient's family may have a history of DI. A history of "water-loving" babies who died early, perhaps with seizures, is sometimes encountered. Laboratory features of DI can include increased P_{osm} (with hypernatremia and hypertonicity), azotemia and hyperuricemia (reflecting volume depletion), and, occasionally, signs of secondary hyperaldosteronism. However, in mild cases all of these markers may be normal. The urinary findings (relatively large urine volumes at a relatively low U_{osm} or low specific gravity) are characteristic only if water intake is unrestricted.

These clinical and laboratory features are characteristic of both CDI and NDI.[185,224] Some points may be gleaned in taking the patient's history (e.g., recent pituitary surgery) that makes CDI more likely; others (e.g., use of demeclocycline) make NDI more likely. Of particular interest, CDI secondary to pituitary dysfunction may be accompanied by an MRI or computed tomography abnormality of the neurohypophysis.[44,146] The distinction between CDI and NDI is made by measuring P_{ADH} levels: in CDI the P_{ADH} is low or undetectable; it is high or normal in NDI. Results of a standard dehydration test present another diagnostic point: there is no response to exogenous ADH in NDI; in CDI response is normal. In addition, DI must be separated from primary polydipsia, which also presents with polydipsia and polyuria, and has laboratory features overlapping those of DI. Again, measurement of ADH levels or a standard dehydration test, performed under appropriate conditions, can identify primary polydipsia: both tests should be normal. ("Differential diagnosis of polyuria," below, details the diagnostic procedures.) Diagnosis may be complicated by several disturbances in water metabolism that may coexist, and by the occurrence of different disturbances in the same patient at different times.

In CDI, serum urea concentrations may be lower after dehydration than before dehydration, suggesting that urea reabsorption occurs mostly in distal, ADH-sensitive tubules, and is influenced by either the presence or absence of ADH.[49] On the other hand, chloride concentrations may be increased in sweat in nephrogenic but not CDI.[67]

The immediate treatment of water deficits in DI or CDI should include oral and/or intravenous administration of solutions containing electrolyte-free water, as would be true for any other "pure" water loss. Following correction of any water deficit and restoration of normal access to water, prevention of recurrence of hypertonicity requires that long-term therapy be instituted.

Calculation of pure water deficits The calculation of a pure water deficit is based on the assumption that the TBS has not changed, and consequently that the hypertonicity is directly proportional only to the deficit in TBW. These relationships are expressed by the following equations:

$$\text{TBS} = \text{TBW} \times P_{osm} \quad (8)$$

$$\text{Normal TBW} \times \text{normal } P_{osm} = \text{present TBW} \times \text{present } P_{osm} \quad (9)$$

In these equations P_{osm} is often replaced by the serum $[Na^+]$ multiplied by 2 (for anions) because the easily obtained value of serum $[Na^+]$ reflects the principal cation contributing to P_{osm} in a pure water deficit. Using $2[Na^+]$ avoids the potential error in tonicity calculations if azotemia is present, because urea (a permeant solute) elevates osmolality but not tonicity. Pure water deficits are always associated with hypertonicity, but not necessarily with hyperosmolality.

Equation 7 can be rewritten as

$$2\,(\text{normal } [Na^+])(\text{normal TBW}) = 2\,(\text{present } [Na^+])(\text{present TBW}) \quad (10)$$

and rearranged, so that:

$$\text{Present TBW} = \frac{\text{normal } [Na^+]}{\text{present } [Na^+]} \times \text{normal TBW} \quad (11)$$

With substitution from Equation 11, the pure water deficit ΔW can be calculated from:

$$\Delta W = \text{normal TBW} - \text{present TBW} \quad (12)$$

For example, consider the case of a patient who normally weighs 70 kg, whose serum $[Na^+]$ is normally 140 meq/liter, but now is 160 meq/liter as a result of pure water losses. Then, from Equation 11,

$$\text{Normal TBW} = 60 \text{ percent of normal body weight} = (0.6)(70) = 42 \text{ liters} \quad (13)$$

$$\text{Normal TBS} = (2)(\text{normal serum } [Na^+])(\text{normal TBW}) = (2)(140)(42) \quad (14)$$

But by hypothesis (pure water loss), there has been no change in TBS; therefore

$$\text{Present TBS} = \text{normal TBS} = (2)(140)(42) \quad (15)$$

However, the present TBS can also be calculated in the following way:

$$\text{Present TBS} = 2(\text{present serum } [Na^+])(\text{present TBW}) = 2(160)(\text{present TBW}) \quad (16)$$

Therefore, Equations 15 and 16 can be set equal to each other, and rearranged to give

$$2(140)(42) = 2(160)(\text{present TBW}) \quad (17)$$

$$\text{Present TBW} = \frac{2(140)(42)}{2(160)} = 36.8 \text{ liters} \quad (18)$$

Since for a pure water deficit, from Equation 12, ΔW = normal TBW − present TBW, in this case:

$$\Delta W = 42 - 36.8 = 5.2 \text{ liters} \quad (19)$$

Note that the calculations can be simplified by factoring if the arithmetic is delayed until the penultimate step (Equation 18).

Calculation of the water deficit is only one step in the management of hypertonic states. The therapy of hypertonicity has three basic objectives: (1) replacement of water deficits (and solute deficits, if any); (2) administration of sufficient water (and solute, if needed) to match continuing losses; and (3) treatment of the underlying disease processes responsible for the hypertonicity. When water deficits are severe (greater than 7 liters), particularly in the presence of hypotension or shock, improvement in EABV should take precedence over improvement in tonicity; thus, the administration of colloid and/or isotonic saline should precede the administration of more hypotonic solutions. The correction of the hypertonicity can be delayed until EABV is restored to safe levels. Some patients may require whole blood or blood products if there are hematological deficiencies. These fluids should receive the highest priority for replacement. Correction of hematological deficits is particularly important in the elderly as anemia may be obscured by dehydration, and excessive fluid replacement might precipitate heart failure.

The rapidity with which water deficits are replaced depends on the patient's symptoms and on the severity of hypertonicity. As discussed above, there is a danger that cerebral edema could be produced if water deficits are replaced too rapidly.[10,79,80] In general, half of the calculated deficit should be replaced within 12 to 24 h; neurological status should be monitored carefully; continuing losses must be replaced. The remainder of the deficit should be replaced slowly during the next 24 to 48 h. As long as the patient is alert and there is little danger of pulmonary aspiration, oral water intake is preferred. Patients with profound water losses prefer drinking cold water; cold water is more effective at satiation of thirst than warm water.[85] It has even been suggested that craving for cold water is a differential point in distinguishing DI (secondary polydipsia) from compulsive water drinking (primary polydipsia), because individuals with the latter disorder do not have a temperature preference for their ingested water. If an intravenous solution is needed, 5 percent dextrose in water can be administered. Pure water can produce dangerous hemolysis when administered intravenously and is contraindicated.

SPECIFIC TREATMENT OF CDI Agents for the treatment of CDI include hormones and hormone analogues, and a variety of nonhormonal drugs.[199] Some drug preparations have intrinsic antidiuretic activity or enhance the action of endogenous ADH; others act by entirely different mechanisms. The characteristics of these agents are summarized in Table 21-4; some additional details about the drugs appear below.

Hormones and hormone analogues *Aqueous vasopressin* (VP) is a water-soluble, posterior pituitary extract comprising a mixture of arginine- and lysine-containing VP (ADH) forms. Intravenous use is usually reserved for investigational purposes. Aqueous VP is often used in diagnostic testing to separate CDI from NDI, and occasionally is used in the short-term treatment of acute CDI. In the latter case (e.g., after head trauma or pituitary surgery) intravenous aqueous VP is useful because its brief duration of action permits frequent reevaluation of the polyuric state, which may be quite variable in its intensity and duration. Aqueous VP has little use in the chronic treatment of CDI because its duration of action is so short. Frequent use of aqueous VP can stimulate the production of VP antibodies, and consequently a diminished diuretic response to the administered hormone.[232]

Vasopressin tannate is an oil-based mixture of Arg-VP and Lys-VP. It has been the standard form of long-acting therapy for complete CDI in the past.[191] The hormone is usually found as a button at the bottom of its container; therefore, the vial must be shaken vigorously, and sometimes also warmed, until the hormone is uniformly dissolved. Failure to dissolve the hormone is the most common cause of therapeutic failure. Because this is a peanut oil-based preparation it should never be given intravenously.

Synthetic 8-lysine-vasopressin is an analogue of Arg-VP with about two-thirds of the potency of the native hormone.[197] Although its short duration of action limits its usefulness in severe or complete CDI, it may obviate the need for injections in some patients, and may be all that is needed in patients with mild or incomplete CDI.

TABLE 21-4 • **Drugs used in treatment of diabetes insipidus**

	Dose	Route	Time for onset of effect, h	Duration, h	Comments
HORMONAL THERAPY					
Aqueous vasopressin (Pitressin) (Arg- and Lys-VP; 20 U/ml)	5–10 U (0.25–0.5 ml)	SC, IM, IV	0.5–1	4–6	IV used primarily for diagnosis, but occasionally for transient CDI (posttrauma, perioperative, etc.)
Vasopressin tannate (Pitressin-in-oil) (Arg- and Lys-VP; 5 U/ml)	2–5 U (0.4–1.0 ml)	SC, IM	2–4	24–72	Emulsion must be shaken and warmed prior to use. Vasoconstriction and smooth muscle contraction are frequent side effects
Synthetic 8-lysine-vasopressin (Lypressin; Diapid) (Lys-VP; 50 U/ml)	5–10 U (1–2 sprays in each nostril)	Nasal spray	0.5–1	4–6	Replaced "pituitary snuff": relatively nonallergenic and nonirritating
DDAVP (Desmopressin) (1-desamino-8-D-Arg-VP; 100 μg/ml)	5–20 μg (1–2 sprays in each nostril)	Nasal spray	0.5–1	12–24	DDAVP is drug of choice for complete CDI. Therapy is usually needed 2× daily
ADJUNCT THERAPY					
Hydrochlorothiazide (Hydrodiuril; 50 mg/tab)	50–100 mg (daily)	PO		12–24	Thiazide side effects may occur. Drug can be used in central or nephrogenic DI
Chlorpropamide (Diabinese; 250 mg/tab)	250–750 mg (daily)	PO		24–36	As single dose: start with 250 mg, add 1 tab every 3–4 days. Hypoglycemia is expected at doses over 500 mg/day. Use only in partial CDI
Clofibrate (Atromid-S; 250 mg/tab)	250–500 mg (every 6–8 h)	PO		6–8	Give frequently. GI distress, myositis, abnormal LFTs may occur. Use only in partial CDI
Carbamazepine (Tegretol; 200 mg/tab)	400–1000 mg (daily)	PO		12–24	Drug may be given as single dose. GI distress, ataxia may occur. Use only in partial CDI

ABBREVIATIONS: VP, vasopressin; SC, subcutaneous; IM, intramuscular; IV, intravenous; PO, per oral, LFTs, liver function tests; CDI, central diabetes insipidus.

The preparation is a nasal spray; it may also be useful with adjunctive therapy which enhances the effectiveness of the hormone, and the combination may be sufficient (see "Nonhormonal agents," below). This nonirritating spray has replaced the use of posterior pituitary powder ("pituitary snuff") as the intranasal agent of choice. The snuff was associated with extreme irritation of the nasal mucosa and allergic pulmonary complications, neither of which seems to occur in response to the spray.

Desmopressin (1-desamino-8-D-argine- vasopressin), or DDAVP, is the newest synthetic analogue of natural Arg-VP, which has increased antidiuretic and decreased pressor activities, a prolonged half-life (t 1/2), and consequently a longer duration of action compared with all previous agents.[45,74,114,191,197,214,241] DDAVP should now be considered the drug of choice for severe or complete CDI, although it usually has to be administered twice a day to achieve good control of symptoms.[42] This analogue can be administered both intranasally and orally.[110,236,238] In addition to the treatment of CDI, DDAVP is used for treating bleeding disorders[121] associated with hemophilia and Von-Willebrand's disease,[104,114] prolonged bleeding times in uremia, nocturnal enuresis,[114] and chronic autonomic dysfunction.[148] Of particular note, the administration of either L-AVP or DDAVP improved short- and long-term memory but did not improve attention span or mental concentrating ability in CDI patients.[134] Another analogue, DGAVP (des-glycinamide^9-(arg)^8-vasopressin), also improved memory in patients with CDI.[135]

Complications of vasopressin therapy Several complications may be encountered in VP therapy. Overdosage is a problem shared by all of these hormonal agents; therefore, careful timing of each dose is important, and it is safest to administer the next dose just as polyuria begins (i.e., when the previous dose is clearly wearing off). VP tannate (pitressin tannate-in-oil) and other VPs administered by the subcutaneous or intramuscular routes may produce local reactions such as rash or vasospasm; occasionally, anaphylactic reactions occur.[136] The peanut oil solvent for VP tannate can induce severe allergic reactions in hypersensitive patients. Pulmonary fibrosis has been reported with intranasal administration of VPs, particularly with the now outmoded pituitary snuff, but has not been reported with either synthetic 8-lysine-vasopressin or DDAVP.[191]

All of these hormonal agents are potential vasoconstrictors, and should be used with caution in patients with coronary artery disease; DDAVP may be the least vasoactive, and is therefore the recommended drug in this setting. Most of these agents also cause smooth muscle contraction and can induce gastrointestinal distress (nausea, cramps); some women experience menstruation-like cramps due to uterine contractions as well. Patients must be carefully instructed about the use of these potent hormonal agents, both in terms of administration techniques and in terms of side effects.

Nonhormonal agents The use of one or more of the *nonhormonal agents* can reduce polyuria and provide an adjunct to hormone therapy in patients with complete or partial CDI. Nonhormonal drugs may be especially valuable when combined with dietary restriction of protein and sodium salts to reduce urinary solute content, and thereby reduce obligatory water excretion. For patients with partial CDI, certain oral agents can enhance the renal effects of the circulating ADH; some may increase the central release of residual ADH. Such agents increase the concentrating capacity of the kidney and decrease polyuria; they may be combined with agents that do not enhance ADH release or action. However, most of these nonhormonal agents are not adequate without hormonal therapy in complete CDI; DDAVP may be the agent of choice in both complete and partial CDI. There remains a limited but definite use for these oral agents when other therapeutic options are contraindicated.

Paradoxically, *diuretic agents* are useful in decreasing the polyuria associated with DI. Although such agents initially increase urine volume by increasing sodium (and water) excretion, the decrease in EABV subsequently reduces the GFR; proximal tubular reabsorption of sodium and water increases. The result is a decrease in the delivery of water to the collecting duct, and therefore a decreased urine volume even if ADH levels are low.[55,56] The reduced urine flow also allows the most efficient water reabsorption by the renal medulla, both in the presence and in the absence of ADH. It is necessary to maintain a state of mild sodium (and EABV) depletion in order to maintain this effect on urine volume; therefore, dietary sodium restriction is also necessary. A typical daily dose of 50 to 100 mg hydrochlorothiazide is usually sufficient; side effects, other than occasional hypokalemia, are uncommon. More potent diuretics, particularly those active at the loop of Henle (e.g., furosemide), are also effective, but they can produce severe electrolyte depletion and are not recommended.

The *sulfonylureas* as a group share three potential sites of action relating to salt and water balance: (1) increasing the CNS release of ADH,[169] (2) enhancing the renal response to ADH,[159] and (3) decreasing the reabsorption of sodium (and water) in the proximal tubule.[162,233] In principle, any of these oral hypoglycemic agents could be net diuretic or antidiuretic, depending on the magnitude of the individual effects for that particular agent.[162,170,233]

The sulfonylurea with those characteristics that seem most useful for the treatment of CDI is *chlorpropamide*.[5,159,162,233] Chlorpropamide stimulates the CNS release of ADH and potentiates the action of ADH on the collecting duct (by inhibiting prostaglandin production; Fig. 21-4); it has little or no effect on the proximal tubule. Recently, studies with Brattleboro rats, which lack ADH, suggested that chlorpropamide increases the electrolyte concentration gradient in the renal medulla, perhaps by increasing NaCl reabsorption in the medullary thick ascending limb, and thereby provides a greater driving force for water reabsorption at any given level of ADH.[27,133] The standard initial dose of chlorpropamide is 250 mg/day; the dose is increased 250 mg every 3 to 4 days until a satisfactory response is reached; the maximum dose is 750 mg/day. Renal response to the drug is dose-related, but doses greater than 500 to 750 mg/day are associated with a substantial incidence of hypoglycemia. The risk of hypoglycemia is particularly important in patients with panhypopituitarism, since these patients cannot mobilize glucose well.[233] Combinations of chlorpropamide and a thiazide diuretic may be very effective in partial CDI; U_{osm} usually rises to equal or slightly exceed P_{osm} if the therapy is effective. Chlorpropamide is not effective in complete CDI, as there is no ADH-release, or in NDI, in which case additional ADH has no impact.[159,170] Other sulfonylureas, for example, tolbutamide, tolazamide, acetohexamide, and glyburide, are either ineffective or inferior to chlorpropamide; they should be not be used.

Clofibrate is an oral hypolipidemic agent which can increase antidiuresis only in patients with partial CDI: its only action is to enhance the CNS release of ADH.[168] The short duration of clofibrate action requires administration 3 to 4 times/day; the need for repeated readministration is a disadvantage when compared with the once-daily dosage of chlorpropamide. Another disadvantage is the seriousness of its potential side effects, which include gastrointestinal and hepatic abnormalities. The advantage of clofibrate is its freedom from complication by the hypoglycemic reactions associated with sulfonylureas. Combinations of clofibrate with thiazides and/or with chlorpropamide are particularly effective. The inconvenient dosage schedule and the side effects make clofibrate a poor initial therapeutic choice in partial CDI.

The anticonvulsant *carbamazepine* was originally developed for the treatment of trigeminal neuralgia (tic douloureux); it was found to increase the CNS release of ADH in partial CDI as a side effect.[230] However, it has few advantages, if any, over clofibrate and chlorpropamide; furthermore, its usefulness is limited by its hematologic toxicity. Therefore, it is not recommended for routine therapy in patients with partial CDI.

Some *analgesic agents* (e.g., aminopyrine and acetaminophen) appear to have intrinsic antidiuretic activity or to sensitize the collecting duct (and/or distal tubule) to the action of ADH.[177] However, their mechanism of action is not well understood; inhibition of prostaglandin synthesis, similar to that described for chlorpropamide, might be important. These agents may be effective adjunctive therapy in partial CDI, but there is little experience with their use for this purpose. They cannot be recommended at this time.

TABLE 21-5 • Renal concentrating defects

ABNORMAL RENAL ANATOMY AND/OR SOLUTE GRADIENT
Acute renal failure
Chronic renal failure
Polycystic renal disease
Obstructive uropathy
Infectious interstitial nephritis
Allergic interstitial nephritis
Vascular disorders (e.g., sickle cell nephropathy)
Amyloidosis
Myeloma renal disease
Sarcoid nephropathy
Sjögren's syndrome
Osmotic diuresis
Prolonged diuretic use
Obesity
NORMAL RENAL ANATOMY AND SOLUTE GRADIENT
Hereditary
Familial
Acquired
Electrolyte disorders:
Hypokalemia
Hypercalcemia
Drug-induced:
Lithium
Demeclocycline
Methoxyflurane
Other

Nephrogenic diabetes insipidus

Disorders in renal concentrating ability may be classified in several ways. One useful classification depends on the normal physiology of the concentrating mechanism, which can be thought of in two large divisions: production and maintenance of the medullary osmotic gradient, and utilization of the gradient under the influence of ADH[26,195,196] (details can be found in Chap. 5). Some physicians include defects in either of these subdivisions as possible causes of NDI.[66,77,120,195,196] Thus, any general tubulointerstitial disorder that interferes with production or maintenance of the osmotic gradient in the renal medulla, and thereby impairs the ability of the kidney to achieve a maximally concentrated urine, could be considered a cause of NDI (Table 21-5). However, these conditions are not associated with a U_{osm} that is much below P_{osm}; many are not commonly associated with polyuria. Therefore, other physicians have restricted the definition of "true" NDI to disorders that specifically affect the ADH-dependent reabsorption of water across the collecting duct in the presence of normal osmotic gradients and P_{ADH} levels. In this chapter we use the more restricted definition of "true" NDI in selecting disorders for more detailed discussion.

Another common classification scheme divides NDI into familial and acquired varieties (Table 21-5). Note that many of the acquired varieties would not be classified as "true" NDI by the restricted definition above, although some of them do fall into the more restricted group (e.g., the NDI associated with certain drugs and electrolyte disorders). All familial forms of NDI are probably "true" NDI because no defects in gradient generation or maintenance have ever been demonstrated in these conditions.

ETIOLOGY OF NDI • *Familial NDI* This congenital disorder presents with polyuria and polydipsia, vomiting and constipation, and recurrent febrile episodes (often with seizures). The fevers appear to correlate with the state of hydration, since body temperature normalizes with rehydration. The diagnosis is frequently missed until early childhood because it is often difficult to detect polyuria and polydipsia in an infant.[176] If adequate caloric intake has been sacrificed to maintain hydration, growth may be impaired as a result of malnutrition. Mental retardation is often found in children surviving infancy, and can run the gamut from minor memory deficits to imbecility. The brain damage is a result of repeated episodes of severe dehydration, cerebral edema following too-rapid rehydration, cerebral hypoxia and recurrent seizures, and/or chronic malnutrition. The most severe cases occur in males, who present with complete NDI; females usually present with partial NDI. This also reflects the pattern of inheritance, which is either an X-linked recessive or an X-linked dominant with variable penetrance in females.[29,171,175,198]

Familial NDI is a heterogeneous disorder associated with a cellular abnormality, either in the renal V_2 receptor (AVP receptor) or in the postreceptor (and Gs activity) cascade of events that mediate VP-induced antidiuresis,[172] resulting in resistance to endogenous or exogenous VP. However, familial NDI is not associated with any structural abnormalities in either the loop of Henle or the collecting duct, and all other renal functions (including renal blood flow, GFR, reabsorption of glucose and phosphate, excretion of hydrogen and ammonia, and overall sodium conservation) seem to be normal.[196] The only consistent abnormality has been the inability to concentrate the urine maximally (abnormally low max U_{osm}). In at least some of these patients urinary cAMP excretion fails to increase in response to addition of exogenous ADH. This implies an inability to generate or maintain an adequate intracellular cAMP level in response to endogenous ADH. Since there is no response to endogenous or exogenous ADH, hormonal therapy is ineffective; therefore, therapy is aimed at reduction of the solute load through sodium and protein restriction, as described for the treatment of CDI.

Drug-induced NDI Table 21-6 details the effects of drugs used to treat NDI at several sites related to the action of ADH.

Polydipsia and polyuria are frequently reported side effects in patients treated with *lithium carbonate* for manic depressive disorders.[18] Although concentrating defects can be demonstrated in many such patients with formal testing, the polyuria (when present) rarely exceeds 3 liters/day, and almost never requires that the drug be discontinued, although dosage reduction may be needed. Lithium affects water metabolism by producing a primary polydipsia, at least in animals, inhibiting CNS release of ADH in some patients, and impairing renal ADH-responsiveness at steps both prior to and after the generation of cAMP. The drug acts by interfering both with ADH-induced adenylate cyclase and with cAMP-dependent protein kinase (Fig. 21- 4).[53,92,99,119,163,188,221] Therefore, lithium usually causes partial NDI, occasionally causes partial CDI, and rarely (if ever) causes primary polydipsia in humans; secondary polydipsia is the rule. Lithium-induced NDI is usually a dose-related, reversible defect in renal water conservation, but the functional defect may persist for months, and possibly indefinitely after the drug is discontinued.[188,220,223] Whether or not lithium causes structural renal damage and/or permanent renal insufficiency is still an open question.[160,223] Lithium has other important effects on the endocrine system in addition to its action on ADH.[204]

Certain tetracyclines, particularly *demeclocycline* (7- chloro-6-demethyltetracycline), produce a dose-dependent, reversible impairment of renal concentrating ability. Demeclocycline impairs ADH-induced water flow by inhibiting both ADH-induced adenylate cyclase and cAMP-induced protein kinase activities.[94,222] In humans, a dose of 900 to 1200 mg/day for several days produces NDI in almost all cases.[164] Polyuria develops gradually and may not be apparent for a week or more.[94,222] When

TABLE 21-6 • Drug-induced nephrogenic diabetes insipidus

	Site(s) of drug-induced interference with ADH action						
	Drug effect on						
DRUG	POLYURIA	ADH RELEASE	PROXIMAL TUBULAR REABSORPTION	ASCENDING LIMB FUNCTION	IN VITRO ADH-INDUCED H_2O FLOW	IN VITRO ADH-STIMULATED ADENYLATE CYCLASE	IN VITRO POST-cAMP FUNCTIONS
Lithium	NDI,CDI?	(↓)	↓	0	↓	↓↓	↓*
Demeclocycline	NDI	(0)	(0)	(0)	↓	↓↓	↓↓*
Methoxyflurane	NDI	0	(0)	(0)	↓	?	(↓)
Glyburide	V	0	(↓)	(0)	↑	0	0
Vasopressinoic acid	0	(0)	(0)	(0)	↓	↓	(0)
Colchicine	0	(0)	(0)	(0)	↓	0	↓**

NOTE: Parentheses indicate function evaluated by indirect means.

ABBREVIATIONS AND SYMBOLS: ↑, Function increased; ↓, function decreased or impaired; ?, unknown; NDI, nephrogenic diabetes insipidus; CDI, central diabetes insipidus; V, urine flow; *, cAMP-dependent protein kinase; **, microtubules.

the drug is discontinued, return of normal concentrating ability may also take weeks. The same steps in the ADH pathway are inhibited by demeclocycline as by lithium. Demeclocycline has been used successfully to treat patients with the syndrome of chronic inappropriate ADH secretion by producing partial NDI, but toxic effects limit its utility in other hyponatremic states.[40,52,64] Other tetracyclines do not produce clinically important defects in water metabolism; there are experimental tetracyclines that lack any antibiotic activity but still impair ADH action.[54]

Certain of the halogenated anesthetics, particularly *methoxyflurane* (1,1-difluoro-2,2-dichloro-ethylmethylether), are associated with the development of acute renal failure and a polyuria that is not responsive to exogenous ADH.[51,115,152-155] The two major metabolites of methoxyflurane, oxalate and inorganic fluoride, are responsible for these disorders. The acute renal failure is definitely associated with deposition of oxalate in the renal medulla, and with acute tubular necrosis. In contrast, the ADH-unresponsiveness appears to be related to the high concentration of inorganic fluoride in the blood and/or urine.[86] Plasma concentrations greater than 90 μmol/liter are associated with polyuria unresponsive to exogenous ADH, but the underlying mechanisms have not been completely defined. Defects in both gradient formation and gradient maintenance have been proposed; such deficits could be due to fluoride-related alterations in renal medullary blood flow. In addition, defects in the cellular response to ADH have been demonstrated, both proximal and distal to the site of generation of cAMP; both adenylate cyclase activity and cellular action of cAMP activity may be inhibited by inorganic fluoride.

Many other agents have been associated with the production of NDI or with lack of responsiveness to ADH in vitro. Certain clinically useful antidiabetic sulfonylureas, such as glyburide, increase urinary volume in normal humans and in patients with CDI.[167] This paradoxical effect can occur in spite of the fact that some sulfonylureas (e.g., chlorpropamide) increase central ADH release, and all sulfonylureas enhance the ADH stimulation of renal water reabsorption. Although part of the increase in urinary volume may be attributable to the direct stimulation of thirst in some cases (e.g., with chlorpropamide), most of the diuresis derives from impaired salt and water reabsorption in the proximal portions of the nephron. Those sulfonylureas, such as glyburide, which have a prominent proximal action of this kind are called diuretic sulfonylureas.

Colchicine impairs ADH-induced water flow in vitro. It does not seem to produce clinical DI in spite of widespread use for the treatment of gout. Colchicine has no effect on the enzymes mediating ADH action in vitro (adenylate cyclase, protein kinase, phosphodiesterase); it seems to act by disrupting the integrity of the intracellular microtubules which are required for transcellular water flow in renal epithelia.[68]

Vasopressinoic acid is an active structural analogue of the arginine form of vasopressin (Arg-VP). It inhibits the action of Arg-VP in vivo and of Lys-VP in vitro. Vasopressinoic acid, and other active structural analogues of ADH, probably act by competing for binding to the ADH receptor sites on renal epithelial membranes. Several of these inactive ADH analogues are under development for the treatment of the syndrome of inappropriate ADH secretion[147,197] (see Chap. 20). Even if free of other side effects, all the inactive VPs would have the potential for producing NDI if administered in an excessive dose. None of these analogues is available for clinical use at this time.

Electrolyte disorders Moderate to severe potassium depletion (where total body potassium deficits are greater than 200 to 300 meq) may be associated with a reversible, ADH-resistant impairment of renal concentrating ability.[190,211] The polyuria and polydipsia are relatively mild or inapparent because the maximal U_{osm} in most patients is equal to or slightly greater than P_{osm}.[22,227] The anatomical lesion most commonly associated with potassium depletion is vacuolization of the proximal tubular epithelium; the relevance of this lesion to the concentrating defect is unclear. There is also evidence that hypokalemia interferes with production and/or maintenance of the osmotic gradient, and produces tubular resistance to the action of ADH.[24,196] (Osmotic gradient deficiencies would not be considered "true" NDI, but resistance of tubules to ADH would so qualify.)

Polyuria and polydipsia occur in many disorders associated with hypercalcemia, with or without hypercalciuria.[101,211] There is considerable evidence that the concentrating defect is multifactorial.[97] Hypercalcemia does interfere with sodium transport, and therefore disturbs the generation and maintenance of the osmotic gradient. Hypercalcemia produces "true" NDI by inhibiting ADH-induced cAMP generation and possibly inhibiting binding of ADH to its renal receptors. These reversible concentrating defects become clinically apparent when the serum calcium concentration exceeds 11 mg/dl. Hypercalcemia may also produce acute renal failure, which may or may not be reversible.

A diminished renal concentrating ability due to a partial unresponsiveness to ADH has been observed in obese individuals after a 14-h fast. Depletion of the osmolar content of the renal medulla has been cited as the probable cause.[128]

Other causes of NDI Some clinical conditions result in significant, generalized renal tubular damage, such that (among various defects) partial or total unresponsiveness to ADH occurs. The damage may affect the loops of Henle or the blood vessels (thereby impairing formation or maintenance of the osmotic gradient) and/or the collecting ducts (thereby impairing utilization of the gradient in the presence of adequate amounts of ADH). In *amyloidosis* abnormal proteins can be deposited in the renal medulla and/or in the collecting ducts. Either problem could produce ADH-unresponsiveness; the latter would be classified as "true" NDI.[39] It is not clear if the abnormal proteins interfere with ADH binding, with the cellular response to ADH, or with the physical permeability to water (by simply thickening the walls of the collecting duct). Bilateral ureteral obstruction with hydronephrosis impairs renal medullary blood flow, flattens the renal papillae, and alters the permeability of the loops of Henle.[218] Which, if any, of these factors is responsible for the insensitivity to ADH is unknown. Other diseases often associated with diffuse medullary and tubular damage, and with lack of ADH responsiveness, include acute tubular necrosis, chronic interstitial nephritis, and diffuse vasculitic or infiltrative diseases.

Clinical presentation of NDI Complete NDI, like complete CDI, is characterized by massive polyuria and polydipsia, in conjunction with an inability to concentrate the urine. However, partial NDI is more prevalent. Many defects that could be classified as partial NDI are asymptomatic and go unrecognized. However, in all other respects, the presentation of NDI is similar to the presentation of CDI. The clinical setting often gives a clue to the specific etiology, but without formal testing it is often impossible to distinguish untreated CDI from untreated NDI.

Diagnosis of NDI The diagnosis of familial NDI is fairly simple if the polyuria and polydipsia are recognized. The disorder presents shortly after birth, and there is usually a strong family history. Acquired NDI can present with polydipsia and polyuria at any time, with clinical and laboratory features similar to those of CDI; however, in NDI there is a lack of responsiveness to exogenous ADH and a normal or increased P_{ADH}. The particular type of acquired NDI present is determined by the clinical setting (e.g., drug use). If water intake is restricted, the risk of profound dehydration with severe hypernatremia and hypertonicity is the same as in CDI. As in CDI, profound dehydration with slow urinary flows can be associated with U_{osm} equal to or slightly greater than P_{osm}, even without response to ADH. The differential diagnosis includes CDI and primary polydipsia; the same tests are used to separate these entities as are described under CDI[185] (see also "Differential diagnosis of polyuria," below).

Treatment of NDI The principles of NDI treatment are identical to the ones governing CDI. Water losses must be replaced (see "Calculation of pure water deficits," above), electrolyte abnormalities must be corrected, and any underlying disorders (such as obstructive nephropathy) should be treated. Dosages of offending or aggravating drugs (e.g., demeclocycline) must be reduced or eliminated. The technique of reducing urine volume by using diuretics combined with solute (sodium and protein) restriction can be used with NDI in the same manner as has been described for CDI.

Specific therapy for VP-resistant DI secondary to lithium has recently been recommended.[16] *Amiloride*, a potassium-sparing diuretic, appears to mitigate lithium-induced polyuria, at least in part by blunting the inhibitory effect of lithium on water transport in the renal collecting tubules.[16,129] *Prostoglandin synthetase inhibitors* have also been recommended for the treatment of NDI. These drugs appear to enhance VP-induced water permeability, and increase maximum urine osmolality after VP.[140]

Of particular note, individuals with NDI raise their plasma levels of factor VIII and VWF factor following a DDAVP infusion indicating no abnormality of the V_1 receptors but only of the V_2 (ADH) receptors.[34]

Primary polydipsia (e.g., psychogenic polydipsia: compulsive water drinking) may be confused with DI because both present with polydipsia and polyuria.[14,234] However, patients with primary polydipsia have a normal to low steady-state P_{osm} (usually below 286 mosm/kg), whereas patients with untreated DI usually have a normal to high P_{osm} (usually 286 to 300 mosm/kg). Furthermore, since patients with primary polydipsia have a tendency to EABV expansion, their BUN and plasma uric acid levels are generally relatively low. Patients with DI have a tendency to EABV contraction, associated with increases in BUN and plasma uric acid levels.

Primary polydipsia is often associated with underlying psychiatric disorders. Such individuals often display (1) an alteration in osmoreceptor function, (2) renal hypersensitivity to ADH, (3) mild but significant defects in urinary dilution after a water load, and (4) an inappropriate thirst response to hypoosmolality.[25,81,102,118]

Dehydration testing can add to the confusion between DI and primary polydipsia. The large urine flows associated with increased water intake in the latter disorder can wash out the renal medullary solute gradient; the loss of the osmotic gradient impairs renal concentrating ability, both with and without the presence of ADH.[161] Therefore, patients with primary polydipsia usually do not achieve a normal maximum urine osmolality after dehydration alone, and do not respond further to exogenous ADH administration. They usually are, however, able to achieve a $U_{osm} > P_{osm}$ with added ADH; in this sense they appear similar to patients with partial NDI. In cases of primary polydipsia with perturbed osmotic gradients, the specific etiology of the polyuria can only be determined after reconstitution of the normal medullary solute gradient. This reconstitution requires both adequate solute intake (sodium chloride, and protein for the generation of urea) and a decrease in the urine volume; the latter can be achieved by administering a long-acting ADH preparation if prolonged water restriction is impossible. Patients with primary polydipsia may become very hyponatremic if water intake is not restricted while they are taking a long-acting ADH preparation; in contrast, patients with NDI may become hypernatremic if water intake *is* greatly restricted. Therefore, frequent measurements of body weight, P_{osm}, U_{osm}, and serum sodium concentration are prudent during the reconstitution process. After reconstitution of the gradient, patients with primary polydipsia should have a normal max U_{osm} after 12 to 14 h of dehydration (i.e., > 850 mosm/kg); as in healthy individuals, these patients should show no further increase in U_{osm} after exogenous ADH administration. In contrast, patients with NDI show no change in their abnormal dehydration tests after reconstitution.

Differential diagnosis of polyuria The approach to the patient with polyuria is important in order to distinguish between DI and other polyuric states, such as solute diuresis and primary polydipsia; the approach must also distinguish between the various kinds of DI (complete versus partial; NDI versus CDI).[152] Although clinical and laboratory features may offer some insights into diagnostic distinctions between polyuric states, in most cases more formal testing is required. Differential diagnosis may be aided by determinations of urinary solutes or their absence, standard dehydration tests, or measurement of plasma ADH levels. These three more formal tests allow for a complete analysis of polyuric states, particularly those associated with water diuresis.

DETERMINATION OF URINARY COMPOSITION The first step in the formal evaluation of a polyuric state should be determining the characteristics of the urine (Fig. 21-12). Measurement of osmolality or specific gravity of urine during polyuria permits immediate differentiation between pure water diuresis and solute diuresis. If the U_{osm} is less than 150 mosm/kg, or the specific gravity is less than 1.005, a relatively pure water diuresis is likely, and one can proceed with the dehydration test described below.

If the U_{osm} is 300 to 400 mosm/kg, or the specific gravity is between 1.008 and 1.012, relatively pure solute diuresis is present. The nature of the solute should then be determined; substantial amounts must be present in the urine to cause the polyuria. If the solute is an electrolyte, it is almost certainly a sodium salt (NaCl or $NaHCO_3$); if the solute is a nonelectrolyte, then it is almost certainly glucose or urea (or some exogenously administered solute, e.g., mannitol or glycerol). With respect to hypotonic states, a solute diuresis may cause polyuria that can be identified with hypernatremias (caused by increased sodium salt intake), hyperglycemias (from diabetes mellitus or glucose administration), azotemic states (e.g., after urea administration), or administration of nonphysiological hypertonic solutes (mannitol, glycerol, etc.).

DEHYDRATION TESTS The "standard" dehydration test is the method traditionally used to evaluate the polyuria due to water diuresis.[161] The test requires 12 to 14 h of dehydration. The complete test has two parts: the first evaluates both the ability of the patient to release ADH in response to hypertonicity and the ability of the kidney to respond to the ADH so released; the second part, which is performed only if a normal max U_{osm} has not already been achieved, evaluates the ability of the kidney to respond to exogenous ADH.

The test procedure is:

1. Baseline values for P_{osm}, U_{osm}, and body weight are obtained. The patient is then allowed no intake for the next 12 to 18 h, or until the test is concluded. (This part of the test is best performed overnight; no intake is allowed after dinner, and breakfast is not allowed the following morning until the test is concluded. Sometimes continuous observation of the patient is required to prevent surreptitious water intake.) Once the test has begun, a urine specimen is obtained every hour, while the patient is awake, and

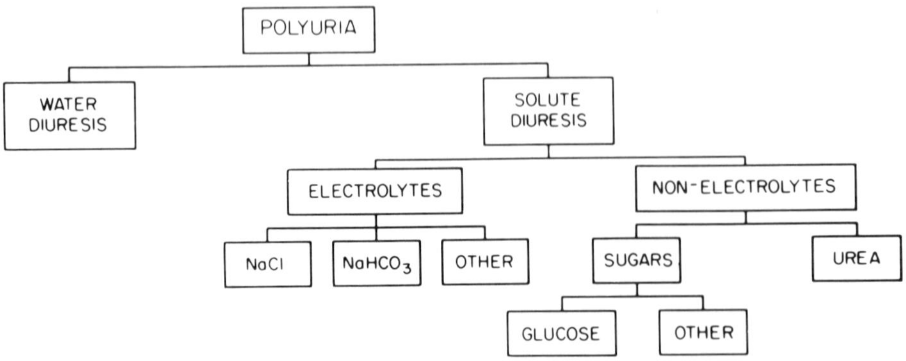

FIGURE 21-12 • Polyuria diagnostic decision tree.

hourly for at least the last 3 h (to ensure that a plateau is reached); both U_{osm} and volume are recorded. A normal individual will experience a decrease in urine flow to < 0.5 ml/min and will achieve a U_{osm} > 850 mosm/kg within 12 to 14 h in part 1 of the test. To be certain that an adequate stimulus to release ADH has been provided, the P_{osm} should reach at least 295 mosm/kg, and/or the body weight should decrease by at least 5 percent; therefore, if a normal U_{max} is not achieved in 12 to 14 h, both P_{osm} and body weight should be checked. The dehydration should be continued until these values have been achieved, and should be terminated only after the U_{osm} reaches a plateau (constant level) on several successive hourly determinations, if these values have not been reached after 14 h. Patients with complete DI will have a U_{max} well below the normal of 850 mosm/kg, usually below 150 mosm/kg; since such patients can become profoundly dehydrated when denied access to water, the test should be terminated as soon as weight loss exceeds 5 percent of their initial body weight (or when P_{osm} > 295 mosm/kg; see below). Some patients with partial DI will have achieved a U_{max} above 200 mosm/kg, but below the normal of 850 mosm/kg, which does not alter with continued dehydration. Other patients with partial DI (partial CDI) will not achieve a normal U_{max} after 14 h of dehydration, in spite of achieving a P_{osm} of 295 mosm/kg (or a 5 percent decrease in body weight), but are clearly having a progressive reduction in urine volume and a progressive increase in successive determinations of U_{osm} when these benchmarks are reached. When the dehydration test is continued, sometimes to 18 h, the urine volumes eventually decrease below 0.5 ml/min, and the U_{osm} eventually rises above 850 mosm/kg. Such patients with partial CDI have a "sluggish" release of endogenous ADH. Since their urine volumes are decreasing and their U_{osm} are increasing at the time the benchmarks are reached, it is safe to continue the dehydration for a few more hours. With the exception of patients with partial CDI caused by "sluggish" ADH release, a failure to have a normal U_{max} after the standard dehydration test does not distinguish CDI from NDI, and part 2 of the test must be performed.

2. In patients who fail to achieve a normal U_{max} after part 1 is completed, exogenous ADH (5.0 U of aqueous VP) is administered subcutaneously, and both urine volumes and U_{osm} are measured for an additional 2 h. Patients with complete CDI will increase U_{osm} in response to exogenous ADH from values much less than P_{osm} to values greater than P_{osm}, although not always to a normal above 850 mosm/kg (see below). Patients with partial CDI may have U_{osm} between 200 and 600 mosm/kg (often above P_{osm}, but below the normal of 850 mosm/kg) after dehydration alone (part I). Exogenous ADH administration substantially increases U_{osm}, often to values well above P_{osm} (often above 850 mosm/kg; see below). Patients with complete or partial NDI will have a U_{osm} similar to patients with complete or partial CDI (respectively) after part 1, but will have no further increase in U_{osm} after exogenous ADH administration in part 2. In other words, the hallmark of NDI is a failure to respond to exogenous ADH. Note that the presence of complete NDI makes the diagnosis of simultaneous CDI impossible without measurements of ADH levels. Also note that the prolonged and profound water diuresis characteristic of complete CDI can wash out the medullary solutes (urea and NaCl) necessary for the maintenance of the osmotic gradient; therefore, exogenous ADH administration may not yield a normal U_{max} in part 2 of the dehydration test unless the test is performed after careful solute replacement for several days.

An alternative dehydration test has recently been developed specifically to identify patients with partial CDI.[161] Patients with mild polyuria begin water deprivation 12 h before specimens are collected to ensure an adequate stimulus to concentrate the urine. Patients with severe polyuria begin on the same day as the test so that they do not lose too much fluid volume. Therefore, patients with mild polyuria begin fluid deprivation at 6 P.M. on the evening before the test, and those with severe polyuria begin at 7 A.M. on the morning of the test. Beginning at 6 P.M. (for patients with mild polyuria) or 8 A.M. (those with severe polyuria), urine specimens are collected hourly for the measurement of U_{osm} and urine volume; blood specimens are collected intermittently for measurement of P_{osm}. When the urine osmolality has become nearly constant (defined as less than a 30 mosm/kg increase between two successive collection periods) the plasma osmolality is again determined and 5 units of aqueous VP are injected subcutaneously. Urine osmolality is then determined 1 h after the VP injection. In addition, all patients are weighed between 6 and 8 A.M. on the morning of the test, and again at the end of the test.

With this procedure, normal individuals achieve a nearly constant U_{osm} in 16 to 18 h, with values ranging from 866 to 1446 mosm/kg (mean: 1068 ± 69 mosm/kg). U_{osm} is always greater than P_{osm} after dehydration in normal individuals. After subcutaneous injection of vasopressin U_{osm} normally falls (to a mean of 978 ± 79 mosm/kg); it should not rise more than 5 percent in individuals with intact neurohypophyseal function. The mean P_{osm} at the time of the max U_{osm} is 290 ± 2 mosm/kg in normal individuals. Patients with primary polydipsia appear normal by this testing procedure, although both their U_{osm} and P_{osm} values are often at the lower end of the normal range. In patients with complete CDI, U_{osm} never exceeds P_{osm}; injection of VP elicits an increase in U_{osm} of greater than 50 percent. The value of U_{osm} usually reaches a plateau in 4 to 18 h in these patients; their mean P_{osm} is 306 ± 3 mosm/kg at the time VP is injected. Patients with values intermediate between those of complete CDI patients and normal individuals are classified as having partial CDI.[161]

Renal function usually decreases as part of the aging process even in individuals classified as normal. The progressive diminution of GFR is usually accompanied by a decrease in renal concentrating ability and an inability to excrete a water load promptly.[20,21,57,60] Thus, elderly patients may not achieve a "normal" max U_{osm} (> 850 mosm/kg), yet they may not show any evidence of a specific previous renal disease. The loss in renal function and concentrating ability has been attributed to progressive vascular disease, with interstitial renal damage and loss of the normal concentration gradient. It is also postulated that the elderly produce an abnormal VP molecule, have abnormal VP receptors or postreceptor responses, and/or have a decreased osmotic gradient in the renal medulla.[20] In addition, healthy elderly individuals deprived of water may not complain of thirst even when they become significantly hyperosmolar.[20,138,182] Impaired AVP secretion associated with hypoangiotensinemia (absolute or relatively low plasma angiotensin II levels and low serum angiotensin I converting enzyme activity) has been reported in hypernatremic, dehydrated elderly patients.[240] Because angiotensin II stimulates thirst, low circulatory levels may predispose the elderly to become hypodipsic.[228] There is, however, little evidence supporting this hypothesis for humans. Elderly individuals (i.e., over the age of 70) may not have a max U_{osm} much greater than 600 mosm/kg; they have a limited ability to conserve water, and this predisposes them to hypernatremia. If the hypothesis above is correct, the loss in concentrating ability should not be classified as "true" NDI (unless the renal deficit is due to amyloidosis, which may develop in elderly individuals; amyloidosis can cause a "true" NDI).

Determination of plasma ADH levels Measurement of ADH concentration in plasma has become feasible with development of reliable radioimmunoassay (RIA) methods.[242] These techniques are often combined with standard dehydration tests and other physiological measurements to permit proper interpretation. They are most helpful in establishing the diagnosis of partial or complete CDI, particularly in the presence of concurrent NDI. Unfortunately, measurements of P_{ADH} may not distinguish primary polydipsia patients from normal individuals or patients with partial CDI; all three may have P_{ADH} values in the normal range because there is marked individual variability among healthy individuals. Not only is the standard dehydration test the best way to make these distinctions, but it usually gives the correct diagnosis in simple CDI as well. Where the diagnosis remains in doubt after all of these tests have been performed, a trial of solute replacement and/or ADH administration can often clarify the nature of the disorder.

Summary: Dehydration tests and ADH levels The principles below govern the interpretation of dehydration tests for the purpose of diagnosing disorders of renal water conservation. Dehydration test results are summarized in Table 21-7.

1. CDI and NDI can be distinguished by the response of the former to exogenous ADH.
2. In patients with complete CDI, U_{osm} increases from $< P_{osm}$ to $> P_{osm}$ after the administration of exogenous ADH. Endogenous ADH levels should be undetectable.
3. In patients with partial CDI, U_{osm} may increase somewhat in part 1 of the dehydration test, but increases further after exogenous ADH is administered in part 2; a normal max U_{osm} is often reached in part 2. Endogenous ADH levels should be low.
4. Patients with complete NDI do not respond to exogenous ADH. Endogenous ADH levels should be elevated.

TABLE 21-7 • Results of dehydration testing (water deprivation test)

	Disorder				
INDICATOR	COMPLETE CDI	PARTIAL CDI	COMPLETE NDI	PARTIAL NDI	PRIMARY POLYDIPSIA
P_{Na}	↑	↑	↑	↑	↓ or normal
P_{osm}	↑	↑	↑	↑	↓ or normal
P_{ADH}	u	↓	↑↑	↑↑	Variable
U_{osm}(−ADH)	$<P_{osm}$	$<P_{osm}$	$<P_{osm}$	$<P_{osm}$	$<P_{osm}$
U_{osm}(+ADH)	$>P_{osm}$	$>P_{osm}$	nr	nr	nr or ↑

SYMBOLS: u, undetectable; $<P_{osm}$, less than P_{osm}; $> P_{osm}$, greater than P_{osm}; nr, no response.

5. Patients with partial NDI may exhibit some increase in U_{osm} in part 1 of the dehydration test; U_{osm} does not increase further after exogenous ADH administration. Endogenous ADH levels should be elevated.
6. Patients with primary polydipsia have a normal or low P_{osm} and an isotonic urine in part 1 of the dehydration test; U_{osm} may not increase in response to exogenous ADH due to medullary solute "washout." Endogenous ADH levels are variable, and may be in the normal range.

Insensible water loss

Insensible fluid losses, primarily from the skin and respiratory tract, average 0.5 to 1.0 liter/day. These fluid losses are hypotonic relative to plasma and therefore tend to elevate P_{osm} and produce hypertonicity if water intake is restricted, even in normal individuals. However, under certain conditions, these losses may increase three- to fivefold; if unmatched by a corresponding increase in water intake, profound hypertonic dehydration can result. Such conditions include hyperthermia (e.g., fever, exposure to high environmental temperatures, thyrotoxicosis), hyperventilation (e.g., septicemia or respiratory tract infection), and skin damage (e.g., burns, exfoliative dermatitis). Certain populations may be expected to be particularly vulnerable to these stresses because their access to water is restricted. They include infants, the elderly, the physically handicapped, the obtunded or comatose, and the mentally ill.[226]

The pathophysiology of this relatively "pure" water loss is shown in Fig. 21-8. It is important to recognize that although only one-twelfth of the volume of "pure" water loss derives from the intravascular compartment, severe or rapid water loss can produce hypotension and shock, as well as seizures and coma. Milder degrees of net water loss may be manifest clinically by increased thirst, dry mucous membranes, and decreased sweating; milder neurological abnormalities, such as confusion, may also ensue. These features may not be present at all times or in all cases. For example, some patients, particularly the elderly, may not exhibit increased thirst and may even have primary hypodipsia.[20] Some patients develop dehydration because of increased sweating (e.g,. in hyperthermia), and their sweating does not decrease until water losses are profound. Still other patients may have normal insensible water losses but coexisting neurological abnormalities may restrict access to water.

The laboratory features of relatively "pure" water loss include hypernatremia (hyperosmolality and hypertonicity), azotemia and hyperuricemia, and evidence of secondary hyperaldosteronism. These clinical and laboratory features are very similar to those of DI, but renal water conservation is normal; urine volumes are therefore small and U_{osm} is high.

The treatment of relatively "pure" water loss has already been discussed in connection with DI (see "Calculation of pure water deficits," above).

Primary hypodipsia

Primary hypodipsia refers to an inadequate sensation of thirst despite the presence of appropriate physiological thirst stimuli. By definition, a "pure" deficit requires that other aspects of osmoregulation and water metabolism be normal. The results of such a "pure" deficit in thirst may then be predicted as follows: the loss of thirst results initially in decreased water intake and a tendency both to hyperosmolality and to reduced EABV. Both changes stimulate ADH release and thereby increase renal water conservation. If the result is sufficient water conservation to balance the decrease in water intake (i.e., if P_{osm} and EABV are returned to near normal), the deficiency in thirst may go unrecognized by the patient. The only changes might be a decrease in the average daily urine volume and an increase in the average daily urine osmolality; neither of these is likely to be noticed.

If the ADH and renal responses are insufficient to compensate for the reduced water intake, symptoms of hyperosmolality and hypovolemia might supervene. Water conservation is limited because insensible water losses (expired and perspired) and renal water losses obligated by the daily solute load (even when excreted at the maximum urine osmolality) continue even at the highest ADH levels.

ETIOLOGY OF PRIMARY HYPODIPSIA Any disorder which affects the CNS can affect the thirst mechanism.[111] In particular, those which involve the hypothalamo-hypophyseal region (the "osmostat" area) and those which involve the higher cortical thirst centers have strong influences on thirst. Hypothalamic syndromes can present with hypernatremia and a variety of other symptoms including periodic spontaneous hypothermia, increased somnolence, hyperphagia, and obesity.[109] In fact, a list of causes of CDI and a list of causes of primary hypodipsia would be very much the same (Table 21-3). Recently an idiopathic variety of hypodipsia in elderly patients has been described. They have no known metabolic or endocrinologic disturbances, but often give a history of previous cerebrovascular accidents.[181] A recent report of a patient with congestive heart failure suggested that zinc deficiency induced a bitter taste for water and, as a result, led to hypernatremia.[124]

CLINICAL PRESENTATION OF PRIMARY HYPODIPSIA The symptoms of primary hypodipsia, as might be expected, are almost the same as those of any form of EABV depletion or dehydration, except for the absence of thirst. In general, for the same degree of water depletion, pure deficits in TBW produce fewer symptoms and signs than combined deficits of total body sodium and water; relatively more water is lost from the extracellular and intravascular compartments in the latter case.

The clinical findings in primary hypodipsia include weakness, fatigue, somnolence, dizziness, confusion, and other nonspecific complaints, but can progress to seizures and coma with severe water depletion (particularly in the very young or the very old). Physical examination may also reveal decreased sweating and tissue turgor, orthostatic hypotension and tachycardia, generalized muscle weakness and hyporeflexia, and other signs of neurological dysfunction. Laboratory findings primarily reflect the decrease in EABV; they include hemoconcentration and leukocytosis, elevation of the BUN out of proportion to any elevation in the serum creatinine concentration, hypernatremia, and hyperosmolality of both plasma and urine. If secondary hyperaldosteronism is well established, hypokalemia may also be present, in addition to relatively high urinary potassium and low urinary sodium concentrations. Levels of both aldosterone and ADH should be elevated.

DIAGNOSIS OF PRIMARY HYPODIPSIA Abnormalities in the sensation of thirst are often very difficult to recognize.[85,194] Failure of thirst perception must be distinguished from failure to provide access to water, a common problem with hospitalized patients and with physically or mentally handicapped outpatients. Primary hypodipsia must also be distinguished from secondary hypodipsia; for example, water administration (because it increases EABV and decreases P_{osm}) would be expected to lead to secondary hypodipsia. Finally, abnormalities in the threshold and/or the sensitivity for thirst perception, in principle, should be distinguishable from each other; it should be possible to separate threshold from sensitivity effects with respect to both "osmolal" and "volumetric" stimuli.

In view of the complex anatomical and physiological interactions, and in view of the uncertainties concerning clinical testing of the thirst sensation, it is not surprising that cases of "pure" primary hypodipsia are difficult to identify. To qualify for this disorder, the patient must have: (1) hypernatremia (increase in P_{osm}) with clinical evidence of EABV depletion, to exclude the diagnosis of essential hypernatremia; (2) free access to water, and the ability to communicate a need for water; and (3) no sensation of thirst (thus permitting exclusion of a diagnosis of water deprivation). The mean U_{osm} must be elevated (usually greater than 700 mosm/kg), and should not increase in response to exogenous ADH (presumably excluding a coincident diagnosis of CDI or NDI). Combinations of CDI and hypodipsia are exceedingly common, as might be expected from the anatomy of the CNS; essential hypernatremia can be viewed as a special case of this combination.

Thirst testing Formal evaluation of thirst deficits is difficult because drinking behavior is influenced by many stimuli unrelated to osmoregulation or volume regulation. Definitive testing for thirst deficits should include both osmolar and volumetric stimuli; usually, only the former is evaluated.[85] Obviously the test subject must be alert, oriented, and able to express whether or not the thirst sensation is present. When studies of osmolar thirst stimuli are performed the subject should be euvolemic, and other dipsogenic stimuli (e.g., hyperthermia, exercise) should be minimized. A commonly used method of testing thirst is to administer hyperosmolal saline (3 percent NaCl) solution at a rate sufficient to elevate the plasma osmolality from the individual's normal level (baseline) to some arbitrary level at least 10 percent above the baseline. The P_{osm} should be determined at the baseline and at frequent intervals (e.g., every 30 min) until the sensation of thirst is reported, or until the P_{osm} has increased by at least 10 percent. This technique will elevate EABV while increasing P_{osm}, but the increasing EABV tends to reduce volumetric thirst stimuli. Moreover, the conclusion of the test is arbitrary if thirst is not elicited; thus, total absence of thirst ("adipsia") can never be defined with certainty.

Dehydration testing (similar to the procedures described above for evaluating ADH release) has often been used to study thirst, but is also subject to some ambiguities. For example, dehydration increases P_{osm} and decreases EABV, which should synergistically increase thirst (and ADH release): if thirst is not elicited a defect is probably present, but the defect cannot be uniquely attributed to either of the two stimuli; if thirst is elicited, a defect in one of the two stimuli may be unrecognized. Finally, there are no well-established clinical tests of pure volumetric stimuli (i.e., elicited by a decrease in EABV with a constant P_{osm}), although trimethapan has been used to produce a 10 mmHg decrease in blood pressure (or a 10 beat per minute increase in heart rate) as a test of volumetric stimuli of ADH release. Others have used thermogenic stimuli[89] or metabolic blocking agents,[89] but in most of these studies the relationship of the stimulus to the normal osmolal and volumetric thirst stimuli is complex, and in some cases,[85] the mechanism of thirst stimulation is entirely unknown.

In recent years, a semiquantitative technique has been developed to evaluate thirst in humans.[84] However, this technique has not yet been applied to clinical problems, so that its potential value in the study of human thirst disorders is uncertain. The technique would have to be combined with the more usual physiological and biochemical measurements (e.g., dehydration testing with measurements of max U_{osm} and P_{ADH}) under carefully controlled conditions (e.g., euvolemia or controlled variations in EABV) to permit rigorous analysis of any abnormalities that might be found.

With these difficulties in interpretation in mind, the lowest P_{osm} at which thirst is reported is usually defined as the "osmolar (osmolal) threshold" for thirst; in humans this is usually 2 to 3 percent above the baseline osmolality (Fig. 21-2). Hypodipsia is usually defined as an elevation in the osmolal threshold for thirst, and "adipsia" as the absence of thirst over the range of osmolality tested. However, this definition of hypodipsia is incomplete; a distinction should be made between the absolute P_{osm} at which thirst is elicited (the osmolal threshold for thirst) and the relative change in plasma osmolality (ΔP_{osm}) from the steady-state baseline which is necessary to elicit thirst (the osmolal sensitivity) at any given baseline value of P_{osm}. Such a distinction is necessary to define the syndrome of "essential hypernatremia" precisely (addressed below). It is theoretically possible to have an abnormal threshold with normal sensitivity, a normal threshold with abnormal sensitivity, or abnormal threshold and sensitivity. All cases of "essential hypernatremia" must have an abnormality in the osmolal threshold for thirst, but may or may not express thirst at still higher plasma osmolalities. Finally, to complete the analogy with defective ADH release, there could be defects in either or both of the two normal physiological thirst stimuli (increasing P_{osm} or decreasing EABV). By definition, patients with essential hypernatremia have intact volumetric stimuli for thirst and ADH release since clinical euvolemia is necessary for the diagnosis of the syndrome. On the other hand, if clinical evidence of a decreased EABV appears in patients with pure hypodipsia, both volumetric and osmolal stimuli must be ineffective, or access to water must be restricted.

TREATMENT OF PRIMARY HYPODIPSIA Water deficits must be replaced, as described earlier (under "Calculation of pure water deficits"), with the appropriate precautions. For long-term management some patients must have water prescribed as if it were a medication. No drugs have been approved for treating primary hypodipsia. Chlorpropamide has been associated with an increase in the sensation of thirst in some patients (in addition to the expected increase in ADH effects), but this action has not been applied to thirst disorders. The phenothiazine thioridazine has also been associated with increased thirst, but is also untested in clinical hypodipsia. A variety of other agents (e.g., lithium, benzodiazepines) may increase water intake, but their mechanism of action is unknown or is too complex to warrant clinical use at this time.[50,223] Clonapramine HCL administration has resulted in increased water intake and normalization of the serum sodium concentration in an individual with the hypothalamic syndrome.[109]

Essential hypernatremia

Essential hypernatremia is a term reserved for selected cases in which hyperosmolality and hypernatremia, euvolemia (by the usual clinical and laboratory findings), and the absence of thirst are all found. Usually a well-defined pathological lesion, often as a result of trauma, tumors, or inflammation (e.g., histiocytosis X) is found. Episodes of encephalopathy, obesity, and anterior-pituitary hypofunction, presumably hypothalamic in origin, occur frequently as well.[98] By definition, this condition represents an upward resetting of the osmolal set point for ADH release and of the osmolal threshold for thirst perception. In some classifications, these two defects would be described as partial CDI and hypodipsia, respectively. But the other volumetric stimuli for ADH and thirst perception must operate at normal or near normal settings to maintain asymptomatic euvolemia by the usual clinical laboratory criteria. In this sense, the syndrome of essential hypernatremia is the hyperosmolal counterpart of the "reset osmostat" syndrome, in which asymptomatic, euvolemic hyponatremia is maintained with a decreased osmolal set point for ADH release and a decreased osmolal threshold for thirst (see Chap. 20). Thus, essential hypernatremia and "reset osmostat" are really upward and downward resetting of the osmostat, respectively.

In some patients in whom the criteria for essential hypernatremia are met, there appears to be abnormal osmolal sensitivity for ADH release, both above and below the elevated set point.[70,98,181] Responses to both dehydration and water loading tests are abnormal, although the patients maintain euvolemic hypernatremia when not so stressed.[1,35,63] In fact, some of these patients excrete dilute urine in response to isotonic saline infusion, suggesting that an increased EABV is capable of further reducing the already subnormal ADH release, even when plasma osmolality is increasing;[63] volumetric stimuli continue to override osmolal stimuli in these patients. In several patients, increased renal sensitivity to VP suggests enhanced end-organ sensitivity and implicates low endogenous ADH levels as the primary defect.[70] Similar osmolal resetting and altered sensitivity may be present for the sensation of thirst,[1,35,122,183] but more careful quantitative studies[35] of the thirst sensation are required. The relationships among the three primary disorders of water metabolism that are usually present with hypernatremia are complex, since many overlapping cases can be found. Nevertheless, it is worth characterizing the "pure" forms of these three disturbances (CDI, primary hypodipsia, and essential hypernatremia or upward resetting of the osmostat) so that more complex circumstances can also

TABLE 21-8 • **Physiological effects of primary disorders of water metabolism**

	Laboratory abnormalities		Abnormal pathways	
DISORDERS	PLASMA OSMOLALITY	URINE OSMOLALITY	ADH RELEASE	THIRST PERCEPTION
Central diabetes insipidus	Increased	Dilute (inappropriate)	Impaired osmoreceptors, baroreceptors	
Primary hypodipsia	Increased or normal	Concentrated (appropriate)		Impaired osmoreceptors
Essential hypernatremia	Increased	Normal (inappropriate)	Impaired osmoreceptors	Impaired osmoreceptors

be recognized. Table 21-8 summarizes criteria for differentiating these three syndromes with respect to their effect on ADH and thirst.

Several cases of "symptomatic" essential hypernatremia have been described. The patients appear to have no symptoms or signs suggesting EABV depletion, are hypodipsic, but also have muscle weakness associated with hypernatremia. Careful review of these cases indicates that when muscle weakness appears in the setting of essential hypernatremia, hypokalemia or total body potassium depletion should be suspected.[1,12,31,62,63,100,103,122,144,145,183]

Hypotonic fluid loss

Clinical hypertonicity occurs most commonly as a result of hypotonic fluid losses (i.e., water losses in excess of electrolyte losses) (Fig. 21-9). In general, clinical findings are similar to, but more severe than, those associated with pure water loss.

Conceptually, hypotonic fluid can be divided into an isotonic portion and an electrolyte-free, pure water portion (Table 21-2). The pure water portion of the hypotonic loss is derived from both ECF and ICF, in proportion to the initial volumes of these two compartments (Fig. 21-8). However, the isotonic (isoelectrolyte) portion comes almost exclusively from the ECF, and therefore produces a much greater reduction in ECF and in intravascular volume than the loss of an equal volume of pure water. Furthermore, since solute is lost in addition to water, the loss of hypotonic solutions produces less hypertonicity than an equal volume of pure water loss (Figs. 21-8 and 21-9).

The following example illustrates these points. If a 70-kg man with a normal 42 liters of TBW loses 5 percent of his body weight (3.5 liters) as pure water, the plasma $[Na^+]$ would rise from 140 to 153 meq/liter (Equation 11), and the intravascular compartment would decrease by one-twelfth of the water loss (292 ml; about the volume of an average blood transfusion). In contrast 3.5 liters of half-isotonic fluids can be thought of as 1.75 liters of pure water and 1.75 liters of isotonic (equivalent to ECF in composition) electrolyte solution. Were the same man to lose 3.5 liters of half-isotonic fluid, as in the first case, one-twelfth of the *pure* water loss ($\frac{1}{12}$ of 1.75 liters, or 146 ml) would be derived from the intravascular compartment; however, an additional one-fourth of the isotonic electrolyte loss ($\frac{1}{4}$ of 1.75 liters = 438 ml) would come from the inravascular compartment, because that compartment represents one-fourth of the original ECF. Therefore, the total loss from the intravascular compartment in this case would be 146 + 438 = 584 ml, which is about twice the intravascular loss occasioned by a pure water loss of the same volume.

The serum $[Na^+]$ would only rise to 146 meq/liter after the hypotonic loss (instead of the 153 meq/liter caused by the loss of an equal volume of pure water). The difference occurs because the loss of isotonic electrolyte (1.75 liters of the total hypotonic loss) would have no effect on the serum $[Na^+]$; and only the 1.75 liters of pure water loss need be considered. However, it must be taken into account before calculating the new TBS that the isotonic loss has reduced the TBW from 42 to 40.25 liters (Equations 8, 9, and 11).

$$\text{TBS} = 2(140)(40.25) \tag{20}$$

This is still the new TBS to be used when calculating the new value for plasma osmolality after the loss of the 1.75 liters of pure water. However, the new TBW has been further reduced from 40.25 to 38.5 liters. Therefore

$$\text{New } P_{osm} = \text{TBS/TBW} = \frac{2(140)(40.25)}{38.5} \tag{21}$$

Since the new serum $[Na^+]$ is one-half of the new P_{osm}

$$\text{New } [Na^+] = \frac{(140)(40.25)}{38.5} = 146 \text{ meq/liter} \tag{22}$$

Thus, patients with hypotonic fluid losses are more likely to become hypotensive due to disproportionate contraction of the ECF, and therefore of EABV, than patients with pure water losses of the same volume. The latter group are more hypertonic and hypernatremic.

Etiology of hypotonic fluid loss

There are many causes of hypotonic fluid losses (Table 21-9). Hypotonic fluid can be lost with such gastrointestinal disorders as recurrent vomiting, prolonged nasogastric suctioning, or profuse diarrhea from gastrointestinal disorders[37,83] or lactulose therapy.[174] In infants, gastroenteritis is the most common cause of hypotonic fluid loss;[47,116] in adults, hypotonic renal losses (e.g., from osmotic diuresis) are more common causes of hypertonicity.[95,149] Osmotic diuresis can produce hypertonicity regardless of whether the solute is permeant (e.g., urea) or impermeant (e.g., glucose, mannitol); although the glomerular filtration of large amounts of solute obligates the urinary excretion of both water and electrolyte, the urinary electrolyte concentration is less than that in plasma water even when the U_{osm} approaches P_{osm}. Clinical examples of hypotonic urinary losses (i.e., losses of relatively electrolyte-free water) include patients with hyperglycemia (and glycosuria); patients on tube feedings with a high protein content (and increased urinary urea);[93] and patients undergoing diuresis after the relief of urinary tract obstruction (and consequent increases in urinary urea). Other examples of hypotonic losses include cutaneous losses from profuse sweating and peritoneal losses during dialysis with hypertonic peritoneal dialysate.[225] In all of these cases, the coexistence of increased pure water intake can mitigate the hypertonicity; intake of pure water can even produce hypotonicity. Such a large increase in water intake might be expected in those circumstances associated with a decreased intravascular volume, and consequently, with an increased *volumetric* stimulus to thirst. Although an increased P_{osm} level also stimulates thirst in hypertonic states, this stimulus should no longer be effective once P_{osm} returns to normal and therefore should not be a cause of hypotonicity.

TABLE 21-9 • Routes of hypotonic fluid loss

- Gastrointestinal
  - Recurrent vomiting
  - Nasogastric suction
  - Severe diarrhea
    - Lactulose
- Renal
  - Osmotic diuretics
  - Urea
    - Following hyperalimentation
    - Postobstructive diuresis
  - Sugars
    - Glucose
    - Mannitol
    - Sorbitol
    - Glycerol
  - Other diuretics
- Cutaneous
  - Hyperthermia
  - Hyperthyroidism
  - Burns
- Peritoneal
  - Peritonitis
  - Peritoneal dialysis

Clinical presentation of hypotonic fluid loss

The clinical presentation of hypotonic losses often includes features of hypertonicity (increased thirst, decreased sweating, dry mucous membranes), and features of decreased EABV (orthostatic hypotension, tachycardia, poor skin turgor). A history of a disorder responsible for hypotonic fluid loss, and an explanation for inadequate water intake, should be sought. The serum $[Na^+]$ is not predictable; the value of serum $[Na^+]$ would reflect the balance between the hypotonic losses and water intake, and the true value might also be obscured (decreased) by the presence of another impermeant solute (e.g., glucose). Except in the presence of renal disease and/or osmotic diuresis, the urine volume is usually reduced, the urine sodium concentration is low, and the U_{osm} is increased. Evidence of secondary hyperaldosteronism, reflecting the decresae in EABV, is provided by the relatively low urinary sodium and high urinary potassium concentrations.

Diagnosis of hypotonic fluid loss

The clinical setting often suggests that a hypotonic fluid loss might have occurred, and the presence of hypernatremia (hypertonicity) combined with EABV depletion strongly suggests this pathophysiological mechanism has been operative. However, hypertonicity is not always present. As discussed above, a substantial decrease in EABV, as expected with hypotonic fluid losses, stimulates thirst even in the absence of hypertonicity; the combination of hypertonicity and decreased EABV is synergistic with respect to both thirst and ADH release. Consequently, many patients with hypotonic fluid losses ingest and retain large amounts of water, and may even become hypotonic (hyponatremic) because the stimulus of a decreased EABV persists even after the P_{osm} has fallen to or below normal (see also "Integration of ADH and thirst," above). Therefore, the presence of both hypertonicity and decreased EABV suggests the patient has some impairment of water intake, as well as loss of hypotonic fluid.[201]

Treatment of hypotonic fluid losses

Replacement of hypotonic fluids can be conceptualized in the same manner as the loss of hypotonic fluids: in both cases the fluids may be considered divisible into isotonic and "pure water" components. However, if there is evidence of EABV depletion, the first priority is to restore the EABV, which is best accomplished with fluids that remain within the extracellular compartment and if EABV is severely depleted with replacement fluids that remain within the intravascular compartment. Isotonic saline (0.9 percent NaCl) solutions are largely restricted to the ECF; various colloid-containing solutions (e.g., albumin, whole blood) are to a great extent further restricted to the intravascular compartment of the ECF. Such colloidal solutuions are most effective when their electrolyte content is isotonic NaCl.

The magnitude of a hypotonic fluid loss can be estimated by physical examination. The usual rule of thumb is that a 3 percent decrease in body weight caused by isotonic NaCl fluid loss produces mild to moderate hypovolemia, characterized by orthostatic hypotension and tachycardia. By the time isotonic losses exceed 5 percent of body weight, the hypovolemia is severe, and is accompanied by marked hypotension, which can lead to irreversible shock if untreated. Thus, a 70-kg individual sustaining a 3 to 5 percent decrease in body weight due to isotonic fluid losses would require 2.1 to 3.5 liters of isotonic NaCl fluid replacement or smaller volume of an albumin-containing NaCl solution to restore the initial EABV.

Restoration of EABV to a safe level takes precedence over correction of any concurrent pure water loss, even if significant hypernatremia exists. Only when blood pressure has been stabilized can consideration be given to the amount of "pure" water needed. The pure water component of the deficit can be calculated from Equation 12. Fluid for replacing lost water can be administered either orally as pure water or intravenously as 5 percent glucose.

Impermeant solute gain

The clinical causes of pure solute gain are usually accidental complications of medical therapy, such as the inadvertent intravenous (instead of intraamniotic) administration of hypertonic saline for therapeutic abortion, or the use of 5 percent NaCl instead of 5 percent dextrose-in-water[41] However, some emergency situations, such as cardiac arrest and severe metabolic acidosis, require the administration of hypertonic solutions (e.g., 7.5 percent, i.e., 893 meq/liter, sodium bicarbonate solution). The osmolal contents of the various solutions that are used in the hospital setting appear in Table 21-10. Many hypertonic solutions that can be found in household and industrial settings are poisons; ingestion of them may lead to a hypertonic state, as well as toxicity.

The laboratory feature of hypertonicity at least partly depends on the impermeant solute involved. The urine is usually isotonic, or nearly isotonic, and contains substantial amounts of the solute responsible for the hypertonicity. Hypernatremia is expected if the added solute is a sodium salt; with other solutes the serum $[Na^+]$ is not easily predicted. Following the acute administration of an

TABLE 21-10 • Therapeutic hypertonic solutions

Solute	Molecular weight	Concentration, mg/dl	Osmolality, mosm/kg water	Typical container size, ml	Use
Sodium chloride	58.5	3	1026	500	Emergency treatment of
		5	1711	500	hypotonic states;
		20	6845	250	intraamniotic instillation for therapeutic abortion
Sodium bicarbonate	84	5	1190	500	Treatment of metabolic
		7.5	1786	50	acidosis, hyperkalemia, cardiopulmonary arrest
Dextrose (glucose) monohydrate	198	10	505	500 and 1000	Caloric supplementation
		20	1010	500	
		50	2525	50 and 500	Treatment of hypoglycemia (50% soln)
Mannitol	182	10	549	500 and 1000	Osmotic diuresis, treat-
		20	1099	250 and 500	ment of acute renal failure,
		25	1374	50	cerebral edema, acute glaucoma
Glycerol	92	50	5435	120	Treatment of cerebral
		75	8152	120	edema, acute glaucoma

SOURCE: Arieff, AI et al: Pathophysiology of hyperosmolar states, in Andreoli TE et al (eds): *Disturbances in Body Fluid Osmolality*. Bethesda, MD, American Physiology Society, 1977.

impermeant solute that is not a sodium salt (e.g., mannitol, glycerol, sorbitol), plasma osmolality rises, but serum [Na^+] falls as water moves from the ICF to the ECF in response to the acute hypertonicity. More prolonged administration of such solutes produces an osmotic diuresis with the loss of urine with an electrolyte concentration lower than that of plasma. In this case, the laboratory findings more closely resemble those obtained in the pathophysiology of hypotonic fluid losses, particularly after the administered impermeant solute has been excreted (see "Hypotonic fluid losses" and "Other impermeant solutes," above).

Hypertonicity due to added sodium salts

ETIOLOGY Acute hypernatremia secondary to solute gain in children is often due to improperly diluted formula, to highly concentrated oral rehydration fluids for diarrhea,[75] to use of baking soda for abdominal pain[186] or to accidental substitution of NaCl for sucrose.[46,82] This pathophysiology rarely occurs in adults, except after the administration of hypertonic sodium-containing solutions, such as accidental intravenous administration of 20 percent NaCl (3448 m*M* or 6896 mosm/liter) during a therapeutic abortion;[65,125] accidental administration of 5 percent NaCl (862 m*M* or 1724 mosm/liter) in place of 5 percent glucose in water; malfunction of the dialysate-proportioning system during hemodialysis; and administration of large quantities of $NaHCO_3$ to correct acidosis during management of a cardiac arrest[150] (each 50-ml ampule of $NaHCO_3$ solution contains either 44 or 50 meq of $NaHCO_3$, that is, approximately 1000 meq/liter, or 2000 mosm/liter). More rarely, accidental poisoning with other sodium salts (e.g., Na_2SO_4) can produce hypernatremia and hyperosmolality by similar mechanisms.

CLINICAL PRESENTATION The two immediate physiological consequences of the abrupt administration of a sodium salt (or another impermeant solute restricted to the ECF) are ECF expansion and ICF contraction (Fig. 21-10). Rapid ECF expansion often results in the development of acute pulmonary edema or other manifestations of congestive heart failure, due to acute expansion of the intravascular compartment. Furthermore, severe cerebral dehydration often occurs because the rapid development of hypertonicity may not permit sufficient time for the brain to produce "idiogenic osmoles" in the ICF[141] (see "Consequences of hypertonicity," above). As a result, neurological abnormalities, especially grand mal seizures, are frequent complications of acute hypertonicity; they may be life-threatening. Other clinical features include vomiting, fever, dyspnea, spasticity, and coma. Infants are particularly susceptible to neurological complications following the cerebral dehydration due to rapid infusions of hypertonic saline; they have a 50 percent mortality, as a result of neurological complications, and those that survive all have residual neurological deficits. Adults are particularly vulnerable to pulmonary and cardiac complications following the rapid expansion of the intravascular compartment.

DIAGNOSIS OF HYPERTONICITY DUE TO SODIUM SALT The patient's history is critical in determining which sodium salt is responsible for the observed hypertonicity. Laboratory findings are often very useful: elevations in chloride or bicarbonate concentration suggest those sodium salts are responsible; any other sodium salt might appear simply as an increase in the "anion gap" (see Chap. 25). However, the clinical presentations of these hypernatremic syndromes, regardless of the specific sodium salt involved, are quite similar. In each case sodium is relatively restricted to the ECF (Fig. 21-10); the intravascular compartment becomes expanded as a result. The consequences of a rapid expansion of the EABV in susceptible individuals might be acute congestive heart failure, accompanied by hypertension and edema (both systemic and pulmonary).

TREATMENT OF HYPERTONICITY DUE TO SODIUM SALTS Despite the presence of hypertonicity, the administration of large amounts of pure water may have adverse medical consequences. Such therapy alone may further expand the ECF, and may possibly worsen already compromised cardiac and pulmonary functions (Fig. 21-10). Therefore, therapy must include both administration of water and removal of excess solute. The theoretical water "deficit" can be calculated to estimate the amount of water needed to "correct" the hypertonicity (i.e., how much water added to the current, increased TBS would restore tonicity to the normal value for P_{osm}).

For example, suppose a normal 70-kg man with a (normal) TBW = 42 liters and a (normal) P_{osm} = 300 mosm/kg is given 1.0 liter of 5 percent saline solution. This solution may be thought of as 1.0 liter of pure water and 1711 mosm of solute (Table 21-10). The new TBS would equal the sum of the normal TBS plus the added solute:

$$\begin{aligned}\text{Normal TBS} &= \text{normal } P_{osm} \times \text{normal TBW}\\ &= (300)(42)\\ &= 12{,}600 \text{ mosm}\end{aligned} \tag{23}$$

$$\begin{aligned}\text{Added solute} &= 1711 \text{ mosm (in 1 liter of 5\% saline)}\\ &= 1711 \text{ mosm}\end{aligned} \tag{24}$$

Therefore, the

$$\begin{aligned}\text{New (present) TBS} &= \text{normal TBS} + \text{added solute}\\ &= 14{,}311 \text{ mosm}\end{aligned} \tag{25}$$

The new TBW would equal the sum of the normal TBW (42 liters) plus the added water (1.0 liter):

$$\begin{aligned}\text{New (present) TBW} &= \text{normal TBW} + \text{added W}\\ &= 42 + 1 = 43 \text{ liters}\end{aligned} \tag{26}$$

The new (present) P_{osm} is given by the ratio of the new TBS to the new TBW:

$$\text{New (present) } P_{osm} = \text{new TBS/new TBW} = \frac{14{,}311}{43} = 333 \text{ mosm/kg} \quad (27)$$

To calculate the amount of water (ΔW) needed to restore a normal P_{osm} (300 mosm/kg) from the present condition, it is assumed that there is no change in the TBS (i.e., that TBS remains at the increased value of 14,311 mosm). The desired (normal) P_{osm} = 300 mosm/kg, and the present TBW = 43 liters. All the necessary data are available:

$$\text{Desired (normal) } P_{osm} = \text{present TBS/desired TBW} \quad (28)$$

$$\text{Desired TBW} = \text{present TBS/desired (normal) } P_{osm} = \frac{14{,}311}{300} = 47.7 \text{ liters} \quad (29)$$

$$\Delta W = \text{desired TBW} - \text{present TBW} = 47.7 - 43.0 = 4.7 \text{ liters} \quad (30)$$

In other words, an addition of 4.7 liters of pure water to the present TBW and TBW would return P_{osm} from its present value (333 mosm/kg) to the desired (normal) value (300 mosm/kg).

The patient has, of course, not "lost" 4.7 liters of pure water; this hypertonic condition was caused by the addition of solute (in excess of water). If this *apparent* deficit were actually restored by pure water administration, further expansion of the ECF would occur, with the potential complications discussed above. In practice, the calculation only serves as a rough guide to the magnitude of "pure water" deficit. The estimated "deficit" should be replaced at 5 percent dextrose in water. Plasma osmolality, the rate of diuresis (urinary solute removal), and, most important, the neurological status of the patient should be monitored during replacement therapy. The neurological symptoms should improve as relatively electrolyte-free solutions are administered slowly; "isotonic water intoxication" and cerebral edema are real dangers if relatively electrolyte-free solutions are administered too rapidly. In most cases, the volume of replacement solutions should not exceed one-half of the apparent deficit in the initial 4 to 6 h of therapy; the remainder of the deficit should be replaced over the next 12 to 48 h. An alternative method is to replace urine output (which contains electrolyte and water) with water alone, on a volume-for-volume basis. This gradually allows the "excess" electrolyte to be excreted with no change in TBW (provided that TBW is nearly normal at the outset, and that additional water is given to account for any nonurinary losses, such as insensible water loss). To avert congestive heart failure and pulmonary edema, it is often desirable to simultaneously administer a diuretic active at the loop of Henle (e.g., furosemide, bumetanide, or ethacrynic acid) to increase solute loss and reduce the ECF volume. However, if renal or cardiac failure are present, phlebotomy or dialysis (particularly, ultrafiltration) or continuous arterio-venous hemofiltration (CAVH)[173] may be needed for solute removal. The removal of solute is the more "physiological" approach since solute gain was responsible for the initial hypertonicity; however, administration of electrolyte-free water is also usually required for immediate treatment of neurological symptoms; the latter alone may be sufficient if cardiac and renal function are good.

Hypertonicity due to glucose

ETIOLOGY Hypertonicity due to hyperglycemia usually occurs in individuals with uncontrolled diabetes mellitus. Occasionally, the same syndrome is observed in nondiabetic patients receiving large amounts of glucose intravenously or during peritoneal dialysis. The pathogenesis of hypertonicity due to hyperglycemia depends on glucose being boh an "effective osmole," that is, a relatively impermeant solute (in the absence of insulin), and an osmotic diuretic.[79,80,96] Thus, hyperglycemia can produce hypertonicity both directly by its presence in the ECF, and indirectly by causing the renal loss of hypotonic fluids during glucose-mediated osmotic diuresis. In addition, although the loss of ECF sodium during the osmotic diuresis tends to reduce ECF volume, the presence of the glucose in the ECF "masks" the contraction; in the absence of insulin, glucose is an effective osmole, causing water to move from the ICF to the ECF and thereby tending to maintain ECF volume even if sodium is depleted (Fig. 21-13). Water deficits can also be "masked" by hyponatremia; the water shift from ICF to ECF compartments decreases the serum sodium concentration, obscuring the magnitude of the water loss. When hyperglycemia develops relatively slowly (over days to weeks), there is more time for water, sodium, and potassium to be depleted, and more time for the generation of "idiogenic osmoles" in the CNS.

Hyperglycemia can exist with hypernatremia, hyponatremia, or a normal serum $[Na^+]$. The serum $[Na^+]$ tends to rise during the hypotonic osmotic diuresis induced by glucosuria, and tends to fall during the shift of water from the ICF to the ECF induced by hyperglycemia. In the latter case, the serum $[Na^+]$ can be "corrected" to account for the fluid shift, and the corrected value might be more easily interpreted in the context of hypotonic fluid losses.

The effect of hyperglycemia on the serum $[Na^+]$ can be estimated by the following approximation: each rise of 100 mg/dl in blood glucose level above normal lowers the serum $[Na^+]$ by 1.6 meq/liter. Symbolically,

$$\Delta[Na^+] \approx \frac{(1.6)[\text{glucose}]}{100} \quad (31)$$

$[Na^+]$ is given in meq/liter and [glucose] is given in mg/dl. If [glucose] = 1000 mg/dl, then Δ [glucose] =

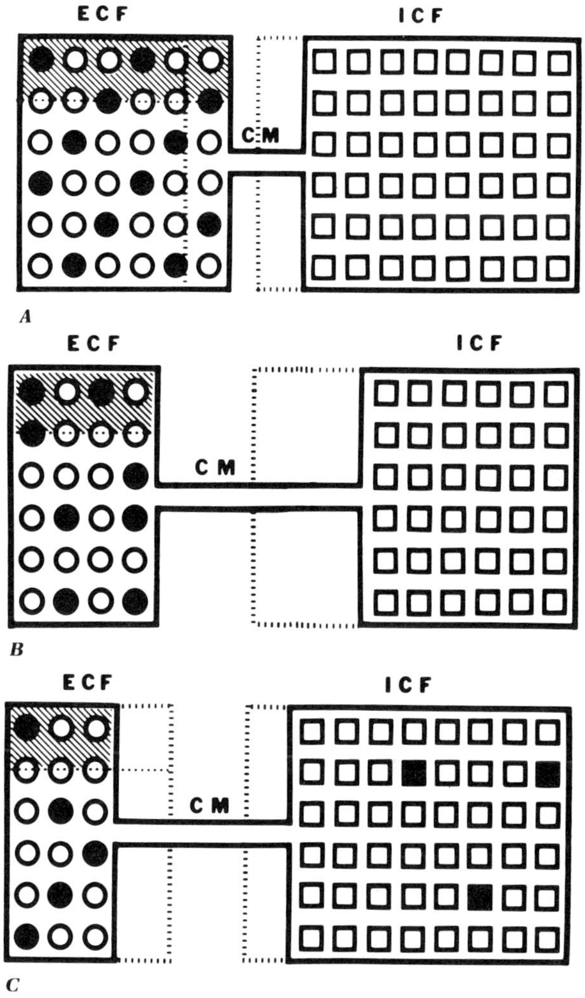

FIGURE 21-13 • Hypertonicity and hyponatremia due to glucose addition (impermeant solute gain). (A) Glucose (solid circles) has been added to the ECF. Since glucose is relatively impermeant in the absence of insulin, it remains restricted to the ECF. The result is an increase in "effective" ECF solute concentration, expansion of the ECF, and contraction of the ICF (water moves from ICF to ECF in response to the osmotic gradient). Note that the nonglucose solute *content* of the ECF (largely sodium salts; open circles) remains the same, but the solute *concentration* decreases (producing hyponatremia). Thus, hyperglycemia can be associated with both hypertonicity and hyponatremia. (B) The alterations in the ECF and ICF as a result of osmotic diuresis with glucose are shown. The osmotic diuresis causes the loss of salt, glucose, and water. The loss of sodium salts (open circles) and glucose (closed circles) from the ECF results in contraction of that compartment. Since the ECF was initially expanded as a consequence of hyperglycemia, the osmotic diuresis returns the volume of this compartment toward normal; glucose (solid circles) contributes significantly to the overall concentration of impermeant ECF solutes. Water losses during the osmotic diuresis are derived from both the ICF (about two-thirds of the loss) and the ECF (about one-third of the loss). Therefore, the ICF, which was already contracted (in A), contracts further, but the ECF volume is maintained as a consequence of the ongoing hyperglycemia. (C) Alterations in ECF and ICF as a result of insulin administration. Insulin administration to treat hyperglycemia in case B above results in the movement of glucose from the ECF to the ICF; eventually, glucose is metabolized to carbon dioxide and water in the ICF. The movement of glucose from the ECF to the ICF is associated with water movement in the same direction as the osmolar gradient changes. As a result the ICF partially reexpands and ECF markedly contracts. The loss of glucose from the ECF, whether by osmotic diuresis or into the cells as a result of insulin administration, thus can produce profound EABV depletion and shock. Infusion of sodium-containing solutions to maintain an adequate circulating volume is necessary prior to the administration of insulin when glucose is the predominant solute supporting the intravascular volume. (Modified, with permission from Feig PU, McCurdy DK: *N Engl J Med* 279:1444, 1977.)

900 mg/dl (i.e., [glucose] is about 900 mg/dl greater than normal). The serum [Na⁺] should decrease by

$$\Delta[\mathrm{Na}^+] = \frac{1.6 \times 900}{100} = 14 \text{ meq/liter} \qquad (32)$$

If the serum $[\mathrm{Na}^+]$ were 142 meq/liter when the [glucose] was 1000 mg/dl, then the "corrected" value for $[\mathrm{Na}^+]$ would be

$$\text{"Corrected } [\mathrm{Na}^+] = 142 + 16 = 158 \text{ meq/liter} \qquad (33)$$

It is important to calculate the value of the "corrected" serum $[\mathrm{Na}^+]$, because this would be the serum $[\mathrm{Na}^+]$ level if [glucose] returned to normal.

If the corrected serum $[\mathrm{Na}^+]$ is above normal, then hypotonic fluid loss has occurred: water and electrolytes have been lost; water loss has been larger than electrolyte loss. In fact, if the uncorrected serum $[\mathrm{Na}^+]$ is normal or elevated in the presence of hyperglycemia, then relatively large water losses must have occurred. In such circumstances, the magnitude of the hypertonic (hypernatremic) state must be "unmasked" by correcting the serum $[\mathrm{Na}^+]$ by applying Equation 31.

If the corrected serum $[\mathrm{Na}^+]$ is normal, then the fluids lost have, on the average, been isotonic rather than hypotonic. If no fluids were lost, then hyperglycemia should be associated with hyponatremia. Equation 31 estimates the magnitude of this expectation. Proper treatment depends heavily on the determination of the magnitude of fluid loss.

CLINICAL PRESENTATION OF HYPERTONICITY DUE TO HYPERGLYCEMIA The typical patient is more than 60 years old, and either is not known to be a diabetic or has very mild diabetes (manageable with diet and/oral hypoglycemia agents). The patient often has a history of recent infection, pancreatitis, or a similar stress. In hospitalized patients, severe hyperglycemia can be precipitated by hyperalimentation[239] or administration of drugs (e.g., steroids, diuretics, phenytoin). In most cases days or weeks of profound polydipsia and polyuria precede the development of coma, sometimes culminating in renal failure and/or severe debility. This syndrome is usually called hyperosmolar (hyperglycemic) nonketotic coma (HNKC).[96,151,184]

Physical findings are determined strongly by the degree of fluid and electrolyte loss, and therefore depend on the length of the hyperglycemic state. After days or weeks of severe polydipsia there is usually evidence of profound reduction of fluid volume, including dry mucous membranes, poor tissue turgor, decreased sweating, hypotension, and tachycardia. However, signs due to EABV depletion of salt and water (hypotension and tachycardia) may be masked, at least partly, by the presence of hyperglycemia (in the manner already discussed). If there is evidence of EABV depletion in the presence of hyperglycemia, then profound losses of TBW and electrolytes have occurred. Evidence of hypertonicity (e.g., acute gastric dilatation with nausea, vomiting, and abdominal pain; focal or generalized neurological findings, such as seizures) is almost always present.

Laboratory evaluation usually reveals hyperglycemia without ketonemia and glycosuria without ketonuria.[151] Fifty percent of HNKC patients have mild metabolic acidosis (see "Diagnosis of HNKC," below, for comparison with diabetic ketoacidosis). Increased triglyceride and cholesterol levels may be associated with the hyperglycemia; hypertriglyceridemia should be suspected if the serum is lactescent. Elevations in the percentage of lipid in a blood sample may result in a false lowering of serum [Na^+] value is usually measured only in the water-containing fraction of the sample; see Chap. 20). The white blood cell (WBC) count may be elevated (>20,000 per cubic millimeter, predominantly polymorphonuclear leukocytes) even in the absence of infection.

DIAGNOSIS OF HNKC Two clinically important hyperglycemic syndromes occur in diabetics: hyperosmolar nonketotic coma (HNKC; also known as hyperglycemic, hyperosmotic, nonketotic coma, or HHNK), and diabetic ketoacidosis (DKA). Although there is substantial overlap of these two conditions, there are also some distinguishing features (Table 21-11) (see Chap. 26). HNKC tends to occur in the neglected patient, i.e., in the very young or very old, in the institutionalized, in the mentally or physically handicapped, and in those who cannot recognize thirst or express their need for water. The blood [glucose] in HNKC is usually greater than 800 mg/dl; P_{osm} is >350 mosm/kg, but there is no ketonemia or ketonuria. However, about half of HNKC patients also exhibit a mild degree of metabolic acidosis (with an anion gap which may represent excess lactic, acetic, or β-hydroxybutyric acids, or uremic acidosis). HNKC is associated

TABLE 21-11 • Features of diabetic ketoacidosis (DKA) and hyperosmolar nonketotic coma (HNKC)

	DKA	HNKC
CLINICAL FEATURES		
Patient characteristics	Young; Type I or brittle diabetic	Old; handicapped; Type II or abn. GTT
Onset	Rapid (hours to days)	Slower (days to weeks)
Symptoms	Polyuria, thirst, high water intake; nausea, vomiting, abdominal pain	Polyuria, (occasionally) thirst, low water intake; confusion, headache
Precipitating factors	Infection; stress; omission of insulin	Infection; stress; glucose load (e.g., peritoneal dialysis, hyperalimentation); drugs (steroids, potassium-wasting diuretics)
Physical findings	Mild volume depletion; Kussmaul respirations; abdominal tenderness; "fruity"-smelling breath	Severe volume depletion; focal neurological abnormalities; seizures; coma
LABORATORY FEATURES		
Blood glucose, mg/dl	<800	>1000
Anion gap, meq/liter*	>20	<17
Osmolality, mosm/kg water	<310	>350
BUN, mg/dl	<60	>60
HCO_3^-, meq/liter	<12	>15
pH (blood)	<7.2	>7.2
Water loss, liters	3–15	6–18

* For DKA, usually acetoacetic acid or other ketones; for HNKC, usually lactic acid.

DEFINITIONS: Brittle diabetes mellitus: frequent bouts of DKA; abn GTT: abnormal glucose tolerance test; Type I: insulin dependent, ketosis prone; Type II: non-insulin dependent, nonketosis prone.

with marked sodium depletion; therefore, hypotension and shock are common. HNKC is also associated with marked water depletion and hypertonicity; making coma and focal neurological impairments common findings.

In contrast, patients with DKA, as a group, are younger, have blood [glucose] levels that are generally less than 800 mg/dl, but have moderate to severe ketoacidosis with ketonuria. However, life-threatening hyperglycemia and hypertonicity develop less commonly in patients with DKA, which distinguishes DKA patients from HNKC patients. Similarly, the volume depletion associated with DKA can be severe but is not usually as profound as in HNKC. Many patients have features of both syndromes; the differing degrees of prominence of various findings allow for classification, and have therapeutic implications.[131]

TREATMENT OF HNKC The treatment of HNKC has five goals: (1) restoring intravascular and ECF volumes, (2) replenishing electrolyte losses, (3) returning tonicity to normal, (4) correcting any associated acid-base or electrolyte disorders, and (5) eliminating precipitating causes, if present. Restoration of the intravascular volume always has the highest priority; blood and/or blood products, albumin or other colloids, and/or isotonic saline may be needed for this correction.[151] Restoring lost electrolytes almost always requires both sodium and potassium salts (and may require bicarbonate, chloride, and/or phosphate). The tonicity is returned to normal by lowering the blood glucose level and by replacing water deficits. It is important to stabilize blood pressure and intravascular volume *before* treating the hyperglycemia. Too rapid lowering of the blood [glucose] removes its "protective" effect in a sodium-depleted patient. Correction of associated acid-base disorders requires attention to both anionic and cationic components of the administered electrolytes, and should be considered conjointly with replacing the electrolyte losses. Precipitating causes, such as drugs or infections, should be sought and eliminated or treated appropriately. In general, isotonic solutions should be used until the blood pressure is controlled; the appropriate hypotonic solutions can follow (as calculated using Equation 31).

The effects of insulin treatment on osmolality can be considered in the context of two theoretical extremes: (1) glucose entry without glucose metabolism, and (2) glucose entry followed by complete glucose metabolism. For example, consider a 70-kg patient with a pretreatment [glucose] of 2000 mg/dl, a pretreatment serum [Na^+] of 120 meq/liter, and an initial ECF volume of 14 liters. Treatment with sufficient insulin to rapidly lower [glucose] to 100 mg/dl would shift about 3 liters of water from the ECF into the ICF in the new steady state after glucose metabolism. A substantial loss of volume from the intravascular compartment, which may already be much smaller than normal due to prolonged hypotonic urinary losses, would result.

If the [glucose] rapidly fell from 2000 to 100 mg/dl *without* glucose metabolism, the shift of glucose (mol wt = 180) into the ICF would represent 1900/18 = 106 mosm/liter. The initial tonicity (effective P_{osm}) can be calculated from Equation 4.

$$\text{Tonicity} = 2(120) + \frac{2000}{18} = 361 \text{ mosm/kg} \qquad (34)$$

Therefore, the osmolar shift is 106/361, or about 30 percent of the initial P_{osm}. About 30 percent of the initial effective ECF solute could abruptly shift to the ICF, and therefore, about 30 percent of the initial ECF water might also shift to the ICF. Of the initial ECF volume of 14 liters, 30 percent (= 4.2 liters) could shift from the ECF to the ICF very rapidly.

However, the rule of thumb, Equation 31, predicts that after intracellular glucose metabolism has taken place, the new steady-state serum [Na^+] would be (1.6 × 19) = 30.4 meq/liter higher than the initial value of 120 meq/liter; therefore, the metabolism of 1900 mg glucose/dl should raise the serum [Na^+] to (120 + 30.4) = 150.4 meq/liter. In the new steady state, the ECF volume will have been proportionally reduced by the solute (glucose) loss:

$$\text{New (steady-state)} = \frac{\text{initial } [Na^+]}{\text{new } [NA^+]} \times \text{initial ECF volume} \qquad (35)$$

$$\text{ECF volume} = \frac{120}{150.4} \times 14 = 11.2 \text{ liters} \qquad (36)$$

Therefore, (14 − 11.2) = 2.8 liters of water will have moved from the ECF to the ICF when the new steady state is reached after metabolism of the glucose. Consequently, if blood or blood products are not required as part of overall management, the initial fluid therapy in HNKC should be intravenous isotonic sodium solution. This solution should be added until the blood pressure, heart rate, urine output, and other findings indicate that ECF volume is no longer a problem. Administration of insulin and hypotonic fluid can then be begun. Extracellular volume should be maintained so that GFR will remain high enough to permit filtration of excess glucose. Loss of glucose by excretion while GFR and EABV are maintained helps substantially in correcting the hyperglycemia.

Patients with HNKC are usually very sensitive to the hypoglycemic action of insulin; small insulin doses should be used initially (e.g., a priming dose of 0.15 unit per kilogram of body weight of regular insulin, intravenously, followed by about 7 U/h. In some cases, hydration alone without insulin reduces the blood sugar; but standard practice is to use small doses of insulin.[235] The blood glucose level should be monitored closely.[151] A mean blood [glucose] of 250 mg/dl is usually achieved in 5 to 6 h by this technique, and larger insulin doses are not usually needed.

Water deficits can be assessed from the corrected serum [Na^+] according to Equations 11 and 12.[59] Since sodium losses are so common in HNKC, it is usually recommended that half-normal saline solutions be used to correct the water deficit. Twice as much half-normal saline is needed to correct a given pure water deficit than if electrolyte-free water were used as the replacement solution. When the blood [glucose] has fallen below 250 mg/dl, 5 percent dextrose in half-normal saline can be used as the replacement solution. It should be remembered that all water deficits should be replaced slowly so that isotonic water intoxication is avoided; the neurological status of the patient should be monitored carefully to prevent the possible development of central pontine myelinolysis.[156,158]

Hypokalemia and total body potassium depletion are often striking in patients with HNKC; they may be either exaggerated or obscured by concurrent acid-base disturbances.[79,80,151] Therefore, potassium should be added to the administered fluids only after it is clear the patient is not hyperkalemic (in spite of possible total body potassium depletion) and is not oliguric (which would result in a tendency to retain potassium). The total body potassium deficits in HNKC can be 5 to 10 meq per kilogram of body weight, and may require days to replace.

Other impermeant solutes

The most common impermeant solutes other than sodium and glucose encountered clinically are mannitol, sorbitol, and glycerol. Mannitol is the most frequently used of these sugars.[13,79,80] It has a molecular weight of 182. For every increment in plasma mannitol concentration of 18.2 mg/dl, the plasma osmolality and tonicity increase by 1 mosm/kg water. Following a mannitol infusion, P_{osm} (and body fluid osmolality everywhere) increases according to the relation:

$$\Delta P_{osm}(\text{mosm/kg}) = \frac{\text{mannitol infused (g)} \times 1000}{\text{TBW (liters)} \times 182} \qquad (37)$$

For example, an infusion of 12.5g of mannitol raises the P_{osm} of a person whose TBW = 42 liters by about 2 mosm/kg. The production of significant hypertonicity thus requires both the administration of large doses of mannitol and the presence of renal insufficiency to prevent rapid excretion. Therefore, the hypertonicity clinically associated with mannitol is not usually due to the mannitol itself, but rather is due to the hypotonic urinary losses induced by the osmotic diuresis.

Sorbitol is only rarely used intravenously in modern clinical medicine, although it once was the osmotic agent found in peritoneal dialysis solutions. Since sorbitol has the same molecular weight as mannitol,[79,80] it has the same osmotic effects and is just as likely to cause hypertonicity in the presence of renal failure (by the same mechanisms as described for mannitol and glucose). Note that oral sorbitol is sometimes used as a carrier for potassium-exchange resins in the treatment of hyperkalemia, and in this setting can induce hypotonic losses through diarrhea. The result can be hypernatremia, hyperosmolality, and hypertonicity, particularly since the exchange resin (administered in the usual sodium form) increases total body sodium substantially.

Glycerol is an impermeant solute used frequently, primarily (like mannitol) to treat cerebral edema or to lower intraocular pressure in glaucoma.[79,80] However, glycerol has a molecular weight of only 92; therefore, glycerol presents twice the osmotic load per administered gram of sugar when compared with glucose, mannitol, or sorbitol. If high doses (greater than 100 g) are used, for example, to treat cerebral edema, significant hypertonicity can result from the hypotonic osmotic diuresis, even in the absence of renal failure.

Replacement of hypotonic water and electrolyte losses induced by the osmotic diuresis (or diarrhea in the case of oral sorbitol) generally corrects the hypertonicity produced by these sugars. However, if large quantities of these impermeant solutes are administered to patients with renal failure, or to individuals with normal renal function at a rate faster than they can be eliminated, severe ECF expansion can result. Additional treatment may then be required, including the use of diuretics and/or dialysis to hasten removal of both the administered solute and the excess ECF volume.

Summary

Many clinical conditions after the homeostatic mechanisms which control the quantity and distribution of TBS and TBW. This chapter emphasized those clinical conditions that result in hyperosmolality with hypertonicity because such conditions may cause severe, yet potentially reversible neurological and/or cardiovascular problems. Neurological findings may range from mild confusion to coma, and may be local or generalized. The cardiovascular symptoms range from marked volume depletion to substantial volume expansion. However, appropriate therapeutic intervention is critically dependent on an understanding of the underlying pathophysiology.

Patients with hyperosmolality, with or without hypertonicity, must be approached in a systematic manner that allows identification of the disturbed physiological mechanisms. The presence of hypertonicity is usually suspected because the serum [Na^+] or the blood [glucose] is elevated. In many cases the initial step in evaluation is a complete medical history, which may identify the etiology (e.g., water deprivation leading to hypernatremia in an elderly patient, or diabetes mellitus leading to hyperglycemia). However, the history may not be readily obtained, particularly if the patient is confused or comatose. The physical examination may be more helpful in some cases: pure water loss usually presents with evidence of cellular dehydration (dry mucous membranes, poor tissue turgor); hypotonic losses present with more evidence of EABV depletion (hypotension, tachycardia); solute gain usually presents with evidence of volume expansion (hypertension, pulmonary edema). In addition to the levels of P_{osm}, serum [Na^+], and [glucose], other helpful laboratory findings include the BUN and blood creatinine concentrations, the serum [Cl^-] and [HCO_3^-], and the urinary osmolality and electrolyte concentration.

With sufficient information derived from history, physical, and laboratory findings, the pathophysiological mechanisms can usually be identified, and the therapeutic interventions can be made judiciously: pure water loss can be replaced by oral water intake or intravenous administration of 5 percent dextrose in water; hypotonic losses can be replaced by a combination of isoelectrolyte and electrolyte-free solutions; solute gains can be treated by diuretic or dialytic solute removal, by hypotonic solution infusion, and, in the case of hyperglycemia, by insulin administration. Correction of hypertonicity must be done relatively slowly to avoid neurological deterioration.[33] The optimal mode of management depends on the specific cause: DDAVP is appropriate long-term replacement for the missing ADH in a patient with CDI, but adequate access to water may be the only treatment needed for an elderly or handicapped patient; yet, both patients may present with hypernatremia. HNKC is a special problem because elements of solute gain (hyperglycemia) and hypotonic loss (osmotic diuresis) may coexist. Maintenance of an adequate circulating volume during correction of the hypertonic state is essential, and it is usually necessary to administer colloid and/or isotonic solutions to maintain EABV before insulin is given for reducing the hyperglycemia and hypertonicity. Thus, a careful description and analysis of the pathophysiology underlying the hypertonic state will almost always identify the correct therapeutic pathway.

REFERENCES

1. Alford FP et al: Symptomatic normovolemic essential hypernatremia. *Am J Med* 54:359, 1973.
2. Andersson B: Regulation of water intake. *Physiol Rev* 58:582, 1978.
3. Andersson B, Rundgren M: Thirst and its disorders. *Annu Rev Med* 33:231, 1982.
4. Ansell J et al: Diabetes insipidus associated with dysplastic pancytopenia. *Am J Med* 83:189, 1987.
5. Arduino FF et al: Antidiuretic action of chlorpropamide in idiopathic diabetes insipidus. *J Clin Endocrinol Metab* 26:1325, 1966.
6. Arem R et al: Selective osmoreceptor dysfunction presenting as intermittent hypernatremia following surgery for a pituitary chromophobe adenoma. *Am J Med* 80:1217, 1986.
7. Arieff AI, Carroll HJ: Non-ketotic hyperosmolar coma with hyperglycemia: Clinical features, pathophysiology, renal function, acid-base balance, plasma cerebrospinal fluid equilibria and the effects of therapy in 37 cases. *Medicine* 51:73, 1972.
8. Arieff AI et al: Brain water and electrolyte metabolism in uremia: Effects of slow and rapid hemodialysis. *Kidney Int* 4:177, 1973.
9. Arieff AI, Guisado R: Effects on the central nervous system of hypernatremic and hyponatremic states. *Kidney Int* 10:104, 1976.
10. Arieff AI et al: Pathophysiology of hyperosmolar states, in Andreoli TE et al (eds): *Disturbances in Body Fluid Osmolality*. Bethesda, MD, American Physiology Society, 1977, p 227.
11. Arieff AI: Osmotic failure: Physiology and strategies for treatment. *Hosp Pract* 23:173, 1988.
12. Avioli LV et al: Chronic and sustained hypernatremia, absence of thirst, diabetes insipidus, and adrenocorticotrophin insufficiency resulting from widespread destruction of the hypothalamus. *Ann Intern Med* 56:131, 1962.
13. Aviram A et al: Hyperosmolality with hyponatremia caused by inappropriate administration of mannitol. *Am J Med* 42:648, 1967.
14. Barlow ED, deWardener HE: Compulsive water drinking. *Q J Med* 28:235, 1959.
15. Barney et al: The effect of acute administration of an angiotensin converting enzyme inhibitor, captopril (SQ 14,225), on experimentally-induced thirst in rats. *J Pharmacol Exp Ther* 212:53, 1980.
16. Battle DC et al: Amelioration of polyuria by amilioride in patients receiving long term lithium therapy. *N Engl J Med* 312:408, 1985.
17. Baxter CF et al: Organic molecules involved in the osmotic regulation of nervous tissue. *Proc Am Soc Neurochem* 7:14, 1976.
18. Baylis PH, Health DA: Water disturbances in patients treated with oral lithium carbonate. *Ann Intern Med* 88:607, 1978.
19. Beasley EW, Phillips LS: Polyuria and refractory hypernatremia after cardiopulmonary arrest. *Am J Med* 82:347, 1987.
20. Beck LH et al: Geriatric hypernatremia. *Ann Intern Med* 107:768, 1987.
21. Beck LH: Kidney function and disease in the elderly. *Hosp Pract* 23:75, 1988.
22. Bennett CM: Urine concentration and dilution in hypokalemic and hypercalcemic dogs. *J Clin Invest* 49:1147, 1970.
23. Berl T et al: Clinical disorders of water metabolism. *Kidney Int* 10:117, 1976.

24. Berl T et al: On the mechanism of polyuria in potassium depletion. *J Clin Invest* 60:620, 1977.
25. Berl T: Psychosis and water balance. *N Engl J Med* 318:441, 1988.
26. Berliner RW: Mechanisms of urine concentration. *Kidney Int* 22:202, 1982.
27. Berndt WO et al: Potentiation of the antidiuretic action of vasopressin by chlorpropamide. *Endocrinology* 84:1028, 1970.
28. Bichet DG et al: Polyuria, dehydration and overhydration in Seldin DW, Giebisch G (eds): *The Kidney: Physiology and Pathophysiology.* New York, Raven Press, 1985, p 951.
29. Bichet DG et al: Hemodynamic and coagulation responses to 1-desamino (8-D-arginine) vasopressin in patients with congenital nephrogenic diabetes insipidus. *N Engl J Med* 318:881, 1988.
30. Bie P: Osmoreceptors, vasopressin, and control of renal water excretion. *Physiol Rev* 60:961, 1980.
31. Blank MS, Farnsworth PB: Idiopathic symptomatic hypernatremia in a 9-year-old boy: A clinical and physiologic evaluation. *J Pediatr* 85:215, 1974.
32. Blasi C et al: Wolfram's syndrome: A clinical, diagnostic and interpretive contribution. *Diabetes Care* 9:521, 1986.
33. Brennan S, Ayus C: Acute versus chronic hypernatremia: How fast to correct ECF volume. *J Crit Illness* 5:330, 1990.
34. Brenner B et al: Normal response of factor VIII and von Willebrand factor to 1-desamino-8-d-arginine vasopressin in nephrogenic diabetes insipidus. *J Clin Endocrinol Metab* 67:191, 1988.
35. Brezis M, Weiler-Ravell D: Hypernatremia, hypodipsia and partial diabetes insipidus: A model for defective osmoregulation. *Am J Med Sci* 279:37, 1980.
36. Brownstein MJ: Biosynthesis of vasopressin and oxytocin. *Annu Rev Physiol* 45:129, 1983.
37. Bruck E et al: Pathogenesis and pathophysiology of hypertonic dehydration with diarrhea. *Am J Dis Child* 115:122, 1968.
38. Cammu H et al: Idiopathic fatty liver of pregnancy associated with transient diabetes insipidus. *Br J Obstet Gynaecol* 94:173, 1987.
39. Carone FA, Epstein FH: Nephrogenic diabetes insipidus caused by amyloid disease: Evidence in man of the role of the collecting ducts in concentrating urine. *Am J Med* 29:539, 1960.
40. Carrillo F et al: Renal failure associated with demeclocycline in cirrhosis. *Ann Intern Med* 87:195, 1977.
41. Cassorla FG et al: Nosocomial hypernatremia. *N Engl J Med* 313:329, 1985.
42. Chanson P et al: Management of early post-operative diabetes insipidus with parenteral desmopressin. *Acta Endocrinol* 117:513, 1988.
43. Cheung WY: Calmodulin: An overview. *Fed Proc* 41:2253, 1982.
44. Chiumello G et al: Magnetic resonance imaging in diabetes insipidus. *Lancet* 1:901, 1989.
45. Cobb WE et al: Neurogenic diabetes insipidus: Management with DDAVP (1-desamino-8-D-arginine vasopressin). *Ann Intern Med* 88:183, 1978.
46. Cockington RA et al: Iatrogenic hypernatremia after oral electrolyte solution. *Med J Aust* 2:715, 1976.
47. Cockington RA et al: Hypernatremia in childhood. *Med J Aust* 1:957, 1977.
48. Coggins CH, Leaf A: Diabetes insipidus. *Am J Med* 42:807, 1967.
49. Comtois R et al: Low serum urea level in dehydrated patients with central diabetes insipidus. *Can Med J* 139:965, 1988.
50. Cooper SJ: Effects of chlordiazepoxide on drinking in rats challenged with hypertonic saline, isoproterenol or polyethylene glycol. *Life Sci* 32:2453, 1983.
51. Cousins MJ, Mazze RI: Methoxyflurane nephrotoxicity: A study of dose response in man. *JAMA* 225:1611, 1973.
52. Cox M et al: Declomycine and therapy of hyponatremia. *Ann Intern Med* 86:113, 1977.
53. Cox M, Singer I: Lithium. Chapter 11, in Bronner F, Coburn JW (eds): *Disorders of Mineral Metabolism.* New York, Academic Press, 1981, vol 1, p 370.
54. Cox M: Tetracycline nephrotoxicity, in Porter G (ed): *Nephrotoxic Mechanisms of Drugs and Environmental Toxins.* New York, Plenum Press, 1982, p 165.
55. Crawford JD, Kennedy GC: Chlorothiazide in diabetes insipidus. *Nature* 183:891, 1959.
56. Crawford JD et al: Clinical results of treatment of diabetes insipidus with drugs of the chlorothiazide series. *N Engl J Med* 262:737, 1960.
57. Crowe MJ et al: Altered water excretion in healthy elderly men. *Age and Ageing* 16:285, 1987.
58. Czernichow P et al: Diabetes insipidus in children: III. Anterior pituitary dysfunction in idiopathic types. *J Pediatr* 106:41, 1985.
59. Daugirdas JT et al: Hyperosmolar coma. *Ann Intern Med* 110:855, 1989.
60. Davis PJ, Davis FB: Water excretion in the elderly. *Endocrinol Clin North Am.* 16:867, 1987.
61. Davison JM et al: Changes in the metabolic clearance of vasopressin and in plasma vasopressinase throughout human pregnancy. *J Clin Invest* 83:1313, 1989.
62. DeRubertis FR et al: "Essential hypernatremia" due to ineffective osmotic and intact volume regulation of vasopressin secretion. *J Clin Invest* 50:97, 1971.
63. DeRubertis FR et al: "Essential" hypernatremia. Report of three cases and review of the literature. *Arch Intern Med* 134:839, 1974.
64. DeTroyer A: Demeclocycline: Treatment for syndrome of inappropriate antidiuretic hormone secretion. *JAMA* 237:2723, 1977.
65. DeVillota ED et al: Hyperosmolal crisis following infusion of hypertonic sodium chloride for purposes of therapeutic abortion. *Am J Med* 55:116, 1973.
66. Dicker SE, Eggleton MG: Nephrogenic diabetes insipidus. *Clin Sci* 24:81, 1963.
67. Doherty-Fuller E, Copeland KC: Sweat tests in patients with diabetes insipidus. *Clin Pediatr* 27:330, 1988.
68. Dousa TP, Barnes LD: Effect of colchicine and vinblastine on the cellular action of vasopressin in mammalian kidney. *J Clin Invest* 54:252, 1974.
69. Dousa TP, Valtin H: Cellular actions of vasopressin in the mammalian kidney. *Kidney Int* 10:46, 1976.

70. Dunger DB et al: Increased renal sensitivity to vasopressin in two patients with essential hypernatremia. *J Clin Endocrinol Metab* 64:185, 1987.
71. Dunger DB et al: The frequency and natural history of diabetes insipidus in children with Langerhans-cell histiocytosis. *N Engl J Med* 321:1157, 1989.
72. Durr JA et al: Diabetes insipidus in pregnancy associated with abnormally high circulating vasopressinase activity. *N Engl J Med* 316:1070, 1987.
73. Durr JA: Diabetes insipidus in pregnancy. *Am J Kidney Dis* 9:276, 1987.
74. Edwards CRW et al: Vasopressin analogue DDAVP in diabetes insipidus: Clinical and laboratory studies. *Br Med J* 3:375, 1973.
75. Elliot EJ et al: Sodium content of oral rehydration solutions: A reappraisal. *Gut* 30:1610, 1989.
76. Epstein AN: The physiology of thirst. *Can J Physiol Pharmacol* 54:639, 1976.
77. Epstein FH: Disturbances in renal concentrating ability, in Andreoli TE et al (eds): *Disturbances in Body Fluid Osmolality*. Bethesda, MD, American Physiology Society 1977, p 255.
78. Feibusch J et al: Tumor-associated nephrogenic diabetes insipidus. *Ann Intern Med* 92:797, 1980.
79. Feig PU, McCurdy DK: The hypertonic state. *N Engl J Med* 297:1444, 1977.
80. Feig PU: Hypernatremia and hypertonic syndromes. *Med Clin North Am* 65:271, 1981.
81. Ferrier IN: Water intoxication in patients with psychiatric illness. *Br Med J* 291:1594, 1985.
82. Finberg L et al: Mass accident salt poisoning in infancy. *JAMA* 184:187, 1963.
83. Finberg L: Hypernatremic (hypertonic) dehydration in infants. *N Engl J Med* 289:196, 1973.
84. Fitzsimons JT: The physiological basis of thirst. *Kidney Int* 10:3, 1976.
85. Fitzsimons JT: Physiological pathology of thirst and sodium appetite, in Selden DW, Giebisch G (eds): *The Kidney, Physiology and Pathophysiology*. New York, Raven Press, 1985, p 885.
86. Frascino JA: Effect of inorganic fluoride on the renal concentrating mechanism: Possible nephrotoxicity in man. *J Lab Clin Med* 79:192, 1972.
87. Fraser CL, Arieff AI: Fatal central diabetes mellitus and insipidus resulting from untreated hyponatremia: A new syndrome. *Ann Intern Med* 112:113, 1990.
88. Fregly MJ (Chairman): Symposium: Angiotensin-induced thirst: Peripheral and central mechanisms. *Fed Proc* 37:2667, 1978.
89. Fregly MJ: Thermogenic drinking: Mediation by osmoreceptor and angiotensin II pathways. *Fed Proc* 41:2515, 1982.
90. Friedler RM et al: Hyponatremia and hypernatremia. *Clin Nephrol* 7:163, 1977.
91. *Frontiers in Hormone Research*. Monograph. Robinson AG, Verbalis J (eds): Karger, Basil, 1985, vol 13.
92. Galla JN et al: Effect of lithium on water and electrolyte metabolism. *Yale J Biol Med* 48:305, 1975.
93. Gault MH et al: Hypernatremia, azotemia and dehydration due to high-protein tube feeding. *Ann Intern Med* 68:788, 1968.
94. Geheb M, Cox M: Renal effects of demeclocycline. *JAMA* 243:2519, 1980.
95. Gennari FJ, Kassirer JP: Osmotic diuresis. *N Engl J Med* 291:714, 1974.
96. Gerich JE et al: Clinical and metabolic characteristics of hyperosmolar non-ketotic coma. *Diabetes* 20:228, 1971.
97. Gill JR, Bartter FC: On the impairment of renal concentrating ability in prolonged hypercalcemia and hypercalciuria in man. *J Clin Invest* 40:716, 1961.
98. Gill G et al: A case of "essential" hypernatremia due to resetting of the osmostat. *Clin Endocrinol* 22:545, 1985.
99. Godinich MJ, Batlle DC: Renal tubular effects of lithium. *Kidney Int* 37(suppl 28):S52, 1990.
100. Goldberg M et al: Asymptomatic hypovolemic hypernatremia: A variant of essential hypernatremia. *Am J Med* 43:804, 1967.
101. Goldfarb S, Agus ZS: Mechanisms of the polyuria of hypercalcemia (review). *Am J Nephrol* 4:69, 1984.
102. Goldman MB et al: Mechanisms of altered water metabolism in psychotic patients with polydipsia and hyponatremia. *N Engl J Med* 318:397, 1988.
103. Golonka JE, Richardson JA: Postconcussive hyperosmolality and deficient thirst. *Am J Med* 48:261, 1970.
104. Grant PJ et al: Effects of physiological concentrations of vasopressin on hemostatic function in man. *Clin Sci* 69:471, 1985.
105. Green JR et al: Hereditary and idiopathic types of diabetes insipidus. *Brain* 90:707, 1967.
106. Griffin KA, Bidani AK: How to manage disorders of sodium and water balance. *J Crit Illness* 5:1054, 1990.
107. Gross PA et al: Prostaglandins and water metabolism: A review with emphasis on in vivo studies. *Kidney Int* 19:839, 1981.
108. Grossman SP: The neuroanatomy of eating and drinking behavior. *Hosp Pract* 12:45, 1977.
109. Gurewitz R et al: Recurrent hypothermia, hypersomnolence, central sleep-apnea, hypodipsia, hypothyroidism, hyperprolactinemia and growth hormone deficiency in a boy—treatment with clomopramine. *Acta Endocrinol* 279(suppl):468, 1986.
110. Hammer M, Vilhardt H: Peroral treatment of diabetes insipidus with a polypeptide hormone analog, desmopressin. *J Pharmacol Exp Ther* 234:754, 1985.
111. Hammond DN et al: Hypodipsia hypernatremia with normal osmoregulation of vasopressin. *N Engl J Med* 315:433, 1986.
112. Handler JS: Vasopressin-prostaglandin interactions in the regulation of epithelial cell permeability to water. *Kidney Int* 19:831, 1981.
113. Handler JS, Orloff J: Antidiuretic hormone. *Annu Rev Physiol* 43:611, 1981.
114. Harris AS: Clinical experience with desmopressin: Efficacy and safety in central diabetes insipidus and other conditions. *J Pediatr* 114(45):711, 1989.
115. Hetrick WD et al: Renal response to light methoxyflurane anesthesia. *Anesthesiology* 38:30, 1973.
116. Hogan G: Hypernatremia—Problems in management. *Pediatr Clin North Am* 23:569, 1976.
117. Hughes JM et al: Recurrent diabetes insipidus associated with pregnancy: Pathophysiology and therapy. *Obstet Gynecol* 73:462, 1989.

118. Illowsky BP, Kirch DG: Polydipsia and hyponatremia in psychiatric patients. *Am J Psychiatry* 145:675, 1988.
119. Jackson BA et al: Lithium-induced polyuria: Effect of lithium on adenylate cyclase and adenosine 3′,5′-monophosphate phosphodiesterase in medullary ascending limb of Henle's loop and in medullary collecting tubules. *Endocrinology* 107:1693, 1980.
120. Jamison RL, Oliver RE: Disorders of urinary concentration and dilution. *Am J Med* 72:308, 1982.
121. Kasper CK: Desmopressin acetate (DDAVP) (editorial). *JAMA* 251:2564, 1984.
122. Kastin AJ et al: Asymptomatic hypernatremia. *Am J Med* 38:306, 1965.
123. Katz MA: Hyperglycemia-induced hyponatremia—Calculation of expected serum sodium depression. *N Engl J Med* 289:843, 1973.
124. Kaufman AM, Kahn T: Congestive heart failure with hypernatremia. *Arch Intern Med* 146:402, 1986.
125. Kerenyi TD: Hypernatremia following intrauterine instillation of hypertonic saline solution: Report of a case and discussion. *Obstet Gynecol* 33:520, 1969.
126. Klee CB et al: Calmodulin. *Annu Rev Biochem* 49:489, 1980.
127. Kleeman CR et al: Urea transport in the central nervous system. *Am J Physiol* 203:739, 1962.
128. Koppeschaar HPF et al: Renal concentrating ability in obesity: Effect of modified fasting and the supplementation of T_3, sodium chloride and carbohydrate. *Metabolism* 34:1066, 1985.
129. Kosten TR, Forrest JN: Treatment of severe lithium induced polyuria with amilioride. *Am J Psychiatry* 143:1563, 1986.
130. Kramer HJ et al: Role of prostaglandins in the regulation of renal water excretion. *Kidney Int* 19:851, 1981.
131. Krane EJ et al: Subclinical brain swelling in children during treatment of diabetic ketoacidosis. *N Engl J Med* 312:1147, 1985.
132. Krege J et al: Transient diabetes insipidus of pregnancy. *Obstet Gynecol Surv* 44:789, 1989.
133. Kusano E et al: Chlorpropamide action on renal concentrating mechanism in rats with hypothalamic diabetes insipidus. *J Clin Invest* 72:1298, 1983.
134. Laczi F et al: Effects of L-AVP and DDAVP on memory in normals and central diabetes insipidus. *Psychoneuroendocrinol* 7:185, 1982.
135. Laczi F et al: Differential effect of desgly-arg VP on cognitive function of central diabetes insipidus and alcoholic patients. *Acta Endocrinol* 115:392, 1987.
136. Lawrence GD et al: Diabetes insipidus with hypersensitivity to pitressin: An immunological study. *Johns Hopkins Med J* 131:172, 1972.
137. Leaf A: Neurogenic diabetes insipidus. *Kidney Int* 15:572, 1979.
138. Leaf A: Dehydration in the elderly (editorial). *N Engl J Med* 311:791, 1984.
139. Lehr D et al: Renin-angiotensin role in thirst: Paradoxical enhancement of drinking by angiotensin converting enzyme inhibitor. *Science* 182:1031, 1973.
140. Libber S et al: Treatment of nephrogenic diabetes insipidus with prostoglandin synthesis inhibitors. *J Pediatr* 108:305, 1986.
141. Lien YHH et al: Effects of hypernatremia on organic brain osmoles. *J Clin Invest* 85:1427, 1990.
142. Lindheimer MD et al: Idiopathic acute fatty liver of pregnancy associates with transient diabetes insipidus. *Br J Obstet Gynaecol* 94:823, 1987.
143. Loeb JN: The hyperosmolar state. *N Engl J Med* 290:1184, 1974.
144. Maddy JA, Winternitz WW: Hypothalamic syndrome with hypernatremia and muscular paralysis. *Am J Med* 51:394, 1971.
145. Mahoney JH, Goodman AD: Hypernatremia due to hypodipsia and elevated threshold for vasopressin release. *N Engl J Med* 279:1191, 1968.
146. Manelfe C et al: Computed tomography in diabetes insipidus. *Front Horm Res* 13:210, 1985.
147. Manning M, Sawyer WH: Antagonists of vasopressor and antidiuretic responses to arginine vasopressin (editorial). *Ann Intern Med* 96:520, 1982.
148. Mathias CJ et al: The effect of desmopressin on nocturnal polyuria, overnight weight loss and morning postural hypotension in patients with autonomic failure. *Br Med J* 293:353, 1986.
149. Mathisen O et al: Mechanisms of osmotic diuresis. *Kidney Int* 19:431, 1981.
150. Matter JA et al: Cardiac arrest in the critically ill: II. Hyperosmolal states following cardiac arrest. *Am J Med* 56:162, 1974.
151. Matz R: Coma in the nonketotic diabetic [Hyperosmolar nonketotic coma (HNKC) in the diabetic] in Ellenberg M, Rifkin H (eds): *Diabetes*, 3d ed. New York, Medical Examination Publishing Co, 1983, p 655.
152. Mazze RI et al: Renal dysfunction associated with methoxyflurane anesthesia. *JAMA* 216:278, 1971.
153. Mazze RI et al: Methoxyflurane metabolism and renal dysfunction: Clinical correlation in man. *Anesthesiology* 35:247, 1971.
154. Mazze RI et al: Dose-related methoxyflurane nephrotoxicity in rats. *Anesthesiology* 36:571, 1972.
155. Mazze RI, Hitt BA: Methoxyflurane metabolism. *Anesthesiology* 44:369, 1976.
156. McComb RD et al: Pontine and extrapontine myelinolysis associated with hypernatremia and hyperglycemia *Neurology* 38(suppl 1)):334, 1988.
157. McCurdy DK: Hyperosmolar hyperglycemic non-ketotic diabetic coma. *Med Clin North Am* 54:683, 1970.
158. McKee AC et al: Central pontine myelinolysis in severely burned patients: Relationship to serum hyperosmolality. *Neurology* 38:1662, 1988.
159. Meinders AE et al: Chlorpropamide treatment in diabetes insipidus. *Lancet* 2:544, 1967.
160. Meyers JB et al: Effects of lithium on the kidney. *Kidney Int* 18:601, 1980.
161. Miller M et al: Recognition of partial defects in antidiuretic hormone secretion. *Ann Intern Med* 73:721, 1970.
162. Miller M, Moses AM: Mechanism of chlorpropamide action in diabetes insipidus. *J Clin Endocrinol Metab* 30:488, 1970.
163. Miller PD et al: Central, renal and adrenal effects of lithium in man. *Am J Med* 66:797, 1979.

164. Miller PD et al: Plasma demeclocycline levels and nephrotoxicity. *JAMA* 243:2513, 1980.
165. Molitch ME, Hedley-Whyte ET: A 33 year old woman with pituitary dysfunction and diabetes mellitus. *N Engl J Med* 312:297, 1985.
166. Morris-Jones PH et al: Prognosis of the neurological complications of acute hypernatremia. *Lancet* 2:1385, 1967.
167. Moses AM et al: Diuretic action of three sulfonylurea drugs. *Ann Intern Med* 78:541, 1973.
168. Moses AM et al: Clofibrate-induced antidiuresis. *J Clin Invest* 52:535, 1973.
169. Moses AM et al: Mechanism of chlorpropamide-induced antidiuresis in man: Evidence for release of ADH and enhancement of peripheral action. *Metabolism* 22:59, 1973.
170. Moses AM: Diabetes insipidus and ADH regulation. *Hosp Pract* 12:37, 1977.
171. Moses AM et al: Marked hypotonic polyuria resulting from nephrogenic diabetes insipidus with partial sensitivity to vasopressin. *J Clin Endocrinol Metab* 59:1044, 1984.
172. Moses AM et al: Two distinct pathophysiological mechanisms in nephrogenic diabetes insipidus. *J Clin Endocrinol Metab* 66:1259, 1988.
173. Moss GD et al: Correction of hypernatremia with continuous arteriovenous hemodiafiltration. *Arch Dis Child* 65:628, 1990.
174. Nelson DC et al: Hypernatremia and lactulose therapy. *JAMA* 249:1295, 1983.
175. Niaudet P et al: Nephrogenic diabetes insipidus: Clinical and pathophysiological aspects (review). *Adv Nephrol* 13:247, 1984.
176. Niaudet P et al: Nephrogenic diabetes insipidus in children (review). *Front Horm Res* 13:224, 1985.
177. Nusynowitz ML, Forsham PH: The antidiuretic action of acetominophen. *Am J Med Sci* 252:429, 1966.
178. Olsen S: The brain in uremia. *Acta Psychiatr Scand* 36(suppl 156):1, 1961.
179. Peden NR et al: Wolfram (DIDMOAD) Syndrome: A complex long-term problem in management. *Q J Med* 58:167, 1986.
180. Pedersen EB et al: Familial central diabetes insipidus—A report of 5 families—genetic, diagnostic and therapeutic aspects. *Q J Med* 57:883, 1985.
181. Perez GO et al: Severe hypernatremia with impaired thirst. *Am J Nephrol* 9:421, 1989.
182. Phillips PA et al: Reduced thirst after water deprivation in healthy elderly men. *N Engl J Med* 311:753, 1984.
183. Pleasure D, Goldberg M: Neurogenic hypernatremia. *Arch Neurol* 15:78, 1966.
184. Podolsky S: Hyperosmolar nonketotic coma in the elderly diabetic. *Med Clin North Am* 62:815, 1978.
185. Price JDE, Lauener RW: Serum and urine osmolalities in the differential diagnosis of the polyuric states. *J Clin Endocrinol Metabol* 26:143, 1966.
186. Puczynski MS et al: Sodium intoxication caused by use of baking soda as a home remedy. *Can Med Assoc J* 128:821, 1983.
187. Pun KK et al: Cranial diabetes insipidus presenting as pyrexia of undetermined origin. *Am J Med* 86:732, 1989.
188. Ramsey TA, Cox M: Lithium and the kidney: A review. *Am J Physiol* 139:443, 1982.
189. Reichlin S: Regulation of the endocrine hypothalamus. *Med Clin North Am* 62:235, 1978.
190. Relman AS, Schwartz WB: The kidney in potassium depletion. *Am J Med* 24:764, 1958.
191. Richardson DW, Robinson AG: Drugs five years later: Desmopressin *Ann Intern Med* 103:228, 1985.
192. Robertson GL et al: The osmoregulation of vasopressin. *Kidney Int* 10:25, 1976.
193. Robertson GL: The regulation of vasopressin function in health and disease. *Recent Prog Horm Res* 33:333, 1977.
194. Robertson GL et al: Neurogenic disorders of osmoregulation. *Am J Med* 72:339, 1982.
195. Robertson GL: Regulation of vasopressin secretion in Seldin DW, Giebisch G (eds): *The Kidney: Physiology and Pathophysiology.* New York, Raven Press, 1985, p 869.
196. Robertson GL, Berl T: Pathophysiology of water metabolism in Brenner BM, Rector FC (eds): *The Kidney*, 3d ed. Philadelphia, Saunders, 1986, p 385.
197. Robertson GL, Harris A: Clinical Use of Vasopressin: Analogues. *Hosp Pract* 24:114, 1989.
198. Robertson MG, Kaplan SA: Inheritance of vasopressin-resistant ("nephrogenic") diabetes insipidus. *Am J Dis Child* 99:164, 1960.
199. Robinson AG, Verbalis JG: Treatment of central diabetes insipidus (review). *Front Horm Res* 13:292, 1985.
200. Robinson IC et al: Familial cerebellar ataxia and diabetes insipidus. *J Neur Neurosurg Pschiatr* 51:1576, 1988.
201. Rosenfeld W et al: Improving the clinical management of hypernatremic dehydration. *Clin Pediatr* 16:411, 1977.
202. Ross EJ, Christie SBM: Hypernatremia. *Medicine* 48:441, 1969.
203. Ross EM, Gilman AG: Biochemical properties of hormone-sensitive adenylate cyclase. *Annu Rev Biochem* 49:533, 1980.
204. Salata R, Klein I: Effects of lithium on the endocrine system: A review. *J Lab Clin Med* 110:130, 1987.
205. Sawyer WH, Manning M: The use of antagonists of vasopressin in studies of its physiological function. *Fed Proc* 44:78, 1985.
206. Scherbaum WA, Bottazo GF: Autoantibodies to vasopressin cells in idiopathic diabetes insipidus: Evidence for an autoimmune variant. *Lancet* 1:897, 1983.
207. Scherbaum WA et al: Diabetes insipidus in children: IV. A possible autoimmune type with vasopressin cell antibodies. *J Pediatr* 107:922, 1985.
208. Scherbaum WA et al: Role of autoimmunity in central diabetes insipidus. *Front Horm Res* 13:232, 1985.
209. Scherbaum WA et al: Autoimmune cranial diabetes insipidus: Its association with other endocrine diseases and with histiocytosis X. *Clin Endocrinol* 25:411, 1986.
210. Schrier RW et al: Osmotic and non-osmotic control of vasopressin release. *Am J Physiol* 236:F321, 1979.
211. Schwartz WB, Relman AS: Effects of electrolyte disorders on renal structure and function. *N Engl J Med* 276:383, 1965.
212. Schwerschlag U et al: Increased PGE_2 excretion by dDAVP in humans depends on state of hydration. *Am J Physiol* 250:F1008, 1986.

213. Seckl JR, Dunger D: Post-operative diabetes insipidus. *Br Med J* 298:2, 1989.
214. Seckl JR et al: Vasopressin antagonist in early post-operative diabetes insipidus. *Lancet* 335:1353, 1990.
215. Shah SV, Thakur VD: Vasopressinase and diabetes insipidus of pregnancy. *Am Intern Med* 109:435, 1988.
216. Shenkin HA, Bouzarth WF: Clinical methods of reducing intracranial pressure. *N Engl J Med* 282:1465, 1970.
217. Sherwood MC et al: Diabetes insipidus and occult intracranial tumors. *Arch Dis Child* 61:1222, 1986.
218. Silverstein E, Tobian L: Pitressin-resistant diabetes insipidus with massive hydronephrosis. *Am J Med* 30:819, 1961.
219. Simmons MA et al: Hypernatremia and intracranial hemorrhage in neonates. *N Engl J Med* 291:6, 1974.
220. Simon NM et al: Persistent nephrogenic diabetes insipidus after lithium treatment. *Ann Intern Med* 86:446, 1977.
221. Singer I et al: Lithium-induced nephrogenic diabetes insipidus: In-vivo and in-vitro studies. *J Clin Invest* 51:108, 1972.
222. Singer I, Rotenberg D: Demeclocycline-induced nephrogenic diabetes insipidus: In-vivo and in-vitro studies. *Ann Intern Med* 79:679, 1973.
223. Singer I: Lithium and the kidney. *Kidney Int* 19:374, 1981.
224. Singer I: Differential diagnosis of polyuria and diabetes insipidus. *Med Clin North Am* 65:303, 1981.
225. Smith RJ et al: Hypernatremic hyperosmolar coma complicating chronic peritoneal dialysis. *Proc Clin Dial Transplant Forum* 4:96, 1974.
226. Snyder NA et al: Hypernatremia in elderly patients: A heterogeneous, morbid and iatrogenic entity. *Ann Intern Med* 107:309, 1987.
227. Stoff JS et al: The concentrating defect of acute potassium depletion in man is independent of renal prostaglandins. *Kidney Int* 16:874, 1979.
228. Stricker EM: The renin-angiotensin system and thirst: Some unanswered questions. *Fed Proc* 37:2704, 1978.
229. Thompson CJ, Baylis PH: Thirst in diabetes insipidus: Clinical relevance of quantitative assessment. *Q J Med* 65:853, 1987.
230. Uhlich F et al: Antidiuretic effects of carbamazine in central diabetes insipidus. *Acta Endocrinol* 159(suppl):51, 1972.
231. Verbalis JG et al: Post-operative and post-traumatic diabetes insipidus (review). *Front Horm Res* 13:247, 1985.
232. Vokes TJ et al: Antibodies to vasopressin in patients with diabetes insipidus: Implications for diagnosis and therapy. *Ann Intern Med* 108:190, 1988.
233. Webster B, Bain J: Antidiuretic effect and complications of chlorpropamide therapy in diabetes insipidus. *J Clin Endocrinol Metab* 30:215, 1970.
234. Wedeen R: Prolonged functional depression of antidiuretic mechanisms in psychogenic polydipsia simulating primary diabetes insipidus. *Ann Intern Med* 54:805, 1961.
235. West ML et al: Quantitative analysis of glucose loss during acute therapy for hyperglycemic hyperosmolar syndrome *Diabetes Care* 9:465, 1986.
236. Westgren U et al: Oral desmopressin in central diabetes insipidus. *Arch Dis Child* 61:247, 1986.
237. Wickramasinghe LSP et al: Cranial diabetes insipidus after upper gastrointestinal hemorrhage. *Br Med J* 296:969, 1988.
238. Williams TDM et al: Antidiuretic effect and pharmacokinetics of oral 1-desamino-8-d-arginine vasopressin: 1. Studies in adults and children. *J Clin Endocrinol Metab* 63:129, 1986.
239. Wolfe BM et al: Complications of parenteral nutrition. *Am J Surg* 152:93, 1986.
240. Yamamoto T et al: Impaired arginine-vasopressin secretion associated with hypoangiotensinemia in hypernatremic dehydrated elderly patients. *JAMA* 259:1039, 1988.
241. Zaloga GP, Chernow B: The use of hormones as therapeutic agents. *Semin Resp Med* 7:39, 1985.
242. Zerbe RL, Robertson GL: A comparison of plasma vasopressin measurements with a standard indirect test in the differential diagnosis of polyuria. *N Engl J Med* 305:1539, 1981.
243. Zerbe RL, Robertson GL: Osmoregulation of thirst and vasopressin secretion in normal subjects: Effects of various solutes. *Am J Physiol* 244:E607, 1983.
244. Zijlstra F et al: Diabetes insipidus associated with dysplastic pancytopenia. *Am J Med* 82:339, 1987.

CHAPTER • 22

Hypokalemic states

G. Gopal Krishna • Susan P. Steigerwalt • Russel Pikus • Rajat Kaul • Robert G. Narins and Kent H. Raymond • Robert T. Kunau

Hypokalemic states are those clinical conditions associated with a low plasma potassium concentration in the presence or absence of depleted total body stores. The initial section of this chapter reviews and compares the current methods used to estimate total body potassium. The second section describes the local and systemic effects of potassium depletion. The final sections present the various disorders associated with hypokalemia followed by a discussion of its clinical evaluation and treatment.

ESTIMATION AND MEASUREMENT OF TOTAL BODY POTASSIUM

Measurement of plasma potassium concentration is the most widely used and readily available test for assessing potassium homeostasis. But, since 98 percent of body potassium is intracellular, any condition stimulating cellular uptake lowers the plasma concentration without affecting total body content. In a practical sense, the plasma potassium concentration does correlate in a general way with total body potassium content in normal subjects (see Fig. 22- 1).[68,498] Patients treated with diuretics show a 10 to 20 percent decrease in total body potassium when the plasma concentration falls by 1 meq/liter.[560] Further, Dyckner and Wester demonstrated a rough correlation between plasma potassium concentration and muscle potassium content.[155] Hypokalemia was predictive of a low muscle potassium content in depleted rats[542] and correlated with leukocyte levels in potassium-depleted rabbits.[409] In a variety of disease states, however, the plasma potassium concentration may be an unreliable indicator of total body potassium.[366]

There are three methods for estimating total body potassium in living subjects, that is, total body counting of naturally occurring radioactive potassium ($^{40}K^+$), determination of total exchangeable potassium, and determination of the tissue content of potassium.[408] Whole body counting was originally described in the 1950s by Sievert [482] and by Burch.[86] The methodology and tech-

The authors acknowledge support from the University Medical Research Foundation.

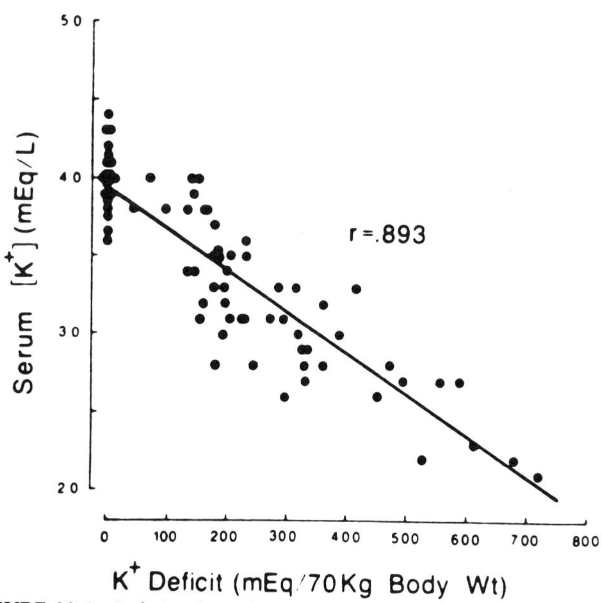

FIGURE 22-1 • Relationship of serum potassium concentration to bodily potassium deficit. The data are derived from 7 metabolic balance studies carried out on 24 subjects depleted of potassium. (From Sterns et al: *Medicine* 60:339, 1981.[498])

nical problems associated with this technique were discussed at an international symposium in 1962[509] and, recently, have undergone further clarification.[71,293,357] The primary isotope of potassium found in humans is $^{39}K^+$, but the presence of a naturally occurring gamma emitter, $^{40}K^+$, allows for total body counting. The test is performed by placing the subject in a large steel-walled chamber wherein $^{40}K^+$ gamma emissions are counted over a given time interval. The method assumes that the proportion of $^{40}K^+$ to $^{39}K^+$ in the body remains constant (0.012 percent of total body potassium consists of $^{40}K^+$). Consequently, total body potassium can be calculated from the results of the measured $^{40}K^+$ content. Although this is a relatively accurate method for estimating total body potassium,[69,108,526] measurement error may be introduced because of differences in body geometry and counting efficiency.[357] The problem with body geometry is seemingly less in children and animals, where a close correlation between chemical determinations and $^{40}K^+$ measurements has been shown.[293,345,452] Given the variation of body geometry in adult humans, it has been necessary to define appropriate reference standards. The importance of sex and age as reference standards was illustrated by Pierson and his coworkers in a study of 3083 normal subjects.[415] The potassium content of fat-free tissue decreased from a mean value of 72 to 50 meq/kg body weight in males and from 60 to 47 meq/kg in females from the ages of 20 to 90 years.[415] Despite the utilization of these reference standards, an error of 10 to 15 percent was encountered when estimating the normal value in a single individual.[415] Interlaboratory reproducibility may also vary considerably.[11] Despite these reservations, this is an accurate and reliable method for estimating total body potassium, measuring potassium depletion, and following individual subjects chronologically, recognizing that adjustments must be made for changes in body composition if subjects are followed for a prolonged period of time.[128]

The isotope dilution method determines the dilution of a known quantity of administered $^{42}K^+$ or $^{43}K^+$. The method assumes that the isotope equilibrates with all the potassium readily available for exchange. Twenty-four to 48 h after administration, samples of plasma or urine are measured for specific activity and an estimate of total body potassium, "exchangeable potassium," is calculated from the dilution of the known original dose after correction for the amount excreted in the urine.[118] Whereas this technique measures 92 to 99 percent of total body potassium at 24 h in normal subjects,[70,506,512] longer equilibration periods may be needed in certain disease states. In uremic patients,[70] exchangeable potassium was only 60 percent of total body potassium at 24 h and in patients with cardiac disease the equilibrium period was as long as 45 h.[138] The importance of methodology has been shown by two studies[274,506] where a marked difference in body potassium content was observed in the same subjects depending on whether urine or plasma specific activity was measured. The variable results generated by this technique were further demonstrated by Price et al. who concluded that a change of 600 meq of body potassium was necessary before the difference was considered significant.[422] These observations are in contrast to the studies of Deuxchaisnes et al.[138] and of Knochel et al.[291] In the latter study, duplicate measurements of total body potassium in a single subject agreed within approximately 200 meq. This variation in reproducibility between laboratories may, in part, relate to the use of the specific activity measured in an ultrafiltrate of the extracellular water where the chemical concentration of potassium is extremely sensitive to small changes in potassium intake during the late stages of a 24- to 72-h equilibration.[416]

Total exchangeable potassium is difficult to interpret in the face of a changing body composition. The relatively selective loss of skeletal muscle rich in potassium[416] or the replacement of muscle by fat which has a low-potassium content[161] are examples of circumstances in which difficulties in interpretation may exist. Total body potassium content as measured by exchangeable potassium is usually slightly lower than that determined by whole body counting.[272] This discrepancy may be due to the fact that either exchangeable potassium measurements were made prior to the plateau of compartmental equilibration, which is especially important in disease states, or that not all tissue compartments participate equally in potassium exchange (e.g., bone).[243]

The third technique frequently used for evaluating total body potassium is the tissue analysis of potassium content, that is, quantity per unit tissue. Skeletal muscle, which contains approximately 60 percent of body potassium,[180] is commonly used for this purpose. Muscle potassium content, however, may not accurately reflect alterations in total body content. The ratio of potassium to nitrogen in muscle tissue is approximately 3 meq of potassium to 1 g of nitrogen.[164] This ratio varies with the nature of the diet ingested.[450] Muntwyler and Griffin studied rats on a low-protein, low-potassium diet for five weeks and could not identify a significant change in muscle potassium content, the latter expressed as milliequivalents per 0.1 kg fat-free dry solids (FFDS).[378] Rats, previously fed a low-potassium, low-protein diet, were given protein supplements. Muscle analysis revealed that potassium content was significantly lower in the rats fed a low-potassium, protein-supplemented diet than in control animals or in animals in which both dietary protein and potassium were restricted. These results could not be attributed to a change in external potassium balance following the assumption of the protein-supplemented diet. The interpretation of muscle potassium content therefore will depend, in part, upon the simultaneous state of protein balance. The nonuniform response to maneuvers that may potentially alter cellular potassium content[6,569] and the variation in potassium content between different sites and muscle groups[47,140,179,484,554] must also be kept in mind when one interprets muscle potassium content. In view of the above remarks, despite the presumption that meaningful data can be obtained from muscle biopsy specimens,[227,391] such information should be examined critically.

Erythrocytes are readily available for study and have proved useful in the study of anion and cation transport.[341,407] Unfortunately, studies that compare red blood cell potassium with other estimates of total body potassium fail to show a high correlation.[17,264,409,542] As suggested by Patrick and Bradford, the leukocyte may be a better indicator of potassium stores.[409] They observed that leukocyte potassium content correlated with external balance studies and with exchangeable potassium in estimating the degree of depletion in both diet and diuretic-induced potassium depletion.[409] Because the metabolic activity of the leukocyte and, thereby, the intracellular electrolyte content may be very sensitive to the external environment, the procedures used to make such determinations must be performed with care.[106,202]

Despite the concerns and limitations expressed above, under appropriate circumstances each of the techniques described may provide meaningful information relating to body potassium stores. The limitations, as well as the strengths, of each technique must, however, be borne in mind.

PATHOPHYSIOLOGICAL CONSEQUENCES OF POTASSIUM DEPLETION

Most of the pathologic consequences accompanying hypokalemia are not a complication of the low-serum concentration but of true total body potassium depletion (Table 22-1). The associated complications include alterations of acid-base balance, metabolic effects, alterations in skeletal, smooth muscle, and renal structure and function, and effects on renin release and prostaglandin production.

TABLE 22-1 • Pathophysiologic consequences of potassium depletion

SYSTEMIC ACID-BASE BALANCE
Metabolic alkalosis or acidosis[201,273]
Respiratory acidosis
METABOLIC EFFECTS
Carbohydrate intolerance[104,110,111,494]
Decreased pancreatic insulin secretion[222,249]
Increased proinsulin secretion[223]
Growth retardation[31,240]
Impaired growth hormone release[419]
Altered protein synthesis[343]
Impaired hepatic glycogen storage and synthesis[65]
SKELETAL MUSCLE EFFECTS
Weakness, fatigue, myalgias, restless leg syndrome
Biochemical derangements[289]
Structural and functional abnormalities[290]
Total paralysis and respiratory arrest[92]
NONVASCULAR SMOOTH MUSCLE
Gastrointestinal and urinary bladder hypomotility[247]
Vascular smooth muscle
Reduced vascular resistance—chronic potassium depletion
Increased vascular resistance—acute potassium depletion
BLOOD PRESSURE
CARDIAC EFFECTS
Electrophysiologic abnormalities[15,41,147,151,156,157,253,261,396,466,491,553]
Contractility abnormalities[11,239,283,292,369]
RENAL EFFECTS
Morphologic changes[1,122,187,374,399,431,562,564]
Functional abnormalities
Reduced glomerular filtration rate[309,377]
Reduced renal blood flow[1]
Impaired urinary concentrating ability[94,176,225,285,344,431]
Increased urinary prostaglandin excretion[195]
Sodium retention[273]
Altered tubular parathyroid hormone respone[39]
Altered P-aminohippurate handling[495]
Increased renin release[475]
HORMONAL EFFECTS
Decreased aldosterone secretion[83,93]

ACID-BASE BALANCE (Table 22-2)

Changes in potassium homeostasis influence systemic acid-base balance by modifying one or more of the following factors: (1) the transcellular distribution of protons, (2) proximal tubular bicarbonate reabsorption, (3) distal nephron proton secretion, (4) renal ammoniagenesis, and (5) aldosterone secretion.[519] The balance struck between these forces ultimately determines the quantitative change in systemic pH. These effects of potassium depletion on systemic pH vary between species. In man and in the rat potassium depletion consistently produces metabolic alkalosis while metabolic acidosis is observed in dogs.[88,201,248,273,519]

Both in vivo microperfusion and free flow micropuncture studies in rats have demonstrated that dietary potassium restriction enhances proximal tubular bicar-

TABLE 22-2 • Mechanism of hyperbicarbonatemia during potassium depletion

1. Enhanced proximal bicarbonate reabsorption
2. Increased renal ammonia synthesis
3. Chloride depletion
4. Intracellular influx of protons in exchange for potassium

bonate reabsorption.[95,519] Potassium depletion also stimulates proton transport in the distal nephron, but it is unknown whether the intracellular pH of the tubular cells is decreased.[519] Increase in ammonium excretion has been observed during potassium depletion in rats, dogs, and humans.[220,517-519] Potassium depletion stimulates ammonium absorption in the medullary thick ascending limb and thereby promotes ammonia recycling and urinary ammonium excretion (see Chap. 10).[220] Microperfusion studies further demonstrate that simultaneously increasing the luminal and bath potassium concentrations inhibits ammonia production in the S_2 segments of mouse, while decreasing the potassium concentrations at these sites has the opposite effect.[380] The increase in ammoniagenesis caused by potassium depletion has been associated with increased activity of renal phosphate-dependent glutaminase.[101] Severe potassium depletion inhibits distal chloride reabsorption in rats.[335,337] It is not known whether the ensuing chloride depletion contributes to the metabolic alkalosis observed during severe hypokalemia. Mild potassium depletion in humans, however, is associated with retention of both sodium and chloride (see below).[299,302,303]

The contribution of potassium depletion to the degree of hyperbicarbonatemia in metabolic alkalosis is markedly influenced by the associated state of ECF volume. In patients with normal extracellular volume, the contribution of hypokalemia is small. In hypovolemic states, however, the hyperbicarbonatemic effects of potassium depletion are markedly exaggerated. Jones et al. observed that modest potassium depletion (300 meq/70 kg) increased plasma bicarbonate concentration by only 2 meq/liter in subjects maintained on a normal salt intake.[273] When the intake of sodium chloride was markedly restricted, plasma bicarbonate rose by 7.5 meq/liter with an equivalent degree of potassium depletion.[248]

MAJOR METABOLIC EFFECTS

Carbohydrate intolerance is the most common metabolic disorder associated with potassium depletion. This complication occurs regardless of whether the deficit accompanies cirrhosis,[109] uremia,[494] Bartter's syndrome,[223] primary hyperaldosteronism,[111] or diuretic therapy.[104] Impairment in glucose tolerance during potassium depletion results from a decrease in insulin secretion.[443]

More recent studies have indicated that thiazide diuretics can impair glucose tolerance by inhibiting peripheral insulin sensitivity.[14] Subjects maintained normal blood sugar levels by a sustained hyperinsulinemia. Gorden and associates found that an increased percentage of the circulating insulin in potassium depletion was in the form of the relatively inactive proinsulin.[223]

The impairment in glucose tolerance observed during chronic diuretic therapy has been ascribed to the accompanying potassium depletion.[236] Potassium supplementation diminishes the glucose intolerance induced by thiazide diuretics.[245] Glucose intolerance in substitution of hypertensives receiving thiazide diuretics is reversed when their serum potassium concentration is normalized by the addition of amiloride.[521] The magnitude of potassium depletion required to induce glucose intolerance is similar to that observed during chronic diuretic therapy.[443] Thus it has been suggested that suppression of insulin secretion induced by potassium depletion mediates the glucose intolerance observed during chronic diuretic therapy. Pollare et al. recently reported that chronic therapy with hydrochlorothiazide lowers insulin sensitivity in hypertensives.[420] Indeed, in this study fasting plasma insulin levels were higher on hydrochlorothiazide compared with the values observed on placebo.[420] It is unknown whether thiazide diuretics directly or indirectly impair peripheral glucose utilization. The relative importance of suppressed insulin secretion and impaired peripheral utilization of glucose requires further study.

Potassium depletion may affect the release of several hormones[350] and the function of numerous enzyme systems through its role as a cofactor.[538] In addition, growth retardation is a known complication of Bartter's syndrome and other potassium-deficiency states.[31,240] The growth retardation may be a consequence of impaired growth hormone release[419] or altered protein synthesis due to relative insulin deficiency.[343] Glycogen storage and synthesis in hepatic and skeletal muscle is impaired during potassium depletion as a result of either insulin deficiency or a decline in glycogen synthetase activity.[65]

SKELETAL MUSCLE

The effects of potassium depletion on skeletal muscle vary with the magnitude of the potassium deficit. Potassium levels of 3.0 to 3.5 meq/liter usually produce no symptoms, while levels below 3.0 meq/liter are often associated with complaints of muscular weakness, general malaise, fatigue, the restless leg syndrome, and occasionally myalgias. When levels fall below 2.5 meq/liter biochemical derangements of muscle enzymes appear, such as elevation of the serum levels of creatinine phosphokinase, aldolase, or glutamic oxaloacetic transaminase.[289] Severe structural and functional abnormalities of muscle with rhabdomyolysis and myoglobinuria may occur when potassium levels fall below 2.0 meq/liter.[290] The severity of muscle weakness can range from a mild decrease in strength to total paralysis and respiratory arrest.[92]

Skeletal muscle weakness is caused by four general defects associated with potassium depletion: a change in transmembrane ion transport, impaired muscle blood flow, a depletion of energy stores, and total loss of cellular integrity resulting in muscle necrosis.[289] The resting transmembrane electrical potential difference of muscle cells rises during early potassium deficiency; however, in humans and dogs, a sharp decline in muscle membrane potential occurs with severe potassium depletion.[62,435] The sharp decline in membrane potential is accompanied by severe muscle weakness and paralysis in dogs.[62] Knochel and Schlein demonstrated that the expected release of potassium and increased blood flow seen in exercising muscle were absent in potassium-deficient dogs.[292] This may have important clincal significance to military recruits and athletes who become potassium-depleted during periods of extreme exertion in hot climates.[291] Glycogen content of muscle is depressed during potassium depletion and may contribute to the impairment of energy production during anaerobic exercise.[48,65] Finally, the culmination of deficient blood flow and lack of energy production can result in loss of cellular integrity and muscle necrosis.[291] In addition to necrosis, histologic examination may show lymphocytic and histiocytic infiltration and the presence of multiple small vacuoles in degenerating fibers.

NONVASCULAR SMOOTH MUSCLE

Gastrointestinal and urinary bladder motility are decreased during periods of potassium depletion. Clinically, intestinal ileus is not an uncommon finding in patients with severe potassium depletion. Henrikson showed that hypomotility of the gastrointestinal tract during potassium deficiency occurs in the absence of histologic changes and promptly improves with the administration of potassium.[247]

BLOOD PRESSURE

Experimental and clinical studies suggest that potassium intake plays a critical role in blood pressure regulation.[303] Epidemiologic surveys conducted in widely divergent geographic locations suggest that populations ingesting diets low in potassium are more susceptible to the development of hypertension. An even more striking correlation has been observed between the ratio of dietary sodium to potassium and the prevalence of hypertension.[266]

Studies in experimental animals on the effect of potassium depletion on blood pressure have yielded divergent responses.[3,43,192,330,394,405,425a] Linas and colleagues observed that potassium depletion lowers blood pressure in normal rats, in rats with renovascular hypertension, and in spontaneously hypertensive rats.[43,330,394,405] The decrease in blood pressure in these rats is accompanied by a decrease in peripheral vascular resistance and an impaired pressor response to the infusion of angiotensin II.[394,405] Potassium depletion in dogs is associated with decreases in cardiac output and blood pressure.[3,304] In contrast to these studies, potassium depletion induced by mineralocorticoid administration is accompanied by an increase in blood pressure.[192] Fujita and Sato demonstrated that amelioration of hypokalemia by the administration of potassium chloride or potassium citrate attenuated the hypertension in uninephrectomized rats receiving deoxycorticosterone acetate.[192]

Several clinical studies demonstrated that potassium depletion is associated with an increase in blood pressure.[279,302-304,316,380] Krishna et al. studied the blood pressure response to dietary potassium depletion in normotensives ingesting normal amounts of sodium.[302] The mean arterial pressure rose after ingesting low-potassium diets for 9 days and was significantly higher than the values noted in the same subjects on normal potassium intakes (Fig. 22-2). Furthermore, potassium depletion sensitized these normotensive subjects to the hypertensive effects of acute sodium loading.[302] Similar increases in blood pressure have been observed in hypertensives ingesting low-potassium diets.[303,305,316] Kaplan et al. observed that amelioration of thiazide-induced hypokalemia potentiated the hypotensive effects of these diuretics.[279] Preliminary studies indicate that potassium supplementation attenuates mineralocorticoid-induced hypertension in humans.[304] Siani and associates observed that dietary potassium supplementation from natural foods reduced the need for antihypertensive medication.[304a] Thus, in humans mild potassium depletion consistently increases blood pressure while potassium supplementation exerts the opposite effect.

The mechanism underlying the increase in blood pressure during potassium depletion is not well understood. Sodium retention, which invariably accompanies potassium depletion (see below), plays an important role. The hypertensive effects of potassium depletion fail to become manifest if sodium intake is curtailed.[299,412] Alterations in the plasma potassium concentration directly influence vascular tone.[10,76] Raij et al. demonstrated that potassium supplementation enhances the endothelium-dependent relaxation of the aorta of hypertensive Dahl

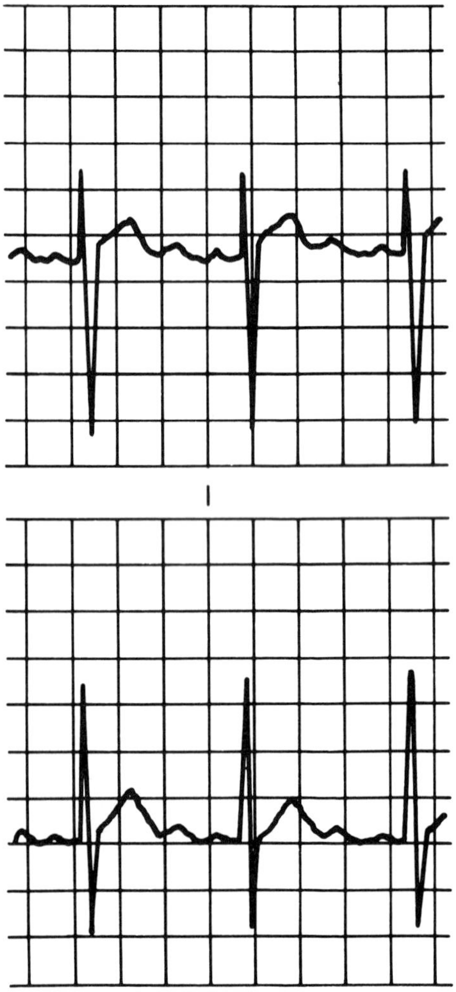

FIGURE 22-2 • The precordial V_2 and V_3 leads of this electrocardiogram show the prominent U waves that are often seen in hypokalemia.

rats.[425a] The role of circulating vasoactive hormones and sympathetic nervous system in mediating potassium-induced changes in blood pressure requires further study.

CARDIAC EFFECTS

The cardiac manifestations of potassium depletion include abnormalities of electrophysiology and contractility. The most serious and potentially fatal complication relates to effects on electrical activity, which is explained by the important role that potassium plays in resting transmembrane potential.[177] Hypokalemia is associated with hyperpolarization of the membrane potential at the end of repolarization, which could lead to increased automaticity, decreased conduction velocity, and shortened refractory period. The electrocardiographic changes in potassium depletion include prolongation of the Q-U interval, widening, flattening, or inverting of the T wave, depression of the S-T segment, prominent U waves, diminished QRS voltage, and increased A-V conduction time[67] (Fig. 22-3).

The potential for a variety of atrial and ventricular arrhythmias is increased during potassium depletion,[396] especially those associated with digitalis. Cardiac sensitivity to digitalis preparations is increased presumably because both a decreased potassium concentration[553] and digitalis itself[131,466] reduce $Na^+ - K^+$ ATPase activity, thus reducing the flux of sodium and potassium ions and providing additional calcium to the contractile proteins.

The potential for serious cardiac arrhythmias secondary to diuretic-induced hypokalemia appears to be substantial, especially in the setting of an acute myocardial infarction. Dyckner et al. studied the effects of the initial serum potassium values on the incidence of cardiac arrhythmias in 444 patients with acute myocardial infarctions and found that certain arrhythmias were significantly overrepresented in hypokalemic patients.[151] Beck and Hockrein[41] and Duke[147] identified an increased incidence of ventricular fibrillation in hypokalemic patients suffering an acute myocardial infarction. The hypokalemia was often associated with diuretic therapy.[147] Solomon and Cole found that diuretic-induced hypokalemia was a clinically significant factor in the development of arrhythmias in 151 patients with acute myocardial infarctions.[491] Hulting studied 1315 patients admitted to a coronary care unit and found the incidence of ventricular fibrillation within 12 h after admission was significantly increased (5.4 percent vs. 1.5 percent) in patients with an initial serum potassium of less than 3.9 meq/liter, including patients without proven myocardial infarctions.[261] Recently, Holland and associates utilized ambulatory Holter monitoring to study the ventricular ectopic activity in 21 hypertensive patients taking hydrochlorthiazide.[253] The results showed the seven of

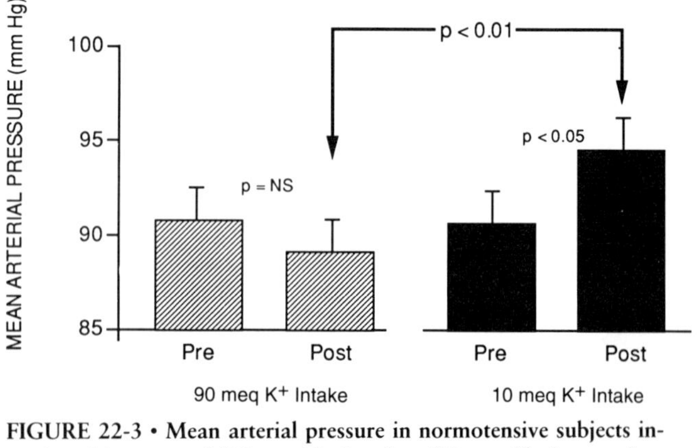

FIGURE 22-3 • Mean arterial pressure in normotensive subjects ingesting either normal (90 meq/day) or low (10 meq/day) potassium for 9 days. Pre and post refer to the measurements obtained at the initiation and termination of study diet. (From Krishna GG et al: *N Engl J Med* 320:1177, 1989.)

21 patients developed ectopic activity and four of the seven developed complex activity, which was more frequent if the serum potassium fell below 3.0 meq/liter. The authors concluded that the hazard of diuretic-induced ventricular ectopic activity warrants correction of hypokalemia and, furthermore, restoration to normokalemia may be required to abolish ectopic activity. In addition, diuretic-induced magnesium depletion must be considered in cases of potassium-resistant cardiac arrhythmias.[156,157]

Cardiac contractility

The effect of potassium depletion on myocardial function varies depending upon the severity of hypokalemia and the species investigated. Abbrecht placed dogs on a low-potassium diet for 30 days and observed a progressive decrease in stroke volume and cardiac output.[3] Potassium repletion reversed these parameters to normal levels. In contrast, Bahler and Rakita induced potassium depletion in dogs by combining low potassium intake with deoxycorticosterone acetate administration over a 2-week period.[24] They observed an increase in cardiac contractility during potassium depletion. Chronic ingestion of a low-potassium diet in young cats has been shown to depress myocardial contractility.[239] Linas et al. observed an increase in cardiac index in rats rendered chronically depleted of potassium.[43,329] Echocardiographic assessment of children suffering from chronic hypokalemia failed to reveal any abnormalities in myocardial function.[400] Morgan et al. in their review of literature found no evidence to implicate diuretic-induced hypokalemia as a cause of heart failure.[369]

In conclusion, chronic potassium depletion can result in several derangements of the cardiovascular system, the most important consequence being an abnormality of cardiac rhythm, especially in association with ischemic myocardial disease and digitalis preparations.

KIDNEY

Morphologic changes

The histologic abnormalities of potassium depletion are variable depending on the species. In humans[374,431] and dogs[1] the characteristic finding is vacuolization of proximal and distal tubular cells. The medullary cytoplasmic droplet that is so characteristic of hypokalemia in rats has only rarely been identified in humans.[187] Cremer and Bock reported on 21 patients with chronic potassium depletion and identified diffuse chronic abacterial interstitial nephritis with glomerular and vascular changes, irrespective of whether the patient had hypertension or not.[122] They concluded that the renal disease is progressive and may terminate in renal failure unless the potasssium depletion is corrected. There were several episodes of urinary tract infections in these patients, but there was no evidence to support an increased susceptibility to infection as has been proposed by others.[564] However, the cause-and-effect relationship between potassium depletion and renal failure remains controversial at this time. Torres et al. recently reported that chronic hypokalemia from hyperaldosteronism is associated with renal cyst formation and interstitial scarring.[524] The number and size of cysts in these patients decreased following correction of hypokalemia.

In rats, the histologic changes are localized to the distal nephron, particularly the collecting ducts, and are characterized by tubular cell hyperplasia and swelling.[399] The aforementioned cytoplasmic droplets are found in the papilla and medulla[399] and contain small vesicles and condensed areas of membrane laminae, the latter being secondary to an increase in medullary phospholipid synthesis.[562] Tolins et al. proposed that increased cortical ammonia levels contribute to the tubular damage resulting from hypokalemia.[522] Sodium bicarbonate supplementation lowered the ammonia production and ameliorated the histologic injury resulting from potassium depletion. It is further suggested that ammonia-mediated activation of the alternate complement pathway may play a role in mediating the renal injury during potassium depletion.

Functional effects

Potassium depletion is responsible for several defects in renal function, including a reduction of glomerular filtration rate (GFR) and renal blood flow, impairment of urinary concentrating capacity, an alteration of renal acidification, and an alteration of the renal handling of sodium.

Studies on GFR in potassium depletion have yielded conflicting results, as some investigators have demonstrated a reduction[309,377] while others have been unable to find any change.[52,469] Abbrecht reported a decrease in renal blood flow in dogs receiving low-potassium diets.[1,3] Linas and Dickman observed that potassium depletion in rats is accompanied by increased renal vascular resistance and a fall in renal blood flow.[329] They attributed the renal hemodynamic alterations to enhanced synthesis of angiotensin II and vasoconstrictor prostaglandins.[329] Mild potassium depletion in humans, however, does not alter renal blood flow or GFRs.[299,302,305]

The potassium-depleted animal is unable to excrete a maximally concentrated urine. The mechanism(s) responsible for this defect have been the subject of a number of studies over the past 30 years. While a defect in antidiuretic hormone release[49,451] could potentially explain the concentrating defect, exogenous vasopressin infusion does not increase the concentration.[431] A number of experiments have demonstrated an abnormal cellular response to vasopressin in renal tubular cells[94,285] and amphibian membranes from potassium-depleted animals.[176] Raymond et al. systematically investigated the mechanism of impaired reponse to vasopressin in potassium-depleted rabbits.[428] Both basal and pitressin-stimulated urinary osmolality were decreased in rabbits following 2 weeks of potassium restriction. Furthermore, the hydraulic conductivity of the cortical collecting tubule in response to vasopressin was significantly depressed in potassium-depleted animals. However, the cAMP-mediated hyperosmotic response was similar between potassium-depleted and control rabbits. These investigators therefore attributed the impaired response to vasopressin to a defect proximal to the activation of the catalytic subunit of adenylate cyclase.

A cardinal feature of the concentrating defect is a reduction in papillary interstitial solute content.[344] The etiology of this decrease in solute content is unclear but may relate to an impairment in solute transport in the thick ascending limb or to a reduction in delivery to this site as suggested by the change in papillary plasma flow seen in this state.[549]

Potassium deficiency also causes primary polydipsia in rats[51] and in humans.[183] A true polyuric state in potassium-deficient humans is likely to be related more to the polydipsia than to the impaired urinary concentrating defect.[448]

Potassium depletion has been associated with increased excretion of urinary prostaglandins in some species[195] but not in others.[257] Certain prostaglandins are known to antagonize the action of vasopressin in vivo[13] and in vitro.[401] Prostaglandin inhibition fails to correct or improve the concentrating defect in rats,[50] dogs,[451] or humans.[441] In contrast, both indomethacin and meclofenamate augment the concentrating ability of potassium-depleted rabbits following vasopressin administration.[429] It is further suggested that prostaglandins impair the vasopressin response of the cortical collecting tubule in potassium-depleted rabbits by activating the guanine nucleotide inhibitory subunits of adenylate cyclase.[429]

Urinary sodium excretion

Changes in external potassium balance produce striking alterations in urinary sodium excretion. Fourman and Harvey observed sodium retention and edema during potassium depletion induced by an exchange resin.[184] Lennon and Lemann induced potassium depletion in normal subjects by ammonium chloride administration and observed retention of both sodium and chloride and an increase in body weight.[321] Krishna et al. investigated the effect of dietary potassium restriction while the sodium intake was kept constant on urinary sodium excretion in normal volunteers and subjects with essential hypertension.[299,302,305] A decrease in sodium excretion was observed within 24 h of restricting potassium intake

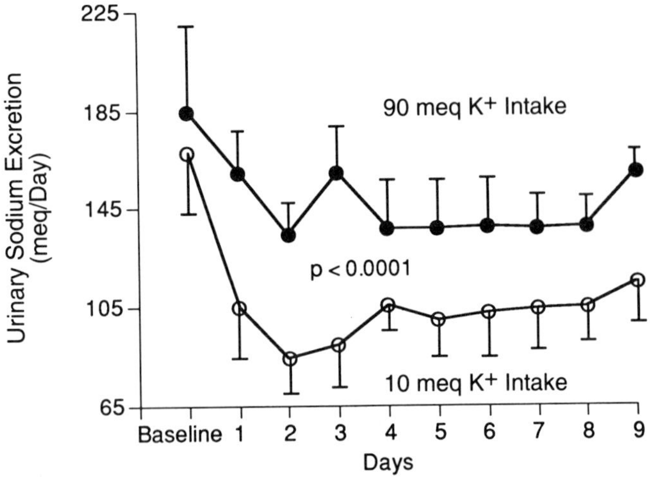

FIGURE 22-4 • Urinary sodium excretion in subjects ingesting either 90 meq/day or 10 meq/day of potassium for 9 days. The sodium intake was kept at normal levels (120 to 200 meq/day). Although the sodium intake varied between subjects, it was kept constant for each subject during both study periods. (From Krishna GG et al: *N Engl J Med* 320:1177, 1989.)

(Fig. 22-4). The sodium-retaining effects of potassium restriction were observed with normal as well as low-sodium intakes.[299,302] It was further observed that potassium depletion impairs the natriuretic response to acute sodium loading.[299,302]

The mechanism by which potassium depletion induces changes in urinary sodium excretion is unknown. This phenomenon occurs independently of changes in catecholamines, aldosterone, and renal hemodynamic changes.[299,302] Potassium depletion may directly influence tubular sodium reabsorption.[308,322] Enhanced proximal tubular sodium reabsorption helps in conserving potassium by limiting distal sodium-potassium exchange. These sodium retentive effects of potassium depletion may play a role in the associated increase in blood pressure (see above).

Recent studies suggest that potassium intake influences the excretion of calcium and phosphorus.[319,476] Increased potassium intake enhances the urinary excretion of these divalent ions while potassium restriction has the opposite effect. Increases in plasma parathyroid hormone levels, perhaps resulting from calcium depletion, have been observed during dietary potassium restriction in hypertensive subjects (unpublished observations, GGK).

Other tubular defects

Potassium depletion is associated with several tubular defects. Parathyroid hormone (PTH)-induced cAMP generation and the PTH-mediated phosphaturic effect are both impaired in hypokalemia.[39] Renal tubular reabsorption and secretion of para-aminohippurate is reduced and aminoaciduria has also been associated with potassium depletion.[495]

Effects on renin

Sealey et al. varied the potassium intake of rats while the sodium intake was kept constant.[475] An inverse relationship was observed between potassium intake and plasma renin activity. Luke et al. similarly detected an increase in plasma renin activity in potassium-depleted rats.[336] Linas et al. noted an increase in plasma renin activity in response to potassium depletion in normal rats and in rats with renovascular hypertension.[43,329,405] Brunner et al. reported an increase in plasma renin activity in normotensive and in hypertensive subjects ingesting low-potassium diets.[83] Bauer and Gaunter studied 20 normal subjects maintained on a potassium intake ranging from 0 to 300 meq/day.[37] Contrasting with earlier studies, these investigators noted a dose-dependent increase in urinary sodium excretion and an increase in plasma renin activity paralleling the increase in potassium intake. Rabelink et al. similarly observed an increase in plasma renin activity following acute potassium loading in healthy subjects and attributed this response to the acute natriuresis induced by potassium.[425] Krishna et al. maintained a group of healthy subjects on a normal or low-potassium intake for a period of 9 days while the sodium intake was kept at normal levels.[303] Plasma renin activity was similar in both groups at the end of 9 days. Similarly, they observed no differences in plasma renin activity when potassium intake was normal or low in subjects maintained on a low-sodium intake.[299] In all these studies potassium restriction was accompanied by a decrease in sodium excretion. Thus, it appears that potassium depletion modifies plasma renin activity by direct stimulation and an indirect suppression through sodium retention. The divergent responses noted in various studies may represent the net effect of these opposing forces. Whether species differences underlie these contrasting effects requires further scrutiny. Generally, studies in humans have investigated the effects of a milder degree of potassium depletion than has been used in the studies in animals.

Effects on prostaglandin production

Clinical and experimental studies investigating the effect of potassium depletion on renal prostaglandin synthesis have yielded a diverse response. Galvez et al. reported that potassium depletion enhances urinary prostaglandin excretion.[195] Raymond et al. observed increases in urinary PGE excretion in rabbits following 2 weeks of potassium depletion.[428] Gullner et al. noted an increase in urinary excretion of 6-keto $PGF_{1\alpha}$ and PGE_2 in rats ingesting low-potassium diets for 9 days.[238] Nasjletti et al. observed that high-potassium intake augments urinary excretion of $PGF_{2\alpha}$ while low-potassium intake increases the excretion of 6-keto $PGF_{1\alpha}$.[388] Excretion of PGE_2 was unchanged by alterations in potassium intake in these studies.[388] Similarly, other studies failed to detect a change in PGE_2 excretion in potassium-depleted rats and humans.[150,257,441,516,573] In vitro studies employing rabbit medullary interstitial cells and papillary slices from rabbits[574] and humans[149] have demonstrated an augmentation of PGE_2 synthesis when the potassium concentration in the medium is reduced. However, Berl et al. found no change in renal medullary prostaglandin content in potassium-depleted rats.[50] Thus, potassium depletion exerts a variable effect on renal prostaglandin synthesis, perhaps determined by the duration and magnitude of hypokalemia and the species investigated.

CLASSIFICATION OF HYPOKALEMIC DISORDERS

Disorders of potassium homeostasis associated with hypokalemia are best classified according to whether there is evidence of decreased intake, redistribution of potassium between intracellular and extracellular fluid compartments, or excessive loss via the renal, gastrointestinal, or integumentary systems. The succeeding sections will discuss in detail those clinical disorders that have been associated with hypokalemia (Fig. 22-4, Table 22-3).

INADEQUATE DIETARY INTAKE

An inadequate dietary intake of potassium is an unusual cause of potassium depletion, but may be an important contributing factor in patients with inappropriate and persistent renal or extrarenal losses. This situation may exist, for example, in patients receiving diuretic therapy or those with mineralocorticoid excess. Nevertheless, modest potassium depletion ensues even in normal subjects maintained on a low-potassium intake.[299,302] Although renal conservation minimizes the net potassium losses, continuing small urinary and stool losses can amount to a substantial cumulative deficit of the cation, if intake is restricted. Elderly subjects and patients suffering from dysphagia may chronically ingest diets very low in potassium and thus become hypokalemic. A diet that is high in carbohydrates but low in potassium-rich foods, such as animal protein, fresh fruits, and vegetables, has been implicated in hypokalemia associated with excessive alcohol consumption.[284,447] In 1959, Elkinton and Huth surveyed 20 patients with anorexia nervosa and found hypokalemia to be a frequent occurrence.[165] Since that time, numerous investigators have verified that the hypokalemia associated with anorexia nervosa often represents total body potassium depletion and not only intracellular shifts secondary to postemetic alkalosis.[96,393,537] Ingestion of certain forms of clay found in the southeast can produce severe hypokalemia.[219,355,478]

TABLE 22-3 • Classification of hypokalemic disorders

1. Inadequate dietary intake
   - High carbohydrate diet
   - Excessive alcohol consumption
   - Anorexia nervosa
   - Clay ingestion
2. Transcellular redistribution
   - Systemic acid-base balance—metabolic and respiratory alkalosis
   - Insulin
   - Mineralocorticoids
   - Sympathomimetic agents
   - Familial hypokalemic periodic paralysis
   - Barium poisoning
   - Rapid cell proliferation, e.g., B_{12} therapy of pernicious anemia rapid tumor growth
3. Excessive renal losses
   - Diuretics
   - Antibiotics
   - Other pharmacologic agents
     - Cisplatinum
     - L-dopa
     - Toleune
     - Lithium
     - Thallium
   - Excessive mineralocorticoid effect
     - Primary hyperaldosteronism
     - Adrenogenital syndromes
     - Cushing's syndrome
     - Corticosteroid excess
     - Hypertensive states—accelerated, malignant, renovascular hypertension
     - Renin-producing tumors
     - Edema-forming states
     - Miscellaneous
       - Acute intermittent porphyria
       - Licorice
       - Carbenoxolone
       - Nasal sprays
   - Intrinsic renal disease
     - Renal tubular acidosis
     - Idiopathic or familial syndromes
       - Bartter's syndrome
       - Bartter-like syndromes
       - Liddle's syndrome
       - Hypomagnesemia—familial and drug-induced
   - Diabetic ketoacidosis
   - Leukemia
   - Hypercalcemia

TABLE 22-3 • *(continued)*

4. Excessive gastrointestinal losses
   - Vomiting
   - Diarrhea
     - Villous adenoma
     - Zollinger-Ellison syndrome
     - Pancreatic cholera
     - Jejunoileal bypass
     - Laxative and enema abuse
     - Infectious etiologies
     - Malabsorption syndromes
     - Fistulas
     - Congenital chloride diarrhea
5. Excessive integumentary losses

Clay entraps potassium in the intestine and prevents its absorption. A history of clay ingestion should be sought out in patients with unexplained hypokalemia, especially if associated with iron deficiency.[355] Iron deficiency results from clay-induced impairment in iron absorption. Interestingly, certain other forms of clay are rich in potassium content, and ingestion of these clays may produce hyperkalemia in patients with renal insufficiency.[207]

REGULATION OF THE TRANSCELLULAR DISTRIBUTION OF POTASSIUM

Stated simply, an increase in the cellular uptake of potassium can potentially induce hypokalemia without a change in total body potassium. Conversely, hyperkalemia can result if the exit of cellular potassium is accelerated. As discussed below, there is a reciprocal relationship between potassium and several regulators of the transcellular distribution of potassium such that the administration of potassium stimulates the release and production of a factor that enhances its cellular uptake. Although this chapter deals with hypokalemia, it is difficult to discuss the regulation of the transcellular distribution of potassium without an appreciation that aberrations of trasncellular potassium regulation can result in hypo- or hyperkalemia. Approximately 60 percent of total body potassium is located in muscle. Consequently, alterations in transcellular potassium distribution in this organ system will be involved in a major way with the regulation of the extracellular potassium concentration. (See also Chap. 6.)

Systemic acid-base balance

It has been generally assumed that there is an inverse relationship between extracellular fluid pH and potassium concentration as a consequence of the reciprocal movement of hydrogen and potassium ions between the intracellular and extracellular compartments. In this context, alkalosis, be it respiratory or metabolic, would be expected to result in hypokalemia. Indeed, it has been implied that this inverse relationship is so precise that it can be stated in mathematical form, for example, a reduction in plasma potassium of 0.6 meq/liter for each 10 mmHg decrease in the arterial P_{CO_2}.[162] The relationship between changes in the extracellular fluid pH and potassium concentration may actually be more complex than originally proposed[53] (see Chap. 6). For example, changes in blood pH in the acidemic direction have a greater effect upon the plasma potassium concentration than do those in the alkalemic direction. The etiology of the acidosis is important in this regard as the administration of organic acids results in a much smaller increase in the plasma potassium concentration than the administration of hydrochloric acid. Metabolic disturbances in acid-base homeostasis induce larger changes in potassium concentration than do respiratory disturbances. Although not uniformly observed, the plasma potassium concentration may vary inversely with the plasma bicarbonate concentration under conditions where the arterial pH is experimentally controlled.[185,186,286,485]

Insulin

Insulin secretion can be induced by potassium loading. If the plasma potassium concentration is increased by 1 to 1.5 meq/liter, peripheral insulin levels increase severalfold.[142,249] On the other hand, insulin enhances the cellular uptake of potassium and thereby aids in the disposal of potassium loads.[135,136,142,249] In fact, insulin secretion need not increase from its basal level to aid in the cellular removal of administered potassium.[136] The ability of insulin to enhance potassium uptake has been demonstrated in a number of tissues, particularly muscle.[53] This effect of insulin is independent of its ability to enhance cellular glucose uptake.[570]

The mechanism(s) by which insulin enhances the cellular uptake of potassium is incompletely defined. Insulin administration causes hyperpolarization of the skeletal muscle membrane before an increase of tissue potassium content occurs.[571] Whether insulin-mediated potassium transport is passively affected by the hyperpolarized state or occurs subsequent to active stimulation of potassium uptake[206,226] is controversial.

Mineralocorticoids

Aldosterone is well recognized as an important regulator of external potassium balance. In the kidney, sweat gland, and colon aldosterone stimulates potassium secretion. The importance of aldosterone as a regulator of the transcellular distribution of potassium is more controversial. Whereas the results of in vitro studies are conflicting,[5,327] data available from in vivo observations suggest that mineralocorticoids may have a marked effect on transcellular potassium regulation. Several of these studies performed in experimental animals have demonstrated that the tolerance to a potassium load and a reduction of the development of hyperkalemia in the anephric state after potassium administration is facilitated by mineralocorticoids.[9,54] The administration of mineralocorticoids to patients with hypoaldosteronism can result in a reduction in the plasma potassium concentration without an increase in urinary or fecal potassium excretion.[134] Thus, intracellular translocation, in addition to the kaliuresis of mineralocorticoid excess, may contribute to the hypokalemia. The relative importance of the former is currently unknown.

Sympathomimetic agents

Catecholamines have direct effects on internal potassium balance. Acute stimulation of alpha-adrenergic receptors results in potassium movement out of cells and hyperkalemia, while beta-adrenergic stimulation increases the inward movement of potassium resulting in hypokalemia. Infusion of epinephrine has a biphasic effect on serum potassium levels. The initial phase is characterized by transient hyperkalemia which is secondary to potassium release from the liver and can be prevented by alpha-adrenergic blockade with dibenamine.[120] This is followed by a prolonged period of hypokalemia which is due to an increased uptake of potassium by cells of both the liver and skeletal muscle. Beta 1 agonists [1-isopropylamino-3- (2-thiazoloxy)-2-propranolol] and beta 2 agonists (salbutamol, soterenol, and terbutaline) facilitate cellular uptake of potassium and this effect is mediated by beta 2 adrenergic receptors. Terbutaline, a beta-adrenergic agonist, has been shown to cause hypokalemia in mongrel dogs approximately 1 to 1½ h after intravenous infusion.[263] The intravenous infusion of terbutaline or ritodrine, a related beta 2 agonist, in obstetrical patients with premature uterine contractions has increased in popularity. Recently, several reports have appeared in the literature documenting hypokalemia following terbutaline administration.[235,367] The increased mortality in asthmatics taking beta 2 agonists (especially fenoterol) may be related to the associated hypokalemia.[121] The hypokalemia complicating theophylline toxicity is likely to be related to the induced increase in adrenal medullary release of epinephrine and the impairment of nonneuronal catechole uptake and metabolism.[282] Theophylline also increases insulin levels.[241a] In addition, numerous other drugs with sympathomimetic activity have been implicated in hypokalemia such as pseudoephedrine and isoxsuprine.[350,398]

Familial hypokalemic periodic paralysis

Familial periodic paralysis is an uncommon disorder characterized by intermittent episodes of muscle weakness and even total flaccid paralysis.[270] The serum potassium is often decreased during attacks, but not always below the normal range. The idiopathic variety of hypokalemic periodic paralysis is inherited as an autosomal-dominant trait that usually becomes symptomatic during the second decade of life.[339] A variant of this disorder, which is strongly associated with thyrotoxicosis, occurs predominantly in orientals and manifests symptoms in the third and fourth decades.[406,417] In addition, Sjögren's syndrome[427] and multiple sclerosis[455] have been associated with hypokalemic periodic paralysis.

The clinical presentation is characterized by generalized muscle weakness, which initially involves proximal muscles before spreading to the distal musculature. The muscles responsible for ventilation, deglutition, and ocular movements are rarely involved. A variety of precipitating factors have been identified, including cold exposure, ingestion of a high-carbohydrate meal, trauma, infections, rest after strenuous exercise, alcohol consumption, obstetric delivery, excessive sodium intake, and insulin administration.[144,270,416,433] The attacks vary in duration, lasting anywhere from a few hours to as long as 24 h.

The pathogenesis of this disorder has not been clearly defined, but several lines of investigation have yielded interesting results. Early observations suggested that the fall in serum potassium concentration was associated with a decrease in urinary potassium excretion, indicating that an internal redistribution of the cation must occur during an attack.[503] Engel and Lambert examined the calcium activation of muscle fibers from hypokalemic periodic paralysis patients and concluded that the critical defect resides in the muscle cell membrane, which becomes electrically unexcitable during attacks.[166] The expected increase in transmembrane potential difference does not occur and, in fact, some studies have shown a fall in the potential difference during symptomatic episodes.[123,434]

Hyperaldosteronism has been implicated in the pathogenesis of this disorder,[114] but levels have not been consistently elevated.[444,528] Interestingly, Streeten and Speller[505] and, most recently, Kabadi[275] have had patients with periodic paralysis whose attacks could be successfully induced only by the administration of ACTH, but not by aldosterone, desoxycorticosterone, or angiotensin II infusions. The reduction or prevention of the ACTH-induced paralysis by metapyrone suggested to these investigators that a mineralocorticoid with hydroxyl radicals at the C-11 and C-18 positions was responsible for the attacks.[505]

Histologic and ultrastructural studies have identified several abnormalities in muscle cells. Platt et al. demonstrated ultrastructural abnormalities of the sarcoplasmic reticulum and transverse tubular system.[417] Buruma et al. examined heart muscle and discovered an unusual amount of intermyofibrillary glycogen, resembling, but to a lesser degree, the increase in glycogen found in the same patient's skeletal muscle biopsy specimen.[89] These structural derangements lend support to earlier studies that suggested that altered muscle organelle function[410] and/or altered carbohydrate metabolism[481] were important pathogenic mechanisms in this disorder.

The pharmacologic administration of acetazolamide, a carbonic anhydrase inhibitor, has been used successfully to treat severe attacks and is more effective than either potassium supplementation or spironolactone.[231,432] Vroom et al. demonstrated that acetazolamide significantly ameliorates the fall in serum potassium induced by the infusion of glucose and insulin in periodic paralysis patients.[532] Johnsen has proposed that the "indirect prophylactic action" of acetazolamide is mediated through a reduction in the levels of insulin and glucose, thus reducing the intracellular flux of potassium during an attack.[269,271] An alternate explanation of acetazolamide's action has been that a mild acidosis develops after administration of the drug thus decreasing the rate of potassium redistribution.[532]

Barium poisoning

The ingestion of soluble barium salts can produce a clinical picture of flaccid skeletal paralysis that resembles hypokalemic periodic paralysis. In addition, barium poisoning can result in respiratory paralysis and death within hours of ingestion. Hypertension, vomiting, diarrhea, and cardiac arrhythmias also may complicate the picture.[372] Hypokalemia has been demonstrated in most of the symptomatic patients.[141] Roza and Berman showed that a significant extracellular to intracellular shift of potassium occurs after barium administration.[446] Nagel demonstrated that barium affects the transcellular shift of potassium by inhibiting potassium conductance.[381]

EXCESSIVE RENAL LOSSES

Diuretics

Hypokalemia is a potential complication of diuretic therapy.[297] This may occur with all of the commonly used diuretics including the thiazides, furosemide, ethacrynic acid, bumetanide, acetazolamide, organomercurials, and osmotic agents.[189] There are several mechanisms responsible for the increased potassium excretion associated with diuretics. Inhibition of sodium reabsorption in the early portion of distal nephron enhances sodium delivery to potassium secretory sites and increases the flow rate in this segment.[515,565] Aldosterone released in response to diuretic-induced hypovolemia further facilitates potassium secretion. Metabolic alkalosis resulting from diuretic therapy contributes to hypokalemia by promoting cellular uptake of potassium and by enhancing urinary losses (see Chap. 29). Hypochloremia decreases filtered chloride and luminal chloride concentration and thereby promotes kaliuresis.[379,515] Magnesium depletion complicating diuretic therapy may contribute to renal potassium losses (see below). Although certain diuretic agents may inhibit potassium reabsorption in the proximal tubule or the loop of Henle, it is not known if this inhibition results in an increase in the amounts excreted in the final urine. Carbonic anhydrase inhibitors, in addition to increasing distal fluid and sodium delivery, can accelerate the peritubular uptake of potassium and, thereby, the secretion of this ion in the distal nephron.[558]

In spite of the various potential mechanisms working to increase potassium excretion during diuretic therapy, the occurrence and severity of either plasma or total body potassium depletion is quite modest.[128,244,513] Morgan and Davidson analyzed publications concerning diuretic-induced hypokalemia and concluded that "50 percent of hypertensive patients taking a thiazide will have a potassium concentration less than 3.5 meq/liter but only 7 percent will be less than 3.0 meq/liter."[368] Among patients taking furosemide, the incidence of values less than 3.5 meq/liter was 5 percent and of those 2 percent had values less than 3.0 meq/liter. Recently, Sandor et al. studied 169 patients with hypertension for 2 years on unrestricted diets taking diuretics, without K^+ supplements, and found a 29 percent incidence of mild hypokalemia (3.0 to 3.3 meq/liter) and a 13 percent incidence of modest hypokalemia (2.6 to 2.9 meq/liter).[457] Only one patient was felt to be symptomatic from the hypokalemia. Interestingly, Lemieux et al. demonstrated that plasma potassium concentration fell during the first 6 weeks of diuretic therapy, seldom to values below 3.5 meq/liter, but then gradually rose to 4.1 meq/liter after 19 months.[320] The magnitude of hypokalemia is greater with such longer-acting (>24 h) diuretics as chlorothalidone, as compared with such short-acting (<6 h) diuretics as furosemide. Administration of a single dose of furosemide induces an acute kaliuresis that lasts for 3 to 4 h and is then followed by potassium retention, thereby returning the body potassium stores to normal.[559] Potassium losses during diuretic therapy are high at the extremes of sodium intake, and minimal at modest sodium restriction (i.e., 80 to 110 meq/day).[379] Thiazide-induced hypokalemia is dose-dependent and is usually observed at high doses (50 to 100 mg/day of hydrochlorothiazide).

Antibiotics: penicillins, amphotericin B, tetracycline, gentamicin, polymixin B, rifampicin

The majority of penicillin derivatives, including sodium penicillin,[82] ampicillin,[212] carbenicillin,[90] nafcillin,[364] oxacillin,[464] and ticarcillin[360] have been implicated as potential causes of hypokalemia. Brunner and Frick suggested two possible mechanisms responsible for the hypokalemic metabolic alkalosis associated with high-dose sodium penicillin.[82] Penicillin (molecular weight of 334) may act as an osmotic diuretic and, since it is a strong organic acid that is completely ionized at any urine pH, it may function as a nonreabsorbable anion. The administration of these antibiotics, especially carbenicillin, is often associated with a large sodium load that further enhances distal tubule flow rate and potassium secretion.[15,251,287,331]

Several other antibiotics also cause hypokalemia by stimulating urinary potassium excretion. Amphotericin B can alter distal tubule permeabililty resulting in potassium loss into the urine.[143,442,561] Similarly, although rarely seen today, large doses of outdated tetracycline can result in a form of proximal renal tubular acidosis and hypokalemia.[233] Gentamicin, a potential renal tubular toxin, can induce hypokalemia, as well as hypomagnesemia, hypocalcemia, and alkalosis.[26] The etiology of the hypokalemia and renal potassium loss is unclear but does not appear to be a consequence of the hypomagnesemia.[124] Rifampicin, an antituberculous agent, was reported to be associated with renal potassium wasting and hypokalemia.[100,389] Another antituberculous agent, para-amino-salicylic acid, may also cause hypokalemia.[354] Polymixin B therapy in febrile leukemic patients has been associated with several plasma electrolyte abnormalities, including hypokalemia.[440]

Other drugs associated with hypokalemia

A number of other drugs have been reported to be associated with hypokalemia. In all cases the mechanism responsible has yet to be clearly elucidated. *Cis*-dichlorodiammineplatinum (cisplatinum), a chemotherapeutic agent, has been associated with hypokalemia, as well as hypomagnesemia.[463,563] In this instance, the hypokalemia is likely due to renal potassium wastage. Of note, the hypokalemia may be resistant to replacement therapy until the magnesium deficiency is corrected.[63] Levodopa (L-dopa), a drug used for the therapy of Parkinson's disease, increases urinary potassium excretion and has been associated with hypokalemia in approximately 10 percent of Parkinsonian patients.[228] This effect can be prevented by peripheral dopa-decarboxylase inhibition.[228] It is of interest that in some instances patients with L-dopa-induced hypokalemia have elevated urinary aldosterone levels.[228] Toluene, an organic solvent inhaled for its effects on the central nervous system, can cause hypokalemia[45,510] as well as alterations in systemic acid-base balance.[178,373] Lithium carbonate toxicity[241] and thallium poisoning[204] have both been reported in association with hypokalemia. Again, the responsible mechanisms are undefined.

Gossypol is a contraceptive medication that reduces male fertility by inducing oligospermia. Hypokalemia is a well-recognized side effect of acute and chronic therapy with this agent.[333,424,536] Although this drug is thought to induce hypokalemia by enhancing urinary losses of potassium, acute reductions in serum potassium concentration have been observed in nephrectomized animals.[514] Thus, gossypol may influence the urinary excretion of potassium as well as its transcellular distribution. Hypokalemia is frequently encountered with *theophylline* intoxication, especially following an acute overdose with this medication.[479]

Excessive mineralocorticoid effect

Primary hyperaldosteronism

In 1955, Conn reported on the first case of a patient with hypertension, episodic muscle weakness, polyuria, tetany, hypernatremia and hypokalemic metabolic alkalosis.[112] The laboratory studies revealed increased aldosterone levels but normal 17-ketosteroids and 17-hydroxycorticosteroids. The abnormal studies and the patient's symptoms remitted following the resection of an adrenal adenoma that contained a large concentration of aldosterone. This initial description of primary hyperaldosteronism, Conn's syndrome, has been followed by numerous reports of similar cases and has resulted in the subdivision of the syndrome of primary hyperaldosteronism into four types: aldosterone producing adenoma (APA), idiopathic hyperaldosteronism (IHA) (adrenocortical hyperplasia, "pseudoprimary" aldosteronism), indeterminate hyperaldosteronism (IndHA), and glucocorticoid remediable hyperaldosteronism. This classification is important because the treatment for each is different, and surgery is indicated for only one type—the APA.

Patients with bilateral adrenal hyperplasia and those with a unilateral, single adenoma (i.e., Conn's syndrome) both present with hypokalemia and hypertension. Because surgery is curative only in those with an adenoma, it is critical to distinguish between these two forms of hyperaldosteronism.[22,59,60,258,334] Several physiologic, pathophysiologic, and biochemical principles have been capitalized upon to identify the anatomic basis of the aldosterone excess.

Two well-known stimuli to aldosterone secretion include postural changes in angiotensin II and the release of ACTH. While adenomatous and hyperplastic tissue can respond to both these stimuli, the former is more responsive to ACTH and the latter is more responsive to angiotensin II. Accordingly, plasma aldosterone levels peak in the early morning in patients with adenomas, paralleling the normal diurnal variation in ACTH secretion. This peak in concentration is minimal to absent in those with hyperplasia. Comparison of plasma aldosterone levels obtained after maintaining a supine posture with those obtained following ambulation shows a clear increase in patients with bilateral adrenal hyperplasia and no change or a reduction in those with adenomas.

Circulating levels of a key precursor of aldosterone biosynthesis, 18-hydroxycorticosterone (18-OHB), are much higher in patients with adenomas than in those with bilateral hyperplasia.[58] Blood levels of 18-OHB greater than 100 ng/dl strongly point to an adenoma. Aldosterone levels also tend to be much higher in patients with an adenoma making it uncertain whether 18-OHB levels enhance our ability to discriminate between adenomas and hyperplasia. Because the 18-OHB levels vary directly with the rate of aldosterone synthesis, they may tell us little more than the plasma concentration of aldosterone. Recent evidence suggests that plasma levels of 19-nordeoxycorticosterone may be significantly higher in patients with adenomas.[18]

Patients with hypertension and unprovoked hypokalemia ($K^+ < 3.5$ meq/liter) and those with diuretic-induced hypokalemia that is not corrected after discontinuation of diuretics and provision of potassium should be screened for primary aldosteronism (see Fig. 22-5). One should first establish that the hypokalemia is associated with renal potassium-wasting. A 24-h collection of urine should be made while the patient ingests at least 100 meq of sodium daily. This salt intake ensures that distal sodium delivery will be sufficient to maximize aldosterone-induced potassium secretion. Conversely, urinary potassium excretion may be very low if subjects ingest sodium-restricted diets, even though extreme hyperaldosteronemia exists. After confirming that a 24-h urine contains >30 meq/day of potassium, and >100 meq/day of sodium, the simplest screening procedure utilizes the ratio of the level of plasma aldosterone to that of renin. Ratios >20 suggest primary aldosteronism. If positive, the diagnosis should be confirmed by obtaining plasma aldosterone levels before and after expanding plasma volume with 2 liters of normal saline infused over 4 h.[79,504] Failure to suppress aldosterone levels to values < 8 ng/ml is suggestive of unregulated hormone secretion. However, aldosterone levels decrease with age, and referral to age-adjusted normal values is important.[244a] Alternately, measurement of 24-h urine aldosterone excretion along with assays of sodium and creatinine have been shown to be both sensitive and specific.[397]

Cushing's syndrome, another cause of hypertension with hypokalemia, should be excluded by a 24-h urine cortisol or a dexamethasone suppression test (see below).

Once the diagnosis of primary aldosteronism is established, a CT scan will identify lesions greater than 4 mm. If the CT scan is equivocal, a radioisotope scan with NP59 (6-beta I^{131} iodomethyl-19 norcholesterol) performed after a 7-day course of dexamethasone can distinguish between an adenoma and hyperplasia. NP59, like 19-iodocholesterol, a radiolabeled precursor of aldo-

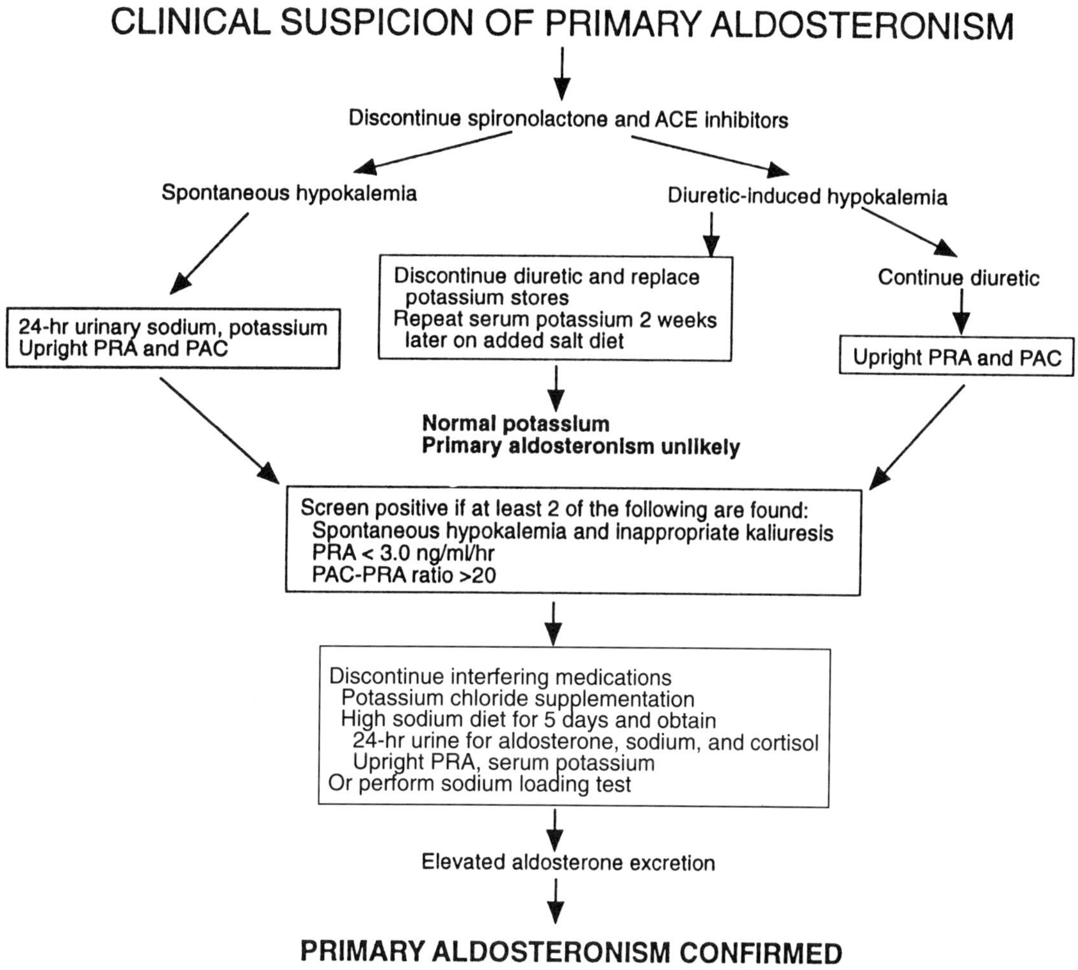

FIGURE 22-5 • Approach to primary aldosteronism (Reproduced with permission from Young WF Jr, et al: Primary aldosteronism: Diagnosis and treatment. *Mayo Clin Proc.*65:96–110, 1990.) Abbreviations: ACE = angiotensin converting enzyme; PAC-plasma aldosterone concentration; PRA = plasma renin activity.

sterone, is taken up preferentially by adenomas, while dexamethasone suppresses its uptake in the remainder of the adrenal gland. Scanning is done over a 3- to 4-day period. A positive scan demonstrates focal increased uptake. Following early diffuse uptake in bilateral hyperplasia, the radiolabel is quickly lost and at no time is focal accumulation noted.[199,550] The syndrome of glucocorticoid remediable hyperaldosteronism (GRH) is a rare autosomal dominant condition associated with enhanced sensitivity of mineralocorticoid production to ACTH. A mutation of a single gene encoding 11-β-hydroxylase and aldosterone synthase is responsible for the syndrome. Instead of normally being restricted to the adrenal's zona glomerulosa—which is essentially unresponsive to ACTH—in GRH, aldosterone synthase is also found in the adjacent. ACTH responsive, zona reticularis. Thus, as with the synthesis and secretion of glucocorticoids, that of aldosterone also becomes responsive to ACTH in this syndrome, thereby increasing its daily secretory rate and violating its normal feedback relationship to extracellular fluid volume.[326] A 7- to 10-day course of dexamethasone cures the hypertension and hypokalemia by suppressing ACTH and thereby the excess aldosterone secretion. Measurement of the urinary metabolites of 18-hydroxy and 18-oxocortisol, which are oversecreted via the cortisol C-18 oxidation pathway, provides an alternate and specific means of diagnosing GRH.[433a]

Hypokalemia in primary aldosteronism is predominantly due to the effects of aldosterone on renal potassium excretion (see Chaps. 7 and 14). The late distal tubule and collecting system are the nephron sites responsive to mineralocorticoid action. In the mineralocorticoid-deficient state, a reduction in potential difference across the entire tubule and the basolateral membrane, a fall in intracellular potassium activity and in luminal membrane permeability are noted.[467,555-557] Consequently, aldosterone has been suggested to accelerate both the uptake of potassium into transporting cells and its removal across the luminal membrane. Presumably, these effects are exaggerated in the presence of aldosterone excess.

In addition to these direct effects of aldosterone on potassium transport, excess hormone may indirectly enhance kaliuresis. The development of a metabolic alkalosis, subsequent to potassium depletion and aldosterone excess, may further enhance renal loss of the cation. Further, the volume-expanded state, associated with aldosterone excess, tends to maintain high delivery rates of sodium and water to the distal nephron thereby enhancing potassium excretion.

Adrenogenital syndromes

Two genetically transmitted adrenal enzyme deficiencies, 11β- and 17α-hydroxylase, are associated with hypokalemia, metabolic alkalosis, and hypertension.[72] In 11β-hydroxylase deficiency, impaired cortisol production results in increased ACTH release and secondarily, in overproduction of the mineralocorticoid, deoxycorticosterone (DOC).[158] The conversion of DOC to corticosterone and its derivatives is impaired, thus producing deficiencies of corticosterone, 18-hydroxycorticosterone, and aldosterone.[389] In addition, the increased ACTH stimulates adrenal androgen production resulting in virilization.[72] In 17α-hydroxylase deficiency, the conversion of DOC to corticosterone is unimpaired, causing 18-hydroxycorticosterone and aldosterone levels to be markedly elevated. The hypermineralocorticoid state and the subsequent development of severe hypokalemia is due to the high levels of all these hormones.[568] In both syndromes, glucocorticoid hormone replacement therapy effectively suppresses ACTH secretion and excessive mineralocorticoid production.[459]

Cushing's syndrome and corticosteroid excess

Cushing's syndrome is characterized by excessive glucocorticoid hormone production that causes obesity, carbohydrate intolerance, muscle wasting, osteoporosis, and mild hirsutism. Hypertension and electrolyte abnormalities are much less frequent in this syndrome than other "hypermineralocorticoid" states. This relates to the weak mineralocorticoid activity of cortisol, which on a comparative basis is only 0.4 percent of aldosterone's activity. However, the plasma levels of cortisol may be of sufficient magnitude to exert a significant mineralocorticoid effect.[38] The differentiation of mineralocorticoid from glucocorticoid hypertension may involve the existence of a third corticosteroid receptor that mediates hypertension and sodium retention under conditions of marked cortisol excess.[106a]

Hypokalemia is seen in a small percentage of patients with Cushing's syndrome.[418] Christy and Larragh identified hypokalemia in 28 percent of their patients and noted that an adrenal adenoma was a much more frequent cause than was adrenal hyperplasia.[105] However, if severe hypokalemia and hypertension are present, a more potent mineralocorticoid than cortisol should be suspected.[459] Deoxycorticosterone and corticosterone have been reported to be elevated in Cushing's syndrome. The increase in these steroids is often associated with an underlying malignancy of the adrenal gland,[492] or as a consequence of the ectopic production of ACTH by such tumors as oat cell or bronchial carcinomas of the lung, thymomas, pancreatic islet cell tumors, pheochromocytomas, ovarian arrhenoblastomas, and medullary carcinoma of the thyroid.[21,117,411,460,499] Recently, Azer and Braunstein reported a patient with hypertension, hypokalemic alkalosis, and elevated DOC associated with a Leydig cell tumor of the testicle that corrected with chemotherapy.[19]

In addition, hypokalemia may be associated with hypermineralocorticoidism from defective peripheral metabolism of cortisol. Ulick et al. described a syndrome characterized by hypertension, hypokalemia, low plasma renin activity, subnormal aldosterone responsiveness to spironolactone, and a decreased rate of conversion of cortisol to cortisone.[527] This appears to be caused by a congenital deficiency of 11-β hydorxysteroid dehydrogenase, the enzyme that catalyzes the renal conversion of cortisol to cortisone (see below). Cortisone has much less mineralocorticoid activity than cortisol. Thus, without the enzyme, cortisol accumulates, stimulating sodium retention and potassium excretion. Hypertension and hypokalemia ensue.[106a]

Hypertension—accelerated, malignant, and renovascular

The majority of hypertensive patients have essential hypertension and normal serum potassium levels.[276] Hypokalemia is much more common in those forms of hypertension associated with high renin-angiotensin-aldosterone levels such as accelerated, malignant, renovascular, and high renin essential hypertension.[84,85,256] In the malignant phase of hypertension, which can develop during the course of all forms of hypertension, the very high levels of plasma renin activity and aldosterone are often associated with hypokalemic alkalosis despite the presence of impaired renal function.[313] In addition to the effects of aldosterone, urinary potassium excretion may be increased due to the severe sodium wasting and polyuria that occurs during the onset of malignant hypertension.[27] Wrong found a serum potassium of less than 3.5 meq/liter in 6 of 14 patients with severe hypertension and papilledema.[566] Hunt and Strong identified hypokalemia in 44 of 214 patients with renal artery stenosis and hypertension.[262] In another large series of renovascular hypertension, potassium concentrations of less than 3.4 meq/liter were found in 17 percent of patients with fibromuscular hyperplasia and in 14 percent of patients witih atherosclerotic renal artery stenosis.[487] Other diseases associated with severe hypertension such as scleroderma crisis[205] and necrotizing vasculitis[552] have been reported to have increased levels of aldosterone and plasma renin activity associated with hypokalemia.

Renin-producing tumors

Juxtaglomerular cell tumors,[32,81,159,436,458] Wilm's tumors,[197,361] and hypernephromas[127,254,317,403] have been associated with the excessive production of renin resulting in hyperaldosteronism, hypertension, and hypokalemia. Conn et al. have shown that the juxtaglomerular cell tumors (hemangiopericytomas) are capable of producing excessive amounts of renin.[113] Selective renal vein sampling may reveal high plasma renin activity on the side of the tumor-laden kidney.[116,127] The hemangiopericytomas are frequently small, but may be visualized on angiography.[113] Baruch et al. described three patients with renin secreting tumors manifesting high plasma renin activity.[32] Although renal venous sampling for renin failed to localize these tumors, renal arteriography revealed avascular areas corresponding to these tumors. The majority of these patients were cured of their hypertension and hypokalemia with resection of their tumors.[32,127,436]

Edema-forming states

Stimulation of aldosterone production has been frequently assumed to exist during the process of edema formation in patients with congestive heart failure, cirrhosis, or nephrosis. Consequently, the hypokalemia occasionally seen in these patients was felt to reflect the increase in aldosterone excretion. Under experimental conditions, in animals[323] and humans,[103] hypokalemia and potassium depletion do not develop despite the presence of aldosterone excretion rates that would be anticipated to enhance renal potassium loss. Undoubtedly, other factors are responsible for the potassium-depleted state. Diuretic therapy[384] and altered acid-base status, for example, acute respiratory[280,376] or metabolic alkalosis,[470] are the major causes of renal potassium losses seen in these patients.

Other conditions associated with mineralocorticoid excess

Farese et al. described a patient with acute intermittent porphyria who presented with hypokalemic metabolic alkalosis, urinary potassium concentration of 50 meq/liter, and secondary hyperaldosteronism.[171]

Hoefnagels et al. reported on five women with hypokalemia and hypertension despite the presence of hypoaldosteronism, hyperreninemia, and normal DOC levels.[250] They postulated that the hypertension and hypokalemia were being maintained by the overproduction of an unknown ACTH-dependent mineralocorticoid. Further, New et al. have suggested that an unidentified mineralocorticoid hormone may also be present in other hypokalemic hypertensive syndromes.[390] The exact identity of these substances remains uncertain.

Drug-induced hypokalemia secondary to excessive mineralocorticoid effect is not an uncommon problem. Licorice, a flavoring commonly found in alcoholic beverages, snuff, chewing tobacco, Lydia Pinkham's Compound, and candies, is associated with a high incidence of hypokalemia if ingested in large amounts.[64,115,311] The active ingredient, glycyrrhizinic acid, produces an aldosterone-like effect on potassium and sodium metabolism. Plasma aldosterone levels and renin activity are suppressed.[115] The clinical manifestations quickly resolve upon discontinuation of licorice ingestion. Several recent studies have explored the mineralocorticoid properties of glycyrrhizic acid and its hydrolytic product, glycyrrhetinic acid.[314,365,500] Monder et al. observed that both these compounds inhibit renal 11β-hydroxysteroid dehydrogenase, an enzyme that catalyzes the conversion of cortisol to cortisone in the human kidney.[365] Since mineralocorticoid receptors in the kidney lack specificity, they bind with cortisol which is abundant in the absence of 11β-dehydrogenase activity.[160,193] This situation is analogous to the congenital absence of 11β-dehydrogenase, also termed "apparent mineralocorticoid excess" (see above).[501] Thus, congenital or acquired deficiency of 11β-dehydrogenase, by impairing the conversion of cortisol to cortisone in the kidney, allows cortisol to function as a mineralocorticoid. Latif et al. reported that glycyrrhetinic acid in addition to its effects on 11β-dehydrogenase also inhibits hepatic enzymes such as Δ^4-5-reductase and 3β-hydroxysteroid dehydrogenase, resulting in an accumulation of aldosterone and 5α-dihydroaldosterone, both of which are potent mineralocorticoids.[314] Salivary extracts from normal subjects who chew tobacco also inhibit Δ^4-5-reductase activity.[370] Carbenoxolone, a derivative of glycyrrhetinic acid used in the treatment of gastric ulcers, has been associated with hypokalemia in approximately 44 percent of patients on long-term therapy.[80,445] This complication occurs with greater frequency in patients older than 60 years of age and appears to be dose related.[196] The administration of steroid compounds with mineralocorticoid activity may result in hypokalemia. Nasal and topical application of 9-alpha-fluoroprednisolone has been associated with hypokalemia, hypertension, metabolic alkalosis with suppressed plasma renin activity and low plasma aldosterone levels.[209,315,346,567] Rare cases of rhabdomyolysis have been reported from prolonged use of these compounds.[315,567]

RENAL TUBULAR ACIDOSIS Hypokalemia secondary to excessive urinary potassium excretion is a common complication of both type I and type II renal tubular acidosis (RTA) (see Chap. 26). However, the pathogenetic mechanisms responsible for the renal potassium wasting differ between the two disorders, thus creating important differences in their therapy.[386]

"Classic," or type I, distal RTA can be differentiated from other varieties of RTA and is characterized by ineffectual distal nephron acidification, the virtually invariable presence of hypokalemia, and an inability to maximally acidify the urine despite systemic acidosis.[34-36] The etiology of the hypokalemia in classic RTA is uncertain, although several studies have suggested a possible mechanism. Patients with this disorder have abnormalities in the renal transport not only of potassium and hydrogen ions but of sodium and chloride as well.[472] This defect is expressed as an inability to establish and maintain a steep gradient in these ions in the distal nephron. If the latter is due to increased membrane permeability, the transport of a number of ions may be affected. Evidence in favor of this possibility is provided by the observation that amphotericin B, a drug reported to induce distal RTA in humans, increases the luminal membrane permeability of the turtle bladder.[497] Secondary hyperaldosteronism may be present in some of these patients,[474] but it is not clear that this is a major contribution to the renal potassium loss.[216] In most patients with distal RTA, potassium supplements are not required to maintain normokalemia when correction of acidosis is sustained.[371] In some patients potassium losses continue despite correction of the acidosis.[371,474]

Type II, or proximal RTA, in adults is usually associated with all of the features of the Fanconi syndrome, including hypokalemia. This is in contrast to the situation in children where an isolated "proximal" RTA without hypokalemia or other features of the Fanconi syndrome is more common. In patients with hypokalemia and proximal RTA, correction of the systemic acidosis with alkali is associated with increased loss of potassium in the urine.[474] The current explanation is that medical treatment with large amounts of bicarbonate overwhelms the diminished proximal reabsorptive capacity, thus resulting in the increased distal delivery of sodium and the relatively impermeant bicarbonate anion. This increase in sodium bicarbonate delivery may result in a more negative intraluminal potential difference in the distal tubule thereby stimulating potassium secretion and ultimately, excretion. Hyperaldosteronism has been reported with proximal RTA and, in some patients, supernormal amounts of dietary sodium fail to lower the aldosterone level.[473] The exact role of aldosterone in this condition is not clear, but it may be a contributing factor to the development of hypokalemia.

Idiopathic or familial causes

BARTTER'S SYNDROME. In 1962, Bartter and associates reported two patients with growth retardation, hypokalemic alkalosis, hyperaldosteronism, hyperreninemia, normal blood pressure, insensitivity to exogenous angiotensin II, and marked hypertrophy and hyperplasia of the juxtaglomerular apparatus.[31] Several additional abnormalities have been noted on occasion since the initial description, including a Pitressin-resistant impairment of urinary concentrating ability,[31,94] insensitivity to exogenous norepinephrine,[213] hypomagnesemia,[338,508] hyperuricemia,[356] erythrocytosis,[167] and increased urinary prostaglandin E_2 excretion.[217] In addition, hypercalciuria with an abnormal serum calcium has been demonstrated in a few patients.[353]

Since 1962, over 100 cases of Bartter's syndrome have been reported in the English literature, making it a rare cause of hypokalemia.[213] The syndrome has been found in blacks,[31] whites,[531] and individuals of Asian origin.[265] There appears to be an increased incidence among females[94] and in certain families.[28,551] An autosomal recessive pattern of transmission has been suggested from a study of consanguineous relationships.[28,508] The majority of patients are children, 50 percent of cases presenting before 5 years of age,[170] but signs and symptoms may not become manifest until the fifth decade.[523]

The most common symptoms and signs among children are failure to thrive, anorexia, salt craving, constipation, polyuria, enuresis, polydipsia, and muscle weakness.[99] Mental retardation has been identified in several patients.[94] In adults, severe proximal muscle weakness is the most common presenting feature and can be quite incapacitating.[523,551] Paralysis is extremely rare but tetany, muscle cramps, and convulsions have been described. In addition to weakness, the physical exam may reveal positive Chvostek's and Trousseau's signs, bradypnea, muscle tenderness, and gouty tophi.[99]

Hypokalemia is the most common laboratory abnormality with values ranging from 1.5 to 2.5 meq/liter in most patients.[31,94,170] Hypochloremic metabolic alkalosis with a serum bicarbonate concentration as high as 40 meq/liter is not uncommon, especially in children.[437] Renal potassium excretion can exceed 300 meq/day despite severe hypokalemia and sodium restriction. The blood urea nitrogen, serum creatinine, creatinine clearance, and renal-diluting capacity are usually normal. Hyperaldosteronism is usually present, but the urinary excretion of 17-ketosteroids and 17-hydroxycorticosteroids are normal, suggesting that adrenal function is normal.[221]

The plasma renin activity is usually very high, but can be appropriately suppressed by volume expansion with saline or hyperoncotic albumin.[221,551] In addition, volume expansion has been shown to enhance the pressor effect of exogenous angiotensin II, a response that is blunted in the basal state.[31,221,278,551] Prostaglandin E excretion is markedly increased in the basal state and may be, in part, responsible for the insensitivity of the vasculature to angiotensin II infusion.[125,217,483] However, inhibition of prostaglandin synthesis fails to increase the low (<0.5) distal fractional reabsorption of chloride, a consistent feature of Bartter's syndrome.[496] The diagnosis of the syndrome hinges on establishing renal potassium and chloride wasting when other causes of renal potassium wasting are carefully excluded. Repeated urinary screening for diuretics is particularly essential to exclude surreptitious diuretic use. Although psychogenic vomiting presents many features similar to Bartter's syndrome, distal fractional reabsorption of chloride is high in this condition.[496]

Radiologic evaluation may reveal nonspecific hydronephrosis and hydroureters in patients with severe polyuria. In addition, retarded bone age[16] and duodenal dilation from hypokalemia-induced ileus has been reported.

The renal biopsy invariably shows hypertrophy and hyperplasia of the juxtaglomerular apparatus, except in early childhood, where the characteristic changes may not become evident until after several years of persistent hypokalemia.[31,99] In addition, glomeruli may appear hypercellular and immature, the glomerular capillary basement membrane thickened, and arterioles narrowed. Renal medullary interstitial cells are often hyperplastic and stain positive with periodic acid-Schiff's reagent, alcian blue, colloidin iron, and Sudan black stains, an observation that has resulted in the postulate that these cells are responsible for the overproduction of prostaglandins and other vasoactive hormones.[529] Other investigators have suggested alternative theories including (1) an aberration in the kallikrein-kinin system, (2) excessive protaglandin production, (3) primary renal potassium wastage, and (4) defective tubular sodium chloride reabsorption. None of the theories readily explains all the features of the syndrome. The syndrome may represent a heterogeneous disorder reflecting several different primary defects, all of which lead to a comon clinical presentation. Although generalized defects in cellular sodium transport have been reported, amelioration of hypokalemia corrects many of these abnormalities.[203,296] The interested reader is referred to a number of publications regarding this perplexing issue.[30,74,94,99,137,191,203,213,214,217,242,296,496,529,530,551]

TREATMENT. The major emphasis in all regimens of therapy is to correct the potassium depletion and its associated symptoms. Potassium chloride replacement, often as much as 200 to 400 meq/day, will usually correct the weakness, tiredness, and easy fatigability, although hypokalemia still persists.[213] Symptoms of gastric irritation may prevent the oral intake of such large doses of potassium, so potassium-sparing diuretics such as triamterene, spironolactone, and amiloride have been utilized, but with varied success.[99,230] Hypomagnesemia should be treated with magnesium supplements. This may improve potassium balance and relieve symptoms of tetany and muscle cramps. Propranolol has resulted in variable effects, plasma renin activity and aldosterone were decreased in some patients[363,490] but not others,[174,468] and it failed to raise serum potassium levels despite a decrease in aldosterone.[363,490] In addition, propranolol may produce symptomatic hypotension and a paradoxical increase in renin and aldosterone; therefore, it is probably not indicated for use in Bartter's syndrome.[174,468] Improvement in plasma potassium levels has been reported with converting enzyme inhibitors, but hypotension can pose a serious problem.[246,461] Prostaglandin synthetase inhibitors, such as indomethacin,[164,217,529] ibuprofen,[217] and aspirin,[395] may only partially correct the hypokalemia, but in combination with potassium supplementation and potassium-sparing diuretics, a greater degree of potassium correction has been made possible.[332] This latter therapy has been shown to stimulate growth and development in children and retard the progression of arteriolar and glomerular disease.[332]

Patients with Bartter's syndrome can become pregnant without untoward effects to the fetus, as the disease will either spontaneously improve or be readily manageable during the pregnancy.[288,502]

BARTTER-LIKE SYNDROMES. Numerous case reports have appeared in the literature describing patients with clinical features that closely resemble Bartter's syndrome. Walker and Firminger reported on two siblings with growth retardation, hypokalemic metabolic alkalosis, and renal sodium and potassium wasting, but both had evidence of renal insufficiency.[535] The renal biopsy revealed immaturity and dysplasia of both the glomeruli and tubules, an abnormality that has been described in Bartter's syndrome, but of less severitiy.[94,535] Potter et al. described two brothers with hypokalemia, hyperreninemia, hyperaldosteronism, and excessive renal sodium and potassium excretion in whom the histologic examination revealed interstitial fibrosis, but no evidence of juxtaglomerular cell hyperplasia.[421] Recently, Bergstein and Weinberger reported on three children with hypokalemia, renal potassium wasting, normotension, and hyperreninemia, but persistently low aldosterone levels despite correction of the serum potassium.[46]

LIDDLE'S SYNDROME. Liddle et al. described in two siblings the clinical findings of hypertension, hypokalemic metabolic alkalosis, abnormal sodium retention, and excessive potassium excretion that strongly suggested the diagnosis of primary aldosteronism.[325] Surprisingly, the excretion rate of aldosterone was markedly low, and inhibition of aldosterone biosynthesis or action did not affect the excretion of sodium or potassium. Subsequent studies in additional family members revealed a similar defect in renal transport properties. Gardner et al. demonstrated altered sodium transport in erythrocytes and proposed that a generalized abnormality of membrane ion transport was present in this disorder.[200] Interestingly, treatment with triamterene, a drug that interferes with distal tubular ion transport independently of aldosterone inhibition, resulted in a natriuresis and decreased potassium excretion.[188,324,370] When combined with a low-salt diet, the blood pressure and electrolytes are restored to normal and remain normal with long-term treatment.

Hypomagnesemia

Magnesium is the second most abundant intracellular cation and the fourth most abundant total body cation. (See Chap. 33.) It serves as a cofactor or coenzyme in over 300 biochemical and physiological reactions, most of which involve the generation of energy and the alteration of membrane properties. Magnesium's importance to the Na^+-K^+ATP-ase pump cannot be overemphasized. This pump ensures constancy of the transcellular electrical gradient by facilitating the active transport of sodium out of and potassium into the cell. Approximately 60 percent of total body magnesium is stored in bone, 35 percent in muscle, and only 1 percent in the extracellular fluid compartment. While many forces are known to influence the internal balance of magnesium, the regulation of its serum level under normal and various pathologic circumstances is currently not well understood. Hence magnesium levels have been notoriously unreliable in predicting the adequacy of total body stores. Normomagnesemia may occasionally occur in both animals and humans despite severe muscle magnesium depletion, and conversely, hypomagnesemia may occur in the setting of normal muscle magnesium stores.[119,453,543,544]

The association of hypokalemia with hypomagnesemia has been well documented.[489a] Cotlove demonstrated that hypokalemia resisted correction in this setting until adequate magnesium replacement was given.[119] Urinary potassium and phosphate wasting are usual concomitants of magnesium depletion.[543] Indeed potassium conservation is impaired despite severe depletion of its body stores.[453] In 1969, Shils induced nutritional magnesium deficiency by restricting nasogastric feeding to a magnesium-deficient diet in seven patients with resected carcinomas of the head and neck.[480] Six of the seven participants experienced refractory hypokalemia that normalized only after magnesium repletion. Whang reported a 42 percent prevalence of hypokalemia in the setting of hypomagnesemia in 106 hospitalized patients.[545,546] Boyd subsequently confirmed that a statistically significant relationship existed between hypokalemia and hypomagnesemia in a study of 421 hospitalized patients.[75] In both studies, the hypokalemia could be corrected only after appropriate magnesium repletion. The surgical, critical care, psychiatric, and cardiological literature have all documented the increased incidence of refractory hypokalemia in the setting of hypomagnesemia.[8,241b,439a,449,541]

Hypokalemia from magnesium depletion is most likely a result of disruption of the Na^+-K^+ATP-ase pump. Bonting demonstrated that magnesium depletion induced a conformational change in the pump, rendering it unable to initiate cellular potassium uptake or sodium removal.[73] Intracellular sodium increases in this setting resulting in cellular swelling and dysfunction. Any tendency for serum potassium concentration to increase because its cellular uptake is impaired is offset by the concomitant kaliuresis. Hypomagnesemia can also alter potassium homeostasis by inducing structural changes in the cell membrane, especially in key phospholipids. Schilling demonstrated that changes in the serum magnesium concentration can alter the surface electrical potential in ascites tumor cells with subsequent loss in cellular potassium.[462]

The most serious consequence of combined hypomagnesemia and hypokalemia is heightened cardiac irritability. Many cardiology, critical care, and surgical studies have documented a higher incidence of malignant arrhythmias and mortality when hypokalemia is associated with hypomagnesemia.[4,8,154,241b] In addition, intracellular magnesium depletion lessens the force of contraction of cardiac muscle by impeding myofibrillar ATP-ase activity, which subsequently impairs the crossbridging between actin and myosin.[488] Also, the kidney may be unable to reclaim potassium in the setting of hypomagnesemia because of disruption of the Na^+-K^+ ATP-ase pump on the proximal tubule border.

In the setting of its severe depletion, the kidney will avidly reclaim magnesium. The typical western diet provides approximately 300 mg of magnesium per day, of which only one-third, or approximately 100 mg, is absorbed, predominantly in the small intestine. The kidney filters approximately 2500 mg of magnesium per day, and reclaims approximately 95 percent of the filtered load. Hence, homeostasis is well maintained by the excretion of 100 to 125 mg of magnesium per day in the urine. In the setting of normal renal function and adequate nutritional intake, a 24-h urinary magnesium collection of less than 25 mg indicates magnesium depletion even in the setting of normomagnesemia. Dyckner and Wester have formulated and utilized the *magnesium retention test* to evaluate magnesium balance.[152] The test requires intravenous loading with magnesium followed by a 24-h urinary collection. Magnesium-deficient individuals will excrete less than 75 percent of the load, assuming normal overall renal function and no tubular defects (see Chap. 33).

Loop diuretics are perhaps the most common iatrogenic cause of refractory hypokalemia in the setting of hypomagnesemia.[139,153,454] Magnesium reabsorption occurs principally in the thick ascending limb of Henle's loop and is inhibited by loop diuretics. Abusers of *alcohol* lose magnesium from gastrointestinal malabsorption or poor nutrition. In addition, acute and chronic alcohol usage increases the filtered load of magnesium, resulting in increased urinary losses. Alcohol also induces an osmotic diuresis and therefore increases urinary loss of both potassium and magnesium.[351] *Osmotic diuresis* is also postulated to be the major mechanism responsible for excessive urinary potassium and magnesium losses observed in diabetic ketoacidosis. Primary *aldosteronism* causes renal magnesium and potassium wastage,[533] and conversely, hypomagnesemia has been reported to cause hyperaldosteronism with resultant hypokalemia. Magnesium is absorbed in the small intestine under the influence of vitamin D in a pattern similar to that of calcium. Hence renal failure or any condition associated with *vitamin D deficiency* can precipitate hypomagnesemia and subsequently, hypokalemia. Other frequent causes of hypokalemia seen in the setting of hypomagnesemia include hypercalcemia,[107] cardiac glycosides,[347] gentamicin,[26] cisplatinum,[463] amphotericin B, chronic interstitial nephritis, the recovery phase of acute tubular necrosis and postobstructive nephropathy, postrenal transplantation, and chronic glomerulonephritis. Tubular dysfunction has also been implicated as a cause of concurrent hypokalemia and hypomagnesemia. Two patterns of tubular dysfunction have been described: (1) an inability to reabsorb both potassium and magnesium, and (2) an inability to reabsorb only magnesium. Gitelman, Graham, and Welt first described three patients who manifested hypokalemic metabolic alkalosis, chronic dermatitis, and excessive renal potassium and magnesium excretion associated with significant hypomagnesemia.[218] Since neither potassium nor magnesium alone corrected the excessive renal losses of these cations, the authors concluded that a familial tubular transport defect was responsible. Subsequent reports have identified familial hypokalemia and hypomagnesemia in children with associated abnormal calcium excretion[493] and an impaired concentrating capacity.[352] Recently, Gullner and associates reported three siblings with familial hypokalemic metabolic alkalosis associated with only magnesium depletion and tubulopathy.[237] They demonstrated a decrease in urinary and fecal potassium excretion and correction of serum potassium after oral magnesium supplementation. Stein and Cushner in independent studies have also demonstrated the association of hypokalemia and hypomagnesemia in *Bartter's syndome*.[126,496] The normal renal response to severe magnesium depletion entails avid reclamation of filtered magnesium with little or no magnesium being detectable in the urine. Significant quantities of magnesium have been measured in the urine of patients with Bartter's syndrome even in the setting of severe magnesium deficiency, implying ongoing tubular dysfunction and magnesuria. Syndrome of inappropriate antidiuretic hormone secretion (SIADH) can cause hypomagnesemia and hypokalemia by decreasing reabsorption secondary to plasma volume expansion.

Because the serum magnesium concentration is not always a reliable index of body magnesium stores, physicians should be aware that hypophosphatemia, hypocalcemia, and hyponatremia are also caused by magnesium depletion and therefore serve as "footprints" of reduced tissue stores of the divalent cation.[545] Magnesium serves as an integral cofactor for parathyroid hormone (PTH) secretion. Acute hypomagnesemia, like acute and chronic hypocalcemia, stimulates PTH secretion. Increased serum PTH levels increase urinary phosphate excretion, causing subsequent hypophosphatemia. As magnesium depletion becomes more chronic, PTH secretion becomes inhibited and hypoparathyroidism develops. The latter impairs calcium absorption causing a calciuresis and hypocalcemia. Interestingly, hyponatremia has been observed in as many as 25 percent of hospitalized patients with hypomagnesemia.[545] The etiology of this association has never been elucidated, and it is not known if this relationship represents true pathology or just an epiphenomenon.

The treatment of hypokalemia as well as hypocalcemia in the setting of hypomagnesemia requires that the latter be corrected first. The urgency and route of magnesium administration depend in large part on the clinical condition of the patient and on the presence or absence of possible ongoing magnesium losses. In the setting of delirium tremens, magnesium should be given intravenously in doses as large as 1 g every 2 to 4 h until clinical improvement is seen (see Chap. 33). In the setting of a cardiac arrhythmia or severe neurologic dysfunction, magnesium can be given as rapidly as 16 to 32 meq in 5 percent dextrose over 10 to 15 min. Ongoing gastrointestinal or renal losses usually require intravenous supplementation as well.

Hypercalcemia

Hypokalemia associated with hypercalcemia has been mentioned sporadically in the literature since 1961[20,173,456,572] (see Chap. 31). Adlinger and Samaan identified hypokalemia in 33 of 103 patients with hypercalcemia.[7] A higher prevalence was found in patients with hypercalcemia associated with malignant disease, 52.3 percent, than in those with primary hyperparathyroidism, 16.9 percent. In addition, the degree and frequency of hypokalemia were greatest at the higher serum calcium levels. Bradley and Sterling reported two cases of tuberculosis complicated by hypokalemia and hypercalcemia.[77] The hypokalemia associated with hypercalcemia is probably due to excessive renal potassium excretion.[77] In animals, several studies have shown increased renal potassium losses associated with elevated serum calcium levels.[172,260] Potassium levels must be measured immediately and monitored continuously during vigorous diuretic treatment of severe hypercalcemia to prevent the development of hypokalemia.

Diabetic ketoacidosis

Diabetic ketoacidosis is a well-known cause of hypokalemia with total body potassium depletion[42] (see Chap. 26). Eskilden and Nerup reported on 24 episodes of diabetic ketoacidosis of which seven episodes, on presentation, were associated with hypokalemia.[168] The potassium depletion is secondary to the kaliuresis caused by the combined osmotic effects of glycosuria and the enhanced excretion of poorly reabsorbed ketoacid anions. Although total body potassium stores are almost always depleted, other associated forces influencing transcellular distribution may prevent the emergence of hypokalemia; indeed, they may occasionally cause hyperkalemia. Azotemia, acidemia, and deficiencies of insulin, catecholamines, and aldosterone all may sustain normo- or hyperkalemia despite depleted stores. Potassium supplementation may be initiated soon after insulin and fluid replacement to prevent sudden dangerous falls in serum potassium levels.[489] Padilla and Loeb reported that hypokalemia during therapy is less frequent during low-dose continuous infusion insulin treatment than during high-dose insulin regimens.[404] The magnitude of total body deficits is usually in the range of 200 to 400 meq but may exceed 600 meq.[42] The greatest fall in serum potassium occurs during the first hour of therapy and warrants careful monitoring of serum potassium levels and electrocardiographic status.

Leukemia

A number of years ago, the association between lysozymuria, hypokalemia, and excessive urinary potassium loss seen in patients with acute myeloid leukemia suggested a causal relationship.[375,402] Further studies have demonstrated that hypokalemia complicates a number of other hematologic malignancies including chronic myelogenous leukemia,[169] chronic lymphocytic leukemia,[438] and acute myeloid leukemia.[312,318] Lysozymuria, however, is not a uniform finding in hypokalemic patients with acute leukemia.[358,359,414,423] Perry et al. observed urinary potassium wastage in patients with acute myelogenous leukemia but could not correlate it with lysozymuria.[413] Other factors that may contribute to the low serum potassium concentration in these patients include vomiting, diarrhea, antibiotic therapy, corticosteroids, hypercalcemia, starvation, blast crisis, and Fanconi's syndrome.[383,438]

EXCESSIVE GASTROINTESTINAL LOSSES

Vomiting and gastric lavage

Vomiting and chronic gastric lavage are common causes of hypokalemia. The concentration of potassium in upper gastrointestinal secretions rarely exceeds 10 meq/liter, indicating that gastric losses of potassium only partially explain the hypokalemia. More important is the associated metabolic alkalosis[208,281] that results in an increase in urinary potassium excretion. The renal mechanism for potassium conservation is sluggish during states of gastrointestinal potassium loss, resulting in a large potassium deficit over the first 2 to 3 days.[342] Transcellular shifts of potassium under these circumstances may also contribute to the decrease in serum potassium concentration.[87] Treatment requires appropriate correction of both the hypokalemia and the hypochloremic metabolic alkalosis with adequate amounts of potassium, sodium chloride, and fluid.

Intestinal losses (see also Chaps. 17 and 35)

The concentration of potassium in lower gastrointestinal secretions approaches 90 meq/liter. The daily excretion of potassium in the stool, on the other hand, in only 5 to 15 meq. As stool water increases in diarrheal states, sodium loss will increase proportionately whereas the change in potassium excretion is less marked.[181]

Diarrhea, due to a multitude of etiologies, can be associated with excessive stool potassium losses and hypokalemia. Classically, profound potassium depletion is seen in patients with diarrhea secondary to colonic villous adenomas, which secrete a profuse amount of watery, potassium-rich mucus.[465] The Zollinger-Ellison syndrome, with the associated intermittent diarrhea, can present with relentless hypokalemia which is corrected by cimetidine and oral potassium supplementation.[102] The Verner-Morrison syndrome, pancreatic cholera, is associated with watery diarrhea, hypochlorhydria, and hypokalemia. Stool potassium losses of 300 meq/day or more can be seen.[267] Vasoactive intestinal polypeptide (VIP), produced by pancreatic islet cell tumors, is thought to be responsible for the manifestations of this syndrome. Ganglioneuromas and oat cell lung carcinomas are capable of producing a similar syndrome with elevated VIP levels.[525] Recently, a patient with a cystadenocarcinoma of the pancreas was described as having hypokalemia and hypoproteinemia secondary to excessive tumor production of mucus that had very high concentrations of potassium and protein.[310]

Jejunoileal bypass, a treatment for morbid obesity, has been associated with numerous metabolic complications including hypokalemia. Campbell et al. identified hypokalemia in 30 of 75 patients with a jejunoileal bypass.[91] The hypokalemia may be difficult to treat unless therapy is also directed toward the coexisting hypomagnesemia.[259]

Laxative and enema abuse are not uncommon causes of diarrhea and hypokalemia.[33,268] In addition, the laxative abuser may ingest excessive amounts of diuretics.[232] Recently, several reports have described severe hypokalemia associated with the chronic use of enemas for "recreational purposes"[486] or as a "natural" form of treatment for cancer.[163] In addition, Forman et al. described a case of severe hypokalemia developing in a child after the use of hypertonic phosphate enemas.[182]

Other causes of diarrhea and hypokalemia include infectious diarrhea,[129,430] malabsorption syndromes,[229] bile, salivary and pancreatic fistulas,[539] appendicovesical fistula,[382] and congenital chloride diarrhea.[255]

EXCESSIVE INTEGUMENTARY LOSSES

Exocrine (sweat) gland secretions have low-sodium but high-potassium concentrations. During heat stress and extreme exercise, several liters of sweat may be produced resulting in potassium depletion and secondary hyperaldosteronism from excessive fluid losses, with concomitant urinary potassium loss.[224]

EVALUATION AND TREATMENT

There are innumerable approaches that can be taken when evaluating a patient with a hypokalemic disorder[385] (Fig. 22-6). The first step is to ensure that a true decrease in the serum potassium concentration exists. The lower limit of normal for potassium in the *serum* is 3.5 meq/liter, but the *plasma* potassium concentration is probably somewhat lower as shown by Kaplan's evaluation of 200 normal medical students and blood donors whose plasma potassium concentrations ranged between 3.0 and 4.8 meq/liter.[277] This is important because many clinical laboratories utilize autoanalyzer systems that measure plasma levels. A thorough understanding of these differences should eliminate laboratory error as a possible etiology of a patient's hypokalemic state.

The next step is to exclude the transcellular redistribution of potassium secondary to alkalosis, insulin excess, periodic paralysis, sympathomimetic agents, barium poisoning, or vitamin B-12 therapy (Fig. 22-5). These disorders are usually associated with a normal total body potassium content as opposed to the remainder of the possible etiologies that are accompanied by total body potassium depletion.

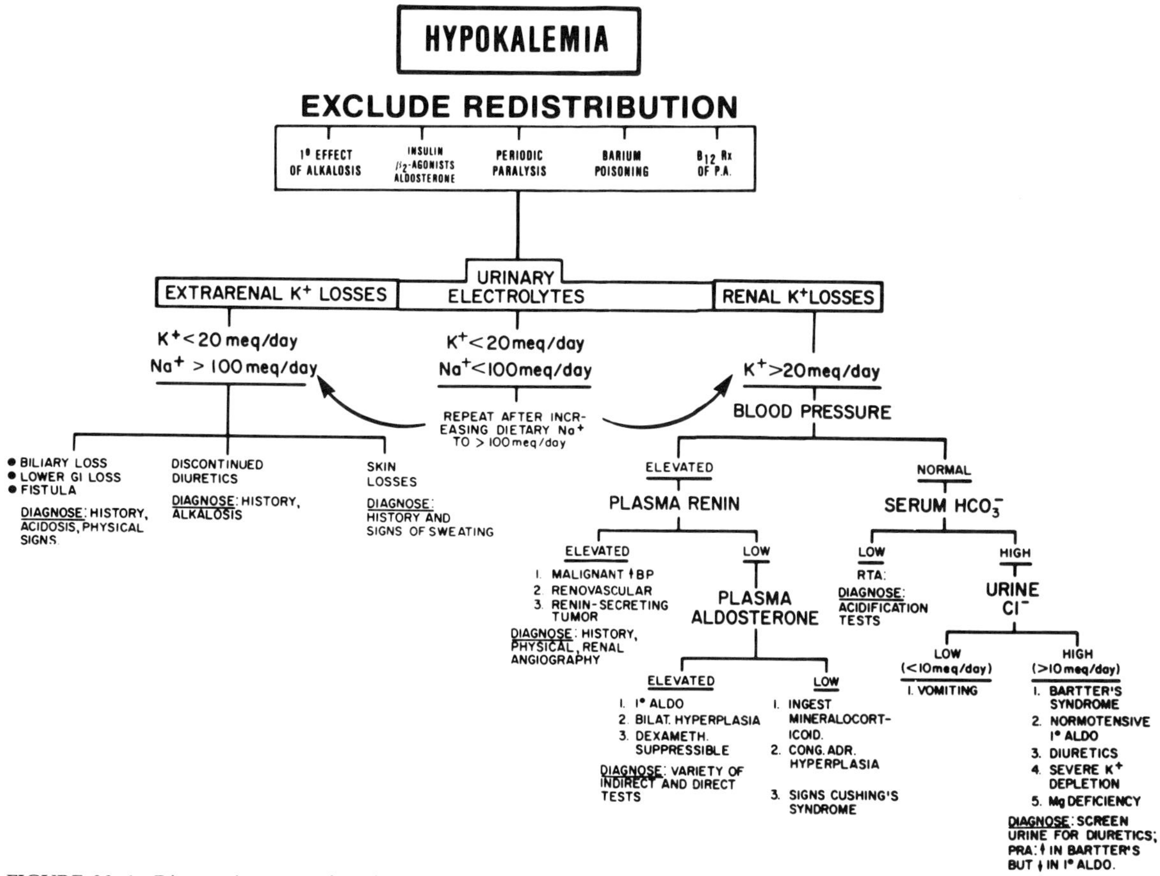

FIGURE 22-6 • Diagnostic approach to hypokalemia: See text for details. (From Narins RG et al: Diagnostic strategies in disorders of fluid, electrolyte and acid-base homeostasis. *Am J Med*, 72:496, 1982.[385])

A careful history and physical examination followed by a few routine laboratory evaluations will successfully identify the etiology in the majority of potassium-depleted patients. The urinary potassium concentration is quite helpful at this juncture for differentiating between renal and extrarenal causes of potassium loss. If the urinary sodium concentration is above 100 meq/day and the urinary potassium concentration is less than 20 meq/day, then extrarenal losses via the gastrointestinal tract or the skin as outlined in the text are the most likely etiologies. Polyuric patients may lose substantial amounts of potassium in the urine even at concentrations well below 20 meq/liter. A 24-h urine sample is preferable in the evaluation of chronic hypokalemia. Gastrointestinal losses of potassium secondary to lower intestinal disorders such as malabsorption, diarrheal states, and fistulas will be accompanied by metabolic acidosis as opposed to the metabolic alkalosis seen with chronic vomiting or gastric lavage. The integumentary system can be implicated through a history or physical signs of excessive sweating.

In contrast, a urinary potassium concentration of greater than 20 meq/day associated with hypokalemia of several days duration strongly suggests excessive renal potassium excretion. The level of blood pressure is helpful at this point in identifying the underlying cause. Hypertension and a high plasma renin activity suggests malignant hypertension, renovascular hypertension, or a renin-secreting tumor and should be further evaluated by a thorough examination of the optic fundus for evidence of retinal hemorrhage followed by the appropriate use of renal sonography, renal isotopic flow scans, computerized axial tomography, and renal angiography.

Hypertension and a low plasma renin activity should be evaluated by an appropriately collected plasma aldosterone level. A high aldosterone level should be further examined to differentiate between the various types of primary hyperaldosteronism while a low aldosterone level may be secondary to ingestion of exogenous "mineralocorticoids," congenital adrenal hyperplasia, or Cushing's syndrome.

The patient with a normal blood pressure should next have a serum bicarbonate determination. A low bicarbonate concentration suggests renal tubular acidosis and appropriate acidification testing will aid in the subclassification (see Chap. 27). The patient with a high serum bicarbonate concentration is best evaluated by testing the urine chloride concentration. A low-urine chloride, less than 10 meq/day, implies that vomiting or excessive gastric lavage has occurred, while a level greater than 10 meq/day is suggestive of Bartter's syndrome, normotensive primary hyperaldosteronism, diuretic ingestion, or severe potassium depletion. In addition, excessive renal potassium losses may be secondary to hypomagnesemia or the effects of several different antibiotics and chemotherapeutic agents, so appropriate tests are indicated under these circumstances.

TREATMENT OF POTASSIUM DEPLETION

The immediate objective of potassium replacement is to prevent life-threatening cardiac complications and the ultimate objective is to replenish total body potassium stores. The rapidity and magnitude of potassium repletion will depend on the estimation of potassium depletion which, as already discussed, is difficult since the serum potassium is a crude indicator of total body stores and can be markedly affected by changes in acid-base and other factors. Although Scribner's early study estimates that the total body deficit in a 70-kg human is approximately 100 to 200 meq when serum potassium falls from 4 to 3 meq/liter,[471] more recent studies suggest that this fall is associated with a 200 to 400 meq total body deficit.[303,304] This appears to be a nonlinear function and as serum potassium continues to fall by 1 meq/liter, the total body deficits increase by 200 to 400 meq.[471]

Transcellular shifts of potassium may further complicate the estimation of a given potassium deficit. In hypokalemic patients with renal tubular acidosis or diarrhea, the serum potassium concentration may underestimate potassium losses. Initiation of bicarbonate therapy may precipitously lower serum potassium concentration by enhancing cellular potassium uptake. In diabetic ketoacidosis, despite substantial depletion of body stores, the decrease in plasma concentration may be minimal because both hyperglycemia and insulinopenia impair cellular potassium uptake.[42] Initiation of therapy with saline and insulin may rapidly lower serum potassium levels by promoting urinary losses and cellular uptake of potassium.

MANAGEMENT OF SEVERE HYPOKALEMIA

Severe hypokalemia (<2.5 meq/liter) can be life-threatening and warrants rapid correction to a safe level, that is, approximating 3.0 to 3.5 meq/liter. Oral replacement is often not feasible in critically ill patients with severe hypokalemia, and large doses of oral supplements are poorly tolerated. If the accuracy of a serum potassium value is in doubt, an ECG should be obtained while a repeat measurement is awaited.

Intravenous potassium administration entails the risk of hyperkalemia and hence should be undertaken with caution. In adults 40 meq of potassium chloride in 1 liter of isotonic or hypotonic saline administered over 1 h is generally considered to be safe. Even if the majority of the infused potassium is transiently retained in the 10 to 15 liters of ECF, the plasma potassium concentration would only increase by approximately 3.0 meq/liter. Severely hypokalemic patients are usually hypovolemic and therefore can usually tolerate the infusion of a large volume of fluid. Often, however, more concentrated solutions are required in patients with compromised cardiac function, hypertensives, and anuric patients. Kruse et al. examined the effect of 20 meq of potassium chloride in 100 ml saline administered over 1 h.[307] An average increment in serum potassium concentration of 0.25 meq/liter was noted. Although in a few instances serum potassium levels rose above 5.0 meq/liter, no life-threatening arrhythmias were encountered. Most importantly, these investigators observed no complications from the administration of potassium chloride through a central venous route. When large amounts of potassium are infused, serum levels must be checked at 30- to 60-min intervals and cardiac rhythm must be continuously monitored. Patients with elevated serum creatinine levels are more likely to become hyperkalemic with a potassium infusion. In patients with hypophosphatemia, part of the infusate can be administered as neutral potassium phosphate. Serum phosphorus and calcium should be closely monitored during potassium phosphate infusion.

MANAGEMENT OF MILD HYPOKALEMIA

Potassium chloride administered in liquid or tablet form is preferred in the majority of hypokalemic states. Diuretic therapy and vomiting are associated with concomitant chloride losses, and chloride salts must be the therapy of choice. Administration of gluconate, phosphate, citrate, or bicarbonate salts would not adequately replete potassium stores. The gluconate and citrate are metabolized to bicarbonate. The filtered bicarbonate and phosphate are not well reabsorbed, and therefore obligate potassium secretion in the distal nephron. Since fruits contain potassium as organic salts, they function as poor sources of potassium for patients receiving diuretics.[295] In the maintenance therapy of hypokalemia associated with distal renal tubular acidosis, potassium bicarbonate can be used for replacement therapy.

The need for routine correction of diuretic-induced hypokalemia is debated. Effort must be made to prevent hypokalemia by using the smallest effective dose of diuretic. Hydrochlorothiazide at doses of 12.5 to 25 mg/day infrequently causes hypokalemia but may still elicit a hypotensive effect. Sodium restriction and concurrent administration of a potassium-sparing diuretic or an angiotensin-converting enzyme inhibitor further limit potassium losses.[300,301] If hypokalemia persists, potassium chloride should be administered to maintain serum K^+ above 3.5 meq/liter. Caution must be exercised in prescribing potassium supplements or potassium-sparing diuretics to patients with compromised renal function.[301]

REFERENCES

1. Abbrecht PH: Effects of potassium deficiency on renal function in the dog. *J Clin Invest* 48:432, 1969.
2. Abbrecht PH, Vander A: Effects of chronic potassium deficiency on plasma renin activity. *J Clin Invest* 49:1510, 1970.
3. Abbrecht PH: Cardiovascular effects of chronic potassium deficiency in dog. *Am J Physiol* 223:555, 1972.
4. Abstracts of the Fifth International Magnesium Symposium, Kyoto, Japan, 1988.
5. Adler S: An extrarenal action of aldosterone on mammalian skeletal muscle. *Am J Physiol* 218:616, 1970.
6. Adler S et al: Intracellular acid-base regulation: I. The response of muscle cells to changes in CO_2 tension or extracellular bicarbonate concentration. *J Clin Invest* 44:8, 1965.
7. Adlinger KA, Samaan NA: Hypokalemia with hypercalcemia. *Ann Intern Med* 84:511, 1977.
8. Aglio LS et al: Hypomagnesemia is common following cardiac surgery. *J Cardiovasc Anesth* 5:201, 1991.
9. Alexander EA, Levinsky NG: An extrarenal mechanism of potassium adaptation. *J Clin Invest* 47:740, 1968.
10. Anderson DK et al: Effect of hypokalemia and hypomagnesemia produced by hemodialysis on skeletal muscle vascular resistance: Role of potassium in active hyperemia. *Circ Res* 31:165, 1972.
11. Anderson EC: Organic scintillation detectors and their use in the study of body composition, in *Body Composition in Animals and Man*. Washington DC, National Academy of Science, 1968, p 266.
12. Anderson J et al: A comparison of the effects of hydrochlorothiazide and of furosemide in the treatment of hypertensive patients. *Q J Med* 40:541, 1971.
13. Anderson RJ et al: Evidence for an *in vivo* antagonism between vasopressin and prostaglandin in the mammalian kidney. *J Clin Invest* 56:420, 1975.
14. Andersson OK et al: Metabolic adverse effect of thiazide diuretics: The importance of normokalemia. *J Intern Med* 229(suppl 2): 89, 1991.
15. Andreol SP et al: Nafcillin, pseudoproteinuria and hypokalemic alkalosis. *J Pediatr* 97:841, 1980.
16. Arant BS et al: Case studies of siblings with juxtaglomerular hyperplasia and secondary aldosteronism associated with severe azotemia and renal rickets—Bartter's syndrome or disease? *Pediatrics* 46:344, 1970.
17. Astrup J: The effect of hypokalemia and of digoxin therapy on red cell sodium and potassium content. *Scand J Clin Lab Invest* 33:11, 1974.
18. Azar ST, Melby JC: 19-Nor-deoxycorticosterone production from aldosterone producing adenomas. *Hypertension* 19:362, 1992.
19. Azer PC, Braunstein GP: Malignant leydig cell tumor. *Cancer* 47:1251, 1981.
20. Azzopardi JG, Whittaker RS: Bronchial carcinoma and hypercalcemia. *J Clin Pathol* 22:718, 1969.
21. Azzopardi JG, Williams ED: Pathology of non-endocrine tumors associated with Cushing's syndrome. *Cancer* 22:274, 1968.
22. Baer L et al: Pseudoprimary aldosteronism. *Circ Res* 26/27(suppl): I-203, 1970.
23. Baertl JM et al: Relation of acute potassium depletion to renal ammonium metabolism in patients with cirrhosis. *J Clin Invest* 42:696, 1963.
24. Bahler RC, Rakita L: Cardiovascular function in potassium-depleted dogs. *Am Heart J* 81:650, 1971.

25. Bank N, Anjedjian HS: A micropuncture study of the renal concentrating defect in potassium depletion. *Am J Physiol* 206:1347, 1964.
26. Bar RS et al: Hypomagnesemic hypocalcemia secondary to renal magnesium wasting: A possible consequence of high-dose gentamicin therapy. *Ann Intern Med* 82:646, 1975.
27. Barraclough MA: Sodium and water depletion with malignant hypertension. *Am J Med* 40:265, 1966.
28. Bartter FC: The syndrome of juxtaglomerular hyperplasia with aldosteronism, hypokalemic alkalosis and normal blood pressure. *Birth Defects* 10:104, 1974.
29. Bartter FC et al: The adrenal cortex and the kidney. *Kidney Int* 6:272, 1974.
30. Bartter FC: On the pathogenesis of Bartter's syndrome. *Miner Electrolyte Metab* 3:61, 1980.
31. Bartter FC et al: Hyperplasia of the juxtaglomerular complex with hyperaldosteronism and hypokalemic alkalosis. *Am J Med* 33:811, 1962.
32. Baruch D et al: Diagnosis and treatment of renin-secreting tumors. Report of three cases. *Hypertension* 6:760, 1984.
33. Basser LS: Purgatives and periodic paralysis. *Med J Aust* 1:47, 1979.
34. Batlle DC: Hyperkalemic, hyperchloremic metabolic acidosis associated with selective aldosterone deficiency and distal renal tubular acidosis. *Semin Nephrol* 1:260, 1981.
35. Batlle DC, Kurtzman NA: Distal renal tubular acidosis: Pathogenesis and classification. *Am J Kidney Dis* 1:328, 1982.
36. Batlle DC et al: Clinical and pathophysiologic spectrum of acquired distal renal tubular acidosis. *Kidney Int* 20:389, 1981.
37. Bauer JH et al: Effect of potassium chloride on plasma renin activity and plasma aldosterone during sodium restriction in normal men. *Kidney Int* 15:286, 1979.
38. Baxter JD et al: Aldosterone receptors and the evaluation of plasma mineralocorticoid activity in normal and hypertensive states. *J Clin Invest* 58:579, 1976.
39. Beck N, Davis BB: Impaired renal response to parathyroid hormone in potassium depletion. *Am J Physiol 228:179, 1975.*
40. Beck N, Shaw JO: Thromboxane B_2 and prostaglandin E_2 in the potassium depleted rat kidney. *Am J Physiol* 240:F151, 1981.
41. Beck OA, Hochrein H: Serum kaliumspiegel and herzrhythmmsstorungem beim akuten myokardinfarkt. *Z Kardiol* 66:187, 1977.
42. Beigelman PM: Potassium in severe diabetic ketoacidosis. *Am J Med* 54:419, 1973.
43. Benedetti RG et al: Effect of potassium deletion on two-kidney, one-clip renal vascular hypertension in the rat. *Kidney Int* 28:621, 1985.
44. Bennett CM et al: Micropuncture study of the proximal and distal tubule in the dog. *Am J Physiol* 213:1254, 1967.
45. Bennett RH, Forman HR: Hypokalemic periodic paralysis in chronic toluene exposure. *Arch Neurol* 37:673, 1980.
46. Bergstein JM, Weinberger MH: Hypokalemia, normal blood pressure and hyperreninemia with hypoaldosteronism. *J Pediatr* 99:561, 1981.
47. Bergström J: Muscle electrolytes in man. *Scand J Clin Lab Invest* 14:(suppl):1, 1962.
48. Bergström J, Hultman E: The effect of thiazides, chlorthalidone and furosemide on muscle electrolytes and muscle glycogen in normal subjects. *Acta Med Scand* 180:363, 1966.
49. Berl T: Water metabolism in potassium depletion. *Miner Electrolyte Metab* 4:209, 1980.
50. Berl T et al: Renal concentrating defect in the hypokalemic rat is prostaglandin independent. *Am J Physiol* 238:37, 1980.
51. Berl T et al: On the mechanism of polyuria in potassium depletion. *J Clin Invest* 60:620, 1977.
52. Beskind H, Mudge GH: Effect of potassium deficiency on renal tubular reabsorption and assimilation of glucose. *Johns Hopkins Med J* 104:252, 1959.
53. Bia MJ, DeFronzo RA: Extrarenal potassium homeostasis. *Am J Physiol* 240:F257, 1981.
54. Bia MJ et al: Chronic adrenal insufficiency causes impaired extrarenal potassium (K) tolerance. *Clin Res* 28:438A, 1980.
55. Biamino G, Wessel HJ: Potassium induced relaxation of vascular smooth muscle: A possible mechanism of exercise hyperremia. *Pflugers Arch* 343:95, 1973.
56. Biava CG et al: Glomerular changes with glomerulodistotubular shunts in patients with Bartter's syndrome. *Lab Invest* 20:575, 1969.
57. Biglieri EG, McIlroy MB: Abnormalities of renal function and circulation reflexes in primary aldosteronism. *Circulation* 33:78, 1966.
58. Biglieri EG, Schambelan M: The significance of elevated levels of plasma 18-hydroxycorticosterone in patients with primary aldosteronism. *J Clin Endocrinol Metab* 49:87, 1979.
59. Biglieri EG et al: Plasma aldosterone concentration. Further characterization of aldosterone-producing adenomas. *Circ Res* 34/35(suppl I):183, 1974.
60. Biglieri EG et al: The intercurrent hypertension of primary aldosteronism. *Circ Res* 26/27(suppl I):195, 1970.
61. Biglieri EG et al: A preliminary evaluation for primary aldosteronism. *Arch Intern Med* 126:1004, 1970.
62. Bilbrey GL et al: Skeletal muscle resting membrane potential in potassium deficiency. *J Clin Invest* 52:3011, 1973.
63. Blachley JD, Hill JB: Renal and electrolyte disturbances associated with cisplatinum. *Ann Intern Med* 95:628, 1981.
64. Blachley JD, Knochel JP: Tobacco chewer's hypokalemia: Licorice revisited. *N Engl J Med* 302:784, 1980.
65. Blachley J et al: Impaired muscle glycogen synthesis and prevention of muscle glycogen supercompensation by potassium deficiency. *Clin Res* 22:517A, 1974.
66. Bland WH, Bassett SH: Potassium deficiency in man. *Metabolism* 2:218, 1953.
67. Blomberg LH, Lindquist T: Electrocardiogram in paroxysmal essential hypopotassemia (periodic paralysis): Report of two cases. *Acta Med Scand* 147:437, 1954.
68. Boddy K et al: The relation between potassium in body fluids and total body potassium in healthy and diabetic subjects. *Clin Sci* 50:455, 1976.
69. Boddy K, King PC: The relationship between total body potassium and exchangeable body potassium measured at 24 and 44 hours after administration of ^{43}K. *Eur J Clin Invest* 3:188, 1973.

70. Boddy K et al: Exchangeable and total body potassium in patients with chronic renal failure. *Br Med J* 1:140, 1972.
71. Boddy K et al: Measurements of total body potassium with a shadow shield whole-body counter. Calibration and errors. *Phys Med Biol* 16:275, 1971.
72. Bongiovanni AM, Root AW: The adrenogenital syndrome. *N Engl J Med* 268:1283; 1342; 1391, 1963.
73. Bonting SL: Magnesium-induced conformational changes in Na-K-ATPase. *Curr Top Membr Transplant* 19:403, 1983.
74. Bourke E, Delaney Y: Bartter's syndrome—a dilemma of cause and effect. *Nephron* 27:177, 1981.
75. Boyd JC et al: Frequency of hypomagnesemia in hypokalemic states. *Clin Chem* 29:178, 1983.
76. Brace RA: Time course and mechanisms of the acute effects of hypokalemia and hyperkalemia on vascular resistance. *Proc Soc Exp Biol Med* 145:1389, 1974.
77. Bradley GW, Sterling GM: Hypercalcemia and hypokalemia in tuberculosis. *Thorax* 33:464, 1978.
78. Brandis M et al: Potassium induced inhibition of proximal tubular reabsorption in rats. *Am J Physiol* 222:421, 1972.
79. Bravo EL et al: The changing clinical spectrum of primary aldosteronism. *Am J Med* 74:641, 1983.
80. Brody SJL et al: Controlled comparison of cimetidine and carbenoxolone sodium in gastric ulcer. *Br Med J* 1:1308, 1979.
81. Brown JJ et al: Hypertension and secondary hyperaldosteronism associated with a renin-secreting renal juxtaglomerular cell tumor. *Lancet* 2:1228, 1973.
82. Brunner FP, Frick PG: Hypokalemia, metabolic alkalosis and hypernatremia to "massive" sodium penicillin therapy. *Br Med J* 4:550, 1968.
83. Brunner HR et al: The influence of potassium administration and potassium deprivation on plasma renin in normal and hypertensive subjects. *J Clin Invest* 49:2128, 1970.
84. Brunner HR et al: Hypertension of renal origin: Evidence for two different mechanisms. *Science* 174:1344, 1971.
85. Brunner HR et al: Essential hypertension: Renin and aldosterone, heart attack and stroke. *N Engl J Med* 286:441, 1972.
86. Burch PRJ, Spiers FW: Measurements of the gamma radiation from the human body. *Nature* 172:519, 1953.
87. Burnell JM et al: The effect in humans of extracellular pH change on the relationship between serum potassium concentration and intracellular potassium. *J Clin Invest* 35:935, 1956.
88. Burnell JM et al: Metabolic acidosis accompanying potassium deprivation. *Am J Physiol* 227:329, 1974.
89. Buruma OJS et al: Heart muscle disease in familial hypokalemic period paralysis. *Acta Neurol Scand* 64:12, 1981.
90. Cabizuca SV, Desser KB: Carbenicillin-associated metabolic alkalosis. *JAMA* 236:956, 1976.
91. Campbell JM et al: Jejunoileal bypass as a treatment of morbid obesity. *Arch Intern Med* 137:602, 1977.
92. Campion DS et al: Rhabdomyolysis and myoglobinuria associated with hypokalemia of renal tubular acidosis. *JAMA* 220:967, 1972.
93. Cannon PJ et al: Relation between potassium balance and aldosterone secretion in normal subjects and in patients with hypertensive or renal tubular disease. *J Clin Invest* 45:865, 1966.
94. Cannon PJ et al: Juxtaglomerular hyperplasia and secondary hyperaldosteronism (Bartter's syndrome): A reevalua tion of the pathophysiology. *Medicine* 47:107, 1968.
95. Capasso G et al: Renal bicarbonate reabsorption in the rat. I: Effects of hypokalemia and carbonic anhydrase. *J Clin Invest* 78:1558, 1986.
96. Carlberger G et al: Severe malnutrition in a middle-aged man with anorexia nervosa. *Nutr Metab* 13:100, 1971.
97. Carney S et al: A study *in vitro* of the concentrating defect associated with hypokalemia and hypercalcemia. *Pflugers Arch* 366:11, 1976.
98. Carey RM et al: Idiopathic hypoaldosteronism. A possible role for aldosterone-stimulating factor. *N Engl J Med* 311:94, 1984.
99. Chan JLM: Bartter's syndrome. *Nephron* 26:155, 1980.
100. Cheng JT et al: Potassium wasting and other renal tubular defects with rifampin nephrotoxicity. *Am J Nephrol* 4:379, 1984.
101. Ching S et al: Renal ammoniagenesis and tissue glutamine, glutamine synthetase and glutaminase I levels in potassium-deficient rats. *J Lab Clin Med* 82:208, 1973.
102. Chisholm JL: Zollinger-Ellison syndrome: Intermittent diarrhea, relentless hypokalemia, and hypergastrinemia. *J Natl Med Assoc* 73:1151, 1981.
103. Chonko AM et al: The role of renin and aldosterone in the salt restriction of edema. *Am J Med* 63:881, 1977.
104. Chowdhury FR, Bleicher SJ: Chlorthalidone induced hypokalemia and abnormal carbohydrate metabolism. *Horm Metab Res* 2:13, 1970.
105. Christy NP, Laragh JH: Pathogenesis of hypokalemia alkalosis in Cushing's syndrome. *N Engl J Med* 265:1083, 1961.
106. Cividalli G, Nathan OG: Sodium and potassium concentration and transmembrane fluxes in leukocytes. *Blood* 43:861, 1974.
106a. Clore J et al: When is cortisol a mineralocorticoid? *Kidney Int* 42:1297, 1992.
107. Coburn JW et al: The effect of calcium infusion on renal handling of magnesium with normal and reduced glomerular filtration rate. *Nephron* 7:131, 1979.
108. Cohn SH, Dombrowski CS: Absolute measurement of whole body potassium by gamma ray spectrometry. *J Nucl Med* 11:230, 1970.
109. Conn HO: Cirrhosis and diabetes: IV. Effect of potassium chloride administration on glucose and insulin metabolism. *Am J Med* 259:394, 1970.
110. Conn JW: Hypertension, the potassium ion and impaired carbohydrate tolerance. *N Engl J Med* 273:1135, 1965.
111. Conn JW: Hypertension, the potassium ion and impaired carbohydrate tolerance. *N Engl J Med* 273:1135, 1965.
112. Conn JW: Presidential address: II. Primary aldosteronism, a new clinical syndrome. *J Lab Clin Med* 45:6, 1955.
113. Conn JW et al: Primary reninism. *Arch Intern Med* 130:682, 1972.
114. Conn JW et al: Intermittent aldosteronism in periodic paralysis: Dependence of attacks on retention of sodium and failure to induce attacks by restriction of dietary sodium. *Lancet* 1:802, 1957.
115. Conn JW et al: Licorice induced pseudoaldosteronism. *JAMA* 205:492, 1968.

116. Connor G et al: Juxtaglomerular cell tumor. *Nephron* 21:325, 1978.
117. Corrall RJM et al: Syndrome of inappropriate ADH secretion concealed by hypokalemia due to ectopic ACTH production. *Acta Endocrinol* 96:182, 1981.
118. Corsa L et al: Measurement of exchangeable potassium in man by isotope dilution. *J Clin Invest* 19:1280, 1950.
119. Cotlove E et al: Effects of electrolyte depletion and acid-base distribution on muscle cations. *Am J Physiol* 167:665, 1951.
120. Craig AB Jr, Mendell PL: Blockage of hyperkalemia and hyperglycemia induced by epinephrine in frog liver and in cats. *Am J Physiol* 197:52, 1959.
121. Crane J et al: Prescribed fenoterol and death from asthma in New Zealand 1981–1983: Case control study. *Lancet* 1:917, 1989.
122. Cremer W, Bock KD: Symptoms and course of chronic hypokalemic nephropathy in man. *Clin Nephrol* 7:112, 1977.
123. Creutzfeldt O et al: Muscle membrane potentials in episodic adynamia *Electroencephogr Clin Neurophysiol* 15:508, 1963.
124. Cronin RE et al: Natural history of aminoglycoside nephrotoxicity in the dog. *J Lab Clin Med* 95:463, 1980.
125. Cunningham RJ et al: Long-term use of propranolol, ibuprofren and spironolactone in the management of Bartter's syndrome. *Pediatrics* 63:754, 1979.
126. Cushner HM et al: Does magnesium play a role in the hypokalemia of Bartter's syndrome? *Am J Kidney Dis* 16:495, 1990.
127. Dahl T et al: Hypernephroma and hypertension. *Acta Med Scand* 209:121, 1981.
128. Dargie HJ et al: Total body potassium in long term furosemide therapy: Is potassium supplementation necessary? *Br Med J* 4:316, 1974.
129. DaSilva OA et al: Hypokalemic respiratory muscle paralysis following strongyloides stercoralis hyperinfection: A case report. *Am J Trop Med Hyg* 30:69, 1981.
130. Davidson C et al: Effect of long-term diuretic treatment on body potassium in heart disease. *Lancet* 2:1044, 1976.
131. Davidson S, Surawicz B: Ectopic beats and atrioventricular corduction disturbances in patients with hypopotassaemia. *Arch Intern Med* 120:280, 1967.
132. Davis BB et al: Hypomagnesemia following the diuresis of post-renal obstruction and renal transplant. *Nephron* 14:275, 1975.
133. Davis JO, Freeman RH: Mechanisms regulating renin release. *Physiol Rev* 56:1, 1976.
134. DeFronzo RA: Hyperkalemia and hyporennemic hypoaldosteronism. *Kidney Int* 17:118, 1980.
135. DeFronzo RA et al: Effect of insulinopenia and adrenal hormone deficiency on acute potassium tolerance. *Kidney Int* 7:586, 1980.
136. DeFronzo RA et al: Influence of basal insulin and glucagon secretion on potassium and sodium metabolism. *J Clin Invest* 61:472, 1978.
137. Delaney V et al: Bartter's syndrome physiologic and pharmacologic studies. *Q J Med* 50:213, 1981.
138. Deuxchaisnes CN et al: Exchangeable potassium in wasting, amyotrophy, heart disease and cirrhosis of the liver. *Lancet* 1:681, 1961.
139. Devane J et al: Dose-dependent reduction in renal magnesium clearance during a furosemide-induced diuresis in rats. *Br J Pharmacol* 80:421, 1983.
140. Dickerson JWT, Widdowson EM: Chemical changes in skeletal muscle during development. *Biochem J* 74:247, 1960.
141. Diengott D et al: Hypokalemia in barium poisoning. *Lancet* 2:343, 1964.
142. Dluhy RG et al: Serum immunoreactive insulin and growth hormone response to potassium infusion in normal man. *J Appl Physiol* 33:22, 1972.
143. Douglas JB, Healy JK: Nephrotoxic effects of amphotericin B, including renal tubular acidosis. *Am J Med* 46:154, 1969.
144. Drake TS et al: Postpartum hypokalemic paralysis. *Obst Gynecol* 54:379, 1979.
145. Drenick EJ et al: Magnesium depletion during prolonged fasting of obese males. *J Clin Endocrinol Metab* 29:1341, 1969.
146. Duarte CG: Effects of ethacrynic acid and furosemide on urinary calcium phosphate and magnesium. *Metabolism* 17:867, 1968.
147. Duke M: Thiazide-induced hypokalemia. Association with acute myocardial infarction and ventricular fibrillation. *JAMA* 239:43, 1978.
148. Dunn MJ: Prostaglandins and Barttter's syndrome. *Kidney Int* 19:86, 1981.
149. Dursing R et al: Renal biosynthesis of prostaglandin E_2 and $F_{2\alpha}$: Dependence of extracellular potassium. *J Lab Clin Med* 92:669, 1978.
150. Dursing R et al: The effect of potassium depletion on urinary prostaglandins in normal man, in Samuelson B et al (eds): *Advances in Prostaglandins and Thromboxane Research*. New York, Raven Press, 1980, p 1189.
151. Dyckner T et al: Initial serum potassium level in relation to early complications and prognosis in patients with acute myocardial infarction. *Acta Med Scand* 197:207, 1975.
152. Dyckner T et al: Magnesium deficiency: Guidelines for diagnosis and substitution therapy. *Acta Med Scand* 66:37, 1981.
153. Dyckner T et al: Intracellular magnesium loss after diuretic administration. *Drugs* 28(suppl 1):161, 1984.
154. Dyckner T et al: Potassium/magnesium depletion in patients with cardiovascular disease. *Am J Med* 82(suppl 3A):11, 1987.
155. Dyckner T, Wester PO: The relation between extra and intracellular electrolytes in patients with hypokalemia and/or diuretic treatment. *Acta Med Scand* 204:268, 1978.
156. Dyckner T, Wester PO: Ventricular extrasystoles and intracellular electrolytes before and after potassium and magnesium infusions in patients on diuretic treatment. *Am Heart J* 97:12, 1979.
157. Dyckner T, Wester PO: Ventricular extrasystoles and intracellular electrolytes in hypokalemic patients before and after correction of the hypokalemia. *Acta Med Scand* 204:375, 1978.
158. Eberlein WR, Bongiovanni AM: Plasma and urinary corticosteroids in hypertensive form of congenital adrenal hyperplasia. *J Biol Chem* 223:35, 1956.

159. Eddy RC, Sanches SA: Renin-secreting renal neoplasm and hypertension and hypokalemia. *Ann Intern Med* 75:725, 1971.
160. Edwards CRW et al: Localisation of 11β-hydroxysteroid-dehydrogenase-tissue specific protector of the mineralocorticoid receptor. *Lancet* 2:986, 1988.
161. Edwards R et al: Needle biopsy for muscle chemistry. *Lancet* 1:736, 1975.
162. Edwards R et al: Acute hypocapneic hypokalemia: An iatrogenic anesthetic complication. *Anesth Analg* 56:786, 1977.
163. Eisele JW, Reay DT: Deaths related to coffee enemas. *JAMA* 244:1608, 1980.
164. Elkinton JR, Danowski TS: *The Body Fluids*. Baltimore, Williams and Wilkins, 1955, p 183.
165. Elkinton JR, Huth EJ: Body fluid abnormalities in anorexia nervosa and undernutrition. *Metabolism* 8:376, 1959.
166. Engel AG, Lambert EH: Calcium activation of electrically inexcitable muscle fibers and primary hypokalemic periodic paralysis. *Neurology* 19:851, 1969.
167. Erkelens DW, Statius van Eps LW: Bartter's syndrome and erythrocytosis. *Am J Med* 55:711, 1973.
168. Eskilden PC, Nerup J: Low-dose insulin treatment of diabetic ketoacidosis. *Acta Med Scand* 202:295, 1977.
169. Evans JJ, Bozdech MJ: Hypokalemia in nonblastic chronic myelogenous leukemia. *Arch Intern Med* 141:786, 1981.
170. Fanconi A et al: Chronic hypokalemia with growth retardation, normotensive hyperrenin-hyperaldosteronism (Bartter's syndrome) and hypercalcuria. *Helv Paediatr Acta* 2:144, 1971.
171. Farese RV et al: Acute intermittent porphyria associated with inappropriate antidiuretic hormone secretion, hypokalemic alkalosis and secondary hyperaldosteronism. *South Med J* 72:1201, 1979.
172. Ferris TF et al: Renal potassium-wasting induced by vitamin D. *J Clin Invest* 41:1222, 1962.
173. Ferris TF et al: Renal tubular acidosis and renal potassium wasting acquired as a result of hypercalemic nephropathy. *N Engl J Med* 265:924, 1961.
174. Fichman MP et al: Role of prostaglandins in the pathogenesis of Bartter's syndrome. *Am J Med* 60:785, 1976.
175. Fichman MP et al: Diuretic-induced hyponatremia. *Ann Intern Med* 75:853, 1971.
176. Finn AT et al: Relation between toad bladder potassium content and permeability response to vasopressin. *Am J Physiol* 210:1279, 1966.
177. Fisch C: Relation of electrolyte disturbances to cardiac arrhythmias. *Circulation* 47:408, 1973.
178. Fischman CH, Oster JR: Toxic effects of toluene: A new cause of high anion gap in metabolic acidosis. *JAMA* 241:713, 1979.
179. Flear CTG et al: Variability in the water sodium, potassium and chloride content of human skeletal muscle. *J Clin Pathol* 18:74, 1965.
180. Forbes GB, Lewis AM: Total sodium, potassium and chloride in adult man. *J Clin Invest* 35:596, 1956.
181. Fordtran JS, Dietschy JM: Water and electrolyte movement in the intestine. *Gastroenterology* 50:263, 1966.
182. Forman J et al: Hypokalemia after hyptertonic phosphate enemas. *J Pediatr* 94:149, 1979.
183. Fourman P: Depletion of potassium induced in man with an exchange resin. *Clin Sci* 13:93, 1954.
184. Fourman P: An experimental study of oedema and potassium deficiency. *Clin Sci* 14:75, 1955.
185. Fraley DS, Adler S: Correction of hyperkalemia by bicarbonate despite constant blood pH. *Kidney Int* 12:354, 1977.
186. Fraley DS, Adler S: Isohydric regulation of plasma potassium by bicarbonate. *Kidney Int* 9:333, 1976.
187. France R: Intracellular granules of the renal medulla in potassium depletion. *Trans Am Clin Climatol Assoc* 74:211, 1962.
188. Frazier HS, Yager H: Drug therapy. The clinical use of diuretics. *N Engl J Med* 288:246, 1973.
189. Frazier HS, Yager H: The clinical use of diuretics. *N Engl J Med* 288:455, 1973.
190. Friedman IM et al: The depressor effect of potassium deprivation on the blood pressure of hypertensive rats. *Am J Physiol* 167:457, 1951.
191. Fujina T et al: The pathogenesis of Bartter's syndrome. Functional and histologic studies. *Am J Med* 63:467, 1977.
192. Fujita T et al: Natriuretic and antihypertensive effects of potassium in DOCA-salt hypertensive rats. *Kidney Int* 24:731, 1983.
193. Funder JW et al: Mineralocorticoid action: Target tissue specificity is enzymes, not receptor, mediated. *Science* 242:583, 1988.
194. Gabuzda GJ, Hall PW III: Relation of potassium depletion to renal ammonium metabolism and hepatic coma. *Medicine* 45:481, 1966.
195. Galvez OG et al: The hemodynamic effects of potassium deficiency in the dog. *Circ Res* 40(suppl I):11, 1977.
196. Ganguli PC, Mohamed D: Long-term therapy with carbenoxolone in the prevention of recurrence of gastric ulcer. Natural history and evolution of important side-effects and measures to avoid them. *Scand J Gastroenterol* 15(suppl):63, 1980.
197. Ganguly A et al: Renin-secreting Wilm's tumor with severe hypertension. *Ann Intern Med* 79:835, 1973.
198. Ganguly A et al: Genetic and pathophysiologic studies of a new kindred with glucocorticoid-suppressive hyperaldosteronism manifest in three generations. *J Clin Endocrinol Metab* 53:1040, 1981.
199. Ganguly A et al: Detection of adrenal tumors by computerized tomographic scan in endocrine hypertension. *Arch Intern Med* 139:589, 1979.
200. Gardner JD et al: Abnormal membrane sodium transport in Liddle's syndrome. *J Clin Invest* 50:2253, 1971.
201. Garella S et al: Alterations of hydrogen homeostasis in pure potassium depletion: Studies in rats and dogs during the recovery phase. *J Lab Clin Med* 93:321, 1983.
202. Garrahan PJ, Glynn IM: The behavior of the sodium pump in red cells in the absence of external potassium. *J Physiol* 192:159, 1967.
203. Garrick R et al: Bartter's syndrome: A unifying hypothesis. *Am J Nephrol* 5:379, 1985.
204. Gastel B: Thallium poisoning. *Johns Hopkins Med J* 142:27, 1978.
205. Gavras H et al: Is elevated plasma renin activity of prog-

nostic importance in progressive systemic sclerosis? *Arch Intern Med* 137:1554, 1977.

206. Gavryck WA et al: Effect of insulin upon membrane bound ($Na^+ - K^+$)-ATPase extracted from frog skeletal muscle. *J Physiol* 252:43, 1975.
207. Gelfand MC et al: Geophagia: A cause of life-threatening hyperkalemia in patients with chronic renal failure. *JAMA* 234:738, 1975.
208. Gennari FJ et al: The nature of the renal adaptation to chronic hypocapnia. *J Clin Invest* 51:1722, 1972.
209. Ghione S et al: Hypertension and hypokalemia caused by 9α-fluoroprednisolone in a nasal spray. *Lancet* 1:1301, 1979.
210. Giebink GS et al: A kindred with familial glucocorticoid suppressive aldosteronism. *J Clin Endocrinol Metab* 36:715, 1973.
211. Giebisch G et al: Renal transport and control of potassium excretion, in Brenner BM, Rector FC Jr (eds): *The Kidney*. Philadelphia, Saunders, 1981, p 408.
212. Gill MA et al: Hypokalemia, metabolic alkalosis induced by high-dose ampicillin sodium. *Am J Hosp Pharm* 34:528, 1977.
213. Gill JR Jr: Bartter's syndrome. *Annu Rev Med* 31:405, 1980.
214. Gill JR Jr, Bartter FC: Evidence for a prostaglandin-independent defect in chloride reabsorption in the loop of Henle as a proximal cause of Bartter's syndrome. *Am J Med* 65:766, 1978.
215. Gill JR Jr, Bartter FC: In J de Graeff, B Leijnse (eds): *Water and Electrolyte Metabolism (II)*. Amsterdam, Elsevier, 1964, p 119.
216. Gill JR Jr et al: Impaired conservation of sodium and potassium in renal acidosis and its correction by buffer anions. *Clin Sci* 33:577, 1967.
217. Gill JR Jr et al: Bartter's syndrome: A disorder characterized by high urinary prostaglandins and a dependence of hyperreninemia on prostaglandin synthesis. *Am J Med* 61:43, 1976.
218. Gitelman HJ et al: A new familial disorder characterized by hypokalemia and hypomagnesemia. *Trans Assoc Am Physicians* 79:221, 1966.
219. Gonzalez JJ et al: Clay ingestion: A rare cause of hypokalemia. *Ann Intern Med* 97:65, 1982.
220. Good DW: Effects of potassium on ammonia transport by medullary thick ascending limb of the rat. *J Clin Invest* 80:1358, 1987.
221. Goodman AD et al: Pathogenesis of Bartter's syndrome. *N Engl J Med* 281:1435, 1969.
222. Gorden P: Glucose intolerance with hypokalemia: Failure of short-term potassium depletion in normal subjects to reproduce the glucose and insulin abnormalities of clinical hypokalemia. *Diabetes* 22:544, 1973.
223. Gorden P et al: Glucose intolerance with hypokalemia. An increased proportion of circulating proinsulin like component. *J Clin Endocrinol Metab* 34:235, 1972.
224. Gordon RS Jr, Cage CW: Mechanism of water and electrolyte secretion by the eccrine sweat gland. *Lancet* 1:1246, 1966.
225. Gottschalk CW et al: Osmolality of renal tubular fluids in potassium-depleted rodents. *Clin Sci* 29:249, 1965.
226. Gourley DRH: Effect of insulin on potassium exchange in normal and ouabain-treated skeletal muscle. *J Pharmacol Exp Ther* 148:339, 1965.
227. Graham JA et al: Muscle biopsy water and electrolyte contents in chronic renal failure. *Clin Sci* 38:583, 1970.
228. Granerus A et al: Kaliuretic effect of L-DOPA treatment in Parkinsonian patients. *Acta Med Scand* 201:291, 1977.
229. Gray GM: Maldigestion and malabsorption: Clinical manifestations and specific diagnosis, in Sleisinger MH, Fordtran JS (eds): *Gastrointestinal Disease*. Philadelphia, Saunders, 1978, p 273.
230. Griffing GT et al: Effect of amiloride on renin-aldosterone system in primary hyperaldosteronism and Bartter's syndrome. *J Clin Pharmacol* 22:505, 1982.
231. Griggs RC et al: Acetazolamide treatment of hypokalemic periodic paralysis. *Ann Intern Med* 73:39, 1970.
232. Gross DJ et al: Edema associated with laxative abuse and excessive diuretic therapy. *Isr J Med Sci* 16:787, 1980.
233. Gross JM: Fanconi syndrome (adult type) developing secondary to the ingestion of outdated tetracycline. *Ann Intern Med* 58:523, 1963.
234. Gross MD, Shapiro B: *Semin Nucl Med* 119:122, 1989.
235. Gross TL, Sokol RJ: Severe hypokalemia and acidosis: A potential complication of beta-adrenergic treatment. *Am J Obstet Gynecol* 138:1225, 1980.
236. Grunfeld C et al: Hypokalemia and diabetes mellitus. *Am J Med* 75:553, 1983.
237. Gullner HG et al: Correction of hypokalemia by magnesium depletion in familial hypokalemic alkalosis with tubulopathy. *Am J Med* 71:578, 1981.
238. Gullner HG et al: Hypokalemia stimulates prostacyclin synthesis in the rat. *Clin Sci* 65:43, 1983.
239. Gunning JF et al: The effects of chronic potassium deficiency on myocardial contractility and oxygen consumption. *J Mol Cell Cardiol* 4:139, 1972.
240. Gustafson AB et al: Protein metabolism *in vivo* in kidney, liver, muscle and heart of potassium deficient rats. *J Lab Clin Med* 82:287, 1973.
241. Habibzadeh MA, Zeller NH: Cardiac arrhythmia and hypopotassemia in association with lithium carbonate overdose. *South Med J* 70:628, 1977.

241a. Hall KW et al: Metabolic abnormalities associated with intentional theophylline overdose. *Ann Intern Med* 101:457, 1984.

241b. Hall RC et al: Refractory hypokalemia secondary to hypomagnesemia in eating disorder patients. *Psychiatry* 29:435, 1988.

242. Haluska PV et al: Bartter's syndrome: Urinary prostaglandin-like material and kallikrein, indomethiacin effects. *Ann Intern Med* 87:281, 1977.
243. Hartsuck JM et al: Potassium in bone: Evidence for a nonexchangeable fraction. *Metabolism* 18:33, 1969.
244. Healy JJ et al: Body composition changes in hypertensive subjects on long-term oral diuretic therapy. *Br Med J* 1:716, 1970.

244a. Hegsted R et al: Ageing and aldosterone. *Am J Med* 74:442, 1983.

245. Helderman JH et al: Prevention of glucose intolerance of thiazide diuretics by maintenance of body potassium. *Diabetes* 32:106, 1983.
246. Hene RJ et al: Correction of hypokalemia in Bartter's syndrome by enalapril. *Am J Kidney Dis* 9:200, 1987.
247. Henrikson HW: Effect of potassium deficiency on gastrointestinal motility in rats. *Am J Physiol* 164:263, 1951.

248. Hernandez RE et al: Dietary NaCl determines severity of potassium depletion-induced metabolic alkalosis. *Kidney Int* 31:1356, 1987.
249. Hiatt M et al: Effect of potassium chloride infusion on insulin secretion *in vivo*. *Horm Metab Res* 4:64, 1972.
250. Hoefnagels WHL et al: Evidence for an unidentified, adrenocorticotrophic hormone-dependent mineralocorticoid maintaining hypertension in young women with hypoaldosteronism. *Clin Sci* 55:272, 1978.
251. Hoffbrand BI, Stewart JDM: Carbenicillin and hypokalemia. *Br Med J* 4:746, 1970.
252. Hogan MJ et al: Concurrent hypercortisolism and hypermineralocorticoidism. *Am J Med* 62:777, 1977.
253. Holland OB et al: Diuretic-induced ventricular ectopic activity. *Am J Med* 70:762, 1981.
254. Hollifield JW et al: Renin-secreting clear cell carcinoma of the kidney. *Arch Intern Med* 135:859, 1975.
255. Holmbert C et al: Congenital chloride diarrhea. *Arch Dis Child* 52:255, 1977.
256. Holten C, Petersen VP: Malignant hypertension with increased secretion of aldosterone and depletion of potassium. *Lancet* 2:918, 1956.
257. Hood VL, Dunn MJ: Urinary excretion of prostaglandin E_2 and prostaglandin $F_{2\alpha}$ in potassium deficient rats. *Prostaglandins* 15:273, 1978.
258. Horton R: Aldosterone: Review of its physiology and diagnostic aspects of primary aldosteronism. *Metabolism* 22:1525, 1973.
259. Houston BD, Turner T: Severe electrolyte abnormalities in a pregnant patient with jejunoileal bypass. *Arch Intern Med* 138:1712, 1978.
260. Howard PJ et al: Localization of renal calcium transport: Effect of calcium loads and of gluconate anion in water, sodium and potassium. *Am J Physiol* 197:337, 1959.
261. Hulting J: Hospital ventricular fibrillation and its relation to serum potassium. *Acta Med Scand* 647(suppl):109, 1981.
262. Hunt JC, Strong CG: Renovascular hypertension: Mechanism, natural history and treatment. *Am J Cardiol* 32:562, 1973.
263. Hurlbert BJ et al: Serum potassium levels during and after terbutaline. *Anesth Analg* 60:723, 1981.
264. Ibsen H: Red blood cell potassium as a measure of body potassium in thiazide-treated patients with essential hypertension. *Scand J Clin Lab Invest* 34:161, 1974.
265. Imai M et al: A case of Bartter's syndrome with abnormal renin response to salt load. *J Pediatr* 74:738, 1969.
266. Intersalt Cooperative Research Group: Intersalt: An international study of electrolyte excretion and blood pressure. Results for 24 hour urinary sodium and potassium excretion. *Br Med J* 297:319, 1988.
267. Jaffe BM et al: Indomethacin-responsive pancreatic cholera. *N Engl J Med* 297:817, 1977.
268. Jimenez RAH, Larson EB: Tumoral calcinosis: An unusual complication of the laxative abuse syndrome. *Am J Med Sci* 282:141, 1981.
269. Johnsen T: Effect upon serum insulin, glucose and potassium concentration of acetazolamide during attacks of familial periodic hypokalemic paralysis. *Acta Neurol Scand* 56:533, 1977.
270. Johnsen T: Familial periodic paralysis with hypokalemia. *Dan Med Bull* 28:1981.
271. Johnsen T: Trial of the prophylactic effect of diazoxide in the treatment of familial periodic hypokalemia. *Acta Neurol Scand* 56:525, 1977.
272. Johnson JE et al: Radio potassium in total body potassium: Studies using ^{43}K and ^{42}K. *Metabolism* 18:663, 1969.
273. Jones JW et al: Systemic and renal acid-base effects of chronic dietary potassium depletion in humans. *Kidney Int* 21:402, 1982.
274. Jones NF: Potassium deficiency: A reappraisal in Slater JDH (ed): *Sixth Symposium on Advanced Medicine*. London, Pitman Medical, 1970, p 203.
275. Kabadi UM: Corticotropin-induced hyperaldosteronism. *NY State J Med* 80:1860, 1980.
276. Kaplan NM: *Clinical Hypertension*. Baltimore, Williams & Wilkins, 1990.
277. Kaplan NM: Secondary aldosteronism: With observations on the definition of hypokalemia. *Am J Clin Pathol* 54:316, 1970.
278. Kaplan NM, Silah JG: The effect of angiotensin II on the blood pressure in humans with hypertensive disease. *J Clin Invest* 43:659, 1964.
279. Kaplan NM et al: Potassium supplementation in hypertensive patients with diuretic-induced hypokalemia. *N Engl J Med* 312:746, 1985.
280. Karetzky MS, Mithoefer JC: The cause of hyperventilation and arterial hypoxia in patients with cirrhosis of the liver. *Am J Med Sci* 254:797, 1967.
281. Kassirer JP, Schwartz WB: The response of normal man to selective depletion of hydrochloric acid. *Am J Med* 40:10, 1966.
282. Kearney TE et al: Theophylline toxicity and the beta-adrenergic system. *Ann Intern Med* 102:766, 1985.
283. Keye JD: Death in potassium deficiency. Report of a case including morphologic findings. *Circulation* 5:766, 1952.
284. Khurana R, Kalyanaraman K: Hypokalemic vacuolar myopathy of chronic alcoholism: A histological and histochemical study. *Dis Nerv Syst* 38:287, 1977.
285. Kim JK et al: Effect of hypokalemia on renal medullary cyclic AMP generation, metabolism and action, abstracted. *Clin Res* 247:420, 1979.
286. Kim WG, Brown EB: Potassium transfer with constant extracellular pH. *J Lab Clin Med* 71:678, 1968.
287. Klastersky J et al: Carbenicillin and hypokalemia. *Ann Intern Med* 78:774, 1973.
288. Klaus D et al: Einfluss der Schwangerschaft auf das Bartter Syndrome. *Klin Wochenschr* 49:1280, 1971.
289. Knochel JP: Neuromuscular manifestations of electrolyte disorders. *Am J Med* 72:521, 1982.
290. Knochel JP: The effect of potassium deficiency on skeletal muscle structure and function. *Cardiovasc Med* 3:247, 1978.
291. Knochel JP et al: Pathophysiology of intense physical conditioning in a hot climate: I. Mechanism of potassium depletion. *J Clin Invest* 51:242, 1972.
292. Knochel JP, Schlein EM: On the mechanism of rhabdomyolysis in potassium depletion. *J Clin Invest* 51:1750, 1972.
293. Kodama Am et al: Accuracy of measurements of potassium content of monkeys by *in vivo* body counting as compared to clinical analysis. *Phys Med Biol* 19:862, 1974.
294. Konold P et al: The effect of potassium on the tone of isolated arteries. *Pflugers Arch* 301:285, 1968.

295. Kopyt N et al: Renal retention of potassium in fruit. *N Engl J Med* 313:582, 1985 (letter).
296. Korff JM et al: Correction of hypokalemia corrects the abnormalities in erythrocyte sodium transport in Bartter's syndrome. *J Clin Invest* 74:1724, 1984.
297. Kosman ME: Management of potassium problems during long-term diuretic therapy. *JAMA* 230:743, 1974.
298. Krakoff LR: Potassium deficiency and cardiac catecholamine metabolism in the rat. *Circ Res* 30:608, 1972.
299. Krishna GG et al: Mild potassium depletion provokes renal sodium retention. *J Lab Clin Med* 109:724, 1987.
300. Krishna GG et al: Hemodynamic consequences of diuretic-induced hypokalemia. *Am J Kidney Dis* 12:329, 1988.
301. Krishna GG et al: Clinical use of potassium-sparing diuretics. *Semin Nephrol* 8:354, 1988.
302. Krishna GG et al: Increased blood pressure during potassium depletion in normotensive men. *N Engl J Med* 320:1177, 1989.
303. Krishna GG: Effect of potassium intake on blood pressure. *J Am Soc Nephrol* 1:43, 1990.
304. Krishna GG et al: Potassium supplementation attenuates mineralocorticoid (MC)-induced hypertension. *J Am Soc Nephrol* 1:508, 1990.
304a. Siani A et al: Increase in dietary potassium intake reduces the need for antihypertensive medication *Ann Intern Med* 115:753, 1991.
305. Krishna GG et al: Potassium depletion induces sodium retention and increases blood pressure in hypertensives. *Kidney Int* 37:277, 1990 (abstract).
306. Kruck F: Disturbances of acid-base balance by diuretics and their prevention. *Acta Cardiol (Brux)* 17(suppl 65):250, 1973.
307. Kruse JA et al: Rapid correction of hypokalemia using concentrated intravenous potassium chloride. *Arch Intern Med* 150:613, 1990.
308. Kunau RT Jr et al: Micropuncture study of proximal tubular factors responsible for the maintenance of alkalosis during potassium deficiency in the rat. *Clin Sci* 34:223, 1968.
309. Kunau RT Jr et al: Characteristics of the relationship between the flow rate of tubular fluid and potassium transport in the distal tubule of the rat. *J Clin Invest* 54:1488, 1974.
310. Kung TM: Cystadenocarcinoma of pancreas with hypokalemia and hypoproteinemia: Case report. *Pathology* 12:479, 1980.
311. Lai F et al: Licorice, snuff and hypokalemia. *N Engl J Med* 303:463, 1980.
312. Lantz B et al: Electrolytes and whole body potassium in acute leukemia. *Acta Med Scand* 206:45, 1979.
313. Laragh JH, Sealey JE: The renin-angiotensin-aldosterone hormonal system and regulation of sodium, potassium and blood pressure homeostasis, in *Handbook of Physiology*, Washington DC, American Physiology Society, 1973, p 831.
314. Latif SA et al: The effects of liquorice derivative, glycyrrhetinic acid, on hepatic 3α- and 3β-hydroxysteroid dehydrogenase and 5α- and 5β-reductase pathways of metabolism of aldosterone in male rats. *Steroids* 55:52, 1990.
315. Lauzurica R et al: Rhabdomyolysis, edema and arterial hypertension: Different syndromes related to topical use of 9α-fluoroprednisolone. *J Human Hypertens* 2:183, 1988.
316. Lawton WJ et al: Effect of dietary potassium on blood pressure, renal function, muscle sympathetic nerve activity, and forearm vascular resistance and flow in normotensive and borderline hypertensive humans. *Circulation* 81:173, 1990.
317. Lebell M et al: Adenocarcinoma of the kidney and hypertension: Report of 2 cases with special emphasis on renin. *J Urol* 118:923, 1977.
318. Ledoux F et al: Long-term hypokalemia in acute myeloid leukemia. *Arch Intern Med* 138:1287, 1978.
319. Lemann J Jr et al: Potassium bicarbonate, but not sodium bicarbonate, reduces urinary calcium excretion and improves calcium balance in healthy men. *Kidney Int* 35:688, 1989.
320. Lemieux G et al: Hypokalemia during the treatment of arterial hypertension with diuretics. *Can Med Assoc J* 122:905, 1980.
321. Lennon EJ et al: The effect of potassium-deficient diet on the pattern of recovery from experimental metabolic acidosis. *Clin Sci* 34:365, 1968.
322. Levine DZ et al: Effects of KCl infusion on proximal tubular function in normal and potassium-depleted rats. *Kidney Int* 4:318, 1973.
323. Levy M: Effects of acute volume expansion and altered hemodynamics on renal tubular function in chronic caval dogs. *J Clin Invest* 51:992, 1972.
324. Liddle GW: Aldosterone antagonists and triamterene. *Ann NY Acad Sci* 139:466, 1966.
325. Liddle GW et al: A familial renal disorder simulating primary aldosteronism but with negligible aldosterone secretion. *Trans Assoc Am Physicians* 79:199, 1963.
326. Lifton RP et al: A chimeric 11β-hydroxylase/aldosterone synthase gene causes glucocorticoid remediable aldosteronism and human hypertension. *Nature* 355:262, 1992.
327. Lim VS, Webster G: The effect of aldosterone on water and electrolyte composition of incubated rat diaphragms. *Clin Sci* 33:261, 1967.
328. Linas SL: Mechanism of hyperreninemia in the potassium-depleted rat. *J Clin Invest* 68:347, 1981.
329. Linas SL et al: Mechanism of the decreased renal blood flow in the potassium-depleted conscious rat. *Kidney Int* 21:757, 1982.
330. Linas SL et al: Potassium depletion ameliorates hypertension in SHR. *Hypertension* 8:990, 1986.
331. Lipner HI et al: The behavior of carbenicillin as a nonreabsorbable anion. *J Lab Clin Med* 86:183, 1975.
332. Littlewood JM et al: Treatment of Bartter's syndrome in early childhood with prostaglandin synthetase inhibitors. *Arch Dis Child* 53:43, 1978.
333. Liu GZ et al: Experiences with Gossypol as a male pill. *Am J Obstet Gynecol* 157:1079, 1987.
334. Luetscher JA et al: Preoperative differentiation of adrenal adenoma from idiopathic adrenal hyperplasia in primary aldosteronism. *Circ Res* 34/35(suppl I):175, 1974.
335. Luke RG et al: Effects of potassium depletion on renal tubular chloride transport in the rat. *Kidney Int* 14:414, 1978.

336. Luke RG et al: Effect of potassium depletion on renin release. *Kidney Int* 21:14, 1982.
337. Luke RG et al: Effect of potassium depletion on chloride transport in the loop of Henle in the rat. *Am J Physiol* 248:F682, 1985.
338. Mace JW et al: Magnesium supplementation in Bartter's syndrome. *Arch Dis Child* 48:485, 1973.
339. MacLachlen TK: Familial periodic paralysis: A description of six cases occurring in three generations of one family. *Brain* 55:47, 1932.
340. MacLeod RM, Fontham EH: Influence of the ionic environment of the *in vitro* synthesis and release of pituitary hormones. *Endocrinology* 86:863, 1970.
341. Maizels M: The anion and cation contents of normal and anaemic bloods. *Biochem J* 30:821, 1936.
342. Malnic G et al: Potassium transport across renal distal tubules during acid-base disturbances. *Am J Physiol* 221:1192, 1971.
343. Manchester KL: Insulin and protein synthesis, in Litwack G (ed): *Biochemical Actions of Hormones*. New York, Academic Press, 1970, vol 1, p 267.
344. Manitius A et al: On the mechanism of impairment of renal concentrating ability in potassium deficiency. *J Clin Invest* 39:684, 1960.
345. Mann MD et al: Total body potassium estimations in young children, the interpretation of results. *Pediatr Res* 8:879, 1974.
346. Mantero F et al: Mineralocorticoid hypertension due to a nasal spray containing 9-fluoroprednisolone. *Am J Med* 71:353, 1981.
347. Martin HE: Clinical magnesium deficiency. *Ann NY Acad Sci* 169:891, 1969.
348. Maronde RF et al: Potassium loss with thiazide therapy. *Am Heart J* 78:16, 1969.
349. Massry SD: Pharmacology of magnesium. *Annu Rev Pharm* 17:67, 1977.
350. McCleave DJ et al: Compartmental shift of potassium: A result of sympathomimetic overdose. *Aust NZ J Med* 8:180, 1978.
351. McCollister RJ et al: Urinary excretion of magnesium in man following the ingestion of ethanol. *Am J Clin Nutr* 12:415, 1963.
352. McCredie DA et al: Potassium-losing nephropathy of childhood. *Med J Aust* 1:129, 1971.
353. McCredie DA et al: Hypercalcuria in potassium-losing nephropathy: A variant of Bartter's syndrome. *Aust Paediatr J* 10:286, 1974.
354. McIntyre PA: Hypokalemia occurring during para-aminosalicyclic acid therapy. *Johns Hopkins Med J* 92:210, 1953.
355. Mengel CE et al: Geophagia with iron deficiency and hypokalemia. *Arch Intern Med* 114:470, 1964.
356. Meyer WJ et al: Gout as a complication of Bartter's syndrome. *Ann Intern Med* 83:56, 1975.
357. Miller CE, Remenchik AP: Problems involved in accurately measuring the K^+ content of the human body. *Ann NY Acad Sci* 110:175, 1963.
358. Mir MA et al: Hypokalemia in acute myeloid leukemia. *Ann Intern Med* 82:52, 1975.
359. Mir MA, Delamore IW: Hypouricemia and proximal renal tubular dysfunction in acute myeloid leukemia. *Br Med J* 3:775, 1974.
360. Mittal VK et al: Use of probenecid in ticarcillin-induced hypokalemia. *Clin Ther* 3:125, 1980.
361. Mitchell JD et al: Renin levels in nephroblastoma (Wilm's tumor). Report of a renin-secreting tumor. *Arch Dis Child* 45:376, 1970.
362. Mitty HA et al: Adrenal venography: Clinical roentgeographic correlation in 80 patients. *Radiology* 119:564, 1973.
363. Modlinger RS et al: Some observations on the pathogenesis of Bartter's syndrome. *N Engl J Med* 289:1022, 1973.
364. Mohr JA et al: Nafcillin-associated hypokalemia. *JAMA* 242:544, 1979.
365. Monder C et al: Liquorice inhibits corticosteroid 11β-dehydrogenase of rat kidney and liver: In vivo and in vitro studies. *Endocrinology* 125:1046, 1989.
366. Moore FD et al: Body sodium and potassium: III. Interrelated trends in alimentary, renal and cardiovascular disease. Lack of correlation between body stores and plasma concentration. *Metabolism* 3: 334, 1954.
367. Moravec MD, Hurlbert BJ: Hypokalemia associated with terbutaline administration in obstetrical patients. *Anesth Analg* 59:917, 1980.
368. Morgan DB, Davidson C: Hypokalemia and diuretics: An analysis of publications. *Br Med J* 280:905, 1980.
369. Morgan DB et al: Potassium depletion in heart failure and its relation to long-term treatment with diuretics: A review of the literature. *Postgrad Med J* 54:72, 1978.
370. Morris BJ et al: Licorice, tobacco chewing and hypertension. *N Engl J Med* 322:849, 1990 (letter).
371. Morris RC Jr et al: Renal acidosis. *Kidney Int* 1:322, 1972.
372. Morton W: Poisoning by barium carbonate. *Lancet* 2:738, 1945.
373. Moss AH et al: Fanconi syndrome and distal renal tubular acidosis after glue sniffing. *Ann Intern Med* 92:69, 1980.
374. Muehrcke RC, Rosen, S: Hypokalemic nephropathy in rat and man. *Lab Invest* 13:1359, 1964.
375. Muggia FM et al: Lysozymuria and renal tubular dysfunction in monocytic and myelomonocytic leukemia. *Am J Med* 47:351, 1969.
376. Mulhausen R et al: Acid-base disturbances in patients with cirrhosis of the liver. *Medicine* 46:185, 1967.
377. Muntwyler E, Griffin GE: Creatinine clearance in normal and potassium deficient rats. *Am J Physiol* 173:145, 1953.
378. Muntwyler E, Griffin GE: Tissue electolyte content of potassium and protein deficient rats. *Proc Soc Exp Biol Med* 89:349, 1955.
379. Nader PC et al: Complications of diuretic use. *Semin Nephrol* 8:365, 1988.
380. Nagami GT: Effect of bath and luminal potassium concentration on ammonia production and secretion by mouse proximal tubules perfused in vitro. *J Clin Invest* 86:32, 1990.
381. Nagel W: Inhibition of potassium conductance by barium in frog skin epithelium. *Biochim Biophys Acta* 552:346, 1979.
382. Naik RB et al: Hypokalemic hyperchloremic metabolic acidosis and vesical stone complicating appendicovesical fistulae. *Br J Urol* 52:274, 1980.
383. Nanji AA, Denegri J: Hypokalemia in leukemia. *Postgrad Med J* 57:482, 1981.

384. Naranjo CA et al: Furosemide-induced adverse reaction in cirrhosis of the liver. *Clin Pharmacol Ther* 25:154, 1979.
385. Narins RG et al: Diagnostic strategies in disorders of fluid, electrolyte and acid-base homeostasis. *Am J Med* 72:496, 1982.
386. Narins RG, Goldberg M: Renal tubular acidosis: Pathophysiology, diagnosis and treatment. *DM* 23:1, 1977.
387. Nasjletti A et al: Interrelations of the renal kallikreinkinin system and renal prostaglandins in the conscious rat. Influence of mineralocorticoids. *Circ Res* 43:799, 1978.
388. Nasjletti A et al: High potassium intake selectively increases urinary PGF_2 excretion in the rat. *Am J Physiol* 248:F382, 1985.
389. Need AG et al: Rifampicin associated renal dysfunction during antituberculous therapy. *Aust NZ J Med* 10:657, 1980.
390. New MI et al: Evidence for an unidentified steroid in a child with apparent mineralocorticoid hypertension. *J Clin Endocrinol Metab* 44:924, 1977.
391. Nichols BL et al: Relationship between muscle potassium and total body potassium in infants with malnutrition. *J Pediatr* 74:49, 1969.
392. Nicolis GL et al: Percutaneous adrenal venography: A clinical study of 50 patients. *Ann Intern Med* 76:899, 1972.
393. Nightingale S et al: Anorexia nervosa, liquorice and hypokalemic myopathy. *Postgrad Med J* 57:577, 1981.
394. Nolan CR et al: Mechanism of antihypertensive effect of potassium depletion in renal vascular hypertension. *Am J Physiol* 223:555, 1972.
395. Norby L et al: Prostaglandins and aspirin therapy in Bartter's syndrome. *Lancet* 2:604, 1976.
396. Nordrehaug JE: Malignant arrhythmias in relation to serum K^+ values in patients with an acute myocardial infarction. *Acta Med Scand* 647(suppl):101, 1981.
397. Noth RH, Biglieri EG: *Med Clin North Am* 72(5):1117, 1988.
398. O'Brien IA et al: Hypokalemia due to salbutamol overdosage. *Br Med J* 282:1515, 1981.
399. Oliver J et al: The renal lesions of electrolyte imbalance: I. The structural alterations in potassium-depleted rats. *J Exp Med* 106:563, 1957.
400. O'Regan S: Echocardiographic assessment of left ventricular function in patients with hypokalemia. *Miner Electrolyte Metab* 11:1, 1985.
401. Orloff J et al: Effect of prostaglandin (PGE_1) on the permeability of toad bladder to vasopressin, theophylline and adenosine 3'-5' monophosphate. *Nature* 205:397, 1965.
402. Osserman EF, Lawlor DP: Serum and urinary lysozyme in monocytic and myelomonocytic leukemias. *J Exp Med* 124:921, 1966.
403. Overgaard, Nielsen H: Arterial hypertension due to a renin-producing renal carcinoma. *Scand J Urol Nephrol* 9:293, 1973.
404. Padilla AJ, Loeb JN: "Low-dose" versus "high-dose" insulin regimens in the management of uncontrolled diabetes. *Am J Med* 63:843, 1977.
405. Paller MS et al: Mechanism of decreased vascular reactivity to angiotensin II in conscious potassium-deficient rats. *J Clin Invest* 73:79, 1984.
406. Papouchado M: Thyrotoxic periodic paralysis. *J R Soc Med* 73:519, 1980.
407. Parker JC, Welt LG: Pathological alterations of cation movements in red blood cells. *Arch Intern Med* 129:320, 1972.
408. Patrick J: Assessment of body potassium stores. *Kidney Int* 11:476, 1977.
409. Patrick J, Bradford BN: A comparison of leukocyte potassium content with other measurements in potassium-depleted rabbits. *Clin Sci* 42:415, 1972.
410. Pearson CM, Kalyanaraman K: Periodic paralysis, in Stanbury JB et al (eds): *The Metabolic Basis of Inherited Disease*. New York, McGraw-Hill, 1972, p 1181.
411. Pentimone F et al: Hypokalemia as the only clinical symptom of ACTH ectopic secretion in a case of small cell carcinoma of the lung with very rapid evolution. *Respiration* 39:114, 1980.
412. Perera GW: Depressor effects of potassium deficient diets in hypertensive man. *J Clin Invest* 32:633, 1953.
413. Perry MC et al: Hypokalemia in acute myelogenous leukemia. *South Med J* 76:958, 1983.
414. Pickering TG, Catovsky D: Hypokalemia and raised lysozyme levels in acute myeloid leukemia. *Q J Med* 42:677, 1973.
415. Pierson RN Jr et al: Total body potassium in health: Effects of age, sex, weight, and fat. *Am J Physiol* 226:206, 1974.
416. Pierson RN Jr et al: Body composition measurements in normal man: The potassium, sodium, sulfate and tritium spaces in 58 adults. *J Chronic Dis* 35:419, 1982.
417. Platt G et al: Thyrotoxic periodic paralysis with upper motor neuron findings. *JAMA* 240:2465, 1978.
418. Plotz C et al: National history of Cushing's syndrome. *Am J Med* 13:597, 1952.
419. Podolsky S et al: Potassium depletion in hepatic cirrhosis: A reversible cause of impaired growth hormone and insulin response to stimulation. *N Engl J Med* 288:644, 1973.
420. Pollare T et al: A comparison of the effects of hydrochlorothiazide and captopril on glucose and lipid metabolism in patients with hypertension. *N Engl J Med* 321:868, 1989.
421. Potter WZ et al: Familial hypokalemia associated with renal interstitial fibrosis. *Am J Med* 57:971, 1974.
422. Price WF et al: Reproductibility of body composition measurements in a single individual. *J Lab Clin Med* 74:557, 1969.
423. Pruzanski W, Platts ME: Serum and urinary proteins, lysozyme and renal dysfunction in mono- and myelomonocytic leukemia. *J Clin Invest* 49:1694, 1973.
424. Qian SZ: Gossypol-hypokalemia inter-relationships. *Int J Andrology* 8:313, 1985.
425. Rabelink TJ et al: Early and late adjustment to potassium loading in humans. *Kidney Int* 38:942, 1990.
425a. Raij L et al: High potassium diet augments endothelium-dependent relaxations in Dahl rats. *Hypertension* 12:562, 1988.
426. Rappaport MI, Hurd HF: Thiazide-induced glucose intolerance treated with potassium. *Arch Intern Med* 113:405, 1964.
427. Raskin RJ et al: Hypokalemic periodic paralysis in Sjogren's syndrome. *Arch Intern Med* 141:1671, 1981.
428. Raymond KH et al: In vivo and in vitro studies of urinary concentrating ability in potassium-depleted rabbits. *J Clin Invest* 76:561, 1985.

429. Raymond KH et al: Prostaglandins and the urinary concentrating defect in potassium-depleted rabbits. *Am J Physiol* 253:F1113, 1987.
430. Reid AC, Draper IT: Flaccid quadriparesis due to salmonella enteritis. *Scott Med J* 25:129, 1980.
431. Relman AS, Schwartz WB: The nephropathy of potassium depletion. *N Engl J Med* 255:195, 1956.
432. Resnick JS et al: Acetazolamide prophylaxis in hypokalemic periodic paralysis. *N Engl J Med* 278:582, 1968.
433. Revers FE: Heeft succus liquiritae een genezende werking op de maagzweer? *Ned Tijdschr Geneeskd* 90:135, 1946.
433a. Rich GM et al: Glucocorticoid-remediable aldosteronism in a large kindred: Clinical spectrum and diagnosis using a characteristic biochemical phenotype. *Ann Intern Med* 116:813, 1992.
434. Riecker G, Bolte HD: Membranpotentiale einzelner skeletuskelzellen bei hypokaliamischer periodischer muskelparalyse. *Klin Wochenschr* 44:804, 1966.
435. Riecker G et al: Hypokallamie und membran-potential. *Reanim Oranges Artif* 1:41, 1964.
436. Robertson PW et al: Hypertension due to a renin-secreting renal tumor. *Am J Med* 43:963, 1967.
437. Robson WL et al: Bartter's syndrome, differentiation into two clinical groups. *Am J Dis Child* 133:636, 1979.
438. Rochman J et al: Adult Fanconi's syndrome with renal tubular acidosis in association with renal amyloidosis. *Arch Intern Med* 140:1361, 1980.
439. Rodriguez M et al: Refractory potassium repletion due to cistplatin-induced magnesium depletion. *Arch Intern Med* 149:2592, 1989.
439a. Rodriguez M et al: Refractory potassium repletion due to cisplatin-induced magnesium depletion. *Arch Intern Med* 149:2592, 1989.
440. Rodriguez V et al: Serum electrolyte abnormalities associated with the administration of polymixin B in febrile leukemic patients. *Clin Pharmacol Ther* 11:106, 1970.
441. Rosa R et al: The renal concentrating defect associated with potassium depletion is independent of prostaglandin E_2. *Am J Kidney Dis* 16:473, 1990.
442. Roscoe JM et al: Effect of amphotericin-B on urine acidification in rats: Implications for the pathogenesis of distal renal tubular acidosis. *J Lab Clin Med* 89:463, 1977.
443. Rowe JW et al: Effects of experimental potassium deficiency on glucose and insulin metabolism. *Metabolism* 29:498, 1980.
444. Rowley PT, Kliman B: The effect of sodium loading and depletion on muscular strength and aldosterone excretion in familial periodic paralysis. *Am J Med* 28:376, 1960.
445. Royston A, Prout BJ: Carbenoxolone-induced hypokalemia simulating Guillain-Barré syndrome. *Br Med J* 2:150, 1976.
446. Roza O, Berman LB: The pathophysiology of barium: Hypokalemic and cardiovascular effects. *J Pharmacol Exp Ther* 177:433, 1971.
447. Rubenstein AE, Wainapel JF: Acute hypokalemic myopathy in alcoholism. *Arch Neurol* 34:553, 1977.
448. Rubini ME: Water excretion in potassium deficient man. *J Clin Invest* 39:2215, 1961.
449. Rude RK: Physiology of magnesium metabolism and the important role of magnesium in potassium deficiency. *Am J Cardiol* 63:31G, 1989.
450. Rudman D et al: Elemental studies during intravenous hyperalimentation of underweight adult subjects. *J Clin Invest* 55:94, 1975.
451. Rutecki G et al: Studies of the diabetes insipidus with K deficiency. *Clin Res* 27:499, 1979.
452. Rutledge MM et al: A longitudinal study of total body potassium in normal breast-fed and bottle-fed babies. *Pediatr Res* 10:114, 1976.
453. Ryan MP et al: Effect of magnesium deficiency on cardiac and skeletal muscle potassium during dietary potassium restriction. *Proc Soc Exp Biol Med* 142:1045, 1973.
454. Ryan MP: Diuretics and potassium/magnesium depletion. *Am J Med* 82(suppl 3):38, 1987.
455. Sadeh M et al: Hypokalemic periodic paralysis associated with multiple sclerosis. *Eur Neurol* 19:252, 1980.
456. Sanderson PH: Renal potassium wasting in hypercalcemia. *Br Med J* 1:679, 1967.
457. Sandor FF et al: Variations of plasma potassium concentrations during long-term treatment of hypertension with diuretics without potassium supplements. *Br Med J* 284:711, 1982.
458. Schambelan M et al: Role of renin and aldosterone in hypertension due to a renin-secreting tumor. *Am J Med* 55:86, 1973.
459. Schambelan M et al: Mineralocorticoid excess and deficiency syndromes, in Brenner BM, Stein JH (eds): *Acid-Base and Potassium Homeostasis.* New York, Churchill Livingstone, 1978, p 232.
460. Schambelan M et al: Mineralocorticoid production in hyperadrenocorticism. Role in pathogenesis of hypokalemic alkalosis. *Am J Med* 51:299, 1971.
461. Scherling B et al: Captopril treatment in Bartter's syndrome. *Scand J Urol Nephrol* 24:123, 1990.
462. Schilling K et al: Effect of magnesium on ATP- generating and ATP-utilizing reactions in Ehrlich ascites tumour cells. *Acta Biol Med Ger* 38:1101, 1979.
463. Schilsky RL, Anderson T: Hypomagnesemia and renal magnesium wasting in patients receiving cisplatinum. *Ann Intern Med* 90:929, 1979.
464. Schlaeffer F: Oxacillin-associated hypokalemia. *Drug Intell Clin Pharm* 22:695, 1988.
465. Schrock LG, Polk HC Jr: Rectal villous adenoma producing hypokalemia. *Am J Surg* 40:54, 1974.
466. Schwartz A: Is the cell membrane Na^+, K^+ ATPase enzyme system the pharmacological receptor for digitalis? *Circ Res* 39:2, 1976.
467. Schwartz GJ, Burg M: Mineralocorticoid effects on cation transport by cortical collecting tubules *in vitro*. *Am J Physiol* 235:576, 1978.
468. Schwartz GJ, Cornfeld D: Propranolol in Bartter's syndrome. *N Engl J Med* 290:966, 1974.
469. Schwartz WB, Relman AS: Effects of electrolyte disorders on renal structure and function. *N Engl J Med* 276:383, 1967.
470. Schwartz WB et al: Role of anions in metabolic alkalosis and potassium deficiency. *N Engl J Med* 179:630, 1968.
471. Scribner BH, Burnell JM: Interpretation of the serum potassum concentration. *Metabolism* 5:468, 1956.
472. Sebastian A et al: Impaired renal conservation of sodium and chloride during sustained correction of systemic aci-

dosis in patients with type I, classic renal tubular acidosis. *J Clin Invest* 58:454, 1976.

473. Sebastian A et al: On the mechansim of renal potassium wasting in renal tubular acidosis associated with the Fanconi syndrome (Type 2 RTA). *J Clin Invest* 50:231, 1971.
474. Sebastian A et al: Renal potassium wasting in renal tubular acidosis (RTA), its occurrence in types 1 and 2 RTA despite sustained correction of systemic acidosis. *J Clin Invest* 50:667, 1971.
475. Sealey JE et al: Potassium balance and the control of renin secretion. *J Clin Invest* 49:2119, 1970.
476. Sebastian A et al: Dietary potassium influences kidney maintenance of serum phosphorus concentration. *Kidney Int* 37:1341, 1990.
477. Seller RH et al: Digitalis toxicity and hypomagnesemia. *Am Heart J* 79:57, 1970.
478. Severance HW Jr et al: Profound muscle weakness and hypokalemia due to clay ingestion. *South Med J* 81:272, 1988.
479. Shannon M et al: Hypokalemia after theophylline intoxication. The effects of acute vs chronic poisoning. *Arch Intern Med* 149:275, 1989.
480. Shils ME: Experimental human magnesium depletion. *Medicine* 48:61, 1969.
481. Shy GM et al: Studies in familial periodic paralysis. *Exp Neurol* 3:53, 1961.
482. Sievert RM: Measurements of gamma radiation from the human body. *ARK FYS* 3:337, 1951.
483. Silverberg AB et al: Resistance to endogenous norepinephrine in Bartter's syndrome. *Am J Med* 64:231, 1978.
484. Sim DW, Wellingtoin GH: Potassium concentration in bovine muscle as influenced by carcass location, breed, sex, energy, intake, age, and shrunk body weight. *J Anim Sci* 42:84, 1976.
485. Simmons DH, Avedon M: Acid-base alterations and plasma potassium concentration. *Am J Physiol* 197:319, 1959.
486. Simodynes E: Preoperative shock secondary to severe hypokalemia and hypocalcemia from recreational enemas. *Anesth Analg* 60:762, 1981.
487. Simon N et al: Clinical characteristics of renal vascular hypertension. *JAMA* 220:1209, 1972.
488. Solaro RJ et al: Modulation of Ca control of dog and rabbit cardiac myofibrils by Mg. *Circ Res* 39:8, 1976.
489. Soler NG et al: Intensive care in the management of diabetic ketoacidosis. *Lancet* 2:951, 1973.

489a. Solomon R: The relationship between disorders of K^+ and Mg^{2+} homeostasis. *Semin Nephrol* 7:253, 1987.

490. Solomon RJ, Brown RS: Bartter's syndrome. *Am J Med* 59:575, 1975.
491. Solomon RJ, Cole AG: Importance of potassium in patients with acute myocardial infarction. *Acta Med Scand* 647(suppl):87, 1981.
492. Solomon SS et al: Feminizing adrenocortical carcinoma with hypertension. *J Clin Endocrinol Metab* 28:608, 1968.
493. Spencer RW, Voyce MA: Familial hypokalemia and hypomagnesemia. *Acta Paediatr Scand* 65:505, 1976.
494. Spergel G et al: The effect of potassium on the impaired glucose intolerance in chronic uremia. *Metabolism* 16:581, 1967.
495. Stanbury SN, McCaulay D: Defects of renal tubular function in the nephrotic syndrome. *Q J Med* 26:7, 1957.
496. Stein JH: The pathogenetic spectrum of Bartter's syndrome. *Kidney Int* 28:85, 1985.
497. Steinmetz PR, Lawson DJ: Defect in urinary acidification induced *in vitro* by amphotericin B. *J Clin Invest* 49:596, 1970.
498. Sterns RH et al: Internal potassium balance and the control of the plasma potassium concentration. *Medicine* 60:339, 1981.
499. Stewart C, Kingston CW: Carcinoid tumor of the thymus with Cushing's syndrome. *Pathology* 12:487, 1980.
500. Stewart PM et al: Mineralocorticoid activity of liquorice: 11β-hydroxy-steroid dehydrogenese deficiency. *Lancet* 2:821, 1987.
501. Stewart PM et al: Syndrome of apparent mineralocorticoid excess: A defect in the cortisol-cortisone shuttle. *J Clin Invest* 82:340, 1988.
502. Stokes GS et al: Bartter's syndrome presenting during pregnancy. *Med J Aust* 2:360, 1974.
503. Streeten DHP: Periodic paralysis, in Stanbury JB et al (eds): *The Metabolic Basis of Inherited Disease*, 2d ed. New York, McGraw-Hill, 1966, p 905.
504. Streeten DHP et al: Reliability of screening methods for the diagnosis of primary aldosteronism. *Am J Med* 67:403, 1979.
505. Streeten DHP, Speller PJ: The role of mineralocorticoids in the pathogenesis of hypokalemic periodic paralysis. *J Clin Endocrinol Metab* 39:326, 1974.
506. Surveyor I, Hughes D: Discrepancies between whole-body potassium contents and exchangeable potassium. *J Lab Clin Med* 71:464, 1968.
507. Sutherland DJA et al: Hypertension, increased aldosterone secretion and low plasma renin activity relieved by dexamethasone. *Can Med Assoc J* 95:1109, 1966.
508. Sutherland LE et al: Bartter's syndrome. *Acta Paediatr Scand* 201(suppl):1, 1970.
509. Symposium: Whole-body counting. Vienna: International Atomic Energy Agency, 1962.
510. Taher G et al: Renal tubular acidosis associated with toluene sniffing. *N Engl J Med* 290:765, 1974.
511. Takeuchi K et al: Plasma aldosterone level in a female case of pseudohyphoaldosteronism (Liddle's syndrome). *Endocrinol Jpn* 36:167, 1989.
512. Talso PJ et al: Exchangeable potassium as a parameter of body composition. *Metabolism* 9:456, 1960.
513. Talso PJ, Carbello AJ: Effects of benzothiadiazines on serum and total body electrolytes. *Ann NY Acad Sci* 88:882, 1960.
514. Tam SC: Acute hypokalemic effect of Gossypol. *Can J Physiol Pharmacol* 64:881, 1986.
515. Tannen RL: Diuretic-induced hypokalemia. *Kidney Int* 28:988, 1985.
516. Tan SY et al: Impaired renal prostaglandin E_2 biosynthesis in human hypertensive states. *Prostaglandins Med* 1:76, 1978.
517. Tannen RL: The effect of uncomplicated potassium depletion on urine acidification. *J Clin Invest* 49:813, 1970.
518. Tannen RL: Relationship of renal ammonia production and potassium homeostasis. *Kidney Int* 11:453, 1977.

519. Tannen RL: Effect of potassium on renal acidification and acid-base homeostasis. *Semin Nephrol* 7:263, 1987.
520. Textor EG et al: Effects of major cations on gastric and mesenteric vascular resistances. *Am J Physiol* 212:569, 1967.
521. Thomas JP et al: Comparison of thiazides and amiloride in treatment of moderate hypertension. *Br Med J* 286:2015, 1983.
522. Tolins JP: Hypokalemic nephropathy in the rat. Role of ammonia in the chronic tubular injury. *J Clin Invest* 79:1447, 1987.
523. Tomko DJ et al: Bartter's syndrome study of a 52-year-old man with evidence for a defect in proximal tubular sodium reabsorption and comments on therapy. *Am J Med* 61:111, 1976.
524. Torres VE et al: Association of hypokalemia, aldosteronism and renal cysts. *N Engl J Med* 322:345, 1990.
525. Trump DL et al: Watery diarrhea syndrome in an adult with ganglioneuroma-pheochromocytoma. *Cancer* 40: 1526, 1977.
526. Tyson I et al: Studies of potassium depletion using direct measurements of total body potassium. *J Nucl Med* 11:426, 1970.
527. Ulick S et al: A syndrome of apparent mineralocorticoid excess associated with defects in the peripheral metabolism of cortisol. *J Clin Endocrinol Metab* 49:757, 1979.
528. Vaughnjones R et al: Periodic paralysis: Sodium metabolism and aldosterone outpout in two cases. *Lancet* 1:177, 1959.
529. Verberckmoes R et al: Bartter's syndrome with hyperplasia of renomedullary cells: Successful treatment with indomethacin. *Kidney Int* 9:302, 1976.
530. Vinci JM et al: The kallikrein-kinin system in Bartter's syndrome and its response to prostaglandin synthetase inhibition. *J Clin Invest* 61:1671, 1978.
531. Visser HKA et al: Mineralocorticoid excess in two brothers with dwarfism, hypokalemic alkalosis and normal blood pressure. *Acta Endocrinol* 55:661, 1967.
532. Vroom FQ et al: Acetazolamide treatment of hypokalemic periodic paralysis. *Arch Neurol* 32:385, 1975.
533. Wacker WEC, Parisi AF: Magnesium metabolism. *N Engl J Med* 278:658, 712, 1968.
534. Wald MK et al: Bartter's syndrome in early infancy. *Pediatrics* 47:254, 1971.
535. Walker SH, Firminger HI: Familial renal dysplasia with sodium wasting and hypokalemic alkalosis. *Am J Dis Child* 127:882, 1974.
536. Wang C et al: Gossypol and hypokalemia. *Contraception* 32:237, 1985.
537. Warren SE, Steinberg SM: Acid-base and electrolyte disturbances in anorexia nervosa. *Am J Psychol* 136:415, 1979.
538. Webster LT Jr: Studies on the acetyl coenzyme, a synthetase reaction. *J Biol Chem* 241:5504, 1966.
539. Webster MW, Carey LC: Fistulae of the intestinal tract, in *Current Problems in Surgery*, XIII. Chicago, Year Book Medical Publication, June 1976, p 1.
540. Weinberger MH et al: Primary aldosteronism: Diagnosis, localization and treatment. *Ann Intern Med* 90:386, 1979.
541. Weisberg LS et al: Disorders of homeostasis in critically ill patients. *Crit Care Clin* 3:835, 1987.
542. Welt LG et al: The prediction of muscle potassium from blood electrolytes in potassium-depleted rats. *Trans Assoc Am Physicians* 71:250, 1958.
543. Whang R et al: Observations in experimental magnesium deficiency. *J Clin Invest* 42:305, 1963.
544. Whang R et al: The influence of continuing magnesium deficiency on muscle Krepletion. *J Lab Clin Med* 70:895, 1967.
545. Whang R et al: Predictors of clinical hypomagnesemia. *Arch Intern Med* 144:1794, 1984.
546. Whang R et al: Frequency of hypomagnesemia and hypermagnesemia. Requested vs routine. *JAMA* 263:3063, 1990.
547. Whang R, Aikawa JK: Magnesium deficiency and refractoriness to potassium depletion. *J Chronic Dis* 30:65, 1977.
548. Whang R et al: Magnesium and potassium interrelationships experimental and clinical. *Acta Med Scand* 647(suppl):139, 1981.
549. Whinnery MA, Kunau RT Jr: Effect of potassium deficiency on papillary plasma flow in the rat. *Am J Physiol* 237:F226, 1976.
550. White EA et al: Use of computerized tomography in diagnosing the cause of primary aldosteronism. *N Engl J Med* 303:1503, 1980.
551. White MG: Bartter's syndrome: A manifestation of renal tubular defects. *Arch Intern Med* 129:41, 1972.
552. White RH, Schambelan M: Hypertension, hyperreninemia and secondary hyperaldosteronism in systemic necrotizing vasculitis. *Ann Intern Med* 92:199, 1980.
553. Whittam R, Ager ME: The connection between active cation transport and metabolism in erythrocytes. *Biochem J* 97:214, 1965.
554. Widdowson EM, Dickerson JWT: The effect of growth and function on the chemical composition of soft tissues. *Biochem J* 77:30, 1960.
555. Wiederholt M et al: Intracellular potassium in the distal tubule of the adrenalectomized and aldosterone treated rat. *Pflugers Arch* 347:117, 1974.
556. Wiederholt M et al: Effect of aldosterone on sodium and potassium transport in the kidney. *J Steroid Biochem* 3:151, 1972.
557. Wiederholt M et al: Mechanism of action of aldosterone on potassium transfer in the rat kidney. *Pflugers Arch* 345:159, 1973.
558. Wiederholt M et al: Transport of potassium and sodium across single distal tubules of amphiyma. *J Gen Physiol* 57:495, 1971.
559. Wilcox CS et al: Factors affecting potassium balance during furosemide administration. *Clin Sci* 67:195, 1984.
560. Wilkinson PR et al: Total body and serum potassium during prolonged thiazide therapy for essential hypertension. *Lancet* 1:759, 1975.
561. Wilson R, Feldman S: Toxicity of amphotericin B in children with cancer. *Am J Dis Child* 133:731, 1979.
562. Wilson H et al: Changes in the kidney medullary phospholipid metabolism in the potassium-deficient rat. *Am J Pathol* 71:295, 1973.
563. Winkler LF et al: Cisplatin and renal magnesium wasting. *Ann Intern Med* 91:402, 1979.

564. Woods JW et al: Susceptibility of rats to experimental pyelonephritis during potassium depletion. *J Clin Invest* 40:599, 1961.
565. Wright FS: Renal potassium handling. *Semin Nephrol* 7:174, 1987.
566. Wrong O: Incidence of hypokalemia in severe hypertension. *Br Med J* 2:419, 1961.
567. Wu SC et al: Severe hypopotassemia and rhabdomyolysis in a normotensive subject after use of nasal spray containing 9 fluoroprednisolone. *Recent Prog Med* 80:195, 1989.
568. Yazaki K et al: Hypokalemic myopathy associated with 17 -hydroxylase deficiency. *Neurology* 32:94, 1982.
569. Young WG et al: Role of intracellular and extracellular electrolytes in cardiac arrhythmias produced by prolonged hypercalcemia. *Surgery* 36:636, 1954.
570. Zierler KL: Effect of insulin on potassium efflux from rat muscle in the absence and presence of glucose. *Am J Physiol* 198:1066, 1968.
571. Zierler KL: Hyperpolarization of muscle by insulin in a glucose-free environment. *Am J Physiol* 197:524, 1959.
572. Zilva JF, Nicholson JP: Plasma phosphate and potassium levels in the hypercalcemia of malignant disease. *J Clin Endocrinol Metab* 36:1019, 1973.
573. Zipser R et al: The prostaglandin and kallikrein-kinin systems in mineralocorticoid escape. *J Clin Endocrinol Metab* 47:996, 1978.
574. Zusman RM, Keiser HR: Prostaglandin E_2 biosynthesis by rabbit renomedullary interstitial cells in culture. Mechanism of stimulation by angiotensin II, bradykinin, and arginine vasopressin. *J Biol Chem* 252:2069, 1977.

CHAPTER • 23

Clinical disorders of hyperkalemia

Ralph A. DeFronzo • J. Douglas Smith

INTRODUCTION

In the most general sense, hyperkalemia can develop either from a defect in renal potassium excretion or from a shift of potassium from the intracellular fluid to the extracellular fluid. In order to establish a framework for the discussion of the clinical disorders of hyperkalemia, we first briefly review normal renal and extrarenal potassium homeostasis.

DISTRIBUTION OF POTASSIUM (See Chap. 6)

In adult human beings the *total body potassium content* is approximately 500 meq/kg body weight or about 3500 meq for an average 70-kg person,[32,119,177,365] most of which is readily exchangeable. The majority of this potassium is located inside cells (Fig. 23-1), primarily in muscle, and the intracellular potassium concentration varies from 140 to 150 meq/liter. Less than 2 percent of total body potassium is located in the extracellular fluid (ECF), its concentration ranging from 3.5 to 5.0 meq/liter. The high intracellular-to-extracellular potassium concentration gradient is regulated by the Na^+,K^+-ATPase pump,[342,346] and this distribution is modulated by a variety of other factors, including hydrogen ion (H^+) balance, plasma tonicity and plasma insulin, epinephrine, and aldosterone concentrations.[55]

This large difference in plasma *potassium concentration across the cell membrane* is the primary determinant of the resting cell membrane potential, which is approximately −90mV. Even small changes in the intra-

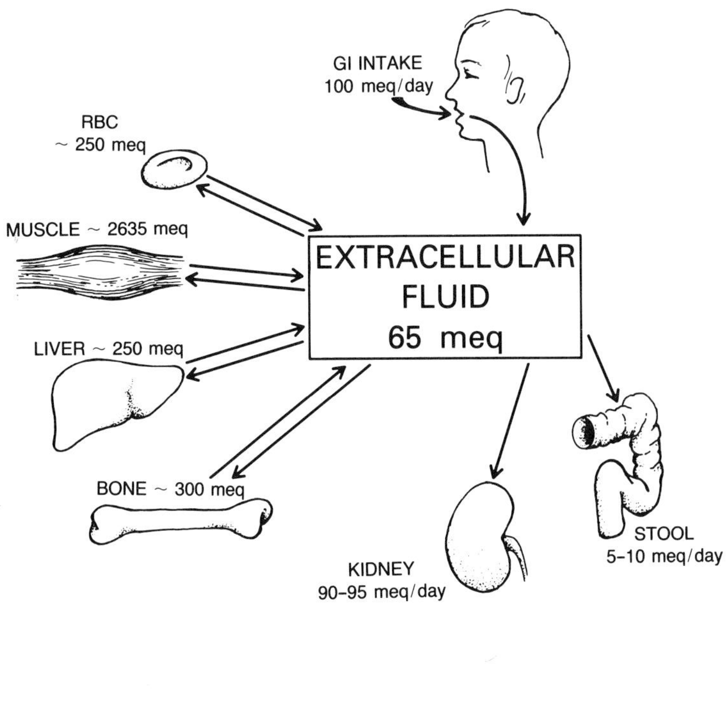

FIGURE 23-1 • Internal and external potassium balance in humans. See text for a more detailed discussion. [Reproduced from Smith JD et al, in Arieff A, DeFronzo RA (eds). *Fluid, Electrolyte, and Acid-Base Disorders*, New York, Churchill Livingstone, 1985, p 413.]

cellular/extracellular potassium ratio can markedly alter this membrane potential and cause severe disturbances in neuromuscular function, particularly of the heart. If renal potassium excretion were impaired and the extracellular potassium content incresed by an amount equal to only 1 percent of the total body potassium content (i.e., 35 meq), the plasma potassium concentration would rise by 50 percent, and this would have pronounced effects on neuromuscular function. Similarly, translocation of a similar amount of potassium from the intracellular (ICF) to the ECF compartment, without net gain or loss of potassium from the body, would have the same effect on neuromuscular excitability. In addition to its vital effect on membrane excitability, cell potassium is important for other fundamental processes. As the major intracellular cation, potassium is an important determinant of the *osmolality* of intracellular fluid. Many *intracellular enzymes* require a high potassium concentration for optimal functioning. *RNA function, protein synthesis, glycogen* formation, and *intracellular pH* have all been shown to have a partial dependence on optimal intracellular potassium concentration in the range of 140 to 150 meq/liter. From these considerations it is obvious that both the total amount of potassium within the body, as well as the distribution of potassium between the ICF and ECF compartments, must be closely regulated within a very narrow range.

Ordinarily the only route of *potassium entry into the body* is via the gastrointestinal tract. The average person consumes approximately 100 meq of potassium per day, and the majority of this is absorbed from the stomach and upper bowel (Fig. 23-1). Approximately 10 meq/day of potassium is excreted in the stool.[265,311] The colonic epithelial cells can secrete potassium, and the factors that regulate potassium secretion by these cells are similar to those which control renal potassium secretion.[35,164] However, their capacity for potassium secretion is limited, and the kidney is the primary organ responsible for the maintenance of *chronic* potassium balance. In contrast, *acute* potassium homeostasis is, in large part, regulated by extrarenal tissues (Fig. 23-2). During the initial 4 to 6 h after potassium administration, only half of the potassium load appears in the urine.[143,145] This is true whether the potassium is given orally[237] or intravenously[143,145,237] and is similar for various species including man,[143,145,237] dog,[143] and rat.[147] If all of the administered potassium that was not excreted was retained within the ECF compartment, the plasma concentration would reach life-threatening levels. This does not occur since the great majority, approximately 80 percent of the retained potassium load, is translocated into the cells. The stimulation of cellular potassium uptake is an intrinsic property of the Na^+,K^+-ATPase pump, which is stimulated by small increases in the plasma potassium concentration.[115,153,154,192,525] Insulin and the sympathetic nervous system also play important roles in regulating the activity of the Na^+,K^+-ATPase pump and in facilitating the movement of potassium into the cell.[115,153,154]

EXTRARENAL POTASSIUM HOMEOSTASIS (See Chap. 6)

As discussed above, nonrenal tissues, primarily muscle and liver, play a major role in the maintenance of acute potassium tolerance because of their enormous capacity to translocate potassium into cellular compartments. The three major factors that regulate normal cellular potassium uptake are *hormones* (insulin, catecholamines, aldosterone), *acid-base status*, and *plasma tonicity*. In

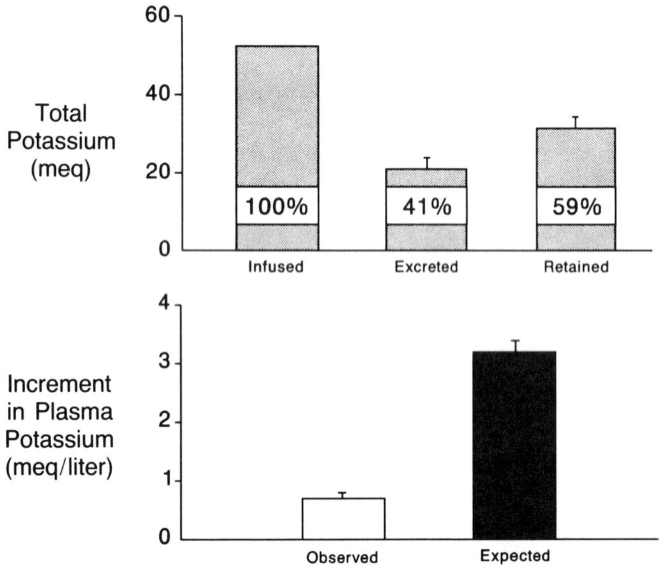

FIGURE 23-2 • Renal and extrarenal distribution of an intravenously infused potassium load (0.75 meq/kg) in healthy young subjects. During the 4 to 6 h following administration of KCl, approximately 40 percent of the infused potassium was excreted. If all of the retained potassium remained in the extracellular fluid compartment, marked hyperkalemia would have ensued. This did not occur since ~75 percent of the retained potassium was translocated into cells. (Drawn from the data presented in DeFronzo RA et al: *J Clin Invest* 61:472, 1978.)

the daily minute-to-minute regulation of potassium distribution among these compartments, only insulin and catecholamines play an important role.[143,147,153,154] However, under pathophysiologic conditions, changes in acid-base status and plasma osmolality can have profound effects on the plasma potassium concentration (see subsequent discussion).

INSULIN

Insulin is the most important regulator of extrarenal potassium homeostasis because of its role in a closed feedback loop that prevents the plasma potassium concentration from rising to excessively high levels (Fig. 23-3). When the plasma potassium concentration increases by more than 1.0 to 1.5 mmol/liter, a twofold to threefold increase in peripheral insulin levels is observed.[162,274,424,472] Consistent with this, in vitro studies have demonstrated that potassium directly stimulates insulin secretion by the pancreas.[173,236,248] If dogs are pancreatectomized before the administration of KCl, a marked deterioration in potassium tolerance and lethal cardiac toxicity ensues.[274,275,424,426,472] If pancreatectomized animals are given exogenous insulin along with the KCl, potassium tolerance is restored to normal.[274,275]

Although smaller, more physiologic increments in the plasma potassium concentration (0.3 to 0.7 mmol/liter) fail to elicit a measurable increase in circulating plasma insulin levels[143,145,147,149,355,401] (Fig. 23-4), the hormone still can be shown to play a permissive role in the basal regulation of extrarenal potassium metabolism.

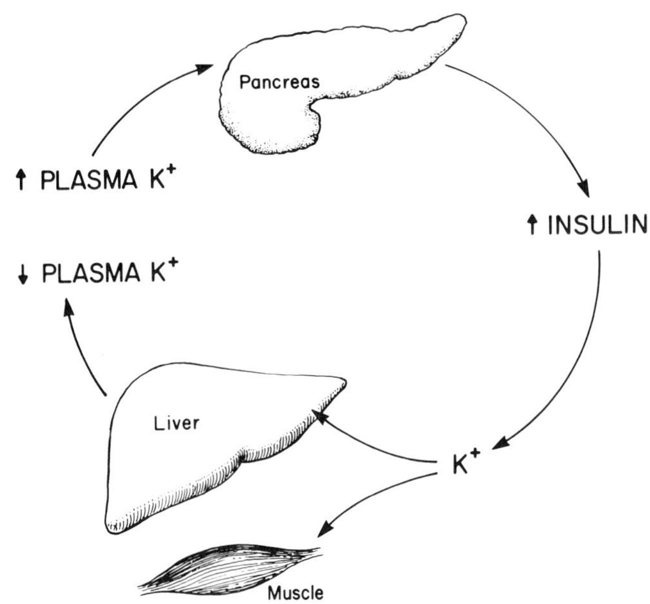

FIGURE 23-3 • Feedback loop relating changes in plasma potassium concentration to changes in insulin secretion by the beta cell. [Reproduced from DeFronzo RA, in Giebisch G (ed): *Current Topics in Membranes and Transport*, 1987, p 299.]

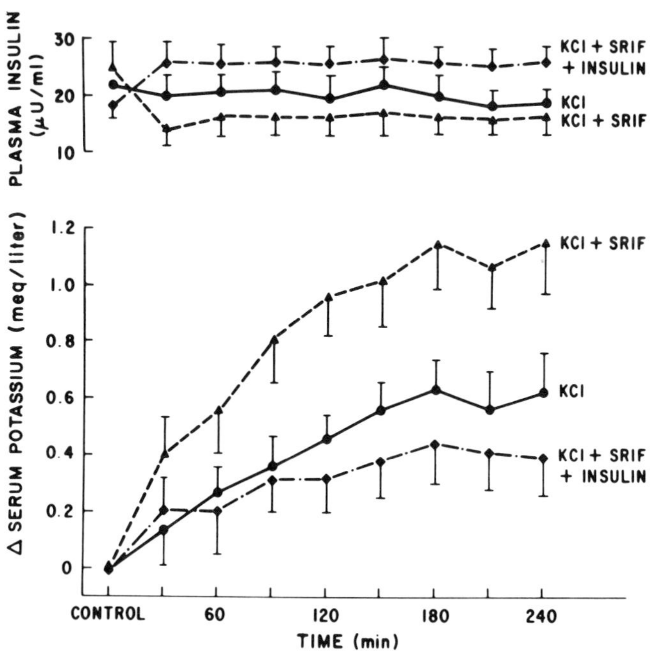

FIGURE 23-4 • The effect of potassium chloride (KCl) infusion alone (solid circles), KCl plus somatostatin (SRIF) infusion (solid triangles), and KCl plus SRIF plus insulin (solid triangles) on the plasma insulin concentration and the change in serum potassium concentration in dogs. (Reproduced from DeFronzo RA et al: *J Clin Invest* 61:472, 1978.)

Thus, if KCl is infused to raise the plasma potassium concentration by only 0.5 to 0.6 mmol/liter while basal insulin secretion is inhibited by somatostatin, the increase in plasma potassium concentration is twofold to threefold greater than if the basal insulin concentration is maintained (Fig. 23-4). Somatostatin infusion with basal insulin replacement restores potassium tolerance to normal (Fig. 23-4). These results emphasize the permissive importance of basal insulin levels in the minute-to-minute regulation of potassium distribution. The role of basal insulin secretion is further emphasized by studies performed in normal humans.[143] When somatostatin is infused to inhibit insulin release, the basal plasma potassium increases by 0.5 to 0.7 mmol/liter, and this is reversed by an exogenous insulin infusion designed to maintain fasting insulin levels constant. These observations have been confirmed both in humans[401] and in dogs,[424] and have been shown to be independent of the kidneys.[143,274,275]

Muscle, liver, and fat represent the major insulin-responsive tissues in human beings. Zierler and Rabinowitz[620] and Andres et al.[16] have shown that both the deep (muscle) and superficial (skin and adipose) forearm tissues in humans participate in potassium uptake following insulin infusion into the brachial artery. Moreover, this effect is independent of glucose uptake. Numerous in vitro and in vivo studies have documented that insulin causes a net uptake of potassium by both skeletal[111,115,244,617,621] and cardiac[115,446,458] muscle, as well as by adipose tissue,[111,115,243] and that this effect of insulin is independent of its effect on glucose metabolism.[98,115,617,621]

As initially demonstrated by Fenn,[189] the liver also plays an important role in potassium disposal following hyperinsulinemia. This effect has been confirmed in subsequent studies using the isolated perfused dog[299] and rat[378] liver. More recently, the important role of the liver in maintaining extrarenal potassium homeostasis has been quantitated in human beings.[146]

The cellular mechanism(s) by which insulin enhances potassium and glucose uptake are depicted in Fig. 23-5. In order for insulin to act, it must first bind to a specific receptor on the cell surface. Prior exposure of cells to the proteolytic enzyme trypsin completely obliterates the effect of insulin on ion transport and membrane potential.[450] Once insulin binds to its receptor, the cell membrane becomes hyperpolarized,[115,153,154,200,617] an effect occurring within seconds to minutes.[624] The change in membrane potential cannot be explained by an increase in ratio of intracellular to extracellular potassium since insulin-induced hyperpolarization precedes any detectable increase in the intracellular potassium concentration.[200,372,618,622] Evidence has been provided to show that the hyperpolarizing action of insulin results both from a decrease in the ratio of sodium to potassium permeability[622] as well as from a stimulation of the Na^+-K^+ pump.[115] The resultant hyperpolarization is sufficient to account for the net cellular accumulation of potassium by passive distribution, in accord with the electrical gradient caused by sodium efflux.

Activation of the Na^+,K^+-ATPase pump is intimately related to insulin's ability to stimulate potassium transport.[115,153,154] However, the second messenger that mediates this effect has yet to be identified. There is no evidence that cyclic adenosine monophosphate (AMP) is involved in this action.[372] This is quite distinct from epinephrine (see subsequent discussion), where it is clear that cyclic AMP generation regulates the catecholamine-mediated increase in potassium transport.[115] The most likely candidate for the second messenger of insulin action is the insulin receptor itself. Recent studies[289,295] suggest that insulin binding is associated with phosphorylation of its own receptor, which, in turn, alters the lipid matrix and fluidity of the plasma membrane[13,303] and stimulates glucose transport. Alternatively, Zierler and others[372,623] have suggested that hyperpolarization per se may account for some of the actions of insulin, including the increase in potassium influx and the stimulation of glucose transport.

CATECHOLAMINES

Studies by DeFronzo et al.,[147,149,153,154] as well as by Rosa et al.[460] and Brown,[89] have emphasized the importance of catecholamines in the normal regulation of extrarenal potassium metabolism in humans. When epinephrine is administered with KCl, the increase in potassium concentration is markedly attenuated (Fig. 23-6).[147,149,460] The effect of epinephrine on extrarenal potassium metabolism can be completely blocked by the simultaneous infusion of propranolol, indicat-

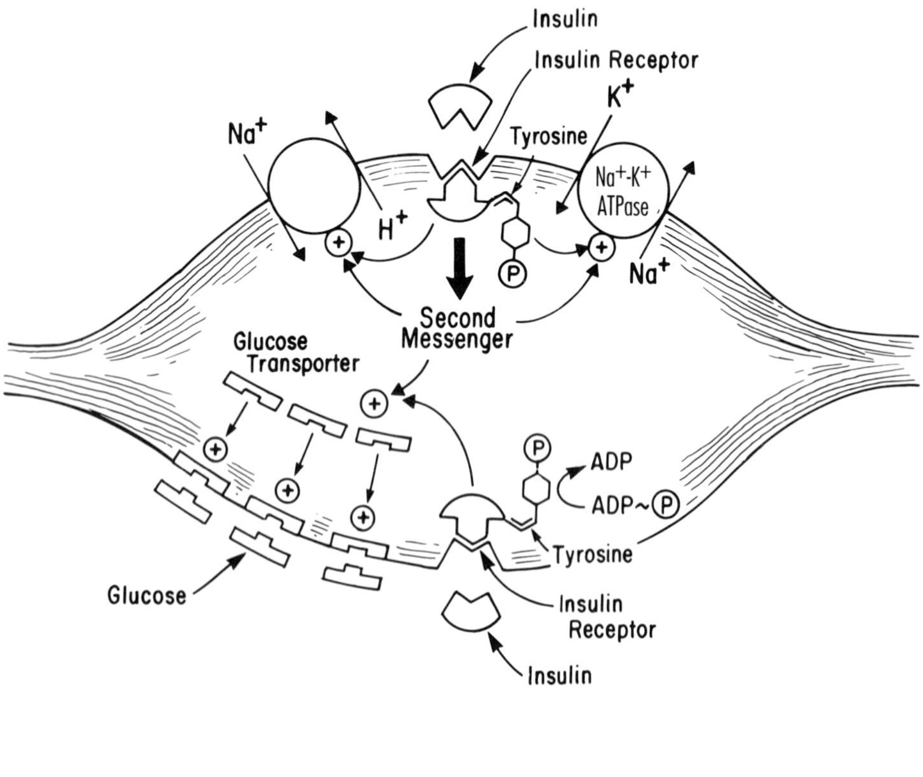

FIGURE 23-5 • Schematic representation of the cellular mechanisms via which insulin stimulates potassium and glucose uptake by extrarenal tissues. [Reproduced from DeFronzo RA, in Giebisch G (ed): *Current Topics in Membranes and Transport*, 1987, p 299.]

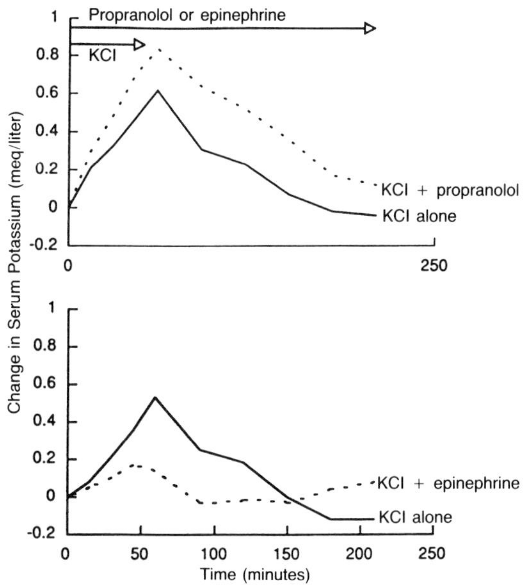

FIGURE 23-6 • Effect of epinephrine and propranolol on the increment in serum potassium during the infusion of potassium chloride (KCl) in normal humans. Beta-adrenergic stimulation blocked the expected rise in serum potassium, whereas beta blockade had the opposite effect. (Redrawn from Rosa RM et al: *N Engl J Med* 302:431, 1980.)

ing that the action of epinephrine is mediated via the beta-receptor.[147,149,460] As with insulin, the simple maintenance of basal epinephrine activity appears to be necessary for the maintenance of normal potassium homeostasis.[147,149,460] If potassium is administered after the beta-adrenergic receptor has been blocked, extrarenal potassium tolerance decreases (Fig. 23-6).[147] These results underscore the important role of catecholamines in the modulation of potassium uptake by extrarenal tissues.

The improvement in extrarenal potassium tolerance following epinephrine results from enhanced muscle[55,112,115,134,170,183,266,335,572] and liver[55,170,335,572] potassium uptake. Epinephrine-mediated potassium uptake by extrarenal tissues can be completely reversed by nonselective beta-blockers or selective beta 2-antagonists.[55,59,102,115,153,154,170,335,554,572] Thus, the stimulatory effect of the beta-adrenergic agonists is mediated via the beta 2 receptor (Table 23-1).[59,102,115,153,154] Beta 1-adrenergic agonists do not affect potassium metabolism by extrarenal tissues.[55,59,153,335,554]

The alpha-adrenergic receptor also plays an important role in extrarenal potassium tolerance.[89,598] Thus, alpha agonists have been shown to impair potassium tolerance without any effect on renal potassium excretion. It is possible that the deleterious effect of beta-adrenergic blockade on potassium metabolism is mediated, in part, by a relative excess of alpha-adrenergic activity.

Recent studies underscore the importance of the adrenergic nervous system in the maintenance of normal extrarenal potassium homeostasis.[56,147,153,154,504,533a] In normal humans,[56,149] inhibition of basal epinephrine activity with propranolol causes a small but significant increase in plasma potassium levels due to impaired extrarenal potassium tolerance, and this effect is accentuated in diabetic[506] and uremic[103] patients. The deleterious effect of beta-blockade on extrarenal potassium metabolism is independent of changes in urinary potassium excretion or plasma aldosterone levels.[59,533a] However, concomitant defects in the secretion and/or action of other hormones (i.e., insulin, aldosterone) involved in extrarenal potassium homeostasis have been shown to amplify any existing deficiency of plasma epinephrine levels.[147,504] This is most likely to occur in the insulin-dependent (type 1) diabetic who may have both autonomic neuropathy (epinephrine and sympathetic nervous system deficiency) and aldosterone deficiency (the syndrome of hyporeninemic hypoaldosteronism) (see subsequent discussion). Likewise, defects in extrarenal potassium homeostasis also commonly occur in individuals who have renal disease and therefore have a limited capacity to excrete potassium. Thus, both diabetic nephropathy and chronic interstitial renal disease[148] commonly are associated with the syndrome of hypoaldosteronism and insulin deficiency and/or resistance; these abnormalities, in concert with the decrease in renal

TABLE 23-1 • Effect of beta- and alpha-adrenergic agonists and antagonists on plasma potassium concentration

Catecholamine specificity	Effect on plasma potassium concentration*
Beta 1 + beta 2 agonist (epinephrine, isoproterenol)	Decrease
Pure beta 1 agonist (ITP)	None
Pure beta 2 agonist (salbutamol, soterenol, terbutaline)	Decrease
Beta 1 + beta 2 antagonist (propranol, sotalol)	Increase; blocks effect of beta agonists
Beta antagonist (practolol, metoprolol, atenolol)	None; does not block effect of beta agonists
Beta 2 antagonist (butoxamine, H 35/25)	Blocks hypokalemic effect of beta agonists
Alpha antagonist (phenoxybenzamine)	None; blocks effect of alpha agonist

* Results refer to the late (after 5 min), sustained effect.
ITP = 1,isopropylamino-3-(2-thiazoloxy)-2-propanol.
SOURCE: Modified from Smith JD et al, in Arieff A, DeFronzo RA (eds): *Fluid, Electrolyte, and Acid-Base Disorders*, New York, Churchill Livingstone, 1985, p 413.

function per se, strongly predispose to episodes of hyperkalemia.

ALDOSTERONE

Aldosterone plays a critical role in the regulation of renal potassium excretion (see review by Young[613]). However, less well appreciated is its effect on extrarenal potassium metabolism. It is well established that the colon responds to mineralocorticoids by increasing potassium secretion.[35,105,164,268,454] When aldosterone is administered to normal human subjects, there is a decrease in sodium concentration and a simultaneous increase in potassium concentration in saliva, sweat, and stool.[105,123,171,507] Although some controversy exists concerning the effect of aldosterone on muscle, a number of in vivo[123,606] and in vitro[2] studies have demonstrated enhanced cellular uptake of potassium in response to mineralocorticoids. Dawborn and Watson[137] in rabbits, Alexander and Levinsky[9] in rats, and Loeb et al.[336] in dogs also have provided evidence for an important role of aldosterone on extrarenal potassium metabolism in vivo. Studies in patients with selective hypoaldosteronism also provide support for an extrarenal effect of mineralocorticoids.[148] The most convincing evidence comes from the studies of Young and Jackson[612,613] in dogs and DeFronzo et al. in rats.[56,147] In an elegant series of studies performed in adrenalectomized dogs, the former investigators demonstrated that for any given level of total body (exchangeable) potassium, the plasma potassium concentration was inversely related to the aldosterone replacement dose (Fig. 23-7); the higher the plasma aldosterone concentration, the greater the amount of the total body potassium that resided within the cells.

HYPERTONICITY (See Chap. 21)

Plasma tonicity plays an important role in maintaining the normal distribution of potassium between intracellular and extracellular compartments,[63,125,301,348,349,373,461,462,499,547,605] and hypertonicity of the ECF is a common cause of hyperkalemia. In principle, an increase in the plasma tonicity could draw potassium out of cells by two interrelated mechanisms. First, as water is forced out of cells by the osmotic pressure gradient, potassium will be entrained in the resulting convective current and will exit cells in proportion to its membrane permeability, given by its reflection coefficient. Second, because the reflection coefficient for potassium is <1, potassium will exit less readily than water. As a result, the intracellular potassium concentration will rise, establishing an outward concentration gradient for potassium exit via diffusion through potassium channels. The impact of changes in the serum tonicity assumes added importance when coexisting abnormalities in potassium homeostatic mechanisms exist, such as insulin or aldosterone deficiency. These clinical syndromes will be discussed in detail below.

Bratusch-Marrain and DeFronzo[75,321] have examined the relationship between the plasma tonicity and plasma potassium levels in healthy young volunteers who participated in three infusion protocols; isotonic saline, isotonic mannitol, and hypertonic mannitol. In the first two studies, plasma tonicity remained constant and plasma potassium levels did not change from baseline (Fig. 23-8). In the third study plasma osmolality increased from 283 to 300 mosm/kg and plasma potassium increased from 4.4 to 5.2 mmol/liter ($p < 0.01$) without any change in circulating insulin levels and despite a marked increase in renal potassium secretion. These results clearly demonstrate that even modest increments in plasma tonicity of a magnitude commonly encountered in clinical practice can have major effects on internal potassium balance.

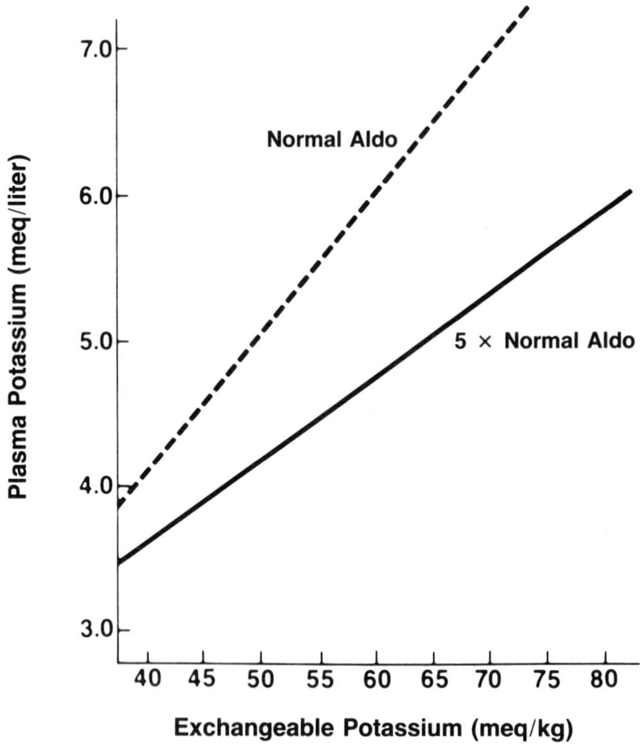

FIGURE 23-7 • Effect of a chronic, sustained increment in plasma aldosterone concentration on total body exchangeable potassium (horizontal axis) and the plasma potassium concentration (vertical axis) in dogs. For any given level of exchangeable potassium, less potassium resided in the extracellular compartment, as demonstrated by a lower plasma potassium concentration. (Reproduced from Young DB: *Am J Physiol* 255:F811, 1988.)

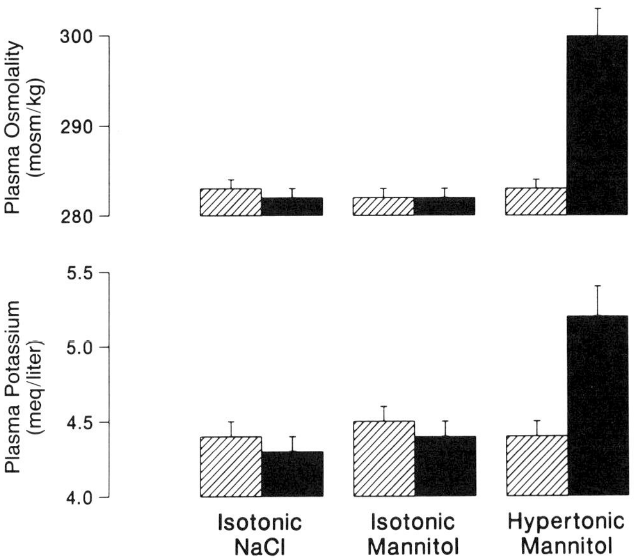

FIGURE 23-8 • Effect of changes in plasma tonicity on the plasma potassium concentration in normal subjects. (Drawn from the data of Bratusch-Marrain P, DeFronzo RA: *Diabetes* 32:1028, 1983 and reproduced from Kurtzman NA et al: *Am J Kidney Dis* 15:333, 1990.)

ACID-BASE BALANCE (See Chap. 24)

Changes in acid-base balance exert a major influence on extrarenal as well as renal potassium homeostasis.[97,505] Metabolic acidosis increases, whereas metabolic alkalosis decreases the plasma potassium concentration. The hyperkalemic effect of metabolic acidosis results from two mechanisms: (1) inhibition of potassium secretion by the distal tubule, by directly reducing the activity of the basolateral Na^+-K^+ ATPase pump, and lowering luminal potassium permeability; and (2) shift of potassium from the ICF to the ECF as H^+ ions move into cells to be buffered.[3,97,505] The same two processes occur in metabolic alkalosis, but in the opposite direction. In contrast to metabolic disturbances, which can elicit a pronounced increase in the potassium concentration (0.5 to 1.2 mmol/liter), respiratory disorders have little effect.[4,491] The reason for this discrepancy is not well understood.

RENAL REGULATION OF POTASSIUM EXCRETION (See Chap. 7)

Micropuncture studies[350,351,447,522,608] have demonstrated that most of the potassium that appears in the final urine is derived from the distal nephron (mid-to-late distal tubule and collecting duct). Although some 600 to 700 meq of potassium are filtered by the glomerulus each day, the majority is reabsorbed and only 10 percent remains by the early distal tubule (Fig. 23-9). This percentage stays constant despite maneuvers that either increase or decrease the rate of final urinary potassium excretion.[223,225,226,522] Approximately 70 to 75 percent of the filtered potassium is reabsorbed by the end of the proximal tubule.[223,225,226,522,608] Under normal conditions alterations in the filtered load of potassium and in proximal tubular potassium reabsorption do not contribute to the regulation of external potassium homeostasis. However, if an osmotic diuresis is induced with either mannitol or glucose, potassium reabsorption by the prox-

FIGURE 23-9 • Schematic representation of the renal tubular handling of potassium. Essentially all filtered potassium is reabsorbed by the early to mid distal tubule. Most of the potassium that appears in the final urine is derived from secretion by the late distal tubule and early collecting tubule. PCT: proximal convoluted tubule. P1, P2, P3: sequential segments of the proximal tubule. LOH: loop of Henle. TAL: thick ascending limb. DCT: distal convoluted tubule. CNT: cortical connecting tubule. CCD: cortical collecting duct. OMCD: outer medullary collecting duct. IMCD: inner medullary collecting duct.

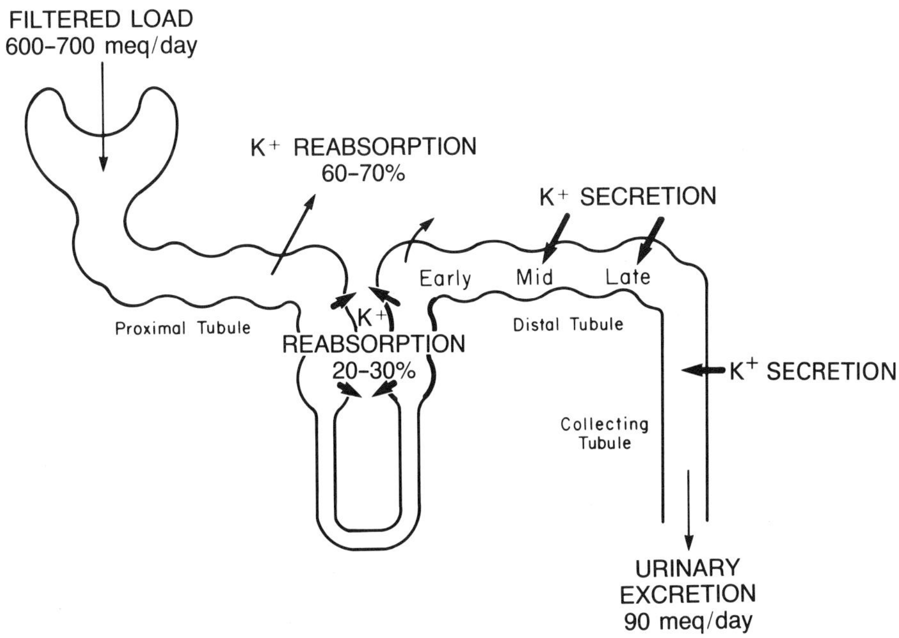

imal tubule is diminished and delivery to the loop of Henle, distal tubule, and collecting tubule is increased.[351,445] This overwhelms the transport capacity of the distal nephron sites where potassium is reabsorbed and a significant kaliuresis results. Micropuncture studies have demonstrated that an additional 20 to 25 percent of the filtered potassium load is reabsorbed by the time the tubular fluid reaches the first accessible segment of the distal tubule. The fraction of filtered potassium reaching the early distal tubule (10 percent) is quite constant despite a 200-fold variation in final urine potassium excretion.[223,225,522] In vitro microperfusion studies have documented that both the proximal straight tubule[93] and thick ascending limb of Henle's loop[94] can reabsorb significant amounts of potassium. Although potassium normally is absorbed by the cortical and medullary segments of the thick ascending limb of Henle, potassium secretion by these segments can be demonstrated following the administration of loop diuretics and after an increase in the potassium concentration in the peritubular fluid.[394,396]

Jamison and colleagues[43,288] have provided evidence that potassium is added to the descending limb of Henle's loop, presumably recycled from interstitial potassium derived from reabsorption across the medullary and papillary collecting ducts.[43,165,288] Stokes has suggested that this high interstitial potassium concentration may serve to block sodium reabsorption in the medullary thick ascending limb, leading to the delivery of more sodium and fluid to those more distal nephron sites which are responsible for potassium secretion.[538]

The late distal nephron segments (late distal tubule, initial collecting tubule, and cortical collecting duct) represent the major sites of potassium addition to the tubular fluid.[223,225,226,350,351,447,522,608] Since cells of the cortical collecting duct are morphologically similar to those of the distal tubule, it is not surprising that both of these nephron segments are capable of net potassium secretion.[223,225,226,246,270,448,449,522,608] Controversy exists concerning the ability of the medullary outer collecting duct to secrete potassium. However, recent studies have indicated that this nephron segment can secrete potassium, albeit at a low rate.[198,222,277,484]

A schematic representation of the cellular mechanisms involved in distal tubular potassium secretion is shown in Fig. 23-10. This diagram represents the composite of data gathered from micropuncture, microperfusion, and other techniques; the reader is referred to several excellent reviews for a more comprehensive treatment of this subject.[222-226,522,526] The salient features of this model are as follows:

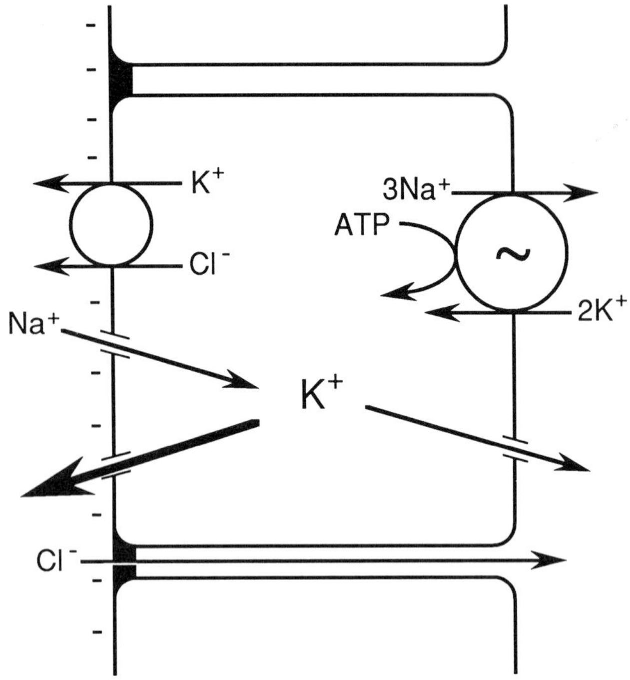

FIGURE 23-10 • **Schematic representation of potassium secretion by an individual principal cell. The tubular lumen is oriented to the left of the diagram. Paracellular chloride reabsorption is shown proceeding through a tight junction. (See text for a more detailed discussion.)**

1. The *luminal (apical) membrane is electronegatively charged* by approximately 50 mV compared with the peritubular (basolateral) membrane. This negative potential is generated by active sodium reabsorption. Sodium transport and the lumen-negative transepithelial voltage are inhibited by amiloride in the tubular fluid and by oubain on the basolateral side.
2. There is an *active pump located in the peritubular membrane* which transports potassium into the cell against a large concentration gradient.
3. Potassium transport by the active pump is coupled to *sodium transport*, and the integrity of the pump is intimately related to the enzyme Na^+,K^+-ATPase.
4. The Na^+,K^+-ATPase pump is strongly dependent upon the *plasma aldosterone* concentration.[192,524,528,529] Aldosterone deficiency impairs potassium secretion while aldosterone excess increases potassium secretion.
5. The activity of the Na^+,K^+-ATPase pump is exquisitely sensitive to small increases in the *potassium concentration* in the surrounding peritubular capillaries;[192,525] hyperkalemia provides a potent stimulus to enhance potassium secretion.
6. The activity of the Na^+,K^+-ATPase pump is directly influenced by changes in *acid-base status. Acute metabolic acidosis* inhibits, whereas acute metabolic alkalosis stimulates potassium secretion. With *chronic metabolic acidosis*,[219] potassium excretion usually increases because of the inhibition of proximal tubular salt and water reabsorption and enhanced sodium and fluid delivery to the distal sites of potassium secretion. If distal tubular flow and sodium delivery rate are held constant, a persistent

inhibitory effect of metabolic acidosis on distal potassium secretion can be demonstrated.[522] *Respiratory acidosis* and *alkalosis* have little effect on potassium secretion by the distal tubule.[352]

7. After *potassium enters the renal tubular cell*, it may either diffuse back into the capillary blood or enter the tubular lumen. The electrical gradient, lumen negative, provides the driving force for the net secretion of potassium into the tubular fluid through specific potassium selective channels.[207,208] If the sodium conductance (which is responsible for the generation of the negative potential) of the luminal membrane is blocked with amiloride, the membrane becomes hyperpolarized and potassium secretion declines.[397,399,526]
8. Potassium also can be secreted by a *paracellular pathway* that is primarily conductive to chloride (Fig. 23-10) and is driven by the lumen-negative transepithelial voltage. However, it is likely that this paracellular pathway accounts for no more than 10 to 15 percent of total potassium secretion, since the majority (85 percent) of potassium secretion can be inhibited by barium, a potent potassium channel blocker.[381]
9. Both increased *sodium delivery*, as well as increased *urine flow*, independent of sodium delivery,[237,300,318,350] stimulate potassium secretion by the distal nephron segments.
10. Potassium secretion by the distal nephron is inhibited by *beta-adrenergic* agonists and stimulated by beta-adrenergic antagonists.[149,151,296] Although epinephrine inhibits potassium secretion by the cortical collecting duct[151] and renal potassium secretion declines,[149] the plasma potassium concentration falls because of the quantitatively greater effect on extrarenal potassium uptake.[59,149]
11. *Arginine vasopressin* augments potassium secretion by the distal nephron,[193,515] but the clinical significance of this is unclear since marked changes in urinary flow brought about by ADH administration have no effect on urinary potassium excretion.
12. A *potassium reabsorptive mechanism* exists in the late distal tubule and/or collecting tubule since urinary potassium excretion can approach zero despite delivery of 5 to 10 percent of the filtered load to the early distal tubule. The cells responsible for potassium reabsorption most likely are different from those which are responsible for potassium secretion. Stimulation of potassium secretion is associated with a marked increase in the basolateral membrane area of the principal cells[523,576] in the initial portion of the cortical collecting tubule, suggesting an increase in the number of Na^+,K^+-ATPase pumps. The cells in the first portion of the cortical collecting tubule are morphologically similar to those in the late distal tubule. Potassium depletion did not affect principal cell histology, but caused a marked increase in the luminal membrane area of the intercalated cells.[523,534] These results suggest that the cells responsible for potassium secretion (principal cells) are different from those that are responsible for potassium reabsorption (intercalated cells). *Insulin* augments renal potassium reabsorption,[468] possibly through an effect on the intercalated cells.

HYPERKALEMIA: CLINICAL DISORDERS (Table 23-2)

Over 90 percent of healthy individuals with normal renal and adrenal function have serum potassium concentrations less than 5.0 meq/liter; values in excess of 5.3 meq/liter are distinctly uncommon.[150,600] Persistently elevated serum potassium levels in excess of 5.3 meq/liter should suggest an abnormality in the mechanisms responsible for the maintenance of normal potassium homeostasis. In two large series of hospitalized patients, 1.2 and 1.4 percent of all admissions had serum potassium concentrations above 6.0 meq/liter, and in 10 percent the level exceeded 5.3 percent at some time during their hospital stay.[403,503]

True hyperkalemia may develop either from a *shift of potassium from intracellular to extracellular compartments* or from a *decreased renal excretion of potassium* (Fig. 23-11). In the presence of normal renal and adrenal function it is distinctly uncommon to observe sustained, chronic hyperkalemia (> 5.3 meq/liter) from an increased input of potassium into the body. The workup of the patient with hyperkalemia can be approached in a logical sequence if one is cognizant of the clinical categories listed in Table 23-2. before an extensive and costly investigation, the serum potassium concentration should be repeated to verify the presence of hyperkalemia. Measurement of the plasma potassium concentration by flame photometry is extremely reliable, and laboratory errors are uncommon. If the repeat potassium concentration is elevated, the more obvious causes of hyperkalemia (1 to 5 in Table 23-2) should be excluded.

PSEUDOHYPERKALEMIA

Pseudohyperkalemia represents an in vitro phenomenon, which results from potassium release by erythrocytes, leukocytes, or platelets during the clotting process.[47,84,201,245,259,264] It may be seen in patients with marked elevations in the circulating white blood cell (> 100,000 per cubic millimeter) or platelet (1,000,000 per cubic millimeter) count. A recent study[245] found significant pseudohyperkalemia in 34 percent of individuals with a platelet count greater than 500,000 per cubic millimeter. The rise in serum potassium concentration

TABLE 23-2 • Etiology of hyperkalemia

1. Factitious
    - Laboratory error
    - Pseudohyperkalemia—in vitro hemolysis, thrombocytosis, leukocytosis, familial
2. Acidemia-metabolic
3. Increased input
    - Exogenous: diet, salt substitutes, low-sodium diet, medications
    - Endogenous: hemolysis, GI bleeding, catabolic states, crush injury, tumorlysis
4. Inadequate distal delivery of sodium and decreased distal tubular flow
5. Renal failure
    - Acute: especially tubulointerstitial disease
    - Chronic: GFR < 15–20 ml/min
6. Impaired renin-aldosterone axis
    - Addison's disease
    - Adrenal enzyme deficiencies (21 hydroxylase, 11 hydroxylase, corticosterone methyl oxidase)
    - Primary hypoaldosteronism (normal renin)
    - Hyporeninemic hypoaldosteronism
    - Angiotensin deficiency or insensitivity
    - Drug-induced (heparin, beta blockers, prostaglandin inhibitors, angiotensin convertying enzyme inhibitors, pentamidine)
7. Primary renal tubular potassium secretory defect
    - Sickle cell disease
    - Systemic lupus erythematosus
    - Postrenal transplantation
    - Obstructive uropathy
    - Tubulointerstitial renal diseases

TABLE 23-2 • *(continued)*

- Pseudohypoaldosteronism
    - Type I pseudohypoaldosteronism of infancy
    - Type II pseudohypoaldosteronism in adults with hypertension
    - Type III pseudohypoaldosteronism in adults without hypertension
    - Hyperkalemic distal renal tubular acidosis
8. Inhibition of tubular secretion
    - Spironolactone
    - Triamterene
    - Amiloride
    - Digitalis
    - Cyclosporine
    - Lithium
9. Abnormal potassium distribution
    - Acidosis-metabolic
    - Insulin deficiency
    - Hypertonicity (hyperglycemia)
    - Aldosterone deficiency
    - Beta-adrenergic antagonists
    - Alpha-adrenergic agonists
    - Exercise
    - Periodic paralysis—hyperkalemic type
    - Tissue damage
    - Succinylcholine
    - Digitalis
    - Arginine hydrochloride, lysine hydrochloride

SOURCE: Modified from Smith JD et al, in Arieff A, DeFronzo RA (eds): *Fluid, Electrolyte, and Acid-Base Disorders*, New York, Churchill Livingstone, 1985, p 413.

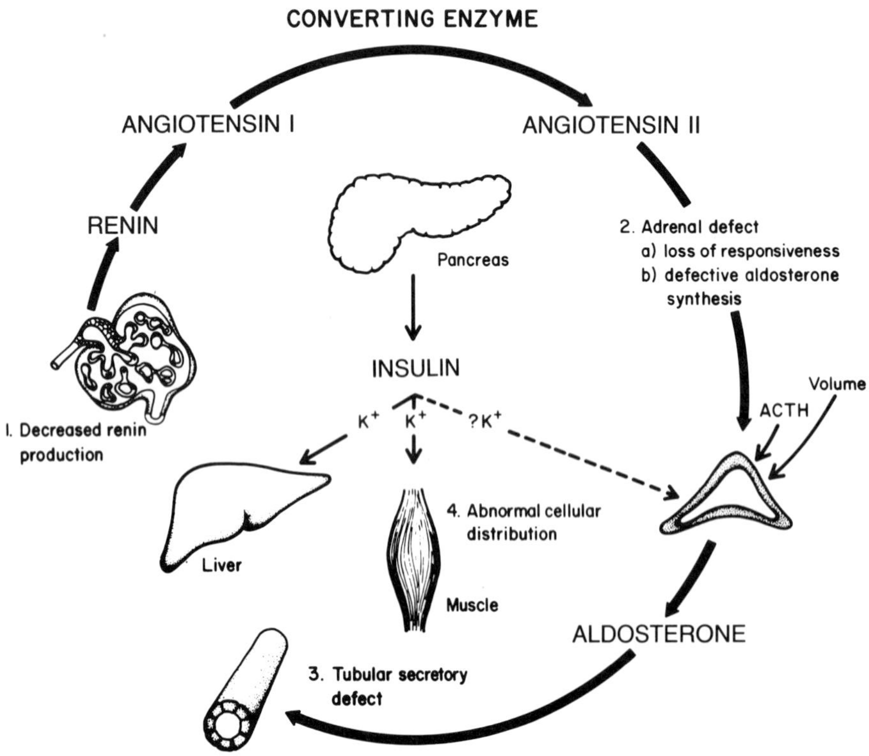

FIGURE 23-11 • Schematic representation of potential hormonal, renal, and extrarenal defects resulting in hyperkalemia. Hyperkalemia may result as a consequence of the following: (1) decreased renin production; (2) decreased aldosterone production despite normal renin secretion (adrenal defect); (3) a renal tubular secretory defect; (4) an abnormal distribution of potassium between intracellular and extracellular fluid compartments. [Reproduced from Smith JD et al, in Arieff A, DeFronzo RA (eds): *Fluid, Electrolyte, and Acid-Base Disorders*, New York, Churchill Livingstone, 1985, p 413.]

was directly related to the increase in platelet count. A similar phenomenon may be observed in patients with increased red blood cell fragility (i.e., hereditary spherocytosis) or abnormalities in the erythrocyte membrane (i.e., acanthocytosis), or with red cell enzyme defects. Simultaneous determination of the plasma (i.e., unclotted) and serum (i.e., clotted) potassium concentration should agree within 0.2 to 0.3 meq/liter. If these determinations differ by more than 0.3 meq/liter, the presence of pseudohyperkalemia should be suspected. Tight tourniquet application in combination with excessive arm exercise prior to venipuncture may also cause a spurious elevation in potassium concentration.[509]

Most recently, pseudohyperkalemia has been described as a familial disturbance characterized by disordered cation transport in erythrocyte membranes.[4,30,68,520] When red blood cells from these patients are left at room temperature, potassium leaks out because of an abnormality in passive potassium and sodium permeability.

ACIDEMIA

Acidemia, especially of metabolic origin, is a well-established cause of hyperkalemia. Two mechanisms are involved: (1) acutely, acidemia directly inhibits potassium secretion by the distal tubule and collecting duct cells.[347,352,367] However, with chronic acidemia proximal tubular fluid and salt reabsorption are inhibited and the resultant increase in urine flow and sodium delivery[225,238] to the distal nephron augments potassium secretion. The net result of these two opposing effects is an increase in distal tubular potassium secretion and a decrease in total body potassium content; (2) nonetheless, unless the magnitude of total body potassium depletion is severe, hyperkalemia will still result from the shift of potassium from the intracellular to the extracellular space as H^+ ions move into cells to be buffered.[3,97,505] Some textbooks state that for every 0.1 unit decrease in blood pH, the serum potassium concentration will increase by 0.5 to 0.6 meq/liter. This relationship was derived from the data of Burnell et al.[97] However, the number of patients in this study was small and the change in serum potassium concentration for each 0.1 unit change in pH was quite variable (0.3 to 1.3 meq/liter), and Burnell and his coworkers warned against generalizing from their results.[97] Some reports[4,419] suggest that the relationship between blood pH and serum potassium concentration during metabolic acidosis is even more variable than initially suggested by Burnell et al.[97] Thus, in some patients marked decreased in blood pH are not accompanied by any change in serum potassium level whereas in other patients much larger increases in serum potassium concentration (1.5 to 2.0 meq/liter) have been reported.[419] These observations indicate that the relationship between changes in blood pH and plasma potassium concentration is complex[3,4,419] and is influenced by a variety of factors (Table 23-3).

The etiology of acidosis, that is, respiratory versus metabolic, is a critical determinant of the magnitude of the resultant hyperkalemia. Respiratory acidosis causes little (0.1 to 0.3 meq/liter) or no increase in the plasma potassium concentration, whereas metabolic acidosis elicits a more pronounced rise in the potassium level (0.5 to 1.2 meq/liter).[4,332,491] The smaller rise in plasma potassium concentration during respiratory acidosis is not well understood.

The nature of the anion that accompanies the increase in H^+ concentration also has been shown to influence the increase in plasma potassium concentration. Hydrochloric acid administration to humans and animals causes marked hyperkalemia,[401,402,553] whereas organic acids (lactic and hydroxybutyric acid), whether infused exogenously or produced endogenously, have a much smaller effect.[401,402,553] In human beings[400] and animals[582] grand mal seizures are associated with severe lactic acidemia yet the plasma potassium does not increase significantly. Similarly, in lactic acidosis[118,211,338] marked hyperkalemia is distinctly uncommon and changes in blood pH correlate poorly with the plasma potassium concentration. The more pronounced hyperkalemia following HCl infusion in vivo cannot be explained by differences in the serum bicarbonate concentration, arterial pH, or urinary potassium excretion. Using the rat hemidiaphragm, Rogers and Wachenfeld[456,457] have made similar observations in vitro. In contrast to hydrochloric acid, both lactic acid and β-hydroxybutyric acid fail to displace potassium from the intracellular compartment.[116,217] The difference between HCl and lactic/β-hydroxybutyric acid is most likely related to the permeability of the accompanying anion. Because chloride is relatively impermeable,[255] each H^+ that enters the cell must be linked to the exit of one potassium or sodium ion to maintain electrical neutrality. In contrast, both lactate[119] and β-hydroxybutyrate[256]

TABLE 23-3. • Factors influencing the effect of acidosis on the plasma potassium concentration

1. Origin of disturbance; metabolic acidosis causes a much greater change in plasma potassium concentration than respiratory acidosis
2. Nature of anion accompanying the increase in hydrogen ion; mineral acids (such as HCl, NH_4Cl) cause a much greater increase in potassium concentration than organic acids (such as ketoacids and lactate)
3. Change in plasma bicarbonate concentration per se
4. Duration of acidosis
5. Extent of intracellular buffering

SOURCE: Reproduced from Smith JD et al, in Arieff A, DeFronzo RA (eds): *Fluid, Electrolyte, and Acid-Base Disorders,* New York, Churchill Livingstone, 1985, p 413.

readily traverse the cell membrane. Since the H^+ that enters the cell is accompanied by an organic anion, electroneutrality is preserved, and potassium does not have to exit. Changes in total body potassium content also will influence the relationship between blood pH and the plasma potassium concentration in patients with organic acidosis.

The average patient admitted with diabetic ketoacidosis has a potassium deficit of 3 to 5 meq/kg of body weight.[315] For a 70-kg adult, this amounts to a deficit of 210 to 350 meq of potassium. The origin of the potassium deficiency is multifactorial and includes osmotic diuresis (secondary to glucosuria and ketonuria), ketonuria which obligates the excretion of cations to maintain electroneutrality, hyperaldosteronism secondary to intravascular volume depletion, intracellular phosphate loss which is associated with potassium exit from the cell, insulin deficiency which leads to decreased cellular (muscle, liver, adipose) potassium stores and an increase in urinary potassium excretion,[468] muscle catabolism associated with insulinopenia and high circulating levels of counterregulatory hormones, and decreased dietary potassium intake. Thus, in patients with diabetic ketoacidosis the effect of elevated H^+ levels to increase the plasma potassium concentration will be offset by a decrease in total body and intracellular potassium content. Not surprisingly, patients admited with diabetic ketoacidosis demonstrate great variability in the plasma potassium concentration, usually ranging from normal to increased on admission.[5,118,211,217,218,315,502,580] In a series containing over 3000 patients with diabetic ketoacidosis, approximatley one-third presented with a potassium concentration above 5.4 meq/liter.[502] As reviewed by Fulop,[211,212] the correlation between blood pH and plasma potassium is poor. Many patients with diabetic,[118,211,217,218,315,502] as well as alcoholic,[127,210,211,212,330] ketoacidosis will have severe acidemia, yet the plasma potassium concentration is not markedly increased and is more often within the normal range. In contrast, patients with hyperosmolar nonketotic coma, who have normal or only slightly decreased blood pH levels, commonly present with severe hyperkalemia.[17,212] These observations suggest that insulin lack[55,143] and hypertonicity,[321,349,373] by causing a shift of potassium from the intracellular to extracellular compartment, are more important determinants of hyperkalemia than acidemia.

A decrease in plasma bicarbonate concentration, independent of changes in blood pH, also has been shown to influence the potassium concentration. If acid is infused to reduce the bicarbonate concentration but the arterial pH is maintained constant by simultaneous reduction of the P_{CO_2},[202,203] the plasma potassium concentration still increases substantially. Moreover, bicarbonate administration lowers the plasma potassium level in hyperkalemic patients even though blood pH remains constant.[203] It should be noted, however, that not all investigators have been able to document an independent effect of bicarbonate.[505]

The *duration of metabolic acidosis* (with both mineral acids and organic acids) and, presumably, the extent of intracellular buffering also affect the plasma potassium concentration.[4,490,505] Immediately following the administration of an acid load, the decline in serum bicarbonate concentration and blood pH is greatest, yet the plasma potassium concentration changes minimally. With time, the plasma bicarbonate and blood pH return to baseline values while plasma potassium concentration rises to its highest level. These observations suggest that it is the magnitude of the H^+ load that is buffered within cells, and not the fall in blood pH or bicarbonate, which determines the rise in serum potassium concentration.

INCREASED POTASSIUM INPUT

Increased potassium influx from either exogenous or endogenous sources can cause a transient increase in the plasma potassium concentration. If sustained, however, an underlying defect in renal potassium handling or extrarenal potassium metabolism should be suspected. In human beings a single oral dose of 0.5 meq/kg (35 meq in a 70-kg person) of potassium produces a minimal increase in serum potassium concentration.[489] Similarly, the intravenous infusion of KCl at 25 meq/h for upward of 4 to 6 h raises the serum potassium concentration by only 0.4 to 0.5 meq/liter.[145] Protection from hyperkalemia is afforded by a combination of enhanced renal potassium excretion and increased cellular potassium influx.[82,143,319] Iatrogenic increases in potassium concentration have been reported in approximately 4 percent of patients receiving potassium chloride supplements.[325] Salt substitutes, which contain 10 to 13 meq of potassium per gram, are also a common source of increased potassium input.[516] Likewise, a low-salt diet is almost by definition a high-potassium diet since potassium-rich foods are commonly substituted for those high in sodium content. A number of studies[70,403,489,501,503] have documented that over 50 percent of hospitalized and outpatient causes of hyperkalemia are iatrogenically induced by potassium supplements. Concomitant use of potassium sparing diuretics, underlying renal disease, advanced age ($>$ 65 years), and diabetes mellitus are present in over half of the patients who develop hyperkalemia during the administration of potassium supplements.

Certain medications such as potassium penicillin (1.7 meq of potassium per million units) contain significant amounts of potassium and can result in acute hyperkalemia if administered in sufficiently high doses.[363] Severe hyperkalemia also has been reported in patients taking potassium salts for purposes other than potassium replacement, such as potassium citrate to alkalinize the urine.[325] Nutritional protein-calorie supplements may be another inadvertent cause of hyperkalemia.[430] Blood that is stored for more than 10 days has a plasma potassium concentration that varies from 7.5 to 13 meq/liter.[364] In addition, lysis of the transfused erythrocytes within a few hours can release significant amounts of potassium. Fatal hyperkalemia has been reported with as little as two units of blood over 1 h.[71] The risk of hyperkalemia and cardiac toxicity rises with massive transfusions, especially when given to patients with diminished renal function. Hypocalcemia, secondary to the use of citrate to anticoagulate blood, decreases cardiac tolerance to hyperkalemia and increases the risk of arrhythmias.[546] The use of Collins solution, which has a potassium concentration of 141 meq/liter and is widely employed in cadaveric renal graft preservation, has been associated with the development of severe hyperkalemia immediately following renal transplantation.[518] This event may be more likely when adult kidneys are transplanted into young recipients.

When the increased potassium input is derived from endogenous sources, the source is ordinarily fairly obvious. The intracellular potassium concentration, approximately 150 meq/liter, greatly exceeds that of plasma. Therefore, tissue damage (rhabdomyolysis, burns, crush injury) may cause cell death and a rapid release of potassium from cells, resulting in marked hyperkalemia. Related causes are rapid tumor dissolution following chemotherapy,[379] intravascular hemolysis,[308] and massive gastrointestinal bleeding. Increased cellular catabolism associated with major surgery and stress is a subtle and commonly overlooked cause of hyperkalemia.

INADEQUATE DISTAL SODIUM DELIVERY AND URINE FLOW

A decrease in sodium delivery to distal potassium secretory sites (i.e., secondary to a reduction in renal plasma flow and/or glomerular filtration rate (GFR) or an increase in sodium reabsorption by the proximal tubule or loop of Henle) is a commonly cited cause of hyperkalemia. However, this situation is unusual unless the rate of urinary sodium excretion is markedly reduced, that is to less than 5 to 10 meq/day. In the rat the sodium concentration in the lumen of cortical distal nephron for the half maximal rate of potassium secretion is 13 meq/liter.[238] Since the majority of potassium secretion occurs in the late distal tubule and early collecting tubule, sodium delivery to these segments is rarely rate-limiting even when dietary sodium intake is markedly decreased.[223,225,226,522,608] Moreover, studies indicate that tubular flow rate, rather than sodium delivery, is the primary determinant of distal potassium secretion.[238] If urine flow is diminished, the potassium concentration in the tubular lumen rises and this inhibits potassium secretion. Although the precise urine flow rate at which potassium secretion becomes impaired has not been determined, it is unusual to observe clinically significant hyperkalemia in individuals with urine outputs in excess of 600 ml/day. The most common clinical situation in which decreased distal sodium delivery and/or diminished urine flow leads to hyperkalemia is acute pulmonary edema, particularly in an individual with underlying renal disease. A second common circumstance is the patient with advanced renal disease who becomes intravascularly volume-depleted. Finally, the Addisonian patient is particularly sensitive to decreases in urine flow and distal sodium delivery. As long as the intravascular volume is maintained, severe hyperkalemia (> 6.0 to 6.5 meq/liter) is unusual even in the complete absence of mineralocorticoid and glucocorticoid activity.[263,383,388,543,550,552,585] If vomiting or diarrhea ensue or if some other complicating illness develops that limits fluid intake, urine output drops, renal potassium secretion becomes impaired, and severe hyperkalemia follows.

RENAL FAILURE

Acute renal failure

In patients who develop acute oligoanuric renal failure, hyperkalemia almost always is observed and is explained by a variety of factors:

1. *Distal sodium delivery and urine flow* are markedly decreased.
2. The *GFR* is often reduced to less than 10 ml/min, and this may of itself become rate-limiting for potassium excretion.
3. The commonest causes of acute renal failure are acute tubular necrosis and interstitial nephritis.[329] In these situations there is widespread damage to the late distal tubule and collecting duct cells, nephron segments that are primarily responsible for *potassium secretion.*
4. The *acuteness* of the renal failure precludes the elapse of sufficient time for the normal renal and extrarenal adaptive mechanisms (see below) to develop. Moreover, the development of these adaptive changes may be impaired in tubular cells that have been damaged by the renal insult.
5. The preceding factors may be coupled with increased *tissue catabolism* (surgery, stress, enhanced steroid secretion) or frank tissue breakdown (rhabdomyolysis, hemolysis, burns, extensive infection) and significant metabolic acidemia, causing the release of potassium into the ECF compartment at a time when renal potassium excretion is markedly compromised.

Chronic renal failure

In stark contrast, patients with chronic renal disease uncommonly display significant hyperkalemia (>5.5 meq/liter) in the basal or fasting state unless the GFR is less than 15 ml/min.[179,237,291,485] Even so, such patients tolerate exogenous potassium loads very poorly.[298,604] This apparent paradox is easily understood if one recognizes that chronic potassium balance and, therefore, the basal plasma potassium concentration are regulated primarily by the kidney. As the renal tubular mass becomes progressively diminished, there is an increase in potassium secretion by the surviving nephrons.[27,237,294,483,485] This phenomenon, known as *renal potassium adaptation*, plays a critical role in maintaining whole body potassium balance and basal plasma potassium levels close to normal. However, the capacity of the remaining nephrons to further augment potassium excretion is limited, and tolerance for an acute potassium challenge becomes compromised in chronic renal failure.[294,298,604]

Studies carried out in dogs demonstrate that an 80 percent reduction in renal mass causes only a transient rise in serum potassium concentration.[294,485] Within several days, the serum potassium level returns to baseline and normal potassium balance is achieved.[294,485] Since the number of functioning nephron units is markedly reduced, yet a normal urinary excretion of potassium is achieved, it follows that the fractional excretion of potassium must have increased markedly; that is, renal potassium adaptation has occurred. However, when the dogs with remnant kidneys received an acute intravenous potassium load, the increment in renal potassium excretion was approximately 50 percent less than in controls, and marked hyperkalemia resulted.[294] Although the rise in potassium excretion correlated closely with the serum potassium concentration in both control and uremic dogs, the relationship was markedly attenuated in dogs with reduced GFR (Fig. 23-12, top panel). Over the 5 h following KCl administration, control animals excreted 65 percent of the potassium load compared with only 35 percent in the remnant group. In the dogs with reduced renal mass, 24 h was required to excrete the entire potassium load. During this time hyperkalemia persisted and was associated with elevated plasma aldosterone levels. It should be noted that not all studies in animals[197,291,483,485] have demonstrated an impaired ability of the diseased kidney to excrete an exogenous potassium load. Indeed, in the dog study just cited, potassium excretion per unit of residual GFR was completely normal (Fig. 23-12, bottom panel). However, in this species as in humans it is clear that exogenous potassium loads are tolerated poorly in the presence of a reduced renal mass in two ways: a longer time is required for the diseased kidney to excrete the infused or ingested potassium, and the plasma potassium level will remain comparatively elevated until the excess is excreted.[298,604]

Aldosterone has a controversial role in this adaptation. Schultze et al.[485] demonstrated that adrenalectomized dogs maintained on a low, fixed dose of mineralocorticoid manifested normal renal potassium adaptation. They concluded that aldosterone plays only a permissive role in this process, and that incremental secretion is not necessary. It is likely, however, that their "low" aldosterone replacement dose actually represented supraphysiologic mineralocorticoid replacement. More recently, Fine et al.[196] have also challenged the importance of aldosterone. They showed that the cortical collecting tubule from adrenalectomized uremic rabbits demonstrated normal potassium adaptation. However, it is likely that the major nephron sites required for adaptation reside more proximally in the late distal tubule and early connecting tubule. Anatomic localization of potassium adaptation has been best characterized in the remnant kidney model, in which increased secretion of potassium is largely accounted for by the activity of these sites (late distal tubule and collecting duct). Tubular hypertrophy, specific proliferation of the basolateral membrane of principal cells, and increased activity of the Na^+,K^+-ATPase pump regularly accompany the increased potassium secretory activity of the remnant model.[27,48,72,160,196,267,319,485,615,616] These structural and functional changes are similar to those observed during chronic deoxycorticosterone acetate (DOCA) administration,[528,530,532,533,576,616] and a high-potassium diet,[532,533,574,615] in which en-

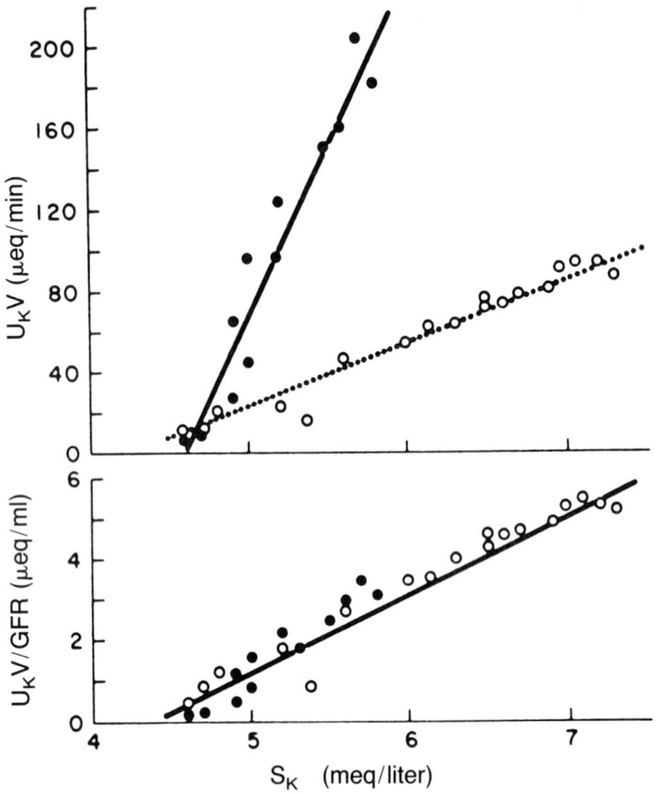

FIGURE 23-12 • Urinary potassium excretion (U_KV) (upper panel) and fractional potassium excretion (U_KV/GFR) (bottom panel) as a function of the serum potassium concentration (S_K) in normal (solid circles) and uremic (open circles) dogs. (Reproduced from Kaplan M et al: *Kidney Int* 19:482, 1981.)

hanced mineralocorticoid activity has been shown to play an important role in augmenting renal tubular potassium secretion.

Although aldosterone is an important regulator of both renal[192,321,524,528,529,613] and extrarenal[55,56,147,153,154,612] potassium homeostasis in humans, little information is available concerning alterations in aldosterone metabolism in patients with renal insufficiency. Considerable controversy exists concerning the plasma aldosterone concentration and aldosterone secretory rate in patients with advanced renal insufficiency. Early studies employing tritium-labeled aldosterone suggested that the hormone secretory rate was increased.[128,231,305] However, considerable overlap was observed between chronic renal failure and control patients. Despite the development of sensitive radioimmunoassay techniques to measure circulating aldosterone levels, controversy still exists and it is not clear whether the plasma aldosterone concentration is increased,[50,271,474,586,591] normal,[86,291,513,586] or decreased[37,148,150,425,474,476,586,591] in uremic subjects. Some of this confusion has arisen because investigators have failed to take into account the prevailing plasma potassium and renin concentrations when interpreting their findings. In many patients with chronic renal insufficiency and hyperkalemia, hyporeninemia is present.[37,148,150,325,425,474,476,511,586,591] In such patients impaired aldosterone secretion and hypoaldosteronism result from the low circulating plasma renin levels. If patients without hyperkalemia and with normal circulating plasma renin levels are studied, the plasma aldosterone concentration has been reported to be, with equal frequency, both normal[86,290,451,597] and increased.[50,271,476,586,591] The study of Hene et al.[271] helps, in part, to clarify these apparently discrepant results. These investigators demonstrated that when the creatinine clearance was greater than 50 to 60 ml/min, the plasma aldosterone concentration (indexed to the plasma renin activity) remained within the normal range. However, when the GFR declined to values less than 50 ml/min, there was a progressive rise in the plasma aldosterone level (Fig. 23-13). Thus, it is likely that some of the discordant results concerning plasma aldosterone values reported in the literature may have resulted from the failure to take into account the prevailing plasma renin activity or the state of total body potassium balance.

Normokalemic patients with normal or elevated aldosterone levels display a normal increase in plasma aldosterone in response to hyperkalemia, adrenocorticotropic hormone (ACTH), and angiotensin II.[37,50,150,290,591,597] Importantly, these normal or elevated levels of aldosterone have been shown to play an important role in the regulation of both sodium and potassium balance in patients with renal insufficiency. Kleeman et al.[305] documented normal basal aldosterone secretory rates in chronic renal failure patients who were ingesting a normal sodium intake. When these same subjects were placed on a restricted sodium intake, aldosterone secretion increased and sodium excretion declined. If spironolactone was administered during the period of sodium restriction, sodium conservation was impaired and hyperkalemia and a hyperchloremic metabolic acidosis developed. Berl et al.[50] also have reported sodium wasting, diminished potassium excretion, and hyperkalemia in normokalemic patients with renal failure who are given spironolactone. The frequent occurrence of hyperkalemia in patients given potassium-sparing diuretics that inhibit aldosterone action underscores these observations.[70,325,403,501,503] The development of hyperkalemia in patients with hyporeninemic hypoaldosteronism[37,148,150,321,425,476] lends further credence to the importance of maintaining aldosterone secretion in patients with progressive renal insufficiency. These results indicate that aldosterone plays an important role in the adaptive response that allows the diseased kidney to maintain normal rates of potassium excretion.

The results of Schambelan et al.[476,498] are particularly instructive. They examined the prevalence of aldosterone deficiency in 31 hyperkalemic patients with diffuse renal parenchymal disease and chronic renal insufficiency (GFR = 10 to 56 ml/min per 1.73 m^2), while ingesting a normal potassium intake. Seven of the 31 subjects had diabetes mellitus and the rest had characteristics consistent with interstitial nephritis. Compared with controls, 14 of 31 patients had overt hypoaldosteronism as determined by the 24-h urinary aldosterone secretory rate. However, when the urinary aldosterone secretory rate was factored by the prevailing serum potassium concentration (to take into account the

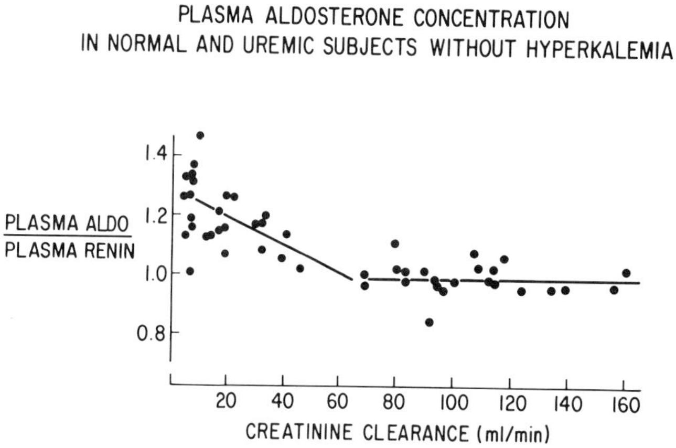

FIGURE 23-13 • Plasma aldosterone (PA) concentration in normal control subjects and in patients with varying degrees of chronic renal insufficiency. On the vertical axis the plasma aldosterone (PA) concentration has been plotted as a function of the plasma renin activity (PRA). Below a GFR (creatinine clearance) of 50 to 60 ml/min, a progressive rise in PA concentration was observed. (Adapted from Hene RJ et al: *Kidney Int* 21:98, 1982.)

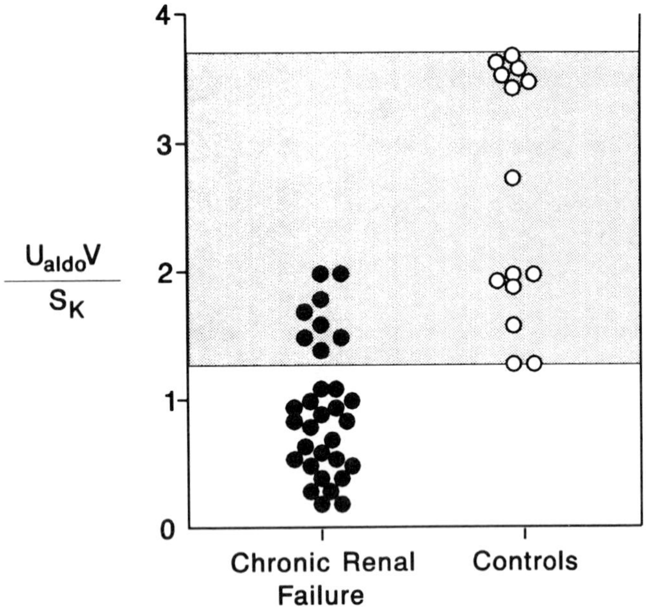

FIGURE 23-14 • The ratio of urinary aldosterone excretion (Ualdo V) to serum potassium concentration (S_K) in 31 hyperkalemic patients with chronic renal failure (solid circles) and in 14 normal subjects (open circles). In 23 patients with renal disease the value for the Ualdo V/S_K ratio fell below the lowest of the controls. The shaded area depicts the normal range. (Redrawn from Schambelan M et al: *Kidney Int* 17:89, 1980.)

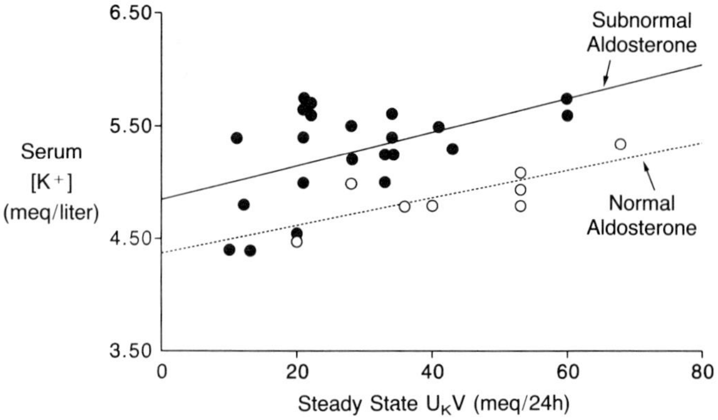

FIGURE 23-15 • Relationship between the serum potassium concentration (S_K) and steady-state 24-h urinary potassium excretion (U_KV) in 23 chronic renal failure (GFR = 32 ml/min) patients with hypoaldosteronism (closed circles) and 8 chronic renal failure (GFR = 28 ml/min) patients without hypoaldosteronism (open circles). For any given rate of potassium excretion, patients with hypoaldosteronism required a higher serum potassium to excrete their daily ingested potassium load. (Redrawn from Schambelan M et al: *Kidney Int* 17:89, 1980.)

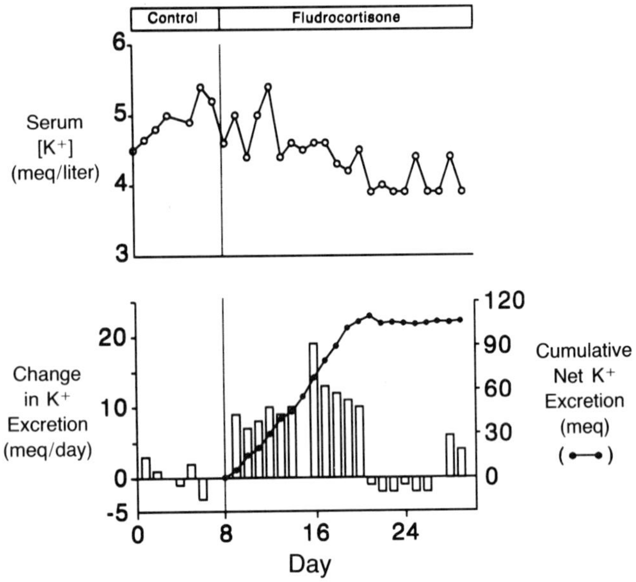

FIGURE 23-16 • Effect of fludrocortisone acetate administration (0.1 to 0.15 mg/day) on serum potassium (open circles) concentration (S_K), change in daily potassium excretion (open bars), and cumulative net potassium excretion (solid circles) in a patient with chronic renal disease and hypoaldosteronism. (Redrawn from Schambelan M et al: *Kidney Int* 17:89, 1980.)

stimulatory effect of potassium on the zona glomerulosa), 23 of 31 patients manifested a deficiency of aldosterone (Fig. 23-14). In both groups (i.e., those with decreased and those with normal aldosterone secretory rates) of patients with chronic renal failure, the serum potassium concentration was closely related to the rate of urinary potassium excretion (Fig. 23-15). However, for any given aldosterone secretory rate patients with hypoaldosteronism excreted significantly less potassium. The role of aldosterone deficiency in the pathogenesis of hyperkalemia in such patients was further examined by administration of fludrocortisone acetate.[495,498] In some patients physiologic amounts of fludrocortisone markedly augmented renal potassium excretion and restored normokalemia (Fig. 23-16), while in others supraphysiologic doses were required. These results suggest that the renal tubular cells in the surviving nephrons of patients with chronic renal disease are often refractory to the potassium secretory effect of mineralocorticoids.

In addition to impaired potassium excretion by the kidney, there also is evidence to suggest that extrarenal potassium metabolism is impaired in uremic humans[179,291,298] and a similar defect in extrarenal potassium tolerance has been demonstrated in rats with chronic renal failure.[27,483] However, Gonick et al.[237] in human beings could not demonstrate a defect in extrarenal potassium tolerance, and Perez et al. have demonstrated normal extrarenal potassium tolerance in dogs with chronic renal insufficiency.[421] The explanation for these apparently discrepant results is not clear. If extrarenal potassium metabolism is indeed impaired in patients with chronic renal failure, this defect is unlikely to be related to decreased fecal potassium excretion, since gastrointestinal potassium secretion is augmented in such patients.[33,265,268,311] It also is unlikely that impaired extrarenal potassium uptake results from excess total body potassium, which secondarily leads to an inability to accept an acute potassium load. Although there is some controversy concerning the best method to quantitate potassium stores,[406] measurements of total body and exchangeable potassium in uremic patients have usually yielded normal values.[51,76,486] In addition, intracellular potassium concentration, determined from muscle biopsies obtained from uremic individuals, has been shown to be normal[79] or reduced.[62] It has been suggested that defects in the secretion and/or tissue sensitivity to insulin, catecholamines, or aldosterone may play a role in the disturbance in extrarenal potassium tolerance.[511] Although this may be true in individual patients, such hormonal abnormalities are unlikely to explain the defects in extrarenal potassium metabolism in the majority of uremic subjects,[511] since both insulin-mediated[12] and adrenergic-mediated[103] changes in extrarenal potassium metabolism do not seem to be impaired in uremic human beings. Similarly, in diabetic patients with modestly reduced GFRs, extrarenal potassium metabolism is not impaired.[514] The finding of low intracellular potassium levels, coupled with impaired sodium efflux (reviewed in reference 292), is consistent with a defect in the Na^+,K^+-ATPase transport pump in the cells of uremic patients. Since this transport defect can be corrected with dialysis, it has been postulated that some uremic toxin(s) is responsible for an alteration in Na^+,K^+-ATPase activity, which results in impaired electrolyte transport in uremic patients.[292] However, most of these studies have been carried out on erythrocytes and white blood cells, which do not play a major role in extrarenal potassium homeostasis. There is little information concerning the Na^+,K^+-ATPase pump in muscle and liver, the major tissues that mediate extrarenal potassium metabolism. In the study by Cotton et al.[131] the muscle of uremic humans was shown to have a decreased resting membrane potential, with a proportional increase in intracellular sodium and decrease in intracellular potassium concentrations. These findings are consistent with a decrease in the Na^+,K^+-ATPase pump in muscle of uremic human beings in the postabsorptive state but do not prove that extrarenal potassium metabolism is impaired under conditions of potassium loading.

In summary, adaptive increases in renal and gastrointestinal excretion of potassium usually suffice to prevent significant hyperkalemia in patients with chronic renal failure as long as the GFR remains above 15 to 20 ml/min and urine flow and distal sodium delivery are maintained. The exception to this is a small group of patients with interstitial nephritis or diabetic nephropathy who may become hyperkalemic early in the course of their renal disease. Such individuals usually turn out to have hypoaldosteronism (see below), which, when superimposed upon a reduction in renal tubular mass, leads to the development of hyperkalemia.

IMPAIRED RENIN-ALDOSTERONE AXIS

Addison's disease

Both aldosterone[192,194,383,436,467,524,528,529,531] and glucocorticoids[1,31,58,192,194,367,436,528,532] have important kaliuretic effects in humans and animals, and both hormones are known to stimulate potassium secretion by the colonic epithelium.[33,35,104,164,268] Aldosterone exerts its action by a direct stimulatory effect on the Na^+,K^+-ATPase pump, whereas the kaliuretic effect of glucocorticoids is an indirect one mediated via increased fluid and sodium delivery to the distal nephron. Therefore, it is not surprising that patients with Addison's disease (combined mineralocorticoid and glucocorticoid deficiency) commonly present with hyperkalemia. In contrast, patients with pituitary disease and ACTH deficiency, in whom aldosterone production is maintained, rarely develop hyperkalemia.[324,444,465] This clinical observation indicates that aldosterone plays a quantitatively more important role than glucocorticoids in the defense of body potassium homeostasis. Recent studies that have examined hormone binding to glucocorticoid and mineralocorticoid receptors[213,323,354] indicate that the ability of "glucocorticoids" to enhance potassium excretion most likely results from overlap binding to the mineralocorticoid receptor. Lan et al.[323] documented that physiologic concentrations of both dexamethasone (considered to be a "pure" glucocorticoid) and cortisol were capable of displacing aldosterone from the mineralocorticoid receptor. Similar results have been reported by Marusic et al.[354] using cytosolic receptors isolated from rat colonic mucosa. In studies combining clearance and micropuncture analysis with renal morphology in adrenalectomized rats, Stanton et al. evaluated the effects of treatment with physiologic doses of aldosterone versus dexamethasone.[527,528] Adrenalectomy was associated with fasting hyperkalemia and a marked impairment in the kidney's ability to excrete an acute potassium load. Aldosterone prevented the development of baseline hyperkalemia and largely restored the ability of the kidney to excrete an acute potassium load. In contrast, dexamethasone failed to correct the basal hyperkalemia and only slightly enhanced the ability of the kidney to excrete an infused KCl load. This slight enhancement in potassium excretion was associated with a large increase in tubular urine flow. When dexamethasone was administered while maintaining distal tubular flow rate constant, no increase in potassium excretion was observed.[192] These results suggest that the small stimulatory effect of dexamethasone to augment renal potassium excretion is indirect and mediated via changes in tubular fluid flow rate. Morphologic analysis is consistent with this hypothesis.[527] Thus, adrenalectomy caused a marked reduction in the basolateral membrane area of the principal cells of the late distal tubule and early collecting duct, and aldosterone restored the basolateral membrane area to normal; in contrast, dexamethasone was without effect. Since the basolateral membrane area of the principal cells has been shown to reflect closely the potassium secretory activity of the late distal nephron, these results favor a primary role for aldosterone (mineralocorticoids) in the renal regulation of potassium secretion. It should be emphasized that nonrenal tissues may have different responses to mineralocorticoids and glucocorticoids. Glucocorticoids enhance colonic sodium reabsorption and stimulate potassium secretion, and these effects are mediated via a specific colonic glucocorticoid receptor.[34]

In 1930, Gutman published his classic monograph reviewing 566 cases of Addison's disease.[250] Sixty-eight percent of the cases were secondary to tuberculosis; only 19 percent resulted from "primary" adrenal atrophy, a disorder now believed to have an autoimmune etiology (Table 23-4). Over the ensuing half century, the spectrum of Addison's disease has changed considerably. In Nerup's review of 108 cases, primary idiopathic adrenal atrophy (66 percent) was the most common cause of Addison's disease.[383] Tuberculosis accounted for less than 20 percent of all casses. As in Gutman's earlier series, all other etiologies are uncommon. Descriptions of the clinical and laboratory presentation of such individuals can be found in any standard textbook of endocrinology and are summarized in Table 23-5.[383] Of particular importance to the present discussion are the frequent disturbances in sodium, acid-base, and potassium metabolism that result from aldosterone deficiency. On presentation, 70 to 80 percent of patients with Addison's disease will be hyponatremic and have an elevated serum urea nitrogen (Table 23-5). Hyperkalemia is less common, occurring in 64 percent of the patients reported by Nerup.[383] Of particular note, the serum potassium concentration was in excess of 6.0 meq/liter in only 14 of 108 patients (13 percent) (Fig. 23-17). The precise incidence of hyperchloremic acidosis is unknown but can be estimated to be about 50 percent.

As discussed previously, aldosterone stimulates potassium secretion by the distal nephron. Not surprisingly, aldosterone deficiency is associated with a decrease in distal tubular fluid potassium concentration.[129,278,279] In addition to their kaliuretic action, mineralocorticoids are also known to augment potassium uptake by extrarenal tissues.[147,151,613] (see previous discussion). Despite these important effects on both renal and extrarenal potassium metabolism, moderate to severe hyperkalemia (> 5.5 to 6.0 meq/liter) is unusual in Addisonian patients with normal renal function as long as the ECF volume does not become contracted.[132,263,388,415,543,550,551,552,585]

TABLE 23-4 • Etiology of Addison's disease

	Gutman (1942) 566 cases (%)	Nerup,[383] 108 cases (%)
Tuberculosis	68	17
Primary atrophy	19	66
Amyloid	1	0
Neoplasm	1	0
Other/unclassifiable*	10	17

* Venous thrombosis, emboli, pressure atrophy, syphilis, hemochromatosis, anticoagulation therapy, hypotensive infarction, meningococcemia.

SOURCE: Reproduced from Smith JD et al, in Arieff A, DeFronzo RA (eds): *Fluid, Electrolyte, and Acid-Base Disorders,* New York, Churchill Livingstone, 1985, p 413.

TABLE 23-5 • Clinical and laboratory features of Addison's disease

Clinical presentation	%	Laboratory data	%
Weakness and easily fatigued	100	Hyponatremia	88
Weight loss	100	Eosinophilia	70–80
Anorexia	100	Neutropenia	70–80
Hyperpigmentation	92	Lymphocytosis	70–80
Hypotension	88	Azotemia	70–80
Gastrointestinal symptoms	56	Hyperkalemia	64
Nervousness and mental symptoms	50	Hypoglycemia	~50
Hypoglycemic symptoms	50	Hyperchloremic acidosis	30–50
Loss of axillary and pubic hair	30	Hypercalcemia	6
Postural dizziness	12		
Muscle pains	6		
Fever	0		

SOURCE: Reproduced from Smith JD et al, in Arieff A, DeFronzo RA (eds): *Fluid, Electrolyte, and Acid-Base Disorders,* New York, Churchill Livingstone, 1985, p 413.

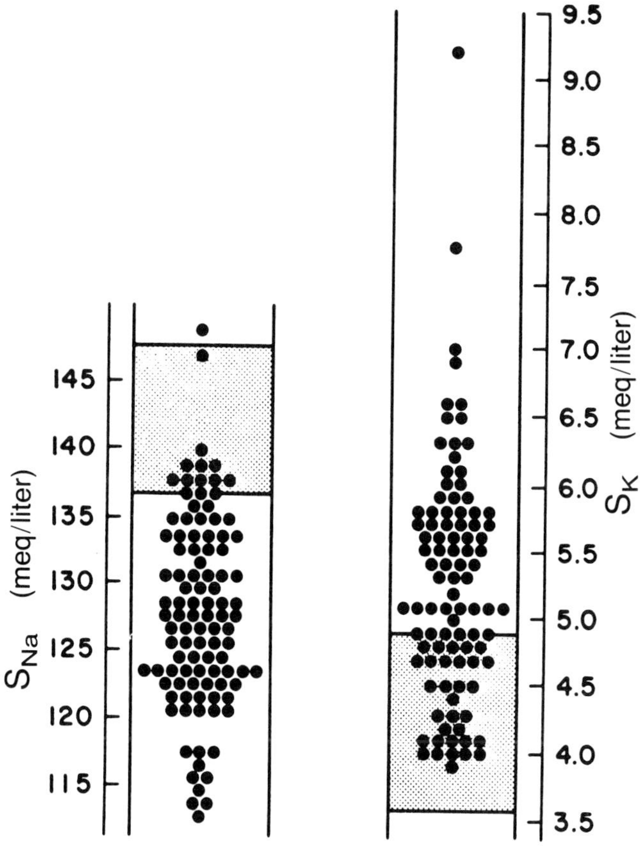

FIGURE 23-17 • Distribution of serum potassium and sodium concentrations at the time of presentation in 108 cases of Addison's disease. Stippled area reflects the normal range. (Adapted from Nerup J: *Acta Endocrinol* 76:127, 1974.)

As long as dietary sodium chloride intake is sufficient to maintain a normal intravascular volume and GFR and to ensure an adequate delivery of fluid and sodium to the distal nephron sites of potassium secretion, the Addisonian patient is able to excrete sufficient amounts of potassium to achieve normal potassium balance. Studies in dogs[262] and humans[132] have shown that following adrenalectomy the maximum urine to plasma potassium concentration ratio is about 10:1. This is in contrast to normal subjects in whom the maximum concentration ratio approximates 40:1. From these considerations it should be obvious that patients with Addison's disease are critically dependent upon urine flow rate. If salt and water intake are inadequate, the intravascular volume becomes contracted and this leads to a reduction in renal plasma flow and GFR and a flow-related decrease in renal potassium secretion. Since aldosterone also stimulates distal H^+ secretion, hyperchloremic metabolic acidosis often coexists.[255] The resultant acidemia will further inhibit renal potassium secretion and cause an increased potassium ion efflux from cells, thereby aggravating the hyperkalemia. The hyperkalemia also inhibits renal ammonia synthesis, which, in turn, reduces net acid excretion.[495]

Once suspected, the diagnosis of Addison's disease is easily established by the findings of low plasma cortisol and urinary 17-hydroxy- and ketosteroids, reduced plasma aldosterone concentration, blunted cortisol and aldosterone response to ACTH, and high plasma renin levels. Adrenal insufficiency secondary to pituitary disease is easily differentiated by normal plasma aldosterone and renin levels, and some combination of low thyroid, growth hormone, and gonadotropin concentrations. If an Addisonian crisis is suspected, the subject should be given 4 mg of dexamethasone intravenously as acute therapy. Simultaneously, an ACTH infusion, 50 units in normal saline given over 8 h, should be started and the plasma cortisol measured before and after ACTH. The bolus of dexamethasone will not affect the adrenal response to ACTH and dexamethasone does not interfere with the determination of plasma cortisol concentration.

The treatment of Addison's disease requires the institution of cortisone acetate, 25 to 37.5 mg/day; a high salt intake also is recommended. In most patients, mineralocorticoid replacement is ordinarily not necessary. This is most likely due to crossover binding of cortisone to the mineralocorticoid receptor.[213,323,354] In occasional patients fludrocortisone acetate (Florinef), 0.1 mg/day, may be needed. It should be remembered that under stress the adrenal glands produce 200 to 400 mg of cortisol per day, and the replacement dose of cortisone acetate should be appropriately adjusted.

Enzyme deficiencies

Aldosterone deficiency can result from a variety of enzymatic defects (Fig. 23-18), of which the most common is 21-hydroxylase deficiency.[45] This enzyme deficiency involves both the zona fasciculata and zona glomerulosa and leads to a combined deficiency of both mineralocorticoid and glucocorticoid function. The clinical presentation is one of renal salt-wasting, hyperkalemia, virilization (due to increased levels of 17-hydroxyprogesterone which result from overproduction of adrenal androgens by the zona fasciculata), and failure to thrive.[45,85,573] The high circulating levels of 17-hydroxyprogesterone and progesterone contribute to the clinical manifestations of mineralocorticoid deficiency since they are mineralocorticoid antagonists that inhibit the renal action of aldosterone. Thus, the mineralocorticoid deficiency is due not entirely to low circulating levels of aldosterone but in part to end-organ resistance to mineralocorticoids. This end-organ resistance may explain the marked variation in renal salt handling that has been described in patients with 21-hydroxylase deficiency, and why some patients with high plasma aldosterone levels are salt wasters.[281,297,312,498]

11 β-Hydroxylase deficiency is the second most frequently encountered adrenal biosynthetic defect and is also associated with an impairment in cortisol and aldosterone secretion.[45,85,198,573] However, in contrast to

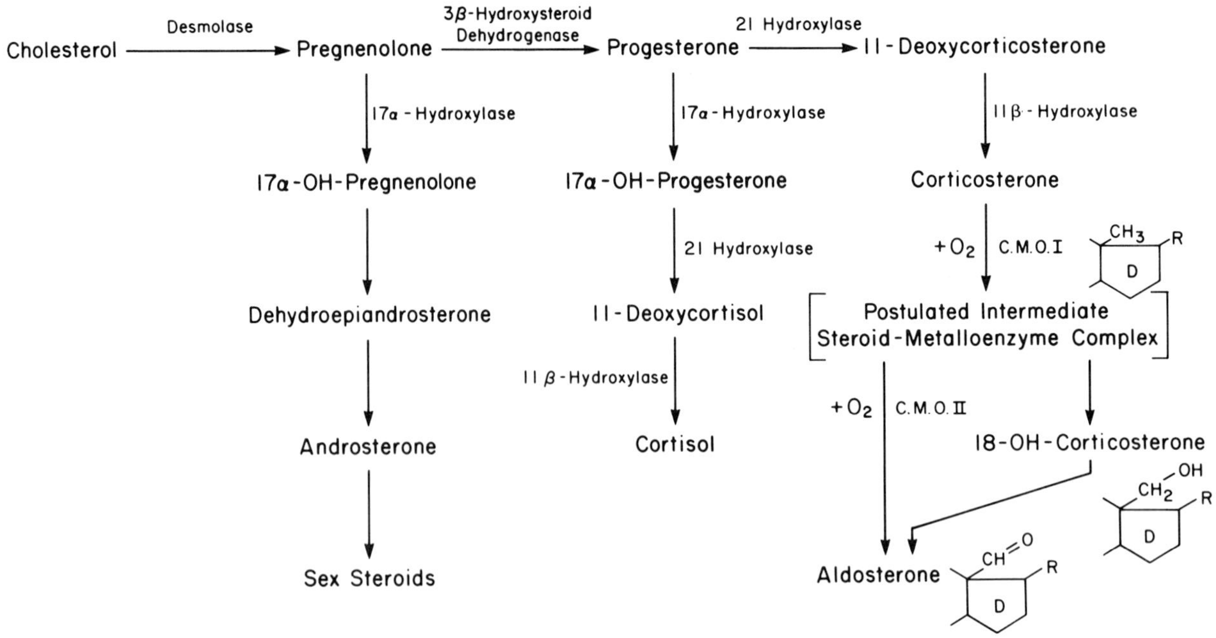

FIGURE 23-18 • Biosynthesis of adrenal steroids. [Reproduced from Smith JD et al, in Arieff A, DeFronzo RA (eds): *Fluid, Electrolyte, and Acid-Base Disorders*, New York, Churchill Livingstone, 1985, p 413.]

21-hydroxylase deficiency, hypertension, sodium retention, and hypokalemia are the classic manifestations. Virilization also is present. Decreased cortisol synthesis enhances ACTH secretion, which in turn stimulates the accumulation of steroids proximal to the block. Deoxycorticosterone (DOC) levels are markedly elevated and promote sodium retention and potassium wasting.

17a-Hydroxylase deficiency also may be associated with decreased circulating plasma aldosterone levels.[45,198] As observed in 11 β-hydroxylase deficiency, hypertension, sodium retention, and hypokalemia are present. The low plasma cortisol levels stimulate ACTH secretion which leads to an increase in DOC, and possibly corticosterone synthesis. These steroids are responsible for the sodium retention and subsequent volume expansion that suppress renin and aldosterone secretion. Evidence of gonadal hypofunction is characteristic and plasma follicle-stimulating hormone (FSH) and luteinizing hormone (LH) levels are elevated.

Recently, specific defects in the aldosterone biosynthetic pathway have been described (Fig. 23-18). The final two steps in the biosynthesis of aldosterone involve mixed function oxidation reactions in which corticosterone is converted to 18-hydroxycorticosterone (type 1 corticosterone methyl oxidase).[562,568] Recent evidence[386,562,568] suggests that 18-hydroxycorticosterone and aldosterone represent two discrete end products derived from a common intermediate. Defects in both the first[156,568] and second[135,443,463,561,567,568] of these enzymatic reactions have been described. Because these enzymes are not necessary for cortisol biosynthesis, evidence of glucocorticoid insufficiency and virilization is not part of the clinical picture. Most patients present in childhood with salt wasting, hyperkalemia, and failure to thrive. The type 2 defect is established by the combination of low plasma aldosterone concentration, increased renin, increased plasma 18-hydroxycorticosterone, and increased urinary excretion of tetrahydro-18-hydroxy-11-dehydrocorticosterone. The plasma aldosterone level may be "normal" in such patients.[463] However, it is quite abnormal when viewed in the context of volume depletion and the marked elevation in plasma renin activity. Although plasma 18-hydroxycorticosterone and corticosterone levels are significantly elevated, and these moieties do possess some mineralocorticoid activity,[124] they are not sufficient to offset the defects in renal potassium secretion and sodium reabsorption that result from aldosterone lack.[463] The type 1 corticosterone deficiency is diagnosed by the finding of low 18-hydroxycorticosterone levels, decreased urinary excretion of tetrahydro-18-hydroxy-11-dehydrocorticosterone, hyperreninemia, and hypoaldosteronism. It is important to recognize that in diabetic patients the corticosterone methyl oxidase deficiency may be an acquired defect that is reversible by improved metabolic control.[74]

Hyporeninemic hypoaldosteronism

Over the last decade a syndrome of hyperkalemia in association with hyporeninemia and hypoaldosteronism has become recognized as a distinct clinical entity. This subject was first reviewed in 1980 by DeFronzo et al.,[148] who reported on 81 cases from the literature. Since this initial review, many more cases have been described, primarily in diabetic patients or in patients with chronic interstitial renal disease.[22,39,40,139,228,406,434,476,558,559]

Clinical syndrome

The clinical presentation is quite typical (Table 23-6). The majority of patients are *elderly* (mean age 65 ± 7 years), and this may be an important contributing factor since both renin and aldosterone secretion decrease with advancing age.[375,590] Most patients (approximately 75 percent) are *free of clinical symptoms* and are diagnosed on routine laboratory screening or during evaluation for some unrelated illness. Only 25 percent of patients present with symptoms attributable to the hyperkalemia, such as muscle weakness or cardiac arrhythmias. A *hyperchloremic metabolic acidosis* is present in more than half of the cases, since aldosterone has an important effect to augment hydrogen ion excretion by the distal nephron and, in its absence, NH_4^+ excretion is impaired. Urine pH in these patients is maximally acidic (see subsequent discussion). Salt wasting is distinctly unusual. Most patients have a partial defect in aldosterone secretion, and the plasma aldosterone level, although decreased, is adequate to maintain sodium balance as long as the individual is consuming a normal sodium intake. If, however, the dietary sodium intake is markedly restricted, negative sodium balance, intravascular volume depletion, and hypotension will ensue. Although the low circulating aldosterone levels are sufficient to maintain normal sodium balance, they are not sufficient to prevent the development of hyperkalemia. Baseline plasma cortisol levels and the cortisol response to ACTH are, by definition, normal in all patients. The majority of patients (approximately 70 to 80 percent) have mild to moderate chronic renal insufficiency. The types of renal disease that have been reported are listed in Table 23-7. Diabetic glomerulosclerosis is the most frequent type of nephropathy and is followed by a variety of diverse interstitial renal diseases including gouty nephropathy, nephrolithiasis, analgesic nephropathy, and urinary tract disease. This syndrome is frequently seen with obstructive uropathy,[40,412] sickle cell disease,[36,148] and systemic lupus erythematosus.[326] Occasional patients with glomerulonephritis also have developed this disorder.[166] Hypertension is present in more than half of the patients,[148,426] and in some nephrosclerosis has been the only renal abnormality described.

TABLE 23-6 • Clinical and laboratory characteristics in 81 patients with the syndrome of selective hypoaldosteronism

1. Mean age = 65 years; range = 32 to 82 years
2. Findings at presentation:
   a. Asymptomatic hyperkalemia (75%)
   b. Muscle weakness (25%)
   c. Cardiac arrhythmia (25%)
   d. Hyperchloremic acidosis (~ 50%)
   e. Salt wasting (unusual)
3. Normal glucocorticoid function
4. Mild to moderate renal insufficiency, 57/81 (70%)
5. Diabetes mellitus, 40/81 (49%)
6. Low or low-normal baseline plasma aldosterone levels: all patients had a subnormal increase following volume contraction, 81/81 (100%)
7. Normal baseline and/or stimulated plasma renin levels, 13/74 (18%)
8. Normal aldosterone response to angiotensin II infusion, 4/27 (15%)
9. Normal aldosterone response to ACTH administration, 7/34 (21%)

SOURCE: Reproduced from Smith JD et al, in Arieff A, DeFronzo RA (eds): *Fluid, Electrolyte, and Acid-Base Disorders*, New York, Churchill Livingstone, 1985, p 413.

TABLE 23-7 • The causes of renal disease in 57 patients with the syndrome of hypoaldosteronism*

Diabetes mellitus	25
Interstitial nephritis (unknown etiology)	7
Hypertension	7
Gout	6
Glomerulonephritis	3
Nephrolithiasis	2
Analgesic nephropathy	1
Urinary tract obstruction	1
Mixed cryoglobulinemia	1
Unknown	4
Obstructive uropathy†	8
Sickle cell disease‡	5

Hypoaldosteronism (either primary or secondary) has been described in a number of other types of renal disease including lead nephropathy, amyloidosis, medullary cystic disease, allergic interstitial nephritis

* Constructed from the data reviewed in DeFronzo RA: *Kidney Int* 17:118, 1980.

† From Batlle DC et al: *N Engl J Med* 304:373, 1981.

‡ From Batlle DC et al: *Am J Med* 72:188, 1981 and DeFronzo et al: *Ann Intern Med* 90:310, 1979.

Hypoaldosteronism

Baseline plasma aldosterone concentrations are low or in the normal range.[148] Following volume contraction, a subnormal increase in plasma aldosterone has been observed in all report cases (Table 23-6).[22,36,39,40,51,139,148,310,426,558,559,564] Although patients may demonstrate some increase in plasma aldosterone concentration following volume depletion, the *absolute* increase is always much less than expected in normal subjects. Two series[157,417] have examined the effect of normalization of the serum potassium concentration (with a Na^+-K^+ exchange resin) on plasma aldosterone secretion. In both reports[157,417] plasma aldosterone levels fell significantly following reduction of the plasma potassium concentration, emphasizing the importance of relating the plasma aldosterone level to the existing plasma potassium concentration.[37,426,476,511] Thus, while occasional patients may have basal plasma aldosterone levels in the normal range, these are clearly subnormal when interpreted in light of the elevated plasma potassium levels.

Renin, acting through angiotensin II, is an important physiologic regulator of aldosterone secretion.[466] In the great majority of patients with selective hypoaldosteronism, the low circulating plasma aldosterone levels can be explained, in large part, by the hyporeninemia.[148,228,271,476] In fact, Schambelan et al.[476] and Hene et al.[271] have provided evidence that the decrease in plasma aldosterone concentration is proportional to the reduction in plasma renin activity in most patients. Studies in anephric patients also provide evidence that links the decrease in plasma renin to the diminished plasma aldosterone levels. In general, baseline plasma aldosterone concentration is reduced in these anephric patients,[46,395,493,579,588,589,597] but in a few series normal basal values[356,368] have been reported. These observations are in keeping with the important physiologic role that renin plays in the regulation of aldosterone secretion. In most series the ability of volume contraction,[25,37,46,228,357,409,588] ACTH,[37,73,357,399,409,435,437] angiotensin II,[37,228,588] and posture[25,37,46,409,476] to stimulate aldosterone secretion is also impaired. Only Mitra et al.[368] have reported consistently normal responses to provocative stimuli in nephrectomized dialysis patients.

As reviewed by Walker and Cooke,[579] the primary regulator of aldosterone secretion in nephrectomized dialyzed patients appears to be the serum potassium concentration. There is an excellent correlation between plasma potassium and aldosterone concentrations. Furthermore, changes in plasma potassium concentration in nephrectomized patients are capable of directly stimulating aldosterone secretion independently of any other known regulatory factors,[46,126] although in the absence of angiotensin II this effect is blunted.[434] Similar findings have been reported in normal control subjects.[136,163,280] Since all patients with the syndrome of hyporeninemic hypoaldosteronism have clinically significant hyperkalemia (serum potassium concentrations often in excess of 6.0 to 6.5 meq/liter), it is surprising that this stimulus does not override the hyporeninemia. Since it does not, it appears that a primary adrenal defect may also contribute to the hypoaldosteronism. Several additional pieces of evidence indicate that factors other than impaired renin secretion per se may play a role in the development of the hypoaldosteronism. First, normal baseline and/or stimulated renin levels have been reported in 13 of 74 (18 percent) patients in whom they were measured (Table 23-6). Similar observations have been made by Schambelan et al.[476] and Hsueh.[228] Second, the aldosterone secretory response to intravenous angiotensin II infusion was normal in only 4 of 27 (15 percent) patients (Table 23-6). Since angiotensin II directly stimulates aldosterone release by the zona glomerulosa cells,[205,257,541] the aldosterone secretory response to angiotensin II should be normal if hyporeninemia were the only defect present. Likewise, the aldosterone response to ACTH, another agent that directly stimulates the adrenal production of aldosterone, was normal in only 7 of 34 (21 percent) patients (Table 23-6). However, these experiments do not unequivocally establish the presence of a primary adrenal defect. More prolonged adrenal stimulation (i.e., several days as opposed to hours) with angiotensin II and ACTH may be necessary for normal aldosterone production because of disuse atrophy of the zona glomerulosa secondary to chronic hyporeninemia.

In a recent report Schambelan et al.[476] studied 14 patients with selective hypoaldosteronism. Following 5 days of salt restriction, plasma renin activity increased from 0.2 to 1.0 ng/ml per hour and corresponding plasma aldosterone values showed a rise from 5.6 to 15.8 ng/dl. The increment in plasma aldosterone concentration was highly correlated with the increase in plasma renin activity, and the slope of the line relating these two variables was not significantly different between hypoaldosteronemic and control subjects. However, the hypoaldosteronemic group was significantly hyperkalemic. Since hyperkalemia per se is known to stimulate aldosterone secretion,[46,126,136,163,280] one would have expected disproportionatley higher aldosterone levels in the study group compared with the controls. It also is noteworthy that despite five days of sodium restriction plasma renin and aldosterone levels could not be increased above baseline recumbent levels observed in normal healthy subjects consuming a normal sodium diet.

All of the studies reviewed above demonstrate that a variety of physiologic stimuli (volume contraction, ACTH, angiotensin II infusion, hyperkalemia) are capable of stimulating aldosterone secretion in patients with hypoaldosteronism, but when viewed in absolute terms, the response is almost universally impaired. Whether this represents a primary defect in aldosterone secretion or represents adrenal atrophy secondary to prolonged hyporeninemia remains to be ascertained. The latter explanation is supported by the observation that the aldosterone response to provocative stimuli often is impaired for a prolonged period following the correction of hyporeninemia in a number of clinical conditions, including 17α-hydroxylase deficiency,[61,234,577] excessive licorice ingestion,[337,542] and removal of aldosterone secreting adenomas.[60,76,519] The most critical study, which involves prolonged (7 to 10 days) adrenal stimulation with angiotensin, has yet to be performed. If plasma aldosterone levels fail to increase normally after prolonged daily angiotensin administration, it must be concluded that secretion of aldosterone is intrinsically impaired within the adrenal gland.

A number of reports have suggested that the terminal enzymatic steps involved in aldosterone biosynthesis may be impaired in some patients with hypoaldosteronism.[157,287,414,417,559,565] Although circulating levels of 18-hydroxycorticosterone or its urinary metabolite were normal, the plasma aldosterone concentration was reduced. Following sodium restriction and angiotensin II or ACTH infusion, the plasma 18-hydroxycorticosterone level increased normally but plasma aldosterone failed to rise. These results suggest an enzymatic block between 18-hydroxycorticosterone and aldosterone. The majority of 18-hydroxycorticosterone is synthesized in the zona glomerulosa. Thus, the acute increase observed following angiotensin II infusion would argue against the presence of zona glomerulosa cell atrophy in these patients. It should be noted, however, that other reports have failed to demonstrate any evidence of impaired aldosterone biosynthesis in patients with selective hypoaldosteronism.[359,362,475] Most of the patients in whom a defect in 18-hydroxylation has been demonstrated are diabetic.[74,77,157,287,414,417,559] Therefore, it could be argued that it is the diabetes per se that is responsible for the abnormality in aldosterone biosynthesis. This seems unlikely since Beretta-Piccoli et al.[49] have demonstrated that in insulin-dependent diabetics, basal plasma 18-hydroxycorticosterone and aldosterone levels are normal and increase appropriately following angiotensin II and ACTH administration.

Insulin deficiency and/or insulin resistance are characteristic of both type I (insulin-dependent) and type II (non-insulin-dependent) diabetes mellitus. Therefore, in the diabetic patient, it is possible that the defect in aldosterone biosynthesis results from insulin lack per se or from some derangement in cellular function that is dependent upon insulin. Indeed, insulin is known to stimulate potassium uptake by a variety of tissues including muscle[16,115,146,622] and liver.[12,146,378] In addition, basal insulin levels have been shown to play an important role in maintaining the normal distribution of potassium between intracellular and extracellular enviornment.[143] In normal and type II diabetic individuals, if basal insulin secretion is inhibited by as little as 50 percent, a predictable rise in plasma potassium concentration of 0.4 to 0.6 meq/liter ensues (Fig. 23-19) and tolerance to exogenously administered potassium becomes markedly impaired.[143] If insulin regulates potassium uptake by adrenal glomerulosa cells as it does by muscle and liver, then a state of intracellular potassium depletion might be present in an insulin-deficient or -resistant state like diabetes. Previous studies[205,541] have shown that the ability of ACTH and angiotensin II to stimulate aldosterone secretion by cultured zona glomerulosa cells is diminished

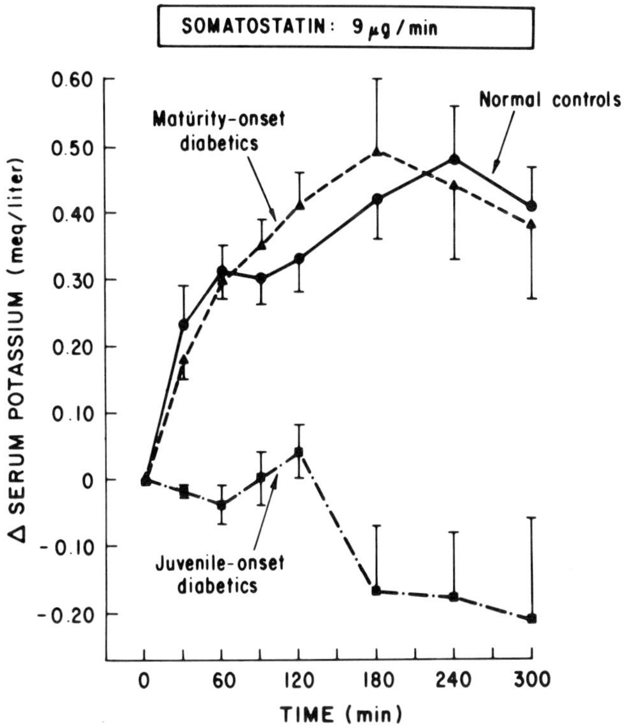

FIGURE 23-19 • Effect of inhibition of basal insulin secretion with somatostatin on the change in plasma potassium concentration in normal controls (solid circles), maturity onset (type II, non-insulin-dependent) diabetics (solid triangles), and juvenile onset (type I, insulin-dependent) diabetics (solid squares). (Reproduced from DeFronzo RA et al: *J Clin Invest* 61:472, 1978.)

in the presence of low potassium concentrations in the incubation medium. These observations are consistent with the known stimulatory effect of potassium on the biosynthetic pathway involving the conversion of cholesterol to deoxycorticosterone as well as corticosterone to aldosterone.[88,257]

Hyporeninism

Many hypotheses have been proposed to explain the defect in renin secretion, yet no single explanation is satisfactory. *Selective damage to the juxtaglomerular apparatus is* possible, especially in diabetic kidneys in which arteriolar sclerosis is regularly observed. However, there are few available data to support this pathogenetic sequence.[426] Several investigators have identified the presence of high concentrations of the biologically inactive renin precursor, "big renin," in association with reduced levels of plasma renin activity in diabetic subjects.[138,157,228,412,494] These observations raise the possibility that hyporeninemia may result from *impaired conversion of pro-renin* (or "big renin") to active renin.[494] A similar defect in nondiabetic patients with selective hypoaldosteronism has not been described, nor is it known how frequently this abnormality occurs in diabetic individuals. Clearly, more work is needed in this area before the pathogenetic significance of elevated levels of big renin can be ascertained.

Decreased circulating *catecholamine* levels and/or autonomic neuropathy also have been suggested to explain the hyporeninemia in diabetic subjects with hypoaldosteronism. Sympathetic nerve terminals are known to innervate the juxtaglomerular apparatus, and epinephrine stimulates renin secretion.[239] Since autonomic neuropathy is a frequent occurrence in diabetes mellitus and since long-standing diabetics may have low circulating catecholamine levels,[108] decreased sympathetic activity has been implicated in the hyporeninemia in diabetic subjects. Support for this hypothesis has been provided by two groups. Tuck et al.[558] found a decreaed plasma renin response to isoproterenol in five hyperkalemic diabetic patients with hyporeninemic hypoaldosteronism and evidence of autonomic and/or peripheral neuropathy. Fernandez-Cruz et al.[191] reported a correlation between stimulated plasma renin activity and the velocity of esophogeal peristalsis in 16 diabetic patients with at most mild renal disease. In contrast, other investigators have described normal plasma and/or urinary catecholamines in six cases of hypoaldosteronism.[87,109,242,565] deChatel et al.[139] failed to find any relationship between decreased plasma epinephrine levels and defects in the reninaldosterone axis in 59 diabetic patients. Although impaired sympathetic nervous system activity and low circulating plasma epinephrine levels may contribute to the hyporeninemia in a minority of diabetics, the high frequency of hyporeninemia remains unexplained. Moreover, there is no evidence that diminished sympathetic activity contributes to the hyporeninemia in nondiabetic subjects with selective hypoaldosteronism.

Low circulating *prostaglandin* levels also have been implicated in the etiology of the hyporeninemia in patients with hypoaldosteronism. Prostaglandins E_2, I_2, and D_2 stimulate renin release,[172,173,174,204,209,614] and inhibition of prostaglandin synthesis with indomethacin or other related drugs impairs renin secretion.[173,204,389,459,544] Prostaglandins E_1 and E_2 also have been shown to augment aldosterone and corticosterone synthesis in vitro.[473] Tan and Mulrow were the first to report clinically significant hyperkalemia in association with hyporeninism and hypoaldosteronism in patients treated with indomethacin[546] (Fig. 23-20). Both the hyperkalemia and the impairment in renin and aldosterone secretion corrected after indomethacin withdrawal and recurred following reinstitution of indomethacin therapy.[546] Since this initial description numerous reports have appeared documenting the development of hyperkalemia and hyporeninemic hypoaldosteronism following indomethacin treatment in both diabetic and nondiabetic patients with and without renal disease.[195,253,343,364,390,545] Other nonsteroidal anti-

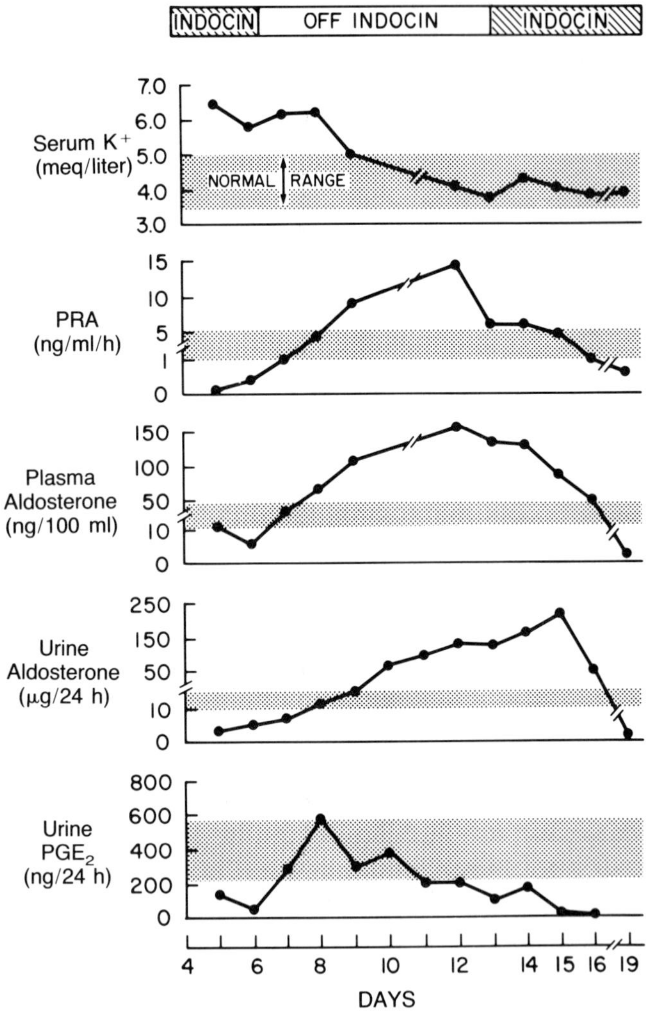

FIGURE 23-20 • Effect of indomethacin administration on the serum potassium (K^+) concentration, plasma renin activity (PRA), plasma aldosterone (aldo) concentration, and urinary excretion of prostaglandin E_2 and aldosterone. (Reproduced from Tan SY et al: *Ann Intern Med* 90:783, 1979.)

inflammatory agents, including ibuprofen, piroxicam, and naproxen, have been implicated in this syndrome.[302,343,366,430,455,487] Thus, it is likely that any agent capable of inhibiting prostaglandin synthesis can produce clinically significant hyperkalemia in susceptible patients. Three studies have documented reduced urinary prostaglandin E_2 levels in some patients with the hyporeninemic hypoaldosteronism syndrome,[390,412,545] but this observation has been challenged by others.[185,253,393] Although the possible association between prostaglandin deficiency and the syndrome of hyporeninemic hypoaldosteronism is an interesting one, further studies are needed to clarify the conflicting reports that have appeared. There is no doubt that treatment with inhibitors of prostaglandin synthesis can produce the syndrome of hyporeninemic hypoaldosteronism and cause life-threatening hyperkalemia, especially in patients with diabetes mellitus, underlying chronic renal disease, or a subclinical defect in the renin-aldosterone axis. However, it remains unclear how often endogenous prostaglandin deficiency contributes to the spontaneous development of hyporeninemic hypoaldosteronism and clinically significant hyperkalemia.

Extracellular fluid volume expansion secondary to sodium retention and hyperglycemia has been reported to cause a state of physiologic renin suppression.[314,393,417,418,426,438,439] However, in none of the studies in which volume contraction was induced with diuretics and/or a low sodium-diet were changes in the plasma potassium concentration or total body potassium stores taken into account. Since hyperkalemia itself suppresses renin secretion,[91,480,492] the simultaneous correction of this abnormality could, in part, have been responsible for the increase in plasma renin activity following volume contraction. Most importantly, even though most patients demonstrated a two- to threefold increase in plasma aldosterone levels in response to volume contraction, the absolute values always were well below those reported in healthy controls with a similar degree of ECF depletion. For example, in the patients reported by Oh et al.[393] plasma renin activity rose into the normal range following prolonged (3 to 6 weeks) volume contraction; plasma aldosterone levels also increased, but still remained low in absolute terms. These discordant responses of renin and aldosterone to volume contraction support the existence of a primary adrenal defect in aldosterone biosynthesis. Nearly identical findings have been reported by Perez et al.[417] and Hsueh et al.[228,235] One could postulate the following pathophysiologic sequence. Plasma levels of aldosterone decline, causing an impairment in renal potassium excretion, and the ensuing hyperkalemia in turn inhibits renin secretion.[91,480,492] In two studies designed to test this hypothesis[475,587] plasma renin activity failed to rise significantly in response to short-term (3 to 4 days) normalization of the plasma potassium concentration. However, concomitant changes in plasma volume and the brief duration of the studies[475,587] introduce difficulties in interpretation.

Finally, a theoretical pathogenetic sequence applicable to the diabetic patient could explain both hyporeninemia as well as *glomerula hyperfiltration*.[80,103a,282,283,284] The normal kidney has a regulatory mechanism (tubuloglomerular feedback) whereby increased delivery of sodium chloride to the macula densa triggers a negative feedback signal that lowers GFR.[481,482,607] Conversely if sodium chloride reabsorption by the macula densa cells is inhibited with furosemide[607,609] or the osmotic agent mannitol,[481,482] the normal tubuloglomerular feedback mechanism is blocked, and single nephron glomerular filtration rate (SNGFR) fails to decline, or even increases. In the diabetic, when the fasting plasma glucose concentration exceeds 160 to 180 g/dl, the large increase in filtered glucose load causes glucosuria and decreased sodium reabsorption by all nephron segments. Glucose, which exerts osmotic effects similar to those of mannitol, should disrupt the normal tubuloglomerular feedback loop. Blantz and Konnen[66] have provided direct experimental evidence to document such a sequence (Fig. 23-21). If the macula densa is perfused with increasing rates of a glucose-free solution, SNGFR drops markedly. If, however, hypertonic glucose is added to the perfusion solution to inhibit sodium reabsorption, the decrease in SNGFR is blunted. The same authors[67,560] have shown that a non-volume-expanding infusion of hypertonic glucose in vivo increases SNGFR despite enhanced tubular flow rate and sodium delivery to the macula densa. The renin-producing cells of the macula densa are strategically placed to participate in tubuloglomerular feedback. Renin release, local generation of angiotensin II, and changes in arteriolar tone and glomerular barrier permeability (K_f) in a direction to lower GFR could ensue following feedback activation. Conversely, disruption of this mechanism by glucosuria could explain the high rates of renal plasma flow and GFR observed early in the course of poorly controlled type I diabetic individuals, as

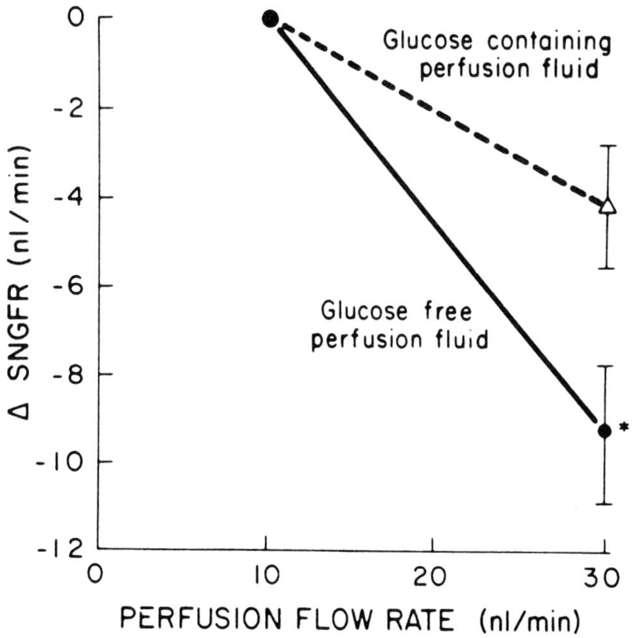

FIGURE 23-21 • Tubuloglomerular feedback-induced changes in single-nephron glomerular filtration rate (SNGFR) using artificial solutions containing no glucose (solid circles) and a solution containing glucose (6 m*M*/liter) and amino acids (6 m*M*/liter) (open triangles). With glucose-free solutions, SNGFR decreased 7 to 10 nl/min when late proximal microperfusion rate was increased from 10 to 30 nl/min (P* < 0.05). When solutions containing glucose and amino acid were used, SNGFR decreased by only 4 nl/min, indicating that addition of these substances decreased tubuloglomerular feedback activity. (Reproduced from Blantz R, Konnen KS: *Kidney Int* 22:5206, 1982.)**

well as the eventual development of hyporeninemia.[369] However, the exact role that the renin-angiotensin system plays in tubuloglomerular feedback is controversial;[46a] although a modulating role appears likely,[428] recent evidence even suggests inhibition of renin secretion when feedback is activated by enhanced sodium chloride delivery to the macula densa.[510] Thus, a causal relationship between glucosuria on the one hand, and suppression of renin production and glomerular hyperfiltration on the other, remains an attractive but unsubstantiated hypothesis.

In summary, there are multiple factors that can impair both renin and aldosterone secretion in diabetic patients, and it is likely that no simple sequence will explain the frequent occurrence of hyporeninemic hypoaldosteronism. The complexity of the alterations in the renin-aldosterone axis in diabetes mellitus is underscored by the findings of deChatel et al.,[139] who characterized renin and aldosterone secretion in 59 normokalemic diabetics (Table 23-8). In 31 of 59 patients (53 percent), both the renin and aldosterone responses during a standardized tilt test were normal. In the other 28 patients a variety of abnormalities were observed. Five (8 percent) had a diminished aldosterone response but a normal renin response, 13 (22 percent) had impaired renin release with a normal aldosterone response, and 10 (17 percent) manifested decreased release of both renin and aldosterone. These results suggest that, at least in the diabetic patient, multiple defects are present in the renin-aldosterone axis and that hyperkalemia is likely to be multifactorial in origin.

Drug-induced causes of hyporeninemic hypoaldosteronism

A variety of drugs have been shown to inhibit the renin-angiotensin-aldosterone axis (Table 23-9). Of these, *prostaglandin inhibitors* (see previous discussion) are the most widely recognized. This class of drugs has been shown to inhibit both renin[173,204,389,459,544] and aldosterone[473] secretion and to cause clinically significant hyperkalemia in the absence of any impairment in renal function.[173,204,253,302,343,361,389,390,430,455,459,487,544,545,546] The hyperkalemia is completely reversible when the prostaglandin inhibitor is discontinued.

Beta-adrenergic antagonists also have been implicated in the development of hyperkalemia, and the disturbance in potassium metabolism is related to both renal and extrarenal mechanisms. Propranolol has been shown to be efficacious in the treatment of high-renin hypertensive states, and its mechanism of action is related to its ability to inhibit renin secretion and secondarily decrease plasma angiotensin II levels and aldosterone secretion. Despite its widespread use, however, few cases of clinically significant hyperkalemia have been reported, and these have primarily occurred in patients who received propranolol prior to cardiopulmonary bypass surgery.[52,422] In most patients who are started on therapy with beta blockers there is a rise in serum potassium concentration, but it is small, on the order of 0.2 to 0.5 meq/liter.[92,168,408,410,556] Individuals with underlying diabetes mellitus[102,610] or chronic renal disease[20,103] are more likely to develop hyperkalemia when treated with a beta-adrenergic antagonist. Whether the hyperkalemia results from inhibition of renin secretion or, as is more likely, from impaired cellular uptake of potassium via the beta-2-adrenergic mechanism[55,59,115,153,321] is not clear. If a beta blocker is needed in a high-risk patient, substitution of metoprolol or atenolol (specific beta-1 antagonists) may be tried,[102,103] since extrarenal potassium metabolism is regulated via the beta-2

TABLE 23-8 • Plasma aldosterone and renin response to tilting in 59 normokalemic diabetic patients

Number	31	5	13	10
Aldosterone	N	↓	N	↓
Renin	N	N	↓	↓
Percentage	53	8	22	17

N = normal
↓ = decreased

SOURCE: Data summarized from deChatel R et al: *Kidney Int* 12:412, 1977.

TABLE 23-9 • Drug-induced hyperkalemia

Impaired renin-aldosterone secretion
- Prostaglandin inhibitors
  - (indomethacin, ibuprofen, piroxicam, aspirin, naproxen, fenoprofen, sulindac)
- Beta-adrenergic antagonists
- Converting enzyme inhibitors
  - (captopril, enalapril, linsinopril)
- Heparin

Inhibitors of renal tubular potassium secretion
- Potassium sparing diuretics
  - (amiloride, spironolactone, triamterene)
- Cyclosporine
- Lithium
- Digitalis

Altered potassium distribution
- Insulin antagonists
  - (somatostatin, diazoxide)
- Beta-adrenergic antagonists
- Alpha-adrenergic agonists
- Hypertonic solutions
  - (glucose, mannitol, saline)
- Digitalis
- Succinylcholine
- Arginine hydrochloride, lysine hydrochloride

receptor.[55,115,153,321] Labetalol, a combined beta-1 and alpha-adrenergic blocker, also has been shown to cause hyperkalemia.[23] Recently, the important role of the beta-2-adrenergic receptor in extrarenal potassium has been used to therapeutic advantage in the treatment of patients with hyperkalemia, by the administration of intravenous or inhalational beta-2 agonists.[10,11,95,140,334,370,371,595]

Captopril, a converting enzyme inhibitor, also has been shown to cause hyperkalemia.[249,584] In a prospective study Textor et al.[549] found that in 23 of 33 hypertensive patients started on captopril the serum potassium concentration rose (increment = 0.8 ± 0.1 meq/liter) in association with a decrease in aldosterone secretion. The rise in serum potassium concentration was inversely related to the GFR, and severe hyperkalemia (> 6.0 meq/liter) was observed only in patients with markedly reduced renal function. Atlas et al.[24] also found a consistent, albeit modest, rise (<1.0 meq/liter) in serum potassium concentration in association with impaired aldosterone secretion in 23 hypertensive patients with reduced GFR. In 400 hypertensive patients with normal renal function who were treated with captopril for 12 weeks, the serum potassium concentration increased significantly but only by 0.11 ± 0.04 meq/liter.[570] These results indicate that captopril therapy in patients with underlying renal disease,[24,549] concomitant treatment with beta-adrenergic antagonists,[249] associated hypertonicity,[440] or renal artery stenosis[8] are at greater risk of developing hyperkalemia. Like captopril, enalapril also has been shown to inhibit aldosterone secretion and to produce mild potassium retention and hyperkalemia during both short-term and prolonged administration.[44,216]

Prolonged, *heparin* administration may cause hyperkalemia.[175,178,345,394,427,602] The deleterious effect of heparin is mediated by inhibition of aldosterone biosynthesis.[229,309] O'Kelly et al.[394] examined the effect of routine heparin therapy on aldosterone secretion in 20 hospitalized patients and found a 50 percent decline in basal plasma aldosterone levels. This decrease was not related to changes in plasma renin activity, which rose threefold following heparin. Unfortunately, plasma potassium concentrations were not reported in this series. On the basis of the magnitude of the decline in plasma aldosterone levels, one would not expect the development of hyperkalemia in patients with otherwise intact potassium homeostatic mechanisms. If, however, a preexisting defect in the renin-aldosterone axis or in potassium metabolism is present (long-standing insulin-dependent diabetes mellitus, concomitant use of converting enzyme inhibitors, chronic renal failure), clinically significant hyperkalemia is a threat.[83,175,178,328]

Recently, the development of severe hyperkalemia has been reported with the use of *pentamidine* to treat pneumocystis carinii infection in patients with acquired immunodeficiency syndrome.[322,413] In 19 of 20 patients treated with pentamidine for more than six days, hyperkalemia (5.1 to 8.7 meq/liter) developed.[322] The concomitant development of a hyperchloremic metabolic acidosis also was observed. Serum potassium and bicarbonate concentrations were normal prior to the start of therapy and returned to normal after discontinuation of pentamidine. In two patients, plasma renin and aldosterone concentrations were reduced.[322] However, this observation is difficult to interpret since the syndrome of hyporeninemic hypoaldosteronism has been reported in patients with AIDS who were not receiving pentamidine.[293] Moreover, the majority of patients treated with pentamidine also develop renal toxicity and a significant reduction in GFR.[322] Therefore, it is possible that the hyperkalemic, hyperchloremic metabolic acidosis was secondary to impaired renal tubular function and not to aldosterone deficiency. The measurement of plasma renin-aldosterone levels and urinary potassium concentration and urine pH could help to distinguish between these two possibilities.

RENAL TUBULAR SECRETORY DEFECT

Over the last decade numerous patients have been described in whom hyperkalemia has been associated with normal or high circulating plasma renin and aldosterone levels and in whom large doses of mineralocorticoid fail to restore normokalemia. These patients are characterized by a defect in the renal tubular secretion of potassium (Fig. 23-11).[22,37,39,148,321,420,498] Varying terminology has been used by different authors for this syndrome, including "renal tubular hyperkalemia," "voltage-dependent renal tubular hyperkalemia," "hyperkalemic distal renal tubular acidosis," and "pseudhypoaldosteronism."[39,321]

Sickle cell disease

DeFronzo et al.[145] studied six young, normokalemic patients with sickle cell disease. All had normal GFRs and normal baseline plasma aldosterone and renin levels. All subjects demonstrated normal increases in aldosterone and renin secretion in response to volume contraction, ACTH, angiotensin II infusion, and upright posture. Nonetheless, the increment in urinary potassium excretion following the administration of intravenous potassium chloride, furosemide, and sodium sulfate was markedly diminished (Fig. 23-22). Impaired potassium secretion with an intact renin-angiotensin-aldosterone axis documents the presence of a primary renal tubular potassium secretory defect. The inability of intravenous sodium sulfate to augment potassium excretion is particularly characteristic of a renal tubular secretory defect. Increased distal delivery of the impermeant sulfate anion stimulates potassium excretion by three mechanisms:

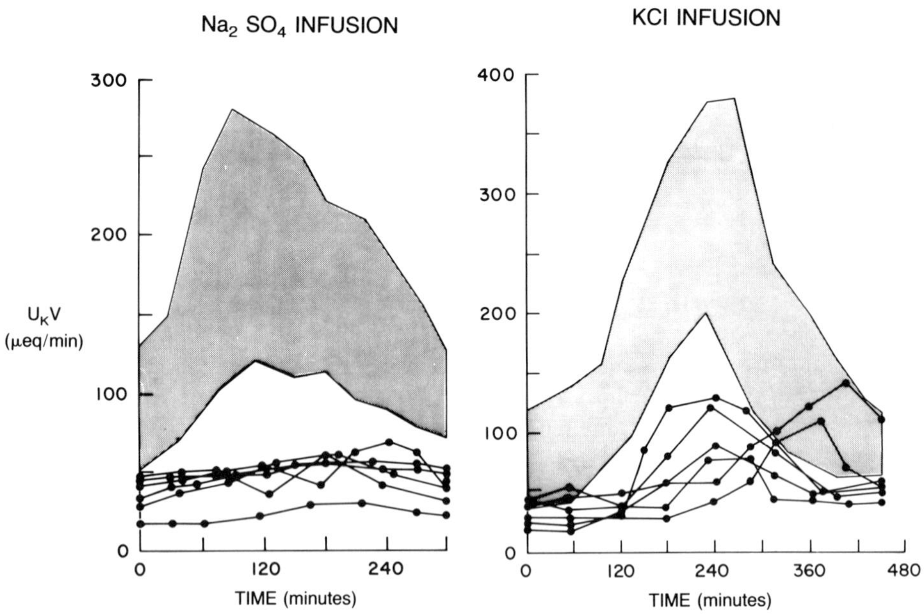

FIGURE 23-22 • (*Left panel*) Urinary potassium excretion (U_KV) after intravenous sodium sulfate administration in subjects with sickle cell disease (closed circles). The shaded area indicates the normal range in control subjects. (*Right panel*) Urinary potassium excretion (U_KV) after intravenous potassium chloride administration in subjects with sickle cell disease (closed circles). The shaded area indicates the normal range in control subjects. (Adapted from DeFronzo RA et al: *Ann Intern Med* 90:310, 1979.)

(1) it augments distal sodium delivery and urine flow;[238,306,318,350] (2) it increases lumen negativity,[110] which enhances distal potassium secretion; and (3) it limits chloride availability, which impairs potassium reabsorption by the distal nephron.[566] The ability of sulfate to stimulate potassium secretion, although somewhat blunted, persists in the absence of aldosterone.[100] Some authors favor the furosemide test over intravenous sodium sulfate as the definitive maneuver to look for a specific renal tubular defect in potassium secretion.[42,321] By increasing distal sodium delivery and urine flow, furosemide should markedly augment renal potassium secretion.

Since the original description of this tubular secretory defect by DeFronzo et al.,[145] a number of cases of life-threatening hyperkalemia have been reported in patients with sickle cell disease.[36,148] Impaired distal potassium secretion also may be observed in patients with sickle cell disease and those with sickle cell trait. It should be emphasized that patients with sickle cell disease also may have a simultaneous defect in the renin-aldosterone axis.[148] The mechanism of the defect in potassium secretion may be related to injury to the distal and collecting tubular cells (secondary to RBC sickling and anoxic damage) or disruption of the normal medullary architecture. In addition, several authors[148,404] have reported the presence of numerous electron-dense deposits within the tubular basement membrane which may represent immune complex formation derived from tubular antigens. These observations suggest the possibility that the defect in renal potassium secretion represents the physiologic counterpart of an immunologic reaction directed at the renal tubular cell.

Systemic lupus erythematosus

Impaired distal hydrogen ion secretion in patients with systemic lupus erythematosus (SLE) has long been recognized.[321,377] An accompanying defect in distal potassium secretion also has been described.[142,169,252,313,326] In the two most extensively studied cases,[142] neither furosemide nor acetazolamide plus bicarbonate was capable of augmenting potassium excretion. Supraphysiologic doses of fludrocortisone acetate also failed to augment potassium excretion despite a normal decline in urinary sodium excretion. Both patients also had a defect in H^+ excretion.[142] A number of investigators[15,81,405] have described a prominent interstitial inflammatory reaction characterized by cellular infiltration, tubular damage, and interstitial fibrosis in patients with SLE. Immunoglobulins, complement, or both, were deposited in tubular basement membrane and interstitial tissue in a granular pattern. Although no physiologic studies were performed in these patients, it is likely that the tubular defects in potassium and H^+ excretion represent the physiologic counterpart of the immunopathologic abnormalities observed.[15,81]

Renal transplantation

Renal transplant patients are at particularly high risk to develop hyperkalemia.[38,141,251] DeFronzo et al.[141] described significant hyperkalemia in 23 of 75 patients (31 percent) during the first three months following renal transplantation. The hyperkalemia was unrelated to kidney rejection, renal failure, oliguria, or acidemia. Six patients studied in detail manifested normal renin-aldosterone responses to volume contraction and upright posture, but did not augment renal potassium excretion in response to furosemide, acetazolamide plus sodium bicarbonate infusion, or fludrocortisone administration. When these patients were reevaluated following spontaneous remission of the hyperkalemia, normal kaliuretic responses to furosemide and fludrocortisone were documented. Although the hyperkalemia could not be related to overt graft rejection, the authors proposed immune injury to renal tubular epithelium as a possible mechanism. In support of this concept, antitubular basement membrane antibodies have been demonstrated in renal transplant patients.[304,601] It is noteworthy that antitubular basement membrane antibodies have been described in patients with sickle cell disease, systemic lupus erythematosus, and postrenal transplantation, and all three disorders have been associated with a renal tubular potassium secretory defect.

Obstructive uropathy

Hyperkalemia is a common feature in animal models of obstructive uropathy.[260] In 1980, Batlle et al. reported hyperkalemia and hyperchloremic metabolic acidosis in 13 patients with obstructive uropathy.[40] In five patients basal plasma aldosterone concentration was normal yet renal potassium excretion failed to increase normally in response to acetazolamide, sodium sulfate, or fludrocortisone. These patients had an isolated renal tubular defect in potassium secretion. The remaining eight patients also failed to increase potassium excretion in response to the standard provocative measures, but in addition had low plasma aldosterone levels. Thus, they had both selective hypoaldosteronism and a renal tubular potassium secretory defect. Similar findings have been noted by others.[412] Recently, Sabatini and Kurtzman[469] have examined both the proton pump and the Na^+,K^+-ATPase pump in microdissected tubules from rats with urinary tract obstruction. Na^+,K^+-ATPase activity was decreased throughout all distal nephron segments while the defect in the proton pump was localized to the collecting tubule. These data indicate that urinary tract obstruction interferes with potassium secretion and acidification by directly inhibiting the potassium and proton pumps, respectively.

Selective hypoaldosteronism

Patients with hypoaldosteronism and hyperkalemia often are treated with a mineralocorticoid, usually fludrocortisone acetate.[148] Most of these patients have diabetes mellitus with renal involvement or chronic interstitial nephritis as the cause of the hypoaldosteronism. In 51 such patients treated with a mineralocorticoid, a reduction in plasma potassium concentration was noted in 43. However, large doses of fludrocortisone, often as high as 0.4 to 1.0 mg daily, were required to reduce the plasma potassium level to normal.[148] These observations indicate that the renal tubular cell is resistant to the action of mineralocorticoids, at least with respect to the effect on potassium secretion. It is likely that this potassium secretory defect is related to the underlying chronic renal disease that is present in most of these patients.

Pseudohypoaldosteronism (Table 23-10)

Renal hyperkalemia also has been described in a variety of diverse clinical situations that have been referred to as "pseudohypoaldosteronism" because the clinical and laboratory presentation is suggestive of mineralocorticoid deficiency, yet circulating plasma aldosterone levels are either normal or increased and treatment with mineralocorticoids does not correct the hyperkalemia. The syndrome is comprised of a variety of disorders including classic pseudohypoaldosteronism of infancy,[106] chronic tubulointerstitial diseases usually associated with renal salt wasting,[563] and 21-hydroxylase deficiency with the accumulation of high levels of endogenous aldosterone antagonists.[281,297] The clinical and laboratory features that distinguish pseudohypoaldosteronism are depicted in Table 23-10.

Type I pseudohypoaldosteronism of infancy

This syndrome was initially reported by Cheek and Perry in 1958 in an infant with marked renal salt wasting.[106] Subsequently, more than 40 cases have been reported and several reviews have been published.[391,441,464] Over 90 percent of the reported cases have been diagnosed in infancy, before the age of 7 months. The major clinical presentation is failure to thrive. Volume contraction, dehydration, and marked electrolyte imbalance are prominent features. All have severe renal salt wasting, impaired potassium excretion, hyperkalemia, and hyperchloremic metabolic acidosis. The plasma cortisol concentration is normal, while plasma aldosterone and renin levels are markedly elevated and there is no kaliuretic response to pharmacologic doses of mineralocorticoids. This constellation of findings documents the presence of resistance to the action of aldosterone. In four patients who had renal biopsies no structural abnormalities were demonstrated. The resistance to aldosterone appears to be shared by multiple target organs, including kidney, colon, sweat glands, and salivary glands.[391] Recently, Armanini et al.[18] have demonstrated a reduction in the number of type I mineralocorticoid receptors on monocytes from three patients with pseudohypoaldosteronism of infancy, including the original case described by Cheek and Perry.[106] Since the mineralocorticoid receptor on monocytes appears to be identical to that on the renal tubular cells, it seems likely that a similar deficiency exists in the

TABLE 23-10 • Clinical and laboratory characteristics of hyperkalemic states associated with renal potassium retention

	GFR	Blood pressure	Salt wasting	Renin	Aldosterone	Plasma HCO_3^-	Plasma Cl^-
Addison's disease	↓,N	↓,N	Yes	↑↑	↓↓	↓	↑
Selective (primary) hypoaldosteronism	↓,N	↑,N	No	N	↓	↓	↑
Hyporeninemic hypoaldosteronism	↓,N	↑,N	No	↓↓	↓	↓	↑
Pseudohypoaldosteronism							
Type I (infancy)*	↓,N	↓,N	Yes	↑↑	↑↑	↓	↑
Type II (adult with hypertension)†	N	↑	No	↓	↓,N	↓	↑
Type III (adult without hypertension)‡	↓	↓,N	Yes	↓,N,↑	↓,N	↓	↑

* Also referred to as classic pseudoaldosteronism of infancy.
† Also referred to as Gordon's syndrome.
‡ Associated with chronic renal failure of the tubulointerstitial variety and distal RTA.
GFR = glomerular filtration rate
N = normal
Number of arrows indicates the magnitude of the increase or decrease

kidney and is responsible for renal salt wasting and hyperkalemia. Whether all cases of pseudohypoaldosteronism of infancy can be explained by the same defect is uncertain at present. Extrapolation of this defect to explain pseudohypoaldosteronism in adults in unwarranted, since the later syndrome is almost always acquired.

Supplementation of the diet with large amounts of sodium chloride greatly improves the hyperkalemia, metabolic acidosis, and hypotension and improves growth velocity. Fortunately, in most affected children the syndrome is self-limiting and sodium supplementation can be discontinued after 1 to 2 years of age.

Type II pseudohypoaldosteronism in adults with hypertension

Patients have recently been described with hyperkalemia, intact renal sodium conservation, normal renal function, hypertension, low plasma renin activity, low to normal plasma aldosterone levels, and a normal antinatriuretic response to mineralocorticoids but absent kaliuretic response.[19,65,76,147,167,186,327,407,435,521,537,596] This constellation of clinical and laboratory features has been referred to as *Gordon's syndrome* in recognition of the original clinical description.[240] Seventeen of the 28 patients reviewed by Gordon[241] came from four families, making a genetic origin likely. However, sporadic cases have been described.[241]

Patients with Gordon's syndrome can be distinguished from those with hyporeninemic hypoaldosteronism by the documentation of normal renal function, absence of any history of diabetes mellitus, uniform presence of hypertension, absence of salt wasting when dietary sodium is restricted, and lack of kaliuretic response to mineralocorticoids. Although the precise nature of the defect in potassium secretion has yet to be delineated, several mechanisms have been postulated. Schambelan et al.[477] suggested that the primary defect may be related to enhanced chloride reabsorption in the early portion of the distal tubule (Fig. 23-23). This limits sodium delivery to the more distal nephron sites of potassium secretion and leads to a decline in lumen negativity with an impairment in potassium secretion due to a voltage-shunting effect. The increase in sodium chloride reabsorption expands the ECF volume, causes hypertension, and suppresses the renin-aldosterone axis. Hyperkalemia also contributes to the inhibition of renin secretion.[471] The plasma aldosterone concentration may be normal or suppressed depending upon the balance between the inhibitory effect of volume expansion and the stimulatory effect of hyperkalemia. Consistent with this thesis, treatment with thiazide or loop diuretics consistently enhances renal potassium and H^+ excretion, corrects the metabolic acidosis and hyperkalemia, normalizes the blood pressure, and returns plasma aldosterone and renin levels to normal.[241,307,331,471,477,498] It should be noted that all of the preceding laboratory abnormalities could be explained equally well by lack of natriuretic or chloriuretic hormone[241,498] or deficiency of E series prostaglandins which are natriuretic.[555] True refractoriness to mineralocorticoids is unlikely since salt restriction corrects all abnormalities.[241,307,331,498] Moreover, administration of fludrocortisone after sodium chloride restriction results in a normal increase in net acid and potassium excretion.[331] Although a primary renal tubular defect in potassium secretion has also been postulated, a normal kaliuretic response to sodium sulfate infusion and furosemide makes this mechanism unlikely.[241,307,331]

Type III pseudohypoaldosteronism in adults without hypertension

In adults a syndrome has been described consisting of hyperkalemia with impaired urinary potassium excretion, high circulating plasma aldosterone levels, and failure of the kidney to respond to exogenous mineralocorticoid administration. This syndrome is usually found in patients with tubulointerstitial renal diseases.[116,339,374,431,437] As reviewed by Uribarri et al.,[563] impaired sodium conservation with frank salt wasting and distal renal tubular acidosis are common accompanying features. As stated above, these patients characteristically have high circulating aldosterone levels, indicating the presence of renal tubular resistance to endogenous mineralocorticoids. Moreover, large doses of exogenous mineralocorticoids fail to correct the hyperkalemia, renal salt wasting, or metabolic acidosis.[563] These patients are truly resistant to the action of aldosterone. Typically, renal histopathology shows chronic tubulointerstitial damage. Most patients have either obstructive uropathy, medullary cystic disease, sickle cell nephropathy, lead nephropathy amyloidosis, or idiopathic interstitial nephritis.[563]

Hyperkalemic distal renal tubular acidosis

The combination of hyperkalemia, impaired renal potassium excretion, hyperchloremic metabolic acidosis, and distal renal tubular acidosis (RTA) (urine pH greater than 5.5 in the presence of systemic acidemia) has recently received much attention.[39,321] It is commonly accompanied by a potassium secretory defect.[22,36,38,39,40,141,142,251,252,377,420,563] Plasma aldosterone and renin concentrations in these patients are normal or increased. Hyperkalemia, and in some cases hyperchloremic metabolic acidosis, are also seen in hyporeninemic hypoaldosteronism. However, in humans[496] and animals[161,558] with hypoaldosteronism, the ability to lower the urine pH is normal, the metabolic acidosis resulting from a defect in ammonium excretion.[161,285,496] By definition, therefore, an inappropriately high urine pH (greater than 5.5) indicates the presence of hyperkalemic distal RTA whether the plasma aldosterone concentration is normal or low.[39,321] It should be noted that hyporeninemic hypoaldosteronism and hyperkalemic distal renal tubular acidosis often coexist.[39,148,321] The patient with hyperkalemic distal RTA is readily distinguished from the person with classic distal RTA by the presence of hypokalemia in the latter.[377,496] The response to sodium sulfate (or furosemide) also helps to differentiate these two groups and provides some insight into the pathogenesis of the two disorders.[39,321] In normal subjects both of these agents augment both distal H^+ and potassium secretion, because the accompanying increase in cortical collecting tubule sodium delivery and reabsorption will enhance luminal electronegativity; an additional effect is provided by the impermeant SO_4^{2-} ion, which in comparison with chloride retards dissipation of the electrical gradient. Consequently, urine pH declines and the fractional excretion of potassium is increased (Fig. 23-24). In patients with classic distal RTA, Na_2SO_4 infusion or furosemide fails to lower the urine pH below 5.5 because of the isolated defect in the H^+-ATPase pump present in intercalated cells, but potassium excretion is increased, because sodium reabsorption and potassium excretion by principal cells is intact (Fig. 23-24). In contrast, in patients with hyperkalemic distal RTA, Na_2SO_4 infusion and furosemide fail to increase either potassium or H^+ excretion.[39,176,321] This could result from separate defects in H^+ and potassium

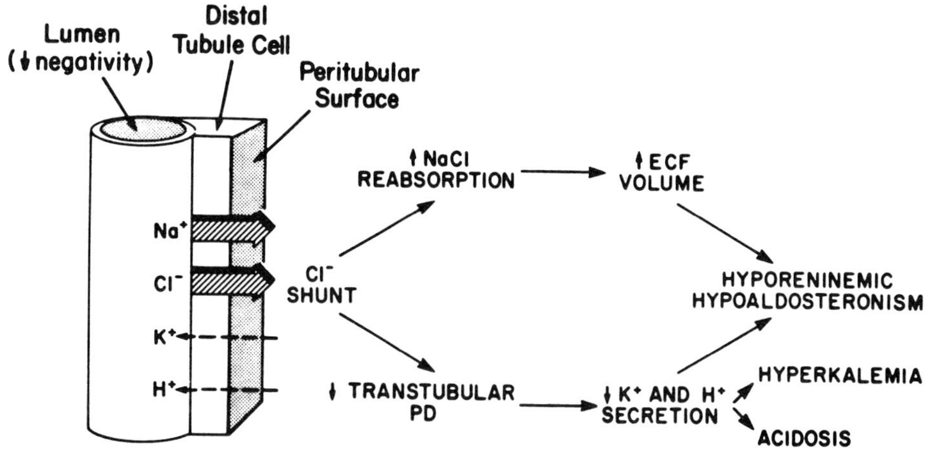

FIGURE 23-23 • Pathophysiologic consequences of enhanced chloride reabsorption by the early distal tubule. (See text for discussion.) [Reproduced from Smith et al, in Arieff A, DeFronzo RA (eds): *Fluid, Electrolyte, and Acid-Base Disorders,* New York, Churchill Livingstone, 1985, p 413, as adapted from Schambelan M et al: *Kidney Int* 19:716, 1981.]

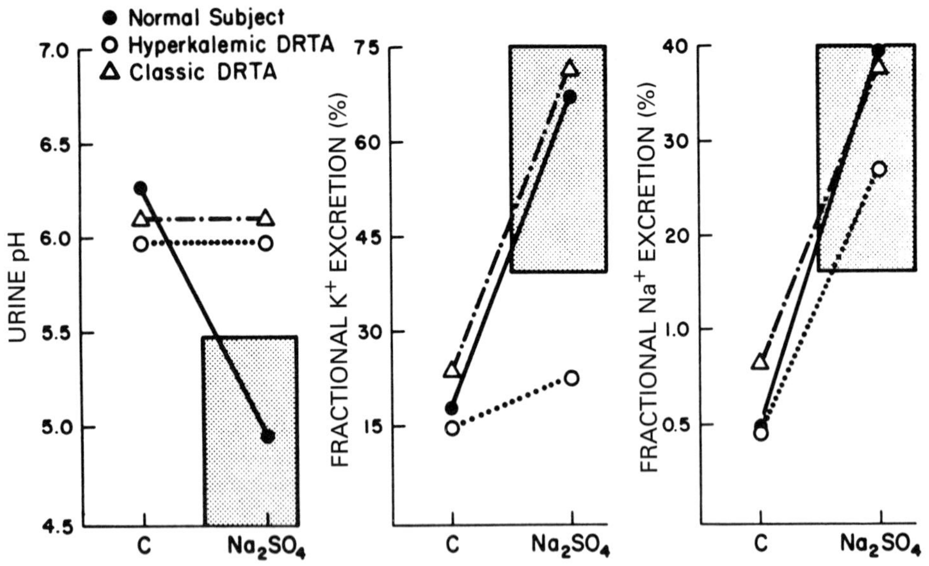

FIGURE 23-24 • Urinary pH, fractional potassium (K) excretion, and fractional excretion of sodium (Na) following Na_2SO_4 infusion into normal subjects (solid circles), subjects with hyperkalemic distal RTA (open circles), and subjects with classical distal RTA (open triangles). Na_2SO_4 fails to lower urine pH or to increase fractional potassium excretion in patients with hyperkalemic distal RTA. In contrast, patients with classical distal RTA increase fractional potassium excretion but cannot lower urine pH normally, indicating the presence of an isolated defect in H^+ secretion. (Adapted from Batlle DC: *Semin Nephrol* 1:260, 1981.)

ion secretion. On the other hand, since both H^+ and potassium secretion in the cortical collecting tubule are dependent upon luminal electronegativity contingent upon sodium reabsorption, it is possible that the primary defect results from impaired renal tubular sodium transport (voltage defect).[39,176,321]

Inhibition of tubular secretion of potassium

Both *spironolactone* and *triamterene* inhibit potassium secretion by the distal tubule. Spironolactone binds competitively to the cytoplasmic mineralocorticoid receptor on the pericapillary side of distal tubular cells, leading to an inhibition of the action of aldosterone.[130] Chronic administration of spironolactone is associated with an increased level of plasma aldosterone and mineralocorticoid resistance.[442] In contrast, inhibition of potassium secretion by triamterene and amiloride is not dependent upon the presence of aldosterone. These agents bind reversibly to the luminal membrane and block sodium entry into the distal tubule cell, thereby reducing luminal negativity and inhibiting potassium secretion.[21,225] Administration of these agents to diabetic patients or patients with renal insufficiency, in whom potassium tolerance is known to be compromised, is particularly hazardous. Life-threatening hyperkalemia also has been described in patients with normal renal function and without diabetes mellitus.[117,188,344,353,578,594] Likewise, with rare exception, potassium salts should not be prescribed for individuals who are ingesting these diuretics.

Massive *digitalis* overdose, as in suicide attempts, also causes potentially lethal hyperkalemia.[64,452,513] The rise in plasma potassium concentration results from a generalized inhibition of membrane Na^+,K^+-ATPase, which leads to a reduction in renal tubular potassium secretion as well as a decrease in potassium uptake by extrarenal tissues. Smith et al.[512] have developed a digoxin specific antibody to rapidly reverse hyperkalemia and arrhythmias in patients with severe digitalis intoxication.

Cyclosporine therapy in patients following renal or cardiac transplantation has been associated with a high incidence of hyperkalemia and hyperchloremic metabolic acidosis.[7,28,247,423] Plasma aldosterone levels are inappropriately low in relation to the degree of hyperkalemia, and urinary acidification is not impaired. However, many patients were on beta blockers for treatment of hypertension and this could have contributed to the blunted rise in plasma aldosterone and hyperkalemia. Since the majority of patients were receiving large doses of prednisone, which should have had crossover binding activity to the mineralocorticoid receptor, one can assume that resistance to endogenously secreted aldosterone also was present. It is likely that some combination aldosterone resistance and deficiency contribute to the development of hyperkalemia in these patients.

In animals, *lithium* intoxication is associated with severe hyperkalemia, but the plasma lithium concentration (>10 meq/liter) at which this is seen is tenfold greater than the normal therapeutic dose in human beings.[258] Voltage-dependent distal RTA also has been described in animals and humans treated with lithium.[41,320] At least one case of hyperkalemia has been reported with plasma lithium levels in the therapeutic range.[230] Since lithium does not impair the renin-aldosterone axis[508] and has been shown to interfere with excretion of a potassium load,[214] direct impairment of tubular potassium secretion probably underlies the hyperkalemia. Since lithium can enter cells and cause the displacement of potassium in vitro, a defect in extrarenal potassium homeostasis also may be present.

ABNORMAL POTASSIUM DISTRIBUTION

Only 2 percent of the total body potassium is located within the ECF compartment. The majority (98 percent) is located within the intracellular space. Thus, a slight imbalance of internal potassium homeostasis may cause profound hyperkalemia (Fig. 23-1).

Metabolic acidosis

Metabolic acidosis is one of the most frequently encountered causes of redistributional hyperkalemia in clinical nephrology. The cellular mechanisms underlying the exchange of H^+ and potassium ions during acidemic states will be discussed in Chap. 27.

Insulin deficiency and hypertonicity

Insulin plays a central role in maintaining the normal distribution of potassium between intracellular and ECF compartments. If basal insulin secretion is halved by somatostatin infusion in humans, plasma potassium will increase by 0.4 to 0.6 meq/liter (Fig. 23-19).[143] If a potassium infusion is added (Fig. 23-4), a marked deterioration in potassium tolerance ensues.[143] Insulin exerts its effect on potassium metabolism by increasing hepatic and muscle cell uptake.[12,16,146,378,622] Insulin deficiency markedly impairs extrarenal potassium tolerance and predisposes the insulin-dependent diabetic to the development of hyperkalemia.[143,144]

Goldfarb et al. were the first to emphasize that hyperglycemia, particularly in diabetics who lack aldosterone, raises the plasma potassium concentration (Fig. 23-25).[233,234] This observation subsequently has been confirmed by numerous other investigators.[14,387,416,418,432,439,540,571] Hyperglycemia increases plasma osmolality, which in turn induces a shift of water and potassium from the intracellular to extracellular space.[63,373,499,547] Bratusch-Marrain and DeFronzo[75,321] have shown that an increase in plasma tonicity by as little as 15 to 20 mosm/kg will raise the plasma potassium concentration by 0.8 meq/liter (Fig. 23-8). In healthy subjects the efflux of potassium from cells is offset by the action of insulin and aldosterone to augment its cellular uptake (Fig. 23-3). If both of these hormones are deficient, clinically significant hyperkalemia may ensue. Replacement of either insulin alone or mineralocorticoid alone is sufficient to prevent the rise in plasma potassium concentration (Fig. 23-25)[14,232,233,540] It should be emphasized that glucose-induced hyperkalemia may occur in diabetic subjects with normal plasma aldosterone levels[14,387,432,439,540] and in nondiabetic individuals with end stage renal failure.[125] Since the syndrome of hyporeninemic hypoaldosteronism most commonly occurs in insulin-dependent (type I) diabetics with renal disease, this group is at particularly high risk to develop hyperkalemia when glycemic control deteriorates. These observations also raise concern about the empiric administration of hypertonic glucose solutions to diabetic patients who are admitted in coma without prior knowledge of the prevailing plasma glucose concentration.

Aldosterone deficiency

The primary action of aldosterone is to enhance renal potassium excretion.[225] However, recent studies have documented an important action of the hormone to enhance extrarenal potassium uptake (Fig. 23-7).[9,55,56,147,148,612] When potassium is administered to chronically adrenalectomized rats, a marked deterioration in potassium tolerance is observed. This impairment in potassium homeostasis cannot be explained by alterations in renal potassium handling and

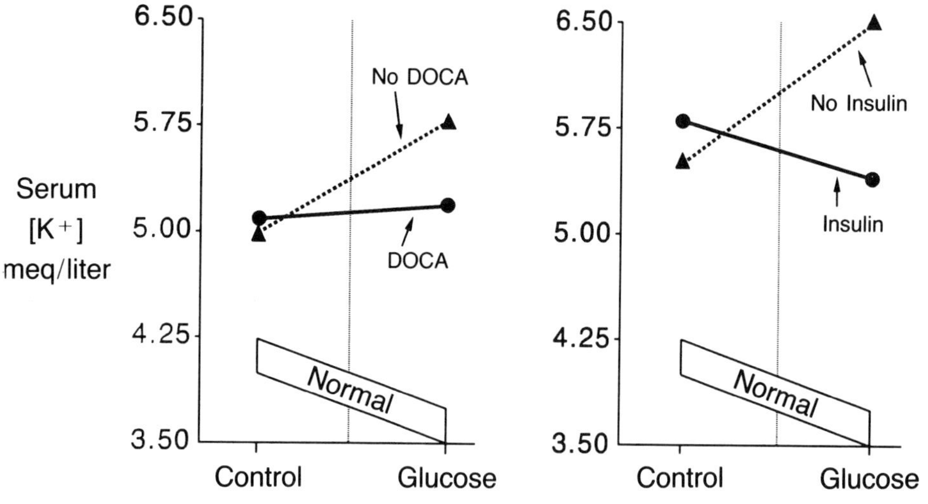

FIGURE 23-25 • Effect of deoxycorticosterone acetate (DOCA) (*left panel*) and insulin (*right panel*) on the serum potassium response to intravenous glucose infusion in diabetic patients with hypoaldosteronism. The normal decline in control subjects is shown for comparison. (Reproduced from Goldfarb S et al: *Ann Intern Med* 84:426, 1976.)

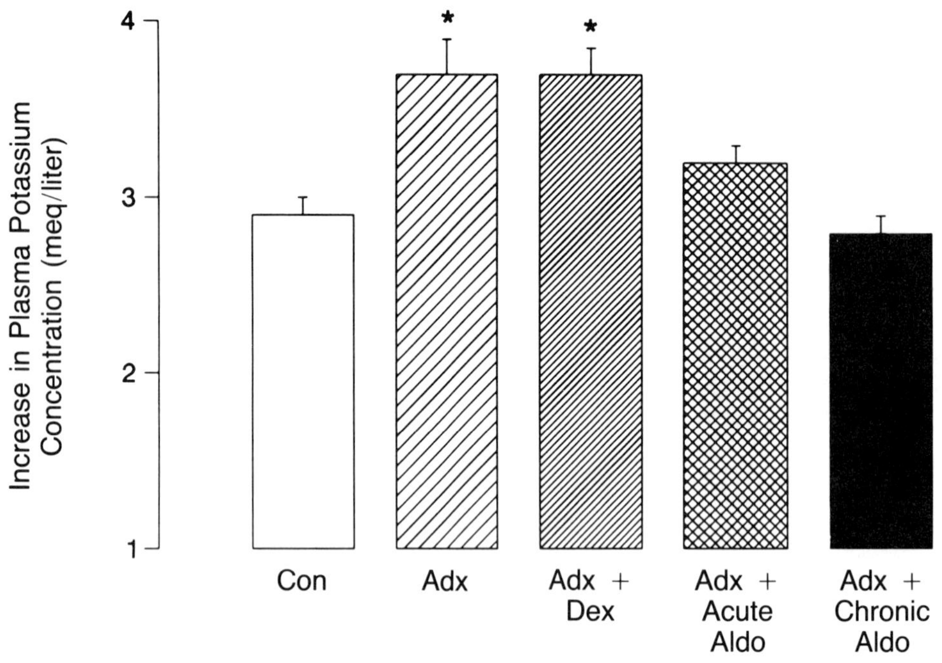

FIGURE 23-26 • Effect of adrenalectomy and adrenal hormone replacement on extrarenal potassium tolerance in rats. Con = control; Adx = adrenalectomy; Dex = dexamethasone; Aldo = aldosterone. (Reproduced from Bia M et al: *Am J Physiol* 242:F641, 1982.)

can be demonstrated in adrenalectomized rats that have been nephrectomized immediately before the administration of the potassium load (Fig. 23-26).[56,147] These results indicate that decreased potassium uptake by nonrenal tissues contributes to the hyperkalemia observed in hypoaldosteronism. In agreement with this concept, mineralocorticoid therapy has been shown to correct hyperkalemia in patients with hypoaldosteronism without any increase in urinary potassium excretion.[29,148,220,392,434] Mineralocorticoids also are effective in treating patients with hyperkalemic periodic paralysis.[539]

Adrenergic antagonists

Catecholamines and beta blockers

As discussed previously, epinephrine enhances potassium uptake by extrarenal tissues,[55,59,149,335,460] and this effect is mediated via the beta 2-adrenergic receptor (Table 23-1). In contrast, nonspecific beta-adrenergic blocking agents such as propranolol inhibit epinephrine-mediated potassium uptake by extrarenal tissues and result in a deterioration of extrarenal potassium tolerance (Table 23- 1).[55,59,149,335,460] Alpha-adrenergic agonists also exert an inhibitory effect on extrarenal potassium homeostasis.[598]

Propranolol enhances the efflux of potassium from muscle,[55,115,134] and this observation explains, in part, the small but significant increase (0.3 to 0.5 meq/liter) in plasma potassium concentration that follows chronic propranolol administration.[410,411,569,575] A similar rise in plasma potassium concentration is observed with all beta-adrenergic blockers that affect the beta-2 receptor.[52,92,408,410,556] Using ^{42}K, Pedersen et al.[411] demonstrated that the rise in plasma potassium concentration during propranolol therapy is not due to retention of potassium within the body but results from a shift from the intracellular to the extracellular compartment. This hyperkalemic effect of propranolol is independent of changes in plasma renin and aldosterone concentration and is not explained by diminished renal potassium excretion. Moreover, both DeFronzo et al.[149] and Rosa et al.[460] have shown that propranolol impairs potassium tolerance despite an augmentation in renal potassium excretion. In clinical situations characterized by impaired renal and/or extrarenal potassium tolerance (i.e., diabetes mellitus, renal disease especially of the interstitial variety, hypoaldosteronism, autonomic insufficiency) or in settings where large potassium loads from either endogenous or exogenous sources (i.e., heavy physical exercise, potassium ingestion, tissue damage) are anticiptaed, the use of beta blocking agents should be undertaken with great caution. It should be remembered that nonspecific beta antagonists also inhibit insulin secretion and thus may remove an important host defense mechanism against hyperkalemia. Despite the deleterious effect of beta blockers, severe hyperkalemia is not commonly encountered, probably because of the potent kaliuretic action of these agents.[296]

Exercise

Exercise is uniformly associated with a rise in the plasma potassium concentration,[75,269] and the magnitude is directly related to the work intensity. In normal subjects the plasma potassium concentration rises to values in excess of 6.0 meq/liter following 10 to 15 min of exhaustive exercise. If the beta-adrenergic nervous system is blocked just prior to the onset of exercise, deterioration in extrarenal potassium tolerance ensues and clinically significant hyperkalemia develops.[101,102,384] If healthy young subjects exercise on a treadmill at 40 to 50 percent of maximum work capacity, the plasma potassium concentration rises by approximatley 0.5 meq/liter, because of a shift from intracellular to extracellular space.[102] If the same exercise is performed following beta blockade with propranolol, the increment in plasma potassium concentration is more than twofold greater, and this effect is magnified in the presence of insulin deficiency.[102] Metoprolol, a beta-1 specific antagonist, does not exacerbate the exercise-induced rise in plasma potassium concentration.[102] A similar deterioration in extrarenal potassium tolerance during exercise has been observed in end stage renal failure patients who are treated with propranolol[103] (Fig. 23-27); metoprolol does not increase the serum potassium beyond that observed with exercise alone. It is noteworthy that heavy exercise, even in the absence of beta-adrenergic agonists, can lead to clinically significant hyperkalemia in hemodialysis patients.[340,341,384]

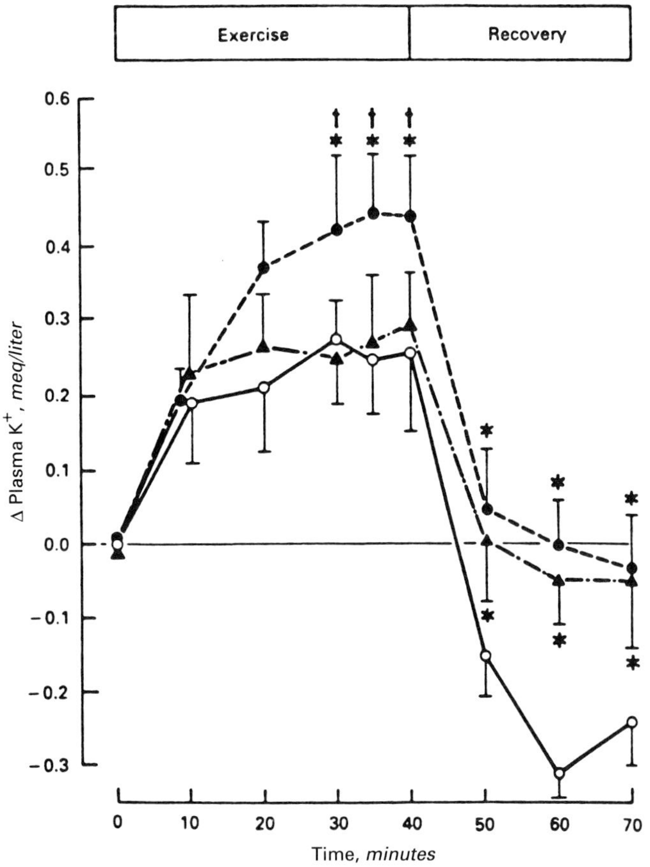

FIGURE 23-27 • Change in plasma potassium concentration (open circles) in patients with end stage renal failure during exercise at 40 percent of their VO_2 max. Propranolol (solid circles), but not metoprolol (solid triangles), caused a signifiant deterioration in extrarenal potassium metabolism. *$P < 0.05$ versus control study. †$P < 0.05$ versus metoprolol study. (Reproduced from Castellino P et al: *Kidney Int* 37:793, 1990.)

Hyperkalemic periodic paralysis

This inherited disorder is transmitted as an autosomal dominant and is characterized by transient attacks of paralysis and hyperkalemia.[55,181,215] Exercise, cold exposure, and potassium administration are known to precipitate attacks. Individuals with this syndrome have normal renal, adrenal, and pancreatic function. During attacks, muscle potassium content decreases as the plasma potassium concentration increases. This causes a marked alteration in the ratio of intracellular to extracellular potassium, an alteration in neuromuscular excitability, and muscle weakness or paralysis. Institution of a high-carbohydrate diet enhances muscle potassium uptake (presumably by causing hyperinsulinemia) and effectively prevents attacks. Thiazide diuretics and acetazolamide, perhaps by increasing the cellular uptake of potassium,[184] also have been employed to decrease the frequency and severity of attacks. Most recently salbutamol, a beta 2-adrenergic agonist, has been shown to be prophylactic in preventing attacks; it also ameliorates the duration and severity of attacks that have already been established.[260,581]

Tissue damage

Significant tissue release of potassium may occur after hemolysis, rhabdomyolysis, burns, major trauma, or tumor lysis.[120,158,380,479,557] Under normal circumstances, the renal tubular cell will respond to the increase in plasma potassium concentration by augmenting secretion. If the tissue destruction is of sufficient magnitude, however, the ability of the kidney to excrete the potassium load may be overwhelmed and hyperkalemia may ensue. If acute renal failure accompanies the tissue damage, hyperkalemia is a common finding and may be life-threatening.

Other causes of cellular potassium redistribution

Digitalis overdose may be accompanied by hyperkalemia, which results from inhibition of the Na^+,K^+-ATPase pump and subsequent release of potassium from cells.[64,115,452,512,513] Use of depolarizing agents, such as *succinylcholine*, during anesthesia or mechanical ventilation may cause a leakage of potassium from cells and lead to hyperkalemia.[316,592,611] *Arginine hydrochloride*, which is used in the treatment of hepatic coma and severe metabolic alkalosis, and as a diagnostic stimulus for the release of growth hormone and insulin, causes efflux of potassium from cells,[159] especially in patients with impaired renal function[273] or liver disease.[99] *Lysine hydrochloride* has a similar hyperkalemic action. *Fluoride* impairs extrarenal potassium uptake, and accidental fluoride poisoning has been reported to cause fatal hyperkalemia in dialysis patients.[360] *Metoclopropamide*, a dopaminergic inhibitor, causes a prompt decline in plasma potassium concentration of 0.2 to 0.4 meq/liter, and *dopamine* has the opposite effect.[53,470] These results indicate that the dopaminergic system plays some role in extrarenal potassium homeostasis, but clinically relevant cases of hyperkalemia related to impaired dopamine receptor function have yet to be reported.

DIAGNOSTIC APPROACH TO HYPERKALEMIC PATIENTS

Once hyperkalemia is discovered, a repeat measurement of the serum potassium concentration should be performed to rule out laboratory error, which is uncommon. Spurious hyperkalemia is readily excluded by simultaneous measurement of the serum and plasma potassium concentrations, which should agree within 0.2 to 0.3 meq/liter (Table 23-11). Metabolic acidosis should be evaluated by blood pH and bicarbonate concentrations. Unless the serum urea nitrogen (>50 to 60 mg/dl) and creatinine (>5 to 6 mg/dl) concentrations are markedly elevated, chronic renal failure per se is unlikely to be the explanation. To define more precisely the level of glomerular function, a 24-h creatinine clearance can be obtained. Hyperkalemia is uncommon with GFRs above 15 to 20 ml/min unless the underlying renal disease is associated with a specific renal tubular defect in potassium secretion or with the syndrome of hyporeninemic hypoaldosteronism, most often encountered in tubulointerstitial renal diseases. In contrast, in acute renal failure, hyperkalemia occurs frequently and often abruptly. Decreased distal sodium delivery and urine flow can be rate limiting for potassium excretion, but not if the daily urine volume is in excess of 800 to 1000 ml and the urine sodium excretion is more than 15 to 20 meq (i.e., urine sodium concentration greater than 15 to 20 meq/liter). Increased potassium input should be considered. It should be remembered, however, that even in the face of an increased potassium load, sustained hyperkalemia (>5.3 meq/liter) is unusual unless there is a concomitant abnormality in renal function and/or in the renin-angiotensin-aldosterone system. A search should be made for drugs that inhibit renin or aldosterone production, block renal tubular potassium secretion, or alter the distribution of potassium between the intracellular and extracellular environment (see Table 23-9). Hyperglycemia (i.e., hyperosmolality) is a common contributory cause of hyperkalemia. If this initial evaluation is not diagnostic, then diagnostic tests aimed at uncovering a defect in the renin-aldosterone axis or a specific renal tubular secretory defect are indicated.

TABLE 23-11 • Diagnostic tests used to evaluate the patient with hyperkalemia*

1. Simultaneous plasma and serum potassium concentrations
2. Blood pH and serum bicarbonate concentration
3. Urine flow rate and sodium excretion
4. Glomerular filtration rate (serum urea nitrogen and creatinine; creatinine clearance)
5. Urine potassium excretion
6. Stimulation of renin secretion
   Volume contraction
   Upright posture
   Epinephrine infusion
7. Stimulation of aldosterone secretion
   Volume contraction
   ACTH
   Angiotensin II
   Hyperkalemia
8. Stimulation of renal tubular potassium secretion
   Diuretics (furosemide)
   Sodium sulfate
   Sodium bicarbonate-acetazolamide
   Mineralocorticoids (DOCA, fludrocortisone acetate)
9. Stimulation of extrarenal potassium uptake KCl infusion

* See text for a more detailed discussion, including doses.

SOURCE: Reproduced from Smith JD et al, in Arieff A, DeFronzo RA (eds): *Fluid, Electrolyte, and Acid-Base Disorders*, New York, Churchill Livingstone, 1985, p 413.

Measurement of urinary potassium excretion is not particularly helpful in evaluating patients with chronic hyperkalemia. By definition, if the hyperkalemia is chronic and stable, potassium balance is neutral; that is, the output must be equal to the input. Whatever the etiology of the hyperkalemia, the plasma potassium concentration will eventually rise to a level that will offset the defect in excretion. Otherwise, progressive hyperkalemia and lethal cardiac toxicity would develop. Also, if the absolute rate of potassium excretion is normal and the serum potassium concentration is elevated, the potassium clearance (i.e., potassium excretion divided by serum potassium concentration) must be reduced. Therefore, in the patient with chronic hyperkalemia, determination of the rate of potassium excretion or the potassium clearance will ordinarily not be helpful in differentiating among a primary renal tubular secretory defect, a defect in the renin-aldosterone axis, or an abnormality in potassium distribution. In all three, absolute potassium excretion will be normal and the potassium clearance will be decreased. Urinary potassium is helpful only if determined at a time when the serum concentration is rising, that is, before balance is established. If potassium excretion is low when the plasma level is rising, a defect is present at the level of the kidney or in the renin-aldosterone axis. Conversely, hyperkalemia resulting from redistribution will augment renal potassium excretion whenever kidney function is intact. However, it is distinctly uncommon to observe the patient during this disequilibrium state.

Recently West and colleagues[182,593] have advocated the transtubular potassium concentration gradient (TTKG) as a semiquantitative index of the activity of the potassium secretory process in the cortical distal nephron:

$$\text{TTKG} = \frac{[\text{K}]_{\text{urine}}/(\text{U/P})_{\text{osm}}}{[\text{K}]_{\text{plasma}}}$$

The numerator in this equation provides an estimate of the potassium concentration in the terminal cortical collecting duct. The term $(\text{U/P})_{\text{osm}}$ compensates for the rise in potassium concentration that occurs secondary to water reabsorption. In the presence of antidiuretic hormone and aldosterone, the potassium concentration and osmolality at the end of the cortical collecting duct are 40 meq/liter and 300 mosm/kg, respectively. This indicates that, when stimulated, the Na^+,K^+-ATPase pump can generate a transtubular potassium gradient of 10:1 (tubular fluid = 40 meq/liter and plasma = 4 meq/liter). In the presence of antidiuretic hormone, water is reabsorbed in the medullary collecting duct and the tubular fluid osmolality can rise to a maximum of approximately 1200 mosm/kg. This will generate a TTKG of 40:1 in the final urine. In normal subjects the TTKG is about 8 and rises to 12 to 13 following fludrocortisone acetate (Florinef) or potassium loading. During potassium deprivation the value declines to 1. The appropriate interpretation of the TTKG is based upon a number of assumptions, and the reader is referred elsewhere for a more detailed discussion.[182,593] Although the concept of TTKG is an important one, the clinical usefulness of the measurement in establishing the etiology of hyperkalemia needs further evaluation.

Categories 1 to 5 in Table 23-2 account for the majority (80 to 90 percent) of cases of hyperkalemia encountered in everyday clinical practice. If these have been excluded, a series of diagnostic studies can be performed to examine: (1) renin secretion, (2) aldosterone secretion, (3) renal tubular potassium secretion, and (4) potassium uptake by extrarenal tissues. For a more detailed description of the provocative tests described below, the reader is referred to previous publications.[36,39,141,142,145,148,321,391,476,546,549]

Renin secretion is best evaluated by volume depletion. This can be achieved by either allow-sodium diet (10 meq/day for 3 to 5 days), diuretic administration (20 to 40 mg of furosemide orally), or the combination. We have routinely utilized the following approach to evaluate renin (and aldosterone) secretion. Subjects are placed on a low-sodium diet (<10 meq/day) in combination with furosemide (40 mg/day) for 3 days. On the morning of the fourth day, baseline plasma renin and aldosterone levels are obtained. Subjects then ambulate continuously for 2 h and the measurement of plasma renin activity and aldosterone concentration is repeated. The combination of volume contraction and upright posture should maximally stimulate renin and aldosterone secretion. Typical values in 10 healthy young subjects are shown in Table 23-12. We have not routinely measured 24-h urinary aldosterone excretion rates, but this can be done before and after 3 days of volume depletion. The patient should be observed closely for signs and symptoms of orthostatic hypotension. If the blood pressure declines by more than 20/10 mmHg or the pulse rate increases by more than 15 to 20 beats per minute upon standing, plasma should be drawn for renin and aldosterone levels and the ECF volume expanded with intravenous sodium chloride.

Like renin, aldosterone secretion can be evaluated following volume contraction and ambulation. Obviously, if the renin response is diminished, the plasma aldosterone response to volume contraction is also likely to be deficient, and one cannot distinguish between the presence of a primary defect in aldosterone secretion, that is, "selective" hypoaldosteronism, versus one that is secondary to renin lack, that is, hyporeninemic hypoaldosteronism. In general, the increment in plasma aldosterone and plasma renin activity should be roughly proportional (see Table 23-12). A large, disproportionate increase in plasma renin compared with aldosterone suggests a primary adrenal defect. Since the zona glomerulosa is directly responsive to ACTH and angiotensin II, these agents can be employed to bypass renin and directly examine aldosterone secretion by the adrenal gland. Cosyntropin is given as a 0.25-mg intravenous bolus, followed by determination of the plasma aldosterone concentration at 30 and 60 min. Angiotensin II is infused at 2 to 4 ng/kg · min for 60 min and the plasma aldosterone level determined at 30 and 60 min. A twofold rise in plasma aldosterone concentration above baseline or an absolute value greater than 15 to 20 mg/dl is normal. If significant adrenal atrophy is present due to renin lack

TABLE 23-12 • Values for plasma renin activity and aldosterone concentration in healthy young subjects

	Plasma renin (ng angiotensin II per ml/per hr)	Plasma aldosterone (ng/dl)
Baseline	0.6 ± 2	13 ± 2
Volume contraction	5 ± 1	26 ± 4
Volume contraction plus upright posture	11 ± 2	66 ± 23

All values represent the mean ± SEM. From DeFronzo RA et al: *Ann Intern Med* 90:310, 1979.

(disuse atrophy), the aldosterone response to all stimuli may be blunted. In such instances, prolonged stimulation (3 to 7 days) may be necessary to assess adrenal responsiveness accurately. Unfortunately, the aldosterone response to ACTH dissipates quickly, and the prolonged angiotensin II infusion is hazardous because of its pressor effect. The newer synthetic angiotensin analogues (e.g., angiotensin III), which have much less pressor activity, may overcome this difficulty.

One of several methods can be employed to test distal tubule potassium secretion. Furosemide, by enhancing both sodium delivery and urine flow to the cortical collecting tubule, is an effective stimulator of potassium secretion. Following an oral dose of 40 to 80 mg (the higher dose is used in patients with chronic renal failure), urinary potassium excretion should increase at least three- to fourfold above baseline.[145,321] In patients with an intrinsic tubular defect in potassium secretion, the kaliuretic response to furosemide is markedly blunted. Agents that increase the luminal negativity of the distal tubule also stimulate potassium secretion. Both sodium sulfate (1.8 mmol/kg infused over 2 h) and combined sodium bicarbonate/acetazolamide infusion have been employed for this purpose.[141,142,145] Urinary potassium excretion should increase two- to threefold in normal subjects.[145] Lastly, the failure of urinary potassium excretion to increase following mineralocorticoid (fludrocortisone acetate or deoxycorticosterone acetate) administration is strongly indicative of a primary secretory defect. Florinef is administered orally in a dose of 0.1 to 0.2 mg/day for 5 to 7 days.

Impaired potassium uptake by extrarenal tissues is the most difficult disorder to evaluate. To establish this diagnosis one must quantitate extrarenal potassium uptake in response to potassium chloride infusion, an undertaking that may entail significant hazard. The plasma potassium concentration should be normalized by dietary means prior to performing this test. We have infused 0.375 meq/kg (26 meq for a 70-kg person) over 2 h.[145] In humans approximately half of the administered load will be excreted via the kidneys over the subsequent 4 to 6 h (Fig. 23-2). Of the remaining half, approximately 80 percent will be translocated from the extracellular to intracellular fluid compartment (Fig. 23-2). Since the total amount of potassium infused and excreted during the study is known, potassium retention can be determined by subtraction. The amount of the potassium load accumulated by the ECF can be estimated as the product of the rise in plasma concentration times the ECF volume (20 percent of body weight). The difference between this value and the amount infused provides a measure of the amount of potassium that has moved from the extracellular to intracellular space. Since hyperkalemia is a potent stimulus for both renal tubular potassium secretion and adrenal aldosterone secretion, this test also can be used to evaluate the potassium secretory capacity of the renal tubular cell and zona glomerulosa function, respectively. Great caution should be employed in carrying out this test. It should *not* be performed unless the plasma potassium concentration has been normalized prior to study. The electrocardiogram and plasma potassium concentration (every 15 min) should be monitored closely throughout the test.

The provocative tests described above are best performed in a controlled environment (such as a clinical research unit) while the patient is receiving a fixed, known potassium and sodium intake. If such a facility is not available, an abbreviated workup can be accomplished by examining the plasma renin and aldosterone response to volume contraction (furosemide and/or a low-sodium diet). Following this, a trial of fludrocortisone acetate (Florinef, 0.1 mg/day for 5 to 7 days) an be instituted. These studies can be performed safely as an outpatient as long as the subject is weighed daily and excessive weight loss or gain (greater than 2 kg) is avoided. These simple maneuvers will define whether one is dealing with a defect in the renin-angiotensin-aldosterone axis or a specific renal tubular secretory disorder.

TREATMENT OF HYPERKALEMIA

The severity and etiology of hyperkalemia, and the presence of neuromuscular symptoms, are the major factors governing choice of treatment. In general, it is less urgent to treat patients with *chronic* hyperkalemia, since cardiac toxicity tends to be less. Whenever a specific cause can be identified, it should be eliminated. Regardless of etiology, certain patients should be treated urgently, particularly when certain clinical manifestations of hyperkalemia are present.

CLINICAL MANIFESTATIONS

The important clinical manifestations of hyperkalemia result from alterations in the membrane potential of excitable tissues. A detailed description of these events is beyond the scope of this review. However, a brief overview of the normal processes that regulate the *generation of a nerve impulse* will serve to emphasize the important role that potassium plays in this process. The resting transmembrane potential difference is approximately −80 mV, with the cell interior negative.[181,221,317,500] The resting potential is primarily determined by the large difference in potassium concentration between the intracellular (approximately 150 meq/liter) and extracellular (3.5 to 5.0 meq/liter) fluid compartments because of the high basal potassium permeability. The large transmembrane potassium gradient (K_i/K_e = 35 to 40:1) is maintained by a membrane-bound Na^+,K^+-ATPase pump, which actively extrudes sodium from the cell in exchange for potassium, in a 3:2 ratio. When the serum potassium concentration rises, K_i/K_e falls and the resting potential becomes less negative; that is, it moves closer to the threshold for excitation, and the cell becomes depolarized (Fig. 23-28). Conversely, if the serum potassium concentration falls, the membrane potential becomes more negative and the cell becomes hyperpolarized.

The electrophysiologic consequences that ensue as a consequence of hyperkalemia, that is, depolarization, are complex, but the end result is a decrease in conduction velocity and an increase in the rate of repolarization.[181,221,317,500]

Cardiac toxicity

Cardiac toxicity is the major source of morbidity and mortality in hyperkalemic patients.[199,306] The earliest electrocardiographic change suggesting hyperkalemia is a symmetrical increase in the amplitude of the T waves ("tented" or "peaked"). This is best observed in the precordial leads and occasionally is associated with some ST depression. These changes result from an increase in the rate of repolarization of the cell membrane and usually become manifest when the serum potassium reaches 5.5 to 6.0 meq/liter. As the serum potassium concentration rises further (6.0 to 7.0 meq/liter), conduction through the His-Purkinje system and ventricular muscle becomes delayed. This is reflected by a lengthening of the PR interval and widening of the QRS complex. With potassium concentrations of 7.0 to 7.5, atrial muscle conduction becomes impaired; there is a progressive flattening of the P wave and continued widening of the QRS complex, and a further delay in A-V conduction. When the potassium concentration exceeds 8 meq/liter, atrial conduction ceases and the P waves disappear. As the QRS complex widens further, it merges with the T wave, producing a sine-wave pattern that is frequently misdiagnosed as ventricular tachycardia. If these ominous changes go unrecognized and appropriate therapy is not begun, ventricular fibrillation or asystole will follow. In addition to the classic sequence of events outlined above, virtually any type of arrhythmia or conduction disturbance may be seen in hyperkalemic patients. Various forms of fascicular and A-V nodal block are particularly common.

Multiple factors can modify the cardiac effects of hyperkalemia. If the hyperkalemia develops slowly (i.e., as occurs in chronic renal failure), cardiac manifestations may be minimal or even absent despite serum potassium concentrations exceeding 7 meq/liter. In contrast, certain metabolic derangements such as hyponatremia, hypocalcemia, and hypomagnesemia, by reducing the threshold potential and moving it closer to the resting potential, will potentiate the myocardial effects of hyperkalemia (Fig. 23-28). Severe cardiotoxicity may then be observed with serum potassium in the range of only 6.0 meq/liter. Lastly, it should be emphasized that cardiac toxicity may develop without any premonitory changes. A normal electrocardiogram may degenerate directly to ventricular tachycardia or fibrillation. This is particularly true in patients with underlying cardiac disease and/or baseline

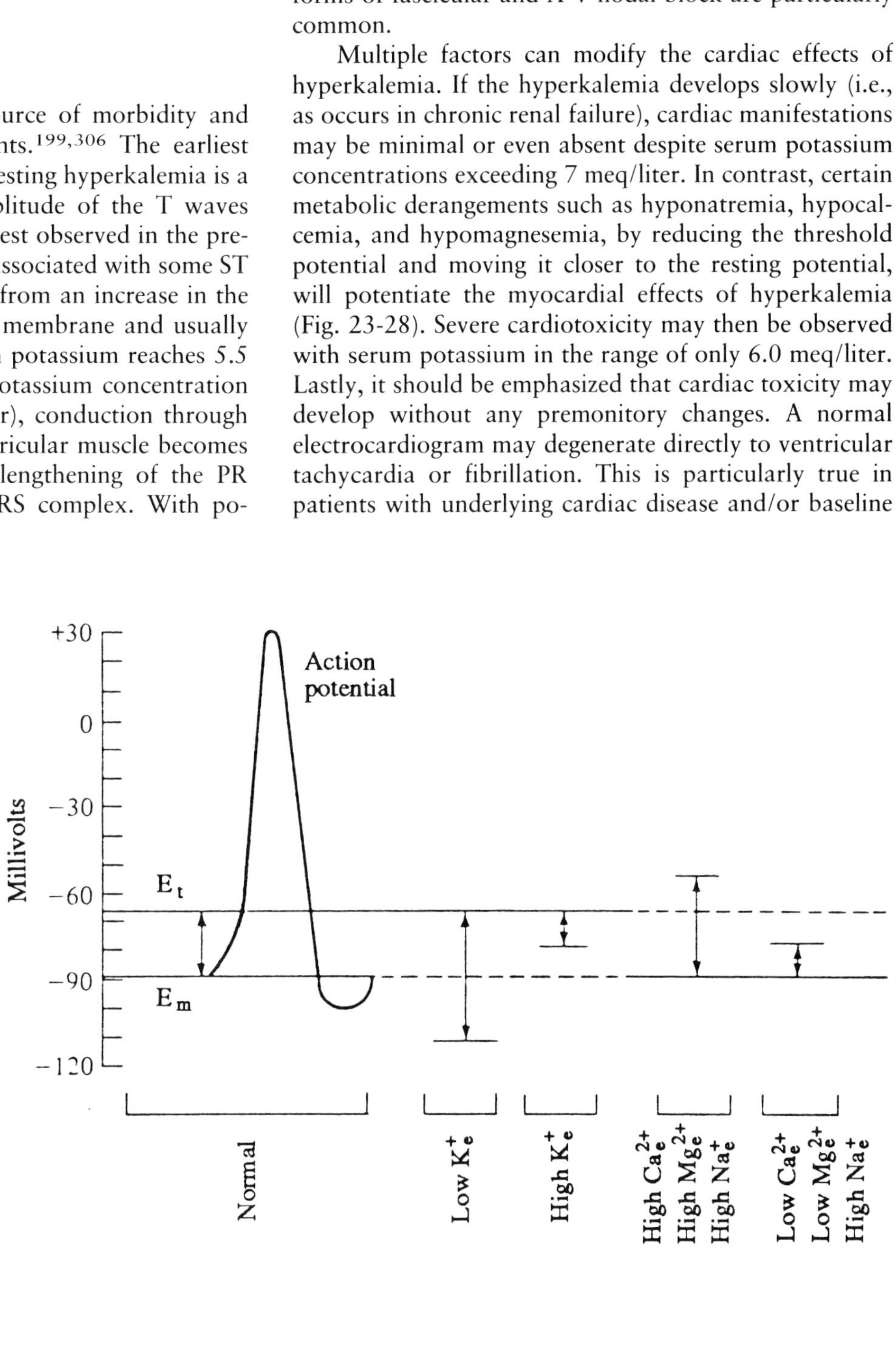

FIGURE 23-28 • Effect of changes in serum electrolyte concentrations on the threshold and resting potential in excitable cells. (See text for a detailed discussion.)

abnormalities in the electrocardiogram. Regardless of the electrical manifestations, therapeutic intervention should be initiated when the serum potassium concentration rises *acutely* to values in excess of 6.0 meq/liter.

Neuromuscular manifestations

The earliest neuromuscular symptoms of hyperkalemia include paresthesias and weakness in the arms and legs.[180,181,429] These are followed by a symmetrical flaccid paralysis of the extremities that ascends toward the trunk and may involve the muscles of respiration, causing hypoxemia and carbon dioxide retention. The deep tendon reflexes are preserved initially, but with worsening muscle paralysis they become progressively depressed. Cranial nerve function usually, but not always, is spared. Sensory changes (diminished vibration, position, and cutaneous sensory perception), when present, are relatively mild compared with the profound muscle weakness.

ACUTE TREATMENT OF HYPERKALEMIA

Treatment of hyperkalemia should be initiated immediately whenever the serum potassium concentration rises acutely to levels exceeding 6.0 meq/liter, or when EKG changes or neuromuscular signs are present. The acute therapy[30,152] of hyperkalemia can be divided into four general categories (Table 23-13). These include measures (1) to oppose the effects of hyperkalemia on the cell membrane, (2) to promote cell uptake of potassium, (3) to remove potassium from the body, and (4) to reverse the specific cause of the hyperkalemia.

Direct antagonism of membrane effects

Calcium

Intravenous calcium infusion immediately antagonizes the effects of hyperkalemia on the heart, even in normocalcemic patients.[152,199,306] Although the calcium ion does not affect the resting membrane potential, it increases the threshold potential at which excitation occurs (Fig. 23-28).[152,221,317] Restoration of the normal difference between the resting and threshold potentials reverses the depolarization blockade that occurs with hyperkalemia. The rise in calcium ion concentration also increases the number of sodium channels within the cell membrane, and this results in faster conduction. Infusion of 10 to 20 ml of 10% calcium gluconate has an immediate onset (1 to 3 min) of action that persists for approximately 30 to 60 min (Table 23-13). If no effect is observed within 5 to 10 min, the dose can be repeated. Failure to respond to the second dose indicates that it is unlikely that additional calcium will be of benefit. If an initial response is seen but the beneficial effect wanes, repeated doses should be given if the electrocardiographic changes of hyperkalemia reappear. When calcium is administered to the patient with hyperkalemia, it is advisable to employ continuous electrocardiographic monitoring. In patients who are taking *digitalis*, calcium should be given cautiously since hypercalcemia potentiates the toxic effects of digitalis on the myocardium. If calcium must be given to patients taking digitalis, it should be added to 100 ml of 5% dextrose in water and infused slowly over 20 to 30 min to allow a more even distribution throughout the extracellular space. Since hypocalcemia potentiates all of the toxic effects of hyperkalemia on neuromuscular function, reestablishing normocalcemia may dramatically reverse the manifestations of cardiac toxicity.

Sodium

Changes in serum sodium concentration (either hyper- or hyponatremia) do not exert a major effect on the heart in the absence of other electrolyte (i.e., potassium, calcium, magnesium) or acid-base disturbances.[199,221,306] In the presence of hyperkalemia the number of sodium channels (which are responsible for the conduction of the electrical impulse once the threshold potential has been reached) is diminished and the decrease in conduction velocity brought about by hyperkalemia is amplified by hyponatremia. Infusion of hypertonic saline (50 to 100 meq of NaCl) may dramatically reverse the cardiotoxicity in this circumstance (Table 23-13).[26,152,199,306] A beneficial action of hypertonic saline is less predictable in patients with a normal serum sodium concentration. Although hypertonic NaCl can effectively reverse the cardiac effects of hyperkalemia, sodium bicarbonate has largely replaced its use because of the additional beneficial effect of the bicarbonate anion per se.

Redistribution of potassium

Sodium bicarbonate

An increase in serum bicarbonate concentration and blood pH will shift potassium into cells even in the absence of acidemia.[221,317,502] However, the effect is greatest when the serum bicarbonate and blood pH are reduced.[16,68,520] Alkalemia will also directly stimulate potassium secretion by the distal tubule. In addition, if the rise in serum bicarbonate concentration exceeds the renal threshold for bicarbonate reabsorption, the excess alkali with its attendant sodium will be delivered to the distal tubule and potassium secretion will be further augmented. Sodium bicarbonate is administered intravenously as a 50-meq bolus over 5 to 10 min (Table 23-13). The onset of action in correcting hyperkalemia is 5 to 10 min, and the effect lasts for approximately 2 h. If no effect is observed within 10 to 15 min, an additional 50 meq can be infused. The major contraindication to sodium bicarbonate therapy is ECF volume

TABLE 23-13 • Acute therapy of hyperkalemia

Therapy	Mechanism	Dose	Onset	Duration of effect
1. Calcium gluconate (10%)	Membrane antagonism	10–20 ml IV	1–3 min	30–60 min
2. Sodium bicarbonate	Membrane antagonism and redistribution	50–100 meq IV	5–10 min	~2 h
3. Sodium chloride (3%)	Membrane antagonism	50–100 meq IV	5–10 min	~2 h
4. Insulin plus glucose	Redistribution	20 units of regular insulin over 30 min with 50 g of glucose IV over 1 h	30 min	4–6 h
5. Albuterol	Redistribution	Nebulized aerosol (10–20 mg)	30 min	2–4 h
		Intravenous (0.5 mg in 100 ml of D5W over 15 min)		
6. Cation exchange resin (Kayexalate)	Excretion	25–50 g PO or per rectum with sorbitol	1–2 h	4–6 h
7. Peritoneal or hemodialysis	Excretion		Within minutes after starting	Until dialysis is completed
8. Diuretics	Excretion		With start of diuresis	Until diuresis ends
Furosemide		40 mg IV		
Ethacrynic acid		50 mg IV		

SOURCE: Modified from Smith JD et al, in Arieff A, DeFronzo RA (eds): *Fluid, Electrolyte, and Acid-Base Disorders,* New York, Churchill Livingstone, 1985, p 413.

expansion and precipitation of congestive heart failure in patients with underlying cardiac disease. Alkalemia may precipitate tetany or seizures in a patient with preexisting hypocalcemia, since the rise in blood pH enhances calcium binding to albumin and further decreases the ionized calcium concentration. Therefore, in hypocalcemic patients it is essential to administer calcium prior to the infusion of bicarbonate. To raise the serum calcium concentration by 1 mg/dl in a 70-kg person, 420 mg of elemental calcium (70 kg × 0.60 × 10 mg/liter) can be added to 100 ml of D5W and infused over 30 to 60 min. Alternatively, one could administer 3% sodium chloride instead of sodium bicarbonate in the hyperkalemic patient with hypocalcemia.

Insulin/glucose

Intravenous insulin stimulates potassium uptake by extrarenal cells, primarily muscle and liver,[16,98,111,146,244,299,620,621] and is an effective means for rapidly lowering the plasma potassium concentration in hyperkalemic patients. The effect of insulin results from its direct action on the cell membrane and is independent of glucose transport or intracellular glucose metabolism.[16,98,111,244,620,621] Glucose is administered with insulin solely for the purpose of preventing hypoglycemia. Glucose should not be given to patients who are hyperglycemic (>200 to 250 g/dl), since the increment in plasma tonicity may pull potassium out of cells and aggravate the hyperkalemia before the insulin has had time to work. When the plasma glucose concentration declines to 150 to 200 g/dl, glucose should be added to the insulin infusion. From the preceding considerations, it also follows that it is unwise to administer the glucose as an acute intravenous bolus since marked hyperglycemia will ensue.

Ten units of insulin is usually given with 50 g of glucose over 60 min (Table 23-13). This may be accomplished by adding the insulin of 500 ml of a 10% glucose solution. The onset of insulin's hypokalemic action is approximately 30 min, and the effect may last for up to 4 to 6 h.[146,152] One can expect the plasma potassium concentration to decrease by 0.5 to 1.2 meq/liter within 1 to 2 h.[146,152] The dose of insulin/glucose can be repeated as frequently as required. The major side effect of insulin therapy is hypoglycemia, but this can be circumvented by infusing the insulin with glucose as previously described. Insulin also reduces the serum phosphate level in a dose-dependent manner, and in the presence of severe hypophosphatemia (<1.0 to 1.5 meq/liter) it may precipitate the phosphate depletion syndrome. Therefore, it is advisable to check the serum phosphate concentration periodically if prolonged insulin therapy is required.

Beta-2-adrenergic agonists

Most recently, selective beta-2-adrenergic agonists have been proposed for the acute management of hyperkalemia.[10,11,95,140,334,370,371,595,603] Stimulation of the beta-2 receptor in muscle and liver enhances cellular potassium uptake via a mechanism that involves the cyclic AMP system and is independent of insulin and aldosterone.[55,59,149,321] *Albuterol* is a selective beta-2 agonist that is available in oral and inhaled (but not parenteral) form in the United States. When given intravenously (0.5 mg in 100 ml of 5% dextrose solution infused over 10 to 15 min), the plasma potassium concentration declines by 0.5 to 1.0 meq/ liter (Table 23-13). The hypokalemic profile of intravenous albuterol is similar to that of insulin. Nebulized albuterol (10 to 20 mg) also has been shown to effectively lower the plasma potassium concentration, with a duration of action of up to 2 h. Although only modest increases in heart rate and blood pressure have been reported when the nebulized form of the drug is employed, caution is warranted in patients with known or suspected coronary heart disease. Recently, ventricular arrhythmias have been reported with the use of beta-2 agonists, and it is our opinion that such therapy should be employed only when other approaches have proved unsuccessful.

Removal of potassium from the body

None of the therapeutic maneuvers discussed above will leaad to a net removal of potassium from the body. Thus, they serve solely as temporizing measures until more definitive therapy can be instituted to diminish the total body potassium content.

Increased renal excretion

Unfortunately, hyperkalemia most frequently is encountered in patients with acute or chronic advanced renal failure and little can be done to enhance renal potassium excretion. However, in the patient with normal kidney function, measures that enhance urine flow and sodium delivery to the distal tubular potassium secretory sites will augment renal potassium excretion. Diuretics that act proximal to the potassium secretory sites, such as furosemide (40 to 80 mg intravenously) and ethacrynic acid (50 to 100 mg intravenously), have proved effective in promoting a kaliuresis and decreasing the total body potassium burden (Table 23-13).

Cation-exchange resins

Cation-exchange resins such as sodium polystyrene sulfonate (Kayexalate) effectively decrease the plasma potassium concentration by promoting the exchange of sodium for potassium within the gastrointestinal tract (Table 23-13). Each gram of resin removes 0.5 to 1 meq of potassium in exchange for 2 to 3 meq of sodium. Significant amounts of calcium and magnesium also may be removed. The usual dose of Kayexalate is 25 g given orally or as a retention enema. Since the resin is constipating, it always should be given with sorbitol (15 ml of 70% sorbitol every 30 min) to induce diarrhea, which can be sustained by administering additional doses every 6 to 8 h. If the patient cannot tolerate oral administration of Kayexalate, 50 g of the resin can be mixed with 50 g of sorbitol and added to 200 ml of 10% dextrose, which is given per rectum with an inflatable rectal catheter. Retention for at least 30 to 60 min is needed to achieve the best therapeutic results. Enemas can be repeated 4 to 6 times per day as necessary. It is important to recognize that Kayexalate's onset of action is relatively slow, in the order of 1 to 2 h. On average, 50 g of Kayexalate will lower the serum potassium concentration by 0.5 to 1.0 meq/liter over the 4 to 6 h period after its administration. The serum potassium concentration should be determined after each enema to guide subsequent therapy. It is noteworthy that in the original studies examining the efficacy of Kayexalate, the administration of oral sorbitol alone was almost as effective as the combination of sorbitol plus Kayexalate in reducing the serum potassium concentration.[478] The major side effects of oral Kayexalate administration are nausea and vomiting. In patients with underlying cardiac disease the increased sodium load may precipitate congestive heart failure.

Dialysis

Both peritonealdialysis[69] and hemodialysis[68,582] are very effective in removing potassium from the body. If acute reduction of the serum potassium concentration is desired, hemodialysis is the preferred choice. With standard dialysis coils (and no addition of potassium to the dialysate), if an individual starts with a plasma potassium concentration of 7 meq/liter, approximately 30 to 40 meq of potassium will be removed during the first hour of dialysis. The plasma potassium concentration will begin to fall within minutes after starting dialysis and the hypokalemic effect will persist for as long as the dialysis is continued. Within the first hour after the initiation of dialysis one can anticipate that the plasma potassium concentration will decline by 1.2 to 1.5 meq/liter.[68,582] The magnitude of the fall correlates with the predialysis plasma potassium level.[187] The major disadvantage of hemodialysis is the time required to prepare the equipment and to insert the catheter. Peritoneal dialysis also is effective in removing potassium from the body, but its hypokalemic effect is significantly slower than with hemodialysis or with cation-exchange resins.[69] If standard 2-liter exchanges are employed, and if each exchange takes 1 h, approximately 5 meq of potassium will be removed each hour. This will have little immediate effect on either the serum potassium concentration or total body potassium content, but over 36 to 48 h about 180 to 240 meq of potassium will be removed and this will have a pronounced potassium lowering effect.

TABLE 23-14 • Treatment of hyperkalemia in patients with chronic hyperkalemia*

1. Eliminate any source of increased potassium intake
2. Low-potassium diet (< 60 meq/day)
3. Avoid drugs that predispose to hyperkalemia (see text)
4. Avoid volume contraction
5. Sodium bicarbonate
6. Diuretics (thiazides)
7. Sodium polystyrene sulfonate (Kayexalate)
8. Mineralocorticoids: 43/51 (84%) responded
   a. Large doses often required
   b. Urinary potassium excretion does not always increase despite normalization of plasma potassium levels

* See text for a more detailed discussion. Data taken from articles reviewed by DeFronzo RA: *Kidney Int* 17:118, 1980.

TREATMENT OF CHRONIC HYPERKALEMIA

After the acute effects of hyperkalemia on cardiovascular and neuromuscular function have been reversed, the precise etiology of the hyperkalemia should be defined (Table 23-2) and more specific therapy instituted to prevent recurrence of the hyperkalemia (Table 23-14). If a reversible cause of the hyperkalemia cannot be identified, more general therapeutic interventions should be initiated. It should be kept in mind that patients with hyperkalemia often are elderly and have other associated medical complications including diabetes mellitus, atherosclerotic cardiovascular disease, chronic renal failure, and hypertension. Therefore, caution should be taken that the side effects of therapy do not outweigh the benefits of correcting the hyperkalemia.

Dietary management

All patients with chronic hyperkalemia should be placed on a diet containing less than 60 meq of potassium per day. In the majority of patients this maneuver alone will suffice to reduce the plasma potassium concentration to an acceptable level. If the hyperkalemia is particularly severe and/or associated with signs of cardiac toxicity, dietery potassium should be decreased to less than 40 meq/day. Foodstuffs that are especially rich in potassium should be avoided. Exogenous and endogenous sources of increased potassium input should be sought out and eliminated. The commonest cause of hyperkalemia in the hospital setting is excessive potassium intake.[403,430,489,501,503] A *low-sodium diet* is by definition high in potassium since the dietitian usually replaces sodium-rich foods with those high in potassium content. Specially prepared low-sodium foods have sodium removed in exchange for potassium. *Salt substitutes* contain 10 to 13 meq of potassium per gram and are a commonly overlooked source of incresed potassium intake. Endogenous input of potassium may be more difficult to recognize. *Rhabdomyolysis*, burns, crush injuries, and chemotherapy are obvious causes. *Chronic hemolysis* and *gastrointestinal bleeding* are less obvious.

Acidemia

It is important to correct any existing metabolic acidemia since both a decrease in blood pH as well as a reduction in the serum bicarbonate concentration, independent of changes in pH, will cause a shift of potassium from the intracellular to the extracellular fluid compartment.[202,203,301] The lower the serum bicarbonate concentration and pH, the greater will be the effect of bicarbonate therapy in reducing the plasma potassium concentration.[16,68] Correction of metabolic acidosis is best accomplished with oral or intravenous sodium bicarbonate, using a bicarbonate distribution space equal to 40 percent of body weight. For example, if a man weighs 70 kg and one desires to raise his serum bicarbonate concentration from 15 to 25 meq/liter,

$$\text{Bicarbonate replacement (meq)} = (70\ \text{kg})(0.40)(25-15\ \text{meq/liter}) = 280\ \text{meq}$$

The major side effect of bicarbonate administration is volume overload. If this is a concern, sodium bicarbonate should be given slowly with a diuretic to promote sodium excretion. Alternatively, calcium carbonate can be substituted. One gram of calcium carbonate contains 10 meq of bicarbonate. Since the calcium ultimately will exchange with bone sodium, significant volume expansion eventually will develop even with calcium carbonate therapy, although the fluid shift will occur more slowly and allow time for cardiovascular compensation to set in.

In some patients receiving bicarbonate, an increase in potassium excretion also may occur. The kaliuresis is multifactorial and results from enhanced distal tubule luminal negativity secondary to the presence of the poorly reabsorbable bicarbonate anion, increased delivery of sodium and fluid to the distal nephron sites of potassium secretion, and a direct stimulatory effect of alkalosis on the distal potassium secretory pump.

Volume expansion

Since both decreased distal sodium delivery and decreased distal tubular urine flow are known to inhibit potassium secretion, care should be taken to maintain normal intravascular volume. In patients with combined cardiac and renal failure, this may be difficult to accomplish. Daily measurement of body weight provides the best assessment of changes in ECF volume in patients who are managed on an outpatient basis.

Specific therapeutic interventions

In the hyperkalemic patient with aldosterone deficiency, physiologic replacement with fludrocortisone acetate (Florinef) is the treatment of choice. The normal replacement dose is 0.1 mg/day orally. In 51 reported cases of hypoaldosteronism who were treated with mineralocorticoids, the plasma potassium concentration decreased significantly in 43, or 84 percent.[148] However, large doses, as much as 0.4 to 1 mg/day, often were required to normalize the plasma potassium concentration, suggesting renal tubular resistance to the action of mineralocorticoids, at least with respect to potassium secretion. Sensitivity to the sodium-retaining effects of fludrocortisone is less affected, and marked sodium retention with edema formation, exacerbation of hypertension, and precipitation of congestive heart failure were common complications of therapy. In many patients addition of a loop diuretic was required to prevent sodium retention. Of note, several patients corrected their hyperkalemia without any increase in urinary or fecal potassium excretion, indicating an extrarenal mechanism or action.[148]

Patients with a primary renal tubular secretory defect are more difficult to treat. If a specific cause (i.e., urinary tract obstruction) can be identified, it should be corrected. Furosemide or the combination of acetazolamide with sodium bicarbonate have been tried with little success. Many patients with a primary renal tubular potassium secretory defect will respond to thiazide diuretics[141,142,477] even though they fail to respond to the more potent diuretics such as furosemide and ethacrynic acid. Occasional patients with a primary renal tubular secretory defect respond to large doses of fludrocortisone acetate (Florinef), 0.4 to 1 mg/day.

If the hyperkalemia fails to correct with fludrocortisone acetate or if the patient responds but excessive sodium retention occurs, one can employ a Na^+-K^+ exchange resin such as Kayexalate. In our experience, however, most patients find this medication difficult to tolerate on a chronic basis and stop taking it. In some patients, particularly those with only mild to moderate hyperkalemia (5.0 to 5.8 meq/liter) and absence of cardiac manifestations, it may be judicious to avoid mineralocorticoid therapy and to check the plasma concentration periodically to ascertain that the hyperkalemia has remained stable.

REFERENCES

1. Adam WR et al: In vivo estimation of changes in distal tubule flow and their role in dexamethasone-induced kaliuresis in control and potassium-adapted rats. *Clin Exp Pharmacol Physiol* 14:47, 1987.
2. Adler S: An extrarenal action of aldosterone on mammalian skeletal muscle. *Am J Physiol* 218:616, 1970.
3. Adler S, Fraley DS: Potassium and intracellular pH. *Kidney Int* 11:433, 1977.
4. Adrogué HJ, Madias NE: Changes in plasma potassium concentration during acute acid-base disturbances. *Am J Med* 71:456, 1981.
5. Adrogué HJ, Madias NE: Changes in plasma potassium concentration during acute acid-base disturbances. *Am J Med* 71:456, 1981.
6. Adrogué HJ et al: Determinants of plasma potassium levels in diabetic ketoacidosis. *Medicine* 65:163, 1986.
7. Adu et al: Hyperkalaemia in cyclosporin-treated renal allograft recipients. *Lancet* 2:370, 1983.
8. Aldigier JC et al: Comparison of the hormonal and renal effects of captopril in severe essential and renovascular hypertension. *Am J Cardiol* 49:1447, 1982.
9. Alexander EA, Levinsky NG: An extrarenal mechanism of potassium adaptation. *J Clin Invest* 47:740, 1968.
10. Allon M et al: Nebulized albuterol for acute hyperkalemia in patients on hemodialysis. *Ann Intern Med* 110:426, 1989.
11. Allon M, Copkney C: Albuterol and insulin for treatment of hyperkalemia in hemodialysis patients. *Kidney Int* 38:869, 1990.
12. Alvestrand A et al: Insulin-mediated potassium uptake is normal in uremia. *Am J Physiol* 246:E174, 1984.
13. Amatruda JM, Finch ED: Modulation of hexose uptake and insulin action by cell membrane fluidity. *J Biol Chem* 254:2619, 1979.
14. Ammon RA et al: Glucose-induced hyperkalemia with normal aldosterone levels. *Ann Intern Med* 89:349, 1978.
15. Andres GA, McCluskey RT: Tubular and interstitial renal disease due to immunologic mechanisms. *Kidney Int* 7:271, 1975.
16. Andres R et al: Effect of insulin on carbohydrate metabolism and on potassium in the forearm of man. *J Clin Invest* 41:108, 1962.
17. Arieff AI, Carroll HJ: Non-ketotic hyperosmolar coma with hyperglycemia. *Medicine* 51:73, 1972.
18. Armanini D et al: Aldosterone-receptor deficiency in pseudohypoaldosteronism. *N Engl J Med* 313:1178, 1985.
19. Arnold JE, Healy JK: Hyperkalemia, hypertension and systemic acidosis without renal failure associated with a

tubular defect in potassium excretion. *Am J Med* 47:461, 1969.
20. Arrizabalaga P et al: Increase in serum potassium caused by beta-2 adrenergic blockade in terminal renal failure: Absence of mediation by insulin or aldosterone. *Proc Eur Dial Transplant Assoc* 20:572, 1983.
21. Arruda JAL et al: Hyperkalemia and renal insufficiency: Role of selective aldosterone deficiency and tubular unresponsiveness to aldosterone. *Am J Nephrol* 1:160, 1981.
22. Arruda JAL et al: Voltage dependent distal acidification defect induced by amiloride. *J Lab Clin Med* 95:407, 1980.
23. Arthur S, Greenberg A: Hyperkalemia associated with intravenous labetalol therapy for acute hypertension in renal transplant recipients. *Clin Nephrol* 33:269, 1990.
24. Atlas SA et al: Interruption of the renin-angiotensin system in hypertensive patients by captopril induces sustained reduction in aldosterone secretion, potassium retention and natriuresis. *Hypertension* 1:274, 1979.
25. Balikian HM et al: Effect of posture on metabolic clearance rate, plasma concentration and blood production rate of aldosterone. *J Clin Endocrinol Metab* 28:1630, 1968.
26. Ballantyne F et al: Cellular basis for reversal of hyperkalemic electrocardiographic changes by sodium. *Am J Physiol* 229:935, 1975.
27. Bank N, Aynedjian HS: A micropuncture study of potassium excretion by the remnant kidney. *J Clin Invest* 52:1480, 1973.
28. Bantle JP et al: Effects of cyclosporine on the renin-angiotensin-aldosterone system and potassium excretion in renal transplant recipients. *Arch Intern Med* 145:505, 1985.
29. Barbour GL, Keller AW: Distal renal tubular acidosis in selective hypoaldosteronism. *South Med J* 71:1397, 1978.
30. Barr G, DeFronzo RA: Treatment of hyperkalemia, in Glassock RJ (ed): *Current Therapy in Nephrology and Hypertension-3*. Philadelphia, Decker, 1991, p 84.
31. Bartter F, Fourman P: The different effects of aldosterone-like steroids on urinary excretion of potassium and acid. *Metabolism* 11:6, 1962.
32. Bartter F, Forbes GB: Correlation of potassium-40 data with anthropometric measurements. *Ann NY Acad Sci* 100:264, 1963.
33. Bastl CP et al: Role of glucocorticoids and aldosterone in maintenance of colonic cation transport. *Am J Physiol* 238:F181, 1980.
34. Bastl CP et al: Glucocorticoid stimulation of sodium absorption in colon epithelia is mediated by corticosteroid IB receptor. *J Biol Chem* 259:1186, 1984.
35. Bastl CP, Sebastian A: Physiologic effects of the endocrine system and gastrointestinal tract, in Maxwell MH et al (eds): *Clinical Disorders of Fluid and Electrolyte Metabolism*. New York, McGraw-Hill, 1987, p 317.
36. Batlle DC et al: Hyperkalemic hyperchloremic metabolic acidosis in sickle cell hemoglobinopathies. *Am J Med* 72:188, 1981.
37. Batlle DC: Hyperkalemic hyperchloremic metabolic acidosis associated with selective aldosterone deficiency and distal renal tubular acidosis. *Semin Nephrol* 1:260, 1981.
38. Batlle DC et al: The pathogenesis of hyperchloremic metabolic acidosis associated with kidney transplantation. *Am J Med* 70:786, 1981.
39. Batlle DC: Hyperkalemic hyperchloremic metabolic acidosis associated with selective aldosterone deficiency and distal renal tubular acidosis. *Semin Nephrol* 1:260, 1981.
40. Batlle DC et al: Hyperkalemic distal renal tubular acidosis associated with obstructive uropathy. *N Engl J Med* 304:373, 1981.
41. Batlle DC et al: Distal nephron function in patients receiving chronic lithium therapy. *Kidney Int* 21:477, 1982.
42. Batlle DC: Segmental characterization of defects in collecting tubule acidification. *Kidney Int* 30:546, 1986.
43. Battilina CA et al: Effect of chronic potassium loading on potassium secretion by the pars recta or descending limb or the juxtamedullary nephron in the rat. *J Clin Invest* 62:1093, 1978.
44. Bauer JH: Role of angiotensin converting enzyme inhibitors in essential and renal hypertension. *Am J Med* 77 (suppl 2A):43, 1984.
45. Baxter JD, Tyrrell JB: The adrenal cortex, in Felig P et al: (eds): *Endocrinology and Metabolism*. New York, McGraw-Hill, 1981, p 447.
46. Bayard RS et al: The regulation of aldosterone secretion in anephric man. *J Clin Invest* 50:1585, 1971.
46a. Bell PD, Navar LG: Intrarenal feedback control of glomerular filtration rate. *Semin Nephrol* 2:289, 1982.
47. Bellevue R et al: Pseudohyperkalemia and extreme leukocytosis. *J Lab Clin Med* 85:660, 1975.
48. Bengele H et al: Tubular sites of potassium regulation in the normal and uninephrectomized rat. *Am J Physiol* 234:F146, 1978.
49. Beretta-Piccoli C et al: Responsiveness of plasma 18-hydroxycorticosterone and aldosterone to angiotensin II or corticotropin in nonazotemic diabetes mellitus. *Diabetes* 32:1, 1983.
50. Berl T et al: Role of aldosterone in the control of sodium excretion in patients with advanced chronic renal failure. *Kidney Int* 14:228, 1978.
51. Berlyne GM et al: Exchangeable potassium and renal potassium handling in advanced chronic renal failure in man. *Nephron* 8:264, 1971.
52. Bethune DW, McKay R: Paradoxical changes in serum potassium during cardiopulmonary bypass in association with non-cardioselective beta-blockade. *Lancet* 2:381, 1978.
53. Bevilacqua M et al: Dopaminergic control of serum potassium. *Metabolism* 29:306, 1980.
54. Bia MJ et al: Chronic adrenal insufficiency causes impaired extrarenal potassium tolerance. *Clin Res* 28:438A, 1980.
55. Bia MJ, DeFronzo RA: Extrarenal potassium homeostasis. *Am J Physiol* 240:F257, 1981.
56. Bia M et al: The effect of dexamethasone on renal electrolyte excretion in the adrenalectomized rat. *Endocrinology* 111:882, 1982.
57. Bia MJ et al: Regulation of extrarenal potassium homeostasis by adrenal hormones in rats. *Am J Physiol* 242:F641, 1982.
58. Bia MJ et al: The effect of dexamethasone on renal po-

tassium excretion and acute potassium tolerance. *Endocrinology* 113:1690, 1983.

59. Bia MJ et al: Beta adrenergic control of extrarenal potassium disposal: A beta-2 mediated phenomenon. *Nephron* 117, 1986.
60. Biglieri EG et al: Postoperative studies of adrenal function in primary aldosteronism. *J Clin Endocrinol Metab* 26:553, 1966.
61. Biglieri EG et al: 17-hydroxylation deficiency in man. *J Clin Invest* 45:1946, 1966.
62. Bilbrey GL et al: Potassium deficiency in chronic renal failure. *Kidney Int* 4:423, 1973.
63. Birhauser M et al: Effect of volume expansion by hyperosmolar and hyperoncotic solutions under constant infusion of angiotensin II on plasma aldosterone in man and its counterbalance by potassium administration. *Eur J Clin Invest* 3:307, 1973.
64. Bismuth C et al: Hyperkalemia in acute digitalis poisoning. Prognostic significance and therapeutic implications. *Clin Toxicol* 6:153, 1973.
65. Blachar Y et al: Pseudohypoaldosteronism. *Clin Nephrol* 11:281, 1979.
66. Blantz RC, Konnen KS: The relation of distal tubular delivery and reabsorptive rate to nephron filtration. *Am J Physiol* 233:F315, 1977.
67. Blantz RC et al: Effect of modest hyperglycemia on tubuloglomerular feedback activity. *Kidney Int* 22:S206, 1982.
68. Blumberg A et al: Effect of various therapeutic approaches on plasma potassium and major regulating factors in terminal renal failure. *Am J Med* 85:507, 1988.
69. Boen ST: Kinetics of peritoneal dialysis. A comparison with the artificial kidney. *Medicine* 40:243, 1961.
70. Borra S et al: Hyperkalemia in an adult hospitalized population. *Mt Sinai J Med* 55:226, 1988.
71. Bostic O, Duvernoy WFC: Hyperkalemic cardiac arrest during transfusion of stored blood. *J Electrocardiol* 5:407, 1972.
72. Bourgoignie JJ et al: Potassium-aldosterone response in dogs with chronic renal insufficiency. *Miner Electrolyte Metab* 11:150, 1985.
73. Boyd GW et al: The role of the renin-angiotensin system in the control of aldosterone in man. *Proc R Soc Biol Med* 62:1253, 1969.
74. Braithwaite SS et al: Acquired partial corticosterone methyl oxidase type II defect in diabetes mellitus. *Diabetes Care* 13:790, 1990.
75. Bratusch-Marrain P, DeFronzo RA: Impairment of insulin-mediated glucose metabolism by hyperosmolality in man. *Diabetes* 32:1028, 1983.
76. Brautbar N et al: Familial hyperkalemia, hypertension, and hyporeninemia with normal aldosterone levels: A tubular defect in potassium handling. *Arch Intern Med* 138:607, 1978.
77. Bravo EL et al: Selective hypoaldosteronism despite prolonged pre- and post-operative hyperreninemia in primary aldosteronism. *J Clin Endocrinol Metab* 41:611, 1975.
78. Brecht HM, Schoeppe W: Increase of total body potassium and decrease of exchangeable sodium after long-term treatment with a beta-receptor-blocking agent (Pindolol) in essential hypertension. *Clin Sci Mol Med* 51 (suppl 3):551, 1976.
79. Brennan LB et al: Total body electrolyte composition and distribution of body water in uremia. *Kidney Int* 17:364, 1980.
80. Brenner BM et al: Dietary protein intake and the progressive nature of kidney disease. *N Engl J Med* 307:652, 1982.
81. Brentjens JR et al: Interstitial immune complex nephritis in patients with systemic lupus erythematosus. *Kidney Int* 7:342, 1975.
82. Bricker NS, Fine LG: The renal response to progressive nephron loss, in Brenner BM, Rector FC (eds): *The Kidney*. Philadelphia, Saunders, 1981, p 1056.
83. Brohee D, Neve P: Heparin side effects. *Arch Intern Med* 144:1693, 1984.
84. Bronson WR et al: Pseudohyperkalemia due to release of potassium from white blood cells during clotting. *N Engl J Med* 274:369, 1966.
85. Brook CGD: Congenital adrenal hyperplasia: Pathology, diagnosis and treatment, in James VHT (ed): *The Adrenal Gland*. New York, Raven Press, 1979, p 243.
86. Brown JJ et al: Hypertension and chronic renal failure. *Br Med Bull* 27:128, 1971.
87. Brown JJ et al: Recurrent hyperkalemia due to selective aldosterone deficiency: Correction by angiotensin infusion. *Br Med J* 1:650, 1973.
88. Brown JJ et al: Site of stimulation of aldosterone biosynthesis by angiotensin and potassium. *J Clin Invest* 51:1413, 1972.
89. Brown RS: Extrarenal potassium homeostasis. *Kidney Int* 30:116, 1986.
90. Browning JJ, Channer KS: Hyperkalaemic cardiac arrhythmia caused by potassium citrate mixture. *Br Med J* 283:1366, 1981.
91. Brunner HR et al: The influence of potassium administration and of potassium deprivation on plasma renin in normal and hypertensive subjects. *J Clin Invest* 49:2128, 1970.
92. Buhler FR et al: Antihypertensive beta blocking action as related to renin and age: A pharmacologic tool to identify pathogenic mechanisms in essential hypertension. *Am J Cardiol* 36:653, 1975.
93. Burg MB: The renal handling of sodium chloride, in Brenner BM, Rector FC Jr (eds): *The Kidney*. Philadelphia, Saunders, 1976, p 272.
94. Burg MB, Bourdeau JE: Function of the thick ascending limb of Henle's loop, in Vogel HG, Ullrich KJ (eds): *New Aspects of Renal Function*. Amsterdam, Excerpta Medica, 1978, vol 6, p 91.
95. Burgess CD et al: A comparison of the extent and duration of hypokalemia following three nebulized beta 2-adrenoceptor agonists. *Eur J Clin Pharmacol* 36:415, 1989.
96. Burl RD, Schambelan M: Hyperkalemia in acute glomerular-nephritis due to transient hyperreninemic hypoaldosteronism. *Kidney Int* 38:1159, 1990.
97. Burnell JM et al: Effect in humans of extracellular pH change in relationship between serum potassium concentration and intracellular potassium. *J Clin Invest* 35:935, 1956.
98. Burton SD et al: Dissociation of potassium and glucose efflux in isolated perfused rat liver. *Am J Physiol* 212:261, 1967.

99. Bushinsky DS, Gennari FJ: Life-threatening hyperkalemia induced by arginine. *Ann Intern Med* 89:632, 1978.
100. Cade R, Shalhoub R: The effect of mineralocorticoids on renal handling of potassium. *J Clin Invest* 40:1028, 1961.
101. Carlsson E et al: Beta-adreno-ceptor blockers, plasma potassium, and exercise. *Lancet* 2:424, 1978.
102. Castellino P et al: Adrenergic modulation of potassium metabolism during exercise in normal and diabetic humans. *Am J Physiol* 252:E68, 1987.
103. Castellino P et al: Adrenergic modulation of potassium metabolism in uremia. *Kidney Int* 27:793, 1990.
103a. Castellino P et al: Hyperfiltration and diabetic nephropathy. Is it the beginning? Or is it the end? *Semin Nephrol* 10:228, 1990.
104. Charney AN et al: Na-K-activated adenosine triphosphatase and intestinal electrolyte transport. *J Clin Invest* 56:653, 1975.
105. Charron RC et al: The effect of adrenal steroids on stool composition as revealed by in vivo dialysis of feces. *Clin Sci* 37:151, 1969.
106. Cheek DB, Perry JW: A salt-wasting syndrome in infancy. *Arch Dis Child* 33:252, 1958.
107. Cheng LC et al: Catechol, a structural requirement for $(Na^+$-$K^+)$-ATPase stimulation in rat skeletal muscle membrane. *Biochem Biophys Acta* 464:338, 1976.
108. Christensen NJ: Plasma catecholamines in long-term diabetes with and without neuropathy and in hypophysectomized subjects. *J Clin Invest* 51:779, 1972.
109. Christlieb A et al: Hypertension with inappropriate aldosterone stimulation. A syndrome. *N Engl J Med* 281:128, 1969.
110. Clapp JR et al: Effect of unreabsorbed anions on proximal and distal transtubular potentials in the rat. *Am J Physiol* 202:781, 1962.
111. Clausen T, Hansen O: Active Na-K transport and the rate of ouabain binding. The effect of insulin and other stimuli on skeletal muscle and adipocytes. *J Physiol* 270:415, 1977.
112. Clausen T, Flatman JA: The effect of catecholamines on Na-K transport and membrane potential in rat soleus muscle. *J Physiol* 270:383, 1977.
113. Clausen T: Adrenergic control of Na^+-K^+ homeostasis. *Acta Med Scand* 672:111, 1983.
114. Clausen T, Flatman JA: Effects of insulin and epinephrine on Na^+K^+ and glucose transport in soleus muscle. *Am J Physiol* 252:E492, 1987.
115. Clausen T, Everts ME: Regulation of the Na, K-pump in skeletal muscle. *Kidney Int* 35:1, 1989.
116. Cogan MC, Arieff AI: Sodium wasting, acidosis, and hyperkalemia induced by methicillin interstitial nephritis. *Am J Med* 64:500, 1978.
117. Cohen AB: Hyperkalemic effects of triameterene. *Ann Intern Med* 65:521, 1961.
118. Cohen AS et al: Diabetic acidosis and evaluation of the cause and course of therapy in 73 cases. *Ann Intern Med* 52:55, 1960.
119. Cohen JJ et al: Disorders of potassium balance, in Brenner BM, Rector FC (eds): *The Kidney*. Philadelphia, Saunders, 1981, p 908.
120. Cohen LF et al: Acute tumor lysis syndrome. *Am J Med* 68:486, 1980.
121. Cohen RD, Iles RA: Lactate acidosis: Some physiological and clinical considerations. *Clin Sci* 53:405, 1977.
122. Cohen RD, Woods HF: *Clinical and Biochemical Aspects of Lactic Acidosis*. Oxford, Blackwell, 1976, p 60.
123. Conn JW: Aldosteronism in man. Some clinical and climatological aspects. *JAMA* 183:775, 1963.
124. Constantopoulos G et al: The mineralocorticoid activity of 18-hydroxy-11-deoxycorticosterone, 11-deoxycorticosterone and aldosterone in the adrenalectomized dog. *Can J Physiol Pharmacol* 57:1407, 1979.
125. Conte G et al: Acute increase in plasma osmolality as a cause of hyperkalemia in patients with renal failure. *Kidney Int* 38:301, 1990.
126. Cooke CR et al: Modulation of plasma aldosterone concentration by plasma potassium in anephric man in the absence of a change in potassium balance. *J Clin Invest* 52:3028, 1973.
127. Cooperman MT et al: Clinical studies of alcoholic ketoacidosis. *Diabetes* 23:433, 1974.
128. Cope CL, Pearson J: Aldosterone secretion in severe renal failure. *Clin Sci* 25:331, 1963.
129. Cortney MA: Renal tubular transfer of water and electrolytes in adrenalectomized rats. *Am J Physiol* 216:589, 1969.
130. Corvol P et al: Mechanism of the antimineralcorticoid effects of spironolactones. *Kidney Int* 20:1, 1981.
131. Cotton JR et al: Resting skeletal muscle membrane potential as an index of uremic toxicity. *J Clin Invest* 63:501, 1979.
132. Culter HH et al: Concentrations of chloride, sodium, and potassium in urine and blood. Their diagnostic significance in adrenal insufficiency. *JAMA* 111:117, 1938.
133. Dagher G et al: Altered erythrocyte cation permeability in familial pseudohyperkalaemia. *Clin Sci* 77:213, 1989.
134. Dahl-Hansen AB, Clausen T: The effect of membrane stabilizers and ouabain on the transport of Na^+ and K^+ in rat soleus muscle. *Biochim Biophys Acta* 318:147, 1973.
135. David R et al: Familial aldosterone deficiency: Enzyme defect, diagnosis, and clinical course. *Pediatrics* 41:403, 1968.
136. Davis JO et al: The effects of alterations of plasma sodium and potassium concentration on aldosterone secretion. *J Clin Invest* 42:597, 1963.
137. Dawborn JK, Watson L: Effect of prolonged administration of aldosterone on potassium and magnesium metabolism in the rabbit. *Med J Aust* 2:304, 1968.
138. Day RP et al: Occurrence of big renin in human plasma, amniotic fluid, and kidney extracts. *J Clin Endocrinol Metab* 40:1078, 1975.
139. deChatel R et al: Sodium, renin, aldosterone, catecholamines, and blood pressure in diabetes mellitus. *Kidney Int* 12:412, 1977.
140. Deenstra M et al: Decrease of plasma potassium due to inhalation of beta-2-antagonists: Absence of an additional effect of intravenous theophylline. *Eur J Clin Invest* 18:162, 1988.
141. DeFronzo RA et al: Investigations into the mechanisms of hyperkalemia following renal transplantation. *Kidney Int* 11:357, 1977.
142. DeFronzo RA et al: Impaired renal tubular potassium secretion in systemic lupus erythematosus. *Ann Intern Med* 86:268, 1977.

143. DeFronzo RA et al: Influence of basal insulin and glucagon secretion on potassium and sodium metabolism. *J Clin Invest* 61:472, 1978.
144. DeFronzo RA et al: Nonuremic diabetic hyperkalemia: Possible role of insulin deficiency. *Arch Intern Med* 137:842, 1979.
145. DeFronzo RA et al: Impaired renal tubular potassium secretion in sickle cell disease. *Ann Intern Med* 90:310, 1979.
146. DeFronzo RA et al: Effect of graded doses of insulin on splanchnic and peripheral potassium metabolism in man. *Am J Physiol* 238:E421, 1980.
147. DeFronzo RA et al: Effect of insulinopenia and adrenal hormone deficiency on acute potassium tolerance. *Kidney Int* 7:586, 1980.
148. DeFronzo RA: Hyperkalemia and hyporeninemic hypoaldosteronism. *Kidney Int* 17:118, 1980.
149. DeFronzo RA et al: The effect of epinephrine on potassium homeostasis. *Kidney Int* 20:83, 1981.
150. DeFronzo RA et al: Clinical disorders of hyperkalemia. *Annu Rev Med* 33:521, 1982.
151. DeFronzo RA et al: Inhibitory effect of epinephrine on renal potassium secretion. A micropuncture study. *Am J Physiol* 245:F303, 1983.
152. DeFronzo RA, Thier SO: Fluid and electrolyte disturbances: Hypo- and hyperkalemia, in Martinez-Maldonado M (ed): *Handbook of Renal Therapeutics*. New York, Plenum, 1983, p 25.
153. DeFronzo RA, Bia M: Extrarenal potassium homeostasis, in Seldin DW, Giebisch G (eds): *The Kidney, Physiology and Pathology*. New York, Raven, p 1179, 1985.
154. DeFronzo RA: Regulation of potassium homeostasis by insulin and catecholamines, in Giebisch G (ed): *Current Topics in Membranes and Transport*. San Diego, CA, Academic Press, 1987, p 299.
155. DeFronzo RA: Hyperkalemic states, in Maxwell MH et al (eds): *Clinical Disorders of Fluid and Electrolyte Metabolism*, 4th ed. New York, McGraw-Hill, 1987, p 547.
156. Degenhart HJ et al: Further investigation of a new hereditary defect in the biosynthesis of aldosterone: Evidence for a defect in 18-hydroxylation of corticosterone. *Acta Physiol Pharmacol Bulg* 14:88, 1966.
157. DeLiefa A et al: Big renin and biosynthetic defect of aldosterone in diabetes mellitus. *N Engl J Med* 295:639, 1976.
158. Demedts W et al: Life-threatening hyperkalemia associated with clofibrate-induced myopathy in CAPD patients. *Peritoneal Dial Bull* 3:15, 1983.
159. Dickerman HW, Walker WG: Effect of cationic amino acid infusion on potassium metabolism in vivo. *Am J Physiol* 206:403, 1964.
160. Diezi J et al: Effects of nephrectomy on renal salt and water transport in the remnant kidney. *Kidney Int* 10:450, 1976.
161. DiTella PJ et al: Mechanism of the metabolic acidosis of selective mineralocorticoid deficiency. *Kidney Int* 14:466, 1978.
162. Dluhy RG et al: Serum immunoreactive insulin and growth hormone response to potassium infusion in normal man. *J Appl Physiol* 33:22, 1972.
163. Dluhy RG et al: Studies of the control of plasma aldosterone concentration in normal man: II. Effect of dietary potassium and acute potassium infusion. *J Clin Invest* 51:1950, 1972.
164. Dobbins J: Gastrointestinal disorders, in DeFronzo RA and Arieff AI (eds): *Fluid, Electrolyte, and Acid-Base Disorders*. New York, Churchill Livingstone, 1985, p 827.
165. Dobyan DC et al: Suppression of potassium recycling in the renal medulla by short-term potassium deprivation. *Kidney Int* 16:704, 1979.
166. Don BR, Schambelan M: Hyperkalemia in acute glomerulonephritis due to transient hyporeninemic hypoaldosteronism *Kidney Int* 38:1159, 1990.
167. Donnell GN et al: Pseudohypoadenalocorticism. *Am J Dis Child* 97:813, 1959.
168. Drayer JM et al: Intrapatient comparison of treatment with chlorothalidone, spironolactone, and propranolol in normoreninemic essential hypertension. *Am J Cardiol* 36:716, 1975.
169. Dreyling K et al: Control of hyperkalemia with fludrocortisone in a patient with systemic lupus erythematosus. *Clin Nephrol* 33:179, 1990.
170. D'Silva JH: The action of adrenaline on serum potassium. *J Physiol* 86:219, 1935.
171. Dulce HJ, Gunther TH: Control of cellular electrolyte and water content by hormones. *Arch Exp Pathol* 238:368, 1960.
172. Dunn MJ, Hood VL: Prostaglandins and the kidney. *Am J Physiol* 2:F169, 1977.
173. Dunn MJ, Zambraski EJ: Renal effects of drugs that inhibit prostaglandin synthesis. *Kidney Int* 18:609, 1980.
174. Dunn MJ: Prostaglandins and Bartter's syndrome. *Kidney Int* 19:86, 1981.
175. Durand D et al: Inducing hyperkalemia by converting enzyme inhibitors and heparin. *Int Soc Nephrol* 34 (suppl 25):S196, 1988.
176. Durtzman NA: Short-circuit distal renal tubular acidosis. *J Lab Clin Med* 95:635, 1980.
177. Edelman IS, Liebman J: Anatomy of body water and electrolytes. *Am J Med* 27:56, 1959.
178. Edes TE, Sunderrajan EV: Heparin-induced hyperkalemia. *Arch Intern Med* 145:1070, 1985.
179. Elkington JR et al: Transfer of potassium in renal insufficiency. *J Clin Invest* 28:378, 1949.
180. Emanuel M, Metcalf RG: Quadriplegia in hyperkalemia. *J Maine Med Assoc* 157:134, 1966.
181. Epstein FH: Signs and symptoms of electrolyte disorders, in Maxwell MH, Kleeman CR (eds): *Clinical Disorders of Fluid and Electrolyte Metabolism*, 3d ed. New York, McGraw-Hill, 1980, p 145.
182. Ethier J et al: The transtubular potassium concentration gradient in patients with hypokalemia and hyperkalemia. *Am J Kidney Dis* 15:309, 1990.
183. Evans RHJ, Smith JW: Mode of action of catecholamines on skeletal muscle. *J Physiol* 232:81, 1973.
184. Ezra D et al: Evidence for an extrarenal action of chlorothiazide on serum potassium. *Am J Nephrol* (in press).
185. Farese RV et al: Urinary prostaglandins following furosemide treatment and salt depletion in normal subjects and subjects with diabetic hyporeninaemic hypoaldosteronism. *Clin Endocrinol* 13:447, 1980.
186. Farfel Z et al: Familial hyperpotassemia and hypertension accompanied by normal plasma aldosterone levels. Possi-

ble hereditary cell membrane defect. *Arch Intern Med* 138:1828, 1978.
187. Feig PU et al: Effect of potassium removal during hemodialysis on the plasma potassium concentration. *Nephron* 27:25, 1981.
188. Feinfeld DA, Carvounis CP: Fatal hyperkalemia and hyperchloremic acidosis: Association with spironolactone in the absence of renal impairment. *JAMA* 240:1516, 1978.
189. Fenn WO: The deposition of potassium and phosphate with glycogen in rat livers. *J Biol Chem* 128:297, 1939.
190. Fernandez J et al: Impaired extrarenal disposal of an acute oral potassium load in patients with end stage renal disease on chronic hemodialysis. *Miner Electrolyte Metab* 12:125, 1986.
191. Fernandez-Cruz A et al: Low plasma renin activity in normotensive patients with diabetes mellitus: Relationship to neuropathy. *Hypertension* 3:87, 1981.
192. Field MJ et al: Differential acute effects of aldosterone, dexamethasone, and hyperkalemia on distal tubular potassium secretion in rat kidney. *J Clin Invest* 74:1792, 1984.
193. Field MJ et al: Influence of ADH on renal potassium handling: A micropuncture and microperfusion study. *Kidney Int* 25:502, 1984.
194. Field MJ, Giebisch G: Hormonal control of renal potassium excretion. *Kidney Int* 27:379, 1985.
195. Findling JW et al: Indomethacin-induced hyperkalemia in three patients with gouty arthritis. *JAMA* 244:1127, 1984.
196. Fine LG et al: Functional profile of the isolated uremic nephron. Potassium adaptation in the rabbit cortical collecting tubule. *J Clin Invest* 64:1033, 1979.
197. Finkelstein FO, Hayslett JP: Role of medullary structures in the functional adaptation of renal insufficiency. *Kidney Int* 6:419, 1974.
198. Finkelstein M, Shaefer JM: Inborn errors of steroid biosynthesis. *Physiol Rev* 59:353, 1979.
199. Fisch C: Electrolytes and the heart, in Hurst JW (ed): *The Heart.* New York, McGraw-Hill, 1982, p 1599.
200. Flatman JA, Clausen T: Combined effects of adrenaline and insulin on active electrogenic Na^+-K^+ transport in rat soleus muscle. *Nature* 281:580, 1979.
201. Fort JA: Thrombocytosis and hyperkalemia revisited. *Am J Pediatr Hematol Oncol* 11:334, 1989.
202. Fraley DS, Adler S: Isohydric regulation of plasma potassium by bicarbonate in the rat. *Kidney Int* 9:333, 1976.
203. Fraley DS, Adler S: Correction of hyperkalemia by bicarbonate despite constant blood pH. *Kidney Int* 12:354, 1977.
204. Franco-Saenz R et al: Prostaglandins and renin production: A review. *Prostaglandins* 20:1131, 1980.
205. Fredlund P et al: Aldosterone production by isolated glomerulosa cells: Modulation of sensitivity to angiotensin II and ACTH by extracellular potassium concentration. *Endocrinology* 100:481, 1977.
206. French W, Manery JF: The effect of aldosterone on electrolytes in muscle, kidney cortex and serum. *Can J Biochem* 42:1459, 1964.
207. Frindt G, Palmer LG: Ca-activated K channels in apical membrane of mammalian CCT and their role in K secretion. *Am J Physiol* 252:F458, 1987.
208. Frindt G, Palmer LG: Low-conductance K channels in apical membrane of rat cortical collecting tubule. *Am J Physiol* 256:F143, 1989.
209. Frohlich JC et al: Renal prostaglandins: Regional differences in synthesis and role in renin release and ADH action, in Karger S (ed): *Proceedings, Seventh International Congress of Nephrology.* New York, 1978, p 107.
210. Fulop M, Hoberman HD: Alcoholic ketosis. *Diabetes* 24:785, 1975.
211. Fulop M: Serum potassium in lactic acidosis and ketoacidosis. *N Engl J Med* 300:1087, 1979.
212. Fulop M: Alcoholism, ketoacidosis, and lactic acidosis. *Diabetes Metab Rev* 5:365, 1989.
213. Funder JW et al: Glucocorticoid receptors in rat kidney: The binding of tritiated dexamethasone. *Endocrinology* 92:1005, 1973.
214. Galla JN et al: Effect of lithium on water and electrolyte metabolism. *Yale J Biol Med* 48:305, 1975.
215. Gamstrop I et al: Adynamia episodica hereditaria: A disease clinically resembling familial periodic paralysis but characterized by increasing serum potassium during the paralytic attacks. *Am J Med* 23:385, 1957.
216. Gavras H et al: Effects of the oral angiotensin-converting enzyme inhibitor MK-421 in human hypertension. *Clin Sci* 61:281S, 1981.
217. Geigelman PM et al: Severe diabetic ketoacidosis. *JAMA* 210:1082, 1969.
218. Geigelman PM: Potassium in severe diabetic ketoacidosis. *Am J Med* 54:419, 1973.
219. Gennari FJ, Cohen JJ: The role of the kidney in potassium homeostasis: Lessons from acid-base disturbances. *Kidney Int* 8:1, 1975.
220. Gerstein A et al: Aldosterone deficiency in chronic renal failure. *Nephron* 5:90, 1968.
221. Giebisch GH, Thier SO: Potassium: Physiological and clinical importance, in Siegel L (ed): *Directions in Cardiovascular Medicine.* Somerville, NJ, Hoechst-Roussel Pharmaceuticals, 1977, p 48.
222. Giebisch GH: The distal tubular potassium transport system, in Vogel HG, Ullrich KH (eds): *New Aspects of Renal Function.* Amsterdam, Excerpta Medica, 1978, vol 6, p 137.
223. Giebisch GH, Stanton B: Potassium transport in the nephron. *Annu Rev Physiol* 41:241, 1979.
224. Giebisch GH: New aspects of renal tubular potassium transport. *Contrib Nephrol* 21:106, 1980.
225. Giebisch GH et al: Renal transport and control of potassium excretion, in Brenner BM, Rector FC Jr (eds): *The Kidney*, 2d ed. Philadelphia, Saunders, 1981, p 408.
226. Giebisch GH: Renal control mechanisms of potassium homeostasis. *Jpn J Nephrol* 23:859, 1981.
227. Gifford J et al: Control of serum potassium during fasting in patients with end stage renal disease. *Kidney Int* 35:90, 1989.
228. Glassock RJ et al: Diabetes mellitus, moderate renal insufficiency and hyperkalemia. *Am J Nephrol* 3:233, 1983.
229. Glaz E, Sugar K: Effect of heparin and heparinoids on the synthesis of aldosterone and corticosterone by the rat adrenal gland. *Endocrinology* 74:159, 1964.
230. Goggans FC: Acute hyperkalemia during lithium therapy of maniac illness. *Am J Psychiatry* 137:869, 1980.
231. Gold EM et al: Sustained aldosterone secretion in chronic renal failure. *Clin Res* 13:135, 1966.

232. Goldfarb S et al: Paradoxical glucose induced hyperkalemia: Combined aldosterone and insulin deficiencies. *Am J Med* 59:744, 1975.
233. Goldfarb S et al: Acute hyperkalemia induced by hyperglycemia: Hormonal mechanisms. *Ann Intern Med* 84:426, 1976.
234. Goldsmith O et al: Hypogonadism and mineralocorticoid excess. The 17-hydroxylase deficiency syndrome. *N Engl J Med* 277:673, 1967.
235. Goldstone R et al: Evidence for two independent mechanisms of juxtaglomerular cell impairment in hyporeninemic hypoaldosteronism. *Clin Res* 31:272A, 1983.
236. Gomez M, Curry DL: Potassium stimulation of insulin release by the perfused rat pancreas. *Endocrinology* 92:1126, 1973.
237. Gonick HC et al: Functional impairment in chronic renal disease. Studies of potassium excretion. *Am J Med Sci* 261:281, 1971.
238. Good DW, Wright FS: Luminal influences on potassium secretion: Sodium concentration and fluid flow rate. *Am J Physiol* 236:F192, 1979.
239. Gordon RD et al: Role of the sympathetic nervous system in regulating renin and aldosterone production in man. *J Clin Invest* 46:599, 1967.
240. Gordon RD et al: Hypertension and severe hyperkalemia associated with suppression of renin and aldosterone and completely reversed by dietary sodium restriction. *Aust Ann Med* 19:287, 1970.
241. Gordon RD: Syndrome of hypertension and hyperkalemia with normal glomerular filtration rate. *Hypertension* 8:93, 1986.
242. Gossain V et al: Impaired renin responsiveness with secondary hypoaldosteronism. *Arch Intern Med* 132:885, 1973.
243. Gourley DRH, Bethea MD: Insulin effect on adipose tissue, sodium and potassium. *Proc Soc Exp Biol Med* 115:821, 1965.
244. Gourley DRH: Effect of insulin on potassium exchange in normal and ouabain-treated skeletal muscle. *J Pharmacol Exp Ther* 148:339, 1965.
245. Graber M et al: Thrombocytosis elevates serum potassium. *Am J Kidney Dis* 8:116, 1988.
246. Grantham JJ et al: The nature of transtubular Na and K transport in isolated rabbit collecting tubules. *J Clin Invest* 49:1815, 1970.
247. Greenberg A et al: Renal failure in heart transplant patients receiving cyclosporin A. *Clin Res* 31:429A, 1983.
248. Grodsky GM, Bennett LL: Cation requirements for insulin secretion in isolated perfused pancreas. *Diabetes* 15:910, 1966.
249. Grossman A et al: Captopril: Reversible renal failure with severe hyperkalaemia. *Lancet* 1:712, 1980.
250. Gutman PH: Addison's disease. *Arch Pathol Lab Med* 10:742, 1942.
251. Györy AZ et al: Renal tubular acidosis, acidosis due to hyperkalemia, disordered citrate metabolism and other tubular dysfunctions following human renal transplantation. *Q J Med* 38:231, 1969.
252. Hadler NM et al: Impaired renal tubular secretion of potassium, elevated sweat sodium chloride concentration and plasma inhibition of erythrocyte sodium outflux as complications of systemic lupus erythematosus. *Arthritis Rheum* 15:515, 1972.
253. Hahn JA et al: Vasoactive systems in hyporeninaemic hypoaldosteronism: Deficiency of kallikrein. *Clin Res* 27:313, 1979.
254. Hahn JR et al: Induction of renin release by exogenous prostaglandins in hyporeninemic hypoaldosteronism. *Prostaglandins* 20:15, 1980.
256. Halperin ML et al: Interpretation of the serum potassium concentration in metabolic acidosis. *Clin Invest Med* 2:55, 1979.
256. Halperin ML et al: Selected aspects of the pathophysiology of metabolic acidosis in diabetes mellitus. *Diabetes* 30:781, 1981.
257. Haning R et al: In vitro effects of ACTH, angiotensin, serotonin and potassium on steroid output and conversion of corticosterone to aldosterone by isolated adrenal cells. *Endocrinology* 87:1147, 1975.
258. Hariharasubramanian N et al: Serum potassium levels during lithium therapy of manic depressive psychosis, in Johnson FN, Johnson S (eds): *Lithium in Medical Practice*. Baltimore, University Press, 1978, p 64.
259. Harman RC et al: Studies on thrombocytosis: I. Hyperkalemia due to release of potassium from platelets during clotting. *J Clin Invest* 37:699, 1958.
260. Harris PM: Salbutamol in hyperkalemic familial periodic paralysis. *Lancet* 1:427, 1976.
261. Harris RH, Yarger WE: Renal function after release of unilateral ureteral obstruction in rats. *Am J Physiol* 227:806, 1974.
262. Harrison HE, Darrow DC: Renal function in experimental adrenal insufficiency. *Am J Physiol* 125:631, 1939.
263. Harrop GA et al: The diagnosis and treatment of Addison's disease. *JAMA* 100:1850, 1933.
264. Hartmann RC, Mellinkoff SM: The relationship of platelets to the serum potassium concentration. *J Clin Invest* 34:938, 1955.
265. Hayes CP et al: An extrarenal mechanism for the maintenance of potassium balance in severe chronic renal failure. *Trans Assoc Am Physicians* 80:207, 1967.
266. Hays ET et al: Epinephrine action on sodium fluxes in frog striated muscle. *Am J Physiol* 227:1340, 1979.
267. Hayslett JP: Functional adaptation to reduced renal mass. *Physiol Rev* 59:137, 1979.
268. Hayslett JP, Binder HJ: Mechanism of potassium adaptation. *Am J Physiol* 243:F103, 1982.
269. Hazeyama Y, Sparks HV: A model of potassium efflux during exercise of skeletal muscle. *Am J Physiol* 236:R83, 1979.
270. Helman SI, O'Neil RG: Model of active transepithelial Na and K transport of renal collecting tubules. *Am J Physiol* 233:F559, 1977.
271. Hene RJ et al: Plasma aldosterone concentrations in chronic renal disease. *Kidney Int* 21:98, 1982.
272. Henquin JC, Lambert AE: Cationic environment and dynamics of insulin secretion: Effect of high concentration of potassium. *Diabetes* 23:933, 1974.
273. Hertz P, Richardson JA: Arginine-induced hyperkalemia in renal failure patients. *Arch Intern Med* 130:778, 1972.
274. Hiatt N et al: Role of insulin in the transfer of infused potassium to tissue. *Horm Metab Res* 5:84, 1973.

275. Hiatt N et al: Necessity for insulin in transfer of excess infused K to intracellular fluid. *Metabolism* 23:43, 1974.
276. Hiatt N et al: Inhibition of transmembrane K transfer in ureter-ligated dogs infused with KC. *Am J Physiol* 231:1660, 1976.
277. Hierholzer K: Secretion of potassium and acidification in collecting ducts of mammalian kidney. *Am J Physiol* 201:318, 1961.
278. Hierholzer K, Wiederholdt M: Some aspects of distal tubulal solute and water transport. *Kidney Int* 9:198, 1976.
279. Hierholzer K et al: Micropuncture study of renal transtubular concentration gradients of sodium and potassium in adrenalectomized rats. *Pfluegers Arch* 285:193, 1965.
280. Himathongkam T et al: Potassium-aldosterone-renin interrelationships. *J Clin Endocrinol Metab* 41:153, 1975.
281. Horner JM et al: The role of renin and angiotensin in salt-losing 21-hydroxylase-deficient congenital adrenal hyperplasia. *J Clin Endocrinol Metab* 48:776, 1979.
282. Hostetter TH et al: Hyperfiltration in remnant nephrons: A potentially adverse response to renal ablation. *Am J Physiol* 241:F85, 1981.
283. Hostetter TH et al: Compensatory renal hemodynamic injury: A final common pathway of residual nephron destruction. *Am J Kidney Dis* 1:310, 1982.
284. Hostetter TH et al: The case for intrarenal hypertension in the initiation and progression of diabetic and other glomerulopathies. *Am J Med* 72:375, 1982.
285. Hulter HN et al: Impaired renal H^+ secretion and NH_3 production in mineralocorticoid-deficient glucocorticoid-replete dogs. *Am J Physiol* 232:F136, 1977.
286. Insel PA: Identification and regulation of adrenergic receptors in target cells. *Am J Physiol* 247:E53, 1984.
287. Jacobs DR, Posner JB: Isolated analdosteronism: II. The nature of the adrenal cortical enzymatic defect, and the influence of diet and various agents on electrolyte balance. *Metabolism* 13:522, 1964.
288. Jamison RL et al: Potassium secretion by the descending limb or pars recta of the juxtamedullary nephron in vivo. *Kidney Int* 9:323, 1976.
289. Kahn CR, White MF: The insulin receptor and the molecular mechanism of insulin action. *J Clin Invest* 82:115, 1988.
290. Kahn T et al: Potassium transport in chronic renal disease. *Clin Res* 24:403A, 1976.
291. Kahn T et al: Factors related to potassium transport in stable chronic renal disease. *Clin Sci* 54:661, 1978.
292. Kaji D, Kahn T: Na^+K^+ pump in chronic renal failure. *Am J Physiol* 252:F785, 1987.
293. Kalin MF et al: Hyporeninemic hypoaldosteronism associated with acquired immune deficiency syndrome. *Am J Med* 82:1035, 1987.
294. Kaplan M et al: Renal handling of potassium in dogs with chronic renal insufficiency. *Kidney Int* 19:46, 1982.
295. Kasuga M et al: Insulin stimulation of phosphorylation of the beta subunit of the insulin receptor. *J Biol Chem* 257:9891, 1982.
296. Katz L et al: Effect of epinephrine on renal potassium excretion in the isolated perfused rat kidney. *Am J Physiol* 247:F331, 1984.
297. Keenan BS et al: Sodium homeostasis and aldosterone secretion in salt-losing congenital adrenal hyperplasia. *J Clin Endocrinol Metab* 48:430, 1979.
298. Keith NM, Burchell HB: Clinical intoxication with potassium: Its occurrence in severe renal insufficiency. *Am J Med Sci* 217:1, 1949.
299. Kestens PJ et al: The effect of insulin on the uptake of potassium and phosphate by the isolated perfused canine liver. *Metabolism* 12:941, 1963.
300. Khuri RN et al: The effects of flow rate and potassium intake on distal tubular potassium transfer. *Am J Physiol* 228:1249, 1975.
301. Kim WG, Brown EB: Potassium transfer with constant extracellular pH. *J Lab Clin Med* 71:678, 1968.
302. Kimberly RP et al: Reduction of renal function by newer non-steroidal anti-inflammatory drugs. *Am J Med* 64:804, 1978.
303. Kimelberg HK: Influence of membrane fluidity on activity of membrane bound enzymes, in Ellis GP, West CG (eds): *Aspects of Cell Surface Organization: Cell Surface Review* 3:205, 1977.
304. Klassen J et al: Tubular lesions produced by autoantibodies to tubular basement membrane in human renal allografts. *Int Arch Allergy Appl Immunol* 45:675, 1973.
305. Kleeman CR et al: The renal regulation of sodium and potassium in patients with chronic renal failure and the effects of diuretics in the excretion of these ions. *Ann NY Acad Sci* 139:520, 1967.
306. Kleeman K, Singh BN: Serum electrolytes and the heart, in Maxwell MH, Kleeman CR (eds): *Clinical Disorders of Fluid and Electrolyte Metabolism*, 3d ed. New York, McGraw-Hill, 1980, p 145.
307. Klemm SA et al: Biochemical correction in the syndrome of hypertension and hyperkalaemia by severe dietary salt restriction suggests renin-aldosterone suppression critical in pathophysiology. *Clin Exp Pharmacol Physiol* 17:191, 1990.
308. Kliger AS, Hayslett JP: Disorders of potassium balance, in Brenner BM, Stein JH (eds): *Acid Base and Potassium Homeostasis*. New York, Churchill Livingstone, 1978, p 168.
309. Kloppenborg PWC et al: Inhibition of adrenal function in man by heparin or heparinoid RO 1-8307. *Acta Med Scand* 197:99, 1975.
310. Knochel JP: The syndrome of hyporeninemic hypoaldosteronism. *Annu Rev Med* 30:145, 1979.
311. Kopple JD, Coburn JW: Metabolic studies of low protein diets in uremia: I. Nitrogen and potassium. II. Calcium, phosphorus, and magnesium. *Medicine* 52:583, 1973.
312. Kowarski A et al: Aldosterone secretion rate in congenital adrenal hyperplasia. A discussion of the theories on the pathogenesis of the salt-losing form of the syndrome. *J Clin Invest* 44:1505, 1965.
313. Kozeny GO et al: Occurrence of renal tubular dysfunction in lupus nephritis. *Arch Intern Med* 147:891, 1987.
314. Krause J et al: Reversibility of hyporeninemia and hypoaldosteronism in chronic hemodialysis patients by correction of fluid excess. *J Lab Clin Med* 96:734, 1980.
315. Kreisberg RA: Diabetic ketoacidosis. New concepts and trends in pathogenesis and treatment. *Ann Intern Med* 88:681, 1978.

316. Krikken-Hogenberk LG et al: Succinylcholine-induced hyperkalemia. *Anesthesiology* 70:553, 1989.
317. Kuffler SW, Nicholls JG: *From Neuron to Brain: A Cellular Approach to the Nervous System.* Sunderland, MA, Sinaver Associates, 1976.
318. Kunau RT et al: Characteristics of the relationship between the flow rate of tubular fluid and potassium transport in the distal tubule of the rat. *J Clin Invest* 54:1488, 1974.
319. Kunau RT, Whinnery MA: Potassium transfer in distal tubule of normal and remnant kidneys. *Am J Physiol* 235:F186, 1978.
320. Kurtzman NA: Nephrology forum. Acquired distal renal tubular acidosis. *Kidney Int* 24:807, 1983.
321. Kurtzman NA et al: A patient with hyperkalemia and metabolic acidosis. *Am J Kidney Dis* 15:333, 1990.
322. Lachaal M, Venuto RC: Nephrotoxicity and hyperkalemia in patients with acquired immunodeficiency symdrome treated with pentamidine. *Am J Med* 87:260, 1989.
323. Lan NC et al: Binding of steroids to mineralocorticoid receptors: Implications for in vivo occupancy by glucocorticoids. *J Clin Endocrinol Metab* 54:332, 1982.
324. Laurado JG: Aldosterone excretion following hypophysectomy in man: Relation to urinary Na/K ratio. *Metabolism* 6:556, 1957.
325. Lawson DH: Adverse reactions to potassium chloride. *Q J Med* 43:433, 1974.
326. Lee FO et al: Mechanism of hyperkalemia in systemic lupus erythematosus. *Arch Intern Med* 148:397, 1988.
327. Lee MR et al: Hypertension and hyperkalemia responding to bendrofluazide. *Q J Med* 48:245, 1979.
328. Leehey P et al: Heparin-induced hypoaldosteronism. *JAMA* 246:189, 1981.
329. Levinsky NG et al: Acute renal failure, in Brenner BM, Rector FC (eds): *The Kidney*, 2d ed. Philadelphia, Saunders 1981, p 1181.
330. Levy LJ et al: Ketoacidosis associated with alcoholism in non-diabetic subjects. *Ann Intern Med* 78:213, 1973.
331. Licht JH et al: Familial hyperkalaemic acidosis. *Q J Med* 213:161, 1985.
332. Liebman J, Edelman IS: Interrelationship of plasma potassium concentration, plasma sodium concentration, arterial pH and total exchangeable potassium. *J Clin Invest* 38:2176, 1959.
333. Lim VA, Webster GD: The effect of aldosterone on water and electrolyte composition of incubated rat diaphragms. *Clin Sci* 33:261, 1967.
334. Lipworth BJ et al: Systemic β-adrenoceptor responses to salbutamol given by metered-dose inhaler alone and with pear shaped spacer attachment: Comparison of electrocardiographic, hypokalaemic and haemodynamic effects. *Br J Clin Pharmacol* 27:837, 1989.
335. Lockwood RH, Lum BKB: Effects of adrenergic agonists and antagonists on potassium metabolism. *J Pharmacol Exp Ther* 189:119, 1974.
336. Loeb RD et al: Electrolyte balance studies in adrenalectomized dogs with particular reference to the excretion of sodium. *J Exp Med* 57:775, 1933.
337. Louis LH, Conn JW: Preparation of glycyrrhizinic acid, the electrolyte active principle of licorice: Its effect upon metabolism and upon pituitary-adrenal function in man. *J Lab Clin Med* 47:20, 1956.
338. Luft D et al: Lactic acidosis in biguanide-treated diabetics. A review of 330 cases. *Diabetologia* 14:75, 1978.
339. Luke RG et al: Hyperkalemia and renal tubular acidosis due to renal amyloidosis. *Ann Intern Med* 70:1211, 1969.
340. Lundborg P et al: Effect of β adrenoceptor blockade on exercise performance and metabolism. *Clin Sci* 61:299, 1981.
341. Lundin AP et al: Fatigue, acid-base and electrolyte changes with exhaustive treadmill exercise in hemodialysis patients. *Nephron* 46:57, 1987.
342. MacKnight ADC: Epithelial transport of potassium. *Kidney Int* 11:391, 1977.
343. Mactier RA, Khanna R: Hyperkalemia induced by indomethacin and naproxen and reversed by fludrocortisone. *South Med J* 81:800, 1988.
344. Maddox RW et al: Extreme hyperkalemia associated with amiloride. *South Med J* 78:365, 1985.
345. Maddox RW: Heparin induced hyperkalemia. *North Carolina Med J* 48:75, 1987.
346. Maffly RH: The body fluids: Volume, composition, and physical chemistry, in Brenner BM, Rector FC (eds): *The Kidney*, 2d ed. Philadelphia, Saunders, 1981, p 76.
347. Mahnensmith R et al: Effect of acute metabolic acidemia on renal electrolyte transport in man. *Metabolism* 28:831, 1979.
348. Makoff DL et al: Hypertonic expansion: Acid-base and electrolyte changes. *Am J Physiol* 218:1201, 1970.
349. Makoff DL et al: On the mechanism of hyperkalemia due to hyperosmotic expansion with saline or mannitol. *Clin Sci* 41:383, 1971.
350. Malnic G et al: Micropuncture study of distal tubular potassium and sodium transport in rat nephron. *Am J Physiol* 211:529, 1966.
351. Malnic G et al: Micropuncture study of renal potassium excretion in the rat. *Am J Physiol* 206:674, 1974.
352. Malnic G et al: Potassium transport across renal distal tubules during acid-base disturbances. *Am J Physiol* 211:1192, 1971.
353. Manning RT, Behrle FC: Use of spironolactone in renal edema; effectiveness and association with hyperkalemia. *JAMA* 176:769, 1961.
354. Marusic ET et al: Corticosteroid binding studies in cytosol of colonic mucosa of the rat. *Am J Physiol* 240:G417, 1981.
355. Massara F et al: Influence of glucagon on plasma levels of potassium in man. *Diabetologia* 19:414, 1980.
356. McCaa RE et al: Increased plasma aldosterone concentration in response to hemodialysis in nephrectomized man. *Circ Res* 31:473, 1972.
357. McCaa RE et al: Relative influence of acute sodium and volume depletion on aldosterone secretion in nephrectomized man. *Circ Res* 33:555, 1973.
358. McCaa RE et al: Role of angiotensin II and potassium in the long term regulation of aldosterone secretion in intact conscious dogs. *Circ Res* 36/37(suppl 1):57, 1975.
359. McGiff JC et al: Interrelationships of renin and aldosterone in a patient with hypoaldosteronism. *Am J Med* 48:247, 1970.
360. McIvor M et al: Hyperkalemia and cardiac arrest from fluoride exposure during hemodialysis. *Am J Cardiol* 51:901, 1983.

361. Meier DE et al: Indomethacin-associated hyperkalemia in the elderly. *J Am Geriatric Soc* 31:371, 1983.
362. Mellinger RC et al: Hyponatremia with low urinary aldosterone occurring in an old woman. *J Clin Endocrinol Metab* 34:85, 1972.
363. Mercer CW, Logic JR: Cardiac arrest due to hyperkalemia following intravenous penicillin administration. *Chest* 64:358, 1973.
364. Michael JM et al: Potassium load in CPD-preserved whole blood and two types of packed red cells. *Transfusion* 15:144, 1975.
365. Miller CE, Remenchik AP: Problems involved in accurately measuring the K content of the human body. *Ann NY Acad Sci* 110:175, 1963.
366. Miller KP et al: Severe hyperkalemia during piroxicam therapy. *Arch Intern Med* 144:2414, 1984.
367. Mills JN et al: The acute effect of hydrocortisone, deoxycorticosterone and aldosterone upon the excretion of sodium, potassium, and acid by the human kidney. *J Physiol* 151:312, 1960.
368. Mitra S et al: Aldosterone secretion in anephric patients. *N Engl J Med* 286:61, 1972.
369. Mogensen CE: Renal functional changes in diabetes. *Diabetes* 25:872, 1976.
370. Montoliu J et al: Treatment of hyperkalaemia in renal failure with salbutamol inhalation. *J Intern Med* 228:35, 1990.
371. Montoliu J et al: Potassium-lowering effect of albuterol for hyperkalemia in renal failure. *Arch Intern Med* 147:713, 1987.
372. Moore RD: Effects of insulin upon ion transport. *Biochem Biophys Acta* 737: 1, 1983.
373. Morena M et al: Increase in serum potassium resulting from the administration of hypertonic mannitol and other solutions. *J Lab Clin Med* 73:291, 1969.
374. Morgan JM: Hyperkalemia and acidosis in lead nephropathy. *South Med J* 69:881, 1976.
375. Morimoto S et al: Reduced aldosterone secretory response to acute ACTH stimulation in sodium restricted elderly subjects. *J Am Geriatr Soc* 28:361, 1980.
376. Morris DJ: The metabolism and mechanisms of action of aldosterone. *Endocr Rev* 2:234, 1981.
377. Morris RC et al: Renal acidosis. *Kidney Int* 1:322, 1972.
378. Mortimore GE: Effect of insulin on potassium transfer in isolated rat liver. *Am J Physiol* 200:1315, 1961.
379. Muggia FM: Hyperkalemia and chemotherapy. *Lancet* 1:602, 1973.
380. Mulligan I et al: Acute haemolysis due to concentrated dialysis fluid. *Br Med J* 284:1151, 1982.
381. Muto S et al: Effects of adrenalectomy on CCD: Evidence for differential response of two cell types. *Am J Physiol* 253:F742, 1987.
382. Nelson DH: The adrenal cortex: Physiological function and disease, in *Major Problems in Internal Medicine*. Philadelphia, Saunders, 1980, vol 18.
383. Nerup J: Addison's disease—Clinical studies. A report of 108 cases. *Acta Endocrinol* 76:127, 1974.
384. Newstead CG et al: Acute hyperkalemia during exercise in haemodialysis patients. *Nephrol Dial Transplant* 3:542, 1988.
385. Newstead CG: Exercise-induced arterial hyperkalaemia in haemodialysis patients. *Nephrol Dial Transplant* 5:400, 1990.
386. Nicolis GL, Ulick S: Role of 18-hydroxylation in the biosynthesis of aldosterone. *Endocrinology* 76:515, 1965.
387. Nicolis GL et al: Glucose-induced hyperkalemia in diabetic subjects. *Arch Intern Med* 141:49, 1981.
388. Nilson HW: Corticoadrenal insufficiency: Metabolism studies on potassium, sodium, and chloride. *Am J Physiol* 118:620, 1937.
389. Norbiato G et al: Effect of prostaglandin synthetase inhibitors on renin and aldosterone in man on a normal or low sodium diet. *Acta Endocrinol* 87:577, 1978.
390. Norby LH et al: Possible role for impaired renal prostaglandin production in the pathogenesis of hyporeninaemic hypoaldosteronism. *Lancet* 2:1118, 1978.
391. Oberfield SE et al: Pseudohypoaldosteronism: Multiple target organ unresponsiveness to mineralocorticoid hormones. *J Clin Endocrinol Metab* 48:228, 1979.
392. Oberleithner H et al: The effect of furosemide on luminal sodium, chloride and potassium transport in the early distal tubule of Amphiuma kidney: Effects of potassium adaptation. *Pflugers Arch* 396:27, 1983.
393. Oh M et al: A mechanism for hyporeninemic hypoaldosteronism in chronic renal disease. *Metabolism* 23:1157, 1974.
394. O'Kelly R et al: Routine heparin therapy inhibits adrenal aldosterone production. *J Clin Endocrinol Metab* 56:108, 1983.
395. Olgaard K, Madsen S: Regulation of plasma aldosterone in anephric and nonnephrectomized patients during hemodialysis treatment. *Acta Med Scand* 201:457, 1977.
396. Oliver J et al: The renal lesions of electrolyte imbalance. I. The structural alterations in potassium depleted rats. *J Exp Med* 106:563, 1957.
397. O'Neil KG: Potassium secretion by cortical collecting tubule. *Fed Proc* 40:2403, 1981.
398. O'Neil RG, Helman SI: Transport characteristics of renal collecting tubules: Influences of DOCA and diet. *Am J Physiol* 233:F544, 1977.
399. O'Neil RG, Boulpaep E: Effect of amiloride on the apical cell membrane cation channels of a sodium-absorbing, potassium-secreting renal epithelium. *J Membr Biol* 50:365, 1979.
400. Orringer CE et al: Natural history of lactic acidosis after grand-mal seizures. *N Engl J Med* 297:796, 1977.
401. Oster JR et al: Relationship between blood pH and potassium and phosphorus during acute metabolic acidosis. *Am J Physiol* 235:F345, 1978.
402. Oster JR et al: Plasma potassium response to metabolic acidosis induced by mineral and nonmineral acids. *Miner Electrolyte Metab* 4:28, 1980.
403. Paice B et al: Hyperkalemia in patients in hospital. *Br Med J* 286:1189, 1983.
404. Pardo V et al: Nephropathy associated with sickle cell anemia. An autologous immune complex nephritis: I. Clinicopathologic study of seven patients. *Am J Med* 59:650, 1975.
405. Pasrk MH et al: Tubulointerstitial disease in lupus nephritis: Relationship to immune deposits, interstitial inflammation, glomerular changes, renal function, and prognosis. *Nephron* 44:309, 1986.

406. Patick J: Assessment of potassium stores. *Kidney Int* 11:476, 1977.
407. Paver WKA, Pauline GJ: Hypertension and hyperpotassaemia without renal disease in a young male. *Med J Aust* 2:305, 1964.
408. Pearson RM et al: Trial of combination of guanethidine and oxeprenolol in hypertension. *Br Med J* 2:933, 1976.
409. Peart WS: Renin and angiotensin in relation to aldosterone. *Am J Clin Pathol* 54:324, 1970.
410. Pedersen EB, Kornerup JH: Relationship between plasma aldosterone concentration and plasma potassium in patients with essential hypertension during aprenolol treatment. *Acta Med Scand* 200:263, 1976.
411. Pedersen G et al: Effect of propranolol on total exchangeable body potassium and total exchangeable body sodium in essential hypertension. *Scand J Clin Lab Invest* 39:167, 1979.
412. Pelleya R et al: Hyporeninemic hypoaldosteronism, sodium wasting and mineralocorticoid-resistant hyperkalemia in two patients with obstructive uropathy. *Am J Nephrol* 3:223, 1983.
413. Peltz S, Hashmi S: Pentamidine and hyperkalemia revisited. *Am J Med* 89:397, 1990.
414. Perez GO et al: Selective hypoaldosteronism with hyperkalemia. *Ann Intern Med* 76:757, 1972.
415. Perez GO et al: Renal acidification in patients with mineralocorticoid deficiency. *Nephron* 17:461, 1976.
416. Perez GO et al: Hyporeninemia and hypoaldosteronism in diabetes mellitus. *Arch Intern Med* 137:852, 1977.
417. Perez GO et al: Effect of alterations of sodium intake in patients with hyporeninemic hypoaldosteronism. *Nephron* 18:259, 1977.
418. Perez GO et al: Potassium homeostasis in chronic diabetes mellitus. *Arch Intern Med* 137:1018, 1977.
419. Perez GO et al: Serum potassium concentration in acidemic states. *Nephron* 27:233, 1981.
420. Perez GO et al: Renal tubular hyperkalemia. *Am J Nephrol* 2:109, 1982.
421. Perez GO et al: Blunted kakiuresis after an acute potassium load in patients with chronic renal failure. *Kidney Int* 24:656, 1983.
422. Petch MC et al: Biochemical effects of beta 2 adrenergic blockade in patients undergoing cardiopulmonary bypass. *Br Heart J* 42:240, 1979.
423. Petersen KC et al: Hyperkalaemia after cyclosporin therapy. *Lancet* 1:1470, 1984.
424. Pettit GW, Vick RL: Contribution of pancreatic insulin to extrarenal potassium homeostasis: A two-compartment model. *Am J Physiol* 226:319, 1974.
425. Phelps KR et al: Pathophysiology of the syndrome of hyporeninemic hypoaldosteronism. *Metabolism* 29:186, 1980.
426. Phelps KR et al: Pathophysiology of the syndrome of hyporeninemic hypoaldosteronism. *Metabolism* 29:186, 1980.
427. Phelps KR et al: Heparin-induced hyperkalemia: Report of a case. *Nephron* 25:254, 1980.
428. Ploth DW et al: Renin angiotensin influences on tubuloglomerular feedback activity in the rat. *Kidney Int* 22:S114, 1982.
429. Pollen RH, Williams RH: Hyperkalemic neuromyopathy in Addison's disease. *N Engl J Med* 263:273, 1960.
430. Ponce SP et al: Drug-induced hyperkalemia. *Medicine* 64:357, 1985.
431. Popovtzer MM et al: Hyperkalemia in salt-wasting nephropathy. Study of the mechanisms. *Arch Intern Med* 132:203, 1973.
432. Popp J et al: Hyperkalemia and hyperglycemic increments in plasma potassium in diabetes mellitus. *Arch Intern Med* 140:1617, 1980.
433. Posner J, Jacobs D: Isolated analdosteronism. I. Clinical entity, with manifestations of persistent hyperkalemia, periodic paralysis, salt-losing tendency, and acidosis. *Metabolism* 13:513, 1964.
434. Pratt JH: Role of angiotensin II in potassium-mediated stimulation of aldosterone secretion in the dog. *J Clin Invest* 70:667, 1982.
435. Proesmans W et al: Pseudohypoaldosteronism, a proximal tubular sodium-wasting disease. *J Pediatr* 92:678, 1978.
436. Rabinowitz L: Model of homeostatic regulation of potassium excretion in sheep. *Am J Physiol* 254:R381, 1988.
437. Rado JP et al: Hyperkalemia unresponsive to massive doses of aldosterone and renal tubular acidosis in a patient with chronic interstitial nephritis: Clinical and experimental studies. *J Med* 7:481, 1976.
438. Rado JP: Glucose-induced paradoxical hyperkalemia in patients with suppression of the renin-aldosterone system: Prevention by sodium depletion. *J Endocrinol Invest* 2:401, 1979.
439. Rado JP: Glucose-induced hyperkalemia in normoaldosteronemic diabetes associated with hyperthyroidism. *Endokrinologie* 78:239, 1981.
440. Rado JP: Glucose-induced hyperkalemia during captopril treatment. *Arch Intern Med* 143:389, 1983.
441. Rampini S et al: Congenital pseudohypoaldosteronism: Case report and review. Effect of indomethacin during sodium chloride depletion. *Helv Paediatr Acta* 33:153, 1978.
442. Ramsay LE et al: Amiloride, spironolactone, and potassium chloride in thiazide-treated hypertensive patients. *Clin Pharmacol Ther* 4:533, 1980.
443. Rappaport R et al: Hypoaldosteronism congenital familial par defaut de la 18-OH-dehydrogenase. *Pediatr Res* 2:456, 1968.
444. Rauschbolb EW et al: Aldosterone secretion after hypophysectomy. *Am J Physiol* 184:55, 1956.
445. Rector FC et al: Proximal tubular reabsorption of potassium during mannitol diuresis in rats. *J Lab Clin Med* 63:100, 1964.
446. Regan TJ et al: Relationship of insulin and strophanthidin to myocardial metabolism and function. *Am J Physiol* 205:790, 1963.
447. Reineck HJ et al: Potassium transport in the distal tubule and collecting duct of the rat. *Am J Physiol* 229:1403, 1975.
448. Reineck HJ et al: Net potassium addition beyond the superficial distal tubule of the rat. *Am J Physiol* 235:F104, 1978.
449. Reineck HJ et al: Nephron heterogeneity in renal excretion of sodium and potassium. *Am J Physiol* 239:F187, 1980.
450. Resh MD et al: Insulin stimulation of Na^+, K^+ adenosine triphosphatase-dependent ^{86}Rb uptake in rat adipocytes. *J Biol Chem* 255:10938, 1980.

451. Reubi FC et al: Interrelationships between sodium clearance, plasma aldosterone, plasma renin activity, renal hemodynamics and blood pressure in renal disease. *Klin Wochenschr* 57:1273, 1979.
452. Reza MJ et al: Massive intravenous digoxin overdosage. *N Engl J Med* 291:777, 1974.
453. Richard JL, Mimran A: Pseudo-hyperkaliemie d'orgine erythrocytaire: Augmentation passive de la permeabilite membranaire du potassium. *Pathol Biol* 31:583, 1983.
454. Richards P: Clinical investigation of the effects of adrenal corticosteroid excess on the colon. *Lancet* 1:437, 1969.
455. Rimmer JM et al: Hyperkalemia as a complication of drug therapy. *Arch Intern Med* 147:867, 1987.
456. Rogers TA: Tissue buffering in rat diaphragm. *Am J Physiol* 191:363, 1957.
457. Rogers TA, Wachenfeld AE: Effect of physiologic acids on electrolytes in rat diaphragm. *Am J Physiol* 193:623, 1958.
458. Rogers WJ et al: Acute effects of glucose-insulin-potassium infusion on myocardial substrates, coronary blood flow, and oxygen consumption in man. *Am J Cardiol* 40:421, 1977.
459. Romero JC et al: The effect of indomethacin and other anti-inflammatory drugs on the renin-angiotensin system in man. *J Clin Invest* 58:282, 1976.
460. Rosa RM et al: Adrenergic modulation of extrarenal potassium disposal. *N Engl J Med* 302:431, 1980.
461. Rosenbaum BJ et al: Acid-base and electrolyte changes induced by acute isotonic saline infusion in the nephrectomized dog. *J Lab Clin Med* 74:427, 1969.
462. Rosenbaum BJ et al: Hypertonic expansion. I. Acid-base and electrolyte changes. *Am J Physiol* 218:1201, 1970.
463. Rosler A et al: The nature of the defect in a salt wasting disorder in Jews of Iran. *J Clin Endocrinol Metab* 44:279, 1977.
464. Rosler A et al: Metabolic responses to the administration of angiotensin II, I and ACTH in two salt-wasting syndromes. *J Clin Endocrinol Metab* 44:292, 1977.
465. Ross EJ et al: Aldosterone excretion in hypopituitarism and after hypophysectomy in man. *Am J Med* 28:229, 1960.
466. Ross EJ: In *Aldosterone and Aldosteronism*. London, Lloyd-Luke, 1975, p 93.
467. Ross EJ: In *Aldosterone and Aldosteronism*. London, Lloyd-Luke, 1975, p 74.
468. Rossetti L et al: Effect of insulin on renal potassium metabolism. *Am J Physiol* 252:F60, 1987.
469. Sabatini S, Kuntzman NA: Enzyme activity in obstructive uropathy: Basis for salt wasting and the acidification defect. *Kidney Int* 37:79, 1990.
470. Sager P, DeFronzo RA: Dopaminergic regulation of extrarenal potassium metabolism in man. *Miner Electrolyte Metab* 13:385, 1987.
471. Sander SE et al: Suppression of plasma renin activity in a boy with chronic hyperkalemia. *Am J Dis Child* 141:922, 1987.
472. Santeusanio R et al: Evidence for a role of endogenous insulin and glucagon in the regulation of potassium homeostasis. *J Lab Clin Med* 81:809, 1973.
473. Saruta T, Kaplan NM: Adrenocortical steroidogenesis: The effects of prostaglandins. *J Clin Invest* 51:2246, 1972.
474. Saruta T et al: Renin, aldosterone, and other mineralocorticoids in hyperkalemic patients with chronic renal failure showing mild azotemia. *Nephron* 29:128, 1981.
475. Schambelan M et al: Isolated hypoaldosteronism in adults—A renin deficiency syndrome. *N Engl J Med* 287:573, 1972.
476. Schambelan M et al: Prevalence, pathogenesis, and functional significance of aldosterone deficiency in hyperkalemic patients with chronic renal insufficiency. *Kidney Int* 17:89, 1980.
477. Schambelan M et al: Mineralocorticoid-resistant renal hyperkalemia without salt-wasting (Type II pseudohypoaldosteronism): Role of increased renal chloride reabsorption. *Kidney Int* 19:716, 1981.
478. Scheer L et al: Management of hyperkalemia with a cation exchange resin. *N Engl J Med* 264:115, 1961.
479. Schilsky RL: Renal and metabolic toxicities of chemotherapy. *Semin Oncol* 9:75, 1982.
480. Schneider EG et al: The effect of potassium infusion on proximal sodium reabsorption and renin release in the dog. *Kidney Int* 2:197, 1972.
481. Schnermann J et al: Regulation of superficial nephron filtration rate by tubuloglomerular feedback. *Pflugers Arch* 318:147, 1970.
482. Schnermann J et al: Tubuloglomerular feedback. Nonlinear relation between glomerular hydrostatic pressure and loop of Henle perfusion rate. *J Clin Invest* 52:862, 1973.
483. Schon DA et al: Mechanism of potassium excretion in renal insufficiency. *Am J Physiol* 227:1323, 1974.
484. Schon DA et al: Role of the medullarly collecting duct in potassium adapted animals. *Kidney Int* 20:655, 1981.
485. Schultze RG et al: On the adaptation in potassium excretion associated with nephron reduction in the dog. *J Clin Invest* 50:1061, 1971.
486. Schultze RG et al: Blood pressure in terminal renal failure. *Nephron* 25:15, 1980.
487. Schwartz AB, Cannon-Babb M: Hyperkalemia due to drugs in diabetic patients. *Clin Pharmacol* 39:225, 1989.
488. Schwartz G, Burg MB: Mineralocorticoid effects on cation transport by cortical collecting tubules in vitro. *Am J Physiol* 235:F756, 1978.
489. Schwartz WB: Potassium and the kidney. *N Engl J Med* 253:601, 1955.
490. Schwartz WB et al: The internal distribution of hydrogen ions with varying degrees of metabolic acidosis. *J Clin Invest* 36:373, 1957.
491. Schwartz WB et al: The response of extracellular hydrogen ion concentration to graded degrees of chronic hypercapnia. The physiologic limits of the defense of pH. *J Clin Invest* 44:291, 1965.
492. Sealey JE et al: Potassium balance and the control of renin secretion. *J Clin Invest* 49:2119, 1970.
493. Sealey JE et al: Studies of plasma aldosterone in anephric people: Evidence for the fundamental role of the renin system in maintaining aldosterone secretion. *J Clin Endocrinol Metab* 47:52, 1978.
494. Sealey JE et al: Prorenin and other large molecular weight forms of renin. *Endocr Rev* 1:365, 1980.
495. Sebastian A et al: Amelioration of metabolic acidosis with fludrocortisone therapy in hyporeninemic hypoaldosteronism. *N Engl J Med* 297:576, 1977.

496. Sebastian A et al: Effect of mineralocorticoid replacement therapy on renal acid-base homeostasis in adrenalectomized patients. *Kidney Int* 18:762, 1980.
497. Sebastian A et al: Disorders of distal nephron function. *Am J Med* 72:289, 1982.
488. Sebastian A, Schambelan M: Renal hyperkalemia. *Semin Nephrol* 7:223, 1987.
499. Seldin DW, Tarail R: Effect of hypertonic solutions on metabolism and excretion of electrolytes. *Am J Physiol* 159:160, 1949.
500. Seldin DW et al: Consequences of renal failure and their management, in Strauss MB, Welt LG (eds): *Diseases of the Kidney*. Boston, Little, Brown, 1971, p 211.
501. Shapiro S et al: Fatal drug reactions among medical inpatients. *JAMA* 216:467, 1971.
502. Sheldon J, Pyke DA: Severe diabetic ketosis. Precoma and coma, in Oakeley WG et al (eds): *Clinical Diabetes and Its Biochemical Basis*. Blackwell, Oxford, 1968, p 420.
503. Shemer J et al: Incidence of hyperkalemia in hospitalized patients. *Isr J Med Sci* 19:659, 1983.
504. Silva P, Spokes K: Sympathetic system in potassium homeostasis. *Am J Physiol* 241:F151, 1981.
505. Simmons DH, Avedon M: Acid-base alterations and plasma potassium concentration. *Am J Physiol* 197:319, 1959.
506. Simonson D et al: Adrenergic blockade alters glucose kinetics during exercise in insulin-dependent diabetes. *J Clin Invest* 73:1648, 1984.
507. Simpson SAS, Tait JF: Recent progress on methods of isolation, chemistry and physiology and aldosterone. *Recent Prog Horm Res* 11:183, 1955.
508. Singer I: Nephrology forum. Lithium and the kidney. *Kidney Int* 19:374, 1981.
509. Skinner SL: A cause of erroneous potassium levels. *Lancet* 1:478, 1961.
510. Skott O, Briggs JP: Direct demonstration of macula densa-mediated renin secretion. *Science* 237:1618, 1987.
511. Smith JD et al: Clinical disorders of potassium metabolism, in Arieff A, DeFronzo RA (eds): *Fluid, Electrolyte, and Acid-Base Disorders*. New York, Churchill Livingstone, 1985, p 413.
512. Smith TW, Willerson JT: Suicidal and accidental digoxin ingestion. Report of five cases with serum digoxin level correlations. *Circulation* 44:29, 1971.
513. Smith TW et al: Treatment of life-threatening digitalis intoxication with digoxin-specific Fab antibody fragments. *N Engl J Med* 307:1357, 1982.
514. Smoller S et al: Blunted kaliuresis after an acute oral potassium load in diabetes mellitus. *Am J Med Sci* 295:114, 1988.
515. Sonnenberg H et al: Effect of vasopressin analogue (dDAVP) on potassium transport in medullary collecting duct. *Am J Physiol* 252:F986, 1987.
516. Sopko JA, Freeman RM: Salt substitutes as a source of potassium. *JAMA* 238:608, 1977.
517. Soudry JF et al: The effect of lumen pH on potassium transport in renal cortical collecting tubules. *Am J Physiol* 230:239, 1976.
518. Soulillou JP et al: Acute hyperkalemic risks in recipients of kidney graft cooled with Collins' solution. *Nephron* 19:301, 1977.
519. Spark RF et al: Activation of aldosterone secretion in primary aldosteronism. *J Clin Invest* 48:96, 1969.
520. Spital A: Bicarbonate in the treatment of severe hyperkalemia. *Am J Med* 86:511, 1989.
521. Spitzer A et al: Short stature, hyperkalemia and acidosis: A defect in renal transport of potassium. *Kidney Int* 3:251, 1973.
522. Stanton BA, Giebisch GH: Mechanism of urinary potassium excretion. *Miner Electrolyte Metab* 5:100, 1981.
523. Stanton BA et al: Structural and functional study of the rat distal nephron: Effects of potassium adaptation and depletion. *Kidney Int* 19:36, 1981.
524. Stanton B, Giebisch G: Effects of pH on potassium transport by renal distal tubule. *Am J Physiol* 242:F551, 1982.
525. Stanton BA, Giebisch GH: Potassium transport by the renal distal tubule: Effects of potassium loading. *Am J Physiol* 243:F487, 1982.
526. Stanton BA, Giebisch GH: Regulation of potassium homeostasis, in Corradino RA (ed): *Functional Regulation at the Cellular and Molecular Levels*. Amsterdam, Elsevier/North Holland, 1982, p 259.
527. Stanton BA et al: Ultrastructure of rat initial collecting tubule: Effect of adrenal corticosteroid treatment. *J Clin Invest* 75:1327, 1984.
528. Stanton B et al: Effects of adrenalectomy and chronic adrenal corticosteroid replacement on potassium transport in rat kidney. *J Clin Invest* 75:1317, 1985.
529. Stanton B et al: Mechanisim and time course of aldosterone-induced stimulation of Na^+ and K^+ transport. *Fed Proc* 44:6761, 1985.
530. Stanton B et al: Ultrastructure of rat initial collecting tubule: Effect of adrenal corticosteroid treatment. *J Clin Invest* 75:1317, 1985.
531. Stanton B: Regulation by adrenal corticosteroids of sodium and potassium transport in loop of Henle and distal tubule of rat kidney. *J Clin Invest* 78:1612, 1986.
532. Stanton B: Renal potassium adaptation: Cellular mechanisms and morphology, in Giebisch G (ed): *Current Topics in Membranes and Transport*. New York, Academic Press, 1987, vol 28, p 225.
533. Stanton B et al: Independent effects of aldosterone and potassium on induction of potassium adaptation in rat kidney. *J Clin Invest* 79:198, 1987.
533a. Sterns RH et al: Role of the adrenergic nervous system in hyperkalemia. *Kidney Int* 23:267, 1983.
534. Stetson DL et al: Morphologic alterations in the rat medullary collecting duct following potassium depletion. *Kidney Int* 17:45, 1980.
535. Stewart GW et al: Familial pseudohyperkalaemia: A new syndrome. *Lancet* 2:175, 1979.
536. Stewart GW, Ellory JC: A family with mild hereditary xerocytosis showing high membrane cation permeability at low temperatures. *Clin Sci* 69:309, 1985.
537. Stokes GS et al: Syndrome of idiopathic hyperkalaemia and hypertension with decreased plasma renin activity: Effects of plasma renin and aldosterone of reducing the serum potassium level. *Med J Aust* 2:1050, 1968.
538. Stokes JB: Consequences of potassium recycling in the renal medulla. *J Clin Invest* 70:219, 1982.
539. Streeten DHP et al: Studies on hyperkalemic periodic paralysis: Evidence of changes in plasma Na and Cl and

induction of paralysis by adrenal glucocorticoids. *J Clin Invest* 50:142, 1971.

540. Sunderlin FS et al: The reninangiotensin-aldosterone system in diabetic patients with hyperkalemia. *Diabetes* 30:335, 1981.
541. Tait JF, Tait SAS: The effect of changes in potassium concentration on the maximal steroidogenic response of purified zona glomerulosa cells to angiotensin II. *J Steroid Biochem* 7:687, 1976.
542. Takeda R et al: Prolonged pseudoaldosteronism induced by glycyrrhizin. *Endocrinol Jpn* 26:541, 1979.
543. Talbott JH et al: Renal function in patients with Addison's disease and in patients with adrenal insufficiency secondary to pituitary pan-hypofunction. *J Clin Invest* 21:107, 1942.
544. Tan SY, Mulrow PJ: Inhibition of the renin-aldosterone response to furosemide by indomethacin. *J Clin Endocrinol Metab* 45:174, 1977.
545. Tan SY et al: Inactive renin and impaired prostaglandin production in hyporeninemic hypoaldosteronism. *Clin Res* 29:452A, 1979.
546. Tan SY et al: Indomethacin-induced prostaglandin inhibition with hyperkalemia. *Ann Intern Med* 90:783, 1979.
547. Tarail R et al: Effects of injection of hypertonic glucose on metabolism of water and electrolytes in patients with edema. *J Clin Invest* 30:1111, 1951.
548. Taylor WC et al: Experimental observations on cardiac arrhythmias during exchange transfusions in rabbits. *J Pediatr* 58:470, 1961.
549. Textor SC et al: Hyperkalemia in azotemic patients during angiotensin-converting enzyme inhibition and aldosterone reduction with captopril. *Am J Med* 73:719, 1982.
550. Thorn GW et al: The effect of cortin on the sodium, potassium, chloride, inorganic phosphorus and total nitrogen balance in normal subjects and in patients with Addison's disease. *Endocrinology* 21:202, 1937.
551. Thorn GW et al: Addison's disease: Evaluation of synthetic deoxycorticosterone acetate therapy in 158 patients. *Ann Intern Med* 16:1053, 1942.
552. Thorn GW: *The Diagnosis and Treatment of Adrenal Insufficiency*. Springfield, Charles C Thomas, 1951.
553. Tobin RB: Varying role of extracellular electrolytes in metabolic acidosis and alkalosis. *Am J Physiol* 195:685, 1958.
554. Todd EP, Vick RL: Kalemotropic effect of epinephrine: Analysis with adrenergic agonists and antagonists. *Am J Physiol* 220:1963, 1971.
555. Tormey WP, Morgan DB: Etiologic considerations in Gordon's syndrome: Possible role of prostaglandins. *Prostaglandins Med* 4:107, 1980.
556. Traub YM et al: Elevation of serum potassium during beta blockade: Absence of relationships to the renin-aldosterone system. *Clin Pharmacol Ther* 28:765, 1980.
557. Trewby PN et al: Heroin and hyperkalaemia. *Lancet* 1:327, 1981.
558. Tuck ML et al: Hyporeninemic hypoaldosteronism in diabetes mellitus. *Diabetes* 28:237, 1979.
559. Tuck ML, Mayes DM: Mineralocorticoid biosynthesis in patients with hyporeninemic hypoaldosteronism. *J Clin Endrocrinol Metab* 50:351, 1980.
560. Tucker BJ et al: Mechanism of diuresis with modest acute hyperglycemia. *Clin Res* 29:478A, 1981.
561. Ulick S et al: An aldosterone biosynthetic defect in a salt-losing disorder. *J Clin Endocrinol Metab* 24:669, 1964.
562. Ulick S: Diagnosis and nomenclature of the disorders of the terminal portion of the aldosterone biosynthetic pathway. *J Clin Endocrinol Metab* 43:93, 1976.
563. Uribarri J et al: Salt-losing nephropathy. *Am J Nephrol* 3:193, 1983.
564. Vaamonde CA et al: Syndromes of aldosterone deficiency. *Miner Electrolyte Metab* 5:121, 1981.
565. Vagnucci AH: Selective aldosterone deficiency. *J Clin Endocrinol Metab* 29:279, 1969.
566. Velaquez H et al: Effects of luminal anion composition and acidity on potassium secretion by renal distal tubule. *Fed Proc* 39:4267A, 1980.
567. Veldhuis JD et al: Inborn error in the terminal step of aldosterone biosynthesis: Corticosterone methyloxidase type II deficiency in a North American pedigree. *N Engl J Med* 303:117, 1980.
568. Veldhuis JD, Melby JC: Isolated aldosterone deficiency in man: Acquired and inborn errors in the biosynthesis of action of aldosterone. *Endocr Rev* 2:495, 1981.
569. Verniory A et al: Effect of sotalol on haemodynamics and renin-angiotensin-aldosterone systems in hypertensive patients. *Clin Sci* 51:9, 1976.
570. Veterans Administration Cooperative Study Group on Antihypertensive Agents: Low-dose captopril for the treatment of mild to moderate hypertension. *Arch Intern Med* 144:1947, 1984.
571. Viberti GC: Glucose-induced hyperkalemia: A hazard for diabetes. *Lancet* 1:690, 1978.
572. Vick RL et al: Epinephrine-induced hypokalemia: Relation to liver and skeletal muscle. *J Pharmacol Exp Ther* 181:139, 1972.
573. Visser KHA: Inherited variation in the biosynthesis of adrenal corticoids in man. *Mem Soc Endocrinol* 15:145, 1967.
574. Waack S et al: Extracellular potassium modifies the structure of kidney epithelial cells in culture. *Am J Physiol* 249:C105, 1985.
575. Waal-Manning HJ: Metabolic effects of beta-adrenoreceptor blockers. *Drugs* II (suppl 1):121, 1976.
576. Wade JB et al: Modulation of cell membrane area in renal collecting tubules by corticosteroid hormones. *J Cell Biol* 81:439, 1979.
577. Waldhausl W et al: Combined 17- and 18-hydroxylase deficiency associated with complete male pseudohermaphroditism and hypoaldosteronism. *J Clin Endocrinol Metab* 46:236, 1978.
578. Walker BR et al: Hyperkalemia after triamterene in diabetic patients. *Clin Pharmacol Ther* 13:643, 1972.
579. Walker GW, Cooke CR: Plasma aldosterone regulation in anephric man. *Kidney Int* 3:1, 1973.
580. Walker M et al: Clinical aspects of diabetic ketoacidosis. *Diabetes Metab Rev* 5:651, 1989.
581. Wang P, Clausen T: Treatment of attacks in hyperkalemic familial periodic paralysis by inhalation of salbutamol. *Lancet* 1:221, 1976.

582. Ward JR, Call LS: Changes in blood chemistry in rats following electrically-induced seizures. *Proc Soc Exp Biol Med* 70:381, 1949.
583. Ward RA et al: Hemodialysate composition and intradialytic metabolic, acid-base and potassium changes. *Kidney Int* 32:129, 1987.
584. Warren SE, O'Connor DT: Hyperkalemia resulting from captopril administration. *JAMA* 244:2551, 1980.
585. Waterhouse C, Kentmann H: Kidney function in adrenal insufficiency. *J Clin Invest* 27:372, 1948.
586. Weidmann P et al: Plasma aldosterone in terminal renal failure. *Ann Intern Med* 78:13, 1973.
587. Weidmann P et al: Syndrome of hyporeninemic hypoaldosteronism and hyperkalemia in renal disease. *J Clin Endocrinol Metab* 36:965, 1973.
588. Weidmann P et al: Dynamic studies of aldosterone in anephric man. *Kidney Int* 4:289, 1973.
589. Weidmann P et al: Control of aldosterone responsiveness in terminal renal failure. *Kidney Int* 7:351, 1975.
590. Weidmann P et al: Effect of aging on plasma renin and aldosterone in normal man. *Kidney Int* 8:325, 1975.
591. Weidmann P et al: Role of the reninangiotensin-aldosterone system in the regulation of plasma potassium in chronic renal disease. *Nephron* 15:35, 1975.
592. Weintraub HD et al: Changes in plasma potassium concentration after depolarizing blockers in anesthetized man. *Br J Anaesth* 41:1048, 1969.
593. West ML et al: New clinical approach to evaluate disorders of potassium excretion. *Miner Electrolyte Metab* 12:234, 1986.
594. Whiting G et al: Severe hyperkalemia with moduretic. *Med J Austr* 1:409, 1979.
595. Whyte KF et al: Salbutamol induced hypokalaemia: The effect of theophylline alone and in combination with adrenaline. *Br J Clin Pharmacol* 25:571, 1988.
596. Wienstein SR et al: Hyperkalemia, acidosis, and short stature associated with a defect in renal potassium excretion. *J Pediatr* 85:355, 1974.
597. Williams GH et al: Studies on the metabolism of aldosterone in chronic renal failure and anephric man. *Kidney Int* 4:280, 1973.
598. Williams ME et al: Impairment of extrarenal potassium disposal by alpha-adrenergic stimulation. *N Engl J Med* 311:145, 1984.
599. Williams ME et al: Catecholamines modulate rapid potassium shifts during exercise. *N Engl J Med* 312:823, 1985.
600. Williams ME et al: Hyperkalemia. *Adv Intern Med* 31:265, 1986.
601. Wilson CB et al: Antitubular basement membrane antibodies after renal transplantation. *Transplantation* 18:447, 1974.
602. Wilson D, Goetz F: Selective hypoaldosteronism after prolonged heparin administration. *Am J Med* 36:635, 1964.
603. Windom H et al: A comparison of the haemodynamic and hypokalaemic effects of inhaled pirbuterol and salbutamol. *N Z Med J* 103:259, 1990.
604. Winkler AW et al: The toxicity of orally administered potassium salts in renal insufficiency. *J Clin Invest* 20:119, 1941.
605. Winters RW et al: The mechanism of acidosis produced by hyperosmotic infusions. *J Clin Invest* 43:647, 1964.
606. Woodbury DM, Koch A: Effects of aldosterone and desoxycorticosterone on tissue electrolytes. *Proc Soc Exp Biol Med* 94:720, 1957.
607. Wright FS, Briggs JP: Feedback control of glomerular blood flow, pressure, and filtration rate. *Physiol Rev* 59:958, 1979.
608. Wright FS, Giebisch GH: Renal potassium transport: Contributions of individual nephron segments and populations. *Am J Physiol* 235:F515, 1978.
609. Wright R, Schnermann J: Interference with feedback control of glomerular filtration rate by furosemide, triflocin, and cyamide. *J Clin Invest* 53:1695, 1974.
610. Yang WC et al: Propranolol-induced hyperkalemia in non-diabetic uremic patients. *Kidney Int* 27:156A, 1985.
611. Yentis SM: Suxamethonium and hyperkalaemia. *Anaesth Intensive Care* 18:92, 1990.
612. Young DB, Jackson TE: Effects of aldosterone on potassium distribution. *Am J Physiol* 243:R526, 1982.
613. Young DB: Quantitative analysis of aldosterone's role in potassium regulation. *Am J Physiol* 255:F811, 1988.
614. Yun J et al: Role of prostaglandins in the control of renin secretion in the dog. *Circ Res* 40:459, 1977.
615. Zalups RK et al: Structural adaptation in initial collecting tubule following reduction in renal mass. *Kidney Int* 27:636, 1985.
616. Zalups RK: Effect of dietary K and 75% nephrectomy on the morphology of principal cells in CCDs. *Am J Physiol* 256:F387, 1989.
617. Zierler KL: Hyperpolarization of muscle by insulin in a glucose-free environment. *Am J Physiol* 197:524, 1951.
618. Zierler KL: Increase in resting membrane potential of skeletal muscle produced by insulin. *Science* 126:1067, 1957.
619. Zierler KL: Effect of insulin on membrane potential and potassium content of rat muscle. *Am J Physiol* 197:524, 1959.
620. Zierler KL, Rabinowitz D: Effect of very small concentrations of insulin on forearm metabolism. Persistence of its actions on potassium and free fatty acids without its effect on glucose. *J Clin Invest* 43:950, 1964.
621. Zierler KL: Effect of insulin on potassium efflux from rat muscle in the presence and absence of glucose. *Am J Physiol* 198:1006, 1968.
622. Zierler KL: Insulin, ions, and membrane potentials, in Greep RO, Astwood EB (eds): *Handbook of Physiology, Endocrinology*. Washington DC: American Physiology Society, 1973, sect 7, vol I, p 347.
623. Zierler K, Rogers EM: Hyperpolarization as a mediator of insulin action: Increased muscle glucose uptake induced electrically. *Am J Physiol* 239:E21, 1980.
624. Zierler K, Rogers EM: Rapid hyperpolarization of rat skeletal muscle induced by insulin. *Biochem Biophys Acta* 640:687, 1981.

CHAPTER • 24

Acid-base disorders: definitions and introductory concepts

Robert G. Narins

With serum concentrations less than three millionths that of sodium, the free, circulating hydrogren ion is truly a trace element. In the face of these vanishingly low concentrations, each day 50 to 100 meq of acid are synthesized and eventually seep into the extracellular fluid (ECF) from cellular sites of production. Thus, over a 24-h period, the ECF is normally inundated with an amount of free protons that exceed the total ECF content of unbound hydrogen ions by more than 100,000-fold. In the face of this minute-to-minute challenge to acid-base homeostasis it must be remembered that many biochemical reactions and organ functions require that ambient acidity barely deviate from normal. The need to maintain the acidity of body fluids within a very narrow range is vital to the host's survival, and indeed, when measured repeatedly over a 24-h period, blood acidity is virtually constant.

The author acknowledges support from the University Medical Research Foundation.

This chapter presents certain selected clinically relevant aspects of this homeostatic system that prevents lethal swings in the acidity of body fluids. Additionally, concepts will be reviewed that bear importantly on the clinical approach to patients with various metabolic and respiratory acid-base disorders. At the outset, it should be appreciated that the control of acid-base homeostasis is predicated on the harmonious interaction of three prime elements: *acid production*, *acid buffering*, and *acid excretion* (Fig. 24-1). Each of these components is separately discussed below.

INTRODUCTORY CONCEPTS AND DEFINITIONS

ACIDITY OF BODY FLUIDS: pH VS. HYDROGEN-ION CONCENTRATION

The acidity of body fluids may be described in terms of ion concentration, i.e., free proton concentration, or in

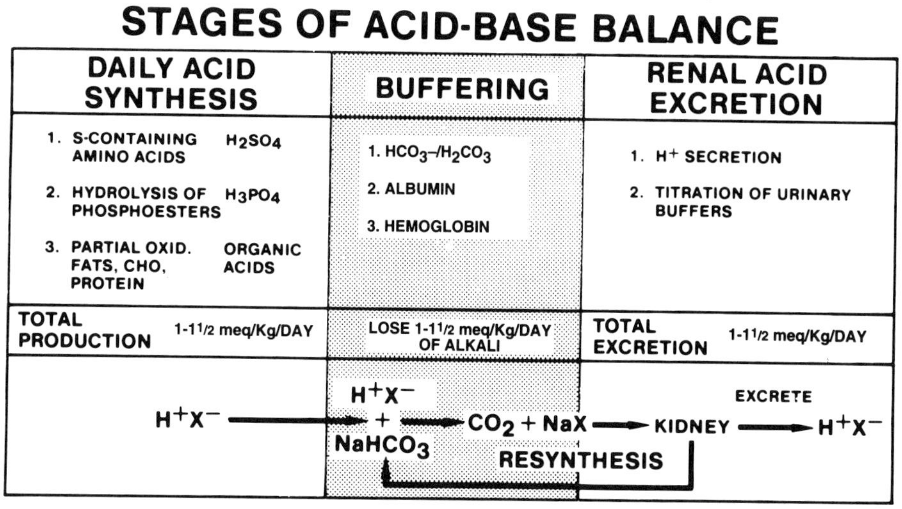

FIGURE 24-1 • Schematic integration of the three phases of acid-base balance. The illustration indicates how renal resynthesis of bicarbonate lost in titrating daily fixed acid production and excretion of this acid sustains normal acid balance. See text for details. Abbreviations: CHO, carbohydrate; HX, generic expression for any fixed acid; S, sulfur.

terms of pH. In many biological fluids the free hydrogen-ion concentration is often a small fraction of the total proton content. The binding of protons by macromolecules accounts for this disparity. Glass electrodes, selectively permeable to free protons, are used to measure the acidity of biological solutions. Under normal conditions the hydrogen-ion concentration of blood is 0.000 000 040 molar, i.e., 40 × $10^{-9}M$ or 40 nmol/liter, or 40 neq/liter. The difficulties encountered with using such small amounts led Sorensen to convert these numbers to their negative logarithms, i.e, the pH:[7]

$$pH = -\log (H^+) \qquad (1)$$

Since the normal proton concentration, $[H^+]$, is 40×10^{-9} *M*, it follows that:

$$pH = -\log [40 \times 10^{-9}]$$
$$-[1.6 + (-9.0)]$$
$$pH = 7.40$$

If the $[H^+]$ *increased* to $60 \times 10^{-9}M$, the pH of this more acid solution would change as follows:

$$pH = -\log [60 \times 10^{-9}]$$
$$= -[1.78 + (-9.0)]$$
$$pH = 7.22$$

If the $[H^+]$ decreased to 20×10^{-9}M, the pH of this more alkaline solution would change as follows:

$$pH = -\log (20 \times 10^{-9})$$
$$= -[1.3 + (-9.0)]$$
$$pH = 7.70$$

Thus, pH and $[H^+]$ vary inversely. As a solution acidifies the $[H^+]$ increases and the pH falls, while alkalinization is defined as a reduction in $[H^+]$ and an increase in pH.

The inverse relationship between pH and $[H^+]$ is depicted in Fig. 24-2. This figure also illustrates certain clinically useful àspects of this mathematical interaction. The normal ranges of hydrogen-ion concentration and pH are 36 neq/liter to 44 neq/liter and 7.44 to 7.36, respectively. Over the range of pH values commonly encountered, i.e., from 7.5 to 7.2, the $[H^+]$ changes by approximately 10 neq/liter for each 0.1 pH unit change. Thus, when the pH acidifies by 0.1 unit, i.e., decreasing from 7.4 to 7.3, the $[H^+]$ increases by 10 neq/liter, from 40 to 50 neq/liter. Conversely, as the pH alkalinizes by 0.1 unit, i.e., an increase from 7.4 to 7.5, the $[H^+]$ declines by approximately 10 neq/liter, from 40 to 32 neq/liter. Another quirk of the mathematical relationship indicates that the $[H^+]$ doubles for each 0.3 unit decrease in pH. On the alkaline side, the $[H^+]$ halves for each 0.3 unit increased in pH (Fig. 24-2). The antilog of 0.3 is 2, accounting for the observed changes. Recognition of this relationship simplifies interconversion of pH and $[H^+]$ as one uses the various formulas and equations that relate to the clinical interpretation of laboratory data (see below).

The terms used to describe blood pH are *acidemia* annd *alkalemia*. The suffix *-emia* refers to the pH of blood. You are alkalemic when your $[H^+]$ decreases to less than 36 neq/liter, corresponding to pH values greater than 7.44. Acidemia obtains when your $[H^+]$ increases to values in excess of 44 neq/liter, corresponding to a pH below 7.36. The term *euphemia* has been used by some to describe the normal range of pH and $[H^+]$, i.e., 7.36 to 7.44, or 36 to 44 neq/liter.

The above definitions are to be contrasted with the terms *acidosis* and *alkalosis*. The suffix *-osis* refers to the pathologic processes that are at work causing acid or alkali to accumulate in body fluid. The acidoses are associated with the generation of either fixed acids or a decrease in the pulmonary clearance of the volatile acid, carbonic acid. The alkaloses cause the accumulation of fixed base or stimulate the increased pulmonary clearance of carbonic acid. Two points regarding the terms acidosis and alkalosis require emphasis. First, these terms imply nothing about blood pH. Indeed, it is quite possible for

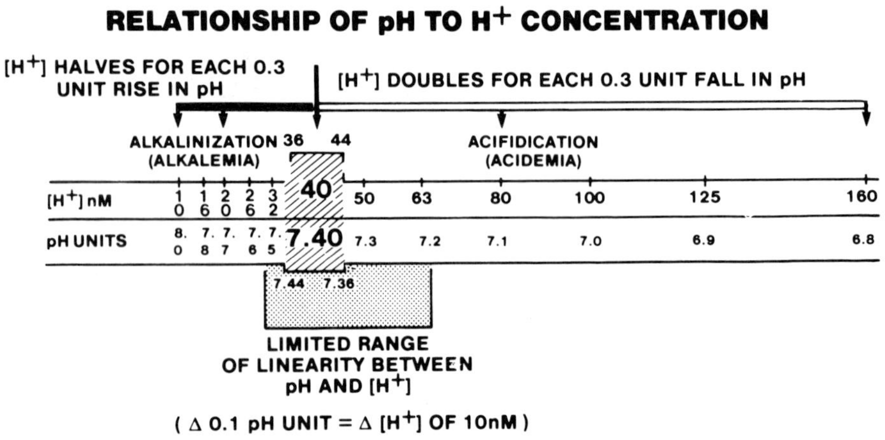

FIGURE 24-2 • Relationship of pH to hydrogen-ion concentration. The line-hatched area emphasizes the normal range of hydrogen-ion concentration, i.e., $[H^+]$ = 36 to 44 nM; this corresponds to a pH range of 7.44 to 7.36. The stippled area highlights the commonly encountered range of pH abnormalities, 7.50 (32 nM) to 7.20 (63 nM). The formula indicates the almost linear, inverse relationship between pH and $[H^+]$ over this biologically important range (see text for details). The top line indicates that as blood is alkalinized, the $[H^+]$ is reduced by one-half for each increment of 0.3 pH units above the normal pH of 7.40. Conversely the $[H^+]$ doubles for each decrement of 0.3 pH units below the normal pH of 7.40.

an acidosis or an alkalosis to be present without acidifying or alkalinizing the blood, i.e., an acidosis without an acidemia or an alkalosis without an alkalemia. The independence of these two events could be brought about because the acidosis or alkalosis is mild, causing the pH to change but still to remain within the relatively broad range of normal. When the acidosis or alkalosis worsens, the pH will eventually move into the pathologic range of alkalemia or acidemia. Second, combinations of pathologic processes may be present simultaneously and exert offsetting effects on blood pH. For example, one may have an acidosis causing fixed acids to accumulate in blood but at the same time have a pathologic pulmonary process that rids the body of excessive amounts of volatile carbonic acid. Thus the combination of pathologic but offsetting processes may allow the pH to remain within the normal range. Examples of mixed acid-base disturbances are discussed in Chap. 31. The terms acidosis and alkalosis always refer to pathologic processes and not to the appropriate, physiologic compensation that normally accompanies primary acid-base disturbances. This point is amplified below.

ACID PRODUCTION

The normal concentration of protons in body fluid is under constant attack from a variety of sources. As lucidly outlined in Chapter 9, children normally produce 1.5 to 2 meq/kg per day and adults 1.0 to 1.5 meq/kg per day of fixed acid. These fixed acids are largely accounted for by the oxidation of sulfur contained in a variety of ingested proteins and amino acids. The partial combustion of dietary fats, carbohydrates, and proteins results in the net generation of such organic acids as lactic acid, citric acid, and ketoacids. The only volatile acid normally produced is carbonic acid. The latter is derived from the catalyzed hydration of CO_2 produced from the complete combustion of organic materials. Approximately 15,000 to 20,000 mmol of carbonic acid are produced daily. The efficient pulmonary clearance of this volatile acid normally maintains its concentration in blood and tissues within very narrow limits. The ventilatory system is sensitive to variations in CO_2 synthesis, such that wide swings in production are met with appropriate changes in ventilation, maintaining the partial pressure of CO_2 (P_{CO_2}) very close to the normal value of 40 mmHg. While the lungs maintain volatile acid balance, the kidneys maintain fixed acid balance. The renal regulation of acid balance has been outlined in Chapter 10.

The primary acid-base disorders are obviously linked to a disruption in the balance normally struck between acid synthesis and excretion. Metabolic (fixed-acid) or volatile-acid accumulation could obviously derive from overproduction or underexcretion of protons. Indeed disorders to be described in the next several chapters are caused by one or both of these pathophysiologic events. Conversely, when fixed- or volatile-acid excretion exceeds production, acid deficit, or alkalinization, develops.

BUFFERING: DEFINITIONS AND DISTRIBUTION

The buffering of protons or alkali plays a central and vital role in the maintenance of acid-base homeostasis[6] (Fig. 24-1). In broad terms, the acids produced via cellular metabolism percolate out of cells and into the extracellular space where they would poisonously disrupt the normal chemical milieu were it not for the presence of buffers. The buffers, in effect, absorb protons, preventing them from fully expressing their physiochemical activity, and innocuously deliver them to the kidney where the acid is transferred to specific renal buffers for excretion. Thus, the 24-h renal excretion of acid rids the body of its daily metabolic production and thereby maintains zero acid balance. The normal close approximation of renal acid excretion with acid production allows for the maintenance of a constant hydrogen-ion concentration in cellular and extracellular body fluids.

Although a variety of buffers exist in the extracellular space, the bicarbonate-carbonic acid buffer pair, by far, plays the largest role. The importance of this buffer system relies on two facts. First, the body content of each member of the buffer pair is plentiful and second, each of the two components is independently but harmoniously regulated by separate organs. The controlled renal excretion of acid simultaneously adds new bicarbonate to blood. Conversely, the regulated renal retention of acid reduces blood bicarbonate concentration when appropriate to the host's needs. The lungs independently regulate P_{CO_2}, futher ensuring stability of acid-base balance.

The transport of CO_2 from its sites of cellular production to the lungs for excretion is described in Chapter 8. Briefly, CO_2 diffuses from cellular areas of high to extracellular areas of lower partial pressure. The gas freely penetrates cell membranes and enters red blood cells (RBC), where it contacts the enzyme carbonic anhydrase which catalyzes CO_2 hydration, forming H_2CO_3, which immediately ionizes to H^+ and HCO_3^-. Hemoglobin absorbs the proton while the bicarbonate exits the RBC in exchange for entering chloride. This *chloride shift* causes reciprocal hypochloremia and hyperbicarbonatemia of venous blood. The increased concentration of fixed alkali partially offsets the acidifying effect of venous hypercapnia. Venous blood entering the lungs is exposed to alveolar air, which is of lower P_{CO_2}, enabling diffusion of CO_2 from the hypercapnic venous circulation down its partial pressure gradient into the alveolus. The fall in pulmonary venous P_{CO_2} reverses the process initiated at the tissue level, causing chloride to reenter the ECF and bicarbonate to reenter the RBC, where CO_2 is reformed preparatory to its excretion by the lungs. Red blood cells entering the arterial circuit have therefore yielded their CO_2 and reduced their venous plasma bicarbonate concentration. It follows that venous blood is slightly more acidified than arterial by consequence of its higher P_{CO_2}.

While the fixed acids leaving cells can be absorbed by a variety of available buffers, the bicarbonate-carbonic acid system is the most important. Buffers have the unique capacity of contributing protons in times of acid deficit and absorbing accumulating hydrogen ions in times of acid surfeit. Equation 2 illustrates this property.

$$\underset{\text{ACID}}{\overset{\text{WEAK}}{\text{HA}}} \; \underset{\text{Reforms to diminish alkalemia}}{\overset{\text{Ionizes to diminish alkalemia}}{\rightleftharpoons}} \; \text{H}^+ + \underset{\text{BASE}}{\text{A}^-} \qquad (2)$$

The equation indicates that if the hydrogen-ion concentration were to increase independently, protons would combine with the base, A^-, thereby reforming HA. This "inactivation" of protons forms the basis of acid buffering. Conversely, if the concentration of protons were to decrease independently, the weak acid, HA, acting as a reservoir, would donate protons to maintain the stability of the ambient hydrogen-ion concentration.

The steady-state acidity of body fluids is maintained and determined by the buffers available to these compartments. Indeed, the ambient $[H^+]$ of a well-mixed compartment can be expressed in terms of any one of the buffer pairs that is in equilibrium with this proton pool.

The *law of mass action* indicates that at equilibrium, when the rates of the forward and backward reactions of an equation (e.g., Equation 2) are equal, the product of the concentrations of H^+ and A^-, when divided by the concentration of the reactant, HA, is equal to a constant:

$$K_{eq} = \frac{[H^+]\,[A^-]}{[HA]} \qquad (3)$$

It follows that the stronger the acid the larger its K_{eq}, i.e., the more easily it relinquishes protons. As with pH, because the ionization constants of many biological acids are quite small, their negative logarithm has been utilized to make the numbers less cumbersome. As with the relationship between pH and hydrogen-ion concentration, the relationship of pK to the K_{eq} is inverse. Thus, the stronger the acid the greater the K_{eq} and the smaller the pK. It turns out that buffers function best when their pK is within one log unit of the ambient pH.[2] Thus, a biologically significant buffer should have its pK close to the ambient pH of blood, i.e., approximately 7.4. Albumin, hemoglobin, and monobasic phosphate ($H_2PO_4^-$) all satisfy this requirement. Since these buffers are not present in abundance, their usefulness, as contrasted with the bicarbonate–carbonic acid pair, is rather limited.

Rearrangement of Equation 3 yields a general expression that defines acidity in terms of any of the buffers that are in equilibrium with the proton pool.

$$[H^+] = \frac{[\text{unionized acid}]}{[\text{base}]} K_{eq} \qquad (4)$$

The use of the monobasic phosphoric acid ($H_2PO_4^-$) and dibasic phosphoric acid (HPO_4^{2-}) buffer pair illustrates the use of this equation. The K_{eq} of $H_2PO_4^-$ is 1.58×10^{-7} (pK = 6.8):

$$H_2PO_4^- \rightleftharpoons H^+ + HPO_4^{2-} \qquad (5)$$

At normal blood pH (7.40, $[H^+] = 40 \times 10^{-9}\ M$) the relationship of the members of the buffer pair is easily illustrated.

$$40 \times 10^{-9} = \frac{[H_2PO_4^-]}{[HPO_4^{2-}]} 1.58 \times 10^{-7}$$

$$25 \times 10^{-2} = \frac{[H_2PO_4^-]}{[HPO_4^{2-}]}$$

Fleshing out Equation 4 with the K_{eq} for $H_2PO_4^-$ at normal pH reveals that the ratio of acid phosphate to basic phosphate is 1:4 (i.e., 0.25, or 25×10^{-2}). Alterations in this ratio define changes in blood acidity. A similar set of equations may be drawn for the $H_2CO_3-HCO_3^-$ buffer pair. The K_{eq} for H_2CO_3 is 2×10^{-4} (pK = 3.8).

$$H_2CO_3 \rightleftharpoons H^+ + HCO_3^- \qquad (6)$$

$$K_{eq} = \frac{[H^+]\,[HCO_3^-]}{[H_2CO_3]} \qquad (7)$$

$$[H^+] = K_{eq}\frac{[H_2CO_3]}{[HCO_3^-]} \qquad (8)$$

The standard *Henderson-Hasselbalch equation* is developed by taking the negative logarithm of both sides of Equation 8. The pH and pK represent the negative logarithms of the $[H^+]$ and K_{eq}, respectively. The negative logarithm of the $[H_2CO_3]/[HCO_3^-]$ ratio is made positive by inverting the ratio.

$$\text{pH} = \text{p}K + \log\frac{[HCO_3^-]}{[H_2CO_3]} \qquad (9)$$

In practical terms, this equation is made cumbersome by the extreme difficulty in measuring the low levels of H_2CO_3 normally present in biological fluids. Under normal conditions, only $6 \times 10^{-6}M$ of H_2CO_3 is found in blood. Utilizing Equation 9 with a pH of 7.40, a HCO_3^- concentration of 24 meq/liter, and carbonic acid's true pK of 3.8 allows one to calculate the actual H_2CO_3 concentration.

In an effort to render Equation 9 more useful and to enable calculation of pH from the $[HCO_3^-]$ and $[H_2CO_3]$, a simple way of defining carbonic acid's concentration had to be developed. Several seemingly disparate observations have been combined, allowing one to comfortably utilize Equation 9.

The CO_2 dissolved in solution is directly proportional to the carbonic acid concentration:

$$CO_2 + H_2O \rightleftharpoons H_2CO_3 \rightleftharpoons H^+ + HCO_3^- \quad (10)$$
(DISSOLVED CO_2)

At equilibrium, the mass action equation for this relationship is as follows:

$$K_{eq} = \frac{[H^+][HCO_3^-]}{[\text{dissolved } CO_2]} \quad (11)$$

This equation indicates that in the steady state, dissolved CO_2 is proportional to the $[H_2CO_3]$ and can be utilized in the denominator of the Henderson-Hasselbalch equation (Equation 9). The dissolved CO_2 can be derived from Henry's law using Bunsen's coefficient. Henry demonstrated that the quantity of gas dissolved in a liquid is directly proportional to the partial pressure of that gas at the surface of the liquid. Bunsen derived the proportionality constant that related carbon dioxide's partial pressure to the amount dissolved. Bunsen's coeffient α for CO_2 indicates that 0.0301 mmol of CO_2 dissolve per liter of fluid per mmHg of CO_2 gas. Thus the product of α and the measured P_{CO_2} yields the concentration of the dissolved gas. Under normal conditions, 1.2 mmol/liter of CO_2 are dissolved in blood (P_{CO_2} 40 mmHg × 0.0301 mmol/liter/mmHg). One last point is required before establishing the Henderson-Hasselbalch equation in its final form. To compensate for inflating the H_2CO_3 concentration by 200 times (increased from its actual value of 0.006 m*M* to 1.2 m*M*, the logarithm of 200,2.3, is added to carbonic acid's true p*K* of 3.8, yielding an apparent p*K* (p*K'*) of 6.1. Thus the Henderson-Hasselbalch equation 12 incorporates an altered p*K* which allows use of the easily measured dissolved CO_2 as a substitute for measured H_2CO_3. The prime sign in the expression p*K'* denotes that this change has been made.

$$pH = pK' + \log\frac{[HCO_3^-]}{\alpha P_{CO_2}} \quad (12)$$

Having already indicated that buffers function best when their p*K* approximates the ambient pH which they protect, the odd fact that the bicarbonate-carbonic acid system is the most effective body buffer but has a p*K'* of only 6.1 seems to belie the above observation. This buffer system owes its effectiveness to the following facts, which have already been alluded to.

Bicarbonate is abundant, achieving a normal concentration of 24 meq/liter in the ECF. Importantly, the base is synthesized in a regulated manner by the kidney. The acid component of the buffer pair, H_2CO_3, is also plentiful and its concentration is under respiratory control. As illustrated below, the independent regulation of each buffer component divorces its buffering capacity from dependence on the inherent strength of the acid, i.e., its p*K*.

As fixed acid (HA) is added to the ECF it is titrated by sodium bicarbonate. Protons combine with and destroy HCO_3^-, forming H_2CO_3, which rapidly dehydrates, yielding CO_2 and H_2O. Thus the addition of fixed acid is initially acidifying by virtue of its simultaneous removal of HCO_3^- and creation of CO_2 gas and H_2CO_3, events that reduce the $HCO_3^-/\alpha P_{CO_2}$ ratio and thereby acidify fluid compartments. This acidification is detected by chemotactic areas in the brainstem and periphery that stimulate ventilation, thereby reducing the P_{CO_2} and lessening the degree of acidification. In time, the kidneys "sense" the acidification and simultaneously excrete the offending acid while resynthesizing lost HCO_3^- (see Chap. 10). Thus buffering and restoration of normalcy depend upon the independent pulmonary-renal regulation of HCO_3^- and P_{CO_2}, respectively. It is also crucial to recognize the critical importance of this "open" buffer system. The pulmonary excretion of CO_2 limits the acidifying effect of the addition of fixed acid. An example of this point follows. Addition of 5 meq/liter of the fixed acid HA to a "closed" (i.e., no pulmonary regulation) buffer system simultaneously reduces the serum bicarbonate concentration from 25 to 20 meq/liter while increasing the H_2CO_3 concentration from 1.2 to 6.2 meq/liter. The change in pH as defined by the Henderson-Hasselbalch equation is illustrated below.

Control (prior to addition of acid):

$$pH = 6.1 + \log (25 \text{ meq/liter})/0.03 (40 \text{ mmHg})$$
$$pH = 7.42$$

Addition of 5 meq/liter of fixed acid to a closed system:

$$pH = 6.1 + \log (20 \text{ meq/liter})/(6.2 \text{ meq/liter})$$
$$pH = 6.61$$

In an "open" buffer system, recognition of this acidification by the afferent limb of the respiratory system not only prevents the CO_2 accumulation but lowers the P_{CO_2} to values below baseline.

Addition of 5 meq/liter of fixed acid to an open system:

$$pH = 6.1 + \log (20 \text{ meq/liter})/0.03 (35 \text{ mmHg})$$
$$pH = 6.1 + \log (20 \text{ meq/liter})/(1.05 \text{ meq/liter})$$
$$pH = 7.38$$

In time, the renal resynthesis of lost HCO_3^- restores normobicarbonatemia, allowing the acid-stimulated respiration once again to normalize. As detailed below, the magnitude of the ventilatory response to this *metabolic acidosis* is dictated by the magnitude of the bicarbonate reduction. Indeed, the lower the bicarbonate concentration, the greater the respiratory stimulation (Table 24-1). This increased ventilation represents the normal, physiologic response to a reduction in bicarbonate concentration and is termed *pulmonary compensation.* It is *not called* respiratory alkalosis; the terms *acidosis* and *alkalosis* are reserved for describing primary pathologic events.

A similar sequence, but opposite in direction, can be described for *metabolic alkalosis.* The primary increase in bicarbonate concentration raises the $HCO_3^-/\alpha P_{CO_2}$ ratio, thereby raising the pH or diminishing the $[H^+]$. This

TABLE 24-1 • Characteristic features of primary acid-base disorders

Primary acid-base disorder	Initiating disturbance	Compensatory response	Limits of compensation
METABOLIC			
Acidosis	↓↓↓[HCO_3^-]	↓↓P_{CO_2}	• P_{CO_2} = 1.5 [HCO_3^-] + 8 ± 2 • Each meq/liter fall in [HCO_3^-] lowers P_{CO_2} by 1-1.3 mmHg • P_{CO_2} = last two digits of pH • P_{CO_2} and last two digits of pH = [HCO_3^-] + 15*
Alkalosis	↑↑↑[HCO_3^-]	↑↑P_{CO_2}	• P_{CO_2} increases by 6 mmHg for each 10 meq/liter increase in [HCO_3^-] • P_{CO_2} and last two digits of pH = [HCO_3^-] + 15*
RESPIRATORY			
Acidosis			
Acute (hours)	↑↑↑P_{CO_2}	↑[HCO_3^-]	• [HCO_3^-] increases 1 meq/liter for each 10 mmHg increase in P_{CO_2}
Chronic (days)	↑↑↑P_{CO_2}	↑↑[HCO_3^-]	• [HCO_3^-] increases 3-3.5 meq/liter for each 10 mmHg increase in P_{CO_2}
Alkalosis			
Acute	↓↓↓P_{CO_2}	↓[HCO_3^-]	• [HCO_3^-] falls 2.5 meq/liter for each 10 mmHg fall in P_{CO_2}
Chronic	↓↓↓P_{CO_2}	↓↓[HCO_3^-]	• [HCO_3^-] falls 5.0 meq/liter for each 10 mmHg fall in P_{CO_2}

* Formula is valid for [HCO_3^-] only in the range of 8 to 40 meq/liter.

wave of alkalinity seeps into the brainstem and slows ventilation; the rising P_{CO_2} attenuates the alkalinizing process. Once again the magnitude of this physiologic, respiratory response is proportional to the magnitude of the hyperbicarbonatemia (Table 24-1).

As detailed in Chaps. 25 and 28, the respiratory compensation for the metabolic acid-base disturbances is highly predictable; indeed, the P_{CO_2} that is appropriate for any given change in serum HCO_3^- concentration can be precisely estimated (Table 24-1). Failure of respiration to properly adapt to hypo- or hyperbicarbonatemia indicates that another primary pathologic process must be acting on the respiratory system, thereby violating the normal compensation. A P_{CO_2} that is too high or too low for a given change in bicarbonate concentration identifies the presence of another primary pathologic process, i.e., respiratory acidosis (P_{CO_2} too high) or respiratory alkalosis (P_{CO_2} too low). Armed with this information, the physician must now identify the pathologic process that is preventing normal compensation. Thus, with knowledge of the narrow limits for respiratory compensation, one can unearth the presence of such disruptive disorders as pneumonia, brainstem lesions, and pulmonary emboli from careful examination of the key acid-base parameters: pH, P_{CO_2}, and HCO_3^- concentration.

Two caveats must be remembered. Although pulmonary compensation begins within minutes of a fall in bicarbonate levels, it takes many hours for the P_{CO_2} to reach its new steady-state level. The formulas predicting what the P_{CO_2} ought to be for a given degree of hypobicarbonatemia are all predicated on stable, steady-state values for serum bicarbonate (see Table 24-1 and Chaps. 25 and 28. Premature use of these formulas, while the bicarbonate concentration and P_{CO_2} are still changing, may lead to the erroneous diagnosis of a mixed metabolic and respiratory acid-base disorder. Generally, steady-state values are achieved in 24 to 36 h. The second caveat is that the compensating event does not normalize pH; it simply lessens its deviation from normal. According to current concepts, it is the abnormal pH that sustains the pulmonary compensation. Thus normalization of pH would remove the stimulus driving the pulmonary response. The steady-state pH in simple metabolic acidosis or alkalosis ought to be acid or alkaline, respectively.

Primary disturbances in P_{CO_2} are the hallmark of the *respiratory acid-base disorders* (Table 24-1). The abnormal P_{CO_2} and the associated disturbance in pH elicit compensatory metabolic changes that alter the bicarbonate concentration such that pH returns toward, but not to, normal. As detailed by Dr. Gennari (Chap. 30), the altered P_{CO_2} provokes tissue and circulating buffers to effect a small change in HCO_3^- concentration, which acts to stabilize pH. In hours to days, salutary changes in renal acid excretion further amend serum bicarbonate concentration, thereby returning pH closer to baseline. This acute and chronic metabolic buffering for respiratory acid-base disturbances returns the displaced $HCO_3^-/\alpha P_{CO_2}$ ratio toward normal by altering the numerator. Thus in respiratory acidosis, the hypercapnia acidifies by decreasing the $HCO_3^-/\alpha P_{CO_2}$ ratio. Early extrarenal and late renal bicarbonate synthesis increases the numerator, thereby reducing the pathologically depressed ratio. Conversely, the hypocapnia of primary respiratory alkalosis raises the $HCO_3^-/\alpha P_{CO_2}$ ratio, thereby alkalinizing blood. Early extrarenal, followed by later renal-induced, bicarbonate consumption diminishes the numerator, returning the alkalemic pH toward, but not to, normal.

The unique "open" nature of the HCO_3^-/H_2CO_3 buffer system allows it to absorb the great bulk of acid added to the ECF, despite the presence of other buffers. In a closed system composed of competing buffer pairs, added protons would be taken up by all the buffer bases. In the ECF, added acid would be absorbed by HCO_3^-, HPO_4^{2-}, and protein$^-$; forming H_2CO_3,$H_2PO_4^-$, and H^+ protein, respectively. Since all buffers are accessible to a homogeneous, well-mixed pool of protons, the final ambient $[H^+]$ will reflect the product of the equilibrium constant and the acid-base ratio for each buffer (Equation 4). As developed in Equations 2 to 4, the $[H^+]$ is determined by and in turn reflects this product. During this brief transient, where carbonic and monobasic phosphoric acids and protonated protein are formed, the $(K_{eq}) \times$ (acid/base) molar ratio for each pair will be equal and so define the final $[H^+]$. Unlike the other buffer pairs, however, the $[H_2CO_3]/[HCO_3^-]$ ratio can continue to decrease, because of stimulated ventilation with reduction of P_{CO_2} and therefore of H_2CO_3 levels. The lowered acid-to-base ratio in turn alkalinizes blood. Confronted with a reduced $[H^+]$, $H_2PO_4^-$ and H^+ protein relinquish protons, reducing their acid-base ratios to match that of H_2CO_3/HCO_3^-. Yielded protons are then titrated by HCO_3^-. Thus added protons are initially distributed to all available buffers, but subsequent to respiratory adjustment of H_2CO_3, hydrogen ions are stripped from other buffers and absorbed by HCO_3^-, and the resulting CO_2 is excreted by the lungs. This passage of protons through the buffer pairs with eventual absorption by bicarbonate ensures that it plays the dominant acid-base role. Bicarbonate's role remains paramount until the most severe degrees of hypobicarbonatemia are reached, at which point the other buffers become increasingly more important.

It has been shown that almost 60 percent of an infused load of fixed acid is absorbed by cells.[3] The fate of these intracellular protons is not well understood. Absorption by intracellular proteins and the metabolic incorporation of protons into neutral products are likely. In this regard, it is well known that alkalinization of cells stimulates production of lactic acid and citric acid,[4] thereby mitigating the alkalinizing process. Conversely, acidification of cells reduces organic acid synthesis, thereby reducing the acidifying process.[4]

Unlike intracelluar and extracellular fluid, the range of pH's achievable in the urine is quite broad, spanning from 4.0 to 8.0, reflecting a 10,000-fold change in hydrogen-ion concentration. The reader should appreciate that when the p*K* of a potential urinary buffer is lower than the ambient pH, the acid will ionize and contribute protons. Conversely when the buffer's p*K* is greater than the ambient pH, the buffer will absorb protons. It follows that the most effective urinary buffers have their p*K*s in the range of 7. Thus, as the urine is acidified the buffers absorb protons and carry out biologically significant amounts of acid into the urine. Strong acids like sulfuric acid and hydrochloric acid have very low p*K*s (in the range of 1) and therefore are totally ineffective as urinary buffers. The prime urinary buffers are monovalent phosphate ($H_2PO_4^-$) and ammonia, molecules with p*K*s of 6.8 and 9.1, respectively. These points have been well described in Chap. 10.

Bicarbonate space

Infusions of alkali or acid are often required by desperately ill patients to alter their serum bicarbonate concentrations therapeutically. To titrate the serum bicarbonate concentration precisely requires knowledge of bicarbonate's space of distribution. An apparent oddity develops as one evaluates data relevant to this determination. Most textbooks suggest that the *apparent bicarbonate space* approximates 50 percent of body weight, or roughly 35 liters in a 70-kg man. It follows that the total body bicarbonate content when the serum level is 25 meq/liter is 875 meq (25 meq/liter × 35 liters). The actual total body bicarbonate content obtained from the *true bicarbonate space* (derived from actual measurements), however, is substantially less than that calculated from the apparent space. The bicarbonate content of the ECF space is also a function of the product of its concentration (25 meq/liter) and volume (20 percent of body weight, or 14 liters). Thus 350 meq reside in the ECF. Estimates of the bicarbonate concentration of intracellular fluid (ICF) indicate that its value approximates 8 meq/liter, with an ICF space of roughly 28 liters. Adding the 224 meq of ICF bicarbonate to the 350 meq in the ECF indicates that the body bicarbonate content is only 574 meq, some 300 meq less than predicted from the apparent space. Interestingly, estimation, on the basis of its apparent space, of the amount of $NaHCO_3$ required to increase the serum bicarbonate concentration by a given amount usually achieves the predicted serum level with a fair degree of accuracy.

The accuracy of the apparent bicarbonate space—despite the differences between it and the measured space—is due to the accessibility of administered bicarbonate to cellular and other nonbicarbonate buffers. A fraction of infused alkali is taken up by cells while another portion is titrated and destroyed by cellular and nonbicarbonate buffers. The remaining alkali is free to distribute in bicarbonate's true space and so to increase its serum concentration.

The apparent bicarbonate space overestimates body bicarbonate content by an amount equal to the dissipation of administered alkali by cellular and nonbicarbon-

ate buffers. It provides a simple, albeit indirect way of estimating the dose of acid or alkali required to change the serum bicarbonate concentration by a given amount.

As metabolic acidosis progresses and the body bicarbonate content wanes, nonbicarbonate buffers take on a progressively more important role (see above). As these nonbicarbonate buffers are titrated, the apparent bicarbonate space expands. Indeed, it takes more and more $NaHCO_3$ to effect a given increment in its serum concentration since a greater fraction of the administered load is spent in titrating the other buffers. For this reason the apparent bicarbonate space may greatly exceed total body water in severe metabolic acidosis. In this situation there is, unfortunately, no way to accurately estimate the new apparent space. Estimates of the dose of alkali required are derived empirically. Bicarbonate infusion rates are keyed to the observed therapeutically induced rates of change in the serum level.

Serum anion gap

The anion gap is a simple tool that affords important insights into the diagnosis and therapy of various metabolic acid-base disorders.[5] In broad view, the anion gap is the difference between the concentrations of measured cations and measured anions in serum. Since the levels of the measured cations normally exceed those of the routinely measured anions, an apparent anion gap is created by the clinical laboratory. The first panel in Fig. 24-3 describes the relationship between the total number of cations and anions present in the ECF. It should be apparent that sodium and potassium account for the vast bulk of extracellular cations whereas chloride and bicarbonate account for a lesser fraction of the anions. The difference between the sum of the levels of measured cations and the sum of the levels of measured anions reflects the presence of the usually *unmeasured* anions, i.e., albumin and various other organic and inorganic (sulfate, phosphate) anions. The clinical laboratory measures sodium and potassium, thereby assaying almost the entire pool of cationic charge. By measuring only chloride and bicarbonate, a substantially smaller fraction of the total anionic charge in the ECF is measured, thereby creating an apparent anion gap. Measured in this way, the normal anion gap is 15 ± 2 meq/liter. Because the absolute meq/liter change in serum potassium concentration in health or in disease is minimal, most laboratories will delete it from the anion gap calculation. Thus, in most centers the anion gap is defined as the difference between the concentration of sodium and the sum of the concentrations of chloride and bicarbonate and averages 12 ± 2 meq/liter. Each hospital and laboratory must develop its own set of normal values since various assay techniques may yield significantly different results.

The importance of the anion gap lies in its utility in diagnosing and treating a variety of metabolic acid-base abnormalities. As illustrated in Fig. 24-4, the addition of a fixed acid to plasma simultaneously destroys bicarbonate as the proton combines with the base, forming CO_2 and water. Loss of bicarbonate leaves sodium's positive charge transiently unbalanced, causing retention of the acid anion. In this example, the titration process allows NaX to replace $NaHCO_3$. If the added acid were HCl, as would occur in diarrheal acidosis, renal tubular acidosis, or with acetazolamide therapy, added protons again destroy bicarbonate and the latter is now replaced by chloride. These hydrochloric acidoses do not significantly alter the anion gap since the fall in bicarbonate con-

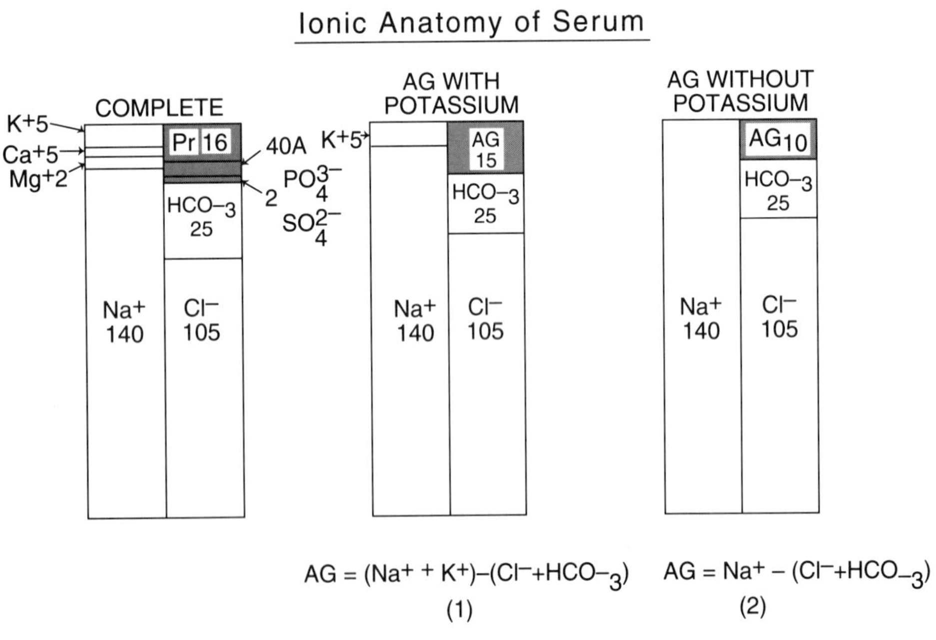

FIGURE 24-3 • Electrolytes: ECF components and the creation of the anion gap (AG). Bar graph on left depicts normal ECF. Middle and rightmost bars indicate that the clinical laboratory routinely measures almost all cations but assays a lesser fraction of the anions. The disparity between measured cations and anions creates the apparent anion gap (see text for details). Abbreviations: OA, organic acid anions; Pr, protein anion. (*Reproduced with permission from Emmett M, Narins RG: Clinical use of the anion gap. Medicine (Baltimore) 56:38, 1977.*)

METABOLIC ACIDOSIS AND THE ANION GAP

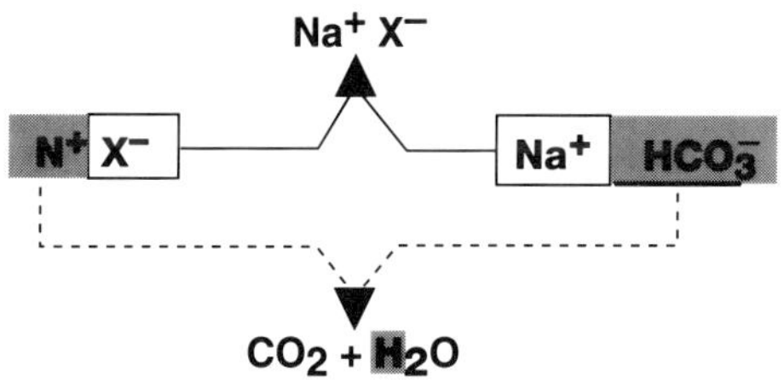

$AG = Na^+ - (Cl^- + HCO_3^-) = 12 \text{ w } 2 \text{ mM}$

METABOLIC ACIDOSIS

	NORMAL	NORMAL AG ACIDOSIS	HIGH AG ACIDOSIS
Na^+	140	140	140
Cl^-	105	115	105
HCO_3^-	25	15	15
AG	10	10	20
ΔHCO_3^-		−10	−10
ΔAG*		0	+10
$LACT.^-$	1	1	11
ΔLACT.*		0	+10

* Δ: CHANGE FROM NORMAL

FIGURE 24-4 • The serum electrolyte pattern in the various forms of metabolic acidosis, schematic representation. The titration of an accumulating generic strong acid (H^+X^-) by sodium bicarbonate is depicted at the top. The effect on the anion gap (AG) of adding HCl or any other biologically available acid is described by the electrolyte patterns on the bottom. (*Modified and reproduced with permission from Emmett M, Narins RG: Clinical use of the anion gap. Medicine (Baltimore) 56:38, 1977.*) See text for details.

centration is counterbalanced by an approximately equal increase in chloride concentration, causing their sum to remain essentially unchanged. The electrolyte pattern created by this hyperchloremic acidosis is illustrated in Fig. 24-4. Addition to blood of any acid other than hydrochloric acid causes the anion gap to increase. For example, the addition of lactic acid causes destruction of bicarbonate and its replacement with the usually unmeasured lactate anion. Thus sodium lactate replaces sodium bicarbonate and the anion gap increases since the fall in bicarbonate concentration is not offset by a similar change in chloride concentration. The electrolyte pattern displayed by the high anion gap acidoses, of which lactic acidosis is one, is shown in the last column in Fig. 24-4.

Thus, in assessing patients with metabolic acidosis, it is quite useful to sort them into normal anion gap and high anion gap groupings. This classification allows one to approach very quickly and efficiently the differential diagnosis of any patient with a metabolic acidosis. As will be discussed in Chap. 25, with a careful history and physical examination and a few simple laboratory tests, one can quickly and precisely diagnose the cause of a given normal or elevated anion gap metabolic acidosis.

An additional diagnostic insight afforded by the anion gap is its use in classifying certain forms of mixed metabolic acid-base disturbances. Returning to Fig. 24-4, the third column to the right illustrates the appropriate relationship between the fall in bicarbonate concentration (ΔHCO_3^-), the change in the anion gap (ΔAG), and the measured change in the concentration of the offending acid anion. In the example cited, the bicarbonate concentration fell by 10 meq/liter, the anion gap increased by 10 meq/liter, and the lactate concentration increased by 10 meq/liter. The thesis illustrated in this figure is that for each meq per liter increase in the acid anion concentration an equal milliequivalent per liter decrease in bicarbonate concentration occurs and the anion gap increases by a like amount. Indeed, the ΔAG is a reasonably precise, albeit indirect measure of the concentration of the acid anion. Figure 24-5 illustrates this concept. The incremental fall in bicarbonate concentration is illustrated on the abscissa and the incremental change in the anion gap is illustrated on the ordinate. A simple high anion gap metabolic acidosis is characterized by a reciprocal fall in bicarbonate concentration and increase in the anion gap, i.e., each meq per liter fall in bicarbonate concentration is associated with an equal rise in the anion gap. This change is portrayed by the line of identity in the illustration (Fig. 24-5). On the other hand, if the patient has a large rise in the anion gap but a much

RELATIONSHIP BETWEEN THE INCREASE IN THE ANION GAP AND THE DECREASE IN THE SERUM HCO_3^- CONCENTRATION (ΔAG, ΔHCO_3^-)

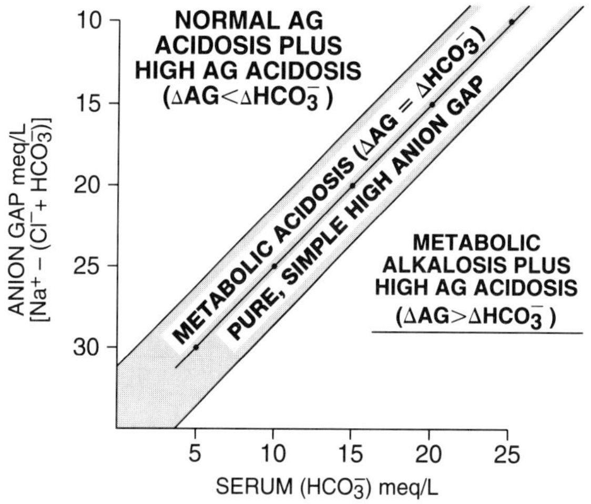

FIGURE 24-5 • The importance of correlating the change in the serum bicarbonate concentration (ΔHCO_3^-) with the change in the anion gap (ΔAG). Any simpe high anion gap acidosis is characterized by inverse numeric equality of the decrease from normal in bicarbonate concentration and the increase from normal in the AG. Failure for such equality to obtain defines the presence of the mixed disturbances shown in the left upper and right lower quadrants of the figure. (*Reproduced with permission from Goodkin D et al: The role of the anion gap in diagnosing mixed metabolic acid-base disorders. Clin Endocrinol Metab 13:333,* 1984.)

smaller fall or even an increase in the bicarbonate concentration, one must say that a mixed metabolic acidosis, metabolic alkalosis is present. The large increase in the anion gap reflects the presence of a large amount of circulating acid that should have destroyed an amount of bicarbonate equal to the increase above normal in the anion gap. Failure of the bicarbonate concentration to fall appropriately indicates that some other source of alkali must be sustaining an inappropriately high level of bicarbonate.

In another setting, suppose the bicarbonate concentration fell by a large amount but was associated with only a small rise in the anion gap. The small increase in the anion gap can account for only a small fraction of the fall in bicarbonate concentration, inferring that a hyperchloremic acidosis must also be present. Thus when the bicarbonate concentration falls substantially more than the anion gap increases, one must diagnosis a mixed high anion gap and normal anion gap metabolic acidosis. These points are further illustrated in Chap 31.

The anion gap also affords therapeutic insights into certain clinical problems. During vigorous alkali therapy of various high anion gap metabolic acidoses the serum bicarbonate concentration may be normalized prior to suppression of the organic acid overproduction. The high bicarbonate concentration would be associated with a continuously increased anion gap. This would alert the physician to the fact that lactic acid or ketoacids were still being overproduced and signal the need for more insulin, better tissue perfusion, etc. When ketoacidosis and lactic acidosis occur simultaneously, the redox potential is such that all ketoacids may be in the form of beta-hydroxybutyric acid, which does not give a positive nitroprusside (ketostix) reaction. In this setting one is confronted by an elevated anion gap acidosis which, in the absence of azotemia or ingestion of a toxin, may be lactic acidosis, beta-hydroxybutyric acidosis, or a combination of the two. Most laboratories can measure serum lactate levels, which when subtracted from the elevated anion gap reveal the component of the acidosis contributed by the ketoacids. For example, if the anion gap were 30 meq/liter with a serum lactate of 10 meq/liter, half of the ΔAG (30 meq/liter − 10 meq/liter = ΔAG of 20 meq/liter) would be lactate and the other half would most likely be beta-hydroxybutyrate. In this way one can diagnosis the presence of mixed ketolactic acidosis.

Table 24-2 illustrates that there are a number of other causes of an elevated anion gap in addition to metabolic acidosis. In general, these other disorders cause trivial elevations and afford little confusion in diagnosing metabolic acidosis. Table 24-3 illustrates the effects of *dehydration on the anion gap*. As shown, loss of water causes proportionate increments in the serum sodium, chloride, and bicarbonate concentration, and thus the anion gap increases by an amount equal to the percentage of dehydration. A 10 percent increase would raise the normal anion gap from 10 to 11 meq/liter. Thus, although water loss increases the anion gap, it is generally trivial. When a significant increase in the anion gap occurs in the face of volume contraction one is more likely dealing with compromised tissue perfusion and a superimposed lactic acidosis. The *infusion of sodium salts of various organic compounds* may occasionally increase the anion gap. This may be seen during the administration of sodium lactate, sodium citrate, or the sodium salts of certain antibiotics, such as carbenicillin or penicillin. Any increment in serum sodium concentration is counterbalanced by the presence of one of the aforementioned unmeasured anions. For these salts to increase the anion gap it is not necessary for the serum sodium concentration to rise. As the sodium salts accumulate in the extracellular space they cause the osmotic withdrawal of cellular water. Translocation of this water to the extracellular space prevents a significant increase in sodium concentration that would otherwise occur, while diluting the concentration of extracellular chloride and bicarbonate. Thus an unchanged serum sodium concentration will be associated with decreased chloride and bicarbonate levels, causing the anion gap to increase. Industrial doses of penicillin (50,000 to 100,000 units daily) or carbenicillin (30 g daily) may increase the anion gap for the same reasons as sodium lactate infusions.

A modest increase in the anion gap may also accompany *magnesium depletion*. Magnesium deficiency engenders hypocalcemia and hypokalemia (see Chap. 34). Reduced concentrations of these three cations cause simultaneous loss of their accompanying chloride anions. Thus hypomagnesemia is associated with hypochloremia. The normal serum sodium concentration in the face of

TABLE 24-2 • Causes of a high anion gap

1. Metabolic acidosis
2. Dehydration
3. Administration of salts of strong acids
4. Certain antibiotics
5. Magnesium deficiency
6. Alkalosis
7. Allopurinol

TABLE 24-3 • Effect of dehydration on the anion gap

Clinical condition	Serum electrolyte (meq/liter)			
	Sodium	Chloride	Bicarbonate	Anion gap
Normal	140	105	25	10
10% loss of body water	154	115.5	27.5	11

hypochloremia causes the anion gap to increase modestly; e.g., 3 to 4 meq/liter increments are commonly seen.

Metabolic and respiratory alkaloses are perhaps the most common nonacidotic cause of an increased anion gap. In our experience, elevations of the anion gap beyond 3 to 5 meq/liter are distinctly unusual for alkaloses. There are two major reasons why the alkaloses increase the anion gap. Metabolic and respiratory alkalosis can stimulate glycolysis, causing a modest accumulation of lactic acid. The overall rate of glycolysis is normally limited by several intervening steps, the most important of which is probably the phosphofructokinase (PFK) reaction. This enzyme is exquisitely sensitive to pH changes, being stimulated by alkalosis and inhibited by acidosis. By deinhibiting PFK, alkalinization enhances conversion of glucose to pyruvate and lactate. Thus alkalosis begets increments in metabolic acid production, thereby lessening the rise in pH. The chemical result of this "metabolic buffering" is a 1 to 3 meq/liter increase in serum lactate concentration, corresponding to a similar increment in the anion gap. Respiratory alkalosis may provoke an even greater effect on glycolysis, lactate production, and the anion gap than does metabolic acidosis. This is presumably due to the greater change of intracellular pH effected by respiratory acid-base changes as compared to metabolic disorders. As bicarbonate accumulates in the extracellular space it is partly titrated by nonbicarbonate buffers. Albumin seems to play a key role in this regard. Equation 13 describes the titration of bicarbonate by protonated albumin.

$$NaHCO_3 + H^+Alb^- \rightarrow Na^+Alb^- + H_2O + CO_2 \quad (13)$$

The bicarbonate associated with sodium is destroyed by the proton relinquished by albumin. Sodium's positive charge is now counterbalanced by the unmeasured anion (albumin). The anion gap increases since the measurable bicarbonate is replaced by the unmeasurable protein. The relationship between alkalosis and the increase in the anion gap may be approached with Equation 14, which defines the interactions of the related parameters.[1]

$$\Delta\text{Protein charge} = S \cdot \Delta\text{pH} \cdot [\text{protein}]p \quad (14)$$

The Δprotein charge defines the increase in the anion gap. S represents the buffering capacity of plasma nonbicarbonate buffers and is 0.11 meq/liter per unit pH change. The increase in the arterial pH and the total protein concentration (in grams per liter) are the remaining components of the equation. Since the changes in protein concentration and the increment in pH are rarely very large, the alkalosis-induced change in the anion gap is usually trivial.

Finally an association has been noted between allopurinol administration to azotemic patients and a spurious increase in the anion gap. When measured on a Kodak electrolyte machine, the chloride concentration was inappropriately low in three azotemic subjects. Analysis of the same samples on a Beckman analyzer revealed the true normochloremia.

Urinary anion gap

Halperin and colleagues described and developed the urinary anion (UAG) as an adjunctive test for defining the etiology and pathophysiology of various forms of metabolic acidosis.[8] While the diagnosis and design of rational therapy for the vast majority of the metabolic acidoses can be established by a careful history and physical examination and by assaying serum electrolytes and arterial blood gases, there are some unusual clinical circumstances where the UAG can "crack open" an otherwise difficult case (see Chap. 28).

Overview

The metabolic acidoses may be broadly classified in terms of acid production, excretion, and loss of base. *Overproduction*: Lactic and ketoacidosis are common examples of this form of metabolic acidosis. The normal kidney responds to the acid overproduction by reclaiming all filtered bicarbonate, acidifying the urine, and increasing its synthesis of ammonia buffer. The increased renal excretion of protonated ammonia (i.e., NH_4^+) simultaneously rids the body of acid while resynthesizing body bicarbonate stores spent in the titration of the accumulating offending acid. Progressive hypobicarbonatemia results when acid production exceeds its renal excretion, yielding a predictable pattern of chemical changes in the blood and in the urine.

Replacement of blood bicarbonates with the usually unmeasured lactate or ketone anions causes the serum anion gap to increase. Although the tubular reabsorptive affinity for lactate and ketone anions differs (see Chap. 28), some filtered sodium lactate, sodium beta-hydroxybutyrate, and sodium acetoacetate will be excreted.

The serum anion gap increases in metabolic acidosis because of the following two interdependent reasons. First, serum bicarbonate is replaced by some anion other than chloride and second, the kidney absorbs this filtered anion along with sodium, thereby sustaining increased plasma levels. However, certain metabolic acidoses are caused by exogenous toxins that generate acids, the anions of which cannot effectively be reabsorbed by the kidney. Prime examples of these acidoses include *toluene* (glue sniffing) and *methionine* exposure. The former generates hippuric acid and the latter generates sulfuric acid.[9,10] The protons from these two acids are titrated by bicarbonate which is then replaced by either hippurate or sulfate. Because these anions are poorly reabsorbed by the kidney, sodium hippurate and sodium sulfate are excreted along with obligate amounts of water. Thus, in both instances, hypobicarbonatemia results from accumulating protons, but the potential substituting anion is lost with sodium and water in the urine. The UAG increases but the serum anion gap does not. Excreted sodium hippurate (or sulfate) with water at once dissipates the high anion gap and causes ECF volume contraction. Because the ECF chloride *content* remains unchanged but is now distributed in a smaller volume, *hyperchloremia* develops. Toluene and methionine toxicity cause overproduction acidoses but cause hyperchloremia because their acid anions are poorly reabsorbed (see Chap. 27).

Underexcretion of acid

When acid excretion decreases to values that are less than the normal acid production, positive proton balance and hypobicarbonatemia ensue. Retained acid anions (sulfate, phosphate, organic anions) raise the serum anion gap. In steady-state chronic renal failure, the excretion of NH_4^+ is reduced as is the excretion of calcium. Dietary restrictions tend to reduce phosphate and sulfate. On balance, these changes in electrolyte excretion tend to modestly reduce the normal UAG.

Loss of base

As described below, loss of alkali equivalents in the stool dramatically reduces the normal UAG and often provokes a negative UAG. The diarrheal acidosis stimulates renal ammoniagenesis and increases the excretion of NH_4Cl while the associated ECF contraction reduces sodium and potassium excretion. A low to negative UAG results (see below) because the urinary concentration of Cl^- exceeds the sum of the concentration of Na^+ and K^+. Distal (type I, classical) renal tubular acidosis (RTA), when causing a hyperchloremic acidosis, generally is associated with a reduction in NH_4Cl excretion but normal to increased sodium and potassium excretion. A mild increase in the UAG may result. Proximal RTA (type II), in steady-state, behaves chemically like type I. When $NaHCO_3$ is administered, it is filtered, not reabsorbed, and is excreted. The increment in excreted sodium and potassium is roughly matched by that of bicarbonate, causing little change in the UAG.

Tools for evaluating the UAG

Whereas potassium adds little to the serum anion gap, it is a major contributor to the UAG. Subjects in external cation balance excrete their ingested load of cations, thereby adding 100 to 200 meq of sodium and 50 to 100 meq of potassium to the urine. When using the UAG to evaluate most metabolic acidoses, the urinary pH is usually well below 7.0, indicating that the bicarbonate concentration must be vanishingly small. Parenthetically, the reason for this can be seen by evaluating the Henderson-Hasselbalch equation for the urine. In this example the urinary pH is 6.1, the apparent pK for the $HCO_3^- - H_2CO_3$ buffer pair is also 6.1, and the urinary P_{CO_2} is 40 mmHg.

$$\text{Urinary pH} = \text{p}K' + \log\frac{(HCO_3^-)}{\alpha P_{CO_2}} \tag{12}$$

$$6.1 = 6.1 + \log\frac{(HCO_3^-)}{0.03(40)} \tag{15}$$

By subtracing the pK' (6.1) from the pH, Equation 15 becomes

$$0 = \log\frac{(HCO_3^-)}{1.2} \tag{16}$$

Taking the antilog of both sides of Equation 16,

$$1 = \frac{1.2}{(HCO_3^-)} \tag{17}$$

Because the antilog of zero is 1, the urinary bicarbonate concentration must be 1.2 meq/liter. Thus, when the urinary pH approaches 6.0, the bicarbonate concentration must be very low.

The other major urinary cation contributing to the UAG, is NH_4^+, a chemical parameter not usually measured by the clinical laboratory. Finally, other contributors to the UAG include the divalent cations Ca^{2+} and Mg^{2+} and the inorganic anions PO_4^{3-} and SO_4^{2-} and a variety of organic anions (e.g., lactate, ketones). The normal net balance between these usually unmeasured divalent cations and the usually unmeasured anions is such that the amount of excreted but *unmeasured* anions exceeds the amount of *measured* cations by 80 meq.[11] Thus the normal UAG approximates

$$(Na^+ + K^+ + NH_4^+) - (Cl^- + HCO_3^-) = 80 \text{ meq/day} \tag{18}$$

It follows that in *diarrheal acidosis*, the loss of alkali equivalents in the stool (see Chap. 36) along with sodium and potassium, causes ECF contraction and a hyperchloremic acidosis. Stimulated by the systemic acidosis, renal synthesis of ammonia buffer increases and NH_4Cl excretion increases. The ECF contraction tends to reduce renal sodium and potassium excretion. Thus the final urine contains reduced amounts of Na^+ and K^+ but is rich in Cl^-. The difference between the sum of sodium and potassium concentration (or content) and that of chloride approaches zero and often becomes negative, reflecting the stimulated excretion of NH_4Cl. If the UAG calculation included values for NH_4^+, the final value would be positive.

In the *overproduction acidoses* [e.g., ketoacidosis, lactic acidosis, or toluene or methionine exposure (see above)] the sodium, potassium, and ammonium salts of the acids are excreted in large amounts. The ECF is often contracted in these settings, stimulating the reabsorption of filtered NaCl. Thus urinary chloride excretion tends to fall while Na^+, K^+, and NH_4^+ excretion increases, thereby raising the UAG.

For further use of urinary acid-base parameters in evaluating clinical disorders, readers are referred to Chaps. 27 and 28 and Ref. 8.

REFERENCES

1. Adrogué HJ et al: Changes in the plasma anion gap during chronic metabolic acid-base disturbances. *Am J Physiol* 235:F281, 1978.
2. Henderson LJ: The theory of neutrality regulation in the animal organism. *Am J Physiol* 21:427, 1908.
3. Kassirer JP, Bleich HL: Rapid estimation of plasma carbon dioxide tension from pH and total CO_2 content. *N Engl J Med* 272:1067, 1965.
4. Mitchell JH et al: The effects of acid-base disturbances on cardiovascular and pulmonary function. *Kidney Int* 1:375, 1972.
5. Narins RG, Emmett M: Simple and mixed acid-base disorders: A practical approach. *Medicine* (Baltimore) 56:161, 1980.
6. Pitts RF: *Physiology of the Kidney and Body Fluids.* Chicago, Yearbook, 1974, chap. 2.
7. Sorensen SPL: Enzymstudien. 2. Mitteilung uber die Messung und die Bedeutung der Wasserstoffonenkonzentration bei enzymatischen Prozessen. *Biochem Z* 21:131, 1909.
8. Halperin ML et al: Use of urine electrolytes and osmolality, in Narins RG (guest ed), Stein JH (series ed): *Contemporary Issues in Nephrology, Diagnostic Techniques in Renal Disease,* vol 25. New York, Churchill Livingstone, 1992, p 1.
9. Carlisle E et al: Glue-sniffing and distal renal tubular acidosis: Sticking to the facts. *J Am Soc Nephrol* 1:1019, 1991.
10. Lemann J Jr, Relman AS: The relation of sulfur metabolism to acid-base balance and electrolyte excretion: The effects of DL-methionine in normal man. *J Clin Invest* 38:2215, 1959.
11. Kamel K et al: Urine electrolytes and osmolality: When and how to use them. *Am J Nephrol* 10:89, 1990.

CHAPTER • 25

The metabolic acidoses

Robert G. Narins • G. Gopal Krishna • Jerry Yee
Daniel Ikemiyashiro • Rebecca J. Schmidt

INTRODUCTORY CONCEPTS

DEFINITIONS

The three prime acid-base parameters include P_{CO_2} and the concentrations of hydrogen ion and bicarbonate. The *Henderson* equation (equation 1) which describes the interrelationship of these three forces was derived in Chap. 24.[136]

$$[H^+] = 24 \frac{P_{CO_2}}{[HCO_3^-]} \qquad (1)$$

The *simple acid-base disorders* may be defined on the basis of this equation. The *respiratory disorders* (Chap. 30) are characterized by an initial abnormality in P_{CO_2}. In respiratory acidosis the P_{CO_2} rises, defining an increase in hydrogen ion concentration; whereas in respiratory alkalosis the P_{CO_2} falls, defining a decrease in hydrogen ion concentration. The *primary change* in P_{CO_2}, and subsequently in the $P_{CO_2}/[HCO_3^-]$ ratio, determines the magnitude of change in the hydrogen ion concentration. A series of *secondary* or *compensating events* occur during the course of acute and chronic respiratory acid-base disorders. These events alter the HCO_3^- concentration, thereby lessening the impact of the primary change in P_{CO_2} on the hydrogen ion concentration. This metabolic buffering increases the HCO_3^- concentration in respiratory acidosis and decreases it in respiratory alkalosis. Thus, respiratory acidosis and alkalosis primarily alter the P_{CO_2}, which, in turn, elicits a compensating change in the bicarbonate concentration, thereby ameliorating the induced change in the $P_{CO_2}/[HCO_3^-]$ ratio and, thereby, in acidity (see Chap. 24).

The *metabolic acid-base disorders* are characterized by primary pathologic changes in the bicarbonate concentration. In metabolic acidosis the bicarbonate concentration diminishes, whereas in metabolic alkalosis the bicarbonate concentration increases. The resulting change in the $P_{CO_2}/[HCO_3^-]$ ratio causes the expected change in hydrogen ion concentration. Compensating or secondary events also occur in the metabolic acid-base disorders that tend to ameliorate the change in hydrogen ion concentration; for example, in metabolic acidosis the resulting decrease in pH stimulates respiration, causing the P_{CO_2} to decline, whereas in metabolic alkalosis the increase in pH depresses respiration, causing the P_{CO_2} also to increase. The change in P_{CO_2} lessens the alteration in hydrogen ion concentration but does not prevent the primary disorder from rendering blood acidity abnormal.

The concentration of hydrogen ion normally present in the extracellular fluid (ECF) is measured in nanomoles per liter and is therefore virtually a trace element. As described in Chaps. 9 and 24, approximately 50 to 100 meq of hydrogen ion is synthesized each day, passing from cells through the extracellular space, eventually to be excreted in the urine. Thus, the daily traffic of acid through the extracellular space is some 200,000 times the total free hydrogen ion content of the entire extracellular space. The exquisite balance struck between acid production, acid buffering, and renal acid excretion maintains the hydrogen ion concentration in the ECF within the very narrow range of normal. Large swings in acid production and accumulation bring about rather small absolute changes in free hydrogen ion concentration, although these changes are translatable into potentially lethal effects in the host. Thus, the ebb and flow of acid production and excretion is like the wind; one does not see the wind but simply its effect (e.g., a flag waving in the breeze). Analogously, one does not routinely directly assay the accumulation of free acid but rather measures the effect of the acid—that is, a change in bicarbonate concentration. As is explained in Chap. 24, bicarbonate serves as the major body buffer of fixed acids, and its increase or decrease reflects the gain and loss of alkali in

The authors acknowledge support from the University Medical Research Foundation.

the extracellular space. Accordingly, the hallmark of metabolic acidosis is the net accumulation of fixed acid, usually made manifest chemically by a fall in bicarbonate concentration. The secondary event in metabolic acidosis is the acidemia-induced increase in ventilation, resulting in hypocapnia, which in turn has an ameliorating effect on the degree of blood acidification. These primary and secondary changes in metabolic acidosis are discussed further below (see also Chap. 8).

The term *metabolic acidosis* refers to the process acting to disrupt the serum bicarbonate concentration. Therefore, any primary pathologic event that lowers serum bicarbonate concentration is called a metabolic acidosis. It turns out that the metabolic acidosis need not be associated with an abnormal blood pH—that is, an acidosis need not be associated with an acidemia (see Chap. 24). There are two reasons for this discordance. First, the range of normal pH is rather broad, from 7.37 to 7.44. In a mild, or in an early, phase of metabolic acidosis, blood pH may fall from the normal 7.43 to the more acid, but still normal, value of 7.38. With greater severity, the acidosis eventually displaces blood pH into the abnormal range. Second, even a severe metabolic acidosis may be associated with a normal pH when other primary acid-base disturbances are superimposed. A classic example of this "mixed acid-base disorder" is seen in patients who are clinically uremic. During the development of chronic progressive renal disease, the kidney becomes increasingly less capable of excreting the daily acid load, and a net accumulation is made manifest by a fall in serum bicarbonate concentration. This is the general sequence seen in a typical uremic acidosis. When the end stages of renal disease are near and the serum bicarbonate concentration has reached distinctly low levels, the clinical syndrome of uremia may develop. Vomiting, a major component of this syndrome, gives rise to metabolic alkalosis. (With the loss of gastric acid, alkali is returned to blood, causing hyperbicarbonatemia.) At this point the patient's acid-base status is being assaulted from two opposite directions: the failing kidney allows acid to accumulate and destroy bicarbonate while the vomiting leads to the synthesis of abnormal amounts of alkali. Depending on which of these two primary acid-base disturbances dominates, the resulting serum bicarbonate concentration may be increased or decreased—or may remain within the normal range. Thus, regardless of what the final bicarbonate concentration is, such a patient clearly manifests two pathologic processes: metabolic acidosis due to renal failure, and a metabolic alkalosis that is painfully obvious from the patient's retching (see Chap. 31).

In summary, a simple metabolic acidosis is characterized chemically by the accumulation of fixed acid, with a resulting decrease in bicarbonate concentration, and by a secondary increase in ventilation, with a resulting decrease in the P_{CO_2}. The resulting pH is a function of the primary fall in bicarbonate concentration, which is then offset by the normal respiratory response. The degree of acidemia will be a function of the severity of the metabolic acidosis and of whether this is a simple or a mixed acid-base disturbance.

PATHOGENIC MECHANISMS UNDERLYING THE METABOLIC ACIDOSES

The pathogenesis of the metabolic acidoses is a direct extension of the dynamics of normal fixed acid metabolism. As discussed in Chaps. 9 and 24, the balance struck between fixed acid production, buffering, and renal excretion maintains normal acid-base balance. It follows that the metabolic acidoses may develop when there is pathologic *overproduction of fixed acid, loss of ECF bicarbonate buffer,* or *failure of normal renal acid excretion.* A general review of these pathogenic forces follows, and the individual disorders are then discussed.

Acid overproduction

As outlined in Chaps. 9 and 24, some 50 to 100 meq of fixed acid is produced daily from the partial combustion of fats, carbohydrates, and protein, and from the oxidative conversion of sulfur-containing amino acids to sulfuric acid. These metabolic acids are titrated in the ECF by bicarbonate, forming the acid salt, CO_2, and water. Filtration of acid anions and their recoupling in the tubular lumen with secreted protons reforms the parent acid, which is then excreted in association with phosphate and ammonia buffers. As previously noted, each milliequivalent of net acid excreted causes one milliequivalent of bicarbonate to be returned systemically, thereby replenishing lost alkali stores.

Pathologic increments in fixed acid production acidify cellular and extracellular fluids and stimulate renal acid excretion. A new steady state is achieved wherein the increased acid produced is excreted, albeit at the expense of a stable but more acid ECF. Thus, the kidney responds to a doubling or tripling of acid production by a quantitatively similar increase in net acid excretion, thereby preventing the progressive accumulation of fixed acid. When acid production exceeds maximal acid excretion, positive acid balance develops, and progressive, life-threatening acidosis ensues.

The two most common examples of endogenous acid overproduction are ketoacidosis and lactic acidosis. A variety of toxins contribute acid while also stimulating poisoned host tissues to overproduce endogenous acids. Such toxins include ethylene glycol, methanol, and aspirin (see below).

Acid underexcretion

The section on uremic acidosis (see below) carefully details the pathophysiologic elements of the acidosis resulting from primary failure of the kidneys to excrete the normal daily acid load. Defects in renal acid excretion—that is, the renal acidoses—may be sub-classified as uremic acidosis and the various forms of renal tubular acidosis.

Uremic acidosis is characterized by concomitant retention of organic and inorganic acid anions, secondary to failure of glomerular filtration, and proton retention, secondary to failure of net tubular acid secretion and excretion. Resulting hydrogen ion accumulation destroys bicarbonate, which is replaced by retained acid anions, causing the anion gap to increase (see Chap. 24). The pathogenesis of the bicarbonaturia and failure of renal buffer synthesis are outlined below.

Renal tubular acidosis describes a group of disorders characterized by failure of tubular acid excretion that develop, at least initially, in the presence of normal glomerular function. The normal glomerular filtration rate (GFR) ensures continued excretion of acid anions. Bicarbonate lost in titration of retained acid is replaced by dietary chloride. The normal anion gap is typical of the renal tubular acidoses. These disorders are thoroughly discussed in Chap. 27.

Bicarbonate wasting

Loss of bicarbonate, a major extracellular buffer, occurs in proximal renal tubular acidosis (Chap. 27) and in diarrheal states (see below and Chap. 36). Excretion of sodium, bicarbonate, and osmotically obligated water causes contraction of the extracellular space. Since the body chloride content remains essentially unchanged but becomes redistributed in a smaller space, hyperchloremia results. Thus, the bicarbonate wasting syndromes typically cause a normal anion gap acidosis; in other terms, lost bicarbonate is replaced with chloride.

RESPIRATORY COMPENSATION FOR METABOLIC ACIDOSIS

Intracellular and extracellular buffer systems other than the bicarbonate/P_{CO_2} system make modest contributions to the stability of blood pH during the course of metabolic acidosis. The hypocapnia resulting from acidemia-induced increases in respiration plays a key role in lessening the acidifying effect of a given degree of hypobicarbonatemia. Within the constraints imposed by the Henderson equation (equation 1), the hydrogen ion concentration increases less if a given decrease in bicarbonate concentration is offset by a reduction in the P_{CO_2}. Indeed, the magnitude of primary hypobicarbonatemia determines the degree of respiratory compensation.[5] The lower the steady-state bicarbonate concentration, the greater the stimulation of ventilation and, of course, the lower the P_{CO_2} (Fig. 25-1). On the basis both of prospective and of retrospective studies of experimentally

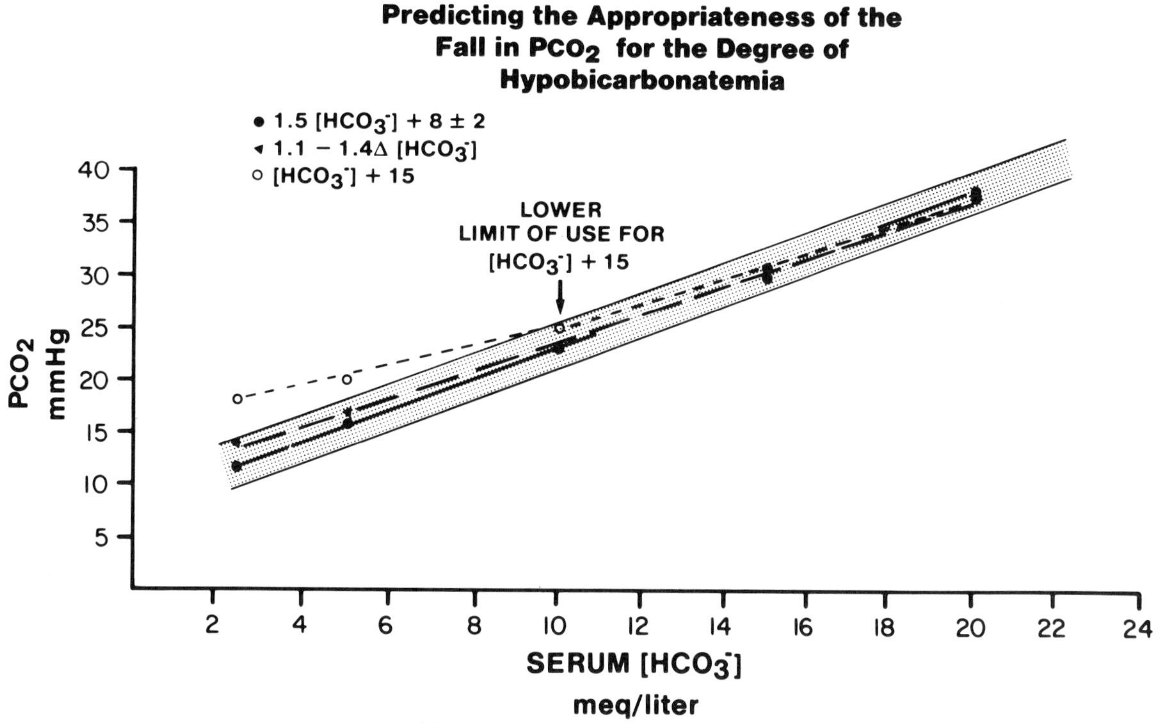

FIGURE 25-1 • Respiratory compensation for metabolic acidosis. The P_{CO_2} falls in a predictable fashion in response to steady-state values of hypobicarbonatemia. The three formulas used to predict the P_{CO_2} for a given serum bicarbonate concentration are shown in the inset. The shaded area defines the 95 percent confidence limits for formula one (1.5 [HCO_3^-] + 8). The P_{CO_2} predicted for a given bicarbonate concentration is plotted for the three formulas. The inaccuracy of the third formula ([HCO_3^-] + 15) becomes unacceptable below bicarbonate concentration of 10 meq/liter (see text for details).

induced and spontaneously occurring metabolic acidosis (Chap. 8), there is a highly predictable degree of respiratory compensation that should be provoked by a given decrease in bicarbonate concentration. If the P_{CO_2} is higher or lower than predicted for a given level of hypobicarbonatemia, a primary respiratory acidosis or alkalosis must be superimposed.

Several formulas are available that accurately predict what the P_{CO_2} should be for a given low bicarbonate concentration.[194] Albert and coworkers found that in stable, steady-state metabolic acidosis the P_{CO_2} appropriate to the degree of hypobicarbonatemia equals 8 plus the product of 1.5 and the serum bicarbonate concentration.[5]

$$P_{CO_2}\,(\text{mmHg}) = 1.5\,[HCO_3^-] + 8 \pm 2 \qquad (2)$$

Although the interval has not been precisely defined, it appears to take 12 to 36 h of stable acidosis for the P_{CO_2} to achieve its nadir.[222] Use of this formula prior to achievement of the steady state—that is, while the bicarbonate concentration is at its nadir but while the P_{CO_2} is still decreasing toward its nadir—gives the false impression that the P_{CO_2} is inappropriately high for the measured serum bicarbonate concentration.

Similar precision in predicting the appropriateness of the P_{CO_2} may be achieved by knowing that in steady-state metabolic acidosis the P_{CO_2} declines by 1.1 to 1.4 mmHg for each 1-meq/liter decrease in serum bicarbonate concentration.[112] Thus, a decline of 10 meq/liter in serum bicarbonate concentration, from the normal value of 25 meq/liter to the abnormal value of 15 meq/liter, should lower the P_{CO_2} by 11 to 14 mmHg (i.e., from the normal value of 40 mmHg to between 26 and 29 mmHg) (Fig. 25-1).

An accidental feature of the mathematics relating P_{CO_2}, $[HCO_3^-]$, and pH is that in steady-state, pure metabolic acidosis the P_{CO_2} (in mmHg) equals 100 times the last two digits of the pH. For example, when the pH is 7.30 the P_{CO_2} will approximate 30 mmHg.

Finally, in steady-state metabolic acidosis, addition of the number 15 to the measured serum bicarbonate concentration yields the P_{CO_2} and the last two digits of the pH.[195] This formulation is accurate over a serum bicarbonate range of 12 to 40 meq/liter.

As outlined in Chap. 31, when the P_{CO_2} is too high or too low for a given low serum bicarbonate concentration, a mixed respiratory-metabolic acid-base disorder must be present. Thus, by knowing what the P_{CO_2} should be for any given degree of metabolic acidosis, the physician can determine whether the respiratory response is appropriate. This powerful diagnostic tool can unveil a primary respiratory acid-base disorder that is superimposed on a primary metabolic acidosis (Chap. 31). Unsuspected

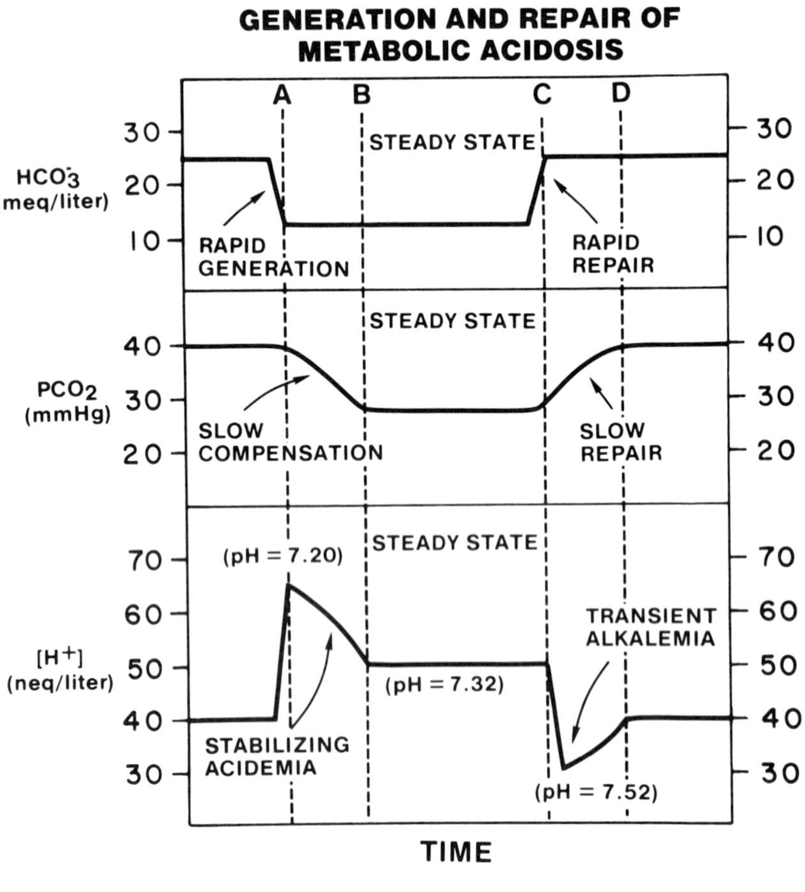

FIGURE 25-2 • Relationship of $[HCO_3^-]$, P_{CO_2}, $[H^+]$, and pH during the generation and repair of metabolic acidosis. (*a*) Precipitous lowering of the serum bicarbonate concentration, before respiratory compensation occurs, causes a precipitous and severe increase in $[H^+]$ (i.e., lowering of pH). (*b*) Evolving respiratory compensation and hypocapnia, for a given low bicarbonate concentration, returns the $[H^+]$ and pH toward more normal values. Steady-state values for P_{CO_2} and pH are predicated on the magnitude of hypobicarbonatemia. (*c*) The bicarbonate concentration is normalized faster than the P_{CO_2}, transiently alkalinizing the blood due to the fall in the $P_{CO_2}/[HCO_3^-]$ ratio (see equation 2). (*d*) As alveolar respiration normalizes the P_{CO_2}, $[H^+]$, and pH also normalize. (See text for further details.) (Modified from Cohen JJ, Kassirer JP, in Maxwell MM, Kleeman CR: *Clinical Disorders of Fluid and Electrolyte Metabolism*, 3d ed. New York, McGraw-Hill, 1980, p 203.)

pneumonia, pulmonary embolus, salicylism, or other causes of respiratory alkalosis or acidosis may be first suspected only after a careful review of the blood gases.

The interplay between the primary change in serum bicarbonate concentration, the secondary change in P_{CO_2}, and the resulting change in pH (H^+ concentration) is illustrated in Fig. 25-2.

According to current concepts, the change in serum bicarbonate concentration is transmitted only slowly to the interstitium of the brainstem, where it signals chemoreceptors located below the surface of the medulla oblongata.[58] Activated receptors translate this chemical message into a change in respiration by signaling other neurons in the medullary respiratory center that in turn alter phrenic nerve activity and, subsequently, alveolar ventilation. The time required to maximize respiration is a function of the speed with which the acidity of plasma can be transmitted to the interstitial fluid of the brainstem. Since changes in systemic bicarbonate concentration are even more slowly transferred to the cerebrospinal fluid, respiration is stimulated and the P_{CO_2} is decreased well before any change in cerebrospinal fluid bicarbonate concentration is measurable. Unlike bicarbonate, which can penetrate the blood-brain barrier only slowly, arterial P_{CO_2} instantaneously makes itself felt in the cerebrospinal fluid. Thus the early stages of systemic acidosis and acidemia cause a *paradoxical alkalinization of the cerebrospinal fluid*, which is due to the asynchronous fall in P_{CO_2} and bicarbonate concentration; that is, the $P_{CO_2}/[HCO_3^-]$ ratio decreases (equation 1). In time, the spinal fluid acidifies as the bicarbonate concentration declines in proportion to that in blood. Although the point is controversial, some authors believe that the respiratory response to metabolic acidosis does not maximize until the initial spinal fluid alkalinization fades.[58] During the reparative phase of metabolic acidosis, when the serum bicarbonate concentration is increasing, a *paradoxical acidification of the cerebrospinal fluid* occurs. The improving bicarbonate concentration signals the medullary respiratory center to reduce the rate of ventilation. Because the increasing P_{CO_2} gains access to the cerebrospinal fluid faster than does bicarbonate, a transient ("respiratory") acidification occurs. Recent studies have suggested that peripheral chemoreceptors in the carotid bodies play a minor role, if any, in mediating the respiratory compensation to metabolic acidosis.[128,132]

SYSTEMIC EFFECTS OF METABOLIC ACIDOSIS (TABLE 25-1)

The pH of the microenvironment surrounding intracellular enzymes, as well as the transport proteins inserted into cell membranes, strongly influences the biosynthetic reactions and accessibility of electrolytes and nutrients to the intracellular milieu.[234] The biosynthetic reactions and transport processes influenced by pH are located throughout the body. It follows that abnormalities of systemic pH may effect wide-ranging changes in tissue and organ function. The symptoms and signs shared by many of the metabolic acidoses relate to these generalized effects; other specific effects of the individual disease entities add to the complexity of presentation.

TABLE 25-1 • Systemic effects of metabolic acidosis

Cardiovascular
Heart: bradycardia; arrhythmias; reduced contractility
Vascular: arteriolar dilatation; increased venous tone
Pulmonary
Ventilation: Kussmaul respiration
Oxygen delivery: increased in acute metabolic acidosis; normal in chronic metabolic acidosis
Gastrointestinal
Gastric distension
Intestinal effects
Renal
Sodium/potassium wasting
Uric acid retention in organic acidoses
Hypercalciuria
Electrolytes
Potassium, calcium, magnesium, phosphorus (see text)
Metabolic/hormonal
Protein wasting
Organic acid synthesis: feedback inhibition (see text)
Catecholamine secretion: increased
Aldosterone secretion: may be increased
Parathyroid hormone: action on bone enhanced; secretion variable (see text)
Vitamin D: activation may be impaired (see text)

The clinical features of the metabolic acidoses are strongly influenced by the rate and magnitude of the fall in pH. As with many metabolic disorders, those developing rapidly are far more likely to produce dramatic signs and symptoms than are the more slowly developing disorders. For example, in chronic renal failure the serum bicarbonate concentration and blood pH progressively decline over months to years, eventually reaching steady-state values of 18 meq/liter and 7.30, respectively. Patients usually show no symptoms of these modest changes. In acute renal failure, however, the same abnormalities may develop over a period of hours to days, in which case symptoms almost always are present. In general, however, when blood pH declines to values below 7.20 most patients are symptomatic.

Cardiac effects

Rate and rhythm

The heart rate responds biphasically to increasing degrees of acidemia. Tachycardia is frequently observed as blood pH falls from 7.40 toward 7.10. This increasing heart rate is caused by the acid-stimulated release of epinephrine from the adrenal medulla.[290] Predictably, the use of β-adrenergic blocking agents prevents the increase in heart rate otherwise seen with progressive acidemia. As blood pH falls below 7.10, the heart rate progressively slows, exacerbated by β-adrenergic blocking drugs.[174,290] The pathogenesis of this bradycardia is uncertain but probably relates to the inhibitory effect of worsening acidemia on the cardiac effects of catecholamines, or to the accumulation of acetylcholine caused by inhibition of acetylcholinesterase by acidemia.[183] Although conflicting reports appear in the literature, on balance it appears that systemic acidosis predisposes to the development of ventricular fibrillation.[92,143] The more malignant ventricular arrhythmias complicating the metabolic acidoses may be related, in part, to associated electrolyte abnormalities (e.g., potassium, magnesium, or phosphorus depletion).

Contractility

Severe acidemia impairs myocardial contractility.[183] Impaired contraction results from the algebraic sum of the opposing actions of acid. Acid exerts both a negative inotropic effect directly on the heart and an indirect positive inotropic effect, by stimulating the release of epinephrine.

The cellular entry of calcium and its interaction with sarcolemmal membranes and proteins plays a central role in the complex function of myocardial contraction. Hydrogen ions at once impair calcium entry via interactions with specific membrane channels and may competitively replace the divalent cation at sarcolemmal binding sites.[197,291] Catecholamines enhance calcium entry into cells, but this adrenergic effect is inhibited by increasing concentrations of protons.[196] Thus the negative inotropic effect of acidemia may well be mediated by acid inhibition of calcium's salutary effect on contraction.

Not surprisingly, the negative inotropic effects of acidosis are more easily and more reproducibly demonstrated with the simpler preparations of heart muscle and the isolated perfused heart than with more complex in-vivo models.[196] Inconsistent effects of acid on in-vivo contractility are most likely related to the offsetting direct inhibitory effect of acid on the heart and acid's stimulation of the secretion of the positive inotrope epinephrine.[196] As blood pH falls from 7.40 toward 7.20, the negative inotropic effect of acid and the positive inotropic effect of released catecholamines offset each other and leave myocardial contraction largely unscathed. As blood pH falls below 7.20, the negative inotropic effect of acidosis becomes progressively more apparent. It remains unproved (though it appears likely) that acute or chronic heart disease sensitizes the myocardium to the detrimental effects of increasing acidemia. On the basis of the aforementioned pathophysiologic principles it appears likely that patients receiving β-adrenergic antagonists or calcium entry blocking drugs would be more sensitive to the negative inotropic effects of acidosis.

Vascular effects

Arteriolar effects of metabolic acidosis

The countervailing effects of low pH and increasing concentrations of catecholamines leave arteriolar tone largely unchanged until pH values below 7.20 are reached.[60,183,290] While a variety of in-vivo and in-vitro systems have been used to demonstrate these aforementioned effects, studies of the perfused human forearm have most convincingly demonstrated the net vasodilatory effect of low pH.[148,196] The hypotension complicating severe metabolic acidosis is frequently characterized by warm, well-perfused peripheral tissues, giving rise to the term *warm shock*.

Venous effects of metabolic acidosis

Advancing acidemia causes sustained venoconstriction.[251] Venous smooth muscle contracts in the presence of increasing concentrations of protons and may persistently respond to catecholamines despite the severe acidemia.[251] Constriction of peripheral veins reduces their reservoir function, forcing more blood centrally and increasing the workload of the heart. Hemodynamic studies in cholera victims have shown clearly that the fraction of total blood volume present in the central circulation increases directly with hydrogen ion concentration.[113] Predictably, therapy with alkali diminishes the elevated pressures in the ventricle and pulmonary artery.[113] This centralization of blood volume from increasing degrees of acidemia adds to the heart's burden when myocardial contraction is impaired. It follows that congestive heart failure is one of the dreaded results of unchecked severe acidemia.

Summary and synthesis of the cardiovascular effects of systemic acidosis

Animal and human data, on balance, indicate that increasing acidemia progressively reduces cardiac output. This appears to be the outcome of decreased myocardial contraction combined with a progressive slowing of heart rate. The exacerbating effects of increasing central blood volume and the tendency to ventricular arrhythmias together cause the lethal hemodynamic effects complicating advanced degrees of metabolic acidosis. In general, it appears that the myocardium is less vulnerable when blood pH is maintained above 7.20, which broadly corresponds to a blood bicarbonate concentration greater than 10 meq/liter (assuming that respiratory compensation is appropriate). Accordingly, in compromised patients with metabolic acidosis, blood pH should be maintained above 7.20 with administration of judicious amounts of alkali.

Pulmonary effects

Ventilation

Increasing degrees of hypobicarbonatemia stimulate respiration, allowing the salutary effect of hypocapnia to mitigate the degree of acidemia (see above). This chronic increase in ventilation is often difficult for even the most careful observer to identify, since small increases in the rate and depth of ventilation enable the lungs to enhance their clearance of CO_2 from the blood. Acute, severe metabolic acidoses, however, cause hyperpnea (i.e., increased tidal volume) and modest degrees of tachypnea (i.e., rapid respiration). Kussmaul first called attention to this pulmonary response in 1874, when he described three cases of what has come to be known as *Kussmaul's air-hunger.*[153]

Tissue oxygen delivery

A variety of metabolic and physicochemical effects of acidosis may strikingly alter the transport and delivery of oxygen to peripheral tissues. Two offsetting and synchronous effects of acidosis are important to tissue oxygenation. The *Bohr effect* describes the interaction of hydrogen ions with hemoglobin.[11] Increased concentrations of protons within the microenvironment of the red blood cell instantaneously decrease the affinity of hemoglobin for oxygen, thereby facilitating tissue oxygenation. Alkalinization has an immediate and opposite effect. An offsetting effect of pH on hemoglobin-oxygen binding is more slowly mediated by induced changes in red blood cell glycolysis. Increasing acidemia slows glycolysis and, over a period of 12 to 36 h, depletes erythrocytes of certain of its glycolytic intermediates, most notably 2,3-diphosphoglyceric acid (DPG).[44] This compound behaves like acid in that it decreases hemoglobin's affinity for oxygen. Alkalinization has an equal and opposite influence on the rate of glycolysis, which is also slowly mediated.

It follows logically that acute acidosis beneficially affects tissue oxygenation by eliciting the Bohr effect. With time, during sustained acidosis, the progressive depletion of red blood cell DPG nullifies this benefit of acidosis. In a similar fashion, acute alkalinization may abruptly depress tissue oxygenation; but in time, increasing red blood cell concentrations of DPG reestablish normal tissue oxygen delivery (Fig. 25-3). The latter effect is caused by the rapid onset of increased hemoglobin affinity for oxygen and the slower buildup of DPG. From the aforementioned observations, it has been argued that the rapid administration of alkali to patients with chronic metabolic acidosis may result in transient tissue hypoxia. The chronically acidotic patient has normal tissue oxygenation, resulting from the offsetting actions of low pH and red blood cell depletion of DPG. Excessively rapid therapy with large amounts of alkali, it is argued, may remove the beneficial Bohr effect while erythrocytes remain depleted of phosphorylated intermediates. During this transient phase, hemoglobin affinity for oxygen may increase to the point of depriving tissues of much-needed oxygen. However, there is currently no clear evidence to justify this conclusion. Indeed, animal studies have not found that alkali therapy of chronic acidosis significantly compromises tissue oxygenation.[28]

Gastrointestinal effects

Experimentally induced systemic acid-base perturbations alter gastrointestinal motility, absorption, secretion, and structural integrity. The difficulties inherent in studying the various functions of the gastrointestinal tract, especially in sick, acidotic patients, have left it uncertain

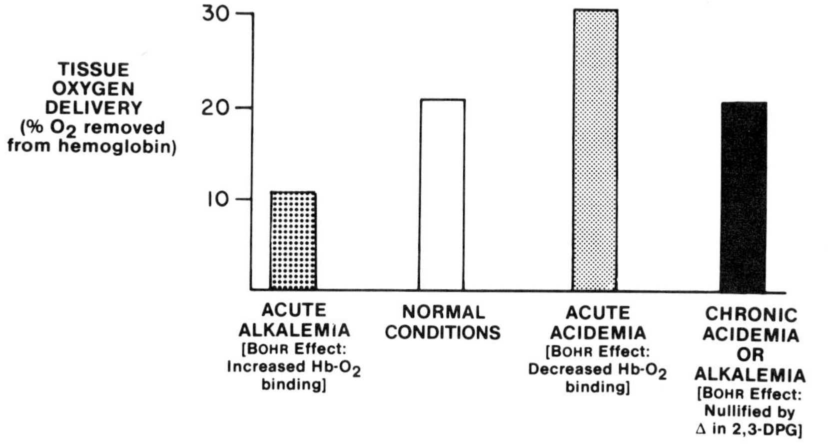

FIGURE 25-3 • Tissue oxygen delivery in acute and chronic acidemia and alkalemia. Tissue oxygen delivery is increased and decreased, respectively, by acute acidemia and alkalemia. Intra-erythrocytic pH changes alter hemoglobin's affinity for oxygen (Bohr effect; see text for details). Chronic acidemia and alkalemia decrease and increase, respectively, intra-erythrocytic 2,3-diphosphoglyceric acid concentrations, which nullifies the Bohr effect, returning oxygen delivery to baseline values. (See text for details.)

whether data derived from animal studies are translatable to humans. Some of these findings are briefly summarized below.

Gastric effects

A variety of functional gastrointestinal complaints and physical findings are seen in up to 50 percent of patients presenting with acute diabetic ketoacidosis.[137] Abdominal pain, distension, nausea and vomiting are often prominent features in this setting. The gastrointestinal findings are occasionally so severe as to suggest the presence of an acute abdominal emergency. These symptoms and signs are quickly reversed by appropriate therapy of ketoacidosis. Since these findings often complicate the initial presentation of type 1 diabetes, it is unlikely to be caused by preexisting neuropathic changes. The ready reversibility of all signs and symptoms also belies the possibility of chronic underlying disease. It is not yet clear whether these symptoms are related to the acidosis itself, the ketogenesis, or other complicating fluid-electrolyte and biochemical changes accompanying the ketoacidosis.

Although much work has been done to define the basis for the negative inotropism and disordered arteriolar and venous muscle tone in severe metabolic acidosis, surprisingly little has been done to clarify the effects of acid-base changes on gastrointestinal tone and motility. Muscle strips from the lower esophagus and stomach, when bathed in acidotic media, demonstrated decreased amplitude and frequency of spontaneous contraction.[243] As with the heart, acidosis may alter the net accumulation of free calcium inside cells and thereby disrupt normal tone and contraction (see above).

Intestinal effects

Intestinal muscle tone and contractility, as in the heart and stomach, appear to be adversely affected by systemic acidosis. Rabbit taenia coli muscle preparations demonstrate decreased sensitivity to cholinergic stimulation when incubated in even mildly acidotic media.[166] Although there are no convincing data to show that these observations also hold for the human colon, it is tempting to speculate that some of the intestinal manifestations of chronic acid-base abnormalities are mediated by such changes.

The effects of systemic acid-base changes on intestinal ion transport and secretion have been studied extensively by Charney and Haskall.[71] These careful studies, which evaluate the independent influences of the various acid-base parameters, demonstrated little effect on net sodium absorption but did show modest changes in potassium, chloride, and bicarbonate transport. The clinical significance of these observations remains uncertain.

Renal effects

Proximal renal tubule sodium chloride reabsorption is impaired by acute metabolic acidosis but is rapidly normalized with repair of the hypobicarbonatemia.[102a] This effect is at least partly due to impairment of the passive portion of proximal renal tubule sodium reabsorption. Under normal conditions filtered sodium bicarbonate is reabsorbed along with isosmotic amounts of water in the earliest segments of the proximal tubule.[146] Because sodium is reabsorbed with proportionate amounts of water while disproportionately more bicarbonate is reabsorbed, the residual tubular filtrate has an unchanged sodium concentration but a lower bicarbonate concentration. Unreabsorbed chloride is now dispersed in a smaller volume of glomerular filtrate, thereby increasing the chloride concentration above that of the parent plasma.[102a] The high chloride concentration and the favorable lumen-to-plasma gradient stimulate the passive absorption of the anion. The positive luminal charge resulting from disproportionate reabsorption of anionic chloride then facilitates passive sodium reabsorption. With acute metabolic acidosis the serum bicarbonate concentration, and therefore the filtered load of bicarbonate, decreases to low levels. Since the filtered load of sodium bicarbonate is diminished, its absolute reabsorption in the earliest portion of the proximal tubule falls, thereby rendering unfavorable the generation of the passive forces required for nonactive sodium chloride reabsorption. Accordingly, more sodium chloride is delivered distally, a portion of which escapes into the final urine, effecting the natriuresis of acute acidosis.

Acute and chronic renal failure alter renal net potassium secretion. This is discussed below.

Lactic acidosis and ketoacidosis are typically associated with increases in the plasma uric acid concentration. Current evidence indicates that the hyperuricemia is due not to overproduction of uric acid but rather to a reduction in renal clearance of the organic acid. Uric acid competes with lactate and ketone anions for the proximally located organic acid transport systems.[96,299] Through competitive inhibition, hyperlactatemia and hyperketonemia effectively reduce uric acid clearance, causing hyperuricemia.

Electrolytes

Potassium metabolism (see Chaps. 6, 7, 22, 23)

Acid-base changes in general, and metabolic acidosis specifically, exert profound effects on the extrarenal and renal handling of potassium.

EXTRARENAL POTASSIUM HANDLING It is now well known that many forces modify internal potassium balance—that is, the distribution of potassium between in-

TABLE 25-2 • Factors determining the cellular uptake of potassium

FACTORS	Net cellular potassium uptake ENHANCED	INHIBITED
Hormones		
Catecholamines		
β-Adrenergic	+	
α-Adrenergic		+
Insulin	+	
Aldosterone	+	
ECF pH		
Acid		+
Alkaline	+	
ECF bicarbonate		
Hypobicarbonatemia		+
Hyperbicarbonatemia	+	
Hyperosmolality		+

tracellular and extracellular fluid (Table 25-2). The hormonal influences include the *catecholamines*, *insulin*, and *aldosterone*, all of which stimulate the cellular uptake of potassium. The first two hormones play the more potent role. Changes in the serum *bicarbonate concentration*, independent of any associated change in blood pH, also influence the transcellular distribution of potassium. In addition, *extracellular fluid volume, osmolality*, and the *availability of oxygen* exert important effects on the serum potassium concentration. Besides changing blood pH and bicarbonate concentration, many of the metabolic acidoses alter these other forces which strongly influence potassium's internal balance.

The old dictum mandating a 0.6-meq/liter increase in serum potassium concentration for each 0.1-unit decrement in pH is no longer tenable. A review of clinical and experimental studies investigating the change in serum potassium concentration for a given degree of acidemia reveals widely disparate results.[99] The highly variable increment in serum potassium concentration in response to metabolic acidosis is undoubtedly related to the unavoidable lack of control of the aforementioned hormonal and chemical influences on serum potassium concentration.

An additional confounding observation has been the lack of change in serum potassium concentration in response to organic acidosis and the much more robust change seen in the inorganic acidoses.[210] Infusion of HCl has repeatedly been shown to cause a rapid and dramatic increase in serum potassium concentration, whereas equimolar infusions of organic acids (lactic acid, ketoacid) barely change serum potassium concentration.[210] Thus organic acidoses like diabetic ketoacidosis and lactic acidosis should not be expected to increase the serum potassium concentration simply on the basis of a fall in blood pH. Nevertheless, it is widely recognized that hyperkalemia is a common complication of these acidoses (see below and Chap. 26). These life-threatening conditions, however, are frequently associated with hyperosmolality, volume contraction, and decreased renal perfusion; diabetics commonly manifest hypoaldosteronemia and hypocatecholaminemia, and, of course, lack insulin activity. Each of these pathophysiologic forces acts to increase the serum potassium concentration, regardless of preexisting blood pH.

The disparate effects of organic and inorganic acidosis on serum potassium concentration, although not precisely determined, are likely related to differences in the cellular penetration of the accompanying acid anion. Ketone and lactate anions freely penetrate cells along with protons, thereby leaving the transcellular electrochemical gradient for potassium unchanged. Infusion of HCl, however, is associated with cellular uptake of positively charged protons while the chloride anion remains imprisoned in the ECF. Due to the cellular gain of positive charges and the accumulation of negative charges in the ECF, a very favorable electrical gradient is created for the outward movement of cationic potassium.

Experiments noting the effect of HCl infusion on serum potassium concentration are not easily related to the human inorganic acidoses. The three major inorganic acidoses—diarrhea, renal tubular acidosis, and uremic acidosis—are all associated with the accumulation of inorganic acids in the ECF, but each condition has an independent effect on serum potassium concentration. Diarrhea and renal tubular acidosis cause intestinal and renal potassium wasting independently of the acid-base status of the patient; and in advanced azotemia, renal potassium handling is, of course, variably compromised.

From the foregoing discussion, it becomes apparent that no simple relationship exists between the change in acid-base balance and the serum potassium concentration. Simple formulas purporting to relate the change in pH to the change in serum potassium concentration are misleading and potentially dangerous; the reader will do well to avoid their use. Figure 25-4 illustrates how misleading these formulas can be. When factored for pH, it appears that a given degree of inorganic metabolic acidosis causes a greater increment in serum potassium concentration than the decrement seen with similar but upward changes in pH in metabolic alkalosis. It turns out that the hydrogen ion concentration increases more for each 0.1-unit change in pH on the acid side than is seen with similar pH changes on the alkaline side. Thus, when one factors the change in serum potassium concentration for the change in hydrogen ion concentration, metabolic acidosis and alkalosis appear to exert similar, but directionally opposite, effects.[99]

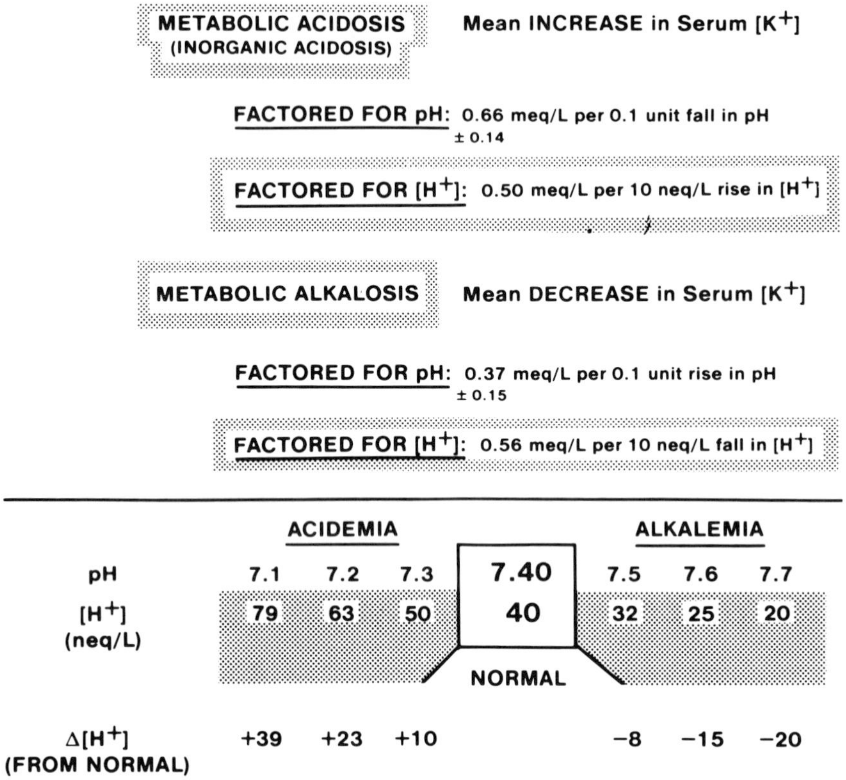

FIGURE 25-4 • Changes in serum potassium concentration in metabolic acidosis and alkalosis. The magnitude of change in the serum potassium concentration, factored for the change in arterial pH and hydrogen ion concentration, is shown for inorganic metabolic acidosis and alkalosis. (See text for details.)

RENAL POTASSIUM HANDLING Net renal potassium excretion is reduced during acute metabolic acidosis, but increases progressively as the chronic stage is achieved.[91] As has been noted, acute metabolic acidosis decreases passive proximal sodium chloride reabsorption, causing more filtered sodium and volume to be delivered to distal potassium secretory sites (see above). Changes in ECF volume, hypertonicity, and hyperkalemia tend to stimulate aldosterone and antidiuretic hormone release; both hormones enhance distal potassium secretion (see Chap. 6). Thus acute metabolic acidosis stimulates a number of potent forces that tend to increase net renal potassium secretion. Conversely, uptake of hydrogen ions by distal tubule epithelial cells displaces potassium from cellular transport sites, thereby diminishing secretion into the distal tubule lumen. The algebraic sum of these opposing forces results in a modest decline in kaliuresis during acute metabolic acidosis. During sustained metabolic acidosis the balance of forces shifts in favor of potassium excretion. Striking kaliureses can become a prominent feature of chronic forms of metabolic acidosis.

Calcium homeostasis

Of the many important effects of metabolic acidosis, none is more complicated than the interplay between metabolic acidosis, serum calcium concentration, and the forces regulating calcium homeostasis. Direct and indirect actions of metabolic acidosis have been shown to influence virtually every step in the accumulation, distribution, and excretion of calcium.[196] There are also important interactions between metabolic acidosis and parathyroid hormone (PTH) and active vitamin D. Thus metabolic acidosis disrupts normal calcium balance, and certain hypercalcemic states tend to cause metabolic acidosis. The elements of this complex interaction are discussed below.

ALTERED CALCIUM METABOLISM IN METABOLIC ACIDOSIS • *Serum calcium concentration* Approximately one-half of circulating calcium is bound to serum albumin and so is biologically inactive (see Chap. 11). Cationic calcium is normally bound to anionic carboxyl groups of various proteins. With increasing degrees of acidemia, protons replace calcium on protein, thereby increasing the ionized, biologically active form of calcium. This ionized fraction is now freely filtered at the glomerulus. Thus, acidemia tends to increase the filtered load of calcium.

Effect of acidosis on calcium regulatory hormones Parathyroid hormone Two well-conducted studies came to opposite conclusions regarding the effect of metabolic acidosis on PTH secretion.[48,286] One group found that acute metabolic acidosis stimulated secretion of the hormone; the other group found no effect. Further studies must be carried out to resolve this important question.

Other authors have shown that PTH plays an important role in mediating bone buffering of accumulating acid loads.[18,81] These workers have shown that parathyroidectomized animals became more hypobicarbonatemic from a given acid load than did intact controls.[18,81] Treatment with exogenous PTH restored normal bone buffering. These studies underscore the importance of PTH and bone in regulating acid-base homeostasis. However, a more recent study that was unable to confirm these results has thrown this issue into some question.[168]

1,25-Dihydroxyvitamin D_3 In-vitro studies have shown clearly that the proximal tubular enzyme 1α-hydroxylase is inhibited by physiologic concentrations of acid.[21,33] This enzyme is required for the activation of vitamin D (see Chap. 12). In-vivo studies, however, have been conflicting.[40,88,286] Part of the conflict may relate to the different species studied, the age of the animal model, and whether the animals had been vitamin D–deficient prior to study. Much more work remains to be done before the pathophysiologic significance of acidosis-induced inhibition of vitamin D activation can be properly interpreted.

Effect of acidosis on bone It is well known that increasing burdens of acid are absorbed and buffered by bone. Pioneering studies by Lemann and coworkers demonstrated that a close stoichiometry existed between positive hydrogen balance and negative calcium balance in human volunteers ingesting excessive acid loads.[160] These studies led to the view that entering hydrogen ions titrated bone carbonates, thereby protecting the serum bicarbonate concentration at the expense of the slow dissolution of bone. In-vitro studies have shown that acidification of the medium results in the dissolution of incubated bone.[41] These data have been further extrapolated to suggest that the chronic metabolic acidosis complicating advanced renal disease plays a significant role in uremic osteodystrophy (see Chap. 41). The mechanism by which acidosis dissolves bone is, in part, a simple physicochemical titration of the otuer shell of bone by accumulating acid, but additional effects have been proposed. The isolated perfused tibia increases its uptake of PTH and formation of cyclic-AMP when perfused with a medium of low pH and low bicarbonate concentration.[175] Other studies have shown that the calcemic action of PTH is enhanced in acidotic animals, further indicating that bone sensitivity to PTH is increased by low bicarbonate concentrations.[26]

Effect of acidosis on kidney It has been clearly shown that acute metabolic acidosis inhibits the tubular reabsorption of calcium and that this effect is independent of the availability of PTH.[61,160,272] The overall effects of acute and chronic metabolic acidosis vary as to the site of this inhibition and whether hypercalciuria results. During acute metabolic acidosis proximal calcium reabsorption is inhibited;[61] but since distal calcium reabsorption is simultaneously stimulated,[272] calcium excretion remains unchanged. During chronic metabolic acidosis the proximal reabsorption of calcium is now stimulated while distal reabsorption is inhibited, resulting in hypercalciuria.[272] Thus some chronic metabolic acidoses are characterized by the increased flow of calcium from bone into the extracellular space, where the low pH causes less calcium to be bound to protein. The increased concentration of ionized calcium, in turn, increases its renal filtration. Since net tubular calcium reabsorption is decreased, the increased filtered load is translated into striking degrees of hypercalciuria. Distal renal tubular acidosis is the major form of chronic metabolic acidosis associated with such large increments in calcium excretion. Although the mechanism by which systemic acidosis impairs calcium absorption is unknown, it appears to be independent of systemic arterial pH.[214]

EFFECTS OF HYPERCALCEMIA ON ACID-BASE BALANCE
Sustained increases in serum calcium concentration can affect acid-base balance in a number of ways. The nonspecific renal damage that occurs from chronic hypercalcemia can result in uremic acidosis.[67] Hypercalcemia has other direct and indirect effects that also profoundly influence acid-base balance. The interaction of PTH and calcium in tubular bicarbonate handling is complex. Many workers have shown that PTH inhibits proximal sodium bicarbonate reabsorption, but with few exceptions the increased distal flow of alkali is readily recaptured by distal bicarbonate-reabsorbing epithelia, preventing bicarbonaturia.[229] Hypercalcemia, on the other hand, stimulates proximal bicarbonate reabsorption.[55] Thus, in states of hyperparathyroidism, the elevated levels of PTH tend to cause bicarbonate wasting and hyperchloremic acidosis. However, the hypercalcemia that characterizes this syndrome offsets the effect of PTH by stimulating bicarbonate reabsorption. Thus a given patient may or may not manifest a hyperchloremic acidosis.

Phosphorus

The interactions of acid-base balance and phosphorus metabolism are discussed thoroughly in Chap. 12.

Magnesium

The interplay of acid-base metabolism and magnesium balance is discussed in Chap. 13.

Metabolic effects

Hormonal effects of acidosis

As has been noted, catecholamine secretion during metabolic acidosis plays a prominent role in the response of myocardial contraction, arteriolar dilatation, and potassium distribution (see above). Increased plasma catecholamine levels not only reflect the general stress of metabolic acidosis but appear to be a specific response elicited by acidified extracellular fluid. When the adrenal gland is perfused with an acidified fluid, catecholamine secretion is specifically stimulated.[192] While aldosterone secretion is clearly increased in metabolic acidosis,[215,216] it is uncertain whether this is a specific effect of acidosis or is secondary to associated hyperkalemia or adrenocorticotropic hormone (ACTH) release. The interactions of acidosis with PTH and 1,25-$(OH)_2D_3$ have been noted above.

Protein wasting

The kidney responds to increases in the daily acid burden by increasing net acid excretion. The increment in acid excreted is largely a function of the kidney's ability to increase its synthesis of ammonia buffer. As discussed in Chap. 10, the kidney extracts amino acid precursors, strips the nitrogen from them, and disposes of the remaining carbon skeleton in the form of CO_2 and glucose. Glutamine serves as the prime renal ammoniagenic precursor. It therefore follows that during periods of acid stress, the kidney's ability to enhance proton excretion will depend on an increasing supply of glutamine and increased renal capacity to extract the glutamine and subsequently convert it to ammonia buffer. Endogenous and exogenous proteins serve as a ready source of glutamine. Hannaford and coworkers have shown that during starvation ketosis, the breakdown of endogenous protein serves as a ready source of nitrogen precursors for the kidney.[110,111] Administration of sodium bicarbonate to the starving ketotic subject reduces the net burden of acid required for excretion and accordingly diminishes the endogenous rate of protein breakdown.[110,111] Thus it appears that acidosis simultaneously stimulates endogenous protein breakdown, ensuring delivery of glutamine to the kidney. Stimulation of renal ammoniagenesis by acidosis then enhances the conversion of the amino acid to the needed ammonia buffer.

Feedback inhibition and stimulation of endogenous acid production

The importance of precise regulation of serum bicarbonate concentration is well recognized. It would make great sense, therefore, if a feedback regulatory system were present to stimulate or inhibit endogenous acid production and thereby sustain an unchanged serum bicarbonate concentration. This possibility was recently studied by Hood and coworkers.[120] Starving obese volunteers were, at different times, fed sodium bicarbonate, sodium chloride, or ammonium chloride to define whether varying loads of exogenous acid and alkali influenced endogenous ketone production during starvation. The authors demonstrated that 24-h urinary excretion of ketones is stimulated by the administration of exogenous alkali and inhibited by exogenous acid.[120] The authors concluded that a feedback regulatory system is in operation. Subsequent studies by the same group have indicated that experimentally induced hypercapnia may also reduce endogenous acid production.[1] Certain states of chronic lactic acidosis—for example, malignancy-associated lactic acidosis—are characterized by increased lactic acid production during exogenous alkali therapy.[80,107] The clinical significance of these observations has yet to be determined.

CLINICAL FEATURES OF HIGH ANION GAP METABOLIC ACIDOSES

As discussed in Chap. 24, the metabolic acidoses are best classified on the basis of their effects on the anion gap. Accordingly, the high anion gap and normal anion gap acidoses are discussed in sequence.

DIFFUSE RENAL FAILURE

Introduction

The unceasing cumulative production of 50 to 100 meq/day of organic and inorganic acid replaces a like amount of bicarbonate, placing the normal host in constant jeopardy of metabolic acidosis. The kidneys interdict the development of acidosis by reabsorbing filtered bicarbonate and by excreting the daily acid load while simultaneously resynthesizing alkali lost in buffering metabolic acids. As explained in Chap. 10, renal bicarbonate reabsorption and synthesis and acid excretion depend on renal epithelial cell synthesis of H_2CO_3 and the regulated exchange of cellular protons for luminal sodium (Fig. 25-5). The immediate ionization of H_2CO_3 formed in proximal epithelial cells yields H^+ and HCO_3^- ions, which are separately transported by luminal and peritubular membranes. Secretion of protons across the luminal membrane in exchange for previously filtered luminal sodium, and the simultaneous secretion of cellular HCO_3^- across peritubular membranes into adjacent capillaries, at once acidifies tubular fluid and alkalinizes peritubular blood. Alkali filtered from blood at the glomerulus creates a bicarbonate-rich proximal tubule fluid, enabling each milliequivalent of secreted proton to destroy a like amount of HCO_3^- by converting it to CO_2

FIGURE 25-5 • Mechanism of sodium bicarbonate reabsorption. The diagram illustrates the interplay between the Na^+/H^+ antiporter, the Na^+-K^+ ATPase, and the epithelial synthesis of H_2CO_3 in bicarbonate reabsorption. (See text for details.)

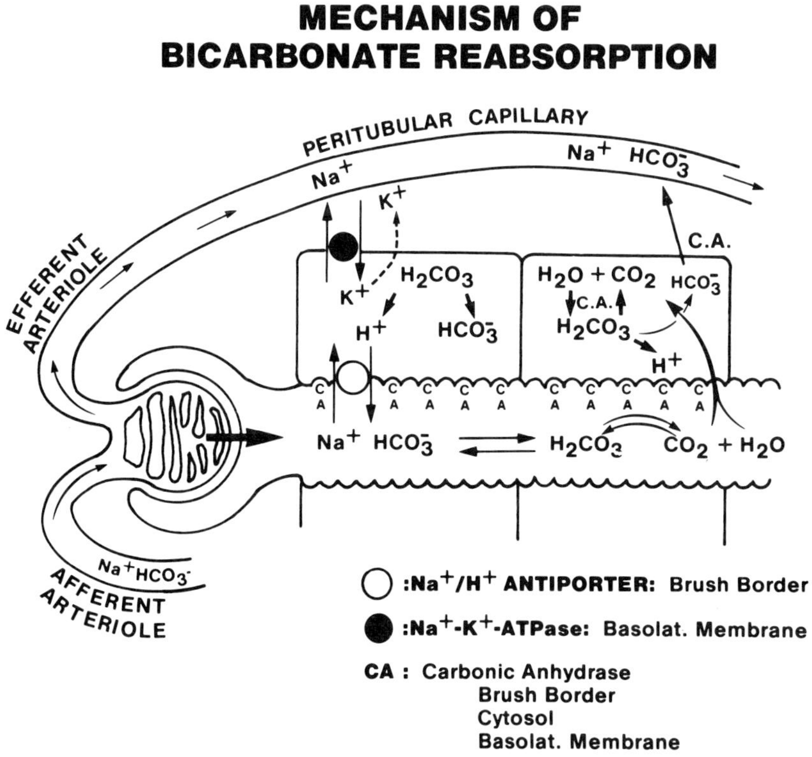

and water. The potential loss of blood HCO_3^- that might otherwise ensue is prevented by the systemic return and replacement of bicarbonate via peritubular transport of alkali. This process ensures that lost luminal bicarbonate is returned to the ECF via the renal venous effluent. Bicarbonate reabsorption is largely a proximal tubule event, the normal regulation of which ensures that 25 meq of alkali is reclaimed from each liter of glomerular filtrate. Bicarbonate present in excess of this concentration is rejected by the tubule. The resulting corrective bicarbonaturia thereby prevents any tendency toward hyperbicarbonatemia. Conversely, proximal tubule reabsorption occurs during hypobicarbonatemia; that is, metabolic acidosis prevents further loss of alkali, thereby stabilizing plasma levels. A variety of factors are known to strongly influence renal bicarbonate reclamation (Table 25-3). When P_{CO_2}, ECF volume, arterial pH, calcium and potassium levels, and PTH are normal, bicarbonate reabsorption also remains normal, and the kidneys sustain a serum HCO_3^- level of 25 meq/liter. Alterations in these factors aid and abet the sustained displacement of serum bicarbonate concentration from normal (see Chap. 29).

Tubular processing ensures the virtual absence of bicarbonate from the glomerular filtrate by the time it reaches the distal nephron. Similar transport of cytosolically derived H^+ and HCO_3^- again renders contents of the lumen acid and the peritubular blood alkaline. Lack of alkali allows secreted protons to acidify the luminal contents quickly. Were buffer not provided to this fluid, the free H^+ concentration would swiftly rise to such levels as to restrict further secretion of protons. The key urinary buffers, ammonia (NH_3) and dibasic phosphates (HPO_4^{2-}), absorb secreted protons, preventing development of concentration gradients that would perniciously restrict further acid secretion. In the absence of luminal bicarbonate, each milliequivalent of protons secreted is bound by a milliequivalent of buffer, and each milliequivalent of titrated butter that is eventually excreted reflects one milliequivalent of HCO_3^- returned to blood. Acid secretion and excretion wax and wane so as to precisely match daily acid production. Since one milliequivalent of HCO_3^- is returned systemically for each proton excreted as titrated buffer, aciduria not only rids the body of acid but also replenishes bicarbonate lost in consequence of the daily addition of strong acids to the ECF.

TABLE 25-3 • Major determinants of renal bicarbonate reabsorption

Stimulates reabsorption	Inhibits reabsorption
ECF contraction	ECF expansion
Hypercapnia	Hypocapnia
Hypokalemia	Hyperkalemia
Hypobicarbonatemia	Hyperbicarbonatemia
Hypercalcemia	Hypocalcemia
Hypoparathyroidism	Hyperparathyroidism

Normally, net acid excretion [i.e., the sum of titrated buffer (NH_4^+ and titratable acid) minus any bicarbonate lost in the urine] exactly matches daily acid production. In renal-metabolic parlance, *zero acid balance* is achieved. Readers should appreciate that urinary protons are found in both free and bound forms. Free protons, "sensed" by pH-sensitive measuring techniques, represent vanishingly small concentrations of acid. For example, a pH of 4.0 corresponds to a hydrogen ion concentration of only 0.1 meq/liter, or a mere 0.1 percent of the daily acid synthesized (i.e., 100 meq). However, excretion of 50 to 100 meq of acid bound to NH_3 or HPO_4^{2-} enables achievement of zero acid balance and thereby avoid metabolic acidosis.

Excretion of the anions generated with the daily acid load is largely a passive glomerular process. Partial reabsorption of sulfate, phosphate, and organic anions that gain access to the tubular lumen via the glomerular filtrate allows excretion of the same number of milliequivalents of anions and protons.

It follows that metabolic acid may be retained when renal bicarbonate reabsorption or synthesis is impaired. Herein follows a discussion of the pathogenesis, clinical features, and therapy of the acidosis that complicates acute and chronic renal failure.

The uremic acidoses

As reviewed above, the kidneys closely monitor and regulate serum bicarbonate concentration. During the course of most forms of severe acute or chronic renal failure this regulatory process becomes compromised, resulting in bicarbonate's replacement with chloride, sulfate, phosphate, or various organic anions. The *renal tubular acidoses* (see Chap. 27) are characterized, at least initially, by more tubular than glomerular damage. Tubular damage results in the retention of acid with resulting hypobicabonatemia. Persistently normal glomerular function rids the acid anions (from sulfuric, phosphoric, and organic acids) while retained dietary chloride replaces lost bicarbonate. Laboratory studies reveal a typical normal anion gap acidosis (Table 25-4). In *diffuse acute and chronic renal diseases*, glomerular and tubular damage advance in proportion, allowing retained sulfate, phosphate, and organic anions to replace bicarbonate. The emerging serum electrolyte pattern reveals a high anion gap acidosis (Table 25-4). Since the rate of tubular damage may exceed that of glomerular damage in some disorders, a mixed pattern of normal and high anion gap acidosis is occasionally found (Table 25-4).

The acidoses that complicate the various forms of acute and chronic renal failure are reviewed separately.

Acute renal failure

Disorders acutely suppressing renal function do so either by severely restricting renal perfusion, profoundly damaging the renal parenchyma, or by obstructing urinary outflow from an otherwise undamaged urinary tract. Accordingly, acute renal failure (ARF) is conveniently classified as (1) *pre-renal ARF*, in which renal perfusion is compromised because of volume contraction, myocardial pump failure, or severe renal vasoconstriction; (2) *intrinsic renal ARF*, in which an acute insult to glomeruli, vasculature, interstitium or tubules impairs overall renal function; or (3) *post-renal ARF*, where an obstructing lesion prevents outflow. These subclasses of ARF are separately discussed below.

PRE-RENAL ARF Renal perfusion may become compromised as a consequence of heart failure or inadequate plasma volume. Reduction of renal blood flow by approximately 30 to 40 percent greatly stimulates the proximal tubules's reabsorption of sodium and water, thereby compromising the delivery of filtrate to the distal tubule. When distal tubule sodium delivery is markedly reduced, the generation of favorable electrical gradients for continued proton secretion becomes further impaired. A form of renal tubular acidosis develops. Reduced renal perfusion may so severely diminish glutamine delivery to the kidney as to impair ammoniagenesis and net acid excretion. This has been seen in salt-avid, hypoalbuminemic subjects with cirrhosis.[32,209,259] When renal perfusion becomes further compromised, the delivery

TABLE 25-4 • Electrolytes in the renal acidoses

	mg/100 ml		meq/liter			
ELECTROLYTE PATTERN	BUN	Cr	Na^+	Cl^-	HCO_3^-	AG
Normal	15	1.0	140	105	25	10
Pure uremic acidosis (UA)	50	5.0	140	105	15	20
Pure hyperchloremic acidosis (HCA)	15	1.0	140	115	15	10
Mixed UA plus HCA	35	3.5	140	110	15	15

Abbreviations: BUN, blood urea nitrogen; Cr, creatinine; AG, anion gap.

of metabolic substrate and oxygen to the kidneys may limit tubular function, resulting in metabolic acidosis with disordered handling of other electrolytes. At this stage, when proportionate failure of glomerular filtration and tubular function occurs, a typical high anion gap metabolic acidosis ensues. The metabolic acidosis complicating prerenal ARF often reflects a complex array of contributing factors. As has been mentioned, the high anion gap acidosis of prerenal ARF may combine with increased lactic acid production from compromised extrarenal tissue perfusion, causing a mixed high anion gap acidosis (see Chap. 31). If the ECF fluid loss was created by various gastrointestinal disorders, the acid-base abnormality may be complicated by gastric alkalosis or diarrheal acidosis. Furthermore, if congestive heart failure is associated, alterations in the pulmonary clearance of CO_2 may be associated. Thus, patients with prerenal ARF often have several coexisting primary acid-base abnormalities. As discussed in Chap. 31, mixed metabolic acidosis, metabolic alkalosis, and respiratory acidosis or alkalosis may combine in various permutations.

INTRINSIC RENAL ARF The acute onset of severe renal parenchymal disease can so compromise function that renal maintenance of the internal milieu is forfeited. Disorders that so afflict that kidney may be categorized in terms of the primary site of histologic damage. Accordingly, intrinsic renal ARF may be due to acute vasculitis, acute glomerulonephritis, acute interstitial nephritis, or acute tubular necrosis. Any of these disorders may so severely damage the kidney that a uremic acidosis soon supervenes.

The acute interstitial nephritides may occasionally injure the tubules more than the glomerulus and result in bicarbonate wasting and a hyperchloremic acidosis. This reaction is certainly the exception to the rule; the more common result of severe acute interstitial nephritis is a uremic, high anion gap acidosis. When renal function is so severely compromised that little urine is produced, given a normal rate of endogenous acid production, the serum bicarbonate concentration diminishes, on average, by 2 meq/liter daily.[160a,231] On the other hand, many of the causes of acute tubular necrosis develop in a setting of sepsis and poor tissue perfusion. The increased tissue catabolism resulting from these systemic effects can strikingly increase the endogenous rate of acid production, resulting in more rapid and profound declines in serum bicarbonate concentration. Indeed, the highest levels of blood sulfate are seen in intrinsic ARF.[83]

Metabolic acidosis from all causes results in tubular epithelial cell damage with consequent inhibition of proximal tubular reabsorption and catabolism of proteins.[42c,166a] Tubular proteinuria may be an early, clinically useful reflection of such damage in the setting of acute renal failure of any etiology and in diabetic ketoacidosis and ammonium chloride loading. In other words, the metabolic acidosis may augment the tubular damage caused by coexisting disorders.

POST-RENAL ARF When the flow of urine is totally occluded, the complete suppression of renal function results in a high anion gap metabolic acidosis. Prolonged backpressure in the distal nephron, from partial urinary tract obstruction, may impair distal tubule proton and potassium secretion. A hyperchloremic and hyperkalemic acidosis may ensue.[24] If urinary tract obstruction has been chronic, the associated interstitial nephritis may impair renal renin secretion, which may, in turn, compromise the secretion of aldosterone—which will, of course, aggravate the hyperkalemia.

Chronic renal failure

It is generally believed that acidosis resulting from chronic renal failure does not become manifest until the GFR is reduced to values below 30 ml/min, and that this acidosis is generally associated with an increased anion gap.[159,259] However, Widmer and coworkers noted significant hypobicarbonatemia and hyperchloremia in the early stages of chronic renal failure.[289] In patients with advanced azotemia the acidosis was mixed—that is, it was only partially accounted for by an increased anion gap. Additional studies are needed to confirm these results. While it is also believed that chronic interstitial nephritides are more likely to cause a hyperchloremic acidosis in early renal failure, recent studies have not convincingly confirmed this impression.[63,64,129] Hypoaldosteronism is being recognized as a complicating feature of many chronic renal diseases, especially in diabetics, making it likely that mixed high anion gap and hyperchloremic acidoses will be seen more frequently.

The acidosis of chronic renal failure has an insidious onset and generally tends to be mild. The serum bicarbonate concentration reaches a nadir of 12 to 18 meq/liter and is steadily maintained at this level unless there is an intercurrent complication. With normal respiratory compensation, arterial pH in uncomplicated chronic renal failure usually does not fall below 7.25. Goodman and coworkers noted that patients with azotemic acidosis with stable bicarbonate levels excreted less acid than they produced metabolically.[100] Since this positive acid balance occurs despite an unchanging serum bicarbonate concentration, an extrarenal, nonbicarbonate buffer must exist to neutralize endogenous acid escaping urinary excretion. Bone has been shown to serve as this important buffer in the acidosis of chronic renal failure.[159] Metabolic balance studies have indicated that the positive acid balance is accompanied by an equivalent degree of negative calcium balance.[159] Retained acid is neutralized by calcium carbonate in bone; thus the serum HCO_3^- concentration is protected, at the expense of osteopenia. Approximately 35,000 meq of carbonate resides in bone.

Chronic acidosis is therefore regarded as a compounding factor in the pathogenesis of renal osteodystrophy (see Chap. 41).[161]

A parallel adverse effect of chronic metabolic acidosis is that seen on muscle tissue, which serves as an additional important source of buffering capacity. Skeletal muscle biopsy studies of patients nearing dialysis-dependence with chronic renal failure and untreated metabolic acidosis reveal the presence of significant intracellular acidosis.[57b] In rats with chronic renal failure, metabolic acidosis appears to mediate, and possibly worsen, derangements of branched-chain amino acid metabolism by oxidative decarboxylation, irrespective of the presence of azotemia.[111b] Defective muscle protein metabolism in chronically uremic rats appears to be secondary to acidosis-induced acceleration of muscle proteolysis along with inhibition of insulin-stimulated muscle protein synthesis; the latter is not acidosis-dependent.[175a] Loss of lean body mass in patients with chronic renal failure may be partly a result of concomitant systemic metabolic acidosis, and hence may be ameliorated by therapy for the same.

PATHOGENESIS OF UREMIC ACIDOSIS Renal acidosis may result from failure to reabsorb filtered bicarbonate, failure to provide buffer appropriate for the daily acid excretion, or failure to acidify the urine.

Bicarbonate reabsorption Normal kidneys respond to metabolic acidosis by excreting an intensely acid, bicarbonate-free urine. An early study of uremic acidosis indicated that three of the four subjects excreted overt quantities of bicarbonate despite the presence of significant hypobicarbonatemia.[244] Bicarbonaturia ceased only when plasma concentrations fell below 20 meq/liter. Since all subjects lost weight during the course of the study, the potential influence of prior ECF volume expansion in lowering bicarbonate reabsorption remains unclear. Slatapolsky and coworkers performed titration studies on azotemic patients with varying GFRs to determine what influence ECF volume expansion exerted on renal bicarbonate reabsorption.[262] They concluded that intrinsic renal disease per se does not depress bicarbonate reabsorption per unit of residual GFR. However, when uremic subjects with stable rates of bicarbonate reabsorption were subjected to acute volume expansion, natriuresis increased strikingly and bicarbonate reabsorption decreased in a corresponding fashion.

Thus bicarbonate reabsorption in uremic subjects is influenced by the concurrent control of sodium excretion. Several studies have attempted to determine the effects of chronic renal failure on bicarbonate reabsorption that are independent of the influence of ECF volume. Arruda and coworkers studied bicarbonate reabsorption in dogs before and after induction of renal failure, produced by unilateral nephrectomy and partial infarction of the remaining kidney.[15] Volume expansion decreased bicarbonate reabsorption in control and uremic groups. At comparable levels of fractional chloride excretion (used as an index of the degree of hypervolemia), bicarbonate reabsorption was significantly greater in azotemic than in control animals. When sodium bicarbonate was administered orally in amounts sufficient to neutralize endogenous acid production, bicarbonate reabsorption remained higher than in nonazotemic control animals. In separate studies of uremic and normal rats the maximal tubular reabsorption of bicarbonate, when factored for GFR (i.e., $TmHCO_3^-/GFR$), was similar despite higher levels of chloride excretion in uremic animals.[17] The ratio of absolute bicarbonate reabsorption (meq/minute) to the absolute sodium reabsorption, a parameter that corrects for the influence of volume, was significantly higher in uremic rats. Similarly, in eight patients with chronic renal failure the ratio of bicarbonate reabsorption to sodium reabsorption rose as GFR fell.[17] This bicarbonate avidity was demonstrated over a wide range of fractional chloride excretion. Schmidt and coworkers also noted an increase in bicarbonate reabsorption in the presence of high fractional excretion rates for sodium, potassium, and phosphate.[241] Thus it is suspected that in chronic renal failure reabsorption of bicarbonate is actually enhanced relative to that of sodium and chloride. More recently Wong and coworkers investigated the tubular handling of bicarbonate in dogs with experimental renal failure.[296] Micropuncture studies were performed to examine segmental reabsorption of bicarbonate and chloride in the remnant kidney of dogs with experimental renal failure. The ratio of absolute bicarbonate reabsorption to absolute sodium reabsorption was found to be increased in both the distal and proximal tubules. Chloride reabsorption was found to be depressed at the late proximal site, resulting in greater delivery to the distal nephron. The distal segment reabsorbed a constant fraction of delivered chloride, resulting in increased fractional chloride excretion. Thus it was suggested that as an adaptation to reduced nephron mass, sodium bicarbonate reabsorption is enhanced and sodium chloride transport is reduced.

Although some studies have demonstrated that bicarbonate wasting may not complicate some experimental forms of renal failure, others have shown that significant numbers of azotemic patients do manifest bicarbonaturia. Several possible mechanisms have been advanced to explain this alkali wasting.

SECONDARY HYPERPARATHYRODISM Several studies have shown that parathyroid hormone (PTH) influences proximal bicarbonate reabsorption.[187,189,200] Parathyroid extract, when infused into dogs, induces transient bicarbonaturia.[135] Bank and Aynedjian performed micropuncture studies of bicarbonate reabsorption in thyroparathyroidectomized rats before and after the administration of PTH.[20] The hormone caused a moderate reduction in proximal tubule bicarbonate reabsorption; however, distal nephron segments reabsorbed the added load. Other studies in dogs have demonstrated that acutely administered PTH does not lower bicarbonate reabsorption enough to cause chemically or clinically significant metabolic acidosis.[229] The potential role of chronically elevated PTH levels in patients with chronic renal failure in mediating acidosis remains unclear. Muldowney has suggested that secondary hyperparathyroidism associated with chronic azotemia and gastrointestinal malabsorption causes significant bicarbonaturia and hypobicarbonatemia.[187] A significant rise in steady-state plasma HCO_3^- values has been documented following elevation of serum calcium levels with vitamin D therapy in patients with chronic renal disease.[187] The reduction in serum PTH levels consequent to normocalcemia may have enhanced the bicarbonate reabsorption. In contrast, neither parathyroidectomy[187] nor proportional reduction of phosphate intake[20] in uremic dogs influenced renal bicarbonate reabsorption. Thus the potential role of secondary hyperparathyroidism in the bicarbonate wasting of uremic acidosis remains unclear.

SOLUTE DIURESIS With progressive reduction in nephron mass there occurs a marked increase in the solute load excreted by each remaining nephron. This solute diuresis may influence the excretion of such anions as chloride and bicarbonate. Increased solute excretion per nephron enhances the delivery of $NaHCO_3$ to the distal tubule, thereby potentially impairing urinary acidification.[249] In this way, renal failure may be similar to the bicarbonaturia induced in normal subjects by infusion of the nonreabsorbable, nonmetabolizable sugar mannitol.[225] Although solute diuresis may play a role under some circumstances, it is unlikely to contribute significantly to bicarbonaturia seen in chronic renal failure. All azotemic subjects undergo this solute diuresis, but few have significant bicarbonaturia.

RELATIONSHIP TO RENAL SODIUM HANDLING As the nephron mass progressively shrinks, maintenance of salt balance in the face of unchanged intake requires that remaining nephrons excrete a steadily increasing amount of sodium. At a constant sodium intake, if the GFR declines from 100 ml/min to 10 ml/min, the fractional sodium excretion has to increase tenfold to maintain external sodium balance. Proximal and distal tubular rejection of sodium participates in this adaptation.[36] Bicarbonaturia accompanies the natriuresis, contributing to the systemic acidosis. If sodium intake were reduced in proportion to the reduction in GFR, less sodium would have to be excreted, and tubular salt transport could remain intact. If bicarbonate "followed" sodium, this manipulation would be expected to prevent the development of bicarbonaturia. Indeed, when this experiment was carried out in rats, the bicarbonate threshold increased and uremic acidosis was markedly attenuated.[70] Consistent with these findings is the observation that salt-retaining edematous subjects with azotemia and nephrotic syndrome manifest increased renal avidity for bicarbonate.[262] Thus fractional bicarbonate excretion appears to be closely linked to sodium excretion.

In summary, at least some patients with chronic renal failure develop bicarbonaturia as renal damage progresses. Solute diuresis and increased fractional sodium excretion play key roles in this bicarbonate wastage. What role the secondary hyperparathyroidism may have in mediating bicarbonaturia of renal failure remains unclear at this time.

Reduced buffer excretion Ammonia excretion in renal failure (see Chap. 27) A major portion of excreted acid is carried by ammonia buffer, which is synthesized by the kidney. Although the entire nephron is capable of generating ammonia, the proximal tubule appears to synthesize the bulk of this key buffer.[275] The medullary trapping of proximally produced ammonia also plays an important role in ammonia excretion (Fig. 25-6).

Proximal epithelial cells, by hydrating CO_2, generate H_2CO_3, which immediately ionizes to H^+ and HCO_3^-. By excreting the proton while retaining the HCO_3^- the kidney effectively synthesizes new base. The tubular cell transports the proton, which is bound to ammonia (NH_4^+), into the lumen of the proximal tubule while separately transporting the $NaHCO_3$ across the basolateral membrane into the blood. Eventual excretion of the NH_4^+ allows for the net addition of bicarbonate to body alkali stores. Were the NH_4^+ subsequently reclaimed, it would eventually be delivered to, and metabolized by, the liver, thereby reforming H^+ while synthesizing urea, and effectively neutralizing accumulating bicarbonate. It follows that in order to realize any net gain of bicarbonate, NH_4^+ must be excreted. An intricate series of transport processes distributed along the length of the nephron combine to prevent excessive reclamation of luminal NH_4^+ and thereby precisely match NH_4^+ excretion with the host's need for alkali.

Proximal Epithelium • Ammonia derived from extracted glutamine combines with protons derived from H_2CO_3 to form NH_4^+. The HCO_3^- derived from H_2CO_3 remains in the cell. The sodium-hydrogen antiporter in the apical membrane exchanges intracellular NH_4^+ for luminal Na^+, at once forming NH_4Cl in the glomerular filtrate and $NaHCO_3$ in the cell. Cellular $NaHCO_3$ reaches peritubular capillaries via the Cl^-- HCO_3^- exchanger situated in the basolateral cell membrane.

Distal Nephron • The bulk of ammonium produced in cortical proximal tubules is added to the medullary interstitium by passive forces acting on the descending limb of Henle's loop and by an active transporter in the thick ascending limb (see Chaps. 10 and 27). The descending limb's permeability to water, but not to

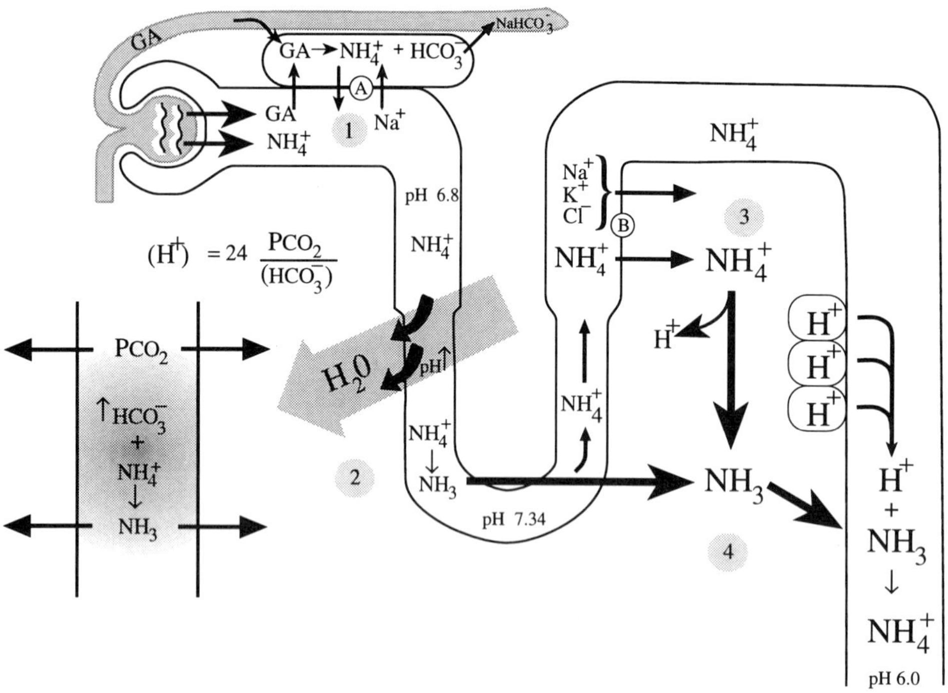

FIGURE 25-6 • Medullary ammonia trapping. The sequential steps required to synthesize and excrete amounts of ammonia appropriate for maintaining acid-base balance are outlined. (1) Proximal epithelial cells obtain glutamine (GA) from the glomerular filtrate and from peritubular blood. The amino acid is converted to NH_4^+ and HCO_3^-. The HCO_3^- and reabsorbed Na^+ are delivered to the peritubular blood, and the NH_4^+ enters the tubular lumen via the Na^+-H^+ antiporter (A). (2) Loss of water from the descending limb of Henle's loop simultaneously concentrates luminal HCO_3^- and CO_2. The diffusibility of CO_2 and bicarbonate's lack thereof raises the pH of the filtrate, converting a small fraction of luminal NH_4^+ to NH_3, which diffuses into the medulla (insert). (3) The bulk of synthesized NH_4^+ enters the medullary interstitium via the Na^+-K^+ $2Cl^-$ transporter (B) located in the thick ascending limb of Henle. (4) Medullary NH_4^+ serves as a source of NH_3, which diffuses down its concentration gradient into the collecting duct (CD). Proton secretion by CD cells maintains reduced luminal NH_3 levels, ensuring the continued net addition of ammonia from the interstitium to the CD (see text for further details).

various solutes, allows the progressive concentration of luminal contents as water moves into the hypertonic medullary interstitium (Fig. 25-6). The freely permeable CO_2 escapes as the luminal HCO_3^- concentration increases, thereby raising the intraluminal pH. The increasing luminal alkalinity titrates NH_4^+ to NH_3 (Fig. 25-6), which rapidly diffuses into the medullary interstitium. The Na^+-K^+-$2Cl^-$ transporter located in the thick ascending limb removes the greatest amount of NH_4^+ from the distal filtrate (Fig. 25-6). As NH_4^+ accumulates in the medullary interstitium, a small but biologically significant amount of NH_3 also accumulates. The latter diffuses into the collecting ducts (Fig. 25-6). Secretion of protons into the lumen of the collecting ducts ensures the trapping of NH_3 by creation of the poorly diffusible NH_4^+ cation. It follows that the rate of proximal ammoniagenesis, the transport of ammonia out of the distal nephron, the concentration of NH_3 (P_{NH_3}) in the medulla, and the secretion of protons by the collecting duct determine the rate of NH_4^+ excretion and, thereby, that of net acid excretion.

The above scenario allows ammonia produced in cortical proximal tubules to move into the descending limb of Henle's loop, to the collecting duct, and then into the final urine, thereby avoiding the need to reenter the cortex. This "medullary detour" allows for excretion of a greater fraction of synthesized NH_3, the importance of which is as follows.

Excretion of H^+ derived from H_2CO_3 (see above) with NH_3 allows the HCO_3^- derived from intracellular H_2CO_3 to replenish body alkali stores. If proximally synthesized ammonia were allowed to reenter the cortex, a significant fraction would be reabsorbed and returned systemically. Reclaimed NH_4Cl would be catabolized by the liver, thereby freeing its proton. Thus, for net alkali to be added to the body, NH_4^+ must be excreted. The medullary trapping of ammonia, therefore, prevents rerouting of buffer from urine to blood and thereby ensures efficient acid excretion and alkali generation.

As renal disease progresses, the amount of ammonia produced per unit of residual tissue is unchanged, but since there is an inexorable shrinkage of tissue mass, less and less ammonia is synthesized each day.[259,298] Simpson and coworkers studied 10 patients with chronic renal disease and confirmed that absolute urinary ammonia excretion was decreased though the fractional excretion was increased.[259] When normalized for the GFR, the production per unit of functional tissue was increased.[259]

As the number of nephrons decreases, there is a compensatory increase in ammonia excretion by the residual tissue. This adaptive increase is the result of both compensatory cellular hypertrophy and increased activity of enzymes concerned with the generation of ammonia.[167,242] As renal failure progresses the total absolute ammonia production steadily falls, thereby decreasing the amount of net acid excreted, eventually causing positive acid balance and hypobicarbonatemia. Disruption of medullary integrity during the course of many chronic renal diseases, especially the interstitial disorders, may well impair medullary trapping of ammonia, thereby worsening the acidosis. Recent micropuncture data confirm this sequence of events.[37a,38,264a] Prostaglandins have been shown to inhibit renal ammoniagenesis.[130] Since the production of certain prostanoids increases during the course of chronic renal disease, it is conceivable that their inhibitory action limits buffer synthesis and thereby contributes to the acidosis of renal failure.

Although glutamine serves as the dominant ammoniagenic precursor under normal conditions, some other, as yet undefined, nitrogen source appears to take on added importance in chronic renal failure.[281] It has been shown in a variety of renal disorders that the amount of ammonia leaving the kidney exceeds that which could possibly be derived from the relatively small amount of glutamine extracted.[281] Renal degradation of circulating low-molecular-weight proteins and increased filtration of albumin with its subsequent catabolism may serve as nitrogen sources.

Titratable acid excretion Although titratable acid excretion is increased per unit of residual GFR, the absolute amount excreted each day remains unchanged in patients with chronic renal failure, as well as in animals with experimentally induced disease.[259] Dietary protein restriction and therapy with aluminum-containing antacid gels limit the availability of dietary phosphate and so may limit buffer availability and acid excretion. Acid retention consequent to a fall in phosphate excretion would normally stimulate ammonia synthesis, thus compensating for the decrease in titratable acid excretion. In advanced renal failure ammonia synthesis is already maximally stimulated, precluding expanded ammoniagenesis from further compensating for diminished phosphate excretion.

Urinary acidification Failure to maximally acidify the urine interferes with the complete titration of the excreted phosphate and ammonia buffers. The ability of patients with renal failure to maximally acidify their urine has been tested by means of the infusion of sodium sulfate.[249] Reabsorption of infused sodium without the nonreabsorbable sulfate anion increases luminal electronegativity, which is a potent stimulus for proton secretion. Patients with renal failure acidify their urine to a degree comparable to that of control subjects.[249] Concomitant distal renal tubular acidosis, or bicarbonate wasting resulting from volume expansion or secondary hyperparathyroidism, may occasionally interfere with this process.

In summary, the progressive loss of ammoniagenic capacity is the central cause of the acidosis of chronic renal failure. This can be worsened by the concomitant decrease in the availability of phosphate buffer as well as the presence of inappropriate bicarbonaturia. Some patients with chronic renal failure waste bicarbonate because of some combination of solute diuresis, high fractional excretion of sodium, and secondary hyperparathyroidism.

THEREAPY OF THE ACIDOSIS OF CHRONIC RENAL FAILURE The acidosis accompanying chronic renal failure tends to be mild and nonprogressive. However, since the bicarbonate reserve is compromised, superimposition of an acute acid load from sepsis, diarrhea, or mild CO_2 retention might more easily lead to an overwhelming degree of acidemia. Metabolic acidosis has been implicated as one of several pathogenic factors in uremic osteodystrophy.[161,234] Since chronic acidosis impairs bone growth in children, alkali therapy is definitely indicated in this setting. Controlled studies evaluating the risks and benefits of alkali therapy in adults with uremic acidosis are lacking. Since most such adults are not overtly symptomatic, and growth is not an issue, many physicians do not routinely administer alkali.

In rats with chronic renal failure, bicarbonate administration has been shown to reduce oxidative decarboxylation of branched-chain amino acids and to correct the increased protein degradation, but not the lower rates of insulin-stimulated protein synthesis, associated with uremia.[175a] Sodium bicarbonate supplements given to patients with chronic renal failure increase arterial pH and bicarbonate levels while decreasing blood urea nitrogen and plasma uric acid levels. In the face of stable urea clearances and stable states of total body water content, these results suggest a significant reduction in muscle protein breakdown.[128a] Thus appropriate correction of metabolic acidosis may be crucial to maximization of positive nitrogen balance and maintenance of lean muscle mass.

The dose of alkali required to maintain plasma bicarbonate concentration at 20 to 23 meq/liter does not usually result in volume overload. Studies by Husted and coworkers show that $NaHCO_3$ is better tolerated than NaCl,[123] weight gain and edema being unusual during alkali therapy. It is suggested that a chloride leak, perhaps from the thick ascending limb of Henle's loop, allows NaCl to be excreted in exchange for retained $NaHCO_3$. Alkali can be administered as $NaHCO_3$, sodium citrate, or calcium carbonate. Each gram of $NaHCO_3$ contains 12 meq of alkali; the usual dose for adults is 2 to 4 g daily. *Shohl's solution* contains 1 meq/ml of sodium citrate and causes less abdominal bloating than $NaHCO_3$. The usual dose of Shohl's solution in adults is 25 to 50 ml daily—that is, 25 to 50 meq of alkali in divided doses. Calcium carbonate is a source of alkali, as well as of needed calcium, but constipation can be an annoying side effect.

Dietary protein restriction along with the administration of phosphate binders may restrict the availability of urinary phosphate and so markedly limit titratable acid excretion. This may impair net acid excretion and worsen acidosis. Patients receiving phosphate binders should be carefully monitored for this complication.

Despite this potential pathophysiologic consequence, the use of low-protein diets for amelioration of the progression of renal failure has become widespread. Protein stores are depleted in experimental uremia. The major cause of this depletion is the inhibition of insulin's normal stimulation of anabolism. Metabolic acidosis and dietary protein restriction may worsen the protein loss.[182a,182b] Others reported that the low protein diet may actually lessen the anti-anabolic effect of acidosis.[102c] Metabolic acidosis was corrected in chronically uremic patients compliant with a low-protein diet supplemented with essential amino acids and ketoanalogues, and renal-function decline was slowed.[22a] While some authors believe that ketoacid supplements slow progressive renal injury,[284a,284c] low nitrogen intake appears protective as well, by virtue of its prevention of tubulointerstitial damage, which occurs as a consequence of increased single-nephron ammonia production.[144a] It is recommended that all chronic renal failure patients on low-protein diets be closely monitored for their acid-base status and that metabolic acidosis be corrected to maximize positive nitrogen balance and maintenance of lean muscle mass.

Development of hyperchloremic acidosis in a uremic patient should alert physicians to the possibility of volume contraction or urinary tract obstruction (see above).[24] Hyperkalemia reduces bicarbonate reabsorption[16,152] and ammonia production.[170,274] Maher and coworkers have shown that correction of hyperkalemia by dietary potassium restriction can result in significant amelioration of metabolic acidosis in patients with chronic renal insufficiency and hyperkalemia.[170]

KETOACIDOSIS

The various forms of ketoacidosis are extensively discussed in Chap. 26.

LACTIC ACIDOSIS

Explosive in onset and often unyielding to therapy, lactic acidosis usually reflects the presence of an underlying disorder that, if left untreated, leads to death. Over the past quarter-century much has been learned regarding cellular intermediary metabolism and the causes of lactic acidosis. This section reviews current concepts of the biochemistry and kinetics of lactate turnover, the disorders that disrupt this homeostatic balance, and the therapies currently available.

The biochemistry of lactate and pyruvate metabolism (Fig. 25-7)

Lactic acid may be considered a metabolic "deadend" in that pyruvic acid, its only immediate precursor, is also its only route of metabolic transformation. Reduced nicotinamide adenine dinucleotide (NADH) undergoes oxidation when pyruvate is converted to lactate; conversely, the lactate dehydrogenase (LDH)–catalyzed conversion of lactate back to pyruvate entails reduction of the cofactor.

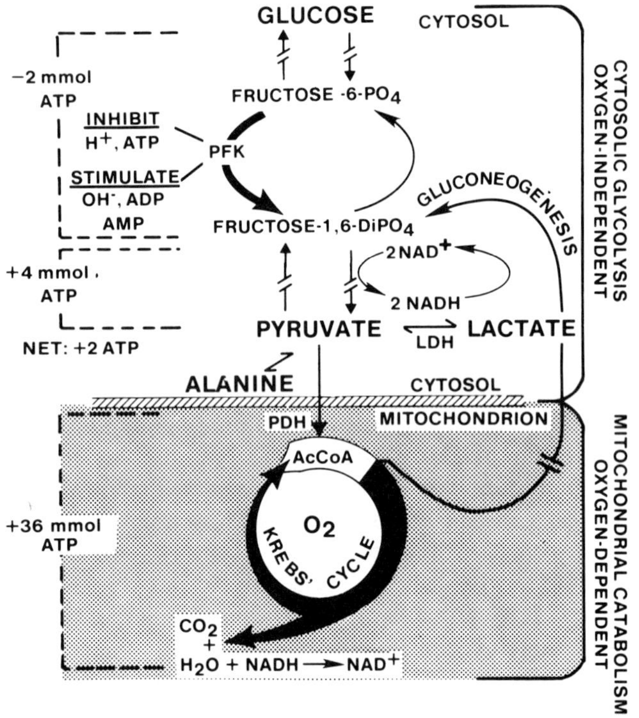

FIGURE 25-7 • Cytosolic and mitochondrial factors influending lactic acid production and utilization. The interplay is shown between the anaerobic glycolytic reactions forming pyruvate and lactate in the cytosol and the aerobic mitochondrial reactions that generate the bulk of high-energy phosphates and reoxidize reduced pyridines. The dynamics of this interaction are detailed in the text. Abbreviations: AcCoA, activated acetate; ADP, adenosine diphosphate; AMP, adenosine monophosphate; NAD+, oxidized nicotinamide adenine dinucleotide; NADH, reduced nicotinamide adenine dinucleotide; PDH, pyruvate dehydrogenase; PFK, phosphofructokinase; PO_4, phosphate.

$$\underset{\text{Pyruvate}}{H_3C{-}\overset{\overset{\displaystyle O}{\|}}{C}{-}\overset{\overset{\displaystyle O}{\|}}{C}{-}O^-} + H^+ + NADH \underset{\text{LDH}}{\rightleftharpoons} \underset{\text{Lactate}}{H_3C{-}\overset{\overset{\displaystyle HO}{|}}{C}{-}\overset{\overset{\displaystyle O}{\|}}{C}{-}O^-} + NAD^+ \quad (3)$$

Clearly, the availability of pyruvate, the pH, and the redox state of the cell are the key determinants of the lactate concentration. The mass action expression for equation 3 allows derivation of K_{eq}, the equilibrium constant (equation 4), which, in turn, yields equation 5 when solved for lactate.

$$K_{eq} = \frac{(\text{Lactate})(NAD^+)}{(\text{Pyruvate})(NADH)(H^+)} \quad (4)$$

$$\text{Lactate} = (K_{eq})\,(\text{Pyruvate})\,\frac{(NADH)}{(NAD^+)}\,(H^+) \quad (5)$$

From equation 5 it follows that three variables dictate the precise concentration of lactate: the pyruvate concentration, the NADH/NAD$^+$ ratio, and the hydrogen ion concentration. While the availability of NADH and protons determines the relative proportions of lactate and pyruvate, it is the net rate of pyruvate formation that ultimately exerts the greatest influence on lactate buildup. The normal lactate and pyruvate concentrations in plasma are 1.0 meq/liter and 0.25 meq/liter, respectively. Thus even the most favorable NADH/NAD$^+$ ratio or availability of protons would scarcely change the lactate concentration, in absolute terms, if the rate of pyruvate formation did not increase in concert with the enhanced conversion of pyruvate to lactate. Conditions that favor the accumulation of pyruvate very often simultaneously induce an increase in the NADH/NAD$^+$ ratio and a decrease in pH, prompting profound surges in lactate production.

Pyruvate is an intermediate compound common to several fundamental metabolic pathways (Fig. 25-7). Glucose and the amino acid alanine are the physiologically significant precursors of pyruvate. Pathological states that stimulate the conversion of glucose or alanine to pyruvate predispose to lactic acidosis. High rates of anaerobic glycolysis are particularly threatening in this regard. Oxygen-independent cytosolic glycolysis yields only 2 mmol of adenosine triphosphate (ATP) when 1 mmol of glucose is converted to 2 mmol of pyruvate (Fig. 25-7). Subsequently, complete mitochondrial oxidation of the 2 mmol of pyruvate generates 36 mmol of additional ATP. The enzyme pyruvate dehydrogenase (PDH) plays an integral role in this process by catalyzing the intramitochondrial conversion of pyruvate to acetyl CoA, thereby providing an entry point to Krebs' cycle and oxidation of pyruvate to CO_2 and water. Disease states such as shock or hypoxia deplete cells of ATP and impair the oxidative functions of the mitochondrion. Low levels of ATP increase glycolysis by deinhibiting such rate-limiting enzymes as phosphofructokinase (PFK) (Fig. 25-7). Without mitochondrial function, however, the rate of anaerobic glycolysis must increase enormously if cellular energy requirements are to be met and ATP stores repleted. Only 2 mmol of the potential 38 mmol of ATP derived from each millimole of glucose is formed anaerobically (Fig. 25-7). Furthermore, conversion of 1 mmol of glucose to 2 mmol of pyruvate generates 1 mmol of H$^+$ and reduces 2 mmol of NAD$^+$ to NADH. Thus anaerobic glycolysis increases the NADH/NAD$^+$ ratio, which, in the absence of aerobic Krebs' cycle activity, can be restored only by converting pyruvate to lactate (equation 3). Disorders impairing oxidative metabolism, therefore, set the stage for lactic acidosis in several ways. Glucose is rapidly catabolized to pyruvate; conversion of this pyruvate to lactate is assured by the accumulation of H$^+$ and the elevated NADH/NAD$^+$ ratio.

Oxidation of acetyl CoA, followed by entry into the Krebs' cycle, is not the sole metabolic fate of pyruvate (Fig. 25-7). This three-carbon intermediate may also be converted into fat or amino acids, or back to glucose (i.e., gluconeogenesis). Forces that prevent such transformations of pyruvate will also predispose to lactic acidosis.

Quantitative aspects of lactate turnover

Approximately 1400 mmol of lactic acid is produced endogenously and consumed daily by a typical human being.[50,52,150,247,295] Diffusion of the 1400 mmol of acid into the ECF destroys 1400 mmol of $NaHCO_3$, converting the alkali to sodium lactate. Hepatic oxidation of extracted sodium lactate regenerates lost bicarbonate in this cyclic process. This prodigious rate of turnover tends to be forgotten, because the normal blood lactate concentration approximates only 1 meq/liter. But if one considers that total daily H$^+$ excretion is normally less than 100 meq, then the great magnitude of lactate-related proton flux becomes clear. The 100 meq of net acid production is only a small fraction of the total traffic in protons. Skeletal muscle, skin, erythrocytes, and brain contribute most of the ongoing lactic acid load, while tissue uptake and catabolism occurs primarily in the liver and kidneys.[50]

The liver is likely to consume more lactate than any other organ. During lactic acidosis in dogs, up to 90 percent of total lactate extraction is effected by the liver.[52] The hepatic contribution to lactate clearance in normal, resting human beings is between 30 and 50 percent.[297] Thus it is not surprising that many patients with liver disease have elevated blood lactate concentrations and almost half of patients with lactic acidosis concomitantly demonstrate hepatic dysfunction.[6] Although these facts clearly underscore the liver's substantial role in lactate homeostasis, it is incorrect to conclude that hepatic failure and lactic acidosis are invariably linked. Kinetic calculations reveal that at a normal rate of lactate production even an abrupt, total cessation of lactate clearance by the liver would not result in a clinically significant acute lactic acidosis.[297] Presumably, enhanced extraction of lactate by extrahepatic tissues compensates for the loss of the liver's normal contribution. Yet lactic acidosis often strikes quickly—in fact, in the absence of toxin exposure, the development of severe acidemia and hypobicarbonatemia of less than 8 meq/liter suggests the presence of lactic acidosis. Only a profound and rapid increase in lactate synthesis can account for such acute hyperlactatemia, though liver disease and decreased utilization certainly would be expected to exacerbate the disorder.

The precise renal contribution to lactate removal in human beings is unknown; the renal contribution in rats has been estimated to be 16 percent.[300] The kidneys dispose of lactate in three ways: urinary excretion, gluconeogenesis, and oxidation. Only 0.4 mmol of lactate is normally excreted in the urine each day.[50] In human beings the threshold for urinary lactate excretion is between 6 and 10 meq/liter. This relatively high reabsorptive maximum ensures retention of synthesized lactate and maintenance of high blood levels. Because many of the experiments done to define the renal lactate threshold were carried out in volume-expanded animals, the threshold may actually be substantially higher.

Skeletal muscle may also dispose of circulating lactate,[4,295] but this hypothesis has been challenged.[52]

The ebb and flow of lactate production and consumption are exquisitely balanced under normal conditions. This potent acid accumulates, however, in disease states characterized by either a frenzied rate of glycolysis and lactic acid synthesis and/or diminished hepatic and renal consumption of the organic acid. Thus hepatic and renal failure may contribute importantly to the severity of lactic acidosis when production is stimulated by some pernicious underlying metabolic process.

Clinical aspects of lactic acidosis

The signs and symptoms resulting from severe acidemia have been described earlier and aptly apply to lactic acidosis.

Laboratory features (Table 25-5)

Lactic acid titration of blood buffers is recognized by its replacement of bicarbonate with lactate. If the clinically measurable bicarbonate is replaced by the usually unmeasured lactate anion, the anion gap increases. In our experience, a stoichiometric fall of bicarbonate and increase in lactate are routinely observed. The increment in blood lactate concentration will be matched by a virtually identical increment in the anion gap and decrement in serum HCO_3^- concentration, until the lactate level exceeds 17 meq/liter.[207] However, interpretation of the blood chemistries is often made more complex in patients sufficiently ill to develop lactic acidosis by the presence of multiple acid-base disorders—for example, concomitant respiratory alkalosis, diarrhea, or ketoacidosis. The reader is referred to Chap. 31 for a more detailed discussion of these mixed disorders. Other authors have claimed that the degree of hypobicarbonatemia often exceeds the increase in the anion gap.[202] For reasons outlined in Chap. 31, this chemical pattern generally suggests the presence of a mixed high- and normal-anion-gap acidosis, the alkali being replaced by a combination of some unmeasured anion and by chloride. Oh and coworkers offered that following titration of HCO_3^-, the lactate anion reentered cells, thereby erasing the increase in the anion gap while leaving the hypobicarbonatemia unchanged.[202]

TABLE 25-5 • Laboratory findings typically associated with lactic acidosis

Elevated anion gap
Hyperuricemia
Hyperphosphatemia
Leukocytosis
Normokalemia

Blood samples for lactate assays should be collected in tubes containing 10 mg of sodium fluoride and 2 mg of potassium oxalate, or rapidly precipitated with perchloric acid, to avoid continued in-vitro lactate synthesis by red blood cells.[240] Samples should be kept on ice until plasma is separated from unprecipitated specimens; this should be done within 15 min of collection. A lactate concentration in excess of 5 meq/liter denotes a significant metabolic perturbation (although *any* increase qualifies as an acidosis, by definition).

One study, in 1971, suggested that patients with lactic acidosis tend to *ventilate* in excess of the expected respiratory compensation for simple metabolic acidosis[233] (see above and Chap. 24). Fulop has convincingly demonstrated, however, that the vast majority of patients with lactic acidosis manifest arterial P_{CO_2} values well within the predicted 95 percent confidence band.[86]

Considerable *hyperuricemia* is often associated with lactic acidosis, because lactate, like other organic anions, competes with urate for secretion by the renal tubules, thereby competitively reducing urate excretion.[193] Another concomitant finding, *hyperphosphatemia*, may reflect widespread cellular phosphate efflux due to persistent, unreplenished ATP hydrolysis and tissue hypoxia.[201,282] Acidemia-induced *catecholamine release* prompts the demargination of white blood cells, causing the *leukocytosis* that so frequently accompanies lactic acidosis.[193,233] Lactic acidosis typically does *not* cause hyperkalemia (see above).[205] Unlike mineral acid anions (e.g., HCl), the lactate anion more readily permeates cell membranes. This cellular entry prevents the development of electrical gradients resulting from the isolated entry of H^+ into cells, which would favor the extrusion of the cationic potassium down its electrochemical gradient (see Chap. 6).[99]

Types of lactic acidosis

The life-threatening nature of lactic acidosis is underscored by the observation that increasing blood lactate concentrations prognosticate progressively higher mortality rates.[6] The physician must uncover the underlying cause of this metabolic derangement from a wide variety of diagnostic possibilities. Cohen and Woods classify the syndromes of lactic acidosis under two broad etiologic categories (types A and B), thereby providing a starting point for differential diagnosis (Table 25-6).[50]

TABLE 25-6 • Causes of lactic acidosis

TYPE A: CLINICALLY APPARENT TISSUE HYPOXIA
Cardiovascular insufficiency
Arterial oxygen desaturation
Profound anemia
Massive catecholamine excess
TYPE B: TISSUE OXYGENATION APPEARS NORMAL
Common disorders
Diabetes mellitus
Hepatic failure
Renal failure
Neoplasia
Seizures
Alkaloses
Drugs/toxins
Biguanide hypoglycemics
Ethanol
Methanol
Fructose
Sorbitol
Xylitol
Cyanide
Carbon monoxide
Streptozotocin
Salicylates
Isoniazid
Congenital enzymatic defects
Glucose-6-phosphatase deficiency
Fructose-1,6-diphosphatase deficiency
Pyruvate carboxylase deficiency
Pyruvate dehydrogenase deficiency
Methylmalonic aciduria
Miscellaneous
D-Lactic acidosis
Hypoglycemia

TYPE A LACTIC ACIDOSIS The term *type A lactic acidosis* refers to states characterized by clinically apparent, profound impairment of tissue oxygenation associated with hypotension, signs of poor tissue perfusion (e.g., cyanosis, cold extremities), or usually obvious arterial oxygen desaturation).[50] As discussed earlier, cellular hypoxia effects ATP depletion and markedly accelerates anaerobic glycolysis; accumulation of pyruvate and lactate shortly follows. Furthermore, dogs in shock states have been shown to increase their metabolism of carbohydrates and certain amino acids, which enhances pyruvate and lactate production.[57] The authors of these studies contend that shock can lead to lactic acidosis by altering intermediary metabolism independently of oxygen deficiency.

When a patient in frank shock develops hyperlactatemia it hardly requires the perspicacity of an Osler to decipher the cause of the disorder. Recognition of *incipient shock* as the cause of increasing blood lactate levels, on the other hand, is less straightforward, though also of considerable import. In this setting, arterial oxygen saturation and blood pressure are maintained within the broad limits of normal, albeit below the subject's basal value, despite tissue hypoperfusion. Peripheral and splanchnic vasoconstriction supports the blood pressure at the expense of tissue oxygen and substrate delivery. Peripheral vasoconstriction explains the increased synthesis of lactate, while the splanchnic vasoconstriction accounts for decreased hepatic clearance of lactate. Hence, when lactic acidosis rapidly unfolds in a seriously ill patient, blood pressure is only tenuously maintained. Physicians should interpret this chemical signal as portending the imminent onset of circulatory collapse. This is especially true for geriatric patients with severe infections. In this setting clinical observation must be intensified and therapy reevaluated.

Acute respiratory failure or sudden hypoxemia may precipitate profound lactic acidosis if the arterial saturation falls below 74 percent.[121] Lactic acidosis is uncommon, however, in chronically hypoxemic patients, because adaptations such as increases in erythrocyte 2,3-diphosphoglycerate (DPG, which facilitates hemoglobin's release of oxygen) and in the number of red blood cells protect against tissue hypoxia. Hyopxemic lung diseases that stimulate hyperventilation and respiratory alkalosis may cause mild increases in blood lactate concentration. The glycolytic enzyme phosphofructokinase (PFK) (Fig. 25-7) is stimulated by alkalosis, thereby increasing glycolysis and inducing a mild type B lactic acidosis (see below).

Severe anemia can cause type A lactic acidosis by impairing oxygen delivery to peripheral tissues and depressing cardiac performance. Anemia per se is a most unusual cause of type A lactic acidosis. In fact, the literature records only one case of lactic acidosis due solely to anemia.[50] *Iron deficiency* may contribute to lactic acidosis by an esoteric mechanism in addition to its role in producing anemia. Depletion of the iron-containing mitochondrial enzyme α-glycerophosphate oxidase impedes oxygen-dependent glycolysis.[78]

Case reports suggest that *catecholamine excess*, in the pharmacologic range, can lead to lactic acidosis. A young man who attempted suicide by intravenous injection of 20 mg of epinephrine was found to be cyanotic, "enormously constricted peripherally," and hyperlactatemic.[147] A patient with adrenaline and noradrenaline elevations 5000 times normal, due to pheochromocytoma, also has been reported with lactic acidosis (blood lactate 18 meq/liter).[141] The authors deemed the latter example a case of type B lactic acidosis on the basis of maintained blood pressure and ventilation. However, we interpret the reported pale skin, cold extremites, and hypertension as signs of peripheral vasoconstriction compatible with a type A diagnosis.

TYPE B LACTIC ACIDOSIS Lactic acidosis in the absence of any physical signs of hypoxemia or circulatory insufficiency is termed *type B*. Such cases were often labeled "spontaneous" or "idiopathic" during the period of Huckabee's pioneering reports in the early 1960s. Since then many specific causes of type B lactic acidosis have been recognized (Table 25-6). In some cases, mechanisms such as defective mitochondrial utilization of normally delivered oxygen and diseased intermediary metabolic pathways have been elucidated. It is instructive to review the most prevalent causes of type B lactic acidosis.

Diabetes mellitus (see Chap. 26) sets the stage for lactate accumulation in several ways. Insulin normally activates pyruvate dehydrogenase, the rate-limiting enzyme for the oxidation of pyruvate (Fig. 25-7). Insulinopenia causes a build-up of pyruvate, which in turn is converted to lactate. Insulin deficiency also provokes muscle catabolism, providing more alanine to serve as additional substrate for pyruvate synthesis. Ten to fifteen percent of acutely ill diabetic patients have blood lactate levels greater than 5 meq/liter,[193] and the diabetic predisposition to lactic acidosis seems particularly heightened during ketoacidotic episodes. Increases in the intracellular $NADH/NAD^+$ ratio, hypoperfusion, and increased H^+ concentration accompany the volume depletion and acidemia of diabetic ketoacidosis (DKA). Volume expansion using an isotonic fructose solution to treat DKA can worsen the lactic acidosis. *Fructose* does not require insulin for cellular uptake and enters the glycolytic pathway downstream from the rate-controlling enzyme, PFK. The resulting marked increase in glycolysis begets an accumulation of pyruvate and lactate, which further lowers serum bicarbonate levels. Lastly, *phenformin* and other biguanide oral hypoglycemic medications interfere with the membrane function of renal and hepatic mitochondria, causing lactic acidosis.[85] Prior to its removal from the market, phenformin was a rather common cause of lactic acidosis.

Patients with *hepatic or renal failure* are at increased risk of lactic acidosis when stressed by pathological lactate burdens. This predisposition is due to limitations on their ability to clear lactate, as discussed earlier. The incidence of net overproduction of lactate increases if a patient with liver failure develops an associated respiratory alkalosis, since the latter stimulates glycolysis via the PFK reaction (see above). Also, advanced stages of kidney and liver failure often lead to sepsis or hypovolemia, with their attendant risks of inadequate tissue perfusion and excess lactate synthesis.

A variety of *malignancies* have been associated with lactic acidosis, including lymphoma, leukemia,[34,76,182] Hodgkin's disease,[191] reticulum cell sarcoma,[131] and oat cell carcinoma of the lung.[265] Chemotherapy of the underlying malignancy often alleviates the lactic acidosis. Neoplasia elicits lactic acidosis by several mechanisms. Although the healthy liver can readily metabolize large infusions of lactate, tumor overproduction of lactate from glucose may prove overwhelming.[34,76,191] Certain neoplasms release tryptophan metabolites that have been postulated to inhibit lactate utilization.[258] Extensive hepatic infiltration by tumor can, of course, interfere with lactate clearance, and other organs may become hypoxic and overproduce lactate when packed with cancerous cells.

Other authors have observed, further, that large soft-tissue tumors may induce striking degrees of *hypoglycemia*, with concomitant lactic acidosis.[77,80,107] The hypoglycemia has been alternately attributed to excess tumor consumption of glucose, diminished glucose release by the liver, tumor elaboration of an insulinlike compound, and tumor-associated glucagon deficiency.[257] The relationship between hypoglycemia and hyperlactatemia, in general, is equally complex. Medalle and coworkers set forth a reasonable explanation, predicated on a setting of liver dysfunction, which we have illustrated in Fig. 25-8.[179] Hypoglycemia can ensue from inadequate caloric intake, once glycogen stores have been depleted. Excessive tumor utilization of glucose and its elaboration of putative inhibitors of gluconeogenesis worsens hypoglycemia. Advancing hepatic decompensation further reduces gluconeogenesis and impairs glycogenolysis, thereby perpetuating the hypoglycemia. Hypoglycemic reduction in liver function also occurs, which further prevents extraction of circulating lactate. The lactate levels are further elevated because hypoglycemia prompts epinephrine secretion, which stimulates extrahepatic lactate production. Hypoglycemia may suppress insulin release and so cause ketoacidosis. The serum bicarbonate concentration then falls, on account of the accumulation

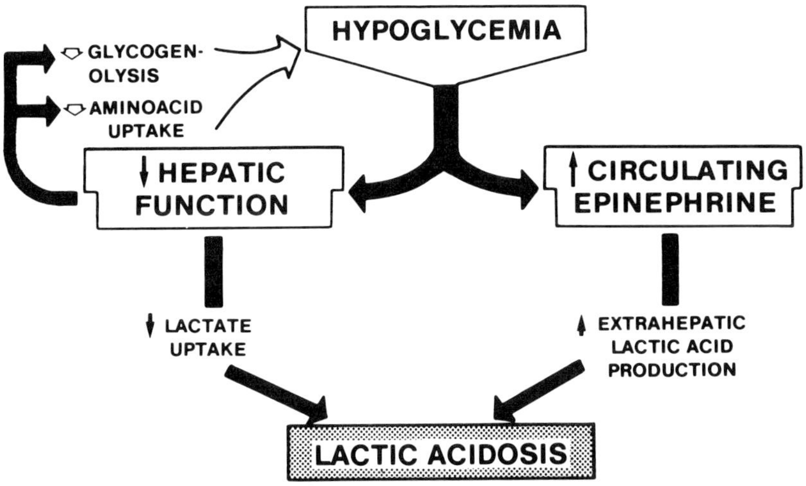

FIGURE 25-8 • Hypoglycemic lactic acidosis. Schematic depiction of how hypoglycemia could facilitate net overproduction of lactic acid. (See text for details.)

of both organic acids. In the absence of cancer, the entire hypoglycemic process may be readily reversed by glucose administration.[169,179] Paradoxically, one case report describes a young woman with a bulky, differentiated carcinoma who developed dramatic lactic acidosis only in response to the administration of hypertonic glucose.[98] It appears that her tumor avidly converted the glucose to lactate. *Acetaminophen* toxicity, especially in patients with preexisting liver disease, is another cause of hypoglycemic lactic acidosis.[193] Prompt therapy with *N*-acetylcysteine can be life-saving in this setting.

Grand mal seizures result in maximal rates of skeletal muscle anaerobic glycolysis. An acute surge of lactate flows from the apneic patient's hypoxic contracting muscles into the blood. The hyperlactatemia lasts only 1 to 2 h in the absence of recurrent seizure activity, because hepatic lactate clearance is brisk. Serum lactate levels and acid-base parameters normalize within 1 h after a single grand mal seizure.[205]

Ingestion of *ethanol* typically does not raise the blood lactate concentration above 3 meq/liter. Hepatic lactate uptake is decreased.[151] Ethanol and *methanol* may produce lactic acidosis via inhibition of gluconeogenesis, with resultant hypoglycemia and peripheral lactate overproduction. Many other drugs and toxins occasionally induce lactic acidosis by interfering with mitochondrial enzyme functions (Table 25-6).

Carbon monoxide (CO) poisoning, usually from smoke inhalation, may lead to clinically inapparent arterial oxygen desaturation, tissue hypoxia, and lactic acidosis. Tissue delivery of oxygen is impaired for two reasons: First, CO's greater affinity for hemoglobin displaces oxygen, thereby decreasing arterial oxygen saturation while the P_{CO_2} remains normal. Second, the accumulation of carboxyhemoglobin causes the oxyhemoglobin dissociation curve to shift to the left (i.e., hemoglobin's affinity for oxygen is increased).[79a,237a] Therapy consists of administering 100% oxygen; hyperbaric oxygen is used in severe cases.[190a] *Cyanide* poisons the mitochondrial cytochrome oxidase system, thereby limiting oxidative metabolism and stimulating glycolysis subsequent to ATP depletion; severe lactic acidosis ensues. Nitroprusside therapy is known to cause cyanide accumulation as a side effect and thus has been tentatively linked to at least one case of lactic acidosis.[122]

The *congenital enzymatic defects* that beget recurrent lactic acidosis are rare pediatric diseases. Their victims must adhere to stringent restrictions of muscular activity or diet because of their limited capacity for carbohydrate metabolism.[37]

Two optical isomers of lactic acid, the D and L forms, are differentiated on the basis of the configuration of the four substituents forming a tetrahedron about the middle carbon atom (Fig. 25-9). The LDH present in mammalian cells synthesizes only the L-isomer. In human beings the trivial quantities of D-lactate that appear in blood and the urine are absorbed from food, produced in the GI tract by certain lactobacilli, or infused intravenously on surgical services where Ringer's lactate (a racemic mixture of D- and L-lactate) abounds.[50] Experimental infusions of the two isomers have revealed that D-lactate is cleared more slowly than its enantiomer and that the presence of the D-isomer significantly prolongs the half-life of the normal L-lactate.[52] Preparations of the pure L-isomer would be preferable to the racemically mixed (i.e., having equal concentrations of the D and L enantiomers) solutions currently administered to patients during peritoneal di-

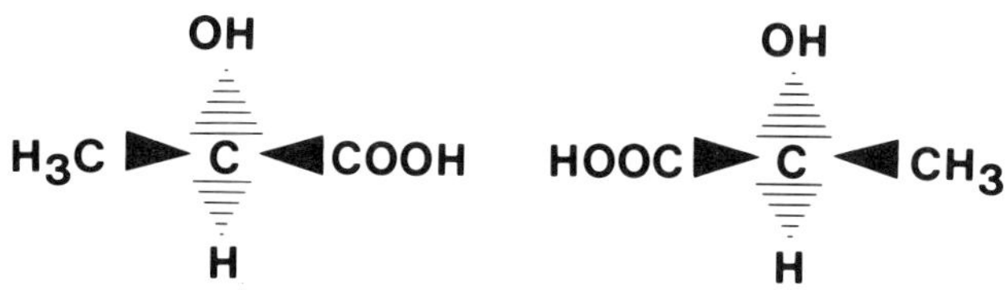

FIGURE 25-9 • Formulas of the D- and L- enantomers of lactic acid. (See text for details.)

alysis and surgical procedures (e.g., Ringer's and Hartman's solutions).

D-*Lactic acidosis* is being detected with increasing frequency in patients with short bowel syndromes who develop overgrowth of D-lactic acid-producing bacteria.[203,217,238,255,270,271] Commonly, these individuals have eaten foods rich in lactobacilli, such as yogurt and sauerkraut (hopefully not both at once). An accompanying neurologic condition tends to distinguish this acidosis. Weakness, ataxia, slurred speech, and confusion are often combined with bizarre behavior. These findings do not necessarily correlate with blood levels of D-lactate. Other absorbed bacterial products may underlie the neuropathology. Routine laboratory lactate assays employ an LDH enzyme that is specific for L-lactate. Therefore, a high-anion-gap acidosis caused by D-lactic acid specifies that measurement with D-LDH is necessary. Oral administration of poorly absorbable antibiotics (e.g., vancomycin) has proved beneficial in eliminating the pathological bacteria, although some authors contend that simply reducing food intake may be adequate treatment.[109] A recent paper indicates that increased urinary D-lactate excretion results from necrotizing enterocolitis in infants, providing a potentially valuable diagnostic test for that disorder.[89]

Treatment of lactic acidosis

To be effective, therapy of all forms of metabolic acidosis must be directed at the underlying cause of acid overproduction or underexcretion, or bicarbonate wasting; at the same time it must supply enough alkali to reduce the disorder's immediate lethality. Merely giving bicarbonate without removing the cause of ongoing lactic acid production would be like treating DKA without insulin, or giving aspirin without antibiotics to febrile septic patients. It cannot be overemphasized that the patient's survival ultimately will depend on diagnosis and therapy of the *underlying cause* of the lactic acidosis. Type A lactic acidosis demands vigorous resuscitation to restore tissue oxygenation, whereas specific therapy of type B lactic acidosis depends on the given diagnosis (e.g., cancer chemotherapy for malignancy associated disease, or antiseizure medications for the acidosis associated with this disorder).

Sodium bicarbonate (for further discussion see Chap. 26)

Arrhythmias and cardiovascular collapse result from severe acidemia (see above). Hence we advocate the use of intravenous $NaHCO_3$ for patients suffering lactic acidosis if the arterial pH decreases to values below 7.20. Bicarbonate administration should be adjusted to maintain arterial pH between 7.20 and 7.25, since the adverse hemodynamic consequences of acidemia emerge at pH values less than 7.20. Lactate production and clearance rates are so unpredictable that alkali titration must be tailored to each individual's needs and reassessed with great frequency. In severely acidemic settings therapy with boluses of sodium bicarbonate is followed by infusions, the rates of which are adjusted on the basis of resulting changes in the patient's acid-base parameters. "Overshoot" alkalosis caused by overzealous $NaHCO_3$ therapy may further stimulate lactate production, lower the seizure threshold, or impair cardiovascular function. It must be avoided. The additive effects of exogenous alkali plus endogenous metabolic conversion of lactate to bicarbonate may cause frank hyperbicarbonatemia. Avoidance of this complication can be achieved by carefully following two key parameters. The increment in the anion gap (ΔAG)—that is, the number of meq/liter) by which the observed anion gap exceeds normal (observed anion gap minus 10 to 12 meq/liter)—closely reflects the circulating concentration of lactate in patients with a pure, simple lactic acidosis. With removal of the stimulus for continuing lactic acid overproduction, the serum lactate (i.e., ΔAG) will be converted to HCO_3. Thus an anion gap of 30 meq/liter corresponds to a ΔAG of approximately 20 meq/liter, the conversion of which to alkali could potentially increase the serum bicarbonate concentration by 20 meq/liter. With appropriate respiratory compensation a serum bicarbonate concentration of 10 meq/liter should sustain an arterial pH of approximately 7.25. We suggest, therefore, that enough alkali be administered to sustain a serum level of only 10 meq/liter. In the reparative phase, endogenous synthesis of 10 to 20 meq/liter of bicarbonate from oxidized lactate will restore a serum bicarbonate level that has been maintained at 10 meq/liter to maximal values of only 20 to 30 meq/liter. In this matter more dangerous degrees of "overshoot" alkalosis are avoided. Potent diuretics are often required to avoid the volume overload resulting from the large quantities of sodium bicarbonate often needed. At times dialysis will be required, and a bicarbonate bath is obviously a superior choice to either lactate or acetate. The latter two anions are poorly metabolized to bicarbonate in this setting. The bicarbonate bath alkalinizes the blood more rapidly and induces hypotension less often than a lactate or acetate bath.

Theoretical objections have been raised to the use of $NaHCO_3$ in treating lactic acidosis. These concerns are largely focused on alkali's potential for further stimulating lactic acid synthesis and on potential adverse end-organ effects of bicarbonate.[13,193] These theoretical issues, derived primarily from rather unique animal models of lactic acidosis, are of interest, but in our opinion they are not likely to have any bearing on the human condition. Pichette and coworkers convincingly argue that the blood lactate concentration can rise by 50 percent solely on the basis of nonionic diffusion, with a lactate *shift* from the ICF to the ECF, following the development of an alkali-triggered favorable pH gradient.[221] Such lactate redistribution by no means represents an increase in net lactate accumulation. It would be expected to elevate blood lactate concentration only temporarily and with no concomitant increase in circulating H^+ concentration.

Mixtures of sodium carbonate and sodium bicarbonate (Carbicarb)

The titration of protons with HCO_3^- generates carbon dioxide.

$$HCO_3^- + H^+ \rightleftharpoons H_2CO_3 \rightleftharpoons CO_2 + H_2O \quad (6)$$

Because CO_2 instantly enters the ICF, whereas HCO_3^- enters more slowly, the increasing bicarbonatemia and CO_2 production that attend alkali therapy may paradoxically, although transiently, acidify the intracellular milieu. With well-preserved cardiopulmonary function, little change in P_{CO_2} accompanies even rapid administration of large quantities of $NaHCO_3$. Nonetheless, many patients with severe lactic acidosis have depressed myocardial function, hypotension, and diminished pulmonary flow. In this setting CO_2 generated from endogenous metabolism and from administered alkali tends to accumulate in the peripheral venous blood.[286a] Indeed, in cardiovascular collapse, the normal disparity in pH, P_{CO_2}, and HCO_3^- concentration between mixed venous blood (i.e., returning from the tissues) and peripheral arterial blood (i.e., oxygenated and cleared of excess CO_2 by passage through the lungs) becomes exaggerated.[286a] For example, during cardiopulmonary resuscitation, simultaneous sampling of mixed venous and femoral arterial blood revealed equivalent and relatively normal concentrations of HCO_3^-; but because the mixed venous P_{CO_2} was approximately twice that in the femoral artery, venous pH was less than 7.15, despite a normal peripheral arterial pH.[3b,3c,286a] The decreased rate of return of venous blood to the lungs allowed the CO_2 to accumulate, whereas the diminished volume of blood passing through the lungs was oxygenated and cleared of CO_2, yielding the more normal chemistries seen in the peripheral arterial blood. Bicarbonate therapy exaggerated these differences.[3b,3c] It follows that in the setting of shock, blood gases from *both* circulations must be assessed to adequately define pulmonary and acid-base status. Furthermore, unless cardiac output can be improved, bicarbonate therapy in this setting may prove detrimental.

Alkali therapy would be improved if its generation of CO_2 could be minimized. Adding Na_2CO_3 to $NaHCO_3$ may accomplish this end.

$$Na_2CO_3 + H_2O + CO_2 \rightleftharpoons 2HCO_3^- + 2Na^+ \quad (7)$$

In effect, the carbonate (CO_3^{2-} "absorbs" CO_2 as it forms bicarbonate. The commercial preparation Carbicarb incorporates equimolar amounts of Na_2CO_3 and $NaHCO_3$ (0.33 *M* of each).[77a] Thus the mixture has the same alkalinizing effect as a 1-*M* $NaHCO_3$ solution but generates only two-thirds as much CO_2. While early observations in experimental acidoses suggest that the mixture may be helpful,[90a] there are not yet enough studies with human beings to justify its widespread use.

Dichloroacetate

Dichloroacetate (DCA) is a potentially important ancillary medication in the therapy of lactic acidosis. PDH activity is stimulated by DCA, leading to the oxidative conversion of pyruvate and lactate to bicarbonate. DCA also brought about a threefold increase in the rate of pyruvate metabolism by cardiac muscle in only 10 min in an in-vitro rat preparation.[288] This may account for the immediate improvement in cardiac output and blood pressure seen in human beings with lactic acidosis upon infusion of DCA. These hemodynamic effects precede any change in serum pH, HCO_3^- concentration, or lactate concentration.[267] The drug markedly lowers the morbidity and mortality of experimental lactic acidosis in dogs.[14,212] In a group of 29 patients with lactic acidosis given DCA, blood lactate levels declined by more than 20 percent in 23 patients. This occurred within 4 to 6 h after therapy.[267] Responders had a 43 percent mortality rate within 48 h of DCA therapy, whereas nonresponders had a 100 percent mortality rate. In the absence of a control group this observation is uninterpretable. It is possible that only persons with more mild disease can respond to DCA. The 43 percent mortality rate increased to 92 percent, with only 2 of 23 responders eventually leaving the hospital.[267] This observation again underscores the importance of treating the precipitating disease in addition to any of its manifestations (e.g., lactic acidosis).

The importance of bicarbonate and DCA therapy is that they may, by diminishing the likelihood of early death from acidemia, give physicians the time needed to effectively treat the potentially lethal disorder causing the acidosis.

Thiamine

Thiamine is a cofactor of PDH. For a patient with lactic acidosis who may be vitamin-deficient (e.g., an alcoholic), thiamine is a safe medication that may provide great benefit. In patients with full-blown Shoshin beriberi, lactic acidosis is common. Here thiamine corrects the metabolic acidosis by improving cardiac output and tissue perfusion, in addition to its fulfilling PDH's need for the cofactor.[19] Finally, thiamine is useful both therapeutically and diagnostically in cases of congenital PDH or pyruvate carboxylase deficiencies.[37]

Insulin

Insulin stimulates the activity of PDH. Furthermore, its anabolic effects include the inhibition of alanine mobilization; this decreases the availability of one substrate for pyruvate and lactate production. Patients with persistent type B lactic acidosis may benefit from low-dose hourly insulin administration with dextrose. However, it is important to avoid loss of glycemic control, which would exacerbate the generation of pyruvate and lactate.

TOXIC INGESTANTS

Salicylates

With more than 200 products on the market that contain salicylates, either as aspirin (acetylsalicylic acid, or ASA) or as one of its congeners, the potential for acute or chronic intoxication with this compound is enormous—especially given its use for many different medical indications.[157a] In light of this enormous consumption and potential for abuse, it is not surprising that salicylate intoxication is a frequently encountered and major cause of drug-induced morbidity and mortality. Toxic manifestations often present as diagnostic challenges, because of the widespread effects of the drug on the CNS, lungs, gastrointestinal mucosa, hemostasis, renal function, and acid-base balance, and the interaction of salicylates with other medications. More recently, salicylates have been implicated in the pathogenesis of Reye's syndrome; however, this remains controversial.[57a,122a]

Pharmacologic and biochemical principles

The gastrointestinal absorption of aspirin depends on several factors. The pH of the stomach, the pK_a of ASA, and the "form" of aspirin—namely, "coated" or "uncoated" tablets—all dictate the rapidity and completeness of absorption. The rate of gastric emptying and the presence of food also determine the degree of absorption. However, the rate of tablet dissolution is the rate-limiting factor. With large ingestions, as may occur in a suicide attempt, aspirin may precipitate into concretions; this slows absorption and delays toxicity. In the acid milieu of the stomach, aspirin is poorly soluble; the pK_a of ASA is only 3.0, which dictates that only 50 percent of an ingested quantity will be in the un-ionized, freely diffusible form. However, rapid and complete absorption may obtain whenever the compound is taken with antacids. In this circumstance absorption proceeds through the mucosa of the small intestine, despite its relatively alkaline environment, because of its large surface area. In blood, in the wall of the gastrointestinal tract, and during passage through the liver ASA is hydrolyzed to acetic and salicylic acids. The hepatic "first-pass" effect is substantial for therapeutic ingestions.[164,266] The short half-life of ASA (15 to 20 min) is prolonged to 2 to 3 h following its conversion to salicylic acid. The latter's half-life is dose-dependent, increasing to 20 h when more than 300 mg is ingested.[164] Virtually all aspirin ingested can be recovered quantitatively from the urine, primarily in the form of aspirin's metabolites.[163] Hepatic metabolism of ASA is important at therapeutic doses; however, renal excretion becomes more important whenever supratherapeutic ingestions occur. ASA's principal metabolite and excretory product is the glycine conjugate, salicyluric acid. Salicylic acid may also combine with glucuronic acid to form salicylphenolic glucuronide or salicylacylglucuronide. A small percentage of salicylic acid is metabolized to gentisic acid. When ASA doses exceed 4 to 6 g/day the glycine and glucuronide detoxification pathways are overwhelmed, allowing salicylic acid to accumulate.[162,164] When low doses of ASA are administered, less than 15 percent is excreted as salicylic acid; but this figure increases to 50 percent when glycine and glucuronide pathways are saturated and salicylate kinetics for disposition switch from first-order to zero-order, allowing salicylic acid to accumulate.[161a,162,164] Additionally, aging decreases the rate of metabolism of salicylates—an effect apparently related to the drug's decreased serum protein binding.[266d,300b]

Unimpeded glomerular filtration followed by tubular reabsorption and secretion characterizes the renal handling of salicylate. Urinary excretion reflects the net balance between tubular reabsorption and secretion. Tubular processing of the drug can be regulated and forms the basis of the therapeutic approach to ASA toxicity (see below). Salicylic acid's pK_a is 3.0, indicating that this strong acid is almost entirely ionized at the relatively alkaline pH of normal blood. Indeed, at pH 7.40, the ratio of ionized to un-ionized aspirin (i.e., of salicylate to salicylic acid) is approximately 25,000 to 1. The acid's state of ionization profoundly changes its ability to permeate cell membranes. The un-ionized species freely penetrates cell membranes and therefore readily undergoes tubular reabsorption. It follows that when ECF and glomerular filtrate are acidified, more salicylate is converted to salicylic acid and therefore more easily passes into tubular cells, leading to renal retention. Systemic and urinary acidification markedly enhances toxicity by reducing excretion and by increasing salicylate's accessibility to intracellular fluid. Conversely, alkalinity affords therapeutic benefit by decreasing the ratio of un-ionized to ionized salicylate, thereby trapping more drug in the ECF and the tubular lumen. Increased salicylate excretion and diminished exposure of intracellular fluid to the drug act to ameliorate toxicity. As urinary pH is progressively increased above 7.00, the rate of salicylate excretion approaches and then exceeds that of filtration, highlighting the stimulation of net secretion by alkalinization.[103]

Uricosuria is mildly inhibited when serum salicylate levels are low (below 5 mg/100 ml), but striking uricosuria occurs with higher drug concentrations. This biphasic response results from the fact that low serum concentrations of salicylate inhibit uric acid secretion, whereas higher salicylate levels inhibit the quantitatively more important reabsorptive process.

In a group of divergent disease states (e.g., cirrhosis, sytemic lupus erythematosus, and chronic renal failure), and in states characterized by decreased effective arterial blood volume,[220,223] maintenance of the GFR becomes increasingly more dependent on enhanced *renal prostaglandin synthesis*.[30,246,301] The vasodilatory prostaglandins offset the vasoconstrictive effects of locally produced angiotensin II, thereby limiting the net vasoconstrictive effect provoked by these disorders.[198] Aspirin, like other nonsteroidal anti-inflammatory drugs, inhibits prostaglandin synthesis, unmasking angiotensin's total vasoactive potential. This effect is mediated by the irreversible acetylation of cyclooxygenase, the pivotal enzyme in the formation of the vasodilatory prostaglandins PGI and PGE.[33a,198a] Renal vascular resistance increases and *GFR may transiently decline*.[30,246,301]

Salicylates may exert either a *hyper-* or a *hypoglycemic* effect in normal and diabetic adults.[22,54,165,250] Other findings include transient abnormalities of *liver function tests*, especially in patients with collagen vascular disorders, and a prolonged bleeding time.[277]

Several disparate effects of salicylate conspire to induce complex *acid-base changes*. In toxic doses aspirin has been shown to strongly influence CO_2 production and excretion and to markedly alter endogenous fixed acid production. Salicylates have been shown to increase ventilation, causing *respiratory alkalosis* by a direct action on the CNS.[278] Injection of aspirin into the cerebrospinal fluid evokes marked degrees of hyperventilation in the absence of measurable arterial concentrations of the drug.[278] This direct action, plus aspirin's enhancement of CNS sensitivity to CO_2, accounts for the hyperventilation seen in salicylate-intoxicated patients.[7] A peripheral chemoreceptor stimulation has been demonstrated in rats.[178a] By uncoupling oxidative phosphorylation, aspirin removes a major restraint on oxygen consumption and CO_2 production that is generally overridden by drug-induced stimulation of alveolar ventilation. The net result of these two offsetting forces is to reduce arterial P_{CO_2}. Paradoxically, *respiratory acidosis* may occur when salicylism develops in patients with preexisting pulmonary disease or in those simultaneously ingesting respiratory depressants. Failure of alveolar ventilation to increase while CO_2 generation increases accounts for this unexpected effect of aspirin.[263]

The *high-anion-gap metabolic acidosis* associated with aspirin overdose is well known, but its pathogenesis has not been well defined. Accumulating salicylate anions account for part of the increased anion gap; the remainder apparently reflects stimulated production of various organic anions. Although no single organic acid has been consistently incriminated, lactate and ketoanions have been shown, on occasion, to play major roles.[261,263,294] It is the toxic effects of salicylate on various enzymes and on oxidative phosphorylation that presumably increase net production of numerous organic acids.[263]

In children the effects of salicylates on acid-base balance are different from those seen in adults. Children, especially those under 6 years of age, are more frequently acidemic and ketonuric.[261,294] The anion gap in children is often elevated to more than 20 meq/liter.[294] As with adults (see below), children receiving CNS depressants along with salicylates have the lowest blood pH values. In a series of 33 children with salicylate intoxication, 4 of 5 with arterial pH below 7.20 had ingested either phenobarbital or phenylsalicylate, or had a primary pulmonary process that compromised ventilation.[294] Adult patients usually have a normal-to-alkaline arterial pH[227]; indeed, in a series of 67 adults a mixed metabolic acidosis–respiratory alkalosis was the most frequently observed acid-base disorder (seen in 56 percent).[87] Twenty-two percent of those ingesting only salicylates developed a pure respiratory alkalosis.[87] When other drugs, especially CNS depressants, were ingested, respiratory alkalosis was less frequent; these patients tended to be more acidemic.[87] Respiratory acidosis occurred only in the group ingesting multiple drugs. Indeed, significant acidemia in an adult with salicylate intoxication usually implies either additional drug ingestion or an underlying disease compromising ventilation.[87,227]

Clinical features of toxicity

The clinical features of aspirin overdose vary according to age and duration of aspirin exposure. The diagnosis of salicylate intoxication in young adults is hardly challenging, since in most cases there is a history of exposure or an evident empty aspirin bottle. In infants and small children, intoxication usually is a complication of overzealous therapy of a febrile illness. This iatrogenically induced disorder is also quite evident. More elusive, however, is the diagnosis of accidental or deliberate intoxication in older patients. These subjects generally have underlying diseases requiring chronic salicylate therapy. The very signs of overdosage may mimic the underlying disease for which aspirin was given. A recent study showed that the diagnosis of salicylate intoxication in the elderly is often delayed for 6 to 72 h (30 percent of cases). The elderly often present with nonfocal neurologic signs such as lethargy, agitation, confusion, and tachypnea, and are often misdiagnosed as having cardiopulmonary insufficiency or an encephalopathy. As one would anticipate, this group manifests higher rates of morbidity and mortality.[9]

With recent ingestion symptoms may be absent at first, but they develop soon and increase in severity with time. Hyperpnea is particularly common. CNS manifestations are nonfocal; they include tinnitus, agitation, lethargy, seizure, and coma, and do not correlate well with blood levels of salicylate.[59,227]

The physical findings of salicylate intoxication vary. Aspirin-induced fever occurs most often in small children. CNS findings are diffuse and may range from disorientation to coma. Asterixis has been noted in some patients.[10] Noncardiogenic pulmonary edema,[102b,116] vomiting, and gastrointestinal hemorrhage may also occur. Acute renal failure is a rare occurrence with acute ingestion.[42] Salicylate-induced clotting abnormalities may cause ecchymoses and mucosal bleeding. Any and all of the above may occur in the setting of Reye's syndrome.

Diagnosis of salicylate intoxication

The diagnosis of salicylate ingestion can be made by the addition of 1 ml of 10% ferric chloride to 3 ml of urine. A purple color develops within 30 min in the presence of salicylates. The test is very sensitive, however, yielding a positive reaction after ingestion of only one 320-mg tablet.[139] The urinalysis may show proteinuria, tubular cells, and granular casts.

Salicylate intoxication should be considered in any patient with a high-anion-gap acidosis of obscure etiology. This is especially true when the acidosis is accompanied by a superimposed respiratory alkalosis—that is, when the P_{CO_2} is lower than predicted by the degree of hypobicarbonatemia (see above and Chap. 31). Note that salicylate levels correlate poorly with the severity of clinical presentation, because of the variable time lag from ingestion to hospitalization. In one series, salicylate metabolism was shown to follow first-order kinetics in 17 previously well patients suffering salicylate intoxication.[59] When peack salicylate levels were calculated, patients could be stratified into separate groups relating symptoms at the time of presentation to peak levels. Peak levels were calculated with the formula:

$$\log S_c = \log S^* + 0.015\,T \qquad (8)$$

where S_c is the peak level, S^* is the level at the time of presentation, and T is time, in hours, post-ingestion. With this calculation it was shown that all fatalities occurred when peak levels exceeded 160 mg/100 ml. However, when peak levels were 100 mg/100 ml, the patients demonstrated severe lethargy, seizures, and coma.[9]

Ingestion of enteric-coated aspirin presents unique diagnostic and therapeutic problems. In this setting initial serum levels may not accurately reflect the severity of toxic exposure. The enteric coating is designed to resist dissolution by stomach acid and to dissolve rapidly when exposed to alkaline intestinal secretions. Because of erratic and delayed gastric emptying, salicylism may develop suddenly when accumulated enteric-coated tablets pass into the alkaline duodenum. Serum kinetics will be grossly different with the new enteric-coated aspirin than with regular tablets, as demonstrated by a recent case report.[154] The use of initial serum levels after ingestion of 30 g of enteric-coated aspirin would have predicted an asymptomatic event. However, peak levels were not reached until more than 24 h after ingestion, and the patient underwent a stormy course belying the benign response predicted by the low salicylate concentrations found early in the course.[154] The formation of gastric concretions, delayed gastric emptying, and delayed salicylate metabolism from hepatic dysfunction may also delay the appearance of maximal serum salicylate levels.[266a]

Assessment of the severity of aspirin intoxication requires careful attention to the quantity ingested, the time elapsed between ingestion and discovery, and whether regular or enteric-coated drug was taken. As always, clinical assessment of the patient is crucial to the evaluation.

Therapy

Therapy should begin with correction of any existing fluid deficits, and *the stomach should be emptied* by induction of emesis in children or by gastric lavage in adults. Because aspirin delays gastric emptying, the stomach should be emptied even if intoxication is discovered 6 to 12 h after ingestion.[162] Since lavage cannot remove small bowel contents, intestinal absorption will continue, causing serum salicylate levels to increase for as long as 24 h after ingestion. To counter this delayed absorption, adults should receive 50 g of *activated charcoal.* Charcoal therapy should be repeated several times at 4-h intervals to help reduce the plasma salicylate's half-life.[118a] A cathartic is recommended by some authors to purge the intestine after charcoal administration.[277] In comatose patients gastric lavage is hazardous without endotracheal intubation.

For overdosage of enteric-coated aspirin tablets, treatment plans have included gastric lavage with a sodium bicarbonate solution. The latter dissolves the tablets in the stomach; the slurry is then removed by lavage.[154] Undissolved tablets form a fringe around the top of the slurry. Indeed, the astute physician will immediately recognize the "slurry with the fringe on top." Other authors point out that this use of enteral bicarbonate may be dangerous, since alkali can enhance salicylate absorption.[64a]

Since urinary excretion affords the only practical route for salicylate elimination, therapies have been developed that enhance renal disposal. Renal drug clearance increased when urinary volume and pH were simultaneously increased.[56,157] The principles of nonionic diffusion (see above) demand that aspirin excretion increase as urinary alkalinity increases. The hypocapnia that usually complicates salicylism reduces tubular bicarbonate reabsorption, ensuring that the fractional excretion of administered alkali is increased. Since the increased urinary pH is a function of the resulting urinary bicarbonate concentration, simultaneous treatment with diuretics may truncate the increase in urinary pH by diluting bicarbonate concentration. The increasing diuresis prevents achievement of the highest urinary concentrations of bicarbonate and thus limits the elevation of pH. A recent study evaluated the use of alkali without diuretics, hoping to capitalize on the fact that urinary pH has a more pronounced effect on salicylate clearance than does urinary volume.[226] The more limited diuresis facilitates urinary alkalinization. Not only did treatment with alkali alone improve salicylate clearance, but it also led to the recovery of more drug than did alkali and diuresis combined. The authors of the study attributed this to the fact that urinary pH could be raised to 8.10 ± 0.5 with alkali alone, as opposed to only 7.30 ± 0.4 with combined alkali and diuresis.[228] The authors administered 1.5 liters of a 150 meq/liter $NaHCO_3$ solution over a 4-h period to those receiving bicarbonate alone. Despite the lack of diuretic therapy, this treatment did not result in the retention of substantial amounts of fluid. Since the acidemia accompanying aspirin toxicity can impair myocardial contraction, and since many of these patients are elderly, it is important to monitor salt and water balance carefully and to avoid volume overload and precipitation of congestive heart failure.

Precisely when to initiate therapy is a clinical judgment that should be based on the quantity of aspirin consumed and the patient's clinical condition. Ingestion of less than 10 g of aspirin (150 mg per kilogram of body weight) by adults usually is well tolerated and generally requires no therapy.[277]

The importance of treating acidosis promptly cannot be overemphasized. Lowering arterial pH from 7.40 to 7.20 doubles the concentration of the non-ionized portion of the salicylate, thereby favoring its entry into cells.[139] The cytotoxic effects of salicylates include impaired glucose, amino acid, and lipid metabolism, and diminished Krebs' cycle activity. Brain glucose content is reduced by salicylate poisoning despite normal serum levels in nonacidemic patients, and the entry of more salicylates into cells can only worsen metabolism.[280] Thus the greatest rates of mortality and CNS depression occur in an acidemic environment.

Carbonic anhydrase inhibitors (e.g., acetazolamide) cause bicarbonaturia, and by virtue of the increased urinary pH they enhance salicylate removal.[75,184] Although this therapy is effective, care must be taken to replace excreted alkali lest hypobicarbonatemia and acidemia develop. As has been noted, a fall in systemic pH increases mortality.[118] This danger has been highlighted by reports of enhanced toxicity in chronic salicylate users beginning carbonic anhydrase therapy for intercedent glaucoma.[8]

Though salicylate can be removed by dialysis, this procedure is generally reserved for intoxicated patients with advanced chronic renal failure or for those who develop acute oliguric renal insufficiency, which precludes initiation of an alkaline diuresis. Dialysis should also be considered in those severely intoxicated patients with an unresponding acidosis, persistent or worsening CNS symptoms, or obvious deterioration despite the taking of other appropriate measures.[292] Seizures portend an unfavorable prognosis and warrant early use of dialysis. Hemodialysis is superior to peritoneal dialysis in removing salicylate[127] and surpasses charcoal perfusion in its ability to correct electrolyte or fluid imbalances present on admission or developing during therapy.[292] Some authors have advocated that dialysis be used when serum salicylate levels surpass 100 to 120 mg/100 ml in cases of acute ingestion, and when they reach 60 to 80 mg/100 ml in the chronic setting.[64a,292] Hemodialysis is more effective than peritoneal dialysis and is always the modality of choice when conservative nondialytic therapy proves inadequate.

The physician should be aware of the side effects of therapy of salicylate intoxication. Cerebral edema,[127] pulmonary edema,[227] fluid retention,[228] and hypokalemia[157] have occurred during forced fluid therapy, and some deaths have resulted.

Gastric lavage, charcoal, and urinary alkalinization are sufficient in most cases of adult salicylate intoxication presenting with normal-to-slightly-elevated blood pH. Despite normal arterial pH, bicarbonate therapy usually is well tolerated, although frequent monitoring of arterial blood gases and electrolytes is recommended.

Ethylene glycol

Ethylene glycol is a clear aliphatic diol with a pleasant odor and a warm, sweet taste. It has been used as a solvent for paints and plastics, in hydraulic brake fluid, in ink, and for softening cellophane; it is the principal component (usually 95 percent) of motor vehicle antifreeze. Because of its ready availability, many cases of ethylene glycol toxicity are seen, especially in desperate alcoholics.

Pharmacologic and biochemical principles

After rapid absorption through the stomach, this highly water-soluble compound distributes evenly throughout bodily tissues. The elimination half-life is 3 to 5 h. In the kidney the compound is filtered and passively reabsorbed, with nearly 20 percent of a dose of 1 mg per kilogram of body weight excreted unchanged in the urine. However, hepatic metabolism accounts for nearly all of the rest of this drug's elimination and is catalyzed by the enzyme alcohol dehydrogenase.[190] Ethylene glycol metabolism may follow several pathways: Small amounts (3 to 10 percent) of oxalic acid are formed, and an even smaller amount of hippuric acid is generated. Formation of oxalic acid proceeds through glycoaldehyde, glycolate, and glyoxylate, with consequent generation of NADH, the reduced form of the pyridine nucleotide NAD^+. These metabolites are more toxic than their parent compound. The increase in the cellular $NADH/NAD^+$ ratio augments lactic acid production from pyruvic acid. Glycolic acid accounts for most of the increment in the anion gap in experimental and human poisonings associated with ethylene glycol.[47,87a,117a]

In the absence of prompt therapy, a lethal dose of ethylene glycol is 1.0 to 1.5 ml per kilogram of body weight, or approximately 100 ml in an average-sized adult.[102] However, there is actually a considerable range of reported lethal doses, and survival of substantially larger ingestions has been documented. Toxic symptoms and the degree of metabolic acidosis most closely parallel the plasma level of glycolic acid.[87a,117a] Hepatic alcohol dehydrogenase's affinity for alcohol is 100 times greater than its affinity for ethylene glycol. Since the enzyme has a greater affinity for the former substrate than for the latter, ethanol therapy has been used to slow ethylene glycol's metabolism to its more toxic byproducts. In fact, concurrent ingestion of ethanol with ethylene glycol may delay the onset of the latter's toxicity.

Clinical features of toxicity

The clinical features of ethylene glycol poisoning are well characterized. Patients tend to pass through three distinct stages of toxicity.[31,84] The initial findings are those of CNS depression, ataxia (which is dose-dependent), slurred speech and stupor (with modest ingestion), and coma and convulsions (when larger quantities have been consumed). This first stage usually lasts for up to 12 h, but may be prolonged for days; it is during this period that metabolic acidosis becomes evident.[218a] Mortality rates tend to be high during this initial phase.[185,224]

Cardiopulmonary failure defines the second stage of toxicity and is characterized by tachypnea, tachycardia, rales, a ventricular gallop rhythm, cyanosis, and even mild hypertension. Whether the pulmonary edema is simply a function of toxic myocardial depression or whether noncardiac causes also contribute has not been clarified.

The last stage is marked by oliguric or anuric acute renal failure and may be heralded by flank pain in awake and responsive patients. Anuria has lasted for as long as 42 days[248] and 50 days.[51] Patients usually recover renal function, although this may take months, and even then renal function may not return to baseline levels.[31,124] Cytotoxic effects of ethylene glycol's metabolites and the deposition of calcium oxalate account for the renal failure. Some patients pass directly from the first to the third stage, completely bypassing the cardiopulmonary disorder.

Ethylene glycol ingestion increases both the anion and osmolal gaps[248] (see equation 9 below). In addition to glycolate, lactate may add to the increased anion gap. Hypoxia, hypotension, and altered tissue redox ratios contribute to the lactic acidosis.[125,218,218a,264] The urinary sediment reveals either the acicular (needle-shaped) crystals of calcium oxalate monohydrate[51,124] or its more familiar octahedrals (i.e., the "envelopes") of calcium oxalate dihydrate. Rarely the monohydrate may take on the shape of a dumbbell.[61b] There may be no crystalluria if the patient presents soon after ingestion, since maximum production of oxalate does not occur until 8 h after ingestion.[293] Repeated urinalyses may be necessary to reveal emerging crystalluria.[283] The degree of hypobicarbonatemia is roughly equal to the circulating level of glycolate and to the increment in the anion gap.[125] Hypocalcemia and leukocytosis are other reported findings. Lumbar puncture usually shows a mild pleocytosis, normal glucose concentration, and mild-to-moderate increases in protein.

Ethylene glycol levels can be roughly approximated from the difference between the measured and calculated serum osmolalities (Fig. 25-10). The electrolyte and nonelectrolyte contribution to normal serum osmolality is almost entirely accounted for by the sum of sodium and its accompanying anions, and by urea and glucose:

$$\text{Serum osm}_{(\text{calc.})} = 2\,[\text{Na}+]\ (\text{meq/liter}) + \frac{\text{BUN (mg/100 ml)}}{2.8} + \frac{\text{glucose (mg/100 ml)}}{18} \tag{9}$$

$$\text{Osmolal gap} = \text{serum osm}_{(\text{meas.})} - \text{serum osm}_{\text{calc.})} \tag{10}$$

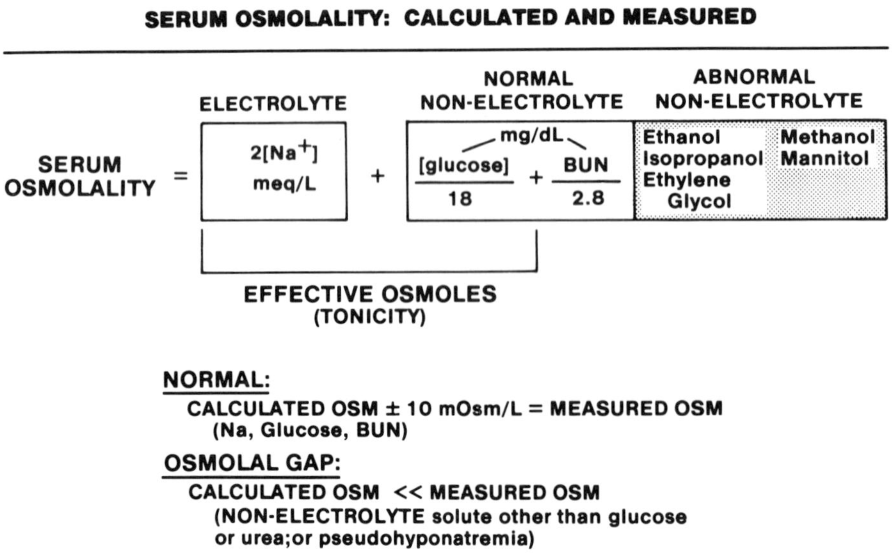

FIGURE 25-10 • Osmolal gap. (See text for details.)

Doubling the serum sodium concentration accounts for the electrolytic component of serum osmolality; dividing the BUN and glucose by 2.8 and 18, respectively, converts them from mass units to milliosmoles per liter. The calculated serum osmolality should agree with the value actually measured to within 10 mosm/liter. To the extent that the measured osmolality exceeds the calculated one by more than 10 mosm/liter, some circulating nonelectrolyte solute *not* accounted for by urea or glucose is causing the disparity. Most drugs do not contribute to an osmolal gap, because they are of high molecular weight and are taken in small amounts. Ethylene glycol, however, can cause this osmolal gap. Since its molecular weight is only 62, each 62 mg/100 ml of circulating ethylene glycol increases the osmolal gap by 10 mosm/liter. It should be remembered that patients may enter the hospital many hours after ingesting ethylene glycol. The parent compound may have been fully catabolized, allowing the blood ethylene glycol level to approach zero while glycolic acid levels remain high. The acid does not add to the osmolal gap, since its proton is lost with HCO_3^- in the titration process; the glycolate simply replaces lost alkali. Thus, at this stage, the osmolal gap is normal, while the anion gap is increased.

Exposure to toxins has most likely occurred when a high-anion-gap acidosis is unassociated with azotemia or with keto- or lactic acidosis. If the osmolal gap is also increased, then ethylene glycol or methanol is most likely the culprit.[66,125]

Thus the typical clinical picture of ethylene glycol toxicity, in the presence of an elevated-anion-gap acidosis and an osmolal gap, is highly characteristic. Demonstration of leukocytosis, hypocalcemia, and calcium oxalate crystalluria, and, finally, the finding of ethylene glycol in the blood, confirm the diagnosis.

Autopsy often reveals calcium oxalate deposition in the vessels and meninges of the brain and kidney tubules.[31,224] In surviving patients calcium oxalate crystals have been shown to persist in the kidney for months.[51,248]

Therapy

Because of the very rapid absorption of ethylene glycol from the stomach, gastric lavage, though it should be attempted, may be of limited benefit.[124,226] Thus therapy is directed at treating the acidemia and preventing further metabolism of ethylene glycol. A loading dose of 0.6 to 1.0 g of *ethanol* per kilogram of body weight should be given over 1 h and should be followed by a sustaining infusion of 10 to 20 g/h. A blood ethanol level of 100 mg/100 ml should be maintained. The rationale for this approach rests on the 100-fold greater affinity of hepatic alcohol dehydrogenase for ethanol than for ethylene glycol.[82,126a,218] Hemodialysis and peritoneal dialysis have both been used to remove these highly dialyzable toxins. Rebound increases in ethylene glycol levels may occur after dialysis is stopped,[269] making it critically important to continue therapy for at least 24 h after plasma levels of ethylene glycol become unmeasurable.[102] To prevent development of dangerous toxicity, hemodialysis should be instituted immediately if there is clinical or laboratory evidence of extreme exposure.[283] Though hemodialysis more efficiently removes ethylene glycol, peritoneal dialysis is an effective alternative and should be initiated if hemodialysis is unavailable.[124,284]

To avoid the difficulties of monitoring and maintaining therapeutic ethanol levels, some authors have recommended adding the alcohol directly to the dialysate bath (100 mg/100 ml).[219] To enhance renal oxalate excretion, the ECF volume should be kept appropriately expanded and diuretics given to achieve and maintain a brisk diuresis.[213,269,283] 4- Methylpyrazole (4-MP) inhibits alcohol dehydrogenase more potently than does ethanol, thereby more effectively preventing the conversion of ethylene glycol to its toxic metabolites. Moreover, the metabolism of ethanol is slower than that of 4-MP; this indicates that the latter has a more rapid onset of action. The metabolism of alcohol is also highly variable, rendering titration of therapeutic levels more difficult. 4-MP has been used effectively in Europe in animals, and its kinetics have been studied in single-dose trials in healthy human volunteers. Demonstrated efficacy has been established in monkeys and in human beings.[24b,45,47]

If the osmolal gap is repeatedly normal in a patient known to have ingested ethylene glycol many hours earlier, one may assume that the blood glycol levels are very low. Ethanol therapy becomes unnecessary at this point, since the alcohol's only therapeutic purpose is to prevent conversion of the parent compound into its more toxic products. Dialysis is still indicated for removal of the toxic metabolites.

Methanol

Pharmacologic and biochemical principles

Methyl alcohol—methanol—is a clear liquid with a molecular weight of 32. Its odor is distinctly different from that of ethanol, but its presence may be masked by impurities added during its production or by the many liquids with which it is miscible. In illicit alcoholic beverages the cheaper methanol may be substituted for the more expensive ethanol. (The recent methanol epidemic from Italian wines came about when vintners added methanol to their product in place of the more expensive sugar, which would have produced ethanol by fermentation.) This toxin is widely available, being found in many solvents, cleaners, shellacs, and varnishes, and is added to industrial ethanol-containing solutions to "denature" them—that is, to render them poisonous. Toxic exposure to methanol can occur by several routes, including ingestion, inhalation, and absorption from the skin. However, with better industrial safety standards, inhalation and skin absorption are now infrequent, and most toxicities derive from ingestion. Despite this, recent reports have documented sporadic cases and outbreaks of methanol intoxication occurring from skin absorption.[133] The application of methanol-soaks to the skin of febrile children has led to fatal toxicity. Inhalation of methanol vapors from the compresses may have played an additional role. Methanol poisoning from ingestion has occurred both sporadically and in epidemics.[29,123a,134,230,273] In addition to denatured alcohol, other sources of methanol include certain antifreeze preparations, car windshield cleaners,[171] Sterno, and, most recently, diluents used for photocopy machines.[123a,273] The most frequently cited lethal dose is 30 ml of absolute methanol,[53] but patients have been known to survive after ingesting 500 ml; others have died after taking as little as 15 ml of a 40% solution.[29,46] Despite aggressive therapy, mortality from methanol poisoning continues to approximate 20 percent and is related to both duration and severity of the ensuing acidosis.[177]

Methanol has an apparent volume of distribution similar to that of ethanol (0.6 to 0.7 liters per kilogram of body weight). It diffuses readily into lipid-containing tissues. The highest concentrations are found within the kidney, liver, and gastrointestinal tract. High concentrations within the optic nerve and the vitreous humor account for one of its major toxicities: visual impairment and blindness. Formate is primarily responsible for the ocular toxicity.[210a] Pulmonary excretion accounts for at least 25 percent of methanol elimination, and animal studies indicate that only 3 to 5 percent is excreted unchanged in the urine.[199,235] Metabolism of methanol occurs mainly in the liver, at a rate that is independent of serum levels and only one-seventh as rapid as that of ethanol.[172] The alcohol dehydrogenase pathway is the principal route of the alcohol's metabolism in human beings, monkeys, and rats.[68,92,264] This enzyme catalyzes methanol's sequential conversion to formaldehyde and formic acid. The latter's oxidation to CO_2 and water is folate-dependent.[68,211,264] Accordingly, specific folate inhibitors such as methotrexate have been shown to increase formate levels by a factor of 3.5 in methanol-treated dogs.[206] In rhesus monkeys, methanol-induced formic acidosis can be prevented by pretreatment with folic acid or 5-formyl-tetrahydrofolate.[177] This vitamin-dependency of formate metabolism has led to speculation that malnourished alcoholics may not readily clear formic acid.[12]

Elimination kinetics depend on the quantity of methanol absorbed. Serum half-life at low dosages is 14 to 20 h, whereas the half-life at higher dosages increases to 24 to 30 h. If alcohol dehydrogenase is blocked by ethanol, the half-life is extended to 30 to 35 h.[237]

Clinical features of toxicity

The by-products of methanol metabolism, principally formaldehyde and formic acid, account for the clinical manifestations of toxicity.[172,264] Unmetabolized methanol exerts little toxic effect. Indeed, despite the fact that peak serum methanol levels occur within 1 to 2 h of ingestion, a lag time of 8 to 30 h obtains from the time of ingestion until the onset of symptoms and signs. This lag time correlates well with the time required for the toxic accumulation of formic acid.

Acutely exposed patients develop symptoms and signs primarily relating to the central nervous and gastrointestinal systems. Headache, confusion, vertigo, and lethargy are common. Blurred vision, blindness, photophobia, and a feeling of "being in a snowfield" are ocular complaints in half of the cases of epidemic toxicity. Dilated pupils, constriction of the visual fields, retinal edema; and hyperemia, blurring, and loss of cupping of the optic disk may be seen. "Ophthalmic tolerance"—that is, normal eyegrounds despite the presence of other toxic manifestations—may result from subtoxic repeated exposures. Euphoria, which frequently accompanies ethanol ingestion, is not a feature of methanol intoxication. Abdominal pain may obtain from pancreatitis, with consequent hyperamylasemia; from mucosal irritation of the gastrointestinal tract; or from swelling of the kidney. Notably, the hyperamylasemia usually represents salivary isoamylase, levels of which are often elevated in alcoholics.[29,61a] CNS symptoms rarely occur at levels below 20 mg/100 ml, but since formate accounts for the bulk of toxicity, peak levels must be gauged with respect to a given individual's symptoms.[192a]

Ocular symptoms usually are not manifest at levels less than 100 mg/100 ml. A peak level of more than 50 mg/100 ml indicates serious poisoning. Fatalities in untreated patients generally occur with levels of 150 to 200 mg/100 ml, but correlate best with the degree of meteabolic acidosis secondary to the acumulation of formic acid—as does ocular toxicity. All signs are potentially reversible with prompt initiation of therapy; however, severe sequelae, such as blindness and parkinsonism, may occur if treatment is delayed.

A high anion gap metabolic acidosis, due to formic acid accumulation, occurs with severe toxicity.[68,173,264,268] A recent study of 11 patients suffering acute methanol intoxication indicated that almost the entire increment in the anion gap was accounted for by accumulated formate.[178] Lactic acidosis and ketoacidosis have also been known, on occasion, to complicate methanol toxicity.[29,178] Formate seems to account for the entire increment in the anion gap in the early stages of the acidosis and in patients with mild exposure. More severely intoxicated patients are likely to develop ketosis and/or lactic acidosis. The purported explanation depends both on the lactic acidosis of respiratory and circulatory failure and on increased lactate production by the liver at very low pH levels.[25,177]

Methanolemia increases the *osmolal gap*.[126,268] Each 100 mg/liter (i.e., each 10 mg/100 ml) of methanol contributes 3.4 mosm/liter.[268] Ethanol levels should be obtained, since ethanol is frequently consumed with methanol and also adds to the osmolal gap. In patients ingesting sufficient ethanol with methanol, the osmolal gap often increases disproportionately more than the increment in the anion gap. This is due to ethanol's slowing of methanol metabolism, which at once maintains a higher methanol level, raising the osmolal gap, while the reduced rate of formate accrual minimizes any increase in the anion gap.[66,125,156] The ethanol, of course, also contributes to the osmolal gap.

The laboratory findings in methanol intoxication include hyperamylasemia, increased circulating levels of various liver enzymes, proteinuria, glycosuria, and, occasionally, hematuria.[144] Autopsy findings have revealed a variety of diffuse multisystemic changes. The CNS pathology includes ganglion cell degeneration of the retina, and cerebral edema and hemorrhage showing a striking predilection for symmetrical involvement of the putamen.[101,125] Miscellaneous changes that are consistently found include pulmonary congestion, fatty lever, hemorrhagic pancreatitis, and acute tubular necrosis.

Therapy

It is generally accepted that both mortality and the potential for irreversible ophthalmopathy parallel both the duration and the severity of the metabolic acidosis. In a large series the mortality rate was 50 percent when the serum bicarbonate concentration was less than 10 meq/liter.[29] Other authors have reported similar outcomes.[101] Additionally, ocular toxicity seems to correlate with the degree of acidosis.[29,177] It is not possible to predict whether acute visual impairment will persist or will improve with therapy. Thus, once the diagnosis is strongly suspected, therapy should be initiated promptly. Gastric lavage and/or administration of ipecac is indicated for patients presenting within 2 h of methanol ingestion, but may be useful after longer periods if the patient has impaired gastrointestinal motility, as may be seen with coma or with coingestion of drugs that impair motility.

Folate, as leucovorin, should be administered intravenously, especially since alcoholic patients often are malnourished and ineffectively utilize folic acid—therapy potentially prolonging the elimination of half-life of formic acid. Sodium bicarbonate should be infused in doses appropriate to sustain the arterial pH above 7.20. The hemodynamic consequences of severe acidosis may impair tissue perfusion, causing lactic acidosis to become superimposed on the methanol-induced formic acidosis (see above). Appropriate alkali therapy in conjunction with ECF volume expansion protects against this vicious circle.

As in the case of ethylene glycol toxicity (see above), ethanol also reduces the rate of methanol metabolism by more aggressively competing for binding to alcohol dehydrogenase. Roe was the first to make the astute observation that patients ingesting ethanol along with methanol manifested milder degrees of toxicity.[236] Thus ethanol therapy should be instituted immediately in patients with metabolic acidosis, methanol levels exceeding 20 to 30 mg/100 ml, or other clinical signs of toxicity.[237]

Dialysis remains one of the mainstays of therapy. Methanol's small molecular size and water-solubility allow for its efficient removal by dialysis.[140,285] The easy dialyzability of formate contributes to the efficacy of dialysis in treating methanol intoxication. Although the clearance of formate is less than that of methanol, its volume of distribution is much less than methanol's. Thus the plasma half-life of formic acid is shorter than that of methanol in a hemodialyzed patient.[173] In a small series comparing hemodialysis to peritoneal dialysis, the latter was found less effective; indeed, all three peritoneally dialyzed patients eventually required hemodialysis.[195] Though hemodialysis is eight times more effective than peritoneal dialysis in clearing methanol, peritoneal dialysis should be used if hemodialysis is unavailable. Endogenous clearance of methanol is equal to one-fifth to one-tenth of peritoneal clearance.[177,237] While methanol is cleared much more rapidly by hemodialysis, care must be taken to avoid using a recirculating dialysis (REDY) system, since the cartridge is quickly saturated with the toxin, rapidly rendering the procedure ineffective.[287] Because ethanol is also cleared with dialysis, infusion rates of ethanol should be increased, or ethanol should be added to the dialysate bath (see "Therapy" under "Ethylene glycol" above).[123a,237]

Dialysis should be initiated for methanol intoxication when any of the following indications obtain: known ingestion of at least 30 ml of absolute methanol; a blood methanol level of 50 mg/100 ml or more; the presence of a high-anion-gap metabolic acidosis; or mental, visual, or funduscopic changes attributable to methanol.[101,171] As has been mentioned, dialysis also clears formate well, thereby removing one of methanol's principal metabolites.[125,173] Dialysis should be continued until the methanol level has been reduced to less than 25 mg/100 ml.[101]

Animal studies suggest that formate is responsible for methanol's toxic manifestations. Accordingly, inhibition of alcohol dehydrogenase by such compounds as pyrazole or 4-methylpyrazole ameliorates the toxicity of methanol in monkeys (see "Therapy" under "Ethylene glycol" above).[177] Studies comparing the efficacy of these drugs versus ethanol in treating human beings have yet to be done.

Paraldehyde

Paraldehyde, which has been used as a sedative for more than a century, is a low-molecular-weight cyclic polyether of polymerized acetaldehyde. It is a colorless liquid with a strong, unpleasant odor. It is prone to spontaneous decomposition when stored unprotected from light and air.

Paraldehyde, still used as a sedative and as an antiseizure medication, may be given orally, parenterally, or rectally. Regardless of its route of administration, 7 percent is excreted by the lungs within 4 h,[95] with an additional 4 to 21 percent eventually being exhaled.[260] The remainder is metabolized chiefly by the liver; little to none appears in the urine. It is catabolized, in sequence, to acetaldehyde, acetic acid, and, finally, CO_2 and water. Liver disease retards this oxidation. Disulfiram administration has been shown to slow paraldehyde metabolism in animals.[104] When phenobarbital was added to rat liver microsomes in vitro, the amount of acetaldehyde produced from paraldehyde was greatly increased,[105] most likely because of interference of cytochrome P-450 function.[300a]

Despite more than a century of use of the substance, paraldehyde-associated acidosis was first recognized only in 1957.[285] Toxicity typically occurred in patients consuming large quantities of ethanol, who were often addicted to paraldehyde as well. It is presumed that a tachyphylaxis to paraldehyde-induced narcosis occurs, allowing patients to remain awake while continuing their ingestion.

Presenting symptoms of intoxicated patients have included nausea and vomiting (oten hematemesis), abdominal pain, and lethargy. Most patients ingested considerable quantities of paraldehyde up to the time of admission, presenting with the unmistakable, offensive odor of the drug.

Paraldehyde administration to ethanol-intoxicated patients can be dangerous, as was shown by one series where nine patients with varying degrees of ethanol intoxication died within 4 h of paraldehyde administration.[39]

Findings on presentation have included mild-to-moderate dehydration, hypotension, Kussmaul respirations, and heme-positive gastric contents or stool. The lungs are usually clear to auscultation, but a case of paraldehyde-induced noncardiogenic pulmonary edema has occurred after repeated parenteral doses of the drug.[186] Fatalities have been reported after paraldehyde administration, and in those cases pulmonary edema was demonstrable at autopsy.[95,149,176] Nonfatal pulmonary congestion was significant morbidity has also been seen;[95,149] direct alveolar capillary membrane toxicity was suspected in these instances.[186]

In these studies the patients often showed hyperkalemia and striking leukocytosis. The laboratory findings have also included acidemia with an increased anion gap. Although acetate, pyruvate, lactate, and the measurable ketone, acetoacetate, have been excluded, the offending acid has not been identified. It is quite possible, if not likely, that β-hydroxybutyric acidosis accounts for the paraldehyde-associated increased anion gap. The oxidation of paraldehyde generates reduced pyridine nucleotide, which in turn stimulates conversion of acetoacetate to the nitroprusside-negative β-hydroxybutyrate. This chemical sequence acts to cloud the diagnosis. Until recently there had been no reported cases of paraldehyde-associated acidosis in more than a decade; it was during that period that we first became aware of the entity of β-hydroxybutyric acidosis. Older literature suggested that the increased anion-gap acidosis was the result of ingestion of the acetic acid formed from decomposed paraldehyde; however, when dogs were fed fresh and decomposed paraldehyde preparations, there was no difference in the otherwise trivial high anion gap acidosis that developed.[27] Despite the proposed accumulation of nitroprusside-negative β-hydroxybutyrate as the unmeasured anion, a patient may in fact show positive ketones in serum. It should be remembered that acetaldehyde gives a false-positive nitroprusside reaction (pseudoketosis); this should be borne in mind when one is considering the significance of ketonemia.[105]

If a normal anion gap acidosis develops, renal tubular acidosis, which has been linked to paraldehyde, should be considered.[62] In addition to the problems associated with acidosis and pulmonary edema, the clinical course of paraldehyde toxicity may be further complicated by acute renal failure.[27,104,105]

Therapy should be directed at the acidosis and hypotension induced by paraldehyde intoxication. Thus treatment consists of intravenous administration of saline solution to correct fluid deficits, and bicarbonate administration to correct acidemia. Removal of paraldehyde by dialysis has not been documented; however, dialysis may be required to treat sodium overload from bicarbonate administration in severely acidemic, oliguric patients.

CLINICAL FEATURES OF NORMAL ANION GAP METABOLIC ACIDOSES

The normal anion gap metabolic acidoses are characterized by the addition of hydrochloric acid (HCl) to body fluid. Each milliequivalent of accumulating H^+ consumes a like amount of HCO_3^-. Since each H^+ is accompanied by one Cl^- anion, each milliequivalent of titrated HCO_3^- is effectively replaced by Cl^-. Given an unchanged Na^+ concentration, the anion gap will, of course, remain unchanged (Fig. 25-11; see also Chap. 24). This view, while clinically useful, may in fact be something of an oversimplification.[2] If bicarbonate were the only available buffer capable of accepting protons, the decrease in the serum concentration of bicarbonate would indeed equal the increase in that of chloride. However, normal polyanionic serum proteins (e.g., albumin) also take part in the buffering process, which at once limits serum acidification and *lowers* the anion gap. A portion of sodium's positive charge is balanced by the negatively charged protein. Protons from accumulating HCl displace Na^+ from the routinely unmeasured protein anion and cause it to reassociate with the measured chlo-

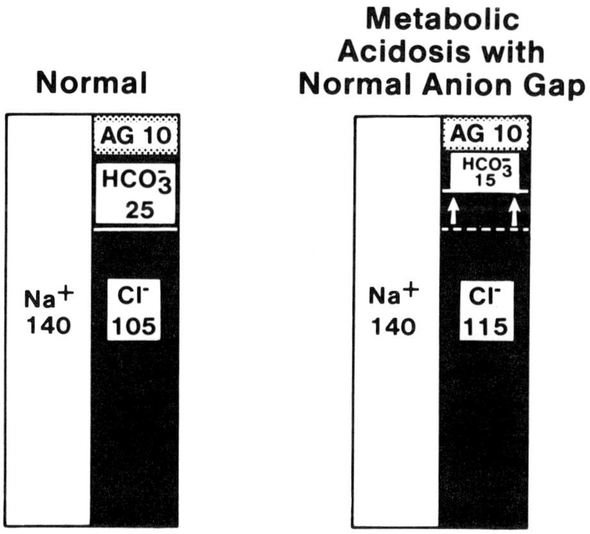

FIGURE 25-11 • Serum electrolyte patterns. Normal baseline and normal anion gap (AG) acidosis. (See text for details.)

ride anion (equation 9). Since a greater fraction of sodium is now associated with a measured anion, the normal anion gap decreases.

$$HCl + Na^+Prot^- \rightarrow NaCl + H^+Prot^- \quad (11)$$

To view it another way: when HCl is buffered by protein, bicarbonate is spared while chloride is increased. The sum of the measured anions, CL^- and HCO_3^-, increases, thereby lowering the anion gap. Because this change is small, the diagnostic significance of this lower anion gap is rather limited.

The hyperchloremia responsible for maintaining the normal anion gap may be manifested by an *absolute* or *relative* increase in serum chloride concentration.[65] The concentrations of serum Na^+ and Cl^- are intimately related to the state of hydration. Since the levels of both Na^+ and Cl^- change proportionately with a given change in body water content, any disproportionate change in chloride concentration relative to that of sodium can be attributed to derangements in the acid-base status. Figure 25-12 illustrates these interrelationships. When overhydration causes the serum sodium and chloride levels to decrease by 10 percent, their respective values fall to 126 meq/liter and 90 meq/liter (Fig. 25-12*b*). Serum bicarbonate concentration is maintained at normal levels by the combined effects of extrarenal (bone and intracellular fluid) buffering (see "Dilutional acidosis" below) and renal bicarbonate synthesis. If a 10-meq/liter "hyperchloremic" metabolic acidosis were not to develop, the electrolyte pattern depicted in Fig. 25-12*c* would then obtain. In this example, the serum Na^+ concentration remains at 126 meq/liter, while Cl^- levels increase to 102 meq/liter. The disproportionate lowering of serum sodium concentration relative to that of chloride should suggest the combined presence of overhydration and an acid-base disturbance. The "hyperchloremic" metabolic acidosis in this example occurs with an apparently normal value for serum chloride concentration. Of course, the serum bicarbonate concentration of 15 meq/liter and the essentially normal anion gap also fit this diagnosis.

Additional examples of the use of relative sodium and chloride concentrations in assessing acid-base and hydration status are given in Table 25-7.[65] A hyperchloremic metabolic acidosis may be caused by any one,

FIGURE 25-12 • Serum electrolyte patterns: normal baseline (*a*), water retention (overhydration), (*b*) and superimposition of a 10 meq/liter acidosis during overhydration (*c*). Increased height of the bars (*b, c*) reflects the volume expansion caused by water retention. (See text for details.)

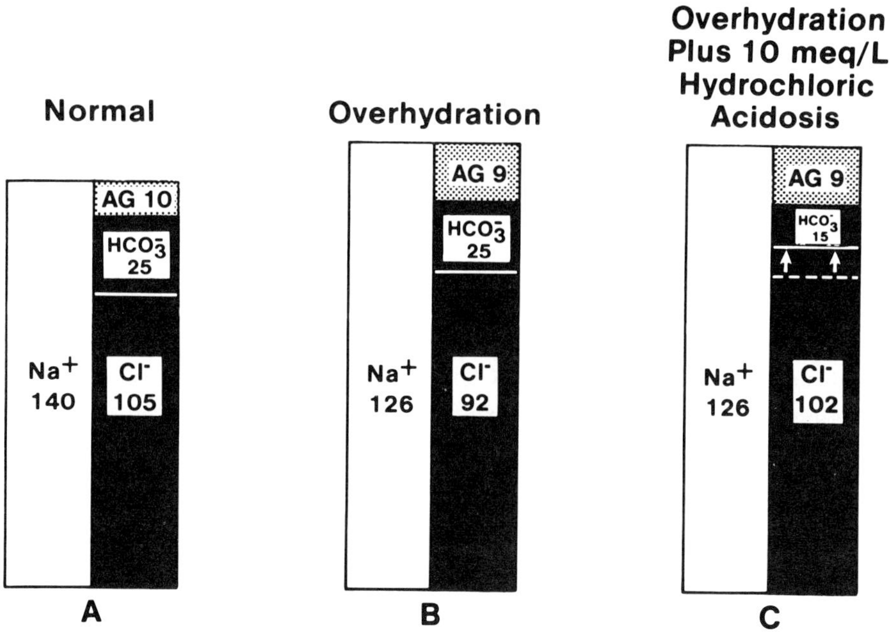

TABLE 25-7 • Assessment of acid-base and hydration status

PROPORTIONATE CHANGES IN [Na] AND [Cl]: ALWAYS DUE TO HYDRATION ALONE

Dehydration
- [Na]: 140 → 154 meq/liter = +14 meq/liter = 10% rise
- [Cl]: 100 → 100 meq/liter = +10 meq/liter = 10% rise

Overhydration
- [Na]: 140 → 126 meq/liter = −14 meq/liter = 10% fall
- [Cl]: 100 → 90 meq/liter = −10 meq/liter = 10% fall

CHANGES IN [Cl] BUT NOT IN [Na]: ALWAYS DUE TO ACID-BASE DISTURBANCES

Respiratory acidosis or metabolic alkalosis
- [Na]: 140 → 140 meq/liter = 0 change
- [Cl]: 100 → 90 meq/liter = −10 meq/liter = 10% fall

Respiratory alkalosis or hyperchloremic alkalosis
- [Na]: 140 → 140 meq/liter = 0 change
- [Cl]: 100 → 110 meq/liter = +10 meq/liter = 10% rise

DISPROPORTIONATE CHANGES IN BOTH [Na] AND [Cl]: DISTURBED HYDRATION AND ACID-BASE BALANCE

Dehydration plus respiratory acidosis or metabolic alkalosis:
- [Na]: 140 → 154 meq/liter = +14 meq/liter = 10% rise
- [Cl]: 100 → 100 meq/liter = 0 change
- ↓ [Na], normal [Cl]: Overhydration plus respiratory alkalosis or hyperchloremic acidosis
- [Na]: 140 → 126 meq/liter = −14 meq/liter = 10% fall
- [Cl]: 100 → 100 meq/liter = 0 change

Dehydration plus respiratory acidosis or metabolic alkalosis
- [Na]: 140 → 154 = +14 meq/liter = 10% rise
- [Cl]: 100 → 75 = −25 meq/liter = 25% fall

Overhydration plus respiratory alkalosis or metabolic alkalosis
- [Na]: 140 → 126 = −14 meq/liter = 10% fall
- [Cl]: 100 → 75 = −25 meq/liter = 25% fall

Dehydration plus respiratory acidosis or metabolic alkalosis
- [Na]: 140 → 168 = +28 meq/liter = 20% rise
- [Cl]: 100 → 110 = +10 meq/liter = 10% rise

or any combination, of four different pathophysiologic mechanisms. The loss of *bicarbonate-rich, chloride-deficient fluid* renders the ECF at once hypobicarbonatemic and hyperchloremic. An unchanged ECF chloride content dispersed in a newly reduced volume of fluid accounts for this concentration change. Diarrheal states and renal acidoses are characterized by electrolyte patterns created in this manner. The *addition of HCl* or of certain related compounds can also cause a hyperchloremic metabolic acidosis by directly destroying bicarbonate while replacing the lost anion with chloride. Rapid *dilution of the ECF* using bicarbonate-free solutions can lead to a transient hypobicarbonatemia. Finally, under special circumstances, certain forms of *high-anion-gap metabolic acidosis* may be transformed into hyperchloremic acidoses. These disorders are all characterized by the accumulation of fixed acids, the anions of which are rapidly cleared by the kidneys. If, for example, HX accumulated in some metabolic acidosis, the acid's titration by $NaHCO_3$ would yield NaX. Replacement of measurable serum HCO_3^- by the usually unmeasured X^- anion would, of course, raise the anion gap. Because X^- is rapidly cleared by the kidneys, excretion of NaX with obligate amounts of water would convert the acidosis from a high-anion-gap form into a normal-anion-gap variant. Excretion of X^- rids the blood of the anion responsible for the increased anion gap, while excretion of sodium with water shrinks the ECF, causing an unchanged body content of Cl^- to be distributed in a smaller space (i.e., hyperchloremia occurs). Examples of such acidoses include toluene ("glue-sniffing") toxicity (see below and Chap. 28),[42a] exposure to excessive amounts of methionine, and, under certain conditions, diabetic ketoacidosis (see Chap. 26). The accumulating acids in toluene and methionine toxicities are hippuric and sulfuric, respectively. Both sodium hippurate and sodium sulfate are rapidly cleared by the kidneys. More detailed discussion of these acidoses follow.

Each of these pathophysiologic mechanisms can disturb potassium homeostasis, but they work in different ways. These differences are exploited to subclassify the hyperchloremic metabolic acidoses into those typically associated with hypokalemia and those more often associated with normal-to-elevated levels of serum potassium (Table 25-8). The discussion that follows uses this classification.

HYPOKALEMIC, HYPERCHLOREMIC METABOLIC ACIDOSES

Diarrhea

Pathophysiology

Diarrhea is perhaps the most frequent cause of hyperchloremic metabolic acidosis. To understand how this occurs, one must first become familiar with aspects of normal gastrointestinal physiology (see Chap. 17). The acidic fluid exiting the stomach is progressively and extensively modified as it passes along the small intestine. Separate intestinal cation and anion exchangers effectively reabsorb luminal sodium chloride without effecting any net change in systemic or luminal acid-base balance. The *cation exchanger* reabsorbs sodium while secreting protons, transiently rendering the lumen more acid and the blood more alkaline. Adjacent anion exchangers reabsorb luminal chloride while, in effect, transporting blood bicarbonate into the intestinal cavity. Addition of blood bicarbonate to the intestinal lumen reverses the tendency toward systemic alkalinization and luminal acidification created by the cation exchanger. The process effectively translocates luminal NaCl to ECF.[79]

TABLE 25-8 • Etiologies of normal-anion-gap metabolic acidosis

Normal-to-high serum potassium	Low serum potassium
Hypoaldosteronism	Gastrointestinal disorders
Primary adrenal disorders	Diarrhea, biliary or pancreatic fistulas, pancreatic transplant
Low renin secretion	Ureteral diversions
Renal tubular resistance to aldosterone	Ureterosigmoidostomy
Early uremic acidosis	Ileal bladder
Hyperalimentation	Renal tubular acidosis (see Chap. 27)
Posthypocapnia	
Dilutional acidosis	
Administration of HCl or related compounds	
NH_4Cl	
$CaCl_2$ (oral)	
Lysine HCl	
Arginine HCl	
Cholestyramine	
Renal tubular acidosis (see Chap. 27)	

The two major anions secreted into the bowel lumen are chloride and bicarbonate; the former is extensively secreted by epithelial cells in the upper small intestine, while the latter is predominantly secreted by the ileum and colon. The secretion of these anions depends on the interaction of three forces: two basolateral transporters, the *Na^+-K^+ ATPase* and the *Na^+-K^+-Cl^- cotransporter*; and the *selective permeability* of the apical membrane to intracellular chloride (Fig. 25-13). The low intracellular sodium concentration created by Na^+-K^+ ATPase activity favors the cellular reentry of Na^+ from the ECF, down its electrochemical gradient (Fig. 25-13*a*, *b*). Sodium entry into the cell via the peritubular membrane is accompanied by K^+ and Cl^-; this cation/anion entry is mediated by the aforementioned cotransporter (Fig. 25-13*b*). Entering Na^+ is actively extruded from the cell while K^+ exits via a specific membrane channel. Only the apical membrane is readily permeable to Cl^-, allowing

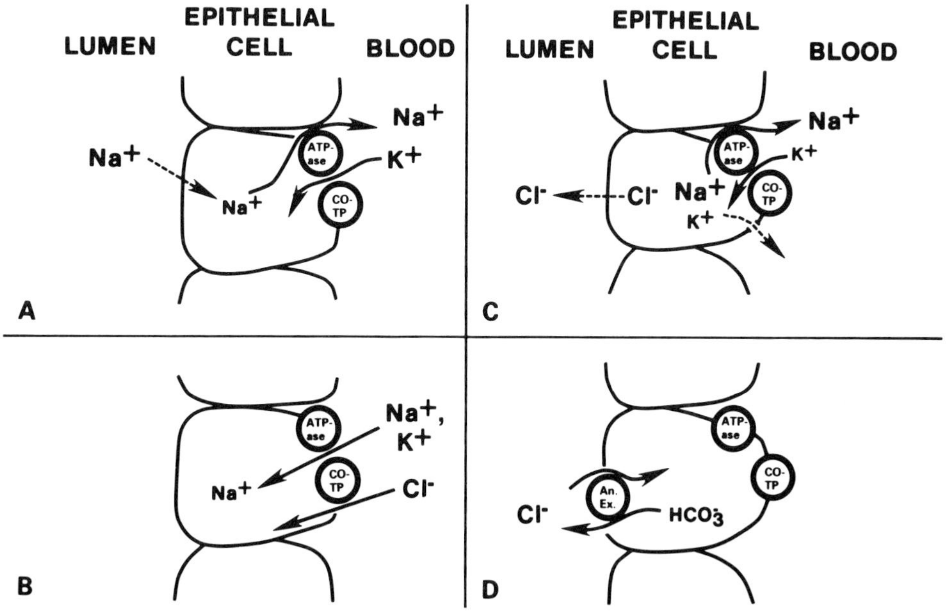

FIGURE 25-13 • Schematic representation of intestinal electrolyte transport. (*a*) Intracellular Na^+ concentration is maintained low by Na^+-K^+ ATPase at the contraluminal border. Luminal Na^+ moves into the cell, down its electrochemical gradient. (*b*) Na^+, K^+, and Cl^- from the extracellular fluid move intracellularly via the contraluminal Na^+-$K^+$$Cl^-$ cotransporter (CO-TP). (*c*) Na^+ is pumped out of cells via the Na^+-K^+ ATPase, while accumulating cellular K^+ exits via K^+ channels in the contraluminal cell membrane. Apical permeability to Cl^- allows the anion to enter the lumen. Thus, steps *a* to *c* effect net Cl^- secretion. (*d*) Secreted Cl^- in the ilcal and colonic lumina is exchanged for cellular HCO_3^-.

this anion to exit into the lumen (Fig. 25-13*c*). Epithelial cells of the ileum and colon have modified this system by consequence of having inserted a *Cl^-/HCO_3^- exchanger* into the apical membrane. Secreted Cl^- is now reabsorbed in exchange for HCO_3^-, effectively alkalinizing the luminal contents while acidifying blood (Fig. 25-13*d*). A more detailed description of this system appears in Chap. 17.

The 600 ml of intestinal fluid reaching the colon each day contains approximately 135 meq/liter of cations (Na^+, 125 meq/liter; K^+, 10 meq/liter) with an equal concentration of measurable anions (HCO_3^-, 75 meq/liter; Cl^-, 60 meq/liter). Colonic reabsorption prevents escape of all but 100 ml of water in the final stool. Sodium reabsorption and net potassium secretion continue as persisting activity of the Cl^-/HCO_3^- exchanger alkalinizes the luminal contents while returning Cl^- to the blood. The emerging stool contains 130 meq/liter of cations (Na^+, 40 meq/liter; K^+, 90 meq/liter), but only 45 meq/liter of measured anions (HCO_3^-, 30 meq/liter; Cl^-, 15 meq/liter).[79] Thus, despite continued secretion of bicarbonate into the colon, its concentration in the final stool is reduced. Additionally, while the sum of measured cations and anions was equal in the terminal ileal fluid, an anion gap develops in stool fluid. The sum of the measured cations—K^+ + Na^+ (90 meq/liter + 40 meq/liter)—minus the sum of the measured anions—HCO_3^- + Cl^- (30 meq/liter + 15 meq/liter)—is 85 meq/liter. The surprisingly low bicarbonate concentration, as well as the increased stool anion gap, is directly attributable to the metabolic activity of colonic bacteria. Bacterial fermentation of unabsorbed carbohydrates generates such organic acids as propionic acid, butyric acid, acetic acid, and lactic acid. The resulting titration converts sodium bicarbonate to sodium butyrate, sodium acetate, and other organic salts (Fig. 25-14). Colonic reabsorption can prevent the loss of alkali by directly reabsorbing bicarbonate and by reclaiming the organic anions (acetate, butyrate, etc.). The latter are delivered to peripheral tissues, especially the liver, where they are metabolically transformed to bicarbonate. Thus stool losses of bicarbonate or organic anions (i.e., potential bicarbonate) cause an alkali deficit and metabolic acidosis. The stool anion gap reflects the organic anion concentration. The amount of actual (30 meq/liter) and potential (85 meq/liter) alkali contained in normal daily stool is 115 meq/liter; in the 100 ml of stool water, only 11.5 meq of alkali is normally excreted.

Diarrheal states increase water and bicarbonate losses. Sodium cannot be efficiently extracted from this unsavory current of rapidly moving stool, resulting in a higher sodium and lower potassium concentration than is found in normal stool fluid. The diarrheal fluid is generally rich in bicarbonate or potential bicarbonate. Because bacterial acid production increases during diarrhea,[73] bicarbonate is more extensively titrated, and its final concentration may approach zero. The resulting increased stool anion gap reflects the loss of organic anion (i.e., potential bicarbonate). Loss of this chloride-free solution results in systemic hyperchloremia. Contraction of ECF in turn stimulates renal retention of ingested NaCl, further augmenting the hyperchloremia. Although diarrheal stool may be markedly acidic, its loss usually generates a systemic acidosis! The acid that lowers stool pH is produced within the colon by luminal bacteria; little, if any, is available systemically. A small amount of organic acid or its sodium salt can be reabsorbed from the colon. Oxidation of the acid yields CO_2 and H_2O, while metabolism of the sodium salt eventually regenerates bicarbonate.

Clinical and laboratory features

The clinical severity of diarrhea depends on its etiology, infectious complications, and extend of fluid, electrolyte, and acid-base abnormalities.

Since the electrolyte concentration of normal or diarrheal stool is usually less than that of normal plasma, its

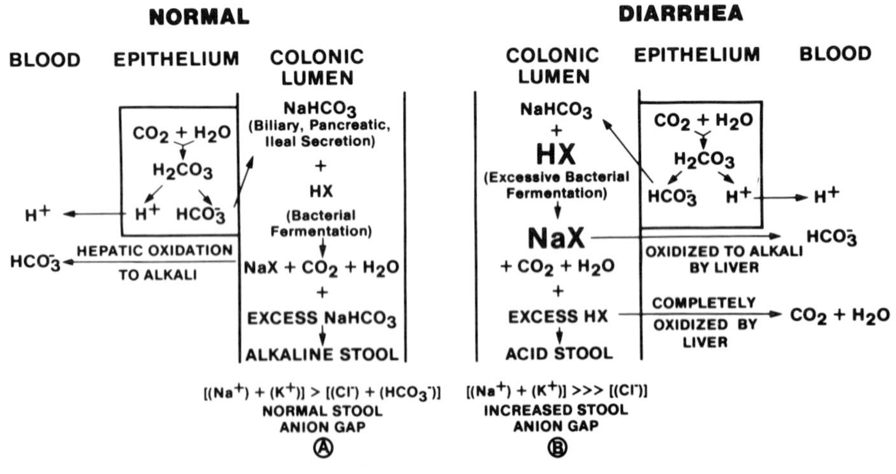

FIGURE 25-14 • Diarrhea: pathogenesis of stool and blood electrolyte and acid-base perturbations. Ileum, pancreas, and biliary tree add HCO_3^- to the lumen. Bacterial fermentation generates organic acids in the lumen, which titrates HCO_3^-. The sodium salt of the organic acid is partially reabsorbed and converted to $NaHCO_3$. In diarrheal state (*b*), organic acid production is excessive. The stool anion gap reflects excreted organic acid anions. (See text for details.)

TABLE 25-9 • **Simple and mixed acid-base disorders associated with diarrhea**

Na+ (meq/liter)	Cl− (meq/liter)	HCO_3^- (meq/liter)	K+ (meq/liter)	AG (meq/liter)	P_{CO_2} (mmHg)	pH	BUN/Cr (mg/100 ml)
UNCOMPLICATED DIARRHEA							
140	115	15	3.0	10	30	7.32	25/1.3
DIARRHEA PLUS LACTIC ACIDOSIS							
140	115	5	3.0	20	15	7.14	40/1.8
DIARRHEA PLUS VOMITING							
140	105	25	2.5	10	40	7.40	35/1.5
DIARRHEA PLUS RESPIRATORY ALKALOSIS							
140	120	10	2.5	10	20	7.32	25/1.3
DIARRHEA, LACTIC ACIDOSIS, RESPIRATORY ALKALOSIS							
140	115	5	3.0	20	10	7.32	40/1.8

Abbreviations: AG, anion gap; BUN, blood urea nitrogen; Cr, creatinine.

excretion represents loss of isotonic fluid and free water. Failure to replace such fluid results in isotonic contraction of ECF, and the loss of electrolyte-free water causes hypernatremia (see Chap. 21). Conversely, if these salt and water losses are replaced with pure tap water, hyponatremia results (see Chap. 20). Hypokalemia typically complicates diarrhea, on account of direct loss of potassium in the stool (see Chap. 22).

Mixed acid-base disorders commonly complicate diarrheal states (Table 25-9) (Chap. 31). *Lactic acidosis* can result from the associated hypovolemia and sepsis. Two distinct acidoses may therefore become superimposed. Since the bicarbonate concentration decreases much more than the anion gap increases, a mixed high anion gap and hyperchloremic acidosis must be present. The small increment in the anion gap reflects the accumulated lactate anion, while the associated proton causes a similar decrease in the bicarbonate concentration. The remainder of the decrement in bicarbonate levels reflects the hyperchloremic component (Table 25-9).

Because viral gastrointestinal illnesses commonly cause vomiting as well as diarrhea, *metabolic alkalosis* frequently coexists with metabolic acidosis. Since one disorder acts to increase serum bicarbonate concentration while the other acts to decrease it, the resulting serum bicarbonate concentration will more closely reflect the dominant process. Hypokalemia may be severe, since colonic losses are compounded by modest gastric losses. Furthermore, renal potassum wasting becomes extensive and worsens the hypokalemia when vomiting predominates and hyperbicarbonatemia prevails (see Chaps. 22 and 29).

Respiratory alkalosis can complicate the metabolic acidosis of diarrhea when endotoxin from gram-negative enteric pathogens is absorbed and carried to the brain, where it profoundly stimulates the respiratory center (Chap. 30). Even in the absence of generalized sepsis, endotoxin from normal colonic flora may gain access to the blood when inflammation disrupts the intestinal permeability barrier.

Thus, although diarrhea usually produces a hyperchloremic metabolic acidosis, commonly associated pathophysiologic events often lead to a more complex acid-base picture.

Treatment

Whenever possible, therapy must be directed at the underlying cause of the diarrhea. In addition, medications that reduce the volume of diarrhea, such as diphenoxylate or bismuth subsalicylate, may be appropriate. Fluid, electrolyte, and alkali losses require judicious replacement. In contrast to the organic acidoses, the accumulating anion in diarrheal acidosis (i.e., chloride) is not metabolizable, and the only endogenous means for restoring normobicarbonatemia requires renal acid excretion and bicarbonate synthesis. This is a relatively slow process and, of course, is significantly impaired by renal insufficiency. Alkali therapy becomes increasingly more important as the pH falls below 7.25 and the serum bicarbonate concentration is reduced below 10 meq/liter. When diarrhea and acute or chronic renal failure coexist, alkali therapy is mandatory, since there is no endogenous means of replenishing lost bicarbonate. When alkali replacement is given, correction of bicarbonate deficits, as well as ongoing losses, must be taken into account.

In the presence of hypokalemia, alkali therapy is not without risk. Since rapid infusions of bicarbonate can drive potassium into cells, preexisting hypokalemia can be worsened. Severe hypokalemia may result in paralysis, occasionally involving the muscles of respiration. The resulting hypercapnea, when superimposed on preexisting hypobicarbonatemia, may abruptly lower arterial pH to potentially lethal levels. Suffice it to say that marked hypokalemia and acidemia often requires intensive-case monitoring for proper treatment. In general, potassium levels should be raised to at least 2.5 to 3.0 meq/liter before vigorous administration of alkali.

Biliary and pancreatic drainage

Biliary and pancreatic secretions are markedly alkaline. Hepatocytes and exocrine pancreatic cells hydrate CO_2 in the presence of carbonic anhydrase to form H_2CO_3, which, in turn, instantaneously ionizes, forming H^+ and HCO_3^-. Secretion of bicarbonate into bile and pancreatic fluid involves a Cl^-/HCO_3^- exchanger and the Na^+-K^+-Cl^- cotransport pathway (see above and Fig. 25-13). Hydrogen ions are added to the blood, but net systemic acidification is prevented by the eventual direct or indirect reabsorption of HCO_3^- from the intestinal lumen.

Bile can contain up to 55 meq/liter of bicarbonate in a total daily volume of as much as 800 ml. External drainage can result in daily bicarbonate losses approximating 45 meq.[69] Similarly, drainage of pancreatic secretions containing up to 150 meq/liter of bicarbonate, in a daily volume of 1 liter or more, can result in external loss of more than 150 meq of alkali per day.[181] Loss of this bicarbonate-rich, chloride-deficient fluid causes hypobicarbonatemia and hyperchloremia. It follows that pancreatic drainage would more often result in an acidosis than would biliary drainage. Furthermore, since intact kidneys can eliminate some or all of this retained acid, clinically significant acidosis most often occurs in the setting of concomitant renal insufficiency. Measurement of daily bicarbonate losses guides rational alkali replacement.

Urinary-intestinal communications

Diversion of urine through a segment of the gastrointestinal tract becomes necessary when the ureters and/or the urinary bladder become irreparably damaged. Procedures have been designed whereby intestinal tissue substitutes for a scarred, ineffective, or excised urinary bladder. The first such procedure, done in 1911,[49] entailed implantation of both ureters into the *sigmoid colon*, creating a new reservoir and outflow tract for the urine. This technique obviates an external drainage site and, by virtue of an intact anal sphincter, affords voluntary control of urinary evacuation. Unfortunately, a high incident of severe and recurrent phylonephritis, often with profound metabolic acidosis, complicates the procedure.[245] Renal infection is related to the high intraluminal pressures created during defecation, which force bacteria-laden sigmoid contents up through the surgically constructed ureterosigmoid valve.

The hyperchloremic, hypokalemic metabolic acidosis derives from events within the bowel lumen as well as from secondary changes within the kidneys. The aforementioned Cl^-/HCO_3^- anion exchanger is quite active in the sigmoid colon. As the diverted urinary stream bathes the intestinal lining, chloride is reabsorbed in exchange for secreted bicarbonate. Because the urine can be voluntarily retained within the bowel lumen for prolonged periods, the extensive contact time increases the magnitude of the acidemia-inducing HCO_3^-/Cl^- exchange. Loss of alkali coupled with chloride accumulation results in a hyperchloremic acidosis. Active sodium reabsorption ensures a favorable electrochemical gradient for potassium secretion, resulting in hypokalemia.

A second mechanism whereby the acidosis is generated involves effective reversal of renal acid excretion (Fig. 25-15). Renal ammonia synthesis normally provides the major buffer required for net acid excretion. As renal tubular cells secrete protons into the tubular lumen, bicarbonate is added to the blood. This bicarbonate may then be secreted into the sigmoid lumen in exchange for chloride derived from urinary NH_4Cl. The secreted alkali then strips NH_4^+ of its proton, forming NH_3 and H_2CO_3.

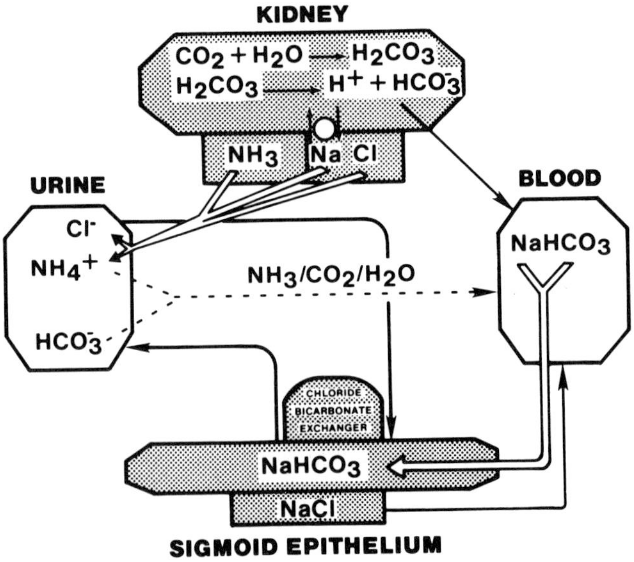

FIGURE 25-15 • Sigmoid bladder: pathogenesis of hyperchloremic acidosis. The kidney effects entry of NH_4Cl into the urine and $NaHCO_3$ into the blood, thereby ridding unwanted acid and replenishing lost HCO_3^-. Blood bicarbonate is secreted by the sigmoid epithelium into the urine in exchange for reabsorbed Cl^-. Alkaline titration of urinary NH_4^+ returns NH_3 to blood. Lost blood HCO_3^- is replaced by Cl^-, causing a hyperchloremic acidosis. (See text for details.)

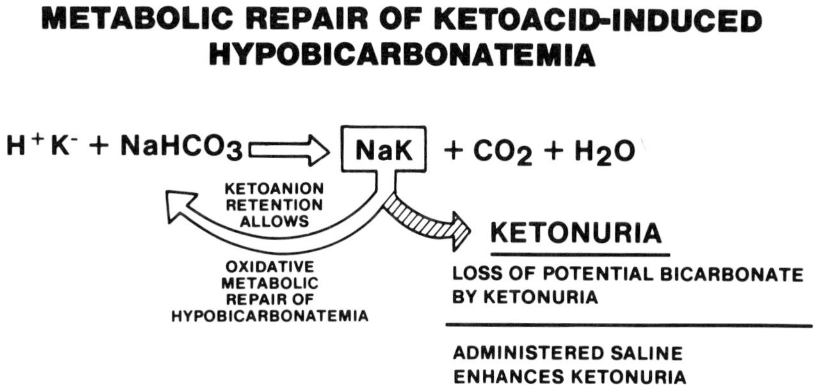

FIGURE 25-16 • Schematic representation of the conversion of ketoanion to bicarbonate. Urinary loss of ketoanion is tantamount to losing alkali. H^+K^-, ketoacid. (See text for details.)

The latter dehydrates to CO_2 and water. The free NH_3 is readily absorbed into the blood. This process can, on occasion, culminate in severe neurologic signs and symptoms from hyperammonemia.[74] Thus protons excreted by the kidney as NH_4^+ are reclaimed by the chemical events occurring in the sigmoid.

Finally, loss of renal mass, secondary to reflux and infection, interferes with renal acid excretion and worsens the degree of hypobicarbonatemia. This reflux and increased ureteral pressure seem to mimic obstructive uropathy, a condition known to stimulate renal production of prostaglandins. These are known to inhibit renal ammoniagenesis and thereby may further impair acid excretion.[130]

Substitution of an ileal for a sigmoid bladder minimizes the above-mentioned complications. One end of an excised segment of *ileum* is closed and anchored to the sacrum; the stoma is then opened to the abdominal wall, and the ureters are implanted into this newly formed bladder. That a bag must be worn over the stoma, to collect the constantly draining urine, constitutes the major disadvantage of this approach. On the other hand, high intraluminal pressures are avoided, the ileal bladder is relatively sterile, and the free drainage shortens contact time between urine and ileal epithelium, thereby limiting the deleterious exchange of bicarbonate for chloride. Metabolic acidosis does not ordinarily occur unless stomal stenosis develops. The narrowed orifice impairs drainage, stretching the bladder, and the resulting urinary stasis and increased mucosal surface area facilitate the exchange of blood bicarbonate for urinary chloride. In fact, new onset or worsening acidosis should prompt a search for stomal outflow obstruction in patients with ileal bladders.

When the ureters are destroyed, other related procedures, such as pyeloileostomy, are required. The renal pelves are anastomosed along one end of an excised segment of ileum, while the other end is exteriorized to the abdominal wall. The pathophysiology of the hyperchloremic acidosis that occasionally complicates this procedure mirrors that of the ileal bladder.

Recovery phase of diabetic ketoacidosis

The metabolic derangements characterizing diabetic ketoacidosis (DKA) are detailed in Chap. 26. Overproduced ketoacids replace consumed bicarbonate with the usually unmeasured ketone anions, thereby increasing the anion gap. Conversion to a hyperchloremic metabolic acidosis with normalization of the anion gap can result by way of any of four different pathophysiologic mechanisms (Figs. 25-16 and 25-17).[202]

Ketone anions are readily filtered at the glomerulus and are poorly reabsorbed by the tubules, causing substantial ketonuria, especially when renal function is well preserved. Ketonuria occurs both during the development of the ketoacidosis and during the early phase of treatment, as restoration of intravascular volume increases GFR. Infused sodium chloride effects replacement of lost ketone anions with chloride. Thus a high anion gap acidosis is converted to a normal anion gap variant. Had all the overproduced organic anion been retained, it would

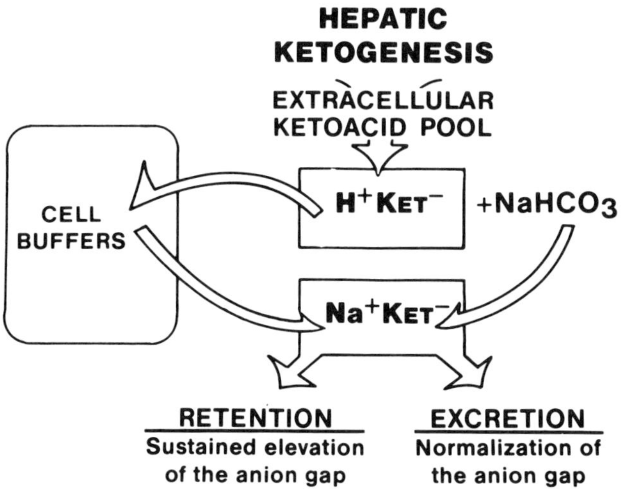

FIGURE 25-17 • Pathogenesis of normal-anion-gap acidosis during the course of ketoacidosis. The importance of back-titrating cell buffers during the reparative phase of acidosis is stressed. (See text for details.)

have been oxidized to bicarbonate during the reparative phase, thereby returning serum bicarbonate levels to baseline values. Thus lost acetoacetate (AcAc) and β-hydroxybutyrate (BHB) represent lost (potential) alkali.

Ketoacidotic patients may also develop a hyperchloremic metabolic acidosis prior to the onset of therapy.[3] It is rare for a pure normal anion gap acidosis to occur at this stage; more commonly, a mixed high anion gap, hyperchloremic acidosis obtains. In this setting the lost bicarbonate is replaced partially with unmeasured anion (ketoacid) and partially with the measured chloride anion. In other terms, the decrement in bicarbonate concentration exceeds the increment in the anion gap (see Chap. 31). The hyperchloremic component of the acidosis becomes more prominent when renal function is well preserved. The prevention of marked intravascular volume depletion and prerenal azotemia by adequate salt and water intake sustains filtration and excretion of ketone anions while ingested chloride is retained. Conversely, with ECF volume contraction, ketone anions are less likely to be filtered and lost; this creates a more typical high anion gap acidosis.

The titration of intracellular buffers and bicarbonate's greater space of distribution vis á vis that of ketoanions are other likely causes of hyperchloremia (Fig. 25-17). The sequence of pathophysiologic events that appears to underlie this aspect of the hyperchloremia proceeds as follows: Ketoacids produced in the liver enter the ECF, and a portion of the acid load remains extracellular and is titrated by bicarbonate. Protons from the remaining fraction of the added ketoacids enter cells without ketoanions. Cellular sodium and potassium enter the ECF in exchange for added protons, and the latter are absorbed by intracellular buffers. Thus extracellular ketoacid salts derive from titration of cellular and extracellular buffers by acetoacetic and β-hydroxybutyric acids. Sodium salts of the ketoacids are added to the ECF, raising the anion gap, but serum bicarbonate levels are unaffected. During the reparative phase of DKA, bicarbonate lost from the ECF must be replaced and alkali must be added to cells to back-titrate intracellular buffers.

Ketoanions are eventually oxidized, largely by muscle, and in the process re-form bicarbonate (see Chap. 26). If all the organic anion added to the ECF were retained and eventually converted to bicarbonate, cellular and extracellular acid-base parameters would be totally restored to normal. To the extent that substantial amounts of sodium and potassium salts of ketoanions are excreted, the pool of potential alkali is reduced. In the reparative phase of DKA, oxidation of the remaining ketoanions will only partially restore alkali losses. If exogenous alkali is not administered, hypobicarbonatemia will be sustained until renal bicarbonate synthesis replenishes lost alkali. The only other biologically available anion that can replace lost bicarbonate is chloride.

Infusion of a large quantity of alkali-free fluid transiently dilutes ECF bicarbonate, causing mild hypobicarbonatemia (see Dilutional Acidosis below).

The final mechanism resulting in hyperchloremic acidosis relates to the large amount of potassium chloride that must often be administered. As the infused potassium moves intracellularly to replenish body stores, sodium and protons exit cells to maintain electroneutrality. Serum bicarbonate is thus lowered, while the infused chloride contributes to the hyperchloremia.

Toluene toxicity

Toluene, variously referred to as "methylbenzene," "toluol," and "methyl benzol," is an aromatic hydrocarbon that, being less toxic than benzene, often is substituted for it. Principally used as a solvent, toluene is found in paint thinners, varnishes, lacquers, solvents, coatings, and glues. It is also used as a pure solvent and is used extensively in the production of chemicals and fuels.

Pharmacologic and biochemical principles

Toluene can be *absorbed* through the gastrointestinal tract, by inhalation, and cutaneously. Absorption after ingestion is presumably complete, and peak blood levels are usually attained within 2 h.[281a] Inhaled doses are retained to a variable extent. At resting tidal volumes, approximately one-half of an inspired dose is retained; however, this proportion may increase with greater minute ventilation.[42b] After ingestion, pulmonary excretion of toluene accounts for nearly 20 percent of its elimination. When inspired air is rich in toluene, pulmonary clearance of blood toluene is reduced, eliminating a major route of the toxin's excretion. The cutaneous absorption of toluene is slow and generally does not produce toxicity.

Toluene is highly lipid-soluble and distributes primarily in elements of the nervous system and other tissues rich in fat. However, toluene does not permeate other organs, including the myocardium, renal parenchyma, and the gastrointestinal tract.

Biliary and renal excretory routes play only a minor role in excreting toluene. The hepatic cytochrome P-450 mixed-function oxidase system initiates detoxification by hydroxylating toluene to benzyl alcohol; this initial step is inhibited by coexposure to other hydrocarbons.[3] Benzyl alcohol is oxidized to benzaldehyde by hepatic alcohol dehydrogenase and then oxidized further to benzoic acid.[27b] The latter compound is primarily conjugated to glycine, which, in turn, is converted to hippuric acid; a smaller portion of glycine is conjugated to glucuronic acid and excreted as benzyl glucuronide. The minor portion of unconjugated benzoic acid is excreted as benzoate in the urine. *Hippuric acid* readily dissociates into a proton and its conjugate base, hippurate. The anion enters the tubule by filtration and epithelial secretion, with its renal clearance approximating that of renal plasma flow.[284a]

Clinical features of toxicity

The acute toxicity of toluene derives principally from its inhalation and relates to the chemical's lipophilic nature. Inhalational toxicity occurs secondarily to either inadvertent occupational overexposure or illicit "solvent abuse." "Paint sniffing" and "glue sniffing" constitute the majority of the latter forms of exposure. In fact, upon presentation, freshly intoxicated patients may "smell like glue."[262a]

Neuropsychiatric symptoms dominate the acute phase of toxicity. Dizziness, fatigue, syncope, generalized skeletal muscular weakness, and even flaccid quadriparesis are early manifestations.[27b,185a,156a] Hallucinations, relaxation, and a "feeling of tranquility" may occur in the intoxicated patient. Cerebellar signs, including titubation (stumbling gait, indicative of midline cerebellar damage) and ataxia, have been reported.[35a,113a,145c,213a]

Gastrointestinal side effects include nausea, abdominal pain, and anorexia.[284a] Hepatotoxicity, with increased levels of the transaminases, may occur with higher levels of exposure.[113a] Jaundice and abnormal coagulation studies developed in an individual who sniffed an 80% solution of toluene; however, chronic hepatotoxicity has not been documented.[213a] Hematologic damage does not occur. Earlier suggestions that leukopenia was a complication were probably based on unsuspected admixture of benzene with toluene. Sudden death from cardiac arrhythmias may develop, possibly secondarily to sensitization of the myocardium to the effects of catecholamines. Toluene impairs contractility and depresses atrioventricular conduction in animals.[275a,300c] Fatal pulmonary edema has been reported.[190b]

Most subjects develop ECF volume contraction and hypokalemia resulting from cationic loses obligated by excretion of the hippurate load. Sodium losses induce a state of secondary hyperaldosteronism and hypokalemia. Indeed, 20 percent of intoxicated patients have had initial serum potassium levels below 2.0 meq/liter.[42a] Hypokalemia may be aggravated by the surge of catecholamines that accompanies this stress. Other significant electrolyte abnormalities include hypocalcemia, hypophosphatemia, and hypouricemia.[185a]

Direct renal effects of toluene poisoning include tubular dysfunction and abnormalities of the urinary sediment.[185a] However, short-term studies lasting several hours revealed no evidence for tubular dysfunction as measured by albumin or β_2-microglobulin excretion.[149a] Scandinavian workers exposed to the putative "safe" limit of 200 ppm of toluene did not develop urinary abnormalities as measured by albumin and β_2-microglobulin excretion.[149a] The same authors concluded that chronic exposure to moderate amounts of organic solvents was not associated with the development of renal lesions.[151a] Nephrolithiasis is rarely associated with chronic inhalation of toluene.[213a] Insufficient numbers of patients prohibit drawing a clearcut relationship between stone formation and solvent abuse. Nephrotic syndrome and glomerulosclerosis[27a,41a,224b,229a] have been proffered as sequelae of chronic toluene exposure in case reports, but proof of causality is lacking.

Flank pain, hematuria, proteinuria, and leukocyturia have been noted in the acute setting.[213a] Acute renal failure may occur. Its pathogenesis may include prerenal azotemia from volume contraction; tubular dysfunction[198a,271a,290a] and rhabdomyolysis.[271a] The latter stems from prolonged muscle compression in those patients who develop syncope secondarily to various electrolyte disturbances.[145a,145b]

While initial reports indicated that toluene poisoning was associated with a normal anion gap acidosis,[273a] Fischman and Oster[78a] described three cases in which the anion gap was increased. Their patients had seven episodes of acidosis with arterial pH levels as low as 6.90. The presenting anion gap varied between 10 and 39 meq/liter, with venous lactate levels less than 2.2 meq/liter. Urinary ketones were absent, virtually excluding the possibility of ketoacidosis. The increased production of hippuric acid and its accumulation accounted for the increased anion gap. ECF volume contraction favored the elevated anion gap by reducing the GFR and effective renal plasma flow (ERPF), thereby limiting hippurate excretion. Reexpansion of the ECF with saline solution, by increasing the GFR and ERPF, would quickly enhance the renal clearance of sodium hippurate, thereby lowering the plasma and raising the urinary anion gap. Infused sodium chloride would then replace the excreted sodium hippurate. In this manner a hyperchloremic acidosis is substituted for a high anion gap acidosis.

The literature clearly and persuasively recognizes that toluene toxicity causes a reversible metabolic acidosis, and that hippuric acid is the offending acidifying agent. Ambiguities have arisen because of variable serum electrolyte patterns associated with this disorder. On balance, the central role of renal hippurate clearance in defining the level of the prevailing anion gap (see above) establishes a uniform and logical approach to the disorder. The anion gap is likely to be normal when the renal clearance of sodium hippurate is unimpeded, whereas acute renal failure—from reduced renal perfusion, intrinsic parenchymal damage, or obstruction—allows hippurate to accumulate, thereby raising the anion gap.[42a] However, very large doses of toluene can impair H^+ secretion in turtle bladders, and a patient has been described in whom toluene was associated with Fanconi syndrome and bicarbonate wasting.[24a,185a] Thus a form of renal tubular acidosis may complicate the course of toluene toxicity.

The issue remains unclear, because these patients are often exposed to many potential renal toxins in addition to toluene. Furthermore, toluene-induced interstitial nephritis[237b] might secondarily alter tubular function. Careful study of more cases should clarify this puzzle.

Chronic organ damage may occur in the nervous system,[145a] kidneys,[213a,273b] heart, and lungs, and in the fetus carried by a pregnant woman. A putative peripheral neuropathy from chronic exposure has been inferred, but clear-cut epidemiologic studies demonstrating a dose-response relationship are lacking. Moreover, the effects of peripheral neuropathy may have been secondary to prolonged coexposure to other organic solvents, such as *n*-hexane. Cerebellar damage from long-term solvent abuse and resulting accumulation of solvents probably has been underreported.[35a] The possibility that toluene may be teratogenic has been recently reviewed, after that the frequency of birth defects was eighty percent in the offspring of mothers who had sniffed glue chronically.[27a]

Diagnosis

Toluene poisoning, like other organic hydrocarbon intoxication syndromes, may present with neurologic changes and metabolic acidosis. The concomitance of skeletal muscle paralysis and cerebellar signs should suggest this diagnosis. The residual smell of glue, a pungent benzene-like odor, may be the only clue to the diagnosis on physical examination. The finding of hippuric acid crystals (needle-shaped) by microscopic analysis is informative. However, urinalyses must be performed repeatedly, because hippurate production is variable, and its excretion may therefore be delayed, depending on the state of induction of the cytochrome P-450 system and alcohol dehydrogenase. An increased urinary anion gap in the presence of a hyperchloremic acidosis is seen only with toluene toxicity or methionine toxicity, or, in some patients, with ketoacidosis. The absence of ketonuria and a history of methionine exposure in patients with this serum and urinary chemical pattern should suggest the diagnosis.

Whenever initial assessments and laboratory data cannot render a diagnosis, more sophisticated techniques should be used. These tests include thin-layer chromatography and high-performance liquid chromatography, which can detect urinary hippurate levels of less than 0.05 mg/ml.[111a] Gas chromatography combined with mass spectrometry can determine the exact composition of toluene metabolites in the serum. With this methodology, Jone and Wu demonstrated the presence of acetoacetic, azelaic, and benzoic acids in large amounts in a patient who had ingested a toluene-containing substance.[129a] This patient had a hippuric acid level that was lower than anticipated.

Therapy

No specific antidote is available for toluene poisoning; treatment is largely supportive. Frequent arterial blood gas monitoring is absolutely critical, since these patients can easily develop ventilatory insufficiency and obtundation. Urgent correction of abnormal electrolyte levels—especially those of potassium and phosphorus—and of the acidosis should obviously be done, as in the forms of intoxication previously discussed.

Renal tubular acidosis

The various forms of renal tubular acidosis are extensively discussed in Chap. 27.

NORMOKALEMIC OR HYPERKALEMIC HYPERCHLOREMIC METABOLIC ACIDOSES

Post-hypocapneic metabolic acidosis

Acute reversal of chronic hypocapnia produces a transient hyperchloremic metabolic acidosis (Table 25-10). Acid released by extrarenal buffers reduces serum bicarbonate concentration, thereby immediately lessening the alkalemia induced by acute respiratory alkalosis

TABLE 25-10 • Pathogenesis of posthypocapneic metabolic acidosis

Blood parameters	Normal		Chronic respiratory alkalosis		Posthypocapneic metabolic acidosis (rapid normalization of P_{CO_2})
Na^+ (meq/liter)	140		140		140
Cl^-	105		115		110
HCO_3^-	24	slowΔ	→ 14	slow Δ	→ 19
AG	11		11		11
P_{CO_2} (mmHg)	40	rapid Δ	→ 20	rapid Δ	→ 40
pH	7.40		7.46		7.30

AG = anion gap.

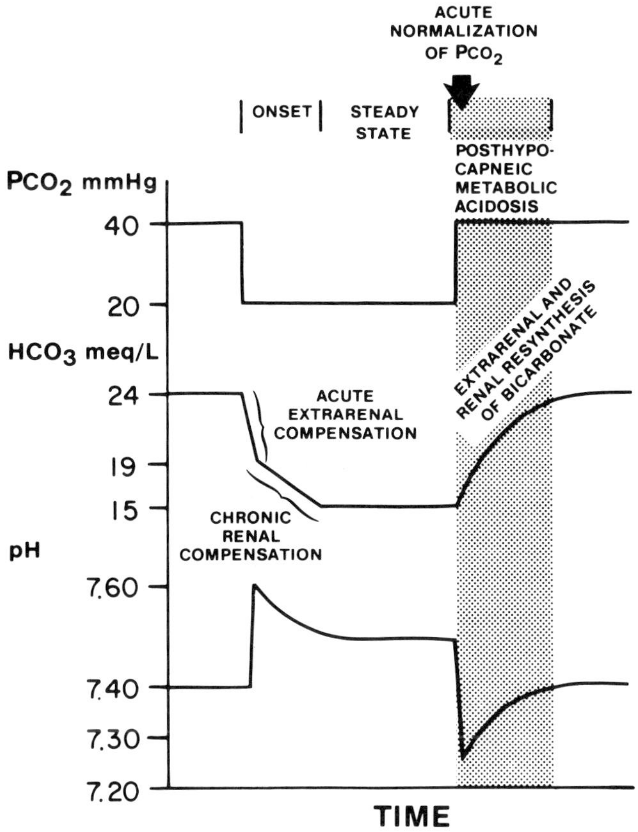

FIGURE 25-18 • Pathogenesis of posthypocapneic metabolic acidosis. Asynchronous normalization of primary hypocapnia and secondary hypobicarbonatemia results in transient hyperchloremic acidosis (shaded area).

(Fig. 25-18). With time, mild bicarbonaturia and renal acid retention further reduce serum bicarbonate levels, returning blood pH to values more closely approximating normal (Chap. 30).

In the reparative phase of respiratory alkalosis, the P_{CO_2} may normalize faster than the serum bicarbonate concentration; during this transient stage of readjustment, the proportionately greater increase in P_{CO_2} than in bicarbonate acidifies the blood (Table 25-10). Such asynchronous changes in P_{CO_2} and bicarbonate concentration may be seen with rapid and ill-advised changes in respirator settings or in rapid defervescence of a pneumonitic or bronchitic process.

Administration of exogenous hydrochloric acid or its equivalent

That direct administration of HCl causes a hyperchloremic acidosis is readily apparent; somewhat less obvious is the way in which certain HCl precursors produce the same result.

Ammonium chloride

Ammonium chloride is used inappropriately as a mild diuretic by some obese persons in desperate attempts to lose weight. The salt is also used therapeutically as an acidifying agent, and is used diagnostically in the evaluation of renal tubular acidosis. It is metabolized in the liver, producing urea and HCl and thereby causing a hyperchloremic metabolic acidosis. Large doses have caused severe metabolic acidosis even in healthy individuals with previously normal renal function.[232]

Intravenous hyperalimentation solutions

These solutions contain a mixture of cationic, neutral, and anionic amino acids. Certain preparations contain a disproportionate number of cationic residues and may therefore produce a normal-anion-gap metabolic acidosis.[117] These positively charged amino acids—lysine, arginine, and histidine—are metabolized to neutral products, and in the process liberate hydrogen ions. Because the anion accompanying these amino acids is chloride, a hyperchloremic metabolic acidosis ensues. If renal function is intact, this acid load is effortlessly excreted. The potential problem that this acidosis creates has been largely eliminated by the addition of counterbalancing amounts of alkali to the solutions. This can be accomplished by adding a sufficient amount of anionic amino acid, which consumes H^+ when metabolized. Another approach is to use histidine- and arginine-free bases and lysine acetate rather than the chloride salts of these cationic amino acids.

Elemental sulfur or sulfur-containing amino acids

Methionine, cystine, and cysteine are sulfer-containing amino acids that are metabolized to sulfuric acid.[158,253] Normally one must ingest large quantities of these amino acids to produce a significant degree of acidosis.[158] Because sulfate is an unmeasured anion, one might expect a high anion gap acidosis to develop. Titration of sulfuric acid by sodium bicarbonate effects replacement of the alkaline salt with sodium sulfate. The sulfate readily undergoes glomerular filtration but is poorly reabsorbed. The ECF volume contraction secondary to the excretion of sodium sulfate and obligate amounts of water stimulates renal retention of dietary sodium chloride.[35,138] The sodium sulfaturia raises the urinary anion gap—that is, $(Na^+ + K^+)\text{-}Cl^-$. The only other hyperchloremic acidoses associated with increased urinary anion gaps are diabetic ketoacidosis (see above) and toluene toxicity (see above). In this manner a hyperchloremic metabolic acidosis is produced.

Elemental sulfur, available without a prescription, is used as a folk remedy for intestinal complaints and dyspnea, and also as a general "tonic."[35] Metabolic production of sulfuric acid from this drug results in a hyperchloremic metabolic acidosis, as described above.

Cholestyramine

Cholestyramine's chloride salt is an anion exchange resin used to bind bile acids in the bowel lumen, in an effort to lower serum cholesterol levels. Given orally, it may be used to treat hypercholesterolemia, and also to treat pruritus associated with partial biliary tract obstruction and cholestatic liver disease.[145]

Because bicarbonate competes with bile acids for binding sites on the resin, some intestinal bicarbonate is taken up in exchange for chloride. The resultant hyperchloremic metabolic acidosis[23] becomes clinically significant only in the setting of acute or chronic renal impairment.

Calcium chloride

Calcium chloride is acidifying only when taken by mouth; parenteral administration does not produce significant acid-base disturbances. The pathogenesis of this oral effect evolves from the following sequence of events:[25] Exocrine pancreatic cells, in the presence of carbonic anhydrase, hydrate CO_2, forming carbonic acid (H_2CO_3), which immediately ionizes to H^+ and HCO_3^-. Cellular transport directs the alkali into the intestine while protons are returned to the general circulation via the venous blood. Sustained systemic acidification is averted by the eventual reabsorption of intestinal bicarbonate. Calcium chloride interrupts the neutralization of acid with absorbed alkali by precipitating the intestinal bicarbonate as the poorly absorbable $CaCO_3$ salt.[106] Oral $MgCl_2$ probably exerts the same effect.[108,208] This intestinal trapping of pancreatic bicarbonate allows for the net addition of acid to blood.

Oral $CaCl_2$ can be used as an acidifying agent instead of ammonium chloride by alkalotic patients with advanced liver disease; this averts the obvious dangers of hyperammonemia.[208]

Dilutional acidosis

Rapid volume expansion with bicarbonate-free solutions causes transient, mild hyperchloremic metabolic acidosis.[254] Dilutional hypobicarbonatemia in the face of a constant P_{CO_2} is mildly acidifying.

Dilutional acidosis is of only minor clinical significance, because rapid intracellular and bone buffering briskly returns the serum bicarbonate concentration toward normal. Renal excretion of the infused fluid and electrolytes eventually normalizes acid-base status. Only under the most extreme circumstances do alkali-free solutions produce clinically significant acidosis.[90]

Early uremic acidosis (see above)

The falling GFR of progressive renal failure leads to accumulation of metabolically produced sulfuric, phosphoric, and organic acids. The unmeasured anions of these acids produce an elevation of the anion gap.

In early renal insufficiency—especially in such processes as tubulointerstitial disease and diabetic nephropathy—disproportionate tubular dysfunction may accompany a relatively well-preserved GFR. The resultant defect in net hydrogen ion excretion may be related to deficient renal ammoniagenesis, hyporeninemic hypoaldosteronism, or, possibly, hyperparathyroidism.[188] The normal-anion-gap metabolic acidosis that ensues is transformed into one with an elevated anion gap as glomerular filtration deteriorates further.[289]

REFERENCES

1. Abu Romeh S, Tannen RL: Amelioration of hypoxia-induced lactic acidosis by superimposed hypercapnia or HCl infusion. *Am J Physiol* 250:F1205, 1986.
2. Adrogué HJ et al: Changes in the plasma anion gap during chronic metabolic acid-base disturbances. *Am J Physiol* 235:F291, 1978.
3. Adrogué HJ et al: Plasma acid-base patterns in diabetic ketoacidosis. *N Engl J Med* 307:603, 1982.

3a. Adrogué HJ et al: Salutary effects of modest fluid replacement in the treatment of adults with diabetic ketoacidosis. Use in patients without extreme volume deficit. *JAMA* 262:2108, 1989.

3b. Adrogué HJ et al: Assessing acid-base status in circulatory failure: Differences between arterial and central venous blood. *N Engl J Med* 320:1312, 1989.

3c. Adrogué HJ et al: Arteriovenous acid-base disparity in circulatory failure: Studies on mechanism. *Am J Physiol* 257:F1087, 1989.

4. Ahlborg G et al: Influence of lactate infusion on glucose and FFA metabolism in man. *Scand J Clin Lab Invest* 36:193, 1976.
5. Albert MD et al: Quantitative displacement of acid-base equilibrium in metabolic acidosis. *Ann Intern Med* 66:312, 1967.
6. Alberti KG, Nattrass M: Lactic acidosis. *Lancet* 2:25, 1977.
7. Alexander JK et al: Modification of the respiratory response to carbon dioxide by salicylate. *J Clin Invest* 34:533, 1955.
8. Anderson CJ et al: Toxicity of combined therapy with carbonic anhydrase inhibitors and aspirin. *Am J Ophthalmol* 86:516, 1978.
9. Anderson RJ et al: Unrecognized adult salicylate intoxication. *Ann Intern Med* 85:745, 1976.
10. Anderson RJ: Asterixis as a manifestation of salicylate toxicity. *Ann Intern Med* 95:188, 1981.
11. Antonini E, Brunori M: Hemoglobin. *Annu Rev Biochem* 39:977, 1970.

12. Aquilonius SM et al: Computerized tomography in severe methanol intoxication. *Br Med J* 2:929, 1978.
13. Arieff AI et al: Effects of $NaHCO_3$ in therapy of experimental lactic acidosis, abstracted. *Proc Annu Meet Am Soc Nephrol* 11:11A, 1978.
14. Arieff AI et al: Treatment of experimental lactic acidosis with dichloroacetate (DCA), abstracted. *Clin Res* 26:410A, 1978.
15. Arruda JAL et al: Bicarbonate reabsorption in chronic renal failure. *Kidney Int* 9:481, 1976.
16. Arruda JAL, Kurtzman NA: Metabolic acidosis and alkalosis. *Clin Nephrol* 7:210, 1977.
17. Arruda JAL et al: Bicarbonate reabsorption in chronic renal failure: Studies in man and rat. *Pflugers Arch* 376:193, 1978.
18. Arruda JAL et al: Parathyroid hormone and extrarenal acid buffering. *Am J Physiol* 239:F533, 1980.
19. Attas M et al: Fulminant beriberi heart disease with lactic acidosis: Presentation of a case with evaluation of left ventricular function and review of pathophysiologic mechanisms. *Circulation* 58:566, 1978.
20. Bank N, Aynedjian HS: A micropuncture study of the effect of parathyroid hormone on renal bicarbonate reabsorption. *J Clin Invest* 58:336, 1976.
21. Baran DT et al: Acidosis-induced stimulation of 25-hydroxy, D-1α-hydroxylase, abstracted. *Sixtieth Proc Annu Meet Endocrinol Soc* Miami, FL, 1978, p 235.
22. Barnett HL et al: Salicylate intoxication in infants and children. *J Pediatr* 21:214, 1942.
22a. Barsotti G et al: Compliance with protein restriction: Effects on metabolic acidosis and progression of renal failure in chronic uremics on supplemented diet. *Contr Nephrol* 81:42, 1990.
23. Bartlett GR: Combustion of C^{14} labeled methanol in intact rat and its isolated tissues. *Am J Physiol* 163:614, 1950.
24. Batlle DJ et al: Hyperkalemic distal renal tubular acidosis associated with obstructive uropathy. *N Engl J Med* 304:373, 1980.
24a. Batlle DC et al: On the mechanism of toluene-induced renal tubular acidosis. *Nephron* 49:210, 1988.
24b. Baud FJ et al: Treatment of ethylene glycol poisoning with intravenous 4-methylpyrazole. *N Engl J Med* 319:97, 1988.
25. Beaudry C et al: Methanol poisoning. Value of hemodialysis in the recovery of visual impairment. *Proc 2nd Int Cong Neuro-genet Neuro-ophthal*, Montreal, September, 1967, p 270.
26. Beck N, Webster SK: Effects of acute metabolic acidosis on parathyroid hormone action and calcium mobilization. *Am J Physiol* 230:127, 1976.
27. Beier LS et al: Metabolic acidosis occurring during paraldehyde intoxication. *Ann Intern Med* 53:155, 1963.
27a. Bengsston U: Glomerulonephritis and organic solvents. *Lancet* 2:566, 1985.
27b. Benignus VA: Health effects of toluene: A review. *Neurotoxicology* 2:567, 1981.
28. Benjamin J et al: Tissue oxygen delivery is stable despite rapid correction of chronic metabolic acidosis (abstract). *Am Soc Nephrol* 136A, 1982.
29. Bennett IL et al: Acute methyl alcohol poisoning: A review based on experiences in an outbreak of 323 cases. *Medicine* 32:431, 1953.
30. Berg KJ: Acute effects of acetylsalicylic acid in patients with chronic renal insufficiency. *Eur J Clin Pharmacol* 11:111, 1977.
31. Berman LB et al: The nephrotoxic lesion of ethylene glycol. *Ann Intern Med* 46:611, 1957.
32. Better OS et al: Defect in urinary acidification in cirrhosis. *Arch Intern Med* 130:77, 1972.
33. Bickie EG, Rasmussen H: The ionic control of 1,25-dihydroxy-vitamin D_3 production in isolated chick renal tubules. *J Clin Invest* 55:292, 1975.
33a. Blasingham MC, Nasjletti A: Differential renal effects of cyclooxygenase inhibition in sodium-replete and sodium-deprived dogs. *Am J Physiol* 239:F360, 1980.
34. Block JB et al: Metabolic abnormalities of lactic acid in Burkitt-type lymphoma with malignant effusions. *Ann Intern Med* 65:101, 1966.
35. Blum JE, Coe FL: Metabolic acidosis after sulfur ingestion. *N Engl J Med* 297:869, 1977.
35a. Boor JW, Hurtig HI: Persistent cerebellar ataxia after exposure to toluene. *Ann Neurol* 2:440, 1977.
36. Bricker NS: Sodium homeostasis in chronic renal disease. *Kidney Int* 21:886, 1982.
37. Brunette MG et al: Thiamine-responsive lactic acidosis in a patient with deficient low-Km pyruvate carboxylase activity in liver. *Pediatrics* 50:702, 1972.
37a. Buerkert J et al: Ammonia handling by superficial and juxtamedullary nephrons in the rat. *J Clin Invest* 70:1, 1982.
38. Buerkert J et al: Effect of reduced renal mass on ammonium handling and net acid formation by the superficial and juxtamedullary nephron of the rat. *J Clin Invest* 71:1661, 1983.
39. Burstein CL: The hazard of paraldehyde administration. *JAMA* 121:187, 1943.
40. Bushinsky D et al: Effects of metabolic acidosis on PTH and $1{,}25(OH)_2D_3$: Response to low calcium diet. *Am J Physiol* 243:F570, 1982.
41. Bushinsky D et al: Cellular contribution to pH- mediated calcium flux in neonatal calvariae. *Am J Physiol* 248:F85, 1985.
41a. Cagnoli L et al: Relation between hydrocarbon exposure and nephrotic syndrome. *Br Med J* 1:1068, 1980.
42. Campbell EJM, Maclaurin RE: Acute renal failure in salicylate poisoning. *Br Med J* 1:503, 1958.
42a. Carlisle E et al: Glue-sniffing and distal renal tubular acidosis: Sticking to the facts. *J Am Soc Nephrol* 1:1019, 1991.
42b. Carlsson A: Exposure to toluene: Uptake, distribution, and elimination in man. *Scand J Work Environ Health* 8:43, 1982.
42c. Carone FA et al: Renal tubular transport, catabolism of proteins and peptides. *Kidney Int* 16:271, 1979.
43. Carr DB et al: D-Lactic acidosis simulating a hypothalamic syndrome after bowel bypass. *Ann Neurol* 11:195, 1982.
44. Chanutin A, Churnish RR: Effect of organic and inorganic phosphates on the oxygen equilibrium of human erythrocytes. *Arch Biochem* 121:96, 1967.
45. Chou JY, Richardson KE: The effect of pyrazole in eth-

ylene glycol toxicity and metabolism in the rat. *Toxicol Appl Pharmacol* 43:33, 1978.
46. Clay KL et al: Experimental methanol toxicity in the primate: Analysis of metabolic acidosis. *Toxicol Appl Pharmacol* 34:49, 1975.
47. Clay KL, Murphy RC: On the metabolic acidosis of ethylene glycol intoxication. *Toxicol Appl Pharmacol* 39:39, 1977.
48. Coe FL et al: Effect of acute and chronic metabolic acidosis on serum immunoreactive parathyroid hormone in man. *Kidney Int* 8:262, 1975.
49. Coffey RC: Physiologic implantation of the severed ureter or common bile duct into the intestine. *JAMA* 56:397, 1911.
50. Cohen RD, Woods HF: *Clinical and Biochemical Aspects of Lactic Acidosis.* Oxford, Blackwell Scientific Publications, 1976.
51. Collins JM et al: Recovery after prolonged oliguria due to ethylene glycol intoxication. *Arch Intern Med* 125:1059, 1970.
52. Connor H, Woods HF: Quantitative aspects of L(+)−lactate metabolism in human beings, in Porter R: *Metabolic Acidosis*: CIBA Foundation Symposium 87. London, Pittman Books Ltd, 1982, p 214.
53. Cooper JR, Kini MM: Biochemical aspects of methanol poisoning, editorial. *Biochem Pharmacol* 11:405, 1962.
54. Cotton EK, Fahlberg VI: Hypoglycemia with salicylate poisoning. *Am J Dis Child* 108:171, 1964.
55. Crumb CK et al: Effects of volume expansion, purified parathyroid extract, and calcium on renal bicarbonate absorption in the dog. *J Clin Invest* 54:1287, 1974.
56. Cumming G et al: Alkaline diuresis in treatment of aspirin poisoning. *Br Med J* 2:1033, 1969.
57. Daniel AM et al: Lactate metabolism in the dog during shock from hemorrhage, cardiac tamponade or endotoxin. *Surg Gynecol Obstet* 143:581, 1976.
57a. Daniels SR et al: Scientific uncertainties in the studies of salicylate use and Reye's syndrome. *JAMA* 249:131, 1983.
57b. Del Canale S et al: Uremic acidosis and intracellular buffering. *Scand J Urol Nephrol* 20:310, 1986.
58. Dempsey JA, Forster HV: Mediation of ventilatory adaptations. *Physiol Rev* 62:262, 1982.
59. Done AK: Salicylate intoxication. Significance of measurements of salicylate in blood in cases of acute ingestion. *Pediatrics* 26:800, 1960.
60. Downing SE et al: Cardiovascular responses to metabolic acidosis. *Am J Physiol* 208:237, 1965.
61. Dubb J et al: Tubular effects of acute metabolic acidosis in the rat. *J Lab Clin Med* 90:318, 1977.
61a. Eckfeldt JH, Kernshaw MJ: Hyperamylasemia following methyl alcohol intoxication: Source and significance. *Arch Intern Med* 146:194, 1986.
61b. Ekins BR et al: Standardized treatment of severe methanol poisoning with ethanol and hemodialysis. *West J Med* 142:337, 1985.
62. Elkinton JR et al: Renal tubular acidosis with organic aciduria during paraldehyde ingestion. *Am J Med* 23:977, 1957.
63. Elkinton JR: Hydrogen ion turnover in health and in renal disease. *Ann Intern Med* 57:660, 1962.
64. Elkinton JR: Clinical disorders of acid-base regulation. *Med Clin North Am* 50:1325, 1966.
64a. Ellenhorn MJ, Barceloux DG: Salicylates, in Ellenhorn MJ, Barceloux DG (eds): *Medical Toxicology: The Diagnosis and Treatment of Poisoning.* New York, Elsevier, 1988, p 560.
65. Emmett M, Seldin DW: Clinical syndromes of metabolic acidosis and metabolic alkalosis, in Seldin DW, Giebisch G (eds): *The Kidney: Physiology and Pathophysiology.* New York, Raven Press, 1985, p 87.
66. Enger E: Acidosis, gaps and poisonings (editorial). *Acta Med Scand* 212:1, 1982.
67. Epstein F: Calcium and the kidney. *Am J Med* 45:700, 1968.
68. Erlanson P et al: Severe methanol intoxication. *Acta Med Scand* 177:393, 1965.
69. Erlinger S: Secretion of bile, in Schiff L, Schiff ER (eds): *Diseases of the Liver.* Philadelphia, Lippincott, 1982.
70. Espinel CH: The influence of salt intake on metabolic acidosis of chronic renal failure. *J Clin Invest* 56:286, 1975.
71. Feldman G, Charney AN: Effect of acute metabolic alkaloses and acidoses on intestinal electrolyte transport in vivo. *Am J Physiol* 239:F427, 1982.
72. Fera RT, Nagaoawa HT: Metabolism of paraldehyde to acetaldehyde by rat liver microsomes. *Res Commun Chem Pathol Pharmacol* 34:531, 1981.
73. Fernandez LB et al: Fecal acidorrhea. *N Engl J Med* 284:295, 1971.
74. Ferris DO, Odel HM: Electrolyte pattern of the blood after bilateral ureterosigmoidostomy. *JAMA* 142:634, 1950.
75. Feuerstein RC et al: The use of acetazolamide in the therapy of salicylate poisoning. *Pediatrics* 25:215, 1960.
76. Field M et al: Significance of blood lactate elevations among patients with acute leukemia and other neoplastic proliferative disorders. *Am J Med* 40:528, 1966.
77. Fields ALA et al: Chronic lactic acidosis in a patient with cancer: Therapy and metabolic consequences. *Cancer* 47:2026, 1981.
77a. Filley GF, Kendig NB: Carbicarb, an alkalinizing ion-generating agent of possible clinical usefulness. *Trans Am Clin Climatol Assoc* 96:141, 1984.
78. Finch CA et al: Lactic acidosis as a result of iron deficiency. *J Clin Invest* 64:129, 1979.
78a. Fischman CM, Oster JR: Toxic effects of toluene: A new cause of high anion gap metabolic acidosis. *JAMA* 241:1713, 1979.
79. Fordtran JS: Speculations on the pathogenesis of diarrhea. *Fed Proc* 26:1405, 1967.
79a. Forster RE: Carbon monoxide and the partial pressure of oxygen in tissue. *Ann NY Acad Sci* 174:233, 1970.
80. Fraley DS et al: Stimulation of lactate production by the administration of bicarbonate in a patient with a solid neoplasm and lactic acidosis. *N Engl J Med* 303:1100, 1980.
81. Fraley DS, Adler S: An extrarenal role for parathyroid hormone in the disposal of acute acid loads in rats and dogs. *J Clin Invest* 63:985, 1979.
82. Freed CR et al: Ethanol for ethylene glycol poisoning. *N Engl J Med* 304:967, 1981.

83. Freeman RM, Richards CJ: Studies on sulfate in end stage renal disease. *Kidney Int* 15:167, 1979.
84. Friedman EA et al: Consequences of ethylene glycol poisoning. *Am J Med* 32:891, 1962.
85. Frommer JP: Lactic acidosis. *Med Clin North Am* 67:815, 1983.
86. Fulop M: Ventilatory response in patients with acute lactic acidosis. *Crit Care Med* 10:173, 1982.
87. Gabow PA et al: Acid-base disturbances in the salicylate intoxicated adult. *Arch Intern Med* 138:1481, 1978.
87a. Gabow PA et al: Organic acids in ethylene glycol intoxication. *Ann Intern Med* 304:21, 1986.
88. Gafter U et al: Effect of metabolic acidosis on intestinal absorption of calcium and phosphorous. *Am J Physiol* 239:G480, 1980.
89. Garcia J et al: Urinary D-lactate excretion in infants with necrotizing enterocolitis. *J Pediatr* 104:268, 1984.
90. Garella S et al: Dilution acidosis and contraction alkalosis: Review of a concept (editorial). *Kidney Int* 8:279, 1975.
90a. Gazmuri RJ et al: Cardiac effects of carbon dioxide-consuming and carbon dioxide-generating buffers during cardiopulmonary resuscitation. *J Am Coll Cardiol* 15:482, 1990.
91. Gennari FJ, Cohen JJ: Role of the kidney in potassium homeostasis: Lessons from acid-base disturbances. *Kidney Int* 8:1, 1975.
92. Gerst PH et al: Increased susceptibility of the heart to ventricular fibrillation during metabolic acidosis. *Circ Res* 19:63, 1966.
92a. Glabman S et al: Micropuncture study of ammonia excretion in the rat. *Am J Physiol* 205:127, 1963.
93. Glasser L et al: Serum osmolality and its applicability to drug overdose. *Am J Clin Pathol* 60:695, 1973.
94. Godolphin W et al: Case 38-1979 ethylene glycol poisoning. *N Engl J Med* 302:465, 1980.
95. Gold JA et al: The effect of intravenous paraldehyde as recorded by the chest X-ray film. *Dis Chest* 37:453, 1960.
96. Goldfinger S et al: Renal retention of uric acid induced by infusion of beta-hydroxybutyrate and acetoacetate. *N Engl J Med* 272:351, 1965.
97. Gonda A et al: Hemodialysis for methanol intoxication. *Am J Med* 64:749, 1978.
98. Goodgame JT Jr et al: Iatrogenic lactic acidosis: Association with hypertonic glucose administration in a patient with cancer. *Cancer* 42:800, 1978.
99. Goodkin DA, Narins RG: Quantitation of serum potassium changes during acute acid-base disturbances, in Whelton PK, Whelton A (eds): *Potassium in Cardiovascular and Renal Medicine*. New York, Marcel Dekker, 1986, p 67.
100. Goodman AD et al: Production, excretion and net balance of fixed acid in patients with renal acidosis. *J Clin Invest* 44:495, 1965.
101. Goodman L, Gilman A: *The Pharmacological Basis of Therapeutics*, 5th ed. New York, MacMillan, 1975, p 131.
102. Gordon HL, Hunter JM: Ethylene glycol poisoning. *Anaesthesia* 37:332, 1982.
102a. Green R, Giebisch G: Ionic requirements of proximal tubular sodium transport: I. Bicarbonate and chloride. *Am J Physiol* 229:1205, 1975.
102b. Greenstein SM: Pulmonary edema and salicylate intoxication. *JAMA* 230:866, 1974.
102c. Grete A et al: A low protein diet protects uremic rats against the negative sequelae of metabolic acidosis. *Nephron* 54:327, 1990.
103. Gutman A et al: A study by simultaneous clearance techniques of salicylate excretion in man. Effect of alkalinization of the urine by bicarbonate administration: Effect of probenecid. *J Clin Invest* 34:711, 1955.
104. Gutman RA et al: Paraldehyde acidosis. *Am J Med* 42:435, 1967.
105. Hadden JW, Metzner RJ: Pseudoketosis and hyperacetaldehydemia in paraldehyde acidosis. *Am J Med* 47:642, 1969.
106. Haldane JBS et al: Calcium chloride acidosis. *J Physiol* 57:20, 1923.
107. Halperin ML: Lactic acidosis and ketoacidosis: Biochemical and clinical complications. *Can Med Assoc J* 116:1034, 1977.
108. Halperin ML: Metabolism and acid-base physiology. *Artif Organs* 6:357, 1982.
109. Halverson J et al: D-Lactic acidosis and other complications of intestinal bypass surgery. *Arch Intern Med* 144:357, 1984.
109a. Hammeke M et al: Hyperchloremic metabolic acidosis in diabetes mellitus: A case report and discussion of the pathoyphysiologic mechanism. *Diabetes* 27:16, 1978.
110. Hannaford MC et al: Role of acidosis in the protein wasting of fasting in the rat and the rabbit. *Can J Physiol Pharmacol* 60:331, 1981.
111. Hannaford MC et al: Protein wasting due to acidosis of prolonged fasting. *Am J Physiol* 243:E251, 1982.
111a. Hansen SH, Dossing M: Determination of urinary hippuric acid and o-cresol, as indices of toluene exposure, by liquid chromatography on dynamically modified silica. *J Chromatog* 229:141, 1981.
111b. Hara Y et al: Acidosis, not azotemia, stimulates branched-chain amino acid catabolism in uremic rats. *Kidney Int* 32:808, 1987.
112. Harrington JT, Cohen JJ: Metabolic acidosis, in Cohen JJ, Kassirer JP (eds): *Acid-Base*. Boston, Little, Brown, 1982, p 128.
113. Harvey RM et al: Hemodynamic effects of dehydration and metabolic acidosis in Asiatic cholera. *Trans Assoc Am Physicians* 79:177, 1966.
113a. Hayden JW et al: Toxicology of toluene (methyl benzene): Review of the literature. *Clin Toxicol* 11:549, 1977.
114. Hayward JN, Boshell BR: Paraldehyde intoxication with metabolic acidosis. *Am J Med* 23:977, 1957.
115. Heath A: Methanol poisoning. *Lancet* 1:1339, 1983.
116. Heffiner JE, Sahn SA: Salicylate-induced pulmonary edema. *Ann Intern Med* 95:405, 1981.
117. Heird WC et al: Metabolic acidosis resulting from intravenous alimentation mixtures containing synthetic amino acids. *N Engl J Med* 287:943, 1972.
117a. Hewlett TP, McMartin KE: Ethylene glycol poisoning. The value of glycolic acid determinations for diagnosis and treatment. *Clin Toxicol* 24:389, 1986.

118. Hill JB: Experimental salicylate poisoning: Observations on the effects of altering blood pH on tissue and plasma salicylate concentration. *Pediatrics* 47:658, 1971.

118a. Hillman RJ, Prescott LF: Treatment of salicylate poisoning with repeated oral charcoal. *Br Med J* 291:1472, 1985.

119. Hodgkinson A, Zarembski PM: Oxalic acid metabolism in man: A review. *Calcif Tissue Res* 2:115, 1968.

120. Hood VL et al: Impact of hydrogen ion on fasting ketogenesis: Feedback regulation of acid production. *Am J Physiol* 242:F238, 1983.

121. Huckabee WE: Relationship of pyruvate and lactate during anaerobic metabolism: III. Effect of breathing low oxygen gases. *J Clin Invest* 37:264, 1958.

122. Humphrey SH, Nash DA Jr: Lactic acidosis complicating sodium nitroprusside therapy. *Ann Intern Med* 88:58, 1978.

122a. Hurwitz ES et al: Public health service study on Reye's syndrome and medications. Report of the pilot phase. *N Engl J Med* 313:849, 1985.

123. Husted RC et al: $NaHCO_3$ and NaCl tolerance in chronic renal failure. *J Clin Invest* 56:414, 1975.

123a. Jacobsen D et al: Studies on methanol poisoning. *Acta Med Scand* 212:5, 1982.

124. Jacobsen D et al: Studies on ethylene glycol poisoning. *Acta Med Scand* 212:11, 1982.

125. Jacobsen D et al: Anion and osmolal gaps in the diagnosis of methanol and ethylene glycol poisoning. *Acta Med Scand* 212:17, 1982.

126. Jacobsen D et al: Toxicokinetics of formate during hemodialysis. *Acta Med Scand* 214:409, 1983.

126a. Jacobsen D et al: Glycolate causes the acidosis in ethylene glycol poisoning and is effectively removed by hemodialysis. *Acta Med Scand* 216:409, 1984.

127. James JA et al: Experimental salicylate intoxication: I. Comparison of exchange transfusion, intermittent peritoneal lavage, and hemodialysis as a means of removing salicylate. *Pediatrics* 29:442, 1962.

128. Javaheri S et al: Ventilatory drive in acute metabolic acidosis. *J Appl Physiol* 45:913, 1979.

128a. Jenkins D et al: The metabolic consequences of the correction of acidosis in uraemia. *Nephrol Dial Transplant* 4:92, 1989.

129. Johnson CW, Morgan JM: Acidosis: A clue to the etiology of renal failure. *South Med J* 58:1513, 1965.

129a. Jone CM, Wu AHB: An unusual case of toluene-induced metabolic acidosis. *Clin Chem* 34:2596, 1988.

130. Jones ER et al: Prostaglandins inhibit renal ammoniagenesis in the rat. *J Clin Invest* 74:992, 1984.

131. Kachel RG: Metastatic reticulum cell sarcoma and lactic acidosis. *Cancer* 36:2056, 1975.

132. Kaehny WD, Jackson JT: Respiratory response to HCl acidosis in dogs after carotid body denervation. *J Appl Physiol* 46:1138, 1979.

133. Kahn A, Blum D: Methyl alcohol poisoning, in an 8 month old boy: An unusual route of administration. *J Pedatr* 94:841, 1979.

134. Kane RL et al: A methanol poisoning outbreak in Kentucky. *Arch Environ Health* 17:119, 1968.

135. Karlinsky ML et al: Effect of parathormone and cyclic adenosine monophosphate on renal bicarbonate reabsorption. *Am J Physiol* 227:1226, 1974.

136. Kassirer SP, Bleich HL: Rapid estimation of plasma carbon dioxide from pH and total carbon dioxide content. *N Engl J Med* 272:1067, 1965.

137. Katz LA, Spiro HM: The gastrointestinal manifestations of diabetes. *N Engl J Med* 275:1350, 1966.

138. Kaye S: *Handbook of Emergency Toxicology*, 2nd ed. Springfield, CC Thomas, 1961, p 214.

139. Kaye S et al (eds): *Clinical Laboratory Methods and Diagnosis*. St. Louis, Mosby, 1963, p 421.

140. Kaye S, Haag H: Study of death due to combined action of alcohol and paraldehyde in man. *Toxicol Appl Pharmacol* 6:316, 1964.

141. Keller U et al: Pheochromocytoma with lactic acidosis. *Lancet* 2:606, 1978.

142. Keplinger ML, Wells JA: Effect of antabuse on the action of paraldehyde in mice and dogs. *Fed Am Soc Exp Biol* 15:445, 1956.

143. Kerber RE et al: The effect of ischemia, hypertrophy, hypoxia, acidosis and alkalosis on canine defibrillation. *Am J Physiol* 244:H825, 1983.

144. Keyvan-Larijarni H, Tannenberg AM: Methanol intoxication: Comparison of peritoneal dialysis and hemodialysis treatment. *Arch Intern Med* 134:293, 1974.

144a. Klahr S, Harris H: Adaptation of remnant nephrons, in Giovanetti S (ed): *Nutritional Treatment of Chronic Renal Failure*. Boston, Kluwer Academic, 1989, p 13.

145. Kleinman PK: Cholestyramine and metabolic acidosis, letter. *N Engl J Med* 290:861, 1974.

145a. Knochel JP, Schlein JM: On the mechanism of rhabdomyolysis in potassium depletion. *J Clin Invest* 51:1750, 1972.

145b. Knochel JP: The pathophysiology and clinical characteristics of severe hypophosphatemia. *Arch Intern Med* 137:203, 1977.

145c. Knox JW, Nelson JR: Permanent encephalopathy from toluene inhalation. *N Engl J Med* 275:1494, 1966.

146. Kokko JP: Proximal tubule potential difference: Dependence on glucose, HCO_3^- and amino acids. *J Clin Invest* 52:1362, 1973.

147. Kolendorf K, Moller BB: Lactic acidosis in epinephrine poisoning. *Acta Med Scand* 196:465, 1974.

148. Kontos H: Vasodilator effect of hypercapnic acidosis on human forearm vessels. *Am J Physiol* 215:1403, 1968.

149. Kotz J et al: Idiosyncrasy to paraldehyde. *JAMA* 110:2145, 1938.

149a. Kraemmer H et al: Renal effects of chronic exposure to organic solvents. *Acta Med Scand* 218:317, 1985.

150. Kreisberg RA et al: Lactate turnover and gluconeogenesis in normal and obese humans: Effect of starvation. *Diabetes* 19:53, 1970.

151. Kreisberg RA et al: Ethanol-induced hyperlacticacidemia: Inhibition of lactate utilization. *J Clin Invest* 50:166, 1971.

151a. Krussel L et al: Renal effects of chronic exposure to organic solvents. *Acta Med Scand* 218:323, 1985.

152. Kurtzman NA et al: Effect of potassium and extracellular volume on renal bicarbonate reabsorption. *Metabolism* 22:481, 1973.

153. Kussmaul A: Concerning a peculiar mode of death in diabetics, concerning acetonemia, the glycerin treatment of diabetes and the injection of diastase into the blood in this disease. *Dsch Arch F Klin Med* XIV:1, 1874.
154. Kwong TC et al: Self-poisoning with enteric-coated aspirin. *Am J Clin Pathol* 80:888, 1983.
155. Lacouture PG, Lovejoy FH Jr: Methanol. *Clin Toxicol Rev* 3:12, 1981.
156. Lang D et al: Rate of pulmonary excretion of paraldehyde in man. *Toxicol Appl Pharmacol* 15:269, 1969.
156a. Lavoie FW et al: Recurrent resuscitation and "no code" orders in a 27-year-old spray paint abuser. *Ann Emerg Med* 16:1266, 1987.
157. Lawson AAH et al: Forced diuresis in the treatment of acute salicylate poisoning in adults. *Q J Med* 38:31, 1969.
157a. Leist ER, Barnwell JG: Products containing aspirin. *N Engl J Med* 291:710, 1974.
158. Lemann J Jr, Relman AS: The relation of sulfur metabolism to acid-base balance and electrolyte excretion: The effects of DL-methionine in normal man. *J Clin Invest* 38:2215, 1959.
159. Lemann J Jr et al: Effects of chronic acid loads in normal man: Further evidence for the participation of bone mineral in the defense against chronic metabolic acidosis. *J Clin Invest* 45:1608, 1966.
160. Lemann J Jr et al: Studies of the mechanism by which chronic metabolic acidosis augments urinary calcium excretion in man. *J Clin Invest* 46:1318, 1967.
160a. Lennon EJ, Lemann J Jr: Defense of hydrogen ion concentration in chronic metabolic acidosis. *Ann Intern Med* 65:265, 1966.
161. Lennon EJ: Metabolic acidosis: A factor in the pathogenesis of azotemic osteodystrophy. *Arch Intern Med* 124:557, 1969.
161a. Levy G, Tsuchiya T: Salicylate accumulation in man. *N Engl J Med* 287:430, 1972.
162. Levy G: Clincal pharmacokinetics of aspirin. *Pediatrics* 62:867, 1978.
163. Levy G: Pharmacokinetics of salicylate in man. *Drug Metab Rev* 9:3, 1979.
164. Levy G: Comparative pharmacokinetics of aspirin and acetaminophen. *Arch Intern Med* 141:279, 1981.
165. Limbeck GA et al: Salicylates and hypoglycemia. *Am J Dis Child* 109:165, 1965.
165a. Lintner CM, Linter SP: Severe lactic acidosis following "paraldehyde" administration. *Br J Psych* 149:650, 1986.
166. Lofquist J, Nillson E: The influence of acid-base ranges on carbachol and potassium induced contractions of taenia coli in the rabbit. *Acta Physiol Scand* 111:59, 1981.
166a. Maack T et al: Renal filtration, transport, and metabolism of low-molecular-weight proteins: A review. *Kidney Int* 16:251, 1979.
167. Maclean AJ, Hayslett JP: Adaptive change in ammonia excretion in renal insufficiency. *Kidney Int* 17:595, 1980.
168. Madias NE et al: Effects of the acute acid buffering response from endogenous parathyroid hormone. *Am J Physiol* 243:F141, 1982.
169. Maguire LC et al: Glucose therapy of recurrent lactic acidosis. *Am J Med Sci* 276:305, 1978.
170. Maher T et al: Amelioration of metabolic acidosis by dietary potassium restriction in hyperkalemic patients with chronic renal insufficiency. *J Lab Clin Med* 103:432, 1984.
171. Makar AB, Mannering JG: Role of the intracellular distribution of hepatic catalase in the peroxidative oxidation of methanol. *Mol Pharmacol* 4:484, 1968.
172. Makar AB, Tephly TR: Methanol poisoning in the folate-deficient rat. *Nature* 261:715, 1976.
173. Marc-Aurele J, Schreiner GE: The dialysance of ethanol and methanol: A proposed method for the treatment of massive intoxication by ethyl or methyl alcohol. *J Clin Invest* 39:802, 1960.
174. Marsiglis JC et al: Relevance of beta receptor blockade to the negative inotropic effect induced by metabolic acidosis. *Cardiovasc Res* 7:336, 1973.
175. Martin KJ et al: The effect of acute acidosis on the uptake of parathyroid hormone and the production of adenosine 3':5'-monophosphate by isolated perfused bone. *Endocrinology* 106:1607, 1980.
175a. May RC et al: Mechanisms for defects in muscle protein metabolism in rats with chronic uremia. *J Clin Invest* 79:1099, 1987.
176. McDougall J, Wyllis AM: A fatal case of paraldehyde poisoning with postmortem findings. *J Ment Sci* 78:374, 1932.
177. McMartin KE et al: Methanol poisoning: I. The role of formic acid in the development of metabolic acidosis in the monkey and the reversal by 4-methylpyrazole. *Biochem Med* 13:319, 1975.
178. McMartin KE et al: Methanol poisoning in human subjects. Role for formic acid accumulation in the metabolic acidosis. *Am J Med* 68:414, 1980.
178a. McQueen DS et al: Arterial chemoreceptor involvement in salicylate-induced hyperventilation in rats. *Br J Pharmacol* 98:413, 1989.
179. Medalle R et al: Lactic acidosis and associated hypoglecemia. *Arch Intern Med* 128:273, 1971.
180. Methanol poisoning, editorial. *Lancet* 1:910, 1983.
181. Meyer JH: Pancreatic physiology, in Sleisenger MH, Fordtran JS (eds): *Gastrointestinal Disease. Pathophysiology, Diagnosis and Management.* Philadelphia, Saunders, 1983, p 125.
182. Mintz U et al: Lactic acidosis and diffuse histiocytic lymphoma (DHL). *Am J Hematol* 4:359, 1978.
182a. Mitch WE et al: Review: Mechanisms for abnormal protein metabolism in uremia. *J Am Coll Nutr* 8(4):305, 1989.
182b. Mitch WE et al: Protein and amino acid metabolism in uremia: Influence of metabolic acidosis. *Kidney Int* 36:S205, 1989.
183. Mitchell JH et al: The effects of acid-base disturbances on cardiovascular and pulmonary function. *Kidney Int* 1:375, 1972.
184. Morgan AG, Polak A: Acetazolamide and sodium bicarbonate in treatment of salicylate poisoning in adults. *Br Med J* 1:16, 1969.

185. Moriarty RW, McDonald RH: The spectrum of ethylene glycol poisoning. *Clin Toxicol* 7:583, 1974.
185a. Moss AH et al: Fanconi's syndrome and distal renal tubular acidosis after glue sniffing. *Ann Intern Med* 92:69, 1980.
186. Mountain R et al: Noncardiac pulmonary edema following administration of parenteral paraldehyde. *Chest* 82:371, 1982.
187. Muldowney FPD et al: Correction of renal bicarbonate wastage by parathyroidectomy. Implications in acid-base homeostasis. *Q J Med* 40:487, 1971.
188. Muldowney FPD et al: Parathyroid acidosis in uremia. Q J Med 38:321, 1972.
189. Muldowney FPD: Renal acidosis, in Black D, Jones NF (eds): *Renal Disease*, 4th ed. Oxford, Blackwell Scientific Publications, 1979, p 588.
190. Mundy RL et al: Pyrazole as an antidote for ethylene glycol poisoning. *Toxicol Appl Pharmacol* 28:320, 1974.
190a. Myers RAM et al: Value of hyperbaric oxygen in suspected carbon monoxide poisoning. *JAMA* 246:2478, 1981.
190b. Musclow CE, Awen CF: Glue sniffing: Report of a fatal case. *Can Med Assoc J* 104:315, 1977.
191. Nadiminti Y et al: Lactic acidosis associated with Hodgkin's disease. *N Engl J Med* 303:15, 1980.
192. Nahas GG et al: Acidemia and catecholamine output of the isolated canine adrenal gland. *Am J Physiol* 213:1186, 1967.
192a. Nanji AA: Absence of symptoms and acidosis in potentially lethal methanol poisoning. *Ann Emerg Med* 13:487, 1984.
193. Narins RG et al: Lactic acidosis and the elevated anion gap. *Hosp Prac* May 1980, p 125 and June 1980, p 91.
194. Narins RG, Emmett M: Simple and mixed acid-base disorders: A practical approach. *Medicine* 56:161, 1980.
195. Narins RG, Gardner LB: Simple acid-base disturbances. *Med Clin North Am* 65:321, 1981.
196. Narins RG et al: Acid-base metabolism, in Gonick HC (ed): *Current Nephrology*. New York, Wiley, 1982, vol 5, p 79.
197. Nayler WG et al: A protective effect of a mild acidosis on hypoxic heart muscle. *J Mol Cell Cardiol* 11:1053, 1979.
198. Negus P et al: Indomethacin potentiates the vasoconstrictor actions of angiotensin II in normal man. *Prostaglandins* 12:175, 1976.
198a. Nielsen HK et al: Renal effects of acute exposure to toluene. *Acta Med Scand* 218:317, 1985.
198b. Oates JA et al: Clinical implications of prostaglandin and thromboxane A_2 formation. *N Engl J Med* 319:689, 1986.
199. Noker PE et al: Methanol toxicity: Treatment with folic acid and 5-formyl tetrahydrofolic acid. *Alcoholism: Clin Exp Res* 4:378, 1980.
200. Nordin BEC: The effect of intravenous parathyroid extract on urinary pH, bicarbonate and electrolyte excretion. *Clin Sci* 19:311, 1960.
201. O'Connor LR et al: Hyperphosphatemia in lactic acidosis. *N Engl J Med* 297:707, 1977.
202. Oh MS et al: Hyperchloremic acidosis during the recovery phase of diabetic ketosis. *Ann Intern Med* 89:925, 1978.
203. Oh MS et al: D-Lactic acidosis in a man with the short bowel syndrome. *N Engl J Med* 301:249, 1979.
203a. Oh MS et al: The mechanism of hyperchloremic acidosis during the recovery phase of diabetic ketoacidosis. *Diabetes* 30:310, 1981.
204. Oh MS et al: Metabolic utilization and renal handling of D-lactate in man. *Metabolism* 34:621, 1985.
205. Orringer CE et al: Natural history of lactic acidosis after grand-mal seizures. *N Engl J Med* 297:796, 1977.
206. Orthner H: Die Methylalkoholvergiftung mit besonderer Berücksichtigung neuaritiger Hirmbefunde: *Monographien aus dem Gesamtgebiet der Neurologie und Psychiatrie*, Heft 74. Berlin, Springer, 1950.
207. Osnes J, Hermansen L: Acid-base balance after maximal exercise of short duration. *J Appl Physiol* 32:59, 1972.
208. Oster JR et al: A short duration renal acidification test using calcium chloride. *Nephron* 14:281, 1975.
209. Oster JR et al: Abnormal renal acidification in alcoholic liver disease. *J Lab Clin Med* 85:987, 1975.
210. Oster JR et al: Relationship between blood pH and potassium and phosphorus during acute metabolic acidosis. *Am J Physiol* 235:F345, 1978.
210a. Osterloh JD et al: Serum formate concentrations in methanol intoxication as a criterion for hemodialysis. *Ann Intern Med* 104:200, 1986.
211. Pappas S, Silverman M: Treatment of methanol poisoning with ethanol and hemodialysis. *Can Med Assoc J* 126:1391, 1982.
212. Park R, Arieff AI: Treatment of lactic acidosis with dichloroacetate in dogs. *J Clin Invest* 70:853, 1982.
213. Parry MF, Wallach R: Ethylene glycol poisoning. *Am J Med* 57:143, 1974.
213a. Patel R, Benjamin J Jr: Renal disease associated with toluene inhalation. *Clin Toxicol* 24:213, 1986.
214. Peraino RA, Suki WN: Urine HCO_3^- augments renal Ca^{2+} absorption independent of systemic acid-base changes. *Am J Physiol* 238:F394, 1980.
215. Perez GO et al: Effect of NH_4Cl on plasma aldosterone, cortisol and renin activity in supine man. *J Clin Endocrinol Metab* 45:762, 1977.
216. Perez GO et al: The effect of acute metabolic acidosis on plasma cortisol, renin activity and aldosterone. *Horm Res* 11:12, 1979.
217. Perlmutler DH et al: D-Lactic acidosis in children: An unusual metabolic complication of small bowel resection. *J Pediatr* 102:234, 1983.
218. Peterson CD et al: Ethylene glycol poisoning: Pharmacokinetics during therapy with ethanol and hemodialysis. *N Engl J Med* 304:21, 1981.
219. Peterson CD et al: Ethanol for ethylene glycol poisoning. *N Engl J Med* 304:977, 1981.
220. Photz pH, Kimberly RP: Acute effects of aspirin and acetaminophen on renal function. *Arch Intern Med* 141:343, 1981.
221. Pichette C et al: Elevation of the blood lactate concentration by alkali therapy without requiring additional lactic acid accumulation: Theoretical considerations. *Crit Care Med* 10:323, 1982.

222. Pierce NF et al: The ventilatory response to acute base deficit in humans. Time course during development and correction of metabolic acidosis. *Ann Intern Med* 72:633, 1970.
223. Planas R et al: Acetylsalicylic acid suppresses the renal hemodynamic effect and reduces the diuretic action of furosemide in cirrhosis with ascites. *Gastroenterology* 84:247, 1983.
224. Pons CA, Custor RP: Acute ethylene glycol poisoning. A clinico-pathologic report of 18 fatal cases. *Am J Med Sci* 211:544, 1946.
225. Poole-Wilson PA et al: Renal excretion of bicarbonate and hydrogen ions: Effects of mannitol diuresis in normal man. *Clin Sci* 43:561, 1972.
226. Prescott LF et al: Diuresis or urinary alkalinization for salicylate poisoning? *Br Med J* 285:1383, 1982.
227. Proudfoot AT, Brown SS: Acidemia and salicylate poisoning in adults. *Br Med J* 2:547, 1969.
228. Prowse K et al: The treatment of salicylate poisoning using mannitol and forced diuresis. *Clin Sci* 38:327, 1970.
229. Puschett JB, Zurbach P: Acute effects of parathyroid hormone on proximal bicarbonate transport in the dog. *Kidney Int* 9:501, 1976.
229a. Raunskov U: Exposure to organic solvents—a missing link—poststreptococcal glomerulonephritis. *Acta Med Scand* 203:351, 1978.
230. Reif G: Uber die Giftigkeit des Methylalkohols. *Dsch Med Wochenschr* 49:183, 1923.
231. Relman AS: Renal acidosis and renal excretion of acid in health and disease. *Adv Intern Med* 12:295, 1964.
232. Relman AS et al: Profound acidosis resulting from excessive ammonium chloride in previously healthy subjects. *N Engl J Med* 264:848, 1966.
233. Relman AS: Lactic acidosis. *Trans Am Clin Climatol Assoc* 82:70, 1971.
234. Relman AS: Metabolic consequences of acid-base disorders. *Kidney Int* 1:347, 1972.
235. Rietbrock N et al: Folat-katalysierte Elimination der Ameisensaure bei Methanvolvergiftung. *Biochem Pharmacol* 20:2613, 1971.
236. Roe O: Methanol poisoning. *Acta Med Scand* 126 (suppl 182):1, 1946.
237. Roe O: The metabolism and toxicity of methanol. *Pharmacol Rev* 7:399, 1955.
237a. Roughton FJW, Darling RC: The effect of carbon monoxide on the oxyhemoglobin dissociation curve. *Am J Physiol* 141:17, 1944.
237b. Russ G et al: Renal failure from glue sniffing. *Med J Aust* 2:127, 1981.
238. Satoh T et al: D-Lactic acidosis in two patients with short bowel syndrome: Bacteriological analyses of the fecal flora. *Eur J Pediatr* 138:324, 1982.
239. Saus J et al: Recovery after potentially lethal amount of methanol. *Lancet* 1:158, 1984.
240. Savoy J, Kaplan A: A gas chromatographic method for the determination of lactic acid in blood. *Clin Chem* 12:559, 1966.
241. Schmidt RW et al: Bicarbonate reabsorption in the dog with experimental renal disease. *Kidney Int* 10:287, 1976.
242. Schoolwerth AC et al: Effects of nephron reduction and dietary protein content on renal ammoniagenesis in the rat. *Kidney Int* 7:397, 1975.
243. Schultz K, Belriweuand-lepsien YG: Depression of mechanical and electrical activity in muscle strips of opossum stomach and esophagus by acidosis. *Gastroenterology* 82:720, 1982.
244. Schwartz WB et al: On the mechanism of acidosis in chronic renal failure. *J Clin Invest* 38:39, 1959.
245. Schwartz WB, Kassirer JP: Effects of ureteral implantation in Strauss MB, Welt LG (eds): *Diseases of the Kidney*. Boston, Little, Brown, 1963, p 578.
246. Seaman WE, Plotz PH: Effect of aspirin on liver function tests in patients with RA or SLE in normal volunteers. *Arthritis Rheum* 19:155, 1976.
247. Searle GL, Cavalieri RR: Determination of lactate kinetics in the human. Analysis of data from single injection vs continuous methods. *Proc Soc Exp Biol Med* 139:1002, 1972.
248. Seeff LB et al: Ethylene glycol poisoning. *Med Ann DC* 39:31, 1970.
249. Seldin DW et al: The effect of Na_2SO_4 on urinary acidification in chronic renal disease. *J Lab Clin Med* 69:893, 1967.
250. Seltzer HS: Drug- induced hypoglycemia: A review based on 473 cases. *Diabetes* 21:955, 1972.
251. Sharpey-Schafer EP et al: Venous constriction after exercise; its relation to acid-base changes in venous blood. *Clin Sci* 29:397, 1965.
252. Shear L et al: Renal tubular acidosis in cirrhosis. *N Engl J Med* 280:1, 1969.
253. Sherman HC, Gettles AO: The balance of acid forming and base forming elements in food and its relation to ammonia metabolism. *J Biol Chem* 11:323, 1912.
254. Shires GT, Tolman J: Dilution acidosis. *Ann Intern Med* 28:557, 1948.
255. Shoorel EP et al: D-Lactic acidosis in a boy with short bowel syndrome. *Arch Dis Child* 55:810, 1980.
256. Sijersted OM et al: Formate concentrations in plasma from patients poisoned with methanol. *Acta Med Scand* 213:105, 1983.
257. Silbert CK et al: Tumor hypoglycemia: Deficient splanchnic glucose output and deficient glucagon secretion. *Diabetes* 25:202, 1976.
258. Silverstein MN et al: Role of tryptophan and its metabolites in hypoglycemia associated with neoplasia. *Clin Res* XVI:357, 1964.
259. Simpson DP: Control of hydrogen ion homeostasis and renal acidosis. *Medicine* 50:503, 1971.
260. Sinal SH, Crowe JE: Cyanosis, cough and hypotension following intravenous administration of paraldehyde. *Pediatrics* 57:158, 1976.
261. Singer RB: The acid-base disturbances in salicylate intoxication. *Medicine* 33:1, 1954.
262. Slatapolsky E et al: On the influence of extracellular fluid volume expansion and of uremia on bicarbonate reabsorption in man. *J Clin Invest* 49:988, 1970.

262a. Smith H et al: The renal clearances of substituted hippuric acid derivatives and other aromatic acids in dogs and man. *J Clin Invest* 24:388, 1945.
263. Smith PK et al: Studies on the pharmacology of salicylates. *J Pharmacol Exp Ther* 87:237, 1946.
264. Smith SR et al: Combined formate and lactic acidosis in methanol poisoning. *Lancet* 2:1295, 1981.
264a. Sonnenberg H et al: Ammonia addition into medullary collecting duct of the rat. *Kidney Int* 19:281, 1981.
265. Spechler SJ et al: Lactic acidosis in oat cell carcinoma with extensive hepatic metastases. *Arch Intern Med* 138:1663, 1978.
266. Spenney JG, Nowell RM: Acetysalicylate hydrolase of rabbit gastric mucosa. Isolation and purification. *Drug Metab Dispos* 7:215, 1979.
266a. Springer DJ, Groll A: Poisoning with enteric coated acetylsalicylic acid complicating gastric outlet obstruction. *Can Med Assoc J* 122:1032, 1980.
267. Stacpoole PW et al: Dichloroacetate in the treatment of lactic acidosis. *Ann Intern Med* 108:58, 1988.
268. Stinebaugh BJ: The use of peritoneal dialysis in acute methyl alcohol poisoning. *Arch Intern Med* 105:613, 1960.
269. Stokes JB, Aueron F: Prevention of organ damage in massive ethylene glycol ingestion. *JAMA* 243:2065, 1980.
270. Stolberg LM et al: Evaluation and treatment of D-lactate acidosis in two patients: A result of abnormal gut colonization. *Clin Res* 29:36A, 1981.
271. Stolberg LM et al: D-Lactic acidosis due to abnormal gut flora. *N Engl J Med* 306:1044, 1982.
271a. Streicher HZ et al: Syndromes of toluene sniffing in adults. *Ann Intern Med* 94:758, 1981.
272. Sutton RAL et al: Effects of metabolic acidosis and alkalosis on sodium and calcium transport in the dog kidney. *Kidney Int* 15:520, 1979.
273. Swartz RD et al: Epidemic methanol poisoning: Clinical and biochemical analysis of a recent episode. *Medicine* 60:373, 1981.
273a. Taher SM et al: Renal tubular acidosis associated with toluene "sniffing." *N Engl J Med* 290:765f, 1974.
274. Tannen RL: Relationship of renal ammonia production and potassium homeostasis. *Kidney Int* 11:453, 1977.
275. Tannen RL: Ammonia and acid-base homeostasis. *Med Clin North Am* 67:781, 1983.
275a. Taylor GJ, Harris WS: Glue sniffing causes heart block in mice. *Science* 170:866, 1970.
276. Temple AW et al: Salicylate poisoning complicated by fluid retention. *Clin Toxicol* 9:61, 1976.
277. Temple AW: Acute and chronic effects of aspirin toxicity and their treatment. *Arch Intern Med* 141:364, 1981.
278. Tenney SM, Miller RM: The respiratory and circulatory actions of salicylate. *Am J Med* 19:498, 1955.
279. Terlinsky AS et al: Monohydrate calcium oxalate crystalluria in ethylene glycol poisoning, letter. *N Engl J Med* 302:922, 1980.
280. Thurston JH et al: Reduced brain glucose with normal plasma glucose in salicylate poisoning. *J Clin Invest* 49:2139, 1970.
281. Tizianello A et al: Renal metabolism of amino acids and ammonia in subjects with normal renal function and in patients with chronic renal insufficiency. *J Clin Invest* 65:1162, 1980.
281a. Toftgard R, Gustafsson JA: Biotransformation of organic solvents. A review. *Scand J Work Environ Health* 6:1, 1980.
282. Tranquada RE et al: Lactic acidosis *Arch Intern Med* 117:192, 1966.
283. Underwood F, Bennett WM: Ethylene glycol intoxication: Prevention of renal failure by aggressive management. *JAMA* 226:1453, 1973.
284. Vale JA et al: Treatment of ethylene glycol with peritoneal dialysis. *Br Med J* 284:557, 1982.
284a. Von Oettingen W et al: The toxicity and potential dangers of toluene. *JAMA* 118:579, 1942.
284b. Von Schule C et al: Nephrotic syndrome due to subacute glomerulonephritis—association with hydrocarbon exposure. *Acta Med Scand* 200:427, 1976.
284c. Walser M et al: Progression of chronic renal failure in patients given ketoacids following amino acids. *Kidney Int* 32:123, 1987.
285. Waterhouse C, Stern E: Metabolic acidosis occurring during administration of paraldehyde. *Am J Med* 23:987, 1957.
286. Weber HP et al: The lack of effect of chronic metabolic acidosis on 25-OH vitamin D metabolism and serum parathyroid hormone in humans. *J Clin Endocrinol Metab* 43:1047, 1976.
286a. Weil MH et al: Difference in acid-base status between venous and arterial blood during cardiopulmonary resuscitation. *N Engl J Med* 315:153, 1986.
287. Whalen JE et al: Inadequate removal of methanol and formate using the sorbent based regeneration hemodialysis delivery system. *Clin Nephrol* 11:318, 1979.
288. Whitehouse S, Randle PJ: Activation of pyruvate dehydrogenase in perfused rat heart by dichloracetate. *Biochem J* 134:651, 1973.
289. Widmer B et al: Serum electrolyte and acid-base composition. *Arch Intern Med* 139:1099, 1979.
290. Wildenthal K et al: Effects of acute lactic acidosis on left ventricular performance. *Am J Physiol* 214:1352, 1968.
290a. Will AM, McLaren EH: Reversible renal damage due to glue sniffing. *Br Med J* 283:525, 1981.
291. Williamson JR et al: Effects of acidosis on myocardial contractility and metabolism. *Acta Med Scand* 587 (suppl):95, 1975.
292. Winchester JF et al: Extracorporeal treatment of salicylate or acetaminophen poisoning. Is there a role? *Arch Intern Med* 141:370, 1981.
293. Winek CL et al: Ethylene and diethylene glycol toxicity. *Clin Toxicol* 13:297, 1978.
294. Winters RW et al: Disturbances of acid-base equilibrium in salicylate intoxication. *Pediatrics* 23:260, 1959.
295. Woll PJ, Record CO: Lactate elimination in man: Effects of lactate concentration and hepatic dysfunction. *Eur J Clin Invest* 9:397, 1979.
296. Wong NLM et al: Tubular handling of bicarbonate in dogs with experimental renal failure. *Kidney Int* 25:912, 1984.
297. Woods HF et al: The role of altered lactate kinetics in the

pathagonesis of Type B lactic acidosis, in Porter R (ed): *Metabolic Acidosis*. CIBA Foundation Symposium 87, Pittman, 1980, p 91.

298. Wrong O, Davies HFF: The excretion of acid in renal disease. *Q J Med* 28:259, 1959.
299. Yü TF et al: Effect of sodium lactate infusion on urate clearance in man. *Proc Soc Biol Exp Med* 96:809, 1957.
300. Yudkin J, Cohen RD: The contribution of the kidney to the removal of a lactic acid load under normal and acidotic conditions in the conscious rat. *Clin Sci* 48:121, 1975.

300a. Zaleska MM, Gassner PK: Metabolism of paraldehyde to acetaldehyde in liver microsomes. *Biochem Pharmacol* 32:3749, 1983.

300b. Zapadniuk VI et al: Age-related characteristics of the pharmacokinetics of acetylsalicylic acid. *Farmakologiia I Toksikologiia* 50:79, 1987.

300c. Zee-Ching CS et al: Toluene sniffing and severe sinus bradycardia. *Ann Intern Med* 103:482, 1985.

300d. Zimmerman SW et al: Hydrocarbon exposure and chronic glomerulonephritis after solvent exposure. *Arch Intern Med* 140:230, 1980.

301. Zipser R et al: Evidence for a critical role of prostaglandins in renin release, vascular reactivity, and renal function in liver disease, abstracted. *Clin Res* 25:305A, 1977.

CHAPTER • 26

Diabetic acidosis and coma

James R. Oster • Nelson P. Kopyt • Charles R. Kleeman • Thomas P. Dunfee • Robert A. Kreisberg • Robert G. Narins

Much has been learned in recent years of the pathogenesis and natural history of the diabetic comas. Translation of these pathophysiologic principles into refined therapeutic prescriptions is slowly taking place and ought to progressively reduce the 5 to 15 percent mortality currently associated with these disorders.[132] A recent review of deaths associated with diabetic ketoacidosis and hyperosmolar coma occurring between 1973 and 1988 at a single institution revealed an overall mortality of 6.2 percent.[125] The mortality for diabetic ketoacidosis was 4.9 percent and that for hyperosmolar coma 14.6 percent.[125]

This chapter reviews and puts into clinical perspective the biochemical and physiologic concepts underlying these diabetic syndromes. A practical diagnostic and therapeutic approach to these disorders is developed. Others have recently reviewed this topic as well.[5,140,161,167,171,312]

INSULIN DEFICIENCY

The fundamental cause of diabetic ketoacidosis, nonketotic hyperosmolar or hyperglycemic coma, and combined diabetic ketoacidosis and lactic acidosis is a relative or absolute deficiency of insulin. While "normal" amounts of insulin (radioimmunoreactive) have frequently been detected in the circulation of these patients, these concentrations are obviously inadequate for the degree of hyperglycemia and/or the deranged metabolic state. The major causes of insulin deficiency are the following:

1. Patients fail to take insulin or fail to take an adequate amount, usually because they lack an understanding of the disease and its treatment, often because of inadequate instruction. Occasionally, patients develop some disorder that causes marked anorexia. Because of this anorexia and the fear of insulin reactions, they stop taking insulin entirely. This, of course, makes little difference in mild to moderate diabetes; however, in severe or moderately severe diabetes, failure to take insulin for 1 to 2 days, particularly when one does not eat, may lead to the rapid development of ketoacidosis.
2. Infections to which the diabetic is susceptible may be obvious at the time of examination or may require special studies, such as blood and urine cultures, for detection. The intelligent, well-trained patient with diabetes often takes additional insulin during an obvious infectious process.
3. Surgical emergency, severe trauma, myocardial infarction, and severe emotional stress represent other frequent precipitating causes. Severe emotional stress is a particularly common cause of uncontrolled diabetes in the juvenile patient.
4. The abrupt onset of failure of insulin formation or secretion in juvenile diabetics leads to severe ketoacidosis or coma as the initial indication of diabetes mellitus.
5. Acute hemorrhagic pancreatitis in the absence of true diabetes mellitus is a rare cause. Mild abnormalities in carbohydrate metabolism are often seen in this disorder, but occasionally pancreatitis may precipitate frank, severe diabetic acidosis.
6. Chronic, severe overinsulinization with repeated hypoglycemic reactions may lead to deglycogenation of the liver and severe ketosis disproportionate to the extent of glycosuria and hyperglycemia.
7. An associated endocrine disorder develops that significantly antagonizes the metabolic effects of insulin (e.g., acromegaly, Cushing's syndrome, thyrotoxicosis, or pheochromocytoma).

Robert G. Narins acknowledges support from the University Medical Research Foundation.

8. In patients with latent or subclinical diabetes, acute deficiency may be produced by massive overeating, particularly of carbohydrates, or by parenteral alimentation exceeding the borderline insulin secretory capacity of the pancreas.
9. In approximately 20 percent of patients with diabetic ketoacidosis, no precipitating factor can be identified.
10. A rare type of severe insulin resistance is due to prereceptor-receptor resistance caused by high-affinity insulin antibodies. This syndrome is identified when the insulin need is greater than 100 units/h and steroid therapy is required. It is interesting that potassium and acid-base responses to insulin occur even though resistance is present to insulin's hypoglycemic action.[214]

The lack of insulin immediately and diffusely impairs glucose utilization and mobilizes long-chain fatty acids from storage in adipose tissue. Concomitantly, there is increased release of glucagon, which stimulates hepatic glucose and ketone production, accentuating the severe elevation of blood glucose and the ketonemia that characterize diabetic ketoacidosis. The altered carbohydrate, fat, and protein metabolism effects predictable changes in acid production and in the distribution and excretion of body water and electrolytes (see below).

THE ROLE OF GLUCAGON

Glucagon, a hormone composed of a 29 amino acid chain, is synthesized as a prohormone and stored in the alpha cells of the pancreas. Its release is prompted by certain amino acids (primarily arginine and alanine) as well as other hormones (i.e., cholecystokinin-pancreozymin). Somatostatin reduces plasma levels of glucagon, resulting in a transiently depressed fasting blood glucose concentration. Glucagon levels also increase in many states of extreme stress, such as trauma, hypoglycemia, infection, exercise, and starvation. Basal levels have been found to be increased in patients with diabetes mellitus, but they can be restored to normal with aggressive insulin therapy. Plasma glucagon concentration is markedly increased in diabetic ketoacidosis.[4,167] It also rapidly increases when diabetics discontinue their insulin therapy.[7,106] However, it is quite clear that there must be a deficiency of insulin for glucagon to cause sustained increases in plasma glucose and ketone concentrations.[83] Pharmacologically induced hyperglucagonemia to three to six times basal levels does not impair glucose tolerance in normal subjects or cause deterioration of diabetic control as long as insulin is available.[83]

When insulin is withdrawn from previously well-controlled insulin-dependent diabetics, hepatic glucose production increases within 2 h, with a concomitant rise in peripheral glucose levels.[199] Over the next 8 h, glucose production gradually declines, perhaps due to depletion of glycogen stores, but remains higher than basal levels. Hyperglycemia persists, however, because of both the decreased peripheral glucose utilization secondary to insulin deficiency and the contraction of the extracellular fluid (ECF) space caused by the osmotic diuresis. If the insulin is withdrawn and somatostatin, an inhibitor of glucagon release, administered, hyperglycemia is less severe.[107] Similarly, administration of somatostatin with insulin to ketoacidotic patients decreases the time required to normalize plasma glucose levels.[115]

The stimulation of hepatic gluconeogenesis by glucagon has been well-defined (Fig. 26-1). Adding glucagon to isolated hepatocytes decreases by more than 90 percent the cellular levels of fructose 2,6-bisphosphate (fructose-2,6-P_2), a key metabolite that controls hepatic glucose metabolism.[255] Phosphofructokinase 2 (PFK_2) is the enzyme that synthesizes fructose-2,6-P_2, while fructose-6-bisphosphatase 2 (FBPase 2) dephosphorylates it.[90]

The activities of PFK_2 and FBPase 2 have been found to occur on the same protein.[79,80] This dimeric enzyme therefore acts as both a kinase (phosphotransferase) and a phosphatase (phosphohydrolase). Cyclic AMP-dependent phosphorylation of the enzyme, triggered by glucagon, switches it from one mode of action to the other.[79] The phosphorylated enzyme acts as a phosphatase (thus decreasing fructose-2,6-P_2 concentration), while the dephosphorylated enzyme acts as a kinase (thus increasing fructose-2,6-P_2 concentration). Therefore, high glucagon levels keep the enzyme phosphorylated and depress fructose-2,6-P_2 levels. Fructose-2,6-P_2 influences hepatic glucose metabolism by activating phosphofructokinase 1 (classical PFK, a key enzyme in the glycolytic pathway, which catalyzes the conversion of fructose-6-phosphate to fructose 1,6-diphosphate), thereby enhancing glycolysis and inhibiting the activity of fructose 1,6-bisphosphatase 1 (a key enzyme in the gluconeogenic pathway).

In summary, insulin deficiency induces hyperglucagonemia, which reduces hepatic fructose-2,6- P_2 levels, and this deinhibits gluconeogenesis while decreasing glycolysis (see above).[90] These effects, coupled with the direct activation of glycogen breakdown by glucagon,[82] stimulate hepatic glucose synthesis.

Catecholamines, cortisol, and growth hormone may play a role in glucose overproduction, but their levels have not been found to be increased in nonstressed diabetics when insulin is removed.[199] Epinephrine has been shown to decrease fructose-2,6-P_2 levels, but much less than does glucagon.[254]

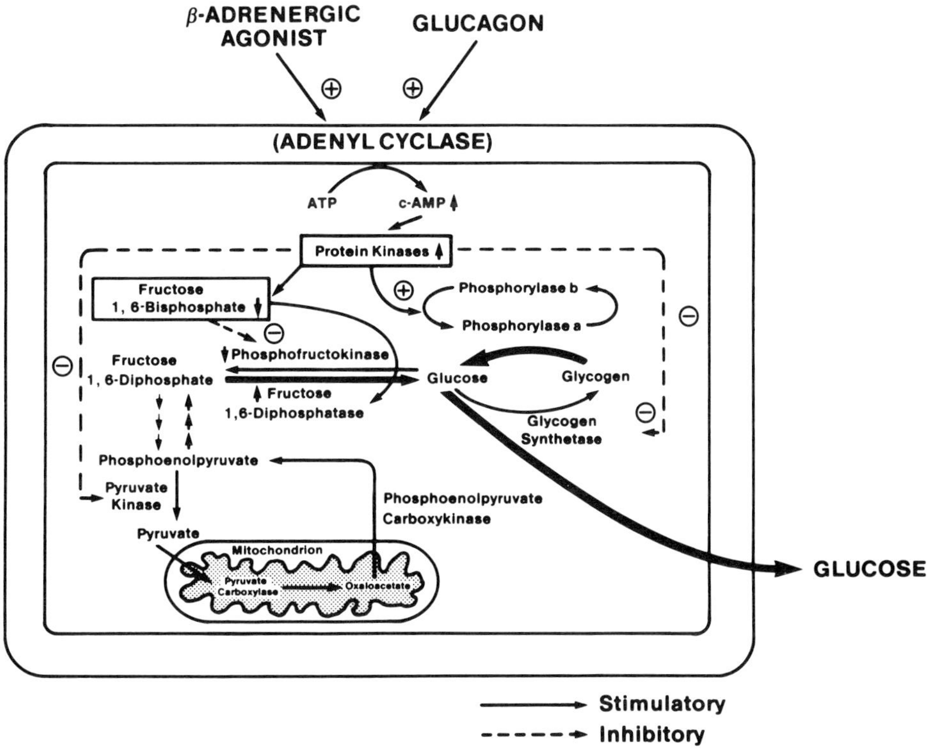

FIGURE 26-1 • Schematic representation of the stimulation of hepatic gluconeogenesis by glucagon.

HYPERGLYCEMIA, HYPEROSMOLALITY, AND INTERNAL SHIFTS OF FLUID

The lack of insulin immediately impairs glucose utilization by most tissues (excluding brain tissue) and causes excessive hepatic production of glucose from noncarbohydrate sources (i.e., gluconeogenesis is stimulated). Both processes, underutilization and excessive production, cause progressive hyperglycemia. In the absence of insulin, the cells are relatively impermeable to glucose, and therefore the increasing hyperglycemia progressively raises the effective osmotic pressure (i.e., tonicity) of the extracellular fluid. The calculation of the osmotic contribution of glucose is presented in Fig. 26-2. As the tonicity of the extracellular fluid increases, water diffuses from the cells to the extracellular compartment, thereby reestablishing transcellular osmotic equivalence. This process progressively dehydrates cells while expanding the ECF. The expansion is limited by the resulting glycosuria and attending salt and water diuresis (see below).

In brief, the increasing concentration of glucose in the blood (ECF) causes water to shift out of the cells; this in turn dilutes the remaining extracellular solutes, the most abundant of which are the sodium salts. This process is illustrated in Fig. 26-3.

Approximately 30 years ago, Welt[319] and Goldberger[109] calculated that sodium concentration would decrease by approximately 2.8 meq/liter for each 100 mg/100 ml rise in glucose above normal. In 1973, Katz[152] rejected their calculations for their failure to take into account the change in intracellular fluid (ICF) volume as intracellular water moves to the extracellular compartment in response to the increasing ECF osmolality. Utilizing this correction, Katz determined that there would be a 1.6 meq/liter decline in sodium concentration for each 100 mg/100 ml increase in glucose concentration. This calculation, however, assumes that the intracellular solute concentration remains constant as the

1. Millimole (mmol) = molecular weight (MW) in milligrams
   MW Glucose = 180
   1 mmol = 180 mg
2. If blood glucose is 180 mg/100 ml, each 100 ml has 180 mg (or 1 mmol) and each liter has 1800 mg (or 10 mmol).
3. Divide blood glucose (mg/100 ml) by 18 to get its osmotic contribution.
4. Since each mmol of glucose accounts for 1 mosm, every 180 mg/100 ml rise of blood glucose causes a 10 mosm/liter rise.

FIGURE 26-2 • Method of calculating the osmotic contribution of glucose to the blood.

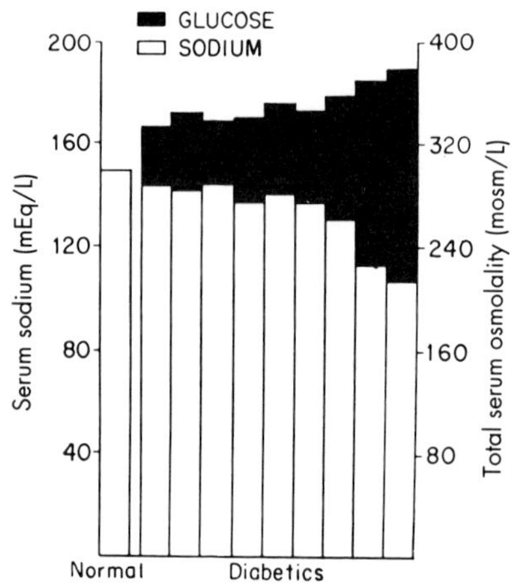

FIGURE 26-3 • Relationship between the concentrations of glucose and sodium and the total serum osmolality in diabetic acidosis. (From Peters JP, *Metabolism* 1:223, 1952. Used by permission.)

extracellular concentration increases during hyperglycemia. Exogenous glucose was added to raise blood sugar in this example. In patients with diabetic ketoacidosis, however, glucose intake is minimal, hyperglycemia resulting from metabolism of intracellular substrates such as glycogen, lactate, pyruvate, glycerol, and amino acids. Synthesized glucose ultimately enters the extracellular compartment. An equation relating the effect of increasing plasma glucose concentration to sodium concentration must therefore take both the fluctuating compartment volumes and solute concentrations into consideration.[207]

Moran and Jamison have derived such an equation and demonstrated that plasma sodium concentration declines nonlinearly by 1.5 to 1.6 meq/liter for each 100 mg/100 ml rise in plasma glucose concentration in a euvolemic 70 kg subject (Fig. 26-4). A similar degree of hyperglycemia in a normonatremic, *volume-expanded* subject causes osmotic withdrawal of somewhat more cellular water, but the expanded ECF is diluted to a lesser extent. Conversely, an equivalent degree of hyperglycemia in a normonatremic, *volume-contracted* subject withdraws somewhat less fluid from cells, but the shrunken ECF space is—on a percentage basis—diluted to a greater extent. Thus, the degree of hyponatremia caused by a given degree of hyperglycemia is dependent on the prevailing volume of the ECF. These relationships are illustrated in Figs. 26-4 and 26-5 (see Chap. 20).[207] The edematous patient with a 15 percent increase in ECF volume would manifest a 1.25 to 1.35 meq/liter decrease in sodium concentration for each 100 mg/100 ml increase in glucose concentration. On the other hand, in the hypovolemic patient with a 10 percent decrease in ECF volume, the ratio would increase so that a fall of 1.8 to 1.9 meq/liter in serum sodium concentration would follow each 100 mg/100 ml increase in blood sugar.

It is apparent from Fig. 26-3 that, although the osmolality of the total body fluid progressively increases during uncontrolled hyperglycemia, the sodium and chloride concentration in the ECF is usually normal or low in the untreated patient. While the chloride level may be further reduced by vomiting, the hyponatremia is a reflection not so much of the loss of salt in excess of water but of dilution of the ECF with sodium-poor ICF. Replacement of ongoing intestinal or renal salt losses with hypotonic solutions worsens the hyponatremia. This phenomenon is the major cause of the hyponatremia and hypochloremia present in diabetic ketoacidosis.

A further contribution to the lowering of the serum sodium concentration may be its movement into the cells as they become progressively depleted of potassium. Rarely, severe hypertriglyceridemia, as is seen in some diabetic patients, may contribute to a spurious, or fictitious, hyponatremia (see Chap 20). Under these circumstances, all the solutes dissolved in the aqueous phase of the blood or plasma are reduced. When a unit volume of

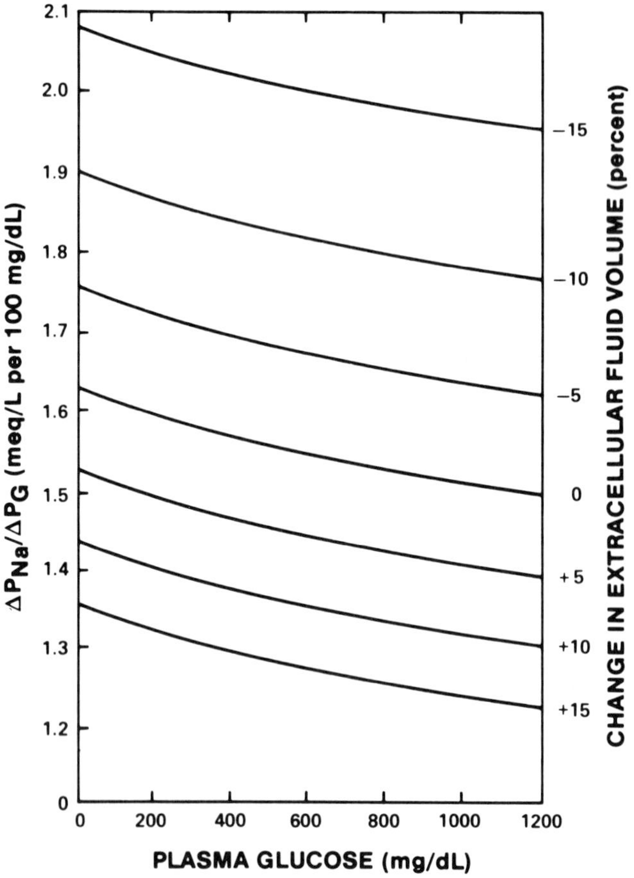

FIGURE 26-4 • The prevailing ECF volume influences the magnitude of the hyponatremic response to a given change in plasma glucose. Depicted is the change in plasma sodium concentration (ΔP_{Na}) for a given change in plasma glucose concentration ($\Delta P_{glucose}$) relative to a given percentage change in ECF volume. See the text for details. (From Moran MS, Jamison RL, *West J Med* 142:49, 1985. Used by permission.)

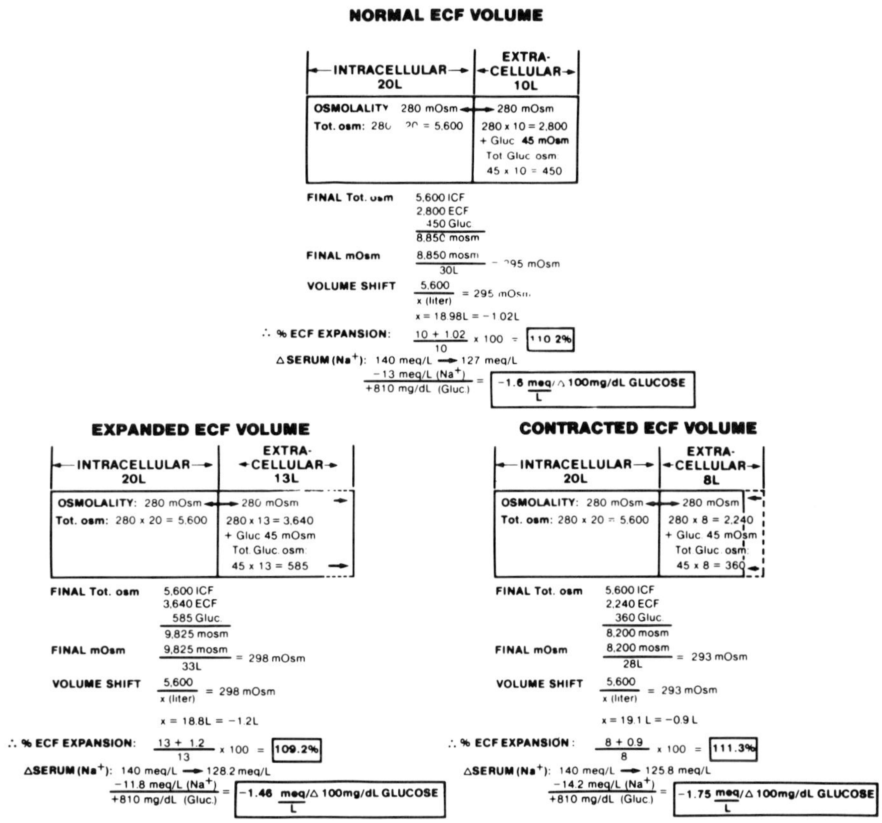

FIGURE 26-5 • Calculation of the serum sodium concentration when the plasma glucose level is raised to 45 mosm and the ECF volume is normal, expanded, or contracted. See the text for details.

plasma or serum contains an abnormally large proportion of lipid, the water phase, with its contained electrolytes, is proportionately reduced. See Chap. 20, "Pseudohyponatremia").

If, despite the hyperglycemia, serum sodium concentration is normal or even elevated, this indicates an even more profound degree of water loss. This is most characteristic of nonketotic hyperosmolal diabetic coma (see below). The combination of hypernatremia and profound hyperglycemia is seen most often in the older patient with uncontrolled diabetes in whom progressive glycosuria and polyuria continue for many days to weeks with minimal, if any, ketonemia and acidosis. Thus, the patient is usually not seen in the hospital until large quantities of water have been lost (see below).

Glucose, sodium and its attendant anions, and urea make up the major solutes of the plasma. From their values, the total osmolality of the body fluids can be calculated:

$$P_{osm} = 2[Na^+] + \frac{\text{blood urea nitrogen mg/100 ml}}{2.8} + \frac{\text{blood glucose mg/100 ml}}{18} \quad (1)$$

The serum osmolality may also be determined directly by measuring the freezing point of the plasma with an osmometer. A measured osmolality that greatly exceeds the calculated osmolality would suggest the possibility of severe hyperproteinemia (e.g., myeloma) or hyperlipemia. The latter, of course, can always be detected by the lactescence of the plasma. This disparity between the calculated and measured osmolalities may also reflect circulating ethanol or other low-molecular weight toxins (see Chap. 25). The authors have found that the direct measurement of the serum osmolality is of great value in calculating the total deficit of body water in patients with diabetic acidosis. The normal osmolality of the body fluids is approximately 285 mosm/liter. If the osmolality of a patient with diabetic acidosis is 314 mosm/liter, this represents a 10 percent increment in solute concentration, or approximately a 10 percent *decrement* in total body water. If the calculated normal total body water is 40 liters, a 10 percent loss would be 4 liters. This calculation assumes that no solute has been lost from the body fluids; this is obviously not true in diabetic acidosis. However, the authors have observed that the positive water balance during the first 48 h of treatment correlates well with the deficit calculated from serum osmolality. This empirical observation suggests that the increment in solute concentration contributed to the body fluids from the elevated blood sugar level approximates the decrement that would occur from the electrolyte loss.

GLYCOSURIA AND RENAL LOSSES OF WATER AND ELECTROLYTES

As the blood sugar increases, the glomerular filtration of glucose increases in parallel, and soon the filtered load exceeds the threshold for its renal tubular reabsorption; glucose then appears in the urine in increasing amounts. This carbohydrate, like any other nonreabsorbed solute (osmotic diuretic), prevents the reabsorption of water and sodium salts, leading to a progressive increase in urine flow. Figure 26-6 illustrates the effect of glycosuria during diabetic acidosis on the rate of urinary flow and electrolyte loss. This osmotic diuresis is the *major* cause of sodium, chloride, and water losses in severe diabetic acidosis. Glycosuria may exceed 50 g/h, or 278 mosm/h (Fig. 26-6). The concentration of sodium and chloride in the urine during this glucose diuresis is usually between 50 and 100 meq/liter but may be as low as 10 to 25 meq/liter if the stimulus for sodium conservation is marked and the simultaneous rate of glomerular filtration is below normal. This is characteristic of the concentration of these electrolytes in the urine during any severe osmotic diuresis. The *hypotonic* nature of the urine with respect to sodium and chloride should be emphasized. The loss of body fluid as a consequence of osmotic diuresis can be visualized as a combination of isotonic saline solution and free water. For example, the loss of 1 liter of urine during an osmotic diuresis can be illustrated diagrammatically as follows:

1.0 liter of 75 meq/liter of Na^+	≅	0.5 liter of 150 meq/liter of Na^+ (Loss of this fluid would not alter ECF [Na^+]).
		0.5 liter of H_2O (The additional loss of this fluid would lead to a rise in the magnitude of ECF [Na^+], which is limited by the continued osmotic loss of intracellular water.)

As volume contraction worsens, glomerular filtration and renal blood flow progressively decrease, and the patient may become oliguric or even anuric in spite of the marked hyperglycemia. In the treatment of the severely dehydrated oliguric patient, fluid replacement reexpands the extracellular volume, improving renal hemodynamics and causing urinary volume to increase progressively. Thus, glycosuria may actually increase despite a falling blood sugar level. Stated differently, as the glomerular filtration rate (GFR) increases, the filtered load of glucose, a function of $P_g \times$ GFR, increases despite a decrease in the concentration of ECF glucose. A corollary

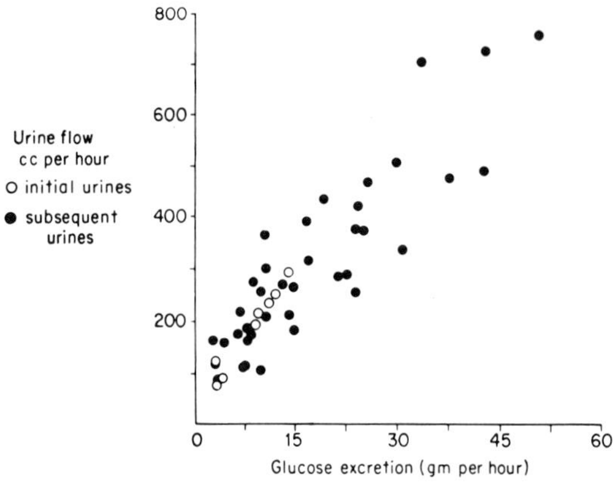

FIGURE 26-6 • The relationship of urinary flow to the excretion rate of glucose during diabetic acidosis. Initial urine samples are those obtained at the beginning of therapy and subsequent ones are those obtained during therapy. (From Seldin DW, Tarail R, *J Clin Invest* 29:552, 1950. Used by permission.)

to this relationship is that the presence of chronic or acute renal disease (e.g., acute tubular necrosis, diabetic glomerulosclerosis, glomerulonephritis, or nephrosclerosis) reduces the GFR per nephron and thus decreases the filtered load of glucose or ketones for any given increase in blood level. Hyperglycemia and ketonemia may exist with little or no sugar or ketones in the urine (i.e., there exists an abnormally high renal threshold for these substances).

POTASSIUM LOSS

Although osmotic diuresis slightly increases the renal excretion of potassium (see Chaps. 6 and 7) this effect is much less than its effect on the excretion of sodium and chloride. The major causes of the loss of potassium in diabetic acidosis are as follows:

1. Lean tissue breakdown, with the liberation of approximately 3 meq of potassium per gram of nitrogen lost. This is due to the starvationlike state created by the intermediary metabolic defect associated with insulin deficiency and the marked hypersecretion of adrenal glucocorticoids that accompanies severe uncontrolled diabetes mellitus.[48,142]
2. The progressive depletion of tissue stores of glycogen. Normally, 1 meq of potassium is "deposited" in the cells with every 3 g of glycogen. As the latter is mobilized and not repleted, the "freed" potassium is excreted. Severe diabetic acidosis in an adult may cause a 200 to 300 g deficit of glycogen, with its accompanying 70 to 100 meq of potassium.
3. The loss of intracellular water (cellular dehydration) is a strong stimulus for the loss or net flux of po-

tassium from body cells[191] and its continued high rate of excretion. Because the sustained hyperglycemia in uncontrolled diabetes causes the continuous withdrawal of cellular water, this stimulus for potassium loss persists until the cellular deficit of water is corrected.

4. The deficiency of insulin may well prevent cells from maintaining the highest or optimal intracellular/extracellular concentration ratio for potassium.[110,131,337] Therefore, potassium may more readily diffuse out of cells down its electrochemical gradient into the ECF and then into the urine. This action of insulin is not dependent on or secondary to its effect on glucose transport.
5. The increased secretion of aldosterone[60] caused by the profound depletion of sodium and extracellular volume enhances the renal loss of potassium for any given metabolic state and rate of sodium excretion.
6. Severe anorexia and vomiting prevent ingestion of potassium-containing foods necessary for the correction of the developing deficit of potassium. Sustained vomiting causes the loss of almost 10 to 20 meq of potassium per liter of vomitus.

In summary, the combination of ongoing cellular losses of potassium and continued renal potassium wasting results in the severe defects observed. Despite the marked deficit of potassium produced by these derangements, the serum potassium level is usually normal or elevated when the patient with untreated diabetic acidosis enters the hospital.[95] The factors that tend to increase the initial level of potassium in the serum are (1) increased plasma glucose concentration,[110,131] with its associated increased osmolality (see Chap. 7);[337] (2) defects in the intermediary metabolic processes (e.g., inadequate tissue oxygenation or impaired generation of ATP for the Na^+-K^+ ATPase) that are essential for the maintenance of the concentration gradient for potassium between the cell and ECF; (3) the deficiency of insulin (see number 4 above); and (4) functional renal impairment due to loss of intravascular volume, hypotension, and marked intrarenal vasoconstriction, which would lower the renal clearance of potassium for any given metabolic setting. A recent study demonstrated a reversible impairment in renal potassium secretion in patients presenting with both diabetic ketoacidosis and hyperglycemic, hyperosmolar syndrome. This effect is therefore not related to ketonemia or ketonuria.[321] The mechanism of this hyperglycemia-induced reversible impairment of potassium secretion is still uncertain. In the latter context, an unusually high serum potassium level should also bring to mind the syndrome of hyporeninemic hypoaldosteronism in the diabetic patient (see Chaps. 23 and 45).[110] While acute *inorganic* acidosis (e.g., with infusions of HCl) causes highly predictable increments in serum potassium concentration, comparable degrees of acute *organic* acidosis do not cause significant hyperkalemia.[228-230] Two important differences exist regarding those acidoses that play upon the transcellular distribution of potassium. Ketoacid anions (β-hydroxybutyrate) stimulate insulin secretion in dogs, which in turn enhances cellular entry of potassium.[228] The cellular penetrability of the acid anion may also play a key role in altering potassium distribution. The electronegativity of the internal milieu plays a major role in preventing loss of cationic cellular potassium. As protons enter the cell, their cationic charge diminishes the transcellular potential. Restriction of negatively charged inorganic anions to the ECF augments the tendency of potassium to exit cells and may account for HCl-incuded hyperkalemia. Since *organic* anions more freely enter cells, the transmembrane potential is unaltered, thereby sustaining normokalemia. The presence of a low serum potassium level prior to therapy therefore indicates an especially profound degree of potassium depletion.

LEAN TISSUE AND NITROGEN LOSS

The patient with uncontrolled diabetes with moderate acidosis often has a progressive loss of appetite, frequently diminishing the caloric intake. This lack of calories, together with the loss of the normal nitrogen-sparing effect of carbohydrates when there is a relative or absolute deficiency of insulin, leads to progressive tissue breakdown and negative nitrogen balance. The increased endogenous production of urea secondary to this tissue breakdown causes an increase in the blood urea nitrogen that is out of proportion to the degree of renal impairment or to the increase in serum creatinine. It also causes a marked increase in the renal excretion of urea, which contributes a further osmotic effect in addition to that of the glycosuria. The destruction of tissue protein is associated with the liberation of intracellular potassium, phosphorus, and magnesium, which are lost from the body through the urine in increasing amounts as diabetic acidosis proceeds and which, of course, must be replenished during treatment and recovery.

KETOGENESIS

The generation and maintenance of net ketoacid production involves the interaction of three basic elements (Fig. 26-7): (1) adipose tissue, (2) the liver, and (3) extrahepatic tissue. Free fatty acids (FFAs), derived from adipose tissue, serve as substrate for hepatic ketogenesis, and the ketones are finally metabolized by such extrahepatic tissues as muscle and brain. In the uncontrolled diabetic state, alterations in each of these elements result

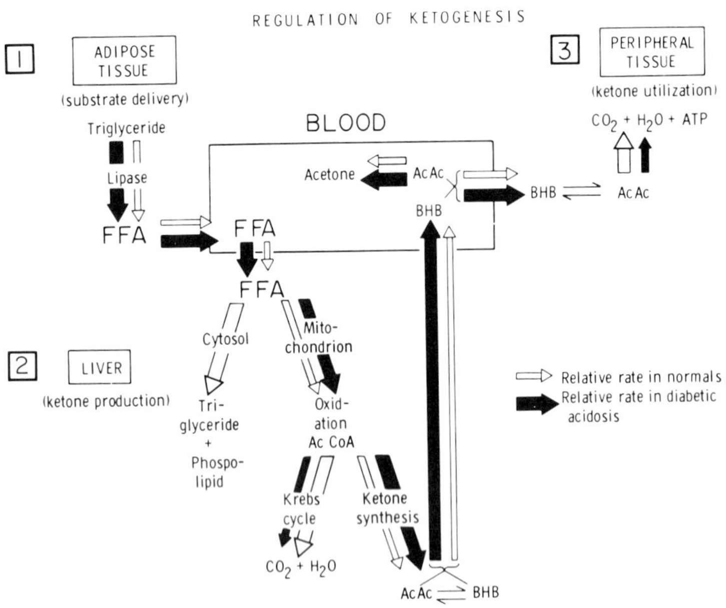

FIGURE 26-7 • Scheme of the three elements of net ketone production. See the text for details. AcAc, acetoacetic acid; AcCoA, acetyl coenzyme A; ATP, adenosine triphosphate; βHB, β-hydroxybutyric acid; FFA, free fatty acids.

in massive overproduction and underutilization of ketone acids, with development of life-threatening ketoacidosis.

The conversion of triglycerides to FFAs by adipose tissue is largely controlled by a hormone-sensitive lipase.[283] Certain hormones (e.g., epinephrine and glucocorticoids) enhance cAMP formation; this, in turn, activates the lipase, resulting in enhanced lipolysis and FFA mobilization. In contrast to the other hormones, insulin impairs lipase activity by inhibiting adenylate cyclase, thereby reducing cAMP. Reduced insulin activity therefore unleashes lipase and allows large amounts of FFAs to gain access to the circulation.

The liver's ability to rapidly metabolize FFAs limits the plasma concentration of these substrates, preventing a significant fall in pH due to FFAs per se. The entry of FFAs into hepatocytes is largely governed by their plasma concentration. Upon entry into the liver cell, rapid conversion to the metabolically active coenzyme A (CoA) derivative occurs in the cytosol. A small fraction of the active fatty acid forms triglyceride and phospholipid, while the remainder is transported into the mitochondrion, where it is oxidized. The primary regulatory site for the β-oxidation of fatty acyl-CoA to ketones is at the inner mitochondrial membrane, where the enzyme carnitine palmitoyl transferase I (CPT I) resides (see Fig. 26-7).[90] This enzyme transesterfies fatty acyl-CoA (which is impermeable to the mitochondrial membrane) with carnitine. The carnitine ester can enter the mitochondrion, possibly via a translocase, where the esterification is reversed by carnitine palmitoyl transferase II. The majority of the reformed fatty acyl-CoA is then oxidized to acetoacetate and β-hydroxybutyrate via the hydroxymethylglutaryl-CoA pathway.[198] High levels of glucagon suppress the production of malonyl-CoA, an inhibitor of CPT I, and also increase carnitine concentrations in the hepatocyte.[90] The hyperglucagonemia that accompanies ketoacidosis may therefore enhance the ketogenic potential of the liver by facilitating the availability of FFAs to the biosynthetic site of ketones.[83,90,198]

Further metabolism of acetyl-CoA is effected by enzymes of the Krebs cycles to carbon dioxide and water or by other intramitochondrial enzymatic pathways to ketone acids. In uncontrolled diabetes mellitus, there is much evidence to suggest that cycle activity is diminished, thereby forcing acetyl-CoA to form ketones.[168] Acetoacetic acid is the first ketone formed from acetyl-CoA and will slowly and non-enzymatically decarboxylate to form acetone (N18; Fig. 26-7). The conversion of the strong acetoacetic acid to the nonacid acetone represents one form of metabolic buffering, since this reaction prevents the hydrogen ion of acetoacetic acid from expressing its physiochemical activity. Since acetone is only partially metabolized and since it is excreted far less efficiently than the other ketones, it may remain in the blood for many hours following the normalization of ketogenesis by insulin. In this setting, acetone may cause positive nitroprusside test results, creating the confusing picture of a treated diabetic whose blood sugar and bicarbonate concentrations have normalized but whose serum ketone levels remain positive. The normal bicarbonate concentration and absence of an elevated anion gap indicate that acetoacetic *acid* is not present and that the positive nitroprusside reaction most likely reflects acetone.

The third ketone body is β-hydroxybutyric acid, which is the reduction product of acetoacetic acid (Fig. 26-7). These two ketones, β-hydroxybutyric and acetoacetic acid, are interconvertible. Their relative concentrations depend upon the availability of reduced pyridine nucleotide ($NADH_2$). The latter, in turn, is regulated by the availability of oxygen to the tissues for reoxidation of $NADH_2$ and/or the rate of $NADH_2$ generation, which is increased in diabetic ketoacidosis from increased FFA metabolism or from concomitant ingestion of alcohol. It follows, therefore, that with tissue hypoxia (e.g., in shock, pneumonia, etc.), when $NADH_2$ is abundant, the β-hydroxybutyric acid/acetoacetic acid ratio will be increased. Since β-hydroxybutyric acid, at any concentration, is nonreactive to nitroprusside, ketosis will be obscured when tissue hypoxia obtains. Thus, hypotensive, acidotic diabetics whose semi-quantitative nitroprusside tests (tablets, powder, or dipsticks) reveal zero to moderate ketosis may actually be "hiding" massive amounts of ketones as the unmeasurable β-hydroxybutyric acid. With fluid and insulin therapy, total ketone production decreases, but increased tissue perfusion and oxygenation drive the β-hydroxybutyric acid to the measurable acetoacetic acid form, giving the false impression of worsening or nonimproving ketosis. Some patients with diabetic ketoacidosis have β-hydroxybutyric acid ketoacidosis in the absence of impaired oxygen delivery to the tissues. The explanation for this is currently unknown.

Since the renal excretion of β-hydroxybutyric acid and acetoacetic acid is extremely efficient, it is common to see ketonuria in the absence of ketonemia in patients with only mild ketosis. The only time the reverse occurs (i.e., ketonemia without ketonuria) is when severe acute or chronic renal failure is present.

The liver, unlike peripheral tissue, is unable to metabolize the ketone acids it synthesizes. The β-hydroxybutyric acid and acetoacetic acid are taken up from the circulation by such tissues as muscle and kidney and oxidized to carbon dioxide and water. Although not well studied in humans, there are substantial data from animal studies to indicate that the peripheral catabolism of ketones is depressed in uncontrolled diabetes.[30] Studies in humans are compatible with this observation.[324]

In summary, the absence of insulin initiates a series of reactions that result in severe overproduction of ketoacids. Increased fat mobilization and glucagon release provide substrate and stimulate the controlling hepatic biosynthetic reactions of ketogenesis. A decreased peripheral utilization may further increase the circulating level of ketoacids. Thus, the diabetic state is associated with the stimulation of all three of the basic elements involved in ketogenesis.

ACID-BASE CHANGES

UNCOMPLICATED

The normal response to ketone acid overproduction is reflected by biochemical changes in plasma and functional alterations in lungs and kidney. Changes in all three areas are directed toward prevention of life-threatening acidosis.

As β-hydroxybutyric acid and acetoacetic acid gain access to the extracellular space, blood buffers are progressively titrated in an effort to limit the acidifying process. Bicarbonate, the most easily measured of the blood buffers, is consumed, and its anionic charge is replaced by the negatively charged β-hydroxybutyrate and acetoacetate. The acidosis is manifested by the fall in bicarbonate and reciprocal rise in the anion gap (AG).[81] The latter represents those anions, other than chloride and bicarbonate, that offset the positive charge of sodium: AG = $Na^+ - (Cl^- + HCO_3^-) = 12 \pm 2$ meq/liter (normal). In pure diabetic ketoacidosis, the increment in the anion gap above normal equals the amount of circulating ketoacid and consequently also equals the decrement in serum bicarbonate concentration.[81] With therapy, the ketones are converted to bicarbonate by muscle, a process that at once normalized the serum bicarbonate concentration and anion gap.

Respiration is stimulated by the acidemia and the consequent decrease in P_{CO_2}, and carbonic acid acts to bring arterial pH back toward normal (see Chaps. 24 and 25). This labored, deep ventilation was first described in 1874 by Kussmaul in his report of an obese, 35-year-old diabetic. She was described as "breathing loud, rapid and the respiratory movements strikingly large. Powerful costal abdominal inspirations alternating with powerful expirations."[190] It takes approximately 12 to 24 h for a given degree of acidosis to elicit a maximal respiratory response.[242] The expected fall in P_{CO_2} appropriate for a given degree of systemic acidosis is defined by the following formula, which relates the observed total CO_2 (or bicarbonate concentration) to the expected arterial P_{CO_2}:[4]

$$P_{CO_2} \text{ (mmHg)} = 1.5 \text{ (total } CO_2) + 8 \pm 2$$

A ketoacidotic patient with a total CO_2 of 10 meq/liter ought to have a P_{CO_2} of 23 (±2) mmHg. If the observed P_{CO_2} were less than 21 or greater than 25 mmHg, a superimposed respiratory disorder would be diagnosed (see Chap. 30).

The renal response to diabetic ketoacidosis is similar to that seen in other metabolic acidoses. The tubules reabsorb all filtered bicarbonate, thereby conserving alkali and acidifying the urine. The major urinary buffers, phosphate and ammonia, are titrated, effecting the excretion of large amounts of acid. Under the stimulus of systemic acidosis, renal synthesis and excretion of ammonia increase markedly, and the combined excretion of titratable acid plus ammonium accounts for the seven- to tenfold increase in acid excretion during severe ketoacidosis.[29] There is some evidence, however, that ketones may suppress renal ammonia synthesis, thereby limiting the maximal increase that could otherwise occur in severe ketoacidosis.[179]

It is important to recognize that it usually takes from many hours to several days for ketoacidosis to develop when insulin is removed.[29] The abrupt onset of acidosis should suggest the possibility of lactic acidosis (see below) or the presence of a toxin.

COMPLICATED (MIXED) ACID-BASE DISORDERS

A number of pathophysiologic changes occur in uncontrolled diabetes that may further complicate acid-base metabolism. When a metabolic alkalosis or respiratory acidosis or alkalosis is superimposed upon ketoacidosis, a "mixed" acid-base disorder is said to exist. An indication that a mixed metabolic disturbance may exist could be inferred from the ratio of the increase in anion gap to the deficit in bicarbonate concentration. As discussed above, in uncomplicated diabetic ketoacidosis, this ratio is equal to 1.0:

$$\frac{\text{Excess anion gap (AG} - 12\text{ meq/liter)}}{\text{Bicarbonate deficit (24 meq/liter} - \text{observed } HCO_3^-)} = 1.0 \qquad (2)$$

The excess anion gap is the increment of the anion gap above normal. This excess is an indirect measure of accumulated acid anions. Since each milliequivalent per liter increment in such acid should reduce the bicarbonate concentration by a like amount, the ratio in equation 2 should be 1.0. A ratio greater than 1 indicates that the plasma bicarbonate concentration has decreased less than expected, given the increment in accumulated acid (as defined by the increment in the anion gap). In other words, some other source of alkali has sustained a more normal bicarbonate concentration. A ratio below 1.0 indicates that the bicarbonate concentration has decreased more than can be accounted for by accumulated unmeasured acid anions (the excess anion gap). This typifies a mixed high anion gap/normal anion gap acidosis (see below). The most common mixed disturbances seen in diabetes are discussed below.

Mixed ketoacidosis and metabolic alkalosis

It is quite common for the vomiting that frequently complicates ketoacidosis to superimpose a metabolic alkalosis on the preexisting ketoacidosis. (see Chap. 31).[111,321] A similar picture may also develop from overzealous therapy with alkali. Table 26-1 outlines the serum electrolytes and acid-base parameters found in this mixed disorder.

Vomiting or alkali therapy, while replenishing circulating bicarbonate, either exerts no effect or may increase ketone anions.[181] Consequently, the pH, P_{CO_2}, and bicarbonate level may normalize, while the anion gap remains elevated. This highlights the importance of the anion gap in diagnosing acid-base disorders.[81] Less severe alkaloses only partially correct the bicarbonate level, in which case the increment in the anion gap exceeds the decrement in the bicarbonate level.

TABLE 26-1 • DKA and coexistent metabolic alkalosis: chemical pattern

Measurement	Normal	DKA	Vomiting or $NaHCO_3$ therapy plus DKA
Na^+, meq/liter	140	140	145
K^+, meq/liter	4	5	4
Cl^-, meq/liter	105	105	95
CO_2, meq/liter	25	10	25
AG, meq/liter	10	25	25
pH	7.40	7.23	7.40
P_{CO_2}, mmHg	40	22	40

ABBREVIATIONS: AG, anion gap; DKA, diabetic ketoacidosis.

With therapy, the ketones are metabolized to alkali, and the final serum bicarbonate concentration will equal the sum of this regenerated bicarbonate plus the additional amount due to vomiting or therapy. Thus, reversal of ketoacidosis unmasks the metabolic alkalosis.

Mixed high anion gap and normal anion gap metabolic acidosis

It is not uncommon for diabetics to develop a hyperchloremic metabolic acidosis with a tendency toward hyperkalemia as their diabetic nephropathy progresses (Chap. 30).[225] This mixed disorder primarily results from the following factors. Functional and/or absolute aldosterone deficiency (i.e., hyporeninemic hypoaldosteronism) and progressive tubulointerstitial disease, as a result of nephrosclerosis or infection, commonly complicate the course of diabetes. Hyperchloremic acidosis results from impaired hydrogen ion secretion and reduced ammonia buffer generation (see Chap. 27). Hyperkalemia, which is common in this setting, impairs ammonia synthesis. As glomerular filtration inexorably declines, phosphate, sulfate, and organic acid anions accumulate, eliciting the well-recognized high anion gap acidosis of uremia.

Diarrhea and hyporeninemic hypoaldosteronism are the most common causes of hyperchloremic acidosis in the nonketotic diabetic patient. The recovery phase of treated diabetic ketoacidosis is also commonly associated with a mixed high anion gap and hyperchloremic acidosis (see Chap. 25).[224] Since the kidney has a relatively low capacity to reabsorb filtered ketoacids, a significant fraction of their filtered load escapes reabsorption. Therefore, sodium salts of ketoacids (potential alkali) escape into the urine, resulting in a hyperchloremic, hypobicarbonatemic serum electrolyte pattern. Lost ketoanion reduces the increased anion gap, while the bicarbonate concentration remains low. Replacement of lost bicarbonate with chloride completes the picture.

Ketoacidotic patients with the most profound intravascular volume depletion are most likely to have a pure high anion gap acidosis.[2,3] With volume depletion, the resultant decrease in GFR reduces the excretion of ketoanions, resulting in an equimolar increase in the anion gap and decrease in the bicarbonate concentration.[3] During the reparative phase, saline expansion of the ECF increases the rate of ketoanion loss and replaces it with the infused chloride. Since retained ketoanions would have been oxidized to bicarbonate, ketonuria sustains the low serum bicarbonate concentration and replaces it with chloride.

Mixed ketoacidosis and respiratory alkalosis

Diabetics have an increased susceptibility to infection, especially pneumonia and gram-negative sepsis, and these infections often precipitate an episode of ketoacidosis. Since pneumonia and endotoxemia cause hyperventilation,[280] it is not uncommon to see respiratory alkalosis superimposed upon diabetic ketoacidosis. These processes have offsetting effects on pH but additive effects on bicarbonate concentration. It is common, therefore, to find a normal pH with a strikingly low serum bicarbonate concentration. An example is shown in Table 26-2. In this example, the severe hyperventilation decreased the serum carbonic acid concentration so markedly that the pH moved toward the frankly alkalemic range. Worsening hypobicarbonatemia, in the face of normalization of pH, emphasizes the fact that the serum bicarbonate concentration by itself does not give enough information to appropriately evalute acid-base disorders.

It is very common to see a similar mixed acid-base disorder develop during the recovery phase of any severe metabolic acidosis, including ketoacidosis. Bicarbonate, P_{CO_2}, and pH all begin to increase as acetoacetate and β-hydroxybutyrate are metabolized to alkali. During this stage, respiratory compensation recovers more slowly than serum bicarbonate concentration, resulting in a sustained lowering of P_{CO_2}, while bicarbonate levels approach normal. In consequence, the pH rapidly normalizes or may even move into the frankly alkaline range. By 12 to 36 h, respiration normalizes and acid-base balance returns. Therapy with $NaHCO_3$ during the acidemic phase tends to worsen this "alkaline overshoot" by further elevating the serum bicarbonate concentration at a time when the P_{CO_2} is inappropriately low. If careful attention has been paid to reexpansion of the ECF volume with saline solution and the needed potassium replacement, it is unlikely that the kidney will retain this additional bicarbonate. In the face of normovolemia, normokalemia, and hypocapnia, the kidney tends to excrete, not retain, bicarbonate.

TABLE 26-2 • DKA and coexistent respiratory alkalosis: chemical pattern

Measurement	Normal	DKA	Respiratory alkalosis plus DKA
Na^+, meq/liter	140	140	139
K^+, meq/liter	4	5	4
Cl^-, meq/liter	105	105	106
CO_2, meq/liter	25	10	8
AG, meq/L	10	25	25
pH	7.40	7.23	7.44
P_{CO_2}, mmHg	40	22	12

ABBREVIATIONS: AG, anion gap; DKA, diabetic ketoacidosis.

CLINICAL EVALUATION OF KETOSIS

A number of semiquantitative tests based on the nitroprusside reaction (e.g., Ketostix and Acetest tablets or powder) are used for the detection of ketosis. The chemical reaction is strongest with acetoacetic acid, weak with acetone, and nonreactive with β-hydroxybutyric acid. The serum acetoacetic acid concentration is high enough in the great majority of patients with diabetic ketoacidosis to give a positive nitroprusside reaction. In the presence of tissue hypoxia or ethanol, however, the severity or even the very presence of ketonemia may go unrecognized because the bulk of ketones reside in the β-hydroxybutyric acid form, which is nitroprusside-negative. Since the β-hydroxybutyric acid/acetoacetic acid ratio is subject to much variability, it is not surprising that a poor correlation exists between the serum nitroprusside test result and the exact quantitative assessment of total ketones.[9]

As previously noted, substantial levels of acetone may remain in the serum following clearing of acetoacetic acid and β-hydroxybutyric acid. The positive nitroprusside reaction in this setting does not reflect ongoing ketosis, which would, of course, signal the need for more insulin, but, rather, indicates the natural evolution of resolving ketosis.[298]

Thus, a positive test result for acetoacetic acid is very helpful in diagnosing ketoacidosis, but a trace positive or negative test does not rule it out. It follows that a negative test result in an acidotic diabetic may reflect either β-hydroxybutyric ketoacidosis, a mixed ketolactic acidosis, or a pure lactic acidosis. In this setting, therapy with insulin should be begun and specific tests for β-hydroxybutyric acid and lactic acid carried out.

During therapy for ketoacidosis, changes occur in the β-hydroxybutyric acid/acetoacetic acid ratio and serum acetone level that impose important restrictions on the interpretation of the degree of positivity of the serum Acetest. Because of these uncertainties, the authors no longer rely on the Acetest, in serial plasma dilution, to dictate insulin needs.

A confusing picture is sometimes presented by patients with "euglycemic diabetic ketoacidosis."[212] This group also presents with severe ketoacidosis, but with a normal to slightly elevated blood sugar (<350 mg/dl). It almost always occurs in known diabetics who are insulin-dependent and who have taken their insulin dose on the day of admission. The pathophysiology of this syndrome is still to be worked out. Therapy is similar to that for hyperglycemic ketoacidosis, but glucose-containing solutions are used from the outset.

It is important to remember that there are other causes of ketosis that must be distinguished from diabetic ketoacidosis and that may stimulate the picture of euglycemic diabetic ketoacidosis (see Table 26-3).

The severe ketoacidosis sets off a chain of aggravating physiologic changes:

1. There is a marked peripheral vasodilatation, in spite of hypotension, causing the cherry-red skin and mucous membranes characteristic of the patient in severe diabetic acidosis. This peripheral vasodilatation leads to increased cutaneous insensible water loss that further aggravates the fluid deficit.
2. Loss of appetite and excessive nausea and vomiting follow the ketoacidosis so that thirst cannot be satisfied.
3. Further sodium chloride, potassium, and water losses occur through the vomitus.

The diffuse and/or localized abdominal pain seen in association with many cases of diabetic acidosis is secondary to the ketoacidosis per se. This abdominal pain has often been misdiagnosed as an acute surgical emergency. An important point that differentiates this from other acute surgical abdominal conditions is that the loss of appetite followed by nausea and vomiting in diabetic acidosis *always* precedes the abdominal pain. This sequence is in contrast to that seen in most surgical emergencies. The characteristic polymorphonuclear leukocytosis, which may be secondary to the dehydration, acidosis, and adrenal cortical stimulation, further confuses the picture and may actually reach leukemoid proportions of 40,000 to 50,000 white blood cells per cubic millimeter of blood. Diabetic acidosis and coma may be precipitated by a fulminant, acute, hemorrhagic pancreatitis. In this situation, the abdominal pain will be persistent and severe. The hypotension will be very resistant to water, electrolytes, and even blood replacement, and the patient will fail to improve during therapy in contrast to the improvement of the patient in the usual diabetic coma.

With respect to the diagnosis of acute pancreatitis associated with diabetic ketosis, plasma amylase levels may be greatly elevated without pancreatic inflammation or any disorder of exocrine function of the pancreas. In fact, Warshaw and associates[319] have recently demonstrated that the elevated serum amylase observed in at least 50 percent of their patients with diabetic ketoacidosis was, in six out of seven cases, of salivary and not pancreatic origin when isoenzyme analysis of the plasma was carried out by polyserylamide-gel electrophoresis. Finn and Cope[85] documented that during recovery the decrease of the amylasemia parallels the fall in blood sugar level, suggesting a relationship between the abnormal carbohydrate metabolism and the elevated serum amylase level. The value of the amylase clearance/creatinine clearance ratio in the diagnosis of true acute pancreatitis in diabetes and in other states with impaired renal function has been documented.[316]

QUANTITATIVE WATER AND ELECTROLYTE LOSSES

Figures 26-8 and 26-9 summarize the characteristics of the water and electrolyte losses in uncontrolled diabetic

TABLE 26-3 • **Causes of ketoacidosis**

Disorder	Degree of ketosis	Blood sugar	Clue to diagnosis
Starvation	+1 - +2	Low-normal	History, serum $HCO_3^- \geq 17$ meq/liter
High-fat diet	+1 - +2	Normal	Dietary history
Drugs/toxins			
Paraldehyde[119]	+1 - +2	Normal	History, paraldehyde odor on breath
Isopropyl alcohol[24]	+1 - +4	Normal-low	Ketosis due to acetone, normal HCO_3^- and anion gap
Alcoholic ketosis[99]	+2 - +4	Low-normal	Recent binge, vomiting
von Gierke's disease[135]	+2 - +4	Low	Hypoglycemia, hepatomegaly

Source	Osmolality	Sodium concentration
Skin and lungs	Distilled water	0
Kidney	Iso- or hypertonic	25–100 meq/liter
Vomitus	Isotonic	50–80 meq/liter

FIGURE 26-8 • Qualitative characteristics of the fluids lost during diabetic acidosis with respect to their total osmolality and sodium concentration.

Substance	Parameter	Range
Water	75–100 ml/kg	
Na^+	8 meq/kg	5–10
Cl^-	5 meq/kg	3–10
K^+	6 meq/liter	3–11
N	0.5 g/kg	

FIGURE 26-9 • Average losses of water, nitrogen, and electrolytes in severe diabetic acidosis; derived from balance studies during the recovery phase. Values represent those available in the literature and from the authors' series.

acidosis.[28,48,49,92,213] It is readily apparent that all avenues of sodium and chloride loss are hypotonic to the normal body fluids (i.e., the water losses are in excess of the simultaneous sodium losses). Thus, the water loss in diabetic acidosis represents the most serious form of hypertonic dehydration and leads to extreme intracellular depletion of fluids. The water losses through the skin, lungs, and gastrointestinal tract are aggravated by the usual inability of the patient to replace water because of anorexia, vomiting, or coma. The extreme depletion of body fluids from all spaces leads to a relentless contraction of the vascular volume, hypotension, and often shock. As in all states associated with a depletion of the vascular volume and increased blood viscosity, there is a progressive reduction in renal blood flow and GFR,[265] which further impairs renal compensatory mechanisms, thus leading to a more rapidly developing and severe acidosis. To emphasize the adverse role of hypovolemia per se, Porte and associates[246] showed that the administration of appropriate salt solutions *without insulin* greatly inhibited the development of ketoacidosis following withdrawal of insulin from insulin-dependent diabetic subjects. Further, it has been shown that hemorrhagic or hypovolemic hypotension and shock can seriously impair the output of insulin from the pancreas and that this is due to norepinephrine or alpha-adrenergic inhibition of insulin secretion.[57,246]

The sustained renal ischemia, even in the absence of acute organic renal failure, may cause transient albuminuria and the appearance of granular casts in the urine, which may be erroneously attributed to an associated acute or chronic renal disease. However, if the severe renal ischemia is sustained, actual acute tubular necrosis may be superimposed upon the prerenal azotemia and will greatly complicate the diagnostic and therapeutic problems. Spurious artifactual increases in serum creatinine are caused by acetoacetate interference with standard colorimetric assays of creatinine.[215] This false "hypercreatininemia" gives the erroneous appearance of worsened renal function.

Figure 26-9 presents average values for water, electrolyte, and nitrogen losses incurred during severe diabetic acidosis.[28,48,49,92,213] These values should be remembered, for they give the physician an empirical starting point in estimating the total deficit that developed prior to the patient's hospitalization. It will be noted that magnesium and phosphate, although lost in large quantities during severe uncontrolled diabetes mellitus, have not been included.

The use of parenteral inorganic phosphorus therapy as a component of the early (first 24 to 36 h) treatment of diabetic acidosis and coma is controversial. In the late 1940s, Franks and associates[92] treated 10 patients with diabetic ketoacidosis with 1.3 to 2.6 g of elemental phosphorus given rapidly during the early hours of parenteral fluid therapy, and they compared this group with patients receiving saline solution only and with another 11 receiving glucose and saline solution. They concluded that "the administration of sodium phosphate was accompanied by (a) a tendency toward improved utilization of carbohydrate, (b) a rise in plasma chloride and in carbon-dioxide combining power, (c) an apparent retention of fluid in the vascular system, (d) a rapid clearing of the mental state, and (e) a statistically significant decrease in fatality rate. The results of this study suggest that the therapeutic regimen in diabetic coma should include the parenteral administration of sodium phosphate 4 to 8 hours after the first dose of insulin." Before Franks' study,[92] Guest and Rapaport[117] had carried out extensive experiments in animals and humans showing the marked derangement in inorganic and organic phosphate metabolism in the red blood cells during diabetic ketoacidosis.

Four recent well-controlled, randomized studies [33,86,156,327] failed to demonstrate a favorable effect of phosphate therapy on the clinical course of diabetic ketoacidosis. One of the studies demonstrated a slight increase in red blood cell 2,3-diphosphoglyceric acid (DPG) content that was not statistically significant in the phosphate-treated group. The avidity of hemoglobin for oxygen remained unchanged in both groups.[86] A recent study showed that intravenous phosphate therapy in severe diabetic ketoacidosis had a small but significant effect on oxygen affinity and DPG levels only after the first 48 h of therapy.[61]

Phosphorus, like potassium, is an integral part of the intracellular milieu, and with increased catabolism during ketoacidosis, there is a shift of phosphorus from the tissue to the extracellular space, making it more available for urinary excretion. Consequently, these patients rarely (~ 11 percent) present with hypophosphatemia despite severe phosphorus deficiency. Almost invariably, however, serum phosphorus levels fall progressively during therapy. Within 4 to 6 h, it may decline to values well below normal, and by 12 to 24 h, it may decrease to as low as one mg/100 ml or less.

Caution must be exercised when intravenously administering phosphate during diabetic ketoacidosis.[329] In one report, 6 of 9 children developed transient hypocalcemia, and 5 of 9 developed transient hypomagnesemia associated with depressed parathyroid hormone levels.[340] One child developed carpopedal spasm. Replacement should not be considered until volume depletion, acidosis, and hyperglycemia have been corrected and renal function has been adequately restored. After normocalcemia has been documented, one can consider replacement therapy if the serum phosphorus level has decreased to levels of 2.0 mg/100 ml or less.

The mean phosphorus deficit in ketoacidosis is 0.5 to 1.5 mmol/kg body weight.[329] The replacement dose then becomes approximately 50 mmol of elemental phosphorus (equivalent to 50 mmol of phosphate or 1600 mg of elemental phosphorus) given intravenously over 24 to 36 h. Oral therapy would, of course, be preferable.

Today it is clear that acute phosphate depletion and severe hypophosphatemia, as seen before and during the treatment of these patients, may produce clinically significant abnormalities in the central and peripheral nervous system, skeletal muscles, oxygen transport by the red cells, and phagocytic and migratory capacity of the white cells (see Chap. 32).[66,163,178] It has also been suggested that severe phosphate depletion may adversely affect respiratory[219] and myocardial[223] function. Despite this, we still cannot routinely recommend the addition of phosphorus to our early parenteral therapy of diabetic acidosis and coma.

Many of our comments regarding phosphorus also apply to the hypomagnesemia and total body depletion of magnesium in uncontrolled diabetes.[213] Evidence that this chemical abnormality requires acute correction is at best uncertain. With rapid repair of diabetic ketoacidosis, most subjects quickly return to a normal diet, which provides adequate magnesium and phosphorus.

TREATMENT

The fundamental physiologic principles that have been presented govern therapy in all cases; however, each case must be individualized. There is no substitute for careful clinical and laboratory observation of each patient. Only through rigorous observation can one properly evaluate the patient's needs and response to therapy. This type of observation is far more important than the slight to moderate differences in the approach to therapy that can be seen from institution to institution or from one "authority" to another. In fact, given the meticulous hour-to-hour care necessary and a few basic principles, the major morbidity and mortality are primarily related to the patient's associated disorders and even the patient's socioeconomic status.

GENERAL POINTS

1. The patient must be examined by the physician frequently and completely for clinical changes. The observation and care of the patient in diabetic acidosis *cannot* be left only to the nursing staff.
2. Diabetic acidosis is never associated with fever unless some complication is present. "Prophylactic" antibiotics should not be used, but antibiotic therapy should be initiated if the patient is febrile and a careful effort, with appropriate cultures, has been made to determine the cause of the fever.
3. Young adults appear much less dehydrated than they actually are. A history of the patient's weight just before the onset of the acute illness is extremely important. Weight loss is a good approximation of the magnitude of fluid loss. Allow for a tissue loss (protein and fat) of 0.5 kg/day for each day that the patient has not eaten prior to admission or 0.25 kg/day if food intake has been curtailed but not been stopped.
4. All deep reflexes should be checked very carefully on the initial physical examination. This and the electrocardiogram are the best methods for following a rapidly decreasing serum potassium concentration. In spite of the marked potassium depletion, the serum potassium level on admission is usually normal or elevated, and the electrocardiogram may show peaking of the T waves, suggestive of potassium intoxication (see above).
5. Serum sodium concentration should be closely scrutinized, as should serum osmolality, in patients presenting with severe hyperglycemia.[71] A normal or increased serum sodium level indicates that significant cellular dehydration has occurred and that the patient should be monitored more closely for neurologic abnormalities. Hyponatremia suggests that total body water may be preserved although displaced from the cellular to the excellular space. The corrected serum sodium level should be calculated in all cases of severe hyperglycemia to rule out a "masked" hypernatremic state.
6. The patient with severe diabetic ketoacidosis is frequently stuporous and relatively unresponsive and at

times in frank coma. It is clear that the level of consciousness is best correlated with the magnitude of hyperglycemia and hyperosmolality of the body fluids noted at the time of the patient's admission (Fig. 26-10; see Chap. 46).[96] This depression of the sensorium is usually readily responsive to the corrective therapy. However, at times after the initial clearing, the patient may once again become stuporous or semicomatose despite biochemical improvement in the metabolic parameters and may follow this same untoward course. Sporadic cases have been described[14,19] where the patient, after initial clearing of the sensorium, suddenly lapsed into deep coma with falling blood pressure, tachycardia, and often fever and shortly thereafter died despite progressive improvement in the abnormal blood chemistry values. Postmortem examination has consistently demonstrated severe cerebral edema.[14,19,87,98,336] Fulop[99] has suggested that before therapy the prolonged hyperglycemia has caused a significant rise in the glucose concentration in the interstitial and intracellular space of the brain, despite the blood-brain barrier. As the blood sugar level falls rapidly during effective therapy, there is a reversal of the gradient of glucose concentration between the blood and the brain, the osmotic pressure of the blood falls below that of the brain, and the water moves into the interstitial and intracellular space of the brain, causing severe cerebral edema. However, increased content of glucose in the brain makes up only a small part of the increase in brain osmolal content during sustained hyperglycemia. The content of glucose has never been reported to exceed 25 percent of plasma glucose levels. When the glucose concentration in the plasma is *rapidly* reduced with insulin to normal or near normal values in animals with experimental diabetic coma, the brain content of glucose falls at the same rate as does the glucose in the plasma with no evidence of retention in the brain.[22,23] Despite this, total brain osmolality falls at a significantly slower rate than does that of the plasma, causing an osmotic gradient between brain and plasma and the rapid development of brain edema. A substantial portion of the increase in total osmolal content of the brain consists of measured solutes such as sodium (11 percent), chloride (8 percent), and potassium (26 percent), but the largest part consists of undetermined or idiogenic osmols (45 percent). This osmolar generation is the direct result of the insulin therapy, for comparably rapid lowering of plasma glucose with peritoneal dialysis does not cause an increase in brain solute content and does not cause cerebral edema.[22,23] In the majority of the reported cases of brain edema complicating treatment of ketoacidosis, blood glucose was rapidly reduced to levels close to 100 mg/100 ml. It may be possible to prevent the effects of insulin leading to brain edema by avoiding overly rapid reduction of blood glucose to normal during the total therapy of diabetic coma. Attempts to treat the cerebral edema with mannitol and glucocorticoids have not been successful.[15] Two recent studies failed to significantly implicate the rate of hydration, tonicity of administered fluids, rate of correction of glycemia, or use of bicarbonate in the incidence of intracerebral crisis in diabetic ketoacidosis.[77,261] One study did demonstrate a weak but possibly significant correlation between the time of onset of herniation and the rate of fluid administration (90 percent of the patients with herniation received >4 liters fluid/m^2 body surface area per day).[77] A correlation between increased blood hydrogen ion concentration and decreased level of consciousness has also recently been demonstrated in diabetic ketoacidosis.[263] Subsequent to this correlation, a hypothesis has been developed that suggests that cytoplasmic acidification may activate the Na^+-H^+ exchanger and in the presence of extracellular sodium may cause cell swelling and cerebral edema.[303]

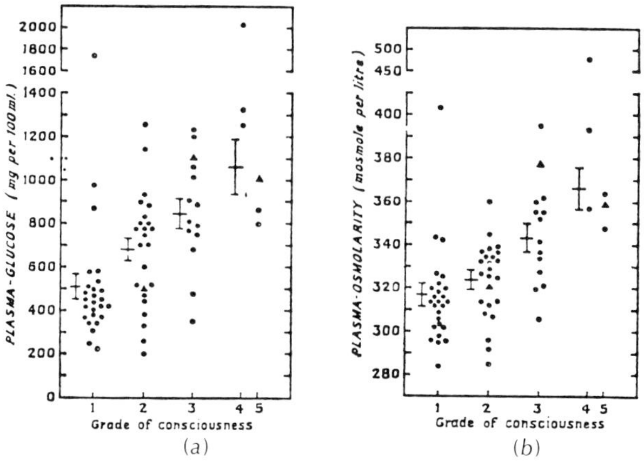

FIGURE 26-10 • (*a*) Relationship between state of consciousness and plasma glucose in 70 episodes of diabetic ketoacidosis. (*b*) Relationship between state of consciousness and calculated plasma osmolalrity in 70 episodes of diabetic ketoacidosis. (From Fulop M et al, *Lancet* 2:635, 1973. Used by permission.)

7. A decision as to catherization of the bladder may be based on the following factors: (a) if the patient is lucid and can void spontaneously and if rectal or vaginal examination discloses no evidence of prostatic enlargement or cystocele, catheterization is not necessary, and the patient should be allowed to void spontaneously; (b) if a large residual urine is suspected in a conscious patient, the patient should void and be immediately catheterized *one time only* to check the residual urine and obtain a urine culture, after which the catheter should be removed; and (c) if the patient is stuporous or if urine specimens cannot

be obtained, an indwelling catheter with a sterile sealed drainage system may be inserted but must be removed as soon as the patient becomes lucid enough to void spontaneously; *the physician should make every effort to avoid catheterizing the patient in diabetic acidosis or coma* because of the danger of causing a urinary tract infection or a serious exacerbation of an already existing one.

8. With respect to the question of admitting the patient with mild ketoacidosis to the hospital, it is always better to err on the side of being overly cautious and to hospitalize. At times the physician may know the patient so well and be so convinced of the patient's intelligence and reliability that the physician may choose to treat mild ketosis and mild dehydration and volume depletion on an ambulatory basis. The patient under the doctor's direction initiates hourly oral feedings with juices, water, salted broth, and dietetic carbonated drinks and hourly subcutaneous injections of 5 to 10 units of regular insulin. Urine is checked hourly for sugar and ketones, and this treatment is continued until ketonuria is cleared and there has been a significant decrease in the degree of glycosuria. The patient can then be placed on a schedule of one dose of regular insulin before each meal for 1 to 2 days before reinstituting the usual insulin regimen. Failure of the patient to respond promptly to such an ambulatory approach should lead to the necessary hospitalization.

INSULIN ADMINISTRATION

Randomized studies have shown that the speed of recovery from ketoacidosis does not correlate with the total dose of insulin used when cumulative doses ranging from 125 to 800 units were studied.[278,282] Nevertheless, physicians continue to treat with large doses, justifying their use in the deep-rooted notion that acidosis and ketosis incude an acute state of insulin resistance.[188,311] Hundreds of units of insulin have been and are still being used in an effort to overcome this presumed resistance, and dosage is often based on complicated formulas that add to the mystique surrounding therapy for ketoacidosis.

Many studies have clearly demonstrated that ketoacidosis may be safely, simply, and effectively treated with cumulative doses of regular insulin well under 100 units.[6,10,53,78,103,127,159,160,208,294] Kitabchi recently presented a comprehensive review of low-dose insulin therapy for diabetic ketoacidosis.[158] Continuous infusion of 4 to 8 units/h or hourly intramuscular or subcutaneous injections of 5 to 10 units have been shown to lower blood sugar smoothly, improve ketosis, and repair acidosis at rates indistinguishable from those achieved with conventional, higher-dose regimens.[6,340] The reason for this is that the mechanism of the insulin effect is an all-or-none phenomenon dependent on the number of insulin receptors that are bound. Studies have shown that hepatic glucose production is maximally inhibited by 100 μU/ml of insulin, peripheral glucose utilization is stimulated to 75 percent of maximal by 100 μU/ml of insulin and maximally stimulated by 200 μU/ml of insulin, and lipolysis is completely inhibited by 50 to 100 μU/ml.[67,73,116,277] Utilization of this low-dose insulin protocol produces plasma insulin levels of 20 to 200 μU/ml,[6,153] thus providing maximal or near maximal effects on both carbohydrate and lipid metabolism. Doses of insulin that produce plasma levels in excess of 1000 μU/ml do not increase its physiologic effect but, rather, prolong its duration of action and predispose patients to a higher incidence of hypoglycemia, hypokalemia, and hypophosphatemia.[159] Table 26-4 is taken from the prospective study of Kitabchi and coworkers,[159] which compared conventional, intermittent high-dose insulin therapy with low-dose intramuscular (IM) therapy. No significant difference in the time required to reverse the

TABLE 26-4 • Comparison of results with high-dose and low-dose insulin therapy

	High-dose	Low-dose	p
Number of patients	24	24	
Glucose ≤ 250 mg/100 ml	4.5 ± 0.8 h	6.7 ± 0.8 h	NS
HCO_3^- > 15 meq/liter	11.6 ± 1.6 h	11.1 ± 1.2 h	NS
pH > 7.3	6.9 ± 1.3 h	8.3 ± 0.9 h	NS
Acetone < 1:2	10.3 ± 1.2 h	12.0 ± 1.8 h	NS
Alertness	11.1 ± 2.6 h	7.5 ± 1.5 h	NS
Insulin given to achieve glucose level of 250 mg/100 ml	263.4 ± 45.3 U	46 ± 5 U	<0.001
Total fluid given during first 6 h	4233.4 ± 284 ml	4006 ± 250 ml	NS
Number of patients with hypoglycemia	6	0	

ABBREVIATION: NS, not significant.
SOURCE: Kitabchi et al.[159]

hyperglycemia, ketosis, or acidosis was observed between the two groups. Six of the 24 high-dose and none of the low-dose subjects became hypoglycemia during therapy. Hypokalemia occurred in 7 subjects from the high-dose group, whereas it developed in only 1 of the low-dose subjects. These data underscore the effectiveness of low-dose therapy and suggest that it may achieve normoglycemia and normokalemia more smoothly than does high-dose therapy.

These levels of plasma insulin (20 to 200 μU/ml) rapidly and effectively reverse the hyperglycemia and ketosis in uncontrolled diabetics, thereby negating the notion that ketosis and/or acidemia commonly induces biologically significant degrees of insulin resistance. Similar conclusions were reached by Hockaday and Alberti,[132] who found no difference in insulin sensitivity in patients whose initial pH ranged from 6.90 to 7.25. Defronzo and Beckles,[73] however, have demonstrated by means of hyperglycemic and euglycemic clamp studies in normal volunteers that abnormal tissue sensitivity to insulin impaired glucose metabolism during metabolic acidosis. Recent studies have shown that low pH accelerates the dissociation of receptor-bound insulin and that the chemical basis of decreased insulin binding during metabolic acidosis may be that the receptor contains a pH-sensitive group. While these biochemical events are of interest, they do not measureably alter our therapeutic approach.[149,196]

Low-dose insulin schedules that have proved effective are outlined below.

Intramuscular and subcutaneous therapy

In normotensive patients, regular insulin therapy is initiated with 0.2 unit/kg given by deep IM injection. Doses of 5 to 10 units are given intramuscularly each hour thereafter until the blood sugar reaches 250 mg/100 ml and the ketoacidosis clears. At this time, further insulin is given every 2 h subcutaneously. Subsequent subcutaneous (SC) doses are based on blood sugar level or on the glucose content of double-voided urine specimens. It is important to underscore the need for repeated tests of the blood sugar level and frequent doses of SC regular insulin. There is a tendency for many physicians to relax their therapy and vigilance once acute ketoacidosis has been reversed. Ketoacidosis and hyperglycemia are quick to return unless the patient's ongoing need for insulin is met. If the patient is hypotensive initially, insulin should be given intravenously, since absorption from hypoperfused muscle may be erratic. Once the blood pressure has stabilized, IM or SC therapy may be used. Following its initial rapid decline, as a consequence of rehydration, the blood sugar level continues to fall by 75 to 100 mg/100 ml per hour.[6,294] The presence of an infection can slow the rate of decline in blood sugar level by 50 percent, to approximately 50 mg/100 ml per hour.[284] This value may be used to anticipate when the blood sugar level will reach 250 mg/100 ml and therapy with glucose-containing solutions should be begun. Blood should be collected for serum enzyme studies prior to initiating IM therapy, since these injections will traumatize muscle and increase serum enzyme levels.

CONTINUOUS INTRAVENOUS THERAPY

The binding of insulin to the glass and plastic used for its infusion potentially decreases the dose delivered to the patient. This binding will not significantly affect delivery, however, if sufficiently high concentrations of regular insulin are used and the tubing is rinsed with the solution. If 100 units of regular insulin is added to 1 liter of normal saline solution and if the tubing is washed out with the first 50 ml, the remaining fluid will accurately deliver the desired dose.[241] This high concentration and the washout procedure apparently saturate the insulin-binding sites. One milliliter per minute of this solution delivers 6 units of insulin per hour, a dose sufficient for most patients. Fluid is best delivered with a infusion pump, but in its absence, a pediatric infusion set may be safely and conveniently employed. As noted with IM therapy, when the blood sugar reaches 250 mg/100 ml and if the ketosis has cleared, one should switch to SC therapy.

The simplicity of low-dose IM, SC, or intravenous therapy, coupled with its ability to effect smooth reversal of the biochemical abnormalities and to minimize hypoglycemia and hypokalemia, make the low-dose regimen more attractive to the authors. Regardless of which therapy and dose of insulin the physician selects—and they may be equally effective[6,153,294]—it is absolutely critical to follow serum electrolyte levels and biochemical parameters. One must be prepared to increase or decrease insulin therapy depending upon the patient's response. The patient who is truly resistant to insulin may require many hundreds of units before a response is obtained. If the blood sugar level has remained unchanged or has increased 1 to 2 h after initiating therapy, as outlined above, the patient should be given 100 units of regular insulin intravenously. The dose may be doubled every 1 to 2 h (100, 200, 400 units, etc.) if no response is obtained. This degree of resistance is rarely met.

A recent study comparing the efficacy of human and porcine insulin in the treatment of diabetic ketoacidosis demonstrated no clinically significant difference between the two.[295]

ALKALI THERAPY

The accession of strong ketone acids to the extracellular space causes progressive loss of bicarbonate, fall in systemic pH, and compensatory decrease in P_{CO_2}, as was previously noted. With therapy, β-hydroxybutyrate and acetoacetate are metabolized to bicarbonate, thereby reversing the ketoacidosis. If the patient retains every millimole of ketone produced, its eventual oxidative conversion to alkali would return the serum bicarbonate concentration to exactly normal. To the extent that sodium β-hydroxybutyrate and sodium acetoacetate are lost in the urine, a true bicarbonate deficit would exist, which could only be replenished by renal synthesis or by exogenous replacement.

Many have argued that, since insulin therapy reverses the biochemical abnormalities, including the bicarbonate deficit, alkali therapy is not only unnecessary but may in fact be detrimental. Others have felt that patients with severe degrees of acidosis and acidemia (i.e., pH <7.15 and bicarbonate ≤ 8 meq/liter) were at substantial risk from their low pH and therefore have advocated early therapy with alkali.[256]

The perceived need for alkali is based on the following observations:

1. Insensitivity of peripheral tissues to insulin occurs in acidosis.[73,149,188,196,311] It might therefore be expected that alkali therapy would allow insulin to exert its full effects more rapidly. As noted above, the physiologic importance of this acid inhibition has been seriously questioned.[127,208]
2. Profound hemodynamic effects of acidosis may lead to life-threatening pulmonary edema, hypotension, and shock.[325] Acidosis directly impairs myocardial contractility but simultaneously causes the release of epinephrine. The positive inotropic effect of the latter largely offsets the inhibitory effects of low pH.[326] However, when the pH falls below 7.20 to 7.15, the catechole effect is inhibited, thereby unmasking the negative inotropic effects of acidosis. These low pHs causes venous constriction and arteriolar dilatation, leading to a decrease in venous capacitance and peripheral vascular resistance. The fall in capacitance forces more blood into the pulmonary circuit, while arteriolar dilatation leads to hypotension. Thus, greater demands are placed on a compromised myocardium, potentially leading to pulmonary edema and to hypotension and shock.
3. Acidosis induces widespread metabolic defects that may disrupt cellular function.[253] Defects in glycolysis and lactate consumption are two such examples.[122,128]

The undesirable effects of alkali therapy have received much attention and are briefly outlined below:

1. In their oft-quoted paper, Posner and Plum[247] describe *two* ketoacidotic diabetes whose mental status worsened during sodium bicarbonate therapy. Their cerebrospinal fluid (CSF) pH fell by 0.15 and 0.12 units, respectively, when their state of consciousness worsened. It has been argued that the increase in ECF pH consequent to alkali therapy acts on peripheral chemoreceptors to diminish alveolar ventilation, thereby raising the P_{CO_2}. Because carbon dixoide, but not bicarbonate, rapidly enters the CSF, the brain is exposed primarily to the acidifying effects of P_{CO_2}. Thus, in the early phase of alkali therapy, when ECF pH is rising, a paradoxical fall in CSF pH alters cerebral function. In time, bicarbonate also enters the CSF and causes its pH to return toward control levels. Thus, on the basis of these two patients, the widespread belief has developed that CSF acidosis and stupor are significant and common complications of alkali therapy. Subsequent studies, however, have shown that CSF pH falls during conventional therapy for ketoacidosis regardless of whether bicarbonate is used.[26,226] In fact, the decline in CSF pH in diabetics treated with bicarbonate (-0.12 ± 0.02) was not significantly different from the decline in those treated without alkali (-0.07 ± 0.05).[26,226] It is of interest that the fall in CSF pH that routinely occurred in diabetics who did not suffer CNS dysfunction closely approximated that of Posner and Plum's two patients. These observations cast serious doubt on the importance of the fall in CSF pH. In the opinion of the authors, the occurrence or worsening of the state of consciousness during alkali therapy is so rare that it should not strongly influence the decision to use bicarbonate.
2. The affinity of hemoglobin for oxygen is greatly influenced by acid-base changes. Low pH decreases affinity (Bohr effect) and thereby enables hemoglobin to unload more oxygen at the tissue level.[276] When the red blood cell glycolytic intermediate 2,3-diphosphoglycerate (2,3-DPG) is abundant, the affinity of hemoglobin for oxygen also falls, whereas affinity rises when a dearth of 2,3-DPG exists.[59] Acidosis, by impairing red blood cell glycolysis, causes the 2,3-DPG content to fall.[50,117,151] Thus, acidosis exerts positive and negative effects of hemoglobin-oxygen binding, and these effects need not occur simultaneously. Although the Bohr effect is induced rapidly, the red blood cell 2,3-DPG content falls slowly (Table 26-5). The predominance of the Bohr effect in early acidosis tends to increase tissue oxygenation, but the fall in 2,3-DPG, which occurs in time, counters the Bohr effect and thereby returns hemoglobin-oxygen affinity to baseline.[34] Rapid normalization of pH during alkali treatment reverses the Bohr effect more rapidly than red blood cell 2,3-DPG can be replenished. During this transient state of imbalance, when 2,3-DPG is low and the Bohr effect is absent, oxygen will be more tightly bound to hemoglobin, and tissue oxygen delivery might suffer. This observation has been used as a caveat to enjoin

TABLE 26-5 • **Effects of acid-base changes on hemoglobin-oxygen affinity**

Stage of acidosis	2,3-DPG	Bohr effect	Net change in hemoglobin-oxygen affinity	Potential effect on tissue oxygenation
Initial acute acidosis	Remains normal	Present	Fall (<basal)	Increased
Steady-state acidosis	Low	Present	Return to basal	Return to basal
Initial response to alkali	Remains low	Absent	Rise	Decreased

ABBREVIATION: 2,3-DPG, 2,3-diphosphoglycerate.

physicians from the injudicious use of bicarbonate. The authors are presently unaware of any evidence that, when critically reviewed, proves that alkali therapy in any way impairs tissue oxygenation in patients. In fact, Munk and colleagues[211] demonstrated that the affinity of hemoglobin for oxygen increased during therapy for juvenile ketoacidosis regardless of whether bicarbonate was given. Rapid correction of chronic metabolic acidosis in rats did not affect exercise tolerance or increase lactate production during exercise,[35] indicating that, in this model, alkali therapy did not impair tissue oxygenation. It is the opinion of the authors that the imperfections in our understanding of how acid-base changes influence tissue oxygenation are presently far too great to justify withholding alkali in diabetics.

3. The "alkaline overshoot" that tends to occur with therapy may be exacerbated by $NaHCO_3$ therapy, as discussed above.
4. In starvation ketosis, alkali therapy without insulin or glucose stimulates ketone synthesis. The 1:1 stoichiometry of added bicarbonate-to-acid produced prevents major increments in serum bicarbonate concentration. This interesting observation should not influence alkaki therapy for diabetic ketoacidosis, since in this setting alkali is given simultaneously with insulin. The overriding effect of the hormone is to reduce ketone synthesis, while the alkali neutralizes the life-threatening effects of acidemia.

One must bear in mind that arterial pH is exquisitely sensitive to small changes in serum bicarbonate concentration in patients with severe diabetic ketoacidosis. The bicarbonate/carbonic acid ratio defines the pH. When low absolute levels of bicarbonate prevail, an additional, even small, change effects large changes in the ratio and thereby in the pH. This point helps to put matters into perspective. As shown in Table 26-6, a further 2.5 meq/liter fall in serum bicarbonate level in a typical patient with severe ketoacidosis would lower the pH from 7.12 to 6.83. Hypotension with lactic acidosis, unchecked ketoacidosis, or even the dilutional acidosis caused by rapid saline infusions could cause this small decline in bicarbonate concentration and thereby precipitate sudden, severe worsening of acidosis. In the same patient, a small, sudden elevation of P_{CO_2} is shown to result in a similar catastrophic fall in pH. It should be obvious that such patients are in precarious balance. This sensitivity to bicarbonate may also be used to the patient's advantage. A small *increase* in bicarbonate from 5.0 to 8.0 meq/liter elevates the pH from the dangerously low value of 7.12 to the far safer figure of 7.32 (Table 26-6). In the authors' opinion, the benefits derived from small doses of bicarbonate far outweigh any theoretical or as yet poorly defined side effect. There is little clinical information documenting adverse effects of reasonable use of bicarbonate therapy. Marr and associates reported that, in 131 children with diabetic ketoacidosis treated over a 21-year period, no adverse effect of bicarbonate therapy was noted.[195]

Sodium bicarbonate is clearly the alkali of choice for parenteral therapy. Other sources of base, such as sodium lactate, must first be metabolized to bicarbonate before becoming effective. As was pointed out by Schwartz and

TABLE 26-6 • **Effects of small changes in serum HCO_3^- and P_{CO_2} on pH in severe DKA**

Measurement	Normal	Severe DKA	Further minimal fall in HCO_3^-	Acute minimal rise in P_{CO_2}	Combined changes in HCO_3^- and P_{CO_2}	Minimal rise in HCO_3^-
HCO_3^-, meq/liter	24	5.0	2.5	5.0	2.5	8.0
P_{CO_2}, mmHg	40	16.0	16.0	30.0	30.0	16.0
pH	7.40	7.12	6.83	6.83	6.54	7.32

ABBREVIATION: DKA, diabetic ketoacidosis.

Waters,[271] one cannot always rely on this metabolic conversion to occur; thus, these indirect forms of alkali are less dependable.

When the initial pH is 7.15 or less and the serum bicarbonate concentration is 10 meq/liter or lower, therapy should begin with 50 to 100 meq of sodium bicarbonate in adults and 0.5 to 1.0 meq/kg in children. Hypotensive patients and those whose bicarbonate concentration is less than 5 meq/liter should be given larger doses based on their deficits.

WATER AND SODIUM REPLACEMENT

It is clear that the net overall loss of salt (NaCl) and water in diabetic ketoacidosis and coma is quite hypotonic to the normal ECF and can be approximated by one-half normal (0.45 %) saline solution or even by more dilute solutions in hyperosmolal ketotic or nonketotic coma. This being the case, the final total mix of the solutions used in therapy must approach this hypotonic deficit. Failure to use hypotonic fluid in the overall replacement therapy of these patients may lead to hyperosmolality, manifested by hypernatremia and hyperchloremia. This may mean that more salt than necessary has been given during the process of total correction of the water deficit. The hypernatremia delays the rehydration of cells, and the renal excretion of any excess salt contributes to a continued osmotic diuresis even after glycosuria has been corrected.

That we have stressed the hypotonic nature of the fluid losses should not be taken to mean that it is best to *initiate* intravenous therapy with hypotonic solutions. The latter, in the form of 0.45% saline solution, can certainly be used even from the beginning in the patient who has no hypotension or signs of shock. However, it must be remembered that isotonic saline solution supports the blood volume far better than does one-half normal saline solution despite the fact that it delays correction of the *intracellular* water deficit. When the more hypotonic solution is given and the blood sugar level is falling in response to effective insulin therapy, the major part of the administered water moves intracellularly, correcting the intracellular dehydration, but at times at the expense of the optimum reexpansion of the plasma volume. Since rapid rehydration of the cells, especially those of the brain, may not be best, and since we have stressed the serious adverse effects of continuing hypovolemia, it seems most rational to administer isotonic saline solution as the initial replacement solution. The rate and amount of replacement depend on the observed state of the circulation. The greater the degree of hypotension, the faster and larger will be this replacement. In general, a rate of 500 to 1000 ml/h is satisfactory, and when the blood pressure and pulse have stabilized, one can switch to the 0.45% saline solution with or without 5% dextrose, depending on whether the blood sugar level has fallen below 250 to 300 mg/100 ml.

BLOOD, PLASMA, AND VOLUME EXPANDERS

Volume expanders, such as blood, plasma, and isooncotic albumin, have a definite place in the treatment of diabetic acidosis. It is imperative that severe hypotension and shock be corrected as rapidly as possible. If, after the first hour of electrolyte and water replacement, sustained hypotension is not ameliorated, blood or plasma should be immediately administered. Shock, secondary to fluid and electrolyte loss, is more rapidly corrected when blood or plasma accompanies the electrolyte and water replacement.[328] It should be stressed that adrenergic substances such as norepinephrine or dopamine are not effective in correcting oligemic shock, and severe acidosis must be corrected to allow the circulatory system to respond to the patient's own endogenously produced catecholamines. Secondary hypotension or shock developing 4 to 8 h after initiating therapy usually indicates (1) rapid development of hypokalemia, (2)myocardial infarction, (3) overwhelming sepsis, or (4) gastrointestinal or internal hemorrhage.

GLUCOSE AND FRUCTOSE ADMINISTRATION

Glucose solutions with or without electrolytes should be initiated when the blood sugar level has fallen to approximately 250 to 300 mg/100 ml. There is little point in administering glucose when the blood sugar level is still markedly elevated, for this will only potentiate the hyperglycemia and cellular dehydration and enhance glycosuria and renal salt and water loss. However, carbohydrate replacement is an integral part of the overall treatment of diabetic acidosis. The total body stores of carbohydrate are markedly diminished in spite of the hyperglycemia. In the average adult suffering severe diabetic acidosis, approximately 50 g of carbohydrate is available in the ECF, whereas the total body depletion of glycogen stores may range from 200 to 400 g. It is not unusual during therapy to see the blood sugar level decrease to hypoglycemic levels *without* an appreciable clearing of the plasma ketonemia. This occurs because, when insulin is administered, the amount of glucose available in the ECF is rapidly utilized for glycogenesis but is inadequate to reverse the process of excessive ketogenesis. Furthermore, reexpansion of the ECF space increases the GFR and consequently also increases the filtered load of glucose. The ensuing glycosuria also dissipates extracellular glucose stores. Approximately 75 percent of the initial decline in blood sugar level is due to renal glucose excretion and dilution from administered fluids and about 25 percent is due to glucose metabolism.

It is appropriate at this point to discuss the present role, if any, of fructose in the treatment of diabetic acidosis.[69,201] This hexose, unlike glucose, does not require insulin for transcellular transport and can be used as a glucose substitute by all tissues, with the exception of the central nervous system. Once inside the cell, fructose enters at an intermediary metabolic point that bypasses some of the early steps of the Emden-Myerhoff pathway. Therefore, fructose can be utilized in a surprisingly normal manner in the insulin-requiring patient with uncontrolled diabetes. However, despite the theoretical benefits, there are five drawbacks to the use of fructose in the treatment of diabetic acidosis:

1. Fructose cannot be utilized by the central nervous system and therefore cannot correct the clinical manifestations of hypoglycemia. If fructose is used early in the course of treatment, it should be replaced by glucose solutions when the blood sugar level has decreased significantly.
2. If fructose is infused at a rate exceeding 1 g/kg body weight per hour, its metabolism rapidly produces lactic and pyruvic acids.[37] When these acids are liberated into the ECF, they may actually potentiate the acidosis in spite of clearing of all the plasma ketones. The authors have observed this phenomenon when treating mild diabetic acidosis with fructose solutions alone. This acidosis may also occur in nondiabetic subjects receiving fructose at the above rate.[37]
3. Fructose is considerably more expensive than glucose as a replacement solution.
4. The two- to three-carbon fragments derived from fructose metabolism in the liver can be rapidly channeled into new glucose molecules, which, in the absence of insulin, can be liberated into the circulation and contribute to the maintenance of hyperglycemia.
5. Fructose may be falsely measured as glucose in many of the presently utilized automated techniques for plasma sugar determination.

In view of these qualifications, there seems no practical or beneficial reason for the use of fructose solutions as replacement therapy.

POTASSIUM REPLACEMENT

Potassium salts should be added when the blood sugar level begins to decrease or when the electrocardiogram, blood pressure, or peripheral deep tendon reflexes suggest a significant decrease in serum potassium concentration (Chap. 22). Occasionally, such signs may occur as early as 2 h after initiation of therapy if the patient shows a very prompt response or rarely may be noted upon examination of the first electrocardiogram or blood specimen if potassium depletion is profound.[1] Under these circumstances, one must be prepared to administer potassium early, particularly if a secondary fall in blood pressure occurs. Thus, it is important to have an initial control electrocardiogram before or shortly after starting treatment in diabetic acidosis. Obviously, if the patient presents with hyperkalemia, potassium supplements ought not be administered until the serum level returns to normal. For normokalemic patients, 10 to 30 meq/h may be administered intravenously, assuming there is an adequate renal function. For severely hypokalemic and potassium-depleted patients, as much as 40 to 80 meq/h may be required. With these large doses, electrocardiographic monitoring is mandatory, as is hourly monitoring of serum potassium concentration. Repletion rates should be appropriately reduced (5 to 15 meq/h) in the presence of persistent oliguria or renal failure.

It is important to remember that potassium depletion itself can produce shock and that a patient in severe diabetic acidosis with anuria may still be profoundly potassium-depleted. Under these circumstances, this ion should still be administered to correct any marked electrocardiographic abnormalities or secondary hypotension if it should occur. Certainly, however, when in doubt one should err on the low side in potassium replacement in the anuric or oliguric patient.

Potassium chloride is the salt that is usually administered in the treatment of diabetic acidosis. At times, as much as 200 to 300 meq is given during the first 24 h of therapy. Since the chloride ion is distributed primarily in the extracellular space, while potassium moves to an intracellular site in exchange for hydrogen ions, potassium can actually potentiate a mild acidosis of a hyperchloremic type even after the ketonemia has been completely corrected. Potassium phosphate or potassium acetate salts do not produce this mild acidosis. The acetate ion is metabolized, and the phosphate ion moves into the intracellular site with potassium to replace the intracellular deficit of phosphate.

ORAL REPLACEMENT

If patients are conscious and lucid, have not been nauseated or been vomiting, and show no evidence of gastric dilatation, they may be carefully started on liquid or soft small feedings and potassium-containing fluids early in the course of therapy; otherwise, it is probably better to wait 12 to 24 h before introducing any form of oral replacement. The authors have not found that gastric aspiration is necessary in every patient with diabetic acidosis or coma. If the patient has shown clinical evidence of gastric dilatation, such as (1) profound vomiting, (2) left upper quadrant tympany with or without an obvious succussion splash, or (3) an emesis that has a coffee-grounds appearance or is oily in consistency but is benzidine- or guaiac-negative, a Levin tube is inserted, the stomach is aspirated as completely as possible, and the tube may be left in place for 12 to 24 h.

MISCELLANEOUS MEASURES

A diabetic coma flow sheet is essential and should be kept by the patient's bedside, and the recorded information should be as complete as possible. Fractional urine specimens are checked at hourly intervals for volume, qualitative sugar, and acetone. One must remember that the urinary acetone level may still be 4+ when the plasma level has decreased virtually to zero by qualitative testing. In following the patient's course, the authors rely much more heavily on blood sugar level, electrolyte levels, and acid-base parameters than on measurements in the urine. The most important reason for collecting urine in diabetic acidosis is to measure its volume, or hourly output. This enables one to evaluate the magnitude of the continued urinary loss of fluid during corrective therapy. It is not unusual for a patient who has a deficit of 6 to 7 liters to receive this volume in the first 12 h of therapy. During this time, the patient may excrete 5 of these 7 liters because of the sustained glycosuria. If this is not known, a false impression of the net magnitude of the replacement will be obtained.

PATHOPHYSIOLOGY AND CLINICAL ASPECTS OF THE HYPERGLYCEMIC, HYPEROSMOLAR SYNDROME

A great variety of terms have been applied to the clinical syndrome characterized by hyperglycemia and hyperosmolality without marked ketoacidosis (see also Chaps. 21 and 46). One of the most commonly used has been hyperglycemic, hyperosmolar, nonketotic coma (often abbreviated as HHNC). Nevertheless, because detectable, albeit relatively mild, ketoacidosis is present in most patients and frank coma is absent in approximately two-thirds, this designation is not entirely appropriate. As early as 1976, the use of the term hyperglycemic hyperosmolar syndrome was suggested,[113] and more recently several additional investigators have argued persuasively for the aptness of this designation.[124,192,320] We agree and will henceforth use the abbreviation HHS, and for simplicity we will not distinguish between the terms hyperosmolarity and hyperosmolality.

HHS appears to have been first described in the 1880s[75] and subsequently in 1925.[313,314] Modern interest in this syndrome was stimulated by a report in 1957.[268] Of interest, the patient described by these investigators was stuporous but not in deep coma despite a blood sugar level of 1548 mg/dl.[268] Since then, an increasing number of patients with marked alteration in sensorium (stupor to coma) and severe hyperglycemia, but without prominent ketoacidosis, have been described.[14,68,87,104,120,141,154,157,165,250,260,264] In a series reported in 1975, 33 percent of the 86 episodes of diabetic coma were of the hyperosmolal variety. The true incidence of HHS is unknown but has been estimated to be one-sixth to one-tenth that of diabetic ketoacidosis.[104] Excellent reviews continue to appear.[308]

Despite the separate discussions in this chapter of diabetic ketoacidosis and HHS, these conditions are best considered as constituting extremes of a spectrum or a continuum of disorders rather than as entirely distinct entities. Although they differ importantly in several clinical features, as discussed below, diabetic ketoacidosis and HHS also have important similarities. Indeed, patients may present with what appears to be a mixture of the two syndromes, and some have been reported to manifest each condition at different times. Furthermore, each disorder may occur in a relatively mild or early form that differs in several respects from the prototypical condition.

CLINICAL ASPECTS

The definition of HHS is somewhat variable with respect to specific criteria. In one study HHS was characterized by hyperglycemia (blood sugar level >600 mg/dl), hyperosmolality (serum osmolality >350 mosm/kg H_2O), serum HCO_3^- levels greater than 15 meq/liter, and qualitative serum ketones values less than 4+ at a 1:1 dilution, with depression of sensorium to at least stupor. Others have suggested that the pH be no less than 7.30 and/or that the serum osmolality be more than 320 to 350 mosm/liter. The majority of patients are elderly, typically either with no previous diagnosis of diabetes[43,44] (i.e., the diabetes is first discovered during the presenting hyperosmolal coma[264]) or with mild maturity-onset diabetes. Nonetheless, HHS has been described on occasion in very young patients as well as in insulin-dependent diabetics with previous episodes of frank ketosis.[165,264] Because a reduced or inadequate fluid intake may be an important pathogenic factor,[32,112] it is not surprising that many patients are demented, infirm, alcoholic, or socially isolated or have an impaired thirst mechanism. Whereas race does not appear to be a predisposing factor, a disadvantaged socioeconomic background may be.[162]

Specific precipitating factors can be identified in approximately 50 percent of patients. As shown in Table 26-7, these factors include various causes of stress, including burns, surgery, infection, and stroke; administration of large amounts of simple carbohydrate, as during hyperalimentation or from ingestion of large amounts of sugar-containing beverages; dialysis using dialysates with

TABLE 26-7 • **Factors predisposing to HHS**

Extensive body burns and glucose administration[222,260]
Heat stroke[206]
Hypothermia
Infections
Surgery
Gastrointestinal bleeding
Myocardial infarction
Cerebrovascular accident[25]
Thyrotoxicosis[143]
Dialysis: hemo-[248] and peritoneal[126]
Intravenous hyperalimentation[299]
Excess sugar-containing beverages[186]
Acute pancreatitis
Severe water restriction
Severe acute hyponatremia[93]
Medications: diuretics,[88] diazoxide, glucocorticoids,[43] phenytoin, propranolol,[243] chlorpromazine, cimetidine, and L-asparaginase

high glucose content; several medications, particularly thiazides, glucocorticoids, and phenytoin; and inadequate fluid intake.

An informative study regarding predisposing factors was reported in 1987.[307] The investigators evaluated the data of 135 patients with HHS and compared them with those of 135 age-matched diabetic control subjects. The HHS patients were more likely to be female (71 versus 53 percent), nursing home residents (28 versus 15 percent), newly diagnosed diabetics (36 versus 7 percent), and demented (18 versus 8 percent) and to have an acute infection (39 versus 19 percent). Of note, however, is the fact that multivariate analysis revealed that only three of these factors were statistically significant predictors of HHS: female gender, newly diagnosed diabetes, and acute infection.

Findings on history and physical examination

Frequently, weakness, fatigue, polyuria, polydipsia, and loss of weight precede or coexist with the gradual development of impairment of consciousness (lethargy to deep coma, depression, irritability, and hallucinations), but these symptoms may be overshadowed by those of the associated illness. The syndrome may occur without excessive glycosuria and polyuria, for example, in burn patients with very large insensible (pulmonary and skin) water loss[222] and in patients with severe chronic renal failure undergoing peritoneal dialysis.[42] With progression, the major clinical manifestations relate to hypovolemia and altered central nervous system function, both resulting from profound dehydration and volume contraction. Fever may occur as a consequence of associated complications[264] and/or the effect on the central nervous system of the hypertonic dehydration per se.

Seizures and focal neurologic signs may provide the first clinical clues to the presence of HHS.[118,291] These signs may be misinterpreted as manifestations of a cerebrovascular accident, but the frequent reversibility of the neurologic symptoms, signs, and electroencephalographic abnormalities upon control of the metabolic imbalance[187] points to a direct relationship between the hyperosmolality and the neurologic abnormalities (Table 26-8).[20,118] Seizures occur in perhaps 20 percent of patients and most often are of the focal motor type. Occasionally, they are repetitive (epilepsia partialis continua),[291,305] with the patient sometimes assuming an unusual posture (e.g., "fencing seizures").[305] Generalized seizures are less common. Typically, HHS-related seizures are refractory to routine pharmacologic therapy but, as mentioned, remit as the metabolic derangements are corrected. It is important to remember that the anticonvulsant phenytoin may itself cause or worsen existing hyperglycemia. At times, intracerebral and subarachnoid bleeding may occur, with or without a generalized hemorrhagic tendency.[260] Such bleeding appears to be due to

TABLE 26-8 • **Neurologic symptoms and signs in hyperglycemic hyperosmolal coma**

Type	Topographical origin	Characteristics
Consciousness: altered or lost; hallucinations and other psychic disturbances often present	Cerebral cortex	Rarely absent; deep coma the rule
Focal dysfunctions: aphasia, hemiparesis, unilateral hyperreflexia, and unilateral Babinski reflex	Cerebral cortex	May be seen independently of seizures; may be prolonged (1 week)
Seizures	Cerebral cortex and/or thalamus	Focal as a rule; common
Hyperthermia	Hypothalamus	Very frequent

SOURCE: Adapted from Maccario.[187]

noninflammatory capillary rupture secondary to the severe cellular dehydration.[84]

Abdominal pain, when present, may be due either to an intraabdominal complication or to the uncontrolled metabolic state, as discussed in the sections on diabetic acidosis. Both the odor of acetone on the breath and Kussmaul's respirations are absent. Air hunger is reported as an unusual presenting symptom and can occur in patients with severe coexistent lactic or uremic acidosis.[70]

Laboratory findings

Marked hyperosmolality attributable to hyperglycemia and, frequently, hypernatremia associated with limited ketoacidosis are the prototypical laboratory features (Table 26-9).

Hyperglycemia

Severe hyperglycemia (>600 mg/dl) is an obligatory finding. Blood sugar levels frequently reach 1000 mg/dl or more; a French patient with a blood sugar level of 4800 mg/dl has been reported.[177] Serum or plasma osmolality may exceed 400 mosm/kg H_2O. If an osmometer is not available, the osmolality of the plasma can be estimated using a simple equation (see equation 1).

Serum sodium

Hypernatremia (serum sodium concentration >145 meq/liter) and hyperchloremia (serum chloride concentration >107 meq/liter) may be present in patients with HHS. Hypernatremia is obviously indicative of a greater degree of water depletion, for, as explained earlier, hyperglycemia per se tends to cause hyponatremia due to osmotic withdrawal of salt-free water from the cells and dilution of the residual sodium in the ECF. A rise of 100 mg/dl in the measured plasma glucose is associated with a decrease in plasma sodium of approximately 1.3 to 1.6 meq/liter (see above). Since the movement of water out of cells to some extent attenuates the rise in the plasma glucose level, a measured increase of 100 mg/dl actually reflects the addition of slightly more glucose to the plasma. Plasma insulin levels in these patients with HHS are generally low and are not significantly different from those observed in diabetic ketoacidosis.[104]

TABLE 26-9 • Clinical and laboratory features distinguishing HHS and DKA

Feature	HHS	DKA
Type of patient	Typically an elderly type II diabetic (or a patient with no prior history of diabetes)	Typically a young type I diabetic
Duration of prodrome	Typically 3 days to 3 weeks	Typically 1–4 days
Precipitating event	More often a serious underlying medical illness[29]	Less often a serious underlying medical illness
Mental status	Typically more depressed than in DKA	Variable, alert to comatose
Seizures	Quite common, typically focal	Uncommon
Kussmaul's breathing	Usually absent (unless there is concomitant severe lactic acidosis)	Often present
Current mortality	~10–20%	<10%
Serum glucose	>600 mg/dl and typically higher	Usually 500–600 mg/dl
Plasma osmolality	Typically >350 mosm/kg H_2O	Usually <335 mosm/kg H_2O
Serum ketones (nitroprusside positive)	<4+ (1:1 dilution)	4+ (1:1 dilution)
Free fatty acids	In general, moderately elevated	Often more elevated than in HHS
Serum Na	On the average, higher than in DKA	Normal, high, or low
Serum K	On the average, lower than in DKA	Low, normal, or, more often, slightly elevated
Anion gap	Frequently elevated, but less so than in DKA	Usually markedly elevated
Blood urea nitrogen and creatinine	Typically more elevated than in DKA and often do not return to normal following treatment of HHS	Modest elevations common
Size of fluid deficit (70-kg man)	Typically 8–9 liters (~25% of total body water)	Not as severe

NOTE: As discussed in the text, the distinction between these two conditions, which are really components of a spectrum, is not absolute, but a matter of degree.

ABBREVIATIONS: DKA, diabetic ketoacidosis; HHS, hyperglycemic hyperosmolar syndrome.

Acid-base variables

Although the absence of severe ketoacidosis is essential for the diagnosis of HHS, it is incorrect to term the condition nonketotic because many, if not most, patients have detectable, albeit limited, degrees of ketosis. Unfortunately, the lack of availability of a quantitative enzymatic test for β-hydroxybutyrate and acetoacetate has resulted in a paucity of precise data. In a very limited number of patients evaluated, β-hydroxybutyrate levels were found to range from 0.8 to 5.2 meq/liter (n = 7; mean, 2.8 meq/liter) and acetoacetate concentrations from 0.28 to 0.83 meq/liter (n = 3; mean, 0.6 meq/liter).[124,318]

Prototypically, the plasma HCO_3 level is usually greater than 15 to 18 meq/liter and the blood pH greater than 7.30.[43,44] Nevertheless, there is evidence that appreciable acidosis occurs in at least 50 percent of patients.[19] Indeed, in one of the seminal papers describing the syndrome, it was reported that the arterial blood pH was 7.35 or less, and the serum bicarbonate level was less than 22 meq/liter in 12 of the 20 patients in whom it was measured.[19] Moreover, marked hemoconcentration tends to raise the blood HCO_3 concentration and perhaps mask the presence of some instances of acidosis. The presence of metabolic acidosis is supported by the finding of many patients with prominently elevated levels of the blood anion gap.[19,60]

It has been postulated that the anion gap elevation in patients with HHS might be attributable to β-hydroxybutyrate (which is not detected by nitroprusside-based tests), lactate, renal failure, or hemoconcentration. Nevertheless, it appears that none of these possibilities, even taken together provides an entirely adequate explanation. Similarly, the suggestion that hyperosmolality per se might result in metabolic acidosis[19] is supported by only limited evidence.[285]

Despite the probability that hypovolemia-related reduction in organ perfusion (kidney, liver, and muscle) might lead to anaerobic metabolism and frank lactic acidosis, we are unaware of any data indicating that clear-cut lactic acidosis is any more frequent in HHS than in diabetic ketoacidosis. For example, although arterial plasma lactate concentrations were elevated in 10 of the 15 patients whose levels were determined in one series, in only 2 patients (both with hypotension) were they in the range seen in frank lactic acidosis.[19] The average plasma lactate concentration for the group was 3.3 meq/liter. The authors interpreted these data as militating against the presence of marked alteration of the reduction-oxidation (redox) state.[19]

Serum potassium, creatinine, and urea nitrogen

As in the case of ketoacidosis, serious potassium depletion, perhaps as much as 400 to 1000 meq,[307] is usually present. Nevertheless, some patients manifest normokalemia and occasionally hyperkalemia. It is likely that hyperosmolality and insulin lack are factors tending to maintain the serum potassium concentration at a higher level than would seem appropriate for the degree of potassium loss.[208] An elevated blood urea nitrogen level may be indicative of chronic or acute reversible reduction of GFR, increased fractional reabsorption of urea related to decreased urine flow rate, and enhanced lean tissue breakdown. Because of these latter two factors, the increase in the blood urea nitrogen level is frequently disproportionate to that of serum creatinine, so that the ratio of these two variables may greatly exceed the normal average value of 10-15:1. Although impaired renal blood flow secondary to dehydration, hemoconcentration, and hypovolemia is a major cause of the reduced GFR, many patients also have preexisting organic renal disease.[19]

Urinalysis and complete blood count

Characteristically, the urine shows 4+ glycosuria with minimal ketonuria. Urinary tract infection is common. The hematocrit, hemoglobin, and white blood cell count are usually increased, the number of leukocytes at times approaching 50,000/mm^3 in the absence of infection. The latter is probably attributable to the demargination of leukocytes.

DIFFERENCES BETWEEN HHS AND DIABETIC KETOACIDOSIS

The principal differences between HHS and diabetic ketoacidosis are outlined in Table 26-9. These differences are relative, rather than absolute, and include, with reference to HHS, older age, greater frequency of serious precipitating factors (particularly infection), greater depression of mental status, less frequent vomiting, higher mortality,[332] longer prodrome, absence of Kussmal's breathing, higher serum sodium concentration, lower serum potassium concentration, less elevated anion gap, higher blood urea nitrogen and serum creatinine levels, and greater fluid deficit.

PATHOGENESIS

Figure 26-11 summarizes the pathogenesis of HHS.

Hyperglycemia and hyperosmolality

The extreme hyperglycemia found in patients with HHS is generally caused by the interaction of several factors: insulin deficiency and/or insulin resistance; enhanced hepatic gluconeogenesis related to inadequate insulin effect and to the increased release of epinephrine, glucagon, cortisol, and growth hormone; increased intake of simple carbohydrate; volume contraction; and decreased urinary glucose excretion.

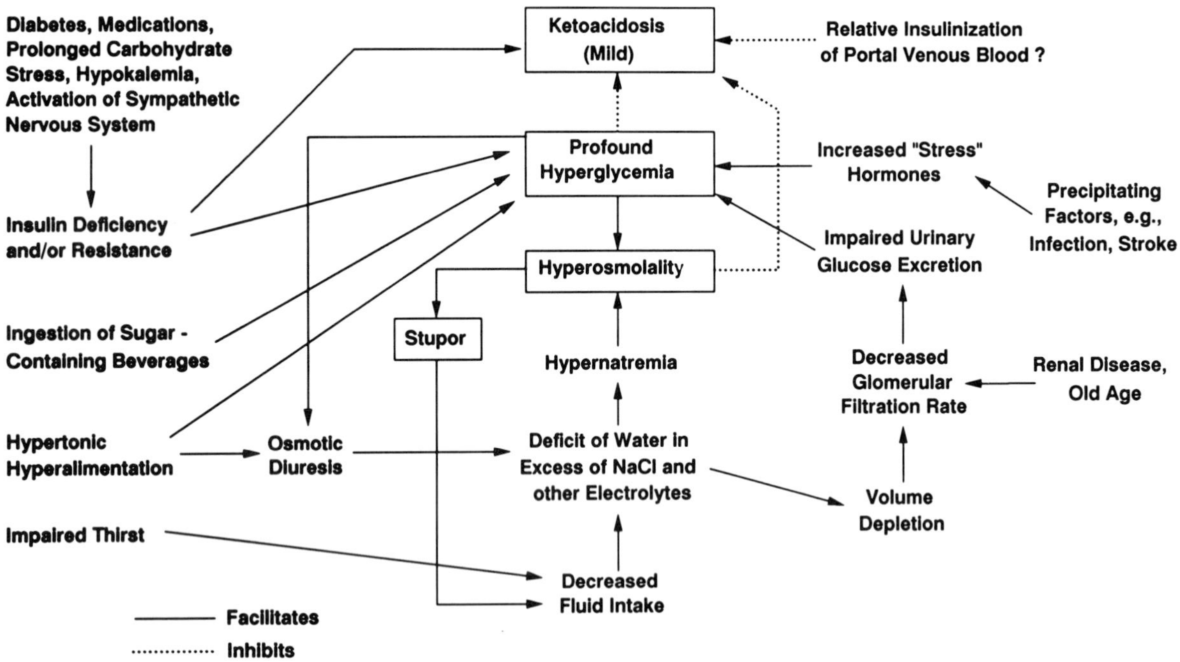

FIGURE 26-11 • Pathogenic schema for the HHS. See the text for details.

In a patient with type II diabetes, a continuous 7-day infusion of glucose, with sustained hyperglycemia, at first causes an increase in plasma insulin, which later declines below the preinfusion concentration.[273] In contrast, normal control subjects maintain their increased levels of insulin throughout the infusion, despite similar degrees of hyperglycemia.[273] This "low insulin reserve" of the patient with adult-onset diabetes most likely contributes to additional hyperglycemia.

One of the factors contributing to, and perhaps necessary for, the profound hyperglycemia in patients with HHS might be the presence of modest ketoacidosis.[124] The postulated mechanism for this is that the observed elevated levels of β-hydroxybutyrate (~3 meq/liter, or 100 times normal) serve as substrate for cerebral caloric needs, thus reducing brain glucose utilization and resulting in higher blood sugar levels.[124]

Certain chemotherapeutic agents[286] and phenytoin[108] predispose to HHS by inhibiting insulin synthesis or secretion; glucocorticoids do so by increasing gluconeogenesis and decreasing peripheral utilization of glucose.

By restricting the urinary excretion of glucose, a reduction in GFR from whatever cause plays an important role in exacerbating hyperglycemia.[172] Indeed, it has been argued that in patients with normal renal function (in the absence of an exogenous source of glucose) the blood sugar level cannot exceed a value of about 500 mg/dl. On the other hand, reductions in GFR permit proportional increments in blood glucose levels. Thus, the glycosuria secondary to the increased filtration of glucose limits further increments in glycemia.

The cause of the hyperosmolal state is virtually identical to that described earlier for diabetic ketoacidosis, although the degree of water depletion, or hypertonic dehydration, is considerably greater with HHS. One reason for this might be that the earlier depression of the sensorium in the generally older patients results in failure of oral ingestion of water to keep up with renal and extrarenal water losses. In some patients with this syndrome, intense thirst leads to excessive use of sugar-containing beverages (e.g., fruit juices), and the blood glucose level rises further. In other instances, extreme hyperglycemia is caused in part by parenteral administration of hypertonic glucose solutions, by dialysis using hypertonic glucose, or by a very high dietary intake of carbohydrate (Fig. 26-12).[260]

In a study of infants and young children, it was found that hypertonic (hypernatremic) dehydration associated with acute gastroenteritis causes hyperglycemia (up to 685 mg/dl) with an inappropriately low insulin response.[193] The blood sugar levels returned to normal after correction of the dehydration. The clinical impression that hyperosmolality might contribute to reduced insulin secretion and/or enhanced insulin resistance is supported by experimental data.[45] Using the euglycemic insulin clamp model, the investigators showed that hypertonicity induced by mannitol significantly reduces insulin-mediated glucose metabolism.[45]

In summary, the profound hyperglycemia of HHS results from an abnormally high rate of hepatic gluconeogenesis, and in some patients, from ingested sugar. The glucose-induced osmotic diuresis causes ECF volume contraction, which, in turn, reduces the

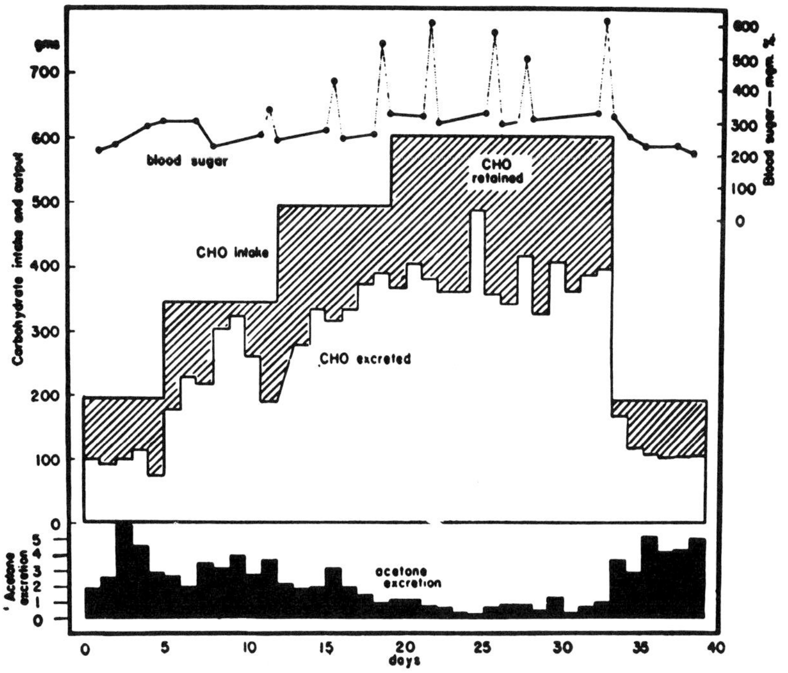

FIGURE 26-12 • Effect of exogenous insulin deprivation and the influence of a high carbohydrate intake in an adult diabetic. The dashed lines off the blood sugar curve refer to the highest blood sugar levels observed during the day. Insulin administration was stopped at zero days.

glomerular filtration rate, thereby eventually uniting the glycosuria.[302]

Limited ketosis

Despite its pathophysiologic importance and the investigation and speculation undertaken, the mechanism whereby ketoacidosis is restrained in patients with HHS remains unclear. The principal postulated factors are listed in Table 26-10. Currently, it seems appropriate to conclude that the determining factors are frequently multiple and may vary from patient to patient. In some patients, mild ketosis may be present but masked by severe volume contraction, impaired oxygen delivery, altered cellular reduction and oxidation, and an increase in β-hydroxybutyrate levels, at the expense of acetoacetate levels.

The absence of moderate to severe ketoacidosis in diabetic patients with marked hyperglycemia must be due to enhanced utilization and/or limited production of ketoacids. The available data favor the latter as the more important factor.[14,19] Similarly, current information indicates that decreased substrate (free fatty acid, or FFA) availability, resulting from decreased lipolysis, is probably a more important pathogenic factor[104,113] than is a specific intrinsic limitation in hepatic ketogenesis. Indeed, using an animal model of HHS, it has been clearly shown that the intragastric instillation of medium-chain triglycerides causes marked enhancement of hepatic ketogenesis.[112] On the other hand, in a small study of 5 HHS and 10 diabetic ketoacidosis patients, it was found that, although the mean level of serum FFA in the former (1.25 mmol/liter) was somewhat lower than that of the latter (1.66 mmol/liter), the levels of FFA were raised in almost all of the HHS patients and were similar to those of many of the patients with diabetic ketoacidosis.[318] Values above 2.9 mmol/liter, however, were seen only with diabetic ketoacidosis. Nevertheless, individual HHS patients with plasma FFA levels in excess of 4 mmol/liter may not manifest prominent ketoacidosis.[89]

Although some of the results of early investigations suggested that serum insulin levels are higher in HHS than in diabetic ketoacidosis and that this might be an explanation for restrained ketosis in the former syndrome, it is now believed that plasma insulin levels are usually similar in both conditions.[104,318] Studies in experimental animals, however, suggest that, despite similar

TABLE 26-10 • Mechanisms postulated for restriction of ketosis in HHS

Limited lipolysis and ketogenesis as a result of hyperosmolality
Moderate increase in plasma FFAs in comparison to DKA (i.e., limited availability of substrate for hepatic ketogenesis)
Relative insulinization of portal blood (in comparison to peripheral blood)
Impairment of hepatic uptake of FFAs
Perturbed intrahepatic handling of FFAs
Availability of carbohydrate (glycogen) in liver
Extreme hyperglycemia permits hepatic glucose utilization (thus inhibiting ketogenesis, even in the absence of insulin)

ABBREVIATIONS: DKA, diabetic ketoacidosis; FFA, free fatty acid; HHS, hyperglycemic hyperosmolar syndrome.

low concentrations in peripheral blood, insulin levels in portal venous blood in HHS are higher than in diabetic ketoacidosis,[145,146] supporting the hypothesis of relative insulinization of the liver in the former condition. The finding of abundant hepatic glycogen in an animal model has also been interpreted as indicative of a "marginally sufficient" amount of portal insulin and of the availability in the liver of carbohydrate as a "fuel" source.[145]

Despite hyperglycemia and very low serum insulin levels, ketosis was not observed in diabetic patients during the continuous infusion of glucose for 7 days.[273] There appears to be a direct relationship between blood glucose level and glucose utilization and an inverse relationship between blood glucose level and blood ketone levels,[203] suggesting that hyperglycemia per se is antiketogenic. Thus, it seems possible that, despite insulin deficiency, marked and prolonged hyperglycemia can cause sufficient glucose utilization to restrain the development of ketosis.[129]

Severe water deprivation in fasted rats, although leading to impaired glucose tolerance and hyperglycemia, also inhibits both FFA mobilization from fat stores and ketone body production.[105] Therefore, in HHS, hyperosmolal dehydration and restricted ketosis, rather than being two independent phenomena, might be partially linked in a cause-and-effect relationship.

Finally, if glucagon resistance occurs in humans, as it does in ob/ob mice,[335] this factor might play a role in the obviation of severe ketosis in patients with HHS.

COMA AND OTHER NEUROLOGIC ABNORMALITIES

The similarity between the neurologic disturbances in hyperglycemic and other hyperosmolal states suggests a common etiologic mechanism. This formulation is supported by the close correlation found between the plasma osmolality (but not the plasma glucose concentration) and depression of the sensorium in 53 patients with HHS.[20] Several other, but not all,[157] investigators have also observed that neurologic abnormalities correlated better with the degree of hyperosmolality than with the level of blood glucose.[97,300] The electron microscopic

TABLE 26-11 • Differentiation of hyperosmolar syndromes based on clinical characteristics and laboratory values

	Corrected* serum sodium concentration			
	Normal	Normal	High	High
Uncorrected serum sodium level	Low	Low	Slightly low, normal, or high	Slightly low, normal, or high
Serum glucose level	High	High	High	High
Rate of onset of hyperglycemia	Hours to days	Minutes	Hours to days	Hours to days
Effective serum osmolality, mmol/kg	High	High	Usually >320	Usually >320
Renal function	Negligible or absent	Usually normal	Negligible or absent	Present
Osmotic diuresis	−	−	−	+
Osmotic ultrafiltration during dialysis	None or limited	NA	Excessive	NA
Brain dehydration	Unlikely	Likely	Likely	Likely
Neurologic abnormalities	Often absent	Present	Present	Present
Patient types	Most dialysis patients with hyperglycemia	Massive accidental parenteral glucose infusion	Dialysis patients exposed to dialysis solution with very high glucose levels	Patients with classic nonketotic hyperosmolar coma Patients receiving total parenteral nutrition Patients with burns

ABBREVIATION: NA, not applicable.
*The corrected serum Na level is calculated by increasing serum Na by 1.3 to 1.6 meq/liter for every 100 mg/dl (5.56 mmol/liter) increment in serum glucose
SOURCE: From Daugirdas JT et al: *Ann Intern Med* 10:855, 1989. Used by permission.

pathologic changes associated with severe hyperosmolal dehydration consist of massive shrinkage of the oligodendroglial cytoplasm, decrease in oligodendroglial processes abutting the vessels, vacuolation of the endothelial cells, and increased density of the nerves.[185]

Daugirdas and associates have stressed the potential value of the "corrected" serum sodium concentration (the measured value adjusted for the degree of hyperglycemia) as a useful index of the state of cerebral cellular hydration, thereby identifying those patients most at risk for neurologic abnormalities.[71] Of course, in the face of severe hyperglycemia, a normal or increased uncorrected serum sodium level indicates that severe dehydration is present, and there is less value in calculating the corrected value. Mild hypernatremia in severely hyperglycemic patients, on the other hand, may be associated with corrected serum sodium values in the very hypernatremic range, indicating increased risk. As shown in Table 26-11, patients with profound hyperglycemia and corrected serum sodium levels in the normal range fall into two subgroups. In the first subgroup, severe reduction of GFR prevented the osmotic diuresis that usually causes much of the water loss. These patients ordinarily manifest no neurologic deficits.[245] In the other subgroup (patients accidentally given massive infusions of glucose), neurologic abnormalities may occur despite the absence of corrected hypernatremia, presumably because of the very rapid development of severe hypertonicity.[71]

The likelihood that multiple interactive factors are necessary for the induction of HHS is supported by work utilizing an experimental animal model.[32,112] In rats rendered diabetic by the administration of either alloxan or streptozotocin, the investigators observed that both corticosteroid administration and water deprivation are necessary for production of the syndrome. This finding indicates that the typical severe dehydration of the patients is a cause as well as a consequence of the extreme hyperglycemia. Similarly, data from an alloxan-diabetic rat model are indicative of a complex pathogenesis.[32,112]

PROGNOSIS

Most of the investigators reporting the initial large series of patients with HHS in the late 1960s and early 1970s emphasized a high mortality rate of approximately 30 to 40 percent or more.[19,104,113,154,197] This rate was considerably in excess of that occurring in patients with classical diabetic ketoacidosis, in whom mortality at that time had been reduced to about 10 to 15 percent. This difference was attributed not only to older age, a greater frequency of serious intercurrent chronic conditions, and various complications in patients with HHS, but to the importance of some of the life-threatening conditions frequently precipitating HHS (e.g., stroke and myocardial infarction). It was postulated that only about one-third of the deaths in HHS were related to the metabolic abnormalities (e.g., hypertonicity and coma) per se.

Currently, with the greater recognition of, and ability to manage, the associated and preexisting conditions and the various fluid and electrolyte abnormalities, the overall mortality of HHS has been reduced to approximately 10 to 20 percent.[54] Nevertheless, this rate remains considerably in excess of that seen today with diabetic ketoacidosis. Most deaths occur in older patients as a result of sepsis, adult respiratory distress syndrome, cardiovascular collapse, and thromboembolic complications.[54,154] Deaths occurring within the first 2 days are most likely to be caused by shock and/or the metabolic derangements per se.

THERAPY

The main aspects of therapy for HHS are outlined in Table 26-12 (Fig. 26-13). Because many of these features (including the need for individualization) are similar to those pertaining to the management of diabetic ketoacidosis, only important differences or special considerations are discussed in the text. The controversy over whether 0.9% saline or 0.45% saline is the preferable initial form of fluid replacement remains unresolved.[45,157] Nonetheless, the extreme salt and water loss present in many patients with HHS jeopardizes their hemodynamic state. The osmotic effect of severe hyperglycemia tends to stabilize ECF volume and thereby to help sustain cardiac output and blood pressure. With insulin therapy, the blood sugar level may decline rapidly from cellular uptake and renal excretion of glucose; consequently unmasking the actual severity of ECF depletion. It therefore makes most sense to initiate therapy with normal saline solution to offset the reentry of ECF into the cells. We would use 0.9% saline solution until the patient's hemodynamic status has been clarified. Liter for liter, half-normal saline solution provides only slightly more than half as much ECF expansion as does normal saline solution. As discussed elsewhere (Chaps. 20 and 21 and below), rapid reduction of ECF osmolality may leave brain cells relatively hypertonic, causing cerebral edema. The latter issue also limits the need for half-normal saline solution. To achieve the same degree of ECF expansion with 0.45% saline solution as occurs with normal saline solution, twice as much electrolyte-free water must be given. Normal saline solution is, of course, relatively hypotonic for most patients with HHS.

Patients with HHS may require a total of as little as 50 or as much as 500 units of regular insulin to reverse their hyperglycemia. Based in part on the very rapid initial decline in blood sugar level observed in some patients, there has been considerable controversy regarding the sensitivity of HHS patients to insulin.[332] Although there may be an important degree of heterogeneity with

TABLE 26-12 • Principal aspects of the early management of patients with HHS

A. Fluid administration[45,51,269,307]
 1. Unless there is evidence of fluid overload, administer 1–2 liters of fluid in the first 2 h, a total of approximately one-half of the estimated fluid deficit (typically 8–9 liters) in first 12 h, and the remainder over the subsequent 24 h. Replacement must be based in part on the clinical response. Elderly patients and those with cardiac disease or renal insufficiency should be treated more cautiously.
 2. Generally, the first 1–2 liters of fluid should be 0.9% saline solution. In some patients with extreme hypertonicity and stable hemodynamics, 0.45% saline solution is justified from the onset (with cautious observation for a falling blood pressure.)[45] If frank hypotension is present and does not respond to 0.9% saline, the infusion of albumin or even whole blood should be considered.
 3. After the initial use of 0.9% saline to stabilize the blood pressure, 0.45% saline in water or in 5% dextrose (depending upon the blood sugar and whether insulin administration is continuing) should be used.
 4. When to begin and how long to continue the intravenous infusion of glucose depends on whether the administration of insulin is continuing. To avoid hypoglycemia, the use of 5% dextrose may be begun when the blood sugar level declines to approximately 250–300 mg/dl. The prolonged infusion of glucose may result in continuing osmotic diuresis and difficulty in correcting either the dehydration or the hyperglycemia.

B. Insulin (all as regular insulin)[192,307]
 1. Following an initial intravenous bolus dose (0.1–0.2 units of regular insulin per kilogram body weight), 0.1 units/kg per hour is administered by constant infusion. Using this regimen, the blood sugar level should fall by approximately 80–100 mg/dl per hour.
 2. If the blood sugar level does not decline as quickly as desired or if it rises, the dose of insulin should be doubled at 2 h intervals.
 3. When the blood sugar level has declined to approximately 250–300 mg/dl, insulin administration should either be stopped or reduced (e.g., 0.5–1 units/h, depending in part on whether infusion of glucose is initiated).

C. Potassium
The rate of potassium (K^+) replacement is based on its concurrent serum level (the electrocardiogram may also be helpful). We agree with the following guidelines[199] for initial administration: 0, 10, 20, or 30 meq/h, respectively, if the corresponding serum potassium level is >5.0, between 4.0 and 5.0, between 3.0 and 4.0 or <3.0 meq/liter, respectively. In general, no more than a total of 40 meq of potassium should be given as the phosphate salt.

D. If possible, treat underlying and precipitating conditions.

TABLE 26-12 • *(continued)*

E. Because of the risk of thrombosis, the use of low-dose heparin administation (e.g., 5000 units given subcutaneously at 12 h intervals) should be strongly considered.

F. Employ usual support measures for coma, if present, including placement of a nasogastric tube after insertion of a cuffed endotracheal tube.*

G. Place a central venous pressure catheter if the patient remains hypotensive after initial fluid challenge or if there is cardiovascular overload.

H. Undertake other general measures, such as administration of oxygen and bladder catheterization, when necessary.

NOTE: The need for frequent, sequential monitoring of serum chemistries is as essential in HHS as it is in diabetic ketoacidosis. The optimal mode of several aspects of therapy (e.g., the type and rate of fluid replacement) remains controversial.
*If cerebral edema occurs, the insertion of an intracranial pressure monitoring device should be considered.

respect to insulin sensitivity, much of the initial decrement in blood glucose level is attributable to marked glucosuria following volume reexpansion. There are data indicating that marked insulin resistance is present in some patients with HHS.[262] Thus, in one study, during the first 7 h of insulin administration, the blood sugar level declined by an average rate of 80 ± 7 mg/dl per hour in 9 patients with HHS in comparison to 508 ± 3 mg/dl per hour in 6 normal subjects made hyperglycemic by combined infusions of somatostatin and glucose.[262] In contrast, in a small series of 17 episodes of HHS compared to 26 episodes of diabetic ketoacidosis, an insulin regimen of 6 to 10 units/hour (after an initial loading dose of 10 or 20 units), resulted in satisfactory reduction of blood sugar levels in the majority of patients in each group, with no evidence of relative insulin resistance in the HHS group.[332]

Because a reduction in GFR is probably an important pathogenic factor contributing to the profound hyperglycemia characteristic of HHS, it is not surprising that much of the decrement in blood sugar occurring after the initiation of fluid replacement is attributable to enhanced glucosuria related to volume expansion.[172,320] Indeed, data obtained from patients not receiving insulin suggest that, during the first 4 h of therapy, most of the reduction in plasma glucose level is produced by glucosuria, dilution, and perhaps lessening of insulin resistance and/or increased insulin secretion.[124,172,320] It has been suggested, therefore, that the most common cause of an early failure of the blood sugar level to fall appropriately is inadequate volume reexpansion.[43,44]

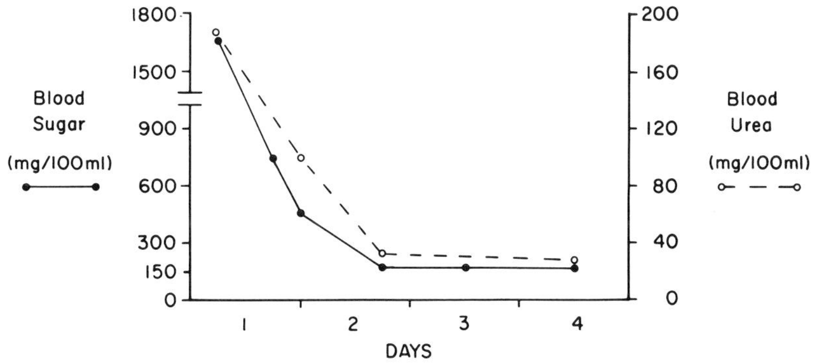

	1	2	3	4
SERUM				
Osmolal. (mOsm/l)	396			
Sodium (mEq/l)	140	138	135	
Potassium (mEq/l)	3.0	3.5	3.5	
Bicarbonate (mEq/l)	20			
Ketonemia	–	–	–	–
URINE				
glycosuria	++++	++++	++	–
ketonuria	–	–	–	–
volume (l/day)	0.5	1	2	
THERAPY				
Insulin (units)	500	300	100	150
Fluid (liters)	8	4	1.5	1.5

FIGURE 26-13 • An example of hyperglycemic coma. A 52-year-old woman not previously known to be diabetic mentioned polyuria and polydipsia for 15 days before admission and an intake of about 5 to 6 liters daily of sugar-containing soft drinks. She had been unconscious for 1 day. On admission she was comatose and extremely dehydrated, and her breathing was not acidotic. Blood pressure was $^{90}/_{50}$ mmHg. Further physical examination was noncontributory. As can be seen in the figure, the patient had on admission severe hypoglycemia and high blood urea levels without acidosis or ketosis. She was treated with hypotonic saline solution (NaCl 0.45%) plus 800 units of regular insulin within the first 48 h. After recovery, the patient was discharged on a low-caloric diet and chlorpropamide (0.5 g/day).

With respect to electrolyte and water replacement, the same principles apply to these patients as to those with diabetic ketoacidosis, with the exception that their average water requirements are typically twice those of the patient with nonhyperosmolal diabetic ketoacidosis. If the patient is conscious, alert, and not vomiting, water may be administered by mouth, but this is rarely advisable or possible. Ten or more liters may be necessary. Until an adequate state of hydration and volume reexpansion is achieved (sometimes requiring 12 to 24 h), the frequently observed oliguria may persist. As mentioned, patients who have not sustained a massive water loss (e.g., those with renal insufficiency) may have corrected serum sodium levels to within the normal range and may be fully alert and without any neurologic manifestations.[71,245] These patients should have less aggressive correction of their hyperglycemia.[245] Likewise, their need for intravenous fluids is generally less than that of patients with the classical form of HHS.[245,267]

After recovering from the acute episode, many patients with HHS return to a state of clinically mild diabetes mellitus, often controlled by diet alone. This indicates that these patients have enough residual insulin secretory reserve to support their usual requirements.[180,222]

COMPLICATIONS

The main complications of HHS are outlined in Table 26-13. They can be subdivided into those caused by HHS per se and those related to therapy. Among the former, the most important are death or irreversible neurologic deficit from brain dehydration and complications resulting from shock (e.g., stroke and myocardial infarction). Rhabdomyolysis[281,330] and disseminated intravascular

TABLE 26-13 • Principal complications of HHS and its treatment

Resulting from the condition itself
Death or permanent neurologic deficit from brain dehydration
Rhabdomyolysis
Stroke or myocardial infarction from hypotension or shock
Thromboembolism from hemoconcentration
Disseminated intravascular coagulation
Gastric stasis and/or ileus
Related to therapy
Cerebral edema from overly rapid reduction in blood sugar and/or osmolality
Hypotension from inadequate or inappropriately slow administration of fluids
Congestive heart failure from overly rapid and/or excessive fluid administration, particularly in older patients
Hypoglycemia from excessive use of insulin or inadequate administration of glucose
Hypokalemia from inadequate administration of potassium
Hypophosphatemia from inadequate repletion of phosphorus

coagulation,[150] which also may occur in diabetic ketoacidosis, are more recently recognized problems. Some investigators believe that subclinical rhabdomyolysis is a common finding and have suggested that preexisting total-body potassium deficiency is a predisposing factor.[281] As shown in Table 26-13, a host of potential complications may occur as a result of therapeutic misadventures, most of which are related to inadequate, inappropriate, or excessive administration of fluids, minerals, and insulin.

Cerebral edema is a rare but often disastrous therapy-associated complication that may occur at a time when most of the metabolic abnormalities have been largely corrected. It has been reported in both children and adults and is said to be more common in the former. Indeed, in the pediatric literature[306] it has been recommended that intracranial pressure be monitored in any comatose patient because of the potentially disastrous results of this complication and its possible reversibility with mannitol.[91] The typical adult patient manifesting this complication is said to be in his or her mid-sixties, and the blood sugar level has been reduced from very high levels (1496 ± 296 mg/dl in a small series of five patients) to less than 250 to 300 mg/dl within the initial 24 h of therapy.[19] In contrast, when insulin administration was discontinued with the plasma glucose level at about 250 mg/dl (a glucose-containing solution was usually begun at this time), neither an increase in cerebrospinal fluid pressure nor clinical evidence of cerebral edema was observed in 53 patients.[74] An overly rapid decrement in plasma osmolality related to a precipitous fall in serum sodium levels can also produce cerebral edema. In both instances, a translocation of water into cerebral cells (osmotic type of cerebral edema) appears to be responsible. Although the optimal rate of correction of hypernatremia remains to be defined precisely, the general rule not to lower the serum sodium level more rapidly than 0.5 to 1.0 meq/liter per hour seems reasonable at this time.

LACTIC ACIDOSIS

The association of diabetes mellitus with lactic acidosis is of considerable interest (see Chap. 25).[70,94,317] In part, this is because of the pathophysiologic implications, which remain controversial, and the potential for diagnostic confusion and therapeutic mismanagement when diabetic ketoacidosis and lactic acidosis coexist. Nevertheless, as discussed below, in the absence of additional specific factors known to perturb lactate metabolism (e.g., the use of phenformin or the presence of hypotension), full-blown lactic acidosis, as opposed to mild increases of plasma lactate levels, is rare, even in the presence of diabetic ketoacidosis.[94,317]

NORMAL AND ABNORMAL LACTATE METABOLISM

Lactate is formed primarily as the end product of the anaerobic metabolism of glucose.[63,170] Each mole of lactate formed is accompanied by the generation of an equivalent quantity of protons. The source of these hydrogen ions is the hydrolysis of adenosine triphosphate (ATP): ATP + $H_2O \rightarrow$ ADP + P_i + H^+.[205,339] ATP turnover by aerobic mechanisms is not acidifying because the protons produced are reutilized when more ATP is formed.[339] Metabolism of lactate either to carbon dioxide and water or to glucose results in an equimolar removal of protons.

The cellular metabolism of lactate is inextricably linked with the metabolism of glucose, pyridine nucleotides (i.e., NAD and $NADH_2$), ATP, and pyruvate (Fig. 26-14). The cellular content of ATP appears to play a central role, and factors altering its level may cause major acid-base changes. Energy released during intermediary metabolism is captured and stored as ATP, which in turn serves as the energy source for many vital cellular functions. The ability of ATP to inhibit several of the key enzymes of energy metabolism allows a negative feedback loop to develop, thereby stabilizing cellular energy reserves. A decrease in ATP levels stimulates metabolic reactions that synthesize more of this high-energy phosphate.

The phosphofrutokinase (PFK) reaction (Fig. 26-14) is a major rate-limiting step in anaerobic glycolysis; its

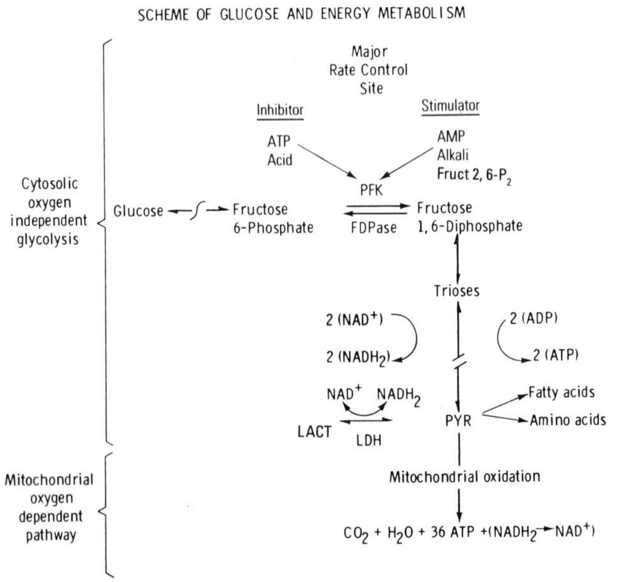

FIGURE 26-14 • Scheme of anaerobic and aerobic glucose metabolism. AMP, adenosine monophosphate; ATP, adenosine triphosphate; FDPase, fructose diphosphatase; Fruct 2,6P_2, fructose-2, 6-bisphosphate; Lact, lactate; LDH, lactate dehydrogenase; NAD^+, nicotine adenine dinucleotide, oxidized form; $NADH_2$, nicotine adenine dinucleotide, reduced form; PYR, pyruvate.

activity increases when cellular ATP stores diminish. The resulting increase in glycolysis generates 2 mmol each of ATP, pyruvate, and reduced pyridine nucleotide ($NADH_2$) for every millimole of glucose catabolized.

In the presence of oxygen and normal mitochondria, pyruvate may be completely oxidized to CO_2 and water. This generates an additional 36 mmol of ATP. Mitochondria also oxidize the $NADH_2$, which ensures a steady supply of oxidized pyridine (NAD), enabling glycolysis to continue unimpaired. Thus, the ATP yield and the efficiency of cellular energy metabolism are greatest in the presence of oxygen, which allows for the use of oxidative mitochondrial reactions.

As the tissue oxygen supply becomes limited, ATP production and $NADH_2$ oxidation switch from the highly efficient but oxygen-requiring mitochondrial processes to the inefficient but oxygen-independent cytosolic reactions. In order to maintain adequate rates of ATP production in this setting, anaerobic glycolysis must increase markedly, thus greatly increasing the synthesis of pyruvate and $NADH_2$. By catalyzing the conversion of pyruvate to lactate, the cytosolic enzyme lactate dehydrogenase (LDH) also oxidizes $NADH_2$, thus providing enough NAD to allow glycolysis to continue unabated. In essence, acidosis is the price that cells must pay in order to stabilize energy stores during hypoxia.

When the tissues are resupplied with oxygen, the LDH reaction regenerates pyruvate and $NADH_2$ from lactate and NAD. Aerobic mitochondrial reactions are now able to oxidize pyruvate and $NADH_2$ and thereby replenish depleted tissue stores of ATP.

Extrahepatic tissues normally produce more pyruvate and lactate than can be catabolized locally. As a consequence, large numbers of protons reach the circulation daily. It is estimated that in humans 1500 to 1900 mmol of lactate are synthesized daily.[173,272] Net lactate production, however, is minimal, since the liver takes up the vast bulk of the organic anion and metabolizes it to CO_2, water, bicarbonate, and glucose. Thus, the alkali consumed in the periphery by the protons produced in association with lactate ions is regenerated by hepatic lactate utilization. The process of peripheral conversion of glucose to lactate and hepatic reconversion of lactate to glucose is referred to as the Cori cycle. This cycle not only plays a major role in glucose homeostasis but also has vital implications for acid-base balance.

Another way to view the Cori cycle is to remember that the source of H^+ during lactate generation is the hydrolysis of ATP.[203,339] When oxidative metabolism is intact, ADP and phosphate reform ATP, a process that consumes protons. Thus, an abnormal Cori cycle implies an imbalance between ATP generation and ATP hydrolysis.[205] It has been suggested that gluconeogenesis buffers H^+ by virtue of the associated generation of ATP and that circumstances in which the capacity for gluconeogenesis decreases (e.g., ethanol intoxication, hepatic failure, or phenformin use) enhance the risk of lactic acidosis.[205]

The effect of very low pH per se on lactate metabolism is complex. Acidemia appears to reduce the rate of glycolysis (and therefore lactate synthesis). Although this pH-related change occurs rapidly and operates to limit further deterioration of acid-base homeostasis, the effect is often small and transitory.[134] The effects of pH on lactate utilization are uncertain.[133,134]

The presence of hyperlactatemia always indicates an imbalance between lactate production and utilization, that is, a disordered Cori cycle. Serum lactate elevation may be caused by an increased rate of production, which overwhelms lactate utilization by the liver and other tissues, or by a failure of utilization with normal production. Combinations of excess production and decreased utilization appear to be the rule.

The etiology and prognosis of hyperlactatemia has been related to prevailing serum lactate/pyruvate (L/P) ratios. As originally proposed by Huckabee,[136] elevations of serum lactate associated with increased serum L/P ratios reflect tissue hypoxia and augur a poor prognosis. This conclusion was based on the following data and assumptions.

Under normal circumstances, the diffusion of pyruvate and lactate into the ECF results in an L/P ratio of 4-10:1.[137] Increments in pyruvate production, unassociated with tissue hypoxia, cause proportionate increases in serum lactate and pyruvate concentrations and a stable L/P ratio. Glucose and pyruvate infusions[137] and acute alkalosis[136] cause such proportionate increases in lactate and pyruvate levels. When hypoxia is present, the associated increase in $NADH_2$ increases the fraction of pyruvate converted to lactate (Fig. 26-14), thereby increasing the L/P ratio. Lactic acidosis caused by hypoperfusion and/or hypoxia is generally far more ominous than the variety associated with normal tissue oxygen utilization.

Except in the differential diagnosis of the various rare enzymatic defects causing lactic acidosis wherein determination of the L/P ratio is of great value,[257] the pathophysiologic implications and practical importance of the L/P ratio are limited.[205] This is because an increased ratio may occur in a variety of situations in which tissue oxygenation is normal, including acidemia itself. Furthermore, the cause of lactic acidosis is usually apparent, and little additional clinical benefit accrues from the measurement of pyruvate and calculation of the L/P ratio.

CAUSES OF LACTIC ACIDOSIS IN DIABETICS

Patients with diabetes mellitus are not immune to any of the causes of lactic acidosis that are detailed in Chap. 25. Whether any metabolic defect exists in diabetes that sensitizes patients to this disorder remains controversial.

Several of the known and postulated mechanisms by

which diabetes might predispose to lactic acidosis are listed in Table 26-14 and include disturbances in perfusion (and rheology) and metabolism. Lactic acidosis can be associated with states of both hyperglycemia and hypoglycemia (Table 26-15). In the case of *hypoglycemia*, the impairment of gluconeogenesis implies reduced utilization of pyruvate (and lactate) at a time when the supply of pyruvate from protein or other sources may be increased. Classically, hypoglycemia is associated with lactic acidosis in patients with the rare condition known as von Gierke's disease. It may also occur in patients with fulminating hepatic failure,[232,249,251] with alcoholic ketoacidosis,[233] and in those receiving biguanides (see below).

Although the mechanism remains unclear, diabetes (along with hepatic and renal insufficiency and some neoplasms) has been considered one of the small number of diseases predisposing to type B lactic acidosis (lactic acidosis not caused by overt shock and/or overt hypoxia).[63,226,239,301] Perhaps 50 percent or more of patients with type B lactic acidosis have diabetes.[232] Nevertheless, biguanide toxicity probably played a role in many, if not most, of these instances. Under certain experimental and clinical circumstances, the diabetic patient may demonstrate a unique biochemical predisposition to the development of lactic acidosis.[101,170]

Insulin seems to be required for normal activity of the pyruvate dehydrogenase (PDH) enzyme complex, which is responsible for the oxidation of pyruvate.[121] It is possible, therefore, that insulin deficiency and/or insulin resistance decreases the metabolic clearance of pyruvate while at the same time increasing the production of pyruvate from protein sources.[121]

Although insulin appears to have a role in the therapy of certain diabetic patients with lactic acidosis (see below), its administration to a diabetic without lactic acidosis may increase serum lactate levels by approximately 25 percent above the mean of control subjects.[221] This effect has been postulated to relate to insulin's inhibition of gluconeogenesis.

Not all available data indicate that lactate metabolism is abnormal in patients with diabetes. In diabetic patients in the steady state, the blood lactate level is typically within the normal range[13,301] and not significantly different from that of control subjects.[301] The rate of disappearance of labeled lactate from the blood is almost the same in diabetic rats as in normal animals, although in the former it appears that more lactate is diverted to glucose formation rather than to oxidation.[279] After the ingestion of sodium lactate, diabetic patients excrete at least as much lactate in the urine as do normal control subjects.[12]

On the other hand, exercising patients with type I diabetes have greater increases in blood lactate levels than do control subjects,[36,305] possibly because of reduced lactate utilization in muscle.[305] One of the experimental animal models of lactic acidosis involves the induction of diabetes in rabbits with alloxan together with the administration of β-hydroxybutyric acid (to convert NAD to $NADH_2$). This is followed by the continuous infusion of sodium bicarbonate (to increase lactate production by stimulating glycolysis).[21] Beta-hydroxybutyric acid and $NaHCO_3$ do not induce lactic acidosis in nondiabetic animals.[21] Streptozotocin, a chemotherapeutic agent used to treat insulinomas, may induce both diabetes and lactic acidosis. The latter may result from impaired gluconeogenesis.[217] Finally, the infusion of glucose may cause minor increases (<2 mmol/liter) in serum lactate levels.[46]

Despite all of the abovementioned considerations, frank lactic acidosis is uncommon in diabetics, even those with diabetic ketoacidosis. The conditions that prototypically may cause clinically significant degrees of lactic acidosis in diabetics are shock and the administration of either fructose or a biguanide-type oral hypoglycemic agent.

TABLE 26-14 • Known and postulated mechanisms by which diabetes might predispose to lactic acidosis

Macrovascular and microvascular disease (e.g., ischemia)
Increased hemoglobin affinity for oxygen
Abnormal platelet function
Altered blood viscosity
Use of biguanide hypoglycemic agents
Impairment of the pyruvate dehydrogenase (PDH) enzyme complex by insulin deficiency and/or insulin resistance

SOURCE: Adapted from Kreisberg.[170]

TABLE 26-15 • Associations between hyperglycemia or hypoglycemia and hyperlactatemia and/or lactic acidosis

With hyperglycemia
Diabetic ketoacidosis
HHS
Biguanide use in diabetic patients
Fructose administration to diabetic patients
Pheochromocytoma[155]
Epinephrine administration and/or toxicity,[55,65,164] particularly in a diabetic[55]
Streptozotocin (may induce both diabetes and lactic acidosis)[217]
With hypoglycemia[200]
Biguanide use in diabetic patients
Acute hepatic failure (concomitant reduction in hepatic utilization of alanine and lactate)
von Gierke's disease
Some patients with alcoholic ketoacidosis
Administration of fructose

Fructose

Unlike glucose, which must pass through the rate-limiting PFK reaction, fructose (after phosphorylation) enters the glycolytic pathway at the triose level (Fig. 26-14). By entering the metabolic pathway at a point beyond the major rate-limiting step, fructose is more freely converted to pyruvate and lactate. Moreover, the rapid phosphorylation of fructose in the liver decreases hepatic ATP levels, resulting in enhanced glycolysis and lactate production.[331] Finally, fructose inhibits gluconeogenesis, causes the accumulation of $NADH_2$, and interferes with lactate utilization. A rise in the blood levels of counterregulatory hormones leads to an increased flux to pyruvate of three-carbon glucose precursors.[170]

When given rapidly (0.5 g/kg per hour), fructose can cause the plasma lactate concentration to increase by 3 to 5 meq/liter. In normal subjects, this will have only minor effects of acid-base balance because serum bicarbonate will fall to only 20 to 22 meq/liter. Patients in profound ketoacidosis, however, are far more sensitive to a similar decline in bicarbonate. A typical patient with severe ketoacidosis may have an initial serum bicarbonate of 5 meq/liter. An additional 3 meq/liter decrease, as a consequence of fructose therapy, would lower such a patient's arterial blood pH to less than 7.0. It has been suggested that the risk of fructose-induced lactic acidosis may be particularly high in patients with HHS (see above).[76] Because of its acidifying potential and for the reasons already stated, the use of fructose as a source of calories in the therapy of diabetic ketoacidosis has fallen into disfavor. We believe that its use is contraindicated.

Hypotension and shock

The acidemia and profound fluid and electrolyte losses that attend diabetic ketoacidosis and HHS commonly cause hypotension. The resulting tissue hypoxia may compromise pyruvate oxidation and induce lactic acidosis. In addition to stimulating lactate production, the change in the oxidation-reduction state associated with tissue hypoxia tends to shift acetoacetate to β-hydroxybutyrate, thereby confounding the diagnosis of ketoacidosis.[233] Finally, the superimposition of lactic acidosis on an established ketoacidosis can acutely lower blood pH to catastrophic levels.

Biguanide therapy

Many well-documented cases of lactic acidosis have been reported in diabetics using oral hypoglycemic biguanides (e.g., phenformin and metformin).[74] The association was so convincing that phenformin was removed from the market in the United States in 1978. Metformin is a far less dangerous drug and has been widely and safely used in Europe. Several of the known and postulated risk factors for biguanide-induced lactic acidosis are listed in Table 26-16. Because the use of biguanides continues in several countries and because of the pathophysiologic and historic importance of the issue, a discussion of the evidence incriminating biguanides is included herein.

TABLE 26-16 • Known and postulated risk factors for biguanide-induced lactic acidosis in diabetic patients

Age >60 years
Underlying diseases: cardiovascular, renal (with decrease in GFR), hepatic, or infectious
Shock
Diabetic ketoacidosis
Surgery
Respiratory insufficiency
Ethanol abuse
Fasting

1. In 34 patients with phenformin-associated lactic acidosis in whom the duration of phenformin therapy was noted, 24 (71 percent) developed lactic acidosis within two months of initiating therapy.[63]
2. A number of reports have shown that an overdose of phenformin can cause severe lactic acidosis even in patients without diabetes.[39,62,72,297]
3. Blood levels of phenformin have been markedly elevated in all acidotic patients in whom they were measured.[27,63] The retention of phenformin is related at least in part to renal insufficiency, which reduces urinary excretion of the medication.
4. Phenformin diminishes lactate tolerance in humans. Therapeutic dosages are associated with elevated fasting blood lactate levels, and this effect is exaggerated after an intravenous glucose load.[304] Furthermore, infusions of sodium lactate or the generation of endogenous lactate with alcohol or exercise results in higher peak serum lactate levels and a slower decline following the ingestion of phenformin.[130]
5. The infusion of phenformin has been successfully employed in dogs to produce an experimental model of full-blown lactic acidosis.[16-18]
6. The large number of cases reported in diabetics with no cause of lactic acidosis other than phenformin ingestion strongly suggested a cause-and-effect relationship.[100]

The mechanism by which phenformin lowers blood sugar levels remains controversial. Three postulates with extensive experimental support are inhibition of oxidative metabolism (the electron transport system), causing a relative rise in $NADH_2$;[74] reduction of gluconeogenesis (the metabolism of pyruvate to glucose); and suppression of gastrointestinal absorption of glucose.[83,121,270,293]

These metabolic derangements could stimulate lactate production by the muscle and impair its utilization by the liver, thereby resulting in elevated serum lactate levels. In addition, there is evidence suggesting that a phenformin-induced reduction of hepatic intracellular pH probably decreases the activity of pyruvate carboxylase, thereby impairing lactate consumption.[16,182] Moreover, based on data from phenformin-induced lactic acidosis in experimental dogs, it appears that this medication markedly increases gut production of lactate.[16] Impairment of cardiac contractility with subsequent reduction in systemic perfusion may also contribute to biguanide-induced lactic acidosis.[18]

COMBINED DIABETIC KETOACIDOSIS-LACTIC ACIDOSIS

Prior to the treatment of typical diabetic ketoacidosis, the average serum lactate level is in the range of approximately 2 to 4 meq/liter.[8,94,224,235,317] The distribution of values tends to be bimodal; for example, in the series of Fulop and coworkers[94] 11 of 39 values were within the range of normal (<1.7 meq/liter), as were 8 of 23 values reported by Watkins and coworkers.[317] In the study of Fulop and colleagues,[94] in which phenformin was a risk factor in an indeterminate number of patients, the mean lactate level was 2.9 meq/liter, and the mean plasma level of β-hydroxybutyrate was 12.4 meq/liter.[94] Of their 11 patients with lactate levels in excess of 4.0 meq/liter, 7 had risk factors predisposing to lactic acidosis, including the use of phenformin, hypotension, hypothermia, hypoxia, gastrointestinal bleeding, and liver disease. Of the 11 patients with weak nitroprusside-based tests for ketones, 6 suffered mainly from lactic acidosis (and 5 of those 6 had received phenformin).[94]

During therapy, increases (usually small) in blood lactate concentration may occur.[8,94,317] The data of Alberti and Hockaday suggest that two groups may be defined by the change in lactate after insulin treatment.[8] Those patients manifesting a decrease in their lactate levels had higher pretreatment values (4.7 ± 1.1 versus 1.8 ± 0.1 meq/liter) and had higher total ketone levels, lower blood pH, and higher blood sugar levels than did the group in whom blood lactate concentration increased. An increase in plasma lactate levels during therapy might be related to an insulin-induced reduction of lactate uptake by the liver. Moreover, as mentioned above, insulin administration would also tend to reduce the lactate level both by decreasing the rate of pyruvate formation from protein and by increasing pyruvate removal by PDH.[121]

Lactate concentrations do not correlate with the severity of the diabetic ketoacidosis as measured by the degree of acidosis (pH and HCO_3^- concentration), the concentrations of β-hydroxybutyrate or glucose, or the P_{CO_2}.[94,317] Thus, despite the hypovolemia and severe metabolic abnormalities, increased lactate production in diabetic ketoacidosis appears to be of limited importance in most patients.[94,169]

Approximately 9 to 15 percent of acutely ill acidotic diabetics have lactate levels in excess of 5 meq/liter. Some of these patients may develop full-blown lactic acidosis.[94,121,194,317] This might relate either to the factors discussed above or to unknown or poorly understood mechanisms, including ethanol abuse.[174,234] Frank lactic acidosis, whether occurring alone or in combination with ketoacidosis, adds significantly to the morbidity and mortality of diabetes.

Sestoft and associates[274,275] divide the course of a patient with severe diabetic ketoacidosis into two phases. The early phase is defined as the period before arterial blood pH declines below 7.1, and the late phase, defined by a pH less than 7.1, is characterized by a decrease in ketogenesis related to lessened hepatic delivery of FFAs and inhibited beta-oxidation. This phase results from failure of homeostatic mechanisms caused in part by reduced hepatic and peripheral blood flow and oliguria. This produces impaired ketoanion oxidation, conversion of hepatic lactate utilization to net production, less urinary acid excretion, and a limited capacity for respiratory compensation.[274,275]

CLINICAL AND LABORATORY FINDINGS

The clinical presentation of lactic acidosis in diabetic patients is similar to that of diabetic ketoacidosis. It is not surprising that much of the data (Table 26-17) are related to biguanide-induced cases.[74,184]

Progressive dyspnea, abdominal pain, nausea, and vomiting with diminishing state of consciousness characterize the clinical picture. These symptoms typically begin within two weeks (in 17 of 34 instances in one series) to two months (in 24 of 34 cases) of the onset of biguanide therapy.[62] Signs of dehydration and ECF volume contraction are found in approximately 50 to 65 percent of patients,[74] but frank shock is absent in the majority of patients at presentation.[100,184] Hypothermia, with rectal temperatures less than 36.5°C, were found in about half of the patients reviewed by Dembo and colleagues.[74] Laboratory data are consistent with a severe high anion gap metabolic acidosis in which arterial pH is commonly below 7.10. The plasma lactate level is generally well in excess of 10 meq/liter, and the L/P ratio often exceeds 50. Serum alanine levels are often elevated because impairment of the metabolism of pyruvate and lactate impedes the utilization of alanine, which is in equilibrium with pyruvate.[74]

The altered redox state may also be associated with elevation of the β-hydroxybutyrate/acetoacetate ratio (see above), making an assessment of the degree of associated ketoacidosis difficult.[94,100,194] Comparison of the

TABLE 26-17 • Clinical and laboratory features of biguanide-induced lactic acidosis in patients with diabetes

Presence of underlying diseases or conditions (other than diabetes), %[184]	
Cardiovascular, 44	Pulmonary, 19
Renal, 35	Hepatic, 15
Anuria, 17	Shock, 24
Infection, 25	
Symptoms or signs prior to diagnosis, %[74,184,*]	
Vomiting, 51	Lethargy, 15
Somnolence, 50	Diarrhea, 14
Nausea, 36	Thirst, 4
Epigastric pain, 35	Kussmaul's respirations, 78
Loss of appetite, 27	Hypothermia, 55
Hyperpnea, 26	ECF contraction, 65
Laboratory findings at time of diagnosis[74,184,*]	
pH, 6.95 ± 0.1	Cl^-, 97 ± 1 meq/liter
P_{CO_2}, 21 ± 1 mmHg	P, 5.9 ± 0.6 mg/dl
HCO_3^-, 6.7 ± 0.2 meq/liter	Glucose, 173 ± 9 mg/dl
Lactate, 16.9 ± 0.5 meq/liter	Osmolality, 318 ± 2 mosm/kg H_2O
Pyruvate, 0.4 ± 0.1 meq/liter	Plasma ketones weakly positive or negative, 97%
Anion gap, 37 ± 1 meq/liter	Unmeasured anions >15 meq/liter in excess of blood lactate, 80%
Creatinine, 3.3 ± 0.2 mg/dl	Blood glucose <100 mg/dl, 46%; <60 mg/dl, 28%
Na^+, 138 ± 1 meq/liter	White blood cell count greater than 12,000/mm³, 80%
K^+, 5.5 ± 0.1 meq/liter	

*From reviews of 330 and 76 case examples, respectively, but n varied considerably among the variables.[74,184]

presumed rise in the anion gap with the measured level of serum lactate may be helpful in this regard.[231] Short of doing a specific test for β-hydroxybutyrate, there may be no way for the clinician to be certain of the absence of a mixed ketolactic acidosis. The blood sugar level is usually normal but occasionally may be frankly low. The white blood cell count is frequently elevated, along with the blood urea nitrogen and serum creatinine levels, as expected in volume-contracted, acidemic patients. Biguanide-induced lactic acidosis is rare in the presence of a normal or near normal GFR.[184] Because the kidney clears ketoacid anions so effectively, the urinary anion gap increases briskly. Lactate clearance is far less than that of ketones, suggesting that the urinary anion gap ought to lower when lactic acidosis dominates (see Chap. 25).

DIAGNOSIS AND PROGNOSIS

The diagnosis of pure lactic acidosis or mixed keto-acidosis-lactic acidosis ultimately depends on demonstration of increased plasma levels of lactate. Because acidosis is defined as a process that generates acid, without regard to the prevailing pH of blood or to the amount of acid accumulated, any increase of plasma lactate concentration represents lactic acidosis. Nevertheless, the strict definition of lactic acidosis (to minimize false-positive and -negative diagnoses) requires specified blood levels of pH, HCO_3^-, and lactate.[63,227,301] In addition, the clinical importance of lactate accumulation, is related to the preexisting level of plasma bicarbonate.

The presence of lactic acidosis may be suspected in severely acidotic diabetics whose serum ketone levels are negative or only weakly positive. As already mentioned, however, the major (or even the sole) metabolic abnormality in such patients may be ketoacidosis (i.e., β-hydroxybutyric acidosis), with lactic acidosis absent or only a minor component. On the other hand, of course, the acidosis of such patients may be partially or predominantly caused by lactic acid. Unfortunately, the diagnosis of patients with a very high anion gap is often difficult.[224] In the absence of renal failure, metabolic acidosis with an increased anion gap is generally considered indicative of organic acidosis, but this is not necessarily the case.[102] In one series, 29 percent of the patients with anion gaps of 20 to 29 meq/liter did not have identifiable organic acidosis.[102] When the investigators tested the usual premise that a high anion gap in the absence of both azotemia and detectable ketonemia usually represents lactic acidosis, it proved incorrect 60 percent of the time.[102] The anion gap has been alleged to have a low sensitivity as a screen to detect hyperlactatemia in critically ill patients.[138] In one series, 6 of 12 patients with blood lactate levels between 5.0 and 9.9 mmol/liter and 26 of 33 of those with levels between 2.5 and 4.9 mmol/liter had anion gaps less than

16 meq/liter.[138] Finally, both the wide prediction interval and volume depletion impair the usefulness of the anion gap as a screen for mixed acid-base disorders in patients with diabetic ketoacidosis.[240] However, as with all tests in medicine, one must understand the various forces that modify the interpretation of results. As discussed in Chap. 24, low albumin levels, hemodilution, and circulating positively charged proteins may reduce the basal anion gap, thereby allowing substantial amounts of acid anion to "hide" behind a relatively low anion gap. When the bicarbonate is higher than the increased anion gap would otherwise allow, one can usually find a cause of metabolic alkalosis (Chaps. 24 and 29).

THERAPY

The general management of a patient with lactic acidosis depends on whether the patient has the type A or type B disorder and on the specific etiology. Thus, patients with type A lactic acidosis might be treated with volume expanders, oxygen, or cardioactive medications, depending on whether they are hypotensive, hypoxic, or in severe congestive heart failure. On the other hand, the treatment of patients with type B lactic acidosis might involve the removal of toxins, chemotherapy for malignancies, or the administration of thiamine (a necessary cofactor of the PDH complex). Because many patients are volume-contracted and hypotensive when initially seen, a component of hypoxic lactic acidosis may be present (irrespective of other pathogenic factors). The judicious use of oxygen and volume expansion with bicarbonate-containing solutions (see below) can be lifesaving at this stage (Table 26-18).

Classically, there have been three main principles underlying the therapy for lactic acidosis: (1) decreasing net lactate production (i.e., restoring the Cori cycle to normal), (2) provision of sufficient alkali to prevent the life-threatening adverse hemodynamic effects of profound acidemia, and (3) prevention, by use of diuretics or dialysis, of the volume overload that often attends $NaHCO_3$ administration. In recent years, the second of these approaches (at least regarding the use of $NaHCO_3$ per se) has become an issue of contention (see below). With rare exceptions, patients with prominent lactic acidosis are best treated in an intensive care unit setting.

Insulin

Although the role of early parenteral insulin in treating the lactic acidosis of patients with diabetes remains uncertain, there is considerable evidence indicating that it may be helpful in many patients. As previously discussed, profound lactic acidosis can mask the presence or the severity of any associated ketosis. Because a significant number of these patients are also ketotic (and some hyperglycemic),[27,100,331] the use of insulin may be important.[74,144] Even if the patient is not ketoacidotic and the elevated anion gap is totally explained by the plasma lactate level, insulin therapy may help to reverse abnormal lactate metabolism, perhaps by decreasing the release of certain amino acids from muscle.[52] Moreover, insulin may also enhance the activity of PDH, thereby stimulating pyruvate and lactate oxidation. Insulin, either exogenous or endogenous, decreases the hyperlactatemia induced in dogs by large doses of phenformin.[183]

The evidence supporting a therapeutic role for insulin in decreasing net lactate production is at present only

TABLE 26-18 • Accepted and controversial aspects of therapy for lactic acidosis in patients with diabetes mellitus

Accepted therapy	Controversial therapy
1. General measures to reverse precipitating factors, such as O_2 for hypoxia, volume expanders for hypotension, etc.	1. Sodium bicarbonate to sustain the serum bicarbonate concentration at 10-12 meq/liter.
2. Insulin (with or without glucose, depending on the blood sugar level) if patient has ketoacidosis	2. Dichloroacetate remains an experimental drug and is of questionable benefit.[290a]
3. Glucose if the patient is hypoglycemic	3. Use of the commercially available agent Carbicarb to replace bicarbonate (Chap. 25).
4. Diuretics (furosemide), if necessary, in patients with sufficient renal function to obviate or reverse volume overload during the administration of sodium bicarbonate.	4. The use of dialysis to remove lactate.
5. Dialysis (either hemodialysis, peritoneal dialysis, or ultrafiltration), to prevent or reverse volume overload and to provide alkali.	
6. Epinephrine, and possibly other catecholamines, should be avoided, if possible, because their metabolic effects tend to worsen lactic acidosis.	

suggestive.[74,144,204] In the review by Dembo and associates[74] of phenformin-associated lactic acidosis, the rate of survival was 17/26 (65 percent) in those patients receiving insulin, in comparison to 19/40 (80 percent) in those treated without insulin. As pointed out by Park and Arieff,[239] however, the multifactorial nature of the therapy for these patients renders it extremely difficult to assess the specific therapeutic benefit of insulin and glucose.

The mortality of full-blown lactic acidosis is so high that the potential benefits of insulin therapy should be considered in diabetic patients regardless of whether ketosis is detected (particularly if the patient is not responding to other measures). Because patients may not be hyperglycemic, sufficient glucose must be given with the insulin to prevent hypoglycemia.

Sodium bicarbonate

The role of bicarbonate in the management of patients with organic acidosis is highly controversial.[64,218,239,266] The problems with the use of $NaHCO_3$ include evidence that its administration might lead to worsening intracellular acidosis and increased lactate production, lack of demonstrable efficacy, and data suggesting that such therapy actually increases mortality.[64,218,239] This issue is discussed in detail in Chap. 25.

Several lines of evidence, both theoretical and experimental, suggest that Carbicarb (see Chap. 25), which is an equimolar solution of sodium carbonate and sodium bicarbonate, has considerable promise in the treatment of severe metabolic acidosis in general and lactic acidosis in particular. In a preliminary trial in an animal model of hypoxic lactic acidosis, the administration of Carbicarb, in contrast to that of $NaHCO_3$, improved arterial blood gas variables, tissue intracellular pH, lactate production, and cardiac hemodynamics.[38] The results of further studies, particularly in humans, are eagerly awaited.

We believe that on balance the data suggest that profound life-threatening acidemia ought to be treated with judicious amounts of $NaHCO_3$.

If sodium bicarbonate is employed, it is generally infused at rates sufficient to maintain the serum HCO_3 concentration at a level of 10 to 12 meq/liter. Assuming normal pulmonary compensation, this should maintain arterial blood pH at or above 7.20 and, potentially, allow time for primary therapeutic measures to become effective. After initial loading doses, a sustaining infusion of approximately 150 meq/liter $NaHCO_3$ (three 50 ml ampules of $NaHCO_3$ [1 meq/ml] added to 1000 ml 5% dextrose in water) is used to maintain the desired pH. Rates of infusion must be individualized, and the physician must be prepared to alter this rate promptly, depending upon sequentially determined values of arterial pH and bicarbonate concentration. It is not unusual for patients to require more than 100 meq of $NaHCO_3$ per hour. Obviously, such rates of administration of sodium may lead to serious, even life-threatening, volume overload.

As net lactate production declines and hourly bicarbonate requirements diminish, it is important to discontinue alkali therapy even though the patient's serum bicarbonate level might have risen to only 10 to 15 meq/liter. The factors that determine the final serum bicarbonate concentration are the continuing rate of acid production, the amount of administered bicarbonate that is retained and the amount of alkali that in effect, is "resynthesized" from lactate. During the induction of acidosis, each milliequivalent of titrated bicarbonate is replaced by one of lactate. If only trivial amounts of lactate are lost in the urine, metabolism of the retained amount should normalize the serum bicarbonate concentration. Thus, a metabolic alkalosis may develop due to additive effects of the administered (and retained) $NaHCO_3$ and that resynthesized from lactate. This alkalosis may be minimized if the administration of exogenous $NaHCO_3$ is discontinued early and patients are allowed to increase their serum bicarbonate concentration by metabolizing lactate. Continued hyperventilation may add a respiratory component to the alkalosis. Occasionally in a volume-expanded patient who develops prominent metabolic alkalosis, the administration of the carbonic anhydrase inhibitor acetazolamide (250 to 500 mg given orally or intravenously) may be helpful in restoring plasma volume and serum bicarbonate to normal levels.

Diuretics

As indicated, volume overload and congestive heart failure may result from the very large loads of $NaHCO_3$ required to treat lactic acidosis. Although the judicious use of potent diuretics may be useful in avoiding or treating this complication, the characteristic hemodynamic abnormalities associated with lactic acidosis often make it impossible to maintain sodium balance with diuretics. Dialysis or hemofiltration may be required in some patients, particularly in those with impaired renal function.

Furosemide should be used only after the physician is certain that initial volume depletion has been repaired. At this point, diuretics should be given in amounts sufficient to cause sodium and water losses equivalent to the quantity being given by vein. Ideally, the NaCl diuresis should assure that sufficient "space" remains available to accommodate the needed alkali. One should anticipate using intravenous doses of 40 to 100 mg of furosemide every 1 to 2 h. Urine flow rates of 0.5 to 1.5 liters/h may result, with levels of sodium of 50 to 100 meq/liter and potassium of 20 to 30 meq/liter. The sodium lost in the urine may be replaced as the bicarbonate salt; urinary potassium losses may be replaced hourly as potassium chloride. Hemodynamic measurements must be followed carefully, along with hourly measurements of serum and urinary electrolytes.

Dialysis

Those patients whose renal failure does not permit the successful use of diuretics may be treated with dialysis. Dialysis should not be used until it becomes apparent that volume overload will develop without it. Fluid may be removed and alkali given via the dialysate, while additional $NaHCO_3$ may be given by vein, as replacement for the fluid removed by dialysis.[176] Obviously dialysis does not remove lactic acid, which cannot exist at physiologic pH; rather, it rids the body of lactate, a metabolizable organic anion, which, as mentioned, is a potential source of alkali. If it is shown in the future that the lactate ion per se is toxic, then the removal from the body of lactate may become a goal of therapy. Finally, although there are presently few data precisely defining the dialyzability of biguanides, it appears that at least some of these medications can be removed by dialysis.[175,176] Thus, early use of this therapeutic modality may indicate if one of these agents is an etiologic factor.

Hemodialysis using a bicarbonate-based dialysate is acceptable if the blood pressure permits it. Frequently, however, hypotension contraindicates this approach, and peritoneal dialysis must be used instead. One of the standard peritoneal dialysis solutions uses lactate as the source of alkali and therefore is inappropriate for the therapy for this disorder. Bicarbonate-containing solutions should be prepared. The hospital pharmacy can be asked to make 2 liter portions of peritoneal dialysis fluid containing 135 meq/liter of sodium, 3 meq/liter of potassium, 98 meq/liter of chloride, 40 meq/liter of HCO_3, and 1.5 to 4.5% glucose. Calcium and magnesium cannot be added because the cations form insoluble salts in the presence of bicarbonate. If this approach is not feasible, an acceptable peritoneal dialysis solution can be made up by mixing 1 liter of 0.9% NaCl in water with 1 liter of 0.45% NaCl in 5% glucose to which 50 to 80 meq of $NaHCO_3$ and the desired amount of KCl are added. This provides a sodium concentration of 141 to 156 meq/liter, an HCO_3 level of 25 to 40 meq/liter, and 2.5% glucose. Magnesium and calcium may have to be given intravenously as needed.

Newer *extracorporeal* therapies in the setting of lactic acidosis have recently received much attention. Continuous arteriovenous hemofiltration (CAVH), continuous veno-veno hemofiltration (CVVHD), and continuous veno-veno hemodiafiltration (CVVHD) are now available. These therapies hold promise in the management of lactic acidosis because they not only provide a mechanism of continuously clearing the excess fluid associated with $NaHCO_3$ therapy but also provide for effective solute clearance enabling one to replace dialyzed chloride with bicarbonate. These therapies because of their low obligate blood flows are in general better tolerated hemodynamically than is conventional hemodialysis.

Dichloroacetate

Dichloroacetate (DCA), still an experimental medication, exerts diverse effects on intermediary metabolism.[287] It facilitates the metabolism of pyruvate and lactate at least in part by inhibiting PDH kinase, thereby stimulating the activity of the PDH enzyme complex.[290,322] Aside from its metabolic effects, there is evidence that it improves cardiac output and systemic hemodynamics, probably by facilitating myocardial metabolism of carbohydrate and lactate.[259,287,289] Thus, the medication is believed to decrease net lactate production by directly facilitating aerobic lactate metabolism as well as by increasing the perfusion and oxygenation of peripheral tissues.[290] DCA appeared to hold promise in many early trials in the management not only of type B lactic acidosis but also in patients and animals with various forms of the type A disorder.[114,259,289] DCA also appears to have a natriuretic effect, the mechanism of which is obscure.[259,287]

DCA has been reported to decrease lactate levels in diabetic patients without lactic acidosis,[288,292] to decrease lactate production in experimental animals given biguanides,[11,238] and to reduce fructose-induced hyperlactatemia in galactosamine-treated rats.[147] In rats with experimental diabetic ketoacidosis, DCA decreases the net release of lactate, pyruvate, and alanine from extrasplanchnic tissues and inhibits ketogenesis.[40] Regarding the diabetic patient with full-blown lactic acidosis, we were able to find only one reported case (biguanide-induced) in which DCA was used, and the patient did not respond.[139]

The results from the recent controlled DCA-L-actic acidosis study group revealed significant but clinically unimportant changes in arterial blood lactate concentrations and pH. These changes failed to alter hemodynamics or survival from lactic acidosis.[290a] Currently DCA in the therapy of lactic acidosis appears to afford little-to-no clinical benefit.

REFERENCES

1. Abramson E, Arky R: Diabetic acidosis with initial hypokalemia. *JAMA* 195:115, 1966.
2. Adrogué HJ et al: Plasma acid-base patterns in diabetic ketoacidosis. *N Engl J Med* 307:1603, 1982.
3. Adrogué HJ et al: Diabetic ketoacodisis: Role of the kidney in acid-base homeostasis reevaluated. *Kidney Int* 25:591, 1984.

4. Albert MS et al: Quantitative displacement of acid-base equilibrium in metabolic acidosis. *Ann Intern Med* 66:312, 1967.
5. Alberti KGMM: Diabetic emergencies. *Br Med Bull* 45:243, 1989.
6. Alberti KGMM et al: Small doses of intramuscular insulin in the treatment of diabetic coma. *Lancet* 2:515, 1973.
7. Alberti KGMM et al: Role of glucagon and other hormones in the development of diabetic ketoacidosis. *Lancet* 2:1307, 1975.
8. Alberti KGMM, Hockaday TDR: Blood lactic and pyruvic acids in diabetic coma. *Diabetes* 21:350, 1972.
9. Alberti KGMM, Hockaday TDR: Rapid blood ketone body estimation in the diagnosis of diabetic ketoacidosis. *Br Med J* 2:565, 1972.
10. Alberti KGMM, Hockaday TDR: Diabetic coma: A reappraisal after five years. *Clin Endocrinol Metab* 6:421, 1977.
11. Alberti KGMM, Holloway PAH: Dichloroacetate and phenformin-induced lactic acidosis (abstract). *Diabetes* 26:377, 1977.
12. Anderson J et al: Pyruvate and lactate excretion in diabetes mellitus after sodium lactate. *Br Med J* 2:1114, 1966.
13. Anderson J, Mazza C: Pyruvate and lactate excretion in patients with diabetes mellitus and benign glycosuria. *Lancet* 2:270, 1963.
14. Arieff AI: Kidney, water, and electrolyte metabolism in diabetes mellitus, in Brenner BM, Rector FC (eds): *The Kidney*. Philadelphia, Saunders, 1976, vol 2, p 1257.
15. Arieff AI: Cerebral edema complicating nonketotic hyperosmolar coma. *Miner Electrolyte Metab* 12:383, 1986.
16. Arieff AI et al: Pathophysiology of experimental lactic acidosis in dogs. *Am J Physiol* 239:F135, 1980.
17. Arieff AI et al: Systemic effects of $NaHCO_3$ in experimental lactic acidosis in dogs. *Am J Physiol* 242:F586, 1982.
18. Arieff AI et al: Lactic acidosis and the cardiovascular system in the dog. *Clin Sci* 64:573, 1983.
19. Arieff AI, Carroll HJ: Nonketotic hyperosmolar coma with hyperglycemia: Clinical features, pathophysiology, renal function, acid-base balance, plasma-cerebrospinal fluid equilibria and the effects of therapy in 37 cases. *Medicine* 51:73, 1972.
20. Arieff AI, Carroll HJ: Cerebral edema and depression of sensorium in nonketotic hyperosmolar coma. *Diabetes* 23:525, 1974.
21. Arieff AI, Kerian A: Lactic acidosis: An experimental model. *Metabolism* 25:307, 1976.
22. Arieff AI, Kleeman CR: Studies on the mechanisms of cerebral edema in diabetic comas: 1. Effect of hyperglycemia and rapid lowering of plasma glucose in normal rabbits. *J Clin Invest* 52:571, 1973.
23. Arieff AI, Kleeman CR: Cerebral edema in diabetic comas: 2. Effects of hyperosmolality, hyperglycemia and insulin in diabetic rabbits. *J Clin Endocrinol Metab* 38:1057, 1974.
24. Ashkar FS, Miller R: Hospital ketosis in the alcoholic diabetic, a syndrome due to isopropyl alcohol intoxication. *South Med J* 64:1409, 1971.
25. Asplund K et al: Hyperosmolar non-ketotic coma in diabetic stroke patients. *Acta Med Scand* 212:407, 1982.
26. Assal J et al: Metabolic effects of sodium bicarbonate in management of diabetic ketoacidosis. *Diabetes* 23:405, 1974.
27. Assan R et al: Phenformin-induced lactic acidosis in diabetic patients. *Diabetes* 24:791, 1975.
28. Atchley DW et al: A detailed study of electrolyte balances following the withdrawal and reestablishment of insulin therapy. *J Clin Invest* 12:297, 1933.
29. Atchley DW et al: On diabetic acidosis. *J Clin Invest* 12:310, 1933.
30. Balasse ED, Havel RJ: Turnover rate and oxidation of ketone bodies in normal and diabetic dogs. *Diabetologia* 6:36, 1970.
31. Baum D, Porte D Jr: Adrenergic regulation of the inhibition of insulin release in hypothermia. *Diabetes* 17(suppl 1):298, 1968.
32. Bavli S, Gordon EE: Experimental diabetic hyperosmolar syndrome in rats. *Diabetes* 20:92, 1971.
33. Becher DJ et al: Phosphate replacement during treatment of diabetic ketosis. *Am J Dis Child* 137:241, 1983.
34. Bellingham AJ et al: Regulatory mechanisms of hemoglobin-oxygen affinity in acidosis and alkalosis. *J Clin Invest* 50:700, 1971.
35. Benjamin J et al: Tissue O_2 delivery is stable despite correction of chronic metabolic acidosis (abstract), *American Society of Nephrology Proceedings*, 1982, p 136A.
36. Berger M et al: Metabolic and hormonal effects of muscular exercise in juvenile type diabetics. *Diabetologia* 13:355, 1977.
37. Bergstrom J et al: Lactic acid accumulation in connection with fructose infusion. *Acta Med Scand* 184:359, 1968.
38. Bersin RM, Arieff AI: Improved hemodynamic function during hypoxia with Carbicarb, a new agent for the management of acidosis. *Circulation* 77:227, 1988.
39. Bingle JP et al: Fatal self-poisoning with phenformin. *Br Med J* 3:752, 1970.
40. Blackshear PJ et al: Metabolic interactions of dichloroacetate and insulin in experimental diabetic ketoacidosis. *Biochem J* 146:447, 1975.
41. Bosanac P et al: Phenformin (DBI) tolerance and its renal tubular secretion in man (abstract). *Am Soc Nephrol* 9:9, 1976.
42. Boyer J et al: Hyperglycemia and hyperosmolality complicating peritoneal dialysis. *Ann Intern Med* 67:368, 1967.
43. Boyer MH: Hyperosmolar anacidotic coma in association with glucocorticoid therapy. *JAMA* 202:95, 1967.
44. Braaten JT: Hyperosmolar nonketotic diabetic coma: Diagnosis and management. *Geriatrics* 42:83, 1987.
45. Bratusch-Marrain, DeFronzo RA: Impairment of insulin-mediated glucose metabolism by hyperosmolality in man. *Diabetes* 32:1028, 1983.
46. Brown RH et al: Caveat on fluid replacement in hyperglycemic, hyperosmolar, nonketotic coma. *Diabetes Care* 1:305, 1978.
47. Bueding E, Goldfarb WJ: Blood changes following glucose, lactate and pyruvate injections in man. *J Biol Chem* 147:33, 1943.
48. Butler AM: Parenteral fluid therapy in diabetic coma. *Acta Paediatr Scand* 38:59, 1949.
49. Butler AM: Diabetic coma. *N Engl J Med* 243:648, 1950.

50. Butler AM et al: Metabolic studies in diabetic coma. *Trans Assoc Am Physicians* 60:102, 1947.
51. Cahill GF Jr: Hyperglycemic hyperosmolar coma: A syndrome almost unique to the elderly. *J Am Geriatr Soc* 31:103, 1983.
52. Cahill GF Jr et al: Insulin and muscle protein, in Steiner DF, Freinkel N (eds): *Handbook of Physiology*, sec 7, vol 1, *Endocrine Pancreas*. Washington, DC, American Physiological Society, 1977, p 563.
53. Campbell LV et al: Routine use of low-dose intravenous insulin infusion in severe hyperglycemia. *Med J Aust* 2:519, 1976.
53a. Canaud B et al: Acute renal failure associated with multiple organ failure: Pump assisted continuous venovenous hemofiltration, the ultimate treatment modality. *Contrib Nephrol* 93, 1991.
54. Carroll P, Matz R: Uncontrolled diabetes mellitus in adults: Experience in treating diabetic ketoacidosis and hyperosmolar nonketotic coma with low-dose insulin and a uniform treatment regimen. *Diabetes Care* 6:579, 1983.
55. Caruso M et al: Lactic acidosis and insulin resistance associated with epinephrine administration in a patient with non-insulin-dependent diabetes mellitus. *Arch Intern Med* 147:1422, 1987.
56. Caspary WF, Crentszfeldt W: Inhibition of intestinal amino acid transport by blood sugar lowering biguanides. *Diabetologia* 9:6, 1973.
57. Cerchio GM et al: Inhibition of insulin release during hypovolemic shock. *Metabolism* 22:1449, 1973.
58. Chaikoff IL, Soskin S: Utilization of acetoacetic acid by normal and diabetic dogs before and after evisceration. *Am J Physiol* 87:58, 1928.
59. Chanutin A, Churnish RR: Effect of organic and inorganic phosphates on oxygen equilibrium of human erythrocytes. *Arch Biochem Biophys* 121:96, 1967.
60. Christlieb AR et al: Plasma renin activity and blood volume in uncontrolled diabetes: Ketoacidosis, a state of secondary aldosteronism. *Diabetes* 24:190, 1975.
61. Clerbaux T et al: Effect of phosphate on oxygen-hemoglobin affinity, diphosphoglycerate and blood gases during recovery from diabetic ketoacidosis. *Intens Care Med* 15:495, 1989.
62. Cohen RD et al: The relation between phenformin therapy and lactic acidosis. *Diabetologia* 9:43, 1973.
63. Cohen RD, Woods HF: *Clinical and Biochemical Aspects of Lactic Acidosis*. Oxford, Blackwell Scientific, 1976.
64. Cooper DJ et al: Bicarbonate does not improve hemodynamics in critically ill patients who have lactic acidosis: A prospective controlled clinical study. *Ann Intern Med* 112:492, 1990.
65. Cori CF, Cori GT: The mechanism of epinephrine action: 4. The influence of epinephrine on lactic acid production and blood sugar utilization. *J Biol Chem* 84:683, 1929.
66. Craddock PR et al: Acquired phagocyte dysfunction: A complication of the hypophosphatemia of parenteral hyperalimentation. *N Engl J Med* 290:1403, 1974.
67. Cristensen NJ, Orskov H: The relationship between endogenous serum insulin concentration and glucose uptake in the forearm muscles of nondiabetics. *J Clin Invest* 47:1262, 1968.
68. Danowski TS, Nabarro JDN: Hyperosmolar and other types of nonketoacidotic coma in diabetes. *Diabetes* 14:162, 1965.
69. Darragh JH et al: Fructose in the treatment of diabetic ketosis. *J Clin Invest* 32:1214, 1953.
70. Daughaday WH et al: Lactic acidosis as a cause of nonketotic acidosis in diabetic patients. *N Engl J Med* 267:1010, 1962.
71. Daugirdas JT et al: Hyperosmolar coma: Cellular dehydration and the serum sodium concentration. *Ann Intern Med* 110:855, 1989.
72. Davidson MB et al: Phenformin hypoglycemia and lactic acidosis. *N Engl J Med* 275:886, 1966.
73. DeFronzo RA, Beckles AD: Glucose intolerance following chronic metabolic acidosis in man. *Am J Physiol* 236:E328, 1979.
74. Dembo AJ et al: Insulin therapy in phenformin-associated lactic acidosis: A case report, biochemical considerations, and review of the literature. *Diabetes* 24:28, 1975.
75. Dreschfeld J: The Bradshawe lecture on diabetic coma. *Br Med J* 2:358, 1886.
76. Druml W et al: Fructose-induced hyperlactemia in hyperosmolar syndromes. *Klin Wochenschr* 64:615, 1986.
77. Duck SC, Wyatt DT: Factors associated with brain herniation in the treatment of diabetic ketoacidosis. *J Pediatr* 113:10, 1988.
78. Dupré J: Insulin therapy: Progress and prospects. *Hosp Pract* April 1983, p 125.
79. El-Mayhrabi MR et al: Cyclic AMP dependent phosphorylation of rat liver 6-phosphorylase 2 kinase/fructose 2,6-bisphosphatase. *Biochem Biophys Res Commun* 106:794, 1982.
80. El-Mayhrabi MR et al: Regulation of rat liver fructose 2,6-bisphosphatase. *J Biol Chem* 257:7607, 1982.
81. Emmett M, Narins RG: Clinical use of the anion gap. *Medicine* 56:38, 1977.
82. Exton JH: The effects of glucogen metabolism and gluconeogenesis, in Unger RH, Ore IL (eds): *Glucagon: Physiology, Pathophysiology, and Morphology of the Pancreatic Alpha-Cells*. New York, Elsevier/North Holland, 1981, p 195.
83. Feng P et al: Insulin, glucagon, and somatostatin in normal physiology and diabetes mellitus. *Diabetes* 25:1091, 1976.
84. Finberg L et al: Pathogenesis of lesions in the nervous system in hypernatremic states. *Pediatrics* 23:46, 1959.
85. Finn R, Cope S: The plasma amylase in diabetic coma. *Diabetes* 12:141, 1963.
86. Fisher JN, Kitabchi AE: A randomized study of phosphate therapy in the treatment of diabetic ketoacidosis. *J Clin Endocrinol Metab* 57:177, 1983.
87. Fitzgerald MG et al: Fatal diabetic ketosis. *Br Med J* 1:247, 1961.
88. Fonseca V, Phear DN: Hyperosmolar non-ketotic diabetic syndrome precipitated by treatment with diuretics. *Br Med J* 284:36, 1982.
89. Foster DW: Insulin deficiency and hyperosmolar coma. *Adv Intern Med* 19:159, 1974.
90. Foster DW, McGarry JD: The metabolic derangements and treatment of diabetic ketoacidosis. *N Engl J Med* 309:159, 1983.
91. Franklin B et al: Cerebral edema and ophthalmoplegia

reversed by mannitol in a new case of insulin-dependent diabetes mellitus. *Pediatrics* 69:87, 1982.
92. Franks M et al: Metabolic studies in diabetic acidosis: II. Effect of administration of sodium phosphate. *Arch Intern Med* 81:42, 1948.
93. Fraser EL, Arieff AI: Fatal central diabetes mellitus and insipidus resulting from untreated hyponatremia: A new syndrome. *Ann Intern Med* 112:113, 1990.
94. Fulop M et al: Lactic acidosis in diabetic patients. *Arch Intern Med* 136:987, 1976.
95. Fulop M: Hypercalcemia in diabetic ketoacidosis. *Am J Med Sci* 299:164, 1990.
96. Fulop M et al: Ketotic hyperosmolar coma. *Lancet* 2:635, 1973.
97. Fulop M et al: Hyperosmolar nature of diabetic coma. *Diabetes* 24:594, 1975.
98. Fulop M: Cerebral edema in severe diabetic ketoacidosis. *N Engl J Med* 276:1445, 1967.
99. Fulop M, Hoberman HD: Alcoholic ketosis. *Diabetes* 24:785, 1975.
100. Fulop M, Hoberman HD: Phenformin-associated metabolic acidosis. *Diabetes* 25:292, 1976.
101. Fulop M, Hoberman HD: Is lactic acidosis spontaneous? *N Y State J Med* January 24, 1977, p 586.
102. Gabow PA et al: Diagnostic importance of an increased serum anion gap. *N Engl J Med* 303:854, 1980.
103. Genuth SM: Constant intravenous insulin infusion in diabetic ketoacidosis. *JAMA* 223:1348, 1973.
104. Gerich JE et al: Clinical and metabolic characteristics of hyperosmolar nonketotic coma. *Diabetes* 20:228, 1971.
105. Gerich JE et al: Effect of dehydration and hyperosmolarity on glucose, free fatty acid and ketone body metabolism in the rat. *Diabetes* 22:264, 1973.
106. Gerich JE et al: Plasma glucagon and alanine responses to acute insulin deficiency in man. *J Clin Endocrinol Metab* 40:526, 1975.
107. Gerich JE et al: Prevention of human diabetic ketoacidosis by somatostatin: Evidence for an essential role of glucagon. *N Engl J Med* 292:985, 1975.
108. Goldberg EM, Sanbar SS: Hyperglycemic, nonketotic coma following administration of Dilantin (diphenylhydantoin). *Diabetes* 18:101, 1969.
109. Goldberger E: *A Primer of Water, Electrolyte and Acid Base Syndromes*. Philadelphia, Lea & Febiger, 1965, p 399.
110. Goldfarb S et al: Acute hyperkalemia induced by hyperglycemia: Hormonal mechanisms. *Ann Intern Med* 84:426, 1976.
111. Goldman JM, Chirboga M: Diabetic ketoacidosis with alkalemia. *J Emerg Med* 7:369, 1989.
111a. Golper TA: Continuous arteriovenous hemofiltration in acute renal failure. *Am J Kidney Dis* 6:373, 1985.
112. Gordon EE, Duga J: Experimental hyperosmolar diabetic syndrome: Ketogenic response to medium-chain triglycerides. *Diabetes* 24:301, 1975.
113. Gordon EE, Kabadi UM: The hyperglycemic hyperosmolar syndrome. *Am J Med Sci* 271:252, 1976.
114. Graf H et al: Effects of dichloroacetate in the treatment of hypoxic lactic acidosis in dogs. *J Clin Invest* 76:919, 1985.
115. Greco AV et al: Somatostatin and insulin infusion in the management of diabetic ketoacidosis. *Horm Metab Res* 13:310, 1981.
116. Guerra SMO, Kitabchi AE: Comparison of the effectiveness of various routes of insulin injection: Insulin levels and glucose response in normal subjects. *J Clin Endocrinol Metab* 42:869, 1976.
117. Guest GM, Rapaport S: Organic acid soluble phosphorus compounds of the blood. *Physiol Rev* 21:41, 1941.
118. Guisado R, Arieff AI: Neurologic manifestations of diabetic comas' correlation with biochemical alterations in the brain. *Metabolism* 24:665, 1975.
119. Hadden JW, Metzner RT: Pseudoketosis and hyperacetaldehydemia and paraldehyde acidosis. *Am J Med* 47:642, 1969.
120. Halmos PB et al: Hyperosmolar non-ketoacidotic coma in diabetes. *Lancet* 1:675, 1966.
121. Halperin ML: Lactic acidosis and ketoacidosis: Biochemical and clinical implications. *Can Med Assoc J* 116:1034, 1977.
122. Halperin ML et al: Factors that control the effect of pH on glycolysis in leukocytes. *J Biol Chem* 244:384, 1969.
123. Halperin ML et al: Quantitative aspects of hyperglycemia in the diabetic: A theoretical approach. *Clin Invest Med* 2:127, 1980.
124. Halperin ML et al: Can marked hyperglycemia occur without ketosis? *Clin Invest Med* 8:253, 1985.
125. Hamblin PS et al: Deaths associated with diabetic ketoacidosis and hyperosmolar coma 1973–1988. *Med J Aust* 151:439, 1989.
126. Handa SP, Cushner GB: Hyperosmolar hyperglycemic nonketotic coma during peritoneal dialysis. *South Med J* 61:700, 1968.
127. Hannan TJ, Stathers GM: Constant low-dose insulin infusion in severe diabetes mellitus. *Med J Aust* 1:11, 1976.
128. Hems R et al: Gluconeogenesis in the perfused rat liver. *Biochem J* 101:284, 1966.
129. Henry DP, Bressler R: Serum insulin levels in nonketotic hyperosmotic diabetes mellitus. *Am J Med Sci* 256:150, 1968.
130. Hermann LS: Biguanide and lactate metabolism, a review. *Dan Med Bull* 20:65, 1973.
131. Hiatt N et al: Necessity for insulin in the transfer of excess infused K^+ to intracellular fluid. *Metabolism* 23:43, 1973.
132. Hockaday TDR, Alberti KGM: Diabetic coma. *Clin Endocrinol Metab* 1:751, 1972.
133. Hood VL, Tannen RL: pH control of lactic acid and ketoacid production. A mechanism of acid-base regulation. *Miner Electrolyte Metab* 9:317, 1983.
134. Hood VA, Tannen RL: Regulation of acid production in ketoacidosis and lactic acidosis. *Diab Metab Rev* 5:393, 1989.
135. Howell RF et al: Glucose-6-phosphatase deficiency glycogen storage disease: Studies on the interrelationships of carbohydrate lipid and purine abnormalities. *Pediatrics* 29:553, 1962.
136. Huckabee WE: Relationships of pyruvate and lactate during anaerobic metabolism: 1. Effects of infusion of pyruvate of glucose and of hyperventilation. *J Clin Invest* 37:244, 1958.

137. Huckabee WE: Abnormal resting blood lactate: 2. Lactic acidosis. *Am J Med* 30:840, 1961.
138. Iberti TJ et al: Low sensitivity of the anion gap as a screen to detect hyperlactatemia in critically ill patients. *Crit Care Med* 18:275, 1989.
139. Irsigler K: Dichloroacetate in biguanide-induced lactic acidosis. *Lancet* 2:1026, 1977.
140. Israel RS: Diabetic ketoacidosis. *Emerg Med Clin North Am* 7:859, 1988.
141. Jackson WPU, Forman R: Hyperosmolar nonketotic diabetic coma. *Diabetes* 15:714, 1966.
142. Jacobs HJS, Nabarro JDN: Plasma II-hydroxycorticosteroid and growth hormone levels in acute medical illnesses. *Br Med J* 2:595, 1969.
143. Jacobson R et al: Hyperglycemia and hyperosmolarity in a brittle diabetic with thyrotoxicosis. *Diabetes* 19:70, 1970.
144. Jensen HA: Treatment of lactic acidosis with insulin and glucose. *Dan Med Bull* 20:16, 1973.
145. Joffe BI et al: Factors in the pathogenesis of experimental nonketotic and ketoacidotic diabetic stupor. *Diabetes* 22:653, 1973.
146. Joffe BI et al: Pathogenesis of nonketotic hyperosmolar diabetic coma. *Lancet* 1:1069, 1975.
147. Johnson GAH, Alberti KGMM: The metabolic effects of sodium dichloroacetate in experimental hepatitis in the rat. *Biochem Soc Trans* 5:1387, 1977.
148. Johnson RD et al: Mechanisms and management of hyperosmolar coma without ketoacidosis in the diabetic. *Diabetes* 18:111, 1969.
149. Jungas PL et al: The chemical basis for the reduction of insulin binding during metabolic acidosis (abstract), in *American Society of Nephrology Proceedings*, 1984, p 186A.
150. Kaneshige H et al: Hyperosmolar nonketotic diabetic state associated with disseminated intravascular coagulation and acute renal failure : A case report. *Takai J Exp Clin Med* 7:81, 1982.
151. Kanter Y et al: 2,3-Diphosphoglycerate, nucleotide phosphate, organic and inorganic phosphate levels during the early phases of diabetic ketoacidosis. *Diabetes* 26:429, 1977.
152. Katz MA: Hyperglycemia-induced hyponatremia calculation of expected serum sodium depression. *N Engl J Med* 289:843, 1973.
153. Kaufman IA et al: Diabetic ketosis and acidosis: The continuous infusion of low doses of insulin. *J Pediatr* 87:846, 1975.
154. Keller U et al: Course and prognosis of 86 episodes of diabetic coma: A five year experience with a uniform schedule of treatment. *Diabetologia* 11:93, 1975.
155. Keller U et al: Phaeochromocytoma with lactic acidosis. *Br Med J* 3:606, 1978.
156. Keller U, Berger W: Prevention of hypophosphatemia by phosphate infusion during treatment of diabetic ketoacidosis and hyperosmolar coma. *Diabetes* 29:87, 1980.
157. Khardori R, Soler NG: Hyperosmolar hyperglycemic nonketotic syndrome: Report of 22 cases and brief review. *Am J Med* 77:899, 1984.
158. Kitabchi AE: Low-dose insulin therapy in diabetic ketoacidosis fact or fiction? *Diabetes Metab Res* 5:337, 1989.
159. Kitabchi AE et al: The efficacy of low-dose vs conventional therapy of insulin for treatment of diabetic ketoacidosis. *Ann Intern Med* 84:633, 1976.
160. Kitabchi AE et al: Diabetic ketoacidosis: Reappraisal of therapeutic approach. *Annu Rev Med* 30:339, 1979.
161. Kitabchi AE, Murphy MB: Diabetic ketoacidosis and hyperosmolar hyperglycemic nonketotic coma. *Med Clin North Am* 72:1545, 1988.
162. Knight G, Leatherdale BA: The role of race and environment in the development of hyperosmolar hyperglycemic non-ketotic coma. *Postgrad Med J* 58:351, 1982.
163. Kock JC et al: Hemolytic anemia and somatic cell dysfunction in severe hypophosphatemia. *Arch Intern Med* 134:360, 1974.
164. Kølendorf K, Møller BB: Lactic acidosis in epinephrine poisoning. *Acta Med Scand* 196:465, 1974.
165. Kolodny HD, Sherman L: Hyperglycemic nonketotic coma in insulin-dependent diabetes mellitus. *JAMA* 203:119, 1968.
166. Kopec B, Fritz IB: Comparison of properties of carnitine palmityltransferase II, and preparation of antibodies to carnitine palmityltransferases. *J Biol Chem* 248:4069, 1973.
167. Krane EJ: Diabetic ketoacidosis: Biochemistry, physiology, treatment, and prevention. *Pediatr Adolescent Endocrinol* 34:935, 1987.
168. Krebs HA: Rate control of the tricarboxylic acid cycle. *Adv Enzyme Regul* 8:335, 1970.
169. Kreisberg RA: Diabetic ketoacidosis: New concepts and trends in pathogenesis and treatment. *Ann Intern Med* 88:681, 1978.
170. Kreisberg RA: Lactate homeostasis and lactic acidosis. *Ann Intern Med* 92:227, 1980.
171. Kreisberg RA: Diabetic ketoacidosis: An update. *Crit Care Clin* 5:817, 1987.
172. Kreisberg RA: Diabetic ketoacidosis revisited again. *Mayo Clin Proc* 63:1144, 1988.
173. Kreisberg RA et al: Lactate turnover and gluconeogenesis in obesity, effect of phenformin. *Diabetes* 19:64, 1970.
174. Kreisberg RA et al: Ethanol-induced hyperlacticacidemia: Inhibition of lactate utilization. *J Clin Invest* 50:166, 1971.
175. Lalau JD et al: Bicarbonate hemodialysis: An adequate treatment for lactic acidosis in diabetics treated by metformin. *Intens Care Med* 13:383, 1987.
176. Lalau JD et al: Hemodialysis in the treatment of lactic acidosis in diabetics treated by metformin: A study of metformin elimination. *Int J Clin Pharmacol Ther Toxicol* 27:285, 1989.
177. Larcan A et al: Non-acidotic metabolic comas in diabetics. *Diabetes* 11:99, 1963.
178. Lee DBN, Kleeman CR: Phosphorus depletion in man, in Banks G (ed): *McGaw Medical Monographs*. November 1976.
179. Lemieux G et al: The effect of ketone bodies on renal ammoniagenesis. *J Clin Invest* 50:1781, 1971.
180. Liberman B et al: Hyperosmolar nonketotic diabetic coma. *Rev Bras Pesqui Med Biol* 1:133, 1968.
181. Lipsky SR et al: The effects of alkalosis upon ketone body production and carbohydrate metabolism in man. *J Clin Invest* 33:1269, 1954.
182. Lloyd MH et al: Effect of phenformin on gluconeogenesis

from lactate and intracellular pH in the isolated perfused guinea pig liver. *Diabetes* 24:618, 1975.
183. Loubatieres A et al: L'insuline exogene et endogene s'opposent a l'hyperlactacidemie produit chez le chein par l'administration de phenformie. *CR Acad Sci Paris* 276:847, 1973.
184. Luft D et al: Lactic acidosis in biguanide-treated cases: A review of 330 cases. *Diabetologia* 14:75, 1978.
185. Luse SA, Harris B: Brain ultrastructure in hydration and dehydration. *Arch Neurol* 4:131, 1961.
186. Macaulay MB: Hyperosmolar non-ketotic diabetes. *Postgrad Med J* 47:191, 1971.
187. Maccario M: Neurological dysfunction associated with nonketotic hyperglycemia. *Arch Neurol* 19:525, 1968.
188. Mackler B et al: Effects of ammonium chloride acidosis on the action of insulin in dogs. *Am J Physiol* 166:191, 1951.
189. Madison LL: Low dose insulin: A plea for caution. *N Engl J Med* 294:393, 1976.
190. Major RH: *Classic Descriptions of Disease.* Springfield, Ill, Charles C. Thomas, 1959, p 247.
191. Makoff DL et al: Hypertonic expansion, acid-base and electrolyte changes. *Am J Physiol* 218:1201, 1970.
192. Malone JK et al: The hyperglycemic hyperosmolar syndrome. *Indiana Med* 81:766, 1988.
193. Mandell F, Fellers FX: Hyperglycemia in hypernatremic dehydration. *Clin Pediatr* 13:367, 1974.
194. Marliss EB et al: Altered redox state obscuring ketoacidosis in diabetic patients with lactic acidosis. *N Engl J Med* 283:978, 1970.
195. Marr TJ et al: The use of sodium bicarbonate in the treatment of diabetic children. *J Kan Med Soc* 82:282, 1981.
196. Marshall S et al: Low pH accelerates dissociation of receptor bound insulin. *Endocrinology* 113:37, 1983.
197. McCurdy DK: Hyperosmolar hyperglycemic nonketotic diabetic coma. *Med Clin North Am* 54:683, 1970.
198. McGarry JD, Foster DW: Ketogenesis and its regulation. *Am J Med* 61:9, 1976.
199. McGarry JD, Foster DW: Regulation of hepatic fatty acid oxidation and ketone body production. *Annu Rev Biochem* 49:395, 1980.
200. Medalle R et al: Lactic acidosis and associated hypoglycemia. *Arch Intern Med* 128:273, 1971.
201. Miles JM et al: Effects of acute insulin deficiency on glucose and ketone body turnover in man: Evidence for the primary production of glucose and ketone bodies in the genesis of diabetic ketoacidosis. *Diabetes* 29:926, 1980.
202. Miller M et al: Metabolism of intravenous fructose and glucose in normal and diabetic subjects. *J Clin Invest* 31:115, 1952.
203. Mirsky IA et al: The role of excessive carbohydrate intake in the etiology of diabetic coma. *J Clin Endocrinol Metab* 1:307, 1941.
204. Misbin RI: Phenformin-associated lactic acidosis: Pathogenesis and treatment. *Ann Intern Med* 87:591, 1977.
205. Mizock BA: Controversies in lactic acidosis: Implications in critically ill patients. *JAMA* 258:497, 1987.
206. Montelenone JA, Keefe DM: Transient hyperglycemia and aketotic hyperosmolar acidosis with heat stroke. *Pediatrics* 44:737, 1969.
207. Moran MS, Jamison RL: The variable hyponatremic response to hyperglycemia. *West J Med* 142:49, 1985.
208. Moreno M et al: Increase in serum potassium resulting from the administration of hypertonic mannitol and other solutions. *J Lab Clin Med* 73:29, 1969.
209. Moseley J: Diabetic crises in children treated with small doses of intramuscular insulin. *Br Med J* 1:59, 1975.
210. Muller WA et al: Hyperglucagonemia in diabetic ketoacidosis. *Am J Med* 54:52, 1973.
211. Munk P et al: Effect of bicarbonate on oxygen transport in juvenile diabetic ketoacidosis. *J Pediatr* 84:510, 1974.
212. Munro JF et al: Euglycemic diabetic ketoacidosis. *Br Med J* 2:578, 1973.
213. Nabarro JDN et al: Metabolic studies in severe diabetic ketosis. *Q J Med* 21:225, 1952.
214. Naghmi R, Kabuor M: Transient severe insulin resistance in diabetic ketoacidosis: A report of four episodes. *Horm Metabol Res* 20:584, 1988.
215. Nanji AA, Campbell DJ: Falsely elevated serum creatinine values in diabetic ketoacidosis, clinical implications. *Clin Biochem* 14:91, 1981.
216. Narins RG: Acid-base metabolism, in Gonick HC (ed): *Current Nephrology.* Los Angeles, Pinecliff Medical, 1977, vol 1, p 127.
217. Narins RG et al: Streptozotocin-induced lactic acidosis: A case report and some experimental observations. *Am J Med Sci* 265:455, 1973.
218. Narins RG, Cohen JJ: Bicarbonate therapy for organic acidosis: The case for its continued use. *Ann Intern Med* 106:615, 1987.
219. Newman JH et al: Acute respiratory failure associated with hypophosphatemia. *N Engl J Med* 296:1101, 1977.
220. Nicolis GL et al: Glucose induced hyperkalemia in diabetic subjects. *Arch Intern Med* 141, 1953.
221. Nosadini R et al: The metabolic and hormonal response to acute normoglycaemia in type 1 (insulin-dependent) diabetes: Studies with a glucose controlled insulin infusion system (artificial endocrine pancreas). *Diabetologia* 23:220, 1982.
222. Oakes DD et al: Hyperglycemic, nonketotic coma in the patient with burns: Factors in pathogenesis. *Metabolism* 18:103, 1969.
223. O'Connor L et al: Effect of hypophosphatemia on myocardial performance in man. *N Engl J Med* 297:901, 1977.
224. Oh MS et al: Hyperchloremic acidosis during the recovery phase of diabetic ketosis. *Ann Intern Med* 89:925, 1978.
225. Oh MS et al: Mechanism of normochloremic and hyperchloremic acidosis in diabetic ketoacidosis. *Nephron* 54:1, 1990.
226. Ohman JL et al: The cerebrospinal fluid in diabetic ketoacidosis. *N Engl J Med* 284:382, 1971.
227. Oliva PB: Lactic acidosis. *Am J Med* 48:209, 1970.
228. Orringer CE et al: Natural history of lactic acidosis after grand mal seizures: A model for the study of an anion gap acidosis not associated with hyperkalemia. *N Engl J Med* 297:769, 1977.
229. Oster JR et al: Relationship between blood pH and potassium and phosphorus during acute metabolic acidosis. *Am J Physiol* 235:F345, 1978.
230. Oster JR et al: Plasma potassium response to acute meta-

bolic acidosis induced by mineral and non-mineral acids. *Miner Electrolyte Metab* 4:28, 1980.
231. Oster JR et al: The use of the anion gap in clinical medicine. *South Med J* 81:229, 1988.
232. Oster JR, Epstein M: Acid-base aspects of ketoacidosis. *Am J Nephrol* 4:137, 1984.
233. Oster JR, Perez GO: Acid-base homeostasis and pathophysiology in liver disease, in Epstein M (ed): *The Kidney in Liver Disease*, 3d ed. Baltimore, Williams & Wilkins, 1988, p 119.
234. Ott A et al: Severe lactic acidosis associated with alcohol for premature labor. *Obstet Gynecol* 48:362, 1976.
235. Owen OE et al: Human splanchnic metabolism during diabetic ketoacidosis. *Metabolism* 26:381, 1977.
236. Padilla AJ, Loeb JN: "Low dose" insulin vs "high dose" insulin regimens in the management of uncontrolled diabetes: A survey. *Am J Med* 63:843, 1977.
237. Park R, Arieff AI: Lactic acidosis. *Adv Intern Med* 25:33, 1980.
238. Park R, Arieff AI: Treatment of lactic acidosis with dichloroacetate in dogs. *J Clin Invest* 70:853, 1982.
239. Park R, Arieff AI: Lactic acidosis: Current concepts. *Clin Endocrinol Metab* 12:339, 1983.
240. Paulson WD: Anion gap-bicarbonate relation in diabetic ketoacidosis. *Am J Med* 81:995, 1986.
241. Peterson L et al: Insulin absorbance to polyvinylchloride surfaces with implications for constant-infusion therapy. *Diabetes* 25:72, 1976.
242. Pierce NF et al: The ventilatory response to acute base deficit in humans. *Ann Intern Med* 72:633, 1970.
243. Podolsky S, Pattavina CG: Hyperosmolar nonketotic diabetic coma: A complication of propranolol therapy. *Metabolism* 22:685, 1973.
244. Pope DW, Dansky D: Hyperosmolar hyperglycemic nonketotic coma. *Emerg Med Clin North Am* 7:849, 1989.
245. Popli S et al: Asymptomatic, nonketotic, severe hyperglycemia with hyponatremia. *Arch Intern Med* 150:1962, 1990.
246. Porte D: Sympathetic regulation of insulin secretion, its relation to diabetes mellitus. *Arch Intern Med* 123:252, 1969.
247. Posner JB, Plum F: Spinal-fluid pH and neurologic symptoms in systematic acidosis. *N Engl J Med* 277:605, 1967.
248. Potter DJ: Death as a result of hyperglycemia without ketosis: A complication of hemodialysis. *Ann Intern Med* 64:399, 1966.
249. Prytz H, Thomsen AC: Acid-base status in liver cirrhosis: Disturbances in stable, terminal, and portacaval shunted patients. *Scand J Gastroenterol* 11:249, 1976.
250. Pyorala K et al: Steroid therapy and hyperosmolar nonketotic coma. *Lancet* 1:596, 1968.
251. Record CO et al: Metabolic studies in experimental liver disease resulting from d(+) galactosamine administration. *Biochem J* 130:37, 1972.
252. Reichard DA et al: Plasma acetone metabolism in the fasting human. *J Clin Invest* 63:619, 1979.
253. Relman AS: Metabolic consequences of acid-base disorders. *Kidney Int* 1:347, 1972.
254. Richards CS, Uyeda IL: Hormonal regulation of fructose 6P, 2-kinase and fructose 2, 6-P_2 by two mechanisms. *J Biol Chem* 257:8854, 1982.
255. Richards CS, Uyeda IL: Changes in concentration of activation factor for phosphofructokinase in hepatocytes in response to glucose and glucagon. *Biochem Biophys Res Commun* 97:1535, 1980.
256. Riley L et al: Alkalai therapy of diabetic ketoacidosis: Biochemical, physiological, and clinical prospectives. *Diabetes Metab Rev* 5:627, 1989.
257. Robinson BH: Lactic acidemia, in Scriver CR et al (ed): *The Metabolic Basis of Inherited Disease*, 6th ed. New York, McGraw-Hill Information Services, 1989, p 869.
258. Rogers TA, Wachenfeld AE: Effect of physiologic acids and electrolytes on rat diaphragm. *Am J Physiol* 193:623, 1958.
259. Romeh SA, Tannen RL: Therapeutic benefit of dichloroacetate in experimentally induced hypoxic lactic acidosis. *J Lab Clin Med* 107:378, 1986.
260. Rosenberg SA et al: The syndrome of dehydration, coma and severe hyperglycemia without ketosis in patients convalescing from burns. *N Engl J Med* 272:931, 1965.
261. Rosenbloom AL: Intracerebral crisis during treatment of diabetic ketoacidosis. *Diabetes Care* 13:22, 1990.
262. Rosenthal NR, Barrett EJ: An assessment of insulin action in hyperosmolar hyperglycemic nonketotic diabetic patients. *J Clin Endocrinol Metab* 60:607, 1985.
263. Rosivial V: The influence of blood hydrogen ion concentration on the level of consciousness in diabetic ketoacidosis. *Ann Clin Res* 19:23, 1987.
264. Rubin HM et al: Hyperosmolality complicating diabetes mellitus in childhood. *J Pediatr* 74:117, 1969.
265. Ruebi FC: Glomerular filtration rate, renal blood flow and blood viscosity during and after diabetic coma. *Circ Res* 1:410, 1953.
266. Ryder REJ: The danger of high dose sodium bicarbonate in biguanide-induced lactic acidosis: The theory, the practice and alternate therapies. *Br J Clin Prac* 41:730, 1987.
267. Ryder REJ, Hayes TM: Normo-osmolar, nonketotic, hyponatremic diabetic syndrome associated with impaired renal function. *Diabetes Care* 6:402, 1983.
268. Sament S, Schwartz MB: Severe diabetic stupor without ketosis. *S Afr Med J* 31:893, 1957.
269. Schade DS et al: *Diabetic Coma: Ketoacidotic and Hyperosmolar*. Albuquerque, University of New Mexico Press, 1981, p 201.
270. Schafer G: Site specific uncoupling and inhibition of energy transfer by biguanides. *Biochem Biophys Acta* 93:279, 1964.
271. Schwartz WB, Waters WC: Lactate vs bicarbonate. *Am J Med* 32:831, 1962.
272. Searle GL, Cavalieri RR: Determination of lactate kinetics in the human analysis of data from single injection vs continuous infusion methods. *Proc Soc Exp Biol Med* 139:1002, 1972.
273. Seltzer HS, Harris VL: Exhaustion of insulogenic reserve in maturity-onset diabetic patients during prolonged and continuous hyperglycemic stress. *Diabetes* 13:6, 1964.
274. Sestoft L et al: Development of diabetic ketoacidosis: Some observations on and deductions about the sources of acid. *Acta Med Scand* (suppl) 639:7, 1980.
275. Sestoft L et al: Acid-base balance in diabetic ketoacidosis, in *Metabolic Acidosis*. London, Pitman, *Ciba Found Symp* 87:254, 1982.

276. Severinghaus JW: Oxyhemoglobin dissociation curve correction for temperature and pH variation in human blood. *J Appl Physiol* 12:485, 1958.
277. Shade DS, Easton RP: Dose response to insulin in man: Differential effects on glucose and ketone body regulation. *J Clin Endocrinol Metab* 44:1038, 1977.
278. Shaw CE Jr et al: A clinical and laboratory study of insulin dosage in diabetic acidosis: Comparison with small and large doses. *Diabetics* 2:23, 1962.
279. Shichiri M et al: Disappearance of DL-lactate-2-C^{14} from blood in normal and diabetic rats. *Proc Soc Exper Biol Med* 125:1238, 1967.
279a. Sigler MH, Teehan BP: Solute transport in continuous hemodialysis: a new treatment for acute renal failure. *Kidney Int* 32:562, 1987.
280. Simmons DH et al: Hyperventilation and respiratory alkalosis as signs of gram negative bacteremia. *JAMA* 197:2196, 1960.
281. Singhal PC et al: Rhabdomyolysis in the hyperosmolal state. *Am J Med* 88:9, 1990.
282. Smith K, Martin HE: Response of the diabetic to various insulin dosages. *Diabetes* 3:287, 1954.
283. Sneyud JGT et al: The role of cyclic AMP in the action of insulin, in Beck N et al (eds): *Pharmacology of Hormonal Polypeptides and Proteins*. New York, Plenum Press, 1968, p 367.
284. Soler NG et al: Comparative study of different insulin regimens in management of diabetic ketoacidosis. *Lancet* 2:1221, 1975.
285. Sotos JF et al: Studies in experimental hypertonicity: 2. Hypertonicity of body fluids as a cause of acidosis. *Pediatrics* 30:180, 1962.
286. Spenney JG et al: Hyperglycemic, hyperosmolar, nonketoacidotic diabetes. *Diabetes* 18:107, 1969.
287. Stacpoole PW: The pharmacology of dichloroacetate. *Metabolism* 38:1124, 1989.
288. Stacpoole PW et al: Metabolic effects of dichloroacetate in patients with diabetes mellitus and hyperlipoproteinemia. *N Engl J Med* 298:526, 1978.
289. Stacpoole PW et al: Treatment of lactic acidosis with dichloroacetate. *N Engl J Med* 309:390, 1983.
290. Stacpoole PW et al: Dichloroacetate in the treatment of lactic acidosis. *Ann Intern Med* 108:58, 1988.
290a. Stacpoole PW et al: A controlled clinical trial of dichloroacetate for treatment of lactic acidosis in adults. *N Engl J Med* 327:22, 1992.
291. Stahlman GC et al: Neurologic manifestations of nonketotic hyperglycemia. *J Tenn Med Assoc* 81:77, 1988.
292. Standl E et al: The effect of a combined therapy with buformin and dichloroacetate on blood lactate concentrations in diabetics. *Klin Wochenschr* 55:969, 1977.
293. Steiner DF, Williams RH: Respiratory inhibition and hypoglycemia by biguanides and decamethylenediguanide. *Biochem Biophys Acta* 30:329, 1958.
294. Stenvert LS et al: Low dose intravenous insulin infusion vs subcutaneous insulin injections: A controlled comparative study of diabetic ketoacidosis. *Pediatrics* 59:733, 1977.
295. Storms FEME et al: Comparison of efficacy of human and porcine insulin in treatment of diabetic ketoacidosis. *Diabetes Care* 10:49, 1987.
296. Strangaard S et al: Blood lactate and ketone bodies in diabetic ketoacidosis. *Acta Med Scand* 190:17, 1971.
297. Strauss FG, Sullivan MA: Phenformin intoxication resulting in lactic acidosis. *Johns Hopkins Med J* 128:278, 1970.
298. Sulway MJ, Malins JM: Acetone in diabetic ketoacidosis. *Lancet* 2:736, 1970.
299. Sypniewski E Jr et al: Hyperosmolar, hyperglycemic, nonketotic coma in a patient receiving home total parenteral nutrient therapy. *Clin Pharm* 6:69, 1987.
300. Tachibana Y et al: Tap-induced blink reflex and central nervous system dysfunction in diabetics with hyperosmolality. *Eur Neurol* 30:145, 1990.
301. Tranquada RE et al: Lactic acidosis. *Arch Intern Med* 117:192, 1966.
302. Unger RH, Foster DW: Diabetes mellitus, in Foster DW, Wilson JD (eds): *Williams Textbook of Endocrinology*, 7th ed. Philadelphia, Saunders, 1985, p 1018.
303. Van der Meulen JA et al: Possible mechanisms for cerebral oedema in diabetic ketoacidosis. *Lancet* Aug 8:306, 1987.
304. Varma SK et al: Hyperlactataemia in phenformin-treated diabetics. *Br Med J* 1:205, 1972.
305. Venna N, Sabin TD: Tonic focal seizures in nonketotic hyperglycemia of diabetes mellitus. *Arch Neurol* 38:512, 1981.
306. Vernon DD, Postellon DC: Nonketotic hyperosmolal diabetic coma in a child: Management with low-dose insulin infusion and intracranial pressure monitoring. *Pediatrics* 77:770, 1986.
307. Vignati L et al: Coma in diabetes, in Marble A et al (eds): *Joslins's Diabetes Mellitus*, 12th ed. Philadelphia, Lea & Febiger, 1985, p 526.
308. Wachtel TJ: The diabetic hyperosmolar state. *Clin Geriatr Med* 6:797, 1990.
309. Wachtel TJ et al: Predisposing factors for the diabetic hyperosmolar state. *Arch Intern Med* 147:499, 1987.
310. Wahren J et al: Splanchnic and leg exchange of glucose, amino acids, and free fatty acids during exercise in diabetes mellitus. *J Clin Invest* 55:1303, 1975.
311. Walker BB et al: Inhibition of insulin by acidosis. *Lancet* 2:964, 1963.
312. Walker BB et al: Clinical aspects of diabetic ketoacidosis. *Diabetes Metab Rev* 5:651, 1989.
313. Warburg E: Diabetic coma with uremia. *Acta Med Scand* 61:301, 1925.
314. Warburg E: Some cases of diabetic coma complicated with uraemia, and some remarks on the previous history of the diabetic coma. *Acta Med Scand* 61:301, 1925.
315. Warshaw AL et al: On the cause of raised serum amylase for diabetic ketoacidosis. *Lancet* 1:929, 1977.
316. Warshaw AL, Fuller AF: Specificity of increased renal clearance of amylase in diagnosis of acute pancreatitis. *N Engl J Med* 292:325, 1975.
317. Watkins PJ et al: Lactic acidosis in diabetes. *Br Med J* 1:744, 1969.
318. Watkins PJ et al: Ketonaemia in uncontrolled diabetes mellitus. *Br Med J* 4:522, 1970.
319. Welt LG: *Clinical Disorders of Hydration and Acid-Base Balance*. Boston, Little Brown, 1959, p 145.
320. West ML et al: Quantitative analysis of glucose loss dur-

ing acute therapy for hyperglycemic hyperosmolar syndrome. *Diabetes Care* 9:465, 1986.

321. West M et al: A renal mechanism limiting the degree of potassium loss in severely hyperglycemic patients. *Am J Nephrol* 8:373, 1988.
322. Whitehouse S et al: Mechanism of activation of pyruvate dehydrogenase by dichloroacetate and other halogenated carboxylic acids. *Biochem J* 141:761, 1974.
323. Wick AN et al: Tissue distribution of C^{14}-labelled beta-phenethylbiguanide. *Diabetes* 9:163, 1960.
324. Wildenhoff KE: Blood ketone body disappearance rate in diabetics and normals after rapid infusion of DL-3-hydroxybutyrate: Studies before and after diabetic treatment. *Acta Med Scand* 200:79, 1976.
325. Wildenthal K: The effects of acid-base disturbances on cardiovascular and pulmonary function. *Kidney Int* 1:375, 1972.
326. Williams RH, Palmer JP: Farewell to phenformin for treating diabetes mellitus. *Ann Intern Med* 83:567, 1975.
327. Wilson HK et al: Phosphate therapy in diabetic ketoacidosis. *Arch Intern Med* 142:517, 1982.
328. Winkler AW et al: Role of colloid and of saline in treatment of shock. *J Clin Invest* 25:220, 1946.
329. Winter RJ et al: Diabetic ketoacidosis: Induction of hypocalcemia and hypomagnesemia by phosphate therapy. *Am J Med* 67:899, 1979.
330. Wood MLB et al: Fatal rhabdomyolysis associated with hyperosmolar diabetic decompensation. *Diabetes Res* 8:97, 1988.
331. Woods HF, Alberti KGMM: Dangers of intravenous fructose. *Lancet* 2:1354, 1972.
332. Wright AD et al: Low-dose insulin treatment of hyperosmolar diabetic coma. *Postgrad Med J* 57:556, 1981.
333. Wyne V: Electrolyte disturbances associated with failure to metabolize glucose during hypothermia. *Lancet* 2:575, 1954.
334. Yalow RS et al: Plasma insulin and growth hormone levels in obesity and diabetes. *Ann N Y Acad Sci* 131:357, 1965.
335. Yen TT et al: Hepatic insensitivity to glucagon in ob/ob mice. *Res Commun Chem Pathol Pharmacol* 30:29, 1980.
336. Young E, Bradley RF: Cerebral edema with irreversible coma in severe diabetic ketoacidosis. *N Engl J Med* 276:12, 1967.
337. Zierler KL: Effect of insulin on potassium efflux from rat muscle in the presence and absence of glucose. *Am J Physiol* 198:1066, 1960.
338. Zierler KL, Rabinowitz D: Roles of insulin and growth hormone, based on studies of forearm metabolism in man. *Medicine* 42:385, 1963.
339. Zilva JF: The origin of the acidosis in hyperlactataemia. *Ann Clin Biochem* 15:40, 1978.
340. Zipf WB et al: Hypocalcemia, hypomagnesemia, and transient hypoparathyroidism during therapy with potassium phosphate in diabetic ketoacidosis. *Diabetes Care* 2:365, 1979.
341. Zonszein J, Baylor P: Diabetic ketoacidosis with alkalemia: A review. *West J Med* 149:217, 1988.

CHAPTER • 27

Renal tubular acidosis

Mitchell L. Halperin • Euan J.F. Carlisle • Sandra Donnelly • Kamel S. Kamel • Somkiat Vasuvattakul

Renal tubular acidosis (RTA) is a generic term encompassing a heterogeneous group of disorders in which there is metabolic acidosis with a normal value for the anion gap in plasma (12 ± 2 meq/liter) and a reduced rate of excretion of net acid (NAE). In these cases, the reduced rate of NAE is not due to renal insufficiency.

This chapter will be divided into three sections to highlight recent advances in the concepts surrounding this disease category. The *first section* summarizes relevant acid-base physiology and provides a historical perspective on RTA. The *second section* reviews the pathogenesis, clinical course, and treatment of the subtypes of RTA. The *third section* provides an approach to metabolic acidosis of renal origin, using the metabolic acidosis associated with toluene abuse as an illustrative example.

PHYSIOLOGY OF ACID-BASE METABOLISM (see Chap. 10)

ACID-BASE BALANCE: AN OVERVIEW

Hydrogen ions (H^+) are formed during normal intermediary metabolism. Some H^+ are removed when their conjugate base is converted to a neutral end product by oxidation (e.g., oxidation of citric acid, equation 1). In more detail (equation 1, lines *i–iv*), citric acid dissociates to yield 3 H^+ when it enters body fluids (equation 1, line *i*). These H^+ are removed from the body by combining with buffers such as bicarbonate, forming CO_2 which is exhaled (equation 1, line *ii*). At this point, there is a gain of citrate anions that is equal, in terms of meq/liter, to the deficit of titrated bicarbonate. Three mmol of bicarbonate will be regenerated when the organic anion, citrate $^{3-}$, plus 3 mmol H^+ are oxidized to water and CO_2 (equation 1, line *iii*). The H^+ that must be consumed during the oxidation of the citrate anion are formed when CO_2 is hydrated, yielding bicarbonate as a product (equation 1, line *iv*). Overall, there is no net gain of H^+ in this metabolic process.[1]

$$\text{Citric acid} \rightarrow \text{Citrate}^{3-} + 3\,H^+ \qquad (i)$$

$$3\,H^+ + 3\,HCO_3^- \rightarrow 3\,CO_2 + 3\,H_2O \qquad (ii)$$

$$\text{Citrate}^{3-} + 3\,H^+ + 4.5\,O_2 \rightarrow 6\,CO_2 + 4\,H_2O \qquad (iii)$$

$$3\,CO_2 + 3\,H_2O \rightarrow 3\,H^+ + 3\,HCO_3^- \qquad (iv)$$

$$\text{Citric acid} + 4.5\,O_2 \rightarrow 6\,CO_2 + 4\,H_2O \qquad (1)$$

Another way that H^+ can be removed is by excretion of an anion in the urine that binds a proton [called *titratable acid* (TA)], as in glomerular filtration of HPO_4^{2-} with subsequent excretion of $H_2PO_4^-$.

In contrast to the above, some H^+ are produced without a "partner anion" that helps to remove protons—that is, the anions cannot be metabolized to neutral end products or excreted as TA. An example of this type of acid is sulfuric acid, which is produced during the oxidation of sulfur-containing amino acids.

H^+ can be removed, or bicarbonate added, during metabolic processes when an organic anion is converted to a neutral end product (see Chap. 28). Examples of such metabolizable anions include the Na^+ or K^+ salts of citrate^{3-}, malate^{2-}, lactate$^-$, glutamate$^-$, and aspartate$^-$. As discussed below, another example is the synthesis and excretion of an anion plus the cation, NH_4^+, in the kidney.

ACID-BASE BALANCE: THE ROLE OF THE KIDNEY

Metabolism of a typical western diet yields a net of 70 mmol of H^+ per day.[2] These H^+ are removed by combining with bicarbonate to form CO_2, which is excreted by the lungs (equation 2). Lost bicarbonate is regenerated by the excretion of 70 mmol of net acid (Fig. 27-1).

$$H^+ + HCO_3^- \leftrightarrow H_2CO_3 \rightarrow CO_2 + H_2O \qquad (2)$$

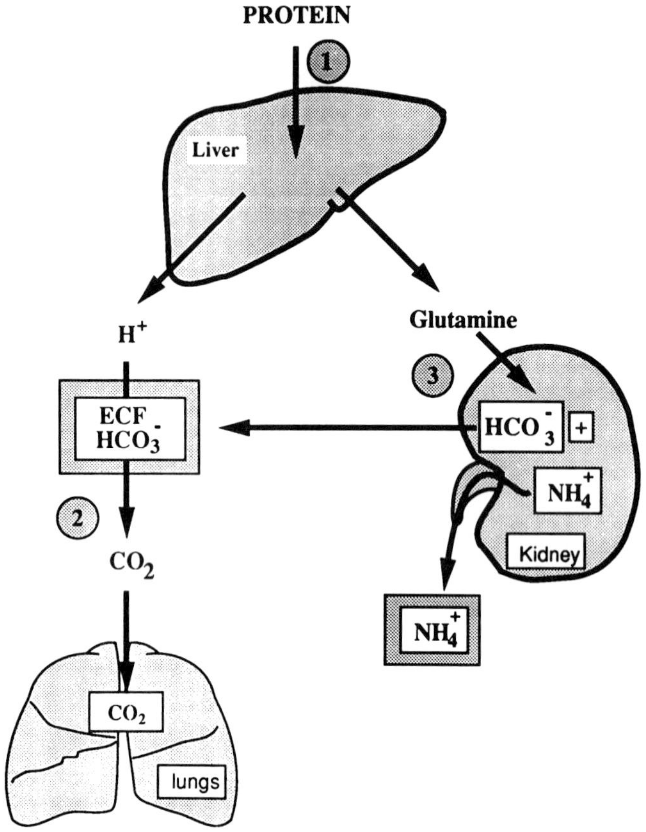

FIGURE 27-1 • Interplay of the liver, lungs, and kidney in acid-base balance. H^+ are formed in the liver, largely via the oxidation of certain amino acids. Glutamine, another amino acid, is partly synthesized in the liver. H^+ are consumed by combining with bicarbonate to form water and CO_2; the CO_2 is excreted by the lungs. The kidney synthesizes new bicarbonate during the metabolism of glutamine, so long as NH_4^+ is excreted in the urine.

The kidney stabilizes the concentration of bicarbonate in plasma in two ways. First, it must reabsorb all the bicarbonate filtered, a task largely performed by the proximal convoluted tubule. This step simply prevents any decrease in the existing concentration of bicarbonate in the plasma, but does not replenish any existing losses. To raise the content of bicarbonate in the body, new alkali must be generated by the kidney, by excretion of either TA (minor component) or NH_4^+ (major component). In this latter process, an organic cation, NH_4^+, is formed along with an organic anion when glutamine is metabolized in the cells of the proximal tubule. The organic anion is metabolized to such neutral end products as glucose or CO_2 and water, thereby generating bicarbonate in the kidney which is subsequently returned to the extracellular fluid (ECF). The NH_4^+ must be excreted in the urine to retain this new bicarbonate (Fig. 27-2). If the NH_4^+ were retained it would be delivered to the liver, where, in combination with the new bicarbonate, urea would be formed. The NH_4^+, therefore, must be excreted if this hepatic dissipation of newly synthesized bicarbonate is to be avoided (equation 3). We wish to emphasize that the excretion of NH_4^+ per se does not generate new bicarbonate[3]; it simply prevents its loss owing to events in the liver (equation 3 and Fig. 27-3).

$$2\ NH_4^+ + 2\ HCO_3^- \leftrightarrow \text{Urea} + CO_2 \qquad (3)$$

Much new information has been gathered concerning the excretion of NH_4^+. In the following section we shall address the physiology of the reabsorption of bicarbonate and the excretion of NH_4^+ in some detail, since both play important roles in the pathogenesis of various forms of RTA.

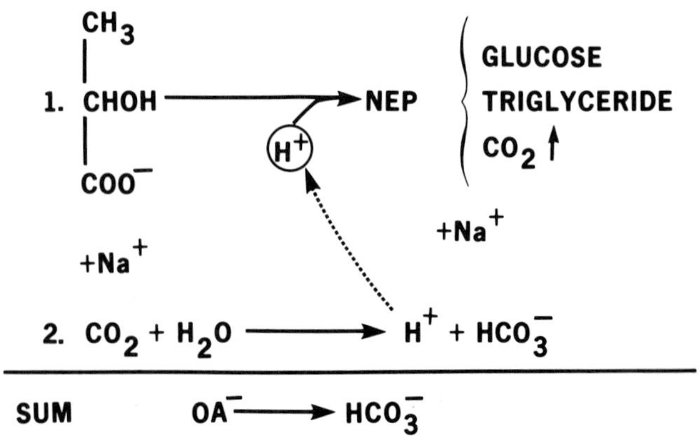

FIGURE 27-2 • Metabolism of an organic anion to yield bicarbonate. The chemical structure is lactate; it is present as the Na^+ salt. For details, see text.

FIGURE 27-3 • Making NH_4^+ an end product of renal metabolism. The cation, NH_4^+, is produced along with the anion 2-oxoglutarate^{2-} in the kidney during the metabolism of glutamine. To gain new bicarbonate, this NH_4^+ must be excreted in the urine (top portion of figure) so that it cannot return to the liver and be made into urea, consuming the new bicarbonate in the process (bottom portion of figure).

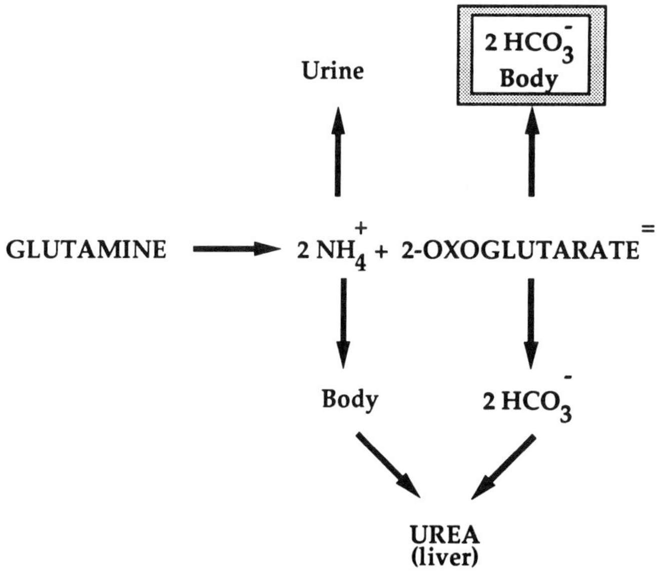

Reabsorption of bicarbonate

Normally, 80 to 90 percent of the filtered bicarbonate is reabsorbed in the proximal tubule (Table 27-1) (see Chap. 10). Secretion of H^+, largely by the *electroneutral Na^+/H^+ antiporter* in the luminal membrane, is thought to underlie this process.[4,5] This transport is driven by the favorable lumen-to-cell electrochemical gradient for Na^+, established by the activity of the *Na^+-K^+-ATPase* on the basolateral membrane of proximal cells (Fig. 27-4). To a lesser extent, H^+ may also gain entry into luminal fluid of the proximal tubule by secretion of protons by *H^+-ATPase*.[6,7] In the lumen, secreted H^+ combine with filtered bicarbonate to form carbonic acid, which is instantly converted to $CO_2 + H_2O$ by a reaction catalyzed by *carbonic anhydrase*, the active site of which faces the lumen. The activity of this carbonic anhydrase is critical to permit rapid rates of reabsorption of bicarbonate. Reabsorbed bicarbonate exits the proximal cell via the *electrogenic $Na(HCO_3)_3^{2-}$ symporter* located at the basolateral surface.[4] These processes must work in a tightly coordinated fashion to maintain a constant pH of the intracellular fluid (see Chap. 10). Factors that increase this reabsorptive process include an increased filtered load of bicarbonate, metabolic acidosis, angiotensin II, hypokalemia, hypercapnea, a low ECF volume, a low level of parathyroid hormone, a slow luminal flow rate, and hypercalcemia.[8]

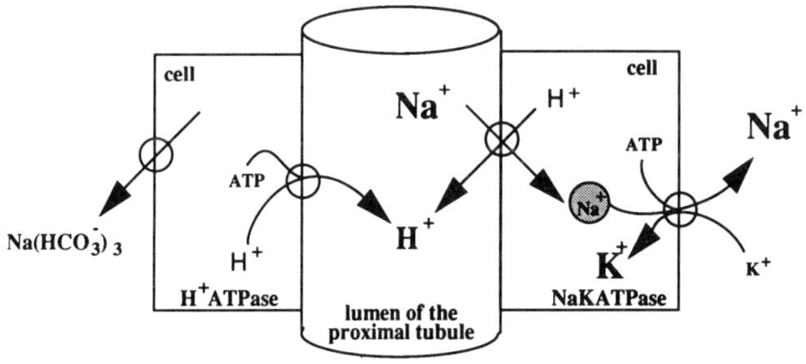

FIGURE 27-4 • Reclaiming bicarbonate in the proximal tubule. The two rectangles represent one proximal cell, drawn twice for simplicity of presentation. The Na^+-H^+ ion antiporter is in the luminal membrane, and the Na^+-K^+-ATPase is in the basolateral membrane; both are depicted in the cell on the right. By keeping intracellular Na^+ concentration very low, the Na^+-K^+-ATPase allows luminal Na^+ to enter the cell down its electrochemical gradient in exchange for H^+ produced in the cell with HCO_3^-. The cell on the left contains the other major transporters, the H^+-ATPase in the luminal membrane, and the bicarbonate exit step in the basolateral membrane.

TABLE 27-1 • Reabsorption of bicarbonate by the kidney

Nephron site	Share of total bicarbonate reabsorption (%)
Proximal tubule	85
Loop of Henle	10
Distal nephron	5

The 15 percent of filtered bicarbonate not recaptured proximally is reabsorbed by more distal nephron segments (Table 27-1). Most of this alkali is reabsorbed in the loop of Henle using a luminal Na^+-H^+ antiporter and a basolateral bicarbonate exit step. That alkali escaping proximal and loop reclamation is reabsorbed via a different mechanism in the more distal nephron. Secretion of H^+ by intercalated cells in the distal nephron is mediated by an *electrogenic H^+-translocating ATPase*[9,10] and by an electroneutral H^+- K^+-ATPase.[11,12] The exit of bicar-

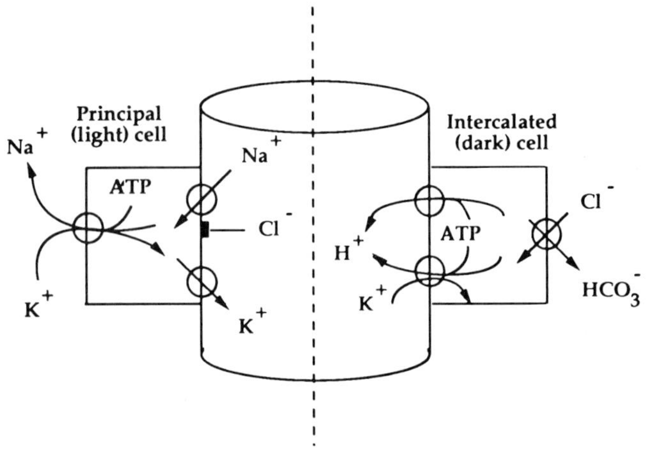

FIGURE 27-5 • Secretion of H^+ in the distal nephron. The energy required by the pumps to secrete H^+ is derived from ATP, whereas the exit step for bicarbonate does not require ATP (intercalated cell). In the cortex, a lumen-negative transepithelial potential difference generated by reabsorption of Na^+ by principal cells can augment the secretion of H^+ by intercalated cells.

bonate from these cells occurs via an electroneutral Cl^-/HCO_3^- exchange[13,14] (Fig. 27-5). The distal proton transport systems are not directly dependent on the reabsorption of Na^+. However, the rate of secretion of H^+ by the H^+-ATPase in the cortical collecting duct can be augmented by the lumen-negative transepithelial voltage generated by Na^+ reabsorption[15] (Fig. 27-5). The inner medullary collecting duct does not generate a lumen-negative transepithelial voltage,[16] rendering secretion of H^+ in this segment unresponsive to the delivery of Na^+.

Aldosterone plays an important role in the regulation of secretion of H^+ by the collecting duct. The hormone acts directly on the *intercalated cells* that secrete H^+.[17] It also stimulates the reabsorption of Na^+ by the *principal cells* of the cortical collecting duct, and hence increases the magnitude of the lumen-negative transepithelial voltage that favors the secretion of H^+.[16]

The cortical collecting duct reabsorbs and secretes bicarbonate, with the acid-base status of the animal determining which process dominates. These separate processes occur in two distinct subtypes of intercalated cells.[18] The precise physiologic role of secretion of bicarbonate and its importance to acid-base balance have yet to be ascertained.

Excretion of net acid

Excretion of titratable acid (TA)

About half of dietary phosphate is in the form of diester-phosphates, the metabolism of which yields HPO_4^{2-} and H^+.[3] The HPO_4^{2-} is then filtered by the kidney, titrated by secreted protons, and excreted as $H_2PO_4^-$. Thus, metabolism of diester-phosphates generates protons and the means for their quantitative excretion (Fig. 27-6). In contrast, when monoester-phosphates are metabolized, HPO_4^{2-} is added to the body without any H^+. Excretion of this portion of TA generates new bicarbonate and accounts for the excretion of approximately 15 mmol H^+ per day (half the TA).

Excretion of TA does not substantially increase in metabolic acidosis, because phosphaturia is not substantially increased in this setting. Given that the p*K* of $H_2PO_4^-$ is 6.8 at the ionic strength of plasma,[19] 90 percent will be titrated at pH 5.8.* Hence, lowering the pH of urine below 5.5 has little quantitative impact on the excretion of TA (a small amount of creatinine and organic anions are titrated in this range). Another point to consider is *where* TA is formed in the nephron. If the pH of fluid leaving the proximal convoluted tubule is 6.5, then two-thirds—or 20 of 30 mmol—of TA has already been formed at this site.[20] This leaves little additional TA to be generated when the filtrate pH is lowered below this value in the collecting duct.[3]

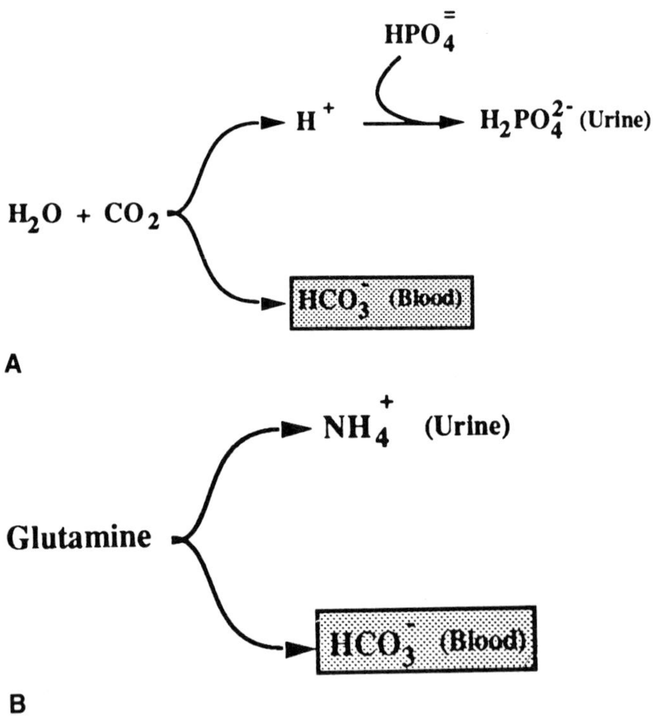

FIGURE 27-6 • Synthesis of new bicarbonate during net acid excretion. The respective mechanisms for the generation of new bicarbonate during the excretion of TA and NH_4^+ differ as shown.

* The p*K* is a measure of the strength with which the anion "holds" the H^+. Strong acids have low p*K*s, reflecting the ease with which they give up their H^+. The concentration of H^+ in the anion's environment must be high (i.e., the pH low) for the anion to retain protons. The p*K* of $H_2PO_4^-$ is 6.8, indicating that at pHs achievable in urine it will remain at least partially undissociated. The pK of SO_4^{2-} is very low (less than 2.0), indicating that even at a pH of 4.0 (the lowest achievable in urine) the SO_4^{2-} will remain almost totally dissociated.

Renal handling of NH_4^+

Before discussing the disorders characterized by a low rate of excretion of NH_4^+, we shall first provide an overview of ammoniagenesis, emphasizing areas where recent advances have been made.

Two major factors influence the rate of excretion of NH_4^+; its rate of production in the proximal tubule and its rate of transfer into the final urine.

PRODUCTION OF NH_4^+ NH_4^+ is produced during the metabolism of glutamine (Fig. 27-3). This metabolism occurs in the proximal tubule and is stimulated by chronic metabolic acidosis and hypokalemia, but a lag period of several days is required before very rapid rates of production can be achieved.[21] When 1 mmol of the amino acid is totally converted to CO_2, 27 mmol of ATP is formed; but only 7 mmol of ATP is formed when 1 mmol of glutamine is converted to glucose.[22] Since the catabolism of glutamine is inextricably linked to the production of ATP, and since accumulating ATP diffusely inhibits various key metabolic reactions, including glutamine catabolism, the nucleotide's concentration must be stabilized and precursors for its synthesis must be abundant if ammoniagenesis is to proceed. It follows that the rate of ammonia synthesis is also modified by the generation of ATP from fuels other than glutamine and the rate of utilization of ATP.[22]

Here we would like to stress the following points concerning the regulation of the production of NH_4^+:

Turnover of ATP No organ, cell, or organelle can synthesize more ATP than it uses to perform biological work, since the availability of ADP, the nucleotide's precursor, is extremely limited.[23] Therefore, production of ATP requires its continued utilization, which liberates the ADP needed for the resynthesis of ATP. The bulk of renal ATP is used to reabsorb filtered Na^+, which, in absolute terms, occurs primarily in the proximal tubule. The presence of the "metabolic machinery" to catabolize glutamine and the ability to limit ATP accumulation make this nephron segment critically important to ammoniagenesis. Experimental data illustrating this tight coupling of ammoniagenesis and the rate of turnover of ATP in proximal tubules of dogs with chronic metabolic acidosis are illustrated in Fig. 27-7.

During chronic metabolic acidosis, adaptive changes in enzyme activity allow the kidney to use glutamine in a preferential way while diminishing its use of other potential fuels. Nevertheless, the rate of synthesis of NH_4^+ is always less than that theoretically achievable by the available enzymes that convert glutamine to its end products, CO_2 and glucose.[21]

When renal mass declines, there are at least two reasons why the rate of excretion of NH_4^+ falls. First, it is

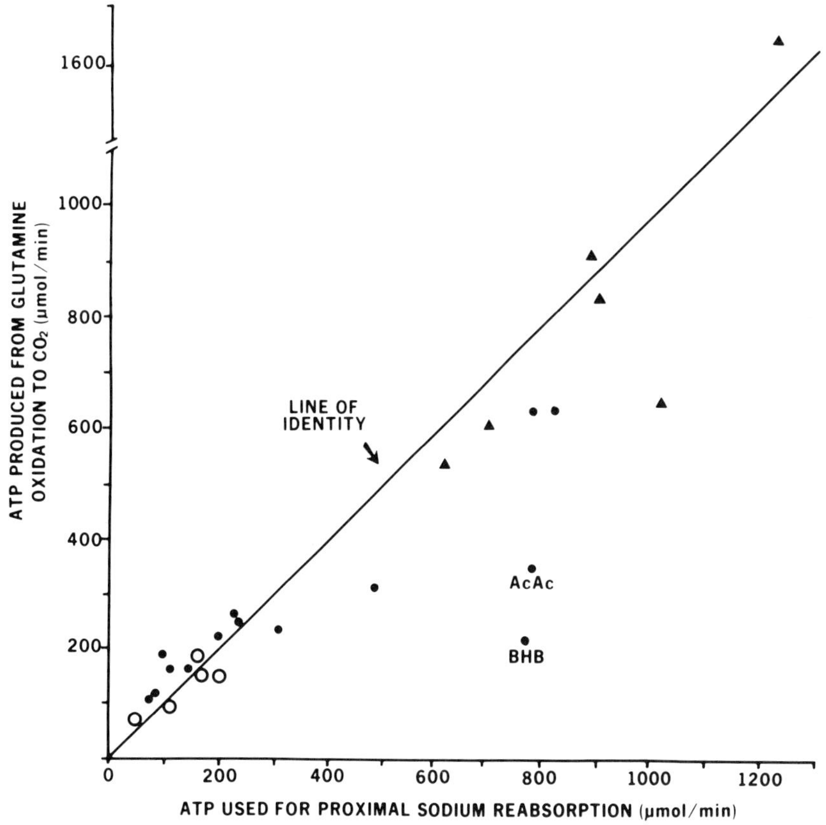

FIGURE 27-7 • Data to illustrate that energy considerations may influence the maximum rate of production of NH_4^+. ATP required for reabsorption of Na^+ in the proximal tubule is shown on the abscissa. The ordinate shows the quantity of ATP formed during the oxidation of glutamine. The solid line is the line of identity for these two parameters. The data from dogs infused with acetoacetate (AcAc) and β-hydroxybutyrate (BHB) do not fall on the line of identity.[22] (See text for details.)

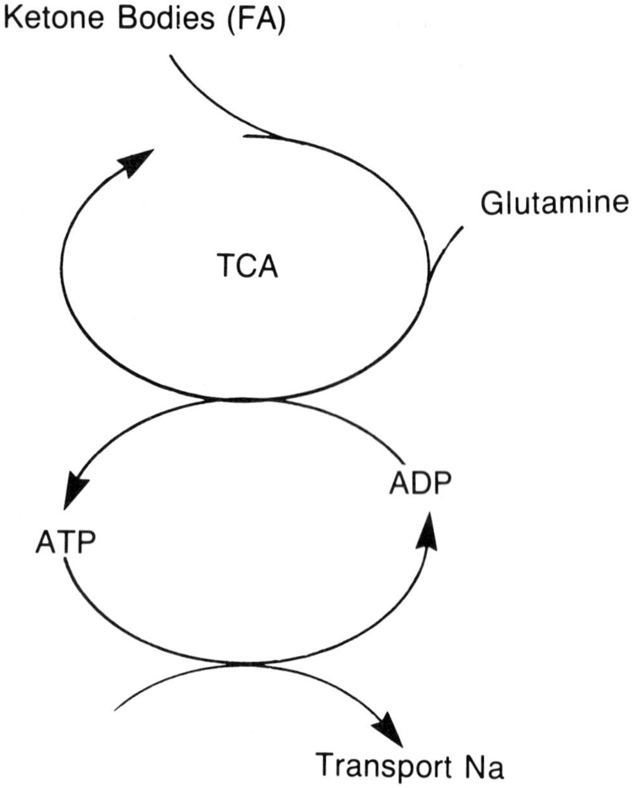

FIGURE 27-8 • Fuel competition and the production of NH_4^+. There are several fuels that can synthesize ATP in proximal tubular cells. During chronic metabolic acidosis, glutamine is the preferred fuel. (See text for details.)

possible that so much renal mass has been destroyed that the maximum capacity to produce NH_4^+ during chronic metabolic acidosis is reduced. Second, it is possible that there is still sufficient enzyme activity to catalyze the synthesis of NH_4^+, but that there is either a lack of substrate (glutamine) or the presence of an inhibitor of this pathway. Inhibition might result from a decrease in the rate of turnover of ATP in cells of the proximal tubule. This decrease in turnover of ATP could be the result of a reduced load of Na^+ to be reabsorbed, which may result from a decline in glomerular filtration rate (GRF).[24] Indeed, the activity of key enzymes (phosphate-dependent glutaminase) and the substrate, glutamine, is sufficient to yield higher rates of production of NH_4^+ in renal insufficiency.[21] Further, when the GFR was reduced acutely in dogs with chronic metabolic acidosis, the rate of production of NH_4^+ declined in parallel with the rate of reduction in GFR.[22] Finally, in most models with chronic metabolic acidosis, the rate of production of NH_4^+, when expressed per unit GFR (or per unit consumption of O_2), is similar despite very wide fluctuations in the GFR.[21]

Fuel competition Glutamine is only one of many fuels that the kidney can metabolize to yield ATP. Thus, at a constant rate of energy turnover, the rate of production of ATP from other fuels must be reduced so that more glutamine can be metabolized (Fig. 27-8). For example, if such non-ammonia-producing fuels as ketoacids,[25] or perhaps those delivered during total parenteral nutrition,[26,27] are oxidized in proximal tubule cells to produce ATP, they will compete with glutamine as potential substrates for the synthesis of ATP and, thereby, reduce the rate of production of NH_4^+.

Inhibition of production It is generally accepted that hyperkalemia inhibits the production of NH_4^+.[28] An alkaline pH of the proximal tubular cells may also inhibit the rate of ammoniagenesis; this has been suggested as a pathogenic feature of isolated proximal RTA.[29]

TRANSFER OF NH_4^+ TO THE URINE Almost all new bicarbonate formed in the kidney by ammoniagenesis is derived from the metabolism of glutamine. Net retention of this bicarbonate requires that NH_4^+ be excreted (see above) (Fig. 27-3). Our understanding of the mechanism of excretion of NH_4^+ has changed markedly over the past five years.[30] Diffusion trapping seems to play a less important role. The major nephron sites where NH_4^+ is added to and reabsorbed from the lumen of the nephron are illustrated in Fig. 27-9. The major components of the new picture of transfer of NH_4^+ into the urine can be summarized as follows:

1. The NH_4^+ formed in the proximal tubule epithelium is preferentially secreted into the lumen. The mecha-

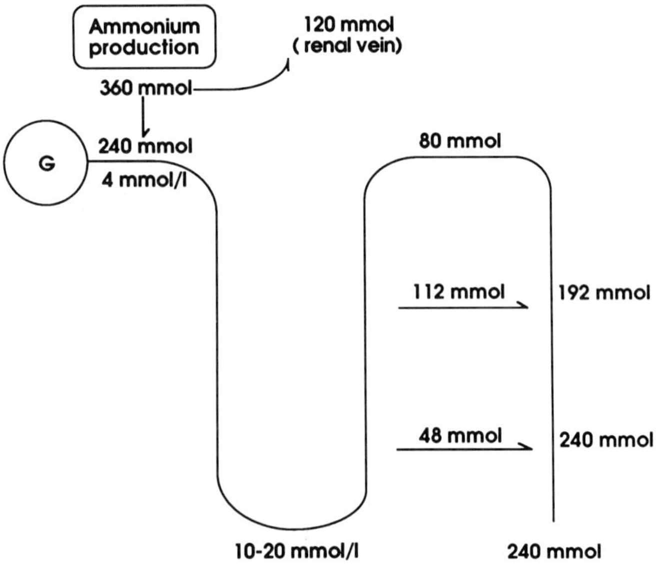

FIGURE 27-9 • Nephron sites where NH_4^+ is added to the urine in chronic metabolic acidosis. The data shown serve only to provide a rough quantitative estimate of events that may occur in a human being, over a 24-h period, with chronic metabolic acidosis. Production data were derived from experiments in dogs,[22] while transport data were derived from experiments in rats.[216] Approximately one-third of the NH_4^+ produced returned to the body via the renal vein. Two-thirds of the NH_4^+ that enters the loop of Henle is "shunted" to the collecting duct, mainly in the cortex.

nism remains uncertain; it is possible that NH_4^+ replaces H^+ on the Na^+-H^+ antiporter.[31,32]

2. Much of the NH_4^+ that enters the loop of Henle is reabsorbed, largely as a result of active transport in the thick ascending limb.[33,34] This reabsorption is likely to occur when NH_4^+ replaces K^+ on the Na^+, K^+, $(Cl^-)_2$ cotransporter.
3. Reabsorption of NH_4^+ by the thick ascending limb represents the "single effect" for a countercurrent multiplication process that results in accumulation of NH_3 in the renal medulla.[35]
4. Accumulation of NH_4^+ in the lumen of the collecting duct is vitally dependent on a favorable medullary interstitium-to-lumen concentration difference for the un-ionized NH_3. The concentration of NH_3 in the medullary interstitium is maximized by the following four forces: high rates of proximal tubule ammoniagenesis; reabsorption of NH_4^+ by the thick ascending limb[34]; a disequilibrium for NH_3 across the lùminal membrane of this nephron segment, owing to the low permeability for NH_3[36]; and an effective countercurrent system. Reduction of the concentration of NH_3 in the lumen of the collecting duct is largely achieved by the secretion of H^+, which converts NH_3 to NH_4^+.[37,38] The high medullary interstitial the low luminal concentrations of NH_3 augment its passive diffusion into the distal nephron. The facilitating effect of collecting duct acidity on diffusion of NH_3 is largely achieved when the pH of the filtrate approximates 6.0. Further declines in distal pH exert little further absolute effect on the concentration of NH_3 in the lumen (Table 27-2).

TABLE 27-2 • Excretion of NH_4^+: Relative importance of urinary pH and medullary NH_3

As the urinary pH falls from close to 6.0, it causes a large *relative* change in the concentration of NH_3 in the lumen (twofold per 0.3 unit ΔpH), but this translates into a small *absolute* change in the difference in concentration between the medullary interstitium and the lumen of the collecting duct. Hence, its effect on the rate of excretion of NH_4^+ becomes less important. Data were obtained in rats with chronic metabolic acidosis.[33] Values for the effect of a change in urinary pH were derived on the assumption that there was no fall in the concentration of NH_3 in the interstitium.

	Fall in pH of fluid in the lumen			
	NONE	0.3	0.6	0.9
$[NH_3]$ (μmol/liter)				
Interstitium	169	169	169	169
Lumen	84	42*	21*	11*
Difference	85	127	148	158
Difference in concentration of NH_3 to drive its diffusion (vs. none), expressed as a % rise	—	50	75	86

* Calculated fall in lumen $[NH_3]$ with the hypothetical fall in lumen pH.

APPLICATION OF THE PHYSIOLOGY OF ACID-BASE METABOLISM TO RTA

Historical perspective of RTA

The discovery that more NH_4^+ exited the kidney than was delivered to it established this organ's fundamental role in the production of NH_4^+.[37] The importance of glutamine as a precursor of NH_4^+ was not reported until 20 years later.[38] The critical role of the excretion of NH_4^+ in the maintenance of acid-base balance was actually recognized over 100 years ago. Walter[39] noted that the administration of relatively small amounts of acid rendered rabbits more seriously ill than dogs, and this is now attributed to the rabbit's low rate of excretion of NH_4^+.[40]

Later, high rates of excretion of NH_4^+ were observed to accompany metabolic acidosis, both in clinical[41] and in experimental settings.[42,43] Studies of the metabolic acidosis complicating renal failure emphasized the key role of an inadequate rate of excretion of NH_4^+.[44] The syndrome of "renal acidosis resulting from tubular insufficiency without glomerular insufficiency" was described by Albright.[43] This was later called "renal tubular acidosis" by Pines and Mudge.[45] The distinction between proximal and distal RTA was not recognized until the 1960s.[46,47]

In the late 1950s, perhaps as a result of the important study of Wrong and Davies,[48] investigators focused on the urinary pH rather than on the rate of excretion of NH_4^+ to diagnose distal RTA.[48-53] So prevalent was this viewpoint that it was claimed that a urinary pH greater than 5.5 was the sine qua non for the diagnosis.[49] As discussed below, under "Laboratory Tests for RTA," this is inappropriate on physiologic grounds. The key points in the issue are these:

1. The quantity of free H^+ excreted in the urine is trivial (less than 0.1 mmol/liter) even when its pH is 4.0.
2. The importance of a urinary pH less than 5.5 in augmenting the excretion of NH_4^+ during chronic metabolic acidosis is marginal (Table 27-2).
3. The rate of NAE hinges on the rate of excretion of NH_4^+, not on that of TA. In chronic metabolic acidosis, the increase in the concentration of NH_3 in the medullary interstitium is more important than the decrease in the concentration of NH_3 in the lumen in

permitting NH_3 to enter the lumen of the collecting duct. NH_3 entering the collecting duct lumen absorbs protons, which in turn tends to alkalinize the urine. Thus, failure to maximally reduce urinary pH may reflect *either* excessive availability of NH_3 or impaired distal H^+ secretion.[54-57]

To summarize, the excretion of NH_4^+ has been known since the beginning of this century to be the critical rectifying response of the kidney to metabolic acidosis. Jimenez-Diaz[58] wrote the following about the acidosis of Addison's disease in 1936: "This failure of ammonia formation (for me the essential fact upon which everything else depends) has been observed by others, but not sufficiently appreciated." We suggest that, unfortunately, this is true even today (Table 27-3).

Classification of RTA

The obvious way to subdivide disorders of NAE is to examine the rate of excretion of the various components of NAE (equation 4).

$$NAE = (NH_4^+ + TA) - HCO_3^- \qquad (4)$$

Impaired reclamation of filtered bicarbonate

The urine should not contain bicarbonate in the presence of metabolic acidosis. Bicarbonaturia in this setting defines a defect in reclaiming or recycling filtered alkali. When present, this defect is in the proximal tubule. It is usually the result of a decreased rate of secretion of H^+ by the Na^+/H^+ antiporter located on the luminal membrane. The disease is called *proximal RTA*; it is not a common disorder.

Impaired generation of new bicarbonate

IMPAIRED EXCRETION OF NH_4^+ After several days of metabolic acidosis, the urine should contain more than 200 mmol of NH_4^+ per day.[56,57] Patients who excrete less than 50 mmol of NH_4^+ per day during sustained metabolic acidosis clearly have "low NH_4^+ excretion disease."[59]

IMPAIRED EXCRETION OF TA This is virtually never a problem. It can occur only if there is a markedly reduced rate of excretion of H^+ acceptors—that is, a low rate of phosphaturia (e.g., ingestion of binders of phosphate in

TABLE 27-3 • Definition of distal renal tubular acidosis

Text Source	Definition
Nephrology	
Brenner, Rector (eds): *The Kidney* 1986[209]	Patients with hyperchloremic, hypokalemic metabolic acidosis that fail to lower the urine pH appropriately (< 5.5) during stable systemic acidosis.
Chan, Gill (eds): *Kidney Electrolyte Problems*, 1990[210]	Distal RTA is characterized by the inability of the distal nephron to maintain the hydrogen ion gradient that a normal nephron can.
Kokko, Tannen (eds): *Fluids and Electrolytes*, 1986[211]	Type I distal RTA is a clinical syndrome of hypokalemic hyperchloremic metabolic acidosis due to an impairment in distal nephron acidification that is manifested by an inability to lower urine pH in the presence of metabolic acidosis.
Schrier, Gottschalk (eds): *Diseases of the Kidney* 1988[212]	The characteristic manifestation of this entity is the inability to lower the urine pH maximally, even in the presence of severe systemic acidosis.
Internal Medicine	
Wyngaarden, Smith (eds): *Cecil Textbook of Medicine*, 1988[213]	Classic distal (type I) RTA is a hypokalemic, hyperchloremic metabolic acidosis due to a selective defect in distal acidification and is characterized by inability to lower the urine pH normally and, therefore, by subnormal urinary net acid excretion.
Kelley (ed): *Textbook of Internal Medicine*, 1989[214]	Distal RTA is characterized by hypokalemia and hyperchloremic metabolic acidosis in association with a urine that is less than maximally acidic.
Weatherall, Ledingham, Warrell (eds): *Oxford Textbook of Medicine*, 1987	This form of RTA is characterized by the inability to generate a normal minimum urinary pH even in the presence of severe systemic acidosis.
Stein (ed): *Internal Medicine*, 1987[215]	Distal RTA is usually characterized by reduced ammonium excretion despite metabolic acidosis, inappropriately high urine pH (usually > 6), and hypokalemia due to renal potassium wasting.

TABLE 27-4 • Classification of renal tubular acidosis

Type	Traditional classification	Pathophysiologic classification
I	Distal or classic RTA (hypokalemic type)	Low excretion of NH_4^+
II	Proximal RTA	Low reabsorption of HCO_3^-
III	Distal RTA with bicarbonate wasting	?
IV	Type IV RTA (hyperkalemic type)	Low excretion of NH_4^+
Other	Incomplete RTA (a problem for any classification)	Occult low NH_4^+ excretion or High availability of NH_3

patients with renal insufficiency). In the absence of renal failure, should the excretion of TA decline, acidosis will be prevented by a corresponding increase in the rate of excretion of NH_4^+. Since TA is a relatively minor contributor, in quantitative terms, to NAE during metabolic acidosis, we shall not consider it further in this chapter.

Classification of RTA; traditional view vs. modified view

The traditional approach to the classification of RTA is outlined in Table 27-4. Although this classification was based on pathophysiology for some of the major subclasses, the hard and fast separations have been modified somewhat. We prefer to return to a strict pathophysiologic classification. Accordingly, a modified classification of RTA based on pathophysiology is presented in Table 27-5; it is based on an NAE formula (equations 5 and 6) that contains all the identified components of renal acid-base handling.[60]

TABLE 27-5 • Classification of renal acidosis based on pathophysiology

Proximal (type II) RTA
Low NH_4^+ excretion disease—can be overt or occult
- Low NH_3 subtype due to:
  - Low production of NH_4^+ due to:
    - Lower turnover of ATP (low GFR)
    - Alkaline pH of proximal tubular cells (e.g., hyperkalemia and/or isolated proximal RTA)
    - Fuel competition (low availability of glutamine, high availability of fuels other than glutamine—e.g., TPN)
  - Low NH_3 in the renal medulla due to:
    - Medullary interstitial diseases
- Low H^+ in the lumen of the collecting duct due to:
  - Decreased secretion of H^+ into the collecting duct
    - H^+ pump problem
    - Voltage defect
    - Backleak

$$NAE = (NH_4^+ + TA) - (HCO_3 + \text{“}HCO_3\text{ equivalents”}) \quad (5)$$

$$NH_4^+ \leftrightarrow NH_3 + H^+ \quad (6)$$

We prefer not to use roman numerals (e.g., “type I”) or casual names (e.g., “classical”); rather, we use the pathophysiologic descriptive terms. We recognize the following groups:

- Disorders associated with reduced reabsorption of bicarbonate.
- Disorders associated with reduced excretion of NH_4^+.
- Disorders associated with increased excretion of “potential bicarbonate.”[61] This subgroup can be viewed as a type of RTA, but we have elected not to discuss it further in this chapter.

LABORATORY TESTS FOR RTA

Several factors must be considered interpreting laboratory tests related to the diagnosis of RTA. At some times, the purpose of testing is to establish the diagnosis; at others, tests are used to establish the underlying cause of RTA. We shall stress only the former aim in this section.

It is obvious that greater weight should be given to tests that reflect more important aspects of the disorder. To interpret results from these tests properly, values obtained must be compared to “expected values,” given the pathophysiologic stimulus. For example, a certain concentration of insulin in plasma may be normal during normoglycemia but abnormal during hypoglycemia. Accordingly, tests will be presented with emphasis on their importance for diagnosis, and will be interpreted in light of their expected values.

At times, it may be inconvenient or too expensive to perform tests with the greatest specificity. Therefore, we shall also describe tests that may be used for screening purposes to identify subjects who merit further study. Examples of the laboratory approach to RTA are depicted in Figs. 27-10, 27-11, and 27-12. These flow

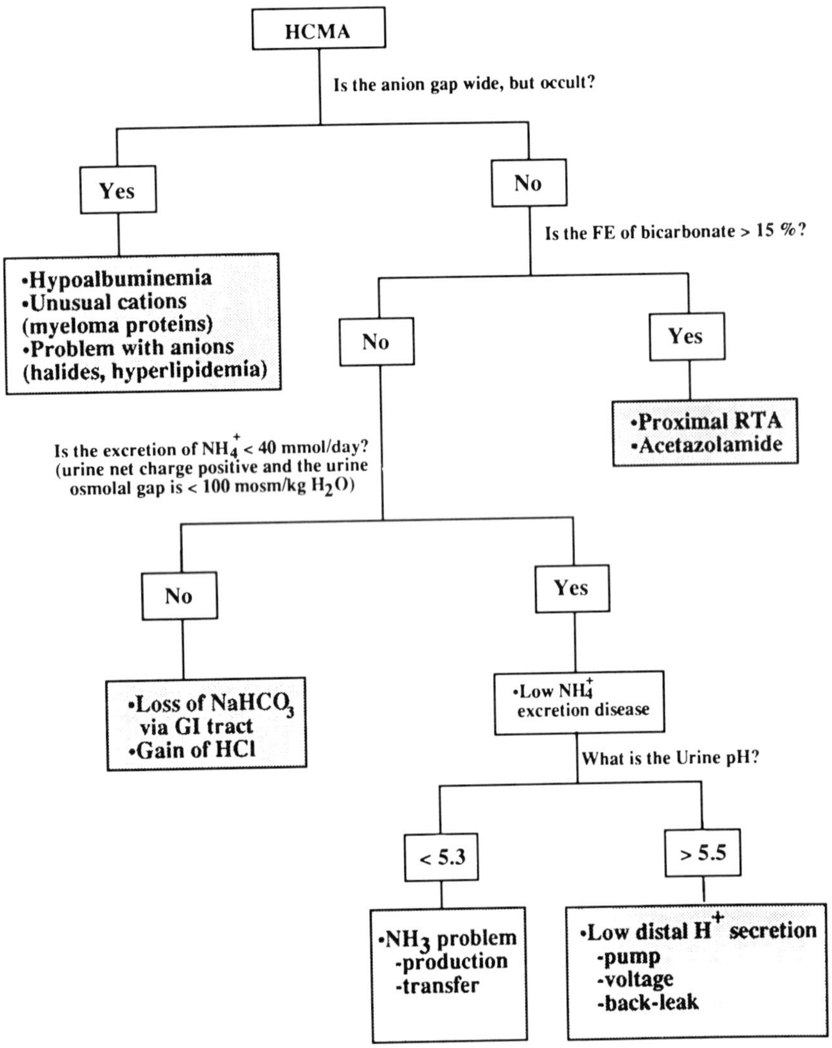

FIGURE 27-10 • Approach to the patient with hyperchloremic metabolic acidosis. The first step is to rule out an "occult" high-anion-gap type metabolic acidosis. The final diagnostic categories are shown in the shaded rectangles. The urinary osmolal gap is useful if NH_4^+ is excreted with an anion other than Cl^-. (FE = fractional excretion.)

charts deal with the clinical approach to three different clinical settings: a patient with hyperchloremic metabolic acidosis (HCMA); a patient who is suspected of having RTA, but who has normal acid-base parameters in blood; and a patient with a pH of urine that is consistently greater than 5.5.

Laboratory tests in a patient with HCMA

Reabsorption of bicarbonate

When this parameter is evaluated, the question asked is, *Can the kidney reabsorb bicarbonate at a normal rate, or is proximal RTA present?* To evaluate bicarbonate reabsorption, sufficient alkali must be given to induce bicarbonaturia without expanding the ECF volume too greatly; also, hypokalemia or hyperkalemia must be avoided. In practice, 2 to 3 mmol of sodium bicarbonate per kg body weight is administered intravenously, using a solution of 700 to 900 mmol/liter. The usual rate of infusion is 1 to 2 mmol per kilogram of body weight per hour; this rate should be increased to 1.5 to 2.5 mmol per kilogram of body weight per hour if the expected rate of rise in the concentration of bicarbonate in plasma (2 mmol/liter per hour) is not observed. The test is adequate if the concentration of bicarbonate in plasma rises to more than 25 mmol/liter and the pH of urine is less than 7.0. Hourly aliquots of urine are collected throughout the study (catheterization is not required); mid-point samples of blood, for measurements of bicarbonate and creatinine, are also obtained. This permits calculation of the fractional excretion of bicarbonate and the quantity of bicarbonate reabsorbed per liter GFR. The *fractional excretion of bicarbonate* is the percentage of filtered bicarbonate that escapes reabsorption. It may be calculated as shown in equation 7. Proximal RTA should be considered when, in the face of a normal plasma bicarbonate level, the fractional excretion of bicarbonate exceeds 15 percent. Should a patient reabsorb at least 24 mmol of bicarbonate per liter GFR (equation 8), proximal RTA

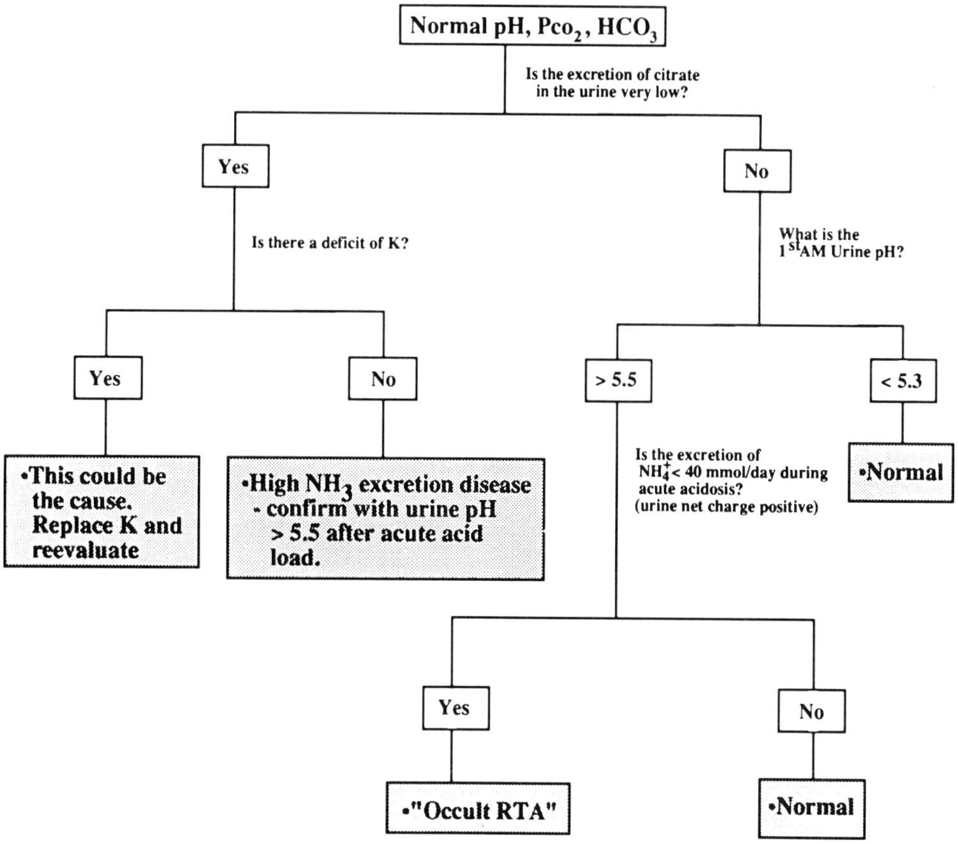

FIGURE 27-11 • Screening for the presumptive diagnosis of incomplete RTA. The starting point is the finding of normal acid-base parameters in plasma. The initial screening test is the rate of excretion of citrate (very low: <1 mmol/day). The final diagnostic categories are shown in the shaded rectangles. *Occult distal RTA*) is a term used to describe the syndrome in which the renal defect of distal RTA (low excretion of NH_4^+) is present in a subject who ingests a net load of alkali. To confirm the diagnosis of "high excretion of NH_3" with the urinary pH, see Fig. 27-10. ("First AM Urine" = first morning urine.)

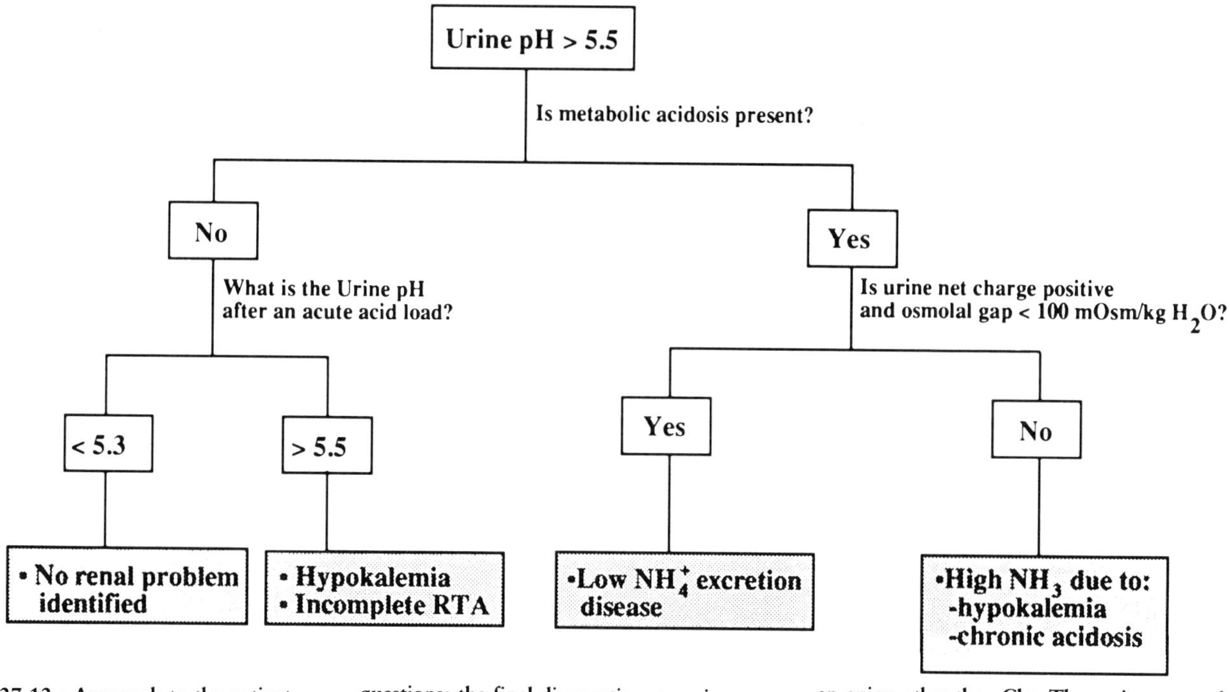

FIGURE 27-12 • Approach to the patient with a high (>5.5) pH of the first morning urine. The options to evaluate are shown as questions; the final diagnostic categories are shown in the shaded rectangles. The urinary osmolal gap is useful if NH_4^+ is excreted with an anion other than Cl^-. The options to evaluate between hypokalemia and incomplete RTA are shown in Fig. 27-10.

has been ruled out.[4] Potential pitfalls to avoid are conditions that increase the capacity to reabsorb bicarbonate (hypokalemia and a contracted ECF volume) and those that decrease it (hyperkalemia, an expanded ECF volume, or the presence of inhibitors of carbonic anhydrase).

$$FE_{HCO_3}\ (\%) = 100 \times ([HCO_3]urine \times [Creatinine]plasma)/([HCO_3]plasma \times [creatinine]urine) \quad (7)$$

$$\text{Reabsorption of bicarbonate (mmol/liter)} = \text{(Filtered-excreted bicarbonate)/GFR} \quad (8)$$

Excretion of NH_4^+

When this parameter is evaluated, the question asked is, *Can the kidney add a sufficient quantity of "new" bicarbonate to the body?* In a patient who has a low rate of excretion of NH_4^+, further investigations are required to delineate whether the problem is that of a low availability of NH_3 in the renal medulla or a low rate of secretion of H^+ in the collecting duct.

In chronic metabolic acidosis, the expected value for the rate of excretion of NH_4^+ is greater than 0.14 mmol/min (i.e., greater than 200 mmol/day).[56,57] Measurements of NH_4^+ may be made on a randomly collected or timed urine specimens. Values may be reported in terms of mmol of NH_4^+ excreted per unit time or per unit of creatinine, because the expected rate of excretion of creatinine is close to 0.2 mmol per kilogram of body weight per day. There is no reliable reference source to consult to evaluate the expected rate of excretion of NH_4^+ when the GFR is slightly to moderately reduced. Nevertheless, when the rate of NH_4^+ excreted in patients with normal GFRs is low enough to cause acidemia (i.e., less than 0.035 mmol/min or less than 50 mmol/day during chronic metabolic acidosis), the diagnosis of RTA is easy to confirm.

Since direct assays for urinary NH_4^+ are not routinely available in most hospital laboratories,[62] indirect methods must be used. The urinary net charge[63] and the urinary osmolal gap[64-66] provide a reasonable estimate of this excretion. In contrast, as discussed below, the pH of the urine does not provide an unambiguous indication of the rate of excretion of NH_4^+.

URINARY NET CHARGE The urinary net charge provides a convenient reflection of the rate of excretion of NH_4^+ in most settings.[63] It is calculated by subtracting the urinary concentrations of Na^+ and K^+ from that of Cl^-. Since the sum of the anions and the cations in the urine must be equal (in meq/liter), it follows that

$$Na^+ + K^+ + 2\,Ca^{2+} + 2\,Mg^{2+} + NH_4^+ = Cl^- + HCO_3^- + H_2PO_4^- + 2\,HPO_4^{2-} + 2\,SO_4^{2-} + \text{organic anions}$$

On a regular diet, the amounts of Ca^{2+} and Mg^{2+} excreted are small, and those of phosphate, sulfate, and organic anions are fairly constant.[67] The difference in rates of excretion of these anions and cations approximates 80 meq of anions per day.[67] Thus the urinary net charge ($Na^+ + K^+ - Cl^-$) reflects the excretion of NH_4^+ the one important urinary cation that is not usually measured. Further, this relationship between the urinary net charge and NH_4^+ is linear in patients with chronic metabolic acidosis, with a slope near unity.[63] Therefore, a random urine specimen with a pH less than 6.5 (equation 9) will hold if the pitfalls outlined below are avoided.

$$NH_4^+ = Cl^- - (Na^+ + K^+) + 80 \quad (9)$$

The urinary net charge should be used in the following way: If the concentration of Cl^- exceeds that of ($Na^+ + K^+$) in the urine, the concentration of NH_4^+ is high enough to exclude a "low NH_4^+ excretion disease" as the sole cause of the acidosis. In contrast, "low NH_4^+ excretion disease" may be present if the summed concentrations of Na^+ and K^+ exceed that of Cl^- in the urine. Further studies may now be indicated to estimate the concentration of NH_4^+ in the urine. This can be obtained directly or by the urinary osmolal gap (see below).[64-66]

There are two potential pitfalls to avoid when evaluating the urinary net charge. First, there are clinical situations where the urine contains an appreciable amount of unusual anions; this will change the normal cation–anion difference from 80 (equation 9) to some other value. The presence of additional unmeasured anions will lead to an underestimation of the excretion of NH_4^+, since NH_4^+ is being excreted with an anion other than Cl^-. This situation may occur with ketonuria (fasting or diabetic ketoacidosis), the excretion of certain drugs (e.g., salicylates or penicillin), or the excretion of unusually large quantities of anions such as hippurate (during toluene sniffing[68]). In contrast, the concentration of anions other than Cl^- decreases when the volume of urine is very large, thereby diminishing the "constant" value of 80 (equation 9). Hence, equation 9 should not be employed in an unmodified form when polyuria is present.†

OSMOLAL GAP IN THE URINE[64-66] The urinary osmolal gap is the difference between the measured osmolality and that calculated from the sum of urea, glucose, and twice the sum of Na^+ and K^+ (all in mmol/liter) in the urine. This test reflects the presence of an NH_4^+ salt. Hence, it provides information superior to the urinary net charge, which reflects only the NH_4^+ excreted with Cl^-.

† While the simple formula for the urinary net charge is usually adequate, one can, if one desires—and especially in the case of a patient with polyuria—gain a closer approximation of the rate of excretion of NH_4^+ in mmol/day using the following formula concentrations in meq/liter:

$$\text{Excretion } NH_4^+ = 0.8\,[Cl^- - (Na^+ + K^+)] \times \text{urine volume (liters/day)} + 80$$

The concentration of NH_4^+ is half the urinary osmolal gap if the anions in the urine are monovalent. A value for the urinary osmolal gap that exceeds 100 reflects the presence of more than 50 mmol of NH_4^+ per liter of urine.

URINARY pH It is important to put into perspective the role played by a low pH of the urine in the excretion of net acid. The lowering of urinary pH is considered a function primarily of the distal nephron. First, the lowest possible pH of the urine can account for only a trivial excretion of protons. For example, the excretion of 2 liters of urine at pH 4.0 translates into the elimination of only 0.2 mmol of H^+. Quantitatively, this represents just 0.25 percent of the normal daily net production of H^+. If it does not account for significant amounts of excretion of H^+, what then is the implication of a low urinary pH? Two commonly held views of its importance are as follows:

First, a low urinary pH is thought necessary to titrate HPO_4^{2-} and other buffers in urine and thereby help excrete a substantial fraction of the daily acid load (70 mmol). The pH of the fluid in the lumen at the most distal portion of the proximal tubule accessible to micropuncture is approximately 6.8.[20] Because the pK of $H_2PO_4^-$ is also 6.8,[19] the Henderson-Hasselbalch relationship requires that more than half of the filtered HPO_4^{2-} remaining in the tubule have been converted to $H_2PO_4^-$. Thus, if the final pH of the urine could be lowered only to 6.8, approximately 15 mmol of H^+ would still be excreted. The cells of the proximal convoluted tubule synthesize virtually all the NH_4^+ produced by the kidney. This cation enters the proximal lumen directly, and since its pK is greater than 9.0, only trace amounts of nonprotonated NH_3 can exist at pH 6.8. Thus, the overwhelming amount of buffer accessible to the urine has already been titrated proximally, thereby minimizing the distal nephron's further role in the titration process.[3]

The second alleged value of a low urinary pH is that it ensures the excretion of a large percentage of the NH_4^+ that was produced in the cells of the proximal tubule. It has been argued that secretion of H^+ in the distal nephron enhances the efficiency of the excretion of NH_4^+. A lower urinary pH diminishes the concentration of NH_3 in the lumen of the collecting duct and thereby favors the net addition of NH_3 and its excretion as NH_4^+. This impact of progressive lowering of the pH of the urine becomes quantitatively less significant at values below 6.0 (Table 27-2). Nonetheless, it is important to discern why this capacity to achieve a low pH in urine is lost in some patients and what role it may play in the natural history of the renal tubular disease.

It should be apparent that if the *capacity* to secrete protons in the distal nephron were limited, regardless of how many H^+ acceptors (NH_3) were made available, net acid excretion must be reduced for want of the new H^+ needed for their conversion to NH_4^+. By limiting net acid excretion to values less than daily acid production, a *rate-limited* (i.e., low capacity) distal H^+ secretory defect would cause H^+ balance to become positive and overt distal RTA to emerge. The clinical scenario that would evolve after the acute onset of rate-limited distal RTA would be as follows: Reduced secretion of H^+ in the distal nephron would diminish net acid excretion, which, in turn, would induce positive balance for H^+. Even though worsening acidosis would stimulate ammoniagenesis,[69] failure to provide protons distally to titrate the burgeoning amounts of the NH_3 could sustain low excretory rates of NH_4^+ and, thereby, net acid.

Notwithstanding, another type of distal proton secretory defect is possible. In this setting the distal capacity to secrete protons is potentially normal as long as the electrochemical gradient for H^+ remains favorable and as long as secreted protons do not leak back from lumen to cell to blood. In this setting, if more H^+ acceptors (NH_3) are present in the lumen, a restriction imposed on net secretion of H^+ by a low luminal pH would no longer be present. Said another way, the enhanced presence of NH_3 in the lumen would absorb and thereby minimize back diffusion of secreted protons, sustaining a favorable concentration gradient for the continued secretion of protons. The clinical scenario emerging after the acute onset of gradient-limited distal RTA would be as follows: Decreased H^+ secretion would transiently develop in the wake of a *gradient-limited secretory defect.* The resulting decrease in net acid excretion would cause a slight fall in serum bicarbonate concentration. The hypobicarbonatemia, in turn, would stimulate ammoniagenesis. The resulting increase in distal NH_3 delivery would then reestablish proton secretion, which allows net acid excretion to normalize, thereby reestablishing zero H^+ balance.

To summarize, in itself, achievement of a very low pH of urine (less than 5.5) endows the host with only minor physiologic advantages. Indeed, very low values for the pH of the urine are not required to achieve very high rates of excretion of $NH_4{}^+$.[69] By itself, impaired lowering of the urine pH due to a gradient-limited distal H^+ secretory defect should not alter serum electrolytes to a major degree. In contrast, a reduced rate of excretion of $NH_4{}^+$ and hypobicarbonatemia would ensue if there is a failure to lower the pH of the urine due to a capacity, rather than a gradient limit to the net secretion of H^+.

In a patient with metabolic acidosis, the inability to lower the pH of the urine below 5.3 has been considered by many authors as central to the diagnosis of distal RTA (Table 27-3). Implicit in this approach is the notion that one can deduce a value for the rate of excretion of NH_4^+ from the pH of the urine. The question, however, is *Does the urine pH provide the clinician with unambiguous information about the rate of excretion of* NH_4^+*?*[55] There are two critical, but rather opposing, sets of data that one

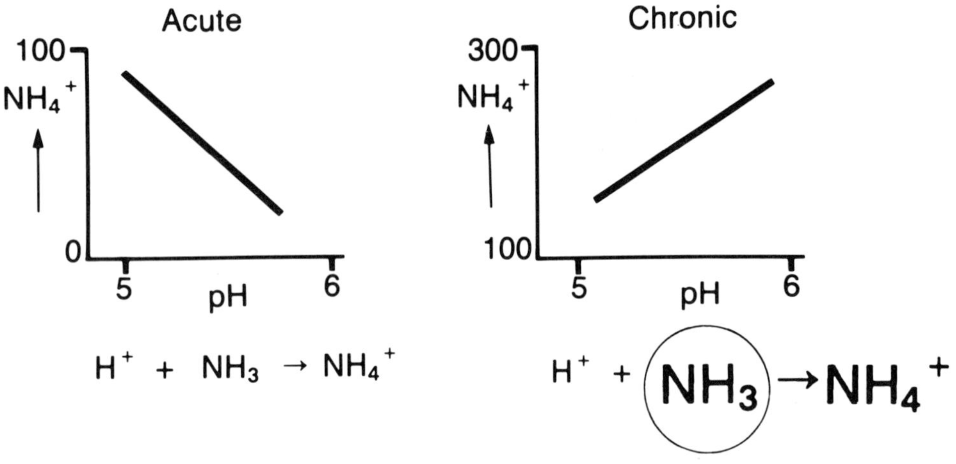

FIGURE 27-13 • Effect of urinary pH on the excretion of NH_4^+. In acute acidosis (left-hand panel), the rate of production of NH_4^+ is increased only to a small extent. The excretion of NH_4^+ is higher when the urinary pH is *lower*, because the increased $[H^+]$ traps more NH_3 in the lumen as NH_4^+. Thus the secretion rate of H^+ exceeds that of NH_3.

In chronic acidosis (right-hand panel), both the H^+ secretory rate and the availability of NH_3 are increased. The increase in NH_3 is due to augmented ammoniagenesis and the trapping of ammonia in the medulla; this is relatively larger than the increment in H^+ secretion. Thus, the rate of excretion of NH_4^+ is increased in conjunction with a *higher* urinary pH.

has to consider to answer this question (Fig. 27-13). When an *acute* acid load is given, the increase in the secretion of H^+ by the distal nephron is not matched by a rise in the availability of NH_3, because of a time lag required to augment renal ammoniagenesis.[69] Hence, *acutely* the pH of the urine is low—characteristically less than 5.3.[48] In contrast, during *chronic* metabolic acidosis, the excretion of NH_4^+ is high. Increased availability of NH_3 in the renal medullary interstitium and the collecting duct reduces the concentration of free H^+ in the urine, and the pH of the urine approximates 6 (Fig. 27-14, line 3). Clearly, the pH of the urine is not a reliable index of the rate of excretion of NH_4^+; hence it should not be the sine qua non for diagnosing distal RTA, which is truly a "low NH_4^+ excretion disease."

The urinary pH is, however, useful once one knows that a patient has metabolic acidosis with a low rate of excretion of NH_4^+. A low urinary pH in this setting suggests a problem with adding NH_3 to the urine (low NH_3 in the renal medullary interstitium—Table 27-5), whereas a high urinary pH suggests that there is a problem adding H^+ to the collecting duct lumen (low distal H^+ secretion subtype—Table 27-5 and Fig. 27-15).

The urinary pH can also provide valuable information in the following settings. It is useful to detect bicarbonate in the urine. Bicarbonate is virtually absent when the pH is less than 6, and is greater than 10 mmol/liter when the pH of urine is greater than 7. Very high concentrations of bicarbonate (i.e., greater than 100 mmol/liter) are not found until the pH of the urine is greater than 7.7.

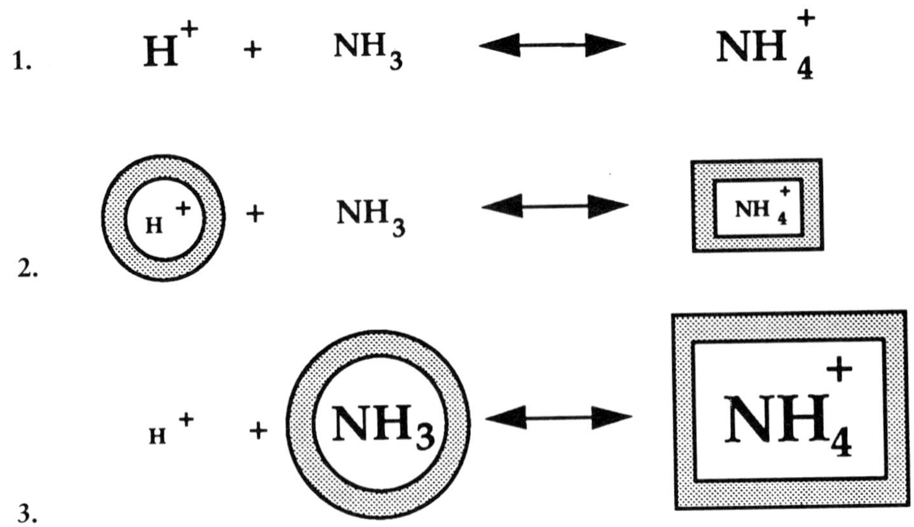

FIGURE 27-14 • Explanation of the high urinary pH. The situation in a normal individual is depicted in line 1. Underlying problems in lines 2 and 3 are shown in the circles; their effects on the rate of excretion of NH_4^+ are shown in the rectangles. In a subject with a reduced rate of secretion of H^+ in the distal nephron, the pH of the urine is high and the excretion of NH_4^+ is low (line 2). In contrast, when the availability of NH_3 is very high, the pH of the urine is also high, but the rate of excretion of NH_4^+ is also high (line 3).

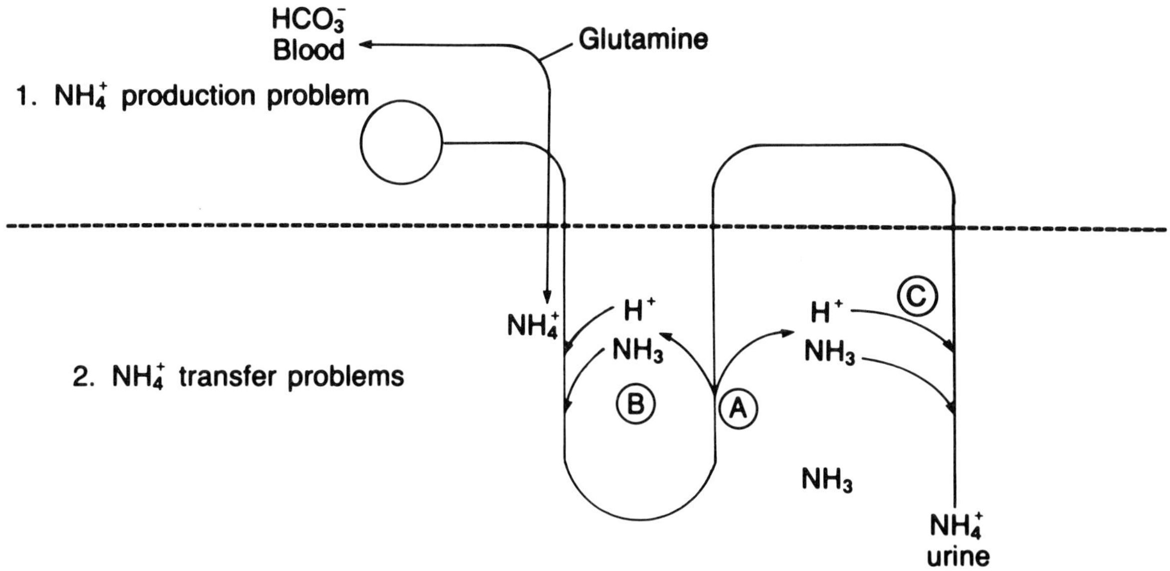

FIGURE 27-15 • Analysis of low excretion of NH_4^+. REDUCED NH_4^+ PRODUCTION: The two major causes are the energy constraints imposed by a low GFR, and hyperkalemia-induced inhibition of ammoniagenesis. REDUCED TRANSFER OF NH_4^+ INTO THE URINE: A low concentration of NH_3 in the medullary interstitium is the main determinant. It may be caused by reduced reabsorption of NH_4^+ in the loop of Henle secondary to hyperkalemia or possibly to aldosterone deficiency (see figure); by impaired countercurrent system due to medullary interstitial disease (see figure); or by impaired trapping of NH_3 in the collecting duct from the various causes of a low rate of H^+ secretion (see figure).

The pH of the urine is also useful in diagnosing *incomplete RTA* (Fig. 27-14, line 3) (see "Clinical Example" below for further discussion).

Laboratory tests in a patient who does not have HCMA

Urinary P_{CO_2} *in alkaline urine*

The difference in P_{CO_2} between urine and blood (U−B P_{CO_2}) during a bicarbonate diuresis was originally proposed as a diagnostic test of distal nephron H^+ secretion in patients with distal RTA.[70] The generation of a high P_{CO_2} in the inner medullary interstitium during a bicarbonate diuresis is caused by the secretion of protons into bicarbonate-rich tubular fluid with subsequent slow dehydration of carbonic acid so generated. The latter process is slow because, unlike the proximal tubule, the distal nephron lacks luminal carbonic anhydrase (Fig. 27-16). While the U-B P_{CO_2} during bicarbonate loading has been criticized on technical and physical-chemical grounds,[71,72] micropuncture studies by DuBose and coworkers[73,74] have demonstrated that the magnitude of the increase in urinary P_{CO_2} is related to the secretion of protons in the distal nephron with the generation of an acid-disequilibrium pH. These observations provide information concerning the pathophysiology of various experimental models of distal RTA. It should be appreciated that the P_{CO_2} of the urine provides the same information as the U-B P_{CO_2} in normocapnic subjects. Only in patients with respiratory acid-base disorders does the P_{CO_2} of the urine have to be interpreted in light of P_{CO_2} of the blood; in this case, there is still some doubt as to which P_{CO_2} one should use for this correction.[75,76]

This test is performed as follows: The patient is given a quantity of sodium bicarbonate sufficient to raise urinary pH to greater than 7.4. The dose of bicarbonate

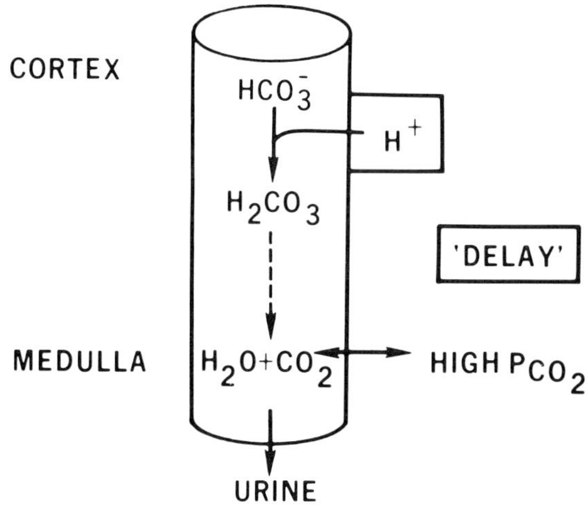

FIGURE 27-16 • The urinary P_{CO_2}. The barrel-shaped structure is the collecting duct. The square represents an intercalated cell in the cortex. Since there is no luminal carbonic anhydrase, the H_2CO_3 formed in the cortex descends into the medullary collecting duct. Sufficient time has elapsed for spontaneous dehydration to CO_2; this gas is in diffusion equilibrium with medullary structures.

required depends on the degree of acidosis; suffice it to say that enough bicarbonate must be administered to achieve an alkaline urine. The first alkaline urine sample is discarded to avoid mixing this urine with previously formed acid urine, which would generate P_{CO_2} in the urinary bladder. Subsequent urine samples are collected with as little agitation of the specimen as possible. The smaller the surface area–to–volume relationship in the container, the more accurate the readings will be. It is not necessary to catheterize the patient to obtain this sample of urine, nor is it necessary to collect the sample under oil if there is no delay in transferring it to a sealed blood gas syringe. By taking care to obtain the sample in the syringe from the *bottom*, rather than the top, of the sample of urine, one avoids the potential error of obtaining an aliquot where there has been significant loss of CO_2 to the air.

Patients with normal rates of distal H^+ secretion should have a urinary P_{CO_2} that is greater than 65 mmHg or a U-B P_{CO_2} that is greater than 25 mmHg. In contrast, patients with certain types of distal RTA (H^+ pump defect or voltage defect) have subnormal values, while those with a gradient or back-leak type of defect (e.g., caused by amphotericin B) have normal values (see below).

Urinary citrate

Changes in systemic acid-base balance cause profound alterations in the rate of excretion of citrate.This rate is increased following a bicarbonate load, whereas it falls to very low levels during most forms of metabolic acidosis.[77] These changes in excretion of citrate may reflect the pH of the proximal convoluted tubule cell.[78,79] While mechanisms have yet to be established, it is possible that a bicarbonate load alkalinizes intracellular pH and inhibits the oxidation of citrate by decreasing its entry into mitochondria on the tricarboxylate carrier.[80] As the intracellular concentration of citrate rises, its rate of cellular uptake diminishes and its rate of excretion increases. The opposite sequence of events occurs in metabolic acidosis. This might also explain the decrease in citraturia during hypokalemia, which acidifies cell pH.[48]

Recent studies, however, have provided a different explanation for the observed changes in the excretion of citrate during metabolic acidosis. Citrate is reabsorbed in the proximal tubule via an Na^+-linked electrogenic transporter that preferentially transports the dicarboxylate form of citrate (citrate^{2-}).[81] The pH dependency of citrate excretion may then be due to changes in the concentration of citrate^{2-} in the lumen. Therefore, the change in the rate of excretion of citrate may reflect changes in luminal, rather than intracellular, pH.

There are certain disease states that break the above "rules" on acid-base status and the excretion of citrate. Patients with the isolated form of proximal RTA have an appreciable degree of citraturia despite the presence of metabolic acidosis.[82] To explain this discrepancy, Halperin and coworkers[29] suggested that the underlying defect in this case might be an alkaline pH of proximal tubule cells. In contrast, patients with incomplete RTA have hypocitraturia despite the absence of systemic acidosis.[83-86] Donnelly and coworkers[87] have suggested that an acidic pH in the cells of the proximal tubule, independent of the prevailing systemic pH, may be the underlying defect to explain this latter discrepancy.

Capacity to excrete NH_4^+

There is no value in giving an acid load to most patients who have metabolic acidosis. In the absence of metabolic acidosis, however, one may wish to examine the capacity to excrete NH_4^+ in the urine. Ideally, the patient should receive enough acid (0.1 g NH_4Cl per kilogram of body weight in three divided doses with meals) to sustain a metabolic acidosis for about 5 to 7 days; at the end of that period the rate of production of NH_4^+ should be assessed. Since one can measure only rates of excretion, expected values should approximate 200 mmol of NH_4^+ per day in the absence of any renal lesion.[56,57] Nevertheless, there are many reasons why such a test is of only academic value: excretion, rather than production, of NH_4^+ is measured; the load of acid is not well tolerated; and the test is potentially dangerous if not well supervised. These problems notwithstanding, all other tests of ammoniagenic potential are far from ideal.

The acute NH_4Cl loading test[48] (or other similar tests, such as calcium chloride loading) does not reflect the capacity to produce NH_4^+ by the kidney, owing to the lag period before this production begins. This test measures the ability to transfer preformed NH_4^+ to the urine. To perform this test, a subject consumes 0.1 g NH_4Cl per kilogram of body weight over 60 min. Venous blood is drawn every 2 h, and hourly urine samples are examined. The end point, a low pH of the urine, may reflect either a changed rate of secretion of H^+ in collecting duct cells that exceeds the supply of NH_3, or normal secretion of H^+ in the face of a low availability of NH_3. Hence, it does not provide information that is sufficiently valuable to be a first-line test in the initial diagnosis of distal RTA (Fig. 27-14).

Other tests

Some authors recommend that phosphate, sulfate, or furosemide be given prior to measurement of the pH or P_{CO_2} of the urine.[50] We do not find these tests particularly helpful, but data from them may be of some use for certain research purposes.

SPECIFIC DISORDERS

PROXIMAL RTA

Definition

The two major features required to establish the diagnosis of proximal RTA are HCMA and a subnormal rate of reabsorption of bicarbonate.[51,88]

Proximal RTA may occur as an isolated entity[89] or as part of a diffuse proximal tubule reabsorptive defect (Fanconi syndrome).[90] The Fanconi syndrome is characterized by abnormalities in the excretion of glucose, phosphate, amino acids, organic anions, and carnitine[91] in addition to bicarbonate.

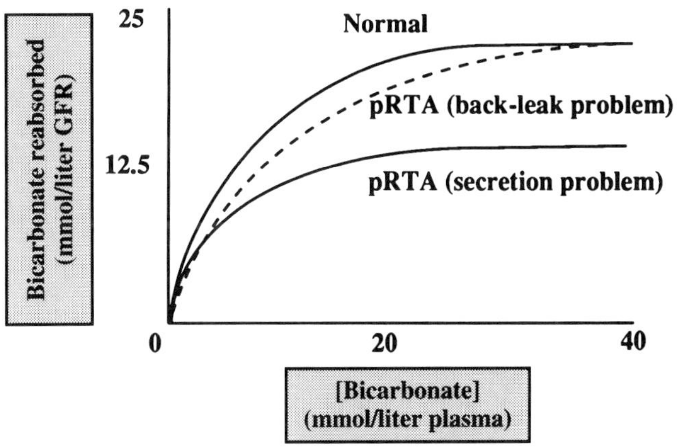

FIGURE 27-17 • Kinetics of the reabsorption of bicarbonate. The data from Table 27-6, for both models of proximal RTA, are presented in graphic form. (For details, see Table 27-6.)

Pathophysiology

Although almost all the transport events in the proximal tubule are linked to Na^+, proposed mechanisms must explain the difference in the pattern of solute wasting observed in Fanconi syndrome and in isolated proximal RTA.

A critique of the proposed pathogenesis of the Fanconi syndrome

If the Fanconi syndrome is present, all the transport events linked to Na^+ in the proximal tubular cell are affected.[90] Explanations of the pathophysiology fall into two major subgroups: those that cite increased backleak as the cause, and those that cite decreased reabsorption of key metabolites from the filtrate.[92]

BACKLEAK PROPOSALS These theories suggest that if the concentration of a given metabolite is lower in the lumen of the proximal tubule than in blood, back-diffusion from blood to lumen will diminish net reabsorption. To test this hypothesis, the kinetics of reabsorption should be examined. When this is done, this theory seems unlikely as a cause of the Fanconi syndrome (Appendix 1 and Fig. 27-17).

MODELS FOR DECREASED REABSORPTION Two major defects have been suggested as the cause of impaired reabsorption of all metabolites linked to that of Na^+: low levels of ATP in proximal cells,[93-96] and diminished activity of the Na^+K^+ATPase in proximal cells.[96]

A limited amount of ATP Many of the animal models of proximal RTA require that various inhibitors of energy metabolism be infused (e.g., maleic acid—Fig. 27-18). These models are all characterized by decreased levels of ATP in cells of the proximal tubule.[93-96] There are, however, conceptual problems with this formulation. If a limited quantity of ATP were the basis of the Fanconi syndrome in human beings, these subjects would have to live very close to their threshold for reabsorbing Na^+ while performing many vital biosynthetic functions. Said another way, they would not have enough ATP to reabsorb Na^+ when the GFR rose or if biological work increased for any reason in the kidney. In quantitative terms, if the GFR rose 25 percent after a meal (from 6 to 7.5 liters per hour), an extra 225 mmol of sodium would be filtered. If even half of this Na^+ were not reabsorbed distally, the net loss of Na^+ would be close to 100 mmol/h; this is not seen in these patients.

Deficiency of Na^+-K^+-ATPase A decrease in the activity (V_{max}) of the Na^+K^+ATPase has been proposed to explain the reduced rate of reabsorption of Na^+ and cotransported metabolites. Indeed, a small decline in this V_{max} was noted in the maleic acid model of proximal RTA.[96] Like the hypothesis of a lack of ATP, this too seems unattractive, because it also requires that patients be in marked jeopardy of Na^+ and nutrient diuresis whenever the GFR rises. The corollary would also be true—that is, the proximal lesions would disappear with a minor reduction in GFR. Again, this is not the common clinical experience.

Alternate proposal to explain the pathophysiology of the Fanconi syndrome The Fanconi syndrome might be brought about if proximal Na^+-K^+-ATPase had a reduced affinity for Na^+. Said another way, If Na^+-K^+-ATPase had a lower affinity for Na^+ (or a higher K_m), less Na^+ would be pumped if the concentration of Na^+ in the cell remained normal. Nevertheless, normal pumping of Na^+ could occur if this low affinity for the cation were counterbalanced by an increased concentration of Na^+ in the cell. A reasonable example that suggests that this K_m can rise is provided by skeletal muscle during potassium

TABLE 27-6 • **Hypothetical data during the fanconi syndrome**

For details, see text. We assume that the GFR is 100 liters per unit time, and 60 liters of this filtrate was reabsorbed isotonically in the proximal tubule. Isotonic reabsorption required that 140 meq of Na and 24 meq of HCO_3^- be reabsorbed with each of the 60 liters of filtrate. Thus, 1440 mmol of HCO_3^- was reclaimed without changing the [HCO_3^-] of the remaining filtrate. Reabsorption of 10 mmol of HCO_3^- from each of the 40 liters remaining reduced the filtrate [HCO_3^-] by 10 mmol/liter. The concentration difference for bicarbonate can only be 10 mmol/liter in the backleak model. The V_{max} for the reabsorption of bicarbonate is 25 mmol/liter GFR and the distal nephron absorbs 200 mmol of bicarbonate (2 mmol/liter GFR).

Bicarbonate						
Concentration in plasma (mmol/liter)	*Filtered* HCO_3^- (mmol)	*Reabsorbed* (mmol)		*Excreted* (mmol)	*Reabsorbed* (mmol per liter GFR)	*Fractional excretion* HCO_3^- (%)
		Proximal	Total			
Rate-limit model						
15	1500	1500	1500	0	15.0	0
24	2400	1500	1700	700	17.0	29
40	4000	1500	1700	2300*	17.0	57.5
Backleak model						
15	1500	1300	1500	0	15.0	0
24†	2400	1840	2040	360	20.4	12.5‡
40	4000	2500	2700	1300	27.0§	32.5

* Higher than V_{max}.

† Sample calculation for the backleak model: When the concentration of bicarbonate in plasma is 24 mmol/liter, the filtered load is 2400 mmol (GFR 100 liter). All the bicarbonate is reabsorbed from 60 liters of filtrate (60 × 24 = 1440 mmol), and 10 mmol is reabsorbed from each of the remaining 40 liters (400 mmol). Thus 1840 mmol of bicarbonate is reabsorbed. Since 200 mmol of bicarbonate can be reabsorbed distally, total reabsorption is 2040 mmol.

‡ Note that this is below 15 percent.

§ Note that this is not low.

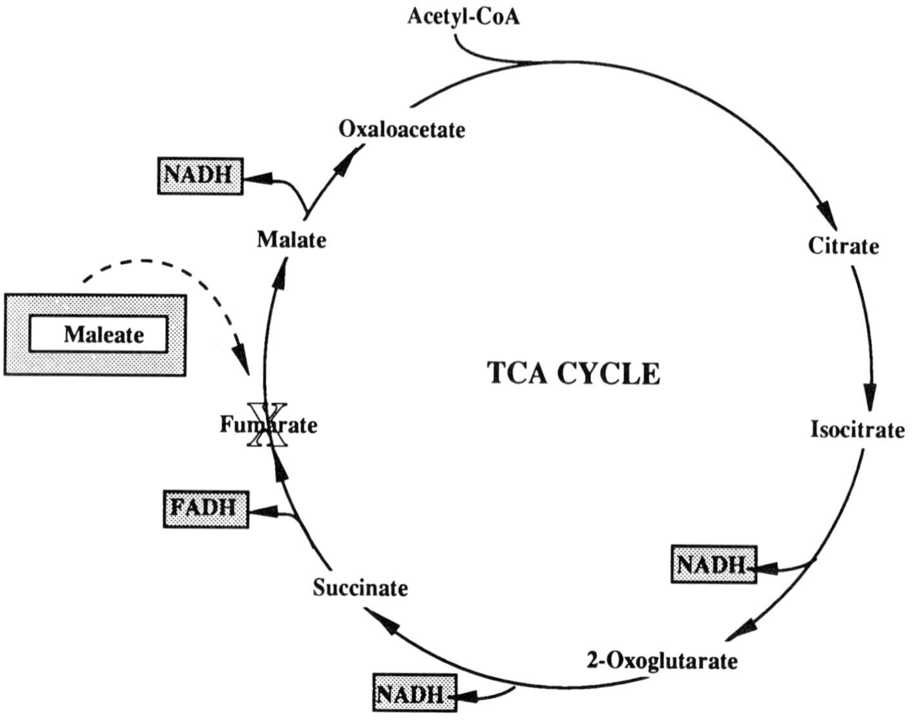

FIGURE 27-18 • Maleic acid and proximal RTA. The site of inhibition of the production of ATP is indicated by the large open X.

deficiency.[97] Thus, a high K_m would lead to a higher steady-state concentration of Na^+ in these cells, but not necessarily to a reduced rate of flux through the Na^+-K^+-ATPase (see Halperin and Rolleston[1] for a simple discussion of kinetics). The higher concentration of Na^+ in the intracellular fluid (ICF) would diminish the difference in concentration of Na^+ between the luminal fluid and the ICF of proximal cells, thereby decreasing the driving force to reabsorb key metabolites such as glucose, and to secrete H^+ on the Na^+-H^+ antiporter. This hypothesis does not require that filtered Na^+ and cotransported metabolites be rejected when there is a rise in the GFR. That notwithstanding, although there is an appropriate animal model (the Basenji dog) to test the above proposed mechanisms, suitable data have not been reported.[98-100]

PROPOSALS TO EXPLAIN THE PATHOPHYSIOLOGY OF ISOLATED PROXIMAL RTA Possible explanations for isolated proximal RTA include decreased activity of the Na^+-H^+ antiporter, the H^+-ATPase, or the $Na(HCO_3)_3^{2-}$ symporter, as well as asynchrony of their activity. One unifying hypothesis that seems attractive to us is the possibility that the pH of proximal cells is more alkaline than normal.[29] This might result from an aberration in any or all of the above-noted components of the reabsorption of bicarbonate. There are two pieces of evidence to support this hypothesis. First, the rate of excretion of citrate in patients with isolated proximal RTA is similar to that in normal subjects,[82] which contrasts with the depressed rates of excretion of citrate seen in other settings of metabolic acidosis.[77] Second, there is a much smaller augmentation of the excretion of NH_4^+ in response to steady-state metabolic acidosis. When these subjects were given a load of NH_4Cl for 3 days, the rate of excretion of NH_4^+ did not increase to the same extent as seen in normal subjects.[101]

Another mechanism that might cause isolated proximal RTA is reduced activity of carbonic anhydrase.[102]

In summary, proximal RTA is believed to result from a lesion affecting the reabsorption of Na^+ by the proximal cell in the Fanconi syndrome, and from an aberration in a process restricted to the reabsorption of bicarbonate in the isolated form. Precise descriptions of the different entities that can generate each of these situations have not been established.

Diagnostic tests

The diagnostic tests warranted in a patient suspected of having proximal RTA fall into three categories:

1. Those that define the acid-base diagnosis.
2. Those aimed at other proximal tubular functions to establish the presence of the Fanconi syndrome.
3. Tests used to determine the underlying cause of the renal defect.

1. Defining the acid-base diagnosis

The diagnosis of proximal RTA is established by the presence of HCMA and a reduced rate of reabsorption of bicarbonate (per liter GFR), or, conversely, an increased fractional excretion of bicarbonate (greater than 15 percent) when the concentration of bicarbonate in plasma is normal (see "Laboratory Tests in a Patient with HCMA" under "Laboratory Tests for RTA" above). Care must be taken to control other factors that influence the rate of reabsorption of bicarbonate—for example, hypokalemia or hyperkalemia, expansion or contraction of the ECF volume, and drugs that inhibit carbonic anhydrase.

TESTS THAT ARE STRONGLY SUGGESTIVE OF PROXIMAL RTA Normocitraturia despite the presence of metabolic acidosis favors the diagnosis of proximal RTA. Although the excretion of citrate is not depressed in either the Fanconi syndrome or isolated proximal RTA, the reasons for its continued excretion may differ. If isolated proximal RTA is caused by an alkaline intracellular pH, the alkalinity or lack of intracellular acidity should lead to normal or reduced catabolism of citrate, and hence should preserve the near-normal or high rate of its excretion.[78] In the Fanconi syndrome the proximal tubule fails to reabsorb citrate, much as it does the other organic anions; hence, relative hypercitraturia is present.

OTHER TESTS • *The* P_{CO_2} *in alkaline urine* The P_{CO_2} in alkaline urine is very high in animal models as well as in human beings with proximal RTA.[103] This test is used to evaluate whether defects in the secretion of H^+ in the proximal and distal nephrons are both present while performing the bicarbonate titration test. It does not test proximal function per se.

Excretion of NH_4^+ Several factors play upon the interpretation of NH_4^+ excretion in proximal RTA. Under steady-state conditions, zero acid balance is reestablished in these patients. At the onset of proximal RTA, bicarbonate wasting and hypobicarbonatemia continue until the reduced filtered load of alkali can once again be reclaimed by the defective proximal tubule. At this point a constant degree of hypobicarbonatemia is associated with a net acid excretion that equals the normal daily production of acid (i.e., zero acid balance).[47,88,89,101] Thus, although ammoniagenesis meets the daily demands of acid production and stabilizes the low concentration of bicarbonate in plasma, it remains unclear why systemic acidosis does not provoke a greater than "normal" synthesis and excretion of NH_4^+. As discussed above,[29] if proximal cell pH were more alkaline than normal, one could explain the bicarbonate wasting and lack of an increased rate of synthesis of NH_4^+. The low concentration of bicarbonate in plasma due to bicarbonaturia would eventually lower the pH in cells of the proximal tubule to normal, and this normal cellular pH would be the proximate cause of the "normal" ammoniagenesis.

Indeed, if production of NH_4^+ exceeded normal, in response to the systemic acidosis, the bicarbonate synthesized in excess of daily acid production would increase its filtered load and cause a persistent bicarbonaturia. Urines with high concentrations of bicarbonate and NH_4^+ are very rare; they occur in alligators[104-106] and in human beings with urinary tract infections caused by urea-splitting organisms.

Tests of proximal tubular function

The Fanconi syndrome is characterized by glycosuria in the absence of hyperglycemia, a generalized amino aciduria, and a reduction of more than 20 percent in the tubular reabsorption of phosphate, organic anions, and carnitine. The Fanconi syndrome may be partially or fully expressed in any given patient. A patient may have a reduction in reabsorption of some, but not all, of the compounds that are cotransported with Na^+ in the proximal tubule at the time of initial evaluation. In time, either a more profound or a more comprehensive reduction of reabsorption of these compounds may become evident. To establish the diagnosis and follow its course, the fractional excretion (or reabsorption) of each of the compounds in question can be measured and this value compared to expected values. The formula for the fractional excretion of bicarbonate (equation 8) can be used for any of the other transported solutes. To interpret the test, the level in plasma should be high enough to permit an adequate rate of excretion. Normal values for these parameters have been widely published.[107,108]

Tests to establish etiology

A clinical evaluation that includes a history taking, physical examination, and laboratory tests addressing the potential secondary causes (Table 27-7) is warranted in patients in whom the diagnosis of isolated proximal RTA or the Fanconi syndrome is established, particularly if there are problems that can be treated successfully.[109]

Clinical Features

The clinical presentation of proximal RTA is distinctive of the population in which it occurs (i.e., pediatric versus adult) and of its association with the Fanconi syndrome. Most cases of proximal RTA are associated with the Fanconi syndrome; indeed, isolated proximal RTA is an uncommon entity. In all situations, the degree of acidosis is usually not severe with typical values for plasma bicarbonate in the range of 18 to 22 mmol/liter.

TABLE 27-7 • **Conditions leading to decreased reabsorption of bicarbonate in the proximal convoluted tubule**

Isolated wasting of bicarbonate
Idiopathic
Genetic
Sporadic
Problem with carbonic anhydrase
Inhibition (acetazolamide, mafenide)
Deficiency (associated with osteopetrosis)
Secondary to hyperkalemia
Generalized proximal tubular defect (Fanconi syndrome)
Hereditary defects
Cystinosis, Wilson's disease, transferase deficiency galactosemia, Lowe's syndrome, hepatorenal tyrosinemia, hereditary fructose intolerance, glycogen storage disease type I
Toxic damage to proximal cells
Heavy metals: lead (acute), cadmium, uranium, mercury, platinum
Drugs: Aminoglycosides, 6-mercaptopurine, methyl-5-chromone, lysol, paraquat, outdated or improperly stored tetracyline
Others: inhibitors of the synthesis of ATP (maleic acid)
Dysproteinemias
Multiple myeloma, amyloidosis, light-chain nephropathy, benign monoclonal gammopathy, hypergammaglobulnemia
Immunologic disorders
Autoimmune diseases (e.g., chronic active hepatitis, Sjögren's syndrome, systemic lupus erythematosus)
Renal transplantation
Interstitial nephritis
Lymphoid malignancy with peritubular infiltrates
High levels of parathyroid hormone
Deficiency of, or resistance to, vitamin D

Isolated proximal RTA

CHILDREN Infants (ages under one year), whose normal threshold for the reabsorption of bicarbonate is lower than that of adults, sustain a bicarbonate concentration in plasma that is close to 20 mmol/liter. During the first decade of life, this threshold rises progressively to adult levels.[108] Infants and children with proximal RTA have a bicarbonate concentration that is usually in the range of 15 mmol/liter in plasma, and they present with failure to grow at a normal rate.[110] The natural history of this proximal RTA is such that it tends to disappear with time. Therapy, if initiated, usually can be discontinued by two years of age. These children usually do not have permanent sequelae.

ADULTS Adults develop isolated proximal RTA uncommonly. A recent search of the literature revealed case reports where this disorder was present in conjunction with chronic active hepatitis,[111] familial normoaldosteronemic hyperkalemia and hypertension,[112] tetralogy of Fallot,[113] and metachromatic leukodystrophy.[114] A familial form of the disease describes a paucity of clinical consequences in adults; the only abnormality was a stunting of growth that is likely due to the effect of acidosis during childhood and adolescent periods.[110] These patients, even at age 72, do not have evidence of bone disease (L. Brenes, personal communication). Rare cases are reported with dental abnormalities.[115] In contrast to patients with distal RTA, proximal RTA is rarely associated with renal stones or nephrocalcinosis.

The most important clinical problem probably derives from aggressive attempts to correct the hypobicarbonatemia with Na^+ bicarbonate or its equivalent, Na^+ citrate, because this may result in very large losses of K^+ in the urine. The major problem with therapy with bicarbonate is that bicarbonaturia can lead to very high rates of excretion of K^+, provided that aldosterone is present in the plasma. This loss of K^+ occurs for two major reasons: a very high transtubular K^+ concentration gradient[116] and an increase in urine flow. Bicarbonaturia induces a large kaliuresis even when Cl^- is present in the urine, in contrast to the effect of other anions, such as sulfate.[116] To avoid large deficits of K^+, a considerable portion of the bicarbonate should be administered as the K^+ salt. Giving such a large quantity of K^+ can be dangerous if there are other factors that limit the excretion of K^+ (e.g., low GFR secondary to loss of Na^+ or the intake of K^+-sparing diuretics).[117] Hence, treatment with bicarbonate may not offer enough advantage in the adult to merit recommending its use.

Patients with proximal RTA are in acid balance, but they have acidemia.[88] It is said that this preservation of acid balance prevents progressive buffering by bones. Perhaps this helps to explain the low incidence of metabolic bone disease in chronic proximal RTA. We believe this last statement to be a "half-truth." Buffering is a physical-chemical process. The law of mass action dictates that the quantity of H^+ buffered depends on the concentration (activity) of H^+ and the pK of the buffer. Since the pK should be constant in vivo, the degree of buffering in steady state is dependent only on the concentration of H^+. Therefore, for a given acid pH under steady-state conditions, a patient with proximal RTA and a patient with renal failure ought to exhibit the same degree of bone buffering, unless other factors are operative. One might imagine that perhaps another consequence of proximal RTA was prevention of loss of bone mass during acidemia, or that there were additional consequences of renal insufficiency (in addition to acidemia) that caused loss of bone mass per se or accelerated the titration of alkaline bone salts during acidemia. In this regard, it is important to emphasize that the bulk of buffering in bone, as indicated by the excretion of calcium, occurs soon after a load of NH_4Cl[118-120] but greatly diminishes during chronic metabolic acidosis.[121] Hence there is still a major problem in determining why loss of bone mass occurs to a major or minor extent in patients with proximal RTA. One might speculate that perhaps osteocytes or osteoclasts share with the proximal epithelial cells an alkaline cell pH. As the concentration of bicarbonate in plasma falls, bone cell pH normalizes. If this scenario were correct, there would not be a stimulus for bone buffering and reabsorption. (R. Narins, personal communication).

Patients with isolated proximal RTA do not develop hypercalciuria. This, in conjunction with their normal rate of excretion of citrate, may explain, in part, their low incidence of nephrocalcinosis and renal stones.

Fanconi syndrome

The generalized dysfunction of the proximal renal tubule leads to impaired reabsorption of bicarbonate, glucose, phosphate, amino acids, carnitine, and urate. In addition to the renal wasting of these solutes, the second component of Fanconi syndrome is a vitamin D–resistant metabolic bone disease. The bone disease presents as rickets in children and as osteomalacia in adults. It results not only from the hypophosphatemia and the metabolic acidosis, but also because of the impaired vitamin D metabolism.[122] The 1-α-hydroxylation of 25-OH-cholecalciferol is impaired in the Fanconi syndrome.[123]

In contrast to the clinical consequence of renal wasting of bicarbonate and phosphate, there are no clinical sequelae from the excretion of glucose, amino acids, or urate lost in the urine. Losses of carnitine in the urine may result in a clinically significant deficiency that should be treated.[91] In addition to the acidemia and metabolic bone disease, other clinical manifestations are determined by the cause of the Fanconi syndrome and are distinct for the pediatric and adult populations.

CHILDREN Children with the Fanconi syndrome present with complex clinical picture that is nonspecific but that results from the renal wasting of the abovementioned solutes as well as loss of fluid and electrolytes. The presenting clinical characteristics are polyuria, polydipsia, hypovolemia, hypokalemia, and acidosis. Growth retardation and the features of vitamin D–resistant rickets are often the presenting signs of the disease.

The most common hereditary form of the Fanconi syndrome is due to *cystinosis*. Cystinosis is an autosomal recessive disease that may present in infancy, adolescence, or early adulthood.[124] It is associated with the intralysosomal accumulation of cystine in numerous tissues throughout the body and is due to a defect in transport of cystine out of the lysosome. In general, the earlier the presentation, the more severe the disease. Only the infantile and adolescent forms are associated with Fanconi syndrome; the adult form is generally benign. The infantile and nephropathic forms are usually evident at between 6 and 12 months of age. They present with the Fanconi syndrome, and progress to end-stage renal disease by the end of the first decade. The Fanconi syndrome is marked by acidosis and hypophosphatemic rickets. The recurrent episodes of vomiting, hypovolemia, and electrolyte abnormalities pose an unrelenting therapeutic challenge. Renal transplantation cures the Fanconi syndrome and its uremic consequences, but this therapeutic accomplishment has permitted a clear recognition of the systemic nature of this illness.[124,125] Oral cysteamine (methenamine), a drug that binds to cysteine, if introduced early, can improve the rate of growth and may delay the decrease in GFR. The Fanconi syndrome, however, is not averted with oral cysteamine.[126] It may be necessary to introduce the drug before the age of 1 year to avoid this complication.[127] The dramatic improvement in the prognosis for patients with nephropathic cystinosis is highlighted by a recent report of a successful pregnancy in an affected individual.[128]

In several other inherited autosomal recessive diseases, the Fanconi syndrome results from a reversible abnormality of renal metabolism. The Fanconi syndrome resolves when fructose, galactose, tyrosine, or copper is restricted or altered in form in the diet of a subject with hereditary fructose intolerance,[46,129] galactosemia,[130] tyroninemia,[131] or Wilson's disease,[132] respectively. Hence, these disorders are not common causes of Fanconi syndrome, but patients may have sporadic episodes depending on dietary indiscretions.

The major clinical manifestations of *Wilson's disease* ensue from accumulation of copper in the CNS, kidneys, and liver. Deposition of copper in the proximal convoluted cells may result in renal acidification problems, aminoaciduria, glucosuria, and rickets.[133] Poor growth and nephrolithiasis may be presenting symptoms.

Oculocerebrorenal (Lowe's) syndrome is a rare and probably X-linked recessive disorder that was originally described by Lowe in 1952.[134] The Fanconi syndrome is marked by severe rickets and retardation of growth. The name derives from the associated cataracts and glaucoma, and severe mental retardation. The specific defect responsible for the syndrome remains unknown. In addition, the large losses of fluid and electrolytes give rise to other clinical manifestations. Infants may present with polydipsia, polyuria, and dehydration. The metabolic acidosis can lead to retardation of growth. Frontal bossing, rachitic rosary, and bowing deformities of the legs may result from hypophosphatemic rickets.

ADULTS In contrast to the importance of hereditary causes of the Fanconi syndrome in children, acquired forms are, obviously, more often seen in adults (Table 27-7). Toxins and dysproteinemias are the most common causes in this group. The clinical features result from dysfunction of the proximal tubule, which is usually reversible if exposure is discontinued.

Occupational or environmental exposure to a number of heavy metals for a prolonged period may result in chronic nephrotoxicity, which may present as the Fanconi syndrome. The toxicity of *cadmium*[135] and *uranium*[136] is felt to be much greater than that of *lead*[137] and *mercury*.[136] In acute lead nephrotoxicity intranuclear inclusion bodies are found in the proximal convoluted tubular cells. They consist of lead bound to a nuclear protein.[137] A degradation product of outdated or improperly stored tetracycline, anhydro-4-epi-tetracycline, induces a reversible form of Fanconi syndrome.[138]

The second important group of disorders causing Fanconi syndrome in adults are the dysproteinemias. *Multiple myeloma* may not be evident initially, but Bence Jones proteinuria is often present. *Amyloidosis*,[139] *light chain nephropathy*,[140] *benign monoclonal gammopathy*,[141] and *nonmyelomatous hypergammaglobulinemia*[142] are other causes of the Fanconi syndrome.

Treatment

The objectives of therapy are again determined by the population at risk as well as by the association with Fanconi syndrome.

Isolated proximal RTA

Isolated proximal RTA in children probably should be treated until the disease resolves. In these subjects, the aim is to achieve a higher (near-normal) concentration of bicarbonate in the plasma, so as to reverse or minimize the retardation of growth that results from systemic acidosis. In adults, on the other hand, treatment of the isolated form of proximal RTA is not necessary, because retardation of growth is not a consideration and there do not appear to be other clinical sequelae (L. Brenes, personal communication).

Some authors recommend that extremely large doses of bicarbonate (6 to 15 mmol per kilogram of body weight per day) be given to children, because of the excessive loss of alkali as normobicarbonatemia is approached (Table 27-6).[88,143] Bicarbonaturia can provoke the loss of large amounts of K^+. Accordingly, the bicarbonate or citrate should be given, in large part, in the form of a K^+ salt. Furthermore, enhancement of proximal reabsorption, in general, by ECF volume contraction can diminish the dose of alkali required to achieve a given plasma level. The use of thiazide diuretics has been suggested in such cases.[144] Finally, the use of nonsteroidal anti-inflammatory drugs to reduce the GFR has been reported to be of some benefit in a subject who experienced gastrointestinal side effects with bicarbonate therapy.[145] By reducing the filtered load of bicarbonate, urinary losses are diminished, thereby allowing a lesser dose to achieve the desired blood bicarbonate levels but at a potentially high price to pay.

Fanconi syndrome

CHILDREN In children with the Fanconi syndrome, the primary aim is to remove metabolites, compounds, and exogenous toxins responsible for the lesion. This largely involves dietary manipulations or drug administration, depending on the specific cause [examples include methenamine for cystinosis, and penicillamine for Wilson's disease; for more detailed information regarding the specific therapies for secondary Fanconi syndrome (see Bergeron and Gougoux)].[109]

The acidosis is treated as described for the isolated form of proximal RTA, again stressing the importance of supplements with K^+. Losses of salt and water with intercurrent illnesses should also be replaced vigilantly. Oral carnitine replacement has been recommended in nephropathic cystinosis[146] and may be considered in other forms of Fanconi syndrome. As in the various forms of vitamin D-deficient rickets, large doses of phosphate (up to 56 mmol in 5 to 6 divided doses) and vitamin D are required.[147] The form of vitamin D to administer is 1,25-$(OH)_2$ vitamin D, because of the possible impaired metabolism of vitamin D in patients with the Fanconi syndrome.[123] The goals of therapy should be to bring the concentrations of phosphate and vitamin D close to the normal range, while monitoring the levels of Ca^{2+} and alkaline phosphatase.

ADULTS In adults, the focus of therapy is on the primary disease. Removal of toxic elements can involve a major change in lifestyle. In addition, specific therapy for the underlying condition, such as multiple myeloma, is of obvious importance. Treatment of the acidosis is not really necessary (nor likely to be successful), since there is no longer a problem with retardation of growth in this population. Phosphate and 1,25-$(OH)_2$ vitamin D may avert potential complications of osteomalacia, as discussed above.

DISEASES WITH A LOW RATE OF EXCRETION OF NH_4^+

Definition

The hallmark, or key pathophysiologic feature, of these disorders is a low rate of excretion of NH_4^+.[43,59] The presence or absence of acidemia is an important but variable characteristic. The relative magnitude of H^+ generation or ingestion and the magnitude of the renal defect in "new" bicarbonate synthesis determine whether the concentration of bicarbonate will change. Hence, hypobicarbonatemia and acidemia may be present (overt) or absent (occult).

Low NH_4^+ excretion disease with overt acidemia

Patients with clinically overt low NH_4^+ excretion disease—that is, classic distal RTA—must have both of the following major features:

1. Metabolic acidosis with a normal anion gap.
2. Low rate of excretion of NH_4^+. All of these patients have a chronic steady-state metabolic acidosis and continue to excrete up to 40 mmol of NH_4^+ per day, while maintaining a low pH in the blood.

Most authorities include a value for the pH of the urine in this definition (Table 27-3). We have not done so because, as discussed under "Physiology of Acid-Base Metabolism" above, the quantity of free H^+ excreted is minuscule and the urinary pH is an unreliable index of the rate of excretion of NH_4^+. Nevertheless, the pH of the urine can be of value when interpreted in conjunction with the quantity of NH_4^+ excreted (see "Pathophysiology" below).

Occult "low NH_4^+ excretion disease" (distal RTA without acidemia)

There is probably a much larger group of patients who have a subnormal rate of excretion of NH_4^+ when faced with a chronic acid load. They may present with overt distal RTA if challenged with an additional net load of acid (i.e., a change in diet from alkaline ash to acid ash[61]). Since the kidney is contributing to the degree of acidemia by excreting less NH_4^+ than expected,[56,57] and since recognition of this fact will influence decisions about therapy, we prefer to include these patients in the category of "low NH_4^+ excretion disease" or define them as having "occult" distal RTA. This diagnosis requires a provocative test to confirm that there is really a low rate of excretion of NH_4^+ (Figs. 27-9, 27-10, and 27-11).

Pathophysiology

The underlying problem in these patients is a low rate of excretion of NH_4^+. Two types of distal RTA are recognized on clinical grounds: the hypokalemic, or classic distal RTA, and the hyperkalemic, or type IV, RTA (Table 27-4). Although this classification has clinical merit, it does not have a strong basis in pathophysiology. For instance, patients with the hyperkalemic variety of RTA might have a defect in the production of NH_4^+, a reduced rate of reabsorption of NH_4^+ in the loop of Henle that leads to a low concentration of NH_3 in the medullary

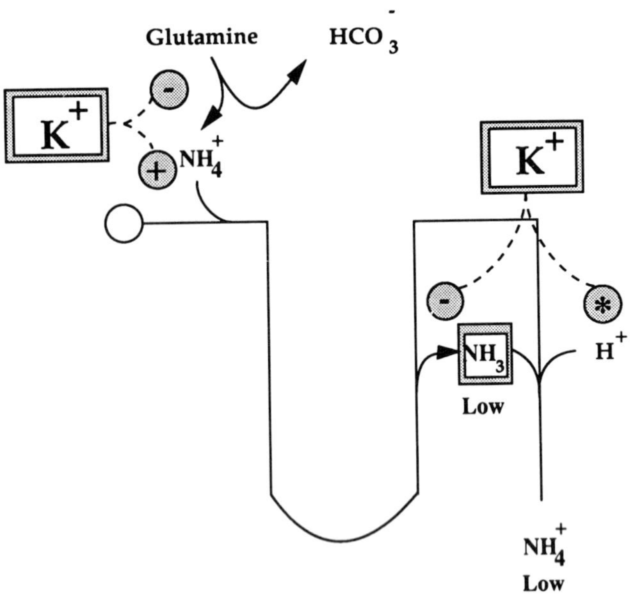

FIGURE 27-19 • Effect of hyperkalemia on the excretion of NH_4^+. Hyperkalemia leads to a reduction in synthesis of NH_4^+, but also to an increase in its transfer into the lumen in the proximal convoluted tubule. It diminishes the concentration of NH_3 in the medullary interstitium (its most important effect), and may inhibit or stimulate the secretion of H^+ in the collecting duct, depending on the cause of hyperkalemia (see * in figure).

interstitium, or a generalized distal nephron dysfunction with a defect in the secretion of H^+ as well (Fig. 27-19).

We find a classification that addresses the pathophysiology of the disorder more appealing than one that is merely descriptive. Accordingly, we prefer to classify the disorders associated with a low rate of excretion of NH_4^+ into those with an *NH_3 defect* and those with an *H^+* defect, as these are the two determinants of the concentration of NH_4^+ in the urine (Table 27-5, above, and equation 10, below). The former group, recognized by a low pH of the urine, includes disorders with a low rate of production of NH_4^+, or with failure to generate a high concentration of NH_3 in the medullary interstitium. The group with an H^+ defect, recognized by a high pH of the urine, includes patients with a decreased net rate of secretion of H^+ in the distal nephron as a result of H^+ pump failure (rate defect), a voltage defect, or a backleak problem (gradient defect).

$$NH_3 + H^+ \leftrightarrow NH_4^+ \quad (10)$$

A low rate of secretion of H^+ in the distal nephron caused by either diminished H^+-ATPase or H^+-K^+-ATPase activity might compromise the net addition of NH_3 to the lumen. Flawed H^+ secretion keeps the luminal NH_3 concentration increased, thereby creating an unfavorable medulla-to-lumen diffusion gradient (Fig. 27-5). This failure of secretion should compromise the excretion of NH_4^+ only to a modest degree, since one might anticipate that production of NH_4^+ in the proximal cell would be stimulated, thereby raising the concentration of NH_3 in the renal medulla. Hence, most persons with this form of distal RTA with severe acidemia probably have an additional component to their disorder, one that limits the rise in NH_3 in the renal medulla. Thus, many patients have a mixed picture (e.g., medullary interstitial disease) that leads to failure to generate a high concentration of NH_3 in the medullary interstitium and to pump sufficient H^+ into the lumen of the collecting duct.

Common underlying causes

NH_3 DEFECT • *Low production of NH_4^+* The two most common reasons for a low rate of production of NH_4^+ in the proximal tubule are a low GFR[22] and hyperkalemia.[28] Each will be discussed below.

Low GFR A low GFR in turn lowers the filtered load of sodium, and hence diminishes the rate of turnover of ATP in the proximal cells. One should also be aware of an occult reduction in the GFR. By this we mean a patient with a low GFR and a confusingly low serum creatinine concentration. Reduced muscle mass and low-protein diets commonly cause this picture.[148]

Hyperkalemia This group is called *type IV RTA* by most nephrologists. It is, in effect, one subtype of "low NH_4^+ excretion disease." An important role for hyperkalemia in decreasing NAE was first demonstrated in 1976, when its correction with an ion exchange resin corrected the metabolic acidosis and increased the excretion of NH_4^+.[149] Clinical and experimental studies have confirmed the importance of K^+ in the regulation of acid-base balance.[150-153] The possible effects of hyperkalemia on the excretion of NH_4^+ are summarized in Fig. 27-19. Hyperkalemia may inhibit the formation of NH_4^+ in the proximal convoluted tubule of the rat.[28] In contrast, K^+ has little effect on the production of NH_4^+ in the dog (Halperin, unpublished observations). There are no data to document the effect of hyperkalemia on the production of NH_4^+ in human beings. Interesting data have been published recently concerning the transfer of NH_4^+ from the cells of the proximal convoluted tubule to the lumen. It now appears that there is enhanced secretion of NH_4^+ during hyperkalemia.[154,155] Hence, because a greater fraction of the reduced production is secreted into the lumen, little change occurs in the delivery of NH_4^+ to the loop of Henle.

Other causes Two other examples of persons with possible decreased NH_4^+ production are patients with a poor nutritional state where the plasma concentration of the NH_4^+ precursor, glutamine, is very low; and subjects infused with a high concentration of fat-derived fuels [as occurs with total parenteral nutrition (TPN)], the oxidation of which generates ATP at the expense of glutamine utilization.[26]

Failure to generate a high concentration of NH_3 in the medullary interstitium A key determinant of the excretion of NH_4^+ is a high concentration of NH_3 in the renal medullary interstitium.[30] Since a normal medullary countercurrent system is required to achieve this level, it follows that a variety of diseases that damage the renal medulla may compromise this function. Low rates of excretion of NH_4^+ complicate many diverse diseases, including various hereditary disorders (e.g., medullary sponge kidney), inflammatory diseases (e.g., pyelonephritis, collagen vascular diseases), disorders characterized by crystalline deposits (e.g., nephrocalcinosis, urate nephropathy), various drugs (e.g., phenacetin), and damage secondary to obstructive diseases. Although the concentration of NH_3 is low in the medulla, it is possible that disorders of secretion of H^+ are also present, owing to nonselective damage to the medullary interstitium. Depending on the relative magnitudes of the defects in NH_3 and H^+, the final pH of the urine may be either lower (predominant impairment generating a high concentration of NH_3) or higher (predominant impairment of H^+ secretion).

Hyperkalemia may lead to a decreased rate of transport of NH_4^+ in the thick ascending limb of the loop of Henle, leading to problems with the generation of a high concentration of NH_3 in the renal medullary interstitium. Apparently, a high concentration of K^+ in the luminal fluid in the thick ascending limb of the loop of Henle inhibits the reabsorption of NH_4^+ by the Na^+-K^+-$(Cl^-)_2$ cotransporter. This, in turn, leads to a low concentration of NH_3 in the renal medulla, which diminishes the transfer of NH_3 to the lumen of the collecting duct (Fig. 27-19).[156] These changes cause elaboration of an acid urine with reduced concentrations of NH_3 and NH_4^+.[154,157] In addition, aldosterone has been shown to stimulate the Na^+, K^+, $(Cl^-)_2$ cotransporter in the thick ascending limb of the loop of Henle in rats. Hence, low levels of circulating aldosterone and/or tubular resistance to the effects of the hormone may reduce the level of NH_3 in the renal medulla.[158,159]

DISORDERS WITH H^+ SECRETORY DEFECT In some patients with distal RTA the primary defect is a low rate of secretion of H^+. Ammonium excretion eventually diminishes. This defect may result from:

1. A reduced number, or reduced activity, of H^+ pumps (e.g., caused by interstitial renal disease).
2. Excessive backleak of normally secreted H^+ (e.g., caused by amphotericin B).
3. A lower voltage in the collecting duct, due to decreased aldosterone bioactivity or the administration of amiloride. Decreased aldosterone bioactivity may be due to low circulating levels of the hormone, or to tubular insensitivity to its action. Modulation of Na^+-dependent secretion of H^+ by mineralocorticoid has been demonstrated in several studies.[16,160-163] By stimulating reabsorption of Na^+ in the cortical collecting duct, aldosterone increases the transepithelial voltage at this site, which, in turn, stimulates the rate of secretion of protons.[159] An aldosterone-mediated increase in H^+ transport, independent of Na^+, was first observed in the turtle bladder.[164] A similar phenomenon was later shown in the medullary collecting duct of the rabbit.[17] Aldosterone is also thought to directly stimulate the H^+-ATPase in this segment of the nephron.

Clinical features • **Natural history** The hallmark of this disorder is a reduced rate of excretion of NH_4^+. Hence, with a constant normal daily acid production of 70 mmol of H^+, an output that is less than 70 mmol/day will eventually lead to metabolic acidosis. In most patients, when the acidosis becomes chronic, the rate of excretion of NH_4^+ increases somewhat and once again matches acid production, but this occurs only at the expense of steady-state metabolic acidosis. Clinical subgroups are listed in Table 27-8.

Symptoms of acidosis The only symptoms specifically attributable to acidosis are those related to hy-

TABLE 27-8 • Causes of distal renal tubular acidosis

NH_3 defect
Problem with ammoniagenesis
Decreased synthesis of ATP in proximal tubule
Low GFR
Inhibition of metabolism of glutamine
Hyperkalemia is most common cause
Decreased availability of glutamine
Malnutrition or gastrointestinal disorder
Fuel competition
Ketoacidosis or total parenteral nutrition
Problem with transfer of NH_3
Interstitial renal diseases and hyperkalemia are likely causes (Examples of renal interstitial disease include infections, such as pyelonephritis; drugs, such as analgesics or methicillin; depositions, such as urate; obstructive disorders; structural damage, such as medullary sponge kidney; autoimmune diseases; and abnormal proteins.)
Defect in H^+ secretion
H^+ Pump defect
Interstitial renal diseases (described above); low aldosterone bioactivity
Voltage defect
Low delivery of Na^+; inhibitors of reabsorption of Na^+, such as amiloride or lithium. Low aldosterone bioactivity usually causes hyperkalemia (see Table 27-9).
H^+ backleak
Hereditary disorders, or drugs such as amphotericin B

For details, see text.

perventilation. Nonspecific symptoms, such as feelings of malaise and weakness, may also be present.

Potassium Hypokalemia is very common in patients with "classic" distal RTA, especially if the acidosis is severe.[165] The mechanisms responsible for the hypokalemia are poorly understood. Each of the following may play a role: high levels of aldosterone secondary to ECF volume contraction; high rates of flow to the distal nephron; and a high transepithelial voltage in the cortical distal nephron, perhaps due to a high concentration of bicarbonate in the distal lumen (secondary to diminished reclamation of the remaining fraction of filtered bicarbonate).[116] Another proposed mechanism to explain the occurrence of hypokalemia and metabolic acidosis is a defect in the H^+-K^+ ATPase in the medullary collecting duct. Nevertheless, appropriate studies [e.g., the transtubular K^+ concentration gradient (TTKG) in conjunction with hormone levels and concentrations of anions in the urine[166]] have not been reported in sufficient numbers of cases to allow the drawing of firm conclusions. Hypokalemia, regardless of its pathogenesis, can be responsible for the majority of the symptoms, the predominant symptom often being extreme weakness. This is particularly important in a patient who must depend on hyperventilation to minimize the threat of acidemia.

Hyperkalemia and HCMA characterize the so-called type IV RTA (Table 27-9). Hyperkalemia may be due to aldosterone deficiency and/or tubular insensitivity to the action of aldosterone.

Bone problems When present, these problems seem to accompany chronic metabolic acidosis, although we cannot explain why dissolution of bone is greater in that setting than in proximal RTA. In addition to loss of calcium secondary to buffering,[167] there can also be reduced levels of active vitamin D or resistance to its actions on bone. Damage to the medullary interstitium, with nephrocalcinosis, is seen in many cases. The latter is likely caused by the hypercalciuria coupled with hypocitraturia. Renal calculi may develop in this milieu, and may be more likely if too much bicarbonate is given as therapy. This potential danger can be avoided by giving an appropriate amount of bicarbonate—less than 40 mmol/day, once the acidosis is corrected—because the diet provides only 70 mmol of H^+ per day, and TA will still be formed (30 mmol/day). There are few data on the incidence of bone disease in type IV RTA; one study suggested that radiologically evident skeletal abnormalities are uncommon.[168]

Polyuria Owing to medullary interstitial damage, or possibly to chronic and severe hypokalemia, the osmolality of the urine is much lower than in normal subjects (close to 300 mosm per kg H_2O). This requires a volume of urine that approaches 3 liters per day with the usual load of osmoles to excrete (close to 900 mosm/day).

TABLE 27-9 • Causes of metabolic acidosis associated with hyperkalemia and decreased rate of excretion of NH_4^+ in the absence of renal failure

- Primary deficiency of aldosterone
  - Combined deficiency of aldosterone and cortisone
    - Addison's disease, idiopathic
    - Bilateral adrenalectomy
    - Bilateral adrenal destruction due to hemorrhage, tumor, infection of infiltration
    - Congenital enzymatic defects
  - Isolated deficiency of aldosterone
    - Familial deficiency of cortisone methyoxidase (types I and II)
    - Transient hypoaldosteronism of infancy
    - Chronic idiopathic hypoaldosteronism
    - Heparin
- Secondary or hyporeninemic hypoaldosteronism
  - Diabetes mellitus
  - Tubulointerstitial nephritis
  - Nephrosclerosis
  - Drugs
- Mineralocorticoid-resistant hyperkalemia
  - Generalized distal nephron dysfunction
    - Obstructive nephropathy
    - Sickle cell disease
    - Interstitial nephritis
    - Amyloidosis
  - Pseudohypoaldosteronism (hypovolemic)
  - Chloride shunt (hypervolemic)
  - Drugs
    - Spironolactone
    - Amiloride
    - Triamterene

Clinical disorders Distal RTA with hypokalemia may occur in the absence of other diseases as a spontaneous or inherited defect. Although most cases are sporadic, families with the disorder have been reported.[92] The mode of inheritance is autosomal-dominant in some families, X-linked in others, and unclear in yet others.

The frequency with which distal RTA with hypokalemia complicates the hyperglobulinemic states is notable.[169] Distal RTA has been reported with Sjögren's syndrome,[170] thyroiditis, primary biliary cirrhosis, chronic active hepatitis,[171] fibrosing alveolitis,[172] cryoglobulinemia, and systemic lupus erythematosus.[173] It is not clear how these conditions result in RTA, but an immunological basis has been suggested.

Several drugs and toxins can result in distal RTA. These include amphotericin B,[174] lithium carbonate,[175,176] and analgesics.

Tubulointerstitial disease, including chronic pyelonephritis, obstructive uropathy, hypercalciuria and nephrocalcinosis, sickle cell disease, and medullary sponge kidney,[177] have been associated with distal RTA.

Diagnostic tests

URINARY NH_4^+ The hallmark for this group of diseases is a reduced rate of excretion of NH_4^+ (see "Physiology of Acid-Base Metabolism" above). To summarize, if a direct assay for NH_4^+ is not available,[62] the urinary net charge[63] or osmolal gap offers indirect means for its estimation.[64-66] If the concentration of Cl^- in the urine is greater than that of $Na^+ + K^+$, substantial amounts of NH_4^+ are present making this diagnosis unlikely as the sole cause of the acidosis; conversely, if the urinary concentration of $Na^+ + K^+$ is greater than that of Cl^-, "low NH_4^+ excretion disease" is present in most, but not all, cases,[68] and its confirmation should be sought with other tests. We prefer to estimate the concentration of NH_4^+ with the urinary osmolal gap.[64-66] A value of less than 100 mosm per kg H_2O in the face of chronic metabolic acidosis strongly suggests the diagnosis of "low NH_4^+ excretion disease." We think that the urinary pH is misleading often enough to rule out its use as a reflection of the rate of excretion of NH_4^+.[55] Obviously, a direct assay for NH_4^+ in the urine is the best test. Even with a direct assay, one must be certain that urea-splitting organisms are not spuriously increasing the urinary NH_4^+ levels. If these organisms are present, the urinary pH and net charge are the best ways to determine how much NH_4^+ in the urine was of renal origin, because when urea is hydrolyzed, NH_4^+ and bicarbonate are produced (there is a high urinary pH, but the concentration of Cl^- does not exceed the sum of concentrations of Na^+ and K^+). If NH_4^+ is excreted with Cl^-, this cannot be NH_4^+ produced from hydrolysis of urea.[63]

TESTS TO CLARIFY THE CAUSE OF REDUCED EXCRETION OF NH_4^+ • *Urinary pH* We utilize the urinary pH to clarify whether the low rate of excretion of NH_4^+ is due primarily to diminished NH_3 availability or to an H^+ secretory defect (Table 27-8).[59] A low pH suggests the former, while a high pH suggests that the H^+ secretory defect is causative. Midrange values (5.3 to 6.0) suggest that both components are defective (usually because of damage to the renal medulla).

Concentration of K^+ in the plasma Hypokalemia most commonly complicates the subgroup with a H^+ secretory defect, whereas hyperkalemia is the most common cause a of low production of NH_4^+ in the absence of a severe degree of renal failure (GFR more than 20 percent or normal). Most patients in this category have a moderate (close to 50 percent) reduction in the GFR (low NH_3 availability subgroup—Table 27-7). This latter aspect is discussed in detail below.

Urinary P_{CO_2} in alkaline urine This test can be utilized to gain independent information concerning the process of secretion of H^+ in the distal nephron, because bicarbonate is virtually the sole acceptor for protons secreted in the distal nephron when the pH of the urine is greater than 7.4 (Fig. 27-15). Low values help to identify low rates of secretion of H^+, while high values may be found in an NH_3 defect or a disorder involving a backleak of H^+ (e.g., resulting from use of amphotericin B).[70]

Treatment

In the interest of brevity, we shall not discuss the treatments for the many disorders that may cause distal RTA (Table 27-8). It is obvious that careful attention must be given to these primary disorders, in hopes of stemming further renal damage and of perhaps reversing existing defects.

ACIDOSIS It is important to correct the acidemia to prevent bone disease, and to minimize the dangers of nephrolithiasis and nephrocalcinosis. Further, in children, correction of the acidosis is important to avoid growth retardation.[110]

There are two features to consider with respect to the acidosis. First, one must give sufficient bicarbonate to correct the acidosis. This is a one-time component of therapy. The quantity of bicarbonate in mmol needed can be estimated by multiplying the reduction in the blood concentration of bicarbonate by 50 percent of the body weight.[178,179] This is a crude estimate, and its efficacy must be evaluated by serial determinations of serum bicarbonate concentration.

The second component of therapy is to provide sufficient bicarbonate to maintain normobicarbonatemia. Usually this should be somewhat less than the rate of excretion of net acid; in fact, only the decrement in the rate of excretion of NH_4^+ should be replaced with oral bicarbonate. Thus, most patients require less than 40 mmol of bicarbonate per day. Two additional features must be considered. More alkali must be given if there is ongoing bicarbonaturia caused by alkaline tide, or improper spacing of the oral bicarbonate supplement; and when bicarbonate is deposited as alkaline bone salts (e.g., in children who are still growing, and in all patients who have healing bone lesions). Similarly, additional alkali are needed if losses of bicarbonate occur via the gastrointestinal tract (diarrhea, ileus), the urine (carbonic anhydrase inhibitors), or an indirect loss of bicarbonate (loss of the conjugate base of an acid with sodium or potassium—Fig. 27-18[61]).

With correction of the metabolic acidosis, hypercalciuria usually disappears and the excretion of citrate may increase. While nephrocalcinosis usually persists, the incidence of nephrocalcinosis may decline unless therapy with alkali is excessive.

POTASSIUM • *Distal RTA with hypokalemia* Treatment of hypokalemia is a critical component of therapy. One must bear in mind, however, that patients taking large supplements of K^+ are at risk of life-threatening hyperkalemia if a drug that blocks the excretion of K^+ is introduced or if a situation arises that compromises the rate of excretion of K^+.[117]

There is one other aspect of therapy with K^+ that is very important. Not infrequently, patients present with extreme weakness owing to hypokalemia. Nevertheless, they need to maintain a very high rate of alveolar ventilation, owing to the metabolic acidosis. If paresis prevents this full respiratory response, life-threatening acidemia may develop, because of the combined metabolic and respiratory acidosis. Administration of bicarbonate to correct the metabolic acidosis will yield a large extra load of CO_2 and demand additional hyperventilation. The alkali therapy can also cause more profound hypokalemia, owing to a shift of K^+ into cells, and thereby exacerbate the weakness. Accordingly, K^+ should be replaced before, or simultaneously with, the bicarbonate load, and the patient should be ventilated promptly if necessary. The dose of K^+ that we think should be administered in a catastrophic situation can be as high as 6 mmol/min for the first minute, followed by a maintenance load of 1 mmol/min until the concentration of K^+ in plasma approaches 3.0 mmol/liter. Obviously this load of K^+ must be administered via a central venous catheter, since K^+ at these concentrations can sclerose small vessels. Detailed explanations can be found in the report of Donnelly and coworkers.[180] This not only prevents life-threatening cardiac arrhythmias, but often also corrects the respiratory component of the acidosis.

Distal RTA with hyperkalemia (see Chap. 23) The most important aspect of therapy is the control of the accompanying hyperkalemia. This not only prevents life-threatening arrhythmias, but also corrects the acidosis. Hyperkalemia may inhibit the production of NH_4^+ by the cells of the proximal tubule; it may also lead to a decreased rate of transport of NH_4^+ in the thick ascending limb of the loop of Henle and, hence, a lower concentration of NH_3 in the renal medullary interstitium.

Dietary restriction of K^+ is advisable, and in itself may be sufficient to correct both the hyperkalemia and the acidosis.[181] Furosemide increases the excretion of both K^+ and net acid, even in patients with moderately advanced renal failure, and has been reported to be both clinically safe and effective;[182,183] large doses of diuretic may be required. Thiazide diuretics are rarely of value, because of the associated renal insufficiency; generally they should be avoided. Fludrocortisone supplements in physiologic doses (0.1 to 0.2 mg) are often disappointing in efficacy, but such supplements in higher doses are sometimes beneficial.[184] This tubular resistance to aldosterone remains unexplained, but underlines the fact that the disturbances in K^+ and acid-base metabolism in type IV RTA are not simply due to low aldosterone levels, despite the commonly used term "hypoaldosteronism." Continued use of mineralocorticoid may lead to significant salt and water retention, even to the point of heart failure; the addition of a diuretic is valuable in such cases.[183] Ion exchange resins are effective, but are poorly tolerated in the long term by most patients. Correction of the acidosis generally follows successful treatment of the hyperkalemia; bicarbonate is rarely needed to correct the acidosis.

INCOMPLETE RTA

Definition

There is a problem for nephrologists who deal with patients who are said to have incomplete RTA. This problem can be illustrated by the example of a patient who is referred because of recurrent nephrolithiasis. The pH of the patient's first morning urine is consistently greater than 6, but acidosis is never present. The question is, *does this patient have incomplete RTA*? There are three major diagnostic possibilities. First, if the pH of the urine falls to less than 5.3 after an acute load of NH_4Cl, the patient probably does not have RTA (Fig. 27-12); probably he or she is normal and consumes a diet with a small net acid load. The other two entities are lumped into the diagnostic category of incomplete RTA. The hallmark of this group of lesions is that the pH of the urine remains above 5.5 following an acute load of NH_4Cl.[48] We recognize the two separate diagnostic categories by examining the rate of excretion of NH_4^+ and the components of net acid excretion. First, this patient may have what we call "occult" distal RTA [a low rate of excretion of NH_4^+ during acidemia, not apparent now because he or she consumes a diet with a very small net acid load (a diet rich in fruits and vegetables) or is being treated with bicarbonate or its equivalent for the nephrolithiasis]. The second diagnostic possibility for the persistently high pH of the urine that fails to decline below 5.5 with an acute load of NH_4Cl is "bonafide" incomplete RTA. These patients do not have a reduced rate of NAE. Nevertheless, the components of NAE in these patients differ from those in normal subjects; these patients excrete more NH_4^+ and less TA.[48] We shall discuss only the bonafide incomplete RTA group, emphasizing the pathophysiology for a relatively high rate of excretion of NH_4^+ at a high pH of the urine.

Clinical features

The diagnosis of incomplete RTA is usually suspected in patients with nephrocalcinosis or nephrolithiasis in whom metabolic acidosis is not present and the urinary pH is persistently high (greater than 5.5).[185,186] Some cases are detected during the screening of the kindred of a proband with established distal RTA.[187-191] The diagnosis is established when the subject fails to excrete urine with a pH less than 5.3 after the administration of an acute acid load.[48] Patients at this stage of their disease do not develop metabolic acidosis of renal origin. It is of interest that patients with incomplete RTA and those with "occult distal RTA" have several features in common (persistently high urinary pH and a low rate of excretion of citrate). Nevertheless, they have one major difference, a difference related to the excretion of NH_4^+. This will be emphasized below.

Pathophysiology

A high urinary pH that fails to decrease in response to an acute acid load can result from either of two major pathophysiologic mechanisms: a low rate of secretion of H^+ or a high availability of NH_3 in the medullary interstitium (Fig. 27-14). These two causes for a high pH of the urine are differentiated by examining the rate of excretion of NH_4^+; it will be low in the case of a reduced rate of secretion of H^+ in the distal nephron (occult distal RTA), and high in the case of a higher availability of NH_3 in the medullary interstitium (incomplete RTA).

We reserve the term *incomplete RTA* for cases in which the subjects have unusually high concentrations of NH_3 in the urine.[87] A high concentration of NH_3 in the urine reflects the net results of two processes. First, the rate of input of NH_3 into the medullary interstitium may be high. This is directly related to the rate of production of NH_4^+ in the proximal tubule,[69] together with its reabsorption and accumulation in the renal medullary interstitium.[30] Second, the rate of transfer of NH_3 from the medullary interstitium to the lumen of the collecting duct reflects in large part, the concentration of H^+ in the lumen. The major pathophysiologic stimuli of NH_4^+ production are acidosis[69] and hypokalemia.[28] In patients with incomplete RTA these two stimuli, acidosis and hypokalemia, are not present. Therefore, to account for the observations of high excretion of NH_3 in the absence of systemic acidosis or hypokalemia, Donnelly and coworkers[87] hypothesized that there was an increased rate of production of NH_4^+ that resulted from an acidified proximal tubular cell. Supporting evidence for this hypothesis was derived from the fact that the rate of excretion of citrate in these patients was low in the absence of acidemia.[79,189]

The natural history of this disorder is interesting. At the earliest stage, patients have persistently high urinary pH together with a rate of excretion of NH_4^+ that is relatively high. The final stage of the disease is characterized by nephrocalcinosis and classic distal RTA with low excretion of NH_4^+. At both stages there is a high pH of the urine, but possibly for different reasons (high NH_3 on the one hand, and low H^+ secretion—due to destruction of the renal medulla—at later stages). The question remains, *How did a disease that starts with high excretion of NH_4^+ lead to one with a low rate of excretion of NH_4^+?* A hypothesis that can explain this scenario begins with an acidified proximal cell. This, in turn, leads to an enhanced rate of production of NH_4^+ and a reduced rate of excretion of citrate. This combination of events may lead to damage of the renal medulla by one or both of two mechanisms:

Damage by a high concentration of NH_3

The high concentration of NH_3 in the medulla may activate complement via the alternate pathway causing a non-immune-mediated interstitial inflammation, as proposed by Nath and coworkers.[192]

Damage by the deposition of calcium

The shunting of NH_4^+ from the loop of Henle to the collecting duct may be associated with a more alkaline medullary interstitium.[3] This alkalinity, in conjunction with the low citrate (or separately from it), may promote the development of nephrocalcinosis and nephrolithiasis that contribute to parenchymal damage.

Once damage to the renal medulla has occurred, the transfer of NH_4^+ to the urine may be compromised.[30] A reduced rate of excretion of NH_4^+ will decrease NAE, which may ultimately give rise to a systemic acidosis. The development of acidosis marks the clinical transformation of high NH_3 disease to overt low NH_4^+ excretion disease.

Diagnostic tests

The tests that are of use in subjects with incomplete RTA are those used to screen patients suspected of having this disorder, and those used to establish the diagnosis. The disease is currently defined by the response to the short NH_4Cl loading test that is associated with a minimum urinary pH that is greater than 5.3. As greater understanding of this entity evolves, however, the role of the high NH_3 in generating this result should be taken into account.

Screening tests include the pH of the first morning urine and the rate of excretion of citrate. A first morning voided urine with a pH greater than 6.0 has been suggested in one report as the most sensitive standard.[187] Other authors have used spot urine citrate concentrations for broad-based population screening.[193] Although preliminary results seem promising, this method has not been subjected to a systematic evaluation.

Treatment

The objective of therapy is to minimize the risk of further episodes of nephrolithiasis and the development of nephrocalcinosis. In so doing, perhaps the natural history of the disease can be favorably modified. We cannot evaluate data in the literature in this regard, since patients with incomplete RTA (high NH_3 in the urine) were not separated from patients with "occult distal RTA" in these reports.

Hypokalemia must be avoided. Indeed, if a 24-h urine collection reveals a diet poor in K^+ (under 50 mmol/day), the effects of an augmented dietary K^+ intake can be easily measured. Furthermore, the finding of hypocitraturia that responds to K^+ citrate therapy also provides a measurable outcome that may be monitored. Other measures are controversial. Therapy with alkali (citrate or bicarbonate) may be of benefit. Such recommendations are tempered by the consideration that a more alkaline urine may increase the tendency to nephrolithiasis or nephrocalcinosis. The K^+, rather than the Na^+, salt of citrate may offer benefits, in that—although both increase the excretion of citrate—only the K^+ salt leads to a decrease in the excretion of calcium and saturation of the urine with calcium oxalate and Na^+ urate.[194]

CLINICAL EXAMPLE

The following example is provided to illustrate that focusing on the urinary pH, rather than on the rate of excretion of NH_4^+ in the urine, may give rise to a very different interpretation of the cause of hyperchloremic metabolic acidosis. The example that we have chosen addresses the association of hyperchloremic metabolic acidosis with exposure to toluene. Judge for yourself the relative merits of each form of analysis.

The association between toluene and hyperchloremic metabolic acidosis was first recognized by Taher and coworkers[195] and was said to be due to distal RTA, on the basis of the presence of metabolic acidosis with a near-normal anion gap and a high urinary pH.[195-206]

Carlisle and coworkers[68] challenged this interpretation of the data. In the 8 patients who abused toluene for whom key data are reported, the excretion of NH_4^+ in the urine was not low in 6 of the 8. One can safely say that 6 of these patients did not have low NH_4^+ excretion disease and that the kidney was not the sole cause of their acidosis. The basis for their hyperchloremic metabolic acidosis seemed to be the conversion of toluene to hippuric acid in the liver; this process adds 1 mmol of H^+ to the body for every 1 mmol of toluene metabolized. This production of acid was substantial, because the excretion of hippurate was as high as 250 mmol/day.[197] Thus the acidosis associated with toluene is due, at least in part (and sometimes exclusively), to the overproduction of hippuric acid.

This metabolic acidosis presents with a normal anion gap, because there is an indirect loss of Na^+ and bicarbonate. This is illustrated in Fig. 27-20. The key components are:

1. Overproduction of a nonvolatile acid (hippuric acid).
2. Titration of endogenous bicarbonate, forming CO_2, which is exhaled. The net result is loss of bicarbonate from the body.
3. Excretion of the conjugate base (hippurate) in the urine at a rate that exceeds the rate of excretion of H^+ and NH_4^+; thus hippurate will be lost with Na^+ or K^+.

Taken together, the above three steps will lead to metabolic acidosis due to overproduction of acid and will be accompanied by a normal anion gap in the plasma.[61] The maintenance of this normal anion gap depends on the near-complete elimination of hippurate in the urine.[207] If the rate of excretion of hippurate falls, hippurate will accumulate in the plasma and the anion gap will be elevated. This might occur with a low GFR or inhibited secretion of hippurate.[199]

The above example emphasizes the limitation of the urinary pH as an initial diagnostic test for RTA. A high rate of excretion of NH_4^+ during metabolic acidosis indicates that distal RTA is not the sole cause of acidosis, even if the urinary pH is not low. For this reason we urge all practitioners, when considering the diagnosis of distal RTA in a patient with metabolic acidosis, to "*R*ecognize *T*he *A*mmonium defect and *pH*orget the urinary pH" as an initial step (Fig. 27-13).[59]

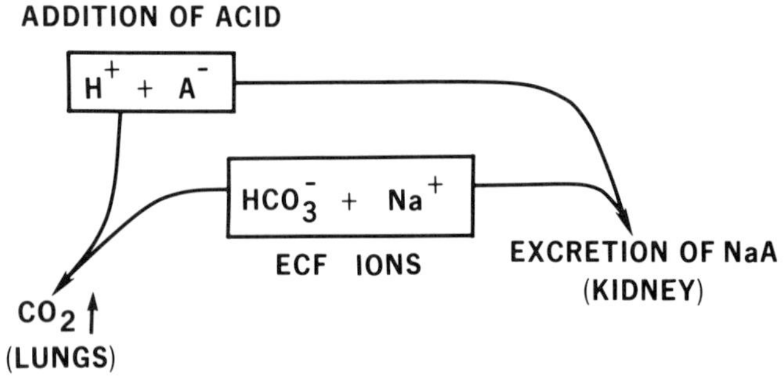

FIGURE 27-20 • "Indirect" loss of sodium bicarbonate. There are two components to the loss of ECF Na^+ and bicarbonate: First, there is production of an acid (H^+) other than carbonic acid (smaller rectangle); second, the anion or conjugate base of that acid (A^-) is excreted in the urine with Na^+ or K^+, not with H^+ or NH_4^+. Thus there is loss of $NaHCO_3$ from the body. (From Halperin ML, Goldstein MB: *Fluid, Electrolyte, and Acid-Base Emergencies.* Philadelphia, Saunders, 1988. Used by permission.)

APPENDIX 1

Consider the filtration and reabsorption of bicarbonate for example (Table 27-6). For ease of calculation, we set the following as constants: GFR is 100 liters per unit time; the concentration of bicarbonate in plasma is either 15 mmol/liter, 24 mmol/liter, or 40 mmol/liter (the latter two figures represent concentrations obtained during an infusion of sodium bicarbonate); the maximum rate of reabsorption of bicarbonate is 25 mmol per liter GFR; bicarbonate will be absorbed in the proximal tubule until its concentration is 10 mmol/liter lower in the lumen than in plasma (owing to backleak of bicarbonate), or until the maximum velocity (V_{max}) of absorption of bicarbonate is reached; and the distal nephron reabsorbs only 2 mmol per liter GFR. As can be seen in Fig. 27-17 and Table 27-6, one would not achieve a constant rate of absorption of bicarbonate per liter GFR that was lower than that in normal subjects during an infusion of bicarbonate in the backleak model; in fact, reabsorption of bicarbonate would rise until the normal V_{max} was achieved. Since there is a lower rate of reabsorption of bicarbonate in subjects with Fanconi syndrome who received a large infusion of bicarbonate,[88,208] we do not think that the backleak model is a likely explanation of the basis of the Fanconi syndrome.

REFERENCES

1. Halperin M, Rolleston F: *Biochemical detective stories: A problem-based approach to clinical cases.* Burlington, North Carolina, Neil Patterson Publications, 1990, pp 25–26, 91–97.
2. Halperin ML, Jungas RL: Metabolism and acid-base physiology. *J Int Soc Art Org* 6:357, 1983.
3. Halperin ML: How much "new" bicarbonate is formed in the distal nephron in the process of net acid excretion? *Kidney Int* 35:1277, 1989.
4. Alperin R: Cell mechanisms of proximal tubule acidification. *Physiol Rev* 70:79, 1990.
5. Murer H et al: Sodium/proton antiport in brush-border-vesicles isolated from rat small intestines and kidney. *Biochem J* 154:597, 1976.
6. Bank N et al: Evidence for a DCCD-sensitive component of proximal bicarbonate reabsorption. *Am J Physiol* 249:F636, 1985.
7. Kinne-Saffran E et al: An ATP-driven proton pump in brush border membranes from the rat renal cortex. *J Membr Biol* 64:67, 1982.
8. Cogan M: Regulation and control of bicarbonate reabsorption in the proximal tubule. *Semin Nephrol* 10:115, 1990.
9. Gluck S et al: The proton translocating ATPase responsible for urinary acidification. *J Biol Chem* 257:9230, 1982.
10. Gluck S, Al-Awqati Q: An electrogenic proton translocating adenosine triphosphatase from bovine kidney medulla. *J Clin Invest* 73:1704, 1984.
11. Garg L, Narang N: Ouabain-insensitive K-adenosine triphosphatase in distal nephron segments of the rabbit. *J Clin Invest* 81:1204, 1988.
12. Wingo C: Active proton secretion and potassium absorption in the rabbit outer medullary collecting duct. *J Clin Invest* 84:361, 1989.
13. Fisher J et al: Chloride dependence of the HCO_3^- exit step in urinary acidification by the turtle bladder. *Am J Physiol* 245:F564, 1983.
14. Stone D et al: Anion dependence of medullary collecting duct acidification. *J Clin Invest* 71:1505, 1983.
15. McKinney T, Burg M: Bicarbonate secretion by rabbit cortical collecting tubule in vitro. *J Clin Invest* 61:1421, 1987.
16. Laski M, Kurtzman N: Characterization of acidification in the cortical and medullary collecting tubule of the rabbit. *J Clin Invest* 72:2050, 1983.
17. Stone D et al: Mineralocorticoid modulation of rabbit medullary collecting duct acidification—a sodium independent effect. *J Clin Invest* 72:77, 1983.
18. Schwartz G, Al-Awqati Q: Two functionally distinct types of mitochondria-rich (MR) cells in cortical collecting tubule (CCT) as determined by changes in cell pH (pH_i) in individually identified cells. *Kidney Int* 27:288, 1984.
19. Bank N, Schwartz WB: Influence of certain urinary solutes on acidic dissociation constant of ammonium at 37°C. *J Appl Physiol* 15:125, 1960.
20. Buerkert J et al: Segmental analysis of the renal tubule in buffer production and net acid formation. *Am J Physiol* 244:F442, 1983.
21. Halperin ML et al: Biochemistry and physiology of ammonium excretion, in Seldin D, Giebisch G (eds): *The Kidney: Physiology and Pathophysiology.* New York, Raven Press, 1991, pp 1471–1489.
22. Halperin ML et al: Regulation of the maximum rate of renal ammoniagenesis in the dog with chronic metabolic acidosis: A quantitative analysis. *Am J Physiol* 248:F607, 1985.
23. Flatt JP: On the maximal possible rate of ketogenesis. *Diabetes* 21:50, 1972.
24. Mandel L, Balaban R: Stoichiometry and coupling of active transport to oxidative metabolism in epithelial tissues. *Am J Physiol* 240:F357, 1981.
25. Lemieux G et al: The effect of ketone bodies on renal ammoniagenesis. *J Clin Invest* 50:1781, 1971.
26. Fraley DS et al: Metabolic acidosis after hyperalimentation with casein hydrolysate. *Ann Intern Med* 88:352, 1978.
27. Vinay P et al: Effect of fatty acids on renal ammoniagenesis in vivo and in vitro studies. *Am J Physiol* 231:880, 1976.
28. Tannen R: Effect of potassium on renal acidification and acid-base homeostasis. *Semin Nephrol* 7:263, 1987.
29. Halperin M et al: What is the underlying defect in patients with isolated, proximal renal tubular acidosis? *Am J Nephrol* 9:265, 1989.
30. Knepper MA et al: Ammonium transport in the kidney. *Am Physiol Soc* 69:179, 1989.
31. Good D, Burg M: Ammonia production by individual segments of the rat nephron. *J Clin Invest* 73:602, 1984.
32. Nagami G: Luminal secretion of ammonia in the mouse

proximal tubule perfused in vitro. *J Clin Invest* 81:159, 1988.

33. Good DW, DuBose TD Jr: HCO_3^- and NH_4^+ transport in rat medullary thick ascending limb: Effects of acid-base and Na^+ balance. *Clin Res* 37:581(A), 1989.
34. Good DW et al: Ammonia and bicarbonate transport by thick ascending limb of rat kidney. *Am J Physiol* 247:F35, 1984.
35. Good DW: Active absorption of NH_4^+ by rat medullary thick ascending limb: Inhibition by potassium. *Am J Physiol* 255:F78, 1988.
36. Kikeri D et al: Cell membranes impermeable to NH_3. *Nature* 339:478, 1989.
37. Nash T, Benedict S: The ammonia content of the blood and its bearing on the mechanism of acid neutralization in the animal organism. *J Biol Chem* 48:463, 1921.
38. Van Slyke D et al: Glutamine as source material of urinary ammonia. *J Biol Chem* 150:481, 1943.
39. Walter F: Untersuchungen uber die wirkung der sauren auf den tierischen organismus. *Arch Expt Pathol Pharmakol* 7:148, 1877.
40. Yu HL et al: Stimulation of ammonia production and excretion in the rabbit by inorganic phosphate. *J Clin Invest* 58:557, 1976.
41. Atchley D et al: A detailed study of electrolyte balances following the withdrawal and reestablishment of insulin therapy. *J Clin Invest* 12:297, 1933.
42. Folling A: On the mechanism of the ammonium chloride acidosis. *Acta Med Scand* 71:221, 1929.
43. Albright F et al: Osteomalacia and late rickets: Various etiologies met in United States with emphasis on that resulting from specific form of renal acidosis, therapeutic indications for each etiological subgroup, and relationship between osteomalacia and Milkman's syndrome. *Medicine* 25:399, 1946.
44. Henderson L, Palmer W: On the several factors of acid excretion in nephritis. *J Biol Chem* 21:37, 1915.
45. Pines K, Mudge G: Renal tubular acidosis with osteomalacia. Report of three cases. *Am J Med* 11:302, 1951.
46. Morris RJ: An experimental renal acidification defect in patients with hereditary fructose intolerance II. *J Clin Invest* 47:1648, 1968.
47. Soriano et al: Bicarbonate reabsorption and hydrogen ion excretion in children with renal tubular acidosis. *J Pediatr* 71:802, 1967.
48. Wrong O, Davies W: The excretion of acid in renal disease. *Q J Med* 23:259, 1959.
49. Batlle D et al: Distal renal tubular acidosis with intact capacity to lower urinary pH. *Am J Med* 72:751, 1982.
50. Kurtzman NA: Renal tubular acidosis: A constellation of syndromes. *Hosp Pract* 22:173, 1987.
51. Morris RJ: Renal tubular acidosis: Mechanisms, classification and implications. *N Engl J Med* 281:1405, 1969.
52. Reynolds T: Observations on the pathogenesis of renal tubular acidosis. *Am J Med* 25:503, 1958.
53. Soriano J, Edelman C: Renal tubular acidosis. *Annu Rev Med* 20:363, 1969.
54. Schloeder FX, Stinebaugh BJ: Defect of urinary acidification during fasting. *Metabolism* 15:17, 1966.
55. Richardson RMA, Halperin ML: The urine pH: A potentially misleading diagnostic test in patients with hyperchloremic metabolic acidosis. *Am J Kidney Dis* 10:140, 1987.
56. Simpson D: Control of hydrogen ion homeostasis and renal acidosis. *Medicine* 50:503, 1971.
57. Madison LL, Seldin DW: Ammonia excretion and renal enzymatic adaptation in human subjects, as disclosed by administration of precursor amino acids. *J Clin Invest* 37:1615, 1958.
58. Jimenez-Diaz C: Death in Addison's disease (functional renal failure). *Lancet* 2:1135, 1936.
59. Carlisle E et al: Renal tubular acidosis (RTA): Recognize The Ammonium defect and pHorget the urine pH. *Pediatr Nephrol* 5:242, 1991.
60. Kamel K et al: The removal of an inorganic acid load in subjects with ketoacidosis of chronic fasting: The role of the kidney. *Kidney Int* 37:507, 1990.
61. Hammeke M et al: Hyperchloremic metabolic acidosis in diabetes mellitus: A case report and discussion of the pathophysiologic mechanisms. *Diabetes* 27:16, 1978.
62. Katagawa K et al: Urinary ammonium measurement by the auto-analyzer method. *Kidney Int* 36:291, 1989.
63. Goldstein M et al: The urine anion gap: A clinically useful index of ammonium excretion. *Am J Med Sci* 292:198, 1986.
64. Dyck R et al: A modification of the urine osmolal gap: An improved method for estimating urine ammonium. *Am J Nephrol* 10:359, 1990.
65. Halperin ML et al: The urine osmolal gap: A clue to estimate urine ammonium in "hybrid" types of metabolic acidosis. *Clin Invest Med* 11:198, 1988.
66. Kamel K et al: Urine electrolytes and osmolality: When and how to use them. *Am J Nephrol* 10:89, 1990.
67. Relman AS et al: Endogenous production of fixed acid and the measurement of the net balance of acid in normal subjects. *J Clin Invest* 40:1621, 1961.
68. Carlisle E et al: Glue-sniffing and distal renal tubular acidosis: Sticking to the facts. *J Am Soc Nephrol* 1:1019, 1991.
69. Brosnan JT et al: Renal ammonium production—une vue Canadienne. *Can J Physiol Pharmacol* 65:489, 1987.
70. Halperin M et al: Studies on the pathogenesis of type I (distal) renal tubular acidosis as revealed by the urinary P_{CO_2} tensions. *J Clin Invest* 53:669, 1974.
71. Arruda et al: The critical importance of urinary concentrating ability in the generation of urinary carbon dioxide tension. *J Clin Invest* 60:922, 1977.
72. Maren T: Carbon dioxide equilibria in the kidney: The problems of elevated carbon dioxide tension, delayed dehydration, and disequilibrium pH. *Kidney Int* 14:395, 1978.
73. DuBose TJ: Hydrogen ion secretion by the collecting duct as a determinant of the urine to blood P_{CO_2} gradient in alkaline urine. *J Clin Invest* 71:55, 1982.
74. DuBose TJ, Caflisch C: Validation of the difference in urine and blood carbon dioxide tension during bicarbonate loading as an index of distal nephron acidification in experimental models of distal renal tubular acidosis. *J Clin Invest* 75:1116, 1985.
75. Adrogue H et al: Decreased distal acidification in acute hypercapnia in the dog. *Am J Physiol* 244:F19, 1983.

76. Batlle D et al: Suppression of distal urinary acidification after recovery from chronic hypocapnia. *Am J Physiol* 245:F433, 1983.
77. Dedmond R, Wrong O: The excretion of organic anion in renal tubular acidosis with particular reference to citrate. *Clin Sci* 22:19, 1962.
78. Simpson D: Citrate excretion: A window on renal metabolism. *Am J Physiol* 244:F223, 1983.
79. Hamm L, Simon E: Roles and mechanisms of urinary buffer excretion. *Am J Physiol* 253:F595, 1987.
80. Robinson B et al: Regulation of citrate transport and pyruvate dehydrogenase in rat kidney cortex mitochondria by bicarbonate. *J Biol Chem* 252:5661, 1977.
81. Brennan S et al: Effect of pH on citrate reabsorption in the proximal convoluted tubule. *Am J Physiol* 255:F301, 1988.
82. Donnelly S et al: Isolated proximal renal tubular acidosis: Dissociation of cellular and systemic pH. *Clin Invest Med* 14:A134, 1991.
83. Preminger GM et al: Prevention of recurrent calcium stone formation with potassium citrate therapy in patients with distal renal tubular acidosis. *J Urol* 134:20, 1985.
84. Buckalew V Jr et al: Incomplete renal tubular acidosis: Physiologic studies in three patients with a defect in lowering urine pH. *Am J Med* 45:32, 1968.
85. Buckalew VMJ Jr: Nephrolithiasis in renal tubular acidosis. *Medicine* 141:731, 1989.
86. Caruana R, Buckalew VMJ Jr: The syndrome of distal (Type 1) renal tubular acidosis: Clinical and laboratory findings in 58 cases. *Medicine* 67:84, 1988.
87. Donnelly S et al: Might distal renal tubular acidosis be a proximal disorder? *Am J Kidney Dis* 19:272, 1992.
88. Soriano et al: Proximal renal tubular acidosis. A defect in bicarbonate reabsorption with normal urinary acidification. *Pediatr Res* 1:81, 1967.
89. Brenes L et al: Familial proximal renal tubular acidosis: A distinct clinical entity. *Am J Med* 63:244, 1977.
90. Fanconi G: Die nicht diabetischen. Glykosurienund hyperglykamien des alteren kindes. *Jahrb f Kinderh* 133:256, 1931.
91. Bernardini I et al: Plasma and muscle free carnitine deficiency due to renal Fanconi syndrome. *J Clin Invest* 75:1124, 1985.
92. DuBose TJ, Alpern R: Renal tubular acidosis, Scriver C et al (eds): *Metabolic Basis of Inherited Disease*, 6th ed. New York, McGraw-Hill, 1989, pp 2539–2568.
93. Angielski S, Rogulski S: Effect of maleic acid on the kidney. I Oxidation of Krebs cycle intermediates by various tissues of maleate intoxicated rats. *Biochem Polonica* 9:357, 1962.
94. Berliner R et al: Effect of maleic acid on renal function. *Proc Soc Exp Biol Med* 75:791, 1951.
95. Gougoux A et al: Maleate-induced stimulation of glutamine metabolism in the intact dog kidney. *Am J Physiol* 248:F585, 1985.
96. Kramer H, Gonick H: Experimental Fanconi syndrome I. Effect of maleic acid on renal cortical Na-K-ATPase activity and ATP levels. *J Lab Clin Med* 76:799, 1970.
97. Akaike N: Regulation of sodium and potassium in muscle of potassium-deficient rats. *News in Physiol Sci* 3:25, 1988.
98. Bovee K et al: Spontaneous Fanconi syndrome in the dog. *Metabolism* 27:45, 1978.
99. Bovee K et al: The Fanconi Syndrome in Basenji dogs: A new model for renal transport defects. *Science* 201:1129, 1978.
100. Easley J, Breitschwerdt E: Glucosuria associated with renal tubular dysfunction in three Basenji dogs. *JAMA* 168:938, 1976.
101. Brenes LG et al: Impaired urinary ammonium excretion in patients with proximal renal tubular acidosis (pRTA). *Kidney Int* 33:183 (abstract), 1988.
102. Kondo T et al: Inactive form of erythrocyte carbonic anhydrase B in patients with primary renal tubular acidosis. *J Clin Invest* 61:610, 1978.
103. Gougoux A et al: Effect of blood pH on distal nephron hydrogen ion secretion. *Kidney Int* 17:615, 1980.
104. Lemieux G et al: Metabolic machinery of the alligator kidney. *Am J Physiol* 247:F686, 1984.
105. Coulson RA, Hernandez T: Source and function of urinary ammonia in the alligator. *Am J Physiol* 197:873, 1959.
106. Lemieux G et al: Net tubular secretion of bicarbonate by the alligator kidney. Antimammalian response to acetazolamide. *Kidney Int* 28:760, 1985.
107. Roth K et al: The Fanconi syndrome and mechanisms of tubular transport dysfunction. *Kidney Int* 20:705, 1981.
108. Edelman C Jr et al: Renal bicarbonate reabsorption and hydrogen ion excretion in normal infants. *J Clin Invest* 46:1309, 1967.
109. Bergeron M, Gougoux A: The renal Fanconi syndrome, in Scriver C et al: (eds): *Metabolic Basis of Inherited Disease*, 6th ed. New York, McGraw-Hill, 1989, pp 2569–2580.
110. McSherry E, Morris R Jr: Attainment and maintenance of normal stature with alkali therapy in infants and children with classic renal tubular acidosis. *J Clin Invest* 61:509, 1978.
111. Puig J et al: Complete proximal tubular acidosis (Type 2, RTA) in chronic active hepatitis. *Clin Nephrol* 13:287, 1980.
112. Farfel Z et al: Proximal renal tubular acidosis. Association with familial normaldosteronemic hyperpotassemia and hypertension. *Arch Intern Med* 138:1837, 1978.
113. Soriano R et al: Proximal renal tubular acidosis in tetralogy of Fallot. *Acta Paediatr Scand* 64:671, 1975.
114. Soriano R et al: Proximal renal tubular acidosis in metachromatic leukodystrophy. *Helv Paediat Acta* 33:45, 1978.
115. Koppang H et al: Dental features in congenital persistent renal tubular acidosis of proximal type. *Scand J Dent Res* 92:489, 1984.
116. Carlisle E et al: Studies on the effects of anion excretion on potassium secretion in man. *Kidney Int* 39:1206, 1991.
117. Ponce S et al: Drug-induced hyperkalemia. *Medicine* 64:357, 1985.
118. Lemann J Jr et al: The effects of chronic acid loads in normal man: Further evidence for the participation of bone mineral in the defence of acidosis. *J Clin Invest* 45:1608, 1966.

119. Lemann J Jr, Lennon E: Role of diet, gastrointestinal tract and bone in acid-base homeostasis. *Kidney Int* 1:275, 1972.
120. Adams N et al: The calciuria of fixed acid production in humans: Evidence against a role of parathyroid hormone and 1,25$(OH)_2$-vitamin D. *Calcif Tissue Int* 28:233, 1979.
121. Oh M: Irrelevance of bone buffering to acid-base homeostasis in chronic metabolic acidosis. *Nephron* 59:7, 1991.
122. Langman C: Calcitriol metabolism during chronic metabolic acidosis. *Semin Nephrol* 9:65, 1989.
123. Brewer E et al: Maleic acid-induced impaired conversion of 25$(OH)D_3$ to 1,25$(OH)_2D_3$: Implications for Fanconi's syndrome. *Kidney Int* 12:244, 1977.
124. Gahl W: Cystinosis: Progress in a Prototypic Disease. *Ann Intern Med* 109:557, 1988.
125. Mahoney C et al: Renal transplantation for childhood cystinosis. *N Engl J Med* 283:397, 1970.
126. Gahl W et al: Cysteamine therapy for children with nephropathic cystinosis. *N Engl J Med* 316:971, 1987.
127. da Silva V et al: Long-term treatment of infantile nephropathic cystinosis with cysteamine. *N Engl J Med* 313:1460, 1985.
128. Reiss R et al: Successful pregnancy despite placental cystine crystals in a woman with nephropathic cystinosis. *N Engl J Med* 319:223, 1988.
129. Richardson R et al: Pathogenesis of acidosis in hereditary fructose intolerance. *Metabolism* 28:1133, 1979.
130. Holzel A et al: Galactosemia. *Am J Med* 22:703, 1957.
131. Kvittingen E: Hereditary tyrosinemia type I. An overview. *Scand J Clin Lab* 46:27, 1986.
132. Morgan H et al: Wilson's disease and the Fanconi syndrome. *Q J Med* 31:361, 1962.
133. Elsas L et al: Wilson's disease with reversible renal tubular dysfunction: Correlation with proximal tubular ultrastructure. *Ann Intern Med* 75:427, 1971.
134. Lowe C et al: Organic-aciduria, decreased renal ammonia production, hydrophthalmos, and mental retardation: A clinical entity. *Am J Dis Child* 83:164, 1952.
135. Adams R et al: The development of cadmium-induced proteinuria, impaired renal function, and osteomalacia in alkaline battery workers. *Q J Med* 38:425, 1969.
136. Clarkson T, Kench J: Urinary excretion of amino acids by men absorbing heavy metals. *Biochem J* 62:361, 1956.
137. Chisolm JJ et al: Amino-aciduria, hypophosphatemia, and rickets in lead poisoning. *Am J Dis Child* 89:159, 1955.
138. Gross J: Fanconi syndrome (adult type) developing secondary to the ingestion of outdated tetracycline. *Ann Intern Med* 58:523, 1963.
139. Rochman J et al: Adult Fanconi's syndrome with renal tubular acidosis in association with renal amyloidosis: Occurrence in a patient with chronic lymphocytic leukemia. *Arch Intern Med* 140:1361, 1980.
140. Smithline N et al: Light-chain nephropathy: Renal tubular dysfunction associated with light-chain proteinuria. *N Engl J Med* 294:71, 1976.
141. Dahlstrom U et al: Occurrence of adult Fanconi syndrome in benign monoclonal gammopathy. *Acta Med Scand* 208:425, 1980.
142. Kamm D, Fischer M: Proximal renal tubular acidosis and the Fanconi syndrome in a patient with hypergammaglobulinemia. *Nephron* 9:208, 1972.
143. Nash M et al: Renal tubular acidosis in infants and children. *J Pediatr* 80:738, 1972.
144. Callis L et al: Effect of hydrochlorothiazide on rickets and on renal tubular acidosis in two patients with cystinosis. *Helv Paediat Acta* 25:602, 1970.
145. Garin E, Scott D: Indomethacin in the treatment of proximal tubular acidosis. *Clin Pediatr* 24:711, 1985.
146. Gahl W et al: Oral carnitine therapy in children with cystinosis and renal Fanconi syndrome. *J Clin Invest* 81:549, 1988.
147. McEnery P, Silverman F: Acceleration of growth with combined vitamin D-phosphate therapy of hypophosphatemic resistant rickets. *J Pediatr* 80:763, 1972.
148. Phelps K, Uribarri J: Metabolic acidosis due to inapparent defects in renal acid excretion in a patient with chronic diarrhea. *Am J Nephrol* 10:37, 1990.
149. Szylman P et al: Role of hyperkalemia in the metabolic acidosis of isolated hypoaldosteronism. *N Engl J Med* 294:361, 1976.
150. Tannen H et al: Renal adaptation to a high potassium intake: The role of hydrogen ion. *J Clin Invest* 52:2089, 1973.
151. Sastrasinh S, Tannen R: Effect of potassium on renal NH_3 production. *Am J Physiol* 244:F383, 1983.
152. Hulter H et al: Impaired renal H^+ secretion and NH_3 production in mineralocorticoid-deficient glucocorticoid-replete dogs. *Am J Physiol* 232:F136, 1977.
153. Hulter H et al: Chronic hyperkalemic renal tubular acidosis induced by KCl loading. *Am J Physiol* 244:F255, 1983.
154. DuBose TD Jr, Good D: Effects of chronic hyperkalemia on renal production and proximal tubule transport of ammonium in the rat. *Am J Physiol* 260:F680, 1991.
155. Nagami GT: Effect of bath and luminal potassium concentration on ammonia production and secretion by mouse proximal tubules perfused in vitro. *J Clin Invest* 86:32, 1990.
156. Good DW: Effect of potassium on ammonia transport by medullary thick ascending limb of the rat. *J Clin Invest* 80:1358, 1987.
157. DuBose TD Jr, Good D: Chronic hyperkalemia impairs ammonium accumulation and transport in the inner medulla of the rat. *J Clin Invest*, 1991.
158. DuBose TD Jr, Caflisch CR: Effect of selective aldosterone deficiency on acidification in nephron segments of the rat inner medulla. *J Clin Invest* 82:1624, 1988.
159. Stanton B: Regulation by adrenal corticosteroids of sodium and potassium transport in loop of Henle and distal tubule of rat kidney. *J Clin Invest* 78:1612, 1986.
160. Schwartz G, Burg M: Mineralocorticoid effects on cation transport by cortical collecting tubules in vitro. *Am J Physiol* 235:F576, 1978.
161. Koeppen B, Helman S: Acidification of luminal fluid by the rabbit cortical collecting tubule perfused in vitro. *Am J Physiol* 242:F521, 1982.
162. Kornandakieti C, Tannen R: H^+ transport by the aldosterone-deficient rat distal nephron. *Kidney Int* 25:629, 1984.
163. Harrington et al: Mineralocorticoid-stimulated renal acid-

ification: The critical role of dietary sodium. *Kidney Int* 30:43, 1986.
164. Al-Awqati Q et al: Characteristics of stimulation of H^+ transport by aldosterone in turtle urinary bladder. *J Clin Invest* 58:351, 1976.
165. Sebastian A et al: Renal potassium wasting in renal tubular acidosis (RTA): Its occurrence in types 1 and 2 RTA despite sustained correction of systemic acidosis. *J Clin Invest* 50:667, 1971.
166. Ethier J et al: The transtubular potassium concentration in patients with hypokalemia and hyperkalemia. *Am J Kidney Dis* 15:309, 1990.
167. Litzow J et al: The effect of treatment of acidosis on calcium balance in patients with chronic azotemic renal disease. *J Clin Invest* 46:280, 1967.
168. Brenner R et al: Incidence of radiographically evident bone disease, nephrocalcinosios, and nephrolithiasis in various types of renal tubular acidosis. *N Engl J Med* 307:217, 1982.
169. Morris R Jr, Fudenberg H: Impaired renal acidification in patients with hypergammaglobulinemia. *Medicine* 46:57, 1967.
170. Talal N: Sjogren's syndrome, lymphoproliferation, and renal tubular acidosis. *Ann Intern Med* 74:633, 1971.
171. Bridi G et al: Glomerulonephritis and renal tubular acidosis in a case of chronic active hepatitis with hyperimmunoglobulinemia. *Am J Med* 52:267, 1972.
172. Mason A et al: Fibrosing alveolitis associated with renal tubular acidosis. *Br Med J* 4:596, 1970.
173. Tu W, Shearn M: Systemic lupus erythematosus and latent renal tubular dysfunction. *Ann Intern Med* 67:100, 1967.
174. McCurdy D et al: Renal tubular acidosis due to amphotericin B. *N Engl J Med* 278:124, 1968.
175. Perez GO: Incomplete syndrome of renal tubular acidosis induced by lithium carbonate. *J Lab Clin Med* 86:386, 1975.
176. Batlle DC et al: Distal nephron function in patients receiving chronic lithium therapy. *Kidney Int* 21:477, 1982.
177. Higashirhara E et al: Medullary sponge kidney and renal acidification defect. *Kidney Int* 25:453, 1984.
178. Garella S et al: Severity of metabolic acidosis as a determinant of bicarbonate requirements. *N Engl J Med* 289:121, 1973.
179. Fernandez P et al: The concept of bicarbonate distribution space: The crucial role of body buffers. *Kidney Int* 36:747, 1989.
180. Donnelly S et al: Hypokalemia, in Glassock R (ed): *Current Therapy in Nephrology and Hypertension*, 3d ed. Philadelphia, BC Decker, 1991, pp 1015–1023.
181. Maher T et al: Amelioration of metabolic acidosis by dietary potassium restriction in hyperkalemic patients with chronic renal insufficiency. *J Lab Clin Med* 103:432, 1984.
182. Rastogi S et al: Effect of furosemide on urinary acidification in distal renal tubular acidosis. *J Lab Clin Med* 104:271, 1984.
183. Sebastian A, Schambelan M: Amelioration of hyperchloremic acidosis with furosemide therapy in patients with chronic renal insuffiency and type IV renal tubular acidosis. *Am J Nephrol* 4:287, 1984.
184. Sebastian A et al: Amelioration of metabolic acidosis with fludrocortisone therapy in hyporeninemic hypoaldosteronism. *N Engl J Med* 297:576, 1977.
185. Backman U et al: Incidence and clinical importance of renal tubular defects in recurrent renal stone formers. *Nephron* 25:96, 1980.
186. Osther P et al: Screening renal stone formers for distal renal tubular acidosis. *Br J Urol* 63:581, 1989.
187. Tannen R et al: Incomplete renal tubular acidosis: Some clinical and physiological features. *Nephron* 15:111, 1975.
188. Nordin B, Smith D: Citric acid excretion in renal stone disease and in renal tubular acidosis. *Br J Urol* 35:438, 1963.
189. Norman M et al: Urinary citrate excretion in the diagnosis of distal renal tubular acidosis. *J Pediatr* 92:394, 1978.
190. Nicar M et al: Low urinary citrate excretion in nephrolithiasis. *Urology* 21:8, 1983.
191. Coe F, Parks J: Stone disease in hereditary distal renal tubular acidosis. *Ann Intern Med* 93:60, 1980.
192. Nath K et al: Pathophysiology of chronic tubulo-interstitial disease in rats. *J Clin Invest* 76:667, 1985.
193. Nilwarangkur S et al: Endemic primary distal renal tubular acidosis in Thailand. *Q J Med* 74:289, 1990.
194. Preminger G et al: Alkali action on the urinary crystallization of calcium salts: Contrasting responses to sodium citrate and potassium citrate. *J Urol* 139:240, 1988.
195. Taher S et al: Renal tubular acidosis associated with toluene "sniffing." *N Engl J Med* 290:765, 1974.
196. Steinmetz P et al: Specialty rounds: Nephrology rounds, University of Iowa Hospitals: Renal tubular acidosis. *Am J Med Sci* 271:40, 1976.
197. Batlle D et al: On the mechanism of toluene-induced renal tubular acidosis. *Nephron* 49:210, 1988.
198. Bennett R, Forman H: Hypokalemic periodic paralysis in chronic toluene exposure. *Arch Neurol* 37:673, 1980.
199. Fischman C, Oster J: Toxic effects of toluene: A new cause of high anion gap metabolic acidosis. *JAMA* 241:1713, 1979.
200. Moss A et al: Fanconi's syndrome and distal renal tubular acidosis after glue sniffing. *Ann Intern Med* 92:69, 1980.
201. Streicher H et al: Syndromes of toluene sniffing in adults. *Ann Intern Med* 94:758, 1981.
202. Patel R, Benjamin J Jr: Renal disease associated with toluene inhalation. *Clin Toxicol* 24:213, 1986.
203. Voigts A, Kaufman C Jr: Acidosis and other metabolic abnormalities associated with paint sniffing. *South Med J* 76:443, 1983.
204. Martinez J et al: Renal tubular acidosis with an elevated anion gap in a "glue-sniffer" *Hum Toxicol* 8:139, 1989.
205. Lavoi F et al: Recurrent resuscitation and "no code" orders in a 27-year-old spray paint abuser. *Ann Emerg Med* 16:1266, 1987.
206. Goodwin T: Toluene abuse and renal tubular acidosis in pregnancy. *Obstet Gynecol* 71:715, 1988.
207. Smith H et al: The renal clearances of substituted hippuric acid derivitives and other aromatic acids in dogs and man. *J Clin Invest* 24:388, 1945.
208. Pitts R, Lotspeich W: Bicarbonate and the renal regulation of acid base balance. 138, 1946.

209. Cogan M, Rector FJ: Acid-base disorders, in Brenner B, Rector FJ (eds): *The Kidney*, 3d ed. Philadelphia, Saunders, 1986, p 481.
210. Klahr S, Weiner I: Disorders of acid-base metabolism, in Chan J, Gill J Jr (eds): *Kidney Electrolyte Disorders*. New York, Churchill Livingstone, 1990, p 18.
211. Toto R: Normal anion gap acidosis, in Kokko J, Tannen R (eds): *Fluids and Electrolytes*. Philadelphia, Saunders, 1986, p 258.
212. Madias N, Perrone R: Acid-base disorders in association with renal disease, in Schrier R, Gottschalk C (eds): *Diseases of the Kidney*. Boston/Toronto, Little, Brown, 1988, p 2959.
213. Cogan M: Specific renal tubular disorders, in Wyngaarden J, Smith LJ (eds): *Cecil Textbook of Medicine*, 18th ed. Philadelphia, Saunders, 1988, p 622.
214. Brazy P, Klotman P: Specific renal tubular transport defects, in Kelley W (ed): *Textbook of Internal Medicine*. Philadelphia, Lippincott, 1989, p 784.
215. Richardson R, Kunau RJ: Disorders of acid-base balance, in Stein J (ed): *Internal Medicine*, 2d ed. Boston/Toronto, Little, Brown, 1987, p 829.
216. Sajo IM et al: Sites of ammonia addition to tubular fluid in rats with chronic metabolic acidosis. *Kidney Int* 20:353, 1981.

CHAPTER • 28

Metabolic aspects of metabolic acidosis and metabolic alkalosis

Kamel S. Kamel • Surinder Cheema-Dhadli • Mitchell L. Halperin

The purpose of this chapter is to emphasize the *metabolic* aspects of acidosis and meteabolic alkalosis. In each section, key principles of metabolism, their physiologic importance, and their clinical implications will be discussed. The approach is based on a quantitative, rather than a qualitative, analysis, emphasizing principles of regulation of metabolism. Such an approach can both improve our understanding of the pathophysiology of metabolic acidosis and alkalosis and aid us in determining where leverage should be exerted on the selection and timing of therapy.

METABOLIC ACIDOSIS

Metabolic acidosis is a disease category that includes a wide variety of clinical conditions. Traditionally, causes are divided into two groups based on whether the anion gap in plasma is increased. We prefer to use a classification based on whether acids are produced at a very rapid rate (Table 28-1), rather than one based on a laboratory test (the anion gap in plasma). With overproduction of acids, two categories are recognized, depending on the fate of the conjugate base. If the anion is retained in the body (not filtered or largely reabsorbed by the kidney), the anion gap in plasma will be increased. On the other hand, in a patient with an acid overproduction type of metabolic acidosis with enhanced excretion of the conjugate base in the urine, the anion gap in plasma may not be increased. Therefore, reliance on a high value of the anion gap in plasma will fail to detect the latter subtype, where there is overproduction of an acid. A clinical example of this subtype is the metabolic acidosis associated with glue sniffing.[6] Toluene, a major component of glue, is converted to hippuric acid in the liver. Because the kidney clears the hippurate anion faster than it replenishes the lost bicarbonate,[76] metabolic acidosis with a normal anion gap in plasma will ensue. On the other hand, patients whose metabolic acidosis is due to renal insufficiency have an increased anion gap in plasma, but an overproduction of acids is not usually present.[53]

TABLE 28-1 • Types of metabolic acidosis

ACID OVERPRODUCTION
L-Lactic acid (hypoxia is the most common cause)
D-Lactic acid (GI disorder: stasis, altered bacterial flora)
Ketoacids: insulin lack due
Diabetes mellitus
Ethanol
Fasting
Hypoglycemia
Intoxicants (e.g., methanol, ethylene glycol, toluene)
NO ACID OVERPRODUCTION
Loss of sodium bicarbonate via
GI tract (diarrhea, ileus, drainage)
Urine (acetazolamide, proximal RTA)*
Failure to excrete normal daily acid load
Low NH_4^+ excretion (distal RTA)
Renal failure (really a failure to excrete NH_4^+)

* RTA = renal tubular acidisis.

At times, the basis of the overproduction of acids is not clear from the clinical setting. An additional test that can help the clinician sort out the pathophysiology is an attempt to deduce the properties of the conjugate base of the acid by examining its renal handling. The test we utilize is the *fractional excretion of anions*.[2] This can be calculated as illustrated in equation 1:

$$100 \times [(\text{anion})_{\text{urine}}/(\text{anion})_{\text{plasma}}]/[(\text{creatinine})_{\text{urine}}/(\text{creatinine})_{\text{plasma}}] \quad (1)$$

The concentration of the anion in plasma is estimated from the anion gap in plasma (including K^+ and an estimate for the anionic charge on albumin, 4 meq/liter for every 10 g/liter of albumin.[83] The concentration of the anion in urine is the difference between the concentration of the major cations in the urine (Na^+, K^+, and NH_4^+) and that of the usual anion in the urine (Cl^-). While the concentrations of Na^+, K^+, and Cl^- are readily measured, that of NH_4^+ can be estimated from the osmolal gap in the urine.[14,37,45] We use the fractional excretion of anions as follows. When this fractional excretion exceeds 100 percent, the anion is not only filtered but also secreted (e.g., hippurate[76]). A fractional excretion of anion that is 10 to 15 percent indicates near-complete renal reabsorption of the anion, the best example being L-lactate. The third group of patients are those who would have a fractional excretion of anions that is 20 to 80 percent. The usual cause of a fractional excretion close to 20 percent is ketoacidosis.[74] When values are in the higher range (40 to 80 percent), a mixture of ketoacidosis and lactic acidosis should be suspected.[2]

Patients with metabolic acidosis without overproduction of acids can be divided into two categories. First, sodium bicarbonate could be lost via the gastrointestinal (GI) tract (patients with diarrhea or ileus) or the urine (patients with proximal renal tubular acidosis or those given acetazolamide). Second, the normal rate of production of acids could obtain where the protons remove bicarbonate ions while the conjugate base (e.g., SO_4^{2-}) is excreted in the urine. To achieve acid-base balance, new bicarbonate must be formed; this occurs when NH_4^+ is excreted (Fig. 28-1). Hence, indirect loss of bicarbonate might occur if there is a low rate of excretion of NH_4^+.

Metabolic acidosis is a component of many clinical situations in which a patient can be in great jeopardy. We recognize four major reasons to make the diagnosis of metabolic acidosis, and to do so quickly (Table 28-2). First, the patient might be at great risk because the net

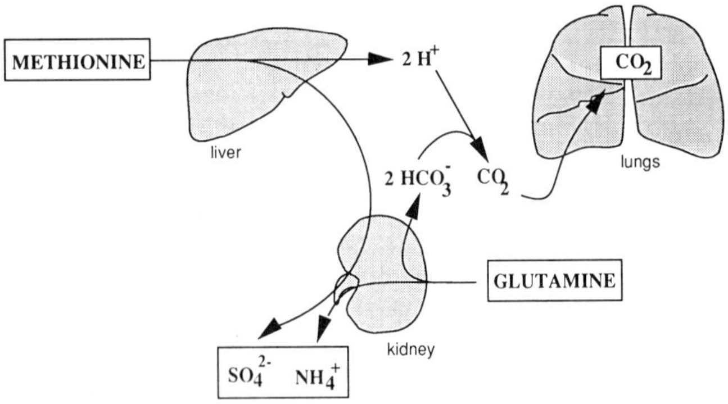

FIGURE 28-1 • Acid-base balance and the kidney. H^+ is produced when a neutral substance (e.g., sulfur-containing amino acids) is converted into anions (SO_4^{2-}) and protons. H^+ is removed when glutamine is converted in the kidney to NH_4^+ and carboxylate anions, with metabolism of the latter to a neutral end product (CO_2 or glucose). NH_4^+ must be excreted in the urine to prevent its conversion in the liver to urea plus H^+.

TABLE 28-2 • Clinical approach to serious threats during increased anion gap metabolic acidosis

Type	Reason for threat	Keys to recognition
Lactic acidosis	• H^+ load: very rapid rate of H^+ production	• Shock • Hypotension
Ketoacidosis	• Relative rate of H^+ production increases in advanced disease • Hyperglycemia • Underlying disease	• History • Serum ketones usually strongly positive • Fluid and electrolyte problems
Intoxications	• Toxic metabolites (formaldehyde, oxalic acid)	• History (methanol, ethylene glycol) • Increased plasma osmolal gap
Renal failure	• Hyperkalemia	• Increased serum creatinine levels • History
D-Lactic acidosis	• Slowly progressive rise in H^+ production • Underlying GI disorder	• Slow GI motility • Altered GI flora (antibiotics) • CNS signs

rate of production of H^+ is so high that death due to acidemia might be imminent. This, in effect, applies to lactic acidosis due to hypoxia or possibly certain cases of ketoacidosis.[32] Second, metabolic acidosis may signal that a patient is at risk from a toxin (e.g., methanol or ethylene glycol). Third, the acidosis might exacerbate the degree of hyperkalemia (e.g., renal failure). Fourth, metabolic acidosis might signal a serious underlying disease (e.g., septicemia or dysfunction of the GI tract).

It is not our intent to discuss even one of the categories in a comprehensive fashion. Rather, we wish to highlight selected metabolic aspects of ketoacidosis and lactic acidosis conditions in which the rate of acid production is very high.

BACKGROUND CONCERNING THE PRODUCTION AND REMOVAL OF H^+ IONS

Production of H^+ ions

In general, metabolism of dietary constituents liberates H^+ ions when a nutrient is converted into a metabolic product that contains a greater net anionic charge (Table 28-3).[28] Thus, oxidation of carbohydrates or triglycerides to exhaled CO_2 and water or the metabolism of most amino acids does not generate H^+ ions because uncharged substrates are converted into uncharged products (equation 2). Exceptions to this generalization are the formation of lactic acid from carbohydrate during states of hypoxia and the formation of ketoacids from fats in states with a relative lack of insulin.

$$\text{Glucose}^0 \rightarrow \text{triglyceride}^0 + H_2O + CO_2 \quad (2)$$

Metabolism of dietary amino acids generates most of the nonvolatile acids (H_2SO_4 and HCl) that normal subjects produce each day. Nonvolatile acids are produced when amino acids that contain sulfur are converted into sulfate anions and protons (equation 3); this results in the generation of 70 mmol/day of H^+ on a typical North American diet.[28]

$$\text{Methionine}^0 \text{ or cysteine}^0 \rightarrow \text{glucose}^0 + \text{urea}^0 + SO_4^{2-} + 2\,H^+ \quad (3)$$

A second type of reaction that generates H^+ is the conversion of cationic amino acids (lysine, arginine, and some histidines) into neutral products (equation 4). The total load of H^+ arising from metabolism of cationic amino acids in the liver is approximately 140 mmol/day.[28]

$$\text{Arginine}^+ \text{ or Lysine}^+ \rightarrow \text{Glucose}^0 \text{ (or triglyceride}^0\text{)} + \text{urea}^0 + H^+ \quad (4)$$

The other major source of the acid load from the diet is the conversion of diesterphosphates to monoesterphosphates (equation 5). Both products of this metabolism can be excreted directly as titratable acid ($H_2PO_4^-$; equation 6). Hence, this process has no major acid-base impact.

TABLE 28-3 • **Diet and the production of acids**

Nutrient	Product	H^+/day, mmol
REACTIONS GENERATING H^+		
Sulfur-containing amino acids	H_2SO_4	70
Cysteine, cystine		
Methionine		
Cationic amino acids	HCl	140
Lysine		
Arginine		
Histidine (½)		
Organic phosphate diesters	$H^+ + H_2PO_4^-$	30
REACTIONS REMOVING H^+		
Anionic amino acids		
Glutamate	HCO_3^-	−70
Aspartate	HCO_3^-	−40
Nonprotein organic anions	HCO_3^-	−60
Organic phosphate monoesters	$H_2PO_4^-$	−30

$$\text{Diester } PO_4^- \rightarrow CO_2^0 + \text{glucose}^0 + HPO_4^{2-} + H^+ \quad (5)$$

$$H^+ + HPO_4^{2-} \text{ (body)} \rightarrow H_2PO_4^- \text{ (urine)} \quad (6)$$

Removal of H^+ ions

Removal of H^+ ions by metabolism:

Metabolism of anions to neutral end products will remove H^+ ions. The typical diet contains anions from two sources. First, approximately 100 mmol of H^+ are removed daily via the metabolism of anionic amino acids (glutamate and asparate, but not their amide derivatives glutamine and asparagine; equation 7):

$$\text{Glutamate}^- \text{ or aspartate}^- + H^+ \rightarrow \text{urea}^0 + CO_2^0 + \text{glucose}^0 \quad (7)$$

The second source of anions is the metabolism of the sodium or potassium salts of dietary organic anions to neutral end products (CO_2, glucose, and triglycerides; equation 8). Examples include acetate, lactate, gluconate, malate, and citrate anions. Although it is difficult to estimate their quantities, a value of 60 meq/day is probably reasonable.[28]

$$\text{Lactate}^- + H^+ \rightarrow CO_2^0 \text{ or glucose}^0 \quad (8)$$

Removal of H^+ ions by the kidney: generation of new bicarbonate

The net result of the production of these strong, nonvolatile acids is a reduction in the concentration of bicarbonate and an elevation in the P_{CO_2} in venous blood. The volatile CO_2 will be excreted via the lungs, but it is the task of the kidney to restore the concentration of bicarbonate in the plasma (Fig. 28-1).[27] Neither sulfuric acid nor hydrochloric acid can be destroyed by metabolic processes, nor can their anions be titrated in the urine. The body, however, can achieve their removal indirectly by using H^+-consuming reactions. This is accomplished by the kidney, which converts glutamine to the cation NH_4^+ and carboxylate anions. The NH_4^+ is excreted in the urine, and carboxylate anions are metabolized to neutral end products, with two protons being removed in the process:

$$\text{Glutamine}^0 \rightarrow 2NH_4^+ + \text{carboxylate}^{2-} \quad (9)$$

$$\text{Carboxylate}^{2-} \rightarrow \text{glucose}^0 \text{ or } CO_2^0 + 2HCO_3^- \quad (10)$$

Although the excretion of NH_4^+ does not directly result in elimination of H^+ generated from amino acid metabolism, it prevents the NH_4^+ from returning to the liver, where formation of urea would liberate protons (or remove bicarbonate; equation 11; Fig. 28-1):[31]

$$2NH_4^+ + 2HCO_3^- \rightarrow \text{urea}^0 + CO_2^0 \quad (11)$$

In quantitative terms, the rate of excretion of NH_4^+ is 0.025 mmol/min in normal subjects,[65] and this rate can rise to 0.20 mmol/min in chronic acidosis.[55,75] Hence, this renal mechanism can only defend against very small acid loads.

Removal of H^+ ions by buffering

To determine how threatening metabolic acidosis might be, it is critical to know the rate of production of H^+ and the capacity of the body to remove this acid via buffering or metabolism. We shall address the issue of buffering here and deal with the rate of removal of H^+ ions via metabolism later (see "Principle 2: The Rate of Production or Removal of H^+ in an Organ Is Determined by the Rate of Turnover of ATP in that Organ").

BUFFERING IN THE EXTRACELLULAR FLUID The major buffer of the extracellular fluid (ECF) is the bicarbonate system. Since the concentration of bicarbonate is normally 25 mmol/liter and the total ECF volume approximates 15 liters in a normal adult, the ECF can buffer only up to 375 mmol of H^+ (25 mmol/liter × 15 liters).

BUFFERING IN THE INTRACELLULAR FLUID There are various ways of gaining quantitative information on the buffer capacity of the ICF. Each method, however, has its limitations. For example, 65 mmol of H^+ are buffered per kilogram of homogenized muscle per unit pH by direct measurements.[3] One must consider, however, which buffers were titrated in a homogenate of muscle. Consider phosphate, for example. Inorganic phosphate is an ideal buffer in that its pK is close to the pH of the ICF. Notwithstanding, there is very little inorganic phosphate (perhaps a few millimoles per liter) available to buffer acid.[86] In contrast, the quantity of organic phosphates is large, but their pKs are too low to make them effective buffers in vivo (4.9 for creatine phosphate and 6.3 for ATP). Homogenized muscle releases inorganic phosphate from two major sources: the products of hydrolysis of creatine phosphate (17 mmol/kg muscle) and ATP (5 mmol/kg muscle, but three phosphates can be liberated in vitro).

The buffer capacity could be deduced if the pH of the ICF and the pK of nonbicarbonate buffers and the total number of these buffers were known with certainty. This, however, is not the case. Therefore, we feel that the most reasonable value to use is the one derived from in vivo studies. For example, Swan and Pitts[81] infused a large quantity of HCl into dogs and determined that 60 percent of buffering occurred in a compartment other than the ECF. In contrast, Vasuvattakul and associates[84] demonstrated that, when a modest acid load was given, most (98 percent) of the buffering was via the bicarbonate buffer system, with little contribution from intracellular nonbicarbonate buffers. Specifically, one-third of this buffering was via intracellular bicarbonate, provided that the appropriate degree of hyperventilation occurred.

Review

Is the retention of H^+ a serious threat in a patient with acute renal failure? We have already established that 70 mmol of $H^+$are produced per day upon metabolism of the usual diet and that 1000 mmol of H^+ can be buffered in total. Thus, with a rate of production of H^+ of 0.05 mmol/min (70 mmol/1440 min), the patient can survive a long time. In fact, the patient's bicarbonate concentration might decline by 2 mmol/liter per day. As discussed, the major threat for a patient with renal failure is hyperkalemia rather than acidosis per se.

PRINCIPLES OF METABOLISM

Four principles of metabolic regulation that are central to our understanding of the metabolic aspects of metabolic acidosis are considered in this section. This discussion can be facilitated by considering the following question: Must the production of β-hydroxybutyric acid be a H^+-producing reaction?

Principle 1: Definition of a metabolic process

To examine the stoichiometry of a series of metabolic reactions, it is only necessary to consider the starting and end points of this sequence. We have called this type of approach a metabolic process type of analysis to distinguish it from the traditional analysis with emphasis on individual metabolic pathways.[29]

Consider the overall process. A person who has not eaten for many days requires a fat-derived, water-soluble fuel to metabolize so that ATP can be regenerated in the brain.[61] That fuel, β-hydroxybutyrate (β-HB^-) (+ H^+), was derived ultimately from the bulk energy store, triglyceride in adipose tissue. The metabolic intermediate, free fatty acid, was delivered to the liver bound to albumin in the circulation and was transformed to β-HB^- (+ H^+), which entered the circulation. The brain extracted and oxidized β-HB^- (+ H^+). The net effect is the transfer of energy from a storage form in one organ (adipose tissue) to a useful product (ATP) in another organ (brain).

Metabolic processes commonly involve more than one organ. In general, the starting points are dietary fuels or metabolic stores (glycogen, triglyceride, or protein); and the end points are ATP, other metabolic stores, or metabolites that accumulate in the body (e.g., β-HB anions when there is a lack of insulin). One only need examine the balanced reactions in each organ of the body to determine its role in acid-base balance; the sum of these components of the metabolic process tells the overall acid-base story. For the production and utilization of ketoacids, events occurred in three organs: the adipose tissue (adipocytes), the liver (hepatocytes), and the brain.

A few H^+ ions were produced in adipose tissue when fatty acid anions were released; many more H^+ ions were produced in the liver when the β-HB^- anion was produced. In contrast, the H^+ ions that were produced in this metabolic process were consumed by the brain when the β-HB^- anion was oxidized to yield ATP, CO_2, and water. Hence, there is no net production or removal of H^+ in the metabolic process.

Let us now apply these principles to answer our question: Must the production of β-hydroxybutyric acid be a H^+-producing reaction? First, let us examine these two metabolic sequences:

$$\underset{\text{neutral compound}}{\text{Triglyceride}} \rightarrow \underset{\text{4 anions}}{4\beta\text{-HB}^-} + 4H^+ \quad (12)$$

$$\underset{\text{2 anions}}{2\text{Acetate}^-} + H^+ \rightarrow \underset{\text{1 anion}}{\beta\text{-HB}^-} \quad (13)$$

In equation 12, the net anionic charge of the product (β-HB^-) exceeds that of the reactants. Thus, in cases where β-HB^- is produced from neutral precursors, H^+ is produced. The situation is different in equation 13. In this case, the net anionic charge of the products (β-HB^-) is less than that of the substrates (two acetate anions). Therefore, H^+ is consumed during this stage of metabolism. Hence, this production of β-hydroxybutyric acid and its removal during dialysis with a bath containing acetate anions is a H^+-removing reaction.[24] It is true that if β-HB^- was not dialyzed from the body but oxidized to a neutral endproduct (CO_2 or fat), more H^+ would be removed. This fact does not detract from the initial interpretation that the production of ketoacids is a H^+-removing process when the substrate has a larger net anionic charge (equation 13).

Principle 2: The rate of production or removal of H^+ in an organ is determined by the rate of turnover of ATP in that organ

ATP is produced or utilized in reactions that produce or remove H^+ (equations 14 through 16). It is important to recognize that reactions that result in the synthesis of ATP can occur only in response to an initial decline in the concentration of ATP.[18,34,35,42]

$$\text{Palmitate} + 6O_2 \rightarrow$$
$$2\beta\text{-HB}^- + 2\text{AcAc}^- \text{ (actoacetate)} + 4H^+ + 27\text{ATP} \quad (14)$$

$$\beta\text{-HB}^- + H^+ + 4.5O_2 \rightarrow 4CO_2 + 4H_2O + 27\text{ATP} \quad (15)$$

$$2\text{ Lactate}^- + 2H^+ + 6\text{ATP} \rightarrow \text{glucose} \quad (16)$$

A basic tenet of energy metabolism is that the *rate of production of ATP in any organ cannot exceed its rate of use because there is a very limited quantity of the precursor of ATP: ADP*. Thus, to continue to produce ATP via the oxidation of an anion, there must be continued hydrolysis of ATP to perform biochemical work. It follows that the rate of fuel consumption is governed by the rate of turnover of ATP.[18,34,35,42] Therefore, an important influence on the rate of production and removal of H^+ is the rate of turnover of ATP. Hence, the rate of production of H^+ during ketogenesis and the rate of removal of H^+ by oxidation of lactate (or gluconeogenesis) is determined by the rate of turnover of ATP in the organs involved. As a corollary, fuels compete for oxidation and production of the requisite ATP. This "fuel selection" can exert a significant influence on acid-base balance (see "Principle 4: Not All Fuels Are Equal in Terms of ATP or H^+ Production and Utilization" for details).

Principle 3: The liver must process diverse fuels and yield universal products

The liver initiates the metabolism of a wide array of fuels. For example, virtually all amino acids and ethanol are converted in the liver to glucose, triglycerides (amino acids and ethanol in the fed state), or ketoacids (ethanol and ketogenic amino acids).[42] In every case, ATP is also synthesized in the liver. The constraints of the turnover of ATP and fuel selection influence the contribution of the liver to acid-base balance (e.g., by determining the maximum rates of synthesis of ketoacids or the maximum rates of removal of lactic acid).

Principle 4: Not all fuels are equal in terms of ATP or H^+ production and utilization

The purpose of oxidizing fuels is to regenerate ATP. Although a small quantity of ATP can be produced without oxygen during anaerobic glycolysis, virtually all ATP is regenerated in normal subjects by aerobic metabolism. Fuels that are oxidized aerobically to regenerate ATP are primarily carbohydrates (glucose) and fat (fatty acids). Complete oxidation of these fuels does not produce or consume H^+, but there can be acid-base effects of this metabolism. The acid-base effect and ATP yields from the oxidation of carbohydrates and triglycerides are summarized in Table 28-4. The following section further discusses the acid-base impact of fuel selection.

CLINICAL APPLICATIONS OF THE PRINCIPLES

In the management of patients with metabolic acidosis, the important question to answer is, How soon might this patient die as a direct consequence of acidemia? We have already established that the capacity to buffer H^+ ions is limited (close to 1000 mmol) and that the kidney at best can handle only a small load of H^+ (200 to 300 mmol/day).[30] The question then becomes, How fast can H^+ be produced or removed by metabolic reactions?

TABLE 28-4 • **Not all fuels are created equal**

	per mmol Substrate					
Substrate	O_2 consumed, mmol	CO_2 formed, mmol	ATP formed, mmol	Ratio ATP/O_2	H+ mmol	CO_2/100 mmol ATP consumed, mmol
Glucose	6	6	36	6	0	16.7
Lactate	3	3	18	6	1	16.7
β-HB	4.5	4	27	6	1	14.8
AcAc	4	4	24	6	1	16.7
Palmitate	23	16	129	5.6	1	12.4
Ethanol	3	2	16	5.3	0	12.5

NOTE: For details, see the text. The stoichiometry of oxygen consumption, ATP formation, and acid-base implications were calculated from equations 15, 21, 24, and 25. The results reported per 100 mmol ATP are shown to illustrate the difference in production of CO_2 factored for ATP turnover.

KETOACIDOSIS

How fast can ketoacids be synthesized?

Ketogenesis occurs in the liver and at appreciable rates only if there is a lack of insulin (i.e., fasting, diabetic ketoacidosis, ethanol intoxication plus contraction of the ECF volume; see Chap. 26). Hence, events in hepatocytes must be examined in detail. It is noteworthy that the liver receives approximately 1 liter of blood per minute and extracts approximately 2 mmol of oxygen per minute.[5]

Regulation of ketogenesis by the supply of substrates to the liver

The three substrates for ketogenesis are fatty acids, oxygen, and ADP. Each is discussed in turn.

Fatty acids

The supply of fatty acids can be important in regulating the maximum rates of production of ketoacids. Typical levels of fatty acids in blood during fasting or diabetic ketoacidosis are close to 1 mmol/liter of plasma (i.e., 0.6 mmol/liter of blood).[61] Since the liver receives approximately 1 liter of blood per minute and since 4 ketoacids are produced by each 16-carbon fatty acid, the maximum yield could be 2.4 mmol of ketoacids per minute if the liver could extract 100 percent of the fatty acids delivered. Since fatty acids are bound to albumin because of their poor water solubility and since they must traverse many water compartments between plasma and hepatic mitochondria, the actual supply of fatty acids may approximate only half of this delivery rate. Hence, based on the rate of supply of fatty acids, the maximum rate of ketogenesis is probably close to 1 mmol/min.

Oxygen

Oxygen is another substrate for ketogenesis. The portal circulation delivers 6 mmol O_2 in each liter of blood.[5] Use of 6 mmol O_2 yields 4 mmol of ketoacids (equation 14), if 100 percent of O_2 is extracted and ketogenesis is the only metabolic pathway that consumes O_2. Thus, the supply of O_2 is unlikely to limit ketogenesis.

ADP

The third substrate for ketogenesis is ADP (said another way, a product of ketogenesis is ATP). Since no organ can synthesize more ATP than it uses for its biological work (or uncoupled metabolism), owing to the very low availability of ADP, it follows that this substrate could impose a limitation on the rate of production of ketoacids by limiting the rate of turnover of ATP in hepatocytes.[18,34] Since the liver extracts only approximately 2 mmol of O_2 per minute to synthesize its requisite ATP,[5] only 1.1 mmol of ketoacid per minute can be generated (Table 28-5). This value is similar to that derived from the rate of delivery of fatty acids to the liver and could also be an important regulator of the maximum rates of ketogenesis. It is important to stress that this rate will be smaller if ketogenesis is not the *only* ATP-forming reaction in these cells.

TABLE 28-5 • **Hepatic oxygen metabolism during chronic fasting**

Parameter	Oxygen metabolism, mmol/day
Oxygen uptake	3000
Oxygen utilized during	
Protein metabolism*	600*
Ketogenesis	2400
Palmitate to ketoacids	400*
Maximum rate of ketogenesis	1600†

* Amino acids to glucose as judged by nitrogen balance data.

† Oxidation of 1 mmol of palmitate to equal proportions of β-HB and AcAc utilizes 6 mmol of oxygen and yields 4 mmol of ketoacids.

This limitation of ketogenesis by the turnover of ATP may be altered in several ways. This rate could be higher if the liver's consumption of oxygen increased secondary to the accelerated utilization of ATP from increased ion (Na^+) pumping, more biosynthesis of glucose (from lactate), the conversion of NH_4^+ to urea, and so on. Uncoupling oxidative phosphorylation or the export of the reducing power of NADH from hepatocytes (during the synthesis of glucose, synthesis of lactate, or conversion of more AcAc to β-HB) may enhance ketogenesis. In contrast, the rate of ketogenesis would decline if the rate of hepatic work declined (less biosynthesis) or if ATP is regenerated from other metabolic processes (gluconeogenesis from amino acids[42] and oxidation of acetyl coenzyme A [CoA] in the citric acid cycle).

How fast can ketoacids be utilized?

Ketogenesis provides a net load of H^+ only if β-HB^- anions accumulate in the body or are excreted in the urine with a cation other than H^+ or NH_4^+. There are two major ways for ketoacids to be removed from the body: by conversion to acetone or metabolism to CO_2 + ATP.

Conversion to acetone occurs spontaneously and has no metabolic significance other than the removal of H^+ (equation 17). The rate is directly proportional to the concentration of $AcAc^-$ and has been estimated to be 0.1 mmol/min during diabetic ketoacidosis.[71]

$$AcAc^- + H^+ \rightarrow \text{acetone} + CO_2 \qquad (17)$$

Ketoacids are oxidized in organs containing mitochondria. Using the two principles of turnover of ATP and fuel selection, one can identify organs that are likely to oxidize these fuels and to estimate the quantitative aspects of the oxidation. First, it is clear that *ketoacids are not oxidized in the liver.* The liver does not have a sufficient quantity of the enzyme that catalyzes the synthesis of acetoacetyl CoA from $AcAc^-$. If ketoacids were oxidized in liver, ATP would be synthesized and the maximum rate of ketogenesis would decline. In quantitative terms, the oxidation of one ketoacid would yield 27 mmol of ATP (equation 15), whereas the production of 1 ketoacid yields close to 7 ATPs when the product is half $AcAc^-$ and half β-HB^- (equation 14). Hence, for balance of ATP, every ketoacid oxidized would reduce by 3 to 4 mmol the quantity of ketoacids that could be synthesized.

Fuel selection seems to work with a hierarchy of fatty acids/β-HB^-/glucose.[29] Hence, muscle oxidizes fatty acids when their concentration is high and consequently rejects the oxidation of ketoacids.[15] Thus, only in organs where there is an appreciable rate of oxidation of glucose (brain) or glutamine plus lactate (proximal cells of the kidney[66]) might one anticipate high rates of oxidation of ketoacids when their levels are high. In fact, the brain and kidneys are the two major sites of oxidation of ketoacids (Table 28-6); oxidation of ketoacids provides 75 to 80 percent of the ATP needed by the brain during fasting.[61] Hence, half the total production of ketoacids, 750 mmol (0.5 mmol/min), is oxidized by the brain to supply almost all the ATP it requires (Tables 28-5 and 28-6). Further, there is little room to increase this rate of removal owing to the constraints on ATP turnover in the brain.

TABLE 28-6 • Ketone body turnover during chronic fasting

Ketone body metabolism	Organ	Turnover
Production	Liver	1500
Conversion to acetone	?	150
Excretion	Kidney	150*
Oxidation	Brain	750†
	Kidney	250‡
	Muscle, etc.	200

NOTE: For details, see the text.

* This excretion obliges NH_4^+ excretion and leads to wasting of lean body mass.

† This oxidation of β-HB spares lean body mass.

‡ This oxidation of β-HB appears to diminish renal glutamine metabolism and thereby spares lean body mass.

The kidney removes approximately 0.25 mmol/min of ketoacids, two-thirds by oxidation and one-third by excretion (as an NH_4^+ salt).[62] Again, the constraints imposed by the turnover of ATP limit the possibility of increasing this rate.[34]

Teleologic explanation for why the rate of ketogenesis approximates one mmol/min in an adult

Ketogenesis is necessary for survival during prolonged fasting because ketoacids are a fat-derived, water-soluble fuel that can be oxidized by the brain. In this setting, the oxidation of ketoacids spares about 1.5 kg of muscle per day.[38]

Given that the buffer capacity is close to 1000 mmol, survival depends on the fact that less than 1000 mmol of H^+ accumulates. In the case of ketoacids, more than 1000 mmol is produced per day during starvation. Hence, survival depends on a matched rate of removal of H^+ in the steady state. The removal of H^+ occurs primarily by oxidation of ketoacids in the brain and the kidney. In both cases, energy constraints imposed by the turnover of ATP and by fuel selection set the upper limit on production, 1500 mmol/day, a rate perfectly matched to limits set by energy constraints in other organs (brain and kidney) on the rate of removal of these ketoacids. It follows that anything that interferes with this delicate balance can have serious acid-base consequences (see "Clinical Implications" for more discussion).

LACTIC ACIDOSIS

How fast can lactic acid be synthesized?

There is no net production of H^+ when carbohydrates are converted to the energy stores, glycogen, or triglyceride or oxidized to CO_2 plus ATP. Nevertheless, H^+ will accumulate during the partial oxidation of glucose (i.e., the conversion of glucose to lactate anions plus ATP; equations 18 through 20).

$$2ATP^{4-} + 2H_2O \rightarrow 2ADP^{3-} + 2Pi^{2-} + 2H^+ + \text{Bioloigcal work} \quad (18)$$

$$\text{Glucose} + 2ADP^{3-} + 2Pi^{2-} \rightarrow 2ATP^{4-} + 2\ \text{lactate}^- \quad (19)$$

$$\text{Sum: Glucose} \rightarrow 2\ \text{lactate}^- + 2H^+ + \text{biological work} \quad (20)$$

During hypoxia, for example, anaerobic glycolysis becomes a critical pathway for the cells to produce the essential metabolite ATP. Despite the fact that anaerobic glycolysis yields only 2 mmol of ATP per mmol of glucose metabolized and complete oxidation of glucose yields 36 to 40 mmol of ATP per mmol of glucose metabolized, the flux in anaerobic glycolysis is much greater than twenty-fold faster than during complete oxidation of pyruvate. This point is immediately obvious when one considers the relative velocity maintained during a 100-m (10 m/s) run relative to that maintained during a 1500-m run (6 m/s).[59] Quantitatively, 1 mmol of H^+ ions is produced for each mmol of ATP regenerated during anaerobic glycolysis from glucose. Because a patient at rest needs to regenerate 72 mmol of ATP per minute, as much as 72 mmol of H^+ could be produced in a minute under conditions of anoxia.

Regulation of glycolysis by the supply of substrates

ADP

The primary regulator of anaerobic glycolysis is the concentration of ADP in tissues. Normally, this concentration is very small; however, if the rate of turnover of ATP rises (to permit biological work), the rate of regeneration of ATP increases in parallel. If the need for ATP cannot be met by aerobic metabolism, ATP will be regenerated via anaerobic glycolysis, and this will develop very quickly, provided that the substrate, glucose (glycogen), is available. This fact has particular relevance in such states of high turnover of ATP as the sprint.[7]

For hypoxic cells to produce ATP anaerobically, sufficient quantities of glucose (glycogen) must be available. Therefore, it is important to determine how much of these substrates can be made available to cells that are hypoxic.

Glucose

If the concentration of glucose in blood is 5 mmol/liter and if hypoglycemia is to be avoided (i.e., levels remain $\geq$ 3 mmol/liter), then only 60 mmol of lactic acid can be produced from glucose in the ECF (2 mmol/liter $\times$ 151 $\times$ 2 mmol lactate per 1 mmol glucose metabolized = 60 mmol). The content of glucose in the ICF is much smaller; it is extremely small in muscle cells, whereas the cummulative amount of glucose in other organs is only approximately 20 mmol.[72] Therefore, in the absence of hypoglycemia, the content of glucose in the ECF and ICF can yield only 100 mmol of lactic acid.

Glucose could be also provided from exogenous sources. It is important to realize that 1 liter of 5% dextrose contains 50 g of glucose and could provide the carbon skeleton for 550 mmol of lactic acid.

Glycogen

The major endogenous precursor of pyruvate is glycogen. Most glycogen in the body is in muscles. Although its content in muscle varies with exercise and with the antecedent diet, in most adults the body content of glycogen approximates 450 g (2500 mmol of glucose). Hence, this glycogen can provide the carbon skeleton for 5000 mmol of lactic acid, more than enough to exceed the buffer capacity of the body (1000 mmol).

The liver is the other major source of glycogen in the body in the fed state. The liver contains about 90 g of glycogen (500 mmol of glucose), the complete conversion of which to lactic acid would produce 1000 mmol of H^+. In the fasting state, however, there is little glycogen available in the liver.

In summary, the rate of production of H^+ during hypoxia is determined by two factors: the need of the hypoxic tissues for ATP and the availability of the carbon precursors, glucose or glycogen. Thus, a fasted and resting subject without muscle hypoxia can only develop a modest degree of acute lactic acidosis owing to a limited availability of carbon precursors.

How fast can lactic acid be removed?

H^+ will be removed when lactate anions are oxidized to CO_2 or are converted to glucose. Each is discussed in turn. Again, the principles of turnover of ATP and selection of fuels will play a key role in determining the quantitative aspects of the rate of removal of H^+.

Oxidation of lactate

The oxidation of lactate removes 1 mmol of H^+ per 1 mmol of lactate oxidized (equation 21). While on inspection of equations 21 and 22 it appears that one achieves balance for H^+ with simultaneous flows in these reactions, this is not true for ATP. The production of lactic acid generated 1 mmol of H^+ per mmol of ATP synthesized (equation 22), whereas oxidation of 1 mmol removed 1 mmol of H^+ and generated 18 mmol of ATP (equation 21). Hence, net removal of H^+ via oxidation of lactate can be achieved only if the rate of turnover of ATP is 18 times higher in organs that are oxidizing lactate than in organs that are producing lactic acid. A corollary of this statement is that drugs cause net removal of H^+ if there is an appreciable ongoing rate of anaerobic glycolysis (see "Clinical Implications" for a discussion of more quantitative aspects).[32]

$$H^+ + \text{lactate}^- + 3O_2 \rightarrow 3CO_2 + 3H_2O + 18\text{ATP} \qquad (21)$$

$$0.5\ \text{Glucose} \rightarrow \text{lactate}^- + H^+ + \text{ATP} \qquad (22)$$

Gluconeogeneis and the removal of H^+ plus lactate

Most gluconeogenesis occurs in the liver and in the renal cortex. Both organs, however, cannot remove lactate anions via gluconeogenesis at a rapid rate, even when the levels of blood lactate are high.[32] We can identify three limits on this process, recognizing that the conversion of 2 mmol of lactate to glucose consumes 6 mmol of ATP (equation 23). Again, the cofactors of ADP and ATP can be ignored in the balanced equations, as these adenine nucleotides will be both synthesized and utilized at equal rates:

$$2\text{Lactate}^- + 2H^+ + 6\text{ATP} \rightarrow \text{glucose} + 6\text{ADP} \qquad (23)$$

Although the following discussion addresses possible limitations of glucogenesis from lactate in the liver, similar constraints also occur in the renal cortex:

1. *Limit by the supply of O_2:* To synthesize 3 mmol of ATP, $\frac{1}{2}$ mmol of oxygen must be consumed (P:O is 3). Since the hepatic blood flow is one liter/min and each liter of portal blood has 6 mmol O_2/liter,[5] the maximum capacity of this gluconeogenesis is 12 mmol/min of lactate (6 mmol O_2 has 12 oxygen atoms).
2. *Limit by the hepatic uptake of oxygen:* The liver only extracts one-third of the oxygen delivered, or 2 mmol/min.[5] This fact could limit the maximum rate of extraction of lactate for gluconeogenesis to 4 mmol/min ($\frac{1}{3} \times 12$).
3. *Other constraints:* To the extent that the liver uses ATP to perform other biological work, there will be less flux in gluconeogenesis unless the rate of consumption of oxygen by the liver increases. Further, there could be constraints on gluconeogenesis owing to limitations imposed by the activities of the rate-limiting steps in gluconeogenesis.[50]

In summary, the rate of production of H^+ in hypoxic lactic acidosis can be very high. Considering the limited buffer capacity and the constraints of ATP turnover on the rate of removal of H^+ via the metabolism of lactate anions (oxidation or gluconeogenesis), a life-threatening situation due to progressive acidosis will ensue rapidly during anoxia.

SOME ACID-BASE ASPECTS OF EXERCISE

Let us consider the following question: If muscles have enough fuel to provide sufficient ATP for 80 s, why can maximum sprinting not be maintained for much longer than 20 s? During short bursts of intensive exercise, anaerobic glycolysis supplies the bulk of the required energy. The maximum rate of utilization of ATP in human muscle is close to 3 mmol/s per kilogram of muscle.[7] Since 1 kg of muscle contains approximately 80 mmol of glycogen and 1 mmol of glycogen yields 3 mmol of ATP via anaerobic glycolysis, it is obvious that there is enough fuel to provide sufficient ATP to maintain maximum sprinting for about 80 s. Sprinting, however, cannot be maintained for much longer than 20 s. Moreover, the time for running a 400-m race is greater than fourfold that for a 100-m sprint.

One possible explanation for this phenomenon is that fatigue might result from a low intracellular pH. Anaerobic glycolysis of 1 mmol of glycogen provides enough energy for the muscle for 1 s but also yields 2 mmol of H^+. The question, then, is, How many seconds of buffer capacity does the muscle have?

Quantitatively, the imidazole groups of histidine are the principal buffers in muscle because no other amino acids (other than the N-terminal) have a pK in the range of ICF pH. We shall assume a mean value of 40 mmol of histidine per kilogram of muscle (proteins contain 20 to 30 mmol of histidine per kilogram of wet weight, and the dipeptides sarcosine plus carnosine contain an additional 10 to 15 mmol of histidine).[12] Since the ICF pH is close to the pK of the imidazole buffer system, only one-half the amount of total histidine would be available for buffering of H^+ (i.e., 20 mmol per kilogram of muscle).

Creatine phosphate can be a proton remover during exercise when it is hydrolyzed and inorganic phosphate is produced. H^+ is removed due to the change of pK of phosphate from 4.5 to 6.8.[73] The concentration of creatine phosphate in human muscle is about 17 mmol/kg.[86] In severe, short-lasting, exhaustive exercise, about 13 mmol of creatine phosphate are consumed.[7] This process provides the needed energy for approximately 4 s and the capacity to buffer approximately another 13 mmol of H^+ once the pH of the ICF declines well below the pK of inorganic phosphate:

$$\text{Creatine phosphate}^{2-} + H^+ \rightarrow \text{creatine}^0 + H_2PO_4^- \qquad (24)$$

Another major intracellular buffer is bicarbonate. The intracellular concentration of bicarbonate in muscle is approximately 10 mmol/liter.[9] Its consumption during buffering requires, however, that CO_2 be removed (i.e., hyperventilation occurs and cardiac output rises).[84] From the information given above, one can calculate that, although the muscle has enough fuel for 80 s of sprinting, its buffer capacity would be titrated in less than 20 s. Obviously the ICF pH of the muscle must fall for this buffering to occur.

Decline in lactate levels after a race

After performing exhaustive anaerobic exercise (a sprint), lactic acid accumulates to very high levels in the circulation (20 to 30 mmol/liter).[7,39] If the sprinter were simply to rest after the race, 1 to 2 h would be required before the concentration of lactate returns to normal. In contrast, jogging after the race leads to a much more rapid decline in lactate. This information illustrates that the nonoxidative pathways for the removal of lactate (i.e., gluconeogenesis) usually proceed at a very slow rate, whereas oxidation of lactate can occur at a more rapid rate during periods when there is accelerated aerobic metabolism.[51]

ACID-BASE ASPECTS OF FUEL SELECTION

The kidney and fuel selection

Despite their large turnover of ATP for the transport of sodium, cells of the proximal tubule always contain a surplus of potential fuels for oxidation, largely due to the reabsorption of glucose, amino acids, lactate, and keto-acid anions from the glomerular filtrate. In addition, nutrients such as glutamine enter these cells via the basolateral membrane.[89] Under normal conditions, lactate is the preferred fuel from which the kidney synthesizes ATP.[66,67] In acidosis, glutamine replaces lactate as the principal fuel for the proximal tubule cells, and this switch permits normal subjects to eliminate an acid load.[68]

To illustrate the acid-base impact of fuel selection by the kidney, we have analyzed renal fuels with respect to production of ATP per bicarbonate synthesized (Table 28-7). Consider the following example. During the ketoacidosis of fasting, if the kidney oxidized sufficient fatty acids to yield 2700 mmol of ATP, this oxidation will yield no new bicarbonate, and it could prevent the complete oxidation of 100 mmol of glutamine (due to ATP balance considerations). Hence, 200 mmol of NH_4^+ and an equal quantity of potential new bicarbonate will not be generated. It is obvious, then, that fuel selection by the kidney has both energy and acid-base implications. Should the oxidation of fat become an important pathway to provide ATP in proximal cells, this would diminish the quantity of glutamine that could be oxidized to provide ATP.[35] This factor could become important if there was high delivery of fat and an acid load (possibly in some cases where total parenteral nutrition is being administered to a patient who has lost sodium bicarbonate via the GI tract).[19,52,85]

Impact of fuel selection under conditions where the supply of oxygen is limited

Individual fuels have various yields of H^+ ions and/or ATP per oxygen consumed, which can be important in patients with a limited supply of oxygen. To illustrate this point, the acid-base and ATP yield from glucose- and fat-derived fuels are summarized in Table 28-8. Oxidation of glucose or fat to CO_2 consumes oxygen but has no direct acid-base impact, provided that the CO_2 can be exhaled.

TABLE 28-7 • Metabolic and acid-base consequences of the metabolism of ammoniagenic and nonammoniagenic substrates by the kidney

Substrate	ATP mol/mol	NH_4^+ mol/mol	HCO_3^- mol/mol	ATP/HCO_3^-
Fatty acids (palmitate) to CO_2	129	0	1	129
β-HB to CO_2	27	0	1	27
Lactate to CO_2	18	0	1	18
Glutamine to				
CO_2	27	2	2*	13.5
Glucose	7	2	2*	3.5
Alanine	9	1	1*	9.0
Lactate	9	2	2*	4.5

NOTE: There are two ways of looking at the synthesis of bicarbonate in the kidney: (1) unique new bicarbonate synthesis during ammoniagenesis and (2) bicarbonate synthesis in the kidney or elsewhere (e.g, the metabolism of the anions fatty acids, lactate, or β-HB to neutral end products).

* This gain of bicarbonate is contingent upon the excretion of the NH_4^+ formed from the metabolism of glutamine. If this NH_4^+ is not excreted, it will return to the liver and be converted to urea, consuming bicarbonate in the process. In normal subjects, approximately one-third of this NH_4^+ is excreted in the urine, whereas two-thirds of the NH_4^+ is excreted during chronic metabolic acidosis.

TABLE 28-8 • ATP balance in the liver during ethanol and fat metabolism

	Moles ATP per mole ethanol
Ethanol conversion to	
Acetic acid	+ 6
$CO_2 + H_2O$	+ 16
β-HB	+ 2.5
Acetoacetate	+ 4
	Moles ATP per mole ketone body
Fatty acid conversion to	
β-HB	+ 5.3
AcAC	+ 8.3
	ATP balance
Lactate release	− 3

NOTE: The assumptions required for these calculations are as follows: each mole of NADH causes 3 moles of ATP to be formed, 2 moles of ATP are used to synthesize the CoA derivatives of acetate and fatty acids, and 1 mole of NADH is used to synthesize β-HB.

H^+ will be removed if lactate replaces fat as a fuel for the same oxygen consumption. Consider the example where there is a limited supply of oxygen (6 mmol) and that 36 mmol of ATP is needed. If glucose is oxidized, all 36 mmol of ATP are supplied, so there is no anaerobic glycolysis. If lactate anions are the fuel, the same amount of ATP will be produced, but 2 mmol of H^+ will be consumed. In contrast, if palmitate is the fuel, only 32.25 mmol of ATP can be generated, as dicated by the stoichiometry of the oxidation of palmitate (equation 26). From an acid-base point of view, only 0.25 mmol of H^+ (and palmitate) ions was consumed. However, because 3.75 mmol of ATP had to be produced by anaerobic glycolysis (as 36 mmol of ATP are required in our example), 3.75 mmol of H^+ had to be produced. Hence, by selecting lactate over palmitate, there was a net removal of 5.5 mmol of H^+. Such a shift could theoretically occur by administering an activator of pyruvate dehydrogenase (PDH), such as dichloroacetate (DCA)[79] or an inhibitor of the oxidation of fatty acids.

The rate of production of CO_2

Hyperventilation is the expected response to metabolic acidosis; thus, control of the arterial P_{CO_2} depends for the most part on the degree of stimulation of alveolar ventilation. In this analysis, the rate of production of CO_2 in metabolic processes is presumed to be constant. We were prompted to reevaluate the importance of various rates of production of CO_2 during metabolic acidosis by a case in which a severely cachetic individual maintained P_{CO_2} at 8 mmHg with severe acidemia (pH, 7.05; bicarbonate, 2 mmol/liter).[25]

Nonmetabolic issues

CO_2 can be produced independently of oxidative metabolism when H^+ is buffered by the bicarbonate buffer system. The question is, How fast is CO_2 produced in this way relative to its usual production via metabolic reactions? As a point of reference, the rate of production of CO_2 from metabolism in a subject at rest is close to 10 mmol/min.[29] Because the net rate of production of H^+ is, with one exception, always less than 1 mmol/min and the bicarbonate buffer system generates abundant quantities of CO_2 only in mild metabolic acidosis,[84] production of appreciable quantities of CO_2 due to buffering is rare. Dealing with the abovementioned exception, a rapid rate of production of H^+ occurs during anaerobic glycolysis, especially if there is a high rate of turnover of ATP (the sprint or finishing kick in a longer race, or fever with shock); further, if acidosis is not yet severe, most of the H^+ will be removed by the bicarbonate buffer system,[84] thereby generating CO_2. Accordingly, nonmetabolic issues can be a rare cause for very high rates of production of CO_2.

Production of CO_2 by metabolism

Three points should be emphasized with respect to the rate of production of CO_2 by metabolism:

1. *Rate of turnover of ATP:* During fever, exercise, and other states (e.g., hyperthyroidism) in which the metabolic work increases or there is exposure to drugs that uncouple oxidative phosphorylation, the rate of production of CO_2 may markedly rise. Conversely, a much lower rate of production of CO_2 will result from a reduced requirement for ATP (e.g., inactivity, hypothermia, hypothyroidism, or low body mass). The latter phenomena can contribute to a lower than expected P_{CO_2} in a patient with metabolic acidosis.
2. *Change in the yield of CO_2 per unit of ATP regenerated:* The oxidation of glucose leads to the production of 26 percent more CO_2 than does the oxidation of fatty acids (Table 28-4).
3. *Fate of the carbon:* When ketoacids are formed during the partial oxidation of fatty acids or ethanol in the liver, O_2 is consumed, with CO_2 being produced. In severe ketoacidosis, the production of ketoacids can supply all the ATP for the liver, consume 20 to 30 percent of the oxygen in the body, and yet yield little or no CO_2 by metabolism or via titration of bicarbonate (see above).

To summarize, a patient with diabetic ketoacidosis (DKA) who is also modestly hypothermic, physically inactive, and comatose and who has a low glomerular filtration rate (GFR; contracted ECF volume) and severe acidosis should achieve a very low P_{CO_2} without massive alveolar ventilation. Thus, factors in addition to the stimulus to the respiratory system might need to be considered with respect to the expected P_{CO_2} in a patient with severe metabolic acidosis.

CLINICAL IMPLICATIONS

KETOACIDOSIS

Possible explanation for the natural history of DKA

The time course of events in patients with DKA (see Chap. 26) has an interesting feature. Toward the end stage, the degree of ketoacidosis becomes more severe very quickly. For ketoacidosis to worsen rapidly, either the rate of production of ketoacids must rise markedly or the rate of utilization of ketoacids must decline appreciably. With respect to production, perhaps a higher level of fatty acids in the circulation or an increased rate of turnover of ATP secondary to enhanced conversion of lactate to glucose in the liver could make some contribution to increased ketogenesis. Notwithstanding, there is little leverage to increase this rate appreciably because of the control exerted by the limited rate of turnover of ATP in hepatocytes. Further, the potential for an increased rate is also offset by the lower rate of delivery of fatty acids (hypovolemia) and the increased production of ATP during the conversion of amino acids to glucose (Table 28-5).[42]

The degree of ketoacidosis can be influenced to a major degree by decreasing the rate of removal of ketoacids rather than by increasing their rate of production. The majority of ketoacids are removed during their metabolism to yield ATP in the brain and kidney (Table 28-6). The presence of semicoma can decrease the demand for the synthesis of ATP in the brain by 50 percent;[49] this is equivalent to the failure to remove close to 400 mmol of ketoacids per day. Similarly, the very low GFR consequent to hypovolemia will decrease the turnover of ATP in the kidney (less reabsorption of sodium).[30] Both of these factors could lead to the failure to remove several hundred millimoles of ketoacids per day. Should general anaesthetics or even sedatives be administered, or if a lesion of the central nervous system (CNS) is present that led to coma for other reasons, the degree of ketoacidosis might be aggravated.

Criteria for the use of bicarbonate in DKA

There is little debate that aggressive therapy with alkali is advisable if the degree of acidemia is truly life-threatening.[57] We shall not consider that issue here. Rather, we would like to add one criterion to the list of considerations for alkali therapy in DKA, a criterion based on the rate of turnover of ATP, which will determine the rate of removal of ketoacids via metabolism. Consider a patient with DKA and quite severe metabolic acidosis who has been comatose. In this case, the brain and the kidneys, owing to hypovolemia, cannot be counted on to remove their usual 0.75 mmol of ketoacid per minute; this rate may decline by 0.5 mmol/min. If it takes several hours before ketogenesis declines (the lag period between the administration of insulin and the decline in ketonemia), there could be the accumulation of 100 mmol more H^+ in a subject with little remaining buffer capacity. Hence, one could make an argument to use exogenous alkali in this metabolic setting to ease the patient through this acid-base emergency.

TREATMENT OF LACTIC ACIDOSIS

Lactic acidosis (see Chap. 25) represents a heterogeneous group of disorders.[54] We shall only consider some issues related to the treatment of the hypoxic variety here. In hypoxic lactic acidosis, increasing the supply of oxygen to the tissues is the best treatment. This will decrease their need for anaerobic glycolysis. The use of bicarbonate and DCA was thought to help buy time while attempting to treat the underlaying etiology. In the following sections, we wish to provide a quantitative analysis of the utility of these agents in the treatment of hypoxic lactic acidosis.

Bicarbonate in the treatment of lactic acidosis

This issue continues to be the subject of a major debate.[40,57,77] We do not intend to consider the pros and cons of using bicarbonate but, rather, to point out to its limited utility. To illustrate this point, consider a situation in which there is a 50 percent deficit of delivery of oxygen to tissues (6 mmol/min). Since the basal rate of consumption of oxygen is close to 12 mmol/min and the P:O ratio is 3, the basal rate of production of ATP will be close to 72 mmol/min ($12 \times 3 \times 2$ oxygen atoms per O_2). If the supply of oxygen was decreased by 50 percent, there would be a deficit of 36 mmol of ATP per minute. To provide 36 mmol of ATP per minute by anaerobic glycolysis, 36 mmol of H^+ per minute would be added to the body. Since the buffer capacity is only approximately 1000 mmol, survival would be less than 30 min in this situation. If the clinician attempted to titrate the production of H^+ with exogenous isotonic sodium bicarbonate, about $\frac{1}{4}$ liter would have to be infused per minute. In a patient with poor cardiac function, this would be disastrous. Thus, in severe hypoxia, arguments about whether to use sodium bicarbonate are not germane. The important thing to do is to enhance the delivery of oxygen to tissues, and to do so as quickly as possible.

There is an additional factor to consider. The body could supply only the glucose needed for lactic acid production from glycogen in liver and muscle. In the fasted patient who is not exercising, hypoglycemia rather than acidosis might be the major problem. If in this setting, the 150 mmol of bicarbonate was dissolved in a liter of 5% dextrose, the glucose (275 mmol) provided could be converted into 550 mmol of H^+, more than negating any acid-base benefit from the administered bicarbonate.

DCA in treatment of lactic acidosis

DCA, an activator of pyruvate dehydrogenase (PDH),[78] is currently under evaluation for the treatment of patients with lactic acidosis. PDH is a key enzyme in the regulation of fuel metabolism (Fig. 28-2). It catalyzes an irreversible reaction in which pyruvate, which can be made into carbohydrates, is converted to acetyl-CoA, which cannot generate glucose. Because carbohydrates and proteins must be preserved during fasting, flux through PDH is always tightly regulated.[17] PDH is regulated by two mechanisms. First, the active enzyme is inhibited by the products of the reaction it catalyzes (i.e., increased ratios of acetyl-CoA:CoA and $NADH^+$:NAD); and, second, the active form of PDH is reversibly inactivated via phosphorylation.[64,69] DCA inhibits PDH kinase (EC 2.7.99) and maintains PDH in its unphosphorylated, active form.[88] DCA has been shown to be effective in lowering the concentration of lactate in experimental models of lactic acidosis[1,26,63] and in some patients with lactic acidosis.[79,80]

DCA could benefit patients with lactic acidosis due to hypoxia if it led to an increase in the delivery of oxygen as a result of increasing the cardiac output. Although DCA has been shown to improve cardiac function in dogs with experimentally induced myocardial ischemia,[56] to stabilize the cardiac index in dogs with experimental lactic acidosis,[63] and to increase myocardial efficiency index in patients with coronary artery disease,[87] the data on the effect of DCA on the cardiac output in patients with lactic acidosis are less clear. While an effect of the drug to increase the cardiac output was suggested in a study by Stacpoole and colleagues,[80] it was not substantiated in a more recent study.[79]

In the absence of an increase in the delivery of oxygen, could DCA be of value in the treatment of lactic acidosis due to hypoxia? Restating this question, Can DCA, for example, ameliorate lactic acidosis due to hypoxia when there is 11, and not the needed 12, mmol of oxygen delivered per minute? Let us imagine that one organ of the body that normally consumes 1 mmol of oxygen per minute has no supply of oxygen. It will synthesize its requisite ATP by anaerobic glycolysis, yielding 6 mmol of H^+ and 6 mmol of lactate anions per minute. If the rest of the body could be "convinced" by DCA to metabolize lactate for all of its needs for ATP, then the consumption of lactate and H^+ would be only 3.67 mmol/min (11 mmol O_2 at 3 mmol O_2 per lactate; equation 21). Thus, it is clear that DCA, at best, can overcome only a small degree of hypoxia if it acts by enhancing the oxidation of lactate. Said another way, because glycolysis yields 18 mmol of H^+ and 18 mmol of lactate anions per 18 mmol of ATP synthesized, whereas oxidation of 1 mmol of lactate anion yields 18 mmol of ATP and removes only 1 mmol of H^+, oxidation of lactate must lose the H^+ battle if it is less than 18-fold greater than the rate of anaerobic glycolysis (5.6 percent hypoxia). This ability to withstand hypoxia is further decreased if fat supplies ATP in any organ of the body.

The foregoing analysis, which suggests a limited role for activating PDH in the treatment of hypoxic lactic acidosis, seems to contradict the results of previous studies. Notwithstanding, conclusions from these studies were based on models in which the net rate of production of lactic acid was low. In a study by Graf and coworkers[26] on the effect of DCA in the treatment of hypoxic lactic acidosis in dogs, the net rate of production of lactic acid was only 1 mmol/min. Since the rate of consumption of oxygen in dogs is close to 5 mmol/min (equivalent to 30 mmol/min ATP), the rate of production of H^+ was very low (equivalent to 3.3 percent hypoxia).

We have recently described an unexpected mechanism of action of DCA.[43] Lactic acidosis was induced in anaesthetized rabbits that were given an overdose of insulin. In this model of lactic acidosis, the supply of oxygen was not limited, and virtually all synthesis of ATP occurred consequent to flux through PDH (respiratory quotient [RQ] = 1; hence, there is little fat oxidation). We therefore expected that an activator of PDH, such as DCA, would have little impact on this lactic acidosis. Nevertheless, there was a rapid removal of lactate, despite the fact that there was no net uptake of lactate across the splanchnic, jugular, and femoral venous drainage systems. A quantitative analysis of the rate of

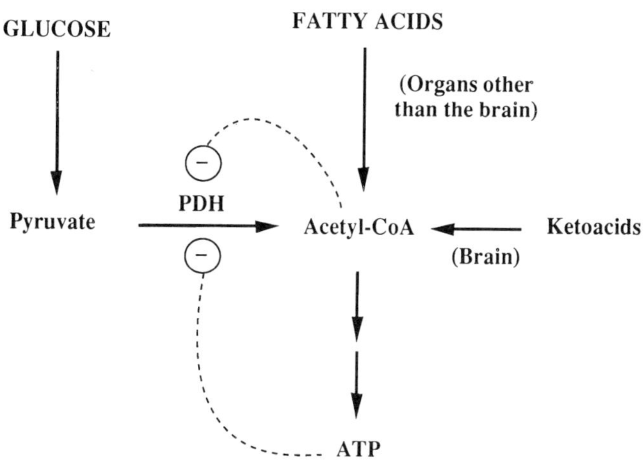

FIGURE 28-2 • Key role of PDH in energy metabolism. PDH catalyzes an irreversible reaction that allows for the irreversible conversion of carbohydrate (or protein) to fatty acids (or CO_2). The reaction is tightly regulated. In essence, oxidation of fatty acids leads to inhibition of PDH. (From Halperin ML, Rolleston FS: *Biochemical Detective Stories: A Problem-Based Approach to Clinical Cases,* Burlington, NC, Neil Patterson, 1990. Used by permission.)

removal of lactate led us to speculate that the effect of DCA to lower the level of lactate in blood was achieved by stimulating gluconeogenesis in the kidney.[43] The results of that study point out the importance of a quantitative analysis and a strict definition of the metabolic setting under which the drug was used to determine its biological effect.

METABOLIC ACIDOSIS IN THE ALCOHOLIC

The two major types of metabolic acidosis specifically related to the metabolism of ethanol are ketoacidosis and lactic acidosis (see Chap. 25). To prepare for a discussion of these disorders in the alcoholic, we shall first review the key features related to the metabolism of ethanol. This review will entail a brief description of the pathway.

Summary of important features of the biochemistry of the metabolism of ethanol

The features that dictate the pathway and regulation of the metabolism of ethanol in vivo are (Fig. 28-3):

1. Initial metabolism of ethanol must occur in the liver because that is the primary location of alcohol dehydrogenase.
2. NADH is a product of alcohol dehydrogenase. Hence, ATP is always a product during the metabolism of ethanol in the liver and may limit the rate of metabolism of ethanol.
3. The metabolic process for the metabolism of ethanol differs in the fed and fasting states. In the fed state, the end products are triglyceride, CO_2, and ATP; hence, it is has no acid-base impact, as both substrates and products are electroneutral. In contrast, ketoacids are produced during the metabolism of ethanol during fasting. We shall soon consider how rapidly this metabolism can occur.
4. The kinetics of alcohol dehydrogenase are such that it is always saturated with its substrate in the alcoholic (K_m 0.4 mmol/liter; the legal limit for intoxication is close to 20 mmol of ethanol per liter). Since this enzyme is not regulated directly, flow through alcohol dehydrogenase is limited by the rate of removal of its product, NADH, in the cytosol or its V_{max}. Its V_{max} is such that it can catalyze the synthesis of sufficient ATP in the liver to match the observed rate of turnover of ATP.[33] K_m equals the concentration of substrate to yield half the maximum velocity (V_{max}) catalyzed by a given amount of enzyme.
5. High concentrations of the products of the metabolism of ethanol stimulate the production of acids from the metabolism of fat (ketoacidosis due to the accumulation of acetyl CoA in hepatic mitochondria) and carbohydrates (lactic acidosis due to the accumulation of NADH; Fig. 28-3). It can also predispose a fasting subject to hypoglycemia.[16,20]

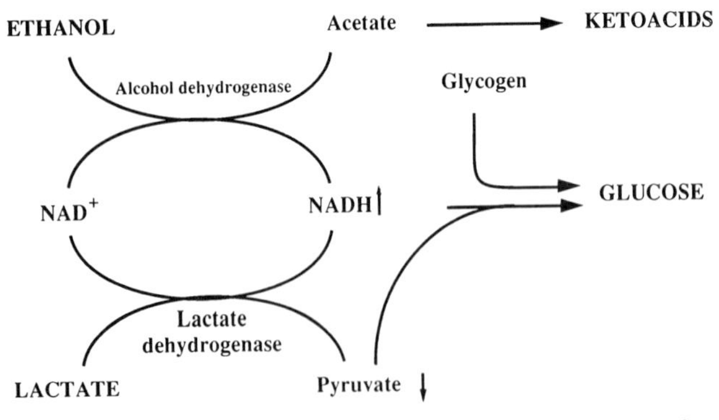

FIGURE 28-3 • Biochemistry of the metabolism of ethanol. For details, see the text.

Ketoacids and ethanol

One of the products of the initial steps in the oxidation of ethanol is NADH; oxidation of NADH yields ATP. Given that the liver consumes 2 mmol/min of oxygen and that this is equivalent to the production of 12 mmol/min of ATP (P:O = 3), the maximum rate of metabolism of ethanol can be calculated based on the turnover of ATP (Table 28-8).[33] If ethanol were fully oxidized in the liver to CO_2, its rate of oxidation would be 0.75 mmol/min (12 mmol/min ATP, 16 mmol ATP/mmol of ethanol; equation 25). This situation would permit clearance of close to 1 mole (1000 mmol) of ethanol (46 g) per day if ethanol provided 100 percent of the ATP for the liver. Similarly, if acetic acid were the product, 2 mol (2000 mmol) (92 g) of ethanol could be utilized per day. Since the observed rate of metabolism of ethanol is close to 250 g/day, ketogenesis must be the major product of the metabolism of ethanol during fasting (equations 25 through 28):

$$2\ \text{Ethanol} + 6O_2 \rightarrow 4CO_2 + 32\text{ATP} \quad (25)$$

$$2\ \text{Ethanol} + O_2 \rightarrow 2\ \text{acetic acid} + 12\text{ATP} \quad (26)$$

$$2\ \text{Ethanol} + O_2 \rightarrow \beta\text{-HB}^- + H^+ + H_2O + 5\text{ATP} \quad (27)$$

$$2\ \text{Ethanol} + 1.5O_2 \rightarrow \text{AcAc}^- + H^+ + 8\text{ATP} \quad (28)$$

If the distribution of ketone acids generated in the liver were 50 percent β-HB and 50 percent AcAc, as it is in DKA,[62] 6.5 mmol of ATP would be generated per millimoles of ketoacid formed. This value is similar to that obtained during the ketoacidosis from endogenous fat. Therefore, all the quantitative issues regarding the ketoacidosis of fasting discussed previously probably pertain to this situation as well. In addition,

1. The rate of ketogenesis might be decreased if the rate of turnover of ATP in the liver were lower, other fuels

provided ATP in the liver, or there was a large degree of damage to the liver secondary to the abuse of alcohol.

2. The rate of utilization of ketoacids might be lower for three reasons. First, sedation of the brain during intoxication might reduce its rate of turnover of ATP, and thereby reduce the rate of oxidation of fuels (β-HB$^-$) in the brain. Second, with marked hypovolemia, there is less sodium filtered and reabsorbed by the kidney and thereby a lower rate of turnover of ATP in that organ.[36] Third, the higher NADH:NAD ratio in the liver might cause the conversion of AcAc to β-HB (equation 29). Only AcAc and not β-HB is converted to acetone (equation 30):

$$AcAc^- + NADH \leftrightarrow \beta\text{-}HB^- + NAD^+ + H^+ \quad (29)$$

$$AcAc^- + H^+ \rightarrow \text{acetone} + CO_2 \quad (30)$$

Other considerations

Although the production of H^+ can be lethal, there are several reasons why generation of ketoacids is not an entirely negative feature in the alcoholic:

1. It permits a higher rate of utlilization of ethanol, the depressant of the CNS, for reasons of turnover of ATP in the liver (equations 25 through 28), up to the V_{max} permitted by alcohol dehydrogenase.
2. It provides a suitable fuel for the brain (β-HB). This helps to spare a considerable quantity of lean body mass (up to 1 kg, owing to the generation of ATP in the brain from the metabolism of ketoacids.)[38] A rise in the NADH:NAD ratio diverts pyruvate to lactate and hence lessens the availability of this carbon source for formation of glucose. In addition, formation of glucose from a variety of amino acids that feed carbon into the gluconeogenic pathway at the level of citric acid intermediates will be diminished due to a fall in oxaloacetate concentration, a gluconeogenic precursor, also because of the high concentration of NADH.
3. Oxidation of a noncarbohydrate fuel in the brain is critical in a subject who has a deficiency of thiamine owing to poor nutrition. Thiamine is a cofactor for pyruvate dehydrogenase.[70] When thiamine is lacking and ketoacids are not available, the generation of ATP occurs only by glycolysis, and therefore excessive quantities of H^+ will be produced in those cells with a high rate of turnover of ATP. This could explain, at least in part, the development of the Wernicke-Korsakoff syndrome in some of these patients. The clinical corollary of this statement is that thiamine (vitamin B_1) should be given at the outset of therapy in alcoholic ketoacidosis (before the levels of ketoacids decline markedly).
4. Ketoacids will be present whether circulating alcohol levels are still high or not. This obtains because the very marked hypovolemia that accompanies this clinical picture leads to very high levels of epinephrine, the alpha-effect of which suppress the release of insulin. Thus, consequent to insulinopenia, an increased release of fatty acids from adipocytes occurs, providing the substrate for a liver that is poised for ketogenesis.
5. It is of interest that ethanol is therapeutic for the severe metabolic acidoses of methanol and ethylene glycol intoxication. The metabolism of ethanol markedly depresses that of methanol and ethylene glycol by more avidly competing for alcohol dehydrogenase and in so doing limits the rate of generation of toxic aldehyes.[33] However, acetic acid is now formed from ethanol. The reason that acetic acidosis is not a problem in this setting is that the acetic acid is oxidized rapidly in muscle, brain, and kidney, thereby making this pathway a metabolic process that does not have the net generation of H^+.

Lactic acid and ethanol

The metabolism of ethanol via alcohol dehydrogenase in the cytosol of hepatocytes leads to an elevated NADH:NAD ratio (Fig. 28-3). Accordingly, pyruvate levels fall and those of lactate rise as their interconversion is catalyzed by lactate dehydrogenase's near-equilibrium reaction:

$$\text{Pyruvate} + NADH \leftrightarrow \text{lactate} + NAD^+ \quad (31)$$

Eventually a new steady state is achieved such that input and output of lactate are equivalent but the concentration of lactate will be higher and that of pyruvate only somewhat lower than normal. Hence, only a modest degree of lactic acidosis is expected. Because lactate anions were derived from neutral precursors (glucose, glycogen, and alanine), this will yield a net load of H^+ ions.

Other factors also contribute to the degree of elevation of the concentration of lactate in this setting. It is important to recognize that there is no direct contribution of ethanol to the NADH:NAD ratio in organs other than the liver, since they do not contain appreciable alcohol dehydrogenase activity. Nevertheless, flux through pyruvate dehydrogenase should be lower in these organs because of the oxidation of ketoacids.[33,61,69,70] These considerations help to explain a modest degree of lactic acidosis. One should also appreciate that other causes of lactic acidosis might also be present in this clinical setting (e.g., shock, sepsis, or thiamine deficiency), and their presence should be suspected in patients with a higher degree of lactic acidosis.

There is another metabolic aspect of the lactic acid and ethanol story. As a result of the increased hepatic cytoplasmic NADH:NAD ratio and the inhibition of pyruvate utilization by the high acetyl-CoA concentration in hepatocytes during the metabolism of ethanol, the carbon from the amino acids that were delivered to the liver will be exported from the liver as lactic acid. Since gluconeogenesis from amino acids is an ATP-producing process,[42] 3 moles of ATP will not be formed in the liver for each mole of lactate released. This will diminish an ATP-mediated constraint on hepatic methanol metabolism. However, this process may have metabolic consequences in the starved patient. The catabolic pathway can be summarized as follows:

$$\underset{\text{muscle}}{\text{Protein}} \rightarrow \text{amino acids} \rightarrow \underset{\text{liver}}{\text{pyruvate}} \rightarrow \underset{\text{liver}}{\text{lactate}} \rightarrow \underset{\text{muscle}}{CO_2} \quad (32)$$

We have calculated that the consumption of 1 mole of lactate (90 g) in this process could lead to the loss of 1 pound of muscle (80 percent water).

Overall, the points to stress regarding the acid-base problems related to the metabolism of ethanol are as follows:

1. ATP balance must be maintained in all organs. The liver can utilize only 18 moles of ATP per day. In the typical patient (fasting with relative insulin deficiency), formation of ketoacids permits the liver to metabolize the largest quantity of ethanol while maintaining ATP balance. In such a patient, this will also provide a fuel for the brain and minimize excessive loss of lean body mass.
2. The degree of acidosis is rarely very severe in the patient with alcoholic ketoacidosis because of the offsetting processes, with respect to pH, of the severe metabolic alkalosis of vomiting and the ketoacidosis. Lactic acidosis will be a life-threatening process only in the presence of other problems, such as shock, sepsis, and thiamine deficiency.
3. There are dangers in therapy if a deficit of thiamine is present and not rapidly replaced.
4. Other issues not discussed in this chapter can be life-threatening: the deficit in potassium, glycemic disorders, underlying or associated diseases, and problems related to the withdrawal of alcohol.

METABOLIC ALKALOSIS

Elevated values for pH and bicarbonate in plasma are the hallmarks for the diagnosis of metabolic alkalosis (Chap. 29).[22,41] The factors responsible for the rise in the concentration of bicarbonate can be evaluated by considering its content in the ECF (numerator) and the volume of the ECF (denominator). Hence, this diagnostic category represents a heterogeneous pathophysiology. By taking a quantitative approach that deals with the ECF, ICF, and the kidney, one can better understand its pathophysiology and the impact of suggestions for its treatment.

Principles pertaining to metabolic alkalosis

Law of electroneutrality

It is obvious that the net charge from anions and cations that are gained or lost in any major compartment of the body must be equal, otherwise sparks fly! This statement does not deny the possibility of generating an electrical gradient across a membrane, since very few ions are involved in this process. Accordingly, when a cation such as K^+ exits from the ICF, either another cation such as Na^+ or H^+ must enter the ICF or an anion such as phosphate must leave to maintain this electroneutrality. There is not a fixed stoichiometry for these processes. The only rule that must be obeyed is the law of electroneutrality. Thus, a shift of cations across the ECF-ICF interface may have a large impact on the degree of metabolic alkalosis and on the pH of ICF.

Examination of acid-base balance in all body compartments

Acid-base events in the ECF may differ in quantity and even in direction from those in the ICF. For example, when there is a large deficit of K^+ ions, most of the K^+ ions were derived from the ICF, and electroneutrality was maintained in both ECF and ICF for the most part by a reciprocal movement of Na^+ and H^+.[10,11] To the extent that H^+ ions are involved, one will not obtain an accurate acid-base evaluation by only examining parameters in the ECF. This shortcoming had led to some of the confusion about overall bicarbonate balance in metabolic alkalosis (expecting a surplus of bicarbonate and a requirement for bicarbonaturia when metabolic alkalosis was corrected; but in reality, a total body deficit of bicarbonate might be present; see below).

Problems associated with the term net acid excretion

Net acid excretion is measured to evaluate the role of the kidney for balance of bicarbonate in the body.[68] Overall balance of bicarbonate is also influenced by the renal handling of anions that could be metabolized to bicarbonate;[44] the latter anions are not considered in the net acid excretion formula. Consider the situation in which there is a high rate of excretion of K^+ salts following a bicarbonate load in an animal that has not consumed food.[13] In this setting, acids such as citric acid are formed and excreted as their K^+ salt; this is equivalent to the loss of bicarbonate ions from the body (Fig. 28-4), a loss that is not detected by the net acid excretion formula. in summary, excretion of NH_4^+ with Cl^- does represent a positive balance for bicarbonate because most Cl^- ions enter the body along with the cation Na^+. In contrast, the excretion of NH_4^+ with endogenously produced citrate

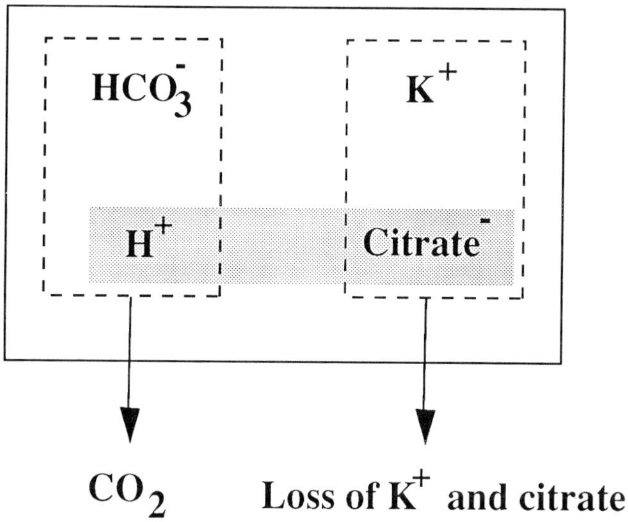

FIGURE 28-4 • Direct and indirect loss of bicarbonate. Bicarbonate ions can be lost directly in the urine along with K^+ (left side of figure). Alternatively, bicarbonate ions and K^+ can be lost indirectly when K^+ is excreted with citrate anions, because citrate anions are produced in metabolic reactions along with H^+.

anions will not lead to a positive balance for bicarbonate, since citrate anions are produced along with protons.

Clinical aspects of metabolic alkalosis

The diagnosis of the so-called Cl^- depletion type of metabolic alkalosis in usually very straightforward.[21,41] Most commonly there will be a history of a loss of Cl^- via the GI tract (usually vomiting) or the urine (usually diuretics). This loss of Cl^- with H^+ in the former instance or with NH_4^+ in the latter leads to an exchange of anions, Cl^- loss, and bicarbonate gain in the ECF. Secondary changes occur thereafter that may alter the picture in terms of overall balance. The negative balance becomes one in which there is an equimolar cumulative loss of K^+ and Cl^- (e.g., the postdrainage period of selective deficiency of HCl).[47,58,82] In this setting, there is no longer a total body surplus of bicarbonate.[13] Specifically, for a loss of K^+ to occur, K^+ must be lost with an anion other than Cl^-. It is unlikely that virtually all these lost anions are accompanied by Na^+ or H^+. Focusing on H^+, given the unchanging size of the bicarbonate pool in the ECF and the need to lose K^+ in the urine, virtually all of the H^+ must be retained in the ICF (Fig. 28-5).

Further support for the idea that there could be a negative balance for bicarbonate and yet a higher concentration of bicarbonate in the ECF during metabolic alkalosis with equimolar losses of K^+ and Cl^- ions was provided in a study where the deficit of KCl was replaced over 8 h by Scheich and associates[13] and during prolonged balance experiments carried out by Bleich and colleagues.[4] When Scheich and coworkers[13] replaced the deficits of K^+ and Cl^- over a very short time period, there was a larger fall in the concentration of bicarbonate in plasma as compared to a control series given equimolar NaCl. This greater fall in bicarbonate could not be explained by a larger rise in ECF volume. Examining other events that could have influenced the concentration of bicarbonate in plasma revealed that events in the kidney were not important (excretion of net acid and the difference in the concentrations of $Na^+ + K^+ - Cl^-$ were small and did not change appreciably following the administration of KCl). Further, the anion gap in plasma was not elevated in the NaCl and KCl groups. Hence, an additional source of H^+ was needed to lower the concentration of bicarbonate in the ECF in the KCl group; this source of H^+ occurred without addition of a conjugate base. These authors speculated that the source of the H^+ was the ICF and represented an exit of H^+ when the administered K^+ entered cells.

Emphasis on the role of the ICF can be illustrated by reexamining the model of metabolic alkalosis initiated by selective depletion of HCl in dogs reported by Bleich and associated.[4] The fact that more H^+ was retained in the ICF than bicarbonate ions were retained in the ECF can be appreciated by considering events in this study in three phases (Fig. 28-5). In the first phase, although metabolic alkalosis was initiated by the selective loss of HCl, there was a spontaneous conversion to a model of near-equimolar losses of K^+ and Cl^- (118 and 110 mmol, respectively) in the postdrainage period.[82] In the second phase, sufficient HCl was administered to correct the metabolic alkalosis in the ECF (bicarbonate fell from 32.4 to 21.2 mmol/liter). There was no significant change in external balance of Na^+ (1 mmol) or Cl^- (−36 mmol). At this point, the deficit of K^+ was not replaced, and the intracellular accumulation of H^+ remained unchanged. In the third phase, the large deficit of K^+ was replaced as their sulfate or phospate salts, which uncovered intracellular events. There was a large increase in the excretion of net acid after giving these K^+ salts; this was equivalent to a gain of 157 mmol of bicarbonate ions, but only close to 30 mmol of this bicarbonate was retained in the ECF (7 mmol/liter × 4 liters, the ECF volume in a 20-kg dog). Accordingly, most was annihilated (combined with H^+ to form $CO_2 + H_2O$). If this loss of bicarbonate ions was attributed to endogenous acid production, there must be retention of an equivalent amount of anions in plasma, or the conjugate base of that acid must be excreted in the urine. Since these extra anions were not detected, it appears that H^+ was exported from the ICF; the driving force for its release was the intracellular accumulation of a near-stoichiometric quantity of K^+ (130 mmol of the 157 mmol that were retained). Accordingly, although the intracellular acidosis and depletion of K^+ from the ICF were corrected in the third phase, metabolic alkalosis was

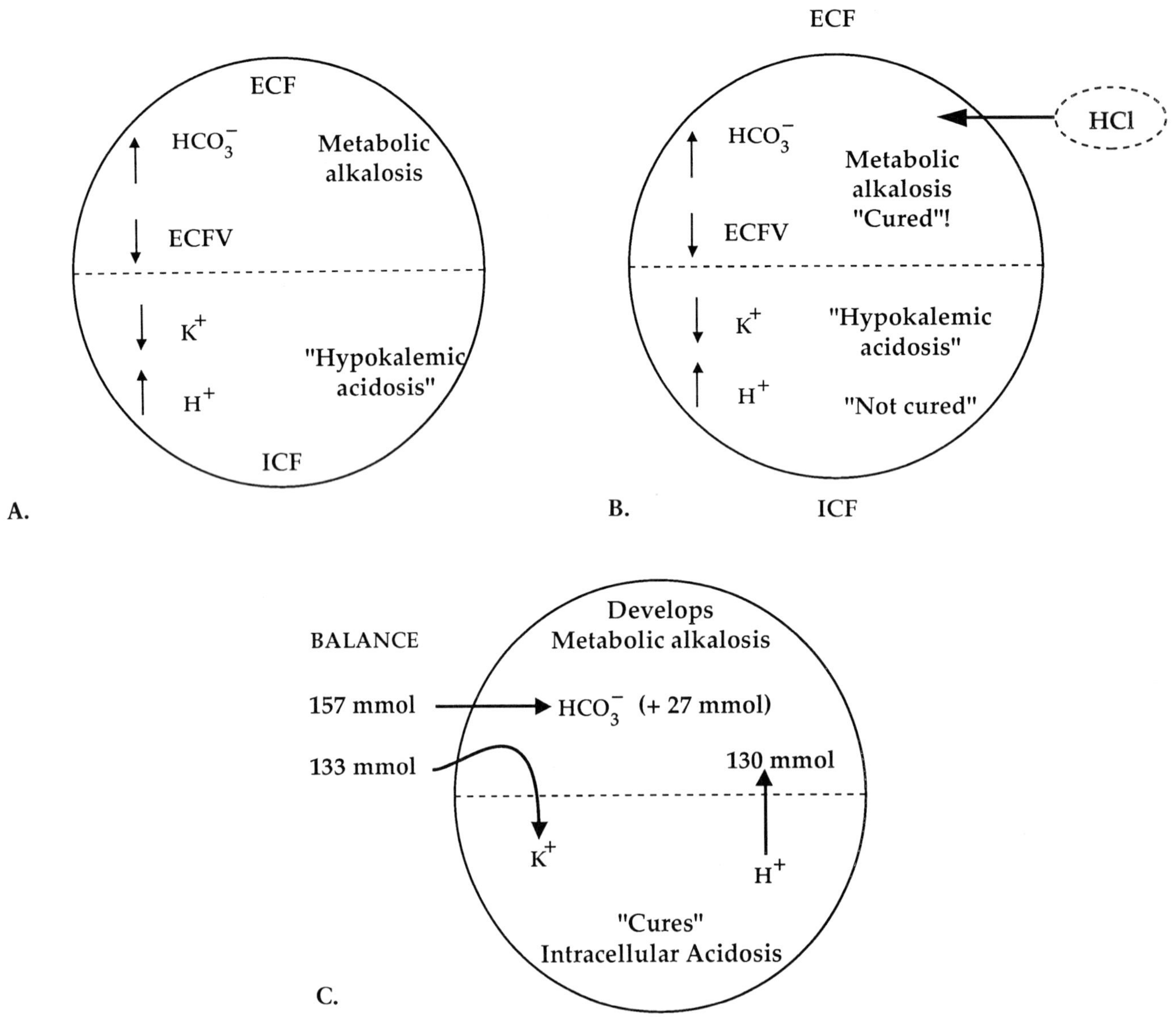

FIGURE 28-5 • Correction of metabolic alkalosis. For details, see the text. Correction of metabolic alkalosis requires an analysis of events in the ECF, ICF, and urine. Data were obtained from the studies of Bleich and coworkers.[4,82] The top portion of the figure represents the infusion of HCl to correct the extracellular component of metabolic alkalosis. The bottom portion of the figure represents the infusion of K^+ as its phosphate or sulfate salt to correct events in the ICF. The key observations are the positive balances for net acid excretion (equivalent to a positive balance of 130 mmol bicarbonate) and K^+ (133 mmol) when the K^+ salts are administered.

produced when viewed in ECF terms (rise in bicarbonate in plasma from 22.1 to 28.4 mmol/liter).

This analysis underlines the importance of addressing events in all three compartments when trying to correct metabolic alkalosis: the ECF requires removal of bicarbonate ions and provision of Cl^- together with a source of NaCl to replace any deficits; the ICF requires provision of K^+ to remove extra H^+ and Na^+ from the ICF plus a source of new bicarbonate to restore whole body bicarbonate balance; and renal events must be restored to normal to complete the correction of this condition.

Given the foregoing discussion, a note of caution should be inserted about the term *correction* of metabolic alkalosis. First, if administered saline solution overexpands the ECF volume,[8,46-48] a dilutional fall in the concentration of bicarbonate will occur. Since this concerns only the ECF and edema is not a desired end point, this is not correction of the underlying metabolic processes, and the metabolic alkalosis is not really saline-sensitive. Second, consider a patient with metabolic alkalosis whose ECF volume is contracted. If an agent that increased the excretion of Na^+ and bicarbonate ions was given, it would undoubtedly cause the concentration of bicarbonate in the ECF to fall, but the degree of contraction of the ECF volume would become more severe. This, again, should not be viewed as correction of the metabolic process, but it is a potential threat to the circulating volume. Third, should organic acids be produced during therapy, the concentration of bicarbonate will again fall, but the underlying metabolic process is not corrected; an example of this sequence of events can be seen in a study by Galla.[23] Accordingly, we think that use of the word *correction* should be restricted to therapy addressing all three compartments: the ECF, the ICF, and the kidney. To correct the ECF, one needs Cl^- and sufficient Na^+ to restore the ECF volume *to normal*. A source of H^+ or a loss of bicarbonate ions is also needed. For the ICF, one needs a source of K^+. To the extent that H^+ exits from the ICF, a source of bicarbonate ions may also be required. Finally, the rates of excretion of NH_4^+ and bicarbonate ions must also be regulated to permit the restoration of a normal concentration of bicarbonate in the ECF.

CONCLUDING REMARKS

Metabolic aspects of metabolic acidosis have been emphasized here. To do this, four general principles related to the regulation of metabolism and acid-base balance were highlighted. It is critical that a quantitative, rather than a qualitative, analysis be performed so that enlightened decisions and rational expectations can be achieved during therapy. Selected aspects of ketoacidosis and lactic acidosis were discussed.

Traditionally, metabolic alkalosis has been described in terms of Cl-depletion[22] or K-depletion,[60] and the therapeutic approach was based on a requirement to induce bicarbonaturia (saline-responsive metabolic alkalosis). This approach seems to fall short for several reasons. First, the pathophysiology of metabolic alkalosis is heterogeneous, may vary over time, and includes important events in the ICF. Second, since metabolic alkalosis might be accompanied by a total body deficit of bicarbonate, bicarbonaturia should not be considered a cornerstone of its correction. Further, the basis of an elevated bicarbonate concentration may change during the natural history of metabolic alkalosis despite unchanging alkalemia. Appropriate attention must be paid to stoichiometry and electroneutrality in order to interpret events in metabolic alkalosis, and the analysis should include a quantitative interpretation of events in three compartments: the ECF, ICF, and the urine.

REFERENCES

1. Abu Romeh S, Tannen RL: Amelioration of hypoxia-induced lactic acidosis by superimposed hypercapnea or hydrochloric acid infusion. *Am J Physiol* 250:F720, 1986.
2. Bayoumi A et al: Deducing the cause of metabolic acidosis from the renal handling of the anion. *Clin Invest Med* 14:A134, 1991.
3. Bettice JA, Gamble JL: Skeletal buffering of acute metabolic acidosis. *Am J Physiol* 229:1618, 1975.
4. Bleich HL: The induction of metabolic alkalosis by correction of potassium deficiency. *J Clin Invest* 45:573, 1966.
5. Brauer RW: Liver circulation and function. *Physiol Rev* 43:115, 1965.
6. Carlisle EJF et al: Glue-sniffing and distal renal tubular acidosis: Sticking to the facts. *J Am Soc Nephrol* 1:1019, 1991.
7. Cheetham ME et al: Human muscle metabolism during sprint running. *J Appl Physiol* 61:54, 1986.
8. Cohen JJ, Ellis JH: Correction of metabolic alkalosis by the kidney after isometric expansion of extracellular fluid. *J Clin Invest* 47:1181, 1968.
9. Conway EJ, Fearon PJ: The acid-labile CO_2 in mammalian muscle and the pH of the muscle fibre. *J Physiol (London)* 103:274, 1944.
10. Cooke R et al: The extrarenal correction of alkalosis associated with potassium deficiency. *J Clin Invest* 31:798, 1952.
11. Cooke R et al: The role of potassium in the prevention of alkalosis. *Am J Med* 180, 1954.
12. Davey CL: The significance of carnosine and anserine in striated skeletal muscle. *Arch Biochem Biophys* 89:303, 1960.
13. Scheich A et al: Can metabolic alkalosis be a disorder with a deficit of bicarbonate? *Clin Invest Med* 15 (in press) 1992.
14. Dyck RF et al: A modification of the urine osmolal gap: An improved method for estimating urine ammonium. *Am J Nephrol* 10:359, 1990.
15. Felig P et al: Amino acid metabolism during prolonged starvation. *J Clin Invest* 48:584, 1969.
16. Field JB et al: Studies on the mechanism of ethanol-induced hypoglycemia. *J Clin Invest* 42:497, 1963.
17. Fields ALA et al: Theoretical aspects of weight loss in patients with cancer. *Cancer* 50:2183, 1982.
18. Flatt JP: On the maximal possible rate of ketogenesis. *Diabetes* 21:50, 1972.
19. Fraley DS et al: Metabolic acidosis after hyperalimentation with casein hydrolysate. *Ann Intern Med* 88:352, 1978.
20. Freinkel N et al: Alcohol hypoglycemia: 1. Carbohydrate metabolism of patients with clinical alcohol hypoglycemia and the experimental reproduction of the syndrome with pure ethanol. *J Clin Invest* 42:1112, 1963.
21. Gallas JH, Luke RG: Chloride transport and disorders of acid base balance. *Annu Rev Physiol* 50:141, 1988.
22. Galla JH et al: Adaptations to chloride-depletion alkalosis. *Am J Physiol* 261:R771, 1991.
23. Galla JH et al: Effects of chloride and extracellular fluid volume on bicarbonate reabsorption along the nephron in metabolic alkalosis in the rat. *J Clin Invest* 80:41, 1987.
24. Gennari FJ: Acid-base balance in dialysis patients. *Kidney Int* 28:678, 1985.
25. Goguen J et al: Can a double shot of vodka produce severe ketoacidosis? *Clin Invest Med,* 1992 (submitted).
26. Graf H et al: Effects of dichloroacetate in the treatment of hypoxic lactic acidosis in dogs. *J Clin Invest* 76:919, 1985.
27. Halperin ML: How much "new" bicarbonate is formed in

the distal nephron in the process of net acid excretion? *Kidney Int* 35:1277, 1989.

28. Halperin ML, Jungas RL: Metabolic production and renal disposal of hydrogen ions. *Kidney Int* 24:709, 1983.
29. Halperin ML, Rolleston FS: *Biochemical Detective Stories: A Problem-Based Approach to Clinical Cases.* Burlington, NC, Neil Patterson, 1990.
30. Halperin ML et al: Biochemistry and physiology of ammonium excretion, in Seldin DW, Giebisch G (eds): *The Kidney: Physiology and Pathophysiology.* New York, Raven Press, 1992, p 2645.
31. Halperin ML et al: Disposal of the daily acid load: An integrated function of the liver, lungs, and kidneys. *Trends Biol Sci* 12:197, 1987.
32. Halperin ML et al: Lactic acidosis, ketoacidosis, and energy turnover: "Figure" you made the correct diagnosis only when you have "counted" on it—quantitative analysis based on principles of metabolism. *M Sinai J Med* 59:1, 1992.
33. Halperin ML et al: Metabolic acidosis in the alcoholic: A pathophysiologic approach. *Metabolism* 32:308, 1983.
34. Halperin ML, Cheema-Dhadli S: Renal and hepatic aspects of ketoacidosis: A quantitative analysis based on energy turnover. *Diabetes Metab Rev* 5:321, 1989.
35. Halperin ML et al: A quantitative analysis of renal ammoniagenesis and energy balance: A theoretical approach. *Can J Physiol Pharmacol* 60:1431, 1982.
36. Halperin ML et al: Regulation of the maximum rate of renal ammoniagenesis in the acidotic dog. *Am J Physiol* 248:F607, 1985.
37. Halperin ML et al: The urine osmolal gap: A clue to estimate urine ammonium in "hybrid" types of metabolic acidosis. *Clin Invest Med* 11:198, 1988.
38. Hannaford MC et al: Protein wasting due to the acidosis of prolonged fasting. *Am J Physiol* 243:E251, 1982.
39. Hermansen L: Lactate removal at rest and during exercise, Howard H, Poortman J (eds): in *Metabolic Adaptation to Prolonged Physical Exercise.* Proceedings of the second international symposium on Biochem. Basel, Switzerland, Birkhauser Verlag, 1975, p 101.
40. Hindman BJ: Sodium bicarbonate in the treatment of subtypes of acute lactic acidosis: Physiologic considerations. *Anesthesiology* 72:1064, 1990.
41. Jacobson HR, Seldin DW: On the generation, maintenance, and correction of metabolic alkalosis. *Am J Physiol* 245:F245, 1983.
42. Jungas RL et al: Quantitative analysis of amino acid oxidation and related gluconeogenesis in humans. *Physiol Rev* 72(2):419, 1992.
43. Kamel KS, Halperin ML: DCA lactic acidosis. 1992 (submitted).
44. Kamel KS et al: The removal of an inorganic acid load in subjects with ketoacidosis of chronic fasting: The role of the kidney. *Kidney Int* 37:507, 1990.
45. Kamel KS et al: Urine electrolytes and osmolality: When and how to use them. *Am J Nephrol* 10:89, 1990.
46. Kassirer JP, Schwartz WB: Correction of metabolic alkalosis in man without repair of potassium deficiency. *Am J Med* 40:19, 1966.
47. Kassirer JP, Schwartz WB: The response of normal man to selective depletion of hydrochloric acid. *Am J Med* 40:10, 1966.
48. Kassirer JP et al: The critical role of chloride in the correction of hypokalemic alkalosis in man. *Am J Med* 38:172, 1965.
49. Kety SS et al: The blood flow and oxygen consumption of the human brain in diabetic acidosis and coma. *J Clin Invest* 27:500, 1948.
50. Krauss-Friedman N: *Hormonal Control of Gluconeogenesis.* Boca Raton, Fla, CRC Press, 1986.
51. Krebs, HA et al: Hyperlactataemia and lactic acidosis, Marks V, Hales C (eds): in *Essays in Medical Biochemistry.* London, William Clowes, 1975, p 81.
52. Lemieux G et al: The effect of ketone bodies on renal ammoniogenesis. *J Clin Invest* 50:1781, 1971.
53. Litzow JR et al: The effect of treatment of acidosis on calcium balance in patients with chronic azotemic renal disease. *J Clin Invest* 46:280, 1967.
54. Madias NE: Lactic acidosis. *Kidney Int* 29:752, 1986.
55. Madison LL, Seldin DW: Ammonia excretion and renal enzymatic adaptation in human subjects, as disclosed by administration of precursor amino acids. *J Clin Invest* 37:1615, 1958.
56. Mjos OD et al: Effects of dichloroacetate on myocardial substrate extraction, apicardial ST-segment elevation, and ventricular blood flow following coronary occlusion in dogs. *Cardiovasc Res* 10:427, 1976.
57. Narins RG, Cohen JJ: Bicarbonate therapy for organic acidosis: The case for its continued use. *Ann Intern Med* 106:615, 1987.
58. Needle MA et al: The effects of selective depletion of hydrochloric acid on acid-base and electrolyte equilibrium. *J Clin Invest* 43:1836, 1964.
59. Newsholme EA, Leech AR: Thermodynamics in metabolism, in *Biochemistry for the Medical Sciences.* Chichester, Wiley, 1983, p 10.
60. Norris SH, Kurtzman NA: Does chloride play an independent role in the pathogenesis of metabolic alkalosis? *Semin Nephrol* 8:101, 1988.
61. Owen OE et al: Brain metabolism during fasting. *J Clin Invest* 46:1589, 1967.
62. Owen OE et al: Liver and kidney metabolism during prolonged starvation. *J Clin Invest* 48:574, 1969.
63. Park R, Arieff AI: Treatment of lactic acidosis with dichloroacetate in dogs. *J Clin Invest* 70:853, 1982.
64. Patel MS, Roche TE: Molecular biology and biochemistry of pyruvate dehydrogenase complexes. *FASEB J* 4:3224, 1990.
65. Pitts RF: Renal production and excretion of ammonia. *Am J Med* 36:720, 1964.
66. Pitts RF et al: Metabolism of glutamine by the intact functioning kidney of the dog. *Am J Physiol* 244:1463, 1973.
67. Pitts RF et al: Relation of renal amino and amide nitrogen extraction to ammonia production. *Am J Physiol* 204:187, 1963.
68. Pitts RF et al: The renal regulation of acid-base balance in man: 1. The nature of the mechanism for acidifying the urine. *J Clin Invest* 26:48, 1947.
69. Randle PJ: Fuel selection in animals. *Biochem Soc. Trans* 14:799, 1986.

70. Reed LJ: Pyruvate dehydrogenase complex, in Horecker B, Stadtman E (eds): *Current Topics in Cellular Regulation.* New York, Academic Press, 1969, p. 233.
71. Reichard GA et al: Ketone body production and oxidation in fasting obese humans. *J Clin Invest* 53:508, 1974.
72. Roscoe JM et al: Hyperglycemia-induced hyponatremia: Metabolic considerations in calculation of serum sodium depression. *Can Med Assoc J* 112:452, 1975.
73. Sahlin K et al: Creatine kinase equilibrium and lactate content compared with muscle pH in tissue samples obtained after isometric exercise. *Biochem J* 152:173, 1975.
74. Sapir DG, Owen OE: Renal conservation of ketone bodies during starvation. *Metabolism* 24:23, 1975.
75. Simpson DP: Control of hydrogen ion homeostasis and renal acidosis. *Medicine* 50:503, 1971.
76. Smith HW et al: The renal clearances of substituted hippuric acid derivitives and other aromatic acids in dogs and man. *J Clin Invest* 24:388, 1945.
77. Stacpoole PW: The case against bicarbonate therapy. *Ann Intern Med* 105:276, 1986.
78. Stacpoole PW: The pharmacology of dichloroacetate. *Metabolism* 38:1124, 1989.
79. Stacpoole PW et al: Dichloroacetate in the treatment of lactic acidosis. *Ann Int Med* 108:58, 1988.
80. Stacpoole PW et al: Treatment of lactic acidosis with dichloroacetate. *N Engl J Med* 309:390, 1983.
81. Swan RC, Pitts RF: Neutralization of infused acid by nephrectomized dogs. *J Clin Invest* 34:205, 1955.
82. Tannen RL et al: The renal response to acid loads in metabolic alkalosis: An assessment of the mechanisms regulating acid excretion. *J Clin Invest* 45:562, 1966.
83. Van Leeuven A: Net cation equivalency ("base binding power") of the proteins. *Acta Med Scand* 422:1, 1969.
84. Vasuvattakul S: Quantitative role of the intracellular bicarbonate buffer system in response to an acute acid load. *Am J Physiol* 262:R305, 1992.
85. Vinay P et al: Effect of fatty acids on renal ammoniagenesis in vivo and in vitro studies. *Am J Physiol* 231:880, 1976.
86. Voet D, Voet JG: *Biochemistry.* New York, Wiley, 1990.
87. Wargovich TJ et al: Myocardial metabolic and hemodynamic effects of dichloroacetate in coronary artery disease. *Am J Cardiol* 61:65, 1988.
88. Whitehouse S, Randle PJ: Activation of pyruvate dehydrogenase in perfused rat heart by dichloroacetate. *Biochem J* 134:651, 1973.
89. Windus DW et al: Glutamine transport in renal basolateral vesicles from dogs with metabolic acidosis. *Am J Physiol* 246:F78, 1984.

CHAPTER 29

Metabolic alkalosis

Sandra Sabatini • Neil A. Kurtzman

Metabolic alkalosis is a primary pathophysiologic event characterized by an increase in bicarbonate concentration or a loss of nonvolatile acid from the extracellular fluid (ECF). The hypoventilation and hypercapnia that characterize the respiratory compensation for metabolic alkalosis *minimize* the degree of alkalemia, but do not fully normalize blood pH. Recognition of coexisting acid-base disorders is discussed in Chap. 31.

This chapter first addresses the factors that control renal bicarbonate reabsorption, then reviews the forces affecting acid excretion, then reviews the forces affecting acid excretion. A discussion of the generation and maintenance of metabolic alkalosis follows, with an illustration of these principles through a selective review of the major disease states that spawn the alkalosis. The chapter concludes with a section on therapy.

FACTORS CONTROLLING RENAL BICARBONATE REABSORPTION

Most of the available evidence suggests that proximal bicarbonate reabsorption is mediated by sodium-hydrogen ion exchange rather than by direct reabsorption[25,37,39,42,44,128,155] (see also Chap. 10). The overall schema is shown in Fig. 29-1. The secreted hydrogen ion derives from the dissociation of the carbonic acid

$$H_2CO_3 \rightarrow H^+ + HCO_3^-$$

formed by the hydration of carbon dioxide and water, end products of intermediary metabolism.

$$CO_2 + H_2O \rightarrow H_2CO_3$$

An alternative—less likely, in our view—is that the ionization of water may contribute protons for secretion [$H_2O \rightarrow H^+$ (secreted) + OH^- (remains in cytosol)]. Secreted protons would convert luminal HCO_3^- to CO_2 and H_2O, while cytosolic OH^- would react with cellular CO_2 to form HCO_3^-. The latter would be returned with reabsorbed sodium to venous blood. The protons are then secreted into the tubular lumen in exchange for sodium. The secreted H^+ reacts with filtered HCO_3^- to form carbonic acid, which in turn dissociates into carbon dioxide and water. The reaction is catalyzed by carbonic anhydrase, an enzyme found inside the cell and on the luminal surface of proximal tubular epithelium.[123,186] Carbon dioxide diffuses into the tubular cell, beginning the cycle again. There is also evidence that carbonic acid may enter the cell directly.[9,10]

The cellular HCO_3^- formed secondary to proton secretion is passively returned to the blood—either by electrically neutral chloride, for HCO_3^- exchange, or by conductive HCO_3^--facilitated diffusion.[183] The source of energy for proton secretion is probably sodium-potassium ATPase (Na^+-K^+ ATPase), an enzyme found in abundance on the basolateral surface of proximal tubular cells.[72,76,98,162] The Na^+- K^+ ATPase generates the elec-

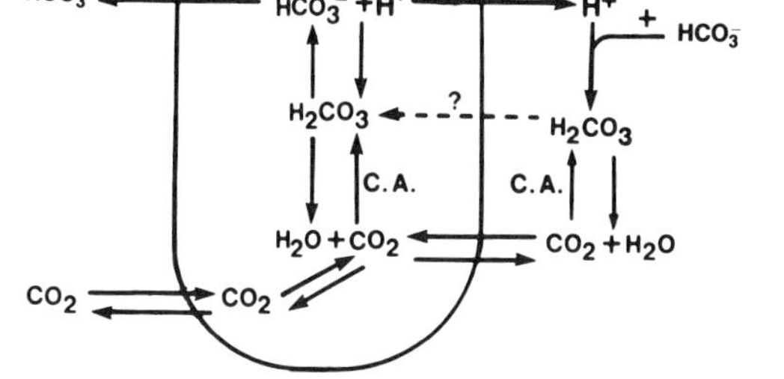

FIGURE 29-1 • Hydrogen ion secretion in the proximal tubule. (CA, carbonic anhydrase.)

This work was supported in part by grants from the National Institutes of Health, No. R01-DK-36119 and No. R01-DK-36199.

trochemical gradient for sodium entry into the cell by maintaining a low cellular sodium concentration. Thus, basolateral sodium transport supplies the energy for luminal sodium/hydrogen exchange. It is possible that a small component of electrogenic non-sodium-coupled proton secretion may occur as well.

Whil this process occurs in both the proximal and the distal nephron, the bulk of this transport takes place at the former location. The proximal tubule (unlike the distal nephron) is a high-capacitance, low-pH gradient system that is affected by many factors (see Table 29-1).

EFFECTIVE ARTERIAL VOLUME

The state of the ECF volume is one of the major factors controlling HCO_3^- reabsorption.[105] When ECF volume is expanded, proximal tubule sodium reabsorption is inhibited; this process secondarily depresses HCO_3^- reabsorption. Conversely, when ECF volume is contracted, sodium reabsorption is enhanced, as is that of HCO_3^-. Bicarbonate reabsorption in normal subjects is complete when the plasma HCO_3^- is 26 meq/liter (the maximum rate of tubule reabsorption, or T_m, of HCO_3^-). In volume-contracted subjects the *Tm* is increased.[105] The *Tm* for HCO_3^- is expressed per unit glomerular filtration rate (GFR) (not per unit time, as is done for glucose, etc.), and defines the maximal rate of reabsorption under the particular set of circumstances in which it is measured. It has been suggested that Cl^- deficiency stimulates HCO_3^- reabsorption.[105,158] Chloride depletion is almost invariably synonymous with salt depletion, and therefore with contraction of the ECF volume. Thus, it is likely that Cl^- depletion enhances HCO_3^- reabsorption through depletion of ECF volume (see below for further discussion of the role of Cl^-). The precise mechanism whereby volume expansion decreases acidification is not completely understood; it is probably linked directly to a change in sodium transport, a discussion of which is beyond the scope of this chapter (see Chap. 10).

TABLE 29-1 • Factors affecting bicarbonate reabsorption by the proximal tubule

Maneuver	Decreases HCO_3^- reabsorption	Increases HCO_3^- reabsorption
Volume expansion	+	
Hyperkalemia	+	
Hypocapnia	+	
Hyperparathyroidism	+	
Phosphate depletion	+	
Hypocalcemia	+	
Hypercalcemia		+
Volume contraction		+
Hypercapnia		+
Hypokalemia		+
Glucose loading		+
Aldosterone	No direct effect	No direct effect

SOURCE: Adapted from Sabatini S et al, *Med Clin North Am* 67:120, 1983.

GLOMERULAR FILTRATION RATE AND FILTERED LOAD OF BICARBONATE

The classic studies of Pitts and colleagues[144,145] demonstrated that HCO_3^- reabsorption varied in proportion with changes in GFR. They also noted that at low levels of filtered load, HCO_3^- reabsorption was complete, with none appearing in the urine. When the plasma HCO_3^- level reached 26 to 28 meq/liter, there was no further increase in HCO_3^- reabsorption, and HCO_3^- began to appear in the urine.

More recently, several investigators have argued that the filtered load of HCO_3^- is a major determinant of HCO_3^- reabsorption. Using clearance techniques in dogs, Langberg and colleagues[113] demonstrated that HCO_3^- reabsorption is a function of filtered HCO_3^- load and pH, and that there was no evidence for special effects of plasma HCO_3^-, P_{CO_2}, or GFR. Using micropuncture techniques, Cogan and colleagues[41] demonstrated a tight relationship in the superficial proximal tubule between HCO_3^- reabsorption and the filtered load in both normal and acidotic rats. There was no inhibitory effect of ECF volume expansion on proximal HCO_3^- reabsorption independent of filtered HCO_3^- load. Substantiating data were presented by Berry and Cogan,[24] using isolated perfused proximal tubules from rabbits, which were subjected to in-vitro volume expansion (induced by changes in protein concentration) and showed no change in HCO_3^- reabsorption while sodium chloride transport was significantly reduced. This observation is in sharp contrast to the earlier work of Cohen,[47] who demonstrated that metabolic alkalosis was corrected in animals during volume expansion when the GFR (and hence the filtered load of HCO_3^-) was kept constant by aortic constriction. The differences between these contrasting data await elucidation.

The resolution of these conflicting studies has major implications for our understanding of the forces that maintain clinical metabolic alkalosis. If the filtered load of HCO_3^- is the main determinant of its excretory rate, then subjects with persistent metabolic alkalosis must have a decline in the filtered load of alkali—which can result only from a decrease in the GFR, since the plasma HCO_3^- concentration is high. Correction of metabolic alkalosis would, therefore, require maneuvers that increase the filtered load of HCO_3^-, thereby causing a corrective bicarbonaturia. Conversely, if Cohen's study[47] bears more keenly on clinical metabolic alkalosis, then correction of metabolic alkalosis should be mediated through changes in volume, potassium homeostasis, or other maneuvers that influence HCO_3^- excretion through mechanisms other than changes in filtered load.

CARBONIC ANHYDRASE

Carbonic anhydrase plays a major role in the renal transport of HCO_3^-.[129,156] Its importance is easily demonstrable by observing the effect of administering enzyme inhibitors. The infusion of such inhibitors as acetazolamide results in a prompt HCO_3^- diuresis. Under normal conditions, approximately 30 percent of filtered HCO_3^- appears in the urine following carbonic anhydrase inhibition.[42,54,124] In the superficial proximal tubule, infusion of such inhibitors decreases HCO_3^- transport by 70 to 100 percent.[42,124] Synthesis of these two observations indicates that whole kidney HCO_3^- reabsorption is affected to a much lesser degree than is that in the superficial proximal tubule. This suggests that there exists, at sites other than the accessible proximal nephron, a major carbonic anhydrase-independent pathway for HCO_3^- reabsorption. The site of this enzyme-independent reabsorption may be the deeper proximal tubules inaccessible to micropuncture, or the more distal segments of the nephron, or both.[62] Administration of amiloride with acetazolamide increases HCO_3^- excretion by an additional 10 percent. Amiloride acts mainly in the cortical collecting tubule,[54] suggesting strongly that there is carbonic anhydrase-independent HCO_3^- reabsorption in this nephron segment.

Finally, if distal nephron acidification is to a large extent dependent upon the presence of carbonic anhydrase activity, one would predict that the infusion of acetazolamide, or a similar inhibitor, would decrease the rate of distal urinary acidification. When acetazolamide is infused to animals under a variety of experimental conditions, it does not decrease urine-blood P_{CO_2} gradient (a marker of distal acidification) (see Chap. 27), suggesting that, in vivo, distal acidification is not inhibited by blocking carbonic anhydrase activity.[149] This is in sharp contradistinction to the affect of amiloride, which consistently lowers the urine-blood P_{CO_2} gradient.[10] This further suggests that there is a large component of distal urinary acidification which is independent of carbonic anhydrase activity. Again, the reasons for the discrepancies between in vivo and in vitro studies remain unclear.

POTASSIUM

It has been known for many years that renal HCO_3^- reabsorption is inversely proportional to the level of body potassium stores.[52,63] In other words, HCO_3^- reabsorption is depressed in potassium-loaded animals and increased in potassium-depleted animals. The demonstration that hypokalemic metabolic alkalosis could be corrected by the administration of sodium chloride alone casts doubt on the role of potassium as a key regulator of HCO_3^- reabsorption.[94] Subsequently, however, it was demonstrated that potassium exerts a regulatory role over HCO_3^- reabsorption which is independent of any effect attributable to volume. Kurtzman and coworkers[109] studied HCO_3^- reabsorption in three groups of dogs: one with potassium depletion (induced by a potassium-free diet and desoxycorticosterone), a second group with hyperkalemia, and a third, normal, group. Bicarbonate reabsorption fell in all three groups following volume expansion with isotonic saline. The higher the fractional Cl^- excretion, the lower the HCO_3^- reabsorption. At any given level of fractional Cl^- excretion, HCO_3^- reabsorption was higher in potassium-depleted animals than in normal animals. Bicarbonate reabsorption was higher in normal animals than in those that were potassium-loaded. When salt excretion was very low—and, by inference, ECF volume markedly contracted—there was no difference in HCO_3^- reabsorption among the three groups. These authors concluded that volume expansion depressed HCO_3^- reabsorption in potassium-loaded, normal, and potassium-depleted animals, but that, independent of volume, the state of body potassium stores affected HCO_3^- reabsorption. It also became clear that volume contraction, a major stimulus to increased HCO_3^- reabsorption, could completely overcome the depressive effect of potassium loading. A micropuncture study by Kunau and coworkers[104] demonstrated a direct effect of hypokalemia on the capacity of the proximal tubule to reabsorb HCO_3^-. It is likely that the effects of potassium on hydrogen ion secretion are mediated by changes in cell pH, such that potassium deficiency causes a decrease in cell pH, which subsequently increases HCO_3^- reabsorption.

CHLORIDE

It is virtually impossible to study the role of Cl^- in proximal HCO_3^- reabsorption without inducing changes in ECF volume. As the primary ECF anion, Cl^- movement across cells can be totally accounted for by the Nernst equation. Therefore, changes in Cl^- alone in vivo cannot be studied without inducing significant changes in other ions. Studies have shown proton secretion to be unaffected when Cl^- ions are removed from the bath and from the perfusate of isolated proximal tubules.

Selective Cl^- depletion in vivo in the face of volume contraction decreases whole kidney GFR and juxtamedullary single nephron GFR (SNGFR).[66] Metabolic alkalosis develops and is maintained until Cl^- is replaced. The fall in whole kidney GFR and SNGFR is greater in chloride-dependent animals than in equally volume-contracted animals with normal Cl^- stores. Since the filtered load of HCO_3^- was the same in both groups, it is not clear whether Cl^- per se plays any role in proximal HCO_3^-, reabsorption other than by reducing the GFR.

ARTERIAL P_{CO_2}, BLOOD pH, AND CELL pH

An acute decrease in P_{CO_2} depresses renal HCO_3^- reabsorption; conversely, an increase in plasma P_{CO_2} enhances HCO_3^- reabsorption.[106] The mechanism underlying these effects may entail either an alteration of cellular pH, a hemodynamic effect, or both.

To examine the first issue, Langberg and coworkers[113] found that the effect of altering P_{CO_2} on HCO_3^- reabsorption was better correlated with a change in extracellular pH than with the change in P_{CO_2} per se. When the P_{CO_2} was changed in proportion to plasma HCO_3^- concentration (such that pH remained constant), HCO_3^- reabsorption remained unchanged. When the pH was allowed to change, HCO_3^- reabsorption varied inversely with the pH.[113] From these studies it was concluded that extracellular pH was a major determinant of HCO_3^- reabsorption. Another explanation, however, is that changes of extracellular pH merely reflect changes in cell pH, and it is the cell pH that is the critical determinant of changes in HCO_3^- reabsorption. Changing pH by altering plasma P_{CO_2} would rapidly change cell pH (as opposed to changing the HCO_3^- concentration), because of the easy diffusibility of CO_2 across cell membranes.

The hemodynamic effect of alterations in P_{CO_2} is well known.[106] An acute increase in the P_{CO_2} causes renal vasodilation and a fall in GFR. Bicarbonate reabsorption rises markedly. If one prevents the fall in GFR, the effect of hypercapnia on HCO_3^- reabsorption is of much lesser magnitude. Thus, the effects of alterations in plasma P_{CO_2} are probably mediated via two mechanisms. The first, and probably most important, is mediated by an alteration of extracellular pH, which, in turn, changes cell pH. The second is modulated by an alteration of renal hemodynamics, which subsequently changes HCO_3^- reabsorption by changing the filtered load.

ANGIOTENSIN II (AII) AND ATRIAL NATRIURETIC FACTOR (ANF)

In-vivo microperfusion studies of the proximal tubule have shown that AII profoundly increases HCO_3^- reabsorption.[119,120] The effect was more marked in the early proximal tubule, a site where AII receptor density is greatest.[120] More important, this occurred at a dose of AII that had no effect on blood pressure. In the proximal tubule AII has receptors on both the apical and basolateral membrane; thus it is uniquely capable of "talking" to both sides of the cell. That the increase in HCO_3^- reabsorption was blocked by amiloride suggests that the Na^+-H^+ antiporter is involved in the response. Angiotensin II decreases cyclic AMP in a number of cells and the AII receptor is functionally coupled to adenylate cyclase by an inhibitory G-protein, G_i. Cyclic AMP inhibits Na^+-H^+ antiporter activity; its absence may stimulate it. This scenario would nicely explain the findings cited above.

Atrial natriuretic factor is a polypeptide known to be released from atrial granules following a variety of stimuli, including volume expansion. The hormone is thought to have both glomerular and tubular effects. In-vivo microperfusion studies similar to those just discussed have revealed that ANF has no effect on basal HCO_3^- reabsorption by proximal tubule.[121] When AII was infused and HCO_3^- reabsorption increased, ANF still was without effect. From this study the precise role, if any, of ANF in proximal HCO_3^- reabsorption is not clear.

ALDOSTERONE

Aldosterone plays no direct role in proximal HCO_3^- reabsorption.[107,125,135] Microchemical and autoradiographic techniques described by Farman and coworkers[60,61] have demonstrated that there is no binding of [^{3}H] aldosterone to proximal convoluted tubules of the rabbit. Rather, specific binding occurred in the distal nephron (cortical collecting tubule). Aldosterone excess enhances acid secretion, thereby causing metabolic alkalosis; aldosterone deficiency is associated with metabolic acidosis.[35,87,107] This effect of aldosterone on acid secretion is probably mediated by a proton-translocating ATPase localized in the distal nephron (see Chaps. 10 and 27).[140]

OTHER

Glucose

Patients returning to a normal diet after prolonged fasting commonly develop metabolic alkalosis.[165] Glucose loading increases HCO_3^- reabsorption in these patients and also enhances HCO_3^- reabsorption in normal dogs.[172] These effects appear to be mediated by a direct action of glucose, since insulin administration does not raise HCO_3^- reabsorption. Glucose loading in human beings also enhances acid excretion.[70]

Parathyroid hormone (PTH), calcium, phosphate, and vitamin D

Acute administration of pharmacologic doses of PTH to dogs and human beings leads to an increase in HCO_3^- excretion.[53,96] The effect of PTH on HCO_3^- reabsorption is of small magnitude despite the high doses used in these studies. Acute hypercalcemia enhances HCO_3^- reabsorption in normal dogs.[53] Since this effect occurs in thyroparathyroidectomized (TPTX) animals, it appears that calcium may increase hydrogen ion secretion independently of its inhibition of PTH secretion. Siegfried and coworkers[160] have shown that vitamin D enhances HCO_3^- reabsorption. Chronic phosphate depletion decreases HCO_3^- reabsorption,[77] apparently by decreasing intracellular hydrogen ion concentration. That acid-base status is not markedly changed is probably the effect of phosphate depletion to increase extrarenal buffering.[13] Whether this effect is mediated through calcium is not known.

In summary (Table 29-1), many factors increase proximal HCO_3^- reabsorption and therefore could sustain a metabolic alkalosis. Volume contraction, hypercapnia, hypokalemia, glucose loading, and acute hypercalcemia enhance HCO_3^- reabsorption. Volume expansion, hyperkalemia, hypocapnia, hyperparathyroidism, and phosphate depletion decrease HCO_3^- reabsorption. While aldosterone has no effect on proximal HCO_3^- reabsorption, the hormone plays a major role in distal urinary acidification.

FACTORS CONTROLLING RENAL ACID EXCRETION

Normal metabolism generates 1 to 1.5 meq/ of hydrogen ion per kilogram of body weight per day[148,161] (see Chap. 9). These hydrogen ions are derived from the metabolism of sulfoproteins and phosphoproteins, which yield sulfuric and phosphoric acids, respectively. The incomplete oxidation of fats and carbohydrates also contributes protons. These acids are neutralized by the buffers in ECF, which, of course, consumes HCO_3^-. It is obvious that there must be a way of replenishing the extracellular HCO_3^- used to neutralize endogenous acid; were there not, metabolic acidosis would inexorably ensue.

Once filtered HCO_3^- reabsorption is essentially complete, each additional meq of hydrogen ion secreted by the kidney generates 1 meq of new HCO_3^-, which is added to the blood (Fig. 29-2).[146] The kidney thus regenerates the HCO_3^- used in neutralizing endogenously produced acid. The net amount of acid excreted daily by the kidney equals the daily production of acid, provided that the subject is in normal acid-base (or zero) balance and is on a constant diet. The renal secretion of hydrogen ions stabilizes serum HCO_3^- concentration by mediating HCO_3^- reabsorption and synthesizing new HCO_3^-. The latter requires that secreted protons be excreted as titratable acid and ammonium.

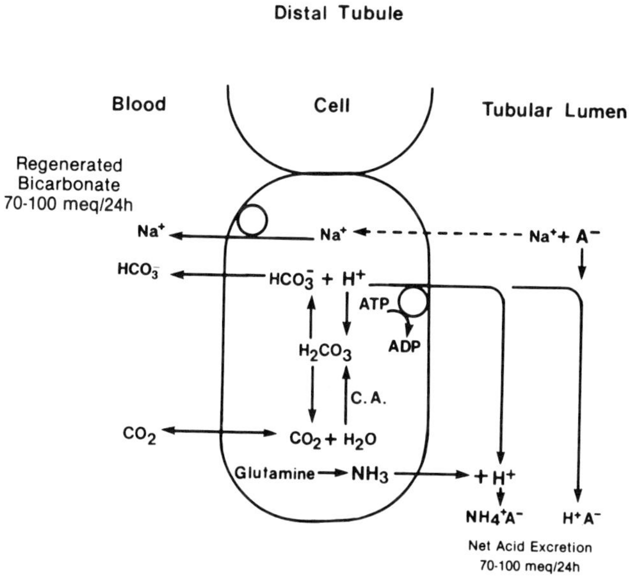

FIGURE 29-2 • Hydrogen ion secretion in the distal nephron. [A, anion (phosphate, sulfate, urate); CA, carbonic anhydrase.]

Reabsorption of HCO_3^- requires that hydrogen ions be secreted. It follows that impaired proton secretion reduces HCO_3^- reabsorption and the resulting bicarbonaturia produces a net gain of hydrogen ions. Measurement of maximal HCO_3^- reabsorption defines total renal hydrogen ion secretion. Maximal HCO_3^- reabsorption, however, mainly assesses reabsorption in the proximal tubule, since the amount of HCO_3^- reabsorbed in the distal nephron is comparatively small.[133]

Net acid excretion is measured by the sum of titratable acid excretion plus ammonium, minus HCO_3^- excretion. Metabolic hydrogen ion production usually approximates 60 to 100 meq per day, thereby requiring the excretion of an identical amount of net acid. If, for example, the kidney excretes 60 meq of HCO_3^- daily when acid production is 60 meq and the sum of excreted ammonium and titratable acid is also 60 meq, then net acid excretion will be zero and the subject will be in positive hydrogen ion balance. This metabolic acidosis will soon lower blood HCO_3^- concentration and pH. Conversely, if the amount of acid excreted by the kidney exceeds that of endogenous hydrogen ion produced, metabolic alkalosis will develop. (See also Chap. 10.)

TITRATABLE ACID

Titratable acid refers to the urinary hydrogen ions associated with weak acid anions (phosphate, creatinine, urate, etc.). Figure 29-2 also shows the schema for the titration of urinary buffers. The following factors influence titratable acid excretion.

pK of the buffer system

According to the Henderson-Hasselbalch equation, $pH = pK + \log A^-/HA$, where A^- is the conjugate base of a weak acid (HA). From this equation it is obvious that the pK of the system equals the pH when the concentration of A^- is equal to the concentration of HA (the log of 1 is 0, and thus pH = pK). This means that at a pH equal to the pK of the buffer system, 50 percent of the buffer pair is in the nonionized form. As the pH increases above the pK, most of the buffer will exist in the ionized form. Conversely, as the pH decreases below the pK, most of the buffer will be in the nonionized form. Thus the buffer system can accept both hydroxyl and hydrogen ions when the pH is close to the pK. Therefore, the ideal buffer has a pK between the blood pH and the final urine pH. If the pK of a substance is at either extreme, it will be a poor buffer. The phosphate system has a pK of 6.8; at a blood pH of 7.4 the molar ratio of Na_2HPO_4 to NaH_2PO_4 is 4:1, whereas at a pH of 6.8 this ratio is 1:1. If one has 1000 μM of phosphate at a blood pH of 7.4, 800 μM will be in the form of Na_2HPO_4 and 200 μM as NaH_2PO_4. At a urine pH of 6.8 there will be 500 μM of Na_2HPO_4 and 500 μM of NaH_2PO_4. Thus, as 1000 μM of phosphate are filtered and appear in the urine, 300 μM of hydrogen ion will be accepted as urine pH is reduced from 7.4 to 6.8. At a urine pH of 5.5 the ratio of Na_2HPO_4 to NaH_2PO_4 is very low; therefore this buffer can accept very few additional hydrogen ions. At a pH of 5.5 other weak acids, such as creatinine (pK = 5.0) and urate (pK = 5.8), are the main titratable acids.[151]

Amount of buffer

It is obvious that the amount of titratable acid excreted is directly related to the amount of buffer excreted. Most of the titratable acid in the urine is excreted as phosphate; creatinine, uric acid, and other organic acids constitute only a small portion of total titratable acid excretion. The amount of phosphate excreted per day is relatively constant, provided the subject is on a normal diet; consequently, the excretion of titratable acid is limited by the amount of phosphate filtered.

Urine pH

The urine pH is also a determinant of titratable acid excretion. The lower the urine pH, the more titratable acid will be present in the urine. Metabolic acidosis lowers urine pH and slightly increases titratable acid excretion; however, this increased titratable acid excretion is limited by the amount of buffer available, as well as by the pK of the buffer. While phosphate is only one component of titratable acid excretion, its pK of 6.8 means that most of the phosphate (about 50 percent) has been titrated by the time the fluid leaves the proximal tubule ($pH \simeq 6.8$).

AMMONIA

Ammonia (NH_3) is a weak base (pK = 9.4) that is freely diffusible across cell membranes. Ammonia can accept a hydrogen ion, forming cationic ammonium (NH_4^+), which, according to present concepts, is thought not to be freely diffusible across cell membranes.[142,143] Thus, the amount of NH_3 present on each side of the membrane depends upon the pH of the two compartments. Ammonia is produced in the renal tubular cells—primarily from the deamidation and deamination of glutamine, and to a much lesser extent from other amino acids—and diffuses into the blood and tubular fluid.[111]

Urine pH is a major factor influencing NH_4^+ excretion. As the urine pH is acutely decreased, more NH_3 is thought to be trapped in the lumen, forming NH_4^+ which is then excreted in the urine. The changes in NH_4^+ excretion, however, may not be related solely to changes in NH_3 distribution and trapping due to urine pH. When NH_4^+ transport is examined in vitro in the isolated nephron or with in-vivo microperfusion, the diffusion trapping model is not completely adequate to explain transport. Gradients of NH_3 exist, and NH_4^+ is secreted by the proximal tubule and reabsorbed by the thick ascending limb. Basal proximal tubular NH_4^+ secretion in the early segment is greater than that in the late segment.[75,101] Chronic metabolic acidosis enhances the secretion of NH_4^+ across the apical membranes of both proximal tubular segments. The exact transport mechanisms stimulated by acidosis are incompletely understood. There may be direct secretion of NH_4^+ as has been shown in some membranes,[10,32,33] or there may be substitution of NH_4^+ for protons on the internal binding site of the Na^+-H^+ antiporter.[99,136]

Following preferential secretion of NH_4^+ by the proximal tubule, 50 percent is reabsorbed by the thick ascending limb.[74] The following two mechanisms may be involved:

1. Passive NH_4^+ reabsorption driven by the lumen positive voltage.
2. Transcellular transport via the Na^+-K^+-$2Cl^-$ cotransporter localized to the apical membrane.

Evidence exists for both mechanisms. Passive flux accounts for about one-half of the NH_4^+ transported. Competition may occur between NH_4^+ and K^+ for the cotransporter on the apical membrane. Predictably, furosemide inhibits NH_4^+ transport in the loop of Henle. Reabsorption of NH_4^+ plus the action of the countercurrent multiplier results in high concentrations of NH_4^+ in the medullary interstitium.

In addition to pH, systemic potassium balance is an important factor affecting renal ammonium excretion. Potassium depletion stimulates NH_4^+ excretion, and hyperkalemia depresses it. The decrease in NH_4^+ seen with hyperkalemia may be due to competition between potassium and NH_4^+ for the transport site on the thick ascending limb Na^+-K^+-$2Cl^-$ cotransporter.[101]

POTASSIUM

Potassium, the primary intracellular cation, is important in many aspects of cell function, particularly in myoneural tissue.[101] The kidney handles potassium by filtration and reabsorption; however, virtually all the potassium found in the urine is there as a result of secretion by the distal nephron (see Chap 7).[92] This was first suggested by Berliner[23] and was found to be true in a variety of microinjection and micropuncture studies.[29,68,127,187] Subsequent studies have suggested that the proximal tubule of the juxtamedullary nephrons may be a site of active potassium secretion.[22,91] Much of our information about the distal nephron comes from isolated tubule studies. These investigations have shown that both the distal convoluted tubule and the cortical collecting duct have the capacity to secrete potassium in amounts sufficient to account for that found in the papillary base and tip.[57,79,140] A low plasma potassium level directly stimulates renin release from the juxtaglomerular cells of the macula densa.[79,92] Its role in acid secretion, independent of any effect on aldosterone, is not known. The rate of potassium secretion is augmented by potassium loading or mineralocorticoid administration. In the medullary collecting tubule, potassium transport appears to be entirely passive. Morphologic evidence suggests that potassium secretion is a function of the principal cells, and that potassium reabsorption is a function of the intercalated cells.[72]

A variety of hormones have been shown to affect plasma potassium and cause intracellular movement of the cation (e.g., insulin) (see Chap. 6). Since potassium depletion combined with aldosterone excess increases distal H^+ secretion, it is likely that these hormones may either directly or indirectly influence distal proton secretion. The zona glomerulosa of the adrenal gland is stimulated directly by hyperkalemia. This stimulates active secretion of both potassium and acid by the cortical and medullary collecting duct. Insulin and beta agonists cause potassium to move into cells and thereby cause redistributional hypokalemia (see Chap. 6). Low plasma potassium concentration inhibits the release of both aldosterone and insulin.[72] Hypokalemia, however, stimulates renin release, which in turn increases angiotensin II levels. In recent studies angiotensin II has been shown to markedly increase proximal HCO_3^- reabsorption at a dose that is below that causing vasoconstriction (see above).[119] Saralasin, the angiotensin II inhibitor, had the opposite effect. The highest receptor density for angiotensin II is found in the early proximal tubule. The action of angiotensin II in this part of the nephron may account for one-third of total renal hydrogen ion secretion.[120]

During potassium depletion there is an increase in NH_4^+ excretion, relative to urinary pH.[174] The enzyme primarily responsible for glutamine metabolism and ammoniagenesis is the phosphate-dependent glutaminase. It has been shown that the enzyme's activity increases in potassium depletion in parallel with the increase in ammoniagenesis.[6,19,22,89,134,141,175] It is thought that the key mechanism underlying these effects relates to intracellular acidosis, although changes in cell phosphate may also be important.[174]

ALDOSTERONE

In general, aldosterone excess favors acid excretion, while aldosterone deficiency reduces it. There are a number of mechanisms whereby aldosterone may modulate distal acidification (see Chaps. 10 and 14). Aldosterone, however, is not required to generate large pH gradients between blood and urine.[11,12,16-20] This can be demonstrated both in vitro and in vivo. In turtle bladder the addition of aldosterone increases proton conductance, but not proton motive force.[5] In dogs, rats, and human beings aldosterone deficiency is associated with acid retention, but with intact ability to lower urine pH during acidemia.[16,18-20,58]

Aldosterone may modulate distal acidification through its effect on sodium transport. Furthermore, if aldosterone deficiency results in salt wastage and volume contraction, distal sodium delivery may be reduced. Increased levels of aldosterone enhance ammoniagenesis, while the reverse is seen in the absence of the hormone.[86] Since aldosterone is a major potassium-regulatory hormone, its effect on potassium may also modulate ammoniagenesis and urinary acid excretion. Finally, if ECF volume is contracted as a consequence of aldosterone deficiency, renal blood flow—and, thus, glutamine delivery—might be reduced, with a further subsequent reduction in ammoniagenesis.

In and of itself, aldosterone probably plays a relatively small role in regulating overall acid excretion. Normal human subjects rendered mineralocorticoid-deficient retain acid, but only for a short period and only in an amount sufficient to lower the serum HCO_3^- concentration by less than 2 meq/liter. This situation, however, is not likely to apply to patients in whom aldosterone deficiency is associated with reduced GFR.[16] Under these conditions, aldosterone may be critical for maintenance of normal acid-base homeostasis.[35]

DISTAL SODIUM DELIVERY

The state of sodium reabsorption by the distal nephron has a major impact on net acidification. This effect is the result of the negative potential difference generated by the active transport of sodium in the distal nephron. The generation of a lumen-negative potential difference accelerates the rate of proton transport regardless of the fact that hydrogen ion secretion occurs in the absence of sodium transport. Thus, factors that interfere with sodium reabsorption, and therefore with the generation of a lumen-negative potential difference, can markedly reduce the overall rate of distal acidification.[10,12,16,18-21] This influence of sodium transport on acidification is clearly illustrated by the effect of the diuretic agent amiloride. In the turtle bladder this drug, the main effect of which is the reduction of the entry of sodium across the luminal membrane, reduces proton secretion only in open-circuited condition.[10] That is to say, amiloride exerts an effect on acidification only when there is a mucosal negative potential difference that the drug reduces to zero. If the potential difference is restored to control values in the continued presence of amiloride, acidification returns to control values.[10] This component of acidification that is reduced by amiloride is the voltage-dependent component of proton secretion. In animals and human beings, distal acidification is inhibited by the administration of amiloride (or lithium), presumably through its effect on the luminal potential difference, although recent enzymatic data suggest that this explanation may be somewhat incomplete.[112] This voltage-dependent component of acidification may, under a variety of normal and abnormal circumstances, be the critical modulator of net acidification. In other words, the overall rate of the proton pump, independent of the effects of sodium, may be relatively constant. The rate of proton transport may respond, in a variety of circumstances, to changes induced secondarily to alterations in sodium transport.

Thus, any event that reduces distal sodium transport, all else being equal, reduces distal acidification. Distal sodium transport may be reduced from an intrinsic abnormality in the capacity of the tubule to transport sodium; from the decreased availability of sodium for transport, as a consequence of decreased distal delivery of the cation; or because of aldosterone deficiency.

NATURE OF THE ANION

The reabsorbability of the anion delivered to the distal nephron may be of importance in modulating acid secretion.[14] Penicillins, especially carbenicillin, and sulfate have been noted to cause metabolic alkalosis.[183] Poorly reabsorbed anions presented to the distal tubule in the face of avid sodium reabsorption markedly increase the lumen-negative potential difference. The enhanced transtubular potential difference creates a favorable gradient for proton (and potassium) secretion, increasing urine acid (and potassium) excretion.[178] This creates a hypokalemic, hypochloremic metabolic alkalosis.

GENERATION OF METABOLIC ALKALOSIS

To generate a metabolic alkalosis, there must be a gain of base or a loss of acid (Table 29-2). The gain of base may result from the administration of alkaline solutions; acid may be lost via the gastrointestinal tract or kidney. For example, depletion of hydrochloric acid from the stomach, as the consequence of vomiting or nasogastric suction, leaves behind large amounts of HCO_3^-. Enhanced renal acid excretion induced by diuretics and aldosterone excess will effect the same result.

To maintain acid-base balance, the kidney must excrete the 60 to 100 meq of acid produced each day. For each meq of net acid excreted, 1 meq of new HCO_3^- is generated and added to the blood. The kidney replaces quantitatively the alkali lost due to the addition of strong acid to the ECF. For the kidney to generate a metabolic alkalosis, net acid excretion must increase, at least transiently, thereby adding amounts of HCO_3^- to blood that exceed the daily loss of alkali.

That new HCO_3^- is added to the blood (regardless of the mechanism) does not necessarily mean that metabolic alkalosis will ensue. The new HCO_3^- may subsequently be excreted by the kidney, thus preventing development of a sustained metabolic alkalosis. Clearly for metabolic alkalosis to be sustained, the excess HCO_3^- generated or administered must be reclaimed by the kidney. An increase in HCO_3^- reabsorptive capacity, unaccompanied by the gain of alkali or loss of acid, cannot by itself generate a metabolic alkalosis.

Metabolic alkalosis must be considered in two phases: the *generation of new* HCO_3^- and the *maintenance of a high plasma* HCO_3 *concentration*, which is accomplished by the increased tubular reabsorption of HCO_3^-. The kidney can generate a metabolic alkalosis if the capacity of the distal nephron to secrete hydrogen ions is increased when there is adequate distal sodium delivery. Aldosterone excess increases both sodium and chloride reabsorption in the distal nephron and enhances potassium excretion. The retained salt expands the ECF volume, which in turn depresses proximal salt reabsorption, thereby increasing distal sodium delivery.

Patients with aldosterone excess commonly have a metabolic alkalosis. This type of metabolic alkalosis is almost invariably accompanied by hypokalemia. Kurtzman and coworkers[107] reported data that suggest both hyperaldosteronism and hypokalemia are required for the kidney to generate a metabolic alkalosis. Dogs were depleted of potassium by the administration of a potassium exchange resin in desoxycorticosterone acetate (DOCA), and their diet contained both sodium chloride and sodium bicarbonate. The animals developed a sustained metabolic alkalosis. When DOCA was discontinued, the metabolic alkalosis was rapidly corrected, despite continued maintenance of the hypokalemia.

TABLE 29-2 • The generation and maintenance of metabolic alkalosis

Generation	Maintenance	Example
LOSS OF ACID FROM THE EXTRACELLULAR SPACE		
Loss via gastric fluid	Reduced EABV	Vomiting
Loss via urine: increased Na^+ delivery in the presence of hyperaldosteronism	1. K^+ depletion + aldosterone excess 2. Diuretic administration	1. Primary aldosteronism 2. Reduced EABV + K^+ deficiency
Loss of acid into cells	Sustained K^+ deficiency	Any cause of K^+ deficiency
Loss of acid via stool	Reduced EABV	Congenital chloride-losing diarrhea
EXCESSIVE HCO_3 LOADS		
Absolute		
1. Oral or parenternal loads of HCO_3^- or alkalinizing salts	1. Reduced EABV, continuous alkali administration, K^+ deficiency	1. $NaHCO_3$ administration, milk-alkali syndrome
2. Metabolic conversion of salts of organic acids (e.g., ketones, lactate) to HCO_3^-	2. Reduced EABV, K^+ deficiency or continuous anion administration	2. Lactate, acetate, citrate administration
Relative		
Alkaline loads in renal failure	Renal failure	Alkali administration to patients with acute or chronic renal failure
POSTHYPERCAPNIC STATE		
	Reduced EABV	Correction of chronic hypercapnia in the presence of a low-salt diet

Abbreviation: EABV, effective arterial blood volume.
SOURCE: Adapted from Sabatini S et al, *Med Clin North Am* 62:1223, 1978.

When DOCA was then restarted in these potassium-depleted animals, metabolic alkalosis immediately redeveloped. Once the metabolic alkalosis returned, sodium bicarbonate was removed from the diet and replaced with equal amounts of potassium bicarbonate. This resulted in the correction of both the potassium depletion and the metabolic alkalosis, even though excessive amounts of DOCA were still being administered. In this animal model of "primary aldosteronism" both the generation and the maintenance of metabolic alkalosis were dependent on the simulatenous presence of potassium depletion and mineralocorticoid excess. Neither factor alone was able to generate or maintain the alkalosis. Thus, the generation and the maintenance of metabolic alkalosis in patients with primary mineralocorticoid excess is likely the consequence of accelerated distal hydrogen ion secretion driven by both steroid excess and potassium depletion.

In normal males, potassium depletion in the face of low renin and aldosterone levels results in mild metabolic acidosis associated with a decrease in net acid excretion and titratable acid and an increase in NH_4^+ excretion.[93] The loss of aldosterone-induced stimulation of net acid excretion causes retention of endogenous protons and a decrease in serum HCO_3^- concentration. A new steady state is achieved by the increase in NH_4^+ excretion that resulted from the potassium depletion and metabolic acidosis.

Potassium depletion decreases intracellular pH in muscle, since protons enter the cell in partial replacement of lost cations.[4,51] While not shown directly, such ion shifts presumably occur also in the renal tubular cells.

MAINTENANCE OF METABOLIC ALKALOSIS

Factors involved in the maintenance of metabolic alkalosis are shown in Table 29-3 and have been reviewed in detail by Sabatini and Kurtzman[152] and by Jacobson and Seldin.[90]

PROXIMAL TUBULE

Volume contraction and reduced filtered load

Cogan and coworkers[41] demonstrated that the change in fractional HCO_3^- reabsorption induced by volume expansion in the superficial proximal tubule in rats with

TABLE 29-3 • Factors that maintain metabolic alkalosis

1. Decreased GFR (prevents elevated plasma HCO_3^- concentration from exceeding T_m, i.e., fractional HCO_3^- reabsorption increases)
2. Volume contraction (stimulates tubular HCO_3^- reabsorption)
3. Hypokalemia
   a. Decreases GFR
   b. Increases tubular HCO_3^- reabsorption
4. Hypochloremia
   a. Decreases GFR
   b. Decreases in distal delivery of Cl^- leads to increased H^+ secretion in the medullary collecting tubule
   c. Increases renin
5. Passive HCO_3^- backflux
6. Aldosterone (increases medullary collecting tubule, sodium-independent H^+ secretion)
7. Continued loss of acid
8. Continued addition of base

normal acid-base status and in animals with metabolic acidosis was secondary to alterations in filtered HCO_3^-. Bicarbonate reabsorption in this nephron segment had a constant relationship to filtered load. No inhibitory effect of volume expansion on proximal HCO_3^- reabsorption, independent of change in filtered HCO_3^-, was discerned.

Studies by Chan and associates[38] using the technique of in-vivo microperfusion yielded results consistent with the notion that the filtered load is the prime determinant of HCO_3^- transport in the proximal tubule. They further demonstrated that HCO_3^- reabsorption in the proximal tubule at any level of perfused load was depressed when the pH was increased. When the pH was held constant, increasing the HCO_3^- concentration of the perfusate increased its absorption at any given load. These data, thus, demonstrate that alkalemia tends to depress proximal HCO_3^- transport, while the presence of a favorable HCO_3^- gradient across the tubule enhances its transport. Using the isolated perfused rabbit proximal tubule, Sasaki and coworkers[153] achieved similar results. A favorable HCO_3^- concentration gradient from lumen to bath stimulated its absorption, while increased bath pH suppressed transport.

In summary, these results indicate that proximal tubule HCO_3^- transport is highly dependent on the filtered load. They further demonstrate that, at any filtered load, HCO_3^- reabsorption can be modified by the presence or absence of favorable concentration gradients and by changes in ECF pH. Studies are not available to define how extracellular pH modulates HCO_3^- transport. The most likely explanation is that changes in extracellular pH are reflected by similar changes in intracellular pH that increase or decrease the availability of protons for secretion.

Using clearance techniques, Langberg and colleagues[113] obtained results consistent with those just described in the proximal tubule. These investigators demonstrated that changes in arterial P_{CO_2} had no effect on HCO_3^- reabsorption in the whole kidney, provided that pH was held constant. The relationship of HCO_3^- reabsorption to filtered load was the same regardless of the P_{CO_2}. On the other hand, when the pH was allowed to change, HCO_3^- reabsorption, at any given filtered load, was significantly greater in animals with a lower pH than in animals with pH values 0.3 units higher. Thus, the intact animal behaves similarly to the isolated proximal tubule.

While it is tempting to invoke changes in the filtered load as the mechanism whereby changes in volume effect alterations in HCO_3^- excretion, there remain contradictory data. In 1970, Cohen[47] demonstrated that metabolic alkalosis could be corrected by the infusion of isometric solutions to dogs with aortic constriction. Metabolic alkalosis was corrected without any change in the filtered load of HCO_3^-. Furthermore, reanalysis of old data from our laboratory, also using the dog as the experimental animal, has shown numerous circumstances in which volume expansion depressed HCO_3^- reabsorption without changes in filtered load.

In sharp contradistinction to these older studies of metabolic alkalosis is a study in the rat by Cogan and Liu.[43] These investigators induced chronic hypokalemic metabolic alkalosis by administering an electrolyte-deficient diet supplemented with sodium sulfate. They also added sodium bicarbonate to the drinking water and injected the animals with DOCA. These alkalotic animals had a marked reduction in single nephron GFR, which resulted in an unchanged filtered load of HCO_3^-. That is to say, GFR diminished and plasma HCO_3^- concentration rose, causing their product to remain unchanged in control and alkalotic animals. Similarly, absolute proximal HCO_3^- absorption in alkalotic animals was the same as in controls, despite the higher luminal HCO_3^- concentration, contracted ECF volume, and potassium depletion. When single nephron GFR was increased by volume expansion, absolute proximal HCO_3^- reabsorption did not change. Bicarbonaturia ensued, in concert with the increase in filtered load. Furthermore, animals were studied before and after the induction of metabolic alkalosis associated with varying amounts of potassium depletion and volume contraction. In all cases, the increase in blood HCO_3^- concentration was inversely proportional to the reduction in GFR, so that the filtered load of HCO_3^- remained unchanged. Thus, in this model, a reduction in GFR is seen as the critical event preventing the excretion of HCO_3^-, allowing the elevated plasma HCO_3^- concentration to be maintained.

The rat and the dog seem to differ with respect to the mechanism whereby changes in volume depress HCO_3^- reabsorption in alkalotic animals and thus correct the alkalosis. A decrease in GFR seems to be the critical event in maintaining metabolic alkalosis in the rat,[43,45] while volume seems to affect HCO_3^- transport through mechanisms independent of changes in filtered load in the alkalotic dog.[47] Studies in human beings are necessary to determine what role changes in effective arterial volume play on bicarbonate transport, independently of alterations in the filtered load.

Potassium

In the 1950s Pitts demonstrated an inverse relationship between HCO_3^- reabsorption and plasma potassium concentration.[143] Studies from our laboratory demonstrated that when ECF volume is contracted, HCO_3^- reabsorption is indistinguishable from that of control animals in both potassium-loaded and potassium-depleted dogs.[109] When volume was expanded, however, HCO_3^- reabsorption was greater in potassium-depleted animals than in normal animals. Bicarbonate reabsorption in the control animals was greater than in the potassium-loaded animals. This effect was not due to differences in filtered load. More recently, Chan and coworkers[38] demonstrated that protracted potassium depletion increased proximal tubular HCO_3^- reabsorption independently of changes in filtered load. There are, however, several micropuncture studies that do not demonstrate any change in proximal acidification in potassium-depleted animals as compared with normokalemic control animals.[116,177]

Because there is no doubt that potassium administration corrects most forms of metabolic alkalosis, and because there are inconsistencies as to the effect of potassium depletion on proximal tubule acidification, additional mechanisms whereby potassium depletion may perpetuate metabolic alkalosis should be invoked. The original postulate linking potassium depletion to the maintenance of metabolic alkalosis required a decrease in intracellular pH.[183] A rise in intracellular proton concentration would favor hydrogen ion secretion and thus would increase HCO_3^- reabsorption. Numerous studies in both the rat and the dog have demonstrated that potassium depletion is associated with a reduction in GFR.[3,34,71,85] Linas and Dickman[118] demonstrated that potassium depletion in the rat caused a marked decrease in renal plasma flow. This hemodynamic effect of potassium depletion was shown to be the result of increased vasoconstriction within the kidney secondary to activation of angiotensin II and thromboxane. The study of Cogan and Liu[43] clearly demonstrated that the GFR was reduced during a hypokalemic metabolic alkalosis. Thus, hypokalemia may be seen as maintaining metabolic alkalosis not only by tending to increase HCO_3^- transport directly, but also by reducing the filtered load of HCO_3^-. Reduction of filtered HCO_3^- in the face of an elevated plasma concentration presents the kidney with a normal filtered load, thereby preventing development of bicarbonaturia. The relative importance of these two mechanisms in the maintenance of metabolic alkalosis in humans has yet to be examined.

Chloride

The work of Galla and associates[64-66,182] suggests that Cl^- depletion per se may also play a role in the maintenance of metabolic alkalosis, albeit through a different mechanism than originally supposed. These workers have presented data that invoke a hemodynamic role for Cl^- depletion in the maintenance of metabolic alkalosis. Hypochloremic metabolic alkalosis was induced using peritoneal dialysis. There was no discernible change in effective arterial blood volume. Provision of Cl^- as either sodium or choline chloride resulted in complete correction of the alkalosis, despite weight loss.

The likely explanation for this effect of Cl^- is as follows: Hypochloremia, without any alteration of volume, stimulates renal renin release, which decreases the GFR.[2,103] The decrease in GFR, when associated with an elevated plasma HCO_3^- concentration, prevents the filtered load of HCO_3^- from exceeding the capacity of proximal tubule to reabsorb it. Thus the role of hypochloremia seems to be mediated by changes in filtered load, as discussed above for volume and potassium depletion.

Passive reabsorption

In 1982 Alpern and colleagues[7] demonstrated that the net flux of total CO_2 in the proximal tubule was a function of mean luminal CO_2 concentration. They further demonstrated a significant component of passive HCO_3^- reabsorption measured in the presence of acetazolamide. This passive component became prominent at luminal HCO_3^- concentrations in excess of 35 meq/liter. Thus, under conditions where proximal tubule HCO_3^- concentration rises to values in excess of those of blood, large amounts of HCO_3^- may passively be returned to the blood. It is conceivable that passive HCO_3^- reabsorption contributes to the maintenance of metabolic alkalosis. The studies of Cogan and Liu,[43] however, fail to show proximal tubule HCO_3^- concentrations sufficiently high to allow for any significant amount of passive backflux. Whether such concentrations may be reached in another animal model, or in clinically relevant settings, is not known.

DISTAL NEPHRON

Mineralocorticoid

Aldosterone has long been known to play a role in the maintenance of metabolic alkalosis.[108,115,154,159] Animals on a normal-salt diet with steroid-induced metabolic alkalosis do not maintain the alkalosis if steroid intake is reduced to physiologic levels.[108] Studies using the perfused collecting tubule have examined the role of aldosterone on acidification.[114,122,131,140] It was found that the baseline rate of hydrogen ion secretion is considerably greater in the medullary collecting tubule than in the cortical collecting tubule. Hydrogen ion secretion in the cortical tubule is sodium-dependent, whereas that in the medullary tubule is not.[170] Aldosterone influences hydrogen ion secretion in the cortex through its effect on sodium transport.[140,168] Sodium transport creates a lumen-negative potential difference that favors proton secretion. In the medullary tubule active sodium transport is absent.[167] The potential difference in this nephron segment is lumen-positive. Aldosterone also increases hydrogen ion secretion at this site. Electrical neutrality is apparently maintained in this circumstance by the passive movement of Cl^- from serosa to mucosa.[169]

While we know that aldosterone-dependent hydrogen ion secretion in the medullary collecting tubule is of greater magnitude than in the cortex, its role in overall acidification is difficult to sort out at present. If the medullary collecting tubule were the dominant site of acidification, circumstances in which large amounts of aldosterone were present and the Cl^- concentration in medullary tubular urine was low should result in a marked acceleration of renal acid excretion. In fact, the opposite prevails. Patients with primary aldosteronism do not develop metabolic alkalosis if salt is removed from their diets.[147,159] This observation suggests that a large distal delivery of sodium under conditions of aldosterone excess accelerates sodium-hydrogen exchange, a process that presumably occurs in the cortical collecting tubule. An alternative explanation might be that hydrogen ion secretion in the medullary tubule is flow-dependent. If this were true, salt restriction might diminish the flow rate in the medullary tubule, with a consequent decrease in acidification.

Another observation that is difficult to fit into models requiring that aldosterone excess stimulate hydrogen ion secretion through a sodium-independent process in the medullary collecting tubule is that potassium repletion in such models corrects metabolic alkalosis in the face of continued steroid excess.[108] It is difficult to see how potassium depletion would influence medullary hydrogen ion secretion although recent enzymatic studies of the H^+-K^+ ATPase data promise to shed some light on this issue.[112] Potassium repletion might decrease acidification in the collecting tubule or might result in an increase in filtered HCO_3^- and decrease proximal tubule HCO_3^- transport, flooding the distal nephron with the anion and overwhelming the acidification process in this segment of the tubule. Additional work is needed to integrate sodium-independent, aldosterone-dependent medullary hydrogen ion secretion into an overall scheme of renal acidification, with special emphasis on its role in the maintenance of metabolic alkalosis.

Potassium depletion

Potassium depletion enhances HCO_3^- reabsorption and thus can maintain metabolic alkalosis.[109] Most cases of metabolic alkalosis can be corrected by volume expansion without repletion of potassium deficits. There are, however, a few cases of metabolic alkalosis associated with severe potassium depletion that are not corrected by saline alone ("saline-resistant metabolic alkalosis"). These cases are usually secondary to primary aldosteronism or Cushing's syndrome, but also can be found in other diseases associated with severe potassium depletion. In patients with primary aldosteronism, metabolic alkalosis is maintained by a distal mechanism. Although these patients are potassium-depleted, they are also volume-expanded. Potassium depletion enhances proximal HCO_3^- reabsorption, whereas volume expansion depresses it. These two mechanism tend to counterbalance each other; therefore, enhanced proximal reabsorption does not seem to play a major role in the maintenance of this type of metabolic alkalosis. This probably explains why saline alone does not correct the metabolic alkalosis.

CONTINUED LOSS OF ACID

Continued gastrointestinal loss of acid generally occurs in prolonged vomiting or nasogastric suction with inadequate fluid replacement. More rarely it can occur in congenital chloride-losing diarrhea, in which copious amounts of acid are lost via the colon. In all these instances the loss of acid is accompanied initially by an increase in urinary sodium and HCO_3^- excretion that is consequent to the rise in plasma HCO_3^- concentration. In essence, these are all volume-contracted states and should be easily corrected with fluid administration.

CONTINUED ADDITION OF HCO_3^-

Addition of base could occur as HCO_3^- directly, or as a precursor of HCO_3^-. Massive intake of alkali in persons with normal renal function may occur in the form of baking soda gluttony, in the milk-alkali syndrome, or in the use of chloride-deficient formulas containing an organic anion. Excessive bone turnover or destruction, subsequently releasing base, could also cause continued addition of HCO_3^- to the ECF. In the usual case, the increase in filtered load of HCO_3^- would be easily excreted by the kidney. In pathologic states (e.g., volume contraction, potassium depletion, aldosterone excess) this will not easily occur.

Table 29-2 lists the general mechanism involved in the generation of metabolic alkalosis. The associated mechanism involved in the maintenance of metabolic alkalosis is given in the middle column. Finally, a clinical example is given in the last column. It is important to recognize that the factor involved in the generation of metabolic alkalosis need be present only transiently. Once the metabolic alkalosis is generated, it may be maintained secondarily by different factors (Table 29-3). Thus the correction of metabolic alkalosis involves correction of both the primary and secondary factors.

PATHOPHYSIOLOGIC STATES ASSOCIATED WITH METABOLIC ALKALOSIS

PRIMARY DISORDERS

Primary aldosteronism

First described by Conn,[48] this disorder is characterized by hypokalemia, hypertension, and metabolic alkalosis. Plasma renin activity is low (Table 29-4). The disease is usually due to a single adenoma of the adrenal cortex. It is less commonly due to bilateral adrenal hyperplasia and is rarely caused by a carcinoma of the adrenal gland[8] (see also Chaps. 14 and 45).

Aldosterone stimulates sodium and chloride reabsorption in the cortical collecting tubule. The chronic salt retention expands extracellular volume, which in turn increases arterial pressure, decreases plasma renin activity, and inhibits salt reabsorption. Suppression of proximal salt reabsorption causes the well-known "escape phenomenon" (see Chap. 18). Thus, while weight increases, there is no edema formation. The collecting tubule continues to reabsorb sodium and secrete potassium and hydrogen at accelerated rates. Aldosterone increases proton secretion by the collecting tubule by at least three mechanisms[82,83,102,122,140,166,173,174]:

1. Aldosterone stimulates sodium reabsorption in the cortical collecting tubule, thus creating a more favorable lumen-negative potential difference for proton secretion.
2. Aldosterone directly stimulates proton secretion by the cortical and medullary collecting tubule.
3. Aldosterone indirectly stimulates ammoniagenesis by enhancing potassium secretion in the collecting tubule (see above). The hypokalemia also increases acid secretion.

Polyuria occasionally occurs as a result of the hypokalemia. Modest degrees of hypernatremia occasionally result from sodium retention and water loss, because of upward resetting of ADH secretion (see Chap. 4). If volume expansion is prevented by administration of a low-sodium diet, metabolic alkalosis is prevented.[159]

The diagnosis of primary aldosteronism is easily made in patients with hypokalemia, metabolic alkalosis, hypertension, low plasma renin, and high plasma aldosterone concentrations.[27,44,48,49,56,95,163] Failure to suppress plasma aldosterone with a sodium chloride infusion further establishes the diagnosis. It is important, of course, to distinguish between a single adenoma and carcinoma, and to recognize the presence of bilateral adrenal hyperplasia.[97] Surgical correction of the latter lesion rarely ameliorates the hypertension. High-resolution computed tomography (CT) is most useful for determining adrenal size. Unilateral adrenal enlargement virtually always signifies a single nodule. Iodocholesterol nuclear scanning can also aid in localization. The distinction between adenoma and carcinoma is made surgically.[84,115] Bilateral adrenal vein catheterization has been largely discarded, because the risk of serious side effects far outweighs that of the CT scan.

Primary aldosteronism resulting from unilateral adenoma is best treated surgically; such treatment often results in complete cure of the disorder. There are patients who respond successfully to spironolactone, a competitive antagonist of aldosterone. If the side effects of this agent are not tolerated (gynecomastia, decreased libido, impotence), then triamterene or amiloride (noncompetitive aldosterone anatagonists) may also be used. Bilateral adrenal hyperplasia is best treated with

TABLE 29-4 • Clinical states associated with metabolic alkalosis

Syndrome	Mineralocorticoid production	Renin production	EABV
1. Primary aldosteronism (hyperplasia, adenoma, carcinoma)	↑	↓	↑
2. Adrenogenital syndrome (11β- and 17α-hydroxylase deficiency)	↑ (DOC)	↓	↑
3. Pseudohyperaldosteronism (Liddle's syndrome, licorice ingestion)	↓	↓	↑
4. Unilateral renal artery stenosis, accelerated hypertension, hemangiopericytoma	↑	↑	↑
5. Congestive heart failure, liver disease, nephrotic syndrome	↑	↑	↓
6. Congenital chloride-losing diarrhea, posthypercapnic alkalosis	↑	↑	↓
7. Vomiting, diuretics, magnesium deficiency (?), Bartter's syndrome	↑	↑	↓

Abbreviations: EABV, effective arterial blood volume; DOC, desoxycorticosterone; ↑, increased; ↓, decreased.

spironolactone (or another potassium-sparing diuretic) in combination with conventional antihypertensive therapy. Glucocorticoid-suppressible hyperaldosteronism may be treated with dexamethasone.

Adrenogenital syndrome

Two forms of adrenogenital syndrome are associated with mineralcorticoid excess.[26,28,31,78,138] In both, the hemodynamic and electrolyte abnormalities are identical to those seen in primary aldosteronism. The excess hormone is desoxycorticosterone (DOC). DOC is the immediate metabolite (via 21-hydroxylation) of progesterone and is central in the formation of glucocorticoid and mineralocorticoid synthesis (see also chap. 45).

11β-hydroxylase deficiency

In this disorder DOC cannot be converted to corticosterone; thus aldosterone levels are very low. There is also a defect in the hydroxylation of 11-deoxycortisol, causing cortisol deficiency. Since the 17α-hydroxylase pathway for sex hormone synthesis is intact, the increase in ACTH secretion resulting form the 11β-hydroxylase deficiency causes virilism in association with hypertension and hypokalemic metabolic alkalosis. The alkalosis is secondary to high levels of DOC. The virilism is striking, allowing early diagnosis of the disorder—often in infancy. Cortisol therapy suppresses ACTH release and thereby corrects all the abnormalities of this syndrome, if started early enough.[31]

17α-hydroxylase deficiency

Unlike the 11β-hydroxylase deficiency, the 17α-hydroxylase deficiency is not associated with virilization.[78] The defect prevents conversion of the precursor pregnenolone to androgens or estrogens; consequently the males are pseudohermaphrodites. Hypogonadism and amenorrhea occur in the female. Hypertension, hypokalemia, and metabolic alkalosis with increased DOC and its metabolite, corticosterone, are found. Low levels of aldosterone and renin occur and are probably secondary to the salt-retaining effect of corticosterone.[28,181] Some authors have postulated an enzymatic defect in the conversion of corticosterone to aldosterone. Again, treatment utilizes 10 to 30 mg/day of cortisol, with particular attention paid to adequate salt intake and potassium repletion.

Cushing's syndrome

This syndrome, characterized by excess cortisol, causes hypertension, hypokalemia, and metabolic alkalosis[40,80] (see also Chap. 45). The metabolic alkalosis is secondary to the mineralocorticoid properties of cortisol. The diagnosis may be easily made by physical examination and the laboratory findings of cortisol excess. The cortisol excess is usually due to bilateral adrenal hyperplasia. Less frequently it is due to a single adenoma, and more rarely to adrenal carcinoma. The distinction between these three forms of glucocorticoid excess may be made with a dexamethasone suppression test. A solitary lesion may be found on high-resolution CT of the adrenal glands.

Pseudohyperaldosteronism

There are two disorders that fall under this category. Both are associated with hypertension, hypokalemia, and metabolic alkalosis in association with very low aldosterone levels.

Liddle's syndrome, first reported in 1963, was described in two siblings.[117] Both patients had salt retention, hypertension, hypokalemia, and metabolic alkalosis, and behaved as though they were in a state of mineralocorticoid excess. However, both aldosterone and renin levels were very low. It is thought that aldosterone levels are low in this syndrome because of the hypokalemia and low renin. This rare disorder of tubular transport responds to triamterene or amiloride, but not to spironolactone, a competitive inhibitor of aldosterone. The favorable response to amiloride and triamterene supports the hypothesis that this syndrome is a defect in tubular transport characterized by enhanced salt reabsorption and accelerated potassium and hydrogen ion secretion. Further studies, showing that aminoglutethimide, an inhibitor of adrenal steroid biosynthesis, has no effect, strongly suggest that steroid biosynthesis is essentially normal. Studies of the kinetics of erythrocyte sodium transport in patients with Liddle's syndrome have shown that sodium influx and efflux are increased.[69]

In 1948 Revers noted that patients with peptic ulcer disease who were treated with an extract of licorice developed edema. A decade later Conn and coworkers showed that 1 to 4 g/day of ammonium glycyrrhizate caused salt retention, hypokalemia, and suppression of renin and aldosterone.[1,50,117] Carbenoxolone, a compound synthesized from the aglycone of glycyrrhizic acid, also useful in peptic ulcer disease, causes a similar metabolic picture. In the isolated toad bladder this compound alone has no effect on sodium transport. When it is combined with suboptimal doses of aldosterone, sodium reabsorption is markedly enhanced. This suggests that carbenoxolone sensitizes the collecting duct to small amounts of aldosterone. Alternatively, it may be that one of the enzymes degrading the compound is altered, resulting in the accumulation of an aldosterone-like metabolite. In recent studies by Stewart and coworkers[164] it has been shown that glycyrrhizic acid inhibits the 11-dehydrogenase enzyme (11-DH) (for an excellent review of corticosteroids and the kidney, see Martin[130]). Normally, 11-DH converts cortisol to corticosterone at the level of the distal tubule. This prevents cortisol from binding to aldosterone receptors to exerting its mineralocorticoid effects. Corticosterone does not bind to these same receptors. Thus, by inhibiting 11-DH, glycyrrhizic acid allows cortisol to become an effective mineralocorticoid. In the United States certain forms of chewing tobacco are treated with licorice; thus hypokalemic metabolic alkalosis may develop in those "chewers" who swallow the tobacco juice.[81]

SECONDARY DISORDERS

Hypertensive states

Accelerated hypertension and renal artery stenosis may produce metabolic alkalosis secondary to high aldosterone levels. In these states plasma renin is always high and secondarily increases aldosterone secretion.[100] Renal underperfusion is responsible for the increased release of renin.

There are rare reports of renal tumors that secrete renin, causing metabolic alkalosis. These tumors are usually hemangiopericytomas, tumors of the capillary pericytes of the juxtaglomerular apparatus. They were first described 25 years ago; there have been only about 30 reported cases to date. The diagnosis is first made by assessing renin activity in both renal veins. Only the involved kidney releases excessive renin. Renal arteriography shows no renal artery stenosis and may reveal a tumor blush on the affected side. Nephrectomy is the treatment of choice.

Nonhypertensive states

Edema-forming states

Of the edema-forming states, liver disease and heart failure are well known to be associated with metabolic alkalosis. While the picture of metabolic alkalosis may be complicated by other factors (diuretics, respiratory alkalosis), the common denominator is a decrease in effective arterial blood volume (EABV). In the case of severe liver disease one may think of the decrease in EABV as resulting from the opening of many arteriovenous fistulae and manifesting itself clinically as ascites, spider angiomata, and the like. In the case of heart failure the decrease in EABV is secondary to the decrease in cardiac contractility with subsequent poor perfusion of the renal bed. In the nephrotic syndrome EABV may also be decreased. If volume is low, renin will be released and the secondary aldosteronism will lead to enhanced proton secretion by the collecting duct. If renal function is impaired, the retention of protons may negate the effect of aldosterone, and a normal metabolic acid-base picture will be present. None of these states of secondary hyperaldosteronism will cause hypokalemic metabolic alkalosis if distal sodium delivery is low. This accounts for the tight association with metabolic alkalosis and diuretic therapy in these patients.

Nonedematous states

VOMITING With vomiting or gastric drainage, profound metabolic alkalosis may occur. Each meq of hydrochloric acid lost from the stomach represents 1 meq of HCO_3^- added to the ECF. As can be seen from Table 29-5, there is little sodium and potassium present in gastric fluid; hence, the profound hypokalemia and volume contraction accompanying gastric alkalosis must occur through a mechanism other than the loss of sodium and potassium in vomitus or gastric drainage per se.[46,105,150,157,158]

The sequence of events is outlined in Fig. 29-3 and is as follows: The loss of hydrochloric acid increases plasma HCO_3^- concentration, with little change in the concentrations of sodium and potassium. When the increase in plasma HCO_3^- concentration raises the filtered load of alkali beyond the reabsorptive capacity of the proximal tubule, HCO_3^- appears in the urine. The HCO_3^- is delivered to the distal nephron as sodium bicarbonate; there some of the sodium is exchanged for potassium. Thus, as shown in Table 29-6, early in the course of vomiting there is a high urine pH, and high urinary sodium and potassium levels. Urine Cl^- is low because of its loss in gastric juice. Overall, this represents the loss of salt and water and causes the EABV to contract. With the contraction of EABV, proximal HCO_3^- reabsorption increases and the generated metabolic alkalosis is thus maintained. Decreased amounts of sodium bicarbonate are then delivered to the distal nephron. Because of the volume contraction, aldosterone is stimulated. As can be seen in Table 29-6, late in vomiting, urine sodium excretion falls and potassium excretion increases. Because of the decrease in distal HCO_3^- delivery, the urine pH falls as HCO_3^- disappears from the urine.

With the development of potassium depletion, aldosterone secretion falls; however, proximal HCO_3^- reabsorption remains high because of volume contraction and hypokalemia. While aldosterone levels are in the

TABLE 29-5 • Composition of gastric fluid

Components of gastric fluid	Concentration	
	Mean	*Range*
Na^+ (meq/liter)	20	10–30
K^+ (meq/liter)	10	5–40
Cl^- (meq/liter)	120	80–170
H^+ (meq/liter)	90	65–150
Volume (ml/24 h)	1000	400–5000

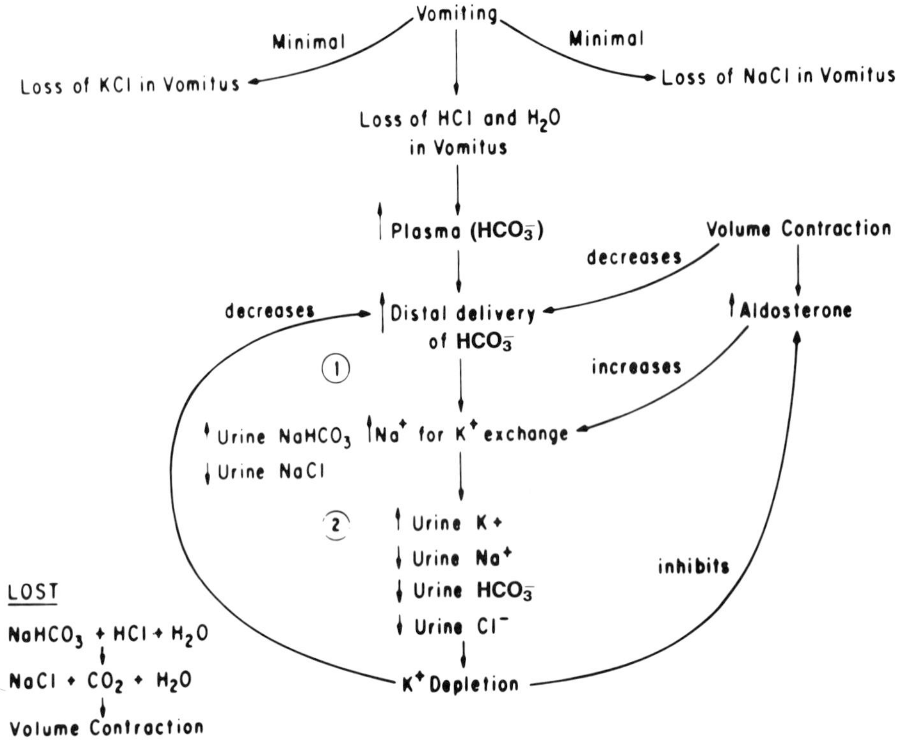

FIGURE 29.3 • Pathophysiology of gastric alkalosis.

"normal range" when corrected for the hypokalemia, it becomes clear that profound secondary hyperaldosteronism exists. Note that, both early and late in gastric alkalosis, urine Cl^- is the only accurate marker of the state of volume. Use of the urine sodium alone may yield incorrect information as regards the state of EABV (Table 29-6).

Therapy is directed toward correction of the sodium, potassium, and water deficits. In patients without severe cardiac or renal disease, the urine Cl^- is used to assess adequate replacement. A urine Cl^- concentration greater than 40 meq/liter usually indicates that sufficient salt has been administered.

DIURETICS ("CONTRACTION" ALKALOSIS) Administration of thiazides, ethacrynic acid, bumetanide, or furosemide is commonly associated with metabolic alkalosis. It has been suggested that ethacrynic acid and furosemide, which act in the loop of Henle, may induce metabolic alkalosis without loss of acid.[36,155] This alkalosis has been called "contraction" alkalosis[36] and is thought to be due to enhanced excretion of sodium and chloride without proportional loss of HCO_3^-. Bicarbonate reabsorption in the loop of Henle is minimal; the chloriuresis and natriuresis without bicarbonaturia acutely diminishes the volume of the ECF compartment without changing total body HCO_3^- content. Consequently, the blood HCO_3^- concentration increases. The P_{CO_2} does not rise to the same degree because it is controlled independently by the respiratory center. It should be pointed out, however, that adrenalectomized dogs treated with maintenance doses of dexamethasone, DOCA, and furosemide failed to develop metabolic alkalosis. When the dogs were volume-contracted as large amounts of DOCA were given, metabolic alkalosis did develop.[108] The generation of this type of metabolic alkalosis is due to enhanced acid excretion brought on by potassium depletion and secondary hyperaldosteronism. Once generated, diuretic-induced metabolic alkalosis is maintained by volume contraction and potassium depletion.[108] "Contraction" per se seems an incomplete explanation for this type of metabolic alkalosis. To increase plasma HCO_3^- from 25 to 30 meq/liter requires contraction of 20 to 25 percent of ECF volume—a devastating hemodynamic situation. Consequently, excess renal acid excretion must occur for substantial degrees of metabolic alkalosis to develop (see Chap. 19).

TABLE 29-6 • Urinary electrolyte excretion in gastric alkalosis

Stage of gastric alkalosis	Na^+	K^+	Cl^-	HCO_3^-	pH
Early	↑	↑	↓	↑	↑
Late	↓	↑	↓	↓	↓

Abbreviations: ↑, increased excretion; ↓, decreased excretion.

BARTTER'S SYNDROME The study of this rare disorder, characterized by metabolic alkalosis, hypokalemia, salt wastage, and juxtaglomerular hyperplasia, has contributed much to our understanding of the pathophysiology of acid-base disturbances.[15] The primary defect appears to be impairment in salt transport in the thick ascending limb of the loop of Henle.[73,110] Such a defect was initially postulated because of the characteristic inability of these patients to excrete urine low in Cl^- concentration, regardless of dietary Cl^- intake.[110] All the features of this disorder can be explained by this defect. The hyperreninemia and hyperaldosteronism result from chronic volume contraction secondary to defective sale transport in the loop of Henle. The metabolic alkalosis results from increased urinary acid excretion secondary to enhanced distal delivery of sodium in the face of increased levels of aldosterone. The hypokalemia can be explained as the result of both impaired potassium reabsorption in the ascending limb of the loop of Henle, secondary to the primary defect, and the kaliuretic effect of hyperaldosteronism. The observation that adrenalectomy and administration of large amounts of spironolactone failed to correct the hypokalemia of these patients is consistent with a primary defect at the level of the loop of Henle.[176]

In 1978 Gill and Bartter provided evidence in favor of a defect in the ascending limb of the loop of Henle.[78] Dysfunction at this site of the nephron is suggested by the finding of impaired diluting and concentrating capacities in patients with Bartter's syndrome. While decreased concentrating capacity can be easily explained by hypokalemia, the presence of impaired diluting capacity may be caused by decreased salt transport by the thick ascending limb of the loop of Henle.

The resistance to the pressor effects of infused AII appears to be the consequence of hypokalemia. Hypokalemia stimulates renal production of prostaglandins by the medullary interstitial cells. The increased levels of prostaglandins stimulate renin pro duction and inhibit the vasoconstrictor effect of AII.[67] Administration of prostaglandin inhibitors decreases plasma renin activity, thus restoring sensitivity to AII.

Another finding in some patients with Bartter's syndrome is hypomagnesemia and renal magnesium wasting. Magnesium is largely reabsorbed by the ascending limb; therefore, a defect at this level of the nephron would also explain the presence of renal magnesium wasting. Magnesium deficiency itself can cause renal potassium wasting and, thus, may contribute to the hypokalemia. In fact, in some patients with Bartter's syndrome, potassium wasting improves with chronic administration of magnesium.[126]

The differential diagnosis of Bartter's syndrome includes chronic diuretic abuse and protracted vomiting. These conditions are associated with hypokalemia, metabolic alkalosis, hyperreninemia, and hyperaldosteronism (Table 29-7). A high urinary excretion of prostaglandins can also occur in these three disorders. The differentiation of these syndromes can be easily accomplished by evaluating the pattern of urinary electrolytes. While urinary levels of sodium and potassium can be increased in these three disorders, the urinary level of Cl^- clearly separates patients with Bartter's syndrome from those with protracted vomiting. In the latter patients, the urinary level of Cl^- is always low (i.e., less than 20 meq/liter), whereas patients with Bartter's syndrome have elevated Cl^- levels even in the face of volume contraction. Patients with protracted diuretic abuse, however, can present with all the features of Bartter's syndrome, including a high urinary Cl^- level. The differential diagnosis can be made by means of a thorough history taking. Because patients who abuse diuretics often deny the abuse, screening for urinary diuretics is useful.

Current treatment of Bartter's syndrome is less than satisfactory. In most patients it is exceedingly difficult to restore serum potassium to normal levels, despite the administration of large amounts of the electrolyte and concomitant treatment with potassium-sparing diuretics. Prostaglandin synthesis inhibitors, such as indomethacin (75 to 150 mg daily), in conjunction with potassium supplements are the treatments of choice.[139,180] This

TABLE 29-7 • Differential diagnosis of Bartter's syndrome, diuretic abuse, and vomiting

	Blood pressure	Hypokalemia	Metabolic alkalosis	Renin	Aldosterone	Prostaglandins	Urinary electrolytes			
							Na^+	*K^+*	*Cl^-*	*Mg^{2+}*
Bartter's syndrome	↓	Present	Present	↑	↑	↑	↑	↑	↑	↑
Diuretic abuse	↓	Present	Present	↑	↑	↑	↑ *	↑	↑ *	↑
Protracted vomiting	↓	Present	Present	↑	↑	↑	↑ +	↑	↓ +	↓

* Urinary levels of sodium and chloride can be low in patients who take diuretics if severe volume contraction has developed.

+ Urinary levels of sodium can be increased or decreased in patients with protracted vomiting but the urinary level of chloride is always low in such patients. Thus, the urinary level of chloride is most useful in the differential diagnosis of these three disorders.

Abbreviations: ↑, increased; ↓, decreased.

mode of treatment does not completely correct the hypokalemia but may render patients asymptomatic.

MAGNESIUM DEFICIENCY AND NONREABSORBABLE ANIONS The effects of magnesium deficiency on acid-base status are controversial. Hypomagnesemia has been reported in some studies to cause metabolic alkalosis by stimulation of the renin-aldosterone axis, whereas others have shown that two months' deprivation of magnesium to pair-fed animals had no effect on acid-base homeostasis.[132] Large amounts of nonreabsorbable anion, such as carbenicillin or sodium sulfate, have been reported to cause metabolic alkalosis, presumably via the anion's stimulation of proton secretion by the distal nephron in response to a favorable lumen-negative potential difference.[14]

OTHER

Excessive bicarbonate loads

Administration of sodium bicarbonate in doses up to 140 g/day (1667 meq) for periods of up to three weeks has been shown to produce metabolic alkalosis with plasma HCO_3^- concentrations ranging between 33 and 36 meq/liter. A linear relationship is noted between the doses of sodium bicarbonate administered and the increase in serum HCO_3^- concentration. If neither volume contraction nor potassium depletion develops, the metabolic alkalosis will correct as soon as HCO_3^- administration ceases, because of the enormous intrinsic capacity of the kidney to excrete HCO_3^-. In renal failure, however, a smaller dose of sodium bicarbonate may produce metabolic alkalosis beause of the limited capacity of the severely diseased kidney to excrete HCO_3^-.

Postfasting metabolic alkalosis

It is well established that fasting patients returning to a normal diet with a high glucose content may develop metabolic alkalosis. HCO_3^- reabsorption in these patients correlates with the sodium balance;[165] it is low in the first week of fasting, when the sodium balance is negative, but high in the second and third weeks, when sodium balance becomes positive. Glucose administration further increases HCO_3^- reabsorption and worsens the metabolic alkalosis. The maintenance of this type of metabolic alkalosis seems to be caused by contracted ECF volume and the effect of glucose to enhance HCO_3^- reabsorption. The mechanism underlying its generation is not clear at present; it may be secondary to increased acid excretion by the distal nephron.

Hypercalcemia and hypoparathyroidism

A few cases of metabolic alkalosis have been reported in association with hypoparathyroidism. Hypercalcemia is more commonly associated with metabolic alkalosis. It is likely that PTH depresses HCO_3^- reabsorption and that the absence of the hormone enhances reabsorption.[53,96] Hypercalcemia increases HCO_3^- reabsorption by supressing PTH secretion and by a direct effect on renal hydrogen ion secretion. Although these observations explain the maintenance of metabolic alkalosis in these conditions, they leave unsolved the question of how metabolic alkalosis is generated. Parathyroid hormone appears to have an inhibitory effect on acid excretion; theoretically, a lack of the hormone could lead to enhanced acid excretion. This, however, has yet to be proved. The generation of metabolic alkalosis secondary to hypercalcemia has been attributed to a greater availability of the buffering capacity of the skeleton secondary either to bone destruction or increased bone turnover. Studies suggest that PTH has a direct effect on the skeleton to mobilize buffer into the ECF compartment.[9,11] In a detailed study, Hulter and coworkers[88] showed the chronic administration of large doses of PTH to intact dogs, or of 1,25-$(OH)_2D_3$ to TPTX dogs, caused metabolic alkalosis without changing net acid excretion (renal and extrarenal in origin). Chronic hypercalcemia in TPTX dogs, induced by feeding or infusing calcium, caused metabolic acidosis with an increase in net acid excretion. This study suggests that metabolic alkalosis or acidosis will occur, depending on the net movement of calcium. Calcium movement into bone or soft tissue results in acidosis, whereas calcium release from bone results in metabolic alkalosis. Thus, patients with hypercalcemia and hyperparathyroidism may develop metabolic alkalosis as a consequence of enhanced transfer of buffer from bone to the circulation. Patients with hypercalcemia alone would develop metabolic acidosis.

Posthypercapnic metabolic alkalosis

Chronic hypercapnia enhances acid and Cl^- excretion. At the same time, it stimulates HCO_3^- reabsorption, maintaining an increased concentration of plasma HCO_3^-. Following the return of the P_{CO_2} to normal, there usually is retention of Cl^- and excretion of HCO_3^- in the urine. If patients with hypercapnia are on a low-salt diet or are treated with diuretics so that volume is contracted, proximal reabsorption will be enhanced and HCO_3^- reabsorption will remain elevated following the return of the P_{CO_2} to normal, resulting in posthypercapnic metabolic alkalosis.[157] Salt administration usually corrects this type of metabolic alkalosis. This syndrome may result if EABV is contracted for any reason, such as congestive heart failure. In this latter instance successful treatment of the heart failure is required to correct the alkalosis; salt administration in this instance is contraindicated.

Congenital chloride-losing diarrhea

Patients with this rare disease have hyperchloremia, a high stool Cl^- concentration, and absence of Cl^- in the urine.[55,59] The stool Cl^- concentration is higher than the sum of the sodium and potassium concentrations. This is in contrast to all other diarrheal states, in which the sum of sodium and potassium concentrations in the stool is higher than the Cl^- concentration. These patients have a defect in chloride-bicarbonate transport in the ileum. They are unable to transport Cl^- against an electrochemical gradient; this defect results in a loss of Cl^- and protons in the stool, which in turn causes metabolic alkalosis.

Severe potassium depletion

In human beings, pure potassium depletion has been shown to cause mild metabolic alkalosis in the absence of excess mineralocorticoid.[93] In rat studies, several, but not all, investigators have shown that dietary potassium restriction alone causes metabolic alkalosis.[115,159,171,173,185,187] In dogs, dietary potassium deprivation has been shown to cause either no change in acid-base status or a hyperchloremic metabolic acidosis.[33,86,179] The mechanism for the acidosis may be due to the effect of low potassium to inhibit aldosterone secretion. Van Ypersele de Strihou and Dieu[179] were unable to show an effect of potassium depletion on aldosterone secretion. Hulter and coworkers[86] showed that hyperkalemic adrenalectomized dogs on a fixed dosage of aldosterone did not develop acidosis.

SYMPTOMS, SIGNS, AND THERAPY OF METABOLIC ALKALOSIS

The most dramatic effects of metabolic alkalosis are on the *central nervous system* (Table 29-8). Mental confusion and obtundation occur secondary to the decrease in cerebral blood flow caused by alkalemia. The seizure threshold is reduced, and paresthesias, cramping, and tetany may occur. Since respiratory compensation for metabolic alkalosis decreases alveolar ventilation, *hypoxemia* and exacerbation of obstructive lung disease may develop. *Cardiac arrhythmias* may occur secondary to hypoxemia and hypokalemia; *congestive heart failure* may be caused by associated hypophosphatemia (see Chap. 33). Severe metabolic alkalosis modestly reduces the ionized fraction of total serum *calcium* by increasing its protein binding and complexing with phosphate, HCO_3^- and other organic anions. The precise way in which metabolic alkalosis affects myocardial calcium handling, an abnormality that may further impair contractility, is not completely clear. *Digitalis toxicity* is increased in the intact animal following HCO_3^- infusion (even when arterial pH remains within the normal range); drug toxicity also persists longer in metabolic alkalosis.[30,184]

The *anion gap* is increased in pure metabolic alkalosis. The precise explanation for this is not clear, since

TABLE 29-8 • Adverse effects of metabolic alkalosis

CENTRAL NERVOUS SYSTEM
Mental confusion, obtundation, delirium
Decrease in seizure threshold
NEUROMUSCULAR
Tetany, increased excitability
Increased release of acetylcholine
CARDIOVASCULAR
Decreased electrical stability, ventricular fibrillation
Increased sensitivity to cardiac glycosides
Hypotension, decreased cardiac output
PULMONARY
Aveolar hypoventilation
METABOLIC
Hypokalemia
Hypophosphatemia
Decrease in ionized calcium
Increase in glycolysis and lactate production
Shift of oxyhemoglobin curve to left

only one-half of the increment can be explained by protein and metabolic buffering. Protons, released primarily from albumin, titrate HCO_3^- thereby mitigating the degree of hyperbicarbonatemia. Alkalosis also stimulates the production of organic acids, further minimizing the increase in serum HCO_3^- concentration. The accumulated lactate and citrate will complex with calcium, which tends to exacerbate the increased neuromuscular excitability.

Acute metabolic alkalosis also decreases the concentration of ionized *magnesium*, presumably by causing the cation to shift intracellularly.[130,132] The extent to which this is important in various clinical abnormalities is not yet known. Magnesium is a critical component of membranes and ATPases; its deficiency causes hypotension, flaccid paralysis, conduction defects with heart block, and cardiac arrest.

Once the pathophysiology of the type of metabolic alkalosis has been delineated, treatment is simple (Table 29-9). If volume contraction is the perpetuating mechanism for hyperbicarbonatremia, normovolemia should be restored. Potassium deficits should be repleted. If primary mineralocorticoid excess is present, it may be antagonized with spironolacotone prior to effecting definitive therapy (e.g., adrenalectomy). Acetazolamide administration induces a prompt HCO_3^- diuresis by inhibiting the enzyme carbonic anhydrase. The drug has little to no value in alkalotic patients who are volume-contracted. It can be very useful, however, in those normovolemic or hypervolemic patients with symptomatic alkaloses (e.g., posthypercapnic metabolic alkalosis, or diuretic-induced alkalosis in congestive heart failure). An

TABLE 29-9 • Acidifying agents used in the treatment of metabolic alkalosis

Agents	Dose (mmol/g)	Routes of administration	Adverse effects
Ammonium chloride	19	Oral, intravenous	↑ BUN, ↑ NH_3
Calcium chloride	9	Oral	↑ Ca^{2+}
Lysine monohydrochloride	5.5	Oral	
Arginine monohydrochloride	5.5	Intravenous	↑ Plasma K^+, ↑ BUN
Hydrochloric acid	28	Intravenous (100–200 meq/liter)	

Abbreviations: ↑, increased; ↓, decreased.

oral or intravenous dose of 250 to 500 mg will begin working rapidly and may be repeated as dictated by the change in serum HCO_3^- concentration and the patient's symptoms and signs. It is important to remember that carbonic-anhydrase inhibitors should be used infrequently and that they are very kaliuretic. Attention to the other aspects of therapy is mandatory in these difficult management cases.

Recently cimetidine, an H_2-histamine receptor blocker, has proved useful in the therapy of gastric alkalosis. Cimetidine (30 mg every 6 h, intravenously) decreases acid secretion by the stomach and minimizes the rate and magnitude of HCO_3^- generation. This should not be used prophylactically, since the drug itself is associated with mental confusion and cramping, particularly in the elderly.

Acid administration may be indicated in patients unresponsive to the above maneuvers who are allergic or resistant to the sulfa-containing carbonic anhydrase inhibitors, or who have renal failure not requiring dialysis (Table 29-9). The most commonly used acidifying salts include ammonium chloride, calcium chloride, lysine, and arginine monohydrochloride. If hydrochloric acid is used, it should be infused into the vena cava. The solution has a pH of about 1, and accordingly should *not* be infused directly into the right atrium. Narins[137] has summarized the use of this approach, citing a number of original references. Hemodialysis using a normal or low-HCO_3^- bath is also a technique that may be used to treat metabolic alkalosis complicating acute or end-stage renal failure. These therapeutic modalities have very precise and limiting indications and may be very hazardous when improperly applied. Their use should be reserved for the physician who is expert in the management of renal disease in general and in acid-base disturbances in particular.

REFERENCES

1. Aarskog D et al: Hypertension and hypokalemic alkalosis associated with underproduction of aldosterone. *Pediatrics* 39:884, 1967.
2. Abboud HE et al: Stimulation of renin by acute selective chloride depletion in the rat. *Circ Res* 44:815, 1979.
3. Abbrecht PH: Effect of potassium deficiency on renal function in the dog. *J Clin Invest* 48:432, 1969.
4. Adler S, Fraley DS: Potassium and intracellular pH. *Kidney Int* 11:433, 1977.
5. Al-Awqati Q et al: Characteristics of stimulation of H+ transport by aldosterone in turtle urinary bladder. *J Clin Invest* 58:351, 1976.
6. Alleyne GAO, Robol A: Renal metabolic processes and acid-base changes. *Med Clin North Am* 59:781, 1975.
7. Alpern R et al: Effect of luminal bicarbonate concentration on proximal acidification in the rat. *Am J Physiol* 243:F53, 1982.
8. Alterman SL et al: Primary adrenocortical carcinoma causing aldosteronism. *Cancer* 24:602, 1969.
9. Arruda JAL et al: Metabolic acidosis and alkalosis. *Clin Nephrol* 7:201, 1977.
10. Arruda JAL, Kurtzman NA: Voltage dependent distal acidification defect induced by amiloride. *J Lab Clin Med* 95:407, 1980.
11. Arruda JAL et al: Parathyroid hormone and extrarenal acid-base buffering. *Am J Physiol* 239:533, 1980.
12. Arruda JAL, Kurtzman NA: Mechanisms and classification of deranged distal urinary acidification. *Am J Physiol* 239:F515, 1982.
13. Arruda JAL et al: Metabolic and hormonal factors influencing extrarenal buffering of an acute acid load. *Miner Electrolyte Metab* 6:22, 1982.
14. Bank N, Schwartz WB: The influence of anion penetrating ability on urinary acidification and the excretion of titratable acid. *J Clin Invest* 39:1516, 1960.
15. Bartter FC et al: Hyperplasia of the juxtaglomerular complex with hyperaldosteronism and hypokalemic alkalosis: A new syndrome. *Am J Med* 33:811, 1962.
16. Batlle DC: Hyperkalemic hyperchloremic metabolic acidosis associated with selective aldosterone deficiency and distal renal tubular acidosis. *Semin Nephrol* 1:260, 1981.
17. Batlle DC et al: The pathogenesis of hyperchloremic metabolic acidosis associated with renal transplantation. *Am J Med* 70:786, 1982.
18. Batlle DC et al: Hyperkalemia distal renal tubular acidosis associated with obstructive uropathy. *N Engl J Med* 304:373, 1981.
19. Batlle DC et al: Clinical and pathophysiological spectrum of acquired distal renal tubular acidosis. *Kidney Int* 20:389, 1981.

20. Batlle DC et al: Hyperkalemic hyperchloremic metabolic acidosis in sickle cell hemoglobinopathies. *Am J Med* 72:188, 1982.
21. Batlle DC, Kurtzman NA: Syndromes of aldosterone deficiency and excess. *Med Clin North Am* 67:879, 1983.
22. Battilana CA et al: The effect of chronic potassium loading on potassium secretion by the pars recta or descending limb of the juxtamedullary nephron in the rat. *J Clin Invest* 62:1093, 1978.
23. Berliner RW: Renal mechanisms for potassium excretion. *Harvey Lect* 55:141, 1961.
24. Berry CA, Cogan MA: Influence of peritubular protein on solute absorption in the rabbit proximal tubule. *J Clin Invest* 68:506, 1981.
25. Bichara M et al: Hydrogen transport in rabbit kidney proximal tubules: Na^+:H^+ exchange. *Am J Physiol* 238:F445, 1980.
26. Biglieri EG: Plasma deoxycorticosterone concentrations in the adrenal enzymatic deficiencies causing hypertension, in New MI, Levine LS (eds): *Juvenile Hypertension*. New York, Raven Press, 1977.
27. Biglieri EG, Forsham PH: Studies on expanded extracellular fluid and responses to various stimuli in primary aldosteronism. *Am J Med* 30:564, 1961.
28. Biglieri EG et al: 17α-Hydroxylation deficiency in man. *J Clin Invest* 45:1946, 1966.
29. Black DAK et al: Renal handling of radioactive potassium in man. *Clin Sci* 15:227, 1956.
30. Bliss HA et al: Effect of alterations of blood pH on digitalis toxicity. *J Lab Clin Med* 62:53, 1963.
31. Bongiovanni AM, Root AW: The adrenogenital syndrome. *N Engl J Med* 268:1283, 1963.
32. Boron WF, Boulapaep EL: Intracellular pH regulation in the renal proximal tubule of the salamander: Basolateral HCO_3 transport. *J Gen Physiol* 81:53, 1983.
33. Boron WF, Boulapaep EL: Intracellular pH regulation in the proximal tubule of the salamander: Na-H exchange. *Gen Physiol* 81:29, 1983.
34. Brunner FP et al: The mechanisms of the urinary concentrating defect in potassium deficient rats. *Pfluegers Arch* 290:202, 1966.
35. Burnell JM et al: Metabolic acidosis accompanying potassium deprivation. *Am J Physiol* 227:329, 1974.
36. Cannon PJ et al: "Contraction" alkalosis after diuresis of edmatous patients with ethacrynic acid. *Ann Intern Med* 62:979, 1965.
37. Chan Y, Giebisch G: The relationship between sodium and bicarbonate ion transport in the rat proximal convoluted tubule. *Am J Physiol;* 240:F222, 1981.
38. Chan YL et al: Control mechanism of bicarbonate transport across the rat proximal convoluted tubule. *Am J Physiol* 242:F532, 1982.
39. Chantrelle BC et al: Relation of Na transport and acidification in the rat proximal convoluted tubule. *Kidney Int* 16:809, 1979.
40. Christy NP, Laragh JH: Pathogenesis of hypokalemic alkalosis in Cushing's syndrome. *N Engl J Med* 265:1083, 1961.
41. Cogan MG et al: Control of proximal bicarbonate reabsorption in normal and acidotic rats. *J Clin Invest* 64:1168, 1979.
42. Cogan MG et al: Effect of acetazolamide on bicarbonate reabsorption in the proximal tubule of the rat. *Am J Physiol* 237:F447, 1979.
43. Cogan MG, Liu FY: Metabolic alkalosis in the rat. *J Clin Invest* 71:1124, 1983.
44. Cogan MG et al: Metabolic alkalosis. *Med Clin North Am* 67:903, 1983.
45. Cogan MG: Regulation and control of bicarbonate reabsorption in the proximal tubule. *Semin Nephrol* 10:115, 1990.
46. Cohen JJ: Correction of metabolic alkalosis by the kidney after isometric expansion of extracellular fluid. *J Clin Invest* 47:1118, 1968.
47. Cohen JJ: Selective Cl retention in repair of metabolic alkalosis without increasing filtered load. *Am J Physiol* 218:165, 1970.
48. Conn JW: Presidential address: II. Primary aldosteronism: A new clinical syndrome. *J Lab Clin Med* 45:6, 1955.
49. Conn JW et al: Suppression of plasma renin activity in primary aldosteronism. *JAMA* 190:213, 1964.
50. Conn JW et al: Licorice-induced pseudoaldosteronism: Hypertension, hypokalemia, aldosteronopenia, and suppressed plasma renin activity. *JAMA* 205:80, 1968.
51. Costa-Silva VL et al: Role of luminal buffers in renal tubular acidification. *J Membr Biol* 63:13, 1981.
52. Cronin RE, Knochel JP: The consequences of potassium deficiency, in Brenner BM, Stein JH (eds): *Acid-base and Potassium Homeostasis, Contemporary Issues in Nephrology*. New York, Churchill Livingstone, 1978, vol 2, p 205.
53. Crumb CK et al: Effects of volume expansion, purified parathyroid extract and calcium on renal bicarbonate absorption in the dog. *J Clin Invest* 54:1287, 1974.
54. Cruz-Soto M et al: Carbonic anhydrase-independent reabsorption in rats with chronic papillary necrosis. *Miner Electrolyte Metab* 10:319, 1984.
55. Darrow DC: Congenital alkalosis with diarrhea. *J Pediatr* 26:519, 1945.
56. Davis WW et al: Bilateral adrenal hyperplasia as a cause of primary aldosteronism with hypertension, hypokalemia, and suppressed renin activity. *Am J Med* 42:642, 1967.
57. De Mello-Aires MG et al: Kinetics of potassium transport across single distal tubules of rat kidney. *J Physiol* 232:47, 1973.
58. DiTella PJ et al: Mechanism of the metabolic acidosis of selective mineralocorticoid deficiency. *Kidney Int* 14:466, 1978.
59. Evansen TM, Stanbury SW: Congenital chloridorrhea or so-called congenital alkalosis with diarrhea. *Gut* 6:29, 1965.
60. Farman N et al: Aldosterone binding in isolated tubules: Biochemical determination in proximal and distal parts of the rabbit nephron. *Am J Physiol* 242:F63, 1982.
61. Farman N et al: An autoradiographic study of concentration dependency in the rabbit nephron. *Am J Physiol* 242:F69, 1982.
62. Frommer P et al: Internephron heterogeneity for carbonic anhydrase-independent bicarbonate reabsorption in the rat. *J Clin Invest* 73:1034, 1984.
63. Fuller GR et al: Influence of potassium salts on the renal

tubular reabsorption of bicarbonate. *Am J Physiol* 182:111, 1955.

64. Galla JH et al: Effects of chloride and extracellular fluid volume on bicarbonate reabsorption along the nephron in metabolic alkalosis in the rat: Reassessment of the classical hypothesis of the pathogenesis of metabolic alkalosis. *J Clin Invest* 80:41, 1987.
65. Galla HJ et al: The correction of acute chloride-depletion alkalosis in the rat without volume expansion. *Am J Physiol* 244:F217, 1983.
66. Galla JH et al: Segmental chloride and fluid handling during correction of chloride-depletion alkalosis without volume expansion in the rat. *J Clin Invest* 73:96, 1984.
67. Galvez OG et al: The hemodynamic effects of potassium deficiency in the dog. *Circ Res* 40:111, 1977.
68. Garcia-Filho E et al: Effects of changes in electrical potential difference on tubular potassium transport. *Am J Physiol* 238:F235, 1980.
69. Gardener JD et al: Abnormal membrane sodium transport in Liddle syndrome. *J Clin Invest* 50:2253, 1971.
70. Garrett ES, Nahmias C: The effect of glucose on the urinary excretion of sodium and hydrogen ion in man. *Clin Sci* 47:589, 1974.
71. Giebisch G et al: The effect of adrenal steroids on renal tubular reabsorption of bicarbonate. *Am J Physiol* 183:377, 1955.
72. Giebisch G et al: Renal transport and control of potassium excretion, in Brenner BM, Rector FC Jr (eds): *The Kidney*, 2d ed. Philadelphia, Saunders, 1981, p. 408.
73. Gill JR, Bartter FC: Evidence for a prostaglandin independent defect in chloride reabsorption in the loop of Henle as a proximal cause of Bartter's syndrome. *Am J Med* 65:766, 1978.
74. Good DW et al: Transepithelial ammonia gradients in inner medulla of the rat. *Am J Physiol* 252:F491, 1987.
75. Good DW, DuBose TD: Ammonia transport by early and late proximal convoluted tubule of the rat. *J Clin Invest* 79:684, 1987.
76. Glynn IM, Karlish SJD: The sodium pump. *Annu Rev Physiol* 37:13, 1975.
77. Gold LS et al: Renal bicarbonate wasting during phosphate depletion. *J Clin Invest* 52:2556, 1973.
78. Goldsmith O et al: Hypogonadism and mineralocorticoid excess: The 17α-hydroxylase deficiency syndrome. *N Engl J Med* 277:673, 1967.
79. Grantham JJ et al: The nature of transtubular Na and K transport in isolated rabbit renal collecting tubules. *J Clin Invest* 49:1815, 1970.
80. Grollman AP, Gamble JL:Metabolic alkalosis, a specific effect of adrenocortical hormones. *Am J Physiol* 196:135, 1959.
81. Gross EG et al: Hypokalemic myopathy with myoglobinuria associated with licorice ingestion. *N Engl J Med* 274:602, 1966.
82. Gross JB et al: A functional comparison of the cortical collecting tubule and the distal convoluted tubule. *J Clin Invest* 55:1284, 1975.
83. Gross JB, Kokko JP: Effect of aldosterone and potassium-sparing diuretics on electrical potential differences across the distal nephron. *J Clin Invest* 59:82, 1977.
84. Hogan MJ et al: Location of aldosterone-producing adenomas with ^{131}I-19-iodocholesterol. *N Engl J Med* 294:410, 1976.
85. Holliday MA, Egan TJ: Change in GFR and CH_2O before and after repair of K deficiency in rats. *Am J Physiol* 202:773, 1962.
86. Hulter HN et al: Pathogenesis of renal hyperchloremic acidosis resulting from dietary potassium restriction in the dog: Role of aldosterone. *Am J Physiol* 238:F79, 1980.
87. Hulter HN et al: Impaired renal H^+ secretion and ammonia production in mineralocorticoid-deficiency glucocorticoid-replete dogs. *Am J Physiol* 232:F136, 1977.
88. Hulter HN et al: Renal and systemic acid base effects of chronic administration of hypercalcemia-producing agents: Calcitriol, PTH, and intravenous calcium. *Kidney Int* 21:445, 1982.
89. Iacobellis M et al: Enzyme concentration changes in the kidneys of protein- and/or potassium-deficient rats. *Am J Physiol* 178:477, 1954.
90. Jacobson HR, Seldin DW: On the generation, maintenance, and correction of metabolic alkalosis. *Am J Physiol* 244:F425, 1983.
91. Jamison RL et al: Potassium secretion by the descending limb of pars recta or juxtamedullary nephron in vivo. *Kidney Int* 9:323, 1976.
92. Jamison RL et al: New pathways for potassium transport in the kidney. *Am J Physiol* 243:F297, 1982.
93. Jones IW et al: Systemic and renal acid-base effects of chronic dietary potassium depletion in humans. *Kidney Int* 21:402, 1982.
94. Kaissirer JP, Schwartz WB: The response of normal man to selective depletion of hydrochloric acid: Factors in the genesis of persistent gastric alkalosis. *Am J Med* 40:10, 1966.
95. Kamm DE, Strope GL: Glutamine and glutamate metabolism in renal cortex, from potassium depleted rats. *J Clin Invest* 224:1241, 1973.
96. Karlinsky ML et al: Effect of parathormone and cyclic adenosine monophosphate on renal bicarbonate reabsorption. *Am J Physiol* 227:1226, 1974.
97. Katz FH: Primary aldosteronism with suppressed plasma renin activity due to bilateral nodular adrenocortical hyperplasia. *Ann Intern Med* 67:1035, 1967.
98. Kinne R et al: The localization of the Na^+-K^+ ATPase in the cells of the rat kidney cortex. *Pfluegers Arch* 329:191, 1971.
99. Kinsella JL, Aronson PS: Properties of the Na/H exchanger in serial microvillus membrane vesicles. *Am J Physiol* 238:F461, 1980..
100. Kliger AS, Hayslett JP: Disorders of potassium balance, in Brenner BM, Stein JH (eds): *Acid-Base and Potassium Homeostasis*. New York, Churchill Livingstone, 1978, p 168.
101. Knepper MA et al: Ammonium transport in the kidney. *Physiol Rev* 69:179, 1989.
102. Koeppen BM, Helman SI: Acidification of luminal fluid by the rabbit cortical collecting tubule perfused in vitro. *Am J Physiol* 242:F521, 1982.
103. Kotchen TA et al: Contribution of chloride to the inhibition of plasma renin by sodium chloride in the rat. *Kidney Int* 13:201, 1978.

104. Kunau RT et al: Micropuncture study of the proximal tubular factors responsible for the maintenance of metabolic alkalosis during potassium deficiency in the rat. *Clin Sci* 34:223, 1968.
105. Kurtzman NA: Regulation of renal bicarbonate reabsorption by extracellular volume. *J Clin Invest* 49:586, 1970.
106. Kurtzman NA: Relationship of extracellular volume and CO_2 tension to renal bicarbonate absorption. *Am J Physiol* 219:1299, 1970.
107. Kurtzman NA et al: Aldosterone deficiency and renal bicarbonate reabsorption. *J Lab Clin Med* 77:931, 1971.
108. Kurtzman NA: Pathophysiology of metabolic alkalosis. *Arch Intern Med* 131:702, 1973.
109. Kurtzman NA et al: The effect of potassium and extracellular volume on renal bicarbonate reabsorption. *Metabolism* 22:481, 1973.
110. Kurtzman NA, Gutierrez LF: The pathophysiology of Bartter's syndrome. *JAMA* 234:758, 1975.
111. Kurtzman NA: Ammonia secretion and urinary acidification. *Semin Nephrol* 2:1, 1982.
112. Kurtzman NA: Disorders of distal acidification. *Kidney Int* 38:720, 1990.
113. Langberg H et al: Filtered bicarbonate and plasma pH as determinants of renal bicarbonate reabsorption. *Kidney Int* 20:780, 1981.
114. Laski ME, Kurtzman NA: Characterization of acidification in the rabbit collecting tubule. *J Clin Invest* 71:400, 1983.
115. Leutscher JA et al: Preoperative differentiation of adrenal adenoma from idiopathic adrenal hyperplasia in primary aldosteronism. *Circ Res* 34/35(suppl 1):1–175, 1974.
116. Levine DZ et al: Effects of KCl infusion on proximal tubular function in normal and potassium-depleted rats. *Kidney Int* 4:318, 1973.
117. Liddle GW et al: A familial renal disorder simulating primary aldosteronism but with negligible aldosterone secretion. *Trans Assoc Am Physicians* 76:199, 1963.
118. Linas SL, Dickman D: Mechanism of the decreased renal blood flow in the potassium-depleted conscious rat. *Kidney Int* 21:757, 1982.
119. Lui FY, Logan MG: Angiotensin II: A potent regulator of acidification in the rat early proximal convoluted tubule. *J Clin Invest* 80:272, 1987.
120. Liu FY, Logan MG: Angiotensin II stimulation of hydrogen ion secretion in the rat early proximal tubule: Modes of action, mechanism, and kinetics. *J Clin Invest* 82:601, 1988.
121. Liu FY, Logan MG: Atrial natriuretic factor does not inhibit basal or angiotensin II-stimulated proximal transport. *Am J Physiol* 255:F434, 1989.
122. Lombard WE et al: Comparison of bicarbonate transport in cortical and medullary collecting tubules: Identification of the major absorptive site. *Am J Physiol* 244:F289, 1983.
123. Lonnerholm G, Ridderstråle Y: Intracellular distribution of carbonic anhydrase in the rat kidney. *Kidney Int* 17:162, 1980.
124. Lucci MS et al: Carbonic anhydrase-dependent bicarbonate reabsorption in the rat proximal tubule. *Am J Physiol* 236:F58, 1979.
125. Lynche RE et al: Absence of mineralocorticoid-dependent sodium reabsorption in dog proximal tubule. *Am J Physiol* 223:40, 1972.
126. Mace JW et al: Magnesium supplementation in Bartter's syndromes. *Arch Dis Child* 48:485, 1973.
127. Malnic G et al: Microperfusion study of distal tubular potassium and sodium transfer in rat kidney. *Am J Physiol* 211:548, 1966.
128. Malnic G, de Mello-Aires M: Kinetics of bicarbonate reabsorption in proximal tubule of the rat. *Am J Physiol* 220:1759, 1971.
129. Maren TH: Current status of membrane bound carbonic anhydrase. *Ann NY Acad Sci* 341:246, 1980.
130. Martin HE: Clinical magnesium deficiency. *Ann NY Acad Sci* 162:891, 1969.
131. Marver D: *Corticosteroids and the Kidney. Seminars in Nephrology.* Philadelphia, Saunders, 1990, vol 10, p 307.
132. Massry SG: Hypomagnesemia and hypermagnesemia, in Massry SG, Ghassock RJ (eds): *Textbook of Nephrology.* Baltimore, Williams & Wilkins, 1989, p 323.
133. McKinney TD, Burg MB: Bicarbonate absorption by rabbit cortical collecting tubules in vitro. *Am J Physiol* 234:141, 1978.
134. Muntwyler E et al: Kidney glutaminase and carbonic anhydrase activities and renal electrolyte excretion in rats. *Am J Physiol* 184:83, 1956.
135. Muryama Y et al: Microperfusion of Henle's loop in the kidney of the adrenalectomized rat. *Jpn J Pharmacol* 18:518, 1968.
136. Nagami GT: Luminal secretion of ammonia in the mouse proximal tubule perfused *in vitro*. *J Clin Invest* 81:159, 1988.
137. Narins RG: Acid-base metabolism, in Gonick HC (ed): *In Current Nephrology.* Pacific Palisades, CA, Pinecliff Medical, 1977, vol 1, p 37.
138. New MI: Male pseudohermaphroditism due to a 17α-hydroxylase deficiency. *J Clin Invest* 49:1930, 1970.
139. Norby L et al: Prostaglandins and aspirin therapy in Bartter's syndrome. *Lancet*, 2:604, 1976.
140. O'Neil RG: Aldosterone regulation of sodium and potassium transport in cortical collecting duct. *Semin Nephrol* 10:365, 1990.
141. Pagliara AS, Goodman AD: Relation of renal cortical gluconeogenesis, glutamate content and production of ammonia. *J Clin Invest* 49:1967, 1970.
142. Pitts RF: Renal production and excretion of ammonia. *Am J Physiol* 36:720, 1964.
143. Pitts RF: *Physiology of the Kidney and Body Fluids.* Chicago, Year Book Medical Publishers, 1974.
144. Pitts RF, Lotspeich WD: Bicarbonate and the renal regulation of acid-base balance. *Am J Physiol* 147:138, 1946.
145. Pitts RF et al: The renal regulation of acid-base balance in man: III. The reabsorption and excretion of bicarbonate. *J Clin Invest* 28:35, 1949.
146. Rector FC Jr: Acidification of the urine, in Orloff MJ, Berliner RW (eds): *Handbook of Physiology.* Baltimore, Williams and Wilkins, 1973, p 431.
147. Relman AS, Schwartz WB: The effect of DOCA on electrolyte balance in normal man and its relation to sodium chloride intake. *Yale J Biol Med* 24:540, 1952.
148. Roth DG, Gamble JL: Deoxycorticosterone induced alkalosis in dogs. *Am J Physiol* 208:90, 1965.

149. Rubinstein H et al: Urinary P_{CO_2} during carbonic anhydrase inhibition. *Miner Electrolyte Metab* 5:49, 1981.
150. Sabatini S: The acidosis of chronic renal failure. *Med Clin North Am* 67:120, 1983.
151. Sabatini S et al: Disorders of acid base balance. *Med Clin North Am* 62:1223, 1978.
152. Sabatini S, Kurtzman NA: The maintenance of metabolic alkalosis. *Kidney Int* 25:357, 1984.
153. Sasaki S et al: Effect of luminal and peritubular HCO_3 concentrations and P_{CO_2} on HCO_3 reabsorption in rabbit proximal convoluted tubules perfused in vitro. *J Clin Invest* 70:639, 1982.
154. Schambelan M et al: Mineralocorticoid excess and deficiency syndromes, in Brenner BM, Stein JH (eds): *Acid-Base and Potassium Homeostasis.* New York, Churchill Livingstone, 1978, vol 2, p 232.
155. Sebastian A et al: Metabolic alkalosis, in Brenner BM, Stein JH (eds): *Contemporary Issues in Nephrology, Acid-base and Potassium Homeostasis.* New York, Churchill Livingstone, 1978, vol 2, p 101.
156. Schwartz JH et al: Carbonic anhydrase function and the epithelial organization of H^+ secretion in turtle urinary bladder. *J Clin Invest* 51:2653, 1972.
157. Schwartz WB et al: Acidification of the urine and increased ammonia excretion without change in acid-base equilibrium: Sodium reabsorption as stimulus to the acidifying process. *J Clin Invest* 34:673, 1955.
158. Schwartz WB et al: Role of anions in metabolic alkalosis and potassium deficiency. *N Engl J Med* 279:630, 1968.
159. Seldin DW et al: The role of sodium salts and adrenal steroids in the production of hypokalemic alkalosis. *Yale J Biol Med* 29:229, 1956.
160. Siegfried D et al: Influence of vitamin D on bicarbonate reabsorption, in Massry SG, Ritz E (eds): *Phosphate Metabolism.* New York, Plenum, 1978, p 395.
161. Simpson DP: Control of hydrogen ion homeostasis and renal acidosis. *Medicine* 50:503, 1971.
162. Skou JC: Enzymatic basis for active transport of Na^+ and K^+ across cell membranes. *Physiol Rev* 45:596, 1965.
163. Spark RF, Melby JC: Hypertension and low plasma renin activity: Presumptive evidence for mineralocorticoid excess. *Ann Intern Med* 75:831, 1971.
164. Stewart PM et al: Mineralocorticoid activity of liquorice: 11β-hydroxysteroid dehydrogenase. *Lancet* 2:821, 1987.
165. Stinebaugh BJ, Schloeder FX: Glucose-induced alkalosis in fasting subjects. *J Clin Invest* 51:1326, 1972.
166. Stokes JB: Ion transport by the cortical and outer medullary collecting tubule. *Kidney Int* 22:473, 1982.
167. Stokes JB: Consequences of potassium recycling in the renal medulla: Effects on ion transport by the medullary thick ascending limb of the loop of Henle. *J Clin Invest* 70:219, 1982.
168. Stokes JB et al: Heterogeneity of the rabbit collecting tubule: Localization of mineralocorticoid hormone action to the cortical portion. *Kidney Int* 20:340, 1981.
169. Stone DK et al: Chloride dependence of medullary collecting duct acidification. *Kidney Int* 23:239, 1982.
170. Stone DK et al: Anion dependence of medullary collecting duct acidification. *J Clin Invest* 71:1505, 1983.
171. Struyvenberg A et al: The role of chloride in hypokalemic alkalosis in the rat. *J Clin Invest* 44:326, 1965.
172. Suki WN et al: Effects of glucose on bicarbonate reabsorption in the dog kidney. *J Clin Invest* 54:1, 1974.
173. Tannen RL: The effect of uncomplicated potassium depletion on urine acidification. *J Clin Invest* 49:813, 1970.
174. Tannen RL: Relationship of renal ammonia production and potassium homeostasis. *Kidney Int* 11:453, 1977.
175. Tannen RL, Kunin AS: Effect of potassium on ammoniagenesis by renal mitochondria. *Am J Physiol* 231:44, 1976.
176. Trygstad CW et al: A sibship with Bartter's syndrome: Failure of total adrenalectomy to correct the potassium wasting. *Pediatrics* 44:234, 1969.
177. Ullrich KJ et al: Renal proximal tubular buffer-(glycodiazine) transport: Inhomogeneity of local transport rate dependence on sodium, effect of inhibitors and chronic adaptation. *Pfluegers Arch* 357:149, 1975.
178. Velasquez H et al: Luminal influences on potassium secretion: Chloride replacement with sulfate. *Am J Physiol* 242:F46, 1982.
179. Van Ypersele de Strihou C, Dieu J: Potassium deficiency acidosis in the dog: Effect of sodium and potassium balance on renal response to a chronic acid load. *Kidney Int* 11:335, 1977.
180. Verberckmoes R et al: Bartter's syndrome with hyperplasia of renal medullary cells: Successful treatment with indomethacin. *Kidney Int* 9:302, 1976.
181. Waldhausl W et al: Combined 17α- and 18-hydroxylase deficiency associated with complete male pseudohermaphroditism and hypoaldosteronism. *J Clin Endocrinol Metab* 46:236, 1978.
182. Wall BM et al: Importance of the correction of chronic metabolic alkalosis in the rat. *Am J Physiol* 253:F1031, 1987.
183. Warnock DG, Rector FC Jr.: Renal acidification mechanisms, in Brenner BM, Rector FC Jr (eds): *The Kidney,* 2d ed. Philadelphia, Saunders, 1981, p 440.
184. Warren MC et al: Digitalis toxicity II: The effect of metabolic alkalosis. *Am Heart J* 75:358, 1968.
185. Welbourne TC, Francoeur D: Influence of aldosterone on renal ammonia production. *Am J Physiol* 233:E56, 1977.
186. Wistrand PJ, Kinne R: Carbonic anhydrase activity of isolated brush-border and basal-lateral membranes of renal tubular cells. *Pfluegers Arch* 370:121, 1977.
187. Wright FS et al: Potassium secretion by distal tubule after potassium adaptation. *Am J Physiol* 221:437, 1971.

CHAPTER 30

Respiratory acidosis and alkalosis

F. John Gennari

The partial pressure of CO_2 (P_{CO_2}) in the body fluids is normally maintained by a precise balance between the body's CO_2 production and CO_2 excretion via the lungs. The regulatory system that maintains arterial P_{CO_2} at approximately 40 mmHg involves chemoreceptors located in the brain stem that perceive changes in pH induced by changes in arterial P_{CO_2}.[21,171] The receptors signal changes in alveolar ventilation ($\dot{V}_E$) via efferent nerves to the muscles of respiration. (See Chap. 8 for a full discussion of this regulatory system.) Minute-to-minute changes in CO_2 production are signaled to this system and appropriate changes in CO_2 excretion occur as a result of changes in alveolar ventilation. When this normal regulatory system is disrupted, arterial P_{CO_2} deviates from normal and the respiratory acid-base disturbances are initiated. Respiratory acidosis is produced by CO_2 retention, leading to *hypercapnia,* i.e., an elevation in arterial P_{CO_2}. Respiratory alkalosis is produced by hyperventilation, leading to a reduction in arterial P_{CO_2} (*hypocapnia*).

When arterial P_{CO_2} increases or decreases, immediate changes in blood pH occur; the acid-base changes titrate body buffers, which results in a change in bicarbonate concentration. This buffer response begins as soon as arterial P_{CO_2} is altered, and its effect on bicarbonate concentration is fully manifest within 15 to 30 min. If the alteration in arterial P_{CO_2} is sustained for more than 6 to 12 h, renal mechanisms induce far larger changes in bicarbonate concentration. The impact of the renal response on bicarbonate levels in the blood is maximal within 3 to 5 days; renal effects lead to production of a new steady state. Because of the two-tiered response to primary alterations in arterial P_{CO_2} (i.e., tissue buffers and renal response), the respiratory acid-base disorders are subdivided into *acute* and *chronic* phases.

Acute respiratory acidosis or alkalosis involves the immediate tissue buffer response to hyper- or hypocapnia; chronic respiratory acidosis or alkalosis involves the renal response. Although both the acute and the chronic response to the respiratory acid-base disturbances normally result in amelioration of the acidemia or alkalemia produced by the primary change in arterial P_{CO_2}, in neither instance is the blood pH returned completely to normal. In respiratory acidosis, acidemia persists; in respiratory alkalosis, alkalemia persists. It should be emphasized that this description of the respiratory acid-base disorders excludes those changes in arterial P_{CO_2} that occur in response to primary changes in plasma bicarbonate concentration (the metabolic acid-base disturbances). The expected changes induced by these disorders are discussed in Chaps. 25 and 29.

RESPIRATORY ACIDOSIS

PATHOPHYSIOLOGY

Respiratory acidosis is initiated by an increase in arterial P_{CO_2}. This change in arterial P_{CO_2} indicates that CO_2 excretion is insufficient to match CO_2 production without an increase in alveolar CO_2 concentration. The excretion of CO_2, which must balance CO_2 production in the steady state, is a function of $\dot{V}_E$ and the alveolar partial pressure of CO_2; CO_2 excreted $= (K)(\dot{V}_E)(P_{CO_2})$ (here, P_{CO_2} = *alveolar* partial CO_2 pressure). From this relationship it can be seen that whenever alveolar ventilation is insufficient to excrete the CO_2 produced by the body, alveolar P_{CO_2} rises until the product $(\dot{V}_E)(P_{CO_2})$ again equals the CO_2 production. Because arterial CO_2 is the source of alveolar CO_2, it follows that alveolar P_{CO_2} rises in parallel with arterial P_{CO_2}. Failure to achieve a new steady state (as, for example, in apnea) results in a relentless increase in arterial P_{CO_2} until lethal hypoxia and acidosis ensue. Thus, sustained hypercapnia represents a new equilibrium between CO_2 production and excretion. In this new steady state, the reduction in alveolar ventilation is offset by an increase in P_{CO_2}.

Hypercapnia occurs most commonly as a result of lung injury and a consequent impairment in CO_2 excretion. However, brain damage or pharmacologic depression, or damage to efferent nerves or to the muscles of respiration, can also lead to impaired CO_2 excretion and respiratory acidosis. Central to all forms of respiratory acidosis is a failure of alveolar ventilation and CO_2 excretion to increase in response to a rise in arterial P_{CO_2}. Increases in CO_2 production alone are not sufficient to overcome the normal ability of the lungs to increase alveolar ventilation.[11,100,247] An increase in CO_2 production in the face of fixed ventilation, however, can result in respiratory acidosis[59,114] (see Causes of Hypercapnia" below).

Failure of the lungs to excrete CO_2 normally can be subdivided into two types of ventilatory disorders.[297] The first, "pure" hypoventilation, occurs as a result of brainstem or neuromuscular dysfunction or restrictive lung disease. In this setting, the lung simply fails to move enough air in and out to exchange CO_2 and oxygen. As a result, arterial oxygen tension falls in proportion to the rise in P_{CO_2}. Usually, however, alveolar hypoventilation is the result of a disequilibrium between perfused and ventilated segments of a damaged lung (*ventilation-perfusion inequality*). In this setting, a fall in arterial P_{O_2} often precedes hypercapnia; when hypercapnia develops the reduction in P_{O_2} is proportionally greater than the rise in P_{CO_2}. With both types of ventilatory defects, however, hypoxemia is a concurrent finding when hypercapnia is present.

Secondary physiologic response

Acute respiratory acidosis

NATURE OF THE ADAPTIVE RESPONSE An increase in P_{CO_2} produces an instantaneous increase in H^+ activity (decrease in pH) in the body fluids. As indicated by a consideration of the Henderson equation (Table 30-1), an increase in P_{CO_2} from 40 to 80 mmHg, in the absence of any change in bicarbonate concentration, doubles blood H^+ activity, from 40 to 80 neq/liter (a decrease in pH from 7.4 to 7.1). Bicarbonate concentration, however, increases within minutes of an increase in P_{CO_2}, because a fraction of the hydrogen ions released by the dissociation of carbonic acid ($H_2CO_3 \rightleftharpoons H^+ + HCO_3^-$) combines with nonbicarbonate buffers, thereby producing new bicarbonate ions[172] (Fig. 30-1). The buffers participating in this reaction include hemoglobin and other intracellular buffers, as well as plasma proteins; of these, hemoglobin predominates. The buffer response of hemoglobin is linearly related to the change in pH induced by hypercapnia; 3 meq of new bicarbonate ions are produced by each millimole of hemoglobin per unit reduction in pH.[172] Plasma proteins have a similarly predictable buffer contribution. Other buffers are available in cells and in bone. In in vitro experiments, bone buffers do not appear to participate in the acute buffer response to respiratory acidosis.[39,40] Because the concentrations and characteristics of other intracellular buffers are not well defined, the buffer response to hypercapnia has been determined empirically from whole-body CO_2 titration curves in human beings and animals.[30,54,131,155]

The acute buffer response to hypercapnia is complete within 10 to 15 min after arterial P_{CO_2} increases; a steady-state response persists for at least 1 h in human beings.[30] In studies of longer duration in dogs, the acute steady-state response persists for 6 h or more.[54] The development of an acute steady state of respiratory acidosis reflects the fact that renal mechanisms require a longer period of time to develop sufficiently to affect serum bicarbonate concentration. Although some investigators have observed a decrease in urine pH and an increase in acid excretion within the first hour of exposure to respiratory acidosis,[18,32,45,86,205] the changes are small and have not uniformly been found to occur.[30,54] In addition to minor changes in acid excretion, acute expo-

TABLE 30-1 • Effect of hypercapnia on acid-base equilibrium

$$[H^+](\text{neq/liter}) = 24\left(\frac{P_{CO_2}\,(\text{mmHg})}{[HCO_3^-](\text{meq/liter})}\right)$$

	[H+], *neq/liter*	*pH*
NORMAL		
P_{CO_2} = 40 mmHg $[HCO_3^-]$ = 24 meq/liter	$24\left(\frac{40}{24}\right) = 40$	7.40
HYPERCAPNIA		
P_{CO_2} = 80 mmHg Immediate impact—no change in $[HCO_3^-]$(theoretical)	$24\left(\frac{80}{24}\right) = 80$	7.10
Acute, steady state	$24\left(\frac{80}{27}\right) = 71$	7.15
Chronic, steady state	$24\left(\frac{80}{38}\right) = 50$	7.30

P_{CO_2} = arterial P_{CO_2}.

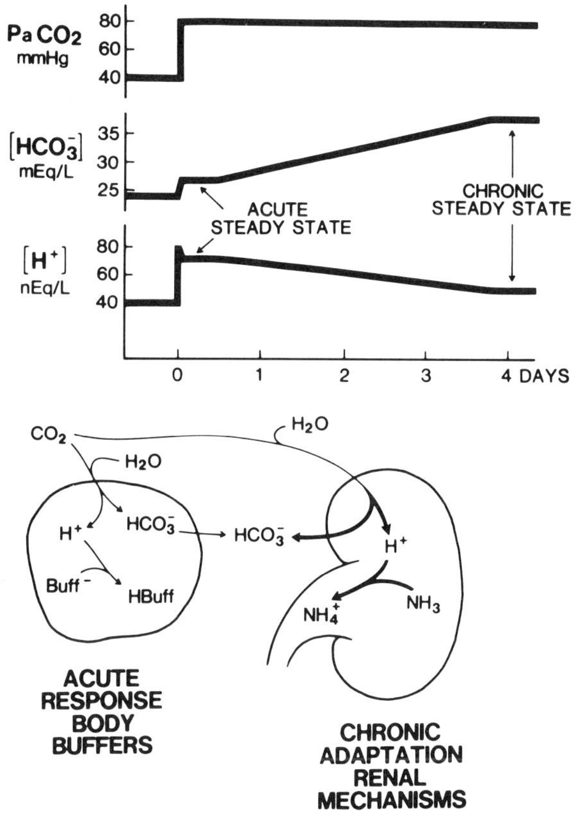

FIGURE 30-1 • Schematic representation of time course and mechanism of bicarbonate generation during adaptation to respiratory acidosis. The acute response is characterized by generation of new bicarbonate from hemoglobin and tissue buffers. During the period of adaptation to sustained hypercapnia, new bicarbonate is generated by increased acid excretion by the kidney.

sure to respiratory acidosis reduces organic acid production.[151] This effect is also minor, and does not contribute significantly to the protection of pH. Thus, the acute steady-state response is produced primarily by the buffer response of the tissues and blood to hypercapnia (Fig. 30-1).

ACUTE STEADY-STATE CHANGES IN PLASMA COMPOSITION In acute respiratory acidosis, blood H^+ activity increases in direct relation to the increase in arterial P_{CO_2}. For each mmHg increase in P_{CO_2}, $[H^+]$ increases by 0.7 to 0.8 neq/liter (Fig. 30-2). This relatively large $[H^+]$ increment reflects the modest increase in HCO_3^- concentration produced by titrating the body's buffers. As can be seen, up to an arterial P_{CO_2} of 90 mmHg, plasma bicarbonate concentration does not exceed 30 meq/liter in acute respiratory acidosis.

The response of the intact organism to acute respiratory acidosis differs notably from that seen when whole bood is titrated in vitro.[172] In vitro titration of blood with CO_2 leads to larger increments in plasma bicarbonate concentration, demonstrating the preponderant role of hemoglobin in buffering the acidity induced by hypercapnia. In the intact organism, the buffer response of hemoglobin is dissipated by diffusion of newly generated bicarbonate out of the vascular compartment into the large poorly buffered interstitial compartment. Although tissues other than red cells normally contribute to the buffer response, their participation does not completely offset the diffusion of hemoglobin-generated bicarbonate into the interstitial compartment.

Aside from the modest increase in bicarbonate concentration that occurs in acute respiratory acidosis, there are no major changes in serum composition. Despite the reduction in pH produced by respiratory acidosis, serum potassium concentration does not increase markedly.[3] Potassium concentration increases by only 0.1 meq/liter for each 0.1-unit decrement in pH in acute respiratory acidosis, a difference that is barely detectable. Thus, the finding of notable hyperkalemia ($[K^+] > 5.0$ meq/liter) in a patient with acute respiratory acidosis should prompt the physician to seek other causes for the high potassium. Respiratory acidosis is associated with a fall in blood lactate concentration and a small increase in plasma phosphorus concentration.[30] Although a small increase in sodium concentration (approximately 2 to 4 meq/liter) has been noted in experimental studies, this change is probably not detectable in the clinical setting. No changes in chloride, magnesium, or calcium concentration occur.

Chronic respiratory acidosis

NATURE OF THE ADAPTIVE RESPONSE The adaptive response to sustained hypercapnia hinges on changes in acid excretion, and on changes in bicarbonate and chloride reabsorption by the kidney. In response to hypercap-

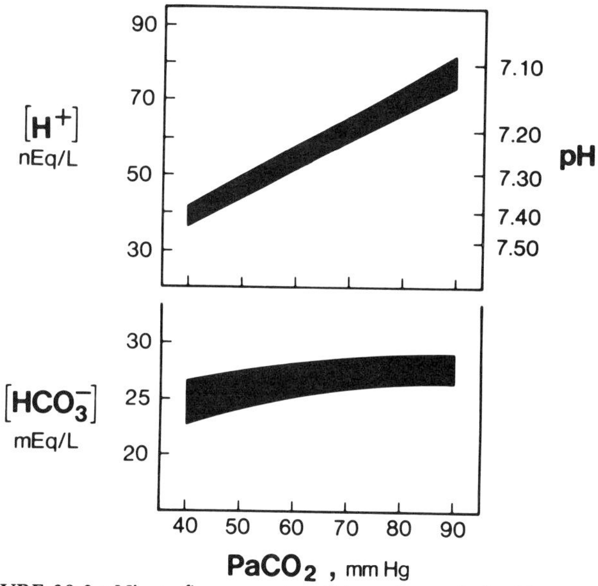

FIGURE 30-2 • Ninety-five percent confidence intervals for H^+ activity and serum $[HCO_3^-]$ in acute respiratory acidosis in human subjects. (From Brackett NC Jr et al: *N Engl J Med* 272:6, 1965.)

nia, the kidney generates HCO_3^- by increasing net acid (particularly ammonium) excretion, and also changes the pattern of bicarbonate reabsorption, so that the newly generated HCO_3^- is all reabsorbed.[53,249,254] This process is associated with a concomitant reduction in Cl^- reabsorption; therefore, Cl^- is lost in the urine during the adaptive process.[254] The mechanism by which these changes in renal function are triggered is unclear; present evidence suggests that hypercapnia per se, rather than acidemia, leads to the renal response.[170,173] Once initiated by hypercapnia, the renal adaptive response is unaffected by dietary sodium intake, by changes in body potassium stores, and by changes in aldosterone release.[162,176,221] In addition, concomitant hypoxemia (P_{O_2} = 45 to 55 mmHg) does not influence the renal response to hypercapnia.[251]

The changes in renal reabsorption and excretion described above are sufficient to exert an impact on plasma composition after 12 to 24 h of hypercapnia, but the full effect of the changes is not manifest until after 3 to 5 days of hypercapnia (Fig. 30-1). At this point a chronic steady-state response develops that persists for up to 2 months.[254] In the chronic steady state, plasma bicarbonate concentration is much higher for any given level of arterial P_{CO_2} than in acute respiratory acidosis. Nonetheless, the increase in plasma bicarbonate concentration is insufficient to return pH to control levels, and a mild acidemia persists.[254] Because renal generation of new bicarbonate is central to adaptation to chronic hypercapnia, the expected response does not occur in patients with end-stage renal disease.[97] As a result, severe acidemia persists with sustained hypercapnia; survival is limited in patients with renal failure.

CHRONIC STEADY-STATE CHANGES IN PLASMA COMPOSITION The steady-state relationship between arterial P_{CO_2} and serum bicarbonate concentration during chronic respiratory acidosis in dogs is shown in Fig. 30-3.[254] As can be seen, over the P_{CO_2} range from 40 to 90 mmHg, serum $[HCO_3^-]$ increases by approximately 3 meq/liter for each 10 mmHg increase in P_{CO_2}. Hydrogen ion activity ($[H^+]$) increases by 0.32 neq/liter for each mmHg increment in P_{CO_2}. Comparable data have been difficult to obtain in human subjects. However, studies of patients with sustained hypercapnia reveal a similar pattern.[31,67,72,76,235,287] In one such study, shown in Fig. 30-4, hydrogen ion activity increased by 0.24 neq/liter per mmHg increase in arterial P_{CO_2}. In contrast to dogs, however, in this study $[H^+]$ values in human beings overlap the normal range up to a P_{CO_2} of 60 to 70 mmHg.

In chronic respiratory acidosis, the increase in serum $[HCO_3^-]$ is coupled with a decrease in $[Cl^-]$. No notable changes occur in $[Na^+]$ or $[K^+]$, a finding which may prove useful for separating chronic respiratory acidosis from metabolic alkalosis. Although both disorders are characterized by an increase in bicarbonate and a decrease in chloride concentration, metabolic alkalosis is virtually always associated with hypokalemia (see Chap. 29). Of course, the pH is alkaline (> 7.45) in the latter disorder, whereas it is slightly acid (< 7.40) in chronic respiratory acidosis. No major changes occur in serum calcium, magnesium, phosphate, or lactate concentrations in chronic hypercapnia.

CLINICAL MANIFESTATIONS OF HYPERCAPNIA

Acute and chronic respiratory acidosis are virtually always associated with other adverse conditions. As noted earlier, hypoxemia invariably accompanies respiratory acidosis. Congestive heart failure, infection, confounding metabolic acid-base disturbances, and the superimposed effects on cardiovascular and cerebral function of a variety of drugs all make it difficult to attribute a particular manifestation of the clinical presentation specifically to hypercapnia. Information concerning the specific effects of hypercapnia comes mainly from studies in normal volunteers and experimental animals exposed to high levels of atmospheric CO_2. For the most part, these studies have been carried out during the acute adaptive response to hypercapnia; experimental data on the clinical effects of chronic hypercapnia are fragmentary.

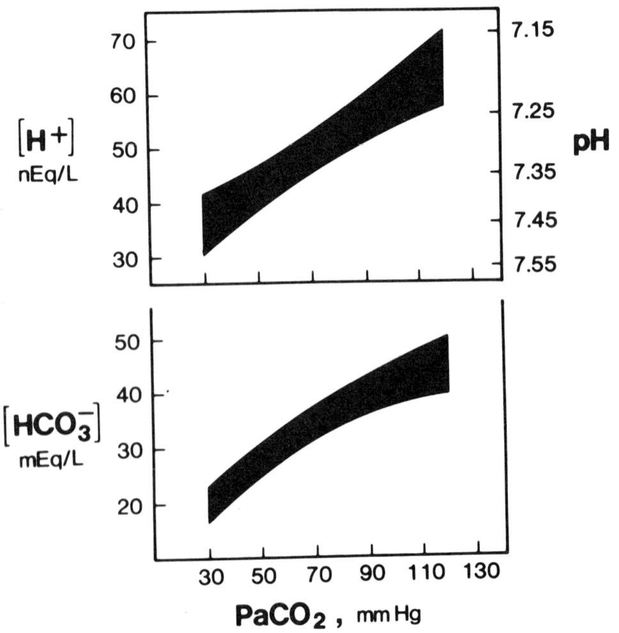

FIGURE 30-3 • Ninety-five percent confidence intervals for H^+ activity and serum $[HCO_3^-]$ in chronic respiratory acidosis in dogs. (From Schwartz WB et al: *J Clin Invest* 44:291, 1965.)

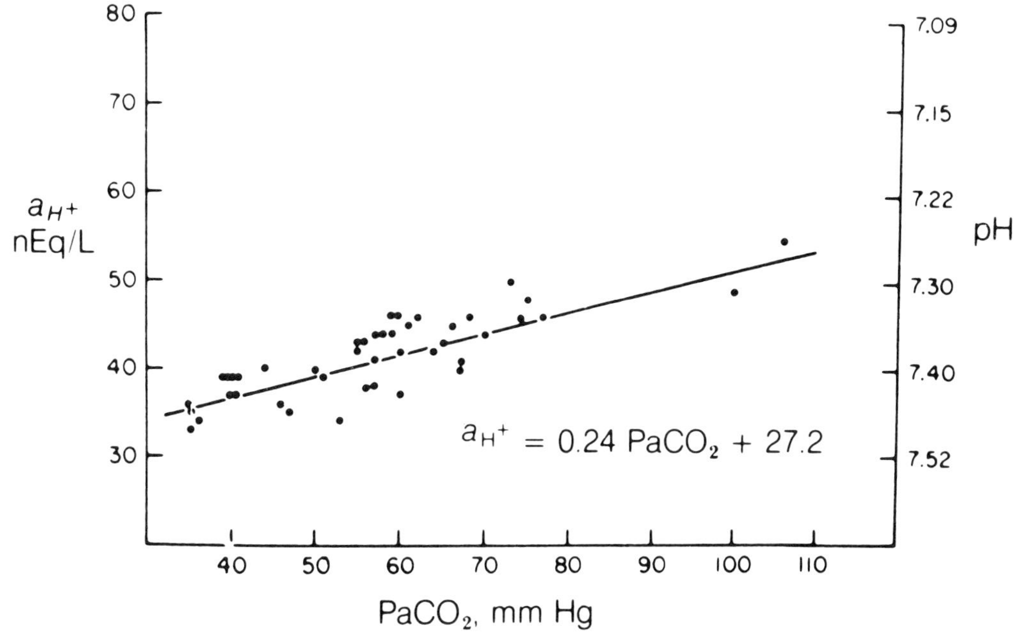

FIGURE 30-4 • Relationship between H^+ activity and serum [HCO_3^-] in chronic respiratory acidosis in human beings. Observations were made on patients with uncomplicated chronic respiratory acidosis. (From Brackett NC Jr et al: *N Engl J Med* 280:124, 1969.)

Acute hypercapnia

Cardiovascular effects

Acute hypercapnia invariably causes blood pressure to rise.[22,30,85,140,143,225,255] In human beings, increased cardiac output contributes variably to hypertension. In some studies, pulse rate and cardiac output increase so that total peripheral resistance actually falls.[225,255] In other studies, cardiac output increases little if at all, and total peripheral resistance increases.[143,225] In anesthetized dogs, acute hypercapnia decreases cardiac contractility, but cardiac output increases nonetheless on account of an increase in heart rate.[289] The latter effect and the increase in cardiac output are results of beta-adrenergic stimulation; they can be blocked by pharmacologic inhibition of the beta-adrenergic system.[9,289] In animal studies, acute hypercapnia increases coronary artery blood flow.[286]

Acute hypercapnia has two opposing effects on peripheral vessels. Hypercapnia leads to vasodilatation by directly influencing vascular smooth muscles; it produces vasoconstriction through stimulation of sympathoadrenal discharge.[147,172,194,225] The net effect of these opposing influences in most vascular beds ranges from mild vasodilatation to mild vasoconstriction.[139,194,225] An important exception is the cerebral vasculature. Cerebral vascular resistance falls and cerebral blood flow increases in direct relation to the increase in arterial P_{CO_2}, at levels up to 100 mmHg (Fig. 30-5).[236] In monkeys, cerebral blood flow doubles when arterial P_{CO_2} increases rapidly from 40 to 100 mmHg.[236] Cerebral blood flow in human subjects increases to a similar degree if arterial P_{CO_2} increases from 40 to 60 mmHg.[140] This marked cerebral vasodilatation may be one factor accounting for the head-

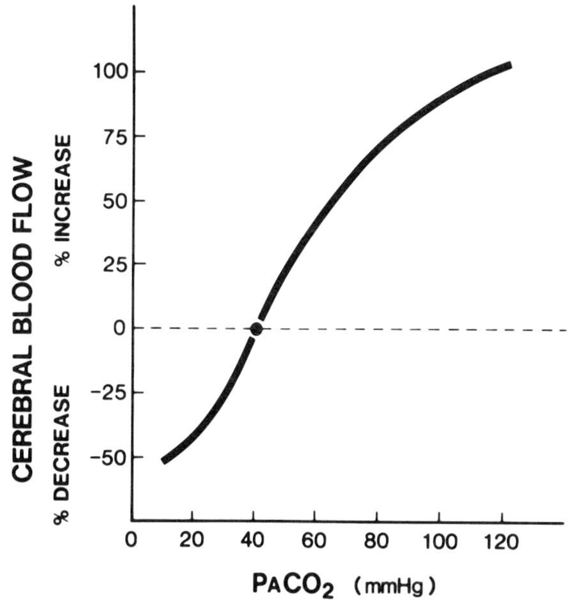

FIGURE 30-5 • Relationship between cerebral blood flow and alveolar P_{CO_2} during acute respiratory acidosis and alkalosis. Observations were made on anesthetized monkeys. (From Reivich M: *Am J Physiol* 206:25, 1964.)

ache that occurs with acute hypercapnia, as well as the occasional presence of papilledema.[178,208]

Renal vascular resistance falls and renal blood flow appears to increase slightly during exposure to low-level hypercapnia, but vascular resistance increases and blood flow falls below control values when arterial P_{CO_2} exceeds 70 mmHg.[22,23,142] Pulmonary vascular resistance is not affected by acute exposure to mild hypercapnia, but increases if arterial P_{CO_2} is abruptly increased to levels above 70 mmHg.[143] In experimental animals, acute hypercapnia results in an increase in blood flow to the gastric mucosa[256] and a decrease in pancreatic blood flow.[34] Hepatic arterial blood flow also drops, but this reduction is offset by an increase in portal venous blood flow.[129]

Endocrine and renal effects

Acute hypercapnia stimulates sympathoadrenal discharge. Receptor response to catecholamines is reduced in acute hypercapnia,[20] but the depressed response is offset by the profuse catecholamine secretion that is engendered.[172,282,302] The plasma concentrations of both norepinephrine and epinephrine increase; plasma corticosteroid levels increase as well.[255,282] Acute hypercapnia stimulates renin release via beta-adrenergic stimulation and results in an increase in aldosterone levels.[9] In addition, hypercapnia stimulates antidiuretic hormone (ADH) release[278] and reduces sodium and water excretion. The water retention is due in part to increased ADH release, but also appears to result from renal adrenergic stimulation.[22]

Central nervous system (CNS) effects

Acute hypercapnia is associated with moderate-to-marked discomfort and a feeling of breathlessness. When arterial P_{CO_2} quickly increases to above 60 mmHg, multiple CNS symptoms develop, including nausea and vomiting, headache, restlessness, confusion, loss of consciousness, and seizures.[30,141,243,255] A fine tremor characteristically develops, but asterixis is also seen.[141,255] These symptoms appear to be independent of hypoxia; they are roughly correlated with the magnitude of the acute rise in arterial P_{CO_2}. However, it should be emphasized that the correlation is weak, and tremendous individual variation is seen in the response. For example, when exposed to similar levels of arterial P_{CO_2}, some individuals become somnolent and others are extremely agitated.

The failure of the CNS to protect against acidity in this disorder is one explanation advanced to account for the notable CNS symptoms. In respiratory acidosis, the fall in arterial pH is closely reflected by a drop in cerebrospinal fluid (CSF) pH.[222,261] Studies in dogs and in human beings, moreover, suggest that the CSF buffer response to acute hypercapnia is, if anything, less than that seen in the blood.[26,243] Because CO_2 readily permeates the blood-brain barrier, elevations in arterial P_{CO_2} are reflected immediately in the CSF. The CSF contains fewer buffer substances than does the blood, and therefore the pH falls to a greater extent until bicarbonate can diffuse in to buffer the resultant acidosis. This process requires several hours.[26,243] Within several hours, CSF pH changes parallel those seen in blood with both acute and prolonged hypercapnia.[26,243,261] Whether changes in CSF pH or other factors are responsible for the CNS symptoms of acute respiratory acidosis, however, is unclear.

The increase in cerebral blood flow induced by acute hypercapnia leads to an increase in intracranial and intraocular hydrostatic pressure.[269] The pressure increases correlate directly with P_{CO_2}. Cerebral vasodilatation is evident in cut sections of the brain as well as with in situ observations of the pia mater.[13,75,294] The increase in blood flow occurs in all segments of the brain [42] and appears to be due solely to acidosis. Return of pH to normal levels by bicarbonate infusion reverses the vasodilatation.[146,294]

Chronic hypercapnia

Cardiovascular effects

Chronic hypercapnia in human beings is so intimately associated with cor pulmonale that it is difficult to obtain data on the isolated effects of sustained hypercapnia. In the few observations available, cardiac output and systemic arterial pressure appear to be in the normal range.[1,78] Pulmonary artery pressure is increased.[78] Few data are available concerning regional blood flow. Cerebral blood flow appears to remain increased, although the vasodilatation is less than is seen with a comparable degree of acute hypercapnia.[158,212]

Supraventricular and ventricular arrhythmias are extremely common in patients with chronic respiratory acidosis,[123,127,260] particularly in association with acute decompensation. With 72-hour monitoring, the incidence exceeded 90 percent in one group of patients with arterial P_{CO_2} levels greater than 50 mmHg.[123] The arrhythmias, however, correlate poorly with the level of P_{CO_2} or acidemia, and are more closely linked to hypoxemia.[127,260] The arrhythmias are probably due to multiple adverse influences, including hypoxemia, underlying heart disease (cor pulmonale), electrolyte abnormalities, sympathetic discharge, and medications (bronchodilators, digitalis). In the absence of heart disease or hypoxemia, even severe abrupt elevations in P_{CO_2} have very little influence on cardiac irritability.[7,30,85,242] Considerable evidence indicates that respiratory failure enhances the ability of digitalis to induce cardiac arrhythmias.[108,172] Again, this enhancement is more likely due to hypoxemia, electrolyte abnormalities, and increased catecholamine levels than to a specific effect of hypercapnia per se.

CNS effects

Chronic stable hypercapnia is associated with far fewer symptoms than acute hypercapnia. Patients with arterial P_{CO_2} levels ranging from 75 to as high as 110 mmHg have been reported to have no CNS signs or symptoms save for a fine tremor.[206] Nonetheless, CNS symptoms do develop in these patients, particularly in the face of superimposed acute changes in P_{CO_2}.[141,243] As in acute hypercapnia, the symptoms range from coma to delirium and correlate poorly with specific level of arterial P_{CO_2}.[141,243] In studies of normal dogs exposed to high atmospheric concentrations of CO_2 for prolonged periods of time, no major problems developed until arterial P_{CO_2} exceeded 100 mmHg.[254] Above this level a slight ataxia developed, and the dogs all refused food. Cerebrospinal fluid pH in chronic hypercapnia falls in parallel with blood pH.[26,243,261] No specific correlation is noted between CSF pH and CNS symptoms in chronic respiratory acidosis.[243]

TABLE 30-2 • Causes of acute respiratory acidosis

Airway obstruction
Aspiration
Laryngospasm
Severe bronchospasm
Obstructive sleep apnea
Circulatory catastrophes
Cardiac arrest
Severe pulmonary edema
Massive pulmonary embolism
CNS depression
General anesthesia
Sedative overdosage
Cerebral trauma or infarct
Central sleep apnea
Neuromuscular impairment
High-cervical cordotomy
Guillain-Barré syndrome
Myasthenic crisis
Botulism; tetanus
Hypokalemic myopathy
Familial hypokalemic periodic paralysis
Drugs and toxins
Ventilatory restriction
Pneumothorax
Hemothorax
Flail chest
Severe pneumonia
Infant/adult respiratory distress syndrome
Mechanical ventilation
Increased CO_2 production with fixed minute ventilation
Parenteral nutrition with high carbohydrate content
Sorbent-regenerative hemodialysis
Iatrogenic mishaps
Anesthesia equipment failures
CO_2 insufflation
Bronchoscopy

TABLE 30-3 • Causes of chronic respiratory acidosis

Airway obstruction
Chronic obstructive pulmonary disease
CNS depression
Chronic sedative overdosage
Methadone/heroin addiction
Primary alveolar hypoventilation (Ondine's curse)
Obesity-hypoventilation syndrome (Pickwickian syndrome)
Brain tumor
Bulbar poliomyelitis
Neuromuscular impairment
Muscular dystrophy
Multiple sclerosis
Amyotrophic lateral sclerosis
Diaphragmatic paralysis
Myxedema
Poliomyelitis
Primary myopathy
Ventilatory restriction
Kyphoscoliosis
Fibrothorax
Hydrothorax
Interstitial fibrosis
Severe chronic pneumonitis
Obesity

CAUSES OF HYPERCAPNIA

The causes of acute and chronic respiratory acidosis are listed in Tables 30-2 and 30-3. These are grouped under four general categories: airway obstruction, respiratory center depression, neuromuscular disorders, and restrictive lung disease. It is obvious, however, that in many instances factors from several of these categories contribute to the production of hypercapnia. The causes of respiratory acidosis are reviewed in depth by Madias and Cohen.[172]

Acute respiratory acidosis

Acute hypercapnia occurring in individuals without preexisting respiratory insufficiency is generally the result of a catastrophic event. Acute airway obstruction, sudden interference with neuromuscular function, overwhelming pneumonia or bronchospasm, pulmonary edema, drug-induced CNS depression, circulatory collapse, and cardiac arrest are examples of such events. In such cases, severe hypoxemia, rather than the acute hypercapnia itself, is the immediate threat to life. With total cessation of ventilation, arterial P_{CO_2} rises by between 3 and 5 mmHg/min.[85] Thus, 10 to 15 min. of apnea is required to develop severe hypercapnia; life-threatening hypoxemia occurs in several minutes. In fact, periods of apnea as long as 30 to 45 min. are tolerated if hypoxemia is prevented by suffusing the bronchial tree with 100% O_2, even when arterial P_{CO_2} rises as high as 250 mmHg.[7,85]

In patients with severe circulatory failure, CO_2 retention can result from an insufficient delivery rate of blood to the lungs. If ventilation is supported mechanically in this setting, assessment of arterial blood may fail to identify the hypercapnia, because the blood reaching the arterial tree will have excreted its excess CO_2.[5,296] The presence of hypercapnia can be readily detected by sampling central venous blood, which will show P_{CO_2} values 30 to 60 mmHg higher than those for arterial blood.[5] Aside from this unusual situation in which cardiovascular collapse is coupled with mechanical ventilatory assistance, arterial blood is the preferred source for assessing acid-base status.[94]

Acute hypercapnia occurring in the setting of pulmonary edema, pneumonia, bronchial asthma, or adult or infantile respiratory distress syndrome is a grave prognostic sign.[2,172,186,234,291] The hypoxemia induced by these problems usually leads to alveolar hyperventilation and hypocapnia (see "Respiratory Alkalosis" below). Drug-induced depression of the respiratory center sufficient to produce acute respiratory acidosis can occur with all general anesthetic agents (although nitrous oxide given alone may be an exception).[181] Fentanyl, a drug used for induction of anesthesia, can produce hypercapnia by inducing truncal rigidity and interfering with ventilator motion.[57] Drug overdosage with barbiturates, opiates, glutethimide, ethchlorvynol, or large quantities of ethanol can result in respiratory depression sufficient to produce hypercapnia.[172] By contrast, most other sedatives and tranquilizers (e.g., meprobamate, benzodiazepines, tricyclic antidepressants, thorazine) do not produce respiratory acidosis in normal individuals even when taken in toxic amounts. However, if these drugs are administered in combination with the first group of drugs they have a significant additive effect; severe respiratory depression may occur with smaller amounts than would otherwise be required to produce respiratory acidosis. In patients with preexisting chronic respiratory acidosis, acute superimposed hypercapnia can occur after the use of any of these sedatives and tranquilizing agents.[46,198,199]

Interference with neuromuscular function can be induced by drugs or toxins, can result from severe neuromuscular disorders, or can come from severe hypokalemia.[56] The administration of paralyzing drugs such as curare or succinylcholine can readily produce respiratory paralysis and apnea. Ingestion of organophosphorus compounds that inhibit cholinesterase activity can produce the same result. In addition, respiratory paralysis has been observed in association with administration of certain antibiotics that block neuromuscular junctions. These include the aminoglycosides, polymyxin, bacitracin, and colistin.[215,303] In virtually all reported cases, however, the antibiotics were only a contributing factor. Underlying myasthenic syndromes or the use of paralyzing agents in anesthesia usually also contributed to the impairment in respiration. Severe hypokalemia (serum potassium less than 2.0 meq/liter) leads to an ascending paralysis which can eventually impede respiration. Although hyperkalemia also interferes with muscle function, cardiac arrhythmias usually intervene before respiratory paralysis occurs. Thus, hypercapnia (except in the setting of cardiac arrest) is not usually a feature of hyperkalemia. An exception to this rule is the patient with end-stage renal disease. In such patients, severe hyperkalemia often presents as an ascending paralysis before any life-threatening cardiac arrhythmia occurs.

Severe neuromuscular disorders such as Guillain-Barré syndrome, myasthenia crisis, and amyotrophic lateral sclerosis can all eventually lead to respiratory acidosis. Head or spinal cord trauma can impede ventilation by CNS depression or interruption of nerve transmission. Damage to the chest wall (flail chest), acute hemothorax or pneumothorax, thermal injury to the airways, and severe smoke inhalation can all impede ventilation and lead to respiratory acidosis.[172]

Patients maintained on mechanical ventilators that are improperly adjusted can, of course, develop respiratory acidosis. Acute respiratory acidosis can also occur in patients whose minute ventilation is fixed by a mechanical ventilator when CO_2 production increases.[59,130] When parenteral nutrition is instituted in such patients, CO_2 production may increase dramatically. Administration of large carbohydrate loads (> 2000 kcal/day) to semistarved patients increases the respiratory quotient from approximately 0.8 to between 1.2 and 1.3. Thus, CO_2 production can increase by as much as 40 to 50 percent even in the absence of an increase in oxygen consumption.[11] In patients who are breathing spontaneously and not severely hypercapnic, this increase in CO_2 production is simply balanced by an increase in alveolar ventilation, with little or no change in arterial P_{CO_2}.[11]

The sorbent regenerative bath used in some forms of hemodialysis is another source of CO_2 that can lead to respiratory acidosis in patients maintained at a fixed alveolar ventilation rate.[114] With sorbent regenerative hemodialysis, fresh dialysis bath fluid is regenerated continuously during dialysis by passage through a cartridge containing urease, anion and cation exchangers, and activated charcoal. Large amounts of CO_2 are produced in the cartridge by the breakdown of urea to ammonium and carbonate, and by the addition of hydrogen ions to the dialysate by cation exchange. The CO_2 crosses the dialysis membrane and enters the venous circulation of the patient. As in the case of increased CO_2 production from carbohydrate feeding, no change in arterial P_{CO_2} occurs in patients dialyzed by this technique whose ventilation can increase normally in response to the added CO_2. Severe respiratory acidosis, however, can ensue rapidly in patients whose alveolar ventilation rate is fixed by a mechanical ventilator.[114]

Malfunction of anesthetic equipment has also led to acute hypercapnia. The disorder is particularly dangerous in this setting because severe acidosis can develop rapidly without any specific symptoms. In one instance, hypercapnia resulted from the use of a rebreathing anesthesia system from which CO_2 was not removed because the sodium hydroxide had been exhausted.[65] In another, the nitrous oxide line had been inadvertently connected to the central CO_2 supply.[145] The use of a bronchoscope large enough, relative to the bronchial tree, to obstruct air flow has also led to hypercapnia in pediatric patients.[229] Peritoneal insufflation with CO_2 for peritoneoscopy transiently increases arterial P_{CO_2} in anesthetized patients as well, on average by about 5 mmHg.[117]

As discussed in Chap. 29, severe metabolic alkalosis can lead to marked hypercapnia. Arterial P_{CO_2} levels in excess of 70 mmHg have been reported in this acid-base disorder.[116] It is occasionally difficult to identify the primary disorder in these patients. The presence of notable alkalemia (pH > 7.45) points to metabolic alkalosis as the problem; it is verified by the restoration of normal arterial P_{CO_2} levels after correction of the metabolic alkalosis. Because hypercapnia is part of the normal adaptive response to metabolic alkalosis, an elevated arterial P_{CO_2} level in this setting is not considered to be respiratory acidosis (see Chap. 29).

Chronic respiratory acidosis

In animals, when hypercapnia is sustained for more than 3 to 5 days, a chronic steady-state response develops.[254] Thus, any of the causes for acute respiratory acidosis discussed above can also cause chronic respiratory acidosis if they produce a sufficiently protracted elevation in P_{CO_2}. The most common cause for chronic respiratory acidosis is chronic obstructive lung disease. In this disorder, respiratory acidosis is the end stage of a long-term process of progressive alveolar destruction.

Hypoxemia always precedes the development of hypercapnia in patients with chronic obstructive lung disease, and is invariably present when respiratory acidosis becomes manifest. Typically, hypercapnia first develops in these patients in the setting of intercurrent infection or congestive heart failure. Once hypercapnia develops, however, it often persists. Sustained hypercapnia eventually results in a decrease in the ventilatory response to inhaled CO_2.[89,118] The depressed response is presumably related to the fact that $[HCO_3^-]$ in the CSF and brain tissue is elevated in chronic hypercapnia. The high intracerebral $[HCO_3^-]$ minimizes the fall in pH induced by a superimposed increase in P_{CO_2}.[118] Because the respiratory center is less sensitive to increments in P_{CO_2}, acute hypercapnia can be induced readily in these patients by the injudicious use of sedatives or oxygen (which removes another stimulus to maintain ventilation, hypoxemia).

Although chronic obstruction by disease is the most common cause of chronic respiratory acidosis, CO_2 retention can also occur in severe long-standing restrictive disease.[172] However, the more common disorder seen in restrictive lung disease is mild chronic respiratory alkalosis (see "Causes of Hypocapnia" under "Respiratory Alkalosis" below).

Primary alveolar hypoventilation (Ondine's curse) and the obesity-hyperventilation syndrome (Pickwickian syndrome) are two unusual causes of chronic hypercapnia. In the first disorder, the responsiveness of the CNS to inhaled CO_2 is lacking.[188,240] In most reported cases, the defect appears to be acquired, usually appearing after the third decade of life.[188,240] In rare instances it occurs in infants.[188] Arterial P_{CO_2} levels in the disorder vary widely, but are generally only midly elevated (50 to 55 mmHg). In Pickwickian syndrome the CNS is again less sensitive to CO_2, but the diminished responsiveness appears to be coupled with impaired chest wall mechanics secondary to obesity. Hypercapnia is generally mild in this disorder as well, although decompensation and severe respiratory acidosis can occur.[191]

Drug-induced respiratory depression can occur as a chronic disorder in individuals on methadone maintenance.[180,250] Arterial P_{CO_2} levels have been demonstrated to be mildly increased prior to ingestion of the daily methadone dose. Similar, although less well documented, chronic respiratory depression probably occurs in heroin and morphine addicts.[252]

Chronic hypercapnia may occur as a complication of a variety of neuromuscular disorders, including poliomyelitis, multiple sclerosis, amyotrophic lateral sclerosis, and muscular dystrophy. Kyphoscoliosis may also produce chronic hypercapnia. Severe uncontrolled myxedema is associated with chronic hypercapnia.[183,293] In this disorder hypercapnia is thought to occur as a result of impairment of chest wall muscle function and a decreased central responsiveness to CO_2.[183]

DIAGNOSIS

Respiratory acidosis may be suspected on clinical grounds, but the diagnosis is dependent on laboratory measurements of arterial pH and P_{CO_2} (or pH and total CO_2 content). The finding of a pH less than 7.4 in conjunction with an elevation in P_{CO_2} establishes the presence of respiratory acidosis. On the basis of experimental observations described earlier, clinical rules of thumb

TABLE 30-4 • **Clinical rules of thumb for evaluating respiratory acid-base disorders**

Disorder	$[H^+]$	$[HCO_3^-]$	Anion gap*
Respiratory acidosis			
Acute	7–8 neq/liter increase per 10 mmHg increment in P_{CO_2}†	Ranges from 24–30 meq/liter	Normal
Chronic	2–3 neq/liter increase per 10 mmHg increment in P_{CO_2}	3–4 meq/liter increase per 10 mmHg increment in P_{CO_2}	Normal
Respiratory alkalosis			
Acute	7–8 neq/liter decrease per 10 mmHg decrement in P_{CO_2}	2 meq/liter decrease per 10 mmHg decrement in P_{CO_2}	Normal
Chronic	Variable; dependent on pre-alkalosis HCO_3^-; normal: 4–5 neq/liter decrease per 10 mmHg decrement in P_{CO_2}	4 meq/liter decrease per 10 mmHg decrement in P_{CO_2}	Increases by 2–4 meq/liter

* $[Na^+] - ([Cl^-] + [HCO_3^-])$; normal value = 7–12 meq/liter.
† P_{CO_2} = arterial P_{CO_2}.

have been developed to evaluate whether acute or chronic respiratory acidosis is present (Table 30-4). Once the presence of respiratory acidosis is established, these rules should be used to determine, for the observed arterial P_{CO_2}, whether the pH and bicarbonate concentration are consistent with simple acute or chronic respiratory acidosis or whether they indicate the presence of a mixed acid-base disturbance (see Chap. 31).

Acute respiratory acidosis

In acute respiratory acidosis, blood H^+ activity increases by 7 to 8 neq/liter for each 10 mmHg increment in P_{CO_2}. Serum $[HCO_3^-]$ increases only slightly; even with severe acute respiratory acidosis, $[HCO_3^-]$ should be less than 30 meq/liter. Evaluating whether the serum bicarbonate concentration is between 24 and 30 meq/liter obviates the need to carry out any mathematical analysis, and is the simplest way to determine whether the acid-base data are consistent with acute respiratory acidosis. As noted earlier, only minor changes occur in serum sodium and potassium concentrations in acute respiratory acidosis. Thus, the concentrations of serum electrolytes, Na^+, K^+, Cl^-, and HCO_3^- should all be essentially within normal limits in this disorder. The unmeasured anion concentration, or "anion gap" ($[Na^+] - ([Cl^-] + [HCO_3^-])$), is also within normal limits. If serum pH and bicarbonate concentration deviate widely from the expected values, or if the anion gap is increased, another acid-base disorder is present (see Chap. 25). The most common disorder occurring in association with acute respiratory acidosis is a metabolic acidosis with an increased anion gap. The presence of this confounding disorder is easily identified if the serum bicarbonate concentration is lower than predicted and the anion gap is increased.

It should be emphasized that the rules of thumb summarized in Table 30-4 are only guides; undue attention should not be given to minor deviations from expected values. In addition, the finding that values lie within the guidelines does not completely exclude the presence of mixed acid-base disturbances. In rare instances, a fortuitous interaction between several coexisting acid-base disturbances can lead to values consistent with a single acid-base disturbance (see "Chronic Respiratory Acidosis" below).[10] Attention should be paid to the clinical setting and the evolution of the disorder as treatment is given.

Chronic respiratory acidosis

In chronic respiratory acidosis, blood H^+ activity increases by 2 to 3 neq/liter and serum $[HCO_3^-]$ increases by 3 to 4 meq/liter for each 10 mmHg increment in arterial P_{CO_2}. The latter rule is the simpler to use because it does not require converting the measured pH to hydrogen ion activity. For example, a patient with an arterial P_{CO_2} of 60 mmHg should have an increase in bicarbonate concentration of 6 to 8 meq/liter in uncomplicated chronic respiratory acidosis. Serum $[Na^+]$ and $[K^+]$ are normal in chronic respiratory acidosis, and the increase in $[HCO_3^-]$ is counterbalanced by a fall in $[Cl^-]$ (Fig. 30-6). The anion gap is normal. If the pH and bicarbonate concentration deviate widely from the expected values, or if the anion gap is increased, then the data cannot be explained by chronic respiratory acidosis alone, and a complicating acid-base disturbance must be present.

Perhaps the most common coexisting acid-base disturbance in patients with chronic respiratory acidosis is superimposed acute respiratory acidosis. Unfortunately, the rules of thumb for acute respiratory acidosis do not strictly apply when an acute increase in P_{CO_2} is added to chronic respiratory acidosis.[105] Because the bicarbonate concentration is higher than normal in chronic respiratory acidosis, the effect of an acute increase in P_{CO_2} on

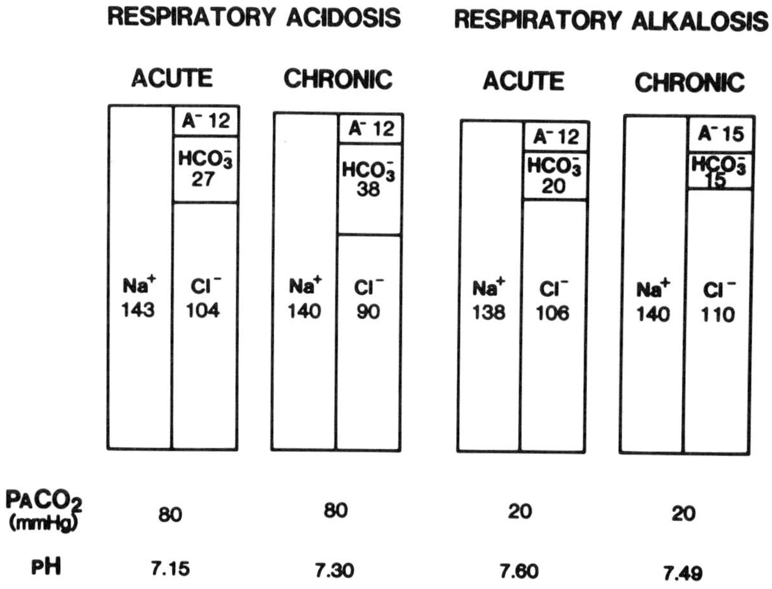

FIGURE 30-6 • Serum electrolytes, pH, and arterial P_{CO_2} (Pa_{CO_2}) in acute and chronic respiratory acidosis and alkalosis.

hydrogen ion activity is less[4,105] (Fig. 30-7). The distinction between acute and chronic components of respiratory acidosis is often difficult to make solely from laboratory data. The specific diagnosis depends on a clinical assessment of the case under consideration.

The nonrespiratory acid-base disorder most commonly associated with chronic respiratory acidosis is metabolic alkalosis.[19] Both disorders increase bicarbonate concentration and decrease chloride concentration, and both are associated with an increase in P_{CO_2}. In metabolic alkalosis, however, the pH is usually greater than 7.45 and hypokalemia is almost invariably present. When chronic respiratory acidosis is complicated by superimposed metabolic alkalosis, the pH rises to normal or to

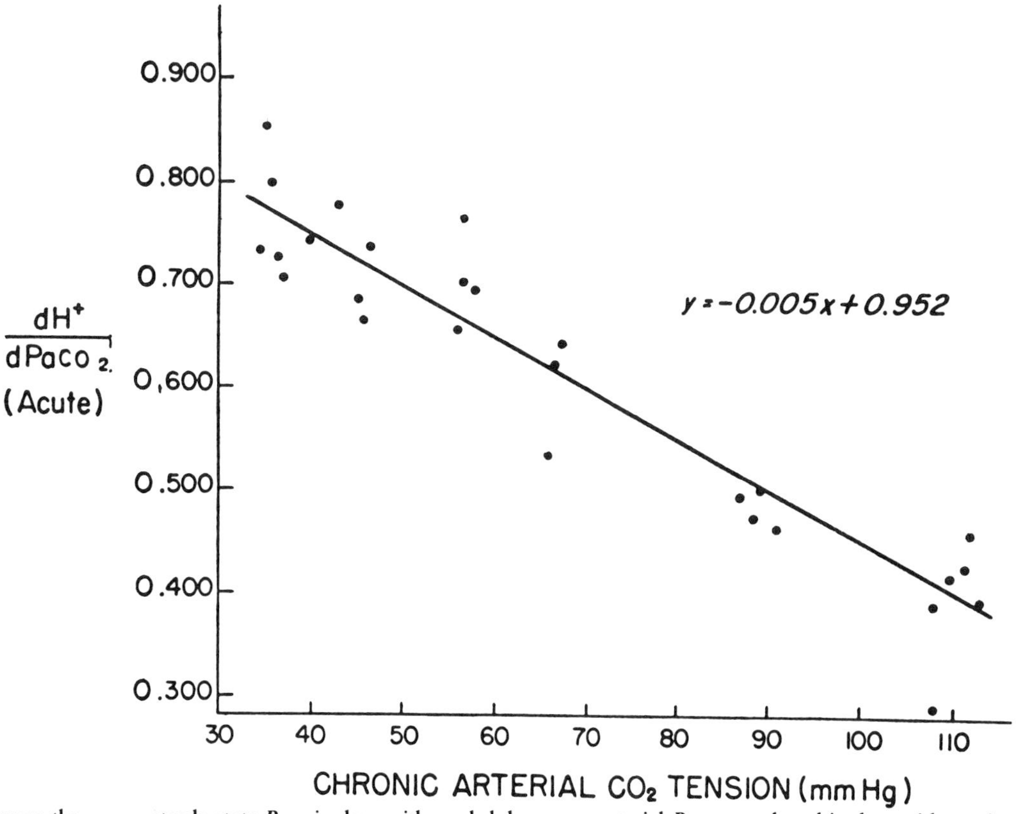

FIGURE 30-7 • Relationship between the change in H^+ activity per unit acute change in arterial P_{CO_2} ($d[H^+]/dPa_{CO_2}$) and chronic steady-state P_{CO_2} in dogs with graded degrees of chronic respiratory acidosis. The acute observations were made 30 to 60 min after arterial P_{CO_2} was altered in dogs with varying degrees of chronic hypercapnia. (From Goldstein MB et al: *J Clin Invest* 50:208, 1971.)

TABLE 30-5 • Evolution of triple acid-base disorder with fortuitous resemblance to chronic respiratory acidosis

1. Chronic respiratory acidosis (CRA)
   P_{CO_2} = 55 mmHg
   $[HCO_3^-]$ = 31 meq/liter
   $[H^+]$ = 43 neq/liter
   pH = 7.37
2. CRA + metabolic alkalosis
   P_{CO_2} = 59 mmHg
   $[HCO_3^-]$ = 38 meq/liter
   $[H^+]$ = 37 neq/liter
   pH = 7.43
3. CRA + metabolic alkalosis + acute respiratory acidosis
   P_{CO_2} = 75 mmHg
   $[HCO_3^-]$ = 38 meq/liter
   $[H^+]$ = 48 neq/liter
   pH = 7.32

Note: P_{CO_2} = arterial P_{CO_2}.

alkaline levels. Identifying the presence of this complicating disorder can sometimes be difficult. Table 30-5 demonstrates that the combined effects of acute and chronic respiratory acidosis coupled with metabolic alkalosis can fortuitously lead to blood acid-base values that are consistent with uncomplicated chronic respiratory acidosis. This combination of events is extremely common in patients with chronic respiratory insufficiency who require hospitalization. This "triple" acid-base disturbance is usually uncovered when arterial P_{CO_2} is reduced to the chronic stable level by therapy.

MANAGEMENT

The primary goal of therapy in respiratory acidosis is to improve alveolar ventilation and thereby to return arterial P_{CO_2} to as near normal as possible. Reducing P_{CO_2} is the most rapid and direct way to correct the associated acidemia; attention should therefore be directed primarily at improving pulmonary function, rather than administering alkali to improve pH. This general approach to management applies to both acute and chronic respiratory acidosis. Because of differences in the adaptive response, however, and the greater difficulty in reducing P_{CO_2} in chronic respiratory acidosis, specific management issues for the two disorders are discussed separately below.

Acute respiratory acidosis

In patients with acute respiratory acidosis, immediate attention to pulmonary function is critical. The physician should determine rapidly whether large airway obstruction is present, and relieve it as promptly as possible. If fluid accumulation or bronchospasm is responsible for the ventilatory impairment, immediate treatment with diuretics or bronchodilators should be instituted. If diuretic therapy is ineffective in removing fluid, treatment with dialysis or isolated ultrafiltration should be undertaken to relieve pulmonary congestion.[98,263] In patients with acute respiratory failure due to chronic bronchitis or asthma, short-term steroid therapy is of proven benefit.[4,79] If pulmonary infection is contributing to respiratory failure, appropriate antibiotic therapy should be started promptly.

As noted earlier, the greatest threat to life in acute respiratory acidosis is hypoxemia and not hypercapnia. Oxygen administration carries no risk of worsening hypercapnia in uncomplicated acute respiratory acidosis (see below for problems in patients with chronic respiratory acidosis), and should be administered immediately if hypoxemia is severe. If conservative means fail to correct hypoxemia and hypercapnia promptly, intubation and external ventilatory assistance are indicated.[172]

Given the body's buffer response to acute hypercapnia, severe acidemia (pH $<$ 7.10) would be expected only if arterial P_{CO_2} exceeds 100 mmHg (see Table 30-1)—a rare event. In one retrospective analysis of acute respiratory failure, pH values below 7.10 occurred in fewer than 1 percent of the cases.[152] Some workers have advocated intravenous bicarbonate administration when acidosis is severe.[152] It is difficult to assess the specific impact of this treatment in the cases in which it has been used, however, because arterial P_{CO_2} was also reduced. If a complicating metabolic acidosis is present, then bicarbonate administration is appropriate. Bicarbonate therapy entails the risk of volume overload and further embarrassment of alveolar ventilation due to fluid accumulation. It is clear that the first approach to therapy should be to reduce P_{CO_2}, if possible.

When severe acute respiratory acidosis occurs as a complication of bronchial asthma (or acute bronchospasm from any cause), bicarbonate administration appears to have a beneficial effect if bronchospasm cannot be relieved promptly with bronchodilator therapy.[196,197] In the cases in which bicarbonate administration has proved helpful, arterial blood pH has generally been below 7.00 and P_{CO_2} has been greater than 100 mmHg. As noted earlier, acidemia blunts the response of tissues to adrenergic stimulation. Administration of sufficient bicarbonate to increase pH to above 7.2 appears to improve the bronchodilatory response to administered epinephrine.[196,197] It cannot be emphasized too strongly, however, that bicarbonate therapy should not be a routine part of the treatment of asthma, since in most instances a respiratory alkalosis is present[185,186,203] (see "Causes of Hypocapnia" under "Respiratory Alkalosis" below). With respiratory alkalosis, bicarbonate administration serves only to exacerbate the existing alkalemia.

Bicarbonate therapy has also been advocated to stabilize pH in patients with status asthmaticus in whom the arterial P_{CO_2} cannot be lowered without risk of serious barotrauma.[189] In such patients bicarbonate administration allows the physician to decrease ventilation and increase P_{CO_2} transiently without exacerbating the acidemia, while other treatment modalities are being used to relieve bronchospasm. There is no evidence that nonbicarbonate buffers, such as tromethamine, have any place in the management of acute respiratory acidosis.[172]

Rapidly reducing P_{CO_2} could theoretically produce a sudden increase in pH that induces CNS complications and cardiac arrythmias.[36] There is no evidence in human beings to indicate that the potential for CNS involvement or arrythmias is a significant risk in the clinical setting of acute respiratory acidosis. Even in cases in which the initial arterial P_{CO_2} is greater than 100 mmHg, rapid correction of P_{CO_2} resulted in no CNS or cardiac complications.[152,197]

Chronic respiratory acidosis

In patients with stable chronic respiratory acidosis, reduction in P_{CO_2} is a long-term management problem. Treatment of fluid accumulation, infection, and bronchospasm is needed continuously in order to maximize the function of the diseased lung. Sedation, even with mild tranquilizers such as diazepam or chlordiazepoxide, should be avoided, as tranquilizers may impair ventilatory drive and exacerbate hypercapnia.[46,198,199] Ventilatory drive may also be impaired and hypercapnia exacerbated by the development of a complicating metabolic alkalosis due to diuretic administration or vomiting.[19,104,193] If fluid accumulation and metabolic alkalosis are concurrent problems, then the use of the diuretic acetazolamide may be helpful.[19,193] This agent is an inhibitor of carbonic anhydrase activity, and results in a sodium bicarbonate diuresis. Thus, acetazolamide decreases plasma bicarbonate concentration and pH as well as extracellular fluid (ECF) volume. The fall in pH should help to stimulate ventilation.[19,104,193] Alternatively, bicarbonate concentration can be reduced by ammonium chloride or arginine monohydrochloride administration. Both carry attendant risks: the first produces gastric irritation and can lead to ammonia toxicity in susceptible individuals; arginine monohydrochloride can produce severe hyperkalemia if hepatic or renal function is impaired.[41] Bicarbonate concentration can be reduced most directly by the administration of hydrochloric acid. The limitation of this approach is the volume of fluid needed to deliver sufficient acid. By using a central vein in an intensive care setting, the concentration of hydrochloric acid can safely be increased to as high as 250 m*M*.[33] In the absence of metabolic alkalosis, however, there is no evidence that acidifying agents have any specific benefit. If a diuretic agent is needed, furosemide, bumetanide, and ethacrynic acid are all more potent diuretics than acetazolamide.

The administration of oxygen at low levels (< 4 liters/min) to patients with stable chronic hypercapnia has become an important adjunct to long-term therapy.[201,206] This treatment, however, has a finite potential for further exacerbating the hypercapnia, particularly in patients whose hypercapnia is, for other reasons, acutely decompensated.[73] As noted earlier, patients with chronic hypercapnia have a blunted (or no) ventilatory response to further increases in P_{CO_2}. During episodes of acute decompensation, it appears that the major stimulus to increased ventilatory drive is the worsening hypoxemia that accompanies the decompensation. Administering oxygen to such patients without providing ventilatory assistance commonly leads to an increase in P_{CO_2},[27,73] and may precipitate coma and respiratory arrest. Patients particularly prone to this complication are those with more severe acidosis and hypoxemia.[27] Thus, oxygen administration without ventilatory support in such patients should be undertaken only if blood gases and ventilatory status are closely monitored.

Rapid reduction in arterial P_{CO_2} to normal levels in patients with moderate or severe chronic respiratory acidosis, or in patients with combined metabolic alkalosis and respiratory acidosis, may produce severe alkalemia. Simple computation, using the Henderson equation, indicates that blood pH exceeds 7.60 whenever the arterial P_{CO_2} falls below the serum bicarbonate concentration. Thus, in patients with bicarbonate levels above 40 meq/liter, abrupt reduction of the P_{CO_2} level to 40 mmHg or less leads to a level of alkalemia at which seizures and cardiac arrythmias may occur. Even if sufficient chloride is available, several hours may elapse before the serum bicarbonate concentration falls in response to the reduction in P_{CO_2}. In patients with a low chloride intake, however, the bicarbonate concentration remains elevated after correction of chronic hypercapnia, and a posthypercapnia metabolic alkalosis develops[253] (see Chap. 29). Abrupt reductions in P_{CO_2} in patients with chronic hypercapnia can also produce hypophosphatemia due to a shift of phosphate into cells, an effect that may contribute to morbidity.[150]

In addition to the use of mechanical ventilators to improve pulmonary function directly, pharmacologic agents have been administered in an attempt to stimulate ventilation. Drugs as diverse as nikethamide, ethamivan, amiphenazole, aspirin, and progesterone have been tried. In general, the results have been disappointing in patients with chronic obstructive lung disease.[172] Doxapram, and more recently almitrine, specific stimulators of chemoreceptors, have provided significant short-term benefit in patients with acute decompensation.[68,202] Medroxyprogesterone has provided encouraging results in patients with primary alveolar hypoventilation and obesity-hypoventilation syndromes.[109,166,276] In addition, a small but significant benefit from this treatment has been found to occur in patients with chronic obstructive pulmonary disease.[267,268] Diaphragmatic pacing has been used in patients with quadriplegia for long-term ventilatory support.[102,103] Because the ventilatory response to an increase in P_{CO_2} is blunted during sleep, nocturnal ventilator therapy has been used with good results in the management of hypercapnia in patients with neuromuscular disease or kyphoscoliosis.[89] Long-term management of patients with these disorders using noninvasive ventilators has led to a fall in both P_{CO_2} and $[HCO_3^-]$; the latter change has increased respiratory sensitivity to subsequent increases in P_{CO_2}.

RESPIRATORY ALKALOSIS

PATHOPHYSIOLOGY

Respiratory alkalosis results from an increase in alveolar ventilation. As discussed earlier (and in detail in Chap. 8), arterial P_{CO_2} is maintained within close limits by appropriate adjustments in alveolar ventilation in response to variations in the rate of CO_2 production. If alveolar ventilation ($\dot{V}_E$) rises out of proportion to CO_2 production, then arterial P_{CO_2} falls. It is apparent from the relationship presented earlier—that is, (K)(alveolar P_{CO_2}) = (CO_2 production/$\dot{V}_E$), that for any given rate of CO_2 production an increase in alveolar ventilation reduces P_{CO_2}. Using this relationship, it can be seen, for example, that P_{CO_2} drops from 40 to 20 mmHg if the alveolar ventilation rate is doubled.

Hyperventilation can result from stimulation of brainstem or peripheral chemoreceptors, from stimulation of nociceptive receptors in the lung, or from signals from higher centers in the brain that override the chemoreceptors. Ventilation is normally regulated by chemoreceptors that respond to changes in pH and O_2 tension. Thus, either a reduction in pH or hypoxemia can produce an increase in ventilation. The first of these, acidemia, occurs either when P_{CO_2} increases (see "Respiratory Acidosis" above) or when serum $[HCO_3^-]$ is reduced by metabolic acidosis (see Chap. 25). In the case of metabolic acidosis, the reduction in P_{CO_2} that ensues is considered to be a normal adaptive response. (The situation is not discussed further here.) Hypoxemia as a cause of respiratory alkalosis is discussed below.

It is easily demonstrable that the normal chemoreceptor regulation of ventilation can be overridden simply by volition. Voluntary hyperventilation demonstrates that higher cortical centers can influence ventilation. The involuntary hyperventilation that occurs in anxiety states and in some forms of CNS disease is another manifestation of this cortical influence. A variety of drugs can stimulate ventilation, either through an action on higher cortical centers or by stimulating the chemoreceptors directly. Finally, a series of nociceptive receptors have been identified in the lung parenchyma with afferent connections to the CNS. In pathologic states these receptors can stimulate the CNS to signal an increase in ventilation independent of oxygen tension, pH, or volition.

Secondary physiologic response

Acute respiratory alkalosis

NATURE OF THE ADAPTIVE RESPONSE A decrease in P_{CO_2} produces an instantaneous fall in H^+ activity (hence, increased pH) in the body fluids. As demonstrated in Fig. 30-8 and Table 30-6, a decrease in arterial P_{CO_2} from 40 to 20 mmHg reduces H^+ activity from 40 to 20 neq/liter (increasing pH from 7.40 to 7.70) in the absence of any change in bicarbonate concentration. Protection against this potentially lethal degree of alkalemia, however, develops rapidly. Within minutes, $[HCO_3^-]$ falls because of the release of H^+ ions from nonbicarbonate buffers.[96] Prediction of the buffer response of these substances was discussed earlier[96] (see "Acute Respiratory Acidosis" above).

Experiments on animals and human beings indicate that only approximately one-third of the buffer response can be attributed to red cell and extra-cellular protein buffering.[10,99] The remainder is the result of the release of hydrogen ions from tissues. The specific mechanisms by which the tissues ameliorate the alkalemia, moreover,

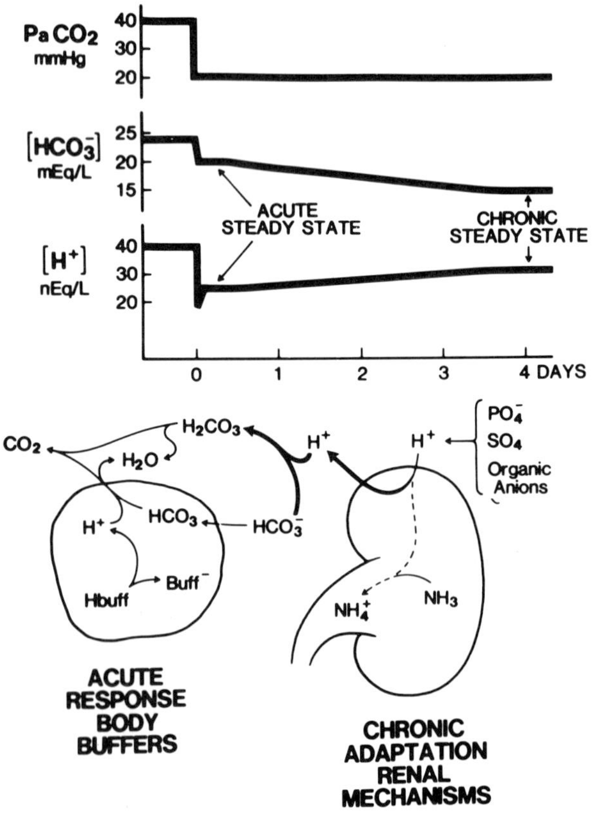

FIGURE 30-8 • Schematic respresentation of the time course and mechanism of bicarbonate loss during adaptation to respiratory alkalosis. In acute adaptation, bicarbonate is consumed by reaction with hydrogen ions released from hemoglobin and other nonbicarbonate tissue buffers. During the chronic adaptive process, bicarbonate is consumed by reactions with hydrogen ions retained as a result of a decrease in renal acid excretion.

TABLE 30-6 • **Effect of hypocapnia on acid-base equilibrium**

	$[H^+]$, *neq/liter*	*pH*
NORMAL		
Arterial P_{CO_2} = 40 mmHg $[HCO_3^-]$ = 24 meq/liter	$24 \times \frac{40}{24} = 40$	7.40
HYPOCAPNIA		
Arterial P_{CO_2} = 20 mmHg Immediate impact—no change in $[HCO_3^-]$(theoretical)	$24 \times \frac{20}{24} = 20$	7.70
Acute, steady state	$24 \times \frac{20}{20} = 25$	7.60
Chronic, steady state	$24 \times \frac{20}{16} = 30$	7.52

may involve more than a simple chemical buffer response. Changes in organic acid production and active transport of hydrogen ions out of cells have been implicated as participants in the tissue "buffer" response.[96] In anesthetized animals subjected to severe hypocapnia (arterial P_{CO_2} < 15 mmHg), 50 to 75 percent of the buffer response is accounted for by an increase in lactic acid production.[61,62,68,88] In awake animals and human beings with milder hypocapnia (arterial P_{CO_2} of 20 to 30 mmHg), however, blood lactate levels increase only slightly (by only 0.5 to 1.5 meq/liter), and the increase is transient.[43,74,280] Thus, the large increase in lactic acid production seen in anesthetized animals is most likely an artifact of the anesthesia coupled with severe passive hyperventilation.[96] In addition to its influence on lactic acid production, acute hypocapnia increases ketoacid levels, and presumably ketoacid production, in conscious rats.[151] This effect is also very minor in terms of titration of body bicarbonate stores. The specific contributions of chemical buffering, changes in H^+ transport, and organic acid production to the protection of extracellular pH in acute respiratory alkalosis remain to be defined.

The acute buffer response to hypocapnia is complete within 15 min; the plasma bicarbonate concentration remains constant for 2 to 5 h if hypocapnia is sustained.[10,43,74,101,179] During this interval changes in renal bicarbonate reabsorption and acid excretion are detectable,[18,273] but their cumulative impact on plasma acid-base composition is negligible. Thus, the acute steady-state response to hypocapnia is produced primarily by buffers and metabolic events.

CHANGES IN PLASMA COMPOSITION IN THE STEADY STATE In acute respiratory alkalosis, blood H^+ activity falls in direct relation to the reduction in arterial P_{CO_2} (Fig. 30-9), by 0.7 to 0.8 neq/liter per mmHg.[10,178] Bicarbonate concentration falls by approximately 2 meq/liter for each 10 mmHg decrease in arterial P_{CO_2}. The alkalemia associated with acute respiratory alkalosis causes only minor transcellular potassium shifts; therefore serum $[K^+]$ falls very slightly (by 0.1 to 0.2 meq for each 0.1 unit change in pH in awake human beings).[3,10,178] Thus, the finding of notable hypokalemia ($[K^+]$ < 3.0 meq/liter) in patients with acute respiratory alkalosis should alert the physician to seek other causes for the low potassium level. In studies in normal human subjects, the serum sodium concentration also falls slightly (approximately 3 meq/liter) during acute respiratory alkalosis.)[10] This small reduction in $[Na^+]$ would probably not be detectable without observations before and during respiratory alkalosis in the same subject. Serum $[Cl^-]$ does not change; the anion gap is not notably increased.[10] Phosphate concentration decreases slightly (0.3 mmol/liter); no changes in total calcium

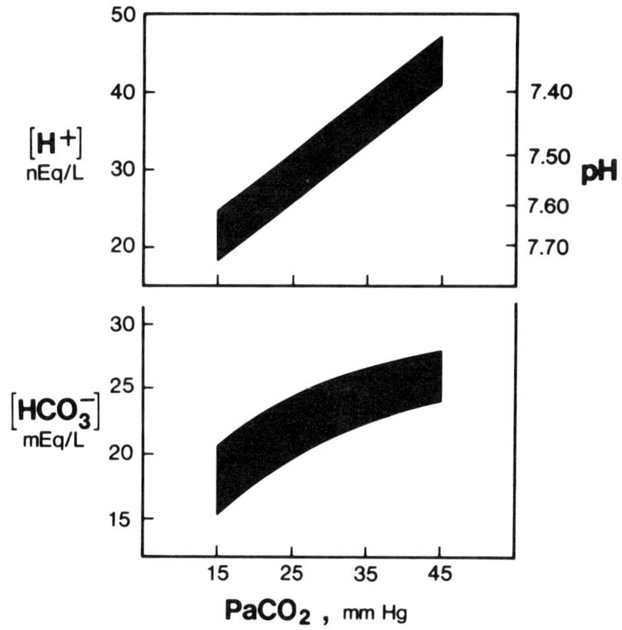

FIGURE 30-9 • **Nintey-five percent confidence intervals for H^+ activity and serum $[HCO_3^-]$ in human acute respiratory alkalosis. (From Arbus GS et al: *N Engl J Med* 280:117, 1969.)**

concentration occur. Serum composition in acute respiratory alkalosis therefore remains essentially normal, save for the small reduction in [HCO_3^-].

Chronic respiratory alkalosis

NATURE OF THE ADAPTIVE RESPONSE When hypocapnia is sustained for more than a few hours, further adaptation occurs as a result of changes in renal bicarbonate reabsorption and acid excretion (Fig. 30-8). Within 30 min of the onset of hypocapnia, urine pH and bicarbonate excretion increase.[18,273] Bicarbonaturia persists very briefly, however; as plasma [HCO_3^-] falls on account of tissue buffering and acid retention, HCO_3^- disappears from the urine and urine pH falls back toward control values. Over the first 24 h of hypocapnia, renal acid excretion falls sufficiently to account for approximately one-half of the total reduction in serum [HCO_3^-].[101,149]

Renal adaptation to hypocapnia returns pH toward control levels and therefore not only reduces [HCO_3^-] but also back-titrates the nonbicarbonate buffers. Within 2 to 3 days of the start of hypocapnia a new steady-state response develops; this state is characterized by a larger reduction in serum bicarbonate concentration than is seen in acute respiratory alkalosis, and by a significant increase in [Cl^-][92,93,149]

The renal response to chronic hypocapnia is not achieved by coupling the decrease in hydrogen ion secretion with a concomitant increase in chloride reabsorption, as might be predicted from the blood composition changes. Sodium is lost in the urine without any chloride, and ECF volume falls; hence chloride concentration rises.[92,101,149] ECF loss is not an obligatory part of the response to hypocapnia; it can be blocked simply by removing sodium from the diet prior to adaptation.[92] This change in diet, however, impairs adaptation slightly.[92] In animals previously placed on a low-salt diet, the reduction in serum [HCO_3^-] is less after adaptation to sustained hypocapnia, the pH is more alkaline, and the serum chloride concentration does not increase. Thus, for optimal adaptation, it appears that sodium chloride intake must be adequate to allow for the development of sodium loss and ECF volume contraction in response to hypocapnia.

The specific mechanisms responsible for the renal adaptive response to hypercapnia remain to be defined. The response, however, appears to be independent of blood or intracellular pH.[50] A sustained reduction in arterial P_{CO_2} reduces serum [HCO_3^-] by about 4 to 5 meq/liter for each 10 mmHg reduction in P_{CO_2}, regardless of the preexisting bicarbonate level.[92,93,96,149] When bicarbonate concentration is reduced in animals by metabolic acidosis, the superimposed hypocapnia-induced [HCO_3^-] reduction in some instances exacerbates the acidemia.[55,169] Such evidence suggests that a reduction in P_{CO_2} signals the kidney directly to reduce hydrogen ion secretion.

In the steady state following renal response to hypocapnia, renal acid excretion returns to control levels. The changes in serum electrolyte composition produced during adaptation are maintained by an increase in Cl^- reabsorption and a reduction in HCO_3^- reabsorption. The steady-state response achieved in the first several days of hypocapnia is maintained for as long as 1 to 2 months of continued hypocapnia (Table 30-7).[61,62] As in the case of respiratory acidosis, the change in bicarbonate concentration induced by prolonged hypocapnia depends on renal function. Thus, severe and sustained alkalemia can result when hypocapnia occurs in patients with end-stage renal disease. Blood pH levels above 7.70 have been found to occur in such individuals.[97,138]

TABLE 30-7 • Studies of adaptation to chronic hypocapnia

Reference	N	Duration, days	P_{CO_2}, mmHg	[HCO_3^-] meq/liter	[H^+], neq/liter	pH	$\Delta HCO_3^- / \Delta P_{CO_2}$	$\Delta H^+ / \Delta P_{CO_2}$
Dempsey et al.[61]	10	45	32	20.5	38	7.42	0.50	0.33
Dempsey et al.[62]	7	21–28	32	20.8	38	7.42	0.40	0.38
Severinghaus et al.[257]	10	8	29	22.2	33	7.48	0.34	0.45
Forwand et al.[84]	22	4	25	18.0	35	7.45	0.50	0.38
Forster et al.[83]	5	10–11	25	17.3	35	7.45	0.48	0.33
Gennari et al.[93]	4	8–11	20	17.1	30	7.53	0.39	0.50
Krapf et al.[149]	4	6	31	21.7	34	7.47	0.41	0.39
							(mean = 0.43)	(mean = 0.39)

Note: Baseline and hypocapnia values were obtained in the same subjects in each study; hypocapnia observations were made after at least 3 days exposure. Hypocapnia was induced by exposure to high altitude, except where controlled ventilation without hypoxemia was used. (Gennari et al.[93])

CHANGES IN BLOOD COMPOSITION IN THE CHRONIC STEADY STATE In chronic respiratory alkalosis, the change in H^+ activity is strongly dependent on the prevailing HCO_3^- concentration prior to adaptation. Studies in normal and acidotic dogs have demonstrated that serum [HCO_3^-] falls by approximately 5 meq/liter for each 10 mmHg reduction in arterial P_{CO_2}, regardless of its influence on pH.[50,55] In dogs with preexisting metabolic alkalosis, induction of sustained hypocapnia causes a slightly larger reduction in bicarbonate concentration; this is most likely due to a small but persistent increase in blood lactate concentration.[174] The bicarbonate concentration in normal dogs is approximately 21 meq/liter. Because of this low starting level and the magnitude of the change in [HCO_3^-], hydrogen ion activity falls by only 0.17 neq/liter for each mmHg reduction in P_{CO_2} in chronic respiratory alkalosis.[92] This rate of change in hydrogen ion activity has been suggested for use in the evaluation of hypocapnia in human beings, but it is inappropriate. In human beings the reduction in hydrogen ion activity induced by sustained hypocapnia is more than twice as great as in dogs, averaging 0.39 neq/liter for each mmHg reduction in P_{CO_2} (Table 30-7).[61,62,83,84,93,126,149,257] The major factor responsible for this difference is the higher normal serum [HCO_3^-] in human beings, 24 meq/liter. In addition, the fall in [HCO_3^-] during human adaptation to chronic hypocapnia is slightly less than in dogs, averaging only 4 meq for each 10 mmHg reduction in P_{CO_2} (Table 30-7).

Figure 30-10 demonstrates that in human beings, as in dogs, the reduction in [HCO_3^-] during sustained hypocapnia is closely linked to the reduction in P_{CO_2}.[93] In four human subjects with [HCO_3^-] ranging from 23 to 28 meq/liter prior to adaptation, bicarbonate fell by virtually identical amounts when arterial P_{CO_2} was reduced from 40 to 20 mmHg and maintained at that level for 1 to 2 weeks. Because of the different starting levels, however, arterial pH differed during chronic hypocapnia, ranging from 7.46 to 7.60.

At a normal arterial [HCO_3^-] of 24 meq/liter, hydrogen ion activity falls by approximately 4 neq/liter for each 10 mmHg fall in arterial P_{CO_2} (Table 30-7). At higher plasma bicarbonate concentrations, the rate of change is affected only slightly, but if bicarbonate concentration is reduced prior to adaptation to chronic hypocapnia, the H^+ activity change per unit P_{CO_2} change is reduced. At a bicarbonate concentration of 17 meq/liter prior to adaptation, for example, the rate of change is predicted to be only 0.15 neq/liter per mmHg decrease in P_{CO_2}.

As noted earlier, plasma [Cl^-] increases significantly in chronic respiratory alkalosis. The increment, however, is less than the fall in [HCO_3^-]. As a result, the anion gap increases by approximately 3 meq/liter when

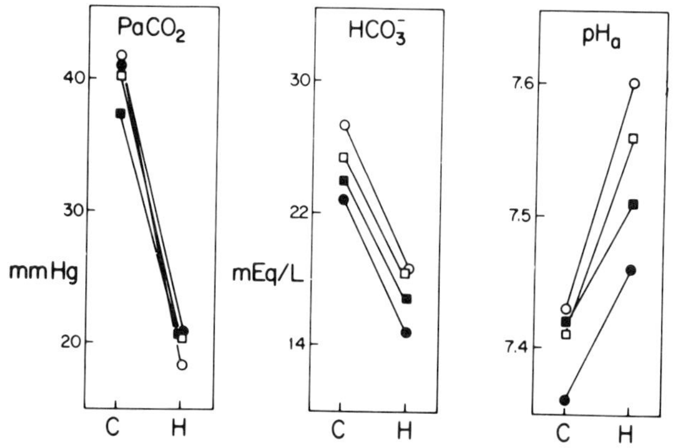

FIGURE 30-10 • Arterial P_{CO_2} (Pa_{CO_2}), serum [HCO_3^-], and arterial pH (pH_a) in four human subjects before (*C*) and during (*H*) a 1- to 2-week period of exposure to hypocapnia. Arterial P_{CO_2} was reduced from 40 to 20 mmHg by increasing minute ventilation. (Data from Gennari FJ et al: *Clin Res* 28:553A, 1980.)

arterial P_{CO_2} drops from 40 to 20 mmHg.[66,92,93] The anion gap increase is not due to increased lactic acid production; blood lactate levels are within normal limits,[62,66,83,92,93,101,149,] even when hypoxemia accompanies hypocapnia.[62,66,83,92,149] The factors responsible for the slight increase in unmeasured anions remain to be defined. A reduction in serum potassium concentration of 0.5 meq/liter (from 4.5 to 4.0 meq/liter) has been noted in normal human subjects after induction of chronic hypocapnia by exposure to high altitude.[149] In contrast, sustained hypocapnia produced at sea level does not appear to affect serum potassium levels.[92,93,101] No other notable abnormalities in blood composition have been identified in chronic respiratory alkalosis. The small changes in sodium and phosphate concentrations observed during acute respiratory alkalosis do not persist.

CLINICAL MANIFESTATIONS OF HYPOCAPNIA

Acute hypocapnia is associated with a characteristic set of signs and symptoms. Chronic hypocapnia, in contrast, is asymptomatic, and its specific effects have not been well characterized. When other disease processes accompany either acute or chronic hypocapnia, their manifestations usually overshadow those of hypocapnia. The clinical manifestations of acute and chronic hypocapnia are discussed separately below.

Acute respiratory alkalosis

Acute respiratory alkalosis typically produces paresthesias of the extremities, tightness in the chest, and a sensation of circumoral numbness.[163,175,238,248] When hypocapnia is severe it is associated with lightheadedness and confusion.[230,248] Formal testing indicates that acute hypocapnia impairs judgment, calculation, and discrimination.[230,248] In rare instances generalized convulsions may occur.[106,230,248] These symptoms and CNS abnormalities are most likely to be present when arterial P_{CO_2} is reduced to below 25 mmHg. Most of these findings can be explained by the cardiovascular, CNS, and metabolic effects of acute hypocapnia (summarized below).

Cardiovascular effects

In awake individuals, acute hypocapnia has no notable effect on cardiac output or blood pressure.[35,38,106,239,246] Pulse rate, however, increases significantly, indicating that stroke volume decreases.[38,140,239] Despite the absence of a change in blood pressure or cardiac output, major changes in regional blood flow develop. Cerebral blood flow varies directly with arterial P_{CO_2} in acute hypocapnia, as it does in acute hypercapnia (Fig. 30-5).[106,140,236,290] Thus, cerebral blood flow falls to less than 50 percent of normal values when P_{CO_2} is abruptly reduced to below 20 mmHg. Direct observation of blood vessels in the pia mater reveals that vasoconstriction involves both small and large vessels.[294] Blood flow to the skin decreases,[51] and blood flow to muscles increases.[38,51,239] The decrease in blood flow to the skin may contribute to the acral paresthesias observed during acute hypocapnia.

It should be noted that the cardiovascular response in anesthetized human beings and animals differs from that in waking subjects with acute hypocapnia. In anesthetized subjects and animals, cardiac output and blood pressure fall during acute hypocapnia.[140,159,226] Peripheral resistance increases; therefore a primary reduction in cardiac function is responsible for the drop in blood pressure.[140,226] In anesthetized dogs subjected to severe hypocapnia, blood pressure falls by as much as 60 mmHg.[159] Part of the difference between awake and anesthetized subjects may be due to the decrease in venous return that occurs as a result of the higher intrathoracic pressure generated by passive hyperventilation in anesthetized subjects.[226] In addition, anesthetized subjects fail to develop the tachycardia seen in awake individuals during acute hypocapnia. Thus, the conpensatory increase in heart rate may be the factor that prevents a decrease in cardiac output in awake individuals.

In normal volunteers subjected to severe acute hypocapnia, cardiac arrhythmias have not been observed. Observations in individuals with underlying coronary artery disease and associated hypocapnia, however, indicate that respiratory alkalosis can be a factor contributing to arrhythmias.[15] In patients with hypocapnia, atrial and ventricular tachyarrhythmias are reversed simply by restoring arterial P_{CO_2} to normal. Acute hypocapnia may produce ST–T wave changes in the ECG that are consistent with myocardial ischemia.[175] These changes occur even in the absence of any demonstrable fixed lesions on coronary angiography.[132,154,187] Although such observations led investigators to conclude that the ECG changes represented false-positives, more recent data indicate that acute hypercapnia can produce significant coronary artery spasm and angina in susceptible patients.[304]

CNS effects

Cerebral blood flow falls dramatically during acute hypocapnia, as a result of cerebral vasoconstriction. The decrease in cerebral blood flow that accompanies acute hypocapnia is associated with a reduction in intracranial and intraocular hydrostatic pressure.[214,269] Cerebral oxygen consumption does not decrease when blood flow is reduced, so oxygen tension falls in the cerebral parenchyma and cerebral veins.[106,140,290] The reduction in cerebral blood flow induced by acute hypocapnia is associated with characteristic EEG changes. These include high-voltage wave forms and generalized slowing.[106] The EEG changes do not correlate with alkalemia; they appear to be closely related to the fall in cerebral venous oxygen tension.[106,277]

The decrease in cerebral blood flow and venous hypoxemia almost certainly contribute to the CNS symptoms of light-headedness and confusion. The development of seizures also appears to be associated with severe cerebral venous hypoxemia.[106] The lactate content of the brain increases to a greater degree than does lactate in systemic blood, and persists at the elevated level[137,218]; central hypoxis is suggested to be responsible. Although it is insufficient to account, alone, for the seizures,[69] calcium binding secondary to alkalemia may contribute to their development. The calcium ion concentration falls by a greater amount in metabolic alkalosis than in respiratory alkalosis, but the occurrence of tetany and seizures is associated only with the latter disorder.[209]

The changes in CSF acid-base composition during acute hypocapnia parallel those seen in systemic blood.[62,63,83,124,136] The degree of alkalinization in CSF is the same as in arterial blood during acute hypocapnia; therefore no acid-base changes unique to CSF are observed.

Other effects

A transient small increase in blood lactate concentration occurs during acute respiratory alkalosis. In human beings, blood lactate concentration rises by less than 1 meq/liter.[74] Presumably, the lactate elevation is a result of increased lactic acid production. Small increases in serum ketoacid levels have been noted as well when acute respiratory alkalosis is induced in animals with high basal ketoacid production, presumably reflecting an increase in ketoacid production.[151] The concentrations of pyruvate, glutamate, citrate, and malate in the brain increase during hypocapnia[157]; whether blood levels increase as well has not been reported.

The alkalemia induced by acute hypocapnia results in increased binding of calcium to albumin. As noted earlier, acute hypocapnia also induces a small shift of sodium and potassium into cells. No information is available concerning changes in hormone levels in acute respiratory alkalosis.

Chronic respiratory alkalosis

Individuals with chronic respiratory alkalosis are asymptomatic, and are usually unaware that they are hyperventilating. Sometimes the increase in minute ventilation is not noticed by the examining physician, because it is accomplished through a combination of slight increases in both the depth and the rate of breathing. Because experimental chronic respiratory alkalosis is induced most readily by the use of a hypoxemic stimulus, the specific manifestations of alkalosis are not easily separated from concurrent effects due only to hypoxemia. Thus, experimental results should be extrapolated only with caution to a clinical setting in which chronic hypocapnia is not accompanied by hypoxemia.

Cardiovascular effects

When hypocapnia persists for more than 8 to 12 h, cardiac output increases and peripheral resistance falls. During exposure to high altitude, cardiac output doubles in the first 3 to 6 days and heart rate increases.[12,126,144,288] Blood pressure does not change, indicating that peripheral resistance falls. With longer exposure (1 to 4 weeks), cardiac output returns to normal or nearly normal, although the pulse rate remains elevated.[12,144,288] At least some of these changes are probably due to the associated hypoxemia. Many of the changes in the distribution of blood flow that develop with acute hypocapnia appear to be sustained during chronic hypocapnia. Blood flow to the skin remains reduced.[156] Although measurements are not available, it is likely that muscle blood flow is increased, given the changes in cardiac output and peripheral resistance. Indirect observations suggest that cerebral blood flow returns toward normal after several days of sustained hypocapnia.[258] Liver blood flow, estimated indirectly from galactose clearance, is 33 percent higher in sojourners at high altitude.[232] Renal plasma flow, at high altitude, is reduced by 10 to 20 percent without any change in GFR[213,237]; this change is almost certainly due to the hypoxemia-induced hematocrit increase.

Plasma and ECF volume fall by 10 to 25 percent during adaptation to chronic hypocapnia.[12,228,262] The decrease in volume is related to the sodium losses that occur as part of the renal adaptive response.[92,101,149] The sodium losses occur whether or not hypoxemia is present; they therefore represent a specific effect of sustained hypocapnia. During prolonged exposure to high altitude, plasma volume remains reduced, although blood volume returns to normal as the result of the red cell mass increase attributable to hypoxemia.[228]

CNS effects

During sustained hypocapnia the CSF pH is normal or nearly normal, and bicarbonate concentration is reduced. In human beings and animals studied after 1 to 2 weeks at high altitude, the changes in CSF pH and bicarbonate concentration parallel the changes in arterial blood[61,62,83,210]; that is, CSF pH increases and $[HCO_3^-]$ falls. If hypocapnia is mild (P_{CO_2} greater than 28 mmHg), the CSF pH returns to baseline levels after several days.[49,257,258] CSF pH is normal as well during the mild chronic hypocapnia that accompanies pregnancy.[168] Thus, the CSF pH rises in chronic hypocapnia but the increase can only be detected if the decrement in P_{CO_2} is sufficiently large. The CSF lactate level remains slightly elevated during sustained hypocapnia, despite the return of arterial lactate to a normal level.[62,83,258]

Other effects

During sustained hypocapnia, few if any other clinical effects are apparent. The transient increase in lactic acid production seen in acute respiratory alkalosis does not persist. The factors contributing to the sustained small increase in unmeasured anions have not been defined. No hormonal abnormalities have been identified. In dogs, chronic hypocapnia results in increased sensitivity (or responsiveness) of the kidney to ADH administration. Water retention exceeds control values, plasma osmolality falls, and the dogs rapidly develop severe hyponatremia.[133] The basis for this abnormality is unknown.

CAUSES OF HYPOCAPNIA

The causes of respiratory alkalosis are listed in Table 30-8. These are grouped under the general headings of hypoxia, CNS disorders, drugs, pulmonary disease, and other causes. With few exceptions, all causes of respiratory alkalosis are associated with both the acute and the chronic form of the disorder. Acute respiratory alkalosis is seen most commonly in the anxiety-hyperventilation syndrome, or in the setting of a serious acute illness such as gram-negative septicemia, pneumonia, pulmonary edema, or pulmonary embolism. Chronic hypocapnia is a much more common finding in patients with CNS disease, hepatic failure, or chronic pulmonary interstitial disease. Adaptation to high altitude produces chronic

TABLE 30-8 • Causes of respiratory alkalosis

- Hypoxia
  - Decreased inspired O_2 tension
  - High altitude
  - Ventilation-perfusion inequality
  - Hypotension
  - Severe anemia
- CNS Disorders
  - Voluntary hyperventilation
  - Anxiety-hyperventilation syndrome
  - Neurologic disease
    - Cerebrovascular accident
    - Infection
    - Trauma
    - Tumor
- Drugs
  - Salicylates
  - Nicotine
  - Dinitrophenol
  - Xanthine family
  - Pressor hormones
  - Progesterone
  - Medroxyprogesterone
- Pulmonary Disease
  - Interstitial lung disease
  - Pneumonia
  - Pulmonary edema
  - Pulmonary embolism
  - Bronchial asthma
- Other
  - Pregnancy
  - Hepatic failure
  - Gram-negative septicemia
  - Heat exposure
  - Mechanical overventilation
  - Recovery from metabolic acidosis

hypocapnia in otherwise normal individuals. It is important to emphasize that in the hospital setting, respiratory alkalosis is generally associated with serious illness. A review of records of 8000 intensive care unit patients indicates that respiratory alkalosis occurred in 45 percent of the cases.[184] Moreover, the presence of respiratory alkalosis was a grave prognostic sign. Mortality correlated with the severity of the respiratory alkalosis, rising to 88 percent in patients with arterial P_{CO_2} levels of 15 mmHg or less.[184] A review of blood gas analyses in hospitalized patients showed a similarly poor prognosis for patients with respiratory alkalosis, as well as a correlation between mortality and the severity of the alkalosis.[8]

Hypoxemia

ADAPTATION TO HIGH ALTITUDE Exposure to an atmosphere at sea level that contains 12 to 13% O_2 or less, or exposure to a reduced atmospheric pressure that produces a similar oxygen tension (as at 9000 to 10,000 ft, or 3000 m, above sea level) produces hyperventilation and hypocapnia.[28,112,113,119,231] The ventilatory response to hypoxemia involves increases in both the rate and the depth of ventilation; rate increases more than depth.[233] A reduction in arterial P_{O_2} to below 60 mmHg appears to be necessary to stimulate ventilation and reduce P_{CO_2} during short-term exposure, but prolonged exposure to a low-oxygen environment yields a more complex response. Remaining at altitudes as low as 4000 to 6000 ft for several days also produces a discernible increase in ventilation and decrease in arterial P_{CO_2}, though P_{O_2} is reduced much less (Fig. 30-11).[231]

Sustained exposure to high altitude produces a progressive increase in ventilation, which reaches a maximum value for a given elevation after 3 to 6 days.[28,63,156,231,257] As a result, arterial P_{CO_2} is 5 to 10 mmHg lower after several days at high altitude than after brief exposure. Moreover, arterial P_{O_2} rises, so that after 1 week at 3000 m, for example, it approaches 70 mmHg, in association with a sustained reduction in P_{CO_2} to 28 to 30 mmHg. The gradual increase in ventilation, although its cause is not clearly defined, seems likely to be due to the gradual reduction in systemic alkalinity that results from the renal adaptive response to hypocapnia. Thus the dampening effect of alkalinity on ventilation, acting through the central chemoreceptors, is gradually eased, allowing hypoxemia to stimulate ventilation more vigorously. Studies in dogs suggest that, for any given level of inspired oxygen tension, a balance is achieved in the steady state between stimulation of ventilation by hypoxemia and inhibition of ventilation by alkalemia.[92]

This steady-state ventilatory response persists for at least several months of residence at high altitude.[61,156] With long-term residence (greater than several years), a different pattern of ventilation develops. In high altitude natives, arterial P_{O_2} is lower and P_{CO_2} higher than in sojourners at the same altitudes.[48,190,259] The difference is not explained by differences in hematocrit or in the oxygen-carrying capacity of the blood. At 3000 to 4000 m above sea level, arterial P_{CO_2} is 5 to 7 mmHg higher in natives than in sojourners, and P_{O_2} is 5 to 7 mmHg lower. The reduction in ventilatory response appears to be due to an acquired insensitivity to hypoxemia of the peripheral chemoreceptors. In individuals residing at high altitude for 4 years or more, the ventilatory response to an acute reduction in P_{O_2} is minimal or absent.[271,295] Ventilatory response to exercise is normal in these individuals, suggesting that central chemoreceptors are unaffected.[295] In both short and long stays at high altitude the pattern of blood pH and $[HCO_3^-]$ is consistent with adaptation to chronic hypocapnia.

OTHER CAUSES OF HYPOXEMIA Hypoxemia due to impaired oxygen transfer across the alveolar membrane produces the same ventilatory response as the hypoxemia that occurs when environmental oxygen tension is reduced. If alveolar reserve is sufficient, hypocapnia develops when arterial P_{O_2} falls below 60 mmHg. Hypocapnia secondary to hypoxemia occurs in pulmonary embolism, pneumonia, pulmonary edema, bronchial asthma, adult respiratory distress syndrome, and diffuse interstitial lung disease.[16,184] Hypocapnia can also develop with these pulmonary diseases independent of hypoxemia, because of stimulation of nociceptive receptors in the lung parenchyma (see "Pulmonary Disease" below).

Hypotension can also lead to hyperventilation and hypocapnia, even when arterial oxygen tension is not markedly reduced.[184,300] Because the peripheral chemoreceptors respond to oxygen delivery rather than oxygen concentration, the hyperventilation that occurs with shock is believed to be mediated by stimulation of these receptors as a result of decreased blood flow. Arterial P_{CO_2} typically falls to 20 to 30 mmHg, but can fall as low as 15 mmHg.[184] Hypocapnia in association with shock occurs most commonly in the setting of sepsis or myocardial infarction. As indicated below, other factors in addition to hypotension may contribute to the hyperventilation seen in these patients.

Hypocapnia has also been reported to occur, albeit rarely, in patients with severe anemia (i.e., with hemoglobin less than 30 percent of normal).[200] Although little information is available concerning the pathogenesis of the hyperventilation that accompanies the anemia in such patients, it is presumed to be due to a decrease in oxygen delivery to the peripheral chemoreceptors.

CNS-mediated hypocapnia

VOLUNTARY HYPERVENTILATION Humans can produce hypocapnia at will. Arterial P_{CO_2} can easily be reduced to below 20 mmHg within minutes. In one study, trained human subjects were able to maintain arterial P_{CO_2} at 30 to 32 mmHg for longer than 24 h by voluntary hyperventilation.[101] Cessation of voluntary hyperventilation does not result in apnea in awake individuals, but in anesthetized human beings and animals (and even in dozing volunteers) breathing ceases until P_{CO_2} rises sufficiently to stimulate ventilation.[81,82,119,217]

ANXIETY-HYPERVENTILATION SYNDROME Hyperventilation occurs as part of a reaction to acute anxiety in susceptible individuals.[163,175] The resultant hypocapnia is often relatively severe (P_{CO_2} < 30 mmHg) and abrupt in onset; thus it is associated with moderately severe alkalemia. Individuals developing the anxiety-hyperventilation syndrome are often unaware that hyperventilation is the inciting event, and appear to be gasping for air. The attacks are usually associated with the characteristic symptoms of acute hypocapnia—circumoral numbness, acral paresthesias, and chest tightness. If the hyperventilation intensifies, patients can appear to be seriously ill; on occasion, overt tetany or loss of consciousness ensues. That hypocapnia is the cause of the entire syndrome has been verified by the demonstration that all symptoms are rapidly reversed by an increase in the P_{CO_2} in the inspired air.[175,238,270]

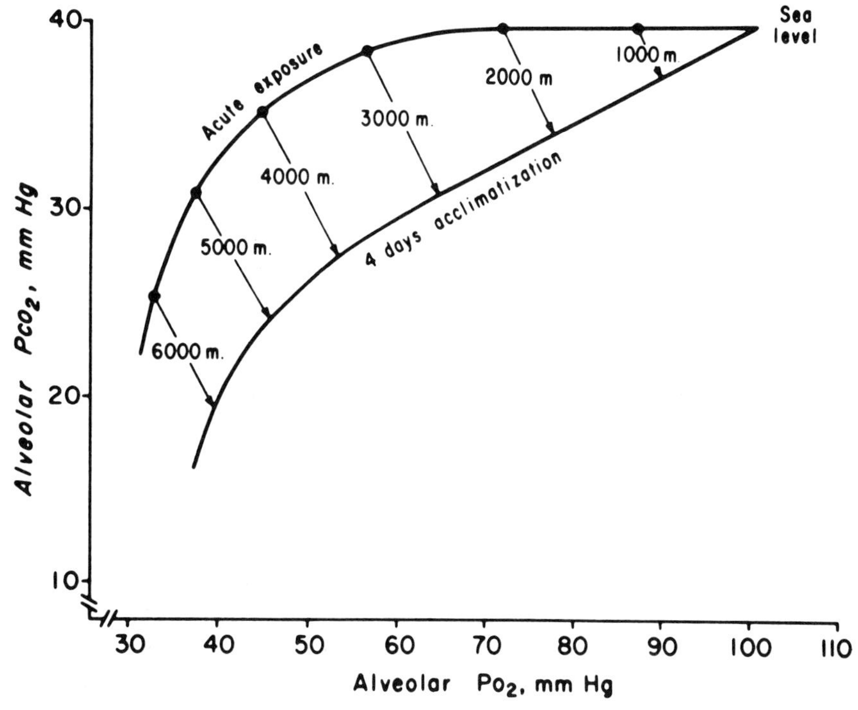

FIGURE 30-11 • Relationship between alveolar P_{O_2} and alveolar P_{CO_2} during exposure to high altitude. Upper line shows changes in alveolar P_{CO_2} that occur in response to hypoxemia during the first several hours at high altitude; lower line shows response after four days of acclimatization. The numbers between the two curves indicate the altitude in meters. (From Lenfant C, Sullivan K: *N Engl J Med* 284:1298, 1971. Adapted from Rahn H, Otis AB: *Am J Physiol* 157:445, 1949.)

CNS DISEASE Hyperventilation and sustained hypocapnia are features of a wide variety of CNS illnesses and injuries. Two distinct breathing patterns have been described in association with hypocapnia: *central hyperventilation* and *Cheyne-Stokes respiration.* In central hyperventilation the pattern of breathing is extremely regular; it has been described as "metronomic."[220] There is a striking increase in both the rate and the depth of breathing. In Cheyne-Stokes respiration, by contrast, periods of hyperventilation alternate with periods of apnea.[37]

Central hyperventilation is associated with injury or disease in the pons or midbrain. Because lesions in these areas usually result in coma and death, this pattern of hyperventilation is usually seen in comatose patients and indicates that prognosis is very poor.[220,245] However, the pattern has also been observed to occur rarely in individuals who are awake and alert, with tumor involvement localized to the pons or midbrain.[153,216] The hypocapnia that occurs with central hyperventilation is usually severe and sustained. These patients typically have arterial P_{CO_2} levels of 25 to 30 mmHg or lower, and the blood acid-base composition is consistent with chronic respiratory alkalosis. Marked hypoxemia is not present.[220] The pathophysiology of central hyperventilation has not been defined, but the hyperventilation presumably is the result either of damage to a normal inhibitory conduction pathway or of damage-induced activation of a normal stimulant pathway.

Cheyne-Stokes respiration occurs in association with clinical evidence of bilateral cortical disease, usually involving the pyramidal or extrapyramidal motor tracts.[37,120,220] In contrast to patients with central hyperventilation, patients with Cheyne-Stokes respiration usually have associated hypoxemia. However, the hypocapnia appears to be unrelated to the hypoxemia, since correction of the latter problem by oxygen administration fails to correct the respiratory alkalosis.[37] In these patients arterial P_{CO_2} is lowest at the onset of apnea and highest at the peak of hyperventilation. Thus, it appears that Cheyne-Stokes respiration represents an exaggerated response of the central chemoreceptors to CO_2, analogous to a peripheral hyperreflexia.[37,120,122] The brisk ventilatory response to an increase in P_{CO_2} in these patients results in an overshoot, reducing P_{CO_2} far below the threshold value; it is followed by apnea until P_{CO_2} rises again to a level to stimulate the chemoreceptors, starting the cycle again. The prolonged apnea that occurs in patients with Cheyne-Stokes respiration when P_{CO_2} is reduced below threshold values is also an abnormal response. It occurs in patients with bilateral cortical brain disease who are otherwise awake and alert, following voluntary hyperventilation[217]; it also occurs in anesthetized human beings and animals.[82] Cheyne-Stokes respiration and respiratory alkalosis in patients with CNS disease is a serious prognostic sign; mortality exceeds 50 percent.[245]

Cheyne-Stokes respiration also has been reported to occur in cardiac failure and in markedly obese patients.[135] The relation between Cheyne-Stokes respiration and respiratory alkalosis in these disorders is not clear. When Cheyne-Stokes respiration is associated with respiratory alkalosis, however, diffuse brain disease is virtually always the underlying cause.[37,135]

Pharmacologic agents

SALICYLATES Salicylates directly stimulate the medullary chemoreceptors to produce hyperventilation. Direct perfusion of the medullary CSF with salicylates increases both the rate and the depth of ventilation in experimental animals, an effect not blocked by vagal interruption, denervation of the carotid chemoreceptors, or decerebration.[52,244,283] In human beings, ingestion of as little as 4 g of aspirin per day produces hyperventilation and notably lowers arterial P_{CO_2}[241]; ingestion of 12 g of aspirin over 24 h reduces arterial P_{CO_2} to 30 mmHg.[80] The respiratory stimulation that occurs after accidental or intentional ingestion of larger amounts of aspirin leads to even greater reductions in P_{CO_2}. Values as low as 10 mmHg have been reported.[265,301] Because aspirin can also produce metabolic acidosis, aspirin intoxication commonly causes a mixed disorder (respiratory alkalosis with metabolic acidosis; see Chaps. 25 and 31). In adults and in children older than 8 to 10 years, respiratory alkalosis usually predominates, yielding an alkaline blood pH; in young children acidosis is predominant, and blood pH can fall to low levels.[88,115] It is important to emphasize, however, that regardless of the initial blood pH, salicylate stimulation of ventilation is independent of the metabolic acidosis. Thus, hyperventilation persists even if the metabolic acidosis is corrected.

OTHER DRUGS Nicotine, dinitrophenol, and the xanthine group of drugs can all stimulate ventilation and lead to hypocapnia. Nicotine stimulates ventilation by acting on both the peripheral and central chemoreceptors.[121,195] At the concentrations normally achieved by smoking cigarettes, the effect of nicotine on ventilation is minor. However, rapid cigarette puffing can result in a reduction in arterial P_{CO_2} to below 30 mmHg.[192] Dinitrophenol acts in a fashion identical to the salicylates. Aminophylline and related xanthine drugs can stimulate ventilation and produce hypocapnia, but the mechanism by which they increase ventilation is unknown. The respiratory alkalosis that follows aminophylline administration in human beings is mild, and can be blocked by CNS-depressant drugs such as meperidine.[292] In a single well-documented case, severe respiratory alkalosis was induced by nortriptyline in a patient with end-stage renal disease.[275] Sustained hypocapnia developed when blood nortriptyline levels were in the therapeutic range on two separate occasions. Whether this report represents an idiosynchratic reaction or a general effect of nortriptyline in this population of patients remains to be determined.

The pressor agents epinephrine, norepinephrine, and angiotensin have all been demonstrated to effect a small reduction in arterial P_{CO_2} (to a level greater than 30 mmHg) when given in large amounts.[17,224,298] Their action is probably due to CNS stimulation. It is unlikely that physiologic fluctuations in any of these hormones play any role in the regulation of ventilation. However, the increase in adrenal medullary hormone secretion in stress states may be a contributor to the hyperventilation and hypocapnia that is seen.

Administration of progesterone or medroxyprogesterone to human subjects reduces arterial P_{CO_2} by 3 to 6 mmHg; the effect develops within 24 h and is sustained for as long as the agent is given.[266,305] The mechanism by which progesterone increases alveolar ventilation is unknown; it is presumed to act centrally.[165,266,305] The stimulatory effect of progesterone on ventilation is almost certainly the basis for the lower P_{CO_2} values found in women,[95] and for the hypocapnia that normally accompanies pregnancy (see below). Studies in women demonstrate that arterial P_{CO_2} falls by 3 to 6 mmHg during the luteal phase of the menstrual cycle; this effect is paralleled by a rise in pH and a fall in renal acid excretion.[168,281] In both pregnant and nonpregnant women P_{CO_2} is inversely related to the blood progesterone level.[168] Because it stimulates ventilation, medroxyprogesterone has been used therapeutically in patients with the sleep apnea syndrome (see "Management" under "Respiratory Acidosis" above).

Pulmonary disease

Hyperventilation and hypocapnia can occur in a variety of pulmonary diseases even in the absence of severe hypoxemia. The hyperventilation in these diseases is signaled to the brain via vagal afferent impulses from nociceptive receptors within the lung parenchyma.[148] At least three separate receptor types have been identified within the lung: stretch receptors, irritant receptors, and J (juxtacapillary) receptors. The irritant receptors are activated by the presence of irritant substances in the small airways; the J receptors are activated by pulmonary capillary congestion.[47,211] The function of the stretch receptors is unclear, but the two nociceptive receptors are thought to be responsible for the hyperventilation that accompanies the pulmonary diseases described below.

PULMONARY EDEMA Respiratory alkalosis unaccompanied by any other acid-base disorder occurs in perhaps 5 to 10 percent of patients with pulmonary edema.[2] Hypoxemia is certainly one factor accounting for the hypocapnia, but experimental evidence indicates that J receptor stimulation also contributes to the hyperventilation.[148] Hypocapnia may also occur in congestive heart failure without pulmonary edema as the result of J receptor stimulation.[44,58] It should be emphasized that metabolic acidosis and respiratory acidosis are more common acid-base disturbances in pulmonary edema.

PULMONARY EMBOLISM Respiratory alkalosis is a diagnostic feature of pulmonary embolism; alkalosis occurs in 80 to 90 percent of cases.[279] Although hypoxemia also occurs commonly, it does not appear to be responsible for the hypocapnia. Hyperventilation persists even when hypoxemia is corrected by oxygen administration.[148] Experimental observations in animals indicate that the hyperventilation is due to vagal afferent signals, presumably from nociceptive receptors in the lung.[125,274]

PNEUMONIA In a fashion similar to pulmonary edema and pulmonary embolism, hypocapnia may accompany pneumonia in the absence of severe hypoxemia.[148] Animal studies have shown that hyperventilation is mediated via vagal afferent signals.[284]

INTERSTITIAL LUNG DISEASE Mild respiratory alkalosis (P_{CO_2} levels 30 to 35 mmHg) is a feature in approximately 20 percent of patients with chronic interstitial lung disease.[160] In a larger fraction, arterial P_{CO_2} levels are at the lower limit of normal.[160] Hypoxemia is not sufficient to account for the hypocapnia. Studies of animals and indirect evidence in human beings suggest that the hyperventilation is mediated by vagal afferent signals.[110,148,160,164]

BRONCHIAL ASTHMA The most common acid-base disorder occurring in patients with acute bronchial asthma is respiratory alkalosis.[186,203] The hypocapnia is due in part to the hypoxemia induced by acute bronchoconstriction and in part to stimulation of pulmonary nociceptive receptors.

Other causes of hypocapnia

PREGNANCY Normal pregnancy is accompanied by a sustained reduction in P_{CO_2}, most likely due to stimulation of ventilation by progesterone (see above). In the first trimester of pregnancy blood pH rises to approximately 7.47 and arterial P_{CO_2} levels fall to about 34 mmHg.[161] This P_{CO_2} level is similar to that observed during the luteal phase of the menstrual period; serum progesterone levels are also similar to those seen in the luteal phase.[168,280] In the second trimester arterial P_{CO_2} falls further, to 32 mmHg on average; in the last trimester, when progesterone levels are at their peak P_{CO_2} drops to 27 to 29 mmHg.[25,95,161,168] The changes in pH and $[HCO_3^-]$ that occur in association with hypocapnia in pregnancy are consistent with adaptation to chronic respiratory alkalosis. In the immediate postpartum period, the P_{CO_2} level returns to about 34 mmHg; this value is consistent with predictions from observed progesterone levels.[168]

HEPATIC FAILURE Chronic hypocapnia is an almost constant feature of end-stage hepatic disease.[167,184,200,227] Patients with hepatic coma often sustain arterial P_{CO_2} levels below 30 mmHg; on occasion, P_{CO_2} levels below 20 mmHg have been reported to occur.[64,285] In patients with hepatic insufficiency without coma, P_{CO_2} values of 30 to 35 mmHg are common. The changes in pH and $[HCO_3^-]$ seen in these patients are consistent with chronic respiratory alkalosis, indicating that hyperventilation is primary. The hyperventilation is not related to hypoxemia. It seems probable that central stimulation of ventilation by some accumulating toxic substance is responsible for the hypocapnia, but no specific substance or substances have been identified. Although abnormal levels of progesterone as well as other substances in the blood have been implicated in causing the hypocapnia, the hypocapnia correlates best with blood ammonia levels.[134,285] Regardless of the cause of the liver disease, the finding of respiratory alkalosis with a P_{CO_2} level below 25 mmHg in a patient with liver disease is a grave prognostic sign; such an individual usually does not survive longer than several months.[184,200]

SEPTICEMIA Hypocapnia has been reported to occur in over 50 percent of patients with gram-negative sepsis.[24,264,300] The respiratory alkalosis is typically moderately severe, with arterial P_{CO_2} between 20 and 30 mmHg; on occasion, P_{CO_2} has been observed to be less than 15 mmHg.[184,264,300] Because the alkalosis is usually acute in onset, pH usually exceeds 7.50. The hypocapnia is unrelated to hypoxemia, hypotension, or acidemia; it is believed to be due to a direct stimulatory effect of bacterial toxins on the central chemoreceptors.[184,264,300] Hyperventilation and hypocapnia persist until appropriate antibiotic therapy is given.[264] Because of the relative frequency of respiratory alkalosis in patients with gram-negative septicemia, the development of unexplained respiratory alkalosis in a hospitalized patient should signal the physician to determine whether bacteremia is present. No specific gram-negative organism has been identified as the cause. Respiratory alkalosis has been observed in infections with organisms as diverse as *Escherichia coli* and *Proteus, Pseudomonas* and *Klebsiella* species.[300] Respiratory alkalosis may also occur in septicemia due to gram-positive organisms,[300] but in this setting hypotension and hypoxemia probably contribute to the hyperventilation.

HEAT EXPOSURE Exposure to high environmental temperatures raises body temperature and produces acute respiratory alkalosis.[14,90,107] Some observers have extrapolated from this observation and concluded that fever produces respiratory alkalosis[70,182]; this inference is not warranted.[96] On the other hand, both heat exhaustion and heat stroke can produce respiratory alkalosis.[29,272] In army troops suffering from heat exhaustion, the predominant acid-base abnormality was severe respiratory alkalosis; over one-half of the subjects had arterial P_{CO_2} levels below 20 mmHg.[29] In heat stroke, metabolic acidosis predominates, but isolated respiratory alkalosis can occur as well.[272] Other hyperpyretic states such as hyperthyroidism and delirium tremens have been implicated in producing respiratory alkalosis, but the association between these states and respiratory alkalosis has not been well documented.

MECHANICAL OVERVENTILATION Devices that automatically control ventilatory depth and rate have the potential to produce respiratory alkalosis in patients with sufficient alveolar reserve. Early on in the development of ventilator therapy, the aggressive use of such machines to raise arterial oxygen tension by increasing minute ventilation led to a high incidence of respiratory alkalosis.[299] Hypocapnia in such patients can easily be corrected by appropriate adjustments in dead space or in the rate or depth of breathing. For most patients who require ventilator therapy, a mixture of machine-initiated and patient-initiated ventilation is now used. Two techniques are currently employed: intermittent mandatory ventilation and controlled/assisted ventilation. With either technique, machine-induced respiratory alkalosis is not a problem.[60,128]

RECOVERY FROM METABOLIC ACIDOSIS Hyperventilation and hypocapnia often persist for as long as 24 to 48 h during recovery from metabolic acidosis. Persistent hypocapnia is more likely to occur when the inciting metabolic acidosis has been severe or lasts more than 24 hours. Because the persistent hypocapnia is coupled with rising blood bicarbonate concentrations during recovery, blood pH can rise to frankly alkaline values. Usually the alkalemia is transitory and requires no specific treatment. It has been postulated that the hypocapnia is due to cerebral interstitial acidemia that persists for some time after blood pH is corrected. Although some pH measurements of lumbar CSF support this view,[219,223] the point has not been completely proven because hyperventilation persists in some instances even after CSF pH returns to normal values.[223]

The common occurrence of delayed recovery of P_{CO_2} during treatment of metabolic acidosis has important therapeutic implications. Overtreatment with bicarbonate should be avoided (see Chap. 25). Attempts to correct plasma $[HCO_3^-]$ completely by rapid bicarbonate administration can produce severe alkalemia. The goal of therapy should be to increase $[HCO_3^-]$ only to an intermediate level, usually 10 to 15 meq/liter.

DELIBERATE INDUCTION OF RESPIRATORY ALKALOSIS Deliberate induction of respiratory alkalosis has been used as a treatment for brain edema in some comatose patients.[111] The major reduction in cerebral blood flow induced by hypocapnia (Fig. 30-5) has been demonstrated to reduce brain edema in patients with head trauma or acute infection. In patients with brain edema secondary to a cerebrovascular accident or severe hypoxia, however, hyperventilation has not generally been successful in reducing swelling, and is not recommended.[111] Hypocapnia has also been used as an adjunct to anesthesia, reducing the total amount of anesthetic agent required.[10,91]

DIAGNOSIS

As is the case with respiratory acidosis, the diagnosis of respiratory alkalosis depends on laboratory measurements of pH and P_{CO_2} (or of pH and total CO_2 content). The finding of a pH greater than 7.40 in conjunction with a reduction in arterial P_{CO_2} to below 35 mmHg establishes the presence of respiratory alkalosis. On the basis of the experimental observations described above, clinical rules of thumb have been developed that allow the physician to evaluate whether the associated changes in pH and bicarbonate concentration are consistent with acute or chronic respiratory alkalosis, or whether a mixed acid-base disturbance is present (Table 30-4). The use of these guidelines is reviewed below for acute and chronic respiratory alkalosis. In addition to analyzing the blood acid-base composition, the physician should pay close attention to the clinical features and history to assist in the correct diagnosis. Although abnormal breathing patterns are often overlooked, careful observation usually can demonstrate their presence in patients with respiratory alkalosis. More frequently, the diagnosis is first suggested by the finding of a reduced total CO_2 content in routine laboratory measurements. The finding of respiratory alkalosis can be an important diagnostic clue to the presence of a serious underlying systemic illness.

Acute respiratory alkalosis

In acute respiratory alkalosis, serum bicarbonate concentration falls by approximately 2 meq/liter and H^+ activity falls by 7 to 8 neq/liter for each 10 mmHg decrement in arterial P_{CO_2} (Table 30-4). From this relationship it is apparent that serum $[HCO_3^-]$ is usually 20 meq/liter or higher, except in severe hypocapnia—that is, with P_{CO_2} below 20 mmHg. Only minor decrements occur in $[Na^+]$ and $[K^+]$; such changes are usually undetectable in the absence of careful paired observations. Thus, with the exception of a slight reduction in $[HCO_3^-]$, the serum electrolyte levels are within normal limits in acute respiratory alkalosis (Fig. 30-6). As discussed earlier, blood lactate rises only slightly. Because bicarbonate and sodium concentrations both fall slightly, the anion gap does not increase. Thus, an increased anion gap or a major abnormality in $[K^+]$ indicates the presence of additional acid-base and electrolyte problems. Acute respiratory alkalosis is sometimes associated with subjective symptoms of paresthesias and confusion. In a patient with clinical manifestations of a systemic disease, the symptoms of that disease usually overshadow any symptoms specific to acute respiratory alkalosis.

The mixed acid-base disturbance most commonly associated with acute respiratory alkalosis is metabolic acidosis with an increase anion gap.[87,204] The coexistence of these two disorders can be identified by the conjunction of a low P_{CO_2} level, a normal or alkaline blood pH, and an increased anion gap.[87] The conjunction of respiratory alkalosis and metabolic acidosis characteristically occurs in patients who have ingested toxic amounts of salicylates, but this combination of acid-base disorders also occurs commonly in gravely ill patients.

Chronic respiratory alkalosis

In chronic respiratory alkalosis the plasma bicarbonate concentration falls by approximately 4 meq/liter for each 10 mmHg decrement in arterial P_{CO_2} (Table 30-4). As noted earlier, pH varies fairly widely in chronic respiratory alkalosis; pH values generally range from 7.45 to 7.55 when P_{CO_2} is reduced to below 30 mmHg. Plasma $[Cl^-]$ increases in chronic respiratory alkalosis, but the increment is smaller than the decrement in $[HCO_3^-]$, and the anion gap increases slightly (Fig. 30-6). When P_{CO_2} has decreased to 20 mmHg the anion gap is elevated by approximately 3 meq/liter. Although a sustained reduction in serum $[K^+]$ has been noted in high altitude studies,[149] hypokalemia is not a feature of chronic respiratory alkalosis in the clinic. No notable change occurs in serum $[Na^+]$.

The electrolyte pattern seen in chronic respiratory alkalosis (increased serum $[Cl^-]$ and decreased $[HCO_3^-]$) is often mistaken for hyperchloremic metabolic acidosis (see Chap. 25). The two disorders can be separated easily by measurement of arterial blood pH. Blood pH is greater than 7.40 if respiratory alkalosis is present. The crucial step in this differentiation is the recognition that respiratory alkalosis is a possibility. It is important to emphasize that the electrolyte changes seen in chronic hypocapnia develop within 3 to 4 days. Thus, "chronic" does not necessarily imply months or years. In addition, chronic respiratory alkalosis is essentially asymptomatic. The hyperventilation is not usually noted by the patient, and it is often overlooked by observers as well.

If the pH is alkaline and the P_{CO_2} is reduced, but the change in bicarbonate concentration is not consistent with the expected changes in acute or chronic respiratory alkalosis, or if the anion gap is markedly increased, then a mixed acid-base disorder is present (see Chap. 31). Chronic respiratory alkalosis is usually unassociated with other acid-base disturbances; metabolic acidosis is probably the most common complication.

TABLE 30-9 • **Fortuitous resemblance of partial recovery from metabolic acidosis to chronic respiratory alkalosis**

METABOLIC ACIDOSIS
P_{CO_2} = 15 mmHg
$[HCO_3^-]$ = 5 meq/liter
$[H^+]$ = 72 neq/liter
pH = 7.14
PARTIAL CORRECTION OF HCO_3^- DEFICIT AND CONTINUED HYPERVENTILATION
P_{CO_2} = 22 mmHg
$[HCO_3^-]$ = 16 meq/liter
$[H^+]$ = 33 neq/liter
pH = 7.48

Note: P_{CO_2} = arterial P_{CO_2}.

It should be emphasized that the finding of laboratory abnormalities consistent with chronic respiratory alkalosis does not completely exclude a complicating acid-base disorder.[10] Complicated acid-base disturbances can fortuitously result in laboratory values consistent with an uncomplicated disorder. An example of this circumstance occurs in the recovery phase of metabolic acidosis. During treatment of diabetic ketoacidosis or salicylate ingestion, $[Cl^-]$ rises and the anion gap falls to normal. Continued hyperventilation produces a respiratory alkalosis. During this phase (Table 30-9) the electrolyte levels are consistent with uncomplicated chronic respiratory alkalosis, although in fact the changes are due to a mixed metabolic acidosis and respiratory alkalosis.

MANAGEMENT

The presence of respiratory alkalosis is a diagnostic clue rather than a treatment problem. Hypocapnia per se poses little threat to the patient's health, and no specific treatment is indicated in most instances. An exception to this rule is the anxiety-hyperventilation syndrome,[163,175] in which an abrupt increase in P_{CO_2} can alleviate the symptoms rapidly. An increase in P_{CO_2} can be achieved simply by having the patient breathe into a paper bag, thereby increasing the amount of inspired CO_2. Metabolic acidosis and hypoxemia should be excluded by clinical assessment, or blood gas measurements, before embarking on this treatment. Moreover, although this maneuver is an excellent short-term treatment, it is not a long-term solution to the underlying problem. Psychological counseling is often necessary for the management of anxiety-hyperventilation syndrome.[163,175]

Another cause of hypocapnia for which treatment is appropriate and beneficial is ventilator-induced hypocapnia. In patients with this disorder, P_{CO_2} can easily be increased by an increase in the dead space, or by decreases in the rate and depth of ventilation. As noted earlier, correction of ventilator-induced hypocapnia, particularly in patients with underlying heart disease, can reduce the incidence of arrhythmias. It should be recalled, however, that in patients on controlled ventilation who are chronically adapted to hypocapnia, an abrupt large increase in P_{CO_2} sharply reduces both arterial and CSF pH.[49] Thus, care should be exercised in the raising of P_{CO_2} in patients in whom ventilation cannot adjust to changes in pH.

REFERENCES

1. Aber GM et al: Inter-relationships between renal and cardiac function and respiratory gas exchange in obstructive airways disease. *Clin Sci* 25:159, 1963.
2. Aberman A, Fulop M: The metabolic and respiratory acidosis of acute pulmonary edema. *Ann Intern Med* 76:173, 1972.
3. Adrogué HJ, Madias NE: Changes in plasma potassium concentration during acute acid-base disturbances. *Am J Med* 71:456, 1981.
4. Adrogué HJ, Madias NE: Influence of chronic respiratory acid-base disorders on acute CO_2 titration curve. *J Appl Physiol* 58:1231, 1985.
5. Adrogué HJ et al: Assessing acid-base status in circulatory failure. *N Engl J Med* 320:1312, 1989.
6. Albert RK et al: Controlled clinical trial of methylprednisolone in patients with chronic bronchitis and acute respiratory insufficiency. *Ann Intern Med* 92:753, 1980.
7. Altschule MD, Sulzbach WM: Tolerance of human heart to acidosis: Reversible changes in RS-T interval during severe acidosis caused by administration of carbon dioxide. *Am Heart J* 33:458, 1947.
8. Anderson LE, Henrich WL: Alkalemia-associated morbidity and mortality in medical and surgical patients. *South Med J* 80:729, 1987.
9. Anderson RJ et al: Mechanism of effect of hypercapnic acidosis on renin secretion in the dog. *Am J Physiol* 238:F119, 1980.
10. Arbus GS et al: Characterization and clinical application of the "significance band" for acute respiratory alkalosis. *N Engl J Med* 280:117, 1969.
11. Askanazi J et al: Respiratory changes induced by the large glucose loads of total parenteral nutrition. *JAMA* 243:1444, 1980.
12. Asmussen E, Consolazio FC: The circulation in rest and work on Mount Evans. *Am J Physiol* 132:55, 1941.
13. Auer LM, Johansson BB: Dilatation of pial arterial vessels in hypercapnia and in acute hypertension. *Acta Physiol Scand* 109:249, 1980.
14. Augustinsson D et al: Influence of heat exposure on acid/base and fluid balance in hyperhydrated goats. *Acta Physiol Scand* 126:499, 1986.
15. Ayres SM, Grace WJ: Inappropriate ventilation and hypoxemia as causes of cardiac arrhythmias. *Am J Med* 46:495, 1969.
16. Ayres SM et al: The lung in shock. *Am J Cardiol* 26:588, 1970.

17. Barcroft H et al: The effect of carbon dioxide on the respiratory response to noradrenaline in man. *J Physiol* 137:365, 1957.
18. Barker ES et al: The renal response in man to acute experimental respiratory alkalosis and acidosis. *J Clin Invest* 36:515, 1957.
19. Bear R et al: Effect of metabolic alkalosis on respiratory function in patients with chronic obstructive lung disease. *Can Med Assoc J* 117:900, 1977.
20. Bendixen HH et al: Influence of respiratory acidosis on circulatory effect of epinephrine in dogs. *Circ Res* 13:64, 1963.
21. Berger AJ et al: Regulation of respiration. *N Engl J Med* 297:92, 194, 1977.
22. Berns AS et al: Effect of hypercapnic acidosis on renal water excretion in the dog. *Kidney Int* 15:116, 1979.
23. Bersentes TJ, Simmons DH: Effects of acute acidosis on renal hemodynamics. *Am J Physiol* 212:633, 1967.
24. Blair E: Acid-base balance in bacteremic shock. *Arch Intern Med* 127:731, 1971.
25. Blechner JN et al: Oxygen, carbon dioxide and hydrogen ion concentrations in arterial blood during pregnancy. *Am J Obstet Gynecol* 100:1, 1968.
26. Bleich HL et al: The response of cerebrospinal fluid composition to sustained hypercapnia. *J Clin Invest* 43:11, 1964.
27. Bone RC et al: Controlled oxygen administration in acute respiratory failure in chronic obstructive pulmonary disease. *Am J Med* 65:896, 1978.
28. Boycott AE, Haldane JS: The effects of low atmospheric pressures on respiration. *J Physiol* 37:355, 1908.
29. Boyd AE, Beller GA: Heat exhaustion and respiratory alkalosis. *Ann Intern Med* 83:835, 1975.
30. Brackett NC Jr et al: Carbon dioxide titration curve of normal man. *N Engl J Med* 272:6, 1965.
31. Brackett NC Jr et al: Acid-base response to chronic hypercapnia in man. *N Engl J Med* 280:124, 1969.
32. Brazeau P, Gilman A: Effect of plasma CO_2 tension on renal tubular reabsorption of bicarbonate. *Am J Physiol* 175:33, 1953.
33. Brimiouille S et al: Hydrochloric acid infusion for the treatment of metabolic alkalosis associated with respiratory acidosis. *Crit Care Med* 17:232, 1989.
34. Broadie TA et al: The effect of hypoxia and hypercapnia on canine pancreatic blood flow. *J Surg Res* 27:114, 1979.
35. Brown EB: Physiological effects of hyperventilation. *Physiol Rev* 33:445, 1953.
36. Brown EB et al: Ventricular fibrillation following a rapid fall in alveolar carbon dioxide tension. *Am J Physiol* 169:56, 1952.
37. Brown HW, Plum F: The neurologic basis of Cheyne-Stokes respiration. *Am J Med* 30:849, 1961.
38. Burnum JF et al: The effect of hypocapnia on arterial blood pressure. *Circulation* 9:89, 1954.
39. Bushinsky DA: Net proton influx into bone during metabolic, but not respiratory acidosis. *Am J Physiol* 254:F306, 1988.
40. Bushinsky DA: Net calcium efflux from live bone during chronic metabolic, but not respiratory acidosis. *Am J Physiol* 256:F836, 1989.
41. Bushinsky DA, Gennari FJ: Life threatening hyperkalemia induced by arginine. *Ann Intern Med* 89:632, 1978.
42. Busija DW, Heistad DD: Atropine does not alleviate cerebral vasodilation during hypercapnia. *Am J Physiol* 242:H683, 1982.
43. Cain SM, Dunn JE: Transient arterial lactic acid changes in unanesthetized dogs at 21,000 feet. *Am J Physiol* 206:1437, 1964.
44. Carroll D: Oxygen tension and acid-base adjustment in cardiac failure. *Johns Hopkins Med J* 103:242, 1958.
45. Carter NW et al: Tissue and renal response to chronic respiratory acidosis. *J Clin Invest* 38:949, 1959.
46. Catchlove RFH, Kafer ER: The effects of diazepam on respiration in patients with obstructive pulmonary disease. *Anesthesiology* 34:14, 1971.
47. Cherniack NS, Von Euler C: Central neural and reflex control of breathing, in Fishman AP (ed): *Assessment of Pulmonary Function*. New York, McGraw-Hill, 1980, p. 69.
48. Chiodi H: Respiratory adaptation to chronic high altitude hypoxia. *J Appl Physiol* 10:81, 1957.
49. Christensen MS: Acid-base changes in cerebrospinal fluid and blood and blood volume changes following prolonged hyperventilation in man. *Br J Anaesth* 46:348, 1974.
50. Clark DD et al: Secondary hypocapnia fails to protect "whole body" intracellular pH during chronic HCl acidosis in the dog. *Kidney Int* 23:336, 1983.
51. Clark RSJ: The effect of voluntary overbreathing on the blood flow through the human forearm. *J Physiol* 118:537, 1952.
52. Cochran JB, Ramsay AG: The hyperpnoea produced by intravenous administration of salicylates. *Br J Pharmacol* 11:364, 1956.
53. Cogan MG: Chronic hypercapnia stimulates proximal bicarbonate reabsorption in the rat. *J Clin Invest* 74:1942, 1984.
54. Cohen JJ et al: The nature of the carbon dioxide titration curve in the normal dog. *J Clin Invest* 43:777, 1964.
55. Cohen JJ et al: Regulation of acid-base equilibrium in chronic hypocapnia. Evidence that the response of the kidney is not geared to the defense of extracellular H^+. *J Clin Invest* 57:1483, 1976.
56. Cohen JJ et al: Disorders of potassium balance, in Brenner BM, Rector FC Jr (eds): *The Kidney*, 2d ed. Philadelphia, Saunders, 1981, p 908.
57. Comstock MK et al: Rigidity and hypercarbia associated with high dose fentanyl induction of anesthesia. *Anesth Analg* 60:362, 1981.
58. Cosby RS et al: Pulmonary function in left ventricular failure including cardiac asthma. *Circulation* 15:492, 1957.
59. Covelli HG et al: Respiratory failure precipitated by high carbohydrate loads. *Ann Intern Med* 95:579, 1981.
60. Culpepper JA et al: Effect of mechanical ventilator mode on tendency toward respiratory alkalosis. *Am Rev Respir Dis* 132:1075, 1985.
61. Dempsey JA et al: Control of exercise hypernea under varying durations of exposure to moderate hypoxia. *Respir Physiol* 16:213, 1972.
62. Dempsey JA et al: Ventilatory acclimatization to moderate hypoxemia in man. *J Clin Invest* 53:1901, 1974.
63. Dempsey JA et al: Effects of moderate hypoxemia and hypocapnia on CSF H^+ and ventilation in man. *J Appl Physiol* 38:665, 1975.

64. Denes AE et al: Severe respiratory alkalosis. Unusual manifestation of viral hepatitis. *Postgrad Med* 63:240, 1978.
65. Detmer MD et al: Occurrence of hypercarbia due to an unusual failure of anesthetic equipment. *Anesthesiology* 52:278, 1980.
66. Dill DB et al: Blood as a physicochemical system: XII. Man at high altitudes. *J Biol Chem* 118:649, 1937.
67. Dulfano MJ, Ishikawa S: Quantitative acid-base relationships in chronic pulmonary patients during the stable state. *Am Rev Respir Dis* 93:251, 1966.
68. Dull WL et al: The pulmonary hemodynamic effects of almitrine infusion in men with chronic hypercapnia. *Clin Sci* 64:25, 1983.
69. Edmondson JW et al: Quantitative interrelationships between calcium and alkalosis. *Am J Physiol* 228:1082, 1975.
70. Eichenholz A: Respiratory alkalosis. *Arch Intern Med* 116:699, 1965.
71. Eichenholz A et al: Primary hypocapnia: A cause of metabolic acidosis. *J Appl Physiol* 17:283, 1962.
72. Eichenholz A et al: The pattern of compensatory response to chronic hypercapnia in patients with chronic obstructive pulmonary disease. *J Lab Clin Med* 68:265, 1966.
73. Eldridge F, Gherman C: Studies of oxygen administration in respiratory failure. *Ann Intern Med* 68:569, 1968.
74. Eldridge F, Salzer J: Effect of respiratory alkalosis on blood lactate and pyruvate in humans. *J Appl Physiol* 22:461, 1967.
75. Ellis EF et al: The effect of O_2 and CO_2 on prostaglandin levels in the cat cerebral cortex. *Circ Res* 51:652, 1982.
76. Engel K et al: Quantitative displacement of acid-base equilibrium in chronic respiratory acidosis. *J Appl Physiol* 24:288, 1968.
77. Engel K et al: Quantitative displacement of blood acid-base status in acute hypocapnia. *Scand J Clin Lab Invest* 23:5, 1969.
78. Enson Y et al: The influence of hydrogen ion concentration and hypoxia on the pulmonary circulation. *J Clin Invest* 43:1146, 1964.
79. Fanta CH et al: Glucocorticoids in acute asthma. A critical controlled trial. *Am J Med* 74:845, 1983.
80. Farber HR et al: The effect of therapeutic doses of aspirin on the acid-base balance of the blood in normal adults. *Am J Med Sci* 217:256, 1949.
81. Fink BR: Influence of cerebral activity in wakefulness on regulation of breathing. *J Appl Physiol* 16:15, 1961.
82. Fink BR et al: Monitoring of ventilation by integrated diaphragmatic electromyogram. Determination of carbon dioxide (CO_2) threshold in anesthetized man. *JAMA* 172:1367, 1960.
83. Forster HV et al: Incomplete compensation of CSF H^+ in man during acclimatization to high altitude (4300m). *J Appl Physiol* 38:1067, 1975.
84. Forwand SA et al: Effect of acetazolamide on acute mountain sickness. *N Engl J Med* 279:839, 1968.
85. Frumin MJ et al: Apneic oxygenation in man. *Anesthesiology* 20:789, 1959.
86. Fuller GR, MacLeod MG: Excretion of titratable acid during acute respiratory disturbances of acid-base balance. *Am J Physiol* 186:505, 1956.
87. Fulop M: Metabolic acidosis with alkalemia. *NY State J Med* 80:1365, 1980.
88. Gabow PA et al: Acid-base disturbances in the salicylate intoxicated adult. *Arch Intern Med* 138:1481, 1978.
89. Garay SM et al: Sustained reversal of chronic hypercapnia in patients with alveolar hypoventilation syndromes. Long-term maintenance with noninvasive nocturnal mechanical ventilation. *Am J Med* 70:269, 1981.
90. Gaudio R, Abramson N: Heat-induced hyperventilation. *J Appl Physiol* 25:742, 1968.
91. Geddes IC, Gray TC: Hyperventilation for maintenance of anaesthesia. *Lancet* 2:4, 1959.
92. Gennari FJ et al: The nature of the renal adaptation to chronic hypocapnia. *J Clin Invest* 51:1722, 1972.
93. Gennari FJ et al: Acid-base response to chronic hypocapnia in man. *Clin Res* 28:533A, 1980.
94. Gennari FJ et al: Measurement of acid-base status, in Cohen JJ, Kassirer JP (eds): *Acid-base.* Boston, Little, Brown, 1982, p 97.
95. Gennari FJ et al: Normal acid-base values, in Cohen JJ, Kassirer JP (eds): *Acid-base.* Boston, Little, Brown, 1982, p 107.
96. Gennari FJ, Kassirer JP: Respiratory alkalosis, in Cohen JJ, Kassirer JP (eds): *Acid-base.* Boston, Little, Brown, 1982, p 349.
97. Gennari FJ, Rimmer JM: Acid-base disorders in end-stage renal disease. Part II. *Semin Dialysis* 3:161, 1990.
98. Gerhardt RC et al: Isolated ultrafiltration in the treatment of fluid overload in cardiogenic shock. *Arch Intern Med* 139:358, 1979.
99. Giebisch G et al: The extrarenal response to acute acid-base disturbances of respiratory origin. *J Clin Invest* 34:231, 1955.
100. Gieseke J et al: Effects of carbohydrate on carbon dioxide excretion in patients with airway disease. *Chest* 71:55, 1977.
101. Gledhill N et al: Renal response to short-term hypocapnia in man. *Kidney Int* 8:376:1975.
102. Glenn WWL et al: Total ventilatory support in a quadriplegic patient with radiofrequency electrophrenic respiration. *N Engl J Med* 286:513, 1972.
103. Glenn WWL et al: Long-term ventilatory support by diaphragm pacing in quadriplegia. *Ann Surg* 183:566, 1976.
104. Goldring RM et al: Respiratory-renal adjustments in chronic hypercapnia in man. *Am J Med* 51:772, 1971.
105. Goldstein MB et al: The influence of graded degrees of chronic hypercapnia on the acute carbon dioxide titration curve. *J Clin Invest* 50:208, 1971.
106. Gotoh F et al: Cerebral effects of hyperventilation in man. *Arch Neurol* 12:410, 1965.
107. Graham G, Poulton EP: Influence of high temperature on protein metabolism with reference to fever. *Q J Med* 6:82, 1912.
108. Green LH, Smith TW: The use of digitalis in patients with pulmonary disease. *Ann Intern Med* 87:459, 1977.
109. Guilleminault C et al: Clinical overview of the sleep apnea syndromes, in Guilleminault C, Dement WC (eds): *Sleep Apnea Syndromes.* New York, Liss, 1978, p 1.
110. Guz A et al: Experimental results of vagal block in cardiopulmonary disease, in Porter R (ed): *Breathing: Hering-Breuer Centenary Symposium.* London, Churchill, 1970, p 315.
111. Haffner JG, Salm SA: Controlled hyperventilation in pa-

tients with intracranial hypertension. Applications and management. *Arch Intern Med* 143:765, 1983.
112. Haldane JS, Poulton EP: The effects of want of oxygen on respiration. *J Physiol* 37:390, 1908.
113. Haldane JS, Priestly JG: The regulation of the lung ventilation. *J Physiol* 32:225, 1905.
114. Hamm LL et al: Sorbent regenerative hemodialysis as a potential cause of acute hypercapnia. *Kidney Int* 21:416, 1982.
115. Harrington JT, Cohen JJ: Metabolic acidosis, in Cohen JJ, Kassirer JP (eds): *Acid-base*. Boston, Little, Brown, 1982, p 121.
116. Harrington JT, Kassirer JP: Metabolic alkalosis, in Cohen JJ, Kassirer JP (eds): *Acid-base*. Boston, Little, Brown, 1982, p 227.
117. Hassan H et al: Hypercapnia and hyperkalaemia. *Anaesthesia* 34:897, 1979.
118. Heinemann HO, Goldring RM: Bicarbonate and the regulation of ventilation. *Am J Med* 57:361, 1974.
119. Henderson Y, Haggard HW: Respiratory regulation of the CO_2 capacity of the blood: III. The effects of excessive pulmonary ventilation. *J Biol Chem* 33:355, 1918.
120. Heyman A et al: Effects of bilateral cerebral infarction on respiratory center sensitivity. *Neurology* 8:694, 1958.
121. Heymans C et al: Sinus carotidien et réflexes respiratoires: III Sensibilité des sinus carotidiens aux substances chimiques. Action stimulante respiratoire reflexe en sulfure de sodium, du cyanure de potassium, de la nicotine et de la lobeline. *Arch Int Pharmacodyn Ther* 40:54, 1931.
122. Hoff HE, Breckenridge CG: Intrinsic mechanism in periodic breathing. *Arch Neurol Psychiatry* 72:11, 1954.
123. Holford FD, Mithoefer JC: Cardiac arrhythmias in hospitalized patients with chronic obstructive pulmonary disease. *Am Rev Respir Dis* 108:879, 1973.
124. Hornbein TF, Pavlin EG: Distribution of H^+ and HCO_3 between CSF and blood during respiratory alkalosis in dogs. *Am J Physiol* 228:1149, 1975.
125. Horres AD, Bernthal T: Localized multiple minute pulmonary embolism and breathing. *J Appl Physiol* 16:842, 1961.
126. Houston CS, Riley RL: Respiratory and circulatory changes during acclimatization to high altitude. *Am J Physiol* 149:565, 1947.
127. Hudson LD et al: Arrhythmias associated with acute respiratory failure in patients with chronic airway obstruction. *Chest* 63:661, 1973.
128. Hudson LD et al: Does intermittent mandatory ventilation correct respiratory alkalosis in patients receiving assisted ventilation? *Am Rev Respir Dis* 132:1071, 1985.
129. Hughes RL et al: Effect of hypercarbia on hepatic blood flow and oxygen consumption in the greyhound. *Br J Anaesth* 51:289, 1979.
130. Hunter FD et al: Metabolic and nutritional evaluation of patients supported with mechanical ventilation. *Crit Care Med* 8:628, 1980.
131. Ichiyanagi K et al: Acid-base changes of arterial plasma during exogenous and endogenous hypercapnia in man. *Respir Physiol* 7:310, 1969.
132. Jacobs WF et al: False positive ST-T wave changes secondary to hyperventilation and exercise: A cineangiographic correlation. *Ann Intern Med* 81:479, 1974.
133. Kaehny WD et al: Influence of steady-state $PaCO_2$ on escape from ADH-induced water retention in the dog. *Am J Physiol* 234:F291, 1978.
134. Karetzy MS, Mithoefer JC: The cause of hyperventilation and arterial hypoxia in patients with cirrhosis of the liver. *Am J Med Sci* 254:797, 1967.
135. Karp HR et al: Cerebral circulation and function in Cheyne-Stokes respiration. *Am J Med* 30:861, 1961.
136. Kazemi H et al: Brain CO_2 buffering capacity in respiratory acidosis and alkalosis. *J Appl Physiol* 22:241, 1967.
137. Kazemi H et al: Brain and cerebrospinal fluid lactate concentration in respiratory acidosis and alkalosis. *Respir Physiol* 6:178, 1969.
138. Kenamond TG et al: Severe recurrent alkalemia in a patient undergoing continuous cycling peritoneal dialysis. *Am J Med* 81:588, 1986.
139. Kendrick JG et al: Regulation of blood flow to respiratory muscles during hypoxia and hypercapnia. *Proc Soc Exp Biol Med* 166:157, 1981.
140. Kety SS, Schmidt CF: The effects of altered arterial tensions of carbon dioxide and oxygen on cerebral blood flow and cerebral oxygen consumption of normal young men. *J Clin Invest* 27:484, 1948.
141. Kilburn KH: Neurologic manifestations of respiratory failure. *Arch Intern Med* 116:409, 1965.
142. Kilburn KH, Dowell AR: Renal function in respiratory failure. *Arch Intern Med* 127:754, 1971.
143. Kilburn KH et al: Effects of breathing 10% carbon dioxide on the pulmonary circulation of human subjects. *Circulation* 39:639, 1969.
144. Klausen K: Cardiac output in man in rest and work during and after acclimatization to 3800 m. *J Appl Physiol* 21:609, 1966.
145. Klein SL, Lilburn JK: An unusual case of hypercarbia during general anesthesia. *Anesthesiology* 53:248, 1980.
146. Koehler RC, Traystman RJ: Bicarbonate ion modulation of cerebral blood flow during hypoxia and hypercapnia. *Am J Physiol* 243:H33, 1982.
147. Kontos HA et al: Roles of hypercapnia and acidosis in the vasodilator response to hypercapnic acidosis. *Am J Physiol* 215:1406, 1968.
148. Kornbluth RS, Turino GM: Respiratory control in diffuse interstitial lung disease and diseases of the pulmonary vasculature. *Clin Chest Med* 1:91, 1980.
149. Krapf R et al: Chronic respiratory alkalosis: The effect of sustained hyperventilation on renal regulation of acid-base equilibrium. *N Engl J Med* 324:1394, 1991.
150. Laaban JP et al: Hypophosphatemia induced by mechanical ventilation in patients with chronic obstructive pulmonary disease. *Crit Care Med* 17:1115, 1989.
151. Lagrange BM, Hood VL: Ketoacid production in acute respiratory and metabolic acidosis and alkalosis in rats. *Am J Physiol* 256:F437, 1989.
152. Lakshminarayan S et al: Bicarbonate therapy in severe acute respiratory acidosis. *Scand J Resp Dis* 54:128, 1973.
153. Lange LS, Laszlo G: Cerebral tumour presenting with hyperventilation. *J Neurol Neurosurg Psychiatry* 28:317, 1965.
154. Lary D, Goldschlarger N: Electrocardiogram changes during hyperventilation resembling myocardial ischemia in patients with normal coronary arteriograms. *Am Heart J* 87:383, 1974.

155. Laszlo G et al: The immediate buffering of retained carbon dioxide in man. *Clin Sci* 37:299, 1969.
156. Lenfant C, Sullivan K: Adaptation to high altitude. *N Engl J Med* 284:1298, 1971.
157. Leusen I, Weyne J: Metabolic processes in the brain during respiratory and non-respiratory alkalosis and acidosis, in Loeschcke HH (ed): *Acid-Base Homeostasis of the Brain Extracellular Fluid and the Respiratory Control System.* Stuttgart, Thieme, 1976, p 27.
158. LeVasseur JE et al: Responses of pial arterioles after prolonged hypercapnia and hypoxia in the awake rabbit. *J Appl Physiol* 46:89, 1979.
159. Little RC, Smith CW: Cardiovascular response to acute hypocapnia due to overbreathing. *Am J Physiol* 206:1025, 1964.
160. Lourenco RV et al: The regulation of ventilation in diffuse pulmonary fibrosis. *Am J Med* 38:199, 1965.
161. Lucius H et al: Respiratory functions, buffer system and electrolyte concentrations of blood during human pregnancy. *Respir Physiol* 9:311, 1970.
162. Luke RG, Levitin H: The renal and electrolyte response to respiratory acidosis in the adrenalectomized rat. *Yale J Biol Med* 39:27, 1966.
163. Lum LC: The syndrome of chronic habitual hyperventilation, in Hill OW (ed): *Modern Trends in Psychosomatic Medicine.* London, Butterworth, 1976, vol 3, p 196.
164. Lynne-Davies P et al: Partitioning of immediate ventilatory stability to added elastic loads in cats. *J Appl Physiol* 30:814, 1971.
165. Lyons HA, Antonio R: The sensitivity of the respiratory center in pregnancy and after the administration of progesterone. *Trans Assoc Am Physicians* 72:173, 1959.
166. Lyons HA, Huang CT: Therapeutic use of progesterone in alveolar hypoventilation associated with obesity. *Am J Med* 44:881, 1968.
167. Lyons JH, Moore FD: Posttraumatic alkalosis: Incidence and pathophysiology of alkalosis in surgery. *Surgery* 60:93, 1966.
168. Machida H: Influence of progesterone on arterial blood and CSF acid-base balance in women. *J Appl Physiol* 51:1433, 1981.
169. Madias NE et al: The maladaptive renal response to secondary hypocapnia during chronic HCl acidosis in the dog. *J Clin Invest* 60:1393, 1977.
170. Madias NE et al: Maladaptive renal response to secondary hypercapnia in chronic metabolic alkalosis. *Am J Physiol* 238:F283, 1980.
171. Madias NE, Cohen JJ: Determinants of arterial carbon dioxide tension and carbon dioxide balance, in Cohen JJ, Kassirer JP (eds): *Acid-base.* Boston, Little, Brown, 1982, p 41.
172. Madias NE, Cohen JJ: Respiratory acidosis, in Cohen JJ, Kassirer JP (eds): *Acid-base.* Boston, Little, Brown, 1982, p 307.
173. Madias NE et al: Regulation of acid-base equilibrium in chronic hypercapnia. *Kidney Int* 27:538, 1985.
174. Madias NE et al: Influence of acute and chronic respiratory alkalosis on preexisting chronic metabolic alkalosis. *Am J Physiol* 258:F479, 1990.
175. Magarian GJ: Hyperventilation syndromes: Infrequently recognized common expressions of anxiety and stress. *Medicine* 61:219, 1982.
176. Makoff D, Rosenbaum BJ: Adaptation to chronic hypercapnia in the potassium depleted dog. *Am J Physiol* 220:1724, 1971.
177. Manfredi F et al: Papilledema in chronic respiratory acidosis. *Am J Med* 30:175, 1961.
178. Manfredi F: Effects of hypocapnia and hypercapnia on intracellular acid-base equilibrium in man. *J Lab Clin Med* 69:304, 1967.
179. Markello R et al: Hyperventilation studies during nitrous oxide-narcotic relaxant anesthesia. *Anesthesiology* 24:225, 1963.
180. Marks C, Goldring R: Chronic hypercapnia during methadone maintenance. *Am Rev Respir Dis* 108:1088, 1973.
181. Marshall BE, Wollman HL: General anesthetics, in Gilman AG et al (eds): *The Pharmacological Basis of Therapeutics*, 6th ed. New York, MacMillan, 1980, p 276.
182. Martinez-Maldonado M, Sanchez-Montserrat R: Respiratory acidosis and alkalosis. *Clin Nephrol* 7:191, 1977.
183. Massumi RH, Wimacker JL: Severe depression of the respiratory center in myxedema. *Am J Med* 36:876, 1964.
184. Mazzara JT et al: Extreme hypocapnia in the critically ill patient. *Am J Med* 56:450, 1974.
185. McCombs RR et al: Myths, morbidity and mortality in asthma. *JAMA* 242:1521, 1979.
186. McFadden ER Jr, Lyons HA: Arteriolar blood gas tensions in asthma. *N Engl J Med* 278:1027, 1968.
187. McHenry PL et al: False positive ECG response to exercise secondary to hyperventilation. Cineangiographic correlation. *Am Heart J* 79:683, 1970.
188. Mellins RB et al: Failure of automatic control of ventilation (Ondine's Curse). *Medicine* 49:487, 1970.
189. Menitove SM, Goldring RM: Combined ventilator and bicarbonate strategy in the management of status asthmaticus. *Am J Med* 74:898, 1983.
190. Milledge JS, Lahiri S: Respiratory control in lowlanders and Sherpa highlanders at altitude. *Respir Physiol* 2:310, 1967.
191. Miller A, Granada M: In-hospital mortality in the Pickwickian syndrome. *Am J Med* 56:144, 1974.
192. Miller LC et al: Potential hazards of rapid smoking as a technique for the modification of smoking behavior. *N Engl J Med* 297:590, 1977.
193. Miller PD, Berns AS: Acute metabolic alkalosis perpetuating hypercarbia. *JAMA* 238:2400, 1977.
194. Mitchell JH et al: The effects of acid-base disturbances on cardiovascular and pulmonary function. *Kidney Int* 1:375, 1972.
195. Mitchell RA et al: Regions of respiratory chemosensitivity on the surface of the medulla. *Ann NY Acad Sci* 109:661, 1963.
196. Mithoefer JC et al: Use of sodium bicarbonate in treatment of acute bronchial asthma. *N Engl J Med* 272:1200, 1965.
197. Mithoefer JC et al: Indication for the use of sodium bicarbonate in the treatment of intractable asthma. *Respiration* 25:201, 1968.
198. Model DG: Nitrazepam induced respiratory failure in chronic obstructive lung disease. *Br J Dis Chest* 67:128, 1973.
199. Model DG, Berry DJ: Effects of chlordiazepoxide in respi-

ratory failure due to chronic bronchitis. *Lancet* 2:869, 1974.

200. Moller B: The hydrogen ion concentration in arterial blood. *Acta Med Scand* 165(suppl 348):11, 1959.
201. Morse JO et al: Effect of long-term continuous oxygen therapy in patients with severe chronic hypercapnia. *Am Rev Respir Dis* 107:1064, 1973.
202. Moser KM et al: Respiratory stimulation with intravenous doxapram in respiratory failure. *N Engl J Med* 288:427, 1973.
203. Mountain RB et al: Acid-base disturbances in acute asthma. *Chest* 98:651, 1990.
204. Narins RG, Emmett M: Simple and mixed acid-base disorders: A practical approach. *Medicine* 59:161, 1980.
205. Narins RG et al: Effects of acute acid-base changes on in vivo total ammonia synthesis in the rat. *Contrib Nephrol* 31:47, 1982.
206. Neff TA, Petty TL: Long-term continuous oxygen therapy in chronic airway obstruction. Mortality and relationship to cor pulmonale, hypoxia and hypercapnia. *Ann Intern Med* 72:621, 1970.
207. Neff TA, Petty TL: Tolerance and survival in severe chronic hypercapnia. *Arch Intern Med* 129:591, 1972.
208. Newton DAG, Bone I: Papilloedema and optic atrophy in chronic hypercapnia. *Br J Dis Chest* 73:399, 1979.
209. Oberleithner H et al: The effect of respiratory and metabolic acid-base changes on ionized calcium concentration: In vivo and in vitro experiments in man and rat. *Eur J Clin Invest* 12:451, 1982.
210. Orr JA et al: Cerebrospinal fluid alkalosis during high altitude sojourn in unanesthetized ponies. *Respir Physiol* 25:23, 1975.
211. Paintal AS: The nature and effects of sensory inputs into the respiratory centers. *Fed Proc* 36:2428, 1977.
212. Patterson JL et al: Cerebral circulation and metabolism in chronic pulmonary emphysema. *Am J Med* 12:382, 1952.
213. Pauli HG et al: Renal function during prolonged exposure to hypoxia and carbon monoxide. *Scand J Lab Clin Invest* 103(suppl):55, 1968.
214. Petounis AD et al: Effect of hypercapnia and hyperventilation on human intraocular pressure during general anesthesia following acetazolamide administration. *Br J Ophthalmol* 64:422, 1980.
215. Pittinger CB et al: Antibiotic-induced paralysis *Anesth Analg* 49:487, 1970.
216. Plum F: Hyperpnea, hyperventilation and brain dysfunction. *Ann Intern Med* 76:328, 1972.
217. Plum F et al: Neurologic significance of post hyperventilation apnea. *JAMA* 191:1050, 1962.
218. Plum F et al: Effect of hyperbaric-hyperoxic hyperventilation on blood, brain and CSF lactate. *Am J Physiol* 215:1240, 1968.
219. Plum F, Price RW: Acid-base balance in cisternal and lumbar cerebrospinal fluid in hospital patients. *N Engl J Med* 289:1346, 1973.
220. Plum F, Swanson AG: Central neurogenic hyperventilation in man. *Arch Neurol Psychiatry* 81:535, 1959.
221. Polak A et al: Effects of chronic hypercapnia on electrolyte and acid-base equilibrium: I. Adaptation. *J Clin Invest* 40:1223,1965.
222. Posner JB et al: Acid-base balance in cerebrospinal fluid. *Arch Neurol* 12:479, 1965.
223. Posner JB, Plum F: Spinal-fluid pH and neurologic symptoms in systemic acidosis. *N Engl J Med* 277:605, 1967.
224. Potter ED, McCloskey DI: Respiratory stimulation by angiotensin II. *Respir Physiol* 36:367, 1979.
225. Price HL: Effects of carbon dioxide on the cardiovascular system. *Anesthesiology* 21:652, 1960.
226. Prys-Roberts C et al: Circulatory influences of artificial ventilation during nitrous oxide anaesthesia in man: II. Results: The relative influence of mean intrathoracic pressure and arterial carbon dioxide tension. *Br J Anaesth* 39:533, 1967.
227. Prytz H, Thomsen AC: Acid-base status in liver cirrhosis. Disturbances in stable, terminal and porta-caval shunted patients. *Scand J Gastroenterol* 11:249, 1976.
228. Pugh LGCE: Blood volumes and haemoglobin concentration at altitudes above 18000 feet (5500 m). *J Physiol* 170:344, 1964.
229. Rah KH et al: Respiratory acidosis with the small Storz-Hopkins bronchoscopes: Occurrence and management. *Ann Thorac Surg* 27:197, 1979.
230. Rahn H et al: The effects of hypocapnia on performance. *J Aviation Med* 17:164, 1946.
231. Rahn H, Otis AB: Man's respiratory response during and after acclimatization in high altitude. *Am J Physiol* 157:445, 1949.
232. Ramsoe K et al: Liver function and blood flow at high altitude. *J Appl Physiol* 28:725, 1970.
233. Rebuck AS et al: Respiratory frequency response to progressive isocapnic hypoxia. *J Physiol* 258:19, 1976.
234. Rebuck AS, Read J: Assessment and management of severe asthma. *Am J Med* 51:788, 1971.
235. Refsum HE: Acid-base status in patients with chronic hypercapnia and hypoxemia. *Clin Sci* 27:407, 1964.
236. Reivich M: Arterial PCO_2 and cerebral hemodynamics. *Am J Physiol* 206:25, 1964.
237. Rennie D et al: Renal oxygenation in male Peruvian natives living permanently at high altitude. *J Appl Physiol* 30:450, 1971.
238. Rice RL: Symptom patterns of the hyperventilation syndrome. *Am J Med* 8:691, 1950.
239. Richardson DW et al: General regional circulatory response to changes in blood pH and carbon dioxide tension. *J Clin Invest* 40:31, 1961.
240. Richter T et al: The syndrome of alveolar hypoventilation and diminished sensitivity of the respiratory center. *N Engl J Med* 256:1165, 1957.
241. Riley DJ et al: Ventilatory response to hypercapnia and hypoxia during continuous aspirin ingestion. *J Appl Physiol* 43:971, 1977.
242. Robertson BJ et al: Enhancement of the arrhythmogenic effect of hypercapnia of surgical stimulation during halothane anesthesia in man. *Can Anaesth Soc J* 28:342, 1981.
243. Roncoroni AJ et al: Acid-base equilibrium of cerebrospinal fluid in chronic respiratory acidosis and provoked hypercapnia in relaxed patients. *Am Rev Respir Dis* 102:790, 1971.
244. Rosenstein R, Borison HL: Actions of carbon dioxide and sodium salicylate on central control of respiration in cats. *J Pharmacol Exp Ther* 139:361, 1963.
245. Rout MW et al: Prognosis in acute cerebrovascular acci-

dents in relation to respiratory pattern and blood gas tension. *Br Med J* 3:7, 1971.

246. Rowe GG et al: Effects of hyperventilation on systemic and coronary hemodynamics. *Am Heart J* 63:67, 1962.
247. Salzman MA, Salzano JV: Effect of carbohydrate metabolism upon respiratory gas exchange. *J Appl Physiol* 30:228, 1971.
248. Saltzman H et al: Correlation of clinical and physiological manifestations of sustained hyperventilation. *N Engl J Med* 268:1431, 1963.
249. Santella RN et al: Delivery dependence of early proximal bicarbonate reabsorption in the rat in respiratory acidosis and alkalosis. *J Clin Invest* 87:631, 1991.
250. Santiago TV et al: Control of breathing during methadone addiction. *Am J Med* 62:347, 1977.
251. Sapir DG et al: The effects of chronic hypoxemia on electrolyte and acid-base equilibrium: An examination of normocapneic hypoxemia and of the influence of hypoxemia on the adaption to chronic hypercapnia. *J Clin Invest* 46:369, 1967.
252. Sapira J: The narcotic addict as a medical patient. *Am J Med* 45:555, 1968.
253. Schwartz WB et al: Effects of chronic hypercapnia on electrolyte and acid-base equilibrium: II. Recovery, with special reference to the influence of chloride intake. *J Clin Invest* 40:1238, 1961.
254. Schwartz WB et al: The response of extracellular hydrogen ion concentration to graded degrees of chronic hypercapnia. The physiologic limits of the defense of pH. *J Clin Invest* 44:291, 1965.
255. Sechzer PH et al: Effect of CO_2 inhalation on arterial pressure, ECG and plasma catecholamines and 17-OH corticosteroids in normal man. *J Appl Physiol* 15:454, 1960.
256. Semb BKA: The effect of hypercarbia on gastric mucosal flow in conscious animals. *Scand J Gastroenterol* 17:657, 1982.
257. Severinghaus JW et al: Respiratory control at high altitude suggesting active transport regulation of CSF pH. *J Appl Physiol* 18:1155, 1963.
258. Severinghaus JW et al: Cerebral blood flow in man at high altitudes, role of cerebrospinal fluid pH in normalization of flow in chronic hypocapnia. *Circ Res* 19:274, 1966.
259. Severinghaus JW et al: Respiratory insensitivity to hypoxia in a chronically hypoxic man. *Respir Physiol* 1:308, 1966.
260. Sideris DA et al: Type of cardiac dysrhythmias in respiratory failure. *Am Heart J* 89:32, 1975.
261. Siesjo BK: The regulation of cerebrospinal fluid pH. *Kidney Int* 1:360, 1972.
262. Siggaard-Andersen J et al: Plasma volume and vascular permeability during hypoxia and carbon monoxide exposure. *Scand J Clin Lab Invest* 103(suppl):39, 1968.
263. Silverstein ME et al: Treatment of severe fluid overload by ultrafiltration. *N Engl J Med* 291:747, 1974.
264. Simmons DH et al: Hyperventilation and respiratory alkalosis as signs of gram-negative bacteremia. *JAMA* 174:2196, 1960.
265. Singer RB: The acid-base disturbance in salicylate intoxication. *Medicine* 33:1, 1954.
266. Skatrud JB et al: Ventilatory response to medroxyprogesterone acetate in normal subjects: Time course and mechanism. *J Appl Physiol* 44:939, 1978.
267. Skatrud JB et al: Determinants of chronic carbon dioxide retention and its correction. *J Clin Invest* 65:813, 1980.
268. Skatrud JB et al: Correction of CO_2 retention during sleep in patients with chronic obstructive pulmonary diseases. *Am Rev Respir Dis* 124:260, 1981.
269. Smith RB et al: Intraocular and intracranial pressure during respiratory alkalosis and acidosis. *Br J Anaesth* 53:967, 1981.
270. Soley MH, Shock NW: The etiology of effort syndrome. *Am J Med Sci* 196:840, 1938.
271. Sorenson SC, Severinghaus JW: Irreversible respiratory insensitivity to acute hypoxia in man born at high altitude. *J Appl Physiol* 25:217, 1968.
272. Sprung CL et al: The metabolic and respiratory alterations of heat stroke. *Arch Intern Med* 140:665, 1980.
273. Stanbury SW, Thomson AE: The renal response to respiratory alkalosis. *Clin Sci* 11:357, 1952.
274. Stein M, Levy SE: Reflex and humoral response to pulmonary embolism. *Prog Cardiovasc Dis* 17:167, 1974.
275. Sunderrajan S et al: Nortriptyline-induced severe hyperventilation. *Arch Intern Med* 145:746, 1985.
276. Sutton FD et al: Progesterone for outpatient treatment of Pickwickian syndrome. *Ann Intern Med* 83:476, 1975.
277. Swanson AG et al: Effects of blood pH and carbon dioxide on cerebral electrical activity. *Neurology* 8:787, 1958.
278. Szatalowicz VL et al: Plasma antidiuretic hormone in acute respiratory failure. *Am J Med* 72:583, 1982.
279. Szucs MM et al: Diagnostic sensitivity of laboratory findings in acute pulmonary embolism. *Ann Intern Med* 74:161, 1971.
280. Takano N: Blood lactate accumulation and its causative factors during passive hyperventilation in dogs. *Jpn J Physiol* 16:481, 1966.
281. Takano N, Kaneda J: Renal contribution to acid-base regulation during the menstrual cycle. *Am J Physiol* 244:F320, 1983.
282. Tenney SM: The effect of carbon dioxide on neurohumoral and endocrine mechanisms. *Anesthesiology* 21:674, 1960.
283. Tenney SM, Miller RM: The respiratory and circulatory actions of salicylate. *Am J Med* 19:498, 1955.
284. Trenchard D et al: Role of pulmonary vagal afferent nerve fibers in the development of rapid shallow breathing in lung inflammation. *Clin Sci* 42:251, 1972.
285. Vanamee P et al: Respiratory alkalosis in hepatic coma. *Arch Intern Med* 97:762, 1956.
286. Vanee JP et al: Response of mean and phasic coronary arterial blood flow to graded hypercapnia in dogs. *Br J Anaesth* 51:523, 1979.
287. van Ypersele de Strihou C et al: The "carbon dioxide response curve" for chronic hypercapnia in man. *N Engl J Med* 275:117, 1966.
288. Vogel JA, Harris CW: Cardiopulmonary response of resting man during early exposure to high altitude. *J Appl Physiol* 22:1124, 1967.
289. Walley KR et al: Acute respiratory acidosis decreases left ventricular contractility but increases cardiac output in dogs. *Circ Res* 67:628, 1990.
290. Wasserman AJ, Patterson JL: The cerebral vascular re-

sponse to reduction in arterial carbon dioxide tension. *J Clin Invest* 40:1297, 1961.
291. Webb AK et al: Severe bronchial asthma requiring ventilation. A review of 20 cases and advice on management. *Postgrad Med J* 55:162, 1979.
292. Wechsler RL et al: The effects of intravenously administered aminophylline on cerebral circulation and metabolism in man. *J Clin Invest* 29:28, 1950.
293. Weg JG et al: Hypothyroidism and alveolar hypoventilation. *Arch Intern Med* 115:302, 1965.
294. Wei EP et al: Role of prostaglandins in pial arterial response to CO_2 and hypoxia. *Am J Physiol* 238:H226, 1980.
295. Weil JV et al: Acquired attenuation of chemoreceptor function in chronically hypoxic man at high altitude. *J Clin Invest* 50:186, 1971.
296. Weil MH et al: Difference in acid-base status between venous and arterial blood during cardiopulmonary resuscitation. *N Engl J Med* 315:153, 1986.
297. West JB: Causes of carbon dioxide retention in lung disease. *N Engl J Med* 284:1232, 1971.
298. Whelan RF, Young IM: The effect of adrenaline and noradrenaline infusions on respiration in man. *Br J Pharmacol* 8:98, 1953.
299. Wilson RF et al: Severe alkalosis in critically ill surgical patients. *Arch Surg* 105:197, 1972.
300. Winslow et al: Hemodynamic studies and results of therapy in 50 patients with bacteremic shock. *Am J Med* 54:421, 1973.
301. Winters RW et al: Disturbances of acid-base equilibrium in salicylate intoxication. *Pediatrics* 23:260, 1959.
302. Wood WB et al: The effects of CO_2-induced respiratory acidosis on the depressor and pressor components of the dog's blood pressure to epinephrine. *J Pharmacol Exp Ther* 139:238, 1963.
303. Wright EA, McQuillen MP: Antibiotic induced neuromuscular blockage. *Ann NY Acad Sci* 183:358, 1971.
304. Yasue H et al: Coronary arterial spasm and Prinzmetal's variant form of angina induced by hyperventilation and trisbuffer infusion. *Circulation* 58:56, 1978.
305. Zwillich CM et al: Effects of progesterone on chemosensitivity in normal men. *J Lab Clin Med* 92:262, 1978.

CHAPTER 31

Mixed acid-base disorders

Michael Emmett • Robert G. Narins

INTRODUCTORY CONCEPTS AND CLASSIFICATION

Diagnosis and classification of the mixed acid-base disturbances require a clear understanding of the compensatory mechanisms that develop in response to the simple acid-base disorders (Table 31-1). The compensatory response may be described in terms of the Henderson equation (equation 1), which depicts the interdependence of the three prime acid-base parameters, hydrogen ion concentration ($[H^+]$), P_{CO_2}, and bicarbonate concentration ($[HCO_3^-]$).

$$[H^+]\ (\text{neq/liter}) = \frac{24\ P_{CO_2}(\text{mmHg})}{[HCO_3^-]\ (\text{meq/liter})} \quad (1)$$

The derivation and use of this equation were extensively discussed in Chap. 24.

Metabolic acid-base perturbations are characterized by primary disturbances in the bicarbonate concentration. The resulting change in the $P_{CO_2}/[HCO_3^-]$ ratio displaces the hydrogen ion concentration from normal. A secondary or compensatory change in P_{CO_2} acts to return the $[H^+]$ toward, but not to, normal. Thus, in metabolic acidosis, the primary reduction in bicarbonate concentration raises the $P_{CO_2}/[HCO_3^-]$ ratio, thereby acidifying blood. Acidemia stimulates respiration and secondarily lowers the P_{CO_2}, thereby ameliorating the initial reduction in pH. Metabolic acidosis is therefore characterized by primary hypobicarbonatemia, secondary hypocapnia, and a low arterial pH. Conversely, the chemical pattern of metabolic alkalosis encompasses primary hyperbicarbonatemia, secondary hypercapnia, and an increased arterial pH (Table 31-1).

Respiratory acid-base disorders primarily alter the P_{CO_2}, and the resulting change in the $P_{CO_2}/[HCO_3{}^-]$ ratio renders arterial pH abnormal. Secondary or compensatory changes in serum $[HCO_3^-]$ lessen the impact of the primary disorder. Thus, respiratory acidosis is characterized by primary hypercapnia, secondary hyperbicarbonatemia, and a low pH. Conversely, respiratory alkalosis displays a primary hypocapnia, secondary hypobicarbonatemia, and high pH. Maximal compensatory changes of $[HCO_3^-]$ develop over many hours to days. Therefore, compensation for respiratory disturbances are divided into *acute* and *chronic* stages.

TABLE 31-1 • Compensating responses to the simple acid-base disorders

Disorder	Primary disturbance	Compensating response	Expected limits of compensation
METABOLIC			
Acidosis	↓↓↓ HCO_3^-	↓↓ P_{CO_2}	$P_{CO_2} = 1.5(HCO_3^-) + 8 \pm 2$
Aklalosis	↑↑↑ HCO_3^-	↑↑ P_{CO_2}	P_{CO_2} increases by 6 mmHg for each 10 meq/liter increase in HCO_3^-
RESPIRATORY			
Acidosis			
Acute	↑↑↑ P_{CO_2}	↑ HCO_3^-	HCO_3^- increases 1 meq/liter for each 10 mmHg rise in P_{CO_2}
Chronic	↑↑↑ P_{CO_2}	↑↑ HCO_3^-	HCO_3^- increases 3.5 meq/liter for each 10 mmHg rise in P_{CO_2}
Alkalosis			
Acute	↓↓↓ P_{CO_2}	↓ HCO_3^-	HCO_3^- decreases 2 meq/liter for each 10 mmHg fall in P_{CO_2}
Chronic	↓↓↓ P_{CO_2}	↓↓ HCO_3^-	HCO_3^- decreases 5 meq/liter for each 10 mmHg fall in P_{CO_2}

Additionally, the expected relationships between changes in the anion gap and the serum bicarbonate concentration permit recognition of a variety of mixed metabolic disturbances (see Chap. 24). The biochemical basis for this diagnostic "tool" is the complex interaction between the accumulating acid and its prime titrant, sodium bicarbonate. For reasons discussed at length in Chap. 24, sodium bicarbonate clearly absorbs the vast bulk, although other buffers are potentially available to titrate accruing fixed acids. This being the case, the following relationship obtains between the change in [HCO_3^-] and the change in the anion gap. Figure 31-1[58] illustrates that a standard set of serum electrolytes provides enough information to diagnose coexisting high anion gap metabolic acidosis and metabolic alkalosis. Serum electrolytes also can reveal the coexistence of a mixed high anion gap and normal anion gap metabolic acidosis. The basis for these observations follows.

Addition of fixed acid to blood requires that entering protons combine with and destroy extracellular bicarbonate. The acid's accompanying anion effectively replaces the HCO_3^-. Hence $NaHCO_3$ is replaced by the sodium salt of the offending acid (Fig. 31-1). Should the added fixed acid be hydrochloric acid, as would occur in such metabolic acidoses as diarrhea and renal tubular acidosis, the anion gap would remain unchanged. Each added HCl molecule removes one bicarbonate anion and substitutes one chloride anion. Thus, the sum of the chloride and bicarbonate concentrations remains unchanged, since one anion (HCO_3^-) decreases by an amount equaling the other's (Cl^-) increase. The normal anion gap acidosis spawned by this titration is illustrated in the middle panel of Fig. 31-1. Should any acid other than hydrochloric acid be added, the anion gap must increase, owing to substitution of the routine measured bicarbonate anion with such usually unmeasured anions as β-hydroxybutyrate, acetoacetate, lactate, and others (see Table 10, Chap. 25). Since the sum of the concentrations of chloride and bicarbonate is reduced while the sodium concentration remains unchanged, the anion gap must increase. Serum electrolytes typical of any organic or inorganic acidosis elevating the anion gap are depicted in the third column of Fig. 31-1. Notice that both the normal and the high anion gap acidoses each reduce the serum bicarbonate concentration by 10 meq/liter. The lost bicarbonate is replaced by chloride in the hyperchloremic acidosis while lactate substitutes for the destroyed alkali in the high anion gap lactic acidosis. Were it to be measured, the serum lactate concentration would increase by 10 meq/liter, rising from 1 meq/liter to 11 meq/liter. Since the bicarbonate concentration fell by 10 meq/liter while the chloride and sodium concentrations remained unchanged, the anion gap had to increase by 10 meq/liter, rising to 20 meq/liter (Fig. 31-1). Although they move in opposite directions, the decrease in serum bicarbonate concentration (ΔHCO_3^-) matches both the increment in serum lactate concentration (Δlactate) and the increment in the anion gap (ΔAG). This

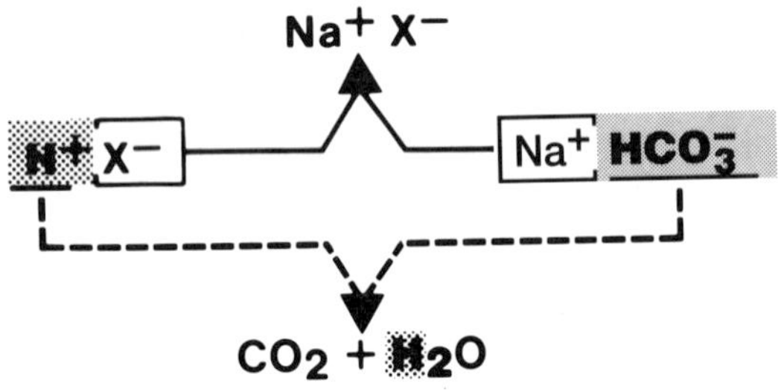

$$AG = Na^+ - (Cl^- + HCO_3^-) = 12 \pm 2 \text{ mM}$$

METABOLIC ACIDOSIS

	NORMAL	NORMAL AG ACIDOSIS	HIGH AG ACIDOSIS
Na^+	140	140	140
Cl^-	105	115	105
HCO_3^-	25	15	15
AG	10	10	20
ΔHCO_3^-*		−10	−10
ΔAG*		0	+10
LACT.$^-$	1	1	11
ΔLACT.*		0	+10

* Δ: CHANGE FROM NORMAL

FIGURE 31-1 • Titration of $NaHCO_3$ with a strong acid. Schematic representation. AG, anion gap; Lact., lactate. (From Narins RG, Emmett M: *Medicine* 59:161, 1980. Used by permission.)

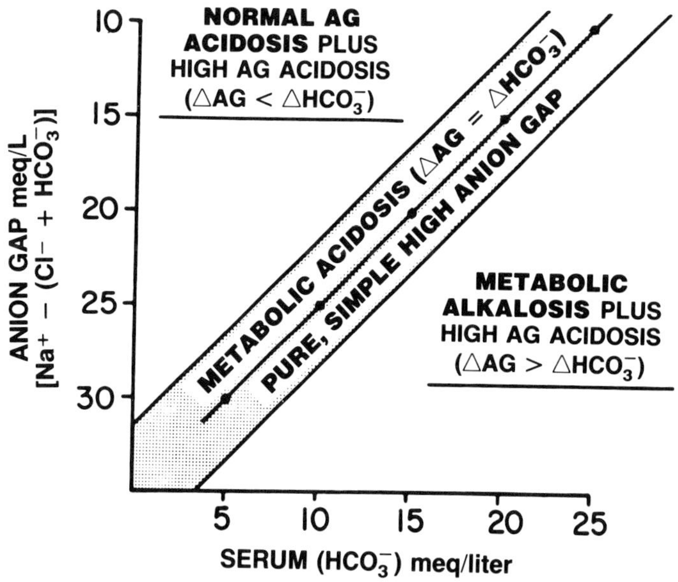

FIGURE 31-2 • Relationship between the anion gap (AG) and serum bicarbonate concentration in simple, high AG metabolic acidosis and in mixed metabolic disorders. See text for details. (From Goodkin et al: *Clin Endocrinol Metab* 13:333, 1984. Used by permission.)

thesis suggests that each meq/liter change in the anion gap (ΔAG) reflects a similar concentration change in serum lactate and the ΔAG (and therefore, the lactate concentration) should precisely equal the ΔHCO_3^- This point is illustrated in Fig. 31-2.[40] The close stoichiometry between the Δlactate and ΔHCO_3^- in exercise-induced acute lactic acidosis is shown in Fig. 31-3. Healthy volunteers with exertional lactic acidosis induced by exercise on a rapidly moving treadmill lowered their ΔHCO_3^- by an amount equal to Δlactate.

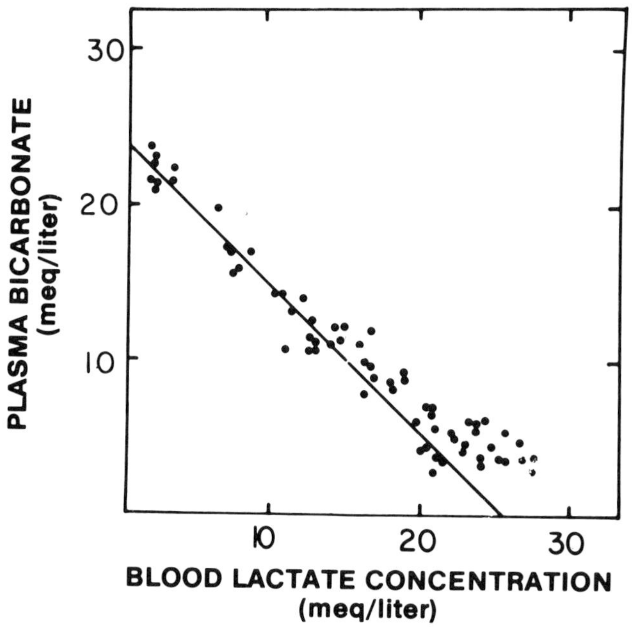

FIGURE 31-3 • Exercise-induced lactic acidosis lowers the serum bicarbonate concentration stoichiometrically. Solid line: line of identity; i.e., if each meq/liter increase in lactate concentration reduced the bicarbonate concentration by a like amount, all points would fall on the line. See text for details. (Modified from Osnes and Hermansen: *J Appl Physiol* 32:59, 1972. Used by permission.)

It follows from this assessment that patients with a pure, simple high anion gap metabolic acidosis ought to have a ΔHCO_3^- equal to their ΔAG. It also follows that a coexisting mixed metabolic acidosis and metabolic alkalosis must be present if a large ΔAG (i.e., a large acid accrual) is associated with a significantly smaller ΔHCO_3^-; that is, a large ΔAG demands that the serum $[HCO_3^-]$ fall by a large amount when an uncomplicated high anion gap acidosis develops. To the extent that $[HCO_3^-]$ falls less than predicted by the large ΔAG, some external or internal source of alkali (e.g., vomiting, diuretics, and so on) must be present to prevent development of the requisite degree of hypobicarbonatemia. This chemical pattern defines a mixed high anion gap metabolic acidosis and metabolic alkalosis.

Similarly, if a patient suffers a large fall in serum $[HCO_3^-]$ but a much lesser ΔAG, a normal and an elevated anion gap acidosis must coexist. In this case the ΔAG accounts for only a fraction of bicarbonate consumed, the remainder reflecting the addition of hydrochloric acid to blood (Fig. 31-1).

Thus, stoichiometric identity between the fall in $[HCO_3^-]$ and increase in the anion gap are chemical changes that typify a pure, simple high anion gap metabolic acidosis. When the ΔAG exceeds the $\Delta[HCO_3^-]$, a mixed metabolic acidosis and metabolic alkalosis must be present. When the ΔHCO_3 exceeds the ΔAG, a mixed high anion gap and a normal anion gap metabolic acidosis are coexistent.

The mixed acid-base disorders are conveniently and practically classifiable on the basis of how the individual primary disorders affect blood pH (Table 31-2). *Additive combinations* include such disorders as mixed metabolic

TABLE 31-2 • Classification of the mixed acid-base disorders

Mixed disorders	Chemical changes
ADDITIVE COMBINATIONS	
Respiratory acidosis and metabolic acidosis	Severe acidemia, low HCO_3^-, increased P_{CO_2}
Respiratory alkalosis and metabolic alkalosis	Severe alkalemia, high HCO_3^-, low P_{CO_2}
COUNTERBALANCING COMBINATIONS	
Respiratory acidosis and metabolic alkalosis	Variable acidity, high HCO_3^-, high P_{CO_2}
Respiratory alkalosis and metabolic acidosis	Variable acidity, low HCO_3^-, low P_{CO_2}
Metabolic acidosis and metabolic alkalosis	Variable acidity, variable HCO_3^-, variable P_{CO_2}. The increment in the anion gap may exceed the decrement in HCO_3^-.
TRIPLE DISORDERS	
Respiratory acidosis, metabolic acidosis, and metabolic alkalosis	Variable HCO_3^- and P_{CO_2}. Final pH is a function of the relative dominance of acidifying and alkalinizing processes in either triple disorder.
Respiratory alkalosis, metabolic acidosis, and metabolic alkalosis	

and respiratory acidosis; that is, both primary disturbances lower blood pH but do so by different mechanisms. *Counterbalancing combinations* include such disorders as metabolic acidosis and respiratory alkalosis, that is, disturbances that individually act to displace blood pH in opposite directions. The final pH reflects the dominant of the two countervailing disorders.

MIXED ACID-BASE DISORDERS

ADDITIVE COMBINATIONS

Metabolic and respiratory acidosis

Primary metabolic acidosis reduces $[HCO_3^-]$ and arterial pH. Appropriate respiratory compensation decreases the P_{CO_2}, which, in turn, minimizes the decline in pH. If respiratory compensation is inadequate, that is, if the P_{CO_2} is higher than it should be for the magnitude of hypobicarbonatemia, a mixed metabolic and respiratory acidosis is diagnosed. Conversely, primary respiratory acidosis elicits a precise increment in $[HCO_3^-]$ for a given rise in P_{CO_2} (Table 31-1). Failure of appropriate metabolic compensation for primary respiratory acidosis also indicates a mixed metabolic and respiratory acidosis.

The disturbances that produce primary respiratory acidosis are identical to those responsible for impairing respiratory compensation for metabolic acidosis. Therefore, the diagnosis of mixed metabolic and respiratory acidosis should prompt consideration of those diseases that can simultaneously produce both primary acid-base disorders. This mixed disorder can also be due to the concomitant occurrence of two independent though not necessarily related diseases, one causing metabolic acidosis and the other respiratory acidosis. A mixed metabolic and respiratory acidosis can also occur when a patient

TABLE 31-3 • A 60-year-old man with chronic obstructive lung disease and CO_2 retention was found to have the pattern of electrolytes and acid-base parameters seen in column A. A second set of chemical studies was obtained after two days of diarrhea (Column B). See text for details

	(A) Chronic respiratory acidosis (CRA)	(B) CRA plus acute metabolic acidosis
Na^+, meq/liter	140	140
K^+	4.5	4.0
Cl^-	95	102
HCO_3^-	32	25
AG	13	13
P_{CO_2}, mmHg	65	65
pH	7.31	7.20

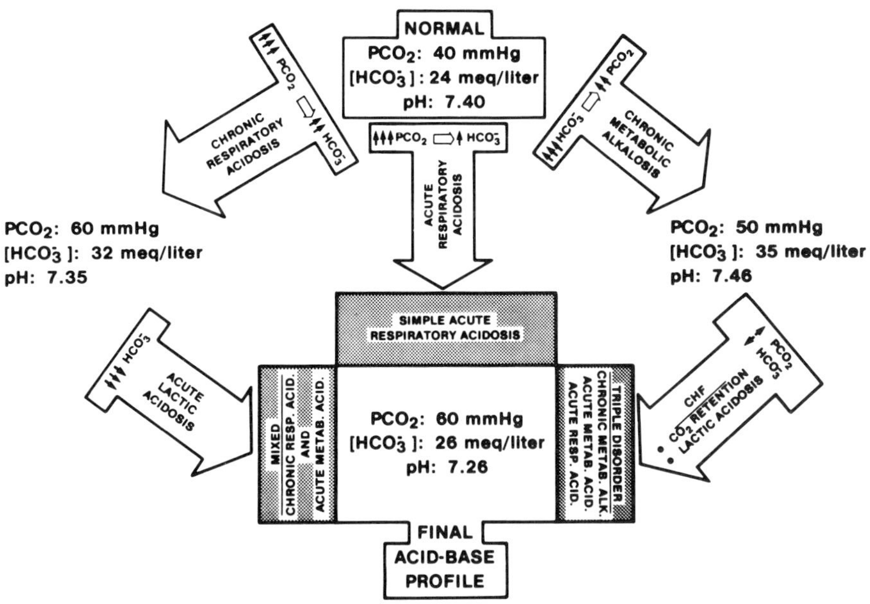

FIGURE 31-4 • A single set of abnormal acid-base parameters may be derived from any one of several possible simple or mixed disorders. The importance of clinical data to the correct interpretation of electrolytes and blood gases is stressed. (See text for details.)

with preexisting chronic respiratory acidosis develops metabolic acidosis (Table 31-3). In this situation, the increased P_{CO_2} is associated with a [HCO_3^-] that is not appropriately increased. In the more extreme case, [HCO_3^-] is in the "normal" range or is reduced. A correct diagnosis requires clinical and historical data because identical laboratory findings may result from uncomplicated acute respiratory acidosis, that is, increased P_{CO_2} with a relatively normal [HCO_3^-] (Fig. 31-4); or an acute exacerbation of chronic respiratory acidosis (increased P_{CO_2} with a lower than expected [HCO_3^-]). For example, if a patient with chronic respiratory acidosis, P_{CO_2} 50 mmHg and [HCO_3^-] 29 meq/liter, suddenly worsens and his P_{CO_2} rises to 60 mmHg, his [HCO_3^-] increases only to 30 meq/liter. Thus the acid-base and electrolyte parameters outlined in column B of Table 31-3 can be spawned by several different clinical situations. This underscores the critical importance of interpreting the chemical results together with the historical and physical findings. One remains clinically blind without both pieces of data.

Mixed metabolic and respiratory acidosis is most pernicious when a frankly high P_{CO_2} and an overtly low [HCO_3^-] coexist. This combination produces severe acidemia, even when the individual metabolic and respiratory disturbances are relatively modest. Table 31-4 illustrates other varieties of mixed respiratory and metabolic acidosis.

One common clinical disorder producing this mixed disorder is *cardiopulmonary arrest.* Simultaneous respiratory and cardiovascular failure couples lactic acidosis due to hypoxemia and decreased tissue perfusion with CO_2 retention. The obvious treatment for this disorder is reinstitution of ventilation and tissue perfusion. Successful cardiopulmonary resuscitation (CPR) can rapidly reverse the respiratory acidosis. Adequate ventilation is also absolutely critical for the treatment of the metabolic component. Exogenous $NaHCO_3$ has little impact on the

TABLE 31.4 • **Mixed metabolic acidosis and respiratory acidosis**

			Mixed metabolic acidosis and respiratory acidosis	
	Normal	Metabolic acidosis	Severe	Mild
Na^+, meq/liter	140	140	140	140
K^+	4	4.5	5.0	4.5
Cl^-	105	105	103	103
HCO_3^-	25	15	17	16
AG	10	20	20	21
P_{CO_2}, mmHg	40	30	50	37
pH	7.40	7.32	7.15	7.26

arterial pH of an inadequately ventilated patient. In such a "closed" system, $NaHCO_3$ cannot function as an effective buffer since its titration by protons merely generates additional CO_2, which is not effectively removed. Although [HCO_3^-] may increase somewhat, the higher P_{CO_2} offsets any beneficial effect on pH. Indeed, the clinical status may worsen.[14,63] Even when ventilation is adequate, excessive use of $NaHCO_3$ may be dangerous.

In the setting of cardiopulmonary arrest, acid-base parameters simultaneously obtained from pulmonary and peripheral arteries may be widely divergent.[85] Mixed venous blood sampled from the pulmonary artery reflects the acid-base status of the tissues, whereas peripheral arterial blood reflects the corrective effects of passing this blood through the lungs. Relative to arterial blood, the mixed venous sample normally has a higher P_{CO_2} and HCO_3^- concentration and a lower pH and PO_2. These changes obviously reflect tissue oxygen consumption and CO_2 formation. Tissue CO_2 enters erythrocytes that generate HCO_3^-, thereby minimizing the mixed venous acidemia. Passage of mixed venous blood through the lungs reduces to normal the P_{CO_2} and HCO_3^- concentration and raises the pH and PO_2; changes that are then reflected in arterial blood samples.

The hypotensive, ventilated patient, having suffered a cardiopulmonary arrest, may strikingly exaggerate the normal mixed venous-peripheral arterial differences in acid-base and blood gas parameters. In this setting the mixed venous P_{CO_2} rises dramatically, for three reasons. First, the impaired cardiac output allows normally generated CO_2 to accumulate, owing to the sluggish return of peripheral venous blood to the lungs. Second, hypoxic tissues overproduce lactic acid, which combines with venous HCO_3^-, generating CO_2 in this titration process. Finally, infused $NaHCO_3$ further stimulates CO_2 production. Since the rate of delivery of CO_2 to the lungs is diminished, the gas accumulates, thereby raising the mixed venous P_{CO_2}. The ventilated lungs, however, clear CO_2 from whatever blood reaches them, thereby ensuring normalcy of the acid-base and blood gas parameters of the blood leaving the lungs via the pulmonary veins, and eventually entering the peripheral arterial circuit. For these reasons mixed venous acidemia may coexist with normal arterial blood gases.

Lessons to be learned from these observations include the following. Normal peripheral arterial blood gases may be misleading in cardiopulmonary arrest, since tissue hypoxia and acidification will be reflected only by mixed venous gases (or from samples taken from a large vein[4]) correction of the underlying tissue hypoxia requires improvement in cardiac output. Finally, $NaHCO_3$ should be used sparingly in this setting. Alkalinizing salts that generate less CO_2 may be advantageous. Carbicarb, a mixture of Na_2CO_3 and $NaHCO_3$, is such an agent, which is currently undergoing investigation.[11,28]

Sodium bicarbonate is most often infused as a hypertonic bolus at a concentration of 880 meq/liter. Excessive use of such hypertonic solutions can produce severe hypernatremia and hypertonicity that elicits cellular dehydration and intravascular volume expansion.[52] Furthermore, administration of large quantities of $NaHCO_3$ during successful cardiopulmonary resuscitation will lead to "rebound" metabolic alkalosis during the recovery phase (see Mixed Metabolic Acidosis and Alkalosis, below). It is now recommended that $NaHCO_3$ be administered cautiously during resuscitation. The dose should be dictated by serial arterial blood gas measurements.

Pulmonary edema decreases lung compliance, producing hypoxemia that stimulates ventilation and usually generates a respiratory alkalosis. However, respiratory acidosis can develop when severe pulmonary edema leads to airway collapse, ventilation-perfusion mismatching, and respiratory muscle fatigue.[1] Hypercarbia is exacerbated by the accelerated CO_2 generation produced by extreme respiratory efforts. When pulmonary edema is associated with left ventricular failure and decreased cardiac output, reduced tissue perfusion may combine with hypoxemia to produce lactic acidosis (see Chap. 25).[30] Therefore, mixed lactic and respiratory acidosis may develop in patients with left ventricular failure and severe pulmonary edema. Although CO_2 retention is a relative contraindication to morphone administration, Aberman and Fulop reported that patients with pulmonary edema and hypercarbia often improve after morphine.[1]

Lactic acidosis is distinctly uncommon in patients with uncomplicated *chronic obstructive pulmonary disease* despite marked hypoxemia.[24] A variety of compensatory mechanisms develop to improve tissue oxygen delivery. These salutary forces include an increased hematocrit, increased oxygen extraction, and a rightward shift in the oxyhemoglobin dissociation curve to facilitate peripheral oxygen release from hemoglobin. These compensating mechanisms develop relatively slowly; therefore, severe *acute hypoxemia* is far more likely to produce lactic acidosis.[44] Patients with chronic obstructive lung disease that is complicated by severe anemia, decreased cardiac output, or hypotension may also develop lactic acidosis. Because metabolic compensation for chronic respiratory acidosis elevates the bicarbonate concentration, superimposition of metabolic acidosis reduces the [HCO_3^-] toward "normal." Therefore, patients with chronic respiratory acidosis whose [HCO_3^-] is "normal" may have a complicating metabolic acidosis. An increased anion gap can be a clue to the presence of this mixed disturbance.

Some forms of metabolic acidosis are frequently complicated by *hypokalemia*. If exogenous $NaHCO_3$ is administered, potassium shifts into cells, further exacerbating the hypokalemia. Glucose infusions produce similar effects. Hypokalemia can produce muscle weakness, which is usually more pronounced in the extremities, especially the quadriceps. Severe potassium depletion, however, can also partially paralyze the diaphragm, intercostal muscles, and accessory muscles of

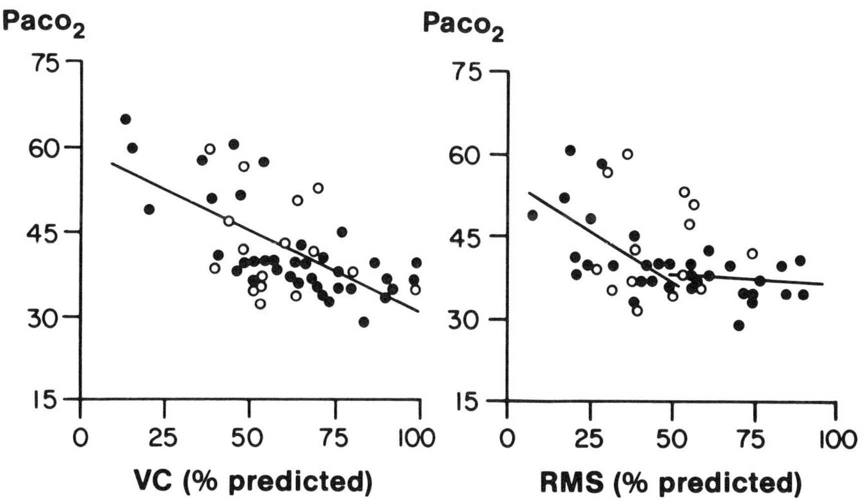

FIGURE 31-5 • Relationship between arterial CO_2 tension (Pa_{CO_2}, in mmHg) and vital capacity (VC) or respiratory muscle strength (RMS) in patients with uncomplicated myopathy (closed circles) and patients with myopathy and chronic lung disease (open circles). (From Braun MNT et al: *Thorax* 38:616, 1983. Used by permission.)

respiration. CO_2 retention and respiratory acidosis ensues and, in combination with the preexisting metabolic acidosis, can cause lethal acidemia.

When *hypophosphatemia* complicates metabolic acidosis it may also contribute to respiratory muscle weakness. This will be exacerbated by intravenous glucose infusions, which cause inorganic phosphate to shift into cells. Acute respiratory failure and respiratory acidosis may thereby be precipitated by hypophosphatemia.[60]

Patients with *primary muscle disorders* such as polymyositis or muscular dystrophy may also develop respiratory acidosis. This may be unmasked when they develop metabolic acidosis and subsequently fail to achieve appropriate respiratory compensation. Figure 31-5 shows the linear relationship between respiratory muscle strength, vital capacity, and the development of hypercarbia in patients with various myopathies.[19]

A variety of *poisons and drug intoxications* can depress the respiratory center, resulting in respiratory acidosis. In some instances, direct pulmonary toxicity exacerbates the respiratory acidosis. In many cases, severe metabolic acidosis also develops; it is usually due to an accumulation of organic acids that are metabolic products of the drug or poison. Examples include the formic acidosis produced by methanol poisoning and the glycolic acidosis caused by ethylene glycol ingestion.[25,35] Other toxins interfere with intermediary metabolism and cause accumulation of endogenous organic acids. Agents having such an effect include salicylate, cyanide, and carbon monoxide. Finally, many drug intoxications and poisonings can eventuate in cardiopulmonary collapse, which produces lactic acidosis.

Metabolic and respiratory alkalosis

An increased arterial pH and [HCO_3^-] with an appropriate compensatory rise in P_{CO_2} characterize the chemical components of metabolic alkalosis (see Chap. 29). If the P_{CO_2} is not appropriately elevated (Table 31-1), or is frankly depressed (less than 40 mmHg) in a patient with metabolic alkalosis, a mixed metabolic and respiratory alkalosis may be diagnosed. Extreme alkalemia develops when a low P_{CO_2} accompanies frank hyperbicarbonatemia; the P_{CO_2}/[HCO_3^-] ratio decreases sharply as the numerator shrinks and the denominator increases (equation 1). Examples of mild and severe metabolic-respiratory alkalosis are illustrated in Table 31-5. In the cited examples, the key difference between the severe and mild

TABLE 31-5 • Chemical changes in simple and mixed alkaloses

		Simple alkaloses		Mixed alkaloses	
	Normal	Metabolic	Respiratory	Severe	Mild
Na^+	139	139	139	139	139
K^+	4	3	3.5	2.8	3.0
Cl^-	105	89	107	92	92
HCO_3^-	24	35	17	32	32
AG	10	15	15	15	15
P_{CO_2}, mmHg	40	47	25	30	39
pH	7.40	7.49	7.45	7.65	7.53

mixed disorders is caused by the P_{CO_2}. In the severe disorder the P_{CO_2} is frankly low; in the mild disorder it is simply not increased to levels normally dictated by the magnitude of the hyperbicarbonatemia.

The prognosis of critically ill patients with combined metabolic and respiratory alkalosis and with severe alkalemia frequently is extremely poor.[5,50,87] There are many reasons underlying this pernicious association. Respiratory alkalosis is a potent cerebral vasoconstrictor and metabolic alkalosis exerts similar, albeit less marked, effects.[13,56] Acute alkalemia also shifts the oxyhemoglobin dissociation curve toward the left, therby increasing the affinity of hemoglobin for oxygen.[29] Because the cerebral demand for oxygen remains stable despite its decreased delivery consequent to the reduced blood flow and increased hemoglobin binding, severe cerebral hypoxia may develop. Ensuing irritability and confusion may progress to seizures and coma.[41,48]

Metabolic and respiratory alkalosis also produce complex cardiovascular effects. The direct cardiac effects of these acid-base disturbances may be partially offset by neurocardiac reflexes and alterations in peripheral vascular resistance.[56,68] Metabolic alkalosis has a mild direct positive inotropic effect.[56] Respiratory alkalosis decreases cardiac output in anesthetized humans[68] but exerts little effect in the awake state.[74] In patients with fixed coronary artery lesions and those susceptible to coronary arterial spasm, respiratory alkalosis may constrict these vessels, precipitating angina and malignant cardiac arrhythmias.[59,90,91] Hypokalemia, hypomagnesemia, and hypocalcemia commonly complicate metabolic and respiratory alkalosis and also contribute to the development of arrhythmias. Although alkalosis induced cardiac arrhythmias are uncommon in otherwise normal individuals, they do occur frequently in patients receiving digitalis or in those with underlying coronary artery disease.[18]

Alkalemia has more specific adverse effects, in certain clinical settings. For example, the neurologic status of patients with severe liver dysfunction may deteriorate with the development of alkalemia.[7] The alkaline pH increases the concentration of the nonionized fraction of ammonia (NH_3) and of other nitrogen-containing compounds. Through nonionic diffusion (see Chap. 2) these uncharged moieties more readily enter brain cells. When alkalosis is associated with hypokalemia, renal ammoniagenesis is also stimulated (Chap. 10), and increases systemic NH_3 levels. Hyperammoniemia together with an alkaline blood pH sharply increases the concentration of uncharged NH_3 and may precipitate hepatic encephalopathy.

In addition to the direct consequences of this combined alkalosis, many of the disorders causing respiratory alkalosis carry a very poor prognosis. Sepsis, pulmonary emboli, severe neurologic damage, and liver failure are common causes of respiratory alkalosis. The poor prognosis in mixed metabolic and respiratory alkaloses is therefore a function of both the often life-threatening underlying cause and the effects of extreme alkalemia.

Lyons and Moore studied critically ill surgical patients and found that 65 percent developed alkalemia during their hospitalization.[50] Most of these patients developed combined metabolic and respiratory alkalosis. Subsequently, Wilson et al. reported that 12 percent of 1415 critically ill surgical patients had an arterial pH of 7.50 or greater while in the intensive care unit.[87] As anticipated, the highest pH developed in those patients with mixed metabolic and respiratory alkalosis. Hypoxemia was frequently the cause of hyperventilation. Many patients requiring respiratory assistance were relatively overventilated. Pain, occurring postoperatively or due to trauma, stimulated respiration and contributed to the respiratory alkalosis. The most common causes of metabolic alkalosis were nasogastric suction and vomiting. Diuretics, high-dose steroid therapy, and exogenous alkali (such as Ringer's lactate, citrated blood products, and intensive antacid therapy) also contributed to the metabolic alkalosis. Wilson et al. also found that mortality approached 65 percent in those whose pH was between 7.60 and 7.64, and exceeded 90 percent when arterial pH was 7.64 or higher.[87] These findings have been confirmed by others.[5]

Transfusion of large amounts of blood and blood products may cause metabolic alkalosis. Blood collected for transfusion is usually mixed with the anticoagulant/preservative, "CPD solution," containing sodium citrate, citric acid, sodium phosphate, and dextrose. The citrate chelates calcium and thereby inhibits coagulation. The other components prolong the shelf life of stored red blood cells. Generally, 450 ml of blood is mixed with 63 ml of CPD solution, which results in a final sodium citrate concentration of 34 meq/liter. The critic acid reacts with HCO_3^- in the freshly collected blood to produce CO_2 and water. Therefore, immediately after collection, bank blood has a reduced [HCO_3^-], increased P_{CO_2} (the generated CO_2 slowly diffuses through the plastic bag), and a high citrate concentration. During storage, anaerobic metabolism generates lactic acid, which consumes additional HCO_3^-. After two weeks of storage, the [HCO_3^-] is approximately 12 meq/liter and the lactate concentration is also 12 meq/liter.[8] Both the lactate and citrate anions represent "potential" HCO_3^- to which they can be metabolically converted. Therefore, the total and "potential" [HCO_3^-] in each unit of blood is approximately 58 meq/liter (the 24 meq/liter of HCO_3^- present in the donoted blood plus the 34 meq/liter of added sodium citrate). Each meq/liter reduction in [HCO_3^-] is matched by an equal increment in lactate concentration. Infused blood has a low pH, low [HCO_3^-] and high P_{CO_2} so that it may be transiently "acidifying." However, it represents a net alkaline load after metabolic generation of alkali from citrate and lactate occurs. Various products derived from whole blood, such as plasma protein fraction, fresh frozen plasma, and packed red blood cells, also contain relatively large quantities of potential alkali.

Consequently, infusion of large quantities of blood or blood products can strikingly increase the [HCO_3^-]. Although patients with normal renal function can excrete such alkali loads, those who require large volumes of blood generally have decreased renal perfusion due to intravascular volume depletion. This impairs the kidney's ability to excrete HCO_3^- (see Chap. 29). Any form of acute or chronic renal failure will also reduce the patient's ability to excrete alkali loads. It follows that severe metabolic alkalosis can develop in patients with renal failure requiring large volumes of blood.[9,48] Metabolic alkalosis may also develop when citrated plasma protein fraction or fresh frozen plasma is used to replace extracellular fluid (ECF) volume during plasmapheresis or thoracic duct drainage in patients with renal disease.[65,71] If dialysis is required, the metabolic alkalosis can be efficiently treated by adjusting the Cl^-/HCO_3 ratio of hemo- or peritoneal dialysis fluid.[6,9,79]

Patients requiring massive transfusions also frequently develop respiratory alkalosis. This results from the combination of catecholamine release, hypoxemia, and noncardiogenic pulmonary edema, which frequently occur. Therefore, mixed metabolic and respiratory alkalosis should be anticipated in these circumstances. Hypotension will also produce lactic acidosis, resulting in a triple disorder (see Triple Acid-Base Disorders, below).

Mixed metabolic and respiratory alkalosis may develop during *pregnancy*. Progesterone, a potent respiratory stimulant, increases the sensitivity of the respiratory center to the stimulatory effects of CO_2.[49] Indeed, the cyclic increases of serum progesterone that occur in normal ovulating women are associated with accelerated minute respiration and decreased P_{CO_2}.[67] Progesterone levels increase further during pregnancy and the P_{CO_2} declines progressively. In the third trimester, the mean P_{CO_2} approximates 30 mmHg.[16,67] As with other chronic respiratory alkaloses, that produced by pregnancy is compensated by a predictable decrement in [HCO_3^-].[47] Metabolic compensation reduces the serum [HCO_3^-] to approximately 20 meq/liter in the third trimester. If a "normal" (i.e., 24 meq/liter) or increased [HCO_3^-] exists late in pregnancy, complicating metabolic alkalosis is likely to be present. When metabolic alkalosis occurs during pregnancy, it is frequently the result of persistent vomiting or the excessive use of diuretics.

Patients with chronic liver disease develop a variety of acid-base disturbances. The most common simple disturbance is respiratory alkalosis[57,69,72] due to an accumulation of respiratory stimulants such as progesterone, ammonia, and other biogenic amines.[45,57,72] Hypoxemia, another respiratory stimulus, occurs commonly in these patients because of ventilation-perfusion mismatching, abnormal pulmonary vascular shunting, and diaphragmatic elevation from ascites.[45,57,72] Cerebral edema may also contribute to accelerated ventilation. Metabolic alkalosis frequently complicates the course of chronic liver disease, usually resulting from vomiting, nasogastric suction, diuresis, and high-dose steroids use. Persistent secondary hyperaldosteronism can also contribute to metabolic alkalosis, especially when diuretic therapy ensures distal delivery of salt and water. Metabolic alkalosis is sustained because "effective" ECF volume is reduced, thereby decreasing renal perfusion. These patients may also develop metabolic acidosis as a result of renal tubular acidosis, lactic acidosis, and/or uremic acidosis. Therefore, triple acid-base disturbances (chronic respiratory alkalosis, metabolic alkalosis, and metabolic acidosis) often occur in patients with severe liver disease.

Patients with chronic respiratory acidosis have an elevated P_{CO_2} and a compensatory increase of serum [HCO_3^-]. If such patients are artificially ventilated, reducing the P_{CO_2} to normal or to frankly low levels, combined metabolic and respiratory alkalosis develop. Typically, these patients are salt-restricted and receive diuretics. Contraction of their intravascular volume impairs normal renal excretion of accumulated HCO_3^-.[75] Cautious administration of salt and readjustment of the ventilator reverses this mixed metabolic-respiratory alkalosis (see Triple Acid-Base Disturbances, below).

Mixed metabolic acidoses

Mixed high anion gap acidoses

A variety of organic acids may accumulate simultaneously. The increased anion gap can therefore encompass several accumulating acid anions. Actually, most common high anion gap metabolic acidoses result from the accumulation of several organic acids. For example, both lactate and pyruvate (albeit to a much smaller degree) account for the increased anion gap in patients with lactic acidosis, while β-hydroxybutyric acid and acetoacetic acid accumulate in the ketoacidoses. Combined ketoacidosis and lactic acidosis (i.e., the accumulation of four organic acid anions) may occur in *decompensated diabetics* with compromised circulatory status, *alcohol binge drinkers*,[22,31] and patients with enzymatic defects such as *glucose-6-phosphatase* and *fructose-1,6-diphosphatase deficiencies*.[64,92] Uremic acidosis is frequently complicated by other forms of high anion gap acidosis, producing a mixed high anion gap acidosis. Often some of the accumulating acid anions cannot be defined.[34]

Mixed hyperchloremic and high anion gap metabolic acidoses

When the hypobicarbonatemia of metabolic acidosis is balanced partially by an increased anion gap and partially by an increased chloride concentration, a mixed high anion gap, hyperchloremic metabolic acidosis exists. However, alternative interpretations must also be considered. For example, patients with chronic respiratory alkalosis have a compensatory decline in HCO_3^- associated with an increase in chloride concentration. Cellular alkalinization stimulates glycolysis and increases the blood levels of several organic acids, including lactic acid.[73] This increases the anion gap slightly. Thus, the resulting electrolyte pattern has a ΔHCO_3^- that exceeds the ΔCl^-. The ΔHCO_3^- equals the $\Delta Cl^- + \Delta AG$. This electrolyte profile could reflect a compensated chronic respiratory alkalosis, or the additive effects of a mixed hyperchloremic and high anion gap metabolic acidosis. The arterial pH will differentiate these diagnostic possibilities.

A mixed high anion gap and hyperchloremic metabolic acidosis may develop in patients with severe *diarrhea*. Loss of $NaHCO_3$ and potential $NaHCO_3$ into the stool produces a hyperchloremic acidosis. This may then be complicated by lactic acidosis and/or uremic acidosis as a result of ECF volume depletion[83] (see Chap. 25). A similar electrolyte pattern may occur in patients with progressive renal failure (see also Chap. 7).[86] Hyperchloremic acidosis is common with *early renal failure*, when renal ammonia synthesis and net acid excretion are reduced more sharply than the GFR. This allows continued anion filtration and excretion. The excretion of these sodium salts stimulates chloride retention and hyperchloremic acidosis develops. In time, with further decline in the glomerular filtration rate (GFR), the hyperchloremic acidosis is replaced by a uremic high anion gap acidosis due to the retention of phosphate, sulfate, and other inorganic and organic acid anions (see Chap. 25).[27,86]

A relatively pure high anion gap metabolic acidosis can be partially, or totally, converted to a hyperchloremic pattern by several mechanisms (see Chaps. 25 and 26). If the kidney excretes the acid anion as a sodium salt, the anion gap decreases as the serum chloride concentration increases. Loss of the sodium salt together with water leaves a fixed quantity of chloride to be distributed in a smaller volume, thereby increasing its concentration. Renal retention of exogenous chloride also contributes to the hyperchloremia. The loss of sodium salts of organic acid anions via the kidney (or GI tract) is equivalent to the loss of "potential" $NaHCO_3$. The effect of such losses on the electrolyte profile is identical to the loss of $NaHCO_3$; that is, a hyperchloremic metabolic acidosis develops. When metabolic acidosis is due to the accumulation of organic acids, or to nonchloride inorganic acids (H_2SO_4, H_2PO_4, etc.), the increased anion gap reflects retention of these anions. If the anion is excreted, or metabolized, the anion gap decreases. If the excreted anion is accompanied by a proton, or metabolism of the organic anion also consumes protons, the metabolic acidosis is reversed, the anion gap decreases, and serum $[HCO_3^-]$ increases. However, excretion of the anion with sodium or potassium does *not* regenerate HCO_3^-. To the extent this occurs the hypobicarbonatemia is sustained while the anion gap normalizes. This latter sequence may develop in patients with diabetic ketoacidosis (see Chaps. 25 and 26). Renal excretion of the sodium or potassium salts of β-hydroxybutyrate and acetoacetate represents lost "potential" HCO_3^- and converts the anion gap ketoacidosis to a hyperchloremic acidosis.[3,36,42,61] This is more likely to occur in patients with ketoacidosis when renal perfusion and glomerular filtration are well preserved. These individuals have high rates of renal ketoacid salt excretion. Reduced glomerular filtration causes greater ketoanion retention and a higher anion gap.[3]

Similar mechanisms are responsible for the conversion of the high anion gap metabolic acidosis caused by sulfuric acid to a hyperchloremic metabolic acidosis.[17] The low renal threshold for sulfate allows rapid excretion of sodium, sulfate, and water and results in hyperchloremia. The hippuric acidosis of toluene toxicity ("glue sniffing") creates a similar electrolyte pattern.[19a]

Mixed respiratory acid-base disorders

Acute respiratory acidosis may complicate the course of chronic respiratory acidosis. For example, patients with chronic obstructive lung disease may suffer an acute pulmonary decompensation due to bronchitis, pneumonia, or congestive heart failure. Blood gas and chemical analysis will then show a very high P_{CO_2} and an increased $[HCO_3^-]$. However, the latter is not increased to the level expected for this degree of chronic hypercarbia.[21] Note that other mixed acid-base disorders may produce identical biochemical parameters. Only careful evaluation of the clinical picture and, when available, sequential biochemical parameters, will ensure a correct diagnosis (Fig. 31-4).

Anxiety, fear, salicylism, and other disorders that cause acute respiratory alkalosis may develop in patients with chronic respiratory alkalosis, thereby acutely exacerbating their preexisting alkalemia (see Chap. 7). A relatively high $[HCO_3^-]$ associated with severe hypocapnia may reflect a mixed acute and chronic respiratory alkalosis, or a mixed respiratory and metabolic alkalosis (see above). Once again, clinical data and sequential biochemical parameters are necessary for correct diagnostic conclusions.

COUNTERBALANCING COMBINATIONS

Mixed metabolic-respiratory disorders

Metabolic alkalosis and respiratory acidosis

This combined disturbance is identified by an increased P_{CO_2} associated with an inappropriately high serum $[HCO_3^-]$. If the hypercapnia is assumed to be the primary defect, the hyperbicarbonatemia exceeds the level ex-

TABLE 31-6 • Mixed metabolic alkalosis and respiratory acidosis

	Normal	Simple chronic respiratory acidosis	Simple metabolic alkalosis	Mixed metabolic alkalosis and resp. acidosis
Na^+, meq/liter	140	140	140	140
K^+	4.0	4.0	3.0	3.5
Cl^-	105	94	92	90
HCO_3^-	25	36	36	40
AG	10	10	12	10
P_{CO_2}, mmHg	40	70	48	67
pH	7.40	7.33	7.49	7.40

pected for normal compensation (Table 31-1). If, on the other hand, the metabolic alkalosis is assumed to be primary, the P_{CO_2} is higher than expected for respiratory compensation (Table 31-1). It may be difficult to determine which disturbance is primary, especially when the resulting arterial pH is near normal. Since compensation for simple acid-base disorders rarely normalizes pH (chronic respiratory alkalosis is the sole exception, see Chap. 30), when the $[HCO_3^-]$ and P_{CO_2} are both abnormal but produce a normal pH, mixed counterbalancing disorders probably exist. Table 31-6 illustrates several examples of mixed metabolic alkalosis and respiratory acidosis.

Patients with chronic obstructive lung disease and CO_2 retention often require treatment with diuretics or glucocorticoids, which can produce metabolic alkalosis. It is important to recognize and treat the excessive $[HCO_3^-]$, since normalization of arterial pH by the superimposed metabolic alkalosis further depresses respiration, worsening CO_2 retention. Correction of the alkalosis may improve ventilation and ameliorate the hypercarbia.[10,55] In one study, the average P_{CO_2} decreased from 61 to 48 mmHg after the metabolic component of mixed respiratory acidosis and metabolic alkalosis was corrected.[10] The metabolic alkalosis may be reversed with acetazolamide, if continued diuresis is necessary, or by cautious volume expansion if the patient can tolerate the additional fluid.

Metabolic alkalosis is often associated with hypokalemia, which when severe may cause weakness of respiratory muscles (see Metabolic and Respiratory Acidosis). When extreme hypokalemic metabolic alkalosis is associated with marked hypercapnia the latter is probably the result of respiratory muscle weakness.[62]

Metabolic acidosis and respiratory alkalosis

Reduced pH and $[HCO_3^-]$ characterize metabolic acidosis. The P_{CO_2} should be reduced to compensate for the primary disturbance. If the P_{CO_2} is depressed below this level (Table 31-1), coexistent respiratory alkalosis is diagnosed. Table 31-7 illustrates several examples of this mixed disturbance.

TABLE 31-7 • Mixed respiratory alkalosis plus metabolic acidosis

	Normal	Metabolic acidosis	Mixed respiratory alkalosis plus metabolic acidosis: Severe	Mild
Na^+, meq/liter	140	140	140	140
K^+	4.0	4.5	3.5	4.0
Cl^-	105	105	13	106
HCO_3^-	25	15	13	14
AG	10	20	20	20
P_{CO_2}, mmHg	40	31	15	24
pH	7.40	7.30	7.56	7.39

One clinical setting in which mixed metabolic acidosis and respiratory alkalosis occurs commonly is *salicylate intoxication* (see Chap. 25). At high concentrations, salicylates uncouple mitochondrial oxidative phosphorylation (similar to 2,4-dinitrophenol) and thereby increase oxygen utilization, heat generation, and the production of lactic acid and CO_2. Despite accelerated CO_2 generation, high salicylate levels simultaneously stimulate the respiratory center in the brain stem, causing hyperventilation and hypocapnia.[80] Intracellular alkalinization stimulates glycolysis and pyruvate generation, which together with uncoupled mitochondrial oxidation, sharply increases lactic acid accumulation. In addition to lactic acidosis, ketoacidosis may develop, especially in children and pregnant women.[33,77] Salicylic acid is itself a strong organic acid and contributes 3 to 5 meq/liter to the increased anion gap. Therefore, the increased anion gap includes lactate, ketone, and salicylate anions. Whether the respiratory alkalosis or the metabolic acidosis is likely to predominate varies with the age of the patient. Infants usually develop severe metabolic acidosis and acidemia, while older children and adults more commonly manifest severe respiratory alkalosis and alkalemia.[33,37,88]

The dominant acid-base disturbance in patients with salicylate toxicity has an important impact on drug-induced morbidity and mortality. Salicylic acid has a low p*K* and is almost entirely ionized in biological fluids. The salicylate anion poorly permeates cell membranes, but the small fraction of unionized salicylic acid readily crosses cell membranes. Therefore, any factor that increases the concentration of the unionized acid species in the blood will increase salicylate penetration into the brain, liver, and other organs. A low systemic pH drives the reaction toward nonionized salicylic acid and increases the burden of drug within cells.[43] This contributes to the worse prognosis of acidemic, salicylate-intoxicated patients. [33,37,43]

The treatment of salicylate intoxication begins with removal of unabsorbed drug from the gastrointestinal tract by inducing vomiting or initiating gastric lavage. Activated charcoal and sorbitol may be administered to decrease gastrointestinal absorption of residual salicylate and accelerate its transit through the gastrointestinal tract. Volume contraction, hypokalemia, and metabolic acidosis must be aggressively corrected. The arterial pH should be maintained in the normal-to-alkaline range to minimize CNS penetration of salicylate. An alkaline diuresis, with urine flow rates of 2 to 3 ml/min, maximizes renal salicylate excretion. The alkaline urine pH traps salicylate by nonionic diffusion (the urine concentration of nonionized salicylic acid is reduced by the high pH so that this moiety moves down a gradient from blood to urine). Systemic administration of alkali and acetazolamide may be used to induce the alkaline diuresis. However, the administration of acetazolamide must be carefully monitored to avoid the production of systemic acidemia, which can have catastrophic consequences.[43]

As previously discussed, respiratory alkalosis is the most common simple acid-base disturbance associated with *severe liver disease* and in this circumstance is frequently complicated by metabolic acid-base disorders. A variety of chronic liver diseases, including primary biliary cirrhosis, autoimmune liver disease, alcoholic cirrhosis, and Wilson's disease, may be associated with renal tubular acidosis.[12,20,38,39] Although the liver is the major site of lactate uptake, severe liver disease alone rarely causes lactic acidosis. However, accelerated lactic acid production resulting from hypoxemia and/or hypotension more readily produces lactic acidosis when it complicates chronic liver disease.[66] Severe liver failure may be complicated by the hepatorenal syndrome and lead to uremic metabolic acidosis.

The frequent development of mixed respiratory and metabolic alkalosis in critically ill surgical patients has already been discussed. Mazzara et al.[53] studied patients in a *medical intensive care unit* and reported a high incidence of respiratory alkalosis and metabolic acidosis. The metabolic acidosis was often due to lactic acidosis. Metabolic alkalosis occurred less frequently than in critically ill surgical patients. Surgical patients may be more likely to develop metabolic alkalosis due to nasogastric suction, vomiting, and high-volume transfusions. Mazzara et al. also found that patients with mixed respiratory alkalosis and metabolic acidosis in the medical intensive care unit had a high mortality rate.[53]

Endotoxin from gram-negative bacteria is a potent central respiratory stimulant.[77] It follows that respiratory alkalosis is a common complication of gram-negative infections. Indeed hyperventilation and respiratory alkalosis—physical and chemical manifestations of endotoxemia—may precede the development of overt sepsis by 24 h.[77] In the appropriate clinical setting, the astute physician can recognize otherwise unexplained respiratory alkalosis as a forerunner of impending sepsis. The hypotension, poor tissue perfusion, or diarrhea associated with various forms of gram-negative sepsis superimposes lactic acidosis or HCO_3^- wasting on the respiratory alkalosis.

Mixed metabolic acidosis and alkalosis

Thus far, we have discussed those mixed acid-base disturbances which combine a primary metabolic disturbance with a primary respiratory disturbance. When one disturbance is diagnosed, the second component is identified as either inadequate or excessive compensation. Inappropriate compensation may not be present when metabolic acidosis and alkalosis coexist. The anion gap is most useful in elucidating the mixed metabolic acid-base disorders. As described in Chap. 24 and in the introduction to this chapter, when the increment in the anion gap (ΔAG) exceeds the decrement in the bicarbonate concentration

TABLE 31-8 • Mixed metabolic acidosis and metabolic alkalosis

				Metabolic alkalosis plus	
	Normal	High AG metabolic acidosis	Normal AG metabolic acidosis	High AG metabolic acidosis	Normal AG metabolic acidosis
Na^+, meq/liter	140	140	140	140	140
K^+	4.0	5.0	5.0	3.5	3.5
Cl^-	105	150	115	95	105
HCO_3^-	25	15	15	25	25
AG	10	20	10	20	10
P_{CO_2}, mmHg	40	31	31	40	40
pH	7.40	7.30	7.30	7.40	7.40

(ΔHCO_3^-), a mixed metabolic acidosis and alkalosis may exist.

As illustrated in Table 31-8, the coexistence of a high anion gap metabolic acidosis and alkalosis is suggested by the loss of stoichiometry between the ΔAG and $\Delta[HCO_3^-]$. When the metabolic alkalosis is more severe than the metabolic acidosis, $[HCO_3^-]$ will rise to supranormal values but the anion gap remains elevated. However, severe metabolic alkalosis can itself increase the anion gap. Extreme alkalemia causes plasma proteins to relinquish bound protons. The released acid decreases the serum $[HCO_3^-]$ while the anionic charge density of plasma proteins increases. Hemoconcentration may also elevate the protein concentration and thereby further increase the anion gap. Extreme alkalosis also slightly increases serum lactate levels.[51] Therefore, the anion gap can increase with metabolic alkalosis in the absence of a true metabolic acidosis.[2,51] However, this effect is generally small and is not usually a significant clinical issue.

Mixed metabolic acidosis and metabolic alkalosis occurs whenever exogenous $NaHCO_3$ is administered to a patient with severe metabolic acidosis. Figure 31-6 illustrates the sequence of events produced by hypertonic $NaHCO_3$ infusions during a successful cardiopulmonary resuscitation. The initial "arrest" results in lactic acidosis which reduces the serum $[HCO_3^-]$ and increases the anion gap, as indicated in panel B. (At this point blood gas analysis would be likely to reveal a mixed metabolic

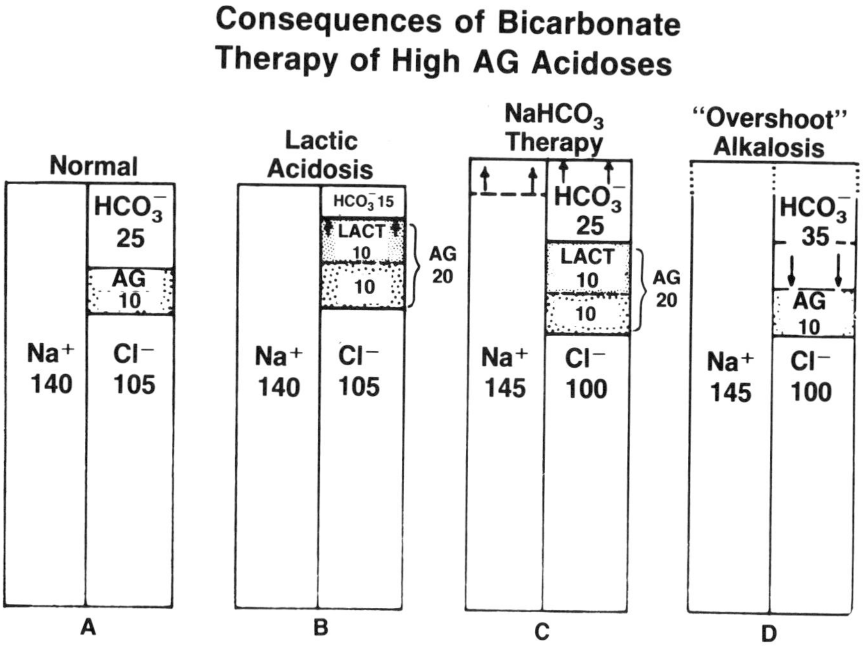

FIGURE 31-6 • Schematic view of serum electrolytes during lactic acidosis, following therapy with sodium bicarbonate, and during the reparative phase. See text for details. (From Emmett M, Narins RG, *Medicine* 56:38, 1977. Used by permission.)

acidosis and respiratory acidosis. The acute respiratory disturbances will have little effect on the serum electrolytes.) With successful resuscitation, accumulated lactate is oxidized, which simultaneously reduces the anion gap and increases [HCO_3^-] (panel B reverts to panel A). If the cardiopulmonary arrrest is prolonged and hypertonic $NaHCO_3$ is infused, a form of iatrogenic metabolic alkalosis is produced, converting the values in panel B to those in C. The [Na^+] and [HCO_3^-] increase while [Cl^-] declines as a result of ECF expansion. The increased anion gap remains stable. At this stage the increased anion gap is accompanied by a relatively normal [HCO_3^-]. These chemistries indicate the presence of a mixed metabolic acidosis and metabolic alkalosis. If the patient is now successfully resuscitated, the accumulated lactate is oxidized and generates HCO_3^-, which, in addition to the administered $NaHCO_3$, produces frank hyperbicarbonatemia. The values in panel C are thus converted to those in panel D. This development is termed "rebound metabolic alkalosis."[54,84] This disturbance may be responsible for intractable cardiac arrhythmias in the postarrest period. Mixed high anion gap metabolic acidosis and metabolic alkalosis also commonly occurs in patients with diabetic and alcoholic ketoacidosis.[23,32,82] The alkalosis most often results from vomiting, but exogenous $NaHCO_3$ loads, diuretics, and increased mineralocorticoid levels may also contribute. When patients with end-stage renal disease develop uremic symptoms and begin to vomit, gastric alkalosis complicates the uremic acidosis.

When hyperchloremic metabolic acidosis coexists with metabolic alkalosis, blood chemistries and blood gas parameters may all normalize. The acidosis causes hyperchloremia and hypobicarbonatemia while the alkalosis exerts opposite effects. If the two disturbances are of similar severity they may totally neutralize each other. When gastroenteritis produces both vomiting and diarrhea, patients may develop this mixed disorder. They may be volume-depleted and hypokalemic but the anion gap, [HCO_3^-] and chloride concentrations may be normal. This mixed disturbance is diagnosed on the basis of history and physical examination. It may be suspected when metabolic acidosis or alkalosis is less impressive than expected from the severity of the vomiting or diarrhea.

Mixed respiratory disorders

Mixed acute respiratory alkalosis and chronic respiratory acidosis

Chronic CO_2 retention is chemically characterized by primary hypercapnia, secondary hyperbicarbonatemia, and an acid pH. A change in clinical states may acutely reduce the P_{CO_2} while the compensatory increase in serum [HCO_3^-] persists (Table 31-9). Returning the P_{CO_2} toward normal increases arterial pH, since the sustained hyperbicarbonatemia results in a fall in the P_{CO_2}/[HCO_3^-] ratio (equation 1 and Table 31-9). This sequence spawns a *posthypercapneic metabolic alkalosis* or a mixed acute respiratory alkalosis and chronic respiratory acidosis. Most commonly this mixed disorder occurs when patients with chronic lung disease and CO_2 retention are placed on respirators and afforded "pulmonary toilet" (Fig. 31-6). Brisk lowering of the P_{CO_2} creates the alkalemic syndrome described. The abrupt, and ill-advised, lowering of the P_{CO_2} may severely alkalinize the central nervous system. Neuromuscular hyperexcitability, tetany, and seizures may develop.[46] Chronic hypercapnia should be corrected slowly. Bicarbonaturia can then correct the acid-base status if potassium stores and ECF volume are adequate. Hypokalemia and hypovolemia will stimulate renal HCO_3^- retention and thereby predispose subjects to posthypercapneic metabolic alkalosis.[75,80] Acetazolamide may be used to correct severe alkalemia, if diuresis is required.

Acute respiratory acidosis and chronic respiratory alkalosis

Chronic respiratory alkalosis is characterized by primary hypocapnia, secondary hypobicarbonatemia, and varying degrees of alkalemia (Table 31-10). If the P_{CO_2} abruptly increases, this will increase the P_{CO_2}/[HCO_3^-] ratio (equation 1) into the acidemic range. This pathophysiologic sequence produces a *mixed acute respiratory acidosis superimposed upon a chronic respiratory alkalosis* or a *posthypocapneic metabolic acidosis* (Table 31-10).

This unusual sequence may develop when patients with cerebral lesions and central hyperventilation or pa-

TABLE 31-9 • Mixed acute respiratory alkalosis and chronic respiratory acidosis

	Normal	Chronic respiratory acidosis (CRA)	Acute respiratory alkalosis plus CRA
P_{CO_2}, mmHg	40	65	45
HCO_3^-, meq/liter	24	35	35
pH	7.40	7.35	7.51

TABLE 31-10 • Mixed acute respiratory acidosis and chronic respiratory alkalosis

	Normal	Chronic respiratory alkalosis (CRALK)	Acute respiratory acidosis plus CRALK
P_{CO_2}, mmHg	40	20	45
HCO_3^-, meq/liter	24	14	14
pH	7.40	7.46	7.11

tients with severe liver disease are placed on a respirator. The P_{CO_2} may precipitously increase if the amount of dead space in the system is excessive or if respirator settings are inappropriately assigned. Any other cause of acute respiratory acidosis may be superimposed on chronic respiratory alkalosis and will then spawn this chemical sequence.

TRIPLE ACID-BASE DISORDERS

Triple acid-base disorders occur when three primary perturbations develop simultaneously or sequentially. Most often metabolic acidosis and alkalosis combine with either respiratory acidosis or alkalosis. The net effect of the opposing metabolic disturbances determines the final serum [HCO_3^-]. If hypobicarbonatemia results, respiratory compensation should reduce the P_{CO_2} appropriately. If HCO_3^- is restored to normal, the P_{CO_2} should be normal. If hyperbicarbonatemia results, respiratory compensation should increase the P_{CO_2}. When the respiratory response is inappropriate for the abnormal [HCO_3^-], a superimposed respiratory disorder exists.

Triple acid-base disorders occur commonly in patients with severe liver disease. Hyperventilation and respiratory alkalosis frequently develop. Often these patients develop GI distress with vomiting and/or require nasogastric suction, which generates a metabolic alkalosis. Finally, they may develop a variety of metabolic acidoses, such as renal tubular acidosis, diarrheal acidosis, uremic acidosis, and lactic acidosis (see above). The approach outlined should permit the logical dissection of these complex acid-base disorders. Therapy is simplified by adhering to several key principles.

Importance of blood pH. One measure of the severity of a given acid-base disorder is the degree to which the pH is displaced from normal. Accordingly, the urgency with which simple or mixed acid-base disorders, including triple disorders, are approached therapeutically is a function of the prevailing pH. Since additive disorders generally have the most abnormal pH, they usually require rapid and aggressive therapy. Counterbalancing disorders may produce a near normal pH, which tempers the need for rapid therapy. When the resulting blood pH is less than 7.20, or greater than 7.50, more urgent therapy is required.

Therapy must be directed at each component of the mixed disorder. Treating only one component of a mixed, counterbalancing disorder unmasks the other opposing disorder. For example, treating only respiratory alkalosis in a patient with a mixed metabolic acidosis-respiratory alkalosis, unmasks and highlights the metabolic component. Conversely, treatment of the metabolic acidosis would allow blood pH to rise rapidly in response to the unopposed respiratory disorder. Similarly, treatment of only one or two components of a triple disorder would allow the second and third disorders to express their effects more fully. Thus, the treatment of mixed disorders must address each component simultaneously. Attention must be directed toward the causes of the respiratory and metabolic disorders.

It is critical to monitor arterial blood gases closely. Since components of a mixed disorder may improve asynchronously, rapid changes in blood pH may occur. The aggressiveness of therapy must be guided by frequent monitoring of blood pH, P_{CO_2}, and HCO_3^-.

Acknowledgment The authors gratefully acknowledge the technical assistance of Ann Drew in the preparation of the manuscript.

REFERENCES

1. Aberman A, Fulop M: The metabolic and respiratory acidosis of acute pulmonary edema. *Ann Intern Med* 76:173, 1972.
2. Adrogué HJ et al: Changes in plasma anion gap during chronic metabolic acid-base disturbances. *Am J Physiol* 235:F291, 1978.
3. Adrogué HJ, Wilson H: Plasma acid base patterns in diabetic ketoacidosis. *N Engl J Med* 307:1603, 1982.
4. Adrogué HJ et al: Assessing acid-base status in circulatory failure: Differences between arterial and central venous blood. *N Engl J Med* 320:1312, 1989.
5. Anderson LE, Henrich WL: Alkalemia-associated morbidity and mortality in medical and surgical patients. *South Med J* 80(6):729, 1987.

6. Ayus JC et al: Alkalemia associated with renal failure. Correction by hemodialysis with low bicarbonate dialysate. *Arch Intern Med* 140:513, 1980.
7. Baertl JM et al: Relation of acute potassium depletion to renal ammonium metabolism in patients with cirrhosis. *J Clin Invest* 42:696, 1963.
8. Bailey DN, Bone JR: Chemical and hematological changes in stored CPD blood. *Transfusion* 15:244, 1975.
9. Barcenas CG et al: Metabolic alkalosis after massive blood transfusion. Correction by hemodialysis *JAMA* 236:953, 1976.
10. Bear R et al: Effect of metabolic alkalosis on respiratory function in patients with chronic obstructive lung disease. *Can Med Assoc J* 117:900, 1977.
11. Bersin RM, Arieff AI: Improved hemodynamic function during hypoxia with carbicarb, a new agent for the management of acidosis. *Circulation* 77:22, 1988.
12. Better OS et al: Defect in urinary acidification in cirrhosis. The role of excessive tubular reabsorption of sodium in its etiology. *Arch Intern Med* 130:77, 1972.
13. Betz E, Heuser D: Cerebral cortical blood flow during changes of acid-base equilibrium of the brain. *J Appl Physiol* 23:726, 1976.
14. Bishop, RL, Weisfeldt L: Sodium bicarbonate administration during cardiac arrest. Effect on arterial pH, PCO_2 and osmolality. *JAMA* 235:506, 1976.
15. Blair E: Acid-base balance in bacteremic shock. *Arch Intern Med* 127:731, 1971.
16. Blechner JN et al: Oxygen, carbon dioxide and hydrogen ion concentrations in arterial blood during pregnancy. *Am J Obstet Gynecol* 100:1, 1968.
17. Blum JE, Coe FL: Metabolic acidosis after sulfur ingestion. *N Engl J Med* 297:869, 1977.
18. Brader DC, Morelli HF: Systemic alkalosis and digitalis related arrhythmias. *Acta Med Scand* 647(suppl):79, 1981.
19. Braun MNT et al: Respiratory muscle and pulmonary function in polymyositis and other proximal myopathies. *Thorax* 338:616, 1983.
19a. Carlisle EJ et al: Glue sniffing and distal renal tubular acidosis: Sticking to the facts. *J Am Soc Nephrol* 1:1019, 1991.
20. Cochrane AMG et al: Lymphocyte cytotoxicity for kidney cells in the renal tubular acidosis of autoimmune liver disease. *Gut* 16 (10):828, 1975.
21. Cohen JJ, Schwartz WB: Evaluation of acid base equilibrium in pulmonary insufficiency. An approach to a diagnostic dilemma. *Am J Med* 41:163, 1966.
22. Cooperman MT et al: Critical studies of alcoholic ketoacidosis. *Diabetes* 23:433, 1974.
23. Cronin JW, Kroop SF: Alkalemia in diabetic ketoacidosis. *Am J Med* 77:192, 1984.
24. Eldridge F: Blood lactate and pyruvate in pulmonary insufficiency. *N Engl J Med* 274:878, 1966.
25. Emmett M, Narins RG: Clinical use of the anion gap. *Medicine* 56:38, 1977.
26. Emmett M, Seldin DW: Metabolic acidosis and alkalosis, in *The Kidney: Physiology and Pathophysiology*. New York, Raven Press, 1985, p 1567.
27. Enia et al: Hyperchloraemia: A non-specific finding in chronic renal failure. *Nephron*, 41:189, 1985.
28. Filley GF, Kindig NB: Carbicarb, an alkalinizing-ion generating agent of possible clinical usefulness. *Trans Am Clin Climatol Assoc* 96:141, 1984.
29. Finch CA, Lenfant C: Oxygen transport in man. *N Engl J Med* 286:407, 1972.
30. Fulop M et al: Lactic acidosis in pulmonary edema due to left ventricular failure. *Ann Intern Med* 79:180, 1973.
31. Fulop M, Hoberman HD: Alcoholic ketosis. *Diabetes* 24:785, 1975.
32. Fulop M: Metabolic acidosis with alkalemia. *NY State J Med* 80:136, 1980.
33. Gabow PA et al: Acid-base disturbances in the salicylate-intoxicated adult. *Arch Intern Med* 138:1481, 1978.
34. Gabow PA et al: Diagnostic importance of an increased serum anion gap. *N Engl J Med* 3030:84, 1980.
35. Gabow PA et al: Organic acids in ethylene glycol intoxication. *Ann Intern Med* 105:16, 1986.
36. Gamblin GT et al: Diabetic ketoacidosis presenting with a normal anion gap. *Am J Med* 80:759, 1986.
37. Ghose RR: The significance of acid-base measurements in the management of salicylate intoxication. *Postgrad Med J* 43:454, 1967.
38. Golding PL, Mason AMS: Renal tubular acidosis and autoimmune liver disease. *Gut* 12:153, 1971.
39. Golding PL: Renal tubular acidosis in chronic liver disease. *Postgrad Med J* 51:550, 1975.
40. Goodkin DA et al: The role of the anion gap in detecting and managing mixed metabolic acid-base disorders. *Clin Endocrinol Metab* 13:333, 1984.
41. Grace WJ, Barr DP: Complications of alkalosis. *Am J Med* 4:331, 1948.
42. Hammeke M, Bear R: Hyperchloremic metabolic acidosis in diabetes mellitus. *Diabetes* 27:16, 1977.
43. Hill JB: Salicylate intoxication. *N Engl J Med* 288:1110, 1973.
44. Huckabee WE: Relationships of pyruvate and lactate during anaerobic metabolism: III. Effect of breathing low-oxygen gases. *J Clin Invest* 37:264, 1958.
45. Karetzky MS, Mithoefer JC: The cause of hyperventilation and arterial hypoxia in patients with cirrhosis of the liver. *Am J Med Sci* 254:798, 1967.
46. Kilburn KH: Shock, seizures, and coma with alkalosis during mechanical ventilation. *Ann Intern Med* 65:979, 1966.
47. Krapf R et al: Chronic respiratory alkalosis: The effect of sustained hyperventilation on renal regulation of acid-base equilibrium. *N Engl J Med* 324:1394, 1991.
48. Litwin MS et al: Metabolic alkalosis following massive transfusion. *Surgery* 45:805, 1959.
49. Lyons HA, Antonio R: The sensitivity of the respiratory center in pregnancy and after the administration of progesterone. *Trans Assoc Am Physicians* 72:173, 1959.
50. Lyons JH Jr, Moore FD: Posttraumatic alkalosis: Incidence and pathophysiology of alkalosis in surgery. *Surgery* 60:93, 1966.
51. Madias NE et al: Increased anion gap with metabolic alkalosis. The role of plasma-protein equivalency. *N Engl J Med* 300:1421, 1979.
52. Mattar JA et al: Cardiac arrest in the critically ill: II. Hyperosmolal states following cardiac arrest. *Am J Med* 56:162, 1974.

53. Mazzara JT et al: Extreme hypocapnia in the critically ill patient. *Am J Med* 56:450, 1974.
54. Medical house Staff, Robin ED: Dynamic aspects of metabolic acid-base disorders. Phenformin lactic acidosis with alkaline overshoot. *Trans Assoc Am Physicians* 85:317, 1972.
55. Miller PD, Berns AS: Acute metabolic alkalosis perpetuating hypercarbia: A role for acetazolamide in chronic obstructive pulmonary disease. *JAMA* 238:2400, 1977.
56. Mitchell JH et al: The effects of acid-base disturbances on cardiovascular and pulmonary function. *Kidney Int* 1:375, 1972.
57. Mulhausen R et al: Acid base disturbances in patients with cirrhosis of the liver. *Medicine* 46:185, 1967.
58. Narins RG, Emmett M: Simple and mixed acid-base disorders: A practical approach. *Medicine* 59:161, 1980.
59. Neill WA, Hattenhauer M: Impairment of myocardial O_2 supply due to hyperventilation. *Circulation* 52:84, 1975.
60. Newman JH, et al: Acute respiratory failure associated with hypophosphatemia. *N Engl J Med* 296:1101, 1977.
61. Oh MS, Carroll HJ: Hyperchloremic acidosis during the recovery phase of diabetic ketosis. *Ann Intern Med* 89:925, 1978.
62. Oliva PB: Severe alveolar hypoventilation in a patient with metabolic alkalosis. *Am J Med* 52:817, 1972.
63. Ostrea EM, Odell GB: The influence of bicarbonate administration of blood pH in a "closed system." *J Pediatr* 80:671, 1972.
64. Pagliara AS et al: Hepatic fructose-1, 6-diphosphatase deficiency. A cause of lactic acidosis and hypoglycemia in infancy.
65. Pearl RG, Rosenthal MH: Metabolic alkalosis due to plasmaphoresis. *Am J Med* 79:391, 1985.
66. Perrett CL et al: Lactic acidosis and liver damage. *Helv Med Acta* 34:377, 1969/1970.
67. Prowse CM, Gaensler EA: Respiratory and acid-base changes during pregnancy. *Anesthesiology* 26:381, 1965.
68. Prys-Roberts C et al: Circulatory influence of artificial ventilation during nitrous oxide anesthesia in man: II. Results: The relative influence of mean intrathoracid pressure and arterial CO_2 tension. *Br J Anaesth* 39:533, 1967.
69. Prytz H, Thomsen AC: Acid-base status in liver cirrhosis. Disturbances in stable, terminal and porta-caval shunted patients. *Scand J Gastroenterol* 11:249, 1976.
70. Rackow EC et al: Myocardial acidosis during cardiopulmonary resuscitation. *Fed Proc* 46:1401, 1987.
71. Rahilly GT, Berl T: Severe metabolic alkalosis caused by administration of plasma protein fraction in end-stage renal failure. *N Engl J Med* 301:824, 1979.
72. Record CO et al: Acid-base and metabolic disturbances in fulminant hepatic falure. *Gut* 16:144, 1975.
73. Relman AS; Metabolic consequences of acid-base disorders. *Kidney Int* 1:347, 1972.
74. Rowe GG et al: Effects of hyperventilation on systemic and coronary hemodynamics. *Am Heart J* 63:67, 1962.
75. Schwartz WB et al: Effects of chronic hypercapnia on electrolyte and acid-base equilibrium: II. Recovery, with special reference to the influence of chloride intake. *J Clin Invest* 40:1238, 1961.
76. Segar WE, Holliday MA: Physiologic abnormalities of salicylate intoxication. *N Engl J Med* 259:1191, 1958.
77. Simmons DH et al: Hyperventilation and respiratory alkalosis as signs of gram negative bacteremia. *JAMA* 74:2196, 1960.
78. Spagrole SV: Cyanosis of cirrhosis. *Med Clin North Am* 59:983, 1975.
79. Swartz RD et al: Correction of postoperative metabolic alkalosis and renal failure by hemodialysis. *Ann Intern Med* 86:52, 1977.
80. Tenney SM, Miller RM: The respiratory and circulatory actions of salicylate. *Am J Med* 19:498, 1955.
81. Turino GM et al: Renal response to mechanical ventilation in patients with chronic hypercapnia. *Am J Med* 56:151, 1974.
82. Walsh CH, Lim KC: Diabetic ketoalkalosis, a readily misdiagnosed entity. *Br Med J* 2:19, 1976.
83. Wang F et al: The acidosis of cholera. Contributions of hyper-proteinemia, lactic acidemia and hyperphosphatemia. *N Engl J Med* 315:1591, 1986.
84. Wang RL: "Bicarbonate overshoot": An indication for acetazolamide therapy. *South Med J* 68:733, 1975.
85. Weil MH et al: Difference in acid-base state between venous and arterial blood during cardiopulmonary resuscitation. *N Engl J Med* 315:153, 1986.
86. Widmer B et al: Serum electrolyte and acid-base composition. The influence of graded degree of chronic renal failure. *Arch Intern Med* 139:1099, 1979.
87. Wilson RF et al: Severe alkalosis in critically ill surgical patients. *Arch Surg* 105:197, 1972.
88. Winters RW et al: Disturbances of acid-base equilibrium in salicylate intoxication. *Pediatrics* 23:260, 1959.
89. Wolfe JD, Tashkin DP: Hypoxemia of cirrhosis. *Am J Med* 63:746, 1977.
90. Yasue H et al: Coronary arterial spasm and Prinsmetal's variant form of angina induced by hyperventilation and tris-buffer infusion. *Circulation* 58:56, 1978.
91. Yasue H et al: Alkalosis-induced coronary vasoconstriction: Effects of calcium diltiazem, nitroglycerine and propranolol. *Am Heart J* 102:206, 1981.
92. Zuppinger K, Rossi E: Metabolic studies in liver glycogen disease with specific reference to lactate metabolism. *Helv Med Acta* 35:406, 1969.

CHAPTER • 32

Disorders of calcium metabolism

Julio E. Benabe • Manuel Martínez-Maldonado

CALCIUM METABOLISM

Calcium is one of the most important divalent cations in humans. It is the third most abundant ion in the body and represents about 2 percent of the body weight.[281] Of the approximately 1400 g of calcium in the adult, 99 percent is found in bone and only 0.03 percent in plasma (Table 32-1).

Plasma calcium concentration normally ranges from 8.5 to 10.5 mg/dl. Approximately 40 percent is bound to plasma proteins, predominantly to albumin. The remaining 60 percent is diffusible; of that, 90 percent occurs in ionized (ultrafilterable) form; the remaining 10 percent is bound to citrate, phosphate, and bicarbonate ions.

Normal plasma calcium concentration is maintained by the close regulation of intestinal calcium absorption, renal calcium reabsorption, and the turnover of skeletal calcium. These three biological processes are regulated by the combined effects of parathyroid hormone (PTH) and cholecalciferol (vitamin D_3).

The general physiology of calcium is treated in Chap. 11.

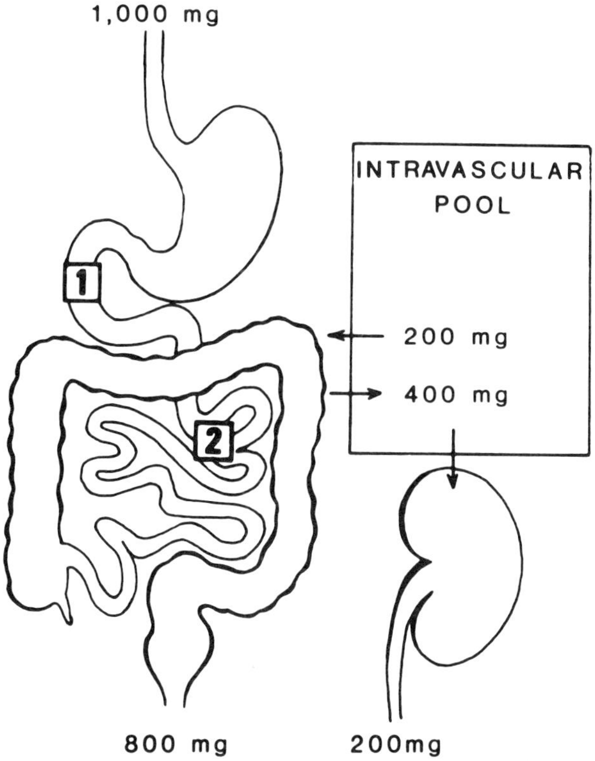

FIGURE 32-1 • Schematic representation of intestinal handling of Ca^{2+}. Approximately 40 percent of ingested Ca^{2+} is absorbed, predominantly in the duodenum (1) and jejunum (2). Calcium secretion has been shown to occur in experimental animals; its physiological significance in humans is unknown.

INTESTINAL ABSORPTION

Most intestinal absorption of calcium occurs in the duodenum and jejunum (Fig. 32-1).[32] Analysis of the absorptive process has shown that it is composed of saturable and nonsaturable components.[134,330,331] The nonsaturable component involves passive diffusion. It depends on and varies linearly with intestinal calcium concentration and is driven by electrical and chemical gradients. Diffusion predominates at luminal calcium concentrations exceeding 2 m*M*;[135,332] it is not influenced by 1α,25-dihydroxycholecalciferol [1α,25-$(OH)_2D_3$] (see Chap. 11). The saturable component, on the other hand, is stimulated by 1α,25-$(OH)_2D_3$. It represents an energy-

TABLE 32-1 • Distribution of Calcium in a 70-kg adult man

Site	Calcium content, g	% of total
Skeleton	1300	98.9
Teeth	7	0.5
Soft tissues	7	0.5
Plasma	0.35	0.04
Extravascular fluid	0.70	0.06
Total	1315	100.00

requiring, carrier-mediated process with a K_m of 1.0 mM.[134] There is also experimental evidence that calcium is secreted into the bowel lumen by a process that can be stimulated by glucose[331] and somatostatin;[136] the physiological significance of such a mechanism in humans and experimental animals is not known.

RENAL HANDLING

By renal reabsorption the organism reclaims ultrafiltered calcium or allows it to be excreted in the urine (Fig. 32-2). Approximately 60 percent of the filtered load is reabsorbed in the *proximal convoluted tubule* (PCT). Reabsorption at this tubule site is largely passive and is proportional to sodium and water reabsorption.[436] Reabsorption in the PCT is enhanced by extracellular fluid (ECF) volume contraction and is diminished by ECF volume expansion.[5,358] In the *proximal straight tubule* (PST) calcium is transported against both electrical and chemical gradients. That suggests the transport process is energy-requiring, active, and dissociable from sodium and water transport.[383,384]

The *thick ascending limb* reabsorbs 20 percent of the filtered calcium.[280] Most studies agree that reabsorption in the medullary portion is passive, sensitive to furosemide, and driven by the positive luminal potential.[41,437] Conflicting results, have been found in the cortical thick ascending limb, however, where passive, electrically driven[41,56,405,438] calcium reabsorption as well as active, cAMP-mediated calcium transport[215,379,384,433,437] have been demonstrated.

Roughly 10 percent of calcium reabsorption in the nephron occurs in the *distal convoluted tubule* (DCT).[90,255] This transport process is active; it occurs against an electrochemical gradient. Reabsorption of Ca^{2+} in the DCT can be dissociated from sodium reabsorption by administering thiazide. Also in this segment PTH enhances calcium reabsorption independent of changes in sodium reabsorption or luminal potential,[91] probably by stimulating adenylate cyclase in the granular cells.[316]

Micropuncture studies of the *collecting tubule* (CT) have shown that 3 to 10 percent of filtered calcium is reabsorbed in this segment.[5,255] Current evidence suggests that calcium reabsorption is active, occurring in the granular cortical collecting tubule, and is independent of electrical potential or sodium transport.[405] Granular cells, which are sensitive to PTH, may be the primary site of transport. These properties are similar to those seen in the DCT. The DCT and CT together could be the final regulators of renal calcium reabsorption. Parathyroidectomy and use of saline for ECF space expansion have been shown to abolish Ca^{2+} reabsorption at sites beyond the late DCT.[5]

In addition to the regulatory effects of hormones and volume status, changes in acid-base balance can also influence calcium homeostasis. Acidosis can increase calcium release from bone[266] and produce calciuria by inhibiting tubular calcium reabsorption.[14,439] In acidosis, binding of calcium to serum proteins is decreased, which

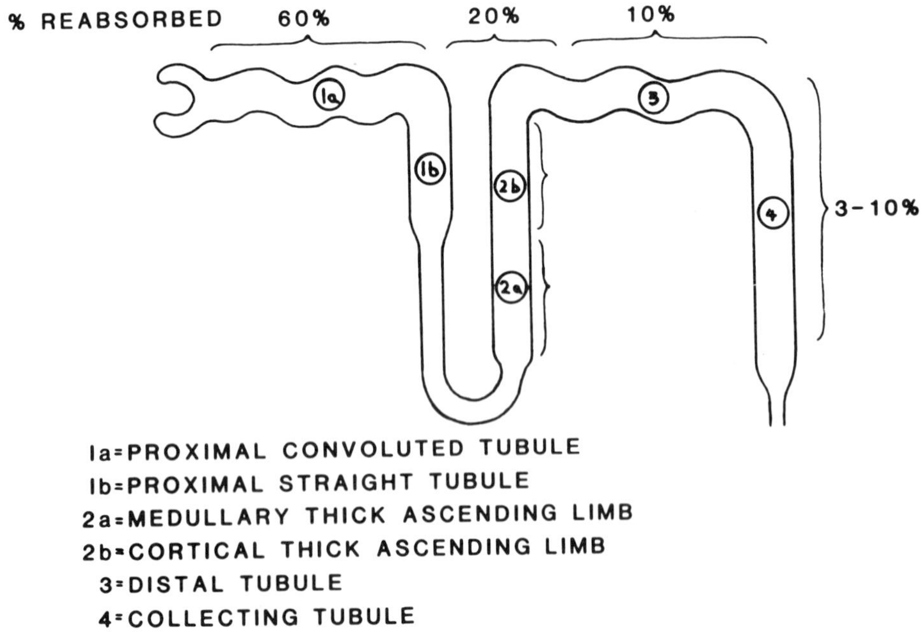

FIGURE 32-2 • Schematic representation of renal handling of Ca^{2+}. Approximately 60 percent of ultrafiltered Ca^{2+} is reabsorbed in the proximal tubule. Reabsorption in the proximal convoluted tubule (1a) is predominantly passive and proportional to sodium reabsorption. In the proximal straight tubule (1b) reabsorption occurs through active transport. Approximately 20 percent of the filtered Ca^{2+} is reabsorbed in the thick ascending limb. Passive reabsorption sensitive to furosemide occurs in the medullary portion (2a) while PTH regulates reabsorption in the cortical portion (2b). PTH also regulates reabsorption in the distal tubule (3), where 10 percent of the filtered Ca^{2+} is reabsorbed. Thiazides can also influence reabsorption in the distal tubule. From 3 to 10 percent of the filtered Ca^{2+} is reabsorbed in the collecting tubule (4), which together with the distal tubule may be the final regulators of Ca^{2+} reabsorption in the kidney.

increases the proportion of ultrafilterable calcium. Alkalosis, on the other hand, increases calcium binding to proteins, decreases free calcium levels, and increases PTH secretion. These effects result in hypocalciuria. It has also been shown that alkalosis enhances renal tubular calcium reabsorption independent of any change in PTH.[114] Acid-base changes can also regulate the synthesis of $1\alpha,25\text{-}(OH)_2D_3$.[261] Acidosis inhibits PTH-dependent adenylate cyclase, which, in the PCT, stimulates 1α-hydroxylase. In a recent study in rats the activity of 1α-hydroxylase was indeed found to be decreased in acidosis.[234]

The effects of vitamin D_3 on the renal handling of Ca^{2+} remain poorly understood. Some studies have shown that vitamin D_3 increases reabsorption; others show that reabsorption is decreased.[268]

Thus reabsorption along the nephron occurs through a heterogeneous set of processes that can be regulated by ECF volume status, various hormones, and acid-base changes.

BONE TURNOVER

The potentially most important activity determining plasma calcium concentration is bone turnover. Calcium is the principal divalent cation in the mineral component of bone. Bone demineralization is mediated by osteoclastic activity or osteocytic osteolysis. The balance between bone formation and bone accretion determines the net calcium turnover in bone.

Several hormones are known to regulate osteocyte and osteoclast activity in bone. PTH (1) increases the rate of osteocytic and osteoclastic bone resorption, (2) increases the conversion of mononuclear cells to osteoclasts, and (3) affects the rate of synthesis of bone collagen. Another hormone known to exert regulatory actions on bone is vitamin D_3. The precise mechanism of this hormone's action on the skeletal system is unknown. Clinical and experimental observations suggest that it may enhance mineralization of osteoid and synthesis of subcellular organelles in osteoblasts and osteocytes.[449,488] Vitamin D_3 also exerts a permissive effect on PTH-stimulated osteoclastic resorption. The most potent metabolite of vitamin D_3 mediating this effect is $1\alpha,25\text{-}(OH)_2D_3$.

Calcitonin is a third hormone that may influence bone calcium turnover. This hormone is known to inhibit osteoclastic bone resorption and induce hypocalcemia; however, its importance in the daily physiological regulation of skeletal calcium is not known.

The coordinated interactions of the hormones controlling intestinal calcium absorption, renal calcium reabsorption, and bone resorption determine daily the plasma calcium concentration.

HYPERCALCEMIA

The prevalence and causes of hypercalcemia are distinctly different among individuals in the general population on the one hand and hospitalized patients on the other. The prevalence in the general population ranges between 0.05 and 0.6 percent;[40,195,296] in the hospital inpatient population the prevalence ranges from 0.6 to 3.6 percent.[144,296]

Malignancy accounts for roughly half of the cases[144,145,499] of hypercalcemia in hospitalized patients. In a recent study of an urban population, primary hyperparathyroidism was found in 54 percent of all hypercalcemic subjects.[325]

In general, malignancy and primary hyperparathyroidism account for up to 70 to 80 percent of all cases of hypercalcemia.[6] These two conditions account for an annual incidence rate of hypercalcemia of approximately 400 new patients per million population per year.[326]

Prompt identification of hypercalcemia and its cause(s) becomes of paramount importance in preventing the morbidity and mortality associated with this metabolic disorder. An algorithm for the diagnostic evaluation of hypercalcemia is shown in Fig. 32-3.

CAUSES AND MECHANISMS

Increased bone resorption

Malignancy

Hypercalcemia is a common complication in patients with cancer. The incidence of this metabolic disorder in malignancies depends on the population of patients studied and on the type of malignancy. In a study of 3969 patients with neoplasms, 9 percent were hypercalcemic.[60] Of all the patients with hypercalcemia and malignancy, 44 percent had hematologic and 41 percent had solid neoplasms. Hypercalcemia complicated 11 percent of all the hematologic neoplasms but only 6 percent of patients with solid neoplasms were hypercalcemic.[60]

In general, the incidence of hypercalcemia in patients with neoplasms is between 10 and 20 percent.[413] The most common malignancies associated with this disorder are breast cancer, lung cancer, and multiple myeloma.[60,144,325,413]

The principal source of calcium in the hypercalcemia of malignancy is the skeletal system. The majority of cases result from osteolytic skeletal metastases, yet a significant number of patients have been recognized with hypercalcemia without bone metastases, *paraneoplastic hypercalcemia*. Patients with primary hyperparathyroidism have a high incidence of associated malignancies. Farr and coworkers[133] reported on the presence of malignancies in 34 of 100 patients with proven primary hyper-

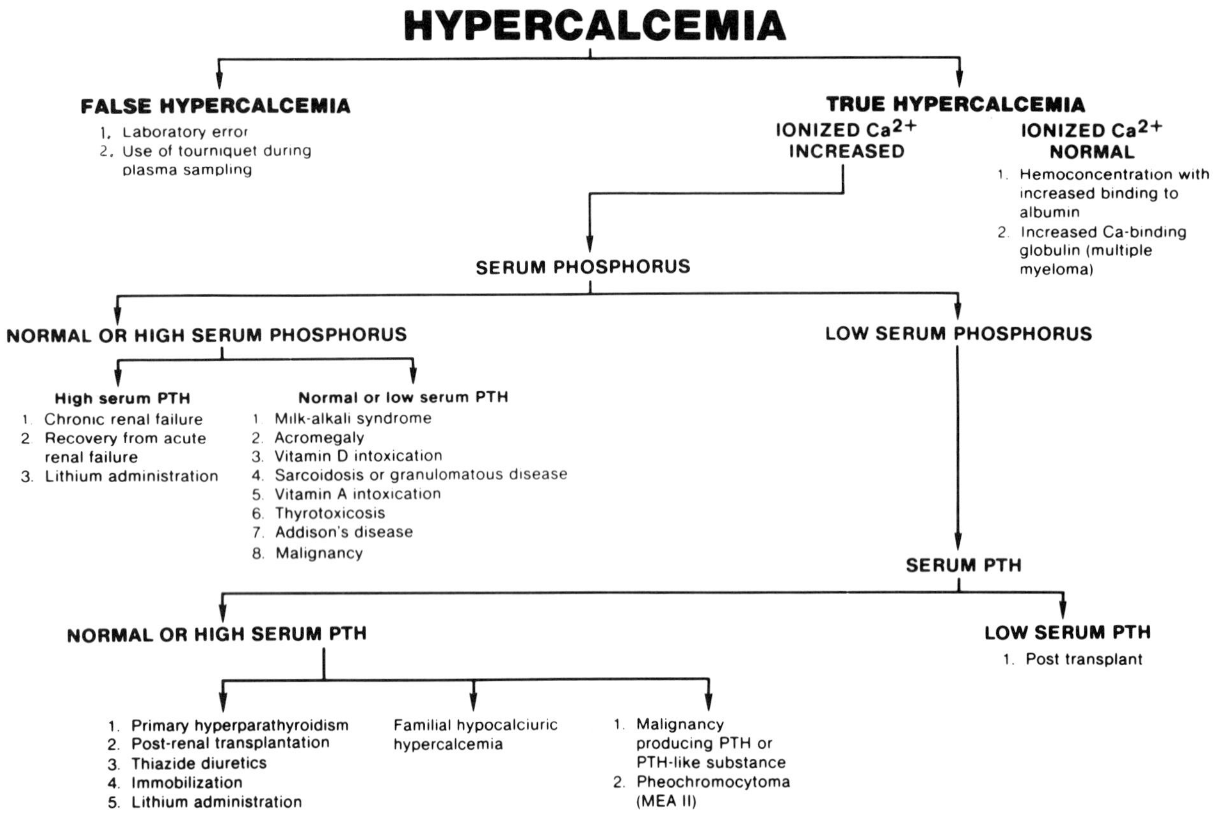

FIGURE 32-3 • Diagnostic steps in the evaluation of hypercalcemia.

parathyroidism. Kaplan et al. reported that 16 percent of patients with parathyroid adenomas had malignancies[230] and Samaan et al. found that 30 percent of patients with primary hyperparathyroidism had malignant tumors.[392] The incidence of cancer in these patients might be overestimated since the statistics come from centers that primarily treat cancer patients. Nevertheless, it is apparent that primary hyperparathyroidism may not be an uncommon condition in hypercalcemic patients with malignancy. In fact, Drezner and Lebovitz found that 6 of 15 patients with paraneoplastic hypercalcemia had high levels of nephrogenous cAMP excretion and in all 6 parathyroid adenomas were discovered at surgery.[111] Larger series report a similar incidence.[417]

Paraneoplastic hypercalcemia results from the production by tumor cells of humoral factors that can stimulate bone resorption.[328] These include (1) PTH secreted by the tumor, (2) a PTH-like substance, immunochemically different from endogenous PTH, (3) prostaglandins (PGs), and (4) osteoclast activating factors (OAF), a series of various cytokines.[320]

Ectopic PTH synthesis by nonparathyroid tumors was initially suggested by Albright in 1941.[9] Evidence for his proposal was first advanced by Tashjian and associates in 1964.[442] Ectopic synthesis of PTH-like material has been demonstrated in various malignancies, including anaplastic carcinomas of the parotids,[407] hepatomas,[243] squamous cell carcinomas,[187] cervical carcinomas,[37,205] transitional cell carcinomas of the bladder,[334] carcinomas of the breast,[204,441] hypernephromas,[38] and leukemia.[256,316,501] Production of PTH by nonparathyroid tumors is uncommon.[408] Simpson and coworkers studied cell lines in tissue culture obtained from tumors that are frequently associated with hypercalcemia. They were not able to detect parathyroid hormone RNA transcripts in mRNA prepared from the tumor cells.[411] Their findings indicate that PTH production by tumors rarely causes hypercalcemia in malignancy.

A PTH-like substance with different immunochemical properties from glandular PTH is frequently synthesized by tumors.[319,440] A study by Stewart et al. of 50 patients with cancer-associated hypercalcemia revealed that nephrogenous cAMP was elevated in 41 patients, reaching values comparable to those seen in patients with proven hyperparathyroidism.[425] The 41 patients had a similar reduction in the tubular reabsorption of phosphate. The patients had lower serum levels of $1\alpha,25\text{-}(OH)_2D_3$ and lower values for immunoreactive PTH (measured by four different radioimmunoassays). Their findings were consistent with a PTH-like substance capable of stimulating proximal tubule adenylate cyclase and inhibiting phosphate reabsorption, but incapable of stimulating 25 hydroxy-vitamin D 1α-hydroxylase. The substance was also immunochemically different from endogenous PTH. Similar findings have been reported in a patient with hypernephroma.[174] A protein factor secreted by renal carcinoma cells in culture has been shown to activate renal adenylate cyclase via the PTH receptor.[430] This protein factor was displaced from the receptor by an analogue of PTH but was not recognized by antisera specific for PTH.[61]

It is known that some solid tumors synthesize and secrete a parathyroid hormone-related peptide (PTH-rP) with striking biological similarities to PTH.[50] The effects of PTH-rP (hypercalcemia, phosphaturia, and elevation of urine cyclic AMP) may be blocked by PTH inhibitors, suggesting a common interaction with the PTH receptor and at least partial homology with the hormone. In fact, purification of PTH-rP and cloning of its gene revealed close sequence homology at the extreme amino-terminal end of the molecule with the first 13 amino acids being virtually identical with authentic PTH.[208] The structural divergence from there on accounts for the incapacity of immunoassays for PTH to recognize PTH-rP.

Immunoradiometric assays for the 1-to-74 fragment of PTH-rP and a radioimmunoassay for carboxyl terminal 109-to-188 showed frequent marked elevations of the peptide in the plasma of patients with malignant hypercalcemia.[50] Moreover, in some patients curative surgery or palliative interventions reduced plasma PTH-rP as calcium levels fell to normal. Since PTH-rP levels are not elevated in primary hyperparathyroidism, and PTH levels not elevated in malignant hypercalcemia, measurement of both peptides may help distinguish the two most common causes of clinical hypercalcemia. This, however, required further study of the PTH-rP control in hyperparathyroidism and clear-cut recognition of malignant hypercalcemia. The latter is particularly taxing, because the clinical diagnosis is frequently imprecise. This is usually the result of failure to measure urine cyclic AMP, a test unavailable in most clinical laboratories.[35] Moreover, there is some evidence that PTH-rP may be responsible for hypercalcemia in benign conditions,[237] a possibility necessitating further study and evaluation. Finally, some patients with cancer do not develop hypercalcemia despite elevations of PTH-rP.[55] Thus, it is still unclear whether the assays for the peptide are imperfect or other factors are needed to act with PTH-rP to induce hypercalcemia.[326a]

Prostaglandins are also potential mediators of hypercalcemia caused by certain malignancies. Prostaglandin-induced bone reabsorption was first demonstrated by Klein and Raisz in 1970.[242] PGE_1 and PGE_2 caused the release of ^{45}Ca from bone to the same extent as did parathyroid hormone. Tashjian and coworkers have examined the role of PGs in the pathogenesis of hypercalcemia associated with tumors. These investigators identified PGE_2 and its metabolite, 13,14-dihydro-15-keto PGE_2, as the factors responsible for bone resorption in the tumor cells. Furthermore, indomethacin reduced in parallel the capacity of tumor cells to resorb bone and their PGE_2 content. The results of these studies provided convincing evidence that PGE_2 was the agent responsible for hypercalcemia.[443-445]

Elevated levels of PGE_2 were first found in a patient with hypercalcemia of malignancy by Robertson et al.[375] Subsequently Seyberth et al. studied 14 hypercalcemic patients with solid tumors. Eight subjects were found to have elevated levels of a metabolite of PGE_2, low levels of PTH, and no evidence of skeletal metastases.[399] High plasma values of PGE_2 have also been reported in some patients with cancer.[100,226,376] The hypercalcemia has been reversed by inhibitors of PG synthesis.[47,312,376, 399]

Production of PGs by bone cells in response to humoral factors has also been found by Minkin et al.[312] These investigators demonstrated that extracts of cancers causing hypercalcemia stimulated bone resorption in vitro but that this effect was abolished by PG inhibition.

Another potential role of PGs in the hypercalcemia of malignancy is its interaction with OAF, lymphokines released by stimulated peripheral blood leukocytes.[209,461] OAF was initially described as a heterogeneous protein with a molecular weight between 13,000 and 25,000.[273,323] Monocytes are necessary for the release of OAF by activated lymphocytes; the permissive effect of monocytes is mediated by prostaglandins.[495,496] OAF has been detected in the supernatant fluid of cultured lymphoid cell lines obtained from patients with multiple myeloma,[320] Burkitt's lymphoma,[321] malignant lymphoma,[321] and lymphosarcoma cell leukemia.[323]

Even though experimental data support the role of prostaglandins as a cause of hypercalcemia in some malignancies, an understanding of their exact role is far from complete.[68,306,377]

Patients with multiple myeloma usually have extensive bone destruction from increased osteoclastic activity. Osteoclasts are stimulated by cytokines produced by the plasma cells. The cytokine lymphotoxin has been found to be the major bone resorbing factor produced in myeloma.[165] Normally, cytokine lymphotoxin is produced by activated T-lymphocytes. It is a member of the same family of immune cell products as tumor necrosis factor (TNF) and interleukin-1, both of which are produced by cells in the monocyte-macrophage lineage. Both of these cytokines stimulate the differentiation of committed osteoclast precursors into mature cells. Moreover, they act on mature multinucleated cells to cause them to form reabsorption lacunae.[454,455]

Other humoral factors (called *osteolysins*) have been implicated in causing the hypercalcemia of malignancy. Epidermal growth factor-like substance and transforming growth factor have received recent attention.[221] Their precise role in producing hypercalcemia and the frequency with which it occurs are unknown. The finding of vitamin D_3 receptors in breast tumor cells[120,121] has also suggested that a potential role is played by vitamin

D_3 in the hypercalcemia of malignancy. Nevertheless, the exact mechanism by which vitamin D_3 in tumor cells causes hypercalcemia remains to be elucidated. A recent report by Breslau and coworkers[49] suggested that in some lymphomatous patients with hypercalcemia the humoral mediator could be $1\alpha,25\text{-(OH)}_2D_3$ produced by the malignancy.

Clearly hypercalcemia in malignancy can result from a variety of mechanisms. Purification of PTH-rP and cloning of its gene is a great advance that may permit prompt diagnosis and more specific modes of treatment.

Primary hyperparathyroidism

Hypercalcemia in primary hyperparathyroidism results from: (1) increased bone resorption, (2) increased intestinal absorption of calcium secondary to a PTH-induced increase in $1\alpha,25\text{-(OH)}_2D_3$ and (3) increased renal reabsorption of calcium mediated by increased PTH. The introduction of automated serum calcium determinations has increased the frequency of diagnosing hypercalcemia and recognizing hyperparathyroidism. Previously, the most common clinical presentation included nephrolithiasis, osteitis fibrosa cystica, and soft tissue calcifications; asymptomatic hypercalcemia is now more frequent.[17] Albright and Reifenstein reported in 1948 that only 2 percent of patients with hyperparathyroidism were asymptomatic.[8] Recent series have disclosed that more than 45 percent of patients with primary hyperparathyroidism were asymptomatic at the time of diagnosis.[251,360]

Single adenomas account for 75 percent of the cases of primary hyperparathyroidism, while multiglandular disease or hyperplasia is found in 25 percent and 1 to 3 percent have parathyroid carcinomas.[6,232]

A syndrome characterized by markedly elevated PTH levels followed by cycles of hypercalcemia, polyuria, dehydration, reduced renal function, and continuously worsening hypercalcemia has been named *acute primary hyperparathyroidism*. The syndrome may be the result of either an adenoma or hyperplasia. Forty-three cases were reported by 1987.[146] Levels of PTH in these individuals can be as high as 20 times normal. There is severe skeletal (53 percent) and renal involvement. The latter is manifested by nephrolithiasis and nephrocalcinosis.[325] In addition to the usual forms of treatment for hypercalcemia (see below), surgical removal of parathyroid tissue will correct the disturbance.[34]

The etiology of primary hyperparathyroidism remains unknown. A possible relation between neck radiation therapy and the development of autonomous hyperparathyroidism has been suggested,[457,458] and support for it has been given by several reports.[77,367,389,448,459] The clinical and biochemical manifestations of radiation-associated hyperparathyroidism are not different from hyperparathyroidism in patients not exposed to radiation. Yet, almost 80 percent of those with radiation exposure had concomitant thyroid disease.[232]

Primary hyperparathyroidism can also be found in patients with multiple endocrine adenomatosis (MEA). *Wermer's syndrome* (MEA type 1) consists of pancreatic and pituitary tumors associated with parathyroid adenomas. The clinical manifestations of this syndrome are also similar to primary hyperparathyroidism.[253]

Pheochromocytomas and medullary carcinoma of the thyroid are found in *Sipple's syndrome* (MEA type 2). This condition is associated with hyperparathyroidism in type 2a or with mucosal neuromas and a Marfan's syndrome-like habitus in type 2b. It has been postulated that a defect in the development of neuroectodermal tissue explains the concurrence of pheochromocytomas and medullary carcinoma. The present evidence suggests that these disorders are inherited as autosomal dominant traits. Except for those cases of MEA syndrome, less than 10 percent of patients with primary hyperparathyroidism have associated endocrine disease.[490]

An interesting recent finding may help shed light on the etiology of primary hyperparathyroidism. Two patients have been studied in whom the parathyroid hormone gene was rearranged to a site adjacent to well-known oncogenes.[17,18] While such an abnormality may be responsible for aberrant growth of the parathyroid cells, the number of cases exhibiting the gene rearrangement is too small for major conclusions to be reached regarding its etiologic role.

The pathophysiology of the deranged PTH production in primary hyperparathyroidism is still unknown. Increased parathyroid mass has been considered to be a contributing factor. However, in a recent study Bellorín-Font and coworkers found altered adenylate cyclase kinetics in parathyroid tissue obtained from 10 patients with hyperfunctioning glands.[29] These investigators found increased affinity of adenylate cyclase for Mg^{2+}, suggesting that alterations in the enzyme may be related to enhanced production of PTH. Although there are reports of correction of hypercalcemia and of decreased PTH production in patients with chronic renal failure treated with propranolol[33,67] or cimetidine,[220,254] these results have not been reproduced by several other investigators.[378,474]

Immobilization

The hypercalcemia of immobilization is the consequence of an imbalance between the rates of bone formation and bone resorption. This process is more conspicuous in patients with Paget's disease or in growing children in whom bone turnover is increased.[160,369,492] The events leading to hypercalcemia in this condition are still unexplained. A study of immobilized patients by Lawrence et al. showed low levels of PTH that returned to normal with correction of the hypercalcemia.[258] On the other hand, Lerman et al. reported elevated PTH levels in two young patients with immobilization hypercalcemia.[267] After mobilization Ca^{2+} and PTH returned to normal. The reason for the differences in these observations is unknown.

Factors that have not been examined and that could contribute to the development of immobilization hypercalcemia include volume contraction, decreased glomerular filtration rate (GFR), and, possibly, malnutrition in the chronically ill and bedridden patient. These factors could contribute to hypercalcemia by augmenting Ca^{2+} retention, impairing the kidney's ability to excrete the increased load of Ca^{2+} coming from bone, and increasing $1\alpha,25\text{-}(OH)_2D_3$ production (due to phosphate depletion from malnutrition. Of interest is that the increase in bone resorption may result in hypercalciuria (resorptive hypercalciuria) and lead to both upper and lower urinary tract nephrolithiasis.[426] Further, if the condition is allowed to continue, osteopenia will result. The exact pathogenesis of immobilization hypercalcemia awaits a better understanding of the renal hemodynamic and metabolic changes induced by immobilization.

Hyperthyroidism

Total serum calcium is increased in 10 to 20 percent of the patients with hyperthyroidism.[25,132] Nevertheless, the frequency of hypercalcemia can be as high as 50 percent if serum $[Ca^{2+}]$ is measured.[58]

The pathogenesis of hypercalcemia in hyperthyroidism can be deduced from the effects of triiodothyroxine (T_4) or triiodothyronine (T_3) on calcium metabolism. Studies have shown that intestinal calcium absorption can be decreased in hyperthyroid subjects.[400,414] The concentration of 25-OH-D_3 in the serum of patients with hyperthyroidism was less than 50 percent of the concentration obtained in age-matched controls.[473] These findings are inconsistent with participation of either intestinal calcium absorption or vitamin D_3 in the hypercalcemia of hyperthyroidism.[350]

The prominence of the role of increased bone resorption in the production of hypercalcemia is supported by both clinical and laboratory findings. Biochemical evaluation of patients with hyperthyroidism has demonstrated hypercalciuria, increased alkaline phosphatase, and increased serum and urinary hydroxyproline.[241,309] Increased osteoclastic bone resorption has been recognized in patients with hyperthyroidism.[149,307] Total body calcium content is reduced by 9 percent; this deficit improves with antithyroid therapy.[84] Studies in vitro have also supported a direct stimulation of bone resorption by both T_4 and T_3.[322] The precise mechanism of this stimulatory effect is not known, but several possibilities have been considered. Increased sensitivity of beta-adrenergic receptors in the hyperthyroid state could enhance bone resorption. This possibility is supported by clinical reports and in vitro studies which show that propranolol can reverse the hypercalcemia of hyperthyroidism.[322,386] Other studies have proposed that PGs[138] or increased OAF production[324] are responsible for the hypercalcemia in this disease, but definite evidence for the role of these substances is lacking. Further studies will be necessary before the exact mechanism of increased bone resorption in hyperthyroidism is unraveled. To date the available information indicates that the increased bone resorption leads to increased Ca^{2+} release from bone, which depresses PTH and vitamin D_3 secretion. These two hormones, in turn, increase urinary Ca^{2+} excretion.

Vitamin A intoxication

Excess vitamin A can increase bone resorption and lead to hypercalcemia. Studies in animals have shown that large doses of vitamin A increase osteoclastic activity.[23] High concentrations of vitamin A disrupt lysosomes and thus release hydrolytic enzymes that may increase bone resorption.[102] In human beings, chronic ingestion of amounts of vitamin A exceeding 50,000 units per day leads to hypercalcemia, bone pain, nephrocalcinosis, and renal insufficiency.[142,151,227,233] In many of the reported cases vitamin D was also ingested with vitamin A; thus a combined effect could have precipitated hypercalcemia. Recently, the widespread use of vitamin A analogues such as *cis*-retinoic acid for the treatment of acne and other dermatological conditions has been occasionally associated with hypercalcemia. The mechanism appears to involve osteoclast-mediated bone resorption.[471]

In vitro studies have shown that vitamin A can augment PTH secretion.[72] In vivo studies found elevated PTH release in response to high doses of vitamin A;[73] however, no evidence has been provided that PTH can be altered by the chronic use of vitamin A in vivo.

Posttransplantation hypercalcemia

After successful renal transplantation hypercalcemia may occur as a result of increased PTH production by hyperplastic parathyroid glands. Typically it disappears within 6 months after transplantation as the gland undergoes involution.[76,96] Occasionally hypercalcemia may last as long as 24 months.[10,292,356,395] Patients with radiological evidence of bone disease and soft tissue calcification during their pretransplant period are more likely to develop posttransplant hypercalcemia, probably from mobilization of calcium present in extraskeletal calcifications.[96,166]

Occasionally, hyperplastic glands persistently secrete PTH even in the presence of hypercalcemia (i.e., the "calcium-stat" is reset). Parathyroidectomy should be considered when serum calcium is persistently higher than 12 mg/dl, particularly if there is evidence of renal graft dysfunction. The glands may be preserved for future autotransplantation to the forearm, since some of these patients may develop persistent hypocalcemia some time after parathyroidectomy.[489,490]

The development of posttransplantation hypercalcemia depends on several other factors besides PTH. These factors include ostomalacia, phosphate depletion, and the use of steroids and diuretics. Osteomalacia may protect from the development of posttransplantation hypercalcemia by providing osteoid in which mineral will deposit.[70,353,424] Patients without evidence of hypocalcemia and/or osteomalacia during the pretransplant period may be more susceptible to developing hypercalcemia.[298]

Steroid therapy can attenuate the stimulus provided by high PTH to 1α,25-$(OH)_2D_3$ synthesis in the transplanted kidney. As steroid administration is gradually reduced the antagonist effect of steroids on the hypercalcemia action of vitamin D_3 can diminish, which contributes to the hypercalcemia. Furthermore, persistent hypophosphatemia due to a phosphate leak in the transplanted kidney can augment the synthesis of 1α,25-$(OH)_2D_3$ and contribute to increased intestinal calcium absorption.[166,381]

We also believe that the use of thiazide diuretics in the posttransplant patient with good graft function may contribute to the development of hypercalcemia, particularly in the presence of high PTH and high vitamin D_3 levels.[310]

Increased intestinal absorption

Vitamin D intoxication

Treatment of hypoparathyroidism, rickets, or osteomalacia with vitamin D is the most common setting for vitamin D intoxication. Not infrequently, correction of the hypocalcemia or of the bone disease is attempted too quickly or adequate follow-up is lacking.[346] The disorder usually arises when serum levels of 25-hydroxycholecalciferol (25-OH-D_3) are very high[93,213] despite low or only slightly elevated levels of 1α,25-$(OH)_2D_3$.[409] It is clear that high levels are not absolutely necessary because intoxication with vitamin D has also been reported in an anephric patient.[93] Further evidence that 25-OH-D_3 is responsible for the hypercalcemia can be deduced from knowledge of the metabolism of vitamin D_3. Reversal of the hypercalcemia seen with vitamin D intoxication is characteristically slow and may take months before serum calcium concentration returns to normal. Reversal of the toxic effects of 25-OH-D_3 occurs in 7 to 30 days;[191] the half-life of the metabolite is from 10 to 20 days. The toxicity of 1α,25-$(OH)_2D_3$ disappears after 2 to 10 days because of its shorter half-life. The incidence of hypercalcemia produced by 1α,25-$(OH)_2D_3$ in patients with chronic renal failure and hypoparathyroidism has risen since the therapeutic use of this compound has become more widespread.[27,191]

Sarcoidosis and other granulomatous diseases

Sarcoidosis was responsible for 0.2 percent[144] and 2.5 percent[499] of the hypercalcemia reported in different series. Hypercalcemia is found in 15 to 20 percent of another set of patients with sarcoidosis;[370] however, hypercalciuria can also occur in sarcoidosis; 50 percent of the patients with sarcoidosis have been reported to be hypercalciuric. The abnormal calcium metabolism in sarcoidosis may be the result of either excessive endogenous production of vitamin D[199] or an abnormal sensitivity to it.[13] Vitamin D provokes increased intestinal absorption of Ca^{2+}, which leads to hypercalcemia and/or hypercalciuria. Papapoulus and coworkers[344] described a patient with sarcoidosis whose episodes of hypercalcemia were confined to the summer months. During those periods he exhibited abnormally high serum 1,25-$(OH)_2D_3$ concentrations in association with hypercalcemia. Treatment with steroids returned serum calcium and 1α,25-$(OH)_2D_3$ levels to normal. Subsequently Bell and coworkers[28] reported that three patients with sarcoidosis and hypercalcemia had increased plasma levels of 1α,25-$(OH)_2D_3$. Furthermore, when vitamin D_2 was given to normal subjects, to subjects with sarcoidosis without hypercalcemia, and to a group who had sarcoidosis and a history of hypercalcemia, the plasma levels of 1α,25-$(OH)_2D_3$ increased above normal only in the patients with a history of abnormal calcium metabolism. Subsequently Koide et al. demonstrated that, consistent with the finding of Bell et al.,[28] patients with sarcoidosis and hypercalcemia had reduced serum immunoreactive PTH levels and inappropriately elevated levels of 1α,25-$(OH)_2D_3$.[245] An anephric patient with sarcoidosis was recently shown to have increased levels of 1α,25-$(OH)_2D_3$ and hypercalcemia, suggesting the vitamin D metabolite had come from an extrarenal source.[20] Furthermore, a patient with surgical hypoparathyroidism in whom sarcoidosis developed was found to have an elevated level of serum 1α,25-$(OH)_2D_3$ but the serum calcium value was normal.[502] The available evidence suggests that hypercalcemia in sarcoidosis is the result of increased 1α,25-$(OH)_2D_3$ levels. The increased synthesis of this metabolite of vitamin D occurs in an extrarenal site and is independent of PTH.

It is now known that elevated plasma levels 1,25$(OH)_2D_3$ in sarcoidosis result from its increased production by the macrophage, a prominent constituent of the sarcoid granuloma.[2,3] These cells contain 25(OH)D_3-1-hydroxylase and this enzyme has a high affinity for its substrate 25(OH)D_3.[2a,217] The 1-hydroxylation reaction in macrophages is inhibitable by glucocorticoids, a finding that explains in part why these agents are the mainstay of therapy of sarcoid-induced hypercalcemia.[412]

Tuberculosis is another granulomatous disease associated with hypercalcemia.[1,44,45,225,401,406] In a series of 50 patients with active tuberculosis 24 were reported to be hypercalcemic.[240] In a recent series of 79 patients with active pulmonary tuberculosis Abbasi and coworkers reported that 22 patients developed hypercalcemia. Furthermore a positive correlation between daily vitamin D supplementation and the degree and duration of hypercalcemia was demonstrated. These features of calcium metabolism in tuberculosis are strikingly similar to sarcoidosis and suggest that a common pathogenetic mechanism may exist for all the granulomatous disorders.

In fact, elevated levels of $1,25(OH)_2D_3$ have also been demonstrated in the serum and pleural fluid of patients with tuberculosis.[22,168]

Other granulomatous diseases associated with hypercalcemia include berylliosis,[428] histoplasmosis,[480] and coccidioidomycosis.[260] The mechanism of hypercalcemia in these conditions is not clear at present. Increased levels of plasma $1,25(OH)_2D_3$ have been found in association with hypercalcemic and/or hypercalciuric patients with leprosy and disseminated candidiasis.[207,229, 391] Granulomas induced by the use of silicone for cosmetic reasons have also been shown to be associated with hypercalcemia and elevated calcitriol.[248]

Milk alkali syndrome

Burnett and coworkers described the milk-alkali syndrome in 1948.[59] This syndrome includes hypercalcemia, metabolic alkalosis, and renal impairment. In a recent review Orwoll described the important elements for the development of the syndrome.[339] The ingestion of large quantities of Ca^{2+}, exceeding 5g/day, leads to increased intestinal absorption, which produces increased serum Ca^{2+} levels. The elevation of serum $[Ca^{2+}]$ suppresses PTH production and thereby decreases the synthesis of $1\alpha,25\text{-}(OH)_2D_3$. Under these conditions increased Ca^{2+} losses due to hypercalciuria can reverse the hypercalcemia. By the same token, ingestion of the alkali alone increases plasma HCO_3^- and expands intravascular volume. These two effects of alkali ingestion may decrease free $[Ca^{2+}]$ by increasing protein binding to Ca^{2+},[315] and by diluting serum Ca^{2+}. As a consequence, PTH secretion increases and renal bicarbonate reabsorption decreases.[197] Bicarbonaturia may then ensue, returning serum $[HCO_3^-]$ to normal. The milk-alkali syndrome develops only when both Ca^{2+} and alkali are ingested together.

Ingestion of large amounts of Ca^{2+} leads to an increase in intestinal intraluminal $[Ca^{2+}]$. This calcium ion concentration elevation enhances reabsorption through a concentration-dependent, nonsaturable, passive mechanism; serum $[Ca^{2+}]$ then rises. The ingestion of alkali, by increasing protein-bound calcium and renal reabsorption of Ca^{2+},[114,315,439] contributes to hypercalcemia. Serum PTH falls, enhancing bicarbonate reabsorption.[94] The persistently high serum $[Ca^{2+}]$ reduces filtration rate,[31] thus limiting the capacity to excrete increased loads of Ca^{2+} and alkali; the hypercalcemia can cause ECF volume contraction, which worsens alkalosis and reduces the capacity to excrete calcium. Extremely severe hypercalcemia can be seen under these circumstances.[153]

Idiopathic infantile hypercalcemia

Lightwood in 1952 described a syndrome comprising hypercalcemia and failure to thrive.[271] Between 1953 and 1955 more than 200 cases were reported in Great Britain, but only 10 cases were reported in the United States. At the time milk in Great Britain was supplemented with five to six times the amount of vitamin D used in America.[137] When the British reduced the vitamin D supplementation hypercalcemia of infancy became a rarity.[85]

Several authors have reported an association of the hypercalcemia of infancy with abnormalities of the great vessels such as supravalvular aortic stenosis and pulmonary artery stenosis.[164,397] A striking facial appearance, the "elfin facies," consisting of low-set ears, receding mandible, depressed nasal bridge, high narrow palate, and prominent upper lip, can also be part of the syndrome. Renal insufficiency can also be present, most likely secondary to hypercalcemia. This syndrome is rarely seen today.

Other causes

Recovery from acute renal failure

The recovery from acute renal failure due to rhabdomyolysis can be complicated by hypercalcemia.[447] Muscle necrosis in the presence of myoglobinuric renal failure causes severe hyperphosphatemia, which initiates Ca^{2+} deposition in soft tissue. Technetium 99m diphosphonate scanning[139,140] has shown widespread Ca^{2+} deposition which disappears upon recovery. Hypocalcemia resulting from the massive Ca^{2+} deposition stimulates PTH secretion that may lead to hyperplasia of the parathyroid glands after 7 to 10 weeks. It has been postulated that during recovery from renal failure mobilization of Ca^{2+} from soft tissues and elevated PTH levels contribute to the development of hypercalcemia. Weinstein et al. reported that blood PTH levels increased during the hypocalcemic period, while serum $25\text{-}OH\text{-}D_3$ concentration remained normal.[486] The authors proposed that the hypercalcemia results from mobilization of muscle Ca^{2+} during the recovery phase. In another report Llach and coworkers studied patients with rhabdomyolysis-induced acute renal failure. All six patients had severe hyperphosphatemia and hypocalcemia associated with low levels of $1\alpha,25\text{-}(OH)_2D_3$ during the oliguric state.[272] Hypercalcemia during early recovery was accompanied by an increase in plasma $1\alpha,25\text{-(OH)}_2D_3$ level and persistent elevation of PTH. The authors proposed the hypercalcemia resulted from increased synthesis of $1\alpha,25\text{-(OH)}_2D_3$, high PTH levels, and recovery of renal function.

Other investigators have reported that large amounts of $25\text{-OH-}D_3$ are released from damaged muscle[139,140] where vitamin D can be stored under normal conditions.[295] The most likely explanation for the hypercalcemia includes contributions of Ca^{2+} mobilization, high [PTH], and excessive vitamin D levels. Knochel has also proposed that the uremic state can interfere with the sodium-calcium exchange system and allow accumulation of Ca^{2+} in tissues.[244] With improvement of the uremic state, Ca^{2+} can be mobilized and returned to the blood, contributing to the hypercalcemia. Thus patients with extensive muscle destruction and prolonged and severe acute renal failure who in addition require frequent treatment for symptomatic hypocalcemia are at a greater risk for developing hypercalcemia during the recovery phase.

Familial hypocalciuric hypercalcemia

Foley et al. described familial hypocalciuric hypercalcemia (FHH) in 1972.[148] The etiology of this condition remains unknown. It is inherited as an autosomal dominant trait with hypercalcemia exhibiting 100 percent penetrance at all ages.[283,286,290] The principal features of this condition include hypercalcemia beginning the first decade of life,[288] low fractional urinary Ca^{2+} excretion when compared to other hypercalcemic states,[347] tendency to develop hypermagnesemia,[284] normal renal function,[288] and failure of hypercalcemia to be corrected by subtotal parathyroidectomy.[286]

It has been estimated that each year in the United States approximately 25 patients with unrecognized FHH are diagnosed as having primary hyperparathyroidism; they are therefore advised to undergo parathyroidectomy, which is unsuccessful. Pathological examination reveals mild hyperplasia;[456] hyperplasia in FHH is distinctly lower in degree compared with primary hyperparathyroidism. When serum immunoreactive PTH is measured in patients with FHH the values can be abnormally high,[98,285] although not as high as in primary hyperparathyroidism. The infusion of PTH in patients with FHH increases nephrogenous cAMP to values higher than in normal patients or subjects with primary hyperparathyroidism.[194,287] Whereas chronic hypercalcemia in primary hyperparathyroidism is commonly associated with severe impairment in urine-concentrating ability, patients with FHH and long-standing hypercalcemia do not display such an impairment.[289] Polyuria and polydipsia are likely to be central effects of the hypercalcemia, or possibly manifestations of a subtle renal defect.[288] Symptoms that are commonly found in hypercalcemic conditions, such as abdominal pain, constipation, and pruritis, are uncommon in patients with FHH.[290] Although hypercalcemia in FHH usually follows a benign course, Marx and coworkers [288,290] have found that among kindreds with FHH those with hypercalcemia had significantly more fatigue, weakness, mental problems, arthralgia, headaches, polydipsia, and polyuria than their normocalcemic kin.[288,290] This has been corroborated in a recent study of 21 families by Law and Heath.[257] It has also been pointed out that chondrocalcinosis occurs more frequently in FHH than in the normal population[290] and pancreatitis, although uncommon, may be fatal when present.[288,290]

The diagnostic signs most helpful in discriminating FHH from primary hyperparathyroidism are the hypercalcemia occurring at an early age and the low urine fractional excretion of calcium (a value below 0.01 suggests FHH is present[284,286]). It should also be pointed out that severe neonatal primary hyperparathyroidism requiring surgery has been associated with FHH.[159,291]

Addison's disease

The hypercalcemia of adrenal cortical insufficiency characteristically responds to small doses of steroids.[106,349] Several factors have been incriminated in causing hypercalcemia. Patients with adrenal insufficiency have volume contraction that is known to enhance tubular calcium reabsorption.[481] Hemoconcentration of plasma proteins also results in an increase in the relative concentration of Ca^{2+} bound to proteins; hyponatremia might also increase the affinity of Ca^{2+} for proteins.[481] The absence of the anti-vitamin D effects of glucocorticoids might also contribute to hypercalcemia. When tuberculosis causes adrenal insufficiency the infection itself may add significantly to the development of hypercalcemia (see Sarcoidosis, above).

Pheochromocytoma

Primary hyperparathyroidism and pheochromocytoma are included in the multiple endocrine adenomatosis syndrome (MEA). In addition, however, other factors may contribute to hypercalcemia in pheochromocytomas. First, catecholamines have been shown to cause PTH release in vivo and in vitro;[52,143] presumably, the effect of catecholamines is exerted through stimulation of adenylate cyclase. Second, in thyroparathyroidectomized animals, infusion of catecholamines leads to hypercalcemia.[236] Clearly, catecholamines can produce hypercalcemia by direct effects on bone resorption or enhanced release of PTH from parathyroid glands.

Another factor that can contribute to the hypercalcemia seen in pheochromocytoma is production of a PTH-like substance by the tumor.[249,427] Nevertheless, excess PTH-like or PTH-related protein secreted by the tumor cannot always explain the hypercalcemia. A patient with low PTH level and high levels of immunoreactive calcitonin (also secreted by the tumor) has been reported.[193] The mechanism by which hypercalcemia occurred in this patient must therefore have involved some of the other factors discussed above.

Acromegaly

Excess production of growth hormone (GH) is associated with increased intestinal absorption of Ca^{2+} and hypercalcemia.[416] It is therefore conceivable that excess $1\alpha,25\text{-}(OH)_2D_3$ production is involved. Eskildsen and coworkers[125] demonstrated increased plasma $1\alpha,25\text{-}(OH)_2D_3$ in acromegalic patients with high levels of GH. When the levels of GH were reduced there was a concomitant decrease in $1\alpha,25\text{-}(OH)_2D_3$ without changes in immunologic PTH (iPTH). Studies of animals have also shown that removal of the hypophysis reduces the production of $1\alpha,25\text{-}(OH)_2D_3$; replacement of GH reestablished production of the vitamin.[150,423]

The levels of $1\alpha,25\text{-}(OH)_2D_3$ are higher in young growing subjects than in older ones; they correlate best with the levels of GH[354] in these two age groups. Thus the available data suggest that GH can enhance the formation of $1\alpha,25\text{-}(OH)_2D_3$ by stimulating 1α-hydroxylation of $25\text{-}OH\text{-}D_3$; this is the expected physiological response to the increased Ca^{2+} needs during growth.

Thiazides

Thiazide diuretics can cause hypercalcemia, particularly when there is an underlying condition that may perpetuate the increase in serum $[Ca^{2+}]$. Studies in human subjects have shown that thiazide administration increases total and ionized calcium in subjects with hyperparathyroidism. In general, a transient increase of serum calcium is provoked in individuals with normal parathyroid function; no change takes place in those with hypoparathyroidism.[357] Severe hypercalcemia has been associated with the combined use of therapeutic calcium carbonate and thiazides.[182] Combined use of lithium and thiazide diuretics has also been reported to induce hypercalcemia.[162]

Thiazide-induced hypercalcemia may be mediated by several mechanisms. Volume contraction may increase renal reabsorption of calcium; associated hyperproteinemia can increase bound calcium concentration. Fluid space contraction can also lead to increased calcium binding of protein by producing metabolic alkalosis. Studies by Constanzo and Windhager[89] have shown a direct effect of thiazides on distal tubular Ca^{2+} reabsorption in the rat.

Because thiazides can produce hypercalcemia in patients with chronic renal failure who are on hemodialysis,[247] a direct effect of thiazides on bone has been suggested. However, studies in vitro have failed to show that thiazides potentiate the effects of PTH on bone.[278]

Lithium administration

Patients with manic-depressive disorders who are treated with lithium have been reported to develop hypercalcemia[162] and high circulating iPTH levels.[78] It has been suggested that lithium can increase the threshold at which serum calcium suppresses PTH secretion.[79] In addition, lithium carbonate can produce hypocalciuria, probably mediated in part by excess PTH secretion or direct enhancement of tubular calcium reabsorption,[311] although the latter seems less likely.

Blue-diaper syndrome and miscellaneous causes

Drummond and coworkers[113] described two siblings with hypercalcemia, nephrocalcinosis, and increased urinary excretion of an oxidation product of indican. A defect in the intestinal absorption of tryptophan has been recognized in this disease. Tryptophan is metabolized by intestinal bacteria, which yields indoles and indicans; increased absorption of these metabolites leads to their excretion in the urine as a blue pigment. Ingestion of a load of tryptophan is associated with increased intestinal Ca^{2+} absorption and hypercalcemia in these patients.

Hyperalimentation may cause hypercalcemia in the presence of phosphate depletion when large quantities of Ca^{2+} are administered.[167,470] The use of *tamoxifen*[262,476] in the treatment of breast cancer, and of *massive plasma infusions* in treating thrombocytopenic purpura[66] have also been associated with hypercalcemia. Patients suffering from theophylline toxicity (18 percent) have been shown to exhibit hypercalcemia.[300] Calcium levels return to normal after the drug levels decrease to therapeutic or subtherapeutic levels. Propanolol abolished the hypercalcemia induced by theophylline in normal volunteers, suggesting a beta-adrenergic regulation of the hypercalcemia.[300] Hypercalcemia without elevation of ionized calcium can be seen in *multiple myeloma*[15] when excess production of a Ca^{2+}-binding immunoglobulin[223] causes total serum calcium to increase. Because the biologically important ionized calcium fraction remains normal, this form of hypercalcemia is asymptomatic and not corrected by hydration or saline diuresis. Reduction of IgG by the chemotherapy directed at the myeloma will eventually normalize serum calcium.[304]

Patients on hemodialysis who suffer from aluminum intoxication may exhibit severe hypercalcemia despite PTH suppression. The condition worsens after removal of the parathyroid glands and thus has been called pseudohyperparathyroidism.[406a]

CONSEQUENCES OF HYPERCALCEMIA

General and central nervous system effects

The clinical manifestations of hypercalcemia are influenced by several factors. The higher the free Ca^{2+} concentration[250] the more intense the symptoms and the faster the evolution and progression of these symptoms. In addition, acute hypercalcemia is more symptomatic than chronic hypercalcemia. Another important factor is the etiology of the hypercalcemia. Malignancies can present with severe hypercalcemia (>15 mg/dl) more commonly than other conditions. Diseases in which hypercalcemia coexists with high iPTH may present symptoms that are absent in other hypercalcemic disorders.

The clinical spectrum of hypercalcemia ranges from the asymptomatic patient found to have hypercalcemia on a routine serum analysis to the patient with hypercalcemic crisis who presents in coma.

Central nervous system (CNS) changes can range from subtle alterations in personality to acute psychosis. Specific manifestations include depression, bizarre behavior, and memory impairment.[352] The mechanism for these disturbances is not clear; increased [Ca^{2+}] in cerebrospinal fluid (CSF) has been alleged to decrease the conduction of nerve terminals.[281] In a prospective study Cogan et al. found brain Ca^{2+} content significantly higher in patients with secondary hyperparathyroidism than it was in normal controls.[83] There were no changes in Mg^{2+} content in the brain tissue.[83] Thus increased cell [Ca^{2+}] in some unknown way may alter brain cell function. Acute hypercalcemia in the patient on hemodialysis can present symptoms suggestive of dialysis dementia such as dysarthria, disorientation, seizures, myoclonic jerks, confusion, and memory defects.[372] Electroencephalographic (EEG) changes can help in establishing the correct diagnosis.[83,372] The EEG and clinical changes reverse when hypercalcemia is corrected promptly.

Other neurological symptoms include muscle weakness and depressed deep tendon reflexes. The cause of these manifestations has also been shown to be related to increased intracellular [Ca^{2+}] in nerve cells[173,276] in the presence of excess PTH.

Cardiovascular and pulmonary effects

Calcium is an important regulator of the excitation-contraction coupling of the heart and of smooth muscle tension in peripheral vessels. The Ca^{2+} ion exerts a positive inotropic effect on the heart and reduces heart rate, similar to the effect of cardiac glycosides. Hypercalcemia has been shown to correlate with shortening of the Q-T interval in the electrocardiogram;[333] the administration of Ca^{2+} to patients taking digitalis must be done therefore with extreme care since it can precipitate severe arrhythmias.

Hypercalcemia can also exert important effects on the systemic vasculature. Hypertension is recognized to occur in about 30 percent of patients with hyperparathyroidism.[115,382] Hypertension may be elicited by an acute infusion of Ca^{2+}.[279] The mechanism for the increase in blood pressure may be multifactorial. Several studies have shown that serum levels of epinephrine and norepinephrine are higher in hypercalcemic subjects than in normocalcemic subjects.[279,478] High Ca^{2+} levels also enhance vascular reactivity to catecholamines[478] as well as to angiotensin II.[479] These findings have also been reported with hypercalcemia in experimental animals.[422] Another factor contributing to the hypertension of hypercalcemia is the renin-angiotensin system. Elevated plasma renin activity has been reported in patients with primary hyperparathyroidism.[479] High renin levels have also been found in conjunction with hypercalcemia induced by malignancy in experimental animals.[421] In addition, in patients with sarcoidosis a positive correlation has been reported between hypercalcemia and serum angiotensin converting enzyme activity, but a similar correlation was not found in patients with other hypercalcemic disorders.[380] It is also recognized that Ca^{2+} may have a direct effect on vascular smooth muscle by activating the actin-myosin interaction, leading to increased muscle tension. Persistent hypercalcemia may result in renal insufficiency that also contributes to hypertension.

Calcification of cardiac valves and narrowing of the coronary arteries may result from calcium deposition when hypercalcemia has become chronic.[373]

Pulmonary damage may also originate with hypercalcemia. Thick bronchial secretions and inhibition of the motion of bronchial cilia may result from a direct effect of Ca^{2+} as well as from the volume contraction that can be associated with high serum [Ca^{2+}]. Extensive pulmonary calcification has been reported in chronic hypercalcemia.[281]

Renal effects

Impairment of renal function can result from either acute or chronic hypercalcemia as a result of decreased renal blood flow and GFR.[31] Humes and coworkers have shown that Ca^{2+}, particularly in the presence of PTH, can reduce the ultrafiltration coefficient (K_f),[214] a major determinant of single nephron filtration rate, which together with afferent arteriolar vasoconstriction may explain the reduction in GFR.

Most patients with symptoms of acute hypercalcemia lose increased amounts of salt and water, which leads to volume contraction. Impairment of sodium reabsorption results from inhibition of Na^+-K^+ ATPase in the thick ascending limb and distal tubules.[122,434] Increased free water losses result from impairment of the renal concentrating capacity. Several factors contribute to this renal defect. Decreased GFR, by decreasing delivery to the distal segments, limits the concentrating capacity. Inhibition of the Na^+ pump in the medullary portion of the kidney[176] diminishes medullary solute concentration;[277] in consequence the kidney becomes unable either to concentrate or dilute the urine. In addition, redistribution of the blood flow to the medulla causes further reduction of the medullary solutes ("washout").[54] Production of PGs is enhanced by hypercalcemia, which may also contribute to the blood flow redistribution.[500] These substances may also impair the capacity to concentrate the urine by direct inhibition of the action of antidiuretic hormone (ADH) on the collecting tubules.[14,175,398] Calcium can also inhibit adenylate cyclase and directly oppose the effects of ADH on water flow.[26,105] Another effect of acute hypercalcemia that may contribute to impairment of the capacity to concentrate the urine is disruption of the assembly of tubulin into cytoplasmic microtubules.[21] Microtubules are necessary for the hydroosmotic effect of ADH both in vitro and in vivo.[105] Ca^{2+} can also interfere with the availability of energy in the form of ATP by inhibiting enzymes in the glycolytic pathway (e.g., phosphofructokinase, pyruvate kinase, and pyruvate carboxylase);[105,123] epithelial cell metabolism is thus limited.

Hypercalcemia in the presence of low iPTH and volume contraction is associated with increased bicarbonate reabsorption. It has been shown that in parathyroidectomized animals high serum [Ca^{2+}] leads to enhanced bicarbonate reabsorption[94,313] as a result of increased hydrogen ion secretion.[340] Inhibition of sodium reabsorption by hypercalcemia, and the subsequent volume reduction, engenders enhanced potassium excretion. Metabolic alkalosis is augmented by the increase in potassium excretion. It should be pointed out that either metabolic acidosis or normal acid-base balance could be present instead of alkalosis. This is a consequence of the direct inhibition of proximal tubule HCO_3^- reabsorption by PTH[197,231] and the increased loss of bicarbonate in the urine. Hypercalcemia may also inhibit ammonia formation[196] and contribute to the development of metabolic acidosis.[475]

Other effects of acute hypercalcemia include hypermagnesuria and attendant hypomagnesemia. These effects result from inhibition of Mg^{2+} reabsorption in the proximal tubule[263] and in the thick ascending limb.[363] Hypophosphatemia can also be found in primary hyperparathyroidism; it results from decreased phosphate reabsorption and hyperphosphaturia.

Hypercalcemia leads to hypercalciuria by increasing the filtered load of Ca^{2+}. Nephrolithiasis as a result of the hypercalciuria is more common in chronic than in acute hypercalcemia.[82,342]

Other manifestations of chronic hypercalcemia include chronic interstitial nephritis[282] and nephrocalcinosis.[318] Both acute and chronic hypercalcemia produce structural changes in the kidney.[200] Focal degenerative and necrotic lesions of the tubular epithelium in the thick ascending limb, distal convoluted tubules, and collecting duct[163] have been described in acute hypercalcemia patients. In chronic hypercalcemia, Ca^{2+} deposition occurs in the interstitium. This leads to a mononuclear interstitial inflammation, scarring, and nephrocalcinosis involving predominantly the medulla and the corticomedullary region. Occasionally the outer cortex may be involved.[393] Calcium deposition in the renal parenchyma results in abnormalities of renal function such as nephrogenic diabetes insipidus, salt-losing nephritis, and distal renal tubular acidosis (RTA).[141] Obstructive nephropathy as a result of nephrolithiasis may also aggravate the functional defects and predispose to bacterial infections and pyelonephritis.[177] Vascular and glomerular calcifications[92] contribute to the renal insufficiency usually seen with chronic interstitial nephritis and nephrocalcinosis. As already mentioned, hypertension may be caused by hypercalcemia, which in turn can produce nephrosclerosis and contribute to renal insufficiency. Nephrocalcinosis in the presence of high PTH can also result in a Fanconi-like syndrome with glucosuria, phosphaturia, and aminoaciduria. Bicarbonaturia may be partly blunted under these circumstances by high serum calcium concentration.

Gastrointestinal, hematological, and musculoskeletal effects

Constipation, nausea, and vomiting are classic symptoms of hypercalcemic states.[127] Constipation results from diminished gastrointestinal motility caused by the action of calcium on smooth muscle and on nerve conduction, as well as from dehydration. Altered gastrointestinal motility and constipation contribute to delayed gastric emptying, anorexia, nausea, and vomiting. Esophageal motility can also be influenced by high Ca^{2+} levels and contribute to the symptoms seen in hypercalcemic states.[95]

Duodenal ulcer disease occurs in 10 to 20 percent of hypercalcemic patients.[198] Increased gastric acid secretion, promoted by a direct effect of Ca^{2+} on parietal cells,[103] and increased gastrin secretion,[24] contribute to the development of duodenal ulcers. Pancreatitis can occur in as much as 35 percent of patients in acute hypercalcemic crisis.[235,259] The mechanism of development of pancreatitis involves intraductal deposition of Ca^{2+} with obstruction of the pancreatic ducts.[89] Moreover, Ca^{2+} activates proteolytic enzymes that digest the pancreatic parenchyma.[171,192]

Hypercalcemia per se is usually not associated with hematological manifestations. Nevertheless, in primary hyperparathyroidism, anemia may result from myelofibrosis produced by the high PTH levels.[43] In a recent in vitro study by Meytes and coworkers[308] it was shown that intact PTH inhibited erythropoiesis. This may explain in part the anemia associated with high-[PTH] states.

The musculoskeletal system can also be involved in producing hypercalcemia, particularly in patients who also have hyperparathyroidism. Proximal muscle weakness,[276] arthritis, and arthralgias[62] are commonly associated with primary hyperparathyroidism. Radiological evidence of chondrocalcinosis in hypercalcemic patients with high PTH is not rare, but the condition usually remains asymptomatic.[359] Almost all patients with hyperparathyroidism have evidence of bone disease when examined with sensitive methods such as photon absorptiometry.[341] Bone pain in hypercalcemic patients may result from osteitis fibrosa cystica in hyperparathyroidism or from metastatic disease in malignancy. Gout and hyperuricemia have also been associated with hyperparathyroidism.[396]

Metabolic effects of hypercalcemia

Glucose-stimulated insulin release takes place when cytosolic Ca^{2+} increases.[410] A study by Kim et al. demonstrated that insulin levels, as well as the response to stimulation of insulin release, are augmented in hyperparathyroidism.[238] Nevertheless, patients with parathyroid disorders usually respond normally in glucose tolerance tests.[494] High insulin levels with normal glucose tolerance occur with peripheral insulin resistance. In hyperparathyroidism, hypophosphatemia can account for peripheral resistance to insulin, because glucose phosphorylation is a necessary step for glucose utilization. A PTH-induced increase in gluconeogenesis and glycogenolysis[212,317] may also contribute to increased serum glucose and high insulin levels.

TREATMENT OF HYPERCALCEMIA

Hypercalcemia can result in significant morbidity and high mortality if adequate treatment is not established promptly. Treatment is aimed at reducing serum $[Ca^{2+}]$ by increasing urinary Ca^{2+} excretion, inhibiting bone resorption, blocking intestinal Ca^{2+} absorption, or enhancing formation of calcium complexes (Table 32-2). Management should be directed at the recognition and treatment of the underlying cause of hypercalcemia.

TABLE 32-2 • Modes of treatment for hypercalcemia

Forced diuresis with furosemide
Mithramycin
Calcitonin
Steroids
Phosophate salts
Bisphosphonates
Dialysis
Inhibitors of prostaglandin synthesis

Forced diuresis with furosemide

Adequate hydration and volume reexpansion should make up the first step in managing hypercalcemia.[211] One or two liters of 0.9 percent (normal) saline must be given hourly. With volume expansion urinary Ca^{2+} excretion increases due to inhibition of proximal reabsorption; distal tubules, however, are not affected. The use of a loop diuretic further augments Ca^{2+} excretion by inhibiting distal Ca^{2+} reabsorption.[116,117,435] An intravenous (IV) dose of 80 to 100 mg furosemide should be given every 1 to 2 h until serum $[Ca^{2+}]$ drops sufficiently. Careful evaluation of fluid balance is essential to sustain the salutary effects of volume expansion. Replacement of sodium, potassium, and magnesium is necessary to avoid volume depletion, hypernatremia, and inadequate circulating levels of each of the ions.[498] If serum calcium is below 15 mg/dl, smaller doses of furosemide (20 to 80 mg IV) can be given every 2 to 4 h, together with isotonic saline to which the appropriate electrolytes have been added.

It should be noted that in an experimental model of Bence-Jones proteinuria with cast nephropathy, furosemide actually accelerates cast formation, presumably by increasing distal tubule luminal NaCl concentration.[39] The presence of cast-forming Bence-Jones proteins could conceivably be a contraindication for furosemide-saline therapy in a hypercalcemic patient with multiple myeloma.

Mithramycin

The antineoplastic antibiotic mithramycin inhibits DNA-dependent RNA synthesis.[224] It lowers serum $[Ca^{2+}]$ by inhibiting osteoclastic bone resorption and by decreasing bone turnover. A mithramycin dose of 25 μg per kilogram of body weight is infused in a 5 percent dextrose solution over a period of 4 to 8 h. A response is usually seen within 24 to 48 h of the infusion. If serum $[Ca^{2+}]$ does not drop, the same dose is repeated for 2 to 4 days. Once a response is obtained the effects may last from 3 to 7 days or even longer in some patients.[281,326]

Side effects associated with mithramycin therapy include anorexia, nausea, vomiting, bone marrow suppression, and a bleeding phenomenon attributable to either thrombocytopenia or thromboasthenia. Special attention is required in patients with renal impairment since mithramycin is largely excreted through the kidneys; toxicity is more likely to occur in patients with renal insufficiency.[244a] Hepatoxicity and nephrotoxicity[390] can also occur; thus evaluation of liver enzymes and renal function is also necessary during therapy with mithramycin. Toxic epidermal necrolysis has also been reported, but only at the high doses used for the treatment of cancer.[362]

Salmon calcitonin

Calcitonin decreases serum Ca^{2+} concentration by inhibiting osteoclast bone resorption.[157] Calcitonin can also increase the urinary excretion of phosphorus and Ca^{2+};[16] however, the phosphaturia and calciuria probably contribute little to the hypocalcemic action of the hormone. Salmon calcitonin is given at a dose of 4 MRC units per kilogram of body weight intravenously, followed by an additional 4 MRC units per kilogram subcutaneously after 12 to 14 h. Rapid loss of the effect of calcitonin can occur after 24 to 72 h of treatment. This abolition of hypocalcemic action has been referred to as the "escape" phenomenon; it can be partly explained by down-regulation of hormone receptors[446] as well as by uncoupling of receptors from adenylate cyclase.[297] The combined use of salmon calcitonin and glucocorticoids has been shown to be effective in preventing the escape from calcitonin in vivo.[36] Occasionally, oral phosphate administration restores responsiveness to calcitonin.[281]

Side effects of calcitonin use include nausea, vomiting diarrhea, and facial flushing. Soreness and inflammation at the site of the injection can also occur. Hypersensitivity reactions have been described, albeit rarely, following the use of calcitonin.[281,326] Development of antibodies to the salmon hormone can be induced after several weeks and may contribute to loss of calcitonin effectiveness.[281,326]

Recent studies have demonstrated that combinations of calcitonin and biphosphonate are quite effective in controlling the hypercalcemia of malignancy.[366] Furthermore, salmon calcitonin administered as suppositories led to fast if short-lived reductions in serum calcium in patients with malignant hypercalcemia.[450,451] Moreover, the combination of a single dose of 3-amino-1-hydroxypropylidene-1-biphosphonate (also known as ADP, AHPrBP, palmidronate disodium) and salmon calcitonin given as suppositories for 3 days corrected hypercalcemia in 17 patients. By contrast, in patients matched for their initial level of hypercalcemia, type of tumor, urinary hydroxyproline levels, and the dose of ADP, only 14 of the 17 patients normalized their serum calcium by day 9. A major effect of calcitonin was to induce hypercalciuria and, as a consequence, plasma calcium levels in the experimental group were lower than in the controls from days 2 to 4. Neither treatment resulted in side effects, and specifically neither flushing nor nausea was observed.[452]

Steroids

Glucocorticoids reduce serum Ca^{2+} in hypercalcemic conditions by inhibiting the vitamin D_3-mediated calcium absorption in the intestine;[152,239] glucocorticoids also inhibit osteoclastic bone resorption.[323,431] They are most efficient in vitamin D intoxication[429] and sarcoidosis but can also be effective in malignancies. The effect of glucocorticoids in the hypercalcemia of malignancy may be mediated through inhibition of OAF, and of osteoclastic bone resorption, and through cytolysis of tumor cells and inhibition of PG synthesis.

Steroid therapy may begin with hydrocortisone 5 mg per kilogram of body weight per day for 2 to 3 days; thereafter dosage is reduced to a maintenance level. Prednisone may be given at a dosage of 40 to 80 mg/day until serum $[Ca^{2+}]$ is controlled.

Complications arising from the use of steroids include infections, peptic ulcer disease, glucose intolerance, hypokalemia, and a cushingoid appearance.

Phosphate salts

Several mechanisms have been suggested to explain why phosphate salts reduce ECF calcium concentration. Phosphate inhibition of bone resorption has been demonstrated both in vivo and in vitro.[364,365] Oral phosphate therapy can inhibit intestinal Ca^{2+} absorption by forming poorly soluble Ca^{2+} salts in the intestinal lumen or by reducing the conversion of 25-OH-D_3 to 1α,25-$(OH)_2D_3$ through inhibition of 1α- hydroxylase.[190] Phosphate can lower serum $[Ca^{2+}]$ by inducing soft tissue calcification; this effect is one of the major drawbacks to the use of phosphate for the treatment of hypercalcemia.

An oral dose of 2 to 4 g of phosphate salts per day, in divided doses, is the therapy usually recommended for hypercalcemia. Intravenous administration is effective[65] but dangerous particularly when serum $[Ca^{2+}]$ is very high, since extensive calcification can occur. Side effects after ingestion of phosphate salts include nausea, vomiting, and diarrhea. Oral phosphate should not be given to a patient with impaired renal function since severe hyperphosphatemia and further impairment in renal function can be provoked.

Bisphosphonates

The Bisphosphonates are a new group of compounds that are synthetic analogues of pyrophosphate and form stable bonds resistant to enzymatic hydrolysis. They inhibit osteoclastic bone resorption and retard the deposition of hydroxyapatite in bone collagen, increase unmineralized osteoid, and inhibit formation of calcium phosphate crystals.[154] The one most recently made available, dichloromethylenebisphosphonate (Cl_2MDP), inhibits bone resorption at doses that do not affect mineralization of osteoid. Recent reports have shown that oral and intravenous Cl_2MDP is effective in the treatment of hypercalcemia in primary hyperparathyroidism,[375,403,404] malignancies,[71,222,228] and Paget's disease.[104] Other bisphosphonates such as ethane-1-hydroxy-1,1-bisphosphonate (EHDP) have been used in the hypercalcemia of malignancy and primary hyperparathyroidism; however, its use is limited by the increase in unmineralized osteoid tissue which may lead to rickets or osteomalacia. Another bisphosphonate with less effect on bone mineralization is 3-amino-1-hydroxypropane-1,1-bisphosphonate (APD). In a clinical study, patients with Paget's disease showed marked improvement when treated with APD, without the amount of unmineralized osteoid changing.[158]

Bisphosphonates are administered by oral or intravenous routes. EHDP is used in a dose of 5 to 10 mg per kilogram of body weight daily. APD can be given in a dose of 500 to 1000 mg/day orally, and intravenously in doses of 45 to 60 mg/24 h. Cl_2MDP can be given orally in a 1600-mg daily dose for as long as 12 weeks; or it can be administered IV over 2 h: 2.5 mg per kilogram is infused on the first day and 5 mg per kilogram for 2 to 7 days thereafter.[403,404] These drugs are felt to be the treatment of choice for tumor-induced hypercalcemia because of their efficacy and good patient tolerance.[452,453] Their onset of action is slow (24 to 48 h) after the initiation of a slow intravenous infusion. Combinations of bisphosphonates (APD specifically) with salmon calcitonin may speed the time and effectiveness of the response.[451]

A series of reports by Warrell et al. have indicated that gallium nitrate may be useful in the treatment of both cancer-related hypercalcemia and parathyroid carcinoma. Intravenous administration of gallium nitrate in daily doses of 200 mg/m^2 reverse refractory hypercalcemia in patients with high PTH levels (10 to 30 times normal) lowered serum calcium, hydroxyproline excretion, and serum PTH in patients with refractory hypercalcemia and parathyroid carcinoma.[482] In a randomized double-blind study, patients with cancer-related hypercalcemia responded better (69 percent) than those receiving calcitonin (19 percent) by achieving normocalcemia.[483] The mechanism of the effect of gallium nitrate appears to involve inhibition of bone resorption.[484]

In a randomized double-blind study, a greater percentage of patients with cancer-related hypercalcemia achieved normocalcemia when treated with gallium nitrate than when calcitonin was administered (69 vs. 19 percent).[483]

Dialysis

Patients with hypercalcemia and renal failure may require dialysis for initial treatment of their hypercalcemia.[201] Normocalcemia attained through peritoneal dialysis is only temporary; additional therapy is required for prolonged control of serum [Ca^{2+}]. Hemodialysis has also been used in the treatment of hypercalcemia in patients with acute renal failure, but its effects are transient unless additional modes of therapy directed at the primary origin of hypercalcemia are also used.[498]

Inhibitors of prostaglandin synthesis

Nonsteroidal anti-inflammatory agents such as indomethacin have been reported to correct hypercalcemia associated with renal cell carcinoma.[47,218,375] Nevertheless, a recent clinical study demonstrated that indomethacin was ineffective in the majority of patients with malignancy-associated hypercalcemia.[327] These findings most likely reflect the fact that PGs are the primary mediators of hypercalcemia only for a select (and small) group of neoplasms.

HYPOCALCEMIA

The hormonal system that controls serum [Ca^{2+}] is made up of PTH, vitamin D_3, and the target organs for these hormones, that is, bone, kidney, and intestine. Despite the close association between PTH and vitamin D_3, hypocalcemic disorders can be classified into a primary deficiency of PTH or a deficiency of vitamin D_3. An algorithm for the diagnostic evaluation of hypocalcemia is shown in Fig. 32-4. The action of PTH depends on vitamin D_3. Thus, hypocalcemia occurs in the absence of vitamin D_3 even when the plasma concentrations of PTH are normal or high.[189] Since the production of biologically active metabolites of vitamin D_3 by the kidney depends on PTH, reduced synthesis of $1\alpha,25\text{-}(OH)_2D_3$ accompanies hypoparathyroidism and thereby worsens the associated hypocalcemia.

CAUSES AND MECHANISMS

Decreased activity of PTH

Hypoparathyroidism

Hypoparathyroidism may be either idiopathic or acquired.[57] Idiopathic hypoparathyroidism is relatively rare. It may be familial or sporadic. The familial form may be subdivided into early and late onset hypoparathyroidism. The distinction is based on whether the disorder starts before or after one year of age. The sporadic form may also present early, associated with congenital absence of the thymus and the parathyroid glands. This disorder is related to cellular immune deficiency and is known as *DiGeorge's syndrome*.[101] Patients with this disorder have normal circulating antibodies yet they usually die, from persistent infection and severe hypocalcemia, during the first two years after birth.

The late forms of both *familial* and *sporadic idiopathic* hypoparathyroidism have been associated with adrenal insufficiency, pernicious anemia, hypothyroidism, and candidiasis. Ovarian failure, vitiligo, cirrhosis, steatorrhea, and myasthenia gravis may also be present. An autoimmune mechanism has been suspected in view of the presence of parathyroid, adrenal, gastric, ovarian, and thyroid antibodies in the plasma of subjects with the disease.[38a]

Hypoparathyroidism may also arise as a consequence of thyroid *surgery*. Characteristically postsurgical hypo-

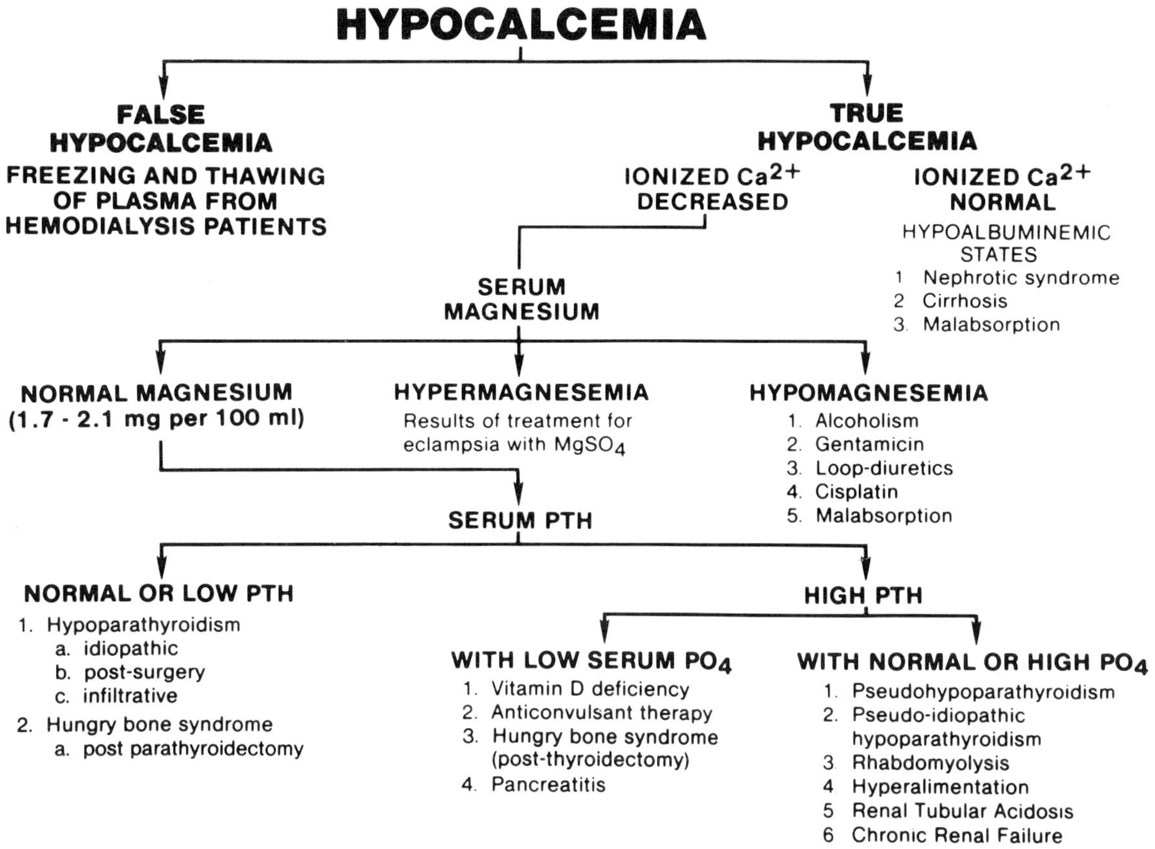

FIGURE 32-4 • Diagnostic steps in the evaluation of hypocalcemia.

calcemia is transient; it has occurred in approximately 17 percent of patients in one series who underwent thyroid surgery.[309] It has been proposed that the hypocalcemia may result when Ca^{2+} is deposited in bone to compensate for preexisting thyrotoxic osteopenia. Intraoperative release of calcitonin has been proposed as another possible mechanism for hypocalcemia that complicates thyroid surgery.[491] In a recent report Watson et al. found a close correlation between the decrements in serum [Ca^{2+}] and the increase in plasma calcitonin;[485] no significant changes in the levels of PTH were observed, suggesting that calcitonin released during surgery accounts for the initial fall in serum [Ca^{2+}]. In addition, it was suggested that interference with normal parathyroid function as a result of trauma to the glands does not allow PTH to increase and that this also contributes to low serum [Ca^{2+}].[485] Once calcitonin levels fall serum [Ca^{2+}] values return to normal.[485] Permanent postsurgical hypoparathyroidism occurs in only a small percentage of cases: the incidence in recent series approximated 3 percent.[179,188] The frequency of this complication depends on variables such as the experience and technical prowess of the surgeon. Extensive neck surgery is also likely to be associated with a high incidence of permanent hypoparathyroidism.[329]

A less frequent cause of hypoparathyroidism is *metastasis* to the parathyroids. While the incidence of parathyroid involvement in widespread metastatic disease can be as high as 5 to 12 percent, hypocalcemia is uncommon.[210] Iron deposition in the parathyroid glands due to *hemochromatosis* can also lead to hypoparathyroidism. It has been speculated that *Wilson's disease* may be associated with hypoparathyroidism in a similar way, by leading to deposition of copper in the parathyroid glands.[69]

Hypomagnesemia

Magnesium depletion and hypomagnesemia (<1 mg/dl) may produce hypocalcemia by several mechanisms. In normal subjects, an acute change in serum magnesium concentration will alter PTH secretion: hypomagnesemia stimulates while hypermagnesemia inhibits secretion of the hormone. During chronic and severe magnesium deficiency, however, PTH secretion is imparied.[11,12,126] In a study by Rude et al., patients with hypomagnesemia and hypocalcemia were found to have low, normal, or even high serum PTH levels.[387] Nevertheless, magnesium replacement provoked increases in serum PTH regardless of the baseline values of the hormone. In hypomagnesemic patients with chronic renal disease, and high PTH, magnesium administration has also been shown to stimulate PTH secretion.[302] These findings indicate that normal or even high PTH values may be inadequate to maintain a normal serum Ca^{2+} in magnesium-depleted subjects.

Skeletal resistance to PTH can also contribute to the development of hypocalcemia in hypomagnesemic states. In a study by Frietag and coworkers using isolated bone perfusion, the uptake of PTH and the formation of cAMP were found to be significantly diminished in perfused bones from hypomagnesemic animals.[155] Correction of hypocalcemia without affecting serum PTH has been described in some patients with renal failure, hypocalcemia, hypomagnesemia, and high PTH who were given magnesium.[264] In some patients with renal insufficiency, therefore, resistance to PTH action may be the result of hypomagnesemia.

Impaired release of PTH and skeletal resistance to the hormone can be assumed to contribute to hypocalcemia in hypomagnesemic conditions. Since Mg^{2+} is an important cofactor for the activation of adenylate cyclase it is possible that severe deficiency may lead to impaired function of the adenylate cyclase-related receptor[219] and account, in part, for the observed derangement in PTH release and for the skeletal resistance during hypomagnesemia. Bellorín-Font and coworkers have provided support for this inference: substitution of Mg^{2+} by Mn^{2+} leads to a progressive decline in the ability of PTH to stimulate adenylate cyclase activity in isolated kidney cortical membranes.[30]

Another mechanism proposed to explain the hypocalcemia of magnesium depletion is that skeletal exchange of Ca^{2+} and Mg^{2+} is reduced, thereby leading to decreased Ca^{2+} resorption from bone. This hypothesis is based on the finding that induction of hypomagnesemia in parathyroidectomized animals leads to a further decrease in serum Ca^{2+}.[180] Direct experimental evidence for this mechanism is not available.

Patients with hypocalcemia due to magnesium deficiency are resistant not only to PTH but also to parenteral calcium and vitamin D therapy. The resistance to vitamin D is probably the result of impaired metabolism since plasma levels of $1,25(OH)_2D_3$ are low.[388]

Excess plasma magnesium may also influence parathyroid function. Experimental[293] and clinical[119] evidence suggests that hypermagnesemia can decrease PTH release and cause hypocalcemia.

Gentamicin

Hypocalcemia produced by gentamicin results from the hypermagnesuria which leads to hypomagnesemia and subsequently to hypocalcemia.[19] Replacement of serum magnesium corrects the hypocalcemia.

Pancreatitis

Hypocalcemia is a common complication of acute pancreatitis; it occurs in 40 to 75 percent of patients with acute pancreatitis.[86,183] Several factors have been identified that can contribute to the decrease in serum $[Ca^{2+}]$ levels. The findings of Ca^{2+} deposition in areas of fat necrosis in the pancreas initially led to the proposal that the formation of calcium soaps was the main cause of the hypocalcemia in pancreatitis.[343,374] It is now clear that diminished secretion of PTH also contributes to the hypocalcemia. Studies of patients with hypocalcemia and pancreatitis have reported inappropriately low levels of PTH[63,216,294,299,374] for the degree of hypocalcemia. Moreover, hypocalcemia can be corrected by the administration of exogenous PTH. Others have reported undetectable plasma PTH levels due to either parathyroid gland exhaustion or destruction of PTH by proteolytic enzymes.[86] Results of some studies suggest that increased glucagon secretion[343] and hypercalcitoninemia[63] may be contributors to the development of hypocalcemia in some patients with pancreatitis. However, elevated levels of these hormones have not consistently been found.[487] Other factors that have been proposed to contribute to the hypocalcemia in pancreatitis include hypomagnesemia,[183] hypoalbuminemia,[216] acute renal failure,[183,294,418] and an as yet unidentified defect of bone metabolism.[487]

Neonatal hypocalcemia

Neonatal hypocalcemia occurs during the first 72 h of life. It is most commonly seen in premature newborns, those born to insulin-dependent diabetic mothers, and infants with asphyxia at birth.[462,464-466] Functional immaturity of the parathyroid glands has often been considered among the pathogenetic mechanisms for the hypocalcemia.[425,462,463] Occasionally, hypercalcemia (from any cause) during pregnancy can suppress fetal parathyroid gland secretion and produce transient hypocalcemia in the newborn.[99]

Hypocalcemia occurring later than the first three days of life can be caused by feeding milk containing a low calcium:phosphorus ratio. A low GFR per body surface area in the newborn combined with high tubular phosphate reabsorption causes hyperphosphatemia; that in turn leads to hypocalcemia. Low serum calcium level can persist until the parathyroid glands function well enough to respond.

Other factors that have been identified as contributing to the hypocalcemia of the newborn are hypomagnesemia,[97,467,469] high calcitonin level,[64] and vitamin D deficiency.[202]

Decreased vitamin D activity

Pseudohypoparathyroidism

Albright et al. reported in 1942 the first three cases of pseudohypoparathyroidism (PHP).[7] Many of the patients with the syndrome exhibited characteristic features including round face, short stature, and obesity. Bone abnormalities are common; they include exostosis and shortening of the metacarpals, metatarsals, and phalanges, particularly of the fourth digit. These somatic features, sometimes called Albright's hereditary osteodystrophy (AHO), are present in most patients with PHP but are not essential to its diagnosis.[48] Hypocalcemia, hyperphosphatemia, and high circulating levels of PTH are present in patients with PHP. Administration of exogenous PTH does not correct the calcium and phosphate abnormalities; the disorder has been postulated to result from resistance to the actions of PTH.[7]

Since Albright's original description, it has become clear that there are several varieties of PHP.[109] Patients with PHP type I have markedly blunted nephrogenous cAMP responses to exogenous PTH, suggesting that the plasma-bound adenyl cyclase complex of renal tubule cells is abnormal. The defect, however, does not seem to be specific for PTH. Some patients with PHP type I display resistance to multiple hormones that activate adenyl cyclase, and express other abnormalities such as hypothyroidism, hypogonadism, mental retardation, impaired olfaction,[131,270] and Albright's hereditary osteodystrophy (see above).

Studies by different investigators have given support to this hypothesis.[130] Drezner and Burch[112] demonstrated that plasma membranes obtained from cells from the renal cortex of a patient with PHP had an abnormal guanine-nucleotide-binding regulatory protein (G protein) in the adenylate cyclase receptor that rendered the receptor refractory to hormone stimulation. These findings have been corroborated by other investigators[42,107,129,269] using different sources of adenylate cyclase. This disorder is now known as PHP type 1a. Patients in this group demonstrate an approximately 50 percent reduction in $G_s\alpha$ activity in plasma membranes from multiple cell types, whereas their membrane levels of $G_i\alpha$ are normal.[108] Recent studies have suggested that in some patients a mutation in the gene encoding the stimulatory G protein of adenyl cyclase is responsible for AHO.[348]

Some patients, however, have been found to have normal $G_s\alpha$ protein activity (PHP type 1b). The cause for the metabolic resistance to the effects of PTH in this group has not been defined. Only a few patients with PHP type 1b manifest the bone abnormalities that are common with PHP type 1a.

A third group of PHP patients has been reported. These individuals respond to exogenous PTH with an increase in urinary cAMP but without phosphaturia.[109] In this group with PHP type 2, a defect distal to the site of formation of cAMP has been postulated. The adenylate cyclase receptor has the normal capability to increase urinary cAMP. Thus, the nature of this defect is unknown.

The information on PHP that has accrued so far is consistent with a disorder of heterogenous pathogenesis and clinical manifestations that exhibits hypocalcemia and hyperphosphatemia with high circulating PTH levels.

Serum 25-OH-D_3 has been found to be normal in patients with PHP. Nevertheless, the combined effects of resistance to PTH and hyperphosphatemia in PHP can lead to suppression of 1α-hydroxylase activity producing 1α,25-$(OH)_2D_3$ deficiency and hypocalcemia.[110,246,252,305]

A rare disorder that resembles PHP has been described in several patients.[335] Subjects affected with this condition have normal to high levels of immunoreactive PTH but respond to exogenous PTH by increasing urinary phosphate and cAMP excretion. The condition is known as pseudo-idiopathic hypoparathyroidism. It is believed to represent formation of defective PTH molecules by the parathyroid glands.

Hyperphosphatemia

Exogenous administration of phosphate can cause hyperphosphatemia and hypocalcemia. This situation commonly develops during hyperalimentation or the treatment of hypercalcemia with oral or IV phosphate. Hyperphosphatemia can also occur as a result of diminished phosphate excretion (e.g., in acute renal failure from rhabdomyolysis and chronic renal failure) or increased endogenous release (e.g., during treatment of certain lymphomas and leukemias of lymphocytic cells).[468] Hyperphosphatemia can cause hypocalcemia by inhibiting 1,α-hydroxylase, which results in diminished 1α,25-$(OH)_2D_3$ formation.[190] Inhibition of bone resorption[364,365] and precipitation of calcium phosphate complexes in soft tissues[65] also occurs.

In patients with or without hyperphosphatemia who are on hemodialysis, refrigeration or freezing of plasma, and refrigeration but not freezing of serums cause a fall in calcium concentration; the calcium loss is abolished if the samples are diluted with a lanthanum solution prior to storage. The mechanism underlying this *false hypocalcemia* is not known. It does not occur in uremic patients who are not on dialysis.[81]

Vitamin D_3 deficiency states

The principal sources of cholecalciferol (vitamin D_3) are the conversion in the skin of 7-hydroxycholesterol to cholecalciferol and from exogenous nutrients. Nutritional deficiency of vitamin D has been largely eliminated by supplementation of dairy products with vitamin D; nevertheless, it can occur in breast-fed infants or in malnourished elderly patients. The minimum daily requirements for vitamin D_3 for children and adults is 2.5 μg (100 IU). The recommended daily dietary allowance is 10 μg (400 IU).

Factors predisposing to nutritional vitamin D_3 deficiency include rapid growth, premature birth, inadequate light exposure, malabsorption, intestinal surgery, and hepatobiliary disease.

Hypocalcemia can also occur in hereditary deficiency of 1α-hydroxylase (vitamin D-dependent rickets). This disease is a rare autosomal recessive disorder[368] in which levels of 1α,25-$(OH)_2D_3$ are very low or undetectable. In contrast to vitamin D-resistant rickets, patients do respond to exogenous vitamin D_3. Brooks and coworkers have described a single patient with vitamin D-dependent rickets and increased serum $1\alpha,25\text{-(OH)}_2D_3$.[51] The patient responded to exogenous vitamin D_3. The authors have suggested therefore that diminished target cell responsiveness to endogenous vitamin D_3 metabolites may have caused the hypocalcemia.[51]

A disorder resembling vitamin D-dependent rickets but in which circulating levels of $1\alpha,25\text{-(OH)}_2D_3$ are normal represents resistance to the actions of the vitamin D_3 metabolite. This is vitamin D-resistant rickets;[368] it is an inherited X-linked condition. Treatment of this condition requires combined use of phosphate and calcitriol.[169,368]

Malabsorption syndromes

Most vitamin D is absorbed in the proximal small intestine. Bile salts play an important role in the absorption of fat-soluble vitamins such as vitamin D. Thus, intestinal absorptive disorders are likely to produce hypocalcemia by decreasing the absorption of vitamin D, bile salts, and calcium. Other factors that can contribute to hypocalcemia in malabsorption syndromes include hypoproteinemia, hypomagnesemia, and the use of drugs that can interfere with Ca^{2+} metabolism (e.g., corticosteroids, cimetidine).

Partial gastrectomy with gastrojejunostomy is among the common causes of vitamin D deficiency in gastrointestinal disease.[415] Hypocalcemia has been found in approximately 7 percent of such patients.[303] Malabsorption of vitamin D can occur as a result of rapid gastric emptying because of duodenal bypass, bacterial overgrowth, or avoidance of fatty foods.[303]

Malabsorption of vitamin D with hypocalcemia can also occur in Crohn's disease, treatment of obesity with jejunoileal bypass, nontropical sprue, pancreatic insufficiency, and hepatobiliary disease.[303]

When chronic diarrhea and hyperchloremic metabolic acidosis accompany the hypocalcemia of a malabsorptive state, rapid correction of the acidosis may precipitate tetany; alkalinization increases binding of protein to Ca^{2+}. Hypomagnesemia, which is prominent in malabsorption, causes resistance of serum calcium level to augmentation by PTH. Hypomagnesemia should thus be corrected prior to or concurrently with correction of acidosis.

Renal tubular acidosis

Classical distal tubular acidosis can cause hypocalcemia, hypophosphatemia, and metabolic bone disease (see Chap. 27). Proximal renal tubular acidosis (RTA) can result in bone disease if the renal wastage of phosphate is severe enough to lead to hypophosphatemia. In distal RTA resulting hydrogen ion retention, hypobicarbonatemia, and acidemia increase bone resorption. As a consequence, serum $[Ca^{2+}]$ increases and PTH level decreases, leading to hypercalciuria.[266] The hypercalciuria is a consequence, in addition to increased Ca^{2+} mobilization from bone,[265] of increased filtered load and decreased renal tubular reabsorption.[441] Metabolic acidosis also decreases the activity of 1α-hydoxylase in the kidney and decreases the production of $1\alpha,25\text{-(OH)}_2D_3$.[493] The combined effects of decreased intestinal Ca^{2+} absorption due to low $1\alpha,25,\text{-(OH)}_2D_3$ and increased urinary Ca^{2+} excretion eventually lead to hypocalcemia. Replacement of $1\alpha,25\text{-(OH)}_2D_3$ and correction of the metabolic acidosis can correct the Ca^{2+} disorder.

Acute and chronic alcoholism

Alcohol abuse can cause hypocalcemia by several mechanisms. Peng et al. demonstrated that the oral administration of alcohol to dogs and rats is followed within minutes by hypocalcemia.[351] The hypocalcemia occurred even after removal of the thyroid and parathyroid glands, suggesting that Ca^{2+} is incorporated into bone or soft tissue; the calcium uptake is independent of changes in PTH or calcitonin.

The acute effects of alcohol on calcium and parathyroid hormone were recently studied in normal men and women.[251a] Ingestion of 1.2 to 1.5 g of alcohol per kilogram of body weight over a 3-h period (doses sufficient to cause acute alcohol intoxication) led to transient hypoparathyroidism as indicated by a reduction in circulating parathyroid hormone concentration of 58 percent at the end of the 3 h. Eight hours after alcohol exposure, serum ionized calcium had fallen to its nadir and urinary calcium excretion increased. In addition, serum magnesium levels rose and hypermagnesiuria supervened. Of interest was the development of rebound hyperparathyroidism during the last 6 h of the study period. These results suggest that significant hypoparathyroidism and hyperparathyroidism may be responsible for some of the long-term effects of alcohol on bone and mineral metabolism.

The hypocalcemia of chronic alcoholism is multifactorial. Chronic alcoholics exhibit low levels of 25-OH-D_3

TABLE 32-3 • Causes of hypocalcemia in alcoholism

Direct effect of ethanol
Low levels of 25-(OH)-D_3
Hypomagnesemia
Hypoalbuminemia
Pancreatitis
Intestinal malabsorption
Alkalosis
Liver cirrhosis

even when the liver is not cirrhotic.[472] Hypomagnesemia appears to occur concomitantly with hypocalcemia. Parenteral administration of vitamin D to alcoholic patients with hypocalcemia and hypomagnesemia does not correct the Ca^{2+} disorder.[126] Responsiveness to PTH and correction of the hypocalcemia are, however, attained with magnesium replacement; magnesium deficiency thus appears to play a central role in this disturbance. Hypocalcemia may also result from hypoalbuminemia, pancreatitis, respiratory or metabolic alkalosis, or intestinal malabsorption (Table 32-3).

Nephrotic syndrome

A decrease in serum albumin concentration is always accompanied by a decrease in total serum calcium. Free $[Ca^{2+}]$ usually does not change, but it may be low in patients with nephrotic syndrome. The low calcium level may not result from hypoalbuminemia itself. Haddad et al. found low levels of vitamin D binding protein in nephrotic patients.[178] Goldstein and coworkers studied 26 patients with nephrotic syndrome who were found to have low levels of 25-OH-D_3.[172] These investigators found an inverse correlation between the levels of 25-OH-D_3 and the degree of proteinuria. They proposed that the low levels of vitamin D in nephrotic patients were due to its excretion in urine; this, in turn, was responsible for the hypocalcemia. Long-term replacement of vitamin D in nephrotic syndrome has been shown to correct the low levels of 25-OH-D_3 as well as those of 1α,25-$(OH)_2D_3$; the effect of this therapy on Ca^{2+} metabolism remains to be completely evaluated.[184]

"Hungry bone" syndrome

Deposition of Ca^{2+} in bone during the healing of osteodystrophies can lead to hypocalcemia. When bone formation exceeds bone resorption, Ca^{2+} deposition may surpass intake and make it difficult to maintain normocalcemia. The hypocalcemia that ensues may be severe enough to impair cell function.[128,477] This syndrome has been observed after *parathyroidectomy* in primary hyperparathyroidism[361] or after *thyroidectomy* for hyperthyroidism.[309] Compared with patients with uncomplicated metabolic responses to parathyroid surgery, patients with hungry bone syndrome are usually older by a mean of 10 years. In addition, they have higher preoperative serum levels of calcium, alkaline phosphatase, N-terminal parathyroid hormone, and blood urea nitrogen. The resected parathyroid adenomata in these individuals are larger.[46]

Increased bone formation and hypocalcemia may also occur during *osteoblastic metastasis* from prostate,[419] breast,[185] and lung[318] malignancies. In rare instances, symptomatic hypocalcemia may occur in calcitonin-producing tumors.[275,301]

Drugs and miscellaneous causes

The *anticonvulsants* phenobarbital and diphenylhydantoin are recognized causes of hypocalcemia. These drugs have been shown to induce hepatic microsomal P450 oxidase activity, which accelerates the rate of metabolism of vitamin D_3 and 25-OH-D_3 into polar, hydroxylated, and biologically inactive products of cholecalciferol.[87,181] Anticonvulsant drugs may also cause hypocalcemia by inhibition of intestinal Ca^{2+} absorption and by reduction of PTH-induced bone resorption.[181]

Cisplatin can also cause hypocalcemia.[274] Renal tubular damage caused by cisplatin can lead to renal magnesium wasting and magnesium depletion.[394] Hypocalcemia may be a consequence of the hypomagnesemia and its correction can be attained by magnesium replacement.[274]

Estrogen therapy is another cause of drug-induced hypocalcemia.[53] Riggs et al. demonstrated that estrogens inhibited bone resorption without changing bone formation in patients with osteoporosis.[371] These effects of estrogen on bone metabolism were associated with a significant fall in serum $[Ca^{2+}]$. Hypocalciuria has been shown to occur in women after menopause;[497] these women tend also to be hypercalcemic relative to premenopausal women. Inhibition of bone resorption may directly cause hypocalcemia during therapy with mithramycin and calcitonin. Excess endogenous production of calcitonin may be a mediating factor, as it is in the hypocalcemia seen in the toxic shock syndrome.[74]

Up to 40 percent of critically ill patients, including those with sepsis and shock, exhibit hypocalcemia.[4] Incidence of hypocalcemia is similar whether the patient has gram-positive or gram-negative infections. In a study of 80 patients the nadir of serum calcium concentration was achieved on days 6 to 8, and was significantly lower in males than in females.[4] Serum calcium concentration did not correlate with serum levels of albumin, transaminase, or creatinine but had an inverse relationship to the degree of fever. The mechanism for the hypocalcemia or bacteremia is not clear, but reduced vitamin D production, increased resistance to PTH, or altered PTH secretion could, individually or in any combination, be responsible.

Hypocalcemia may also arise following the use of *citrate-buffered blood*,[203,338] presumably due to binding of free Ca^{2+} with citrate. This has also been observed during plasmapheresis and exchange transfusions utilizing citrated blood.[460] Treating hypercalcemia by *infusing phosphate* salts or sodium *EDTA* to chelate calcium can also lead to hypocalcemia.

Enhanced Ca^{2+} excretion induced by *loop diuretics* may precipitate hypocalcemia, particularly in patients with hypoparathyroidism. Volume reduction and alkalosis resulting from the use of these diuretics increases concentrations of serum proteins and protein-bound calcium and decreases free $[Ca^{2+}]$.[161]

TABLE 32-4 • Drugs associated with hypocalcemia

Gentamicin	Propylthiouracil
Cimetidine	Glutethimide
Estrogens	Furosemide
Heparin	Cisplatin
Mithramycin	Dilantin
Phosphate salts	Phenobarbital

Other drugs presumed to cause hypocalcemia include propylthiouracil,[402] glutethimide (with chronic abuse),[336] and cimetidine[118] (Table 32-4). Spurious hypocalcemia due to in vitro formation of calcium soaps in blood samples has been reported in hemodialysis patients after heparinization.[170]

CONSEQUENCES OF HYPOCALCEMIA

General, neurological, and neuromuscular effects

The most important clinical manifestations of hypocalcemia are those related to the neuromuscular and central nervous systems. Tetany, the classic manifestation of neuromuscular irritability in hypocalcemia, can be elicited by tapping the facial nerve and producing a contraction of the facial muscles (Chvostek's sign) or by inflation of a blood pressure cuff above systolic pressure for 3 min to observe if carpopedal spasm develops (Trousseau's sign). Chvostek's sign is present in 25 percent of normal adults;[206] it is not, therefore, specific for hypocalcemia. Trousseau's sign is equally nonspecific; neither is it sensitive, occurring in 4 percent of the normal population, and may be negative in 30 percent of subjects with latent tetany.[281]

Seizures are another important neurological manifestation of hypocalcemia. The precise mechanism involved is not known, but high [Ca^{2+}] in the CSF has been shown to have an anticonvulsive action.[503] Thus, it is intuitively reasonable to expect that low CSF calcium concentration may predispose to seizures in hypocalcemic disorders.

Hypocalcemia may also lead to extrapyramidal manifestations. These include parkinsonian tremors, dystonia, ataxia, hemiballismus, and choreoathetosis.[420] There are calcifications of the basal ganglia in long-standing hypocalcemic disorders. These, however, are believed not to cause the extrapyramidal symptoms, since treatment of the hypocalcemia corrects the symptoms without changing the basal ganglia calcifications.

Hypocalcemia may also impair higher cerebral functions. In adults depression, emotional instability, confusion, anxiety, or even frank psychosis may be the primary manifestation of hypocalcemia.[124,418]

Proximal muscle weakness is another important and potentially disabling manifestation of hypocalcemia, particularly in vitamin D_3 deficiency states. Absence of vitamin D_3 has been shown to have important effects on skeletal muscle calcium metabolism. Pleasure and coworkers[355] have shown that mitochondria isolated from skeletal muscle of vitamin D_3-deficient chicks with muscle weakness contain significantly less calcium than normal mitochondria. Correction of serum calcium in these animals by oral calcium administration does not reestablish the normal mitochondrial calcium level and does not improve the muscle weakness. However, treatment with vitamin D_3 increases mitochondrial calcium content and the muscle weakness improves. These findings suggest that vitamin D_3 deficiency alone, rather than the hypocalcemia, accounts for the muscle weakness.

Cardiovascular, ectodermal, and gastrointestinal effects

Calcium ions play an important role in the contraction of cardiac muscle. Clinical and experimental studies have shown that hypocalcemia induced by transfusions of citrated blood results in cardiac index, stroke volume, and left ventricular stroke work values that are significantly lower than during normocalcemia.[338,432] Congestive heart failure that is refractory to treatment with digitalis can occasionally result from hypocalcemia.[75,88]

Electrocardiographic manifestations of hypocalcemia include prolongation of the Q-T interval and nonspecific T wave changes that revert to normal upon correction of the hypocalcemia.

Long-standing hypocalcemia is known to cause ectodermal defects. Children with hypoparathyroidism may exhibit failure of teething, dental hypoplasia, or carious teeth.[156] Coarse, dry, and scaly skin has also been described in hypocalcemic patients. Their nails are brittle with transverse grooves; thin brittle, sparse hair, and, frequently, scanty eyelashes and eyebrows, and absence of axillary or pubic hair are also observed after prolonged hypocalcemia.

Psoriasis and eczema can be exacerbated by hypocalcemia. Bilateral cataracts may also occur; their progression can be avoided by normalizing serum calcium concentration. The gastrointestinal manifestations of hypocalcemia include severe diarrhea with or without steatorrhea,[80] gastric achlorhydria,[103] and malabsorption of vitamin B_{12}.[186]

TREATMENT OF HYPOCALCEMIA

Acute

Acute symptomatic hypocalcemia requires immediate correction to avert serious complications. Adults requiring emergency treatment can be given 10 to 20 ml of 10 percent calcium gluconate (one 10-ml ampule contains 90 mg of elemental calcium) intravenously. The infusion rate should not exceed 2 ml/min. Patients receiving digitalis should be monitored by ECG during the infusion since administration of calcium may produce fatal arrhythmias if the infusion is given rapidly. In severe hypocalcemia a continuous intravenous infusion of calcium gluconate may be necessary. Between 15 and 20 mg of elemental Ca^{2+} per kilogram of body weight can be given in 4 to 8 h as needed. Other available calcium salt preparations are shown in Table 32-5.

TABLE 32-5 • **Calcium preparations for clinical use**

Compound	Dosage	Content	Indications	Mechanisms	Complications
Calcium carbonate*	1–2 g three times daily	260 mg elemental calcium per 650-mg tablet	Mild hypocalcemia Osteomalacia Osteporosis Renal osteodystrophy	Converted in stomach to soluble calcium salt by HCl; ineffective in patients with achlorhydria	Hypercalcemia after long-term therapy, particularly if vitamin D given concurrently
Calcium chloride	5–10 ml of 10% solution given slowly IV (rarely given orally because of irritation of GI tract)	360 mg per 10-ml ampule	Severe hypocalcemia	Rapidly increases Ca^{2+}	Irritant to veins and subcutaneous tissue if extravasated Hypercalcemia during long-term therapy, particularly if given with vitamin D
Calcium gluceptate (glucoheptate)	5–10 ml solution, IV. In newborn infants, 0.5 ml after every 100 ml in exchange transfusion; 2 to 5 mg IM in gluteal region	220 mg/ml or 80 mg/ml of calcium per 5-ml container	Severe hypocalcemia Exchange transfusion	Increases Ca^{2+}	Transient tingling and metallic taste after IV infusion Enhanced digitalis effect in the heart, precipitating arrhythmia
Calcium gluconate	20 ml of 10% solution injected slowly, followed by slow infusion of 30–40 ml of 10% solution in 500 ml or 1 liter of 5% glucose or 0.9% NaCl over a 4-h period Children should receive 500 mg/kg body weight daily in divided doses Adults, 15g daily in divided doses	90 mg elemental calcium per 10-ml ampule 90 mg elemental calcium per 1-g tablets	Severe hypocalcemia, IV Mild hypocalcemia, oral	As above	As above
Calcium lactate	Adults, 1.5–3.0 g 3x daily with meals Children should receive 500 mg/kg body weight orally in divided doses	60 mg elemental calcium per 300-mg tablet	Mild hypocalcemia and maintenance therapy	As above	As above

* Calcium should not be mixed with any solution containing bicarbonate because of the possibility of precipitation.

TABLE 32-6 • Dose requirements of vitamin D and metabolites

	Daily dose for hypoparathyroidsim, μg	Time to achieve normocalcemia, weeks	Maximal effect, weeks*	Duration of effect after cessation, weeks
Vitamin D_2 (ergocalciferol)	750–3000	4–8	4–10	6–18
DHT	250–1000	1–2	2–4	0.5–1
25-OH-D_3	50–200	2–4	4–20	0.5–1
1α,25-$(OH)_2D_3$	0.5–2.0	0.5–1	4–12	0.5–1

* Earliest times for maximal effect uncertain.

SOURCE: Adapted from Martinez-Maldonado M, Garcia A, chap 3: Hypo- and hypercalcemia, in Martinez-Maldonado M (ed), *Handbook of Renal Therapeutics*. New York, Plenum, 1983.

Chronic

Long-term treatment of hypocalcemia is required most commonly in hypoparathyroidism or in chronic vitamin D deficiency states. The initial treatment includes oral administration of 2 to 4 g of elemental calcium per day. The addition of a vitamin D preparation is necessary in most cases, particularly when serum calcium has been less than 7.5 mg/dl before treatment is initiated. The optimal dose of vitamin D varies according to the preparation used (Table 32-6) and the condition requiring treatment.[189,337]

In hypoparathyroidism 25-OH-D_3 can maintain serum calcium within a narrower range than vitamin D_3 or dihydrotachysterol (DHT).[345] Exogenous 25-OH-D_3 can also be advantageous in conditions associated with external losses of 25-OH-D_3 such as hepatobiliary disease, intestinal bypass surgery,[415] or nephrotic syndrome. Neonatal hypocalcemia has also been shown to respond to 25-OH-D_3.[64,147] 1α,25-dihydroxycholecalciferol can be useful when 1α hydroxylase activity is low or absent such as in renal disease, vitamin D-dependent rickets, or pseudohypoparathyroidism.

Ergocalciferol (vitamin D_2) and DHT have also been used in the treatment of chronic hypocalcemia. The doses of vitamin D_2 or DHT required are generally higher than with the vitamin D_3 derivatives, but treatment with D_2 is less expensive than with the calciferol derivatives.

When hypomagnesemia is the cause, magnesium can be replaced by the administration of $MgSO_4 \cdot 7H_2O$ either intramuscularly or intravenously. Because of the painful effects of intramuscular medication, a continuous intravenous infusion of 48 meq/24 h may be preferable (see Chap. 34 for further details of treatment of hypomagnesemia).

Hypercalciuria usually ensues when serum calcium returns to normal. This increases the risk of nephrolithiasis and nephrocalcinosis. Treatment with a low-salt diet and thiazide diuretics may help to diminish hypercalciuria and avoid its consequences.

REFERENCES

1. Abbasi AA et al: Hypercalcemia in active pulmonary tuberculosis. *Ann Intern Med* 90:324, 1979.
2. Adams JS et al: Metabolism of 25-hydroxyvitamin D_3 by alveolar macrophages in sarcoidosis. *Clin Res* 31:499A, 1983.
2a. Adams JS et al: Isolation and structural identification of 1,25-dihydroxyvitamin D_3 produced by cultured alveolar macrophages in sarcoidosis. *J Clin Endocrinol Metab* 60:72, 1985.
3. Adams JS et al: Characterization of 1α-hydroxylation of vit D_3 sterols by cultured alveolar macrophages from patients with sarcoidosis. *J Exp Med* 161:755, 1985.
4. Aderka D et al: Bacteremic hypocalcemia: A comparison between the calcium levels of bacteremic and nonbacteremic patients with infection. *Arch Intern Med* 147:232, 1987.
5. Agus ZS et al: Regulation of urinary calcium excretion in the rat. *Am J Physiol* 232:F545, 1977.
6. Agus ZS et al: Disorders of calcium and phosphate balance. Chapter 19 in Brenner BM, Rector FC Jr (eds): *The Kidney*, 2d ed. Philadelphia, Saunders, 1981, p 940.
7. Albright F et al: Pseudohypoparathyroidism—An example of "Seabright-Bantam Syndrome." *Endocrinology* 30:922, 1942.
8. Albright F, Reifenstein EC, Jr.: *The Parathyroids and Metabolic Bone Disease*, 1st ed. Baltimore, Williams and Wilkins Co, 1948, p 46.
9. Albright F: Case records of the Massachusetts General Hospital. *N Engl J Med* 225:789, 1941.
10. Alfrey AC et al: Resolution of hyperparathyroidism, renal osteodystrophy and metastatic calcification, after renal homotransplantation. *N Engl J Med* 279:1349, 1968.
11. Anast CS et al: Evidence for parathyroid failure in magnesium deficiency. *Science* 177:606, 1972.
12. Anast CS et al: Impaired release of parathyroid hormone in magnesium deficiency. *J Clin Endocrinol Metab* 42:707, 1976.
13. Anderson J et al: Effect of cortisone on calcium metabolism in sarcoidosis and hypercalcemia, possible antag-

onistic action of cortisone and vitamin D. *Lancet* 2:720, 1954.
14. Anderson RJ et al: Evidence for an in vivo antagonism between vasopressin and prostaglandin in the mammalian kidney. *J Clin Invest* 56:420, 1975.
15. Annesley TM et al: Artifactual hypercalcemia in multiple myeloma. *Mayo Clin Proc* 57:572, 1982.
16. Ardaillou R et al: Renal excretion of phosphate, calcium and sodium during and after a prolonged thyrocalcitonin infusion in man. *Proc Soc Exp Biol Med* 131:56, 1969.
17. Arnaud CD, Stewler GJ: Primary hyperparathyroidism. *Semin Nephrol* 1:376, 1981.
17a. Arnold A et al: Monoclonality and abnormal parathyroid hormone genes in parathyroid adenomas. *N Engl J Med* 318:658, 1988.
18. Arnold A et al: Molecular cloning and chromosomal mapping of DNA rearranged with the parathyroid hormone gene in a parathyroid adenoma. *J Clin Invest* 83:2034, 1989.
19. Bar RS et al: Hypomagnesemic hypocalcemia secondary to renal magnesium wasting. A possible consequence of high dose gentamycin therapy. *Ann Intern Med* 82:646, 1975.
20. Barbour GL et al: Hypercalcemia in an anephric patient with sarcoidosis: Evidence for extrarenal generation of 1,25-dihydroxyvitamin D. *N Engl J Med* 305:440, 1981.
21. Barnes LD et al: Studies on in vitro polymerization of tubulin from renal medullary extracts. *Biochim Biophys Acta* 405:422, 1975.
22. Barnes LD et al: Transpleural gradient of 1,25-dihydroxyvitamin D in tuberculous pleuritis. *J Clin Invest* 83:1527, 1989.
23. Barnicot NA, Datta SP: Vitamin A and bone, in *The Biochemistry and Physiology of Bone. Physiology and Pathology*, vol 2, 1st ed. Bourne GH (ed). New York, Academic Press, 1972, p 197.
24. Barreras RF, Donaldson RM Jr: Role of calcium in gastric hypersecretion, parathyroid adenoma and peptic ulcer. *N Engl J Med* 276:1122, 1967.
25. Baxter JD, Bondy PK: Hypercalcemia of thyrotoxicosis. *Ann Intern Med* 65:429, 1966.
26. Beck N et al: Pathogenic role of cyclic AMP in the impairment of urinary concentrating ability in acute hypercalcemia. *J Clin Invest* 54:1049, 1974.
27. Bell NH et al: Hypercalcemia during long-term treatment with 1,25-dihydroxyvitamin D_3 in hypoparathyroidism. *N Engl J Med* 301:1183, 1979.
28. Bell NH et al: Evidence that increased circulating 1,25-dihydroxyvitamin D is the probable cause for abnormal calcium metabolism in sarcoidosis. *J Clin Invest* 64:218, 1979.
29. Bellorín-Font E et al: Altered adenylate cyclase kinetics in hyperfunctioning human parathyroid glands. *J Clin Endocrinol Metab* 52:499, 1981.
30. Bellorín-Font E et al: Regulation of PTH receptor-adenylate cyclase system of canine kidney: Influence of Mn^{2+} on effects of Ca^{2+}, PTH and GTP. *Am J Physiol* 242:F457, 1982.
31. Benabe JE, Martínez-Maldonado M: Hypercalcemic nephropathy. *Arch Intern Med* 138:777, 1978.
32. Benabe JE, Martínez-Maldonado M: Disorders of calcium metabolism, Maxwell MH et al (eds): *Clinical Disorders of Fluid and Electrolyte Metabolism*, 4th ed. New York, McGraw-Hill, 1987, p 759.
33. Besarab A et al: Suppression of secondary hyperparathyroidism by propranolol in renal failure patients. *Nephron* 27:127, 1981.
34. Bilezikian JP: The medical management of primary hyperparathyroidism. *Ann Intern Med* 96:198, 1982.
35. Bilezikian JP: Parathyroid hormone-related peptide in sickness and in health. *N Engl J Med* 322:1151, 1990.
36. Binstock ML, Mundy GR: Effect of calcitonin and glucocorticoids in combination on the hypercalcemia of malignancy. *Ann Intern Med* 93:269, 1980.
37. Birge S et al: Malignant hypercalcemia: Clinicopathological conference. *Am J Med* 67:486, 1979.
38. Blair AJ et al: Ectopic hyperparathyroidism in a patient with metastatic hypernephroma. *Metabolism* 22:147, 1973.
38a. Blizzard RM et al: The incidence of parathyroid and other antibodies in the sera of patients with idiopathic hypoparathyroidism. *Clin Exp Immunol* 1:119, 1966.
39. Booker BB, Sanders PW: Furosemide aggravates intranephronal obstruction from human Bence-Jones proteins (BJP). *Clin Res* 38:985A, 1990.
40. Boonstra CE, Jackson CE: Serum calcium survey for hyperparathyroidism: Results in 50,000 clinic patients. *Am J Clin Pathol* 55:523, 1971.
41. Bourdeau JE, Burg MB: Voltage dependence of calcium transport in the thick ascending limb of Henle's loop. *Am J Physiol* 236:F357, 1979.
42. Bourne HR et al: Fibroblast defect in pseudohypoparathyroidism, type I: Reduced activity of receptor-cyclase coupling protein. *J Clin Endocrinol Metab* 53:636, 1981.
43. Boxer M et al: Anemia in primary hyperparathyroidism. *Arch Intern Med* 137:588, 1977.
44. Bradley GW, Sterline GM: Hypercalcemia and hypokalemia in tuberculosis. *Thorax* 33:464, 1978.
45. Braman SS et al: Steroid responsive hypercalcemia in disseminated bone tuberculosis. *Arch Intern Med* 132:269, 1973.
46. Brasier AR, Nussbaum SR: Hungry bone syndrome: Clinical and biochemical predictors of its occurrence after parathyroid surgery. *Am J Med* 84:654, 1988.
47. Brereton HD et al: Indomethacin-responsive hypercalcemia in a patient with renal cell adenocarcinoma. *N Engl J Med* 291:83, 1974.
48. Breslau NA, Pak CYC: Hypoparathyroidism. *Metabolism* 28:1261, 1979.
49. Breslau NA et al: Hypercalcemia associated with increased calcitrol levels in three patients with lymphoma. *Ann Intern Med* 100:1, 1984.
50. Broadus AE et al: Humoral hypercalcemia of cancer: Identification of a novel parathyroid hormone-like peptide. *N Engl J Med* 319:556, 1988.
51. Brooks MH et al: Vitamin D-dependent rickets type II: Resistance of target organs to 1,25-dihydroxyvitamin D. *N Engl J. Med* 298:996, 1978.
52. Brown EM et al: Beta-adrenergic stimulation of cyclic AMP content and parathyroid hormone release from

isolated bovine parathyroid cells. *Endocrinology* 100:1696, 1977.

53. Burckhardt P et al: Estrogen-induced tetany in idiopathic hypoparathyroidism. *Horm Res* 6:321, 1975.
54. Brunette MG et al: Hyposthenuria in hypercalcemia: A possible role of intrarenal blood flow redistribution. *Pflugers Arch* 350:9, 1974.
55. Budayr AA et al: Increased serum levels of a parathyroid-hormone-like protein in malignancy-associated hypercalcemia. *Ann Intern Med* 111:807, 1989.
56. Burg MB: Thick ascending limb of Henle's loop. *Kidney Int* 22:454, 1982.
57. Burckhardt P: Idiopathic hypoparathyroidism and autoimmunity. *Horm Res* 16:304, 1982.
58. Burman KD et al: Ionized and total serum calcium and parathyroid hormone in hyperthyroidism. *Ann Intern Med* 84:668, 1976.
59. Burnett CH et al: Hypercalcemia without hypercalciuria or hypophosphatemia, calcinosis and renal insufficiency: A syndrome following prolonged intake of milk and alkali. *N Engl J Med* 240:787, 1949.
60. Burt ME, Brennan MF: Incidence of hypercalcemia and malignant neoplasm. *Arch Surg* 115:704, 1980.

60a. Burtis WJ et al: Humoral hypercalcemia of malignancy. *Ann Intern Med* 1008:454, 1988.

61. Burtis WJ et al: Immunochemical characterization of circulating parathyroid hormone-related protein in patients with humoral hypercalcemia of cancer. *N Engl J Med* 322:1106, 1990.
62. Bywaters EGL et al: Joint lesions of hyperparathyroidism. *Ann Rheum Dis* 22:171, 1963.
63. Canale DD et al: Hypercalcitoninemia in acute pancreatitis. *J Clin Endocrinol Metab* 40:738, 1975.
64. Cannanozzi DB et al: Hypercalcitonemia in infancy. *Clin Chim Acta* 66:387A, 1976.
65. Carey RW et al: Massive extraskeletal calcification during phosphate treatment of hypercalcemia. *Arch Intern Med* 122:150, 1968.
66. Carmosino LS, Feffer SE: Hypercalcemia associated with plasma therapy for thrombotic thrombocytopenic purpura. *N Engl J Med* 307:1454, 1982.
67. Caro JF, Besarab A: propanolol therapy for hyperparathyroidism? *Lancet* 1:827, 1978.
68. Caro JF et al: Prostaglandin E and hypercalcemia in breast carcinoma: Only a tumor marker? *Am J Med* 66:337, 1979.
69. Carpenter TO et al: Hypoparathyroidism in Wilson's disease. *N Engl J Med* 309:873, 1983.
70. Carroll RNP et al: The effect of renal transplantation on renal osteodystrophy. *Proc Eur Dial Transplant Assoc* 10:446, 1973.
71. Chapuy MC et al: Effects of disodium dichloromethylene diphosphonate on hypercalcemia produced by bone metastases. *J Clin Invest* 65:1243, 1980.
72. Chertow BS et al: The interactions between vitamin A, vinblastin, and cytochalasin B in parathyroid hormone secretion. *Proc Soc Exp Biol Med* 147:16, 1974.
73. Chertow BS et al: Vitamin A stimulation of parathyroid hormone: Interactions with calcium, hydrocortisone and vitamin E in bovine parathyroid tissues and effects of vitamin A in man. *Eur J Clin Invest* 7:307, 1977.
74. Chesney RW et al: Pathogenic mechnaisms of the hypocalcemia of the staphylococcal toxic-shock syndrome. *J Lab Clin Med* 101:576, 1983.
75. Chopra D et al: Insensitivity to digoxin associated with hypocalcemia. *N Engl J Med* 296:917, 1977.
76. Christensen MS et al: Hypercalcemia and parathyroid function after renal transplantation. *Acta Med Scand* 201:35, 1977.
77. Christensoon T: Hyperparathyroidism and radiation therapy. *Ann Intern Med* 89:216, 1978.
78. Christansen C et al: Lithium, hypercalcemia and hyperparathyroidism. *Lancet* 2:144, 1976.
79. Christansen C et al: Lithium, hypercalcemia, hypermagnesemia and hyperparathyroidism. *Lancet* 2:969, 1976.
80. Clarkson B et al: Clinical and metabolic study of a patient with malabsorption and hypoparathyroidism. *Metabolism* 9:1093, 1960.
81. Coburn JW et al: The physiochemical state and renal handling of divalentions in chronic renal failure. *Arch Intern Med* 124:302, 1969.
82. Coe FL: Idiopathic hypercalciuria. Chapter 4 in Coe FL (ed): *Nephrolithiasis: Pathogenesis and Treatment.* Chicago, Year Book Medical Publishers, Inc, 1978.

82a. Coe FL, Parks JH: Familial (idiopathic) hypercalciuria, in Coe FL, Parks JH (eds): *Nephrolithiasis: Pathogenesis and Treatment*, 2d ed. Chicago, Year Book Medical Publishers, Inc, 1988, p 168.

83. Cogan MG et al: Central nervous system manifestations of hyperparathyroidism. *Am J Med* 65:963, 1978.
84. Cohn SH et al: Alterations in elemental body composition in thyroid disorders. *J Clin Endocrinol Metab* 36:742, 1973.
85. Committee Report: Hypercalcemia in infants and vitamin D. *Br Med J* 1:149, 1956.
86. Condon JR et al: The etiology of hypocalcemia in acute pancreatitis. *Br J Surg* 62:115, 1975.
87. Conney AH: Pharmacologic implications of microsomal enzyme induction. *Pharmacol Rev* 19:317, 1967.
88. Connor TB et al: Hypocalcemia precipitating congestive heart failure. *N Engl J Med* 307:869, 1982.
89. Cope O et al: Pancreatitis, a diagnostic clue to hyperparathyroidism. *Ann Surg* 145:857, 1957.
90. Costanzo LS, Windhager EE: Calcium and sodium transport by the distal convoluted tubule of the rat. *Am J Physiol* 235:F492, 1978.
91. Costanzo LS, Windhager EE: Effects of PTH, ADH, and cyclic AMP on distal tubular Ca and Na reabsorption. *Am J Physiol* 239:F478, 1980.
92. Cotran RS: Tubulointerstitial diseases. Chapter 29 in Brenner BM, Rector FC (eds): *The Kidney*, 2d ed. Philadelphia, Saunders, 1981, p 1633.
93. Counts SJ et al: Vitamin D intoxication in an anephric child. *Ann Intern Med* 82:196, 1975.
94. Crumb CK et al: Effects of volume expansion, purified parathyroid extract and calcium on renal bicarbonate absorption in the dog. *J Clin Invest* 54:1287, 1974.
95. Danielides IC, Mellow MH: Effect of acute hypercalcemia on human esophageal motility. *Gastroenterology* 75:1115, 1978.
96. David DS et al: Hypercalcemia after renal transplantation. *N Engl J Med* 289:398, 1973.

97. David L, Anast CS: Calcium metabolism in newborn infants. The interrelationship of parathyroid function and calcium, magnesium and phosphorus metabolism in normal "sick" and hypocalcemic newborns. *J Clin Invest* 54:287, 1974.
98. Davies M et al: Familial hypocalciuric hypercalcemia and acute pancreatitis. *Br Med J* 282:1029, 1981.
99. Delmonico FL et al: Hyperparathyroidism during pregnancy. *Am J Surg* 131:328, 1976.
100. Demers LM et al: Plasma prostaglandins in hypercalcemic patients with neoplastic disease. *Cancer* 39:1559, 1977.
101. Di George AM: Congenital absence of thymus and its immunologic consequences: Concurrence with congenital hypoparathyroidism. *Birth Defects* 4:116, 1968.
102. Dingle JH: Action of vitamin A on the stability of lysosomes, in *Ciba Symposium on Lysosomes*. Boston, Little, Brown, 1963, p 384.
103. Donegan WL, Spiro HM: Parathyroids and gastric secretion. *Gastroenterology* 38:750, 1960.
104. Douglas DL et al: Effect of dichloromethylene disphosphonate in Paget's disease of bone and in hypercalcemia due to primary hyperparathyroidism or malignant disease. *Lancet* 1:1043, 1980.
105. Dousa TP, Valtin H: Cellular actions of vasopressin in the mammalian kidney. *Kidney Int* 10:46, 1976.
106. Downie WW et al: Hypercalcemic crisis as presentation of Addison's disease. *Br Med J* 1:145, 1977.
107. Downs RW Jr et al: Deficient adenylate cyclase regulatory protein in renal membranes from a patient with pseudohypoparathyroidism. *J Clin Invest* 71:231, 1983.
108. Downs RW Jr et al: The inhibitory adenyl cyclase coupling protein in pseudohypoparathyroidism. *J Clin Endocrinol Metab* 61:351, 1985.
109. Drezner MK et al: Pseudohypoparathyroidism type II: A possible defect in the reception of the cyclic-AMP signal. *N Engl J Med* 289:1056, 1973.
110. Drezner MK et al: 1,25-dihydroxycholecalciferol deficiency: The probable cause of hypocalcemia and metabolic bone disease in pseudohypoparathyroidism. *J Clin Endocrinol Metab* 42:621, 1976.
111. Drezner MK, Lebovitz HE: Primary hyperparathyroidism in paraneoplastic hypercalcemia. *Lancet* 1:1004, 1978.
112. Drezner MK, Burch WM: Altered activity of the nucleotide regulatory site in the parathyroid hormone sensitive adenylate cyclase from the renal cortex of a patient with pseudohypoparathyroidism. *J Clin Invest* 62:1222, 1978.
113. Drummond KP et al: The blue-diaper syndrome—familial hypercalcemia with nephrocalcinosis and indicanuria: A new familial disease with definition of the metabolic abnormality. *Am J Med* 37:928, 1964.
114. Dubb J et al: Tubular effects of acute metabolic acidosis in the rat. *J Lab Clin Med* 90:318, 1977.
115. Earll JM et al: Hypercalcemia and hypertension. *Ann Intern Med* 64:378, 1966.
116. Editorial: Management of hypercalcemic crisis. *Lancet* 2:617, 1978.
117. Editorial: Management of severe hypercalcemia. *Br Med J* 280:204, 1980.
118. Edwards H et al: Effect of cimetidine on serum calcium levels in an elderly patient. *Arch Surg* 116:1088, 1981.
119. Eisenbud E, LoBue CC: Hypocalcemia after therapeutic use of magnesium sulfate. *Arch Intern Med* 136:688, 1976.
120. Eismen JA et al: Normal and malignant breast tissue is a target organ for 1,25-$(OH)_2$ vitamin D_3. *Clin Endocrinol* 13:267, 1980.
121. Eisman JA et al: Frequency of 1,25-dihydroxyvitamin D_3 in human breast cancer. *Cancer Res* 41:5121, 1981.
122. Epstein FH, Whittam R: The mode of inhibition by calcium of cell-membrane adenosine-triphosphatase activity. *Biochem J* 99:232, 1966.
123. Epstein FH: Calcium and the kidney. *Am J Med* 45:700, 1968.
124. Eraut D: Idiopathic hypoparathyroidism presenting as dementia. *Br Med J* 1:429, 1974.
125. Eskildsen PC et al: Acromegaly and vitamin D metabolism. *J Clin Endocrinol Metab* 49:484, 1979.
126. Estep H et al: Hypocalcemia due to hypomagnesemia and reversible parathyroid hormone unresponsiveness. *J Clin Endocrinol Metab* 29:842, 1969.
127. Eversmann JJ et al: Gastrointestinal manifestations of hyperparathyroidism. *Arch Intern Med* 119:605, 1967.
128. Falko JM et al: Case report. Congestive heart failure complicating the hungry-bone syndrome. *Am J Med Sci* 271:85, 1976.
129. Farfel Z et al: Defect of receptorcyclase coupling protein in pseudohypoparathyroidism. *N Engl J Med* 303:237, 1980.
130. Farfel Z, Bourne HR: Pseudohypoparathyroidism: Mutation affecting adenylate cyclase. *Miner Electrolyte Metab* 8:227, 1982.
131. Farfel Z, Friedman E: Mental deficiency in pseudohypoparathyroidism type 1 is associated with Ns-protein deficiency. *Ann Intern Med* 105:197, 1986.
132. Farnsworth AW, Dobyns BM: Hypercalcemia and thyrotoxicosis. *Med J Aust* 2:782, 1974.
133. Farr HW et al: Primary hyperparathyroidism and cancer. *Am J Surg* 126:539, 1973.
134. Favus MJ: Transport of calcium by intestinal mucosa. *Semin Nephrol* 1:306, 1981.
135. Favus MJ et al: Kinetic characteristics of calcium absorption and secretion by rat colon. *Am J Physiol* 240:G350, 1981.
136. Favus MJ et al: The effects of somatostatin on intestinal calcium transport in the rat. *Am J Physiol* 241:G215, 1981.
137. Fellers FX, Schwarts R: Etiology of the severe form of idiopathic hypercalcemia of infancy. *N Engl J Med* 258:1050, 1958.
138. Feinblatt JD et al: Secretion of a bone resorbing factor by chick thyroid glands in organ culture. *Endocrinology* 99:1363, 1976.
139. Feinstien EI et al: Hypercalcemia and acute widespread calcifications during the oliguric phase of acute renal failure due to rhabdomyolysis. *Miner Electrolyte Metab* 2:193, 1979.
140. Feinstein EI et al: Delayed hypercalcemia with acute renal failure associated with non-traumatic rhabdomyolysis. *Arch Intern Med* 141:753, 1981.

141. Ferris T et al: Renal tubular acidosis and renal potassium wasting acquired as a result of hypercalcemic nephropathy. *N Engl J Med* 265:924, 1961.
142. Fisher G, Skillern PG: Hypercalcemia due to hypervitaminosis A. *JAMA* 227:1413, 1974.
143. Fisher JA et al: Acute parathyroid hormone response to epinephrine in vivo. *J Clin Invest* 52:2434, 1973.
144. Fisken RA et al: Hypercalcemia—A hospital survey. *Q J Med* 49:405, 1980.
145. Fisken RA et al: Hypercalcemia in hospital patients. Clinical and diagnostic aspects. *Lancet* 1:202, 1981.
146. Fitzpatrick LA, Bilezikian JP: Acute primary hyperparathyroidism. *Am J Med* 82:275, 1987.
147. Fleischman AR et al: 25-Hydroxyvitamin D. Serum levels and oral administration of calcifediol in neonates. *Arch Intern Med* 138:869, 1978.
148. Foley TP Jr et al: Familial benign hypercalcemia. *J Pediatr* 81:1060, 1972.
149. Follis RH: Skeletal changes associated with hyperthyroidism. *Johns Hopkins Med J* 92:405, 1953.
150. Fontaine O et al: 25-Hydroxycholecalciferol metabolism in hypophysectomized rats. *Endocrinology* 102:1822, 1978.
151. Frame B et al: Hypercalcemia and skeletal effects of chronic hypervitaminosis A. *Ann Intern Med* 80:44, 1974.
152. Frame B, Parfitt AM: Corticosteroid responsive hypercalcemia with elevated serum 1-alpha, 25 dihydroxyvitamin D. *Ann Intern Med* 93:449, 1980.
153. Frame B et al: Acute severe hypercalcemia a la Münchausen. *Am J Med* 70:316, 1981.
154. Francis MD et al: Diphosphonates inhibit formation of calcium phosphate crystals in vitro and pathological calcification in vivo. *Science* 165:1264, 1969.
155. Freitag JJ et al: Evidence for skeletal resistance to parathyroid hormone in magnesium deficiency: Studies in isolated perfused bone. *J Clin Invest* 64:1238, 1979.
156. Frensilli JA et al: Dental changes of idiopathic hypoparathyroidism. *J Oral Surg* 29:727, 1971.
157. Friedman J et al: Response of fetal rat bone to thyrocalcitonin in tissue culture. *Endocrinology* 82:149, 1968.
158. Frijlink WB et al: Treatment of Paget's disease with (3-amino-1-hydroxy propylidene) -1,1-bisphosphonate (APD). *Lancet* 1:799, 1979.
159. Fujita T et al: Familial hypocalciuric hypercalcemia involving four members of a kindred including a girl with severe neonatal primary hyperparathyroidism. *Miner Electrolyte Metab* 9:51, 1983.
160. Fuss M et al: Hypercalcemia due to immobilization in Paget's disease of bone. *Lancet* 2:941, 1978.
161. Gabow PA et al: Furosemide-induced reduction in ionized calcium in hypoparathyroid patients. *Ann Intern Med* 86:579, 1977.
162. Gammon GD, Docherly JP: Thiazide induced hypercalcemia in a manic-depressive patient. *Am J Psychiatry* 137:1453, 1980.
163. Ganote CE et al: Acute calcium nephrotoxicity: An electron microscopical and semiquantitative light microscopical study. *Arch Pathol Lab Med* 99:650, 1975.
164. García RE et al: Idiopathic hypercalcemia and supravalvular aortic stenosis. *N Engl J Med* 271:117, 1964.
165. Garrett RI et al: Production of lymphotoxin, the bone-resorbing cytokine lymphotoxin by cultured human myeloma cells. *N Engl J Med* 317:526, 1987.
166. Geis WP et al: The diagnosis and treatment of hyperparathyroidism after renal homotransplantation. *Surg Gynecol Obstet* 117:997, 1973.
167. Gilligan JE et al: Hypercalcemia associated with parenteral amino acid and dextrose infusion. *Am J Clin Nutr* 35:993, 1982.
168. Gkonos PJ et al: Hypercalcemia and elevated 1,25-hydroxyvitamin D levels in a patient with end-stage renal disease and active tuberculosis. *N Engl J Med* 311:1683, 1984.
169. Glorieux FH et al: Bone response to phosphate salts, ergocalciferol and calcitriol in hypophosphatemic vitamin D resistant rickets. *N Engl J Med* 303:1023, 1980.
170. Godolphin W et al: Spurious hypocalcemia in hemodialysis patients after heparinization: In vitro formation of calcium soaps. *Am J Clin Pathol* 71:215, 1979.
171. Goebell H et al: Stimulation of pancreatic secretion of enzymes by acute hypercalcemia in man. *Eur J Clin Invest* 3:98, 1973.
172. Goldstein DA et al: Blood levels of 25-hydroxyvitamin D in nephrotic syndrome. Studies in 26 patients. *Ann Intern Med* 87:664, 1977.
173. Goldstein DA et al: Effect of parathyroid hormone and uremia on peripheral nerve calcium and motor nerve conduction velocity. *J Clin Invest* 62:88, 1978.
174. Gottleib S et al: Humoral hypercalcemia of malignancy: A syndrome in search of a hormone. *Am J Med* 73:751, 1982.
175. Grantham JJ, Orloff J: Effects of prostaglandin E, on the permeability response of the isolated collecting tubule to vasopressin, adenosine 3′, 5′-monophosphate and theophylline. *J Clin Invest* 47:1154, 1968.
176. Guignard J-P et al: Effect of brief hypercalcemia on free water reabsorption during solute diuresis: Evidence for impairment of sodium transport in Henle's loop. *Clin Sci* 39:337, 1970.
177. Guillenwater JY: Clinical aspects of urinary tract obstruction. *Sem Nephrol* 2:46, 1982.
178. Haddad JG Jr, Walgate J: Radioimmunoassay of the binding protein for vitamin D and its metabolites in human serum. *J Clin Invest* 58:1217, 1976.
179. Haff RC: Technical factors influencing morbidity in thyroid operation. *Am J Surg* 126:383, 1973.
180. Hahn TJ et al: Effects of magnesium depletion on responsiveness to parathyroid hormone in parathyroidectomized rats. *J Clin Invest* 51:886, 1972.
181. Hahn TJ: Drug-induced disorders of vitamin D and mineral metabolism. *Clin Endocrinol Metab* 9:107, 1980.
182. Hakin R et al: Severe hypercalcemia associated with hydrochlorothiazide and calcium carbonate therapy. *Can Med Assoc J* 121:591, 1979.
183. Haldimann B et al: Renal function and blood levels of divalent ions in acute pancreatitis: A prospective study in 99 patents. *Miner Electrolyte Metab* 3:190, 1980.
184. Haldimann B, Trechsel U: Vitamin D replacement therapy in patients with the nephrotic syndrome. *Miner Electrolyte Metab* 9:154, 1983.
185. Hall TC et al: Hypocalcemia—An unusual complication of breast cancer. *N Engl J Med* 275:1474, 1966.
186. Halmos V et al: Idiopathic hypoparathyroidism with im-

paired vitamin B absorption. *Can Med Assoc J* 87:173, 1962.
187. Hamilton JW et al: Synthesis of parathyroid hormone-like peptides by a human squamous cell carcinoma. *J Clin Endocrinol Metab* 45:1023, 1977.
188. Hans SS, Lee TP: Post-thyroidectomy hypoparathyroidism. *Am Surg* 42:930, 1976.
189. Haussler MR, McCain TA: Basic and clinical concepts related to vitamin D metabolism and action. *N Engl J Med* 297:1041, 1977.
190. Haussler MR, McCain TA: Basic and clinical concepts related to vitamin D metabolism and action. *N Engl J Med* 297:974, 1977.
191. Haussler MR, Cordy PE: Metabolites and analogues of vitamin D: Which for what? *JAMA* 247:841, 1982.
192. Haverback BJ et al: Trypsin, trypsinogen and trypsin inhibitor in human pancreatic juice. Mechanism for pancreatitis associated with hyperparathyroidism. *Am J Med* 29:424, 1960.
193. Heath H III, Edis AJ: Pheochromocytoma associated with hypercalcemia and ectopic secretion of calcitonin. *Ann Intern Med* 91:208, 1979.
194. Heath H III, Purnell D: Urinary cyclic 3′,5′-adenosine monophosphate responses to exogenous and endogenous parathyroid hormone in familial benign hypercalcemia and primary hyperparathyroidism. *J Lab Clin Med* 96:974, 1980.
195. Heedman PA, Stenstrom G: Clinical findings in patients with hypercalcemia. A preliminary investigation based on biochemical screening. *Acta Med Scand* 193:167, 1973.
196. Heinemann HO: Reversible defect in renal ammonium excretion in patients with hypercalcemia. *Metabolism* 12:792, 1963.
197. Hellman DE et al: Evidence for a direct effect of parathyroid hormone on urinary acidification. *Am J Physiol* 209:643, 1964.
198. Hellstrom J: Hyperparathyrodism and gastroduodenal ulcer. *Acta Chem Scand* 116:207, 1959.
199. Henneman PH et al: The cause of hypercalciuria in sarcoid and its treatment with cortisone and sodium phytate. *J Clin Invest* 35:1229, 1956.
200. Heptinstall RH: Calcium and the kidney. Chapter 28 in Heptinstall RH (ed): *Pathology of the Kidney*, 2d ed. Boston, Little, Brown, 1974.
201. Heyburn PJ et al: Peritoneal dialysis in the management of severe hypercalcemia. *Br Med J* 280:525, 1980.
202. Hillman LS, Haddad JG: Human perinatal vitamin D metabolism: II. Serial 25-hydroxyvitamin D concentrations in sera of term and premature infants. *J Pediatr* 86:928, 1975.
203. Hinkle JE, Cooperman LH: Serum ionized calcium changes following citrated blood transfusion in anesthetized man. *Br J Anesth* 43:1108, 1971.
204. Hirshorn JE et al: Carcinoma of the breast associated with hypercalcemia and the presence of parathyroid hormone-like substances in the tumor. *J Clin Endocrinol Metab* 48:217, 1979.
205. Hoeg JM, Slatopolsky E: Cervical carcinoma and ectopic hyperparathyroidism. *Arch Intern Med* 140:569, 1980.
206. Hofmann E: The Chvostek sign: A clinical study. *Am J Surg* 96:33, 1958.
207. Hoffman VN, Korzeniowski OM: Leprosy, hypercalcemia, and elevated serum calcitriol levels. *Ann Intern Med* 105:890, 1986.
208. Horiuchi N et al: Similarity of synthetic peptide from human tumor to parathyroid hormone in vivo and in vitro. *Science* 238:1566, 1987.
209. Horton JE et al: Bone resorbing activity in supernatant fluid from cultured human peripheral blood leukocytes. *Science*, 177:793, 1972.
210. Horwitz CA et al: Secondary malignant tumors of the parathyroid glands: Report of two cases with associated hypoparathyroidism. *Am J Med* 52:797, 1972.
211. Hosking DJ et al: Rehydration in the treatment of severe hypercalcemia. *Q J Med* 50:473, 1981.
212. Hruska KA et al: Effects of intact parathyroid hormone in hepatic glucose release in the dog. *J Clin Invest* 64:1016, 1979.
213. Hughes MR et al: Radioligand receptor assay for 25-hydroxyvitamin D_2/D_3 and 1,25-dihydroxyvitamin D_2/D_3. *J Clin Invest* 58:61, 1976.
214. Humes HD et al: Evidence for a parathyroid hormone-dependent influence of calcium on the glomerular ultrafiltration coefficient. *J Clin Invest* 61:32, 1978.
215. Imai M: Calcium transport across the rabbit thick ascending limb of Henle's loop perfused in vitro. *Pflugers Arch* 374:255, 1978.
216. Imrie CW et al: Hypocalcemia of acute pancreatitis. The effect of hypoalbuminemia. *Curr Med Res Opin* 4:101, 1976.
217. Insogna KL et al: Enhanced production rate of 1,25-dihydroxyvitamin D in sarcoidosis. *J Clin Endocrinol Metab* 66:72, 1988.
218. Ito H et al: Indomethacin-responsive hypercalcemia. *N Engl J Med* 293:558, 1975.
219. Iyengar R, Birnbaumer L: Hysteretic activation of adenlyate cyclase I. Effect of Mg ion on the rate of activation by guanine nucleotides and fluoride. *J Biol Chem* 256:11036, 1981.
220. Jacob AI et al: Reduction by cimetidine of serum parathyroid hormone in uremic patients. *N Engl J Med* 302:671, 1980.
221. Jacobs JW et al: Identification of transforming growth factors associated with the humoral hypercalcemia of malignancy. *Clin Res* 31:502A, 1983.
222. Jacobs TP et al: Hypercalcemia of malignancy: Treatment with intravenous dichloromethylene diphosphonate. *Ann Intern Med* 94:312, 1981.
223. Jaffe JP, Mosher D: Calcium binding by a myeloma protein. *Am J Med* 67:343, 1979.
224. Jarbro JW et al: Mithramycin inhibition of ribonucleic acid synthesis. *Cancer Res* 26:36, 1966.
225. Johnson N McI, Shneerson G: Hypercalcemia and hypercalciuria associated with pulmonary tuberculosis. *Br J Dis Chest* 74:201, 1980.
226. Josse RG et al: Hypercalcemia with ovarian carcinoma: Evidence of a pathogenetic role for prostaglandins. *Cancer* 48:1233, 1981.
227. Jowsey J, Riggs BL: Bone changes in patient with hypervitaminosis A. *J Clin Endrocrinol Metab* 228:1833, 1968.
228. Jung A et al: Parenteral diphosphonates for treating malignant hypercalcemia. *Cancer* 48:1922, 1981.

229. Kantarjian HM et al: Hypercalcemia in disseminated candidiasis. *Am J Med* 74:721, 1983.
230. Kaplan L et al: Malignant neoplasma and parathyroid adenoma. *Cancer* 28:401, 1971.
231. Karlinsky M et al: Effect of parathormone and cyclic adenosine monophosphate on renal bicarbonate reabsorption. *Am J Physiol* 227:1226, 1974.
232. Katz A, Braunstein GD: Clinical, biochemical and pathologic features of radiation-associated hyperparathyroidism. *Arch Intern Med* 143:79, 1983.
233. Katz CM, Tzagournis M: Chronic adult hypervitaminosis A with hypercalcemia. *Metabolism* 21:1171, 1972.
234. Kawashima H et al: Metabolic acidosis suppresses 25-hydroxyvitamin D_3-1α-hydroxylase in the rat kidney: Distinct site and mechanism of action. *J Clin Invest* 70:135, 1982.
235. Kelly RT, Falor WH: Hyperparathyroid crisis associated with pancreatitis. *Ann Surg* 168:917, 1968.
236. Kenny AD: Effect of catecholamines on serum calcium and phosphorus levels in intact and parathyroidectomized rats. *Naunym-Schmiedbergs Arch Pharmacol* 248:144, 1964.
237. Khosla S et al: Parathyroid hormone-related protein and hypercalcemia secondary to massive mammary hyperplasia. *N Engl J Med* 322:1157, 1990.
238. Kim H et al: Plasma insulin disturbances in primary hyperparathyroidism. *J Clin Invest* 50:2596, 1971.
239. Kimberg DB et al: Effect of cortisone treatment on the active transport of calcium by the small intestine. *J Clin Invest* 50:1309, 1971.
240. Kitrou MP et al: Hypercalcemia in active pulmonary tuberculosis. *Ann Intern Med* 96:255, 1982.
241. Kivirikko KT et al: Value of urine and serum hydroxyproline in the diagnosis of thyroid disease. *J Clin Endocrinol Metab* 25:1347, 1965.
242. Klein DC, Raisz LG: Prostaglandins: Stimulation of bone resorption in tissue culture. *Endocrinology* 86:1436, 1970.
243. Knill-Jones RP et al: Hypercalcemia and increased parathyroid-hormone activity in primary-hepatoma: Studies before and after hepatic transplantation. *N Engl J Med* 282:704, 1970.
244. Knochel JP: Serum calcium derangements in rhabdomyolysis. *N Engl J Med* 305:161, 1981.
244a. Kofman S et al: Mithramycin in the treatment of embryonal cancer. *Cancer* 17:938, 1964.
245. Koide Y et al: Increased 1,25-dihydroxycholecalciferol as a cause of abnormal calcium metabolism in sarcoidosis. *J Clin Endocrinol Metab* 52:494, 1981.
246. Kooh SW et al: Treatment of hypoparathyroidism and pseudohypoparathyroidism with metabolites of vitamin D: Evidence for impaired conversion of 25-hydroxyvitamin D to 1α,25-dihydroxyvitamin D. *N Engl J Med* 293:840, 1975.
247. Koppel MH et al: Thiazide-induced rise of serum calcium and magnesium in patients on maintenance hemodialysis. *Ann Intern Med* 72:895, 1970.
248. Kozeny GA et al: Hypercalcemia associated with silicone-induced granulomas. *N Engl Med* 311:1103, 1984.
249. Kukreja SC et al: Pheochromocytoma causing excessive parathyroid hormone production and hypercalcemia. *Ann Intern Med* 79:838, 1973.
250. Ladenson JH et al: Relationship of free and total calcium in hypercalcemic conditions. *J Clin Endocrinol Metab* 48:393, 1979.
251. Lafferty FW: Primary hyperparathyroidism. Changing clinical spectrum, prevalence of hypertension and discriminant analysis of laboratory test. *Arch Intern Med* 141:1761, 1981.
251a. Laitinen K et al: Transient hypoparathyroidism during acute alcohol intoxication. *N Engl J Med* 324:721, 1991.
252. Lambert PW et al: Demonstration of a lack of change in serum 1α,25-dihydroxyvitamin D in response to parathyroid extract in pseudohypoparathyroidism. *J Clin Invest* 66:782, 1980.
253. Lamers CBHW, Froeling PGAM: Clinical significance of hyperparathyroidism in familial multiple endocrime adenomatosis Type 1 (MEA I). *Am J Med* 66:422, 1979.
254. Lanier D Jr et al: Cimetidine therapy for severe hypercalcemia in two chronic hemodialysis patients. *Ann Intern Med* 93:573, 1980.
255. Lassiter WE et al: Micropuncture study of tubular reabsorption of calcium in normal rodents. *Am J Physiol* 204:771, 1963.
256. Laugen RH et al: Hypercalcemia associated with chronic lymphocytic leukemia. *Arch Intern Med* 139:1307, 1979.
257. Law WM, Heath H: Familial benign hypercalcemia (hypocalciuric hypercalcemia): Clinical and pathogenetic studies in 21 families. *Ann Intern Med* 102:511, 1985.
258. Lawrence MGD et al: Immobilization hypercalcemia: Some new aspects of diagnosis and treatment. *J Bone Joint Surg* 87:55A, 1973.
259. Layer P et al: Effects of experimental chronic hypercalcemia on feline exocrine pancreatic secretion. *Gastroenterology* 82:309, 1982.
260. Lee JC et al: Hypercalcemia in disseminated coccidioidomycosis. *N Engl J Med* 297:431, 1977.
261. Lee SW et al: 25-Hydroxycholecalciferol to 1,25-dihydroxycholecalciferol: Conversion impaired by systemic metabolic acidosis. *Science* 195:994, 1977.
262. Legha SS et al: Tamoxifen-induced hypercalcemia in breast cancer. *Cancer* 47:2803, 1981.
263. LeGrimellec C et al: Simultaneous Mg, Ca, P, K, Na, and Cl analysis in rat tubular fluid: III. During acute Ca plasma loading. *Pflugers Arch* 346:171, 1974.
264. Lein JWK: Hypomagnesemic hypocalcemia in renal failure. *Br Med J* 2:1400, 1978.
265. Lemann J Jr, Lennon EJ: Role of diet, gastrointestinal tract and bone in acid-base homeostasis. *Kidney Int* 1:275, 1972.
266. Lemann J Jr et al: The effects of chronic acid loads in normal man: Further evidence for the participation of bone mineral in the defense against chronic metabolic acidosis. *J Clin Invest* 45:1608, 1966.
267. Lerman S et al: Parathyroid hormone and the hypercalcemia of immobilization. *J Clin Endrocrinol Metab* 45:425, 1977.
268. Levine BS et al: Does vitamin D affect the renal handling of calcium and phosphorus? *Miner Electrolyte Metab* 1:295, 1978.
269. Levine MA et al: Deficient activity of guanine nucleotide

regulatory protein in erythrocytes from patients with pseudohypoparathyroidism. *Biochem Biophys Res Commun* 94:1319, 1980.
270. Levine MA et al: Resistance to multiple hormones in patients with pseudohypoparathyroidism association with deficient activity of guanine nucleotide regulatory protein. *Am J Med* 74:545, 1983.
271. Lightwood R: Idiopathic hypercalcemia with failure to thrive. *Proc R Soc Lond* 45:401, 1952.
272. Llach F et al: The pathophysiology of altered calcium metabolism in rhabdomyolysis induced acute renal failure. *N Engl J Med* 305:117, 1981.
273. Luben RA et al: Partial purification of osteoclast-activating factor from phytohemagglutinin-stimulated human leukocytes. *J Clin Invest* 53:1473, 1974.
274. Lyman NW et al: Cisplatin-induced hypocalcemia and hypomagnesemia. *Arch Intern Med* 140:1513, 1980.
275. Maguire PJ, MacDonald JS: Hypocalcemia associated with a calcitonin-producing hepatocellular carcinoma. *Arch Intern Med* 141:687, 1981.
276. Mallette LE et al: Neuromuscular disease in secondary hyperparathyroidism. *Ann Intern Med* 82:474, 1975.
277. Manitius A et al: On the mechanism of impairment of renal concentrating ability in hypercalcemia. *J Clin Invest* 39:693, 1960.
278. Marcus R et al: Thiazide diuretics do not potentiate cAMP response to parathyroid hormone. *Metabolism* 27:701, 1978.
279. Marone C et al: Acute hypercalcemic hypertension in man: Role of hemodynamics, catecholamines and renin. *Kidney Int* 20:92, 1980.
280. Martínez-Maldonado M et al: Diuretics in nonedematous states. *Arch Intern Med* 131:797, 1973.
281. Martínez-Maldonado M, García A: Hypo- and hypercalcemia. Chapter 3 in Martínez-Maldonado M (ed): *Handbook of Renal Therapeutics*. New York, Plenum Press, 1983.
282. Martínez-Maldonado M et al: Acute renal failure associated with tubulo interstitial disease including papillary necrosis. Chapter 16 in Brenner BM, Lazarus JM (eds): *Acute Renal Failure*. Philadelphia, Saunders, 1983.
283. Marx SJ et al: Family studies in patients with primary parathyroid hyperplasia. *Am J Med* 62:698, 1977.
284. Marx SJ et al: Divalent cation metabolism: Familial hypocalciuric hypercalcemia versus typical primary hyperparathyroidism. *Am J Med* 65:235, 1978.
285. Marx SJ et al: Circulating parathyroid hormone activity: Familial hypocalciuric hypercalcemia versus typical primary hyperparathyrodism. *J Clin Endocrinol Metab* 47:1190, 1978.
286. Marx SJ: Familial hypocalciuric hypercalcemia. *N Engl J Med* 303:810, 1980.
287. Marx SJ et al: Adenosine 3′, 5′-monophosphate response to parathyroid hormone: Familial hypocalciuric hypercalcemia versus typical primary hyperparathyroidism. *J Clin Endocrinol Metab* 50:546, 1980.
288. Marx SJ et al: The hypocalciuric or benign variant of familial hypercalcemia: Clinical and biochemical features in fifteen kindreds. *Medicine* 60:397, 1981.
289. Marx SJ et al: Maximal urine concentrating-ability: Familial hypocalciuric hypercalcemia versus typical primary hyperparathyroidism. *J Clin Endocrinol Metab* 52:736, 1981.
290. Marx SJ et al: Familial hypocalciuric hypercalcemia: The relation to primary parathyroid hyperplasia. *N Engl J Med* 307:416, 1982.
291. Marx SJ et al: An association between neonatal severe primary hyperparathyroidism and familial hypocalciuric hypercalcemia in three kindreds. *N Engl J Med* 306:257, 1982.
292. Massry SG et al: Secondary hyperparathyroidism in chronic renal failure. The clinical spectrum in uremia, during hemodialysis and after renal transplantation. *Arch Intern Med* 124:931, 1969.
293. Massry SG et al: Evidence for suppression of parathyroid gland activity by hypermagnesemia. *J Clin Invest* 49:1619, 1970.
294. Massry SG et al: Skeletal resistance to parathyroid hormone in renal failure. Study in 105 human subjects. *Ann Intern Med* 78:357, 1973.
295. Mawer EB et al: The distribution and storage of vitamin D and its metabolites in human tissues. *Clin Sci* 43:413, 1972.
296. Mays ET, Weakley SD: Serum multichannel autoanalyzers in the detection of hypercalcemia and hyperparathyroidism. *Surg Gynecol Obstet* 133:603, 1971.
297. Mazzuoli GF et al: Il fenomeno escape e plateu: Studi su la desensibilizzazione precoce alla calcitonina in vivo, in Gennari C, Segree G (eds): *The Effects of Calcitonin in Man*. Milano, Masson Italia Editori, 1983, p 60.
298. McIntosh DA et al: Autonomy of parathyroid function after renal homotransplantation. *Ann Intern Med* 65:900, 1966.
299. McMahon MJ et al: The nature of hypocalcemia in acute pancreatitis. *Br J Surg* 65:216, 1978.
300. McPherson ML et al: Theophylline-induced hypercalcemia. *Ann Intern Med* 105:52, 1986.
301. Melvin KEW, Tashjian AH: The syndrome of excessive thyrocalcitonin produced by medullary carcinoma of the thyroid. *Proc Natl Acad Sci USA* 59:1216, 1968.
302. Mennes P et al: Hypomagnesemia and impaired parathyroid hormone secretion in chronic renal failure. *Ann Intern Med* 88:206, 1978.
303. Meredith SC, Rosenberg IH: Gastrointestinal-hepatic disorders and osteomalacia. *Clin Endocrinol Metab* 9:131, 1980.
304. Merlini G et al: A human immunoglobulin G binding four moles of calcium associated with asymptomatic hypercalcemia. *J Clin Immunol* 4:185, 1984.
305. Metz SA et al: Selective deficiency of 1,25- dihydroxycholecalciferol: A cause of isolated skeletal resistance to parathyroid hormone. *N Engl J Med* 297:1084, 1977.
306. Metz SA et al: Prostaglandins as mediators of paraneoplastic syndromes: Review and update. *Metabolism* 30:299, 1981.
307. Meunier PJ et al: Bony manifestations of thyrotoxicosis. *Orthop Clin North Am* 3:745, 1972.
308. Meytes D et al: Effect of parathyroid hormone on erythropoiesis. *J Clin Invest* 67:1263, 1981.
309. Michie W et al: Mechanism of hypocalcemia after thyroidectomy for thyrotoxicosis. *Lancet* 1:508, 1971.
310. Middler S et al: Thiazide diuretics and calcium metabolism. *Metabolism* 22:139, 1973.

311. Miller PD et al: Hypocalciuric effect of lithium in man. *Miner Electrolyte Metab* 1:3, 1978.
312. Minkin C et al: Bone resorption and humoral hypercalcemia of malignancy: Stimulation of bone resorption in vitro by tumor extracts is inhibited by prostaglandin synthesis inhibitors. *J Clin Endocrinol Metab* 53:941, 1981.
313. Mitnick P et al: Effects of two models of hypercalcemia on renal acid base metabolism. *Kidney Int* 21:613, 1982.
314. Moore EW: Ionized calcium in normal, serum ultrafiltrates and whole blood determined by ion-exchange electrodes. *J Clin Invest* 49:318, 1970.
315. Morel F et al: Functional segmentation of the rabbit distal tubule by micro determination of hormone dependent adenylate cyclase activity. *Kidney Int* 9:264, 1976.
316. Motokura T et al: Parathyroid hormone-related protein in adult T-cell leukemia-lymphoma. *Ann Intern Med* 111:484, 1989.
317. Moxley MA et al: Parathyroid hormone stimulation of glucose and urea production in isolated liver cells. *Am J Physiol* 227:1058, 1974.
318. Muggia FM, Hansen HH: Osteoblastic metastasis in small cell (oat cell) carcinoma of the lung. *Cancer* 30:801, 1972.
319. Mundy GF: The hypercalcemia of malignancy revisited. *J Clin Invest* 82:1, 1988.
320. Mundy GF et al: Evidence for the secretion of an osteoclast stimulating factor in myeloma. *N Engl J Med* 291:1041, 1974.
321. Mundy GF et al: Bone resorbing activity in supernatants from lymphoid cell lines. *N Engl J Med* 290:867, 1974.
322. Mundy GR et al: Direct stimulation of bone resorption by thyroid hormones. *J Clin Invest* 58:529, 1976.
323. Mundy GR et al: Pathogenesis of hypercalcemia in lymphosarcoma cell leukemia. Role of an osteoclast activating factor-like substance and a mechanism of action for glucocorticoid therapy. *Am J Med* 65:600, 1978.
324. Mundy GR, Raisz LG: Thyrotoxicosis and calcium metabolism. *Miner Electrolyte Metab* 2:285, 1979.
325. Mundy GR et al: Primary hyperparathyroidism: Changes in the pattern of clinical presentation. *Lancet* 1:1317, 1980.
326. Mundy GR, Martin TJ: The hypercalcemia of malignancy: Pathogenesis and management. *Metabolism* 31:1247, 1982.
326a. Mundy GF et al: The hypercalcemia of cancer: Clinical implications and pathogenic mechanisms. *N Engl J Med* 310:1718, 1984.
327. Mundy GR et al: Comparative study of available medical therapy for hypercalcemia of malignancy. *Am J Med* 74:421, 1983.
328. Mundy GR, Yates AJP: Recent advances in pathophysiology and treatment of hypercalcemia of malignancy. *Am J Kidney Dis* 14:2, 1989.
329. Nagant de Deuzchaisnes C, Krane SM: Hypoparathyroidism, in Avioli LV, Drane SM (eds): *Metabolic Bone Disease*. New York, Academic Press, 1978, vol 2, p 620.
330. Nellans HN, Kimberg DV: Cellular and paracellular calcium transport in rat ileum: Effects of dietary calcium. *Am J Physiol* 235:E726, 1978.
331. Nellans HN, Kimberg DV: Anomalous calcium secretion in rat ileum: Role of paracellular pathway. *Am J Physiol* 236:E473, 1979.
332. Nellans HN, Goldsmith RS: Transepithelial calcium transport by rat cecum: High-efficiency absorptive site. *Am J Physiol* 240:G424, 1981.
333. Nierenberg DW, Ransil BJ: Q-T interval as a clinical indicator of hypercalcemia. *Am J Cardiol* 44:243, 1979.
334. Notman DD et al: Fulminating hypercalcemia and markedly increased nephrogenous cyclic AMP in a patient with transitional cell carcinoma of the bladder. *Am J Med* 66:870, 1979.
335. Nusynowitz MC, Klein MH: Pseudoidiopathic hypoparathyroidism. Hypoparathyroidism with ineffective parathyroid hormone. *Am J Med* 55:677, 1973.
336. Ober KP et al: Severe hypocalcemia associated with chronic glutethimide addiction: A case report. *Am J Psychiatry* 138:1239, 1981.
337. Okano K et al: Comparative efficacy of various vitamin D metabolites in the treatment of various types of hypoparathyroidism. *J Clin Endocrinol Metab* 55:238, 1982.
338. Olinger GN et al: Acute clinical hypocalcemic myocardial depression during rapid blood transfusion and postoperative hemodialysis. *J Thorac Cardiovasc Surg* 72:503, 1976.
339. Orwoll ES: The milk alkali syndrome: Current concepts. *Ann Intern Med* 97:242, 1982.
340. Oster JR et al: A short duration renal acidification test using calcium chloride. *Nephron* 14:281, 1975.
341. Pak CYC et al: Photon absorptiometric analysis of bone density in primary hyperparathyroidism. *Lancet* 2:7, 1975.
342. Pak CYC: Pathogenesis, consequences, and treatment of the hypercalciuric states. *Semin Nephrol* 1:356, 1981.
343. Paloyan E et al: Glucagon-induced hypocalcemia. *Metabolism* 16:35, 1967.
344. Papapoulus SE et al: 1,25-Dihydroxycholecalciferol in the pathogenesis of the hypercalcemia of sarcoidosis. *Lancet* 1:627, 1979.
345. Parfitt AM: Adult hypoparathyroidism. Treatment with calcifediol. *Arch Intern Med* 138:874, 1978.
346. Paterson CR: Vitamin D poisoning: Survey of causes in 21 patients with hypercalcemia. *Lancet* 1:1164, 1980.
347. Paterson CR, Gunn A: Familial benign hypercalcemia. *Lancet* 2:61, 1981.
348. Patten JL et al: Mutation in the gene encoding the stimulatory G protein of adenylate cyclase in Albright's hereditary osteodystrophy. *N Engl J Med* 322:1412, 1990.
349. Pedersen KO: Hypercalcemia in Addison's disease. Report on two cases and review of literature. *Acta Med Scand* 181:691, 1967.
350. Peerenboom H et al: The defect in intestine calcium transport in hyperthyroidism and its response to therapy. *J Clin Endocrinol Metab* 59:936, 1984.
351. Peng TC et al: The hypocalcemic effect of ethyl alcohol in rats and dogs. *Endocrinology* 91:586, 1972.
352. Petersen P: Psychiatric disorders in primary hyperparathyroidism. *J Clin Endocrinol Metab* 28:1491, 1968.
353. Pierides AM et al: Assessment of renal osteodystrophy following renal transplantation. *Proc Eur Dial Transplant Assoc* 11:481, 1974.
354. Pike JW et al: Circulating 1α-25-$(OH)_2D$ during physiological states of calcium stress, in Norman AW et al (eds): *Vitamin D: Biochemical, Chemical and Clinical*

Aspects Related to Calcium Metabolism. Berlin, W de Gruyter, 1977, p 187.
355. Pleasure D et al: Skeletal muscle calcium metabolism and contractile force in vitamin D-deficient chicks. *J Clin Invest* 64:1157, 1979.
356. Pletka PG et al: Secondary hyperparathyroidism in human kidney transplant recipients. *Nephron* 17:371, 1976.
357. Popovtzer MM et al: The acute effect of chlorothiazide on serum ionized calcium: Evidence for a parathyroid hormone dependent mechanism. *J Clin Invest* 55:1295, 1975.
358. Poujeol P et al: Influence of extracellular fluid volume expansion on magnesium, calcium and phosphate handling along the rat nephron. *Pflugers Arch* 365:203, 1976.
359. Pritchard MH, Jessop J: Chondrocalcinosis in primary hyperparathyroidism. Influence of age, metabolic bone disease and parathyroidectomy. *Ann Rheum Dis* 36:146, 1977.
360. Purnell DC et al: Primary hyperparathyroidism: A prospective clinical study. *Am J Med* 50:670, 1971.
361. Purnell DC et al: Treatment of primary hyperparathyroidism. *Am J Med* 56:800, 1974.
362. Purpora D et al: Toxic epidermal necrolysis after mithramycin. *N Engl J Med* 299:1412, 1978.
363. Quamme GA, Dirks JH: Magnesium transport in the nephron. *Am J Physiol* 239:F393, 1980.
364. Raisz LG, Niemann I: Effect of phosphate, calcium and magnesium on bone resorption and hormonal responses in tissue culture. *Endocrinology* 85:446, 1969.
365. Raisz LG: Physiologic and pharmacologic regulation of bone resorption. *N Engl J Med* 282:909, 1970.
366. Ralston SH et al: Comparison of aminohydroxypropylidene diphosphonate, mithramycin and corticosteroids/calcitonin in treatment of cancer-associated hypercalcemia. *Lancet* 2:207, 1985.
367. Rao SD et al: Hyperparathyroidism following head and neck irradiation. *Arch Intern Med* 140:205, 1980.
368. Rasmussen H, Anast C: Familial hypophosphatemic (vitamin D-resistant) rickets and vitamin D-dependent rickets, in Stanbury JB, Wyngaarden JB (eds): *The Metabolic Basis of Inherited Disease*, 4th ed. New York, McGraw-Hill, 1978, p 246.
369. Reifenstein EC Jr, Albright F: Paget's disease: Its pathologic physiology and the importance of this in the complications arising from fracture and immobilization. *N Engl J Med* 231:343, 1944.
370. Reiner M et al: Abnormal calcium metabolism in normocalcemic sarcoidosis. *Br Med J* 2:1473, 1976.
371. Riggs BL et al: Effect of sex hormones on bone in primary osteoporosis. *J Clin Invest* 48:1065, 1969.
372. Rivera-Vázquez AB et al: Acute hypercalcemia in hemodialysis patients: Distinction from "dialysis dementia." *Nephron* 25:243, 1980.
373. Roberts WC, Waller BF: Effect of chronic hypercalcemia on the heart: An analysis of 18 necropsy patients. *Am J Med* 71:371, 1981.
374. Robertson GM Jr et al: Inadequate parathyroid response in acute pancreatitis. *N Engl J Med* 294:512, 1976.
375. Robertson RP et al: Elevated prostaglandins and suppressed parathyroid hormone associated with hypercalcemia and renal cell carcinoma. *J Clin Endocrinol Metab* 41:164, 1975.
376. Robertson RP et al: Plasma prostaglandin E in patients with cancer with and without hypercalcemia. *J Clin Endocrinol Metab* 43:1330, 1976.
377. Robertson RP: Prostaglandins and hypercalcemia of cancer. *Med Clin North Am* 65:845, 1981.
378. Robinson MF et al: Failure of cimetidine to affect calcium homeostasis in familial primary hyperparathyroidism. *J Clin Endocrinol Metab* 51:912, 1980.
379. Rocha AS et al: Calcium and Phosphate transport in isolated segments of rabbit Henle's loop. *J Clin Invest* 59:975, 1977.
380. Romer FK: Angiotensin-converting enzyme in hypercalcemic disorders. *Acta Med Scand* 211:31, 1982.
381. Rosenbaum RW et al: Decreased phosphate reabsorption after renal transplantation: Evidence for a mechanism independent of calcium and parathyroid hormone. *Kidney Int* 19:568, 1981.
382. Rosenthal FD, Roy S: Hypertension and hyperparathyroidism. *Br Med J* 4:396, 1972.
383. Rouse D et al: Calcium transport in the pars recta and thin descending limb of Henle of the rabbit, perfused in vitro. *J Clin Invest* 65:37, 1980.
384. Rouse D, Suki WN: Calcium and the kidney. *Semin Nephrol* 1:295, 1981.
385. Rouse D, Suki WN: Renal control of extracellular calcium. *Kidney Int* 38:700, 1990.
386. Rude RK et al: Treatment of thyrotoxic hypercalcemia with propranolol. *N Engl J Med* 294:431, 1976.
387. Rude RK et al: Parathyroid hormone secretion in magnesium deficiency. *J Clin Endocrinol Metab* 47:800, 1978.
388. Rude RK et al: Low serum concentration of 1,25-dihydroxyvitamin D in human magnesium deficiency. *J Clin Endocrinol Metab* 761:933, 1985.
389. Russ JE et al: Parathyroid adenomas following irradiation. *Cancer* 43:1078, 1979.
390. Ryan WG et al: Mithramycin in Paget's disease of bone. *JAMA* 213:1153, 1970.
391. Ryzen E et al: Hypercalcemia and abnormal 1,25-dihydroxyvitamin D concentrations in leprosy. *Am J Med* 84:325, 1988.
392. Samaan NA et al: Hypercalcemia in patients with known malignant disease. *Surgery* 80:382, 1976.
393. Scarpelli DG: Experimental nephrocalcinosis: A biochemical and morphological study. *Lab Invest* 14:123, 1965.
394. Schilsky RL, Anderson T: Hypomagnesemia and renal magnesium wasting in patients receiving cisplatin. *Ann Intern Med* 90:929, 1979.
395. Schwarts GH et al: Hypercalcemia after renal transplantation. *Am J Med* 49:42, 1970.
396. Scott JT et al: Association of hyperuricemia and gout with hyperparathyroidism. *Br Med J* 1:1070, 1964.
397. Seeling MS: Vitamin D and cardiovascular, renal and brain damage in infancy and childhood. *Ann NY Acad Sci USA* 147:539, 1969.
398. Serros ER, Kirschenbaum MA: Prostaglandin-dependent polyuria in hypercalcemia. *Am J Physiol* 241:F224, 1981.
399. Seyberth HW et al: Prostaglandins as mediators of hypercalcemia associated with certain types of cancer. *N Engl J Med* 293:1278, 1975.
400. Shafer RB, Gregory DH: Calcium malabsorption in hyperthyroidism. *Gastroenterology* 63:235, 1972.

401. Shai F et al: Hypercalcemia in mycobacterial infection. *J Clin Endocrinol* 34:251, 1972.
402. Shambaugh GE III et al: Hypocalcemia accompanying agranulocytosis during propylthiouracil therapy. *Ann Intern Med* 91:576, 1979.
403. Shane E et al: Effects of dichloromethylene diphosphonate on serum and urinary calcium in primary hyperparathyroidism. *Ann Intern Med* 95:23, 1981.
404. Shane E et al: Therapy of hypercalcemia due to parathyroid carcinoma with intravenous dichloromethylene diphosphonate. *Am J Med* 72:939, 1982.
405. Shareghi GR, Stoner LC: Calcium transport across segments of the rabbit distal nephron in vitro. *Am J Physiol* 235:F367, 1978.
406. Sharma OP et al: Hypercalcemia and tuberculosis. *JAMA* 222:582, 1972.
406a. Sherrard DJ et al: Pseudohyperparathyroidism: Syndrome associated with aluminum intoxication in patients with renal failure. *Am J Med* 79:127, 1985.
407. Sherwood LM et al: Production of parathyroid hormone by non-parathyroid tumors. *J Clin Endocrinol Metab* 27:140, 1967.
408. Sherwood LM: The multiple causes of hypercalcemia in malignant disease. *N Engl J Med* 303:1412, 1980.
409. Shetty KR et al: Protracted vitamin D intoxication. *Arch Intern Med* 135:986, 1975.
410. Siegel EG et al: Evidence for the involvement of Na/Ca exchange in glucose-induced insuline release from rat pancreatic islets. *J Clin Invest* 66:996, 1980.
411. Simpson EL et al: Absence of parathyroid hormone messenger RNA in non-parathyroid tumors associated with hypercalcemia. *N Engl J Med* 309:325, 1983.
412. Singer FR, Adams JS: Abnormal calcium homeostasis in sarcoidosis. *N Engl J Med* 315:755, 1986.
413. Singer FR et al: Pathogenesis of hypercalcemia in malignancy. *Miner Electrolyte Metab* 2:161, 1979.
414. Singhelakis P et al: Intestinal calcium absorption in hyperthyroidism. *Metabolism* 23:311, 1974.
415. Sitrin M et al: Vitamin D deficiency and bone disease in gastrointestinal disorders. *Arch Intern Med* 138:886, 1978.
416. Sjoberg HE: Retention of oral^{47} calcium in acromegaly. *Horm Metab Res* 1:136, 1969.
417. Skrabanek P et al: Tumor hypercalcemia and "ectopic hyperparathyroidism." *Medicine* 59:262, 1980.
418. Slyter H: Idiopathic hypoparathyroidism presenting as dementia. *Neurology* 29:393, 1979.
419. Smallridge RC et al: Hypocalcemia with osteoblastic metastasis in a pateint with prostate carcinoma: A cause of secondary hyperparathyroidism. *Am J Med* 71:184, 1981.
420. Soffer D et al: Paroxysmal choreoathetosis as a presenting symptom in idiopathic hypoparathyroidism. *J Neurol Neurosurg Psychiatry* 40:692, 1977.
421. Sowers JR et al: Hypereninemic hypoaldosteronism in association with neoplasia induced hypercalcemia in the Fischer rat. *Metabolism* 30:987, 1981.
422. Sowers JR, Barrett JD: Hormonal changes associated with hypertension in neoplasia-induced hypercalcemia. *Am J Physiol* 242:E330, 1982.
423. Spencer EM, Tobiassen O: The effects of hypophysectomy on 25-hydroxyvitamin D_3 metabolism in the rat, in Normal AW et al (eds): *Vitamin D—Biochemical, Chemical, and Clinical Aspects Related to Calcium Metabolism*, 1st ed. Berlin, W de Gruyter, 1977, p 197.
424. Stanbury SW: Bone disease in uremia. *Am J Med* 44:714, 1968.
425. Stewart AF et al: Biochemical evaluation of patients with cancer-associated hypercalcemia: Evidence for humoral and nonhumoral groups. *N Engl J Med* 303:1377, 1980.
426. Stewart AF et al: Calcium homeostasis in immobilization: An example of resorptive hypercalciuria. *N Engl J Med* 306:1136, 1982.
427. Stewart AF et al: Hypercalcemia in pheochromocytoma: Evidence for a novel mechanism. *Ann Intern Med* 102:776, 1985.
428. Stoeckle JD et al: Chronic beryllium disease. Long term follow-up of sixty cases and selective review of the literature. *Am J Med* 46:545, 1969.
429. Streck WF et al: Glucocorticoid effects in vitamin D intoxication. *Arch Intern Med* 139:974, 1979.
430. Strewler GJ et al: Human renal carcinoma cells produce hypercalcemia in the Nude mouse and a novel protein recognized by parathyroid horome receptors. *J Clin Invest* 71:769, 1983.
431. Strumpf M et al: Effect of glucocorticoid on osteoclast activating factor. *J Lab Clin Med* 92:772, 1978.
432. Stulz PM et al: Ventricular pump performance during hypocalcemia: Clinical and experimental studies. *J Thorac Cardiovasc Surg* 78:185, 1979.
433. Suki WN, Rouse D: Hormonal regulation of calcium transport in thick ascending limb renal tubules. *Am J Physiol* 241:F171, 1981.
434. Suke WN et al: The renal diluting and concentrating mechanism in hypercalcemia. *Nephron* 6:50, 1969.
435. Suki WN et al: Acute treatment of hypercalcemia with furosemide. *N Engl J Med* 283:836, 1970.
436. Suki WN: Calcium transport in the nephron. *Am J Physiol* 237:F1, 1979.
437. Suki WN et al: Calcium transport in the thick ascending limb of Henle: Heterogeneity of function in the medullary and cortical segments. *J Clin Invest* 66:1004, 1980.
438. Suki WN, Rouse D: Mechanism of calcium transport. *Miner Electrolyte Metab* 5:175, 1981.
439. Sutton RAL et al: Effects of metabolic acidosis and alkalosis on sodium and calcium transport in the dog kidney. *Kidney Int* 15:520, 1979.
440. Suva LJ et al: A parathyroid hormone-related protein implicated in malignant hypercalcemia: Cloning and expression. *Science* 237:745, 1987.
441. Sztern M et al: Hypercalcemia in carcinoma of the breast without evidence of bone destruction: Beneficial effect of hormonal therapy. *Cancer* 48:2383, 1981.
442. Tashjian AH Jr et al: Immunochemical identification of parathyroid hormone in non-parathyroid neoplasms associated with hypercalcemia. *J Exp Med* 119:467, 1964.
443. Tashjian AH Jr et al: Evidence that the bone resorption stimulating factor produced by mouse fibrosarcoma cells is prostaglandin E_2—A new model for hypercalcemia of cancer. *J Exp Med* 136:1329, 1972.
444. Tashjian AH Jr et al: Effects of hydrocortisone on the hypercalcemia and plasma levels of 13, 14-dihydro-15-

keto-prostaglandin E_2 in mice bearing the HSDM, fibrosarcoma. *Biochem Biophys Res Commun* 74:199, 1977.
445. Tashjian AH Jr: Role of prostaglandins in the production of hypercalcemia by tumors. *Cancer Res* 38:4138, 1978.
446. Tashjian AH Jr et al: Calcitonin binding sites in bone: Relationship to biological response and escape. *Recent Prog Horm Res* 34:285, 1978.
447. Tavill AS et al: Idiopathic paroxysmal myoglobinuria with acute renal failure and hypercalcemia. *N Engl J Med* 271:283, 1964.
448. Taylor DA et al: Neck radiation and hyperparathyroidism. *Ann Intern Med* 89:1012, 1978.
449. Teitelbaum SL: Morphological effects of vitamin D and its analogues on bone. *Am J Clin Nutr* 29:1300, 1976.
450. Thiebaud D et al: Effectiveness of salmon calcitonin administered as suppositories in tumor-induced hypercalcemia. *Am J Med* 82:745, 1987.
451. Thiebaud D et al: Fast and effective treatment of malignant hypercalcemia. *Arch Intern Med* 150:2125, 1990.
452. Thiebaud D et al: A single day treatment of tumor-induced hypercalcemia by intravenous amino-hydroxypropylidene biphosphonate. *J Bone Miner Res* 1:555, 1989.
453. Thiebaud D et al: Comparison of oral versus intravenous AHPrBP(APD) in tumor-induced hypercalcemia. *Bone* 7:247, 1986.
454. Thomson BM et al: Tumor necrosis factor alpha and beta induce osteoblastic cells to stimulate osteoclastic bone resorption. *J Immunology* 138:775, 1987.
455. Thomson BM et al: Osteoblasts mediate interleukin-1 stimulation of bone resorption by rat osteoclasts. *J Exp Med* 164:104, 1986.
456. Thorgeirsson U et al: The parathyroid glands in familial hypocalciuric hypercalcemia. *Hum Pathol* 12:229, 1981.
457. Tisell LE et al: Kan stralterapi inducera hyperparathyroidism? *Svensk Kurugi* 32:83, 1975.
458. Tisell LE et al: Autonomous hyperparathyroidism. A possible late complication of neck radiotherapy. *Acta Chir Scand* 142:367, 1976.
459. Tisell LE et al: Hyperparathyroidism in persons treated with x-rays for tuberculous cervical adenitis. *Cancer* 40:846, 1977.
460. Tofalletti J et al: Influence of continuous infusion of citrate on response to immunoreactive PTH, calcium, magnesium components, and other electrolytes in normal adults during plasmapheresis. *J Clin Endocrinol Metab* 60:874, 1985.
461. Trummel CL et al: Release of osteoclast activating factor by normal human peripheral blood leukocytes. *J Lab Clin Med* 85:1001, 1975.
462. Tsang RC et al: Possible pathogenetic factors in neonatal hypocalcemia of prematurity. *J Pediatr* 82:423, 1973.
463. Tsang RC et al: Neonatal parathyroid function: Role of gestational age and postnatal age. *J Pediatr* 83:728, 1973.
464. Tsang RC et al: Neonatal hypocalcemia in infants with birth asphyxia. *J Pediatr* 84:428, 1974.
465. Tsang RC et al: Parathyroid function in infants of diabetic mothers. *J Pediatr* 86:399, 1975.
466. Tsang RC et al: Calcium physiology and pathology in the neonate. *Pediatr Clin North Am* 23:611, 1976.
467. Tsang RC et al: Hypomagnesemia in infants of diabetic mothers: Perinatal studies. *J Pediatr* 89:115, 1976.
468. Tsokos GC et al: Renal and metabolic complications of undifferentiated and lymphoblastic lymphomas. *Medicine* 60:218, 1981.
469. Turner TL et al: Magnesium therapy in neonatal tetany. *Lancet* 1:283, 1977.
470. Ulstrom RA, Brown DM: Hypercalcemia as a complication of parenteral alimentation. *J Pediatr* 81:419, 1972.
471. Valente JD et al: Hypercalcemia associated with oral isotretinoin in the treatment of severe acne. *JAMA* 250:1899, 1983.
472. Valentzas C et al: Abnornal vitamin-D levels. *Ann Intern Med* 86:198, 1977.
473. Valentzas C et al: Vitamin D levels in thyrotoxicosis. *Lancet* 1:370, 1977.
474. Vanherweghem JL et al: Cimetidine and parathyroid hormone levels. *N Engl J Med* 303:395, 1980.
475. Vavatsi-Manos O, Preuss HG: The effects of high calcium concentrations on renal ammoniagenesis by rat kidney slices. *Nephron* 17:474, 1976.
476. Villalon AH et al: Hypercalcemia after tamoxifen for breast cancer: A sign of tumor response? *Br Med J* 2:1329, 1979.
477. Vincent RG et al: Abnormal behavior following parathyroidectomy. *JAMA* 180:372, 1962.
478. Vlachakis ND et al: Sympathetic system function and vascular reactivity in hypercalcemic patients. *Hypertension* 4:452, 1982.
479. Waeber B et al: Hypertention in a patient with hypercalcemia. *Arch Intern Med* 142:143, 1982.
480. Walker JV et al: Histoplasmosis with hypercalcemia, renal failure and papillary necrosis: Confusion with sarcoidosis. *JAMA* 237:1350, 1977.
481. Walser M et al: The hypercalcemia of adrenal insufficiency. *J Clin Invest* 42:456, 1963.
482. Warrell RP et al: Gallium nitrate for treatment of refractory hypercalcemia from parathyroid carcinoma. *Ann Intern Med* 107:683, 1987.
483. Warrell RP et al: Gallium nitrate for acute treatment of cancer-related hypercalcemia: A randomized, double-blind comparison to calcitonin. *Ann Intern Med* 108:669, 1988.
484. Warrell RP et al: Gallium nitrate inhibits calcium resorption from bone and is an effective treatment for cancer-related hypercalcemia. *J Clin Invest* 73:1487, 1984.
485. Watson CG et al: The role of calcitonin and parathyroid hormone in the pathogenesis of post-thyroidectomy hypocalcemia. *Metabolism* 30:588, 1981.
486. Weinstein RS, Hudson JB: Parathyroid hormone and 25-hydroxycholecalciferol levels in hypercalcemia of acute renal failure. *Arch Intern Med* 140:410, 1980.
487. Weir GC et al: The hypocalcemia of acute pancreatitis. *Ann Intern Med* 83:185, 1975.
488. Weisbrode SE et al: Influence of parathyroid hormone on ultrastructural and enzymatic changes induced by vitamin D in bones of thyroparathyroidectomized rats. *Lab Invest* 30:786, 1974.
489. Wells SA Jr et al: Parathyroid autotransplantation in primary parathyroid hyperplasia. *N Engl J Med* 295:57, 1976.
490. Wells SA Jr et al: Primary hyperparathyroidism. *Curr Probl Surg* 17:398, 1980.

491. Wilkin TJ et al: Post-thyroidectomy hypocalcemia: A feature of the operation or the thyroid disorders? *Lancet* 1:621, 1977.
492. Wolf AW et al: Immobilization hypercalcemia. *Clin Orthop* 118:124, 1976.
493. Won-Lee S et al: 25-Hydroxycholecalciferol to 1,25-dihydroxycholecalciferol: Conversion impaired by systemic metabolic acidosis. *Science* 195:994, 1977.
494. Yasuda K et al: Glucose tolerance and insuline secretion in parathyroid disorders. *N Engl J Med* 292:501, 1975.
495. Yoneda T, Mundy GR: Prostaglandins are necessary for osteoclast activating factor (OAF) production by activated peripheral blood leukocytes. *J Exp Med* 149:279, 1979.
496. Yoneda T, Mundy GR: Monocytes regulate osteoclast activating factor production by releasing prostaglandins. *J Exp Med* 150:338, 1979.
497. Young MM, Nordin BEC: Effects of natural and artificial menopause on plasma and urinary calcium and phosphorus. *Lancet* 2:118, 1967.
498. Zawada ET Jr et al: Management of hypercalcemia. *Postgrad Med* 66:105, 1979.
499. Zawada ET Jr et al: Causes of hypercalcemia. *Postgrad Med* 66:91, 1979.
500. Zenser TV, Davis BB: Effects of calcium on prostaglandin E_2 synthesis by rat inner medullary slices. *Am J Physiol* 235:F213, 1978.
501. Zidar BL et al: Acute myeloblastic leukemia and hypercalcemia. A case of probable ectopic parathyroid hormone production. *N Engl J Med* 297:692, 1976.
502. Zimmerman J et al: Normocalcemia in a hypoparathyroid patient with sarcoidosis: Evidence for parathyroid-hormone-independent synthesis of 1,25-dihydroxyvitamin D. *Ann Intern Med* 98:338, 1983.
503. Zuckerman EC, Glaser GH: Anticonvulsive action of increased calcium concentration in cerebrospinal fluid. *Arch Neurol* 29:245, 1973.

CHAPTER • 33

Hypophosphatemia and hyperphosphatemia: clinical and pathophysiologic aspects

Barton S. Levine • Charles R. Kleeman

HYPOPHOSPHATEMIA

THE EVOLUTION OF HYPOPHOSPHATEMIA AND PHOSPHATE DEPLETION AS A MAJOR CLINICAL ENTITY

The earliest description of the potential hazards of hypophosphatemia in man may have been provided by Joseph Flavius when he described the horrors of the siege of Jerusalem. "Some of the deserters . . . fled to the Romans. Their fate was worse than if they had stayed in the city and the hunger they had left behind was as they discovered less lethal than the plenty that the Romans provided. They arrived blown up by starvation as if by dropsy, then stuffed their empty bellies non-stop till they burst—except for those who were wise enough to restrain their appetite and take the unaccustomed food a little at a time."[164]

In more recent times, detailed descriptions of clinical phosphorus depletion were provided by veterinarians studying the disease in livestock.[17,86,104] Early hypophosphatemia in livestock was followed by decreased appetite, weight, and milk production and by infertility or breeding difficulties. When phosphorus deficiency became chronic, the animals suffered from muscle stiffness, joint swelling, osteomalacia, and, in some studies, severe muscle weakness and inability to walk. The mortality rate was high; over a 40-month period, 66 percent of the cattle not supplemented with bone feed died, whereas only 9 percent of their supplemented mates succumbed.[104] Causes of death included cachexia and fractures. Chronic borderline phosphorus deficiency resulted in the more subtle manifestation of growth retardation.

Progressive difficulty in walking was reported in young rats fed a phosphate-deficient diet.[86] Initial slow growth was followed by loss of weight and, finally, death. Other manifestations included cyanosis, swelling of the extremities, priapism, polydipsia, and increased stool bulk. Phosphorus deficiency in growing pigs led to "chronic diffuse nephritis of parenchymatous type" and "widely distended uriniferous tubules with flattened epithelial cells."[86,104]

Human beings rarely develop spontaneous phosphorus depletion. Large populations in Europe were deprived of phosphorus during World War II. During the five years of German occupation in France, phosphorus use by French farmers was reduced to one-fifth of what it had been before the war. The supply of phosphorus in the immediate postwar period remained low because of transport difficulties. Large tracts of French soil were completely deprived of phosphorus fertilizers between 1943 and 1947. The incidence of bone fractures, dental decay, vertebral decalcifications, and spinal curvature markedly increased. Such disorders became far less common after 1947, when phosphate-containing fertilzers once again became plentiful.

HYPOPHOSPHATEMIA, DIETARY PHOSPHATE DEPRIVATION, AND PHOSPHORUS DEPLETION

It is important to distinguish between hypophosphatemia, phosphorus deprivation, and phosphorus depletion. *Hypophosphatemia* simply means that serum phosphorus concentration is below the range found in the normal population. As discussed in a subsequent section, there are myriad situations whereby hypophosphatemia may occur in the absence of phosphorus depletion or deprivation.

Phosphorus deprivation is the omission of phosphorus from the diet. This should be differentiated from *complete starvation*, which is total caloric deprivation. Starvation leads to a catabolic state with loss of water, nitrogen, potassium, phosphorus, and magnesium from cells in a proportional manner. The phosphorus content of the remaining tissue would be expected to be normal. The consequences of acute dietary phosphorus deprivation were described by Dominguez and coworkers in healthy volunteers fed a low-phosphate diet.[97] Urinary phosphate disappeared after 12 to 24 h, with a marked hypercalciuria and magnesuria apparent at 24 to 36 h (Figs. 33-1 to 33-5). Serum magnesium decreased in 24 to 48 h, without a significant change in serum calcium concentration. These changes could be reversed by ingestion of a normal-phosphate diet. The biochemical changes of acute dietary phosphate deprivation (skeletal and muscular changes) are similar to the phosphate depletion syndrome, without the cellular abnormalities.

Phosphorus depletion indicates a state in which a specific reduction in body phosphorus stores occurs, or in which new protoplasm is formed without adequate phosphate. The distinction between phosphorus deprivation and phosphorus depletion is important because many changes attributed to phosphorus depletion may in fact develop within hours of selective removal of phosphorus from the diet—that is, long before net phosphorus loss from the body could have taken place.

CLASSIFICATION AND INCIDENCE OF HYPOPHOSPHATEMIA

Hypophosphatemia may be moderate, arbitrarily defined as a serum phosphorus level of 1.0 to 2.5 mg/100 ml (see the Appendix to this chapter for conversion to m*M* and meq); or severe, defined as a serum phosphorus level below 1.0 mg/100 ml.

The degree of hypophosphatemia on a daily or chronic basis cannot be established on the basis of a single plasma sample. When Portale and coworkers[266] measured serum phosphorus in normal subjects throughout the day, the levels were low in the morning following the overnight fast and reached a nadir by 11 A.M. Levels then rose to a plateau at 4 P.M. They increased further during the evening and reached a peak value at 1 A.M. With phosphate depletion of 10 days, fasting serum phosphate was lower than with the normal intake of phosphate; but the difference was most dramatic at 4 P.M., when serum phosphate was actually lower than the fasting values. Thus, the degree of hypophosphatemia may fluctuate during the day and may not be reflected by a single fasting blood specimen (Fig. 33-6).

Hypophosphatemia is relatively common in the hospital setting.[142] In a retrospective study of a large general hospital population the incidence of hypophosphatemia was approximately 0.4 percent; 20 percent of the cases of hypophosphatemia were severe (defined as a serum phos-

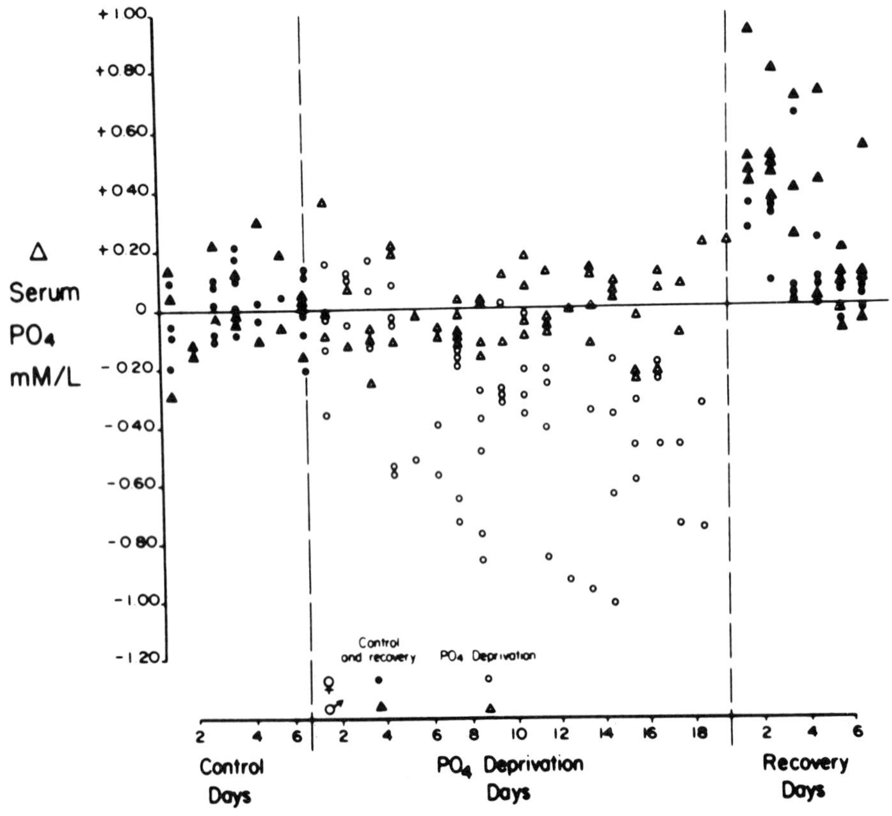

FIGURE 33-1 • Changes in serum phosphorus concentration in normal volunteers during pretreatment period, dietary phosphorus deprivation, and recovery phase. (From Dominguez JH et al: *J. Clin Endocrinol Metab* 48:1056, 1976, with permission.)

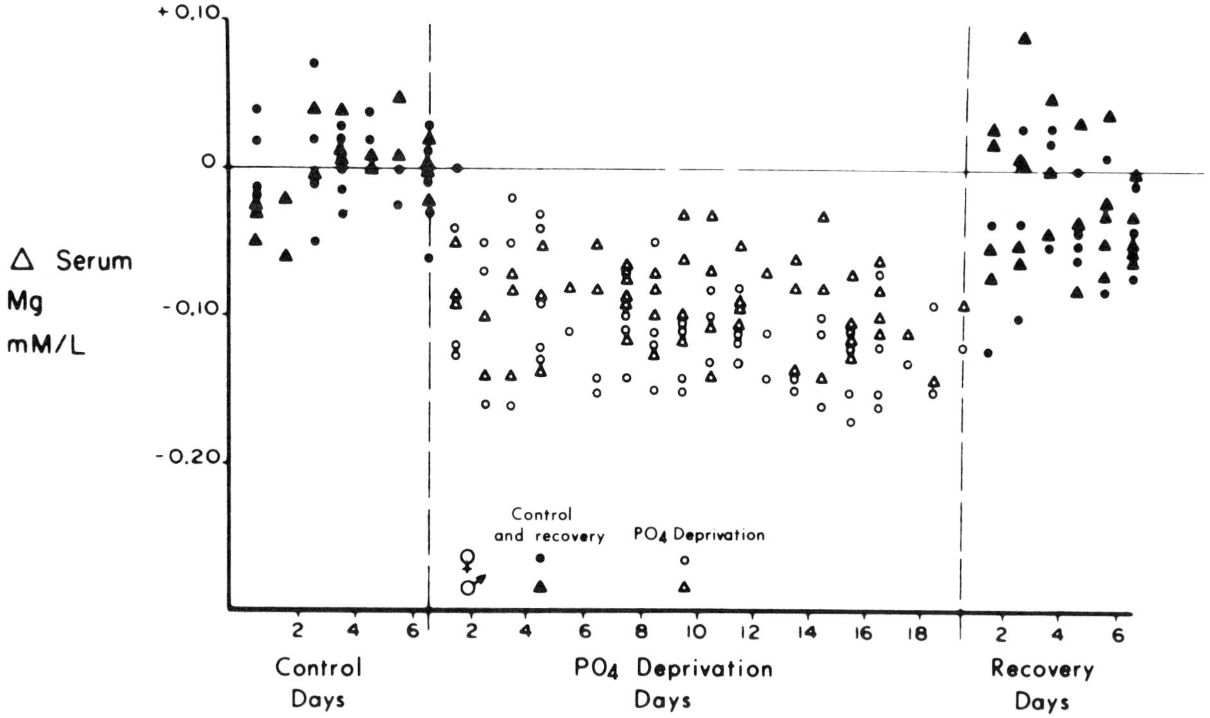

FIGURE 33-2 • Changes in serum magnesium concentration in normal volunteers during pretreatment period, dietary phosphorus deprivation, and recovery phase. (From Dominguez JH et al: *J Clin Endocrinol Metab* 48:1056, 1976, with permission.)

FIGURE 33-3 • Changes in urinary excretion of phosphorus in normal volunteers during pretreatment period, dietary phosphorus deprivation, and recovery phase. Triangles, males; circles, females. (From Dominguez, JH et al: *J Clin Endocrinol Metab* 48:1056, 1976, with permission.)

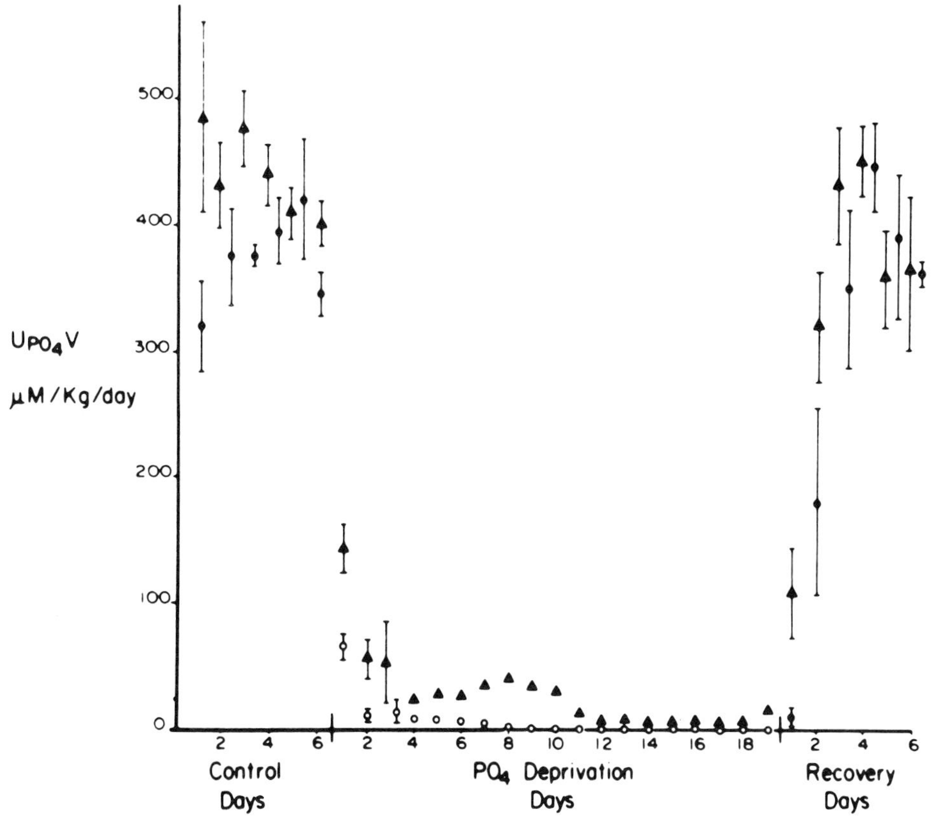

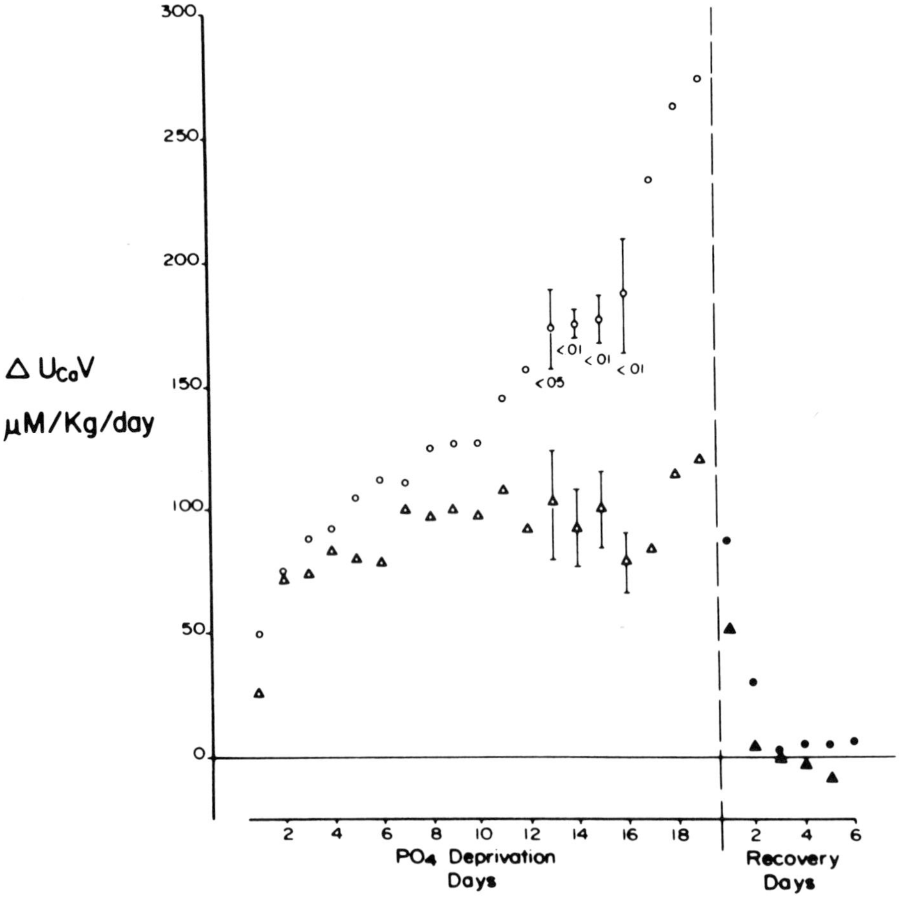

FIGURE 33-4 • Changes in urinary calcium excretion in normal volunteers during dietary phosphorus deprivation and recovery phase. Triangles, males; circles, females. (From Dominguez JH et al: *J Clin Endicrinol Metab* 48:1056, 1976, with permission.)

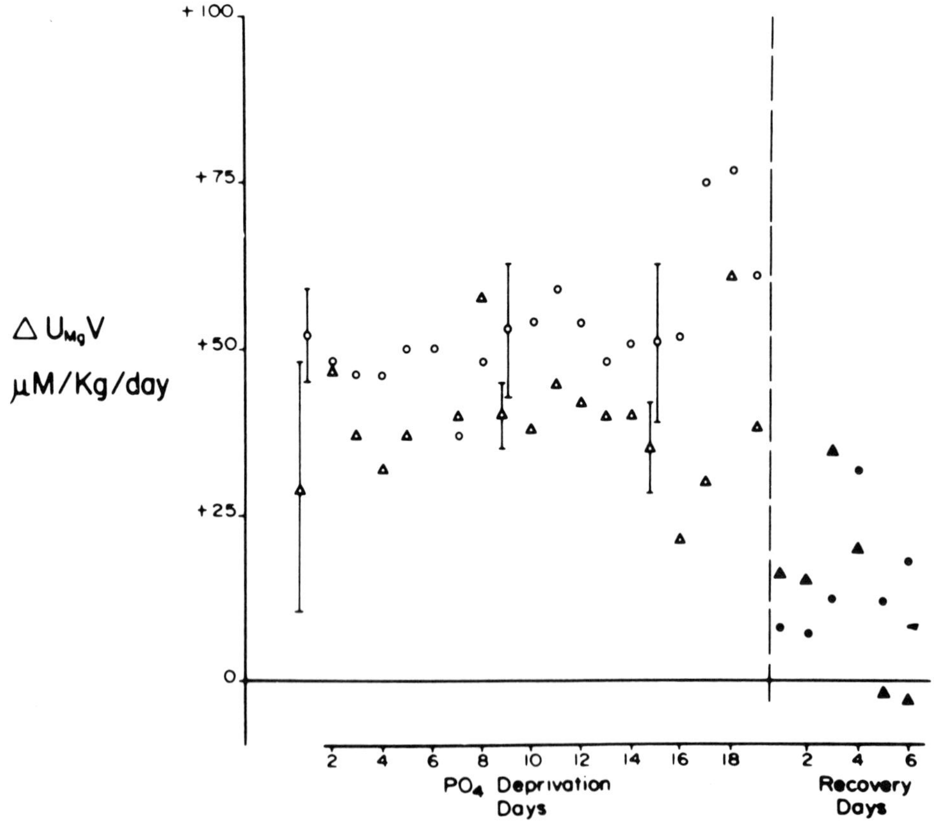

FIGURE 33-5 • Changes in urinary magnesium excretion in normal volunteers during dietary phosphate deprivation and recovery phase. Triangles, males; circles, females. (From Dominguez JH et al: *J Clin Endocrinol Metab* 48:1056, 1976, with permission.)

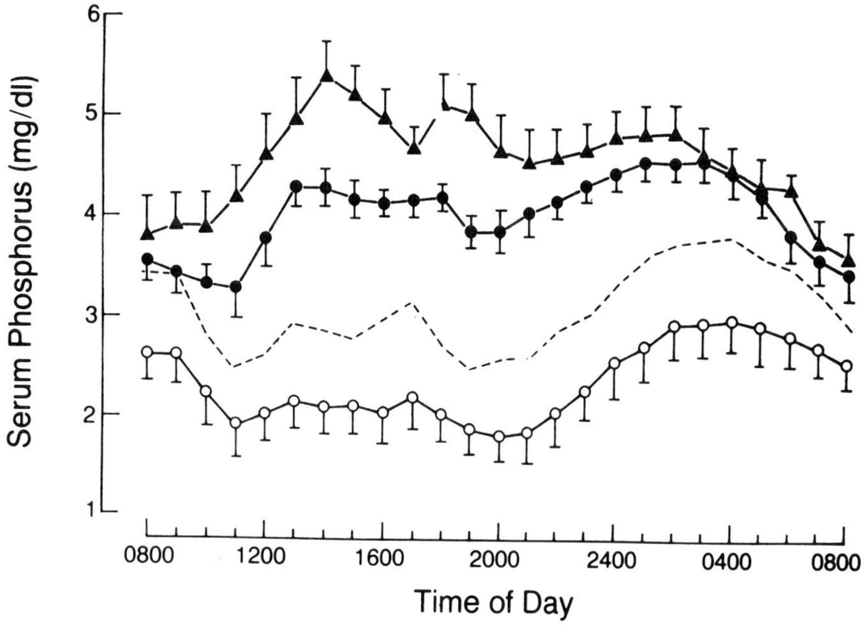

FIGURE 33-6 • The effect of dietary phosphorus on serum phosphorus concentration in normal males. (●) = serum phosphorus after receiving normal phosphorus intake for 9 days; (--) = serum phosphorus after receiving restricted intake of phosphorus (<500 mg/day) for 1 day; (○) = serum phosphorus after receiving restricted intake of phosphorus for 10 days; (▲) = serum phosphorus after dietary phosphorus supplementation (3000 mg/day) for 10 days. Values are mean ± sem. (From Portale A et al: *J Clin Invest* 80:1149, 1987, by copyright permission of the American Society of Clinical Investigation).

phate level below 1.0 mg/100 ml.[142] Similar data were obtained in a prospective screening of more than 16,000 blood samples in a general hospital where the incidence of severe hypophosphatemia (defined as a serum phosphate level below, or equal to, 1.0 mg/100 ml) was 0.22 percent.[72]

CAUSES OF HYPOPHOSPHATEMIA

There are three basic mechanisms underlying the development of hypophosphatemia and/or phosphate-depletion: (1) decreased gastrointestinal absorption of phosphorus, due either to the absence of dietary phosphorus or to decreased phosphate absorption; (2) a net flux of phosphate into non-extracellular sites; and (3) renal loss of phosphate, or loss through extracorporeal dialysis. Either singly or in various combinations, these three mechanisms are responsible for the hypophosphatemia occurring in myriad situations (Table 33-1 and Fig. 33-7). In the absence of at least one of these basic mechanisms a spurious (pseudo-) hypophosphatemia should be suspected when one is confronted with a "low" serum phosphorus measurement.

Pseudohypophosphatemia

Pseudohypophosphatemia may occur in patients receiving large doses of mannitol.[98,106] Mannitol binds to the molybdate used in the colorimetric assay for phosphorus,

TABLE 33-1 • **Clinical conditions associated with hypophosphatemia**

Moderate
Renal phosphate loss
Hyperparathyroidism
Sodium bicarbonate infusion
Volume expansion
Hypokalemia
Hypomagnesemia
Corticosteriod administration
Diuretic therapy
Renal tubular defects (acquired and congenital)
Gastrointestinal phosphate loss
Malabsorption syndromes
Vitamin D deficiency
Shifts of phosphorus from blood to soft tissue and bone
Gram-negative bacteremia
Salicylate poisoning
Acute gout
Fructose or glucose administration
Insulin administration
Excess catecholamine secretion
Severe
Chronic alcoholism
Alcohol withdrawal
Excessive use of pharmacologic phosphate binders
Uncontrolled diabetic ketoacidosis
Hyperalimentation
Respiratory alkalosis
Excess catecholamine secretion

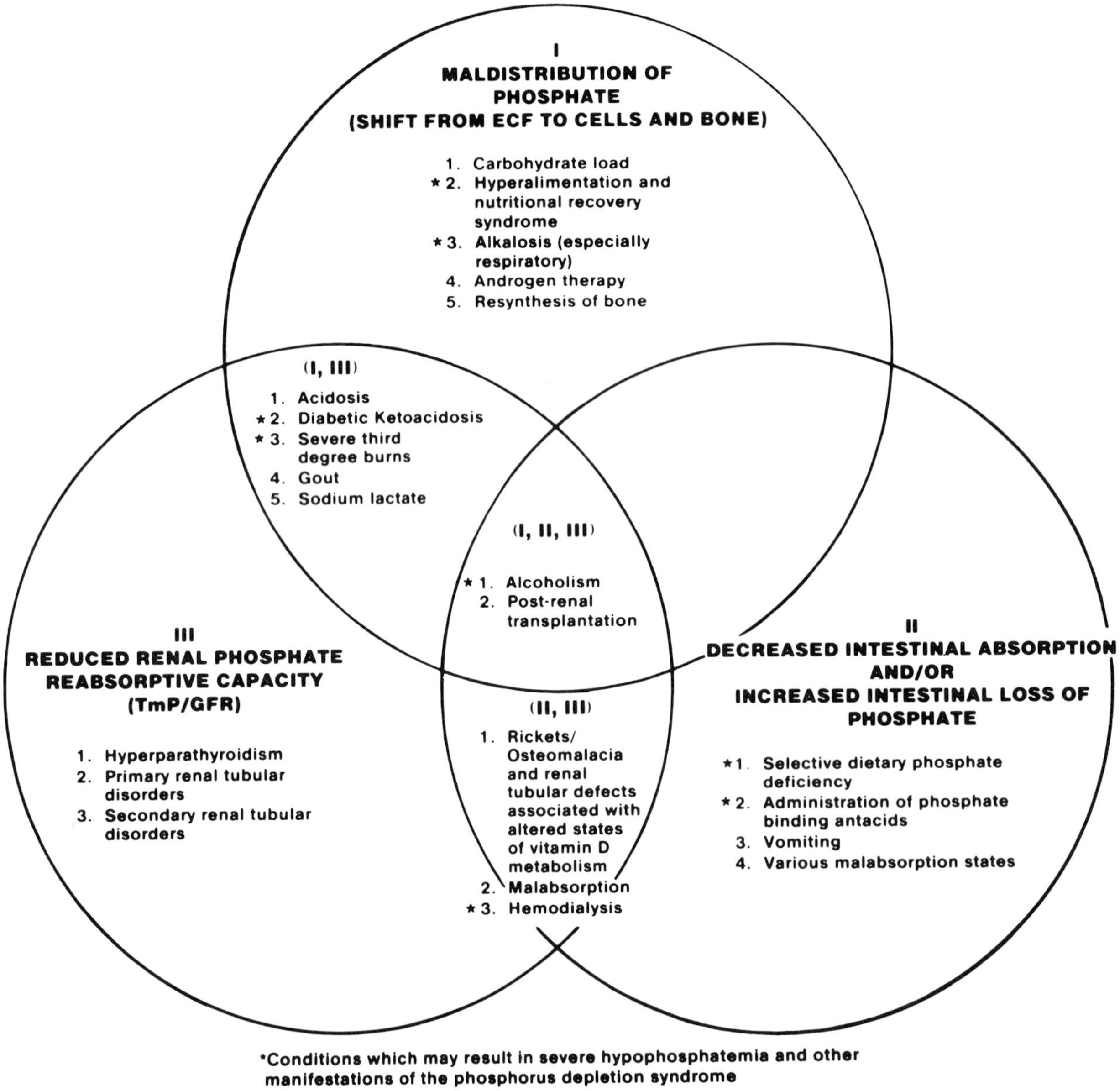

FIGURE 33-7 • Clinical disorders associated with hypophosphatemia, classified according to mechanism. (From Lee DBN et al: Disorders of phosphorus metabolism, in Bronner F, Coburn JW (eds): *Disorders of Mineral Metabolism*, New York, Academic Press, 1981, vol III, p 284. Used by permission.)

resulting in a falsely low value. This tends to occur in assays using relatively low concentrations of molybdate.

Hypophosphatemia caused by redistribution of phosphorus

Redistribution of phosphorus from the extracellular space into cells and bone is a frequent cause of hypophosphatemia and may occur by various mechanisms including: elevated levels of insulin and/or glucose; elevations in circulating catecholamine levels; respiratory alkalosis; increased cell production or anabolism; and rapid bone remineralization.

Insulin/glucose

There are several clinical situations whereby increased glucose loads or elevated insulin levels may produce hypophosphatemia. In several large surveys, a common contributing factor to acute hypophosphatemia in hospitalized patients, particularly alcoholics, was the intravenous administration of glucose-containing solutions.[29] A lesser effect has been observed following the oral intake of a carbohydrate load.[11] The use of glucose-insulin-potassium infusions to prevent myocardial ischemia invariably produces hypophosphatemia, which may be severe.[226] Plasma insulin may increase with quinine infusions and may contribute to the hypophosphatemia reported to occur in patients suffering from malaria.[207] Whatever the cause, elevated levels of insulin promote the transfer of both glucose and phosphate into skeletal muscle and liver. As one might expect, glucose-induced hypophosphatemia is diminished in diabetics and in patients with severe muscle disease.[82,118]

The rapid infusion of fructose is even more pernicious than that of glucose, since it may effect severe degrees of hypophosphatemia while also reducing the intracellular content of inorganic phosphate; depletion of the intracellular nucleotide pool results.[34] The rapid intracellular phosphorylation of fructose coupled with the relatively slow dephosphorylation of fructose-1-phosphate acts to "fix" free cytosolic phosphorus.[34]

Cell growth

Situations in which cell growth or repletion of cell phosphate stores is enhanced may produce significant hypophosphatemia. Profound, and sometimes fatal, hypophosphatemia can develop in animals and humans receiving total parenteral nutrition (TPN) when the hyperalimentation fluid has not been sufficiently supplemented with phosphate[294,295] (see Chap. 44). Rapid refeeding of severely starved prisoners of war has elicited a similar response. The morbidity of this "nutritional recovery syndrome" was reduced by replacing simple carbohydrates with skim milk. Skim milk is rich in phosphorus and potassium, suggesting that these supplements are important during the refeeding period.[234,310] More recently, hypophosphatemia has been associated with refeeding of patients suffering from anorexia nervosa.[78] Anabolic steroids may have a similar effect by stimulating cell growth.

Hypophosphatemia may occur with rapidly growing tumors such as Burkitt's lymphoma[334] and hairy cell leukemia; in the latter case, the hypophosphatemia may resolve with splenectomy, lending support to the postulate that rapidly dividing leukemic cells may produce hypophosphatemia.[23]

Bone mineralization

Incorporation of phosphate into bone in the "hungry bone syndrome" may lead to a decrease in serum phosphorus. This may occur following parathyroidectomy in patients with end-stage renal disease, although frank hypophosphatemia is uncommon. The more severe the preoperative hyperphosphatemia, the greater the decrease in serum phosphorus after surgery. Farrington and coworkers studied 13 patients with chronic renal failure who developed severe hypophosphatemia 3 to 52 weeks after parathyroidectomy.[112] Before surgery, patients who went on to develop postparathyroidectomy hypophosphatemia had higher alkaline phosphatase activity and greater bone resorption activity, as measured by iliac crest bone biopsy, than patients who remained normophosphatemic after parathyroidectomy.

Several possible mechanisms underlie the postoperative decrease in plasma phosphorus concentration. Mobilization of bone phosphorus is reduced because of surgical reduction in circulating parathyroid hormone (PTH). Increased accretion of phosphate by healing bone may also occur. In patients developing hypophosphatemia while receiving dialysis, other factors may also be important. Phosphate-binding antacids, low dietary phosphate intake, repeated dialysis with phosphate-free dialysate, and reduced absorption of phosphate due to the use of oral calcium supplements may all play roles.

Chronic hypophosphatemia after parathyroidectomy may lead to delayed healing of bone lesions. Therefore, careful postoperative monitoring of plasma phosphate and calcium concentrations is necessary in these patients so that appropriate treatment may be instituted. In many patients, when tissue and/or bone demands are great, addition of phosphate to the dialysis fluid does not prevent persistent hypophosphatemia, and oral phosphate supplements may be necessary.

Respiratory alkalosis

A common denominator of many of the clinical situations associated with hypophosphatemia, such as sepsis, alcoholism, pancreatitis, salicylate intoxication, and gout, is an associated respiratory alkalosis. Respiratory alkalosis can produce severe hypophosphatemia. Mosteller and Tuttle documented serum phosphorus concentrations as low as 0.3 mg/100 ml and the virtual disappearance of phosphorus from the urine in normal subjects with acute respiratory alkalosis.[242] In contrast, similar degrees of metabolic alkalosis only modestly reduced serum phosphorus concentration, from 3.5 to 3.0 mg/100 ml.[242] Although the mechanism underlying the effect of respiratory alkalosis is unknown, it probably results from the stimulation of glycolysis by the alkaline intracellular pH. The formation of phosphorylated intermediates increases, thereby drawing more phosphorus into cells; hypophosphatemia results. In hyperventilated dogs, development of acute hypophosphatemia was associated with marked increases in skeletal muscle glucose-6-phosphate, total phosphorus, and inorganic phosphorus content[46]—changes consistent with increased skeletal muscle glycolytic activity and increased incorporation of phosphorus into phosphorylated organic intermediates (Figs. 33-8 and 33-9).

The more profound effect of respiratory alkalosis on serum phosphorus, compared with that of metabolic alkalosis, suggests that an increase in intracellular pH is a critical factor in producing the hypophosphatemia. Because carbon dioxide and carbonic acid penetrate cell membranes more readily than does bicarbonate, for a

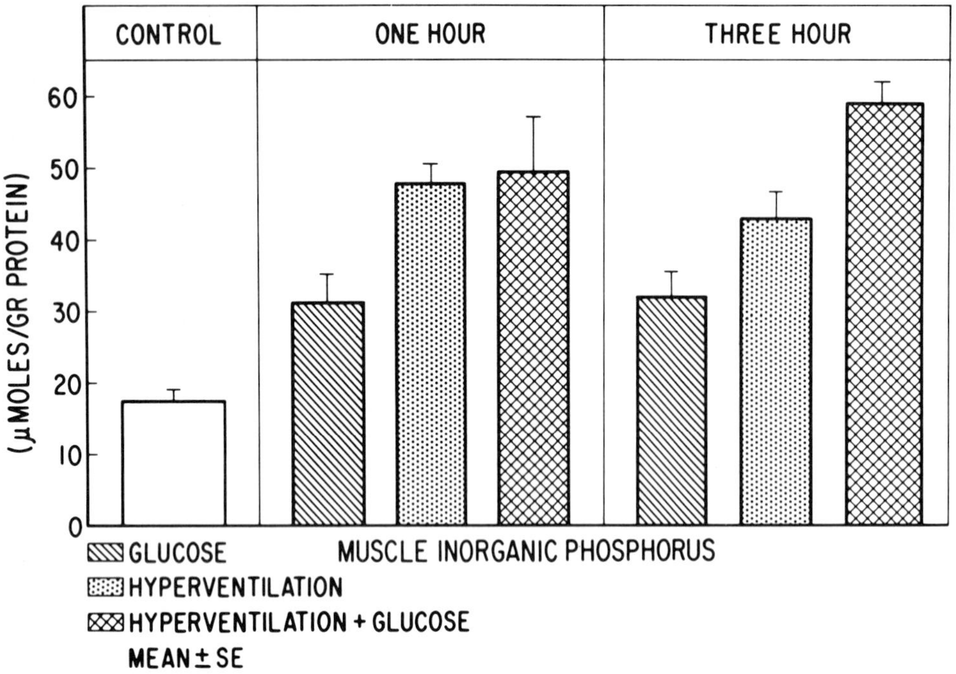

FIGURE 33-8 • Changes in skeletal muscle inorganic phosphorus content during experimental hyperventilation in dogs. (From Brautbar N et al: *Mineral Electrolyte Metab* 9:115, 1983, with permission.)

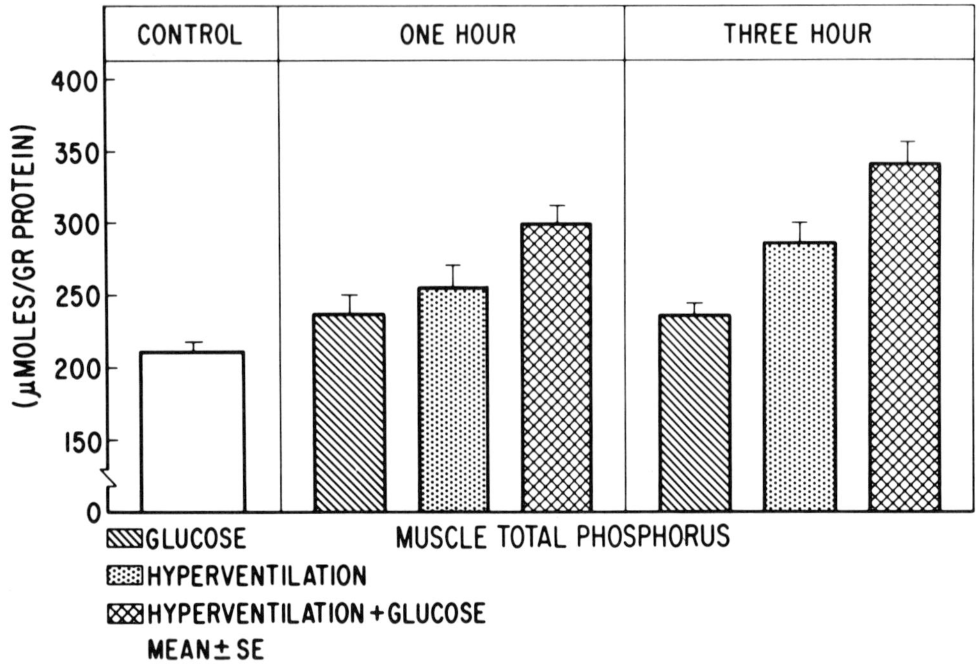

FIGURE 33-9 • Changes in skeletal muscle total phosphorus content during experimental hyperventilation in dogs. (From Brautbar N et al: *Mineral Electrolyte Metab* 9:115, 1983, with permission.)

given extracellular pH, respiratory alkalosis raises intracellular pH more than similar degrees of metabolic alkalosis.[279]

That intracelllular pH, rather than extracellular pH, is important is further suggested by the hypophosphatemia observed in patients with respiratory failure occurring concomitantly with resolution of their respiratory acidosis. Thus, hypophosphatemia, at times severe, has been reported to occur following mechanical ventilation of patients suffering from severe asthmatic attacks or decompensated chronic obstructive pulmonary disease (Fig. 33-10). The patients presented with significant respiratory acidosis and, at times, with hyperphosphatemia. However, after initiation of mechanical ventilation a significant hypophosphatemia ensued despite the fact that arterial pH was never above normal.[182,303] These studies suggest that a high extracellular pH, per se, is not a prerequisite for developing hypophosphatemia, and emphasize the importance of changes in intracellular pH and its impact on cell glycolysis.

A significant incidence of hypophosphatemia occurs in patients suffering from panic disorder; this may result from the intermittent hypocapnia occurring in at least a subgroup of these patients.[20,135] The physiologic significance of the low serum phosphorus in this disorder is speculative. Gorman and coworkers[135] have hypothesized that hypophosphatemia may have value in predicting which patients suffering from panic disorder will have a panic response to lactate infusions. Other mechanisms postulated to produce the hypophosphatemia in this setting are elevated catecholamine levels and abnormalities in ionized plasma calcium with resultant increases in PTH and phosphaturia.[1]

The hypophosphatemia occurring with gram-negative bacteremia and acute salicylate intoxication may be the result of the associated hyperventilation. In addition, hyperventilation may develop as a complication of severe phosphate depletion per se, further aggravating the already profound hypophosphatemia.

Hypophosphatemia may complicate acute pancreatitis, usually in association with respiratory alkalosis. However, hypophosphatemia has also been reported to occur with acute idiopathic pancreatitis in the absence of respiratory alkalosis[184]—perhaps because of increased catecholamine discharge, alterations in circulating insulin or glucagon, or intravenous administration of glucose.

Catecholamines

Epinephrine may play an important role as a mediator of redistributional hypophosphatemia.[35] Insulin-induced hypoglycemia, a potent stimulus to endogenous epinephrine secretion, decreased serum phosphorus concentrations in six healthy volunteers by 0.9 ± 0.1 mg/100 ml while causing lesser increments in concentrations of serum magnesium and total and ionized calcium. Plasma immunoreactive parathyroid hormone (iPTH) concentration decreased and plasma immunoreactive calcitonin (iCT) concentration increased in a predictable fashion. To determine whether these effects of insulin required catecholamine mediators, epinephrine was infused over 60 min without insulin in doses effecting steady-state plasma epinephrine concentrations of 52 to 945 pg/ml (levels spanning the physiologic range). Serum ionized calcium, iPTH, and iCT concentrations were unaltered by these physiologic elevations. The catecholamine infusion, however, resulted in dose-dependent decrements in serum phosphate concentration; a fall of 0.6 ± 0.1 mg/100 ml was noted at the highest epinephrine infusion rate. The plasma threshold concentration of epinephrine for this hypophosphatemic effect was approximately 50 to 100 pg/ml. Thus, the sensitivity of the hypophosphatemic response to epinephrine is comparable to that of the cardiac chronotropic, systolic pressor, and lipolytic responses to epinephrine, and considerably greater than that of the diastolic depressor, glycogenolytic, glycolytic, and ketogenic responses to the hormone in human beings. In view of its rapidity and the absence of associated phosphaturia, the authors attributed epinephrine's hypophosphatemic effect to a net shift of phosphate from the extracellular to the intracellular compartment.[35] This effect was obviously not mediated by PTH or calcitonin (CT). Subsequent studies by Ljunghall and coworkers[213] demonstrated that the hypophosphatemic effect of epinephrine was blunted with the administration of propranolol, suggesting that beta-adrenergic stimulation was important in the hypophosphatemic response to catecholamines.

These studies have important clinical implications and may explain, in part, the hypophosphatemia of sepsis, acute myocardial infarction, toxic shock syndrome, thyrotoxicosis, burn injury, and other conditions associ-

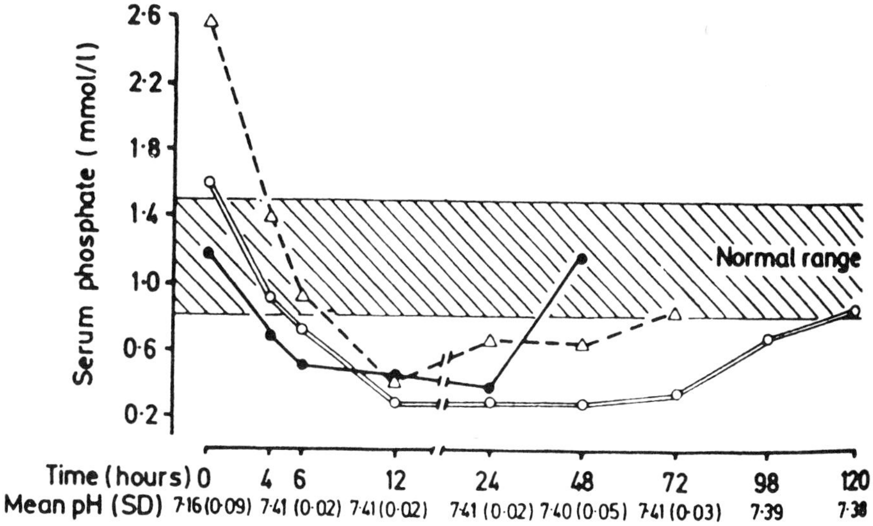

FIGURE 33-10 • Changes in serum phosphate in three patients with chronic obstructive pulmonary disease and acute respiratory acidosis after the initiation of mechanical ventilation. (From Storm TL: *Br Med J* 289:456, 1984, with permission.)

ated with increased epinephrine release. In thyrotoxic patients, preoperative hypophosphatemia was blunted by betablockers; and in a parallel study of experimental animals, the first phase of posttraumatic hypophosphatemia was prevented by the beta-blocking agent propranolol.[41,217]

Excess catecholamines may produce hypophosphatemia in other clinical settings. Normally serum phosphate increases with exercise, particularly in runners in excellent condition—presumably because of lactic acidosis or, perhaps, a failure of oxidative phosphorylation. However, hypophosphatemia has been observed in poorly conditioned runners who have collapsed after a "fun run."[80] A shift of phosphate intracellularly has been postulated as the mechanism for the hypophosphatemia, this may result from an increase in catecholamine release and the relative $beta_2$-selectivity of epinephrine.[56]

The potential role of catecholamines in the development of hypophosphatemia is further illustrated by clinical situations involving the administration of sympathomimetic agents. Both hypophosphatemia and hypokalemia have been reported to follow overdoses of sympathomimetic agents.[229] Nebulized salbutamol, a sympathomimetic agent, may produce a fall in plasma phosphate within 20 min;[56] while in patients wih respiratory failure, plasma levels of theophylline correlated with the development of hypophosphatemia following treatment of respiratory failure.[38]

Thus, epinephrine may be a key mediator of hypophosphatemia. However, studies with alpha-adrenergic blockers are still required in order to define the full spectrum of catecholamine effects of phosphate transport.

Hypophosphatemia caused by reduced intestinal phosphorus absorption

Hypophosphatemia due to a selective deficiency in dietary phosphorus is rare in the clinical setting. Low-birth-weight infants may develop hypophosphatemia when fed human milk rather than cow's milk. The development of low serum phosphorus correlated with lower vitamin D intakes during this period.[143]

A more common cause of decreased intestinal absorption of phosphate is excessive use of phosphate-binding antacids.[33,216] As described by Lotz and coworkers,[216] phosphate-binding antacids produce a syndrome characterized by severe hypophosphatemia, marked hypophosphaturia, and hypercalciuria. This can occur even in patients with end-stage renal disease, a condition usually characterized by phosphate retention. Signs and symptoms may include muscle weakness, malaise, bone pain, anorexia, and rickets or osteomalacia. The hypophosphatemia need not be severe[237]; often it may be difficult to elicit a history of ingestion of large amounts of phosphate-binding antacids. On the other hand, ingestion of small amounts of antacid (see "Treatment of Hypophosphaturia" below) may have little impact on phosphate balance. Spencer and coworkers found no difference in phosphate balance between a control group and patients on low-dose antacids.[302] Thus, in general, low doses of antacids should be used whenever possible to prevent the development of phosphate depletion.[237,282]

Hypophosphatemia also may develop as a consequence of sustained vomiting or of various malabsorptive diseases, especially when the latter are severe.

Hypophosphatemia caused by phosphaturia

Primary and secondary hyperparathyroidism

Primary and secondary forms of hyperparathyroidism cause hypophosphatemia by impairing renal tubular reabsorption of phosphorus. The mechanisms underlying this effect of PTH are fully discussed in Chap. 12.

Renal tubular dysfunction

Renal phosphate wasting may occur with volume expansion,[212] with Fanconi syndrome,[281] with obstructive uropathy,[109] and during the diuretic phase of acute tubular necrosis. Various drugs may induce renal phosphate wasting. Phosphaturia may result from aggressive doxycyline therapy of SIADH, with acetaminophen poisoning,[162] or following chemotherapy with ifosfamide; the latter has been associated with rickets in children.[246,298]

Diuretics, particularly thiazide diuretics and the newer diuretic indapamide, may produce an increase in the renal clearance of inorganic phosphorus and hypophosphatemia.[158,262] The mechanism may involve a direct effect of the diuretic on distal renal tubular reabsorption of phosphate, as well as changes in potassium homeostasis (see below).

The administration of large doses of estrogens in patients with metastatic prostatic carcinoma have been reported to produce hypophosphatemia.[67,68] Similar observations have been made following mestranol therapy in oophorectomized women.[4] The mechanism appears to be a decrease in renal phosphate reabsorption due to a decrease in the phosphate threshold clearance, or *T*mP/GFR (see Chap. 12). Although plasma levels of calcitriol increase with estrogen administration, recent studies suggest that the hypophosphatemia resulting from estrogen therapy produces the rise in calcitriol, rather than the sterol's causing the hypophosphatemia.[255]

Hypophosphatemia associated with increased renal phosphate clearance has been reported in patients with hypokalemia and potassium depletion.[10] In these patients the serum phosphorus level returns to normal with potassium repletion. Recent studies by Sebastian and coworkers[291] suggest that changes in dietary potassium within the normal range may have an impact on renal phosphate excretion through unknown mechanisms.

Magnesium depletion can also lead to phosphate depletion due to renal phosphate wasting, but hypophosphatemia itself is rare.[174]

Hyperthermia can produce a dramatic lowering of serum phosphorus, which is associated with a decrease in the *T*mP/GFR. The changes in phosphate homeostasis appear to be independent of circulating levels of PTH and arterial carbon dioxide tension.[141]

Oncogenic hypophosphatemia

Hypophosphatemia in the absence of hypercalcemia may occur in association with several different types of tumors, but most commonly with mesenchymal tumors.[3] This syndrome may also occur sporadically,[257,315] in association with fibrous dysplasia and neurofibromatosis,[153] with the sebaceous nevus syndrome,[60] and with melorheostosis,[194] a rare congenital mesenchymal disorder of unknown etiology. The patients develop severe osteomalacia, with muscle weakness, that is often resistant to normal doses of calcitriol. In many of these patients, renal phosphate excretion is high, *T*mP/GFR is low, PTH levels are normal, and calcitriol levels are decreased, despite the low serum phosphorus levels. The clinical findings do not improve with massive doses of vitamin D and phosphate supplements, whereas complete surgical removal of the tumor results in the restoration of normal mineral homeostasis. The low serum concentration of calcitriol and the finding of improvement after administration of calcitriol suggests that production of the compound is impaired. Therefore, therapeutic levels of calcitriol may not be achieved despite large doses of vitamin D_3.[83]

The impairment in calcitriol production may be attributable to elaboration of a humoral substance by the tumor, which then acts on the renal tubular cells to inhibit both calcitriol production and renal tubular phosphate reabsorption; several studies provide support for the existence of such a humoral factor. Thus, phosphaturic activity has been found in saline extracts of such tumors.[14,187,264] Miyauchi and coworkers[232] transplanted a hemangiopericytoma excised from a patient with tumor-induced osteomalacia into mice and noted a marked increase in urinary phosphate excretion. Tumor extracts added to primary cultures of renal tubular cells inhibited renal 25-hydroxyvitamin D_1alpha-hydroxylase activity. The factor(s) responsible for producing the phosphaturia and the suppression of calcitriol levels remains to be identified. Interestingly, transforming growth factor alpha has been shown to inhibit sodium-dependent phosphate uptake by opossum kidney cells in culture via a mechanism independent of that of PTH-related peptide.[260] Whether this factor or a similar growth factor is responsible for the phosphate wasting in oncogenic osteomalacia remains to be determined.

A therapeutic regimen for patients with this syndrome should be designed with several goals in mind: increasing serum phosphate concentration by increasing gastrointestinal absorption; preventing secondary hyperparathyroidism; suppressing PTH, if possible; and providing levels of calcitriol sufficient to promote bone healing. The ideal therapy probably includes the administration of calcitriol, calcium, and phosphate. A combination of 3 μ/day of calcitriol and 2 g/day of oral phosphorus may completely heal the histologic abnormalities.[102] With this regimen, levels of calcitriol increase above normal. For complete healing of bone disease normal levels of serum phosphorus are probably necessary, which in the presence of a renal transport defect may require a marked increase in intestinal phosphate absorption. The therapeutic regimen, therefore, must include both phosphate and large doses of calcitriol.

Hypophosphatemia resulting from more than one mechanism

The etiology of hypophosphatemia is usually multifactorial, particularly in the hospital setting;[142,172] at least two, and often all three, of the basic mechanisms producing hypophosphatemia are present in a given patient.

Metabolic acidosis

The association between acidosis and increased phosphate excretion has long been recognized.[139] Acidosis induces decomposition of intracellular organic compounds with release of inorganic phosphate, which is subsequently excreted in the urine. Furthermore, renal proximal tubular reabsorption of phosphate is decreased. Recent studies have shown that chronic metabolic acidosis inhibits the sodium-dependent phosphate transporter located on the renal proximal tubular brush-border membrane,[169,200] an effect related to elevated levels of glucocorticoids.[36]

The increased net loss of phosphate from cells is sometimes associated with a reduction in GFR, and may actually raise the plasma phosphate level during the acidotic state. During the reparative phase of acidosis cellular organic phosphates are resynthesized, causing extracellular phosphorus to move into cells, resulting in hypophosphatemia. This sequence of hyperphosphatemia on initial presentation and subsequent hypophosphatemia is commonly seen during therapy of patients with previously uncontrolled diabetes mellitus (see below) and in patients with lactic or respiratory acidosis. These examples stress the importance of monitoring serum phosphate levels under these clinical settings to avoid the late complication of severe hypophosphatemia.

It has been known for many decades that diabetics formed the second largest group of hypophosphatemic patients; uncontrolled diabetes mellitus and *diabetic ketoacidosis* cause urinary phosphate wasting and, thus, marked loss of body phosphorus with relatively inadequate phosphorus intake. Serum phosphorus is usually normal when diabetes is adequately controlled.[206] However, hypophosphatemia of varying degrees may develop in patients with uncontrolled diabetes mellitus, especially when the latter is complicated by ketoacidosis.[15,120]

Several mechanisms may underlie the hypophosphatemia in patients with diabetes mellitus. Osmotic diuresis, metabolic acidosis, and insulin therapy may all contribute to the genesis of hypophosphatemia (Fig. 33-11). Total body phosphorus deficit has been estimated in patients with diabetic ketoacidosis by "reverse balance" studies in which the net quantity of phosphorus retained was measured over a period of several weeks. Initial net phosphorus losses were often substantial, ranging up to 400 mmol.

Gout

The hypophosphatemia of untreated gout has also been attributed to respiratory alkalosis produced by pain-induced hyperventilation, and to the reduced ability of renal tubules to reabsorb phosphate.[90] Sodium lactate infusion may cause hypophosphatemia through both reduced phosphate reabsorption, from ECF expansion, and enhanced movement of phosphate into cells. The latter may result from alkalosis consequent to hepatic conversion of lactate into glucose and bicarbonate. The infusion of lactate may induce hyperventilation and respiratory alkalosis in patients suffering from panic disorder, thereby producing hypophosphatemia.

Essential hypertension

A "relative hypophosphatemia" may occur in patients with essential hypertension.[173] Several studies have shown that serum PTH levels are higher in hypertensive than in normotensive subjects and that the degree of elevation may be exacerbated by a high salt intake.[340,341] Circulating catecholamines may be elevated in hypertensive persons and may contribute to the relative hypophosphatemia observed, presumably by shifting phosphate intracellularly.[173] Finally, postprandial levels of insulin may be elevated in hypertensive persons, especially in those who are obese.[276] A higher level of insulin may result in a greater shift of phosphate intracellularly, either directly or by stimulating catecholamine discharge.

Alcoholism

Hypophosphatemia and phosphate depletion commonly develop with chronic alcoholism and with acute alcohol intoxication, delirium tremens, decompensated cirrhosis, and hepatic coma.[119,306] Hypophosphatemia was found during the second to fifth hospital days in 30.4 percent of male alcoholic patients admitted to medical wards, but is only 1.8 percent of matched nonalcoholics.[283] The mechanisms underlying the hypophosphatemia have not been extensively studied; likely possibilities are outlined in Fig. 33-12.[174,227] Possible causes include (1) decreased intestinal phosphate absorption due to diarrhea, vomiting, and routine use of antacids; (2) repeated bouts of β-hydroxybutyric acidosis and lactic acidosis, with loss of organic phosphate from cells and excretion in the urine;

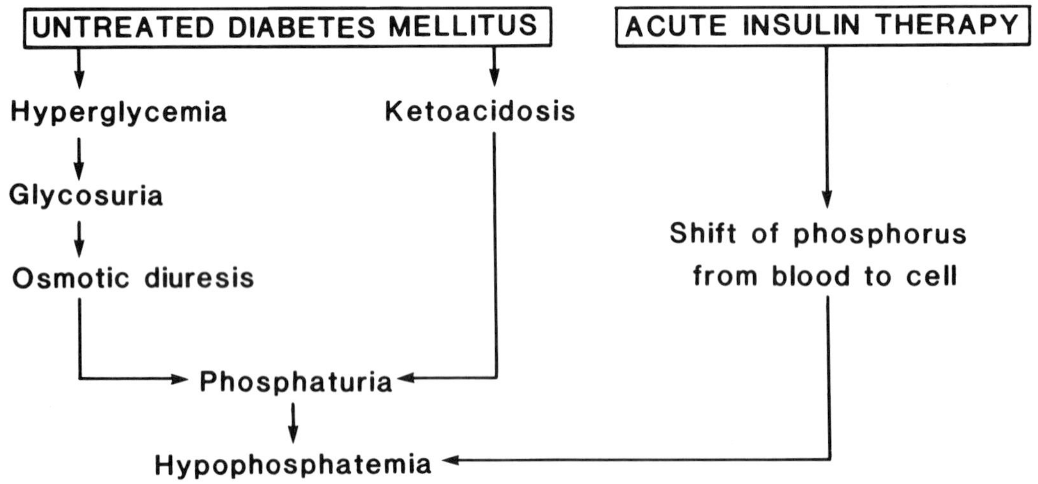

FIGURE 33-11 • Mechanism of hypophosphatemia in patients with untreated, uncontrolled diabetes mellitus. (From Massry SG: *Adv Exp Med Biol* 103:301, 1978, with permission.)

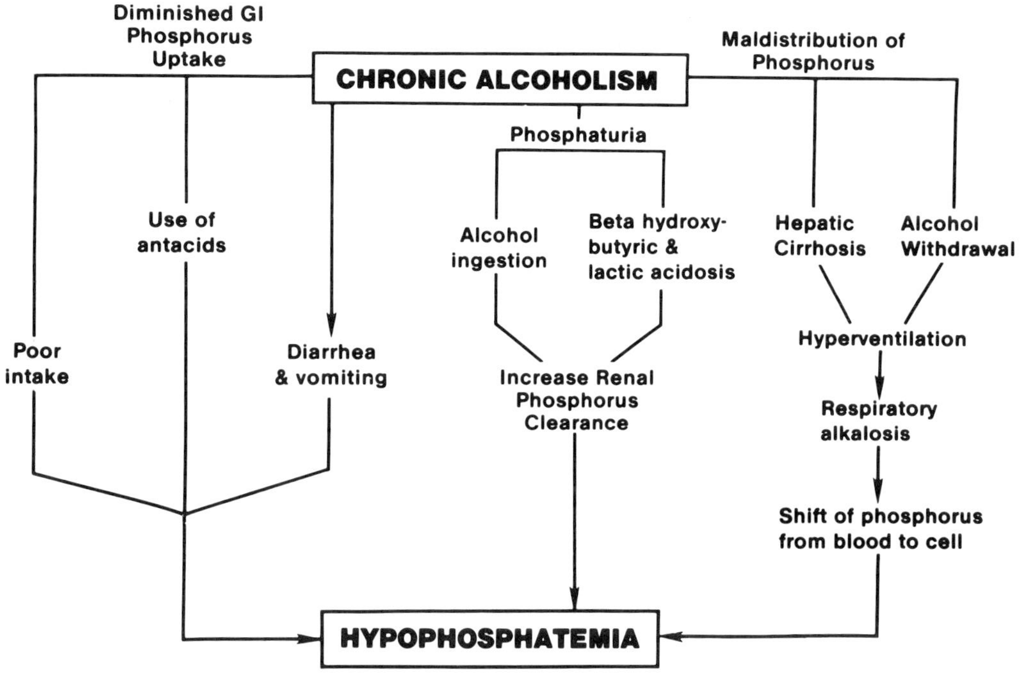

FIGURE 33-12 • Mechanism of hyperphosphatemia in alcoholic patients. (From Massry SG: *Adv Exp Med Biol* 103:301, 1978, with permission.)

(3) migration of phosphate into cells secondary to glucose infusion and respiratory alkalosis; and (4) renal phosphate wasting as a result of tubular dysfunction associated with hypomagnesemia or with alcohol per se.[183]

Surgery

In a hospital survey about 43 percent of the cases of severe hypophosphatemia occurred in the surgical population, particularly in patients undergoing surgical procedures involving the gastrointestinal tract.[142] The decrement in serum phosphate in these patients was thought to be related to a lack of dietary intake of phosphate coupled with the use of glucose-containing intravenous solutions during the postoperative period.

In patients undergoing colorectal surgery, Rasmussen and coworkers[274] found that the mode of administration of intravenous glucose solutions contributed to the degree of hypophosphatemia postoperatively. Hypophosphatemia was less severe when patients received an infusion of 10% glucose over a 5-h period than when they were given a constant infusion of 4% glucose. Although the patients in both treatment groups received the same amount of glucose daily, renal reabsorption of phosphate and *T*mP/GFR were reduced in patients receiving the constant glucose infusion.

Another mechanism that may contribute to hypophosphatemia in the postoperative state is incorporation of phosphate into cells following significant ischemia. Andersen and coworkers[9] noted moderate degrees of hypophosphatemia in patients 2 to 4 days after abdominal aortic bypass surgery. Significant tissue ischemia was induced by cross-clamping the aorta; it was postulated that regeneration of ATP and creatine phosphate in the postischemic period contributed to the development of the hypophosphatemia. Finally, increased catecholamine secretion may also contribute to this postsurgical hypophosphatemia.

Post–renal transplantation

A moderate degree of hypophosphatemia is relatively common following renal transplantation, even with normal allograft function. Garabedian and coworkers reported that 60 percent of children with a transplanted kidney develop hypophosphatemia during the immediate posttransplant period.[125] The hypophosphatemia usually is transient, but may persist.

Posttransplant hypophosphatemia usually is moderate, is well tolerated, and correlates with a tubular phosphate leak and a decreased *T*mP/GFR.[125] Persistence of secondary hyperparathyroidism is a primary contributor to the renal phosphate wasting, since calcium infusions normalize serum phosphate levels and nearly correct the renal excretion of phosphate. Glucocoticoid administration is another contributing factor to the phosphate wasting, particularly during the early period after transplantation;[150] large doses of vitamin D have been advocated to correct the steroid-induced phosphate malabsorption. Interestingly, serum calcitriol levels are often low or "inappropriately" normal in the kidney transplant patients despite their hypophosphatemia. Thus, reduced intestinal absorption of phosphate arising from calcitriol deficiency may conribute to the phosphorus depletion.[101,125,325] Excessive antacid use may also lower the intestinal absorption of phosphate in this setting.

As prolonged hypophosphatemia is a serious risk factor for the development of osteomalacia, it is recommended that the mechanisms be evaluated in each transplant patient and that therapy be planned accordingly.

Burn injury

Severe burn injury is commonly associated with hypophosphatemia, which usually reaches its nadir by the fourth to fifth day after the burn occurs. The hypophosphatemia may contribute to burn-associated fatalities. The mechanism by which the hypophosphatemia develops is not known; several investigators have suggested that respiratory alkalosis secondary to gram-negative septicemia may be a cause. Lennquist and coworkers measured urinary and serum phosphorus levels, blood CT and PTH levels, and urinary epinephrine and norepinephrine levels in 33 patients.[195] In all patients serum phosphorus concentration decreased significantly to 0.74 m*M* (2.3 mg/100 ml) on the fourth postburn day and gradually returned to normal thereafter. The duration of the hypophosphatemia varied from 2 to 10 days, with a mean of 3 days. Serum PTH levels were normal, whereas CT concentration was markedly elevated. Urinary phosphate excretion decreased, reaching its nadir on the seventh day after injury; thereafter, it returned to normal levels. Urinary epinephrine was usually increased, and urinary norepinephrine was markedly elevated. The failure of marked hypophosphatemia to eliminate phosphate from the urine suggests that renal phosphate wasting occurred. The authors attributed this inappropriate phosphaturia to increased circulating CT levels. The roles of respiratory alkalosis, hyperalimentation, and excess catecholamine and cortisol secretion in generating hypophosphatemia in these patients have not been examined; they may well be important contributors.

Vitamin D deficiency

Deficiency of vitamin D is associated with hypophosphatemia and urinary phosphate loss.[236,289] The hallmarks of vitamin D deficiency are reduced intestinal absorption of calcium and reduced ionized calcium concentration. As a result of the decrease in blood ionized calcium, secretion of PTH is increased, producing a decreased *T*mP/GFR and hypophosphatemia. A decrease in intestinal phosphate absorption may also be a contributing factor to the hypophosphatemia, since calcitriol enhances the intestinal absorption of phosphate.[115,204]

Vitamin D-dependent rickets

There are several familial disorders associated with a tubular defect in the reabsorption of phosphate (Table 33-2) and hypophosphatemia.[121] In most of these, abnormal vitamin D metabolism occurs; in which case abnormal intestinal phosphate absorption may contribute to the hypophosphatemia. One such entity, vitamin D-dependent rickets, exists in two forms: type I, in which the production of calcitriol is defective; and type II, in which a tissue resistance to calcitriol exists. Vitamin D-dependent rickets type I represents an inborn error of metabolism. Increased plasma levels of 25-OH-D and decreased levels of calcitriol have been reported by sev-

TABLE 33-2 • Characteristics of familial rickets

	VDDR				
	Type I	Type II	VDRR	HHRH	HBD
Characteristics					
Genetics	Autosomal dominant	Autosomal recessive	X-linked	Autosomal recessive	Autosomal dominant
Radiologic bone disease	+	+	+	+	±
Serum phosphorus	↓	↓	↓	↓	↓
Serum calcium	↓	↓	←→	←→	←→
PTH	↑	↑	←→	↓	←→
Calcitriol	↓	↑	←→ or ↓	↑	?
Urinary calcium	↓	↓	↓	↑	?
Treatment					
Calcitriol	Small	Large	Large	None	Normal
Phosphate	None	None	Yes	Yes	No

VDDR = vitamin D-dependent rickets; VDRR = vitamin D-resistant rickets; HHRH = hereditary hypophosphatemic hypercalciuric rickets; HBD = hypophosphatemic bone disease.

eral investigators. The observation that only physiologic doses of calcitriol are needed to effect rapid correction of the biochemical abnormalities, while pharmacologic doses of vitamin D_3 or D_2 or 25-OH-D are required to achieve therapeutic responses, is compatible with the notion that type I vitamin D-dependent rickets is due to an inborn error in the conversion of 25-OH-D to calcitriol.

In contrast to type I, in type II vitamin D-dependent rickets circulating levels of calcitriol are elevated. The defect in type II vitamin D-dependent rickets appears to be an end-organ resistance to calcitriol. In a study of seven related families suffering from this syndrome, Malloy and coworkers[223] demonstrated that skin fibroblasts and Epstein-Barr virus-transformed cells of affected family members failed to bind radiolabeled calcitriol and had undetectable vitamin D receptors as well as undetectable messanger RNA for such receptors; obligate heterozygotes had half the expected number of receptors. The data suggest that a point mutation has occurred within the steroid-binding domain of the receptor.

Hydroxylation defects may occur in type II patients. Zerwekh and coworkers described a 28-year-old patient with hypocalcemia, hypophosphatemia, secondary hyperparathyroidism, and biopsy-proven osteomalacia with no response to vitamin D.[342] Treatment with 25-$(OH)_2D_3$ corrected the hypocalcemia, hyperparathyroidism, and osteomalacia; yet circulating levels of calcitriol were persistantly elevated. The decreased intestinal absorption of calcium and the osteomalacia suggested that end-organ refractoriness to calcitriol existed. In addition to the end-organ resistance to calcitriol, the patient displayed impaired hydroxylation of vitamin D to 25-OH-D_3. Since the osteomalacia responded to therapy with 25-OH-D_3, part of the bone disease seems to have resulted from the 25-hydroxylation defect. Liberman and coworkers described a patient with rickets resistant to the administration of high doses of vitamin D, calcitriol, and 1α-OH-D_3.[209] The high circulating levels of calcitriol and the presence of osteomalacia and hypocalcemia pointed to end-organ resistance to the action of calcitriol. Blood levels of 24,25-$(OH)_2D$ were low and the patient responded to the administration of 24,25-$(OH)_2D$, conditions compatible with a defect in the synthesis of this metabolite. Thus, patients with a clinical syndrome similar to vitamin D-dependent rickets but with elevated levels of calcitriol and multiple defects in synthesis of vitamin D metabolites are part of the clinical spectrum of this syndrome. The treatment of choice for these patients will be to supplement the missing vitamin D metabolite(s)—namely, calcitriol or 24,25-$(OH)_2D_3$, or both.

Familial X-linked hypophosphatemic rickets

Familial X-linked hypophosphatemic rickets (FHR), or vitamin D-resistant rickets, is characterized by a low serum phosphorus concentration, decreased TmP/GFR, decreased intestinal absorption of calcium and phosphate, growth retardation, and rickets or osteomalacia of variable severity. Genetic mapping of families suffering from the disorder suggests that the gene responsible for it is located on the distal short arm of the X chromosome.[221]

The pathogenesis of this disorder is incompletely understood. The renal phosphorus threshold is invariably low; current evidence implicates a defect in proximal tubule phosphate transport. Despite the hypophosphatemia, the cardinal features of phosphorus depletion—myopathy and bone resorption with hypercalciuria—are not seen in FHR.[272,308] The reasons for the absence of symptoms and signs are unclear. Recent studies have found concentrations of calcitriol to be normal or low-normal,[43,74,97,191] even though hypophosphatemia is regularly associated with elevated circulating levels of calcitriol. Similarly, in X-linked hypophosphatemic mice, calcitriol levels were found to correlate directly with serum phosphorus, emphasizing the presence of a deranged vitamin D homeostatic mechanism in this disorder.[337] Furthermore, the renal response to phosphorus deprivation is impaired in subjects with FHR.[157] After 4 days of dietary phosphorus restriction, subjects with FHR excreted more than five times as much phosphorus after 72 to 96 h of deprivation as did control subjects (176 ± 61 versus 33 ± 11 mg/24 h, $p < .05$). Despite these striking differences in phosphorus excretion, the change in serum phosphorus concentration was not significantly different between controls and FHR subjects (1.8 ± 0.1 versus 1.6 ± 0.1 mg/100 ml). Parathyroid hormone activity was not elevated in individuals with FHR and activity was not changed by phosphate deprivation. Thus, patients with FHR do not usually manifest signs or symptoms of hypophosphatemia, but may be predisposed to developing the syndrome if subjected to a low-phosphate diet or exposed to causes of renal or gastrointestinal phosphorus wasting.

Hypophosphatemic bone disease

Scriver and coworkers[290] described a group of children with severe hypophosphatemia and only modest bone disease. Serum levels of calcitriol were normal—a factor that may have ameliorated the bone disease. This disorder has been termed *hypophosphatemic bone disease.*

Hereditary hypophosphatemic rickets and hypercalciuria

Recently a new syndrome has been added to this category of hypophosphatemia: *hereditary hypophosphatemic rickets and hypercalciuria* (HHRH). Serum phosphate is only moderately decreased in HHRH, yet these subjects often have bone disease, suggesting that under certain circumstances hypophosphatemia of only moderate degree may lead to a significant alteration in bone metabolism.[319,320] Closely related family members of subjects with HHRH have a modified form of the disease, with biochemical abnormalities intermediate between normal persons and those with HHRH; they lack bone disease. Furthermore, a strong inverse correlation exists between levels of serum phosphate and circulating calcitriol levels, suggesting the importance of serum phosphate in modulating calcitriol production.

REGULATORY AND ADAPTIVE RESPONSES TO CHANGES IN PHOSPHATE LOADS

With hypophosphatemia, phosphate deprivation, or phosphate depletion, homeostatic mechanisms are activated in an attempt to maintain normal phosphate balance. Most likely, the maintenance of some component(s) of intracellular phosphate is the primary goal of the adaptive process. The mechanisms underlying phosphate homeostasis have been extensively studied, but clear insight is still needed into the elements of the phosphorus regulatory circuit: the afferent limb, which "senses" changes in phosphorus "load" and generates a message; the integrating center, which translates the "message(s)" from the afferent limb; and the efferent limb, which receives these signals and in turn alters an absorptive, distributional, or excretory function so as to effect a salutary change in phosphorus regulation. One difficulty in defining the various elements of the homeostatic process is the probability that the components of the various limbs of the regulatory process are not static; factors important during the initial stages of phosphorus deprivation may no longer play a critical role during chronic phosphate depletion.

Afferent limb

Little is known about the afferent limb of the regulatory process. One potential "signal" in the afferent limb is a change in serum phosphorus concentration pe se. Serum phosphorus levels decrease within 1 h after administration of a diet low in phosphorus to rats; this precedes changes in phosphate transport by the renal proximal tubular brush-border membrane.[201] The decrease in serum phosphate concentration may result from a redistribution of phosphate intracellularly due to increased plasma levels of insulin. Conversely, an infusion of phosphate raises serum phosphorus levels, within 1 h sodium-dependent phosphate transport by renal proximal tubule brush border membranes decreases. Furthermore, sodium-dependent phosphate transport is enhanced in cells exposed to phosphate-free media, and uptake is diminished in cells exposed to media containing high concentrations of phosphate.[31,61] Although serum phosphorus has been "normal" in some studies of chronic phosphate depletion,[97] these observations are not necessarily incompatible with an important role for the serum phosphorus concentration. Thus, changes in serum phosphorus levels may be critical during the early stages of adaptation but not with established phosphate depletion. Alternatively, the serum phosphorus concentration may be an important signaling mechanism in both early and late phases of adaptation, and the normal levels of serum phosphorus noted in some studies may not be representative of serum phosphorus levels throughout the day.[266] Furthermore, in an adaptive process one would expect the level of a regulated factor to be near normal if the adaptive process were functioning appropriately.

Integration center

There is also a paucity of data regarding the presence of a "central" integration center. Again, in vitro studies in cell cultures suggest that a given cell may contain all the necessary elements to integrate information from a given signal, such as a change in extracellular phosphate concentration. Therefore, the existence of a "central" integration center is conjectural.

Studies by Allon and coworkers[8] suggest that the pancreas may serve an integration center in early phosphate deprivation. Insulin levels were found to be higher in rats 45 min after receiving a diet low in phosphate compared to control animals, while infusion of somatostatin blunted both the rise in insulin and the renal adaptive response. Insulin has been shown to increase renal phosphate reabsorption and sodium-dependent phosphate uptake by isolated proximal tubule brush-border membrane vesicles.[140,144] Again, in vitro studies in cultured cells suggest that changes in phosphate transport following exposure to phosphate-free medium can occur without changes in insulin levels. Furthermore, insulin secretion is blunted with chronic phosphate deprivation[343] and, therefore, appears not to be critical in the later stages of adaptation.

Efferent limb

Much more information is available regarding the changes occurring in the target organs of the adaptive process. The final response to selective acute and chronic dietary phosphate deprivation consists of several components: (1) virtual elimination of phosphorus from the urine, and reduction in its fecal excretion to less than 5 percent of the normal value; (2) growth cessation, reducing the metabolic need for phosphorus; and (3) mobilization of phosphate from bone to satisfy the needs of various soft tissues in which life-sustaining processes occur.

Kidney and intestine

One of the most striking and consistent renal responses to dietary phosphate deprivation is profound hypophosphaturia. This "adaptive" change occurs within 2 to 24 h of the placement of rats, dogs, or human beings on a phosphate-deficient diet. The remarkable rapidity with which the urine is cleared of phosphorus cannot be the result of phosphorus depletion.[42] Studies by Moser and coworkers[258] suggested that the changes in urinary phosphate were primarily the result of the rapid fall in serum phosphate and, thus, of the decrease in filtered load that occurred in the first 24 h of phosphate deprivation. More recent studies using isolated brush-border membranes from the renal cortex have demonstrated that the rate of transport of phosphate across this membrane is increased within 2 to 4 h of dietary phosphate deprivation,[62,199,201] suggesting that the kidney adapts rapidly; a decrease in filtered load of phosphate alone does not account for the hypophosphaturia observed in the early stages of phosphate deprivation.

The mechanism for the adaptation remains unclear. In studies using isolated renal proximal tubule brush-border membrane preparations the maximal capacity of the phosphate transporter (V_{max}) is increased with phosphate deprivation, while the affinity of the carrier for phosphate (K_t) is unchanged—suggesting that the number or rate of carrier movement across the membrane is increased. Recent studies in rats have suggested that with chronic phosphate deprivation, the cholesterol in the renal proximal tubular brush-border membrane is decreased and that there is an associated increase in membrane fluidity. Increased membrane fluidity may allow the phosphate carrier to move more rapidly across the membrane, resulting in enhanced phosphate uptake.[197,198,233] More recent studies by Levine and coworkers[202] failed to demonstrate any changes in renal proximal tubular brush-border membrane fluidity during the early stages of adaptation, despite dramatic changes in phosphate transport—suggesting that changes in brush-border membrane fluidity are not critical for initial adaptive changes in phosphate transport. Further studies are needed to determine whether the changes in brush-border membrane fluidity are critical for chronic adaptation or are merely an epiphenomenon.

The phosphaturic response to PTH is blunted with phosphate depletion.[305,318] Studies in dogs suggest that the PTH receptor-adenylate cyclase unit is uncoupled by phophate depletion.[26]

Although phosphorus depletion is associated with virtual elimination of phosphate from the urine, phosphorus debt is generally incurred because of continued phosphorus loss through fecal excretion.[86] However, evidence from animal studies suggests that there is intestinal adaptation to phosphorus deprivation. Phosphorus depletion in young rats is consistently associated with increased in vitro [^{32}P]phosphate uptake by the duodenal and jejunal segments[69,326] and by very low fecal phosphorus excretion. Caverzasio and coworkers[62] have shown that changes in dietary phosphorus can increase sodium-dependent uptake of phosphate by isolated intestinal brush-border membranes within hours, and Lee and coworkers[193] have shown that changes in extracellular phosphate levels can produce changes in serosa-to-mucosa flux of phosphate.

Bone mineralization

A number of observations lend support to the thesis that phosphate removed from bone is used to replenish soft tissue during phosphate depletion. Several studies have demonstrated that, with the exception of blood and its components, the total phosphorus content of nonskeletal tissues is normal in phosphorus-depleted rats.[113] The analysis of total tissue phosphorus, however, does not answer the more critical questions on the possible changes in the inorganic and various organic phosphorus fractions and their distribution in the subcellular fractions. Brautbar and coworkers observed that myocardial and skeletel muscle inorganic phosphorus content decreased after 4 weeks of phosphate depletion, while ATP levels were normal.[45] These data further support the concept of mobilization of bone phosphorus stores to replenish soft tissue in order to maintain vital functions of the organism in the face of severe depletion of phosphorus.

Growth rate

The observation that experimental phosphate depletion is difficult to achieve in adults and in nongrowing animals—whereas in young, growing, animals the syndrome develops within 1 to 3 days of the initiation of depletion—suggests that a link exists between the tissue requirement for phosphate and the severity of the syndrome. Indeed, development of the biochemical features of phosphate depletion syndrome in acutely anabolic patients (e.g., nutritional recovery syndrome and recovery from burn injury) demonstrates the existence of this relationship between tissue metabolic demands and total body phosphate balance. Experimental studies have validated this concept. Growing rats require a phosphorus-enriched diet. When fed a diet "normal" in phosphate content, growing rats, for unexplained reasons, undergo an accelerated rate of growth and develop the biochemical syndrome of phosphate depletion. The authors concluded that the syndrome evolves as a result of increased metabolic demand for phosphorus in the rapidly growing tissue. Indeed, the animals fed the normal-phosphate diet displayed avid renal tubular reabsorption of phosphate and normal soft tissue total phosphorus levels, whereas bone phosphorus was reduced. These changes were comparable to the changes displayed by rats fed a low-phosphate diet, suggesting that renal conservation of phosphate and mobilization of phosphate were supplementing metabolic demands of soft tissue.

If this relationship is indeed a major determinant in the development of the biochemical effects of phosphate depletion, decreasing soft tissue or body demands for phosphorus should abolish the biochemical changes. Indeed, on evaluation of the effects of growth retardation in hypophysectomized rats, the hypophosphatemia, hypophosphaturia, and hypercalciuria of phosphate depletion were observed to be blunted.[43,191] Retardation of growth by means of hypophysectomy decreased the metabolic demands for phosphate. Copp, in his early classic studies, demonstrated that these typical biochemical changes in the phosphate-depleted rat were completely eliminated by fasting the animal for as little as 48 h;[74] the soft tissue breakdown liberated enough phosphorus to correct or eliminate the residual tissue demands for phosphorus. Striking clinical demonstrations of this concept include recent observations showing that premature infants with incompletely developed soft and osseous tissues, when fed breast milk low in phosphate, may develop a full-blown, even hypercalcemic, phosphate depletion syndrome with classic rickets. These studies clearly demonstrate that total body phosphorus balance and the renal and intestinal handling of phosphate are closely interrelated and that any clinical condition that imposed an increased demand relative to supply can trigger several adaptive mechanisms aimed at the maintenance of vital soft tissue metabolic activities.

CLINICAL MANIFESTATIONS AND BIOLOGICAL CONSEQUENCES OF HYPOPHOSPHATEMIA AND PHOSPHATE DEPLETION

The biochemical and clinical consequences of acute hypophosphatemia are, in part, a function of total body phosphorus stores. A recent case report illustrates the importance of this concept:[277]

> Two weeks after admission to the hospital, a 53-year-old woman with regional enteritis developed restlessness, paresthesias, weakness, abdominal distension, and hyperventilation.
>
> The patient had been well until 2 years before admission, when she began vomiting daily. One year before admission she developed intermittent abdominal pain without relation to food intake or bowel movements. She began to lose weight and was admitted to another hospital. Anorexia nervosa was diagnosed. Prior to the admission described here, weight loss accelerated; the patient's weight fell from 55 kg to 40 kg. On admission to the hospital, she appeared markedly malnourished with diffuse muscle wasting. Laboratory findings were remarkable for: serum calcium, 3.3 meq/liter (6.6 mg/100 ml); serum phosphorus, 2.8 to 3.7 mg/100 ml; total serum protein, 3.0 to 3.8 g/100 ml; plasma urea nitrogen, 9 mg/100 ml; plasma creatinine, 0.6 mg/100 ml. A gastrointestinal evaluation was compatible with malabsorption.
>
> The patient failed to gain weight; therefore, on the 13th hospital day, parenteral nutrition was initiated. The patient received 418 g of glucose per 24 h, synthetic L-amino acids (8.03 g alpha-amino nitrogen per 24 h), xylitol (100 g per 24 h), lactate (1 mmol per 24 h), acetate (59 mmol per 24 h), regular insulin (24 U per 24 h), sodium (75 mmol per 24 h), potassium (65 to 145 mmol per 24 h), and phosphate (9 mmol per 24 h).
>
> On the 19th hospital day, 6 days after the hyperalimentation was started, the patient became progressively restless and complained of peripheral tingling and numbness. She was lethargic and slightly disoriented, but otherwise mentation was normal. Serum calcium was 3.1 meq/liters; serum phosphorus was 0.25 mg/100 ml.

Several important findings in this case illustrate the interplay between body demands for phosphorus and phosphorus supply. The patient's plasma phosphorus level was 2.9 mg/100 ml on admission, before initiation of parenteral hyperalimentation. Of major importance were the low but detectable amounts of phosphate in the urine on the first day of hyperalimentation (124 mg per 24 h). These serum and urine biochemical findings suggest that the patient was not phosphate-depleted, since one of the most pronounced and earliest findings in depletion is the virtual absence of phosphate from the urine. The low but substantial urinary phosphorus excretion, despite the malabsorption and decreased intake of phosphate prior to admission, indicates that the patient's total body phosphorus stores were not reduced. Her phosphorus requirements were reduced by the lower metabolic demand for the mineral because of her decreased caloric intake; the release of phosphorus from muscle and bone caused by her catabolic state met the decreased demand. That it took 5 to 6 days for parenteral hyperalimentation to provoke the clinical manifestations of acute hypophosphatemia also argues against preexisting phosphorus depletion; almost all patients with preexisting phosphorus depletion develop clinical signs and symptoms within 1 to 2 days of the initiation of parenteral hyperalimentation.

Renal consequences

A list of renal abnormalities occurring in phosphate-depleted and hypophosphatemic patients and animals appears in Table 33-3.

Hypercalciuria

A well-known biochemical characteristic of phosphorus deprivation is the striking increase in excretion of calcium, which begins within hours. It is clear that the elevated calcium excretion and renal clearance is caused by release of calcium from the skeleton, a process that begins within hours of withdrawal of phosphate from the diet.[42,324]

Several observations suggest that a tubular defect in calcium transport may contribute to the hypercalciuria. Micropuncture studies in phosphate-depleted rats dem-

TABLE 33-3 • Renal consequences of phosphorus depletion and hypophosphatemia

Urinary changes
GFR decrease
Hypercalciuria
Hypermagnesuria
Hypophosphaturia
Decreased *Tm* for bicarbonate; bicarbonaturia
Decreased *Tm* for glucose; glycosuria
Uricosuria
Amino aciduria
Reduced titratable acid excretion
Decreased ammonia production and acquired distal renal tubular acidosis
Decreased proximal reabsorption of sodium with natriuresis
Blunted phosphaturic response to PTH and volume expansion
Altered renal metabolism
Decreased renal content of inorganic phosphorus
Decreased renal content of adenine nucleotides (prolonged phosphorus depletion)
Decreased renal gluconeogenesis
Decreased intracellular [H^+]
Impaired phospholipid synthesis

onstrated that the greatest inhibition of calcium reabsorption occurs in the proximal tubule.[186] Meyer-Sabellek and coworkers noted that thiazides blunted the hypercalciuria (Fig. 33-13), underscoring the importance of renal tubular transport changes in the genesis of this effect.[231] The authors also noted a marked hypercalcemic effect of thiazide diuretics in phosphate-depleted rats. Because thiazide diuretics have been shown to enhance bone resorption directly, the authors suggested that part of the thiazide-augmented hypercalcemia in these animals was from the action of the diuretic on the skeleton. These observations suggest that phosphate depletion in human beings receiving thiazide diuretics might induce hypercalcemia.

Increased intestinal absorption of calcium may contribute slightly to hypercalciuria; however, removal of calcium from the diet of phosphorus-depleted animals reduces urinary calcium only minimally.[76]

Increased levels of calcitriol have been found in patients[97,265] and animals[189] with phosphate depletion. Since calcitriol has been shown to cause increased bone mobilization of calcium, hypercalcemia, and hypercalciuria, increased levels of the vitamin may be responsible for the hypercalciuria of phosphate depletion. However, it has been shown that vitamin D–deficient, phosphate-depleted rats develop hypercalcemia and hypercalciuria;[40] the importance of calcitriol in this setting is, thus, questionable.

Phosphate depletion suppresses PTH secretion,[44,192] which may also contribute to the hypercalciuria; physiologic doses of exogenous PTH given to phosphate-depleted thyroparathyroidectomized dogs reduced the magnitude of the associated hypercalciuria, suggesting that hypoparathyroidism indeed may contribute.

In summary, it seems that at least three mechanisms contribute to the hypercalciuria of phosphate depletion: (1) mobilization of bone calcium, (2) a tubular defect in calcium transport, and (3) hypoparathyroidism.

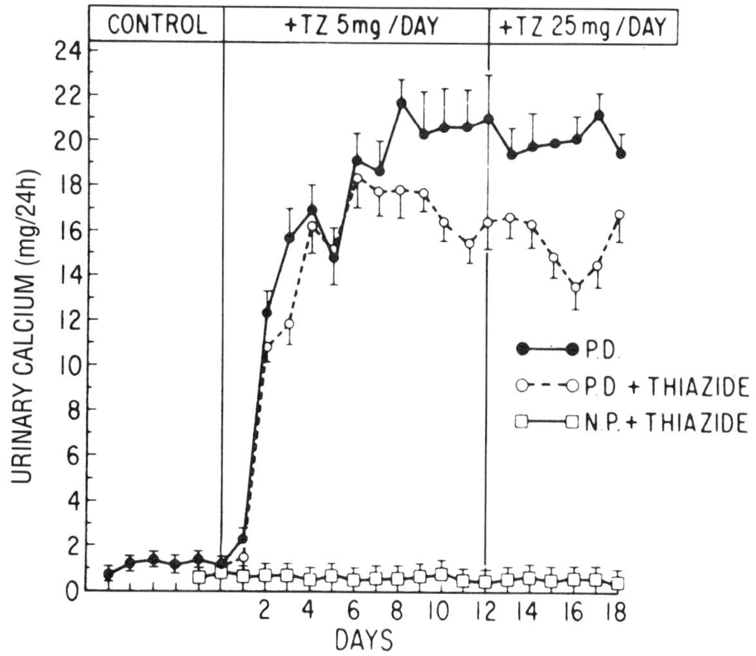

FIGURE 33-13 • Effects of thiazide diuretics on the hypercalciuria of phosphate depletion. ***NP,*** **normal-phosphate diet; PD, phosphate depletion. (From Meyer-Sabellek W et al: *J Lab Clin Med* 96:830, 1980, with permission.)**

Hypermagnesuria

Hypermagnesuria commonly complicates phosphate depletion in human beings and experimental animals. Two major mechanisms probably underlie this finding: increased mobilization of bone magnesium and a tubular defect in magnesium transport. Brautbar and coworkers demonstrated that hypermagnesuria and negative magnesium balance developed in rats within several days of phosphate depletion; bone content of magnesium was simultaneously reduced.[39] The urinary and bone changes (Fig. 33-14) clearly implicate bone magnesium mobilization in the magnesuria of phosphate depletion. A tubular defect in magnesium transport is implicated by the marked hypermagnesuria that both human volunteers and animals develop on low-phosphate diets despite the resulting hypomagnesemia. This hypomagnesemia was shown to be corrected by supplementation of the diet with magnesium.[39]

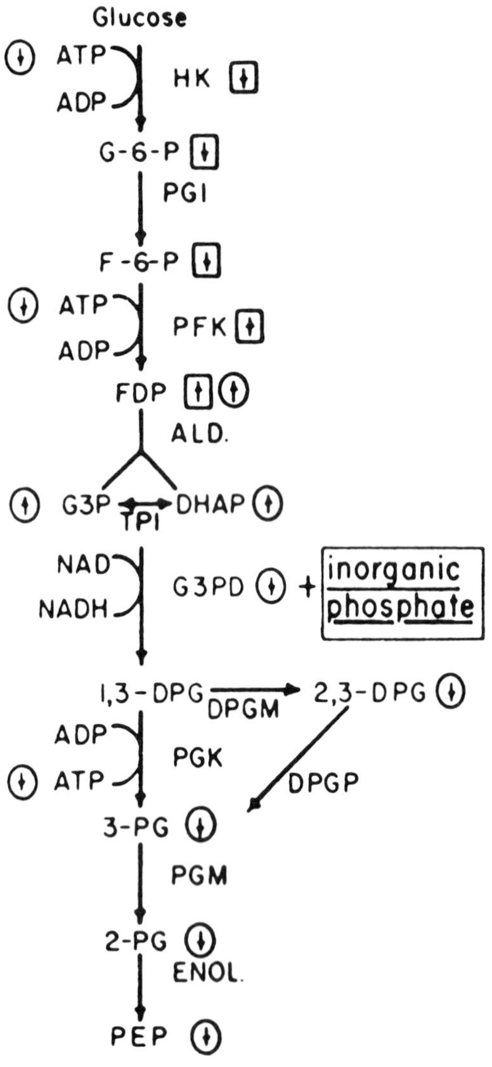

FIGURE 33-14 • Effects of inorganic phosphorus on the glycolytic cycle (adapted from effects of inorganic phosphorus on red blood cell glycolytic activity). (From Knochel JP: *Arch Intern Med* 137:203, 1977, with permission.)

Defective proximal bicarbonate reabsorption and distal hydrogen ion secretion

Gold and coworkers evaluated the renal handling of bicarbonate in phosphate-depleted dogs.[132] They found that the fall in bicarbonate levels correlated with the fall in serum phosphorus, and bicarbonate wasting occurred in the proximal tubule. Since PTH levels in phosphate depletion are low, the authors concluded that the altered acid-base homeostasis resulted from phosphate depletion and not from PTH.

Because phosphate depletion causes bone resorption and bone contains large quantities of alkali, it became evident that the interplay between bone and kidney could influence the acid-base balance induced by phosphate depletion. Emmett and coworkers showed that acid-base balance in phosphate-depleted rats was dictated by the algebraic sum of two opposing forces:[107] bicarbonaturia developed, with its potential for hypobicarbonatemia and systemic acidification; however, the release of alkali from bone acted to offset the renal defect.[107] In early phosphate depletion these countervailing forces cancelled one another; systemic acid-base parameters, therefore, did not change. With prolonged phosphate depletion, however, depletion of bone alkali reserves was followed by metabolic acidosis. Arruda and coworkers infused HCl into phosphate-depleted and control animals; the fall in blood pH and bicarbonate concentration was clearly blunted in the phosphate-depleted animals, supporting the role played by extrarenal buffering of acid in phosphate depletion. Thus, the acid-base changes complicating phosphate depletion in animals are dictated by the duration and severity of the phosphate loss.

The distal tubule influences acid-base homeostasis in an important way by actively secreting H^+, maximally acidifying the glomerular filtrate, and thereby titrating the major urinary buffers, while the proximal tubule is largely responsible for the bulk of ammonia buffer synthesized by the kidney.[53,285] Ammoniagenesis is vitally related to the activity of phosphate-dependent glutaminase, a site at which phosphate depletion might impair synthesis of this key buffer. Studies by Arruda and coworkers demonstrated that phosphate-depleted rats are unable to maximally lower urinary pH in response to prolonged ammonium chloride administration.[13] Severe phosphate depletion also reduces ammoniagenesis.

It is clear from the above studies that phosphate depletion is associated with three major alterations in renal acid-base regulation: (1) proximal tubular bicarbonate wasting, (2) impaired distal acidification, and (3) decreased buffer excretion secondary to hypophosphaturia and diminished renal ammoniagenesis.

Acid-base stability is generally well preserved in most patients suffering from phosphate depletion, because of the balance of acidifying and alkalinizing forces. However, prolonged and severe phosphate depletion may exhaust bone stores of alkali, thereby allowing metabolic acidosis to become manifest. Because pure phosphate depletion is rare, many patients have accompanying disorders of vitamin D and calcium metabolism, which additionally influence acid-base homeostasis.

Other renal effects

Gold and coworkers showed that the maximal rate of glucose transport (*T*mG) and its relationship to glomerular filtration rate, *T*mG/GFR, is reduced in phosphate-depleted dogs.[132] Similarly, aminoaciduria has been shown to occur in rats with phosphate depletion of 5 weeks.[79]

The effect of phosphate depletion on renal sodium and fluid reabsorption remains unclear. Proximal tubular fluid reabsorption is reduced in phosphate-depleted dogs[134] but is unchanged in phosphate-depleted rats.[243] Glomerular filtration rate is not altered by phosphorus depletion in either experimental animal. Clinical expressions of the above renal abnormalities are minimal.

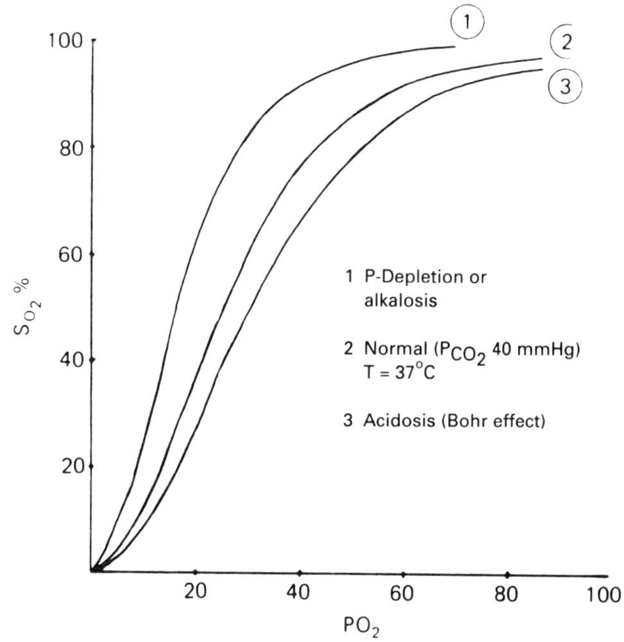

FIGURE 33-15 • Oxygen dissociation curve, illustrating effects of phosphate depletion.

Hematopoietic System

Red Blood cells (RBCs)

Phosphate depletion reduces RBC levels of 2,3-diphosphoglycerate (2,3-DPG) and ATP. Travis and coworkers measured the concentrations of RBC glycolytic intermediates in five hypophosphatemic patients.[321] They demonstrated that the triose phosphates, dihydroxyacetone phosphate and glyceraldehyde-3-phosphate, increased from normal values of 8 mmol/ml to concentrations of 200 to 600 mmol/ml (Fig. 33-14). This accumulation of intermediates was attributed to a deficiency in inorganic phosphate. The relative lack of inorganic phosphate reduces the activity of glyceraldehyde-3-phosphate dehydrogenase, which catalyzes the conversion of the triose phosphates to 1,3-diphosphoglycerate. Consequently, formation of glycolytic intermediary products distal to this step is suppressed, limiting the formation of 2,3-DPG and ATP (Fig. 33-14). Similarly, exposure of RBCs to a phosphate-free balanced salt solution depletes the cells of 2,3-diphosphoglycerate.[168]

The effect of phosphate depletion on 2,3-DPG levels of RBCs may affect oxygen delivery to tissues. Release of oxygen from hemoglobin is strongly influenced by 2,3-DPG, which reduces the affinity of hemoglobin for oxygen by two mechanisms: first, it binds preferentially to deoxyhemoglobin and thereby alters the equilibrium between oxygen and hemoglobin; second, increased erythrocyte 2,3-DPG levels reduce intraerythrocyte pH, which decreases hemoglobin-oxygen affinity by the Bohr effect.[27]

Changes in the oxyhemoglobin dissociation curve are expressed in terms of P_{50}, the oxygen tension (P_{O_2}) that causes 50 percent desaturation of hemoglobin. Hypophosphatemia may reduce P_{50} from a normal value of 27 mmHg to 16 mmHg. Thus, instead of yielding 50 percent of its bound oxygen at a P_{O_2} of 27 mmHg, hypophosphatemia requires that the P_{O_2} fall to 16 mmHg to similarly supply the tissues with oxygen. Values for P_{50}, RBC 2,3-DPG level, and plasma phosphorus concentration are related in patients with diabetic ketoacidosis[96] and on total parenteral nutrition.[321] Even during severe hypophosphatemia, RBC levels of 2,3-DPG generally do not fall below 40 percent of normal; at this level oxygen release may be reduced approximately 15 percent when arterial P_{O_2} values are between 60 and 100 mmHg. Although such changes would be relatively inconsequential in healthy subjects, they may play a critical role in the decompensation of severely hypophosphatemic patients (Fig. 33-15).

The normal RBC concentration of ATP, 1 to 1.5 mmol/liter, may be reduced to 60 to 80 percent in severe hypophosphatemia. The critical role of ATP in maintaining the integrity of cell structure and function is well known. In one study, induction of hypophosphatemia by hyperalimentation of previously starved dogs caused RBCs to become spheroidal, abnormally rigid, and more easily trapped and destroyed by the spleen.[338] The changes were prevented or reversed in vivo by the provision of phosphate supplements or in vitro by brief incubation of the cell with adenosine and phosphate.[338] Reversible hemolytic anemia has also been described in severe hypophosphatemia in human beings.[161] These changes in red cells are probably related to a deficiency of ATP-dependent, actin- or myosin-like contractile proteins, which are important in the maintenance of RBC shape and viability.[27] Hemolytic anemia secondary to hypophosphatemia and ATP depletion is not common and generally occurs only if plasma phosphorus levels fall below 0.5 mg/100 ml or erythrocyte [ATP] decreases to values below 0.2 mmol/liter. The ATP also promotes oxygen release from hemoglobin, although its effect is much less than that of 2,3-DPG. Theoretically, the rigid, nondeformable RBC in hemolytic anemia should perfuse tissue capillaries less readily, compounding the tissue hypoxia that results from the increase in binding of oxygen by hemoglobin.

Although not rigorously studied, many of the clinical features of phosphate depletion may result from, or be aggravated by, tissue hypoxia caused by RBC dysfunction. Hypoxia, per se, may lead to hyperventilation, respiratory alkalosis, and more profound hypophosphatemia; it can also cause lactic acidosis, which may further deplete RBC 2,3-DPG.[27]

White blood cells (WBCs)

Chemotaxis, phagocytosis, bactericidal activity, and ATP levels were depressed in granulocytes from dogs made severely hypophosphatemic by TPN. In-vivo phosphate repletion or in-vitro incubation of the defective WBCs with adenosine and phosphate increased ATP content and corrected the motility defect.[75] In the same study, similar findings were documented in one patient with TPN-associated hypophosphatemia. Garner and associates found that guinea pigs infected with salmonella organisms developed hypophosphatemia before death.[126] When the animals were supplemented with phosphate, mortality was markedly reduced and the number of organisms found in tissues decreased.

The mechanism of WBC dysfunction in severe hypophosphatemia is not clearly understood. It is probably related to reduced ATP synthesis which leads secondarily to impaired formation of proteins and other products important in regulating the mechanical and functional properties of the phagocyte.

Platelets

Yawata and coworkers found a host of platelet abnormalities in hypophosphatemic dogs, including thrombocytopenia, shortened life span, megakaryocytosis of the bone marrow, and impaired clot retraction.[338] These findings were associated with a tendency toward hemorrhage into the gastrointestinal tract and skin. Platelet ATP content was reduced by about 50 percent. These abnormalities were not observed in dogs supplemented with phosphate. Although mild mucosal bleeding has been reported in a few hypophosphatemic patients, platelet abnormalities have not been systematically investigated in human beings. Preliminary studies, however, indicate that phosphorus deficiency may lead to decreased platelet synthesis of ATP. This abnormality may be reversed by in-vivo or in-vitro phosphorus repletion.

Skeletal muscle

Phosphate depletion is commonly associated with proximal muscle weakness, muscle pain, impaired resting membrane potential, and mild elevation of serum levels of creatine phosphokinase (CPK) and aldolase.[174] Similar changes occur in experimental phosphorus depletion.[288] Resting muscle membrane potential and muscle content of potassium and total phosphorus fall, while sodium, chloride, and water content rise, in skeletal muscles of phosphate-depleted dogs[123] (Fig. 33-16). Serum CPK activity, however, remains normal in these animals. All abnormalities return to, or toward, normal with phosphate repletion.

Knochel and coworkers[177] have suggested that changes in the phosphorylation potential of the muscle cell constitute a major mechanism mediating the myopathy of hypophosphatemia. The phosphorylation potential, defined biochemically as $([ATP]/[ADP]) \times [P_i]$, is altered with changes in ATP, ADP, or inorganic phosphorus content. If the value for phosphorylation potential decreases secondarily to reduced intracellular inorganic phosphate concentration, the capacity of the cell to synthesize energy (ATP) is compromised. Furthermore, a low inorganic phosphate level activates AMP deaminase and 5′-nucleotidase, resulting in a loss of adenylic acid—an important precursor from which ATP is synthesized. The net result is an inability to generate ATP, which can have an important impact on cell integrity. Furthermore, abnormalities in the creatine phosphate energy shuttle required for cellular energy transport, in mitochondrial oxidative phosphorylation, and in myofibrillar energy utilization, have all been found in experimental phosphate depletion, associated with a marked reduction in cellular inorganic phosphorus stores.[45]

Structural changes in the skeletal muscle cells may also occur with phosphate depletion. In hypophosphatemic rats, electron microscopic studies indicated the presence of immature muscle fibers associated with mitochondrial and neurogenic dysfunction.[248]

Prior subclinical injury may enhance the susceptibility of the muscle cell to phosphate depletion. Thus, severe acute hypophosphatemia produced in subclinically phosphorus-depleted dogs by TPN with a phosphate-deficient solution brought about clinical, biochemical, and histological signs of rhabdomyolysis.[177] The resemblance between these experimental models and the

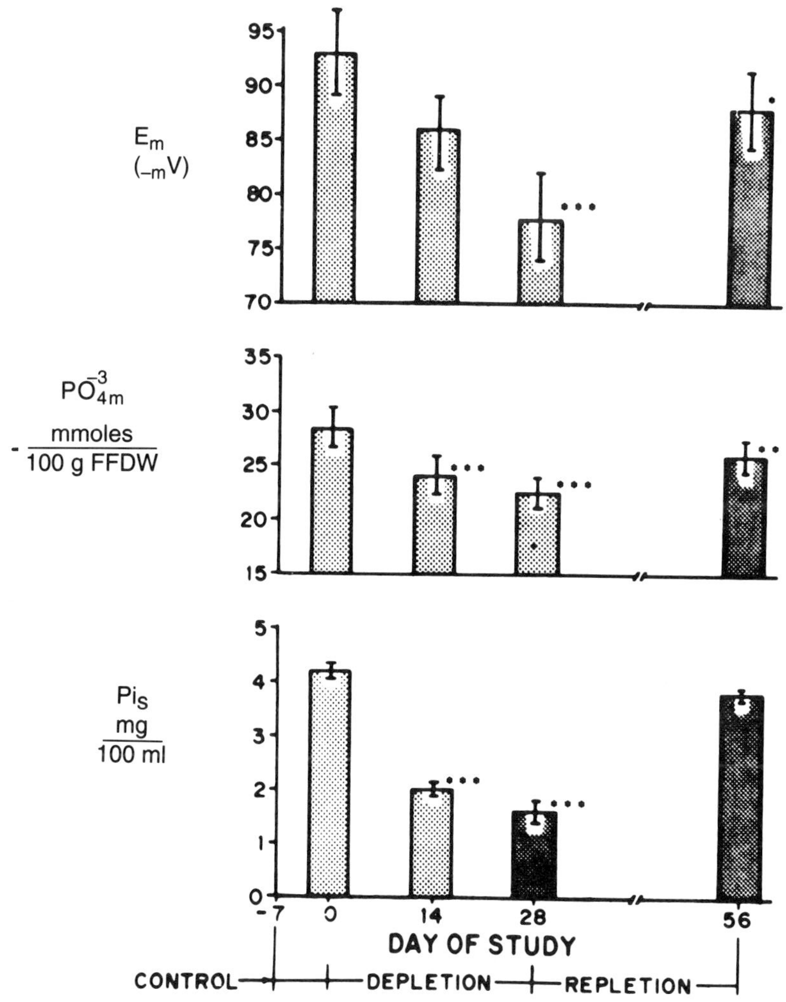

FIGURE 33-16 • Effects of experimental dietary phosphorus deprivation on skeletal muscle resting membrane potential (*Em*) (*upper panel*), total phosphorus content by fat-free day weight (*FFDW*) (*middle panel*), and serum phosphorus concentration (PO_4^{3-}) (lower panel), in dogs. (From Fuller TJ et al: *J Clin Invest* 57:1019, 1976, with permission.)

clinical rhabdomyolysis seen in malnourished chronic alcoholics is striking. Such patients are usually given large amounts of carbohydrates and other nutrients following hospitalization. Within a few days they develop muscle pain and profound weakness associated with severe hypophosphatemia and gross elevations in CPK and aldolase (Fig. 33-17).

Alcohol, per se, may increase the susceptibility of the skeletal muscle to phosphate depletion.[237] Structural, electrochemical, and biochemical abnormalities of skeletal muscle are common in alcoholic patients. Ferguson and coworkers fed alcohol to dogs over a prolonged period while avoiding malnutrition.[115] After 1 month, skeletal muscle phosphorus and magnesium content had declined markedly despite unchanged serum levels. Intracellular sodium and chloride concentrations, transmembrane potential difference (E_m), and Na^+-K^+ ATPase activity increased significantly. These data suggest that alcohol has a direct effect on skeletal muscle membrane and the muscle's ionic content. Whether these abnormalities are mediated via primary changes in intracellular phosphorus cannot be answered from this study, since inorganic phosphorus was not measured. (Total phosphorus measurement does not represent inorganic phosphorus.) However, the biochemical changes induced by alcohol may make the development of rhabdomyolysis more likely to occur after acute phosphate deprivation.

Muscles of respiration

Several studies in adult patients have shown that pulmonary muscle weakness may occur as a consequence of hypophosphatemia.[247] Planas and coworkers assessed pulmonary function and respiratory muscle performance during experimental phosphate depletion.[261] The authors demonstrated that no change in basal pulmonary muscle function occurred in phosphate-depleted dogs, but performance following fatiguing stimulation of the diaphragm dropped markedly.

Gravelyn and coworkers[137] found that 16 of 23 hypophosphatemic patients (defined as having a serum phosphorus level below 2.5 mg/100 ml) exhibited respiratory muscle weakness, defined as a maximal inspiratory pressure less than 40 mmH_2O or a maximal expiratory

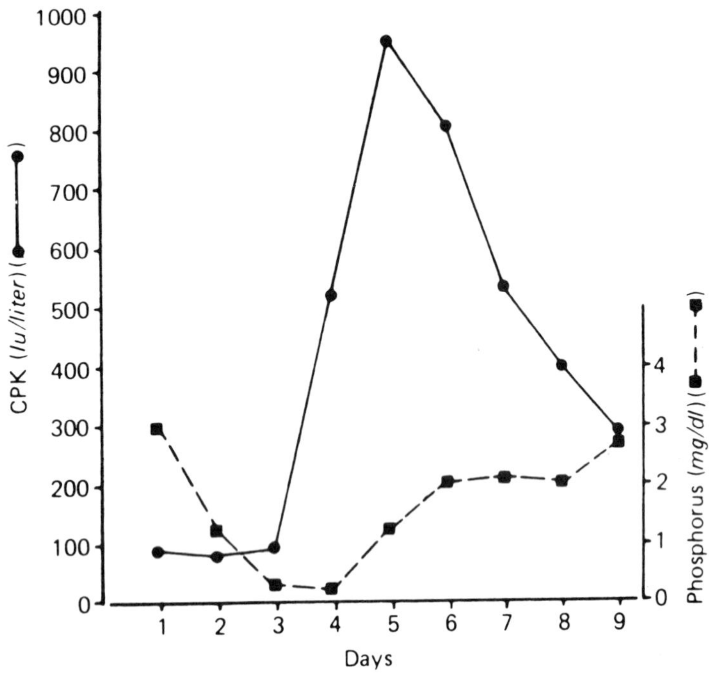

FIGURE 33-17 • Relationship between hypophosphatemia and elevation of creatine phosphokinase activity. (From Knochel JP, *Arch Intern Med* 137:203, 1977, with permission.)

pressure of less than 70 mmH_2O. These parameters improved with phosphate repletion. A nuclear magnetic resonance study of a patient with hypophosphatemic respiratory failure demonstrated a defect in muscle metabolism, including sharp drops in intracellular pH and in the ratio of phosphocreatine/(phosphocreatine + P_i), that took several weeks to completely resolve.[208] Such observations may have important clinical implications, since many individuals who are hypophosphatemic are either poorly nourished alcoholics with recurrent pulmonary infections or patients with uncontrolled diabetes who are immunocompromised and thus have a greater tendency to develop pulmonary infections.

Phosphate depletion may not only produce respiratory failure, but may also impede the weaning of patients from ventilators.[55,309] In some cases patients can be removed from the ventilator soon after phosphate repletion.

Cardiac and vascular muscle

O'Connor and coworkers reported that phosphate depletion reduced stroke work and left ventricular stroke volume, and increased pulmonary artery wedge pressure, in seven patients.[251] Phosphate repletion rapidly corrected these effects. Fuller and coworkers studied cardiac function in dogs before and during selective dietary phosphate depletion.[124] Stroke volume, maximum ascending aortic blood flow, and maximum left ventricular rate of pressure change decreased significantly with depletion. These changes also disappeared after phosphate repletion.

In contrast to these findings, other investigators using echocardiography, radionucleotide ventriculography, and impedance cardiography were unable to demonstrate myocardial dysfunction in hypophosphatemic patients.[273,323] The discrepancies between the various clinical studies may reflect the varying degrees of phosphate depletion present in the study populations. Thus, Davis and coworkers,[84] using systolic time interval measurements to assess myocardial performance, found that the ratio PEP/LVET (pre-ejection period/left ventricular ejection time) improved with phosphate repletion in patients with severe hypophosphatemia, but not in those with moderate hypophosphatemia—suggesting that abnormal myocardial performance occurred only with severe hyphosphatemia.

Biochemical studies of the phosphate-depleted myocardium have shown that mitochondrial oxygen consumption is impaired and that myofibrillar energy utilization and energy transport via the creatine phosphate shuttle are both reduced.[15] In addition to the effects of phosphate depletion on myocardial energy metabolism, recent studies have demonstrated additional abnormalities in fatty acid oxidation and cellular membrane phospholipid synthesis by the myocardium.[48] It is of interest that all the above abnormalities were related to the changes in intracellular inorganic phosphorus content rather than changes in high-energy nucleotide concentration (Figs. 33-18–33-20).

Phosphate depletion may also be associated with a decreased sensitivity to inotropic and vasoconstrictive agents. Kreusser and coworkers examined the effects of experimental phosphate depletion on myocardial hemo-

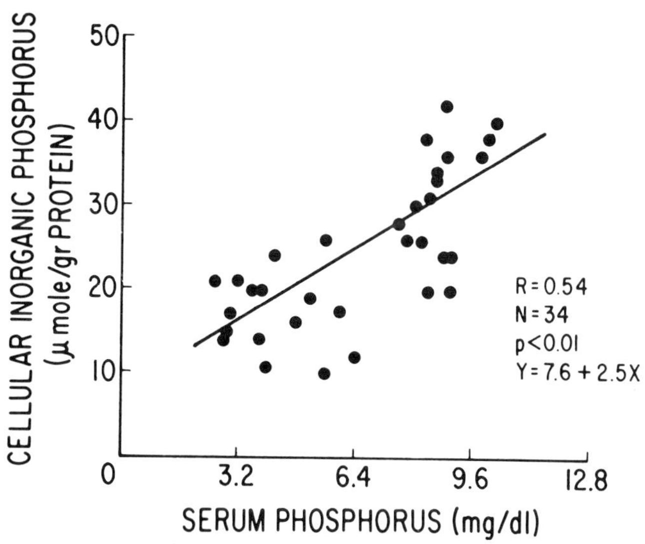

FIGURE 33-18 • Relationship between changes in serum phosphorus and cellular inorganic phosphorus concentrations in myocardium. (From Brautbar N et al: *Am J Physiol* 242:F699, 1982, with permission.)

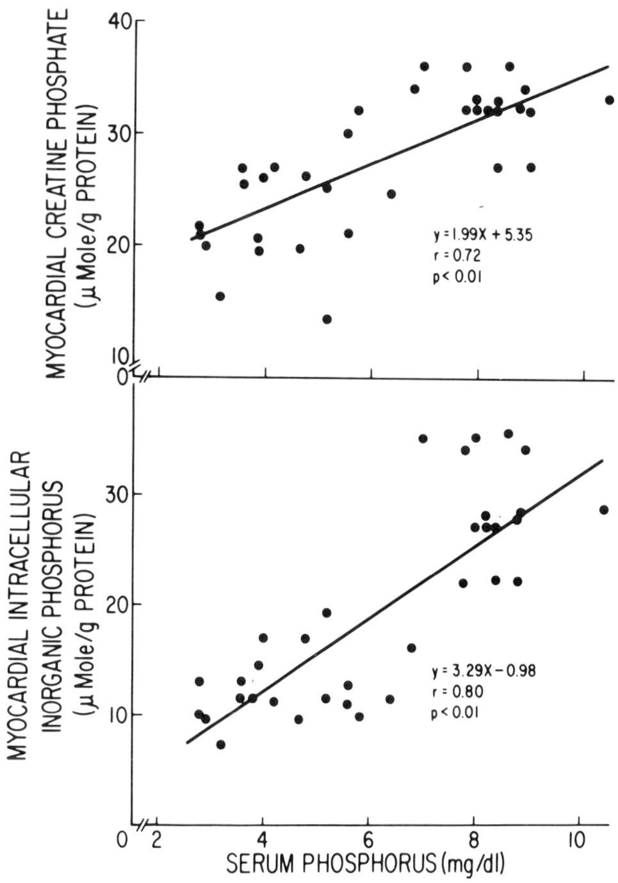

FIGURE 33-19 • Correlation between serum phosphorus concentration and myocardial creatine phosphate content. (From Brautbar N et al: *Am J Physiol* 242:F699, 1982, with permission.)

dynamics and metabolism; they discovered impairment of contractile force, inotropic response to catecholamines, and vasoconstrictor response to angiotensin II.[180] These hemodynamic changes were associated with reduced cardiac muscle content of ATP, creatine phosphate, and total phosphorus. Thus, in addition to a reduction in myocardial performance during phosphate depletion, a reduced vascular response to pressor agents was evident. Indeed, Saglikes and coworkers recently reported finding a lower resting mean arterial blood pressure in phosphate-depleted rats, as well as resistance to the pressor effects of angiotensin II and catecholamines.[57]

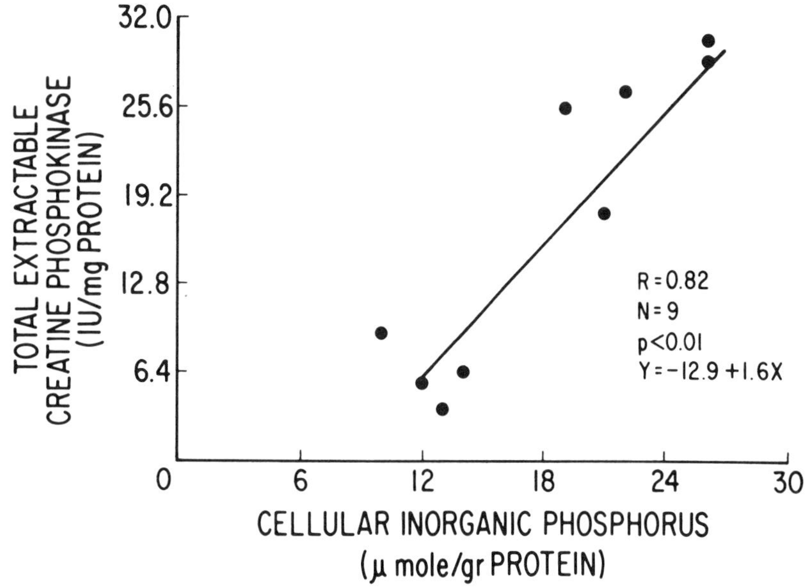

FIGURE 33-20 • Effects of experimental phosphorus deprivation on creatine phosphokinase (CPK) activity. Correlation between cellular inorganic phosphorus concentration and total extractable CPK. (From Brautbar N et al: *Am J Physiol* 242:F699, 1982, with permission.)

These arterial changes were associated with markedly reduced arterial wall ATP, creatine phosphate, and inorganic phosphate levels.

The clinical importance of these findings is not yet known. The extent to which phosphate depletion and hypophosphatemia are responsible for the refractory congestive heart failure in patients with reduced dietary intake of phosphate and increased use of phosphate-binding antacids needs further exploration.

Hypophosphatemia may also be associated with an increased incidence of cardiac arrythmias. In a prospective study, Venditti and coworkers[322] evaluated the effects of hypophosphatemia as the sole electrolyte abnormality on cardiac rhythm. An increased incidence of ventricular arrythmias, including ventricular tachycardia, was noted in hypophosphatemic patients compared to a control group admitted for syncope. Furthermore, treatment of the hypophosphatemia resulted in improvement of the abnormal heart rhythm. It is of interest that, when the subjects with hypophosphatemia were divided into those with and those without a significant ventricular arrythmia, the serum phosphorus levels were similar between groups (1.6 ± 0.13 mg/100 ml without arrythmia, versus 1.8 ± 0.09 mg/100 ml with arrythmia). With phosphate repletion, however, the rise in serum phosphate and the increase in urinary phosphate excretion were less in the group with the arrythmias, suggesting a greater degree of phosphate depletion.

Serum phosphorus levels tend to be lower in patients with essential hypertension, leading to the speculation that disordered phosphate metabolism may contribute to the elevated blood pressure in this disorder. If intracellular phosphate is also lower in hypertensives, then Na^+-K^+ATPase in vascular smooth muscle cells may be inhibited, producing a rise in intracellular sodium and a subsequent elevation in intracellular calcium .[155,276] A rise in intracellular calcium might then increase vascular smooth muscle contractility directly or increase the sensitivity of the vascular smooth muscle cell to an agonist such as norepinephrine. In either case, increased contractility might lead to an increase in systemic vascular resistance and hypertension. Although there is some evidence that intracellular calcium increases with chronic phosphate depletion, at least in some cells,[228,343] studies demonstrating a decrease in blood pressure with phosphate depletion in rats and a decrease in the vascular response to norepinephrine[284] are difficult to reconcile with the postulate that hypophosphatemia plays a causative role in hypertension.

Central nervous system

The neuroencephalopathy associated with phosphate deficiency has protean manifestations. Irritability and apprehensiveness may progress to confusion, obtundation, convulsion, coma, and death. Other clinical features may include numbness, paresthesias, tremors, lack of coordination, ballismus, nystagmus, unequal pupils, and ataxia. Bulbar involvement also occurs, causing dysarthria, dysphagia, and shallow respiration. Acute respiratory failure, requiring emergency tracheostomy and assisted respiration, has also been described.[247] The EEG may show diffuse abnormalities characteristic of metabolic encephalopathy; the cerebrospinal fluid (CSF) protein content is generally elevated. The CNS syndrome may mimic, or coexist with, disorders such as delirium tremens and Guillain-Barré syndrome.[151] In experimental phosphate deficiency with neuroencephalopathy, autopsy examinations have revealed diffuse hemorrhages in the white matter, cerebral edema, and intracellular acidosis.[280] Interestingly, on autopsy the inorganic phosphorus content of the brain tissue was normal.[280]

The basic mechanism causing the CNS disturbances in phosphorus depletion is not clear. Decreased phosphate availability may impair glucose utilization, which in turn would be expected to reduce ATP synthesis in the brain. Glucose oxidation and ATP production may also fall because of a deficiency in 2,3-DPG and hypoxia. However, early reports of decreased ATP levels in the brain of phosphorus-depleted dogs could not be confirmed in subsequent studies.[116] Experimental phosphate depletion in rats produced a significant reduction in dopamine, norepinephrine, and epinephrine concentrations in various parts of the brain.[30] Whether these alterations in catecholamine concentrations play a role in altered CNS function in human beings with phosphate depletion is unknown.

Elevated levels of intracellular free cytosolic calcium have been found in synaptosomes prepared from rats depleted of phosphate for 6 weeks.[228] Since free cytosolic calcium is a critical second messenger in cell function, the abnormal levels could have a profound effect on CNS function. ATP levels were low in the synaptosomes prepared from phosphate-depleted rats, but not when the rise in cytosolic calcium was prevented by treatment with nifedipine—suggesting a cause-and-effect relationship between the changes in cytosolic calcium and changes in ATP levels. Whether altered levels of cytosolic calcium are important in phosphate depletion in human beings remains to be determined.

Early observations suggested that hypophosphatemia leads to intracellular edema.[254,296,336] More recent studies, however, have failed to demonstrate an increase in cerebral water content; in fact, brain water has been shown to decrease.[91-93]

A similarity between the CNS syndrome of phosphate depletion and Wernicke's encephalopathy has been suggested.[24] The latter disorder is related to thiamine deficiency[259] and has occurred with the refeeding of starved patients.[100] It appears unlikely that thiamine deficiency plays a role in the hyperalimentation syndrome; a large quantity of thiamine has been present in the infusion in all of the animals studied, and the majority of the patients described have had thiamine supplements.

Studies by Silvis and coworkers demonstrated that neurological symptoms and hypophosphatemia may be induced by oral intake in both human beings and experimental animals.[297] A common denominator was severe malnutrition, predisposing the patients and dogs to hypophosphatemia and neurological symptoms with the administration of enteric alimentation. Animals that had not been starved or calorically deprived did not develop the syndrome. These observations suggest that acute hypophosphatemia is more apt to cause neurological damage in a "sick" cell—that is, one previously subjected to caloric deprivation, as already described for muscle cells.[235]

Another clinical situation where hypophosphatemia may have an additive effect in producing cerebral dysfunction is liver failure. Anecdotal reports have suggested that hypophosphatemia may precipitate or aggravate hepatic encephalopathy; phosphate repletion or correction of hypophosphatemia appeared to improve the comatose state in patients with hepatic encephalopathy.[82a] Further studies are needed to examine the energy state and cellular inorganic phosphate content of these cells in order to further evaluate the cellular mechanisms mediating the neurological symptoms associated with phosphate depletion.

Bone

Phosphate depletion is associated with a rapid and severe breakdown of bone, much more so than severe hypocalcemia or vitamin D depletion. Bone loss leads to the development of rickets and osteomalacia in animals and human beings.[86,317] Baylink and coworkers, using quantitative histomorphometry, found that bone resorption was markedly increased in phosphate-depleted rats.[25] Endosteal resorbing surface was enlarged, indicating enhanced osteoclast activity. The magnitude of the increase in bone resorption did not differ between thyroparathyroidectomized and untreated rats, suggesting that neither PTH nor CT was involved in the observed changes. A negative correlation was found between serum phosphorus concentration and percent endosteal resorbing surface. This inverse relationship appeared to hold for levels of serum phosphorus concentration both above and below normal. Although superimposed vitamin D deficiency blunted the magnitude of the bone resorption rate, it did not normalize it, indicating that the elevated calcitriol level of phosphate depletion is not primarily responsible for the abnormally rapid bone turnover.[25] In severely hypophosphatemic rats, bone formation was also reduced.[159] This was reflected by a decrease in matrix formation as well as osteoid maturation and mineralization. All these observations clearly account for the reduced bone content of calcium, magnesium, and phosphorus in phosphate-depleted rats (Fig. 33-21).

In contrast to the findings of Baylink and coworkers, Harrison and coworkers[145] noted an increase in linear

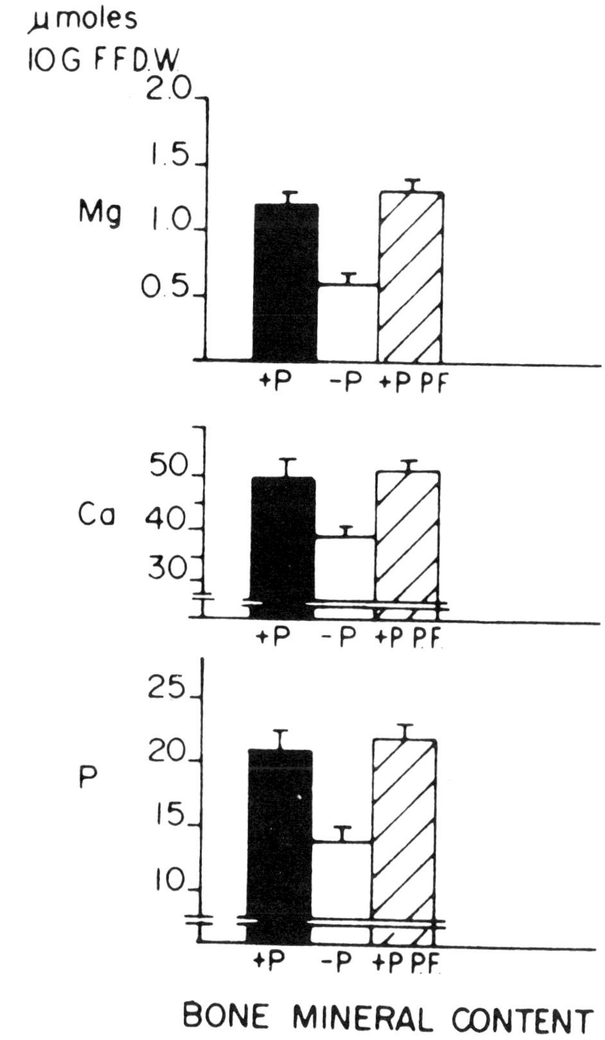

FIGURE 33-21 • Changes in bone minerals during phosphorus deprivation in the rat. (From Brautbar N et al: *Am J Physiol* 237:E152, 1979, with permission.)

bone apposition rate with phosphate depletion in weanling rats that was dependent on vitamin D intake but independent of plasma levels of calcitriol. The discrepancy between the two studies may reflect differences in the degree and duration of phosphate depletion, or differences in bone labeling techniques.

Chronic hypophospatemia may also produce marked changes in bone histomorphometry in humans, but the extent may vary depending on the clinical situation. Nineteen patients with hypophosphatemia secondary to renal phosphate wasting were examined with bone histomorphometry by de Vernejoul and coworkers.[94] The patients displayed decreased osteoblastic surface area with normal resorption surfaces, osteoid volume, and calcification front. There was no correlation between serum phosphate level and histomorphometric parameters. The authors concluded that hypophosphatemia in adults does not always lead to osteomalacia but may produce an unusual osteopenia due to an isolated decrease in bone formation. Felsenfeld and coworkers[114] studied the effect of long-term hypophosphatemia in renal transplant recipients and also found no evidence of osteomalacia. In contrast to these findings, patients with HHRH or antacid-induced hypophosphatemia of only moderate severity may have significant degrees of osteomalacia on bone biopsy.[59,65,131,319,320] Therefore, chronic phosphate depletion and hypophosphatemia should be excluded in any patient presenting with unexplained bone pain or fractures—particularly with a history of chronic antacid consumption.

Another osseous abnormality that may occur with phosphate depletion is bone proliferation at sites of ligament, tendon, joint capsule, and interosseous membrane attachment (enthesopathic changes). These changes may be seen in adults with long-standing hypophosphatemic osteomalacia and may produce musculoskeletal symptoms.[54] The severity of changes may vary; any such changes noted radiologically should be recognized as possible signs of hypophosphatemic osteomalacia.

The gastrointestinal tract

Calcium absorption

Phosphorus depletion can lead to increased intestinal calcium absorption and subsequent renal calcium wasting both in human beings[97] and in animals.[238,316] In human beings this increase in intestinal calcium absorption is associated with an accelerated turnover of the plasma pool of 25-hydroxyvitamin D_3 (25-OH-D_3) because of increased renal synthesis of calcitriol.[97] Studies by Portale and coworkers[266] in normal male subjects showed that phosphate depletion of 10 days increased the production rate of calcitriol and increased its circulating levels by 80 percent. In patients with hypophosphatemia due to HHRH, plasma levels of calcitriol and intestinal calcium absorption are increased;[65,319] in relatives with a phenotypically milder expression of this disorder, levels of plasma calcitriol are lower, as is urinary calcium excretion.[320] These data are consistent with the interpretation that phosphorus depletion increases calcium absorption in human beings and animals at least in part because of an alteration in the renal synthesis or metabolism of calcitriol.

In contrast to these findings, Lee and coworkers reported that net intestinal calcium absorption, as determined by balance techniques, was unchanged or decreased in phosphorus-depleted rats, even though in-vitro uptake studies had shown an increase.[190] It is possible that different degrees of phosphorus deprivation lead to different responses in calcium absorption. Clark and Rivera-Cordero measured calcium, magnesium, and phosphorus balances in intact and parathyroidectomized adult male rats placed on diets with constant calcium content (0.4 percent) and varying levels of phosphorus (0.2 to 9.2 percent).[69] Calcium absorption increased as dietary phosphorus content was reduced to 0.31 percent. A further reduction of dietary phosphorus was followed by a decrease, rather than an increase, in calcium absorption. It is possible, therefore, that intestinal calcium absorption would increase under progressive phosphorus restriction until a critical degreee of phosphorus deficiency was attained; thereafter, calcium absorption would decrease as phosphorus was further depleted. The reduction in fecal calcium observed in human subjects undergoing dietary phosphate restriction may be accounted for by the low level of phosphorus deficiency attained.[97] The interrelationship of low-phosphate diet, vitamin D metabolism, and intestinal calcium absorption awaits further definition.

An important unanswered question is whether dietary phosphorus deprivation leads to increased intestinal levels of calcitriol in humans. In phosphorus-deprived chicks the increase in calcium absorption is paralleled by an increase in both calcium-binding proteins[21] and calcitriol[105] in the intestinal epithelium. The mechanism responsible for this increased intestinal accumulation of calcitriol is not clear.

Magnesium absorption

Dietary phosphorus deprivation in human beings is associated with increased net magnesium absorption when measured in balance studies.[97] This adaptation compensates for the associated hypermagnesuria, thereby maintaining magnesium balance. In young rats the fraction of dietary magnesium absorbed may not be altered; this, coupled with the marked hypermagnesuria, can lead to negative magnesium balance.[39]

Liver

Anecdotal reports have suggested that the hypophosphatemia often occurring with liver failure may aggravate the severity of liver dysfunction.[85] Kurokawa and coworkers[181] found that modest phosphorus deficiency in rats produced a decrease in total phosphorus and adenine nucleotide content of the liver. In contrast, studies in dogs were unable to find any changes in phosphate content of the liver despite severe phosphate depletion.[175]

Severe hepatocellular injury may occur with fructose administration in association with hypophosphatemia. Fructose, after entering the liver cell, is incorporated into fructose-1-phosphate. Fructose-1-phosphate does not inhibit fructokinase, the enzyme responsible for this phosphorylation reaction. Inorganic phosphate is "trapped" by fructose binding, resulting in activation of AMP-deaminase and ATP depletion of the cell.[175] Aside from this condition, the role of phosphate deficiency in liver failure remains anecdotal and requires further study.

Pancreas

As already mentioned, phosphate depletion of several weeks in rats can lead to decreased pancreatic release of insulin in response to a glucose load.[343] Concomitant in-vitro studies showed that the ATP/ADP ratio in the pancreatic cell was low and resting free cytosolic calcium levels were elevated in the basal state; with exposure to ionomycin the cytosolic calcium increased but did not return to baseline in normal fashion, suggesting an abnormality in the plasma membrane calcium pump mechanism, which extrudes calcium from the cell. It is postulated that the low ATP levels may alter ATP-dependent potassium channels, thereby affecting insulin release.

EFFECTS OF PHOSPHATE DEPLETION ON INTERMEDIARY METABOLISM

Carbohydrate metabolism

Phosphate is essential for cellular glucose uptake, and glycolysis is stimulated by high concentrations of intracellular inorganic phosphorus and inhibited by low concentrations (Fig. 33-22). It is reasonable, therefore, to suspect that an abnormality in carbohydrate metabolism would complicate phosphate depletion. Indeed, the early studies of Gold and coworkers and Harter and coworkers demonstrated hyperglycemia in the face of hyperinsulinemia in phosphate-depleted dogs.[133,146] The authors suggested that insulin resistance occurred because of hypophosphatemia. Studies by Allon and coworkers[8] demonstrated that insulin resistance could occur within hours of feeding in a rat whose diet was low in phosphorus, suggesting that phosphate depletion per se is not necessary to the development of insulin resistance. In addition to insulin resistance, prolonged phosphate depletion may decrease pancreatic insulin secretion.[343]

Glucose metabolism is abnormal in several tissues of phosphate-depleted animals. Davis and coworkers found that acute hypophosphatemia had no effect on rat skeletal muscle glucose uptake, whereas chronic hypophosphatemia inhibited uptake; a direct linear correlation was found between glucose uptake and plasma phosphorus concentration.[83] These data were recently confirmed in hypophosphatemic patients.[87]

Brautbar and coworkers examined glucose and glycogen metabolic pathways in liver, skeletal muscle, and heart from normal and phosphate-depleted rats.[41,47] The hypophosphatemia was associated with a marked and significant reduction in intracellular inorganic phosphorus, glucose-6-phosphate, fructose-1-phosphate, and glycogen concentrations. The changes in glycogen and glucose-6-phosphate concentrations correlated with the changes in intracellular inorganic phosphorus concentration (Figs. 33-22 and 33-23). These data demonstrate that glycolytic activity is reduced in these animals by a fall in intracellular inorganic phosphorus concentration. Horle and coworkers have corroborated these findings by showing reduced glycogen content and glycogen synthetase activity, and increased glycogen phosphorylase activity, in the hearts of phosphate-depleted animals.[154] Phosphate depletion has also been shown to inhibit gluconeogenesis by renal proximal tubules.[179]

The above findings may have important clinical implications. Impaired gluconeogenesis and hypoglycemia have been reported in patients with phosphate depletion who also developed liver dysfunction. The resistance to insulin and impairment of carbohydrate metabolism seen in phosphate depletion may also exacerbate metabolic abnormalities in uncontrolled diabetes.

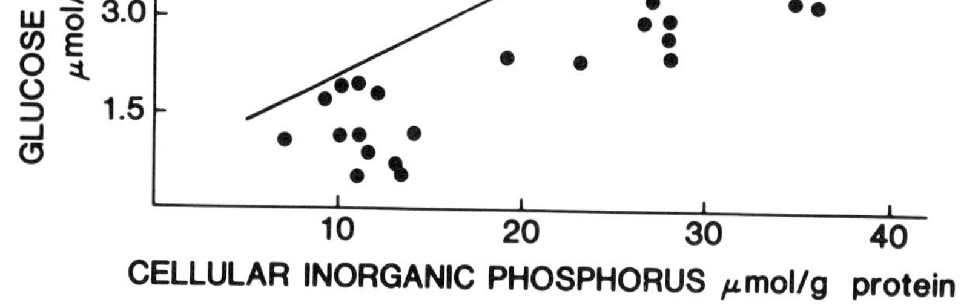

FIGURE 33-22 • Correlation between skeletal muscle inorganic phosphorus and glucose-6-phosphate concentrations. (From Brautbar N et al: *Kidney Int* 24:53, 1983, with permission.)

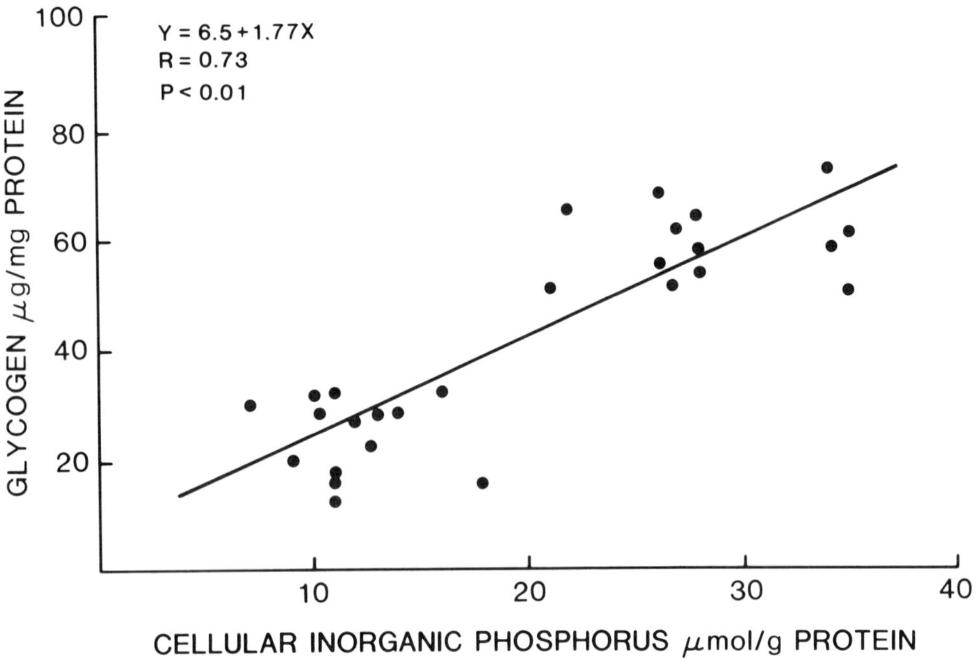

FIGURE 33-23 • Correlation between skeletal muscle inorganic phosphorus and glycogen concentration. (From Brautbar N et al: *Kidney Int* 24:53, 1983, with permission.)

Lipid metabolism membrane integrity

Ramsay and Douglas recently found decreases in total lipids, sterol esters, triacyl glycerol, and phosphatidylserine in cell walls of bacteria grown on a phosphate-free medium.[269] Brautbar and coworkers showed that a marked reduction in amounts of acid-extractable, water-soluble phospholipids occurred in kidney, liver, and cardiac muscle, but not in skeletal muscle, in the phosphorus-depleted state.[41] Phospholipid biosynthesis in the myocardium was studied during short-term (4-week) and long-term (8- to 12-week) dietary phosphate depletion.[48] Analysis of major cellular phospholipids showed markedly lower content of phosphatidylcholine and phosphatidylethanolamine as a consequence of impairment of various steps in phospholipid biosynthesis (Fig. 33-24).

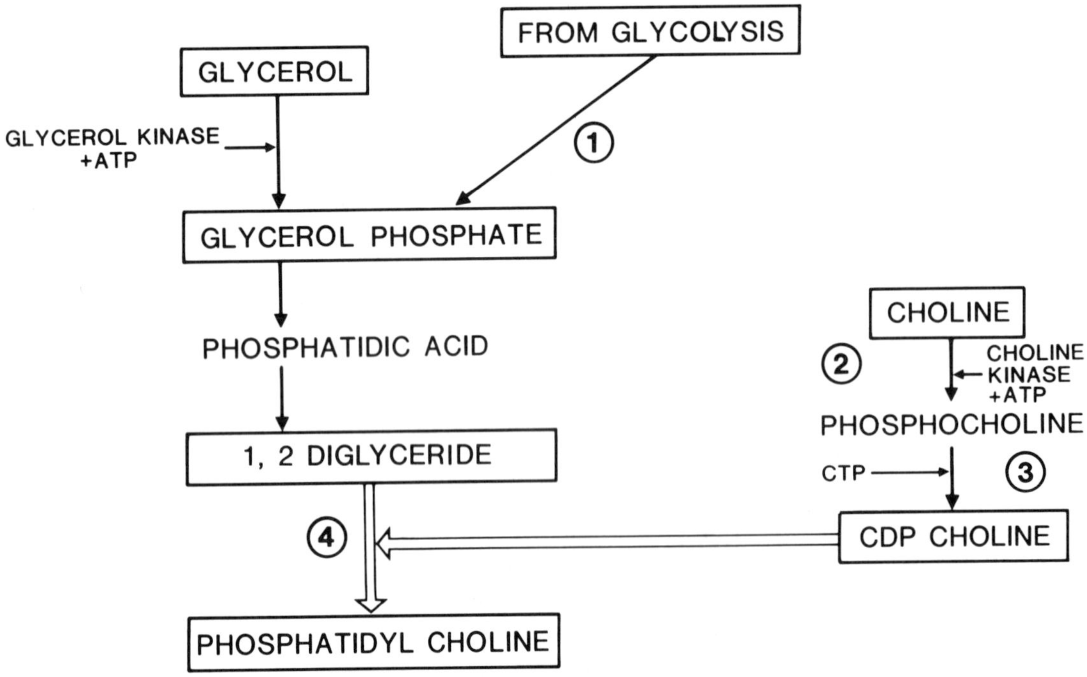

FIGURE 33-24 • Major pathways of phospholipid biosynthesis.

Also, as we have already said, fatty acid oxidation by heart mitochondria obtained from phosphate-depleted rats is markedly impaired.[48]

Studies by Molitoris and coworkers[233] suggest that the changes in membrane phospholipid content do not occur rapidly. In rats fed a low-phosphate diet for 7 to 9 days, both renal proximal tubular brush-border membrane and basolateral membrane phospholipid content were unchanged compared to values obtained in rats fed a normal diet.

Several investigators[197,198,202,233] have demonstrated that cholesterol levels in the renal proximal tubular brush-border membrane are decreased in rats after 7 to 14 days of phosphate restriction. The change in cholesterol content of membranes can have a major impact on the structural integrity of the membrane as well as on various transport processes occurring across the membrane, as already discussed.

MECHANISMS OF CELLULAR INJURY IN PHOSPHATE DEPLETION

Combined phosphate depletion and hypophosphatemia can result in severe cellular damage. Whether hypophosphatemia independent of phosphate depletion can induce cellular damage is unclear; several clinical and experimental studies suggest that when severe cellular damage occurs, both mechanisms are involved. In most instances where severe hypophosphatemia has been associated with either clinical or biochemical abnormalities, chronic phosphate depletion is present. These abnormalities include impaired myocardial function, respiratory muscle paralysis, central nervous system disorders, and skeletal muscle changes. Skeletal muscle or myocardial dysfunction and biochemical abnormalities develop during experimental phosphate depletion only after dietary phosphate depletion and hypophosphatemia of 4 to 8 weeks' duration.[45,47,123,124] Since hypophosphatemia develops within 2 to 5 days, these observations suggest that the cellular injury must be mediated partly by changes in intracellular phosphorus stores.

Changes in cellular inorganic phosphorus may influence the cell via several mechanisms:

Phosphorylation state of cellular ATP

The supply of inorganic phosphorus in the cytosol plays a major regulatory role in mitochondrial respiration, glycolysis, and oxidative ATP synthesis. Recent studies have shown that prolonged hypophosphatemia is associated with reduced intracellular phosphate concentration; these changes trigger abnormalities in mitochondrial respiration and energy production, transport, and utilization. It is possible that the fall in cellular inorganic phosphorus reduces ATP synthesis, causing cellular injury. This notion is compatible with the hypothesis that the phosphorylation potential represents the energy store of the cell and, in turn, regulates cellular respiration.

Another factor that may affect ATP production is the level of free intracellular cytosolic calcium. As we have said, cytosolic calcium is increased in the pancreas[343] and synaptosomes[228] of rats after 6 weeks of phosphate depletion. Intracellular ATP levels were also low. Treatment with nifedipine prevented the elevation in cytosolic calcium with phosphate depletion, and intracellular ATP levels were normal. These studies suggest that cytosolic calcium abnormalities may be a critical factor in the lower ATP levels observed with prolonged phosphate depletion.

The creatine phosphate shuttle and creatine phosphokinase isoenzymes

The creatine phosphate shuttle is an additional mechanism triggered by reduced intracellular phosphorus stores that must be of major importance in the regulation of cellular respiration and bioenergetics. Studies by Brautbar and coworkers and Saglikes and coworkers showed that cardiac output is reduced in experimental phosphate depletion and that this reduction is associated with a fall in cellular inorganic phosphate, but with no change in ATP concentration.[45,283a] However, creatine phosphate concentration fell markedly, and myofibrils were unable to use energy for contraction. These observations suggest that decreased ATP content and altered phosphorylation potential may develop late in the course of phosphate depletion and that they are only partly responsible for the cellular injury.

The currently accepted scheme for myocardial and skeletal muscle bioenergetics is outlined in Fig. 33-25. Energy, in the form of ATP, is produced in the mitochondria as a result of oxidative phosphorylation. The mitochondrial creatine phosphokinase (CPK) isoenzyme then transfers the high-energy phosphate bond from ATP to creatine, forming creatine phosphate. The latter then diffuses to the myofibrils and sarcoplasmic reticulum, phosphorylating the myofibrillar ADP to form ATP.[296] This step is regulated and facilitated by the myofibrillar isoenzyme of CPK.[28,286] This energy shuttle is called the *creatine phosphate shuttle* and is regulated by the CPK isoenzymes.[222,292] It has been shown that a fall in cellular inorganic phosphorus reduces the activity of both mitochondrial and myofibrillar CPK isoenzymes; these changes occur earlier than the fall in ATP.[45] It is possible, therefore, that the creatine phosphate shuttle in myocardial and in skeletal muscle is a sensitive system affected early in phosphate depletion.

Changes in the creatine phosphate shuttle with phosphate depletion may have important clinical consequences. Using nuclear magnetic resonance spectroscopy, Lewis and coworkers[208] found that phosphocreatine lev-

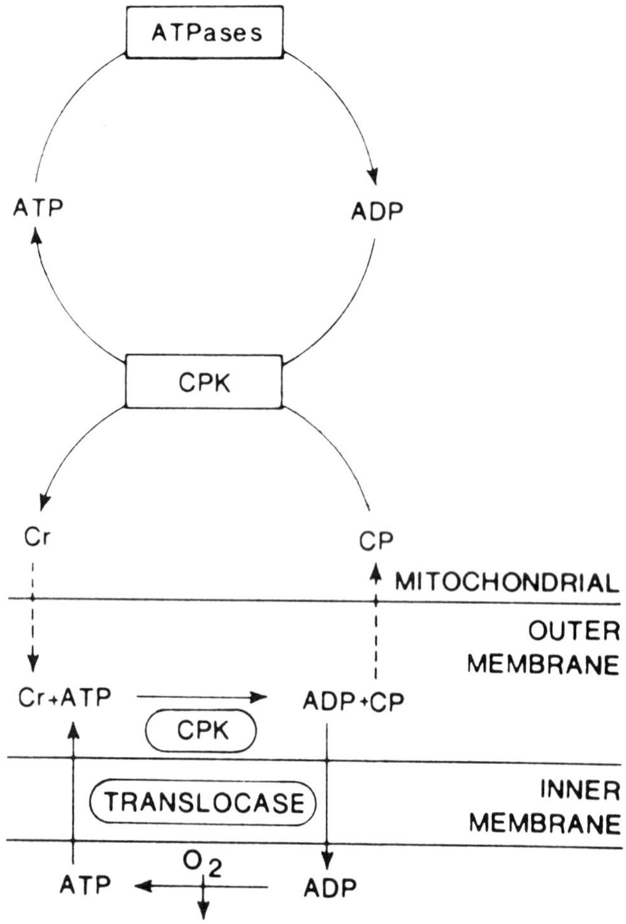

FIGURE 33-25 • Regulation of skeletal muscle and myocardial energy production, transport, and utilization.

els decreased rapidly with mild exercise in a patient with hypophosphatemia and respiratory failure, suggesting that an abnormality in the phosphocreatine pathway may play a role in the clinical presentation of patients with hypophosphatemia. The defect in phosphocreatine metabolism required several weeks of therapy to resolve, suggesting that the effects of severe hypophosphatemia may linger after correction of the serum levels.

The mechanism by which a fall in intracellular phosphate concentration inhibits the activity of the CPK isoenzyme is not known; reduced synthesis, as well as altered phosphorylation of the enzymes, is possible. The CPK system is peculiar to skeletal muscle, myocardium, and brain. It may be a mechanism by which cellular injury in phosphate depletion occurs in these organ systems.

The adenine nucleotides and AMP deaminase

Cytosolic inorganic phosphorus content is an important regulator of the overall size of the adenine nucleotide pool. A marked reduction in intracellular phosphate content accelerates the degradation of AMP by relieving the inhibition of AMP deaminase, which leads, in turn, to a reduction in the size of the adenine nucleotide pool. Phosphorus depletion stimulates the sequence:

$$2\text{ADP} \rightarrow \text{ATP} + \text{AMP}$$

$$\text{AMP} \underset{\text{AMP deaminase}}{\rightarrow} \text{IMP} \rightarrow \text{Reduction in adenine nucleotide pool}$$

This mechanism may play a role in cell injury only in situations where hypophosphatemia develops rapidly and where there is intracellular "trapping" of free inorganic phosphate, as seen in acute hyperalimentation or fructose administration. Studies of hyperventilated and chronically phosphate-depleted animals have found no changes in AMP levels or increases in IMP levels in skeletal or cardiac muscle.

Cellular membrane abnormalities

Abnormalities in cellular membrane biochemical integrity occur with phosphate depletion which may also partly mediate injury to cells in phosphate depletion. The possibility of functional and/or structural abnormalities in cell membranes of phosphate-depleted animals was suggested by Fuller and coworkers.[123] The authors demonstrated that membrane resting potential was decreased in skeletal muscle from phosphate-depleted dogs. The integrity of the cell membrane depends partly on normal phospholipid and cholesterol metabolism; as we have said, the membrane content of these lipids is abnormal with chronic phosphate depletion. Cell energy metabolism is regulated partly by membrane-bound kinases, and energy compartmentation is of major importance to the preservation of cell integrity. Therefore any abnormality in the cellular and subcellular membranes, by impairing these functions, causes cellular injury.

No single mechanism can explain the cell injury of phosphate depletion in all tissues; one or more of the mechanisms described above may operate in several tissues.

TREATMENT OF HYPOPHOSPHATEMIA

General considerations

Should hypophosphatemia be treated? This question is somewhat controversial, because carefully controlled studies have not been performed. Data from a study of Halevy and coworkers[142] suggest that the presence of hypophosphatemia augurs a poor prognosis. The mortality rate for patients with hypophosphatemia was over 20 percent, but whether the low levels of serum phosphate were causative or produced any untoward side effects was not directly addressed. In contrast, the effects of severe hypophosphatemia appeared to be minimal when evaluated prospectively by King and coworkers,[172] and levels of serum phosphate increased to 2 mg/100 ml or greater with minimal amounts of phosphate supplementation (50 percent of patients required less than 25 mmol of replacement therapy); in some cases no intervention was required. However, the lack of clinical sequelae, despite the low levels of serum phosphate in this study, may have reflected the early recognition and prompt treatment of the hypophosphatemia.

Although we lack definitive evidence that the treatment of hypophosphatemia is beneficial, in various clinical settings it appears judicious to reverse, at least partially, the hypophosphatemia or phosphate depletion. This categorical statement is based on the numerous clinical studies in the literature in which one or more of these abnormalities is reversed or cured only by phosphorus replacement and correction of the profound hypophosphatemia. Many of these patients have associated electrolyte, acid-base, and nutritional abnormalities, which are often simultaneously corrected; very few controlled studies with and without phosphorus administration are available. However, in most of the experimental and clinical studies reported there is such a strong probability that phosphorus administration is primarily responsible for correction of the specific disorder that the basic correctness of this conclusion seems acceptable.

In most of the reported cases, the dysfunction caused by phosphate depletion is serious enough that replacement therapy cannot justifiably be withheld. However, randomized studies with and without phosphorus therapy are still necessary.

Various factors should be taken into account in deciding whether it is necessary to treat a patient with hypophosphatemia. A prime consideration is whether the patient manifests any of the signs or symptoms of hypophosphatemia. One should also factor in the anticipated duration of the hypophosphatemia. Thus, in patients with uncomplicated diabetic ketoacidosis it may not be necessary to treat the hypophosphatemia per se, since these patients often start eating normal diets almost immediately. This point is illustrated by a study of Keller and Berger, who randomly assigned 40 patients to receive either conventional treatment alone or standard treatment in combination with infusions of phosphate from the beginning of therapy.[170] The initial serum concentration of inorganic phosphate was normal or elevated in almost every patient. In those receiving phosphorus it fell to a low of 2.8 to 3 mg/100 ml within 8 h, while in the control group a low of 1.8 mg/100 ml was attained; these values persisted over the next 24 to 48 h. Food was permitted ad libidum in both groups after the second day of treatment. The conclusion drawn from this study was that phosphate therapy did not have a demonstrably favorable effect on the clinical course of diabetic ketoacidosis or hyperosmolar coma. That profound hypophosphatemia almost always develops during recovery from these conditions is well known; yet the vast majority of clinical centers have not given parenteral phosphorus replacement during the past four or five decades. Most likely, the failure to see the complications of severe hypophosphatemia in this setting is attributable to the initiation of oral intake of phosphorus-containing nutrients early in the course of treatment, usually by the end of the first 24 h.

The severity of the hypophosphatemia should also be a determining factor in the decision whether to initiate treatment. Hypophosphatemia in the absence of phosphate depletion rarely produces symptoms before levels fall below 1 mg/100 ml. With levels below 1 mg/100 ml, even in the absence of phosphate depletion, various complications can occur, including hemolysis, respiratory failure, neuromuscular complications, and impairment of oxygen delivery. Therefore, it is imperative to treat hypophosphatemia when levels are below 1 mg/100 ml, particularly if the condition is prolonged. Treatment should be initiated at higher levels of serum phosphorus in patients with other debilitating problems that may be aggravated by the hypophosphatemia. Rubin and Narins[282] recommend parenteral treatment of persistent hypophosphatemia of less than 2 mg/100 ml in patients unable to eat appropriately.

Prevention of hypophosphatemia

There are several clinical situations where the development of hypophosphatemia can be anticipated, allowing prophylactic therapy. One such situation is during the administration of *TPN*, particularly when therapy is superimposed on a background of phosphate depletion or severe malnutrition. In a non-phosphate-depleted patient the serum phosphate level may fall at a rate of 0.3 mg/100 ml per day with TPN; this rate is often accelerated in a phosphate-depleted and/or malnourished patient.[103,282] The addition of phosphate to the TPN solution can prevent any significant decline in serum phosphate, but the necessary amount is highly variable. Currently it is recommended that phosphate be given as neutral phosphate, 300 mg/1000 kcal,[293] while serum phosphate is closely monitored.

Another clinical situation in which the development of hypophosphatemia can be anticipated is that of *administration of antacids*.[216] The potential to develop hypophosphatemia can be monitored via measurement of daily urinary output of phosphate by a patient receiving a given amount of antacid; if the urinary excretion of phosphate is maintained between 250 and 500 mg/day, the development of significant phosphate depletion is unlikely.[282] If the urinary excretion of phosphate falls below 250 mg/day then the dosage of antacid can be lowered, or the antacid can be given between meals to decrease the amount of phosphate bound; and the patient can be treated with alternate forms of therapy, such as H_2

antagonists. If the clinical situation precludes alternate forms of therapy, supplemental phosphate may be provided with meals to maintain urinary phosphate between 250 and 500 mg/day. Empirically one can administer 250 to 500 mg of phosphate for each 100 ml of antacid.[282]

Alcoholics often develop hypophosphatemia shortly after admission to the hospital. The hypophosphatemia is usually associated with other electrolyte abnormalities—including hypocalcemia, hypokalemia, and hypomagnesemia—which may contribute to the development of phosphate depletion and may make the patient refractory to supplemental phosphate therapy. As we have said, there are anecdotal reports suggesting that phosphate depletion in the alcoholic setting may accentuate the liver disease per se, as well as the coma associated with liver failure. Hence, prevention and treatment of hypophosphatemia in this setting is advisable. Since hypocalcemia may be accentuated by failure to treat the concomitant hypomagnesemia often present in alcoholic patients, it is recommended that an "infusion cocktail" be used, which will provide supplementation of each of these ions. The cocktail should include (per liter of 5% dextrose in 0.5 *N* saline solution): neutral potassium phosphate (4:1 mixture of K_2HPO_4 and KH_2PO_4), 20 mmol; KCl, 20 meq; and $MgSO_4$, 16 meq. One liter of this solution should be given every 8 h for several days and the amount adjusted by careful monitoring of the electrolyte status of the patient.[282]

Patients presenting in *diabetic* ketoacidosis may develop severe hypophosphatemia within 24 to 48 h after admission, despite normal or even elevated levels of serum phosphorus on admission. As we have said, in the uncomplicated setting the hypophosphatemia will reverse when the patient begins eating a normal diet. Treatment of hypophosphatemia should be initiated, however, if significant deleterious conditions coexist that may be aggravated by severe phosphate depletion, such as sepsis or respiratory failure. Rubin and Narins[282] advocate the use of 1 to 2 g/day of elemental alkaline phosphate salts during the first few days of admission in an effort to maintain serum phosphorus in the range of 2 to 3 mg/100 ml.

Treatment modalities for severe hypophosphatemia

Phosphate may be administered either orally or parenterally. Intravenous phosphate is indicated only during extreme hypophosphatemia associated with life-threatening complications, such as rapidly advancing seizures or coma, skeletal or myocardial dysfunction, or respiratory muscle paralysis. Parenteral phosphate administration is also indicated for phosphorus-depleted patients who are unable to tolerate or absorb oral feedings. In almost all other situations, oral phosphate supplementation is the therapy of choice.

Oral phosphate treatment

Skim or lowfat milk is a safe and desirable form of phosphate supplement. Every quart of milk contains 1 g each of phosphorus and calcium. A buffered laxative (e.g., Phospho-Soda) may be used for phosphate repletion. Each 100 ml contains 48 g NaH_2PO_4 and 18 g Na_2HPO_4, providing a total of 16.4 g of elemental phosphorus. Other oral phosphate supplements are available; generally they are sodium or potassium salts, or a mixture of both.

It is preferable to initiate oral treatment with no more than the equivalent of 3 g/day of elemental phosphorus in divided doses. The schedule can then be modified according to laboratory and clinical response as well as to the patient's tolerance. Mild diarrhea is an anticipated side effect.

Parenteral phosphate treatment

Parenteral phosphate should be administered to phosphate-depleted patients with caution. The clinician should be familiar with usual dosages for intravenous administration of phosphate salts. Intravenous phosphate preparations may vary in composition between different hospitals. Since this route of administration may lead to detrimental side effects, the user should be familiar with the potential side effects and contraindications. If the patient is oliguric then sodium salts, rather than potassium salts, should be administered. A 1-liter solution composed of 80 mmol Na_2HPO_4 and 20 mmol NaH_2PO_4 delivers 701 mg of elemental phosphate. In most situations the neutral phosphate preparations are preferable unless a given acid-base disturbance dictates the use of an acidic or alkaline preparation.

Phosphate-depleted patients are extremely hypophosphaturic and remain so for quite some time, despite normalization of serum phosphate. Thus, urinary loss of acutely administered phosphate may be ignored.

The amount of parenteral phosphate needed to treat a given patient with hypophosphatemia must, of necessity, be decided empirically. Since phosphate is primarily in bone and intracellular fluid, the space of distribution of a given phosphate load is difficult to estimate. In normal subjects, Hebert and coworkers found the distribution space to be approximately 40 percent. The latter figure would most likely be an underestimate of the space of distribution in a patient with phosphate depletion. Furthermore, the distribution of phosphate between intracellular and extracellular compartments is complicated and greatly influenced by prevailing pH, blood glucose concentration, and insulin availability. To avoid iatrogenic hyperphosphatemia, the ultraconservative assumption should be made that administered phosphate is restricted to the extracellular space. Since a significant fraction of the phosphate provided enters cells, the maximal serum level is never quite achieved.

An excessive increase in serum phosphate concentration causes a decrease in serum calcium levels that may be profound. Thus, in a matter of hours, phosphate depletion may be transformed into phosphate "excess," with hazardous consequences. Reduced renal clearance of phosphate sensitizes the phosphate-depleted patient to hyperphosphatemia during aggressive phosphate replenishment. Under most circumstances, therefore, elemental phosphate should not be infused at rates greater than 1 g/24 h; serum phosphorus concentration and the rate of rise in urinary phosphorus should be followed closely.

Possible complications of parenteral phosphate administration include soft tissue calcification, hypocalcemia, hypomagnesemia, hypotension, and renal failure. The diuresis associated with phosphate administration can also lead to dehydration, hypokalemia, and hypernatremia. On the other hand, hyperkalemia may result from excessive administration of potassium phosphate. Serious complications are most apt to develop when phosphate is given intravenously, or when it is given to patients with impaired renal function.

HYPERPHOSPHATEMIA

CAUSES OF HYPERPHOSPHATEMIA

A dynamic term for the plasma phosphate concentration can be derived from the formula expressing the steady-state relationship between daily urinary phosphate excretion and the difference between the filtered load of phosphate and renal tubular reabsorption of phosphate:[192,278]

$$UpV = FLp - T_pP = (PLp \times GFR) - T_P$$

where Up is the concentration of phosphate in the urine, V is urine volume, FLp is the filtered load of phosphate, T_P is the rate of tubular reabsorption of phosphate and PL_p is plasma phosphate. Since tubular reabsorption of phosphate is usually at or near its maximal capacity, the term TmP can be substituted for T_P, and, by rearrangement of the formula, an expression for plasma phosphate can be obtained:

$$PLp = UpV/GFR + T_mP/GFR$$

Under steady-state conditions, UpV represents primarily the amount of phosphate absorbed by the intestine in the nonfasted state.[278] Under various pathophysiologic conditions the load may come from other sources, such as bone or the intracellular pool. The T_mP/GFR is a theoretical plasma concentration of phosphate below which all of the FLp is reabsorbed and at which the Tm, or maximal tubular capacity to reabsorb phosphate, is reached and phosphate appears in the urine. This formula basically states that PLp is proportional to the sum of the phosphate load (normally intestinal absorption and the tubular reabsorption of phosphate) and is inversely related to the GFR. Under normal circumstances the GFR is the primary regulator of plasma phosphate; but as GFR decreases, the load factor and tubular reabsorption becomes more important.[32] As the load (UpV) increases one can expect an increase in PLp, unless one of the other terms in the formula changes concomitantly—for example, if renal adaptation occurs to decrease the reabsorption of phosphate (T_mP/GFR decreases), or if GFR increases. If the T_mP/GFR increases, perhaps because of lower levels of PTH, one can expect an increase in PLp.

The formula for plasma phosphorus provides a framework for approaching the differential diagnosis of hyperphosphatemia (Table 33-4): (1) hyperphosphatemia resulting from an *increase in the phosphate load* (increased UpV); (2) hyperphosphatemia due to a *decrease in GFR*; and (3) hyperphosphatemia resulting from an *increase in the renal phosphate threshold*, or T_mP/GFR. In addition, various combinations of these factors may occur. One must also be aware that a high level of serum phosphorus may be *factitious*. Unrecognized pseudohyperphosphatemia might lead to unnecessary treatment.

Pseudohyperphosphatemia

Pseudohyperphosphatemia may occur in *hyperglobulinemic*[2] and *hyperlipidemic*[339] states. Most autoanalyzers measure phosphorus by adding phosphomolybdic acid and a reducing agent to a deproteinized specimen. There ensues a color change that is proportional to the phosphorus content of the specimen. Protein present in the sample produces turbidity when exposed to the reagents used in some assays. The turbidity may interfere with the color reaction, resulting in a factitious elevation in the phosphorus level.[329] Generally, either of two methods is employed to deproteinize the specimen. In one the protein is removed by dialysis; in the other the protein is diluted by the additon of reagents. In the face of markedly elevated protein levels the latter method may not adequately prevent interference from protein. Adler and coworkers[2] noted an elevated level of serum phosphorus in several patients with dysproteinemia when measured by the dilutional method, but not when the specimens were dialyzed or deproteinized using sulfosalicylic acid. It appears that specific characteristics of the protein may be important as well, since not all subjects with equivalent elevations in serum protein had pseudohyperphosphatemia.

A similar phenomenon may occur when plasma lipid levels are elevated. Yudis and coworkers[339] reported a case of apparent hyperphosphatemia in a subject with only mild azotemia whose triglyceride levels were

TABLE 33-4 • Causes of hyperphosphatemia

Decreased GFR
Renal failure
Chronic
Acute
Increased phosphate loads
Exogenous
Enteric
Oral ingestion
Increased phosphorus absorption, e.g., in vitamin D intoxication
Phosphorus-containing laxatives or enemas
Parenteral
Intravenous phosphorus
Transfusion of old blood
Cutaneous
White phosphorus burns
Endogenous
Phosphorus redistribution between cells and ECF
Respiratory acidosis
Diabetic ketoacidosis
Lactic acidosis and tissue ischemia
Cell destruction
Rhabdomyolsis
Malignant hyperpyrexia
Neoplastic disease treated with cytotoxic therapy
Hemolysis
Increased T_mP/GFR
Hypoparathyroidism
PTH resistance
Pseudohypoparathyroidism
Transient resistance of infancy
Abnormal PTH (?)
Other endocrine disorders
Hyperthyroidism
Acromegaly
Juvenile hypogonadism
Postmenopausal state
Ambient high temperature
Disodium etidronate
Miscellaneous
Magnesium deficiency
Volume decrease
Tumoral calcinosis
Cortical hyperostosis
Familial intermittent hyperphosphatemia
Factitious hyperphosphatemia

1300 mg. Adding Liposol to the serum to remove the lipids lowered the phosphorus level to normal. The exact mechanism for the false elevation in phosphorus with hyperlipidemia is unknown. Finally, a false elevation in plasma phosphorus can result from in-vitro hemolysis.[29]

Hyperphosphatemia due to increased phosphate load (UpV)

With normal renal function, an increase in the phosphate load can raise plasma phosphorus significantly only if the load is introduced rapidly and is of a large magnitude. With a decrease in renal function the rise in plasma phosphorus is magnified; the severity of the hyperphosphatemia is determined by the imbalance between the kidney's capacity to excrete phosphorus and the rate at which phosphorus enters the ECF and plasma. The phosphate load can be introduced from an exogenous or an endogenous source.

Exogenous load

A common exogenous route is via the gastrointestinal tract. Ingestion of large amounts of phosphate has been reported to raise serum phosphorus, particularly when vitamin D is taken concomitantly.[192] *Vitamin D intoxication* itself may be associated with hyperphosphatemia, presumably from enhanced intestinal phosphate absorption and increased bone resorption. Patients treated with *milk* for peptic ulcer disease have been reported to have significant elevations in plasma phosphorus.[29] Hyperphosphatemia has occurred in infants fed unadapted cow's milk, which has a higher concentration of phosphate than human milk or adapted cow's milk.[253] Infants may also be more susceptible to the development of hyperphosphatemia if a simultaneous resistance to parathyroid hormone is present.[211] Although under normal circumstances little, if any, phosphate is absorbed by the large intestine, hyperphosphatemia has been reported to occur with the use of *enemas* containing high concentrations of phosphate.[16,225,270] A rise in plasma phosphate is more likely to occur if a defect in the bowel mucosa is present, as may occur in subjects who abuse enemas[270] or in subjects with Hirschsprung's disease, in whom retention time is lengthened by the presence of the aganglionic colon.[240] Phosphate-containing enemas can produce hyperphosphatemia in infants and in normal subjects during routine preparation for barium enemas;[16,225] hyperphosphatemia may also occur following the *infusion of phosphate-containing solutions*. This typically occurs during treatment of hypophosphatemia, a situation in which the kidney is set to retain nearly all the filtered phosphate. Blood transfusions, infusions of lipid emulsions for total parenteral nutrition, and heparin infusions have also been reported to produce hyperphosphatemia.[129,152]

White phosphorus burns, a common injury during the Korean War, are associated with elevations in plasma phosphorus.[37] Similar burns induced in rabbits were associated with severe hyperphosphatemia, hypocalcemia, and death.[37]

Endogenous load

An increase in phosphate load from an endogenous source may result from a shift of phosphate from *intracellular stores*, or from a release of phosphate from cells following *tissue necrosis*. Hyperphosphatemia is a common occurrence with *metabolic acidosis*, particularly organic acidosis. O'Connor and coworkers[252] measured serum phosphorus levels in patients with diabetic or lactic acidosis and found significant elevations in serum phosphorus in both groups, particularly those with lactic acidosis. The mean serum phosphorus concentration was over 9.0 mg/100 ml in those with lactic acidosis and 5.5 mg/100 ml in those with diabetic ketoacidosis. Since ketones (acetoacetate, acetone) falsely elevate the serum creatinine level, and since plasma phosphorus was higher with lactic acidosis, the phosphate/creatinine ratio was found to increase with lactic acidosis relative to diabetic ketoacidosis; a ratio greater than 3.0 was highly suggestive of lactic acidosis. However, the difference in serum phosphorus between lactic and ketoacidosis may not be real. Kebler and coworkers[167] evaluated serial serum phosphorus levels in 69 episodes of ketoacidosis in 48 diabetic patients. The incidence of hyperphosphatemia was 94.7 percent with a mean value of 9.2 mg/100 ml on initial evaluation (a value similar to that in patients with lactic acidosis in the study by O'Connor and coworkers[251] However, within 12 h plasma phosphorus levels fell to a mean of 2.8 mg/100 ml. Therefore, the level of serum phosphorus measured with diabetic ketoacidosis is time-dependent, and a single value will not reflect its dynamic nature.

Lactic acidosis may contribute to the hyperphosphatemia reported to occur with major abdominal or thoracic surgery, although other factors, such as tissue breakdown and hemolysis, are important as well.[70]

Strenuous *exercise* may result in significant elevations in serum lactate levels associated with marked elevations in serum potassium and phosphorus. Ljunghall and coworkers[213] evaluated changes in lactate levels, pH, and electrolytes following intense ergometric exercise. There was a close correlation between the reduction in pH and the increase in plasma phosphorus, suggesting that the change in pH may contribute to the rise in plasma phosphorus. Furthermore, the oxygen deficit associated with vigorous exercise may result in a failure of oxidative phosphorylation. Inorganic phosphate may accumulate intracellularly and eventually leak from muscle cells. Despite the fact that an infusion of epinephrine normally decreases the plasma phosphorus level, adrenergic stimulation may also contribute in some manner to the elevation in plasma phosphorus with strenuous exercise, since beta blockade partially blunts the rise in serum phosphorus with exertion.

Serum phosphorus levels increase rapidly following the induction of *respiratory acidosis* but return toward normal with chronic respiratory acidosis.[138,192,203] The rapid rise in serum phosphorus with acute respiratory acidosis is thought to result from a decrease in intracellular pH, which inhibits glycolysis. The rate of incorporation of inorganic phosphate into organic compounds decreases and the concentration of free intracellular inorganic phosphate rises, resulting in an increase in the efflux of phosphate into the extracellular space.

Marked elevations in plasma phosphorus may occur following tissue damage. The *tumor lysis syndrome*, which occurs following chemotherapy for various malignancies, is associated with hyperkalemia, hyperuricemia, and hyperphosphatemia.[7] Tumors where the elevation in plasma phosphorus may be particularly dramatic include acute lymphoblastic leukemia and Burkitt's lymphoma.[49,345] Hyperphosphatemia may also occur spontaneously in some leukemic patients without any apparent predisposing cause.[163]

Acute hemolysis may be associated with hyperphosphatemia; elevations in serum phosphorus have been reported to occur with thalassemia and paroxysmal nocturnal hemoglobinuria.[29]

Rhabdomyolysis is associated with hyperkalemia, hyperuricemia, hyperphosphatemia, and acute renal failure. The hyperphosphatemia is often out of proportion to the degree of renal dysfunction and can lead to severe hypocalcemia.[178] The hyperphosphatemia associated with *malignant hyperthermia* (see Chap. 47) may be attributed, in part, to rhabdomyolysis. Malignant hyperthermia occurs during the induction of general anesthesia. The onset is heralded by fever, profuse sweating, and progressive rigidity.[88,263] During the second phase body temperature rises more dramatically, and anhydrosis develops. Severe metabolic and respiratory acidosis ensue; bradycardia and cardiac arrest may occur. The bradycardia may respond to the infusion of calcium, suggesting that hypocalcemia may be the cause. In some cases there may be a genetic basis for the development of this syndrome.[89] Elevated levels of CPK were found in a patient who survived an episode of malignant hyperpyrexia and in several of his family members, some of whom had a mild myopathy.

Hyperphosphatemia due to a decrease in GFR

Hyperphosphatemia occurs with both acute and chronic renal failure.[29] With chronic renal failure, various adaptive mechanisms prevent a significant rise in plasma phosphorus until the GFR is below 25 ml/min.[299] As GFR decreases, PTH levels increase; circulating levels of calcitriol decrease; and intrinsic tubular adaptation occurs. All of these changes may decrease the fraction of phosphate reabsorbed. In parathyroidectomized animals, adaptation to nephron loss also occurs, albeit at a higher level of plasma phosphorus.[63,313] Other factors that blunt the rise in plasma phosphorus with nephron loss include volume expansion and the development of acidemia, both of which are phosphaturic. These adaptive mechanisms result in a dramatic increase in the fractional excretion of phosphate. Eventually, however, the loss in GFR dominates, and hyperphosphatemia develops. Furthermore, factors previously preventing the rise in plasma phosphorus may now augment the rise; with loss of renal function, the phosphaturic effects of PTH and metabolic acidosis are diminished relative to their effects on bone resorption.[224,304]

With progression of renal failure, the effect of a phosphate load on plasma phosphorus is magnified. If one looks at the above formula for plasma phosphorus concentration, it is apparent that changes in phosphate load will have only a minor effect on plasma phosphorus under steady-state conditions in the presence of normal renal function. For instance, if GFR is 100 ml/min, intestinal absorption of phosphorus is 1000 mg/day, and T_mP/GFR is 3.0 mg/100 ml, then the plasma phosphorus level is approximately 3.07 mg/100 ml. If one doubles the phosphorus load while the other parameters remain constant, then plasma phosphorus increases to 3.14 mg/100 ml. With a GFR of 5 ml/min, an intestinal absorption of 1000 mg/day, and the same T_mP/GFR, the plasma phosphorus is 4.4 mg/100 ml. This figure increases to 5.8 mg/100 ml with a doubling of the phosphate load. Thus, wider swings in the plasma phosphorus will occur as the GFR declines.

Hyperphosphatemia secondary to an increase in T_mP/GFR

Disorder of parathyroid hormone (PTH)

A relatively common cause of hyperphosphatemia in this category is the absence of PTH (hormonopenic hypoparathyroidism), or resistance to PTH (hormonoplethoric hypoparathyroidism).[250] Typical features of *hypoparathyroidism* include hypocalcemia, hyperphosphatemia, tetany, cataracts, basal ganglia calcification, and decreased bone mineralization without evidence of rickets or osteomalacia. A decline in circulating levels of PTH may occur following surgical removal of parathyroid glands during thyroid or parathyroid surgery or during radical neck surgery.[250] Less common causes include ^{131}I irradiation therapy, drugs (such as as L-asparaginase), metastatic carcinoma, and hemochromatosis.[250]

Various congenital or familial causes of hypoparathyroidism occur. Branchial dysembryogenesis (*DiGeorge syndrome*) results from abnormal development of neural crest tissue and may be either complete or incomplete.[128] In the complete form the thymus and parathyroid glands are absent. Cardiac abnormalities occur, including truncus arteriosus and interrupted aortic arch, along with immunoregultory disturbances. The pattern of inheritance of this disorder is not clear; the degree of penetrance may vary. Hypoparathyroidism may be idiopathic, with two modes of transmission—one unknown, the other sex-linked. Occasionally an infusion of ethylenediamine tetraacetic acid (EDTA) may be necessary to unmask latent symptoms of hypoparathyroidism in less severely affected individuals.[128]

The term *pseudohypoparathyroidism* encompasses a wide range of disorders associated with abnormal calcium and phosphorus metabolism. The syndrome, first described by Fuller Albright in 1942, is characterized by several somatic anomalies, including stocky build, short neck, round face, and shortening of the metatarsals and metacarpals. Biochemical abnormalities include hypocalcemia, hyperphosphatemia, and elevated PTH levels.[5] An increased incidence of hypertension occurs in subjects with this syndrome.[51] Both a skeletal and renal resistance to PTH are present. Chase and coworkers[64] observed that the rise in urinary cAMP following a PTH infusion was blunted in subjects with pseudohypoparathyroidism, demonstrating that a resistance to the renal effects of PTH was present. Subsequently, several cases have been described in which the appropriate rise in urinary cAMP occurs after a PTH infusion but the phosphaturic response is blunted (type II), suggesting that a defect distal

TABLE 33-5 • Classification and characteristics of pseudohypoparathyroidism

			Response to PTH			
	GNRP	Albright's hereditary osteodystrophy	*cAMP*	*Phosphate*	Osteitis fibrosa	Multiple hormone resistance
Type Ia	Low	Variable	Impaired	Impaired	Variable	Variable
Type Ib	Normal	Variable	Impaired	Impaired	Variable	Variable
Type II	Normal	Absent	Normal	Impaired	Variable	Absent

SOURCE: Adapted from Kerr and Hosking,[171] with permission.

to the generation of cAMP exists.[101] Patients with the defect proximal to cAMP generation are now said to have *type I* pseudohypoparathyroidism; *type II* pseudohypoparathyroidism is distinguished by a defect distal to the generation of cAMP (Table 33-5).

Type I pseudohypoparathyroidism is not a homogeneous disorder. Its sufferers can be divided into those subjects with both the somatic and biochemical alterations of pseudohypoparathyroidism (*type Ia*) and those who manifest only the biochemical abnormalities (*type Ib*).[99,205] The majority of subjects with the somatic abnormalities have a decrease in guanine nucleotide regulatory protein (GNRP) activity in several types of cells, including platelets, fibroblasts, red cells, and renal membranes;[99,205] generally, those with type Ib have normal levels of this protein.

Multiple endocrinologic defects would be predicted if the activity of GNRP, an element common to many hormonal systems, were decreased. Indeed, multiple endocrine abnormalities have now been described in type I patients, such as a blunted cAMP response to glucagon or ACTH infusions, primary hypothyroidism, and gonadal dysfunction. Unexpectedly, multiple endocrinologic defects may also occur in type Ib patients, although GNRP levels are normal in this group.

Several variants of pseudohypoparathyroidism exist. Some manifest a renal resistance to PTH alone; others have only a skeletal resistance to PTH. These syndromes may or may not be associated with somatic anomalies. Whether these differences reflect a heterogeneity in etiology or are related to a difference in the degree of secondary events, such as changes in calcitriol levels, remains to be determined.[171]

Nysnowitz and Klein[249] described a patient with the biochemical parameters of hypoparathyroidism but with normal or high levels of iPTH, depending on the assay used. Other causes of hypocalcemia and hyperphosphatemia were ruled out, and bone biopsy showed low bone formation rate and decreased mineralization. A PTH infusion produced a rise in urinary cAMP and a phosphaturia. The authors termed this syndrome *pseudo-idiopathic hypoparathyroidism* and postulated that the subject's own parathyroid gland was producing defective PTH.

Other hormones

Hyperphosphatemia has also been reported in *acromegaly* and *hyperthyroidism*. Both disorders appear to be associated with an increased T_mP/GFR.[29] Growth hormone administration in human beings decreases phosphate excretion within 24 h, and plasma phosphorus concentrations are increased. An elevation in plasma phosphorus may occur with juvenile hypogonadism, or with low levels of estrogen resulting from ovariectomy or following menopause. In contrast, *estrogen replacement therapy* lowers the serum phosphorus levels when administered to women with osteoporosis.[4,244] Whether the action of estrogens on renal phosphate excretion is direct or occurs via their effects on other factors, such as vitamin D metabolism, is unclear. Growth hormone levels may also be elevated following menopause; this may contribute to the hyperphosphatemia.

Hyperphosphatemia may be a manifestation of glucocorticoid withdrawal. Glucocorticoids have been shown to inhibit sodium-dependent phosphate uptake by renal proximal tubular brush-border membranes.[36] Hyperphosphatemia occurred in five patients who had undergone unilateral adrenalectomy for resection of a crotisol-producing adenoma. The increase in serum phosphorus was accompanied by an increase in the T_mP/GFR from 2.6 ± 0.2 mg/100 ml to 7.4 ± 0.4 mg/100 ml. Changes in other electrolytes were not significant. Takuwa and coworkers[314] noted similar changes in three patients following unilateral adrenalectomy, despite replacement therapy with hydrocortisone. Hyperphosphatemia developed 3 to 7 weeks after surgery while the patients were receiving 20 to 25 mg/day of hydrocortisone; two patients demonstrated clinical manifestations of glucocorticoid deficiency.

Miscellaneous disorders

An increase in T_mP/GFR is also thought to produce the hyperphosphatemia associated with *tumoral calcinosis* and *hyperostosis*. These rare syndromes are similar in their manifestations. Both are associated with hyperphosphatemia, normocalcemia, and normal levels of PTH. Tumoral calcinosis is characterized by calcium phosphate deposits in periarticular soft tissue, a normal GFR, normal-to-increased levels of calcitriol, and a familial distribution. Inheritance may be either autosomal recessive or autosomal dominant, with variable clinical expression.[220a] The disorder is more common in blacks. Hyperostosis, in contrast, is associated with episodes of painful swelling of long bones. Rarely the two syndromes have been reported to occur in a single subject.[332a]

The etiology of the renal retention of phosphate in these syndromes remains to be determined. Studies by Wilber and coworkers[331] and Balderson and coworkers[19] have shown that the tubular response to a PTH infusion, or to endogenous PTH released following an EDTA infusion, is intact in subjects with this disorder. The absence of a phosphaturic response to acetazolamide administration suggests the presence of an intrinsic proximal tubular defect that allows enhanced phosphate reabsorption.[19]

Prince and coworkers reported that calcitriol levels were elevated in two patients with hyperphosphatemic tumoral calcinosis, while PTH and 25-OH-D_3 levels were significantly decreased.[267] The investigators suggested that a failure of the feedback mechanism normally regulating the enzyme 25-hydroxy-1α-hydroxylase may be the mechanism responsible. Lufkin and coworkers examined this mechanism in two patients with hyperphosphatemic tumoral calcinosis who were put on a low-phosphate diet.[219] Phosphate depletion was accompanied by a fall in serum phosphorus concentration from 6.1 mg/100 ml to 2.6 mg/100 ml and by rises in plasma 25-OH-D_3 and calcitriol. These data confirm the previous observations of abnormally high calcitriol levels in the face of hyperphosphatemia but normal response to dietary phosphate depletion. Further studies are needed to determine the exact causes of the increase in T_mP/GFR in these two rare disorders and the possible role of calcitriol.

Iwanami and coworkers demonstrated that plasma phosphorus concentration rises from 4.0 mg/100 ml in winter to 6.2 mg/100 ml in summer in a population of normal Japanese; corresponding changes in T_mP/GFR occurred.[160] Plasma phosphorus concentration and *ambient temperature* throughout the year were closely correlated.

Etidronate disodium, an accepted therapeutic agent in the treatment of Paget's disease, may produce hyperphosphatemia. Its hyperphosphatemic effect appears to be dose-dependent; no change in plasma phosphorus concentration was observed with a dose below 5 mg/per kilogram of body weight per day.[95] The associated rise in T_mP/GFR is not accompanied by concomitant changes in circulating levels of PTH, growth hormone, cortisol, or thyroxine. Nephrogenous cAMP excretion and the phosphaturic response to exogenous PTH are also normal. Other diphosphonates have similar effects on serum phosphorus, but not to the same degree. McCloskey and coworkers[230] examined the effects of three diphosphonates (etidronate, clodronate, and aminohexane diphosphonate) in patients with Paget's disease or hypoparathyroidism. All three diphosphonates raised serum phosphorus levels and renal absorption of phosphorus in patients with Paget's disease, but the effect of etidronate was of greater magnitude and duration. The differences in the effects of the diphosphonates on the magnitude and duration of the increase in serum phosphorus may stem from their varying effects on PTH. Unlike etidronate, clodronate and aminohexane diphosphonate produced a decrease in serum and urinary calcium and a homeostatic increase in iPTH. In hypoparathyroid patients with an inability to raise PTH levels, the effect of clodronate on serum phosphorus was exaggerated. Finally, an infusion of PTH produced a phosphaturic response in etidronate-treated patients.

Hyperphosphatemia has been described in cases of experimentally induced *magnesium depletion* and hypomagnesemia. The applicability of these observations is not clear, since almost all clinically apparent conditions of magnesium depletion and hypomagnesemia result from both phosphorus and magnesium losses; most of the patients are hypophosphatemic as well as hypomagnesemic.

Acute loss of volume resulting from *furosemide administration* causes a transient increase in the concentration of plasma phosphorus of about 0.6 to 1.0 mg/100 ml.[147] This increase lasts only a few hours and has been attributed to a combination of reduced GFR and increased tubular phosphate reabsorption.

CONSEQUENCES OF HYPERPHOSPHATEMIA

Signs and symptoms of hyperphosphatemia

Progressive hyperphosphatemia that develops rapidly (i.e., within hours or days) is followed by the "phosphate excess" syndrome. The symptoms and signs are due to the induced hypocalcemia (serum calcium concentration below 7 mg/100 ml, or 3.5 meq/liter) and/or the rapid deposition of amorphous calcium phosphate salts in organs and tissues (Table 33-6). These $Ca_3(PO_4)_2$ deposits can be clinically identified by technetium polyphosphonate scanning of the soft tissues.

Rapid metastatic calcification may cause serious physiologic dysfunction in many organs and tissues. *Acute renal failure* may be caused by an oral, parenteral, or endogenous load of phosphate.[18,58] The loss of GFR results from intratubular precipitation of calcium and phosphorus. The loss of renal function may exacerbate the hyperphosphatemia and the other signs and symp-

TABLE 33-6 • Effects of hyperphosphatemia

Organ or tissue	Symptoms and/or signs
Heart	Conduction disturbances; arrhythmias; forward and backward pump failure leading to progressive hypotension, pulmonary congestion, and shock
Kidneys	Oliguria leading to anuria and progressive azotemia
GI tract	Severe anorexia; nausea; vomiting; paralytic ileus; hematemesis and melena
Lungs and alveolar lining	Dyspnea; impaired O_2 diffusion leading to hypoxemia
Cornea and conjunctiva	Haziness of cornea; conjunctival inflammation producing pain, discomfort, and red eyes
Skin and subcutaneous vessels	Papular eruptions; ischemic necrosis of fingers, toes, and skin at any site

toms already mentioned. *Arrythmias* may occur, and cardiac arrest has been reported.[245] Finally, severe *tetany* and convulsions may accompany the hypocalcemia.

While severe hypocalcemia and tetany usually result from hyperphosphatemia, serum phosphorus and calcium concentrations may rise together if rapid bone breakdown is the basic cause. In this setting the soft tissue deposition of amorphous calcium phosphate is even more severe. The combined increase in divalent ions can then spawn the aforementioned changes without tetany.

Biochemical and metabolic effects

Bone

Phosphate retention induced by increased feeding or decreased excretion of phosphate causes osteodystrophy. Thus, secondary hyperparathyroidism and bone disease occur in response to augmented phosphate feeding in animals with normal renal function. Increased ingestion of phosphate in human volunteers is also associated with elevated blood PTH levels.[268] The mechanism for the development of secondary hyperparathyroidism is discussed under "Serum Calcium and PTH" below.

Soft tissue

The effects of excess phosphate on soft tissue are a broad and complex subject. One of the most serious side effects of phosphate treatment for hypercalcemia is the possible occurrence or worsening of extraskeletal precipitation of calcium. Because soft tissue calcification can be found in untreated hypercalcemic patients, it has been difficult to determine if such calcifications are produced or aggravated by phosphate administration in clinical practice. Laboratory studies, however, have shown that inorganic phosphate treatment of hypercalcemia leads to calcium deposition in heart, kidney, and other tissues.[287] Oral phosphate administration in experimental hypercalcemia has been shown to accelerate calcium sequestration in soft tissue.[301] In one study, only those hypercalcemic rats that were treated with phosphate died. Extensive soft tissue calcification has also been described in rabbits given oral phosphate therapy.[287]

Metastatic calcification is common in uremic patients. The alteration most frequently associated with metastatic calcification is elevation of the plasma calcium-phosphorus product. Since the majority of uremic patients are hypocalcemic, the increase in calcium-phosphorus product is mainly the result of hyperphosphatemia. The product in normal subjects is approximately 40 $mg^2/(100\ ml)^2$ (i.e., 10 mg/100 ml × 4 mg/100 ml). Precipitation of calcium phosphate occurs in vitro when the product exceeds a critical level. In uremic patients with metastatic calcification, the product usually exceeds 70 $mg^2/(100\ ml)^2$.[129,215] The tendency toward development of extraosseous calcification in uremic patients has been attributed to a number of other factors, including azotemia, age, hyperparathyroidism, and increased sensitivity to calcification.

The effects of metastatic calcification in uremic patients can be dramatic and life-threatening. Calciphylaxis is a syndrome occurring in uremic patients that is associated with medial calcinosis of medium- and small-sized arteries.[129] Typically the patients have had long-standing uremia and develop ulcerating lesions in both upper and lower extremities, which can result in autoamputation and even death. Several factors may contribute to this syndrome, including hyperphosphatemia, hypercalcemia, and secondary hyperparathyroidism.

Hyperphosphatemia or phosphate retention in renal failure may exacerbate the rate of decline in renal function; dietary phosphate restriction has been reported to ameliorate the decline in renal function in experimental renal disease.[156] This may well be a secondary effect of decreased phosphate retention and soft tissue calcification.[185] Control of hyperphosphatemia by dietary phosphate restriction and use of enteric phosphate binders has led to improvement in extraosseous calcification in chronic renal failure.

Red blood cells

Erythrocytes from uremic patients exhibit increased rates of glycolysis; their content of 2,3-diphosphoglycerate (DPG) and ATP is also increased. The increases have been attributed to the hyperphosphatemia of chronic renal failure.[210] However, Barcenas and associates demonstrated that the increases in red cell 2-3-DPG and ATP persist even after successful renal transplantation and in the face of hypophosphatemia. The stable elevation in these phosphorus compounds may be a result of steroid treatment: increased erythrocyte 2,3-DPG content has been found in acid citrate dextrose blood incubated with hydrocortisone or methylprednisolone in vitro.[258]

Serum calcium and PTH

Although the calcium and phosphate concentrations in plasma do not conform to a fixed solubility product ratio, a rise in plasma phosphate is often followed by a fall in plasma calcium. Although direct precipitation of mineral in the blood or soft tissues should not occur until plasma phosphate concentration rises to at least 6 mg/100 ml or higher, a much smaller increase produced by phosphate administration actually suffices to lower ionized calcium. Part of this fall is due to increased formation of $CaHPO_4$ ion-pair complexes in plasma, but increases in plasma phosphate concentration are also transmitted to the extra- and intracellular fluid of the bones. Whatever the true composition of the fluid, amorphous mineral is immediately deposited at the bone surface, and the concentration of ionized calcium in the bone fluid drops. As a result, the concentration of Ca^{2+} in the plasma decreases. If parathyroid function is normal, appropriate changes in PTH secretion restore the ionized calcium level to normal. Therefore, for any given metabolic or hormonal setting, any factor that causes a rise in plasma or extracellular fluid (ECF) phosphate concentration lowers ionized calcium concentration.

A reduction in urinary calcium excretion occurs following phosphate administration. This has been attributed to an increase in PTH secretion. However, the hypocalciuric effect may persist after PTH levels return to normal, and can also occur in hypoparathyroid patients.[256] The mechanism of this PTH-independent hypocalciuric effect is unknown.

Hyperphosphatemia has long been thought to play a critical role in the development of secondary hyperparathyroidism associated with chronic renal failure. The decrease in ionized plasma calcium associated with hyperphosphatemia has long been thought to play a central role.[50] It has been hypothesized that with nephron loss a small rise in serum phosphorus occurs, which results in a small, undetectable decrease in serum calcium. The latter stimulates PTH secretion, which returns serum calcium and phosphorus levels to normal—but at the expense of an elevated serum level of PTH. This scenario repeats itself as more nephrons are lost; eventually a state of severe secondary hyperparathyroidism develops. However, several lines of evidence make the role of hyperphosphatemia in the pathogenesis of secondary hyperparathyroidism dubious.[214] Several studies failed to demonstrate an elevated level of fasting serum phosphorus with renal failure. Greater doubt has been established by careful measurements of serum phosphorus throughout the day in subjects with moderate renal failure. Portale and coworkers[265] measured serum phosphorus hourly in a group of control subjects and children with moderate renal failure (mean GFR 45 $\pm$ 4 ml/min) and elevated levels of PTH. Fasting serum phosphorus levels were actually lower in children with renal failure, and were never higher than in control subjects throughout the day. Wilson and coworkers[332] administered an oral phosphate load to control subjects and patients with mild renal insufficiency. The two groups showed similar rises in serum phosphorus following the oral load. These observations provide a strong argument against the role of hyperphosphatemia in the development of secondary hyperparathyroidism with early-to-moderate renal failure. Alterations in phosphate metabolism per se may play a critical role in the development of secondary hyperparathyroidism independent of serum phosphorus. Thus there appears to be a correlation between dietary intake of phosphate and secondary hyperparathyroidism. This effect may be due to phosphate retention and an increase in intracellular phosphate, which in turn may suppress the production of calcitriol;[214] the latter hormone has been shown to increase with phosphate restriction in both adults and children with moderate renal failure. It is also clear that the development of hyperphosphatemia can aggravate the degree of secondary hyperparathyroidism, and that hyperparathyroidism may be ameliorated or prevented by restriction of dietary phosphate and judicious use of phosphate binding antacids.

TREATMENT OF HYPERPHOSPHATEMIA

The treatment of hyperphosphatemia is aimed both at prevention and at the removal of phosphate from the circulation.

Prevention

Prevention includes the elimination of exogenous or endogenous phosphate sources in patients with impaired renal function and, importantly, the maintenance of renal function. Thus, in patients with the tumor lysis syndrome, prevention of uric acid nephropathy may prevent the development of significant hyperphosphatemia in many cases, despite an increased phosphate load from cell breakdown. The avoidance of nephrotoxic agents under these circumstances is also helpful.

Phosphate removal

In patients with severe hyperphosphatemia whose calcium-phosphate product is dangerously high, removal of phosphate from the body is indicated. Dialysis in combination with the use of large doses of intestinal phosphate binders reduces serum phosphorus levels rapidly (12 to 35 h). For patients with chronic renal failure, oral therapy and eventual dialysis are also critical modalities in the control of phosphate homeostasis.

Hemodialysis

During hemodialysis all substances freely filterable through cellophane membranes have thresholds determined conjointly by the volume and composition of the bath fluid and the blood and body fluids. The rate of excretion at any instant is proportional to the concentration gradient between plasma and body fluid at that instant. Phosphate is a poorly diffusible ion; its diffusion coefficient is 0.31 (compare to the coefficient of 1.0 for potassium, a highly diffusible ion).[333] Hemodialysis using a large-surface, high-efficiency dialyzer removes approximately 400 to 600 mg in a 4-h dialysis.[6] Relative to the dietary intake of phosphate, which ranges from 1.0 to 1.5 g/24 h, the dialysis may not seem to provide a marked improvement. However, if 600 mg of phosphate removed by dialysis is expressed as milligrams of phosphate per 100 milliters of blood, then 600 mg of phosphate removed, divided by 11 liters (plasma water plus interstitial water), represents an approximate reduction in serum phosphate of 5.5 mg/100 ml. The only problem with this calculation is that serum phosphate rebounds to predialysis levels at 6 to 10 h post-dialysis, even in the absence of an additional phosphate load; the reequilibration of intracellular phosphate stores reestablishes hyperphosphatemia. Thus, frequent hemodialysis treatment may be necessary in the treatment of severe hyperphosphatemia in a patient whose renal function has deteriorated, particularly when a large exogenous or endogenous source for phosphate persists.

Various factors may have an impact on the effectiveness of hemodialysis in lowering serum phosphorus. In addition to the removal of phosphate from the blood, dialysis may affect the volume through which phosphate is distributed. Indeed, Wathen and coworkers recently suggested that the hypophosphatemia and hypokalemia that arise during hemodialysis result from a redistribution of phosphate and potassium ions. That redistribution, they suggested, is produced by the sharp changes in cellular intermediary metabolism that are brought on by the acetate dialysate.[328]

The type of dialysis membrane used may be critical. Polycarbonate membranes readily clear compounds of high molecular weight and have very high ultrafiltration rates. Polycarbonate membranes capped with conventional cellophane membranes provide markedly higher phosphate clearance.[117] Other studies suggest that the type of membrane used for dialysis may not be as critical as the available surface area during conventional dialysis. Also, biofiltration may have a greater phosphate clearance than conventional dialysis; and the use of bicarbonate rather than acetate is associated with a lesser rise in serum phosphorus following dialysis.[344]

Oral phosphate binders

Oral administration of phosphate-binding antacids has been shown to lower serum phosphorus levels effectively, and aluminum-containing gels have been a cornerstone in the treatment of hyperphosphatemia. The latter act by binding intestinal phosphate and rendering the ion nonabsorbable. In addition to preventing dietary phosphate absorption, intestinal phosphate binders disrupt the reabsorption of endogenous phosphate, which is excreted normally via the parotid glands and pancreatic fluid. Two commonly used phosphate binders are aluminum hyroxide gel and aluminum carbonate gel. Liquid gels are generally most effective. Metabolic balance studies have shown that the ingestion of 75 to 200 ml/day of aluminum hydroxide gel can enhance fecal loss of phosphorus by 30 to 144 percent. With the ingestion of aluminum hydroxide gel and the maintenance of dietary phosphate intake at 1.0 g/day, fecal phosphorus output exceeded the dietary intake, suggesting that phosphorus was actually lost. When dietary intake increased to 2.0 g/day, phosphate balance was positive despite the administration of aluminum hydroxide gel. Thus, a certain degree of dietary phosphate restriction should accompany the administration of aluminum hydroxide gels.[282]

The optimal time to administer phosphate binders is with meals. The dose should be proportional to the size of the meal; if the largest intake of phosphate occurs with dinner, more binder should be given with this meal.[300]

The use of aluminum-containing antacids, which have been the primary phosphate binders used for many years, leads to a significant degree of aluminum absorption, resulting in aluminum overload with severe clinical sequelae.[72,73] Therefore, measures have been sought to prevent the consequences of aluminum intoxication including the use of calcium and magnesium containing phosphate binders. These are discussed in detail in Chap. 41.

Other treatment modalities

In patients with end-stage renal failure and severe intractable hyperphosphatemia—particularly if calciphylaxis occurs—parathyroidectomy may be indicated to reduce the bone and hyperphosphatemic effects of PTH by shifting phosphorus from bone to the circulation. Treatment of tumoral calcinosis may include surgical removal of tumor masses; more recently, though, the use of phosphate-binding antacids has proved efficacious in conjunction with dietary protein restriction.[82b]

APPENDIX

"NEUTRAL" PHOSPHATE

The salts used in therapy are derived from phosphoric acid (H_3PO_4), which ionizes according to the following equation:

$$H_3PO_4 = H^+ + H_2PO_4^- = H^+ + HPO_4^{2-} = H^+ + PO_4^{3-}$$

The parent compound, H_3PO_4, is far too strong an acid to exist as such at physiologic pH; it therefore exists only in its ionized forms. The end product, PO_4^{3-}, is far too strong a base to exist as such at physiologic pH; that is, there is always too much H^+ present in biological solutions to allow free PO_4^{3-} to exist. Therefore, only $H_2PO_4^-$ and HPO_4^{2-} exist in biological fluids.

The Henderson-Hasselbalch equation is used to define the relationship of the acid dihydrogen phosphate ($H_2PO_4^-$) to its salt, monohydrogen phosphate (HPO_4^{2-}). The negative logarithm of the ionization constant (i.e.,

pK_a) of $H_2PO_4^-$ is 6.8. Thus, in "neutral" serum where pH = 7.40, the acid and its salt obey the following relationship:

$$pH = pK + \log \frac{[salt]}{[acid]}$$

$$7.40 = 6.8 + \log \frac{[HPO_4^{2-}]}{[H_2PO_4^-]}$$

$$0.60 = \log \frac{[HPO_4^=]}{[H_2PO_4^-]}$$

Taking the antilog of both sides gives

$$4 = \frac{[HPO_4^{2-}]}{[H_2PO_4^-]}$$

Thus, at neutral serum pH, 4 mmol of phosphate is in the divalent (HPO_4^{2-}) form for each 1 mmol in the monovalent ($H_2PO_4^-$) form. It follows that any phosphate solution containing a mixture of HPO_4^{2-} and $H_2PO_4^-$ in the proportion of 4 mmol HPO_4^{2-} to 1 mmol $H_2PO_4^-$ must have the pH of normal serum—that is, 7.40. Phosphate solutions are prepared and given in the neutral form in order to preserve acid-base balance.

RELATIONSHIP OF MILLIMOLES TO MILLIEQUIVALENTS TO MILLIGRAMS

To express a given quantity of a substance in terms of *millimoles*, divide the formula weight, in milligrams by the molecular weight. Consider, for example, 13.92 g of K_2HPO_4. The constituent atomic weights are K = 39, H = 1, P = 31, O = 16. 13.92 g = 13,920 mg; 13,920/174 = 80 mmol.

The *milliequivalent* relates to combining power with H^+. Since the salt of HPO_4^{2-} is divalent and the acid is univalent, neutral phosphate may be redefined as 4 mmol HPO_4^{2-} and 1 mmol $H_2PO_4^-$; that is, 4 mmol HPO_4^{2-} = 8 meq; 1 mmol $H_2PO_4^-$ = 1 meq. The mean apparent valency of neutral phosphate is −1.8 (see below).

Determining the number of milligrams of elemental phosphorus

First, the percentage of phosphorus in the salt is defined by means of atomic and molecular weights. For example, how much elemental phosphorus is contained in 80 mmol of K_2HPO_4?

$$MW = 174$$

$$\text{atomic weight of P} = 31$$

$$\text{percentage P} = \frac{31}{174} = 0.18$$

$$80 \text{ mmol } K_2HPO_4 \times 0.18 = 14.25 \text{ mmol P} = 441.8 \text{ mg}$$

How much elemental phosphorus is contained in 20 mmol of KH_2PO_4?

$$MW = 136 \text{ percentage P} = 0.23$$

$$20 \text{ mmol } K_2HPO_4 \times 0.23 = 4.6 \text{ mmol P} = 143 \text{ mg}$$

Thus 1 liter of neutral phosphate, containing 80 mmol K_2HPO_4 and 20 mmol KH_2PO_4, has 160 meq of HPO_4^{2-} and 20 meq of $H_2PO_4^-$. This (neutral) solution contains 442 + 143 = 585 mg of elemental phosphorus.

Converting mmol/liter of serum phosphorus to meq/liter

The average valency of circulating phosphorus is 1.8. The figure 1.8, which is used to calculate number of milliequivalents, is derived as follows. At neutral pH each 5 mmol of phosphorus can be subdivided into

$$4 \text{ mmol } HPO_4^{2-} = 8 \text{ negative charges}$$

$$1 \text{ mmol } H_2PO_4^- = 1 \text{ negative charge}$$

$$\text{Total} = 9 \text{ negative charges}$$

Therefore, 9 negative charges are distributed among 5 mmol, giving an average value of 1.8 negative charges per mmol. It follows that 1 mmol/liter of serum phosphorus equals 1.8 meq/liter (since mmol × valency = meq).

Finding the potassium content of a solution

The potassium content of a solution of 100 mmol of potassium mono- and dihydrogen phosphate at pH 7.4 is determined by

$$80 \text{ mmol } K_2HPO_4 = 160 \text{ mmol K}$$

$$20 \text{ mmol } KH_2PO_4 = \underline{20 \text{ mmol K}}$$

$$\text{Total} = 180 \text{ mmol K}$$

REFERENCES

1. Aalbers C et al: Serum phosphate and anxiety in major depression. *Psychiatry Res* 31:217, 1990.
2. Adler SG et al: Hyperglobulinemia may spuriously elevate measured serum inorganic phosphate levels. *Am J Kidney Dis* 10:260, 1988.
3. Agus ZS: Oncogenic hypophosphatemic osteomalacia. *Kidney Int* 24:113, 1983.
4. Aitken JM et al: The effect of long-term mestranol administration on calcium and phosphorus homeostasis in oophorectomized women. *Clin Sci* 41:233, 1971.
5. Albright F et al: Pseudohypoparathyroidism: An example of the Seabright-Bantam syndrome. *Endocrinology* 30:922, 1942.
6. Albright R et al: Potassium and phosphate removal with bicarbonate hemodialysis. *Trans Am Soc Nephrol*, 15th annual meeting, 1982, p 48A.
7. Allon M et al: Hyperphosphatemia, hypocalcemia, and renal failure in a patient with acute leukemia. *Am J Kidney Dis* 11:442, 1988.
8. Allon M et al: Insulin in the acute renal adaptation to

dietary phosphate restriction in the rat. *Kidney Int* 37:14, 1990.
9. Andersen PT et al: Severe hypophosphatemia following elective abdominal aortic bypass grafting. *Acta Chir Scand* 153:641, 1987.
10. Anderson J, Foster JB: Effect of cortisone on urinary phosphate excretion in man. *Clin Sci* 18:437, 1959.
11. Annino JS, Relman AS: The effect of eating on some of the clinically important chemical constituents of the blood. *Am J Clin Pathol* 31:155, 1959.
12. Ando M et al: Generation of hypophosphatemia in rats by continuous oral administration of cadmium. *Toxicology* 53:1, 1988.
13. Arruda JAL et al: Distal acidification defect induced by phosphate deprivation. *Metabolism* 29:826, 1980.
14. Aschinberg LC et al: Vitamin D resistant rickets associated with epidermal nevus syndrome. Demonstration of a phosphaturic substance in the dermal lesions. *J Pediatr* 91:56, 1977.
15. Atchley DW et al: On diabetic acidosis. A detailed study of electrolyte balances following the withdrawal and reestablishment of insulin therapy. *J Clin Invest* 12:287, 1933.
16. Atkins CE: Sodium phosphate enemas: How to kill cats, cause cardiac arrest, and cure eye rolling at Stanford. *JAMA* 257:258, 1987.
17. Aubel CE: The effects of low phosphorus rations on growing pigs. *J Agric Res* 52:149, 1936.
18. Ayala G et al: Acute hyperphosphatemia and acute persistent renal insufficiency induced by oral phosphate therapy. *Ann Intern Med* 83:520, 1975.
19. Baldersson H et al: Tumoral calcinosis with hyperphosphatemia: A report of a family with incidence in four siblings. *J Bone Joint Surg* 51A:913, 1969.
20. Balon JM et al: Relative hypophosphatemia in patients with panic disorders. *Arch Gen Psychiatry* 45:294, 1988.
21. Bar A, Wasserman RH: Control of calcium absorption and intestinal calcium binding protein synthesis. *Biochem Biophys Res Commun* 54:191, 1973.
22. Barcenas CG et al: Erythrocyte adenosine triphosphate and 2,3-diphosphoglycerate after human renal transplantation: Dissociation from hypophosphatemia. *Clin Sci* 52:413, 1977.
23. Bar-Khayim Y et al: Transient hypophosphatemia associated with hairy-cell leukemia. *Harefuah* 118:83, 1990.
24. Baughman FA Jr, Papp JP: Wernicke's encephalopathy with intravenous hyperalimentation: Remarks on similarities between Wernicke's encephalopathy and the phosphate depletion syndrome. *Mt Sinai J Med* 43:48, 1976.
25. Baylink D et al: Formation, mineralization and resorption of bone in hypophosphatemic rats. *J Clin Invest* 50:2519, 1971.
26. Bellorin-Font E et al: Uncoupling of the parathyroid hormone receptor-adenylate cyclase system of canine kidney during dietary phosphorus deprivation. *Endocrinology* 115:544, 1984.
27. Benesch B, Benesch RE: The effects of organic phosphates from human erythrocytes on the oxygen equilibrium of human erythrocytes. *Biochem Biophys Res Commun* 26:162, 1967.
28. Bessman SP, Geiger PJ: Transport of energy in muscle: The phosphorylcreatine shuttle. *Science* 211:448, 1981.
29. Betro MG, Pain RW: Hypophosphatemia in hospital population. *Br Med J* 1:273, 1972.
30. Bhaskaran D et al: Effect of hypophosphatemia on brain catecholamines content in the rat. *Miner Electrolyte Metab* 13:469, 1987.
31. Biber J et al: Na-P_i cotransport in LLC-PK_1 cells: Fast adaptive response to P_i deprivation. *Am J Physiol* 249:C430, 1985.
32. Bijvoet OLM: The importance of the kidneys in phosphate homeostasis, in Avioli L et al (eds): *Phosphate Metabolism, Kidney and Bone,* Paris, Nouvelle Imprimerie Fournie, 1975, p 42.
33. Bloom WL, Finchum D: Osteomalacia with pseudofractures caused by the ingestion of aluminum hydroxide. *JAMA* 174:181, 1960.
34. Bode JC et al: Depletion of liver adenine phosphates and metabolic effects of intravenous infusion of fructose or sorbitol in man and in the rat. *Eur J Clin Invest* 3:436, 1973.
35. Body JJ et al: Epinephrine is a hypophosphatemic hormone in man. Physiological effects of circulating epinephrine on plasma calcium, magnesium, phosphorus, parathyroid hormone and calcitonin. *J Clin Invest* 71:572, 1983.
36. Boross M et al: Glucocorticoids and metabolic acidosis-induced renal transports of inorganic phosphate, calcium and NH_4. *Am J Physiol* 250:F827, 1986.
37. Bowman TE et al: Sudden death after phosphorus burns: Experimental observations of hypocalcemia by phosphatemia and electrocardiographic abnormalities following production of a standard white phosphorus burn. *Ann Surg* 174:779, 1971.
38. Brady HR et al: Hypophosphatemia complicating bronchodilator therapy of acute severe asthma. *Arch Intern Med* 149:2367, 1989.
39. Brautbar N et al: Influence of dietary magnesium in experimental phosphate depletion: Bone and soft tissue mineral changes. *Am J Physiol* 237:E152, 1979.
40. Brautbar N et al: Interactions between vitamin D deficiency and phosphorus depletion in the rat. *J Clin Invest* 63:335, 1979.
41. Brautbar N et al: Effects of phosphate depletion on cell membrane phospholipids and glucose pathways in liver, kidney and skeletal muscle. *Trans Am Soc Nephrol*, 13th annual meeting, 1980, p 2A.
42. Brautbar N et al: Normophosphatemic phosphate depletion in the growing rat. *Am J Physiol* 236:E282, 1979.
43. Brautbar N et al: Soft tissue and bone mineral changes in experimental phosphate depletion: The role of growth and growth hormone. *Miner Electrolyte Metab* 5:304, 1981.
44. Brautbar N et al: The divalent ions, in Freinkel N (ed): *Contemporary Metabolism.* New York, Plenum Press, 1982, p 441.
45. Brautbar N et al: Impaired energy metabolism in rat myocardium during phosphate depletion. *Am J Physiol* 242:F699, 1982.
46. Brautbar N et al: On the mechanism of hypophosphatemia during acute hyperventilation. *Miner Electrolyte Metab* 9:115, 1983.

47. Brautbar N et al: Impaired skeletal muscle energetics in phosphate depleted rats. *Kidney Int* 24:53, 1983.
48. Brautbar N et al: Impaired lipid metabolism in phosphate depletion. *Kidney Int* 26:18, 1984.
49. Brereton HD et al: Hyperphosphatemia and hypercalcemia in Burkitt lymphoma. Complications of therapy. *Arch Intern Med* 135:307, 1975.
50. Bricker NS: On the pathogenesis of the uremic state: An exposition of the "Trade-off Hypothesis." *N Engl J Med* 286:1093, 1972.
51. Brickman AS et al: Hypertension in pseudohypoparathyroidism Type I. *Am J Med* 85:785, 1988.
52. Brown EL, Jenkins BAG: A case of respiratory failure complicated by acute hypophosphatemia. *Anaesthesia* 35:42, 1980.
53. Burch HB et al: Distribution along the rat nephron of three enzymes of gluconeogenesis in acidosis and starvation. *Am J Physiol* 253:F246, 1978.
54. Burnstein MI et al: The enteropathic changes of hypophosphatemia osteomalacia in adults: Radiologic findings. *Am J Roentgenol* 153:785, 1989.
55. Bushe CJ: Low phosphate levels in ventilated patients. *Lancet* 2:579, 1987.
56. Bushe CJ: Profound hypophosphatemia in patients collapsing after a "fun run." *Br Med J* 292:898, 1986.
57. Campese VM et al: Effect of phosphate depletion in blood pressure. *Proc Am Soc Nephrol*, 15th Annual Meeting, 1982, p 4A.
58. Carey RW et al: Massive extraskeletal calcification during phosphate treatment of hypercalcemia. *Arch Intern Med* 122:150, 1968.
59. Carmichael KA et al: Osteomalacia and osteitis fibrosa in a man ingesting aluminum hydroxide antacid. *Am J Med* 76:1137, 1984.
60. Cary DE et al: Hypophosphatemic rickets/osteomalacia in linear sebaceous nevus syndrome: A variant of tumor-induced osteomalacia. *J Pediatr* 109:994, 1986.
61. Caverzasio J et al: Adaptation of phosphate transport in phosphate deprived LLC-PK_1 cells. *Am J Physiol* 248:F122, 1985.
62. Caverzasio J et al: Adaptation of phosphate transport to low phosphate diet in renal and intestinal brush border membrane vesicles: Influence of sodium and pH. *Eur J Physiol* 409:333, 1987.
63. Caverzasio J et al: Parathyroid hormone independent adaptation of the renal handling of phosphate in response to renal mass reduction. *Kidney Int* 21:471, 1982.
64. Chase LR et al: Pseudohypoparathyroidism: Defective excretion of 3′,5′-AMP in response to parathyroid hormone. *J Clin Invest* 48:1832, 1969.
65. Chen C et al: Hypercalciuric hypophosphatemic rickets, mineral balance, bone histomorphometry, and therapeutic implications of hypercalciuria. *Pediatrics* 84:276, 1989.
66. Chordiker BN et al: Hyperphosphatemia in infantile hypophosphatasia: Implications for carrier diagnosis. *Am J Hum Genet* 46:280, 1990.
67. Citrin DL et al: Estramustine affects bone mineral metabolism in metastatic prostate cancer. *Cancer* 58:2208, 1986.
68. Citrin DL et al: Decreased serum phosphate levels after high-dose estrogens in metastatic prostate cancer. *Am J Med* 76:787, 1984.
69. Clark L, Rivera-Cordero F: Effects of endogenous parathyroid hormone on calcium, magnesium and phosphate metabolism in rats: II. Alterations of dietary phosphate. *Endrocrinology* 95:360, 1974.
70. Clowes GHA et al: Acute hypocalcemia in surgical patients. *Ann Surg* 146:530, 1970.
71. Coburn JW et al: Intestinal absorption of calcium, phosphorus and magnesium in chronic renal insufficiency, in David DS (ed): *Calcium Metabolism in Renal Failure.* New York, Wiley, 1977, p 79.
72. Coburn J: Aluminum metabolism and the clinical features of aluminum toxicity, in Cecchittin M et al (eds): *Calciotoropic Hormones and Calcium Metabolism.* Verona, Bitgi, 1988, p 115.
73. Coburn JW et al: Toxic effects of aluminum in end-stage renal disease: Discussion of a case. *Am J Kidney Dis* 12:171, 1988.
74. Copp DH, Suiker AP: Study of calcium kinetics in calcium and phosphorus deficient rats with the aid of radiocalcium, in McLean FC et al (eds): *Radioisotopes and Bone.* Oxford, Blackwell, 1962, p 1.
75. Craddock PR et al: Acquired phagocyte dysfunction. A complication of the hypophosphatemia of parenteral hyperalimentation. *N Engl J Med* 290:1403, 1974.
76. Cuisinier-Gleizes P et al: Effet ostéolytique du régime pauvre en phosphore chez le rat, in Hioco DJ (ed): *Phosphate et Metabolisme Phosphocalcique.* Paris, Editions Sandoz, 1971, p 117.
77. Cuisinier-Gleizes P et al: Homeostasis and P and Ca in phosphorus deprivation, in Avioli L et al (eds): *Phosphate Metabolism, Kidney and Bone*, Paris, Nouvelle Imprimerie Fournie, 1975, p 381.
78. Cumming AD et al: Refeeding hypophosphatemia in anorexia nervosa and alcoholism. *Br Med J* 295:490, 1987.
79. Dabbagh S et al: Effect of vitamin D deficiency on amino acid excretion in the phosphate-depleted rat. *Miner Electrolyte Metab* 15:283, 1989.
80. Dale G et al: Fitness, unfitness and phosphate. *Br Med J* 294:939, 1987.
81. Danowski TS: *Clinical Endocrinology.* Baltimore, Williams & Wilkins, vol III.
82. Danowski TS et al: Muscular dystrophy. Blood sugar and serum electrolytes following insulin and dextrose, alone or in combination. *Am J Dis Child* 91:429, 1956.
82a. Davenport A et al: Hypophosphatemia in acute liver failure. *Br Med J* 296:131, 1988.
83. Davis JL et al: Acute and chronic phosphate depletion as a modulator of glucose uptake in rat skeletal muscle. *Life Sci* 24:629, 1979.
84. Davis SV et al: Reversible depression of myocardial performance in hypophosphatemia. *Am J Med Sci* 295:183, 1988.
85. Dawson DJ et al: Hypophosphatemia in acute liver failure. *Br Med J* 295:1312, 1987.
86. Day HG, McCollum EV: Mineral metabolism, growth, symptomatology of rats on diet extremely deficient in phosphorus. *J Biol Chem* 130:269, 1939.

87. Defronzo RA, Lang R: Hypophosphatemia and glucose intolerance: Evidence for tissue insensitivity to insulin. *N Engl J Med* 303:1259, 1980.
88. Denborough MA et al: Biochemical changes in malignant hyperpyrexia. *Lancet* 2:1137, 1970.
89. Denborough MA et al: Myopathy and malignant hyperpyrexia. *Lancet* 2:1138, 1970.
90. De Oliveira HD, Lans-Filhot A: Letter—Hypophosphatemia in gout. *Lancet* 2:215, 1961.
91. Derr RF, Zieve L: Etiology of hyperalimentation coma. *N Engl J Med* 288:1080, 1973.
92. Derr RF, Zieve L: Effect of carbohydrate load by intravenous infusion in fasted rats on liver glucose-6-phosphate dehydrogenase and malic enzyme. *J Nutr* 104:65, 1974.
93. Derr RF, Zieve L: Weakness, neuropathy and coma following total parenteral nutrition in underfed or starved rats: Relationship to blood hyperosmolarity and brain water loss. *J Lab Clin Med* 42:521, 1978.
94. de Vernejoul CM et al: Nonosteomalacic osteopathy associated with chronic hypophosphatemia. *Calcif Tissue Int* 34:219, 1982.
95. DeVries HR, Bijvoet OLM: Results of prolonged treatment of Paget's disease of bone with disodium ethane-1-hydroxy-1,1-diphosphonate (EHDP). *Neth J Med* 17:281, 1974.
96. Ditzel J: Effect of plasma inorganic phosphate on tissue oxygenation during recovery from diabetic ketoacidosis. *Adv Exp Med Biol* 37A:163, 1971.
97. Dominguez JH et al: Dietary phosphate deprivation in women and men: Effects on mineral and acid balances, parathyroid hormone and the metabolism of 25-OH-vitamin D. *J Clin Endocrinol Metab* 42:1056, 1976.
98. Donhowe JM et al: Factitious hypophosphatemia related to mannitol therapy. *Clin Chem* 27:1765, 1981.
99. Downs RW et al: Deficient adenylate cyclase regulatory protein in renal membranes from a patient with pseudohypoparathyroidism. *J Clin Invest* 71:231, 1983.
100. Drenick EJ et al: Occurrence of acute Wernicke's encephalopathy during prolonged starvation for the treatment of obesity. *N Engl J Med* 274:937, 1966.
101. Drezner MK et al: Pseudohypoparathyroidism type II: A possible defect in the reception of the cyclic AMP signal. *N Engl J Med* 289:1056, 1973.
102. Drezner MK et al: Evaluation of a role for 1,25-di-hydroxyvitamin D-3 in the pathogenesis and treatment of X-linked hypophosphatemic rickets and osteomalacia. *J Clin Invest* 66:1020, 1980.
103. Dudrick SJ et al: Parenteral hyperalimentation—metabolic problems and solutions. *Ann Surg* 176:259, 1972.
104. Dutoit PJ, Bisschop THR: The breeding of cattle on phosphorus-deficient veld. *Rep Dir Vir Serv Anim Ind Onderstepoort* 15:1050, 1929.
105. Edelstein SA et al: The functional metabolism of vitamin D in chicks fed low calcium and low phosphorus diets. *Biochim Biophys Acta* 385:438, 1976.
106. Eisenbrey AB et al: Mannitol interference in an automated serum phosphate assay. *Clin Chem* 33:2308, 1987.
107. Emmett M et al: The pathophysiology of acid-base changes in chronically phosphate-depleted rats. Bone-kidney interaction. *J Clin Invest* 59:291, 1977.
108. Errcinsk M et al: Regulation of cellular metabolism by intracellular phosphate. *Biochim Biophys Acta* 462:20, 1977.
109. Falls WF et al: Postobstructive diuresis. *Am J Med* 54:404, 1973.
110. Farber E: ATP and cell integrity. *Fed Proc* 32:1534, 1973.
111. Farrington K et al: Dissociation of absorption of calcium and phosphate after successful cadaveric renal transplantation. *Br Med J* 17:712, 1979.
112. Farrington K et al: Hypophosphatemia after parathyroidectomy in chronic renal failure. *Br Med J* 284:856, 1982.
113. Feaster JP et al: 32-P distribution and excretion in rats fed vitamin D-free and low phosphorus diets. *J Nutr* 51:381, 1953.
114. Felsenfeld AJ et al: Hypophosphatemia in long-term renal transplant recipients: Effects on bone histology and 1, 25-dihyroxycholecalciferol. *Miner Electrolyte Metab* 12:333, 1986.
115. Ferguson ER et al: Experimental alcoholism induced phosphorus and magnesium deficiency in skeletal muscle, in Massry SG et al (eds): *Advances in Experimental Biology and Medicine*. New York, Plenum Press, 1982, p 291.
116. Fitzgerald FT: Hypophosphatemia. *Adv Intern Med* 23:137, 1978.
117. Fleming LW et al: Improved phosphate clearances with polycarbonate membranes. *Clin Exp Dialysis Apheresis* 6:211, 1982.
118. Forsham PH, Thorn GW: Changes in inorganic serum phosphorus during intravenous glucose tolerance test as an adjunct to the diagnosis of early diabetes mellitus. *Proc Am Diab Assoc* 9:101, 1949.
119. Frank BW, Kern F Jr: Serum inorganic phosphorus during hepatic coma. *Arch Intern Med* 110:865, 1962.
120. Franks M et al: Metabolic studies in diabetic acidosis: II. The effect of administration of sodium phosphate. *Arch Intern Med* 81:42, 1948.
121. Fraser D, Scriver CR: Familial forms of vitamin D-resistant rickets revisited. X-linked hypophosphatemia and autosomal recessive vitamin D dependency. *Am J Clin Nutr* 29:1315, 1976.
122. Fujita T et al: Adult-onset vitamin D-resistant osteomalacia with the unresponsiveness to parathyroid hormone. *J Clin Endocrinol Metab* 50:927, 1980.
123. Fuller TJ et al: Reversible changes of the muscle cell in experimental phosphorus deficiency. *J Clin Invest* 57:1019, 1976.
124. Fuller TJ et al: Reversible depression in myocardial performance in dogs with experimental phosphorus deficiency. *J Clin Invest* 62:1194, 1978.
125. Garabedian M et al: Chronic hypophosphatemia in kidney transplanted children and young adults, in Massry SG et al (eds): *Phosphate and Minerals in Health and Disease*. New York, Plenum Press, 1979, p 249.
126. Garner GB et al: Dietary phosphorus and salmonellosis in guinea pigs. *Fed Proc* 26:799, 1967.
127. Gertner JM et al: Mineral metabolism in diabetes mellitus: Changes in accompanying treatment with a probable subcutaneous insulin infusion system. *J Clin Endocrinol Metab* 50:862, 1980.

128. Gidding SS et al: Unmasking of hypoparathyroidism in familial partial DiGeorge syndrome by challenge with disodium edetate. *N Engl J Med* 319:1589, 1988.
129. Gipstein RM et al: Calciphylaxis in man. A syndrome of tissue necrosis and vascular calcification in patients with chronic renal disease. *Arch Intern Med* 136:1273, 1976.
130. Glorieux FH et al: Bone response to phosphate salts, ergocalciferol and calcitriol in hypophosphatemic vitamin D-resistant rickets. *N Engl J Med* 303:1023, 1980.
131. Godsall JW et al: Vitamin D metabolism and bone histomorphometry in a patient with antacid-induced osteomalacia. *Am J Med* 77:747, 1984.
132. Gold LW et al: Renal bicarbonate wasting during phosphate depletion. A possible cause of altered acid-base homeostasis in hyperparathyroidism. *J Clin Invest* 52:2556, 1973.
133. Gold LW et al: Effect of phosphate depletion in renal tubular reabsorption of glucose. *J Lab Clin Med* 89:554, 1977.
134. Goldfarb S et al: Renal tubular effects of chronic phosphate depletion. *J Clin Invest* 59:770, 1977.
135. Gorman JM et al: Blood gas changes and hypophosphatemia in lactate-induced panic. *Arch Gen Psychiatry* 43:1067, 1986.
136. Grabie M et al: The role of parathyroid hormone in the hypercalciuria of chronic phosphate depletion. *Miner Electrolyte Metab* 1:279, 1978.
137. Gravelyn TR et al: Hypophosphatemia-associated respiratory muscle weakness in a general inpatient population. *Am J Med* 84:870, 1988.
138. Gray SP et al: Renal handling of calcium, magnesium and inorganic phosphate and hydrogen ions during prolonged exposure to elevated carbon dioxide concentrations. *Clin Sci Mol Med* 45:751, 1973.
139. Guest GM: Organic phosphates of the blood and mineral metabolism in diabetic acidosis. *Am J Dis Child* 64:410, 1942.
140. Guntapalli J et al: Effect of insulin on renal phosphorus handling in the rat: Interaction with PTH and nicotinamide. *Am J Physiol* 249:F610, 1985.
141. Guntupalli KK et al: Effects of induced total-body hyperthermia on phosphorus metabolism in humans. *Am J Med* 77:250, 1984.
142. Halevy J et al: Severe hypophosphatemia in hospitalized patients. *Arch Intern Med* 148:153, 1988.
143. Hall RT et al: Hypophosphatemia in breast-fed low birthweight infants following initial hospital discharge. *Am J Dis Child* 143:1191, 1989.
144. Hammerman MR et al: Insulin stimulates P_i transport in brush border vesicles from proximal tubular segments. *Am J Physiol* 247:E616, 1984.
145. Harrison JE et al: The relationship between bone apposition rate and vitamin D activity in phosphate-deficient rats. *Metabolism* 35:126, 1986.
146. Harter HR et al: The relative role of calcium, phosphorus and parathyroid hormone in glucose and tolbutamide mediated insulin release. *J Clin Invest* 58:359, 1976.
147. Haug TO: Time course of changes in concentration of some plasma components after furosemide. *Br Med J* 3:622, 1976.
148. Hayek ME: Severe hypophosphatemia following the institution of enteral feedings. *Arch Surg* 124:1325, 1989.
149. Herrath DV et al: Calcium-Ketovalin (KV), a new, very effective aluminum-free phosphate binder. *Kidney Int* 35:388, 1989.
150. Higgins RM et al: Hypophosphatemia after renal transplantation: Relationship to immunosuppressive drug therapy and effects on muscle detected by ^{31}P nuclear magnetic resonance spectroscopy. *Nephrol Dial Transplant* 5:62, 1990.
151. Hoff SD et al: Guillain-Barré syndrome due to hypophosphatemia following intravenous hyperalimentation. *JPEN* 12:414, 1988.
152. Hoff SD et al: Hyperphosphatemia from lipid emulsion in a patient on total parenteral nutrition. *JPEN* 1:84, 1988.
153. Hogan DB et al: Hypophosphatemic osteomalacia complicating von Recklinghausen's neurofibromatosis: Increase in spinal density on treatment. *Bone* 7:9, 1986.
154. Horle WH et al: Abnormalities of glycogen metabolism in cardiomyopathy of phosphorus depletion, in Massry SG et al (eds): *Phosphate and Minerals in Health and Disease.* New York, Plenum Press, 1979, p 343.
155. Huang W et al: Regulation of (Na^+ + K^+)-ATPase by inorganic phosphate: pH dependence and physiological implications. *Biochem Biophys Res Commun* 123:438, 1984.
156. Ibels LS et al: Preservation of function in experimental renal disease by dietary restriction of phosphate. *N Engl J Med* 298:122, 1978.
157. Insognia KA et al: Impaired phosphorus conservation and 1,25-dihydroxyvitamin D generation during phosphorus deprivation in familial hypophosphatemic rickets. *J Clin Invest* 71:1562, 1983.
158. Itescu SH: Thiazide induced clinically significant hypophosphatemia. *Clin Nephrol* 27:161, 1987.
159. Ivey J et al: The effect of phosphate depletion on bone, in Massry SG et al (eds): *Homeostasis of Phosphate and Other Minerals.* New York, Plenum Press, 1978, p 373.
160. Iwanami M et al: Seasonal variations in serum inorganic phosphate and calcium with special reference to parathyroid activity. *J Physiol* 149:23, 1959.
161. Jacob HS, Amsden T: Acute hemolytic anemia with rigid red cells in hypophosphatemia. *N Engl J Med* 385:1446, 1971.
162. Jones AF et al: Hypophosphatemia and phosphaturia in paracetamol poisoning. *Lancet* 2:608, 1989.
163. Jordan GW: Serum calcium and phosphorus abnormalities in leukemia. *Am J Med* 41:381, 1966.
164. Josephus R, Williams GA (trans): *The Jewish War.* UK Harmondwsorth, Penguin Books, 1959, p 300.
165. Jowsey J, Balasurbramanian P: Effect of phosphate supplements on soft tissue calcification and bone turnover. *Clin Sci* 42:289, 1972.
166. Kanter Y et al: 2,3-diphosphoglycerate, nucleotide phosphate, and organic and inorganic phosphate levels during the early phases of diabetic ketoacidosis. *Diabetes* 26:429, 1977.
167. Kebler R et al: Dynamic changes in serum phosphorus levels in diabetic ketoacidosis. *Am J Med* 79:571, 1985.
168. Kemp GJ et al: Regulation of phosphate metabolism in human red cells following prolonged incubation to steady state in vitro. *Biochem Biophys ACTA* 969:139, 1988.

169. Kempson SA: Effect of metabolic acidosis on renal brush border membrane adaptation to low phosphorus diet. *Kidney Int* 22:225, 1982.
170. Keller U, Berger W: Prevention of hypophosphatemia by phosphate infusion during treatment of diabetic ketoacidosis and hyperosmolar coma. *Diabetes* 29:87, 1980.
171. Kerr D et al: Pseudohypoparathyroidism: Clinical expression of PTH resistance. *Q J Med* 247:889, 1987.
172. King AL et al: Severe hypophosphatemia in a general hospital population. *South Med J* 80:831, 1987.
173. Kjeldsen SE et al: Decreased serum phosphate in essential hypertension related to increased sympathetic tone. *Am J Hypertens* 1:403, 1988.
174. Knochel JP: The pathophysiology and clinical characteristics of severe hypophosphatemia. *Arch Intern Med* 137:203, 1977.
175. Knochel JP et al: Selective phosphorus deficiency in the hyperalimented hypophosphatemic dog and phosphorylation potentials in the muscle cell in Massry SG et al (eds): *Phosphate and Minerals in Health and Disease.* New York, Plenum Press, 1979, p 323.
176. Knochel JP et al: Hypophosphatemia and rhabdomyolysis. *J Clin Invest* 62:1240, 1978.
177. Knochel JP: Does hypophosphatemia play a role in acute liver failure? *Hepatology* 9:504, 1989.
178. Koffler A et al: Acute renal failure due to nontraumatic rhabdomyolysis. *Ann Intern Med* 85:23, 1976.
179. Kreusser WJ et al: Effect of phosphate depletion on renal gluconeogenesis. *Miner Electrolyte Metab* 3:312, 1980.
180. Kreusser W et al: Haemodynamics and myocardial metabolism of phosphorus depleted dogs: Effect of catecholamines and angiotensin II. *Eur J Clin Invest* 12:219, 1982.
181. Kurokawa K et al: Phosphate depletion and adenine nucleotide metabolism in kidney and liver, in Massry SG et al: *Homeostasis of Phosphate and Other Minerals.* New York, Plenum Press, 1978, p 327.
182. Laaban J et al: Hypophosphatemia complicating management of acute severe asthma. *Ann Intern Med* 112:68, 1990.
183. Labib M et al: Hypophosphataemic osteomalacia and alcoholism: A possible link. *Alcohol Alcohol* 23:111, 1988.
184. Lachter J et al: Hypophosphatemia and idiopathic pancreatisis. *N Engl J Med* 81:1221, 1986.
185. Lau K: Phosphate excess and progressive renal failure: The precipitation-calcification hypothesis. *Kidney Int* 36:918, 1989.
186. Lau K et al: Renal tubular sites of altered calcium transport in phosphate-depleted rats. *J Clin Invest* 64:1681, 1979.
187. Lau K et al: Evidence for a humoral phosphatemic factor in oncogenic hypophosphatemic osteomalacia. *Clin Res* 27:421A, 1979.
188. Leaf A: The syndrome of osteomalacia, renal glycosuria, aminoaciduria, and hyperphosphaturia (the Fanconi syndrome), in Stanbury JB et al (eds): *The Metabolic Basis of Inherited Disease*, 2d ed. New York, McGraw-Hill, 1966, p. 1205.
189. Lee DBN et al: The biochemical indices of experimental phosphorus depletion. A re-examination of their physiological implications, in Massry SG et al: (eds): *Homeostasis of Phosphate and Other Minerals.* New York, Plenum Press, 1978, p. 382.
190. Lee DBN et al: Effects of phosphorus depletion on intestinal calcium and phosphorus absorption. *Am J Physiol* 236:E451, 1979.
191. Lee DBN et al: The role of growth hormone in experimental phosphatae depletion. *Calcif Tissue Int* 32:105, 1980.
192. Lee DBN et al: Disorders of phosphorus metabolism, in Bronner F, Coburn JW (eds): *Disorders of Mineral Metabolism.* New York, Academic Press, 1981, vol III, p. 284.
193. Lee DBN et al: Jejunal phosphate transport is not regulated by the PTH-adenylate cyclase system. *Miner Electrolyte Metab* 12:293, 1986.
194. Lee SH et al: Case report: Hypophosphataemic rickets and melorheostosis. *Clin Radiol* 40:209, 1989.
195. Lennquist S et al: Hypophosphatemia in severe burns. *Acta Chir Scand* 145:1, 1979.
196. Levi J et al: Hypocalcemia in magnesium depleted dogs: Evidence for reduced responsiveness to parathyroid hormone and relative failure of parathyroid gland function. *Metabolism* 23:323, 1974.
197. Levi M et al: Cholesterol modulates rat renal brush border membrane phosphate transport. *J Clin Invest* 85:231, 1990.
198. Levi M et al: Role of lipid composition and fluidity in impaired renal P_i transport in aged rat. *Am J Physiol* 256:F85, 1989.
199. Levine BS et al: Early renal brush border membrane adaptation to dietary phosphorus. *Miner Electrolyte Metab* 10:222, 1984.
200. Levine BS et al: Effect of metabolic acidosis on phosphate transport by the renal brush border membrane. *Biochim Biophys ACTA* 727:7, 1983.
201. Levine BS et al: Renal adaptation to phosphorus deprivation: Characterization of early events. *J Bone Miner Res* 1:33, 1986.
202. Levine BS et al: Renal adaptation to dietary phosphate deprivation: Role of proximal tubule brush-border membrane fluidity. *Am J Physiol* 260:F613, 1991.
203. Levine BS et al: Effect of acute acidemia on phosphate uptake by renal proximal tubular brush-border membranes. *Am J Physiol* 251:F889, 1986.
204. Levine BS et al: The effects of vitamin D sterols and diet magnesium on calcium and phosphorus homeostasis. *Am J Physiol* 241:E35, 1981.
205. Levine MA et al: Resistance to multiple hormones in patients with pseudohypoparathyroidism: Association with deficient activity of guanine nucleotide regulatory protein. *Am J Med* 74:545, 1983.
206. Levy J et al: Plasma calcium and phosphate levels in an adult noninsulin-dependent diabetic population. *Calcif Tissue Int* 39:316, 1986.
207. Lewis DJM: Hypophosphatemia: A feature of malaria? *Br Med J* 295:416, 1987.
208. Lewis JF et al: Hypophosphatemia and respiratory failure: Prolonged abnormal energy metabolism demonstrated by nuclear magnetic resonance spectroscopy. *Am J Med* 83:1139, 1987.
209. Liberman UA et al: End-organ resistance to 125-hydroxycholecalciferol. *Lancet* 1:504, 1980.

210. Lichtman MA, Miller DR: Erythrocyte glycolysis, 2,3-diphosphoglycerate and adenosine triphosphate concentration in uremic subjects: Relationship to extracellular phosphate concentration. *J Lab Clin Med* 76:267, 1970.
211. Linarelli LG et al: Newborn urinary cyclic AMP and developmental renal responsiveness to parathyroid hormone. *Pediatrics* 50:14, 1972.
212. Liput J et al: Inhibition of volume expansion of phosphate uptake by the renal proximal tubule brush border membrane. *Biochem Pharmacol* 38:321, 1989.
213. Ljunghall S et al: Plasma potassium and phosphate concentrations—influence of adrenaline infusion, beta-blockade and physical exercise. *Acta Med Scand* 221:83, 1987.
214. Llach F et al: On the mechanism of secondary hyperparathyroidism in moderate renal insufficiency. *J Clin Endocrinol Metab* 61:601, 1985.
215. Logan MA: Recent advances in the chemistry of calcification. *Physiol Rev* 20:522, 1940.
216. Lotz M et al: Evidence for phosphorus depletion syndrome in man. *N Engl J Med* 278:409, 1968.
217. Loven L et al: Effect of beta blocking on preoperative changes in serum phosphate. *Acta Chir Scand* 148:339, 1982.
218. Loven L et al: Traumatically induced hypophosphatemia in anesthetized pigs. *Acta Chir Scand* 148:21, 1982.
219. Lufkin EG et al: Phosphorus excretion in tumoral calcinosis: Response to parathyroid hormone and acetazolamide. *J Clin Endocrinol Metab* 50:648, 1980.
220. Lyles KW et al: The efficacy of vitamin D-2 and oral phosphate therapy in X-linked hypophosphatemic rickets and osteomalacia. *J Clin Endocrinol Metab* 54:307, 1982.
220a. Lyles KW et al: Genetic transmission of tumoral calcinosis: Autosomal dominant with variable clinical expressivity. *J Clin Endocrinol Metab* 60:1093, 1985.
221. Machler M et al: X-linked dominant hypophosphatemia is closely linked to DNA markers DXS41 and DXS43 at Xp22. *Hum Genet* 73:271, 1986.
222. Mahler M: Progressive loss of mitochondrial creatine phosphokinase activity in muscular dystrophy. *Biochem Biophys Res Commun* 88:895, 1979.
223. Malloy PJ et al: The molecular basis of hereditary 1,25-dihydroxyvitamin D_3 resistant rickets in seven related families. *J Clin Invest* 86:2071, 1990.
224. Marchi SD et al: More on the role of metabolic acidosis in causing uremic hyperphosphatemia. *Miner Electrolyte Metab* 13:67, 1987.
225. Martin RR et al: Fatal poisoning from sodium phosphate enema: Case report and experimental study. *JAMA* 257:2190, 1987.
226. Marwich TH et al: Severe hypophosphatemia induced by glucose- insulin-potassium therapy. A case report and proposal for altered protocol. *Int J Cardiol* 18:327, 1988.
227. Massry SG: The clinical syndrome of phosphate depletion. *Adv Exp Med Biol* 103:301, 1978.
228. Massry SG et al: Phosphate depletion increases cytosolic calcium of brain synaptosomes. *Am J Physiol* 260:F12, 1991.
229. McCleave D: Compartmental shift of potassium—a result of sympathomimetic overdose. *Aust N Z J Surg* 8:180, 1978.
230. McCloskey EV et al: Diphosphonates and phosphate homeostasis in man. *Clin Sci* 74:607, 1988.
231. Meyer-Sabellek W et al: Effect of thiazides on the hypercalciuria of phosphate depletion. *J Lab Clin Med* 96:830, 1980.
232. Miyauchi A et al: Hemangiopericytoma-induced osteomalacia: Tumor transplantation in nude mice causes hypophosphatemia and tumor extracts inhibit renal 25-hydroxyvitamin D-1α-hydroxylase activity. *J Clin Endocrinol Metab* 67:46, 1988.
233. Molitoris BA et al: Renal apical membrane cholesterol and fluidity in regulation of phosphate transport. *Am J Physiol* 249:F12, 1985.
234. Mollison PL: Observations on cases of starvation at Belsen. *Br Med J* 1:4, 1946.
235. Montanari A et al: Skeletal muscle cell abnormalities in acute hypophosphaturia during parenteral nutrition. *Miner Electrolyte Metab* 10:52, 1984.
236. Morgan DB: Calcium and phosphorus transport across the intestine, in Girdwood RH, Smith AN (eds): *Malabsorption*. Edinburgh, University Press, 1969, p 73.
237. Morris RCJ: "Moderate" hypophosphatemia—Not always an innocent bystander. *West J Med* 147:577, 1987.
238. Morrisey RL, Wasserman RH: Calcium absorption and calcium binding protein in chicks in differing calcium and phosphorus intakes. *Am J Physiol* 220:1509, 1970.
239. Mosel PK, Segar WE: Fluid and serum electrolyte disturbances as a complication of enema in Hirschsprung's disease. *Am J Dis Child* 115:714, 1968.
240. Moseley PK et al: Fluid and serum electrolyte disturbances as a complication of enema in Hirschsprungs's disease. *Am J Dis Child* 115:714, 1968.
241. Moser S et al: On the mechanism of hypophosphaturia during acute and chronic dietary phosphate restriction. *Miner Electrolyte Metab* 5:39, 1981.
242. Mostellar ME, Tuttle EP Jr: The effects of alkalosis on plasma concentration and urinary excretion of phosphate in man. *J Clin Invest* 43:138, 1964.
243. Muhlbauer RC et al: Tubular localization of adaptation to dietary phosphate in the rat. *Am J Physiol* 233:F342, 1977.
244. Nassim JR et al: Effect of stilbestrol on urinary phosphate excretion. *Clin Sci* 15:367, 1956.
245. Nemer WF et al: Cardiac arrest after acute hyperphosphatemia. *South Med J* 81:1068, 1988.
246. Newbury-Ecob RA et al: Hypophosphatemic rickets after ifosfamide treatment. *Br Med J* 299:258, 1989.
247. Newman JH et al: Acute respiratory failure associated with hypophosphatemia. *N Engl J Med* 297:1101, 1977.
248. Nishimura N: Histological study of muscle in the experimental hypophosphatemic rat. *J Jpn Orthop Assoc* 61:39, 1987.
249. Nusynowitz ML et al: Pseudoidiopathic hypoparathyroidism. *Am J Med* 55:677, 1973.
250. Nusynowitz ML et al: The spectrum of the hypoparathyroid states. A classification based on physiologic principles. *Medicine* 55:105, 1976.
251. O'Connor LR et al: Effect of hypophosphatemia on myocardial performance in man. *N Engl J Med* 291:901, 1977.
252. O'Connor LR et al: Hyperphosphatemia in lactic acidosis. *N Engl J Med* 297:707, 1977.
253. Oppe TE et al: Calcium and phosphorus levels in healthy

newborn infants given various types of milk. *Lancet* 1:1045, 1968.
254. O'Tauma LA et al: Raised intracranial pressure after hyperalimentation. *Lancet* 2:1101, 1973.
255. Packer E et al: Effects of estrogen on daylong circulating calcium, phosphorus, 1,25-dihydroxyvitamin D, and parathyroid hormone in postmenopausal women. *J Bone Miner Res* 5:877, 1990.
256. Parfitt AM, Frame B: Phosphate loading and depletion in vitamin D treated hypoparathyroidism, in Avioli L et al (eds): *Phosphate Metabolism, Kidney and Bone*. Paris, Armour Montagu, 1975, p 179.
257. Pettifor JM et al: Acquired hypophosphataemic vitamin D resistant rickets in black children. *Bone Miner* 1:307, 1986.
258. Petty C. Bageanat T: In vitro manipulation of 2,3-diphosphoglycerate levels in acid-citrate-dextrose blood with steroids. *Life Sci* 14:1279, 1974.
259. Phillips GB et al: A study of the nutritional defect in Wernicke's syndrome. The effect of a purified diet, thiamine, and other vitamins on the clinical manifestations. *J Clin Invest* 31:859, 1952.
260. Pizurki L et al: Effect of transforming growth factor-alpha and parathyroid hormone-related protein on phosphate transport in renal cells. *Am J Physiol* 259:F929, 1990.
261. Planas RF et al: Effects of hypophosphatemia on pulmonary muscle performance, in Massry SG et al (eds): *Advances in Experimental Biology and Medicine*. New York, Plenum Press, 1981, p 283.
262. Plante GE et al: Effect of indapamide on phosphate metabolism and vascular reactivity. *Am J Med* 84(suppl 1B):26, 1988.
263. Pollock RA, Watson RL: Malignant hyperthermia associated with hypocalcemia. *Anesthesiology* 34:188, 1971.
264. Popovitzer MM: Tumor induced hypophosphatemic osteomalacia: Evidence for a phosphaturic cyclic AMP-dependent action of tumor extract. *Clin Res* 21:418A, 1981.
265. Portale AA et al: Effect of dietary phosphorus on circulating concentrations of 1,25-dihydroxyvitamin D and immunoreactive parathyroid hormone in children with moderate renal insufficiency. *J Clin Invest* 73:1580, 1984.
266. Portale AA et al: Dietary intake of phosphorus modulates the circadian rhythm in serum concentration of phosphorus: Implications for the renal production of 1,25-dihyroxyvitamin D. *J Clin Invest* 80:1147, 1987.
267. Prince MJ et al: Hyperphosphatemic tumoral calcinosis. Association with elevation of serum 1,25-dihydroxycholecalciferol concentration. *Ann Intern Med* 96:586, 1982.
268. Raisz LG: The effect of factors implicated in osteopenia on bone formation and resorption in tissue culture, in Barzel US (ed): *Osteoporosis*. New York, Grune & Stratton, 1970, p 174.
269. Ramsay AM, Douglas LJ: Effects of phosphate limitation of growth on the cell-wall and lipid composition of Saccharomyces cerevisiae. *J Gen Microbiol* 110:185, 1979.
270. Rao KJ et al: Hypocalcemic tetany. Result of high phosphate enema. *NY State J Med* 76:968, 1976.
271. Raskin P, Pak CYC: The effect of chronic insulin therapy on phosphate metabolism in diabetes mellitus. *Diabetologia* 21:50, 1981.
272. Rasmussen H, Anast C: Familial hypophosphatemic (vitamin D-resistant) rickets and vitamin D-dependent rickets, in Wyngaarden JB, Frederickson DC (eds): *The Metabolic Basis of Inherited Disease*, 4th ed. New York, McGraw-Hill, 1974, p 1537.
273. Rasmussen A et al: Postoperative myocardial performance during glucose-induced hypophosphatemia. *Acta Chir Scand* 313:13, 1985.
274. Rasmussen A et al: Severity of postoperative hypophosphatemia in relation to glucose administration and renal handling of phosphate. *Acta Chri Scand* 154:617, 1988.
275. Rasmussen H et al: Calcium in the regulation of aldosterone secretion and vascular smooth muscle contraction. *Hypertension* 10:123, 1987.
276. Reaven GM et al: Hypertension as a disease of carbohydrate and lipoprotein metabolism. *Am J Med* 87:2S, 1989.
277. Ritz E: Acute hypophosphatemia. *Kidney Int* 22:84, 1982.
278. Robertson WG: Plasma phosphate homeostasis, in Nordin BEC (ed): *Calcium, Phosphorus and Magnesium Metabolism*. Edinburgh, Churchhill Livingstone, 1976, p 217.
279. Roos A, Boron WF: Intracellular pH. *Physiol Rev* 61:296, 1981.
280. Rosen R et al: Central nervous system dysfunction and hypophosphatemia (HP). *Kidney Int* 12:460, 1977.
281. Roth KS et al: The Fanconi syndrome and mechanisms of tubular dysfunction. *Kidney Int* 20:705, 1981.
282. Rubin MF et al: Hypophosphatemia: Pathophysiological and practical aspects of therapy. *Semin Nephrol* 10:536, 1990.
283. Ryback R et al: Clinical relationship between serum phosphorus and other blood chemistry values in alcoholics. *Arch Intern Med* 140:673, 1980.
283a. Saglikes Y et al: Effects of phosphate depletion on blood pressure. *J Clin Invest* (in press).
284. Saglikes Y et al: Effect of phosphate depletion on blood pressure and vascular reactivity to norepinephrine and angiotensin II in the rat. *Am J Physiol* 248:F93, 1985.
285. Sajo IM et al: Studies of ammonia addition to tubular fluid in rats with chronic metabolic acidosis. *Kidney Int* 20:353, 1981.
286. Saks VA et al: Studies of energy transport in heart cells. *J Biol Chem* 255:755, 1980.
287. Schneeberger EE, Morrison AB: Increased susceptibility of magnesium-deficient rats to a phosphate induced nephropathy. *Am J Pathol* 50:549, 1967.
288. Schnieder H. Steenbock H: A low phosphate diet and the response of rats to vitamin D. *J Biol Chem* 128:159, 1939.
289. Scriver CR: Rickets in the pathogenesis of impaired tubular transport of phosphate and other solutes. *Am J Med* 57:43, 1966.
290. Scriver CR et al: Hypophosphatemic nonrachitic bone disease: An entity distinct from X-linked hypophosphatemia in the renal defect, bone involvement and inheritance. *Am J Med Genet* 1:101, 1977.
291. Sebastian A et al: Dietary potassium influences kidney maintenance of serum phosphorus concentration. *Kidney Int* 37:1341, 1990.
292. Seraydarian MW, Artaza L: Regulation of energy metabolism by creatine in cardiac and skeletal muscle cells in culture. *J Mol Cell Cardiol* 8:669, 1976.
293. Sheldon BF et al: Phosphate depletion and repletion:

Relation to parenteral nutrition and oxygen transport. *Ann Surg* 182:683, 1975.
294. Silvis SE, Paragas PV Jr: Fatal hyperalimentation syndrome. Animal studies. *J Lab Clin Med* 78:918, 1971.
295. Silvis SE, Paragus PD Jr: Paresthesias, weakness, seizures and hypophosphatemia in patients receiving hyperalimentation. *Gastroenterology* 62:513, 1972.
296. Silvis SE et al: Cerebral edema occurs in hyperalimentation syndrome. *Gastroenterology* 64:803, 1973.
297. Silvis SE et al: Hypophosphatemia and neurological changes secondary to oral caloric intake. *Am J Gastroenterol* 73:215, 1980.
298. Skinner R et al: Hypophosphatemic rickets after ifosfamide treatment in children. *Br Med J* 298:1560, 1989.
299. Slatopolsky E et al: Control of phosphate excretion in uremic man. *J Clin Invest* 47:1865, 1968.
300. Slatopolsky E et al: Long-term effects of calcium carbonate and 2.5 mEq/liter calcium dialysate on mineral metabolism. *Kidney Int* 36:897, 1989.
301. Spaulding SW, Walser M: Treatment of experimental hypercalcemia with oral phosphate. *J Clin Endocrinol Metab* 31:531, 1970.
302. Spencer H et al: Effect of small doses of aluminum containing antacids on calcium and phosphorus metabolism. *Am J Clin Nutr* 36:32, 1982.
303. Squara P et al: Hypophosphatemia during mechanical ventilation for chronic obstructive pulmonary disease. *Presse Med* 14:1225, 1985.
304. Stanbury SW et al: Elective subtotal parathyroidectomy for renal hyperparathyroidism. *Lancet* 1:793, 1970.
305. Steele TH: Renal resistance to parathyroid hormone during phosphorus deprivation. *J Clin Invest* 58:1461, 1976.
306. Stein JH et al: Hypophosphatemia in acute alcoholism. *Am J Med Sci* 252:78, 1966.
307. Sterling MA: Diabetic ketoacidosis in childhood. *Pediatr Clin North Am* 26:152, 1979.
308. Stickler GB et al: Vitamin D-resistant rickets: Clinical experience with 41 typical familial hypophosphatemic patients and 2 atypical non-familial cases. *Mayo Clin Proc* 45:197, 1970.
309. Storm TL: Severe hypophosphatemia during recovery from acute respiratory acidosis. *Br Med J* 289:456, 1984.
310. Strickler JC et al: Micropuncture study of inorganic phosphate excretion in the rat. *J Clin Invest* 43:1596, 1964.
311. Stubbs M et al: Control of the redox state of nicotineamide-adenine nucleotide couple in rat liver cytoplasm. *Biochem J* 126:59, 1972.
312. Suzuki K et al: Hyperphosphatemia as a detectable laboratory manifestation of glucocorticoid withdrawal syndrome. *Bone Miner* 1:51, 1986.
313. Swenson RS et al: Evidence that parathyroid hormone is not required for phosphate homeostasis in renal failure. *Metabolism* 24:199, 1975.
314. Takuwa Y et al: Hyperphosphatemia after surgical correction of hypercortisolism. *Miner Electrolyte Metab* 12:119, 1986.
315. Tan TT et al: Sporadic adult-onset hypophosphatemic osteomalacia—a report of two cases. *Singapore Med J* 30:410, 1989.
316. Tanaka Y, De Luca HF: Intestinal calcium transport: Stimulation by low phosphorus diets. *Science* 181:564, 1973.
317. Theiler A, Green HH: Aphosphorosis in ruminants. *Nutr Abstr Rev* 1:359, 1932.
318. Thode J et al: Parathyroid hormone and hypophosphatemia. *Ann Intern Med* 108:641, 1988.
319. Tieder M et al: Hereditary hypophosphatemic rickets with hypercalciuria. *N Engl J Med* 312:611, 1985.
320. Tieder M et al: "Idiopathic" hypercalciuria and hereditary hypophosphatemic rickets: Two phenotypical expressions of a common genetic defect. *N Eng J Med* 316:125, 1987.
321. Travis SF et al: Alterations of red cell glycolytic intermediates and oxygen transport as a consequence of hypophosphatemia in patients receiving intravenous hyperalimentation. *N Engl J Med* 285:763, 1971.
322. Venditti FJ et al: Hypophosphatemia and cardiac arrhythmias. *Miner Electrolyte Metab* 13:19, 1987.
323. Vered Z et al: Left ventricular function in patients with chronic hypophosphatemia. *Am Heart J* 107:796, 1984.
324. Voltin RF et al: Prevention of the fatal hyperalimentation syndrome. *Clin Res* 23:501, 1975.
325. Walker GS et al: Factors influencing the intestinal absorption of calcium and phosphorus following renal transplantation. *Nephron* 26:225, 1980.
326. Walling MW: Effects of 1-alpha-25-dihydroxyvitamin D-3 on active intestinal inorganic phosphate absorption, in Norman AW et al (eds): *Vitamin D. Biochemical, Chemical and Clinical Aspects Related to Calcium Metabolism.* Berlin, de Gruyter, 1977, p 321.
327. Wardrop CAJ: Oxygen availability from the blood and the effect of phosphate replacement on erythrocyte 2,3-diphosphoglycerate and haemoglobin-oxygen affinity in diabetic ketoacidosis. *Diabetologia* 15:381, 1978.
328. Wathen RL et al: Acid-base and metabolic responses to anion infusion in the anesthetized dog. *Kidney Int* 21:592, 1982.
329. Weinberg J et al: Spurious hyperphosphatemia in patients with dysglobulinemia. *Miner Electrolyte Metab* 15:185, 1989.
330. Whang R, Welt LG: Observations in experimental magnesium depletion. *J Clin Invest* 42:305, 1962.
331. Wilber JF et al: Hyperphosphatemia and tumoral calcinosis. *Ann Intern Med* 68:1044, 1968.
332. Wilson L et al: Altered divalent ion metabolism in early renal failure: Role of 1,25-$(OH)_2D$. *Kidney Int* 27:565, 1985.
332a. Wilson MP et al: Hyperphosphatemia associated with cortical hyperostosis and tumoral calcinosis. *J Pediatr* 114:1010, 1989.
333. Wolf AV et al: Artificial kidney function: Kinetics of hemodialysis. *J Clin Invest* 40:1062, 1961.
334. Wollner A et al: Tumor genesis syndrome. Hypophosphatemia accompanying Burkitt's lymphoma cell leukemia. *Miner Electrolyte Metab* 12:173, 1986.
335. Woods HF et al: The cause of hepatic accumulation of fructose-1-phosphate on fructose loading. *Biochem J* 119:504, 1970.
336. Wright PD: Intravenous feeding. *Lancet* 2:1335, 1973.
337. Yamaoka K et al: Abnormal relationship between serum phosphate concentration and renal 25-hyroxycholecal-

ciferol-1-alpha-hydroxylase activity in X-linked hypophosphatemic mice. *Miner Electrolyte Metab* 12:194, 1986.

338. Yawata Y et al: Blood cell abnormalities complicating the hypophosphatemia of hyperalimentation: Erythrocyte and platelet ATP deficiency associated with hemolytic anemia and bleeding in hyperalimented dogs. *J Lab Clin Med* 84:643, 1974.
339. Yudis M et al: Pseudohyperphosphatemia secondary to hypertriglyceridemia. *Kidney Int* 31:362, 1987.
340. Zemel MB et al: Saline infusion causes rapid increase in parathyroid hormone and intracellular calcium levels. *Am J Hypertens* 2:185, 1989.
341. Zemel MB et al: Erythrocyte cation metabolism in salt-sensitive hypertensive blacks as affected by dietary sodium and calcium. *Am J Hypertens* 1:386, 1988.
342. Zerwekh JE et al: A unique form of osteomalacia associated with end organ refractoriness to 1,25-dihydroxyvitamin D and apparent defective synthesis of 25-hydroxy-vitamin D. *J Clin Endocrinol Metab* 49:171, 1979.
343. Zhou X et al: Phosphate depletion impairs insulin secretion by pancreatic islets. *Kidney Int* 39:120, 1991.
344. Zucchelli P et al: Inorganic phosphate removal during different dialytic procedures. *Int J Artif Organs* 10:173, 1987.
345. Zusman J et al: Hyperparathyroidism, hyperphosphatemia, hyperphosphaturia and hypocalcemia in acute lymphoblastic leukemia. *N Engl J Med* 289:1335, 1973.

CHAPTER • 34

Hypomagnesemia and hypermagnesemia

Zalman S. Agus • Shaul G. Massry

DISTRIBUTION OF MAGNESIUM

Body magnesium is distributed in three major compartments: (1) extracellular fluid, 1.3 percent; (2) intracellular fluid, 13 percent; and (3) bone, 67 percent. Thus, magnesium is mainly located in areas that are poorly accessible to study: the intracellular and bony compartments. Unfortunately, most of the available data on magnesium metabolism are derived from measurements of the blood concentration of magnesium. Recently, however, new methods have been developed that allow measurement of free magnesium. The data indicate that while total magnesium may approximate 8 to 10 m*M*, the free magnesium concentration is only in the range of 0.4 to 0.6 m*M*.[9,115,128] Chapter 13 presents a detailed discussion of the factors regulating serum magnesium concentration and cellular bone and magnesium content.

TABLE 34-1 • Daily requirements for magnesium

	Age (years)	Daily need mg (meq)
Infants	0.25–0.5	50 (4.2)
	0.5–1.0	70 (5.8)
Children	1–3	150 (12.5)
	4–6	200 (16.6)
	7–10	250 (20.8)
Males	11–14	350 (29.2)
	15–18	400 (33.3)
	19 on	350 (29.2)
Females	11–14	300 (25.0)
	15 on	300 (25.0)
	Pregnancy	450 (37.5)
	Lactation	450 (37.5)

SOURCE: Flink.[65] Reprinted by permission.

MAGNESIUM BALANCE

Reviews of magnesium requirements have concluded that 5–6 mg/kg per day is necessary to maintain magnesium balance.[65,144] The Food and Nutrition Board of the National Academy of Sciences recommends an intake of 300–350 mg/day for adult females and males, or approximately 5 mg/kg per day.[114] The requirement for magnesium may increase in pregnant women or adolescents. Table 34-1 shows magnesium requirements for various age groups.

From the magnesium content of food, as calculated from tables of food consumption and from chemical analysis, it is clear that, in a mixed general American diet, the intake of magnesium is closely correlated with the calories consumed.[65] This is true as long as the calories are not consumed in the form of alcohol or sugar, since both have little or no mineral content and may also cause renal wasting of magnesium. Magnesium is found in high concentration in nuts, green vegetables, soybeans, chocolate, and whole cereal grains. In some areas, the drinking water contains some magnesium, depending on the hardness of the water.

HYPOMAGNESEMIA AND MAGNESIUM DEPLETION

DEFINITIONS

Hypomagnesemia can develop without concomitant magnesium losses,[98] and cellular magnesium depletion can occur in the presence of normomagnesemia.[67,100] Since magnesium is primarily an intracellular cation, it is sometimes extremely difficult to precisely judge body magnesium content in clinical reports and experimental studies that measure only the serum levels. However, with all its limitations, serum magnesium concentration remains the prime clinical diagnostic tool. If patients are found to be hypomagnesemic, it is safe to state that in most cases the condition will be associated with some degree of magnesium depletion. Special care and a high index of suspicion should be used for patients whose clinical condition (e.g., chronic diarrhea) suggests the presence of magnesium depletion but whose serum magnesium may be normal or very slightly reduced. In these special cases the physician should look for other laboratory and clinical findings associated with magnesium depletion.

Several investigative tools are available to aid in the diagnosis of magnesium depletion. The *magnesium retention test* has been used in the study of magnesium depletion and in the evaluation of magnesium balance. The test is relatively easy to perform and requires the intravenous loading of magnesium and collection of urine.[57] In a normal subject, 75 to 80 percent of an administered load will be excreted in the urine within 24 h. In a magnesium-deficient individual, less than 75 percent of the administered magnesium will be excreted, provided no tubular defect in magnesium reabsorption is present. Dyckner and Wester[57] have used this test for the diagnosis of magnesium depletion (Fig. 34-1). They administered 30 mmol of magnesium in a solution of 5% dextrose intravenously over 12 h, with the measurement of 24-h urinary magnesium excretion before and after the test. Retention of less than 20 percent indicates that magnesium depletion is unlikely.

THE PREVALENCE OF MAGNESIUM DEPLETION

Earlier studies by Jackson and Meier found the prevalence of hypomagnesemia (serum magnesium below 1.53 meq/liter) among 5100 consecutive ambulatory and hospitalized patients to be 10.2 percent.[90] Subsequent studies confirm that the prevalence in the outpatient and hospitalized population approximates 6 to 12 percent.[171,172,175] In hypokalemic patients the incidence rises markedly to 42 percent[172] and rises even higher, to between 60 and 65 percent, in patients in an intensive care setting,[36,49,143] where nutrition, diuretics, hypoalbuminemia, and aminoglycosides may play important roles. Thus, although criteria for the severity of hypomagnesemia may vary from study to study, and other parameters of magnesium depletion were not studied, it is clear that hypomagnesemia—and possibly magnesium depletion—is a common clinical problem.

CAUSES OF HYPOMAGNESEMIA AND MAGNESIUM DEPLETION

The causes and disease entities where magnesium depletion and hypomagnesemia are common are shown in Table 34-2.

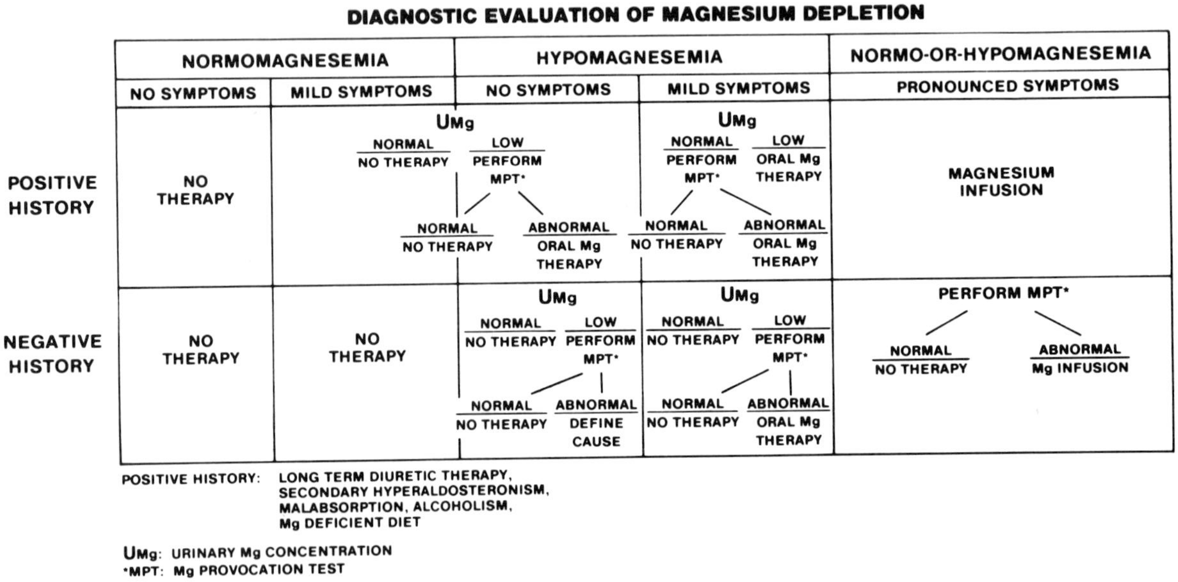

FIGURE 34-1 • A schematic representation of the diagnostic evaluation of magnesium depletion. The role of magnesium infusion. (From Dyckner T, Webster PO: *Acta Med Scand* 66:37, 1981.)

TABLE 34-2 • Causes of hypomagnesemia and magnesium depletion

DECREASED INTAKE
Protein-calorie malnutrition
Starvation
Prolonged intravenous therapy
DECREASED INTESTINAL ABSORPTION
Malabsorption syndromes, including nontropical sprue
Massive surgical resection of the small intestine
Neonatal hypomagnesemia with selective malabsorption of magnesium
EXCESSIVE LOSSES OF BODY FLUIDS
Prolonged nasogastric suction
Excessive use of purgatives
Intestinal and biliary fistulas
Severe diarrhea, as in ulcerative colitis and infantile gastroenteritis
Rarely, prolonged lactation
EXCESSIVE URINARY LOSSES
Diuretic therapy (especially "loop" agents)
Diuretic phase of acute renal failure
Chronic alcoholism
Primary aldosteronism
Hypercalcemic states: malignancy, hyperparathyroidism, and vitamin D excess
Renal tubular acidosis
Diabetes, especially during and following treatment of acidosis
Hyperthyroidism
Idiopathic renal magnesium wasting
Chronic renal failure with renal magnesium wasting
Gentamicin toxicity
Tobramycin nephrotoxicity
Cisplatinum nephrotoxicity
MISCELLANEOUS
Idiopathic hypomagnesemia
Acute pancreatitis
Porphyria with inappropriate secretion of antidiuretic hormone
Multiple transfusions or exchange transfusions with citrated blood
Bartter's syndrome

Hypomagnesemia with no net magnesium losses: redistribution of magnesium

Hypomagnesemia with no net total body magnesium loss occurs as a result of maldistribution from blood to the intracellular, bone, and soft tissue compartments. This occurs, for example, in refeeding after starvation. Such hypomagnesemia is due to increased trapping of the cation in newly formed tissue. The same mechanism is responsible for the development of hypomagnesemia in patients maintained with intravenous feedings containing glucose, amino acids, and inadequate amounts of magnesium.[57] Potts and Roberts[126] found that hypomagnesemia commonly develops following parathyroidectomy for hyperparathyroidism. This reduction in serum levels was attributed to the fall in circulating parathyroid hormone (PTH) levels and the restoration of normal cellular function. The hypomagnesemia complicating acute *pancreatitis* is most likely due to deposition of magnesium in injured tissues.[69,162]

Hypomagnesemia due to reduced dietary intake

Reduced oral intake of magnesium in adults has been associated with hypomagnesemia and evidence of magnesium depletion. As described elsewhere, the defense against negative magnesium balance is the ability of the kidney, specifically the ascending limb of the loop of Henle, to augment magnesium absorption markedly when the serum magnesium concentration falls. Gastrointestinal secretory losses are not similarly regulated; hypomagnesemia can develop with very severe dietary deprivation of magnesium. Stool losses of magnesium continue despite the lack of ingestion. The rapidity with which hypomagnesemia develops with relatively small negative balances reflects the fact that the acutely exchangeable pool for magnesium is principally the extracellular fluid. Bone and soft tissue do not buffer the hypomagnesemia acutely; days to weeks are required for equilibration to occur. Shils[150] studied the effect of dietary magnesium restriction in eight patients for a period of 42 to 266 days. Indications of hypomagnesemia such as Trousseau sign, abnormal skeletal muscle electromyograms, and spasticity developed as early as 42 days after initiating dietary restriction. Both plasma and red blood cell magnesium levels were significantly reduced by 7 days of dietary magnesium restriction. All the clinical findings were reversed after administering magnesium salts. These studies clearly show that hypomagnesemia and magnesium depletion can develop when magnesium intake is severely reduced.

Relatively reduced magnesium intake in settings in which magnesium requirements are increased (pregnancy and infancy) may also result in magnesium depletion. The formation of new tissue in pregnancy requires that dietary magnesium be higher than in nonpregnant women of the same age. Coons and Blunt[45] studied magnesium balance in pregnant women and found a negative magnesium balance, despite an intake of 400 mg/day. Indeed, pregnant women have a tendency to develop hypomagnesemia. Bogert and Acass[21] examined serum magnesium levels in 40 pregnant women at various times during pregnancy and found a decline toward the end of pregnancy.

Protein calorie malnutrition is commonly associated with magnesium depletion.[32] Reduced urinary magnesium excretion, negative magnesium balance, and reduced red blood cell magnesium content have been described. The mechanism is related to both reduced intake and reduced intestinal absorption of magnesium.

Hypomagnesemia with net loss of total body magnesium

Gastrointestinal losses

Increased intestinal loss is a common cause of magnesium depletion and hypomagnesemia, especially in disease entities that produce *steatorrhea*, such as nontropical sprue, short-bowel syndrome, and malabsorption secondary to inflammation of the intestinal wall or pancreatic insufficiency. Booth and coworkers[24,25] reported hypomagnesemia in 36 percent of patients with malabsorption syndrome. Hypomagnesemia develops secondary to the formation of intestinal soaps due to the malabsorption of fat and the binding of magnesium to these soaps. Although net magnesium loss most commonly causes hypomagnesemia, the possibility of tissue magnesium depletion in the face of normal serum magnesium levels should always be considered. Indeed, Lim and Jacob[100] have shown reduced skeletal muscle magnesium levels in patients with chronic diarrhea, in the face of normal serum magnesium levels.

Primary hypomagnesemia is a rare and genetically determined disorder that presents early in infancy with convulsions and tetany. Magnesium balance in a 4-year-old patient was negative and was due to the fecal losses of magnesium.[112] Luminal perfusion studies of the intestine demonstrated net loss of magnesium into the intestinal lumen when perfusion concentrations of magnesium were low (1 to 2 mmol/liter) in contrast to control subjects in whom no such loss occurred. At high concentrations of luminal magnesium (10 mmol/liter) net absorption took place at similar rates in control subjects and patients with primary hypomagnesemia. These data suggest that in primary hypomagnesemia magnesium malabsorption is due to a defect in carrier-mediated magnesium transport. The non-carrier-mediated transport remains intact, as shown by the correction of hypomagnesemia with a high intake of magnesium salts.

Hallberg examined magnesium metabolism in 191 patients before and after *bowel resection* for the treatment of morbid obesity.[80] During the first postoperative year, 50 percent of the patients developed hypomagnesemia. It is of interest that oral administration of magnesium acetate corrected the hypomagnesemia. In 12 patients studied, muscle magnesium content was low and rose to normal levels after intravenous administration of 30 mmol $MgSO_4$.

An interesting entity associated with decreased intestinal absorption of magnesium is *idiopathic hypercalciuria and nephrolithiasis*. Although no data are available to support or rule out evidence for magnesium depletion in patients with this condition, clinical studies have shown reduced urinary excretion of the cation. Both intestinal perfusion and metabolic balance studies demonstrate impaired absorption of magnesium and negative balance. It is of interest to note that the impaired absorption is the result of the carrier-mediated transport, and can be overcome by the administration of high magnesium diets.

Biliary fistulas and *prolonged nasogastric suction* with the administration of *magnesium-free parenteral fluids* are commonly associated with hypomagnesemia and magnesium depletion.

Acute pancreatitis is not infrequently associated with hypocalcemia and hypomagnesemia. The mechanism is not clear but is at least partially attributed to the deposition of magnesium within the fatty soaps of injured tissues in and around the pancreas.

Reduced intestinal absorption of magnesium has been described in subjects on a *low protein diet.*[109] Several studies suggest a correlation between dietary carbohydrates and magnesium absorption.[5,68] Increased dietary glucose has been shown to reduce intestinal magnesium absorption, an effect that can be reversed by the administration of 2,4-dinitrophenol.[2] Increased dietary fat reduces absorption of magnesium, while reduced dietary fat increases its absorption and the concentration of serum magnesium.[24]

Renal losses

Magnesium depletion, hypomagnesemia, and negative magnesium balance can result from impaired renal reabsorption of the cation. The renal response to magnesium deficiency reduces urinary excretion to less than 1 meq/day. Renal magnesium wasting, as defined by continued urinary magnesium excretion in the face of hypomagnesemia, can be due to renal or extrarenal causes (Table 34-3).

Diuretics can cause renal magnesium wasting. Of 33 patients treated with "loop" diuretics, severe hypomagnesemia (0.8 ± 0.13 mg/100 ml) was present in all.[58] This was associated with a marked reduction in muscle potassium content that was not improved by potassium supplementation but was reversed after intravenous magnesium administration.

Studies by Leary and Reyes[97] and by Ryan and coworkers[139] support the notion that biologically important magnesium losses may result from chronic adminstration of diuretics, with loop diuretics causing more profound depletion than thiazides. Most studies, however, suggest that long-term thiazide treatment can be

TABLE 34-3 • Conditions associated with renal wasting of magnesium

Primary renal magnesium wasting
Loop diuretic administration
Diabetic ketoacidosis (osmotic diuresis)
Bartter's syndrome
Hyperaldosteronism
Syndrome of inappropriate ADH secretion
Alcoholism
Hypercalciuria or salt-wasting states
Amphotericin toxicity
Aminoglycoside (gentamicin) administration
Cisplatinum administration

SOURCE: Dirks.[51] Reprinted with permission.

associated with hypomagnesemia.[52,87,95] Administration of piretanide (a thiazide) to nine patients for twelve weeks resulted in a marked fall in serum magnesium concentration. The addition of 10 mg per day of amiloride to hydrochlorothiazide (100 mg daily) administered to 15 hypertensive subjects blunted the fall in serum magnesium concentration.[139] This observation underscores the importance of adding potassium- and magnesium-sparing substances to diuretics employed in chronic diuretic therapy. Indeed, Widman and coworkers[174] were able to prevent the fall in muscle content of magnesium with the addition of amiloride or triamterene.

Cisplatinum administration is associated with nephropathy and hypomagnesemia secondary to hypermagnesuria.[101,148] The pathogenic factor responsible for the magnesium wasting is not clear. The possible mechanisms to be considered include (1) a direct effect of cisplatinum on the renal absorption of magnesium, and (2) interstitial nephritis due to cisplatinum with damage to the loop of Henle and, in turn, reduced magnesium absorption.

Aminoglycosides are associated with nephrotoxicity and urinary magnesium wasting.[15] Although the precise mechanism underlying the magnesuria is not known, some indirect information is available. The nephrotoxic effect of aminoglycosides is exerted mainly on the proximal tubule.[51] It is possible that inhibition of proximal magnesium transport leads to increased magnesium delivery to the loop of Henle, exceeding the loop's reabsorptive capacity, resulting in magnesuria. A possible direct effect on the loop of Henle cannot be ruled out.

Other toxic agents, such as *cyclosporine*[18] and *amphotericin B*,[17] have been associated with renal magnesium wasting.

Inborn defects in tubular magnesium reabsorption, although not common, should be carefully looked for in any patient with unexplained hypomagnesemia and hypermagnesuria. Two types are known: (1) impaired renal conservation of magnesium and potassium, and (2) isolated impairment in renal conservation of magnesium. The first is characterized by hypokalemia, hypomagnesemia, metabolic alkalosis, and inappropriately high urinary magnesium and potassium levels.[75,120] When placed on low magnesium or low potassium diets, these patients cannot conserve magnesium and potassium. Repletion with potassium does not correct the renal magnesium wasting; therefore, it seems that the defect is not related to the hypokalemia. There is no evidence of impaired sodium reabsorption, and the excretion of amino acids and phosphorus is normal. It seems that this is an isolated tubular defect in magnesium and potassium reabsorption. Renal biopsy in one of the patients has shown normal renal tissue.[120] The renin-aldosterone axis is normal and the renal response to spironolactone and mineralocorticoids is intact. These observations suggest that potassium transport at the distal nephron is normal. Patients with this syndrome suffer from spontaneous muscle weakness, tetany, and sometimes convulsions.[10] The genetics of the disorder have not been clarified. While some authors describe an autosomal recessive pattern of inheritance, others describe variable penetrance of the gene.

Isolated renal magnesium wasting is an unusual disorder that may present sporadically or as a familial disorder.[23,62,72,136] It usually first appears in childhood with symptomatic hypocalcemia. Since automated techniques have allowed more frequent measuring of serum magnesium levels, it is likely that acquired renal magnesium wasting due to aging and mild interstitial renal disease will become a more commonly recognized syndrome. In the familial syndrome there is an increased incidence of hypercalciuria and nephrocalcinosis.[62] The diagnosis is made by the demonstration that significant amounts of magnesuria (over 1.5 meq/day) occur despite the presence of hypomagnesemia and the absence of magnesuric drugs.

Phosphate depletion is commonly associated with hypomagnesemia and renal magnesium wasting.[41] The magnesuria is correlated with the degree of hypophosphatemia, and the administration of phosphate corrects the abnormality. *Calcium infusion* impairs the renal reabsorption of magnesium and results in hypomagnesemia.[127] Inappropriate secretion of ADH (SIADH) is associated with hypomagnesemia and urinary magnesium wasting. The volume expansion associated with SIADH reduces net renal magnesium reabsorption.[85,117]

Hypokalemia and potassium depletion can be associated with hypomagnesemia secondary to impaired renal magnesium conservation.[119] The hypomagnesemia and magnesium wasting associated with primary hyperaldosteronism are the results of volume expansion rather than direct effects of aldosterone on magnesium transport.[105] *Bartter's syndrome* is also associated with hypomagnesemia and increased urinary magnesium excretion.[155]

Alcohol ingestion, both acute and chronic, is associated with renal magnesium losses. Muscle biopsy specimens from alcoholic patients have shown significant reduction in cellular magnesium content.[99] Interestingly enough, the tissue magnesium depletion occurred in the face of normal serum magnesium levels in 56 percent of the patients studied. Alcohol has direct renal tubular effects. Acute ingestion of alcohol is associated with a marked increase in the urinary excretion of magnesium.[92,111] A major contributing factor in this scenario is the high incidence of chronic diarrhea and gastrointestinal magnesium loss. Sullivan and coworkers[160] reported that 30 percent of all patients with alcoholism have evidence of hypomagnesemia.

Hypomagnesemia due to renal wasting has also been observed following the diuresis that may follow the relief of urinary tract obstruction.[48]

SYMPTOMS AND SIGNS OF MAGNESIUM DEPLETION

As symptomatic magnesium depletion is often associated with multiple biochemical abnormalities such as hypokalemia, alkalosis, and hypocalcemia, it is difficult to ascribe specific manifestations to isolated changes in magnesium balance (Table 34-4). In 1960, Vallee and coworkers[168] reported 5 patients with symptoms considered to be typical of magnesium depletion, including tetany, positive Chvostek and Trousseau signs, and generalized convulsions. Shils[150] induced magnesium deficiency in volunteers and observed similar findings, including generalized weakness, anorexia, hypokalemia, hypocalcemia, and positive Trousseau and Chvostek signs. The underlying mechanism of hypomagnesemic tetany is unclear, but it can occur in the absence of hypocalcemia or alkalosis and is presumably due to lowering of the threshold for nerve stimulation.[70] Abnormalities of cardiac function have also been described. In moderate magnesium depletion, widening of the QRS complex and peaking of T waves have been noted,[145] while with more severe depletion there is prolongation of the PR interval, progressive widening of the QRS complex and diminution of the T wave,[145] and an apparent increased incidence of ventricular arrthymias.[88,96] The mechanism underlying some of these effects is discussed below.

TABLE 34-4 • Clinical and laboratory effects of magnesium depletion

BIOCHEMICAL

Hypomagnesemia
Hypocalcemia
Hypophosphatemia
Hypokalemia
Hypocalciuria
Hypomagnesuria

CARDIOVASCULAR

Electrocardiographic changes
Increased myocardial irritability
Increased incidence of digitalis intoxication
Reduced myocardial contractility
Hypertension

MUSCULOSKELETAL

Abnormal skeletal muscle function
Myopathic EMGs
Muscle fibrillation

BONE

Resistance to the calcemic action of PTH
Increased incidence of osteoporosis

CENTRAL NERVOUS SYSTEM

Hyperreflexia
Tetany
Ataxia
Vertigo
Carpopedal spasm
Irritability
Depression
Psychosis

ENDOCRINE

Reduced PTH secretion
Resistance to the calcemic action of PTH
Increased renin and aldosterone secretion
Reduced lipolytic activity

EFFECTS OF MAGNESIUM DEPLETION ON ORGAN SYSTEMS

Bone and calcium metabolism

The most classic sign of severe hypomagnesemia (magnesium concentration below 1 meq/liter) is hypocalcemia. Early in vitro studies showed that reduction of magnesium, in the absence of changes in calcium, stimulated parathyroid hormone secretion. In contrast, measurements of immunoreactive parathyroid hormone levels in most hypomagnesemic-hypocalcemic patients have been found to be normal or undetectable.[35,43,135] Parenteral administration of magnesium rapidly raises parathyroid hormone levels suggesting that in most patients hypomagnesemia suppresses the hormone's secretion.[11,35] Levels are normal in some patients, however, indicating that secretory failure cannot explain the hypocalcemia in all patients and that bone resistance to parathyroid hormone may play a role. Estep and coworkers[61] and Muldowney and coworkers[113] presented evidence of resistance to the calcemic effects of parathyroid extract in hypocalcemic, hypomagnesemic patients. In vitro studies are consistent with these observations. Thus, Freitag and coworkers[73] showed that isolated tibias from magnesium-depleted dogs generated less cyclic AMP in response to perfusion with parathyroid hormone than tibias obtained from normal animals. The mechanism responsible for this finding is not currently understood. It is possible that severe hypomagnesemia may interfere with G protein activation in response to parathyroid hormone, causing less stimulation of adenylate cyclase and cyclic AMP production.

Heart and cardiovascular system

Magnesium has been shown to affect a number of cardiac cellular systems. Most of these changes have been ascribed to altered cytosolic magnesium activity. Unfortunately, little is known concerning the regulation and modulation of cytosolic magnesium; as yet there has been no documentation of reduced intracellular free magnesium levels in hypomagnesemic or magnesium depletion states. The clinical disturbance of most interest and potential importance is the association of hypomagnesemia with ventricular arrhythmias, particularly during myocardial ischemia.[86] A derivative relationship that is receiving increasing attention is the prophylactic use of parenteral magnesium, in the absence of documented hypomagnesemia, in the first 24 to 48 h following an ischemic event. It is hoped that this therapy will reduce mortality, presumably by reducing life-threatening ventricular arrhythmias. In the sections that follow we will review what little is known about the regulation of cytosolic magnesium concentration; the effects of cytosolic magnesium on ion channel function, excitation-contraction coupling, and bioenergetics; and the association of magnesium with arrhythmias and with protection during ischemia.

Cellular magnesium stores and cytosolic magnesium activity

The total intracellular magnesium content approximates 8 to 10 m*M*. Most is bound to ATP and other intracellular nucleotides and enzyme complexes. The reported concentration of free ionized magnesium varies, depending on the method of measurement. Earlier studies using microelectrodes and ^{31}P nuclear magnetic resonance suggested values ranging between 1.5 and 6 m*M*.[29,42,122] But more recent studies, using refined microelectrode measurements and magnesium-sensitive dyes based on the FURA compound, indicate that the free cytosolic concentration in heart (and probably most organ systems) is more likely in the range of 0.4 to 0.6 m*M*.[9,115,116,128]

Changes in plasma magnesium levels alter cellular magnesium content slowly. Polimeni and Page[122] measured the specific activity of radioactive magnesium in the heart and blood after injection of the isotope in vivo, and demonstrated that maximal accumulation occurred at 3 h. The accumulation of magnesium exceeds unity only after 3 h and reaches a peak at 9 to 10 h. These data indicate that the effect of blood magnesium levels on myocardial magnesium concentration is a relatively slow process. The mechanisms that regulate cell magnesium concentration are not yet clear. Although it is clear that cardiac muscle cells are permeable to magnesium, it is not known by what pathways magnesium ions enter the cells. There is no evidence for magnesium entry through a channel or other electrogenic mechanism. Since the intracellular free magnesium activity is significantly below that expected at electrochemical equilibrium, however, there must be some type of energy-dependent extrusion mechanism. An ATP-dependent Na/Mg exchanger has been described in squid axon and in red blood cells,[50,74] but little evidence for such a mechanism has been found in cardiac tissue.[115] It should be pointed out, however, that, given the kinetics of such systems in other tissues, it would be very difficult to detect such a system in the types of acute experiment that have been performed to date.

Ion channel modulation

Recent studies have provided abundant new information on the effects of cytosolic free magnesium on calcium and potassium channels in mammalian cardiac myocytes. Increasing cytosolic magnesium above the normal range produces marked inhibition of the inward calcium current, which is responsible for the plateau phase of the action potential and inhibits the normal augmentation of this channel current by cyclic AMP and beta-adrenergic agents. Lowering of magnesium concentration below the normal range has opposite effects, producing marked augmentation of the calcium channel current and potentiating the response to cyclic AMP.[3,173] The physiologic significance of these effects are not known. It is known that cytosolic magnesium concentration rises during ischemia, reflecting the fall in ATP levels.[116] Inhibition of calcium channel current by the increased magnesium may reduce the excitability of the cell and exert a protective effect during ischemia. The inwardly rectifying potassium channel is responsible for maintenance of the normal resting membrane potential at close to electrochemical equilibrium for potassium. The rectification is produced by magnesium's moving into the channel at depolarizing voltages and completely blocking outward potassium movement. The K_D is extremely low for this effect (0.17 μM).[4,173] Cytosolic magnesium also modulates the delayed rectifier current. This channel, which passes outward potassium current and is an important component of repolarization, is very sensitive to magnesium within the physiologic range. Thus, lowering cytosolic magnesium from 0.8 to 0.4 m*M* doubles the outward potassium current, while an increase to 1.6 m*M* markedly inhibits the current and prevents enhancement by beta-adrenergic agents.[4] The mechanisms of these effects of magnesium are unclear, but they may have profound clinical significance. Thus, increasing outward potassium currents would significantly shorten the action potential, may alter intracellular potassium concentration, and may increase susceptibility to arrhythmias.[4]

Other cellular effects of magnesium

Hormonal activation of second messenger systems such as adenylate cyclase involves activation by the hormone-receptor complex of a G (guanine nucleotide regulatory) protein. G proteins can be stimulatory or inhibitory and can have direct effects on channel function as well as alter adenylate cyclase activity. This activation is magnesium-dependent, with affinity depending on the hormone-receptor interaction and the type of G protein involved. Magnesium may modulate calcium uptake by Ca-ATPase in the sarcoplasmic reticulum and, in high concentration, may also interfere with mitochondrial calcium intake.

Effects on cellular bioenergetics

Myocardial bioenergetics depends on the normal interplay between mitochondria, cytosol, and myofibrils. The mitochondrial redox state is controlled by the cytoplasmic phosphorylation state of the adenine nucleotides, the *phosphorylation potential.* These variables were measured in rats raised on magnesium-deficient or control diets.[27] A marked reduction in myocardial inorganic phosphorus levels was found after eight weeks of magnesium depletion. Creatine phosphate levels were significantly higher in magnesium depletion, while ADP and ATP levels were reduced by 50 percent and 20 percent, respectively. Total adenine nucleotides and total phosphorus (i.e., total organic and inorganic phosphorus) were also markedly reduced. There was a marked fall in tissue magnesium content at four weeks and eight weeks of magnesium depletion. It is of interest that a significant fall in tissue magnesium content was found only after four weeks of magnesium depletion, despite the early occurrence of hypomagnesemia. Since the ionized fraction represents only a small portion of the total magnesium, these data probably reflect the changes in adenine nucleotides (which bind most of the intracellular magnesium) rather than changes in free magnesium.

Effects on contractility

We have examined the effects of magnesium depletion on myocardial contractility. Serum magnesium levels fell from 1.8 mg/100 ml to 0.6 mg/100 ml in rats raised on a low magnesium diet for eight weeks. There was a 50 percent reduction in the development of tension in the myocardium from magnesium-depleted rats. Pretreatment of magnesium-depleted rats with intraperitoneal magnesium 4 h prior to the experiment normalized the development of myocardial tension. In contrast, the addition of magnesium in vitro to the contracting atria did not improve the contractility. The observation that only in vivo administration of magnesium normalized the tension development suggests that the serum magnesium level by itself is not a primary mediator of the impaired contractility. In contrast to these chronic effects, Shine and Douglas[151,152] found that increasing magnesium concentration rapidly decreased tension development in isolated perfused rat intraventricular septa. They suggested that this effect of magnesium may be due to interference with calcium entry into the cell.

Magnesium and ischemic heart disease

Life-threatening arrhythmias, corrected by magnesium therapy, have been described in individuals with hypomagnesemia,[89] but most of the circumstantial evidence associating magnesium deficiency with arrhythmias has been described in patients with ischemic heart disease. Several investigators have demonstrated that a relationship exists between decreased magnesium content of the myocardium and coronary arteries and increased mortality from nonocclusive coronary artery disease. The incidence of the disease is highest in geographic areas with soft drinking water or soil poor in magnesium.[146] The observation that there is a significantly reduced magnesium level in heart tissue and coronary vessels of patients who experience sudden death from nonocclusive coronary heart disease suggests a contributing role for chronic hypomagnesemia in the morbidity and mortality of coronary artery disease. Manthey and coworkers[102] measured serum levels of magnesium in 106 patients undergoing coronary angiography. Patients with severe coronary heart disease had lower mean serum magnesium and higher serum copper and manganese concentrations than those without the vasculopathy. Dyckner and coworkers[54] showed a 46 percent incidence of hypomagnesemia in 342 patients with acute myocardial infarction and demonstrated that these patients had a threefold greater frequency of ventricular arrhythmias. Kafka and coworkers[91] found that patients with acute myocardial infarction who were hypomagnesemic had a 50 percent greater frequency of ventricular arrhythmias than normomagnesemic patients, although some of the symptomatic patients were also hypokalemic. It is well documented that immediately after the onset of myocardial infarction there is a sharp fall in magnesium levels and a sharp rise in free fatty acid levels.[66] For these reasons it seems prudent to prevent hypomagnesemia in patients with coronary artery disease. The use of parenteral magnesium prophylactically in the management of patients with acute ischemic injury is currently receiving attention.[134,153] Abraham and coworkers[1] found a reduction in potentially lethal arrhythmias during the first 24 h after admission in patients given a single intravenous dose of 2.4 g of magnesium sulfate, compared to placebo-treated patients. Similarly, two other large placebo-controlled studies[130,131,153] using different dosage regimens suggest that magnesium administration seems to be associated with improved mortality due, at least in part, to reduced incidence of arrhythmias. Finally, the most striking antiarrhythmic effects of magnesium have been demonstrated in patients with torsade de pointes.[167] It is clear that large, well-designed studies are now indicated to determine whether magnesium is indicated routinely in the management of patients with acute ischemic injury.

Skeletal muscle

The myopathy of chronic alcoholism resembles the morphologic changes described in experimental magnesium deficiency in the rat. Stendig-Lindberg and coworkers[156] examined 10 patients with hypomagnesemia and myopathic symptoms, seven of whom were chronic alcoholics and three of whom had hypomagnesemia secondary to malabsorption syndrome. In the hypomagnesemic patients, muscle strength was significantly reduced, as was muscle creatine phosphate content. Anderson and coworkers[12] evaluated skeletal muscle total phosphorus and magnesium content in 13 patients with acute alcoholic myopathy. Total muscle phosphorus and magnesium content were significantly reduced. These findings suggest that the myopathy of alcoholism results, in part, from chronic magnesium depletion.

The effects of magnesium depletion on skeletal muscle function and structure are difficult to study, since severe isolated magnesium deficiency is commonly associated with hypokalemia, hypophosphatemia, and hypocalcemia. Cronin and coworkers[47] examined the effects of magnesium depletion on transmembrane electrical potential difference of skeletal muscle and muscle cell morphology in magnesium-deficient dogs. The magnesium content of skeletal muscle fell only modestly despite prolonged magnesium deficiency (ten weeks). The most pronounced muscle compositional change was a marked loss of muscle total phosphorus and gain of calcium, sodium, and chloride with no changes in cellular potassium levels and only a slight change in magnesium levels. Muscle histology showed areas of focal necrosis in four of nine dogs, with muscle cell hyperpolarization developing after ten weeks of magnesium depletion. The authors concluded that the skeletal muscle abnormalities complicating magnesium depletion are primarily due to the associated deficiency of muscle phosphorus. Interestingly, serum phosphorus levels were normal in these dogs, while muscle total phosphorus content was reduced. Several major problems exist, however, with the interpretation of these studies:

1. The results of skeletal muscle content of the various electrolytes were expressed per dry weight but not per milligram of protein or DNA. Since it is not possible to rule out an effect of magnesium depletion on protein synthesis, which would further change the distribution of magnesium and phosphorus in the cell, it is possible that, if expressed per milligram protein, there might be no fall in magnesium or phosphorus.
2. Analysis of total phosphorus does not relate to either inorganic phosphorus or nucleotide phosphorus. A reduction in total phosphorus may be limited to changes in total nucleotide phosphorus or protein phosphorus with no change in cellular inorganic phosphorus.
3. The observation that muscle magnesium declined only slightly may not be relevant, since most of the active cell magnesium is unbound and cannot be detected by tissue-ashing methods.

Potter and coworkers[125] have reviewed magnesium's role in the regulation of muscle contraction, focusing on the cation's effects on the cellular calcium-binding proteins troponin, parvalbumin, myosin, and calmodulin. The major effect of magnesium is to greatly reduce the rate of calcium binding to sites that bind magnesium and calcium competitively. Thus, during a transient increase in magnesium (similar to that seen during muscle activation) these sites would bind very little calcium. These data indicate a role for intracellular magnesium in the regulation of the high-affinity calcium-binding proteins and suggest a mechanism by which magnesium depletion may affect muscle function.

Studies by Stephenson and coworkers[158] and Hasselbach and coworkers[82] suggest that the initial event in magnesium depletion is an impairment in the uptake of calcium by the sarcoplasmic reticulum that, in turn, inhibits the excitation-contraction coupling of muscle.

Blood vessels and hypertension

Acute hypomagnesemia in animals and humans is often associated with increases in blood pressure and elevation in peripheral vascular resistance in a variety of regions of the circulation. Several disease entities associated with hypomagnesemia are commonly associated with elevated blood pressure—for example, diabetes mellitus, alcoholism, and essential hypertension. Hypermagnesemia has been associated with reduction in blood pressure levels, and early studies by Hazard and Wurmser[83] have shown that acute elevations of serum magnesium are associated with hypotension. Recent in vitro studies of blood vessel contractility and reactivity indicate that hypermagnesemia induces rapid vasodilatation and depresses reactivity to contractile agonists.[8] Lowering magnesium levels increases reactivity to pressor agonists. In addition to modulating drug- and hormone-induced contraction by smooth muscle cells, magnesium can also alter the basal tension or tone.[8] Magnesium was also shown to directly influence the uptake, content, binding, and distribution of calcium in smooth muscle cells.[8]

Diabetes mellitus is commonly associated with marked hypomagnesemia and a high incidence of hypertension. Recent in vitro experiments in alloxan diabetic rats[163,165,166] suggest that the altered vascular tone noted in these experimental animals may in part be due to modification in the Mg-Ca exchange sites at the vascular smooth muscle cell membranes.

A role for hypomagnesemia in essential hypertension has been suggested (see Chap. 48). Recent in vitro experiments in rats with spontaneous hypertension have shown impaired vascular smooth muscle responsiveness to vasopressors and to removal or administration of magnesium.[8,165,166] Both clinical and experimental evidence suggest that verapamil and other calcium channel blockers can produce peripheral vasodilatation, decrease arterial blood pressure, and lower systemic vascular resistance. The basic mechanism mediating these effects is thought to be inhibition of calcium influx into the vascular smooth muscle. Turlapaty and coworkers[164] examined the possible interactive effects of verapamil and magnesium on tone and contractility of vascular smooth muscle. Thoracic aorta and portal vein were examined in vitro. The authors demonstrated that magnesium and verapamil have synergistic effects on the amplitude of contraction via the effects on inhibition of calcium fluxes and probably by decreasing cytosolic calcium content. These data are consistent with the effects of cytosolic magnesium concentration on calcium channel function as described above.[3] These observations have important clinical implications for treatment of hypertensive and cardiac patients who are simultaneously treated with magnesium-wasting diuretics and verapamil.

Studies by Resnick and coworkers[133] have examined the relationship between serum magnesium and hypertension. Blood magnesium and plasma renin activity were measured in 102 normotensive and 98 hypertensive subjects. The authors found a strong negative correlation between the degree of blood pressure elevation and the reduction in blood magnesium levels.

Population studies in the United States evaluating magnesium consumption and high blood pressure are not available. McCarron,[110] in a survey of calcium and nutrition, found a difference in magnesium consumption between normotensive patients and hypertensive patients, but the difference was not statistically significant.

A possible role for magnesium in the development of the hypertension seen with hypercalcemia has been suggested.[177] Future metabolic balance studies in large population groups in the United States may uncover a possible role for reduced dietary magnesium in the development of essential hypertension. At this point the data are experimental and cannot be applied clinically.

INTERRELATIONSHIP BETWEEN MAGNESIUM AND POTASSIUM

Magnesium is second only to potassium as the most abundant intracellular cation. The metabolism of both ions has been shown to be closely interrelated. Specifically, evidence from both experimental animals and clinical observations suggests that magnesium plays a major role in potassium homeostasis. The following observations support the existence of this interaction:

1. Magnesium deficiency is associated with a widely distributed loss of cellular potassium.
2. Combined magnesium and potassium deficiencies result in greater losses of cell potassium than occur in simple potassium deficiency.
3. In the combined cation deficiency, even parenteral administration of large doses of potassium will not correct deficits until magnesium losses have been eliminated. The kaliuresis caused by magnesium depletion prevents the retention of administered potassium.

Cotlove and coworkers, in 1951,[46] described a significant loss of skeletal muscle potassium in magnesium-deficient rats. Loss of cellular potassium has also been documented in cardiac tissue and in renal tissue in experimental rats made magnesium-deficient.[103,112,147] Ryan and coworkers[138] examined the ability of ascites tumor cells to grow and maintain potassium levels in magnesium-deficient mice. There was significant reduction in potassium levels in the ascites tumor cells taken from magnesium-deficient mice. The cell potassium loss during magnesium deficiency is accompanied by a decrease in magnesium concentration and an increase in sodium and calcium concentrations.

Magnesium also plays a major role in restoring potassium loss from skeletal muscle cells. Ryan and coworkers[137] and Ryan and Hingerty[141] compared the restoration rate of red muscle potassium and sodium in potassium-depleted rats and in combined magnesium- and potassium-depleted rats following intraperitoneal injections of KCl. Within several hours of receiving an intraperitoneal injection of KCl, the potassium-depleted group had restored muscle potassium content to normal, while sodium extrusion took approximately 7 h. In marked contrast, the combined magnesium- and potassium-depleted group did not restore either muscle potassium or sodium after the intraperitoneal injection of only KCl. Several direct and indirect mechanisms have been suggested as mediators of this effect of magnesium depletion on potassium homeostasis.

Indirect mechanisms

Hyperaldosteronism has accompanied magnesium deficiency in rats, and several investigators have suggested that the hormone-induced kaliuresis accounts for the negative potassium balance.[33,59] Countervailing data also exist. A recent micropuncture study, for example, found that although dietary magnesium restriction reduced total body magnesium by 30 percent and total body potassium by 10 percent, renal potassium excretion was not altered.[34] The authors concluded that the reduction in cellular potassium content during magnesium deficiency in the presence of normal plasma potassium concentration is a reflection of the cell's inability to maintain an appropriate potassium gradient.

Direct mechanisms

Several lines of evidence suggest that lack of magnesium has a direct effect on cellular potassium transport. Incubation of diaphragm muscle in magnesium-free solutions resulted in loss of muscle potassium.[176] Arnold and Ryan[13] reported that isolated rat soleus muscle was unable to replenish its potassium when incubated in potassium-enriched medium unless magnesium was present. Work on ascites tumor cells in vitro also confirmed a magnesium requirement for maintenance of cell potassium.[138]

As discussed above, intracellular magnesium modulates potassium channels in cardiac myocytes.[4] Recent evidence suggests that potassium channels in the cortical thick ascending limb of Henle's loop are also sensitive to cytosolic magnesium activity and inhibited by increased magnesium levels.[93] Other portions of the distal nephron have not yet been directly studied. It is possible, therefore, that renal potassium wasting in hypomagnesemic states reflects increased potassium channel conductance consequent to reduced cytosolic magnesium activity in Henle's loop and distal portions of the nephron.

Reviews of magnesium's role in the regulation of cellular Na^+-K^+ ATPase indicate that the enzyme has an unequivocal and absolute requirement for the cation.[22,60,64] It is not clear, however, that cytosolic magnesium activity ever falls sufficiently in hypomagnesemia to alter Na^+-K^+ ATPase activity.

Many clinical studies and observations are compatible with the notion that magnesium plays a major role in the regulation of cellular potassium homeostasis and of body potassium balance. Dunn and Walser[53] studied magnesium-depleted patients and found that hypokalemia, alkalosis, and reduced muscle potassium content were common. Haijama and MacDowall[79] measured the distribution of magnesium, potassium, sodium, and calcium in extracellular and intracellular compartments during magnesium depletion in infants with primary hypomagnesemia. The hypomagnesemia was associated with hypokalemia and hypocalcemia, while intracellular potassium decreased and intracellular sodium increased. Shils,[150] in his classic study, examined patients who had undergone radical head and neck surgery while they were ingesting a low magnesium diet. The hypomagnesemia was associated with reduced total body potassium. Administration of KCl did not correct the hypokalemia or the reduced total body potassium unless magnesium was replenished. Stewart and Fleming[159] studied the relationship between plasma and erythrocyte magnesium and potassium concentration in subjects during an 18-day fast. Erythrocyte potassium concentration decreased by 9 percent in hypomagnesemic patients, but did not fall in patients given magnesium supplements. These observations suggested a role for extracellular magnesium concentration in intracellular potassium balance.

Ryan and coworkers[140,142] found that potassium administration did not effectively reverse hypokalemia in patients with congestive heart failure who had high aldosterone levels, hypomagnesemia and reduced lymphocyte magnesium and potassium content. However, magnesium sulfate administration, either intravenous or intramuscular, produced significant increases in both lymphocyte magnesium and potassium. Dyckner and Wester[55,56] demonstrated that the administration of magnesium to patients with cardiac arrhythmias and reduced muscle potassium content induced restoration of normal potassium concentration and control of arrhythmias.

Potassium depletion resistant to even parenteral therapy, may, in many cases, be secondary to an underlying but undetected magnesium deficiency. It is therefore prudent for physicians confronted with resistant cardiac arrhythmias or resistant hypokalemia and potassium depletion to examine magnesium in blood and erythrocytes, or perform a magnesium loading test (see above).

THERAPY OF MAGNESIUM DEPLETION AND HYPOMAGNESEMIA

The elements or stages of magnesium therapy are conveniently divided into the following categories: prevention of depletion in high risk groups; replenishment of established depletion; and emergency therapy of dangerously symptomatic depletion. First, we shall review terms used in the quantification of magnesium.

RELATIONSHIP BETWEEN MILLIMOLES AND MILLIEQUIVALENTS OF PHOSPHATE

Terms describing the quantification of magnesium include milligrams, millimoles, and milliequivalents. Familiarity with these terms and their interconversions is of obvious importance to the interpretation of serum levels, balance data, and the administration of magnesium. In mass terms, magnesium is most commonly quantified in milligrams. Dividing the number of milligrams by the cation's atomic weight of 24 yields millimoles (mmol). Thus, 24 mg of magnesium constitutes 1 mmol. Milliequivalents (meq) are derived by multiplying the millimoles by magnesium's valence of 2. Thus, 1 mmol of magnesium is synonymous with 2 meq, while 1 meq is equal to 0.5 mmol, or 12 mg.

The number of milligrams of elemental magnesium provided by 1 g of the commonly used salt, $MgSO_4 \cdot 7H_2O$, is determined as follows. The molecular weight of $MgSO_4 \cdot 7H_2O$ is calculated by summing the atomic weights of its components: Mg, 24; S, 32; 4 O, each 16 (total 64); 14 H, each 1 (total 14); 7 O, 112; grand total: 246. Thus, 1 g of $MgSO_4 \cdot 7H_2O$ provides 4.065 mmol (1000 ÷ 246), and since magnesium comprises 24/246 or 9.76 percent of the salt, 1 g provides 97.6 mg, 4 mmol, or 8 meq of elemental magnesium.

PREVENTION OF MAGNESIUM DEPLETION IN HIGH RISK GROUPS

This category includes the following clinical groups: (1) patients receiving total parenteral nutrition; (2) patients with chronic diarrheal disorders and intestinal magnesium wasting; (3) patients with renal magnesium wasting, either primary or diuretic-induced; and (4) lactating females and growing children.

Both oral and intravenous magnesium supplementation can be used in these subjects. In groups 1 and 2, magnesium is best administered parenterally, via deep intramuscular injection or intravenously. In these patients, 5 to 25 mmol (120 to 600 mg) per day of magnesium should adequately prevent depletion. The larger doses are given to patients wasting more generous amounts of the cation.

In groups 3 and 4, oral intake of magnesium is most convenient. Magnesium gluconate tablets (500 mg) deliver 1.2 mmol of elemental magnesium per tablet, whereas each 15 g of magnesium sulfate powder provides 61.2 mmol of magnesium. Each tablet of magnesium hydroxide, $Mg(OH)_2$, provides 400 mg of the salt with 3.5 mmol of elemental magnesium. In our experience, oral therapy with magnesium gluconate is better tolerated than $MgSO_4$ powder; diarrhea and abdominal cramps are more common with the latter. Because of the risks of hypermagnesemia (see below) during preventive and replacement therapy, physicians must make certain that renal function is normal and adequate to excrete the excess magnesium administered. When renal function is impaired in patients receiving magnesium daily, blood levels should be monitored, and, in general, the intravenous dose should be appropriately adjusted.

REPLENISHMENT OF ESTABLISHED MAGNESIUM DEPLETION

It is important to recall that the primary regulator of renal magnesium transport is the plasma magnesium level (possibly via its influence on intracellular activity). In hypomagnesemia, therefore, renal excretion is appropriately reduced. If, during therapy, plasma levels are increased abruptly prior to replenishment of tissue stores, renal tubular transport will be reduced and urinary excretion will increase, resulting in loss of some of the administered magnesium into the urine. In the absence of clinical symptoms of hypomagnesemia, therefore, it is prudent to administer magnesium orally, using sustained-release tablets to provide slow, sustained intake without acute increases in plasma levels.

In patients manifesting clinical and chemical evidence of magnesium depletion, the intravenous administration of magnesium is indicated. Alcoholics and diabetics in ketoacidosis most often require this kind of rigorous therapy. If renal function is normal and the patient is not symptomatically hypomagnesemic, replacement of 50 to 100 meq (600 to 1200 mg) of magnesium daily, for several days, is generally adequate to restore body deficits. Additional cation should be added to replace ongoing losses. Since renal excretion of parenterally administered magnesium normally develops prior to replenishment of body stores, one should give several hundred milliequivalents over several days, to replace the average 50 to 150-meq deficit.

EMERGENCY ADMINISTRATION

Symptomatic patients manifesting dangerous signs of increased neuromuscular excitability and cardiac ectopy or dysrhythmias should receive large intravenous doses of magnesium. Life-threatening ventricular arrhythmias often require infusion of 16 to 32 meq of magnesium (4 to 8 ml of 50 percent magnesium sulfate) in 100 to 500 ml of 5% dextrose, given over a 10- to 15-min period. Continuous ECG monitoring and repeated analysis of serum magnesium levels are obviously required. The patient's response to therapy dictates the quantity of additional doses.

HYPERMAGNESEMIA AND MAGNESIUM TOXICITY

Since large loads of magnesium can easily be eliminated in the urine when renal function is normal, it is unusual to encounter hypermagnesemia in the absence of azotemia. Some of the conditions in which hypermagnesemia have been noted include (1) acute and chronic renal failure, (2) adrenal insufficiency, (3) magnesium therapy for eclampsia (the hypermagnesemia also affecting the infant), and (4) during the administration of pharmacologic doses of magnesium and use of magnesium-containing oral purgatives, rectal enemas, or antacids, especially in patients with impaired renal function. Absolute magnesium excretion falls as the GFR declines; this may result in hypermagnesemia. As long as the patient remains on a normal diet, the serum levels of magnesium will stabilize at approximately 2.5 meq/liter. However, when patients with chronic renal failure are treated with magnesium-containing antacids, the plasma level can reach 4 to 6 meq/liter, a value often associated with signs and symptoms of toxicity.

Elderly subjects are more likely to develop magnesium toxicity, because renal function declines with age and magnesium-containing antacids or vitamins are commonly consumed by this group.

The principal sources of magnesium in medications can be classified as antacids, laxatives, and urologic irrigation solutions. Table 34-5 lists the most commonly used prescriptions associated with magnesium toxicity in patients with reduced renal function.

Signs and symptoms

The signs and symptoms of hypermagnesemia reflect the ion's action on the nervous and cardiovascular systems. Deep tendon reflexes are usually lost when blood magnesium concentration exceeds 6 meq/liter. Respiratory paralysis, narcosis, hypotension, and a prolonged P-R interval with abnormal cardiac conduction may occur as blood levels of magnesium approach 10 meq/liter, and complete heart block may occur at levels approaching 15 meq/liter.

Several reports have suggested a relationship between the blood levels of magnesium and symptoms. However, there seems to be a great deal of individual variability. While some patients have reported drowsiness and altered levels of consciousness at levels of 5 meq/liter, others reported normal mental and CNS responses during mild hypermagnesemia.[129,154,158] The most common clinical signs and symptoms described in patients whose blood magnesium increased to 4 meq/liter were drowsiness, lethargy, and diaphoresis.

Treatment

Discontinuation of the patient's exposure to magnesium, coupled with the intravenous administration of calcium compounds, is the initial step in treating symptomatic hypermagnesemia. The administration of 5 to 10 meq (100 to 200 mg) of elemental calcium may be adequate to reverse the manifestations of hypermagnesemia, but greater amounts may be required. Peritoneal dialysis or hemodialysis may be needed to lower the concentration of blood magnesium in patients with severe hypermagnesemia.

MAGNESIUM METABOLISM IN RENAL FAILURE

Renal failure may be associated with disturbances in several aspects of magnesium metabolism. These include the renal handling of magnesium, its concentration in blood, tissue content, intestinal absorption, and overall balance.

RENAL HANDLING OF MAGNESIUM IN RENAL FAILURE

The daily urinary excretion of magnesium is usually reduced in patients with advanced renal failure.[123,129,157,169] In 50 patients with creatinine clearance of 1 to 30 ml/min studied in our laboratory, the urinary excretion of magnesium per 24 h ranged between 12 and 133 mg with a mean of 57 ± 31 (SD) mg. Only two-thirds of the patients had significant reduction in their excretory rates; the other one-third had either normal or increased excretion of magnesium.[123] In patients with uremia and salt wasting, such as those with chronic interstitial nephritis, the 24-h urinary excretion of magnesium may be normal or high,[123] and renal magnesium wasting has been reported in few such patients.[129]

The fraction of filtered magnesium excreted (fractional excretion) increases as renal failure progresses[40,78,123,124,157]; the increment is more marked when the GFR is less than 10 ml/min. It is important to consider the changes in the fractional excretion of magnesium in terms of the renal handling of sodium, since in tubular reabsorption these two ions are interrelated.[30,51,104] Indeed, there is a positive and significant correlation between the fractional excretion of magnesium and that of sodium in patients with GFRs below

TABLE 34-5 • Medications containing magnesium

Brand name	Magnesium salt(s)	Amount of elemental magnesium per dosing unit (mg*)
ANTACIDS		
Aludrox suspension	Magnesium hydroxide	42.9
Aludrox tablets	Magnesium hydroxide	35
A-M-T tablets	Magnesium trisilicate	30
Camalox suspension	Magnesium hydroxide	83.4
Camalox tablets	Magnesium hydroxide	83.4
Creamalin tablets	Magnesium hydroxide	32.3
Delcid suspension	Magnesium hydroxide and citrate	302
Di-Gel liquid	Magnesium hydroxide	36
Di-Gel tablets	Magnesium hydroxide	50
Gelusil liquid	Magnesium hydroxide	82
Gelusil II liquid	Magnesium hydroxide	164
Gelusil-M liquid	Magnesium hydroxide	82
Kolantyl liquid	Magnesium hydroxide	63
Kolantyl wafers	Magnesium hydroxide	71.4
Kolantyl tablets	Magnesium oxide	111.5
Maalox suspension	Magnesium hydroxide	83.4
Maalox Plus suspension	Magnesium hydroxide	83.4
Maalox No. 1 tablets	Magnesium hydroxide	83.4
Maalox No. 2 tablets	Magnesium hydroxide	166.8
Maalox Plus tablets	Magnesium hydroxide	83.4
Mylanta liquid	Magnesium hydroxide	83.4
Mylanta tablets	Magnesium hydroxide	83.4
Mylanta II liquid	Magnesium hydroxide	166.8
Mylanta II tablets	Magnesium hydroxide	166.8
Riopan suspension	Magaldrate	93
Riopan tablets	Magaldrate	93
Riopan Plus suspension	Magaldrate	103
Riopan Plus chew tablets	Magaldrate	103
Silain-Gel liquid	Magnesium hydroxide	119
Simeco suspension	Magnesium hydroxide	125
Trisogel liquid	Magnesium trisilicate	108
Trisogel Pulvules	Magnesium trisilicate	50
WinGel liquid	Magnesium hydroxide	69
WinGel tablets	Magnesium hydroxide	69
		Magnesium content per unit
LAXATIVES		
Citrate of magnesia	Magnesium citrate	3.26 g/300 ml
Haley's M-O	Magnesium hydroxide	379 mg/15 ml
Milk of magnesia	Magnesium hydroxide	498 mg/15 ml
UROLOGIC IRRIGATING SOLUTIONS		
Suby's solution G	Magnesium oxide	
McGaw	420 mg/100 ml	253 mg/100 ml
Cutter	384 mg/100 ml	231.6 mg/100 ml
Abbott	384 mg/100 ml	231.6 mg/100 ml

* Per tablet or per 5 ml of liquid.

SOURCE: Ratzan.[132] Reproduced with permission.

40 ml/min.[124] A similar relationship was observed in dogs with experimental renal failure.[78]

We have evaluated the renal handling of magnesium during the diuretic phase of acute renal failure in 10 patients. The fractional excretion of magnesium is increased, and there is a positive and significant correlation between it and that of sodium.

SERUM MAGNESIUM IN RENAL FAILURE

Acute renal failure

The effect of acute renal failure on the blood concentration of magnesium was studied by Massry and coworkers[108] in 10 patients. Hypermagnesemia was present in all but one patient during the oliguric phase. The highest values ranged between 2.2 and 4.6 mg/100 ml. During the diuretic phase the levels fell to normal or slightly below normal. The magnesium concentration in serum was normal after recovery.

Chronic renal failure

The concentration of magnesium in blood is usually normal in patients with early renal failure, but hypermagnesemia is common in patients with advanced renal failure.[40] The relation between serum magnesium concentration and the level of renal function in a large number of patients with creatinine clearance rates below 30 ml/min is presented in Fig. 34-2. The percentage of serum magnesium not bound to protein was 76 ± 8 percent, not different from the value of 75 ± 9 percent observed in normal subjects.[40] Abrupt increases in serum magnesium can occur when patients consume magnesium-containing antacids or laxatives.[129] Hypomagnesemia has been reported in some patients with renal failure.[81,154,170]

The levels of serum magnesium in patients undergoing hemodialysis are clearly related to the concentration of magnesium in the dialysate, as well as the dietary intake of this ion. It is known that magnesium readily crosses the dialysis membrane and that its movement depends on the gradient between the concentration of diffusible magnesium in blood and the concentration of magnesium in the dialysate.[118] Schmidt and coworkers[149] reported total magnesium losses as high as 700 mg per dialysis when the dialysate magnesium concentration was 0.27 mg/100 ml. The importance of dialysate magnesium levels in determining the predialysis blood magnesium concentrations is demonstrated by observations in patients treated in two separate dialysis centers, one using dialysate with 0.6 mg/100 ml of magnesium and the other 1.8 mg/100 ml. Predialysis blood magnesium levels ranged from 1.7 to 2.5 mg/100 ml and from 3.0 to 5.0 mg/100 ml in the two centers, respectively.[40] Similar observations were reported by other authors.[20]

An abrupt rise in the serum magnesium concentration may acutely inhibit the release of PTH.[31,76,106] Indeed, acute hypermagnesemia, produced either by intravenous infusion of magnesium or by increasing the magnesium concentration of dialysate, was associated with a fall in the blood levels of PTH in patients undergoing regular hemodialysis.[71,121] Whether chronic hypermagnesemia, such as that observed in advanced uremia, may alter the function of parathyroid glands is unknown.

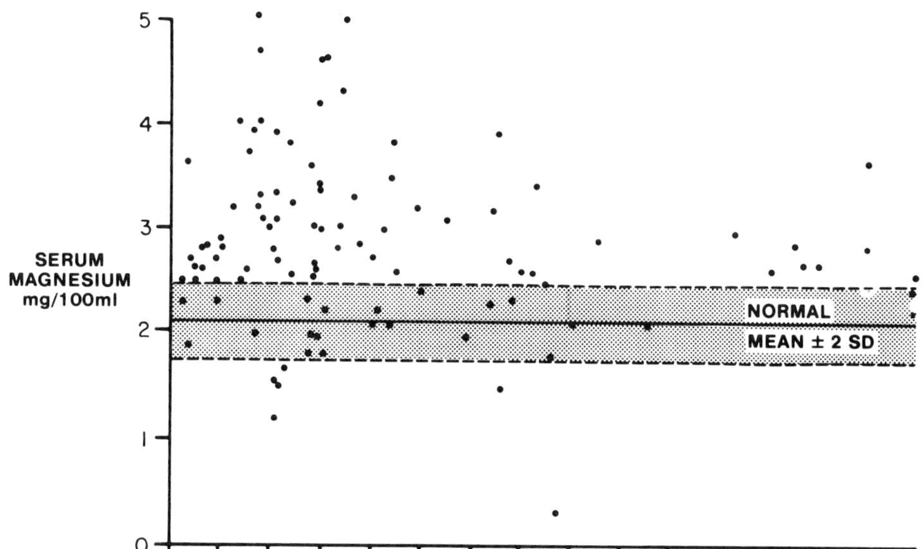

FIGURE 34-2 • Relationship between serum magnesium concentration and creatinine clearance rates in patients with chronic renal disease. Each symbol represents a single patient. (From Coburn JW et al: *Arch Int Med* 124:302, 1969.)

TISSUE CONTENT OF MAGNESIUM IN RENAL FAILURE

Red blood cells (RBCs)

The RBC magnesium content in uremic patients undergoing treatment with hemodialysis is usually higher than that of normal persons.[149] The content of magnesium in RBCs in these patients correlates well with the concentration of magnesium in their serum.[20]

Skin

The magnesium content of the skin in patients undergoing maintenance hemodialysis is affected by the concentration of magnesium in the dialysate. The magnesium content of skin was evaluated in two populations of patients treated with hemodialysis for periods of 2 months to 5 years with dialysate containing magnesium in concentrations of either 1.8 or 0.6 mg/100 ml. Although there was an overlap between the individual values, the skin content of magnesium was significantly higher ($p < .01$) in the group treated with dialysate containing 1.8 mg/100 ml.[107]

Muscle

The magnesium content of muscle in patients with renal failure may be low, normal, or evaluated.[44,100] Thus, Lim and coworkers[98] found that the mean magnesium content in the muscles of nine uremic patients [55.03 ± 7.4 (SE) meq per kg of dry fat-free solids] is significantly lower ($p < .05$) than that of normal subjects (71.80 ± 2.5 meq per kg of dry fat-free solids). The magnesium content in the muscle of patients treated with dialysis was not different from that observed in the nondialyzed patients. On the other hand, Contiguglia and coworkers[44] reported that the magnesium content figures for muscle from normal and uremic patients did not differ—75 ± 8.6 and 80.9 ± 14.3 meq/kg fat-free dry solids, respectively. The reasons for these contrasting findings are not clear.

Bone

The magnesium content of bone is increased in advanced renal failure. Contiguglia and coworkers[44] found that the magnesium content of both cortical and trabecular bone was increased by 66 percent. These observations were confirmed later by Berlyne and coworkers.[19] Alfrey and Miller[7] found that bone contains at least two distinct magnesium pools. One is rapidly exchangeable and constitutes 30 percent of total bone magnesium. The other is a nonexchangeable pool. In patients with advanced renal failure, the excess magnesium in bone is distributed in both pools. The most probable cause for the increase in bone magnesium in patients with chronic renal failure is the hypermagnesemia usually present in these patients.

Intestinal absorption of magnesium in renal failure

The fraction of dietary magnesium absorbed by the GI tract varies from 25 to 60 percent of that ingested. This estimation is based on data from fecal magnesium levels, which range between 40 and 75 percent of the amount ingested,[53,94,144] and on observations indicating that the part of fecal magnesium contributed by endogenous intestinal secretion is very small (12 to 24 mg/day).[14] In human beings, most magnesium absorption occurs in the small intestine,[77] but magnesium can also be absorbed by the large intestine[63] (see Chap. 13).

There are no convincing data to show that an adaptation occurs in renal failure in terms of the dietary intake and absorption of magnesium or of the body's need for the cation. Under normal conditions excess dietary magnesium is readily absorbed, and any surfeit is normally excreted by the kidney.[37,51] Conversely, the kidney efficiently conserves magnesium when dietary intake of this mineral is reduced.[6,16,150] With impaired renal function, the kidney's capacity to excrete a magnesium load is impaired, making it apparent why marked alterations in magnesium homeostasis may occur in advanced renal failure.

Data from human beings suggest that diets rich in calcium reduce intestinal absorption of magnesium. Heaton and coworkers[84] found that an increase in calcium intake from 1500 to 3800 mg/day was associated with a 25 percent increase in fecal magnesium and a 15 percent decrease in urinary magnesium excreted. Clarkson and coworkers[39] found similar effects of high dietary calcium.

The effect of vitamin D on intestinal absorption of magnesium in human beings is not well studied. Heaton and coworkers found that fecal magnesium was reduced in four of six patients treated with either vitamin D_2 or dihydrotachysterol.[84] On the other hand, Brickman and coworkers[28] reported that administration of 1,25-$(OH)_2D_3$, 0.7 to 1.7 μg/day for 10 days, to three normal subjects led to a significant decrease in fecal magnesium in only one case, despite a substantial effect on calcium absorption in all three.

Observations on the effect of PTH on intestinal absorption of magnesium in human beings are also limited. King and Stanbury[94] found that fecal magnesium tends to be lower in patients with primary hyperparathyroidism ingesting a diet with a high magnesium content as compared to that of normal individuals. These data suggest that PTH may enhance intestinal absorption of magnesium in human beings.

Data are not adequate on intestinal absorption of magnesium in patients with renal failure. Clarkson and coworkers[38] studied six patients with creatinine clearances less than 30 ml/min and noted that the fractional absorption of magnesium varied from 0.16 to 0.47. Evaluation of the available data indicates that net magnesium absorption figures, in relation to dietary intake, in normal subjects and uremic patients do not differ. However, Brannan and coworkers[26] showed, in studies using the jejunal perfusion technique, that magnesium absorption is reduced in uremic patients. These data suggest that although intestinal magnesium absorption may be impaired in one segment of the intestine in patients with chronic renal failure, overall magnesium absorption is not reduced. Thus, this ion continues to be readily absorbed by these patients despite the presence of hypermagnesemia.

REFERENCES

1. Abraham AS et al: Magnesium in the prevention of lethal arrhythmias in acute myocardial infarction. *Arch Intern Med* 147:753, 1987.
2. Acoor TAM, Moore EW: Magnesium absorption by everted sacs of rat intestine and colon. *Gastroenterology* 59:745, 1970.
3. Agus ZS et al: Cytosolic magnesium modulates calcium channel activity in mammalian ventricular cells. *Am J Physiol* 256:C452, 1989.
4. Agus ZS, Morad M: Modulation of cardiac ion channels by magnesium, in Hoffman JF, DeWeer P (eds): *Annual Review of Physiology*. Palo Alto, Annual Reviews, Inc, 53:299, 1991.
5. Aikawa JK et al: Magnesium metabolism in rabbits using ^{28}Mg as a tracer. *Am J Physiol* 197:97, 1959.
6. Alcock N, MacIntyre I: Interrelation of calcium and magnesium absorption. *Clin Sci* 22:185, 1962.
7. Alfrey AC, Miller N: Bone magnesium pools in uremia. *J Clin Invest* 52:3019, 1973.
8. Altura BM, Altura BT: Magnesium ion and contraction of vascular smooth muscles: Relationship to some vascular diseases. *Fed Proc* 40:2672, 1981.
9. Alvarez-Leefman FJ et al: Intracellular free magnesium in excitable cells—its measurement and its biologic significance. *Can J Physiol Pharmacol* 65:915, 1987.
10. Anast CS, Gardner WD: Magnesium metabolism, in Bronner F, Coburn JW (eds): *Disorders of Mineral Metabolism*. New York, Academic Press, 1981, vol III, p 423.
11. Anast CS et al: Impaired release of parathyroid hormone in magnesium deficiency. *J Clin Endocrinol Metab* 42:707, 1976.
12. Anderson R et al: Skeletal muscle phosphorus and magnesium deficiency in alcoholic myopathy. *Min Elect Metab* 4:106, 1980.
13. Arnold OF, Ryan MP: The effect of magnesium on potassium transport in isolated rat soleus muscle, in Durlac J (ed): *Proc First Int Symp Magnesium Deficit in Human Pathology*. Vittel, France, Springer-Verlag, 1973, p 63.
14. Avioli LV, Berman J: Mg^{28} kinetics in man. *J Appl Physiol* 21:1688, 1966.
15. Bar RS et al: Hypomagnesemia, hypocalcemia secondary to renal magnesium wasting. *Ann Intern Med* 82:646, 1975.
16. Barnes BA et al: Magnesium conservation in human beings on low magnesium diet. *J Clin Invest* 37:430, 1958.
17. Barton CH et al: Renal magnesium wasting associated with amphotericin B therapy. *Am J Med* 77:471, 1984.
18. Barton CH et al: Hypomagnesemia and renal magnesium wasting in renal transplant recipients receiving cyclosporine. *Am J Med* 83:693, 1987.
19. Berlyne GM et al: Increase in bone magnesium content in renal failure. *Nephron* 9:90, 1972.
20. Bloomfield J et al: Control of the hypermagnesemia of renal failure by maintenance haemodialysis. *Med J Aust* 1:854, 1970.
21. Bogert LT, Acass ED: Placental transmission. I: The calcium and magnesium content of fetal and maternal blood serum. *J Biol Chem* 56:299, 1923.
22. Bonting SL et al: Magnesium-induced conformational changes in Na-K-ATPase. *Curr Top Membr Trans* 19: 403, 1983.
23. Booth BE, Johanson A: Hypomagnesemia due to renal tubular defect in reabsorption of magnesium. *J Pediatr* 85:350, 1975.
24. Booth CC et al: Incidence of hypomagnesemia in intestinal malabsorption. *Br Med J* 2:141, 1963.
25. Booth CC: The metabolic effects of intestinal rejection in man. *Postgrad Med J* 37:725, 1961.
26. Brannan PG et al: Magnesium absorption in the human small intestine. Results in patients with absorptive hypercalciuria. *J Clin Invest* 57:1412, 1976.
27. Brautbar N: Cellular injury in phosphate depletion: Pathogenesis and mechanisms in the myocardium. *Adv Exp Med Biol* 194:451, 1986.
28. Brickman AS et al: Action of 1,25$(OH)_2$ and 1-alpha-(OH)-vitamin D_3 on magnesium metabolism in man. *Clin Res* 23:315, 1975.
29. Brierley GP et al: Studies on ion transport. II: The accumulation of inorganic phosphate and Mg ions by heart mitochondria. *J Biol Chem* 238:3482, 1963.
30. Brunette M et al: Micropuncture study of magnesium reabsorption in the proximal tubule of the dog. *Am J Physiol* 216:1510, 1969.
31. Buckle RM et al: The influence of plasma magnesium concentration on parathyroid hormone secretion. *J Endocrinol* 42:529, 1968.
32. Caddell JL: Studies in protein-calorie malnutrition. I: *N Engl J Med* 276:533, 1967.
33. Cantin M: Relationship of juxtaglomerular apparatus and adrenal cortex to biochemical and extracellular fluid volume changes in magnesium deficiency. *Lab Invest* 22:558, 1970.
34. Carney SL et al: Effects of magnesium deficiency and excess on renal tubular potassium transport in the rat. *Clin Sci* 60:549, 1981.
35. Chase LR, Slatopolsky E: Secretion and metabolic efficiency of parathyroid hormone in patients with severe hypomagnesemia. *J Clin Endocrinol Metab* 28:363, 1974.

36. Chernow B et al: Hypomagnesemia in patients in post-operative intensive care. *Chest* 95:391, 1989.
37. Chesly LC, Teffer I: Some effects of magnesium loading upon renal excretion of magnesium and certain other electrolytes. *J Clin Invest* 37:1362, 1958.
38. Clarkson EM et al: Magnesium metabolism in chronic renal failure. *Clin Sci* 28:107, 1965.
39. Clarkson EM et al: The effect of high intake of calcium on magnesium metabolism in normal subjects and patients with chronic renal failure. *Clin Sci* 32:11, 1967.
40. Coburn JW et al: The physicochemical state and renal handling of divalent ions in chronic renal failure. *Arch Intern Med* 124:302, 1969.
41. Coburn JW, Massry SG: Changes in serum and urinary calcium during phosphate depletion. Studies on mechanisms. *J Clin Invest* 49:1073, 1970.
42. Cohen SM, Burt CT: ^{31}P nuclear magnetic relaxation studies of phosphocreatine in intact muscle: Determination of intracellular free magnesium. *Proc Natl Acad Sci USA* 74:4271, 1977.
43. Connor TB et al: Parathyroid function during chronic magnesium deficiency. *Johns Hopkins Med J* 131:100, 1972.
44. Contiguglia SR et al: Total body magnesium excess in chronic renal failure. *Lancet* i:1300, 1972.
45. Coons CM, Blunt K: The retention of nitrogen, calcium, phosphorus and magnesium by pregnant women. *J Biol Chem* 86:1, 1930.
46. Cotlove E et al: Effects of electrolyte depletion and acid-base disturbances on muscle cations. *Am J Physiol* 167:6665, 1951.
47. Cronin RE et al: Skeletal muscle injury after magnesium depletion in the dog. *Am J Physiol* 243:F113, 1982.
48. Davis BB et al: Hypomagnesemia following the diuresis of post-renal obstruction and renal transplant. *Nephron* 14:275, 1975.
49. Desai TK et al: Prevalence and clinical implications of hypocalcemia in acutely ill patients in a medical intensive care setting. *Am J Med* 84:209, 1988.
50. Di Polo R, Beauge L: An ATP-dependent Na^+/Mg^{2+} countertransport is the only mechanism for Mg extrusion in squid axons. *Biochim Biophys Acta* 946:424, 1988.
51. Dirks JH: The kidney and magnesium regulation. *Kidney Int* 23:771, 1983.
52. Dorup J et al: Reduced concentration of potassium, magnesium, and sodium-potassium pumps in human skeletal muscle during treatment with diuretics. *Br Med J* 296: 455, 1988.
53. Dunn MJ, Walser M: Magnesium depletion in normal man. *Metabolism* 15:884, 1966.
54. Dyckner T: Serum magnesium in acute myocardial infarction. Relation to arrhythmias. *Acta Med Scand* 207:59, 1980.
55. Dyckner T, Wester PO: The relation between extra and intracellular electrolytes in patients with hypokalemia and/or diuretic treatment. *Acta Med Scand* 204:269, 1978.
56. Dyckner T, Wester PO: Ventricular extrasystoles and intracellular electrolytes before and after potassium and magnesium infusion in patients on diuretic treatment. *Am Heart J* 97:12, 1979.
57. Dyckner T, Wester PO: Magnesium deficiency: Guidelines for diagnosis and substitution therapy. *Acta Med Scand* 66:37, 1981.
58. Dyckner T, Wester PO: Intracellular magnesium loss after diuretic administration. *Drugs* 28:161, 1984.
59. Elin RL et al: Adrenal gland factors in magnesium-deficient rats. *Proc Soc Exp Biol Med* 134:542, 1970.
60. Ellory JC et al: Inhibition of red cell sodium and potassium transport by divalent cations. *J Physiol* 340:1, 1983.
61. Estep H et al: Hypocalcemia due to hypomagnesemia and reversible parathyroid hormone unresponsiveness. *J Clin Endocrinol Metab* 29:842, 1969.
62. Evans RA et al: The congenital "magnesium-losing kidney." *Q J Med* 1:39, 1981.
63. Fawcett DW, Gens JP: Magnesium poisoning following enema of epsom salt solution. *JAMA* 123:1028, 1943.
64. Flatman PW, Lew VL: The magnesium dependence of sodium:potassium and sodium:sodium exchange mediated by the sodium pump in intact human red cells. *J Physiol* 287:33, 1979.
65. Flink EB: Nutritional aspects of magnesium metabolism. *West J Med* 133:304, 1980.
66. Flink EB et al: Alternations of long chain free fatty acid and magnesium concentration in acute myocardial infarction. *Arch Intern Med* 141:441, 1981.
67. Fourman P, Morgan DB: Chronic magnesium deficiency. *Proc Nutr Soc* 21:34, 1962.
68. Forbes GB: Sodium, in Comar CL, Bronner F (eds): *Mineral Metabolism.* New York, Academic Press, 1962, p 1.
69. Foster GV: Magnesium metabolism, in Dyke SC et al: *Recent Advances in Clinical Pathology,* 2d ed. New York, Churchill Livingstone, 1969, p 131.
70. Frankenhauser B, Meves H: Effect of magnesium and calcium on frog myelinated nerve fiber. *J Physiol* 142:360, 1958.
71. Freeman RM, Deftos LJ: Parathyroid hormone response to magnesium infusion in man, in Frame B, Parfitt A, Duncan H (eds): *Clinical Aspects of Metabolic Bone Disease.* Amsterdam, Excerpta Medica, 1973, p 582.
72. Freeman RM, Pearson E: Hypomagnesemia of unknown etiology. *Am J Med* 41:645, 1966.
73. Freitag JJ et al: Skeletal resistance to parathyroid hormone in magnesium deficiency. Studies in isolated perfused bone. *J Clin Invest* 64:1238, 1979.
74. Frenkel EJ et al: ATP requirement of the sodium-dependent magnesium extrusion from human red blood cells. *J Physiol* 414:385, 1989.
75. Gitelman HJ et al: A new familial disorder characterized by hypokalemia and hypomagnesemia. *Trans Assoc Am Physicians* 79:221, 1966.
76. Gitelman HJ et al: Inhibition of parathyroid gland activity by hypermagnesemia. *Am J Physiol* 215:483, 1968.
77. Graham LA et al: Gastrointestinal absorption and excretion of ^{28}Mg in man. *Metabolism* 9:646, 1960.
78. Gutman FD et al: The correlation of fractional excretion of sodium and magnesium in the chronically diseased kidney of dog and man. *J Lab Clin Med* 74:642, 1969.
79. Haijama H, MacDowall IG: Distribution of divalent cations at the cellular level during primary hypomagnesemia in infancy. *Acta Paediatr Scand* 61:591, 1972.

80. Hallberg DAG: Magnesium problems in gastroenterology. *Acta Med Scand* 661:62, 1981.
81. Hanna S: Plasma magnesium in health and disease. *J Clin Pathol* 14:410, 1961.
82. Hasselbach W et al: Magnesium dependence of sarcoplasmic reticulum calcium transport. *Fed Proc* 40:2657, 1981.
83. Hazard R, Wurmser L: Action des sels de magnésium sur les vasoconstricteurs rénaux. *C R Soc Biol* 110:525, 1932.
84. Heaton FW et al: Observations in the relationship between calcium and magnesium metabolism in man. *Clin Sci* 27:31, 1964.
85. Hellhan ES et al: Abnormal electrolyte and water metabolism in acute intermittent porphyria. Transient inappropriate secretion of antidiuretic hormone. *Am J Med* 32:734, 1962.
86. Hollenberg NK, Hollifield JW (eds): Symposium on potassium/magnesium depletion: Is your patient at risk of sudden death? *Am J Med* 82 (Suppl 3A), 1987.
87. Hollifield JW: Magnesium depletion, diuretics and arrhythmias. *Am J Med* 82:30, 1987.
88. Iseri LT: Magnesium and cardiac arrhythmias. *Magnesium* 5:111, 1986.
89. Iseri LT, Bures AR: Serious ventricular arrhythmias due to magnesium deficiency, in Cantin M, Seelig MS (eds): *Magnesium in Health and Disease.* New York, Spectrum, 1980, p 559.
90. Jackson CE, Meier DW: Routine serum magnesium analysis: Correlation with clinical state in 5100 patients. *Ann Intern Med* 69:743, 1968.
91. Kafka H et al: Serum magnesium and potassium in acute myocardial infarction. *Arch Intern Med* 147:465, 1987.
92. Kalbfleisch JM et al: Effect of ethanol administration on urinary excretion of magnesium and other electrolytes in alcoholic and normal subjects. *J Clin Invest* 42:1471, 1965.
93. Kelepouris E: Cytosolic Mg^{2+} modulates whole cell K^+ and Cl^- currents in cortical thick ascending limb cells of rabbit kidney. *Abstracts Am Soc Nephrol* 22:376A, 1989.
94. King RG, Stanbury SW: Magnesium metabolism in primary hyperparathyroidism. *Clin Sci* 39:218, 1970.
95. Kroenke K et al: The value of serum magnesium determination in hypertensive patients receiving diuretics. *Arch Intern Med* 147:1553, 1987.
96. Kurnick BRC et al: Hypomagnesemia-induced cardiomyopathy. *Magnesium* 7:49, 1988.
97. Leary WR, Reyes AT: The magnesium effects of a single dose of hydrochlorothiazide in healthy adults. *Curr Therapy Res* 32:425, 1982.
98. Lim P et al: Intracellular magnesium depletion in chronic renal failure. *N Engl J Med* 280:981, 1965.
99. Lim P, Jacob E: Magnesium status of alcoholic patients. *Metabolism* 21:1045, 1972.
100. Lim P, Jacob E: Tissue magnesium levels in chronic diarrhea. *J Lab Clin Med* 80:313, 1977.
101. Lyman NW et al: Cisplatin-induced hypocalcemia and hypomagnesemia. *Arch Intern Med* 140:1513, 1980.
102. Manthey J et al: Magnesium and trace methods: Risk factors for coronary heart disease? *Circulation* 64:722, 1981.
103. Martindale L, Heaton FW: Magnesium deficiency in the adult rat. *Biochem J* 92:119, 1964.
104. Massry SG et al: Effect of NaCl infusion on urinary $Ca^{++}$and Mg^{++} during reduction in their filtered loads. *Am J Physiol* 213:1218, 1967.
105. Massry SG et al: Effects of long term desoxycorticosterone acetate administration on renal excretion of calcium and magnesium. *J Lab Clin Med* 71:212, 1968.
106. Massry SG et al: Evidence for suppression of parathyroid glands by hypermagnesemia. *J Clin Invest* 49:1619, 1970.
107. Massry SG et al: Mineral content of human skin in uremia: Effect of secondary hyperparathyroidism and haemodialysis. *Proc Eur Dial Transplant Assoc* 7:146, 1970.
108. Massry SG et al: Divalent ion metabolism in patients with acute renal failure: Studies on the mechanism of hypocalcemia. *Kidney Int* 5:437, 1974.
109. McCance RZ et al: Effect of protein intake on absorption of calcium and magnesium. *Biochem J* 36:686, 1942.
110. McCarron DA: Divalent cations, anions and blood pressure. *Ann Intern Med* 98:800, 1983.
111. McCollister RJ et al: Urinary magnesium excretion in man following ingestion of ethanol. *Am J Clin Nutr* 12:415, 1963.
112. Milla PJ et al: Studies in primary hypomagnesemia: Evidence for defective carrier mediated small intestinal transport of magnesium. *Gut* 20:1028, 1979.
113. Muldowney FP et al: Parathormone-like effects of magnesium replenishment in steatorrhea. *N Engl J Med* 282:61, 1970.
114. Food and Nutrition Board: *Recommended Dietary Allowances,* 9th ed, Washington, D.C.: National Academy of Science, 1979. Cited in Munro HN: Nutritional requirements for health: Their relevance to tissue function in renal failure. *Am J Clin Nutr* 33:1555, 1980.
115. Murphy E et al: Monitoring cytosolic free magnesium in cultured chicken heart cells by use of the fluorescent indicator Furaptra. *Proc Natl Acad Sci USA* 86:2981, 1989.
116. Murphy E et al: Cytosolic free magnesium levels in ischemic rat heart. *J Biol Chem* 264:5622, 1989.
117. Nielsen B: Correlation between antidiuretic hormone effect and renal excretion of magnesium and calcium in man. *Acta Endocrinol* 45:151, 1964.
118. Ogden DA, Holmes JH: Changes in total and ultrafiltrable plasma calcium and magnesium during hemodialysis. *Trans Am Soc Artif Intern Organs* 12:200, 1966.
119. Parfitt AM, Kleerekoper M: Clinical disorders of calcium, phosphorus and magnesium metabolism, in Maxwell MH, Kleeman CR (eds): *Clinical Disorders of Fluid and Electrolyte Metabolism,* 3d ed. New York, McGraw-Hill, 1979, p 947.
120. Paunier L, Sizomenko PC: Asymptomatic chronic hypomagnesemia and hypokalemia in a child. A cell membrane disease? *J Pediatr* 88:51, 1976.
121. Pletka P et al: Effect of magnesium on parathyroid hormone secretion during chronic hemodialysis. *Lancet* 2:462, 1971.
122. Polimeni P, Page E: Magnesium in heart muscle. *Circ Res* 33:367, 1973.
123. Popovtzer MM et al: Interrelationship between sodium,

calcium and magnesium excretion in advanced renal failure. *J Lab Clin Med* 73:763, 1969.
124. Popovtzer MM et al: Divalent ion excretion in chronic kidney disease: Relation to degree of renal insufficiency. *Clin Sci* 38:297, 1970.
125. Potter JD et al: Magnesium and the regulation of muscle contraction. *Fed Proc* 40:2653, 1981.
126. Potts JT, Roberts B: Clinical significance of magnesium deficiency and its relation to parathyroid disease. *Am J Med Sci* 235:205, 1958.
127. Quamme GA, Dirks JH: Magnesium transport in the nephron. *Am J Physiol* 8:393, 1980.
128. Raju B et al: A fluorescent indicator for measuring cytosolic free magnesium. *Am J Physiol* 256:C540, 1989.
129. Randall RE et al: Hypermagnesemia in renal failure. Etiology and toxic manifestations. *Ann Intern Med* 61:73, 1964.
130. Rasmussen AS et al: Intravenous magnesium in acute myocardial infarction. *Lancet* i:234, 1986.
131. Rasmussen HS et al: Magnesium infusion reduces the incidence of arrhythmias in acute myocardial infarction: A double blind study. *Clin Cardiol* 10:351, 1987.
132. Ratzan RM et al: Uncovering magnesium toxicity. *Geriatrics* 12:75, 1980.
133. Resnick LM et al: Divalent ions in essential hypertension. *N Engl J Med* 309:888, 1983.
134. Roden DM: Magnesium treatment of ventricular arrhythmias. *Am J Cardiol* 63:43G, 1989.
135. Rude RK et al: Functional hypoparathyroidism and parathyroid hormone and organ resistance in human magnesium deficiency. *Clin Endocrinol* 5:209, 1976.
136. Runeberg et al: Hypomagnesemia due to renal disease of unknown etiology. *Am J Med* 59:873, 1975.
137. Ryan MP et al: Effect of magnesium deficiency on cardiac and skeletal muscle potassium during dietary potassium restriction. *Proc Soc Exp Biol Med* 143:1045, 1973.
138. Ryan MP et al: Effects of magnesium and potassium deficiencies on composition and growth of ascites tumor cells in vivo. *Life Sci* 8:485, 1969.
139. Ryan MP et al: Effects of diuretics on the renal handling of magnesium. *Drugs* 28:167, 1984.
140. Ryan MP et al: The effect of diuretics on lymphocyte magnesium and potassium. *Acta Med Scand* 647:153, 1981.
141. Ryan MP, Hingerty D: Effects of magnesium deficiency on restoration of potassium and sodium levels in potassium-depleted muscle. *Ir J Med Sci* 2:137, 1969.
142. Ryan MF, Ryan MP: Lymphocyte electrolyte alterations during magnesium deficiency in the rat. *Ir J Med Sci* 148:108, 1979.
143. Ryzen E: Magnesium homeostasis in critically ill patients. *Magnesium* 8:201, 1989.
144. Seelig MS: Requirement of magnesium by normal adults: Summary and analysis of published data. *Am J Clin Nutr* 14:242, 1964.
145. Seelig MS: Magnesium deficiency and cardiac dysrhythmia, in Seelig MS (ed): *Magnesium Deficiency in Pathogenesis of Disease*. New York, Plenum, 1980, p 219.
146. Seelig MS, Heggtvest HA: Magnesium interrelationship in ischemic heart disease: A review. *Am J Clin Nutr* 27:59, 1974.
147. Seta K et al: Myocardium and plasma electrolytes in dietary magnesium and potassium deficiency in the rat. *J Nutr* 87:179, 1965.
148. Schilsky RL, Anderson T: Hypomagnesemia and renal magnesium wasting in patients receiving cisplatin. *Ann Intern Med* 90:929, 1979.
149. Schmidt P et al: Magnesium metabolism in patients on regular dialysis treatment. *Clin Sci* 41:131, 1971.
150. Shils ME: Experimental human magnesium depletion. *Medicine* 118:61, 1969.
151. Shine KI, Douglas AM: Magnesium effects on ionic exchange and mechanical function in rat ventricle. *Am J Physiol* 227:317, 1974.
152. Shine KI, Douglas AM: Magnesium effect on rabbit ventricle. *Am J Physiol* 228:1545, 1975.
153. Smith LF et al: Intravenous infusion of magnesium sulfate after acute myocardial infarction. Effects on arrhythmias and mortality. *Int J Cardiol* 12:175, 1986.
154. Smith WO, Hammarstein JF: Serum magnesium in renal diseases. *Arch Intern Med* 102:5, 1958.
155. Sutherland LE et al: Bartter's syndrome. Report of four cases, including three in one sibship, with comparative histologic evaluation of the juxtaglomerular aparatuses and glomeruli. *Acta Paediatr Scand* 201 (suppl):1, 1970.
156. Stendig-Lindberg et al: Hypomagnesemia, muscle electrolytes and metabolites. *Acta Med Scand* 201:273, 1977.
157. Steele TH et al: The contribution of chronically diseased kidney to magnesium homeostasis in man. *J Lab Clin Med* 71:455, 1968.
158. Stephenson E: Magnesium effect on activation of skinned fibers from striated muscle. *Fed Proc* 40:2662, 1981.
159. Stewart WK, Fleming LW: Relationship between plasma and erythrocyte magnesium and potassium concentrations in fasting obese subjects. *Metabolism* 22:535, 1973.
160. Sullivan JF et al: Serum magnesium in chronic alcoholism. *Lancet* ii:802, 1962.
161. Tansy MF et al: Alterations in gastrointestinal function in the magnesium-deficient rat, in Cantin M, Seelig H (eds): *Magnesium in Health and Disease*. New York, Spectrum, 1980, p 137.
162. Thoren L: Magnesium metabolism. *Prog Surg* 9:131, 1971.
163. Turlapaty PDMV et al: Ca uptake and distribution in alloxan diabetic rat arterial and venous smooth muscle. *Experientia* 36:1298, 1980.
164. Turlapaty PDMV et al: Interactions of magnesium and verapamil on tone and contractility of vascular smooth muscle. *Eur J Pharmacol* 76:268, 1981.
165. Turlapaty PDMV, Altura BM: Magnesium deficiency produces spasms of coronary arteries: Relationship to etiology of sudden death ischemic heart disease. *Science* 208:198, 1980.
166. Turlapaty PDMV, Altura BM: Magnesium ions and contractions of alloxan diabetic vascular muscle artery. *Artery* 6:375, 1980.
167. Tzivoni D et al: Magnesium therapy for Torsades de Pointes. *Am J Cardiol* 53:528, 1984.
168. Vallee B et al: The magnesium deficiency tetany syndrome in man. *N Engl J Med* 262:155, 1960.
169. Wallach S et al: Magnesium transport in normal and uremic patients . *J Clin Endocrinol Metab* 26:1069, 1966.

170. Walser M: Invited discussion. *Arch Intern Med* 124:292, 1969.
171. Whang R et al: The need for routine serum magnesium determination. *Clin Res* 12:154A, 1977.
172. Whang R et al: Predictors of clinical hypomagnesemia—hypokalemia, hypophosphatemia, hyponatremia and hypocalcemia. *Arch Intern Med* 144:1794, 1984.
173. White RE, Hartzell HC: Magnesium ions in cardiac function. Regulator of ion channels and second messengers. *Biochem Pharmacol* 38:859, 1989.
174. Widman L et al: Effects of moduretic and aldactone on electrolytes in skeletal muscle in patients on long term diuretic therapy. *Acta Med Scand* 661:35, 1981.
175. Wong ET et al: A high prevalence of hypomagnesemia and hypermagnesemia in hospitalized patients. *Am J Clin Pathol* 79:348, 1983.
176. Woodward DL, Reed DJ: Effects of magnesium deficiency on electrolyte distribution in the rabbit. *Am J Physiol* 217:1477, 1969.
177. Zawada ET, Brautbar N: The possible role of magnesium in hypercalcemic hypertension. *Magnesium* 3:132, 1984.

SECTION II-2

MEDICAL AND SURGICAL CONDITIONS ASSOCIATED WITH FLUID AND ELECTROLYTE DISORDERS

CHAPTER • 35

Fluid and electrolyte metabolism during pregnancy

Mark S. Paller • Thomas F. Ferris

HEMODYNAMIC CHANGES DURING PREGNANCY

Pregnancy provides a unique opportunity to witness extraordinary alterations in cardiovascular physiology for a relatively prolonged period. Cardiac output increases in the first trimester and reaches a maximum of 30 to 40 percent above the nonpregnant level by the twenty-fourth week of gestation.[89,143] The increase in cardiac output early in pregnancy is due to an increase in stroke volume; as pregnancy advances, heart rate increases and stroke volume falls to nonpregnant levels. The cause of the increase in cardiac output may be the decrease in peripheral vascular resistance that occurs early in pregnancy. The fall in vascular resistance is not due to an increased metabolic demand of the mother or fetus, since the arteriovenous oxygen difference declines early in pregnancy.[104] Nor can it be explained by the increase in uterine blood flow acting as an arteriovenous fistula, since vascular resistance is lowest early in pregnancy, when minimal change in uterine blood has occurred, and when uterine blood flow is at its maximum, late in the third trimester, peripheral vascular resistance increases.[7] Peripheral vasodilation is often clinically evident in the palmar erythema and spider telangiectasis that develop during pregnancy.

Both plasma and red blood cell volume increase early in pregnancy;[19,74,112] the greater increase in plasma than in red blood cell volume results in the physiologic anemia of pregnancy, with hematocrits ranging from 33 to 38 percent and hemoglobin concentration from 11 to 12 g/100 ml during pregnancy. Plasma volume increases approximately 48 percent in women with single pregnancies and 67 percent in women with twin pregnancies and increases more in multiparous than in primiparous women.[121] The hormonal factors that cause these striking changes in extracellular volume and vascular capacity during pregnancy have been extensively studied but have not been elucidated.

RENAL BLOOD FLOW

A striking increase in renal blood flow occurs early in pregnancy (Fig. 35-1).[2] In one woman studied before and after conception, renal plasma flow increased 45 percent by the ninth week of pregnancy.[130] A review of the four published studies of the serial changes in renal plasma flow, utilizing para-aminohippuric acid (PAH) clearance, throughout pregnancy reveals a mean renal plasma flow of 809 ml/min in the first trimester, 695 ml/min the last 10 weeks of pregnancy, and 482 ml/min following delivery.[6,33,36,130] Although it has been suggested that reduction in renal blood flow in late pregnancy was due to measurements being obtained with the patient in the supine position, which might cause a spurious reduction in renal plasma flow because of compression of the inferior vena cava by the uterus, two studies have been unable to demonstrate such positional effects.[35,130] Thus, it seems that a reduction in renal plasma flow in late pregnancy does occur.

The cause of the rise in renal blood flow during pregnancy is not clear. Although an increase in cardiac output of approximately 40 percent occurs as early as the

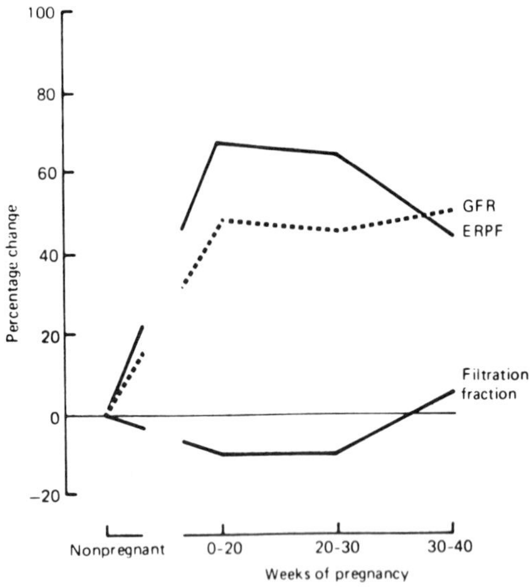

FIGURE 35-1 • Effect of pregnancy on renal blood flow (ERPF, effective renal plasma flow), glomerular filtration rate (GFR), and filtration fraction. (From Davison JM, Dunlop W: *Kidney Int* 18:152, 1980. Used by permission.)

first trimester, blood flow to all regional beds does not increase uniformly; no increase in cerebral or hepatic blood flow has been detected in pregnancy. A decrease in renal vascular resistance accounts in large measure for the increase in renal blood flow. Filtration fraction, the percentage of renal plasma flow filtered by the glomeruli, also decreases in early pregnancy, reflecting a fall in postglomerular efferent arteriolar resistance. One can calculate the change in renal vascular resistance occurring with pregnancy from the published data on renal plasma flow during and after pregnancy. Assuming a blood pressure of 120/80 (mean arterial pressure, or MAP, 93 mmHg) and a hematocrit of 40, renal blood flow (renal plasma flow 482 × 1.4) is 675 ml/min after pregnancy, and renal resistance (MAP/renal blood flow) is 0.138 mmHg/ml. Assuming a blood pressure of 100/70 (MAP, 80 mmHg) during pregnancy and a hematocrit of 30, renal blood flow (809 × 1.3) is 1052 ml/min in the first trimester, and renal resistance is 0.076 mmHg/ml, approximately half that in nonpregnant women. The cause of the decrease in renal vascular resistance is unclear, but observations indicating that urinary excretion of prostaglandin E_2 (PGE_2) and 6-keto $PGF_{1\alpha}$, the major metabolite of prostacyclin (PGI_2) are elevated in pregnancy might be of significance.[11,91] Infusions of PGE_2 and PGI_2 into the renal circulation decrease renal vascular resistance and increase renal blood flow, whereas drugs inhibiting prostaglandin synthesis, such as indomethacin or aspirin, reduce renal blood flow in certain experimental and clinical circumstances. Whether an increase in renal prostaglandin synthesis during pregnancy is the cause of the decreased renal vascular resistance is, however, speculative at this time.

Human growth hormone is known to cause a modest increase in renal blood flow.[24] Although growth hormone levels are normal during pregnancy, human placental lactogen, which is immunologically and chemically similar to human growth hormone, increases as early as the sixth week of gestation.[132] Whether placental lactogen has an effect similar to that of growth hormone is not known. Placental lactogen also increases with a hydatidiform mole and choriocarcinoma, but no increase in renal blood flow has been documented in these clinical circumstances. Therefore, placental lactogen does not appear to be a major factor in the increase in renal blood flow that occurs during normal pregnancy.

GLOMERULAR FILTRATION RATE

Smith stated, "A pregnant woman is a very interesting phenomenon. I do not know of any other way to increase glomerular filtration rate [GFR] by 50 percent or better for prolonged periods.[131] The increase in glomerular filtration, like the increase in renal blood flow, occurs early in pregnancy.[6,28,33,130] In a study of eight women, creatinine clearance was found to be significantly increased within 4 weeks of the last menstrual period.[28] As shown by inulin clearance, the mean GFR in four published studies rose from 96 ml/min in nonpregnant women to 143 ml/min in the first trimester of pregnancy and remained at that level throughout the remainder of the pregnancy.[28a] The increase in GFR in pregnancy is reflected by the low blood urea nitrogen (8.7 ± 1.5 mg/100 ml) and serum creatinine (0.46 ± 0.13 mg/100 ml) in pregnant women compared with nonpregnant values of 13 ± 3 mg/100 ml and 0.67 ± 0.14 mg/100 ml, respectively.[130]

The increase in GFR in pregnancy is probably due to the increase in glomerular plasma flow that occurs. In micropuncture studies of pregnant rats, one group found that the rise in superficial single-nephron GFR was due to both an increase in glomerular plasma flow and an increase in effective filtration pressure, caused by a higher glomerular hydrostatic capillary pressure in the pregnant animals.[27] In contrast, in another study no rise in glomerular capillary pressure was found, although single-nephron GFR increased because of a rise in glomerular plasma flow.[12] In both studies, renal resistance at the afferent and efferent arteriole was reduced. It is interesting to find that the increase in GFR can be induced in rats for up to 9 days by pseudopregnancy.[13] Pseudopregnancy is induced by mating with a sterile male and occurs without the development of a fetus or placenta. Therefore, the increase in GFR seen in pseudopregnancy is the result of maternal rather than placental factors. It is also interesting to note that plasma volume increases in pseudopregnant rats (Fig. 35-2). In pregnant women, GFR, estimated from creatinine clearance, varies directly with dietary protein.[129] This effect is most likely caused by dietary protein-induced increases in renal plasma flow.[117]

The increase in GFR occurs despite a fall in filtration fraction, which has been found to average 0.20 in nonpregnant women, 0.18 in the first 30 weeks of pregnancy, and 0.22 in the last 10 weeks of pregnancy.[28a] In late pregnancy, the rise in filtration fraction that occurs may have multiple causes, including efferent arteriolar constriction as well as a fall in plasma oncotic pressure. Serum protein concentration falls approximately 1 g/100 ml in late pregnancy, which diminishes plasma oncotic pressure by approximately 7 mmHg.[118] This change in oncotic pressure would increase filtration fraction by increasing the proportion of glomerular plasma flow that is filtered.

SODIUM METABOLISM DURING PREGNANCY

GENERAL CONCEPTS

Mean weight gain in pregnant women on an unrestricted diet is 12.5 kg,[139] with a cumulative sodium retention of between 500 and 900 meq,[74,96,100] which occurs gradually at the rate of 20 to 30 meq/week.[67] It has been estimated that 300 to 400 meq of this retained sodium is stored in maternal extracellular space, while the rest is stored in the fetus, placenta, and amniotic fluid.[74]

Retention of sodium during pregnancy requires a resetting of those factors controlling extracellular volume. Extracellular volume is determined by both afferent signals coming to the kidney from various volume receptors in the vascular system and efferent factors within the

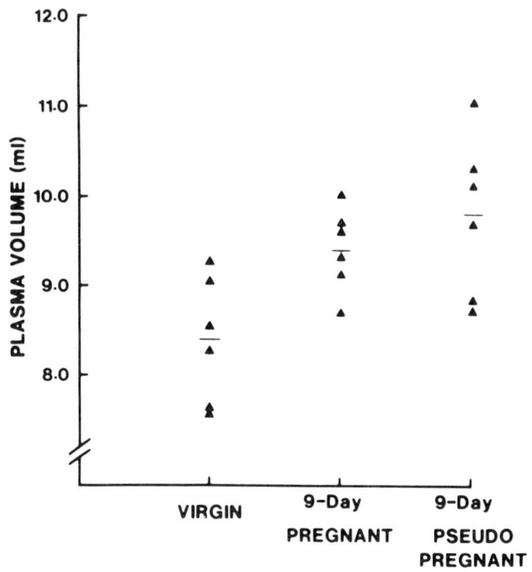

FIGURE 35-2 • Plasma volume measurements in virgin, pregnant, and pseudopregnant rats. (From Baylis C, *Am J Physiol* 234:F300, 1982. Used by permission.)

kidney that modulate sodium excretion. Since peripheral vascular resistance falls early in pregnancy, low vascular resistance[74,101] and low blood pressure cause an increase in vascular capacity, which results in underfilling of the circulation. Thus, the "effective" blood volume, the measure of how well the arterial blood volume fills the capacity of the arterial circulation, falls, and renal sodium excretion is diminished. Underfilling of the circulation results in stimulation of baroreceptors in the cartoid sinus and aortic arch, which increases sympathetic nerve activity to the kidney, increase levels of circulating catecholamines and probably other vasoactive substances, and activate the renin-angiotensin system, all of which decrease renal sodium excretion.[126]

During pregnancy, plasma levels of PGI_2 and PGE_2 are elevated,[11,91,152] and a striking resistance to the pressor effects of angiotensin II develops.[1,14,21,58] Whether the increased synthesis of vasodilating prostaglandins is also the cause of the increased capacitance of the circulation in pregnancy is not clear. The elevated plasma renin activity (PRA), angiotensin II, and plasma aldosterone in pregnancy support the concept of vascular underfilling. When pregnant baboons were studied serially with Swan-Ganz catheters from the onset of pregnancy, decreases in right atrial, systemic, and pulmonary arterial pressure and systemic and pulmonary vascular resistance were found by the fourth week of gestation.[111] PRA and aldosterone concentration were elevated at that time, and stroke volume was increased, but plasma volume was not observed to be expanded until 8 weeks later. Cardiac filling pressure was never increased during middle or late pregnancy. Therefore, these serial studies in pregnant primates suggest that, as a consequence of peripheral vasodilatation, there is vascular underfilling, with a stimulation of the renin-angiotensin system and subsequent plasma volume expansion.

In late pregnancy, decreased venous return to the heart as a result of uterine compression of the inferior vena cava,[82,102] and hypoalbuminemia[118] would also contribute to the decreased filling of the thoracic vascular compartment. During pregnancy, standing and lying supine result in a greater decrease in sodium excretion than in nonpregnant women,[94,116] but these postural factors are probably more important in altering the circadian rhythm of sodium excretion[80] than in overall sodium balance and may be responsible for the nocturia that occurs with pregnancy.

However, the increase in cardiac output, renal blood flow, and GFR during pregnancy argue against underfilling of the circulation. Central blood volume increases during pregnancy,[122] and PRA and plasma aldosterone are responsive to changes in sodium intake.[11] Studies of arginine vasopressin (AVP) release in the rat also indicate that nonosmotic AVP secretion in response to blood volume depletion is similar in pregnant and nonpregnant animals.[10] Atrial naturetic peptide (ANP) levels in the plasma are also believed to be indicators of plasma volume. In volume-expanded states, ANP levels are increased, whereas in volume-depleted states, ANP levels are low. Most studies of normal pregnant women have found either normal or increased plasma ANP levels.[52,105,109,135,138] In pregnant rats, the renal naturetic response to ANP was not altered.[83] These responses of ANP argue against underfilling of the circulation in pregnancy. Thus, there are features of pregnancy that are not consistent with vascular underfilling, suggesting a renal cause of the sodium retention.

An increase in GFR per se would tend to enhance excretion of sodium by increasing its filtered load. Both fractional and absolute sodium reabsorption increase dramatically in pregnancy to maintain sodium balance and prevent the natriuresis that would otherwise occur. The magnitude of this increase in tubular reabsorption can be assessed by calculating the increase in sodium reabsorption neessitated by a 50 percent increase in GFR. Assuming a sodium concentration of 140 meq/liter in glomerular filtrate and a GFR of 100 ml/min, the daily filtered sodium is approximately 20,160 meq. An increase in GFR to 150 ml/min would increase daily sodium filtration to 30,240 meq; in other words, the renal tubules must reabsorb 10,080 meq more sodium than in the nonpregnant state if sodium wasting is not to occur.

When placed on a 10-meq sodium intake, pregnant women reduce urinary sodium excretion as readily as nonpregnant women without excess weight loss. (Fig. 35-3).[11] After 7 days both pregnant and nonpregnant women were in sodium balance and had lost 1.5 kg, with

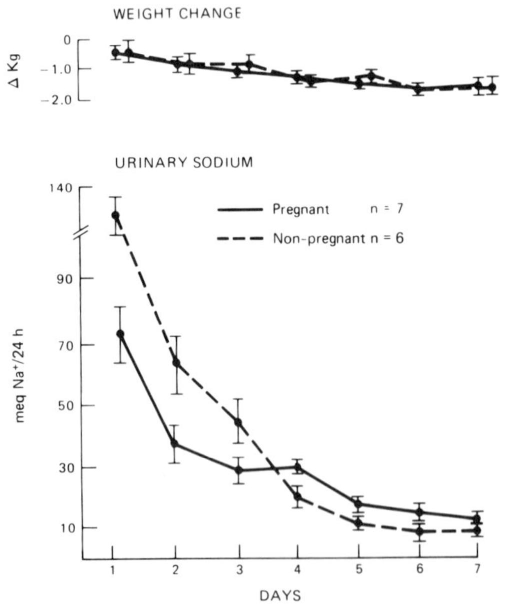

FIGURE 35-3 • Weight changes and urinary sodium excretion in pregnant and nonpregnant women on a 10-meq sodium diet. (From Bay WH, Ferris TF: *Hypertension* 1:410, 1979. Used by permission.)

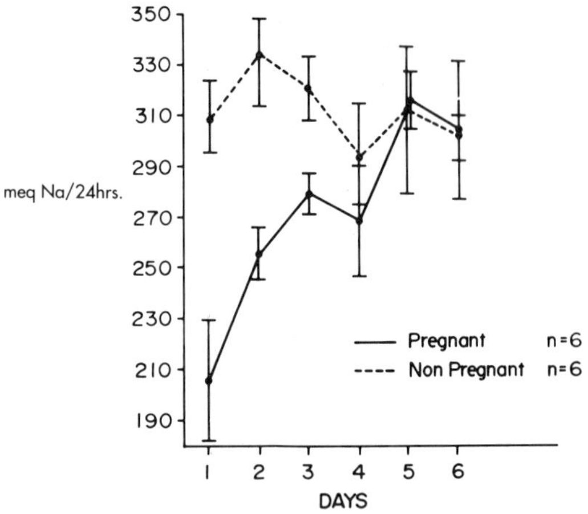

FIGURE 35-4 • Urinary sodium excretion in pregnant and nonpregnant women on a 300-meq sodium diet. (From Bay WH, Ferris TF: *Hypertension* 1:410, 1979. Used by permission.)

net sodium loss similar in both groups. When placed on a 300-meq sodium intake, pregnant women came into balance after 4 days, although more sodium was retained than in nonpregnant women (Fig. 35-4). Excretion of an acute intravenous sodium load has been found to be as rapid in pregnant as in nonpregnant women.[20,94] These studies demonstrate that during pregnancy the ability to conserve or excrete sodium when intake is dramatically altered is not changed in spite of the 50 percent increase in filtered sodium that occurs. Pregnancy is a dramatic example of the importance of glomerular tubular balance in maintenance of sodium balance. Since postglomerular Starling forces are important modifiers of proximal tubular sodium handling, one would expect the fall in filtration fraction with pregnancy to decrease proximal tubular sodium reabsorption by decreasing postglomerular plasma protein concentration and oncotic pressure.[17] That this does not happen indicates that in pregnancy, as in so many other clinical circumstances, as yet undefined factors must be influencing renal sodium metabolism.

Micropuncture studies of pregnant rats demonstrate no difference in proximal fractional sodium reabsorption.[45] Because sodium transport in the kidney is mediated in part by Na^+-K^+ ATPase, located on the basal and lateral membranes of renal tubular cells, it is of note that in the pregnant rat renal cortical Na^+-K^+ ATPase activity increases in late pregnancy.[93]

Recently, the interesting observation was made that red blood cells from pregnant women have an increased rate of sodium-lithium countertransport.[97,153] The importance of this observation is not immediately apparent, since Na^+-Li^+ countertransport is equivalent to Na^+-Na^+ exchange, which would not alter intracellular Na^+ concentration.[4] However, it has been suggested that the increase in Na^+-Li^+ countertransport during pregnancy might be a marker for increased proximal tubule

Na^+-H^+ exchange and therefore increased proximal tubule Na^+ reabsorption beyond the site available for micropuncture.[47] The finding of an increase in proximal tubular length during pregnancy in the rat is also compatible with this hypothesis.[59]

HORMONAL EFFECTS

Renin-aldosterone

A striking increase in renin secretion occurs during the first trimester of pregnancy.[148,150] The increase in renin secretion is unusual in that high secretory rates persist throughout pregnancy despite expansion of the extracellular fluid volume; increased renal blood flow; increased GFR; and, because of the increased glomerular filtration, presumably increased delivery of sodium to the macula densa. Various suggestions have been made to explain the rise in renin secretion during pregnancy. One suggestion is that it is due to a salt-losing tendency caused by both the increase in GFR and increased progesterone secretion. Progesterone secretion increases early in pregnancy[86,88] and is a competitive antagonist at the mineralocorticoid receptor in the renal tubule.[87,106,127] However, there is no evidence that pregnant women cannot conserve sodium normally. As noted above, when pregnant women are placed on a 10 meq sodium intake, urinary sodium falls to the same level as in nonpregnant women,[11] and because pregnancy is associated with retention of approximately 900 meq of sodium to provide for the needs of the expanded vascular space and the fetus, it is hard to see evidence of salt wasting in pregnancy.

We found that pregnant women in the third trimester had supine PRA of 12 ± 3 ng/ml per hour, compared to values of 2.4 ± 0.9 ng/ml per hour in nonpregnant women, and with standing, PRA increases to 18 ± 3 ng/ml per hour, compared to 4 ± 0.08 ng/ml per hour in nonpregnant control subjects.[11] Accompanying the increase in PRA was an increase in plasma aldosterone. Supine plasma aldosterone was 20 ± 3 ng/100 ml and increased to 36 ± 7 ng/100 ml with standing in pregnant women, compared to values of 6.3 ± 1 ng/100 ml and 7.7 ± 8 ng/100 ml, respectively, in nonpregnant women. Urinary aldosterone excretion in pregnant women was 66 ± 10 μg/24 h, compared to less than 18 μg in nonpregnant women.[11]

Although a three- to fourfold increase in renin substrate concentration accounts in part for the increase in PRA, plasma renin concentration is approximately eight times higher in pregnant that in nonpregnant women, and plasma angiotensin is 78 ± 24 pg/ml in pregnant women, compared to a range of 5 to 35 pg/ml in nonpregnant women.[18,149] The cause of the increase in renin secretion is not known, but it does respond to change in sodium intake. After 7 days of a 10-meq sodium intake, we found that PRA rose appropriately to 59.6 ± 11 ng/ml per hour (Fig. 35-5), and after a 300-meq sodium intake for 7 days, PRA decreased to 10.2 ± 1.4 ng/ml per hour, compared to 1.5 ± 0.3 ng/ml per hour in nonpregnant women (Fig. 35-6). Thus, although PRA responds to change in sodium intake, it remains higher at all levels of sodium intake than in nonpregnant women.[11] Plasma aldosterone also responds to these changes in PRA and is also higher at all levels of sodium intake.

Renin is present in high concentration in the uterus of pregnant women and animals.[49,68,134,137] The high renin concentration in human amniotic fluid is in the form of prorenin, an inactive form that is activated by incubation at acid pH.[125] The role of these larger renin molecules is unknown; they may not have a physiologic importance. Uterine renin, however, might be involved in the regulation of uterine blood flow. Angiotensin increases uterine blood flow in the pregnant rabbit,[50] dog,[8] and monkey[55] by decreasing uterine vascular resistance. Since angiotensin also increases uterine vein PGE_2 concentration,[55] an increase in uterine prostaglandin synthesis may be the cause of the decrease in uterine vascular resistance and the increase in flow with angiotensin. Prostaglandin synthesis inhibitors such as indomethacin decrease uterine blood flow,[145] and the angiotensin I-converting enzyme inhibitor, captopril, causes uterine vein PGE_2 concentration and uterine blood flow to fall concomitantly.[48] Thus, the maintenance of uterine blood flow may be dependent upon a cybernetic system involving local synthesis of angiotensin II and PGE_2.

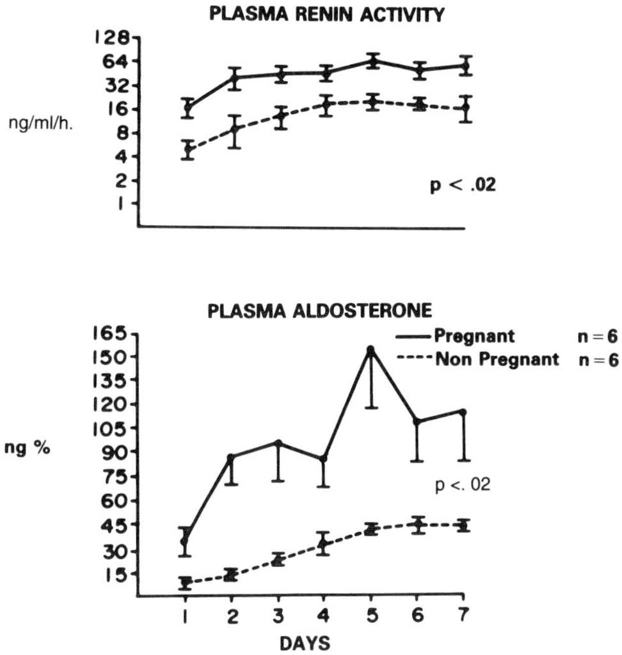

FIGURE 35-5 • Plasma renin activity and aldosterone levels in pregnant and nonpregnant women on a 10-meq sodium diet. (From Bay WH, Ferris TF: *Hypertension* 1:410, 1979. Used by permission.)

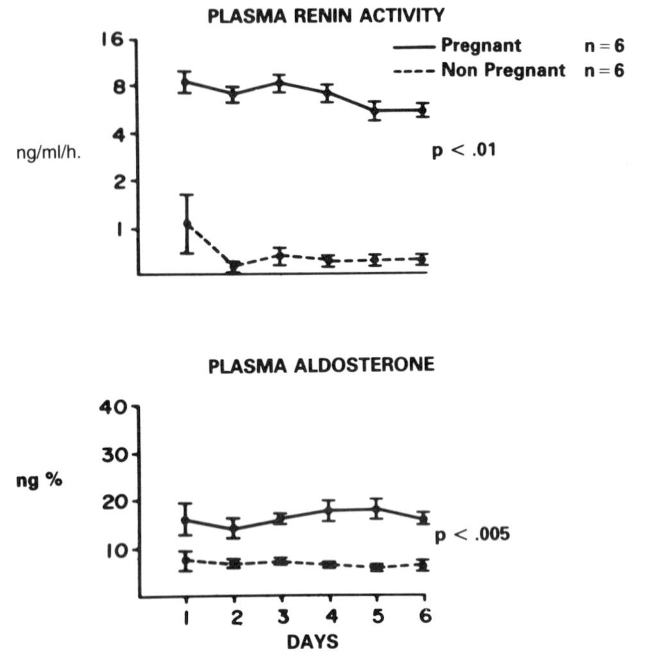

FIGURE 35-6 • Plasma renin activity and aldosterone levels in pregnant and nonpregnant women on a 300-meq sodium diet. (From Bay WH, Ferris TF: *Hypertension* 1:410, 1979. Used by permission.)

Prostaglandin synthesis

Extraordinary concentrations of PGE_2, approximately 150 ng/ml, are found in the uterine vein of pregnant rabbits.[145] Uterine vein PGE_2 falls following use of cyclooxygenase inhibitors, with a concomitant reduction in uterine blood flow. An increase in plasma and urinary PGE_2 and plasma and urinary 6-keto $PGF_{1\alpha}$ occurs with human pregnancy.[11,91,152] Whether the uterus is the source of the high plasma PGE_2 is not clear. Approximately two-thirds of PGE_2 injected into the right ventricle is metabolized to inactive prostaglandins in a single passage through the pulmonary circulation.[63] Urinary PGE_2 excretion is thought to represent renal synthesis, since PGE_2 injected into the renal artery does not increase urinary excretion.[57] The high plasma 6-keto $PGF_{1\alpha}$ may indicate increased PGI_2 synthesis in all blood vessels throughout pregnancy.

Pregnancy has certain similarities to Bartter's syndrome. Resistance to angiotensin II develops early in pregnancy, and this resistance is reversed by administration of indomethacin.[42] However, unlike Bartter's syndrome, the increase in urinary PGE_2 excretion with pregnancy is not associated with urinary potassium wasting, and normal free water clearance and maximum urinary concentration exist in pregnancy.[78,94] Although urinary PGE_2 excretion reflects renal synthesis of PGE_2, the site in the kidney that contributes to urinary PGE_2 is not exactly clear. The medullary interstitial cells are known to contain large concentrations of arachidonic acid as well as the cyclooxygenase enzyme necessary for prostaglandin synthesis, but renal cortical and medullary collecting tubules, endothelial cells of the renal vasculature, and glomerular mesangial cells are also capable of synthesizing prostaglandins.[136] PGE_2 is synthesized in the cells of the collecting tubule and mesangium, whereas PGI_2 is synthesized in the renal interlobular arteries and afferent arterioles. Thus, measurement of urinary PGE_2 excretion could reflect contributions from various cellular sites and account for the striking difference in the renal manifestations of Bartter's syndrome and pregnancy. However, the combination of insensitivity to angiotensin II and increased prostaglandin synthesis in both conditions is striking.

Estrogens

Because both estrogen and progesterone secretion increase with the onset of pregnancy, both hormones have been evaluated concerning their possible role in the changing hemodynamics of pregnancy. It was noted over 50 years ago that pregnancy protected adrenalectomized animals against volume depletion,[120] which raised the possibility that progesterone, estrogen, or both had a mineralocorticoid effect during pregnancy. In 1938, Thorn and Engle observed enhanced sodium and water reabsorption in male dogs given crude preparations of estrogen.[140] Since sodium retention also occurred in adrenalectomized animals, the effect was thought to be a primary antinatriuretic action of estrogen. In studies of humans, estradiol, in doses of 10 to 20 mg/day, decreased urinary sodium excretion for a 9- to 10-day period.[115] In female dogs, Johnson and coworkers have demonstrated that both estradiol and estriol cause sodium retention, which seemed independent of aldosterone, since no change in potassium excretion occurred during the sodium retention.[76] Unlike the sodium retention seen with most mineralocorticoids, blood pressure did not rise. Whether the action of estrogen on sodium reabsorption is a direct tubular effect remains unclear; the observation that 17β-estradiol increases the short-ciruit current in frog skin suggests that estrogen might have a direct effect upon sodium transport.[142] However, the effect of estrogen on sodium reabsorption may be extrarenal, mediated by an increase in vascular capacity. It is known that administration of estrogen to apes and monkeys causes salt and water retention, primarily in sexual skin,[9] and vasodilation in estrogen-responsive tissues. Estrogen does not prevent the normal escape from mineralocorticoids, but it can produce further sodium retention in dogs that have escaped from deoxycorticosterone acetate (DOCA).[76]

It has been speculated that estrogen might cause sodium retention through an effect on renin and aldosterone secretion. Estrogen increases renin substrate concentration by its stimulation of hepatic synthesis of proteins, but the subsequent rise in plasma angiotensin II normally suppresses renin secretion. Aldosterone secretion is not uniformly elevated in women taking estrogen-containing contraceptives or estrogen for postmenopausal symptoms.[124] Ethinyl estradiol, at a dose of 0.5 mg/day, may increase urinary excretion of aldosterone during the first several days of administration, but no uniform increase in aldosterone excretion occurs with chronic administration.[99] There is evidence, however, that prolonged intake of oral contraceptives may result in expansion of extracellular fluid volume.[26] However, the finding that estrogens caused sodium retention in at least one addisonian patient[141] and in adrenalectomized dogs on glucocorticoid replacement indicates that an increase in aldosterone secretion is not necessary for estrogen-induced sodium retention.[76]

For estrogen to have an effect on the renal handling of sodium and water, there would have to be responsive receptor sites somewhere along the nephron. Specific estradiol macromolecular complexes in the cytosol and nuclei of fetal guinea pig kidneys have been described, and these receptors appear to be distinct from other hormonal receptors.[110] In rat kidney, a low concentration of 17β-estradiol receptor located in nuclear chromatin has been reported.[34] Estrogen receptors seem to reside primarily in the proximal tubule but have a far lower affinity for estrogen than other tissues, such as uterus, mammary gland, and pituitary. How binding of estrogen to a cytosolic protein receptor would induce biochemical changes in protein synthesis in the nucleus, causing change in sodium absorption, is unknown. However, there is no evidence to suggest that the estrogen receptors found in the kidney play any role in mediating estrogen-induced changes in sodium and water reabsorption.

Progesterone

Progesterone increases sodium absorption in adrenalectomized ferrets and mice[60,61] and has been reported to decrease sodium excretion in adrenalectomized dogs.[140] However, subsequent studies in dogs have failed to demonstrate an antinatriuretic effect of progesterone, and in rats the results have been conflicting.[75,95] In humans, there is a uniform decrease in sodium reabsorption during progesterone administration,[107] and the mechanism is thought to be antagonism of aldosterone at the renal tubule receptor. There is no evidence to suggest that there are progesterone receptors in renal tissue, but progesterone in high doses can displace aldosterone from binding sites in the toad bladder and antagonize the effect of aldosterone on sodium transport.[128] Physiologic doses of progesterone do not significantly influence aldosterone-mediated sodium transport in the toad bladder.[114] It appears that in some species, when progesterone binds to mineralocorticoid receptors, it acts as an agonist, but in humans the hormone acts as a competitive inhibitor of aldosterone. This competitive inhibition is thought to be the cause of the increase in aldosterone secretion that occurs during the luteal phase of the menstrual cycle, when progesterone secretion is increased. Some have suggested that part of the natriuretic action of progesterone was independent of aldosterone inhibition, since progesterone causes a similar natriuresis in humans on a low- or high-sodium diet.[107] Progesterone, by competitively inhibiting the effect of aldosterone, attenuates the kaliuretic action of mineralocorticoids.[40] This may be the reason that patients with primary aldosteronism become normokalemic during pregnancy, although hypertension usually persists.[15]

A feature of pregnancy is the absence of a kaliuresis despite high aldosterone secretion and normal sodium intake. Administration of high doses of mineralocorticoid also fails to induce a kaliuresis in pregnancy. Ehrlich and associates administered DOCA, 20 mg/day intramuscularly, to women in the third trimester and noted sodium retention but no kaliuresis.[41] Since 100 mg daily of progesterone administered to a man also prevented kaliuresis during DOCA administration, the failure to increase potassium excretion was attributed to the increase in progesterone secretion that occurs with pregnancy. Although serum progesterone increases early in pregnancy and parallels the increase in plasma aldosterone, there are several features about the lack of a mineralocorticoid-induced kaliuresis that are difficult to reconcile with competitive inhibition of aldosterone. Pregnant women can vary their secretion of aldosterone with change in sodium intake; plasma aldosterone ranges from 22 ± 3 ng/100 ml after 7 days on a 300-meq sodium intake to 127 ± 27 ng/100 ml after 6 days on a 10-meq sodium diet,[11] but progesterone secretion does not change as dietary sodium is altered.[147] During administration of DOCA to pregnant women, urinary aldosterone excretion falls to only 25 μ/24 h, compared to levels below 10 μ/24 h in nonpregnant subjects,[41] and on a high-sodium diet, plasma aldosterone was found to be 22 ± 3 ng/100 ml in pregnant women, compared to 3.9 ± 0.04 ng/100 ml in nonpregnant women.[51] Thus, although plasma and urinary aldosterone respond to changes in sodium intake in pregnancy, neither is suppressed to the same extent as in nonpregnant women on a high-sodium intake or following DOCA administration. This would suggest that factors other than the presence of a competitive inhibitor of mineralocorticoid are the cause of the increased aldosterone secretion in pregnancy.

In addition to high plasma aldosterone, plasma deoxycorticosterone is elevated, ranging from 50 to 70 ng/100 ml in pregnant women, compared to levels in nonpregnant women of approximately 10 ng/100 ml.[41] Plasma deoxycorticosterone, like progesterone, is also not influenced by variations in salt intake, again making it difficult to explain the absence of a mineralocorticoid-induced kaliuresis by a fixed progesterone secretion, if the effect is one of competitive inhibition. Of further interest is the observation that the increase in sodium retention without a kaliuresis seen in pregnant women following administration of DOCA differs from findings in men given progesterone and DOCA. In men, there is neither a kaliuresis nor increased sodium reabsorption. Women with primary aldosteronism have correction of the hypokalemia but persistent hypertension during pregnancy.[3,15] Because spironolactone, a progestational agent that is a competitive inhibitor of mineralocorticoid activity, corrects both the hypertension and the potassium wasting of primary aldosteronism,[133] the rather specific antagonism to the kaliuretic effect of mineralocorticoids during pregnancy may reflect more than simple progesterone antagonism.

The different response in pregnancy to mineralocorticoid suppression has also been demonstrated by the use of a heparinoid compound in a third-trimester, pregnant woman. Heparin and related compounds selectively inhibit aldosterone secretion, but when they are given during pregnancy, urinary sodium increases without change in urinary potassium excretion, unlike the situation in nonpregnant women, in whom urinary potassium falls and serum potassium rises.[38,39] The antagonism to mineralocorticoid responsiveness of the renal tubule during pregnancy may be explained in part by an increase in progesterone secretion, but other, undefined factors seem to be involved.

POTASSIUM

During pregnancy, there is cumulative retention of approximately 350 meq of potassium. This retained potassium is stored in the fetus and also in the uterus, placenta, breasts, and red blood cells.[74] As noted above, potassium retention occurs despite increased circulating levels of mineralocorticoids and increased delivery of sodium to the distal nephron resulting from the increase in GFR.

WATER METABOLISM

Pregnant women are capable of attaining both normal maximal and normal minimal urinary osmolality. In a study of 75 normotensive pregnant women, maximum osmolality after water deprivation averaged 900 mosm/kg of water, a value not different from that in nonpregnant women.[78] Thus, in spite of increased renal blood flow and decreased renal vascular resistance, there is no evidence that papillary osmolality is reduced. Since urinary PGE_2 is also elevated in pregnancy, the normal capacity for urine concentration is all the more interesting. In vitro, PGE_2 is known to antagonize the effect of antidiuretic hormone in causing water movement across the isolated collecting tubule.[66] The failure to demonstrate a defect in maximum urine concentration despite increased renal synthesis of PGE_2 makes speculations about the physiologic importance of renal PGE_2 synthesis based upon in vitro observation difficult.

Minimal urine osmolality following a water load is also normal in pregnancy. Urinary osmolalities ranged between 25 and 88 mosm/kg, values similar to those obtained for nonpregnant women.[94] The rate of excretion of a water load may, however, be slower in late pregnancy,[73,106] especially when the woman is supine.[82,116]

In spite of the normal ability to dilute the urine in pregnancy, serum sodium falls approximately 5 meq/liter during late pregnancy, with a fall in serum osmolality of approximately 10 mosm/kg H_2O.[99] Hyponatremia and hypoosmolality are caused by changes in the osmotic regulation of thirst as well as changes in the osmotic regulation of AVP release from the pituitary gland.[30,31] Nonpregnant women secrete AVP when plasma osmolality exceeds 285 mosm/kg H_2O, whereas pregnant women secrete AVP when plasma osmolality exceeds 276 to 278 mosm/kg H_2O (Fig. 35-7). Although the threshold (or set point) for AVP release is decreased in the pregnant state, the sensitivity (or gain) of AVP release in response to changes in osmolality is not dramatically altered. Thus, pregnant women behave as if they have a "reset osmostat" and secrete AVP to maintain a lower plasma osmolality.

Although a change in the osmotic threshold for AVP release is one factor that contributes to the hypoosmolality in pregnancy, other factors also exist, since pregnant Brattleboro rats, which have congenital lack of AVP, also develop hypoosmolality.[38] In these rats, fluid intake is increased during pregnancy. Pregnant women also demonstrate increased thirst, with 24-h urine volumes approximately 25 percent greater than in nonpregnant women.[28] To maintain hypoosmolality, the osmotic threshold for thirst needs to be diminished, or pregnant women would merely have higher plasma AVP levels but normal plasma osmolality. Whereas nonpregnant women have an osmotic thirst threshold (derived from analogue scales relating the desire to drink water to plasma osmolality) of 290 mosm/kg H_2O and perceive thirst (conscious desire to drink) at 298 mosm/kg H_2O, pregnant women have an osmotic thirst threshold of 280 mosm/kg H_2O and perceive thirst at 288 mosm/kg H_2O.[31] The decrease in osmotic thirst threshold may actually precede the change in threshold for AVP release. Thirst threshold reaches its minimal level within 5 to 8 weeks of pregnancy, whereas the decreased threshold for AVP release reaches its minimum at 10 to 12 weeks of pregnancy.

The mechanisms responsible for resetting thirst control and AVP secretion have not been revealed.[54] Studies in pregnant rats revealed that in response to volume

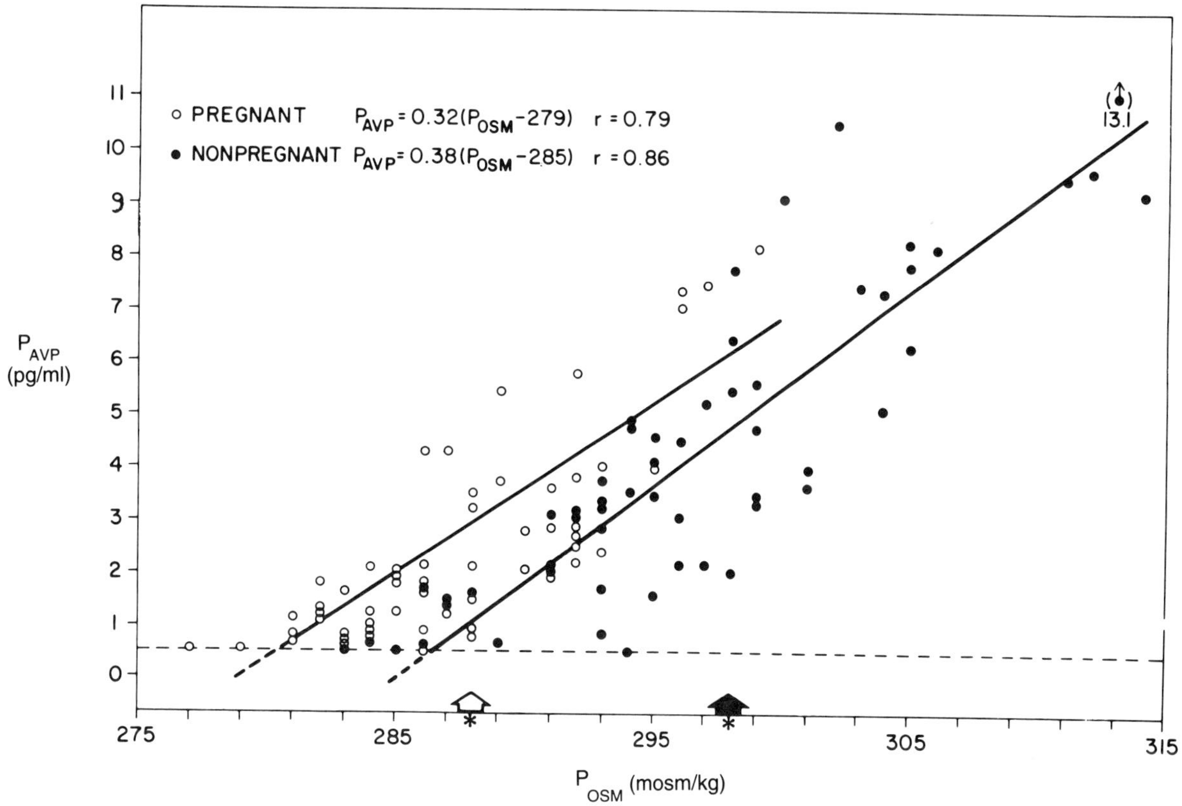

FIGURE 35-7 • Relationship between P_{osm} and P_{avp} when osmolality was altered by infusion of 5% saline in pregnant and nonpregnant women. Arrows represent thirst thresholds. (From Davison JM et al: *Am J Physiol* 246:F105, 1984. Used by permission.)

depletion, AVP secretion was similar to that seen in nonpregnant animals.[10] Studies in pregnant women employing head-out water immersion to reversibly increase central blood volume also demonstrated that changes in plasma volume did not affect AVP release or the osmotic threshold for thirst.[32] Therefore, the increased plasma volume of pregnancy is sensed as normal, and the nonosmotic secretion of AVP is similar to that of nonpregnant subjects. One potential candidate for the mediator of reset thirst and AVP release in pregnancy is human chorionic gonadotropin (hCG).[32] Nonpregnant women infused with hCG had decreases in plasma osmolality, thirst, and AVP release thresholds similar to that which occur in pregnant women. On the other hand, men infused with hCG had no changes. Thus, hCG, perhaps acting in concert with other ovarian factors, may mediate altered osmotic regulation in pregnancy.

PLASMA GLUCOSE AND GLUCOSURIA

Although the increase in GFR does not compromise the pregnant woman's ability to maintain sodium balance, pregnancy is frequently associated with glucosuria, which is due to the inability of some women to increase glucose reabsorption in parallel with the increase in glucose filtration. A reduction in the renal threshold for glucose in pregnancy has been observed: 155 ± 17 mg/100 ml, compared to 194 ± 6 mg/100 ml in nonpregnant women.[22] However, the tubular maximum for glucose transport (Tm_G), a measure of the capacity of the tubules to reabsorb glucose in a given time, was the same in pregnant and control women. This study was interpreted to indicate that the reduced threshold was due to the increase in filtered glucose. Although the concept of Tm_G is an oversimplification, since many factors affect glucose transport in the proximal tubule, it does provide a method of comparing the changes in glucose reabsorption in pregnant women with glucosuria. In 29 pregnant women, 16 without and 13 with glucosuria, GFR was the same in both groups, but Tm_G was significantly lower in pregnant women with glucosuria (310 ± 18 mg/min), compared to those without glucosuria (378 ± 18 mg/min) or in a nonpregnant control group (366 ± 16 mg/min).[151] There is a normal increase in Tm_G with an increase in GFR, but pregnancy displaces the slope of the regression line of Tm_G on GFR to the right, and pregnant women with glucosuria have an even greater reduction in Tm_G relative to GFR (Fig. 35-8). Thus, the increase in the filtered load of glucose is not associated with as great an increase in glucose reabsorption in pregnant as in non-

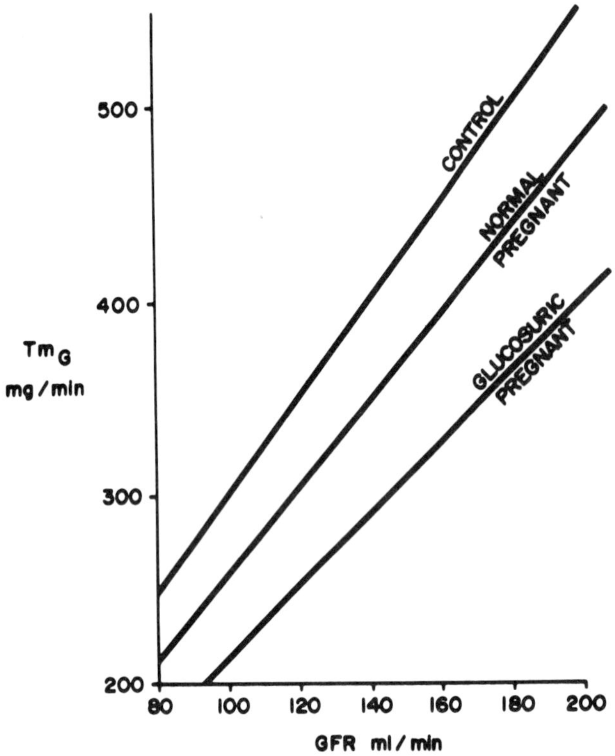

FIGURE 35-8 • Relationship between maximum tubular glucose absorption (Tm_G) and GFR in pregnant women with and without glucosuria and nonpregnant controls. (Adapted from Welsh GW, Sims EAH in Burrow GN, Ferris TF: *Medical Complications during Pregnancy*, Philadelphia, Saunders, 1982. Used by permission.)

Pregnancy is associated with striking changes in glucose metabolism. Plasma glucose and amino acids are reduced, and levels of free fatty acids, ketones, and triglycerides are increased.[56] As early as the fifteenth week of gestation, plasma glucose, after an overnight fast, is 15 to 20 mg/100 ml lower than in nonpregnant women,[45] and glucose levels are significantly lower during sleep in the second and third trimester, compared to nonpregnant women.[25] This tendency to fasting hypoglycemia with pregnancy results in exaggeration of fasting ketosis, with blood levels of β-hydroxybutyric acid and acetoacetic acid two to four times higher in pregnancy after an overnight fast.[45] The cause of fasting hypoglycemia in pregnancy is not due to inadequate glucose production, since studies have demonstrated a 16 percent greater glucose production in pregnant than in nonpregnant women.[79] Glucose and amino acid utilization by the fetus contributes to the hypoglycemia of pregnancy, but other factors are undoubtedly at play,[44] since fasting also induces lower blood sugar in nonpregnant women than in men.[103] The fasting hypoglycemia of pregnancy may be

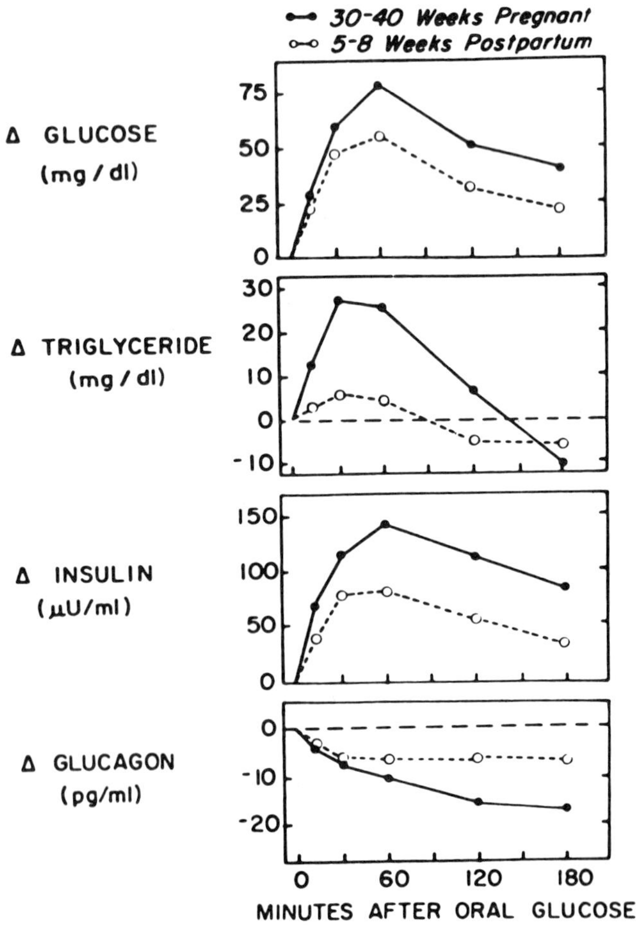

FIGURE 35-9 • Effect of an oral glucose load on plasma glucose, triglyceride, insulin, and glucagon in pregnancy. Data are expressed as changes from basal values. (From Freinkel N: *Diabetes* 29:1023, 1980. Used by permission.)

pregnant women, so all pregnant women have a propensity to develop glucosuria. In a comparison of the renal handling of glucose in late pregnancy and 8 to 12 weeks after delivery, the reabsorption of glucose was shown to be decreased in all pregnant women compared to individual postpartum values.[29] Moreover, women with glucosuria had lower fractional glucose reabsorption both during and after pregnancy. In women who had glucosuria greater than 150 mg/day during pregnancy, the disappearance of glucosuria postpartum was due to diminished filtration of glucose as GFR returned to nonpregnant levels. Women who had greater degrees of glucosuria during pregnancy demonstrated diminished reabsorption of glucose after pregnancy. These studies confirm earlier findings that glucosuria in pregnancy is due to an increase in filtered glucose in women who have a diminished capacity for glucose reabsorption in the nonpregnant state.[151]

Micropuncture studies have demonstrated that the distal tubule reabsorbs glucose and that glucose reabsorption is reduced at that site in pregnant rats.[16] Hormonal changes occurring with pregnancy seem to be the most likely cause of these changes in reabsorption, but no convincing evidence that estrogen or progesterone alters the tubular reabsorption of glucose has been provided.

an exaggeration of hormonal differences existing between females and males. These factors are probably of importance in the tendency of pregnant diabetics to develop severe ketoacidosis in the absence of marked increase in plasma glucose.

The response of a pregnant woman to a glucose load is different than that of a nonpregnant woman and is characterized by hyperglycemia, hyperinsulinemia, hypertriglyceridemia, and diminished sensitivity to insulin (Fig. 35-9).[56] The hyperinsulinemic response to feeding is most marked in the third trimester, and insulin levels are higher even when blood glucose is similar to that of nonpregnant women. Thus, there appears to be a change in the responsiveness of the beta cells to glucose, which is supported by the finding of hypertrophy and hyperplasia of the beta cells of the pancreas during pregnancy.[144]

In spite of the hyperinsulinemia, the blood glucose response to an oral carbohydrate load is higher than in nonpregnant women,[108] which is the result of insulin resistance by the liver during pregnancy.[46] A diminished response to intravenous insulin administration is also seen in pregnancy, which suggests that peripheral tissues, such as adipose tissue and muscle, share in this resistance to insulin. Studies using the glucose clamp technique indicate that tissue sensitivity to insulin is reduced by as much as 80 percent in pregnancy.[53] Since glood glucose levels stay within a range that is only modestly increased above nonpregnant levels, the increased insulin level counteracts the decreased sensitivity. The cause of the diminished insulin sensitivity in pregnancy is not clear. A variety of hormones secreted by the placenta, including progesterone, estrogen, and human placental lactogen, have been suggested to result singly or synergistically in the abnormal glucose metabolism in pregnancy.

AMINO ACID REABSORPTION

In addition to glucosuria, aminoaciduria occurs during pregnancy. Excretion of many amino acids is increased, with corresponding reduction in their plasma levels.[23,146] The fractional reabsorption of histidine is decreased. Indeed, an increase in urinary histidine was first proposed as a test for pregnancy in 1929 and services as the basis for one such commercial test. It is interesting that cortisone administration causes a pattern of aminoaciduria similar to that seen in pregnancy, and the aminoaciduria of pregnancy has been interpreted as indicating an increased cortisol effect on the renal tubules.[154] Glycine, histidine, threonine, serine, and alanine excretion increases early in pregnancy, and by term the urinary loss of these amino acids can be substantial. In one study, up to 20 percent of the filtered glycine and histidine was excreted daily in some pregnant women,[72] which indicates a decrease in the reabsorptive capacity for these two amino acids. There is not a uniform increase in excretion of amino acids during pregnancy; for instance, excretion of glutamic acid and methionine does not increase at any time during pregnancy.

URIC ACID

Uric acid, the end product of purine metabolism, is freely filtered by the glomerulus and actively reabsorbed in the proximal tubule. Urate clearance, which is approximately 10 percent of the creatinine clearance, is the net result of reabsorption of filtered urate and secretion of urate into the tubule at a site distal to the reabsorptive site. Men and women excrete between 500 and 800 mg of urate daily in the urine, and there is no evidence that this is increased during pregnancy. There is, however, an increase in urate clearance in pregnancy; the mean serum urate level in pregnancy is 3 ± 0.17 mg/100 ml, compared to 4.2 ± 1.2 mg/100 ml in nonpregnant women.[37] The estimation of the contribution of glomerular filtration, tubular secretion, and reabsorption to urate clearance has been difficult to determine and has depended on inferences made in humans based on changes in urate clearance following the administration of pyrazinamide, a drug known to inhibit urate secretion. Since these studies suggest that urinary urate largely represents the effect of tubular secretion, the rise in urate clearance in pregnancy might be the result of the increase in renal plasma flow with delivery of greater urate to the tubular secretory site. As pregnancy progresses, serum uric acid concentration gradually rises, so that by late pregnancy the serum urate concentration is similar to that in nonpregnant women. The decrease in urate clearance in late pregnancy may be the result of the decrease in renal plasma flow and the increase in filtration fraction that occur. It has been demonstrated that administration of angiotensin or norepinephrine decreases renal plasma flow, increases the filtration fraction, and decreases urate clearance.[47] This decrease in urate clearance during maintenance of GFR has been thought to be the result of diminished postglomerular blood flow. A similar change in renal hemodynamics and urate clearance occurs with volume depletion, with salt depletion, and following the use of diuretics.

The characteristic decrease in urate clearance that occurs with the development of toxemia may be due to a decrease in renal plasma flow. A similar decrease in urate clearance has been observed in essential hypertension, when renal plasma flow is reduced. Studies of renal blood flow depend upon para-aminohippuric acid (PAH) clearance, which is unreliable during the conditions of low urine flow that have been present in the published studies of renal hemodynamics during toxemia.

Toxemia, like other hypertensive states, is associated with diminished plasma volume and hemoconcentration, and this, as well as other, undefined hypertension-induced changes in the renal circulation, undoubtedly plays a role in the diminished urate clearance. Saline loading in normotensive pregnant women in the third trimester does not increase urate clearance, but this does not clarify why urate clearance is reduced with toxemia. Urate clearance is decreased by organic acids, such as lactate or ketoacids, but no consistent elevation in either has been noted in toxemia.[43,62,69]

ACID-BASE BALANCE

Pregnancy is associated with a compensated respiratory alkalosis, which begins early in pregnancy and continues to term.[92] Arterial P_{CO_2} decreases from 40 mmHg to approximately 30 mmHg during gestation, and pregnant women have an arterial pH of 7.44 ± 0.003, compared to the normal value of 7.40.[92] The alkalosis is thought to be due to an effect of progesterone on the central nervous system, causing hyperventilation.[98] The renal compensation for a chronic respiratory alkalosis results in a decrease in plasma bicarbonate concentration to 18 to 20 meq/liter, compared to 24 to 28 meq/liter in nonpregnant women. Since their total buffering capacity is reduced, pregnant women are more prone to develop severe acidosis with either ketoacidosis or lactic acidosis. Acid excretion by the kidney is unchanged in pregnancy; studies have demonstrated normal excretion of both titratable acid and ammonium following ammonium chloride loading.[5]

CALCIUM METABOLISM

A nonpregnant woman requires about 0.5 g/day of calcium to maintain normal calcium balance, whereas a pregnant woman requires 1.5 to 2 g. The fetal requirement of 25 to 30 g of calcium is retained mostly during the second half of pregnancy. Calcium balance is achieved by an increase in intestinal absorption caused by increased plasma 1α,25-dihydroxyvitamin D [1α,25-$(OH)_2D_3$] levels.[70,84] Under normal circumstances, calcium balance in pregnancy is easily maintained by a normal diet.

Total serum calcium concentration begins to fall during the second or third month of gestation and reaches its nadir between the twenty-eighth and thirty-second weeks.[113] This decrease in serum calcium is due to the normal hypoalbuminemia that occurs in pregnancy;[81] serum ionized calcium concentration remains unchanged. Despite hypocalcemia and diversion of calcium to the fetus, urinary excretion of calcium is increased in pregnant women.[65] This increase has been attributed to increased glomerular filtration, but the increase in calcium intake with pregnancy is the probable cause, since in patients not receiving calcium supplementation the urinary excretion of calcium decreases between early gestation and the month prior to term.[64]

The occurrence of maternal parathyroid hyperplasia during normal pregnancy suggests increased hormone production. Serum parathyroid hormone (PTH) values rise progressively throughout pregnancy,[113] but there is no correlation between the total serum calcium concentration and serum PTH, and normal serum PTH concentrations during the last trimester have been reported.[71] No differences in PTH have been found between maternal and cord blood at term.[90] Serum calcitonin concentrations have been found to be elevated during pregnancy in some, but not all, studies.[71,123] Calcitonin may be of importance during pregnancy in inhibiting PTH-induced bone resorption and in conserving skeletal calcium.

Plasma 1α,25$(OH)_2D_3$ levels are elevated in the first trimester of pregnancy and continue to rise during gestation. Since the increase in 1α,25$(OH)_2D_3$ and intestinal calcium absorption may precede the increase in plasma PTH, stimuli other than PTH must be active. Estrogens, progesterone, and human placental lactogen have all been suggested as possible mediators of the increased synthesis of vitamin D.[85] In late pregnancy, PTH is likely to play a role.

The diagnosis of hyperparathyroidism is difficult to make during pregnancy because of the decrease in total calcium concentration. In pregnant patients with hyperparathyroidism, serum calcium levels range from 9.5 to 20.6 mg/100 ml.[77] Although 27 of 30 patients have a serum calcium value greater than 12 mg/100 ml, the diagnosis may be missed in some pregnant patients if the usual value of 10.6 mg/100 ml for nonpregnant patients is taken as the upper limit of normal. Other tests of parathyroid function, such as serum phosphate concentration and tubular reabsorption of phosphate, may be helpful, but serum calcium concentration remains the best single test.

MAGNESIUM METABOLISM

Serum magnesium decreases by 6 to 9 percent in pregnancy, reaching its lowest value in the second trimester.[113,119] Plasma volume expansion and decreased plasma protein binding, rather than true magnesium deficiency, are the probable causes of this decrease in serum magnesium. Urinary magnesium excretion, fractional magnesium excretion, and the ratio of magnesium clearance to sodium clearance are not altered by pregnancy.[119]

REFERENCES

1. Abdul-Karim R, Assali NS: Pressor response to angiotensin in pregnant and nonpregnant women. *Am J Obstet Gynecol* 82:246, 1971.
2. Alexander EA et al: Renal hemodynamics and volume homeostasis during pregnancy in the rat. *Kidney Int* 18:173, 1980.
3. Aoi W et al: Primary aldosteronism aggravated during the peripartum period. *Jpn Heart* 19:946, 1978.
4. Aronson PS: Red-cell sodium-lithium countertransport and essential hypertension. *N Engl J Med* 307:317, 1982.
5. Assali NS et al: Renal responses to ammonium chloride acidosis in normal and toxemic pregnancies. *J Appl Physiol* 7:367, 1955.
6. Assali NS et al: Renal function in human pregnancy: Effects of venous pooling on renal hemodynamics and water, electrolyte and aldosterone excretion during normal gestation. *J Lab Clin Med* 54:394, 1959.
7. Assali NS et al: Measurements of uterine blood flow and metabolism: 8. Uterine and fetal blood flow and oxygen consumption in early human pregnancy. *Am J Obstet Gynecol* 79:86, 1960.
8. Assali NS et al: Regional blood flow and vascular resistance of the fetus in uterine action of vasoactive drugs. *Am J Obset Gynecol* 83:809, 1962.
9. Aykroyd OE, Zuckerman S: Factors in sexual skin edema. *J Physiol* 94:13, 1938.
10. Barron W et al: Role of volume in the regulation of vasopressin secretion during pregnancy in the rat. *J Clin Invest* 73:923, 1984.
11. Bay WH, Ferris TF: Factors controlling plasma renin and aldosterone during pregnancy. *Hypertension* 1:410, 1979.
12. Baylis C: The mechanism of increased glomerular filtration rate in the twelve-day pregnant rat. *J Physiol* 305:405, 1980.
13. Baylis C: Glomerular ultrafiltration in the pseudopregnant rat. *Am J Physiol* 234:F300, 1982.
14. Berssenbrugge AD et al: The effect of pregnancy on the angiotensin II pressor response in the rabbit. *Am J Obstet Gynecol* 136:762, 1980.
15. Biglieri EG, Slaton PE: Pregnancy and primary aldosteronism. *J Clin Endocrinol Metab* 27:1628, 1967.
16. Bishop JHV, Green R: Effects of pregnancy on glucose handling by distal segments of the rat nephron. *J Physiol* 289:98P, 1978.
17. Brenner BM, Troy JL: Postglomerular vascular protein concentration: Evidence for a causal role in governing fluid reabsorption and glomerulotubular balance by the renal proximal tubule. *J Clin Invest* 50:336, 1971.
18. Broughton-Pipkin F, Symonds EM: Angiotensin II levels in normal and hypertensive primigravid pregnancy. *Br J Obstet Gynaecol* 81:1003, 1974.
19. Chesley LC: Plasma and red cell volumes during pregnancy. *Am J Obstet Gynecol* 112:440, 1972.
20. Chesley LC et al: Excretion of sodium loads by nonpregnant and pregnant normal, hypertensive and preeclamptic women. *Metabolism* 7:575, 1958.
21. Chesley LC et al: Vascular reactivity to angiotensin II and norepinephrine in pregnant and nonpregnant women. *Am J Obstet Gynecol* 91:837, 1965.
22. Christensen PJ: Tubular reabsorption of glucose during pregnancy. *Scand J Clin Lab Invest* 10:364, 1958.
23. Christensen PJ et al: Amino acids in blood plasma and urine during pregnancy. *Scan J Clin Lab Invest* 9:43, 1957.
24. Corvilain J, Abramov M: Some effects of human growth hormone on renal hemodynamics and on tubular phosphate transport in man. *J Clin Invest* 41:1230, 1962.
25. Cousins L et al: The 24-hour excursion and diurnal rhythm of glucose, insulin and c-peptide in normal pregnancy. *Am J Obstet Gynecol* 136:483, 1980.
26. Crane MG, Harris JJ: Plasma renin activity and aldosterone excretion rate in normal subjects: 1. Effects of ethinyl estradiol and methoxyprogesterone acetate. *J Clin Endocrinol* 29:550, 1969.
27. DalCanton A et al: Effects of pregnancy on glomerular dynamics: Micropuncture study in the rat. *Kidney Int* 22:608, 1982.
28. Davison JM: Changes in renal function and other aspects of homeostasis in early pregnancy. *Br J Obstet Gynaecol* 81:1013, 1974.
28a. Davison JM, Dunlop W: Renal hemodynamics and tubular function in normal human pregnancy. *Kidney Int* 81:152, 1980.
29. Davison JM, Hytten FE: The effect of pregnancy on the renal handling of glucose. *Br J Obstet Gynaecol* 82:374, 1975.
30. Davis JM et al: Altered osmotic thresholds for vasopressin secretion and thirst in human pregnancy. *Am J Physiol* 246:F105, 1984.
31. Davison JM et al: Serial evaluation of vasopressin release and thirst in human pregnancy: Role of human chorionic gonadotrophin in the osmoregulatory changes of gestation. *J Clin Invest* 81:798, 1988.
32. Davison JM et al: Influence of humoral and volume factors on altered osmoregulation of normal human pregnancy. *Am J Physiol* 258:F900, 1990.
33. DeAlvarez RR: Renal glomerulotubular mechanisms during normal pregnancy: 1. Glomerular filtration rate, renal plasma flow and creatinine clearance. *Am J Obset Gynecol* 75:931, 1958.
34. DeVries JR et al: Estradiol renal receptor molecules and estradiol-dependent antinatriuresis. *Kidney Int* 2:95, 1972.
35. Dunlop W: Investigations into the influence of posture on renal plasma flow and glomerular filtration rate during late pregnancy. *Br J Obstet Gynaecol* 83:17, 1976.
36. Dunlop W: Renal physiology in pregnancy. *Postgrad Med J* 55:329, 1979.
37. Dunlop W, Davison JM: The effect of normal pregnancy upon the renal handling of uric acid. *Br J Obstet Gynaecol* 84:13, 1977.
38. Durr JA et al: Osmoregulation during pregnancy in the rat: Evidence for resetting of the threshold for vasopressin secretion during gestation. *J Clin Invest* 68:337, 1981.
39. Ehrlich EN: Heparinoid induced inhibition of aldosterone secretion in sodium conservation during normal pregnancy. *Am J Obstet Gynecol* 109:963, 1971.
40. Ehrlich EN, Lindheimer MD: Effect of administered mineralocorticoid or ACTH in pregnant women. *J Clin Invest* 51:1301, 1972.

41. Ehrlich EN et al: Mineralocorticoids in normal pregnancy, in Lindheimer MD et al (eds): *Hypertension in Pregnancy*. New York, Wiley, 1976, p 217.
42. Everett RB et al: Effect of prostaglandin synthetase inhibition on pressor response to angiotensin II in human pregnancy. *J Clin Endocrinol Metab* 46:1007, 1978.
43. Fadel HE et al: Hyperuricemia in pre-eclampsia: A reappraisal. *Am J Obstet Gynecol* 125:640, 1976.
44. Felig P: Body fuel metabolism and diabetes mellitus in pregnancy. *Med Clin North Am* 61:43, 1977.
45. Felig P, Lynch V: Starvation in human pregnancy: Hypoglycemia, hypoinsulinemia, and hyperketonemia. *Science* 170:990, 1970.
46. Felig P et al: Influence of oral glucose ingestion on splanchnic glucose and gluconeogeneic substrate metabolism. *Diabetes* 24:468, 1975.
47. Ferris TF, Gorden P: Effect of angiotensin and norepinephrine upon urate clearances in man. *Am J Med* 44:359, 1968.
48. Ferris TF, Weir EK: Effect of captopril on uterine blood flow and prostaglandin E synthesis in the pregnant rabbit. *J Clin Invest* 71:809, 1983.
49. Ferris TF et al: Rabbit uterus as a source of renin. *Am J Physiol* 212:698, 1967.
50. Ferris TF et al: Uterine blood flow and uterine renin secretion. *J Clin Invest* 51:2828, 1972.
51. Ferris TF et al: Studies of the mechanism of sodium retention in idiopathic edema. *Trans Assoc Am Physicians* 86:310, 1973.
52. Fievet P et al: Atrial natriuretic factor in pregnancy-induced hypertension and preeclampsia: Increased plasma concentrations possibly explaining these hypovolemic states with paradoxical hyporeninism. *Am J Hypertens* 1:16, 1988.
53. Fisher PM et al: Insulin response to glucose infusion in normal human pregnancy. *Diabetologia* 19:15, 1980.
54. Fitzsimmons JT: The physiological basis of thirst. *Kidney Int* 10:3, 1976.
55. Franklin GO et al: The effect of angiotensin II intravenous infusion on plasma renin activity and prostaglandin A, E, and F levels in the uterine vein of the pregnant monkey. *Prostaglandins* 6:271, 1974.
56. Freinkel N: Of pregnancy and progeny. *Diabetes* 29:1023, 1980.
57. Frohlich JC, Wilson TW: Urinary prostaglandins: Identification and origin. *J Clin Invest* 55:763, 1975.
58. Gant NF et al: The nature of pressor responsiveness to angiotensin II in human pregnancy. *Obstet Gynecol* 43:854, 1974.
59. Garland HO et al: Changes in body weight, kidney weight and proximal tubular length during pregnancy in the rat. *Renal Physiol* 1:42, 1978.
60. Gaunt R, Hays HW: Life maintaining effect of crystalline progesterone in adrenalectomized ferrets. *Science* 88:576, 1938.
61. Gaunt R et al: Cortical hormone-like action of progesterone and non-effect of sex hormones on water intoxication. *Proc Soc Exp Biol Med* 39:319, 1938.
62. Goldfinger S et al: Renal retention of uric acid induced by infusion of beta-hydroxybutyrate and acetoacetate. *N Engl J Med* 272:351, 1965.
63. Golub M et al: Metabolism of prostaglandins A_1 and E_1 in man. *J Clin Invest* 56:1401, 1975.
64. Goss DA: Renal conservation of calcium during pregnancy. *Obstet Gynecol* 20:199, 1962.
65. Graham WP et al: Effect of pregnancy and of the menstrual cycle on hypoparathyroidism. *J Clin Endocrinol Metab* 24:512, 1964.
66. Grantham JJ, Orloff J: Effect of prostaglandin E_1 on the permeability response of the isolated collecting tubule to vasopressin, adenosine 3′,5′-monophosphate, and theophylline. *J Clin Invest* 47;1154, 1968.
67. Gray MJ, Plentl AA: The variations of the sodium space and the total exchangeable sodium during pregnancy. *J Clin Invest* 33:347, 1954.
68. Gross F et al: A renin-like substance in the placenta and uterus of the rabbit. *Lancet* 1:914, 1964.
69. Handler JS: The role of lactic acid in the reduced excretion of uric acid in toxemia of pregnancy. *J Clin Invest* 39:1526, 1960.
70. Heany RP, Skillman TG: Calcium metabolism in normal human pregnancy. *J Clin Endocrinol Metab* 33:661, 1971.
71. Hillman LS et al: Perinatal vitamin D metabolism: 4. Maternal and cord serum 24,25-dihydroxyvitamin D concentrations. *J Clin Endocrinol Metab* 47:1073, 1978.
72. Hytten FE, Cheyne GA: The aminoaciduria of pregnancy. *Br J Obstet Gynaecol* 79:424, 1972.
73. Hytten FE, Klapper AI: Response to a water load in pregnancy. *Br J Obstet Gynaecol* 70:811, 1963.
74. Hytten FE, Leitch I: *The Physiology of Human Pregnancy*, 2d ed. Oxford, Blackwell Scientific, 1971.
75. Johnson JA et al: Effect of estrogen and progesterone on electrolyte balances in normal dogs. *Am J Physiol* 219:1691, 1970.
76. Johnson JA et al: Effects of estradiol on sodium and potassium balances in adrenalectomized dogs. *Am J Physiol* 223:194, 1972.
77. Johnstone RE et al: Hyperparathyroidism during pregnancy. *Obstet Gynecol* 40:580, 1972.
78. Katz AL: Urinary concentrating ability in pregnant women with asymptomatic bacteriuria. *J Clin Invest* 49:1331, 1961.
79. Kalhan SC et al: Glucose production in pregnant women at term gestation. *J Clin Invest* 63:388, 1979.
80. Kalousek G et al: Circadian rhythyms of creatinine and electrolyte excretion in healthy pregnant women. *Am J Obstet Gynecol* 103:856, 1969.
81. Kerr C et al: Calcium and phosphorous dynamics in pregnancy. *Am J Obstet Gynecol* 83:2, 1962.
82. Kerr MG: The mechanical effects of the gravid uterus in late pregnancy. *Br J Obstet Gynaecol* 72:513, 1965.
83. Kristensen CG et al: Effect of atrial natriuretic factor in pregnancy. *Am J Physiol* 250:R589, 1986.
84. Kumar R et al: Elevated 1,25(OH)D_3 levels in normal human pregnancy and lactation. *J Clin Invest* 63:342, 1979.
85. Kumar R et al: Vitamin D and calcium hormones in pregnancy. *N Engl J Med* 302:1143, 1980.
86. Laidlaw JC et al: The influence of estrogen and progesterone on aldosterone excretion. *J Clin Endocrinol Metab* 22:161, 1962.

87. Landau RL, Lugibihl K: Inhibition of sodium-retaining influence of aldosterone by progesterone. *J Clin Endocrinol Metab* 18:1237, 1958.
88. Ledoux F et al: Plasma progesterone and aldosterone in pregnancy. *Can Med Assoc J* 112:943, 1975.
89. Lehtovirta P: Hemodynamic effects of combined estrogen-progesterone oral contraceptives. *Br J Obstet Gynaecol* 81:517, 1974.
90. Lequin RM et al: A radioimmunoassay for parathyroid hormone in man: 2. Measurement of parathyroid concentrations in human plasma by means of radioimmunoassay for bovine hormone. *Acta Endocrinol* 63:655, 1970.
91. Lewis PJ et al: Prostacyclin in pregnancy. *Br Med J* 280:1581, 1980.
92. Lim VS et al: Acid-base metabolism in pregnancy. *Am J Physiol* 231:1764, 1976.
93. Lindheimer MD, Katz AI: Kidney function in the pregnant rat. *J Lab Clin Med* 78:633, 1971.
94. Lindheimer MD, Weston PV: Effect of hypotonic expansion on sodium, water and urea excretion in late pregnancy: The influence of posture on these results. *J Clin Invest* 48:947, 1969.
95. Lindheimer MD et al: Renal function in normal and hypertensive pregnant rats, in Lindheimer MD et al (eds): *Hypertension in Pregnancy.* New York, Wiley, 1976, p 217.
96. Little B: Water and electrolyte balance during pregnancy. *Anesthesiology* 26:400, 1965.
97. Logan A et al: Sodium-lithium countertransport and passive cation permeability abnormalities in erythrocytes of pregnant women. *Kidney Int* 23:173, 1983.
98. Lyons HA, Antonio R: The sensitivity of the respiratory center in pregnancy and after the administration of progesterone. *Trans Assoc Am Physicians* 72:173, 1959.
99. MacDonald HN, Good W: The effect of parity on plasma sodium, potassium, chloride and osmolality levels during pregnancy. *Br J Obstet Gynaecol* 79:441, 1972.
100. MacGillivray I, Buchanan TJ: Total exchangeable sodium and potassium in nonpregnant women and in normal and pre-eclamptic pregnancy. *Lancet* 2:1090, 1958.
101. MacGillivray I et al: Blood pressure survey in pregnancy. *Clin Sci* 37:395, 1969.
102. McLennan CE: Antecubital and femoral venous pressure in normal and toxemic pregnancy. *Am J Obstet Gynecol* 45:568, 1943.
103. Merimee TJ, Tyson JE: Stabilization of plasma glucose during fasting: Normal variation in two separate studies. *N Engl J Med* 291:1275, 1974.
104. Metcalfe J, Ueland K: Maternal cardiovascular adjustments to pregnancy. *Prog Cardiovasc Dis* 16:363, 1974.
105. Miyamoto S et al: Circadian rhythm of plasma atrial natriuretic peptide, aldosterone, and blood pressure during the third trimester in normal and preeclamptic pregnancies. *Am J Obstet Gynecol* 158:393, 1988.
106. Oelkers W et al: Effects of progesterone and four synthetic progesterones on sodium balance and the renin-aldosterone system in man. *J Clin Endocrinol Metab* 39:882, 1974.
107. Oparil S et al: Effects of progesterone on renal sodium handling in man: Relation to aldosterone excretion and plasma renin activity. *Clin Sci* 49:139, 1975.
108. O'Sullivan JB, Mahan CM: Criteria for the oral glucose tolerance test in pregnancy. *Diabetes* 13:278, 1964.
109. Otsuki Y et al: Changes in concentration of human atrial natriuretic peptide in normal pregnancy and toxemia. *J Endocrinol* 114:325, 1987.
110. Pasqualini JR et al: Steroid hormone receptors in fetal guinea pig kidney. *J Steroid Biochem* 5:977, 1974.
111. Phippard AF et al: Circulatory adaptation to pregnancy: Serial studies of hemodynamics, blood volume, renin and aldosterone in the baboon (*Papio hamadryas*). *J Hypertens* 4:773, 1986.
112. Pirani BBK et al: Plasma volume in normal first pregnancy. *Br J Obstet Gynaecol* 80:884, 1973.
113. Pitkin RM et al: Calcium metabolism in normal pregnancy: A longitudinal study. *Am J Obstet Gynecol* 133:781, 1979.
114. Porter GA et al: On the mechanism of action of aldosterone on sodium transport: The role of RNA synthesis. *Proc Natl Acad Sci U S A* 52:1326, 1964.
115. Preedy JRK, Aitken EH: The effect of estrogen on water and electrolyte metabolism. *J Clin Invest* 35:423, 1956.
116. Pritchard JA et al: The effect of the supine position on renal function in the near-term pregnant woman. *J Clin Invest* 34:777, 1955.
117. Pullman TN et al: The influence of dietary protein on specific renal functions in normal man. *J Lab Clin Med* 44:320, 1954.
118. Robertson EG: Increased erythrocyte fragility in association with osmotic changes in pregnancy serum. *J Reprod Fertil* 16:323, 1968.
119. Roelofsen JMT et al: Urinary excretion rates of calcium and magnesium in normal and complicated pregnancies. *Eur J Obstet Gynecol Reprod Biol* 27:227, 1988.
120. Rogoff JM, Stewart GN: Studies on adrenal insufficiency: 3. The influence of pregnancy upon the survival period of adrenalectomized dogs. *Am J Physiol* 79:508, 1927.
121. Rovinsky JJ, Jaffin H: Cardiovascular hemodynamics in pregnancy: 1. Blood and plasma volumes in multiple pregnancy. *Am J Obstet Gynecol* 93:1, 1965.
122. Rovinsky JJ, Jaffin H: Cardiovascular hemodynamics in pregnancy: 3. Cardiac rate, stroke volume, total peripheral resistance and central blood volume in multiple pregnancy: Synthesis of results. *Am J Obstet Gynecol* 95:787, 1966.
123. Samaan NA et al: Immunoreactive calcitonin in medullary carcinoma of the thyroid and in maternal and cord serum. *J Lab Clin Med* 81:671, 1973.
124. Saruta T et al: A possible mechanism for hypertension induced by oral contraceptives. *Arch Intern Med* 120:621, 1974.
125. Sealey JE et al: Prorenin and other large molecular weight forms of renin. *Endocr Rev* I:365, 1980.
126. Seely JF, Levy M: Control of extracellular fluid volume, in Brenner BM, Rector FC Jr (eds): *The Kidney,* 2d ed. Philadelphia, Saunders, 1981, p 371.
127. Sharp GWC, Leaf A: Mechanism of action of aldosterone. *Physiol Rev* 46:593, 1966.
128. Sharp GWG et al: Studies on the binding of aldosterone in the toad bladder. *J Clin Invest* 45:450, 1966.

129. Shiffman RL et al: Effect of dietary protein on glomerular filtration rate in pregnancy. *Obstet Gynecol* 73:47, 1989.
130. Sims EA, Krantz KE: Serial studies of renal function during pregnancy and the puerperium in normal women. *J Clin Invest* 37:1764, 1958.
131. Smith H: Summary of observation of renal hemodynamics in pre-eclampsia, in Fomon SJ (ed): *Report of First Ross Obstetric Research Conference*. Ohio, Ross Laboratories, 1956, p 75.
132. Soler NG et al: Serial determinations of human placental lactogen in the last half of normal and complicated pregnancies. *Am J Obstet Gynecol* 120:214, 1974.
133. Spark RF, Melby JC: Aldosteronism in hypertension: The spironolactone response test. *Ann Intern Med* 69:685, 1968.
134. Stakemann G: A renin-like pressor substance found in the placenta of the cat. *Acta Pathol Microbiol Scand* 50:350, 1960.
135. Steegers EA et al: Plasma atrial natriuretic peptide in late pregnancy and puerperuim. *Eur J Obstet Gynecol Reprod Biol* 26:213, 1987.
136. Sun FF et al: Metabolism of prostaglandins in the kidney. *Kidney Int* 19:760, 1981.
137. Symonds EM et al: Production of renin by in vitro cultures of human chorion and uterine muscle. *Nature (London)* 217:1152, 1968.
138. Thomsen JK et al: Atrial natriuretic peptide concentrations in preeclampsia. *Br Med J* 294:1508, 1987.
139. Thomson AM, Billewicz WZ: Clinical significance of weight trends during pregnancy. *Br Med J* 1:243, 1957.
140. Thorn GW, Engle LL: The effect of sex hormones on renal excretion of electrolytes. *J Exp Med* 68:299, 1937.
141. Thorn GW et al: A study of the mechanism of edema associated with menstruation. *Endocrinology* 22:155, 1938.
142. Tomlinson RWS: The action of progesterone derivatives and other steroids on the sodium transport of isolated frog skin. *Acta Physiol Scand* 83:407, 1971.
143. Ueland K et al: Maternal cardiovascular dynamics: 4. The influence of gestational age on the maternal cardiovascular response to posture and exercise. *Am J Obstet Gynecol* 104:856, 1969.
144. Van Aasche FA, Aerts L: Morphologic and ultrastructure modifications in the endocrine pancreas in pregnant rats, in Camerini-Davalos RA, Cole HS (eds): *Early Diabetes in Early Life*. New York, Academic Press, 1975, p 333.
145. Venuto R et al: The effect of prostaglandin inhibition on uterine blood flow. *J Clin Invest* 55:193, 1975.
146. Wallraff EB et al: Urinary excretion of amino acids in pregnancy. *J Clin Invest* 29:1542, 1950.
147. Wambach G et al: Regulation of serum progesterone in patients with essential hypertension. *Acta Endocrinol* 95:207, 1980.
148. Weinberger MH et al: Sequential changes in the renin-angiotensin and plasma progesterone concentration in normal and abnormal human pregnancy, in Lindheimer MD et al (eds): *Hyptertension in Pregnancy*. New York, Wiley, 1976, p. 263.
149. Weir RJ et al: Plasma renin, renin substrate, angiotensin II, and aldosterone in hypertensive disease of pregnancy. *Lancet* 1:291, 1973.
150. Weir RJ et al: Studies of the renin-angiotensin-aldosterone system, cortisol, DOC, and ADH in normal and hypertensive pregnancy, in Lindheimer MD et al (eds): *Hypertension in Pregnancy*. New York, Wiley, 1976, p 251.
151. Welsh GW, Sims EAH: The mechanisms of renal glucosuria in pregnancy. *Diabetes* 9:363, 1960.
152. Whalen JB et al: Plasma prostaglandins in pregnancy. *Obstet Gynecol* 51:52, 1978.
153. Worley RJ et al: Increased sodium-lithium countertransport in erythrocytes of pregnant women. *N Engl J Med* 307:412, 1982.
154. Zinneman HH et al: Urinary amino acids in pregnancy, following progesterone and estrogen. *J Clin Endocrinol Metab* 27:397, 1967.

CHAPTER 36

Small and large intestinal disorders: associated fluid and electrolyte complications

Sidney F. Phillips

The physiologic basis of intestinal secretion and absorption of water and electrolytes (Chap. 17) has evolved from a considerable body of experimental work. Although information on the pathophysiology of these systems in disease is accumulating, much of it as yet is incomplete or has not been integrated fully into the clinical sciences. The subject of fluid and electrolyte disorders in intestinal disease is best approached by an overview of the physiology in intact human beings.

NORMAL PHYSIOLOGY

The gastrointestinal tract is a large body compartment that normally contains isotonic solutions of electrolytes. Intestinal contents differ in composition from extracellular fluid because of the various mucosal membranes that are interposed and that actively modify equilibrium between the two. Mucosal secretion and absorption can greatly influence body water and electrolyte content, since the magnitudes of the exchanges involved far exceed those of other systems; with normal fluid intake and normal endogenous secretion of fluids, some 9 liters enters the upper intestine daily. During passage through the bowel the mixture is selectively altered and then so efficiently conserved that 200 ml or less is excreted in the feces.

The major physiologic functions of the gastrointestinal tract are motility, for propulsion and mixing of foodstuffs; secretion, whereby fluids of widely differing electrolyte composition are added to the intestinal contents; digestion, a sequence of physicochemical reactions that break down dietary components to simpler compounds that can be absorbed; and selective absorption of the products of digestion and of water and electrolytes.

Most of these functions are relatively quiescent under basal circumstances, variably stimulated by sensory (cephalic) activators, and evoked specifically by the ingestion of food. The concept that different organs and functions are normally integrated by hormonal, paracrine, and neural mechanisms into a precisely coordinated whole is central to an understanding of how localized disease can derange water and electrolyte metabolism throughout the system. Nevertheless, each specialized region of the gastrointestinal tract must be considered separately to be understood as a part of the whole.

ENTEROSYSTEMIC CYCLING OF WATER AND ELECTROLYTES

A large proportion of the extracellular fluid enters the alimentary canal daily (Fig. 36-1). For example, in a 70-kg adult, about half the extracellular fluid volume is secreted into the upper gastrointestinal tract—far more fluid than is added normally through the diet. An average daily intake of sodium (150 meq), potassium (50 meq), and chloride (200 meq) is similarly trivial compared with the amounts secreted into the intesinal lumen in 24 h (Table 36-1).

Food entering the upper gastrointestinal tract promotes simultaneous or sequential secretions of saliva, gastric juice, bile, and pancreatic juice; these fluids contain widely varying concentrations of sodium, potassium, chloride, bicarbonate, and hydrogen ions (Table 36-1). Mixing, propulsion, digestion, and progressive equilibration toward the physiologic extracellular pH and os-

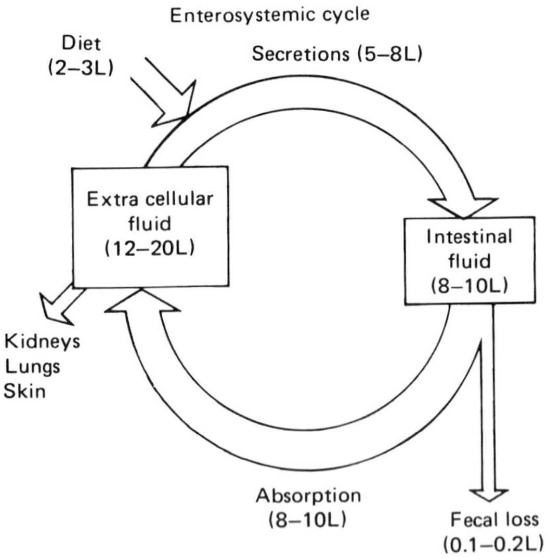

FIGURE 36-1 • Cycling of water and electrolytes between the alimentary canal and ECF is represented by entry into the bowel (diet and secretions) and exit from the bowel (absorption and fecal loss).

molality occur in the stomach and duodenum. In the small intestine, an uncertain volume of isotonic, neutral, small bowel secretion (succus entericus) is added to the contents. In the jejunum this fluid is rich in chloride; in the ileum, bicarbonate is the predominant anion (Fig. 36-2).

Absorption of different nutrients begins in the duodenum and peaks, in most persons, in the proximal jejunum. The jejunum receives 8 to 10 liters of isotonic electrolyte solution per 24 h; reabsorption in the proximal bowel preserves 6 to 8 liers of water, more than 500 meq each of sodium and chloride, 200 meq of bicarbonate, and 100 meq of potassium. Absorption of water and electrolytes continues in the ileum and is completed in the colon, where each day 1 to 2 liters of semiliquid material is progressively desiccated to feces. Some 500 ml of water and 100 meq of cation per 24 h is simultaneously recycled through the enterohepatic circulation.

The stomach has a primary function of secretion, although it is also capable of limited absorption (e.g., of water, some drugs, and alcohol). The small and large intestines are primarily areas for absorption, but are capable of secretion under pathophysiologic circumstances. The normal processes of secretion are stimulated mainly by the intake of food, and absorption is believed to be largely obligatory; thus, homeostasis of the whole organism must be adjusted through changes in renal, and not gastrointestinal, function.

SECRETION, ABSORPTION, TRANSIT

Secretion

Biliary secretion

Bile contains water, electrolytes, bilirubin, neutral fat, cholesterol, lecithin, and bile salts.[16] Secretion of bile involves several different active and passive mechanisms that transport the various constituents from liver cells into the biliary ductules. Neutral, humoral, and chemical mechanisms control secretion. Of these, the choleretic effects of secretin, released from the small intestinal mucosa, and of bile salts, reabsorbed actively from the ileum, are most important. Secretin increases the volume and bicarbonate concentration of bile, which may in-

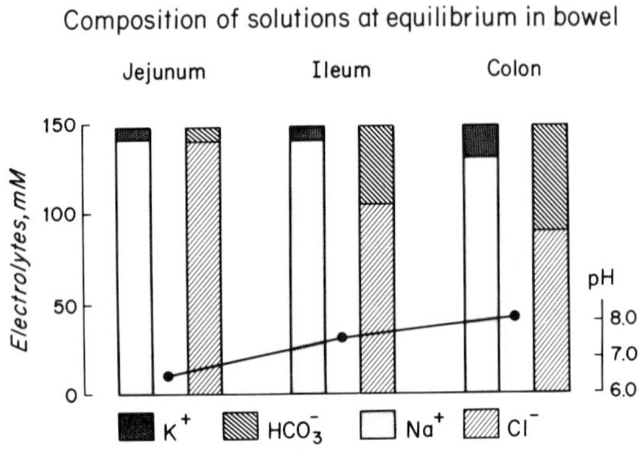

FIGURE 36-2 • Composition of isotonic electrolyte solutions that develop and equilibrate in the small and large bowel. These compositions approximate those of chyme or fasting intestinal content at the same sites.

TABLE 36-1 • Approximate composition of diet and gastrointestinal secretions per 24 H

	Content, meq/volume					Concentration, meq/liter				
	FLUID (LITER)	Na^+	K^+	Cl^-	HCO_3^-	Na^+	K^+	Cl^-	HCO_3^-	pH
Diet	2–3	150	50	200						
Saliva	1.0	50	20	40	50	20–80	10–20	20–40	20–60	7.0–8.0
Gastric juice	1–2	40–160	15	200	—	20–100	5–10	120–160	—	1.0–7.0
Bile	1.0	100	5	40	40	150–250	5–10	40–80	20–40	7.0–8.0
Pancreatic juice	1.0–2.0	150	5	40	120	120	5–10	10–60	80–120	7.0–8.0
Succus entericus	1.0–2.0	140–280	5–10	variable	variable	140	5	variable	variable	7.0–8.0

crease to 60 meq/liter (pH 8) and thus help neutralize acid gastric contents. During fasting, bile is stored in the gallbladder, since resting common bile duct pressure is low and does not overcome the resistance of the sphincter of Oddi. Active and passive absorption of sodium and water by the gallbladder concentrates the bile fivefold. Contraction and emptying of the gallbladder is induced through vagal innervation and by cholecystokinin-pancreozymin (CCK), which is secreted from the small intestinal mucosa in response to the products of fat and protein digestion.

Pancreatic secretion

Pancreatic juice has two components with different functions and cellular origins. The components vary reciprocally according to the nature of the stimulus to secretion. One, an alkaline watery fluid containing a high concentration of bicarbonate, is derived from the ductular cells; these remove carbon dioxide from arterial blood and hydrate it to carbonic acid, which dissociates into hydrogen and bicarbonate ions.[33] Cations in this secretion are in concentrations similar to those in the plasma. The second component, a more viscous secretion of acinar cells, contains digestive enzymes including trypsin, amylase, and lipase. A small, continuous, basal secretion of pancreatic juice occurs during fasting, and a cephalic phase of secretion mediated through the vagus has been demonstrated. Hormones released from the mucosa of the upper small intestine are the major controls of pancreatic secretion. Secretin is released particularly through acidification of duodenal contents and promotes secretion of water and bicarbonate. CCK promotes simultaneous output of digestive enzymes.

Succus entericus

In health, the intestine continuously secretes small volumes (probably 50 ml/h or less) of an isotonic, alkaline mixture of goblet-cell mucus, intestinal (Brunner's) gland secretions, desquamated epithelium containing intracellular enzymes, and an untrafiltrate of plasma. The contribution of this secretion, called *succus entericus*, to the normal enterosystemic cycle is uncertain, since accurate measurements of its volume and composition are not available for healthy human beings. Diseases are known, however, in which the volume increases to many liters per day.[30]

Intestinal secretion

Intestinal secretion (Table 36-2) has already been discussed in Chap. 17. The phenomenon can be summarized as a state in which the mucosa of the small and/or large bowel ceases to function in an absorptive mode. Rather, an active secretion of chloride ions leads to an accumulation in the lumen of an isotonic solution of electrolytes and water, adding to the volume of "succus." This phenomenon is now recognized to be an important mechanism of fluid loss and diarrhea.[30] Among the diverse stimuli to intestinal secretion can now be included:

1. Bacterial enterotoxins (as in Asiatic cholera, toxigenic *Escherichia coli* infections, and numerous other intestinal infections).
2. Humoral stimulation of the bowel (Zollinger-Ellison and Verner-Morrison syndromes).
3. Malabsorption (where dihydroxy bile acids and/or fatty acids act as luminal secretagogues).
4. Miscellaneous stimuli such as drugs (many laxatives) and mechanical obstruction.

TABLE 36-2 • Intestinal secretion and diarrhea

Disorder	Secretory stimulus
Asiatic cholera, staphylococcal and clostridial food poisoning, *E. coli* diarrheas ("turista")	Bacterial enterotoxins (heat-stable and heat-labile forms have been described)
Islet-cell tumors (pancreatic cholera, WHDA)	Gastrointestinal hormones [vasoactive intestinal polypeptide (VIP) possibly others]
Medullary thyroid cancer	Calcitonin
Steatorrhea	Long-chain fatty acids
Ileal resection	Dihydroxy bile acids
Laxative abuse	Anthraquinone cathartics
Intestinal obstruction	Stimulus unknown

Absorption

Absorption moves nutrients, ions, and water from the lumen of the bowel into portal venous blood and the abdominal lymphatics via a variety of passive and active transport systems (see Chap. 17). Most important nutrients are absorbed by active mechanisms, which require specific mucosal "carriers." Passive transport of ions is determined by relative chemical (concentration) and electrical (mucosal-serosal potential difference) forces across the mucosa. Active transport involves movement not explicable by, and sometimes against, electrochemical gradients. Absorption may be modified also by "solvent drag"—that is, incorporation of solute into the bulk flow of water. Solvent drag is related to the particulate size of solutes in solution relative to hypothetical, water-filled "pores" through which solvent moves. Diamond[11] has described the functional variability of "pores" at different intestinal loci. It appears that epithelial surfaces vary greatly in their degree of "tightness" or "leakiness," reflecting the functional size of "pores," which are localized to the junctions between epithelial cells.

Absorption of sodium is considered central to the absorption of water, other electrolytes, and certain nutrients throughout the intestines. Sodium transport is active throughout the small and large intestines, and inhibition of active sodium absorption leads to net accumulation of sodium in the lumen, which in turn creates an osmotic gradient along which water flows. An ATP-dependent "sodium pump," which normally transports sodium from lumen to blood across the basolateral surface of enterocytes, is sensitive to a variety of toxic, humoral, or mechanical insults. Inhibition of active Na^+ transport can "unmask" a simultaneous mechanism for loss of sodium from extracellular fluid into the lumen. There is evidence that mucosal villi are the prime site of fluid absorption and that crypts are the source of secretions. Several additional factors influence the transport of water and electrolytes in the intestines. Glucocorticoids, mineralocorticoids, gastrointestinal hormones (gastrin, secretin, and CCK), and other active neuropeptides (VIP, enkephalins) alter absorption and/or secretion of electrolytes and water. Overproduction of peptides is thought to be pathogenic in the secretory diarrheas associated with nonislet cell tumors of the pancreas.[30]

Absorption in the jejunum

Sodium is absorbed actively against small electrochemical gradients and also moves with bulk flow of water through the relatively large mucosal "pores" of the proximal bowel. Glucose, other actively absorbed monosaccharides, amino acids, and bicarbonate ions all enhance sodium absorption; sodium in turn augments glucose and amino acid transport. Water transport is considered to be passive and to depend on osmotic forces. Potassium also moves across the mucosa following its concentration gradient between the lumen and blood, modified by the small negative electric potential of jejunal mucosa. Chloride mostly follows sodium, to preserve electrical neutrality in the lumen. Bicarbonate disappears rapidly from the lumen by a mechanism involving either active ionic absorption or neutralization of bicarbonate by hydrogen ions secreted by the mucosa.[37]

Absorption in the ileum

Each day, 2 to 3 liters of neutral, isotonic chyme passes through the ileum. The ileal mucosa is less permeable than the jejunal to simple diffusion of ions; however, sodium is absorbed actively against larger electrochemical gradients, and water follows.[19,38] Movement of potassium across the mucosa of the ileum can be explained by electrochemical gradients, but the mechanisms of anion movement are more complex. Absorption of chloride and secretion of bicarbonate are coupled by a process that may involve active transport of one or both ions. It follows that pH and bicarbonate concentrations increase in the distal small bowel (Fig. 36-2), and losses from the distal small bowel are more likely to result in metabolic acidosis.

Absorption in the colon and rectum

Highly efficient mechanisms for absorption of water and electrolytes are present in the colon; 1 to 2 liters of liquid ileal contents is converted to formed feces every 24 h, and more than 90 pecent of the sodium and chloride entering the cecum is absorbed.[9,10] Sodium transport is active and occurs against very large concentration gradients; chloride is absorbed simultaneously by a passive process, thereby establishing osmotic gradients necessary for passive absorption of water. Active bicarbonate secretion occurs in the colon; part of this appears to be exchanged for chloride absorption.[8,10] Organic acids are also major constituents of colonic content, and they modify the intraluminal pH and ionic exchanges between the lumen and circulation. These compounds ("short-chain fatty acids," or SCFAs) are generated in the colon by anaerobic metabolism by fecal bacteria of unabsorbed carbohydrates from the diet and other endogenous sources (mucus, glycoproteins). Butyrate, propionate, and acetate are the major products;[24] all are well absorbed by the colon,[31] and their absorption may even promote absorption of other ions (e.g., sodium). The presence of SCFAs in fecal fluid is to be anticipated in any patient taking oral nutrients, and their excretion in excess quantities should be considered only as a marker, not an etiology, of diarrhea. Though the colon absorbs potassium in health, small amounts may be secreted under certain circumstances (see Chap. 14). The secretory process is predominantly passive; potassium diffuses along the electric gradient created by the highly negative colonic mucosa. In addition, potassium may be secreted in the mucus discharged by the abundant goblet cells of the colon. This loss contributes to potassium depletion in villous adenoma and other diseases characterized by excess loss of intestinal mucus.[32,34]

Normally, feces contain approximately 100 ml water and less than 5 meq sodium per day. Conservation of sodium by the colon is particularly important, since the small intestine cannot absorb sodium sufficiently well to maintain sodium balance on diets greatly restricted in sodium. Thus, subjects with ileostomies are particularly sensitive to sodium depletion.[20]

Transit

The integration of propulsion and absorption is important to the subsequent handling of water and electrolytes by the gastrointestinal tract. Duodenal function is coordinated by the fine control of gastirc emptying which is evoked by the entrance of food into the duodenum. Emptying of gastric contents into the duodenum is slow and intermittent; in the antrum, both propulsion and retropulsion occur. Osmolality of the duodenal contents exerts a major control of gastric emptying through osmoreceptors in the duodenal wall. Neural impulses carried by the vagi mediate and integrate both the release of the peptides and the contractile response of the stomach.

Fasting and postcibal motility

The fasting bowel is not quiescent but exhibits cycles of contractility, which are interrupted by food.[40] With a periodicity of approximately 2 h, an intense burst of motor activity begins in the stomach; at this time every "pacesetter potential" (slow wave) has an action potential associated with it, and the antrum contracts powerfully at its maximal rate of 3 contractions per minute. This wave of intense motor activity passes caudally through duodenum, jejunum, and ileum. The velocity of the "front" is such that on its reaching the terminal ileum another "migrating motor complex" originates in the stomach. At any single locus the cycle lasts approximately 2 h during fasting, each intense burst of motility lasting 5 to 15 min. The remainder of the 2-h cycle is taken up with relative quiescence (lasting approximately 5 to 30 min.—phase I of the cycle), intermittent contractile activity (about 100 min—phase II), and then the migrating complex (phase III). The migrating complex has been described as the "interdigestive housekeeper." The function proposed is to sweep secretions, desquamated cells, and food residues distally, in preparation for another meal. Food interrupts the cycle, replacing it with the "fed pattern" of intermittent contractions (similar to phase II) that last for 4 to 10 h. Whereas transit is rapid in phase III of fasting, it is slower after a meal.

Control of gastrointestinal motility

The cholinergic system exercises important control over the proximal gut. Vagal denervation impairs receptive relaxation of the stomach and, by reducing gastric accommodation to large volumes, speeds the emptying of liquids. Vagal denervation also impairs the duodenal "brake" on gastric emptying. On the other hand, antral contractions are also weakened by vagotomy, and hence the grinding and emptying of solids are reduced. More rapid emptying of liquids and delayed emptying of solids characterize the postvagotomy state. The sympathetic nervous system becomes more important in the distal bowel, particularly in the coordination of rectal contractions and relaxation of the anal sphincters. A third autonomic system ("noncholinergic, nonadrenergic") also exists, but the mechanism of neurotransmission is as yet unclear. Among the candidates are ATP ("purinergic"), dopaminelike compounds, and the gastrointestinal polypetides (neuropeptides such as vasoactive intestinal polypeptide, neurotensin, substance P, and enkephalins). Some gastrointestinal hormones or neuropeptides may act locally on adjacent epithelial cells or nervous tissue, exhibiting a so-called "paracrine" function. Somatostatin is of special interest, since it augments solute and water absorption, blocks the secretion of other gut peptides, and provides a novel therapeutic approach (see under "Treatment" below). Although clinical associations between disorders of motility and abnormal water and electrolyte metabolism are often striking, the normal relationships between motility, secretion, and absorption of electrolytes in the intestine are still poorly understood.

PATHOPHYSIOLOGY

Water and electrolyte metabolism can become deranged when intestinal motility, digestion, or absorption is altered by disease (Table 36-3). Mismanaged fluid is either lost to the outside or sequestered inside the body. Vomiting, diarrhea, and fistulas are routes of external loss; internal loss by sequestration is characteristic of obstruction, ileus, and peritonitis (Fig. 36-3). The fluid lost is usually isotonic, and in most instances the major deficits are of water and sodium. In addition, potassium depletion can be expected in chronic or severe diarrhea, and alkalosis may be superimposed when vomiting, with loss of acid gastric secretion, has been prominent. These characteristic patterns depend on the source and duration of fluid loss. However, variations are common, since often more than one problem is present. For example, obstruction of the small bowel may result in both intestinal sequestration of fluid and massive vomiting.

Loss of isotonic fluid diminishes the plasma volume and may precipitate hypovolemic shock. Usually plasma concentrations of electrolytes are initially preserved, but if the patient drinks large amounts of electrolyte-free water, the plasma will become progressively dilute, with hyponatremia. Compensatory or aggravating disorders of fluid, electrolyte, or acid-base balance may be superimposed on gastrointestinal disease when changes in renal, cardiac, or pulmonary function result from alterations in the extracellular fluid volume, its pH, or its electrolyte composition.

The effects of disease on the normal functions of the gastrointestinal tract and their integration remain mostly conjectural. For example, the effect of intestinal obstruction on secretion in the proximal intestine is largely unknown. The major reasons for our ignorance are the

TABLE 36-3 • Precipitating factors and treatment of common metabolic disorders

Metabolic disorder	Common precipitating factors	Treatment
Volume depletion	Severe vomiting, diarrhea, or sequestration	Sodium chloride or colloids
Sodium depletion with "dilutional hyponatremia"	Diarrhea, obstruction, peritonitis, ileostomy	Sodium chloride
Potassium depletion	Diarrhea (severe or chronic), vomiting	Potassium chloride
Alkalosis	Vomiting, diarrhea	Ammonium chloride, lysine monohydrochloride
Acidosis	Diarrhea, obstruction, ileus, drainage or fistulas of pancreaticobiliary system, urinary diversions, short bowel (lactic)	Sodium lactate or bicarbonate, antibiotics
Sodium excess	Sodium chloride overload	Stop fluids; give diuretics
Water excess	Overload with sodium-poor fluids	Stop fluids; if severe, use hypertonic saline solution
Calcium depletion	Malabsorption, acute pancreatitis	Parenteral or oral gluconate, calcium, vitamin D
Magnesium depletion	Prolonged parenteral feeding, ileal disease, diarrhea	Parenteral magnesium sulfate

difficulties of applying more sophisticated investigative techniques to seriously ill patients.

DIARRHEA

Definition and basic mechanisms

Diarrhea is characterized by increased frequency and excess water content of the stools. Individual bowel habits vary, but more than four soft or watery bowel movements each 24 h is abnormal. Diarrheal fluid is often isotonic with extracellular fluid; sodium, chloride, inorganic anions, and potassium are the predominant solutes. Bicarbonate may also be lost from the body, but is not often recovered in stools as such. SCFAs are generated in the lumen, especially when oral intake continues; they neutralize bicarbonate and are the major fecal anions. Diarrhea results from impaired absorption or excessive secretion of solute, usually sodium; the excess water follows solute along osmotic gradients.

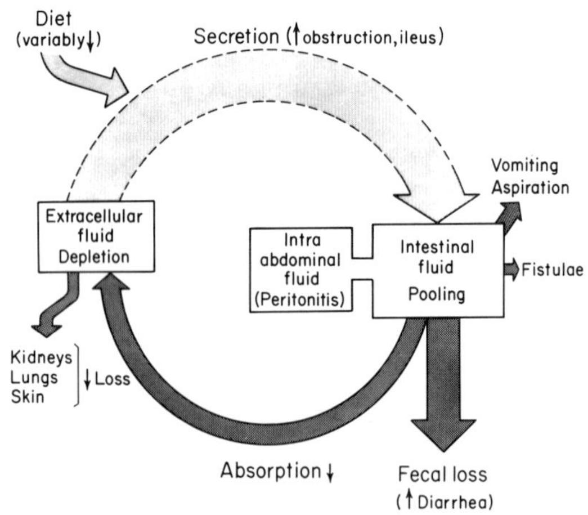

FIGURE 36-3 • Disturbances of the enterosystemic cycle of electrolytes and water produced by disease and resulting in external loss or internal sequestration of fluid.

Pathophysiology

Diarrhea can be caused by excessive intake, maldigestion, malabsorption, abnormal fluid secretion (including exudation), and changes in intestinal motility.

Excessive intake

This rarely causes diarrhea in health, since the capacity of the intestines for absorption of water and solute is great, and volumes that exceed it are usually rejected by vomiting. Occasionally, excessive intake of fat can cause steatorrhea. Certain laxatives (those containing polyvalent, slowly absorbed ions such as $MgSO_4$) act by osmotic effects and, when taken in excessive amounts, can produce diarrhea. Osmotic diarrhea can also follow the ingestion of poorly absorbed carbohydrates such as mannitol, lactose, or lactulose.

Maldigestive diarrhea

When normal digestion is impaired, adsorption of nutrients is decreased and osmotic diarrhea results. The most common cause of steatorrhea are digestive defects: pancreatic insufficiency; bile acid deficiency due to hepatobiliary diseases; and the consequences of gastric surgery, when mixing of digestive secretions and nutrients is poorly coordinated. Carbohydrate absorption is decreased when the brush border enzymes that hydrolyze disaccharides to monosaccharides are deficient.[5] For example, lactase deficiency is extremely common in some ethnic groups (Asians, blacks), and diarrhea should be anticipated in such patients if they ingest lactose (milk sugar). Maldigestive diarrhea is closely related to malabsorptive diarrhea and resembles it.

Malabsorptive diarrhea

This results from mucosal or submucosal diseases that impair absorption by the small or large intestine. Loss of mucosal surface area, as with resection of the bowel or certain fistulas, has the same result. Mucosal disease may impair sodium transport mechanisms directly, or the presence of unabsorbed dietary or digestive components (such as fat or bile acids) may inhibit sodium absorption in the colon. Deficiency of a mucosal cell active transport system (as for monosaccharides) rarely causes an osmotic diarrhea.

Structural changes usually result in generalized exudation. For example, in ulcerative colitis, diffuse mucosal ulceration permits blood, mucus, protein, and electrolytes to exude into the bowel. The normal mechanisms for sodium reabsorption are also disturbed; excessive losses of sodium and chloride are common with generalized colitis.

Secretory diarrhea

Increased secretion of water and electrolytes, without structural change in the intestine, is also a common cause of diarrhea.[30] The ability of intestinal mucosa to secrete isotonic fluid has been known for many years, but has been largely ignored. The stimuli known to evoke intestinal secretion are diverse (Table 36-2). Certain baterial enterotoxins, such as those of *Vibrio cholerae* and *E. coli*, induce secretion by increasing cyclic nucleotides (cAMP or cGMP) in mucosal cells. These systems, together with intracellular levels of calcium ions, have been studied intensively and are conceived of as "intracellular messengers" for the process of secretion. "Traveler's diarrhea" is due to enterotoxigenic strains of *E. coli* in one-third to one-half of cases.

Partial or recently relieved intestinal obstruction is often associated with diarrhea. Obstruction appears to impair normal absorption and to increase proximal secretion as well. The diarrhea that accompanies steatorrhea appears to have a secretory component. The dietary fatty acid, oleic acid, is chemically similar to ricinoleic acid (the active principle of castor oil) and shares with it the property of stimulating intestinal fluid secretion in the small and large bowel. Bile acid malabsorption is often associated with steatorrhea, usually when the underlying disease involves the ileum. Bile acids are mucosal secretagogues; when excess bile acids enter the colon, they act as endogenous cathartics.

Hormones may also stimulate small bowel secretion of fluids. Certain neoplasms (pancreatic islet-cell tumors, bronchogenic carcinomas, and ganglioneuromas) produce peptides (e.g., VIP) that dramatically increase small intestinal secretion. The diarrhea of the Zollinger-Ellison syndrome probably involves several mechanisms, most of them dependent on hypersecretion of gastric fluid. Excessive acid in the small intestine damages the mucosa and also leads to steatorrhea, because lipase and bile acids are inactivated at a low pH. It has also been suggested that hypergastrinemia may directly stimulate bowel secretion.

The experimental observation that glucose absorption and glucose-stimulated sodium absorption continue despite marked secretion of electrolytes and fluid has led to the use of oral glucose-electrolyte solutions in the treatment of cholera and other secretory diarrheas. It is clear that such therapy can reduce the volume of intestinal fluid loss by promoting the absorption of fluid.[15,26,30]

Metabolic consequences

Severe diarrhea can lead to a daily loss of 2 to 10 liters of fluid together with large amounts of sodium, potassium, and bicarbonate (Fig. 36-4). Dehydration, decreased body sodium, hypokalemia, and, usually, acidosis result. Hyponatremia may be secondary to the ingestion of sodium-free liquids or parenteral replacement of water in excess of sodium. In some osmotic diarrheas, water may be lost in excess of sodium, since solutes other than sodium (e.g., disaccharides, organic acids) also trap water in the lumen. Disproportionate loss of water can lead to hypernatremic dehydration, which may be aggravated by the use of replacement fluids rich in solutes, especially sodium.[15] This "hypertonicity syndrome" is seen particularly in young children (under 2 years of age) and requires cautious and appropriate fluid replacement (see also Chap. 21). Clinically significant depletion of total body potassium is to be expected only in severe or chronic diarrhea. Rarely, massive secretion of colonic mucus may occur. Hypokalemia characterizes some islet-cell tumors ("pancreatic cholera") and severe laxative abuse. Prolonged hypokalemia may also injure the renal medulla in

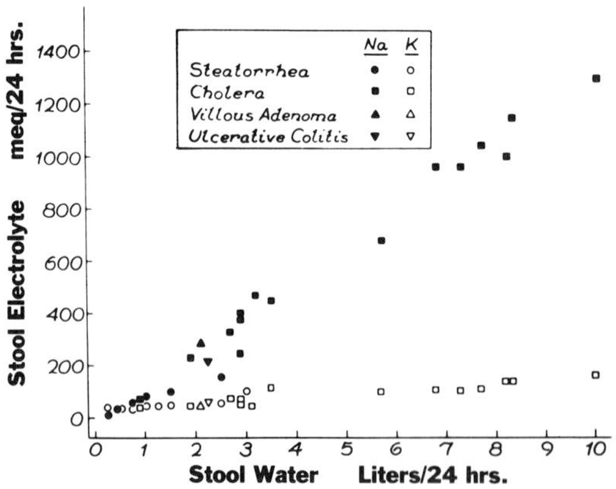

FIGURE 36-4 • **Relationship between fecal losses of electrolytes and water in certain diarrheal diseases. Note that sodium loss increases with greater loss of volume, whereas potassium loss remains constant despite fecal volumes of 5 to 10 liter/day. (From Fordtran JS, Dietschy JM: *Gastroenterology* 50:263–285, 1966. By permission of The Williams & Wilkins Company, Baltimore.)**

such a way that urinary concentrating ability is impaired (see also Chap. 22).

The anions in stool are bicarbonate and organic radicals derived from the fermentative action of colonic bacteria. The relative excretion of acid or base in the stools can be estimated from fecal concentrations of sodium, potassium, and chloride. When the sum of sodium and potassium exceeds the fecal chloride plus the plasma bicarbonate concentration, bicarbonate (or its organic equivalent) is being excreted to excess, and acidosis may be predicted. Bacterial-derived organic acids convert colonic sodium bicarbonate to the acid salt, CO_2, and water. Net loss of alkali is avoided because the salt of the organic acid is normally absorbed and metabolically converted (oxidized) to bicarbonate. Fecal loss of organic anions, therefore, represents loss of potential alkali. However, great deviations from normal acid-base balance are unusual in diarrhea. Additional information can be gained from the comparison of the osmolality of stool water with the concentrations of constituent ions.[25] They can give indications of the nature of the diarrheal mechanism, especially the distinction between secretory and osmotic diarrheas. When secretion is the major mechanism, the osmotic gap (osmolality minus twice the sum of sodium and potassium concentrations) is less than 60 to 80 mosm. Osmolar gaps in excess of 60 to 80 mosm indirectly identify the presence of osmotically active particles not accounted for by sodium, potassium, and their attendant anions. Several fresh samples should be analyzed; if stools are sufficiently fluid, a simple contrifugate will suffice for analysis. A second clinical point to note is the effect on stool volumes to a 48-h fast, supplemented by basal parenteral replacement therapy. Secretory diarrheas continue, with a minimal reduction of stool volumes; osmotic and malabsorptive diarrheas are markedly reduced.

The metabolic consequences of diarrhea at their most acute and extreme develop in infantile diarrhea and Asiatic cholera (Fig. 36-5). In the latter, 10 to 20 liters of isotonic fluid may be lost per day. Each liter of stool contains 100 to 140 meq of sodium, 20 to 40 meq of potassium, 80 to 100 meq of chloride, and 30 to 50 meq of bicarbonate, with insignificant protein, fat, and sugar. Dehydration, acidosis, and hypokalemia develop rapidly, and acute renal failure may be an early complication.

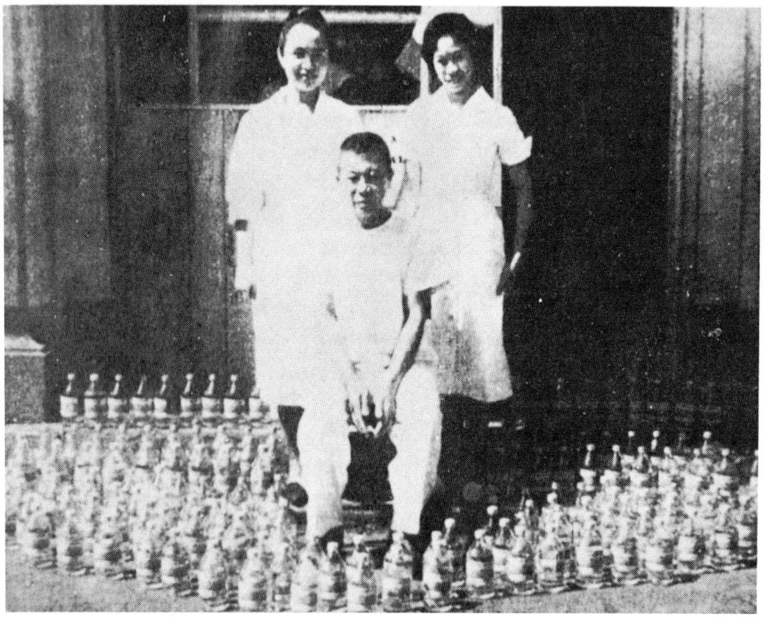

FIGURE 36-5 • **Patient after recovery from Asiatic cholera. This 53-kg human required 60 liters intravenous fluid replacement during 5 days of acute symptoms. (From Phillips RA: *Fed Proc,* 23:705–712, 1964. By permission of the Federation of American Societies for Experimental Biology.)**

Adequate therapy often requires an initial 3 to 6 liters of fluid given intravenously, followed by continuous replacement of subsequent losses.

The incidence of disorders of acid-base balance in patients with severe diarrhea is 70 percent or more. The entire spectrum of disturbances may be found, since respiratory and renal homeostatic responses modify the picture. Acidosis is the more common disorder and is seen especially in pediatric patients, in secretory diarrheas, and in patients with infectious diarrheas. Active secretion produces large volumes of fluid rich in sodium and chloride in the small bowel. During passage of this fluid through the ileum and colon, its composition is altered, leading to major fecal losses of bicarbonate (or its organic equivalent) and potassium, causing metabolic acidosis. Alkalosis is reported in other patients; its pathogenesis remains uncertain.[4]

Two special circumstances of excessive chloride loss need to be mentioned. *Congenital chloridorrhea* is a rare, congenital condition of ileocolonic transport in which voluminous diarrhea occurs.[7] Chloride concentrations in stool water are very high (up to 150 meq/liter), and defects of ileocolonic electrolyte transfer have been demonstrated by intraluminal perfusions of electrolyte solutions.[1,17,22] Although the stomach and proximal small bowel appear to function normally, the distal bowel is unable to reabsorb chloride which cannot be exchanged for bicarbonate. Sodium is absorbed normally; hydrogen ions accompany some of the secreted chloride, neutralizing bicarbonate and acidifying the contents. Together with the renal compensation for contraction of the extracellular volume, a profound alkalosis can develop. The initial description of the condition was "congenital alkalosis with diarrhea."[7]

Villous adenomas of the upper rectum and sigmoid colon may also produce voluminous watery secretions with losses of potassium, sodium, and water. Variable patterns of acid-base imbalance have been reported; hypokalemia is usual and often extreme; acidosis and azotemia are also usually present, although, in some patients, fecal losses of chloride are extremely high and a metabolic alkalosis develops.[14,21,32,34]

INTESTINAL FISTULAS AND RESECTION OF THE INTESTINES

Definition and basic mechanisms

Fistulas are abnormal communications between the bowel and the skin (external fistula) or another hollow viscus (internal fistula). Fistulas arise spontaneously, as a result of gastrointestinal disease, or are created surgically as stomas. The same disturbances of absorption may develop with either form. Loss of absorptive surface, from either resection or short-circuiting, and contamination of the proximal bowel with fecal organisms (as in the blind-loop syndrome) account for most of the problems. Some bacteria deconjugate and dehydroxylate bile acids, precipitating them in the lumen, where they cannot form micelles with fat. Maldigestion of fat with steatorrhea and loss of sodium, water, and other ions—including calcium and magnesium—follow. Bypass or resection of the terminal ileum causes unique problems. Absorption of bile acids at the normal site in the ileum is impossible, and bile acids are lost into the colon. Depletion of the bile acid pool may be severe, impairing digestion of fat in the proximal small intestine and leading to steatorrhea. The presence of excessive amounts of bile acids in the colon blocks sodium and water absorption and adds a watery component to the steatorrhea.

After ileal resection or bypass, a syndrome of hyperoxaluria and renal calculi may develop.[12] This syndrome is produced by increased absorption of dietary oxalate, due to increased passive permeability of colonic mucosa to oxalate and to the binding of calcium ions in the bowel lumen by ionized fatty acids; the reduction of "free" intraluminal calcium increases oxalate solubility. When ileal bypass is performed for obesity, two additional complications may occur: hepatic steatosis, which can lead to coma and death; and a migratory polyarthralgia.

Clinical causes

Spontaneous fistulas are usually complications of peptic ulcer, neoplasia, inflammatory bowel disease, or pancreatitis. Fistulas may also result from trauma. Postoperative fistulas, which usually follow leakage from anastomoses, are numerically important. Intestinal resections are usually performed for inflammatory, vascular, or malignant disease of the bowel. Ileal bypass procedures are sometimes recommended in the treatment of morbid obesity or hyperlipidemia.

Metabolic consequences

External gastric, duodenal, and jejunal fistulas

These can discharge up to 5 liters of fluid daily.[13] The fluid is isotonic and contains high concentrations of sodium; dehydration and sodium depletion are, therefore, common. The anions lost depend on the exact site of the fistua. Acidosis may develop if the primary loss is of duodenal secretion; alkalosis may develop if the loss is mainly gastric. Pancreatic enzymes may digest the abdominal wall. Fistulas of the jejunum are not common and rarely cause severe electrolyte disturbance; however, in approximately 15 percent of cases, enough fluid is lost to produce dehydration. Normal acid-base balance is usually preserved, since the effluent has a nearly neutral pH.

Biliary and pancreatic fistulas

Sodium and water are lost through a biliary fistula, but the loss does not usually create a problem. Pancreatic fistulas are more serious: the loss of fluid can amount to 1 liter daily, acidosis may result from the loss of bicarbonate, and the condition is often complicated by severe autolysis of the abdominal wall from pancreatic enzymes.

Fistulas of the ileum or colon

These seldom produce serious disorders of water and electrolyte metabolism unless the rest of the intestine is diseased, as, for example, with Crohn's disease. A patient with an ileostomy constantly loses excessive water and electrolytes from the bowel and may be chronically water- and sodium-depleted.[20] Sodium balance may be precarious even when stomal function appears normal, since the colon, which normally preserves sodium, is nonfunctional. Consequently, ileostomies may discharge up to 100 meq of sodium each day, regardless of the state of body sodium balance. The water content (up to 1 liter daily) is also greater than that of feces. Since the patient tends toward a low body water and has an obligatory loss via the ileostomy, urine volume is usually low; this may contribute to the increased incidence of urinary calculi following such operations. Development of novel surgical approaches to proctocolectomy has seen the advent of the Kock pouch (continent ileostomy) and ileal pouch–anal anastomosis. Metabolically, these operations should be considered as identical with conventional ileostomies.

Internal fistulas

A fistula between the upper and lower intestine reroutes intestinal contents past some of the mucosa available for absorption. Bacterial overgrowth in the upper intestine often contributes to symptomatology. Inadvertent gastroileostomy is most serious, since inadequately digested food is delivered from the stomach directly to the distal small bowel. In most other circumstances, relatively little food is short-circuited; gastrocolic fistulas, for example, cause malabsorption and diarrhea as a consequence of contamination of the upper intestine by fecal bacteria.

Anastomoses between ureters and bowel

Ureterosigmoidostomy was performed often in the 1950s, but the procedure was superseded by various forms of the ileal conduit when metabolic acidosis, hyperchloremia, and azotemia became recognized as predictable sequelae of this iatrogenic fistula.[6] The metabolic consequences of ureterosigmoidostomy have a logical pathophysiologic basis. Bathing of colonic mucosa with urine rich in chloride and urea will lead to (1) avid reabsorption of chloride ions, some of which will be exchanged for secreted bicarbonate, and (2) bacterial ureolysis with absorption of ammonium. Incomplete drainage of the "colonic bladder" and urinary stasis often resulted in ascending infection, with a further compromise of renal function. Although ileal mucosa also has the potential for chloride-bicarbonate exchange, hyperchloremic metabolic acidosis is less of a problem after fashioning of ileal conduits; more attention is now also given to avoiding stasis.[2]

Short-bowel syndrome

After massive intestinal resection, usually for mesenteric vascular disease or regional enteritis, a syndrome of chronic "intestinal insufficiency" may develop, with multiple disturbances of nutrition, hydration, and electrolyte metabolism. As little as 12 in. of the duodenojejunal segment may barely support life, but a patient with less than 50 in. of small intestine usually needs specific therapy to combat the malabsorptive effects of a minimal absorptive surface, hypermotility and rapid transit of nutrients, reduced bile acid pool, lack of gastrointestinal mucosal hormones, bacterial colonization of the small bowel, and poor digestion. Some of these unfortunate patients can now be managed with total parenteral nutrition (see also Chap. 44).

Metabolic acidosis with the predominant anion being D-lactate has been described in patients with the short-bowel syndrome and after jejunoileal bypass[29,36] (see also Chap. 25). An analogous syndrome, in ruminants overfed with grains, is well recognized in the veterinary literature. Bacterial fermentation of carbohydrate moieties that reach the colon in malabsorptive states produces large quantities of both D- and L-lactic acid. However, only the D form accumulates, because the L form is metabolized efficiently after absorption. Neurologic manifestations are prominent. Bizarre behavior, slurred speech, and ataxia have been noted. Treatment with antibiotics has been associated with correction of acidosis and the neurologic abnormalities.

INTESTINAL SEQUESTRATION: OBSTRUCTION AND ILEUS

Definition and basic mechanisms

Mechanical obstruction or atonic arrest of the intestine (ileus) has characteristic consequences.

In mechanical obstruction, distal progress of air, food, and secretions ceases. The proximal bowel distends and becomes compromised; prolonged obstruction can lead to net secretion of fluid.[35] In experimental obstruction of the canine small intestine, absorption from distended bowel segments diminishes after 6 to 12 h and is replaced by secretion of sodium and water. Increased intraluminal pressure, elevation of portal venous and lymphatic pressures, ischemia, and the toxic effects of rapid bacterial multiplication in the involved segment are among the mechanisms proposed to account for these changes.

Once obstruction is established, edema, petechial hemorrhages, and, finally (if the condition has gone untreated), necrosis and gangrene develop in the bowel wall. These changes are most pronounced when occlusion or strangulation of the vasculature occurs, or in closed-loop obstruction, which produces exceedingly high intraluminal pressures. Excessive permeability of the damaged intestinal mucosa allows loss of proteins from the blood to the intestinal lumen, while bacteria and their toxins move simultaneously in the opposite direction. Peritonitis, therefore, frequently complicates untreated obstruction. Additional injury to ischemic mucosa may be caused by compounds in the intestinal lumen, including pancreatic enzymes, bile acids, and bacterial exotoxins. However, the sequence whereby untreated obstructions leads to irreversible shock and death is uncertain. Volume depletion, free perforation of the bowel, bacterial toxins, gram-negative septicemia, and splanchnic vasoconstriction have been implicated. The general role of bacteria is well established experimentally, since mortality from obstruction is reduced in newborn and in germ-free animals, and in those that have previously received broad-spectrum antibiotics.

Functional obstruction of the bowel (ileus) occurs most frequently in association with peritonitis. The pathogenesis of ileus is unknown, but the condition has conventionally been subdivided into two entities. In spastic ileus, a ring of muscle, constricted because of altered autonomic innervation through the celiac ganglion, is thought to occlude the bowel. Adynamic ileus is postulated to result from neural inhibition of coordinated motor activity, producing atony of the entire small intestine and large bowel. Ileus may complicate spinal injuries and can be induced by ganglionic blocking agents. Hypokalemia is thought to produce adynamic ileus by decreasing the contractibility of smooth muscle. The metabolic consequences of ileus are the same whatever the source, and it is hard to justify the maintenance of two different classifications.

Pseudoobstruction[3,18] is clinically similar to ileus. It is believed to be a manifestation of chronic neuromuscular disease of the gastrointestinal tract. Pathogenic mechanisms are thought to include autonomic denervation (diabetic visceral neuropathy), replacement of smooth muscle by connective tissue (systemic sclerosis and other connective tissue disease), and incoordination of muscular contraction or relaxation (the aganglioneurosis of congenital megacolon).

Clinical causes

Mechanical obstruction of the bowel is caused either by lesions involving the entire circumference of the intestine (as with volvulus, certain congenital malformations, hernias, and adhesive bands) or by lesions that encroach on the lumen (usually tumors or inflammatory disease). Less often, foreign bodies may occlude the bowel by impaction. Ileus (atonic obstruction) is often a temporary reaction to laparotomy. Several intraabdominal diseases, especially pancreatitis, peritonitis, intraabdominal hemorrhage, and occlusive vascular disease, constitute the majority of other instances. Ileus may also occur during the course of systemic disorders, including uremia and septicemia, in which it may have a neurogenic basis.

Metabolic consequences

Hypovolemia, hyponatremia, and hypochloremia are the major abnormalities observed in most cases. During the course of obstruction or ileus, several liters of extracellular fluid may become sequestered in the intestine. With 24 h of experimental obstruction of the distal small bowel, 50 percent or more of the plasma volume has been thus lost.[27] Additional amounts may accumulate in the peritoneal cavity. The degree of total fluid loss varies with the site, duration, and degree of obstruction; the loss may be sufficiently acute and extensive to precipitate hypovolemic shock. Plasma concentrations of electrolytes are initially preserved, since the fluid lost is isotonic; but the patient usually becomes thirsty and drinks sodium-poor fluid, so that he or she is often hyponatremic when first seen. Body chloride is depleted through vomiting. Loss of bicarbonate, impairment of renal function due to hypovolemia, and starvation with consequent ketosis may individually or collectively produce mild acidosis. Alkalosis may be prominent and, early in obstruction of the upper intestine, associated with severe vomiting; but when reflex vomiting is associated with distal obstruction, acidosis is to be expected. The outcome of relieved obstruction is largely determined by the presence of complications: gram-negative sepsis, peritonitis, bowel perforation, and acute renal failure.[27]

PERITONITIS

Definition and basic mechanisms

Peritonitis is an inflammation of the peritoneal membrane due to bacterial or chemical injury. When acute and generalized, it leads to major metabolic disorders and changes in intestinal function. Normally, the large surface area of the peritoneum mediates rapid transport of water and electrolytes between the peritoneal cavity and the circulation. In disease, impairment of these transport mechanisms leads to sequestration of fluid and electrolytes within the peritoneal cavity; the amount may be augmented by the osmotic effects of concomitant exudation of protein.

Clinical causes

Acute peritonitis is usually a complication of either intra-abdominal or pelvic disease. Perforation of the intestine or gallbladder, pancreatitis, penetrating wounds (including laparotomy), and pelvic infections account for most cases. Primary peritoneal infection with pyogenic organisms occurs rarely in children. Tuberculous peritonitis is now uncommon but may manifest as ascites.

Metabolic consequences

Peritonitis primarily causes loss of sodium and water into the peritoneal cavity, but the condition is often complicated by perforation of a viscus or by ileus. Reflex hypotension and shock may predominate immediately after perforation. As large volumes of fluid accumulate, hypovolemia, hyponatremia, acidosis, and renal failure may develop.

IATROGENIC DISORDERS

Iatrogenic disturbances of water and electrolyte metabolism are common in gastrointestinal disease, particularly after abdominal surgery (see also Chaps. 43 and 45). Excessive replacement of fluid and electrolytes, especially as parenteral sodium chloride solutions but also as enemas containing absorbable sodium, represents the most common problem. The decreased ability of the kidneys to excrete sodium in the immediate postoperative period is often the precipitating factor. Fluid overload leading to water intoxication, or sodium retention leading to pulmonary edema or cardiac failure may result—especially in patients with coexistent cardiopulmonary or renal disorders. Depletion of fluid and electrolytes may be produced by prolonged suction of the stomach or intestines if parenteral replacement is inadequate or inappropriate. Certain diets and medication may also produce characteristic syndromes affecting water and electrolyte metabolism. The milk-alkali syndrome, usually found when compulsive patients with peptic ulcer follow an overrigorous therapeutic program, develops from absorption of excessive calcium (prescribed as milk or as an antacid) and absorbable alkali. Alkalosis and hypercalcemia result; later developments include nephrocalcinosis, metastatic calcification, and, ultimately, renal failure. Vomiting is common and may aggravate the alkalosis, dehydration, and impairment of renal function. Anticholinergic drugs, if given to patients with incipient pyloric obstruction, may initiate or aggravate vomiting and cause "gastric alkalosis." Diarrhea, sometimes with dehydration and hypokalemic alkalosis, is a feature of laxative abuse and of prolonged use of enemas. It may occur acutely or as a late chronic complication in patients receiving radiotherapy.

TREATMENT

GENERAL PRINCIPLES

In most instances, the history and physical examination, at best, will yield only a rough approximation of the amount of fluid and the nature of the electrolytes required for managing any clinical problem. Usually it is possible to await the results of appropriate laboratory investigations before embarking on a specific course of therapy. The questions immediately posed revolve around the need to give fluids, the route whereby fluids should be administered, and whether, in addition, aspiration of the gastrointestinal tract should be performed. At the same time, one prepares for rapid delivery of specific therapy for the causative lesion, if such is available. When early, but not emergency, surgical treatment of the condition is needed, effective intestinal intubation and preoperative correction of water, electrolyte, and acid-base disorders should be completed within 24 h or, at the most, 48 h.

The oral route provides the simplest way of replacing fluid and electrolytes. However, it is often contraindicated, most commonly by vomiting, suspicion of certain lesions (such as perforation or complete bowel obstruction), the possibility of early abdominal surgical treatment, or the presence of hypovolemic shock. In such instances, or if dehydration is clinically apparent and thus consistent with a volume deficit of 5 liters or more in an adult, the parenteral route for fluid replacement is preferred. Under rare circumstances, fluid can be administered by other methods, including the peritoneal, rectal, and even subcutaneous routes. Alternatives to oral or intravenous fluid replacement are, in general, unsatisfactory, and secure placement of a needle in an adequate vein is a prime objective.

The decision to intubate the gastrointestinal tract should be made thoughtfully. Continued vomiting, abdominal distension (especially if fluid levels are visible in distended bowel on radiologic examination), obstruction, ileus, and suspected perforation of a viscus are common indications for intubation and aspiration. Both are usually required as preoperative measures when obstruction, ileus, or perforation is suspected or proved. Once the decision to intubate the gastrointestinal tract beyond the stomach has been made, the tip of the tube should be advanced to a point just proximal to the site of the lesion, with the guidance of a radiologist and under fluoroscopic control. Much time and frustration can be saved by this approach, especially when the tube is traversing the gastroduodenal area. Once securely placed in the second part of the duodenum, the tube may be advanced at intervals from the bedside. Periodic fluoroscopic monitoring is essential. A wide variety of tubes and suction instruments is available. We prefer a sumptype tube for aspiration of the stomach, and employ an elongated version for more distal lesions.

If cardiac, pulmonary, and renal functions are satisfactory, normal saline solution is usually a good choice. If hypovolemia or shock predominates, colloidal solutions (blood, plasma, or dextran) are preferred. When laboratory and other data become available, therapy can be appropriately modified. After adequate replacement of the initial deficit is achieved, as judged by the clinical condition, vital signs, and urine flow, further replacement of losses is dictated by the fluid balance and evolving clinical findings.

The amount and nature of replacement therapy cannot be specified in advance. Each patient presents an individual problem, often involving a combination of disorders. In each case an approach based on an appreciation of the pathophysiology, evaluation of all information, and response to initial therapy is essential.

MANAGEMENT OF CHARACTERISTIC COMBINED DISORDERS

Hypokalemic, hypochloremic alkalosis

This sequence results most often from prolonged vomiting or aspiration of gastric contents and reflects predominant loss of hydrochloric acid. Fluid replacement can be mainly sodium chloride, and provided the output of urine is adequate (greater than 600 ml/day), potassium chloride (40 to 100 meq/day) can be added. The degree of alkalosis and its response to treatment determine whether acidifying agents (such as ammonium chloride, 1% solution), combination solutions (containing sodium, potassium, ammonium, and chloride), or lysine monohydrochloride should be used. During the administration of acidifying agents, blood pH or bicarbonate content should be monitored daily. Simultaneously, the serum potassium concentrations serve as a guide to the need for continuing potassium replacement. Since complete pyloric obstruction is unusual, and as continuous aspiration of gastric contents aggravates the loss of electrolytes and alkalosis, the stomach should be aspirated as infrequently as possible. Serial measurements of the volumes recovered reflect the degree of obstruction and its response to conservative treatment (see also Chaps. 22 and 29).

Hyponatremic, hypokalemic acidosis

Loss of isotonic fluid into distended loops of obstructed bowel, from fistulas, or in diarrhea leads to progressive hypovolemia and, when diarrhea is prominent, may also produce acidosis and hypokalemia (see also Chaps. 22 and 25). Initially, replacement of plasma volume with isotonic sodium chloride may be urgent, and in adults 4 to 6 liters can be required to restore the blood pressure and urine output. Acidosis can be treated with 0.6 *M* sodium lactate, or solutions containing bicarbonate (50 to 80 meq/liter with sodium chloride). In less severe examples, orally administered fluids may facilitate resorption of intestinal secretions, as shown in cholera or infantile gastroenteritis when glucose taken by mouth reduces the volume of stools.

The major physiologic differences between infants and adults must be kept in mind when one is considering the ideal composition of oral replacement fluids.[28] As discussed earlier, the efficacy of such therapy depends on preservation of glucose-linked sodium absorption, so all fluids contain sodium, chloride, usually potassium and bicarbonate (which facilitates jejunal absorption of sodium), and a source of glucose (glucose, sucrose, or a glucose polymer). However, children have greater obligatory turnovers of water per kilogram, and in infants the normal response to thirst may not come into play. It has been suggested that there may be a single solution for all forms of oral rehydration, and approaches have been made to the composition of an "ideal" solution.

However, use of the "WHO cholera" solution (90 meq/liter sodium) would be expected to result in serious hypernatremia in some dehydrated infants.[38] Several commercial products contain much less sodium (35 to 45 meq/liter). Field trials have suggested that polymeric glucose (e.g., in the form of rice powder), by providing glucose without hyperosmolality, is of additional benefit.[15,26] Currently, a universal solution cannot be recommended, at least not for infants; but the "ideal" or the "WHO cholera" solution should be satisfactory for most adults (Table 36-4).

Short bowel syndrome; hyponatremia and malnutrition

Treatment should be based on the oral intake of rapidly absorbed nutrients, including artificial dietary supplements. Steatorrhea can be lessened by replacement of dietary fat with medium-chain triglycerides; fat-soluble vitamins may be required; and partially or completely hydrolyzed carbohydrates and protein can be prescribed as peptides, oligosaccharides, glucose, or amino acid mixtures. Sodium, potassium, calcium, and anion supplements may also be needed and can be given in a form convenient for absorption as an oral supplement of iso-

TABLE 36-4 • Compositions of oral rehydration solutions

Solution	Na^+	K^+ meq/liter	HCO_3^-	Glucose, mg/100 ml
"Ideal"	90	20	30	110
"WHO, Cholera"	120	25	48	110
Infants	24	28	31	280

tonic electrolytes with glucose. Acute derangements, usually involving sodium and water balance, may necessitate treatment with intravenous solutions. Magnesium depletion, which may be recurrent and severe, requires therapy with regular parenteral magnesium sulfate.

When total parenteral nutrition is being considered, several well-known complications must be kept in mind before proceeding with the therapy. These include (1) mechanical complications of the catheter (pneumothorax, catheter emboli, etc.); (2) infections; and (3) metabolic disturbances, including hyperosmolar coma, azotemia, hyperammonemia, hypercalcemia, hypophosphatemia, and deficiencies of trace metals, vitamins, and essentially fatty acids.

Fluid balance may be helped by inhibition of gastric acid production; H_2 blockers have reduced stomal outputs in short-bowel syndrome.[23] Also important has been the development of stable, long-acting somatostatin analogs. As well as being effective in "hormonal diarrhea" (e.g., carcinoid syndrome, Verner-Morrison syndrome), these agents have reduced stomal outputs.[39]

REFERENCES

1. Bieberdorf FA et al: Pathogenesis of congenital alkalosis with diarrhea: Implications for the physiology of normal ileal electrolyte absorption and secretion. *J Clin Invest* 51:1958, 1972.
2. Burnham JP, Farrer JA: A group experience with uretero-ileal-cutaneous anastomosis for urinary diversion: Results and complications of the isolated ileal conduit (Bricker procedure) in 96 patients. *J Urol* 83:622, 1960.
3. Camilleri M, Phillips SF: Acute and chronic intestinal pseudoobstruction, in Stollerman E (ed): *Advances in Internal Medicine*, vol 36. St Louis, MO, Mosby-Year Book, 1991, p 287.
4. Caprilli R et al: Faecal excretion of bicarbonate in ulcerative colitis. *Digestion* 35:136, 1986.
5. Caspary WF: Diarrhea associated with carbohydrate malabsorption, in Krejs GJ (ed): *Clinics in Gastroenterology*, vol 15. Philadelphia, Saunders, 1986, pp. 631–656.
6. Clark BG, Leadbetter WF: Ureterosigmoidostomy: Collective review of results in 2897 cases. *J Urol* 73:999, 1955.
7. Darrow DC: Congenital alkalosis with diarrhea. *J Pediatr* 26:519, 1945.
8. Davis G et al: Evaluation of chloride/bicarbonate exchange in the human colon in vivo. *J Clin Invest* 71:201, 1983.
9. Debongnie JC, Phillips SF: Capacity of the human colon to absorb fluid. *Gastroenterology* 74:698, 1978.
10. Devroede GJ, Phillips SF: Conservation of sodium, chloride and water by the human colon. *Gastroenterology* 56:101, 1969.
11. Diamond JM: Tight and leaky junctions of epithelia: A perspective on kisses in the dark. *Fed Proc* 33:2220, 1974.
12. Dobbins JW, Binder HJ: Derangements of oxalate metabolism in gastrointestinal disease and their mechanisms, in Glass GBJ (ed): *Progress in Gastroenterology*, vol 3. New York, Grune and Stratton, 1977, p 505.
13. Edmunds LH et al: External fistulas arising from the gastrointestinal tract. *Ann Surg* 152:445, 1960.
14. Eisenberg HL et al: Villous adenoma of the rectum associated with electrolyte disturbance. *Ann Surg* 159:604, 1964.
15. Elliott EJ et al: Sodium content of oral rehydration solutions. A reappraisal. *Gut* 30:1610, 1989.
16. Erlinger S: Bile Flow, in Arias I et al (eds): *The Liver*. New York, Raven Press, 1982, p 407.
17. Evanson JM, Stanbury SW: Congenital chloridorrhea or so-called congenital alkalosis with diarrhoea. *Gut* 6:29, 1965.
18. Faulk DL et al: Chronic intestinal pseudo-obstruction. *Gastroenterology* 74:922, 1978.
19. Fordtran JS et al: The mechanisms of sodium absorption in the human small intestine. *J Clin Invest* 47:884, 1968.
20. Hill GL: Ileostomy *Surgery, Physiology and Management*. New York, Grune and Stratton, 1976.
21. Hodin E. Remington JH: Villous adenoma with severe electrolyte depletion: Report of a case. *Dis Colon Rectum* 12:36, 1969.
22. Holmberg C et al: Colonic electrolyte transport in health and in congenital chloride diarrhea. *J Clin Invest* 56:302, 1975.
23. Jacobson D et al: Effect of cimetidine on jejunostomy effluents in patients with severe short-bowel syndrome. *Scand J Gastroenterol* 21:824, 1986.
24. Kamath PS et al: Short chain fatty acids stimulate ileal motility in humans. *Gastroenterology* 95:1496, 1988.
25. Ladefoged K et al: Faecal osmolality and electrolyte concentrations in chronic diarrhoea: Do they provide diagnostic clues? *Scand J Gastroenterol* 22:813, 1987.
26. Mehta MN, Subramaniam S: Comparison of rice water, rice electrolyte solution, and glucose electrolyte solution in the management of infantile diarrhoea. *Lancet* i:843, 1986.
27. Moore FD: *Metabolic Care of the Surgical Patient*. Philadelphia, Saunders, 1959.
28. Nalin DR et al: Comparison of sucrose with glucose in oral therapy of acute diarrhoea. *Lancet* ii:277, 1978.
29. Oh MS et al: D-lactic acidosis in a man with short-bowel syndrome. *N Engl J Med* 301:249, 1979.
30. Powell DW: Intestinal water and electrolyte transport, in Johnson LR (ed): *Physiology of the Gastrointestinal Tract*. New York, Raven Press, 1987, p 1267.
31. Ruppin H et al: Absorption of short-chain fatty acids by the colon. *Gastroenterology* 78:1500, 1980.
32. Shrock LG, Polk HC Jr: Rectal villous adenoma producing hypokalemia. *Am J Surg* 40:54, 1974.
33. Schulz I: Electrolyte and fluid secretion in the exocrine pancreas, in Johnson LR (ed): *Physiology of the Gastrointestinal Tract*. New York, Raven Press, 1987, p 1147.
34. Shnitka TK et al: Villous tumours of the rectum and colon characterized by severe fluid and electrolyte loss. *Surg Gynecol Obstet* 112:609, 1961.
35. Taylor AR, Shields R: Electrolyte and metabolic disturbances in surgical gastrointestinal emergencies, in Barany FR et al (eds): *Gastrointestinal Emergencies* 2. New York, Pergamon, 1980, p 35.
36. Traube M et al: D-lactic acidosis after jejunoileal bypass: Identification of organic anions by nuclear magnetic resonance spectroscopy. *Ann Intern Med* 98:171, 1983.

37. Turnberg LA et al: Mechanism of bicarbonate absorption and its relationship to sodium transport in the human jejunum. *J Clin Invest* 49:548, 1970.
38. Turnberg LA et al: Interrelationships of chloride, bicarbonate, sodium and hydrogen transport in the human ileum. *J Clin Invest* 49:557, 1970.
39. Williams NS et al: Use of long acting somatostatin analogue in controlling life threatening ileostomy diarrhea. *Br Med J* 238(2):1027, 1984.
40. Wingate DL: Backwards and forwards with the migrating complex. *Dig Dis Sci* 26:641, 1981.

CHAPTER • 37

Electrolyte, water, mineral, and acid-base disorders in liver disease

Robert J. Anderson

INTRODUCTION

An association between edema formation and the presence of liver disease has been observed for more than three decades. Renal retention of salt and water occurs in patients with severe liver disease and is central to the maintenance of this edematous state. In addition, potassium, acid-base, and mineral metabolism is often disturbed in patients with advanced liver disease. A rational approach to the management of the fluid-electrolyte and acid-base disturbances must be based on an understanding of the pathophysiology of these disorders. In this chapter, we will first review the mechanism involved in the fluid and electrolyte disorders that occur in patients with liver disease. The clinical manifestations and therapeutic modalities of these disorders will be discussed subsequently. Because fluid and electrolyte disturbances appear to be rare and of little clinical significance in uncomplicated acute liver disease, most of our discussion will focus on forms of acute fulminant and chronic progressive liver disease.

SODIUM RETENTION AND EDEMA FORMATION IN LIVER DISEASE

STIMULUS FOR SODIUM AND WATER RETENTION

The traditional view of the pathogenesis of edema formation in hepatic cirrhosis is depicted in Fig. 37-1. According to this view, liver disease results in hepatic venous obstruction, which increases hepatic venous hydrostatic pressure.[107,158] This increase in hydrostatic pressure results in movement of plasma from the vascular space to the lymphatics of the hepatic sinusoids. When the formation of hepatic lymph exceeds the rate of lymph removal, lymph "spills" into the peritoneal cavity and ascites develops. Thus, thoracic duct lymphatic flows as high as 20 liters/day have been documented in cirrhosis.[197] The spillage of hepatic lymph decreases plasma volume, which then stimulates renal sodium and water reabsorption. In addition, splanchnic venous pooling (resulting from portal hypertension) and hypoalbuminema may also contribute to the contraction of plasma volume. Finally, the peripheral vasodilatation commonly observed in cirrhosis increases vascular capacitance, potentially further decreasing the "effective" plasma volume.

Evidence supporting this traditional "underfill" theory includes the fact that expansion of plasma volume, either by administration of saline solution or albumin (which causes peritoneovenous shunting) or by water immersion to the neck, significantly increases renal salt and water excretion in ascitic, cirrhotic patients.[15,55,56,193] Moreover, increased activity or con-

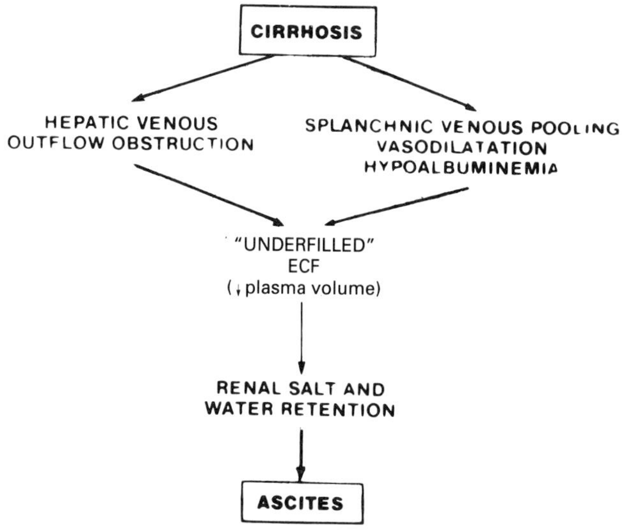

FIGURE 37-1 • Traditional "underfill" theory of ascites formation.

centrations of humoral markers of volume depletion (plasma renin activity, norepinephrine, aldosterone, and vasopressin) are often present in cirrhotic patients with ascites.[17-19] In these patients, water immersion to the neck significantly increases cardiac index, excretion of a water load, and the fractional excretion of sodium. The improvement in renal excretion of salt and water is associated with significant decreases in plasma concentrations of renin, aldosterone, vasopressin, and norepinephrine.[17-19] Taken together, these observations give strong support to the traditional "underfill" view.

A more recent theory proposed by Lieberman and colleagues suggests that liver disease somehow directly induces renal sodium retention (Fig. 37-2).[112-114] The increase in extracellular fluid volume results in an "overfilled" plasma volume, which then spills into the peritoneal cavity under the influence of altered Starling forces. This view leaves unanswered the mechanism of the primary increase in renal tubular sodium reabsorption. In support of this theory, Lieberman and Reynolds measured plasma volume in cirrhotic patients with and without ascites.[112-114] Total plasma volume was found to be expanded, not contracted. Other authors have reported a similar increase in plasma volume.[23,149] Two points about these plasma volume measurements deserve emphasis: First, the formation of cirrhotic ascites and edema is likely to be a dynamic process; thus, measurements of plasma volume carried out after significant salt and water retention has occurred are not likely to demonstrate persisting hypovolemia. Second, Lieberman and coworkers[149] equate measured plasma volume with the "effective circulating plasma volume." It seems more appropriate to define effective plasma volume as the ratio of the nonportal plasma volume to the nonportal vascular holding capacity. This is important, since most patients with advanced liver disease show a decrease in systemic vascular resistance. Despite these objections, it should be noted that low plasma uric acid and urea concentrations and enhanced renal uric acid and urea clearances have been found in edematous, cirrhotic patients.[43] Since plasma volume expansion increases uric acid and urea clearance, these findings support the "overfill" view. From these studies it appears that an underfilled volume is hard to demonstrate in ascitic patients with cirrhosis.

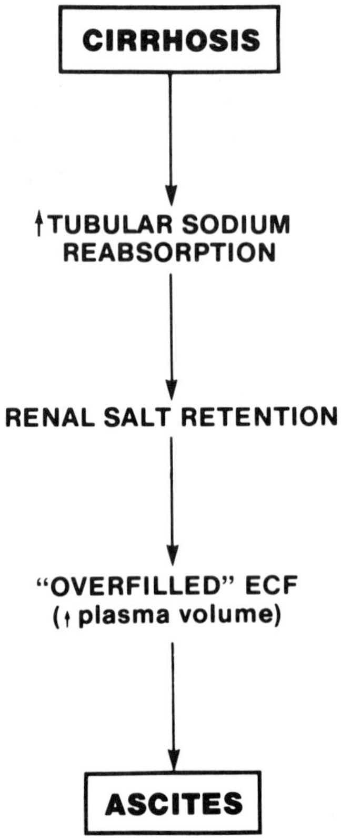

FIGURE 37-2 • "Overfill" theory of ascites formation.

The overfill hypothesis is also supported by animal experiments.[108-111,117,118] Dogs fed the potent hepatotoxin dimethylnitrosamine develop hepatic cirrhosis over 2 months. The cirrhosis is characterized by ascites, portal venous hypertension, porta-systemic collateral formation, hepatic encephalopathy, and gastrointentinal bleeding. In this model, urinary sodium retention precedes the formation of ascites by approximately 10 days.[108] Sodium retention also preceded any change in cardiac output or peripheral vascular resistance.[109] Similar results have been reported in rats made cirrhotic with carbon tetrachloride inhalation and oral phenobarbital.[117] Together, these observations suggest that renal sodium retention precedes the development of ascites in animal models of cirrhosis.

In summary, neither the underfill nor the overfill theory adequately explains all aspects of ascites formation in patients with cirrhosis.[158,167] However, the issue of whether the plasma volume is underfilled or overfilled is an important consideration in the selection of diuretic therapy in this disorder. Thus, if underfilled, diuretic therapy might lead to a further decrease in organ perfusion. In contrast, if overfilled, it should be relatively easy to diurese the cirrhotic patient.[53] The classic studies of Shear and the more recent studies of Pockros and Reynolds suggest that, from a clinical perspective, the patients with cirrhotic ascites and edema behave as if they were in an overfilled state and can safely undergo a diuresis of greater than 1 to 2 kg/day. By contrast, patients with cirrhotic ascites without edema behave as if they were in an underfilled state. Thus, in such nonedematous patients, diuresis rates of less than 0.75 kg/day are indicated.[141,171] Regardless of whether the overfill or the underfill theory is correct, it is apparent that renal salt and water retention play a central role in cirrhotic edema formation.

EFFECTOR MECHANISM FOR SODIUM AND WATER RETENTION

Nephron sites of sodium retention

The glomerular filtration rate (GFR) and filtered load of sodium are reduced in many salt-retaining patients with cirrhosis.[7] However, some salt-retaining cirrhotic patients have normal GFRs, demonstrating that enhanced tubular sodium reabsorption plays a significant role in their salt retention.[136] There is indirect evidence for both enhanced proximal and distal tubular sodium reabsorption in cirrhotic human beings. The following findings support enhanced proximal tubular reabsorption in hepatic cirrhosis:

1. Maneuvers that expand plasma volume and increase delivery of fluid distally (i.e., water immersion and infusion of saline or mannitol) result in increased renal sodium excretion and free water formation independent of changes in GFR.[17,56,65]
2. Suppression of antidiuretic hormone (ADH) secretion during water loading minimizes distal tubular water reabsorption, allowing the rate of urine formation to approximate the rate of distal delivery of glomerular filtrate. At comparably low urinary osmolalities, some water-loaded cirrhotic patients have lower urine flow rates than similarly treated subjects.[97,104] In some clinical studies, calculated distal nephron sodium reabsorption is lower in cirrhotic patients than controls.[7]
3. Patients with cirrhosis and ascites may have a decreased clearance of exogenous lithium.[7] Since lithium is reabsorbed primarily in the proximal tubule, these findings suggest enhanced proximal tubule solute reabsorption in cirrhosis.
4. Enhanced proximal reabsorption of tubular fluid has been found in micropuncture and clearance studies of dogs and rats with chronic bile duct ligation, as well as in rats with cirrhosis secondary to carbon tetrachloride exposure.[10,14,118]

Evidence for enhanced distal nephron sodium reabsorption comprises the following observations:

1. Water-loaded patients with sodium retention and cirrhosis with minimal urinary osmolalities often have urine flow rates (an index of proximal reabsorption) comparable to those in normal control subjects.[35]
2. Water-loaded cirrhotic patients with minimal urine osmolalities have increased calculated distal fractional sodium reabsorption after receiving hypotonic saline infusions.[35]
3. Acetazolamide, a diuretic acting at the proximal tubule, produces a significant natriuresis in cirrhotics only when there is concomitant distal nephron blockade of sodium reabsorption with ethacrynic acid.[168]
4. A phosphaturic response to head-out water immersion occurs in cirrhotic patients independently of any accompanying natriuresis.[58] The implication is that immersion impairs both sodium and phosphorus reabsorption proximally. Failure of sodium to reach the urine indicates that it must be avidly reabsorbed distally.
5. Micropuncture studies in the dimethylnitrosamine and bile duct ligated models of cirrhosis demonstrate enhanced distal nephron sodium reabsorption.[108,118]

In summary, clinical and experimental studies suggest that both the proximal and the distal nephron participate in enhanced renal tubular sodium reabsorption in cirrhosis.

Mechanisms of enhanced tubular sodium reabsorption

As noted previously, a decrease in GFR and thus in the filtered load of sodium often accompanies the sodium retention seen in many cirrhotic patients.[7,136] The mechanisms responsible for enhanced sodium reabsorption at both proximal and distal sites have not been defined clearly and may be multifactorial. A decrease in GFR is not observed in many sodium-retaining cirrhotic patients, suggesting that sodium retention can occur independently of a decrease in GFR.[97,103] An increase in renal vascular resistance and in filtration fraction is often seen in decompensated cirrhosis.[17-19,56] Thus, *peritubular physical forces* (decreased hydrostatic pressure and increased oncotic pressure) may act to enhance proximal tubular sodium reabsorption in cirrhosis. Recently, elevated plasma levels of *norepinephrine* have been observed in cirrhotic patients with ascites.[9,17] Plasma norepinephrine levels correlated positively with plasma vasopressin concentrations and with plasma renin activity, and negatively with urinary sodium excretion.[9,17] These findings suggest that increased activity of the sympathetic nervous system and renal nerves may also result in enhanced renal sodium reabsorption in cirrhosis.

There have been reports of natriuresis occurring after either adrenalectomy or treatment with spironolactone[48,74] a competitive inhibitor of *aldosterone*. In fact, in the majority of ascitic cirrhotic patients a diuresis can be established with spironolactone alone. However, inhibition of aldosterone synthesis with either aminoglutethimide[74] or adrenalectomy[160] did not restore renal sodium excretion entirely to normal in some patients. Moreover, water immersion of patients with cirrhosis results in natriuresis even in the presence of pharmacologic doses of mineralocorticoids.[56] Finally, in one study of cirrhotic patients given excess sodium intake, 5 of 11 patients had suppressed levels of plasma renin activity and aldosterone and yet gained approximately 1 kg body weight per day.[37] These patients retained as much sodium as the 6 patients who had persistently elevated plasma aldosterone levels.[47] Thus it is clear that aldosterone is not the sole factor responsible for sodium retention in cirrhosis. However, the near-uniform response to spironolactone suggests that the high plasma levels of aldosterone frequently seen in cirrhotic patients contribute to increased distal sodium reabsorption.

Sodium retention in cirrhosis has also been postulated to be due to the lack of a yet-unidentified *natriuretic factor* in plasma.[99] The observation that cirrhotic patients without ascites fail to "escape" from the sodium-retaining effects of administered mineralocorticoids[195] has been attributed to the absence of such a natriuretic factor. In a few studies, bioassays of plasma or urine from cirrhotic patients have supported the notion that cirrhotics lack a natriuretic substance that normal subjects have.[63,133] Further work will be needed to isolate, identify, and convincingly demonstrate that liver disease results in a diminished ability to elaborate this natriuretic factor.

The recent discovery of atrial natriuretic factor (ANF) has prompted several studies on the role of this substance in the pathogenesis of sodium retention in advanced liver disease.[28,60,61,86,94,102,129,164,175] Most studies demonstrate normal plasma levels of ANF in cirrhosis without ascites, while high plasma concentrations of ANF are usually present in cirrhosis with ascites.[60,61,86,94,129,175] In cirrhotic patients with ascites undergoing manipulations that increase central blood volume (e.g., water immersion to the neck and/or peritoneovenous shunting), plasma ANF concentrations increase in a fashion comparable to that of control subjects.[28,60,61] Together, these observations do not suggest that a deficiency of ANF contributes to sodium retention in advanced liver disease. In fact, recent studies suggest that an impairment in the renal natriuretic response to exogenously infused ANF occurs in cirrhotic patients.[61,102,175] The site and mechanism of renal tubular hyporesponsiveness to ANF in cirrhosis remain debated. Plasma concentrations of ANF and urinary excretion of cyclic GMP (the putative second messenger of the ANF response) increase comparably in cirrhotic patients with and without a natriuretic response to water immersion.[175] These findings support a postcyclic GMP site to explain the renal tubular resistance to ANF that occurs in some cirrhotic patients.

Finally, several recent studies suggest that other humoral substances, such as *bradykinin*[138,199,202] and *eicosanoids*,[9,24,54,140,152,201,203] may play an effector role in modulating renal sodium excretion in cirrhosis. Whether these agents act by directly affecting tubular sodium transport or by influencing renal hemodynamic function remains to be determined. In summary, the effector mechanisms involved in renal salt retention in cirrhosis are likely multifactorial.

THERAPY OF CIRRHOTIC ASCITES AND EDEMA

Specific considerations for the cirrhotic patient

Shear and associates (in 1970) and Pockros and Reynolds (more recently) have performed careful measurements of ascites fluid kinetics and clinical responses in ascitic, cirrhotic patients with and without edema.[141,171] These studies indicate that ascitic fluid is a separate and relatively nonmobilizable compartment of extracellular fluid with a maximum safe rate of ascitic fluid removal of about 750 ml/day.[141,171] These studies provide some general guidelines for diuretic therapy and suggest that a daily diuresis of 0.75 kg/day in the absence of edema, or 2.0 kg/day in the presence of edema, can usually be safely tolerated.[141,171]

General principles

The general principles underlying the therapy of ascites in cirrhosis are outlined in Table 37-1.[87] Careful evaluation for reversible factors leading to hepatic dysfunction should be undertaken. Active diuretic therapy should be delayed until clinical and biochemical stability of the patient is documented. The rate of diuresis needs to be monitored carefully. Moderate dietary sodium restriction remains the cornerstone of therapy, since 5 to 15 percent of decompensated cirrhotic patients can be successfully managed by a trial of bed rest and moderate dietary sodium restriction.[41,153]

Pharmacologic agents

An approach to the use of diuretic agents in cirrhosis is outlined in Table 37-2[39,87] (see Chap. 19).

Spironolactone and spironolactone plus furosemide are the most widely used diuretic regimens in patients

TABLE 37-1 • General principles in the treatment of ascites

1. Adequate evaluation and treatment of the primary disease process.
2. Frequent clinical and biochemical monitoring.
3. Active drug therapy should not be undertaken unless liver and renal function are stable.
4. The goals of diuresis should be a daily weight loss of 1.0 to 2.0 kg in ascites with edema and 0.25 kg in ascites without edema.
5. The end point of therapy should be maximum patient comfort with minimal drug-induced complications. This may occasionally require a slight liberalization of sodium intake at the expense of an increased dosage of diuretics and the maintenance of some residual ascites in selected patients.

TABLE 37-2 • General approach in the prescription of diuretics in decompensated cirrhotic patients

1. If no diuresis is observed after 2 to 4 days of sodium restriction, spironolactone should be added. The dose may be increased from 50 to 100 mg/day every 3 to 5 days, to a total daily dose of 400 mg. This results in an adequate diuresis in at least 50 percent of the patients.
2. If no diuresis ensues, add furosemide: 20 to 80 mg, twice daily.
3. If no diuresis is observed on this regimen, or if an intital diuresis is aborted, consider the causes of resistance to diuretics (Table 37-3). Additional furosemide and/or consideration of adding metolazone is appropriate at this point.
4. Consider large-volume (2- to 5-liter) paracentesis.
5. Consider performing a LeVeen shunt.

with decompensated liver disease.[29,67] These diuretics are able to decrease ascites and peripheral edema in the majority of patients treated. High-dose spironolactone (300 to 600 mg/day) used alone is almost uniformly effective in cirrhotic patients with relatively refractory ascites.[29]

To compare the efficacy of three commonly used diuretic regimens in the treatment of ascites, 90 patients were recently randomized to three treatment groups: sequential spironolactone (spironolactone followed by furosemide if necessary); combination (spironolactone and furosemide together); and furosemide alone.[67] All diuretics were begun at a low oral dose and the dosage increased until a daily weight loss 0.4 to 0.8 kg was achieved. The three regimens achieved comparable rates of diuresis, but larger doses of furosemide were necessary to achieve a significant diuresis in the furosemide-alone group. The incidences of encephalopathy, hepatorenal syndrome, and marked electrolyte abnormalities were similar for the three treatment groups, except that hyperkalemia was more frequent on combination therapy. This study clearly demonstrates the beneficial effect of spironolactone alone and of spironolactone plus furosemide in cirrhotic ascites. Other prospective studies support the contention that careful use of an aldosterone inhibitor with another diuretic agent results in a satisfactory diuresis in most cirrhotic patients.[77,139]

Patients should be considered resistant to diuretics if they do not lose weight on the above protocol or if they stop losing weight after an initial period of diuresis. At this point, causes of drug-resistant edema should be considered (Table 37-3). Two common processes that may lead to diuretic resistance in cirrhotic patients are spontaneous bacterial peritonitis and gastrointestinal bleeding. In addition, medication noncompliance, continued high sodium intake, and concomitant use of nonsteroidal anti-inflammatory agents can all result in a picture of "diuretic resistance."

In the drug-resistant patient, it is useful to consider the hemodynamic influences of ascites on cardiac function. Guazzi and coworkers,[78] as well as other researchers,[96,174] have demonstrated that tense ascites can adversely affect ventricular function. During graded paracentesis (up to 5 liters) in 21 patients, these investigators were able to demonstrate a significant increase in cardiac output, stroke volume, right and left ventricular stroke work, and mean rate of systolic ejection.[78] These workers postulated that the increased intraabdominal hydrostatic pressure impaired venous return to the heart.

Other studies have also noted a beneficial hemodynamic effect of modest paracentesis in some patients with tense ascites.[96,144,174] Recently, large-volume (4 to 6 liters) paracentesis with or without concomitant intravenous albumin infusion (40 grams using a 25% solution) has been advocated as an effective mode of therapy of ascites.[71,73,96,144,163,174] In prospective trials, the rate of disappearance of ascites with paracentesis approaches 100 percent and is higher than that achieved with diuretics. Also, paracentesis appears to be associated with a shortened hospital stay and fewer complications than diuretic therapy.[72,144] The role of concomitant albumin infusions in paracentesis therapy of ascites has recently been investigated.[73] In patients receiving albumin, paracentesis was not associated with changes in blood urea nitrogen, serum sodium or creatinine concentrations, plasma renin activity, or plasma aldosterene concentration.[73] In contrast, significant increases in blood urea nitrogen, plasma renin activity, and plasma aldosterone, and small but significant decreases in serum sodium concentration, occurred in those not receiving albumin. Surprisingly, biochemical changes were identical in patients who did not receive albumin regardless of the presence or absence of edema. In this study, biochemical and clinical complications in patients undergoing paracentesis occurred in 17 percent of those receiving albumin and 30 percent of those who did not receive albumin.[73] In summary, large-volume paracentesis with an albumin infusion, using strict aseptic techniques, is a safe form of removal of ascitic fluid. This form of therapy should be used with caution in patients with either renal dysfunction or a plasma sodium concentration less than 130 meq/liter. Diuretic therapy is invariably required to subse-

TABLE 37-3 • Diuretic resistance in cirrhosis

1. Patient noncompliance
   A. Not taking diuretic agents
   B. Continued high salt and water intake
2. Inadequate treatment of the primary disorder
3. Intravascular volume depletion
4. Decreased glomerular filtration rate
5. Nonsteroidal anti-inflammatory agents

quently maintain neutral sodium balance. Unfortunately, about 50 percent of patients so treated will require readmission for reaccumulation of ascites within 25 weeks. Some patients appear to have ascites intractable or unresponsive to diuretics and/or paracentesis. In such patients, consideration may be given to the placement of a peritoneovenous (LeVeen) shunt. As recently reviewed in detail, LeVeen shunts result in a significant diuresis in many diuretic-resistant patients.[22,57,59,181] However, formidable complications may occur after the placement of such shunts (e.g., infection, mechanical failure, coagulopathy); this treatment should not be used indiscriminately.

The results of a large, multicenter prospective study comparing peritoneovenous shunting with medical therapy in patients with alcoholic liver disease and massive ascites were recently reported.[181] In this study the mean time to resolution of ascites was 5.4 weeks with diuretic therapy and 3.0 weeks for shunted patients. The time to recurrence of ascites was 4 months in diuretic-treated patients and 18 months in shunted patients. The duration of hospitalization in shunted patients averaged 40 percent less than in medically treated patients. Mortality during initial hospitalization, long-term survival, and frequency of complications (infections, bleeding, and encephalopathy) did not differ when the two groups were compared. These results indicate that peritoneovenous shunting is an effective form of therapy that may offer some advantages over medical treatment. Unfortunately, shunting does not improve survival. In other smaller studies, shunting was associated with a higher frequency of complications than medical therapy.[22,59]

RENAL WATER RETENTION AND HYPONATREMIA IN CIRRHOSIS

MECHANISM OF WATER RETENTION

When a low plasma sodium concentration is obtained in a patient with cirrhosis, laboratory error, hyperglycemia, and hyperlipidemia should be considered first (see Chap. 18).[6,84] If these entities are not present, true hyponatremia, due to impaired renal ability to excrete water and continued water intake, occurs in substantial numbers of patients with cirrhosis of the liver (Table 37-4).[6,8,19,20,51,137,183] Decompensated cirrhotic patients with ascites and/or edema have an abnormal response to water administration; cirrhotic patients without ascites or edema usually excrete water normally.[19,51,183] Thus, as depicted in Table 37-4, hyponatremia is common in patients with decompensated and/or terminal liver disease.

There are three potential mechanisms for this inability to excrete free water: (1) either a decrease in GFR or derangement in renal hemodynamics with decreased fluid delivery to the distal nephron, (2) an extrarenal mechanism involving arginine vasopressin (AVP) release, and (3) use of diuretic agents, such as thiazides, that impair solute transport in the thick ascending limb of Henle, thereby preventing maximal dilution of tubular fluid.[185] Maneuvers that improve distal fluid delivery—such as infusion of mannitol,[165] saline,[165] saline plus albumin,[190] and ascitic fluid,[200] as well as water immersion[17]—improve urinary dilution and water excretion in cirrhosis. These maneuvers also increase central blood volume and may improve water excretion by suppressing baroreceptor-mediated vasopressin release. In this regard, administration of either alcohol, to suppress vasopressin release,[183] or demeclocycline, to antagonize vasopressin action,[45,127] improves water excretion in cirrhosis, also suggesting a role for vasopressin. In addition, we have recently studied four experimental models of altered liver function.[4,5,12,15] In each of these experimental models, a predominant role of vasopressin in the impairment of water excretion was demonstrated. However, in each case, there was also evidence that diminished fluid delivery to the distal diluting segment contributed slightly to the abnormal water excretion.

Recent studies in patients with cirrhosis also point to nonosmotic release of AVP as a major factor responsible for water retention in cirrhosis.[6,115,145] Bichet and co-

TABLE 37-4 • Prevalence of hyponatremia and hypokalemia in liver disease

	Read[146]	De Deuxchaisnes[44]	Schwartz[169]	Hecker[81]	Casey[33,34]
Hyponatremia (<135 meq/liter)					
Stable cirrhosis	5/14	2/10	—	—	—
Decompensated cirrhosis	—	8/17	14/28	8/9*	—
Hypokalemia (<3.5 meq/liter)					
Stable cirrhosis	1/14	0/10	—	—	4/20
Decompensated cirrhosis	—	8/17	10/27	3/8*	3/20

* Terminal

workers[18,19] studied 26 cirrhotic patients who received a standard waterload (20 ml per kilogram of body weight). "Excretors" cleared 80 percent of the water load; "nonexcretors" cleared lesser fractions of the load. Nonexcretors had lower serum sodium concentrations and higher plasma vasopressin levels after the waterload. These nonexcretors also had higher pulse rates, lower plasma albumin levels, and higher plasma renin, aldosterone, and norepinephrine levels than excretors.[18,19] Expansion of the central blood volume by water immersion suppressed vasopressin release and improved water excretion.[19] Finally, it should be noted that a diminution in metabolic clearance rate of vasopressin occurs in cirrhosis.[176] This decrease in AVP clearance, when coupled with continued AVP secretion, further elevates plasma AVP. In summary, experimental and clinical evidence suggests that the impairment in water excretion in association with cirrhosis is mediated predominantly by persistent nonosmotic release of AVP; diminished distal delivery of tubular fluid to the diluting segment of the nephron may also contribute. This diminished renal water excretion, if combined with significant water intake, results in hyponatremia.

THERAPY OF HYPONATREMIA AND WATER RETENTION

Is mild (~125 meq/liter) chronic hyponatremia harmful to the cirrhotic patient?[137] On the one hand, such hyponatremia may result in cell swelling with increased intracranial pressure, thereby contributing to encephalopathy and perhaps lowering the seizure threshold.[137] It is of interest that plasma sodium concentration tends to be lowest in comatose patients[169] and in patients with the greatest degree of respiratory alkalosis.[194] On the other hand, most cirrhotic patients appear to tolerate mild chronic hyponatremia without symptoms. In this regard, Ring-Larson utilized peritoneal dialysis to raise plasma sodium in comatose patients with liver disease. Despite correction of plasma sodium, encephalopathy did not improve.[154] Thus, with mild-to-moderate (>120 meq/liter) hyponatremia, water restriction (to less than 500 to 750 ml/day) will usually result in either stabilization or a slight increase in plasma sodium concentration. As noted previously, demeclocyline (Declomycin), a pharmacologic agent that inhibits the renal hydroosmotic effect of vasopressin, can induce a water diuresis with a resultant increase in plasma sodium concentration in hyponatremic patients with cirrhosis.[45,127] Demeclocycline should be used with special caution in the presence of liver disease, since it accumulates in patients with liver disease and can induce acute renal failure.[127]

Often, the development of mild-to-moderate hyponatremia (120 to 134 meq/liter) occurs shortly after institution of diuretic therapy.[64,146] In such cases, moderate sodium supplementation combined with correction of hypokalemia increases the plasma sodium concentration. Water restriction and use of the lowest dose of diuretic that effects fluid loss usually prevent the development of severe hyponatremia. In addition, replacement of agents such as thiazides (which impair urinary diluting capacity) with loop diuretics may improve plasma sodium concentration.[185]

In rare instances, symptomatic hyponatremia complicates cirrhosis, causing confusion, lethargy, coma, or seizures. In most cases of symptomatic hyponatremia, the serum sodium concentration either declined rapidly, or its final value was very low. In such symptomatic cases, hypertonic saline will acutely increase plasma sodium concentration.[67] If a brisk diuresis can be established with furosemide, replacement of urinary electrolyte losses with small volumes of hypertonic saline will also acutely increase the plasma sodium concentration.[79] Dialytic therapy is an effective means of treating severe symptomatic hyponatremia in patients who cannot tolerate saline or who are unable to establish a diuresis.

DISTURBANCES OF POTASSIUM METABOLISM IN LIVER DISEASE

Plasma potassium concentration varies widely in patients with liver disease. For example, in one large series of patients with advanced hepatic disease, serum potassium concentrations spanned from 2.5 to 8.0 meq/liter.[34] Potential causes of these abnormalities are outlined in Tables 37-4 to 37-6.

HYPOKALEMIA

Hypokalemia is encountered frequently in patients with decompensated cirrhosis (see Chap. 22) (Table 37-4). However, hypokalemia is not usually seen in patients with stable chronic liver disease not receiving diuretic agents and without ascites or edema. Potential causes of hypokalemia are shown in Table 37-5. In many patients with liver disease, a combination of low dietary po-

TABLE 37-5 • Hypokalemia in liver disease

1. Low dietary intake
2. Intracellular shift of extracellular potassium can be induced by alkalemia; insulin and glucose infusion; cellular incorporation of potassium as occurs with treatment of megaloblastic anemia or alimentation
3. Loss of potassium
   - A. Renal loss as caused by diuretics, hyperaldosteronism, magnesium depletion, vomiting, acidosis, renal tubular acidosis
   - B. Gastrointestinal losses

TABLE 37-6 • Causes of true hyperkalemia in patients with liver disease

1. Extracellular shift of intracellular potassium is caused by acidemia, digitalis poisoning, hyperglycemia, deficiency of insulin or catecholamines, hemolysis, rhabdomyolysis
2. Potassium loading
   A. Blood transfusions
   B. Intravenous solutions containing potassium
   C. Salt substitutes (4 to 13 meq/g)
   D. Potassium penicillin (1.7 meq/10^6 units)
3. Diminished potassium excretion
   A. Potassium-sparing diuretics: amiloride, spironolactone, triamterene
   B. Renal failure
   C. Mineralocorticoid deficiency

tassium intake and accelerated urinary or gastrointenstinal loss contributes to total body depletion.[155] Three studies have established that total body potassium (measured by isotope counting) is significantly decreased in patients with liver disease.[34,44,155] Reductions (30 to 40 percent) both in total exchangeable potassium and in milliequivalents of potassium per unit of body weight were demonstrated in these patients. These decrements either exceeded or were equivalent to those found in other patients with chronic debilitating diseases.[34,44,155] Interestingly, the decrement in total body potassium was not different when patients with compensated liver disease (i.e., no ascites, edema, or encephalopathy) were compared with patients having decompensated disease. However, a strong correlation between exchangeable potassium and serum albumin was present.[34] These data establish clearly that patients with chronic liver disease often have a deficiency of potassium.

Renal loss of potassium induced by diuretic agents is one of the most common causes of hypokalemia in patients with liver disease.[146] For example, Sherlock reported that 66 to 64 percent of cirrhotic patients treated with either chlorothiazide or furosemide developed a serum potassium level of less than 3.1 meq/liter.[172] The use of any diuretic that acts proximally to the distal tubular potassium secretory site (i.e., thiazides, furosemide, ethacrynic acid, metolazone, bumetanide) can potentially induce marked renal potassium wasting. The severity of diuretic-induced hypokalemia depends on the magnitude of natriuresis, the degree of hyperaldosteronism, and the body stores of potassium. As will be discussed below, renal tubular acidosis (RTA), which rarely accompanies some forms of chronic liver disease, can lead to significant renal potassium wasting. Magnesium deficiency, a condition frequently associated with chronic alcoholic liver disease, also causes kaliuresis and hypokalemia.[68,125] This potassium wasting does not improve until magnesium stores are normalized. In rats, the urinary potassium loss caused by magnesium deficiency is dependent on aldosterone.[68] Finally, gastrointestinal loss of potassium often contributes to hypokalemia in patients with liver disease.

Does hypokalemia predispose the patient with liver disease to hepatic encephalopathy? Read and coworkers found that chlorothiazide treatment induced hypokalemia and worsened hepatic encephalopathy (as assessed clinically and by EEG).[146] Prevention of hypokalemia with potassium supplementation prevented chlorothiazide-induced encephalopathy. Moreover, potassium depletion induced by oral potassium exchange resins also precipitated encephalopathy.[146] These results suggest that potassium depletion can induce hepatic encephalopathy.

In order to determine the mechanism of this effect, Gabuzda and Hall induced potassium depletion with the diuretic mercuhydrin in patients with liver disease.[71] As serum potassium declined from 4.4 to 2.9 meq/liter, blood ammonium rose from 71 to 131 μg/100 ml. In additional studies, acute intravenous administration of potassium caused urinary and renal venous ammonium concentrations to fall. In more recent studies by Casey and coworkers,[33] intravenous chlorothiazide increased arterial blood ammonium (90 to 121 μg/100 ml) and decreased urine ammonium (23 to 7 meq/liter). As will be discussed below, it is also possible that alkalemia, which often accompanies diuretic-induced hypokalemia, may predispose to hepatic encephalopathy by increasing tissue concentrations of ammonia. Additional adverse effects of hypokalemia include muscle weakness, ileus, myocardial irritability, polyuria, and polydipsia.

In view of potential adverse effects of hypokalemia in patients with liver disease, careful attention must be paid to serum potassium concentration before and during diuretic therapy.

Prospective trials have demonstrated that careful use of diuretic agents usually results in a diuresis without hypokalemia.[1,67,77,139] In this regard, the initial use of spironolactone, alone or in combination with other diuretic agents, usually protects against the development of hypokalemia (Table 37-2). If therapy with a kaliuretic agent (furosemide, metalazone, ethacrynic acid, thiazides, or bumetanide) is undertaken without concomitant use of a potassium-sparing agent (spironolactone, amiloride, triamterene), plasma potassium should be closely monitored; potassium chloride supplementation (20 to 80 meq/day) will be necessary in most cases.

HYPERKALEMIA

Hyperkalemia occasionally complicates chronic liver disease.[34] Potential causes of hyperkalemia in this setting are outlined in Table 37-6 (see Chap. 23). Hyperkalemia is most commonly caused by potassium-sparing diuretics (spironolactone, amiloride, triamterene).[67,70] These agents diminish distal nephron potassium secretion.

Thus, when these agents are used in association with diminished GFR or diminished distal tubular delivery of sodium, or under conditions of potassium loading, hyperkalemia often occurs. In several patients with end-stage cirrhosis, the combination of progressive azotemia, hyponatremia, and hyperkalemia has been observed.[143,188] In these patients, hyperkalemia is due to impaired renal potassium excretion. In other patients, the complications of alcoholism may increase susceptibility to rhabdomyolysis, hemolysis, and gastrointestinal bleeding resulting in endogenous potassium loads and potential hyperkalemia.[69] As arterial pH declines, an increase in serum potassium (due to a shift of potassium from intra- to extracellular sites) may be observed. Thus, severe acidosis, often occurring in terminal cirrhosis,[143] has been shown to be associated with hyperkalemia. The administration of the acidifying agent arginine monohydrochloride may result in life-threatening hyperkalemia in patients with liver disease.[26]

Cessation of potassium supplements and potassium-sparing diuretics should be undertaken if serum levels exceed 5.5 meq/liter. Higher values of potassium mandate careful clinical observation and repeated monitoring of the ECG. If dangerous hyperkalemia is present, the following therapies should be undertaken: infusion of calcium gluconate (10% solution, 10 to 30 ml) to antagonize the membrane effects of hyperkalemia; administer insulin (10 U regular), glucose (10% solution), and bicarbonate (1 to 3 ampules containing 44.6 meq per ampule) to redistribute potassium to intracellular fluid. Subsequently, potassium removal from the body with either an exchange resin [Kayexalate (sodium polystyrene sulfonate) 20 to 50 g with 200 ml of 70% sorbitol] or dialysis should be considered.

CALCIUM, PHOSPHORUS, AND MAGNESIUM METABOLISM IN LIVER DISEASE

Abnormalities in calcium, phosphorus, and magnesium metabolism are commonly encountered in patients with chronic liver disorders (see Chaps. 32 to 34). For example, Long and coworkers found that 25 percent of 32 patients with chronic liver disease (25 biliary cirrhosis, 7 hepatocellular disease) had plasma calcium concentrations less than 8.5 mg/100 ml.[116] In most of these subjects the low serum calcium concentration reflected a low serum albumin concentration. Mild decreases in serum concentrations of phosphorus and magnesium were also observed.[116]

CALCIUM

Most information regarding calcium metabolism in patients with liver disease involves patients with biliary cirrhosis. The resultant cholestasis with decrease in intestinal fat absorption would be expected to diminish vitamin D and calcium absorption, thereby leading to hypocalcemia. Indeed, intestinal calcium absorption has been demonstrated to be diminished in biliary cirrhosis.[95,116] This diminished calcium absorption increased with vitamin therapy in some,[92,95] but not all,[116] studies. With regard to plasma vitamin D, decreased concentrations of plasma 25-hydroxy and 24,25-$(OH)_2D_3$ have been reported in most patients with biliary cirrhosis.[92,95,116,150] and in patients with chronic alcoholic liver disease.[116] Plasma concentrations of 1,α25-$(OH)_2D_3$, however, are usually normal in patients with biliary cirrhosis.[116,122,150] Plasma concentrations of the fat-soluble vitamins A and E also tend to be low, particularly in patients with advanced biliary cirrhosis.[92a,127a] Parathyroid hormone concentrations are normal for the prevailing serum calcium concentrations in patients with alcoholic and biliary cirrhosis.[116,122,150]

Other reasons for a decreased serum calcium level in patients with liver disease include poor dietary intake, concomitant pancreatitis, and magnesium depletion. Thus, severe hypomagnesemia may decrease secretion of parathyroid hormone as well as inhibit bone responsiveness to parathyroid hormone.[36,161,162] Acute severe hyperphosphatemia, as occurs in rhabdomyolysis with massive tissue phosphorus leak, may lower serum calcium. Diminished renal function (serum creatinine level greater than 3 to 4 mg/100 ml) also causes hyperphosphatemia and hypocalcemia.[69] Finally, thyrocalcitonin-secreting hepatic neoplasms may also result in hypocalcemia.[119]

With regard to bone disease occurring in the setting of chronic liver disease, 20 of 32 patients with biliary cirrhosis and hepatocellular disease had either bone pain or recent fractures.[116] Bone biopsies in 22 patients revealed 5 with osteomalacia, 7 with combined osteomalacia and osteoporosis, 5 with osteoporosis, and 5 normal. In other studies of patients with biliary cirrhosis, both osteoporosis and osteomalacia have been found.[38,92,95,122,150] By contrast, another study found that histologic evidence of bone disease was virtually nonexistent when bone biopsies were done at the time of presentation in patients with primary biliary cirrhosis.[127a] Osteomalacia appears to respond to oral vitamin D therapy, but the osteoporosis does not.[92,95,122,156] Bone disease also occurs in patients with chronic alcoholic liver disease.[116] However, the frequency, cause, and type of bone disease in this population remain to be defined.

Tetany, paresthesias, muscle spasms, and cramps, often with a characteristic carpopedal distribution, are the hallmarks of hypocalcemia. Latent tetany may be diagnosed if a twitch is produced by tapping over the facial nerve (Chvostek's sign) or if carpal spasm results when a blood pressure cuff is inflated above systolic pressure for 3 min (Trousseau's sign).

Acute symptomatic hypocalcemia requires immediate therapy because of the possibility of spasm of the glottis, hypotension, and ventricular arrhythmias. Treatment should provide 200 to 300 mg of calcium and should be continued until tetany is controlled. Administration of 20 to 30 ml of 10% calcium gluconate (93 mg of elemental calcium per 10-ml ampule) or 10% calcium chloride (360 mg per 10-ml ampule) will usually reverse neuromuscular hyperexcitability. If symptoms persist or recur, a slow intravenous infusion of 15 mg of elemental calcium per kilogram of body weight over 4 to 6 h will help. Chronic hypocalcemia should be treated with 2 to 4 g per day of calcium as calcium lactate (60 mg of elemental calcium per 300-mg tablet), calcium gluconate (90 mg per 1-tablet), or calcium carbonate (260 mg per 650-mg tablet). If vitamin D deficiency is present, therapy must be individualized. In malabsorption, vitamin D requirements vary markedly; in patients with very large requirements, magnesium depletion should be considered. Measurements of 25-OH-D_3 levels are useful in assessing the adequacy of replacement therapy.

MAGNESIUM

Hypomagnesemia commonly complicates acute and chronic alcoholism. Reduced serum and muscle magnesium levels have been found in patients symptomatic from alcohol withdrawl.[62,66,80,91,121] The many factors contributing to the hypomagnesemia include poor intake and gastrointestinal losses from diarrhea. Renal magnesium excretion is increased by acute elevation of blood alcohol levels, but the excessive magnesuria does not usually persist in the steady state.[2] The early rise in urinary magnesium excretion may persist, however, if starvation and metabolic acidosis are present. On entry to the hospital, acute ethanol withdrawl, intravenous glucose therapy, and respiratory alkalosis may all further reduce extracellular fluid magnesium levels. These reductions in serum magnesium levels, combined with associated hypokalemia, hypocalcemia, and metabolic alkalosis, may result in profound neurologic disturbances. Intestinal malabsorption of magnesium, phosphate depletion, and diuretic therapy all contribute to the hypomagnesemia found in this setting.[89,125,173,198]

Shils' classic study showed that dietary deprivation of magnesium led to a syndrome characterized by personality change, tremor, fasciculations, carpopedal spasm, and generalized spasticity. Biochemical changes included hypomagnesemia, hypocalcemia, and hypokalemia.[173] As discussed previously, magnesium depletion results in renal potassium wasting with hypokalemia and impairs the secretion and action of parathyroid hormone, causing hypocalcemia.[36,161,162] Restoration of dietary magnesium resulted in prompt remission of abnormal signs and symptoms. The onset of symptoms correlated best with the nadir in serum magnesium concentration. Generally, symptoms are not seen unless serum values are 0.5 to 0.75 meq below the normal value of 1.78 ± 0.15 meq/liter.

Most patients with hypomagnesemia can be treated simply by the provision of a normal diet. If urinary or stool losses continue, magnesium supplementation becomes necessary. Renal function should be evaluated prior to therapy. Since approximately 50 percent of an administered dose of magnesium is normally excreted in the urine, renal failure dictates that therapeutic doses be reduced. Symptomatic magnesium deficits are usually between 1 and 2 meq per kilogram of body weight. If oral magnesium therapy is indicated, magnesium oxide, 250 mg (12.5 meq of magnesium) to 500 mg four times daily, is generally well tolerated, with 25 to 50 percent of the total dose being absorbed. If parenteral therapy is required, 12 ml of 50% magnesium sulfate (49 meq) in 1000 ml of glucose is infused over 3 h and 80 meq in 2,000 ml given over the remainder of the first 24-h period. An additional 49 meq/day can be given over the next 3 days.[65]

PHOSPHORUS

Chronic alcoholism is usually the major factor associated with hypophosphatemia. Stein and coworkers found that 15 percent of alcoholic patients admitted to a Veterans Administration hospital had a serum phosphorus concentration of less than 2 mg/100 ml.[182] Territo and Tanaka encountered 12 chronic alcoholics with an admission serum phosphorus concentration of less than 1.8 mg/100 ml; 10 of these patients had phosphorus concentrations of less than 0.9 mg/100 ml.[187]

Other factors contribute to hypophosphatemia in patients with liver disease. Intestinal malabsorption as well as respiratory alkalosis resulting from alcohol withdrawal may contribute to hypophosphatemia.[182] Administration of intravenous glucose and refeeding of the malnourished patient also result in hypophosphatemia.[66,125,182] Rarely, proximal renal tubular dysfunction with phosphaturia and hypophosphatemia occurs in the setting of chronic active hepatitis.

Since phosphorus plays a critical role in cell membrane structure (phospholipids) and energy production (ATP), acute severe hyposphosphatemia may result in marked cellular dysfunction. Clinically significant dysfunction of platelets, white and red blood cells, central nervous system, and skeletal and cardiac muscle have been reported in association with severe phosphate depletion. Confusion, disorientation, and muscular weakness are the most prominent manifestations of severe hypophosphatemia. Hemolytic anemia, rhabdomyolysis, liver function abnormalities, and cardiac dysfunction may occur.

Recently, severe hypophosphatemia was found in about 30 percent of patients with acute liver failure due to acetaminophen.[42,98] In this study, glucose administration and respiratory alkalosis appear to be potential causes of the hypophosphatemia. Although there was no relation between the degree of hypophosphatemia and mortality, a possible contributing role of phosphate depletion in hepatocellular necrosis was raised by the authors.[42]

Patients with mild hypophosphatemia can often be treated with increased dietary phosphate intake (e.g., milk, potassium, and sodium phosphate). When the enteral route is not available, or when hypophosphatemia is severe (less than 1.0 mg/100 ml), intravenous phosphate must be given. This can be administered as either the sodium or potassium salt.[106] Current data suggest that 2.5 to 5.0 mg per kilogram body weight can be given as an initial dose over 6 h.[106] Serum phosphorus concentration should be closely monitored and the intravenous dosage adjusted accordingly.

Hyperphosphatemia in the setting of chronic liver disease suggests the presence of either diminished phosphate excretion (renal failure, hypoparathyroidism) or a high phosphate load; the latter may result from endogenous release of phosphorus by muscle (rhabdomyolysis) or from the exogenous administration of phosphate.[177]

ACID-BASE BALANCE IN LIVER DISEASE

Major acid-base abnormalities are frequently encountered in patients with liver disease (Table 37-7). Stable, noncomatose patients with cirrhosis often have no major acid-base abnormality. However, with increasing severity of cirrhosis and in patients with fulminant liver failure an acid-base disturbance is usually present. Respiratory alkalosis is the disorder encountered with greatest frequency (Table 37-7). For example, in a study of 91 patients with portal cirrhosis of varying severity, 64 percent had respiratory alkalosis.[132] In addition, metabolic acidosis [13] and metabolis alkalosis,[21] as well as respiratory acidosis, are seen in patients with liver disease[132] (see Chaps. 25, 29, and 30).

ALKALEMIA

Respiratory alkalosis

Respiratory alkalosis is encountered in all forms of liver disease (Table 37-7). In general, the degree of respiratory alkalosis increases with increasing severity of underlying liver disease.[132] Significant alkalemia (pH greater than 7.50) is seen most often in patients with hepatic coma and/or fulminant hepatitis (Table 37-7). Prolonged hyperventilation may reduce plasma bicarbonate levels to values as low as 16 meq/liter.[142] In several studies a positive correlation between increasing severity of respiratory alkalosis and decreasing mental status has been observed.[142,143,180,189]

The cause of the respiratory alkalosis seen in liver disease has not been ascertained. Early studies by Heinemann and coworkers established that respiratory alkalosis in patients with liver disease could be demonstrated in the absence of anemia, fever, cardiopulmonary disease, and increased oxygen consumption.[82] A significant inverse relationship between ammonia concentration and P_{CO_2} has been found by Casey and coworkers.[33]

TABLE 37-7 • Occurrence of alkalosis and acidosis in various forms of liver disease

		Alkalosis		Acidosis			
	No Abnormality*	Resp.	Metab.	Resp.	Metab.	Alkalemia (pH > 7.47)	Acidemia (pH > 7.37)
Stable cirrhosis							
Posner et al.[142] (n = 6)	17	83	0	0	0	67	0
Rodman et al.[159] (n = 20)	40	50	5	5	0	20	0
Snell et al.[179] (n = 8)	38	0	25	0	38	13	13
Prytz et al.[143] (n = 55)	49	25	16	2	7	2	7
Unstable cirrhosis, coma							
Vanamee et al.[189] (n = 29)	0	72	14	14	0	72	0
Posner et al.[142] (n = 18)	0	78	17	0	0	83	0
Snell et al.[179] (n = 7)	0	86	14	0	0	29	0
Fulminant liver failure, coma							
Record et al.[148] (n = 28)	0	54	36	0	11	71	11
Prytz et al.[143] (n = 12)	0	0	8	0	92	8	75

* Percent involvement

In addition, hyperventilation follows nonacidifying infusion of ammonia into dogs,[156] mice,[157] and human beings.[120] Although these observations suggest that ammonia may increase ventilation, other studies have not corroborated these findings.[146,188] Moreover, ammonia salts infused either intravenously into human beings or into the carotid artery of dogs produce either no change or only a mild increase in ventilation.[49,196] It appears unlikely that an increase in blood ammonia is the sole factor responsible for respiratory alkalosis in hepatic disease.

Arterial oxygen desaturation has been recognized as an accompaniment of hepatic cirrhosis since 1935.[179] This hypoxemia has been proposed to play a pathogenetic role in respiratory alkalosis. The cause of the hypoxemia remains unclear. The oxyhemoglobin dissociation curve appears normal in most cirrhotic patients.[159] The fact that inhalation of 100% oxygen results in a deficit of physically dissolved oxygen in arterial blood in patients with cirrhosis suggests a shunting of venous blood to the arterial circulation. Although tense ascites and pleural effusions may occasionally result in pulmonary perfusion without ventilation,[82] hypoxemia has been observed in the absence of pulmonary function abnormalities, suggesting a nonpulmonary site of arterial-venous blood admixture.[82,148,159,180] Earlier studies suggest that admixture between the portal and pulmonary venous systems (through paraesophageal, mediastinal, and azygous veins) occurs.[27] Does the arterial hypoxemia that occurs in patients with chronic liver disease contribute to respiratory alkalosis? The degree of hypoxemia is mild, with fewer than 10 to 20 percent of patients exhibiting arterial oxygen saturations below 90 percent.[142,159] Moreover, a strong relationship between either P_{O_2} or arterial oxygen saturation and P_{CO_2} is not present in most cirrhotic patients.[82,142,148,159,180] Together, these observations suggest that hypoxemia does not play a critical role in the pathogenesis of respiratory alkalosis in liver disease.

It is possible that a humoral factor, such as progesterone, may contribute to hyperventilation in cirrhosis. This hormone, a respiratory stimulant in humans, is degraded by the liver.[184] Another view on the cause of respiratory alkalosis has been presented by Bittar and coworkers.[21] These workers suggested that intracellular acidosis occurs in the brainstem of patients with liver disease, despite extracellular alkalosis. Advanced liver disease probably disrupts Krebs' cycle, since increased concentrations of pyruvate and glutamate have been found in cerebrospinal fluid (CSF).[3,50] Such a disruption of cell metabolism might lead to intracellular accumulation of hydrogen ions. If such an intracellular acidosis existed, chronic hyperventilation and an increased ventilatory response to inhaled CO_2 would be anticipated; indeed, this was observed by Karetzky and coworkers.[93] Unfortunately, methodologic limitations have not allowed further exploration of this potential mechanism in humans. Finally, it should be noted that other well-recognized causes of respiratory alkalosis (sepsis, salicylate ingestion, CNS disease, cardiopulmonary disease, and mechanical overventilation) may be operative in selected patients with liver disease and respiratory alkalosis.

Is respiratory alkalosis harmful to the patient with liver disease? The p*K* of ammonia is 8.9 at 37° C. Thus, in normal blood, most ammonia is present in the form of the ammonium ion (NH_4^+) and only a small part as un-ionized ammonia (NH_3). It is only the un-ionized NH_3 that can diffuse into cells. The small fraction of ammonia normally present in diffusible form can be readily altered by changes in blood pH. In mice, for example, an increase in blood pH dramatically lowers the dose of ammonia required to cause death. Furthermore, the neurotoxicity of ammonia varies directly with blood pH.[192] It has been shown that alkalemic enhancement of neurotoxicity is associated with a striking increase in the ratio of brain tissue to arterial blood ammonia.[192] Other studies have also demonstrated that blood alkalinization increases brain and liver ammonia uptake in dogs.[32] Studies in human beings also examined the effect of changes in blood pH on CSF ammonia concentration.[191] In six patients with hepatic coma, 0.2*N* hydrochloric acid (HCl) infused intravenously reduced CSF/arterial ammonia ratio by 40 percent.[191] Thus, alkalemia enhances, and acidemia inhibits, cellular uptake of ammonia by brain and other issues.

Posner and Plum examined the effect of acutely correcting systemic pH on CNS function in patients with respiratory alkalosis and hepatic cirrhosis.[142] Lowering arterial pH acutely with either 5% CO_2 inhalation or intravenous acetazolamide worsened the neurologic status of encephalopathic patients. This worsening occurred despite a decrease in arterial ammonia concentration. Thus, therapeutic efforts directed at treating respiratory alkalosis of liver disease are not advisable.[142]

Metabolic alkalosis

Metabolic alkalosis occurs in many patients with liver disease, and diuretic therapy is most often responsible. In a survey of 64 cirrhotic patients treated with thiazide and loop active diuretics, Sherlock found a 20 percent prevalence of severe metabolic alkalosis.[172] Several mechanisms contribute to diuretic-induced metabolic alkalosis: (1) increased renal secretion of hydrogen ion; (2) loss of chloride-rich, bicarbonate-poor fluid, with resultant "contraction" around existing bicarbonate stores; and (3) a possible shift of hydrogen ions into the intracellular space.

Loop-active and mercurial diuretics typically increase renal acid excretion by 100 to 250 meq over the first week of their administration. This degree of acid loss, however, does not fully account for the hyperbicarbonatemia.[30] Moreover, thiazide diuretics can cause metabolic alkalosis without significantly increasing renal acid excretion. The mechanism whereby thiazides increase net acid excretion is not known with certainty. It is generally thought that increased renal tubular sodium reabsorption and hydrogen ion secretion, due at least in part to aldosterone, increases acid excretion. Increased sodium avidity, hypochloremia, and hypokalemia sustain the alkalosis as long as the diet remains low in potassium and chloride, despite discontinuation of diuretics. Early administration of potassium chloride or use of triamterene, spironolactone, or amiloride will prevent or reduce the alkalosis. Three prospective randomized trials have demonstrated that careful use of combined spironolactone and either a thiazide or a loop-active diuretic rarely leads to significant hypolakemic alkalosis in edematous cirrhotic patients.[1,67,77]

Nasogastric suctioning and/or vomiting are also common causes of metabolic alkalosis in patients with liver disease. The loss of gastric juice can substantially deplete hydrogen ion, water, and electrolyte stores. The severity of the resulting alkalosis depends on the quantity and composition of the shed gastric fluid. Bicarbonaturia occurs during and immediately after acid loss.

Other causes of metabolic alkalosis in patients with liver disease include alkali loading from such sources as citrate from blood transfusions and from antacids. High-dose corticosteroid therapy may also induce metabolic alkalosis. Finally, a recent study of patients with fulminant hepatic failure due to either acetaminophen or viral infection demonstrated a high prevalence (36 percent) of metabolic alkalosis.[148] Only one of these patients received nasogastric suctioning. No cause for the alkalosis could be detected.

The use of certain precautionary measures can effectively prevent development of metabolic alkalosis. When a patient is losing large amounts of gastric fluid, analysis of the fluid is a useful guide to replacement therapy. The histamine-blocking agent cimetidine reduces the quantity of acid lost in gastric fluid.[11] Since cimetidine may accumulate in hepatic failure, thereby worsening encephalopathy, dosage modification may be necessary.[166] Intravenous sodium chloride and potassium chloride are usually needed to correct existing metabolic alkalosis. In patients with fluid overload or compromised renal and/or cardiac function, intravenous 0.1*N* HCl, or an HCl precursor such as arginine monohydrochloride, will effectively lower blood pH. Arginine monohydrochloride should be used with caution, however, since it may exert a hyperkalemic effect in patients with liver and kidney disease.[26] Induction of a bicarbonate diuresis with the carbonic anhydrase inhibitor acetazolamide will reduce plasma bicarbonate and pH in metabolic alkalosis. This therapy, however, may result in profound loss of potassium in the urine as well. Hemodialysis is rarely required to correct severe metabolic alkalosis in patients with liver and renal disease.

ACIDEMIA

High anion gap metabolic acidosis

Elevated anion gap metabolic acidoses have been observed in 10 to 20 percent of patients with chronic liver disease (Table 37-8).

A number of observers have suggested that patients with severe liver disease are susceptible to lactic acidosis.[46] Removal of lactic acid normally occurs via three pathways: (1) oxidation via the tricarboxylic acid cycle, (2) gluconeogenesis, and (3) renal excretion.[100] The liver plays an important role in the first two of these pathways.[100] Each of these disposal routes simultaneously eliminates lactic acid and regenerates alkali. In addition to impaired acid removal and bicarbonate resynthesis, the patient with severe liver disease may also be susceptible to increased lactic acid production. Hypotension due to sepsis or GI hemorrhage can stimulate such synthesis. Several studies on lactic acid metabolism in patients with liver disease have been published.[16,83,101,132,143,148,151] In general, patients with chronic, stable hepatic cirrhosis do not demonstrate a defect in basal hepatic lactate extraction and have normal or minimally elevated plasma lactic acid concentrations. With more advanced liver disease—particularly in the setting of a superimposed hypotensive insult (i.e., sepsis or hemorrhage)—increasing blood lactic acid concentrations and decreasing pH can occur. Usually, the sicker the patient, the higher the lactic acid level. In patients with terminal cirrhosis, up to 30 to 40 percent will have mild-to-moderate lactic acidosis.[143] Increasing blood lactic acid levels correlate inversely with the prognosis in patients with liver disease. Lactic acidosis can complicate the clinical course of up to 20 to

TABLE 37-8 • Causes of high anion gap metabolic acidosis

1. Lactic acidosis
2. Ketoacidosis
   A. Alcoholic
   B. Diabetic
   C. Starvation
3. Toxin ingestion
   A. Methanol
   B. Ethylene glycol
   C. Paraldehyde
   D. Salicylate
4. Renal failure

40 percent of patients with acute fulminant hepatitis.[16,101,148]

Ketoacidosis may arise from a variety of causes in patients with liver disease. Starvation may contribute to ketosis, and diabetic ketoacidosis may occur, especially in patients with pancreatic damage. Alcohol-induced ketoacidosis appears to be especially common in patients with Laennec's cirrhosis. This disorder probably results from a combination of insults including starvation, dehydration, and alcohol-induced impairment in gluconeogenesis and stimulation of lactic acid generation.[40] Ketoacidosis and lactic acidosis typically reduce plasma bicarbonate by 7 to 10 meq/liter. Since most of the acidosis is due to accumulated β-hydroxybutyrate, the nitroprusside reaction may be negative or only weakly positive initially (see Chap. 26). An unusual feature of this illness is the clinical stability of the patient and the relative ease of therapy. Thus, modest amounts of saline solution and glucose usually result in rapid correction of the acidosis.

Ingestion of acid-producing substances can result in high anion gap metabolic acidosis. This is especially common in patients with alcoholic liver disease. In this regard, we continue to see three to five patients per year with metabolic acidosis caused by either methanol or ethylene glycol ingestion (see Chap. 25). Many of these patients are alcoholics with chronic liver disease. Methanol is a common industrial solvent; ethylene glycol is used as an antifreeze (e.g., radiator fluid or windshield wiper fluid). Both agents have intoxicating properties. Thus, both accidental overdose and intentional ingestion of these compounds are seen. These agents may result in significant morbidity and death if their intake is left untreated. The diagnosis of these intoxications requires a high index of suspicion and should be considered if other causes of metabolic acidosis can be excluded. Patients with methanol poisoning may have abdominal and visual disturbances and noncardiac pulmonary edema. Methanol and ethylene glycol can often be rapidly measured by direct blood analysis. Another clue to diagnosis of these disorders is the presence of an "osmolar gap" (i.e., a difference between directly measured plasma osmolality and osmolality as calculated from measurements of plasma sodium, glucose, urea nitrogen, and alcohol levels).[90] The presence of numerous calcium oxalate crystals in the urine is a frequent, but not uniform, accompaniment of ethylene glycol poisoning.

Rapid diagnosis is critically important in these intoxications to prevent significant morbidity and mortality. Prompt removal of these drugs from the body (hemodialysis) and correction of acidemia is needed. Administration of ethanol may prevent degradation of methanol and ethylene glycol to toxic metabolites. Thus, a blood ethanol level of 100 mg/100 ml should be maintained, and careful clinical monitoring and supportive care are essential (see Chap. 25).

Additional causes of high anion gap metabolic acidosis in patients with liver disease include salicylate and paraldehyde intoxication and renal failure. Indeed, Prytz and Thomson found that renal failure was a major contributing factor to high anion gap metabolic acidemia in patients with end stage cirrhosis.[143]

Normal anion gap metabolic acidosis

The causes of normal anion gap (hyperchloremic) metabolic acidosis in the setting of liver disease are listed in Table 37-9. Loss of bicarbonate-rich stool via severe diarrhea is a relatively common cause of hyperchloremic metabolic acidosis in the general population. The diarrhea associated with lactulose therapy may result in a mild hyperchloremic acidosis. Loss of a number of other bicarbonate-rich fluids, as well as administration of hydrochloric acid analoguges (e.g., arginine monohydrochloride), can also produce hyperchloremic acidosis in the setting of liver disease (Table 37-9).

In recent years much attention has been focused on the relationship between renal tubular acidosis (RTA) and liver disease (see Chap. 27). An association between a renal acidification defect (i.e., RTA) and liver disease was first suggested by McCune and coworkers in 1943.[124] In this report, 7 of 12 patients with the Fanconi syndrome (generalized proximal tubular dysfunction) were found to have liver disease at autopsy (2 cirrhosis, 4 focal necrosis, 1 fatty infiltration). In 4 patients cystine crystals were observed in the liver; it was likely that cystinosis was

TABLE 37-9 • Causes of normal anion gap metabolic acidosis in liver disease

I. Diarrhea
II. Renal tubular acidosis
  A. Systemic disorders involving kidney and liver
    1. Wilson's disease
    2. Galactosemia
    3. Cytinosis
    4. Glycogen storage disorders
    5. Amyloidosis
  B. Chronic Liver Disorders
    1. Chronic active hepatitis
    2. Biliary cirrhosis
    3. Cryptogenic cirrhosis
    4. Alcohol-related liver disease
    5. Hepatoma
  C. Drug-induced
    1. Carbonic anhydrase inhibitors
    2. Toluene inhalation
    3. Spironolactone, amiloride, triamterene
III. Addition of hydrochloric acid (arginine, lysine, NH_4Cl)
IV. Miscellaneous (small bowel fluid loss, ileal loop, ureterosigmoidostomy, renal failure, adrenal insufficiency)

TABLE 37-10 • Prevalence of renal tubular acidosis in chronic liver disease

	Cause of cirrhosis			
	Alcohol	Chronic hepatitis	Cryptogenic	Bilary
Read et al., 1968[147]	—	3/81 (3 overt)	—	—
Shear et al., 1969[170]*	9/15 (2 overt)	—	—	—
Better et al., 1972[12]	2/9	—	—	—
Golding, 1975[75]	1/15	15/48 (4 overt)	5/25 (1 overt)	17/29 (6 overt)
Oster et al., 1975[134]	9/22	—	—	—
Caregaro et al., 1981[31]	15/31	1/13	1/7	—

* Some patients were "selected" because of hypokalemia.

responsible for both renal tubular defects and liver dysfunction. Subsequently, an association between abnormalities in renal tubular function and liver disease has been established for several systemic conditions that involve simultaneously the liver and kidney. These disorders include Wilson's disease, galactosemia, amyloidosis, glycogen storage diseases, heavy metal intoxication, and hydrocarbon inhalation.[52,88,105,108,128] These rare disorders typically result in hepatic dysfunction and generalized defects in proximal renal tubular function. Thus, bicarbonate wasting, aminoaciduria, renal glycosuria, and hyperuricosuria are seen. Clinically, a moderate normal anion gap metabolic acidosis diminishes bicarbonate levels to 12 to 20 meq/liter. The chloride concentration is proportionately increased, while hypokalemia, hypophosphatemia, and low plasma uric acid levels are often present.

Since the 1960s, several studies have raised the possibility that liver disease per se results in impaired renal acidification. For example, in 1963, Read and coworkers found overt RTA in 3 of 81 patients with chronic active hepatitis.[147] This association was confirmed subsequently by other reports.[25,75,76,130,178] In the most extensive studies reported to date, Golding has examined urinary acidification and proximal tubular function in 102 patients with chronic liver disease[75,76] (Table 37-10). A mild renal acidification defect following acid loading was present in 31, 20, and 59 percent of patients with chronic active hepatitis, cryptogenic cirrhosis, and biliary cirrhosis, respectively.[75,76] Most cases were occult, manifesting only impaired lowering of urinary pH after acid loading. Overt RTA was encountered in only 7 percent of all patients, most of whom had minor renal acidification defects typical of distal RTA with intact proximal tubular function. A minority of patients with overt RTA and non-alcoholic-related chronic hepatic disease appear to have generalized proximal tubular dysfunction and nephrocalcinosis.[75,76]

What is responsible for the renal tubular dysfunction in patients with chronic hepatitis and biliary cirrhosis? Ten patients with either chronic hepatitis-related liver disease or biliary cirrhosis have undergone renal biopsy. Marked renal interstitial nephritis with tubular damage was observed in 9 of these 10 patients.[25,75,76] These observations suggest that tubulointerstitial injury is responsible for the tubular dysfunction. Hypergammaglobulinemia is another factor that may contribute to the renal tubular dysfunction in the setting of chronic hepatitis and biliary cirrhosis.[130] In summary, decreased renal acidification is present in many patients with chronic hepatitis and either cryptogenic or biliary cirrhosis. However, overt RTA of both the distal and proximal variety is seen in only 1 to 10 percent of patients with these disorders.

Is the overt RTA that may be encountered in patients with chronic hepatitis and biliary cirrhosis harmful? The concomitant renal potassium wasting and resultant hypokalemia is a potentially serious consequence. Hypercalciuria may predispose to renal stones, and the metabolic acidosis to osteopenia. Thus, potassium and alkali replacements are often indicated.

Studies by Owen and coworkers[135] suggest that the alkaline urine of RTA may also predispose to hepatic encephalopathy. These workers studied 11 patients with chronic liver disease who underwent renal vein catheterization. Acetazolamide (500 mg intravenously), a carbonic anhydrase inhibitor, was given; this acutely increased urine pH to greater than 7.0, causing a twofold increase in the ammonia released into the renal veins. The increase in renal venous ammonia was maintained throughout the 60 min of observation and progressively increased arterial blood ammonia following administration of the drug. Alkalinization of the urine causes redistribution of ammonia exiting the kidney; the addition to the renal vein might induce, or worsen, encephalopathy.

Is alcohol-related liver disease associated with a renal acidification defect? This possibility was first suggested by Shear and coworkers in 1969.[170] These observers found that 9 of 15 patients with alcohol-related cirrhosis were unable to reduce urine pH to less than 5.58 in response to an oral acid challenge (calcium chloride). The acidification defect seen in these patients was characterized by a decrease in urinary titratable acidity, with ammonium accounting for an increased percentage of total urinary hydrogen ion excretion. These findings suggest the presence of a "distal" RTA. Six of these nine patients had renal potassium wasting.

Other workers have further examined the relation between alcohol-related liver disease and a renal acidification defect. As shown in Table 37-10, 27 of 77 patients with alcohol-related cirrhosis were found to be unable to lower urinary pH to values below 5.60 in response to an acid load.[13,31,75,76,134,170] None of these 77 patients had overt RTA. Thus, plasma sodium, potassium, and bicarbonate levels in patients with the acidification defect could not be distinguished from those in patients who were able to acidify their urine. The mechanism of the distal renal acidification defect seen in alcohol-related liver disease has not been ascertained. The defect can occur independently of hypergammaglobulinemia, or hypokalemia.[13,31,75,76,134,170] Renal biopsy results are not available; however, renal blood flow and its distribution, as assessed and labeled ^{131}xenon, do not differ when patients with alcohol-induced liver disease with and without RTA are compared. Two recent clinical studies suggest that enhanced proximal tubular sodium reabsorption, with less sodium delivered to distal nephron Na^+-H^+ exchange sites, is responsible for this complication.[13,134] Thus, increasing distal delivery of sodium by spontaneous or pharmacologic diuresis, mannitol infusion, and infusion of sodium salts of phosphate and sulfate lowers urinary pH and restores the diminished titratable acidity.

In summary, alcohol-related cirrhosis may be associated with an inability to lower urinary pH in response to an acid challenge. This disorder, however, generally does not appear to lead to any change in plasma electrolyte composition, and is of little clinical significance.

It is also of interest that proximal renal tubular dysfunction may be encountered rarely in patients with alcohol-related liver disease.[85,123,126] Thus, renal phosphate, glucose, and uric acid wasting, along with hypercalciuria, have been well documented in the setting of alcohol-related liver disease.[85,123,126] The mechanism and frequency of these defects in proximal tubular function in alcohol-related liver disease remain to be determined. In the few cases studied, the defect resolved 3 to 4 weeks after admission.

A study by Gabow and coworkers has elucidated another mechanism of hyperchloremic metabolic acidosis in patients with chronic liver disease.[70] In these studies, six alcoholics with cirrhosis developed reversible metabolic acidosis (HCO_3^- decreased from 18 to 11 meq/liter, pH 7.29) and hyperkalemia (5.0 meq/liter) following spironolactone therapy. Neither the frequency nor the mechanism of these effects of aldosterone inhibition was determined. However, this report clearly demonstrates that spironolactone can worsen or induce metabolic acidosis in patients with alcoholic chronic liver disease. As noted in Table 37-9, toluene inhalation can occasionally result in severe proximal and distal tubular dysfunction and mild liver abnormalities.[131,186]

Finally, it should be noted that respiratory acidosis has been reported in some patients with cirrhosis.[91,157] This acidemia may be due to the presence of associated lung disease. More commonly, it occurs in association with worsening hepatic encephalopathy and excessive sedative-hypnotic drug administration.

A practical approach to the diagnosis of acid-base

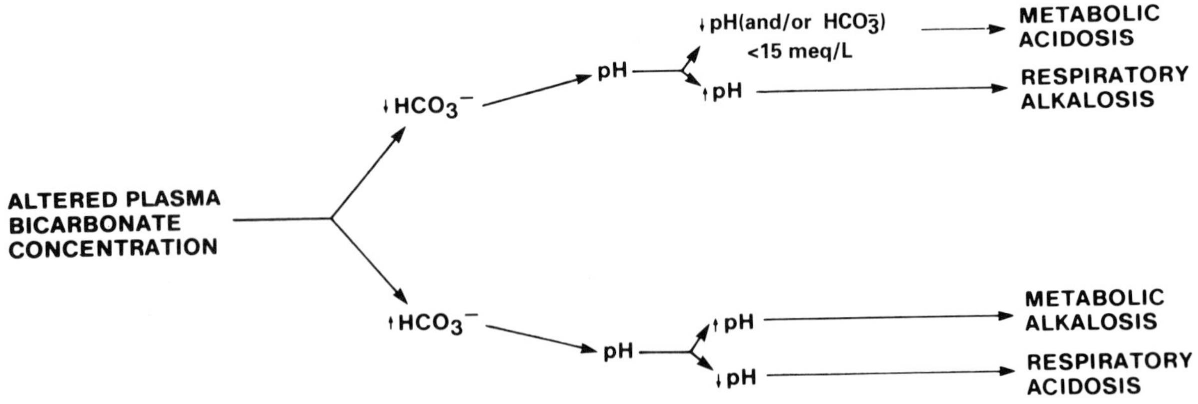

FIGURE 37–3 • Practical approach to the diagnosis of metabolic acid-base disorders.

disorders presenting as alterations in plasma bicarbonate concentration in patients with liver disease is depicted in Fig. 37-3.

REFERENCES

1. Abshagen U et al: Disposition kinetics of spironolactone in hepatic failure and single doses and prolonged treatment. *Eur J Clin Pharmacol* 11:169, 1977.
2. Aikawa JK: Biochemistry and physiology of magnesium. *World Rev Nutr Diet* 28:112, 1978.
3. Amatuzio DS, Nesbitt S: A study of pyruvic acid in the blood, spinal fluid and urine of patients with liver disease with and without hepatic coma (abstract). *J Clin Invest* 29:796, 1950.
4. Anderson RJ et al: Mechanism of effect of thoracic inferior vena cava constriction on renal water excretion. *J Clin Invest* 54:1473, 1974.
5. Anderson RJ et al: Mechanism of portal hypertension induced alterations in renal hemodynamics, renal water excretion and renal secretion. *J Clin Invest* 58:964, 1976.
6. Anderson RJ et al: Hyponatremia: A prospective analysis of the epidemiology and the pathogenetic role of vasopressin. *Ann Intern Med* 102:164, 1985.
7. Angeli P et al: Tubular site of renal sodium retention in ascitic liver cirrhosis evaluated by lithium clearance. *Eur J Clin Invest* 20:111, 1990.
8. Arroyo V et al: Prognostic value of spontaneous hyponatremia in cirrhosis with ascites. *Dig Dis Sci* 21:249, 1976.
9. Arroyo V et al: Sympathetic nervous activity, renin-angiotension system and renal excretion of prostaglandin E_2 in cirrhosis. *Eur J Clin Invest* 13:272, 1982.
10. Bank N, Aynedjian HS: A micropuncture study of renal salt and water retention in chronic bile duct obstruction. *J Clin Invest* 55:994, 1975.
11. Barton CH et al: Cimetidine in the management of metabolic alkalosis induced by nasogastric drainage. *Arch Surg* 114:70, 1979.
12. Better OS et al: Role of antidiuretic hormone in impaired urinary dilution associated with chronic bile duct ligation. *Clin Sci* 58:493, 1980.
13. Better OS et al: Defect in urinary acidification in cirrhosis. *Arch Intern Med* 130:77, 1972.
14. Better OS, Massry SG: Effect of chronic bile duct obstruction on renal handling of salt and water. *J Clin Invest* 51:402, 1972.
15. Better OS, Schrier RW: Disturbed volume homeostasis in patients with cirrhosis of the liver. *Kidney Int* 23:303, 1983.
16. Bihari D et al: Tissue hypoxia during fulminant hepatic failure. *Crit Car Med* 13:1034, 1985.
17. Bichet DG et al: Mechanisms of improvement of water and sodium excretion by enhancement of central hemodynamics in decompensated cirrhotic patients. *Kidney Int* 24:788, 1983.
18. Bichet DG et al: Role of vasopressin in abnormal water excretion in cirrhotic patients. *Ann Intern Med* 96:413, 1982.
19. Bichet DG et al: Potential role of increased sympathetic activity in impaired sodium and water excretion in cirrhosis. *N Engl J Med* 307:1552, 1982.
20. Birchard WH et al: Diuretic responses to oral and intravenous waterloads in patients with hepatic cirrhosis. *J Lab Clin Med* 48:26, 1956.
21. Bittar EE et al: The pH of muscle in Laennec's cirrhosis and uremia. *Clin Sci* 23:265, 1962.
22. Bories P et al: The treatment of refractory ascites by the LeVeen shunt: A multicentre controlled trial (57 patients). *J Hepatol* 3:212, 1986.
23. Bosch J et al: Hepatic hemodynamics and the renin-angiotensin-aldosterone system in cirrhosis. *Gastroenterology* 78:92, 1980.
24. Boyer TD et al: Effect of indomethacin and prostaglandin A_1 on renal function and plasma renin activity in alcoholic liver disease. *Gastroenterology* 77:215, 1979.
25. Bridi GS et al: Glomerulonephritis and renal tubular acidosis in a case of chronic active hepatitis with hyperimmunoglobulinemia. *Am J Med* 52:267, 1972.
26. Bushinsky DA, Gennari FJ: Life-threatening hyperkalemia induced by arginine. *Ann Intern Med* 89:632, 1978.
27. Calabresi P, Abelmann WH: Porto-caval and porto-pulmonary anastomoses in Laennec's cirrhosis and in heart failure. *J Clin Invest* 36:1257, 1957.
28. Campbell PJ et al: Acute effects of peritoneovenous shunting on plasma atrial natriuretic peptide in cirrhotic patients with massive refractory ascites. *Am J Med* 84:112, 1988.
29. Campra JL, Reynolds T: Effectiveness of high-dose spironolactone therapy in patients with chronic liver disease and relatively refractory ascites. *Dig Dis Sci* 23:1025, 1978.
30. Cannon PJ et al: "Contraction" alkalosis after diuresis of edematous patients with ethacrynic acid. *Ann Intern Med* 62:979, 1965.
31. Caregaro L et al: Distal renal tubular acidosis in hepatic cirrhosis: Clinical and pathogenetic study. *Clin Nephrol* 15:143, 1981.
32. Carter CC et al: Organ uptake and blood pH and concentration effects of ammonia in dogs determined with ammonia labeled with 10 minute half-lived nitrogen 13. *Neurology* 23:204, 1973.
33. Casey TH et al: Body and serum potassium in liver disease: II. Relationships to arterial ammonia, blood pH, and hepatic coma. *Gastroenterology* 18:208, 1965.
34. Casey TH et al: Body and serum potassium in liver disease: I. Relationship of hepatic function and associated factors. *Gastroenterology* 18:198, 1965.
35. Chaimovitz C et al: Mechanism of increased renal tubular sodium reabsorption in cirrhosis. *Am J Med* 52:198, 1972.
36. Chase LR, Slatopolsky E: Secretion and metabolic efficacy of parathyroid hormone in patients with severe hypomagnesemia.
37. Chonko AM et al: The role of renin and aldosterone in the salt retention of edema. *Am J Med* 63:881, 1977.
38. Compston HE et al: Treatment of osteomalacia associated with primary biliary cirrhosis with parenteral vitamin D_2 or oral 25-hydroxyvitamin D_3. *Gut* 20:133, 1979.
39. Conn HO: Diuresis of ascites: Fraught with or free from hazards. *Gastroenterology* 73:619, 1977.

40. Cooperman MT et al: Clinical studies of alcoholic ketoacidosis. *Diabetes* 23:433, 1974.
41. Davidson CS: Cirrhosis of the liver treatment with prolonged sodium restriction. *JAMA* 159:1257, 1955.
42. Dawson DJ et al: Hypophosphataemia in acute liver failure. *Br Med J* 295:1312, 1987.
43. Decaux G et al: High uric acid and urea clearance in cirrhosis secondary to increased "effective vascular volume." *Am J Med* 73:328, 1982.
44. De Deuxchaisnes CN et al: Exchangeable potassium in wasting, amyotrophy, heart-disease, and cirrhosis of the liver. *Lancet* 1:7179, 1961.
45. deTroyer A et al: Demeclocycline treatment of water retention in cirrhosis. *Ann Intern Med* 85:336, 1976.
46. Dölle W: Störungen des Saure-Basenstoffwechsels bei chronisch Leberkranken, in Martini GA (ed): *Aktuelle Probleme der Hepatologie*. Stuttgart, George Thieme Verlag, 1962, p. 128.
47. Dominguez JA et al: Dietary phosphate deprivation in women and men: Effects on mineral and acid balances, parathyroid hormone and the metabolism of 25-OH-vitamin D. *J Clin Endocrinol Metab* 43:1056, 1976.
48. Eggert RC: Spironolactone diuresis in patients with cirrhosis and ascites. *Br Med J* 4:401, 1970.
49. Eiseman B, Clark GM: Studies in ammonia metabolism: III. The experimental production of coma by carotid arterial infusion of ammonium salts. *Surgery* 3:476, 1958.
50. Eiseman B et al: The role of ammonia in the production of hepatic coma. *Surg Forum* 6:369, 1955.
51. Eisenmenger WJ et al: Electrolyte studies on patients with cirrhosis of the liver. *J Clin Invest* 292:1491, 1950.
52. Elsas LJ et al: Wilson's disease with reversible renal tubular dysfunction. *Ann Intern Med* 75:427, 1971.
53. Epstein FH: Underfilling vs overflow in hepatic ascites. *N Engl J Med* 307:1577, 1982.
54. Epstein M: Characterization of renal prostaglandin E responsiveness in decompensated cirrhosis: Implications for renal sodium handling. *Clin Sci* 63:555, 1982.
55. Epstein M: Deranged sodium homeostasis in cirrhosis. *Gastroenterology* 76:622, 1979.
56. Epstein M et al: Determinants of deranged sodium and water homeostasis in decompensated cirrhosis. *J Lab Clin Med* 87:822, 1976.
57. Epstein M: The peritoneovenous shunt in the management of ascites and the hepatorenal syndome. *Gastroenterology* 82:790, 1982.
58. Epstein M et al: Interrelationship of renal sodium and phosphate handling in cirrhosis. *Mineral Electrolyte Metab* 7:305, 1982.
59. Epstein M: Treatment of refractory ascites. *N Engl J Med* 321:1675, 1989.
60. Epstein M et al: Relationship between plasma ANF responsiveness and renal sodum handling in cirrhotic humans. *Am J Nephrol* 9:133, 1987.
61. Epstein M: Atrial natriuretic factor in patients with liver disease. *Am J Nephrol* 9:89, 1989.
62. Fankushen D et al: The significance of hypomagnesemia in alcoholic patients. *Am J Med* 37:802, 1964.
63. Favre H: Role of the natriuretic factor in the disorders of sodium balance, in Hamburger J et al (eds): *Advances in Nephrology*. Chicago, Year Book Medical Publishers, 1981, p 187.
64. Fichman MP et al: Diuretic-induced hyponatremia. *Ann Intern Med* 75:853, 1971.
65. Flink EB: Therapy of magnesium deficiency. *Ann NY Acad Sci* 162:901, 1969.
66. Flink EB et al: Magnesium deficiency after prolonged parenteral fluid administration and after chronic alcoholism complicated by delirium tremens. *J Lab Clin Med* 43:169, 1954.
67. Fogel MR et al: Diuresis in the ascitic patient: A randomized controlled trial of three regimens. *J Clin Gastroenterol* 3(suppl 1):73, 1981.
68. Francisco LL et al: Mechanism of negative potassium balance in the magnesium-deficient rat (41291). *Proc Soc Exp Biol Med* 168:382, 1981.
69. Gabow PA et al: The spectrum of rhabdomyolysis. *Medicine* 61:141, 1982.
70. Gabow PA et al: Spironolactone-induced hyper-chloremic acidosis in cirrhosis. *Ann Intern Med* 90:338, 1979.
71. Gabuzda GJ, Hall PW: Relation of potassium depletion to renal ammonium metabolism and hepatic coma. *Medicine* 45:481, 1966.
72. Gines P et al: Comparison of paracentesis and diuretics in the treatment of cirrhotics with tense ascites. *Gastroenterology* 93:234, 1987.
73. Gines P et al: Randomized comparative study of therapeutic paracentesis with and without intravenous albumin in cirrhosis. *Gastroenterology* 94:1493, 1988.
74. Giuseffi J et al: Effect of bilateral adrenalectomy in a patient with massive ascites and post-necrotic cirrhosis. *N Engl J Med* 257:796, 1957.
75. Golding PL: Renal tubular acidosis in chronic liver disease. *Postgrad Med J* 51:550, 1975.
76. Golding PL, Mason ASM: Renal tubular acidosis and autoimmune liver disease. *Gut* 12:153, 1971.
77. Gregory PB et al: Complications of diuresis in the alcoholic patient with ascites: A controlled trial. *Gastroenterology* 73:534, 1977.
78. Guzaai M et al: Negative influences of ascites on the cardiac function of cirrhotic patients. *Am J Med* 59:165, 1975.
79. Hantman D et al: Rapid correction of hyponatremia in the syndrome of inappropriate secretion of antidiuretic hormone. *Ann Intern Med* 78:870, 1973.
80. Heaton FW et al: Hypomagnesaemia in chronic alcoholism. *Lancet* 2:802, 1962.
81. Hecker R: Electrolyte and circulatory changes in terminal liver failure. *Lancet* 2:1121, 1956.
82. Heinemann HO et al: Hyperventilation and arterial hypoxemia in cirrhosis of the liver. *Am J Med* 28:239, 1960.
83. Heinig RE et al: Lactic acidosis and liver disease. *Arch Intern med* 139:1229, 1979.
84. Heckman PE et al: Pseudohyponatremia and primary biliary cirrhosis. *J Clin Pathol* 42:167, 1989.
85. Higuchi T et al: Enhanced renal clearance of uric acid in hepatic cirrhosis. *Isr J Med Sci* 17:1015, 1981.
86. Henriksen JH et al: Circulating atrial natriuretic peptide and central blood volume in cirrhosis. *Liver* 6:361, 1986.
87. Hura CE et al: Use of diuretics in salt-retaining states. *Seminars Nephrol* 8:318, 1988.
88. Huth EJ et al: The renal excretion of hydrogen ion in renal tubular acidosis: III. An attempt to detect latent cases in a

family: Comments on nosology, genetics and etiology of the primary disease. *Am J Med* 28:586, 1960.
89. Iseri LT et al: Magnesium deficiency and cardiac disorders. *Am J Med* 58:837, 1975.
90. Jacobsen D: Anion and osmolal gaps in the diagnosis of methanol and ethylene glycol poisoning. *Acta Med Scand* 212:17, 1982.
91. Kalbfleisch JM et al: Effects of ethanol administration on urinary excretion of magnesium and other electrolytes in alcoholic and normal subjects. *J Clin Invest* 42:1471, 1963.
92. Kaplan MM et al: Effect of 25-hydroxyvitamin D_3 on vitamin D metabolites in primary biliary cirrhosis. *Gastroenterology* 81:681, 1981.
92a. Kaplan MM et al: Fat-soluble vitamin nutritive in primary biliary cirrhosis. *Gastroenterology* 95:787, 1988.
93. Karetzky MS, Mithoefer JC: The cause of hyperventilation and arterial hypoxia in patients with cirrhosis of the liver. *Am J Med Sci* 254:979, 1967.
94. Kawasaki H et al: Plasma levels of atrial natriuretic peptide in patients with chronic liver disease. *Am J Gastroenterol* 83:727, 1987.
95. Kehayoglou AK et al: Bone disease and calcium absorption in primary biliary cirrhosis. *Lancet* 1:715, 1968.
96. Kellerman PS, Linas SL: Large-volume paracentesis in treatment of ascites. *Ann Intern Med* 112:889, 1990.
97. Klinger EL Jr et al: Renal function changes in cirrhosis of the liver. *Arch Intern Med* 125:1010, 1970.
98. Knochel JP: Does hypophosphatemia play a role in acute liver failure? *Hepatology* 9:504, 1989.
99. Kramer HJ: Natriuretic hormone—its possible role in fluid and electrolyte disturbances in chronic liver disease. *Postgrad Med J* 51:532, 1975.
100. Kreisberg RA: Lactate homeostasis and lactic acidosis. *Ann Intern Med* 92:227, 1980.
101. Kruse JA et al: Significance of blood lactate levels in critically ill patienets with liver disease. *Am J Med* 83:77, 1987.
102. Haffi G et al: Renal hemodynamic and natriuretic effects of human atrial natriuretic factor infusion in cirrhosis with ascites. *Gastroenterology* 96:167, 1989.
103. Lancestremere RG et al: Simultaneous determination of cardiac output and renal function in patients with Laennec's cirrhosis during the administration of the pressor amine metaraminol. *J Lab Clin Med* 61:820, 1963.
104. Laragh JH et al: Angiotensin II, norepinephrine and renal transport of electrolytes and water in normal man and in cirrhosis with ascites. *J Clin Invest* 42:1179, 1963.
105. Len ML et al: Renal function in Wilson's disease: Response to penicillamine therapy. *Am J Med Sci* 260:381, 1970.
106. Lentz RD et al: Treatment of severe hypophosphatemia. *Ann Intern Med* 89:941, 1978.
107. Levy M: Pathophysiology of ascites formation, in Epstein M (ed): *The Kidney in Liver Disease,* 3d ed. New York, Elsevier, 1982, p 245.
108. Levy M: Sodium retention and ascites formation in dogs with experimental portal cirrhosis. *Am J Physiol* 233:F575, 1977.
109. Levy M, Allotey JBK: Temporal relationship between urinary salt retention and altered systemic hemodynamics in dogs with experimental cirrhosis. *J Lab Clin Med* 92:560, 1978.
110. Levy M, Wexler MJ: Renal sodium retention and ascites formation in dogs with experimental cirrhosis but without portal hypertension or with increased splanchnic vascular capacity. *J Lab Clin Med* 91:520, 1978.
111. Levy M et al: Sodium retention in dogs with experimental cirrhosis following removal of ascites by continuous peritoneovenous shunting. *J Lab Clin Med* 94:933, 1979.
112. Lieberman FL et al: Effective plasma volume in cirrhosis with ascites. Evidence that a decreased value does not account for renal sodium retention, a spontaneous reduction in glomerular filtration rate (GFR) and a fall in GFR during drug-induced diuresis. *J Clin Invest* 48:975, 1969.
113. Lieberman FL, Reynolds TB: Plasma volume in cirrhosis of the liver: Its relation to portal hypertension, ascites and renal failure. *J Clin Invest* 46:1297, 1967.
114. Lieberman FL et al: The relationship of plasma volume, portal hypertension, ascites and renal sodium retention in cirrhosis: The overflow theory of ascites formation. *Ann NY Acad Sci* 170:202, 1970.
115. Linas SL et al: The role of vasopressin in the impaired water excretion in the conscious rat with experimental cirrhosis. *Kidney Int* 29:173, 1981.
116. Long RG et al: Clinical, biochemical and histological studies of osteomalacia, osteoporosis, and parathyroid function in chronic liver disease. *Gut* 19:85, 1978.
117. Lopez-Novoa JM et al: Dynamics of ascites formation in rats with experimental cirrhosis. *Am J Physiol* 238:F353, 1980.
118. Lopez-Novoa JM et al: A micropuncture study of salt and water retention in chronic experimental cirrhosis. *Am J Physiol* 232:F315, 1977.
119. Maguire PJ, MacDonald JS: Hypocalcemia associated with a calcitonin-producing hepatocellular carcinoma. *Arch Intern Med* 141:687, 1981.
120. Marossero F et al: Studio sperimentale dell'azione del cloruro d'ammonio per iniezione endovenosa rapida sui potenziali corticali di tipo convulsivo. *Boll Soc Ital Biol Sper* 8:913, 1958.
121. Martin HE et al: Electrolyte disturbances in acute alcoholism. *Am J Clin Nutr* 7:191, 1959.
122. Matloff D et al: Effects of 25-OH vitamin D treatment on calcium metabolism and bone disease in primary biliary cirrhosis (PBC) (abstract). *Gastroenterology* 78:1313, 1980.
123. Matz R et al: Renal tubular dysfunction associated with alcoholism and liver disease. *NY State J Med* 69:1312, 1969.
124. McCune DJ et al: Intractable hypophosphataemic rickets with renal glycosuria and acidosis: Report of a case and a review of the literature. *Am J Dis Child* 65:81, 1943.
125. Mendelson JH et al: Effects of alcohol ingestion and withdrawal on magnesium states of alcoholics: Clinical and experimental findings. *Ann NY Acad Sci* 162:918, 1969.
126. Michelis MF et al: Hypouricemia and hyperuricosuria in Laennec cirrhosis. *Arch Intern Med* 134:681, 1974.
127. Miller PD et al: Plasma demeclocycline levels and nephrotoxicity correlation in hyponatremic cirrhotic patients. *JAMA* 243:2513, 1980.
127a. Mitchison HC et al: Metabolic bone disease in primary

biliary cirrhosis at presentation. *Gastroenterology* 94:463, 1988.
128. Morgan HG et al: Wilson's disease and the Fanconi syndrome. *Q J Med* 31:361, 1962.
129. Morgan TR et al: Plasma human atrial natriuretic factor in cirrhosis and ascites with and without functional renal failure. *Gastroenterology* 95:1641, 1988.
130. Morris RC Jr, Fudenberg HH: Impaired renal acidification in patients with hypergammaglobulinemia. *Medicine* 46:57, 1967.
131. Moss AH et al: Fanconi's syndrome and distal renal tubular acidosis after glue sniffing. *Ann Intern Med* 92:69, 1980.
132. Mulhausen R et al: Acid-base disturbances in patients with cirrhosis of the liver. *Medicine* 46:185, 1967.
133. Naccarata et al: Renal handling of sodium and water in early chronic liver disease. *Gastroenterology* 81:205, 1981.
134. Oster JR et al: Abnormal renal acidification in alcoholic liver disease. *J Lab Clin Med* 85:987, 1975.
135. Owen EE et al: The kidney as a source of blood ammonia in patients with liver disease: The effect of acetazolamide. *J Clin Invest* 39:228, 1960.
136. Papadakis MA, Arieff AI: Unpredictability of clinical evaluation of renal function in cirrhosis—a prospective study. *Am J Med* 82:945, 1987.
137. Papadakis MA et al: Hyponatremia in patients with cirrhosis. *Q J Med* 76:675, 1990.
138. Perez-Ayuso RM et al: Renal kallikrein excretion in cirrhotics with ascites: Relationship to renal hemodynamics. *Hepatology* 4:247, 1984.
139. Perez-Ayuso RM et al: Randomized comparative study of efficacy of furosemide versus spironalactone in nonazotemic cirrhosis with ascites: Relationship between the diuretic response and the activity of the renin-aldosterone system. *Gastroenterology* 84:961, 1983.
140. Planes R et al: Acetylsalicylic acid suppresses the renal hemodynamic effect and reduces the diuretic action of furosemide in cirrhosis with ascites. *Gastroenterology* 84:247, 1983.
141. Pockros PJ, Reynolds TB: Rapid diuresis in patients with ascites from chronic liver disease: The importance of peripheral edema. *Gastroenterology* 90:1227, 1986.
142. Posner JB, Plum F: The toxic effects of carbon dioxide and acetazolamide in hepatic encephalopathy. *J Clin Invest* 39:1246, 1960.
143. Prytz H, Thomsen AG: Acid-base status in liver cirrhosis. Disturbances in stable, terminal and porta-caval shunted patients. *Scand J Gastroenterol* 11:249, 1976.
144. Quintero E et al: Paracentesis versus diuretics in the treatment of cirrhosis with tense ascites. *Lancet* 1:611, 1985.
145. Ralli EP et al: Studies of the serum and urine constituents in patients with cirrhosis of the liver during water tolerance tests. *Am J Med* 11:157, 1951.
146. Read AE et al: Neuropsychiatric complications following chlorothiazide therapy in patients with hepatic cirrhosis: Possible relation to hypokalemia. *Clin Sci* 18:409, 1959.
147. Read AE et al: Active juvenile cirrhosis considered as part of a systemic disease and the effect of corticosteroid therapy. *Gut* 4:378, 1963.
148. Record CO et al: Acid-base and metabolic disturbances in fulminant hepatic failure. *Gut* 16:144, 1975.
149. Rector WG, Hossock KF: Pathogenesis of sodium retention complicating cirrhosis: Is there room for diminished "effective" arterial blood volume? *Gastroenterology* 95:1658, 1988.
150. Reed JS et al: Bone disease in primary biliary cirrhosis: Reversal of osteomalacia with oral 25-hydroxyvitamin D. *Gastroenterology* 78:512, 1980.
151. Reichle FA et al: Hepatic metabolism in patients with alcoholic cirrhosis. *Surgery* 84:33, 1978.
152. Reynolds TB, Boyer TD: Prostaglandin insufficiency: A role in the hepatorenal syndrome? *Gastroenterology* 71:A-6/899, 1976.
153. Reynolds TB et al: Spontaneous decrease in portal pressure with clinical improvement in cirrhosis. *N Engl J Med* 263:734, 1960.
154. Ring-Larsen H et al: Peritoneal dialysis in hyponatremia due to liver failure. *Scand J Gastroenterol* 8:33, 1972.
155. Roberti A et al: Etude de Na et du K échangeable et des liquid extracellidaires dans les cirrhosis ethylique. *Sem Hop Paris* 42:1714, 1966.
156. Roberts KE et al: Respiratory alkalosis accompanying ammonium toxicity. *J Appl Physiol* 9:367, 1956.
157. Roberts KE et al: Electrolyte alterations in liver disease and hepatic coma. *Med Clin North Am* 40:901, 1956.
158. Rocco VK, Ware AJ: Cirrhotic ascites. *Ann Intern Med* 105:573, 1986.
159. Rodman T et al: Arterial oxygen unsaturation and the ventilation-perfusion defect of Laennec's cirrhosis. *N Engl J Med* 263:73, 1960.
160. Rosoff L et al: Studies of renin and aldosterone in cirrhotic patients with ascites. *Gastroenterology* 69:698, 1975.
161. Rude RK et al: Parathyroid hormone secretion in magnesium deficiency. *J Clin Endocrinol Metab* 47:800, 1978.
162. Rude RK et al: Functional hypoparathyroidism and parathyroid hormone end-organ resistance in human magnesium deficiency. *Clin Endocrinol* 5:209, 1976.
163. Salerno EF et al: Repeated paracentesis and IV albumin infusion to treat tense ascites in cirrhotic patients: A Safe alternative therapy. *J Hepatol* 5:102, 1987.
164. Salerno EF et al: Atrial natriuretic factor in cirrhotic patients with tense ascites. *Gastroenterology* 98:1063, 1990.
165. Schedl HP, Bartter FC: An explanation for and experimental correction of the abnormal water diuresis in cirrhosis. *J Clin Invest* 39:248, 1960.
166. Schentag JJ et al: Pharmacokinetic and clinical studies in patients with cimetidine-associated mental confusion. *Lancet* 1:177, 1979.
167. Schrier RW: Body fluid volume regulation in health and disease: A unifying hypothesis. *Ann Intern Med* 113:155, 1990.
168. Schubert J et al: The renal mechanism of sodium reabsorption in cirrhosis (abstract). *Am Soc Nephrol* 3:58A, 1969.
169. Schwartz R et al: Blood ammonia and electrolytes in hepatic coma. *J Lab Clin Med* 42:499, 1953.
170. Shear L et al: Renal tubular acidosis in cirrhosis. A determinant of susceptibility to recurrent hepatic precoma. *N Engl J Med* 208:1, 1969.
171. Shear L et al: Compartmentalization of ascites and edema

in patients with hepatic cirrhosis. *N Engl J Med* 282:1391, 1970.

172. Sherlock S: Ascites formation and its management. *Scand J Gastroenterol* 7(suppl):9, 1970.
173. Shils ME: Experimental human magnesium depletion. *Medicine* 48:61, 1969.
174. Simon DM et al: Effects of therapeutic paracentesis on systemic and hepatic hemodynamics and on renal and hormonal function. *Hepatology* 7:423, 1987.
175. Skorecki KL et al: Role of atrial natriuretic peptide in the natriuretic response to central volume expansion induced by head-out water immersion in sodium-retaining cirrhotic subjects. *Am J Med* 85:373, 1988.
176. Skowsky R et al:: Arginine vasopressin kinetics in hepatic cirrhosis. *Clin Res* 24:101A, 1976.
177. Slatopolsky E et al: Hyperphosphatemia. *Clin Nephrol* 7:138, 1977.
178. Smith PM et al: Renal tubular acidosis and cirrhosis. *Postgrad Med J* 43:439, 1967.
179. Snell AM: Effects of chronic disease of liver on composition and physiochemical properties of blood: Changes in serum proteins: Reduction in oxygen saturation of arterial blood. *Ann Intern Med* 9:690, 1935.
180. Snell RE, Luchsinger PC: The relation of arterial hypoxemia to the hyperventilation of chronic liver disease. *Am J Med Sci* 245:289, 1963.
181. Stanley MM et al: Peritoneovenous shunting as compared with medical treatment in patients with alcoholic cirrhosis and massive ascites. *N Engl J Med* 321:1632, 1989.
182. Stein JH et al: Hypophosphatemia in acute alcoholism. *Am J Med Sci* 252:78, 1966.
183. Strauss MP et al: Correction of impaired water excretion in cirrhosis of the liver by alcohol ingestion or expansion of extracellular fluid volume: The role of antidiuretic hormone. *Trans Assoc Am Physicians* 39:222, 1956.
184. Sutton F et al: Progesterone for outpatient treatment of Pickwickian syndrome. *Ann Intern Med* 84:476, 1975.
185. Szatalowicz V et al: Comparative effects of diuretics on renal water excretion in hyponatremic edematous disorders. *Clin Sci* 62:235, 1982.
186. Taher SM et al: Renal tubular acidosis associated with toluene "sniffing." *N Engl J Med* 290:765, 1974.
187. Territo MC, Tanaka KR: Hypophosphatemia in chronic alcoholism. *Arch Intern Med* 134:445, 1974.
188. Tyor MP, Sieker HO: Biochemical, blood gas and peripheral circulatory alterations in hepatic coma. *Am J Med* 27:50, 1959.
189. Vanamee P et al: Respiratory alkalosis in hepatic coma. *Arch Intern Med* 97:762, 1956.
190. Vlachcevic ZR et al: Renal effects of acute expansion of plasma volume in cirrhosis. *N Engl J Med* 272:387, 1965.
191. Warren KS et al: Effect of alterations in blood pH on distribution of ammonia from blood to cerebrospinal fluid in patients in hepatic coma. *J Lab Clin Med* 56:687, 1960.
192. Warren KS, Nathan DG: The passage of ammonia across the blood-brain barrier and its relation to blood pH. *J Clin Invest* 37:1724, 1958.
193. Welt LG: The influence of disease on the renal excretion of water. *Yale J Biol Med* 29:299, 1956.
194. Wilder CE et al: Relationship between serum sodium and hyperventilation in cirrhosis. *Am Rev Respir Dis* 97:971, 1967.
195. Wilkinson SP et al: Studies on mineralocorticoid "escape" in cirrhosis. *Clin Sci* 56:401, 1979.
196. Wilson WP, Tyor MP: Electroencephalographic observations during experimental hyperammonemia. *Neurology* 8:913, 1958.
197. Witte MH et al: Progress in liver disease: Physiological factors involved in the causation of cirrhotic ascites. *Gastroenterology* 61:742, 1971.
198. Wolfe SM, Victor M: The relationship of hypomagnesemia and alkalosis to alcohol withdrawal symptoms. *Ann NY Acad Sci* 162:973, 1969.
199. Wong P: Kallikrein-kinin and renin angiotensin systems in functional renal failure of cirrhosis of the liver. *Gastroenterology* 73:1114, 1977.
200. Yamahiro HS, Reynolds TB: Effects of ascitic fluid infusion on sodium excretion, blood volume and creatinine clearance in cirrhosis. *Gastroenterology* 40:497, 1961.
201. Zipser RD et al: Prostaglandins: Modulators of renal function and pressor resistance in chronic liver disease. *J Clin Endocrinol Metab* 48:894, 1979.
202. Zipser RD et al: Renal kallikrein excretion in alcoholic cirhosis. *Am J Gastroenterol* 75:183, 1981.
203. Zipser RD et al: Urinary thromboxane B_2 and prostaglandin E_2 in the hepatorenal syndrome: Evidence for increased vasoconstrictor and decreased vasodilator factors. *Gastroenterology* 84:697, 1983.

CHAPTER • 38

Acute renal failure: fluid and electrolyte and acid-base complications

Stanley S. Franklin • Keith L. Klein

Acute renal failure refers to the clinical syndrome of an abrupt, frequently reversible impairment or cessation of renal function that is usually, but not always, manifested by oliguria, or anuria. This syndrome encompasses many different entities. The taxonomy in three areas pertaining to acute renal failure should be clarified at the outset:

- *Presentation.* Acute renal failure most often presents as a sudden onset of azotemia in patients with previously normal renal function. It can occur as a rapid, progressive worsening of renal function without known previous renal disease. Occasionally acute impairment of renal function is superimposed on well-documented chronic renal failure, so-called *acute-on-chronic* renal failure. Infrequently, a patient with acute renal failure may present with what is mistaken as end-stage chronic renal disease.
- *Urine output.* Although decreased urine volume is most characteristic of acute renal failure, urine output varies from total anuria to polyuria. Specific categories are defined as follows: *total anuria,* zero urine output; *anuria,* $<$ 50 to 100 ml/day; *oliguria,* $<$ 400 ml/day; *nonoliguria,* 400 to 1000 ml/day; and *polyuric renal failure,* greater than 1000 to 2000 ml/day.
- *Anatomical site of involvement.* *Prerenal* refers to renal hypoperfusion that results in acute azotemia without associated renal parenchymal damage. *Postrenal* refers to outflow obstruction distal to the tubular site of urine formation. Renal sites of involvement may be subdivided into primary vascular, glomerular, interstitial, and tubular; some overlap of pathologic involvement occurs as a secondary event (see Table 38-1).

The most common cause of acute renal failure involving the tubules is an entity that has been termed *acute tubular necrosis* (ATN). ATN is a pathologic term and may not accurately reflect underlying pathogenesis in all cases. The term ATN is used in this chapter, however, because other names (such as lower nephron nephrosis, tubulointerstitial nephritis, and vasomotor nephropathy) have not gained general acceptance.

ATN is a syndrome rather than a distinct clinical entity, and probably accounts for more than 70 percent of all patients with acute renal failure. The syndrome of ATN may involve various modes of initiation and maintenance and may take different clinical courses. Although there are multiple etiologies of ATN, only a few pathogenic events initiate renal damage. These include ischemia, disseminated intravascular coagulation (DIC), and endogenous and exogenous nephrotoxicity (see Table 38-2).

The persistence of reduced renal function, often with associated oliguria, may be ascribed to many possible causes. Vasomotor shunting of blood away from the glomerulus, altered glomerular permeability, abnormal back-diffusion through injured tubular epithelium, obstructed tubules, or a combination of these events may serve to maintain the impairment. One hallmark of ATN is inviolate: the inability to restore renal function by manipulating extracellular factors such as fluid volume, neurogenic tone, or vasoactive substances.

Typically, the oliguria of ATN lasts one to two weeks, followed by the onset of diuresis and the return of renal function to almost normal values. However, the oliguric phase may be absent or permanent or may last from one to six weeks before the onset of diuresis. Similarly, renal function may return only partially or remain

TABLE 38-1 • Differential diagnosis of acute renal failure

PREGLOMERULAR

1. Low perfusion pressure (shock or hypotension)
2. Absolute hypovolemia (dehydration, hemorrhage, burn)
3. Defective cardiac function (CHF, myocardial infarction, tamponade)
4. Acute hypoadrenal crises
5. Hepatorenal syndrome

POSTRENAL OBSTRUCTIVE

1. Low ureteral obstruction (cancer, calculi, ligation, hematoma, edema)
2. Mid-ureteral obstruction (retroperitoneal fibrosis, aneurysm)
3. High ureteral obstruction (hyperuricemia, hypercalcemia, calculi)

VASCULAR

1. Bilateral renal vein thrombosis (dehydration, sickle cell disease, hypernephroma)
2. Bilateral renal artery occlusion (thrombosis, embolism, aneurysm)
3. Malignant nephrosclerosis (essential hypertension, renal hypertension, renovascular hypertension)
4. Scleroderma
5. Hemolytic-uremic syndrome, renal cortical necrosis

GLOMERULAR

1. Acute proliferative glomerulonephritis
2. Rapidly progressive glomerulonephritis
3. Lupus nephritis
4. Polyarteritis nodosa
5. Allergic vasculitis
6. Wegener's granulomatosis
7. Henoch-Schölein purpura
8. Goodpasture's syndrome
9. Postinfectious nephritis (bacterial endocarditis, arteriovenous shunt infections, visceral abscesses)

INTERSTITIAL

1. Fulminant pyelonephritis with or without abscess formation
2. Papillary necrosis (phenacetin, alcoholic, diabetes, obstruction)
3. Acute interstitial nephritis [leptospirosis, idiopathic, drug-induced (methicillin, other penicillins, rifampin, sulfa, anti-inflammatory agents)]

TUBULAR

1. Nephrotoxic acute tubular necrosis
2. Ischemic acute tubular necrosis

totally absent, requiring permanent hemodialysis therapy. Nonoliguric or polyuric forms of ATN may occur in association with progressive azotemia. The incidence of polyuric ATN was once thought to be low, but has been reported to account for 20 to 30 percent of all cases of ATN in two recent series.[1,2]

The mechanism of polyuric and oliguric ATN has been examined in experimental rats with *Escherichia coli* bacteremia.[3] Early polyuria, at 3 to 6 h, was associated with normal creatinine clearance (GFR) but decreased Na^+-K^+ ATPase activity, suggesting deterioration of proximal tubular function. In contrast, late-stage oliguria, at 12 h, was associated with severely depressed GFR.[3]

In humans the etiology varies widely with polyuric ATN, and results frequently from the use of nephrotoxins such as aminoglycosides and amphotericin B. ATN from radiocontrast media administration or trauma rarely involves polyuria. Prophylactic use of mannitol, loop diuretics, and vasodilators and calcium blockers partly explains the high incidence of nonoliguric ATN in conjunction with high-risk surgery or in the treatment of burns. Nonoliguric ATN is generally associated with less renal injury and azotemia and a better overall prognosis. Urinalysis (see below) in patients with polyuric or nonoliguric acute renal failure shows significantly lower urinary sodium concentration and fractional excretion of sodium.

This chapter deals chiefly with fluid, electrolyte, and acid-base abnormalities that are related to the cause, natural history, or therapy of patients with acute renal failure. A list of fluid and electrolyte abnormalities underlying acute renal failure is presented in Table 38-3.

FLUID AND ELECTROLYTE DISORDERS

DISORDERS OF EXTRACELLULAR FLUID VOLUME AND SODIUM CONCENTRATION

General patterns of change in acute renal failure

As a consequence of oliguria or anuria, the two main functions of the kidneys, that is maintenance of a constant composition and volume of body water and electrolytes, and excretion of the catabolic end products of protein breakdown, are both disrupted. Since the aim of therapy in acute renal failure is to maintain the internal environment in as normal a state as possible until the kidneys resume function, it is necessary to delineate and understand the changes that occur in the untreated patient.

In a normal 70-kg male, insensible water loss by vaporization from the skin and lungs is 12 ml per kilogram of body weight, or about 850 ml/day. This is a fixed loss that entails no loss of accompanying electrolytes; it may be modified by rate and depth of respiration, fever and ambient temperature, humidity, and active sweating. In the absence of water intake, insensible water loss is partially compensated by endogenous water of oxidation, formed from the catabolism of body fat and protein (1.07 ml of water per gram of fat and 0.41 ml of water per

TABLE 38-2 • Classification of etiologies and agents of acute tubular necrosis

ACUTE ISCHEMIC RENAL FAILURE

Surgery:
- Major abdominal surgery (2) (1)
- Aortic surgery (1) (2)
- Open-heart surgery (1) (2) (3)
- Transurethral prostatectomy (water irrigation) (3)

Diagnostic radiology (2)

Obstetrics:
- Septic abortion (5) (2) (4)
- Postpartum hemorrhage (1) (2)
- Placenta previa (1) (2)
- Abruptio placenta (1) (2)
- Uterine rupture (1) (2)
- Intrauterine fetal death (1) (2) (4)
- Severe toxemia (1) (2) (4)

Trauma
- Crush injuries (2) (3) (1) (4)
- Fractures (1) (2)
- Hemoglobin release: (3)
  - Infections (septicemia, endotoxins, *Clostridium welshii,* (1) (2) (4) (5), epidemic hemorrhagic fever, (2) (4) (5), malaria (1) (4) (5)
- Mismatched transfusion (3) (4)
- Hemolytic-uremic syndrome (4)
- Glucose-6-phosphate dehydrogenase deficiency (2) (1) (5)
- Valvular heart disease (2) (4)
- Venomous snake bites (2) (1) (4)
- Glycerol therapy (3) (4)
- Fresh water submersion (1) (2) (3)

Myoglobin release:
- Rhabdomyolysis (excessive exercise* (2) (1) (4), crush injury (2) (1) (4), electric shock, burns (2) (3) (1) (4), heatstroke (2) (4), Hoff's disease (epidemic myoglobinuria) (2), potassium depletion (2), idiopathic, primary, paroxysmal (2), acute polymyositis (2))
- McArdel's syndrome (2)

Proteinuria:
- Multiple myeloma with Bence-Jones proteinuria (2) (1)
- Waldenström's macroglobulinemia (2) (1)
- Nephrotic syndrome (2) (1)
- Low molecular weight dextran therapy (2) (1)

Miscellaneous:
- Major hemorrhage (2)
- Vomiting or diarrhea (severe) (2)
- Myocardial infarction (1)
- (?) Hepatorenal syndrome (2) (4)

ACUTE NEPHROTOXIC RENAL FAILURE

Heavy metals
- Mercury (organic and inorganic), bismuth, uranium, cadmium, arsenic, arsine, lithium

Organic solvents:
- Carbon tetrachloride, tetrachoroethylene, ethoxyethanol, methanol, toluene, chloroform, trichloromethane, trichloroethylene

Glycols:
- Ethylene glycol, diethylene glycol, diglycolic acid, oxalic acid

Antibiotics:
- Neomycin, kanamycin, gentamicin, polymyxin, colistin, bacitracin, phenazophyridine, co-trimoxazole, amphotericin, rifampin

Chlorinated hydrocarbon pesticides: Chlordane, paraquat

Miscellaneous:
- Carbon monoxide, mushroom poison, creosol, aniline and other methemoglobin-producing chemicals, phenylbutazone, lysol, phenols, sodium chlorate, diesel fuel, methoxyflurane

Note: Numbers in parentheses indicate contributing factors, in order of importance: (1) hypotension, (2) ECF loss, (3) release of pigments (hemoglobin, myoglobin), (4) DIC, (5) infection.

* Includes march myoglobinuria, anterior tibia syndrome, karate.

gram of protein). The water of oxidation made available in this manner in a 70-kg man in a fasting state is ordinarily about 300 ml/day, or one-third of the insensible loss; in calculations of water balance, water of oxidation must be considered as intake.[4]

In the oliguric patient with acute renal failure, a concatenation of events, physiologic and iatrogenic, usually results in a large relative excess of body water. This has been verified by measurements of total body water with heavy water, D_2O.[5] The setting in which renal damage occurs is usually a very stressful one. In acutely ill or traumatized patients, the catabolism of both fat and protein is markedly increased. It has been shown, for example, that fat utilization in a patient with acute renal failure, as in the postoperative or traumatic injury patient, may be twice normal; these patients, therefore, produce far more endogenous water of oxidation than does the normal individual.[6]

The rate of water production from cellular breakdown is influenced by the intensity of the "stress response" and by size of muscle mass, prior state of nutrition, extent of necrotic tissue or collections of blood within the body, and presence of infection or fever. In addition, carbohydrate depletion accentuates tissue breakdown, and permits the accumulation of ketone bodies from the oxidation of fat.

TABLE 38-3 • **Fluid and Electrolyte abnormalities associated with acute renal failure**

Anatomic Classification	Etiologies	Fluid/electrolyte abnormality
Prerenal	Hemorrhage, GI loss, burns, trauma, sepsis, diabetic ketoacidosis	Hypovolemia, hypotension
	CHF, nephrotic syndrome, hepatorenal syndrome	Hypervolemia, edema
Postrenal	Postobstructive diuresis	Polyuria, hypovolemia, hypernatremia
Renal:		
Vascular	One-kidney renovascular hypertension, malignant hypertension, scleroderma kidney, polyarteritis, cholesterol emboli, nonsteriodal antiinflammatory agents, cyclosporin A therapy	Hypervolemia, hypertension hyponatremia, hypokalemia
Glomerular	Acute nephrotic syndrome, rapidly progressive glomerulonephritis	Hypervolemia, hypertension, edema
Tubular:		
Ischemic ATN	DIC, sepsis, heatstroke	Severe hyperkalemia, severe anion gap metabolic acidosis, respiratory alkalosis, hypophosphatemia
	Cardiac arrest	Hypernatremia
	Severe hyperglycemia	Hypo-, or hypernatremia
	Acute hemorrhagic pancreatitis	Severe hypocalcemia and high anion gap metabolic acidosis
	Hepatorenal syndrome	Respiratory alkalosis, renal tubular acidosis
Endogenous nephrotoxins	Rhabdomyolysis (myoglobin)	Hyperphosphatemia, hypo- or hypercalcemia, servere high anion gap metabolic acidosis
	Myeloma	Hypercalcemia, renal tubular acidosis, Fanconi syndrome
	Solid tumors	Hypercalcemia
	Acute lymphatic leukemia, lymphosarcoma, Burkitt's lymphoma	Hyperphosphatemia, hypocalcemia
Exogenous nephrotoxins	Heavy metals (Hg, Bi, U)	Renal tubular acidosis, Fanconi syndrome
	Methoxyflurane	Hypernatremia, polyuria
	Amphotericin B	Hypokalemia
	Polymyxin B	Normal anion gap metabolic acidosis
	Streptozotocin	Renal tubular acidosis, Fanconi syndrome
	Mithromycin	Hypocalcemia
	Cisplatin	Hypomagnesemia
	Cyclosporin A	Hyperkalemia
	Glycols, snake venom	Severe high anion gap metabolic acidosis

During the oliguric period, caloric intake is seldom adequate, so that most patients lose 0.3 to 0.4 kg of lean body mass per day.[7] In maintaining a normal ratio between water and the decreasing quantity of fat-free solids, a proportionate amount of tissue water is freed, providing still another source of endogenous fluid. Unfortunately, excessive ingestion or administration of fluids is the rule rather than the exception during the first few days of acute renal failure. Voluntary fluid intake is largely a matter of habit rather than thirst, and patients often continue to drink the usual amounts of water, coffee, and other beverages although they are producing less urine. There also may be an element of thirst resulting from the hypovolemia that is frequently present during the initiating events associated with ATN. Furthermore, the physician may administer parenteral fluids in a vain attempt to "flush out the kidneys." If no salt is given this excess water is distributed between the extracellular and intracellular fluid compartments, decreasing the osmolality of body fluids; hyponatremia results. If saline solution is given, it remains largely extracellular. Thus, intracellular volume expansion and/or extracellular edema may be produced.

The state of fluid balance during the diuretic period is variable, depending on the previous state of hydration and on replacement therapy during diuresis. Because tubular reabsorption of water may be impaired, and the functioning nephrons are under a high osmotic load, large volumes of hypotonic urine are frequently excreted.[8] The danger, therefore, is from rapid contraction of body fluid compartments and unrestricted loss of individual electrolytes. This excretory pattern during the diuretic period can be partially or totally modified by antecedent hemodialysis which minimizes both excess body water and excess osmotic load.

Specific disorders of volume

Hypovolemia: prerenal azotemia

Early diagnosis and therapy of prerenal azotemia may prevent the development of ATN. The usual homeostatic response in a normal subject with pure water depletion is an increase in secretion of antidiuretic hormone (ADH), resulting in production of urine of small volume, high specific gravity, and high urea content. The extent of oliguria depends largely upon the water requirements for obligatory solute excretion. At a maximal urinary concentration of 1200 mosm, excretion of the 600 mosmoles of solute generated by a normal diet requires that the urine volume be no less than 500 ml/day. The minimum urinary volume may be even smaller if the intake of protein and salt has been low and a high rate of tissue breakdown is not present. When hypovolemia with a reduced effective blood volume develops in association with hemorrhage, diarrhea, severe sweating, severe burns, or sepsis, other factors come into play. Aldosterone secretion occurs in response to increases in renin and angiotensin II levels, and the urinary concentration of sodium markedly diminishes. In addition, the decreased renal blood flow resulting from renal vasoconstriction is associated with further diminution in the excretion of sodium and water. Because of the virtually complete tubular reabsorption of salt, urinary osmolality is largely accounted for by urea.

When renal ischemia is severe enough to cause a measureable reduction in the glomerular filtration rate (GFR), there is a decreased filtered load and an increased tubular reabsorption of urea, so that azotemia results. In most clinical situations in which this occurs, the patient is usually hypotensive or shows clinical evidence of severe dehydration, that is poor skin turgor, dry axillae, shriveled tongue, and soft eyeballs.

It is obvious that the causes and mechanisms of prerenal azotemia are identical to some of those which result in ATN; the only differences are the lack of organic parenchymatous kidney damage and the potential for rapid reversibility of prerenal azotemia. When the renal ischemia resulting from dehydration or circulatory insufficiency is prolonged and/or severe, ATN may ensue. Frequently, however, in the transition from prerenal oliguria to complete ATN, there is an intermediate phase called partial ATN. In this transitional phase, there may be sufficient reduction in renal blood flow and GFR to impair concentrating ability significantly, as well as to cause varying degrees of azotemia. The reason for making this distinction is that proper therapy during the transition phase may prevent further progression to complete ATN with its obligatory period of severe oliguria unresponsive to therapy. Successfully treated incipient or partial ATN can be likened to nonoliguric ATN, in which there is a modest rise in blood area nitrogen (BUN) and serum creatinine levels, indicating parenchymal renal damage despite normal or even increased urine output.

Prerenal hypovolemia, that is, renal circulatory insufficiency, can arise from a number of clinical states including diminished perfusion pressure secondary to shock, absolute hypovolemia with or without normal blood pressure, low cardiac output states, diminished adrenal function in the setting of hypovolemic crisis, and hepatorenal syndrome where there is a shunting of blood away from the kidney. These diagnoses can usually be made clinically but occasionally require the aid of central venous or pulmonary wedge pressure monitoring (Table 38-4).

A variety of simple renal function tests may be useful in distinguishing between prerenal hypovolemia and acute renal failure (Table 38-5):

- The *urine/plasma (U/P) osmolality* ratio is usually greater than 2:1 in prerenal oliguria, and decreases toward the ratio of 1.1:1 with varying degrees of partial to complete ATN. In contrast, complete ATN has a ratio of less than 1.1:1.[9]
- *Urine sodium concentration* is usually <20 meq/liter in prerenal oliguria, and >40 meq/liter in complete ATN; frequently it is as high as 60 to 80 meq/liter.[10] Persistently lower urinary sodium concentrations despite all the other stigmata of ATN have been noted in nonoliguric renal failure and renal failure associated with severe hypovolemia.[11,12] This finding suggests that tubule function is relatively intact in the nephrons which are forming urine and they are responding to a hypovolemic stimulus.
- The *U/P urea concentration* ratio is usually more than 20:1 in prerenal oliguria, and much below this value in ATN.[13] Similarily, the *U/P creatinine concentration ratio* is usually more than 40:1 in prerenal oliguria. The U/P creatinine ratio has proved to be somewhat more reliable than the U/P urea ratio, because creatinine does not back-diffuse and therefore is a truer estimate of water reabsorption across the nephrons.
- The *fractional excretion of sodium* (Fe_{Na}) is a better index of states of renal hypoperfusion. This calculation is made by dividing the clearance of sodium by the clearance of creatinine. Since the time of urine collection appears in both the numerator and denominator, they cancel out and a spot urine specimen can be used to make this calculation.
- The *renal failure index* gives additional resolution of prerenal oliguria from acute intrinsic renal failure and is similar in value to the Fe_{Na}. The index is obtained by dividing the urinary sodium concentration by the U/P creatinine ratio.[1,14,15,16]

TABLE 38-4 • Renal circulatory insufficiency without acute renal failure

Specific cause	Diagnostic indication	Therapy
↓ Perfusion pressure	↓ BP, ↑ pulse rate	Correct systemic hypotension
Absolute hypovolemia	Normal or ↓ BP Weight loss Negative fluid balance Fluid sequestration ↓ Tissue turgor Hematocrit change	Fluid, crystalloid, colloid, or blood administration
↓ Cardiac function	↑ Central venous or Swan-Ganz pressures Edema, S_3 gallop	Loop diuretic, inotrope Decrease cardiac afterload
↓ Adrenal function	↓ BP, weight loss ↓ P_{Na}, ↑ P_K ↑ U_{Na}, ↓ U_K ↓ P cortisol	Glucocorticoid Volume replacement
↓ Hepatic function	Normal or ↓ BP Ascites Abnormal liver function tests	Volume and/or vasopressors

Note: Clinical renal circulatory insufficiency in the absence of acute renal failure is generally diagnosed on the basis of elevations in BUN/creatine ratio, U/P creatinine, and U/P osmolality, and lowered excretion of urinary sodium. Specific causation is best assessed by indicators shown in center column, using therapeutic modalities in last column for correction.

Symbols: U, urine; P, plasma; ↓, decreased, ↑, increased; BP, blood pressure

Misleading results are occassionally obtained in the above tests when urine has remained in the bladder for several hours before being examined. Moreover, the prior use of diuretics may render the urinary sodium concentration invalid. Claims have been made that prerenal oliguria can be distinguished from ATN by a diuretic response in the former following treatment with mannitol or loop diuretics (furosemide or ethacrynic acid).[17,18,19,20] This contention has, however, been disputed.[21]

The correlation of renal biopsies with Fe_{Na} values was examined in a large series of patients with acute renal failure.[22] In oliguric ATN, Fe_{Na} was almost always elevated and correlated with severe morphological tubular damage on renal biopsy. In contrast, nonoliguric ATN, with milder morphologic damage, had Fe_{Na} elevated in less than half. Furthermore, patients with acute glomerulonephritis had both low and high Fe_{Na} values and thus could not be distinguished from those patients with ATN.[22]

Pseudo-prerenal azotemia is a term used to describe an increase in BUN in association with gastrointestinal hemorrhage. However, the production of urea from bacterial action or digestive breakdown of intraluminal blood should not cause any greater elevation of BUN than is noted from absorption of other high-protein foodstuffs.[23] Indeed, blood is a major dietary constituent of the Masai tribe, and is consumed in many countries as

TABLE 38-5 • Laboratory aids in the diagnosis of acute renal failure*

	Prerenal oliguria	Partial acute renal failure	Complete acute renal failure
U/P osmolality	>2	1.1–1.9	<1.1
Urine sodium concentration, meq/liter	<20	20–40	>40
U/P urea	>20	20–10	<10
U/P creatinine	>40	20–15	<15
U_{Na}/(U/P creatinine)	<1.0	1–5	>5

* Characteristic of ATN but also indistinguishable from obstructive, vascular, or interstitial disease. Only acute glomerulopathies may present with urinary findings suggestive of prerenal oliguria during the early phase; later, the urinary findings may merge with those of acute renal failure.

Symbols: U, urine concentration; P, plasma concentration

blood sausage without any evidence of significantly elevated BUN. Therefore, the azotemia seen with gastrointestinal hemorrhage must be secondary to the absence of blood from the vasculature (hypovolemia) rather than caused by its presence in the gut.[23] When blood is introduced into the gut in quantities that overwhelm its digestive and absorptive capacities, the excess blood stimulates peristalsis and is osmotically active, not unlike a saline cathartic; the result is diarrhea and subsequent removal from the body of a significant percentage of blood and blood breakdown products. Continued BUN elevation cannot be dismissed as related to "blood in the gut." It must be regarded as evidence of continued hypovolemic impairment of renal function, probably indicative of continued bleeding or inadequate replacement.

Spurious serum creatinine elevations have been described in diabetic ketoacidosis.[24,25] Diabetic ketoacidosis is usually accompanied by dehydration, with resulting prerenal azotemia in which BUN is elevated out of proportion to serum creatinine.[25] Occasionally the spurious elevation of serum creatinine due to interference by acetoacetate in the automated assays for serum creatinine reverses the high BUN/creatinine ratio.[24] It has also been reported with *cefoxitin*, which interferes with the Jaffe reaction used in assaying creatinine. The timing of the blood drawing in relation to the last dose of cefoxitin is crucial. *Cimetidine*, which interferes with tubular secretion of creatinine, has been reported to produce elevations of creatinine without causing underlying renal disease. Azotemic patients with preexisting mild elevations of creatinine will have more pronounced increases in creatinine in response to cimetidine.

Rhabdomyolysis produces exaggerated increases in serum creatinine due to the sudden release of massive amounts of muscle creatine phosphate that is rapidly and nonenzymatically converted to creatinine. In this setting the serum creatinine increases disproportionately more than the BUN.[26]

It should be borne in mind that ATN may coexist with hypovolemia if rehydration during the oliguric phase of ATN is incomplete or if fluids and electrolytes are not completely replaced during the diuretic phase. The latter may be associated with a delay in improvement in renal function or an actual reversal with further rise in BUN and creatinine during the diuretic phase.

Hypervolemia

EDEMA/CONGESTIVE HEART FAILURE Prerenal azotemia, frequently with oliguria, may be associated with severe congestive heart failure (CHF) and low cardiac output states. Most commonly, this occurs with advanced CHF with marked right-sided failure and severe passive congestion of the liver and kidneys. On rare occasions, an acute viral pericarditis with tamponade can also present with prerenal azotemia and oliguria. Similarly, an acute myocardial infarction with low cardiac output can be associated with peripheral edema, hypotension, and azotemia. More often than not, such patients are elderly and have a decreased renal reserve or mild frank renal insufficiency; they therefore seem to be more vulnerable to the oliguric prerenal azotemia accompanying low cardiac output syndromes. The urinary studies usually show low concentrations of sodium and high concentrations of creatinine with variable osmolality reflecting a physiologically ischemic kidney in the setting of massive volume overload. The urine indices describe prerenal parameters while the patient is massively fluid overloaded. These patients do not respond to continued volume expansion; rather they need efforts directed at improving cardiac output without further increasing filling pressures. Aggressive diureses usually further aggravate the prerenal condition, causing further increments in the BUN and creatinine. Persisting renal ischemia may culminate in ATN. The chronic passive congestion of the kidneys complicating right-sided heart failure usually produces mild to moderate proteinuria, several red and white blood cells per high-power microscopic field, and many hyaline casts.

On rare occasions, when right-sided CHF is severe and abrupt, ATN may result. This succession has been described with giant cell myocarditis.[27] When an infectious or inflammatory process involves the heart diffusely, signs of right ventricular failure predominate over left ventricular failure because the right ventricle is weaker, thinner, and far more vulnerable to the effects of disease.

ATN secondary to myocardial infarction occurs very rarely, perhaps in approximately 1 percent, usually in association with severe CHF and cardiogenic shock.[28] The associated finding of increased serum fibrin degradation products with normal fibrinogen levels strongly suggests intravascular coagulation in the renal circulation. Occasionally, acute renal failure occurs in association with an acute myocardial infarction as a result of embolization to the kidney from multiple cardiac mural thrombi.[29]

The infrequency of ATN in the presence of acute myocardial infarctions contrasts with its occurrence with the nephrotic syndrome. In the presence of severe hypoalbuminemia and reduced circulating blood volume together with peripheral edema, nephrotic syndrome is associated with a high incidence of ATN.[30] ATN complicating the nephrotic syndrome is most commonly associated with anesthesia and surgery involving compromise of circulating blood volume, radiologic procedures in which contrast material is administered, and associated gram-negative or gram-positive sepsis. On rare occasions, the nephrotic syndrome can present with acute renal failure in association with bilateral renal vein thrombosis, perhaps as a complication of a hypercoagulable state secondary to the hemoconcentration of coagulation factors that occurs in the presence of severe hypoalbuminemia.[31]

Iatrogenic hypervolemia can complicate acute renal failure as a consequence of overzealous administration of crystalloid, colloid, or blood. Whereas aggressive treatment of hypovolemia with appropriate increases in volume is correct management for prerenal oliguria, excessive administration of fluids may lead to hypervolemia, edema, and frank CHF in the presence of oliguric ATN. Excessive administration of intravenous mannitol in the presence of ATN may cause a drastic shift of water from the cellular to the extracellular space resulting similarly in frank edema and CHF. Characteristically, hypervolemia secondary to excess mannitol administration occurs after prerenal oliguria has advanced to frank ATN so that renal excretion of mannitol becomes negligible; when this occurs there is an increase in plasma volume by approximately 1 to 3 ml per kilogram of body weight for each 5 g of mannitol retained.[32]

EDEMA AND HYPERTENSION When acute renal failure occurs in association with moderate or severe hypertension and frequently with edema, the differential diagnosis must include a variety of glomerulopathies and vasculopathies. Acute nephritic syndrome is characterized by acute renal insufficiency, some degree of oliguria, peripheral edema, hypertension, and frequently CHF, which is especially evident in the very young and very old. Laboratory features that support a diagnosis of nephritic syndrome include hematuria (in virtually 100 percent of patients), leukocyturia, and cylinduria (hyaline, granular, and red blood cell casts). Proteinuria is usually present but excretion is usually less than 2 g/m^2 in 24 h. The BUN/creatinine ratio is often elevated.

Edema in the setting of acute glomerulonephritis results from a reduction in GFR secondary to a decrease in glomerular ultrafiltration coefficient despite normal or even increased renal plasma flow; filtration fraction is therefore decreased.[33] The increased renal plasma flow and glomerular hydrostatic pressure are consequences of increased circulating blood volume. Occasionally elements of the nephrotic syndrome complicate the nephritic syndrome, in which case heavy proteinuria and hypoalbuminemia are associated with the other findings of the acute nephritic syndrome.

Patients who present with acute renal failure in the setting of acute nephritic syndrome have either acute or rapidly progressive glomerulonephritis. The former is more often reversible than is the latter. Oliguria is most common with acute glomerulonephritis, whereas anuria suggests a more serious underlying renal abnormality such as rapidly progressive glomerulonephritis. The most common etiology of oliguric acute renal failure secondary to glomerulopathy is poststreptococcal glomerulonephritis, which is more common in adults; the course is more ominous in adults than in children. In the elderly, acute glomerulonephritis may present with unexplained CHF as the intitial manifestation, later progressing to oliguric acute renal failure.[34] These initial findings in the elderly can also result from acute glomerulonephritis due to acute or subacute bacterial endocarditis.[35] Fever and positive blood cultures may be absent in such a setting, because of right-sided cardiac involvement. The presence of suspicious heart murmurs and evidence of DIC with thrombocytopenia provides evidence of the existence of endocarditis. The finding of hypocomplementemia (low C3, C4, and total hemolytic complement) is commonly found in both acute poststreptococcal glomerulonephritis and bacterial endocarditis. The occurrence of systemic symptoms in association with acute nephritic syndrome and renal failure points to a variety of generalized diseases such as lupus erythematosus, Henoch-Schönlein's purpura, Wegener's granulomatosis, polyarteritis, Goodpasture's syndrome, or mixed cryoglobulinemia.[36]

The occurrence of acute renal failure associated with edema, hypertension, and active urinary sediment suggests the presence of glomerulonephritis. Other diagnostic possibilities should also be considered[29,37,38] (Table 38-1). In most cases, a renal biopsy can establish the cause.

Disorders of sodium concentration

Hypernatremia

Hypernatremia occasionally is associated with acute renal failure. Hyperosmotic nonketotic diabetic coma (see Chap. 26), invariably associated with prerenal azotemia, can on occasion go on to frank ATN in the presence of severe hypovolemia with associated hypernatremia.[39] Because the hyperglycemia of uncontrolled diabetes usually lowers the plasma sodium concentration as a result of movement of sodium-free cellular water into the extracellular space, the finding of significant hypernatremia in association with uncontrolled diabetes indicates that water losses have far exceeded sodium losses. Severe dehydration with impaired renal function limits or totally prevents glycosuria leading to glucose retention and worsening hyperglycemia. The frequent association of coma correlates with with the extremely high serum osmolality. Indeed, obtundity or frank coma contributes to the hypernatremia by limiting the perception of and response to thrist. (Chapter 21 presents more information on hypernatremia.)

On occasion, acute renal failure can be complicated by iatrogenic hypernatremia. The relief of obstructive uropathy may result in postobstructive water diuresis which, if not corrected with sufficient fluid replacement, can produce hypernatremia.[40] Insufficient water replacement during the early diuretic phase of ATN may also be associated with hypernatremia, but rarely. The excessive use of sodium bicarbonate during therapy for cardiac arrest ATN may produce significant hypernatremia.[41]

Hypertonic hemodialysis or peritoneal dialysis fluid can result in an excessive loss of water and an excessive sodium level with the subsequent development of hypernatremia. In general, failure to replace ongoing water losses results in hypernatremia.

Severe hyperglycemia resulting from peritoneal dialysis osmotically shifts water from the ICF to the ECF. As glucose is metabolized upon discontinuation of the peritoneal dialysis, water shifts back into the cells. Sodium, which has equilibrated during the dialysis at approximately 140 meq/liter, increases postdialysis.

Total parenteral nutrition (TPN) formulations given in acute or chronic renal failure will often cause hypernatremia. The use of TPN in these situations requires close, constant monitoring. Correction of sodium concentration can be achieved with both dialysis and by altering the sodium concentration in the TPN.

Hyponatremia

So-called pseudohyponatremia has been described with myeloma kidney in association with very high serum globulin levels; the water content of the serum, therefore, is reduced and calculation of serum sodium may be erroneously computed as excessively low.[42] Prerenal azotemia associated with hyponatremia is typical of the excessive salt wasting of adrenal insufficiency, the excessive water retention of CHF, or the hepatorenal syndrome. Proposed mechanisms for the development of hyponatremia in these clinical settings include increased vasopressin secretion and decreased delivery of sodium and water to the distal diluting segment of the nephron. Studies in CHF patients who are hyponatremic have shown a correlation between the presence of hyponatremia, prerenal azotemia, and increased plasma renin activity (see also Chap. 20).[43]

The prerenal azotemia associated with diabetic hyperglycemia is usually associated with hyponatremia, in that glucose is largely confined to the extracellular space where it osmotically draws sodium-free water from the intracellular space. The original suggestion by Katz that there is a decrement in sodium concentration of 1.6 meq/liter for each increment of 100 mg/dl in glucose concentration has been found to be only a rough approximation. The decrease in plasma sodium concentration in response to hyperglycemia is variable and depends on several factors.[44] In the edematous patient with excess extracellular fluid, hyperglycemia produces smaller decrements in serum sodium concentration, whereas in the volume-depleted hypovolemic patient whose volume deficiency is of extracellular fluid, hyperglycemia is associated with an even greater hyponatremic response than predicted by the Katz formula. However, a greater discrepancy in the predicted degree of hyponatremia is associated with excess urinary loss of water over sodium; in this clinical state, severe hyperglycemia may be associated with either normal or elevated serum sodium concentrations.[44]

In the absence of hyperglycemia, hyponatremic acute renal failure is most often a reflection of antecedent hypovolemia and excessive free water administration. The finding of hyponatremic acute renal failure with adrenal insufficiency is occasionally observed in patients infected with the human immunodeficiency virus (HIV) and most often with associated acquired immune deficiency syndrome (AIDS).[45]

Hyponatremia in association with acute renal failure is most commonly of iatrogenic origin. Hyponatremia develops in ATN when osmotically active mannitol is retained in the extracellular space.[46] If the underlying setting for ATN is severe dehydration, excessive administration of water and insufficient administration of crystalloids may produce hyponatremia. Moreover, hyponatremia that is not present at the onset of ATN but develops subsequently is an indication that excessive free water is being administered.

Management of sodium and water disorders in acute renal failure

OLIGURIC PHASE • (1) *Fluids* In the calculation of fluid balance, the production of endogenous water (see above) must be taken into account, so that replacement of insensible fluid loss requires a total fluid intake of approximately 400 ml/day in the average 70-kg man. When there is excessive tissue catabolism, as in traumatic injury or superimposed sepsis, the acceptable total fluid intake may be less 400 ml/day; unusual circumstances, such as severe sweating or diarrhea, of course, will modify the required intake accordingly. Error in calculating fluid intake should be in the direction of too little rather than too much. Inadvertent mild dehydration does not prevent or delay the onset of diuresis. The most accurate and simplest daily check on overall fluid balance is the weight of the patient; 0.2 to 0.5 kg should be lost per day. Insensible loss may be greater in febrile patients or less in intubated patients. Insensible losses increase by approximately 13 percent for each degree Celsius that the patient's temperature rises. Urinary output should be taken into consideration in calculating daily water requirements according to the formula.

$$\text{Daily water intake} = \text{insensible loss} - \text{water from metabolism} + \text{urine output}$$

In centers with a policy of early and frequent dialysis therapy, resulting in a net fluid loss, a more liberal fluid intake is of course permissible.

(2) *Sodium* Generally sodium requirements range from zero in the anuric patient to more than 130 meq/day in the nonoliguric patient. In the absence of diarrhea, vomiting, or large volumes of tube drainage, virtually all

sodium loss is urinary and can be calculated by measuring urinary sodium concentration and volume. When hyponatremia is present, it usually represents serum dilution from excessive body water as noted above. The proper treatment is water restriction, not the administration of sodium salts. However, symptomatic hyponatremia must be partially corrected. For this purpose, parenteral hypertonic solutions of 3 or 5% sodium chloride can be used. Dialysis therapy, however, is frequently the treatment of choice for this complication. When hemodialysis is not feasible because of hemodynamic instability in critically ill patients, continuous arteriovenous hemofiltration (CAVH) can be an effective alternative method of treatment.[47]

DIURETIC PHASE During early diuresis, the kidneys have, in effect, lost all flexibility. Because of a continued high osmotic load, there is a fairly constant and unregulated concentration of electrolytes in the urine which are excreted independent of serum levels or intake. The urine is generally hypotonic; concentrations of sodium chloride are approximately 50 meq/liter.

Because of this inability to conserve water or electrolytes by the usual mechanisms and a common tendency by physicians to continue restricting salt and protein intake, severe dehydration or salt depletion, or a combination of the two, may ensue. The ideal way to determine replacement therapy is to measure urinary electrolyte concentrations. This need not be done daily since the concentrations remain relatively constant during the early diuretic period; if accurate records of urine volume are maintained, the electrolyte losses can be calculated from the preceding day.

It has already been pointed out that for various reasons, most patients have an excess of salt and water at the end of the oliguric period. Unless rigid fluid restriction has been maintained from the time of the initial episode, or a fixed excess has been prevented by the removal of fluids by repeated dialysis procedures, quantitative replacement perpetuates the obligatory water and salt loss. Therefore, intake of more than 3500 ml of fluid should seldom be allowed daily. A weight loss of several pounds is expected during the diuresis. On the other hand, when salt and water overload and inordinate elevations in the blood urea level have been prevented by repeated dialysis therepy, it is not unusual to see a gradual improvement in renal function in the absence of large diuresis.

In acute renal failure secondary to obstruction, a phenomenon known as "postobstructive diuresis" may occur. Intense diuresis frequently ensues which was believed to result primarily from tubular damage. The majority of studies, however, demonstrate that the postobstructive diuresis is either an appropriate excretion of excess total body sodium and water, and/or a urea solute diuresis. When volume increase resolves and BUN falls to less than 40 mg/dl, polyuria usually ceases. Truly inappropriate sodium and water loss following release of obstruction is rare.

POTASSIUM DISORDERS

General pattern of change during acute renal failure

The major clinical electrolyte disorder in acute renal failure is hyperkalemia, due to an inability to excrete a normal potassium load. The cation load may derive from either exogenous or endogenous sources. The principal endogenous source of potassium is protein catabolism. This in turn is influenced by the intensity of the "stress response," size of muscle mass, prior state of nutrition, extent of necrotic tissue or collection of blood within the body, and the presence of infection or fever. The magnitude of hyperkalemia depends on whether the patient is oliguric or nonoliguric and on the catabolic rate.

The catabolic response is best defined clinically by azotemia, which progresses most rapidly during the first few days of oliguria.[5] Urea is freely diffusible throughout the entire body, causing no transcellular osmotic gradients to develop. BUN rises by 25 to 35 mg/dl per day during the first three to five days of the anuric period.[5] This phase of rapid increase reflects the underlying catabolic events that may have precipitated acute renal failure. In young, muscular males undergoing severe trauma, the rate of catabolism may produce a daily increment in BUN of 50 mg/dl or more, with a urea production rate as great as 30 g/day. This corresponds to the destruction of 90 g of protein or some 400 g of tissue. Following the third to fifth day of anuria, there is usually a reduction in the rate of urea accumulation, conforming to a decrease in tissue catabolism. BUN may then increase by 10 to 20 mg/dl per day, in association with the production of an average of 5 to 6 g of urea per day.[5] Carbohydrate-rich diets may slow the rate of rise of urea nitrogen, whereas intercurrent infections, reabsorption of hematoma, or the persistence of devitalized tissue increase the appearance of BUN.

The same factors that determine the rate of rise of urea nitrogen also determine the rate of increase in serum of potassium, uric acid, and phosphorus concentrations and the decrease of bicarbonate levels. The general biochemical guidelines for determining whether a patient is catabolic or noncatabolic are listed in Table 38-6.

Hyperkalemia is a major cause of death in acute renal failure. Cessation of regulated renal potassium excretion concomitant with continuous breakdown of muscle protein leads to dangerous accumulation of potassium. Hyperkalemia usually develops during the oliguric phase; in the absence of specific preventive therapy this becomes life-threatening in about one-third of cases. When hyper-

TABLE 38-6 • Biochemical indicators of hypercatabolic acute renal failure

Marker	Daily change, mg/dl
BUN	>25–30
Serum creatinine	> 1–1.5
Serum uric acid	>10–15
Serum phosphate	> 8–10
Serum potassium	> 1–1.5*
Serum bicarbonate	> 2–3*

* meq/liter.

kalemia is not observed in acute renal failure, the patient usually has a urine volume of 1 liter/day or greater and/or there is extrarenal loss of potassium.

The untoward effects of alterations of potassium on neuromuscular contraction and, more important, on the myocardium, correlate better with serum K^+ levels than with total body content. It also must be emphasized that cardiac changes, as reflected in the electrocardiogram, represent a summation of the influences of various other extracellular electrolytes and of pH.[48] Hyponatremia, hypocalcemia, and acidosis enhance the deleterious effects of hyperkalemia. It has been noted that a serum potassium concentration of 8.5 meq/liter when the serum sodium concentration is 140 meq/liter may be more benign than a K^+ level of 7 meq/liter with serum Na^+ level = 120 meq/liter. For these reasons, the electrocardiogram is a better clinical index of serious potassium intoxication than is the serum level, although both should be obtained.

Progressive electrocardiographic changes follow a definite pattern (Fig. 38-1).[49] In sequence, these are: (1) tall, peaked T waves with a relatively narrow base (the amplitude of the T wave must be correlated with the amplitude and configuration of the QRS complex in the specific lead under consideration); (2) depressed RST segments; (3) decreased amplitude of the R wave and increased depth of the S wave; (4) prolonged PR interval, followed by the disappearance of the P wave; (5) progressive widening of the QRS complex with prolongation of the QT interval, eventually merging with the T wave in a sine-wave configuration. These changes are most apparent in the precordial leads. Ectopic ventricular beats, bradycardia, or other arrhythmias may appear at this time. Death is usually from ventricular fibrillation.

Although a "syndrome" of potassium intoxication has been described, clinical symptoms have been observed to be preceded by electrocardiographic changes, or are minor, atypical or difficult to attribute specifically to hyperkalemia. Sometimes, however, paresthesias or numbness, particularly of the mouth, hands, and feet, may be present, or there may be a progressive increase in

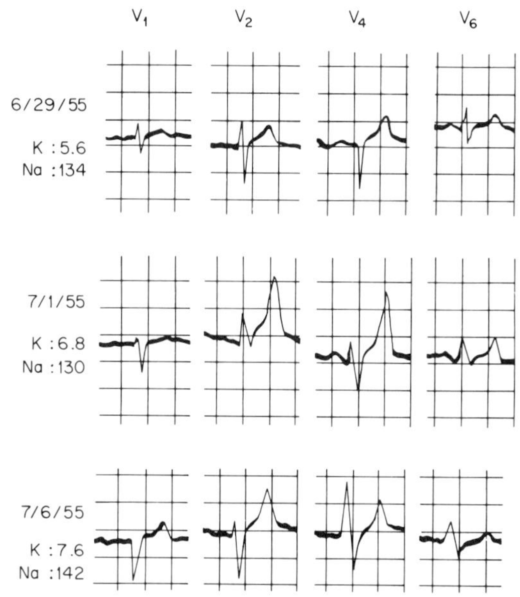

FIGURE 38-1 • Electrocardiographic changes of hyperkalemia. The typical alterations are best seen in leads V_2 and V_4. With increasing serum potassium, the following occur in sequence: T-wave peaking, prolonged PR interval, prolonged QRS complex.

generalized weakness resulting in severe paresis of the extremities or muscles of respiration, restlessness, apprehension with sweating and faint heart sounds, falling blood pressure, bradycardia, or arrhythmias.

(A full treatment of potassium disorders may be found in Chaps. 22 and 23.)

Specific patterns of serum potassium disturbances in acute renal failure

HYPOKALEMIA On occasion, patients may present with acute renal failure in association with hypokalemia or normokalemia, seemingly inappropriate to their oliguria and increased catabolism. These situations give a clinical clue to the possible etiology (see Chap. 22). Prerenal azotemia with hypokalemia can be associated with hepatorenal syndrome; indeed, potassium depletion may be a precipitating cause for the onset of this syndrome with rapidly increasing azotemia. Metabolic alkalosis, with shifts of potassium from the extracellular into the intracellular space, may be a concurrent abnormality that brings on the hepatorenal syndrome. Similarly, hypokalemia may be associated with excessive diuresis in patients with CHF, leading to hypovolemia, prerenal azotemia, and secondary hyperaldosteronism with excessive urinary potassium loss. Other causes of secondary hyperaldosteronism with hypokalemia in association with severe hypertensive states and acute renal failure have been described with scleroderma kidney, polyarteritis nodosa, and rapidly progressive glomerulonephritis.[50,51,52]

ATN presenting with hypokalemia, at least at the onset, has been described in nontraumatic rhabdomyolysis secondary to severe potassium depletion[53,54] and in severe heat stroke with respiratory alkalosis.[55] Despite the high catabolic rate in heat stroke, hypokalemia may be noted early, but it frequently disappears as acute renal failure progresses; hyperkalemia is a late manifestation if oliguria is present and prolonged. Acute nephrotoxicity from amphotericin B therapy of fungal disease has also been associated with marked hypokalemia, in the presence of nonoliguric ATN.[56]

HYPERKALEMIA OUT OF PROPORTION TO THE DEGREE OF RENAL FAILURE In contrast, there are times when hyperkalemia is out of proportion to the duration and severity of acute renal failure. This is characteristic of patients with adrenal insufficiency and severe salt and water depletion. Similarly, patients with stable chronic renal insufficiency given nonsteroidal anti-inflammatory agents can develop severe hyperkalemia in association with nonoliguric worsening of azotemia.[57] Presumably these agents suppress the actions of prostaglandins which are necessary for optimal renin and aldosterone secretion in the presence of chronic renal failure. Cyclosporin-induced acute renal failure in transplant patients is frequently associated with hyperkalemia out of proportion to the degree of renal insufficiency; the mechanism may involve altered renal hemodynamics rather than direct nephrotoxicity of the drug.[58]

The development of severe hyperkalemia in acute renal failure may also be associated with drugs that interfere with normal potassium homeostatic mechanisms. These drugs include digoxin which acts on Na^+-K^+ ATPase; ACE inhibition, which reduces aldosterone secretion; and beta-adrenergic blockers, which impair the effects of epinephrine.

In patients with ATN, the rapid onset of severe hyperkalemia is most frequently seen with hyperacute catabolic responses, for example, in patients with crush syndrome, rhabdomyolysis, or sepsis, especially in well-muscled individuals. Metabolic acidosis frequently complicates hyperacute catabolic renal failure. This syndrome has been described in patients with AIDS who are receiving pentamidine for *Pneumocystis carinii* infection.[59] Finally, overzealous use of mannitol, in a mistaken attempt to provoke diuresis, can produce hyperkalemia by osmotic withdrawal of potassium from cells, especially in diabetics.[60]

THERAPY OF HYPERKALEMIA • *Oliguric phase* Potassium intoxication (Table 38-7) often requires immediate and at times heroic therapy. It has already been stressed that the immediate cause of death from hyperkalemia is disruption of cardiac conduction and that the electrocardiogram, which reflects the summed effects of various ions on the heart, is a better guide to therapy than any single serum electrolyte determination. Daily, or even twice daily, electrocardiograms should be obtained; the graphs should be left in the patient's room for comparison with the previous day's tracings. In addition, when feasible, daily serum potassium and sodium levels should be obtained. Potassium accumulation may be prevented or retarded by meticulous attention to the prophylactic measures already discussed, that is, treatment of infections, debridement of necrotic tissue, drainage of accumulations of blood, prohibition of potassium intake, and provisions for nonprotein calories in the form of glucose and fat.

Additional prophylaxis against potassium intoxication may be accomplished by the use of ion-exchange resins like sodium polystyrene sulfonate (Kayexalate).[61] When feasible, these exchange resins may be given by mouth in doses of 15 g twice or three times daily. Since obstipation or even intestinal obstruction has been reported with the use of these resins, sorbitol, a poorly absorbed, osmotically active alcohol, can be added in sufficient quantity to produce mild diarrhea. If the resin cannot be taken by mouth, it is often useful to combine it with sorbitol and administer as a high-retention enema. This should be retained for a least 1 to 2 h for effective removal of potassium. Thereafter, a flushing enema can be given to facilitate the removal of the previously administered resins prior to instillation of another retention enema.

The most effective means of removing excess potassium from the body and preventing or reversing hy-

TABLE 38-7 • Treatment of hyperkalemia

Severity (serum K^+, meq/liter)	Agent	Onset	Duration	Mechanism
Mild (5.5–6.5)	Decreased intake	Variable	Variable	Restriction
	K^+ exchange resin	1–2 h	4–6 h	Excretion
Moderate (6.5–7.5)	Glucose and insulin	10–30 min	2–4 h	Redistribution
Severe (>7.5)	Sodium bicarbonate	≤1 h	1–2 h	Redistribution, antagonism
	Calcium gluconate	<5 min	30–60 min	Antagonism
	Hemodialysis	<5 min	Variable	Excretion

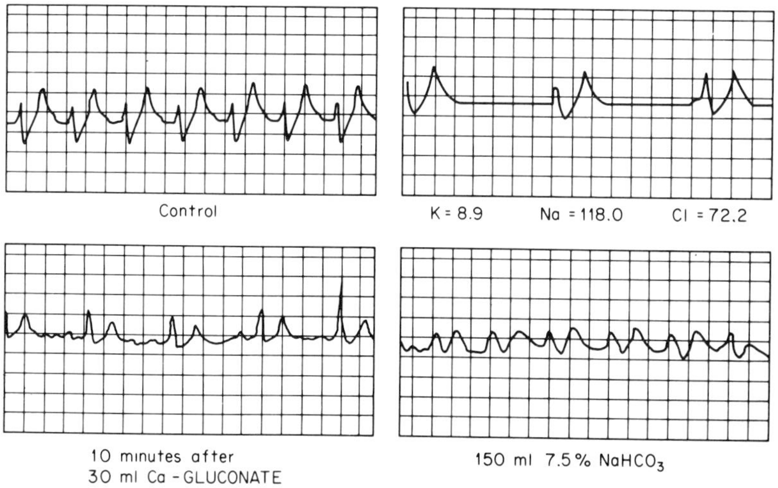

FIGURE 38-2 • Rapid movement seen in electrocardiogram following intravenous administration of calcium in the presence of hyperkalemia: *upper right,* 1 P.M.; *lower left,* 1:10 P.M.; *lower right,* 2:25 P.M. Intravenous calcium gluconate rapidly reversed the sine-wave configuration caused by hyperkalemia. Hypertonic sodium was not as effective.

perkalemia is hemodialysis. This should be used if hyperkalemia recurs or is accompanied by other indications for dialysis, or if ion-exchange resins are ineffective.

In the presence of advanced hyperkalemia, that is, with a serum potassium level of 7 meq/liter or greater, and/or significant changes on the electrocardiogram (see above), treatment that rapidly lowers serum potassium level is indicated. Such emergency treatment includes:

1. Dextrose and insulin, which lowers extracellular K^+ levels by transferring potassium into the cells. Continuous intravenous 50% dextrose infusion (see below) is instituted if the patient is not already receiving it; crystalline insulin is added to the infusate in a ratio of one unit of insulin to 5 g dextrose. This form of treatment may take from 30 to 60 min but usually lasts for several hours (Table 38-7). Once begun, dextrose-insulin therapy should not be discontinued until total body potassium has been reduced by other means because of the danger of rapid intracellular-to-extracellular potassium shifts and the return of dangerous levels of hyperkalemia.
2. Intravenously administered calcium (Fig. 38-2) does not alter potassium levels but rapidly antagonizes its effects on the heart. With continuous electrocardiographic monitoring, 10 to 20 ml of 10% calcium gluconate can be given by syringe at a rate of 2 ml/min, followed by addition of calcium to the infusion of hypertonic glucose and insulin.
3. Correction of acidosis by the rapid infusion of sodium bicarbonate (44 meq per ampule) not only provides Na^+ for antagonizing the cardiac effects of potassium but also deposits potassium intracellularly as a result of correction of the acidosis. It must be remembered that these effects are short-lived (1 to 2 h) and must be reinforced by exchange resins and dialysis.
4. Inhaled isoproterenol, which acutely shifts potassium intracellularly.

The foregoing emergency measures have been lifesaving at times, and they must temporarily take precedence over all other considerations, such as fluid restriction and sodium overload.

Diuretic phase During the diuretic phase of acute renal failure, the majority of patients have a normal serum potassium concentration. On occasion, especially with marked or persistent polyuria, there may be excessive urinary losses leading to hypokalemia. Potassium excretion should be monitored during the recovery phase, and on occasions when serum potassium drops to 3.5 meq/liter or less, supplements should be administered. Within a period of several days, progressive stabilization and normalization of urine volume and renal function results, so that prolonged potassium therapy is usually not required.

ACID-BASE ABNORMALITIES

(Topics covered in the following sections can be explored further in Chaps. 24–31.)

General patterns of acid-base disturbances in acute renal failure

The kidneys normally excrete nonvolatile acids produced at a rate of approximately 1 meq per kilogram of body weight per day.[62] Owing to buffers other than bicarbonate (e.g., hemoglobin and bone), the apparent bicarbonate space is 40 percent of body weight. That is, any addition of acid or base respectively decreases or increases the serum bicarbonate concentration as if bicarbonate were distributed over a body weighing 40 percent of actual body weight. In the absence of renal excretion, the 70 meq of acid produced per day by a 70-kg person diminishes serum bicarbonate by approximately 1 to 2 meq/liter per day in acute renal failure.

There are several factors that determine both the severity and the type of metabolic acidosis that develops in acute renal failure. In general, patients developing acute renal failure have a diminished ability to excrete an acid load due to the marked decrease in GFR, rather than have bicarbonate wasting secondary to abnormal tubular function. The uremic metabolic acidosis of acute renal failure, therefore, is characterized by an increased anion gap due to failure to filter and excrete the unmeasured anions of metabolic acidosis, such as sulfate and phosphate. It is important to realize that the metabolic acidosis in this situation is not due to the retention of these anions, but rather to a decrease in bicarbonate concentration. The removal of the abnormal anions by renal excretion without regeneration or administration of bicarbonate does not correct acidosis; it merely restores the anion gap to normal. Furthermore, the increase in anion gap may be much greater than the decrease in bicarbonate concentration, if bicarbonate is regenerated or administered while abnormal anions are retained.

In general, the rate of development of metabolic acidosis in acute renal failure is greater in patients with oliguric ATN than in nonoliguric patients and those with long-standing oliguria. Most important, the rate is related to the rate of catabolism; that is, patients with hypercatabolic acute renal failure have a daily decrease in serum bicarbonate of greater than 2 or 3 meq/liter. The increased anion gap associated with the metabolic acidosis of acute renal failure is almost invariably less than 30 meq/liter unless the illness is complicated by an organic acidosis superimposed on the inorganic acidosis.[63] The typical acid-base abnormality of acute renal failure, as outlined above, may be complicated by a variety of mixed acid-base disturbances; when analyzed carefully, these acid-base abnormalities may give a clue to the underlying cause of acute renal failure, as well as to a better understanding of possible complications.

Increased anion gap metabolic acidosis complicated by partial nonanion gap acidosis

During the early phase of acute renal failure, relative or absolute hyperchloremia, together with high anion gap acidosis, is not unusual.[64,65] This can occur from a variety of clinical situations. First, if there is severe ECF depletion that is corrected with isotonic sodium chloride, hyperchloremia may develop. Second, hyperchloremic acidosis can occur from loss of bicarbonate in association with severe diarrheal illnesses which can result in acute renal failure. If the loss of sodium bicarbonate exceeds that of water, hyponatremia results and normal chloride concentration represents relative hyperchloremia. Subsequent administration and retention of sodium chloride restores serum sodium concentration to normal and produces absolute hyperchloremia. Third, if acute renal failure develops in a patient with hypoalbuminemia, the anion gap may be reduced; the serum electrolyte pattern may then suggest absolute or relative hyperchloremic acidosis, that is, metabolic acidosis with normal anion gap.

Renal tubular acidosis may occur in conjunction with nephrotoxic acute renal failure. For example, ATN secondary to toxicity from bismuth, mercury, or uranium may be associated with Fanconi syndrome, including proximal renal tubular acidosis, hypophosphatemia, glycosuria, and hypokalemia.[66] Streptozotocin, a nitrosourea that has been used in the treatment of pancreatic islet cell tumors, can cause ATN with associated renal tubular acidosis and a florid Fanconi syndrome.[67] Multiple myeloma with nephrotoxic light-chain proteinuria has been noted to cause both proximal and distal renal tubular acidosis.[68] Finally, type IV renal tubular acidosis has been associated with severe liver disease and development of hepatorenal syndrome, as well as with the acute renal failure resulting from the use of nonsteroidal anti-inflammatory agents.[69] With the subsequent development of more severe ATN of the oliguric variety, any early evidence of normal anion gap acidosis is lost because loss of glomerular function predominates over the loss of tubular function with associted retention of sulfates and phosphates.

Anion gap increase out of proportion to the degree of metabolic acidosis and/or acute renal failure

The most common cause of a high anion gap out of proportion to the degree of renal failure is that seen with the organic acidosis of diabetic ketoacidosis or lactic acidosis. Acute renal failure associated with rhabdomyolysis, DIC, and sepsis, can be related to lactic acidosis.[63] This is especially common in the very young, the very old, pregnant women, and patients with such miscellaneous disorders as acute pancreatitis and snake venom toxicity.[70] Renal sepsis may lead to acute renal failure and secondary papillary necrosis.[71] In contrast, a substantial incidence exists of acute cortical necrosis in the presence of DIC; it frequently presents with anuria and irreversible renal failure and subsequent development of renal calcifications.[72] Phenol toxicity, another rare cause of acute cortical necrosis, was associated with lactic acidosis, aminoaciduria, and glycosuria.[73]

Acute renal failure secondary to glycol intoxication, most commonly ethylene glycol (antifreeze) intoxication, can produce an extremely high anion gap acidosis.[74] Ethylene glycol ATN should be strongly suspected when the patient appears inebriated but carries no odor of alcohol and metabolic acidosis is present together with a large anion gap out of proportion to the degree of renal failure, no evidence of diabetic ketosis, and when a urinalysis has revealed massive calcium oxalate crystalluria. An additional characteristic laboratory finding is a significant increase in delta osmolality, that is, a great increase in measured serum osmolality over what can be calculated from serum electrolytes.[75] The profound acidosis of ethylene glycol intoxication is due to both the metabolic derangements caused by the toxic metabolites and the breakdown products themselves.

Anion gap decrease in association with metabolic acidosis

This rare event can occur during the early phase of acute renal failure secondary to multiple myeloma (IgG, IgM variants). The antibiotic polymyxin B, used against gram-negative bacilli, can produce nephrotoxic ATN in association with an increase in serum chloride levels and a decrease in the anion gap.[76]

Metabolic and respiratory alkalosis associated with acute renal failure

Metabolic alkalosis is an unusual occurrence and is entirely iatrogenic. It has been described in ATN associated with open heart surgery when multiple transfusions have resulted in excessive blood citrate levels.[74,77] The subsequent metabolism of citrate to bicarbonate produces the metabolic alkalosis. Similarly, metabolic alkalosis can develop when excess sodium bicarbonate is administered during a cardiac arrest or to correct severe acidemia in association with diabetic ketoacidosis. Alcohol-induced rhabdomyolysis may result in ATN with mixed metabolic and respiratory alkalosis and is occasionally also complicated by lactic acidosis.[78] Finally, metabolic alkalosis may occur in patients with acute renal failure and associated severe emesis or excessive nasogastric drainage. If the acute renal failure is oliguric, hypercatabolic, and of long duration, a rapid correction of metabolic alkalosis and the ultimate substitution of metabolic acidosis can be expected. In contrast, it is possible to observe a respiratory alkalosis in association with metabolic acidosis in acute renal failure secondary to heatstroke, sepsis, and liver failure.[64,79,80]

General management of metabolic acidosis in acute renal failure

During the course of acute renal failure most patients have an established high anion gap uremic acidosis that is relatively mild and, in the absence of active catabolic events, is not progressive. Serum bicarbonate concentrations of 15 to 20 meq/liter with arterial pH values of greater than 7.25 are the general rule. This degree of metabolic acidosis usually does not require any specific treatment. However, rapid decrements in pH or even slow declines to values below 7.15 may lead to symptomatic discomfort. Such acidemic patients are also more susceptible to the hemodynamic consequences of metabolic acidosis, including a depression of myocardial contractility and a tendency toward serious arrhythmias. Generally, a serum bicarbonate level of less than 15 meq/liter is sufficiently severe to warrant treatment. The base deficit (in meq) is given by body weight × 0.45 × [normal serum bicarbonate concentration minus current serum bicarbonate concentration]. A maximum of 50 percent of the deficit should be replaced over 12 h. To minimize the risk of volume overload, therapy should be restricted to that amount of base necessary to maintain a serum bicarbonate concentration at approximately 20 meq/liter. If metabolic acidosis is corrected too rapidly or excessively, the result may be tetany and/or seizures, hypokalemia, hypoventilation, hypernatremia, or overshoot alkalosis. Often, by the time alkalosis is severe enough so that sodium overload from bicarbonate is a problem, dialysis with low-bicarbonate dialysate may be indicated.[81]

When severe metabolic acidosis is associated with acute uremia, hemodialysis is the treatment of choice. Recent studies have established the superiority of baths containing bicarbonate rather than acetate when treating critically ill, acute renal failure patients with severe metabolic acidosis.[82-84]

DIVALENT ION DISORDERS

(Details of phosphorus, magnesium, and calcium disorders may be found in Chaps. 32–34, 41.)

General pattern of change in acute renal failure

Disturbances in divalent ion metabolism occur early and often in patients with acute renal failure.[85] Hyperphosphatemia and hypermagnesemia are almost invariably present during the oliguric phase of acute renal failure. Elevated serum phosphate and magnesium concentrations result from retention of these ions consequent to the failing kidney's inability to excrete them. In general, the severity of hyperphosphatemia varies from 5 to 8 mg/dl, but on occasion can be as high as 15 to 18 mg/dl (especially in tumor-lysis syndromes). Hypermagnesemia is usually mild to moderate with levels as high as 5.0 mg/dl. Since there is no alteration in the binding of magnesium to serum proteins the fraction of diffusible magnesium remains normal, but the absolute values of diffusible magnesium increases.

Hypocalcemia is invariably present during the oliguric phase of acute renal failure. It may be noted as early as one to two days after the onset of renal failure, with Ca^{2+} concentrations as low as 7.5 to 5.0 mg/dl.[85] There is no difference between normal subjects and patients with acute renal failure in the ratio of ionized to total calcium, but the absolute value of the ratio in each group is lower than normal.

The etiology of hypocalcemia in acute renal failure is multifactorial. There is a poor correlation between hypocalcemia and the degree of hyperphosphatemia. Indeed, hypocalcemia may be observed with low, normal, or elevated serum phosphate levels. The prime cause for hypocalcemia of acute renal failure is probably skeletal resistance to the calcemic action of parathyroid hormone (PTH);[86] hypoalbuminemia, reduced levels of 1α,25-dihydroxyvitamin D_3 (1α,25-$(OH)_2D_3$) and severe hyperphosphatemia may also contribute to the severity of the hypocalcemia.

With the onset of the diuretic phase of acute renal failure, there is an increased fractional excretion of calcium, sodium, magnesium, and phosphorus. In many patients, hypomagnesemia and hypophosphatemia develop ("overshoot") during the diuretic phase. This is usually of short duration and of no clinical significance. Deviations from the usual pattern of divalent ion abnormalities seen during the oliguric and diuretic phase of acute renal failure are not uncommon. Moreover, specific deviations in divalent ion metabolism have a direct bearing on the specific etiology of acute renal failure and, therefore, are of particular clinical relevance.

Specific patterns of divalent ion abnormalities in acute renal failure

Hypocalcemia out of proportion to the duration and severity of acute renal failure

A pattern of early decreased serum Ca^{2+} level, excessive with respect to the deficit in renal function, is characteristic of ATN secondary to rhabdomyolysis.[87] The marked serum phosphate elevation in patients with ATN of this etiology probably enhances deposition of calcium in injured muscles, leading to more severe hypocalcemia. Indeed, there is often evidence of calcification of damaged muscles in these patients. Acute pancreatitis is another cause of ATN in which severe hypocalcemia may occur.[88] When ATN complicates body burns, early and severe hypocalcemia and hypophosphatemia may occur along with metabolic alkalosis.[89] The incidence of hypocalcemia in acute pancreatitis appears to be directly related to the incidence of severe hemorrhagic pancreatitis with associated hypoalbuminemia and hypoparathyroidism, which may contribute to the severity of the hypocalcemia in these patients. Moreover, specific nephrotoxins such as glycols, methoxyflurane, and mithramycin have been associated with excessive degrees of hypocalcemia in relation to the degree of renal insufficiency.

Hypercalcemia associated with acute renal failure

Hypercalcemia occurs commonly during the diuretic phase of ATN; it may be present, infrequently, during the oliguric phase.[87] The majority of patients with hypercalcemia during the diuretic phase of ATN have underlying rhabdomyolysis. The most plausible explanation for the development of hypercalcemia in this setting is the mobilization of calcium previously deposited in damaged muscles into the extracellular space. Elevated blood levels of 1α,25-$(OH)_2D_3$ have been reported in some of these patients and may contribute to the hypercalcemia.[86]

The presence of hypercalcemia during the oliguric phase of ATN is especially hazardous because of associated hyperphosphatemia. The high-calcium phosphorus product may therefore lead to widespread calcium deposition in soft tissues, involving vital organs such as the heart and lungs. Hypercalcemia in this setting, therefore, represents a medical emergency that requires immediate dialysis with calcium-free dialysate. In contrast, the hypercalcemia of the diuretic phase is more benign because it occurs in the setting of rapidly decreasing serum phosphate levels; hypercalcemia during this phase, however, often requires therapy.

On rare occasions, especially sudden and severe hypercalcemia can precipitate acute renal failure. Multiple myeloma is perhaps the most common neoplasm leading to acute renal failure, occurring in approximately 10 to 20 percent of cases.[90,91] The association of light-chain proteinuria interacting with Tamm-Horsfall protein may be important in the pathogenesis of nephrotoxicity in multiple myeloma; other specific host factors include the state of hydration, acid-base balance, and hypercalcemia. Whereas acute renal failure and light-chain proteinuria are frequently associated with hypercalcemia, the initial factor leading to hypercalcemia is increased bone resorption.[92] In this setting, the onset of severe hypercalcemia is more likely to be due to acute renal failure and associated decreased renal excretion of resorbed Ca^{2+} than to any primary etiologic factor in the production of renal failure. In contrast, another important and relatively unappreciated cause of high serum calcium in asymptomatic patients with multiple myeloma is an abnormally extensive binding of calcium to paraprotein.[93,94] Patients have been described with multiple myeloma and total calcium levels above normal but whose free of diffusible calcium concentration is normal.

Other neoplastic diseases reported associated to severe hypercalcemia and renal failure are solid tumors of the breast, lungs, and kidney, as well as leukemias and lymphomas.[95,96] More often, chronic renal failure is seen with these neoplastic diseases but on occasion, especially with the onset of dehydration secondary to nausea and vomiting, hypercalcemia can rapidly become severe and contribute to the production of acute renal failure.

Hyperphosphatemia out of proportion to the duration and severity of acute renal failure

Phosphate concentrations in serum that exceed 8 to 10 mg/dl, frequently associated with severe hypocalcemia in which serum Ca^{2+} levels are below 6 mg/dl, characterized hypercatabolic ATN. Hyperphosphatemia is most commonly noted in ATN resulting from rhabdomyolysis where it is also associated with excessive hyperuricemia and an increase in the rate of rise of serum creatinine in relationship to serum urea nitrogen.[87] Phosphate leakage from damaged muscle cells causes hyperphosphatemia and in turn provokes precipitation of calcium and phosphorus in soft tissues and blood vessels. Causes of nontraumatic rhabdomyolysis are shown in Table 38-8.

Recent reports have described an association of acute renal failure with rapid and severe onset of hyperphosphatemia in patients with acute lymphoblastic leukemia, lymphosarcoma, and Burkitt's lymphoma.[97,98,99] Hyperphosphatemia in patients with these lymphoproliferative disorders can occur as a result of rapid cell lysis after the start of the chemotherapy. Sometimes there is associated severe hyperuricemia which can itself produce acute renal failure; more often than not, however, hyperuricemia is modest, so severe onset of hyperphosphatemia with precipitation of calcium phosphate into soft tissue is the most likely etiologic agent of acute renal failure in this setting.

TABLE 38-8 • Occult myoglobinuric acute tubular necrosis

METABOLIC
Hypokalemia
Hypophosphatemia
Diabetic nonketotic coma
Diabetic ketotic coma
DRUG-INDUCED
Heroin
Ethanolism
Amphetamine
Carbon monoxide
Prolonged drug coma
Succinylcholine
PHYSICAL
Heatstroke
Hyperpyrexia
Grand mal seizures
Vascular occlusions
Strenuous exercise in presence of:
Poor conditioning
Sickle cell trait
McArdle's syndrome
Heat excess
Potassium depletion

Hypophosphatemia in association with acute renal failure

Although hypophosphatemia is rare in acute renal failure, on occasion it can be strikingly present in association with advanced renal insufficiency. Characteristically, it is seen in two specific settings associated with acute renal failure: (1) septicemia and heatstroke,[79,80] both of which are associated with marked hyperventilation and the development of respiratory alkalosis, which tends to shift phosphorus from the extracellular to the intracellular space; (2) rarely, a Fanconi syndrome can occur secondary to heavy metal intoxication, streptozotocin chemotherapy, or multiple myeloma;[66-68] in this case the acute renal failure is nonoliguric.

Management of divalent ion disorders

The infrequency of frank hypocalcemic tetany or seizures in uremia is usually attributed to the concomitant acidosis which increases the concentration of the ionized fraction of calcium. By the same reasoning, the appearance of tetany during administration of alkali to correct acidosis has been attributed to a decrease in the fraction of ionized calcium accompanying the rise in plasma pH. Studies of ultrafilterable calcium (used as an index of ionized calcium fraction) with alterations in plasma pH tend to discredit this hypothesis, since even extreme changes in pH alter the ultrafilterable calcium by less than 5 percent. However, it is difficult to explain the alleviation of alkali-induced tetany by calcium administration in any other way. It may be that the heightened neuromuscular irritability of hypocalcemia is partially offset by the CNS effects of hypermagnesemia. At present, the benignity of hypocalcemia associated with acute uremia cannot be entirely explained. Of more importance in acute renal failure is the exacerbation of the cardiac effects of hyperkalemia by concurrent hypocalcemia (see above).

Hypermagnesemia and hyperphosphatemia occurring during the course of acute renal failure are generally driven further upward by the use of magnesium-containing antacids and laxatives or phosphate-containing enemas (e.g., Fleet's); none of these should be used during acute renal failure. Food intake during the course of acute renal failure is usually poor, and thus hyperphosphatemia occurs less severely in association with renal failure than might be expected. The exception to this observation is rhabdomyolysis-induced acute renal failure, in which severe hyperphosphatemia is the rule.

Unlike sodium and potassium, diets cannot be sufficiently phosphorus-restricted to maintain normal serum levels and still be nutritionally adequate. Thus, when the patient is able to eat, phosphorus-rich foods should be restricted, primarily milk products; serum phosphorus should never be controlled solely by limiting overall nutrition. In other words, the patient should be encouraged to eat whatever he or she can, even at the expense of elevating serum phosphorus.

In chronic renal failure, hyperphosphatemia is treated with phosphate-binding antacids, primarily aluminum hydroxide. During acute renal failure, most patients are confined to bed and constipation or obstipation often results from the use of phosphate-binding antacids in this setting. The negative effects of severe constipation, such as heightened anorexia and hyperkalemia, outweigh the risk of transient mild to moderate hyperphosphatemia. Thus, unless serum phosphorus concentration is greater than 8 mg/dl, aluminum hydroxide antacids should not be given. In those rare circumstances in which aluminum hydroxide must be given, a non-magnesium-containing laxative, for example, 70% sorbitol, should be started at the same time, unless diarrhea is already present. The control of gastric acid secretion is limited by the frequent inability to give or undesirability of oral antacids in patients with acute renal failure. Therefore, histamine H_2 receptor blockers are the treatment of choice for hyperacidity.[100,101]

Hypomagnesemia and hypophosphatemia may occur during acute renal failure, primarily during TPN. Hypomagnesemia may occur during nonoliguric acute renal failure induced by cisplatin.[102] In such an unusual situation, parenteral magnesium may be replaced either intravenously by addition to the TPN solution or by infusion in 5% dextrose, or by the intramuscular route. Magnesium should be administered cautiously in renal failure; the concentration should rarely exceed 25 meq/liter by the intravenous route, and total parenteral magnesium should rarely exceed 75 meq/day. More rapid infusion should only be given for severe symptomatic hypomagnesemia, and should be accompanied by frequent monitoring of serum levels. Phosphorus replacement may be given intravenously as either sodium or potassium neutral phosphate (50 or 25 meq/liter, depending on the extent of the deficit). As with magnesium, more rapid replacement requires more frequent monitoring.

REFERENCES

1. Anderson RJ et al: Nonoliguric acute renal failure. *N Engl J Med* 296:1134, 1977.
2. Seguro AC et al: Acute renal failure of leptospirosis: Nonoliguric and hypokalemia forms. *Nephron* 55:146, 1990.
3. Shimahara Y et al: Pathophysiology of acute renal failure following living Escherichia coli injection in rats: High-energy metabolism and renal functions. *Circ Shock* 21:197, 1987.
4. Ashley BC, Whyte HM: Practical methods for estimating the basic water requirements during oliguric renal failure. *Aust Ann Med* 12:127, 1963.
5. Bluemle LW Jr et al: Changes in body composition in acute renal failure. *J Clin Invest* 35:1094, 1956.
6. Teschan PE et al: Posttraumatic renal insufficiency in military casualties: I. Clinical characteristics. *Am J Med* 18:172, 1955.
7. Bywaters EGJ, Beall D: Crush injuries with impairment of renal function. *Br Med J* 1:427, 1941.
8. Swann RC, Merril JP: The clinical course of acute renal failure. *Medicine* 32:215, 1953.
9. Eliahou HE, Bota A: The diagnosis of acute renal failure. *Nephron* 2:287, 1965.
10. Bull GN et al: Renal function studies in acute tubular necrosis. *Clin Sci* 9:379, 1950.
11. Graber IG, Sevitt S: Renal function in burned patients and its relationship to morphological changes. *J Clin Pathol* 12:25, 1959.
12. Verrel RM, Knochel JP: Nonoliguric acute renal failure. *JAMA* 200:118, 1967.
13. Perlmutter M et al: Urine-serum urea nitrogen ratio. *JAMA* 170:1533, 1959.
14. Espinel CH: The FE_{Na} test—Use in the differential diagnosis of acute renal failure. *JAMA* 236:579, 1976.
15. Handa SP, Morrin PAF: Diagnostic indices in acute renal failure. *Can Med Assoc J* 96:78, 1967.
16. Swenson RS et al: Differential diagnostic indices in early acute renal failure (ARF), abstracted. *Clin Res* 23:122A, 1975.
17. Augur R et al: Use of ethacrynic acid in mannitol-resistant oliguric renal failure. *JAMA* 206:891, 1968.
18. Barry KG et al: Mannitol infusion: II. The Prevention of acute functional renal failure during resection of an aneurysm of the abdominal aorta. *N Engl J Med* 264:967, 1961.
19. Eliahou HE: Mannitol therapy in oliguria of acute onset. *Br Med J* 1:807, 1964.
20. Levinsky NG, Alexander EA: Acute renal failure in Brenner BM, Rector FC Jr (eds): *The Kidney.* Philadelphia, Saunders, 1976, p 809.
21. Levinsky NG et al: Mannitol and diuretics in acute renal failure, in Brenner BM, Lazarus JM (eds): *Acute Renal Failure.* Philadelphia, Saunders, 1983, p 712.
22. Saha H et al: Limited value of the fractional excretion of sodium test in the diagnosis of acute renal failure. *Nephrol Dial Transplant* 2:79, 1987.
23. Moss G: Cause of azotemia after GI hemorrhage, examining an old wives tale. *Am J Surg* 3:269, 1975.
24. Molitch ME et al: Spurious serum creatinine elevations in ketoacidosis. *Ann Intern Med* 93:280, 1980.
25. Trever RW, Cluff LE: The problem of increasing azotemia during management of diabetic acidosis. *Am J Med* 24:368, 1958.
26. Ward MM: Factors predictive of acute renal failure in rhabdomyolysis. *Arch Intern Med* 148(7):1553, 1988.
27. Case records of the Massachusetts General Hospital, (case 32-1972). *N Engl J Med* 287, 1972.
28. Krug H et al: Intravascular coagulation in acute renal failure after myocardial infarction. *Ann Clin Med* 81:494, 1974.
29. Lessman RK et al: Renal artery embolism: Clinical fea-

tures and long-term follow-up of 17 cases. *Ann Intern Med* 89:477, 1978.

30. Chamberlain MJ et al: Oliguric renal failure in the nephrotic syndrome. *Q J Med* 35:215, 1966.
31. Arneil GC et al: Renal venous thrombosis. *Clin Nephrol* 1:119, 1973.
32. Nissenson AR et al: Mannitol. *West J Med* 131:277, 1979.
33. Westen F, Baranowski RL: Hemodynamic consequences of immunologic glomerular injury. *Plasma Ther Transfus Technol* 5:447, 1984.
34. Murphy TR, Murphy FD: The heart in acute glomerulonephritis. *Ann Intern Med* 41:510, 1954.
35. Gutman RA et al: The immune-complex glomerulonephritis of bacterial endocarditis. *Medicine* 51:1, 1972.
36. Couser WG et al: Acute renal failure associated with renal-vascular disease, vasculitis, glomerulonephritis, and nephrotic syndrome, in Brenner BM, Lazarus JM (eds): *Acute Renal Failure*. Philadelphia, Saunders, 1983, p 333.
37. Glassock RJ: Renal arterial thrombosis and embolism, in Massry SG, Glassock RJ (eds): *Textbook of Nephrology*. Baltimore, Williams & Wilkins, 1984, vol 6, p 263.
38. Linton AL et al: Acute interstitial nephritis due to drugs. *Ann Intern Med* 93:735, 1980.
39. Arieff AI, Carroll HJ: Nonketotic hyperosmolar coma with hyperglycemia. *Medicine* 51:73, 1972.
40. Earley LE: Extreme polyuria in obstructive uropathy. *N Engl J Med* 255:600, 1956.
41. Mattar JA et al: II. Cardiac arrest in the critically ill. *Am J Med* 45:162, 1974.
42. Tarial RK et al: Misleading reductions of serum sodium and chloride: Association with hyperproteinemia in patients with multiple myeloma. *Proc Soc Exp Bio Med* 110:145, 1962.
43. Schaer GL et al: Association of hyponatremia with increased renin activity in chronic congestive failure: Impact of diuretic therapy. *Am J Cardiol* 51:1635, 1983.
44. Moran SM, Jamison RL: The variable hyponatremic response to hyperglycemia. *West J Med* 142:49, 1985.
45. Green LW et al: Adrenal insufficiency as an complication of acquired immune deficiency syndrome. *Ann Intern Med* 101:497, 1984.
46. Columbos JT et al: Effect of osmotic (mannitol) diuresis on electrolyte and water excretion in ascites, cirrhotic patients. *Clin Res* 11:69, 1963.
47. Schetz M et al: The use of continuous arteriovenous hemofiltration in intensive care medicine. *Acta Anaesthesiol Belg* 35(1): 67, 1984.
48. Surawicz B: Electrolytes and the electrocardiogram. *Mod Concepts Cardiol Dis* 33:875, 1964.
49. Merrill JP et al: Clinical recognition and treatment of acute potassium intoxication. *Ann Intern Med* 33:797, 1950.
50. Cannon PJ et al: The relationship of hypertension and renal failure in scleroderma. *Medicine* 5311, 1974.
51. Mattern WD et al: Oliguric acute renal failure in malignant hypertension. *Am J Med* 52:187, 1972.
52. Zawada ET et al: Clinical course of patients with scleroderma renal crises treated with captopril. *Nephron* 27:74, 1981.
53. Knochel JP, Schlein EM: On the mechanism of rhabdomyolysis in potassium depletion. *J Clin Invest* 51:1750, 1972.
54. Singhal PC et al: Rhabdomyolysis in the hyperosmolal state. *Am J Med* 88(1):9, 1990.
55. Knochel JP et al: Heat stress, exercise, and muscle injury. *Ann Intern Med* 81:321, 1974.
56. Butler WT et al: Nephrotoxicity of amphotericin B, early and late effects in 81 patients. *Ann Intern Med* 61:175, 1964.
57. Tan SY et al: Indomethacin-induced prostaglandin inhibition with hyperkalemia: A reversible cause of hyporeninemic hypoaldosteronism. *Ann Intern Med* 90:783, 1979.
58. Shulman H et al: Nephrotoxicity of cyclosporin after allogenic marrow transplantation. *N Engl J Med* 305:1392, 1981.
59. Lachaal M, Vento RC: Nephrotoxicity and hyperkalemia in patients with acquired immunodeficiency syndrome treated with pentamidine. *Am J Med* 87(3):260, 1989.
60. Makoff DL et al: On the mechanism of hyperkalemia due to hyperosmotic expansion with saline or mannitol. *Clin Sci* 41:383, 1971.
61. Flinn RB et al: Treatment of the oliguric patient with a new sodium-exchange resin and sorbitol. *N Engl J Med* 264:111, 1961.
62. Narins RG: The renal acidoses, in Brenner BM, Stein JH (eds): New York, Churchill Livingston, 1978, p 30.
63. Gabow PA et al: Diagnostic importance of an increased serum anion gap. *N Engl J Med* 303:854, 1980.
64. Narins RG, Emmett M: Simple and mixed acid-base disorders: A practical approach. *Medicine* 59:161, 1980.
65. Oh MS, Carrol HJ: The anion gap. *N Engl J Med* 297:814, 1977.
66. Urizar R, Vernier RL: Bismuth nephropathy. *JAMA* 198:187, 1966.
67. Sadoff L: Nephrotoxicity of streptozotocin (NSC-85998). *Can Chem Rep* (Part I) 54:457, 1970.
68. Lazar GS, Feinstein DI: Distal renal tubular acidosis in multiple myeloma. *Arch Intern Med* 144:655, 1981.
69. Clive DM, Stoff JS: Renal syndrome associated with nonsterodial anti-inflammatory drugs. *N Engl J Med* 310, 1984.
70. Kaplinsky C et al: Disseminated intravascular clotting and renal cortical necrosis: Complications of a snake bite. *Clin Pediatr* 19:229, 1980.
71. Harvald B: Renal papillary necrosis: A clinical survey of sixty-six cases. *Am J Med* 35:481, 1963.
72. Matlin RA, Gary NE: Acute cortical necrosis. Case report and review of the literature. *Am J Med* 56:110, 1974.
73. Foxall PJ et al: Acute renal failure following accidental cutaneous absorption of phenol: Application of NMR urinalysis to monitor the disease process. *Hum Toxicol* 8(6):491, 1989.
74. Parry MF, Wallach R: Ethylene glycol poisoning. *Am J Med* 57:143, 1974.
75. Emmett M, Narins RG: Clinical use of the anion gap. *Medicine* 56:38, 1977.
76. O'Connor DT, Stone RA: Hyperchloremia and negative anion gap associated with polymyxin B administration. *Arch Intern Med* 138:478, 1978.

77. Barcenas CG et al: Metabolic alkalosis after massive blood transfusion. *JAMA* 236:953, 1976.
78. Pitts TO, Van Thiel DM: Disorders of the serum electrolytes, acid-base balance, and renal function in alcoholism. *Recent Dev Alcohol* 4:311, 1986.
79. Chesney RW et al: Renal manifestations of the toxic-shock syndrome. *Am J Med* 71:583, 1981.
80. Knochel JP, Caskey JH: The mechanism of hypophosphatemia in acute heat stroke. *JAMA* 238:425, 1977.
81. Ayus JC et al: Alkalemia associated with renal failure: Correction by hemodialysis with low bicarbonate dialysate. *Arch Intern Med* 140:513, 1980.
82. Huyghebaert MF et al: Bicarbonate hemodialysis of patients with acute renal failure and severe sepsis. *Crit Care Med* 13(10):840, 1985.
83. Leunissen KM et al: Acetate versus bicarbonate hemodialysis in critically ill patients. *Nephron* 42(2):146, 1986.
84. Lalau JD et al: Bicarbonate haemodialysis: An adequate treatment for lactic acidosis in diabetics treated by metformin. *Intensive Care Med* 13(6):383, 1987.
85. Massry SG et al: Divalent ion metabolism in patients with acute renal failure. *Kidney Int* 5:437, 1974.
86. Llach F et al: The pathophysiology of altered calcium metabolism in rhabdomyolysis-induced acute renal failure. *N Engl J Med* 305:117, 1981.
87. Koffler A et al: Acute renal failure due to nontraumatic rhabdomyolysis. *Am Intern Med* 85:23, 1978.
88. Gordan D, Calne RY: Renal failure in acute pancreatitis. *Br Med J* 3:801, 1972.
89. Vanholder R et al: Renal function in burns. *Acta Anaesthesiol Belg* 38(4):367, 1987.
90. DeFronzo RA et al: Acute renal failure in multiple myeloma. *Medicine* 54:209, 1975.
91. Ganeval D et al: Kidney involvement in multiple myeloma and related disorders. *Contrib Nephrol* 33:210, 1982.
92. Heyburn PJ et al: Relative importance of renal failure and increased bone resorption in the hypercalcemia of myelomatosis. *J Clin Pathol* 34:54, 1981.
93. Jaffee JP, Mosher DF: Calcium binding by a myeloma protein. *Am J Med* 67:343, 1979.
94. Ladensen JH, McDonald JM: Multiple myeloma and hypercalcemia (Washington University Case Conference). *Clin Chem* 25:1821, 1979.
95. Garnick MB, Mayer RJ: Acute renal failure associated with neoplastic disease and its treatment. *Semin Oncol* 5:155, 1978.
96. Glassock RJ et al: Kidney and electrolyte disturbances in neoplastic diseases. *Contrib Nephrol* 7:2, 1977.
97. Cadman EC et al: Hyperphosphatemia and hypocalcemia accompanying rapid cell lysis in a patient with Burkitt's lymphoma and Burkitt cell leukemia. *Am J Med* 62:283, 1977.
98. Kaplan BS et al: Acute renal failure induced by hyperphosphatemia in acute lymphoblastic leukemia. *Can Med J* 124:429, 1981.
99. Zushman J et al: Hyperphosphatemia, hyperphosphaturia, and hypocalcemia in acute lymphoblastic leukemia. *N Engl J Med* 289:1335, 1973.
100. Doherty CC et al: Cimetidine for duodenal ulceration in patients undergoing hemodialysis. *Br Med J* 2:1506, 1977.
101. Vaz AJ: Clinical use of cimetidine in acute renal failure after resection of abdominal aneurysms. *South Med J* 73:1028, 1980.
102. Schilsky RL, Anderson T: Hypomagnesemia and renal magnesium wasting in patients receiving cisplatin. *Ann Intern Med* 90:929, 1979.

CHAPTER • 39

Electrolyte disorders in chronic renal failure

Philip J. Tuso • Allen R. Nissenson • Gabriel M. Danovitch

The most remarkable feature of chronic renal failure (CRF) is the failing kidney's ability to maintain the volume and content of the extracellular fluid (ECF). This chapter emphasizes abnormalities in electrolye metabolism in CRF, but readers should remember how close to "normal" plasma electrolyte levels and fluid compartment volumes remain.

Seventy consecutively studied patients with end-stage renal failure who were about to commence dialysis therapy had normal serum sodium and potassium levels.[1] The most common electrolyte abnormality found in these patients was a mild hyperchloremia with a normal anion gap. Twenty percent had normal concentrations of sodium, potassium, chloride, and bicarbonate. These patients had far advanced renal disease with mean serum creatinine levels greater than 10 mg/dl. The frequency of totally normal serum electrolyte values is likely to increase with lesser degrees of functional impairment and nephron loss.

Clinical experience in human renal failure indicates that typically, in the absence of heart failure, hepatic failure, and hypoalbuminemia, there are no clinically detectable abnormalities in ECF volume until renal failure is far advanced. For a variety of technical reasons it has proved difficult to measure body compartment volumes in CRF accurately, but the available studies reveal no consistent pattern of alteration.[2] Thus, ECF volume is probably normal or mildly elevated in the majority of stable patients. Estimates of total body sodium have tended to show only mild increases.[2]

These observations attest to a remarkable capacity of surviving nephrons to undergo adaptive changes as renal disease progresses. The adaptations, though effective, have their limitations, beyond which emerge many of the familiar clinical features of end-stage renal disease.

RENAL ADAPTATION TO NEPHRON LOSS

The concept that remaining nephrons of the diseased kidney alter their functions to maintain the normalcy of the volume and content of body fluids was proposed 40 years ago by Robert Platt.[3,4] He observed that balance for urea and creatinine was maintained in advanced renal failure, albeit at elevated plasma levels of these solutes, and he was the first to identify that fractional excretions of sodium, potassium, and water were increased in CRF. Bricker and colleagues in series of studies using animal models of renal failure provided a convincing explanation of these clinical findings. The experimental model that was used was an innovative one.[5] Renal disease was induced by infarcting or surgical ablating one kidney while the other remained intact. The intact kidney allowed the function of the diseased or the so-called *remnant kidney* to be studied in a nonuremic environment. Upon removal of the normal kidney the experimental animal became uremic, and repeated studies of the remnant kidney allowed for differentiation between those abnormalities that were intrinsic and those which were manifestations of the uremic state.[5]

Solute handling by the tubules of the remnant and control kidneys, when normalized for differences in glomerular filtration rate (GFR), did not significantly differ. A normal relationship existed between tubular and glomerular functions in the diseased kidney. This orderly relationship in nephron function led to the formulation of the so-called *intact nephron hypothesis*.[6] Simplistically expressed, a kidney working at 25 percent of function has 25 percent of its remaining nephrons working normally—albeit in a uremic environment, rather than all of its remaining nephrons working at 25 percent function.

Nephron loss leads to adaptive changes that alter single nephron GFR (SNGFR) in the surviving glomeruli. The pattern of SNGFR from nephron to nephron differs depending on the nature of the underlying disease. In experimental models of glomerulonephritis there is a net overall decrease in total GFR, but among the surviving glomeruli the filtration rate varies from low to supernormal.[7] In tubulointerstitial nephritis there is also an overall net decrease in GFR, but individual surviving nephrons show uniformly increased filtration, with a broadening of the narrow gaussian distribution of SNGFR that characterizes the normal kidney.[8] It is remarkable that despite this wide variation in SNGFR, glomerular-tubular balance remains intact. The fact that only minor differences in tubular function are clinically detectable in primary interstitial and primary glomerular diseases[9] attests to the uniformity and effectiveness of the adaptive processes for solute balance.

PATTERNS OF THE ADAPTATION TO THE NEPHRON LOSS

It is possible to define three basic patterns of renal adaptation to nephron loss that alter solute excretion in advanced CRF (Fig. 39-1). The plasma concentrations of urea and creatinine, for example, are represented by *curve A*. Tubular secretion of these solutes is minimal and their excretion is largely the result of glomerular filtration. As the GFR falls the BUN and creatinine levels rise. A new filtered load is established and urinary excretion increases until solute balance is again reached and maintained at the new elevated plasma level, unless the GFR falls further and the cycle is repeated. The familiar hyperbolic relationship between these solutes and GFR is thus produced. Teleologically speaking, since BUN and creatinine themselves are only minimally toxic, there is no biologic necessity to adjust their excretion to maintain serum levels or total body content at a fixed level.

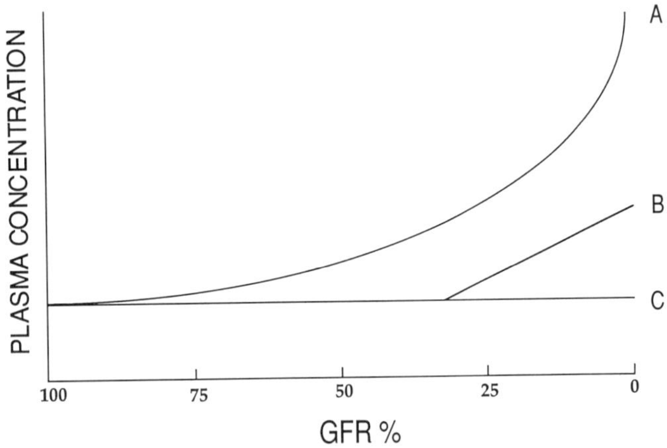

FIGURE 39-1 • Patterns of adaptation for different solutes in chronic renal disease. *Curve A* shows no regulation of solute concentration, which rises progressively as glomerular filtration rate (GFR) falls. *Curve B* shows that this rise occurs only when GFR approaches 24 percent of normal. *Curve C* represents perfect regulation of solute balance. [From Bricker NS, Fine LG: The renal response to progressive nephron loss, in Brenner BM, Rector FC, Jr (eds): *The Kidney*. Philadelphia, Saunders, 1981, p 1058.]

For certain solutes effective adaptive mechanisms take place in the early phase of CRF but homeostasis becomes impaired in the advanced stages. Phosphate, uric acid, and hydrogen ions are good examples of this phenomenon and are represented by *curve B*. In the cases of sodium and potassium, for example, maintenance of normal balance is critical and indeed their balance is maintained fairly precisely until the final stages of renal failure (*curve C*).

Despite much research it remains unclear to what extent adaptive processes in glomerular and tubular function are extrinsic to the kidney or whether they represent intrinsic renal alterations. Adaptive processes for individual solutes are discussed below. There is no evidence to suggest that homeostatic mechanisms in CRF are intrinsically different from those that maintain homeostasis in normal kidneys. In the case of sodium, for instance, despite intensive efforts, it has not proved possible to convincingly identify a unique natriuretic hormone to account for the increasing fractional excretion in CRF. Homeostatic mechanisms are not necessarily solely renal and in the case of potassium the gastrointestinal (GI) tract plays an increasingly more important role in excretion as renal function deteriorates (see below).

LIMITATIONS IN RENAL ADAPTATION

The patient with advancing CRF can indeed maintain sodium balance and ECF volume; however, there are important quantitative limitations on these processes imposed by renal failure. These limits may have dramatic clinical manifestations.

LIMITATION IN SODIUM EXCRETION

A normal subject can maintain sodium balance over a very wide range of intakes. In the absence of dietary sodium, the normal kidney can excrete a virtually sodium-free urine yet when challenged with a salt load sodium excretion can reach hundreds of milliequivalents per day. The latter is accomplished by virtue of small changes in fractional sodium excretion. The normal kidney can thus be said to have a low salt "floor" and a high salt "ceiling." In CRF there is typically a *salt losing* tendency that prevents the elaboration of a salt-free urine in response to a sudden reduction in sodium intake. This

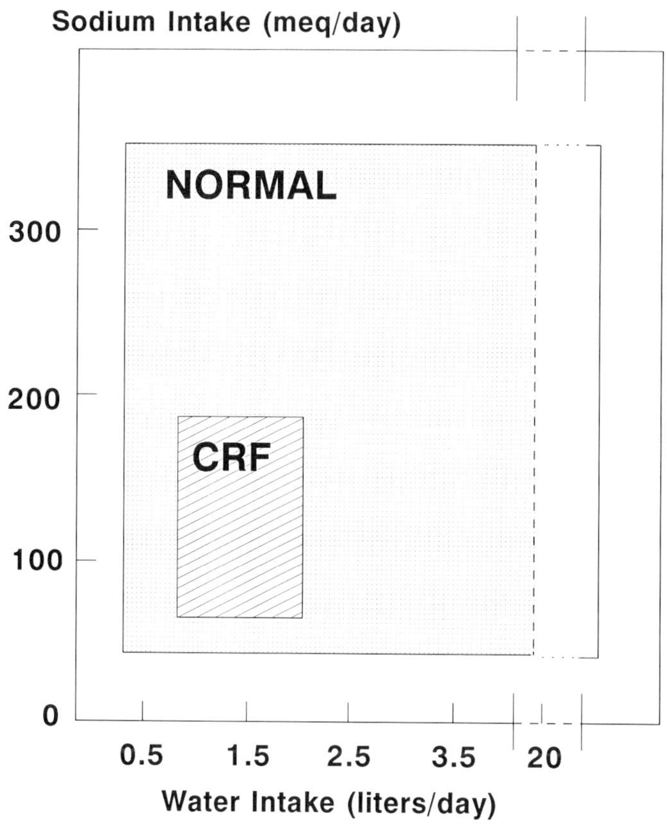

FIGURE 39-2 • Sodium and water intake in a chronic renal failure (CRF) patient compared with patients with normal renal function. Patients with CRF have restrictions on both water and fluid intake, whereas patients with normal renal function can handle large loads of sodium and water.

salt-losing tendency, the mechanism of which is discussed below, varies in severity but typically leads to the persistent excretion of 40 to 50 meq of sodium daily even when sodium balance has been negative. The salt floor can thus be said to be elevated above normal (Fig. 39-2). At a very low GFR the total filtered load of sodium may be only a few hundred milliequivalents (i.e., at a GFR of 3 liters daily and a plasma sodium concentration of 140 meq/liter the filtered sodium load will be 420 meq daily). Even though the fractional excretion of sodium rises in CRF there is still obligatory reabsorption of more than 50 percent of the filtered sodium together with other solutes so that the net maximal capacity to excrete sodium daily may be limited to 100 to 200 meq. The salt ceiling can be said to be reduced (Fig. 39-2). The lower the GFR the narrower the gap tends to become between the elevated floor and the lowered ceiling.

The diminished salt ceiling can be illustrated by the experimental technique of water immersion. Isothermic upright water immersion results in the central redistribution of intravascular volume and induces a natriuresis that tends to return the intravascular volume to preimmersion levels. In normal subjects the natriuresis induced by immersion is approximately equivalent to the infusion of 2 liters of normal saline.[10] In patients with CRF the natriuresis induced by immersion is only approximately 50 percent of the normal response. This blunted natriuretic response tends to delay the correction of the ECF volume expansion induced by immersion (and presumably by a saline infusion or high-salt diet).

A patient with advanced CRF eating a typical or mildly salt restricted diet of 100 to 150 meq daily can usually maintain balance. If, however, sodium intake falls below the salt floor, negative sodium balance ensues. If salt intake exceeds the salt ceiling, positive balance ensues. Clinically, this is expressed as episodes of volume contraction on the one hand and edema, hypertension, and heart failure on the other. Both situations may produce further deterioration in renal function, perpetuating a vicious cycle characterized by worsening perfusion due to volume contraction or volume expansion with congestive heart failure. Salt balance becomes more abnormal and renal function and sodium regulation deteriorate further. It follows that when assessing deteriorating renal function assiduous attention must be given to ECF volume.

Dietary recommendations for salt intake in CRF must also take into account these limitations in sodium excretion. Euvolemic patients with CRF should generally not be placed on strict salt limitation (i.e., less than 40 meq daily). If such a sodium intake is prescribed for patients with clinical evidence of ECF volume overload, assiduous attention must be directed to the monitoring of clinical parameters of ECF volume, for example, body weight, postural hypotension, venous pressure, and renal function. The upper limit of salt intake will depend on the individual patient's GFR and capacity to excrete a sodium load. A euvolemic, normotensive patient need not limit salt intake. A tendency to hypertension and fluid retention is very common in CRF and for these patients moderate limitation of sodium intake (i.e., 80 to 100 meq daily) is appropriate.

LIMITATIONS IN WATER EXCRETION

The extremes of urinary osmolality that can be achieved by the normal kidney approximate 50 to 1200 mosm/kg of water (see Chap. 5). Maintenance of solute balance on a typical North American diet requires the excretion of at least 600 mosm daily. When challenged by a water load, these 600 mosm of solute may be excreted in 12 liters of urine, yielding an osmolality of 50 mosm/kg. When thirsting, these 600 mosm of solute may be excreted in as little as 0.5 liter, yielding an osmolality of 1200 mosm/kg. The capacity to dilute and concentrate the urine is a reflection of the *free water clearance*, which is, in turn, determined by the capacity of the thick ascending limb of Henle's loop and cortical portions of the distal nephron to actively transport sodium chloride without water. The glomerular filtrate is thus diluted and may then be excreted as such or concentrated during passage through more distal segments of the nephron. The capacity to dilute and concentrate the urine is dependent on the number of functioning nephrons.

In a patient with a full complement of nephrons, the maximal free water clearance can reach levels as high as 15 ml/min. At a GFR of 50 percent of normal this will be approximately 7.5 ml/min, which represents approximately 10 liters of water daily and is still far above typical water intake. At a GFR of 10 percent of normal, however, total free water clearance may reach only 2 liters of water, and such a patient may develop positive water balance and hyponatremia at "normal" levels of water intake. The capacity to concentrate the urine is similarly impaired, and as end-stage renal failure is approached the urine is typically isosmolal with a constant osmolality of approximately 300 mosm/kg, though the capacity to dilute the urine tends to be maintained somewhat longer than the concentrating capacity. Since urine osmolality is fixed, urine volume and hence water excretion is determined by solute excretion rather than by the necessities of water balance as in normal people.[11]

The impairment of urinary concentration and dilution is reflected in the diurnal volume of urine. Consider an individual with normal renal function who maintains solute balance excreting 600 mosm of solute daily. If his or her day is divided into an awake period of 16 h and a sleep period of 8 h, 400 mosm of solute will be excreted during the waking hours in a urine volume that will reflect the intake minus any insensible water loss. At night, when there is presumably no water intake, the urine is concentrated maximally and 200 mosm of solute will be excreted at an osmolality of approximately 1000 mosm/kg, requiring approximately 200 ml. This volume approximates the smallest amount that triggers the sensation of fullness in the normal bladder, signaling the need for urination. Thus, the need to urinate at night is not normally sensed, while approximately 200 ml of concentrated urine is passed each morning.

A patient with CRF tends to pass urine with a fixed osmolality of approximately 300 mosm/kg. The necessity to excrete 600 mosm of solute will thus require 2 liters of urine, which will be excreted at a steady rate over 24 h. During the 8 h of sleep period, 600 to 700 ml of urine will be formed, which, if bladder capacity and function are normal, leads to nocturia, with the passage of urine two or three times nightly. The clinical impact of the limitations in the adaptive processes for water excretion in CRF are not just reflected in the inconvenience of nocturia. A patient with CRF whose water intake exceeds the capacity for free water clearance will develop positive water balance and hyponatremia. Water deprivation will lead more rapidly to hypernatremia and volume contraction in a patient with an impaired capacity to concentrate the urine (Fig. 39-2).

LIMITATION IN POTASSIUM AND PHOSPHATE EXCRETION

The renal excretion of these solutes is discussed below and in Chap. 5. As noted above, serum potassium levels remain close to normal in CRF, yet life-threatening hyperkalemia may result from a potassium load that could otherwise be excreted without difficulty by a normal kidney. Hyperphosphatemia tends to develop as GFR falls to below 25 percent of normal and may become exaggerated if the patient is faced with a sudden phosphate load.

HOMEOSTASIS OF SPECIFIC SOLUTES IN CHRONIC RENAL FAILURE

SODIUM

INTRACELLULAR FLUID SPACE

The ionic composition of the intracellular fluid compartment is altered in end stage renal disease (ESRD). The sodium content of erythrocytes is increased, the potassium content is decreased, and there is a decreased activity of ouabain-sensitive Na^+K^+ATPase.[12,13] The actual number of Na,K pumps on erythrocytes is reduced in CRF,[14-16] a finding that is reversed by hemodialysis and transplantation. These uremic defects have also been described in other cell types including leukocytes, neurons, and skeletal muscle.[17,18] It has been suggested that these widespread abnormalities in membrane transport may underlie some of the unexplained clinical manifestations of uremia. It has also been suggested that a circulatory plasma factor responsible for the adaptive alterations in intrarenal sodium handling might also produce the intracellular abnormalities found in CRF.[19] No such factor has yet been convincingly demonstrated.

EXTRACELLULAR FLUID HOMEOSTASIS

As with the normal kidney, the maintenance of sodium homeostasis by the failing kidney serves to stabilize ECF volume. The numerical considerations related to the maintenance of sodium balance with a varying sodium intake are shown in Table 39-1. In Table 39-1 we see the quantitative aspects of sodium excretion at three levels of renal function and at two levels of dietary sodium intake. Note the "magnification" of percent Na^+ excreted ($FENa^+$) with falling renal function and increased so-

TABLE 39-1 • Magnification of sodium excretion with advancing renal failure

	Normal kidney	Moderate renal failure	Advanced renal failure
Sodium intake (meq)	120	120	120
GFR (ml/min)	120	30	5
GFR (liter/day)	173	43	7
Serum Na^+ (meq/liter)	140	140	140
Filtered Na^+ (meq/day)	24,192	6048	1008
Excreted Na^+ (meq/day)	120	120	120
% Na^+ excreted	**0.5**	**2.0**	**12**
Sodium intake (meq/day)	240	240	240
Excreted Na^+ (meq/day)	240	240	240
% Na^+ excreted	**1.0**	**4.0**	**24**

dium intake. At each step it is presumed that sodium balance is maintained. As described above, as renal failure advances the limits of sodium homeostasis become narrower.

The term *salt-losing* was coined to describe the fact that patients with advanced CRF were typically unable to reduce their daily urine sodium content to less than 30 to 40 meq daily. It was originally presumed that this phenomenon was a reflection of an intrinsic defect in tubular function. Danovitch et al.[20] showed that when the sodium intake of a group of patients with CRF was gradually reduced over weeks to months, the patients were, in fact, able to reduce their urinary sodium excretion to less than 10 meq daily and maintain balance on a sodium intake of as low as 5 meq daily (Fig. 39-3). These studies indicated that the salt-losing tendency was not an intrinsic tubular defect but rather a potentially reversible adaptive phenomenon. A "natural" experiment that supported these observations came in the form of a patient with CRF from polycystic kidney disease who had persistent gastrointestinal sodium losses from an ileostomy. His urine sodium excretion remained very low despite CRF. Since the bulk of his sodium excretion was extrarenal, his diseased kidney had not been required to develop an adaptive natriuresis in the remaining nephrons.[21]

REGULATION OF TUBULAR SODIUM EXCRETION IN CHRONIC RENAL FAILURE

Studies in experimental models of chronic renal disease suggest that despite wide variations in SNGFR there is remarkable consistency in glomerular-tubular balance. Thus, despite delivery to different nephrons of a highly variable amount of filtrate, a consistent percentage is reabsorbed by the proximal tubules, thereby stabilizing the delivery to the distal nephron where the final determination of sodium excretion takes place. Collecting duct reabsorption of sodium is markedly diminished in the remnant kidney and likely accounts for much of its increased fractional excretion.

HORMONAL CONTROL OF SODIUM EXCRETION IN UREMIA

It is unlikely that a single overriding hormonal mechanism accounts for sodium balance in CRF. Rather, it appears that balance is maintained, as in health, by integrating the effects of several hormones. Several studies have suggested that circulating natriuretic agents might be responsible for the increase in fractional sodium that is so typical of CRF.[22] Attempts at identifying a hormone unique to chronic renal failure, however, have been unsuccessful.

Atrial natriuretic factor (ANF) is an important modulator of sodium excretion in health and may have a role in the maintenance of sodium homeostasis in CRF. Plasma ANF levels are typically elevated in CRF[23,24] and respond to alteration in sodium balance. In both humans and experimental animals with renal impairment, restriction of sodium intake reduced ANF levels, saline infusions elevated them,[24] and infusions of ANF induced a natriuresis.[25] The latter observation suggests that ANF levels are not just passive reflections of volume status, since the hormone modifies sodium excretion.

Patients with CRF have elevated levels of *aldosterone,* though this hormone is probably more important with respect to potassium excretion in CRF (see below) than sodium excretion.[26] Sodium homeostasis can be maintained in adrenalectomized uremic animals with fixed or high levels of mineralocorticoid administration,[27] though spironolactone, a specific inhibitor of al-

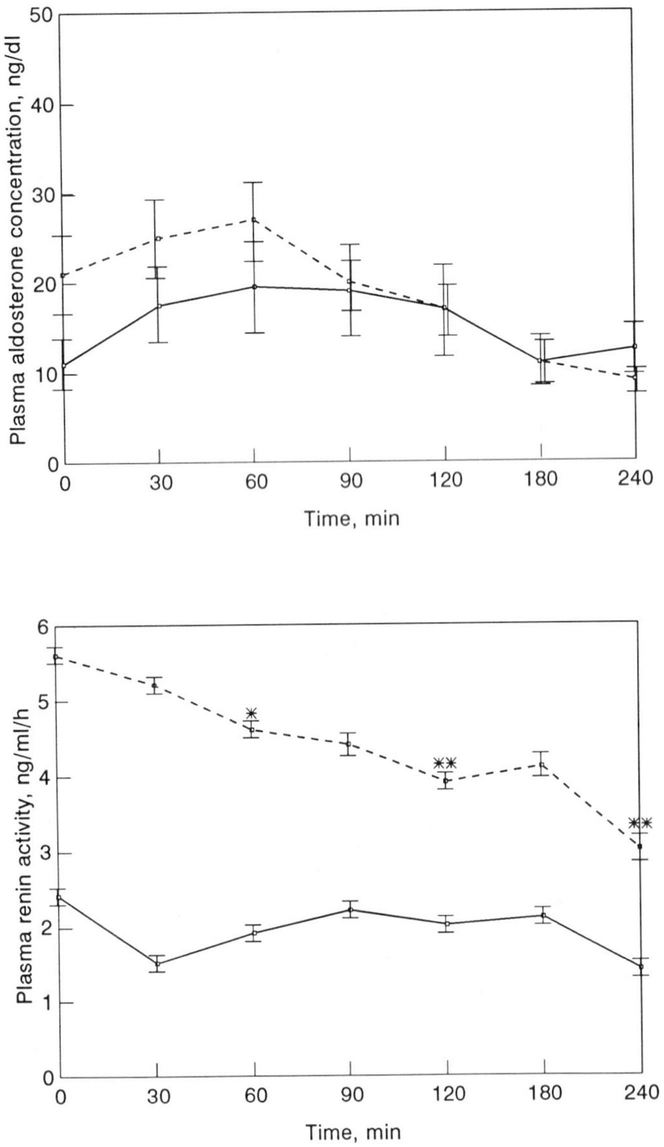

FIGURE 39-3 • Mean plasma aldosterone levels and plasma renin activity before (0 time) and after administration of KCl in control subjects (open circles, dashed lines) and patients (closed circles, uninterrupted lines). For plasma aldosterone (top panel) the asterisks denote changes significantly different ($P < 0.025$ or less) from baseline. There were no differences between the hourly values of patients and control subjects. For plasma renin activity the asterisks denote changes significantly different from baseline (*$P < 0.05$; ** $P < 0.005$). The differences between the two groups were statistically significant during the first 2 h after KCl ($P < 0.05$ or less). (Reprinted from Perez et al.[49])

dosterone, does induce a natriuresis in patients with CRF.

A consistent pattern of alteration of renin levels in CRF has been difficult to identify; moreover plasma *renin* levels may not reflect intrarenal activation of the renin-angiotensin system. Angiotensin converting enzyme (ACE) inhibitors may have important effects on glomerular hemodynamics in CRF, yet a clear-cut effect on sodium excretion has not been recognized.[26]

Norepinephrine levels tend to be elevated in CRF, although the cardiovascular sensitivity to the infused hormone may be less.[28] Epinephrine and dopamine levels are unchanged. The elevated norepinephrine levels may be a reflection of diminished autonomic function in CRF, but it is unclear if there is any significant role in sodium homeostasis.

In the normal kidney locally produced *prostaglandins* may have important effects on glomerular hemodynamics and sodium and water excretion. In CRF renal blood flow and GFR may become increasingly dependent on prostaglandin mediated vasodilation, an effect that is manifested clinically by the decline in these indexes when prostaglandin inhibitors are administered.[29]

POTASSIUM

The threat of potentially fatal degrees of hyperkalemia renders the regulation of serum potassium levels in CRF extremely important (see Chaps. 7 and 23). Since only about 1 to 2 percent of total body potassium resides in the ECF space,[30] small shifts in potassium from the ICF to ECF may result in significant hyperkalemia. Despite this, most patients initiating dialysis therapy for ESRD have normal potassium levels. Wallia et al. reviewed 70 ESRD patients about to receive their first dialysis and found serum potassium levels to be within normal limits despite differences in acid-base status.[1] These data indicate that despite severe renal failure, normal serum potassium levels can still be maintained. The critical adaptations responsible for this vital phenomenon are discussed below.

The factors that regulate the distribution of potassium between ICF and ECF have been well studied in subjects with normal renal function. *Acidosis,*[30–32] *high-potassium diets,*[33,34] *low aldosterone levels,*[35] *digoxin toxicity,*[36] *beta-adrenergic receptor blockade,*[37] and *hyperosmolality*[38] all may cause hyperkalemia. In addition, several systemic diseases have been associated with hyperkalemia in patients with CRF (see Table 39-2). Some of these include sickle cell disease,[39] systemic lupus erythematosus,[40] renal transplantation,[41] and obstructive uropathy.[42] Impairment of potassium secretion in *sickle cell disease* was first reported by De Fronzo et al.[39] These patients were shown to have diminished abilities to excrete potassium after its intravenous administration or in response to furosemide despite having normal GFRs and renal blood flow (RBF). In addition, they found an inability to increase potassium secretion after administration of sodium sulfate. These findings are consistent with a renal tubular potassium secretory defect. Hyperkalemia

TABLE 39-2 • Hyperkalemia in patients with impaired renal function

1. Systemic disorders
   - Sickle cell disease
   - Systemic lupus erythematosus
   - Following renal transplantation
   - Obstructive uropathy
   - Amyloidosis
2. Hereditary disorders
   - Pseudohypoaldosteronism type I
   - Pseudohypoaldosteronism type II
3. Hyporeninemic hypoaldosteronism
   - Diabetes mellitus
   - Mixed cryoglobulinemia
   - Analgesic nephropathy
   - Interstitial nephritis
4. Primary adrenal disease
   - Addison's disease
   - Acquired isolated aldosterone deficiency
   - Hereditary enzymatic defects
     - 3-B-0l-dehydrogenase deficiency
     - C-21 hydrolase deficiency
5. Increased potassium load
   - Rhabdomyolysis
   - Gastrointestinal bleeding
   - Tumorlysis syndrome
   - Hemolysis

in patients withi *systemic lupus erythematosus* (SLE) has been attributed to tubular dysfunction and impaired renin and aldosterone release in response to volume depletion. These defects can increase the likelihood of hyperkalemia after initiation of certain drugs that impair potassium secretion (Table 39-3). Recently, fludrocortisone (< 0.2 mg/day) has been reported to control hyperkalemia in these patients, apparently by overcoming the deficiencies in aldosterone release.[43]

The *renal transplant* patient is at significant risk to develop high potassium levels. Immediate postoperative management of these patients should include blood potassium levels assayed every 4 to 6 h. These patients can develop hyperkalemia from cyclosporin A, anesthetics, blood transfusions, and intravenous fluid that contains KCl. After stabilization of renal function, these patients may have episodes of hyperkalemia out of proportion to decreases in GFR, rejection, or acidosis.[44] Management includes the use of loop diuretics, a low-potassium diet, and avoidance of high cyclosporin A levels. Hyperkalemic *distal renal tubular acidosis* (type IV RTA) is the classic metabolic abnormality associated with obstructive uropathy.[45] This syndrome is also associated with Addison's disease, KCl administration, the use of potassium-sparing diuretics, prostaglandin inhibitors, and isolated aldosterone deficiency.[46,47] The etiology of the syndrome in patients with obstructive uropathy is poorly understood but may be related to defects in urinary acidification.

Patients with CRF are more likely to develop hyperkalemia than are normal individuals when exposed to conditions that cause ECF shifts of potassium or an increased potassium load. Hyperkalemia is obviated in patients with normal renal function by shifting potassium into cells and increasing renal excretion. Therefore, as GFR decreases, the ability of the body to eliminate potassium is impaired. On a normal potassium diet, hyperkalemia is rarely seen until the GFR < 5 to 10 ml/min (Table 39-4). When patients with impaired renal function (GFR < 20 ml/min) develop hyperkalemia, the clinician is obligated to review the case for secondary causes of hyperkalemia. Examples include acute renal failure, various medications (Table 39-3), and an increase in the daily potassium load (diet, gastrointestinal bleeding, rhabdomyolysis, hemolysis).

Once hyperkalemia develops, and the underlying cause is not established or reversed, patients can be managed with loop or thiazide diuretics and potassium exchange resins. Moderate elevations in serum potassium levels (4.5 to 5.5 meq/liter) can be monitored monthly. Potassium levels greater than 5.5 meq/liter should be

TABLE 39-3 • Hyperkalemia in CRF

Three major adaptations to prevent hyperkalemia	Causes of impaired adaptation
Cellular shift: ECF K^+ shifts to the ICF	FAVORS SHIFT OF K^+ TO ECF
	Acidosis
	Hyperosmolality
	Beta-adrenergic blockade
	Digitalis intoxication
	Succinylcholine
	Fluoride intoxication
	Arginine HCl
Increased fractional excretion of K^+ (FE_{K^+})	DECREASES FE_{K^+}
	Prostaglandin inhibitors
	ACE inhibitors
	Heparin
	Cyclosporine
	Spironolactone
	Triamterene
	Amiloride
Increased colonic K^+ secretion	DECREASES SECRETION
	Potassium load
	Digitalis intoxication
	Constipation

TABLE 39-4 • Clinical and biochemical data from patients with renal insufficiency and healthy control subjects

Patient No.	Diagnosis	Serum K (mmol/liter)	PAC* (nmol/liter)	CrCl† (ml/min)
1	Polycystic disease	4.0	0.07	13
2	Diabetes mellitus	5.8	0.10	11
3	Unknown	4.3	0.13	17
4	Glomerulonephritis	5.1	0.15	10
5	Glomerulonephritis	5.4	0.17	7
6	Nephrolithiasis	4.9	0.21	9
7	Analgesic nephropathy	5.0	0.24	30
8	Analgesic nephropathy	5.3	0.39	4
9	Reflux nephropathy	4.3	0.40	12
10	Analgesic nephropathy	4.7	0.53	7
11	Chronic pyelonephritis	4.2	0.94	6
Mean values		4.8 ± 0.6	0.23 ± 0.27	10 ± 6
Controls (mean values, n = 7)		4.1 ± 0.3	0.13 ± 0.07	120 ± 20

* PAC = plasma aldosterone concentration.
† CrCl = creatinine concentration.
SOURCE: Adapted from Hene et al.[54]

monitored closely, that is, at least twice monthly. Hyperkalemia is a serious problem even after patients with CRF start dialysis. The United States Renal Data System reported that 2.2 percent of all dialysis deaths in nonrenal transplant patients were caused by hyperkalemia.[48] Despite severe inability to excrete potassium, most renal patients do not develop hyperkalemia. The adaptive mechanisms that prevent hyperkalemia in chronic renal insufficiency will be discussed below.

PATHOGENESIS OF HYPERKALEMIA

In renal failure, the body protects itself from life-threatening hyperkalemia by *translocating potassium into cells, increasing the fractional urinary excretion of potassium, and increasing the colonic secretion of potassium* (Table 39-3). Impairment in these adaptive mechanisms results in hyperkalemia. The mechanisms underlying these adaptations are currently not well understood. Perez et al.[49] evaluated renal handling and plasma potassium and aldosterone response to an acute oral potassium load in patients with impaired renal function (GFR 32 ± 5 ml/min) and in patients with normal renal function (GFR 123 ± 5 ml/min). Before administration of a potassium load, the two groups had similar plasma potassium concentrations and abilities to excrete potassium in the urine. Following a potassium load, patients with impaired renal function had increments in plasma aldosterone levels that exceeded those of controls despite having significantly lower plasma renin activity (Fig. 39-3). Plasma potassium concentration and the amount of potassium translocated into the intracellular space were significantly higher in patients than in controls. The results of this study indicate that an impaired response to an oral potassium load in CRF is related to defects in renal rather than extrarenal adaptations.

Alvo et al.[50] studied the effect of simultaneous potassium and carbohyddrate loading in patients with CRF. They found that only 59 percent of the potassium load was translocated to the ICF space compared with 81 percent in the controls with normal renal function. Unlike the conclusions of Perez et al., Alvo et al. suggested that patients with CRF have impaired extrarenal handling of potassium. The reasons for the differences in results of these two studies are unclear, but it appears that there is impairment in both renal and extrarenal handling of potassium in patients with CRF.

CELLULAR SHIFT

Tzamaloukas et al.[51] found that most episodes of prehemodialysis hyperkalemia were associated with metabolic acidosis (T_{CO_2} < 15 mmol/liter), azotemia (BUN > 40 mmol/liter), and hyperglycemia (in diabetics). Half of the episodes of hyperkalemia were related to diet, and patients complying with low- potassium diets, even though they were anuric or taking drugs that predisposed to hyperkalemia, were not at increased risk for developing this chemical abnormality. Based on predialysis blood samples, only 10 percent of patients were found to develop severe hyperkalemia (K^+ > 6 meq/liter). Thus, most patients were able to overcome their metabolic abnormalities to maintain normal potassium levels. However, the data suggest that cellular shifts of potassium from acidosis and hyperglycemia are important factors in the development of hyperkalemia. This has been substantiated by studies that have shown that hyperkalemia is associated with low serum insulin levels and hyperglycemia.[52] Transcellular shifts of potassium are also regulated by beta-adrenergic activity. Beta-agonists stimulate cAMP-mediated activation of Na^+-K^+ ATPase that results in the movement of potassium from the ECF to ICF. Therefore, beta-blockers can cause hyperkalemia without impairment in renal function. Special attention should be given to patients receiving beta-blockers and digitalis. These patients are at increased risk of hyperkalemia from the ability of these drugs to block Na^+-K^+ ATPase activity further.

DECREASED FRACTIONAL EXCRETION OF POTASSIUM

Hyperkalemia in CRF has been associated with a variety of drugs that can reduce urinary potassium excretion. *Angiotensin converting enzyme (ACE)* inhibition in patients with hypertension and varying degrees of azotemia causes serum potassium levels to rise.[53] The increment correlates with the degree of azotemia. The rise in serum potassium levels results from the lowering of aldosterone levels due to ACE inhibition.

Hene et al.[54] have shown that plasma aldosterone concentrations are elevated in some patients with GFRs < 50 ml/min (Table 39-4). Other investigators[55] have demonstrated in the rat that an increase in aldosterone reactivity in animals is associated with an increase in fractional excretion of potassium after a potassium load. One of the protective mechanisms in preventing hyperkalemia in patients with a rising serum creatinine is an increase in the effectiveness of aldosterone. As the number of functional nephrons declines, compensatory changes take place in the remaining kidney that maintain potassium homeostasis. Examples include increasing potassium excretory capacity and increasing cortical and medullary Na^+-K^+ ATPase activity.[56] The net result is an increase in the fractional excretion of potassium per functioning nephron with the total daily excretion of potassium equaling the quantity absorbed from the diet (Fig. 39-4).

Diseases associated with low aldosterone levels or drugs that block the effect or release of aldosterone can impair renal excretion of potassium. *Aldosterone deficiency* can be the result of a primary adrenal disease, hyporeninemic hypoaldosteronism, or drugs. Addison's disease, isolated aldosterone deficiency, and hereditary enzymatic defects in the adrenal can be associated with hyperkalemia. Most patients with these disorders can maintain normal potassium levels if their diet is high in sodium and if they avoid volume depletion. Potassium excretion can be impaired in low-salt-intake states and hypovolemia because of decreased delivery of sodium to the distal tubule, the site of sodium-potassium exchange.

Hyporeninemic hypoaldosteronism is most commonly seen in patients with tubulointerstitial disease and diabetes mellitus. Adequate control of hyperkalemia and acidosis in these patients can be achieved by administration of mineralocorticoids and potassium-wasting diuretics. Drugs that can cause hypoaldosteronism and hyperkalemia include heparin, ACE inhibitors, cyclosporin A, and *prostaglandin synthesis inhibitors*. Heparin causes hypoaldosteronism by inhibiting the formation of aldosterone in the adrenal gland. ACE inhibitors block the formation of angiotensin II and therefore decrease the stimulatory effect this hormone has on the adrenal gland. Prostaglandin inhibitors and cyclosporin A decrease renal prostaglandin levels and thereby decrease the production of renin.

The evaluation of patients with hyperkalemia who are thought to have defects in potassium excretion can be accomplished by obtaining a 24-h urine for creatinine and potassium and by measuring plasma renin and aldosterone while the patient is upright. Urine potassium reflects oral intake. Patients ingesting high-potassium diets generally excrete 24-h urines that are rich in potassium. The fractional excretion of potassium can be calculated and will indicate whether the kidney's ability to excrete potassium is proportionate to the degree of renal insufficiency. A high fractional excretion of potassium should obtain in hyperkalemia. Finally, renin and

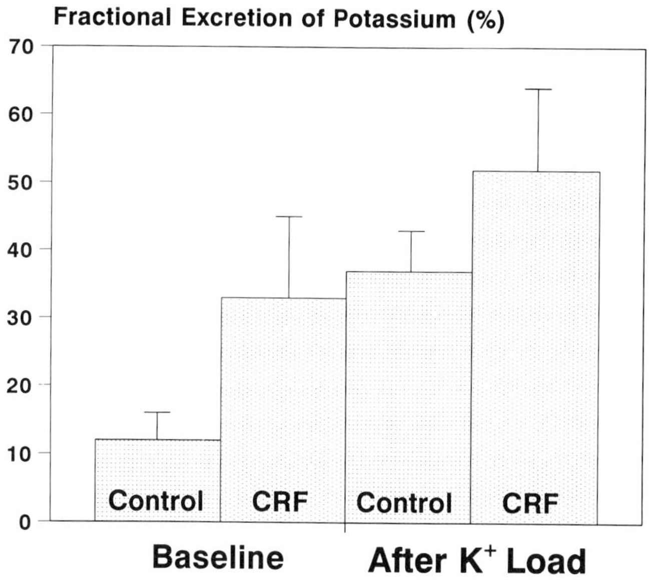

FIGURE 39-4 • Fractional excretion of potassium in patients with CRF following an oral potassium load. Compared with control patients, those patients with CRF have fractional excretions of potassium that are higher at baseline and following a load of potassium. (Adapted from Perez et al.[49])

aldosterone levels will be useful in evaluating hyperkalemic patients. A high renin but low aldosterone level suggests impaired release of aldosterone from the adrenal gland. A low renin and low aldosterone level suggests impaired release of renin from the kidney. An associated adrenal defect must also be present because hyperkalemia should directly stimulate aldosterone release (see Chap. 14). Both conditions can be associated with primary organ disease or drugs.

INCREASED COLONIC POTASSIUM SECRETION

Intestinal potassium excretion has been shown to increase in patients with CRF.[57,58] The fraction of dietary potassium recovered in feces can rise from 12 percent in patients without renal failure to 35 percent in patients with CRF. Data by Martin et al. suggest that augmented intestinal potassium excretion in patients with renal insufficiency is caused by net potassium secretion in the large intestine and not by significant decreases in intestinal potassium reabsorption. Enhanced potassium secretion by the colon may be inhibited by *constipation* and *Na^+-K^+ ATPase inhibition.* Constipation is common in CRF because of the use of large doses of phosphate binders taken by these patients. Constipation inhibits the elimination of the potassium that is secreted in the bowel. As a result, a protective mechanism is lost and serum potassium levels rise. Theoretically, digoxin toxicity could cause inhibition of Na^+-K^+ ATPase in the colon, resulting in a decreased exchange of sodium for potassium and consequently cause hyperkalemia.

CLINICAL MANIFESTATIONS

The clinical manifestations of hyperkalemia are the result of an increase in the ratio of extracellular to intracellular potassium. Cardiac and neuromuscular abnormalities are the two most important findings in a patient with hyperkalemia. When taking the history it is extremely important to probe for the following possibilities. Has the patient been exposed to hyperkalemia-producing medications? Has the patient suffered recent trauma? Key questions regarding pertinent endocrine deficiencies should be asked as well as any knowledge of personal or familial renal insufficiency. The physical examination may be remarkable for abnormalities in pulse and blood pressure. Careful attention should be directed to the neuromuscular examination because patients with hyperkalemia may have weakness, paralysis, fasciculations, myotonia, hyperreflexia, or aflexia.[59] Myalgias are not common. An EKG is crucial in the evaluation of the hyperkalemic patient. EKG changes consistent with hyperkalemia include peaked symmetrical T waves followed by prolongation of the PR interval and by eventual widening of the QRS complex. In severe hyperkalemia the rhythm may deteriorate to ventricular fibrillation. Rarely, the EKG can be normal in severe hyperkalemia.[60]

TREATMENT

Factors seen in CRF that promote the translocation of potassium from the ICF to the ECF include *acidosis, beta-adrenergic receptor antagonists,* and *lack of insulin.* Accordingly, various proposed treatments for hyperkalemia in this setting have included intravenous sodium bicarbonate, beta-adrenergic agonists, and insulin (Table 39-5). Blumberg et al.[61] studied the various effects that these therapeutic modalities have on the acute management of hyperkalemia in patients with CRF. They concluded that patients with renal failure undergoing chronic hemodialysis respond quickly and reliably to *insulin* and *glucose* given intravenously. Infused bicarbonate was ineffective and unreliable in lowering serum potassium quickly.

Albuterol is a beta-agonist than is often used as a bronchodilator. Because albuterol sulfate causes less cardiac irritation than the other agents used in the treatment of bronchospasm, it is the preferred bronchodilator in patients with cardiovascular disease. In a study by Montoliu et al.,[62] albuterol (0.5 mg given intravenously) was shown to increase cellular potassium uptake without significant side effects. Because albuterol can also be given via an aerosolized inhaler (2.5 to 5 mg in normal saline), this treatment can be initiated quickly and does not depend on vascular access.

Patients with mild hyperkalemia may be treated with *cation-exchange resins* that can be given either orally (20 g every 4 to 6 h) or rectally (50 g every 4 to 6 h). This method of treatment relies on the sodium and potassium pumps that exist in the colon. When these pumps are exposed to high concentrations of sodium, they exchange potassium for sodium, resulting in a large transfer of potassium ions into the bowel. When given orally, each gram of kayexalate removes 1 meq of potassium. Rectal administration removes 0.5 meq potassium per gram of kayexalate. These resins are usually given with substances such as sorbitol which will allow rapid expulsion of bowel contents. Potential problems with this type of medication include fluid overload from significant sodium absorption. Caution should obviously be taken when giving this medication to oliguric patients with a history of congestive heart failure. Enhanced urinary or stool excretion of potassium can be accomplished with fludrocortisone (0.1 to 0.2 mg/day), loop diuretics (40 to 60 mg/day or more as needed intravenously or by mouth) or sodium-potassium cation-exchange resins (30 to 50 g in sorbitol, given eveyr 3 to 4 h). Fludrocortisone and loop diuretics potentiate renal potassium excretion. Adjust-

TABLE 39-5 • **Treatment of hyperkalemia**

Treatment	Dose	Onset	Duration	Side effects
Insulin and glucose	10 units regular insulin (IV) + 10–20 g glucose (IV)	15–45 min	4–6 h	Hypoglycemia
Calcium gluconate	10 ml of 10% solution IV over 2–3 min	1–5 min	30 min	May exacerbate digitalis intoxication
Sodium bicarbonate	90–100 meq over 5 min IV	1–5 min	5–10 min	Alkalosis fluid overload
Kayexalate	Oral: 20 g with 20% sorbitol (50 ml) Rectal: 50 g with 20% sorbitol (200 ml) by retention enema	30–60 min	4–6 h	Salt and fluid overload
Furosemide	40–60 mg IV or orally	15–30 min	4 h	Hypotension, volume depletion
Fludrocortisone	0.1–0.2 mg/day	Hours	1–2 days	Sodium retention
Albuterol sulfate	0.5 mg IV or 2.5 mg inhaler	15–30 min	2–4 h	Tachycardia
Hemodialysis	Bath K^+ 0–2 meq/liter	Immediate		May exacerbate digitalis intoxication

ment in the dose of diuretics may be required in patients with decreasing creatinine clearances.

Rapid treatment of hyperkalemia in CRF may be accomplished with insulin and glucose. Five units of regular insulin are given with each 10 g of glucose. This regimen can be repeated every 15 min as indicated. Glucose and potassium levels should be measured hourly until severe hyperkalemia has resolved and EKG changes monitored closely. Albuterol sulfate (0.5 mg intravenously or 2.5 mg by aerosolized inhaler) can be given as needed or in situations when an intravenous access has not yet been established. Intravenous bicarbonate (90 meq given intravenously over 5 min) is less effective and may lead to significant alkalosis and fluid overload.

Life-threatening hyperkalemia ($K^+ > 6.5$ meq/liter) associated with arrhythmias should be treated immediately with intravenous calcium gluconate (10 to 30 ml of 10 percent solution). A repeat dose should be given in 5 to 10 min if there has been no improvement in EKG abnormalities. If severe hyperkalemia persists despite aggressive therapy, the patient should be considered for hemodialysis.

HYDROGEN ION

The kidneys are crucial for the preservation of normal acid-base homeostasis (see Chaps. 10 and 25). The daily production of 1 meq per kilogram of body weight of nonvolatile acids from endogenous catabolism is normally excreted in the urine.[63,64] Acid is excreted in the form of titratable acidity (primarily inorganic phosphate) and ammonium. Ammonia production is critically dependent on the mass of functioning renal tubular epithelial cells, and total production becomes inadequate as CRF progresses.

Hydrogen-ion secretion occurs in the proximal tubule predominantly by a sodium-hydrogen antiporter system that is electrically neutral. In addition, ammonium is secreted into the proximal tubular lumen, probably through the Na/NH_4 antiporter, and contributes most importantly to net acid excretion.[65] In the distal nephron hydrogen-ion secretion occurs down its electrochemical gradient. Reabsorption of filtered bicarbonate, dependent on proximal Na^+- H^+ exchange and carbonic anhydrase activity, is increased in patients with CRF. The latter increase is probably mediated by stimulated Na-H antiporter activity in this setting. Distal bicarbonate reabsorption is also mediated by hydrogen-ion secretion and carbonic anhydrase activity. The distal reclamation can result in a bicarbonate-free urine.[63,66,67]

The urine pH in patients with CRF is acid. Final acidification of the urine depends on distal hydrogen-ion secretion and the availability of titrable acids and ammonia. As the latter become scarcer as CRF progresses, urinary pH remains acid as free hydrogen-ion concentration remains constant or rises.

PATHOGENESIS OF METABOLIC ACIDOSIS

Metabolic acidosis occurs when the renal excretory mechanisms can no longer keep pace with daily acid

TABLE 39-6 • Pathogenesis of metabolic acidosis in CRF

Decreased buffer excretion
Reduced tubular NH_3 production
Reduced excretion of titratable acid
Decreased proton excretion
Increased bicarbonate excretion
Renal tubular acidosis (as a cause of CRF)
PTH effect
Extrarenal bicarbonate loss
Biliary or pancreatic fistula
Urinary diversions
Diarrhea
Increased acid generation
Dietary protein
Increased catabolism

production (Table 39-6). This generally occurs when the GFR falls to less than 30 percent of normal. A decrease in total kidney ammonia production is the most important contributor to this failed acid excretion, although a decrease in the excretion of other buffers, an impaired ability to secrete protons, and increased bicarbonate excretion may also play roles.

DECREASED BUFFER EXCRETION

Ammonia is the major urinary buffer required for the excretion of hydrogen ions. Ammoniagenesis occurs primarily in proximal tubular epithelium.[68] Once ammonia diffuses or ammonium is secreted into the proximal tubule it is delivered to the loop of Henle, where it is actively reabsorbed in the medullary thick ascending limb (MTAL). This transport process occurs by substitution of ammonium for potassium on the Na, K (2 Cl) cotransport system located on the apical surface of MTAL epithelial cells.[69] The efficacy of this process is enhanced by the low permeability of this nephron segment to NH_3, thus limiting the backflux of NH_3 into the tubular lumen.[70]

As a result of the active reabsorption of NH_4^+ by the MTAL, countercurrent multiplication of ammonium occurs, resulting in a corticomedullary concentration gradient for ammonium. The resulting high concentrations of ammonium in the medullary interstitium favor ammonium secretion into the collecting ducts (Fig. 39-5).

As CRF progresses, total renal ammonia synthesis falls, although the production per nephron unit is supernormal. Eventually absolute ammonia excretion falls sufficiently to decrease net acid excretion and leads to a decrease in serum bicarbonate concentration.[71,72] Tubulointerstitial renal diseases may also disrupt medullary ammonia trapping and further compound the metabolic acidosis.

In addition to ammonia, titratable acid excretion falls in far advanced CRF.[73] Decreased phosphate intake with restricted protein diets and the use of phosphate binding gels limit the amount of available buffer and thus contribute to the metabolic acidosis.

DECREASED URINARY PROTON CONCENTRATION

In the absence of renal tubular acidosis, patients with CRF are able to maximally lower urine pH. This has been documented with sodium sulfate infusions.[74] Reabsorption of sodium with exclusion of the nonresorbable anion sulfate results in luminal electronegativity, which, in turn, stimulates proton secretion. Patients with CRF acidify their urine after such a challenge to the same extent as normal controls.[75] The presence of renal tubular acidosis, not uncommon in CRF, may impair this ability, however, and should be considered in any patient with CRF and a urine pH > 5.5. It should be kept in mind, however, that solute diuresis and a high urine volume may also raise urinary pH.

INCREASED BICARBONATE EXCRETION

Several studies have shown that the tubular reabsorption of bicarbonate is increased when acute infusions of sodium bicarbonate are given to animals or patients with CRF. Clearly, volume expansion increases bicarbonate excretion in renal failure patients as in normal subjects.

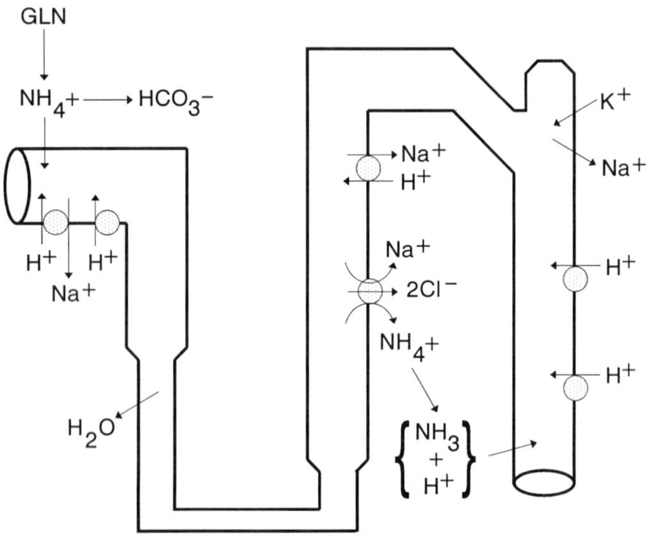

FIGURE 39-5 • Pathways of ammonium excretion. See text for explanation. (Reprinted with permission from Ref. 65.)

Studies by Arruda et al.[76,77] and Schmidt et al.[78] demonstrated that at high solute (Na, K, phosphate) excretion rates bicarbonate reabsorption is enhanced independent of volume status. Thus, an intrinsic adaptation of the renal tubule seems to occur in patients with CRF leading to enhanced bicarbonate reabsorption. Recent micropuncture studies suggest that this adaptation occurs in both proximal and distal nephron segments.[79]

Some patients with CRF, however, clearly waste bicarbonate in the urine. Lameire and Matthys studied 17 uremic patients with CRF with both NH_4Cl and intravenous bicarbonate loading tests.[80] They showed that when mild acidosis is present in CRF patients, considerable bicarbonate wasting can occur. This bicarbonate loss is closely linked to urinary sodium losses and can be reversed by dietary salt restriction.

In addition to urinary sodium excretion, secondary hyperparathyroidism may also lead to enhanced renal bicarbonate excretion.[81–83] Transient and mild hyperchloremic metabolic acidosis occurs following acute PTH administration.[84] More prolonged administration has been reported to increase net acid excretion and lead to mild metabolic alkalosis.[85] No systematic change in acid-base status has been reported in patients with CRF following parathyroidectomy, although most such patients are generally already on dialysis. The precise role of hyperparathyroidism in renal acidosis remains to be clarified.

CLINICAL FEATURES

The acidosis of CRF is generally mild, with serum bicarbonate rarely falling below 15 meq/liter. Arterial pH is maintained at 7.25 to 7.35 unless intercurrent respiratory or diarrheal disease is present. Hyperchloremic acidosis with a normal anion gap was commonly considered typical of tubulointerstitial diseases, while advanced CRF was thought to be associated with an increased anion gap.[86] Widmer et al., however, showed that hyperchloremia was common at all stages of CRF and was independent of the etiology of CRF.[87] Although this study included a highly selected patient population, these findings have been confirmed by other investigators[88] in more carefully designed studies. Enia et al. studied 155 patients with CRF and found that hyperchloremia was common at all stages of CRF and in patients with tubulointerstitial diseases (45 percent) as well as those with chronic glomerulonephritis (39 percent). Those with hyperchloremia had more severe metabolic acidosis than those who were normochloremic.[88]

More recently, Hakim and Lazarus analyzed biochemical parameters in 911 patients with CRF followed for up to 7 years.[89] This study was retrospective but is the only one available that examined serial values in the same

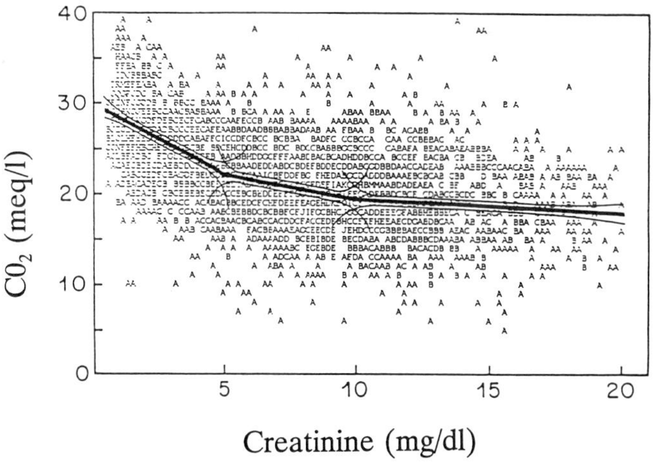

FIGURE 39-6 • The change in total Co_2 (meq/liter) as a function of the rising creatinine (mg/dl). The figure contains approximately 4000 data points. (A = one point, B = two points, C = three points, etc). The line is drawn from the slope of CO_2 vs. creatinine, for three ranges of creatinine: creatinine < 5 mg/dl, creatinine between 5 and 10 mg/dl, and creatinine > 10 mg/dl. The 95 percent confidence limit of the slope is shown around each line. (Reprinted with permission from Ref. 89.)

patients as CRF progressed. The rate of change of total CO_2 was -1.68 meq/liter for each 1 meq/liter rise in serum creatinine during early renal failure (Fig. 39-6). This rate decreased to -0.19 meq/liter in advanced renal failure. Chloride concentration rose during early renal failure and then steadily fell (Fig. 39-7). The anion gap therefore tended to remain normal in early renal failure and to widen as renal failure progressed, in keeping with earlier studies (Fig. 39-8). In addition, a higher serum phosphate, in patients with advanced renal failure, was associated with a lower total CO_2, possibly reflecting the

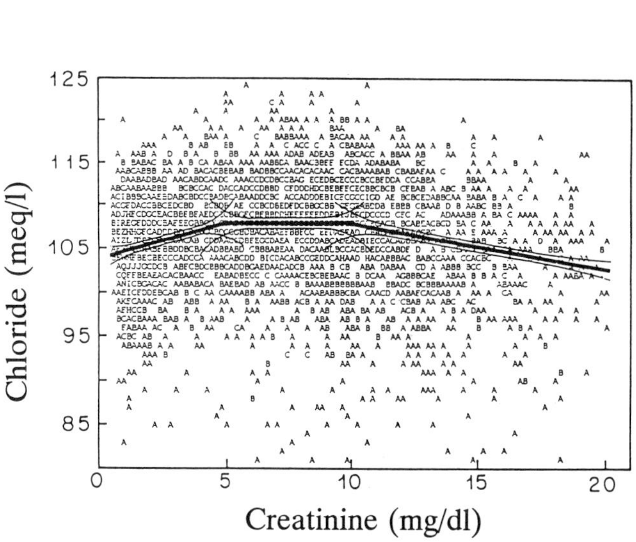

FIGURE 39-7 • The change of chloride concentration (meq/liter) as a function of the rising serum creatinine (mg/dl) level. Other notations are similar to Fig. 39-6. (Reprinted with permission from Ref. 89.)

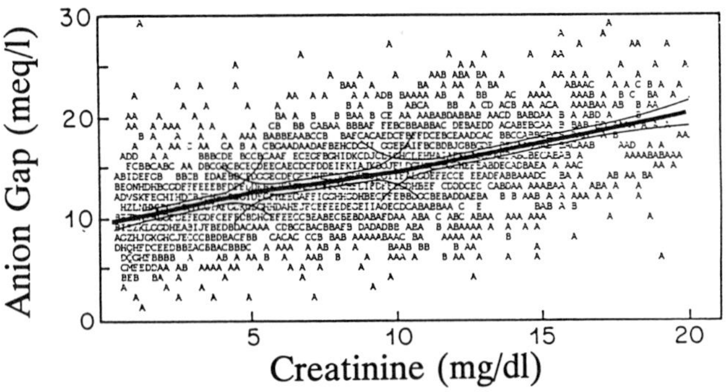

FIGURE 39-8 • Calculated anion gap [(Na^+ − (Cl^- + HCO_3^-)] meq/liter as a function of creatinine (mg/dl). Note that the slope is positive throughout the range of creatinine levels. Other notations are similar to Fig. 39-6. (Reprinted with permission from Ref. 89.)

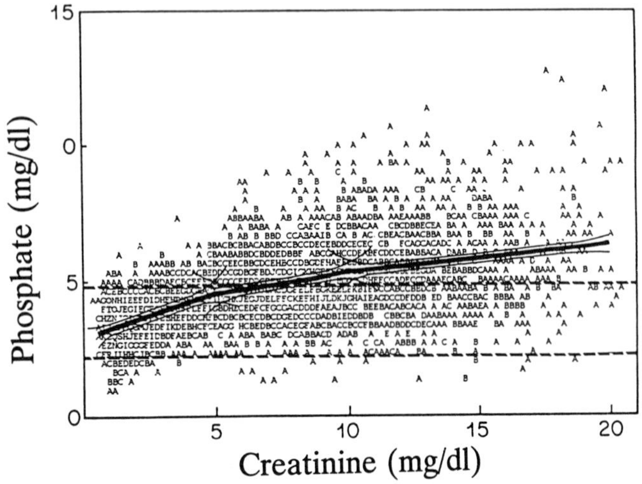

FIGURE 39-9 • The change in inorganic phosphate (mg/dl) as a function of the serum creatinine (mg/dl) concentration. The dotted line is the range of normal values for phosphate. Other notations are similar to Fig. 39-6. (Reprinted with permission from Ref. 89.)

effects of hyperparathyroidism on bicarbonate excretion (Fig. 39-9).

Patients with CRF are in chronic positive proton balance. Since pH and bicarbonate remain stable, additional buffering must be occurring and is thought to take place in bone. Buffering of hydrogen ions by bone carbonate leads to calcium loss from bone, hyperphosphatemia, and osteopenia.[90,91] The precise contribution of uremic acidosis to uremic osteodystrophy, however, remains unclear. Studies describing this relationship have been complicated by the presence of renal tubular acidosis or poor documentation of the histological improvement after alkali replacement. In addition, most current data relate to the effect of mineral acidosis on bone. The acidosis of CRF is more complex, however, with an important contribution not only of sulfuric and phosphoric acid retention but also their resultant impact on PTH secretion and bone metabolism.[91] Additional effects of the acidosis of CRF on bone include a reduction in GI calcium absorption[92] and a release of bone phosphate, both potentially aggravating secondary hyperparathyroidism. Although metabolic acidosis has been reported to suppress 1-alpha hydroxylase activity and thus 1, 25,$(OH)_2$vitamin D production,[93,94] The experimental designs used may have confounded the results. More recent studies[95] in patients have not confirmed these findings.

Other clinical consequences of chronic metabolic acidosis include reduced respiratory reserve with chronic hyperventilation and exhaustion of body buffer stores. Both of these phenomena could make the CRF patient with metabolic acidosis exquisitely sensitive to intercurrent illness—that is, to an additional cause of metabolic acidosis or to the development of respiratory disease. To avoid this, bicarbonate replacement therapy should be given to maintain serum bicarbonate at approximately 18 meq/liter or higher.

Finally, chronic metabolic acidosis may reduce Na^+-K^+ ATPase activity in red-blood cells and myocardial cells.[96,97] In the latter case this may lead to an alteration in the responsiveness of vascular smooth muscle as well as to a decrease in myocardial contractility.[98] Congestive heart failure in CRF patients may improve markedly with treatment of metabolic acidosis.

THERAPY

The goal of therapy is to improve the metabolic acidosis while minimizing the volume expansion associated with sodium bicarbonate administration. Although considerably less volume expansion occurs with sodium bicarbonate compared with sodium chloride, this is still an important concern.[99] Most patients require 50 to 100 meq of bicarbonate daily. This can be given as sodium citrate (Shohl's) solution (1 meq bicarbonate/ml) or as sodium bicarbonate tablets (1.2 g or 14 meq bicarbonate). Sodium citrate should not be used concomitant with aluminum-containing phosphate binders, since citrate markedly increases aluminum solubility and absorption.

Limiting dietary protein intake may also minimize acidosis. Approximately 1 meq of acid is generated per gram of dietary protein ingested independent of the source of protein. Modest protein restriction may therefore minimize the need for bicarbonate replacement.

Finally, avoidance of bicarbonate-wasting diuretics (e.g., acetazolamide) and prompt treatment of diarrhea with its accompanying GI bicarbonate loss should help to minimize bicarbonate replacement needs. If sodium retention does begin to occur and cannot be easily managed with diuretics, dialysis should be initiated.

REFERENCES

1. Wallia R et al: Serum electrolyte patterns in end stage renal disease. *Am J Kidney Dis* 8:98, 1986.
2. Mitch WE, Wilcox CS: Disorders of body fluids, sodium and potassium in chronic renal failure. *Am J Med* 72:536, 1982.
3. Platt R: Renal failure. *Lancet* 1:1239, 1951.
4. Platt R: Structural and functional adaptation in renal failure. *Br Med J* 1:1313, 1952.
5. Bricker NS et al: Renal function in chronic disease. *Medicine* 44:263, 1965.
6. Bricker NS et al: The pathologic physiology of chronic Bright's disease: An exposition of the intact nephron hypothesis. *Am J Med* 28:77, 1960.
7. Allison NEM et al: Pathophysiology of experimental glomerulonephritis in rats. *J Clin Invest* 53:1402, 1974.
8. Wen SF et al: Micropuncture studies of sodium transport in the remnant kidney of the dog. The effect of graded volume expansion. *J Clin Invest* 52:386, 1973.
9. Eknoyan G et al: Chronic tubulointerstitial nephritis: Correlation between structural and functional findings. *Kidney Int* 38:736, 1990.
10. Epstein M et al: Comparison of water immersion and saline infusion as a means of inducing volume expansion in man. *J Appl Physiol* 39:66, 1975.
11. Feinfeld D, Danovitch GM: Solute excretion and urine volume in chronic renal failure. *Am J Kidney Dis* 10:231, 1987.
12. Welt LG et al: An ion transport defect in erythrocytes from uremic patients. *Trans Assoc Am Physicians* 77:169, 1964.
13. Welt LG et al: Membrane transport defect: The sick cell. *Trans Assoc Am Physicians* 80:217, 1967.
14. Patrick J, Jones NF: Cell sodium, potassium and water in uremia and the effects of regular dialysis on the leukocyte. *Clin Sci Mol Med* 46:583, 1974.
15. Patrick J et al: Leukocyte potassium in uremia: Comparisons with erythrocyte potassium and total exchangeable potassium. *Clin Sci* 43:669, 1972.
16. Yoon YS et al: Erythrocyte sodium transport in dialized uremic patients. *Korean J Intern Med* 4:9, 1989.
17. Patrick J, Jones NF: Cell sodium, potassium and water in uremia and the effects of regular dialysis on the leukocyte. *Clin Sci Mol Med* 46:583, 1974.
18. Patrick J et al: Leukocyte potassium and in uremia: Comparison with etythrocyte potassium and total exchangeable potassium. *Clin Sci* 43:669, 1972.
19. Bricker NS: On the pathogenesis of the uremic state: An exposition of the "trade-off hypothesis." *N Engl J Med* 286:1093, 1972.
20. Danovitch GM et al: The reversibility of the "salt losing" tendency of chronic renal failure. *N Engl J Med* 296:14, 1977.
21. Danovitch GM et al: Absence of salt losing tendency in chronic renal failure. *Am J Nephrol* 1:173, 1981.
22. Bourgoignie JJ et al: A natriuretic factor in the serum of patients with chronic uremia. *J Clin Invest* 51:1514, 1972.
23. Woolf AS: Atrial natriuretic peptide and renal disease. *Neph Dial Transplant* 4:1008, 1989.
24. Smith S et al: Role of atrial natriuretic peptide in adaptation of sodium excretion with reduced renal mass. *J Clin Invest* 77:1395, 1986.
25. Woolf AS et al: The effect of low dose intravenous 99-126 atrial natriuretic factor in patients with chronic renal failure. *Postgrad Med J* 65:362, 1989.
26. Keane WF et al: Angiotensin converting enzyme inhibitors and progressive renal insufficiency. *Ann Intern Med* 111:503, 1989.
27. Slobody J et al: Acid-base, elctrolyte, urea and creatinine changes following nephrectomy after adrenalectomy and after infrarenal vena cava ligation in rats. *Acta Chir Scand* 140(7):551, 1974.
28. Schohn D et al: Norepinephrine related mechanism in hypertension accompanying renal failure. *Kidney Int* 28:814, 1985.
29. Niwa T et al: Urinary prostaglandin thromboxane in patients with chronic glomerulonephritis. *Nephron* 46:281, 1987.
30. De Fronzo RA et al: Clinical disorders of hyperkalemia. *Annu Rev Med* 33:521, 1982.
31. Malnic G et al: Potassium transport across renal distal tubules during acid-base disturbances. *Am J Physiol* 221:1192, 1971.
32. Boudry JF et al: The effect of lumen pH on potassium transport in renal cortical collecting tubules. *Am J Physiol* 230:239, 1976.
33. Adler S, Fraley DS: Potassium in intracellular pH. *Kidney Int* 11:433, 1977.
34. Lawson DH: Adverse reactions to potassium chloride. *Q J Med* 43:433, 1974.
35. Sopko JA, Freeman RM: Salt substitutes as a source of potassium. *JAMA* 238:608, 1977.
36. Don BR, Schambelan M: Hyperkalemia in acute glomerulonephritis due to transient hyporeninemic hypoaldosteronism. *Kidney Int* 38:1159, 1990.
37. Waal-Manning HJ: Metabolic effects of beta-adreno-receptor blockers. *Drugs II* 86(suppl):121, 1976.
38. Conte G et al: Acute increase in osmolality as a cause of hyperkalemia in patients with renal failure. *Kidney Int* 38:301, 1990.
39. DeFronzo RA et al: Impaired renal tubular potassium secretion in sickle cell disease. *Ann Intern Med* 90:310, 1979.
40. DeFronzo RA et al: Impaired renal tubular potassium secretion in systemic lupus erythematosus. *Ann Intern Med* 86:268, 1977.
41. Gyory AZ et al: Renal tubular acidosis, acidosis due to hyperkalemia, disordered citrate metabolism and other tubular dysfunction following human renal transplantation. *Q J Med* 38:231, 1969.
42. Batlle DC: Hyperkalemic distal tubular acidosis associated with obstructive uropathy. *N Engl J Med* 304:373, 1981.
43. Dreyling KW et al: Control of hyperkalemia with fludrocortisone in a patient with systemic lupus erythematosus. *Clin Neph* 33:179, 1990.
44. DeFronzo RA et al: Investigations into the mechanisms of hyperkalemia following renal transplantation. *Kidney Int* 11:357, 1977.
45. Batlle DC et al: Hyperkalemic distal renal tubular acidosis associated with obstructive uropathy. *N Engl J Med* 304:373, 1981.

46. Arruda JAL et al: Hyperkalemia (HK) in renal insufficiency (RI): Role of aldosterone deficiency and renal tubular dysfunction. *Clin Res* 27:624A (abs), 1979.
47. DeFronzo RA: Hyperkalemia and hyporeninemic hypoaldosteronism. *Kidney Int* 17:118, 1980.
48. United States Renal Data System's 1990 Annual Report. *Am J Kidney Dis* 26:S2, 44, 1990.
49. Perez GO et al: Blunted kaliuresis after an acute potassium load in patients with chronic renal failure. *Kidney Int* 24:656, 1983.
50. Alvo M et al: Effect of a simultaneous potassium and carbohydrate load on extrarenal K homeostasis in end stage renal failure. *Nephron* 53:133, 1989.
51. Tzamaloukas A, Avasthi PS: Temporal profile of serum potassium concentration in nondiabetic and diabetic outpatients on chronic dialysis. *Am J Nephrol* 7:101, 1987.
52. Gifford JD et al: Control of serum potassium during fasting in patients with end-stage renal disease. *Kidney Int* 35:90, 1989.
53. Textor SC et al: Hyperkalemia in azotemic patients during angiotensin-converting enzyme inhibition and aldosterone reduction with captopril. *Am J Med* 73:719, 1982.
54. Hene RJ et al: Effect of high-dose aldosterone infusions on renal electrolyte excretion in patients with renal insufficiency. *Am J Nephrol* 7:33, 1987.
55. Adam WR, Founder JW: Increased renal sensitivity to aldosterone in the rat: Induction by a high potassium diet. *Clin Exp Pharmacol Physiol* 4:283, 1977.
56. Schon DA et al: Mechanism of potassium excretion in renal insufficiency. *Am J Physiology* 227:1323, 1974.
57. Martin RS et al: Increased secretion of potassium in the rectum of humans with chronic renal failure. *Am J Kidney Dis* 8:105, 1986.
58. Sandle GI et al: Enhanced rectal potassium secretion in chronic renal insufficiency: Evidence for large intestinal potassium adaptation in man. *Clin Sci* 71:393, 1986.
59. Knochel JP: Neuromuscular manifestations of electrolyte disorders. *Am J Med* 72:521, 1982.
60. Szerlip HM et al: Profound hyperkalemia without electrocardiographic manifestations. *Am J Kidney Dis* 7:462, 1986.
61. Blumberg A et al: Effect of various therapeutic approaches on plasma potassium and major regulating factors in terminal renal failure. *Am J Med* 85:507, 1988.
62. Montoliu J et al: Potassium-lowering effect of albuterol for hyperkalemia in renal failure. *Arch Intern Med* 147:713, 1987.
63. Halperin M, Jungas R: Metabolic production and renal disposal of hydrogen ions. *Kidney Int* 24:709, 1983.
64. Arruda JAL: Acidosis of renal failure. *Semin Nephrol* 1:275, 1981.
65. DuBose TD et al: Ammonia transport in the kidney: New physiological concepts and their clinical implication. *J Am Soc Nephrol* 1:1193, 1991.
66. Cogan M et al: Acid-base disorders, in Brenner B, Rector F (eds): *The Kidney* 2d ed. Philadelphia, Saunders, 1981, p 841.
67. Warnock D, Rector F: Renal acidification mechanisms, in Brenner B, Rector F (eds): *The Kidney*, 2d ed. Philadelphia, Saunders, 1981, p 440.
68. Tannen RL: Ammonia and acid-base homeostasis. *Med Clin North Am* 67:781, 1983.
69. Garvin JL et al: Active NH_4^+ absorption by the thick ascending limb. *Am J Physiol* 255:F57, 1988.
70. Kikeri D: Cell membranes impermeable to NH_3. *Nature (Lond)* 339:478, 1989.
71. Welbourne T et al: The effect of glutamine administration on urinary ammonium excretion in normal subjects and in patients with renal disease. *J Clin Invest* 51:1852, 1972.
72. Schoolwerth A et al: Effects of nephron reduction and dietary protein content on renal ammoniagenesis in the rat. *Kidney Int* 7:397, 1975.
73. Simpson DP: Control of hydrogen ion homeostasis and renal acidosis. *Medicine* 50:503, 1971.
74. Seldin DW et al: The effect of Na_2SO_4 on urinary acidification in chronic renal disease. *J Lab Clin Med* 69:893, 1967.
75. Schwartz W et al: On the mechanism of acidosis in CRF. *J Clin Invest* 38:39, 1959.
76. Arruda JAL et al: Bicarbonate reabsorption in chronic renal failure. *Kidney Int* 9:481, 1976.
77. Arruda JAL et al: Bicarbonate reabsorption in chronic renal failure: Studies in man and rat. *Pflugers Arch* 376:193, 1978.
78. Schmidt RW et al: Bicarbonate reabsorption in the dog with experimental renal disease. *Kidney Int* 10:287, 1976.
79. Wong NLM et al: Tubular handling of bicarbonate in dogs with experimental renal failure. *Kidney Int* 25:912, 1984.
80. Lameire N, Matthys E: Influence of progressive salt restriction on urinary bicarbonate wasting in uremic acidosis. *Am J Kidney Dis* 8:151, 1986.
81. Crumb C et al: Effects of volume expansion, purified parathyroid extract and calcium on renal bicarbonate reabsorption in the dog. *J Clin Invest* 54:1287, 1974.
82. Karlinsky M et al: Effect of parathyroid hormone and cAMP on renal bicarbonate reabsorption. *Am J Physiol* 227:1226, 1974.
83. Bank N, Aynedjian H: A micropuncture study of the effect of parathyroid hormone on renal bicarbonate reabsorption. *J Clin Invest* 58:336, 1976.
84. Karlinsky ML et al: Effect of parathormone and cyclic adenosine monophosphate on renal bicarbonate reabsorption. *Am J Physiol* 227:1226, 1974.
85. Hulter HN, Peterson JC: Acid-base homeostasis during chronic PTH excess in humans. *Kidney Int* 28:187, 1985.
86. Simpson DP: Control of hydrogen ion homeostasis and renal acidosis. *Medicine* 50:503, 1971.
87. Widmer B et al: Serum electrolyte and acid-base composition. *Arch Intern Med* 139:1099, 1979.
88. Enia G et al: Hyperchloremia: A non-specific finding in chronic renal failure. *Nephron* 41:189, 1985.
89. Hakim RM, Lazarus JM: Biochemical parameters in chronic renal failure. *Am J Kidney Dis* 11:238, 1988.
90. Lemann J Jr et al: Effects of chronic acid loads in normal man: Further evidence for the participation of bone mineral in the defense against chronic metabolic acidosis. *J Clin Invest* 45:1608, 1966.
91. Green J, Kleeman CR: Role of bone in regulation of systemic acid-base balance. *Kidney Int* 39:9, 1991.
92. Greenberg A et al: Metabolic balance studies in primary

renal tubular acidosis: Effects of acidosis on external calcium and phosphorus balance. *J Pediatr* 69:610, 1966.
93. Lee SW et al: 25-hydroxycholecalciferol conversion impaired by systemic metabolic acidosis. *Science* 195:994, 1977.
94. Kawashima H et al: Metabolic acidosis suppresses 25-hydroxyvitamin D_3-1 hydroxylase in the rat kidney. *J Clin Invest* 70:135, 1982.
95. Kraut JA et al: Effect of chronic metabolic acidosis on vitamin D metabolism in humans. *Kidney Int* 24:644, 1983.
96. Levin M et al: The effects of chronic hypokalemia, hyponatremia and acid-base balance alteration on erythrocyte sodium transport. *Clin Sci* 43:251, 1972.
97. Brown R et al: The interactions of protons, calcium and potassium ions on cardiac purkinje fibres. *J Physiol* 282:345, 1978.
98. Mitchell J et al: The effects of acid-base disturbances on cardiovascular and pulmonary function. *Kidney Int* 1:375, 1972.
99. Husted FC et al: $NaHCO_3$ and NaCl tolerance in chronic renal failure. *J Clin Invest* 56:414, 1975.

CHAPTER • 40

Fluid and electrolyte complications of dialysis

Michael R. Rudnick • Jeffrey S. Berns • Raphael M. Cohen • Louis J. Riley, Jr.

In 1960, Quinton, Dillard, and Scribner described a technique that permitted prolonged cannulation of peripheral blood vessels, thereby allowing for extracorporeal circulation through an artificial kidney.[947] Previously, hemodialysis techniques were restricted to the therapy of acute, potentially reversible renal failure. The Quinton-Scribner arteriovenous shunt made repetitive maintenance hemodialysis feasible and the long-term treatment of irreversible renal insufficiency a reality.

The role of peritoneal dialysis in the treatment of irreversible renal insufficiency has evolved similarly. For many years, peritoneal dialysis was used solely to treat acute renal failure.[337,859] With the development of a permanent indwelling peritoneal catheter by Tenckhoff in 1968, peritoneal dialysis became an accepted alternative to hemodialysis for treating chronic renal insufficiency.[1139]

As a result of these and other developments, more than 110,000 patients in the United States who otherwise would have died from terminal renal failure are currently being maintained by one of the above-mentioned methods of dialysis (Table 40-1).[1171]

Maintenance dialysis, however, has not been without complications. Indeed, dialysis patients can develop treatment-related manifestations affecting virtually every organ system. Dialysis therapy requires not only substitution for impaired renal capacity to excrete metabolic waste products but also maintenance of body fluid, electrolyte, and acid-base homeostasis.

TABLE 40-1 • Distribution of end-stage renal disease patients in the United States treated by dialysis (December 31, 1988)

Treatment modality	No. of patients	Percent of total
Hemodialysis		
Center	83,410	75.6
Home	2,757	2.5
Center, self-assisted	1,125	1.0
Subtotal	87,292	79.1
Peritoneal dialysis		
CAPD	11,683	10.6
CCPD	907	0.8
Other	2,328	2.1
Subtotal	14,918	13.5
Unknown	8,043	7.3
Total	110,253	100

SOURCE: From U.S. Renal Data System: *USRDS 1990 Annual Report,* Bethesda, Md, National Institutes of Health, National Institute of Diabetes and Digestive and Kidney Diseases, 1990.

TRANSPORT PRINCIPLES OF DIALYSIS

Dialysis may be defined as the differential transfer of solutes and water through a passive porous membrane placed as a barrier between two solutions. More detailed discussions of the process may be found in several excellent reviews.[198,467,933,1031] The rate of transfer for any given solute is largely determined by its relative concentration in each solution. When these concentrations are equal, dialyzable solutes pass through the pores of the dialyzing membrane in both directions at equal rates, and there is no net transfer of the solute. The rate of net diffusion depends upon the magnitude of an established concentration gradient between the solutions. Diffusion is also influenced by the molecular radius of each solute particle in relation to the cross-sectional size of the pores in the membrane. In clinical dialyzing techniques in which one of the solutions is the patient's blood, the dialyzing membrane (an artificial membrane in hemodialysis or the peritoneum in peritoneal dialysis) must be selectively semipermeable; that is, it must have a pore size large enough to transmit potentially toxic solutes and electrolyte components of plasma water but small enough to be impermeable to serum proteins and other colloidal solutes, as well as the formed cellular components of the blood.

In contrast to solute transport, the movement of water between solutions separated by a semipermeable dialyzing membrane is effected by establishing either a *hydrostatic* (for hemodialysis) or an *osmotic* (for peritoneal dialysis) pressure gradient. These gradients result in *ultrafiltration*. Hydrostatic pressure gradients are established by the application of positive pressure on the blood compartment of the membrane and/or negative pressure on the dialysis solution compartment. Osmotic pressure gradients are established by the addition of dextrose to the dialysis solution. *Solvent drag* refers to the carriage of solute with ultrafiltered water, a process formally termed *convective transport*. These aspects of dialysis transport are illustrated in Fig. 40-1.

If uremic blood represents one of the solutions, the other solution, known as the *dialysate*, can be specifically designed to correct abnormalities in the concentration of toxic diffusible molecules in the uremic patient's blood. Urea, phosphate, potassium, uric acid, creatinine, and other solutes diffuse from the uremic plasma, where they are present in high concentrations, across the dialyzing membrane into the dialysate, which is free of these solutes, thereby maximizing the blood-dialysate concentration gradient. The electrolyte composition of dialysate is designed to approximate that of normal serum, thereby allowing diffusion to correct any marked abnormalities in the concentration of blood electrolytes. Water flux (ultrafiltration) can be regulated by controlling either hydrostatic or osmotic gradients. Ultrafiltration also augments solute removal by solvent drag (convective transport) and in some dialysis systems (e.g., continuous arteriovenous hemofiltration, discussed below) is the primary transport mechanism for solute removal.

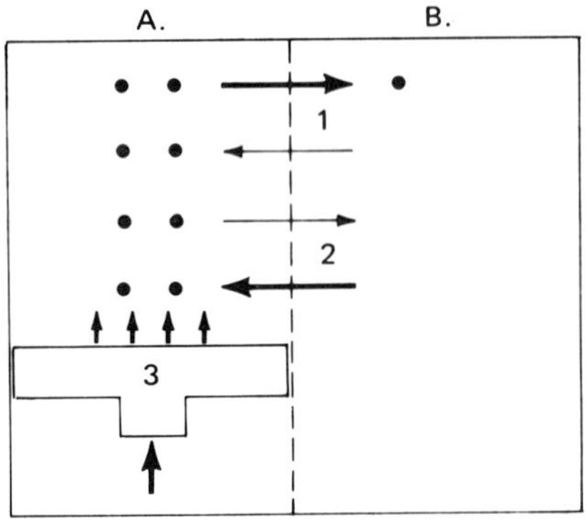

FIGURE 40-1 • Diagrammatic representation of two solutions separated by a porous semipermeable membrane into two compartments. The transport processes of diffusion, osmosis, and ultrafiltration are shown. (*1*) In diffusion there is a net movement of permeable solute (black dots) from the solution of high solute concentration (compartment A) to the one of lower solute concentration (compartment B). (*2*) In osmosis, the transmembrane movement of water occurs from the solution with lower solute concentration or osmolality (compartment B) to the solution with higher solute concentration or osmolality (compartment A). (*3*) Water and solute movement across the semipermeable membrane may also occur by ultrafiltration, the application of external hydrostatic forces to one solution (compartment A); the hydrostatic pressure "squeezes" water and solute through the pores in the membrane into the other solution (compartment B).

In order to draw up a rational "dialysis prescription" for the patient with end-stage renal disease (ESRD) or to meaningfully evaluate and compare various dialysis membranes and systems, it is necessary to quantify the net effects of diffusion, convection, and ultrafiltration on solute and water removal during dialysis.[467] Wolf suggested the term *dialysance* to evaluate hemodialyzer performance.[1256] He defined dialysance as the "*minute rate of net exchange of a substance between blood and bath fluid per unit blood-bath concentration gradient.*"[467,1256] The mathematical expression of dialysance is

$$\text{Dialysance} = \frac{Q_B(C_{Bi} - C_{Bo})}{(C_{Bi} - C_{Di})} \quad (1)$$

where Q_B = blood flow rate through hemodialyzer
C_{Bi} = concentration of solute in blood entering hemodialyzer
C_{Bo} = concentration of solute in blood leaving hemodialyzer
C_{Di} = concentration of solute in dialysis fluid entering hemodialyzer

The term $Q_B(C_{Bi} - C_{Bo})$ is a measure of the *mass transfer rate* for the solute, that is, the absolute amount of solute removed from the blood in a given period of time. The term $(C_{Bi} - C_{Di})$ expresses the concentration gradient for the solute between incoming blood and dialysate. In early systems, dialysis solution was recirculated at high flow rates around and through coil-designed dialyzers; this process is the basis of the *recirculated single-pass (RSP) system*. The inclusion of the term C_{Di} in the dialysance formula was necessary because solute extracted by the recirculated system rapidly accumulates in the recirculating reservoir, affecting the gradient across the dialysis membrane. Newer hemodialysis systems operate under a *single-pass system*; the dialysis solution entering the dialyzer is always fresh, thus ensuring maximal solute concentration gradients. In this situation, $C_{Di} = 0$, and the dialysance expression can be rewritten as[467]

$$\text{Dialysance} = \frac{Q_B(C_{Bi} - C_{Bo})}{C_{Bi}} \quad (2)$$

Equation 2 is similar to the clearance formula used to express the functional capacity of the human kidney for the excretion of any given solute:[467]

$$\text{Clearance} = \frac{UV}{P} \tag{3}$$

where U = concentration of solute in excreted urine
V = amount of urine excreted per unit time
P = serum concentration of solute

In these equations, the terms $Q_B(C_{Bi} - C_{Bo})$ and UV represent the total amount of solute removed by the hemodialyzer or kidney per unit time: the mass transfer rate. Because of these similarities, the term *clearance* is often applied instead of *dialysance* for hemodialyzer transport when the system used has $C_{Di} = 0$ (i.e., for a single pass system).

Dialysance and clearance formulas are practical; they consider, however, only the factors of blood flow, mass transfer rates, and concentration gradients. They do not take into consideration a variety of other factors that modify hemodialyzer performance, such as dialyzer membrane properties, functional surface area, and blood and dialysate flow characteristics.[198,467,1031]

The rate of removal of excess water, the *ultrafiltration rate*, can also be quantified. The ultrafiltration rate, Q_F (in milliliters per hour) for any given dialyzer can be expressed as[1031]

$$Q_F = K_{UF}(P_{\overline{M}}) \tag{4}$$

where K_{UF} = dialyzer ultrafiltration coefficient (ml/h per mmHg)
$P_{\overline{M}}$ = mean transmembrane hydraulic pressure gradient (mmHg)

The *ultrafiltration coefficient* (K_{UF}) is a function of the dialyzer membrane hydraulic permeability and functional surface area. The *mean hydraulic pressure gradient* is the difference between the hydrostatic pressure in the blood compartmetn (P_B) and the hydrostatic pressure in the dialysate compartment (P_D) (i.e., $P_{\overline{M}} = P_B - P_D$). Normally, the minimum hydrostatic pressure in the blood compartment is determined by the blood flow rate and the total resistance to blood flow through the hemodialysis circuit.[409] Usually the area of greatest resistance is at the site where blood is returned to the patient (venous segment of the angioaccess). To increase P_B, and hence ultrafiltration, the venous blood line can be partially clamped. Alternatively, the transmembrane pressure gradient ($P_{\overline{M}}$) can be increased by applying negative hydrostatic pressure to the dialysate compartment. *To determine the transmembrane pressure gradient needed for any given hemodialysis treatment*, the required ultrafiltration rate, Q_F (milliliters per hour) is first determined by dividing the total amount of fluid that is to be removed during the dialysis treatment (milliliters) by the duration of the dialysis treatment (hours). Once Q_F is determined, and since K_{UF} is known for the particular dialyzer being used, the amount of transmembrane pressure ($P_{\overline{M}}$) needed for the desired ultrafiltration rate can be calculated according to equation 4.

The same clearance concepts used to quantitate the efficacy of hemodialysis are also applicable to *peritoneal dialysis*:[467]

$$\text{Clearance} = \frac{C_D Q_D}{C_P} \tag{5}$$

where C_D = concentration of solute in the drained dialysis fluid (mg/ml)
Q_D = volume of peritoneal dialysis fluid per exchange (ml/min)
C_P = plasma solute concentration (mg/ml, measured at midpoint of exchange)

It should be understood that this calculation of peritoneal clearance is an average determination for the entire exchange period; it does not provide an exact clearance determination for any given time period during the exchange.[467]

HEMODIALYSIS

PRINCIPLES, SYSTEM, AND TECHNIQUE

Blood is removed from the patient's circulation (through the arterial line) with the assistance of a blood pump and enters the *hemodialyzer*, which contains the semipermeable membrane (Fig. 40-2).[564,567] Continuous or intermittent infusion of heparin into the arterial line is used to sustain anticoagulation. In high-risk patients, protamine can be administered into the venous line to reverse the anticoagulant effect of heparin (*regional heparinization*). However, use of *low-dose heparin or heparin-free dialysis* appears to be at least as effective in preventing clotting of the extracorporeal circuit and in minimizing hemorrhagic complications.[168,663,1054,1131] Low–molecular weight heparin may offer some advantages in terms of reduced risk of bleeding[72,496] but is not generally available. Regional anticoagulation using *sodium citrate* also avoids systemic anticoagulation.[340,670,926] Sodium citrate is infused into the arterial line while using calcium-free dialysate. Calcium chloride is infused into the venous line to reverse the anticoagulant effect and to restore the plasma calcium concentration. Metabolic alkalosis, hypercalcemia, hypocalcemia, need for increased volume removal during dialysis (due to the additional volumes of the citrate and calcium infusions), hypernatremia, and excessive circulating citrate may complicate this procedure.[555,670,926,1091,1205]

In order to prevent air embolism, a bubble trap in the venous line captures any air that may have come out of

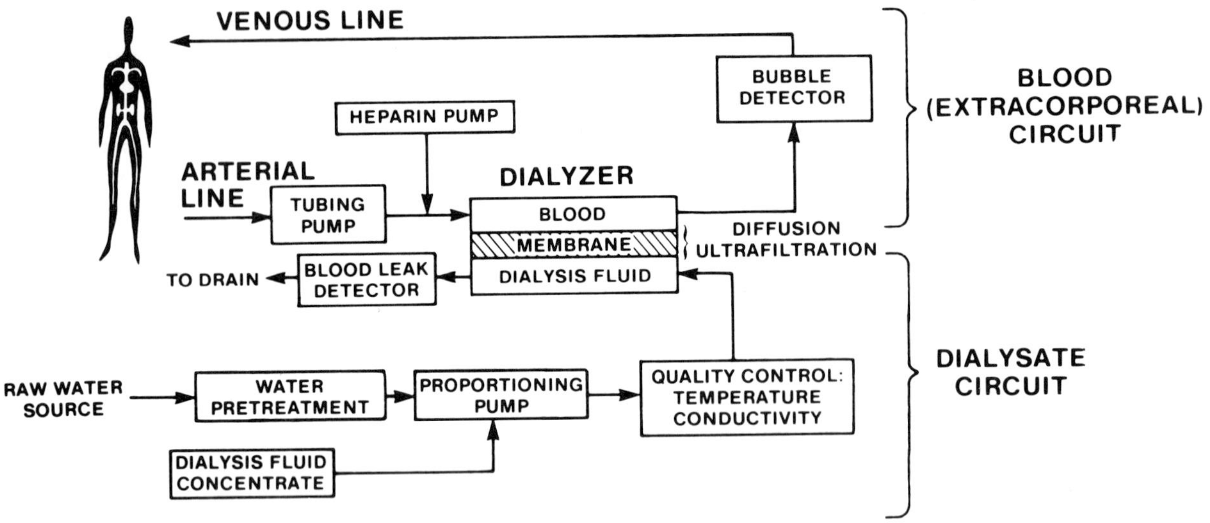

FIGURE 40-2 • Major components of a standard hemodialysis system. (From Colton CK, Lowrie EG, in Brenner BM, Rector FC Jr, eds: *The Kidney*, 2d ed, Philadelphia, Saunders, 1981. Used by permission.)

the blood as it passed through the hemodialyzer. An air sensor detects bubbles or foam in the blood. Pressures are monitored in both the arterial and venous limbs of the blood circuit. Blood flow rates through the extracorporeal circuit approximate 225 to 350 ml/min for conventional hemodialysis but may exceed 400 to 500 ml/min with *high-flux* or *high-efficiency dialysis* (see "Dialysis Membranes and Dialyzers").

Dialysis solution (dialysate) flows through the hemodialyzer at a rate of approximately 500 ml/min for conventional hemodialysis and 700 to 1000 ml/min for high-flux and high-efficiency dialysis in a countercurrent direction to blood flow. The dialysis solution for the entire treatment can be prepared at the outset by mixing a concentrated dialysis solution with water in a large tank (*batch system*). Much more commonly, a *proportioning system* is used whereby concentrated dialysate solution is continuously mixed by a proportioning pump with water, in a ratio of 1:35, to create dialysate with the required electrolyte composition.[420] Untreated tap water may be used for either system, but more commonly, unwanted and potentially dangerous particulate matter, organic material, minerals, electrolytes, and endotoxins are removed prior to the final preparation of the dialysate.[565] Before it enters the hemodialyzer, the final mixed dialysate solution is monitored for temperature and proper electrolyte concentration (conductivity). After passing through the hemodialyzer, the now "soiled" dialysis solution is generally discarded (single-pass system), although a portion of it may be recirculated again through the hemodialyzer (RSP system). The dialysate effluent is monitored for the presence of blood by a photoelectric cell to ensure early detection of any ruptures in the hemodialyzer membrane.

WATER PURIFICATION SYSTEM

During the early experience with hemodialysis, untreated tap water was used in the preparation of the dialysis solution. However, the close physical relationship between the patient's blood and dialysate, separated by only a thin semipermeable membrane, and the large quantities of dialysate required for the hemodialysis treatment (about 400 to 600 liters/week) create the potential for both immediate and long-term adverse effects from contaminants, microbial pathogens, and toxins present in the water used to prepare the dialysis solution.[565] In an effort to minimize or prevent such adverse effects, the Association for the Advancement of Medical Instrumentation (AAMI) has developed standards that define the maximal allowable concentrations permissible for contaminants in such water (Table 40-2).[59]

A variety of pretreatment methods are currently employed to remove contaminants from tap water used for hemodialysis.[565] The type of water pretreatment system selected depends on the specific contaminants found in the facility's regional water, the type of hemodialysis system used, and economic considerations. A brief description of the components commonly used in water pretreatment systems follows.[565,570,1199]

Sediment filters, with pore sizes ranging between 1 and 5 μm, remove particulate matter that can damage other dialysis water treatment equipment. Microbial contamination of sediment filters necessitates regular disinfection to avoid pyrogenic reactions. *Carbon filters* consisting of granular activated charcoal provide a high absorptive capacity for removal of chlorine, chloramines, pyrogens, and other organic materials. Chloramines, which are often used instead of chlorine as bactericidal

TABLE 40-2 • AAMI standards for hemodialysis water quality

Contaminants	Maximum allowable concentration, mg/liter
DESCRIBED IN HEMODIALYSIS LITERATURE	
Fluroide	0.2
Chlorine	0.5
Chloramine	0.1
Nitrate (N)	2
Sulfate	100
Copper	0.1
Zinc	0.1
Aluminum	0.01
NORMALLY INCLUDED IN DIALYSIS*	
Calcium	2 (0.1)
Magnesium	4 (0.3)
Sodium†	70 (3.0)
Potassium	8 (0.2)
DESCRIBED IN DRINKING WATER LITERATURE AND SUBJECT TO EPA REGULATION	
Arsenic	0.005
Lead	0.005
Silver	0.005
Barium	0.1
Cadmium	0.001
Chromium	0.014
Selenium	0.09
Mercury	0.0002

* Numbers in parentheses are activities in meq/liter.

† 230 mg/liter (10 meq/liter) where sodium concentration in dialysate concentrate has been reduced to compensate for excess sodium in water, provided conductivity of the water is continuously monitored.

SOURCE: *American National Standard for Hemodialysis Systems,* Arlington, Va, 1981, p 3, and Keshaviah P and Luehmann DA: Overview of the FDA contract report: Investigation of the risks and hazards associated with hemodialysis devices, in *Issues in Hemodialysis,* Arlington, Va, Association for the Advancement of Medical Instrumentation, 1981, p 8. Used by permission.

agents in municipal water supplies, can cause hemolysis and methemoglobinemia in hemodialysis patients if present in even relatively low levels in dialysate. The importance of adequate carbon filtration is highlighted by a recent episode in which over 40 percent of patients in one hemodialysis center experienced transfusion-requiring hemolytic anemia due to chloramine exposure when the center increased the capacity of its water treatment system without making necessary changes in the carbon filter system.[39,756,1145,1199] It is recommended that at least two activated carbon filters in series be used in hemodialysis water treatment systems.[59,124,295,589,1199,1266] Inadequate removal of sodium hydroxide used to regenerate carbon filters has been reported to result in dialysate of high pH and sodium content.[570] *Water softeners* are commonly used in geographic areas where the water is "hard" (i.e., of high mineral content). These devices are cationic resins that exchange sodium for calcium, magnesium, and other polyvalent cations present in the tap water.* Removal of these cations prevents scaling of reverse osmosis membranes in the water treatment system (see below), which would decrease their performance and life span.[348,565,1199] Failure to use a water softener or inadequate regeneration of the resin may also cause a constellation of clinical symptoms in the hemodialysis patient known as the *hard water syndrome* (see "Calcium," under "Hemodialysis Solutions").[282,354] Periodically, the exchange resin must be regenerated with brine (NaCl). Hypernatremia may occur if, during the regeneration procedure, brine is allowed to contaminate the treated water.[818] A bypass valve will prevent incoming water from entering the softener resin during brine regeneration and prevent this complication.

Deionizers are frequently used in water pretreatment systems to remove dissolved inorganic ions. Cations and anions in the tap water are exchanged for hydrogen and hydroxyl ions, which in turn combine to form water. This exchange process occurs in tanks containing cationic and anionic resins in either a single vessel (mixed bed) or separate vessels (dual bed). Continued operation of the deionizer after exhaustion of the anionic resin bed, which usually has an ion-exchange capacity less than that of the cationic resin, results in the production of highly acidic water from ongoing cation (H^+) release. The acidic water (with pH as low as 2.9) leaches copper from pipes and heating coils in the hemodialysis system, causing severe hemolysis, nausea, vomiting, diarrhea, and abdominal pain, which in some instances has been fatal.[294,519,725,743] To prevent this problem, copper piping and heating elements have been eliminated from hemodialysis systems.[570] Acidification of dialysate water also diminishes the anticoagulant effect of heparin, causing dialyzer clotting.[294,1055,1056] Deionizer exhaustion may also cause elution of large amounts of previously removed fluoride, which may contribute to osteomalacia.[532] Adverse events resulting from exhaustion of deionizer tanks can be prevented by careful monitoring of indicator lamps, which go out when water resistivity falls.[570] Carbon filtration before water enters the deionizer is necessary to prevent the possible formation of carcinogenic nitrosamines by the resin after contact with chlorine.[347,584]

Reverse osmosis, which removes 85 to 95 percent of dissolved ions, is one of the most popular and effective methods of pretreating dialysate tap water.[565,614] Partic-

* The amount of sodium exchanged can be determined from the following relationship: Na^+ (meq/liter) = $CaCO_3$ (mg/liter)/50.[200]

ulate matter, bacteria, pyrogens, and dissolved organic and inorganic solutes are also removed by reverse osmosis. This process subjects impure tap water on one side of a membrane to a hydrostatic pressure gradient that exceeds the opposing osmotic pressure gradient and pushes water across the membrane, leaving the contaminants behind. Water flow occurs in the direction opposite to that predicted by the osmotic gradient, hence the term reverse osmosis.

Additional problems may arise from contaminated dialysis water treatment systems. Leaching of zinc from galvanized iron water tanks or nickel from nickel-plated stainless steel water tanks may lead to hemolysis and cause various gastrointestinal symptoms.[363,922,1224] Contamination of water by nitrates can cause methemoglobinemia and hypotension.[163] Sulfate contamination has been reported to cause nausea, vomiting, and metabolic acidosis.[201] Inadequate rinsing after water treatment system disinfection with hydrogen peroxide may result in hemolysis.[405] Sodium azide contamination of a water treatment system has caused an epidemic of hypotension, headache, vomiting, blurry vision, and syncope in a hemodialysis unit.[39,406]

The recent development of synthetic hemodialyzer membranes with increased hydraulic and solute permeabilities has caused concern that water purity standards that were adequate for standard hemodialysis may be inadequate for *high-flux dialysis* treatments.[81,771] In 1989, nearly 25,000 patients were receiving high-flux or high-efficiency hemodialysis in the United States.[26] Although one recent nationwide survey found that patients treated with high-flux dialysis were at increased risk for dialysis-related pyrogenic reactions,[26] a study from the Centers for Disease Control did not find an increased risk for pyrogenic reactions in patients on high-flux or high-efficiency hemodialysis.[407] The reasons for this apparent discrepancy are unclear, but heightened attention to water quality, particularly regarding microbial and endotoxin contamination, is suggested for patients exposed to these highly permeable dialyzer membranes. Of concern has been a phenomenon termed *back filtration*, in which dialysate, driven by oncotic and hydrostatic pressure gradients, flows across these membranes into blood.[81,993,1043,1120] Use of strict water treatment system disinfection procedures and ultrafiltration methods, including microbial filters, should allow for the routine production of bacteriologically safe, pyrogen-free dialysate.[73,771,1020]

DIALYSIS MEMBRANES AND DIALYZERS

Hemodialysis requires the use of a semipermeable membrane, interposed between the dialysis solution and the patient's blood, to accommodate the transport processes of diffusion and ultrafiltration. The membranes initially used in clinical hemodialysis were composed of *cellophane*.[2,597,1141] Clinically suitable dialysis membranes must be nontoxic, easily manufactured, inexpensive, sterilizable, and resistant to tearing when handled or subjected to the pressures required for ultrafiltration. They must permit the effective movement of uremic solutes and water by differential diffusion and ultrafiltration. These criteria are adequately fulfilled by cellulose-based membranes (regenerated or modified cellulose, cellulose acetate, or saponified cellulose ester), which were being used for 80 percent of hemodialysis patients in a recent survey of hemodialysis facilities in the United States.[26] In recent years, synthetic dialyzer membranes have been manufactured of *polyacrylonitrile (PAN)*, *polysulfone*, *polycarbonate*, and *polymethylmethacrylate*.[75,892,944,1037,1092] Conventional cellulose-based hemodialyzers have in vitro ultrafiltration coefficients (K_{UF}) of about 3 to 6.5 ml/h per mmHg transmembrane pressure. The newer synthetic membranes are increasingly being used for high-efficiency dialysis (ultrafiltration coefficients of 8 to 19 ml/h per mmHg) or high-flux dialysis (ultrafiltration coefficients $\geq$ 20 ml/h per mmHg). Twenty percent of hemodialysis patients in the United States are being treated with these new membranes.[26] The high ultrafiltration coefficients of these synthetic membranes require use of hemodialysis systems capable of precise automatic ultrafiltration control to avoid excessively rapid fluid removal and hypotension.[494,593,727,798,1082]

Theoretically, the maximal achievable solute clearance in a hemodialysis system is equal to the blood flow rate. For any given blood flow rate in a system that maintains optimal solute concentration gradients, the major resistance to mass transfer of the solute is offered by the dialyzing membrane. Currently available clinical hemodialysis systems approach the attainment of maximal blood-dialysate concentration gradients (e.g., single-pass dialysate flow systems). Therefore, the failure to obtain optimal clearance is related primarily to features of dialyzer design and properties of the dialyzer membrane.

Currently there are two hemodialyzer designs in widespread use: *flat plates* (or parallel plates) and *hollow fibers*.[198,494] Coil dialyzers and nondisposable flat-plate dialyzers are rarely, if ever, used any longer. Figure 40-3 depicts these hemodialyzer designs with their blood and dialysate pathways.[198] The total membrane area of various clinical hemodialyzers varies from approximately 0.76 m^2 to 2.5 m^2, comparing favorably with the estimated 0.76 m^2 filtering area of the human kidney. Not all of the membrane area is effective dialyzing area, however, because there may be areas of dead space with poor blood and/or dialysate flow. By proper choice of channel geometry and membrane-supporting structures, such dead space can be minimized, and optimal blood film thickness can be approached.[494]

Resistance to the passage of solute and water is dependent upon the membrane's thickness and pore size, as well as other physicochemical features related to the

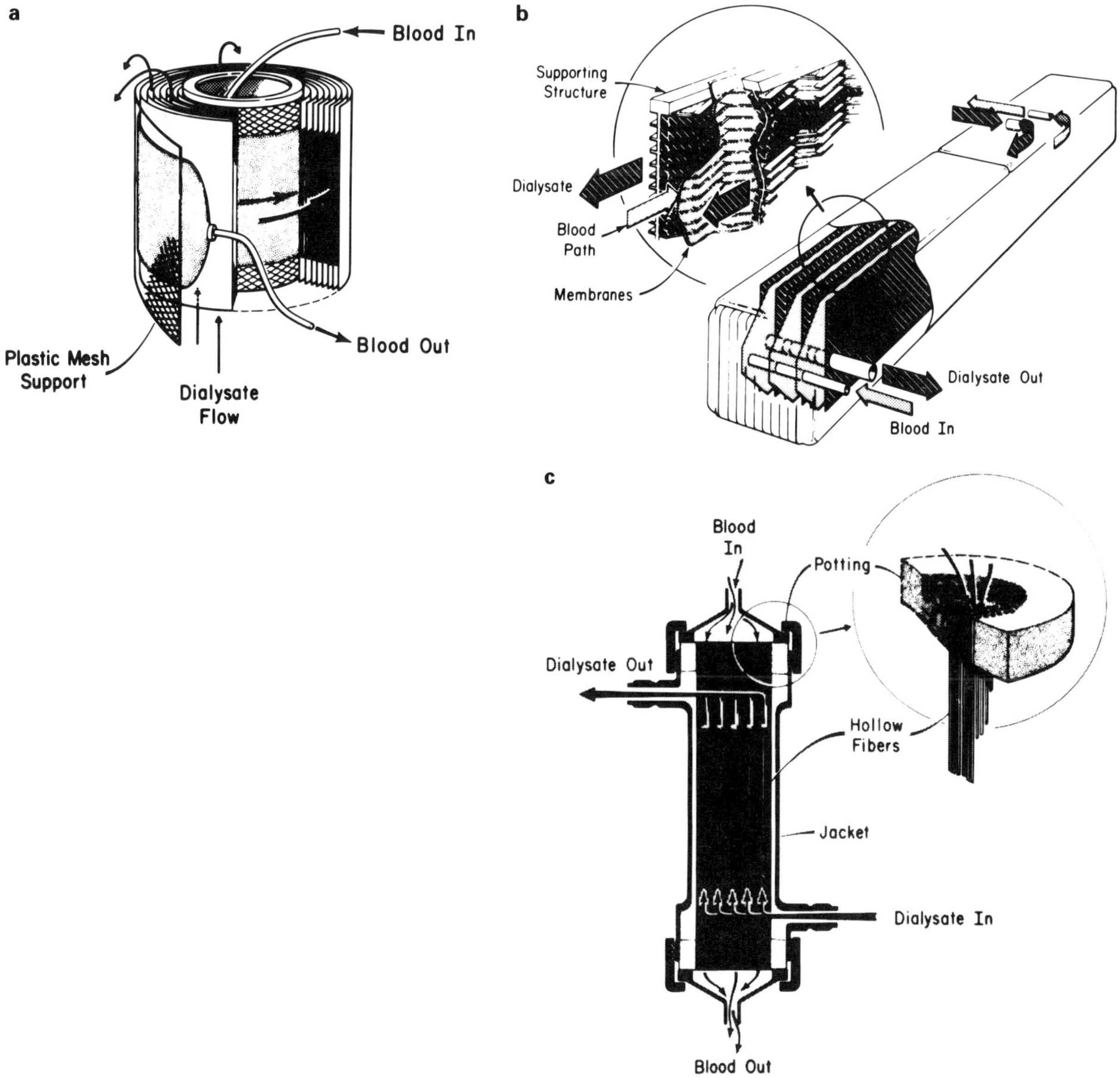

FIGURE 40-3 • Dialyzers with dialysate and blood-flow paths: (*a*) coil, (*b*) parallel-plate, and (*c*) hollow-fiber designs. (From Colton CK, Lowrie EG in Brenner BM, Rector FC Jr, eds: *The Kidney*, 2d ed, Philadelphia, Saunders, 1981. Used by permission.)

chemical nature of the membrane or the manufacturing process itself.[798] Resistance to solute transfer that occurs at the interfaces of dialysate and blood with the membrane can be minimized by optimizing dialyzer design and maximizing dialysate and blood flow rates. Standard cellulose-based hemodialyzers typically have a surface area of about 0.8 to 1.5 m^2, a membrane thickness of 7 to 30 μm, and a K_{UF} ranging from 2.5 to 7 ml/h per mmHg. At a blood flow rate of 200 ml/min and a dialysate flow rate of 500 ml/min, urea clearances approximate 125 to 195 ml/min, and creatinine clearances are typically between 90 and 160 ml/min. High-efficiency and high-flux dialyzers are manufactured with synthetic membranes with surface areas of 1.0 to 1.9 m^2 and a membrane thickness of 20 to 55 μm. The K_{UF} of these membranes may be as high as 40 to 60 ml/h per mmHg. At a blood flow rate of 200 ml/min and dialysate flow rate of 500 ml/min, urea clearances are 150 to 190 ml/min, and creatinine clearances are 130 to 190 ml/min. Although they have substantially higher K_{UF}, the clearances of low–molecular weight solutes such as urea and creatinine are only slightly higher with the high-efficiency or high-flux dialyzers than with conventional hemodialyzers. Urea clearances for conventional hemodialyzers plateau at blood and dialysate flow rates approximating 200 to 250 ml/min, whereas some high-efficiency and high-flux dialyzers may plateau at 275 to 320 ml/min.[494,529,798,1082]

The recent use of recombinant human erythropoietin (EPO) to maintain higher hematocrit levels in hemodialysis patients raised concern that dialysis efficiency, particularly with the shortened treatment times of high-efficiency and high-flux dialyzers, would be reduced.[1083,1201] In fact, urea clearance remains unchanged or decreases slightly (7 to 12 percent). Creatinine, phosphorus, and potassium clearances may be more significantly reduced, although resulting changes in serum levels are minimal. However, dialysis time may need to be increased in some patients.[9,239,651,895,1174,1181]

Certain unidentified *middle molecules*, with molecular weights of 300 to 2000, which are poorly dialyzed with conventional cellulose-based hemodialysis membranes, may be of pathogenetic significance in the uremic syndrome.[67,87] PAN, polycarbonate, polymethylmethacrylate, and polysulfone membranes achieve clearances for solutes in the molecular weight range of vitamin B_{12} (1355) and inulin (5200), which are two- to fivefold greater than clearances achieved with conventional cellulose-based membranes. Utilizing these high-flux membranes, transport characteristics for middle–molecular weight species approach those of urea.[474,944,1092] Augmentation of middle–molecular weight solute transfer has also been achieved by the use of conventional hemodialysis membranes with larger surface areas (e.g., 2.5 m^2) or use of two hemodialyzers in series.[1202]

In addition to the higher hydraulic permeability and solute clearance of these synthetic membranes, they may also be more *biocompatible* than conventional cellulose-based dialyzers, with less complement activation, less interleukin-1 and interleukin-2 production, less protein catabolism, and improved clearance of beta-2 microglobulin.[183,271,430,432,440,529,592,664,919,920,1274] Anaphylactoid reactions, however, have been reported in patients receiving angiotensin-converting enzyme inhibitors when dialyzed with PAN high-flux dialyzers.[1144,1191]

The number of hours per week required for hemodialysis varies, depending on the efficiency of the hemodialyzer, the patient's rate of "uremic toxin" generation, salt and water accumulation, and the physician's definition of adequate dialysis. The definition and determinants of adequacy of dialysis continue to be widely debated, in large part due to the failure to precisely define the specific toxins responsible for the uremic syndrome.[51,67,98,466,673,674,736] Efforts to quantify precisely the prescription of hemodialysis treatments have been stimulated by the National Collaborative Dialysis Study,[411,672,673] a trend toward shortened treatment times with conventional dialysis,[195,196,362,463,1030] and increasing use of high-efficiency, high-flux dialysis. Given the ease of measuring urea and its relationship to protein metabolism, *urea kinetic modeling* has evolved as the principal means of quantitatively assessing dialysis treatment.[8,249,408,410,435,643,664,665] Despite an ongoing debate regarding the methods[221,222,239,504,671] and appropriateness[247,505] of this analysis, kinetic modeling standards are being incorporated into quality assurance medical review criteria by ESRD Network organizations and the Health Care Financing Agency (HCFA). In general, most patients receive three hemodialysis treatments per week, with each treatment lasting 3 to 4 h.[1030]

A more detailed description of the principles, systems, and techniques of hemodialysis can be found elsewhere.[198,357,467,701,719,739]

HEMODIALYSIS SOLUTIONS

In general, although hemodialysis solutions are designed to approximate the ionic composition of normal extracellular fluid (ECF), significant modifications have been made to provide optimal correction of the common fluid, electrolyte, and acid-base disorders that accompany acute and chronic renal failure. The composition of hemodialysis solutions and the range of concentrations commonly employed for each component are listed in Table 40-3.

Sodium

Sodium is the major cation and determinant of osmolality in dialysate. During the early era of hemodialysis, dialysate containing low concentrations (<130 meq/liter) of sodium was commonly used to create a concentration gradient that favored diffusive transport of sodium from the patient.[909] Ultrafiltration of interdialytic fluid accumulation was achieved by osmotically induced water movement by using dialysate with a high glucose concentration. Today, improved dialyzer designs allow high hydrostatic transmembrane pressure gradients to be generated without fear of membrane rupture, eliminating the need for glucose-mediated osmosis.[909] The use of hydrostatic ultrafiltration, with its attendant convective transport, results in the removal of a substantial quantity of sodium during the hemodialysis treatment without reliance on diffusion-based gradients. Thus, the removal of 2 liters of ultrafiltrate during a hemodialysis treatment effects the loss (by convective transport) of 260 meq of sodium, which approximates the average sodium gain between dialyses.[850,909] Quantitatively, the majority of sodium removed during hemodialysis is the result of con-

TABLE 40-3 • Composition of hemodialysis solutions

Component	Range of concentrations, meq/liter
Sodium	130–145
Potassium	1.5–4
Calcium	2.5–4
Magnesium	0.5–1.5
Chloride	96–110
Acetate	33–41
Glucose (g/liter)	0–2.5

vective transport, with diffusive transport playing a minor role except when dialysate is significantly hyponatric.[122,668] Therefore, the necessity for low-sodium dialysate today is less critical. Most dialysis facilities now employ dialysate with sodium concentrations closer to those of normal serum.[117,909,1116, 1118]

In evaluating sodium flux across the dialyzer membrane, it is necessary to appreciate that the plasma sodium available for diffusion (i.e., the plasma sodium activity) is not equivalent to the plasma sodium concentration.[25,666] A portion of the plasma sodium is complexed to proteins and thus not diffusible (Gibbs-Donnan effect).[667] This protein-sodium complex causes ultrafiltrate sodium concentration to be less than plasma water sodium concentration during convective transport.[667] Because proteins occupy volume, plasma water sodium concentration is higher than the measured total plasma sodium concentration.[25] The plasma sodium available for diffusion can be calculated from the plasma concentrations of sodium and protein.[122]

It is currently accepted that the dialysate sodium concentration can effect symptoms of dialysis disequilibrium and hypotension. Uremic serum has an osmolality of approximately 310 mosm/liter before dialysis.[486] During hemodialysis with low-sodium (130 meq/liter) dialysate, removal of urea and sodium reduces the ECF osmolality by 22 mosm/liter.[485,486] This reduction of ECF osmolality is often associated with headaches, nausea, vomiting, muscle cramps, and hypotension.[44,588] The decrease of ECF osmolality is not immediately accompanied by a similar fall in intracellular fluid (ICF) osmolality; thus, an osmotic disequilibrium occurs, causing plasma water to shift into cells, simultaneously reducing the plasma volume (PV) and expanding the ICF compartment. Initially, the osmotic disequilibrium observed with hyponatric dialysate was believed to result from changes in the plasma concentration of sodium and not urea, since urea is freely diffusible across cell membranes.[25,341,1178] However, with the current use of high-efficiency hemodialysis, a urea gradient across cell membranes can develop and contribute to an osmotic disequilibrium.[462] Cerebral edema may develop as a consequence of these events and is believed to be responsible for many of the disequilibrium symptoms. If ultrafiltration is also performed during the hemodialysis treatment, the PV becomes further compromised, and the risk of hypotension increases (see "Hypotension").

Patients otherwise intolerant of volume removal during routine hemodialysis can comfortably sustain losses of large amounts of ultrafiltrate (e.g., 4 liters) if ultrafiltration is performed sequentially, rather than concurrently, with hemodialysis (Figs. 40-4 and 40-5).[86,516,1081] With sequential ultrafiltration, the desired amount of ultrafiltrate can be removed either immediately before or after the hemodialysis treatment (during which time no additional ultrafiltration occurs).

The fall in PV during isolated ultrafiltration is due solely to fluid removal across the dialyzer membrane. In contrast, when ultrafiltration and hemodialysis are performed concurrently, PV is simultaneously diminished by water movement from the ECF to the ICF as a result of an osmotic disequilibrium and by ultrafiltrate removal across the dialyzer (Figs. 40-4 and 40-5).[86] It has also been suggested that declining serum osmolality during hemodialysis may affect vascular reactivity by reducing peripheral vascular resistance.[86,486,1228] A disadvantage of sequential ultrafiltration is that it reduces critical dialysis diffusion time and is inconsistent with the current trend toward shorter hemodialysis treatments.

The role of osmolar shifts is further supported

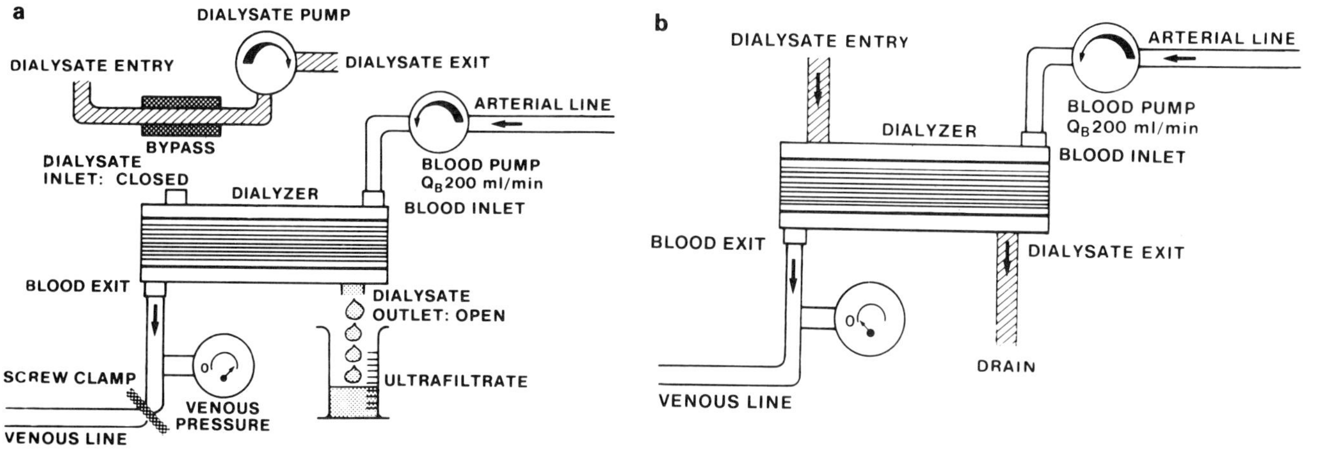

FIGURE 40-4 • (*a*) Isolated ultrafiltration versus (*b*) diffusion dialysis. In isolated ultrafiltration, dialysate flow bypasses dialyzer. An ultrafiltrate is formed as a result of hydrostatic pressure gradients across the dialyzer membrane. These gradients are created by the application of positive pressure in the blood compartment (shown) or negative pressure in the dialysate compartment (not shown). During diffusive hemodialysis, dialysate enters the dialyzer, and solute transport occurs by diffusion. In the absence of hydrostatic pressure gradients, ultrafiltration does not occur. (Modified from Lynggaard F et al: *Dial Transport* 7:1106, 1978. Used by permission.)

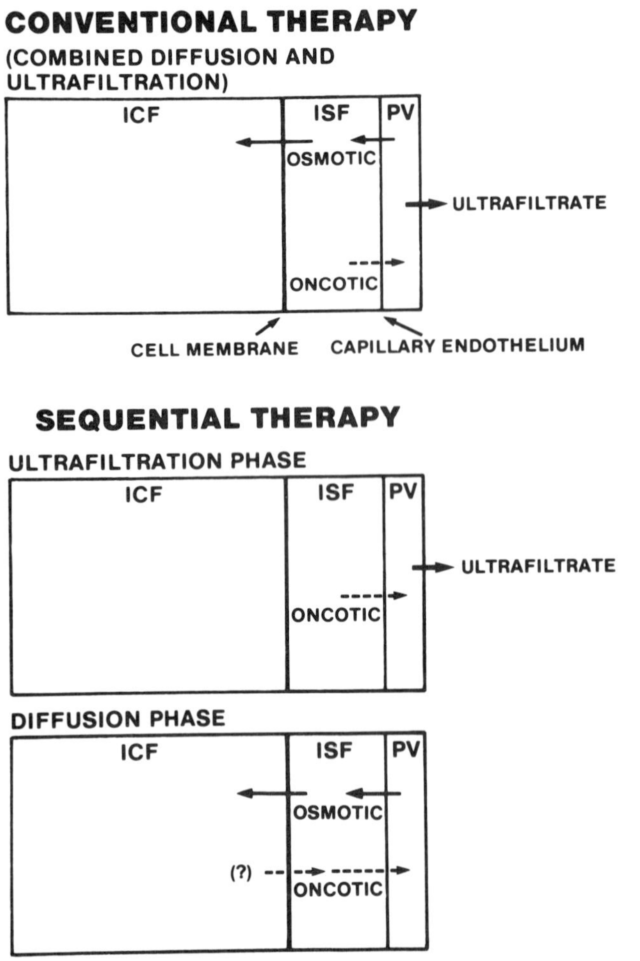

FIGURE 40-5 • Transcompartmental fluid shifts during conventional dialysis therapy, which combines diffusion and ultrafiltration (top panel), ultrafiltration alone (middle panel), and diffusion alone (bottom panel). Solid and broken arrows represent shifts induced by osmotic and oncotic gradients, respectively. The small arrow shows ultrafiltrate loss from PV to the dialysate side of the membrane by hydrostatic pressure gradients. Note that during conventional therapy, PV is depleted by both ultrafiltration and osmotic shifts; during sequential therapy, these forces act alone. During ultrafiltration, PV losses are offset by the oncotic movement of fluid from the ISF as a result of the loss of a protein-free ultrafiltrate (see the text). ICF, intracellular fluid; ISF, interstitial fluid; PV, plasma volume. (Modified from Keshaviah P, Shapiro FI: *Am J Kidney Dis* 2:290, 1982. Used by permission.)

by observations that the use of intravenous hypertonic mannitol, glucose, or saline solution during the hemodialysis treatment is effective in diminishing the symptoms of osmotic disequilibrium and hypotension.[433,486,525,811,958,991] However, mannitol may be toxic with prolonged use,[43,1128] and hypertonic glucose could result in significant hyperglycemia. High dextrose concentrations or glycerol in the dialysate may be useful.[43,283,639,991]

Thus, higher dialysate sodium concentrations eliminate many of the adverse symptoms attending dialysis-induced decreases in serum osmolality.[17,1118,1177] With dialysate sodium concentrations ranging from 140 to 155 meq/liter, increased rates of ultrafiltration during hemodialysis are better tolerated.[25,97,117,213,485,644,668,669,800,865,937,953,1118,1129,1178,1190,1228] As expected, reductions in ECF volumes are less with higher (e.g., 145 meq/liter versus 130 meq/liter) dialysate sodium concentrations.[361] Hypernatric dialysate increases ECF osmolality, causing water to shift from the ICF to the ECF, while hyponatric dialysate has the opposite effect.[122,341,579] Continuous measurements of ICF and ECF volumes during hemodialysis with a noninvasive conductivity technique verify that these predicted fluid shifts actually occur.[253] Sequential ultrafiltration dialysis is better tolerated with higher dialysate sodium concentrations.[52,1228] Hemodialysis machines that employ a conductivity-regulated 1:35 proportioning system to control the final dialysate electrolyte composition may not produce a high sodium dialysate concentration, despite additional sodium in the dialysate concentrate, unless the conductivity limits of the machine are readjusted.[1078]

The advantages of higher dialysate sodium concentrations notwithstanding, there remains a concern that postdialysis hypernatremia may lead to increased thirst, weight gain, hypertension, and pulmonary congestion during the interdialytic period.[213,987,1247] Because predialysis serum sodium concentrations are similar to those in patients dialyzed against low-sodium dialysate, increased water intake in the interdialytic period must occur.[122,213] This premise is supported by several studies that have noted greater interdialytic weight gain in patients treated with high-sodium dialysate.[213,1027] However, the increased ultrafiltration capability afforded by high-sodium dialysate allows for the easy removal of these excess fluid gains.[25] Although the risk of new-onset hypertension from high-sodium dialysate appears to be minimal, caution should be exercised in patients with preexisting hypertension, which may be aggravated by hypernatric dialysate.[25,213]

One method of obviating such concerns is to use specially adapted hemodialysis machines that allow the dialysate sodium concentration to be varied during the hemodialysis treatment, a procedure known as *sodium-gradient hemodialysis,* or *sodium modeling.* High-sodium dialysate concentrations are used during the initial period of the hemodialysis treatment to maximize ultrafiltration and then are lowered toward the end of the treatment to avoid postdialysis hypernatremia, thus preventing excessive thirst and interdialytic weight gains.[180,229,253,289,695,782,800,951,1042] This technique does not appear to offer any significant advantage over the use of a fixed high-sodium dialysate.[25,229] Computer models have been developed to predict the magnitude of transcellular fluid shifts induced by hemodialysis, as well as the postdialysis serum sodium concentration, thus potentially allowing the selection of a dialysate sodium concentration that would eliminate interdialytic problems.[462,580] Finally, a single study has suggested that administration of converting enzyme inhibitors will diminish interdialytic weight gains, presumably by decreasing levels of the dipsogen angiotensin II.[877]

Potassium

Despite an enhanced gastrointestinal elimination of potassium,[452,731,1029] the patient with ESRD depends on hemodialysis as the primary route for potassium removal.[573] The optimal dialysate concentration depends on a variety of clinical and treatment factors, including the predialysis serum potassium concentration, dietary potassium intake, duration of the treatment, efficiency of the hemodialyzer, and associated acid-base changes.[909] Adequate control of the serum potassium concentration is usually achieved with dialysate potassium concentrations between 1.5 and 3.0 meq/liter, although occasionally, concentrations above or below this range are required.

The amount of potassium removed during a hemodialysis treatment has been reported to be as little as 48 meq and as much as 220 meq, reflecting loss from both extracellular and intracellular sites.[108,872,1059] Typically, the amount of potassium removed during a single treatment is between 50 and 80 meq,[573,1107] with intracellular stores contributing from 53 to 72 percent of the amount removed.[1217] The higher the predialysis serum or the lower the dialysate potassium concentration, the greater the cation's removal.[325,498] Serum potassium concentration falls significantly during the early phase of the treatment, with further reductions being minimal in the later stages of dialysis.[498,1107,1250]

In patients with identical predialysis serum and dialysate potassium concentrations who are dialyzed under similar conditions, the amount of potassium removed during the dialysis treatment has been demonstrated to vary by an average of 71 percent.[1076] Because the majority of potassium removed during dialysis is derived from ICF stores,[873] this observed variability implies significant differences among patients in factors that control the movement of potassium from the ICF to the ECF in response to a decrement in ECF potassium.[1076] These factors include insulin, pH, catecholamines, and Na^+-K^+ ATPase.[573] Not only do these factors vary from patient to patient, but they can also be affected by the hemodialysis prescription. For example, dialysis employing a glucose-free dialysate has been demonstrated to result in greater potassium removal.[1076,1217] The lower serum insulin levels[1222] effected by glucose-free dialysate allow more potassium to move from the ICF to the ECF, making it more accessible to the hemodialysis process.[1076] Although the choice of acetate or bicarbonate as the dialysate buffer does not appear to affect the removal of potassium by dialysis,[573,1217,1250] the patient's predialysis acid-base status may play a role in the amount of potassium removed during the hemodialysis treatment.[1246] Correction of predialysis metabolic acidosis could shift potassium to the ICF, thus limiting its removal from the ECF during dialysis.[787]

Immediately following the hemodialysis treatment, the serum potassium concentration is usually normal or low. However, it is common for the postdialysis potassium concentration to rebound to a higher value 2 to 5 h after hemodialysis is terminated.[325,498,573,787] This rebound phenomenon reflects a more rapid removal of potassium from the ECF than the rate of potassium movement from the ICF to the ECF. Thus, a low postdialysis serum potassium concentration does not necessarily require that supplemental potassium be given, although it may signify a risk period for cardiac arrhythmias in susceptible patients (e.g., those on digoxin).[325,573] Conversely, if hemodialysis was intended to correct a state of hyperkalemia, a normal postdialysis serum potassium concentration does not always imply complete correction, since rebound hyperkalemia may still occur several hours later.

Potassium-free dialysate has been used by some investigators in home hemodialysis patients, permitting such patients to enjoy a more liberal dietary potassium intake (60 to 80 meq/day).[248,534,873] In these studies, the average pre- and postdialysis serum potassium concentrations have been found to be 4.6 and 3.0 meq/liter, respectively. In contrast, it has been demonstrated that 40 percent of patients dialyzed against a zero-potassium dialysate had a decrease in serum potassium concentration to less than 3.0 meq/liter at the end of dialysis.[498] Due to the potential of hypokalemia to induce intra- and postdialysis cardiac arrhythmias, the routine use of potassium-free dialysate cannot be recommended.[498] The occasional use of zero- or low-potassium dialysate may be appropriate in patients with known dietary indiscretion or a prolonged interval between dialysis treatments.[498]

Maintenance hemodialysis patients may have low total body potassium stores, possibly from a combination of reduced dietary intake and dialytic potassium removal.[90,152,909] The selection of an optimal dialysate potassium concentration is further complicated by the failure of serum levels to correlate with total body potassium content, although persistently low serum potassium concentrations usually indicate that body stores are depleted.[90,909] In contrast, total body potassium, although initially low in some uremic patients, can be increased once hemodialysis therapy is initiated, provided that the dialysate potassium concentration exceeds 1.5 meq/liter.[90,108,305,787,909,1053]

Calcium

The optimal calcium concentration of dialysate remains undefined, as evidenced by the wide range (between 1.25

and 2.0 mmol/liter) in dialysate calcium concentrations used by most hemodialysis facilities.* The dialysate calcium concentration selected should maintain the plasma calcium level in the normal range, correct any negative calcium balance, and avoid clinically significant postdialysis hypo- or hypercalcemia.[909] During hemodialysis, calcium flux between dialysate and blood depends on the concentration gradient between the ultrafilterable calcium (free calcium ions and calcium ions complexed to anions) in plasma (approximately 60 percent of total calcium) and the ionized calcium in dialysate.[392,552,866] For example, dialysate calcium concentrations of 1.25 to 1.5 mmol/liter and 1.75 to 2.0 mmol/liter effect net transfer of calcium to blood of approximately 2.8 mmol/liter and 14.5 mmol/liter, respectively, during a 6-h hemodialysis treatment.[166,394,909] There is, however, a significant amount of patient-to-patient variation in the net transfer of calcium for a given dialysate calcium concentration.[166] Additional factors that affect calcium transport during hemodialysis include increased plasma protein binding of calcium (caused by an increase in pH or the removal of an inhibitor of protein binding), hemoconcentration of protein-bound calcium, and phosphate removal during the dialysis treatment.[53,165,540,866] Increases in plasma protein concentration and protein-bound calcium from ultrafiltration (hemoconcentration) can account for 46 percent of the rise in serum calcium observed during dialysis.[165] The increased serum calcium concentration following phosphate removal may be due to calcium efflux from bone as phosphate moves from bone to ECF in response to a reduction in the serum phosphate level.[165] Finally, minor variations (about 5 percent) in the dialysate manufacturer's stated calcium concentration can cause significant changes in the mass transfer of calcium during the hemodialysis treatment.[166]

In general, favorable diffusion gradients and hemoconcentration cause increases in the serum calcium concentration following hemodialysis, with dialysate calcium concentrations ranging from 1.3 to 2.9 mmol/liter.[53,166,322,497,531,540,963] Dialysate calcium concentrations of 1.25 mmol/liter or less may be associated with unchanged or decreased serum levels.[531,963] Dialysate calcium concentrations between 1.5 and 1.75 mmol/liter usually cause normal pre- and postdialysis serum calcium values, while concentrations of 2 mmol/liter or more often cause postdialysis hypercalcemia.[531]

When a calcium-free bicarbonate dialysate is employed, 10% calcium chloride is infused into the venous blood line.[550] Calcium-free dialysate has been shown to be advantageous for delivery of bicarbonate dialysate with a single-proportioning hemodialysis machine (see "Alkali" under "Dialysis Solutions"), during regional citrate anticoagulation and when replacement of a specific amount of calcium is desired (e.g., treatment of hypercalcemia).[550] Using this technique, intravenous calcium infusion rates of 10 and 13.3 mmol/h produced changes in calcium balance, ionized serum calcium levels, and parathyroid hormone (PTH) levels that were similar to those effected by standard bicarbonate dialysate with calcium concentrations of 1.5 and 1.75 mmol/liter, respectively.[549]

A positive transfer of calcium is necessary during hemodialysis to replace various ongoing calcium losses. During the hemodialysis treatment, calcium is lost in the ultrafiltrate as a result of convective transport. A loss of 2 liters of ultrafiltrate in a patient with a serum ultrafilterable calcium concentration of 1.5 mmol/liter results in a 3-mmol calcium loss, or 9 mmol/week if a three treatment per week schedule is followed.[552,909] In addition, the impaired calcium absorption of uremia, when coupled with endogenous intestinal calcium secretion, may cause negative calcium balance and culminate in daily gastrointestinal calcium losses of up to 5 mmol.[552,909,1253]

The presence of renal osteodystrophy may also influence the dialysate calcium concentration selected. Until recently, there had been a trend to increase dialysate calcium concentrations for both prevention and therapy of renal osteodystrophy.[54,393] For example, Johnson and coworkers recommended a dialysate calcium concentration of 1.75 mmol/liter to normalize serum calcium levels, balance fecal losses, and improve renal osteodystrophy.[531] Another benefit of a higher dialysate calcium concentration (1.85 mmol/liter) may be improved cardiac contractility during the hemodialysis treatment.[172,483]

High dialysate calcium concentrations may cause hypercalcemia, transient nausea, vomiting, headache, acute pancreatitis, and hypertension,[292,310,530,866,1231,1253,1276] as well as neurologic symptoms that must be differentiated from dialysis encephalopathy.[983] Untreated tap water may contain up to 1.5 mmol/liter of calcium, which adds to the calcium concentration of the dialysate, causing the aforementioned symptoms, and is known as the hard water syndrome.[282,354] Most hemodialysis units now treat their water with reverse osmosis and/or water softening units, thereby eliminating this problem.

During the past few years, there has been an increasing trend to use the carbonate and acetate salts of calcium instead of aluminum hydroxide as oral phosphorus binders, in hopes of eliminating aluminum accumulation (see Chap. 41).[20,184,185,1036,1099] In addition, 1,25-dihydroxycholecalciferol has been widely employed as an effective therapy for secondary hyperparathyroidism.[35,737,1100] These therapies, alone or in combination, may increase the serum calcium concentration, which may reach hypercalcemic values.[35,488,687,710,762,1033,1099] Treatment of hypercalcemia by reducing the amount of calcium containing phosphorus binders or

* [Ca^{2+}]: 1 mmol/liter = 2 meq/liter = 4 mg/dl.

vitamin D may cause hyperphosphatemia and worsening of secondary hyperparathyroidism. Another approach to preventing hypercalcemia in this setting is to use dialysate with a reduced calcium concentration.[687,1033,1098] Dialysate calcium concentrations between 1.05 and 1.35 mmol/liter can often, but not always,[214] prevent hypercalcemia despite the oral administration of 25 to 180 mmol of calcium per day.[687,1033,1098] A dialysate calcium concentration of 1.25 mmol/liter effects the average removal of 5.8 mmol of calcium during a 4-h dialysis treatment and in some cases causes postdialysis asymptomatic hypocalcemia.[497] A 1.25-mmol/liter dialysate calcium concentration has been reported to produce no significant changes in either predialysis serum calcium concentrations or calcium fluxes during dialysis.[497]

In summary, it is reasonable to use calcium dialysate concentrations between 1.5 and 1.75 mmol/liter in patients not receiving large amounts of oral calcium salts as phosphorus binders and/or high doses of vitamin D. These concentrations will prevent calcium loss in hemodialysis patients and in most instances result in a small calcium gain. In patients receiving large amounts of oral calcium salts or high doses of vitamin D, a dialysate calcium concentration between 1.5 and 1.35 mmol/liter may be necessary to avoid hypercalcemia.

Magnesium

As with calcium, no unanimity of opinion exists with respect to what the standard dialysate magnesium concentration ought to be. Because the kidney is the primary determinant of the serum magnesium level, the prevention of hypermagnesemia has been a major concern in dialysis patients. Several studies have demonstrated that the magnesium content of erythrocytes and other tissues is higher in uremic patients than in normal control subjects.[101,205,398,738,909] At serum magnesium concentrations of 6 meq/liter (3 mmol/liter) deep tendon reflexes may be lost, while respiratory paralysis, central nervous system (CNS) changes, abnormal cardiac conduction, and hypotension emerge at serum levels above 10 meq/liter.[735] In addition, hypermagnesemia in patients with chronic renal failure may contribute to renal osteodystrophy and soft tissue calcification.[21,132,141,147,939] Conversely, others have suggested that hypermagnesemia may protect against these bony complications.[757] Although some studies suggest that high serum magnesium levels may inhibit PTH secretion in hemodialysis patients,[821,910,929,938] others have been unable to demonstrate any consistent influence of dialysate magnesium concentration or serum magnesium levels on PTH levels.[398,400,562]

Serum magnesium concentrations normally range from 1.5 to 2.0 meq/liter, with 25 percent being protein-bound and 75 percent in an ultrafilterable form.[735] Chronic renal insufficiency does not change these percentages.[187] The hemodialysis patient's serum magnesium concentration is dictated by the dialysate magnesium concentration.[739,866] For example, predialysis serum magnesium concentrations of 1.5 to 2.2 meq/liter and 2.5 to 4.5 meq/liter have been found when dialysate concentrations have been 0.5 and 1.5 meq/liter, respectively.[147,186,187,398] Dialysate magnesium concentrations below 0.5 meq/liter have caused hypomagnesemia following dialysis, which eventually normalizes or increases to the high-normal range prior to the next treatment.[170,535,562,909,1117]

A 6-h hemodialysis treatment using a magnesium-free dialysate removes 250 mg of magnesium and can correct a positive magnesium balance.[909,1045] Dietary magnesium is absorbed normally in dialysis patients.[1044] Most hemodialysis facilities, however, prescribe a dialysate magnesium concentration between 1.0 and 1.6 meq/liter.[909] Advocates of lower dialysate concentrations (0 to 0.4 meq/liter) claim that improvements occurred in peripheral neuropathy,[13,1119] pruritus,[415,821] and renal osteodystrophy.[147] Magnesium-free dialysate has also been advocated for patients receiving magnesium salts as oral phosphorus binders (see "Disturbances of Serum Phosphate").[141,863] Others, however, argue that magnesium dialysate concentrations between 0.5 and 1.4 meq/liter protect against renal osteodystrophy, metastatic calcification, peripheral neuropathy, and cramping.[562,910] At present, there appears to be a downward trend in dialysate magnesium concentrations, especially in view of the increasing popularity of shortened treatment times.[909] Frequent monitoring of the serum magnesium level is still suggested to detect both hypermagnesemia from indiscrete use of magnesium-containing antacids and laxatives, and hypomagnesemia resulting from significant dietary restrictions.

Alkali: Acetate, bicarbonate, and lactate

In early hemodialysis systems, bicarbonate was added to dialysate to correct the metabolic acidosis of uremia. Precipitation of bicarbonate with the calcium and magnesium additives of dialysate was prevented by bubbling 5 to 10% CO_2 through the dialysate, thus lowering its pH. The *batch-type dialysate* preparation systems used during this period later became impractical for providing the larger dialysate volumes required with the newer *single-pass dialysate* flow systems. Thus, new techniques called *proportioning dialysate preparation systems* were developed for the continuous production of dialysate by mixing fixed proportions of water with a specially prepared liquid dialysate concentrate.[420] However, in these proportioning systems, bicarbonate could not be mixed with the calcium and magnesium salts in the concentrate without producing a precipitate. To eliminate this problem, Mion and associates in 1964 successfully substituted the more soluble acetate for bicarbonate as the principal alkali in dialysate concentrate.[774] Because acetate is less permeable than bicarbonate, a dialysate acetate concentration of 35 to 40 mmol/liter was chosen to ensure an influx of acetate into the patient that slightly exceeded the loss of bicarbonate during the hemodialysis treatment.[774,1254] Following Mion's report, acetate became the primary buffer employed in the hemodialysis procedure. More recently, however, there has been increasing evidence that acetate contributes significantly to the morbidity of the hemodialysis treatment (see below), prompting a renewed interest in bicarbonate or alternative buffers as the primary alkali in dialysate solutions.

The metabolism of acetate during hemodialysis has been extensively studied and is the subject of several excellent reviews.[1187,1196] Briefly, approximately 90 percent of acetate infused during the hemodialysis procedure is metabolized (indirectly) to bicarbonate.[1146] Acetate combines with coenzyme A (CoA) for form acetyl CoA in the heart, liver, and skeletal muscles. This reaction is mediated by the enzyme acetyl CoA synthetase and consumes a hydrogen ion in the process.[594] The source of the hydrogen ion is carbonic acid, which becomes bicarbonate. The majority of acetyl CoA formed undergoes oxidation in the Krebs cycle to CO_2 and water.[1097] A smaller proportion of acetyl CoA can be metabolized to ketone bodies and free fatty acids.[788,1089,1196] The latter metabolic pathway has raised concern that the use of acetate dialysate on a long-term basis may contribute to the hyperlipidemia and arteriosclerotic complications commonly seen in hemodialysis patients.[427] The majority of studies addressing this issue, however, have not demonstrated any significant differences in lipid levels between acetate- and bicarbonate-treated hemodialysis patients.[60,595,716,789,790,854,1039]

The success of acetate hemodialysis in maintaining acid-base balance depends on its rapid metabolic conversion to bicarbonate during the hemodialysis procedure. Normal individuals are able to metabolize acetate at a rate approximating 300 mmol/h.[610,676,977,1196] The rate of acetate metabolism in chronic hemodialysis patients is slightly less, at 250 mmol/h.[538,610,1146,1196,1207] When standard-sized dialyzer membranes and a dialysate acetate concentration of 35 to 40 mmol/liter are used in the hemodialysis procedure, the rate of acetate transfer approximates the maximal rate of acetate metabolism, which is sufficient to offset bicarbonate losses during the dialysis treatment.[1195,1196] Under these circumstances, serum acetate levels initially increase to 2 to 4 mmol/liter and continue at this level for the remainder of the hemodialysis treatment.[538,855,1146,1195] Following the hemodialysis treatment, the accumulated acetate is metabolized, resulting in a delayed increase of 2 to 4 mmol/liter in the serum bicarbonate concentration.

If the rate of acetate influx during hemodialysis exceeds the maximal rate of acetate metabolism or if the rate of acetate metabolism in a given patient is depressed, serum acetate levels will rise to values greater than usual.[1196] This increase may be associated with symptoms of weakness, hypotension, nausea, vomiting, and headaches and has been termed *acetate intolerance* (see "Hypotension"). With high-efficiency or high-flux hemodialysis systems, which use high blood and dialysate flow rates, and dialyzers that have greater acetate permeability than conventional dialyzers, the rate of acetate influx exceeds the maximal endogenous rate of acetate metabolism, producing acetate intolerance.[252,401,416,538,645,724,854,855,1146] Furthermore, these systems promote a rate of bicarbonate efflux across the dialyzer membrane that exceeds the metabolic conversion rate of acetate to bicarbonate, resulting in a fall in the serum bicarbonate concentration during the hemodialysis treatment. Arterial pH values remain stable, however, because of the hypocapnia caused by CO_2 losses across the dialyzer membrane.[401,416,854,855,1146] For these reasons, bicarbonate dialysate is generally used with high-efficiency and high-flux dialysis. The acid-base changes occurring during hemodialysis with acetate and bicarbonate are discussed in detail later in this chapter.

As noted, acetate intolerance can also occur in patients with a decreased capacity to metabolize acetate. Vinay and colleagues demonstrated that approximately 10 percent of hemodialysis patients were unable to metabolize acetate efficiently.[1195] Factors associated with decreased acetate metabolism include diminished muscle mass, as seen in those with small body size, women, the elderly, or cachectic patients, and reduced muscle perfusion secondary to poor cardiovascular function. The presence of alternative oxidizable substrates, as seen in diabetics with hyperglycemia and ketone bodies, patients with lactic acidosis from hypotension, proteolysis induced by steroids or sepsis, and parenteral hyperalimentation during hemodialysis, also impair acetate oxidation.[219,1196] Patients demonstrating any of these factors are at increased risk for acetate intolerance and should be hemodialyzed with bicarbonate dialysate.

It has been well documented that arterial oxygen levels fall during dialysis with acetate, but not usually with bicarbonate, dialysate.[148,300,368,524,1185,1196] The principal mechanism for this arterial hypoxemia is a reduction in pulmonary ventilation secondary to the loss of dissolved CO_2 and bicarbonate into the dialysate and, to a lesser extent, from CO_2 fixation during acetate metabolism.[694,869,1196,1216] High dialysate bicarbonate levels (37 mmol/liter) can also produce hypoxemia, possibly due to a decrease in minute ventilation from a more marked increase in pH.[954] Other adverse complications of acetate metabolism include the generation of interleukin-1, accumulation of inorganic intracellular phosphate, uncoupling of oxidative phosphorylation, reduction of intracellular ATP levels and increase in intracellular AMP levels, increased production of adenosine, and depletion of mitochondrial CoA.[1187,1196] Some of the possible clinical consequences of these biochemical derangements include depressed myocardial contractility, vasodilation, hyperphosphatemia poorly corrected by dialysis, and hypoxemia.[225,1124,1187,1196] A more comprehensive discussion of the adverse biochemical effects of acetate metabolism can be found elsewhere.[1187,1196] Finally, the literature contains a few case reports of acetate dialysate hypersensitivity reactions.[365,901]

The documented morbidity from acetate has renewed interest in bicarbonate as the principal alkali in dialysate fluids. As noted above, rapid or high-flux hemodialysis actually requires bicarbonate dialysate.[568]

Earlier technical limitations on the continuous production of bicarbonate dialysate were overcome with the development in 1977 of a dual-proportioning dialysate delivery system that allows separate bicarbonate and acid (divalent ion) concentrates to be mixed simultaneously with pretreated water to produce a final bicarbonate dialysis solution without precipitation.[564,1032] The bicarbonate concentrate contains all of the bicarbonate and 25 percent of the sodium chloride required in the dialysate.[1032] The acid concentrate contains small amounts of acetic acid; all of the calcium, magnesium, and potassium; and the remaining sodium chloride required for the dialysate, and has a final pH that is very low. Correct mixing of the final dialysate is monitored by a conductivity meter and in some instances a pH electrode.

Bicarbonate dialysate can be prepared from a prepackaged powder or liquid concentrate.[240,824,864,1204] An alternative (but currently uncommon) method of preparing bicarbonate dialysate using less expensive single-proportioning hemodialysis machines has been described.[550,729] In this method, calcium is deleted from the bicarbonate concentrate but is separately infused as 10% calcium chloride through the venous blood line during the hemodialysis treatment. The attractiveness of bicarbonate dialysate as a more physiologic and better-tolerated buffer notwithstanding, the use of this alkali requires more costly hemodialysis delivery systems, is more expensive than acetate dialysate, may suffer from chemical instability or inadequate mixing of powdered preparations, and is susceptible to bacterial contamination.[99,296,372,715,824] The latter problem, however, can be avoided by using water treatment systems designed to eliminate bacterial contamination and using commercially prepared sterile bicarbonate dialysate.[73,771,1019]

Lactate recently has been proposed as an alternative alkali to acetate or bicarbonate in hemodialysis solutions.[223] Lactate has been used successfully for years as the principal alkali in peritoneal dialysate and in replacement fluids for hemofiltration. The attractiveness of lactate as the principal alkalai for hemodialysis solutions is that it may eliminate many of the adverse symptoms commonly seen with acetate dialysate, without the increased technologic requirements, cost, and potential for the bacterial contamination associated with bicarbonate dialysate.[223] Preliminary studies indicate that hemodialysis with lactate-buffered dialysate (either as the sole buffer or mixed in equal amounts with acetate) is associated with significantly less hypotension, vomiting, and headaches than with acetate dialysate.[215,216,1149] Adverse changes in cardiac output and total peripheral resistance during lactate dialysis are less common than seen with acetate.[215] In addition, lactate is capable of satisfactorily correcting the metabolic acidosis of chronic renal failure.[215,1149]

In summary, there remain a significant proportion of hemodialysis patients for whom the use of acetate dialysate continues to be acceptable and well-tolerated.[254,854,1195] Bicarbonate dialysate should be used in selected stable chronic hemodialysis patients who demonstrate intolerance to acetate, as well as in acutely ill patients requiring hemodialysis.[254,1195] It should be noted, however, that some investigators advocate the routine use of bicarbonate dialysate for all hemodialysis patients.[771] At present, despite its potential advantages and until additional studies are performed, lactate-buffered dialysate cannot be recommended as an acceptable replacement for the current standards of acetate and bicarbonate dialysate.[215,1149]

Chloride

The primary determinant of the chloride concentration in the dialysate is the necessity for maintaining electroneutrality.[909] Normally, the physician selects the desired sodium, potassium, calcium, magnesium, and alkali concentrations for the dialysis solution. The chloride concentration for the solution is then simply the difference between the selected concentrations for these cations and the alkali concentration. Most dialysis solutions have a chloride concentration between 92 and 111 mmol/liter.[909]

Dextrose

The only nonelectrolyte component of dialysate is dextrose. During the early years of hemodialysis, high dextrose concentrations in the dialysate provided high osmotic pressure gradients for ultrafiltration.[761] With today's improved dialyzers, it is possible to generate transmembrane hydrostatic pressure gradients sufficient to meet the ultrafiltration goals, obviating the need for high dialysate dextrose concentrations.[909]

Currently, most hemodialysis centers use dextrose concentrations ranging from 100 to 220 mg/dl (5.55 to 12.2 mmol/liter).[909,1115] Dextrose concentrations in this range can provide a small amount of calories for the patient. The inclusion of 182 to 200 mg/dl of dextrose in the dialysate provides approximately 16 to 20 g of dextrose to the patient during the hemodialysis treatment; a dextrose-free treatment results in a loss of 26 to 30 g.[1217,1222] The presence of dextrose in the dialysate may have certain disadvantages, such as promoting bacterial growth and interfering with simple tests for residual formaldehyde. Dextrose-free dialysate has been used safely without causing clinically significant hypoglycemia.[248,965,1217,1222] However, development of electroencephalographic abnormalities and a more profound fall in serum osmolality have been reported with the use of dextrose-free dialysate.[965] It would appear prudent to avoid dextrose-free dialysate in patients at risk for developing dialysis disequilibrium (see "Dialysis Disequilibrium"). The presence of dextrose in the dialysate has been reported to have both beneficial and deleterious effects on amino acid losses, gluconeogenesis, generation of ketoacids, and lipid metabolism during the hemodialysis treatment.[606,909,965,1127,1217] Dextrose-free dialysate also enhances potassium removal but appears to be without effect on acid-base changes during dialysis.[1217] In summary, the balance of evidence suggests that the addition of dextrose to the dialysate is beneficial to minimize losses of organic anions (which ultimately are metabolized to bicarbonate), symptoms of disequilibrium, and the potential for hypoglycemia in glycogen-depleted patients.[606,965,1115,1217]

HYPERTENSION

Hypertension is present in about 70 to 90 percent of long-term dialysis patients[10,709,1104,1230] and may be an important contributor to the cardiovascular complications that are highly prevalent among these patients.[653,1198] Hypertension is strongly associated with left ventricular hypertrophy, which has been shown to be an important risk factor for cardiovascular mortality in dialysis patients.[907,1090] Significant hypertension appears to be more common among patients with underlying vascular or glomerular disease than in those with ESRD due to tubulointerstitial disease.[1230] The pathogenesis of hypertension in patients with ESRD has often been categorized as being either volume-dependent or renin-dependent.[1192,1232] Blood pressure can be normalized or significantly improved by adequate salt and water removal during hemodialysis in about 90 percent of chronic dialysis patients, whereas similar degrees of ultrafiltration are ineffective in other patients, thought to have primarily renin-dependent hypertension.[1192,1232] In the past, renin-dependent hemodialysis patients were often subjected to bilateral nephrectomy as a last recourse in controlling their hypertension.[631,754,880] Although effective for controlling blood pressure, this often resulted in a worsening of anemia, hemodialysis hypotension, and renal osteodystrophy due to the loss of residual endocrine functions of these patients' end-stage kidneys.[970,1114] Because of these complications and the increased availability of more effective antihypertensive medications, such as minoxidil, beta blockers, angiotensin-converting enzyme (ACE) inhibitors, and calcium channel blockers, bilateral nephrectomy is rarely performed today.[142,661,785,1184] The ACE inhibitors should be used with caution in patients dialyzed with PAN dialyzers, however, because anaphylactoid reactions have been reported in these patients.[1144,1191]

More recent investigations suggest that this traditional categorization of hypertensive dialysis patients into volume- and renin-dependent groups is probably an oversimplification.[10] In a majority of dialysis patients, renin secretion appears to be inappropriately increased with respect to ECF volume status and thus may be a more important factor in the pathogenesis of hypertension than previously thought.[10,649,1038,1221,1229,1230] Although less well studied, factors other than volume and renin may also be important.[491,648] These putative factors include elevated levels of plasma catecholamines,[302,520,751] hemodynamic factors,[10,491] enhanced sensitivity of blood pressure to sodium,[742] and increased pressor responses to calcium.[1231] An abnormal diurnal pattern of blood pressure has been reported in chronic dialysis patients based on 24-h ambulatory recordings, with an absence or blunting of the normal nocturnal decline of blood pressure.[82,997] Accidental hypercalcemia has been reported to cause hypertension in hemodialysis patients.[1086] Pseudohypertension may also occur in some hemodialysis patients.[521] This phenomenon is attributable to extensive arteriosclerotic disease with "pipestem" calcifications of peripheral arteries, which decreases arterial compressibility by the blood pressure cuff, preventing accurate auscultation of the Korotkoff sounds.[763] In patients with extensive atherosclerotic disease, both hypertension and end-stage kidney failure may be due to atherosclerotic renovascular disease.[522,856] In selected patients, renal artery revascularization may result in improvement of hypertension, recovery of renal function, and better survival.[553,856]

As many as 25 to 35 percent of chronic hemodialysis patients treated with recombinant human EPO may develop significant worsening of their baseline hypertension or new hypertension.[155,308,642] In a few patients, particularly within the first few months of EPO treatment or with very rapid increases in hematocrit, severe uncontrolled hypertension has been associated with seizures,[307,308,948] although a specific causal relationship has not yet been proven. Mechanisms that have been implicated in the development of hypertension in dialysis patients receiving EPO include rheologic factors (increased blood viscosity), reduction of anemic-hypoxic peripheral vasodilatation, and increased binding of nitric oxide (an endothelium-derived relaxing factor) to hemoglobin.[496,642,730,748,949] Heidenreich and colleagues have also demonstrated a direct endothelial-dependent vasopressor effect of EPO using in vitro isolated renal and mesenteric arterial segments.[459]

HYPOTENSION

Hypotension during hemodialysis is one of the most common adverse reactions associated with this therapeutic modality and has been the subject of several reviews.[220,441,464a,482,569,1071,1281] Approximately 25 percent of hemodialysis treatments are complicated by hypotension, which is often accompanied by symptoms of weakness; cramps in the legs, back, and abdomen; headache; chest pain; nausea and vomiting; dizziness; and sometimes loss of consciousness.[238,464a] Hypotension during hemodialysis may arise from a variety of factors (Table 40-4) that can act singly or in combination to lower blood pressure.[220,441,464a,482,569,1071,1281]

Reduction of the expanded ECF space during dialysis may decrease the PV to a level that results in hypotension.[578] It has been proposed that the hypotension associated with a gradual decline in PV is due to an abrupt failure of compensatory blood pressure support mechanisms, in contrast to settings where a sudden excessive decrease in blood volume overwhelms the compensatory pressure support mechanisms.[694] Unacceptable decreases in blood pressure from excessive depletion of the PV can be avoided by establishng an appropriate dry weight for each patient (i.e., the weight of the patient below which further ultrafiltration will result in hypotension). Blood pressure stability during hemodialysis depends not only on the amount of ultrafiltrate removed but also on the rate of its removal.[464a] As PV falls, salt and water move from the interstitial fluid space to the plasma in response to increases in the plasma oncotic pressure that result from the loss of protein-free plasma water (ultrafiltrate).[321] The magnitude of this plasma "refilling" is such that only minor decreases in PV may occur despite dramatic ultrafiltrate losses[1119a] and is directly correlated with the degree of initial tissue hydration.[598] If the rate of removal of plasma water exceeds the rate of refilling of the PV, then hypotension occurs more rapidly.[598] Priming with albumin during hemodialysis allows for higher ultrafiltration rates without hemodynamic instability.[523] The recent trend toward high-efficiency dialyzers and shorter treatment times exaggerates the ICF/ECF osmotic disequilibrium (see below) created during the dialysis process, which in turn limits the compensatory effect of "refilling."[1071]

TABLE 40-4 • Factors contributing to hemodialysis hypotension

Hypovolemia
Absolute volume
Rate of fluid removal
Decreased serum osmolality
Sequential ultrafiltration and diffusion
Dialysate sodium concentration
Vasodilatation
Acetate versus bicarbonate dialysate
Autonomic dysfunction
Catecholamine abnormalities
Hypoxemia
Membrane-blood interactions
First-use syndrome
Dialysate temperature
Anemia
Ionized calcium concentration
Postprandial hemodynamic alterations
Vasoactive hormone abnormalities
Cardiac dysfunction
Antihypertensive medication

SOURCE: Modified from Keshaviah PR, Shapiro FL: *Am J Kidney Dis* 2:290, 1982. Used by permission.

Blood pressure reductions during hemodialysis can be affected by other factors besides the amount and rate of PV depletion. Bergström in 1976,[86] and subsequently others,[268,447,1005,1065,1227] have demonstrated that greater volumes and rates of ultrafiltration can be achieved without precipitating hypotension if the ultrafiltration component of the hemodialysis treatment is temporally separated from the diffusive component. This technique is known as *isolated*, or *sequential, ultrafiltration*. This process is carried out by applying hydrostatic gradients to a dialyzer that has been bypassed from dialysis solution (Fig. 40-4).[86]

Several mechanisms may account for the improved blood pressure stability with isolated ultrafiltration compared to routine hemodialysis (in which ultrafiltration and diffusion occur simultaneously). Serum osmolality remains stable during isolated ultrafiltration but falls as a result of loss of solutes (urea and sodium) by diffusion during routine hemodialysis. This phenomenon suggests that decreases in serum osmolality play a role in the development of hemodialysis hypotension.[86] Bergström postulated that the fall in osmolality during diffusive hemodialysis resulted in hypotension through an effect on the carotid bodies, vasomotor center, or efferent sympathetic pathways, preventing normal compensatory vasoconstriction.[86] However, hypotension from a decrease in serum osmolality may also occur by an effect on fluid shifts that alter the volumes of body water compartments.[566] Earlier studies of diffusive hemodialysis using hypotonic dialysate demonstrated the occurrence of a significant fluid shift (1.0 to 1.5 liters) from the ECF to the ICF compartment in response to an osmotic gradient (disequilibrium) between these two compartments that was created by the more rapid loss of osmotically active solutes from the ECF.[315,872] Based on these and their own observations, Keshaviah and colleagues have proposed the following model to explain the role of osmolality changes (diffusive solute transport) in hemodialysis hypotension (Fig. 40-5).[569,571,572] During isolated ultrafiltration, the PV is reduced only by the removal of ultrafiltrate. The loss of protein-free ultrafiltrate raises the oncotic pressure in the plasma, resulting in its refilling from the other body water compartments. In routine hemodialysis, both diffusive transport and ultrafiltration occur simultaneously. In this setting, the PV decreases from both a loss of ultrafiltrate across the dialyzer and from the movement of water down its osmotic gradient from the ECF to the ICF. The latter movement occurs in response to the osmotic disequilibrium (ICF > ECF) generated by the loss of osmotically active ECF solutes (urea and sodium) during diffusion hemodialysis. Although urea is presumed to be present in equal concentrations in the ECF and ICF, diffusion hemodialysis more rapidly removes this solute from the ECF due to an equilibration lag for urea across the cell membrane.[464a,1152] A meaningful osmotic role for urea is questionable, however, given the observation that in uremic animals a rapid dialytic reduction in urea levels does not impair the hemodynamic response to volume depletion.[228] The use of dialysate having a sodium concentration less than that of serum only serves to magnify the potential for osmotic disequilibrium. Thus, it is not surprising that the use of higher dialysate sodium concentrations is associated with a lower incidence of hypotension (see "Sodium" under "Hemodialysis Solutions").[25,97,117,213,485,644,668,669,865,937,952,953,991,1085,1116,1118,1129,1178,1190,1228]

Differences in hemodynamic measurements during isolated ultrafiltration and diffusive hemodialysis help to further clarify mechanisms for the contrasting effects these two techniques have on blood pressure stability. During diffusive hemodialysis without ultrafiltration, decreases in blood pressure are associated with an increase in cardiac output (primarily from increased heart rate) and a fall in total peripheral resistance (TPR).[1065] In contrast, during isolated ultrafiltration, cardiac output falls as a result of decreased filling pressures, but TPR increases and thus maintains blood pressure.[581,1227] In addition, venous dilatation, which could contribute to hypotension by reducing capillary filling pressures,[130,693] increases with combined ultrafiltration and diffusive hemodialysis but remains stable during isolated ultrafiltration.[129]

The uptake of acetate during diffusive hemodialysis, but not during isolated ultrafiltration, may also increase susceptibility to hypotension. Acetate has been shown to have both vasodilatory properties[80,225,226,360,780,878] and a direct myocardial depressant effect,[19,583,1018,1197] although the latter effect is debated.[566,723] Several studies have in fact demonstrated that acetate is associated with a positive inotropic effect,[33,179,582,634,647,721,758,826,1257] which may be due either to a direct myocardial effect or to afterload reduction from acetate-induced vasodilatation.[178,227] In these studies, despite a fall in TPR, blood pressure is often maintained by an increased cardiac output.[18,179,227,447,586,647] If reductions in cardiac preload or underlying primary cardiac disease prevent the expected increase in cardiac output, blood pressure falls from unopposed, acetate-induced vasodilatation.[566] In contrast, compensatory increases in TPR have been demonstrated during bicarbonate hemodialysis (see below).[445,446] Acetate, in contrast to bicarbonate, dialysis causes venodilatation[640,1096] and impairs plasma refilling.[500,600a,711,1071] The latter observation has not been confirmed by other investigators.[340a,991a] In another study, acetate and bicarbonate dialysis were demonstrated to be equal in increasing venodilatation.[130]

Studies comparing the effects of acetate and bicarbonate as causes of hemodialysis hypotension are difficult to evaluate because of differences in patient populations, rates of solute flux and ultrafiltrate removal, dialysate sodium concentrations, definition of hypotension, and various metabolic factors.[120,286] A decreased incidence of hypotension and other symptoms of dialysis disequilibrium during bicarbonate hemodialysis have been demonstrated by the majority of investigators.[89,178,416,438,445,446,518,616,624,641,716,722,740a,802,855,874,897,955,957,1042,1058,1110,1170,1180,1197,1228] However, other studies have not been able to demonstrate a signficiant beneficial effect on blood pressure with bicarbonte dialysate.[19,120,169,484,695a,724,1040,1175,1226] Furthermore, although some reports have maintained that serum acetate levels correlate with blood pressure reduction[587,1260] or changes in TPR,[1049] others have been unable to demonstrate such relationships.[120,156,169,479,724,897]

In some instances of hemodialysis hypotension, it remains unclear whether the decrease in blood pressure was due to negative cardiovascular effects of acetate or to a fall in serum osmolality.[566] Wehle and colleagues showed that the incidence of hypotension is lower with bicarbonate than with acetate hemodialysis using low-sodium (hypotonic) dialysate but found no difference between these two buffers when hemodialysis was performed with high-sodium (isotonic) dialysate.[1228] Similar findings have also been noted by other investigators.[89,484,518,955,1189,1190,1226] Keshaviah has suggested that hypotension during the early period of the hemodialysis treatment is due to the effects of acetate, while serum osmolality changes may be responsible for hypotension that occurs later in the treatment.[566]

In summary, the available data, on balance, support a trial of bicarbonate hemodialysis for patients with frequent and significant hemodialysis-associated hypotension. This is especially true in the settings of hypotonic dialysate or high-efficiency hemodialysis and in patients with compromised cardiac reserve or metabolic conditions that could impair their ability to normally metabolize acetate.[254,286] However, for the majority of patients undergoing acetate hemodialysis without significant hypotensive problems, conversion to bicarbonate hemodialysis does not appear to be necessary.[254,854,1195]

There were several recent reviews on the role of autonomic system dysfunction in hemodialysis hypotension.[220,1151,1281] As noted, in some patients with hemodialysis hypotension, heart rate and TPR fail to increase as expected.[181,447,1227] Furthermore, some hemodialysis patients have abnormal responses to the Valsalva maneuver, decreased baroreceptor sensitivity, impaired blood pressure responses to hand-grip exercise, and defective function of sweat glands, all of which suggest that autonomic dysfunction plays a role in the pathogenesis of hemodialysis hypotension.[115,154,220,231,311,458,481,482,563,650,712,752,1121,1151,1239,1281,1284] Abnormalities in cardiopulmonary baroreceptor reflexes in diabetics, the elderly, and patients with hypertension or congestive heart failure make it more difficult to determine a specific role for uremia as a cause of autonomic dysfunction.[220] Several investigators have even questioned whether autonomic dysfunction is a factor in hemodialysis hypotension.[620,803,805,820] During isolated ultrafiltration, TPR rose in the same patients in whom it fell during conventional hemodialysis. This outcome is contrary to expectation if autonomic dysfunction is the cause of hemodialysis hypotension.[569,1227,1253]

Included in the evaluation of the role of autonomic nervous system dysfunction in dialysis hypotension are measurements of plasma catecholamines. It has been observed that plasma catecholamine levels are increased in patients with advancing renal failure not yet on dialysis and in ESRD patients receiving routine hemodialysis.[302,652] It has been proposed that baroreceptor dysfunction observed in these patients results in a loss of tonic sympathetic inhibition (*deafferentation*), with consequent overactivity of the efferent limb of the autonomic system.[231] This overactivity causes maximal vasoconstriction and an inability to respond further when volume depletion occurs.[220,650,1151] Elevated levels of PTH blunt the pressor effect of norepinephrine, possibly by stimulating prostaglandin release.[197] Not all investigators, however, have been able to confirm that plasma catecholamines are increased in hemodialysis patients, raising questions regarding the correctness of a "sympathetic hyperactivity hypothesis".[220,1278] A loss of norepinephrine across the dialyzer membrane has also been proposed as a cause of hemodialysis hypotension.[134,160] The rate of removal appears to be greater with regular hemodialysis than with isolated ultrafiltration.[441] Furthermore, isolated ultrafiltration is associated with a greater rise of plasma norepinephrine levels than seen with regular hemodialysis.[441,486]

It is well-established that arterial hypoxia occurs during routine hemodialysis.[1185] Hemodialysis hypoxemia has been suggested as a cause of hypotension because improved bood pressure stability may occur when supplemental nasal oxygen is used.[14,480] More recently, a beneficial effect of oxygen supplementation on blood pressure stability has been questioned.[335] Hypoxemia may partly underlie the role of acetate in vascular instability. Several investigators have demonstrated hypoxemia during hemodialysis with acetate, but not bicarbonate, dialysate,[63,301,484,502,634,823,956,1170,1179] although others have not been able to demonstrate any difference in P_{O_2} levels between these two buffers.[6,120,413] Mechanisms by which acetate could cause hypoxemia have been discussed above.

First-use syndrome is a group of symptoms and signs that occur between 10 min and 2 h after the initiation of hemodialysis; it is believed to be caused by an allergic reaction to a new dialyzer.[473,513] First-use syndrome may cause hypotension, agitation, nausea, weakness, flushing, pruritus, dyspnea, chest pain, and tachycardia.[513] Hypotension from first-use syndrome can sometimes be distinguished from other causes of hemodialysis hypotension due to its early onset and occurrence in the same subset of patients.[473] More subtle blood-membrane interactions during hemodialysis may also affect blood pressure stability. It has been suggested that commonly used dialysis membranes, such as cuprophane, can result in pulmonary sequestration of leukocytes, causing pulmonary hypertension and decreased cardiac filling.[439,1071,1213] Both reprocessed and more biocompatible dialysis membranes have been associated with less hemodialysis hypotension,[175,985] although this observation has been challenged by some investigators.[1096]

It has been suggested that cooling of the dialysate may decrease the incidence of hemodialysis hypotension. During isolated ultrafiltration, in contrast to routine hemodialysis, blood is not warmed by heated dialysate as it passes through the dialyzer; thus, it returns to the patient at a lower temperature (33.1°C) than does returning blood in routine hemodialysis (37.2°C). It has been suggested that this may partially account for the improved blood pressure stability noted with use of isolated ultrafiltration.[698] Studies of routine hemodialysis in which dialysate has been cooled to between 34.0 and 35.6°C demonstrate that the incidence of symptomatic hypotension is lower.[194,585,660,696-698,705,1077,1079] Long-term observations have shown sustained benefits of cooling.[726] Although not all hemodialysis patients will experience less hypotension with cooler dialysate, those patients who are most frequently hypotensive appear to benefit the most.[889] In addition, if blood is rewarmed to 37°C before being returned to the patient in isolated ultrafiltration, the incidence of hypotension rises to the frequency seen with routine hemodialysis.[696,698] A possible explanation of these events is that blood warmed by heated dialysate produces a heat load that provokes compensatory vasodilation, which in turn counteracts the vasoconstriction needed to maintain blood pressure during ultrafiltration.[230,698] Norepinephrine may participate in this mechanism: cold exposure increases catecholamine secretion, and plasma norepinephrine levels have been found to be increased when cold, instead of warm, dialysate is used.[630,705]

Anemia, almost universally present in ESRD patients, can affect peripheral vascular resistance and thus could play a role in hemodialysis hypotension.[814,1071] Transfusion of packed red blood cells has been shown to decrease the frequency of dialysis hypotension.[1073] It remains unclear whether the recent widespread use of recombinant human EPO to correct the anemia associated with renal disease[308] will reduce the incidence of dialysis hypotension. Changes in the serum calcium concentration during the hemodialysis treatment may affect blood pressure by direct actions on vascular tone or left ventricular contractility (see "Calcium" under "Hemodialysis Solutions").[327,483,1276] High-calcium dialysate increases serum ionized calcium concentration, improves left ventricular performance,[327,483] and causes a smaller reduction in mean arterial pressure during the hemodialysis treatment than does low-calcium dialysate.[749,1075] Despite these observations, the frequency of symptomatic hypotensive episodes in patients (even those at increased risk for hypotension) dialyzed against both high (1.75 mmol/liter) and low (1.25 mmol/liter) calcium dialysate concentrations has been shown to be similar.[1075] Furthermore, correction of chronic hypocalcemia by vitamin D metabolites does not increase predialysis blood pressures.[1080]

Blood pressure can significantly fall postprandially in some elderly people and in patients with autonomic nervous system dysfunction, suggesting that a similar relationship may obtain in hemodialysis patients.[1074,1279] Studies have demonstrated a greater fall in blood pressure, as well as more frequent episodes of symptomatic hypotension, when hemodialysis patients are fed intradialytically than when they fast.[1074,1279] The mechanism responsible is probably splanchnic dilatation mediated by the release of gastrointestinal hormones or insulin. Glucose has also been shown to impair baroreceptor sensitivity.[220] Hemodialysis patients with autonomic dysfunction would be expected to be the most susceptible to postprandial hypotension.[1074,1279] These observations support a policy of not feeding patients, especially those prone to hypotension, during the hemodialysis treatment period.

There has been recent interest in the role of eicosanoids and other vasoactive hormones in blood pressure regulation during hemodialysis.[220,1051] Both in vitro and in vivo studies have demonstrated the release of vasoactive hormones when anticoagulated whole blood is exposed to specific dialyzer membranes. In addition, it has been proposed that dialysate pyrogens can trigger the release of interleukin-1, which stimulates arachidonic acid release, resulting in hypotension.[472] Clinical studies investigating the role of eicosanoids in blood pressure changes during hemodialysis have been few. In one study, administration of indomethacin tended to increase mean arterial pressures pre- and postdialysis despite greater ultrafiltration rates, although these changes were not significantly different than those seen during a placebo period.[118] Another study was able to demonstrate a relationship between plasma protaglandin E_2 (PGE_2) levels and hypotension in patients hemodialyzed with low-sodium dialysate.[1052] Hypotensive dialysis patients have been shown to have increased plasma renin and angiotensin II levels and to be resistant to the pressor effects of angiotensin II.[786,1106a] Vasopressin levels increase in some, but not all, hemodialysis patients during volume reduction.[524] Furthermore, atriopeptin,[1084] PTH, and calcitonin gene-related peptide[857] levels are increased in uremia, and all have vasodilator activity. The role, if any, of these vasoactive hormones in blood pressure regulation during hemodialysis remains unclear.[220]

Finally, underlying cardiac disease and/or use of antihypertensive medications predispose to hemodialysis hypotension by preventing normal compensation of ECF volume losses from ultrafiltration.[441] Hemodialysis patients are subject to several disturbances that can adversely affect cardiac function. These disturbances include accelerated arteriosclerosis, hypertension, pericardial effusions, hypertrophic cardiomyopathy, metastatic myocardial calcification, high-output states from arteriovenous fistulas and anemia, and electrolyte disturbances.[441,591] Recently it has been demonstrated that the hemodialysis treatment impairs early diastolic and compensatory late atrial-assisted filling of the left ventricle, resulting in hypotension.[1007] The high prevalence of hypertension in hemodialysis patients and the failure of some of these patients to judiciously avoid excess salt and water frequently dictate a requirement for antihypertensive medications. These drugs, however, may also impair the cardiac (beta-blockers and calcium channel blockers) and peripheral vascular (vasodilators, calcium channel blockers, and centrally acting agents) compensation needed to maintain blood pressure during the dialysis treatment.[441]

DIALYSIS DISEQUILIBRIUM SYNDROME

The intermittent nature of hemodialysis therapy results in rapid and wide swings of the patient's biochemical blood markers (e.g., blood urea nitrogen, or BUN). These abrupt biochemical changes have been implicated in the production of a constellation of symptoms and signs known as the dialysis disequilibrium syndrome (DDS). The syndrome can occur both during and up to 24 h after the hemodialysis treatment. The clinical findings of DDS are listed in Table 40-5.[353a,746,921,998,1161,1210] Generalized seizures are one of the more common and serious manifestations of this syndrome.[1161] The syndrome is more likely to occur during the initiation of hemodialysis at a time when predialysis BUN values exceed 150 mg/dl or when the hemodialysis treatment is performed under conditions resulting in maximal solute transport. Characteristic electroencephalographic findings of DDS are a predominance of slow-wave activity, increased delta and

TABLE 40-5 • Signs and symptoms of dialysis disequilibrium syndrome

Nausea and/or vomiting
Headache
Mental clouding, disorientation
Anxiety and/or agitation
Weakness, "washed-out" feeling
Visual blurring
Muscle cramps
Peripheral paresthesias
Hyperventilation
Chest pain
Convulsions
Coma

theta waves, and loss of alpha activity.[44,445a,560,1161] In chronically dialyzed patients, changes in the electroencephalogram during hemodialysis have not been found.[78a] Due to the nonspecific nature of the signs and symptoms (Table 40-5), DDS must be differentiated from other neurologic and metabolic disturbances that can present similarly in the hemodialysis patient.[44,353a]

The clinical findings of DDS have been attributed to cerebral edema and increased cerebrospinal fluid (CSF) pressures, both of which are consistently seen in DDS.[44,618] Initially, the cerebral edema was believed to result from an osmotic disequilibrium created by the more rapid removal of urea from blood than from the brain and CSF, which caused water to shift from the ECF to the hyperosmolar CNS.[561,921] This phenomenon has been termed the *reverse urea shift* to contrast these events with the infusion of urea by neurosurgeons to reduce cerebral edema.[559,560] Support for this theory was provided by studies demonstrating that, during hemodialysis, CSF pressures rose and urea levels and osmolality fell to a lesser extent than in blood.[44,382,559,561,998,1095] Use of dialysate containing urea at concentrations similar to those in the patient's blood prevented the usual increase in CSF pressure.[382]

Subsequent reports, however, have questioned whether reverse urea shifts are responsible for DDS. A definite correlation between the electroencephalographic findings of DDS and urea shifts cannot be established.[444] In addition, larger osmotic gradients than those generated by the small differences in urea concentration between blood and cerebral tissue are usually necessary in order to produce the amount of cerebral edema seen in this syndrome.[49,906] Finally, CSF pressures have been shown to rise independently of the presence of dialysis disequilibrium (or cerebral edema).[44,46]

In uremic dogs, Arieff showed that a rapid lowering of blood urea levels was associated with development of cerebral edema, while similar blood urea level reductions with slow hemodialysis were not.[44,46] However, evidence that differences in blood and brain urea concentrations are not the primary cause of cerebral edema was provided by a demonstration that (1) urea concentration differences between cerebral cortex and blood were similar with both rapid and slow hemodialysis; (2) the osmotic gradient from differences in urea concentrations alone was not of sufficient magnitude to cause cerebral edema; and (3) the osmolality of the brain was greater after rapid than after slow hemodialysis, a finding unexplained by the urea concentrations. In addition, although removal of urea from the CSF was impaired during hemodialysis, removal of urea from brain tissue was more rapid and similar to urea removal from blood. Since electrolyte alterations also could not account for the increased cerebral osmolality in the rapid hemodialysis group, it is postulated that the high cerebral osmolalities observed were due to the formation of idiogenic osmoles.[43] Subsequent studies of rapid hemodialysis disequilibrium showed that intracellular cerebral cortex pH and CSF pH fell despite a rise in plasma pH.[45] Values of pH in brain and CSF of dogs who were slowly hemodialyzed and did not develop cerebral edema were significantly higher than values in the rapid hemodialysis comparison group.[45] Arieff has postulated that the increased hydrogen ion activity resulted from an increase in intracellular accumulation of organic acids (by unknown mechanisms), which directly or indirectly increased brain osmolality, causing cerebral edema and disequilibrium.

Other causes of DDS have been postulated, including hyponatremia, hypoglycemia, paradoxical acidosis, and cerebral hypoxemia.[44,981,1211] However, substantial evidence in support of these etiologies has not been presented.[44]

Since the more severe manifestations of DDS occur in patients with a high predialysis BUN concentration (usually > 150 mg/dl) and are more likely with rapid hemodialysis, the risk of DDS can be minimized by modifying the first several hemodialysis treatments in susceptible patients in a manner designed to reduce dialysis efficiency.[44] This result can be accomplished by shortening the duration of hemodialysis, using a small-surface area dialyzer, and decreasing the rate of dialysate and/or blood flow. Osmotically active substances have been used as an adjunct to prevent dialysis disequilibrium.[44] The addition of urea,[533] glucose,[431] sodium,[937,1118] or glycerol[43] to dialysate has been recommended, but benefits have been inconsistent.[44] Intravenous infusions of fructose, glycerol, and mannitol have also been tried. In general, with the exception of intravenous mannitol infusion,[433,540,991] osmotic adjuncts are unnecessary as long as appropriate measures to decrease hemodialysis efficiency are taken. When intravenous mannitol is used, a dose of 1 g/kg body weight given by continuous infusion over the entire hemodialysis treatment has been recommended,[991] although intermittent bolus infusions can also be used successfully. Mannitol use should be restricted to the first few treatments to prevent accumulation.[991] Some nephrologists have prescribed prophylactic anticonvulsants (e.g., diphenylhydantoin), but their use is of questionable benefit. Initiation of renal replacement therapy with peritoneal dialysis has been employed in the past, taking advantage of the lower clearances of urea and other solutes with this technique. However, there have been rare reported cases of disequilibrium even with peritoneal dialysis.[768]

Less serious disequilibrium symptoms, such as headache, muscle cramps, nausea, and vomiting, probably result from small osmotic shifts and occur even during therapy in stabilized chronic hemodialysis patients.[44] These symptoms can be minimized or eliminated by increasing the dialysate sodium concentration (see "Sodium" under "Hemodialysis Solutions"),[1118] using a bicarbonate-buffered dialysate (see "Alkali: Acetate, Bicarbonate, and Lactate" under "Hemodialysis Solutions"),[416] substituting isolated ultrafiltration techniques when appropriate, and administering hypertonic mannitol, saline solution, or glucose.[433,486,525,769,811,958,991]

ACID-BASE DISTURBANCES

Stability of the serum bicarbonate level, despite ongoing acid production in ESRD patients, has been proposed to result from participation by nonbicarbonate buffers, primarily calcium carbonate in bone.[551,638] The recent observation that acetazolamide administration results in more severe metabolic acidosis in hemodialysis patients than in healthy control subjects has been interpreted as further evidence of bone buffering.[244,245] The long-term effects of this buffering by the bone may contribute to renal osteodystrophy. In this regard, Lefebvre and coworkers have demonstrated that patients with increased bone formation rates hemodialyzed with a high-bicarbonate dialysate designed to normalize their predialysis serum bicarbonate values had no progression of their secondary hyperparathyroidism, unlike patients hemodialyzed with standard bicarbonate dialysate.[637] Not all investigators agree, however, that bone is a critical buffer in the acidosis of chronic renal disease.[867] A more extensive discussion of the role of bone buffering in uremic acidosis can be found in several recent reviews.[244,418,867]

One of the primary goals of hemodialysis is to correct uremic acidosis. This is accomplished by the addition of alkali to the dialysate, which in turn diffuses into the patient's blood during the dialysis treatment. During the early period of hemodialysis, dialysate contained bicarbonate in concentrations between 27 and 35 meq/liter.[107,208,478,1234] The final mixture had a pH of approximately 7.4, which was achieved by equilibrating the solution with 5 to 10% CO_2, thus preventing precipitation of bicarbonate with calcium and magnesium in the dialysate. The effectiveness of bicarbonate in these initial studies was evidenced by the demonstration that postdialysis serum pH measurements were alkaline and bicarbonate values were normal. It was further shown that, despite dialytic correction of ECF acidemia, CSF acidemia persisted because the blood-brain barrier prevented rapid bicarbonate equilibration.[208] This event maintained predialytic compensatory hyperventilation, thus accounting for the alkalemic pH and low P_{CO_2} values noted after hemodialysis in these early studies.

As discussed previously, Mion and associates in 1964 substituted acetate for bicarbonate as the alkali in dialysate so that hemodialysis solutions could be prepared by proportioning dialysate systems, without precipitating bicarbonate with calcium or magnesium (see "Alkali: Acetate, Bicarbonate, and Lactate" under "Hemodialysis Solutions").[774] Using an acetate concentration of 35 meq/liter, these investigators observed that bicarbonate levels fell slightly during the first 30 min and then rose into the normal range after 6 to 10 h of hemodialysis.[774] Following this report, acetate became the principal alkali used in dialysis solutions (at concentrations of 35 to 40 meq/liter) to replenish bicarbonate losses that resulted from buffering of endogenous acids produced in the interdialytic period and from diffusion into bicarbonate-free dialysate during hemodialysis (see below).[1219]

One of the earlier and more detailed descriptions of acid-base changes during hemodialysis using acetate dialysate was reported by Rosenbaum and colleagues.[999] Their long-term hemodialysis patients received twice-weekly treatments, each lasting 6 to 9 h. Predialysis arterial blood gas values demonstrated either simple metabolic acidosis with respiratory compensation or a mixed disturbance of metabolic acidosis and respiratory alkalosis. Interpretation of arterial blood gas data by these investigators as well as others is guided by the observation that the ventilatory response to metabolic acidosis is normal in patients with ESRD.[151] Predialysis pH values exceeded 7.32 (range, 7.29 to 7.46) in the majority of patients and in each case rose immediately following hemodialysis.[999] The mean serum bicarbonate value rose from 20 meq/liter predialysis to 26 meq/liter postdialysis. Although the majority of patients demonstrated maximal serum bicarbonate values at the termination of the hemodialysis treatment, in some patients bicarbonate values continued to rise (1.7 to 5.1 meq/liter) following the hemodialysis treatment, suggesting delayed metabolism of acetate. Values for P_{CO_2} were mildly depressed before dialysis and did not change significantly in either the intradialytic or interdialytic periods.[999]

Subsequent studies have demonstrated greater variations in the acid-base parameters of patients receiving hemodialysis with acetate dialysate. These variations result from differences between the rate of acetate influx and its metabolism to bicarbonate and the rate of efflux of bicarbonate and CO_2 across the dialyzer membrane.[1146] The net effect of these separate processes dic-

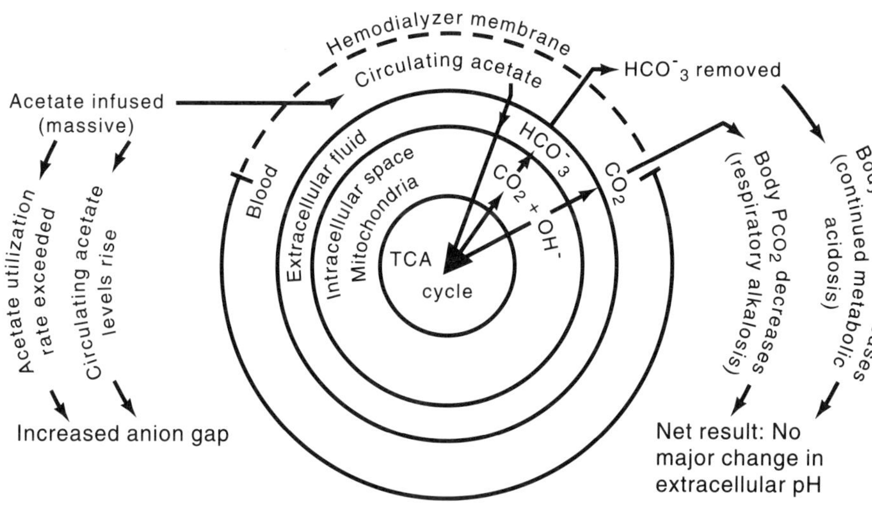

FIGURE 40-6 • Acid-base kinetics during hemodialysis with high mass transfer hemodialysis. Bicarbonate losses across the dialyzer exceed the metabolic conversion of acetate to bicarbonate, worsening metabolic acidosis. No changes occur in pH because of losses of CO_2 across the dialyzer. (From Tolchin N et al: *Kidney Int* 11:366, 1977. Used by permission.)

tates the acid-base changes that occur during and following the hemodialysis treatment (Fig. 40-6).[1146] Several of these subsequent studies have confirmed Rosenbaum's findings of increasing bicarbonate and pH values during hemodialysis,[999] supporting the concept that the rate of influx and metabolic conversion of acetate to bicarbonate exceeds the rate of bicarbonate loss.[90,401,484,758,952,957,1179,1207] In these studies, P_{CO_2} values remained stable or changed only minimally.[120,401,484,758,952,957,999,1179,1207] In all of these reports, standard surface area dialysis membranes and hemodialysis techniques were used.

With the larger-surface area dialysis membranes and increased blood flow rates for high-efficiency or high-flux hemodialysis, a different acid-base pattern was observed during the hemodialysis treatment. In most of these studies, acidosis was exacerbated by the hemodialysis treatment, as evidenced by lower serum bicarbonate values immediately after hemodialysis.[416,538,758,855,1146,1197] Blood pH remained stable or fell slightly, due to a concomitant fall in P_{CO_2} resulting from CO_2 losses across the dialyzer. Following the hemodialysis treatment, serum bicarbonate values were observed to rise slowly, accompanied by increases in pH and P_{CO_2}.[416,538,1146] The explanation of these events is as follows: During high-efficiency hemodialysis, the rate of bicarbonate loss across the dialyzer membrane exceeds the metabolic conversion rate of the infused acetate, resulting in a fall in serum bicarbonate as the hemodialysis treatment proceeds (Fig. 40-6). The gradual rise in serum bicarbonate following the hemodialysis treatment is due to the ongoing metabolic conversion of the retained acetate to bicarbonate. In several of these studies, acetate levels were measured and found to increase during the hemodialysis treatment, subsequently decreasing in the postdialytic period. An additional mechanism that may contribute to the reduction in serum bicarbonate concentration observed in some patients receiving acetate hemodialysis has been suggested by Bosch and colleagues.[123] These investigators, using a gas extraction technique combined with mass balance measurements, demonstrated that CO_2 recovered in dialysate during the hemodialysis treatment exceeded the amount of CO_2 that left the blood during the same period. These observations suggest that, as they passed through the dialyzer, red blood cells generated CO_2, which in turn was lost to the dialysate, resulting in a net gain of hydrogen ions by the patient. In vitro studies have also demonstrated that uremic red blood cells can generate CO_2 when exposed to a low P_{CO_2} and/or low bicarbonate concentrations.[123]

An example of acid-base changes during high-efficiency hemodialysis with acetate (35 meq/liter) dialysate is provided by Mehta and colleagues.[758] In patients receiving hemodialysis with a standard 1-m^2 dialyzer, pre- and post-dialysis values were pH, 7.38 and 7.42, respectively; P_{CO_2}, 33 and 33 mmHg, respectively; and bicarbonate, 19 and 21 meq/liter, respectively. When the same patients underwent hemodialysis using a high-efficiency 2.5-m^2 dialyzer, pre- and postdialysis values were pH, 7.40 and 7.44, respectively, P_{CO_2} 34 and 28 mmHg, respectively; and bicarbonate, 21 and 17 meq/liter, respectively. In another study of high-efficiency hemodialysis, similar acid-base findings were associated with a calculated bicarbonate loss of 47.5 μmol/kg body weight per minute, which exceeded the metabolic conversion rate of acetate to bicarbonate of 42.9 μmol/kg body weight per minute during the hemodialysis treatment.[1146] Although the intensification of metabolic acidosis was not associated with any significant pH changes in these studies because of the reduction of P_{CO_2}, the potential exists for clinically significant acidemia to arise if acetate dialysate is used with high-efficiency hemodialysis techniques in patients whose predialysis bicarbonate levels are markedly depressed.[1146]

In addition to differences in acetate and bicarbonate transport resulting from variations in hemodialysis technique, the potential for worsened metabolic acidosis during acetate hemodialysis depends on the individual patient's capacity to metabolize acetate to bicarbonate. In patients with a relatively low acetate metabolic conversion rate, serum acetate levels rose, and bicarbonate levels fell during acetate hemodialysis.[1207] In contrast, for patients who metabolized acetate more rapidly under similar hemodialysis conditions, bicarbonate levels increased, and acetate levels remained low during the hemodialysis treatment.[1207] Vinay and colleagues have proposed a simple method of identifying patients who do not metabolize acetate optimally.[1195] Using this method, these investigators retrospectively analyzed their acetate dialysis population over a 10-year period and determined that 10 percent were acetate-intolerant, and, of this group, 87 percent were women. If dialysate acetate levels were increased or larger–surface area membranes were used, the percent of acetate-intolerant patients would be expected to increase. To validate their methods, these investigators prospectively studied 60 patients on acetate hemodialysis and measured postdialysis serum acetate levels. In patients classified as acetate-tolerant, postdialysis acetate levels were minimal: 1.75 meq/liter in men and 2.72 meq/liter in women. Patients classified as acetate-intolerant had significantly higher postdialysis serum acetate levels: 8 meq/liter in men and 7.69 meq/liter in women. Factors potentially associated with decreased acetate metabolism have been previously reviewed (see "Alkali: Acetate, Bicarbonate, and Lactate," under "Hemodialysis Solutions").[286,1195]

Because of these and other adverse effects of acetate accumulation and metabolism (see "Alkali: Acetate, Bicarbonate, and Lactate" under "Hemodialysis Solutions"; "Hypotension"; and "Dialysis Disequilibrium"), there has been renewed interest in bicarbonate as the principal alkali used in dialysate. Earlier technological limitations on the preparation and delivery of bicarbonate dialysate have been eliminated by the development of dual-proportioning delivery systems.[1032] Studies of acid-base changes during bicarbonate hemodialysis, regardless of the efficiency of the dialytic technique, have demonstrated progressive increases in serum bicarbonate and pH values throughout the dialysis treatment.[120,178,416,484,758,897,952,957,1146,1179,1197] Values for P_{CO_2} usually remain stable or increase slightly. In general, use of bicarbonate dialysate results in higher pre- and postdialysis values for serum bicarbonate and pH than are seen with acetate dialysate; postdialysis serum bicarbonate levels are more often in the normal range.[120,178,416,437,446,484,624,716,758,825,897,952,1146,1179,1197,1217]

Acid-base parameters were measured in a group of stable dialysis patients after one week of bicarbonate (35 meq/liter) and then one week of acetate (35 meq/liter) dialysis with standard membranes and treatment times.[1217] During acetate hemodialysis, pre- and postdialysis values were pH, 7.35 and 7.42, respectively; P_{CO_2}, 36 and 31 mmHg, respectively, and bicarbonate, 20 and 19 meq/liter, respectively. In contrast, during bicarbonate hemodialysis, pre- and postdialysis values were pH, 7.38 and 7.48, respectively; P_{CO_2}, 38 and 39 mmHg, respectively; and bicarbonate, 22 and 28 meq/liter, respectively. Acid-base parameters were unaffected by the presence or absence of glucose in the dialysate. In a study by Hakim and associates, acid-base determinations in stable patients hemodialyzed for one month each with acetate (41 meq/liter) and then bicarbonate (36 meq/liter) dialysates, significant differences in predialysis values for pH, P_{CO_2}, and bicarbonate were not demonstrable.[437] However, postdialysis values for P_{CO_2} (34 versus 31 mmHg) and bicarbonate (24 versus 22 meq/liter) were higher during the bicarbonate than during the acetate treatment period. Data from Gennari and Rimmer illustrate the ability of bicarbonate dialysate to effect higher predialysis serum bicarbonate values than acetate dialysate in stable chronic dialysis patients.[374] For their patients receiving bicarbonate hemodialysis, the mean predialysis serum bicarbonate value was 21 ± 2 meq/liter (range, 17 to 27 meq/liter), while for patients receiving acetate hemodialysis, the mean bicarbonate value was 17 ± 1 meq/liter (range, 15 to 20 meq/liter).[374]

The effects of acetate and bicarbonate hemodialysis on the electrolyte pattern and anion gap have recently been characterized.[191,890] In a population of stable patients chronically hemodialyzed with acetate dialysate, the distribution of the predialysis electrolyte patterns was pure high anion gap, 30 percent; hyperchloremic, 24 percent; and mixed, 46 percent.[191] The electrolyte pattern of metabolic acidosis varied not only in the hemodialysis population but also in individual patients from month to month. Similar to the results of studies in ESRD patients before the institution of maintenance hemodialysis,[709,1214] the finding of a hyperchloremic or mixed electrolyte pattern in 70 percent of patients was in contrast to the previously held opinion that a pure high anion gap pattern would be present in most of these dialysis patients. Postdialysis, the distribution of electrolyte patterns was hyperchloremic, 48 percent; mixed, 33 percent; and high anion gap, 19 percent.[191] Thus, during acetate hemodialysis, there was a shift from a predominantly mixed to a hyperchloremic electrolyte pattern. This change reflects a loss from the serum during hemodialysis of unmeasured anions (primarily phosphate and sulfate) at a rate that exceeds correction of the bicarbonate deficit. In a related study, Oster and colleagues characterized the electrolyte pattern in a group of stable patients receiving chronic bicarbonate (35 meq/liter) hemodialysis.[890] The average predialysis serum anion gap and bicarbonate levels were 16 ± 0.13 meq/liter and 22 ± 0.17 meq/liter, respectively. The authors noted that the average predialysis anion gap value they observed was similar to that reported by other investigators in undialyzed patients with ESRD, but the average serum bicarbonate value was

2 to 3 meq/liter higher.[436,890,1214,1245] Seventy-one percent of patients demonstrated an increased anion gap either alone or with hyperchloremia (a pure high anion gap pattern was found in 36 percent of the patients). This distribution of electrolyte patterns was similar to that observed predialysis in acetate dialyzed patients.[191] In contrast, the percent of patients with an increased anion gap (pure and mixed pattern) was greater than observed in undialyzed ESRD patients, possibly reflecting a greater residual glomerular filtration rate (GFR) in the latter group, which would minimize the accumulation of acid anions.[890,1214] In the study by Oster and colleagues, changes in the anion gap during bicarbonate hemodialysis were also evaluated.[890] The average fall in the anion gap was 1.6 ± 0.3 meq/liter, while the average increase in the serum bicarbonate level was 3.6 ± 0.5 meq/liter. These findings suggest that bicarbonate influx occurred more rapidly that the efflux of unmeasured anions (although other explanations for maintaining the anion gap relatively constant during dialysis are also possible) and are in contrast to the changes in anion gap and serum bicarbonate levels seen during acetate dialysis, in which the fall in the anion gap was greater than the rise in serum bicarbonate concentration.[191]

Based on the foregoing observations, it is apparent that the use of bicarbonate dialysate corrects uremic acidosis in a more physiologic and complete manner than the delayed and often incomplete correction seen with acetate dialysate. This impression is further supported by the results of Gotch and colleages, who carefully studied hydrogen ion (H^+) balance in a group of stable long-term hemodialysis patients dialyzed for one week each with acetate (40 meq/liter) and bicarbonate (36 meq/liter) dialysate.[412] The amount of H^+ gained during the interdialytic period was approximately 50 meq/day, calculated from the rate of protein catabolism. Hydrogen ion balance during an acetate hemodialysis treatment was equivalent to the net difference between the rates of influx of acetate and efflux of bicarbonate and organic anions. In this study, only 11 percent of the acetate entering the patient added "new" base, since 79 percent of the acetate influx was needed to replace bicarbonate and organic anion efflux during the hemodialysis treatment. Similar findings have also been reported by Vremon and coworkers.[1207] The inclusion of organic anion efflux in the balance equation is necessary, since these anions, if not removed, will ultimately be metabolized to bicarbonate. In this regard, it has been demonstrated that during acetate, but not bicarbonate, hemodialysis, there are significant increases in such metabolites as citrate, acetoacetate, and β-hydroxybutyrate.[1217] In bicarbonate hemodialysis, H^+ balance during hemodialysis is simply equal to the rate of bicarbonate influx.

Hydrogen ion balance in the study by Gotch and colleagues was almost zero during acetate hemodialysis (7 meq H^+ lost per week) and was markedly negative during bicarbonate hemodialysis (175 meq H^+ lost per week); negative H^+ balance is equivalent to gain of base.[412] During bicarbonate hemodialysis, only 30 percent of the base gained could be accounted for by a rise in serum bicarbonate levels; 70 percent of the gain most likely replenished intracellular buffers, probably in bone. Gotch and coworkers postulated that intracellular bone buffers may be depleted by long-term acetate hemodialysis, which is inadequate for correcting H^+ accumulation.[412] Although, in their study, acetate hemodialysis resulted in marginal net hydrogen loss, it is conceivable that under different conditions a small hydrogen ion gain may occur that would become significant on a cumulative basis. This postulate is supported by the findings of Ward and associates, who evaluated changes in serum bicarbonate levels after 12 weeks of bicarbonate hemodialysis in patients who previously received at least one year of acetate hemodialysis.[1218] In this study, as the cumulative time on bicarbonate hemodialysis increased, there were progressive increases in intradialytic serum bicarbonate concentrations accompanied by progressive decreases in H^+ ion activity. These observations were interpreted as being consistent with a significant depletion of intracellular buffers at the initiation of bicarbonate hemodialysis; with time, buffer depletion decreased as intracellular reserves were replaced allowing more of the infused bicarbonate to remain in the ECF. Based on these findings, the authors caution that if long-term bicarbonate hemodialysis is initiated, dialysate bicarbonate may have to be progressively decreased over time to avoid significant postdialysis alkalemia.[1218] In contrast, other investigators have not found a progressive rise in intradialytic serum bicarbonate concentrations after long-term conversion of patients from acetate to bicarbonate hemodialysis.[461] The reasons for these disparate findings are not clear.

In contrast to the studies of Gotch[412] and Ward,[1218] which suggest progressive H^+ accumulation and ICF buffer depletion, Gennari has proposed a theoretical model that states that net H^+ balance is zero with long-term hemodialysis therapy.[373] In this model, during acetate hemodialysis, the amount of acetate influx (and its metabolism to bicarbonate) is constant, while bicarbonate efflux during the hemodialysis treatment is directly proportional to the predialysis serum bicarbonate concentration. Thus, the higher the predialysis serum bicarbonate concentration, the greater the amount of bicarbonate efflux. The net transfer of alkali (amounts of acetate influx minus bicarbonate efflux) during the hemodialysis treatment will vary inversely with the predialysis serum bicarbonate concentration. Net alkali gained during the hemodialysis treatment may or may not be sufficient to balance H^+ gain from endogenous acid production in the interdialytic period and organic anion loss during the hemodialysis treatment itself. If net alkali gain during a given hemodialysis treatment is less than that required to maintain acid balance, the next predialysis serum bicarbonate concentration will be lower due to retained H^+, resulting in a greater net alkali gain during the subsequent dialysis treatment. Conversely, if net alkali gain during the hemodialysis treatment exceeds that required to maintain acid balance, the next predialysis serum bicarbonate concentration will be higher, resulting in a smaller net alkali gain during the subsequent dialysis treatment. Over time, net alkali gain and inter- and intradialytic acid accumulation will equilibrate, resulting in a predialysis serum bicarbonate concentration at which net alkali gain during dialysis will equal acid gain, and hence acid balance will be zero. Under stable conditions, once this point is reached, cumulative H^+ retention should not occur. Table 40-6 quantitates these principles in a theoretical patient receiving acetate hemodialysis. Using similar principles for net alkali transfer during dialysis and interdialytic acid gain, zero acid balance will also eventually occur with chronic bicarbonate hemodialysis (see Table 40-6). Gennari has suggested that this model of neutral acid-base balance with chronic acetate or bicarbonate hemodialysis is analogous to the absence of continued acid retention that occurs with proximal renal tubular acidosis.

Any evaluation of acid-base balance during acetate or bicarbonate hemodialysis must also consider the amount of bicarbonate lost by convective transport whenever ultrafiltration is applied. During the hemodialysis treatment itself, convective losses of bicarbonate will not result in any change in the serum bicarbonate concentration. However, during the interdialytic period, retention of alkali-free fluids will cause the serum bicarbonate concentration to fall further than it does simply from bicarbonate buffering of the daily H^+ load.[374] For example, in one study, a decrease in the interdialytic weight gain by 0.9 kg resulted in a rise in the predialysis serum bicarbonate level of 1.67 meq/liter.[312]

Serum bicarbonate concentrations following hemodialysis are also dependent on the concentration of acetate or bicarbonate in the dialysate solution. Dialysate buffer concentrations of 38 meq/liter result in postdialysis serum bicarbonate concentrations of 24 to 27 meq/liter, compared to 20 meq/liter when the buffer concentration in dialysate is 30 meq/liter.[96,952] Normalization of the serum bicarbonate concentration during the entire interdialytic period has been achieved with a dialysate bicarbonate concentration of 40 meq/liter. However, buffer concentrations of this magnitude can result in immediate

TABLE 40-6 • Acid balance in hemodialysis patients: Theoretical considerations

Acid addition	
From diet	420 mmol/week
Organic anion loss during dialysis	300 mmol/week
Total	720 mmol/week
Alkali required: three dialysis treatments per week	240 mmol/dialysis
Dialysis specifications	
Duration	4 h
Buffer concentration	
Acetate	37 mmol/liter
Bicarbonate	32 mmol/liter
Dialysance	
Acetate	120 ml/min
Bicarbonate	150 ml/min

	Acetate hemodialysis		Bicarbonate hemodialysis	
Predialysis plasma HCO_3, meq/liter	Net alkali, mmol	Alkali − 240, mmol	Net alkali, mmol	Alkali − 240, mmol
16	377	137	360	120
18	305	65	315	75
19	269	29	—	—
20	233	−7	270	30
22	161	−79	225	−15
24	—	—	180	−60

SOURCE: Modified from Gennari FJ: *Kidney Int* 28:678, 1985. Used by permission.

postdialysis bicarbonate values of 29 to 32 meq/liter, with a pH value of 7.52.[15] Alkalemic pH values following hemodialysis may have adverse effects due to tissue hypoxia resulting from a left shift of the oxygen dissociation curve (i.e., the Bohr effect).[298,1061,1148,1262] The occurrence of postdialysis alkalemia can be minimized by utilizing an optimal bicarbonate dialysate concentration for each patient.[461] The dialysate bicarbonate concentration selected will depend on the amount of interdialytic endogenous H^+ produced, the dialysance of bicarbonate, and the amount of ultrafiltration required. Oral base supplements have been used to achieve relatively normal interdialytic serum bicarbonate and pH values without producing postdialysis alkalemia.[1176] This therapy, however, has been associated with reductions in the ionized serum calcium concentration and increases in PTH levels.[167]

Gennari and Rimmer have recently presented a diagnostic approach for simple and mixed acid-base disturbances in patients with ESRD.[374,375] In their schema, it is assumed that under steady state hemodialysis and dietary conditions, stable bicarbonate, pH, and P_{CO_2} levels are achieved.[373] These values can be used as guides to indicate whether additional simple or mixed acid-base disorders are superimposed on the metabolic acidosis of chronic renal failure. In this regard, an abrupt fall of more than 4 meq/liter from a patient's usual serum bicarbonate value suggests the presence of a new metabolic acidosis.[374] The possibility of a fall in the serum bicarbonate level as a renal compensatory response to respiratory alkalosis need not be considered in these functionally anephric patients.[374] Although patients with ESRD are susceptible to all the usual causes of a high anion gap metabolic acidosis, there are some unique considerations in this patient population.[374] For example, in some forms of high anion gap metabolic acidosis (i.e., ketoacidosis), once the excess production of organic acids is halted, patients with ESRD may have an advantage over those with normal kidney function in that the entire amount of organic anions produced are retained and will eventually regenerate all of the bicarbonate that was consumed. In contrast, in metabolic acidosis secondary to toxic ingestion (e.g., methanol), the toxic organic acids produced cannot be eliminated by renal mechanisms, and immediate hemodialysis will be required. Most of the usual causes of hyperchloremic metabolic acidosis are not applicable in the patient with ESRD, with the exception of gastrointestinal losses of alkali.[374] The replacement of bicarbonate-rich ultrafiltrate in the interdialytic period with alkali-free fluids will also result in a dilutional hyperchloremic metabolic acidosis.[374] A unique, but fortunately uncommon, cause of severe metabolic acidosis in hemodialysis patients may occur during dialysis if acid dialysate concentrate used to prepare bicarbonate dialysate (see "Alkali: Acetate, Bicarbonate, and Lactate" under "Hemodialysis Solutions") is mistakenly used instead of acetate dialysate concentrate.[140,375]

Gennari and Rimmer further suggest that an increase in the serum bicarbonate concentration of at least 4 to 5 meq/liter from its equilibrium value should suggest the presence of a metabolic alkalosis.[375] In contrast to individuals with normal renal function, patients with ESRD require only the addition of exogenous alkali or the loss of endogenous acid (e.g., through vomiting) to generate and sustain an increase in the serum bicarbonate concentration.[375] Again, because of the absence of renal compensatory responses, the possibility of chronic respiratory acidosis as the cause of a substantial increase in the serum bicarbonate concentration need not be considered in patients with ESRD. In addition, causes of metabolic alkalosis, such as mineralocorticoid excess, that depend on increased renal bicarbonate synthesis are not pertinent in this patient population. Loss of gastric acid is probably the most common cause of metabolic alkalosis in patients with ESRD.[65,375,946,1132] As previously discussed, metabolic alkalosis can also result from dialysate buffer concentrations that are too high. Other sources of exogenous alkali need to be considered as well.[375] Coadministration of nonabsorbable antacids (aluminum or magnesium hydroxide) with either the cation exchange resin sodium polystyrene sulfonate (Kayexelate) or neutral phosphate has been reported to cause metabolic alkalosis in hemodialysis patients.[692] In the stomach, the magnesium or aluminum forms insoluble complexes with the resin or phosphate that are eliminated in the stool. This interaction prevents aluminum or magnesium from combining with intestinal bicarbonate to form insoluble carbonate salts, as they normally do; the bicarbonate is therefore free to be reabsorbed into the blood. The presence of renal failure prevents the excess bicarbonate from being excreted by the kidneys, and hence metabolic alkalosis results.

Regional citrate infusion is used as an alternative to heparin for anticoagulation during hemodialysis in patients who are at high risk of bleeding.[926] Metabolic alkalosis may result from entry into the systemic circulation of citrate not removed by the dialyzer and its subsequent metabolism to bicarbonate. Most patients undergoing regional citrate hemodialysis do not develop a significant postdialysis alkalemia, although the rise in the serum bicarbonate concentration may be greater with regional citrate anticoagulation than during dialysis with heparin anticoagulation.[1091,1205] In some cases, however, the rise is considerable, with postdialysis serum bicarbonate concentrations ranging from 30 to 38 meq/liter.[555,1091]

The presence of metabolic alkalosis in ESRD patients presents unique treatment considerations. Conventional therapy with saline solution or potassium chloride is usually not possible, due to a severely impaired GFR.

Administration of acidifying agents undesirably adds further volume and nitrogen (in the form of ammonium chloride and arginine hydrochloride).[1132] In most ESRD patients, elevations of the serum bicarbonate concentration above 40 meq/liter are unusual, since standard hemodialysis procedures remove bicarbonate when the serum level equals or exceeds this value.[375] Usually, all that is required for correction of metabolic alkalosis is an elimination of the alkali source. If a more rapid reduction in the serum bicarbonate concentration is required, hemodialysis using a low acetate or bicarbonate (18 to 20 meq/liter) and high chloride dialysate can be used.[1132]

Patients with ESRD who develop a primary respiratory acidosis or alkalosis are able to generate an acute compensatory buffer response, but this response will not change the serum bicarbonate concentration by more than 2 to 4 meq/liter.[375] Because the quantitatively more important renal compensatory responses are absent in this patient population, ESRD patients are more susceptible to extreme pH changes as a result of a primary respiratory acid-base disturbance.[375] If the underlying cause of the respiratory acid-base disturbance cannot be corrected, the best approach is to tailor the hemodialysis prescription in such a manner as to produce serum bicarbonate concentrations that will counter the primary respiratory acid-base disturbance. For example, in primary respiratory acidosis, bicarbonate hemodialysis would be preferred over acetate hemodialysis, while with primary respiratory alkalosis the reverse would be true.[375] One unusual cause of respiratory acidosis in the ESRD population results from the use of bicarbonate dialysate with an acid pH to avoid calcium precipitation. Since the bicarbonate concentration is above normal, it is not surprising that these solutions also have extremely high P_{CO_2} values.[1209] Although most hemodialysis patients are capable of eliminating any CO_2 transferred across the dialyzer membrane, in some patients arterial P_{CO_2} values above 60 mmHg have been recorded.[1209] Thus, special attention should be given to the final pH of bicarbonate dialysate in patients whose respiratory drive is impaired (e.g., ventilator-dependent patients). Because of reactions within the sorbent cartridge, hemodialysis with the REDY (from REcirculation DialYsis) sorbent dialysis system results in a dialysate characterized by low pH and high P_{CO_2} values[976] and has also caused respiratory acidosis in susceptible patients (see "Sorbent Regeneration Dialysis").[443]

ELECTROLYTE DISTURBANCES

The patient with ESRD on maintenance hemodialysis can experience a wide array of electrolyte abnormalities. With the progression of chronic renal insufficiency, adaptations by the diseased kidneys allow balance to be maintained for water and various solutes.[126] Thus, normal body homeostasis, including normal concentration in ECF, is preserved for sodium, potassium, calcium, magnesium, bicarbonate, and other solutes, despite a fall in GFR. These compensatory adjustments are achieved by a variety of physical, neural, and hormonal factors that affect residual glomerular and tubular function.[126] However, with continued loss of glomerular filtration, adaptive control systems begin to fail, and disturbances in homeostasis ensue.

Electrolyte disturbances that arise as a consequence of complications in routine hemodialysis therapy will be considered next.

Disturbances of serum sodium concentration

Hypernatremia

As renal insufficiency progresses to the point that the patient requires dialysis therapy, the role of the kidney in sodium and water balance becomes negligible. In this setting, predialysis serum sodium concentration depends primarily on the relative proportions of salt and water ingestion during the interdialytic period.

Because of the high diffusibility of sodium across the dialyzer membrane, the serum sodium concentration following a hemodialysis treatment reflects the dialysate sodium concentration.[122,579] Dialysate sodium concentrations in excess of 140 meq/liter not only result in postdialysis hypernatremia but may cause significant thirst and interdialytic weight gain, with the potential for worsening of hypertension and congestive heart failure.[213,987,1027,1247]

Accidents in the dialysate delivery system may cause hypernatremia.[570] This condition may result from malfunction of the proportioning pump used to mix concentrated dialysate and water; a leaky valve in a batch system, allowing delivery of incompletely diluted concentrate; and inaccurate conductivity meters.[102,570,654] Hypernatremia from accidents in the water purification system has previously been discussed (see "Water Purification Systems").[818] Regional anticoagulation with trisodium citrate has been reported to cause mild hypernatremia when higher than usual citrate concentrations are used.[926]

Hyponatremia

The most common cause of hyponatremia in hemodialysis patients is the indiscrete ingestion of water during the interdialytic period. Impaired water excretion was probably responsible for the observation that 27 percent of patients with ESRD were found to be hyponatremic at the initiation of chronic hemodialysis therapy.[709] The ability of dialysate with a low sodium concentration to cause postdialysis hyponatremia was previously discussed.[122,1116] Malfunction of the dialysate delivery system may also produce hyponatric dialysate, which may cause massive hemolysis in addition to other systemic symptoms.[570,1024] Prevention of hypo- and hypernatremia resulting from problems in the dialysate delivery and water treatment systems require careful surveillance of the equipment involved. The final conductivity of the dialysate must be monitored prior to and during the hemodialysis treatment.[570]

Disturbances of serum potassium concentration

Hypokalemia

Predialysis hypokalemia is infrequently observed in hemodialysis patients due to the absence of normal renal excretory mechanisms. The ESRD patient nonetheless may develop hypokalemia and/or total body potassium depletion as a result of dietary potassium restriction, gastrointestinal losses, or frequent dialysis treatments with a low potassium dialysate concentration, although the occasional use of potassium-free dialysate is unlikely to cause significant hypokalemia (see "Potassium" under "Hemodialysis Solutions").[498] In addition, dialysis may induce respiratory alkalosis and at times metabolic alkalosis. These disorders could result in the movement of potassium from the ECF to the ICF, thereby causing hypokalemia without affecting total body potassium content.[293,787,999]

Dialysis-mediated worsening of hypokalemia has been described in some chronic renal failure patients who present with hypokalemia and metabolic acidosis.[1246] Hemodialysis with dialysate potassium concentrations exceeding predialysis serum potassium concentrations and administration of supplemental sodium bicarbonate unexpectedly resulted in postdialysis serum potassium levels that were lower than predialysis values by an average of 20 percent; in some cases, profound hypokalemia (potassium ≤2.6 meq/liter) developed. It was suggested that these patients were initially depleted of total body potassium; with correction of the metabolic acidosis by hemodialysis and the supplemental sodium bicarbonate, ECF potassium moved into cells at a rate that exceeded the diffusion of potassium from dialysate to blood.[1246]

Hemodialysis-mediated hypokalemia can result in hypotension, fatigue, and muscular weakness. Of greater concern, however, is the potential for cardiac arrhythmias. Morrison and associates demonstrated that some patients develop an increased frequency of premature ventricular contractions or complex ventricular arrhythmias during hemodialysis.[793] Differences in pre- and postdialysis potassium levels may not distinguish patients who would develop arrhythmias from those who would not.[793,966] Weber and coworkers, however, demonstrated that patients with premature ventricular contractions had lower postdialysis serum potassium concentrations than did patients who were arrhythmia-free.[1223] In Morrison's study, increasing the dialysate potassium concentration from 2.0 to 3.5 meq/liter reduced the frequency of arrhythmias in patients who experienced arrhythmias with the lower dialysate potassium concentration, although at the expense of a higher predialysis serum potassium level.[793] Others have suggested that the rapidity of serum potassium reduction during dialysis is more important in the pathogenesis of intradialytic arrhythmias than is the postdialysis serum potassium concentration.[573] Bicarbonate hemodialysis has been associated with less frequent ventricular arrhythmias and higher postdialysis intraerythrocyte potassium levels than has acetate hemodialysis, possibly due to improved correction of acidosis.[316] Although these reports suggest that potassium plays a major role in the genesis of arrhythmias during hemodialysis, other factors have also been shown to be of pathogenetic significance.[426,579a,793,966] Patients on digitalis who received dialysis with low-potassium dialysate experienced a greater incidence of arrhythmias than that recorded after the digitalis was discontinued.[793] Thus, higher dialysate potassium concentrations are recommended for hemodialysis patients receiving digitalis preparations. Finally, not all investigators have demonstrated serious ventricular arrhythmias during hemodialysis, even with very low to absent dialysate potassium concentrations.[498,613,1223,1255]

Hyperkalemia

Along with total body potassium excess, hyperkalemia is a common accompaniment of acute or chronic oliguric renal failure. In one study, 25 percent of ESRD patients were found to be hyperkalemic at the time of initiation of maintenance hemodialysis therapy.[709] Because of its cardiac toxicity, hyperkalemia can be life-threatening and still contributes to the mortality of long-term hemodialysis therapy.[144] Most hyperkalemia in hemodialysis patients is due to inadequate dietary restrictions and/or dialytic removal of potassium.[1168] Generally, it is necessary to restrict the dietary intake of potassium to 40 to 60 meq/day. Particular attention must be given to avoidance of foods high in potassium content. Assuming satisfactory patient compliance, a significant portion of the 280 to 420 meq of potassium ingested weekly must be removed by hemodialysis to prevent hyperkalemia (see "Potassium" under "Hemodialysis Solutions"). Enhanced gastrointestinal excretion and residual urine output also contribute to maintenance of normal serum potassium concentrations in patients with ESRD.[1107] The observation that spironolactone administration to anephric hemodialysis patients significantly increases the serum potassium level supports the importance of extrarenal potassium elimination.[904]

Other factors common to hemodialysis patients

that may cause hyperkalemia include increased catabolism, metabolic acidosis, hyperosmolar states, and hemolysis.[807] Hyperosmolar states that have caused hyperkalemia in patients with renal failure include hyperglycemia,[784,1168] excessive mannitol use,[119] and the infusion of hypertonic saline solution.[204] The mechanism appears to be a redistribution of potassium from the ICF to the ECF that accompanies the fluid shifts induced by ECF hyperosmolality. Hemolysis has been reported during hemodialysis following accidental exposure to sodium hypochlorite, formaldehyde, overheated or hyper- or hypotonic dialysate, and excess chloramines.[499,570,679,780,1050]

Use of specific drugs has been associated with hyperkalemia in hemodialysis patients. The ACE inhibitors have been reported to increase serum potassium levels,[903] although this has not been a universal observation.[62] As noted above, spironolactone has caused hyperkalemia in hemodialysis patients, including patients who are anephric.[904] Massive ingestion of digoxin is a well-recognized cause of hyperkalemia.[1248] This phenomenon has also been observed in an ESRD patient who ingested therapeutic amounts of digoxin with only a modest increase in the serum digoxin level.[902] The digoxin-induced hyperkalemia in this case may have been enhanced by the concomitant use of propranolol (see below). The administration of recombinant human EPO to correct anemia of renal failure has been associated with a rise in the serum potassium concentration in some patients, sometimes to dangerous levels.[309,1277] Increased appetite and protein intake and decreased hemodialytic clearance of potassium have been suggested as possible mechanisms.[7]

Hemodialysis patients using beta-blockers may be more susceptible to hyperkalemia. Stimulation of beta 2–adrenergic receptors has been shown to facilitate intracellular movement of potassium.[88,1263] Blockade of these receptors with propranolol and other beta-blockers has been reported to increase serum potassium levels in hemodialysis patients by an average of 0.7 to 1.0 meq/liter.[48,894,1263] Thus, if beta-blockers are required in ESRD patients, the use of cardioselective agents may be preferable,[48,894,1263] although hyperkalemia has been reported with these drugs as well.[58] Particular attention should be given to hemodialysis patients using beta-blockers who exercise, because exercise-induced increases in serum potassium concentration[627,675,816] are significantly enhanced by beta 2–receptor blockade.[164,1107]

Less common causes of hyperkalemia in hemodialysis patients have also been reported. McIvor and colleagues described a patient hemodialyzed with fluoride-contaminated dialysate who developed cardiopulmonary arrest associated with severe hyperkalemia.[753] Experimentally, administration of fluoride to animals results in hyperkalemia, with peaked T waves and ventricular fibrillation.[71] This may be due to a toxic effect of fluoride on cell membranes, allowing potassium to leak out. Both geophagia and cautopyreiophagia (ingestion of burnt match heads) have been reported to cause severe hyperkalemia in dialysis patients.[5,371] It has also been suggested that hyperkalemia may be more common in hemodialysis patients who have had a colectomy, which entails loss of a potential extrarenal site of potassium elimination.[452,962]

Elucidation of the relationship between beta-adrenergic receptors and the transcellular movement of potassium[88] has resulted in the demonstration that ESRD patients with hyperkalemia can be treated by beta 2-adrenergic stimulation. Albuterol, a selective beta 2 sympathomimetic agonist, has been shown to significantly lower serum potassium concentrations in hyperkalemic dialysis patients when administered intravenously (0.5 mg)[783] or inhaled in a nebulized preparation (10 or 20 mg).[24] With nebulized administration, the fall in serum potassium occurs by 30 min and persists for at least 2 h. The combination of aerosolized albuterol and intravenous glucose and insulin has a greater potassium-lowering effect than with either therapy alone.[23] Recently, the efficacy of a variety of therapies purported to correct hyperkalemia in hemodialysis patients was evaluated.[103] Intravenous sodium bicarbonate failed to demonstrate any potassium-lowering effect, and only a 50 percent response rate was observed after intravenous epinephrine. Others have also demonstrated that the potassium-lowering effect of beta 2–adrenergic stimulation in patients with ESRD was not uniform.[24,1263] The use of intravenous insulin and glucose or hemodialysis with a 1 meq/liter potassium dialysate have been shown to be the most effective treatments for correcting hyperkalemia in terms of magnitude, uniformity, and rate of response.[103]

Disturbances of serum calcium concentration

Hypocalcemia

Hypocalcemia is an anticipated consequence of the altered divalent ion metabolism that characterizes chronic renal insufficiency. In the uremic milieu, vitamin D deficiency, phosphate retention, and PTH resistance all contribute to a low serum calcium concentration. In one study, 40 percent of uremic patients had serum calcium levels below the normal range.[150] Both total and ionized calcium levels may be depressed; the magnitude of these reductions correlates with the severity of the renal insufficiency.[150,734] Serum calcium levels tend to be lower when primary osteomalacia accounts for the renal osteodystrophy.[734,1112] In general, severe hypocalcemia ($<$6.5 mg/dl, or $<$1.62 mmol/liter) from renal failure per se is unusual.[734] Hypocalcemic patients usually become normocalcemic upon initiation of hemodialysis, while no significant changes are seen in patients whose serum calcium values were not initially depressed.[734]

Parathyroidectomy for severe secondary hyperparathyroidism has been frequently performed in the hemodialysis population. Acute hypocalcemia is common following surgury and may be due to the excess removal of parathyroid tissue, transient hypofunction of an autotransplanted parathyroid gland, or avid skeletal uptake of calcium by poorly mineralized bone ("hungry bone syndome").[233,262,287] Serious postoperative hypocalcemia can be prevented by the use of high calcium concentrations in the dialysate and calcium and vitamin D supplements.

Heparinized plasma stored for several hours at room temperature may falsely lower serum calcium values in hemodialysis patients.[95,188,387,879] Heparin activation of lipoprotein lipase hydrolyzes triglycerides to free fatty acids, which in turn combine with calcium to form an insoluble soap.[387] The use of oral alkali therapy to correct metabolic acidosis in dialysis patients decreases ionized calcium concentrations (total calcium levels remain unchanged) and thereby increases PTH.[167] Regional citrate anticoagulation in dialysis patients at high risk for bleeding can cause hypocalcemia.[792] Current techniques for citrate anticoagulation employ calcium-free dialysate to minimize citrate requirements. This method results in the return of calcium-depleted blood to the patient due to dialytic removal of the calcium-citrate complex.[926] Hypocalcemia is prevented by the infusion of supplemental calcium into the venous blood line, which in some cases may cause mild postdialysis hypercalcemia.[670] More recently, a modification of this technique has been associated with cardiac arrest presumed to be secondary to hypocalcemia from citrate toxicity.[176]

Hypercalcemia

Hypercalcemia may result from high calcium concentrations in dialysate or from contamination of dialysate with water containing significant amounts of calcium ("hard water syndrome"; see "Water Purification System"). High dialysate calcium concentrations and the use of calcium salts and vitamin D metabolites for treatment of renal osteodystrophy are the most common causes of hypercalcemia in hemodialysis patients (see below). Spontaneous hypercalcemia has been observed in dialysis patients with aluminum-induced osteomalacia.[127,189,928] Although the majority of hemodialysis patients with secondary hyperparathyroidism do not have elevated serum calcium levels, this condition can occasionally cause frank hypercalcemia.[28] This phenomenon has been referred to as tertiary hyperparathyroidism and is the result of parathyroid hyperplasia, as well as an altered set point for PTH secretion and an inability to reduce parathyroid cell PTH secretion below a basal level. Under these circumstances, parathyroidectomy had been the indicated treatment.[760] However, many of these patients have coexistent aluminum-induced osteomalacia, and parathyroidectomy in this setting has been demonstrated to worsen the osteomalacia component of the bone disease.[328]

Vitamin D therapy, commonly prescribed for hemodialysis patients, may cause hypercalcemia. Hypercalcemia is more protracted when caused by vitamin D_3 or 25-hydroxyvitamin D_3 than when caused by 1,25-$(OH)_2D_3$ because of the longer half-lives of the first two compounds. Approximately 30 to 67 percent of patients treated with oral 1,25-$(OH)_2D_3$ develop hypercalcemia, which is more common with dosages of 1.0 μg/day, or more.[737] An increased sensitivity to hypercalcemia from vitamin D therapy is seen in patients with severe secondary hyperparathyroidism[737] or pure osteomalacia.[189,493]

The use of the calcium salts of carbonate, citrate, or acetate as oral phosphorus binders is commonly complicated by the development of hypercalcemia, which is usually asymptomatic.[38,214,350,399,488,687,710,762,791,1099] The frequency of hypercalcemia in dialysis patients receiving oral calcium carbonate has been estimated to range from 25 to 33 percent.[38,762] Hypercalcemia in these patients is probably due to gastrointestinal absorption of the large amounts of calcium ingested.[967,1068] As previously discussed (see "Calcium" under "Hemodialysis Solutions"), this phenomenon is more likely to occur with dialysate calcium concentrations of 1.5 mmol/liter or more. Other risk factors for the development of hypercalcemia with these agents include coadministration of vitamin D metabolites, decreased physical activity, and renal osteodystrophy that is aluminum-related or associated with low bone turnover rates.[399,488,762,1099] Serial measurements of the serum calcium concentration are obviously essential for diagnosing and initiating treatment for hypercalcemia. If hypercalcemia from calcium carbonate therapy is to occur, it does so soon after initiating treatment.[762] The hypercalcemia can be corrected by reducing the dose of calcium salt, which may necessitate decreasing the dietary phosphorus load and prescribing aluminum or magnesium hydroxide to prevent recurrent hyperphosphatemia. A more ideal approach, however, is a reduction in the dialysate calcium concentration to less than 1.5 mmol/liter (see "Calcium" under "Hemodialysis Solutions"). In patients with aluminum-induced osteomalacia, chelation treatment for deferoxamine may allow the reinstitution of oral calcium salts without recurrence of hypercalcemia.[488]

Hypercalcemia in hemodialysis patients has also been reported to occur from the treatment of hyperkalemia with calcium-containing ion exchange resins[905] and with severe hypophosphatemia.[109] A few patients have been described who developed significant hypercalcemia after initiation of hemodialysis therapy.[530] Although the mechanism is unclear, hypercalcemia in this instance does not appear to be due to excess PTH, vitamin D or calcium ingestion, severe hypophosphatemia, or high dialysate calcium concentrations. Finally, the ESRD patient is, of course, equally susceptible to nondialysis-related causes of hypercalcemia (see Chap. 32).

Disturbances of serum phosphate concentration

Hyperphosphatemia

Elevation of the serum phosphate concentration in hemodialysis patients is common and has been clearly demonstrated to contribute to the pathogenesis of renal osteodystrophy (see Chap. 41). Methods used to maintain the serum phosphate concentration in the normal range in these patients include reduction of dietary phosphorus intake, hemodialysis, and use of oral phosphorus binders.[328]

Dietary phosphorus is derived primarily from dairy products and protein. In North America, the average daily intake of phosphorus ranges between 1400 and 2000 mg.[487,796] Hemodialysis patients may ingest somewhat less phosphorus; one study found that intake ranged from 650 to 1400 mg/day (mean, 940 ± 46 mg), with the largest amount ingested at dinner.[1098] Protein reduction to 40 g/day can decrease the daily phosphorus intake to 790 mg.[796] The intestinal absorption of phosphorus is highly efficient in normal subjects, who absorb 80 percent of an oral phosphorus load.[967] Hemodialysis patients absorb phosphorus somewhat less efficiently (i.e., 60 percent of an oral load).[186,967]

During hemodialysis, the clearance of phosphate across the dialyzer is only 30 percent of the clearance of urea[1256] but is still adequate to remove a significant amount (600 to 1000 mg).[93,497] The amount of phosphorus removed during dialysis is directly correlated with the predialysis serum phosphate concentration[165,397,497,930,1283] and inversely correlated with the hematocrit value.[397] The clearance of phosphorus can be increased by larger-surface area dialyzer membranes and ultrafiltration but is unaffected by membrane composition.[796,1283] Some investigators have demonstrated greater phosphate removal with bicarbonate than with acetate dialysis,[741] while others have not found any difference between these two buffers.[767]

Unlike the exponential falls in serum urea and creatinine levels during hemodialysis, serum phosphate levels fall during the first half but then remain stable or even rebound to higher levels during the second half of the dialysis treatment.[497,713,930,1124,1283] Thus, an increase in treatment time will not enhance phosphate removal. Predialysis serum phosphate levels are reached by approximately 10 h following the hemodialysis treatment. This rebound phenomenon is greater with acetate than with bicarbonate dialysate and could potentially modify the predialysis serum phosphate concentration.[1283] The amount of phosphorus removed during the hemodialysis treatment exceeds the loss of phosphorus predicted by the decline in the serum phosphate concentration during dialysis.[165] These observations suggest that the ECF phosphate concentration is significantly modulated by such intracellular phosphate compartments as bone.[930]

Due to the limitation of dietary phosphorus restriction, the efficient intestinal absorption rate, and limited clearance by hemodialysis, most dialysis patients require the use of oral phosphorus binders to prevent positive phosphorus balance and hyperphosphatemia.[497,796,987] Aluminum-containing compounds, aluminum hydroxide and aluminum carbonate, have been successfully used for years to prevent hyperphosphatemia. These compounds can result in intestinal losses of phosphorus that exceed intake when the daily dietary load of phosphorus is 1 g or less.[186,796] Another aluminum-containing preparation, sucralfate, has been shown to be as effective as aluminum hydroxide as an oral phosphorus binder, but its greater expense limits its usefulness.[1006] As previously stated, aluminum accumulation from these compounds can result in significant skeletal, neurologic, and hematologic abnormalities (see Chap. 41).[20,184,185] As a result, there has been increasing usage of nonaluminum compounds as oral phosphorus binders. Studies evaluating the efficacy of the hydroxide and carbonate salts of magnesium as oral phosphorus binders have produced mixed results.[428,527,862,863] The use of these compounds is limited by the occurrence of hypermagnesemia and diarrhea (see "Magnesium" under "Hemodialysis Solutions" and "Hypermagnesemia" under "Disturbances of Serum Magnesium").[428]

The carbonate, citrate, and acetate salts of calcium have become increasingly popular as nonaluminum-containing phosphorus binders, with the largest experience being reported with calcium carbonate.[38,214,350,399,488,687,710,791,1033,1099] The daily dose of calcium carbonate required to prevent hyperphosphatemia has ranged from 1 to 20 g.[1036] Calcium carbonate decreases phosphorus absorption as effectively as aluminum hydroxide.[967] Although calcium citrate has also been shown to be an effective oral phosphorus binder,[212,817] citrate increases aluminum absorption from the gastrointestinal tract, limiting the clinical utility of this compound as a phosphorus binder.[779] Most recently, calcium acetate has been demonstrated to be a more efficient phosphorus binder than either calcium carbonate or citrate.[304,707,1035,1068] Unlike calcium carbonate, calcium acetate remains effective at high gastric pH values and is less likely to cause hypercalcemia (see above).[304,707,1035,1068] All of the calcium salts may cause hypercalcemia, diarrhea, and soft tissue calcification from the insolubility of calcium-phosphate complexes. Finally, preliminary data suggest that calcium-containing polymers of uronic acid[487,812] and ketoacids[1035,1206] can be effective oral phosphorus binders. However, there is no evidence that these compounds are more effective than calcium carbonate or acetate, but they are more expensive.

Noncompliance with dietary phosphorus restriction and oral phosphorus binders are, not unexpectedly, the most common causes of hyperphosphatemia in hemodialysis patients. Inadequate dialysis can also result in elevated serum phosphate levels, despite increased use of phosphorus-binding antacids.[449] Vitamin D and its metabolites have variable effects on serum phosphate levels. Increases in the serum phosphate level can occur from enhancement of gastrointestinal absorption of phosphorus by vitamin D, while decreases may result from the vitamin's ability to suppress hyperparathyroidism.[186,737,967] Severe secondary hyperparathyroidism can aggravate hyperphosphatemia that is unresponsive to phosphorus-binding antacids by accelerating bone reabsorption and releasing phosphate into the circulation.[740] Metabolic acidosis in ESRD patients can aggravate or cause hyperphosphatemia.[77,246] Correction of metabolic acidosis will lower the serum phosphate concentration without any change in the total body pool of phosphorus, suggesting that acidosis favors a movement of phosphate from ICF to ECF.[77] Further support of this relationship is provided by the observation of an inverse correlation between serum phosphate and bicarbonate concentrations.[280] Laxatives containing phosphate salts (commonly given in preparation for radiologic bowel procedures or endoscopy) should be avoided in ESRD patients because they can cause both severe hyperphosphatemia and hypocalcemia, even in patients with normal renal function.[182,750,893,1241] Hemolysis from damage to erythrocytes during centrifugation may falsely elevate the serum phosphate level.[1101]

Hypophosphatemia

Noniatrogenic causes of hypophosphatemia are unusual in hemodialysis patients. Hypophosphatemia in this population is most commonly due to excessive doses of phosphorus-binding compounds,[3] often in association with a decrease in the phosphorus content of the diet. Patients with acute renal failure receiving parenteral nutrition frequently develop profound hypophosphatemia.[607] Hypophosphatemia can also occur following parathyroidectomy due to the rapid bone remineralization that occurs in the immediate postoperative period ("hungry bone syndrome").[262,319,636,740] Less commonly, some hemodialysis patients may demonstrate a low predialysis phosphate level despite a normal diet and the absence of phosphate-binding antacids. This may be due to a marked decrease in intestinal phosphorus absorption.[1064]

It has been suggested the hypophosphatemia in dialysis patients can cause osteomalacia.[186,706,925] Because of the correlation between predialysis phosphate levels and the dialytic removal of phosphorus, the critical predialysis phosphate concentration necessary to avoid postdialysis hypophosphatemia can be predicted.[1212] Several techniques have been described for adding phosphate to the dialysis solution for correction of hypophosphatemia.[512,548,925] These techniques may require supplemental dialysate calcium to avoid hypocalcemia.[548]

Disturbances of serum magnesium concentration

Hypermagnesemia

It is not surprising that, with the loss of renal function, patients with severe chronic renal insufficiency not yet receiving hemodialysis therapy commonly manifest mild asymptomatic hypermagnesemia (about 1.96 meq/liter; see also Chap. 34.)[187,398,733a] In addition to the effects of chronic renal insufficiency and the selection of dialysate with relatively high magnesium concentrations,[733a] other mechanisms may cause hypermagnesemia in the hemodialysis population. The accidental use of dialysate with a magnesium concentration of 15 meq/liter has been reported to have resulted in flushing, muscular weakness, hyporeflexia, ataxia, and blurred vision.[414] Hypermagnesemia may also result from the "hard water syndrome." This syndrome, described earlier, is usually characterized by excessive calcium concentrations in the tap water used for dialysis. However, modest amounts of magnesium are also present and may contribute to the clinical manifestations of this syndrome.[282,354] The occurrence of hypertension, nausea, and vomiting has been attributed to calcium, whereas magnesium has been implicated in the development of CNS disturbances and hypotension.

Symptomatic hypermagnesemia may occur in patients with chronic renal insufficiency who consume magnesium-containing antacids or laxatives.[101,330,794,969] Recently, magnesium hydroxide has been recommended as an oral phosphorus binder in the hope of decreasing aluminum toxicity.[428,527,862,863] Dosages of magnesium hydroxide varying between 0.75 and 3.0 g/day resulted in mild hypermagnesemia (mean value, 3.6 meq/liter), although in some patients serum magnesium concentrations exceeded 4.5 meq/liter (see "Magnesium" under "Hemodialysis Solutions").[428]

Hypomagnesemia

Due to the loss of renal magnesium excretion, hypomagnesemia is unusual in hemodialysis patients.[738,807] Potential causes of hypomagnesemia include intracellular accumulation from hyperalimentation, rapid bone accretion following parathyroidectomy, and gastrointestinal losses.[807] Hypomagnesemia may contribute to cardiac arrhythmias during dialysis, especially if the patient is receiving digoxin.[171]

Disturbances of serum glucose concentration

Hyperglycemia

The early use of high dialysate glucose concentrations for ultrafiltration[761] occasionally caused severe hyperglycemia[940] and postdialysis hypoglycemia, the latter from an insulin overshoot effect.[41,431] Smaller increases in dialysate glucose concentrations used to minimize osmolarity changes during hemodialysis may cause mild hyperglycemia. In one report, a dialysate glucose concentration of 400 mg/dl resulted in a mean blood glucose level of 151 mg/dl.[639] Severe hyperglycemia in diabetic patients receiving maintenance hemodialysis therapy results in pathophysiologic disturbances different from the effects in patients with intact renal function.[1162,1164,1169] The usual osmotic diuresis consequent to hyperglycemia, leading to volume contraction and hypertonicity with neurologic manifestations in nonuremic individuals, obviously cannot occur in the ESRD population.[1169] Instead, these patients present with evidence of volume expansion (circulatory overload), which can be corrected solely by the administration of insulin. In addition, the hyperglycemia results in intense thirst, which explains the normal to slightly increased ECF (effective) osmolality (reflecting excess total body water) observed in many of these patients upon presentation.[1169] In these cases, correction of hyperglycemia will expose persistent hyponatremia and may require immediate hemodialysis to avoid symptoms of water intoxication.[1164]

Hypoglycemia

Significant hypoglycemia has been frequently reported in hemodialysis patients.[37,64,74,100,135,320,360,366,632,918,1022,1240] Conversely, renal failure is one of the most common factors contributing to hypoglycemia in hospitalized patients.[41,338] Low blood sugar levels in patients with ESRD may result from spontaneous hypoglycemia of uremia (SHU) or uremic hypoglycemia, rather than from a specific drug, illness, or the hemodialysis process itself. In patients with SHU, the low blood sugar is usually transient but on occasion can be severe and prolonged, with single or recurrent episodes. Usually neuroglycopenic symptoms, and not those mediated by catecholamines, predominate.[41] The occurrence of this entity carries a poor prognosis, with a mortality rate of at least 50 percent.[41] Hypoglycemia itself, however, is not the immediate cause of death in most patients.[1150] The diagnosis of SHU should be made only after drug effects, overt liver disease, sepsis, and endocrine abnormalities such as adrenal insufficiency, hypopituitarism, and an insulinoma are excluded.[37,41] Although the cause of SHU remains unclear, impaired gluconeogenesis and glycogenolysis, hepatic dysfunction, diminished caloric intake, reductions in insulin degradation, and decreased counterregulatory hormonal responses are likely contributors.[41,366,918,964,1275] A recent review of this entity has questioned the appropriateness of the terms SHU and uremic hypoglycemia.[1150] In the opinion of the authors, uremia alone rarely results in significant hypoglycemia. Instead, it is suggested that most patients diagnosed with this entity had other associated factors—malnutrition, drugs, infection, glucose-free dialysate, and multiorgan failure—any one of which could adequately explain the hypoglycemia.[1150]

In most patients with ESRD, hypoglycemia is secondary to a drug or associated illness known to decrease blood glucose even in patients with normal renal function.[41] Nonetheless, in many of these instances, impaired renal function is a predisposing factor. Insulin therapy is one of the most common causes of hypoglycemia in patients with renal insufficiency due to impaired degradation and clearance of the hormone.[41,207,338] Sulfonylureas, especially first-generation agents such as chlorpropamide, tolbutamide, and acetohexamide, are frequently observed to cause hypoglycemia in diabetic patients with renal failure.[41,1060] As with insulin, the mechanism for hypoglycemia is a prolonged duration of action as a result of the requirement for renal elimination of these drugs or their metabolites. Second-generation sulfonylureas, such as glyburide or glipizide, are primarily metabolized in the liver and thus less likely to cause hypoglycemia in patients with impaired renal function.[41,69,914] Other drugs implicated in hypoglycemia in ESRD patients include propoxyphene, sulfonamides, salicylates, disopyramide, and beta-blockers.[40,41,232,359,945]

The use of the beta-blocking agent propranolol for the treatment of hypertension in hemodialysis patients has been associated with several reports of hypoglycemia.[64,417,528,1028,1275] Propranolol alone is capable of interfering with several metabolic processes that defend against a low blood sugar level (e.g., hepatic glycogenolysis, glucagon release, and lipolysis).[1275] Thus, it is not surprising that hypoglycemia can result when these effects of beta-adrenergic blockade are superimposed on the impaired glucose metabolism seen in uremia. The treatment of hyperkalemia in hemodialysis patients with intravenous insulin and dextrose (10 units regular insulin and 25 g dextrose) also has been reported to cause significant hypoglycemia in a large number of patients.[24,103] Since this is a highly effective therapy for hyperkalemia, smaller doses of insulin than previously recommended should be used. Hemodialysis during parenteral hyperalimentation using solutions with high dextrose concentrations and insulin has been reported to cause hypoglycemia due to selective diffusion of glucose from blood to dialysate.[766] Severe hypoglycemia has also occurred with medication errors, such as the mistaken substitution of chlorpropamide (Diabinese) when the phosphorus binder aluminum hydroxide (Dialume) was prescribed.[190] Hypoglycemia has also been reported in a chronic hemodialysis patient after parathyroidectomy.[801] This case was associated with hyperinsulinemia, and possibly related to changes in PTH, vitamin D, and calcium levels. A more extensive discussion of hypoglycemia in renal failure can be found in the excellent review by Arem.[41]

PERITONEAL DIALYSIS

The concept that the peritoneum might clinically function as a dialyzing membrane dates back to the early 1920s.[364,813,941] Confirmation of the potential value of peritoneal dialysis in the treatment of uremia soon followed, but technical difficulties and frequent complications limited acceptance of the technique.[1,250,337,352,422,858] In 1959, Maxwell and colleagues[747] and Doolan and associates,[278] by virtue of technical improvements consisting of the design of a semirigid nylon catheter, standardized and commercially available dialyzing solutions, and a closed system of dialysate flow, established peritoneal dialysis as an effective, simple, and relatively safe therapeutic procedure.[149]

During this period, peritoneal dialysis was used primarily for the treatment of acute renal failure.[112] Widespread application in the treatment of chronic renal failure was limited by the need to puncture the peritoneum for catheter placement with each treatment, a relatively high rate of peritonitis, and the inconvenience of performing the dialysis exchanges manually.[255] However, with the development of a permanent silicone peritoneal catheter by Tenckhoff in 1968[1139] and automated peritoneal dialysis machines,[626,1137,1138] both of which minimized the potential for bacterial peritonitis, peritoneal dialysis became an acceptable alternative treatment to hemodialysis for ESRD. The introduction of ambulatory peritoneal dialysis techniques and equipment in the late 1970s[886,934,935] led to a tremendous growth of this therapy in the 1980s. At present, chronic peritoneal dialysis is practiced in more than 50 countries, maintaining more than 50,000 chronic renal failure patients worldwide.[389,827] The proportions of patients treated with peritoneal dialysis versus hemodialysis vary widely from country to country.[770,781] In the United States in 1991, 19,000 patients, approximately 17 percent of the dialysis population, were practicing chronic peritoneal dialysis.[827]

PRINCIPLES OF PERITONEAL DIALYSIS

Clearance

The two processes—diffusion and osmotic ultrafiltration—that largely govern peritoneal dialysis occur across a semipermeable dialyzing membrane,[700] the peritoneum, the size of which is thought to be equal to the total body surface area (1.8 m^2 for a 70-kg individual)[1225] or the area of the glomerular capillaries,[768] although only a fraction of the peritoneum is probably functionally available for dialysis transport.[468] Peritoneal clearance rates for small solutes such as urea are about one-sixth of those achieved during hemodialysis. However, the peritoneum is more permeable than hemodialysis membranes to solutes in the middle-molecular weight range (500 to 5000),[66,468,476] an observation that may have clinical relevance.[67,1137] The small but finite permeability of the peritoneum to large solutes results in the loss of approximately 10 g of protein per day in patients receiving chronic peritoneal dialysis.[105,288,554,1014]

Factors governing the peritoneal transport of solutes and water have been extensively reviewed.[113,600,683,700,704,828,845,848,932,1140,1153a] Increasing the volume of a given exchange increases net removal of small and large solutes by increasing drain volume, but infusate volume is limited by patient tolerance of peritoneal filling. The rate of equilibration of a solute between dialysate and plasma depends on its molecular weight and charge. Most small-molecular weight substances (e.g., urea) equilibrate completely within 4 to 6 h, whereas large solutes continue to equilibrate at an almost linear rate throughout the peritoneal dwelling of dialysate. Thus, large solute removal depends, not on the dialysate flow rate, but, rather, on the permeability and surface area of the peritoneum, along with the volume of dialysate and the net time spent in dwell. The higher permeability (as measured by the mass transfer area coefficient)[932,976,1153a] of small molecules imposes a greater dialysate flow limitation on their clearances. Therefore, when the dialysate flow rate is altered by modifying the frequency of exchanges, short dwells augment small molecule clearances, with little impact on large solute clearances. Alternatively, long-dwell peritoneal dialysis increases the clearance of large solutes out of proportion to the clearance of small-molecular weight solutes. Although the clearance of smaller solutes can be increased by more rapid exchanges, the intrinsic mass transfer area coefficient and the progressively lower proportion of effective dwell time during the exchange ultimately become limiting factors for net transport. Thus, average urea clearances of 10 to 12 and 18 to 20 ml/min are obtained at dialysate flow rates of 1 and 2 liter/h, respectively, but clearances plateau more abruptly at dialysate flow rates greater than 3.5 liter/h, and urea clearances reach a maximum of 35 to 40 ml/min at dialysate flow rates between 10 and 12 liter/h.[112,113,683,828,1140]

Osmolality of the dialysate influences solute clearance[476,600,683] both by affecting convective capture of solutes and by altering peritoneal blood flow and permeability. To lesser extents, dialysate pH and temperature may also alter solute transport.[507,600,828,1153a] Intrinsic patient characteristics also play a kinetic role; peritonitis enhances solute clearance,[600,1012] while lymphatic absorption of peritoneal fluid may reduce net solute clearance by 15 to 20 percent.[681,686,689]

Peritoneal capillary circulation is the major source of the solutes and fluid removed during peritoneal dialysis.[828] Total splanchnic blood flow approximates 1.2 liters/min,[208] but only a fraction of this flow participates in solute exchange.[828] Nonetheless, peritoneal blood flow rates are significantly higher than maximal clearance rates achieved for solutes such as urea.[828] Thus, small solute removal is not limited by solute delivery (i.e., by blood flow rate) but, rather, by a diffusion barrier composed of fluid films in blood and dialysate, endothelial and mesothelial cells, basement membrane, and interstitial fluid.[700,704,828,832,848,1153a] This diffusion barrier determines the individual's mass transfer area coefficient and permeability of the peritoneal dialyzing membrane. In this respect, peritoneal dialysis differs from hemodialysis, since clearance rates of small solutes with the latter technique have been shown to be strongly blood flow–dependent.[467]

Although the effect of a variety of pharmacologic agents on peritoneal transport has been examined[255,600,828,1008] and some have been found to augment clearances, none is in common clinical use.

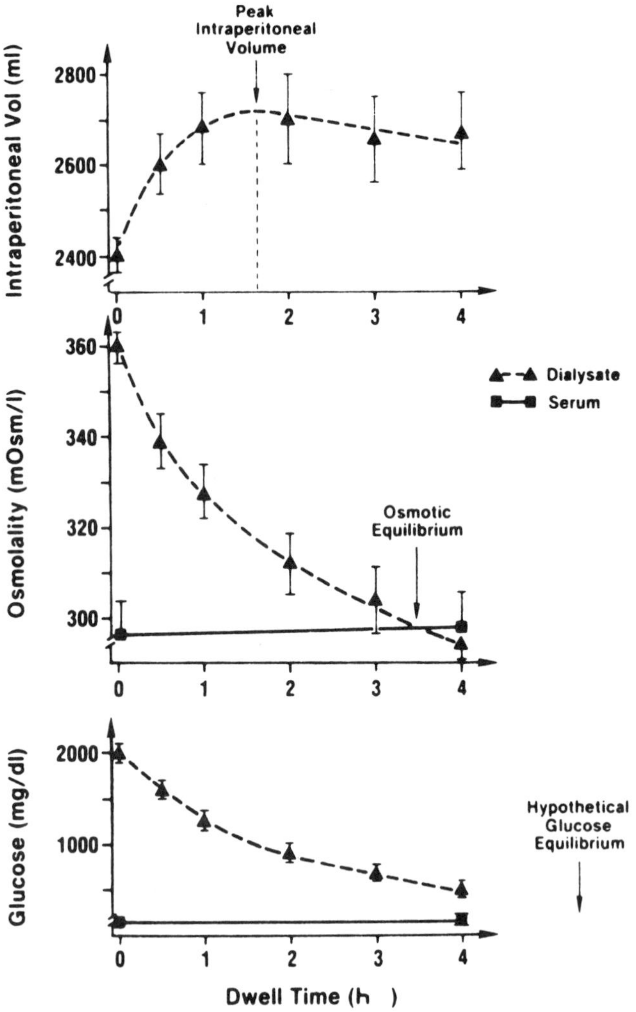

FIGURE 40-7 • Intraperitoneal volume, serum and dialysate osmolarity, and serum and dialysate glucose concentration (mean ± SEM) during 4-h exchanges using 2-liter, 2.5% glucose dialyzer solution ($n = 10$). Arrows indicate peak intraperitoneal volume, osmotic equilibrium, and hypothetical glucose equilibrium. (From Mactier RA et al: *J Clin Invest* 80:1311, 1987. By copyright permission of the American Society of Clinical Investigation.)

Ultrafiltration

Ultrafiltration across the peritoneal membrane[471,683,700,828,830,1153a] is achieved by osmotic equilibration between plasma and dialysate containing a slowly diffusable solute. The source of the ultrafiltrate has been attributed to transcapillary and predominantly intercellular fluid movement.[600,700,841] Typical net ultrafiltration profiles evoked by glucose in the dialysate have been characterized[683,942,1154a,1156] and depend on the hydraulic permeability of the peritoneal membrane and the effective osmotic gradient. This osmotic gradient itself falls exponentially during an exchange as glucose is simultaneously absorbed and diluted by the hypotonic ultrafiltrate (Fig. 40-7). Opposing the net accumulation of intraperitoneal volume from transcapillary ultrafiltration is the isotonic absorption of peritoneal fluid with all its constituents via peritoneal lymphatics.[575,681,683,686,689,828,832,835,1153a] This absorption occurs at a more constant rate (40 to 100 ml/h) than does ultrafiltration during an exchange. Thus, intraperitoneal volume peaks occur when the rate of transcapillary ultrafiltration declines to that of lymphatic absorption. Beyond that point, intraperitoneal volume progressively diminishes as the transcapillary ultrafiltration rate falls below the lymphatic absorption rate, and with prolonged cycles, drained volume can fall below the infusate volume. Transcapillary ultrafiltration ceases when the tonicity of plasma and dialysate equalize. This equalization of tonicities occurs after osmolar equilibration has been achieved because the total osmolality of the dialysate is composed of a greater percentage of effective osmoles (i.e., glucose; Fig. 40-8). The loss of intraperitoneal volume by lymphatic reabsorption reduces net ultrafiltration and clearances in peritoneal dialysis, having a greater impact on long-dwell regimens, in patients with hyperpermeable membranes (who rapidly lose their osmotic gradient) and in children.[574] Even in adults whose peritoneal transport properties are normal, an average of 387 ml of fluid is absorbed during a 4-h exchange, reducing the gross transcapillary ultrafiltration volume by 58 percent and the urea and creatinine clearances by 15 percent.[686,689,835]

Net ultrafiltration in peritoneal dialysis[683,700,1016] can be augmented by increasing the concentration of the osmotically active solute. The transcapillary ultrafiltration rate increases; generating later and higher peaks of intraperitoneal volume. Simply prolonging dwell time

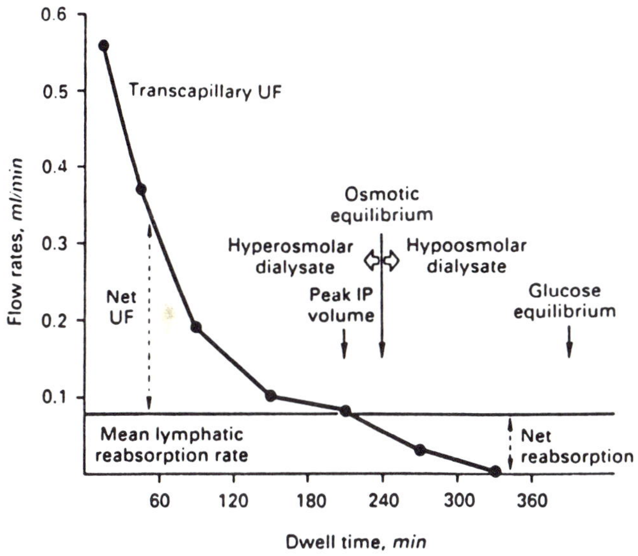

FIGURE 40-8 • Transcapillary ultrafiltration rate profile in a rat model of peritoneal dialysis in relation to lymphatic absorption, osmolar and glucose equilibrium points, and peak intraperitoneal (IP) volume. (From Nolph KD et al: *Kidney Int* 32:219, 1987. Used by permission.)

will achieve progressively smaller net increments in ultrafiltration and, with prolonged exchanges, net reabsorption may occur, causing fluid balance to become positive. Instilling a larger volume of dialysate yields a larger drain volume and increases net ultrafiltration, but this occurs at the expense of an increased glucose load (see below). Net ultrafiltration rates tend to fall transiently during peritonitis.[1012,1013] More persistent ultrafiltration failure (see below) has prompted investigation into other pharmacologic means of manipulating transperitoneal ultrafiltration,[269,492,603,683,690] although the role of such agents in long-term peritoneal dialysis patients awaits clarification.

Although solutes can accompany water flow during ultrafiltration by solvent drag (convective transport), the degree to which this occurs depends on the relative permeability (given by the sieving coefficient) of the solute across the membrane. In peritoneal dialysis, sodium and potassium removal during ultrafiltration are significantly limited, resulting in an ultrafiltrate in which the concentrations of these ions are lower than normally measured in the ECF.[828,841] This contrasts to the more nearly isotonic ultrafiltrate formed in hemodialysis.

APPLICATIONS OF PERITONEAL DIALYSIS

Although the hardware and regimens used in peritoneal dialysis have evolved over time,[55,56,255,281,564,770,883] the basic techniques are similar to those described in the early application of peritoneal dialysis for the treatment of acute renal failure.[747] Sterile dialysate from commercially prepared bags of variable volume is delivered into the peritoneal cavity by gravity flow through connecting tubing that attaches to the indwelling peritoneal dialysis catheter. The latter may be a rigid tube for short-term, acute use, but more commonly a softer silicone tube of variable design is implanted surgically or percutaneously for long term use. The exchange cycle includes an inflow period, followed by a dwell period of variable length, and then an outflow period of gravity drainage through tubing connected to a drain bag. The exchange may be performed manually or with the help of assist devices. Rapid-cycling dialysis techniques frequently use automated cycler machines. The peritoneal dialysis regimen[1153b,1154b] may be intermittent (IPD), in which treatments are performed during several daytime or night-time sessions each week, or continuous, in which, aside from inflow and outflow, dialysate is continuously in contact with the peritoneal membrane 7 days per week.

IPD[225,770,1154] via rigid catheters was first employed in therapy for acute renal failure. The development of permanent peritoneal catheters and automated peritoneal dialysis machines resulted in the more widespread application of IPD for the treatment of chronic renal failure.[112,149,747] When used in this setting, 10 to 12-h periods of dialysis were typically used at a frequency of three to four times per week. Flow rates in IPD are relatively rapid, with typical exchanges of 2 liters every 30 to 60 min yielding peritoneal urea and creatinine clearances of 20 to 25 and 12 to 20 ml/min, respectively. IPD became widely embraced as a therapeutic modality for treating chronic renal failure in the 1970s.[111,261,266,544] In long-term studies, however, IPD patients manifested signs of underdialysis, including malnutrition, anemia, metabolic acidosis, and inadequate volume and blood pressure control. In the absence of residual renal function, it became clear that the cumulative weekly treatment times required for adequate clearance became prohibitive. Increased mortality rates by the third and fourth years were noted, with the majority of patients transferring back to maintenance hemodialysis.[6,381,989,1045] IPD, as described above, still has limited application in patients with acute renal failure, chronic patients with below-average clearance requirements (e.g., small adults with good dietary compliance or patients with residual renal function), or patients awaiting imminent transplantation or vascular access.

To increase the total weekly time and clearance of standard IPD, nightly home IPD (NPD),[255,770,1138,1154,1158a] employing 8- to 10-h nightly sessions of home cycling at high flow rates (2 liters per 30 to 60 min, utilizing 20 to 26 liters per night), has been devised. Although providing satisfactory clearances for patients with high peritoneal permeabilities and those with residual renal function, this mode of therapy still provides relatively low clearances of urea and creatinine for patients with average peritoneal permeability.

A second approach to maximizing IPD clearance efficiency is through the recently described modification of tidal peritoneal dialysis (TPD).[255,770,1154,1155,1158] In this technique, increased contact time between dialysate and peritoneum, despite the same duration and volume of dialysis, is achieved by leaving in the peritoneal cavity a constant residual volume to which a fixed tidal volume is infused and drained, as in standard NPD. Small-molecule clearances equal or surpass those of continuous peritoneal dialysis regimens, although again at the expense of relatively large volumes of dialysate and with the requirement for highly specialized volume-controlled automated cyclers. Larger–molecular weight clearances remain below those of continuous peritoneal dialysis techniques.

In 1976, Popovich and colleagues conceived the idea of equilibration peritoneal dialysis with a low-flow continuous peritoneal dialysis technique,[934,935] which has become known as continuous ambulatory peritoneal dialysis (CAPD). In CAPD,[255,770,934] long dwells punctuated by relatively brief periods of filling and draining are continuously maintained 24 h a day, 7 days a week. Typically, the patient performs 3 to 5 daily exchanges of 2 to 3 liters of dialysate, with dwell times of 4 to 6 h during the day and 6 to 8 h during a single night-time exchange.[845] Small molecules (molecular weight < 100) reach virtual equilibration well within 5 h (Fig. 40-9), but the continuous nature of CAPD compensates for the "wasted" dwelling time beyond equilibration, allowing weekly clearances of small molecules to exceed those in IPD (e.g., cumulative urea clearances of 84 liters/week).[849] Middle–molecular weight substances (e.g., vitamin B_{12} and inulin) achieve dialysate-plasma distribution ratios of 0.5 by 5 h (Fig. 40-9), while large molecules equilibrate linearly and indefinitely during prolonged dialysate-peritoneum contact time. Thus, CAPD achieves weekly middle- and large-molecular weight clearances greater than those in hemodialysis.

With the replacement of bottled dialysate with plastic bags of dialysate in the late 1970s[886,887] and the subsequent development of "disconnect" or bagless systems,[536] CAPD saw rapid and enthusiastic growth as a therapeutic modality for chronic renal failure in the 1980s. Reviews of extended experiences with CAPD in chronic renal failure have variably reported technical and clinical success rivaling that of maintenance hemodialysis.[177,356,389,682,708,782,827,829,831,834,836,931,934,1002,1249] More recently, an in-hospital modification of CAPD has been applied to the treatment of acute renal failure as well.[1113]

Shortly after the introduction of CAPD, another version of prolonged continuous peritoneal dialysis, known as continuous cyclic peritoneal dialysis, or CCPD was developed.[255,256,263,264,265,804] In CCPD, the dialysis cycle is like a mirror image of that on CAPD, with the patient performing 3 to 4 2-liter exchanges while asleep at night via a cycler and leaving 2 liters in the peritoneum during the daytime. Because the shorter nocturnal cycles do not as fully equilibrate for even most small molecules, small-solute clearances on CCPD are somewhat lower than with CAPD using the same net daily dialysate flow rate.[255,256,260] Middle-molecule clearances are similar to those on CAPD because the prolonged daytime dwell allows more complete removal of these compounds. Notwithstanding the detracting effects of lymphatic reabsorption, the prolonged daytime dwell contributes up to 20 percent of urea clearance, 25 percent of creatinine

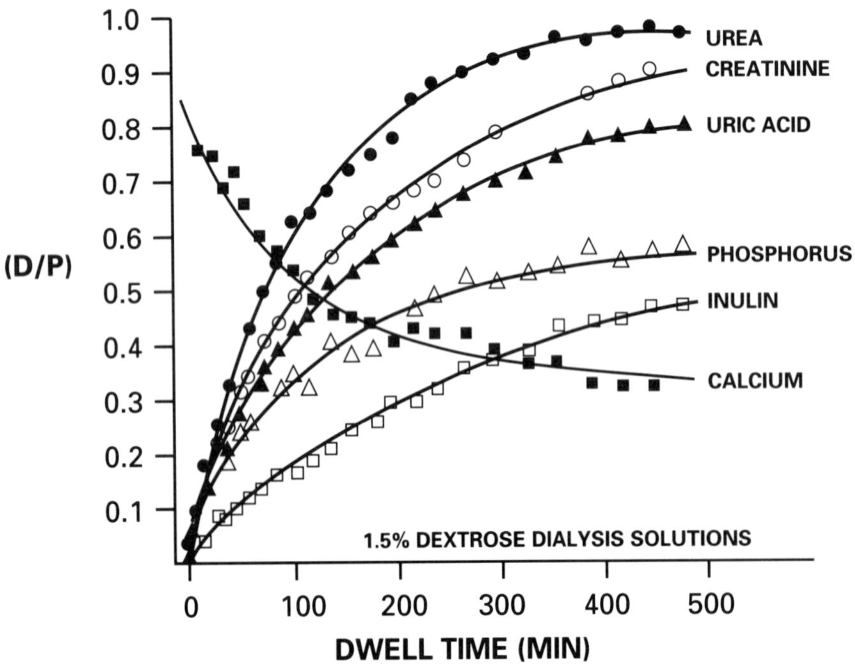

FIGURE 40-9 • Equilibrium curves of various solutes during long-dwell peritoneal dialysis exchanges. D/P, dialysate-plasma concentration ratios. (From Nolph KD et al: *J Lab Clin Med* 93:246, 1979. Used by permission.)

TABLE 40-7 • Typical solute clearances by various dialytic techniques

Modality schedule	Clearance (liters/week)			
	Urea	Creatinine	Vitamin B_{12}	Inulin
Native kidney	600–750	1000–1250	1000–1250	1000–1250
Standard hemodialysis, three 4-h treatments per week, cuprophane membrane	90–140	80–120	30–40	4–6
IPD, 2 liters/h × 40 h/week	40–60	25–40	16–20	12–15
NPD, 24 liters/night × 7 days/week	50–60	35–45		
TPD, 24 liters/night × 7 days/week	60–72	40–46		
CAPD, 8 liters/day × 7 days/week	58–74	45–55	35–45	25–45
CCPD, 8 liters/day × 7 days/week	55–65	40–44	45–50	

ABBREVIATIONS: IPD, intermittent peritoneal dialysis; NPD, nightly peritoneal dialysis; TPD, tidal peritonal dialysis; CAPD, continuous ambulatory peritoneal dialysis; CCPD, continuous cyclic peritoneal dialysis.

clearance, and an even greater percentage of middle- and large-molecular weight clearance during CCPD.[259,260] Despite the potential for lower peritonitis rates, greater patient freedom, and reports of satisfactory clinical experience with CCPD,[255,256,261,263] CCPD has not grown as fast as CAPD, perhaps because of the deterrent of higher costs. Ninety percent of chronic peritoneal dialysis patients in the United States use CAPD.[256,827] However, CCPD may be the preferable mode of peritoneal dialysis for patients who require assistance with exchanges, such as elderly patients and children.

The availability of hemodialysis and multiple techniques for chronic peritoneal dialysis provides clinicians with a variety of alternative ESRD treatments.[93,255,770] The regimen chosen ultimately reflects an interplay of logistical considerations such as cost, patient preference, and access availability. Additional medical considerations include the clearance and ultrafiltration needs of the patient in relation to the transport features of the various regimens (Table 40-7) and the unique kinetic properties of the individual's peritoneal membrane.[1157]

DIALYSIS SOLUTIONS

The composition of peritoneal dialysis solutions has evolved gradually[110] from the use of isotonic saline solution by Ganter[364] to the addition of glucose by Heusser[489] and the inclusion of a base by Rhoads.[973] Currently available solutions[255,256,464,747,770,1008,1193] are similar to those introduced over 30 years ago (Table 40-8). To satisfy the growth of peritoneal dialysis, the variation of regimens, and use in more diverse patient populations, commercial dialysate is now available in both bottled and plastic containers ranging in size from 0.25 to 5 liters. In the sections that follow, the evolution and rationale for the major constituents of dialysate are reviewed, although it should be realized that other additives (such as the preservative sodium bisulfite in concentration less than 0.1 mmol/liter) and other contaminants may be present and that deviations from the labeled concentrations may occur.[94,297] Moreover, the nature of many of the components is now being reevaluated in the face of greater understanding of peritoneal transport physiology[828] and a greater appreciation of the potentially toxic effects of dialysate on the peritoneal milieu.[429,717,1147,1173,1183]

Sodium

The sodium concentration of premixed, commercially available peritoneal dialysis solutions varies between 130 and 140 meq/liter.[772] Concentrations as low as 118 meq/liter can be achieved with dialysate prepared by automated proportioning peritoneal dialysis machines.[1069] Low-sodium dialysate (130 meq/liter) has been recommended to enhance sodium removal, achieve better blood pressure control, and prevent hypernatremia from excessive losses of hyponatric ultrafiltrate.[1193] However, patients receiving prolonged peritoneal dialysis maintain sodium balance primarily through sodium losses during ultrafiltration. For example, patients receiving CAPD

TABLE 40-8 • Composition of commercially available peritoneal dialysis solutions

Component	Range of concentrations, meq/liter
Sodium	130–135
Potassium	0
Calcium	2.5–3.5
Magnesium	0.5–1.5
Lactate	35–45
Chloride	95–106
Glucose (g/dl)	1.5, 2.5, 3.5, 4.25
Osmolarity (mosm/liter)	346, 396, 447, 485

have a net loss of 57 to 127 meq of sodium with each liter of ultrafiltrate removed when 4.25 percent glucose dialysate is used.[842,843] Thus, the removal of 2 liters of ultrafiltrate per day is usually adequate for eliminating the daily dietary sodium intake. If necessary, additional sodium can be removed with low-sodium dialysate.[159] For the special case of correction of fluid overload in patients with insufficient ultrafiltration, removal of sodium by using dialysate with "ultra-low" sodium concentrations (e.g., 98 meq/liter) has been reported to be safe.[805a] Nomograms have been developed for CAPD that predict the amount of sodium removed per day as a function of both the serum sodium concentration and the amount of ultrafiltrate formed.[843]

Potassium

Commercially prepared peritoneal dialysis solutions do not contain any potassium. In IPD, individualization of potassium removal is achieved by the addition of potassium chloride to the dialysate at the time of the dialysis treatment. The average potassium clearance during a 1-h exchange using 2 liters of potassium-free, 1.5% glucose dialysate is 16.8 ml/min.[139] As with sodium, sieving restrictions result in a potassium concentration in ultrafiltrate lower than the concentration in ECF. Since dialysate potassium equilibrates with that in the ECF and not with intracellular potassium, the quantity of potassium that can be removed per 2-liter exchange is minimal. Significantly greater rates of potassium removal can be achieved with hemodialysis (potassium clearances of 100 ml/min can be achieved with potassium-free dialysate) and with the enterally administered sodium polystyrene sulfonate (30 g can remove 30 meq/h).[139] Nonetheless, the serum potassium concentration can be gradually lowered with peritoneal dialysis through cumulative potassium losses, correction of acidosis, and metabolism of glucose.

In view of these considerations, it is not unusual to perform IPD with either no added potassium or with potassium dialysate concentrations below normal serum levels, especially in patients with predialysis hyperkalemia. Boen has reported that when potassium-free dialysate was used for periods of 28 to 59 h, the lowest final serum potassium concentration observed was 3.4 meq/liter.[112] However, in patients with a normal or low predialysis serum potassium concentration, supplemental potassium chloride can be added in a concentration (usually not exceeding 4 meq/liter) that reflects the final serum concentration desired. Oral potassium supplements are more readily used (to avoid hypokalemia-mediated arrhythmias) in peritoneal dialysis patients receiving digoxin. In CAPD patients, potassium is generally not added to the dialysate both because of the increased risk of bacterial contamination and because dietary potassium intake is usually adequate to prevent hypokalemia.[842] For example, with 10 liters of CAPD drainage per day in a patient with a serum potassium of 5.0 meq/liter, the maximum amount of potassium that can be lost per day would be 50 meq. If hypokalemia does develop in a patient receiving CAPD, it can be corrected with oral potassium supplements. As with sodium, nomograms have been developed for CAPD that allow a determination of the average amount of potassium lost per day as a function of the serum potassium level and the quantity of ultrafiltrate formed.[843]

Calcium

Net mass transfer of calcium in peritoneal dialysis is determined by diffusive movement of ionized or ultrafiltrable calcium down concentration gradients between dialysate and blood and convective losses of calcium into the dialysate with ultrafiltration (see the footnote under "Calcium" under "Hemodialysis Solutions"). Thus, the net calcium balance across the peritoneum will vary from patient to patient, depending on individual membrane characteristics, the amount of ultrafiltrate generated by the patient, and the serum calcium concentration, which is also dependent on other sources of external calcium intake. The interpretation of transport data from a number of studies is unclear because of uncertainties regarding the ionized and ultrafilterable calcium levels in some[556,795] and the complete absence of reported serum levels of calcium in others. Moreover, Kwong and associates[611] have pointed out that the dialysate ionized calcium may not be the same as the total dialysate calcium secondary to the complexing of calcium with dialysate anions. Studies comparing net transperitoneal calcium transfer with 1.5% and 4.25% glucose solutions at a constant dialysate calcium concentration of 3.5 meq/liter uniformly find a greater net absorptive balance with the 1.5% solution (with net loss of calcium into hypertonic dialysate noted in some studies).[243,609,611,908] Parker and coworkers,[908] for example, found that 4.6 meq of calcium was absorbed during a 6-h exchange with the 1.5% solution versus 3.2 meq absorbed with the more hypertonic solution. Delmez and associates[243] noted that 0.5 meq of calcium was absorbed during a 6-h exchange with the 1.5% solution versus a negative balance of 1.05 meq with the more hypertonic solution. Kwong and colleagues[611] reported that, using 8-h cycles, 1.45 meq was absorbed from the 1.5% solution, and a net of 0.3 meq was lost into dialysate with the more hypertonic exchange.

In IPD, daily net calcium uptake occurs from 3.5 meq/liter calcium dialysate solution.[32,369] In CAPD,[242] Delmez noted a 4.2 meq/day uptake when using a 4.0-meq/liter calcium dialysate in patients with a mean serum ionized calcium level of 2.4 meq/liter, compared to a net uptake of only 1.85 meq/day with 3.5-meq/liter dialysate, depsite lower serum ionized calcium levels of 2.36 meq/liter. With 3.5-meq/liter calcium dialysate, the same group[243] had previously noted a 2.4 meq/day uptake of calcium by patients with hypocalcemia (mean ionized serum calcium concentration <2.2 meq/liter). In the same study, hypercalcemic patients (mean serum ionized calcium concentration >2.5 meq/liter) lost 3.85 meq of calcium per day into the dialysate. In studies not reporting serum calcium levels, absorption from 3.5-meq/liter calcium dialysate has ranged from 4.2 meq to 15 meq/day[104,842,886,908] while Calderaro[153] noted loss of up to 2.5 meq/day with 3.0-meq/liter dialysate.

As peritoneal dialysis solutions evolved in the 1970s and early 1980s, the goal was to correct the hypocalcemia of chronic renal insufficiency and suppress the attendant osteitis fibrosa.[234] Based on the data summarized above, it was felt that raising the dialysate calcium above a normal (2.5 meq/liter) ionized serum calcium to 3.5 meq/liter would allow diffusive uptake to offset convective loss and permit enough positive transperitoneal calcium balance to suppress secondary hyperparathyroidism.[234,358] High-normal ranges of serum calcium were targeted, since an altered set point for calcium regulation of PTH secretion in chronic renal failure became recognized.[137] However, even in the early 1980s, whole-body balance studies[104] suggested that, when dietary calcium exceeded 36 meq/day, external calcium balance was always positive with 3.5-meq/liter dialysate. Later in the 1980s, more aggressive vitamin D supplementation was urged to suppress parathyroid gland function,[1100] and aluminum-containing phosphorus binders were being phased out and replaced with calcium-containing compounds.[797] It was then calculated that the net calcium balance (36 meq/day of gastrointestinal calcium absorption from 6.25 g/day of calcium carbonate)[733] would be positive enough to increase the frequency of hypercalcemia. Recommendations for lowering dialysate calcium to 2.5 meq/liter began to appear.[241,733,797,1072] Initially, commercial dialysate suppliers provided 2.5 meq/liter calcium only in the 1.5% glucose solutions, but now 2.5 meq/liter calcium is available in all dialysate tonicities and volumes, largely becoming the standard calcium concentration.

Magnesium

As with calcium, the magnesium content of peritoneal dialysate solutions continues to evolve. Transperitoneal magnesium flux depends on transperitoneal concentration gradients of the unbound cation and convective losses. During short-term peritoneal dialysis, magnesium-free dialysate has been used without adverse consequences.[113] In 1973, a dialysate magnesium concentration of 1.5 meq/liter was recommended.[1193] In CAPD, such dialysate with 1.5% glucose has been reported to result in both a small positive (0.44 meq per 6-h exchange)[842,908] and a small negative (0.25 to 0.50 meq per 6-h exchange)[243,611] magnesium balance. However, use of 4.25% glucose dialysate with a similar magnesium concentration results in a greater net negative magnesium balance (0.22 to 1.5 meq magnesium lost per 6- to 8-h exchange)[243,611,908] due to greater ultrafiltrate losses of magnesium. Using the 1.5-meq/liter magnesium dialysate, net positive external magnesium balances have been noted despite daily transperitoneal removal of 2.6 to 3.8 meq.[104,243,908] Stimulated largely by concerns that accumulating magnesium might be contributing to renal osteodystrophy,[133] interest in lowering dialysate magnesium was expressed in the 1980s.[718,840] Shah and associates[1063] demonstrated daily transperitoneal magnesium removal rates of 3.8, 5.5, and 7 meq in a group of CAPD patients using successively, over several weeks, dialysates with magnesium concentrations of 1.5, 0.5, and 0 meq/liter, respectively, despite falling serum magnesium levels at all three dialysate concentrations.

Commercial dialysis solutions are currently available in both 1.5 and 0.5 meq/liter magnesium concentrations. With the reconsideration of magnesium-based phosphorus binders as alternatives to aluminum,[797] further reductions may be in the offing. Jennings and coworkers [527] noted rising serum magnesium levels in seven CAPD patients receiving magnesium hydroxide while using 1.5-meq/liter magnesium dialysate. Shah and colleagues[1063] on the other hand, found more acceptable serum levels (<2.1 meq/liter) in nine patients utilizing the magnesium-free dialysate even while receiving magnesium hydroxide.

Alkali

As in hemodialysis, repletion of body buffer stores with peritoneal dialysis is accomplished by the diffusion and net absorption of base from the peritoneal dialysate. Bicarbonate was used initially as the base,[113] but its precipitation of calcium and magnesium salts in premixed commercial fluid plus the need for an acidic solution to prevent glucose caramelization during sterilization[255,1216] led to the necessary replacement of bicarbonate with acetate or lactate. The lower pK_a of these buffers allows for the acidification of these dialysates to pH 5.0 to 5.8 with small amounts of hydrochloric acid, without generating the high P_{CO_2} levels that diffuse out of the bags of bicarbonate solutions, causing progressive alkalinization of stored dialysate. The low nonphysiologic pH of acetate- and lactate-based dialysates has occasionally been blamed for "inflow pain" occurring in some patients.[12,915] Retitration of dialysate with small amounts of sodium bicarbonate or sodium hydroxide to adjust the pH to 6 to 7 has been said to improve these symptoms.[145,224]

Some investigators have recommended acetate instead of lactate as the alkali of choice in peritoneal dialysis solutions (see above).[772] One (poorly documented) report suggests that acetate may correct metabolic acidosis better than lactate in settings of impaired oxidative metabolism, such as with severe hepatic or circulatory insufficiency.[451] However, any impairment in oxidative metabolism probably equally affects both lactate and acetate conversion to bicarbonate; the reported superiority of acetate as a buffer in these setting is therefore questionable. It has also been claimed acetate dialysate has antibacterial activity not seen with lactate[772,899,978,979] and that lower rates of peritonitis obtain with acetate.[91] When instilled into the peritoneal cavity, acetate solutions take longer to reach physiologic pH than do lactate dialysates.[210,915,986] This longer exposure to a lower pH may impair phagocytic function[646] and has also been blamed for the reports of abdominal pain and chemical peritonitis with the use of acetate-based dialysate.[12,145,915] More serious concern has focused on the effect of long-term acetate exposure on peritoneal morphology and function. Acetate has been implicated in causing loss of peritoneal ultrafiltration, peritoneal sclerosis, and, more rarely, sclerosing peritonitis.[314,379,380,509,612,819,837,838,884,1023,1102,1103] Although the association of acetate use with these problems and others[545,839,1003] is controversial, commercial peritoneal dialysate in North America has shifted almost exclusively to the use of lactate.

From a functional standpoint, peritoneal dialysis with lactate is similar to that with acetate in terms of peritoneal solute clearances and protein losses.[822,846,1015] Treatment with either anion appears equally effective in correcting uremic acidosis during routine dialysis.[615,986,1136,1216] Lactate concentrations of 35 to 45 meq/liter are commonly employed in dialysate solution, consisting of the racemic mixture of the D- and L-isomers. Although one study[1011] suggested more efficient absorption and utilization of the naturally occurring L-isomer, most other studies indicate equally effective uptake across the peritoneum and metabolism of the D-isomer, as measured by its disappearance from dialysate and lack of rise of serum levels.[272,336,617,831,980,1136,1216] The effective utilization of D-lactate from peritoneal dialysate is consistent with the successful clinical use of racemic Ringer's lactate solution and the observation of minimal differences between the metabolism of infused D- and L-lactate.[202,336,810,868] Similar absorption and metabolic rates for D- and L-lactate and equivalent acid-base changes have been noted in tidal peritoneal dialysis comparing dialysates containing racemic lactate to those with L-lactate alone.[831] Although in vivo isomerization of D-lactate to L-lactate has been conjectured,[501,1216] the action of a D-2-hydroxyacid dehydrogenase that has been demonstrated in mammalian tissues to convert D-lactate to pyruvate seems the most plausible explanation for the metabolic clearance of D-lactate in the absence of D-lactate dehydrogenase (D-LDH).[199,1153,1216] Thus, both L- and D-lactate are metabolized predominantly in the liver to pyruvate, which can then enter metabolic pathways, including the Kreb's cycle, gluconeogenesis, and lipogenesis.[1216] Sixty to 80 percent of dialysate lactate is absorbed in short-cycle IPD, while 75 to 90 percent of lactate is utilized during a 4- to 6-h CAPD exchange.[272,617,822,986,1136] Studies of TPD using L-lactate alone have demonstrated that more than 300 meq of L-lactate can be disposed of over 8 h without overloading the metabolic pathways,[831] which are normally felt to handle 15 to 20 meq/kg per day of endogenous L-lactate turnover.[606] The calculated metabolizable load of infused D-lactate (2500 meq/day for a 70 kg man)[868] would also imply that toxicity from D-lactate absorption in peritoneal dialysis regimens would have to involve a defect in the normal utilization of this isomer. The increase in bicarbonate generation achieved by dialysates with higher lactate concentrations and at higher dialysate flow rates, in the face of normal serum lactate and pyruvate levels in most patients on IPD and CAPD, further demonstrates that the input of convertible base is less than the maximum metabolic rate.[272,313,617,831,980,1011,1136] However, hepatic dysfunction and glucose loading can limit the metabolic reserve for lactate and lead to rising serum levels with inefficient bicarbonate generation.[633,1216,1261]

Despite the usually adequate base repletion with acetate and lactate, use of these anion-containing dialysates has been criticized as being unphysiologic in terms of their vasoactive effects, induction of abnormal patterns of intermediary metabolism, and adverse effects on peritoneal and white blood cell function.[332,717,765,1015,1017,1187] These objections have prompted efforts to reintroduce bicarbonate dialysate. In acute peritoneal dialysis (e.g., for critically ill patients with lactic acidosis), manual preparation of bicarbonate-based dialysate has been described.[349,809,815,1070,1186] In these situations, in order to avoid divalent cation precipitation, intraperitoneal calcium and magnesium can be deleted and replaced with intravenous supplementation, or a bicarbonate solution and a separate saline solution containing divalent cations can be sequentially infused manually or mixed by automated cyclers immediately prior to intraperitoneal installation. With the use of these automated delivery systems, bicarbonate-based dialysate has also been prepared for chronic IPD and home CCPD by on-line mixing of the separate constituents.[79,508-511,514,515,1272] Practical application to the more widely employed CAPD has been difficult. Feriani and colleagues[331,333,334,508] have devised a system using a double-lined, partitioned plastic bag in which an upper compartment containing an "acid" solution with divalent ions is separated from a lower compartment with the basic solution. Prior to use, the partition is broken and the contents of the two chambers mix, generating a high P_{CO_2}, which is trapped long enough to prevent extreme alkanization and salt precipitation before installation.

More recently, a less complicated bicarbonate-based CAPD solution buffered at pH 7.35 by glycylglycine has been successfully tested in animals.[1265]

Chloride

As with hemodialysis solutions, the concentration of chloride in peritoneal dialysate is adjusted to maintain electroneutrality and is determined by the difference between the selected concentrations of cations (sodium, calcium, and magnesium) and buffer anions.

Osmotic agents

In peritoneal dialysis, movement of fluid across the peritoneal membrane occurs down the osmotic gradient created by the addition of osmotically active constituents to the dialysate. Huesser,[489] and later Odel,[858] first used glucose to achieve such ultrafiltration, and historically glucose has become the standard osmotic agent in commercial dialysate because it is effective in generating ultrafiltration, safely metabolized, and relatively inexpensive. Commercially premixed dialysate is currently available with glucose monohydrate (molecular weight, 198) concentrations of 1.5% (1.36% anhydrous glucose; net, 346 mosm/liter), 2.5% (2.27% anhydrous glucose; net, 396 mosm/liter), 3.5% (3.18% anhydrous glucose; net, 477 mosm/liter), and 4.25% (3.86% anhydrous glucose; net, 485 mosm/liter; Table 40-8). Glucose concentrations of 7% (net, 675 mosm/liter) used in the past have been discontinued[1193] because of an increased incidence of problems with hyperglycemia, hypernatremia, and hypotension.[370,1193]

The ultrafiltration and osmotic profiles of glucose-based solutions manifest a rapid exponential decline in ultrafiltration with time in response to a parallel fall in the osmotic gradient.[604,845,942,1016,1156] Osmotic equilibration with plasma occurs within 2 to 3 h with 1.5% dialysate and within 4 to 6 h with 4.25% glucose solutions. Typical ultrafiltration rates and volumes during CAPD are shown in Table 40-9.[942] The more hypertonic glucose solutions enhance transperitoneal solute clearances beyond their augmentation of drainage volumes.[136,469,702] These hypertonic solutions also exacerbate protein losses during peritoneal dialysis.[1014] The exponential fall in dialysate glucose concentration with time is due to intraperitoneal dilution by ongoing but diminishing ultrafiltration and by glucose absorption.[845,942,1016] Net glucose absorption is highly dependent on dialysate concentration, flow rates, and duration of dialysis[421,852] as well as individual peritoneal permeability properties.[421,1156] Thus, in IPD, 5 to 10 g/h of glucose may be absorbed from 2 liters of 1.5% solution and 35 to 40 g/h from 2 liters of 4.25% solution.[31,852] In high-flow hypertonic IPD used in certain situations of acute renal failure, absorption of greater than 500 g/day of glucose has been reported.[720] In CAPD, with 60 to 80 percent of infused glucose absorbed during prolonged dwells,[421] 6-h cycles cause the uptake of 15 to 22 g of glucose from a 1.5% solution, 24 to 40 g from a 2.5% solution, and 45 to 60 g from a 4.25% solution.[421] On a daily basis, 100 to 200 g of glucose is typically absorbed from the dialysate in a CAPD patient,[251,421] but this is highly variable, ranging from 50 to 316 g/day.[421,1156] Although transperitoneal glucose kinetics tend to be constant for a given patient, some individuals may demonstrate progressive increases in glucose absorption, leading to type I ultrafiltration failure.[30,838,839] In general, for a given patient, a typical CCPD regimen will result in less glucose absorption than a CAPD schedule for the same amount of net ultra-filtration.[1158a,1158b] Transperitoneal glucose kinetics are not affected by intraperitoneal insulin.[1010] However, peritonitis results in significant transient enhancement of glucose absorption and other solute clearances.[912,1012,1013]

TABLE 40-9 • Ultrafiltration parameters in continuous ambulatory peritoneal dialysis

Parameter	Dialysate dextrose concentration	
	1.5%	4.25%
Maximum ultrafiltration volume, ml	331 ± 187	1028 ± 258
Time required to form maximum volume, min	140 ± 48	247 ± 61
Maximum ultrafiltration rate, ml/min	11.7 ± 13	16.6 ± 7.7
Reabsorption rate, ml/min	0.68 ± 0.61	0.87 ± 0.55

NOTE: Mean ± SD; $n = 4$.

SOURCE: Adapted from Pyle WK et al in Moncrief JW, Popovich RP (eds): *CAPD Update: Continuous Ambulatory Peritoneal Dialysis*, New York, Masson, 1981, p 35. Used by permission.

Transperitoneal glucose uptake can thus account for 15 to 30 percent of the daily caloric intake in a CAPD patient,[421] although it has been suggested that a spontaneous reduction in oral carbohydrate intake compensates for the intraperitoneal load.[68] In addition to its impact on carbohydrate metabolism (see below), the caloric load has also been implicated in the tendency toward worsened hypertriglyceridemia and obesity frequently observed in CAPD patients.[38,125,173,421,457,577,621,655,658,968,1008,1009] In high-flow IPD, excessive glucose absorption can lead to hepatic steatosis and high respiratory quotients (RQ), with increased CO_2 production and the potential for hypercarbic respiratory failure in patients with borderline pulmonary reserve.[192,720]

In addition to the adverse effects of dialysate glucose on intermediary metabolism, other concerns are the apparent inhibition of the phagocytic function of white blood cells caused by the hyperosmolality of dialysate and the low pH required to prevent caramelization of glucose during sterilization (achieved by addition of hydrochloric acid to lower solution pH to less than 5.5).[236,290,1183,1259] The worrisome possibility of damaging effects of long-term hypertonic glucose exposure on the peritoneal membrane itself has also been raised.[273,891]

The potential problems with glucose as the osmotic agent in peritoneal dialysis have prompted a search for alternative osmotic agents.[255,275,388,434,775,776,1008,1158b] Low-molecular weight osmotic agents that utilize metabolic pathways different from those utilized by glucose have been examined. Sugars and sugar alcohols have been found either to accumulate in plasma, leading to hyperosmolar syndromes because absorption exceeds metabolism (e.g., fructose),[959,990] sorbitol,[92,961,1264] mannitol,[275,923,1215] and xylitol[83] or to enter detrimental metabolic pathways of their own (e.g., polyol pathways for fructose and sorbitol,[275,1215] and lactic acidosis and hyperuricemia for xylitol).[83] Glycerol seemed more attractive than glucose because it is metabolized without the need for insulin, it is stable at a more physiologic pH, and its lower molecular weight generates a higher osmolality for a given number of grams.[775,1158b] However, even more rapid absorption prevents glycerol from translating its higher osmolarity into greater ultrafiltration,[218,456,457,656] and the risk of a hyperosmolar syndrome[745] offsets the marginal benefits described in trials with diabetics.[744]

In view of ongoing amino acid losses into standard glucose-based dialysate[277,288,389] and the frequent protein malnutrition complicating CAPD,[1041] interest is currently focusing on amino acid-based dialysates. Gjessing[384] first suggested that intraperitoneal amino acids could act as osmotic agents and nutritional supplements. Pilot studies[576,881,1251] showed that amino acid–based dialysates (which cannot be prepared together with glucose because of potential chemical interaction during sterilization) were well-tolerated over short periods while providing adequate ultrafiltration and clearances. Over the short term, plasma amino acid levels could be normalized. Subsequent clinical studies[42,143,157,267,276,329,916,1269,1270] extending over periods of 2 to 6 months involving small numbers of patients receiving one to two exchanges per day of various amino acid-based solutions have only inconsistently demonstrated positive nitrogen balance with as yet no supportive anthropometric data to demonstrate benefit. Reversal of hyperlipidemia with reduced carbohydrate loading has also not been consistently borne out, while most of the studies have noted mildly worsened azotemia and metabolic acidosis.

Another approach that continues to be explored in the search for the ideal osmotic agent is the use of large-molecular weight compounds.[775,776,847,1158b,1159] Despite the lower osmolarity of such solutions, the very slow solute absorption (predominantly by lymphatics) in long-dwell CAPD would allow for ongoing ultrafiltration. Dextrans proved toxic, as did polyelectrolytes.[217,275,383,1160] Glucose polymers have been tested[425,777,778] in animals, but maltose accumulation may limit their application. Charged gelatin has been proposed,[275,1159] but viscosity and potential immunogenicity have prevented progress. Most recently, dialysate containing both small- and large-molecular weight agents to provide a "bimodal osmotic profile" and yet avoid some of the toxicities of high concentrations of these agents has been suggested.[775] The osmotic properties of peritoneal dialysate remain an evolving area in the field of peritoneal dialysis.[775] At present, glucose-based solutions remain the standard.

HYPERTENSION AND HYPOTENSION

The mechanisms responsible for hypertension in patients receiving peritoneal dialysis are the same as those previously discussed for hemodialysis patients. The technique of CAPD has been shown to be extremely effective in controlling hypertension, with the majority of patients exhibiting normal blood pressures and a reduction in the requirement for antihypertensive agents.[159,256,386,844,1111,1258,1271] Although it has been suggested that removal of vasoactive molecules may be of therapeutic significance,[849] plasma levels of renin, aldosterone, vasopressin, catecholamines, and endothelin in peritoneal dialysis patients are greater than or equal to those of hemodialysis patients.[386,619,1267,1273] The excellent control of hypertension of CAPD patients is primarily due to continuous and adequate ultrafiltration, with more complete normalization of ECF volume.[657,900] Thus, the early experience of less consistent hypertension control with IPD than with CAPD was attributed to the greater incidence of hypernatremia and increased thirst.[1154] Similarly, instances of poorly controlled hypertension in CAPD are usually related to volume overload.[388,770] Volume overload may be due to actual reduction in net drainage volumes resulting from mechanical catheter malfunction or fluid leakage transdiaphragmatically or into the abdominal wall. Truly diminished net ultrafiltration may be due to excessive lymphatic reabsorption, although this is a rarely described clinical entity.[688] In practice, net ultrafiltration failure has been due to hyperpermeability of the peritoneum, with rapid loss of osmotic gradient (type I ultrafiltration failure) or, less commonly, to progressive loss of surface area of the peritoneal membrane associated with both reduced solute clearances and ultrafiltration (sclerosing peritonitis, or type II ultrafiltration failure).[76,314,450,460,509,545,683,830,838,839,994,1102] Prolonged exposure to various constituents in dialysate (e.g., hypertonic glucose and acetate) has been suspected to induce morphologic and functional peritoneal changes.[270,273] Clinical evaluation and standardized peritoneal kinetic testing[1154a,1156] can help sort out these causes of ultrafiltration failure, allowing correction of mechanical factors or alteration in the dialysis prescription to improve volume homeostasis and blood pressure control.

The precipitous falls in blood pressure that are often seen during hemodialysis rarely occur with peritoneal dialysis. Absence of an extracorporeal blood circuit, gradual ultrafiltration and osmolality reduction, and a slow absorption of vasoactive buffers undoubtedly account for the greater stability of blood pressure observed during peritoneal dialysis. However, hypotension may gradually develop in IPD if cumulative fluid losses become excessive.[179] Postural hypotension is not uncommon in CAPD, especially during the first few weeks of treatment.[76,159,770] Excessive ultrafiltration culminating in hypovolemia, possibly as a result of a failure to recognize the rapid increases in "dry weight" after beginning CAPD, appears to be responsible.[76,728] Hypoproteinemia, characteristic of the population receiving CAPD, may also contribute to the postural hypotension. Increasing sodium intake usually corrects this problem,[635,728] but patients with underlying autonomic insufficiency, particularly diabetics, may continue to suffer from orthostatic hypotension.[256,971] High intraperitoneal volume only rarely impairs cardiac output enough to affect blood pressure in patients with severe cardiomyopathy or left ventricular hypertrophy.[353]

ACID-BASE DISTURBANCES

It is well established that uremic acidosis can be either totally or partially corrected by peritoneal dialysis using acetate or lactate as the buffer source.[272,617,1000] However, the acid-base changes during peritoneal dialysis may vary, depending on the specific chronic peritoneal dialysis technique used, the concentration of base in the dialysate, and in some cases the dialysate buffer chosen. Ultimately, acid-base balance in peritoneal dialysis patients depends on the net effects of dietary H^+ retention and base gains and losses during dialysis.[615,1136,1216]

The loss of nonbicarbonate buffer anions from plasma into the dialysate of a CAPD patient is usually low (approximately 4 mmol/day),[1136] while mass transfer coefficients for lactate and bicarbonate are similar;[980] thus, net fluxes of alkali are determined by the prevailing dialysate lactate and serum bicarbonate concentrations. Since transcapillary ultrafiltration results in a convective bicarbonate loss, the steady state acid-base status of a patient will be mainly determined by the dialysate concentration of buffer base and the ultrafiltration requirements of the individual.[374,615,1216]

During an 8-h IPD treatment with flow at 5 liters/h and zero dwell time, similar increases occur in blood pH and bicarbonate concentration using either acetate (41.5 meq/liter) or lactate (43.5 meq/liter) dialysate, indicating that the rate of uptake for either of these bicarbonate precursors (0.9 to 1.0 meq/min of dialysis) is greater than the rate of bicarbonate loss from blood to dialysate.[617] Net weekly transperitoneal buffer base balance in lactate-based IPD patients has varied from 240 to 1100 meq/week,[272,617,980] although these studies have been inconsistent in documenting a steady-state and accounting for convective bicarbonate losses and diffusional organic anion losses. In longer-term evaluations of IPD, however, acid-base balance has been generally felt to be inadequately controlled.[255]

In lactate-based CAPD exchanges of 4 to 8 h, 75 to 100 percent of lactate is taken up from the dialysate, while bicarbonate equilibration occurs by 6 h.[986,1136] Robson and coworkers failed to take into account the contribution of D-lactate to bicarbonate generation and hence calculated no net alkali uptake during a CAPD exchange.[986] Teehan and colleagues,[1136] using a CAPD solution with 36 meq/liter lactate, demonstrated that the loss of bicarbonate into the dialysate (192 meq/day) essentially equaled lactate uptake from the dialysate (212 mmol/day). When dietary H^+ accumulation and organic acid anions (base precursors) lost into the dialysate were also measured, the net base balance amounted to a loss of 26.4 meq/day. This net loss of base was associated with average blood gas values of pH 7.36, a P_{CO_2} of 34 mmHg, and a bicarbonate level of 20 meq/liter. The observation that the serum bicarbonate levels remained stable despite a daily negative base balance suggests the presence of ongoing intracellular buffering, possibly by bone.[1136] Based on these findings, the authors recommended either a higher dialysate lactate concentration or oral alkali supplementation for CAPD patients. These conclusions have been supported by other reports in both CAPD and CCPD patients that suggest that, in order to reliably maintain serum bicarbonate in the normal range, dialysate lactate concentration must be in the 38 to 45 meq/liter range.[822,1216] In one study, after initiation of CAPD using a lactate-buffered dialysate, (45 meq/liter) depressed serum bicarbonate levels rose into the normal range by the second to the fourth month of treatment.[986] Mandelbaum and associates, comparing dialysate concentrations of 35 and 40 meq/liter, found that the average serum bicarbonate level was 19 meq/liter (range, 14 to 22 meq/liter) with the former dialysate and 26 meq/liter (range, 20 to 31 meq/liter) with the latter.[718] Nolph and colleagues[840] were similarly able to maintain serum bicarbonate concentrations at 24 to 27 meq/liter in CAPD patients using a 40-meq/liter dialysate, while 38 percent of their patients had serum bicarbonate concentrations of less than 22 meq/liter when using a dialysate with 35 meq/liter lactate. Nissenson[822] was able to raise the steady-state serum bicarbonate from 22 to 26 meq/liter by changing dialysate lactate concentration from 35 to 40 meq/liter. Similarly, in CCPD patients, a dialysate lactate concentration of 35 meq/liter was unable to achieve "normal" acid-base balance.[146]

Effects of bicarbonate-based maintenance peritoneal dialysis on acid-base status are not well characterizied. Feriani and associates[331] evaluated bicarbonate kinetics using bicarbonate solutions (35 meq/liter and 27 meq/liter) in a CAPD regimen. They found that the higher bicarbonate concentration resulted in a steady-state metabolic alkalosis (pH, 7.50; serum bicarbonate level, 30 meq/liter), while the lower bicarbonate concentration reduced serum bicarbonate levels to 21.5 meq/liter, suggesting that the steady state serum bicarbonate level was 5 meq/liter below the dialysate bicarbonate concentration.

Acetate-based maintenance peritoneal dialysis, which is rarely any longer utilized in North America, appears to be as effective as lactate-based dialysis in achieving acid-base balance. While serum lactate levels are usually in the normal range with lactate dialysate,[272,617,840,986] acetate dialysate more commonly raises serum levels of acetate in CAPD patients,[617] although the degree of hyperacetatemia does not approach that seen in hemodialysis patients with "acetate intolerance." In lactate-buffered CAPD, the serum anion gap generally tends to be in the normal range.[374]

Long-term observations suggest that standard lactate-buffered (≥38 meq/liter) CAPD provides a more complete and smoother steady-state correction of uremic acidosis than do either hemodialysis or intermittent peritoneal dialysis regimens.[374,615,1216] In addition, the capacity of CAPD patients to buffer an exogenous acid load is superior to that of chronic hemodialysis patients, despite similar baseline serum pH and bicarbonate levels.[1093,1094]

Despite the effectiveness of standard peritoneal dialysis in treating uremic acidosis, certain acid-base disorders may be exacerbated by peritoneal dialysis or require modifications of the dialytic prescription. In patients with severe hepatic failure or those with lactic acidosis, the metabolic conversion of lactate to bicarbonate may be impaired.[149,203,349,451,537,633,806,809,1000,1070,1172,1186] Inadequate metabolism of lactate, along with loss of bicarbonate into the dialysate, can exacerbate the lactic acidosis.[1186] In these instances, use of specially prepared bicarbonate dialysate is recommended.[334,349,451,537,633,809,1070,1186] There is also one report of an unsubstantiated case of D-lactate acidosis in a diabetic receiving peritoneal dialysis. Marked encephalopathy in the setting of severe respiratory alkalosis characterized this patient's syndrome.[1188]

Gault and coworkers[370] and Vaamonde and coworkers[1172] have described metabolic alkalosis, which may be severe (pH, 7.60), in patients receiving intermittent peritoneal dialysis. This abnormality appears to be more common in patients with only slightly abnormal predialysis serum bicarbonate levels or when peritoneal dialysis treatment is prolonged over several days. Volume reduction, low diffusibility of bicarbonate from blood to dialysate, and a dialysate lactate concentration of 45 meq/liter are suggested causes.[370] Correction of high blood glucose levels in diabetic patients on CAPD has also been reported to cause contraction metabolic alkalosis if serum bicarbonate levels are normal during the period of hyperglycemia.[367,1163] In addition, the use of dialysate containing high concentrations of lactate (e.g., ≥40 meq/liter) has occasionally caused mild metabolic alkalosis.[840] However, the dialytic process, including peritoneal dialysis, is by nature autoregulatory in terms of metabolic acid-base balance: the higher the prevailing serum bicarbonate concentration, the greater the bicarbonate efflux during nonbicarbonate dialysis or the smaller the influx during bicarbonate-based dialysis, thus limiting alkalinization.

Severe alkalemia can develop in peritoneal dialysis patients with respiratory alkalosis, since the expected renal metabolic compensation does not occur.[858]

Uremic acidosis is characterized by a low bicarbonate concentration and an appropriate compensatory decrease in P_{CO_2}. Normally, there is a lag in the correction of the hypocapnia after the bicarbonate has been normalized. Because hemodialysis rapidly corrects hypobicarbonatemia, the sustained hypocapnia causes a transient alkalemia. The slower correction of bicarbonate by CAPD keeps pace with the slow correction of hypocapnia, thereby minimizing the degree of alkalemia that often complicates repair of metabolic acidosis.[76]

Peritoneal dialysis may also be used for correcting metabolic alkalosis from other causes in patients with renal failure. In this setting, the dialysate is modified to a low-buffer, high-chloride solution.[506,1194]

Although the mild reduction in lung volumes induced by peritoneal dialysis is associated with minimal respiratory complications,[76,235] the metabolic demands imposed by increased glucose and lactate handling do augment oxygen consumption and carbon dioxide generation. Thus, increased ventilation is the normal response to peritoneal dialysis,[300] but with borderline respiratory reserve or with exaggerated carbohydrate loading with high-flow hypertonic peritoneal dialysis, carbon dioxide retention and respiratory acidosis may occur.[92,720]

Insulin-dependent diabetics on peritoneal dialysis who become severely hyperglycemic do not seem particularly prone to develop ketoacidosis.[1166]

ELECTROLYTE DISTURBANCES

Like hemodialysis patients, those receiving peritoneal dialysis are also subject to a variety of electrolyte disturbances. This section describes electrolyte changes or abnormalities that result directly from the technique of peritoneal dialysis. Disturbances that result solely from loss of renal function per se have already been discussed under "Hemodialysis."

Unique to peritoneal dialysis is the ability to determine selected biochemical parameters by measuring their concentrations in residual dialysate that has been allowed to equilibrate intraperitoneally for prolonged periods. In patients on maintenance IPD, measurements of sodium, potassium, bicarbonate, BUN, creatinine, uric acid, and phosphorus concentrations in residual dialysate from 1 to 4 days since the last treatment were virtually identical to their simultaneously measured respective serum concentrations.[557] However, significant differences were found between serum and peritoneal fluid concentrations for other routine biochemical determinations (e.g., chloride, glucose, and calcium) due to alterations caused by the Gibbs-Donnan effect, protein binding, metabolism, and permeability limitations. This observation may help to eliminate some venipunctures in selected patients on chronic peritoneal dialysis.

Disturbances of serum sodium concentration

Hypernatremia

Elevated serum sodium concentrations have been frequently reported as a complication of IPD,[128,370,768,853,960,974,1105] with approximately 8 percent of patients developing serum sodium concentrations greater than 150 meq/liter.[1172] The most severe hypernatremia occurred with use of the now abandoned 7% glucose dialysate. Mild-to-moderate hypernatremia, however, can still occur with currently used dialysate preparations and may be responsible for increased thirst and excessive weight gains in the interdialytic period.[1069] The dialysate glucose concentration and the length of the dwell period appear to be the two major factors governing this complication. Two mechanisms have been proposed to account for hypernatremia caused by high glucose concentrations. It has been suggested that hyperglycemia from reabsorption of intraperitoneal glucose creates an osmotic gradient that causes water to shift from the ICF to the ECF compartment, thus producing dilutional hyponatremia. This hyponatremia in turn could then lead to diffusion of sodium from dialysate to blood. With subsequent metabolism of blood glucose, water would shift back into the ICF space, leaving behind an increased quantity of sodium in a smaller ECF volume.[370]

Alternatively, and perhaps more likely, hypernatremia may result from generation of a low-sodium ultrafiltrate due to glucose-induced osmotic ultrafiltration.[11,853,960] Indeed, short dwell periods have been shown to predispose to hypernatremia.[960] With longer dwell periods, there is greater opportunity for diffusion of sodium from plasma to dialysate, which tends to counterbalance the effects of formation of low-sodium ultrafiltrate. Hypternatremia is rarely seen in CAPD patients because of both the longer dwell times and the tendency of these patients to ingest adequate amounts of hypotonic fluids.[842] Use of current peritoneal dialysate solutions with a sodium concentration of 130 to 135 meq/liter, rather than the 140 to 142 meq/liter in earlier preparations, also reduces any tendency for development of hypernatremia.[11,370,1069,1193]

Hyponatremia

Hyponatremia in peritoneal dialysis patients usually results from excessive ingestion of water. In this setting, pulmonary edema may develop if a favorable diffusion gradient for sodium from dialysate to blood results in a large net positive sodium balance, such as in patients in whom little volume is removed by ultrafiltration.[1126] Hyponatremia may occur in peritoneal dialysis patients with hyperglycemia as a result of osmotic flux of water from the intracellular to the extracellular compartment.[1164,1165,1169] It is interesting to note that the change in serum sodium concentration in response to hyperglycemia in peritoneal dialysis patients differs from the response in chronic hemodialysis patients.[1169] In hemodialysis patients and peritoneal dialysis patients, the normally occurring osmotic diuresis in response to hyperglycemia is absent, and thirst mechanisms remain intact. In hemodialysis patients, this results in a greater decrease in serum sodium concentration for a given degree of hyperglycemia than that predicted for normal individuals.[546,1169] In peritoneal dialysis patients, the degree of hyponatremia more closely parallels that seen in normal individuals. In these patients, water intake appears to be counterbalanced by ongoing removal of hypotonic fluid from the extracellular compartment by peritoneal dialysis.[1169]

Disturbances of serum potassium concentration

Hyperkalemia and Hypokalemia

Hyperkalemia in patients receiving chronic peritoneal dialysis is uncommon but may develop with an increase in dietary intake or in catabolic states. Hyperkalemia can result from the peritoneal dialysis treatment per se if excessive potassium chloride has been added to the dialysate. Mild increases of the serum potassium concentration in diabetic CAPD patients have been attributed to hyperglycemia and can be managed with intraperitoneal insulin or other means of improved blood glucose control.[22,678] Hyperkalemia that has occasionally been noted after termination of peritoneal dialysis may be related to breakdown of stored glycogen.[113]

Hypokalemia requiring potassium supplementation has been noted in about 10 to 20 percent of CAPD patients.[885,1108] It can result when zero or at least insufficient amounts of potassium are added to the dialysate in patients whose initial serum potassium concentration is low, normal, or even slightly elevated. Such hypokalemia is most likely to occur in patients beginning IPD, as a result of glucose-associated cellular potassium uptake and rapid correction of metabolic acidosis.[113,936] For this reason, addition of KCl to at least the first few IPD exchanges should be considered in patients with low or normal potassium concentration. Severe hypokalemia has also been reported in a CAPD patient during a period of diminished dietary intake and increased gastrointestinal losses of potassium.[1001]

Addition of up to 20 meq/liter of KCl to the peritoneal dialysate in a small number of CAPD patients increases the plasma potassium by 0.44 meq/liter within 2 to 3 h.[1108] Sixty-six to 79 percent of the intraperitoneal potassium dose was absorbed via this route. A higher potassium concentration (40 meq/liter) was associated with severe abdominal pain and cramping.

Disturbances of serum calcium, phosphorus, and magnesium

Hypercalcemia

Use of dialysate containing 3.5 meq/liter of calcium in IPD patients in the early 1980s[32,324] caused hypercalcemia. The incidence of this complication became more frequent in CAPD as the use of more vitamin D and calcium carbonate-containing phosphorus binders became commonplace. As many as 40 to 90 percent of patients followed over one to two years may develop hypercalcemia, with an average of one to two episodes per patient per year.[34,279,488,795,1025,1026] In these reports, the hypercalcemia has usually been mild (total serum calcium <5.75 meq/liter, or 11.5 mg/dl) and has often been overlooked if not screened for by measuring ionized calcium concentrations. These high levels typically normalized over one to three weeks following an adjustment of oral calcium and vitamin D doses. The reduction of dialysate calcium to 2.5 meq/liter appears to be reducing the frequency of hypercalcemia in the CAPD-CCPD population, although not yet eliminating it because oral calcium and vitamin D administration is increasing.[503,547,795,927] The problem may ultimately be resolved by the use of phosphate binders with lower potential for calcium absorption[911] or peritoneal dialysate with even lower calcium content. In the extreme, calcium-free dialysate has been used in the past to treat hypercalcemia from various causes, including vitamin D toxicity and malignancy,[234,390,442,490,764,851,1122] but this technique requires the time-consuming manual preparation of dialysate from calcium-free salt and glucose solutions. On the other hand, resistant hypocalcemia following parathyroidectomy has been treated by increasing the dialysate calcium concentrations.[85,326,1143]

Hyperphosphatemia

More effective prevention of hyperphosphatemia is obtained with CAPD than with IPD or maintenance hemodialysis.[104,158,390,391,844,886,1285] The mean amount of phosphorus removed daily in CAPD is approximately 10 mmol (310 mg).[104,243] Removal of phosphorus is augmented when ultrafiltration is increased or when serum phosphate levels are elevated.[243] However, with the dietary protein requirements of CAPD, phosphorus absorption, estimated at 20 to 25 mmol/day (600 to 750 mg/day) exceeds dialytic removal,[104,241] and variable doses of supplemental phosphorus binders are usually required.

As with hemodialysis patients, hypophosphatemia can develop on a multifactorial basis in peritoneal dialysis patients,[996] and in certain situations, neutral phosphate addition to dialysate has provided an intraperitoneal route for the treatment of severe hypophosphatemia.[291,351]

Hypermagnesemia

The combination of nonfunctioning kidneys and the use of dialysate containing 1.5 meq/liter magnesium occasionally produces hypermagnesemia (mean magnesium concentration, 2.8 meq/liter) from the failure to remove interdialytic gains.[104,243,718,844,908] Serum magnesium concentrations approach normal (average, 2.0 meq/liter) when dialysate magnesium concentrations of 0.5 meq/liter are used.[718,840,1063] It should be noted, however, that the clinical significance of mild hypermagnesemia has not been clarified in the peritoneal dialysis population. A muscle biopsy study demonstrated normal-to-low intracellular magnesium concentrations despite mild hypermagnesemia.[657] Hypermagnesemia was correlated to a lesser progression of arterial calcification in a long-term study of CAPD patients.[757]

Disturbances of serum glucose concentration

Hyperglycemia

The ultimate effect of peritoneal dialysis on serum glucose depends on its impact on carbohydrate tolerance and metabolism and the absorbed load of glucose. After a single CAPD exchange with 4.25% glucose, peak blood sugar and stimulated insulin levels occur within 45 to 90 min.[48,251,457,1243] These findings are similar to those observed after an oral glucose load in CAPD patients.[658,659,1242] Intrinsic carbohydrate tolerance in CAPD patients has been reported to remain unchanged[68,455,658,699,1243] or to improve,[455,1046,1047] as shown by the blood glucose and insulin response to an oral glucose tolerance test. On the other hand, Spitz and associates[1109] suggested that rapid IPD caused transient beta cell exhaustion, with a diminished insulin response to an oral glucose challenge that lasted for several days after the IPD session. Armstrong,[48] in an uncontrolled study, noted that glucose tolerance deteriorated and insulin secretion diminished over time in CAPD patients. Weisinger[1233] demonstrated in vitro that peripheral insulin resistance increased in CAPD. However, the effect of weight gain on insulin sensitivity must also be considered in assessing the diabetogenic stress of CAPD.[237,608,655]

Significant hyperglycemia occurs more commonly in IPD than in CAPD, by virtue of more rapid glucose loading and hypotonic ultrafiltration in the former setting. IPD is more frequently used to treat hospitalized acute renal failure patients, who usually have other catabolic stresses that accentuate their glucose intolerance, resulting in a 10 to 15 percent incidence of significant hyperglycemia in this setting.[1130,1172] Hyperglycemic hyperosmolar coma has been frequently described as a complication of IPD.[31,128,138,370,448,852,990,1164,1169,1210,1238] This untoward metabolic complication was more common prior to the discontinuation of 7 percent glucose solutions[1193] and is now rarely seen in the CAPD population.[22,303,852] Hemodialysis patients often have lower serum sodium levels than equally hyperglycemic patients with normal renal function. This effect results from the failure to excrete ingested water and the absence of hypotonic losses secondary to glycosuria. Peritoneal dialysis patients with hyperglycemia tend to become less hyponatremic than equally hyperglycemic hemodialysis patients because of transperitoneal ultrafiltration of hypotonic fluid.[1169] Peritoneal dialysis patients with severe neurologic symptoms from hyperglycemia are predominantly those with serum tonicities greater than 320 mosm/liter. Peritoneal dialysis patients with marked hyperglycemia but lower serum tonicity because of greater hyponatremia usually tolerate the metabolic disorder much better.[22,605,1166,1169] IPD treatments that cause hyperglycemia also produce convective sodium losses, thereby causing signs of significant ECF volume depletion.[31,370,448,1164] Less hypertonic patients, despite similar blood sugars, demonstrated little change in ECF size.[22,605,1164] Episodes of pulmonary edema, sometimes reversible with insulin alone (allowing fluid to shift back from ECF to ICF), have been reported.[539,1164] Ketoacidosis is also an unusual concomitant of uncontrolled hyperglycemia in CAPD patients.[1166]

Insulin can be administered intraperitoneally in dialysate to achieve smooth serum glucose control in diabetics[209,342,345] without an increased incidence of antibody formation.[423] The fact that insulin absorption rates exceed blood-to-dialysate clearance rates of native insulin[1244] suggests that lymphatic absorption plays a major role in insulin absorption. Although only a small portion of the peritoneal insulin is ultimately absorbed,[28,274,699,1062,1244] protocols for CAPD and CCPD patients utilizing two to four times the effective subcutaneous doses[61,70,84,206,255,344,685,1235] have been devised. Many claim this regimen provides better glycemic control than does subcutaneously administered insulin.[29,70,343,691,1004] Tzamaloukas[1167] claimed that only 1.5 percent of diabetic peritoneal dialysis patients have elevated fasting blood sugars.

Hypoglycemia

Hypoglycemia has been reported in patients receiving IPD and CAPD.[100,359,419,1103,1135] Most of these patients had so-called spontaneous hypoglycemia of uremia due to imparied gluconeogenesis. In one report, however, it was suggested that postdialysis hypoglycemia resulted from a hyperinsulinemic state induced by hyperglycemia during the treatment.[419] For patients receiving insulin during IPD, it has been suggested that insulin not be placed intraperitoneally in the last several exchanges or that a 4.25% glucose solution be left dwelling. Subcutaneous doses of insulin should be stopped 4 to 6 h before terminating dialysis.[770] Conversely, peritoneal dialysis has been used as a source of glucose in treating such hypoglycemic states as that due to oral hypoglycemic agents[622] and in glycogen storage disease.[1182]

ADDITIONAL DIALYSIS TECHNIQUES

Sorbent regeneration dialysis

Need for an independent, mobile, and compact dialysate supply for hemodialysis stimulated creation of a sorbent-based dialysate regenerative system.[404] The REDY system (from REcirculation DialYsis)[888] has found its largest application in acute hemodialysis, although it has also been used for chronic dialysis therapy.[106,317] The method employs a recirculation of dialysate at flow rates of 200 to 250 ml/min from a 6-liter dialysate reservoir, with regeneration of the effluent dialysate by passage through a five-layered sorbent cartridge (Fig. 40-10) and the constant infusion of calcium, magnesium, and potassium salts into the dialysate. This small dialysate volume contrasts markedly with the 120 to 150 liters of dialysate required in a standard hemodialysis system. The low dialysate flow rates (in comparison to flow rates of 500 ml/min in standard single-pass hemodialysis systems) are necessary for adequate regeneration of the dialysate but result in a slight (10 to 15 percent), clinically unimportant decrease in the clearance of urea, creatinine, and other small-molecular weight substances. The clearance of middle-molecular weight substances remains unaltered.[284,465,860,1066]

The first layer in the cartridge (Fig. 40-10), containing hydrous zirconium oxide and activated carbon, removes particulate matter and heavy metals. Oxidizing substances such as chlorine, hypochlorite, and chlo-

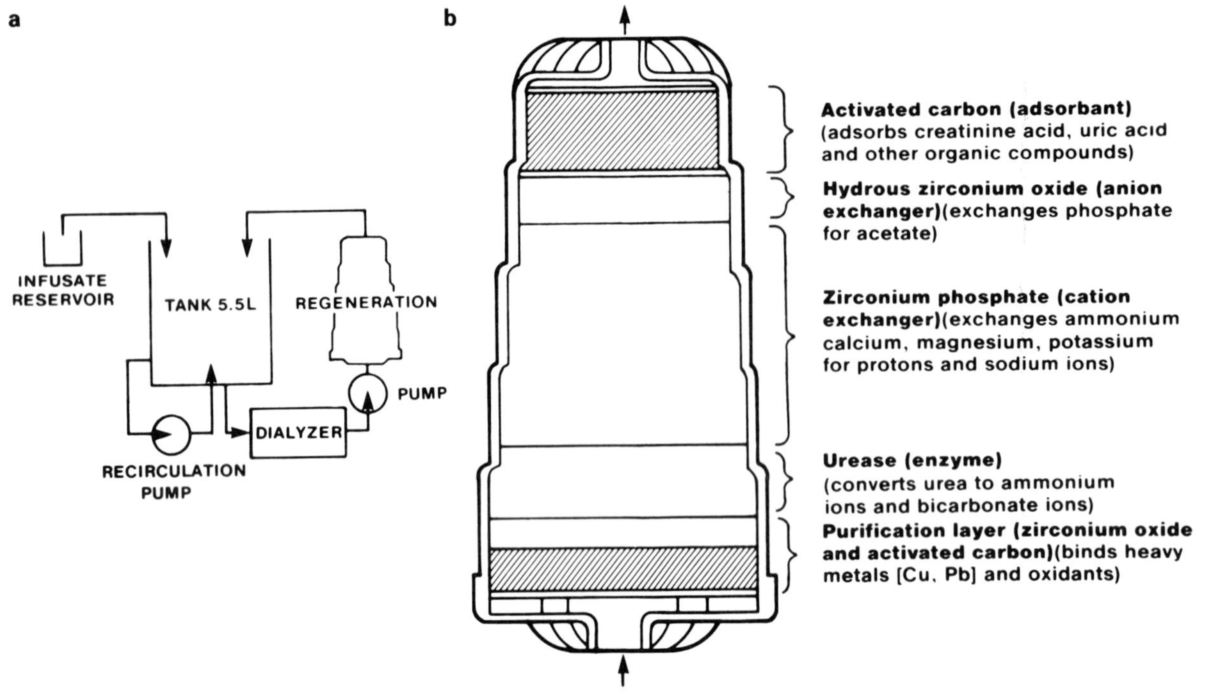

FIGURE 40-10 • (*a*) Dialysate flow path of REDY system. (*b*) Component layers of REDY sorbent cartridge. (Modified from Wing AJ et al in Drucker W et al, eds: *Replacement of Renal Function by Dialysis*, 2d ed., Boston, Martinus Nijhoff, 1983. Used by permission.)

ramines, which inactivate the urease present in the next layer, are also removed. In the second layer, urease catalyzes the conversion of urea in the effluent dialysate to ammonium and carbamic acid, which subsequently generate carbonate, bicarbonate, and hydroxyl ions:[284]

$$H_2N—CO—NH_2 + 2H_2O \xrightarrow{\text{urease}} NH_4^+ + \underset{\text{carbamic acid}}{NH_2COO^-} + H_2O$$

$$NH_4^+ + NH_2COO^- + H_2O \rightleftharpoons 2NH_4^+ + CO_3^{2-}$$

$$2NH_4^+ + CO_3^{2-} \rightleftharpoons NH_4^+ + NH_3 + HCO_3^-$$

$$NH_3 + H_2O \rightleftharpoons NH_4^+ + OH^-$$

Hydrogen and sodium forms of the cation exchanger zirconium phosphate in the third layer adsorb the urease-generated ammonium, as well as the calcium, magnesium, and potassium present in the dialysate fluid in exchange for sodium and hydrogen ions. Because the zirconium phosphate is also a buffer, the ratio of H^+/Na^+ released depends on the pH of the system and the other anions (bicarbonate and acetate) present in the dialysate. The release of sodium ions from the zirconium phosphate results in a gradual increase in dialysate sodium concentration during dialysis. The released hydrogen ions titrate the carbonate generated by the urease reaction and any HCO_3^- that is present, forming CO_2, water, and, to a lesser extent, additional bicarbonate. A limited adsorptive capacity for ammonium limits the amount of urea that can effectively and safely be removed by a single cartridge. The Sorb D-3160 cartridge can remove the ammonium ions generated from 20 g of urea nitrogen, and the Hisorb D-3260 cartridge can remove the ammonium from about 30 g of nitrogen.[888]

The fourth layer consists of hydrous zirconium oxide, which acts as an anion exchanger, removing phosphate and fluoride ions and releasing acetate. Aluminum, iron, lead, and mercury are also adsorbed. Sulfate is not removed.

Activated carbon in the fifth layer adsorbs organic metabolites such as creatinine, uric acid, and other nitrogenous wastes. The adsorptive capacity for such compounds (e.g., 10 g for creatinine) does not present limitations to adequate dialysis. This layer also (variably) removes drugs, but low-molecular weight hydroxyl compounds (e.g., ethanol and ethylene glycol) and amino acids are poorly adsorbed.[1237] Glucose is adsorbed, but the cartridge rapidly becomes saturated with glucose, and the cartridge and dialysate equilibrate with plasma.

The constant addition of a solution of potassium, calcium, and magnesium salts in adjustable concentrations to the dialysate reservoir replenishes the cations removed by the zirconium phosphate layer. These cations are usually administered as the acetate salts, although chloride salts may be used in patients with severe alkalosis. Usually, the initial dialysis solution contains none of these cations, but the constant infusion brings them to the desired steady-state dialysate concentrations within 30 to 60 min of initiating dialysis.

Due to the dynamic interplay of the cartridge's removal of certain solutes and the addition of others by the cartridge and infusate, the dialysate composition does not remain constant during sorbent hemodialysis. However, since the bath is roughly one-seventh to one-fifth the volume of a patient's body water compartment, relatively large changes in dialysate solute concentrations will effect rather small and gradual changes in the patient's serum solute concentrations. However, the dynamics of the system demand—perhaps more than in standard single-pass hemodialysis systems—attention to matching the cartridge and dialysate prescription to individual patient problems and needs.

For example, the initial dialysate prescribed for most patients contains 100 to 110 meq/liter of sodium. Upon beginning dialysis, additional sodium enters the dialysate by diffusion from the priming saline solution across the dialyzer and from loosely bound sodium in the cartridge, increasing the dialysate sodium concentration by 10 to 15 meq/liter. Thereafter, exchange of ammonium for sodium from zirconium phosphate releases approximately 70 to 140 meq of sodium, thus increasing the dialysate sodium concentration by another 13 to 25 meq/liter. Finally, the exchange of sodium for calcium, magnesium, and potassium ions raises the dialysate sodium concentration by approximately 10 meq/liter per hour. Thus, over a 4-h treatment, 360 to 480 meq of sodium (assuming a standard urea load) is added to the dialysate, raising the final sodium concentration to 145 to 160 meq/liter. From this dialysate sodium profile, it can be seen that, in the early period of the dialysis treatment, the serum sodium concentration drops slightly (by 1 to 3 meq/liter, assuming a normal initial serum sodium concentration) as sodium is transferred to the dialysate. The drop is greater for a very small patient or if the initial dialysate sodium concentration is lower (as low as 85 meq/liter can be prepared to treat hypernatremia). The later rise in the dialysate sodium concentration ultimately results in diffusion of sodium from the dialysate to blood and produces a small rise in the serum sodium concentration. The elevation of the dialysate sodium concentration toward the end of the treatment is claimed to reduce late dialytic hypotension and disequilibrium.[888] Although the high-sodium dialysate may result in a modest sodium uptake (up to 100 meq), hypertension and other clinical manifestations of sodium overload are prevented by concurrent convective losses of sodium during ultrafiltration.[284,1252] In view of these dialysate sodium changes, the treatment of severely hyponatremic or hypernatremic patients requires that the starting dialysate be adjusted to provide an appropriately higher or lower sodium concentration, respectively. Alternative methods have been described to maintain the dialysate sodium concentration constant.[984]

After the first hour of treatment, dialysate potassium concentration is essentially set by the infusate additive. However, in the first hour, the dialysate potassium concentration ranges between that in the starting bath reservoir and the infusate concentration, sometimes obligating the physician to use a different infusate concentration during this period.

If bicarbonate is used rather than acetate as the dialysis buffer, it can then diffuse into the dialysate from the patient's blood. Reaction of protons with the carbonate ions produced from urea degradation can also add bicarbonate to the dialysate. Large quantities of CO_2 are produced from hydrogen ions and bicarbonate as the dialysate passes through the cartridge. The P_{CO_2} in the dialysate cartridge effluent can reach levels of 200 to 300 mmHg in both acetate and bicarbonate sorbent dialysis. In bicarbonate treatments using hollow-fiber dialyzers, the P_{CO_2} in the effluent from the dialysate cartridge starts at this level and slowly declines to approximately 160 to 180 mmHg after 4 h. In acetate-based treatments, dialysate P_{CO_2} is initially less than 10 mmHg but increases during the first 2 h to over 200 mmHg.[443] Thus, compared to standard acetate single-pass dialysis, in which there is constant CO_2 loss across the dialyzer, sorbent dialysis causes CO_2 gain.[992] Largely from the hypercapnia, the pH of returning venous blood can be as much as 0.5 pH units lower than that of the blood entering the dialyzer.[917] Hyperventilation during both acetate and bicarbonate sorbent dialysis induced by this CO_2 load prevents significant changes in the arterial P_{CO_2}.[975,992] However, severe respiratory acidosis during sorbent dialysis has been reported in a patient with fixed mechanical ventilation using bicarbonate-based dialysate.[443] Limiting the initial dialysate bicarbonate concentrations to 100 meq/liter or less when planning a bicarbonate treatment (in patients with severe metabolic acidosis) and the use of degassing and agitation techniques should limit the peak P_{CO_2} attainable in the system.[888] Caution is still advised for patients on respirators and those with little ventilatory reserve.

The elevated P_{CO_2} and diminished pH in venous blood from the dialyzer should not obscure the beneficial uptake of base from the dialysate. Although sorbent dialysis results in roughly the same net anion gain by the patient as does standard acetate dialysis (250 to 350 meq), the means of achieving this differs (see "Acid-Base Disturbances" under "Hemodialysis"). In sorbent acetate dialysis, the initial dialysate bath contains about 25 to 28 meq/liter acetate and no bicarbonate. Thus, early in this treatment, the patient also loses bicarbonate to the bath. As noted above, however, the cartridge progressively generates bicarbonate and some acetate (in exchange for anions in the zirconium oxide layer).

Therefore, the rate of acetate uptake progressively falls due to dissipation of its diffusion gradient, but the rate of bicarbonate loss also decreases. The posttreatment dialysate contains 15 to 20 meq/liter acetate and about 15 meq/liter bicarbonate. Overall, a patient may gain 200 to 400 meq acetate and lose less than 100 meq bicarbonate (in a standard acetate hemodialysis system the patient loses about 400 to 700 meq of bicarbonate and gains 700 to 1000 meq of acetate in a 4-h treatment).[284,957] Therefore, compared to standard single-pass acetate hemodialysis, sorbent acetate dialysis results in considerably less acetate uptake and bicarbonate loss by the patient. However, the pattern of arterial blood gas changes during sorbent dialysis is similar to that seen in standard acetate dialysis.[976,1207]

Bicarbonate dialysis with the sorbent system still provides more than half of the patient's net base gain from the acetate derived from anion exchange in the zirconium oxide layer of the cartridge and from the infusion of acetate salts.[376,984] The use of standard sorbent cartridges in patients with minimal urea loads (e.g., treatment of drug overdose) may aggravate metabolic acidosis due to inadequate production of bicarbonate by the cartridge and loss of bicarbonate across the dialyzer membrane.[284]

With recent concerns about aluminum toxicity, it is worth noting that aluminum-induced osteomalacia and dialysis dementia have been reported in patients maintained by sorbent dialysis.[773,924] In vitro, aluminum in concentrations often exceeding 50 μg/liter can be leached from the aluminum oxide stabilizing agent in the cartridges, especially early in dialysis. Bicarbonate dialysate enhances this phenomenon due to a pH effect on aluminum solubility.[131] Newer versions of sorbent cartridges contain less aluminum oxide, resulting in much lower rates of aluminum leakage, although substantial aluminum leakage may still occur, particularly at the start of dialysis.[211,284,285,861,1066,1067] Deferoxamine does not enhance aluminum release from the cartridge.[211] It should also be noted that the anion exchange layer in the cartridge binds sulfate poorly. Higher serum sulfate concentrations have been noted in patients treated chronically with the sorbent system than in those treated with standard single-pass systems.[353b,755] Thus, there is the potential for producing sulfate complexes with calcium, with lowering of the serum calcium concentration.[355] A potential role for hypersulfatemia in renal osteodystrophy has been suggested.[1236]

Another potential problem unique to sorbent regenerative dialysis is ammonia toxicity. The cation exchange resin in the cartridge has a limited ammonia adsorptive capacity, equivalent to 20 or 30 g of urea nitrogen. If more ammonium is generated by the urease than can be adsorbed, it can be transferred to the patient, a phenomenon known as "ammonia breakthough."[403] Ammonium intoxication may result and can produce acute symptoms of metabolic encephalopathy.[161] In clinical practice, it is recommended that the maximum anticipated urea removal be estimated before treatment and that the cartridge effluent be checked with ammonia test paper toward the end of dialysis. The cartridge should be replaced if the effluent ammonia concentration is greater than 2 μg/dl.[888] Use of continuous ammonium monitoring for sorbent hemodialysis has been reported.[57]

Since the sorbent cartridges do not adsorb much glucose, a large glucose load is delivered to the patient from the dialysate and may result in mild-to-moderate hyperglycemia, especially in diabetic patients.[888]

Citrate regional anticoagulation should not be used with sorbent hemodialysis. Citrate uncouples urease from its alumina medium and complexes with aluminum. Aluminum citrate is formed and then released into the circulation. Citrate also competes with the urease for binding to hydrated zirconium oxide. The free urease in dialysate degrades urea and generates ammonia, which enters blood returning to the patient. A venous-arterial NH_3 difference of over 1000 mmol has been reported in this setting.[1124a]

Hemofiltration

This technique evolved largely as an outgrowth of the belief that middle-molecular weight solutes were uremic toxins that were inefficiently removed by standard diffusive hemodialysis. Renal replacement therapy that more closely mimicked actual glomerular filtration, with its convective removal of water and solute, it was reasoned, would more effectively remove these putative toxins.[475,477] With the introduction of membranes with high hydraulic conductivity and high sieving coefficients for compounds up to 6000 daltons came the clinical application of hemodiafiltration, later termed *hemofiltration*.[474,944] Primarily due to economic considerations, however, clinical application of hemofiltration has been limited to a relatively small number of patients treated in European centers. The principles and clinical applications of hemofiltration and related dialysis methods may be found elsewhere.[162,470,640,714,943,1021,1034,1282]

Continuous arteriovenous hemofiltration and hemodialysis

Despite the lack of enthusiasm in North America for maintenance hemofiltration, modifications of this form of therapy, continuous arteriovenous hemofiltration (CAVH), continuous arteriovenous hemodialysis (CAVH-D),[378,601,602,896,1088] and other related continuous dialytic modalities[174,542,680,1123,1134,1268] have gained clinical acceptance in the United States for the treatment of oliguric acute renal failure.[78,396,543,629,1048,1133] For both CAVH and CAVH-D, a small volume, low-resistance hemofilter with high

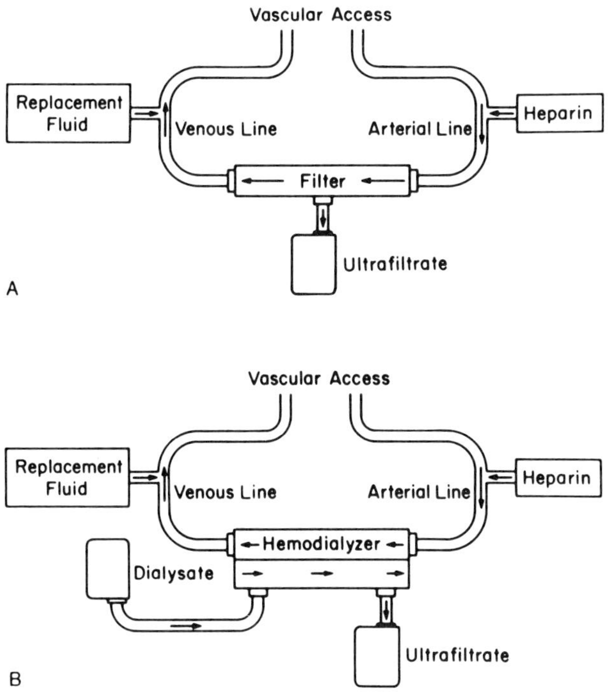

FIGURE 40-11 • Schematic representation of (*a*) continuous arteriovenous hemofiltration and (*b*) continuous arteriovenous hemodialysis. (From Nahman NS, Middendorf DF: *Med Clin North Am* 74:975, 1990. Used by permission.)

water permeability and high sieving coefficients for compounds up to molecular weights of 6000 is perfused by the patient's own arteriovenous (AV) pressure gradient (Fig. 40-11). This allows for continuous bedside ultrafiltration that can be continued for days to weeks to treat fluid overload or maintain fluid balance in oliguric patients requiring large volumes of parenteral fluid. The rate of ultrafiltration depends on the following factors: the blood flow rate, which, in turn, is a function of the patient's mean arterial blood pressure, the type of vascular access, the size of the arterial cannula, and the size of the vessel cannulated; the transmembrane hydraulic and hydrostatic pressure gradients which are dependent on the AV pressure drop across the hemofilter and the height of the ultrafiltrate collection line; the patient's hematocrit; and the plasma protein concentration (Fig. 40-12).[121,299,629,875] Spontaneous ultrafiltration rates of 4 to 15 ml/min (5 to 20 liters/day) have been reported,[543,629,1133] with filtration fractions (ultrafiltration rate/plasma flow) ranging from about 10 to 35 percent. Interposition of a blood pump can increase the rate of fluid removal to 40 ml/min.

The CAVH ultrafiltrate composition reflects that of plasma water, modified by Gibbs-Donnan constraints and the physicochemical characteristics of each solute, and is nearly protein-free (Table 40-10). A Ringer's lactate-type solution is suitable replacement fluid for most patients.[543,1133] However, in patients with lactic acidosis or severe liver dysfunction, bicarbonate-containing replacement fluids may be preferred. Substitution of saline or other solutions without bicarbonate or bicarbonate equivalents will cause a dilutional hyperchloremic metabolic acidosis.[374,396,543,876] When bicarbonate is chosen as the infusate base, calcium- and magnesium-containing saline solutions must be kept separate from bicarbonate solutions until immediately prior to their infusion to avoid precipitation. This can be accomplished by alternating infusions of bicarbonate and nonbicarbonate fluids or with simultaneous infusion of separate solutions.[396] Careful monitoring of plasma electrolytes during CAVH and CAVH-D is essential. Adjustments in replacement fluid composition or in other intravenous fluids should be made as indicated. Hyponatremia is common in patients with oliguric acute renal failure and

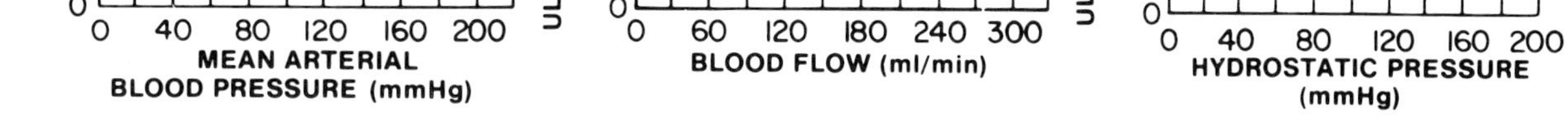

FIGURE 40-12 • Variables affecting ultrafiltration rate in continuous arteriovenous hemofiltration. (*a*) Relationship of blood-flow rate and mean arterial pressure with type of access. Femoral artery cannulation was done with either a 14-gauge(*) or 16-gauge catheter. (*b*) Relationship between ultrafiltration and blood-flow rates. Blood flow rates above 90 ml/min were obtained with use of a blood pump. (*c*) Relationship of ultrafiltration rate and transmembrane hydrostatic pressure gradient with plasma protein concentration. Hydrostatic pressure gradients above 80 mmHg were obtained with use of a blood pump. (From Lauer A et al: *Ann Intern Med* 99:455, 1983. Used by permission.)

TABLE 40-10 • **Continuous arteriovenous hemofiltration**

Component	Plasma (P)	Ultrafiltrate (Uf)	Uf/P ratio
Sodium, meq/liter	136.2 ± 10.4	135.3 ± 11.2	0.99
Potassium, meq/liter	4.1 ± 0.7	4.1 ± 0.7	0.99
Chloride, meq/liter	99.3 ± 10.8	103.7 ± 9.6	1.05
Carbon dioxide, meq/liter	19.8 ± 4.7	22.1 ± 5.1	1.12
Urea nitrogen, mg/dl	79.1 ± 36.1	82.9 ± 38.4	1.05
Creatinine, mg/dl	6.5 ± 3.9	6.6 ± 4.0	1.02
Uric acid, mg/dl	7.4 ± 3.0	7.5 ± 3.3	1.02
Phosphorus, mg/dl	3.9 ± 1.1	4.2 ± 1.3	1.04
Glucose, mg/dl	164.5 ± 76.6	173.0 ± 84.5	1.04
Total proteins, g/dl	6.2 ± 0.3	0.1 ± 0.1	0.02
Albumin, g/dl	2.7 ± 0.5	0.02 ± 0.04	<0.01
Calcium, mg/dl	8.1 ± 0.6	5.1 ± 0.4	0.64
Total bilirubin, mg/dl	12.1 ± 9.5	0.4 ± 0.6	0.03
Direct bilirubin, mg/dl	7.4 ± 5.9	0.3 ± 0.3	0.03

SOURCE: From Kaplan et al: *Ann Intern Med* 100:358, 1984. Used by permission.

can be managed by increasing the sodium concentration of the CAVH replacement solution.[396,625] Potassium, calcium, magnesium, and phosphate levels likewise need to be monitored. Replacement fluids may be administered into the arterial (predilution) or venous (postdilution) lines. Predilution increases filtration rates and solute clearances, while postdilution requires substantially less replacement fluid volume.[541,543] The temptation to simply increase the infusion rate of intravenous hyperalimentation fluid to replace the ultrafiltration losses must be resisted unless the typical composition of these fluids (a low sodium concentration with high concentrations of potassium, phosphate, and magnesium) has been considerably modified.

It is somewhat surprising that hypotension complicating the removal of large volumes of fluid by ultrafiltration with CAVH has not been a particularly common problem.[596,628] When hyypotension does develop in patients during CAVH, in addition to assessing intravascular volume status, patients should also be thoroughly evaluated for cardiac dysfunction, hemorrhage, and sepsis. In a recent study, Lauer and colleagues found that, despite a mean reduction in body weight of 7 kg and a mean net sodium deficit of greater than 1000 meq with CAVH, the cardiac index rose and total vascular resistance was stable or fell in eight of nine patients.[628] The authors attributed the absence of hemodynamic instability to a net negative fluid removal rate (100 ml/h) lower than the rate at which intravascular refilling occurs from the interstitium. Even more rapid removal of large volumes of ultrafiltrate has been accomplished without adverse hemodynamic consequences.[517,982,1125]

Continuous arteriovenous hemodialysis (CAVH-D) combines the convective solute transport of CAVH with diffusion (dialysis) to enhance solute clearance (Fig. 40-11).[377,378,913,995,1087,1088,1200] A dialysis fluid (either peritoneal dialysis solution or commercially available CAVH-D solution) is infused countercurrent to blood flow at about 1 liter/h (16.6 ml/min). The resulting urea clearance due to the combined effects of convection and diffusion reaches 20 to 25 ml/min, which is about $1\frac{1}{2}$ to 2 times that of standard hemodialysis (averaged over a 7-day period), acute peritoneal dialysis, or CAVH (Table 40-11).[1087,1088] Above a blood flow rate of 60 ml/min, diffusive clearance of urea and creatinine is independent of blood flow rate but is equal to, and increases linearly with, dialysate inflow rates up to approximately 26 ml/min. Above this dialysate flow rate, equilibration of blood with dialysate is incomplete, and diffusive clearance increases less than does dialysate flow rate.[116,898,995,1087] Increased dialysate flow rate does not reduce the ultrafiltration rate,[116,395,1087] except perhaps at flows greater than 100 to 150 ml/min.[995]

TABLE 40-11 • **Urea clearance with CAVH, CAVH-D, and other methods of dialysis, ml/min**

CAVH	HD	APD	CAVH-D
10	15.4	17	21

ABBREVIATIONS: HD, hemodialysis with urea clearance of 216 ml/min for 4 h three times per week, expressed as ml/min averaged over 1 week; APD, acute peritoneal dialysis with dwell time of 30 min and cycle time of 1 h.

SOURCE: From Sigler MH, Teehan BP, in Nissenson AR et al (eds): *Clinical Dialysis,* 2d ed, Norwalk, Ct, Appleton & Lange, 1990, p 720. Used by permission.

Substantial phosphate removal necessitates monitoring of the serum phosphorus concentration, with repletion as indicated. An ionized calcium concentration gradient favoring diffusion from dialysate to blood is opposed by a larger convective movement of calcium from blood to dialysate. At a mean ultrafiltration rate of about 8 ml/min, there results a net loss of approximately 13.8 mmol (550 mg) of calcium per day. At lower ultrafiltration rates, calcium losses become negligible. Potassium loss is influenced by the plasma concentration, ultrafiltration rate, and dialysate concentration. With potassium-free dialysate, approximately 130 meq/day can be removed. Glucose extraction from dialysate is dependent on blood flow and can serve as a significant source of calories but may produce hyperglycemia requiring insulin treatment. Net sodium transfer is determined almost entirely by convection, since diffusive transport is limited by a usual dialysate sodium concentration of 132 to 140 meq/liter. Net sodium losses exceeding 1000 to 1500 meq/day at typical ultrafiltration rates may result in a substantial cumulative deficit if the losses are not at least partially replaced. Hyponatremia frequently develops from administration of hypotonic intravenous fluids, hyperalimentation, and dialysate.[1087,1200] Bicarbonate removal (approximately 0.5 meq/min) is generally balanced by lactate or acetate transfer from dialysate to blood; thus, serum bicarbonate concentration remains stable or increases. Metabolic alkalosis (and hypocalcemia) may develop if regional citrate anticoagulation, rather than heparin, is used.[759] Bicarbonate-based dialysate may also be specially prepared for use in patients with severe metabolic acidosis.[526]

The ability to achieve high urea, creatinine, middle-molecule, and electrolyte clearances by combining dialysis with the ultrafiltration capabilities of CAVH makes CAVH-D a particularly useful dialytic therapy. This is especially true in critically ill patients with acute renal failure who are typically catabolic and may have multiorgan failure. Limiting factors for CAVH and CAVH-D include the need for arterial access and anticoagulation as well as a substantial amount of nursing time.

REFERENCES

1. Abbott WE, Shea P: Treatment of temporary renal insufficiency (uremia) by peritoneal lavage. *Am J Med Sci* 211:312, 1946.
2. Abel JJ et al: The removal of diffusible substances from the circulating blood by means of dialysis. *Trans Assoc Am Physicians* 28:51, 1913.
3. Abrams DE et al: Antacid induction of a phosphate depletion syndrome in renal failure. *West J Med* 120:157, 1974.
4. Abu-Hamdan DK et al: Cautopyreiophagia: Cause of life-threatening hyperkalemia in a patient undergoing hemodialysis. *Am J Med* 79:517, 1985.
5. Abu-Hamdan DK et al: Hypoxemia during hemodialysis using acetate versus bicarbonate dialysate. *Am J Nephrol* 4:248, 1984.
6. Acchiardo SR, Hayden AJ: Is Na^+ modeling necessary in high-flux dialysis? *Trans Am Soc Artif Intern Organs* 37:M135, 1991.
7. Acchiardo SR et al: Evaluation of hemodialysis patients treated with erythropoietin. *Am J Kidney Dis* 17:290, 1991.
8. Acchiardo SR et al: Morbidity and mortality in hemodialysis patients. *Trans Am Soc Artif Intern Organs* 36:M148, 1990.
9. Acchiardo SR et al: Are high flux dialysis and erythropoietin on a collision course? *Trans Am Soc Artif Intern Organs* 35:308, 1989.
10. Acosta JH: Hypertension in chronic renal disease. *Kidney Int* 22:702, 1982.
11. Ahearn DJ, Nolph KD: Controlled sodium removal with peritoneal dialysis. *Trans Am Soc Artif Intern Organs* 18:423, 1972.
12. Ahlman J et al: Abdominal pains during CAPD with acetate buffered dialysate (letter to editor). *Lancet* 2:1247, 1983.
13. Ahmad R: Magnesium-induced neuropathy in patients undergoing haemodialysis. *Br Med J* 288:1654, 1984.
14. Ahmad S et al: Effects of oxygen administration on the manifestation of acetate intolerance in dialysis patients. *Am J Nephrol* 2:256, 1982.
15. Ahmad S et al: Effect of the normalization of acid-base balance on post-dialysis plasma bicarbonate. *Trans Am Soc Artif Intern Organs* 26:318, 1980.
16. Ahmad S et al: Intermittent peritoneal dialysis: Status reassessed. *Trans Am Soc Artif Intern Organs* 25:85, 1979.
17. Aizawa Y et al: A fall of plasma osmolality created at dialyzer and its possible effect on circulating blood volume. *Clin Nephrol* 12:269, 1979.
18. Aizawa Y, Shibata A: Hemodynamic effects of acetate in man. *J Dial* 2:235, 1978.
19. Aizawa Y et al: Depressant action of acetate upon the human cardiovascular system. *Clin Nephrol* 8:477, 1977.
20. Alfrey AC: Aluminum intoxication (editorial). *N Engl J Med* 310:1113, 1984.
21. Alfrey AC, Miller NL: Bone magnesium pools in uremia. *J Clin Invest* 52:3019, 1973.
22. Al-Kudsi RR: Extreme hyperglycemia in dialysis patients. *Clin Nephrol* 117:228, 1982.
23. Allon M et al: Albuterol and insulin for treatment of hyperkalemia in hemodialysis patients. *Kidney Int* 38:869, 1990.
24. Allon M et al: Nebulized albuterol for acute hyperkalemia in patients on hemodialysis. *Ann Intern Med* 110:426, 1989.
25. Almeida A, Van Stone JC: Dialysate sodium. *Semin Dial* 2:176, 1989.
26. Alter MJ et al: National surveillance of dialysis-associ-

ated diseases in the United States, 1989. *Trans Am Soc Artif Intern Organs* 36:M148, 1991.
27. Alvarez UF et al: Hemodialysis bone disease: Correlation between clinical, histologic, and other findings. *Kidney Int* 16:68, 1978.
28. Amidon P et al: Adsorption of insulin to the polyvinyl chloride surface of CAPD solution containers. *Proc Clin Dial Transplant Forum* 10:296, 1980.
29. Amir P et al: Continuous ambulatory peritoneal dialysis in diabetics with end-stage renal disease. *N Engl J Med* 306:625, 1982.
30. An international cooperative sutdy, second report: A survey of ultrafiltration in chronic ambulatory peritoneal dialysis. *Perit Dial Bull* 4:137, 1984.
31. Anderson A et al: Glucose absorption from the dialysis fluid during peritoneal dialysis. *Scand J Urol Nephrol* 5:77, 1971.
32. Anderson KEH: Calcium transfer during intermittent peritoneal dialysis. *Nephron* 29:63, 1981.
33. Anderson LE et al: Effects of acetate and bicarbonate dialysate on left ventricular performance. *Am J Kidney Dis* 10:350, 1987.
34. Andreoli S et al: Calcium carbonate is an effective phosphorus binder in children with chronic renal failure. *Am J Kidney Dis* 9:206, 1987.
35. Andress DL et al: Intravenous calcitrol in treatment of refractory osteitis fibrosis of chronic renal failure. *N Engl J Med* 321:274, 1989.
36. Anelli A et al: Substitution of calcium carbonate for aluminum hydroxide in patients on hemodialysis: Effects on acidosis, on parathyroid function, and on calcemia. *Nephron* 52:125, 1989.
37. Anonymous: Uraemic hypoglycemia (editorial). *Lancet* 1:660, 1986.
38. Appel G et al: Lipid abnormalities in renal disease. *Kidney Int* 39:169, 1991.
39. Arduino MJ et al: Adverse patient reactions due to chemical contamination of hemodialysis fluids. *Dial Transplant* 18:655, 1989.
40. Arem R et al: Sulfonamide-induced hypoglycemia in chronic renal failure. *Arch Intern Med* 143:827, 1983.
41. Arem R: Hypoglycemia associated with renal failure. *Endocrinol Metab Clin North Am* 18:103, 1989.
42. Arfeen S et al: The nutritional/metabolic and hormonal effects of 8 weeks of continuous ambulatory peritoneal dialysis with a 1% amino acid solution. *Clin Nephrol* 33:192, 1990.
43. Arieff AI et al: Experimental dialysis disequilibrium syndrome: Prevention with glycerol. *Kidney Int* 14:270, 1978.
44. Arieff AI, Massry SG: Dialysis disequilibrium syndrome, in Massry SG, Selbers AL (eds): *Clinical Aspects of Uremia and Dialysis*. Springfield, Ill, Charles C. Thomas, 1976, p 34.
45. Arieff AI et al: Central nervous system pH in uremia and the effects of hemodialysis. *J Clin Invest* 58:306, 1976.
46. Arieff AI et al: Brain water and electrolyte metabolism in uremia. Effects of slow and rapid hemodialysis. *Kidney Int* 4:177, 1973.
47. Arieff AI et al: Brain tissue osmolality: Method of determination and variations in hyper- and hypo-osmolar states. *J Lab Clin Med* 79:334, 1972.
48. Armstrong VW et al: Effect of dialysate glucose load on plasma glucose and glucoregulatory hormones in CAPD patients. *Nephron* 39:141, 1985.
49. Arrizabalaga P et al: Increase in serum potassium caused by beta-2 adrenergic blockade in terminal renal failure: Absence of mediation by insulin or aldosterone. *Proc Eur Dial Transplant Assoc* 20:572, 1983.
50. Arruda JAL: Acidosis of renal failure. *Semin Nephrol* 1:275, 1981.
51. Asaba H et al: Clinical implications of uremic middle molecules in regular hemodialysis patients. *Clin Nephrol* 19:179, 1983.
52. Asaba H et al: Sequential ultrafiltration and diffusion as an alternative to conventional hemodialysis. *Proc Clin Dial Transplant Forum* 6:129, 1976.
53. Asad SN et al: Plasma calcium fraction dynamics in uremic patients undergoing haemodialysis. *Miner Electrolyte Metab* 10:333, 1984.
54. Asad SN et al: Changes in total body calcium on prolonged maintenance hemodialysis with high and low dialysate calcium. *Nephron* 23:223, 1979.
55. Ash SR: Chronic peritoneal dialysis catheters: Effect of catheter design materials and location. *Semin Dial* 3:39, 1990.
56. Ash SR et al: Peritoneal access devices: Hydraulic function and biocompatibility, in Nissenson AR et al(eds): *Clinical Dialysis*, 2d ed. Norwalk, Ct, Appleton & Lange, 1990, p. 212.
57. Ash SR et al: Clinical trials of the BioLogic-HD: Automated single access, sorbent-based dialysis. *Trans Am Soc Artif Intern Organs* 33:524, 1987.
58. Ashouri OS: Metaprolol-induced hyperkalemia in a diabetic with advanced renal failure (letter to editor). *Arch Intern Med* 145:578, 1985.
59. Association for the Advancement of Medical Instrumentation. *American National Standard for Hemodialysis Systems*. 1982, Arlington, Va.
60. Assomull VM et al: Evidence that acetate in dialysate does not stimulate lipid synthesis. *Proc Clin Dial Transplant Forum* 9:73, 1979.
61. Aujla NS et al: An intraperitoneal insulin regimen for diabetics on continuous cyclic peritoneal dialysis. *Trans Am Soc Artif Intern Organ* 36:119, 1990.
62. Aurell M et al: Captopril treatment in hypertensive dialysis patients. *Scand J Urol* 16:251, 1982.
63. Aurigemma NM et al: Arterial oxygenation during hemodialysis. *N Engl J Med* 297:871, 1977.
64. Avram MM et al: Uremic hypoglycemia: A preventable life threatening complication. *N Y State J Med* 84:593, 1984.
65. Ayus JC et al: Alkalemia associated with renal failure: Correction by hemodialysis with low- bicarbonate dialysate. *Arch Intern Med* 140:513, 1980.
66. Babb AL et al: Bi-directional permeability of the human peritoneum to middle molecules. *Proc Eur Dial Transplant Assoc* 10:247, 1973.
67. Babb AL et al: The genesis of the square meter-hour hypothesis. *Trans Am Soc Artif Intern Organs* 17:81, 1971.

68. Baeyer H et al: Adaptation of CAPD patients to the continuous peritoneal energy uptake. *Kidney Int* 23:29, 1983.
69. Balant L et al: Pharmacokinetics of glipizide in renal insufficiency. *Diabetologia* 9(suppl):331, 1973.
70. Balducci A et al: Intraperitoneal insulin in uraemic diabetics undergoing chronic ambulatory peritoneal dialysis. *Br Med J* 283:1021, 1981.
71. Baltazar RF et al: Acute fluoride poisoning leading to fatal hyperkalemia. *Chest* 78:660, 1980.
72. Bambauer R et al: Comparison of low molecular weight heparin and standard heparin in hemodialysis. *Trans Am Soc Artif Intern Organs* 36:M646, 1990.
73. Bambauer R et al: Ultrafiltration of dialysis fluid to obtain a sterile solution during hemodialysis. *Blood Purif* 8:309, 1990.
74. Bansal VK et al: Intractable hypoglycemia in a patient with renal failure. *Arch Intern Med* 139:100, 1979.
75. Barbour BH et al: Clinical use of NISR polycarbonate membrane for hemodialysis. *Trans Am Soc Artif Intern Organs* 21:144, 1975.
76. Bargman JM, Oreopoulos DG: Complications other than peritonitis or those related to the catheter and the fate of uremic organ dysfunction in patients receiving peritoneal dialysis, in Nolph KD (ed): *Peritoneal Dialysis*, 3d ed. Boston, Kluwer Academic, 1989, p 289.
77. Barsotti G et al: The role of metabolic acidosis in causing uremic hyperphosphatemia. *Miner Electrolyte Metab* 12:103, 1986.
78. Bartlett RH et al: Continuous arteriovenous hemofiltration for acute renal failure. *Trans Am Soc Artif Intern Organs* 34:67, 1988.
78a. Basile C et al: The effects of dialysis on brain water and EEG in stable chronic uremia. *Am J Kidney Dis* 9:462, 1987.
79. Basioli S et al: Buffers in peritoneal dialysis. *Int J Artif Organs* 10:3, 1987.
80. Bauer W, Richards JW: A vasodilator action of acetate. *J Physiol* 66:371, 1928.
81. Bauermeister U et al: Dialysate contamination and back filtration limit the use of high-flux dialysis membranes. *Trans Am Soc Artif Intern Organs* 35:519, 1989.
82. Baumgart P et al: Blood pressure elevation during the night in chronic renal failure, hemodialysis and after renal transplantation. *Nephron* 57:293, 1991.
83. Bazzato G et al: Xylitol as osmotic agent in CAPD: An alternative to glucose for uremic diabetic patients? *Trans Am Soc Artif Intern Organs* 28:280, 1982.
84. Beardsworth SF et al: Intraperitoneal insulin: A protocol for administration during continuous ambulatory peritoneal dialysis and review of published protocols. *Perit Dial Int* 8:145, 1988.
85. Benz RL et al: Successful treatment of postparathroidectomy hypocalcemia using continuous ambulatory intraperitoneal calcium (CAIC) therapy. *Perit Dial Bull* 9:285, 1989.
86. Bergström J et al: Dialysis, ultrafiltration, and blood pressure. *Proc Eur Dial Transplant Asosc* 13:293, 1976.
87. Bergström J et al: Uremic middle molecules exist and are biologically active. *Clin Nephrol* 11:229, 1979.
88. Bia MJ, DeFronzo RA: Extrarenal potassium homeostasis. *Am J Physiol* 240:F257, 1981.
89. Bijaphala S et al: Comparison of high and low sodium bicarbonate and acetate in 5 stable chronic hemodialysis patients. *Clin Nephrol* 23:179, 1985.
90. Bilbrey GL et al: Potassium deficiency in chronic renal failure. *Kidney Int* 4:423, 1973.
91. Binswanger U et al: Peritonitis during continuous ambulatory peritoneal dialysis: Improving patient defense by type of buffer of dialysate. *Nephron* 28:300, 1981.
92. Bischel MD, Barbour BH: Peritoneal dialysis with sorbitol versus dextrose dialysate. *Nephron* 12:449, 1974.
93. Bishop MC et al: Phosphate deficiency in hemodialyzed patients. *Proc Eur Dial Transplant Assoc* 8:106, 1971.
94. Bisson PG et al: Sodium in peritoneal dialysis solutions. *Br Med J* 5:1372, 1979.
95. Biswas CK et al: Heparin effect on ionized calcium concentration. *Clin Chim Acta* 11:343, 1981.
96. Bjaeldager PAL et al: Improved effect of hemodialysis on acidemic patients from an acetate concentration of 38 mmol/L. *Nephron* 27:142, 1981.
97. Bjaphala S et al: Comparison of high and low sodium bicarbonate and acetate dialysis in stable chronic hemodialysis patients. *Clin Nephrol* 23:179, 1985.
98. Blagg CR: Adequacy of dialysis. *Am J Kidney Dis* 4:218, 1984.
99. Bland LE et al: Potential bacteriologic and endotoxin hazards associated with liquid bicarbonate concentrate. *Trans Am Soc Artif Intern Organs* 33:542, 1987.
100. Block MB, Rubenstein AH: Spontaneous hypoglycemia in diabetic patients with renal insufficiency. *JAMA* 215:117, 1971.
101. Blomfield J et al: Control of the hypermagnesemia of renal failure by maintenance hemodialysis. *Med J Aust* 1:854, 1970.
102. Bluemle LW Jr: Current status of chronic hemodialysis. *Am J Med* 44:749, 1968.
103. Blumberg A et al: Effect of various therapeutic approaches on plasma potassium and major regulating factors in terminal renal failure. *Am J Med* 85:507, 1988.
104. Blumenkrantz MJ et al: Metabolic balance studies and dietary protein requirements in patients undergoing continuous ambulatory peritoneal dialysis. *Kidney Int* 21:849, 1982.
105. Blumenkrantz MJ et al: Protein losses during peritoneal dialysis. *Kidney Int* 19:593, 1981.
106. Blumenkrantz M et al: Applications of the REDY sorbent system to hemodialysis and peritoneal dialysis. *Artif Organs* 3:230, 1979.
107. Blumentals AS et al: Acid-base balance changes during hemodialysis. *Metabolism* 14:667, 1965.
108. Boddy K et al: Total body potassium in non-dialyzed and dialyzed patients with chronic renal failure. *Br Med J* 1:771, 1972.
109. Boelens PA et al: Hypophosphatemia with muscle weakness due to antacids and hemodialysis. *Am J Dis Child* 120:350, 1970.
110. Boen ST: History of peritoneal dialysis, in Nolph KD (ed): *Peritoneal Dialysis*, 3d ed. Boston, Kluwer Academic, 1989, p 1.

111. Boen ST: Overview and history of peritoneal dialysis. *Dial Transplant* 6:12, 1977.
112. Boen ST: *Peritoneal Dialysis in Clinical Medicine.* Springfield, Ill, Charles C Thomas, 1966.
113. Boen ST: Kinetics of peritoneal dialysis: A comparison with the artificial kidney. *Medicine* 40:243, 1961.
114. Boen ST et al: Periodic peritoneal dialysis in the management of chronic uremia. *Trans Am Soc Artif Intern Organs* 8:256, 1962.
115. Bondia A et al: Autonomic nervous system in hemodialysis. *Nephrol Dial Transplant* 2:174, 1988.
116. Bonnardeaux A et al: Solute clearances with different dialysate flow rates and glucose absorption from the dialysate in continuous arteriovenous hemodialysis (CAVHD) (abstract). *J Am Soc Nephrol* 1:349, 1990.
117. Boquin E et al: Crossover study of the effect of different dialysate sodium concentrations in large surface area short-term dialysis. *Proc Clin Dial Transplant Forum* 7:48, 1977.
118. Borges HF, Kjellstrand CM: The effect of prostaglandin inhibition on the clinical course of chronic hemodialysis. *Nephron* 42:120, 1986.
119. Borges HF et al: Mannitol intoxication in patients with renal failure. *Arch Intern Med* 142:63, 1982.
120. Borges HR et al: Hypotension during acetate and bicarbonate dialysis in patients with acute renal failure. *Am J Nephrol* 1:24, 1981.
121. Bosch JP, Ronco C: Continuous arteriovenous hemofiltration (CAVH) and other continuous replacement therapies: Operational characteristics and clinical use, in Maher JF (ed): *Replacement of Renal Function by Dialysis*, 3d ed. Dordrecht, The Netherlands, Kluwer Academic, 1989, p. 347.
122. Bosch JP et al: Sodium fluxes during hemodialysis. *Nephron* 45:86, 1987.
123. Bosch JP et al: Carbon dioxide removal in acetate hemodialysis: Effects on acid-base balance. *Kidney Int* 25:830, 1984.
124. Botella J et al: Chloramines, an aggravating factor in the anemia of patients on regular dialysis treatment. *Proc Eur Dial Transplant Assoc* 14:192, 1977.
125. Bouma SF et al: Glucose absorption and weight change on 18 months of CAPD. *J Am Dial Assoc* 84:194, 1984.
126. Bourgoigne JJ et al: Water, electrolyte, and acid-base abnormalities in chronic renal failure. *Semin Nephrol* 1:91, 1981.
127. Boyce BF et al: Hypercalcemic osteomalacia due to aluminum toxicity. *Lancet* 2:1009, 1982.
128. Boyer J et al: Hyperglycemia and hyperosmolality complicating peritoneal dialysis. *Ann Intern Med* 67:568, 1967.
129. Bradley JR et al: Comparison of vascular tone during combined hemodialysis with ultrafiltration and during ultrafiltration followed by hemodialysis: A possible mechanism for dialysis hypotension. *Br Med J* 300:1312, 1990.
130. Bradley JR et al: Is dialysis hypotension caused by an abnormality of venous tone? *Br Med J* 296:1634, 1988.
131. Branger B et al: Aluminum transfer in bicarbonate dialysis using a sorbent regeneration system: An in vitro study. *Proc Eur Dial Transplant Assoc* 17:213, 1980.
132. Brautbar N, Kleeman CR: Disordered divalent ion metabolism in kidney disease: Comments on pathogenesis and treatment. *Adv Nephrol* 8:179, 1979.
133. Brautbar N et al: Magnesium and bone disease. *Nephron* 44:1, 1986.
134. Brecht HM et al: Plasma noradrenaline levels in regular hemodialysis patients. *Proc Eur Dial Transplant Assoc* 12:281, 1976.
135. Brivet F et al: Hemodialysis hypoglycemia (letter to editor). *Nephrol Dial Transplant* 3:482, 1988.
136. Brown EA et al: Effect of hypertonic dialysate on clearances in the rat. *Kidney Int* 13:271, 1978.
137. Brown EM et al: Abnormal regulation of parathyroid hormone release by calcium in secondary hyperparathyroidism due to chronic renal failure. *J Clin Endocrinol Metab* 54:172, 1982.
138. Brown JD et al: Glucose absorption and hyperglycemia during peritoneal dialysis. *Aust N Z J Med* 1:1, 1973.
139. Brown ST et al: Potassium removal with peritoneal dialysis. *Kidney Int* 4:67, 1973.
140. Brueggemeyer CD, Ramirez G: Dialysate concentrate: A potential source for lethal complications. *Nephron* 46:397, 1987.
141. Brunner FP, Thiel G: The use of magnesium-containing phosphate binders in patients with end-stage renal disease on maintenance hemodialysis. *Nephron* 32:266, 1982.
142. Brunner HR et al: Inappropriate renin secretion unmasked by captopril (SQ 14225) in hypertension of chronic renal failure. *Lancet* 2:704, 1978.
143. Bruno M et al: CAPD with an amino acid dialysis solution: A long term cross-over study. *Kidney Int* 35:1189, 1989.
144. Brynger H et al: Combined report on regular dialysis and transplantation in Europe: 10, 1979. *Proc Eur Dial Transplant Assoc* 17:4, 1980.
145. Bunchman TE: Treatment of inflow pain by pH adjustment of dialysate in peritoneal dialysis. *Perit Dial Int* 11:179, 1991.
146. Burgess WP et al: Observations on inadequate buffer concentration in peritoneal dialysis solution for CCPD. *Trans Am Soc Artif Intern Organs* 29:58, 1983.
147. Burnell JM, Teubner E: Effects of decreasing dialysate magnesium in patients with chronic renal failure (abstract). *Proc Clin Dial Transplant Forum* 5:191, 1976.
148. Burns CB, Scheinhorn DJ: Hypoxemia during hemodialysis. *Arch Intern Med* 142:1350, 1982.
149. Burns RO et al: Peritoneal dialysis: Clinical experience. *N Engl J Med* 267:1060, 1962.
150. Burritt MF et al: Comparative studies of total and ionized serum calcium values in normal subjects and patients with renal disorders. *Mayo Clin Proc* 55:606, 1980.
151. Bushinsky DA et al: Arterial P_{CO_2} in chronic metabolic acidosis. *Kidney Int* 22:311, 1982.
152. Butkus DE et al: Tissue potassium in chronic dialysis patients. *Nephron* 13:314, 1974.
153. Calderaro V et al: The evaluation of renal osteodystrophy in patients undergoing chronic ambulatory peritoneal dialysis. *Proc Eur Dial Transplant Assoc* 17:533, 1980.

154. Campese VM et al: Mechanisms of autonomic nervous system dysfunction in uremia. *Kidney Int* 20:246, 1981.
155. Canadian Erythropoietin Study Group: Effect of recombinant human erythropoietin on blood pressure in hemodialysis patients. *Am J Nephrol* 11:23, 1991.
156. Canella G et al: Interrelationships between blood pressure, blood gases and plasma acetate concentrations during conventional hemodialysis. *Int J Artif Organs* 5:357, 1982.
157. Canepa A et al: Continuous ambulatory peritoneal dialysis (CAPD) of children with amino acid solution: Technical and metabolic aspect. *Perit Dial Int* 10:215, 1990.
158. Cannata JB et al: Comparison of control of serum phosphate levels during continuous ambulatory peritoneal dialysis and during hemodialysis. *Perit Dial Bull* 3:97, 1983.
159. Cannaud B et al: Blood pressure control in patients treated by continuous ambulatory peritoneal dialysis, in Legrain M (ed): *Continuous Ambulatory Peritoneal Dialysis*. Amsterdam: Excerpta Medica, 1980.
160. Cannella G et al: Blood pressure behaviors during dialysis and ultrafiltration: A pathogenetic hypothesis on hemodialysis-induced hypotension. *Int J Artif Organs* 1:69, 1978.
161. Canzanello V et al: Hyperammonemic encephalopathy during dialysis. *Ann Intern Med* 99:190, 1983.
162. Capelli G et al: Effects of biofiltration versus hemofiltration in the treatment of chronic uremia. *Int J Artif Organs* 9:21, 1986.
163. Carlson DJ, Shapiro FL: Methemoglobinemia from well water nitrates: A complication of home hemodialysis. *Ann Intern Med* 73:757, 1970.
164. Carlsson E et al: β-adrenoreceptor blockers, plasma potassium and exercise. *Lancet* 2:424, 1978.
165. Carney SL, Gilles AHG: Acute dialysis hypercalcemia and dialysis phosphate loss. *Am J Kidney Dis* 11:377, 1988.
166. Carney SL, Gilles AHG: Effect of an optimum dialysis fluid calcium concentration on calcium mass transfer during maintenance hemodialysis. *Clin Nephrol* 24:28, 1985.
167. Caruana RJ et al: Effects of oral base therapy on serum ionized calcium, phosphorus and parathryoid hormone in chronic hemodialysis patients. *Int J Artif Organs* 12:778, 1989.
168. Caruana RJ et al: Heparin free dialysis: Comparative data and results in high risk patients. *Kidney Int* 31:1351, 1987.
169. Castellani A et al: No relationship between acetate and hypotension in a standard dialysis schedule. *Proc Eur Dial Transplant Assoc* 19:340, 1982.
170. Catto GRD et al: The effect of low magnesium dialysate on plasma, ultrafiltrable, erythrocyte and bone magnesium concentrations from patients on maintenance hemodialysis. *Nephron* 13:372, 1974.
171. Chachati A et al: Importance of dialysate magnesium in the pathogenesis of cardiac arrhythmias in chronic dialysis patients (abstract). *Proceedings Tenth Int Congr Nephrol*, 1987, p. 130.
172. Chaignon M et al: Acute effects of hemodialysis on echographic-determined cardiac performance: Improved contractility from serum increased calcium with reduced potassium despite hypovolemic-induced cardiac output. *Am Heart J* 103:374, 1982.
173. Chan MK et al: Hyperlipidemia in patients on maintenance hemo- and peritoneal dialysis: The relative pathogenetic role of triglyceride production and triglyceride removal. *Clin Nephrol* 17:183, 1984.
174. Chanard et al: Ultrafiltration-pump assisted continuous arteriovenous hemofiltration (CAVH). *Kidney Int* 33(suppl 24):S157, 1988.
175. Chanard J et al: Long-term results of dialysis therapy with a highly permeable membrane. *Int J Artif Organs* 6:261, 1982.
176. Charney DI, Salmond R: Cardiac arrest after hypertonic citrate anticoagulation for chronic hemodialysis. *Trans Am Soc Artif Intern Organs* 36:M216, 1990.
177. Charytan C et al: A comparative study of continuous ambulatory peritoneal dialysis and center hemodialysis. *Arch Intern Med* 146:1138, 1986.
178. Chen TS et al: Hemodynamic changes during hemodialysis: Role of dialysate. *Clin Nephrol* 20:190, 1983.
179. Chen TS et al: Hemodynamic changes during dialysis. *Proc Clin Dial Transplant Forum* 9:66, 1979.
180. Chen WT et al: Hydrostatic ultrafiltration during hemodialysis using decreasing sodium dialysate. *Artif Organs* 4:187, 1980.
181. Chen WT et al: Hemodynamics of post-dialysis hypotension (abstract). *Kidney Int* 12:493, 1977.
182. Chesney RW, Haughton PB: Tetany following phosphate enemas in chronic renal disease. *Am J Dis Child* 127:584, 1974.
183. Cheung AK: Biocompatibility of hemodialysis membranes. *J Am Soc Nephrol* 1:150, 1990.
184. Coburn JW, Salusky IB: Control of serum phosphorus in uremia. *N Engl J Med* 320:1140, 1989.
185. Coburn JW et al: Role of aluminum accumulation in renal osteodystrophy, in Robinson RR (ed): *Nephrology*, New York, Springer-Verlag, 1984, vol 2, p 1383.
186. Coburn JW, Llach F: Renal osteodystrophy and maintenance dialysis, in Drukker W et al (eds): *Replacement of Renal Function by Dialysis*, 2d ed. Boston, Martinus Nijhoff, 1983.
187. Coburn JW et al: The physio-chemical state and renal handling of divalent ions in chronic renal failure. *Arch Intern Med* 124:302, 1969.
188. Coburn JW et al: Spurious hypocalcemia in patients undergoing maintenance hemodialysis. *Am J Clin Pathol* 52:572, 1969.
189. Cochran M et al: Spontaneous hypercalcemia in maintenance dialysis patients: An association with atypical osteomalacia and fractures. *Miner Electrolyte Metab* 5:280, 1981.
190. Cohen DJ et al: Diabinese and Dialume (letter to editor). *Ann Intern Med* 97:285, 1982.
191. Cohen E et al: Patterns of metabolic acidosis in patients with chronic renal failure: Impact of hemodialysis. *Int J Artif Organs* 11:440, 1988.
192. Cohn J et al: Dialysis induced respiratory acidosis. *Chest* 98:1285, 1990.
193. Coles GA et al: When should chronic peritoneal dialysis

be recommended over hemodialysis. *Semin Dial* 2:213, 1989.

194. Coli U et al: Cold as cardiovascular stabilizing factor in hemodialysis: Hemodynamic evaluation. *Trans Am Soc Artif Intern Organs* 29:71, 1983.
195. Collins AJ et al: Shortening of the hemodialysis procedure and mortality in "healthy" dialysis patients. *Trans Am Soc Artif Intern Organs* 36:M145, 1990.
196. Collins AJ, Keshaviah PR: Are there limitations to shortening dialysis treatment? *Trans Am Soc Artif Intern Organs* 34:1, 1988.
197. Collins J et al: Parathyroid hormone and the altered vascular response to norepinephrine in uremia. *Am J Nephrol* 5:110, 1985.
198. Colton CK, Lowrie EG: Hemodialysis: Physical principles and technical considerations, in Brenner BM, Rector FC Jr (eds): *The Kidney*, 2d ed. Philadelphia, Saunders, 1981.
199. Commack R: Assay, purification and properties of a mammalian D-2-hydroxyacid dehydrogenase. *Biochem J* 115:55, 1969.
200. Compty CM, Shapiro FL: Pretreatment and preparation of city water for hemodialysis, in Drukker W et al (eds): *Replacement of Renal Function by Dialysis*, 2d ed. Boston, Martinus Nijhoff, 1983, p 197.
201. Compty CM et al: Prescription water for chronic hemodialysis. *Trans Am Soc Artif Intern Organs* 20:189, 1974.
202. Connor H et al: Comparison of the kinetics and utilization of D(−) and L(+) sodium lactate in normal man. *Ann Nutr Metab* 27:481, 1983.
203. Conte F et al: Lactic acidosis coma in continuous ambulatory peritoneal dialysis (letter to editor). *Nephron* 43:148, 1986.
204. Conte G et al: Acute increase in plasma osmolality as a cause of hyperkalemia in patients with renal failure. *Kidney Int* 38:301, 1990.
205. Contiguglia SR et al: Total body magnesium excess in chronic renal failure. *Lancet* 1:1300, 1972.
206. Copley JB et al: Insulin: Its use in patients on peritoneal dialysis. *Semin Dial* 1:143, 1988.
207. Corvilain J et al: Labeled insulin catabolism in chronic renal failure and in the anephric state. *Diabetes* 20:467, 1971.
208. Cowie J et al: The influence of extracorporeal dialysis on the acid-base composition of blood and cerebrospinal fluid. *Clin Sci* 23:397, 1962.
209. Crossley K, Kjellstrand CM: Intraperitoneal insulin for control of blood sugar in diabetic patients during peritoneal dialysis. *Br Med J* 1:269, 1971.
210. Cullom ET et al: pH equilibration with acetate and lactate solutions during peritoneal dialysis. *Perit Dial Bull* 5:123, 1985.
211. Culpepper C et al: Aluminum kinetics of the REDY system: A study of the impact of desferoxamine therapy. *Trans Am Soc Artif Intern Organs* 29:76, 1983.
212. Cushner HM et al: Calcium citrate, a nonaluminum-containing phosphate-binding agent for the treatment of CRF. *Kidney Int* 33:95, 1988.
213. Cybulsky AVE et al: Effects of high sodium dialysate during maintenance hemodialysis. *Nephron* 41:57, 1985.
214. Daelemans R et al: Calcium carbonate as a phosphate binder in patients on low-calcium dialysate. *Am J Nephrol* 9:348, 1989.
215. Dalal SP et al: L-Lactate high-efficiency hemodialysis: Hemodynamics, blood gas changes, potassium/phosphorus, and symptoms. *Kidney Int* 38:896, 1990.
216. Dalal SP et al: L-Lactate for high-efficiency hemodialysis: Feasibility studies and a randomized comparison with acetate and bicarbonate. *Int J Artif Organs* 2:611, 1989.
217. Daniels F et al: A macromolecular polyelectrolyte (Gelifundol) as an osmotic agent (abstract). *Kidney Int* 29:230, 1986.
218. Daniels FH et al: Glucose and glycerol compared as osmotic agents for peritoneal dialysis. *Kidney Int* 25:20, 1984.
219. Danielsson A et al: Patient-related factors influencing the plasma acetate concentration during haemodialysis. *Nephrol Dial Transplant* 2:526, 1987.
220. Daugirdas JT: Dialysis hypotension: A hemodynamic analysis. *Kidney Int* 39:233, 1991.
221. Daugirdas JT: Bedside formulas for *Kt/V*: A kinder, gentler approach to urea kinetic modeling. *Trans Am Soc Artif Intern Organs* 36:M362, 1990.
222. Daugirdas JT: Rapid methods of estimating *Kt/V*: Three formulas compared. *Trans Am Soc Artif Intern Organs* 35:336, 1989.
223. Daugirdas JT et al: An alternative base for hemodialysis: The promise of L-lactate. *Semin Dial* 2:137, 1989.
224. Daugirdas JT et al: Alkalinization of peritoneal dialysis solution with sodium hydroxide and sodium bicarbonate. *Artif Organs* 12:203, 1988.
225. Daugirdas JT et al: Acetate causes endothelium- independent increases in cyclic AMP in rat caudal artery. *Am J Physiol* 255:H1378, 1988.
226. Daugirdas JT et al: Acetate relaxation of isolated vascular smooth muscle. *Kidney Int* 32:39, 1987.
227. Daugirdas JT et al: Hemodialysis hemodynamics in an animal model: Effect of using an acetate-buffered dialysate. *J Lab Clin Med* 107:517, 1986.
228. Daugirdas JT et al: Ultrafiltration hemodynamics in conscious uremic dogs: Effects of a decreasing plasma urea level. *Miner Electrolyte Metab* 11:79, 1985.
229. Daugirdas JT et al: A double-blind evaluation of sodium gradient hemodialysis. *Am J Nephrol* 5:163, 1985.
230. Daugirdas JT et al: Ultrafiltration haemodynamics in conscious, uremic dogs: Effect of extracorporeal blood temperature. *Trans Am Soc Artif Intern Organs* 29:688, 1983.
231. Daul AE et al: Arterial hypotension in chronic hemodialysis patients. *Kidney Int* 32:728, 1987.
232. David DS et al: Aspirin induced hypoglycemia in a patient on hemodialysis. *Lancet* 1:1092, 1971.
233. Dawborn JK et al: Parathyroidectomy in chronic renal failure. *Nephron* 33:100, 1983.
234. Dawborn JK et al: Peritoneal dialysis: Calcium, phosphate, and bone disease, in Atkins RC et al (eds): *Peritoneal Dialysis*. Edinburgh, Churchill Livingstone, 1981, p 406.
235. DeBroe ME et al: Pulmonary aspects of dialysis patients, in Maher JF (ed): *Replacement of Renal Function by Dialysis*, 3d ed. Boston, Kluwer Academic, 1989, p 827.

236. Defilter C et al: Glycerol versus glucose containing peritoneal dialysis fluid (PDF): Its impact on peritoneal macrophage function in vivo (abstract). *Perit Dial Int* 11(suppl 1):63, 1991.
237. DeFremont JP et al: Metabolic tolerance in chronic ambulatory peritoneal dialysis (CAPD), in Gahl GM et al (eds): *Advances in Peritoneal Dialysis*. Amsterdam, Excerpta Medica, 1981, p. 446.
238. Degoulet P et al: Epidemiology of dialysis induced hypotension. *Proc Eur Dial Transplant Assoc* 18;133, 1981.
239. Delano et al: Dialyzer urea and creatinine clearances are not significantly altered in erythropoietin treated maintenance hemodialysis patients. *Trans Am Soc Artif Intern Organs* 36:36, 1990.
240. Delin K et al: A clinical test of a new device for on-line preparation of dialysis fluid from bicarbonate powder: The Gambro bicart. *Dial Transplant* 17:468, 1988.
241. Delmez J: Control of mineral metabolism in CAPD patients. *Blood Purif* 7:167, 1989.
242. Delmez J: Renal osteodystrophy and aluminum bone disease in CAPD patients, in Khanna R et al (eds): *Advances in Chronic Ambulatory Peritoneal Dialysis*. Toronto, University of Toronto Press, 1987, p 38.
243. Delmez JA et al: Minerals, vitamin D, and parathyroid hormone in continuous ambulatory peritoneal dialysis. *Kidney Int* 21:862, 1982.
244. De Marchi S, Cecchin E: Bone buffering and acidosis in end-stage renal disease. *Semin Dial* 4:148, 1991.
245. De Marchi S et al: Severe metabolic acidosis and disturbances of calcium metabolism induced by acetazolamide in patients on haemodialysis. *Clin Sci* 78:295, 1990.
246. De Marchi S, Cecchin E: More on the role of metabolic acidosis in causing uremic hyperphosphatemia. *Miner Electrolyte Metab* 13:67, 1987.
247. DePalma JR: High-flux revisited, and, who needs *Kt/V?* *Contemp Dial Nephrol* August:28, 1990.
248. DePalma JR et al: Home hemodialysis using glucose and potassium-free dialysate. *Proc Int Congr Nephrol* 4:55, 1969.
249. Depner TA (ed): Prescribing hemodialysis: A guide to urea modeling. Boston, Kluwer Academic, 1991.
250. Derot M: Le dialyse peritoneale: Sa place dans le traitement de l'uremie aigue. *Sem Hôp Paris* 25:3508, 1949.
251. DeSanto NG et al: Glucose utilization from dialysate in patients on chronic ambulatory peritoneal dialysis (CAPD). *Int J Artif Organs* 2:119, 1979.
252. Desch G et al: Plasma acetate levels during hemodialysis. *Clin Chim Acta* 85:231, 1978.
253. De Vries PMJM et al: The influence of dialysate sodium and variable ultrafiltration on fluid balance during hemodialysis. *Trams Am Soc Artif Intern Organs* 36:821, 1990.
254. Diamond SM, Henrich WL: Acetate dialysate versus bicarbonate dialysate: A continuing controversy. *Am J Kidney Dis* 9:3, 1987.
255. Diaz-Buxo JA: Clinical use of peritoneal dialysis, in Nissenson AR et al (eds): *Clinical Dialysis*, 2d ed. Norwalk, Ct, Appleton & Lange, 1990, p. 256.
256. Diaz-Buxo JA: Continuous cyclic peritoneal dialysis, in Nolph KD (ed): *Peritoneal Dialysis*, 3d ed. Boston, Kluwer Academic, 1989, p 169.
257. Diaz-Buxo JA: Current status of continuous cyclic peritoneal dialysis (CCPD). *Perit Dial Int* 9:9, 1989.
258. Diaz-Buxo JA: CCPD is even better than CAPD. *Kidney Int* 28(suppl 17):S26, 1985.
259. Diaz- Buxo JA et al: CCPD: Wet is better than dry. *Perit Dial Int* 7:S22, 1987.
260. Diaz-Buxo JA et al: Comparison of kinetics of CAPD and CCPD. *Perspect Perit Dial* 3:37, 1985.
261. Diaz-Buxo JA et al: Experience with intermittent peritoneal dialysis and continuous cyclic peritoneal dialysis. *Am J Kidney Dis* 7:242, 1984.
262. Diaz-Buxo JA et al: Total parathyroidectomy and autotransplantation. *Clin Nephrol* 16:276, 1981.
263. Diaz-Buxo JA et al: Continuous cyclic peritoneal dialysis. *Trans Am Soc Artif Intern Organs* 27:51, 1981.
264. Diaz-Buxo JA et al: Continuous cyclic peritoneal dialysis (CCPD). *Kidney Int* 19:145, 1981.
265. Diaz-Buxo JA et al: Continuous cyclic peritoneal dialysis: A preliminary report. *Artif Organs* 5:137, 1981.
266. Diaz-Buxo JA et al: Impact of peritoneal dialysis on renal replacement therapy. *Dial Transplant* 8:1061, 1979.
267. Dibble JB et al: Amino acid based continuous ambulatory peritoneal dialysis (CAPD) fluid over twelve weeks: Effects on carbohydrate and lipid metabolism. *Perit Dial Int* 10:71, 1990.
268. DiMaggio A et al: Plasma volume changes induced by sequential ultrafiltration-hemodialysis and sequential hemodialysis-ultrafiltration. *Int J Artif Organs* 10:291, 1987.
269. DiPaolo N et al: Improvement of impaired ultrafiltration after addition of phosphatidylcholine in patients on CAPD (letter to editor). *Perit Dial Bull* 6:44, 1986.
270. DiPaolo N et al: Morphology of the peritoneal membrane during CAPD. *Nephron* 44:204, 1986.
271. DiRaimondo CR, Pollak VE: β_2-Microglobulin kinetics in maintenance hemodialysis: A comparison of conventional and high-flux dialyzers and the effects of dialyzer reuse. *Am J Kidney Dis* 13:390, 1989.
272. Dixon SR et al: Changes in acid-base balance during peritoneal dialysis with fluid containing lactate ions. *Clin Sci* 39:51, 1970.
273. Dobbie JW: New concepts in molecular biology and ultrastructural pathology of the peritoneum: Their significance for peritoneal dialysis. *Am J Kidney Dis* 15:97, 1990.
274. Dolgos ET et al: Plasma insulin and glucose levels in diabetic patients undergoing chronic ambulatory peritoneal dialysis using insulin only in the dialysate. *Cleveland Clinic Q* 51:611, 1984.
275. Dolkart RE et al: Alternative osmotic agents to glucose for chronic ambulatory peritoneal dialysis. *Perit Dial Bull* 7:4, 1987.
276. Dombros N et al: Six-month overnight intraperitoneal amino acid infusion in continuous ambulatory peritoneal dialysis (CAPD) patients: No effect on nutritional status. *Perit Dial Int* 10:79, 1990.
277. Dombros N et al: Plasma amino acid profile and amino acid loss in patients undergoing CAPD. *Perit Dial Bull* 2:27, 1982.
278. Doolan PD et al: An evaluation of intermittent peritoneal lavage. *Am J Med* 26:831, 1959.
279. Dratwa M et al: Dialysate composition: To change or not to change. *Perit Dial Int* 11(suppl 1):71, 1991.

280. Dratwa M et al: Serum bicarbonate (HCO_3) and phosphorus (P) levels: Striking correlation in hemodialysis (HD) patients (abstract). *Kidney Int* 31:231, 1987.
281. Drukker W: Peritoneal dialysis: A historical review, in Maher JF (ed): *Replacement of Renal Function by Dialysis*, 3d ed. Boston, Kluwer Academic, 1989, p 475.
282. Drukker W: The hard water syndrome. A potential hazard during hemodialysis. *Proc Eur Dial Transplant Assoc* 5:284, 1968.
283. Drukker W: Dialysate glucose concentration and plasma osmolality during haemodialysis in acute renal failure. *Proc Eur Dial Transplant Assoc* 2:7, 1965.
284. Drukker W, van Doorn AWJ: Dialysate regeneration, in Maher JF (ed): *Replacement of Renal Function with Dialysis*, 3d ed. Boston, Kluwer Academic, 1989, p 417.
285. Drury PJ et al: Aluminum release from the Sorbsystem D-3160 and D-3260 cartridges. *Life Support Syst* 4:1986, 211.
286. Duarte RR: The rebirth of bicarbonate. *Int J Artif Organs* 6:57, 1983.
287. Dubost C et al: Total parathyroidectomy followed by parathyroid autotransplantation in the secondary hyperparathyroidism of chronic renal failure, in Hamburger J et al (eds): *Advances in Nephrology*. Chicago, Year Book Medical, 1982, vol 2.
288. Dulaney JT et al: Peritoneal dialysis and loss of protein: A review. *Kidney Int* 26:253, 1984.
289. Dumler F et al: Sequential high/low sodium hemodialysis: An alternative to ultrafiltration. *Trans Am Soc Artif Intern Organs* 25:351, 1979.
290. Duwe AK et al: Effect of the composition of peritoneal dialysis fluid on chemiluminescence, phagocytosis and bacterial activity in vitro. *Immunity* 33:130, 1981.
291. Dy G et al: Treatment of severe hypophosphatemia with intraperitoneal phosphate. *Perit Dial Int* 10:304, 1990.
292. Earle JM et al: Hypercalcemia and hypertension. *Ann Intern Med* 64:378, 1966.
293. Earnest DL et al: Acid-base balance in chronic hemodialysis. *Trans Am Soc Artif Intern Organs* 14:434, 1968.
294. Eastwood JB et al: Heparin inactivation, acidosis, and copper poisoning due to presumed acid contamination in a hemodialysis unit. *Clin Nephrol* 20:197, 1983.
295. Eaton JW et al: Chlorinated urban water: A cause of dialysis-induced hemolytic anemia. *Science* 181:463, 1973.
296. Ebben JP et al: Microbiologic contamination of liquid bicarbonate concentrate for hemodialysis. *Trans Am Soc Artif Intern Organs* 33:269, 1987.
297. Ebben J et al: Volume and chemical errors in peritoneal dialysate. *Dial Transplant* 10:876, 1981.
298. Egger U et al: Acid-base balance and oxygen affinity of hemoglobin in patients on maintenance dialysis. *Clin Nephrol* 1:70, 1973.
299. Eisenhauer T: Development and actual performance of continuous arteriovenous hemofiltration (CAVH), in *Continuous Arteriovenous Hemofiltration: International Conference on CAVH, 1984*. Basel, Karger, 1985, p 1.
300. Eiser AR: Pulmonary gas exchange during hemodialysis and peritoneal dialysis: Interaction between respiration and metabolism. *Am J Kidney Dis* 6:131, 1985.
301. Eiser AR et al: Contrasting alterations in pulmonary gas exchange during acetate and bicarbonate hemodialysis. *Am J Nephrol* 2:123, 1982.
302. Elias AN et al: Plasma norepinephrine, epinephrine, and dopamine levels in end-stage renal disease: Effect of hemodialysis. *Arch Intern Med* 145:1013, 1985.
303. Emder PJ et al: Nonketotic hyperosmolar diabetic precoma due to pancreatitis in a boy on chronic ambulatory peritoneal dialysis. *Nephron* 44:355, 1986.
304. Emmett M et al: Calcium acetate control of serum phosphorus in hemodialysis patients. *Am J Kidney Dis* 17:544, 1991.
305. Ericson F, Carlmark B: Potassium in whole body, skeletal muscle, and erythrocytes in chronic renal failure. *Nephron* 33:173, 1983.
306. Ericson F: Intracellular potassium in man: A clinical and methodological study using whole body counting and muscle biopsy techniques. *Scand J Clin Lab Invest* 42(suppl):1, 1982.
307. Eschbach JW et al: New insights into the treatment of the anemia of chronic renal failure with erythropoietin. *Semin Dial* 3:112, 1990.
308. Eschbach JW et al: Recombinant human erythropoietin in anemic patients with end-stage renal disease: Results of a phase III multicenter clinical trial. *Ann Intern Med* 111:992, 1989.
309. Eschbach JW et al: Correction of the anemia of end-stage renal disease with recombinant human erythropoietin: Results of a combined phase I and II clinical trial. *N Engl J Med* 316:73, 1987.
310. Evans DB, Slapak M: Pancreatitis in the hard water syndrome. *Br Med J* 3:748, 1975.
311. Ewing DJ, Winney R: Autonomic function in patients with chronic renal failure on intermittent hemodialysis. *Nephron* 15:424, 1975.
312. Fabris A et al: The importance of ultrafiltration on acid-base status in a dialysis population. *Trans Am Soc Artif Intern Organs* 34:200, 1988.
313. Fabris A et al: Buffer metabolism in continuous ambulatory peritoneal dialysis (CAPD): Relationship with respiratory dynamics. *Trans Am Soc Artif Intern Organs* 28:270, 1982.
314. Faller B, Marichal JF: Loss of ultrafiltration in continuous ambulatory peritoneal dialysis: A role for acetate. *Perit Dial Bull* 4:10, 1984.
315. Falls WF Jr et al: Dialysis induced changes of extracellular fluid volume in man. *Proc Clin Dial Transplant Forum* 2:155, 1972.
316. Fantuzzi S et al: Hemodialysis-associated cardiac arrhythmias: A lower risk with bicarbonate? *Nephron* 58:196, 1991.
317. Farrell PG et al: Clinical evaluation of a dialysate regeneration system for maintenance dialysis. *Aust N Z J Med* 6:292, 1976.
318. Farrington K et al: Vitamin A toxicity and hypercalcemia in chronic renal failure. *Br Med J* 282:1999, 1981.
319. Farrington K et al: Hypophosphatemia after parathyroidectomy in chronic renal failure. *Br Med J* 284:856, 1982.
320. Fassett RG et al: Hypoglycemia in end-stage renal disease. *Dial Transplant* 12:543, 1983.

321. Fauchald P: Transcapillary colloid osmotic gradient and body fluid volumes in renal failure. *Kidney Int* 29:895, 1986.
322. Fauchald P et al: Immunoreactive parathyroid hormone and calcitonin in plasma and ultrafiltrate before and after haemodialysis. *Scand J Clin Med Invest* 45:229, 1985.
323. FDA Drug Bulletin: *Preventing Chloramine Contamination of Renal Dialysate Solutions*. Rockville, Md, US Food and Drug Administration, August 1988, p 20.
324. Feest TG et al: Idiopathic hypercalcemia of chronic dialysis. *Proc Eur Dial Transplant Assoc* 19:248, 1982.
325. Feig PU et al: Effect of potassium removal during hemodialysis on the plasma potassium concentration. *Nephron* 27:25, 1981.
326. Feldman AM et al: Congestive cardiomyopathy in patients on CAPD. *Am J Kidney Dis* 11:76, 1988.
327. Fellner SK et al: Physiological mechanisms for calcium-induced changes in systemic arterial pressure in stable dialysis patients. *Hypertension* 13:213, 1989.
328. Felsenfeld AJ et al: Osteomalacia after parathyroidectomy in patients with uremia. *Ann Intern Med* 94:629, 1982.
329. Fenton S et al: Low protein catabolic role (PCR): Can it be corrected with intraperitoneal (IP) amino acid (AA) supplements (abstract). *Peritoneal Dial Int* 11(suppl): 79, 1991.
330. Ferdinandus J et al: Hypermagnesemia as a cause of refractory hypotension, respiratory depression, and coma. *Arch Intern Med* 141:669, 1981.
331. Feriani M et al: Acid-base correction in bicarbonate CAPD patients. *Adv Perit Dial* 5:191, 1989.
332. Feriani M et al: The Krebs cycle derangements in CAPD patients. *Perit Dial Bull* 7:S30, 1987.
333. Feriani M et al: Substitution of sodium bicarbonate for sodium acetate/lactate in CAPD fluid, in Khanna R et al (eds): *Advances in Continuous Ambulatory Peritoneal Dialysis: 1986*. Toronto, Peritoneal Dialysis Bulletin, 1986, p 16.
334. Feriani M et al: Bicarbonate buffer for CAPD solution. *Trans Am Soc Artif Intern Organs* 31:668, 1985.
335. Fijiwara Y et al: Hypoxemia and hemodialysis-induced symptomatic hypotension. *Clin Nephrol* 24:9, 1985.
336. Fine A: Metabolism of D-lactate in the dog and in man. *Perit Dial Int* 9:99, 1989.
337. Fine J et al: The treatment of acute renal failure by peritoneal irrigation. *Ann Surg* 124:857, 1946.
338. Fischer KF et al: Hypoglycemia in hospitalized patients: Cause and outcomes. *N Engl J Med* 315:1245, 1986.
339. Flanigan MJ et al: Quantitating hemodialysis: A comparison of three kinetic models. *Am J Kidney Dis* 17:295, 1991.
340. Flanigan MJ et al: Reducing the hemorrhagic complications of hemodialysis: A controlled comparison of low-dose heparin and citrate anticoagulation. *Am J Kidney Dis* 9:147, 1987.
340a. Fleming SJ et al: Blood volume changes during isolated ultrafiltration and combined ultrafiltration-dialysis. *Nephrol Dial Transplant* 3:272, 1988.
341. Fleming SJ et al: Effect of dialysate composition on intercompartmental fluid shift. *Kidney Int* 32:267, 1987.
342. Flynn CJ et al: Advantages of continuous ambulatory peritoneal dialysis to the diabetic with renal failure. *Proc Eur Dial Transplant Assoc* 16:184, 1976.
343. Flynn CT: The diabetic patient on continuous ambulatory peritoneal dialysis. *Perit Dial Bull* 3(suppl 1):S16, 1983.
344. Flynn CT: The Iowa Lutheran Protocol. *Perit Dial Bull* 6:106, 1981.
345. Flynn CT et al: Intraperitoneal insulin with continuous ambulatory peritoneal dialysis: An artificial pancreas. *Trans Am Soc Artif Intern Organs* 25:114, 1979.
346. Foley RJ, Hamner RW: Hyperthyroidism in end-stage renal disease. *Am J Nephrol* 5:292, 1985.
347. Food and Drug Administration: Water treatment, in Vlcheck DL et al (eds): *Quality Assurance Guidelines for Hemodialysis Devices*. Rockville, Md, 1991, p 3-1.
348. Food and Drug Administration: Water purification equipment, in Luehmann DA et al (eds): *A Manual on Water Treatment for Hemodialysis*. Rockville, Md, 1989, p 57.
349. Foulks CJ, Wright LF: Successful repletion of bicarbonate stores in ongoing lactic acidosis: A role for bicarbonate-buffered peritoneal dialysis. *South Med J* 74:1162, 1981.
350. Fournier A et al: Calcium carbonate, an aluminum-free agent for control of hyperphosphatemia, hypocalcemia, and hyperparathyroidism in uremia. *Kidney Int* 29(suppl 18):S114, 1986.
351. Frajewicki V et al: Intraperitoneal phosphate administration in hungry bone syndrome. *Clin Nephrol* 34:223, 1990.
352. Frank HA et al: Treatment of uremia after acute renal failure by peritoneal irrigation. *JAMA* 103:703, 1946.
353. Franklin JO et al: Effect of increasing intraabdominal pressure and volume on left ventricular function in continuous ambulatory peritoneal dialysis (CAPD). *Am J Kidney Dis* 12:291, 1988.
353a. Fraser CL, Arieff AI: Nervous system complications in uremia. *Ann Intern Med* 109:143, 1988.
353b. Freeman RM, Richards CJ: Studies on sulfate in end-stage renal disease. *Kidney Int* 15:167, 1979.
354. Freeman RM et al: Hard water syndrome. *N Engl J Med* 276:1113, 1976.
355. Friedlander M et al: The effect of sulfate on serum ionized calcium. *Am J Kidney Dis* 2:660, 1983.
356. Friedman EA: Critical appraisal of continuous ambulatory peritoneal dialysis. *Annu Rev Med* 35:233, 1984.
357. Friedman EA: *Strategy in Renal Failure*. New York, Wiley, 1978.
358. Frifelt JJ et al: CAPD using a higher calcium concentration, in Maher JF, Winchester JF (eds): *Frontiers in Peritoneal Dialysis*. New York, Field, Rich and Associates, 1986, p 265.
359. Frizzell M et al: Spontaneous hypoglycemia associated with chronic renal failure. *Diabetes* 22:493, 1973.
360. Frolich ED: Vascular effects of the Krebs intermediate metabolites. *Am J Physiol* 208:149, 1965.
361. Funck-Bretano JL: Ultrafiltration and diffusion techniques with the polyacrylonitrile membrane dialyzer. *Proc Renal Physicians Assoc* 2:9, 1978.

362. Galen M: Reasonably short hemodialysis time can be achieved without ultra-high efficiency dialyzers and without ultrafiltration-controlled delivery systems. *Trans Am Soc Artif Intern Organs* 35:255, 1989.
363. Gallery EDM et al: Acute zinc toxicity in hemodialysis. *Br Med J* 4:331, 1973.
364. Ganter G: Uber die Beseitigung giftiger Stoffe aus dem Blute durch Dialyse. *Munch med Wochenschr* 70:1478, 1923.
365. Garavaca F et al: Hypersensitivity reactions related to acetate dialysate and cellulose acetate membrane. *Nephron* 45:158, 1987.
366. Garber AJ et al: Hypoglycemia in compensated chronic renal insufficiency: Substrate limitation of gluconeogenesis. *Diabetes* 23:982, 1974.
367. Garella S: Contraction alkalosis in patients on CAPD (letter to editor). *Perit Dial Bull* 4:187, 1984.
368. Garella S, Chang BS: Hemodialysis-associated hypoxemia. *Am J Nephrol* 4:273, 1984.
369. Garrett JJ, Cuddihe RE: Calcium absorption during peritoneal dialysis. *Trans Am Soc Artif Intern Organs* 14:372, 1968.
370. Gault MH et al: Fluid and electrolyte complications of peritoneal dialysis: Choice of dialysis solutions. *Ann Intern Med* 75:253, 1971.
371. Gelfand MC et al: Geophagia: A cause of life-threatening hyperkalemia in patients with chronic renal failure. *JAMA* 234:738, 1975.
372. Gelfman N: Ultrasonic bicarbonate preparation for dialysis. *Dial Transplant* 19:657, 1990.
373. Gennari FJ: Acid-base balance in dialysis patients. *Kidney Int* 28:678, 1985.
374. Gennari FJ, Rimmer JM: Acid-base disorders in end-stage renal disease: 1. *Semin Dial* 3:81, 1990.
375. Gennari FJ, Rimmer JM: Acid-base disorders in end-stage renal disease: 2. *Semin Dial* 3:161, 1990.
376. Gentile D et al: Use of bicarbonate in dialysate of the Sorbent delivery system (abstract). *Trans Am Soc Artif Intern Organs* 6:26, 1977.
377. Geronemus RP: Slow continuous hemodialysis. *Trans Am Soc Artif Intern Organs* 34:59, 1988.
378. Geronemus R, Schneider N: Continuous arteriovenous hemodialysis: A new modality for treatment of acute renal failure. *Trans Am Soc Artif Intern Organs* 30:610, 1984.
379. Ghandi VC et al: Sclerotic thickening of the peritoneal membrane in maintenance peritoneal dialysis. *Arch Intern Med* 140:1201, 1980.
380. Ghandi VC et al: Thickened peritoneal dialysis membrane in maintenance peritoneal dialysis patients. *Kidney Int* 14:675, 1979.
381. Ghantous WN et al: Limitations of peritoneal dialysis (PD) in the treatment of ESRD patients. *Trans Am Soc Intern Organs* 25:100, 1979.
382. Gilliland KG, Hegstrom RM: The effect of hemodialysis on cerebrospinal-fluid pressure in uremic dogs. *Trans Am Soc Artif Intern Organs* 9:44, 1963.
383. Gjessing J: The use of dextran as a dialyzing fluid in peritoneal dialyzing fluid in peritoneal dialysis. *Acta Med Scand* 185:237, 1969.
384. Gjessing J: Addition of amino acids to peritoneal dialysis fluid. *Lancet* 2:812, 1968.
385. Gkonos PJ et al: Hypercalcemia and elevated 1,25-dihydroxyvitamin D levels in a patient with end-stage renal disease and active tuberculosis. *New Engl J Med* 311:1683, 1984.
386. Glasson P et al: Response of blood pressure and the renin-angiotensin-aldosterone system to chronic ambulatory peritoneal dialysis in hypertensive end-stage renal failure. *Clin Sci* 63:207S, 1982.
387. Godolphin W et al: Spurious hypocalcemia in hemodialysis patients after heparinization: In vitro formation of calcium soaps. *Am J Clin Pathol* 71:215, 1979.
388. Gokal R: Continuous ambulatory peritoneal dialysis, in Maher JF (ed): *Replacement of Renal Function by Dialysis*, 3d ed. Boston: Kluwer Academic, 1989, p 590.
389. Gokal R: Continuous ambulatory peritoneal dialysis (CAPD): Ten years on. *Q J Med* 63:465, 1987.
390. Gokal R: Calcium and phosphate control in patients on continuous ambulatory peritoneal dialysis, in Legrain M (ed): *Continuous Ambulatory Peritoneal Dialysis*. Amsterdam, Excerpta Medica, 1980, p 283.
391. Gokal R et al: Histologic renal osteodystrophy, and 25 hydroxycholecalciferol and aluminum levels in patients on continuous ambulatory peritoneal dialysis. *Kidney Int* 23:15, 1983.
392. Goldsmith RS et al: Calcium flux during hemodialysis. *Nephron* 20:132, 1978.
393. Goldsmith RS, Johnson WJ: Role of phosphate depletion and high dialysate calcium in controlling dialytic renal osteodystrophy. *Kidney Int* 4:154, 1973.
394. Goldsmith RS et al: Control of secondary hyperparathyroidism during long-term hemodialysis. *Am J Med* 50:692, 1971.
395. Golper TA, Leone M: Backtransport of dialysate solutes during in vitro continuous arteriovenous hemodialysis. *Blood Purif* 7:223, 1989.
396. Golper TA et al: Continuous arteriovenous hemofiltration in acute renal failure. *Am J Kidney Dis* 6:373, 1985.
397. Gonella M: Serum phosphate concentration with relation to the hematocrit value in uremic patients on chronic hemodialysis. *Int J Artif Organs* 7:341, 1984.
398. Gonella M: Plasma and tissue levels of magnesium in chronically hemodialyzed patients: Effects of dialysate magnesium levels. *Nephron* 34:141, 1983.
399. Gonella M et al: Effects of high $CaCO_3$ supplements on serum calcium and phosphorus in patients on regular hemodialysis treatments. *Clin Nephrol* 24:147, 1985.
400. Gonella M et al: Serum levels of PTH, Mg, Ca, inorganic phosphorus, and alkaline phosphatase in uremic patients on differential Mg dialysis. *Proc Eur Dial Transplant Assoc* 17:362, 1980.
401. Gonzales FM et al: On the effects of acetate during hemodialysis. *Trans Am Soc Artif Intern Organs* 20:169, 1974.
402. Goodman AD et al: Production, excretion, and net balance of fixed acid in patients with renal acidosis. *J Clin Invest* 44:495, 1965.
403. Gordon A et al: Clinical maintenance hemodialysis with a sorbent-based low-volume dialysate regeneration system. *Trans Am Soc Artif Intern Organs* 17:253, 1971.
404. Gordon A et al: A sorbent-based low volume recirculating dialysate system. *Trans Am Soc Artif Intern Organs* 15:347, 1969.

405. Gordon SM et al: Hemolysis associated with hydrogen peroxide at a pediatric dialysis center. *Am J Nephrol* 10:123, 1990.
406. Gordon SM et al: Epidemic hypotension in a dialysis center caused by sodium azide. *Kidney Int* 37:110, 1990.
407. Gordon SM et al: The incidence of pyrogenic reactions in patients receiving conventional, high-efficiency, or high-flux dialysis using bicarbonate dialysate (abstract). *Kidney Int* 37:298, 1990.
408. Gotch FA: Kinetic modeling in hemodialysis, in Nissenson AR et al (eds): *Clinical Dialysis*, 2d ed. Norwalk, Ct, Appleton & Lange, 1990, p 118.
409. Gotch FA: Hemodialysis: Technical and kinetic considerations, in Brenner BM, Rector FC Jr (eds): *The Kidney* Philadelphia, Saunders, 1976.
410. Gotch FA et al: A kinetic survey of US hemodialysis prescriptions. *Am J Kidney Dis* 15:511, 1990.
411. Gotch FA, Sargent JA: A mechanistic analysis of the National Cooperative Dialysis Study (NCDS). *Kidney Int* 28:526, 1985.
412. Gotch FA et al: Hydrogen ion balance in dialysis therapy. *Artif Organs* 6:388, 1982.
413. Gotch FA, Sargent J: Measurement of H^+ balance (H^+b) during acetate and bicarbonate dialysis therapy (abstract). *Kidney Int* 16:887, 1979.
414. Govan JR et al: Acute magnesium poisoning as a complication of chronic intermittent hemodialysis. *Br Med J* 2:279, 1968.
415. Graf H et al: Disappearance of uremic pruritus after lowering dialysate magnesium concentration. *Br Med J* 2:1478, 1979.
416. Graeffe U et al: Less dialysis induced morbidity and vascular instability with bicarbonate in dialysate. *Ann Intern Med* 88:332, 1978.
417. Grajower MM et al: Hypoglycemia in chronic hemodialysis patients: Assocation with propranolol use. *Nephron* 26:126, 1980.
418. Green J, Kleeman CR: Role of bone in regulation of systemic acid-base balance. *Kidney Int* 39:9, 1991.
419. Greenblatt DJ: Fatal hypoglycemia occurring after peritoneal dialysis. *Br Med J* 2:270, 1972.
420. Grimsrud L et al: A central system for the continuous preparation and distribution of hemodialysis fluid. *Trans Am Soc Artif Intern Organs* 10:107, 1964.
421. Grodstein GP et al: Glucose absorption during continuous ambulatory peritoneal dialysis. *Kidney Int* 19:564, 1981.
422. Grollman A et al: Intermittent peritoneal lavage in nephrectomized dogs and its application to the human being. *Arch Intern Med* 87:379, 1951.
423. Groop LC et al: Intraperitoneal insulin administration does not promote insulin antibody production in insulin-dependent diabetes mellitus patients on dialysis. *Diabetes Nephrol* 4:80, 1985.
424. Gross M, McDonald HP Jr: Effect of dialysate temperature flow rate on peritoneal clearance. *JAMA* 202:363, 1967.
425. Gross ML et al: A comparison of glucose polymer and dextrose containing dialysate in CAPD patients. *Trans Am Soc Artif Intern Organs* 30:483, 1984.
426. Gruppo Emodialisi Patologie Cardiovascularie: Multicentre, cross-sectional study of ventricular arrhythmias in chronically haemodialyzed patients. *Lancet* 2:305, 1985.
427. Guarniere GF et al: Acetate intolerance in chronic uremic patients. *Nephron* 24:212, 1979.
428. Guillot AP et al: The use of magnesium-containing phosphate binders in patients with end-stage renal disease on maintenance hemodialysis. *Nephron* 30:114, 1982.
429. Gupta DK et al: Superoxide generation by neutrophils after exposure to a contaminated peritoneal dialysis solution for different time periods. *Intern J Artif Organs* 13:228, 1990.
430. Gutierrez A et al: Effect of in vivo contact between blood and dialysis membranes on protein catabolism in humans. *Kidney Int* 38:487, 1990.
431. Gutman RA et al: Failure of high dialysis fluid glucose to prevent the disequilibrium syndrome. *Lancet* 1:295, 1967.
432. Haeffner-Cavaillon N et al: In vivo induction of interleukin-1 during hemodialysis. *Kidney Int* 35:1212, 1989.
433. Hagstam KE et al: Mannitol infusion in regular dialysis treatment for chronic renal insufficiency. *Scand J Urol Nephrol* 3:257, 1969.
434. Hain H et al: Aspects of new solutions for peritoneal dialysis. *Nephrol Dial Transplant* 2:67, 1987.
435. Hakim RM: Assessing the adequacy of dialysis. *Kidney Int* 37:822, 1990.
436. Hakim RM, Lazarus JM: Biochemical parameters in chronic renal failure. *Am J Kidney Dis* 11:238, 1988.
437. Hakim RM et al: Effects of acetate and bicarbonate dialysate in stable chronic dialysis patients. *Kidney Int* 28:535, 1985.
438. Hakim RM et al: Effects of acetate and bicarbonate dialysate in stable chronic dialysis patients. *Kidney Int* 28:535, 1985.
439. Hakim RM et al: Complement activation and hypersensitivity reactions to dialysis membranes. *N Engl J Med* 311:878, 1984.
440. Hakim RM et al: Biocompatibility of dialysis membranes: Effects of chronic complement activation. *Kidney Int* 26:194, 1984.
441. Hakim RM, Lazarus JM: Complications during hemodialysis, in Nissenson AR et al (eds): *Clinical Dialysis.* Norwalk, Ct, Appleton-Century-Crofts, 1984.
442. Hamilton JW et al: Peritoneal dialysis in the treatment of severe hypercalcemia. *J Dial* 4:129, 1980.
443. Hamm L et al: Sorbent regenerative hemodialysis as a potential cause of acute hypercapnea. *Kidney Int* 21:416, 1982.
444. Hampers CL, Schupak E: *Long-Term Hemodialysis.* New York, Grune & Stratton, 1967, p 119.
445. Hampl H et al: Haemodynamic state in severe chronic renal failure: Pathophysiological aspects of cardiovascular function and the importance of bicarbonate dialysis. *Nephron* 39:102, 1985.
445a. Hampl H et al: Electroencephalogram investigations of the disequilibrium syndrome during bicarbonate and acetate dialysis. *Proc Eur Dial Transplant Assoc* 19:351, 1982.
446. Hampl H et al: Advantages of bicarbonate hemodialysis. *Artif Organs* 6:410, 1982.

447. Hampl H et al: Hemodynamic changes during hemodialysis, sequential ultrafiltration, and hemofiltration. *Kidney Int* 18:S-83, 1980.
448. Handa SP, Cushner GB: Hyperosmolar hyperglycemia nonketotic coma during peritoneal dialysis. *South Med J* 61:700, 1968.
449. Harter HR et al: Effects of dialysis prescription on bone and mineral metabolism: The National Cooperative Dialysis Study. *Kidney Int* 23(suppl 13):S-73, 1983.
450. Hasbargen JA et al: Ultrafiltration failure at the initiation of CAPD. *Perit Dial Bull* 6:46, 1986.
451. Hayat JC: The treatment of lactic acidosis in the diabetic patient by peritoneal dialysis using sodium acetate: A report of cases. Diabetologia 10:485, 1974.
452. Hayes CP et al: An extrarenal mechanism for the maintenance of potassium balance in severe chronic renal failure. *Trans Assoc Am Physicans* 80:205, 1967.
453. *Health Devices Alert: Improper Dialysate.* Plymouth Meeting, Pa, ECRI, 1983, vol 12.
454. Heaton A et al: Evaluation of glycerol as an osmotic agent for continuous ambulatory peritoneal dialysis in end stage renal disease. *Clin Sci* 70:23, 1986.
455. Heaton A et al: Twenty-four hour hormonal and metabolic profiles in uremic patients before and during treatment with chronic ambulatory peritoneal dialysis. *Clin Sci* 69:449, 1985.
456. Heaton A et al: Short term studies on the use of glycerol as an osmotic agent in chronic ambulatory peritoneal dialysis (CAPD). *Clin Sci* 67:121, 1984.
457. Heaton A et al: Carbohydrate and lipid metabolism during chronic ambulatory peritoneal dialysis (CAPD): The effect of a single dialysis cycle. *Clin Sci* 65:539, 1983.
458. Heber ME et al: Baroreceptor, not left ventricular dysfunction, is the cause of hemodialysis hypotension. *Clin Nephrol* 32:79, 1989.
459. Heidenreich S et al: Direct vasopressor effect of recombinant human erythropoietin on renal resistance vessels. *Kidney Int* 39:259, 1991.
460. Heimberger O et al: Peritoneal transport in CAPD patients with permanent loss of ultrafiltration capacity. *Kidney Int* 38:495, 1990.
461. Heineken FG et al: Prescribing dialysate bicarbonate concentrations for hemodialysis patients. *Int J Artif Organs* 11:45, 1988.
462. Heineken FG et al: Intercompartmental fluid shifts in hemodialysis patients. *Biotech Prog* 3:69, 1987.
463. Held PJ et al: Mortality and duration of hemodialysis treatment. *JAMA* 265:871, 1991.
464. Henderson IS: Composition of peritoneal dialysis solutions: Potential hazards. *Blood Purif* 7:86, 1989.
464a. Henderson LW: Symptomatic hypotension during hemodialysis. *Kidney Int* 17:571, 1980.
465. Henderson LW: Redy or not? *Am Soc Artif Intern Organs J* 2:1979, 49.
466. Henderson LW: Middle molecules re-examined. *Nephron* 22:146, 1978.
467. Henderson LW: Hemodialysis: Rationale and physical principles, in Brenner BM, Rector FC Jr (eds): *The Kidney*. Philadelphia, Saunders, 1976.
468. Henderson LW: The problem of peritoneal membrane area and permeability. *Kidney Int* 3:409, 1973.
469. Henderson LW: Peritoneal ultrafiltration dialysis: Enhanced urea transfer using hypertonic peritoneal dialysis fluids. *J Clin Invest* 45:950, 1966.
470. Henderson LW et al (eds): *Hemofiltration.* New York, Springer-Verlag, 1986.
471. Henderson LW et al: Ultrafiltration with peritoneal dialysis, in Nolph KD (ed): *Peritoneal Dialysis*, 3d ed. Boston, Kluwer Academic, 1989, p 117.
472. Henderson LW et al: Hemodialysis hypotension: The interleukin hypothesis. *Blood Purif* 1:3, 1983.
473. Henderson LW et al: Choosing a membrane. *Am J Kidney Dis* 3:5, 1983.
474. Henderson LW et al: Clinical experience with intermittent hemodiafiltration. *Trans Am Soc Artif Intern Organs* 19:119, 1973.
475. Henderson LW et al: Uremic blood cleansing by diafiltration using a hollow fiber ultrafilter. *Trans Am Soc Artif Intern Organs* 16:107, 1970.
476. Henderson LW, Nolph KD: Altered permeability of the peritoneal membrane after using hypertonic peritoneal dialysis fluid. *J Clin Invest* 118:992, 1969.
477. Henderson LW et al: Blood purification by ultrafiltration and fluid replacement. *Trans Am Soc Artif Intern Organs* 13:216, 1967.
478. Henderson LW et al: Factors influencing blood pH changes during extracorporeal dialysis in patients with chronic renal failure. *Trans Am Soc Artif Intern Organs* 12:193, 1966.
479. Heneghan WF: Acetate, bicarbonate, and hypotension during hemodialysis. *Am J Kidney Dis* 2:302, 1982.
480. Heneghan WF et al: Dialysis hypoxemia causes hypotension (abstract). *Kidney Int* 21:169, 1982.
481. Hennessy WJ, Siemsen AW: Autonomic neuropathy in chronic renal failure. *Clin Res* 16:385, 1968.
482. Henrich WL: Hemodynamic instability during hemodialysis. *Kidney Int* 30:605, 1986.
483. Henrich WL et al: Increased ionized calcium and left ventricular contractility during hemodialysis. *N Engl J Med* 310:19, 1984.
484. Henrich WL et al: High sodium bicarbonate and acetate hemodialysis: Double-blind crossover comparison of hemodynamic and ventilatory effects. *Kidney Int* 24:240, 1983.
485. Henrich WL et al: The chronic efficacy and safety of high sodium dialysate: Double-blind crossover study. *Am J Kidney Dis* 2:349, 1982.
486. Henrich WL et al: Role of osmolality in blood pressure stability after dialysis and ultrafiltration. *Kidney Int* 18:480, 1980.
487. Hercz G, Coburn JW: Prevention of phosphate retention and hyperphosphatemia in uremia. *Kidney Int* 32(suppl 22):S215, 1987.
488. Hercz G et al: Use of calcium carbonate as a phosphate binder in dialysis patients. *Miner Electrolyte Metab* 12:314, 1986.
489. Heusser H et al: Untersuchungen uber peritoneal dialyse. *Beitr Z Klin Chir* 141:38, 1927.
490. Heyburn PH et al: Peritoneal dialysis in the management of severe hypercalcemia. *Br Med J* 281:525, 1981.
491. Heyka RJ, Paganini EP: Blood pressure control in chronic dialysis patients, in Maher JF (ed): *Replacement*

of Renal Function by Dialysis, 3d ed. Dordrecht, The Netherlands, Kluwer Academic, 1989, p 772.
492. Hirszel P et al: Pharmacologic alteration of peritoneal transport rates, in Nolph KD (ed): *Peritoneal Dialysis*. Boston, Kluwer Academic, 1989, p 169.
493. Hodsman AB et al: Vitamin D resistant osteomalacia in hemodialysis patients lacking secondary hyperparathyroidism: Description of the syndrome in 19 patients. *Ann Intern Med* 94:629, 1981.
494. Hoenich NA et al: Dialyzers, in Maher JF (ed): *Replacement of Renal Function by Dialysis*, 3d ed. Dordrecht, The Netherlands, Kluwer Academic, 1989, p 144.
495. Hori K et al: Hemodynamic and volume changes by recombinant human erythropoietin (rHuEPO) in the treatment of anemic hemodialysis patients. *Clin Nephrol* 33:293, 1990.
496. Hory B: Hemodialysis with low-molecular-weight heparin in high-risk hemorrhagic patients with acute renal failure (letter to editor). *Am J Med* 84:566, 1988.
497. Hou SH et al: Calcium and phosphorus fluxes during hemodialysis with low calcium dialysate. *Am J Kidney Dis* 18:217, 1991.
498. Hou S et al: Safety and efficacy of low-potassium dialysate. *Am J Kidney Dis* 13:137, 1989.
499. Hoy RH: Accidental systemic exposure to sodium hypochlorite (Chlorox) during hemodialysis. *Am J Hosp Pharm* 38:1512, 1981.
500. Hsu CH et al: Bicarbonate hemodialysis: Influence on plasma refilling and hemodynamic stability. *Nephron* 38:202, 1984.
501. Huennekens FM et al: Studies on the cyclophorase system: 17. The occurrence and properties of an L-hydroxy acid racemase. *Arch Biochem* 30:77, 1951.
502. Hunt JM et al: Gas exchange during dialysis: Contrasting mechanisms contributing to comparable alteration with acetate and bicarbonate buffers. *Am J Med* 27:255, 1984.
503. Hutchinson AS et al: Low calcium dialysate with oral calcium carbonate in CAPD. *Peritoneal Dial Int* 11(suppl 1):116, 1991.
504. Ijelu G et al: Various methods for the calculation of *Kt/V*: A clinical comparison. *Trans Am Soc Artif Intern Organs* 36:M363, 1990.
505. Ijelu G et al: *Kt/V* and hemodialysis morbidity revisited. *Trans Am Soc Artif Intern Organs* 36:M152, 1990.
506. Inagaki Y et al: Peritoneal dialysis as therapy for electrolyte and acid-base disorders. *Int J Artif Organs* 12:632, 1989.
507. Indrapasit S et al: Effect of dialysate temperature on peritoneal clearances. *Nephron* 34:45, 1983.
508. Ing TS et al: Bicarbonate-buffered peritoneal dialysis. *Int J Artif Organs* 8:121, 1985.
509. Ing TS et al: Peritoneal sclerosis in peritoneal dialysis patients. *Am J Nephrol* 4:173, 1984.
510. Ing TS et al: Peritoneal dialysis using bicarbonate buffered dialysate (letter to editor). *Int J Artif Organs* 7:166, 1984.
511. Ing TS et al: Preparation of bicarbonate-containing dialysate for peritoneal dialysis. *Int J Artif Organs* 6:217, 1983.
512. Ing TS et al: Preparation of phosphate-containing dialysate for use in hemodialysis and peritoneal dialysis. *Int J Artif Organs* 6:321, 1983.
513. Ing TS et al: First-use syndrome with cuprammonium cellulose dialyzers. *Int J Artif Organs* 6:235, 1983.
514. Ing TS et al: Peritoneal dialysis using bicarbonate-containing dialysate produced by on-line method. *Artif Organs* 6:457, 1982.
515. Ing TS et al: Peritoneal dialysis using bicarbonate containing dialysate produced by automated dialysate delivery system. *Artif Organs* 6:67, 1982.
516. Ing TS et al: Fluid removal with negative-pressure hydrostatic ultrafiltration using a partial vacuum. *Nephron* 14:451, 1975.
517. Inoue T et al: Effectiveness of continuous arteriovenous hemofiltration for patients with refractory heart failure. *Jpn Heart J* 29:595, 1988.
518. Iseki K et al: Comparison of hemodynamics induced by conventional acetate hemodialysis, bicarbonate hemodialysis and ultrafiltration. *Clin Nephrol* 14:294, 1980.
519. Ivanovich P et al: Acute hemolysis following hemodialysis. *Trans Am Soc Artif Intern Organs* 15:316, 1969.
520. Izzo JL Jr, Sterns RH: Abnormal epinephrine release in uremia. *Kidney Int* 24(suppl 16):S-221, 1983.
521. Jacobs LJ et al: Pseudohypertension due to diffuse vascular calcification in chronic renal failure. *Ann Intern Med* 90:353, 1979.
522. Jacobson HR: Ischemic renal disease: An overlooked clinical entity? *Kidney Int* 24:729, 1988.
523. Jardin F et al: Hemodialysis in septic patients: Improvement in tolerance of fluid removal with concentrated albumin as the priming fluid. *Crit Care Med* 10:650, 1982.
524. Jawadi MH et al: Regulation of plasma arginine vasopressin in patients with chronic renal failure maintained on hemodialysis. *Am J Nephrol* 6:175, 1986.
525. Jenkins PG, Dreher WH: Dialysis-induced muscle cramps: Treatment with hypertonic saline and theory as to etiology. *Trans Am Soc Artif Intern Organs* 21:479, 1975.
526. Jenkins RD et al: Benefit of bicarbonate dialysis during CAVHD. *Trans Am Soc Artif Intern Organs* 36:M465, 1990.
527. Jennings AE et al: Use of magnesium hydroxide and low magnesium dialysate does not permit reduction of aluminum hydroxide during continuous ambulatory peritoneal dialysis. *Am J Kidney Dis* 8:192, 1986.
528. Jensen HA et al: Hypoglycemia in propanolol-treated dialysis patients. *Lancet* 1:368, 1976.
529. Jindal et al: A study of the basic principles determining the performance of several high-flux dialyzers. *Am J Kidney Dis* 14:507, 1989.
530. Johnson WJ: Persistent severe hypercalcemia during maintenance hemodialysis. *Ann Intern Med* 93:272, 1980.
531. Johnson WJ: Optimum dialysate calcium concentration during maintenance hemodialysis. *Nephron* 17:241, 1976.
532. Johnson WJ, Taves DR: Exposure to excessive fluoride during hemodialysis. *Kidney Int* 5:451, 1974.
533. Johnson WJ et al: Effects of urea loading in patients with far advanced renal failure. *Mayo Clin Proc* 47:21, 1972.

534. Johnson WJ et al: Potassium balance in patients maintained by long-term hemodialysis against potassium-free dialysate (abstract), in Alwall N et al (eds): *Proc Fourth Int Congr Nephrol*, Basel, S Karger, 1969, vol 4, p 303.
535. Johny KV et al: Effect of hemodialysis on erythrocyte and plasma potassium, magnesium, sodium, and calcium. *Nephron* 8:81, 1971.
536. Junor BJR: CAPD disconnect systems. *Blood Purif* 7:156, 1989.
537. Jurgesen JC: Dialysis for lactic acidosis. *N Engl J Med* 278:1350, 1968.
538. Kaiser BA et al: Acid-base changes and acetate metabolism during routine and high-efficiency hemodialysis in children. *Kidney Int* 19:70, 1981.
539. Kaldany A et al: Reversible acute pulmonary edema due to uncontrolled hyperglycemia in diabetic individuals with renal failure. *Diabetes Care* 5:506, 1982.
540. Kancir CB et al: Ionized and total calcium variations induced by haemodialysis. *Nephron* 48:319, 1988.
541. Kaplan AA: Predilution versus postdilution for continuous arteriovenous hemofiltration. *Trans Am Soc Artif Intern Organs* 31:28, 1985.
542. Kaplan AA: Clinical trials with predilution and vacuum suction: Enhancing the efficiency of the CAVH treatment. *Trans Am Soc Artif Intern Organs* 32:49, 1986.
543. Kaplan AA et al: Continuous arteriovenous hemofiltration: A report of 6 months' experience. *Ann Intern Med* 100:358, 1984.
544. Karanicolas S et al: Home peritoneal dialysis: 3 years experience in Toronto. *Can Med Assoc J* 116:266, 1977.
545. Katirtzoglou A et al: Is peritoneal ultrafiltration influenced by acetate or lactate buffers?, in Maher JF, Winchester JF (eds): *Frontiers in Peritoneal Dialysis*. New York, Field, Rich and Associates, 1986, p 270.
546. Katz MA: Hyperglycemia-induced hyponatremia: Calculation of the expected sodium depression. *New Engl J Med* 289:843, 1973.
547. Kawanishi H et al: Low calcium peritoneal dialysate (2.5 meq/L) and its clinical applications (abstract). *Perit Dial Int* 11(suppl 1):130, 1991.
548. Kaye M et al: Correction of hypophosphatemia in patients on hemodialysis using a calcium-free dialysate with added phosphate. *Clin Nephrol* 35:130, 1991.
549. Kaye M, Fischer D: Changes in intact parathyroid hormone levels during hemodialysis following exposure to either differing dialysate calcium concentrations or calcium-free dialysis with varying calcium infusion rates. *Clin Nephrol* 34:84, 1990.
550. Kaye M et al: Calcium-free dialysate: Development and applications. *Clin Nephrol* 31:132, 1989.
551. Kaye M et al: A study of vertebral bone powder from patients with chronic renal failure. *J Clin Invest* 49:442, 1970.
552. Kaye MR et al: Studies in calcium metabolism in patients on chronic hemodialysis. *Proc Eur Dial Transplant Assoc* 3:17, 1966.
553. Kaylor WM et al: Reversal of end-stage renal failure with surgical revascularization in patients with athersclerotic renal artery occlusion. *J Urol* 141:486, 1989.
554. Kaysen A et al: Albumin homeostasis in patients undergoing CAPD. *Kidney Int* 25:107, 1984.
555. Kelleher SP, Shulman G: Severe metabolic alkalosis complicating regional citrate hemodialysis. *Am J Kidney Dis* 9:235, 1987.
556. Kelly PM et al: Comparison of serum calcium fractions during haemodialysis and peritoneal dialysis. *Ann Clin Biochem* 24:585, 1987.
557. Kelton JG et al: Comparison of chemical composition of peritoneal fluid and serum: A method for monitoring dialysis patients and a tool for assessing binding to serum proteins in vivo. *Ann Intern Med* 89:67, 1978.
558. Kenamond T et al: Severe recurrent alkalemia in a patient undergoing cyclic peritoneal dialysis. *Am J Med* 81:548, 1986.
559. Kennedy AC et al: The pathogenesis and prevention of cerebral dysfunction during dialysis. *Lancet* 1:790, 1964.
560. Kennedy AC et al: Electroencephalographic changes during hemodialysis. *Lancet* 1:408, 1963.
561. Kennedy AC et al: Urea levels in cerebrospinal fluid after haemodialysis. *Lancet* 1:410, 1962.
562. Kenny MA et al: Magnesium, calcium and PTH relationships in dialysis patients after magnesium repletion. *Nephron* 46:199, 1987.
563. Kersch ES et al: Autonomic insufficiency in uremia as a cause of hemodialysis-induced hypotension. *N Engl J Med* 290:650, 1974.
564. Keshaviah PR: Equipment for hemodialysis and peritoneal dialysis, in Nissenson AR et al (eds): *Clinical Dialysis*, 2d ed. Norwalk, Ct, Appleton & Lange, 1990, p 45.
565. Keshaviah PR: Pretreatment and preparation of city water for dialysis, in Maher JF (ed): *Replacement of Renal Function with Dialysis*, 3d ed. Dordrecht, The Netherlands, Kluwer Academic, 1989, p 189.
566. Keshaviah PR: The role of acetate in the etiology of symptomatic hypotension. *Artif Organs* 6:378, 1982.
567. Keshaviah PR, Shaldon S: Hemodialysis monitors and monitoring, in Maher JF (ed): *Replacement of Renal Function with Dialysis*, 3d ed. Dordrecht, The Netherlands, Kluwer Academic, 1989, p 276.
568. Keshaviah P et al: Technical requirements for rapid high-efficiency therapies. *Artif Organs* 10:189, 1986.
569. Keshaviah PR, Shapiro FL: A critical examination of dialysis-induced hypotension. *Am J Kidney Dis* 2:290, 1982.
570. Keshaviah PR et al: *Investigation of the Risks and Hazards Associated with Hemodialysis Devices*, Technical report, Rockville, Md, U.S. Food and Drug Administration, Department of Health, Education, and Welfare, 1980.
571. Keshaviah PR et al: Transcompartmental fluid shifts induced by ultrafiltration (UF) and diffusion (D) (abstract). *Kidney Int* 14:677, 1978.
572. Keshaviah PR et al: Mechanisms and control of fluid removal by ultrafiltration. *Proc Eleventh Annu Contractor's Conf*, Artificial Kidney Program, National Institute of Arthritis, Metabolism, and Digestive Diseases, 1978, p 124.
573. Ketchersid TL, Van Stone JC: Dialysate potassium. *Semin Dial* 4:46, 1991.
574. Khanna R et al: Why is ultrafiltration lower in children on CAPD? *Kidney Int* 33:247, 1988.

575. Khanna R et al: Peritoneal cavity lymphatics. *Perit Dial Bull* 6:113, 1986.
576. Khanna R et al: Use of amino acid solutions in CAPD patients. *Perit Dial Bull* 4(suppl 121):S125, 1984.
577. Khanna R et al: Lipid abnormalities in patients undergoing chronic ambulatory peritoneal dialysis. *Perit Dial Bull* 3(suppl 1):S13, 1983.
578. Kim KE et al: Blood volume changes and hypotension during hemodialysis. *Trans Am Soc Artif Intern Organs* 16:1508, 1970.
579. Kimura G: Quantitative assessment of sodium and water metabolism in hemodialyzed patients. *Int J Artif Organs* 12:744, 1989.
579a. Kimura KI et al: Cardiac arrhythmias in hemodialysis patients: A study of incidence and contributing factors. *Nephron* 53:201, 1989.
580. Kimura G et al: A simulation study on transcellular fluid shifts induced by hemodialysis. *Kidney Int* 24:542, 1983.
581. Kinet JP et al: Hemodynamic study of hypotension during hemodialysis. *Kidney Int* 21:868, 1982.
582. Kirkendol PL et al: Cardiac and vascular effects of infused sodium acetate in dogs. *Trans Am Soc Artif Intern Organs* 24:714, 1978.
583. Kirkendol PL et al: A comparison of the cardiovascular effects of sodium acetate, sodium bicarbonate, and other potential sources of fixed base in hemodialysis solutions. *Trans Am Soc Artif Intern Organs* 23:399, 1977.
584. Kirkwood R et al: Generation of the precarcinogen dimethyl nitrosamine (DMNA) in dialysate water. *Trans Am Soc Artif Intern Organs* 27:168, 1981.
585. Kishimoto T et al: Cardiovascular stability in low-temperature dialysis. *Dial Transplant* 15:329, 1986.
586. Kishimoto T et al: Acetate intolerance in hemodialysis. *Trans Am Soc Artif Intern Organs* 29:402, 1983.
587. Kishimoto T et al: Morbidity, instability, and serum acetate level during hemodialysis (abstract). *Int Soc Artif Organs Second Annu Meeting* 3:22, 1979.
588. Kjellstrand CM: Osmolar changes during dialysis. *Int J Artif Organs* 3:251, 1980.
589. Kjellstrand CM et al: Hemolysis in dialyzed patients caused by chloramines. *Nephron* 13:427, 1974.
590. Kjellstrand CM et al: Technical advances in hemodialysis of very small pediatric patients. *Proc Clin Dial Transplant Forum* 1:124, 1971.
591. Klein J et al: Hypertrophic cardiomyopathy: An acquired disorder of end stage renal disease. *Trans Am Soc Artif Intern Organs* 29:120, 1983.
592. Klinke B et al: Transmembranous transport and adsorption of beta-2-microglobulin during hemodialysis using polysulfone, polyacrylonitrile, polymethylmethacrylate and cuprammonium rayon membranes. *Int J Artif Organs* 12:697, 1989.
593. Klinkmann H et al: Development and assessment of new cellulose membranes for blood purification. *Kidney Int* 18(suppl 10):S-26, 1980.
594. Knowles SE et al: Production and utilization of acetate in mammals. *Biochem J* 142:401, 1974.
595. Kobayashi N et al: Effect of dialysis on lipid metabolism in chronic renal failure: Acetate versus bicarbonate. *Int J Artif Organs* 6:187, 1983.
596. Kohen JA et al: Continuous arteriovenous hemofiltration: A comparison with hemodialysis in acute renal failure. *Trans Am Soc Artif Intern Organs* 31:169, 1985.
597. Kolff WJ: *New Ways of Treating Uremia*. London, J & A Churchhill, 1947.
598. Koomans HA et al: Plasma volume recovery after ultrafiltration in patients with chronic renal failure. *Kidney Int* 26:848, 1984.
599. Kopple JD et al: Plasma amino acid levels and amino acid losses during continuous ambulatory peritoneal dialysis. *Am J Clin Nutr* 36:295, 1982.
600. Korthuis RJ et al: Role of the peritoneal microcirculation in peritoneal dialysis, in Nolph KD (ed): *Peritoneal Dialysis*, 3d ed. Boston, Kluwer Academic, 1989, p 28.
600a. Kouw PM et al: Interstitial correction of blood volume decrease during hemodialysis. *Int J Artif Organs* 12:626, 1989.
601. Kramer P et al: Intensive care potential of continuous arteriovenous hemofiltration. *Trans Am Soc Artif Intern Organs* 28:78, 1982.
602. Kramer P et al: Arteriovenous haemofiltration: A new and simple method of treating overhydrated patients resistant to diuretics. *Klin Wochenschr* 55:1121, 1977.
603. Krediet RT et al: Fluid and solute transport across the peritoneum during continuous ambulatory peritoneal dialysis (CAPD). *Perit Dial Int* 9:15, 1989.
604. Krediet RT et al: The relationship between peritoneal glucose absorption and body fluid loss by ultrafiltration during continuous ambulatory peritoneal dialysis. *Clin Nephrol* 27:51, 1987.
605. Krediet RT et al: Hyponatremia in chronic ambulatory peritoneal dialysis patients with diabetic nephropathy during hyperglycemic episodes. *Transplant Proc* 28:1702, 1986.
606. Kreisberg RA: Lactate homeostasis and lactic acidosis. *Ann Intern Med* 92:227, 1980.
607. Kurtin P, Kouba J: Profound hypophosphatemia in the course of acute renal failure. *Am J Kidney Dis* 10:346, 1987.
608. Kurtz SB et al: CAPD: Three years' experience at the Mayo Clinic. *Mayo Clin Proc* 58:633, 1983.
609. Kurtz SB et al: Hypercalcemia in chronic ambulatory peritoneal dialysis (CAPD) patients: Observations on parameters of calcium metabolism, in Gahl G et al (eds): *Advances in Peritoneal Dialysis*. Amsterdam, Excerpta Medicina, 1981, p 467.
610. Kveim M, Nesbakken R: Utilization of exogenous acetate during hemodialysis. *Trans Am Soc Artif Intern Organs* 21:138, 1975.
611. Kwong M et al: Transperitoneal calcium and magnesium transfer during an 8 hour dialysis. *Perit Dial Bull* 7:85, 1987.
612. Kwong M et al: Effect of the peritoneal dialysate buffer on ultrafiltration: Studies in normal rabbits. *Perit Dial Bull* 5:182, 1985.
613. Kyriakidis M et al: Cardiac arrhythmias in chronic renal failure: Holter monitoring during dialysis and everyday activity at home. *Nephron* 38:26, 1984.
614. LaBarge SJ: Reverse osmosis: How does it figure into a dialysate water system? *Contemp Dial Nephrol* Sept 32, 1990.

615. LaGreca A et al: Acid-base homeostasis in clinical dialysis, in Maher JF (ed): *Replacement of Renal Function by Dialysis*, 3d ed. Boston, Kluwer Academic, 1989, p 808.
616. LaGreca G et al: Effects of acetate and bicarbonate dialysate on vascular stability: A prospective multicenter study. *Int J Artif Organs* 10:157, 1987.
617. LaGreca G et al: Acid-base balance on peritoneal dialysis. *Clin Nephrol* 16:1, 1981.
618. LaGreca G et al: Brain density studies during dialysis. *Lancet* 2:582, 1980.
619. Lai KN et al: Vasoactive hormones in uremic patients on CAPD. *Clin Nephrol* 35:215, 1991.
620. Lamas S et al: Autonomic neuropathy and symptomatic hypotension in hemodialysis patients. *Nephron* 46:107, 1987.
621. Lameire N et al: Effects of long-term CAPD on carbohydrate and lipid metabolism. *Clin Nephrol* 30(suppl 1):S53, 1988.
622. Lampe WT: Hypoglycemia due to acetohexamide. *Arch Intern Med* 120:239, 1967.
623. Lamperi S et al: Calcium antagonists improve ultrafiltration in patients on continuous ambulatory peritoneal dialysis. *Trans Am Soc Artif Intern Organs* 33:657, 1987.
624. Landwehr DM, Okusa MD: The effect of acetate and bicarbonate dialysis on orthostatic blood pressure reductions. *Artif Organs* 6:417, 1982.
625. Larner AJ et al: Correction of severe hyponatremia by continuous arteriovenous hemofiltration before liver transplantation. *Br Med J* 297:1514, 1988.
626. Lasker N et al: Chronic peritoneal dialysis. *Trans Am Soc Artif Intern Organs* 12:94, 1966.
627. Latos DL et al: Acid-base and electrolyte changes following maximal and submaximal exercise in hemodialysis patients. *Am J Kidney Dis* 10:439, 1987.
628. Lauer A et al: Hemodynamic consequences of continuous arteriovenous hemofiltration. *Am J Kidney Dis* 12:110, 1988.
629. Lauer A et al: Continuous arteriovenous hemofiltration in the critically ill patient: Clinical use and operational characteristics. *Ann Intern Med* 99:455, 1983.
630. LeBlanc J et al: The sympathetic nervous system in short-term adaptation to cold. *Can J Physiol Pharmacol* 49:97, 1971.
631. Lee CL et al: Bilateral nephrectomy for hypertension in patients with chronic renal failure on a dialysis program. *J Urol* 119:20, 1978.
632. Lee DU, Toth EL: Death due to "spontaneous" hypoglycemia in a 28-year-old woman with chronic renal failure. *Clin Invest Med* 12(suppl):R-126, 1989.
633. Lee HA et al: Lacticacidemia in peritoneal dialysis. *Proc Eur Dial Transplant Assoc* 4:150, 1967.
634. Leenen FHH et al: Hemodynamic changes during acetate and bicarbonate hemodialysis. *Artif Organs* 8:411, 1984.
635. Leenen FHH et al: Hypotension on CAPD: An approach to treatment. *Perit Dial Bull* 3(suppl):S33, 1983.
636. Lefavour GS et al: Persistent hypophosphatemia following parathyroidectomy in end-stage renal disease: Report of three patients. *Clin Nephrol* 13:40, 1980.
637. Lefebvre A et al: Optimal correction of acidosis changes progression of dialysis osteodystrophy. *Kidney Int* 36:1112, 1989.
638. Lemann J Jr et al: The effects of chronic acid loads in normal man: Further evidence for the participation of bone mineral in the defense against chronic metabolic acidosis. *J Clin Invest* 45:1608, 1966.
639. Leski M et al: Glucose-enriched dialysate and tolerance to maintenance hemodialysis. *Nephron* 24:271, 1979.
640. Leunissen KML et al: Pathophysiologic aspects of plasma volume preservation during dialysis and ultrafiltration. *Contrib Nephrol* 78:201, 1990.
641. Leunissen KML et al: Acetate versus bicarbonate hemodialysis in chronically ill patients. *Nephron* 42:146, 1986.
642. Levin N: Management of blood pressure changes during recombinant human erythropoietin therapy. *Semin Nephrol* 9:16, 1989.
643. Levine J, Bernard DB: The role of urea kinetic modeling, TAC_{urea}, and *Kt/V* in achieving optimal dialysis: A critical reappraisal. *Am J Kidney Dis* 15:285, 1990.
644. Levine T et al: Effects of varying dialysate sodium using large surface area dialyzers. *Trans Am Soc Artif Intern Organs* 24:139, 1978.
645. Lewis EJ et al: High mass-transfer hemodialysis and acetate metabolism. *Proc Renal Physicans Assoc* 1:10, 1977.
646. Lewis S et al: Host defense mechanisms in the peritoneal cavity of continuous ambulatory peritoneal dialysis patients. *Perit Dial Int* 11:14, 1991.
647. Liang CS, Lowenstein JM: Metabolic control of the circulation: Effects of acetate and pyruvate. *J Clin Invest* 62:1029, 1978.
648. Lifschitz MD et al: Hypertension in chronic renal failure, in Brenner BM, Stein JM (eds): *Contemporary Issues in Nephrology*. New York, Churchill Livingstone, 1981, vol 8, p 223.
649. Lifschitz MD et al: Effect of saralasin in hypertensive patients on chronic hemodialysis. *Ann Intern Med* 88:23, 1978.
650. Lilley LJ et al: Adrenergic regulation of blood pressure in chronic renal failure. *J Clin Invest* 57:1190, 1976.
651. Lim VS et al: Effect of hematocrit on solute removal during high efficiency hemodialysis. *Kidney Int* 37:1557, 1990.
652. Lindberg JS et al: Lysine vasopressin in the treatment of refractory hemodialysis-induced hypotension. *Am J Nephrol* 10:269, 1990.
653. Linder A et al: Accelerated atherosclerosis in prolonged maintenance hemodialysis. *N Engl J Med* 290:697, 1974.
654. Linder A et al: Accidental mass hypernatremia during hemodialysis. *Nephron* 9:99, 1972.
655. Lindholm B et al: Nutritional management of patients undergoing peritoneal dialysis, in Nolph KD (ed): *Peritoneal Dialysis*, 3d ed. Boston, Kluwer Academic, 1989, p 230.
656. Lindholm B et al: Kinetics of peritoneal dialysis with glycerol and glucose as osmotic agents. *Trans Am Soc Artif Intern Organs* 33:19, 1987.
657. Lindholm B et al: Muscle water and electrolytes in pa-

tients undergoing chronic ambulatory peritoneal dialysis. *Acta Med Scand* 219:323, 1986.
658. Lindholm B et al: Serum lipids and lipoproteins during chronic ambulatory peritoneal dialysis. *Acta Med Scand* 220:143, 1986.
659. Lindholm T et al: Glucose metabolism in patients on chronic ambulatory peritoneal dialysis. *Trans Am Soc Artif Intern Organs* 17:58, 1981.
660. Lindholm T et al: Temperature and vascular stability in hemodialysis. *Nephron* 39:130, 1985.
661. Lindner A et al: Propranolol effects in long-term hemodialysis patients with renin-dependent hypertension. *Ann Intern Med* 88:457, 1978.
662. Lindsay RM et al: Urea monitoring during dialysis: The wave of the future. *Trans Am Soc Artif Intern Organs* 37:49, 1991.
663. Lindsay RM et al: Practical use of anticoagulants, in Maher JF (ed): *Replacement of Renal Function with Dialysis*, 3d ed. Dordrecht, The Netherlands, Kluwer Academic, 1989, p 246.
664. Lindsay RM, Spanner E: A hypothesis: The protein catabolic rate is dependent upon the type and amount of treatment in dialyzed uremic patients. *Am J Kidney Dis* 13:382, 1989.
665. Lindsay RM, Henderson LW: Adequacy of dialysis. *Kidney Int* 33(suppl 24):S92, 1988.
666. Locatelli F et al: Sodium kinetics and dialysis performances. *Contrib Nephrol* 70:260, 1989.
667. Locatelli F et al: Sodium kinetics across dialysis membranes. *Nephron* 88:174, 1984.
668. Locatelli F et al: Physiological and pharmacological dialysate sodium concentrations. *Int J Artif Organs* 5:17, 1982.
669. Locatelli F et al: Ultrafiltration and high sodium concentration dialysis: Pathophysiological correlation. *Proc Eur Dial Transplant Assoc* 15:253, 1978.
670. Lohr JW et al: Safety of regional citrate hemodialysis in acute renal failure. *Am J Kidney Dis* 13:104, 1989.
671. Lowrie EG, Lew NL: The urea reduction ratio (URR): A simple method for evaluating hemodialysis treatment. *Contemp Dial Nephrol* February:11, 1991.
672. Lowrie EG, Teehan BP: Principles of prescribing dialysis therapy: Implementing recommendations from the National Cooperative Dialysis Study. *Kidney Int* 23(suppl 13):S113, 1983.
673. Lowrie EG et al: Effect of the hemodialysis prescription on patient morbidity: Report from the National Cooperative Dialysis Study. *N Engl J Med* 305:1176, 1981.
674. Luke RG: Uremia and the BUN (editorial). *N Engl J Med* 305:1213, 1981.
675. Lundin AP et al: Fatigue, acid-base and electrolyte changes with exhaustive treadmill exercise in hemodialysis patients. *Nephron* 46:57, 1987.
676. Lundquist F: Production and utilization of free acetate in man. *Nature (London)* 193:579, 1962.
677. Lyman DT: Membranes, in Drukker W et al (eds): *Replacement of Renal Function by Dialysis*, 2d ed. Boston, Martinus Nijhoff, 1983, p 97.
678. Lyman N et al: Glucose-K^+ relationships during continuous ambulatory peritoneal dialysis: Effects of intraperitoneal insulin. *Kidney Int* 21:172, 1982.
678a. Lynggaard F et al: One year's experience with sequential filtration/hemodialysis. *Dial Transplant* 7:1106, 1978.
679. Lynn KL et al: Hemolytic anemia caused by overheated dialysate. *Br Med J* 1:306, 1979.
680. Macias WL et al: Continuous venovenous hemofiltration: An alternative to continuous arteriovenous hemofiltration and hemodiafiltration in acute renal failure. *Am J Kidney Dis* 18:451, 1991.
681. Mactier RA et al: Peritoneal cavity lymphatics, in Nolph KD (ed): *Peritoneal Dialysis*. Boston, Kluwer Academic, 1989, p 48.
682. Mactier RA et al: CAPD: After the first ten years. *Blood Purif* 7:65, 1989.
683. Mactier RA et al: Influence of dwell time, osmolality, and volume of exchanges on solute mass transfer and ultrafiltration in peritoneal dialysis. *Semin Dial* 1:40, 1988.
684. Mactier RA et al: Influence of phosphatidylcholine on lymphatic absorption during peritoneal dialysis in the rat. *Perit Dial Int* 8:186, 1988.
685. Mactier RA et al: Intraperitoneal insulin in diabetic CAPD patients. *Int J Artif Organs* 11:9, 1988.
686. Mactier R et al: Role of peritoneal cavity lymphatic absorption in peritoneal dialysis. *Kidney Int* 32: 165, 1987.
687. Mactier RA et al: Calcium carbonate is an effective phosphate binder when dialysate calcium concentration is adjusted to control hypercalcemia. *Clin Nephrol* 28:222, 1987.
688. Mactier RA et al: Ultrafiltration failure in continuous ambulatory peritoneal dialysis due to excessive peritoneal cavity lymphatic absorption. *Am J Kidney Dis* 10:461, 1987.
689. Mactier RA et al: Contribution of lymphatic absorption to loss of ultrafiltration and solute clearance on CAPD. *J Clin Invest* 80:1311, 1987.
690. Mactier RA et al: Neostigmine increases ultrafiltration and solute clearances in peritoneal dialysis by reducing lymphatic drainage. *Perit Dial Bull* 7:S50, 1987.
691. Madden MA et al: Chronic ambulatory peritoneal dialysis in diabetes mellitus: The risks and benefits of intraperitoneal insulin. *Am J Nephrol* 2:133, 1982.
692. Madias NE, Levey AS: Metabolic alkalosis due to absorption of "non-absorbable" antacids. *Am J Med* 74:155, 1983.
693. Maeda K et al: Mechanism of dialysis-induced hypotension. *Trans Am Soc Artif Intern Organs* 35:245, 1989.
694. Maeda K et al: Role of hypovolemia in dialysis-induced hypotension. *Artif Organs* 12:116, 1988.
695. Maeda K et al: Hemodiafiltration with sodium concentration-controlled dialysate. *Artif Organs* 4:121, 1980.
695a. Maggiore Q et al: Bicarbonate dialysis: *Con. Int J Artif Organs* 10:151, 1987.
696. Maggiore Q et al: Influence of blood temperature on vascular stability during hemodialysis and isolated ultrafiltration. *Int J Artif Intern Organs* 8:175, 1985.
697. Maggiore Q et al: Blood temperature and vascular stability during hemodialysis and hemofiltration. *Trans Am Soc Artif Intern Organs* 28:523, 1982.

698. Maggiore Q et al: Effect of extracorporeal blood cooling on dialytic arterial hypotension. *Proc Eur Dial Transplant Assoc* 18:597, 1981.
699. Maher JF: Modifications of endocrine and metabolic abnormalities of uremia by chronic ambulatory peritoneal dialysis. *Am J Nephrol* 10:1, 1990.
700. Maher JF: Physiology of the peritoneum: Implications for peritoneal dialysis. *Med Clin North Am* 74:985, 1990.
701. Maher JF (ed): *Replacement of Renal Function by Dialysis*, 3d ed. Dordrecht, The Netherlands, Kluwer Academic, 1989.
702. Maher JF et al: The mechanism of dextrose-enhanced transport rates. *Kidney Int* 28:16, 1985.
703. Maher JF et al: Ultrafiltration by hyperosmotic peritoneal dialysis fluid excludes intracellular solutes. *Am J Nephrol* 4:169, 1984.
704. Maher JF: Characteristics of peritoneal transport: Physiological and clinical implications. *Miner Electrolyte Metab* 5:201, 1981.
705. Mahida BH et al: Effect of cooled dialysate on serum catecholamines and blood pressure stability. *Trans Am Soc Artif Intern Organs* 29:384, 1983.
706. Mahony JF et al: Hypophosphatemic osteomalacia in patients receiving hemodialysis. *Br Med J* 2:142, 1976.
707. Mai ML et al: Calcium acetate, an effective phosphorus binder in patients with renal failure. *Kidney Int* 36:690, 1989.
708. Maiorca R et al: A six-year comparison of patient and technique survivals in CAPD and hemodialysis. *Kidney Int* 34:518, 1988.
709. Malangone JM et al: Clinical and laboratory features of patients with chronic renal disease at the start of dialysis. *Clin Nephrol* 31:77, 1989.
710. Malberti F et al: Efficacy and safety of long-term treatment with calcium carbonate as a phosphate binder. *Am J Kidney Dis* 12:487, 1987.
711. Malberti F et al: The influence of dialysis fluid composition on dialysis tolerance. *Nephrol Dial Transplant* 2:93, 1987.
712. Mallanaci F et al: Autonomic function in uremic patient treated by hemodialysis on CAPD and in transplant patients. *Clin Nephrol* 25:175, 1986.
713. Man NK et al: Phosphate removal during hemodialysis, hemodiafiltration, and hemofiltration. *Trans Am Soc Artif Intern Organs* 37:M463, 1991.
714. Man NK et al: Renal biofiltration. *Trans Am Soc Artif Intern Organs* 35:8, 1989.
715. Man NK et al: Dialysis-associated adverse reactions with high-flux membranes and microbial contamination of liquid bicarbonate concentrate. *Contrib Nephrol* 62:24, 1988.
716. Man NK et al: Effect of bicarbonate-containing dialysate on chronic hemodialysis patients: A comparative study. *Artif Organs* 6:421, 1982.
717. Manahan FJ et al: Effects of bicarbonate-containing versus lactate-containing peritoneal dialysis solutions on superoxide production by human neutrophils. *Artif Organs* 13:495, 1989.
718. Mandelbaum JL et al: Six months' experience with PD-2 solution. *Dial Transplant* 12:259, 1983.
719. Manis T, Friedman EA: Dialytic therapy for irreversible uremia: 1 and 2. *N Engl J Med* 310:1260, 1321, 1979.
720. Manji N et al: Peritoneal dialysis for acute renal failure: Overfeeding resulting from dextrose absorbed during dialysis. *Crit Care Med* 18:29, 1990.
721. Mansell MA et al: Effects of acetate or bicarbonate hemodialysis on cardiocirculatory function and acid-base balance. *Contrib Nephrol* 44:380, 1984.
722. Mansell MA, Wing AJ: Acetate or bicarbonate for hemodialysis? *Br Med J* 287:308, 1983.
723. Mansell MA et al: The effect of hyperacetatemia on cardiac output during regular hemodialysis. *Clin Nephrol* 18:130, 1982.
724. Mansell MA et al: Incidence and significance of rising blood acetate levels during hemodialysis. *Clin Nephrol* 12:22, 1979.
725. Manzler AD, Schreiner AW: Copper-induced acute hemolytic anemia: A new complication of hemodialysis. *Ann Intern Med* 73:409, 1970.
726. Marcen R et al: Hemodialysis with low-temperature dialysate: A long-term experience. *Nephron* 49:29, 1988.
727. Markle R et al: Development of improved membranes for artificial kidney dialysis. *Trans Am Soc Artif Intern Organs* 10:22, 1964.
728. Marquez-Julio A et al: Hypotension in patients on continuous ambulatory peritoneal dialysis, in Legrain M (ed): *Continuous Ambulatory Peritoneal Dialysis*. Amsterdam, Excerpta Medica, 1980.
729. Martens J et al: Bicarbonate dialysis using a single concentrate. *Nephron* 39:400, 1985.
730. Martin J, Moncada S: Blood pressure, erythropoietin, and nitric oxide. *Lancet* 2:644, 1988.
731. Martin RS et al: Increased secretion of potassium in the rectum of humans with chronic renal failure. *Am J Kidney Dis* 8:105, 1986.
732. Martin-Malo A et al: Sequential hypertonic dialysis. *Nephron* 40:458, 1985.
733. Martis L et al: Calcim carbonate as a phosphate binder: Is there a need to adjust peritoneal dialysate calcium concentrations for patients using calcium carbonate. *Perit Dial Int* 9:325, 1989.
733a. Massry SG: Magnesium homeostasis in patients with renal failure. *Contrib Nephrol* 38:175, 1984.
734. Massry SG: Divalent ion metabolism and renal osteodystrophy, in Massry SG, Glassock RJ (eds): *Textbook of Nephrology*, 2d ed. Baltimore, Williams & Wilkins, 1989, p 1278.
735. Massry SG: The clinical pathophysiology of magnesium. *Contrib Nephrol* 14:64, 1978.
736. Massry SG, Kopple JD (guest eds): Symposium on uremic toxins, in Kurtzman NA (ed): *Seminars in Nephrology*. New York, Grune & Stratton, 1983, vol 3, p 73.
737. Massry SG et al: Current status of the use of $1,25(OH)_2$-D_3 in the management of renal osteodystrophy. *Kidney Int* 18:409, 1980.
738. Massry SG, Seelig MS: Hypomagnesemia and hypermagnesemia. *Clin Nephrol* 7:147, 1977.
739. Massry SG, Sellers AL: *Clinical Aspects of Uremia and Dialysis*. Springfield, Ill, Charles C. Thomas, 1976.
740. Massry SG et al: Secondary hyperparathyroidism in

chronic renal failure: The clinical spectrum in uremia during hemodialysis and after renal transplantation. *Arch Intern Med* 124:431, 1969.

740a. Mastrangelo F: Bicarbonate dialysis: Pro. *Int J Artif Organs* 10:145, 1987.

741. Mastrangelo F et al: Favorable effects of bicarbonate dialysis on the body pool and phosphate. *Proc Eur Dial Transplant Assoc Eur Renal Assoc* 21:215, 1984.

742. Matsuoka H et al: Normalization of increased sodium sensitivity by maintenance hemodialysis. *Am J Hypertens* 3:628, 1990.

743. Matter BJ et al: Lethal copper intoxication in hemodialysis. *Trans Am Soc Artif Intern Organs* 15:309, 1969.

744. Matthys E et al: Extended use of glycerol-containing dialysate in diabetic CAPD patients. *Perit Dial Bull* 7:10, 1987.

745. Matthys E et al: Potential hazards of glycerol dialysate in diabetic CAPD patients. *Perit Dial Bull* 7:16, 1987.

746. Mawdsley C: Neurologic complications of hemodialysis. *Proc R Soc Lond* 65:871, 1972.

747. Maxwell MH et al: Peritoneal dialysis: 1. Technique and application. *JAMA* 176:917, 1959.

748. Mayer G et al: Hemodynamic effects of partial correction of chronic anemia by recombinant human erythropoietin in patients on dialysis. *Am J Kidney Dis* 17:286, 1991.

749. Maynard JC et al: Blood pressure response to changes in serum ionized calcium during hemodialysis. *Ann Intern Med* 104:358, 1986.

750. McConnell T: Fatal hypocalcemia from phosphate absorption from laxative preparation. *JAMA* 216:147, 1971.

751. McGrath BP et al: Catecholamines in peripheral venous plasma in patients on chronic hemodialysis. *Clin Sci* 55:89, 1978.

752. McGrath BP et al: Autonomic blockade and the Valsalva maneuver in patients on maintenance hemodialysis: A hemodynamic study. *Kidney Int* 12:294, 1977.

753. McIvor M et al: Hyperkalemia and cardiac arrest from fluoride exposure during hemodialysis. *Am J Cardiol* 51:901, 1983.

754. Medina A et al: Changes in blood pressure, renin, and angiostensin after bilateral nephrectomy in patients with chronic renal failure. *Br Med J* 4:694, 1972.

755. Meeham C et al: Plasma sulfate levels in hemodialysis patients with sorbent regeneration. *Aust N Z J Med* 8:235, 1978.

756. Meeks JN: Chloramines and carbon demystified: 1. *Contemp Dial Nephrol* July:18, 1988.

757. Meema HE et al: Serum magnesium level and arterial calcification in end-stage renal disease. *Kidney Int* 32:388, 1987.

758. Mehta BR et al: Effects of acetate and bicarbonate hemodialysis on cardiac function in chronic dialysis patients. *Kidney Int* 24:782, 1983.

759. Mehta RL et al: Regional citrate anticoagulation for continuous arteriovenous hemodialysis in critically ill patients. *Kidney Int* 38:976, 1990.

760. Memmos DE et al: The role of parathyroidectomy in the management of hyperparathyroidism in patients on maintenance haemodialysis and after renal transplantation. *Nephron* 30:143, 1982.

761. Mendelssohn S et al: High glucose concentration dialysate in chronic hemodialysis. *Trans Am Soc Artif Intern Organs* 13:249, 1967.

762. Meric F et al: Etiology of hypercalcemia in hemodialysis patients on calcium carbonate therapy. *Am J Kidney Dis* 16:459, 1990.

763. Messerli FH et al: Osler's maneuver and pseudohypertension. *New Engl J Med* 312:1548, 1985.

764. Miach PJ et al: Management of hypercalcemia of malignancy with peritoneal dialysis. *Am J Med* 21:782, 1975.

765. Miller FN et al: Hyperosmolality, acetate and lactate: Dilatory factors during peritoneal dialysis. *Kidney Int* 20:397, 1981.

766. Miller JD et al: Severe hypoglycemia due to combined use of parenteral nutrition and renal dialysis. *Br Med J* 285:9, 1982.

767. Miller JH et al: Studies of inorganic phosphate removal during acetate and bicarbonate dialysis. *Proc Am Soc Artif Intern Organs Abstr Book* 12:57, 1983.

768. Miller RB, Tassistro CR: Peritoneal dialysis. *N Engl J Med* 281:945, 1969.

769. Milutinovich J et al: Effect of hypertonic glucose on the muscular cramps of hemodialysis. *Ann Intern Med* 90:926, 1976.

770. Mion CM: Practical use of peritoneal dialysis, in Maher JF (ed): *Replacement of Renal Function by Dialysis*, 3d ed. Boston, Kluwer Academic, 1989, p 537.

771. Mion CM et al: Sterile and pyrogen-free bicarbonate dialysate: A necessity for hemodialysis today. *Adv Nephrol* 19:275, 1990.

772. Mion CM: Practical use of peritoneal dialysis, in Drukker W et al (eds): *Replacement of Renal Function by Dialysis*, 2d ed. Boston, Martinus Nijhoff, 1983.

773. Mion CM et al: Dialysis fracturing osteomalacia without hyperparathyroidism in patients treated with bicarbonate rinsed REDY cartidge. *Trans Am Soc Artif Intern Organs* 27:634, 1981.

774. Mion CM et al: Substitution of sodium acetate for sodium bicarbonate in the bath fluid for hemodialysis. *Trans Am Soc Artif Intern Organs* 10:110, 1964.

775. Mistry CD et al: New osmotic agents for peritoneal dialysis: Where are we and where we're going. *Semin Dial* 4:9, 1991.

776. Mistry CD et al: Alternative osmotic agents. *Blood Purif* 7:109, 1989.

777. Mistry CD et al: The use of glucose polymers (GP) in CAPD: A seven-day study. *Perit Dial Bull* 7:S54, 1987.

778. Mistry CD et al: Ultrafiltration with an isosmotic solution during long peritoneal dialysis exchanges. *Lancet* 2:178, 1987.

779. Molitoris BA et al: Citrate: A major factor in the toxicity of orally administered aluminum compounds. *Kidney Int* 36:949, 1989.

780. Molnar JI et al: Local effects of various anions and H^+ on dog limb and coronary vascular resistance. *Am J Physiol* 203:125, 1963.

781. Moncrieff JW et al: Continuous ambulatory peritoneal dialysis, in Nolph KD (ed): *Peritoneal Dialysis*, 3d ed. Boston, Kluwer Academic, 1989, p 152.

782. Moncrieff JW et al: Continuous ambulatory peritoneal dialysis: Best treatment for end-stage renal disease. *Kidney Int* 28(suppl 17):S23, 1985.
783. Montoliu J et al: Potassium-lowering effects of albuterol for hyperkalemia in renal failure. *Arch Intern Med* 147:713, 1987.
784. Montoliu J, Revert L: Lethal hyperkalemia associated with severe hyperglycemia in diabetic patients with renal failure. *Am J Kidney Dis* 5:47, 1985.
785. Moore SB, Goodwin FJ: Effects of beta-adrenergic blockage on plasma-renin activity and intractable hypertension in patients receiving regular dialysis. *Lancet* 2:67, 1976.
786. Moore TJ et al: Reduced angiotensin receptors and pressor responses in hypotensive hemodialysis patients. *Kidney Int* 36:696, 1989.
787. Morgan AG et al: Potassium balance and acid-base changes in patients undergoing regular hemodialysis therapy. *Br Med J* 1:779, 1970.
788. Morin RJ, Davidson WD: Conversion of acetate to CO_2, lipids, proteins, and lipoproteins during hemodialysis in humans. *Uremia Invest* 8:61, 1984–1985.
789. Morin RJ et al: Effect of acetate vs bicarbonate on plasma lipid and lipoprotein levels in uremic patients. *J Dial* 4:9, 1980.
790. Morin RJ et al: Lipid metabolism in non-uremic and uremic dogs during and after hemodialysis with acetate. *J Dial* 2:113, 1978.
791. Moriniere P et al: Comparison of 1α-OH-vitamin D and high doses of calcium carbonate for the control of hyperparathyroidism and hyperaluminemia in patients on maintenance hemodialysis. *Nephron* 39:309, 1985.
792. Morita Y et al: Regional anticoagulation during hemodialysis using citrate. *Am J Med Sci* 242:32, 1961.
793. Morrison G et al: Mechanism and prevention of cardiac arrhythmias in chronic hemodialysis patients. *Kidney Int* 17:811, 1980.
794. Morton AR: Severe hypermagnesemia after magnesium sulphate enemas. *Br Med J* 291:516, 1985.
795. Morton AR et al: Hypercalcemia in CAPD: Diagnosis, frequency and related bone disease (abstract). *Perit Dial Int* 11(Suppl 1):183, 1991.
796. Morton AR et al: Control of hyperphosphatemia in chronic renal failure. *Semin Dial* 3:219, 1990.
797. Morton AR et al: Control of hyperphosphatemia in chronic renal failure. *Semin Dial* 3:219, 1990.
798. Mujais SK et al: Membranes for extracorporeal therapy, in Maher JF (ed): *Replacement of Renal Function with Dialysis*, 3d ed. Dordrecht, The Netherlands, Kluwer Academic, 1989, p 181.
799. Mulligan I et al: Acute haemolysis due to concentrated dialysis fluid. *Br Med J* 284:1151, 1982.
800. Murisasco A et al: Sequential sodium therapy allows correction of sodium volume balance and reduces morbidity. *Clin Nephrol* 24:201, 1985.
801. Nadkarni M et al: Hypoglycemia with hyperinsulinemia in a chronic hemodialysis patient following parathyroidectomy. *Nephron* 60:100, 1992.
802. Nagai K et al: The influence of acetate vs bicarbonate on patient symptomatology during dialysis. *Proc Eur Dial Transplant Assoc* 16:122, 1979.
802a. Nahman NS, Middendorf DF: Continuous arteriovenous hemofiltration. *Med Clin N Am* 74:975, 1990.
803. Naik RB et al: Effects of hemodialysis on the control of the circulation in patients with chronic renal failure. *Am J Nephrol* 5:96, 1985.
804. Nakagawa D et al: Continuous cycling peritoneal dialysis: A viable option in the treatment of chronic renal failure. *Trans Am Soc Artif Intern Organs* 27:55, 1981.
805. Nakashima Y et al: Localization of autonomic system dysfunction in dialysis patients. *Am J Nephrol* 7:375, 1987.
805a. Nakayama M et al: Effect of ultra low sodium concentration dialysate in patients with ultrafiltration loss. *Perit Dial Int* 4:187, 1991.
806. Naparstek Y et al: Lactic acidosis and peritoneal dialysis. *Isr J Med Sci* 18:513, 1982.
807. Narins RG et al: Diagnostic strategies in disorders of fluid, electrolyte, and acid-base homeostasis. *Am J Med* 72:496, 1982.
808. Narins RG: The renal acidoses, in Brenner BM, Stein JH (eds): *Contemporary Issues in Nephrology*. New York, Churchill Livingstone, 1978, p 48.
809. Nash MA et al: Neonatal lactic acidosis and renal failure: The role of peritoneal dialysis. *J Pediatr* 91:101, 1977.
810. Nawab ZM et al: Use of lactate as a base in hemodialysis. *Am J Nephrol* 7:434, 1987.
811. Neal CR et al: Treatment of dialysis-related cramps with hypertonic dextrose. *Arch Intern Med* 141:171, 1981.
812. Nebeker HG et al: A nonaluminum-containing phosphate binder: Polyuronic acid. *Kidney Int* 27:147, 1985.
813. Necheles H: Uber Dialysieren des stromenden Blutes am Lebenden. *Klin Wochenschr* 2:1257, 1923.
814. Neff MS et al: Hemodynamics of uremic anemia. *Circulation* 48:876, 1971.
815. Neilan GE et al: Simplified method of preparing lactate-free peritoneal dialysis solution. *Am J Hosp Pharm* 41:1994, 1984.
816. Newstead CG: Exercise-induced arterial hyperkalemia in hemodialysis patients. *Nephrol Dial Transplant* 5:400, 1990.
817. Neylan JF et al: The effectiveness of calcium citrate as a phosphate binder in dialysis patients. *Kidney Int* 31:239, 1987.
818. Nickey WA et al: Hypernatremia from water softener malfunction during home dialysis. *JAMA* 214:915, 1970.
819. Nielsen LH et al: Sclerosing peritonitis in CAPD: The acetate-lactate controversy. *Kidney Int* 27:183, 1985.
820. Nies AS et al: Hemodialysis hypotension is not the result of uremic peripheral autonomic neuropathy. *J Lab Clin Med* 94:395, 1979.
821. Nilsson P et al: Magnesium studies in hemodialysis patients before and after treatment with low-dialysate magnesium. *Nephron* 37:25, 1984.
822. Nissenson AR: Acid-base homeostasis in peritoneal dialysis patients. *Int J Artif Organs* 7:175, 1984.
823. Nissenson AR: Prevention of dialysis induced hypoxemia by bicarbonate dialysis. *Trans Am Soc Artif Intern Organs* 26:339, 1980.

824. Nissenson AR et al: Stable liquid bicarbonate hemodialysate (LBD). *Dial Transplant* 14:78, 1985.
825. Nissenson AR et al: Acid-base homeostasis in dialysis patients, in Nissenson AR et al (eds): *Clinical Dialysis.* Norwalk, Ct, Appleton-Century-Crofts, 1984.
826. Nitenberg A et al: Analysis of increased myocardial contractability during sodium acetate infusion in humans. *Kidney Int* 26:744, 1984.
827. Nolph KD: Continuous ambulatory peritoneal dialysis as a long-term treatment of end-stage renal disease. *Am J Kidney Dis* 17:154, 1991.
828. Nolph KD: Peritoneal anatomy and transport physiology, in Maher JF (ed): *Replacement of Renal Function by Dialysis*, 3d ed. Boston, Kluwer Academic, 1989, p 516.
829. Nolph KD: Comparison of continuous ambulatory peritoneal dialysis and hemodialysis. *Kidney Int* 33(suppl 24):S123, 1988.
830. Nolph KD: Factors affecting ultrafiltration in continuous ambulatory peritoneal dialysis. *Perit Dial Bull* 4:14, 1984.
831. Nolph KD et al: Tidal peritoneal dialysis with racemic or L-lactate solutions. *Perit Dial Int* 10:161, 1990.
832. Nolph KD et al: The peritoneal dialysis system, in Nolph KD (ed): *Peritoneal Dialysis*, 3d ed. Boston, Kluwer Academic, 1989, p 13.
833. Nolph KD et al: Continuous ambulatory peritoneal dialysis. *N Engl J Med* 318:1595, 1988.
834. Nolph KD et al: Factors associated with morbidity and mortality among patients on dialysis. *Trans Am Soc Artif Intern Organs* 33:52, 1987.
835. Nolph KD et al: The kinetics of ultrafiltration during peritoneal dialysis: Role of lymphatics. *Kidney Int* 32:219, 1987.
836. Nolph KD et al: Continuous ambulatory peritoneal dialysis in the United States: A three-year study. *Kidney Int* 28:198, 1985.
837. Nolph KD et al: Factors affecting ultrafiltration in continuous ambulatory peritoneal dialysis: First report of an international cooperative study. *Perit Dial Bull* 4:14, 1984.
838. Nolph KD et al: Loss of peritoneal ultrafiltration: An international detective story. *Perit Dial Bull* 4:128, 1984.
839. Nolph KD et al: A survey of ultrafiltration in chronic ambulatory peritoneal dialysis: An international cooperative study, second report. *Perit Dial Bull* 4:137, 1984.
840. Nolph KD et al: Multicenter evaluation of a new peritoneal dialysis solution with a high lactate and low magnesium concentration. *Perit Dial Bull* 3:63, 1983.
841. Nolph KD et al: An hypothesis to explain the ultrafiltration characteristics of peritoneal dialysis. *Kidney Int* 20:543, 1981.
842. Nolph KD, Parker A: The composition of dialysis solutions for continuous ambulatory peritoneal dialysis, in Legrain M (ed): *Continuous Ambulatory Peritoneal Dialysis.* Amsterdam, Excerpta Medica, 1980, p 341.
843. Nolph KD et al: Autoregulation of sodium and potassium removal during continuous ambulatory peritoneal dialysis. *Trans Am Soc Artif Intern Organs* 26:334, 1980.
844. Nolph KD et al: Continuous ambulatory peritoneal dialysis: Three-year experience at one center. *Ann Intern Med* 92:609, 1980.
845. Nolph KD et al: Equilibration of peritoneal dialysis solution during long-dwell exchanges. *J Lab Clin Med* 93:246, 1979.
846. Nolph KD et al: Peritoneal clearances with three types of commercially available peritoneal dialysis solutions. *Nephron* 24:35, 1979.
847. Nolph KD et al: Polymer-induced ultrafiltration in dialysis: High osmotic pressure due to impermeant polymer sodium. *Trans Am Soc Artif Intern Organs* 24:162, 1978.
848. Nolph KD et al: Determinants of low clearance of small solutes during peritoneal dialysis. *Kidney Int* 13:117, 1978.
849. Nolph KD et al: Theoretical and practical implications of continuous ambulatory peritoneal dialysis. *Nephron* 21:117, 1978.
850. Nolph KD et al: Differences in solute sieving with osmotic vs. hydrostatic ultrafiltration. *Trans Am Soc Artif Intern Organs* 22:618, 1976.
851. Nolph KD et al: Calcium-free peritoneal dialysis treatment of vitamin D intoxication. *Arch Intern Med* 128:809, 1971.
852. Nolph KD et al: Peritoneal glucose transport and hyperglycemia during peritoneal dialysis. *Am J Med Sci* 259:272, 1970.
853. Nolph KD et al: Peritoneal sodium transport during hypertonic peritoneal dialysis: Physiologic mechanisms and clinical implications. *Ann Intern Med* 70:931, 1969.
854. Novello A, Kjellstrand CM: Is bicarbonate dialysis better than acetate dialysis? *Trans Am Soc Artif Intern Organs* 6:103, 1983.
855. Novello A et al: Acetate intolerance during hemodialysis. *Clin Nephrol* 5:29, 1976.
856. Novick AC et al: Revascularization to preserve renal function in patients with atherosclerotic renovascular disease. *Urol Clin North Am* 11:477, 1984.
857. Odar-Cederlöf I et al: Is calcitonin gene-related peptide (CGRP) a regulator of blood pressure in hemodialysis patients. *Int J Artif Organs* 13:134, 1990.
858. Odel HM et al: Peritoneal lavage as an effective means of extrarenal excretion. *Am J Med* 9:63, 1950.
859. Odel HM et al: Clinical considerations of the problem of extrarenal excretion: Peritoneal lavage. *Med Clin North Am* 32:989, 1948.
860. Odell RA : Sorbent dialysis, in Nissenson AR et al (eds): *Clinical Dialysis*, 2d ed. Norwalk, Ct, Appleton & Lange, 1990, p 712.
861. Odell R et al: Aluminum kinetics during sorbent (REDY) dialysis. *Contemp Dial* 3:57, 1982.
862. O'Donovan R et al: Substitution of aluminum salts by magnesium salts in control of dialysis hyperphosphatemia. *Lancet* 1:880, 1986.
863. Oe PL et al: Long-term use of magnesium hydroxide as a phosphate binder in patients on hemodialysis. *Clin Nephrol* 28:180, 1987.
864. Oettinger CW, Oliver JC: An economical new process for in-center bicarbonate dialysis production: Comparison with acetate in a large dialysis population. *Artif Organs* 13:432, 1989.
865. Ogden DA: A double-blind crossover comparison of

high and low sodium dialysis. *Proc Clin Dial Transplant Forum* 8:157, 1978.

866. Ogden DA, Holmes JA: Changes in total and ultrafiltrable plasma calcium and magnesium during hemodialysis. *Trans Am Soc Artif Intern Organs* 12:200, 1966.
867. Oh MS: Irrelevance of bone buffering to acid-base homeostasis in chronic metabolic acidosis. *Nephron* 59:7, 1991.
868. Oh MS et al: Metabolic utilization and renal handling of D-lactate in man. *Metabolism* 34:621, 1985.
869. Oh MS et al: A mechanism of hypoxemia during hemodialysis: Consumption of CO_2 in metabolism of acetate. *Am J Nephrol* 5:366, 1985.
870. Oh MS et al: Consumption of CO_2 in metabolism of acetate as an explanation for hypoventilation and hypoxemia during hemodialysis. *Proc Clin Dial Transplant Forum* 9:226, 1979.
871. Oh MS, Carroll HJ: The anion gap. *N Engl J Med* 297:814, 1977.
872. Oh MS et al: Content and distribution of water and electrolytes in maintenance hemodialysis. *Nephron* 14:421, 1975.
873. Oh MS et al: Content and distribution of water and electrolytes in maintenance hemodialysis. *Nephron* 14:421, 1975.
874. Okusa MD et al: Comparison of blood pressure stability with acetate and bicarbonate hemodialysis. *Trans Am Soc Artif Intern Organs* 28:518, 1982.
875. Olbricht CJ et al: Continuous arteriovenous hemofiltration: In vivo functional characteristics and its dependence on vascular access and filter design. *Nephron* 55:49, 1990.
876. Olbricht C et al: Treatment of acute renal failure in patients with multiple organ failure by spontaneous hemofiltration. *Trans Am Soc Artif Intern Organs* 28:33, 1982.
877. Oldenberg B et al: Controlled trial of enalapril in patients with chronic fluid overload undergoing dialysis. *Br Med J* 296:1089, 1988.
878. Olinger GN et al: Vasodilator effects of the sodium acetate in pooled protein fraction. *Ann Surg* 190:305, 1979.
879. Olthuis FMFG et al: Interference of free fatty acids with the determination of calcium in serum. *Clin Chim Acta* 49:123, 1973.
880. Onesti G et al: Bilateral nephrectomy for control of hypertension in uremia. *Trans Am Soc Artif Intern Organs* 14:361, 1968.
881. Oren A et al: Effective use of amino acid dialysate over four weeks in CAPD patients. *Perit Dial Bull* 3:66, 1983.
882. Oreopoulos DG: Peritoneal dialysis solutions. *Perit Dial Bull* 4:70, 1984.
883. Oreopoulos DG et al: Peritoneal catheters and exit-site practices: Current recommendations. *Perit Dial Bull* 7:130, 1987.
884. Oreopoulos DG et al: Sclerosing obstructive peritonitis after CAPD. *Lancet* 2:409, 1983.
885. Oreopoulos DG et al: Continuous ambulatory peritoneal dialysis, 1981. *Nephron* 30:293, 1982.
886. Oreopoulos DG et al: Continuous ambulatory peritoneal dialysis: A new era in the treatment of chronic renal failure. *Clin Nephrol* 11:125, 1979.
887. Oreopoulos DG et al: A simple and safe technique of continuous ambulatory peritoneal dialysis. *Trans Am Soc Artif Intern Organs* 24:484, 1978.
888. Orgagnon Teknika Corporation: *Guide to Custom Dialysis*. Oklahoma City, 1984.
889. Orofino L et al: Epidemiology of symptomatic hypotension in hemodialysis: Is cool dialysate beneficial for all patients? *Am J Nephrol* 10:177, 1990.
890. Oster JR et al: The anion gap of patients receiving bicarbonate maintenance hemodialysis. *Trans Am Soc Artif Intern Organs* 35:800, 1989.
891. Ota K et al: Functional deterioration of the peritoneum: Does it occur in the absence of peritonitis. *Nephrol Dial Transplant* 2:30, 1987.
892. Ota K et al: Polymethylmethacrylate capillary kidney highly permeable to middle molecules. *Proc Eur Dial Transplant Assoc* 12:559, 1975.
893. Oxnard SC et al: Severe tetany in an azotemic child related to sodium phosphate enemas. *Pediatrics* 53:105, 1974.
894. Ozuer M et al: Effects of cardioselective (β_1) and nonselective (both β_1 and β_2) adrenergic blockade on serum potassium in patients with chronic renal failure undergoing hemodialysis (abstract). *Kidney Int* 26:584, 1984.
895. Paganini EP et al: Practical considerations of recombinant human erythropoietin therapy. *Am J Kidney Dis* 14:19, 1989.
896. Paganini E, Nakamoto S: Continuous slow ultrafiltration in oliguric acute renal failure. *Trans Am Soc Artif Intern Organs* 26:201, 1980.
897. Pagel MD et al: Acetate and bicarbonate fluctuations and acetate intolerance during dialysis. *Kidney Int* 21:513, 1982.
898. Pallone TL et al: Blood-dialysate equilibration during continuous arteriovenous hemodialysis. *Trans Am Soc Artif Intern Organs* 34:512, 1988.
899. Panzetta G et al: Effects of various peritoneal dialysis solutions on bacterial growth in vitro. *Perit Dial Bull* 4:27, 1984.
900. Panzetta G et al: Body fluid spaces in patients on CAPD. *Int J Artif Organs* 7:89, 1984.
901. Papadakis JT et al: Hypersensitivity reactions during hemodialysis related to the use of acetate dialysate: A case report. *Clin Nephrol* 35:224, 1991.
902. Papadakis MA et al: Hyperkalemia complicating digoxin toxicity in a patient with renal failure. *Am J Kidney Dis* 5:64, 1985.
903. Papadimitriou M et al: Alarming hyperkalemia during captopril administration in patients on regular hemodialysis. *Dial Transplant* 14:473, 1983.
904. Papadimitriou M et al: The effect of spironolactone in hypertensive patients on regular haemodialysis and after renal allotransplantation. *Life Support Syst* 1:197, 1983.
905. Papadimitriou M et al: Hypercalcemisa from calcium-ion exchange resins in patients on regular hemodialysis. *Lancet* 2:948, 1968.
906. Pappius HM et al: The effects of rapid hemodialysis on brain tissues and cerebrospinal fluid of dogs. *Can J Physiol Pharmacol* 45:129, 1967.

907. Parfrey PS et al: The clinical course of left ventricular hypertrophy in dialysis patients. *Nephron* 55:114, 1990.
908. Parker A, Nolph KD: Magnesium and calcium net mass transfers during CAPD. *Trans Am Soc Artif Intern Organs* 26:194, 1980.
909. Parsons FM, Stewart WK: The composition of dialysis fluid, in Drukker W et al (eds): *Replacement of Renal Function by Dialysis*, 2d ed. Boston, Martinus Nijhoff, 1983.
910. Parsons V et al: The long-term effects of lowering dialysate magnesium on circulating parathyroid hormone in patients on regular hemodialysis therapy. *Acta Endocrinol* 93:455, 1980.
911. Passlick J et al: Calcium alginate, an aluminum-free phosphate binder in patients on CAPD. *Clin Nephrol* 32:96, 1989.
912. Passlick J et al: Alterations in glucose absorption during peritonitis and its effects in diabetic and nondiabetic patients undergoing CAPD (abstract). *Perit Dial Bull* 4(suppl):S48, 1984.
913. Pattison ME et al: Continuous arteriovenous hemodiafiltration: An aggressive approach to the management of acute renal failure. *Am J Kidney Dis* 11:43, 1988.
914. Pearson JG: Pharmacokinetics of glyburide. *Am J Med* 79:67, 1985.
915. Pedersen FB et al: Acetate versus lactate in peritoneal dialysis solutions. *Nephron* 39:55, 1985.
916. Pedersen F et al: Alternative use of amino acid and glucose solutions in CAPD. *Perit Dial Bull* 5:215, 1985.
917. Pedersen F, Christiansen E: On acid-base problems in REDY dialysis. *Scand J Urol Nephrol* 30(suppl):28, 1976.
918. Peitzman SJ, Agarwal BN: Spontaneous hypoglycemia in end-stage renal failure. *Nephron* 19:131, 1977.
919. Petersen J et al: The effects of reprocessing cuprophane and polysulfone dialyzers on β_2-microglobulin removal from hemodialysis patients. *Am J Kidney Dis* 17:174, 1991.
920. Petersen J et al: Evaluation of dialyzers used in shortened dialysis. *Trans Am Soc Artif Intern Organs* 35:338, 1989.
921. Peterson H, deC Swanson AG: Acute encephalopathy occurring during hemodialysis. *Arch Intern Med* 113:877, 1964.
922. Petrie JJB, Row PG: Dialysis anemia caused by subacute zinc toxicity. *Lancet* 1:1178, 1977.
923. Phanichphant S et al: Short-term effect of 4% hypertonic glucose as compared to 4% mixed hypertonic mannitol solution in conventional peritoneal dialysis. *Nephron* 40:322, 1985.
924. Pierides AM, Frohnert P: Aluminum-related dialysis osteomalacia and dementia after prolonged use of the REDY cartridge. *Trans Am Soc Artif Intern Organs* 27:629, 1981.
925. Pierides AM et al: The need and use of a phosphate-enriched dialysate during regular hemodialysis. *Trans Am Soc Artif Intern Organs* 23:376, 1977.
926. Pinnick RV et al: Regional citrate anticoagulation for hemodialysis in the patient at high risk for bleeding. *N Engl J Med* 308:252, 1983.
927. Piraino BM et al: 2.5 meq/L calcium dialysate (D) vs 3.5 meq/L calcium dialysate and aluminum in PD patients (abstract). *Perit Dial Int* 11(suppl):208, 1991.
928. Piraino BM et al: Spontaneous hypercalcemia in patients undergoing dialysis: Etiologic and therapeutic consideration. *Am J Med* 80:607, 1986.
929. Pletka P et al: Effect of magnesium on parathyroid hormone secretion during chronic hemodialysis. *Lancet* 2:462, 1971.
930. Pogglitsch H et al: Phosphorus kinetics during haemodialysis and haemofiltration. *Proc Eur Dial Transplant Assoc Eur Renal Assoc* 21:461, 1984.
931. Pollock CA et al: Continuous ambulatory peritoneal dialysis: Eight years of experience at a single center. *Medicine* 68:293, 1989.
932. Popovich RP et al: Transport kinetics, in Nolph KD (ed): *Peritoneal Dialysis*, 3d ed. Boston, Kluwer Academic, 1989, p 96.
933. Popovich RP et al: Kinetics of peritoneal transport, in Nolph KD (ed): *Peritoneal Dialysis*. The Hague, Martinus Nijhoff, 1981, p 12.
934. Popovich RP et al: Continuous ambulatory peritoneal dialysis. *Ann Intern Med* 88:449, 1978.
935. Popovich RP et al: The definition of a novel portable/wearable equilibrium peritoneal dialysis technique (abstract). *Trans Am Soc Artif Intern Organs* 5:64, 1976.
936. Port FK: Fluid and electrolyte disorders in dialysis, in Kokko JP, Tannen RL (eds): *Fluids and Electrolytes*. Philadelphia, Saunders, 1986, p 593.
937. Port FK et al: Prevention of dialysis disequilibrium syndrome by use of high sodium concentration in the dialysate. *Kidney Int* 3:327, 1973.
938. Posen GA, Kaye M: Magnesium metabolism in patients on chronic dialysis. *Proc Eur Dial Transplant Assoc* 4:224, 1967.
939. Posner AS et al: Role of ATP and Mg in the stabilization of biological and synthetic amorphous calcium phosphates. *Calcif Tissue Res* 22(suppl):208, 1977.
940. Potter DJ: Death as a result of hyperglycemia without ketosis: A complication of hemodialysis. *Ann Intern Med* 64:399, 1966.
941. Putnam TJ: The living peritoneum as a dialyzing membrane. *Am J Physiol* 63:547, 1922–1923.
942. Pyle WK et al: Peritoneal transport evaluation in CAPD, in Moncrief JW, Popovich RP (eds): *CAPD Update: Continuous Ambulatory Peritoneal Dialysis*. New York, Masson, 1981, p 35.
943. Quellhorst E: Cardiovascular problems in end-stage renal failure: Hemofiltration. *Contrib Nephrol* 78:212, 1990.
944. Quellhorst E et al: Treatment of chronic uraemia by an ultrafiltration kidney-first clinical experience. *Proc Eur Dial Transplant Assoc* 13:314, 1976.
945. Quevedo SF et al: Fasting hypoglycemia secondary to disopyramide therapy: Report of two cases. *JAMA* 245:2424, 1987.
946. Quintanilla A, Singer I: Metabolic alkalosis in the patient with uremia. *Am J Kidney Dis* 17:591, 1991.
947. Quinton W et al: Cannulation of blood vessels for prolonged hemodialysis. *Trans Am Soc Artif Intern Organs* 6:104, 1960.
948. Raine AEG: Seizures and hypertension events. *Semin Nephrol* 10(suppl 1):40, 1990.

949. Raine AEG: Hypertension, blood viscosity, and cardiovascular morbidity in renal failure: Implications of erythropoietin therapy. *Lancet* 1:97, 1988.
950. Raja R et al: Comparison of continuous arteriovenous hemofiltration and continuous arteriovenous dialysis in critically ill patients. *Trans Am Soc Artif Intern Organs* 32:435, 1986.
951. Raja RM et al: Sequential changes in dialysate sodium during hemodialysis. *Trans Am Soc Artif Intern Organs* 29:649, 1983.
952. Raja RM et al: Hemodialysis with various dialysate bicarbonate concentrations. *Trans Am Soc Artif Intern Organs* 28:514, 1982.
953. Raja RM et al: High sodium dialysate with addition of chloride, acetate, and bicarbonate. *Trans Am Soc Artif Intern Organs* 27:36, 1981.
954. Raja RM et al: Hemodialysis-associated hypoxemia: Role of acetate and pH in etiology. *Trans Am Soc Artif Intern Organs* 27:180, 1981.
955. Raja RM et al: Prevention of hypotension during iso-osmolar hemodialysis with bicarbonate dialysate. *Trans Am Soc Artif Intern Organs* 26:375, 1980.
956. Raja RM et al: Dialysis hypoxemia with varying dialyzers and dialysate: Role of acetate in etiology (abstract). *Am Soc Artif Intern Organs* 9:60, 1980.
957. Raja RM et al: Improved dialysis tolerance using REDY sorbent system with bicarbonate dialysate in critically ill patients. *Dial Transplant* 8:241, 1979.
958. Raja RM et al: Use of mannitol in hemodialysis. *Dial Transplant* 6:32, 1976.
959. Raja RM et al: Peritoneal dialysis with fructose dialysate. *Ann Intern Med* 79:511, 1973.
960. Raja RM et al: Sodium transport during ultrafiltration peritoneal dialysis. *Trans Am Soc Artif Intern Organs* 18:429, 1972.
961. Raja RM et al: Hyperosmotic coma complicating peritoneal dialysis with sorbitol dialysate. *Ann Intern Med* 73:993, 1970.
962. Raju SF et al: Hyperkalemia in a hemodialysis patient without a colon. *Dial Transplant* 9:1086, 1980.
963. Raman A et al: Effects of varying dialysate calcium concentrations on the plasma calcium fraction in patients on dialysis. *Nephron* 16:181, 1976.
964. Ramirez G et al: Aldosterone response to insulin-induced hypoglycemia in hemodialysis patients. *Am J Nephrol* 9:215, 1989.
965. Ramirez G et al: The role of glucose in hemodialysis: The effects of glucose-free dialysate. *Am J Kidney Dis* 7:413, 1986.
966. Ramirez G et al: Cardiac arrhythmias on hemodialysis in chronic renal failure patients. *Nephron* 36:212, 1984.
967. Ramirez JA et al: The absorption of dietary phosphorus and calcium in hemodialysis patients. *Kidney Int* 30:753, 1986.
968. Ramos JM et al: Sequential changes in serum lipids and their subfractions in patients receiving chronic ambulatory peritoneal dialysis. *Nephron* 35:20, 1983.
969. Randall RE et al: Hypermagnesemia in renal failure: Etiology and toxic manifestations. *Ann Intern Med* 61:73, 1964.
970. Rao TKS et al: Continuing high morbidity during maintenance hemodialysis consequent to bilateral nephrectomy. *Trans Am Soc Artif Intern Organs* 19:340, 1973.
971. Ratge P et al: Plasma catecholamines and alpha and beta adrenoreceptors in circulating blood cells in patients on continuous ambulatory peritoneal dialysis. *Clin Nephrol* 28:15, 1987.
972. Relman AS: Renal acidosis and renal excretion of acid in health and disease. *Adv Intern Med* 12:295, 1964.
973. Rhoads TE: Peritoneal lavage in the treatment of renal insufficiency. *Am J Med Sci* 192:642, 1938.
974. Ribot S et al: Complications of peritoneal dialysis. *Am J Med Sci* 252:505, 1966.
975. Richards C et al: Bicarbonate haemodialysis using a sorbent regenerative system. *Clin Nephrol* 2:289, 1979.
976. Richards C et al: Acetate-free hemodialysis with a sorbent regenerative system. *Proc Clin Dial Transplant Forum* 8:104, 1977.
977. Richards RH et al: Acetate metabolism in normal human subjects. *Am J Kidney Dis* 2:47, 1982.
978. Richardson JA et al: Antibacterial effect of different dialysates (letter to editor). *Br Med J* 2:468, 1972.
979. Richardson JA, Borchardt KA: Adverse effect on bacteria of peritoneal dialysis solutions that contain acetate. *Br Med J* 3:749, 1969.
980. Richardson RMA et al: Bicarbonate, L-lactate and D-lactate balance in intermittent peritoneal dialysis. *Perit Dial Bull* 6:178, 1986.
981. Rigg GA, Beron BA: Hypoglycemia: A complication of hemodialysis. *N Engl J Med* 277:1139, 1967.
982. Rimondini A et al: Hemofiltration as short-term treatment for refractory congestive heart failure. *Am J Med* 83:43, 1987.
983. Rivera-Vasquez AB et al: Acute hyperglycemia in hemodialysis patients: Distinction from "dialysis dementia." *Nephron* 25:243, 1980.
984. Roberts M, Daugirdas JT: REDY sorbent hemodialysis, in Daugirdas JT, Ing TS (eds): *Handbook of Dialysis*. Boston, Little, Brown 1988, p 146.
985. Robson MD et al: Effect of first and subsequent use of hemodialyzers on patient well-being. *Am J Nephrol* 6:101, 1986.
986. Robson MD et al: The metabolism of lactate and bicarbonate in CAPD, in Atkins RC et al (eds): *Peritoneal Dialysis*. Edinburgh, Churchill Livingstone, 1981, p 102.
987. Robson MD et al: Dialysate sodium concentration, hypertension, and pulmonary edema in hemodialysis patients. *Dial Transplant* 7:678, 1978.
988. Robson MD, Oreopoulos DG: Continuous ambulatory peritoneal dialysis: A revolution in the treatment of chronic renal failure. *Dial Transplant* 7:999, 1978.
989. Robson MD et al: Comparison of intermittent with continuous peritoneal dialysis. *Proc Eur Dial Transplant Assoc* 15:197, 1978.
990. Robson MD et al: Hyperglycaemia and hyperosmolarity in peritoneal dialysis: Its prevention by use of fructose. *Proc Eur Dial Transplant Assoc* 6:300, 1969.
991. Rodrigo F et al: Osmolality changes during hemodialysis: Natural history, clinical correlations, and influence of dialysate glucose and intravenous mannitol. *Ann Intern Med* 86:554, 1977.
991a. Rodriguez M et al: Effect of dialysis and ultrafiltration

on osmolality, colloid osmotic pressure and vascular refilling rate. *Kidney Int* 28:808, 1985.
992. Rohmer D et al: A comparison of the respiratory dynamics during hemodialysis using acetate and bicarbonate dialysate in a sorbent regenerative system. *Trans Am Soc Artif Intern Organs* 27:176, 1981.
993. Ronco C: Backfiltration in clinical dialysis: Nature of the phenomenon, mechanisms and possible solutions. *Int J Artif Organs* 13:11, 1990.
994. Ronco C et al: Pathophysiology of ultrafiltration in peritoneal dialysis. *Perit Dial Int* 10:119, 1990.
995. Ronco C et al: Arteriovenous hemodiafiltration associated with continuous arteriovenous hemofiltration: A combined therapy for acute renal failure in the hypercatabolic patient. *Blood Purif* 5:33, 1987.
996. Roodhooft AM et al: Hypophosphatemia in infants on chronic ambulatory peritoneal dialysis. *Clin Nephrol* 34:131, 1990.
997. Rosansky SJ: Nocturnal hypertension in patients receiving chronic hemodialysis. *Ann Intern Med* 114:96, 1991.
998. Rosen SM et al: Hemodialysis disequilibrium. *Br Med J* 2:672, 1964.
999. Rosenbaum BJ et al: Acid-base status during the interdialytic period in patients maintained with chronic hemodialysis. *Ann Intern Med* 71:1105, 1969.
1000. Rossen B, Ladefoged J: A comparison between the effects of acetate and lactate in peritoneal dialysis solutions. *Scand J Urol Nephrol* 16:279, 1982.
1001. Rostand SG: Profound hypokalemia in continuous ambulatory peritoneal dialysis. *Arch Intern Med* 143:377, 1983.
1002. Rotellar C et al: Ten years' experience with continuous ambulatory peritoneal dialysis. *Am J Kidney Dis* 17:158, 1991.
1003. Rottembourg J et al: Severe abdominal complications in patients undergoing continuous ambulatory peritoneal dialysis. *Proc Eur Dial Transplant Assoc* 20:236, 1983.
1004. Rottembourg J et al: Is continuous ambulatory peritoneal dialysis the best dialysis choice for insulin-dependent diabetics. *Proc Eur Dial Transplant Assoc* 19:215, 1982.
1005. Rouby JJ et al: Hemodynamic changes induced by regular hemodialysis and sequential ultrafiltration hemodialysis: A comparative study. *Kidney Int* 17:801, 1980.
1006. Roxe DM et al: Phosphate-binding effects of sucralfate in patients with chronic renal failure. *Am J Kidney Dis* 13:194, 1989.
1007. Rozich JD et al: Dialysis-induced alterations in left ventricular filling: Mechanisms and clinical significance. *Am J Kidney Dis* 17:272, 1991.
1008. Rubin J: Comments on dialysis solution, antibiotic transport, poisonings and novel uses of peritoneal dialysis, in Nolph KD (ed): *Peritoneal Dialysis*, 3d ed. Boston, Kluwer Academic, 1989, p 199.
1009. Rubin J et al: Diabetes, dialysate losses and serum lipids during continuous ambulatory peritoneal dialysis. *Am J Kidney Dis* 10:104, 1987.
1010. Rubin J et al: Effect of intraperitoneal insulin on solute kinetics in CAPD: Insulin kinetics in CAPD. *Am J Med Sci* 291:81, 1986.
1011. Rubin J et al: Stereospecific lactate absorption during peritoneal dialysis. *Nephron* 31:224, 1982.
1012. Rubin J et al: Peritoneal abnormalities during infectious episodes of continuous ambulatory peritoneal dialysis. *Nephron* 29:124, 1981.
1013. Rubin J et al: Peritoneal dialysis during peritonitis. *Kidney Int* 19:460, 1981.
1014. Rubin J et al: Protein losses in chronic ambulatory peritoneal dialysis. *Nephron* 25:218, 1981.
1015. Rubin J et al: Comparison of the effects of lactate and acetate on clinical peritoneal clearances. *Clin Nephrol* 12:145, 1979.
1016. Rubin J et al: Drainage volumes during continuous ambulatory peritoneal dialysis. *Trans Am Soc Artif Intern Organs* 2:54, 1979.
1017. Rubin J et al: Clinical studies with a nonvasoactive peritoneal dialysis solution. *J Lab Clin Med* 93:910, 1979.
1018. Ruder MA et al: Comparative effects of acetate and bicarbonate hemodialysis on left ventricular function. *Kidney Int* 27:768, 1985.
1019. Ruderman MA et al: Preparation of bacteriologically safe bicarbonate concentrate for hemodialysis. *Trans Am Soc Artif Intern Organs* 34:606, 1988.
1020. Ruderman MA et al: Preparation of bacteriologically safe bicarbonate concentrate for hemodialysis. *Trans Am Soc Artif Intern Organs* 34:606, 1988.
1021. Rudnick MR et al: Fluid-electrolyte complications of dialysis, in Maxwell MH et al (eds): *Clinical Disorders of Fluid and Electrolyte Metabolism*, 4th ed. New York, McGraw-Hill, 1987, p 1053.
1022. Rutsky EA et al: Spontaneous hypoglycemia in chronic renal failure. *Arch Intern Med* 138:1364, 1978.
1023. Sabatier J et al: Sclerosing obstructive peritonitis after continuous ambulatory peritoneal dialysis in 3 patients (letter to editor). *Clin Nephrol* 23:266, 1985.
1024. Said R et al: Acute hemolysis due to profound hyposmolality: A complication of hemodialysis. *J Dial* 1:477, 1977.
1025. Salusky IB et al: High-dose calcitriol for control of renal osteodystrophy in children on CAPD. *Kidney Int* 32:89, 1987.
1026. Salusky IB et al: Effects of oral calcium carbonate on control of serum phosphorus and changes in plasma aluminum levels after discontinuation of aluminum-containing gels in children receiving dialysis. *J Pediatr* 108:767, 1986.
1027. Samar RE: Dialysate sodium concentrations in hemodialysis. *Contemp Dialysis* 2:40, 1981.
1028. Samii K et al: Severe hypoglycemia due to beta blocking drugs in hemodialysis patients. *Lancet* 1:545, 1976.
1029. Sandle GI et al: Enhanced rectal potassium secretion in chronic renal insufficiency: Evidence for large intestinal adaptation in man. *Clin Sci* 71:393, 1986.
1030. Sargent JA: Shortfalls in the delivery of dialysis. *Am J Kidney Dis* 15:500, 1990.
1031. Sargent JA, Gotch FA: Principles and biophysics of dialysis, in Maher JF (ed): *Replacement of Renal Function by Dialysis*, 3d ed. Dordrecht, The Netherlands, Kluwer Academic, 1989, p 87.
1032. Sargent JA et al: Technical aspects of on-line proportioning of bicarbonate dialysate. *Proc Clin Dial Transplant Forum* 7:109, 1977.

1033. Sawyer N et al: High-dose calcium carbonate with stepwise reduction in dialysate calcium concentration: Effective phosphate control and aluminum avoidance in hemodialysis patients. *Nephrol Dial Transplant* 4:105, 1989.
1034. Schaefer K, van Herrath D: High-efficiency therapies for clinical dialysis, in Nissenson AR et al (eds): *Clinical Dialysis*, 2d ed. Norwalk, Ct, Appleton & Lange, 1990, p 697.
1035. Schaefer K et al: New hope in the treatment of uremic hyperphosphatemia? *Semin Dial* 3:65, 1990.
1036. Schaefer K et al: Treatment of uremic hyperphosphatemia: Is there still a need for aluminum salts? *Am J Nephrol* 8:173, 1988.
1037. Schaefer K et al: Chronic hemofiltration: A critical evaluation of a new method for the treatment of blood. *Artif Organs* 2:386, 1978.
1038. Schalekamp MA et al: Hypertension in chronic renal failure: An abnormal relationship between sodium and the renin-angiotensin system. *Am J Med* 55:379, 1973.
1039. Scheppach W et al: Effects of acetate during regular hemodialysis. *Clin Nephrol* 29:19, 1988.
1040. Schick EC et al: Comparison of the hemodynamic response to hemodialysis with acetate or bicarbonate. *Trans Am Soc Artif Intern Organs* 29:25, 1983.
1041. Schilling H et al: Nutritional status of patients on long-term CAPD. *Perit Dial Bull* 5:12, 1985.
1042. Schilling H et al: Studies on circulatory stability during bicarbonate hemodialysis with constant dialysate sodium versus acetate hemodialysis with sequential dialysate sodium. *Artif Organs* 9:17, 1985.
1043. Schmidt M et al: Backfiltration in hemodialyzers with highly permeable membranes. *Blood Purif* 2:108, 1984.
1044. Schmidt P et al: Magnesium metabolism in patients on regular dialysis treatment. *Clin Sci* 41:131, 1971.
1045. Schmidt RW, Blumenkrantz MJ: IPD, CAPD, CCPD, CRPD—peritoneal dialysis: Past, present, and future. *Int J Artif Organs* 4:124, 1981.
1046. Schmitz O et al: Insulin-mediated glucose uptake in nondialyzed and dialyzed uremic insulin-dependent diabetic subjects. *Diabetes* 34:1152, 1985.
1047. Schmitz O et al: Aspects of glucose homeostasis in uremia as assessed by hyperinsulinemic euglycemic clamp technique. *Metabolism* 34:465, 1985.
1048. Schneider NS, Geronemus RP: Continuous arteriovenous hemodialysis. *Kidney Int* 24(suppl):S159, 1968.
1049. Schohn DC et al: Correlation between plasma sodium acetate concentration and systemic vascular resistances. *Proc Eur Dial Transplant Assoc* 18:160, 1981.
1050. Schuett H, Port FK: Hemolysis in hemodialysis patients. *Dial Transplant* 9:345, 1980.
1051. Schultze G: Eicosanoids and blood pressure during hemodialysis. *Int J Artif Organs* 13:145, 1990.
1052. Schultze G et al: Prostaglandin E_2 promotes hypotension on low-sodium hemodialysis. *Nephron* 37:250, 1984.
1053. Schultze G et al: Restoration of total body potassium in the course of long-term hemodialysis treatment. *Miner Electrolyte Metab* 6:139, 1981.
1054. Schwab SJ et al: Hemodialysis without anticoagulation: One-year prospective trial in hospitalized patients at risk for bleeding. *Am J Med* 83:405, 1987.
1055. Schwartz WB et al: On the mechanism of acidosis in chronic renal failure. *J Clin Invest* 38:39, 1959.
1056. Schwarzbeck A et al: pH-Dependent heparin inactivation during hemodialysis. *Dial Transplant* 7:740, 1978.
1057. Schwarzbeck A et al: Clotting in dialyzers due to low pH of dialysis fluid. *Clin Nephrol* 7:125, 1977.
1058. Scribner BH: Substitution of bicarbonate for acetate in the dialysate for care of a critically ill patient. *Dial Transplant* 6:26, 1977.
1059. Seedat YK: Total body potassium and chronic renal failure. *Br Med J* 2:405, 1972.
1060. Seltzer HS: Drug-induced hypoglycemia: A review based on 473 cases. *Diabetes* 21:955, 1972.
1061. Severini G et al: Conventional haemodialysis and ultrafiltration: Effects of erythrocyte 2,3-diphosphoglycerate and oxygen affinity in patients with uraemia. *Clin Sci* 59:143, 1980.
1062. Seveso M et al: Insulin absorption to peritoneal dialysate bags. *Perit Dial Bull* 7:S68, 1987.
1063. Shah GM et al: Effects of magnesium-free dialysate on magnesium metabolism during chronic ambulatory peritoneal dialysis. *Am J Kidney Dis* 10:268, 1987.
1064. Shah S et al: Persistent hypophosphatemia in patients on chronic hemodialysis without phosphate binding gels (abstract). *Kidney Int* 10:526, 1976.
1065. Shaldon S: Sequential ultrafiltration and dialysis. *Proc Eur Dial Transplant Assoc* 13:300, 1976.
1066. Shapiro WB: The current status of sorbent hemodialysis. *Semin Dial* 3:40, 1990.
1067. Shapiro W et al: Aluminum leakage from REDY sorbent cartridge. *Kidney Int* 23:536, 1983.
1068. Sheikh MS et al: Reduction of dietary phosphorus absorption by phosphorus binders: A theoretical, in vitro, and in vivo study. *J Clin Invest* 83:66, 1989.
1069. Shen FH et al: Thirst, relative hypernatremia, and excessive weight gain in maintenance peritoneal dialysis. *Trans Am Soc Artif Intern Organs* 24:142, 1978.
1070. Sheppard JM et al: Lactic acidosis: Recovery associated with the use of peritoneal dialysate. *Aust N Z J Med* 4:389, 1972.
1071. Sherman RA: The pathophysiologic basis for hemodialysis-related hypotension. *Semin Dial* 1:136, 1988.
1072. Sherman RA: On lowering dialysate calcium. *Semin Dial* 1:78, 1988.
1073. Sherman RA et al: The effect of red cell transfusion on hemodialysis-related hypotension. *Am J Kidney Dis* 11:33, 1988.
1074. Sherman RA et al: Postprandial blood pressure changes during hemodialysis. *Am J Kidney Dis* 12:37, 1988.
1075. Sherman RA et al: The effect of dialysate calcium levels on blood pressure during hemodialysis. *Am J Kidney Dis* 8:244, 1986.
1076. Sherman RA et al: Variability in potassium removal by hemodialysis. *Am J Nephrol* 6:284, 1986.
1077. Sherman RA et al: Amelioration of hemodialysis-associated hypotension by the use of cool dialysate. *Am J Kidney Dis* 5:124, 1985.
1078. Sherman RA et al: Ineffectiveness of adding salt to concentrate in raising dialysate sodium levels. *Dial Transplant* 14:298, 1985.
1079. Sherman RA et al: Effect of variations in dialysate tem-

perature on blood pressure during hemodialysis. *Am J Kidney Dis* 4:66, 1984.
1080. Shimamatsu K et al: Does 1α $(OH)D_3$ treatment affect blood pressure levels in maintenance hemodialysis patients. *Am J Nephrol* 8:471, 1988.
1081. Shinaberger JH: Dialysis. *Curr Nephrol* 1:314, 1977.
1082. Shinaberger JH et al: Short treatment in Maher JF (ed): *Replacement of Renal Function with Dialysis*, 3d ed. Dordrecht, The Netherlands, Kluwer Academic, 1989, p 360.
1083. Shinaberger JH et al: Erythropoietin alert: Risks of high-hematocrit hemodialysis. *Trans Am Soc Artif Intern Organs* 34:179, 1988.
1084. Shiota J et al: Plasma atrial natriuretic peptide during hemodialysis with or without fluid removal. *Nephron* 55:283, 1990.
1085. Shumizu AG et al: Reducing patient morbidity from high-efficiency hemodialysis: A double-blind crossover trial. *Trans Am Soc Artif Intern Organs* 29:666, 1983.
1086. Sica DA et al: Hypercalcemic hypertension in hemodialysis. *Clin Nephrol* 22:102, 1984.
1087. Sigler MH, Teehan BP: Continuous arteriovenous hemodialysis (CAVHD): An improved technique for treating acute renal failure in critically ill patients, in Nissenson AR et al (eds): *Clinical Dialysis*, 2d ed. Norwalk, Ct, Appleton & Lange, 1990, p 720.
1088. Sigler MH, Teehan BP: Solute transport in continuous hemodialysis: A new treatment for acute renal failure. *Kidney Int* 32:562, 1987.
1089. Sigler MH et al: Acetate and energy metabolism during hemodialysis. *Kidney Int* 24(suppl 16):S97, 1983.
1090. Silberberg JS et al: Impact of left ventricular hypertrophy on survival in end-stage renal disease. *Kidney Int* 36:286, 1989.
1091. Silverstein FJ et al: Metabolic alkalosis induced by regional citrate hemodialysis. *Trans Am Soc Artif Intern Organs* 35:22, 1989.
1092. Silverstein MD et al: Response to rapid removal of intermediate molecular weight solutes in uremic man. *Trans Am Soc Artif Intern Organs* 20:614, 1974.
1093. Singh S et al: Comparison of buffering capacity in patients on hemodialysis and continuous ambulatory peritoneal dialysis. *Nephron* 42:29, 1986.
1094. Singh S et al: Responses to acid loading in patients on hemodialysis and continuous ambulatory peritoneal dialysis. *Perit Dial Bull* 4:S92, 1984.
1095. Sitprija U, Holmes JH: Preliminary observations on the change in intracranial pressure and intraocular pressure during hemodialysis. *Trans Am Soc Artif Intern Organs* 10:323, 1962.
1096. Skroder R et al: Biocompatibility of dialysis membranes is of no importance for objective or subjective symptoms during or after hemodialysis. *Trans Am Soc Artif Intern Organs* 36:M637, 1990.
1097. Skutches CL et al: Plasma acetate turnover and oxidation. *J Clin Invest* 64:708, 1979.
1098. Slatopolsky E et al: Long-term effects of calcium carbonate and 2.5 meq/liter calcium dialysate on mineral metabolism. *Kidney Int* 36:897, 1989.
1099. Slatopolsky E et al: Calcium carbonate as a phosphate binder in patients with chronic renal failure undergoing dialysis. *N Engl J Med* 315:157, 1986.
1100. Slatopolsky E et al: Marked suppression of secondary hyperparathyroidism by intravenous administration of 1,25- dihydroxycholecalciferol in uremic patients. *J Clin Invest* 74:2136, 1984.
1101. Slatopolsky E et al: Hyperphosphatemia. *Clin Nephrol* 7:138, 1977.
1102. Slingeneyer A et al: Permanent loss of ultrafiltration capacity of the peritoneum in long-term peritoneal dialysis: An epidemiological study. *Nephron* 33:133, 1983.
1103. Slingeneyer A et al: Progressive sclerosing peritonitis: A late and severe complication of maintenance peritoneal dialysis. *Trans Am Soc Artif Intern Organs* 29:633, 1983.
1104. Smith MC, Dunn MJ: Hypertension in renal parenchymal disease, in Laragh JH, Brenner BM (eds): *Hypertension Pathophysiology, Diagnosis, and Management*. New York, Raven Press, 1990, p 1583.
1105. Smith RJ et al: Hypernatremic hyperosmolar coma complicating chronic peritoneal dialysis. *Proc Clin Dial Transplant Forum* 4:96, 1974.
1106. Smithard D et al: Spontaneous hypoglycemia during continuous ambulatory peritoneal dialysis (CAPD). *Perit Dial Bull* 3:191, 1983.
1106a. Sorensen SS et al: Hypotension in end-stage renal disease: Effects of postural change, exercise, and angiotensin II infusion on blood pressure and plasma concentrations of angiotensin II, aldosterone, and arginine vasopressin in hypotensive patients with chronic renal failure treated by dialysis. *Clin Nephrol* 26:288, 1986.
1107. Spital A, Sterns RH: Potassium homeostasis in dialysis patients. *Semin Dial* 1:14, 1988.
1108. Spital AS, Sterns RH: Potassium supplementation via the dialysate in continuous ambulatory peritoneal dialysis. *Am J Kidney Dis* 6:173, 1985.
1109. Spitz T et al: The effect of dialysis on the carbohydrate tolerance of chronic renal failure. *Horm Metab Res* 2:86, 1970.
1110. Spongano M et al: Continuous computerized monitoring of hemodynamic parameters during acetate dialysis, bicarbonate dialysis, and acetate-free biofiltration. *Artif Organs* 12:476, 1988.
1111. Stableen DM et al: The effect of CAPD on hypertension control: A report of the national CAPD registry. *Perit Dial Int* 8:191, 1988.
1112. Stanbury SW, Lumb GA: Parathyroid function in chronic renal failure. *Q J Med* 35:1, 1966.
1113. Steiner RW: Continuous equilibration peritoneal dialysis in acute renal failure. *Perit Dial Int* 9:5, 1989.
1114. Stenzel KH et al: Clinical effect of bilateral nephrectomy. *Am J Med* 58:69, 1975.
1115. Stewart WK: The composition of dialysis fluid, in Maher JF (ed): *Replacement of Renal Function by Dialysis*, 3d ed. Dordrecht, The Netherlands, Kluwer Academic, 1989, p 199.
1116. Stewart WK et al: Is hyponatremic dialysis appropriate? A survey of dialysate sodium concentration in the United Kingdom. *Dial Transplant* 6:9, 1977.
1117. Stewart WK, Fleming LW: The effect of dialysate magnesium on plama and erythrocyte magnesium and po-

tassium concentration during maintenance hemodialysis. *Nephron* 10:222, 1973.
1118. Stewart WK et al: Benefits obtained by the use of high sodium dialysate during maintenance hemodialysis. *Proc Eur Dial Transplant Assoc* 9:111, 1972.
1119. Stewart WK et al: Changes in plasma electrolytes and nerve conduction velocities during chronic hemodialysis without magnesium. *Proc Eur Dial Transplant Assoc* 4:285, 1967.
1119a. Stiller S et al: Characteristic profiles of circulating blood volume during dialysis therapy. *Trans Am Soc Artif Intern Organs* 35:530, 1989.
1120. Stiller S et al: Backfiltration in hemodialysis with highly permeable membranes. *Contrib Nephrol* 46:23, 1985.
1121. Stojceva-Taneva O et al: Autonomic nervous system dysfunction and volume-nonresponsive hypotension in hemodialysis patients. *Am J Nephrol* 11:123, 1991.
1122. Stoltz ML et al: Factors affecting calcium removal with calcium free peritoneal dialysate. *J Lab Clin Med* 78:389, 1971.
1123. Storck M et al: Comparison of pump-driven and spontaneous continuous haemofiltration in postoperative acute renal failure. *Lancet* 337:452, 1991.
1124. Sugisaki H et al: Dynamic behavior of plasma phosphate in chronic dialysis patients. *Trans Am Soc Artif Intern Organs* 28:302, 1982.
1124a. Suki WN et al: Citrate for regional anticoagulation: Effects on blood P_{O_2}, ammonia, and aluminum. *Trans Am Soc Artif Intern Organs* 34:524, 1988.
1125. Susini G et al: Isolated ultrafiltration in cardiogenic pulmonary edema. *Crit Care Med* 18:14, 1990.
1126. Swales JD: Sodium uptake in peritoneal dialysis. *Br Med J* 3:345, 1967.
1127. Swamy AP et al: Long-term effect of dialysate glucose on the lipid levels of maintenance hemodialysis patients. *Trans Am Soc Artif Intern Organs* 22:54, 1976.
1128. Swamy AP, Cestero RVM: Mannitol and maintenance hemodialysis. *Artif Organs* 3:116, 1979.
1129. Swartz RD et al: Preservation of plasma volume during hemodialysis depends on plasma osmolality. *Am J Nephrol* 2:189, 1982.
1130. Swartz RD et al: Complications of hemodialysis and peritoneal dialysis in acute renal failure. *Am Soc Artif Intern Organs J* 3:98, 1980.
1131. Swartz RD, Port FK: Preventing hemorrhage in high-risk hemodialysis: Regional versus low-dose heparin. *Kidney Int* 16:513, 1979.
1132. Swartz RD et al: Correction of post-operative metabolic alkalosis and renal failure by hemodialysis. *Ann Intern Med* 86:52, 1977.
1133. Synhaivsky A et al: Acute renal failure treated by slow continuous ultrafiltration. *Mayo Clin Proc* 59:729, 1983.
1134. Tam PY-W et al: Slow continuous hemodialysis for the management of complicated acute renal failure in an intensive care unit. *Clin Nephrol* 30:79, 1988.
1135. Tchetagni J et al: Fatal hypoglycemia during CAPD in a young diabetic not receiving insulin. *Perit Dial Bull* 7:109, 1987.
1136. Teehan BP et al: Acid-base studies in continuous ambulatory peritonal dialysis, in Moncrief JW, Popovitch RO (eds): *CAPD Update: Continuous Ambulatory Peritoneal Dialysis*. New York, Masson, 1981, p 95.
1137. Tenckhoff H, Curtis FK: Experience with maintenance peritoneal dialysis in the home. *Trans Am Soc Artif Intern Organs* 16:90, 1970.
1138. Tenckhoff H et al: A home peritoneal dialysis delivery system. *Trans Am Soc Artif Intern Organs* 15:103, 1969.
1139. Tenckhoff H, Schechter H: A bacteriologically safe peritoneal access device. *Trans Am Soc Artif Intern Organs* 14:181, 1968.
1140. Tenckhoff H et al: The influence of dialysate volume and flow rate on peritoneal clearance. *Proc Eur Dial Transplant Assoc* 2:113, 1965.
1141. Thalheimer W: Experimental exchange transfusions for reducing azotemia: Use of artificial kidney for this purpose. *Proc Soc Exp Biol Med* 37:641, 1937.
1142. The Bergamo Group: Blood pressure and symptoms during polysulfone vs cellulose dialysis: A double-blind study. *Kidney Int* 28:375, 1985.
1143. Thompson TJ et al: Intraperitoneal calcium for resistant hypocalcemia after parathyroidectomy in chronic renal failure. *Br Med J* 296:896, 1988.
1144. Tielemans C et al: Anaphylactoid reactions during hemodialysis on AN69 membranes in patients receiving ACE inhibitors. *Kidney Int* 38:982, 1990.
1145. Tipple MA et al: Investigations of hemolytic anemia after chloramine exposure in a dialysis center. *Trans Am Soc Artif Intern Organs* 34:1060, 1988.
1146. Tolchin N et al: Metabolic consequences of high mass transfer hemodialysis. *Kidney Int* 11:366, 1977.
1147. Topleny N et al: The effect of dialysate on peritoneal phagocyte oxidative metabolism. *Kidney Int* 34:404, 1988.
1148. Torrance JD et al: Changes in oxygen delivery during hemodialysis. *Clin Nephrol* 3:54, 1975.
1149. Torrente J et al: Partial substitution of sodium lactate for sodium acetate in the bath fluid for hemodialysis. *Artif Organs* 14:2, 1990.
1150. Toth EL, Lee LW: "Spontaneous"/uremic hypoglycemia is not a distinct entity: Substantiation from a literature review. *Nephron* 58:325, 1991.
1151. Travis M, Henrich W: Autonomic nervous system and hemodialysis hypotension. *Semin Dial* 2:158, 1989.
1152. Tsang HK et al: Urea dynamics during and immediately after dialysis. *Am Soc Artif Intern Organs J* 8:251, 1985.
1153. Tubbs P: The metabolism of D-hydroxyacids in animal tissues. *Ann N Y Acad Sci* 119:920, 1965.
1153a. Twardowski ZJ: Physiology of peritoneal dialysis, in Nissenson AR et al (eds): *Clinical Dialysis*, 2d ed. Norwalk, Ct, Appleton & Lange, 1990, p 240.
1153b. Twardowski ZJ: Peritoneal glossary III. *Perit Dial Int* 10:173, 1990.
1154. Twardowski ZJ: New approaches to intermittent peritoneal dialysis therapies, in Nolph KD (ed): *Peritoneal Dialysis*, 3d ed. Boston, Kluwer Academic, 1989, p 133.
1154a. Twardowski ZJ: Clinical value of standardized equilibration tests in CAPD patients. *Blood Purif* 7:95, 1989.

1154b. Twardowski ZJ: Peritoneal glossary II. *Perit Dial Int* 8:15, 1988.
1155. Twardowski ZJ et al: Chronic nightly tidal peritoneal dialysis. *Trans Am Soc Artif Intern Organs* 36:M584, 1990.
1156. Twardowski ZJ et al: Peritoneal equilibration test. *Perit Dial Bull* 7:139, 1987.
1157. Twardowski ZJ et al: Choice of peritoneal dialysis regimen based on peritoneal transfer rates. *Perit Dial Bull* 7:S79, 1987.
1158. Twardowski ZJ et al: Eight-hour tidal peritoneal dialysis matches 24-hour CAPD and surpasses 8-hour nightly intermittent peritoneal dialysis clearances (abstract). *Perit Dial Bull* 7(suppl 2):S79, 1987.
1158a. Twardowski ZJ et al: Daily clearances with continuous ambulatory and nightly peritoneal dialysis. *Trans Am Soc Artif Intern Organs* 32:575, 1986.
1158b. Twardowski ZJ et al: Osmotic agents and ultrafiltration in peritoneal dialysis. *Nephron* 42:93, 1986.
1159. Twardowski ZJ et al: Polymers as osmotic agents in peritoneal dialysis. *Perit Dial Bull* 4(suppl 3):S125, 1984.
1160. Twardowski ZJ et al: Polyanions and glucose as osmotic agents in simulated peritoneal dialysis. *Artif Organs* 7:420, 1983.
1161. Tyler HR: Neurologic disorders in renal failure. *Am J Med* 44:734, 1968.
1162. Tzamaloukas AH: Characterization of the state of body fluids in anuric hyperglycemic humans. *Miner Electrolyte Metab* 13:126, 1987.
1163. Tzamaloukas AH: Contraction alkalosis during treatment of hyperglycemia in CAPD patients. *Perit Dial Bull* 3:196, 1983.
1164. Tzamaloukas AH: Hyperglycemia in advanced renal failure: Sodium and water metabolism. *Nephron* 31:40, 1982.
1165. Tzamaloukas AH, Kapsner CO: Diagnosis and management of hypertonicity in peritoneal dialysis. *Perit Dial Bull* 8:235, 1988.
1166. Tzamaloukas AH et al: Acid-base disorders in hyperglycemia of insulin-dependent diabetic patients on chronic dialysis. *J Diabet Complications* 2:75, 1988.
1167. Tzamaloukas AH et al: Management of diabetics on chronic ambulatory peritoneal dialysis with subcutaneous insulin, in *Advances in Chronic Ambulatory Peritoneal Dialysis, 1988*. Proceedings of the Eighth Annual CAPD Conference. Toronto, University of Toronto Press, 1988, p 126.
1168. Tzamaloukas AH, Avasthi PS: Temporal profile of serum potassium concentration in nondiabetic and diabetic outpatients on chronic dialysis. *Am J Nephrol* 7:101, 1987.
1169. Tzamaloukas AH, Avasthi PS: Effect of hyperglycemia on serum sodium concentration in outpatients on chronic dialysis. *Am J Kidney Dis* 7:477, 1986.
1170. Uldall PR et al: A double-blind controlled trial of acetate versus bicarbonate dialysate. *Proc Clin Dial Transplant Forum* 10:220, 1980.
1171. US Renal Data System: *USRDS 1990 Annual Data Report*. Bethesda, Md, National Institutes of Health, National Institute of Diabetes and Digestive and Kidney Diseases, August 1990.
1172. Vaamonde CA et al: Complication of acute peritoneal dialysis. *J Chron Dis* 28:637, 1975.
1173. Van Bronswijk H et al: Cytotoxic effects of commercial continuous ambulatory peritoneal dialysis (CAPD) fluids and of bacterial exoproducts on human mesothelial cells in vitro. *Perit Dial Int* 9:197, 1989.
1174. Van Geelen JA et al: Influence of erythropoietin treatment on urea kinetic parameters in hemodialysis patients. *Clin Nephrol* 35:165, 1991.
1175. Van Geelen JA et al: Bicarbonate versus acetate hemodialysis in ventilated patients. *Clin Nephrol* 28:130, 1987.
1176. Van Stone JC: Oral base replacement in patients on hemodialysis. *Ann Intern Med* 101:199, 1984.
1177. Van Stone JC et al: The effect of dialysate sodium concentration on body fluid compartment volume, plasma renin activity, and plasma aldosterone concentration in chronic hemodialysis patients. *Am J Kidney Dis* 2:58, 1982.
1178. Van Stone JC et al: The effect of dialysate sodium concentration on body fluid distribution during hemodialysis. *Trans Am Soc Artif Intern Organs* 26:383, 1980.
1179. Van Stone JC, Cook J: The effect of bicarbonate dialysate in stable chronic hemodialysis patients. *Dial Transplant* 8:703, 1979.
1180. Van Stone JC, Cook J: The effect of replacing acetate with bicarbonate in the dialysate of stable chronic hemodialysis patients. *Proc Clin Dial Transplant Forum* 9:103, 1978.
1181. Van Wyck DB: Impact of erythropoietin on the dialysis prescription. *Am J Kidney Dis* 18(suppl 1):71, 1991.
1182. Vandepitte K et al: Continuous ambulatory peritoneal dialysis (CAPD) in a patient with glucose-6-phosphatase deficiency. *Perit Dial Int* 9:111, 1989.
1183. Vas SI et al: Natural defense mechanisms of the peritoneum: The effect of peritoneal fluid on polymorphonuclear cells, in Atkins RC et al (eds): *Peritoneal Dialysis*. Edinburgh, Churchill Livingstone, 1981.
1184. Vaughan ED et al: Hemodialysis-resistant hypertension: Control with an orally active inhibitor of angiotensin-converting enzyme. *J Clin Endocrinol Metab* 48:869, 1979.
1185. Vaziri ND: Dialysis induced hypoxemia. *Int J Artif Organs* 5:8, 1982.
1186. Vaziri ND et al: Bicarbonate-buffered peritoneal dialysis: An effective adjunct in the treatment of lactic acidosis. *Am J Med* 67:392, 1979.
1187. Veech RL: The untoward effects of the anions of dialysis fluids. *Kidney Int* 34:587, 1988.
1188. Veech RL et al: Cerebral dysfunction and respiratory alkalosis during peritoneal dialysis with D-lactate-containing dialysis fluids (letter to editor). *Am J Med* 82:572, 1987.
1189. Velez RL et al: Acetate and bicarbonate hemodialysis in patients with and without autonomic dysfunction. *Kidney Int* 26:59, 1984.
1190. Velez RL et al: Acetate and bicarbonate hemodialysis in

patients with and without autonomic dysfunction. *Kidney Int* 26:59, 1984.
1191. Verresen L et al: Angiotensin-converting-enzyme inhibitors and anaphylactoid reactions to high-flux membrane dialysis. *Lancet* 336:1360, 1990.
1192. Vertes V et al: Hypertension in end-stage renal disease. *N Engl J Med* 280:978, 1969.
1193. Vidt DG: Editorial note: Recommendation of choice of peritoneal dialysis solution. *Ann Intern Med* 78:144, 1973.
1194. Vilbar RM et al: Treatment of metabolic alkalosis with peritoneal dialysis in a pateint with renal failure. *Artif Organs* 2:421, 1978.
1195. Vinay P et al: Acetate metabolism and bicarbonate generation during hemodialysis: 10 years of observation. *Kidney Int* 31:1194, 1987.
1196. Vinay P et al: Acetate metabolism during hemodialysis: Metabolic considerations. *Am J Nephrol* 7:337, 1987.
1197. Vincent JL et al: Acetate-induced myocardial depression during hemodialysis for acute renal failure. *Kidney Int* 22:653, 1982.
1198. Vincenti F et al: The role of hypertension in hemodialysis-associated atherosclerosis. *Am J Med* 68:363, 1980.
1199. Vlchek DL: Staying tuned in to the high-tech world: 3. Water-treatment update. *Dial Transplant* 19:119, 1990.
1200. Voerman HJ et al: Continuous arterial-venous hemodiafiltration in critically ill patients. *Crit Care Med* 18:911, 1990.
1201. Von Albertini B: Effect of hematocrit on solute removal during hemodialysis (abstract). *Trans Am Soc Artif Intern Organs* 17:62, 1988.
1202. Von Albertini B et al: High-flux hemodiafiltration: Under six hours/week treatment. *Trans Am Soc Artif Intern Organs* 30:377, 1984.
1203. Von Albertini B et al: Changes in P_{CO_2} during and after hemodialysis. *Proc Clin Dial Transplant Forum* 6:199, 1976.
1204. Von Brecht JH: Liquid bicarbonate dialysate: Interdialytic and storage characteristics. *Dial Transplant* 14:75, 1985.
1205. Von Brecht JH et al: Regional anticoagulation: Hemodialysis with hypertonic trisodium citrate. *Am J Kidney Dis* 8:196, 1986.
1206. Von Herrath D et al: Calcium-ketolavin, a new, very effective aluminum-free intestinal phosphate binder. *Kidney Int* 35:388, 1989.
1207. Vreman HJ et al: Acetate metabolism and acid-base homeostasis during hemodialysis: Influence of dialyzer efficiency and rate of acetate metabolism. *Kidney Int* 18(suppl 10):S62, 1980.
1208. Wade OL et al: The effect of exercise on the splanchnic blood flow and splanchnic blood volume in normal man. *Clin Sci* 15:457, 1956.
1209. Wagner L et al: Side effects in bicarbonate dialysis due to low dialysate pH. *Proc Eur Dial Transplant Assoc* 19:346, 1982.
1210. Wakim KG: The pathophysiology of the dialysis disequilibrium syndrome. *Mayo Clin Proc* 44:406, 1969.
1211. Wakim KG: Predominance of hyponatremia over hypoosmolality in simulation of the dialysis equilibrium syndrome. *Mayo Clin Proc* 44:433, 1969.
1212. Walker GS, Davison AM: Prediction of postdialysis hypophosphatemia. *Br Med J* 2:1060, 1977.
1213. Walker JF et al: A sheep model to examine the cardiopulmonary manifestations of blood-dialyzer interactions. *Am Soc Artif Intern Organs J* 6:123, 1983.
1214. Wallia R et al: Serum electrolyte patterns in end-stage renal disease. *Am J Kidney Dis* 8:98, 1986.
1215. Wang YM et al: Nutritional significance of fructose and sugar alcohols. *Annu Rev Nutr* 1:437, 1981.
1216. Ward RA: Acid-base homeostasis in dialysis patients, in Nissenson AR et al (eds): *Clinical Dialysis*, 2d ed. Norwalk, Ct, Appleton & Lange, 1990, p 330.
1217. Ward RA et al: Hemodialysate composition and intradialytic metabolic, acid-base, and potassium changes. *Kidney Int* 32:129, 1987.
1218. Ward RA et al: Effects of long-term bicarbonate hemodialysis (BHD) on acid-base balance status. *Trans Am Soc Artif Intern Organs* 28:295, 1982.
1219. Ward RA, Wathen RL: Utilization of bicarbonate for base repletion in hemodialysis. *Artif Organs* 6:396, 1982.
1220. Warnock DG: Uremic acidosis. *Kidney Int* 34:278, 1988.
1221. Warren DJ, Ferris TF: Renin secretion in renal hypertension. *Lancet* 1:159, 1970.
1222. Wathen RL et al: The metabolic effects of hemodialysis with and without glucose in the dialysate. *Am J Clin Nutr* 31:1870, 1978.
1223. Weber H et al: Chronic hemodialysis: High-risk patients for arrhythmias? *Nephron* 37;180, 1984.
1224. Webster JD et al: Acute nickel intoxication by dialysis. *Ann Intern Med* 9:631, 1980.
1225. Wegner G: Chirurgishe Bemerkungen uber die Peritinealhohle, mit besonderer Berucksichtigung der Ovariotomie. *Arch F Chir* 20:51, 1877.
1226. Wehle B et al: The influence of dialysate composition on cardiovascular function in isovolaemic haemodialysis. *Proc Eur Dial Transplant Assoc* 18:153, 1981.
1227. Wehle B et al: Hemodynamic changes during sequential ultrafiltration and dialysis. *Kidney Int* 15:411, 1979.
1228. Wehle B et al: The influence of dialysis fluid composition on the blood pressure response during dialysis. *Clin Nephrol* 10:62, 1978.
1229. Weidmann P et al: Hypertension in terminal renal failure. *Kidney Int* 9:294, 1976.
1230. Weidmann P, Maxwell MH: The renin-angiotensin aldosterone system in terminal renal failure. *Kidney Int* 8:S219, 1975.
1231. Weidmann P et al: Blood pressure effects of acute hypercalcemia: Studies in patients with chronic renal failure. *Ann Intern Med* 76:741, 1972.
1232. Weidemann P et al: Plasma renin activity and blood pressure in terminal renal failure. *N Engl J Med* 285:757, 1971.
1233. Weisinger JR et al: Insulin binding and glycolytic activity in erythrocytes from dialyzed and underdialyzed uremia patients. *Nephron* 48:190, 1988.
1234. Weller JM et al: Changes in acid-base balance of uremic patients during hemodialysis. *J Clin Invest* 32:729, 1953.
1235. Werb R et al: Intraperitoneal insulin in diabetics on continuous ambulatory peritoneal dialysis. *Perit Dial Bull* 7:S83, 1987.

1236. Whalen JE et al: Elevated serum alkaline phosphatase in patients receiving sorbent cartridge hemodialysis. *Am Soc Artif Intern Organs J* 4:9, 1981.
1237. Whalen J et al: Inadequate removal of methanol and formate using sorbent-based regenerated hemodialysis system. *Clin Nephrol* 11:318, 1979.
1238. Whang R: Hyperglycemic nonketotic coma induced by peritoneal dialysis. *Lancet* 87:453, 1967.
1239. Whele B et al: Carotid baroreflexes during hemodialysis. *Clin Nephrol* 19:236, 1983.
1240. White MG, Kurtzman NA: Hypoglycemia in diabetes with renal insufficiency. *JAMA* 215:117, 1971.
1241. Wiberg JJ et al: Effect of phosphate or magnesium cathartics on serum calcium: Observations in normocalcemic patients. *Arch Intern Med* 138:1114, 1978.
1242. Wideroe TE et al: Plasma concentrations and transperitoneal transport of native insulin and C-peptide in patients on chronic ambulatory peritoneal dialysis. *Kidney Int* 25:82, 1984.
1243. Wideroe TE et al: Glucose, insulin, and C-peptide kinetics during chronic ambulatory peritoneal dialysis. *Proc Eur Dial Transplant Assoc* 20:195, 1983.
1244. Wideroe TE et al: Intraperitoneal (^{125}I)-insulin absorption during intermittent and continuous peritoneal dialysis. *Kidney Int* 23:22, 1983.
1245. Widmer B et al: Serum electrolyte and acid-base composition: The influence of graded degrees of chronic renal failure. *Arch Intern Med* 139:1099, 1979.
1246. Wiegrand CF et al: Severe hypokalemia induced by hemodialysis. *Arch Intern Med* 141:167, 1981.
1247. Wilkinson R et al: Cramps, thirst, and hypertension in hemodialysis patients: The influence of dialysate sodium concentration. *Clin Nephrol* 7:101, 1977.
1248. Willerson JT, Smith TW: Massive digoxin ingestion: Clinical experience and principles of management. *Clin Med* 81:29, 1981.
1249. Williams AJ et al: Continuous ambulatory peritoneal dialysis and haemodialysis in the elderly. *Q J Med* 74:215, 1990.
1250. Williams AJ et al: Effect of dialysate buffer on potassium removal during hemodialysis. *Proc Eur Dial Transplant Assoc Eur Renal Assoc* 21:209, 1984.
1251. Williams PF et al: Amino acid absorbtion following intraperitoneal administration in CAPD patients. *Perit Dial Bull* 2:124, 1982.
1252. Wing AJ et al: Dialysis regeneration, in Drukker W et al (eds): *Replacement of Renal Function by Dialysis*, 2d ed. Boston, Martinus Nijhoff, 1983, p 206.
1253. Wing AJ: Optimum calcium concentration of dialysis fluid for maintenance hemodialysis. *Br Med J* 4:145, 1968.
1254. Wingert KJ, Weiner MW: Acetate transfer across membranes of artificial kidneys in vitro. *Kidney Int* 15:593, 1979.
1255. Wizemann V et al: Dialysis induced cardiac arrhythmias: Fact or fiction? *Nephron* 39:356, 1985.
1256. Wolf AV et al: Artificial kidney function: Kinetics of hemodialysis. *J Clin Invest* 30:1062, 1951.
1257. Wolff J et al: Effects of acetate and bicarbonate dialysis on cardiac performance, transmural myocardial perfusion, and acid-base balance. *Int J Artif Organs* 9:105, 1986.
1258. Wu G: Cardiovascular deaths among CAPD patients. *Perit Dial Bull* 3:S23, 1983.
1259. Wu G: Osmotic agents for peritoneal dialysis solutions. *Perit Dial Bull* 2:151, 1982.
1260. Yamakawa M et al: Serum levels of acetate and TCA cycle intermediates during hemodialysis in relation to symptoms: Comparative study between hemodialysis with acetate dialysis versus bicarbonate dialysis. *Nephron* 32:155, 1982.
1261. Yamamoto T et al: The interrelationship of dialysate, glucose and lactate in continuous ambulatory peritoneal dialysis. *Trans Am Soc Artif Intern Organs* 31:595, 1985.
1262. Yamamoto T et al: The effect of sodium acetate: Comparison of red-cell 2,3-diphosphoglycerate (2,3-DPG) between acetate and bicarbonate dialysis. *Trans Am Soc Artif Intern Organs* 28:291, 1982.
1263. Yang W et al: Beta-adrenergic mediated extrarenal potassium disposal in patients with end-stage renal disease: Effect of propanolol. *Miner Electrolyte Metab* 12:186, 1986.
1264. Yatuc W et al: Substitution of sorbitol for dextrose in peritoneal irrigation fluid: A preliminary report. *Trans Am Soc Artif Intern Organs* 13:168, 1967.
1265. Yatzidis H: A new stable bicarbonate dialysis solution for peritoneal dialysis: Preliminary report. *Perit Dial Int* 11:224, 1991.
1266. Yawata Y et al: Abnormal red cell metabolism causing hemolysis in uremia: A defect potentiated by tap water hemodialysis. *Ann Intern Med* 79:362, 1973.
1267. Yombissi J et al: Blood pressures in CAPD: Relationship to sodium status renin and aldosterone compared to hemodialysis, in Maher JF, Winchester JF (eds): *Frontiers in Peritoneal Dialysis*. New York, Field Rich and Associates, 1986, p 40.
1268. Yorgin PD: Continuous venovenous hemofiltration. *Pediatr Nephrol* 4:640, 1990.
1269. Young GA et al: The use of amino acid-based CAPD over 12 weeks. *Nephrol Dial Transplant* 4:185, 1989.
1270. Young GA et al: A longitudinal study of the effect of amino acid based CAPD fluid on amino acid retention and protein losses. *Nephrol Dial Transplant* 4:900, 1989.
1271. Young MA et al: Antihypertensive drug requirements in continuous ambulatory peritoneal dialysis. *Perit Dial Bull* 4:85, 1984.
1272. Yu AW et al: Peritoneal dialysis using bicarbonate-containing solution sterilized by ultrafiltration. *Int J Artif Organs* 14:463, 1991.
1273. Zabetakis PM et al: Increased levels of plasma renin, aldosterone, catecholamines and vasopressin in continuous ambulatory peritoneal dialysis (CAPD) patients. *Clin Nephrol* 28:147, 1987.
1274. Zaoui P et al: Hemodialysis with cuprophane membrane modulates interleukin-2 receptor expression. *Kidney Int* 39:1020, 1991.
1275. Zarate A et al: Propranolol-associated hypoglycemia in patients on maintenance hemodialysis. *Int J Artif Organs* 4:130, 1981.
1276. Zawada ET Jr et al: Serum calcium in blood pressure regulation during hemodialysis. *Arch Intern Med* 141:657, 1981.

1277. Zehnder C et al: Human recombinant erythropoietin in anemic patients on maintenance hemodialysis: Secondary effects of the increase in haemoglobin. *Nephrol Dial Transplant* 3:657, 1988.
1278. Ziegler MG et al: Norepinephrine clearance, chromografin A, and dopamine beta-hydroxylase in renal failure. *Kidney Int* 37:1357, 1990.
1279. Zoccali C et al: Postprandial alterations in arterial pressure control during hemodialysis in uremic patients. *Clin Nephrol* 31:323, 1989.
1280. Zoccali C et al: Parasympathetic function in hemodialysis patients. *Nephron* 44:351, 1986.
1281. Zucchelli P: Hemodialysis-induced symptomatic hypotension: A review of pathophysiological mechanisms. *Int J Artif Organs* 10:139, 1987.
1282. Zucchelli P et al: Acetate-free biofiltration: Hemodiafiltration with base-free dialysate. *Blood Purif* 8:14, 1990.
1283. Zucchelli P, Santoro A: Inorganic phosphate removal during different dialytic procedures. *Int J Artif Organs* 10:173, 1987.
1284. Zucchelli P et al: Dysfunction of the autonomic nervous system in patients with end-stage renal failure. *Contrib Nephrol* 45:69, 1985.
1285. Zucchelli P et al: Renal osteodystrophy in CAPD patients. *Miner Electrolyte Metab* 10:326, 1984.

CHAPTER • 41

Renal osteodystrophy

Francisco Llach • Jack W. Coburn

INTRODUCTION

The relationship between renal disease, skeletal abnormalities, and parathyroid hyperplasia has been known for many years.[10,183,415] The studies of Stanbury and Lumb and of Dent and coworkers opened extensive investigation into the basic processes leading to abnormalities of divalent ion metabolism, parathyroid structure and function, vitamin D metabolism, and bone in patients with renal insufficiency.[533]

The lives of patients with end-stage renal failure are now prolonged by better conservative therapy, maintenance dialysis, and successful renal transplantation; consequently, the morbidity due to disordered divalent ion metabolism, soft tissue calcification, and osseous pathology is clinically significant. The clinical features of renal osteodystrophy are well defined, and rational approaches to the prevention and treatment of renal osteodystrophy have been developed. The term *renal osteodystrophy* is used here to include various skeletal diseases reported in patients with renal failure—specifically, retardation of growth, osteomalacia, osteitis fibrosa, adynamic or aplastic bone disease, osteosclerosis, and osteoporosis.

PATHOGENESIS

Many data have accumulated to further our knowledge of the mechanisms underlying altered divalent ion metabolism in renal insufficiency.[114,145,232,290,301,310,314] Nonetheless, there is uncertainty about the initial steps in the pathogenesis of secondary hyperparathyroidism and altered metabolism of vitamin D and the degree of interaction between various pathogenic factors. The processes that cause secondary hyperparathyroidism probably become operative in the early stages of renal insufficiency and continue throughout the life of the patient. Maintenance dialysis leads to improvement of some of the clinical and biochemical manifestations of uremia; however, various pathogenic factors that can aggravate the skeletal disease may persist, and new problems, such as aluminum accumulation, may arise.

Supported in part by a merit-review grant from the Research Funds from the Veterans Administration.

SECONDARY HYPERPARATHYROIDISM

Parathyroid hyperplasia and high circulating levels of parathyroid hormone (PTH) are among the most consistent abnormalities of divalent ion metabolism present in patients with renal function that is only slightly decreased, as shown in Fig. 41-1.[27]

The main factor increasing PTH secretion and causing hyperplasia of the parathyroid glands in uremic patients has been thought to be low levels of ionized calcium. Studies in patients with early renal insufficiency have failed to show a decrease in the total serum calcium level.[318] Nevertheless, when oral physiologic doses of calcitriol are given to the patients, a significant increase in serum calcium is observed.[571] However, it is likely that factors other than hypocalcemia may also be at work. This is suggested by the observation of Lopez and coworkers that secondary hyperparathyroidism can develop in dogs with 70 percent reduction of glomerular filtration rate (GFR) without a decreased, or even with an increased, serum ionized calcium concentration.[322] Kaplan and coworkers also demonstrated increases in serum ionized calcium levels in uremic dogs as compared with control dogs.[270] Factors that can lead to actual hypocalcemia in renal failure include (1) phosphate retention, with increased serum phosphorus concentration and a reciprocal decrease in serum calcium concentration; (2) altered vitamin D metabolism, with intestinal malabsorption of calcium; (3) decreased calcemic response to PTH; (4) altered degradation of PTH; and (5) altered feedback relationship between serum calcium and secretion of PTH

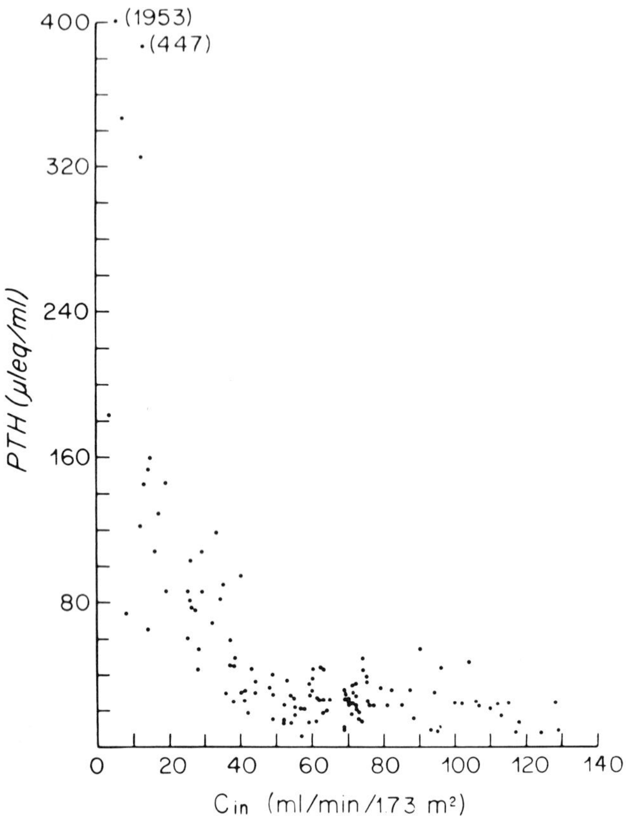

FIGURE 41-1 • Relationship between renal clearance of insulin and serum level of parathyroid hormone in patients with varying levels of renal function. Immunoassay of PTH used antiserum that recognizes entire (84-residue) PTH peptide and its carboxy-terminal fragments. (From Arnaud CD: *Kidney Int* 4:89, 1973. Used by permission.)

("set point" for calcium), which may be related, in part, to abnormal vitamin D metabolism. These factors may be interrelated, but it is likely that one factor may exert a more prominent role than the others at certain stages of renal insufficiency.

Phosphate retention

The role of phosphate retention as a major factor in the pathogenesis of secondary hyperparathyroidism has been emphasized by Slatopolsky and colleagues.[516,517] As the phosphate retention theory was initially proposed, a transient and possibly undetectable increase in serum phosphorus concentration was believed to occur in early renal failure as a result of a small decrement in renal function.[517] The transient hyperphosphatemia was believed to temporarily reduce the concentration of blood ionized calcium, which in turn stimulated PTH secretion. The higher levels of PTH would reduce tubular reabsorption of phosphorus, cause phosphaturia, and return both serum phosphorus and calcium concentrations toward normal, but at the expense of a higher level of circulating PTH.

Considerable evidence supports an important role of phosphate retention in producing secondary hyperparathyroidism. Reiss and coworkers demonstrated that a large oral phosphorus load led to an increase in serum phosphorus concentration, a fall in blood ionized calcium concentration, and an increase in serum PTH level in normal human beings.[454] Others have shown that the long-term feeding of a high-phosphate diet to animals caused parathyroid hyperplasia, high levels of PTH, and mild hypocalcemia.[259,292] Studies with experimentally induced renal failure have shown that reducing the dietary phosphate intake in proportion to the decrease in GFR could largely prevent the development of secondary hyperparathyroidism in dogs with uremia of both 2 months'[516] and 2 years' duration[476] (Fig. 41-2). When dietary phosphate intake was reduced and aluminum hydroxide gel was given to patients with more advanced renal insufficiency (creatinine clearance rate 22 to 63 ml/min), serum PTH concentration fell substantially but the values remained greater than normal.[485] Studies have shown that serum PTH levels correlate positively with the degree of hyperphosphatemia in patients undergoing dialysis, providing support for a role of marked hyperphosphatemia in causing PTH hypersecretion, particularly in patients with advanced uremia.[187,188]

However, recent data suggest that hyperphosphatemia may not play a role in the early stages of renal insufficiency. Low serum phosphorus levels have been reported in patients with early to moderate renal failure.[111,318,319] These observations indicate that a slight decrease in serum calcium levels, which sometimes occurs in such patients, cannot arise as a direct conse-

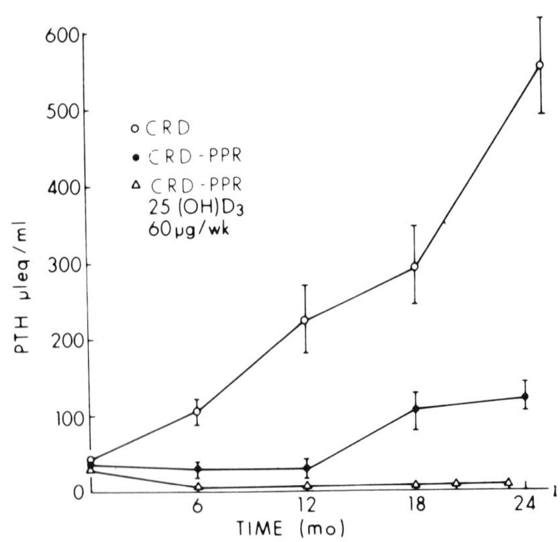

FIGURE 41-2 • Serial values of PTH concentration in dogs with chronic renal insufficiency (mean ± s.e.). Dogs received either a normal, constant-phosphate diet (○), diet with phosphate content reduced in proportion to the decrease in GFR (●), or diet with a proportional reduction in phosphate content plus 60 μg/week 25-hydroxyvitamin D_3 (25-OH-D_3) (Δ). (Reprinted, by permission, from Rutherford WE et al: *J Clin Invest* 60:332, 1977.)

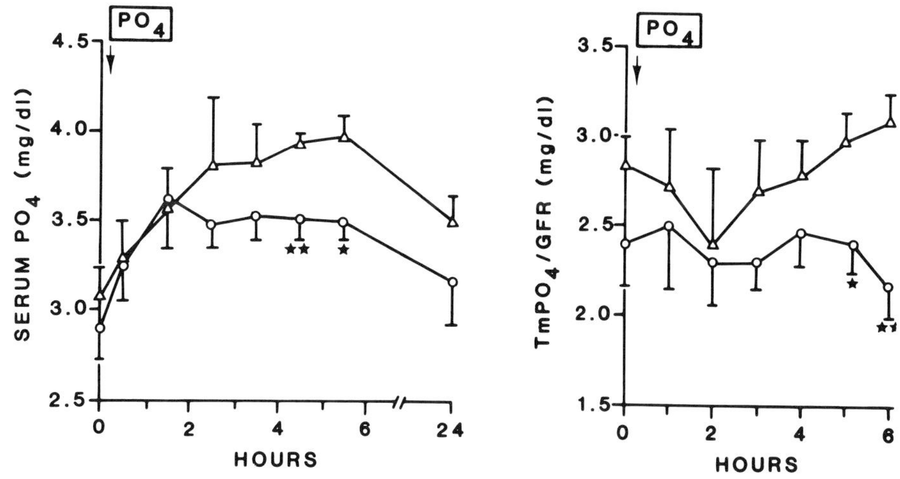

FIGURE 41-3 • Mean values (± s.e.) of serum phosphorus concentration and Tm_{PO_4}/GFR in patients with early renal failure (open circles) and normal subjects (open triangles) during phosphate load test prior to 1α,25-$(OH)_2D_3$ therapy.*, $p < 0.05$;**, $p < 0.01$. (From Wilson L et al: *Kidney Int* 21:65, 1982. Used by permission.)

quence of hyperphosphatemia.[111] To explain the pathogenesis of this hypophosphatemia, Slatopolsky and coworkers have suggested that postprandial hyperphosphatemia may occur and then stimulate PTH secretion, leading to low fasting serum phosphorus levels.[521] Thus, serum phosphorus concentration should be higher in azotemic patients than in normal subjects after a phosphate-containing meal; recent data do not support this. Portale and coworkers measured serum phosphorus and PTH concentrations after hourly meals in children with early renal insufficiency; they were unable to detect any changes in serum phosphorus concentration in the postprandial period.[438] Furthermore, recent studies in patients with early renal failure (GFR 40 to 80 ml/min) who received an oral phosphate load have shown that, rather than hyperphosphatemia and evidence of renal phosphate retention, more rapid excretion of the phosphate load, as compared with control subjects, was exhibited[571] (Fig. 41-3). These patients, interestingly, excreted a phosphate load in a manner similar to patients with primary hyperparathyroidism.[311] Maschio and coworkers demonstrated an impairment in phosphorus excretion following an oral phosphate load in patients with more advanced renal insufficiency; moreover, hyperphosphatemia was found to develop, usually, as renal disease advanced and the GFR fell below 25 ml/min.[207] Thus, in advanced renal failure and during dialysis, hypocalcemia can be shown to be directly related to the marked elevation of serum phosphorus concentration.[344] Recently, we have observed worsening of hyperparathyroidism in patients receiving intravenous calcitriol. This was most likely a consequence of significant hyperphosphatemia due to poor dietary compliance. Some of the factors that aggravate the degree of hyperphosphatemia in advanced renal failure and in patients treated with hemodialysis are noted in Table 41-1.

TABLE 41-1 • Factors influencing serum phosphorus levels in patients with renal failure

Dietary phosphorus intake
Residual renal function
Ingestion of phosphate-binding compounds
Secretion of PTH; responsiveness of the skeleton to PTH
Balance between degradation and synthesis of protoplasm
Extent of vitamin D deficiency and treatment with active vitamin D compounds
Rate of skeletal accretion (i.e., healing of osteomalacia or osteitis fibrosa)
Hypomagnesemia
Parenteral alimentation
Intake of large amounts of supplemental calcium
Phosphate-containing enemas
Frequency, duration, and efficiency of dialysis

SOURCE: Modified from Coburn JW, Llach F, in Drukker W et al (eds): *Renal Osteodystrophy and Maintenance Dialysis*, The Hague, Nijhoff, 1983, p 679. (Used by permission.)

Impaired calcemic response to PTH

A decreased response to the calcemic action of PTH is another cause of hypocalcemia in patients with renal insufficiency. Evanson noted that the calcemic response to an infusion of parathyroid extract (PTE) was significantly lower in hypocalcemic patients with renal failure than in normal subjects or in patients with hypoparathyroidism.[171] Subsequently, Massry and coworkers found that the calcemic response to a standardized infusion of PTE in patients with early renal failure (creatinine clearance of 27 to 87 ml/min) was significantly lower than in normal individuals.[349] This reduced calcemic response was unrelated to the initial levels of serum calcium, phosphorus, or PTH. Llach and coworkers found a delayed recovery from induced hypocalcemia in patients with early renal insufficiency and creatinine clearances of 34 to 93 ml/min compared to normal subjects, despite a greater augmentation in serum PTH levels in the former.[319] A later study confirmed these data.[571] Such observations indicate that the impaired calcemic response to PTH appears early in the course of renal insufficiency. Thus, a greater concentration of circulating PTH may be required to maintain a normal serum calcium level in patients with renal failure. Data from studies of dogs with short-term renal failure indicate that restricting dietary phosphorus intake in proportion to the fall in GFR prevented a rise in serum PTH, while the skeletal resistance to the calcemic action of PTH persisted.[270] It was concluded that the blunted calcemic response to PTH could not be the factor primarily responsible for the secondary hyperparathyroidism of uremia. In contrast to these data, Llach and Massry observed that dietary phosphate restriction in patients with mild renal insufficiency improved the calcemic response to a standardized infusion of PTH.[318]

The factors responsible for skeletal resistance to the calcemic action of PTH are, at present, undefined. Rats with chronic renal failure exhibit a blunted calcemic response to PTE; the administration of 1α,25-dihydroxyvitamin D_3 [1α,25-$(OH)_2D_3$] partly corrects this impaired calcemic response.[527] Administration of 0.5 μg per day of 1α,25-$(OH)_2D_3$ for six weeks similarly improved the calcemic response to PTH in human beings with early renal failure (Fig. 41-4).[510] Such data support the possibility that altered vitamin D metabolism plays a role in the impaired calcemic response to PTH. In dogs with acute renal failure[527] and rats with chronic renal failure, treatment with calcitriol resulted in a partial improvement in the calcemic response to PTH.

Hyperphosphatemia may also be responsible for the impaired calcemic response.[526] Sommerville and Kaye, in an experimental rat model of renal failure, demonstrated that the correction of hyperphosphatemia significantly improved the calcemic response. Recent studies have shown, in dogs with advanced renal failure, that parathyroidectomy restored the calcemic response to normal.[527] The authors suggested that the presence of high PTH levels in the uremic animal desensitizes the skeleton to the action of PTH ("down regulation" of bone receptors).

We have recently evaluated the role of endogenous calcitonin production in the calcemic response to PTH in the rat with chronic renal failure.[466] We observed that in the absence of calcitonin these rats had a significant improvement in the calcemic response to PTH.

Alterations in vitamin D metabolism

Abnormal conversion of vitamin D_3 to its active form probably plays a fundamental role in the development of secondary hyperparathyroidism in early renal failure. The evidence that vitamin D metabolism is altered in advanced renal failure is most convincing. Intestinal absorption of calcium is diminished and poorly responsive to

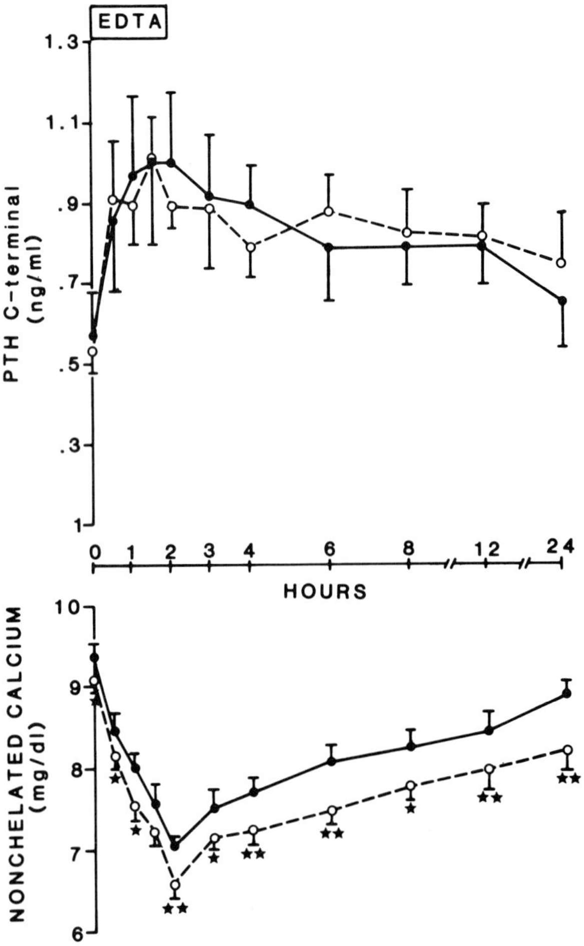

FIGURE 41-4 • Mean values (± s.e.) of serum PTH and nonchelated calcium concentrations during EDTA-induced recovery from hypocalcemia (open circles) and after 1α,25-$(OH)_2D_3$ therapy (closed circles).*, $p < 0.05$;, $p < 0.01$. (Reprinted, by permission, from Wilson L et al: *Kidney Int* 21:65, 1982.)**

vitamin D.[307] In patients with advanced renal insufficiency, metabolic balance studies reveal that fecal calcium excretion is equal to, or even greater than, dietary intake of calcium.[149,285,532] Radioisotopic methods indicate that intestinal absorption of calcium is reduced in most patients with advanced uremia.[71,112] Liu and Chu found no improvement of osteomalacia or calcium balance in uremic patients treated with usual oral doses of vitamin D.[307] These workers suggested that uremia impairs the response to vitamin D. It was shown that the intestinal malabsorption of calcium could be overcome by the administration of vitamin D in doses of 100,000 to 300,000 IU/day.[149,532] With such treatment, calcium absorption increased and rickets or osteomalacia healed.

The kidney is the principal or only organ responsible for converting 25-hydroxyvitamin D_3 [25-OH-D_3] to 1α,25-$(OH)_2D_3$.[189] This discovery provided the framework for the hypothesis that vitamin D metabolism is altered in uremia. Anephric rats are unable to produce

1α,25-$(OH)_2D_3$ from its precursor[215]—an observation that led to speculation that impaired renal production of 1α,25-$(OH)_2D_3$ accounts for impaired calcium absorption and osteomalacia in uremia. Several observations support this premise. Mawer and coworkers, and Schaefer and coworkers, gave radioactive vitamin D_3, labeled both with ^3H on C-1 and C-25 and with ^{14}C at the 4 position, to patients with nutritional vitamin D deficiency and normal renal function.[357] They observed considerable displacement or "loss" of tritium compared to ^{14}C. On the other hand, no loss of tritium was observed in anephric or uremic individuals. Such data provided indirect evidence for the failure of uremic patients to hydroxylate 25-$(OH)_2D_3$ at the 1α position and produce 1α,25-$(OH)_2D_3$. With the development of a receptor assay using nuclear chromatin from the intestine, Brumbaugh and coworkers were able to measure plasma levels of 1α,25-$(OH)_2D_3$.[75] The levels of 1α,25-$(OH)_2D_3$ have been uniformly found to be decreased in patients with advanced renal failure.[101,164,232,251,345]

The nature of the response to replacement with various vitamin D metabolites also supports the view that impaired conversion of 25-OH-D_3 to 1α,25-$(OH)_2D_3$ is of importance in renal failure. Thus, 1α,25-$(OH)_2D_3$ in doses of 0.6 to 1.0 μg/day can increase ^{47}Ca absorption to normal in uremic patients,[66,67] while the quantity of 25-OH-D_3 needed to augment calcium absorption in uremia is 100 to 500 μg;[476] the amount of vitamin D_3 needed is even greater.[111] The relative effect of these vitamin D sterols on calcium absorption is shown in Fig. 41-5. Though the levels of 1α,25-$(OH)_2D_3$ have been found to be low in patients with advanced uremia, recent data indicate that abnormalities in its production may occur even in early and moderate renal insufficiency.[571]

The consequences of reduced generation of 1α,25-$(OH)_2D_3$ in early renal insufficiency deserve consideration. The problems that may arise from a deficiency of this active form of vitamin D include decreased intestinal absorption of calcium, reduced calcemic action of PTH on the skeleton, and increased PTH secretion for any given level of serum calcium concentration.

When in the course of progressive renal insufficiency does the abnormality of vitamin D metabolism occur? Slatopolsky and coworkers, in observations of patients with serum creatinine concentrations ranging from 1.5 to 3.5 mg/100 ml, reported normal 1α,25-$(OH)_2D_3$ levels.[519] Detailed observations by Portale and coworkers in children with moderate renal insufficiency (creatinine clearance rate 25 to 50 ml/min per 1.73 m^2 of body surface) have indicated that 1α,25-$(OH)_2D_3$ levels are reduced 40 percent.[439] When analyzed over the range spanning normal to severely impaired renal function, the PTH values in these children correlated inversely with their 1α,25-$(OH)_2D_3$ levels (Fig. 41-6). Chesney and coworkers have also reported finding low levels of 1α,25-$(OH)_2D_3$ in patients with early renal failure whose creatinine clearance rates were greater than 75 to 80 ml/min.[99] In addition, a significant correlation was found between the creatinine clearance rates and the 1α,25-$(OH)_2D_3$ levels. Likewise, Juttman and coworkers have observed subnormal levels of 1α,25-$(OH)_2D_3$ in patients with creatinine clearance rates between 40 and 50 ml/min.[260] Wilson and coworkers have recently reported low levels of 1α,25-$(OH)_2D_3$ in patients with GFRs be-

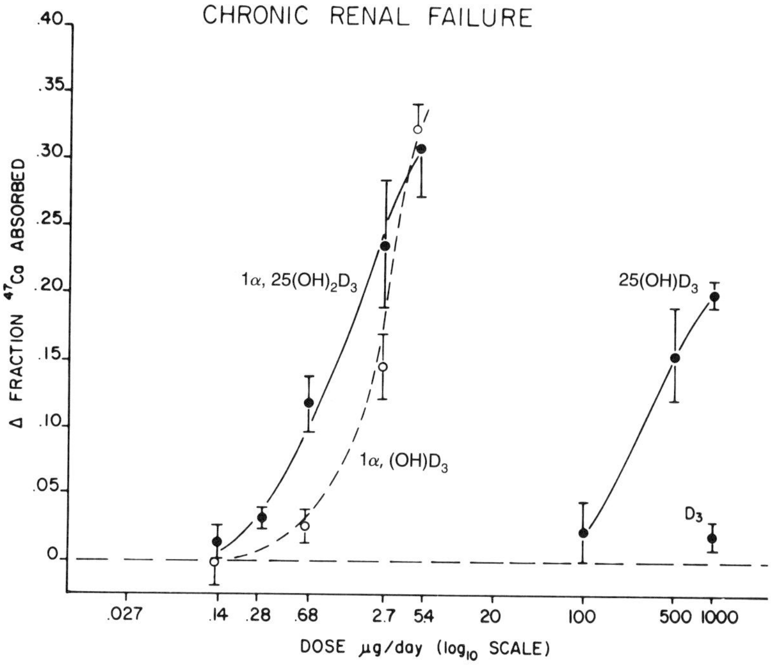

FIGURE 41-5 • Changes (Δ) in the fraction of ^{47}Ca absorbed before, vs. 8 to 10 days after, treatment in patients given different doses of various vitamin D sterols. Values are mean ± s.e. (Data adapted, by permission, from Coburn JW et al: *Kidney Int* 3:264, 1973; Brickman AS et al: *Am J Clin Nutr* 30:1064, 1977; and Colodro IH et al: *Metabolism* 27:745, 1968.)

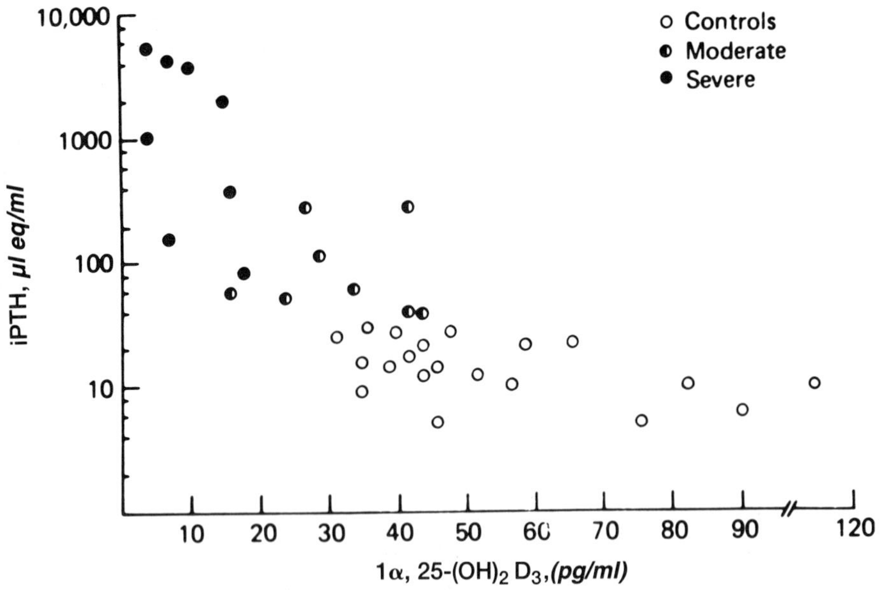

FIGURE 41-6 • Relationship between plasma PTH concentration and 1α,25-$(OH)_2D$ over entire range of renal function, from normal (in controls) to moderate and severe impairment. Correlation is inverse and significant ($r = -0.816$, $p < 0.001$). (From Portale AP et al: *J Clin Invest* 73:1580, 1984. Used by permission.)

tween 50 and 80 ml/min.[571] Thus, the available data suggest that patients with early to moderate renal failure have low levels of 1α,25-$(OH)_2D_3$. Recently, the role of 1α,25-$(OH)_2D_3$ has been evaluated in the pathogenesis of abnormal divalent ion metabolism in patients with early renal failure.[571] The calcemic response to PTH was studied along with the handling of an oral phosphate load both before and after 6 weeks of therapy with 1α,25-$(OH)_2D_3$. Twelve patients with early renal failure and six normal volunteers were studied. As compared with normal subjects, patients with mild renal disease had low serum phosphorus concentrations and low urinary calcium excretion, low serum 1α,25-$(OH)_2D_3$ and high plasma PTH levels, and high levels of urinary cAMP. With EDTA infusion, an impaired calcemic response to PTH was observed in patients with early renal failure but not in normal individuals. These patients demonstrated an increased ability to excrete a phosphate load (Fig. 41-3). After therapy with 1α,25-$(OH)_2D_3$, significant increases in serum phosphorus concentration and urinary calcium excretion and a decrease in level of urinary cAMP were observed in the patients with early renal failure. Furthermore, the impaired calcemic response to PTH improved significantly, the renal handling of phosphate became normal (Fig. 41-7), and the low baseline levels of plasma 1α,25-$(OH)_2D_3$ concentration increased to normal after therapy with 1α,25-$(OH)_2D_3$. In addition, a significant correlation between levels of 1α,25-$(OH)_2D_3$ and creatinine clearances was observed in both patients and normal subjects. These data suggest that a mild deficiency of 1α,25-$(OH)_2D_3$ is present in patients with early renal insufficiency and that the administration of this sterol results in substantial improvement in several biochemical parameters.

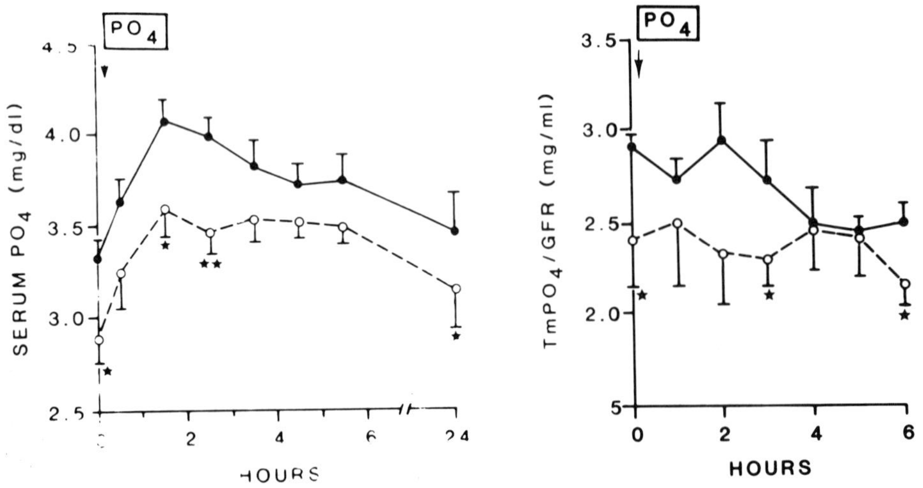

FIGURE 41-7 • Mean values (± s.e.) of serum phosphorus concentration and ratio of phosphate transport rate to GFR (Tm_{PO_4}/GFR) during phosphate load test in patients with early renal failure before (open circles) and after (closed circles) therapy with 1α,25-$(OH)_2D_3$. Differences were significant: *, $p < 0.05$; **, $p < 0.01$. (From Wilson L et al: *Kidney Int* 21:65, 1982. Used by permission.)

The cause of reduced $1\alpha,25\text{-}(OH)_2D_3$ synthesis has not yet been defined. It is possible that $1\alpha,25\text{-}(OH)_2D_3$ systhesis by the kidney is related to the functional state of the proximal renal tubules. Since the GFR reasonably reflects functional renal mass, a decrement in $1\alpha,25\text{-}(OH)_2D_3$ may occur slowly and progressively as glomerular filtration declines in patients with chronic renal insufficiency. In support of this notion are the observations by Kawaguchi and coworkers in the rat: following graded reductions in renal mass, sterol synthesis progressively declined.[272] Portale and coworkers postulated that the intracellular concentration of phosphorus may increase in early renal insufficiency.[438] This, in turn, could reduce the activity of 1α-hydroxylase and decrease the synthesis of $1\alpha,25\text{-}(OH)_2D_3$. Recent observations in four patients with early renal insufficiency who were given phosphate-restricted diets under metabolic conditions bear this out:[318] phosphate excretion decreased, intestinal absorption of phosphate rose, and PTH concentration decreased. Most important, there was a significant increase in the plasma $1\alpha,25\text{-}(OH)_2D_3$ level following phosphate restriction. These events occurred in the absence of significant changes in serum phosphorus concentration and net external balance of phosphorus. Children with moderate renal insufficiency were given a reduced-phosphate diet in recent studies by Portale and coworkers. Plasma levels of $1\alpha,25\text{-}(OH)_2D_3$ again increased, despite a decrease in PTH levels (Fig. 41-8), and a significant decrease in fractional excretion of phosphate occurred.[438] Thus, a disorder of phosphate metabolism within the renal tubular cells may lead to decreased synthesis of $1\alpha,25\text{-}(OH)_2D_3$. Regardless of the cause of decreased secretion of $1\alpha,25\text{-}(OH)_2D_3$, the pathophysiologic consequences of this deficiency may be important. Thus, the low levels of this sterol in early renal insufficiency may impair intestinal absorption of calcium and decrease the calcemic response to PTH, thereby contributing to hypocalcemia.

A final pathophysiologic consequence of a partial deficiency of $1\alpha,25\text{-}(OH)_2D_3$ may be the absence of a modulating inhibitory action of the sterol on PTH secretion, leading to secondary hyperparathyroidism. Recently, Booth and coworkers have provided evidence that parathyroid activity is increased, and stimulation of 1α-hydroxylase activity diminished, in early vitamin D deficiency.[59] Observations of Oldham and coworkers in vitamin D-deficient puppies suggest that the parenteral administration of $1\alpha,25\text{-}(OH)_2D_3$ could enhance the suppression of serum PTH by increasing blood calcium levels.[405] Madsen and coworkers reported that injections of $1\alpha,25\text{-}(OH)_2D_3$ reduce serum PTH levels in patients with acute renal failure independently of a change in serum calcium concentration; PTH secretion may also be modified.[327] Silver and coworkers have shown a significant suppression by $1\alpha,25\text{-}(OH)_2D_3$ of cytoplasmic mRNA coding for pre-proparathyroid hormone in bovine parathyroid cell cultures.[512] Also, Slatopolsky and coworkers have provided evidence for a direct suppressive effect of intravenously administered $1\alpha,25\text{-}(OH)_2D_3$ on PTH secretion in hemodialysis patients.[524] Later, Delmez and coworkers evaluated the inhibitory effect of intravenous calcitriol in dialysis patients with secondary hyperparathyroidism.[144] Serum ionized calcium and PTH (aminoterminal fragment) were determined before and after two weeks of intravenous calcitriol. Despite no significant changes in ionized Ca, PTH levels fell by 22 percent ($p < 0.001$). Recently we have evaluated the direct inhibitory effect of calcitriol on parathyroid function in nine dialysis patients with severe hyperparathyroidism.[155] They received intravenous calcitriol, 2 μg at the end of each dialysis for 10 weeks. In order to avoid hypercalcemia, the dialysate calcium concentration was reduced to 2.5 meq/liter. The basal PTH (intact molecule) fell from 902 ± 126 pg/1 ml to 466 ± 152 pg/ml after 10 weeks of therapy. This occurred in the absence of any

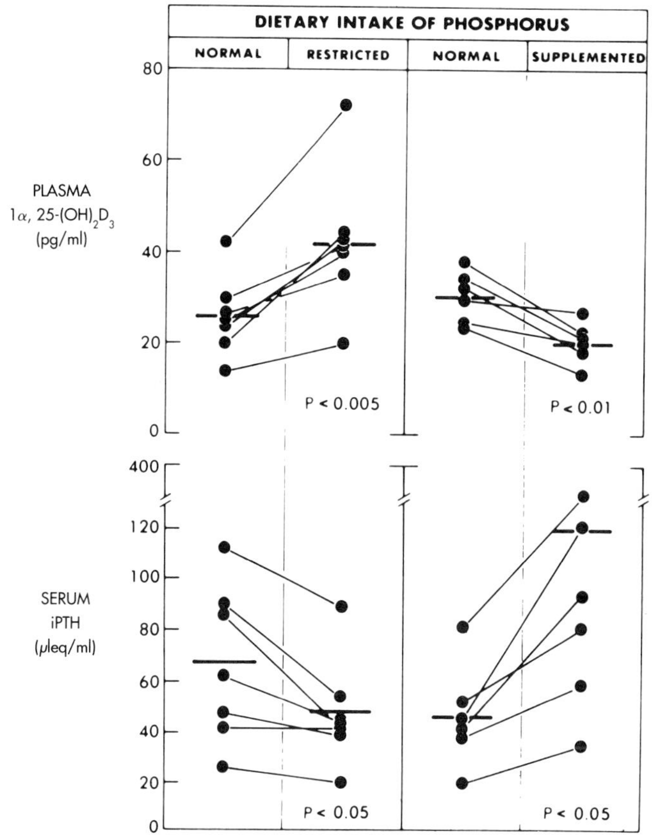

FIGURE 41-8 • Effect of restriction and augmentation of dietary phosphorus intake on plasma levels of $1\alpha,25\text{-}(OH)_2D$ and immunoreactive PTH concentration in children with moderate renal insufficiency (creatinine clearances 25 to 50 ml/min per 1.73 m² of body surface area). With phosphate restriction, plasma $1\alpha,25\text{-}(OH)_2D$ levels rose significantly despite a decrease in serum PTH concentration. Plasma $1\alpha,25\text{-}(OH)_2D$ levels *fell* with phosphate supplementation despite rise in serum PTH concentration. (Reprinted, by permission, from Portale AP et al: *Kidney Int* Z1:627, 1982.)

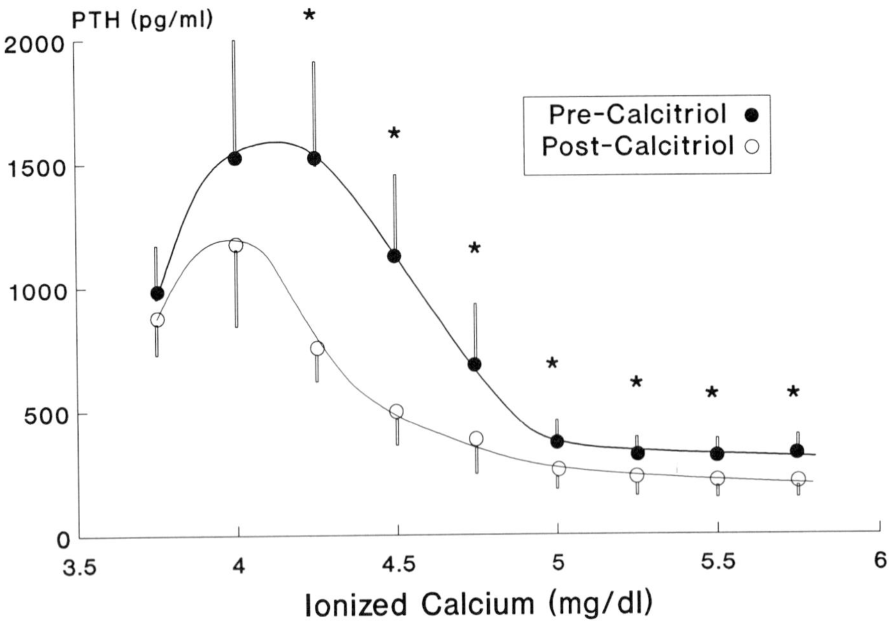

FIGURE 41-9 • The sigmoidal serum ionized calcium-PTH curve before (closed circles) and after (open circles) ten weeks of intravenous calcitriol therapy is shown. The set point is represented by a solid square before, and an open square after, calcitriol. (Reprinted, by permission, from Dunlay R et al: *Kidney Int* 36:1093, 1989.)

significant changes in total serum Ca concentration (Fig. 41-9).

Further study has revealed that the reduction in prepro-PTH mRNA occurs primarily at the transcriptional level.[511] Silver and coworkers have shown that the administration of calcitriol to rats has a profound suppressive effect on in-vivo PTH synthesis. Thus it seems that the major action of calcitriol on PTH secretion may occur as a result of inhibition of the hormone's synthesis. In view of these data, it is possible that an absolute or relative deficiency of $1\alpha,25\text{-}(OH)_2D_3$ may lead to secondary hyperparathyroidism without the involvement of hypocalcemia.

Altered degradation of PTH

It has been generally accepted that an increased rate of secretion of PTH is the major mechanism responsible for high plasma levels of PTH in renal insufficiency. Considerable evidence demonstrates that the kidney plays an important role in the degradation of PTH and that the metabolic clearance of PTH is reduced in renal failure.[512] Reduced renal degradation of PTH may contribute to the hyperparathyroid state in uremia. A brief review of PTH metabolism is in order.

Berson and Yalow reported immunochemical heterogeneity of PTH in the plasma of uremic patients; they suggested that the presence of more than one peptide fragment of PTH and altered metabolism of the hormone could account for the heterogeneity.[47] This initial discovery has been followed by extensive research into the biochemistry and metabolism of PTH.[26,227]

Intact PTH is secreted from the parathyroid gland into the circulation as a 9500-dalton, 84-amino acid peptide chain; its biologic activity resides in the amino-terminal, 1-34 amino acids. The peptide molecule is rapidly degraded, the amino-terminal portion is cleaved, and several inactive fragments from the carboxy-terminal fraction of the peptide appear in the serum. Because of the shorter half-life of both intact PTH and the amino-terminal fragment, the carboxy-terminal fragments become the predominating PTH peptides in the circulation. The intact parent peptide is rapidly degraded in the peripheral tissues, particularly in the kidney and the liver.[87] The liver has a large capacity to degrade the peptide, but it may not play an important role in degradation of either the carboxy- or the amino-terminal fragments.[342] By contrast, the kidney can extract and degrade the intact 84-residue molecule and both the carboxy- and amino- terminal fragments.[249,250,341] In the presence of chronic renal disease, PTH metabolism is altered and degradation of PTH and its fragments is decreased. Such mechanisms may additionally account for the elevated PTH levels seen in patients with renal failure.

There is clear evidence for the role of decreased renal degradation of PTH as a cause of high circulating levels of PTH, particularly when the latter is measured with a carboxy-terminal or midregion antiserum. First, plasma PTH levels are much higher in patients with secondary hyperparathyroidism due to chronic renal failure than in those with primary hyperparathyroidism.[193] Second, PTH disappears from the circulation after parathyroidectomy much more slowly in patients with chronic renal failure than in patients with primary hyperparathyroidism.[193] Third, renal transplantation results in the disappearance of PTH from the circulation at a rate significantly greater than that observed after parathyroidectomy in a dialysis patient.[193] Studies of the turnover of intact (parent) PTH have generally been obtained with the infusion of exogenous bovine PTH, because of the very low levels of the compound normally circulating. Papapoulos and coworkers studied the metabolic clearance rate of bovine PTH; a somewhat lower clearance of the hormone was found in patients with chronic renal failure than in normal individuals.[414] However, there was considerable variation in clearance rate, and some uremic patients had clearance rates within the normal range. The clearance of PTH containing the amino-terminal region was much more rapid than the clearance of the carboxy-terminal fragments in patients with chronic renal failure.

Knowledge of the rates of degradation of various circulating forms of PTH is important, both because biologic activities of different PTH fragments vary and because various antisera used to measure PTH recognize different parts of the molecule. Many immunoassays use antisera directed toward the carboxy-terminal fragments; the values obtained with this assay are often markedly elevated in uremia. Different specificities of antisera probably account for the variability of PTH levels reported from various laboratories.[208] The advent of immunoradiometric assays (IRMA) using antibodies directed toward the intact PTH molecule has profoundly changed our approach to patients with renal bone disease. It has made the diagnosis of secondary hyperparathyroidism easier and more accurate. At present there are excellent data correlating levels of "intact" PTH, as measured by the IRMA and various bone histomorphometric parameters characteristic of osteitis fibrosa.

Abnormal set point for calcium

Studies of the regulation of PTH secretion by calcium indicate a sigmoidal relationship between PTH secretion and plasma calcium concentration over a narrow range of the latter.[224] Recently, it has been shown that isolated parathyroid cells from uremic patients require higher extracellular calcium concentrations than normal cells in order to suppress the secretion of PTH.[73,74] Thus the "set point" for calcium—that is, the concentration of calcium required to produce a 50 percent decrease in maximal PTH release—is shifted upward. This abnormality may be an important factor in the pathogenesis of secondary hyperparathyroidism.

Uremia may alter the release of PTH from parathyroid cells by several mechanisms: (1) increasing tissue mass, via hypertrophy and/or hyperplasia; (2) altering the set point for calcium level needed to suppress PTH secretion; and (3) changing the slope of the suppression line. These mechanisms are diagrammatically illustrated in Fig. 41-10.[392] Thus, with each cell operating in a normal manner, the increased number of cells can cause hyperparathyroidism without any alteration in the calcium set point (panel **A**). A second possibility is that both an increase in parathyroid gland size and a change in the secretion rate, due to an increased set point for calcium, occur (panel **B**); the slope of the curve for calcium suppression then remains normal. Thus the degree of hyperparathyroidism is a product of both increased tissue mass and failure to normally suppress PTH secretion when extracellular calcium concentration is in the normal range. A third possibility is the existence of an increase in tissue mass, an elevation of set point for calcium, and a change in the slope between calcium concentration and rate of PTH secretion (panel **C**). This might occur because of heterogeneity of the set points for suppressibility by calcium among different populations of parathyroid cells.

The earliest evidence suggesting an abnormal set point for calcium was presented by Voigts and coworkers in a report on dialysis patients with significant hyperparathyroidism.[557]

During acute hypocalcemia produced by a low-calcium dialysate, patients exhibited a marked increase in

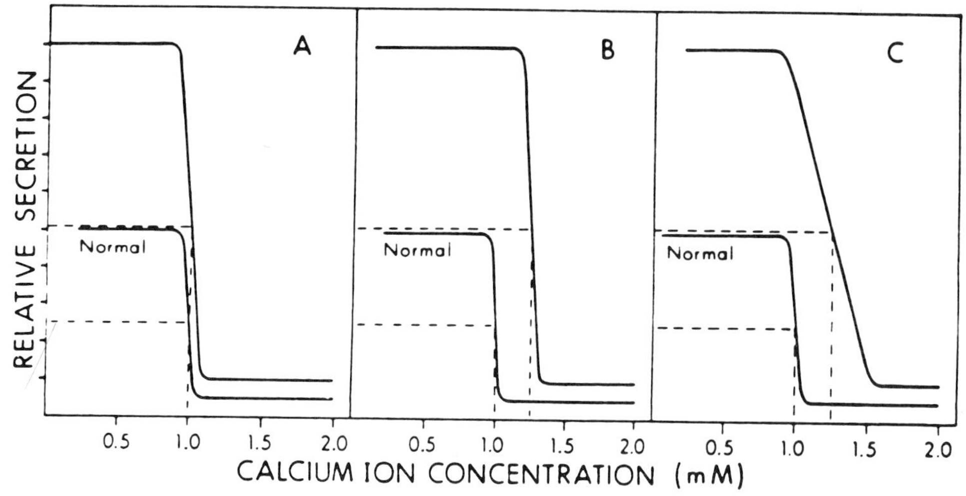

FIGURE 41-10 • Diagrammatic representation of relative rates of PTH secretion with respect to ionized calcium concentrations in normal state used with secondary hyperparathyroidism, with three theoretical considerations. Set point for calcium indicated by vertical broken lines. [Reprinted, by permission, from Morrisey J et al: *Kidney Int* 29(suppl):541, 1986.]

concentrations of carboxy- and amino-terminal PTH when the serum calcium level was falling but was greater than 9 mg/100 ml. Thus it is possible that the set point for calcium is altered, possibly in connection with a partial deficiency of calcitriol. Later, Delmez and associates demonstrated in dialysis patients that the administration of calcitriol for two weeks returned the abnormal set point for calcium toward normal. However, the set point of calcium was estimated as a 50 percent decrease from basal levels of PTH, rather than from maximal PTH stimulation.[144] Recently we have assessed parathyroid gland function in nine patients with significant hyperparathyroidism.[155] This was evaluated by inducing hypo- and hypercalcemia using a low- and a high-calcium dialysate during two separate dialyses performed 1 week apart. PTH values after dialysis-induced hypo- and hypercalcemia were plotted against ionized calcium for each patient, and the actual set point for calcium (i.e., the level of serum calcium that induces a 50 percent inhibition of maximal PTH stimulation) was determined. As can be appreciated from Fig. 41-9, the ionized calcium–PTH sigmoidal curve was abnormally shifted toward the right, resembling the curve observed by Brown and coworkers in in-vitro studies.[74] However, after 10 weeks of intravenous calcitriol therapy (2μg at the end of each dialysis), the curve was shifted back toward the left, to a more physiologic range. Thus the maximal PTH response during hypocalcemia decreased, after calcitriol therapy, from 1661 ± 485 pg/ml to 1031 ± 280 pg/ml ($p < 0.05$). The slope of the curve ranged from -2125 ± 487 to -1563 ± 385 ($p < 0.05$). The set point for calcium, though borderline, did not change significantly after calcitriol. However, if a noncompliant patient who had persistent hyperphosphatemia is excluded, there is a significant change in the set point for calcium. These results demonstrate an abnormal sigmoidal curve in dialysis patients, which is dramatically changed with calcitriol therapy.

In summary, the relative roles of phosphate retention, altered vitamin D metabolism, impaired calcemic response to PTH, and altered degradation and metabolism of PTH in the pathogenesis of hypocalcemia and secondary hyperparathyroidism in renal failure are uncertain. In early renal failure, serum calcium levels and values for intestinal calcium absorption have generally been normal, while serum phosphorus concentrations are either normal or low. Rather than hyperphosphatemia, patients with early renal failure may have an increased ability to excrete a phosphate load, similar to that in patients with primary hyperparathyroidism. Serum PTH levels are commonly increased, but may be normal when an amino-terminal antiserum or an intact PTH molecule assay is used. Restriction of dietary phosphate intake early in the course of renal failure can greatly reduce the magnitude of secondary hyperparathyroidism and largely restore the responsiveness of the skeleton to PTH, indicating that phosphate per se may be an important pathogenic factor. However, the normal or low concentrations of serum phosphorus in early renal failure suggest that the hypocalcemia leading to secondary hyperparathyroidism must be mediated by mechanisms other than hyperphosphatemia. It is possible that an increase in intracellular phosphate concentration in proximal tubular cells may lead to a relative deficit of calcitriol, which in turn may lead to increased PTH secretion by altering the set point for calcium.

DEFECTIVE MINERALIZATION (LOW-BONE-TURNOVER STATES)

Another feature of skeletal disease in patients with advanced renal failure is defective mineralization or, in its severe form, osteomalacia. In contrast to the large amount of experimental and clinical data concerned with the causes of secondary hyperparathyroidism in renal failure, there are fewer data on the pathogenesis of impaired skeletal mineralization. It was initially thought that impaired mineralization resulted from altered vitamin D metabolism; but other pathogenic factors, including aluminum accumulation, are now implicated.

The role of vitamin D

Despite the observations that plasma levels of $1\alpha,25\text{-(OH)}_2D_3$ are low in almost all uremic patients and that intestinal calcium transport is abnormal in uremia,[112,554] overt osteomalacia, or even the histologic features of impaired mineralization, is found in only a fraction of patients with end-stage renal failure.[460,500] Moreover, osteomalacia is often absent in anephric patients.[61] Several factors may affect the frequency of osteomalacia in uremic patients. Impaired mineralization may arise because of factors unrelated to the absence of $1\alpha,25\text{-(OH)}_2D_3$, and it is now known that aluminum accumulation impairs bone mineralization and leads to osteomalacia in patients with renal failure.

Defective skeletal mineralization may have been more common in the United Kingdom than in North America. Eastwood and coworkers noted that uremic osteomalacia correlated with decreased plasma levels of $25\text{-OH-}D_3$;[162] the latter reflect total vitamin D production and intake. Thus, relative vitamin D deficiency is more common in the United Kingdom and Europe than in the United States because of less sunlight exposure and because the fortification of foods with vitamin D is not extensive in the former areas. It is not surprising that vitamin D deficiency leads to greater impairment of skeletal minerealization in patients with renal failure. Low plasma levels of $25\text{-OH-}D_3$ are not infrequent in patients with uremia,[404] and plasma level of $25\text{-OH-}D_3$ was correlated with the protein content of the diet. Under such conditions, low levels of 25-OH-D_3 probably reflect reduced dietary intake of vitamin D. Enhanced renal losses of 25-OH-D_3 can occur with the marked proteinuria of the nephrotic syndrome[490]; this mechanism may contribute to low levels of 25-OH-D_3 in azotemic patients with significant proteinuria.

The mechanism whereby the absence of vitamin D or a related sterol impairs the mineralization of bone is poorly understood. Whether vitamin D (or 1α,25-$(OH)_2D_3$) directly stimulates bone mineralization, or whether it merely leads to bone mineralization by increasing the plasma levels of calcium and phosphorus,[40,248] remains controversial.

Aluminum accumulation

Until the past 15 years aluminum was believed to have no biologic effect. However, convincing data indicate that accumulation of aluminum can cause osteomalacia, hypercalcemia, encephalopathy, and anemia in patients with renal failure.[12,570] Outbreaks of "dialysis osteomalacia" were first reported from dialysis centers in the United Kingdom and also in areas where encephalopathy was common.[420,564] It was first postulated that this "fracturing" bone disease arose from fluoride accumulation[530] or from phosphate depletion,[434] despite the rarity of hypophosphatemia in uremic patients. The hypothesis that aluminum might cause bone disease was raised because aluminum levels were increased in the brains of patients dying with dialysis encephalopathy[14] and because epidemiologic data showed a correlation between the incidence of osteomalacia and high concentrations of aluminum in water used for dialysate.[420] Refractory osteomalacia was observed only sporadically in North America, and cases occurred in centers not using water contaminated with aluminum[246] and when encephalopathy was generally absent. For these reasons, an etiologic role of aluminum was not initially accepted in the United States.

The aluminum content of bone was found to be increased in most dialysis patients, whether measured by neutron activation,[166] electron probe,[128] atomic absorption spectroscopy,[245] or a histochemical staining method.[340] Bone aluminum levels were found to be markedly elevated in patients with refractory osteomalacia[245] (Fig. 41-11), and the aluminum content of bone correlated directly with the extent of osteomalacia in these patients.[245] Moreover, the aluminum was found to localize along the mineralization front.[129,340] Little or no tetracycline was incorporated, indicating absent bone formation, along the surfaces with heavy aluminum staining and the extent of surface aluminum staining correlated inversely with bone formation rate.[340]

In dialysis patients showing bone biopsy features of osteitis fibrosa, mixed features of osteomalacia plus osteitis fibrosa, or "mild" disease, bone aluminum content was often above normal, but the values were generally less than those in patients with dialysis osteomala-

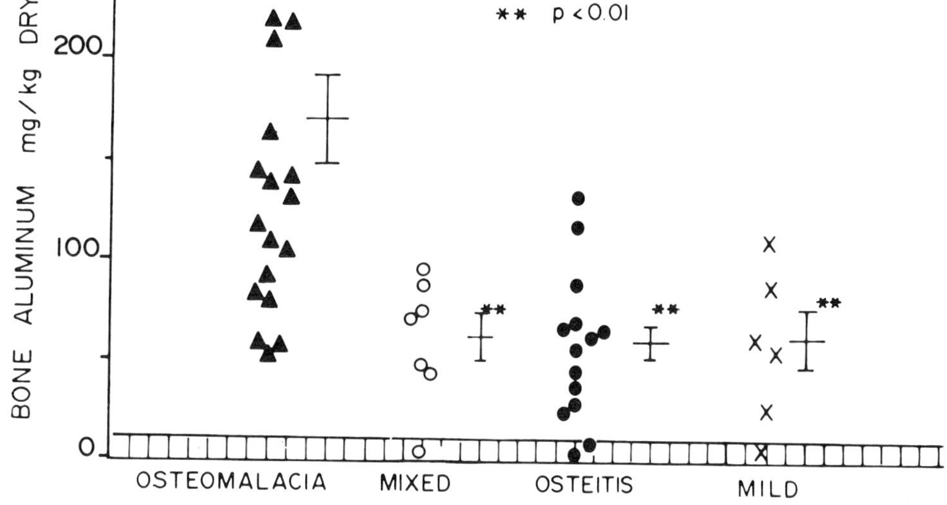

FIGURE 41-11 • Bone aluminum content in patients with symptomatic renal osteodystrophy. Disorders are classified as osteomalacia, osteitis fibrosa, mixture of features of both osteomalacia and osteitis fibrosa, and "mild" bone disease. Significance (p) values refer to group differences from the osteomalacia category. Each symbol represents a different patient; normal range indicated by lower vertically hatched area (Adapted, by permission, from Hodsman AB et al: *J Clin Endocrinol* 54:539, 1982.)

cia.[129,340,421] A subgroup of dialysis patients was identified with bone biopsies showing only mild histiologic features, but these patients had fractures and bone pain similar to those of patients with osteomalacia.[503] Bone biopsies showed reduced numbers of both osteoblasts and osteoclasts; positive surface staining for aluminum; and a markedly reduced rate, or the absence, of bone formation, as measured by double tetracycline labeling. Some of these patients showed patchy areas of wide osteoid. This subgroup has been termed "aplastic"[335] or adynamic bone disease.[503] In some patients, serial bone biopsies have shown the evolution from an aplastic state to osteomalacia, suggesting that the aplastic lesion can be a precursor to more typical osteomalacia.

Other metals can also produce osteomalacia, but this is rare.[428] Staining for both iron and aluminum at the mineralization front is observed in some patients,[430] and some patients have only iron staining in association with osteomalacia.[428] It has been suggested that silicon and sulfur may accumulate at the mineralization front and cause osteomalacia,[72] but such observations have not been confirmed.

Refractoriness to treatment with the active vitamin D sterols is another feature of aluminum-related osteomalacia. When dialysis patients with symptomatic aluminum-related bone disease are treated with the active vitamin D sterols, calcitriol (1α,25-$(OH)_2D_3$ or 1α-OH-D_3, they generally had no change in symptoms nor improvement of bone disease. However, hypercalcemia often developed despite administration of only low doses of the vitamin D sterols.[63,120,246]

The clinical features of aluminum-related bone disease include progressive bone pain, proximal muscle weakness, and fractures of the ribs, vertebrae, pelvis, and hips. Disability and skeletal deformities can be marked.[246] Serum calcium levels may be normal or slightly increased; serum phosphorus concentration does not differ from that in other patients with advanced renal failure, and plasma levels of 25-OH-D_3 are not depressed. Some patients develop spontaneous hypercalcemia; in others hypercalcemia occurs during immobilization, during treatment with vitamin D or oral calcium-based phosphate binders, or with the use of high dialysate calcium concentrations.[63] Parathyroidectomies have been performed unnecessarily in these patients with hypercalcemia, fractures, and bone pain because of suspected secondary hyperparathyroidism, a syndrome called "pseudohyperparathroidism."[502]

Normal plasma alkaline phosphatase levels were reported in patients from the United Kingdom,[18] while elevated levels have been common in patients in the United States.[245,246,400] Serum levels of 1α,25-$(OH)_2D_3$ are low, as expected with end-stage renal disease. Serum levels of PTH often are lower than is usual for dialysis patients[245,246] and fail to increase normally after the induction of hypocalcemia.[20,289] Serum PTH levels may be low because of aluminum accumulation per se, because of the slight increase in blood calcium concentration, or because of both effects. The parathyroid glands can accumulate aluminum preferentially;[84] aluminum added in vitro can inhibit PTH release by parathyroid cells.[392] Indeed, it is possible that aluminum itself inhibits PTH release, thereby lowering bone turnover and rendering the bone more susceptible to the development of osteomalacia.[81] Aluminum-related bone disease has become manifest following parathyroid surgery and after high PTH levels are reduced by treatment with the active vitamin D sterols, 25-OH-D_3 or 1α,25-$(OH)_2D_3$.[176,544] Indeed, there is evidence that high levels of PTH can "protect" from the development of osteomalacia.[165] The pattern of localization of aluminum in the bones of patients with osteitis fibrosa may differ from that seen in patients with osteomalacia. In the former, the aluminum is diffusely distributed in bone; it is localized at the bone surface in osteomalacia.[129] The surface localization of aluminum often increases after parathyroidectomy,[22] and a reduction in PTH levels can predispose to the appearance of osteomalacia. It should be noted that aluminum-related bone disease occasionally occurs in patients with markedly elevated serum PTH levels.[400]

The histologic features of aluminum-related osteomalacia can improve substantially after the removal of only modest amounts of aluminum following infusions of deferoxamine and with only slight increments in serum PTH concentration.[411] The mechanism whereby PTH modifies the features of aluminum-related bone disease remains unknown.

Several experiments in animals have shown that parenteral aluminum loading can reduce bone formation and produce osteomalacia. Ellis and coworkers first reported that parentera injections of aluminum inhibited mineralization in the epiphyseal cartilage of rats.[166] Other investigators have demonstrated more typical lesions of osteomalacia in trabecular bone of rats, dogs, and pigs receiving parenteral aluminum.[92,212,463,495] A reduction of renal function can increase the susceptibility to osteomalacia, because the kidney provides the major route for the removal of aluminum from the body.[92,463] Goodman and coworkers observed reduced mineralization of cortical bone without the appearance of wide osteoid in rats after short-term aluminum loading; such a lesion may be analogous to the "aplastic" lesion observed with renal failure.[211] These observations certainly indicate that parenteral aluminum loading, elevating bone aluminum content to a level similar to that observed in clinical cases, can induce a bone disease similar to that seen in humans. Thus, with regard to the pathogenicity of aluminum, Koch's postulates, as they might be adapted to a noninfectious agent, seem to be fulfilled.

The case for the pathogenic role of aluminum is strengthened by the finding of osteomalacia or "aplastic" bone disease and aluminum staining in patients with near-normal renal function who received long-term parenteral nutrition solutions containing aluminum-contaminated casein hydrolysate.[571]

The view that aluminum itself is pathogenic has been challenged.[448,449] Quarles and coworkers suggested, from observations in vitamin D-deficient dogs, that the aluminum deposited at the mineralization front may not be pathogenic, but rather may represent an epiphenomenon related to the osteomalacic state.[448] In dogs with osteomalacia due to vitamin D deficiency, the administration of aluminum led to its deposition at the mineralization front. When the animals were then treated with vitamin D, the skeletal abnormalities reversed despite the continued administration of aluminum, albeit at a lower dose. It is probable that the osteomalacia of vitamin D deficiency differs from that occurring either in aluminum-loaded animals or in dialysis patients with aluminum-related bone disease.

The mechanism whereby aluminum produces its effect on bone is uncertain. The finding of aluminum along the mineralization front in affected cases has led to the view that the aluminum prevents mineralization;[129,172,340] indeed, aluminum added in vitro can both prevent the generation of hydroxyapatite crystals and retard their growth.[53] Others suggest that aluminum citrate is a factor that inhibits crystal formation.[375] The occurrence of aluminum staining on the cement lines of bone indicates that mineralization has occurred over sites with the earlier deposition of aluminum.[340] Osteomalacia caused by vitamin D deficiency and aluminum loading can be healed by administering vitamin D, indicating that aluminum deposition at the mineralization front does not necessarily impair mineralization.[448] Other observations indicate that aluminum can inhibit the activity of osteoblasts.[302] Conversion of the "aplastic" lesion to true osteomalacia suggests that the earliest abnormality may be inhibition of osteoid synthesis, and that osteoid synthesis is impaired to a greater degree than is mineralization. Also, aluminum can inhibit certain enzymes of the osteoblast,[302] and "inclusion bodies" containing aluminum have been found within active osteoblasts.[128] As noted earlier, aluminum may directly inhibit PTH secretion[289,392] and can also reduce the synthesis of 1,25-dihydroxyvitamin D_3.[212] Both of these features may contribute to abnormal mineralization.

These possible pathogenic mechanisms of impaired mineralization or reduced osteoblast function are not mutually exclusive. Inhibition of the osteoblast may be a first step that reduces matrix synthesis; it may be followed by inhibition of crystal growth and mineralization as increased amounts of aluminum are localized at the mineralization front. Also, aluminum may be more toxic when PTH levels are low and osteoblasts are inactive or absent.

The first cases of dialysis osteomalacia occurred in dialysis units using water with aluminum concentrations above 100 μg/liter;[420] however, a high incidence of bone disease has occurred with dialysate aluminum levels near 50 μg/liter.[456] Since 80 to 90 percent of aluminum in plasma is protein-bound, aluminum is transferred into the patient from the dialysate when the dialysate aluminum concentration exceeds the level of ultrafiltrable aluminum in blood. Aluminum may come from other sources: the cartridges used in the past for the regeneration of dialysate (Redy) released aluminum into dialysate;[384] preparations of peritoneal dialysate have had high concentrations of aluminum on occasion,[130] although samples of peritoneal dialysate evaluated more recently have all had aluminum concentrations less than 5 to 7 μ/liter.[483] On the basis of this experience, it is now recommended that dialysate aluminum levels be lower than 10 meq/liter, and preferably below 5 meq/liter. Significant amounts of aluminum were found in parenteral albumin solutions[383] and in certain other constituents of parenteral solutions.[431]

Aluminum can accumulate in the body via oral absorption. This was first suggested by Berlyne and coworkers,[45] but the warning was largely overlooked. Studies in normal subjects ingesting aluminum hydroxide indicate that small amounts of aluminum are absorbed;[262] since the kidney is the sole route for the excretion of aluminum, the absorbed aluminum will accumulate in patients with renal failure. The aluminum-related bone disease in uremic patients who have never undergone dialysis but who ingest aluminum hydroxide clearly indicates that aluminum toxicity can accumulate from an oral source.[23,175,274] Moreover, close correlation has been noted between plasma aluminum concentration, which probably indicates recent loading with aluminum, and the amount of aluminum-containing gels ingested by children undergoing continuous ambulatory peritoneal dialysis (CAPD)[483,575] (Fig. 41-12). After use of aluminum-containing gels is discontinued in dialysis patients, plasma aluminum levels fall substantially, providing additional evidence for the contribution of oral absorption.[236,241,482,523]

The knowledge that oral absorption of aluminum is a major factor leading to aluminum accumulation in renal failure has led to a consideration of the factors that augment its intestinal uptake. Many renal failure patients can ingest aluminum gels for long periods with little risk, while others develop aluminum loading within a few months after they are given large doses of aluminum gels. Both PTH and vitamin D have been implicated as increasing the intestinal absorption of aluminum;[147,359] however, the effects of vitamin D either were found to be small or could not be documented,[398] and most information indicates little or no effect of PTH. Indeed, patients with high PTH levels seem protected from toxic effects of aluminum.[165] The presence of uremia somehow increases aluminum absorption,[254] although the mechanism for this effect is uncertain. The ingestion of aluminum com-

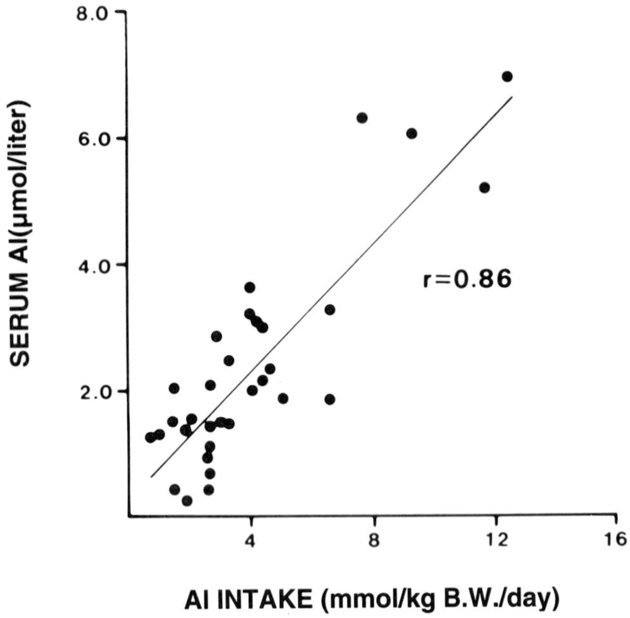

FIGURE 41-12 • Relationship between serum aluminum concentration and total daily ingestion of aluminum in phosphate binders (in mmol per kilogram of body weight; 1 mol Al-27 g) by children undergoing continuous ambulatory peritoneal dialysis (CAPD). Each symbol represents a separate determination in one patient; each patient was studied on two occasions, 6 to 10 months apart. (Reprinted, by permission, from Salusky IB et al: *J Pediatr* 108:767, 1986.)

pounds in conjunction with sodium citrate/citric acid can have a profound effect to enhance aluminum absorption.[515] In certain of the cases with severe aluminum toxicity developing before the need for dialysis, the patients were receiving aluminum gels for hyperphosphatemia and citric acid/sodium citrate (Shohl's solution) to correct acidosis.[33] Indeed, fatal acute aluminum toxicity has been reported in a number of predialysis uremic patients who received this combination.[33,282] Marked enhancement of aluminum absorption has been shown during the ingestion of calcium citrate.[116]. This compound should be used with great care. Moreover, certain over-the-counter compounds (Alka-Seltzer) contain citrate and can augment aluminum absorption.[499] The solubility of many aluminum compounds increases substantially as the pH falls, raising the possibility that gastric pH may modify aluminum absorption substantially. However, prospective studies have shown only modest modification of aluminum absorption by drugs, such as ranitidine, that reduce gastric acid secretion.[118]

The absorption of aluminum from other aluminum-containing compounds has received attention. Aluminum toxicity and aluminum absorption can occur with the ingestion of sucralfate;[464] also, evidence of brain accumulation of aluminum was reported in premature infants who had ingested a low-protein, low-phosphate formula that is often recommended for infants with renal failure.[194] A subsequent prospective study failed to find any evidence of aluminum accumulation in 14 children who ingested this formula for up to 18 months, even though many had consumed sodium citrate/citric acid while ingesting the low-protein infant formula.[483]

Of considerable interest are the host factors that may make certain individuals more susceptible to the toxic effects of aluminum; these include (1) prior parathyroidectomy, (2) earlier rejected renal transplantation, (3) diabetes mellitus, (4) a reduction of PTH levels with active vitamin D sterols, and (4) bilateral nephrectomy.[400]

Reduced plasma phosphorus levels

A low plasma phosphorus concentration may be the cause of impaired mineralization in uremic patients, although such hypophosphatemia is rare. Stanbury and Lumb found an association between the presence of osteomalacia and low plasma calcium-phosphorus product in patients with moderate-to-advanced renal failure.[533] Kanis and coworkers found an inverse relationship between the number of osteoid lamellae, an index of osteomalacia, and the predialysis plasma phosphorus levels in a large group of hemodialysis patients[263] (Fig. 41-13). Evidence for a mineralization defect was common in pa-

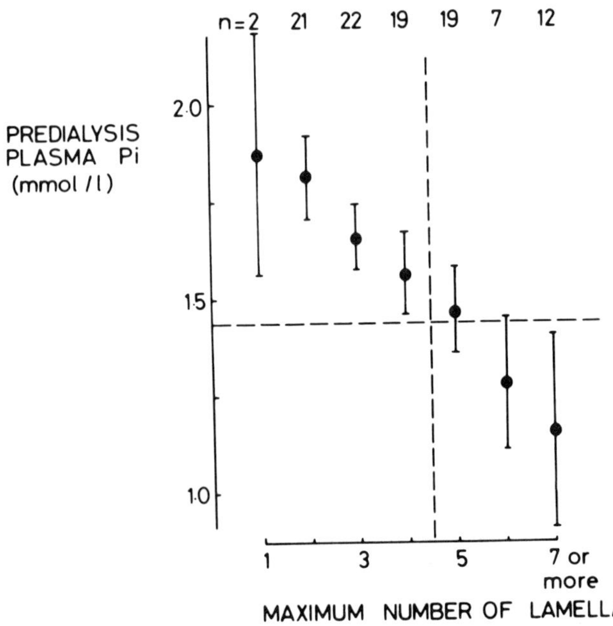

FIGURE 41-13 • Relationship between mean predialysis plasma phosphorus concentration (Pi) and maximum number of lamellae seen on bone biopsy, as an index of osteomalacia, in a large group of patients undergoing regular hemodialysis. Osteomalacia (five or more lamallae) was uncommon in patients with high levels of plasma phosphorus, while there was evidence for impaired mineralization in many patients whose plasma phosphorus concentration lay below the upper limits of normal (horizontal dashed line). (Reprinted, by permission of Walter de Gruyter, from Kanis et al.[263])

tients whose mean plasma phosphorus concentration was below the lower limit of normal. Thus the development of osteomalacia in human beings may require both a lack of vitamin D and the presence of hypophosphatemia, although the latter may be the more important determinant.

Low serum PTH values

A potential contribution of low serum immunologically assayable hormone (iPTH) values to an excessive reduction in bone turnover has been raised. It has been found that a small but growing fraction of dialysis patients have subnormal rates of bone formation but no increase in osteoid (i.e., features of aplastic or "adynamic" bone).[240,242,389] In previous observations, such patients with "aplastic bone disease" had significant surface staining with aluminum and were thought to have aluminum-related bone disease. More recently, a growing number of patients have been identified with histomorphometric and dynamic features of aplastic bone disease on bone biopsy, and yet these patients have lacked significant surface staining for aluminum[240,242] or for iron. Although described among hemodialysis patients,[481] this "disorder" is more common among those treated with long-standing CAPD.[242] The biochemical parameters of serum calcium and phosphorus do not identify patients with low bone turnover, but serum iPTH levels have been lower than those observed in patients with features of osteitis fibrosa or mild hyperparathyroid bone disease, although the values with the intact IRMA have been in the upper range of normal or slightly above. The likely reason for the lower iPTH levels is the combined use of calcium-containing phosphate binders and a dialysate calcium concentration that raises the blood calcium level. During CAPD, the continuous exposure to a calcium concentration of 3.5 meq/liter in peritoneal dialysate may raise ionized serum Ca and inhibit PTH secretion. Further studies are needed to identify other factors that may contribute to this process and to clarify the natural history of the disorder. The substitution of peritoneal dialysate with a calcium concentration reduced to 2.5 meq/liter was associated with a rise in serum iPTH level and a shift in bone formation rate toward normal.[242]

Altered collagen synthesis and maturation

The formation of bone requires both the generation and the maturation of collagen. Without maturation of collagen and the development of specific cross-linkages between collagen molecules, mineral deposition may not proceed normally. There is evidence of an abnormality in collagen synthesis and maturation in uremia. Rats with experimental uremia fail to develop mature, insoluble collagen and exhibit a preponderance of immature and soluble collagen that fails to mineralize normally.[162] The underlying mechanism is unknown, but similarities exist between the abnormalities of collagen maturation observed in uremia and those found in vitamin D deficiency.[364,473] Russell and Avioli found that treatment of uremic animals with 25-OH-D_3 largely restored collagen maturation toward normal, providing additional evidence that altered vitamin D metabolism plays a role in defective collagen maturation.[472] Such abnormal collagen synthesis and maturation may contribute to impaired mineralization of bone in uremic patients.

Maturation of bone crystals

The formation of mineralized bone involves the initial precipitation of amorphous calcium phosphate and its subsequent transformation into crystalline hydroxyapatite. This transformation and maturation of bone is required for the formation of bone of high structural integrity. One characteristic of immature bone is the presence of large quantities of amorphous calcium phosphate, identifiable because of its low density. The evaluation of animals with chronic uremia has revealed a correlation between the skeletal content of amorphous calcium phosphate and the quantity of immature, soluble collagen.[474] In bone material obtained postmortem or by biopsy from uremic human beings the presence of more severe renal osteodystrophy was associated with a decrease in bone density and a decrease in the carbonate content of the skeleton.[77,426]

The reason for the delay in the maturation of bone mineral in uremia is uncertain; several factors may contribute. These include increased bone magnesium content, elevated pyrophosphate content, and diminished carbonate level. Alfrey and coworkers, and Burnell and coworkers, found elevated magnesium content in bone from uremic patients;[15,77] Alfrey and coworkers found a close correlation between bone magnesium content and serum magnesium levels.[15] Alfrey and Solomon noted a fourfold increase in pyrophosphate content and an associated increase in magnesium in bone samples obtained from uremic patients, as compared to nonuremic control subjects.[16] Alfrey and Solomon suggested that pyrophosphate may exist in a transphosphorylated form that is resistant to breakdown.[16] This pyrophosphate may impair the normal conversion of amorphous calcium phosphate to crystalline apatite.[546] Thus, an increase in bone pyrophosphate might contribute to altered crystal maturation.[16] Alfrey and coworkers suggested that pyrophosphate may exist in the form of a magnesium salt and hence may be less susceptible to degradation by naturally occurring pyrophosphatases.[16] In support of a role of magnesium, Kaye found that the rate of bone crystal maturation could be modified by altering the intake of magnesium.[273]

Thus, several features of uremia, which include abnormal vitamin D metabolism, aluminum accumulation, decreased bone carbonate content, increased skeletal magnesium content, and increased pyrophosphate level, may contribute to impaired collagen maturation and/or defective bone crystal development. (Factors related to acidosis are discussed below.) A possible role of some toxic factor related to uremia per se has not been excluded. The role of these factors in contributing to symptomatic bone disease in patients with chronic renal failure remains poorly understood; starting regular dialysis can introduce additional pathogenic factors (see below).

The role of acidosis

The contribution of metabolic acidosis to the pathogenesis of mineral abnormalities in patients with renal failure has yet to be clarified. A number of metabolic studies carried out in patients with uremia implicate acidosis in leading to negative calcium balance and thereby contributing to skeletal disease in renal failure. Patients with stable chronic renal failure can maintain a stable serum bicarbonate concentration despite continued dietary acid loading and reduction in renal acid excretion;[210] this suggests that hydrogen ions continue to be buffered by the body, particularly in bone. Litzow and coworkers found that alkali treatment of azotemic patients with chronic acidosis reduced both urinary and fecal losses of calcium, causing the net balance for calcium to be indistinguishable from zero but failing to induce calcium retention.[306]

Observations on the role of bone in buffering the continued acid load in uremia have been derived from analysis of the mineral content of bone obtained at postmortem or by biopsy. It has been suggested that hydrogen ion accumulates in bone in association with the loss of calcium carbonate from bone.[425] However, the existence of crystalline calcium carbonate itself in bone is a matter of controversy. During short-term acid infusion, carbonate is lost from bone in association with sodium rather than calcium. Burnell and coworkers suggested that carbonate and sodium exist in the hydration shell.[77] Although bone may buffer an acid load through the release of carbonate (or bicarbonate), hydrogen ions are accepted in association with bone resorption and apatite dissolution, no matter what causes bone resorption. Metabolic acidosis induces an increase in bone resorption and a decrease in bone formation in parathyroidectomized rats,[288] but there is more buffering provided by bone during acidosis in animals with intact parathyroid glands than in those with parathyroidectomy—presumably because bone turnover is more rapid.[397] Acidosis can enhance bone resorption in vitro. The calcium release from bone in organ culture is augmented by metabolic acidosis,[79] with cellular activity making an important contribution to this enhanced resorption.[78] Such action may be related to increased osteoclastic resorptive activity that has been observed when the pH in the medium is reduced.[28]

Pellegrino and Biltz[425] found the reduction in carbonate and calcium content in uremic bone at autopsy to be proportional to the duration of uremia; on the other hand, Burnell and coworkers reported no correlation between the degree of acidosis and the quantity of bone carbonate in dialysis patients.[77] Pellegrino and coworkers found an increase in phosphate content of bone in patients treated with dialysis,[425] but Burnell and coworkers found no change in phosphate content except a decrease in phosphorus in patients with marked osteitis fibrosa.[77] Kaye and coworkers reported that bone phosphorus content increased in association with a decrease in carbonate in postmortem material.[276] On the basis of the reciprocal relationship between changes in phosphate and bicarbonate, Kaye and coworkers suggested that apatite that is deficient in carbonate forms in uremia, with phosphate substituted for carbonate; they suggested that this change may occur with only minimal alteration in crystal symmetry and size.[276] The failure of Burnell and coworkers to find an increase in phosphorus content despite reduced carbonate content suggests that the loss of carbonate may not require replacement with phosphate; the data may also reflect a different degree of renal failure and duration of dialysis treatment in the patients studied in Seattle by Burnell and coworkers.[77] The role of bone in the control of systemic acid-base status is considered in a recent review.[217]

Certain observations point to a minor role of acidosis in leading to bone disease in uremia. Alkali therapy of patients suffering from overt renal osteodystrophy failed to produce healing of the bone lesion.[149,532] On the other hand, pharmacologic doses of vitamin D lead to healing even in the presence of acidosis.[529] Moreover, long-term acid feeding of animals produces skeletal lesions more akin to osteoporosis, with a decrease in both bone mineral content and bone matrix, rather than producing secondary hyperparathyroidism.[39]

A combination of renal failure and acidosis may have effects different from those of acidosis per se. The situation may be more complex in dialysis patients, because restoration of body and bone buffer may be incomplete with the usual concentration of buffer, usually acetate, in dialysate. Bone carbonate content is generally reduced. Burnell suggested that the carbonate in bone may affect crystal growth and maturation, thereby providing a mechanism whereby acidosis indirectly affects the skeleton.[77] In normal individuals with metabolic acidosis there is evidence of increased bone resportion[4] but no evidence of increased PTH secretion.[4,287,298] Lefebre and coworkers[296] noted that lower doses of a vitamin D sterol were required to maintain normal serum calcium levels in the dialysis patients whose mild metabolic acidosis was corrected.

In the abovementioned prospective study, which was done to evaluate the role of acidosis among dialysis patients, Lefebvre and coworkers[296] followed a control group of dialysis patients with a dialysate bicarbonate of

33 mmol/liter and an "acidosis-corrected group" with dialysate bicarbonate increased by 7 to 15 mmol/liter to maintain the predialysis plasma bicarbonate level at 24 meq/liter. In the control group, midregion PTH rose progressively, while the PTH values were stable in the "acidosis-corrected" group. Bone biopsies done at the outset and after 18 months of the study revealed a progressive increase of osteoid surface and osteoblast surface in the control patients; these abnormalities did not worsen in the "acidosis-corrected" group. In patients who entered the study with elevated rates of bone formation, the supranormal plasma osteocalcin levels rose even further in the control group but were stable in the "acidosis-corrected" group. Thus there was evidence of progressive secondary hyperparathyroidism in the group using a standard bicarbonate level in the dialysate, while the disease process was arrested with correction of metabolic acidosis. The investigators suggested that acidosis might enhance bone resorption and thereby release more phosphate into extracellular fluid, with the latter being responsible for the worsening of secondary hyperparathyroidism. Further prospective studies of the effect of correcting mild metabolic acidosis are needed to clarify how acidosis can modify the courses of the various types of uremic bone disease.

The role of calcitonin

Plasma levels of calcitonin measured by radioimmunoassay have been found to be increased in patients with acute or chronic renal failure.[243,295] Evidence exists for immunological heterogeneity of circulating plasma immunoreactive calcitonin (iCT), which may account for wide differences in values reported from different laboratories. Lee and coworkers suggested that a different chromatographic pattern of iCT may be found in patients with chronic renal failure compared to individuals with medullary carcinoma of the thyroid.[295] In the uremic patients, a much greater fraction of iCT was present in a high-molecular-weight species, which differed from intact calcitonin. The high-molecular-weight species contained a small fraction of the immunoreactivity. Immunoassays may detect inactive forms of calcitonin; the different forms found in chronic renal failure probably are not biologically active.

The biological significance of increased levels of calcitonin in uremia remains undetermined, although the reports by the groups of Heynen and Kanis suggest the relationship between serum iCT and PTH levels in uremic patients with features of renal osteodystrophy is different from the relationship in those without.[244,265] Dialysis patients were separated into two groups on the basis of a bimodal distribution of plasma alkaline phosphatase activity. The patients with normal alkaline phosphatase activity levels had mean values of serum PTH concentration that were lower, and serum iCT concentration levels that were higher, than values observed in dialysis patients with elevated alkaline phosphatase activities; the serum levels of calcium and phosphorus did not differ between the two groups. A positive correlation was noted between plasma PTH and plasma iCT in uremic patients with normal alkaline phosphatase levels, and also in normal subjects. On the other hand, in the patients with elevated alkaline phosphatase activity serum PTH and iCT were negatively correlated, with higher serum PTH levels and lower iCT values; the result was a higher ratio of PTH to iCT. These authors suggested that high iCT levels in patients with normal alkaline phosphatase levels may have inhibited or blocked the action of PTH on bone. Thus normal alkaline phosphatase activity may occur because of the ability of calcitonin to block the rapid turnover of bone associated with high PTH levels. Patients with elevated alkaline phosphatase activities and overt renal osteodystrophy may have high levels of circulating PTH accompanied by a relative deficiency of calcitonin. The reason for such an apparent deficiency of calcitonin is unclear; these authors suggested it could represent either a lack of adequate stimulus for calcitonin secretion or a failure of normal calcitonin synthesis and secretion in response to an appropriate stimulus. In another group of patients under treatment with regular hemodialysis, Kanis and coworkers noted a fall in plasma alkaline phosphatase activity, a decrease in the number of osteoblasts in biopsied bone, a decrease in plasma phosphorus concentration, and a rise in plasma iCT following bilateral nephrectomy; plasma calcium and PTH concentrations were unchanged.[266] Kanis and coworkers suggested that the rise in plasma calcitonin may be responsible for the transient decrease in bone turnover observed following bilateral nephrectomy. Such observations provide some additional support for their contention that low levels of calcitonin may contribute to increased bone turnover in uremic patients.

In the rat, as was mentioned earlier, the absence of calcitonin improves the calcemic response to PTH.[466] PTH-induced hypercalcemia markedly increases plasma calcitonin in chronic-renal-failure rats with intact thyroid glands; the calcitonin, in turn, impairs the calcemic response to PTH (Fig. 41-14). Whether these observations have any clinical relevance remains to be proved.

Histologic features of bone

The histologic and histochemical evaluation of bone has extended understanding of the pathophysiology and rational management of renal osteodystrophy. The techniques for obtaining, preparing, and interpreting microscopic sections of bone have improved, and laboratories that are specialized for the processing and preparing of undecalcified sections of bone are now available. The systemic use of tetracycline labeling has allowed dynamic evaluation of bone mineralization rate. The development of a staining method by Maloney and coworkers to determine bone aluminum deposits has aided in the under-

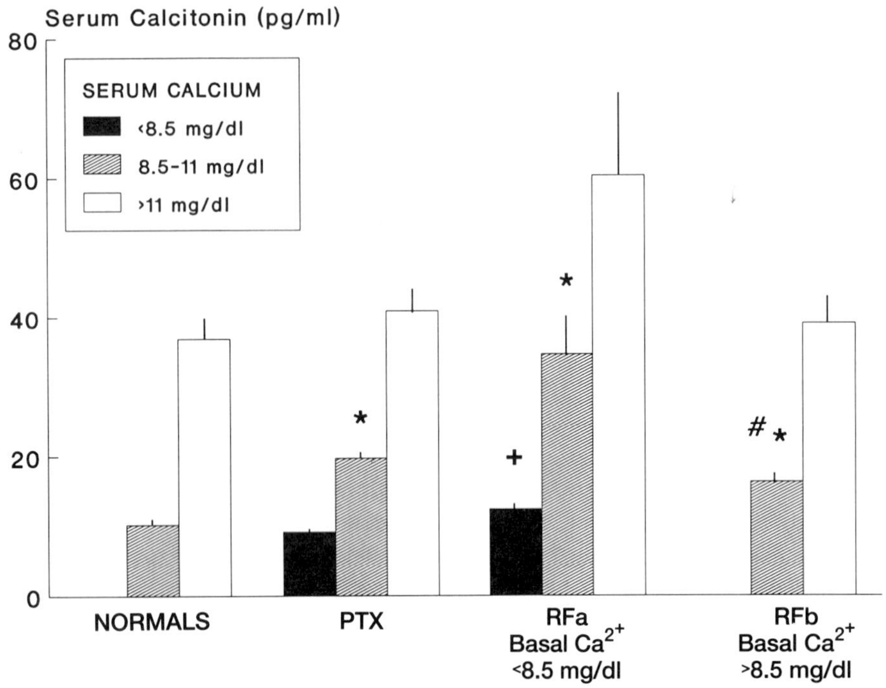

FIGURE 41-14 • The stimulation of serum calcitonin by increases in the serum calcium is shown in four groups: normals, parathyroidectomy (PTX), and the two renal failure groups, RF_a and RF_b. The serum calcitonin level is shown for each range of serum calcium: (■) < 8.5 mg/dl, (□) 8.5 to 11 mg/dl, and (□) > 11 mg/dl. In each group, the serum calcitonin level was significantly greater than the calcitonin level at the previous range of serum calcium. $^*p < 0.05$ as compared with normals; $+p < 0.05$ as compared with PTX; $\#p < 0.05$ as compared with RF_a.

standing of aluminum-induced bone disease.[340] These techniques have been applied widely and with considerable safety in patients with renal osteodystrophy studied in various centers throughout the world.[60,167,177] The incidences of various bone lesions vary from center to center according to multiple factors such as diet, vitamin D intake, primary renal disease, aluminum concentration in water, etc.

The majority of patients with advanced renal disease have osteitis fibrosa characterized by increased bone resorption, extensive osteoclastic and osteoblastic activity, and progressive increase in endosteal fibrosis. When quantitative bone histomorphometric analysis is performed, the amount of endosteal fibrosis and active bone resorption (defined by the presence of osteoclasts at the bone interface) correlates with plasma levels of carboxyterminal PTH.[174,176] Osteoblastic activity is extensive; it correlates with active resorption. The number of osteoclasts is markedly increased in osteitis fibrosa; the osteoclasts are frequently multinucleated and large. In addition to extensively increased surface resorption, there are numerous dissecting cavities through which the osteoclasts tunnel into the bodies of individual trabeculae (Fig. 41-15).

The presence of endosteal fibrosis is characteristic of osteitis fibrosa; the fibrosis can first be appreciated in the resorption lacunae. With continued stimulation, the endosteal fibrosis extends beyond the resorption cavities in a narrow band along the peritrabecular surface (Fig. 41-16). The next stage of extension is represented by bridging of fibrosis between spicules. Finally, the fibrosis may occupy a large, contiguous area of marrow space (Fig. 41-17). Bone mineralization, as assessed by tetracycline labeling, may be increased or normal, although there may be abundant osteoid containing many active osteoblasts (Fig. 41- 18).

Another feature of osteitis fibrosa is the alignment of strands of collagen in an irregular, haphazard, woven pattern, which contrasts with the normal parallel alignment of strands of collagen in lamellar bone (Fig. 41-19).

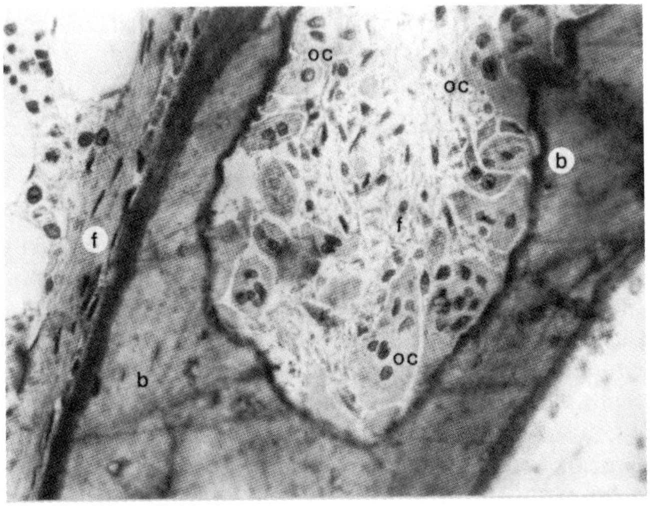

FIGURE 41-15 • Dissecting area of resorption in a patient with chronic renal failure and osteitis fibrosa. Multinucleated osteoclasts (*oc*) have tunneled through trabecular bone (*b*). Endosteal fibrosis can be seen both within dissection cavity and along lateral trabecular surface. (× 375) (From Felsenfeld and Llach: *Mineral Electrolyte Metab* 10:166, 1984. Used by permission.)

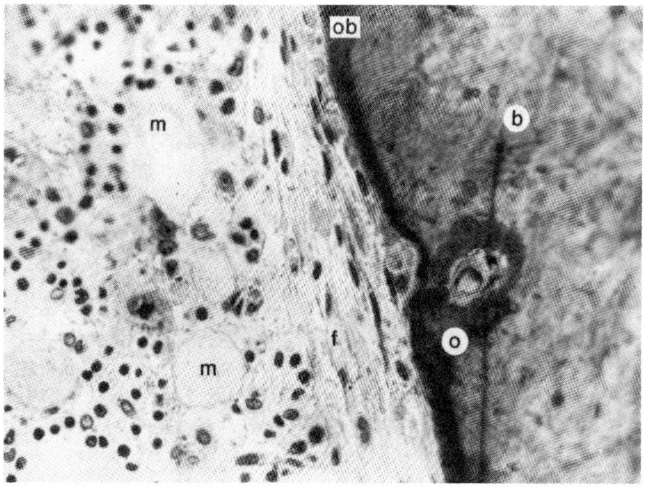

FIGURE 41-16 • Peritrabecular fibrosis in a chronic renal failure patient. Endosteal fibrosis (*f*) visible adjacent to trabecular bone (*b*) and osteoid (*o*) with overlying osteoblasts (*ob*); normal marrow (*m*) also present. (× 375) (From Felsenfeld and Llach: *Mineral Electrolyte Metab* 10:166, 1984. Used by permission.)

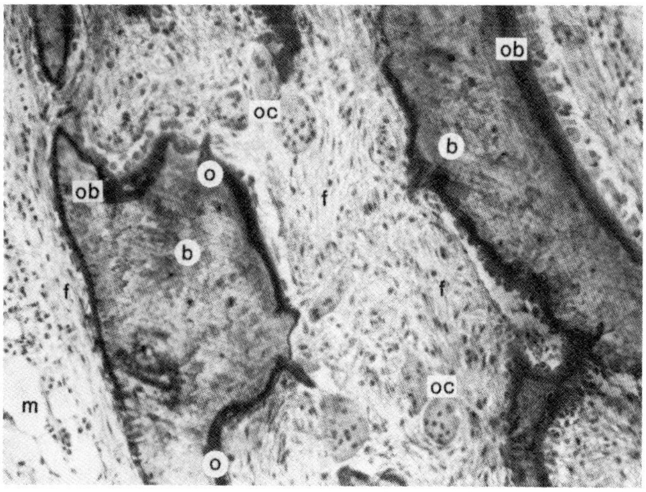

FIGURE 41-17 • Diffuse endosteal fibrosis of marrow space. Endosteal fibrosis (*f*) occupies large, contiguous areas of marrow. Many giant multinucleated osteoclasts (*oc*) are visible. Osteoid (*o*) and osteoblastic osteoid (*ob*) cover much of trabecular bone (*b*) surface. Normal marrow (*m*) is seen in one small area. (× 150) (From Felsenfeld and Llach: *Mineral Electrolyte Metab* 10:166, 1984. Used by permission.)

This disorganized structure of collagen in woven bone may lead to defective physical properties of bone in response to stress. Woven osteoid is capable of becoming mineralized in the absence of vitamin D; however, the calcium is often deposited as amorphous calcium phosphate rather than as hydroxyapatite. Such deposition in woven osteoid may explain the presence of osteosclerosis.[459]

Another major bone lesion observed in uremic patients is osteomalacia; it is characterized by an excess of unmineralized osteoid, providing an increase in osteoid width (Fig. 41-20). The osteoid arises from impaired mineralization of the protein matrix bone. Tetracycline labeling identifies a marked decrease or absence of mineralization. Characteristic features of osteomalacia are the absence of both cell activity and endosteal fibrosis. The presence of increased unmineralized osteoid does not itself imply the presence of a mineralization defect; increased quantities of unmineralized osteoid appear in any condition associated with high rates of skeletal turnover, and mineralization can lag behind the synthesis of matrix. In these situations tetracycline labeling can identify the presence of active or normal mineralization.

A

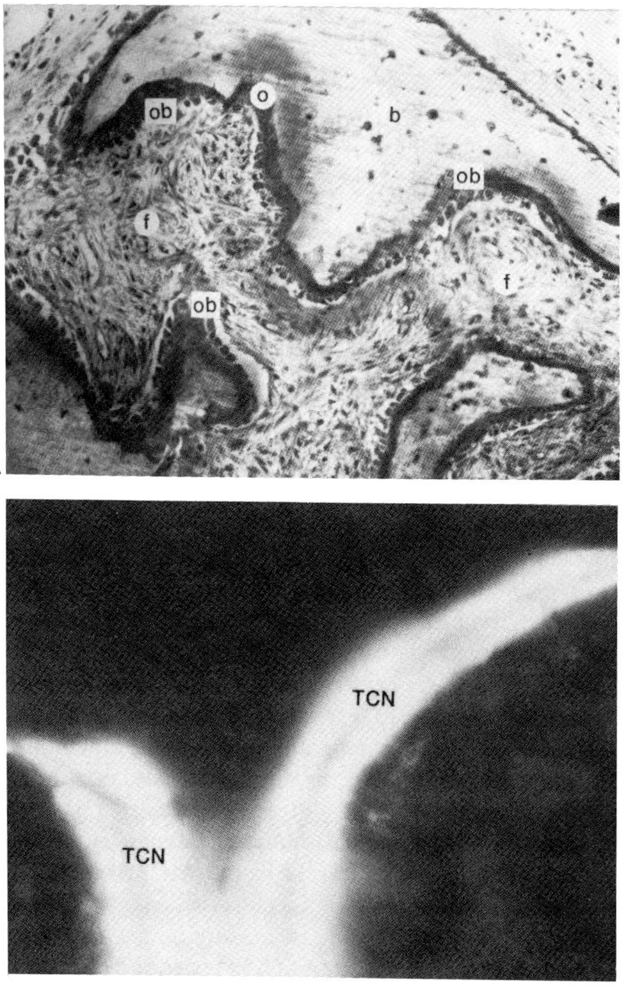

B

FIGURE 41-18 • Osteoblastic osteoid and bone mineralization in osteitis fibrosa. (*A*) Despite presence of abundant osteoid (*o*) in osteitis fibrosa, existence of many active osteoblasts (*ob*) suggests that mineralization is proceeding. (*B*) Mineralization in osteitis fibrosa as assessed by double tetracycline label (*TCN*). Extent of mineralization and bone appositional rate (distance between labels divided by time) are normal. (× 375) (From Felsenfeld and Llach: *Mineral Electrolyte Metab* 10:166, 1984. Used by permission.)

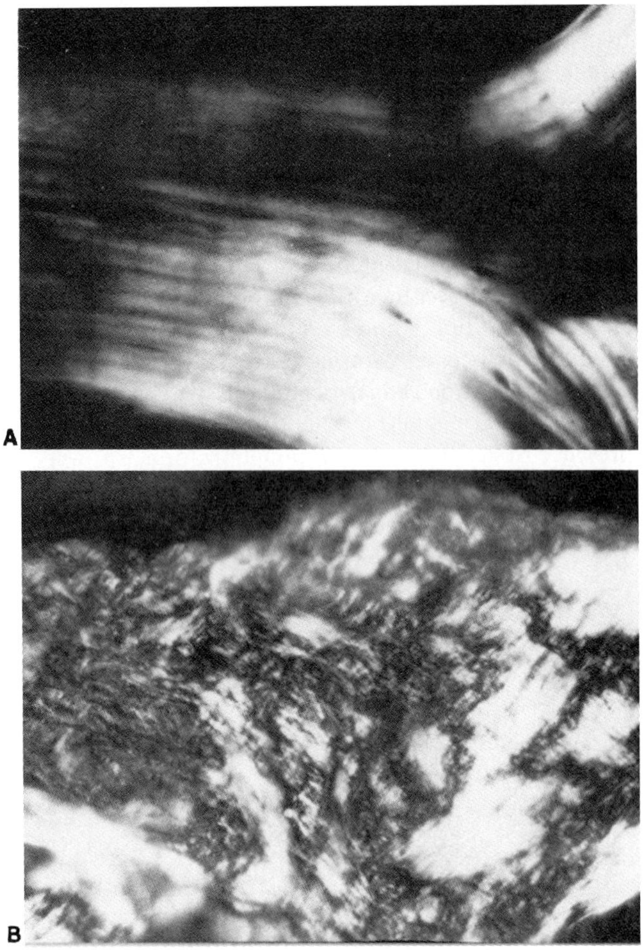

FIGURE 41-19 • Lamellar and woven bone (*A*) Normal bone possesses a lamellar pattern when viewed under polarized light. (× 150) (*B*) Bone of osteitis fibrosa when viewed with polarized light displays a woven (disorganized) pattern. (× 150) (From Felsenfeld and Llach: *Mineral Electrolyte Metab* 10:166, 1984. Used by permission.)

The frequency of osteomalacia appears to have a marked geographic variation. Osteomalacia was initially seen in patients receiving maintenance dialysis.[315,420] Recently, patients with osteomalacia have been reported prior to the initiation of dialysis.[175,274] Epidemiologic evidence has implicated the presence of aluminum in the water, since the incidence of osteomalacia has increased greatly in areas where the aluminum content of the water is high.[565] Pretreatment of the water with reverse osmosis has reduced the incidence of osteomalacia.[184] With the advent of the Maloney stain for aluminum, it has been shown that the great majority of osteomalacic dialysis patients have large deposits of aluminum in the bone.[340] The characteristic pattern in a linear deposition of aluminum along the interface between trabecular bone and osteoid.[299,340] The degree of osteomalacia has been found to correlate closely with bone aluminum content, whether the latter is analyzed biochemically or histologically.[245,340]

Another type of bone lesion observed in dialysis patients is aplastic bone disease.[503] This entity is characterized by features similar to those observed in osteomalacia; the major difference is the absence of large osteoid seams. These patients also have a deficiency of cellular activity and absence of endosteal fibrosis; aluminum deposits are present both at the osteoid-bone interface and on the surface of trabecular bone. It seems that aluminum may be toxic to bone by simultaneously affecting bone formation and remodeling. Thus aplastic bone disease may be a variant of osteomalacia, both being caused by aluminum accumulation.

Because the incidence of aluminum-induced bone disease is steadily decreasing, a new form of aplastic or adynamic bone disease has surfaced. The histologic fea-

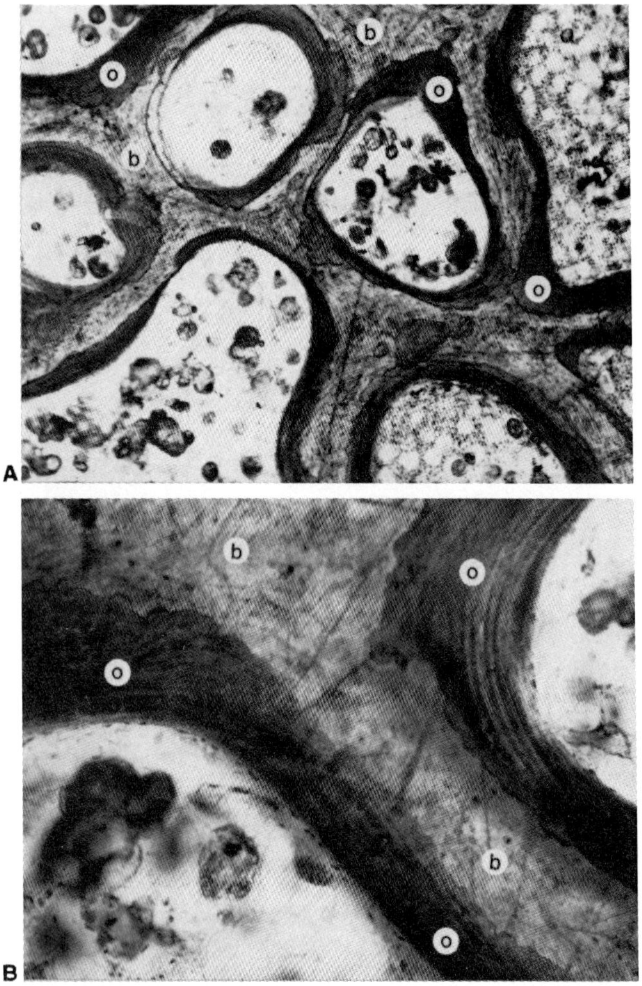

FIGURE 41-20 • Osteomalacia of renal failure. (*A*) Large irregular deposits of osteoid (*o*) cover almost entire surface of trabecular bone (*b*). Osteoblasts, osteoclasts, and endosteal fibrosis are absent. (× 150) (*B*) Excessively wide, scalloped osteoid (*o*) seam covers surface of trabecular bone (*b*). Note the irregularity of bone-osteoid interface. This feature is commonly observed in osteomalacia of renal failure. (× 375) (From Felsenfeld and Llach: *Mineral Electrolyte Metab* 10:166, 1984. Used by permission.)

tures of this entity are similar to those of the abovementioned form; however, aluminum deposits are not present. This lesion has been observed with increasing frequency in diabetic patients as well as CAPD patients.[242]

Mild renal failure

Malluche and coworkers carried out bone biopsies in 22 patients with rates of creatinine clearance between 40 and 117 ml/min per 1.73 m^2 body surface area.[337] Among those patients having a creatinine clearance rate above 60 ml/min, 40 percent exhibited an increase in woven osteoid, which probably indicates the previous existence of increased osteoclastic resorption and high bone turnover. Both the fraction of surface showing active osteoclasts and osteoid volume were normal in these patients. Evidence of a mineralization defect, although present in some patients with creatinine clearance rates above 40 ml/min per 1.73 m^2, was unusual; moreover, a severe mineralizing defect was seen only in patients with more advanced renal failure. Malluche and coworkers interpreted their findings in early renal failure as consistent with excess PTH acting on bone.[336]

Advanced renal failure

As renal failure progresses, overt skeletal disease is more common. There appears to be considerable variation in the incidence and severity of bone disease from one part of the world to another. Although it is not certain whether histologic features of uremia are necessarily different in dialysis patients compared with those in patients with stable, advanced renal failure, certain investigators have suggested that differences do occur. Some investigators have found it convenient to divide patients with advanced renal failure into several groups according to category of skeletal disease;[500] others favor evaluating patients as a single group.[316] Stanbury and coworkers recommended that uremic patients be grouped according to the presence of divergent forms of skeletal disease.[534] One group exhibits a preponderance of osteomalacia; others have features of secondary hyperparathyroidism. The latter patients generally exhibit a higher product of calcium × phosphorus in serum. In these patients, active resorption surface, the number of osteoclasts, and/or increased fibrosis each have been correlated with parathyroid gland weight and serum levels of PTH.[60,235]

Other patients have shown a preponderance of a mineralizing defect. Any of these patients may exhibit features characteristic of secondary hyperparathyroidism as well, with increased areas of fibrosis and resorptive surface.[167] These patients usually have a tendency toward hypocalcemia and a low calcium-phorphorus product.[155] Sherrard and coworkers found that bone turnover rate, as studied by double tetracycline labeling, is increased in patients with osteitis fibrosa but is slowed in patients showing a pure mineralizing defect of osteomalacia.[500]

There is clearly great variation in the type of skeletal disease seen in different geographic locations. In Israel, Italy, and certain parts of the United Kingdom the preponderant bone disease may be osteomalacia;[44,168,343] investigators in Germany,[459] the Netherlands,[157] and the United States,[5] have found lesions of secondary hyperparathyroidism to be more common. A lower incidence of osteitis fibrosa has been attributed to lower dietary phosphorus intake in Israel and Italy; intake of diets low in protein and phosphorus may increase the frequency of osteomalacia.[178] Differences in latitude and climate are known to have major effects on vitamin D production, as measured by plasma levels of 25-OH-D_3;[320] also, the foods that are fortified with vitamin D differ. Such additions are extensive in the United States, where milk, other dairy products, and bread have vitamin D added. In the United Kingdom, however, only margarine has vitamin D added. Such factors may contribute to differences in the types of skeletal disease seen in various parts of the world. Dietary calcium intake varies depending on cultural circumstances, providing yet another possible factor. Data on differences in dietary intake cannot be obtained under comparable circumstances for all places around the world; hence it is difficult to be conclusive. Isolated reports of patients showing osteomalacia secondary to phosphate depletion have also been clearly documented.[6,32]

Patients undergoing regular dialysis

There is disagreement about whether dialysis treatment can lead to specific qualitative differences in the skeletal disease present or whether dialysis merely prolongs the lives of patients with end-stage uremia, thereby exposing them to the various pathogenic factors for a longer period. Certain incriminating factors are unique to dialysis patients, such as administration of heparin,[255] exposure to fluoridated water, exposure to high concentrations of acetate, periodic removal of bicarbonate, exposure to varying concentrations of calcium and magnesium in dialysate, and the presence of aluminum, trace elements, and other substances in dialysate. The most important and toxic factor may be increased aluminum exposure.

From their observations on patients studied in Heidelberg, Ritz and coworkers concluded that there are no qualitative differences between the findings in bones of patients undergoing dialysis compared with those in patients with stable advanced uremia.[459]

Workers in Newcastle, as well as Coburn and Llach, identified a subgroup of dialysis patients exhibiting only osteomalacia or a mineralizing defect that is associated with little or no evidence of secondary hyperparathyroidism.[168,120,315,564] Such patients fail to improve following treatment with 1α-OH-D_3 or $1\alpha,25$-$(OH)_2D_3$, which suggests that there is little or no relationship between their bone disease and altered vitamin D metabolism. This subgroup of patients was later discovered to show associated aluminum toxicity, believed to have arisen from an increased aluminum concentration of water used for dialysate (see above). Originally it was thought that this syndrome occurred only in dialysis patients. However, several investigators have described osteomalacia with bone aluminum deposits in patients with chronic renal failure prior to the commencement of hemodialysis, suggesting that there are sources of aluminum other than the dialysate.[175] In many of these cases the use of aluminum-containing phosphate binders, together with the ingestion of citrate-containing solutions, may have played an important pathogenic role.

It has become apparent that the incidence of aluminum-related osteomalacia is higher than previously thought. Llach and coworkers have evaluated the prevalence of the types of bone lesions in a large, unselected dialysis population coming from the same geographic region; osteitis fibrosa was present in 88 of the 131 patients studied.[315] Osteomalacia was present in 31 patients (23 percent) and aplastic bone disease with aluminum deposits was present in 12 patients (9 percent). Thus osteomalacia was observed frequently in patients originally asymptomatic, but over a period of three years more than one-third became symptomatic.[315] In comparison with patients with osteitis fibrosa, these patients had higher serum calcium levels, lower concentrations of plasma PTH, higher serum aluminum levels, and marked deposits of aluminum at the interface between trabecular bone and osteoid tissue. Most of these patients were dialyzed with dialysate containing a low concentration of aluminum, suggesting that the aluminum burden arose from other sources, most likely aluminum-containing phosphate binders.

BIOCHEMICAL FEATURES OF ALTERED DIVALENT ION METABOLISM

Despite evidence that the pathophysiologic alterations develop early in the course of renal insufficiency, signs and symptoms due to altered calcium homeostasis generally appear only in patients with advanced uremia. In part, this may occur because some symptoms, such as muscle weakness, are so insidious in their appearance that they are not even noticed by the patient. Moreover, many symptoms may be attributed to "uremia" per se. In contrast to the late appearance of symptoms, a number of biochemical alterations regularly appear early in the course of progressive renal insufficiency. The evaluation of altered calcium homeostatis and osteodystrophy is often made from biochemical measurements. Hence, the biochemical parameters are reviewed first; clinical signs and symptoms are considered thereafter.

SERUM PHOSPHORUS LEVELS

Serum phosphorus levels are usually slightly lower than normal[113,319] or normal in the early stages of renal failure.[205,566] Hyperphosphatemia is generally absent until renal function falls to 20 to 30 percent of normal.[117,205] In patients with creatinine clearance rates below 20 ml/min, serum phosphorus levels show wide variation, ranging from 2.5 to 15 mg/100 ml in individual patients.

Serum phosphorus is sharply affected by dietary intake of phosphorus, which causes an increase in serum level, and by the intake of carbohydrate-rich foods, which lowers serum phosphorus levels. Slatopolsky and coworkers suggested that postprandial levels of serum phosphorus may show a marked rise in uremic patients compared to normal subjects.[521] However, available data indicate that there is little difference in serum phosphorus concentration after a phosphorus load in normal individuals compared to patients with renal failure.[355]

Some factors that can affect the serum phosphorus level in patients with renal insufficiency are shown in Table 41-1. Dietary phosphorus intake and fraction of phosphorus absorbed from the intestinal tract have an important effect on blood phosphorus levels, particularly with advanced renal failure. In advanced renal failure, net intestinal absorption of phosphorus is minimally reduced, as determined from metabolic balance studies and from studies using radiophosphate.[82,111,307,532] The relationships between daily fecal phosphorus loss and dietary phosphorus intake in patients with advanced renal failure and in normal subjects are shown in Fig. 41-21. Many observations on fecal phosphorus excretion in patients with renal failure lie above the mean regression line for normal subjects or beyond the normal limits, indicating reduced net absorption of phosphorus. The factors responsible for this mildly impaired phosphorus absorption include altered vitamin D metabolism and increased endogenous fecal phosphate losses; the latter may arise because of hyperphosphatemia, but Kopple and Coburn found no relationship between fecal phosphorus excretion and level of serum phosphorus;[285] such observations suggest that endogenous fecal losses of phosphorus are so small in relation to total fecal phosphorus that the total loss is not modified by serum phosphorus levels. Calcitriol or 1α-25-$(OH)_2D_3$ stimulates phosphorus absorption in the intestine,[560] impaired absorption of phosphorus in uremia may arise from the same abnormality in vitamin D metabolism that impairs calcium absorption.

The dietary content of phosphorus is a major determinant of serum phosphorus levels in patients with renal failure, and the intake of phosphorus can vary consider-

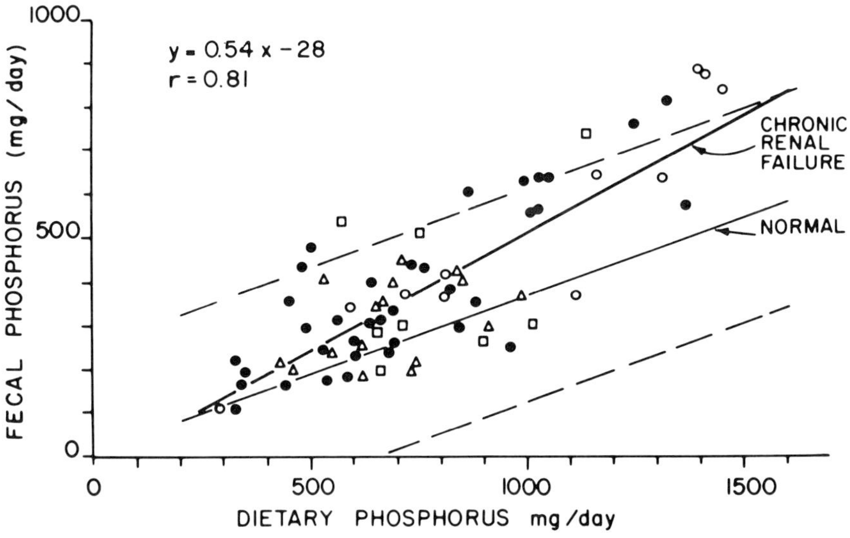

FIGURE 41-21 • Relationship between daily fecal phosphorus excretion and dietary intake of phosphorus in patients with advanced renal failure. (Regression line for normal subjects adapted from Stanbury;[532] other data collected from the literature by Coburn et al.[111]) Interrupted lines indicate 95 percent confidence limits for data for normal subjects; solid heavy line indicates regression slope for data in patients with chronic renal failure. (Reproduced, by permission of John Wiley & Sons, from Coburn et al.[111])

ably in different parts of the world. In the United States and Canada, dietary intake of phosphorus is higher than in many other parts of the world, and it is not uncommon for normal individuals to ingest 1500 to 2000 mg of phosphorus per day. In patients treated with dialysis, this quantity can fall to 1000 to 1500 mg/day, but some degree of dietary restriction is needed to reduce phosphorus intake below this level. With very low-protein diets, dietary phosphorus intake can decrease to 300 to 400 mg/day.[285] Low-protein diets, as have been instituted for the management of uremia in Italy and Germany [a substantial fraction of calories are supplied as pasta in Italy and as potatoes in Germany[178,244]] contain low amounts of phosphorus.

Calcium salts (calcium carbonate or calcium acetate) or the aluminum-containing gels, which bind phosphate in the intestine and render it nonabsorbable, are commonly employed to reduce the absorption of phosphorus in uremia. The compounds most frequently used are calcium carbonate, calcium acetate, and aluminum hydroxide or aluminum carbonate.[329,391] Because of the risk of aluminum toxicity with the long-term ingestion of aluminum gels, it would seem prudent to recommend a calcium salt, calcium carbonate or calcium acetate, as the phosphate binder of choice. A prospective comparative study of Salusky and coworkers[485] in uremic children under therapy with peritoneal dialysis showed evidence of aluminum accumulation developing in the group receiving a low and "safe" dose of aluminum-containing phosphate binder (less than 30 mg per kilogram of body weight, as recommended by Sedman and coworkers);[496] moreover, 1 of 7 children developed bone biopsy evidence of aluminum toxicity. In a study in adults, Jenkins and coworkers[257] found positive staining for aluminum in 2 of 16 patients who had received a mean dose of aluminum hydroxide capsules of 2.6 g/day for 29 to 84 months; moreover, these two patients had plasma aluminum levels as high as 116 and 205 μg/liter. The studies of the relative effectiveness of various phosphate binders carried out by Shiekh and coworkers[498] and by Mai and coworkers[329] indicate small, but probably significant, differences in the effectiveness in phosphate binding of calcium carbonate, calcium acetate, aluminum carbonate, and calcium citrate; calcium acetate and calcium carbonate were the most effective. The liquid aluminum gels are more effective in binding phosphate than are dried aluminum powders.[475] However, the liquid aluminum-containing gels are unpalatable, and compliance with the treatment regimen is difficult to achieve. The appropriate dose of calcium carbonate or aluminum hydroxide for satisfactory control of serum phosphorus levels is determined empirically, by adjustment of the dosage.

The data on the effect of these compounds collected through metabolic balance studies indicate that 75 to 200 ml/day of aluminum hydroxide gel can enhance fecal loss of phosphorus by 30 to 144 percent.[105,530] However, there was a weak relationship between the quantity of aluminum hydroxide gel taken and either the net or relative increases in fecal phosphorus excretion. When dietary phosphorus intake was below 1.0 g/day, fecal phosphorus loss exceeded dietary intake as aluminum hydroxide was added. However, with dietary phosphorus intake above 2.0 g/day, fecal phosphorus excretion was less than dietary intake despite ingestion of aluminum hydroxide gel. Thus, intake of a diet high in phosphorus content can overcome the effect of ingesting substantial amounts of a phosphate binder. Dietary phosphorus restriction in conjunction with regular ingestion of a phosphate binder is needed to prevent hyperphosphatemia in most patients with advanced renal failure and in those undergoing regular dialysis.

The effect of PTH on serum phosphorus levels is

dependent on the degree of renal insufficiency. With mild or only moderate impairment of renal function, an increase in the secretion of PTH decreases renal tubular phosphate reabsorption; serum phosphorus levels are normal or even low. However, as glomerular insufficiency progresses, the renal capacity to excrete phosphorus becomes more limited, even in the face of very high levels of PTH. The PTH continues to act on the bone, causing osteoclastic bone resorption with the release of phosphorus and calcium into the extracellular fluid. Thus PTH can increase the serum phosphorus concentration in patients with advanced renal failure and serum phosphorus levels are often higher in uremic patients with overt secondary hyperparathyroidism than in other patients with equal degrees of renal insufficiency but less-marked secondary hyperparathyroidism.[50,561] The surgical removal of the parathryoid glands in patients with advanced renal failure and overt hyperparathyroidism is almost invariably associated with a marked decrease in concentrations of both serum phosphorus and serum calcium. The serum phosphorus levels can be markedly altered in patients with little or no residual renal function by events that lead to a change in the balance between bone formation and bone resorption. The initial healing of osteomalacia or osteitis fibrosa is often associated with a fall in serum phosphorus concentration; this occurs when bone formation and the deposition of calcium and phosphorus in the skeleton are increased out of proportion to the rate of bone resorption.

The administration of active forms of vitamin D, and probably the status of body stores of vitamin D (i.e., vitamin D deficiency), can affect the serum phosphorus levels. Active forms of vitamin D can change serum phosphorus levels directly by influencing phosphorus homeostasis or indirectly through the mediation of PTH. Studies employing pharmacologic doses of vitamin D, dihydrotachysterol, or calcitriol indicate that intestinal absorption of phosphorus can be increased.[69,530,532] Stanbury and Lumb suggested that there are equimolar increments in the intestinal absorption of calcium and phosphorus in uremic patients with osteomalacia during treatment with vitamin D,[532] and it was suggested that vitamin D augments the absorption of phosphorus indirectly by affecting calcium absorption. However, studies in experimental animals clearly indicate that $1\alpha,25\text{-}(OH)_2D_3$ can augment intestinal transport of phosphorus, even in the absence of calcium in the lumen.[560] Studies with $1\alpha,25\text{-}(OH)_2D_3$ in human beings suggest that the stimulated absorption of calcium and phosphorus is not equimolar[69] (Fig. 41-22). Studies in animals indicate that phosphorus transport is stimulated by $1\alpha,25\text{-}(OH)_2D_3$ in segments of the intestine where it has little or no effect on calcium.[560] Since one action of vitamin D on phosphorus homeostasis is to enhance phosphorus absorption, serum phosphorus might be anticipated to increase following the administration of $1\alpha,25\text{-}(OH)_2D_3$ to uremic patients. However, the administration either of vitamin D in pharmacologic amounts or of $1\alpha,25\text{-}(OH)_2D_3$ often suppresses secondary hyperparathyroidism in uremic patients; this leads to reduced bone resorption with increased net deposition of calcium and phosphorus in bone. Thus the healing of vitamin D-deficiency osteomalacia is often associated with a transient decrease in serum phosphorus levels. Serum phosphorus concentration sometimes drops and a need for phosphate binders is less during the first 2 to 3 months of treatment of uremic patients with $1\alpha,25\text{-}(OH)_2D_3$; later,

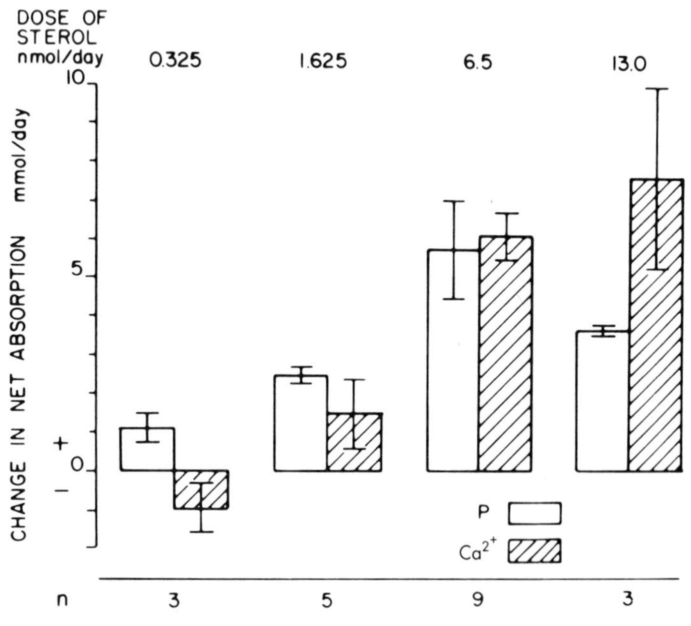

FIGURE 41-22 • The effect of $1\alpha,25\text{-}(OH)_2D_3$ or $1\alpha,25\text{-}OH\text{-}D_3$ on net absorption of calcium and phosphorus in patients with advanced reanl failure studied on a metabolic balance ward (values shown are mean ± s.e.; number of observations *n* shown below). The daily doses of $1\alpha,25\text{-}(OH)_2D_3$ of 0.325, 1.625, 6.5, and 13 nmol/day correspond to 0.13, 0.68, 2.7 and 5.4 μg/day, respectively. (Reprinted, by permission of Plenum Press, from Coburn et al.[111])

serum phosphorus levels may increase.[108] This may occur when the period of rapid skeletal remineralization is complete. If treatment with $1\alpha,25\text{-(OH)}_2D_3$ is then discontinued abruptly, serum phosphorus levels often fall.

Another mechanism whereby vitamin D may affect serum phosphorus concentration is by enhancing the intracellular flux of inorganic phosphate; thus, in vitamin D-deficient animals the administration of either vitamin D_3 or 25-OH-D_3 leads to the movement of phosphate into cells.[49] Whether this effect is important in uremic human beings in unknown.

Serum phosphorus level is also influenced by the balance between synthesis and degradation of body proteins. Thus, marked hyperphosphatemia can appear during a hypercatabolic state. Such an effect is magnified in a patient with markedly decreased renal function; even a mild infection may be associated with disproportionate increases in serum urea nitrogen and phosphorus levels compared to serum creatinine concentration. In an opposite way, periods of increased protein anabolism may be associated with the development of hypophosphatemia due to the intracellular deposition of phosphate. Hypophosphatemia may occur with refeeding following starvation or protein depletion. The administration of diets markedly restricted in protein and containing only small quantities of essential amino acids and reduced quantities of phosphate may be associated with the appearance of marked hypophosphatemia and even of hypercalcemia.[107]

The treatment of uremic patients with a protein-restricted diet containing natural foods rarely leads to hypophosphatemia, despite the limitation of phosphorus intake to 300 to 400 mg/day.[285] The administration of a diet comprising essential amino acids may stimulate protein anabolism to a degree not seen with a low-protein diet composed of natural foods, thereby decreasing serum phosphorus concentration even further. During the infusion of amino acids and hypertonic glucose for total parenteral nutrition, a substantial decrease in serum phosphorus concentration is common unless phosphorus is added to the parenteral solution (see Chap. 44). The ingestion of calcium-containing compounds may suppress PTH secretion, which can reduce the serum phosphorus levels; the phosphate-binding effect of calcium compounds is an important mechanism leading to a reduced serum phosphorus concentration.

Uremic patients generally exhibit an increase in net phosphorus absorption as dietary phosphorus content is increased. A small fraction of uremic or dialysis patients exhibit normal or slightly low levels of plasma phosphorus concentration although they ingest a normal diet and no phosphate-binding agents.[6] The reason for this is uncertain; some patients may have a greater degree of malabsorption of phosphorus than occurs in most uremic patients.[569] Osteomalacia may be more common in uremic patients fed a low-phosphate diet or given aluminum hydroxide;[178] serum phosphorus levels must be monitored during phosphate restriction.

It is apparent that several factors may have long-term or short-lived effects on serum phosphorus levels in uremic patients. Other events that can affect serum phosphorus concentration in nonuremic patients, such as acute respiratory alkalosis or metabolic alkalosis, may have an effect in uremia, but they have not been studied extensively. Whether abrupt changes in acid-base status have significant effects on serum phosphorus level in uremic patients is also unknown.

The important role of phosphate retention and hyperphosphatemia in causing or aggravating secondary hyperparathyroidism in renal insufficiency has been discussed. Hypophosphatemia may also occur and may predispose to impaired skeletal mineralization. Attention must be given to preventing both hyperphosphatemia and hypophosphatemia. Kanis and coworkers found that the number of osteoid lamellae, an index of osteomalacia, correlated inversely with the level of serum phosphorus in a large population of dialysis patients[263] (Fig. 41-13).

No data are available to indicate whether phosphate depletion ever occurs without a fall in serum phosphorus concentration to subnormal levels. Patients with stable chronic uremia and those undergoing dialysis can be in negative balance and yet exhibit modest hyperphosphatemia.[285] The negative phosphorus balance of uremic patients does not correlate with the balance of either nitrogen or calcium, suggesting that excess phosphorus is deposited in soft tissues.[285] Body composition data from neutron activation studies provide support for this view.[299,300]

A possible role of hyperphosphatemia and phosphate retention in either accelerating or aggravating the progression of renal failure itself has been suggested from observations in experimental animals.[252] The use of a very low-phosphate diet in partially nephrectomized rats is associated with little or no progression of renal insufficiency, whereas renal failure progressed in animals receiving normal dietary levels of phosphate.[252] However, very low-phosphate diets lead to reduced intake of food and protein, and it was difficult to separate an effect of dietary phosphate restriction from the effect of a reduction in protein intake in initial studies. More recently, other data indicate that the inhibition of dietary phosphate absorption independent of protein can retard the progression of renal insufficiency in rats following partial nephrectomy.[325] The tissue levels of calcium and phosphorus in the kidney are increased compared to the levels in other tissues from patients with advanced renal failure, raising the possibility that the accumulation of calcium and phosphorus within renal tissue may be one mechanism for the progression of renal damage.[325] In the study of Lumlertgul and coworkers[325] noted above, phosphate absorption was reduced by giving dihydroxyaluminum aminoacetate to the phosphate-restricted rats, while the phosphate-replete group received glycine; the groups were pair-fed to ensure similar intakes of total calories, protein, carbohydrate, vitamins, and minerals. The tissue content of calcium in the heart, aorta, and kidneys was higher in the phosphate-replete group than in the phosphate-restricted animals; however, there was more glomerular sclerosis, interstitial inflammation with fibrosis, and greater tubular atrophy in the phosphate-replete rats. In clinical studies, Barsotti and coworkers[37] prospectively compared two groups of patients with moderate renal insufficiency who were placed on low-protein diets, one group receiving a low-phosphate diet that provided phosphorus, 6.5 mg per kilogram of body weight, while the other group consumed a diet with 12 mg phosphorus per kilogram of body weight per day. The rate of progression of renal failure, as judged by either the rate of increase in serum creatinine with time or the decrease in creatinine clearance, was greater in the group ingesting the higher phosphorus intake. Thus these data suggest that there may be some benefit in reducing phosphate intake, with regard to the progression of renal failure; further experience with this approach will be needed.

HYPOCALCEMIA

A fall in total serum calcium concentration occurs, but not invariably, in patients with advanced renal failure. Although both the mean total serum calcium level and the ionized calcium level are significantly lower in patients with advanced renal failure (creatinine clearance 5 to 20 ml/min) than in normal subjects, total serum calcium levels were below normal (that is, below the lower limits of normal) in only 40 percent of uremic patients.[117] Moreover, levels below 7.5 mg/100 ml were infrequent. The fraction of complexed calcium is increased in patients with advanced uremia because of increased binding of calcium to various anions.[561] If the fraction of complexed calcium increases substantially, the level of ionized blood calcium may be normal despite a normal total serum calcium level. A similar phenomenon can occur immediately after hemodialysis as hemoconcentration increases the protein-bound calcium component.[450] Acidosis can decrease the degree of protein binding, and marked acidosis—present in some uremic patients—may induce this effect in vivo.

The value of measuring the ionized calcium in patients with renal disease is exemplified by the results in patients with the nephrotic syndrome. A low total serum calcium level would be expected in such patients because of the very low level of serum albumin, although it might be assumed that the ionized calcium level is normal in such patients. However, the measurement of ionized calcium with an ion-specific electrode has revealed a decreased level of ionized calcium in such patients.[209]

Decreases in the levels of total and ionized calcium are observed in stable chronic uremia in persons with markedly increased serum creatinine concentration; however, the range of individual values was wide. The initiation of regular hemodialysis is often associated with an increase in total serum calcium concentration toward normal.[107,573] This increase in serum calcium concentration has been observed despite persistent hyperphosphatemia and during the use of dialysate calcium of 2.5 meq/liter.[107] This observation, made several years ago when the control of hyperphosphatemia was poor, points to the existence of some unknown factor, related to dialysis per se, that promotes correction of uremic hypocalcemia. When dialysis is carried out with more modern techniques, the incidence of hypocalcemia is quite low and hypercalcemia becomes a more common problem.[508]

HYPERCALCEMIA IN CHRONIC RENAL FAILURE

Hypercalcemia occurs in patients with renal failure, particularly those undergoing hemodialysis. The recognized causes of hypercalcemia in patients with advanced renal failure are listed in Table 41-2. A greater degree of symptoms of hypercalcemia may occur in these patients than in patients with normal renal function. The cause of hypercalcemia in a patient with renal insufficiency should be delineated; in particular, aluminum toxicity and low bone turnover disease must be separated from overt secondary hyperparathyroidism as the cause, since the management can be so different.

Transient hypercalcemia can occur in uremic patients who ingest large quantities of calcium carbonate or calcium acetate during treatment with vitamin D sterols, and in some, but not all, dialysis patients after the prolonged

TABLE 41-2 • Conditions associated with hypercalcemia in patients with renal failure

Severe secondary hyperparathyroidism
Aluminum-related bone disease
Low bone turnover (even without aluminum bone deposits)
High calcium intake (as phosphate binders)
Treatment with vitamin D sterols
Use of high-calcium dialysate (particularly CAPD)
Phosphate restriction and hypophosphatemia
Immobilization (often associated with the first three items above)
Administration of thiazide diuretics
Use of calcium-cycle ion exchange resins
Use of low-protein or amino acid diets (usually low in phosphate)
Coexistence of other diseases causing hypercalcemia (e.g., multiple myeloma, malignancy)
High calcitriol levels (sarcoidosis, tuberculosis, etc.)
Recovery phase of acute renal failure
After successful renal transplantation

use of dialysate with a calcium concentration of 7 to 8 mg/100 ml (3.0 to 4.0 meq/liter). Hypercalcemia can occur in patients with severe or "overt" secondary hyperparathyroidism; such hypercalcemia may appear within weeks to months after hemodialysis has been initiated. Such hypercalcemia probably occurs because of a marked shift in the "set point" for suppression of PTH by calcium.

In the absence of high serum PTH levels or radiographic or histologic evidence of osteitis fibrosa, high levels of PTH cannot be assumed to be responsible for elevated serum calcium concentration. Persistent elevation of serum calcium levels is not uncommon among dialysis patients with aluminum accumulation and aluminum-related bone disease. X-rays may show only "osteopenia," but subperiosteal erosions may persist from earlier hyperparathyroidism that failed to mineralize when the PTH levels were lowered with the development of aluminum accumulation.[506] The hypercalcemia associated with aluminum accumulation may appear or become worse when these patients receive oral calcium salts and/or small doses of vitamin D sterols, are treated with dialysate containing a calcium concentration of 3.5 meq/liter or higher, or are immobilized.[63,400] The mechanism for the hypercalcemia in patients with aluminum-related bone disease has been evaluated by Rodriguez and coworkers. Thus, aluminum increases calcium binding in the plasma and decreases the concentration of ionized calcium, which in turn mobilizes calcium from bone and interstitium into the vascular space, leading to an increase in total calcium concentration.[465]

Hypercalcemia can occur during treatment with calcium carbonate[241,483,522] or calcium acetate,[487] with the use of a calcium-containing exchange resin,[413] in association with marked phosphate restriction and hypophosphatemia,[107] in conjunction with immobilization, and during the ingestion of thiazide diuretics.[284] Uremic patients may also develop hypercalcemia due to associated illnesses—for example, multiple myeloma or malignancy. They may develop hypercalcemia due to uncontrolled extrarenal synthesis of calcitriol—for example, in sarcoidosis[35] or tuberculosis.[173] The hypercalcemia may also be prolonged and more difficult to treat in uremic patients because the absence of renal function eliminates the body's ability to excrete the calcium mobilized from bone, absorbed through the intestine, or entering from dialysate.

HYPERMAGNESEMIA

Serum magnesium levels are commonly elevated in patients with advanced renal insufficiency. The homeostasis of magnesium in renal failure has received less attention than has the study of calcium or phosphorus metabolism. Normally the kidney provides for the regulation of body magnesium; hence, the loss of renal excretory capability leads to altered homeostasis for this major intracellular cation. Studies of Mg^{2+} balance suggest that its net absorption does not deviate markedly from normal in patients with advanced renal failure,[111] although the absorption may be modestly decreased.[65] With normal intestinal absorption and reduced renal excretion, a tendency to develop hypermagnesemia can be readily understood.

Serum magnesium levels generally are normal unless the creatinine clearance rate is below 30 ml/min.[117] At a further level of deficit in renal function, a larger number of uremic patients exhibit increased serum magnesium concentrations. Approximately 20 percent of magnesium is bound to albumin, a fraction that is unchanged in renal failure despite an increase in total serum magnesium level.[15,117] The increase in serum magnesium levels is associated with an increase in skeletal magnesium content;[15,117] this may have an adverse effect on crystal formation in bone.[17]

There is little evidence that intracellular stores of magnesium are altered in uremia. A reduced cellular magnesium concentration is commonly associated with malnutrition and diminished intracellular potassium concentration.[15]

Whether intestinal handling of magnesium may be altered in uremia is controversial. Its net absorption has been normal, and yet the jejunal and ileal transport of magnesium has been reported to be reduced in uremic patients, as studied by perfusion of different intestinal segments. Treatment with calcitriol restores the magnesium transport of a perfused intestine to normal,[554] and yet there has been no detectable effect of either $1\alpha,25\text{-(OH)}_2D_3$ or $1\alpha\text{-OH-}D_3$ on net intestinal absorption[111] (Fig. 41-23). The reasons for discrepancies between results from intestinal perfusion studies and those from metabolic balance conditions have not been determined. It is possible that magnesium transport is impaired in one portion of the intestine while it is normal or even increased in others, resulting in normal net magnesium absorption through the entire gut.

A small increase in magnesium intake in patients with advanced renal failure generally leads to an equal increase in urinary excretion of magnesium, suggesting that patients accumulate magnesium only very slowly.[285] In the usual patient with advanced renal failure who is not under treatment with dialysis, the major factor that affects serum magnesium level and produces hypermagnesemia is an increase in dietary magnesium intake. With the intake of magnesium-containing antacids or magnesium-containing cathartics, abrupt and marked hypermagnesemia may occur. An increase in magnesium concentration may also occur when magnesium-containing enemas are given. In uremic patients undergoing dialysis, the level of magnesium in the dialysate is a major factor influencing serum magnesium level. Based on tradition, many dialysis centers have used dialysate which contains magnesium in a concentration of 1.5 meq/liter, a

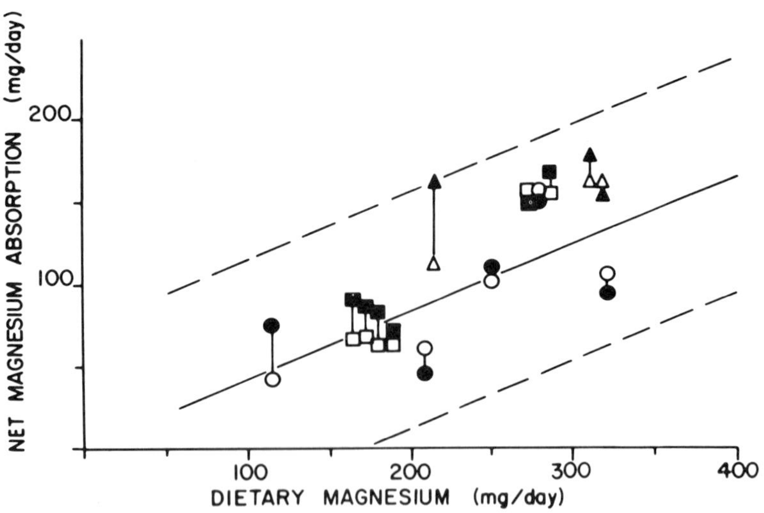

FIGURE 41-23 • The effect of 1α,25-$(OH)_2D_3$ and 1α,-OH-D_3 on net intestinal magnesium absorption in normal individuals (*triangles*) and patients with stable advanced renal failure (*circles, squares*). Open symbols, pretreatment values; closed symbols, measurements taken during treatment. Patients with renal failure received either 1α25-$(OH)_2D_3$ (○) or 1α-OH-D_3 (□); normal subjects received 1α,25-$(OH)_2D_3$. Solid line and interrupted lines represent slope of regression line and 95 percent confidence limits for net magnesium absorption in normal individuals. (Reprinted, by permission of Wiley, from Coburn et al.[111])

value similar to the non-protein-bound or diffusible level in normal serum. With use of this dialysate magnesium concentration, elevated blood magnesium levels of 2.5 to 4.0 meq/liter are common.[117] The use of dialysate that contains magnesium in a concentration of 0.5 to 0.7 meq/liter results in serum magnesium concentrations close to normal in most dialysis patients.[76]

The clinical consequences of hypermagnesemia and increased skeletal content of this cation in uremia have not been resolved. Most uremic patients exhibit no known sequelae from the steady-state moderate hypermagnesemia, although the hypothermia of uremia has been attributed, in part, to magnesium retention.[190] When the serum magnesium concentration is increased to levels above 3.5 to 5.0 meq/liter, flushing and burning of the skin may occur. Such symptoms have developed when the water purification system used for preparing dialysate has suddenly failed.[191] An abrupt and marked elevation of serum magnesium can suppress the secretion of PTH.[226,348] However, no convincing data are available to suggest that long-standing hypermagnesemia can reduce PTH secretion; moreover, any suppressive effect of hypermagnesemia on PTH secretion would be completely and rapidly offset by the stimulation of the parathyroid glands produced by hypocalcemia.

When patients with renal insufficiency also have intestinal malabsorption, poor nutritional intake, or marked renal magnesium wasting, hypomagnesemia can develop. Such hypomagnesemia impairs the secretion of PTH, with resultant marked hypocalcemia.[374]

PLASMA ALKALINE PHOSPHATASE, HYDROXYPROLINE, cAMP, AND GLA-PROTEIN

Alkaline phosphatase

Serum alkaline phosphatase is made up of iso-enzymes that arise from the intestine, liver, kidney, and bone. Despite the heterogeneity of this enzyme, the measurement of total alkaline phosphatase activity can provide a rough indication of increased osteoblastic activity; moreover, studies of isoenzymes have shown that the increased alkaline phosphatase in uremia arises most commonly from bone.[395,514] Serum total enzyme levels have been found to be commonly increased in association with osteitis fibrosa, osteomalacia, or mixed lesions, although markedly elevated levels are said to be more characteristic of osteitis fibrosa with its high rate of bone turnover.[18] Nonetheless, the serial measurement of plasma alkaline phosphatase activity can provide a useful clinical guide for monitoring the therapy of skeletal disease with calcium compounds and/or vitamin D sterols. Serial measurements can also identify the slow progression of skeletal disease, particularly osteitis fibrosa, in a uremic patient. It should be kept in mind that uremic patients can have significant and overt skeletal disease and yet have normal plasma alkaline phosphatase levels. Thus, a major pitfall to avoid is the assumption that normal alkaline phosphatase activity indicates the absence of significant skeletal disease in any individual patient. In studies of large numbers of patients, alkaline phosphatase activities correlate with skeletal histologic features of secondary hyperparathyroidism; thus, alkaline phosphatase activity correlates positively with percentage of osteoblastic surface and percent of active resorption surface.[158,458] Plasma alkaline phosphatase levels in patients with aluminum-related bone disease (osteomalacia or aplastic bone disease) were normal in some reports despite the presence of severe disease,[18,436] but elevated alkaline phosphatase activities were reported by other authors.[245,246] For this reason, the alkaline phosphatase may not discriminate between aluminum-related bone disease and osteitis fibrosa.

Hepatic abnormalities are common in patients undergoing regular dialysis, and it is essential that liver disease be excluded as a cause of an elevated alkaline phosphatase activity. Isoenzymes of alkaline phosphatase can allow identification of such sources other than bone,[514] but these determinations may not be readily available. A practical clinical approach is to measure the γ-glutamyl transferase (GGT) or leucine aminopeptidase activity when the alkaline phosphatase is elevated. The finding of a normal value for the activity of one of these enzymes of hepatic origin can largely exclude the liver as the source of elevated alkaline phosphatase levels.

Hydroxyproline and cAMP

Peptides containing both peptide-bound and free hydroxyproline are released with the degradation of bone collagen; normally, both the free and peptide-bound hydroxyproline are excreted in the urine.[447] In patients with impaired urinary excretion due to renal failure, the plasma levels of both free and peptide-bound hydroxyproline are elevated. With any increase in bone resorption and collagen degradation plasma levels of hydroxyproline will increase even further.[286] Varghese and colleagues reported that total plasma hydroxyproline can provide a valuable index to assess the extent of bone resorption and to evaluate the response to therapy.[552] The plasma levels of hydroxyproline fell in association with improvement of skeletal disease that followed partial parathyroidectomy or treatment with $1\alpha,25\text{-}(OH)_2D_3$. Hart and coworkers have noted that the plasma concentration of free, but not peptide-bound, hydroxyproline correlates with bone histologic features that suggest increased bone resorption.[230] Despite these claims for its utility, the determination of hydroxyproline has not gained wide popularity.

Plasma levels of cAMP can be increased in uremic patients; normally, the plasma levels of cAMP reflect the activity of PTH.[229] However, no correlation has been found between plasma cAMP levels and the degree of secondary hyperparathyroidism, and the levels can remain elevated for some time after parathyroidectomy.[229] The reason for the presence of elevated levels of cAMP in patients with renal failure is unknown; it may be related to catecholamines or other peptide hormones.

Osteocalcin (bone GLA-protein)

Osteocalcin, or bone GLA-protein (BGP or α-carboxyglutamic acid), is an abundant noncollagenous protein from bone that appears in the plasma.[446] Its concentrations in plasma reflect bone turnover,[143,525] but the plasma levels are also increased when renal function is impaired due to reduced plasma clearance of the BGP.[142,225] In a study of 30 patients undergoing regular dialysis, good correlations were found between the plasma levels of bone GLA-protein and histologic parameters of bone turnover and the degree of peritrabecular fibrosis.[334] The osteocalcin levels averaged 8 times the normal value in the dialysis patients with "low-turnover renal bone disease," but the values were increased to greater than 40 times normal in all the patients with "high-turnover bone disease." The level of osteocalcin did provide a better separation of the two disorders than either alkaline phosphatase or N-terminal PTH. In another study of 42 patients with mild to severe chronic renal failure [serum creatinine 4.3 ± 2.0 mg/dl (mean ± SD)] the levels of osteocalcin were above normal in over 80 percent of the patients.[121] There was a direct relationship between serum osteocalcin levels and the serum creatinine level, pointing out an important role of renal function in determining the level of this peptide. In addition, there was a progressive rise in osteocalcin levels with time in the patients who were not treated with calcitriol. In the latter group the osteocalcin levels either stabilized or fell. These observations indicate that the levels of osteocalcin may identify different conditions affecting bone in patients with renal failure. But the degree of renal insufficiency affects the osteocalcin level, and it is not yet possible to identify an individual renal patient as having a specific condition with a high or low bone turnover from the results of serum osteocalcin levels.

SERUM PTH

Serum PTH levels, as noted earlier, are commonly elevated in patients with renal insufficiency; the degree of elevation may be striking. Serum levels are dramatically elevated when measured with an anti-serum directed primarily toward the midregion or the carboxy terminus of the PTH molecule, while the degree of elevation is far less when PTH concentration is measured with an antiserum directed toward the amino terminus.[520] With the advent of sensitive- immunoradiometric assays (IRMA) for the secreted intact PTH molecule, the evaluation of dialysis patients with secondary hyperparathyroidism is easier and in many instances the performance of bone biopsy may be avoided. In the past the conventional radioimmunoassay of PTH was limited by the measurement of biologically inactive midterminal and carboxyterminal fragments generated by the metabolism of the hormone; this is even more important in patients with renal insufficiency, since these fragments are cleared via the kidney. The IRMA assays for PTH have high specificity and sensitivity as well as excellent precision, allowing measurement within and below the normal range. In addition to the diagnostic value, the IRMA assays have helped in the evaluation of parathyroid function of dialysis patients.[155]

However, a large number of commercially available conventional radioimmunoassays (RIA) for serum PTH provide no information about the predictive value of a given serum PTH level with regard to the severity of osteitis fibrosa present. Thus, the discrimination between RIA-measured PTH levels in normal subjects from values in patients with primary hyperparathyroidism[19] provides little or no information about the meaning of a PTH level so measured in a patient with end-stage renal disease. Fortunately, the IRMA assays provide correlative data between serum PTH levels and histologic features of bone disease in uremic patients.

Although pathogenic mechanisms responsible for elevating serum PTH levels exist in all patients with reduced renal function, serum PTH levels are sometimes normal or undectectable. Such a finding may occur in uremic patients with hypomagnesemia;[374] also, low or normal levels of serum PTH are often found in dialysis patients with aluminum-related bone disease.[19,315]

It has been popular to consider that in certain uremic patients with marked hyperplasia secretion of PTH is "autonomous;" however, most evidence suggests that serum PTH levels do fall during either a calcium infusion or dialysis using a high calcium level in the dialysate. It is often necessary for serum calcium concentration to be raised to hypercalcemic levels before PTH falls. The two factors that contribute to this are massive hyperplasia and a change in the set point for PTH suppression by calcium. Massive hyperplasia of the parathyroid glands often exists; serum PTH concentration may rise as a consequence of the increased parathyroid gland mass for any serum calcium level, since basal secretion of PTH continues despite hypercalcemia.[74] Parathyroid hyperplasia per se increases this basal secretion in proportion to the increased number of cells. A change in the set point of extracellular calcium concentration needed to reduce the PTH secretion of parathyroid cells by 50 percent is of even greater consequence.[74] Recent data discussed earlier demonstrate that dialysis patients with secondary hyperparathyroidism have a significant shift of the set point for calcium to the right.[155]

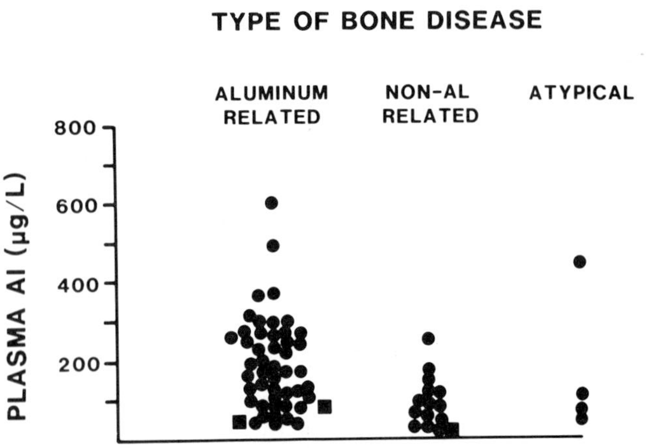

FIGURE 41-24 • Plasma aluminum levels in patients with bone biopsies done because of suspected renal osteodystrophy. Aluminum-related disorders comprise osteomalacia or aplastic disease; non-aluminum-related diseases include other types of bone disease with no aluminum staining. Each symbol represents one patient (Modified from Milliner et al: *Ann Intern Med* 101:775, 1984. Used by permission.)

PLASMA ALUMINUM LEVELS AND THE DESFERRIOXAMINE INFUSION TEST

Endothermal atomic absorption spectroscopy provides an accurate means to measure plasma aluminum levels, although substantial differences in normal serum values have been reported from one laboratory to another. The use of an international quality assessment program has improved the precision and accuracy of aluminum measurement in Europe.[222] Tissue and plasma aluminum levels are substantially above normal in most patients with end-stage renal disease, particularly those who have taken phosphate binders containing aluminum.[12,565] Plasma aluminum concentration laregly reflects the recent "load" of aluminum, and the plasma concentration does not correlate highly with tissue stores.[11,575] However, most patients with aluminum-related bone disease have markedly elevated plasma aluminum concentrations (e.g., $>$ 40 to 75 μg/liter, compared to levels of 2 to 8 μg/liter in normal patients) (Fig. 41-24). Also, patients with markedly elevated plasma aluminum levels (e.g., values above 150 to 200 μg/liter) are very likely to develop aluminum-related bone disease and/or encephalopathy if the exposure to aluminum continues.[575] In a large population study[429] there were higher alkaline phosphatase levels and lower erythrocyte cell volume in dialysis patients with plasma aluminum levels above 100 μg/liter compared to the group with levels below 100 μg/liter. In yet another study, electroencephalographic features of encephalopathy were found in 8 of 27 patients with plasma aluminum levels above 100 μg/liter compared to none among 24 patients with plasma aluminum below 50 μg/liter.[470] It is of interest that only 5 of the 8 patients had any clinical manifestations of encephalopathy. In the former group, with plasma aluminum levels above 100 μg/liter, the 8 patients with abnormal EEGs had higher plasma levels than the 19 patients with normal EEGs.

In patients who have been totally withdrawn from aluminum-containing binders for six months or longer, the plasma aluminum levels are far less helpful in identifying those with clinically significant aluminum accumulation (e.g., greater than 25 percent surface stainable aluminum and subnormal bone formation rate). We have seen plasma aluminum levels as low as 21 μg/liter in a patient with biopsy evidence of aluminum-related bone disease when the ingestion of all aluminum-containing binders was discontinued 18 months earlier.[402]

There has been some uncertainty about the value of monitoring plasma aluminum concentrations at regular intervals in dialysis patients. Measuring plasma aluminum every 3 to 4 months has been recommended by some authors.[575] Marked elevation of plasma aluminum levels (e.g., above 40 to 75 μg/liter) in the majority of patients in a dialysis unit indicates that there has been exposure to unacceptably high concentrations of aluminum in the dialysate. This may arise because the water treatment system has malfunctioned at some time in the recent past. Since aluminum contamination may vary from time to time, the concentration of aluminum in water or dialysate may be normal or acceptable when water or dialysate is sampled. When only a few patients exhibit plasma aluminum levels above 75 to 100 μg/liter, those who are ingesting excessive amounts of aluminum-containing gels or absorbing excess aluminum from the phosphate binders can be identified.

Measurement of the increment in plasma aluminum concentration following a standardized infusion of the chelating agent desferrioxamine has been proposed as a method to recognize dialysis patients with increased aluminum stores and a greater risk of aluminum-related bone disease[382] (Fig. 41-25). The relationship between the increment in plasma aluminum following an infusion of desferrioxamine and the total aluminum content in bone is closer than that between the basal plasma aluminum and the bone aluminum content. However, not all patients with elevated tissue levels of aluminum have evidence of aluminum-related bone disease;[245] aluminum may not be distributed in tissues similarly in all patients, and a given quantity of aluminum in a tissue may not always be pathogenic. Other observations indicate that results may be helpful as a screening test, but they are not highly specific. When there has been total withdrawal from aluminum exposure (dialysate aluminum concentration below 10 μg/liter and all aluminum-containing phosphate binders withdrawn), the increment in plasma aluminum after desferrioxamine falls substantially. Nonetheless, such patients can show features of aluminum toxicity, with significant aluminum staining and reduced bone formation rate. Thus a certain pool of bone aluminum may be very resistant to removal, or is removed very slowly.[551] The latter is particularly likely in a patient who has had prior parathyroidectomy and in whom serum iPTH levels remain low. Several factors may account for the variable results with the use of the desferrioxamine infusion test in the recognition of aluminum toxicity. The initial studies were done in patients with marked aluminum loading and severe symptomatic aluminum toxicity; moreover, the patients continued either to be exposed to inappropriately elevated dialysate aluminum levels or to ingest aluminum-containing gels.

Studies in patients with mild aluminum toxicity indicate that the rise in plasma aluminum after desferrioxamine correlates well with bone aluminum content but less well with bone histology.[137] A recent report of the combined use of results of an intact PTH assay (IRMA) and the desferrioxamine infusion test may provide the optimal means to identify patients with aluminum-related bone disease: The finding of an intact PTH level (IRMA) below 160 pg/ml and an increment of plasma aluminum, after desferrioxamine infusion of 100 μg/liter provided a positive predictive value of 86 percent, a specificity of 97 percent (i.e., only 3 percent false-positive), and a sensitivity of 50 percent.[424] It is apparent that in certain instances a bone biopsy is required for the diagnosis.

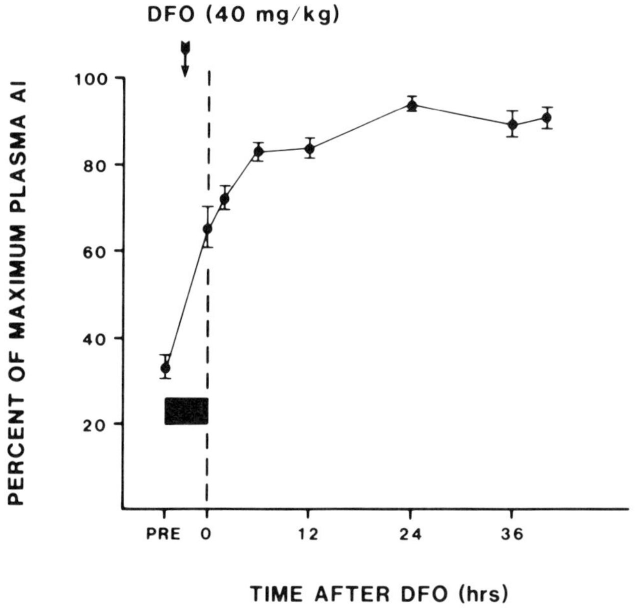

FIGURE 41-25 • Changes in plasma aluminum concentration with time after standardized infusion of 40 mg of deferoxamine (DFO) per kilogram of body weight, given after hemodialysis to patients with proven aluminum-related bone disease. Values are expressed as percent of maximum value; peak levels occurred by 24 h. (Adapted from Milliner et al: *Ann Intern Med* 101:775, 1984, by permission.)

CLINICAL SIGNS AND SYMPTOMS OF OSTEODYSTROPHY

The symptoms that appear in association with osteodystrophy are usually subtle and insidious in their onset. Although fortunately not common, bone pain may develop and slowly progress to produce total disability.[577] This can occur independently of skeletal pathology, whether primarily osteitis fibrosa, osteomalacia, or a mixture of both. The pain is generally vague and deep-seated and may be located in the low back, hips, knees, or legs. It often varies in intensity and is often aggravated by weight bearing or by sudden movement or pressure. Occasionally pain is localized around the knee, ankle, or heel, and it may be of such sudden appearance as to suggest acute arthritis. Pain in the low back may arise from collapse of a vertebral body; sharp chest pain may be the first indication of a rib fracture that has occurred during a cough, sneeze, or even during normal breathing. A change in position, such as sitting up from the supine position or spontaneous rolling over during sleep, may evoke generalized pain throughout the back, hips, and chest. The pain is not relieved by massage or local heat, and the patient usually perceives it as being more deeply seated than in the joints or muscles.

The severity of symptoms often does not correlate closely with radiologic or histologic changes. Thus, severely abnormal skeletal x-rays or bone biopsies may be found in patients who are totally asymptomatic. Patients undergoing regular hemodialysis who are normally active and totally without symptoms may develop, within several weeks to months, such severe pain as to make walking across a room difficult. Others experience such slow and gradual progression of symptoms that little notice is given until total debility has occurred.

Physical findings are frequently lacking; occasionally, localized tenderness may be apparent with pressure on the chest wall or lateral compression of the pelvis; tenderness may also be localized over the vertebral spinous processes or rib.

MYOPATHY AND MUSCLE WEAKNESS

Muscular weakness, largely limited to the proximal musculature, can be a serious and debilitating problem in patients with renal osteodystrophy. The afflicted patient may be confined to a wheelchair or may be unable to hold his or her arms above the head because of shoulder-girdle weakness. This myopathy resembles in many ways the muscle weakness reported in vitamin D deficiency.[49,494] In both forms of myopathy plasma levels of muscle enzymes, such as creatine phosphokinase, are usually normal, and electromyographic abnormalities are either absent or nonspecific. The muscle weakness appears slowly, with the patient unable to climb stairs easily or to rise from a sitting position without help. The gait may become abnormal so that the patient waddles from side to side in a "penguin" style.

Proximal muscle weakness can be caused by secondary hyperparathyroidism, abnormal metabolism of vitamin D, or aluminum loading.[332] Striking improvement in muscle weakness has been observed in some uremic patients following the administration of either 1α,25-$(OH)_2D_3$ (1 to 5 μg/day) or 25-OH-D_3 (10 to 100 μg/day).[70,234] Muscle biopsy, carried out in selected patients, has revealed mild, nonspecific myopathic alterations by light microscopy and severe degenerative changes by electron microscopic examination.[182] In three patients with mild to severe muscle weakness, electron micrographs revealed localized areas of severe disorganization of the myofibrils, with dispersion of Z band materials; the latter reverted to normal following treatment with 25-OH-D_3.[493]

Not all muscle abnormalities present in uremia can be attributed to altered vitamin D metabolism, because features of protein-calorie malnutrition are common in uremia; decreases in alkali-soluble protein, as described in muscle from uremic patients, may contribute to muscle dysfunction.[141] It has been suggested that muscular weakness may arise in secondary hyperparathyroidism on a neuropathic basis; uremic polymyopathy, whatever its pathogenesis, may contribute to muscular weakness.[256,332] Muscle weakness in uremic patients can promptly improve following treatment with 1α,25-$(OH)_2D_3$ before serum PTH levels fall, or with doses that are too low to reduce serum PTH;[70,234] this points to a role of altered vitamin D metabolism rather than secondary hyperparathyroidism in certain patients. However, muscle weakness may be profound in patients with aluminum-related bone disease; moreover, striking improvement has occurred after aluminum removal with desferrioxamine, with little change in PTH status and without vitamin D therapy.[396]

PRURITUS

Itching, a common symptom in patients with advanced renal failure, often improves and may disappear following initiation of regular hemodialysis. However, pruritus sometimes persists and is of such intensity that it prevents sleep and interferes with a patient's normal activities. Pruritus can be severe in patients with clinically evident secondary hyperparathyroidism; pruritus may improve or, indeed, totally disappear within a few days after partial parathyroidectomy.[354] The mechanism whereby secondary hyperparathyroidism can lead to pruritus is uncertain. Elevated levels of calcium in the skin have been reported in such patients.[354] However, the increased calcium content in the skin probably is not responsible for the itching, because the symptom improves within a few days following surgery, while much more time is required before the skin calcium falls. Moreover, reversible itching may develop in uremic patients with the administration of pharmacologic doses of vitamin D and during infusions of calcium; such observations suggest that an elevated concentration of ionic calcium in the ECF may be an important factor contributing to pruritus. Observations that uremic pruritus may be relieved following the intravenous injection of lidocaine,[541] irradiation with ultraviolet light,[199] or ingestion of activated charcoal[423] point to the fact that uremic pruritus is multifactorial in its cause. In the absence of specific evidence of secondary hyperparathyroidism—i.e., very high levels of PTH, radiographic evidence of erosions, and/or bone biopsy features of osteitis fibrosa—parathyroid surgery should not be done. However, the presence of refractory pruritus in a patient with renal failure should direct a clinician to seek evidence of overt and severe secondary hyperparathyroidism.

CALCIPHYLAXIS

The occurrence of an unusual clinical entity, typified by peripheral ischemic necrosis, vascular calcification, and cutaneous ulcerations, has been noted for many years in isolated patients with chronic renal failure.[202,351] This syndrome usually appears in patients with end-stage renal disease and is usually associated with a long-standing history of renal failure, although patients have developed the syndrome following successful renal transplantation. The syndrome has been observed in association with renal diseases of varying causes; there has been no predilection for a specific age or sex.

The skin lesions make their appearances as superficial violacious discolorations in a mottled, circumscribed pattern involving the tips of the toes or fingers or occurring about the ankles, thighs, or buttocks. The lesions are often accompanied by pain. As the lesions progress, they become hemorrhagic with ischemic, "dry" necrosis. Frequently, boring ulcerations and eschar formation occur; lesions of the terminal phalanges are often clearly demarcated and toe or fingertips may even fall off (Fig. 41-26). Such lesions resemble those that accompany vasculitis; however, biopsy specimens fail to show fibrinoid necrosis or granulomatous inflammation. All patients with these lesions have demonstrated evidence of medical calcinosis of small- and medium-sized arteries; skin biopsies generally reveal the presence of medial calcification and intimal thickening. Ischemic myolysis, ischemic cardiac disease, and hemorrhagic panniculitis have been reported in individual cases.

The pathogenesis of this syndrome is uncertain. Extensive medial calcinosis of arteries can occur in patients with renal failure and yet not lead to gangrene and ulceration; however, the possibility has been considered that calcium deposition may give rise to mechanical obstruction. The favorable response of some patients within several days of parathyroidectomy suggests that mechanical obstruction cannot totally explain the ischemia. Vascular spasms related to either hypercalcemia[567] or an effect of PTH itself[96] may be implicated. The occurrence of such lesions after renal transplantation in patients receiving glucocorticoids raises the possibility that steroids may play a role.[202] Selye showed that this syndrome was more common in animals if they had been given large doses of glucocorticoids.[497]

Most uremic patients presenting with this syndrome either previously had, or now have, evidence of overt secondary hyperparathyroidism;[202] most patients have shown substantial improvement following partial parathyroidectomy. Without treatment the lesions often progress with varying degrees of rapidity; a number of afflicted patients have died, usually from secondary infection.[202] Because of the poor prognosis, partial parathyroidectomy is recommended when such lesions appear in conjunction with evidence of secondary hykperparathyroidism (i.e., high serum PTH concentration and gone erosions).[202] Severe phosphate restriction may be useful in the absence of evidence of hyperparathyroidism.[202]

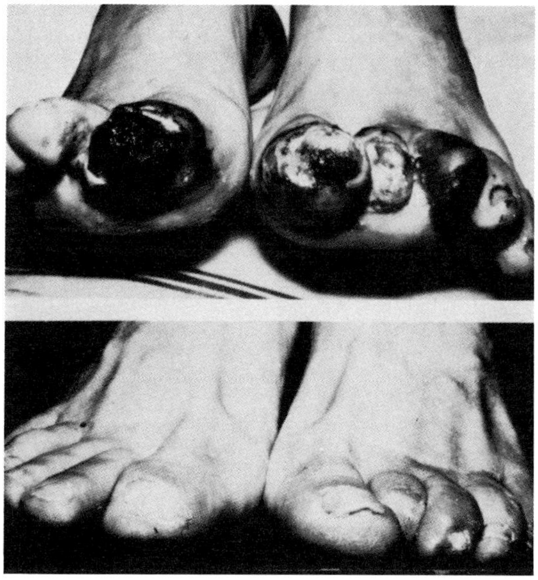

FIGURE 41-26 • Ischemic and necrotic lesions of the feet which appeared after successful renal transplantation (*top*) in a patient with hypercalcemia due to secondary hyperparathyroidism. The lesions healed within 3 to 4 months following partial parathyroidectomy (*bottom*). (Reprinted, by permission, from Massry SG et al: *Arch Intern Med* 124:431, 1969.)

PERIARTHRITIS

Acute pain, redness, and swelling around one or more joints can develop due to altered metabolism of calcium and phosphorus in uremia. Rarely, pain may occur in the ankle or foot without local signs except for vague tenderness and can be associated with radiographic changes of subperiosteal resorption and/or periosteal new bone formation.[320] This syndrome probably reflects overt secondary hyperparathyroidism; the affected patients usually have high levels of serum alkaline phosphatase activity, calcium-phosphorus product, and PTH levels compared with other dialysis patients.[320] Further evidence that such symptoms are related to secondary hyperparathyroidism is provided by the observation that such discomfort can disappear completely within 1 to 2 weeks following partial parathyroidectomy.

Occasionally, calcium deposits may be observed radiographically about the affected joints. Synovial biopsy may reveal crystals that, when studied by x-ray diffraction, are characteristic of hydroxyapatite. This syndrome must be differentiated from pseudogout or gouty arthritis; the last two are characterized by a true monoarticular arthritis and can be differentiated by the identification of specific crystals of either urate or calcium pyrophosphate within the synovial fluid.[320] In general, this syndrome responds well to treatment with anti-inflammatory agents such as indomethacin; parathyroidectomy, as mentioned above, may lead to marked improvement.

SPONTANEOUS TENDON RUPTURE

Spontaneous tendon rupture also occurs in patients with long-standing renal failure; it is usually associated with evidence of marked secondary hyperparathyroidism.[324] The syndrome has been reported in association with primary hyperparathyroidism and other causes of secondary hyperparathyroidism;[103,444,445] it has been suggested that an abnormality of collagen metabolism, as exists in the bone, may occur in the tendon and cause weakening.[29,103] An effect of systemic acidosis causing elastosis of the involved tendon has also been proposed as a pathogenic mechanism.[394] The histologic finding on biopsy specimens of excised quadriceps suggested that repeated minor fractures of the bone cortex had occurred at the site of tendon insertion and preceded the final total tendon rupture. It was concluded that osteitis fibrosa was responsible for the minor fractures;[478] the slow progressive rise in alkaline phosphatase over the preceding four to five years provided evidence for uncontrolled secondary hyperparathyroidism.

Rupture occurs most commonly in the quadriceps tendons, triceps tendons, or in extensor tendons of the fingers. Typically, the quadriceps tendon ruptures while the patient is walking or descending stairs, or after stumbling. Patients are usually unable to extend the affected leg; a palpable gap and ecchymoses above the tendon are characteristic. Surgical treatment with slow rehabilitation has had satisfactory results.[444] The secondary hyperparathyroidism should be treated aggressively.

SKELETAL DEFORMITIES

True deformities of bone are quite common in uremic children, in whom the bone undergoes growth, modeling, and remodeling. Skeletal deformities can, and occasionally do, occur in adults; such deformities arise from abnormalities of skeletal remodeling and from recurrent fractures. The deformities commonly observed in children include bowing of the tibia and femur and defects arising from slipped epiphyses.[369] Most commonly, slipped epiphyses become manifest in preadolescence. The hip is the most common site afflicted, followed by the radius and ulna; lower humeral, lower femoral, and lower tibial sites are more rarely involved.[371] With hip involvement a limp is common and pain is often absent. When the radius and ulna are involved, local swelling and ulnar deviation of the hands appear. The histologic abnormalities associated with slipped epiphyses are those of secondary hyperparathyroidism. The radiolucent zone between the epiphyseal ossification and the metaphysis arises because of an accumulation of poorly mineralized woven bone and/or fibrous tissue and not from an excess of cartilage and chondroosteoid, as is typical of true vitamin D-deficient rickets.[369]

Rarely, children with "renal rickets" exhibit the typical radiographic findings of vitamin D deficiency.[531] Bowing of the long bones may occur in early childhood but generally is not severe until adolescence. Chronic renal insufficiency is a common cause of adolescent "knock-knee," or genu valgum.[418] This can appear within a few months; the presenting symptoms are difficulty in walking and pain in the knees.

In adults with renal failure, particularly those with aluminum-related osteomalacia, skeletal deformities can be marked. Lumbar scoliosis, thoracic kyphosis, and recurrent rib fracture may cause marked deformities to develop over 1 to 2 years in dialysis patients (Fig. 41-27).

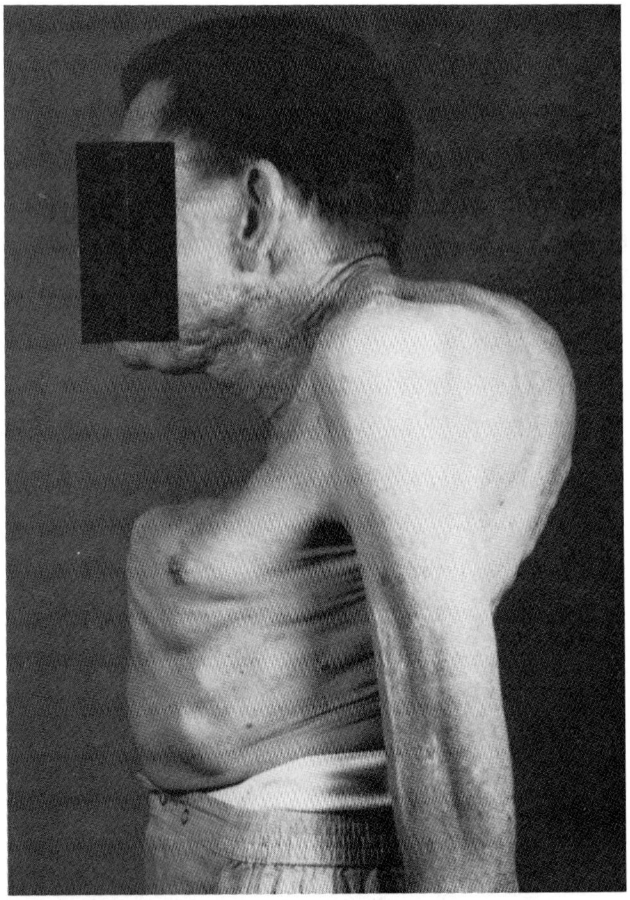

FIGURE 41-27 • Marked kyphoscoliosis in patient undergoing regular hemodialysis who developed osteomalacia associated with normal levels of PTH; the osteomalacia was unresponsive to treatment with $1\alpha,25\text{-}(OH)_2D_3$. Deformity developed over a 2-year period following rejection of a renal homograft; subsequent staining of bone showed evidence of marked aluminum accumulation along mineralization front.

RETARDATION OF GROWTH

Growth retardation is very common in children with chronic renal insufficiency, both before and during management with maintenance hemodialysis or with CAPD.[442,488] Before dialysis, one-third to one-half of children with a "preterminal" stage of chronic renal failure had heights below the third percentile;[488] growth velocity was below normal limits for age in two-thirds of children under treatment with dialysis.[94] Chronic acidosis, malnutrition, renal osteodystrophy, and low levels of somatomedin are some of the factors that have been implicated in leading to this complex problem.[95,363,479] The correction of certain of these abnormalities has been associated with improved growth velocity; however, this does not occur in all cases. Improved or even catch-up growth has been observed in a few children after treatment with calcitriol,[100] but the number of patients studied was small, and subsequent reports in larger numbers of patients have not confirmed the original findings.[94,484] The more recent observations of strikingly improved growth velocity of children with renal failure during therapy with supraphysiologic amounts of human growth hormone are of interest. The improvement is more pronounced before ages 8 to 10 years, and such treatment is associated with markedly increased plasma alkaline phosphatase activities, suggesting that there is increased osteoblastic activity.[283,370,548] The mechanism whereby growth hormone can produce this effect is uncertain.

OTHER UREMIC SIGNS AND SYMPTOMS AND SECONDARY HYPERPARATHYROIDISM

A number of nonskeletal symptoms that commonly coexist in uremic patients with overt renal osteodystrophy may arise as a consequence of a common pathogenic mechanism leading to both the skeletal disease and the nonskeletal manifestations. An opinon has been voiced that PTH, when present in great excess, may be a uremic toxin.[346,353] Some features of the uremic state that may be related to the marked secondary hyperparathyroidism are shown in Table 41-3.

There is evidence that the secondary hyperparathyroidism of experimental acute renal failure can lead to increased calcium content of the brain in association with an abnormal EEG.[24,224] Probable relevance of these animal experiments to acute renal failure in humans has been established by Cooper and coworkers, who found that EEG abnormalities, increased levels of PTH, and increased brain-calcium content occur early in the course of acute renal failure in human beings.[124] During the diuretic and recovery phases, serum PTH decreases to normal and the EEG becomes normal.

A role for high PTH levels in altering CNS function in chronic renal failure and dialysis patients is less well established. The EEG abnormalities of uremia may revert toward normal with regular and adequate dialysis;[281] moreover, brain calcium levels were normal in most patients with chronic renal failure who were tested.[124] Anecdotal experience has shown rather striking improvement of behavioral abnormalities following partial parathyroidectomy in some uremic patients with secondary hyperparathyroidism, which may indicate that a significant neurotoxic role is played by PTH in certain patients.[34]

It has been suggested that peripheral neuropathy may occur with greater frequency in uremic patients with secondary hyperparathyroidism,[30] although this supposition has been challenged.[25] Arieff and Schmidt, for instance, found motor nerve conduction velocity was not associated with PTH levels.[25] In an experimental study of acute uremia, increased nerve content of calcium and slowed motor nerve conduction velocity were reported to be related to increased parathyroid activity.[208] Available information provides support for the view that PTH acts as a neurotoxin in the CNS in acute renal failure; whether it plays a role in peripheral neuropathy remains unsettled.[25]

The possibility that secondary hyperparathyroidism contributes to impotence in patients with end-stage renal failure has also been suggested.[346] In one prospective study, the administration of $1\alpha,25\text{-}(OH)_2D_3$ was associated with an increase in potency in two of seven dialysis patients; a concomitant fall in plasma luteinizing hormone occurred in one of the two, and a rise in plasma testosterone in the other.[394] In another study there was no benefit of $1\alpha,25\text{-}(OH)_2D_3$ administration.[51] Thus the impotence of chronic uremia is probably of multifactorial origin, but excess PTH may play a role in its genesis in certain cases.

TABLE 41-3 • Symptoms, signs, and other features in uremic patients possibly related to parathyroid hormone

? Abnormal carbohydrate metabolism
Acute periarthritis
Anemia and pancytopenia
Bone pain
Central nervous system abnormalities—abnormal EEG
Fractures
? Hyperlipidemia and arteriosclerosis
Hypertension
? Impotence
Ischemic skin ulcers (calciphylaxis)
Muscular weakness
? Myocardial failure
? Peripheral neuropathy
Pruritus
Pseudogout
Skeletal deformities
Spontaneous tendon rupture

Extensive marrow fibrosis and sclerosis of bone can develop in uremic patients as a consequence of secondary hyperparathyroidism; such alterations may contribute to the hematologic abnormalities present in uremia. An association between renal osteodystrophy, myelofibrosis, and abnormal hematopoiesis was reported by Weinberg and coworkers;[567a] they noted that patients with leukopenia, thrombocytopenia, and severe anemia were more likely to have overt bone disease than other dialysis patients. They suggest that splenomegaly may arise in certain uremic patients as a compensatory mechanism in response to the replacement of normal erythroid tissue by osteitis fibrosa. An increased incidence of anemia has been reported in patients with primary hyperparathyroidism[62a] and correlates with the extent of marrow fibrosis. Also, the hematocrit may increase in uremic patients with secondary hyperparathyroidism following partial parathyroidectomy.[308,309] It seems logical that PTH may suppress erythropoietic function through local factors produced by marrow fibrosis. However, a direct effect of PTH on red blood cells is also possible. Meytes and coworkers examined the in-vitro effects of intact PTH and some of its fragments on erythroid colony formation in human peripheral blood and mouse bone marrow.[378] They observed that intact PTH and its carboxy-terminal fragment exert an inhibitory effect on erythropoiesis that might be overcome by increased erythropoietin levels. These observations are complemented by those of Zevin and coworkers, who demonstrated inhibition of RNA and heme synthesis by PTH extracts.[578] Bogin and coworkers examined the effects of PTH on osmotic fragility of human erythrocytes.[56] They noted that the amino-terminal (34-residue) peptide of PTH can induce hemolysis of red blood cells. Thus, an excess of PTH could contribute to the shortened life span of red blood cells noted in uremia.

Inhibition of platelet function occurs in uremia; Remuzzi and coworkers have demonstrated an inhibitory effect of PTH on platelet aggregation.[455] PTH was shown to stimulate platelet cAMP, which may reduce platelet aggregation and cause vasodilatation. Thus it is possible that secondary hyperparathyroidism is a factor in the bleeding tendency of uremia.

Elevated blood concentrations of triglycerides have been reported in a substantial fraction of patients with advanced uremia.[31] Cantin reported that parathyroidectomy partially inhibits the increase in lipids observed after bilateral nephrectomy, while the administration of PTE restores the hyperlipidemia in parathyroidectomized uremic rats.[86] Such data provide support for the possibility that the hyperlipidemia of uremia has some relationship to secondary hyperparathyroidism. Other observations suggest that the resistance to insulin action and hyperglycemia observed in uremia may be related to the presence of secondary hyperparathyroidism.[305]

Uremic patients often have cardiomyopathy. Uremia is associated with an increase in the calcium content of the myocardium; these changes may be due to excess PTH. Bogin and coworkers examined the in-vitro effects of PTH on cultured isolated heart cells.[57] Both PTH fragments caused a significant increase in number of beats per minute, and the cells died earlier than control cells. In addition, sera from uremic parathyroidectomized rats did not affect heart rate, but sera from uremic rats had effects similar to those of PTH. Furthermore, observations of Drueke and coworkers have shown a marked improvement in left ventricular function after parathyroidectomy.[154]

Aluminum may also affect myocardial function in patients with end-stage renal failure. Thus a high mortality from cardiac failure, often accompanied by cardiac arrhythmias, was noted by Llach and coworkers[315] and also by Chazan and coworkers[97] in dialysis patients with evidence of aluminum overload, as determined by bone biopsy[315] or from results of a desferrioxamine infusion test.[97] Preferential accumulation of aluminum has been noted in the myocardium of uremic patients,[12] and an association between left ventricular dysfunction or myocardial hypertrophy and the ultrastructural findings of aluminum accumulation has been reported.[468,547] London and coworkers, in a population study, evaluated left ventricular function by echocardiography in relation to aluminum stores, as assessed by a bone biopsy and from the increment in plasma aluminum following an infusion of desferrioxamine.[321] The patients without aluminum accumulation had significantly lower left ventricular mass and an increased rate of myocardial fiber shortening compared to those with evidence of aluminum accumulation. Moreover, for the entire population the quantitative assessment of aluminum stores correlated with increased left ventricular mass. Thus, these observations suggest that in uremic patients, left ventricular hypertrophy may be linked in some way to increased aluminum stores.

RADIOGRAPHIC FEATURES OF RENAL OSTEODYSTROPHY

Both the types of radiographic abnormality encountered and the incidence of specific radiographic alterations of bone vary considerably in reports from different centers that have evaluated patients with advanced renal failure.[418] Such differences probably reflect some variation in the type of skeletal disease encountered. Also, it is likely that differences both in the radiographic techniques employed, including type of film used, and in the interest of the radiologist are important. The x-ray film and automatic film developing procedures currently in use result in radiographs of much poorer quality than those available 25 to 30 years ago.[150] Sensitive x-rays are particularly useful for radiographic views of the hands, and so should be done with fine-grain film (e.g., Kodak M industrial film or mammography film); manual rather than automatic film developing should be used, and grid or screen techniques should be omitted. Magnification techniques can add further to the sensitivity. Meema and coworkers found the phalanges to be normal in 67 percent of uremic patients using x-ray films obtained and viewed with conventional techniques, and only 8 percent showed subperiosteal erosions.[367] With the introduction of better film and use of magnification techniques, only 26 percent appeared normal, while 29 percent exhibited subperiosteal erosions. There is a danger of overreading films when using these magnification techniques; familiarity with normal variation is required.[462]

RADIOGRAPHIC CHARACTERISTICS OF SECONDARY HYPERPARATHYROIDISM

One of the principal radiographic features of secondary hyperparathyroidism is the presence of *resorption* or *erosions*, which may occur on the subperiosteal, intracortical, and endosteal surface of cortical bone. Another radiographic feature of excess parathyroid activity in azotemic patients is new bone formation at the periosteal surface, a process termed *periosteal neostosis* by Meema and coworkers.[368] Alterations of the trabecular volume of spongy bone may lead to osteosclerosis or osteopenia.

Erosions occurring in conjunction with new bone formation may take the form of *cysts* or osteoclastomas (brown tumors), although these occur less commonly in secondary than in primary hyperparathyroidism.[418] Occasionally, cystic lesions or brown tumors are accompanied by pain; they may alter the configuration of the teeth when they occur in the jaw. Subperiosteal erosions almost invariably accompany such lesions. With healing, the cystic areas may be replaced by areas of sclerosis.

Subperiosteal erosions of the phalanges identified with the use of fine-grain radiographs of the hands are the most sensitive radiographic sign that secondary hyperparathyroidism exists.[152] Abnormalities have been found on radiographs in approximately 40 to 50 percent of the patients who show increased resorptive surfaces on bone biopsy[151,152,367,462] this frequency can be increased with magnification of radiographs. The appearance of bone erosions has been shown to correlate reasonably well with serum PTH levels.[462]

The earliest lesions usually appear on the radial surface of the middle phalanges of the second or third digits of the dominant hand; they first appear as slight irregularities near either the proximal or distal shoulder formed by the metaphysis of the phalanx.[418] As the lesions progress the erosions extend along a greater length of the radial surface of the phalanx (Fig. 41-28) and involve other digits and adjacent proximal and distal phalanges; erosions eventually appear on the ulnar border. The evolution of such lesions has been described in detail by Parfitt.[418] Although such erosions are generally asymptomatic, they occasionally produce erosive synovitis, which leads to soft tissue swelling, pain, and stiffness.

The tufts of the terminal phalanges of the second or third digit commonly show areas of resorption. Because of the natural occurrence of irregularities of the tuft, recognition of loss of the cortical margin may be difficult. Nonetheless, it has been possible to quantify and grade the extent of such erosions.[462] When the erosion of a terminal tuft is severe, marked loss of its structure may result, leading to collapse of the soft tissues; this can change the contour of the fingers to such an extent that they appear to show "clubbing."[160] Healing of erosions of the tuft and phalanges is believed to occur initially with replacement of poorly mineralized fibrous tissue and woven bone. Despite successful treatment and healing, the shape of the bone may not revert to normal.[203] When aluminum overload occurs in conjunction with the presence of significant subperiosteal erosions, remineralization and normalization of radiographs may not occur when secondary hyperparathyroidism is reversed by treatment with an active vitamin D sterol or by parathyroidectomy.[506] Thus, some caution must be exercised in interpreting the presence of subperiosteal erosions as specific radiologic signs of osteitis fibrosa and secondary hyperparathyroidism.

Other skeletal sites commonly showing subperiosteal erosions include the upper end of the tibia, the neck of the femur and humerus, the lower end of the radius and ulna, and the lower surface of the medial end of the clavicle. The predilection for subperiosteal erosions to occur near the junction of the metaphysis with the shaft (Fig. 41-29) is believed to occur because bone modeling during growth into a normal triangular shape with typical metaphyseal flaring requires that surplus bone on the outer cortex be removed. Consequently, the precursor cells of mesenchymal origin are more prone to differentiate into osteoclasts at this site. Such areas are often the first site of subperiosteal resorption in uremic children.[371] Typical resorption of the phalanges may be uncommon in very young children, but it does occur in older adolescents and young adults; it is also less common in uremic patients over 40 years old.[542] Resorption can be seen in the skull, leading to a mottled, lucent appearance; this is commonly associated with areas of osteosclerosis (see below).

Erosions in the lamina dura are frequently seen in primary hyperparathyroidism, but are less commonly observed there in uremic secondary hyperparathyroidism.[443] With secondary hyperparathyroidism, increased resorption of bone also occurs in intracortical bone or in

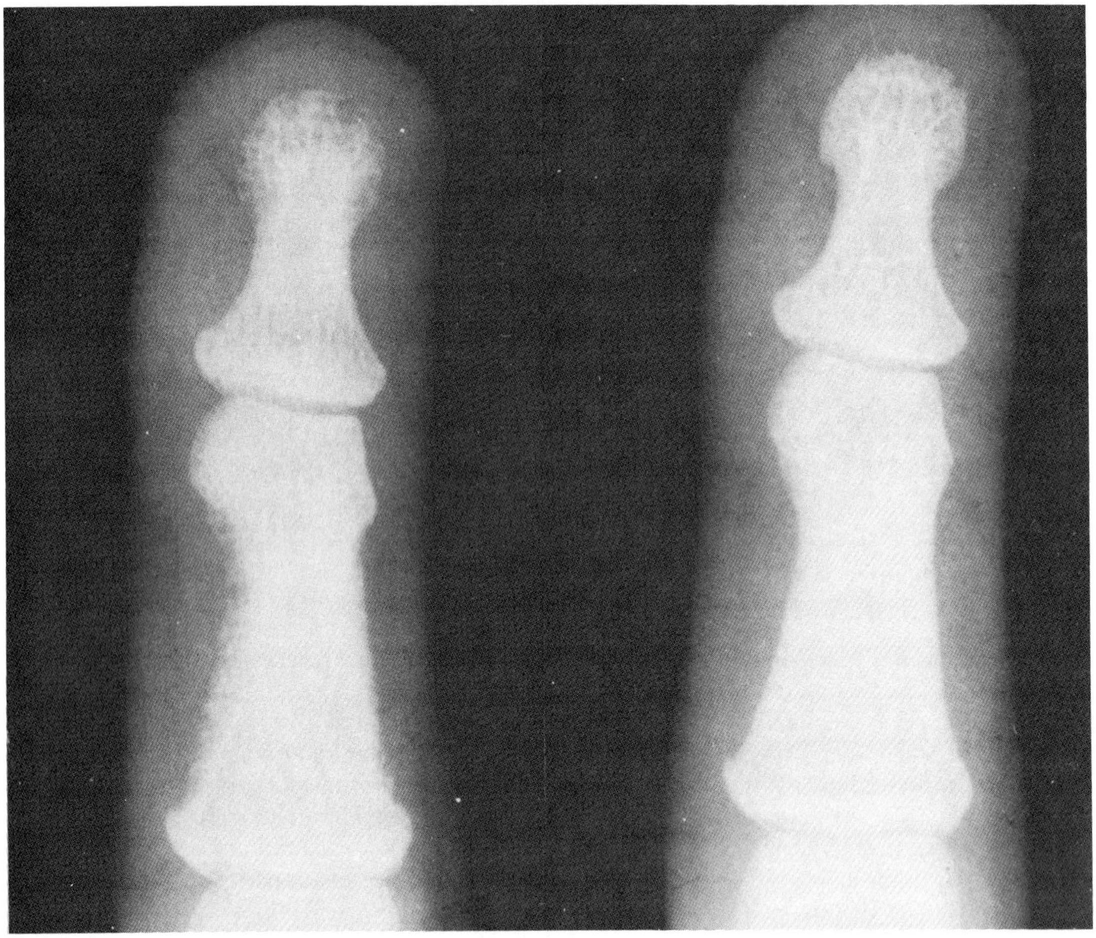

FIGURE 41-28 • Middle and distal phalanx of third digit of a patient with osteodystrophy (*left*); the same digit after treatment with $1\alpha,25\text{-}(OH)_2D_3$ (*right*). Subperiosteal erosions are much more marked on the radial (left) surface of the middle phalanx, although they are also present on the ulnar surface in this patient. Marked erosions are also evident in the distal phalanx.

the Haversian canals. The latter gives rise to increased intracortical striations on radiographs. These cortical striations occur in a number of pathophysiologic processes associated with increased bone turnover: hyperthyroidism, acromegaly, and rapid growth spurt at adolescence. The striations are less specific for hyperparathyroidism than are subperiosteal erosions.[366] Increased endosteal resorption also occurs as a manifestation of secondary hyperparathyroidism; this may produce scalloping of the endosteal surface or widening of the central canals of long bones.

Periosteal neostosis, new woven bone arising within fibrous tissue overlying the periosteum, is separated from existing bone by a radiolucent area that represents the interposed area of fibrous tissue.[368] As the process progresses, the fibrous tissue may calcify and the lucent zone disappear, and the existence of such new bone formation may be distinguished from an increased outer bone diameter (Fig. 41-30).

Osteosclerosis arises because of an increase in the thickness and number of trabeculae in spongy bone. It is generally apparent only in skeletal areas composed largely of cancellous bone with little contribution of compact bone; these areas include the vertebrae, pelvis, skull, clavicle, proximal humerus, and proximal and distal femur and tibia. In the spine, osteosclerosis may lead to a characteristic "rugger jersey" appearance.

Radiographic alterations of the skull have been classified into four types;[169] (1) a diffuse "ground glass" appearance, with loss of sharp margins at the vascular grooves and diploic venous channels; (2) a diffuse mottled or granular appearance (the most frequent type), probably arising from a network of enlarged resorption spaces within the tables of the skull; (3) focal lucent defects, 1 to 3 cm in diameter, which may be present with or without a "ground glass" or mottled appearance of surrounding areas; and (4) focal areas of sclerosis. The lesions may be confused with those of Paget's disease or multiple myeloma. These abnormalities of the skull may disappear after appropriate treatment (Fig. 41-31).

Although radiographic changes may correlate roughly with histology in iliac crest bone biopsy, the relationship may not be close in an individual patient. Such lack of association may be related, in part, to the fact that radiographic abnormalities are most easily seen in cortical bone, while the bone biopsy primarily evaluates trabecular bone. Also, the presence of aluminum-related osteomalacia may prevent healing of erosions as secondary hyperparathyroidism is reversed.[506]

RADIOGRAPHIC FEATURES OF OSTEOMALACIA

The radiographic features of osteomalacia are far less distinctive than those of secondary hyperparathyroidism. Once the epiphyses have closed, the typical radiographic findings of rickets, i.e., widening and splaying of the epiphyseal growth plate, do not occur. The only pathognomonic finding of osteomalacia present in adults is the *Looser zone* or pseudofracture. The Looser zone is a straight, wide band of radiolucency that abuts the cortex and is usually perpendicular to the long axis of the bone;

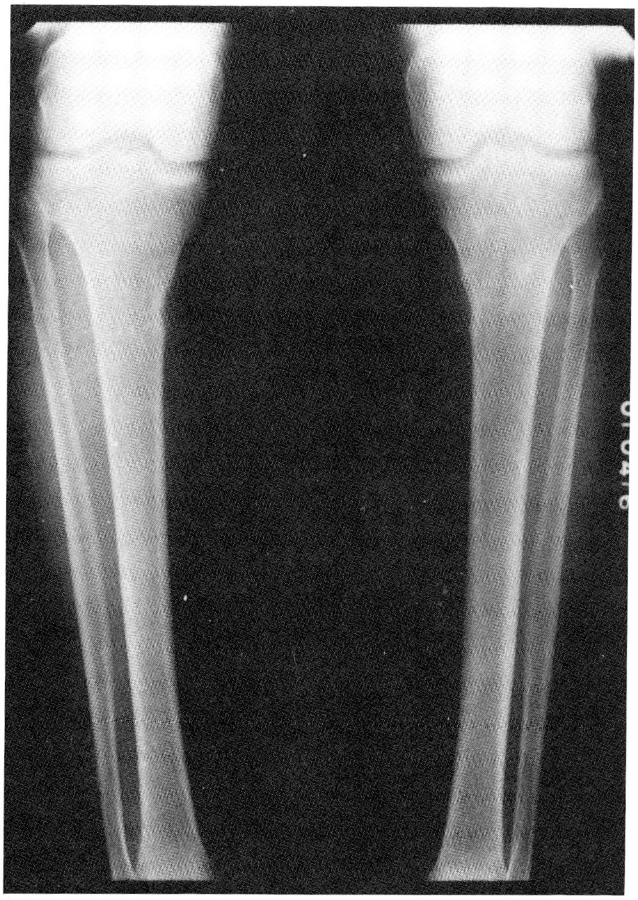

FIGURE 41-29 • Subperiosteal erosions occurring bilaterally near the junction of the metaphysis with the shaft of the tibia, a site sometimes involved with severe osteitis fibrosa (see text).

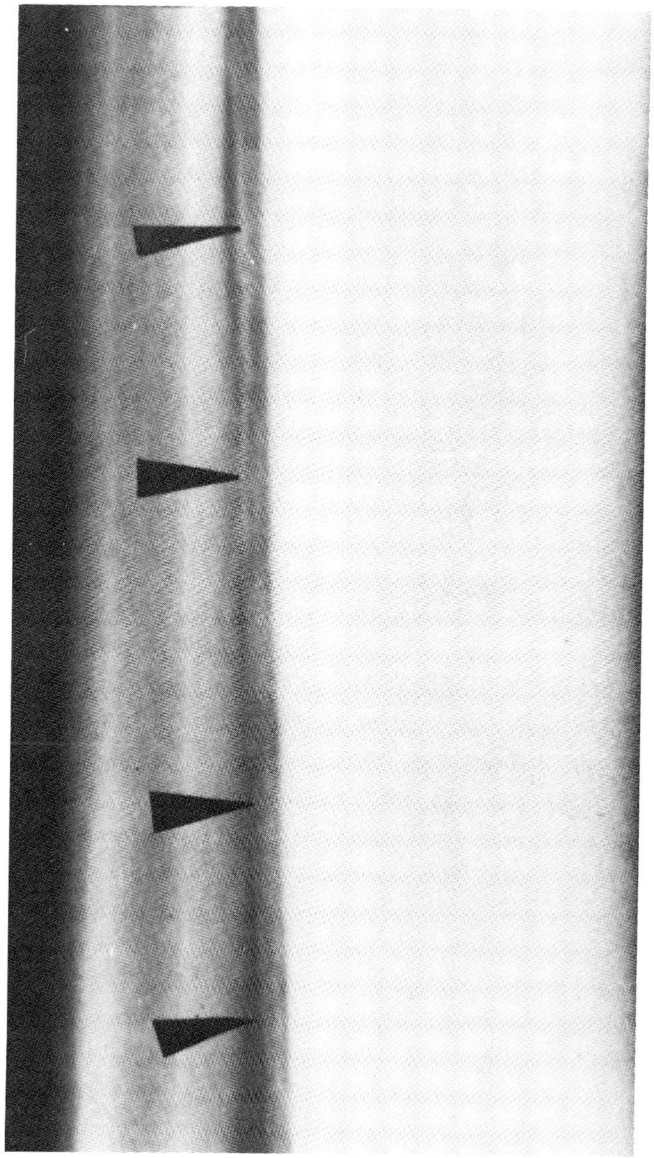

FIGURE 41-30 • Area of periosteal new bone formation (periosteal neostasis) along the tibia in a patient undergoing regular hemodialysis.

it may be bilateral and symmetrical and may or may not be accompanied by a narrow area of sclerosis or a small, poorly mineralized callus.[89,418] Healing or callus formation is usually minimal unless specific treatment is given. The means for distinguishing a Looser zone from a stress fracture have been outlined by Parfitt.[418] One important difference is that the initial hairline break of a stress fracture does not enlarge, but heals with minimal callus formation. In uremic patients spontaneous stress fractures commonly occur in the metatarsals or ribs with variable degrees of pain; these fractures tend to heal spontaneously but slowy with good callus formation. With mechanical stress or when vitamin D deficiency is very severe and prolonged, the Looser zone, like stress

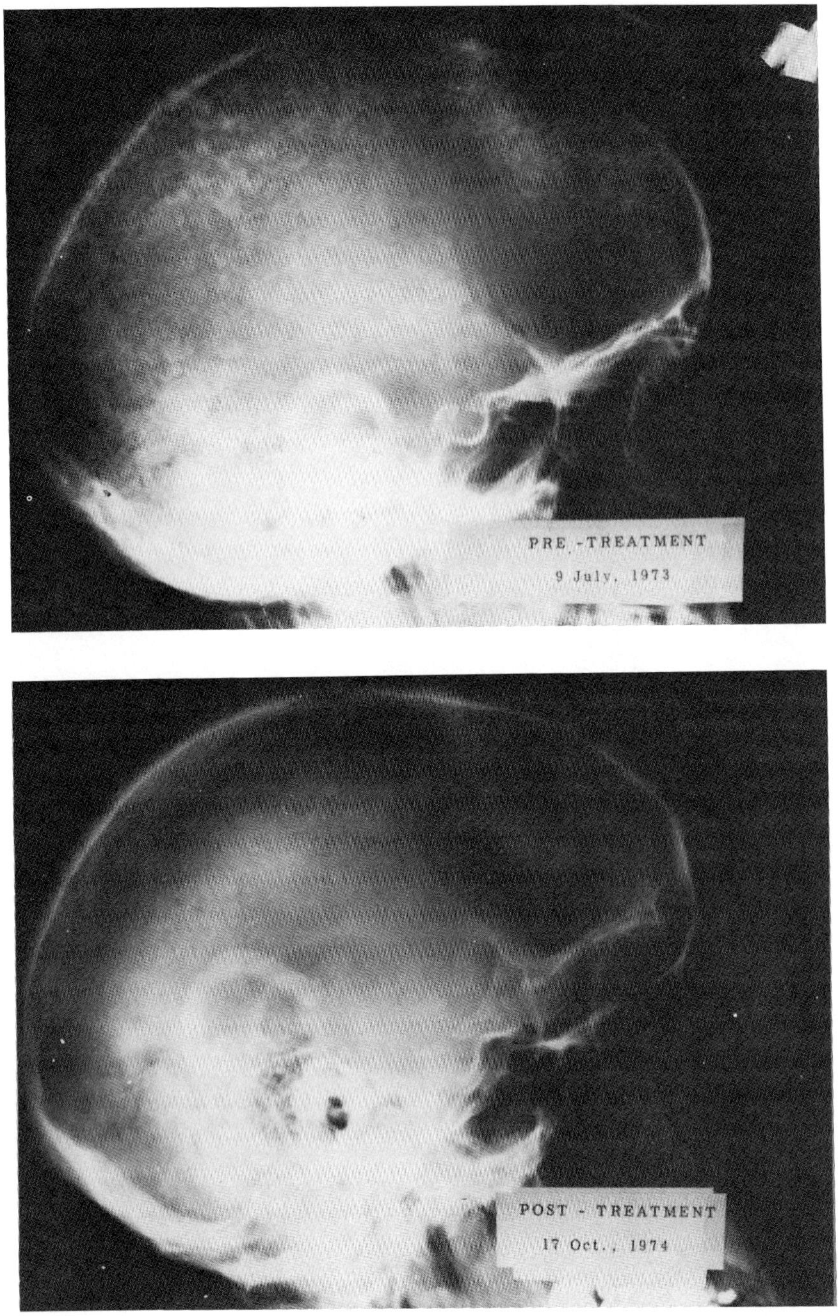

FIGURE 41-31 • Radiographs of the skull in patients with overt renal osteodystrophy. *Upper panel,* areas of modeling, granularity, and increased sclerosis; *lower panel,* appearance after 10 months of treatment with $1\alpha,25\text{-}(OH)_2D_3$. [Reprinted, by permission of the publisher, from Coburn JW, Llach F: *Renal osteodystrophy and maintenance dialysis,* in Drukker W et al (eds): *Renal Osteodystrophy and Maintenance Dialysis.* The Hague, Nijhoff, 1983, p 679.]

fractures, may extend across the full width of bone to produce a true fracture with displacement of the fragments.[89] Looser zones have appeared remarkably infrequently in the authors' experience. Fewer than 2 percent of German dialysis patients exhibited Looser zones,[457] although they were reported in 20 percent of uremic patients with symptomatic osteodystrophy in Australia.[418] They can occur with osteomalacia due to aluminum accumulation, but are infrequent; true fractures may be seen more commonly.

Protusio acetabuli, identified as a convex bulging into the pelvis over the acetabulum, may be a specific feature of osteomalacia.[399] Skeletal demineralization occurs with osteomalacia but is nonspecific. Features such as increased haziness or coarsening of the trabeculae, biconcavity of the vertebral bodies (particularly in association with normal bone density), and bending deformities of long bones are said to be typical of osteomalacia; however, few radiologists can make such distinctions.[150] Uremic patients with osteomalacia may also have secondary hyperparathyroidism, and bone erosions commonly coexist. Thus the features of osteomalacia are predominantly microscopic, and this diagnosis can only be verified by bone histology.

OSTEOPENIA OR OSTEOPOROSIS

A common radiographic feature of patients with advanced renal failure is decreased density of bone, which can arise from either secondary hyperparathyroidism or osteomalacia and therefore is nonspecific. Parfitt and coworkers applied the term "dialysis osteopenia" to a syndrome characterized by a substantial reduction in bone density with an incidence of bone pain and fractures that is increased out of proportion to the radiographic and histologic evidence for either osteomalacia or osteitis fibrosa.[419] The radiographic findings have been likened to those seen in the idiopathic osteoporosis of young adults. Features include loss of cortical bone from the endosteal surface, periarticular rarefaction, loss of trabecular bone with a honeycomb or fishnet pattern, and fractures that are somewhat intermediate in appearance between stress fractures and the typical Looser zones. Unfortunately, histologic studies with radiologic correlations in patients with this syndrome are not available; it is most likely that this syndrome is the radiologic counterpart of aluminum-related bone disease with osteomalacia or aplastic bone disease.

QUANTITATIVE MEASUREMENTS OF BONE MINERAL

The *metacarpal index* can be obtained by measuring the dimensions of the cortex of a metacarpal bone on x-ray film using magnification and a special caliper.[197] Normal data are available for the second left metacarpal, and the metacarpal index is the ratio of cortical to total bone width. On the basis of the assumption that this bone is a perfect cylinder, the ratio of cross-sectional cortical area to total cross section can be calculated.[197] The metacarpal index has been validated by direct comparison to measurement of bone ash.[221] Observations in primary hyperparathyroidism patients have suggested that total bone area is increased while the cortical area is reduced.[417] In patients with chronic renal failure not treated with dialysis, the metacarpal index was found to be reduced in 20 to 40 percent.[366,367] One study suggested that the metacarpal index progressively decreases with duration of dialysis.[58]

Photon absorptiometry

Another noninvasive method for the serial evaluation of the skeleton is photon absorptiometry, in which the absorption of photons emitted from an isotopic source is used to assess the mineral content of bone. The isotopes employed, either ^{125}I or ^{241}Am, emit photons of specific, narrow wavelengths and low energy.[80] Such measurements are taken over the phalanges, the radius and ulna, and the femur. Hahn and coworkers measured both the distal radius, which comprises primarily trabecular bone, and the midshaft of the radius, which represents compact bone; this has enabled them to evaluate the ratio of these two types of bone, which have different turnover rates.[228] Griffiths and coworkers found the mineral content of the mid-radius and ulna to be lower in dialysis patients than in age-matched controls; they also observed a progressive loss of bone with increasing duration of treatment in a dialysis center using a dialysate calcium level of 5.3 mg/100 ml.[218] In a subsequent study they reported that most women on dialysis maintained a stable bone mineral content, whereas 44 percent of males lost bone mass.[219] Photon absorptiometry appears to be more accurate than the methods that measure bone density from radiographs; however, the measurements are limited to certain sites of the skeleton that primarily comprise cortical bone.

It should be noted that bone mineral content can be reduced as a result of several causes: (1) primary reduction in volume of bone tissue, (2) increase in intracortical porosity as a consequence of enlarged Haversian canals, or (3) replacement of normally mineralized bone by unmineralized osteoid or poorly mineralized woven bone.[418] The measurement of bone density by photon absorptiometry does not allow distinction between these causes; the technique is best used when serial measurements are obtained for quantifying bone mineral and the results are evaluated in conjunction with findings on fine-detail radiographs.

Dual-beam photon absorptiometry uses two separate isotopes, permitting the subtraction of overlying soft tissue mass from that of bone. The technique can thus be used to measure the mineral content of sites of the skeleton lying deep within tissues; it is useful for assessing the mineral content of vertebral bodies and the femoral neck. With the advent of *dual energy x-ray bone absorptiometry*, a more precise and complete evaluation of bone mineral content can be obtained. Preliminary observations with this more advanced technique suggest that it may be valuable in the follow-up of dialysis patients with bone disease.

Neutron activation

Neutron activation provides a more accurate method for measuring total calcium or bone mineral content either in the entire body or in isolated parts of the skeleton. This technique requires the availability of a neutron source, for the activation of calcium and other elements in the skeleton, and immediate access to a whole-body counter, for measuring the short-lived radionuclides. This technique has proved useful in research studies of bone mineral content in uremic patients, and it may be particularly useful when serial measurements are used to evaluate the effects of a specific treatment modality.[148]

Scintiscan

Skeletal *scintigraphy* using ^{99m}Tc pyrophosphate provides a sensitive method for the detection of skeletal alterations in patients with renal failure. The technique allows for noninvasive follow-up evaluation of the response to treatment. Although the mechanism responsible for the accumulation of pyrophosphates in bone has not been elucidated, evidence indicates that the pyrophosphate accumulates in areas of increased bone turnover.[180] Rosenthal and Kaye suggested that pyrophosphate accumulates in skeletal areas with abnormal collagen metabolism, including either osteitis fibrosa or osteomalacia.[467] From evaluation of the uptake of the isotopes over the distal femur, Lien and coworkers calculated the bone: soft tissue ratio of isotope uptake.[303] Abnormal uptake was found in 78 percent of long-term dialysis patients and in a similar proportion of patients with chronic renal failure who were not undergoing regular dialysis. On the basis of correlation between bone uptake of ^{99m}Tc pyrophosphate and urinary excretion of hydroxyproline, Lien and coworkers concluded that increased skeletal uptake in uremia is related to the presence of immature collagen.[303] Others have found abnormal scintiscans in 13 of 14 patients undergoing dialysis.[540] Symmetrically increased activity was noted over the skull, mandible, sternum, shoulders, vertebrae, and distal aspects of the femur and tibia. Uptake of the labeled pyrophosphate over certain areas, such as the mandible, was pronounced and appeared before radiographic abnormalities. Olgaard and coworkers found that 90 percent of patients undergoing regular dialysis had pathologic pyrophosphate accumulation on scintigrams, while radiographic abnormalities were present in only one-third[407] (Fig. 41-32). In the presence of osteomalacia or aluminum-related bone disease, bone scintiscans may reveal increased uptake at sites of either true fractures or pseudofractures, particularly the ribs, pelvis, and scapulae; these may be seen on scintiscans at a time when they cannot be detected by radiography.[577] In general, however, pyrophosphate uptake may be reduced in patients with aluminum-related osteomalacia, and uptake can increase strikingly during chelation therapy.

Abnormal scintigrams are more common in dialysis patients who previously received renal homografts; intensive glucocorticoid treatment may aggravate the abnormalities responsible for an abnormal scintiscan. The diphosphate scintiscan can be used to detect soft tissue calcification, particularly in the lungs.[135]

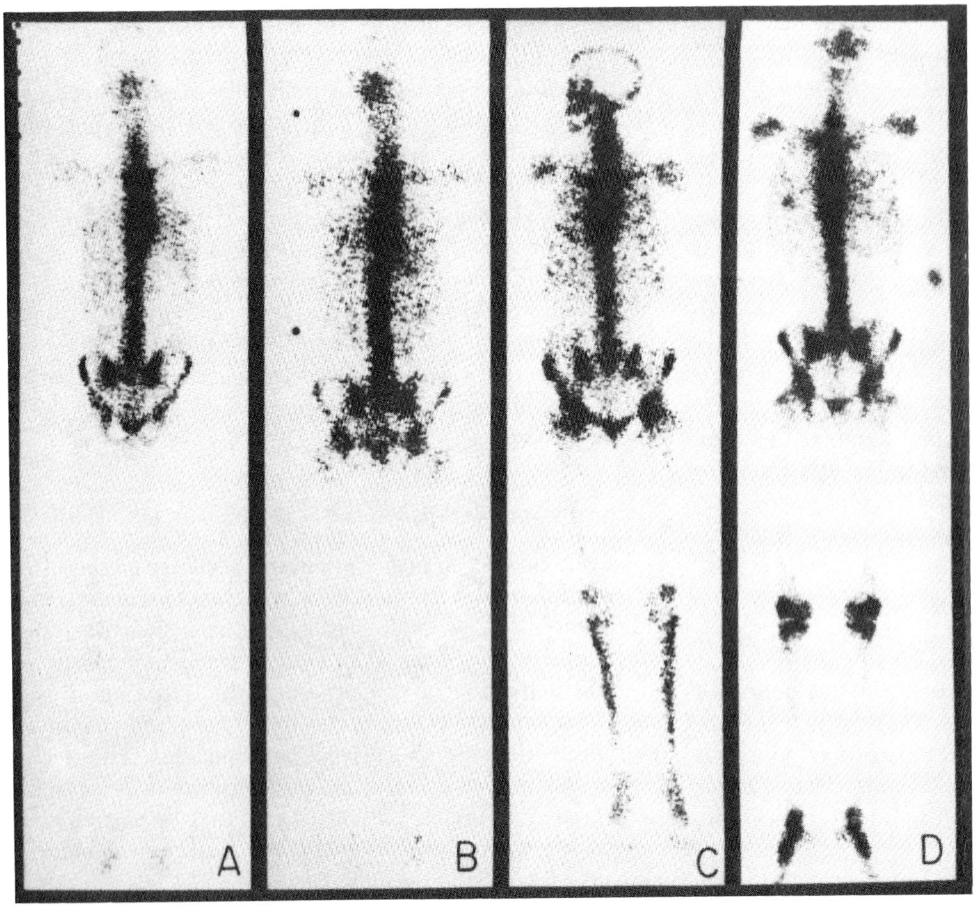

FIGURE 41-32 • Bone scintigrams with technetium-labeled pyrophosphate in a normal subject (*A*) and in patients with renal failure (*B–D*). Grading of severity of abnormality: *A*, grade 0, normal scintigram; *B*, grade 1, scintigram showing normal uptake in femoral heads with extension into femoral neck and trochanter region; *C*, grade 2, scintigram showing abnormal uptake in femoral head and neck and in proximal half of tibial shaft; *D*, grade 3, scintigram showing extensive uptake in femoral head and marked uptake in femoral and tibial condyles, tarsis, and proximal part of the metatarsis. (Reproduced, by permission, from Olgaard K et al: *Nephron* 17:325, 1976.)

Computed tomography

Computed tomography has been applied to measure the mineral content of the lumbar vertebral bodies.[83] It is of value in conditions, such as osteoporosis, that primarily affect the trabecular bone and axial skeleton. It has not been applied widely to renal osteodystrophy, nor have results with this technique been correlated with other methods, particularly bone histology.

EXTRASKELETAL CALCIFICATIONS

Soft tissue calcifications of several distinct types are common in patients with end-stage renal disease. The factors which predispose to their development include an increase in the calcium-phosphorus product of plasma, the degree of secondary hyperparathyroidism, the level of blood magnesium, alkalosis, and local tissue injury.[416] Three major clinical varieties of extraskeletal calcifications occur in uremia: (1) calcification of medium-sized arteries; (2) periarticular or tumor calcifications; and (3) visceral calcifications, which can involve the heart, lung, and kidney. Parfitt has further separated periarticular calcifications into three types:[416] *periarticular chondrocalcinosis*, which can occur in both primary and secondary hyperparathyroidism; *calcific periarthritis*, with associated calcifications similar to those of typical dystrophic calcification; and *tumoral calcinosis*, which was common in early hemodialysis but is now unusual.[258]

Periarticular calcifications remain a problem in dialysis patients. Early reports from dialysis patients noted a prevalence as high as 52 percent.[258] Though more effective control of hyperphosphatemia may have ameliorated this problem, it is still observed in 7.5 to 45 percent of hemodialysis patients.[36,41,102,280,471] Table 41-4 shows recent observations made by various authors in regard to the frequency of periarticular calcifications. This is also a problem in CAPD patients, who have a frequency varying from 12.5 to 22 percent according to recent reports.[36,471]

Occasionally, pain, stiffness, and soft tissue swelling may be associated with calcific periarthritis. Calcifications involving the eye may cause band keratopathy when the sclerae are involved,[43] or may cause the "red eye" of uremia when conjunctival deposits induce acute inflammation due to phagocytosis of crystals.[46] A rise in local pH due to the loss of CO_2 into the air may predispose to ocular calcifications.

The appearance of uremic arterial calcifications can be distinctive (Fig. 41-33): They are diffuse and continuous along the contour of the vessel; they also involve the media. This appearance contrasts with the dense, irregular, and discrete appearance of calcifided intimal plaques. Vascular calcifications may be first detected as a "ring" or "tube" in the dorsalis pedis artery where it descends between the first and second metatarsals.[542] Other common sites are the ankles, feet, pelvis, hands, and wrists. Arterial calcifications often occur without any symptoms; however, the consequent rigidity and lack of compressibility of the vessel may make it difficult to palpate pulses or hear the Korotkov's sounds; also, vascular access for dialysis may be difficult to achieve. Occasionally, extensive vascular calcifications are associated with ischemic lesions and the syndrome of calciphylaxis.[202]

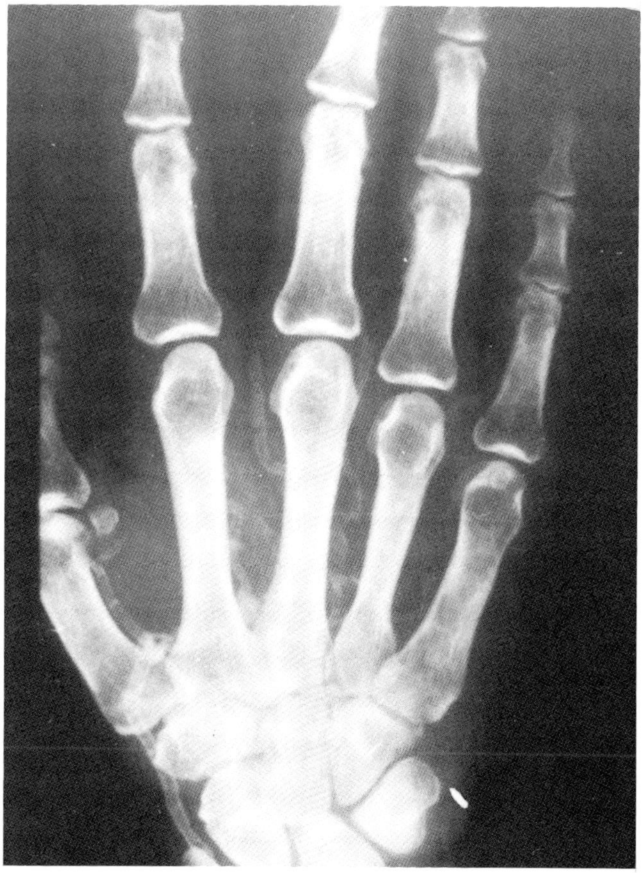

FIGURE 41-33 • Radiograph of hand showing extensive calcification of radial artery and various digital vessels. Features characteristic of calcification involving media of artery are apparent (see text).

TABLE 41-4 • The frequency of periarticular calcifications in dialysis patients

Author	Patients	Age (range or mean)	Calcifications
Rubin et al[47]	59	54	7 (12%)
Chou et al[102]	68	51	5 (7.5%)
Benhamou et al[41]	72	56	32 (44%)
Bardim et al[36]	37	32–70	17 (45%)
Kessler et al[280]	171	59	33 (19%)

An evaluation of the incidence of vascular calcifications suggests that they are age-related; vascular calcifications were found in 50 percent of dialysis patients aged 40 to 50, compared with 30 percent in the 15- to 30-year age group. Vascular calcifications are quite uncommon in children with renal failure.[461] Meema and coworkers documented the occurrence of calcifications in 36 percent of uremic patients not treated with dialysis, 19 percent of those treated with peritoneal dialysis, 13 percent of patients who had received a renal transplant, and 8 percent of those undergoing hemodialysis.[365]

The pathogenesis of these different types of extraskeletal calcification may vary; thus, visceral calcifications can occur in patients totally lacking arterial and periarticular calcification, and the converse also occurs. Most authors agree that periarticular or tumoral calcifications can be reversed by phosphate restriction with a reduction of the calcium-phosphorus product in plasma.[13] However, in other series of dialysis patients, the serum calcium-phosphorus product did not correlate with the extent of periarticular calcifications.[416] Thus, though such calcifications may be releated to the solubility product of calcium phosphate, other possibilities exist; thus, PTH may enhance the accumulation of calcium in soft tissues,[354] or poorly identified inhibitors of crystalization may be lacking. A direct role of PTH is difficult to assess, since overt hyperparathyroidism is usually associated with a high calcium-phosphorus product. Furthermore, though parathyroidectomy may lead to improvement of soft tissue calcification,[139] regression of this calcification does not always occur.[139] Aluminum-related bone disease was noted in 8 out of 12 dialysis patients with tumoral calcinosis,[127] suggesting that aluminum intoxication may play a pathogenic role. Finally, duration of dialysis may play a role: Tatler noted that the frequency of calcification increased with time during a 10-year period of hemodialysis treatment, despite the maintenance of an average serum phosphorus concentration and a calcium-phosphorus product below 70 mg/100 ml.[542]

Contiguglia and coworkers separated visceral calcifications from arterial and periarticular calcifications on the basis of their chemical characteristics.[123] Visceral calcification exists as amorphous calcium phosphate. Usually, amorphous calcium phosphate is rapidly converted to apatite at a physiologic pH; the lack of such conversion led to the interference that increased pyrophosphate content of bone and serum might account for the occurrence of visceral calcifications.[16,17] Contrary to the idea that soft tissue calcification may be associated with secondary hyperparathyroidism, Contiguglia and coworkers found that the degree of secondary hyperparathyroidism, based on either parathyroid size at autopsy or serum calcium-phosphorus product, was not related to the extent of soft tissue calcifications found in uremic patients at autopsy.[123]

Visceral calcification may give rise to serious symptoms, depending on the organ involved. Thus, heart block may occur on account of deposition of calcium in the cardiac conduction system; cardiac failure has been related to the extensive replacement of myocardium with calcification.[123,153] Extensive pulmonary calcification

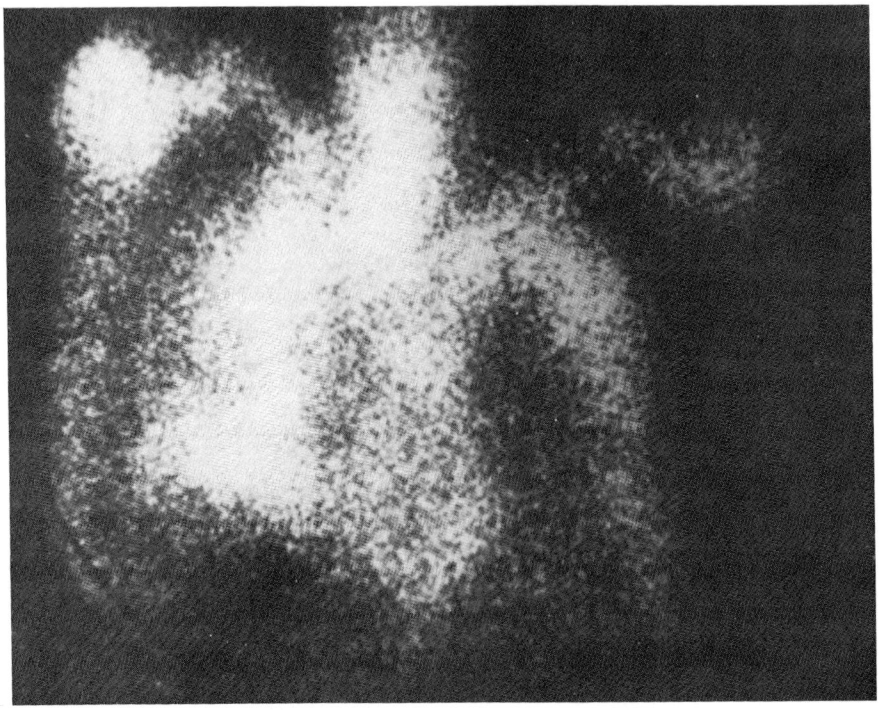

FIGURE 41-34 • Scintiscan of chest showing severe pulmonary calcification in a patient with advanced uremia. (Reprinted, by permission, from Devacaanthan K et al: *Clin Nephrol* 6:488, 1976.)

may lead to diffuse thickening of alveolar septae. Such calcification is only rarely extensive enough to be seen by radiography.[122] Various alterations of pulmonary function, including reduced vital capacity, reduced carbon monoxide diffusion, and low P_{O_2} have been found after death in patients subsequently shown to have severe pulmonary calcification. Such pulmonary calcification may be detected with the technetium pyrophosphate scan[135] (Fig. 41-34). Kuzela and coworkers found morphologic evidence of visceral calcification in 6 of 56 patients dying with chronic renal failure.[291] Such calcifications were more common in patients who had been treated with dialysis than in uremic patients who had not undergone dialysis.

EFFECT OF DIALYSIS ON DIVALENT ION METABOLISM

Hemodialysis itself has several effects upon mineral metabolism in patients with advanced renal failure (see Chaps. 39 and 40).[308] Among the dialysis-related factors that can affect divalent ion homeostasis are the following: (1) the concentration of aluminum, and possibly other trace substances, in water used for dialysate; (2) the concentrations of calcium and magnesium in dialysate; (3) the efficiency of the dialyzer, which can affect the rate of movement of various ions across the membrane, and the duration and frequency of dialysis; (4) periodic fluctuations of blood phosphorus and calcium concentrations and pH, and decreases in the levels of various uremic "toxins" during each dialysis (any of which may modify skeletal responsiveness to PTH, improve intestinal calcium absorption, and modify the flux of calcium and phosphorus from one body compartment to another);[93] (5) the effect of glucose, which is often added to dialysate, on plasma levels of magnesium and phosphorus; (6) a possible effect of heparin, which is given during each hemodialysis; and (7) the effect of a general and gradual improvement of uremia, which occurs following the initiation of regular hemodialysis. No physiologic conditions mimic the sawtooth pattern of certain biochemical parameters, such as phosphorus, magnesium, and H^+ concentrations, that is produced by the intermittency of hemodialysis. Whether such intermittent variations have any effect on divalent ion homeostasis is unknown.

Within a few months after initiation of regular hemodialysis, the concentration of serum calcium generally increases to between 9.0 and 10.0 mg/100 ml. Thus an increase in the serum calcium level generally occurs in patients who were previously hypocalcemic, while little or no change occurs in patients with initial serum calcium levels near normal.[271,378,413,573] Such increments in serum calcium levels can occur with initiation of hemodialysis despite hyperphosphatemia or the use of dialysate with a calcium level lower than that in blood. The mechanism responsible for this increase in serum calcium concentration is unknown; no improvement of the calcemic response to PTH has been detected with the initiation of dialysis.[356] Initiation of regular hemodialysis produces little or no change in intestinal calcium absorption,[113] although a transient increase immediately after dialysis has been reported.[93] With regular dialysis using dialysate with a calcium level of 6 to 7 mg/100 ml, predialysis serum calcium levels are frequently normal; patients with normal or increased serum calcium concentration are found more frequently when dialysate magnesium is reduced so that the serum magnesium concentration can be lowered.[117] In a few patients, overt and persistent hypercalcemia appears some time after the initiation of hemodialysis.[271]

The total serum calcium level almost invariably increases during the dialysis procedure. This may occur because of an increase in albumin level as a consequence of the ultrafiltration and hemoconcentration that accompanies hemodialysis; the affinity of plasma albumin for calcium may also be increased as a result of a rise in blood pH. Studies carried out with calcium-specific electrodes indicate that the ionized blood calcium concentration can fall during hemodialysis with a dialysate calcium level of 2.5 meq/liter even as total blood calcium level *increases.*[450] However, more recent studies have failed to show a specific effect of hemoconcentration or change in pH on calcium binding to serum albumin.[465] In addition, the decrease of ionized blood calcium using a dialysate calcium level of 2 meq/liter has not been confirmed using modern dialysis techniques as well as "state-of-the-art" calcium-specific electrodes. When the same evaluation is made during dialysis with a dialysate calcium level of 6.0 to 7.0 mg/100 ml, the ionized calcium level increases.[385] Other studies show a sharp decrease in PTH concentration, but the decrease in PTH level produced may be transient and PTH concentration may increase to predialysis levels before the next dialysis.[62]

It is likely that with a dialysate calcium concentration of either 3 or 3.5 meq/liter, patients receive inappropriately large amounts of calcium with each dialysis. With the availability of calcitriol, either orally or intravenously administered, an increase in gut absorption of calcium, as well as direct suppression of PTH secretion, can be effectively achieved. In this situation, a lower dialysate calcium concentration may be advisable. Furthermore, recent studies evaluating the long-term effect of calcium carbonate and 2.5 meq/liter calcium dialysate in 21 hemodialysis patients have demonstrated not only that serum phosphorus is well controlled and serum aluminum fell significantly, but also that serum calcium increased and PTH decreased by 20 percent after 7 months of therapy[523]—clearly suggesting the absence of a negative calcium balance. The addition of calcitriol to the majority of patients with secondary hyperparathyroidism will further correct the hyperparathyroidism and promote a more positive calcium balance.

The concentration of Mg^{2+} in dialysate has a major influence on serum magnesium levels in dialysis patients; serum magnesium concentration ranged from 1.5 to 2.4 meq/liter when a dialysate magnesium concentration of 0.5 meq/liter was used; on the other hand, serum levels of magnesium were 2.5 to 4.5 meq/liter in patients using a dialysate magnesium level of 1.5 meq/liter.[117] Burnell and Teubner reported that lowering the dialysate magnesium concentration from 1.0 to 0.5 meq/liter resulted in the slow reduction of predialysis plasma magnesium concentration to values nearer normal[76] (Fig. 41-35).

Serum phosphorus concentration is rapidly decreased by 60 to 70 percent during the early period of each dialysis procedure; the rate of dialysance of inorganic phosphorus is 40 to 50 percent of the rate for urea.[8,538] In some patients, the postdialysis serum phosphorus level rapidly rebounds so that it returns close to the predialysis value within 12 to 18 h after completion of dialysis.[507] The total amount of phosphorus removed during dialysis is determined primarily by the concentration of plasma phosphorus. The quantity removed may be 600 to 800 mg during a standard dialysis. A patient eating 800 to 1000 mg/day of phosphorus with net absorption of 45 percent can be in neutral or positive phosphorus balance unless intestinal absorption of phosphorus is curtailed.[250]

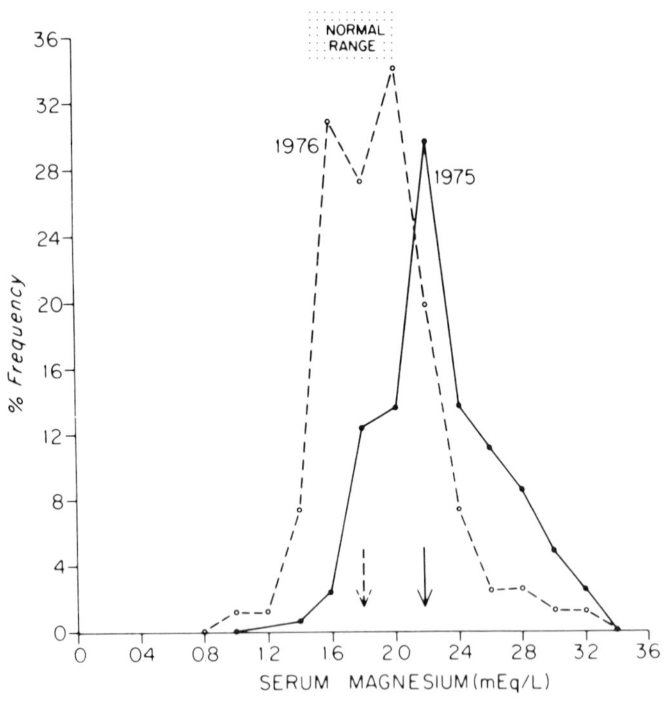

FIGURE 41-35 • Frequency distribution of serum magnesium levels in patients undergoing regular dialysis under care of the Northwest Kidney Center (Seattle, Wash.). Dialysate magnesium concentration was 1.0 meq/liter in 1975 (n = 109) and 0.5 meq/liter in 1976 (n = 81). Arrows indicate mean values for the two groups. (Reproduced, by permission, from Burnell JM, Teubner E: *Proc Clin Dial Transplant Forum* 5:191, 1976.)

With the widespread use of calcitriol, hyperphosphatemia has become an important contraindication for vitamin D therapy. Thus, new attempts have been aimed at enhancing removal of phosphorus during hemodialysis. Unfortunately, the main factor in phosphorus removal is the predialysis serum phosphorus level, and shift of phosphorus from sources other than the extracellular compartment is slow. New dialyzer membranes have been used to improve phosphorus removal. The clearance ratios of plasma phosphorus to urea of cellulose and polycarbonate membrane are similar—that is, 64 to 78 percent.[181] High-flux hemodiafiltration improves the ratio to only 30 percent.[8] It is not surprising that the mass removal rates of phosphorus are similar regardless of the membrane used. For example, the total phosphorus removed during 4 h of hemodialysis using a cuprophan membrane with a mean blood flow of 227 ml/min was 597 + 61 mg per dialysis, while high-flux hemodiafiltration, at a blood flow rate of 504 ml/min, removed 721 + 53 mg per dialysis.[8] Recently it has been suggested that carbonate, rather than acetate, may increase the intracellular pool of phosphorus and thus decrease the serum concentration. However, a recent study comparing dialysates containing the two buffers noted no significant differences in the transfer of phosphorus.[380]

It is absolutely necessary that the water used to prepare dialysate be purified to remove aluminum if the aluminum concentration in the water exceeds 10 μg/liter. Aluminum is bound to transferrin and albumin with high affinity, with only 10 to 20 percent of plasma aluminum being ultrafilterable.[549] Therefore, aluminum will enter plasma from dialysate and accumulate during dialysis when the dialysate aluminum concentration exceeds the ultrafilterable level in plasma.[214,261] Deionization and treatment with reverse osmosis are both effective methods for aluminum removal.[565] However, reverse osmosis is inadequate as a sole purification method when the aluminum concentration of water exceeds 200 to 300 μg/liter, as might arise when a municipal water treatment system uses alum (aluminum sulfate) for the flocculation of water as part of its water treatment. Substantial variations in the aluminum concentration in municipal water supplies can occur over short periods of time, making it difficult to carry out adequate monitoring of tap water for aluminum contamination. Periodic sampling of plasma aluminum levels in a population of patients in a dialysis unit may provide the best indication of intermittent contamination of water with aluminum.[575]

The presence of significant concentrations of fluoride in the tap water used for preparing dialysate results in the movement of significant quantities of fluoride into the patient;[543] the content of fluoride in blood, tissues, and bone increases to very high levels following repeated dialysis with fluoride-containing dialysate,[440] since such patients lack the normal mechanism for renal excretion of fluoride.[562] In a controlled prospective study, Oreopoulos and coworkers failed to detect a difference in the rate of progression of skeletal disease between patients treated with dialysate prepared from fluoridated water and other patients treated with dialysate lacking fluoride.[409] The incidence of osteosclerosis was higher in the fluoridated dialysate group, and this was attributed to fluoride. The high incidence of symptomatic bone disease reported in the past from several dialysis centers employing fluoridated water is likely to have arisen from the presence of aluminum as well as fluoride in the water used for the preparation of dialysate.[126] Appropriate purification of the water would result in the removal of both aluminum and fluoride, substantially reducing the incidence of aluminum-related bone disease and encouraging the erroneous conclusion that fluoride was the cause of bone disease.

Patients undergoing regular dialysis receive periodic injections of heparin; clinical and experimental studies suggest that heparin, when given repeatedly, is associated with decreased skeletal mineralization and may predispose to fractures in patients without renal disease. In one study of bone mineral content in which hand radiographs were analyzed, a positive correlation was noted between rate of decrease in bone mass and the regular dosage of heparin given to dialysis patients.[233] Osteoporosis has been reported in patients receiving 15,000 to 30,000 units of heparin per day over long periods of time;[218] multiple fractures and pseudoarthrosis have also been reported.[255,535] Osteoporosis did not develop in patients receiving lower doses (i.e., 10,000 units/day), and dialysis patients may not receive quantities of heparin large enough to cause difficulties.[218] With the use of efficient dialyzers and shorter duration of dialysis, the quantity of heparin given is less, and the potential for any adverse effect of heparin on the skeleton may be reduced. Since it is not possible at present to carry out regular hemodialysis without using heparin, it is impossible to test the hypothesis that heparin administration plays a role in the pathogenesis of bone disease in dialysis patients.

EFFECTS OF CONTINUOUS AMBULATORY PERITONEAL DIALYSIS

Certain effects of CAPD on mineral homeostasis may differ from those of hemodialysis, although the differences may be quantitative rather than qualitative.[323] The high permeability of the peritoneal membrane to larger molecules probably leads to measurable but insignificant loss into the dialysate of PTH and its important fractions. A small but significant amount of the plasma vitamin D binding protein is lost, with a concomitant loss of 25-OH-D_3.[323] Indeed, both low and normal levels of 25-OH-D_3 have been reported,[204,228,478] and patients may require supplements of vitamin D_3 or 25-OH-D_3. The losses of 1,25-$(OH)_2D_3$ are quite small.[568]

Serum phosphorus levels may be more easily controlled with CAPD than with hemodialysis, but controlled evidence in support of this view is limited. Metabolic studies have demonstrated that phosphate-binding agents are required by male patients treated with CAPD.[52] At comparable plasma aluminum levels, CAPD more effectively removes aluminum than does hemodialysis. The greater aluminum clearance by CAPD is probably related to the greater quantities of protein lost during CAPD than during hemodialysis.[239]

ALTERED MINERAL METABOLISM IN ACUTE RENAL FAILURE

A number of abnormalities of calcium and phosphorus homeostasis occur in patients with acute renal failure (see Chap. 38). Hypocalcemia, hyperphosphatemia, and elevated levels of PTH have been observed in the oliguric phase.[347] The degree of hypocalcemia is variable, but high serum calcium concentration develops within the first few days of acute renal failure and often persists into the diuretic period when serum phosphorus levels often fall to, or below, normal. Serum levels of phosphorus and calcium are uncorrelated, implying that hypocalcemia is not directly caused by hyperphosphatemia. An inverse correlation between serum calcium and PTH levels is observed, indicating that response of PTH secretion to hypocalcemia is appropriate. Nonetheless, infusion of PTE into patients with acute renal failure failed to raise plasma calcium levels appropriately during both the oliguric and diuretic periods.[347] These observations are consistent with the development of skeletal resistance to the calcemic action of PTH early in the course of acute renal failure.[347] Also, it has been shown that the administration of calcitriol to dogs made acutely uremic by bilateral nephrectomy partially restored the calcemic response to PTH.[356] It was suggested that renal production of calcitriol may decrease with the development of acute renal failure, and the reduced skeletal response to PTH could arise from such a deficiency of calcitriol. However, in rats with acute renal failure, treatment with calcitriol failed to restore a normal calcemic response to PTH;[527] in addition, Sommerville and Kaye, using rats with experimentally induced acute renal failure, reported convincing evidence that the reduced calcemic response to PTH is caused by hyperphosphatemia per se.[526] Thus, the mechanism underlying the decrease in calcemic response to PTH remains controversial.

Pietrek and coworkers reported a rapid fall in the plasma levels of 25-OH-D_3 during the course of acute renal failure, which suggests that turnover of 25-OH-D_3

may be enhanced.[435] To date, these observations have not been confirmed; nevertheless, a decrease in the plasma level of 25-OH-D_3 may limit the amount of substrate available for the generation of calcitriol by the damaged kidney.

Elevated plasma levels of PTH may contribute to certain uremic symptoms noted in patients with acute renal failure. The brain's calcium content was found to increase in association with the appearance of an abnormal EEG pattern in an experimental animal with acute renal failure; this increase in brain calcium content and the abnormal EEG could be prevented by parathyroidectomy.[24] Observations in patients with acute renal failure support a pathogenic role of PTH in cerebral dysfunction.[124]

Abnormalities in mineral metabolism in acute renal failure due to rhabdomyolysis have been described by several investigators.[317] This syndrome is characterized by severe muscle necrosis and deterioration of renal function. The biochemical features of the syndrome, which are uncommon when acute renal failure is due to other causes, include marked elevations in the plasma levels of muscle enzymes, severe hyperphosphatemia, and striking hyperuricemia. Abnormalities of calcium and phosphate metabolism are more frequent and pronounced than in patients with acute renal failure that is due to other causes. Hypocalcemia and hyperphosphatemia are usually severe in the oliguric phase, and hypercalcemia is common in the early phase, and hypercalcemia is common in the early polyuric phase. The severe hyperphosphatemia probably plays a role in causing profound hypocalcemia. The hyperphosphatemia arising from the release of phosphate compounds from damaged muscles may facilitate the deposition of calcium and phosphate in soft tissues and in the damaged muscles. Widespread soft tissue calcification within a short time after the onset of renal failure has been described in the lungs, heart, peripheral arteries, conjunctivas, and skin in patients with rhabdomyolysis. Both conventional and electron radiography, as well as technitium 99m disphosphonate scans, have revealed extensive soft tissue calcifications in the early phase of the syndrome.[7]

Figure 41-36 displays the course of clinical status and biochemical parameters in six patients with rhabdomyolysis-induced acute renal failure during the early oliguric and late polyuric phases of the syndrome.[317] On admission, all of the patients had marked hyperphosphatemia, hypocalcemia, and low plasma levels of calcitriol. During the early polyuric phase, moderate hypercalcemia was accompanied by marked elevations in the plasma levels of calcitriol and PTH (both the amino- and carboxy-terminal fragments). Plasma levels of 25-OH-D_3 were normal.

Both the marked hyperphosphatemia and reduced levels of calcitriol observed in these patients have probably contributed to the genesis of the hypocalcemia. Fur-

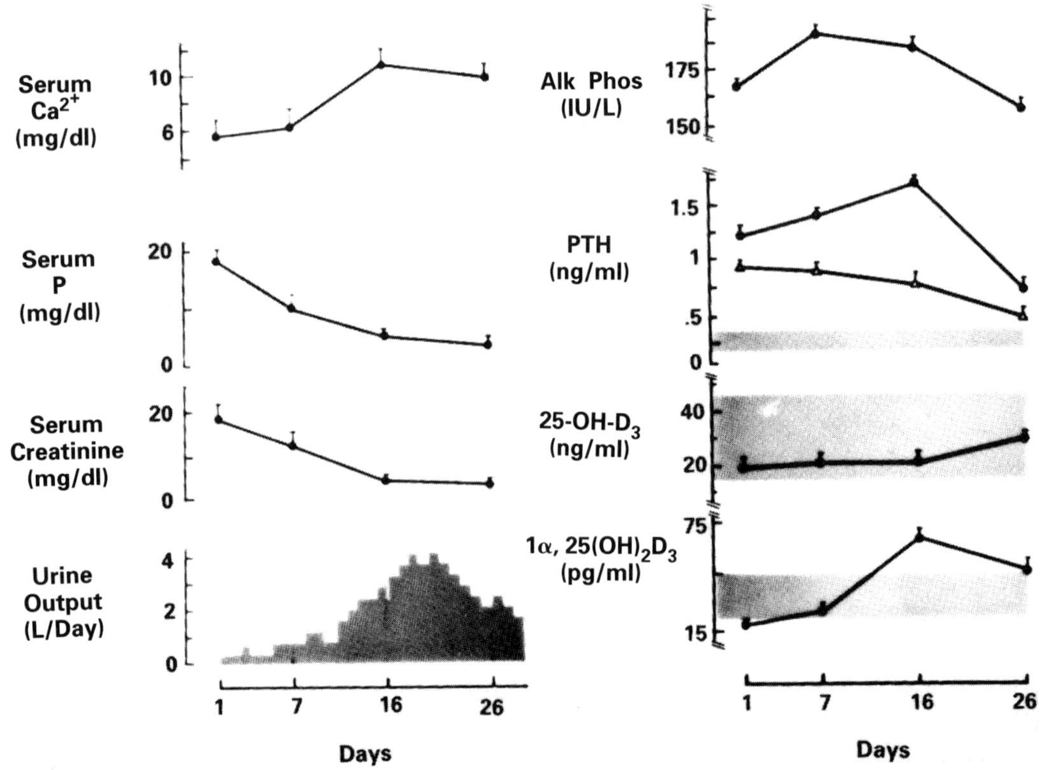

FIGURE 41-36 • Biochemical values on admission and during oliguric, early polyuric, and late polyuric phases of acute renal failure in six patients with acute renal failure due to rhabdomyolysis. (From Llach F et al: *N Engl J Med* 305:117, 1981. Used by permission.)

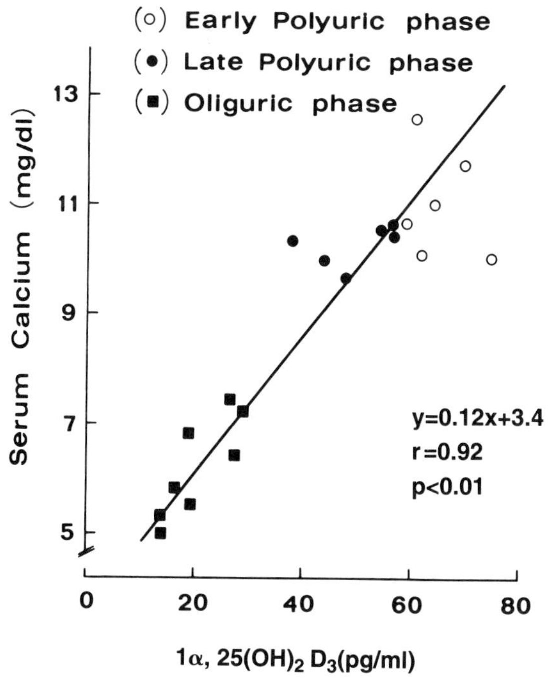

FIGURE 41-37 • Relationship between serum levels of calcium and 1α,25-$(OH)_2D_3$ during oliguric, early polyuric, and late polyuric phases of acute renal failure due to rhabdomyolysis. Each point represents a single measurement. (From Llach F et al: *N Engl J Med* 305:117, 1981. Used by permission.)

thermore, given the important role of serum phosphorus concentration in affecting synthesis of calcitriol it is likely that hyperphosphatemia contributed directly to the low levels of calcitriol. Since calcitriol is an important hormone for calcium homeostasis, its reduced plasma levels early in acute renal failure may cause a decrease in the calcemic response to the action of PTH and depression of intestinal calcium absorption—events that certainly can exacerbate hypocalcemia. That this may be the case is suggested by the significant correlation observed between the levels of serum calcium concentration and calcitriol (Fig. 41-37). It is possible that the marked elevation in plasma levels of calcitriol observed during the diuretic phase of rhabdomyolysis-induced acute renal failure are due to the high PTH levels, and both may contribute to the hypercalcemia.

During the diuretic phase, serum phosphorus concentration often falls to normal or lower. Serum phosphorus concentration may fall as urinary phosphorus excretion increases, because of osmotic diuresis, an increment of extracellular volume, and high circulating levels of PTH. Although the hypercalcemia observed in acute renal failure may be transient and resolve within a few days, serum calcium levels of 13 to 15 mg/100 ml may persist for 3 to 4 weeks.[379] Treatment with saline infusions and furosemide may be necessary.[539] It is unwise to administer phosphate salts, either by mouth or parenterally, unless the serum phosphorus level is low or normal; this is particularly true if renal function has not yet returned to normal. Glucocorticoids should also be given with caution, because of the high catabolic rate that already exists in these patients.

PREVENTION AND MANAGEMENT

The objectives of management of altered divalent ion metabolism and osteodystrophy in patients with renal failure are (1) to keep the blood concentrations of calcium and phosphorus as near normal as possible; (2) to prevent the development of hyperplasia of the parathyroid glands, or, if this has already occurred, to suppress parathyroid secretion and hyperplasia; (3) to restore the skeleton to normal; and (4) to prevent and reverse extraskeletal calcification.

The intensity of treatment and the specific treatment modality must vary depending on the stage of renal insufficiency, the presence or absence of evidence of overt osteodystrophy, and whether regular dialysis has been initiated. Some specific means for the management of renal osteodystrophy are given in Table 41-5, with details provided in the text.

PREVENTION OF PHOSPHATE RETENTION AND HYPERPHOSPHATEMIA

Phosphate retention and hyperphosphatemia both are major factors responsible for the development and maintenance of secondary hyperparathyroidism in renal failure. Slatopolsky and coworkers, and Rutherford and coworkers, have demonstrated that reducing dietary phosphorus intake in proportion to the decrease in GFR in uremic dogs can largely prevent the development of secondary hyperparathyroidism.[476,517,518] Data from a study of human subjects indicate that a reduction in dietary phosphorus intake in proportion to the decrease in GFR in patients with mild renal insufficiency and secondary hyperparathyroidism can reduce the plasma PTH concentration, improve the calcemic response of the skeleton to parathyroid extract, and improve intestinal absorption of calcium.[318] The mechanism for this effect of phosphate retention in the moderate and early phases of renal failure appears to be reduced synthesis of 1α,25-$(OH)_2D_3$.[438] In patients treated with regular dialysis, high plasma levels of phosphorus contribute to the development of extraskeletal calcification—in particular, tumoral and periarticular calcifications. Thus the restriction of dietary phosphorus intake and prevention of hyperphosphatemia are of great importance in the treatment of renal osteodystrophy.

The available options for reducing the phosphate load include reducing the intake of dietary phosphate,

TABLE 41-5 • Guidelines for management of renal osteodystrophy

CONTROL OF SERUM PHOSPHORUS

Restrict dietary phosphorus intake to 0.7 to 0.9 g/day
Give phosphate-binding agents: aluminum hydroxide, aluminum carbonate, or calcium carbonate
Avoid hypophosphatemia and marked elevation of serum aluminum

DIETARY CALCIUM SUPPLEMENTS

Give oral calcium to supply 1 g/day, but only if serum phosphorus concentration is controlled
Use 6.0 to 6.5 mg/100 ml calcium (3.0 to 3.25 meq/liter) in dialysate

VITAMIN D STEROLS

Indications for use: hypocalcemia, hyperparathyroidism (high PTH level, bone erosions) with serum calcium < 11.0 mg/100 ml, osteomalacia (with secondary hyperparathyroidism), chronic renal failure in children, concurrent anticonvulsant therapy (and prophylaxis?)
Vitamin D_2 or D_3, 10,000 to 20,000 IU/day (0.25 to 5 mg)
Dihydrotachysterol, 0.25 to 2.0 mg/day
25-OH-D_3 (calcifediol), 25 to 100 μg/day
1α,25-$(OH)_2D_3$ (calcitriol), 0.25 to 1.0 μg/day
1α-OH-D_3, 0.5 to 2.0 μg/day

PARATHYROIDECTOMY

Indications: evidence of secondary hyperparathyroidism (erosions, increased PTH) after exclusion of aluminum-related bone disease, persistent hypercalcemia (serum calcium levels > 11.5 to 12.0 mg/100 ml), progressive extraskeletal calcification, persistent elevation of serum calcium-phosphorus product, pruritus unresponsive to medical treatment, calciphylaxis (ischemic ulcers, necrosis), symptomatic hypercalcemia after renal transplantation

OTHER FACTORS

Dialysate magnesium concentrations 0.7 to 1.2 mg/100 ml (0.6 to 1.0 meq/liter)
Water treatment: maintain < 20 μeq/liter aluminum and remove excess fluoride, calcium, and magnesium in dialysate
Avoid concurrent treatment with barbiturates, phenytoin, or glutethimide
Normalize or improve acid-base status

inhibiting the absorption of phosphate with phosphate-binding agents, and enhancing the removal of phosphate from the body through more efficient dialysis in patients undergoing regular dialysis.[119] The dietary intake of phosphorus depends primarily on consumption of meat and dairy products. The usual intake of phosphorus by normal adults in the United States varies between 1.5 and 2.0 g/day. Theoretically, the dietary intake of phosphate could be reduced in proportion to the decrease in GFR in patients with mild chronic renal insufficiency. With elimination or restriction of dairy products and rigid limitation to 40 g of protein per day, the dietary intake of phosphorus ranged from 650 to 1000 mg/day—a quantity that is approximately 60 percent of normal intake.[285] With a more restricted protein diet (e.g., 20 g of high biological value protein per day), the dietary phosphorus intake ranged from 450 to 700 mg/day. With the preparation of very special diets, utilizing pasta products made from starch and egg white and with prolonged boiling and washing of certain foods to remove phosphate, Barsotti and coworkers lowered the phosphorus intake to 350 to 450 mg/day (6 mg/per kilogram of body weight).[37,38] Thus, it is possible to reduce phosphate intake substantially by modifying dietary intake, but this is very difficult to achieve in practice. Moreover, when patients enter onto dialysis and are prescribed diets with greater protein intake, the phosphorus intake also rises. In the United States, the average dietary intake of phosphorus in 162 hemodialysis patients who entered the National Cooperative Dialysis Study (NCDS) was 879 ± 248 (s.d.) mg/day; this indicates that substantial numbers of Americans ingest more than 1000 mg/day.[492] Moreover, with a protein intake of 1.0 per kilogram of body weight in patients on CAPD, the measured phosphorus intake ranged from 920 to 1200 mg/day, and when dietary protein was increased even higher, to 1.4 per kilogram of body weight, the phosphorus intake was 1700 to 2400 mg/day.[52]

Because it is difficult to achieve adequate dietary restriction of phosphate, particularly in dialysis patients ingesting more protein, phosphate-binding agents are required by most patients with end-stage renal failure and by many patients with advanced renal failure.[187,188] A mathematical consideration of the mass balance for phosphorus in dialysis patients is given in Table 41-6. The fraction of phosphate that is absorbed in dialysis patients is only slightly lower than the fraction absorbed by normal subjects; thus, Ramirez and coworkers[451] found that 70 and 81 percent of the phosphate was absorbed from a single meal, and Kaye and coworkers estimated that 61 ± 9 percent was absorbed, based on fecal recovery. Even with the intake of aluminum hydroxide in doses ranging from 3.4 to 15 g/day, Blumenkrantz and coworkers[52] found that the net absorption of phosphorus was 55 ± 14 percent of the intake in 13 long-term metabolic balance studies done in patients treated with CAPD.

The amount of phosphorus removed during hemodialysis varies with the predialysis serum phosphorus level and with the efficiency of the dialyzer being used. Kaye and coworkers[278] found that the net phosphate removal was 600 to 750 mg over 4 h of dialysis utilizing a 1.2 m^2 Cuprophan dialyer when the predialysis serum phosphorus level varied from 5.0 to 7.0 mg/100 ml; another study found that phosphate removal was 587 ±

61 mg during 4 h of dialysis and 721 ± 53 mg with high-flux hemodiafiltration carried out for 2 h with a blood flow of 500 ml/min.[8,9] With the application of dialysis that was designed to achieve optimal urea removal (e.g., Kt/V above 1.05), Shinaberger and coworkers[508] found the net removal of phosphorus to be 500 to 600 mg during 4 h of conventional dialysis, and to increase only to 600 to 700 mg per dialysis during 3 h of high efficiency or high flux dialysis using cellulose acetate, polysulfone, and other highly permeable membranes. Several explanations account for the rather poor mass transfer of phosphorus: (1) The dialyzer clearances of phosphate are somewhat lower than urea, although this difference is less with polysulfone dialyzers (however, the differences become greater when blood flow is increased); (2) there is little or no removal of phosphate from the erythrocyte and only plasma phosphate is cleared by the dialyzer; and (3) the equilibration between the pool of plasma phosphate and phosphate in a pool, or pools, outside of ECF is retarded. Thus it is known that the serum phosphorus level falls rapidly over the first 30 to 45 min of dialysis, and the levels may fall to values below 3.0 mg/100 ml. This last factor results in a very low gradient between plasma and dialysate, with less efficient mass transfer as the length of dialysis is extended. This last consideration accounts for the greater efficiency of phosphate removal during peritoneal dialysis, compared to hemodialysis.[238] Thus the phosphorus removal during CAPD averaged 324 ± 23 mg per 24 h, with mean serum phosphorus levels of 4.0 and 4.8 mg/100 ml. From these observations and the mass balance calculations, it is apparent why phosphate binders are required by almost all patients treated with hemodialysis and many of those managed with CAPD.

TABLE 41-6 • Some considerations regarding phosphorus removal and balance in dialysis patients with three different diets: 900 mg daily phosphorus intake (moderate compliance to low-phosphate diet); 1200 mg (occasional noncompliance with dialysis diet); and 1500 mg (more "normal" North American diet)

	Dietary phosphorus intake		
Intake (mg/day)	900	1200	1500
Absorbed (60%)*	540	720	900
Hemodialysis removal (mg/day) (700 mg per 4 h dialysis, 3x/week)†	300	300	300
Balance (mg/day)	+240	+420	+600
Binder needed for "zero" balance (Ca^{2+} acetate tabs/day)‡	8	14	20

* May be as high as 70%; other patients as low as 50%; augmented slightly by vitamin D sterols.
† With serum [P] of 6.0 mg/100 ml; increases moderately as serum [P] rises.
‡ These figures are only approximate, but *relative* figures are correct.

Aluminum-containing phosphate binders

Aluminum gels were the standard phosphate binders prescribed for patients with end-stage renal failure prior to 1985, when nephrologists first appreciated the risk of aluminum toxicity and the important role of oral aluminum intake in its pathogenesis. When aluminum gels are ingested, considerable data indicate that capsules or tablets are less effective than the liquid suspensions;[475] however, patient compliance is generally better with capsules than with the liquid forms. Constipation, which commonly accompanies their ingestion, is the most troublesome side effect limiting compliance with these agents. Because of wide variation in the individual patient's preference and "taste" for different preparations, it is difficult to identify one preparation that satisfies all patients; some patients prefer liquid gels, others insist on tablets, and still others want to sprinkle powdered calcium carbonate on their food. Hence, efforts should be made to find a *specific* preparation that is suitable for each patient.

Are there safe quantities of aluminum gels? It was suggested that there was little or no risk with the ingestion of up to six capsules or tablets of aluminum hydroxide per day by adults with renal failure;[575] it was also suggested that doses below 30 mg per kilogram of body weight had little risk in children with end-stage renal disease.[496] The prospective study of Salusky and coworkers[485] in children undergoing peritoneal dialysis provided evidence of aluminum accumulation even though the dosage of aluminum gels did not exceed 30 mg per kilogram of body weight. They observed a progressive increase of mean plasma aluminum from 22 to 59 μg/liter in the children and young adults assigned to aluminum hydroxide, compared to a significant fall of plasma aluminum in the patients ingesting calcium carbonate. Moreover, one of seven patients developed histologic evidence of skeletal aluminum toxicity after receiving this "low" dose of aluminum hydroxide for one year. The control of hyperphosphatemia and hyperparathyroidism was poorer with the restricted doses of aluminum gel than in the group assigned to calcium carbonate. In a population study in adults who were limited to 6 tablets of aluminum hydroxide per day or 30 ml/day of a liquid suspension (maximum, 2.85 g aluminum hydroxide per day), Jenkins and coworkers found significant aluminum staining on bone biopsies in 2 of 16 adult hemodialysis patients.[257] Thus a certain fraction of dialysis patients who ingest aluminum hydroxide, even in modest doses, will develop clinical evidence of aluminum loading. Doses of aluminum hydroxide larger than those used by Jenkins and coworkers[257] are generally required in adult patients; thus the doses required to prevent serum phosphorus from rising in the National Cooperative Dialysis Study ranged from 3.5 to 4.9 g/day in the two major treatment groups with dialysis treatment schedules that resulted in the best survival and least morbidity.[231] *For the reasons noted above, we recommend that aluminum gels not be the primary phosphate-binding agents prescribed for patients with renal failure.* Aluminum gels will be needed in patients with intolerance to calcium carbonate or calcium acetate because of side effects or when a calcium salt alone is inadequate. The latter patients often require a combination of either calcium carbonate or calcium acetate with an aluminum-based phosphate binder.[522]

Calcium carbonate and calcium acetate as phosphate-binding agents

It was known many years ago that large doses of calcium carbonate were effective in reducing the absorption of phosphorus from the gastrointestinal tract.[106] A number of clnical studies have subsequently shown that calcium carbonate is an effective phosphate-binding agent in dialysis patients.[186,241,331,391,483,486,522] However, calcium carbonate was not without side effects; these include hypercalcemia and various gastrointestinal symptoms. The latter include constipation, diarrhea, changes in bowel habits, and vague abdominal discomfort or dyspepsia. Occasionally these symptoms are so profound that patients have difficulty complying with the prescribed dosages of calcium carbonate. Episodes of hypercalcemia have occurred in a substantial fraction of patients;[241,391,483,486,522] occasionally the hypercalcemia is severe enough to cause symptoms that require dialysis with a lowered calcium level in dialysate. When ionized serum calcium was measured serially in dialysis patients started on calcium carbonate, the mean level increased significantly in a group of dialysis patients.[486] In the United States most patients undergo dialysis with a dialysate calcium concentration of 3.0 to 3.5 meq/liter, and a positive balance for calcium is induced by dialysis with a dialysate calcium of 3.0 meq/liter or higher.[536] Because of this and the development of hypercalcemia, the dialysate calcium has been reduced in certain trials with the use of calcium carbonate as a phosphate binder.[326,486,523] Thus, dialysate calcium was lowered from 3.5 to 2.5 meq/liter by Slatopolsky and coworkers[523] in a total group of dialysis patients receiving 1.5 to 18g/day of calcium carbonate; they successfully managed hyperphosphatemia, and the incidence of hypercalcemia was substantially reduced compared with their historical comparison with another group receiving calcium carbonate and employing a dialysate calcium level of 3.5 meq/liter. Sawyer and coworkers[486] utilized a stepwise reduction in dialysate calcium based on the serum ionized calcium when they initiated therapy with calcium carbonate; they lowered the dialysate calcium first to 2.7 meq/liter, and then, if necessary, to 2.1 meq/liter. In a large group of hemodialysis patients, they avoided hypercalcemia, achieved adequate phosphate control, and noted a significant fall in intact PTH levels.

Quantitation and comparison of phosphate-binders

Most observations with phosphate-binding agents have been clinical trials with dosage adjustment to achieve adequate serum phosphorus levels; controls have been either historical observations of the same or other patients while receiving aluminum hydroxide, or a relatively brief control period with no binder ingested. Only a few studies have addressed the question of how much of a phosphate binder is required to bind the phosphate in a diet. In metabolic balance studies, the administration of 100 ml/day of aluminum hydroxide gel caused a decrease in net absorption of phosphate from 463 ± 108 mg/day to 128 ± 68 mg day in five patients who ingested a diet containing 1135 ± 246 mg of phosphorus per day.[105] In two other patients with dietary phosphorus intake below 700 mg/day, the dietary fecal losses of phosphorus exceeded the amount in the diet. In a few studies with the dosage of aluminum gel at 75 or 150 ml per day, the reduction of phosphorus absorption was similar to that with 100 ml per day.[105] Fortran, Emmett, and their collaborators carried out systematic comparisons of the effect of various phosphate-binding agents on phosphorus absorption from a single meal that provided 320 to 370 mg of phosphorus.[329,451,489,498] In normal subjects the ingestion of 50 meq of aluminum carbonate, calcium carbonate, calcium citrate, and calcium acetate were compared, with the doses of calcium salts or aluminum-containing preparations based on the dosage of calcium or aluminum provided. In normal subjects, the administration of calcium carbonate containing 1000 mg of calcium decreased the average net absorption from the meal with 342 mg phosphorus from 263 mg to 151 mg, an average reduction in net absorption of 110 mg. The reduction of absorption with calcium acetate was 174 mg; with aluminum carbonate suspension, 202 mg; and with calcium citrate, 92 mg. The degrees of reduction with calcium acetate and aluminum carbonate were not different, but each was more effective than both calcium citrate and calcium carbonate.[498] In yet another study in normal subjects, the administration of 50 meq of calcium acetate reduced the mean net absorption of phosphorus from a similar meal by 150 to 170 mg per meal[505] when the agent was taken either immediately before or immediately after a meal, or was divided before and after; and there were no differences. However, there was a significant reduction of the amount of phosphate bound to 65 mg when the calcium acetate was taken 2 h after the meal. When Ramirez and coworkers[451] compared the effect of either calcium carbonate or aluminum hydroxide capsules (75 meq) in patients with end-stage renal disease, they found mean reductions of phosphorus absorption of 45 and 55 mg per meal. In a separate comparison of calcium carbonate (40 percent calcium) and calcium acetate (25 percent calcium), 50 meq per dose, in dialysis patients, there were mean reductions of phosphorus absorption of 43 and 106 mg per meal, respectively;[329] moreover, the calcium acetate was more effective on the basis of its calcium content. In addition, these authors observed less calcium absorption from the calcium acetate than from calcium carbonate.[329] It should be noted that the dose of 75 meq taken with each meal required the ingestion of five capsules of aluminum hydroxide powder (Dialume), four capsules of aluminum carbonate (Basaljel), 25 ml of aluminum carbonate suspension (Basaljel), six tablets of calcium carbonate (625 mg per tablet), and nine tablets of calcium acetate (Phos-Lo). For the 50-meq dosages the dose of aluminum hydroxide would be reduced only by one capsule, and six calcium acetate tablets (Phos-Lo) would be needed. These observations point to the importance of "titrating" the dose appropriately; they also emphasize that large doses of binders may be required, particularly if there is an increase in dietary phosphate. Thus it is important to maintain the dietary phosphorus as low as possible rather than merely increasing the dose of a phosphate binder. The average daily doses of calcium carbonate employed in trials in dialysis patients have been 8.5 g (range 2.5 to 17 g),[522] 5.1 ± 2.5 g,[483] and 5.8 ± 2.5 g[241] in trials in the United States; reports in Europe described adequate control with use of 2.48 g (range 1 to 6 g)[486] and 2.57 g/day (range 1 to 6 g);[331] it is likely that such variations exist because of differences in dietary intake of phosphate in Europe compared to the United States.

Other phosphate-binding agents

Several other phosphate-binding agents have been used but have certain disadvantages or have not been *widely* used. These include calcium citrate,[132] magnesium hydroxide or magnesium oxide,[223,403] and calcium and iron salts of polyuronic acid.[491] Although calcium citrate is as effective a phosphate binder as calcium carbonate, its use should be limited to certain specific situations, because calcium citrate, like other citrate salts,[388,515] markedly augments the absorption of aluminum.[116] Since some dialysis patients must take a small dose of aluminum gel with the calcium salt,[522] there is a major risk of severe, acute aluminum toxicity—a condition with a very high mortality.[33,282] Magnesium salts have been reported to be effective in one trial from the United Kingdom;[403] however, other trials with magnesium salts showed these salts to be ineffective and to lead to significant diarrhea and substantial hypermagnesemia.[223] When constipation accompanies the use of either aluminum-based phosphate binders or calcium salts, the use of lower-magnesium dialysate, combined with a modest ingestion of magnesium salt—such as magaldrate—may be useful. Thus, Moriniere and coworkers have had success combining calcium carbonate with small doses of magnesium salts in long-term management of their patients.[390] The polyuronic acid derivatives are not available in the United States and have not been widely employed in Europe. At this writing, we believe that the use of these three categories of agents should be limited to patients who are totally intolerant of calcium acetate or calcium carbonate or any of the phosphate-binding aluminum gels.

The fall in serum phosphorus level during dietary phosphate restriction and therapy with phosphate binders is often associated with a rise in serum calcium concentration.[105,350] If the magnitude of the rise in serum calcium is adequate, the blood levels of PTH may decrease;[105] this may contribute to the maintenance of the serum phosphorus level at a lower value, because a high PTH level contributes to the elevated serum phosphate levels in advanced renal failure.

It is equally important to avoid lowering the concentration of serum phosphorus to levels lower than normal, to avoid phosphate depletion in uremic patients. A few patients require no phosphate-binding agents; others require larger doses. Even in patients with renal failure, the overzealous use of phosphate binders can produce hypophosphatemia and phosphate depletion; moreover, worsening of bone disease and osteomalacia may result.[32,328]

NUTRITIONAL CALCIUM SUPPLEMENTS

Calcium carbonate or calcium acetate can be given as described above, as a phosphate binder, and can also be used as a nutritional source for additional calcium. When either calcium carbonate or calcium acetate is given orally as a phosphate binder, some calcium is absorbed, despite efforts to minimize absorption. Also, phosphate binding occurs when calcium is given as a nutritional supplement.

The addition of calcium is important in patients with advanced chronic renal failure and those undergoing dialysis because, first, intestinal absorption of calcium is impaired in these patients; second, the diets generally consumed by uremic patients contain reduced amounts of dairy products and, consequently, low quantities of calcium. The dietary calcium intake in patients with advanced renal failure was found to be 400 to 700 mg/day;[285] a neutral or positive balance for calcium can be achieved in uremic patients by supplementation of the diet with calcium carbonate, calcium citrate, or calcium lactate,[106] to increase the total intake of calcium to 1.5 g or more per day.[104,285,361] When, during the course of renal failure, is the best time to add calcium supplements has not been resolved. Coburn and coworkers found normal intestinal calcium absorption in male patients with serum creatinine levels below 2.5 mg/100 ml,[113] while Malluche and coworkers found intestinal calcium absorption to be decreased in certain patients with GFRs of 20 to 50 ml/min.[339] Patients with more advanced renal failure are more prone to develop hypercalcemia with oral calcium supplementation, since they lack the renal avenue for calcium excretion should net calcium absorption increase more than is anticipated.

Effects of long-term calcium supplementation in patients with advanced renal failure have been reported. Makoff and coworkers gave 4 to 10 g of calcium carbonate per day to uremic patients not on dialysis. They observed a reduction of serum phosphorus concentration, a slight rise in serum calcium level, and a small increase in serum bicarbonate level.[330] Meyrier and coworkers gave 5 to 20 g of calcium carbonate per day to one group of hemodialysis patients and compared them to other patients receiving no calcium carbonate.[377] In the former group, bone biopsies showed less resorptive activity, radiographs showed less evidence of skeletal disease, and fewer fractures, episodes of pseudogout, and extraskeletal calcifications were found. Hypercalcemia, which was sometimes profound, resolved upon reduction of the dosage. Curtis and coworkers found plasma alkaline phosphatase activity and serum PTH concentration to decrease in uremic patients with overt secondary hyperparathyroidism given supplements of either calcium carbonate or, in those with low blood phosphorus levels, calcium phosphate.[131] Eastwood and coworkers compared bone biopsies from uremic patients with renal osteodystrophy treated with vitamin D with those from similar patients treated with calcium carbonate.[159,160] In patients receiving calcium carbonate, diffuse patchy deposition of calcium in osteoid was observed, and a distinct calcification front did not develop; but such a front was regularly seen in biopsies from the patients given vitamin D. This study provides evidence that vitamin D is more effective than calcium supplementation in reversing the overt skeletal disease of uremia.

Treatment with oral calcium supplements is not free of risk. Large amounts of oral calcium compounds should be used cautiously in patients with marked hyperphosphatemia, because of the risk of elevating the calcium-phosphorus product and thereby predisposing to extraskeletal calcification. Hypercalcemia may develop in uremic patients, as in patients with normal renal function, during therapy with large quantities of oral calcium salts.[201,330,362,377] Hypercalcemia may be more common in patients with serum phosphorus concentrations below 3 mg/100 ml.[107] Some uremic patients who have mild hypercalcemia (11 to 12 mg/100 ml) are asymptomatic; others may exhibit symptoms despite only modestly elevated serum calcium levels. In addition to nausea, anorexia, vomiting, mental confusion, and lethargy, patients with advanced renal failure may develop pruritus, acute conjunctivitis, and a sharp elevation in blood pressure.[567]

In patients with advanced renal failure and GFR below 10 ml/min, and in patients undergoing regular hemodialysis, calcium supplements should be given—or phosphate binders, as described above.

CONCENTRATION OF CALCIUM IN DIALYSATE

There is growing evidence that when calcium salts—either calcium carbonate or calcium acetate—are used as phosphate binders, the calcium content of dialysate should be reduced to 2.5 meq/liter.[326,486,523] It is not quite certain whether the concentration should be reduced for all patients, as was done by Slatopolsky and coworkers,[523] or whether the concentration should be reduced in patients showing some rise in serum calcium concentration.[326,486] Moreover, there are a few patients who will become hypercalcemic as a result of calcium carbonate or calcium acetate despite the use of a dialysate calcium level of 2.5 meq/liter; in such patients concentrations as low as 2.0 meq/liter have been used.[326,486] Reduction of the concentration to below 2.0 meq/liter may increase the risk of hypotension as a direct consequence of the lowered ionized calcium level.[293] Another advantage of the use of lower calcium levels in dialysate is the greater flexibility in the use of active vitamin D sterols, which are more effective in suppressing the overactive parathyroid glands than a rise in serum calcium per se.[524]

In patients not taking calcium salts as a phosphate binder, a number of studies have evaluated the effect of various levels of calcium in dialysate; these are reviewed elsewhere.[314] The use of dialysate calcium concentrations below 3.0 to 3.25 meq/liter was associated with more rapid loss of bone mineral than the use of dialysate calcium levels of 3.25 to 3.5 meq/liter.[58,148,206] Under these circumstances serum PTH levels have often slowly risen despite the increase in serum calcium concentration.[436] There was little to indicate that dialysate calcium concentrations of 3.25 to 3.5 meq/liter could prevent the development of bone disease,[393,453,542] but the use of a lower concentration of 2.5 meq/liter may be associated with more rapid progression of the bone disease when neither calcium carbonate nor calcium acetate is being given.[88,386] When one employs a dialysate calcium concentration of 2.5 meq/liter, it is important to be certain that the patient remains compliant with his or her prescribed calcium-containing phosphate binding agents; otherwise, progressive negative calcium balance and bone loss may ensue.

USE OF VITAMIN D STEROLS

Despite their adherence to therapy with appropriate dietary phosphate restriction, adequate intake of phosphate binders, appropriate levels of calcium in dialysate, and adequate dietary intake of calcium, significant numbers of patients with advanced renal failure develop secondary hyperparathyroidism and disabling bone disease. The clarification of the role of the kidney in generating calcitriol, the active hormonal form of vitamin D, has prompted the use of vitamin D in treating such patients.[145] In view of recent data, a theoretical case can be made in support of the use of vitamin D sterols early in the course of renal insufficiency; data are limited, however, regarding the use of vitamin D sterols in a prophylactic manner in patients with renal failure. In the clinical trials of one of the vitamin D analogues employed for the management of bone disease in uremic patients, each patient has served as his or her own control, and each study usually involved only one form of vitamin D. Few data comparing the efficacy of different vitamin D sterols are available.[318,571] Nevertheless, during the past decade most studies on the use of various analogs of vitamin D have shown great efficacy. It is our belief that the widespread and appropriate use of vitamin D therapy is the most important single factor in the marked decrease in the numbers of parathyroidectomies performed over the past few years.

When uremic patients exhibit evidence of secondary hyperparathyroidism with bone erosions, high blood levels of PTH, and elevated plasma alkaline phosphatase activity, treatment with an adequate quantity of one of the various forms of vitamin D usually leads to improvement. Pharmacologic doses of vitamin D_2 itself,[556,558] dihydrotachysterol,[545,556] 25-OH-D_3 (calcifediol),[558] $1\alpha(OH)D_3$,[91] and $1\alpha,25\text{-}(OH)_2D_3$[66,67,558] have each led to improvement of symptoms, improvement of x-rays toward normal, amelioration of bone disease, and a fall in plasma alkaline phosphatase activity and serum PTH concentration.

Although vitamin D_2 or D_3 and dihydrotachysterol have been available for a long time, there are only a few well-documented reports on their efficacy.[277,307] Vitamin D has been reported to induce more nearly normal bone mineralization than occurs following calcium supplementation.[307] Stanbury and Lumb, and Dent and coworkers, have shown that vitamin D_2 at a dosage of 50,000 to 200,000 IU/day improves overt skeletal disease in patients with advanced renal failure.[149,532] However, the responsiveness of individual patients varies greatly. Lumb and coworkers reported improvement of radiographic evidence of bone disease in children given 30,000 to 50,000 IU/day of vitamin D for 5 to 13 months.[275]

The principal hazard in the use of vitamin D is hypercalcemia; resolution may require several weeks. When hypercalcemia occurs, it arises as a consequence of high blood levels of 25-OH-D_3; the levels of calcitriol are generally not increased.[558]

Vitamin D or other vitamin D sterols should not be used when serum phosphorus levels are markedly elevated, because an increase in the calcium-phosphorus product can lead to the development of extraskeletal calcification.[333] Treatment with vitamin D, when carried out in conjunction with adequate control of hyperphosphatemia, may be associated with regression of extraskeletal calcifications, including those in blood vessels.[553]

During the last few years, several highly active, naturally occurring forms of vitamin D, 25-OH-D_3, calcitriol, and $24,25\text{-}(OH)_2D_3$ have been evaluated in clinical trials.[556,558] Also, several synthetic analogues have been introduced that bypass the need for renal 1-hydroxylation. These include 1α-OH-D_3, 5,6-*trans*-25-OH-D_3, and 5,6-*trans*-vitamin D_3. Of these, 25-OH-D_3, calcitriol, and 1α-OH-D_3 have had the widest use (see below).

Calcifediol

Despite the availability of 25-OH-D_3 for investigational use since 1969, there are few reports of its use in patients with renal osteodystrophy.[553] Intestinal absorption of calcium can be increased with 100 μg of 25-OH-D_3 per day, while 20 μg/day augments calcium absorption in normal subjects.[146] However, recent data indicate that uremic patients respond favorably to treatment with doses below 100 μg/day. Teitelbaum and coworkers treated five patients with 40 μg/day for 3 to 9 months; serum PTH concentration and alkaline phosphatase activity decreased, and serial bone biopsies showed decreased numbers of osteoclasts, size of osteoid surface covered with active osteoblasts, and marrow fibrosis.[545] Witmer and colleagues treated nine uremic children with 25-OH-D_3.[576] Five had severe osteodystrophy that had previously failed to respond to 350 to 700 μg of vitamin D per day (13,000 to 27,000 IU/day) before 25-OH- D_3 was given. Osteitis fibrosa decreased, number of osteoblasts dropped, and marrow fibrosis decreased in these five children with 25 to 200 μg of 25-OH-D_3 per day. Other children, with normal or near-normal skeletal x-rays at the initiation of hemodialysis, were given either 25 to 50 μg/day of 25-OH-D_3 plus an oral calcium supplemenet or else oral calcium alone. Bone lesions progressively worsened in the group receiving only oral calcium, but skeletal biopsies showed improved mineralization and decreased fibrosis in those given 25-OH-D_3. Fournier and coworkers noted a rise in plasma alkaline phosphatase activity and an increase in the active formation surface area of trabecular bone in three patients given 200 to 300 μg of 25-OH-D_3 three times per week for 4 to 8 weeks.[185] These effects differed from those observed in other patients given 1α-OH-D_3 over the same period. Results from a five-center study have been summarized by Recker and colleagues.[452] These hemodialysis patients received 200 μg three times weekly for 29 weeks, with the dose adjusted to avoid hypercalcemia; the final dose averaged 46 μg/day. As a group the patients noted a significant improvement in symptoms, with decreased bone pain and tenderness and a better overall clinical

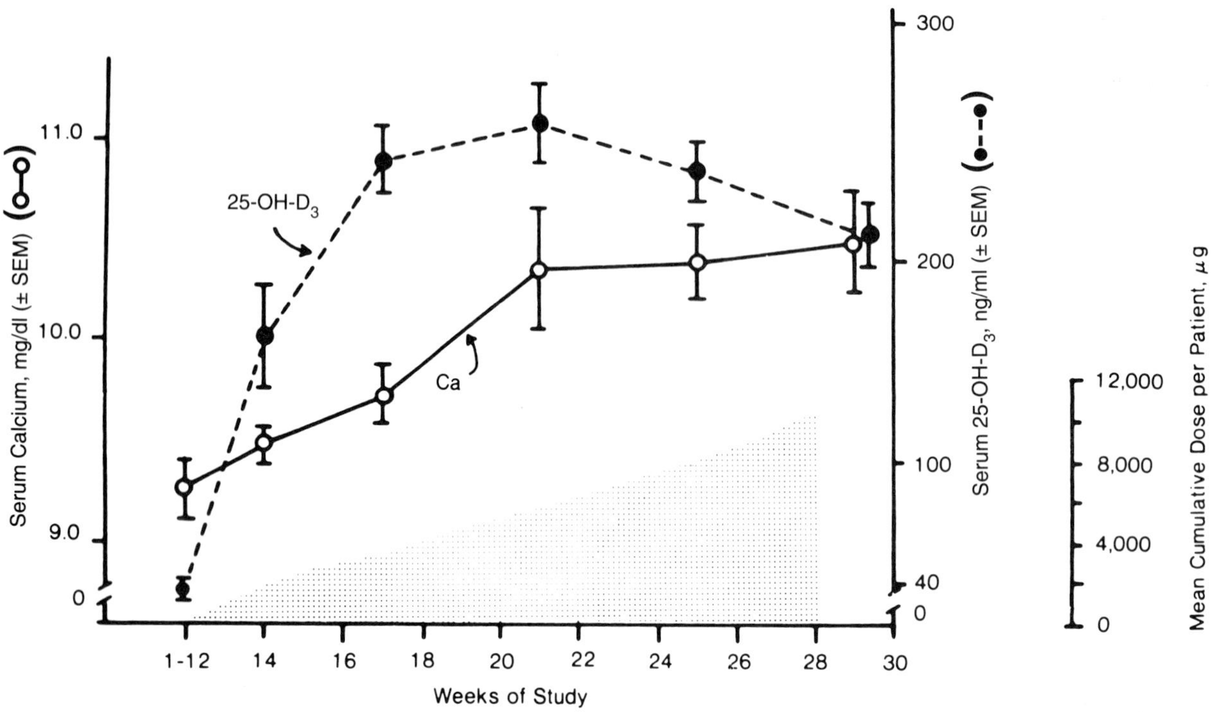

FIGURE 41-38 • Levels of calcium and 25-OH-D$_3$ (mean ± s.e.) in 44 patients with renal osteodystrophy undergoing long-term hemodialysis and treatment with 25-OH-D$_3$. Cumulative dose of 25-OH-D$_3$ shown in stippled area. (Reprinted, by permission, from Recker R et al: *Arch Intern Med* 138:857, 1978.)

status. Small increases in serum calcium and phosphorus concentrations were found, and serum alkaline phosphatase activity fell. Plasma PTH concentration for the entire group was not changed, although individual patients exhibited significant decreases. Bone biopsies disclosed increases in resorption surface area in conjunction with decreased fibrosis. Plasma levels of 25-OH-D$_3$ rose to 200 to 300 ng/100 ml concurrently with the maximum elevation of serum calcium concentration (Fig. 41-38). In each of the series reported, several patients developed hypercalcemia.

Calcitriol

In several clinical trials, calcitriol has proved efficacious for treatment of patients with renal osteodystrophy. In an early study Brickman and coworkers reported observations in eight patients given 0.14 to 0.68 µg of calcitriol per day by mouth for 2 to 4 months. Patients with secondary hyperparthyroidism and osteitis fibrosa showed decreases in serum PTH concentration, marrow fibrosis, and resorption surface area.[42,170] Patients with muscle weakness observed an increase in muscle strength. There was some improvement in the abnormal mineralization front in those with osteomalacia. Similar observations were reported by Henderson and coworkers, and by Silverberg and coworkers.[234,513] Eastwood and coworkers gave 0.54 to 1.35 µg of calcitriol per day IV to five patients for 4 weeks and noted better bone mineralization with an improved calcification front in three patients.[163] Pierides and coworkers noted improvement in secondary hyperparathyroidism as evidenced by changes in bone histology, skeletal x-ray appearance, serum PTH concentration, and alkaline phosphatase activity.[430] Electromyographic improvement was also noted, with an increase in duration of action potential. A series of 40 patients from Los Angeles, Seattle, and Hawaii were treated with calcitriol at an average dose of 0.62 µg/day for 4 to 90 weeks.[108] Bone pain improved in 71 percent and muscle weakness in 85 percent. In patients with elevated serum PTH levels, these levels often decreased and alkaline phosphatase activity declined toward normal. Bone biopsies improved; close correlation was observed between improvement in the degree of osteitis fibrosa and reduction in serum PTH levels.[501] A subgroup with refractory osteomalacia developed hypercalcemia while receiving low doses of calcitriol; these patients were subsequently identified as having aluminum-related bone disease.[410] Similar findings were reported by Pierides and coworkers in patients treated with calcitriol.[431]

In many patients showing a favorable response, serum phosphorus concentration dropped during the first 1 to 3 months of treatment; subsequently, serum phosphorus concentration often increased. Sherrard and colleagues evaluated pre- and posttreatment bone biopsies in uremic patients treated with calcitriol and two control groups of patients undergoing dialysis using either 6.0 or

8.0 mg/100 ml calcium in dialysate and receiving 500 IU of vitamin D_3 per day.[501] The pretreatment bone biopsies showed more extensive osteitis fibrosa in the group given calcitriol. Nonetheless, there was a marked decrease in fibrosis in 10 of 11 patients with osteitis fibrosa, and increased mineralization in 16 of 17 patients treated with calcitriol. The patients treated with calcium in dialysate showed little or no improvement. It was concluded that calcitriol was more effective than adding calcium to dialysate in improving mineralization and reversing secondary hyperparathyroidism.

The studies reviewed above were carried out in patients with advanced renal insufficiency and evidence of overt skeletal disease. Several controlled prospective studies have also been carried out in dialysis patients, including those without symptoms of osteodystrophy.

In a controlled double-blind study of 31 dialysis patients, Berl and coworkers gave either calcitriol, in an average dose of 0.82 μg/day, or vitamin D_3, in a dose of 400 IU/day, for 12 weeks.[42] They noted an increase in serum calcium concentration from 9.05 ± 0.15 to 10.25 ± 0.20 mg/100 ml in those receiving calcitriol; serum calcium levels did not change in those receiving vitamin D_3. Serum PTH concentration fell significantly in 11 of 13 patients receiving calcitriol; this response reverted toward basal levels after vitamin D_3 was substituted for the calcitriol. Bone biopsies showed improvement of osteitis fibrosa in patients given calcitriol, but no change in those receiving vitamin D_3; osteomalacia failed to improve in patients receiving calcitriol.

Maxwell and coworkers followed a similar protocol in a controlled study.[358] They noted a significant decrease in plasma alkaline phosphatase activity in those receiving calcitriol, but no change in those receiving vitamin D_3. Hypercalcemia in patients taking calcitriol rapidly reversed itself after withdrawal of the drug.

In a double-blind trial Memmos and coworkers gave either 0.5 μg/day of calcitriol or a placebo to asymptomatic patients who had been on hemodialysis for at least one year; the trial lasted one to two years.[358] At the end of one year 16 of the 30 patients receiving placebo, but only 1 of 27 patients receiving calcitriol, showed deterioration in hand x-rays. Among the patients who entered the trial with abnormal skeletal x-rays, none of the 16 patients receiving placebo showed improvement after two years, compared to 5 of 11 given calcitriol. Serum PTH levels, which were closely related to the severity of radiographic evidence of hyperparathyroidism, showed a slight increase in the placebo group and fell in the calcitriol-treated patients. Plasma alkaline phosphatase activity fell significantly in the patients with abnormal x-rays who received calcitriol, but in the other groups activity did not change.

In a controlled study in asymptomatic dialysis patients with normal skeletal radiographs and good biochemical control of calcium and phosphorus levels, the frequency of new or worsened erosions was lower in patients given up to 1.0 μg/day of calcitriol, compared to placebo-treated patients.[373] Serum PTH concentration was suppressed in a larger fraction of the patients treated with calcitriol, while PTH concentration more often rose in the control subjects. Analysis of the data in these patients disclosed considerable heterogeneity in the suppressibility of the parathyroid glands; a serum calcium concentration of 10.0 to 10.8 mg/100 ml was needed in many patients to reduce serum PTH levels.[110] Such observations are consistent with an increase in set point so that a higher calcium concentration is required to suppress parathyroid gland activity.

In uremic children overt skeletal disease has a very high incidence compared with adults. Children with advanced renal failure who received calcitriol have responded quite favorably. Improvement in growth or catch-up growth was initially reported in children receiving calcitriol,[100] although subsequent observations have not confirmed such a beneficial effect.[98] More recent observations in children undergoing treatment with CAPD suggest that the maintenance of normal serum calcium concentration during treatment with calcitriol may not invariably lead to reversal of the features of secondary hyperparathyroidism.[421] Indeed, raising the serum calcium concentration to levels slightly above normal has resulted in more consistent reversal of the features of secondary hyperparathyroidism.[484]

In general, the trials with calcitriol and 1α-OH-D_3 suggest that these sterols are most effective in treating patients with secondary hyperparathyroidism, particularly when serum calcium concentration is normal or decreased; when osteomalacia and secondary hyperparathyroidism coexist, a favorable response is usual (Fig. 41-39). Under some circumstances the bone can be restored largely to normal, but in other settings the elevated serum PTH levels persist and treatment with calcitriol is not successful in reversing the secondary hyperparathyroidism. In this situation, as we will discuss later, intravenous administration of calcitriol may be helpful (see below). When severe osteitis fibrosa exists, treatment with calcitriol in doses as high as 1.0 to 2.0 μg/day may be needed for 6 to 18 months; then hypercalcemia may appear rather suddenly, usually when serum alkaline phosphatase activity has returned to normal. This chemical sequence probably signifies completion of a period of rapid healing and remineralization of bone. From this time onward, lower doses of calcitriol should be used, because of a risk of recurrent hypercalcemia.

The administration of calcitriol may help to identify patients with aluminum-related bone disease and those with marked parathyroid hyperplasia where either the large mass of glandular hyperplasia or a marked shift in set point may necessitate intravenous calcitriol therapy, or even parathyroid surgery.[109] Patients with mild skel-

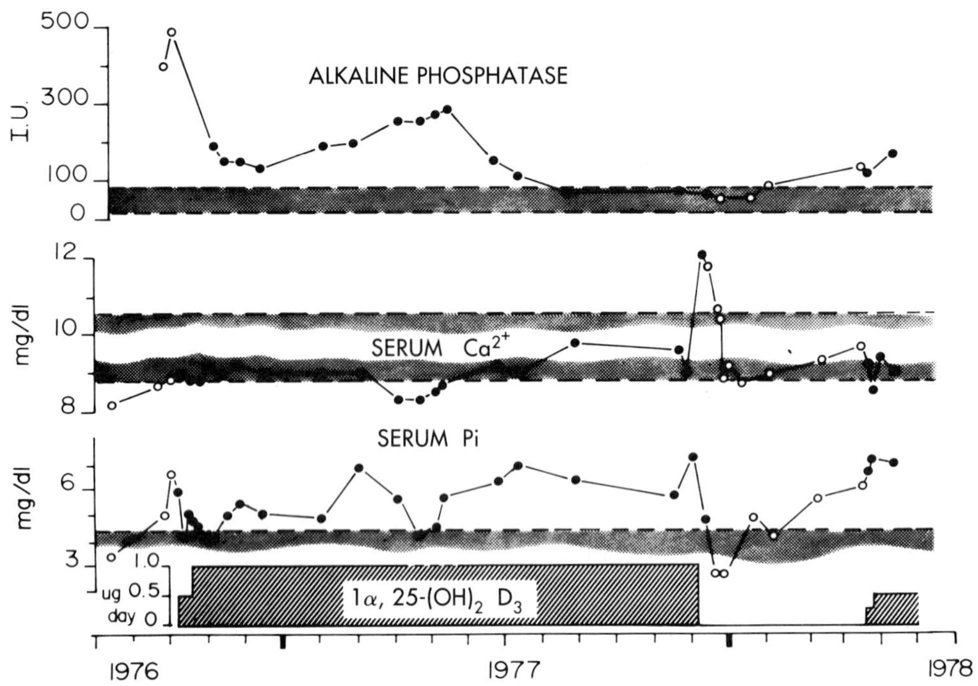

FIGURE 41-39 • Course of overt renal osteodystrophy due to marked secondary hyperparathyroidism in one patient. Serial values of serum alkaline phosphatase activity, calcium concentration, and inorganic phosphorus (P_1) concentration are shown in relation to daily dose of 1α,25-$(OH)_2D_3$. After 14 months, during which the patient received 1.0 μg/day, abrupt hypercalcemia occurred. Hypercalcemia dissipated following withdrawal of treatment; patient was subsequently free of hypercalcemia while receiving 0.5 μg/day. (Winkler and Coburn, unpublished observations.)

etal disease are more prone to develop episodes of hypercalcemia.[574]

Prophylactic treatment of dialysis patients with calcitriol may retard the development of secondary hyperparathyroidism, although there is some disagreement about the cost-benefit ratio of such therapy.[48] Preliminary data have suggested that the administration of calcitriol to patients with early to moderately developed renal insufficiency may reverse and/or prevent the development of secondary hyperparathyroidism without any detrimental effect on renal function.[352] Thus such therapy could prove efficacious in preventing the development of overt, nonsuppressible secondary hyperparathyroidism in patients with more advanced renal failure. The recent demonstration that the intravenous administration of calcitriol to dialysis patients is uniformly effective in reducing serum PTH levels provides additional data demonstrating a direct effect of calcitriol on the parathyroid glands.[155,327] It may also indicate that intravenous calcitriol is a potential alternative to the surgical management of secondary hyperparathyroidism.

Recent in-vitro and in-vivo studies have shown that intravenous calcitriol exerts a direct inhibitory effect on PTH secretion. Recently, we and others have shown the beneficial effect of intravenous calcitriol. Andress and coworkers studied 12 hemodialysis patients with severe hyperparathyroidism refractory to oral calcitriol therapy.[21] They were treated with intravenous calcitriol, 1 to 2.5 μg at the end of each dialysis, for a 14-month period. The researchers noted a mild increase in serum ionized calcium, from 2.5 to 2.6 mmol/liter, a significant decrease in PTH, from 172 to 69 pg/liter; and a marked improvement in bone histology in the second bone biopsy, performed 14 months later. Norris and coworkers also treated 10 patients with overt secondary hyperparathyroidism with intravenous calcitriol.[401] These patients received from 1 to 5 μg three tmes a week, at the end of each dialysis, for 13 months. There was a significant decrease in serum PTH (42 percent) and alkaline phosphatase (62 percent); serum calcium increased from 10.1 to 11.2 mg/100 ml. Dressler and coworkers have recently evaluated 12 hemodialysis patients with severe secondary hyperparathyroidism receiving intravenous calcitriol for 14 months.[294] Patients were selected for the presence of persistent or progressive hyperparathyroidism despite oral calcitriol therapy. The severity of bone disease was estimated by symptoms and by levels of alkaline phosphatase and PTH (determined by IRMA assay). The mean intravenous calcitriol dose administered was 4.4 μg, given at the end of dialysis, three times per week. By the end of the study there was significant clinical improvement in all patients. In addition, PTH decreased from 1179 to 159 pg/ml ($p < 0.05$). Neither serum calcium nor phosphorus changed after vitamin D therapy.

In summary, the available data on intravenous calcitriol strongly suggest that it is a desirable alternative in patients with overt hyperparathyroidism. Also, its use has potential merits in noncompliant dialysis patients.

1α-Hydroxyvitamin D_3

This synthetic analogue of calcitriol undergoes 25-hydroxylation in the liver to calcitriol prior to exerting its action. It is very active in patients with advanced uremia; the dose required to increase intestinal calcium absorption is only 1.5 to 2 times that needed for calcitriol.[68] Both short-term and long-term clinical trials have shown 1α-OH-D_3 to have effects in patients with renal failure that are very similar to those described for calcitriol;[42,68,90,91] the results of one study are summarized in Fig. 41-40.[422] 1α-OH-D_3 is widely used in Europe, Canada, and Japan, but only short-term trials have been carried out in the United States.[68] The improvement of hyperparathyroid bone disease and reversal of other features of secondary hyperparathyroidism following its use are similar to results reported for calcitriol.[422] Patients subsequently shown to have aluminum-related osteomalacia also failed to respond to 1α-OH-D_3,[431] as did those treated with calcitriol.[109]

The importance of concurrent use of phosphate binders to control serum phosphorus concentration was shown by the results of Davison and coworkers. Twenty patients receiving 1α-OH-D_3 and no aluminum hydroxide were compared with a group given aluminum hydroxide to reduce serum phosphorus concentration to below 5.0 mg/100 ml before treatment with 1α-OH-D_3 was initiated.[136] In the former group the incidence of corneal calcifications, pruritus, and radiographic evidence of soft extraskeletal calcifications was higher. Bone erosions resolved in equal numbers of patients in both groups, but there was a higher incidence of periosteal new bone formation in the group not given phosphate-binding gels. Preliminary (and uncontrolled) data have suggested that treatment with 1α-OH-D_3 may be associated with an increase in plasma aluminum levels.[185] However, plasma aluminum levels tend to increase with time in dialysis patients ingesting aluminum hydroxide;[279] hence, carefully controlled observations are needed to determine whether vitamin D sterols do actively increase the need for phosphate binders and/or augment the absorption of aluminum.

Recent observations by Brandi and coworkers have described the effect of intravenous administration of 1α-OH-D_3 for 12 weeks to patients on chronic hemodialysis.[64] They observed a marked suppression of PTH and only a slight increase in serum ionized calcium. Similar observations have been made by Lind and coworkers.[304] Thus intravenous administration of 1α-OH-D_3 seem to have an inhibitory effect on PTH secretion similar to that of calcitriol.

Other vitamin D sterols and general considerations regarding vitamin D use

In addition to the 1α-hydroxylated sterols discussed above, several other synthetic sterols have been introduced for brief trials. Several of these sterols have the A ring of the steroid molecule rotated 180° about the 5,6 double bond; this converts the orientation from a cis to a

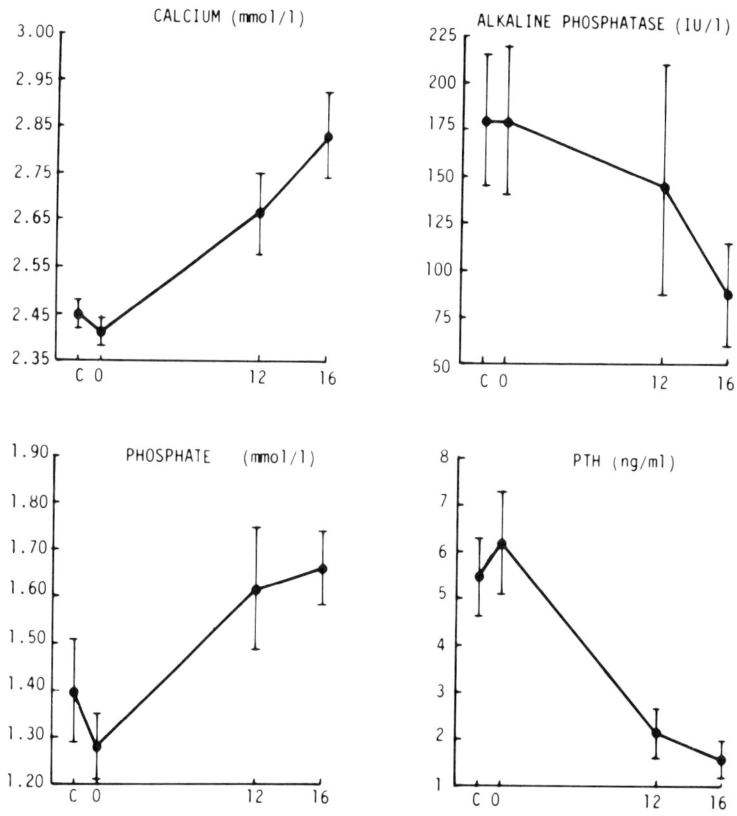

FIGURE 41-40 • Mean values of plasma calcium and phosphorus concentrations, alkaline phosphatase activity, and serum PTH concentration in 10 dialysis patients according to duration (in months) of treatment with 1α,25-OH-D_3. Initial dose was 1.0 μg/day; dosage was adjusted in each patient during trial. [Reproduced, by permission of the publisher, from Papapoulos SE et al: The effect of 1α-hydroxycholecalciferol on secondary hyperparathyroidism of chronic renal failure, in Norman AW et al (eds): *Vitamin D: Biochemical, Chemical and Clinical Aspects Related to Calcium Metabolism.* Berlin, de Gruyter, 1977, p 693.]

trans configuration, with the normal 3-hydroxyl group assuming a geometric position equivalent to that of the 1α-hydroxyl moiety of calcitriol. This may be referred to as a "pseudo 1α-hydroxyl" configuration. Some such compounds can enhance calcium absorption in uremic patients;[220,477] these include 5,6-*trans*-vitamin D_3 and 5,6-*trans*-25-OH-D_3.[220,477] These agents have been given to dialysis patients in Europe. It is not clear that these compounds have any advantage over the natural 1-hydroxylated sterols or dehydrotachysterol itself, which is also active by virtue of its pseudo 1α-hydroxyl characteristics.

One major feature of calcitriol and 1α-OH-D_3 is their relatively rapid turnover compared to vitamin D itself. Brickman and coworkers found the half-time of reversal of hypercalciuria to be approximately 50 to 75 percent greater for 1α-OH-D_3 than for calcitriol.[68] Kanis and Russell evaluated the rate of reversal of hypercalcemia or hypercalciuria induced by vitamin D_3, dihydrotachysterol, 1α-OH-D_3, and calcitriol.[267] The half-time for reversal of the effects was shorter after discontinuing calcitriol than was the case for 1α-OH-D_3, vitamin D_3, or dihydrotachysterol; the differences were independent of the dose given or the length of treatment. Thus calcitriol shows the most rapid dissipation of effect, a useful feature should toxicity occur. In addition, in several documented cases a response to calcitriol, 25-OH-D_3, or 1α-OH-D_3 was elicited after no response to vitamin D_3 or dihydrotachysterol.[172,576]

One consideration in the choice of either 1α-OH-D_3 or dihydrotachysterol is their lack of 25-hydroxyl group; hepatic 25-hydroxylation is necessary before they act. Simultaneous treatment with a drug such as phenobarbital, phenytoin, or glutethimide, which may impair hepatic 25-hydroxylation, may result in impaired action of the vitamin D sterol.[432,441] Pierides and coworkers have reported that anticonvulsant therapy prevented a favorable response to 1α-OH-D_3.[433]

Another question raised is whether the active vitamin D compounds have a significant effect on magnesium homeostasis in uremic patients. Sörenson and coworkers suggested that these active sterols might induce magnesium intoxication.[528] However, Kanis and coworkers, and the authors, have carried out metabolic balance studies in uremic patients treated with calcitriol or 1α-OH-D_3 and found little or no effect of these sterols on serum magnesium level or magnesium balance.[268,269]

One vitamin D sterol whose effects have not been ascertained in patients with end-stage renal failure is 24,25-$(OH)_2D_3$. Kanis and coworkers, and Llach and coworkers, reported finding qualitative differences between the effect of 24,25-$(OH)_2D_3$ and that of calcitriol in patients with renal failure.[264,313] There has also been a report of favorable responses in a small number of patients whose osteomalacia was refractory to therapy with calcitriol alone but who responded to 24,25-$(OH)_2D_3$ combined with calcitriol.[247] Subsequently these patients were found to have aluminum-related osteomalacia,[245] and their favorable responses have been less consistent.[412] Other reports have suggested that 24,25-$(OH)_2D_3$ may have a suppressive effect on the parathyroid glands,[85] although subsequent studies in patients with secondary hyperparathyroidism and in dogs with experimental uremia failed to demonstrate any such effect.[195,406] Nevertheless, recent observations strongly suggest that this sterol, unlike calcitriol, specifically inhibits bone resorption, and that this effect is independent of PTH secretion. Thus, Dunstan and coworkers evaluated 29 dialysis patients treated either with calcitriol or 24,25-$(OH)_2D_3$ alone; a third group was treated with bone sterols together. Bone biopsies were performed in all patients before and after 8 months of therapy.[156] While calcitriol inhibited PTH secretion, 24,25-$(OH)_2D_3$ decreased bone resorption and formation without any change in PTH levels. More important, the administration of both sterols together resulted in greater improvement in bone resorption. Popovtzer et al, in a multicenter controlled trial, have evaluated the effect of 24,25-$(OH)_2D_3$ together with 1,α-$(OH)D_3$ in 58 dialysis patients.[437] Bone biopsies were performed before and after 12 months of 1,α-$(OH)D_3$ alone or together with 24,25-$(OH)_2D_3$. Osteoclastic resorption and bone mineralization improved significantly only in the group receiving both sterols. Thus these studies strongly suggest that combined treatment with 24,25-$(OH)_2D_3$ and 1,α-$(OH)D_3$ or calcitriol may result in a greater improvement in the bone lesions of dialysis patients.

PARATHYROID SURGERY

The medical modalities described can often produce suppression of the parathyroid glands and improvement of symptoms and bone disease in uremic patients. However, these measures may not succeed, and the appearance of certain manifestations of secondary hyperparathyroidism may necessitate parathyroid surgery. The clinical presentations that indicate the need for subtotal parathyroidectomy include unequivocal evidence of hyperparathyroidism in conjunction with (1) hypercalcemia, particularly when it produces symptoms; (2) severe and intractable pruritus that does not respond to dialysis or other medical treatment, and that occurs in association with evidence of secondary hyperparathyroidism (bone erosions and high serum PTH concentration); (3) serum calcium-phosphorus product that consistently exceeds 75 to 80 (in mg/100 ml × mg/100 ml) and is accompanied by progressive extraskeletal calcifications; (4) severe or progressive skeletal and articular pain; (5) calciphylaxis (i.e., ischemia and necrosis of soft tissues with vascular calcifications;[134,139] and (6) exclusion of aluminum toxicity or severe aluminum accumulation.

Persistent, significant hypercalcemia (serum calcium concentration greater than 11 mg/100 ml) is occasionally seen in patients with end-stage renal failure under treatment with regular dialysis. The appearance of hypercalcemia with clinical signs and symptoms (e.g., peptic ulcer disease, nausea, and vomiting) may indicate a need for treatment. It should be remembered that hypercalcemia can occur in uremia in the absence of secondary hyperparathyroidism, and aluminum-related bone disease is not uncommon as a cause of hypercalcemia in dialysis patients in the United States.[115] Therefore, parathyroid surgery for hypercalcemia should not be done in the absence of unequivocal evidence of secondary hyperparathyroidism (i.e., a bone biopsy showing osteitis fibrosa and markedly elevated serum levels of PTH). In the past it was thought that radiographic evidence of erosions is specific; however, it is now apparent that such erosions may persist and still be present when the patient develops aluminum-related osteomalacia. Significant hypercalcemia also may appear in patients with successfully functioning renal transplants and may also necessitate parathyroid surgery (see above).

The occurrence of sufficiently high plasma calcium and phosphate levels to produce a calcium-phosphorus product that consistently exceeds 75 to 80 (in mg/100 ml × mg/100 ml) is often associated with progressive extraskeletal calcifications and/or rapidly progressive skeletal disease. When a persistently elevated calcium-phosphorus product does not respond to aggressive treatment with dialysis, dietary control, and treatment with phosphate-binding gels; serum PTH level is markedly elevated; intravenous administration of appropriate doses of calcitriol does not decrease PTH levels; and there is osteitis fibrosa on bone biopsy, a physician must consider the need for parathyroidectomy. After successful surgery the serum concentrations of calcium and phosphorus both decrease, and extraskeletal calcifications may resolve.

Severe pruritus that is unresponsive to aggressive dialysis and medical treatment is occasionally an indication for parathyroidectomy.[354] In some patients with features of severe osteitis fibrosa, pruritus can disappear or improve within 24 to 48 h after parathyroidectomy; however, other patients show no response. Lidocaine, 200 mg given intravenously, may effectively suppress pruritus in some dialysis patients;[541] this effect of lidocaine persists for 2 to 3 days, and the agent has few side effects. The beneficial effect of activated charcoal, 2 g twice daily, has also been reported.[423] Other authors have reported successful treatment of pruritus by phototherapy with ultraviolet light: eight exposures of the entire skin to long-wave ultraviolet light over a 4-week period were said to produce prolonged relief of pruritus.[199] From available information, partial parathyroidectomy is not recommended for pruritus unless unequivocal evidence of severe secondary hyperparathyroidism (bone erosions, osteitis fibrosa on biopsy, and very high plasma PTH concentration) exists; even then, efforts should be made to suppress parathryoid hyperplasia with the methods noted above.

Occasionally, severe skeletal and articular pain occur because of osteitis fibrosa; these symptoms may incapacitate the patient. Such symptoms may disappear or improve within a few days, or several weeks, after parathyroidectomy.

The syndrome of calciphylaxis, with ischemic lesions of soft tissue leading to ulcerations and necrosis, is a serious complication in patients with end-stage chronic renal failure (Fig. 41-26); this may progress and lead to death from sepsis unless it is appropriately treated. Often, other medical treatment has been unsuccessful; parathyroidectomy has been effective in reversing this serious complication. Ulcerative lesions have slowly healed over a period of days to weeks in the majority of cases reported.[202] In some patients serum PTH levels are found to be low; rigid phosphate restriction may be attempted in the hope of reversing this deficiency.[202]

A situation creating a difficult therapeutic dilemma for the physician is the occurrence of marked hyperphosphatemia and overt secondary hyperparathyroidism in a noncompliant patient. Such patients often have marked hyperphosphatemia, extraskeletal calcifications, bone erosions, and high plasma PTH levels. The serum calcium level may be normal or even slightly elevated. Under such conditions, parathyroid surgery may permit reduction of blood phosphorus concentration and resolution of ectopic calcifications. However, unless the patient then follows the prescribed treatment with dietary phosphate restriction and phosphate binders, the problem is likely to recur.

Two accepted surgical procedures for management of overt secondary hyperparathyroidism are subtotal parathyroidectomy and total parathyroidectomy with parathyroid autotransplantation. Each procedure has its advocates;[309] clearly the most important factor is a surgeon who is highly skilled and experienced with parathyroid surgery. Furthermore, recent observations surveying several hundred cases have clearly demonstrated that similar results are obtained with either treatment.[309] Substantial numbers of patients may have recurrence of hyperparathyroidism after either surgical procedure;[125,469] a major advantage of total parathyroidectomy with forearm autotransplantation is avoidance of the high morbidity associated with reexploration of the neck. With either procedure, cryopreservation of parathyroid tissue is of value in case of devascularization of the residual tissue in the neck (in the case of subtotal parathyroidectomy or failure of function of implanted tissue in the forearm).[509]

At surgery, it is imperative that *all* the parathyroid glands be identified. The number of glands normally varies from two to six;[200] failure to recognize sites of normal fifth and sixth glands is a common cause of failure of parathyroid surgery.[563] When subtotal parathyroidectomy is being performed, it is important that the most suitable gland be identified. Usually the gland that appears least hyperplastic but has an adequate blood supply is the best to partially resect; 40 to 60 mg of tissue should be left. After visually ascertaining that a satisfactory blood supply is preserved in the parathyroid fraction that is to remain in place, the surgeon can totally excise the other glands. The residual parathyroid tissue sometimes undergoes hyperplasia, necessitating a second surgical procedure; therefore, it is recommended that the remaining gland be marked by a metal clip and/or a long, black silk suture.[198,213] When only two or three parathyroid glands in the neck or the upper anterior thorax are accessible at the time of neck exploration, the removal of all three glands is recommended under an assumption that the fourth gland is located elsewhere. Tissues should be maintained by cryopreservation in case permanent hypoparathyroidism develops.[509] This indicates that only two or three glands exist; more commonly the overt hyperparathyroidism is only partially corrected. Good judgment and, even more important, extensive experience of the parathyroid surgeon are clearly important for the identification and management of atypical cases.

For parathyroid transplantation, parathyroid tissue, which has been identified by frozen section, is placed in chilled culture medium; then slices are implanted in multiple pockets in muscle on the lateral aspect of the flexor surface of the forearm of the nondominant arm.[509] Nonabsorbable suture is used to secure the slices in the muscle pockets and to provide a marker for subsequent identification should surgical resection be required. Technical problems during the surgical procedure should be few, and blood loss should be minimal. Usually the patient can leave the hospital within a week. A dialysis patient should be treated with dialysis 1 day prior to surgery.

The typical problem encountered in the postoperative period is prevention and management of severe hypocalcemia. Blood calcium levels almost invariably fall after removal of parathyroid tissue; the degree of hypocalcemia is related to the severity of histologic factors of osteitis fibrosa.[174] Profound and persistent hypocalcemia is more common in patients with x-ray evidence of skeletal erosions and marked elevation of alkaline phosphatase activity. When even modest hyperkalemia occurs in a dialysis patient during the immediate postoperative period, substantial electrocardiographic abnormalities may occur on account of the rise in potassium concentration and the concomitant hypocalcemia. To minimize the postoperative hypocalcemia, 0.5 to 1.0 μg of calcitriol may be given per day for 1 to 2 days before surgery and immediately after it; also, oral calcium carbonate is given to provide 1000 to 2000 mg of elemental calcium. The serum phosphorus levels usually diminish after surgery as well, although hyperphosphatemia may return and contribute to the decrease in serum calcium concentration.

Tetany may occur in such patients during the postoperative period; hemodialysis, perhaps from its alkalinizing effect, may predispose to this problem. The quantity of oral calcium needed is often quite large; the calcium dosage can be increased 0.5 to 1.0 g/day at intervals of 3 to 7 days until serum calcium concentration begins to increase. If the concentration of serum calcium falls below 7.5 mg/100 ml, or if tetany appears, intravenous calcium should be given as well. With such therapy, careful monitoring of serum calcium concentration is mandatory, and administration of phosphate-binding compounds should be adjusted to maintain serum phosphorus concentration in the range of 3.5 to 5.0 mg/100 ml. Tetany occurring in a uremic patient with severe bone disease may be catastrophic; the simultaneous fracture of scapula, clavicle, and both femoral necks has been reported during an episode of tetany during dialysis.[312] Major fractures have been observed (e.g., a spiral fracture of the femur or femoral neck fracture) in three patients after parathyroid surgery; the fractures occurred 1 to 3 weeks after surgery. Interestingly, each occurred late during the hemodialysis procedure itself. In the postoperative management of patients with marked periarticular calcifications, it may be wise to maintain modest hypocalcemia—i.e., serum calcium concentration of 8.0 to 9.0 mg/100 ml—until the ectopic calcifications have resolved.

In patients with very marked skeletal disease, hypocalcemia may occasionally persist for 2 to 3 months after parathyroidectomy. Large amounts of oral calcium supplement and appropriate doses of calcitriol usually are successful in correcting the hypocalcemia. Serum levels of phosphorus and magnesium concentration may also decrease during this time. If the serum magnesium concentration falls below 1.5 mg/100 ml (1.2 meq/liter), supplemental magnesium can be given by mouth. Administration of phosphate salts aggravates hypocalcemia; an increase in the calcitriol dosage may be needed. If the serum phosphorus concentration falls below 2.5 mg/100 ml, administration of phosphate binders should be reduced or stopped, but no effort should be made to increase the phosphorus concentration above 3.5 to 4.0 mg/100 ml.

Failure of serum calcium concentration to decrease significantly after surgery may indicate either that too much residual parathyroid tissue is left behind or that the major skeletal pathology in the patient is not severe osteitis fibrosa. Another postoperative complication of parathyroidectomy is the development of aluminum-related osteomalacia following total or subtotal parathyroidectomy.[22,176] The mechanism responsible for this is unclear; most likely, substantial accumulation of aluminum in bone had developed prior to the parathyroidectomy, and the presence of either high PTH levels or an increased rate of bone turnover had somehow protected the bone from the deleterious effect of aluminum. After parathyroid surgery, bone turnover decreases markedly and aluminum becomes deposited on the mineralization front.[176] The existence of symptomatic osteomalacia after parathyroidectomy indicates that the parathyroid surgery was unnecessary in the presence of hypercalcemia due to preexisting aluminum-related bone disease. Furthermore, in the absence of PTH, removal of aluminum deposits with deferoxamine is more difficult.

During the period of hypocalcemia, remineralization of the skeleton is usually occurring; the blood calcium concentration starts to rise and the requirement for calcium and vitamin D decreases markedly once the "hungry bones" have reached, or neared, calcium saturation. If the doses of calcium and vitamin D are not reduced, hypercalcemia may ensue. The fall of a markedly elevated plasma alkaline phosphatase level to near normal may indicate that the bone is reaching a stage where healing is largely completed; when this occurs, the calcium supplements and vitamin D dosage should be reduced.

New insight into the role of vitamin D and active vitamin D sterols in the regulation of PTH secretion and the availability of highly active forms of vitamin D for the management of uremic patients may make the management of secondary hyperparathyroidism easier in patients with end-stage renal failure; thus there should be less need for parathyroid surgery in these patients. It is our impression that with appropriate early calcitriol therapy, both significant parathyroid hyperplasia and osteitis fibrosa are prevented.

Treatment of bone disease due to aluminum accumulation

Patients with profound aluminum toxicity were initially difficult to manage. Hemodialysis employing aluminum-free water brings about the removal of only small quantities, because of substantial binding of aluminum to transferrin and other plasma proteins;[381,431] and most dialysis units have continued to give aluminum gels as they initiate their water treatment. The management of aluminum-loaded patients with aluminum-free dialysate failed to produce clinical improvement in one study when the patients continued to ingest aluminum-containing phosphate binders.[246] Thus, prevention of this disease, which results from the use of contaminated water, is most important. The finding of several patients with aluminum-related bone disease in a single dialysis unit should prompt reevaluation of the adequacy of the method used for water purification.

The substitution of calcium carbonate or calcium acetate for the aluminum gels, in conjunction with the use of aluminum-free dialysate, can result in the healing of aluminum-related bone disease. Freemont and coworkers reported the improvement of bone biopsies 5 years after initiation of water purification combined with either withdrawal of aluminum hydroxide treatment or reduction of its dosage.[192] In both a well-documented case report and a small series of patients, Hercz and coworkers[236,237] reported substantial improvement of the histologic features of aluminum-related bone disease by 11 to 12 months after the afflicted patients had the total withdrawal of aluminum-containing gels and while they continued to undergo hemodialysis with very low aluminum concentrations (less than 10 μg/liter) in their dialysate baths. They observed an increase in osteoblastic osteoid and a rise in bone formation rates to normal in most patients' bone biopsies. Moreover, these changes in dynamic parameters correlated with the decrease in surface-stainable aluminum on bone biopsy and the substantial lowering of serum aluminum levels.

Ackrill and coworkers first reported that the chelating agent deferoxamine was effective for the removal of aluminum in a dialysis patient with encephalopathy; substantial improvement of both the neurologic features and the patient's musculoskeletal symptoms arising from osteomalacia was observed following treatment with multiple infusions of deferoxamine.[3] Subsequently, this agent, which has a very high affinity for aluminum as well as for iron, was given to dialysis patients with aluminum-related bone disease; favorable responses have been reported.[2,338,411]

Deferoxamine augments the removal of aluminum in two ways: it mobilizes aluminum from tissue stores, thereby increasing the plasma concentration of aluminum, and it increases the fraction of plasma aluminum that is ultrafilterable (Fig. 41-41). Both factors act to increase aluminum removal during hemodialysis or peritoneal dialysis. The quantities of aluminum removed by

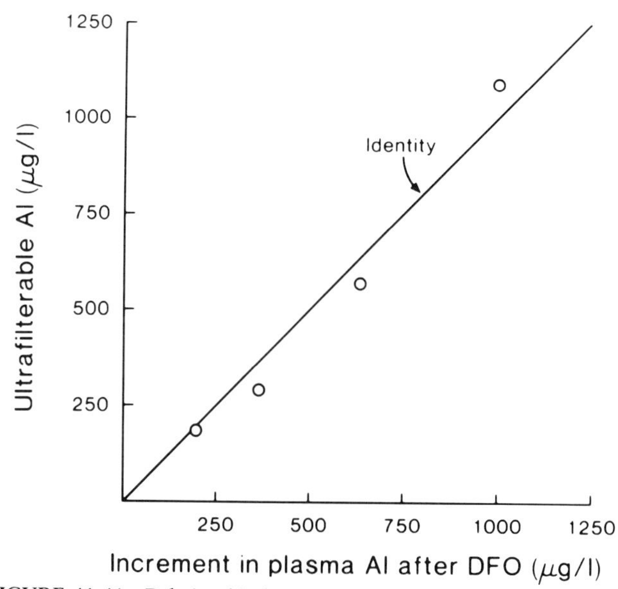

FIGURE 41-41 • Relationship between maximal increment of plasma aluminum concentration following infusion of deferoxamine (DFO) and simultaneous ultrafilterable aluminum concentration. Values fall near to line of identity indicating that increment in ultrafilterable aluminum can be accounted for by increase of plasma aluminum concentration induced by DFO. (Reprinted, by permission, from Milliner DS et al: *Ann Intern Med* 101:775, 1984.)

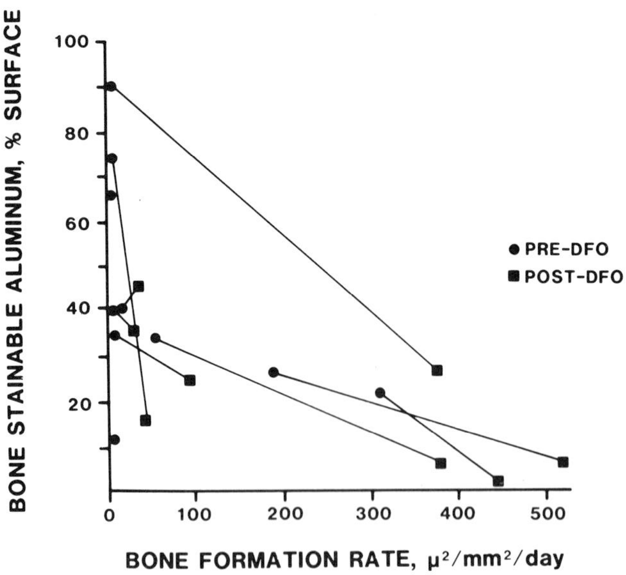

FIGURE 41-42 • Relationship between bone formation rate and stainable bone aluminum in patients with aluminum-related bone disease before and 6 to 10 months after treatment with weekly infusions of deferoxamine (DFO). Each line connects values obtained in one patient. [Adapted, with permission, from Ott SM et al: *Kidney Int* 29(suppl): S108, 1986.]

standard dialysis during hemodialysis using standard cuprophane membranes can increase 50 to 100 times after the infusion of deferoxamine.[381,537] Repeated infusion of deferoxamine, at 1.0 to 6.0 g/week, given to hemodialysis patients with aluminum-related bone disease were associated with substantial clinical improvement.[396,411] A modest reduction of serum calcium concentration was observed, and increments in plasma alkaline phosphatase levels occurred after 4 to 12 weeks of treatment; these observations are consistent with remineralization of bone. Moreover, bone biopsies have shown improvement with reduced aluminum staining and increased bone formation rate (see Fig. 41-42).[411] Malluche and coworkers noted improved bone histology and an increase in the mineralization rate in three patients with mixed bone disease that was characterized by aluminum staining and yet normal bone formation.[338] All the results reported indicate that the removal of aluminum with repeated infusions of deferoxamine can be effective in treating renal patients with aluminum-related bone disease.

As these beneficial effects of therapy with deferoxamine were being noted, a significant number of serious side effects of this agent have been recognized. There were instances of visual and auditory toxicity,[196,408,427] thrombocytopenia,[559] hypotension, and the precipitation of serious and even fatal encephalopathy.[504] In addition, mucormycosis, an infection that is commonly fatal, was appearing among dialysis patients receiving long-term treatment with deferoxamine.[54,55,572] In general, infections with the saprophytic fungi that cause mucormycosis have been associated with diabetic ketoacidosis, immunosuppressive therapy, iron overload, and certain malignancies, particularly lymphomas and leukemias.[297,376] Among the dialysis patients receiving deferoxamine, these predisposing conditions were generally absent;[54] moreover, two independent studies of mucormycosis in experimental animals have documented a role of deferoxamine in enhancing the pathogenicity of the causative fungi.[1,550] Among dialysis patients who developed mucormycosis associated with deferoxamine therapy, the infection was most commonly disseminated; frequently followed a rapidly fatal course; and was not suspected during life, but was recognized only upon postmortem examination.[54]

With regard to the probable pathogenic mechanism, it is likely that deferoxamine, which is a microbial siderophore, stimulates the growth and pathogenicity of certain species of the order Mucorales—the fungi responsible for mucormycosis—by making environmental iron more available to the organism.[550] This may occur as a result of receptors on the fungi for the deferoxamine-iron complex (feroxamine), which then facilitates the uptake of iron by the microorganism.[54] The iron and aluminum complexes of deferoxamine are both cleared from the body largely by the kidneys; therefore, these complexes have a much longer circulation time in dialysis patients than in patients with normal renal function. This may account for the relative rarity of mucormycosis in patients without renal disease who receive deferoxamine for iron overload associated with various hematologic disorders.[133]

The prevalence of mucormycosis among dialysis patients being treated with deferoxamine is unknown; the infection probably is more common than suspected, because it is rapidly fatal and because cultures of blood and other body fluids may not be positive even in cases of histologically proven infection. Because of the seriousness of this potential complication, and because it can appear after treatment for only a few weeks and with relatively low doses,[54] it seems that deferoxamine therapy should be limited to dialysis patients with proven aluminum encephalopathy or those with severe, symptomatic aluminum-related bone disease that has failed to respond to management with total withdrawl of aluminum-containing gels and the elimination of exposure to aluminum-contaminated dialysate. When deferoxamine must be used, it should be given in the lowest doses possible (e.g., 0.5 to 1.0 g every 7 to 10 days), and the dialysis that is done after the treatment should use a highly permeable dialysis membrane that permits the rapid clearance of deferoxamine complexes of iron and aluminum.[387] Moreover, treatment should be discontinued as soon as there is adequate clinical improvement. This very serious potential complication of therapy for aluminum toxicity underscores the importance of prevention of aluminum toxicity by avoidance of exposure to aluminum, whether from dialysate or from ingestion of aluminum-containing gels.

OTHER TREATMENT CONSIDERATIONS

Other management considerations, some of which have been referred to above, depend on the specific circumstances encountered. Loss of skeletal carbonate (or bicarbonate) may be another factor with a deleterious effect on the skeleton; in totally refractory bone disease, a therapeutic trial with dialysate of increased bicarbonate content may be reasonable. Treatment with a beta-adrenergic blocking drug, such as propanolol, or with cimetidine has not been proved to have therapeutic value.

Calcitonin may be useful in certain cases where the secondary hyperparathyroidism is inoperable or where it cannot be managed with a vitamin D sterol because of hypercalcemia.[244,265] Calcitonin can act to suppress certain effects of excess PTH, but one report of its short-term administration in uremic patients indicated it had very little overall effect.[140]

Finding an appropriate means for managing extraskeletal calcifications when they do not respond to control of serum phosphorus level or parathyroidectomy has been a serious dilemma. Zucchelli and coworkers reported treating nine dialysis patients with the diphosphonate compound sodium etidronate; 7.5 to 10 mg per kilogram of body weight was given for 5 to 9 months to patients who had a well-controlled serum phosphorus concentration but persistent ectopic calcification.[580] No change was seen in six patients, but two showed regression of the ectopic calcification, and another showed reduced arterial calcification. Bone biopsies after sodium etidronate treatment revealed a significant increase in osteoid volume and osteoid surface without modification of the calcification front. Slight increases in serum alkaline phosphatase levels were found in most patients. The sodium etidronate was well tolerated; however, a risk of osteomalacia is carried by such treatment.[480] Its use should therefore be limited to cases with severe extraskeletal calcification that is posing a serious threat to the patient and in which all other therapeutic modalities have failed.

Management of fractures

Rib fractures, probably the most frequent fractures in uremic patients, usually heal slowly over a period of several months. Usually they are asymptomatic and require little specific treatment. Traumatic fractures of the long bones and of the femoral neck may have a poor union even after several months. When fractures occur in patients with marked secondary hyperparathyroidism the appropriate surgical repair should be considered, since prolonged immobilization can create even greater complications in such patients. In some patients with fractures due to aluminum-related osteomalacia, slow healing may occur even though aluminum accumulation has not been specifically treated. In other such patients non-union of the fracture occurs, but the fracture then heals after initiation of chelation therapy with deferoxamine to remove excess aluminum.

The successful use of femoral head prostheses has been reported in patients with end-stage uremia and in those on dialysis.[579] When secondary hyperparathyroidism exists in a patient with a fracture, it seems preferable to treat initially with calcitriol, rather than parathyroidectomy, because of the risk of tetany, seizures, and further fractures.[480]

REFERENCES

1. Abe F et al: Effects of iron and desferrioxamine on Rhizopus infection. *Mycopathologia* 110:87, 1990.
2. Ackrill P et al: Treatment of fracturing renal osteodystrophy with desferrioxamine. *Proc Eur Dial Transplant Assoc* 19:223, 1982.
3. Ackrill P et al: Successful removal of aluminum from patients with dialysis encephalopathy. *Lancet* 2:692, 1980.
4. Adams ND et al: The calciuria of increased fixed acid production in humans: Evidence against a role for parathyroid hormone and 1,25 vitamin D. *Calcif Tissue Int* 28:233, 1979.
5. Agus ZS et al: Effects of parathyroid hormone on renal tubular reabsorption of calcium, sodium and phosphate. *Am J Physiol* 224:1143, 1973.
6. Ahmed KY et al: Persistent hypophosphatemia and osteomalacia in dialysis patients not on oral phosphate binders: Response to dihydrotachysterol therapy. *Lancet* 2:439, 1976.
7. Akmal M et al: Resolution of muscle calcification in rhabdomyolysis and acute renal failure. *Ann Intern Med* 89:928, 1978.
8. Albertini BV et al: High flux hemodiafiltration: Under six hours/week treatment. *Trans Am Soc Artif Intern Organs* 30:227, 1984.
9. Albertini BV et al: Performance characteristics of the hemoflow F60 in high-flux hemodiafiltration. *Contrib Nephrol* 46:169, 1985.
10. Albright F et al: Renal osteitis fibrosa cystica: Report of case with discussion of metabolic aspects. *Johns Hopkins Med J* 60:377, 1937.
11. Alfrey AC: Aluminum. *Adv Clin Chem* 21:69, 1983.
12. Alfrey AC et al: Metabolism and toxicity of aluminum in renal failure. *Am J Clin Nutr* 33:1509, 1980.
13. Alfrey AC et al: Resolution of hyperparathyroidism after renal transplantation. *N Engl J Med* 279:1349, 1968.
14. Alfrey AC et al: The dialysis encephalopathy syndrome. Possible aluminum intoxication. *N Engl J Med* 294:184, 1976.
15. Alfrey AC et al: Evaluation of body magnesium stores. *J Lab Clin Med* 84:153, 1974.

16. Alfrey AC et al: Bone pyrophosphate in uremia and its association with extraosseous calcification. *J Clin Invest* 57:700, 1976.
17. Alfrey AC et al: Extraosseous calcification. Evidence for abnormal pyrophosphate metabolism in uremia. *J Clin Invest* 57:692, 1976.
18. Alvarez-Ude F et al: Hemodialysis bone disease: Correlation between clinical, histologic and other findings. *Kidney Int* 14:68, 1978.
19. Andress DL et al: Comparison of parathyroid hormone assays with bone histomorphometry in renal osteodystrophy. *J Clin Endocrinol* 63:1163, 1986.
20. Andress DL et al: Parathyroid hormone response to hypocalcemia in hemodialysis patients with osteomalacia. *Kidney Int* 24:364, 1983.
21. Andress DL et al: Intravenous calcitriol in the treatment of refractory osteitis fibrosa of chronic renal failure. *N Engl J Med* 321:274, 1989.
22. Andress DL et al: Effect of parathyroidectomy on bone aluminum accumulation in chronic renal failure. *N Engl J Med* 312:468, 1985.
23. Andress DL et al: Plasma insulin-like growth factors and bone formation in uremic hyperparathyroidism. *Kidney Int* 36:471, 1989.
24. Arieff AI et al: Calcium metabolism of brain in acute renal failure. *J Clin Invest* 53:387, 1974.
25. Arieff AI et al: Parathyroid hormone as a uremic neurotoxin. *N Engl J Med* 299:362, 1978.
26. Arnaud CD: Parathyroid hormone: Coming of age in clinical medicine. *Am J Med* 55:577, 1973.
27. Arnaud CD: Hyperparathyroidism and renal failure. *Kidney Int* 4:89, 1973.
28. Arnett TR et al: Effect of pH on bone resorption by rat osteoclasts in vitro. *Endocrinology* 119(1):119, 1986.
29. Avioli LV: Collagen metabolism, uremia and bone. *Kidney Int* 4:105, 1973.
30. Avram MM et al: Search for the uremic toxin: Decreased motor nerve conduction velocity and elevated parathyroid hormone in uremia. *N Engl J Med* 298:1000, 1978.
31. Bagdade JD et al: Hypertriglyceridemia: A metabolic consequence of chronic renal failure. *N Engl J Med* 279:181, 1968.
32. Baker LRI et al: Iatrogenic osteomalacia and myopathy due to phosphate depletion. *Br Med J* 3:150, 1974.
33. Bakir AA et al: Acute fatal hyperaluminemic encephalopathy in undialyzed and recently dialyzed patients. *Trans Am Soc Artif Intern Organs* 32:171, 1986.
34. Ball JH et al: The many facets of secondary hyperparathyroidism. *Arch Intern Med* 131:746, 1973.
35. Barbour GL et al: Hypercalcemia in an anephric patient with sarcoidosis: Evidence for extrarenal generation of 1,25 dihydroxyvitamin D. *N Engl J Med* 305:440, 1981.
36. Bardin T et al: Etude prospective de l'atteinte articulaire des malades hemodialyses depuis plus de 10 ans. *Rev Rheum* 55:131, 1988.
37. Barsotti G et al: The decline of renal function slowed by very low phosphorus intake in chronic renal patients following a low nitrogen diet. *Clin Nephrol* 21:54, 1984.
38. Barsotti G et al: Reversal of hyperparathyroidism in severe uremics following very low-protein and low-phosphorus diets. *Nephron* 30:310, 1982.
39. Barzel US et al: The effects of chronic acid and alkali administration on bone turnover in adult rats. *Clin Sci* 36:517, 1969.
40. Baylink DJ et al: Formation, mineralization and resorption of bone in vitamin D deficient rats. *J Clin Invest* 49:112, 1970.
41. Benhamou CL et al: Arthropathies des membres chez les insuffisants renaux dialyses. *Presse Med* 16:119, 1987.
42. Berl T et al: 1,25 dihydroxycholecalciferol effects in chronic dialysis. A double-blind-controlled study. *Ann Intern Med* 88:774, 1978.
43. Berlyne GM: Microcrystalline conjunctival calcification in renal failure: A useful clinical sign. *Lancet* 2:366, 1968.
44. Berlyne GM et al: Rarity of renal osteodystrophy in Israel due to low phosphorus intake. A natural experiment. *Nephron* 10:141, 1973.
45. Berlyne GM et al: Hyperaluminaemia from aluminium resins in chronic renal failure. *Lancet* 2:494, 1970.
46. Berlyne GM et al: Red eyes in renal failure. *Lancet* 1:4, 1967.
47. Berson SA et al: Immunochemical heterogeneity of parathyroid hormone in plasma. *J Clin Endocrinol* 28:1037, 1978.
48. Binswanger U et al: 1,25-dihydroxycholecalciferol in patients with renal failure: The case against its prophylactic use, in Narins RG (ed): *Controversies in Nephrology and Hypertension*. New York, Churchill-Livingstone, 1984, p 523.
49. Birge SJ: Vitamin D, muscle and phosphate homeostasis. *Mineral Electrolyte Metab* 1:57, 1978.
50. Blair HC et al: Macrophage mediated bone resorption occurs in an acidic environment. *Calcif Tissue Int* 37:547, 1985.
51. Blumberg A et al: Influence of 1,25-dihydroxycholecalciferol on sexual dysfunction and related endocrine parameters in patients on maintenance hemodialysis. *Clin Nephrol* 13:208, 1980.
52. Blumenkrantz MJ et al: Metabolic balance studies and dietary protein requirements in patients undergoing continuous peritoneal dialysis. *Kidney Int* 21:849, 1982.
53. Blumenthal NC et al: In vitro model of aluminum induced osteomalacia: Inhibition of hydroxyapatite formation and growth. *Calcif Tissue Int* 36:439, 1984.
54. Boelaert JR et al: Deferoxamine therapy and mucormycosis in dialysis patients: Report of an international registry. *Am J Kidney Dis* 18:660, 1991.
55. Boelaert JR et al: The role of desferrioxamine in dialysis associated mucormycosis. *Clin Nephrol* 29:261, 1988.
56. Bogin E et al: Effect of parathyroid hormone on osmotic fragility of human erythrocytes. *J Clin Invest* 69:1017, 1982.
57. Bogin E et al: Effect of parathyroid hormone on heart cells. *J Clin Invest* 67:1215, 1981.
58. Bone JM et al: Role of dialysate calcium concentration in osteoporosis in patients on hemodialysis. *Lancet* 1:1047, 1972.
59. Booth BE et al: Vitamin D status regulates 25-hydroxyvitamin D_3-1αhydroxylase and its responsiveness to parathyroid hormone in chick. *J Clin Invest* 75:155, 1985.
60. Bordier PJ et al: Evolution of renal osteodystrophy: Correlation of bone histomorphometry and serum mineral

and immunoreactive parathyroid hormone values before and after treatment with calcium carbonate or 25 hydroxycholecalciferol. *Kidney Int* 7:S102, 1975.

61. Bordier PJ et al: Lack of histological evidence of vitamin D abnormality in the bones of anephric patients. *Clin Sci* 44:33, 1973.
62. Bouillon R et al: Influence of dialysate calcium concentration and vitamin D on serum parathyroid hormone during repetitive dialysis. *Kidney Int* 7:422, 1975.
63. Boyce BF et al: Hypercalcemia osteomalacia due to aluminum toxicity. *Lancet* 2:1009, 1982.
64. Brandi L et al: Effects of intravenous $1\alpha(OH)D_3$ on secondary hyperparathyroidism in chronic uremic patients on maintenance hemodialysis. *Nephron* 53:294, 1989.
65. Brannan PG et al: Magnesium absorption in the human small intestine: Results in patients with absorptive hypercalciuria. *J Clin Invest* 57:1412, 1976.
66. Brickman AS et al: 1,25 dihydroxyvitamin D_3 in normal man and patients with renal failure. *Ann Intern Med* 80:161, 1974.
67. Brickman AS et al: Action of 1,25 dihydroxycholecalciferol, a potent, kidney produced metabolite of vitamin D_3 in uremic man. *N Engl J Med* 287:891, 1972.
68. Brickman AS et al: Comparison of effects of 1-α-hydroxyvitamin D_3 and 1,25-dihydroxy-vitamin D_3 in man. *J Clin Invest* 57:1540, 1976.
69. Brickman AS et al: Actions of 1 hydroxyvitamin D_3 and 1,25 dihydroxyvitamin D_3 on mineral metabolism in man. I. Effects on net absorption of phosphorus. *Am J Clin Nutr* 30:1064, 1977.
70. Brickman AS et al: 1,25 dihydroxycholecalciferol: Effect on skeletal lesions and plasma parathyroid hormone in uremic osteodystrophy. *Arch Intern Med* 134:883, 1974.
71. Brown DJ et al: D-resistant osteomalacia in dialysis patients: Bone collagen and mineral content and treatment with desferrioxamine and calcitriol, in Norman AW et al (eds): *Vitamin D: Chemical, Biochemical and Clinical Endocrinology of Calcium Metabolism*. Berlin: Walter de Gruyter, 1982, p. 873.
72. Brown DJ et al: Treatment of dialysis osteomalacia with desferrioxamine. *Lancet* 2:343, 1982.
73. Brown EM: Set point for calcium: Its role in normal and abnormal secretion, in Cohn DV et al (eds): *Hormonal Control of Calcium Metabolism*. Amsterdam, Excerpta Medica, 1981, p 35.
74. Brown EM et al: Abnormal regulation of parathyroid hormone release by calcium in secondary hyperparathyroidism due to chronic renal failure. *J Clin Endocrinol* 54:172, 1982.
75. Brumbaugh PF et al: Radio receptor assay for 1,25-hydroxyvitamin D_3. *Science* 183:1089, 1974.
76. Burnell JM et al: Effects of decreasing magnesium in patients with chronic renal failure. *Proc Clin Dial Transplant Forum* 5:191, 1976.
77. Burnell JM et al: Bone crystal maturation in renal osteodystrophy in humans. *J Clin Invest* 53:52, 1974.
78. Bushinsky DA et al: Cellular contribution to pH mediated calcium flux in neonatal mouse calvaria. *Am J Physiol* 248:F785, 1985.
79. Bushinsky DA et al: Effect of pH on bone calcium and proton fluxes in vitro. *Am J Physiol* 245:F205, 1983.
80. Cameron JR et al: Precision and accuracy of bone mineral determination by direct photon absorptiometry. *Invest Radiol* 3:9, 1968.
81. Canata JB et al: Effect of acute aluminum overload on calcium and parathyroid hormone metabolism. *Lancet* 1:501, 1983.
82. Caniggia A et al: Intestinal absorption of radiophosphate after physiologic doses of $25(OH)D_3$ in normals, liver cirrhosis and chronic renal failure patients, in Norman AW et al (eds): *Vitamin D: Biochemical, Chemical and Clinical Aspects Related to Calcium Metabolism*. Berlin, de Gruyter, 1977, p 755.
83. Cann CE et al: Spinal mineral losses in oophorectomized women. *JAMA* 244:2056, 1980.
84. Cann CE et al: Aluminum uptake by the parathyroid glands. *J Clin Endocrinol Metab* 49:543, 1979.
85. Canterbury JM et al: Inhibition of parathyroid hormone secretion by 25-hydroxycholecalciferol and 24,25-dihydroxycholecalciferol in the dog. *J Clin Invest* 61:1375, 1977.
86. Cantin M: Kidney, parathyroid and lipemia. *Lab Invest* 14:1691, 1965.
87. Catherwood BD et al: Sites of clearance of endogenous parathyroid hormone in the vitamin D deficient dog. *Endocrinology* 98:228, 1976.
88. Catto GRD et al: Haemodialysis therapy and changes in skeletal calcium. *Lancet* 1:1150, 1973.
89. Chalmers J et al: Osteomalacia—A common disease in elderly women. *J Bone Joint Surg* 49B:403, 1967.
90. Chalmers TM et al: 1αHydroxycholecalciferol as a substitute for the kidney hormone 1,25 dihydroxycholecalciferol in chronic renal failure. *Lancet* 2:696, 1973.
91. Chan J et al: 1α-hydroxyvitamin D_3 in chronic renal failure: A potent analogue of the kidney hormone 1,25 hydroxycholecalciferol. *JAMA* 234:47, 1975.
92. Chan Y et al: The effect of aluminum on normal and uremic rats: Tissue distribution, vitamin D metabolites and quantitative bone histology. *Calcif Tissue Int* 35:344, 1983.
93. Chanard J et al: Rapid method for measurement of fractional intestinal absorption of calcium. *J Nucl Med* 15:369, 1974.
94. Chantler C et al: Combined report on regular dialysis and transplantation of children in Europe. *Proc Eur Dial Transplant Assoc* 16:74, 1979.
95. Chantler C et al: Growth in children with renal disease, with special reference to the effects of caloric malnutrition: A review. *Clin Nephrol* 1:230, 1973.
96. Charbon GA: Parathormone: A selective vasodilator, in Talmage RV et al (eds): *Parathyroid Hormone—Thyrocalcitonin (Calcitonin)*. Amsterdam, Excerpta Medica, 1969, p 475.
97. Chazan J et al: Plasma aluminum levels (unstimulated and stimulated): Clinical and biochemical findings in 185 patients undergoing chronic hemodialysis for 4 to 95 months. *Am J Kidney Dis* 13:284, 1989.
98. Chesney RW et al: Influence of long term oral 1,25 dihydroxyvitamin D in childhood renal osteodystrophy. *Contrib Nephrol* 18:55, 1980.
99. Chesney RW et al: Circulating vitamin D metabolite con-

centrations in childhood renal diseases. *Kidney Int* 21:65, 1982.

100. Chesney RW et al: Increased growth after longterm oral 1,25-vitamin D_3 in childhood renal osteodystrophy. *N Engl J Med* 298:238, 1978.
101. Cheung AK et al: Determinants of serum 1,25 $(OH)_2D$ levels in renal disease. *Kidney Int* 24:104, 1983.
102. Chou CT et al: Muskuloskeletal manifestations in hemodialysis patients. *J Rheumatol* 12:1149, 1985.
103. Cirincione R et al: Tendon rupture with secondary hyperparathyroidism. *J Bone Joint Surg* 57:852, 1975.
104. Clarkson EM et al: Net intestinal absorption of calcium in patients with chronic renal failure. *Kidney Int* 3:258, 1973.
105. Clarkson EM et al: The effect of aluminum hydroxide on calcium, phosphorus and aluminum balances, the serum parathyroid hormone concentration and the aluminum content of bone in patients with chronic renal failure. *Clin Sci* 43:519, 1972.
106. Clarkson EM et al: The effect of a high intake of calcium carbonate in normal subjects and patients with chronic renal failure. *Clin Sci* 30:425, 1966.
107. Coburn JW et al: Medical treatment in primary and secondary hyperparathyroidism. *Semin Drug Treat* 2:117, 1972.
108. Coburn JW et al: Clinical efficacy of 1,25 dihydroxyvitamin D_3 in renal osteodystrophy, in Norman AW et al (eds): *Vitamin D: Biochemical, Chemical and Clinical Aspects Related to Calcium Metabolism*. Berlin, de Gruyter, 1977, p 657.
109. Coburn JW et al: Use of $1,25(OH)_2$vitamin D_3 to separate "types" of renal osteodystrophy. *Proc Eur Dial Transplant Assoc* 14:442, 1977.
110. Coburn JW et al: Prospective, double blind trial with calcitriol in the prophylaxis of bone disease in asymptomatic dialysis patients, in Norman AW et al (eds): *Vitamin D: Chemical, Biochemical and Clinical Endocrinology of Calcium Metabolism*. Berlin, de Gruyter, 1982, p 833.
111. Coburn JW et al: Intestinal absorption of calcium, magnesium, and phosphorus in chronic renal insufficiency, in David DS (ed): *Calcium Metabolism in Renal Failure and Nephrolithiasis*. New York, Wiley, 1977, p 77.
112. Coburn JW et al: Intestinal absorption of calcium and the effect of renal insufficiency. *Kidney Int* 4:96, 1973.
113. Coburn JW et al: Study of intestinal absorption of calcium in patients with renal failure. *Kidney Int* 3:264, 1973.
114. Coburn JW et al: Renal osteodystrophy, in Maxwell MH et al (eds): *Clinical Disorders of Fluid and Electrolyte Metabolism*. New York, McGraw-Hill, 1987, p 985.
115. Coburn JW et al: Rapid appearance of hypercalcemia with initiation of hemodialysis. *JAMA* 210:2276, 1969.
116. Coburn JW et al: Calcium citrate markedly enhances aluminum absorption from aluminum hydroxide. *Am J Kidney Dis* 17:708, 1991.
117. Coburn JW et al: The physiochemical state and renal handling of divalent ions in chronic renal failure. *Arch Intern Med* 124:302, 1969.
118. Coburn JW et al: Effect of ranitidine on aluminum absorption in man. *Kidney Int* 35:398, 1989 (abstract).
119. Coburn JW et al: Control of serum phosphorus in uremia. *N Engl J Med* 320:1140, 1989.
120. Coburn JW et al: A skeletal mineralizing defect in dialysis patients: A syndrome resembling osteomalacia but unrelated to vitamin D. *Contrib Nephrol* 18:172, 1980.
121. Coen G et al: Bone GLA protein in predialysis chronic renal failure: Effects of $1,25(OH)_2D_3$ administration in a long-term follow-up. *Kidney Int* 28:783, 1985.
122. Conger JD et al: Pulmonary calcification in chronic dialysis patients. Clinical and pathologic studies. *Ann Intern Med* 83:330, 1975.
123. Contiguglia S et al: Nature of soft tissue calcification in uremia. *Kidney Int* 4:229, 1973.
124. Cooper JD et al: Neurodiagnostic abnormalities in patients with acute renal failure. Evidence for neurotoxicity of parathyroid hormone. *J Clin Invest* 61:1448, 1978.
125. Cordell L et al: Parathyroidectomy in chronic renal failure. *Am J Surg* 138:951, 1979.
126. Cordy P et al: Fluoride and hemodialysis. *Trans Am Soc Artif Intern Organs* 20:197, 1974.
127. Cornelis F et al: Rheumatic syndromes and beta 2 microglobulin amyloidosis in patients receiving long term peritoneal dialysis. *Arthritis Rheum* 47:450, 1989.
128. Cournot-Witmer G et al: Effect of aluminum on bone and cell localization. *Kidney Int* 29(suppl):S37, 1986.
129. Cournot-Witmer G et al: Aluminum localization in bone from hemodialyzed patients: Relationship to matrix mineralization. *Kidney Int* 20:376, 1981.
130. Cumming AD et al: Acute aluminum intoxication in patients on continuous ambulatory peritoneal dialysis. *Lancet* 1:103, 1982.
131. Curtis JR et al: The use of calcium carbonate and calcium phosphate without vitamin D in the management of renal osteodystrophy. *Proc Eur Dial Transplant Assoc* 7:141, 1970.
132. Cushner HM et al: Calcium citrate, a non aluminum containing phosphate binding agent for treatment of CRF. *Kidney Int* 35:95, 1988.
133. Daly A et al: Mucormycosis: Association with deferoxamine therapy. *Am J Med* 87:468, 1989.
134. David DS: Calcium Metabolism in Renal Failure and Nephrolithiasis, in David DS (ed): *Calcium Metabolism in Renal Failure and Nephrolithiasis*. New York, Wiley, 1977, p 145.
135. Davis B et al: Scanning for uremic pulmonary calcifications. *Ann Intern Med* 85:132, 1976.
136. Davison AM et al: Phosphate and 1-alpha-hydroxyvitamin D_3 therapy in haemodialysis patients. *Clin Endocrinol* 7(suppl):91S, 1977.
137. de Vernejoul MC et al: Deferoxamine test and bone disease in dialysis patients with mild aluminum accumulation. *Am J Kidney Dis* 14:124, 1989.
138. de Vernejoul MC et al: Increased bone aluminum deposition after subtotal parathyroidectomy in dialyzed patients. *Kidney Int* 785:2791, 1989.
139. DeFrancisco AM et al: Parathyroidectomy in chronic renal failure. *Q J Med* 55:289, 1985.
140. Delano BG et al: A trial of calcitonin therapy in renal osteodystrophy. *Nephron* 11:287, 1973.
141. Delaporte C et al: Variations in muscle cell protein of severely uremic children. *Kidney Int* 10:239, 1976.
142. Delmas PD et al: Effect of renal function on plasma levels of bone Gla-protein. *J Clin Endocrinol* 57:1028, 1983.

143. Delmas PD et al: Assessment of bone turnover in postmenopausal osteoporosis by measurement of serum bone Gla-protein. *J Lab Clin Med* 102:470, 1983.
144. Delmez JA et al: Parathyroid hormone suppression by intravenous 1,25 dihydroxyvitamin D—A role for increased sensitivity to calcium. *J Clin Invest* 83:1349, 1989.
145. DeLuca HF: Vitamin D endocrine system. *Adv Clin Chem* 19:125, 1977.
146. DeLuca HF et al: Treatment of renal osteodystrophy with 25-hydroxycholecalciferol. *Arch Intern Med* 126:896, 1970.
147. Demontis R et al: 1α(OH)vitamin D_3 increases plasma aluminum in hemodialyzed patients taking $Al(OH)_3$. *Clin Nephrol* 29:146, 1986.
148. Denney JD et al: Total body calcium and long term calcium balance in chronic renal disease. *J Lab Clin Med* 82:226, 1973.
149. Dent CE et al: Treatment of renal glomerular osteodystrophy. *Q J Med* 30:1, 1961.
150. Dent CE et al: Radiological changes associated with certain metabolic bone diseases. *Br J Radiol* 27:605, 1954.
151. Doyle F et al: Bone resorption in chronic renal failure: A comparison of radiological and histological assessments. *Br Med Bull* 28:225, 1972.
152. Doyle FH: Radiological patterns of bone disease associated with renal glomerular failure in adults. *Br Med Bull* 28:220, 1972.
153. Dreher W et al: Atrioventricular block in a long term dialysis patient. Reversal after parathyroidectomy. *JAMA* 234:954, 1975.
154. Drueke T et al: Effects of parathyroidectomy on left ventricular function in hemodialysis patients. *Lancet* 1:112, 1980.
155. Dunlay R et al: Direct inhibitory effect of calcitriol on parathyroid function (sigmoidal curve) in dialysis patients. *Kidney Int* 36:1093, 1989.
156. Dunstan CR et al: Treatment of hemodialysis bone disease with $24{,}25(OH)_2D_3$ and $1{,}25(OH)_2D_3$ alone or in combination. *Mineral Electrolyte Metab* 11:358, 1985.
157. Duursma SA et al: A quantitative histological study of bone in 30 patients with renal insufficiency. *Calcif Tissue Res* 9:216, 1972.
158. Duursma SA et al: Serum alkaline phosphatase: Its relation to bone cells and its significance as an indicator for vitamin D treatment in patients with renal insufficiency, in Norman AW et al (eds): *Vitamin D and Problems Related to Uremic Bone Disease*. Berlin, de Gruyter, 1975, p 167.
159. Eastwood JB et al: Comparison of the effect of vitamin D and calcium carbonate in renal osteomalacia. *Q J Med* 40:569, 1971.
160. Eastwood JB et al: Some biochemical, histological, radiological and clinical features of renal osteodystrophy. *Kidney Int* 4:128, 1973.
161. Eastwood JB et al: The effect of 25-hydroxyvitamin D_3 in osteomalacia of chronic renal failure. *Clin Sci* 52:499, 1977.
162. Eastwood JB et al: Vitamin D deficiency in the osteomalacia of chronic renal failure. *Lancet* 2:1209, 1976.
163. Eastwood JB et al: Biochemical and histological effects of 1,25 dihydroxycholecalciferol in the osteomalacia of chronic renal failure, in Norman AW et al (eds): *Vitamin D and Problems Related to Uremic Bone Disease*. Berlin, de Gruyter, 1975, p 595.
164. Eisman JA et al: 1,25 dihydroxyvitamin D in biological fluids: A simplified and sensitive assay. *Science* 193:1021, 1976.
165. Ellis HA: Aluminum and osteomalacia after parathyroidectomy. *Ann Intern Med* 96:533, 1982.
166. Ellis HA et al: Bone aluminum in hemodialysed patients and in rats injected with aluminum chloride: Relationship to impaired bone mineralization. *J Clin Pathol* 32:832, 1979.
167. Ellis HA et al: Azotemic renal osteodystrophy: A quantitative study on iliac. *J Clin Pathol* 26:83, 1973.
168. Ellis HA et al: Histopathology of renal osteodystrophy with particular reference to the effects of 1 hydroxyvitamin D_3 in patients treated by long-term hemodialysis. *Clin Endocrinol* 7:32S, 1977.
169. Ellis K et al: The skull in hyperparathyroid bone disease. *Am J Roentgenol* 83:732, 1960.
170. Evans RA et al: The use of high calcium dialysate in the treatment of renal osteomalacia. *Aust NZ J Med* 6:10, 1976.
171. Evanson JM: The response to the infusion of parathyroid extract in hypocalcemic states. *Clin Sci* 31:63, 1966.
172. Faugere MC et al: Stainable aluminum and not aluminum content reflects bone histology in dialyzed patients. *Kidney Int* 30:717, 1986.
173. Felsenfeld AJ et al: Hypercalcemia and elevated calcitriol in a maintenance dialysis patient with tuberculosis. *Arch Intern Med* 146:1941, 1986.
174. Felsenfeld AJ et al: Postparathyroidectomy hypocalcemia as an accurate indicator of preparathyroidectomy bone histology in the uremic patient. *Mineral Electrolyte Metab* 10:166, 1984.
175. Felsenfeld AJ et al: Osteomalacia in chronic renal failure: A syndrome previously reported only with maintenance dialysis. *Am J Nephrol* 2:147, 1982.
176. Felsenfeld AJ et al: Osteomalacia after parathyroidectomy in patients with uremia. *Ann Intern Med* 96:34, 1984.
177. Felsenfeld AJ et al: The evolution of osteomalacia (OM) with acute aluminum (AL) toxicity. *Kidney Int* 29:158, 1986.
178. Fiaschi E et al: Low protein diets and bone disease in chronic renal failure. *Kidney Int* 12(suppl):S79, 1978.
179. Fleisch H et al: Diphosphonate treatment in bone disease. *N Engl J Med* 289:1419, 1973.
180. Fleish H et al: Experimental clinical studies with pyrophosphate and diphosphonates, in David DS (ed): *Calcium Metabolism in Renal Failure and Nephrolithiasis*. New York, Wiley, 1977 p 293.
181. Fleming LW et al: Improved phosphate clearances with polycarbonate membranes. *Clin Exp Dialysis Apheresis* 6:211, 1982.
182. Floyd M et al: Myopathy in chronic renal failure. *Q J Med* 43:509, 1974.
183. Follis RH et al: Renal osteomalacia and osteitis fibrosa in adults. *Johns Hopkins Med J* 72:232, 1943.
184. Fotino S et al: Phosphate excretion in chronic renal failure: Evidence for a mechanism other than circulating parathyroid hormone. *Clin Nephrol* 8:499, 1977.

185. Fournier AE et al: 1α-Hydroxycholecalciferol and 25-hydroxycholecalciferol in renal bone disease. *Proc Eur Dial Transplant Assoc* 12:227, 1976.
186. Fournier AE et al: Calcium carbonate, an aluminum free agent for control of hyperphosphatemia, hypocalcemia, and hyperparathyroidism. *Kidney Int* 29(suppl):S114, 1986.
187. Fournier AE et al: Etiology of hyperparathyroidism and bone disease during chronic hemodialysis. II. Factors affecting serum immunoreactive parathyroid hormone. *J Clin Invest* 50:599, 1971.
188. Fournier AE et al: Etiology of hyperparathyroidism and bone disease during chronic hemodialysis. I. Association of bone disease with potentially etiologic factors. *J Clin Invest* 50:592, 1971.
189. Fraser DR et al: Unique biosynthesis by kidney of a biologically active vitamin D metabolite. *Nature* 228:764, 1970.
190. Freeman RM: The role of magnesium in the pathogenesis of azotemic hypothermia. *Proc Soc Exp Biol Med* 137:1069, 1971.
191. Freeman RM et al: Hard water syndrome. *N Engl J Med* 276:1113, 1967.
192. Freemont AJ et al: Water treatment alone allows removal of aluminum from bone and reversal of the calcification defect in aluminum-related osteodystrophy. *Abstracts, IXth Internat Congr Nephrol*, 1984, p 48A.
193. Freitag JJ et al: Impaired parathyroid hormone metabolism in patients with chronic renal failure. *N Engl J Med* 298:29, 1978.
194. Freundlich M et al: Infant formula as a cause of aluminum toxicity in neonatal uremia. *Lancet* 2:527, 1985.
195. Friedlander MA et al: Absence of effect of 24,25 dihydroxycholecalciferol on serum immunoreactive PTH in patients with persistent hyperparathyroidism after renal transplantation. *Clin Nephrol* 22:206, 1984.
196. Gallant S et al: Serial studies of auditory neurotoxicity in patients receiving deferoxamine therapy. *Am J Med* 83:1085, 1987.
197. Garn S et al: Bone measurement in the differential diagnosis of osteopenia and osteoporosis. *Radiology* 100:509, 1971.
198. Geis WP et al: The diagnosis and treatment of hyperparathyroidism after renal homotransplantation. *Surg Gynecol Obstet* 117:997, 1973.
199. Gilchrest B et al: Relief of uremic pruritus with ultraviolet phototherapy. *N Engl J Med* 297:136, 1977.
200. Gilmour JR: The gross anatomy of the parathyroid glands. *J Pathol Bacteriol* 46:133, 1938.
201. Ginsberg DS et al: Hypercalcemia after oral calcium carbonate therapy in patients on chronic hemodialysis. *Lancet* 1:1271, 1973.
202. Gipstein R et al: Calciphylaxis in man: A syndrome of tissue necrosis and vascular calcification in 11 patients with chronic renal disease. *Arch Intern Med* 136:1273, 1976.
203. Glassford D et al: Hyperparathyroidism in the maintenance dialysis patient. *Surg Gynecol Obstet* 142:328, 1976.
204. Gokal R et al: Histological renal osteodystrophy and 25 hydroxycholecalciferol and aluminum levels in patients on continuous ambulatory peritoneal dialysis. *Kidney Int* 23:1521, 1983.
205. Goldman R et al: Phosphorus excretion in renal failure. *J Clin Invest* 33:1623, 1954.
206. Goldsmith RS: The effects of calcium and phosphorus in hemodialysis. *Ann Rev Med* 27:181, 1976.
207. Goldsmith RS et al: Etiology of hyperparathyroidism and bone disease during chronic hemodialysis: III. Evaluation of parathyroid suppressibility. *J Clin Invest* 52:173, 1973.
208. Goldstein DA et al: Effect of parathyroid hormone and uremia on peripheral nerve calcium and motor nerve conduction velocity. *J Clin Invest* 62:88, 1978.
209. Goldstein DA et al: Blood levels of 25 hydroxyvitamin D in nephrotic syndrome: Studies in 26 patients. *Ann Intern Med* 87:664, 1977.
210. Goodman AD et al: Production, excretion and net balance of fixed acid in patients with renal acidosis. *J Clin Invest* 44:495, 1965.
211. Goodman WG et al: Short term aluminum administration in the rat. *J Clin Invest* 73:171, 1984.
212. Goodman WG et al: Parenteral aluminum administration in the dog: II. Induction of osteomalacia and effect on vitamin D metabolism. *Kidney Int* 25:370, 1984.
213. Gordon HE et al: Surgical management of secondary hyperparathyroidism. *Arch Surg* 104:520, 1972.
214. Graf H et al: Aluminum removal by hemodialysis. *Kidney Int* 19:587, 1981.
215. Gray RW et al: Vitamin D metabolism: The role of kidney tissue. *Science* 172:1232, 1971.
216. Gray RW et al: The importance of phosphate in regulating plasma 1,25 vitamin D levels in humans: Studies in healthy subjects, in calcium stone formers, and in patients with primary hyperparathyroidism. *J Clin Endocrinol* 45:299, 1977.
217. Green Jacob et al: Role of bone in regulation of systemic acid-base balance. *Kidney Int* 39:9, 1991.
218. Griffith GC et al: Heparin osteoporosis. *JAMA* 195:1089, 1966.
219. Griffiths HJ et al: The user of photon absorptiometry in the diagnosis of renal osteodystrophy. *Radiology* 109: 277, 1973.
220. Grigoleit H-G et al: Clinical efficacy of 5,6-trans-25-OHCC in chronic renal failure, in Norman AW et al (eds): *Vitamin D: Biochemical, Chemical and Clinical Aspects Related to Calcium Metabolism.* Berlin, de Gruyter, 1977, p 701.
221. Gryfe CI et al: Determination of the amount of bone in the metacarpal. *Age Ageing* 1:213, 1972.
222. Guillard O et al: An international quality assessment program for measurement of aluminum in human plasma: A progress report. *Clin Chem* 34:1603, 1988.
223. Guillot A et al: The use of magnesium containing phosphate binders in patients with end stage renal disease on maintenance hemodialysis. *Nephron* 30:114, 1982.
224. Guisado R et al: Changes in the electroencephalogram in acute uremia: Effects of parathyroid hormone and brain electrolytes. *J Clin Invest* 55:738, 1975.
225. Gundberg CM et al: Osteocalcin: Isolation, characterization and detection, in Moldave K (ed): *Methods in Enzymology, 107.* New York, Academic Press, 1984, p 516.

226. Habener JF et al: Relative effectiveness of magnesium and calcium on the secretion and biosynthesis of parathyroid hormone in vitro. *Endocrinology* 98:197, 1976.
227. Habener JF et al: Biosynthesis of parathyroid hormone. *N Engl J Med* 299:580, 1978.
228. Hahn TJ et al: Osteopenia in patients with rheumatic diseases: Principles of diagnosis and therapy. *Semin Arthritis Rheum* 6:165, 1976.
229. Hamet P et al: Studies of the elevated extracellular concentration of cyclic AMP in uremic man. *J Clin Invest* 56:339, 1975.
230. Hart W et al: The hydroxyproline content of plasma of patients with impaired renal function. *Clin Nephrol* 4:104, 1975.
231. Harter HR et al: Effects of dialysis prescription on bone and mineral metabolism: The National Cooperative Dialysis Study. *Kidney Int* 23(suppl 13):S73, 1983.
232. Haussler MR et al: Basic and clinical concepts related to vitamin D metabolism and action. *N Engl J Med* 297:974, 1977.
233. Henderson RG et al: Loss of metacarpal and iliac bone in chronic renal failure: Influence of haemodialysis, parathyroid activity, type of renal disease, physical activity and heparin consumption. *Clin Sci* 56:317, 1979.
234. Henderson RG et al: Effects of 1,25 dihydroxycholecalciferol on calcium absorption, muscle weakness, and bone disease in chronic renal failure. *Lancet* 249:83, 1974.
235. Henry HL et al: Studies on the mechanism of action of calciferol VII. Localization of 1,25 dihydroxyvitamin D in chick parathyroid glands. *Biochem Biophy Res Commun* 62:781, 1975.
236. Hercz G et al: Reversal of aluminum-related bone disease after substituting calcium carbonate for aluminum hydroxide. *Am J Kidney Dis* 11:70, 1988.
237. Hercz G et al: Improved bone formation in dialysis patients after substitution of calcium carbonate for aluminum gels. *Trans Assoc Am Physicians* 100:139, 1987.
238. Hercz G et al: Prevention of phosphate retention and hyperphosphatemia in uremia. *Kidney Int* 32(suppl 22):S215, 1987.
239. Hercz G et al: Effects of intraperitoneal and intravenous desferrioxamine on aluminum removal during CAPD. *Kidney Int* 27:180, 1985.
240. Hercz G et al: Low turnover bone disease without aluminum in dialysis patients. *Kidney Int* 35:378, 1989.
241. Hercz G et al: Use of calcium carbonate as a phosphate binder in dialysis patients. *Mineral Electrolyte Metab* 12:314, 1986.
242. Hercz G et al: Aplastic osteodystrophy: Role of suppressed parathyroid hormone levels. *Abstracts, XIth Internat Congr Nephrol*, 1990, p 402A.
243. Heynen G et al: Human calcitonin radioimmunoassay in normal and pathologic conditions. *Eur J Clin Invest* 4:213, 1974.
244. Heynen G et al: Evidence that endogenous calcitonin protects against renal bone disease. *Lancet* 2:1322, 1976.
245. Hodsman AB et al: Bone aluminum and histomorphometric features of renal osteodystrophy. *J Clin Endocrinol* 54:539, 1982.
246. Hodsman AB et al: Vitamin D resistant osteomalacia in hemodialysis patients lacking secondary hyperparathyroidism. *Ann Intern Med* 94:629, 1981.
247. Hodsman J et al: Preliminary trials with 24,25 dihydroxyvitamin D_3 in dialysis osteomalacia. *Am J Med* 74:407, 1983.
248. Howard GA et al: Human bone cells in culture metabolize 25 hydroxy vitamin D to 1,25 dihydroxyvitamin D and 24,25 dihydroxyvitamin D. *J Biol Chem* 256:7738, 1981.
249. Hruska KA et al: Metabolism of immunoreactive parathyroid hormone in the dog. The role of the kidney and the effects of chronic renal disease. *J Clin Invest* 56:39, 1975.
250. Hruska KA et al: Degradation of parathyroid hormone and fragment production by the isolated perfused dog kidney. The effect of glomerular filtration rate and perfusate Ca concentrations. *J Clin Invest* 60:501, 1977.
251. Hughes MR et al: Radioligand receptor assay for 25 hydroxyvitamin D_2D_3. *J Clin Invest* 58:61, 1976.
252. Ibels LS et al: Preservation of function in experimental renal disease by dietary restriction of phosphate. *N Engl J Med* 298:122, 1991.
253. Ichikawa I et al: Influence of parathyroid hormone on glomerular filtration in the rat. *Am J Physiol* 3:F393, 1978.
254. Ittel TH et al: Enhanced gastrointestinal absorption of aluminum in uremic rats. *Kidney Int* 32:821, 1987.
255. Jaffe MD et al: Multiple fractures associated with long term sodium heparin therapy. *JAMA* 193:152, 1965.
256. Jebsen R et al: Natural history of uremic polyneuropathy and effects of dialysis. *N Engl J Med* 277:327, 1967.
257. Jenkins DA et al: Can low-dosage aluminum hydroxide control the plasma phosphate without bone toxicity? *Nephrol Dial Transplant* 4:51, 1989.
258. Johnson C et al: Roentgenographic manifestations of chronic renal disease treated by periodic hemodialysis. *Am J Radium Ther Nucl Med* 101:915, 1967.
259. Jowsey J et al: Long term effects of high phosphate intake on parathyroid hormone levels and bone metabolism. *Acta Orthop Scand* 45:801, 1974.
260. Juttmann JR et al: Serum concentrations of metabolites of vitamin D in patients with chronic renal failure (CRF). Consequences for the treatment with 1 hydroxy-derivatives. *Clin Endocrinol* 14:225, 1981.
261. Kaehny WD et al: Aluminum transfer during hemodialysis. *Kidney Int* 12:361, 1977.
262. Kaehny WD et al: Gastrointestinal absorption of aluminum from aluminum containing antacids. *N Engl J Med* 296:1389, 1977.
263. Kanis JA et al: Vitamin D, osteomalacia and chronic renal failure, in Norman AW et al (eds): *Vitamin D: Biochemical, Chemical and Clinical Aspects Related to Calcium Metabolism*. Berlin, de Gruyter, 1977, p 671.
264. Kanis JA et al: Is 24,25 dihydroxycholecalciferol a calcium regulating hormone in man? *Br Med J* 1:1382, 1978.
265. Kanis JA et al: The possible role of calcitonin deficiency in the development of bone disease due to chronic renal failure. *Calcif Tissue Res* 22(suppl):147, 1977.
266. Kanis JA et al: Changes in histological and biochemical indexes of bone turnover after bilateral nephrectomy in patients on hemodialysis: Evidence for a possible role of endogenous calcitonin. *N Engl J Med* 19:1073, 1977.

267. Kanis JA et al: Rate of reversal of hypercalcemia and hypercalciuria induced by vitamin D and its 1α-hydroxylated derivatives. *Br Med J* 1:78, 1977.
268. Kanis JA et al: Effect of 1α hydroxycholecalciferol on magnesium metabolism in chronic renal failure. *Br Med J* 2:878, 1976.
269. Kanis JA et al: Magnesium intoxication during 1-α-hydroxycholecalciferol treatment. *Br Med J* 2:878, 1976.
270. Kaplan MA et al: Effect of dietary phosphorus (P) in the phosphaturic and calcemic response to parathyroid hormone (PTH) in the uremic dog. *Kidney Int* 18:77, 1977.
271. Katz A et al: Secondary hyperparathyroidism and renal osteodystrophy in chronic renal failure. *Medicine* 48:333, 1969.
272. Kawaguchi Y et al: Graded mass reduction and renal synthesis of 1,25 dihydroxyvitamin D_3 in the rat. *Metab Bone Dis Rel Res* 4:333, 1983.
273. Kaye M: Magnesium metabolism in the rat with chronic renal failure. *J Lab Clin Med* 84:536, 1974.
274. Kaye M: Oral aluminum toxicity in a non-dialyzed patient with renal failure. *Clin Nephrol* 20:208, 1983.
275. Kaye M et al: Arrest of hyperparathyroid bone disease with dihydrotachysterol in patients undergoing chronic hemodialysis. *Ann Intern Med* 73:225, 1970.
276. Kaye M et al: A study of vertebral bone powder from patients with chronic renal failure. *J Clin Invest* 49:442, 1970.
277. Kaye M et al: Effect of dihydrotachysterol on calcium absorption in uremia. *Metabolism* 21:815, 1972.
278. Kaye M et al: Aluminum and phosphate. *Kidney Int* 33(suppl 24):S172, 1988.
279. Kerr DNS et al: Aluminum induced dialysis osteodystrophy: The demise of "Newcastle Bone Disease". *Kidney Int* 28(suppl):S558, 1986.
280. Kessler M et al: Arthropathie du dialyse: Resultats d'une étude multicentrique réalisée chez 171 malades hémodialysés depuis plus de 10 ans, in Gaucher A et al (eds): *Actualités en physiopathologie et pharmacologie acticulaires.* Paris, Masson, 1989, p 272.
281. Kiley JE et al: Evaluation of encephalopathy by EEG frequency analysis in chronic dialysis patients. *Clin Nephrol* 5:245, 1976.
282. Kirshchbaum BB et al: Acute aluminum toxicity associated with oral citrate and aluminum containing antacids. *Am J Med Sci* 297:9, 1989.
283. Koch VH et al: Accelerated growth after recombinant human growth hormone treatment of children with chronic renal failure. *J Pediatr* 115:365, 1989.
284. Koppel MH et al: Thiazide induced rise in serum calcium and magnesium in patients on maintenance hemodialysis. *Ann Intern Med* 72:895, 1970.
285. Kopple JD et al: Metabolic studies of low protein diets in uremia. II. Calcium, phosphorus and magnesium. *Medicine* 52:597, 1973.
286. Kowalewski J et al: The elimination of free, peptide bound and protein bound hydroxyproline into dialysate during peritoneal dialysis in patients with renal failure. *Clin Chim Acta* 34:123, 1971.
287. Kraut JA et al: Effect of chronic metabolic acidosis on vitamin D metabolism in humans. *Kidney Int* 24:644, 1983.
288. Kraut JA et al: The effects of metabolic acidosis on bone formation and bone resorption in the rat. *Kidney Int* 30:694, 1986.
289. Kraut JA et al: Parathyroid gland responsiveness to acute hypocalcemia in dialysis osteomalacia. *Kidney Int* 23:725, 1983.
290. Kumar R: The metabolism of 1,25 dihydroxyvitamin D_3. *Physiol Rev* 64:478, 1984.
291. Kuzela D et al: Soft tissue calcification in chronic dialysis patients. *Am J Pathol* 86:403, 1977.
292. LaFlame GH et al: Bone and soft tissue changes with oral phosphate supplements. *J Clin Invest* 51:2834, 1972.
293. Lang RM et al: Left ventricular contractility varies directly with blood ionized calcium. *Ann Intern Med* 108:424, 1988.
294. Laut J et al: Long term effects of intravenous calcitriol in patients with end-stage renal disease and secondary hyperparathyroidism. *Abstracts, Internat Symp Renal Bone Disease*, 1990, p 13.
295. Lee JC et al: Immunochemical heterogeneity of calcitonin in renal failure. *J Clin Endocrinol* 45:528, 1977.
296. Lefebvre A et al: Optimal correction of acidosis changes progression of dialysis osteodystrophy. *Kidney Int* 36:1112, 1989.
297. Lehrer RI et al: Mucormycosis. *Ann Intern Med* 93:93, 1980.
298. Lemann J Jr et al: The effects of chronic acid loads in normal man: Further evidence for the participating of bone mineral in the defense against chronic metabolic acidosis. *J Clin Invest* 45:1608, 1966.
299. Letteri JM et al: Altered calcium metabolism in chronic renal failure. *Kidney Int* 6:45, 1974.
300. Letteri JM, Cohn SH: Total body neutron activation: Analysis in the study of mineral homeostasis in chronic renal disease, in David DS (ed): *Calcium Metabolism in Renal Failure and Nephrolithiasis.* New York, Wiley, 1977, p 249.
301. Levine BS et al: Effects of vitamin D and diet magnesium on magnesium metabolism. *Am J Physiol* 239:E515, 1980.
302. Lieberherr M et al: In vitro effects of aluminum on bone phosphatases: Possible interaction with PTH and vitamin D_3 metabolites. *Calcif Tissue Int* 34:280, 1982.
303. Lien JW et al: Abnormal Tc time pyrophosphate bone scans in chronic renal failure. *Clin Nephrol* 6:509, 1976.
304. Lind L et al: Suppression of serum parathyroid hormone levels by intravenous alphacalcidol in uremic patients on maintenance hemodialysis. *Nephron* 48:296, 1988.
305. Lindall A et al: Insulin hypersecretion in patients on chronic hemodialysis. Role of parathyroids. *J Clin Endocrinol* 32:653, 1971.
306. Litzow JR et al: The effect of treatment of acidosis on calcium balance in patients with chronic azotemic renal disease. *J Clin Invest* 46:280, 1967.
307. Liu SH et al: Studies of calcium and phosphorus metabolism with special reference to pathogenesis and effects of dihydrotachysterol (A.T. 10) and iron. *Medicine* 22:103, 1943.
308. Llach F: Effects of renal failure and dialysis on divalent ion metabolism, in Brenner BM et al (eds): *Divalent Ion*

Homeostasis. Contemporary Issues in Nephrology, vol 11. New York, Churchill Livingstone, 1983, p 291.
309. Llach F: Parathyroidectomy in chronic renal failure: Indications, surgical approach and the use of calcitriol. *Kidney Int* 38:S62, 1990.
310. Llach F: Pathogenesis of secondary hyperparathyroidism in early renal failure. (in press)
311. Llach F et al: Phosphate loading as a test for primary hyperparathyroidism, in Avioli L et al (eds): *Phosphate Metabolism Kidney and Bone*. Paris, Nouvelle Imprimerie Fournie, 1975, p 171.
312. Llach F et al: Unique effects of 24,25-dihydroxyvitamin D_3 in uremic patients. *Contrib Nephrol* 18:212, 1980.
313. Llach F et al: 24,25 dihydroxycholecalciferol, a vitamin D sterol with qualitatively unique effects in uremic man. *Metab Bone Dis Rel Res* 2:11, 1979.
314. Llach F et al: Renal osteodystrophy and maintenance dialysis, in Maher JF (ed): *Replacement of Renal Function by Dialysis*, 3rd ed. Boston, Klewer Academic Publishers, 1989, p 911.
315. Llach F et al: The natural course of dialysis osteomalacia. *Kidney Int* 29:S74, 1986.
316. Llach F et al: Prevalence of various types of bone disease in dialysis patients, in Robinson RR (ed): *Nephrology: Proceedings of the Xth International Congress of Nephrology*. New York, Springer-Verlag, 1984, p 1375.
317. Llach F et al: Pathophysiology of altered calcium metabolism in rhabdomyolysis induced acute renal failure. *N Engl J Med* 305:117, 1981.
318. Llach F et al: On the mechanism of the prevention of secondary hyperparathyroidism in moderate renal insufficiency. *J Clin Endocrinol* 61:601, 1985.
319. Llach F et al: Skeletal resistance of endogenous parathyroid hormone in patients with early renal failure. A possible cause for secondary hyperparathyroidism. *J Clin Endocrinol* 41:338, 1975.
320. Llach F et al: Acute joint syndrome and maintenance hemodialysis. *Proc Clin Dial Transplant Forum* 9:17, 1979.
321. London G et al: Association between aluminum accumulation and cardiac hypertrophy in hemodialyzed patients. *Am J Kidney Dis* 13:75, 1989.
322. Lopez-Hilker S et al: Hypocalcemia may not be essential for the development of secondary hyperparathyroidism in chronic renal failure. *J Clin Invest* 78:1097, 1986.
323. Loschiavo C et al: Effects of continuous ambulatory peritoneal dialysis (CAPD) on renal osteodystrophy. *Peritoneal Dialysis Bull* 5:53, 1985.
324. Lotem M et al: Spontaneous rupture of tendons: A complication of hemodialyzed patients treated for renal failure. *Nephron* 21:201, 1978.
325. Lumlertgul D et al: Phosphate depletion arrests progression of chronic renal failure independent of protein intake. *Kidney Int* 29:658, 1986.
326. Mactier R et al: Calcium carbonate is an effective phosphate binder when dialysate calcium concentration is adjusted to control hypercalcemia. *Clin Nephrol* 28:220, 1987.
327. Madsen S et al: Suppressive effect of 1,25 dihydroxyvitamin D_3 on circulating parathyroid hormone in acute renal failure. *J Clin Endocrinol* 53:823, 1981.
328. Mahoney J et al: Hypophosphataemic osteomalacia in patients receiving hemodialysis. *Br Med J* 2:142, 1976.
329. Mai M et al: Calcium acetate, an effective phosphorus binder in patients with renal failure. *Kidney Int* 36:690, 1989.
330. Makoff DL et al: Chronic calcium carbonate therapy in uremia. *Arch Intern Med* 123:15, 1969.
331. Malberti F et al: Efficacy and safety of long term treatment with calcium carbonate as a phosphate binder. *Am J Kidney Dis* 12:487, 1988.
332. Mallette LE et al: Neuromuscular disease in secondary hyperparathyroidism. *Ann Intern Med* 82:474, 1975.
333. Mallick N et al: Arterial calcification after vitamin D therapy in hyperphosphatemic renal failure. *Lancet* 2:1316, 1968.
334. Malluche HH et al: Plasma levels of bone Gla-protein reflect bone formation in patients on chronic maintenance dialysis. *Kidney Int* 26:869, 1984.
335. Malluche HH et al: Renal osteodystrophy. *N Engl J Med* 321:317, 1989.
336. Malluche HH et al: Bone histology in incipient and advanced renal failure. *Kidney Int* 9:355, 1976.
337. Malluche HH et al: Bone mass in maintenance haemodialysis. Prospective study with sequential biopsies. *Eur J Clin Invest* 6:265, 1976.
338. Malluche HH et al: The use of desferrioxamine in the management of renal patients with bone aluminum accumulation. *N Engl J Med* 311:140, 1984.
339. Malluche HH et al: Intestinal absorption of calcium and whole body calcium retention in incipient and advanced renal failure. *Mineral Electrolyte Metab* 1:264, 1978.
340. Maloney NA et al: Histologic quantitation of aluminum in iliac bone from patients with renal failure. *J Lab Clin Med* 99:206, 1982.
341. Martin KJ et al: The renal handling of parathyroid hormone: Role of peritubular uptake and glomerular filtration. *J Clin Invest* 60:808, 1977.
342. Martin KJ et al: Selective uptake of intact parathyroid hormone by the liver. Differences between hepatic and renal uptake. *J Clin Invest* 58:781, 1976.
343. Maschio G et al: Biochemical and morphological aspects of bone tissue in chronic renal failure. *Nephron* 12:347, 1974.
344. Maschio G et al: Early dietary phosphorus restriction and calcium supplementation in the prevention of renal osteodystrophy. *Am J Clin Nutr* 33:1546, 1980.
345. Mason RS et al: Vitamin D metabolites and their relationship to azotemic osteodystrophy. *Clin Endocrinol* 13:375, 1980.
346. Massry SG: Parathyroid hormone as a uremic toxin, in Massry SG et al (eds): *Textbook of Nephrology*, 2d ed. Baltimore, Williams & Wilkins, 1989, p 1126.
347. Massry SG et al: Divalent ion metabolism in patients with acute renal failure: Studies on the mechanism of hypocalcemia. *Kidney Int* 5:437, 1974.
348. Massry SG et al: Evidence for suppression of the parathyroid gland by hypermagnesemia. *J Clin Invest* 40:1619, 1970.
349. Massry SG et al: Skeletal resistance to parathyroid hormone in renal failure: Study in 105 human subjects. *Ann Intern Med* 78:357, 1973.

350. Massry SG et al: Secondary hyperparathyroidism in chronic renal failure: The clinic spectrum in uremia, during hemodialysis and after renal transplantation. *Arch Intern Med* 124:431, 1969.
351. Massry SG et al: Abnormalities of the musculoskeletal system in hemodialysis patients. *Semin Arthritis Rheum* 4:321, 1975.
352. Massry SG et al: Use of 1,25(OH)$_2$D$_3$ in the treatment of renal osteodystrophy in patients with moderate renal failure, in Frame B et al (eds): *Clinical Disorders of Bone and Mineral Metabolism*. Amsterdam, Excerpta Medica, 1983, p 260.
353. Massry SG et al: Role of parathyroid hormone in uremic toxicity. *Kidney Int* 13(suppl):S39, 1978.
354. Massry SG et al: Intractable pruritus as a manifestation of 2° hyperparathyroidism in uremia. Disappearance of itching following subtotal parathyroidectomy. *N Engl J Med* 279:697, 1968.
355. Massry SG et al: Role of phosphate in the genesis of secondary hyperparathyroidism of renal failure. *Nephron* 18:77, 1977.
356. Massry SG et al: Skeletal resistance to the calcemic action of parathyroid hormone in uremia: Role of 1,25 (OH)$_2$D$_3$. *Kidney Int* 9:467, 1976.
357. Mawer EB et al: Failure of formation of 1,25 dihydroxycholecalciferol in chronic renal insufficiency. *Lancet* 1:626, 1973.
358. Maxwell D et al: Calcitriol in dialysis patients. *Clin Pharmacol Ther* 23:515, 1978.
359. Mayor GH et al: Aluminum absorption and distribution: Effect of parathyroid hormone. *Science* 197:1187, 1977.
360. Mazess RB et al: Total body mineral and lead body mass by dual photon absorptiometry. *Calif Tissue Int* 33:361, 1981.
361. McDonald SJ et al: The effect of a large intake of calcium citrate in normal subjects and patients with chronic renal failure. *Clin Sci* 26:27, 1964.
362. McMillan DE et al: The milk alkali syndrome: A study of the acute disorder with comments on the development of the chronic condition. *Medicine* 44:485, 1965.
363. McSherry E et al: Attainment and maintenance of normal status with alkali therapy in infants and children with classic renal tubular acidosis (RTA). *J Clin Invest* 61:509, 1978.
364. Mechanic GL et al: Quantitative changes of bone collagen cross-links and precursors in vitamin D deficiency. *Biochem Biophys Res Commun* 47:760, 1972.
365. Meema HE et al: Arterial calcifications in severe chronic renal disease and their relationship to dialysis treatment, renal transplant, and parathyroidectomy. *Radiology* 121:315, 1976.
366. Meema HE et al: Comparison of microradioscopic and morphometric findings in the hand bones with densitometric findings in the proximal radius in thyrotoxicosis and in renal osteodystrophy. *Invest Radiol* 7:88, 1972.
367. Meema HE et al: Improved roentgenologic diagnosis of osteomalacia by microradioscopy of hand bones. *Am J Roentgenol* 125:925, 1975.
368. Meema HE et al: Periosteal new bone formation (periosteal neostasis) in renal osteodystrophy. *Radiology* 110:513, 1974.
369. Mehls O et al: Slipped epiphysis in renal osteodystrophy. *Arch Dis Child* 50:545, 1975.
370. Mehls O et al: Improvement of growth and food utilization by human recombinant growth hormone in uremia. *Kidney Int* 33:45, 1988.
371. Mehls O et al: Roentgenological signs in the skeletons of uremic children. An analysis of the anatomical priniciples underlying the roentgenological changes. *Pediatr Radiol* 1:183, 1973.
372. Melick R et al: Parathyroid hormone metabolism in man: Effect of nephrectomy. *Clin Sci* 37:667, 1969.
373. Memmos D et al: Double-blind trial of oral 1,25-dihydroxy vitamin D$_3$ versus placebo in asymptomatic hyperparathyroidism in patients receiving maintenance haemodialysis. *Br Med J* 282:1919, 1981.
374. Mennes P et al: Hypomagnesemia and impaired parathyroid hormone secretion in chronic renal disease. *Ann Intern Med* 88:206, 1978.
375. Meyer JL et al: Aluminum and aluminum complexes. Effect of calcium phosphate precipitation. *Kidney Int* 29(suppl):S20, 1986.
376. Meyer RD et al: Phycomycosis complicating leukemia and lymphoma. *Ann Intern Med* 77:871, 1972.
377. Meyrier A et al: The influence of a high calcium carbonate intake on bone disease in patients undergoing hemodialysis. *Kidney Int* 4:146, 1973.
378. Meytes D et al: Effects of parathyroid hormone on erythrocytes. *J Clin Invest* 67:1263, 1981.
379. Miach P et al: Prolonged hypercalcemia following acute renal failure. *Clin Nephrol* 4:32, 1975.
380. Miller JH et al: Studies of inorganic phosphate removal during acetate and bicarbonate dialysis. *Proc Am Soc Artif Intern Organs* 12:57, 1983.
381. Milliner DS et al: Clearance of aluminum by hemodialysis. Effect of desferrioxamine. *Kidney Int* 20(suppl 18):S100, 1986.
382. Milliner DS et al: Deferoxamine infusion test for diagnosis of aluminum related osteomalacia. *Ann Intern Med* 101:775, 1984.
383. Milliner DS et al: Inadvertent aluminum administration during plasma exchange due to aluminum contamination of albumin-replacement solutions. *N Engl J Med* 312:165, 1985.
384. Mion C et al: Dialysis fracturing osteomalacia without hyperparathyroidism in patients treated with HCO$_3$ rinsed Redy cartridge. *Trans Am Soc Artif Intern Organs* 27:634, 1981.
385. Mirahmadi KS et al: Calcific periarthritis and hemodialysis. *JAMA* 229:548, 1973.
386. Mirahmadi KS et al: A controlled evaluation of clinical and metabolic effects of dialysate calcium levels during regular dialysis. *Trans Am Soc Artif Intern Organs* 17:118, 1971.
387. Molitoris BA et al: Rapid removal of DFO-chelated aluminum during hemodialysis using polysulfone dialyzers. *Kidney Int* 34:98, 1988.
388. Molitoris BA et al: Citrate: A major factor in the toxicity of orally administered aluminum compounds. *Kidney Int* 36:949, 1989.
389. Moriniere P et al: Disappearance of aluminic bone disease in a long term asymptomatic dialysis population restrict-

ing $Al(OH)_3$ intake: Emergence of an idiopathic adynamic bone disease not related to aluminum. *Nephron* 53:93, 1989.
390. Moriniere P et al: Calcium carbonate and magnesium hydroxide in the prevention of renal osteodystrophy or the demise of aluminum toxicity in uremia. *Contrib Nephrol* 64:58, 1988.
391. Moriniere PG et al: Substitution of aluminum hydroxide by high doses of calcium carbonate in patients on chronic hemodialysis: Disappearance of hyperaluminemia and equal control of hyperparathyroidism. *Proc Eur Dial Transplant Assoc* 19:784, 1982.
392. Morrissey J et al: Effect of aluminum on parathyroid hormone secretion. *Kidney Int* 29(suppl):S41, 1986.
393. Mountokalakis T et al: Bone loss in chronic renal failure. *Lancet* 1:363, 1977.
394. Murphy KJ et al: Tears of major tendons in chronic acidosis with elastosis. *J Bone Joint Surg* 53:510, 1971.
395. Naik RB et al: Comparative study of alkaline phosphatase isoenzymes, bone histology, and skeletal radiography in dialysis bone disease. *Br Med J* 1:1307, 1977.
396. Nebeker HG et al: Clinical response of aluminum-related osteomalacia to desferrioxamine. *Abstracts, IXth International Congress Nephrology*, 1984, p 115A.
397. Nichols G et al: Effect of parathyroidectomy on content and availability of skeletal sodium in the rat. *Am J Physiol* 198:749, 1960.
398. Nordal KP et al: Low dose calcitriol versus placebo in patients with predialysis chronic renal failure. *J Clin Endocrinol* 67:929, 1988.
399. Norfray J et al: Renal osteodystrophy in patients on hemodialysis as reflected in the bony pelvis. *Am J Roentgenol* 125:352, 1975.
400. Norris KC et al: Clinical and laboratory features of aluminum related bone disease: Differences between sporadic and "epidemic" forms of the syndrome. *Am J Kidney Dis* 6:342, 1985.
401. Norris KC et al: Intravenous calcitriol for severe secondary hyperparathyroidism in dialysis patients. *Kidney Int* 27:158, 1985.
402. Norris KC et al: Symptomatic renal bone disease: Non-invasive parameters for diagnosis. *Abstracts, XIth Internat Congr Nephrol*, 1990, p 405A.
403. O'Donovan R et al: Substitution of aluminum salts by magnesium salts in control of dialysis hyperphosphataemia. *Lancet* 1:880, 1986.
404. Offerman G et al: Serum 25 hydroxycholecalciferol in uremia. *Nephron* 13:269, 1974.
405. Oldham SB et al: The acute effects of 1,25 dihydroxycholecalciferol on serum immunoreactive parathyroid hormone (iPTH) in the dog. *Endocrinology* 104:248, 1979.
406. Olgaard K et al: Effect of 24,25 dihydroxy-vitamin D_3 on PTH levels and bone histology in dogs with chronic uremia. *Kidney Int* 25:791, 1984.
407. Olgaard K et al: Scintigraphic skeletal changes in uremic patients on regular hemodialysis. *Nephron* 17:325, 1976.
408. Oliveri NF et al: Visual and auditory neurotoxicity in patients receiving subcutaneous deferoxamine. *N Engl J Med* 314:868, 1986.
409. Oreopoulos DG et al: Fluoride and dialysis osteodystrophy: Results of a double blind study. *Trans Am Soc Artif Intern Organs* 20:203, 1974.
410. Ott SM et al: The prevalence of bone aluminum deposition in renal osteodystrophy and its relation to the response to calcitriol therapy. *N Engl J Med* 307:709, 1982.
411. Ott SM et al: Desferrioxamine therapy in patients with aluminum-related osteodystrophy. *Kidney Int* 29(suppl): S108, 1986.
412. Ott SM et al: Vitamin D therapy in aluminum related osteomalacia. *Kidney Int* 32:107, 1983.
413. Papadimitriou M et al: Hypercalcemia from calcium ion exchange resins in patients on regular hemodialysis. *Lancet* 2:948, 1968.
414. Papapoulos SE et al: Clearance of exogenous parathyroid hormone in normal and uraemic man. *Clin Endocrinol* 7:211, 1977.
415. Pappenheimer AM et al: Enlargement of the parathyroid glands in renal disease. *Am J Pathol* 11:73, 1935.
416. Parfitt AM: Soft tissue calcification in uremia. *Arch Intern Med* 124:544, 1969.
417. Parfitt AM: The actions of parathyroid hormone on bone: Relation to bone remodeling and turnover, calcium homeostasis and metabolic bone disease. III. PTH and osteoblasts, the relationship between bone turnover and bone loss, and the state of the bones in primary hyperparathyroidism. *Metabolism* 25:1003, 1976.
418. Parfitt AM: Clinical and radiographic manifestations of renal osteodystrophy, in David DS (ed): *Calcium Metabolism in Renal Failure and Nephrolithiasis.* New York, Wiley, 1977, p 150.
419. Parfitt AM et al: Osteopenia and fractures occurring during maintenance hemodialysis. A "new" form of renal osteodystrophy. *Clin Orthop* 87:287, 1972.
420. Parkinson IS et al: Fracturing dialysis osteodystrophy and dialysis encephalopathy: An epidemiological survey. *Lancet* 1:406, 1979.
421. Paunier L et al: Renal osteodystrophy in children undergoing continuous ambulatory peritoneal dialysis. *Pediatr Res* 18:742, 1984.
422. Peacock M: The Clinical Uses of 1 Hydroxyvitamin D_3. *Clin Endocrinol* 7:1977.
423. Pederson JA et al: Relief of idiopathic generalized pruritus in dialysis patients with activated oral charcoal. *Ann Intern Med* 93:446, 1980.
424. Pei Y et al: Non-invasive prediction of aluminum bone disease in hemo- and peritoneal dialysis patients. *Kidney Int* 41:1374, 1992.
425. Pellegrino ED et al: The composition of human bone in uremia. *Medicine* 44:397, 1965.
426. Pellegrino ED et al: Interrelationships of carbonate, phosphate, monohydrogen phosphate, calcium, magnesium and sodium in uraemic bone: Comparison of dialyzed and nondialyzed patients. *Clin Sci Molec Med* 53:307, 1977.
427. Pengloan J et al: Ocular toxicity after a single intravenous dose of desferrioxamine in 2 hemodialyzed patients. *Nephron* 46:211, 1987.
428. Phelps KR et al: Histological demonstration of iron but not aluminum in a case of dialysis associated osteomalacia. *Am J Med* 84:775, 1988.
429. Piccoli A et al: Serum aluminum level in the Veneto

chronic haemodialysis population: Cross-sectional study on 1,026 patients. *Nephron* 51:482, 1989.
430. Pierce-Myli M et al: Iron and aluminum osteomalacia during hemodialysis: A new syndrome. *Kidney Int* 25:153, 1984 (abstract).
431. Pierides AM et al: Variable response to long term 1α-hydroxycholecalciferol in haemodialysis osteodystrophy. *Lancet* 1:1092, 1976.
432. Pierides AM et al: Barbiturate and anticonvulsant treatment in relation to osteomalacia with haemodialysis and renal transplantation. *Br Med J* 1:190, 1976.
433. Pierides AM et al: 1 hydroxycholecalciferol in hemodialysis renal osteodystrophy. Adverse effects of anticonvulsant therapy. *Clin Nephrol* 5:189, 1976.
434. Pierides AM et al: Haemodialysis encephalopathy: Possible role of phosphate depletion. *Lancet* 1:1234, 1976.
435. Pietrek J et al: Serum 25-hydroxyvitamin D and parathyroid hormone in patients with acute renal failure. *Kidney Int* 13:178, 1978.
436. Pletka P et al: Effects of magnesium on parathyroid hormone secretion during chronic hemodialysis. *Lancet* 2:462, 1971.
437. Popovtzer MM et al: The future of $24,25(OH)_2D_3$ in the treatment of uremic bone disease, in Llach F (ed): *Renal osteodystrophy*. London, Oxford University Press, 1993. (in press)
438. Portale AP et al: Effect of dietary phosphorus on circulating concentrations of 1,25 dihydroxyvitamin D and immunoreactive parathyroid hormone in children with moderate renal insufficiency. *J Clin Invest* 73:1580, 1984.
439. Portale AP et al: Reduced plasma concentration of 1,25 dihydroxyvitamin D in children with moderate renal insufficiency. *Kidney Int* 21:627, 1982.
440. Posen GA et al: Renal osteodystrophy in patients on long-term hemodialysis with fluoridated water. *Fluoride* 4:114, 1971.
441. Postlethwaite RJ et al: Bone disease in children with chronic renal failure: Therapy with 1α-hydroxyvitamin D_3. *Clin Endocrinol* 7(suppl):117S, 1977.
442. Potter D et al: The treatment of chronic uremia in childhood. *Pediatrics* 45:432, 1970.
443. Prager P et al: Diagnostischer Stellenwert der Lamina dura dentium beim sekundaren Hyperparathyreoidismus. *Fortschr Röntgenstrl* 129:237, 1978.
444. Preston E: Avulsion of three major tendons. *JAMA* 221:406, 1972.
445. Preston F et al: Hyperparathyroidism with avulsion of three major tendons. *N Engl J Med* 266:968, 1962.
446. Price PA et al: Origin of the vitamin D-dependent bone protein found in plasma and its clearance by kidney and bone. *J Biol Chem* 256:12760, 1981.
447. Prockop D et al: Relationship of hydroxyproline excretion in urine to collagen metabolism. *Ann Intern Med* 66:1243, 1967.
448. Quarles LD et al: Aluminum deposition in bone: An epiphenomenon of the osteomalacic state. *Clin Res* 32:522A, 1984.
449. Quarles LD et al: Aluminum induced de novo bone formation in the beagle: A parathyroid hormone dependent event. *J Clin Invest* 83:1644, 1989.
450. Raman A et al: Effects of varying dialysate calcium concentration on the plasma calcium fractions in patients on dialysis. *Nephron* 16:181, 1976.
451. Ramirez JA et al: The absorption of dietary phosphorus and calcium in hemodialysis patients. *Kidney Int* 30:753, 1986.
452. Recker R et al: The efficacy of calciferol in renal osteodystrophy. *Arch Intern Med* 138:857, 1978.
453. Regan RJ et al: Effect of dialysate calcium concentration on bone disease in patients on hemodialysis. *Kidney Int* 10:246, 1976.
454. Reiss E et al: The role of phosphate in the secretion of parathyroid hormone in man. *J Clin Invest* 49:2146, 1970.
455. Remuzzi G et al: Parathyroid hormone inhibits human platelet function. *Lancet* 2:1321, 1981.
456. Ricanati ES et al: Evaluation of bone in dialysis patients exposed to aluminum in dialysate. *Kidney Int* 21:176, 1982.
457. Ritz E et al: Skeletal abnormalities in chronic renal insufficiency before and during maintenance hemodialysis. *Kidney Int* 4:116, 1973.
458. Ritz E et al: Metabolic bone disease in patients on maintenance hemodialysis. *Nephron* 12:393, 1974.
459. Ritz E et al: Bone histology in renal insufficiency, in David DS (ed): *Perspectives in Nephrology and Hypertension*. New York, Wiley, 1977, p 197.
460. Ritz E et al: Calcium metabolism in renal failure, in Bronner F et al (eds): *Disorders of Mineral Metabolism*. New York, Academic Press, 1981, vol III, p 151.
461. Ritz E et al: Vascular calcifications under maintenance hemodialysis. *Klin Wochenschr* 55:375, 1977.
462. Ritz E et al: Skeletal x-ray findings and bone histology in patients on hemodialysis. *Kidney Int* 13:316, 1978.
463. Robertson JA et al: Animal model of aluminum induced osteomalacia: Role of chronic renal failure. *Kidney Int* 23:327, 1983.
464. Robertson JA et al: Sucralfate, intestinal aluminum absorption, and aluminum toxicity in a patient on dialysis. *Ann Intern Med* 111:179, 1989.
465. Rodriguez M et al: The role of aluminum in the development of hypercalcemia in the rat. *Kidney Int* 31:766, 1987.
466. Rodriguez M et al: Calcitonin, an important factor in the calcemic response to parathyroid hormone in the rat with renal failure. *Kidney Int* 40:219, 1991.
467. Rosenthal L, Kaye M: Observations on the mechanism of ^{99m}Tc-labeled phosphate complex uptake in metabolic bone disease. *Nucl Med* 5:59, 1976.
468. Roth A et al: Multiorgan aluminum deposits in a chronic haemodialysis patient. Electron microscope and microprobe studies. *Virchows Arch (Pathol Anat)* 405:131, 1984.
469. Rothmund M et al: Re-operations for persistent and recurrent secondary hyperparathyroidism. *Ann Surg* 207:310, 1988.
470. Rovelli E et al: Correlation between serum aluminum concentration and signs of encephalopathy in a large population of patients dialyzed with aluminum free fluids. *Clin Nephrol* 29:294, 1988.

471. Rubin LA et al: Erosive azotemic osteoarthropathy. *Arthritis Rheum* 27:1086, 1984.
472. Russell JE et al: 25 Hydroxycholecalciferol enhanced bone maturation in the parathyroprivic state. *J Clin Invest* 56:792, 1975.
473. Russell JE et al: The nature of the collagen cross links in bone in the chronic uraemic state. *Biochem J* 145:119, 1975.
474. Russell JE et al: Abnormal bone mineral maturation in the chronic uremic state. *J Clin Invest* 52:2848, 1973.
475. Rutherford WE et al: An evaluation of a new and effective phosphorus binding agent. *Trans Am Soc Artif Intern Organs* 19:446, 1973.
476. Rutherford WE et al: Phosphate control and 25 hydroxycholecalciferol administration in preventing experimental renal osteodystrophy in the dog. *J Clin Invest* 60:332, 1977.
477. Rutherford WE et al: The effect of 5,6-trans vitamin D_3 on calcium absorption in chronic renal disease. *J Clin Endocrinol* 40:13, 1975.
478. Ryuzaki M et al: Spontaneous rupture of the quadriceps tendon in patients on maintenance hemodialysis-report of three cases with clinicopathological observations. *Clin Nephrol* 32:144, 1989.
479. Saenger P et al: Somatomedin and growth after renal transplantation. *Pediatr Res* 8:163, 1974.
480. Sakai S et al: Bone injuries due to tetany or convulsion during hemodialysis. *Clin Orthop* 118:118, 1976.
481. Salusky IB et al: Bone disease in pediatric patients undergoing dialysis with CAPD/CCPD. *Kidney Int* 33:975, 1988.
482. Salusky IB et al: Effects of oral calcium carbonate on control of serum phosphorus and changes in plasma aluminum levels after discontinuation of aluminum-containing gels in children receiving dialysis. *J Pediatr* 108:767, 1986.
483. Salusky IB et al: Prospective evaluation of aluminum loading from formula in infants with uremia. *J Pediatr* 116:726, 1984.
484. Salusky IB et al: "High dose" calcitriol for control of renal osteodystrophy in children on CAPD. *Kidney Int* 32:89, 1987.
485. Salusky IB et al: Aluminum accumulation from recommended doses of aluminum hydroxide in dialyzed children. *N Engl J Med* 324:527, 1991.
486. Sawyer N et al: High dose calcium carbonate with stepwise reduction in dialysate calcium concentration: Effective phosphate control and aluminum avoidance in haemodialysis patients. *Nephrol Dial Transplant* 3:1, 1988.
487. Schaefer K et al: Control of serum phosphorus and the use of phosphate binders, in Llach F (ed): *Renal osteodystrophy*, London, Oxford University Press, 1993. (in press)
488. Scharer K et al: Growth in children with chronic renal failure, in Friedman EA, Giordano C (eds): *Uremia. Kidney Int* (suppl 8):S68, 1978.
489. Schiller L et al: Effect of the time of administration of calcium acetate on phosphorus binding. *N Engl J Med* 320:1110, 1989.
490. Schmidt-Gayk H et al: Hydroxyvitamin D in nephrotic syndrome. *Lancet* 2:105, 1977.
491. Schneider HW et al: In vitro and in vivo studies with a non-aluminum phosphate-binding compound. *Kidney Int* 29(suppl 18):S120, 1986.
492. Schoenfeld P et al: Assessment of nutritional status of the national cooperative dialysis study population. *Kidney Int* 23:580, 1980.
493. Schoenfeld PJ et al: Amelioration of myopathy with 25-hydroxyvitamin D_3 therapy ($25(OH)D_3$) in patients on chronic hemodialysis, in *Third Workshop on Vitamin D, Book of Abstracts*. Asilomar, Riverside, Univ Calif Riverside Press, 1977, p 160.
494. Schott GD et al: Muscle weakness in osteomalacia. *Lancet* 1:626, 1976.
495. Sedman AB et al: Tissue and cellular basis for impaired bone formation in aluminum related osteomalacia in the pig. *J Clin Invest* 79:86, 1987.
496. Sedman AB et al: Evidence of aluminum loading in infants receiving intravenous therapy. *N Engl J Med* 312:1337, 1985.
497. Selye H: *Calciphylaxis*. Chicago, Univ of Chicago Press, 1962.
498. Sheikh MS et al: Reduction of dietary phosphorus absorption by phosphorus binders: A theoretical, in vitro and in vivo study. *J Clin Invest* 83:66, 1989.
499. Sherrard DJ: Aluminum: Much ado about something. *N Engl J Med* 324:558, 1991.
500. Sherrard DJ et al: Quantitative histological studies on the pathogenesis of uremic bone disease. *J Clin Endocrinol* 39:119, 1974.
501. Sherrard DJ et al: Skeletal response to treatment with 1,25 dihydroxyvitamin D in renal failure. *Contrib Nephrol* 18:92, 1980.
502. Sherrard DJ et al: Pseudohyperparathyroidism: A syndrome associated with aluminum intoxication in chronic renal failure. *Am J Med* 79:127, 1985.
503. Sherrard DJ et al: Uremic osteodystrophy: Classification, cause and treatment, in Frame B et al (eds): *Clinical Disorders of Bone and Mineral Metabolism*. Amsterdam, Excerpta Medica, 1983, p 254.
504. Sherrard DJ et al: Precipitation of dialysis dementia by deferoxamine treatment of aluminum related bone disease. *Am J Kidney Dis* 12:126, 1988.
505. Shiller LR et al: Effect of the time of administration of calcium acetate on phosphorus binding. *N Engl J Med* 320:1110, 1989.
506. Shimada H et al: Influence of aluminum on the effect of $1\alpha(OH)D_3$ on renal osteodystrophy. *Nephron* 35:163, 1983.
507. Shinaberger JH et al: Studies of phosphate removal in clinical dialysis (abstract). *Kidney Int* 25:193, 1984.
508. Shinaberger JH et al: Characteristics of available dialyzers, in Nissenson AR et al (eds): *Clinical Dialysis*. Norwalk, Appleton-Century-Crofts, 1984, p 99.
509. Sicard GA, Wells SA Jr: Surgical treatment of secondary hyperparathyroidism, in Kaplan EL (ed): *Surgery of the Thyroid and Parathyroid Glands*. Edinburgh, Churchill Livingstone, 1983, p 243.
510. Siddiqui JY et al: Fluoride and bone disease in patients on

regular haemodialysis. *Proc Eur Dial Transplant Assoc* 8:149, 1971.
511. Silver J et al: Regulation by vitamin D metabolites of parathyroid hormone gene in vivo by the rat. *J Clin Invest* 78:1296, 1986.
512. Silver J et al: Regulation by vitamin D metabolites of messenger ribonucleic acid for preproparathyroid hormone in isolated bovine parathyroid cells. *Proc Natl Acad Sci USA* 82:4270, 1985.
513. Silverberg DS et al: Effect of 1,25 dihydroxycholecalciferol in renal osteodystrophy. *Can Med Assoc J* 112:190, 1975.
514. Skillen AW et al: Serum alkaline phospohatase isoenzyme patterns in patients with chronic renal failure. *Clin Chim Acta* 80:339, 1977.
515. Slanina P et al: Dietary citric acid enhances absorption of aluminum in antacids. *Clin Chem* 32:539, 1986.
516. Slatopolsky E et al: The role of phosphorus restriction in the prevention of secondary hyperparathyroidism in chronic renal disease. *Kidney Int* 4:141, 1973.
517. Slatopolsky E et al: On the prevention of secondary hyperparathyroidism in experimental chronic renal disease using "proportional reduction" of dietary phosphorus intake. *Kidney Int* 2:147, 1972.
518. Slatopolsky E et al: On the pathogenesis of hyperparathyroidism in chronic experimental renal insufficiency in the dog. *J Clin Invest* 50:492, 1971.
519. Slatopolsky E et al: Low serum levels of $1,25(OH)_2D_3$ are not responsible for the development of secondary hyperparathyroidism in early renal failure. *Kidney Int* 14:733, 1978.
520. Slatopolsky E et al: Parathyroid hormone: Alterations in chronic renal failure, in Robinson RR (ed): *Nephrology*, vol. II, *Proc IXth Internat Congr Nephrol.* New York, Springer-Verlag, 1984, p 1292.
521. Slatopolsky E et al: How important is phosphate in the pathogenesis of renal osteodystrophy? *Arch Intern Med* 138:848, 1978.
522. Slatopolsky E et al: Calcium carbonate as a phosphate binder in patients with chronic renal failure undergoing dialysis. *N Engl J Med* 315:157, 1986.
523. Slatopolsky E et al: Long term effects of calcium carbonate and 2.5 mEq/liter calcium dialysate on mineral metabolism. *Kidney Int* 36:897, 1989.
524. Slatopolsky E et al: Marked suppression of secondary hyperparathyroidism by intravenous administration of 1,25 dihydroxycholecalciferol in uremic patients. *J Clin Invest* 74:2136, 1984.
525. Slovik DM et al: Clinical evaluation of bone turnover by serum osteocalcin measurements. *Calcif Tissue Int* 34:S15, 1982.
526. Somerville PJ et al: Resistance to parathyroid hormone in renal failure: Role of vitamin D metabolites. *Kidney Int* 14:245, 1978.
527. Somerville PJ et al: Evidence that resistance to the calcemic action of parathyroid hormone in rats with acute leukemia is caused by phosphate retention. *Kidney Int* 16:552, 1979.
528. Sorenson E et al: Iatrogenic magnesium intoxication during 1α-hydroxycholecalciferol treatment. *Br Med J* 2:215, 1976.
529. Stanbury SW: Bone disease in uremia. *Am J Med* 44:714, 1968.
530. Stanbury SW: The phosphate ion in chronic renal failure, in Hioco DJ (ed): *Phosphate Inorganique, Biologie et Physiopathologie. International Symposium.* Paris, Sandoz, 1970, p 187.
531. Stanbury SW: The role of vitamin D in renal bone disease. *Clin Endocrinol* 7:25S, 1977.
532. Stanbury SW et al: Metabolic studies of renal osteodystrophy. I. Calcium, phosphorus and nitrogen metabolism in rickets, osteomalacia, and hyperparathyroidism complicating chronic uremia and in the osteomalacia of the adult Fanconi syndrome. *Q J Med* 35:1, 1966.
533. Stanbury SW et al: Parathyroid function in chronic renal failure: A statistical survey of the plasma biochemistry in azotaemic renal osteodystrophy. *Q J Med* 35:1, 1966.
534. Stanbury SW et al: Osteodystrophy developing spontaneously in the course of chronic renal failure. *Arch Intern Med* 124:274, 1969.
535. Stinchfield FE et al: The effect of anticoagulant therapy on bone repair. *J Bone Joint Surg* 35A:270, 1956.
536. Strong HE et al: Measurement of dialysance and bi-directional fluxes of calcium, in vivo, using radiocalcium. *Trans Am Soc Artif Intern Organs* 17:108, 1971.
537. Stummvoll H et al: Effect of desferrioxamine on aluminum kinetics during hemodialysis. *Mineral Electrolyte Metab* 10:263, 1984.
538. Sugisaki H et al: Phosphate in dialysis patients. *Trans Am Soc Artif Intern Organs* 29:38, 1983.
539. Suki W et al: Acute treatment of hypercalcemia with furosemide. *N Engl J Med* 283:836, 1970.
540. Sy W et al: Bone scan in chronic dialysis patients with evidence of secondary hyperparathyroidism and renal osteodystrophy. *Br J Radiol* 48:878, 1975.
541. Tapia L et al: Parenteral lidocaine in treatment of pruritus in dialysis patients. *N Engl J Med* 296:261, 1977.
542. Tatler GL et al: Evolution of bone disease over 10 years in 135 patients with terminal renal failure. *Br Med J* 4:315, 1973.
543. Taves DR et al: Use of fluoridated water in long term hemodialysis. *Arch Intern Med* 115:167, 1965.
544. Teitelbaum SL et al: Do parathyroid hormone and 1,25 dihydroxyvitamin D modulate bone formation in uremia? *J Clin Endocrinol* 51:247, 1980.
545. Teitelbaum Sl et al: Calcifediol in chronic renal insufficiency: Skeletal response. *JAMA* 235:164, 1976.
546. Termine JD et al: Amorphous/crystalline interrelationships in bone mineral. *Calcif Tissue Res* 1:8, 1967.
547. Timsit F et al: Cardiomyopathie aluminique chez un hémodialysé chronique. *Nephrologie* 6:263, 1985 (abstract).
548. Tonshoff B et al: Growth-stimulating effect of recombinant human growth hormone in children with end-stage renal disease. *J Pediatr* 116:561, 1990.
549. Trapp GA: Plasma aluminum is bound to transferrin. *Life Sci* 33:311, 1983.
550. Van Cutsem J et al: Effects of deferoxamine, feroxamine and iron on experimental mucormycosis (zygomycosis). *Kidney Int* 36:1061, 1989.
551. Vargas J et al: Metabolic bone disease associated with total parenteral nutrition: Course after reducing alumi-

num content in parenteral solutions. *Am J Clin Nutr* 48:1070, 1988.
552. Varghese Z et al: Plasma hydroxyproline in renal osteodystrophy. *Proc Eur Dial Transplant Assoc* 10:187, 1973.
553. Verberckmoes R et al: Disappearance of vascular calcifications during treatment of renal osteodystrophy. *Ann Intern Med* 82:529, 1975.
554. Vergne-Marini P et al: Jejunal and ileal calcium absorption in patients with chronic renal disease: Effect of 1α-hydroxycholecalciferol. *J Clin Invest* 57:861, 1976.
555. Versieck J et al: Measuring aluminum levels. *N Engl J Med* 302:468, 1980.
556. Voigts A et al: The effects of calciferol and its metabolites on patients with chronic renal failure. I. Calciferol, dihydrotachysterol and calcifediol. *Arch Intern Med* 143:960, 1983.
557. Voigts A et al: Parathyroid hormone and bone histology: Response to hypocalcemia in osteitis fibrosa. *Kidney Int* 25:445, 1984.
558. Voigts A et al: The effects of calciferol and its metabolites oñ patients with chronic renal failure. II. Calcitriol, hydroxyvitamin D and 24,25 dihydroxyvitamin D. *Arch Intern Med* 143:1205, 1983.
559. Walker JA et al: Thrombocytopenia associated with intravenous desferrioxamine. *Am J Kidney Dis* 6:254, 1985.
560. Walling MW: Intestinal Ca and phosphate transport: Differential responses of vitamin D metabolites. *Am J Physiol* 133:3488, 1977.
561. Walser M: The separate effects of hyperparathyroidism, hypercalcemia of malignancy, renal failure and acidosis on the state of calcium phosphate and other ions in plasma. *J Clin Invest* 41:1454, 1962.
562. Walser M et al: Renal tubular transport of fluoride compared with chloride. *Am J Physiol* 210:1290, 1966.
563. Wang C et al: Hyperfunctioning supernumerary parathyroid glands. *Surg Gynecol Obstet* 148:711, 1979.
564. Ward MK et al: Osteomalacic dialysis osteodystrophy: Evidence for a waterborne etiological agent, probably aluminum. *Lancet* 1:841, 1978.
565. Ward KM, Parkinson LS: Aluminum toxicity in renal failure, in Drukker W et al (eds): *Replacement of Renal Function by Dialysis,* 2d ed. Boston, Martinus Nijhoff, 1983, p 811.
566. Weeke E et al: Serum fractions of calcium and phosphorus in uremia. *Acta Med Scand* 189:79, 1971.
567. Weidmann P et al: Effect of acute hypercalcemia on blood pressure in patients with chronic renal failure. *Ann Intern Med* 76:741, 1972.
568. Wen-tse C et al: Evaluation of vitamin D-binding protein and vitamin D metabolite loss in children on continuous ambulatory peritoneal dialysis. *Bone Mineral,* 1992 (in press).
569. Wiegmann TB et al: Malabsorption of calcium and phosphate in chronic renal failure: ^{32}P and ^{45}Ca studies in dialysis patients. *Clin Nephrol* 34:35, 1990.
570. Wills MR et al: Aluminum poisoning: Dialysis encephalopathy, osteomalacia, and anaemia. *Lancet* 2:29, 1983.
571. Wilson L et al: Altered divalent ion metabolism in early renal failure: Role of 1,25 $(OH)_2D$. *Kidney Int* 21:65, 1982.
572. Windus DW et al: Fatal rhizopus infections in hemodialysis patients receiving deferoxamine. *Ann Intern Med* 107:678, 1987.
573. Wing AJ et al: Transient and persistent hypercalcaemia in patients treated by maintenance haemodialysis. *Br Med J* 4:150, 1968.
574. Winkler S et al: Hypercalcemia during treatment of uremic patients with $1{,}25(OH)_2D_3$: Analysis of 30 cases. *Kidney Int* 14:667, 1978 (abstract).
575. Winney RJ et al: The role of plasma aluminum in the detection and prevention of aluminum toxicity. *Kidney Int* 29(suppl 18):S91, 1986.
576. Witmer G et al: Effects of 25 hydroxycholecalciferol on bone lesions of children with terminal renal failure. *Kidney Int* 10:395, 1976.
577. Wright RS et al: Musculoskeletal manifestation of chronic renal failure, dialysis and transplantation, in Bacon P et al (eds): *Renal Manifestations in Rheumatic Disease.* London, Butterworth, 1982, p 352.
578. Zevin D et al: Effect of parathyroid hormone and 1,25-dihydroxyvitamin D_3 on RNA and heme synthesis by erythroid precursors. *Mineral Electrolyte Metab* 6:125, 1981.
579. Zingraff J et al: Bilateral fracture of the femoral neck complicating uremic bone disease prior to chronic hemodialysis. *Clin Nephrol* 2:73, 1974.
580. Zuchelli P et al: Treatment of ectopic calcification in uremia. *Kidney Int* 13(suppl 8):S86, 1978.

CHAPTER • 42

Kidney transplantation: associated physiologic, fluid, electrolyte, and acid-base abnormalities

Mario F. Rubin • John Badalamenti • William M. Bennett

INTRODUCTION

The first recorded kidney transplantation was performed in 1906. The last few decades have seen the rapid development of transplantation, which has now become accepted as the most successful form of treatment for patients with end-stage renal disease (ESRD). As a result, increasing numbers of rehabilitated transplanted patients are now followed by nephrologists, internists, and general practitioners.

It is important to note that modern kidney transplantation not only improves the quality of life of patients suffering from chronic renal disease but also provides a scientific opportunity to enhance our understanding of alloimmunity and of renal physiology (e.g., the role of the renal nerves, the renal adaptation to uninephrectomy).

This chapter describes the physiologic changes (circulatory, glomerular, and tubular) that follow the surgical placement of a renal allograft as well as the electrolyte and acid-base abnormalities that are frequently observed in transplant recipients. The reader should keep in mind that the complexity of the clinical setting in which renal transplantation is performed is such that it is often difficult to differentiate between the functional responses attributable to renal allografting and rejection per se and those renal functional patterns that are ascribable to superimposed conditions such as ischemic, nephrotoxic, vascular, and/or mechanical injury.

RENAL CIRCULATION AND GLOMERULAR FILTRATION RATE

The unpredictable recovery of allograft function and of the multiple pretransplant variables associated with cadaveric kidney transplantation has precluded a satisfactory study of the hemodynamic changes that follow engraftment. In fact, most of the presently available information derives from the study of both living related and living unrelated kidney transplants.

Animal and human studies show a decrease in both the glomerular filtration rate (GFR) and the renal plasma flow (RPF) immediately after engraftment.[34,115] The depressed RPF begins to normalize within 12 h following transplantation while the GFR increases at a slower pace, and both reach stable values within 7 to 10 days. These hemodynamic changes account for the low filtration fraction (FF) that is characteristic of living donor kidney transplantation.[115]

The pathophysiology of these circulatory changes is incompletely understood. Autotransplanted animal kidneys show a reduction of superficial cortical blood flow relative to medullary perfusion with normalization of renal blood flow (RBF) distribution in 24 to 48 h.[68,228,249] Data derived from measurements of RBF in experimental canine models of renal ischemia, denervation, and autotransplantation suggest that ischemia is the major factor in the alterations in the distribution of RBF.

A creative animal experimental design by Lackner and McKay reveals that the immediate decreases in RBF are due to ischemia (ischemic and autotransplant models) and are modified following in situ denervation.[140] Morphologic and micropuncture studies performed in isograft rat transplant models by Norlen and colleagues[189] strongly support the role of ischemia. A prolonged cold ischemia time was associated with a greater degree of morphologic and physiologic heterogeneity—dilated tubules without filtration due to a high intratubular pressure with probable obstruction in the late proximal tubule or loop of Henle, collapsed tubules secondary to glomerular ischemia, and normal tubules with decreased glomerular capillary pressure.

The decreased allograft function (GFR and RBF) observed in clinical circumstances is, in general, proportional to the length of total (cold and warm) pretransplant ischemia (see below). As long as neither immunologic (rejection) nor nephrotoxic insults supervene, the long-term function of a kidney transplant is excellent. [82,193] As shown in Figs. 42-1 and 42-2, long-term measurements (34 months) of kidney function (GFR and RPF) in recipients of living donor kidneys show values similar to those of the remaining kidney in the donor. The evaluation of GFR by inulin clearance, was 75.5 ml/min in the donor and 65.8 ml/min in the recipient. Para-aminohippurate (PAH) clearances were 348 and 309 ml/min in the donor and recipient, respectively. Measurements of filtration fraction (FF) were 0.22 percent in both.[193] In summary, a conventionally treated (azathioprine and prednisone) allograft undergoes, with time, the same compensatory changes (e.g., renal growth) that are seen in uninephrectomized donors.

The introduction of *cyclosporine* to the clinical practice of kidney transplantation improved allograft survival but at the expense of increased nephrotoxicity.[38] The renal toxicity of cyclosporine can be both acute and chronic. The pathologic manifestations of cyclosporine toxicity are vascular (concentric medial hypertrophy of small arteries), tubular (isometric vacuolization, giant mitochondria, and microcalcifications of proximal tubular cells), and interstitial (stripped fibrosis).[170,259,271] During the first 6 months of cyclosporine therapy a reversible form of acute renal failure, fundamentally due to vasoconstriction, is usually seen. Improvements in RBF following the conversion of cyclosporine treated patients (for a mean period of 6 months) to azathioprine also point to a reversible form of renal dysfunction.[52] Continuation of cyclosporine beyond this period of time is characterized by an increased incidence of ischemic glomerulopathy, tubular atrophy, and irreversible interstitial fibrosis with progression, in some cases, to end-stage renal disease (Fig. 42-3). A reduced RFB and GFR [the latter due to a reduction in the glomerular capillary hydraulic pressure and permeability coefficient (Kf)] are the pathogenetic mechanisms responsible for the acute renal dysfunction induced by cyclosporine.

Micropuncture studies of rats acutely infused with cyclosporine demonstrate a decline in single nephron GFR and Kf, and an increase in arteriolar resistance.[16,233] Fractional dextran clearance data obtained in heart transplant recipients[185] and morphologic animal studies[74] point to "glomerular afferent arteriolar constriction" as the cause of the increased arteriolar resistance observed during cyclosporine therapy. The combination of this vascular mechanical hindrance to glomerular perfusion (decreased intraglomerular hydraulic pressure) and a decrease in the glomerular capillary surface area (cyclosporine induced mesangial contraction) account for the reduction in GFR.

The cellular and molecular pathogenetic mechanisms of cyclosporine nephrotoxicity are not yet fully understood. The abnormalities in the renin-angiotensin system described in animal models (i.e., activation and increased production of renin by renal cortical slices)[71,129,208,210] are not a feature of cyclosporine treated human trans-

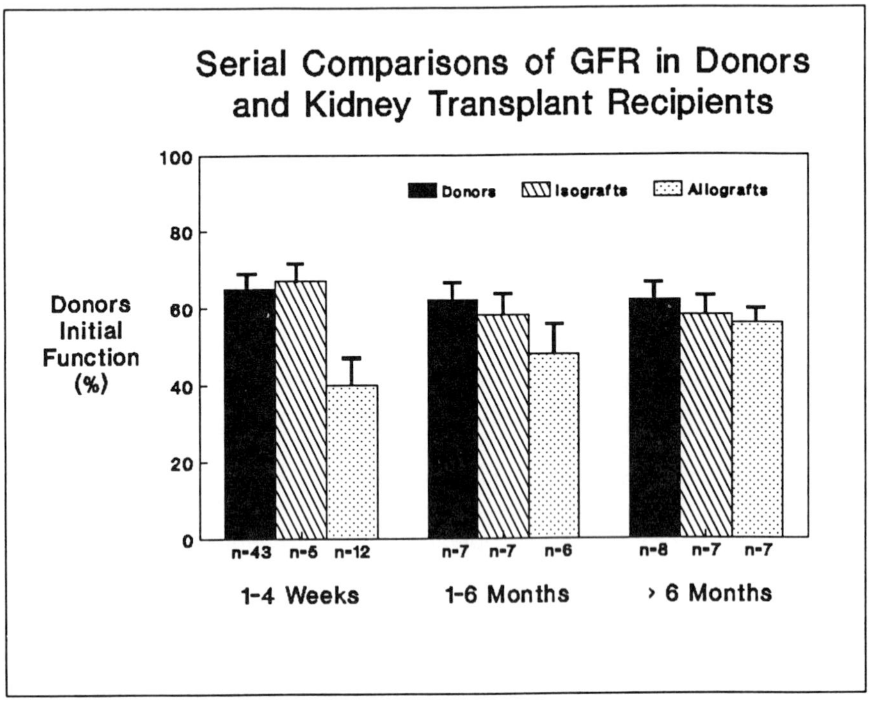

FIGURE 42-1 • Serial comparisons of glomerular filtration rate (GFR) in donors and kidney transplant recipients. (Reproduced with permission of *The American Journal of Surgery* 116:788, 1968.)

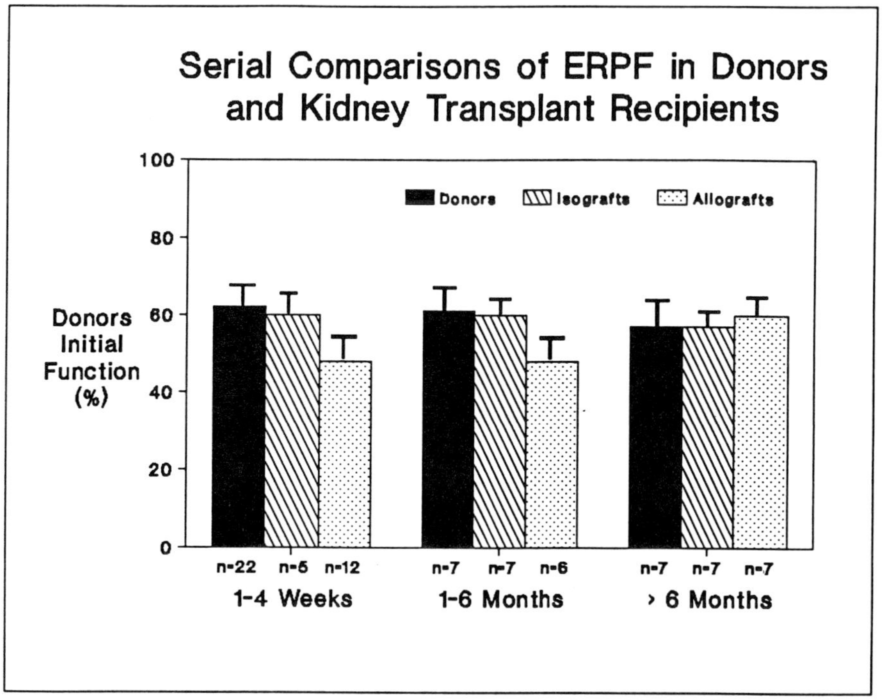

FIGURE 42-2 • Serial comparisons of effective renal plasma flow (ERPF) in donors and kidney transplant recipients. (Reproduced with permission of *The American Journal of Surgery* 116:788, 1968.)

plant recipients.[14,186] The development of volume expansion as a result of cyclosporine therapy (see below) appropriately lowers renin levels. Furthermore, as discussed below, some patients have, at the site of the juxtaglomerular apparatus, an inability to convert prorenin to renin.[184] The administration of angiotensin converting enzyme inhibitors (CEI) to cyclosporine treated patients has failed, with very few exceptions,[15] to improve the renal hemodynamics of the allograft.[92,104,173]

Additionally, caution is recommended when using CEI in cyclosporine treated patients, as some cases of acute renal failure, usually reversible, have been known to occur even in the absence of renal artery stenosis.[4,182]

The increased incidence of cyclosporine nephrotox-

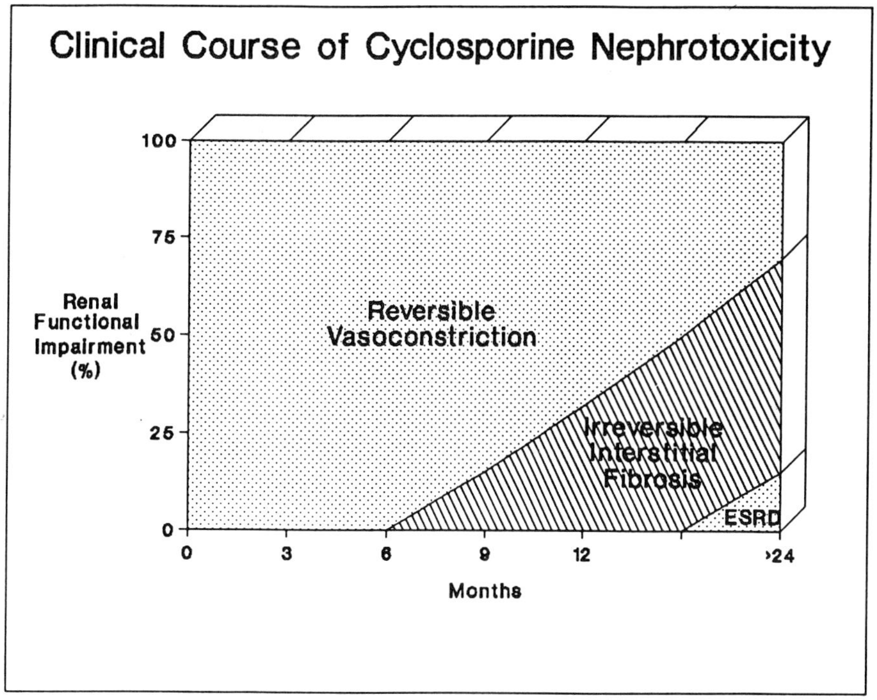

FIGURE 42-3 • Clinical course of cyclosporine nephrotoxicity. (Adapted with permission of *The Journal of the American Society of Nephrology* 1:162, 1990.)

icity following nonrenal transplants (e.g., heart, heart-lung, liver, pancreas, and bone marrow) drew attention to the role of the *autonomic nervous system* as a potential mediator of the toxicity. As opposed to kidney transplant recipients (e.g., denervated allografts), recipients of extrarenal organs retain the innervation of their native kidneys. The increased vascular response to catecholamines in cyclosporine treated animal models[178,181] has not proved to be a consistent feature of human cyclosporine nephrotoxicity.[14,186] Alpha-adrenergic blocking agents have failed to correct cyclosporine-induced hemodynamic abnormalities.[15] The failure to discern the mediator(s) of cyclosporine nephrotoxicity led to the investigation of other potential pathogenetic systems such as the *prostaglandins* (PGs), intracellular calcium, and more recently, the powerful vasoconstrictor endothelin. Cyclosporine treated animals consistently show an increase in the urinary excretion of the vasoconstrictor thromboxane with variable effects on vasodilatory PGs.[76,208-210,214] Pharmacologic manipulation of the PG system has provided interesting pathophysiologic results. Randomized clinical trials in cyclosporine-treated renal allograft recipients have shown improvements in GFR and RBF following the administration of PGE1 analogs and fish oil supplements.[176,253] Similar results have been obtained in pilot studies utilizing thromboxane synthetase inhibitors.[135] In addition, several animal studies have shown that the use of cyclooxygenase inhibitors potentiates the vasoconstrictive effects of cyclosporine.[76,181]

Increased cytosolic *calcium* concentration has been demonstrated in several tissues during cyclosporine therapy, and it has been proposed to account for the drug-induced vascular and mesangial contraction.[169] Cyclosporine may increase plasma membrane calcium permeability and may also spark the release of calcium from intracellular pools.[97,169] Based upon these experimental animal observations, several transplant centers are using calcium blocking agents, particularly in hypertensive cyclosporine-treated patients. Their clinical advantages reside on their effects on glomerular hemodynamics (e.g., preferential afferent arteriolar vasodilatation) and on the immune system (e.g., Ca^{2+} entry is required for lymphocyte activation). The clinician should remember that some calcium channel antagonists (e.g., diltiazem, verapamil) are known to affect cyclosporine metabolism[247,248] and that an adjustment in cyclosporine dosage will therefore be required. Preliminary experimental data in animals suggest that cyclosporine increases the release of *endothelin* from vascular smooth muscle. Antiendothelin monoclonal antibody improved glomerular hemodynamics in cyclosporine-treated animals.[134] Further research into endothelial factors is needed to characterize the intricate mechanism of cyclosporine-mediated vascular damage.

Based upon this information, it is best to avoid the administration of PG inhibitors in the setting of cyclosporine therapy. It remains to be ascertained whether or not the use of PG analogs (e.g., misoprostol) and/or different cyclosporine vehicles (e.g., fish oil) will have a beneficial long-term effect on allograft function.

TUBULAR FUNCTION

The capacity of the transplanted kidney to reabsorb and secrete various solutes and maintain acid-base homeostasis and serum osmolality has been the subject of extensive investigation. The proximal and distal tubular transport abnormalities responsible for the immediate posttransplant polyuric state and the failure to reabsorb bicarbonate and/or to secrete hydrogen and potassium ions in response to hormonal stimuli (see below) are for the most part short-term phenomena that tend to disappear within days. Long-term paired donor-recipient studies have shown normal tubular and hormonal (renin-aldosterone) responses to changes in sodium intake.[29] The generation of solute-free water (CH_2O) and/or reabsorption of solute-free water (TCH_2O) in response to changes in serum tonicity are also intact. On the other hand, some transplant recipients exhibit high plasma antidiuretic hormone (ADH) levels for a given change in serum osmolality and a sluggish tubular concentrating response to water deprivation.[203-205]

It is useful to separate those pathophysiologic events which unfold in the immediate postoperative period from those that develop months or years later. The latter will be more frequently encountered in clinical practice.

IMMEDIATE POSTTRANSPLANT PERIOD

A variety of renal functional patterns (Table 42-1) have been observed during the first 24 to 72 h following transplantation. These patterns range from a total absence of function (primary nonfunction) to one or more selected functional defects. Some allografts with primary nonfunction recover after a period of weeks or months while others, of course, never resume function.

Posttransplant acute tubular necrosis (delayed graft function)

Posttransplant delayed graft function (DGF) commonly occurs in cadaveric transplantation with an incidence that can be as high as 60 percent.[146,192] As shown in Table 42-2, it correlates with several factors such as donor characteristics, harvesting and preservation techniques, and the early use of cyclosporine.[160,184,192]

The *condition of the donor* prior to kidney procurement has been shown to be extremely important. The presence of infection and/or cardiovascular instability

TABLE 42-1 • Renal functional patterns in the immediate posttransplant period

- Primary nonfunction
- Posttransplant acute tubular necrosis (DGF)*
- Posttransplant polyuria

* Delayed graft function.

TABLE 42-2 • Causes of posttransplant acute tubular necrosis (DGF)*

- *Donor factors*
  Premorbid infection
  Prolonged hypotension
  Need for vasopressor drugs
  Advanced age
  Oliguria
- *Surgical and preservation techniques*
  Multiorgan harvesting techniques
  Prolonged cold and/or warm ischemic times
  Difficult ureteroneocystostomy
- *Early cyclosporine administration*

*Delayed graft function.

(e.g., hypotension, nephrotoxic antibiotics, vasopressor drugs) has an adverse effect on immediate graft function. The utilization of kidneys from older donors is also associated with a higher incidence of immediate acute renal failure (ARF) (perhaps as a result of their increased susceptibility to ischemia).[265] The early identification of potential cadaver donors and the prompt correction of premorbid electrolyte and acid-base abnormalities are extremely important measures that have been reported to improve immediate graft function.[17,162,188] Most cadaver donors are intravascularly depleted, in part related to prior administration of mannitol for cerebral edema or the presence of diabetes insipidus. Therefore, recognition and appropriate management of the type of fluid and electrolyte losses lead to restoration of isotonicity, normalization of intravascular volume, and increased urine output.

The tendency to develop ARF following transplantation may also be influenced by *the manner in which the kidney is harvested, preserved, and transported* between donor and recipient. The lower incidence of oliguria following the use of organs from living donors as compared with cadaver donors is in great part due to the minimal ischemic time (cold and warm) in the former (~ 30 to 60 min). The warm ischemia time (the period between low or absent blood supply and cooling of the organ) tends to be much longer in cadaveric transplantation, since these kidneys cannot be harvested until actual cardiac standstill has occurred. Furthermore, with the development of the multiorgan harvesting approach (heart, liver, pancreas, etc.), the harvesting of kidneys is usually relegated to last place.

Lastly, and as previously discussed, *the immediate use of cyclosporine* is associated with an increased incidence of posttransplant acute tubular necrosis (ATN). Indeed, the syndrome of cyclosporine induced early renal dysfunction is much more likely to occur in the setting of renal ischemia, and most transplant centers therefore delay its administration for a variable period of time (hours to days) after engraftment.

Posttransplant ARF can last anywhere from 24 h to several weeks. The electrolyte and acid-base abnormalities found with DGF are the same as those seen in patients with ARF of other causes and will not be discussed here, as they are thoroughly considered in Chap. 38.

We would like to stress that DGF is a diagnosis of exclusion and that prerenal (volume and vascular) and postrenal (obstruction, urinary leakage) causes must always be taken into account. In addition, the possibility of an underlying accelerated rejection process must also be an important consideration. As the presently available noninvasive methodology is neither sensitive nor specific for the diagnosis of rejection, a more diligent search for this entity (e.g., fine needle aspiration and/or allograft biopsy) is needed. This is especially true when other correctable causes (see above) are absent or when the duration of DGF is prolonged (> 7 days).

Posttransplant diuresis

Posttransplant diuresis is a rather characteristic functional syndrome that usually begins in the operating room (at the time of vascular anastomosis) or shortly thereafter. The magnitude, composition, and duration of posttransplant diuresis have been partially defined (primarily in cases of living donor transplants), but its etiology remains unclear. It is first manifested by the prompt excretion of urine that is usually clear but at times may be bloody.[145] The urine volume progressively increases, peaking at about 12 h after surgery, and gradually declines over the next several hours. Urinary volumes as high as 24 liters a day have been reported; therefore, rational replacement therapy during and following the diuresis should depend upon the composition of the urine formed and the mechanisms responsible for its formation.

The nature of the living-donor renal posttransplant polyuria has been characterized as an osmotic diuresis. Henderson and Ogden[115,194] have described the results of renal function studies (in living-donor transplants), performed 2 and 5 h after surgery, respectively, and continued for 7 days. Both studies showed a high fractional excretion of sodium (Fe_{Na} 13 to 21 percent), a lower than expected fractional excretion of potassium relative to urine flow and sodium delivery (Fe_K 5 to 10 percent), and a slighly hypotonic or isotonic urine (Uosm/Posm = 0.76 to 1.0). The ratio of electrolyte osmolal clearance to total osmolal clearance exceeded 50 percent in the majority of the patients, and urinary urea was less than 28 percent of the total urine solute at maximum flow rates.

The pathophysiology of posttransplant diuresis remains unclear. We will briefly discuss the major theories purporting to explain the etiology of this disorder (Table 42-3).

Expansion of the extracellular fluid (ECF) volume is associated with alterations in peritubular capillary physical forces and hormonal changes (increased natriuretic peptide, decreased renin-aldosterone levels) leading to natriuresis as a result of decreased tubular reabsorption. Since most transplant recipients come to surgery with an expanded ECF, it was postulated that the immediate posttransplant diuresis was an expected physiologic response to volume expansion.[244] As discussed below, the clinical observation that spontaneous reductions in fractional sodium excretion and urine volume occur during posttransplant diuresis (in spite of meticulous fluid replacement) is seemingly inconsistent with this overfill theory.[114,115]

The possibility of *urea-induced diuresis* was suggested because of the similarities between posttransplant diuresis and the polyuria following relief of urinary tract obstruction (postobstructive diuresis). However, in posttransplant diuresis the major urinary solute is sodium, not urea.[115,194]

What role, if any, *renal denervation* plays in the etiology of posttransplant diuresis remains unclear. Several animal[140,220,274] and human studies[33,91,266] support the possibility of a denervation-induced natriuresis. However, it is unlikely that denervation is the only cause of this phenomenon since the decrease in posttransplant natriuresis usually takes place shortly after engraftment (24 to 48 h). Since renal denervation extends well beyond these 2 days, its role in the diuresis must be minimal.[88]

The findings of increased water clearance, glucosuria, and aminoaciduria suggest that an important factor in posttransplant diuresis is *proximal tubular dysfunction*.[115] However, the presence of glucosuria and aminoaciduria has not been consistently found in all studies.[137,194] In addition, this theory requires the participation of a reset tubuloglomerular feedback (TGF) mechanism to explain a rise in GFR, rather than a fall, since distally displaced solute loads reach the macula densa where the feedback response is initiated.

TABLE 42-3 • Pathophysiology of posttransplant polyuria

- Preoperative overexpansion of the ECF volume
- Urea osmotic diuresis
- Denervation natriuresis
- Proximal tubular dysfunction
- Resetting of tubuloglomerular feedback
- Medullary ischemia

The importance of *altered TGF* is supported by the data of Muller-Suur and colleagues obtained from rats undergoing orthotopic kidney transplantation.[180] Using micropuncture (stop flow) techniques, these authors found that TGF was intact in the transplanted kidney while the contralateral native kidney was in place. In this setting, the transplanted kidney's GFR diminished appropriately when distal solute delivery was increased.[28] After the removal of the contralateral native kidney, increasing the distal delivery of solute (particularly chloride) in the transplanted kidney no longer normally reduced the GFR because of a shift in the TGF set point. The mediators of this resetting (presently unknown) were thought to be related to the demonstrated increased renal interstitial pressure.

More recently, attention has focused on the role of *medullary ischemia* as an important contributor to posttransplant polyuria. There is mounting experimental evidence to show that the renal medulla is most sensitive to ischemic damage.[154] Micropuncture data showing comparable tubular fluid to plasma insulin ratios (2:1) in the proximal and distal tubules of transplanted and normal kidneys, suggest that the nonfunctional ischemic renal medulla is responsible for the polyuria observed.[180]

In summary, while the exact cause of posttransplant diuresis remains elusive, fluid replacement for living-donor renal transplantation (in the absence of diuretic administration and/or glucosuria) should consist of hypotonic solutions (0.45% normal saline). Potassium administration is hardly ever necessary in the immediate posttransplant period, and its use should be guided by frequent determinations of its serum levels. However, the development of posttransplant hyperglycemia with glucosuria, hypermagnesiuria, and/or the administration of diuretics will require a change in the therapeutic strategy according to the type of losses being generated. For many years, it has been customary to measure the central venous pressure and to replace fluid losses according to the readings being obtained in order to avoid volume depletion. Furthermore, the traditional approach has been to match intake with output. Henderson and associates[115] found that despite strict replacement of fluid and electrolytes, the urine output spontaneously decreased as the fractional excretion of sodium (Fe_{Na} = 0.01 to 0.05 percent) fell. A randomized study of intravenous fluid replacement (without diuretic administration) following living-donor renal transplantation with short ischemia time (< 90 min) also concluded that there was no difference in ultimate allograft function when a "fixed" (125 ml/h) versus "tailored" (total volume of urine output + 30 ml/h) replacement program was used.[114]

Therefore, for most cases of living-donor posttransplant polyuria, a preset rate (~150 to 250 ml/h) of intravenous fluid administration will prove to be adequate. However, this clinical approach should never replace the close monitoring and appropriate treatment of the hemodynamic and homeostatic changes that may develop if this "generic recipe" proves inappropriate for a given patient. The management of the posttransplant diuresis that follows cadaveric renal transplantation is, for several reasons, not as simple. First, the high incidence of delayed or impaired early graft function (~ 50 percent) precludes the routine administration of a predetermined quantity of intravenous fluids. Second, the characteristics of this type of diuresis have not been satisfactorily studied, and finally, the need to administer diuretics (usually mannitol and/or furosemide) introduces multiple variables that hinder an accurate understanding of the pathophysiologic processes involved. However, it is our experience that the administration of hypotonic solutions tailored to urinary losses is most effective.

RENAL TUBULAR AND METABOLIC DEFECTS DEVELOPING LATER IN THE POSTTRANSPLANTATION PERIOD

Abnormalities in sodium and water metabolism

With the exception of the *adrenergic nervous system* (ANS), all other participating elements in the regulation of the ECF volume appear to be functionally intact following renal transplantation.

There is unquestionable histochemical evidence that within 4 weeks of renal transplantation, adrenergic reinnervation occurs in both animals[190,191] and humans.[88] Despite this evidence it must be shown that the functional integrity of the nerve and its innervated tissue is reestablished. Tissue levels of the neurohormone norepinephrine correlate poorly with physiologic responses and so shed little light on this issue.[133] Graded degrees of direct adrenergic electrical stimulation should elicit proportionate vasoconstrictor responses in the normally innervated kidney.[63-65] Unfortunately no such studies have been done in the transplanted kidney. Furthermore, the inability of transplant recipients (without native kidneys) to increase plasma renin activity after standing (a neural-dependent phenomenon) suggests that functional adrenergic reinnervation of the juxtaglomerular apparatus does not occur for periods of up to 60 months after engraftment.[51] The functional consequences of the lack of physiologic renal innervation in the responses of the allograft to changes in sodium intake appear to be of little significance in the overall maintenance of salt and water balance.[29]

Even though the functional capacity of the allograft to maintain salt and water balance is intact, hyponatremic and hypernatremic states can develop in short-term as well as long-term allograft recipients.

Three different types of hyponatremias can be observed in kidney transplant recipients (Fig. 42-4).

Posttransplant pseudohyponatremia (hyponatremia with isoosmolality) can present in association with hyperlipidemia and hyperproteinemia. Hyperlipidemia is a

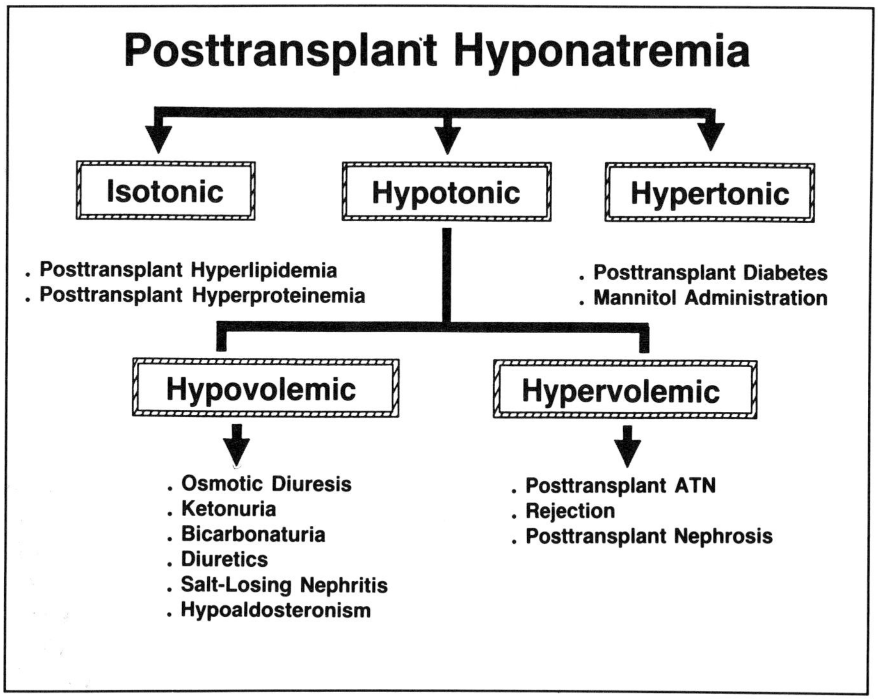

FIGURE 42-4 • Posttransplant hyponatremia.

long recognized, difficult, and common problem following organ transplantation. The cause of posttransplant hyperlipidemia remains unclear. Hypertriglyceridemia is more often seen in conventionally treated patients (azathioprine and prednisone) while hypercholesterolemia occurs much more frequently in the cyclosporine treated group.[27,152,256] The development of posttransplant nephrotic syndrome (e.g., transplant glomerulopathy, recurrence of original glomerular disease), uncontrolled diabetes, and the requirement for parenteral nutrition (e.g., intravenous fat emulsions) are the usual clinical circumstances in which a spurious hyponatremia can be found.

The incidence of monoclonal gammopathies in transplant recipients has increased with cyclosporine therapy. Hyperproteinemia, as seen in multiple myeloma, is yet another cause of pseudohyponatremia. Failure to recognize the true etiology of this type of disorder could result in unnecessary and potentially dangerous therapeutic approaches (e.g., water restriction and/or saline administration). Treatment of the hyperlipidemic state should consist of dietary calorie and fat restriction, supplementation with soluble fiber, and if necessary, cautious use of lipid lowering agents. The treatment of a hyperproteinemic state usually requires the discontinuation of immunosuppressive therapy and appropriate chemotherapy.

Posttransplant hypertonic hyponatremia is usually a short-term phenomenon which occurs more commonly in association with posttransplant oliguria. It is usually the result of hyperglycemia (see below) and/or mannitol administration. A nonfunctioning allograft prevents the development of an osmotic diuresis, and the consequent buildup of effective osmoles in the ECF draws sodium-free water from the intracellular compartment to reestablish osmotic equilibrium. Hence, the maintenance of ECF isotonicity is accomplished at the expense of a dilutional hyponatremia.

Posttransplant hypotonic hyponatremias (particularly the hypovolemic and hypervolemic varieties) are frequently encountered in clinical practice. The most common *hypovolemic* forms are those caused by an osmotic diuresis (glucose, urea, mannitol), ketonuria, bicarbonaturia (renal tubular acidosis, bladder drainage of pancreas transplants), diuretic administration, salt-losing nephritis, and mineralocorticoid deficiency.

The obligate cation excretion induced by an osmotic diuresis can result in hyponatremia. This phenomenon is frequently encountered in the immediate posttransplant period and usually in association with posttransplant polyuria. Replacement of urinary losses with dextrose containing intravenous solutions (particularly to diabetic transplant recipients) in the face of the concurrent administration of large doses of steroids frequently leads to hyperglycemia and glucosuria. A more severe form of glucosuria is seen in association with the development of a hyperosmolar nonketotic state (e.g., pulse steroid therapy, infections, and posttransplant pancreatitis). In addition, the administration of mannitol and/or loop diuretics at the time of vascular anastomosis and the magnitude of urea-induced diuresis are potentially important contributory factors.

The best form of therapy is preventive. Frequent monitoring of serum chemistries and close attention to the type of urinary losses being generated with tailored replacement therapy is strongly encouraged.

The occurrence of posttransplant bicarbonaturia with obligatory excretion of sodium can be the result of either a renal tubular acidosis (see below) or the development of a metabolic alkalosis. A much more common cause of this phenomenon has developed as a result of the surgical technique employed for the drainage of exocrine pancreatic allograft secretions. Massive urinary losses of sodium bicarbonate are usually seen after pancreas transplantation.[237] Failure to provide adequate sodium bicarbonate therapy may result in profound degrees of acidemia, hyponatremia, hypovolemia, and hypotension.[221] Sporadic cases of posttransplant salt-losing nephritis[138] have been described in association with nephrocalcinosis[22,79] idiopathic tubular sodium wasting,[75] and tubular resistance to aldosterone.[252]

The most common *hypervolemic hyponatremic* states are those that occur in association with posttransplant ATN, acute and/or chronic rejection, and posttransplant nephrotic syndrome.

Posttransplant hypernatremia is a rare phenomenon. It has been described in the immediate posttransplant period in association with a large osmotic (urea-induced) diuresis, as a result of the inability of the nonfunctioning renal medulla to concentrate the urine.[219]

ABNORMALITIES IN POTASSIUM METABOLISM

Many of the systemic and renal physiologic forces that influence potassium balance become altered following kidney transplantation. Several of the drugs administered to these patients also alter serum potassium levels. It therefore follows that disturbances in potassium homeostasis are commonly found in kidney transplant recipients.

Hypokalemia

Posttransplant hypokalemia can be the result of transcellular potassium shifts and of gastrointestinal and renal losses (Fig. 42-5). (See Chaps. 6, 7, 22.)

Redistribution of K^+ may develop as a result of alkalemia and/or of the administration of insulin. Increases in serum HCO_3^- concentration are commonly seen following the administration of antacids, sodium bicarbon-

FIGURE 42-5 • Posttransplant hypokalemia.

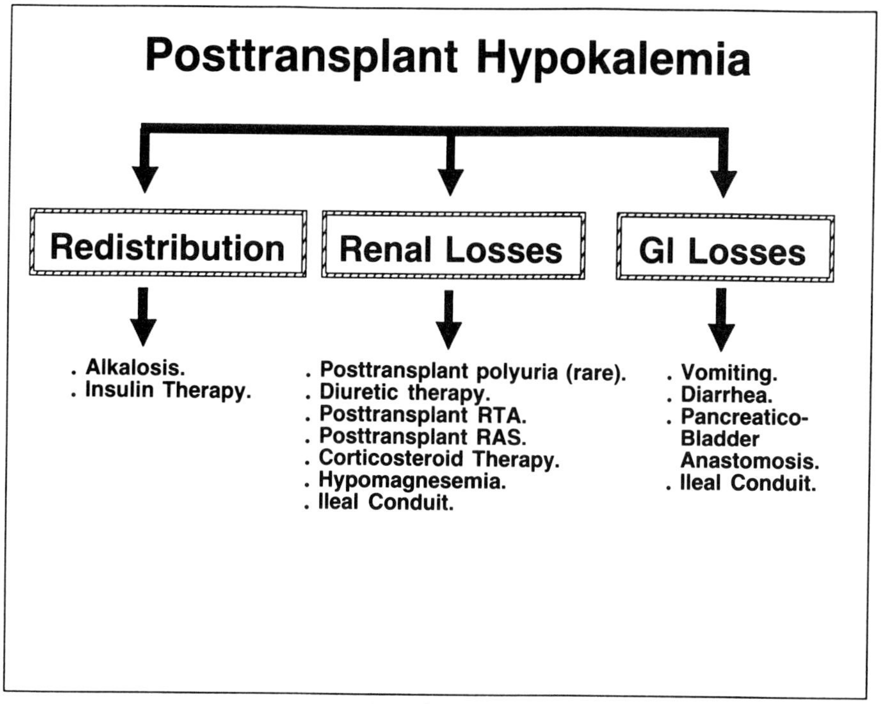

ate (e.g., replacement of fluid losses following pancreas transplantation, management of posttransplant renal tubular acidosis), and corticosteroids. Extracellular alkalinity will promote (perhaps via stimulation of the Na^+/H^+ exchanger and the Na^+K^+ATPase) the intracellular accumulation of potassium. The hypokalemia associated with insulin administration (a common phenomenon in posttransplant diabetes) has also been linked to stimulation of the same transporters.[36]

Gastrointestinal potassium losses (e.g., vomiting, diarrhea, bladder drainage of exocrine pancreatic allograft secretions) are a frequent occurrence in transplant recipients. The low K^+ concentration in gastrointestinal secretions (~5 to 15 meq/liter) requires massive losses of fluid (e.g., after pancreas transplantation) to substantially lower K^+ stores. In fact, stimulation of the renin-angiotensin-aldosterone axis and ADH secretion (from the resulting hypovolemia) are the pathophysiologic processes responsible for the hypokalemia observed (e.g., increased renal tubular K^+ secretion).[80]

Renal potassium losses are usually the result of diuretic therapy (with or without associated hypomagnesemia), but they can also occur in association with posttransplant renal tubular acidosis (RTA), posttransplant renal artery stenosis, glucocorticoid therapy, and mineralocorticoid excess.[24]

The widespread use of cyclosporine (with its associated salt and water retention) requires, in the majority of the cases, concomitant diuretic therapy (e.g, furosemide). As long as salt intake is restricted and hypomagnesemia is corrected, the decreases in serum K^+ levels are mild and usually self-limited.[245] Even though hypokalemia is a frequent finding in patients with distal RTA, the majority of renal transplant acidification defects (see below) tend to disappear with time, and RTA is therefore a rare cause of decreased serum K^+ following transplantation. Posttransplantation renal artery stenosis (RAS) is a variable phenomenon that predominantly develops after living-donor transplantation. The initial increases in the levels of renin-angiotensin-aldosterone are very promptly suppressed by the development of ECF volume expansion (e.g., 1 kidney, 1 clip Goldblatt model of renovascular hypertension). Therefore, in contradistinction to the findings of the national cooperative renovascular hypertension study (e.g., 16 percent incidence of hypokalemia),[159] hypokalemia is seldom the result of posttransplant RAS.

Lastly, the association between posttransplant hypertension and hypokalemia can be the result of the ongoing corticosteroid administration or, very infrequently, an adrenal adenoma.[46]

Hyperkalemia

The incidence of hyperkalemia following kidney transplantation may be as high as 30 percent in conventionally immunosuppressed patients (i.e., azathioprine plus prednisone)[62] but has become an even more common problem in the cyclosporine era (see below). (See Chap. 23.) Posttransplant hyperkalemia can be the result of increased K^+ intake, redistribution, and decreased excretion by the renal allograft (Fig. 42-6).

The routine *administration of* K^+ supplements during the immediate posttransplant period can result in dangerous degrees of hyperkalemia. Physicians should

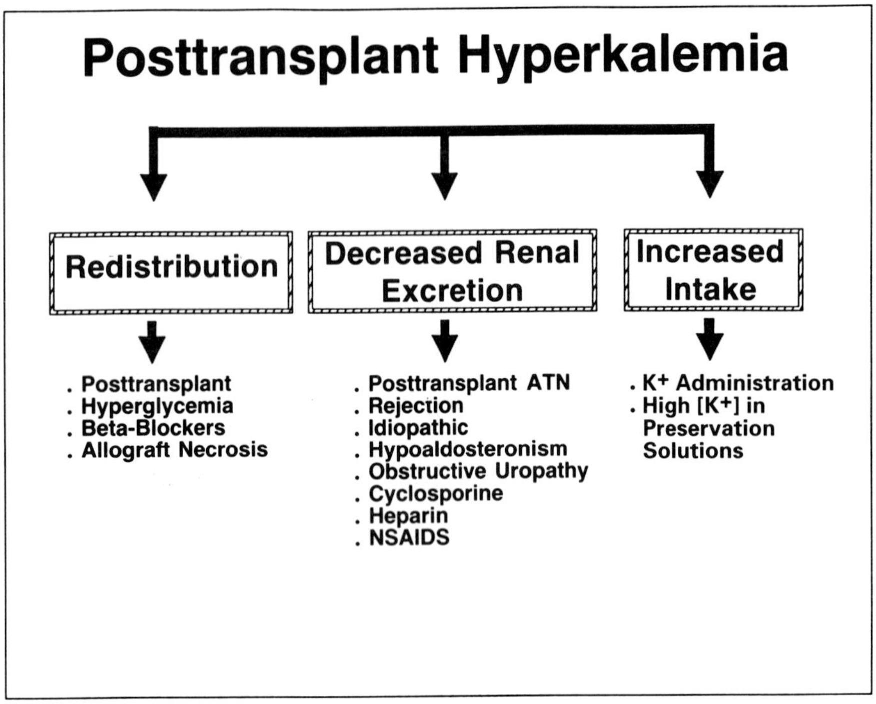

FIGURE 42-6 • Posttransplant hyperkalemia.

keep in mind that, in spite of increased distal sodium delivery (see below), tubular K^+ secretion during the first 48 h after transplantation is impaired. Renal preservation solutions rich in potassium (e.g., Collins solution containing 141 meq/liter K^+) may cause life-threatening degrees of hyperkalemia. Engraftment of cadaver kidneys incompletely flushed of their preservation solution can cause fatal hyperkalemia. Cardiac arrest has occurred from the rapid rise in serum potassium concentration following vascular anastomosis of the kidney allograft.[119,120,240] When such preservation solutions are used, intraoperative measurement of serum potassium levels is mandatory. Some of the newer more widely used preservation solutions (e.g., University of Wisconsin's solution) contain minimal amounts of potassium, thereby removing the potential threat of hyperkalemia.

Posttransplant redistributional hyperkalemia is much more common in diabetic recipients and results from hyperglycemia with insulinopenia and/or the administration of beta-blockers for the management of posttransplant hypertension. The routine measurement of blood glucose levels has significantly decreased the incidence of this problem, particularly during the immediate posttransplantation period. In addition, hyperkalemia may be the first sign of allograft infarct and is due to the massive cellular release of potassium. It is usually the consequence of clotting of the large renal vessels (artery and/or vein) as a result of mechanical obstruction and/or severe rejection leading to cortical necrosis.

A major cause of posttransplant hyperkalemia is related to *decreased distal renal tubular potassium secretion*. This failed secretion occurs despite increased distal delivery of sodium[62,89,115] and nonreabsorbable anions.[62] The cause of this temporary phenomenon[62] has remained elusive despite several well-designed studies.

A number of investigators have demonstrated that plasma aldosterone increases normally in response to such diverse stimuli as upright posture,[21,47,103,161] dietary salt restriction,[47,62,103] ACTH administration,[225] furosemide administration,[62] and angiotensin II infusion.[161] Notwithstanding, some patients have manifested hypoaldosteronism after kidney transplantation,[207,252] and this probably relates to a concurrent hyporeninemia; in addition, there are instances of dissociation between plasma renin activity and aldosterone.[21,62] The distal tubular response to 9-alpha-fludrocortisone in such cases has been variable. The patients studied by DeFronzo[62] failed to exhibit a kaliuresis in response to the exogenous mineralocorticoid, but they responded (by an unknown mechanism) to thiazide diuretics, while the two patients studied by Roll and colleagues[226] exhibited a decrease in urinary sodium with an increased urinary potassium. The introduction of cyclosporine to clinical transplantation has led to an increased incidence of hyperkalemia.[3,13,14,273] The vasoconstrictor properties (see above) of this cyclic undecapeptide[74,181,233] involve preglomerular vessels, which decreases RBF and peritubular capillary hydrostatic pressure. The enhanced proximal tubular reabsorption of sodium and water[142] leads to an expanded ECF volume with a consequent physiologic decrease in renin levels.[13] Studies performed in heart transplant recipients suggest that, in addition, cyclosporine decreases the conversion of prorenin to renin and/or impairs renin release.[187] Aldosterone levels are similar to those found in conventionally treated patients; however, kaliuresis is impaired.[13] The proposition derived from animal studies that cyclosporine induces a distal tubular unresponsiveness to aldosterone is in conflict with the findings of increased kaliuresis observed by increasing distal sodium delivery and/or adding an exogenous mineralocorticoid.[213] The frequent development of hypertension (~80 percent) in cyclosporine treated patients precludes the administration of an exogenous mineralocorticoid. Restrictions in dietary K^+ intake, use of cation-exchange resins (e.g., sodium polystyrene sulfonate), and/or administration of diuretics are the therapeutic maneuvers most commonly employed in the management of cyclosporine induced hyperkalemia.

ABNORMALITIES OF ACID-BASE METABOLISM

The acid-base abnormalities seen following renal transplantation fall into two categories, those that develop in any postoperative setting (e.g., respiratory acidosis and alkalosis) and those that are intrinsically related to the transplant, allograft rejection, and the drugs administered. Simple and mixed acid-base disorders are not uncommon, and their recognition is a powerful clinical tool (e.g., distal renal tubular acidosis as a prelude of chronic rejection).

Metabolic alkalosis

The incidence of posttransplant metabolic alkalosis is not yet known in spite of the interplay of several potential triggering mechanisms. (See Chaps. 29, 31.)

An increased intake of alkali is a frequent occurrence. The common practice of prescribing antacids during the first 3 months posttransplant (e.g., to aid in the prevention of gastrointestinal disease during a period of large steroid intake) represents, if absorbable alkali preparations are used, a source of bicarbonate gain. Surprisingly, very few cases of metabolic alkalosis have been described as a result of this therapeutic modality. A review of the metabolic complications of 297 heart and heart-lung transplant recipients who consumed 4 to 10 g/day of elemental calcium (in the form of calcium carbonate) revealed that 31 patients (10.4 percent) became alkalotic.[128] It is important to note that of the 297 patients, 37 developed hypercalcemia and impaired renal function, which required, in some instances, intravenous hydration and forced diuresis. The incidence of this pathophysiologic mechanism will likely increase as the number of combined pancreas-kidney transplant recipients who take large doses of sodium bicarbonate continues to increase (see below).

Upper gastrointestinal hydrogen-ion losses (e.g., nasogastric suction, vomiting) and *steroid and diuretic therapy* are common causes of acid depletion which are seen in the transplant recipient. Gastric losses are usually seen in diabetic recipients during the immediate posttransplant period as a result of postoperative ileus (e.g., intraperitoneal placement of pancreas-kidney allografts) and/or diabetic gastoparesis. The failure to identify and properly correct this problem may result in severe volume depletion and electrolyte abnormalities with the development of hypotension and maintenance of the alkalotic state.

Metabolic acidosis

Even though an increased anion gap metabolic acidosis can develop in the posttransplant setting (e.g., diabetic ketoacidosis, lactic acidosis secondary to sepsis, and/or cardiovascular collapse following monoclonal-polyclonal antibody administration), the most common acid-base disorder encountered in the posttransplant period is a hyperchloremic, normal anion gap metabolic acidosis (Fig. 42-7). (See Chap. 25.)

Extrarenal forms of normal anion gap hyperchloremic metabolic acidosis occurring in diarrheal states and gastrointestinal-ureteral-bladder connections can frequently develop in the kidney and/or kidney-pancreas transplant recipient. A urinary diversion procedure is usually performed in transplant recipients with either a nonfunctioning or anatomically abnormal urinary bladder. The anastomosis of the transplant ureter to a previously created ileal loop (ileal conduit) may lead, in approximately 10 percent of the cases, to a hyperchloremic-hypokalemic, normal anion gap metabolic acidosis. The presence of an anion exchanger (Cl^-/HCO_3^-) in the ileal luminal mucosa accounts for the absorption of chloride in exchange for bicarbonate secretion. The concomitant excretion of potassium (to preserve electroneutrality) is the basis for the associated hypokalemia. The severity of the acidosis is determined by the length of time that the urine is in contact with the ileal mucosa; therefore, whenever this disturbance is diagnosed, an obstruction of the ileal conduit must be excluded.

The recently adopted pancreatico-duodenal-bladder anastomosis as the preferred surgical method for the elimination of exocrine pancreatic allograft secretions poses a serious threat to electrolyte and acid-base homeostasis. The well-functioning transplanted pancreas restores euglycemia via the secretion of insulin but, at the same time, squanders sodium and bicarbonate (Na^+ 115 to 155 meq/liter; Cl^- 55 to 95 meq/liter; HCO_3^- 95 to 110 meq/liter). The failure to provide prophylactic sodium bicarbonate therapy in adequate amounts will result in hyponatremia (see above) and severe acidemia.

The ability of the transplanted kidney to acidify the urine has been the subject of several investigations. All

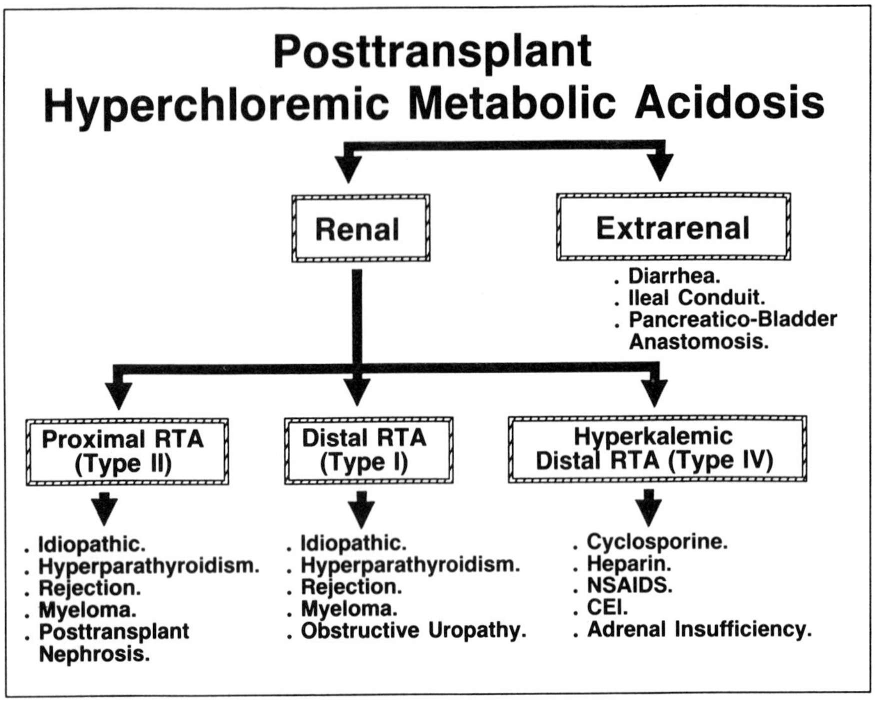

FIGURE 42-7 • Posttransplant hyperchloremic metabolic acidosis.

forms of renal tubular acidosis (RTA) may develop following transplantation.[157] (See Chap. 27.)

Posttransplant proximal RTA (type II) is a form of bicarbonate wastage which may develop in as many as 19 percent of the cases during the first 3 months following renal transplantation.[108,267] The nature of the defect in bicarbonate transport underlying this form of RTA is not known. On the other hand, its early appearance following engraftment and its disappearance with time suggests a causal relationship with other entities (e.g., secondary hyperparathyroidism, ischemia) that have a similar natural course. Its onset in the late posttransplant period (> 2 years) should alert the clinician to the possibility of allograft rejection[84] and/or the development of a monoclonal gammopathy.

Posttransplant distal RTA (type I) is a very frequent acidification defect found in up to 43 percent of kidney transplant recipients.[267] It may present as early as the first trimester[267] and last as long as 9 years after transplantation.[20] Most patients who exhibit a distal RTA also have manifestations of chronic rejection such as hypertension, proteinuria, and increased serum creatinine. Nevertheless, the association between a distal RTA and allograft rejection remains purely conjectural.[174] Even though morphologic findings of a rejection process have been found to coexist with a type I RTA,[20] other reports stress the improvement in tubular acidification capacity 14 to 16 months after transplantation even in the presence of chronic rejection.[25] Studies performed by Batlle and associates strongly suggest that the pathogenesis of the distal type of RTA seen following transplantation is related to a secretory abnormality of hydrogen ion (H^+).[20] Six kidney transplant patients who had a spontaneous normal anion gap acidemia (pH 7.31 ± 0.01) underwent metabolic studies and were compared with four transplant recipients who had no evidence of an acid-base disorder and served as controls. Following the infusion of neutral phosphate and sodium sulfate and/or acetazolamide administration, the study patients failed to increase their U-B pCO_2 (see Chap. 27) and/or decrease their urinary pH, which remained at 6.03 ± 0.2. These studies are indicative of a distal H^+ secretory defect in spite of a favorable electrochemical gradient.

Posttransplant type IV RTA has become a fairly common event following the introduction of cyclosporine therapy. Hyperkalemic metabolic acidosis associated with selective aldosterone deficiency was a rare event with conventional therapy.[20] The pathogenesis of cyclosporine-induced type IV RTA is related, in part, to the decreased distal delivery of sodium and to the functional suppression of the renin-aldosterone system. Its functional nature is demonstrated by its disappearance when patients are switched to azathioprine.[242] It remains to be established if this type of RTA is just the result of a voltage secretory defect or, in addition, decreased ammoniagenesis as a result of the superimposed hyperkalemia.

Patients with persistent distal RTA should receive

alkali therapy because the development of hypercalciuria (from the effects of acidosis) may perpetuate the already present secondary hyperparathyroid state (see below).

ABNORMALITIES IN MAGNESIUM METABOLISM

Hypermagnesemia (see Chap. 34) (resulting from the administration of magnesium containing antacids to patients with allograft dysfunction) was described 30 years ago by Alfrey and associates.[9] At the time of presentation, all three reported cases had severely compromised renal function with creatinine clearances of 3 to 12 ml/min. Magnesium-containing antacids (e.g., Riopan®, Maalox®, Gelusil®, Aludrox®, Amphogel®, Basaljel®) may produce not just hypermagnesemia (e.g., inadvertent administration during posttransplant ATN and/or rejection) but also alkalosis (see above) and hypophosphatemia (see below).

Hypomagnesemia (see Chap. 34) is a more frequent occurrence than hypermagnesemia in the posttransplant setting. Prior to the use of cyclosporine most cases of magnesium depletion were ascribed to increased urinary excretion as a result of hypercalcemia, hypophosphatemia, RTA, diuretics, and/or posttransplant diuresis.[59,222] Several reports have found a correlation between cyclosporine therapy and the development of hypomagnesemia.[18,109,127] To examine the association between cyclosporine and hypomagnesemia, Barton and colleagues carried out a prospective study in cyclosporine ($n = 27$) and azathioprine ($n = 17$) treated patients. In the azathioprine group the serum magnesium levels were at the upper limits of normal (2.3 ± 0.4 mg/dl) during the 6-month observation period. On the other hand, all the cyclosporine treated patients became hypomagnesemic within 2 weeks after transplantation (1.8 ± 0.4 mg/dl), reaching a nadir by the third week (1.6 ± 0.2 mg/dl). In spite of receiving magnesium supplementation (750 to 1500 mg/day of magnesium oxide), 5 of the 27 cyclosporine treated patients developed symptomatic hypomagnesemia with serum magnesium values as low as 0.9 mg/dl. The urinary excretion of magnesium remained inappropriately high (115 ± 75 mg/24 h) throughout the study period despite persistent hypomagnesemia. This renal magnesium wasting took place independently of osmotic diuresis, diuretic administration, hypercalcemia, hypophosphatemia, or acidosis.[18] A positive correlation between cyclosporine blood levels and the development of low magnesium levels has also been described.[109,127] The renal magnesium wasting induced by cyclosporine[19] appears to be a transient phenomenon since it is not found in long-term studies.[139] Its pathogenesis has not yet been characterized. Decreased renal tubular magnesium reabsorption as a result of cyclosporine-induced ECF volume expansion remains an attractive but unproved possibility.

Although posttransplant hypomagnesemia is usually asymptomatic and the cases of neurotoxicity (e.g., convulsions) described in bone marrow transplant patients are usually not seen in kidney transplant recipients,[125,126,246] it is the authors' opinion that, in view of the widespread use of cyclosporine, the potential cardiovascular (e.g., arrhythmias, hypertension) and electrolyte abnormalities (e.g., hypokalemia, hypocalcemia) associated with hypomagnesemia warrant the measurement, on a routine basis, of serum magnesium levels.

ABNORMALITIES IN PHOSPHORUS METABOLISM

Hyperphosphatemia

Posttransplantation hyperphosphatemia is a very rare and brief laboratory finding that can be seen during the first 48 h following transplantation (see Chap. 33). It is among the first manifestations of the pretransplant uremic state which normalizes after engraftment. The resolution of hyperphosphatemia is the result of the restoration of kidney function, normalization of $1,25(OH)_2$ vitamin D production, and/or the effects of the medications being administered (see below). Its appearance in the late posttransplant period is usually the result of allograft function deterioration (e.g., chronic rejection) with the reestablishment of an abnormal parathyroid hormone (PTH)-vitamin D axis.

Hypophosphatemia

Posttransplant hypophosphatemia (serum phosphorus < 2.5 mg/dl) is, on the other hand, a very common phenomenon (80 percent of the cases) following kidney transplantation.[101] (See Chap. 33.) This chemical abnormality is seen in recipients of cadaver[175] and living-donor kidneys.[116,117] It can develop both acutely (within the first 2 weeks after transplantation)[108] and chronically (delayed until more than 6 months after transplantation).[101,175,177,263] The etiology of the hypophosphatemia is related to either a renal phosphate leak and/or gastrointestinal losses (Fig. 42-8).

The mechanisms leading to the hyperphosphaturia have been traced to PTH dependent and independent processes. The association of hypophosphatemia with a low tubular reabsorption of phosphate and elevated parathyroid hormone levels is indicative of a *PTH-dependent process*. Even though serum concentrations of PTH decrease rapidly after transplantation, reaching 20 percent of pretransplant values within 24 h,[153] normalization of PTH levels may take, in some cases, a longer period of

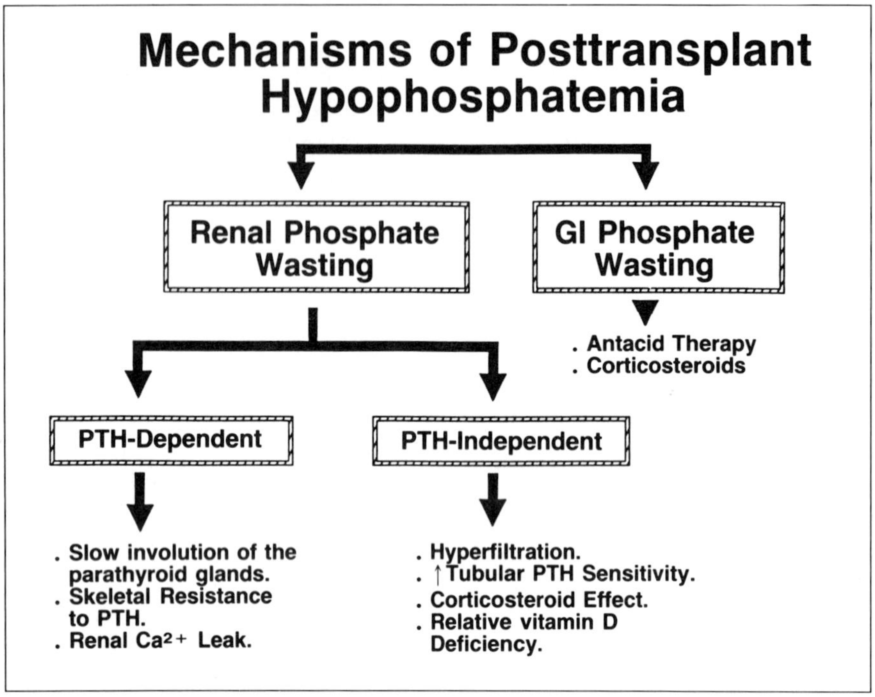

FIGURE 42-8 • Mechanisms of posttransplant hypophosphatemia.

time.[7,198] As discussed below, the persistent posttransplantation elevation of PTH levels may be the result of the slow involution of hyperplastic parathyroid glands, skeletal resistance to the action of PTH,[155] and/or persistence of a negative calcium balance.[234] Studies performed by Pabico and colleagues revealed an incidence of hyperparathyroidism of 58 percent with a mean maximum tubular phosphate reabsorptive rate per unit volume of GFR (TmPi/GFR) (see Chap. 12) of 1.0 mg/dl (normal 2.5 to 4.0).[196] All six subjects responded to an intravenous calcium infusion with reductions in PTH values, decrease in phosphate clearance, and an increase in TmPi/GFR.

The association of mild increases or normal PTH levels, a low tubular reabsorption of phosphorus relative to serum phosphate concentrations, and a decreased TmPi/GFR are suggestive of a *PTH-independent tubular phosphate leak*.[86,87,100,101,200,229,234] The etiology of a putative renal phosphate leak remains incompletely understood. The phosphaturia that develops in these patients takes place in association with a stable GFR. Furthermore, their creatinine clearances are higher (82 ± 8 ml/min) than those measured in normophosphatemic recipients (68 ± 4 ml/min).[229] A low TmPi/GFR in transplant donors with compensatory increases in single-kidney GFR[197] was entertained as a plausible mechanism for the tubular phosphate leak. Measurements of TmPi/GFR in transplant donors revealed a significant difference between the values obtained before (3.1 ± 0.1 mg/dl) and after nephrectomy (2.7 ± 0.1 mg/dl). On the other hand, and with a comparable GFR, the TmPi/GFR was even lower in hypophosphatemic transplant recipients (2.2 ± 0.2 mg/dl).[229] Therefore, the hyperfiltration theory does not explain in its entirety the phosphate tubular leak phenomenon. The possibility of an increased renal tubular sensitivity to PTH was studied by Rosenbaum and colleagues in two groups of patients. Following a calcium infusion, one group (responders) decreased their urinary phosphorus excretion while the other (nonresponders) did not. The nonresponder group was felt to have a state of PTH hyperresponsiveness, since, in the face of similar urinary excretion of cyclic AMP for both groups, they had lower PTH blood levels. However, the similar decreases in cyclic AMP following calcium infusions, in association with different antiphosphaturic responses, is evidence against increased tubular sensitivity to PTH in the nonresponder group.[229]

The suggestion that corticosteroids may contribute to a renal phosphate leak[11,12,224] has not been documented in normal volunteers receiving prednisone therapy (20 mg/day for 2 weeks). No significant differences in serum phosphorus, PTH, and/or TmPi/GFR were found in subjects on or off steroids.[229] It could be argued that the duration of prednisone administration to these normal volunteers was too short and, therefore, by no means resembled the transplant milieu. Furthermore, corticosteroids may indeed have a role in inducing a tubular phosphate leak via their effects on vitamin D metabolism. The spuriously normal levels of vitamin D (in spite of hypophosphatemia) and the improvement of phosphate tubular reabsorption observed with vitamin D therapy suggest a disordered sterol metabolism as the causative agent of this problem.[86,87,100]

Posttransplant gastrointestinal losses of phosphorus are commonly the result of antacid intake.[8,250] In addition, gastrointestinal absorption studies indicate that even though good graft function is established, during the first 2 years after transplantation there is a predominant effect of steroids that causes calcium and phosphorus malabsorption.[261] The effects of corticosteroids on phosphorus absorption may be partly explained by their interference with vitamin D metabolism (see above). However, the malabsorption of phosphorus may persist even though the absorption of calcium returns to normal.[77]

It is important to point out that the abnormalities in phosphorus metabolism described above are those seen with conventional immunosuppressive therapy. At present, the information on the effects of cyclosporine on phosphorus homeostasis is scanty. Theoretically speaking, the reduced creatinine clearance (~50 ml/min) observed in the majority of the cyclosporine-treated cases could result in a persistent hyperparathyroid state and possibly a lower incidence of PTH-independent phosphaturia. Moreover, some of the corticosteroid-related effects (see above) are likely to decrease as a result of the reduced doses being employed in conjunction with cyclosporine therapy.

Even though the clinical manifestations of hypophosphatemia in the transplant recipient are the same as those seen in nontransplant patients,[231] some of them deserve special consideration.

The capacity of the renal allograft to acidify the urine may be seriously compromised as a result of the impairment in ammoniagenesis induced by hypophosphatemia. In addition, hypophosphatemia can have an adverse impact on posttransplant bone healing because it not only increases the urinary excretion of calcium and magnesium but also mobilizes bone carbonates. Even though there is morphologic evidence to indicate that long-term transplant patients (8 years) with persistent hypophosphatemia (< 2.5 mg/dl) have no evidence of osteomalacia by bone biopsy,[78] other authors point to an increased susceptibility to aseptic bone necrosis.[73,202] Whether or not hypophosphatemia enhances the severity of posttransplant diabetes (e.g., insulin resistance), infectious complication, and/or cyclosporine neurotoxicity (e.g., tremors) remains to be determined.

The treatment of posttransplant hypophosphatemia should be based on the underlying pathogenetic mechanism. Gastrointestinal losses can be decreased by reduc-

TABLE 42-4 • Phosphate preparations for parenteral or oral use

Preparations	Pi(mg/ml)	Na^+(meq/ml)	K^+(meq/ml)	Comments
PARENTERAL				
Sodium phosphate (Abbott, Abbott Park, IL)	93	4	—	Comes in 15-ml vial; 10.75 ml deliver 1000 mg Pi with 43 meq Na^+
Potassium phosphate (Abbott)	93	—	4	Comes in 5- and 15-ml vials; 10.75 ml deliver 1000 mg Pi with 43 meq K^+
Hyper-Phos-K (Hoyt, Canton, MA)	67	—	3.3	15 ml deliver 1000 mg Pi and 50 meq K^+
In-Phos (Hoyt)	25	1.6	0.2	40 ml deliver 1000 mg Pi, and 65 meq Na^+, and 8 meq K^+
ORAL				
Fleets Phospho Soda (CB fleet Co., Lynchburg, VA)	149 mg/ml	6 meq/ml	—	6.7 ml deliver 1000 mg Pi and 40 meq K^+
Neutra-Phos (Willen Drug Co., Baltimore, MD)	250 mg/capsule	7 meq/capsule	7 meq/capsule	4 capsules deliver 1000 mg Pi, 28 meq K^+ and 28 meq Na^+
Neutra-Phos-K (Willen Drug Co.)	250 mg/capsule	—	14 meq/capsule	4 capsules deliver 1000 mg Pi and 56 meq K^+
K-Phos (Beach Pharm., Tampa, FL)	114 mg/tablet	—	3.68 meq/tablet	9 tablets provide 1000 mg Pi, 33 meq K^+, and 26 meq H^+
K-Phos-Neutral tablet (Beach)	250 mg/tablet	12 meq/tablet	2 meq/tablet	4 tablets provide 1000 mg Pi, 48 meq Na^+, and 8 meq K^+
Skim milk	1 mg/ml	0.022 meq/ml	0.036 meq/ml	1 liter provides 1000 mg Pi, 22 meq Na^+, and 36 meq K^+

Reproduced with permission of *Seminars in Nephrology* 10:536, 1990.

ing or substituting antacids for agents that protect the GI mucosa (e.g., sulcralfate) or appropriate inhibitors of gastric acid secretion (e.g., histamine H_2 blockers).

Persistent posttransplant hyperparathyroidism (normocalcemic or mildly hypercalcemic) can be managed with oral phosphorus supplementation. The intake of skim milk (1 g of phosphorus per liter) is the easiest and more cost-effective way of replacing phosphorus. Whole milk is best avoided because its large content of fat may not only induce an osmotic diarrhea but also worsen posttransplant hyperlipidemia. Phosphosoda is a hyperosmolar (8240 mosmol) and acidic preparation (pH, 4.8) which may induce not only diarrhea but also an acidosis. Physicians should keep in mind that acidification defects are common in the early period following transplantation and, therefore, they should be extremely cautious with unnecessary acid loads. In addition, it should be stressed that cyclosporine-treated patients retain salt and some of them have an inability to excrete potassium (see above). Therefore, knowledge of the sodium and potassium content of oral phosphate preparations (Table 42-4) is of crucial importance.

Patients with persistent hyperparathyroidism and severe hypercalcemia should undergo a subtotal parathyroidectomy, as this degree of hypercalcemia has adverse effects on allograft function (see below).

Patients with hypophosphatemia secondary to a PTH-independent tubular phosphate leak should receive a trial of $1,25(OH)_2$ vitamin D therapy (particularly those with either low or spuriously normal vitamin D levels).

ABNORMALITIES IN CALCIUM METABOLISM

Hypocalcemia

Hypocalcemia is a much less frequent finding than hypercalcemia in patients with a functioning allograft. (See Chap. 32.) As shown in Fig. 42-9, besides the apparent hypocalcemia due to hypoalbuminemia, a decrease in serum calcium concentration may result from several other pathogenetic mechanisms.

Reductions in serum albumin concentration may be encountered in association with increased losses, impaired synthesis, and/or increased catabolism (e.g., poor nutrition, posttransplant surgical complications, intercurrent infections, malignancy). Urinary losses of albumin are frequently observed in patients with posttransplant nephrotic syndrome (e.g., transplant glomerulopathy secondary to chronic rejection, recurrence of the original glomerular disease). Measurements of ionized serum calcium and/or appropriate correction of the total calcium level for the degree of hypoalbuminemia are measures that will unveil the presence of true hypocalcemia.

Surgical hypoparathyroidism is a frequent cause of posttransplant hypocalcemia. It usually follows the sur-

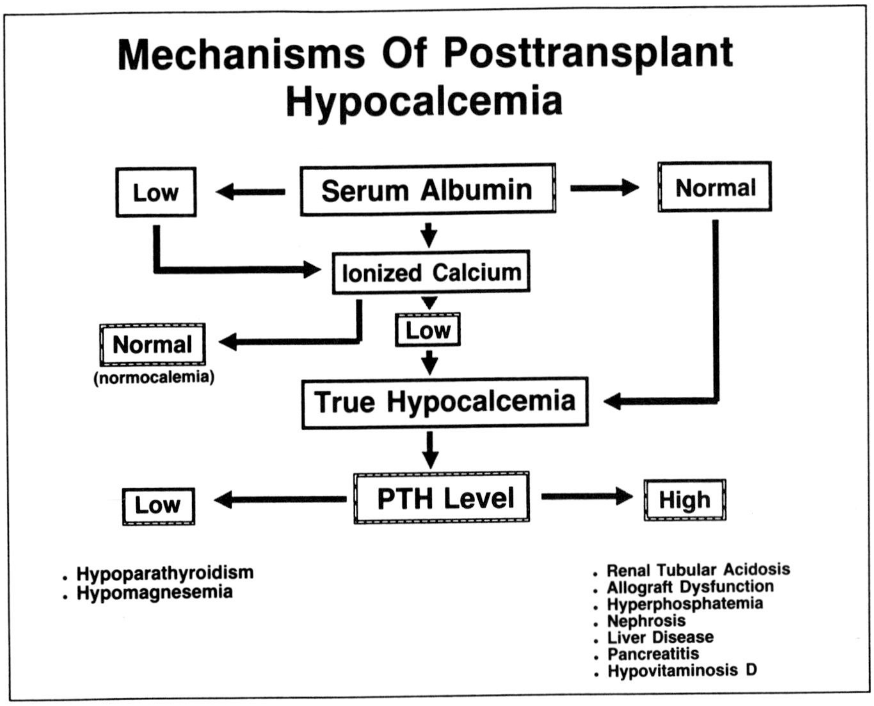

FIGURE 42-9 • Mechanisms of posttransplant hypocalcemia.

gical removal of the parathyroid glands for the treatment of either pretransplantation osteitis fibrosa cystica or posttransplantation hypercalcemia (see below). Moreover, profound hypocalcemia with hypophosphatemia and hypomagnesemia ("hungry bone" syndrome) may complicate the postoperative course of these patients. This syndrome is a medical emergency, and it usually requires aggressive therapy with parenteral calcium and vitamin D preparations.

Posttransplant hyperphosphatemia may cause hypocalcemia via decreased production of calcitrol, inhibition of bone resorption, enhancement of bone formation, and precipitation of calcium phosphate in soft tissues. As previously discussed, it can be the result of allograft dysfunction (acute or chronic), injudicious administration of phosphate, and transcellular shifts. A potentially lethal form of phosphate cellular leak is posttransplant rhabdomyolysis. A nontraumatic variant of this entity may occur as a result of the combined use of cyclosporine with lipid-lowering agents such as HMG-coA reductase inhibitors. Therefore, caution is recommended when the use of these two medications is deemed necessary.

Posttransplant hypomagnesemia (see above) may induce hypocalcemia as a consequence of decreased PTH synthesis and release as well as skeletal resistance to PTH action.[155,156] It is important to recognize this association, as it is refractory to the administration of calcium and/or vitamin D therapy.

Posttransplant RTA may induce hypocalcemia via different pathogenetic mechanisms. Proximal RTA is associated with hypophosphatemia and abnormalities in vitamin D metabolism as a result of acidemia, impaired 1-hydroxylation of 25(OH) vitamin D, or low phosphate levels. The short duration of posttransplant proximal acidification defects (see above) most likely accounts for the low incidence of hypocalcemia in association with a type II RTA. Furthermore, hypercalciuria is a rare phenomenon, perhaps as a result of the distal delivery of large quantities of bicarbonate (a known stimulant of distal calcium reabsorption). On the other hand, a major determinant of hypercalciuria in patients with distal RTA is the degree of acidemia. The buffering of the ongoing acid load by bone carbonates induces the release of calcium into the blood with consequent increases in its filtered load. However, as serum bicarbonate levels increase above 21 meq/liter, urinary calcium excretion returns to normal values. This underscores the need for alkali therapy in this setting.

Posttransplant nephrosis may lead to pseudo-hypocalcemia (see above) and true hypocalcemia via the loss of 25(OH) vitamin D in the urine and, presumably, the vitamin D–binding protein.

Posttransplant liver disease may spawn hypocalcemia as a result of impaired 25-hydroxylation of vitamin D, limitation of bile salt formation with vitamin D malabsorption, and decreased production of vitamin D–binding protein. Viral and/or toxic forms of liver injury are common in transplant recipients and account for significant morbidity and mortality, particularly in long-term survivors.

Posttransplantation pancreatitis (secondary to immunosuppression therapy, viral infections, etc.) may be complicated by hypocalcemia as a result of the precipitation of calcium soaps and decreased PTH levels.

Hypercalcemia

Posttransplantation hypercalcemia[50] is a relatively frequent laboratory finding with an incidence that ranges between 9 and 66 percent.[7,23,41,43,44,57,90,113,122,168,216,218,239] (See Chap. 32.) The main mechanisms (Fig. 42-10) leading to elevations of serum calcium after engraftment are persistent secondary hyperparathyroidism, mobilization of metastatic calcifications, phosphate deficiency, and abnormalities in vitamin D metabolism.[56,61,149-151,223,251]

Secondary hyperparathyroidism is the most common cause of posttransplant hypercalcemia. It correlates with several other variables such as the level of PTH,[43,49,55,130,163,164,260] the duration of dialysis prior to transplantation,[44,49,260,268] and the presence and severity of pretransplant renal osteodystrophy.[49,239] Furthermore, the development of hypercalcemia has been linked to the posttransplant occurrence of other manifestations of secondary hyperparathyroidism, such as hypophosphatemia,[43,44,49,57,90,122,123,168,216] hyperphosphaturia,[7,49,90,113,168,260] posttransplant renal osteodystrophy,[44,57] hypercalciuria,[49,122,260] nephrogenic cyclic adenosine monophosphate generation,[130,163] and alkaline phosphatase levels.[44,48,113] However, it must be emphasized that not all studies have observed these correlations and, as a result, other factors have been postulated or identified (see below). The incidence of posttransplant hyperparathyroidism (as measured by the elevation of PTH levels) ranges from approximately 35[44] to 70 percent[218] and is more frequently (~ 80 percent) found within the first 6 months following transplantation.[218] The presence of a functioning allograft leads to a rapid decrease of PTH levels after transplantation (20 percent of pretransplant values are usually reached within 24 h) and 50 percent of patients have normal PTH levels at the end of 3 years.[153,215] On the other hand, in half of the patients, serum PTH levels may remain elevated indefinitely after successful engraftment. In fact, according to Bigos and collaborators,[26] complete posttransplant involution of the parathyroid glands as defined by a normal Ca^{2+} and PTH axis has been documented in only a very small percentage of cases (6 out of 127 patients).[26,123,124,227,239]

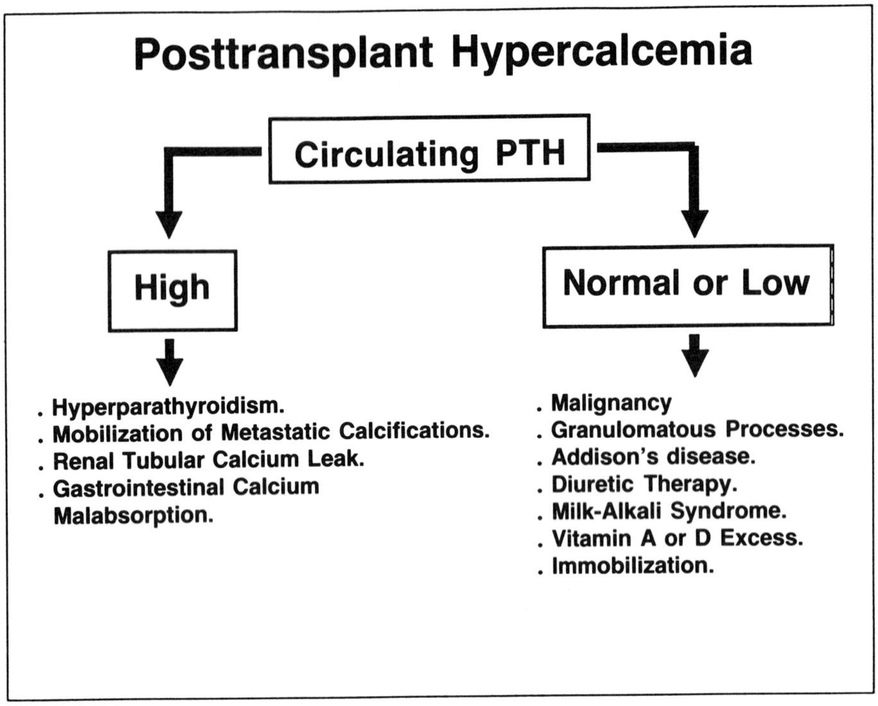

FIGURE 42-10 • Posttransplant hypercalcemia.

The slow involution of the hyperplastic parathyroid glands was initially thought to represent a state of "glandular autonomy" or so-called tertiary hyperparathyroidism.[67] However, this concept appears to be no longer tenable as the sensitivity of the parathyroid glands to either calcium infusion or the induction of hypocalcemia appears to be intact, albeit at a reset set point.[23,43,163,164,183] The slow involution of the parathyroid glands may be simply explained by a persistent increase in the number of otherwise normally responsive chief cells which cannot reduce PTH secretion to zero even in the presence of an elevated serum calcium. This hypothesis is supported by the data from Gittes and Radde, who observed both increased serum PTH and hypercalcemia in rats that were transplanted with normal parathyroid glands.[96] Hyperparathyroidism was not influenced by prior renal failure and persisted in previously uremic animals with a functioning renal allograft. Therefore, the ability of normal parathyroid tissue to produce hypercalcemia may be explained by an obligate minimal secretion of PTH by individual hyperplastic parathyroid cells.[199] In addition to the increase in the number of normally responsive parathyroid cells, the failure of the typical kidney transplant recipient to achieve a positive calcium balance may contribute to the persistent stimulation of PTH synthesis and secretion. A suboptimal gastrointestinal absorption of calcium (in spite of a rise in $1{,}25(OH)_2$ vitamin D levels) and a renal tubular calcium leak have been described in some patients even 24 months after transplantation.[234]

Although the underlying pathogenetic mechanism(s) of such a phenomenon is still unknown, there is some evidence to suggest that steroid therapy may play a contributory role. Corticosteroids induce a dose-related decrement in the serum levels of 25(OH) vitamin D which results in decreased gastrointestinal calcium absorption. Furthermore, low levels of vitamin D contribute to the skeletal resistance to PTH. Therefore, low levels of ionized calcium account for the persistent stimulation of the parathyroid glands.[110,132,155,156]

Mobilization of metastatic calcifications (calcium phosphate deposits in medium-sized arteries and different viscera) is mainly attributed to the posttransplant improvement of uremic secondary hyperparathyroidism.[166,258] The pretransplant mineral deposition correlates with an abnormal calcium-phosphate product, the degree of secondary hyperparathyroidism, the level of blood magnesium, the degree of acidosis, and the presence of local tissue injury.[201] Transplantation candidates with evidence of skin necrosis,[95] heart block,[69] and/or radiologic findings of pulmonary calcification[45] are among those prone to develop this syndrome after engraftment. In addition, the syndrome of calciphylaxis has been reported to develop after transplantation, perhaps as a result of the concomitant steroid therapy.[95,136] The posttransplant finding of skin necrosis and hypercalcemia (particularly in the face of elevated PTH levels) is an indication for parathyroidectomy.

Hypophosphatemia resulting from increased urinary and/or gastrointestinal phosphate losses stimulates the activity of the renal cortical enzyme 1-alpha-hydroxylase. The resulting increased levels of $1,25(OH)_2$ vitamin D lead to increased bone resorption (in conjunction with PTH) and increased gastrointestinal calcium absorption.

In addition, particularly since transplant recipients are immunosuppressed, a diligent search for neoplasia and granulomatous disease (e.g., fungal, viral, and mycobacterial infections) that may induce hypercalcemia must be conducted, particularly when high calcium levels are found in association with normal (or mildly elevated) PTH levels.[1,144,262,272] Less common causes of hypercalcemia such as glucocorticoid deficiency (Addison's disease), diuretic therapy, calcium carbonate administration, and vitamin A or D intoxication should also be considered.

Posttransplant hypercalcemia, as reviewed by Parfitt,[199] can manifest in three distinctive patterns: (1) early posttransplant hypercalcemia; (2) transient posttransplant hypercalcemia; (3) persistent posttransplant hypercalcemia. Although the basis of each entity is the continued secretion of PTH in the face of restored renal function, the specific presentation of these entities brings to light secondary factors that may influence the time course to developing hypercalcemia.

Early posttransplant hypercalcemia usually appears in the initial days or weeks posttransplant and is usually severe (>12.5 mg/dl). It is usually associated with increased morbidity as a result of allograft dysfunction,[57,90,215,254] calciphylaxis with soft tissue metastatic calcifications,[72,93,94,112,166,172,212] gastrointestinal side effects (gastritis, peptic ulcerations, pancreatitis),[83,206,235,236] and it therefore frequently requires parathyroidectomy.[57,165] The severity of the hypercalcemia correlates with its time of onset,[57,168,239] renal allograft function,[57] development of hypophosphatemia,[57,239] and subsequent resolution of metastatic calcifications.[121] Patients with clinical evidence of hyperparathyroid bone disease prior to transplantation are much more likely to develop this marked hypercalcemia once they receive a functioning allograft.[113,239] Over the past several years, the incidence of immediate posttransplant hypercalcemia has declined predominantly as a result of the better understanding and management of secondary hyperparathyroidism (use of calcium-based phosphate binders, vitamin D therapy, and higher dialysate calcium concentrations).

Hypercalcemia of later onset (1.5 to 6 months) has been termed *transient posttransplant hypercalcemia*.[7,41,53,57,66,143,218] The degree of serum calcium elevation is usually mild to moderate (rarely above 12.5 mg/dl), and its association with secondary hyperparathyroidism remains undisputed.[7,113,123,131,255] On the other hand, its temporal relationship to the placement of an allograft suggests that other factors, besides hyperparathyroidism, have a potential causative role. The pathogenetic potential of conditions such as hypophosphatemia and abnormalities of vitamin D metabolism has been the subject of extensive consideration. It is quite likely that the development of this entity is dependent upon the interplay of several factors. The decreased number of cases being reported and the short duration of the hypercalcemic state (weeks to a few months) may be related to the present use of lower steroid dosages and non-phosphate-binding antacids as well as better pretransplant control of hyperparathyroidism.[41,43,199]

Persistent posttransplant hypercalcemia is defined as elevations in serum calcium of greater than 1 year in duration.[41] Measurements of ionized calcium levels suggest that this entity occurs in as many as 66 percent of successful transplant recipients[260] and not in just up to 29 percent of the cases, as previously reported.[7,41,43,57,113,215,216] These data are certainly in agreement with the long-term finding of persistently elevated PTH levels in as many as 50 percent of transplant recipients (see above). Furthermore, a recent study of 41 patients followed for a mean period of 47 months[260] revealed a striking correlation between persistent posttransplant hypercalcemia and several other variables such as increased serum PTH levels, duration of pretransplant dialysis, hypophosphatemia, and hypercalciuria.

It should be stressed that with the exception of severe hypercalcemia (Ca^{2+}> 13 mg/dl), there is no evidence to support an adverse effect of high serum calcium levels on allograft function.[57] Furthermore, documented progression of renal bone disease due to the posttransplant hyperparathyroid environment has been rare.[10] In fact, symptoms of bone pain, lesions of osteitis fibrosa cystica,[7,113,269] and even aluminum-induced osteomalacia[217] have significantly improved within the first year following successful transplantation despite evidence of continued PTH release and progression of bone demineralization.[42,81,99] This phenomenon, that is, the healing of renal osteodystrophy in the face of elevated serum PTH levels, suggests that other unknown factors may play a critical role in the progression of renal bone disease.[199] Consequently, it must be stressed that the management of mild to moderate posttransplant hypercalcemia must be conservative (e.g., phosphate, magnesium, and vitamin D therapy as necessary depending upon the individual case),[102] and parathyroidectomy[6,30,39] should be reserved for those cases of severe hypercalcemia associated with either allograft dysfunction, calciphylaxis, and/or medically refractory gastrointestinal manifestations such as gastrointestinal bleeding, recurrent pancreatitis, and/or peptic ulcer disease.

ABNORMALITIES OF URIC ACID METABOLISM

Asymptomatic hyperuricemia is a well-known complication of azathioprine and cyclosporine therapy. However, gouty arthritis is extremely unusual in azathioprine-treated patients.[147,264] The incidence of hyperuricemia ranges from 13 to 55 percent with azathioprine[98,243] and increases to 51 to 84 percent with cyclosporine therapy.[147,243] Uric acid values greater than 14 mg/dl have been reported only in association with cyclosporine administration. The majority (55 to 80 percent) of hyperuricemic patients have values ranging between 8 and 14 mg/dl.[98] Hyperuricemia commonly develops during the first 3 months after transplantation and, as expected, is much more frequent in patients taking diuretics (Fig. 42-11).[147] Its incidence bears no relationship to kidney function and/or cyclosporine blood levels. On the other hand, it may disappear following withdrawal of cyclosporine therapy.[40] The mechanism of cyclosporine-induced hyperuricemia has been the subject of several studies. Lin and associates measured purine metabolite levels, the activity of enzymes involved in purine metabolism, and the renal clearance of urate in azathioprine ($n = 2$) and cyclosporine ($n = 6$) treated patients and compared them with controls. Even though the number of study patients was small, the results indicate that the predominant mechanism of cyclosporine-induced hyperuricemia is decreased renal excretion of urate.[147] The rates of urate turnover were similar in all three groups, but the urate renal clearance (Fig. 42-12) was much lower in cyclosporine-treated patients (2.7 ± 0.3 ml/min/1.73 m^2) than the one observed in the azathioprine-treated group (5.7 ml/min/1.73 m^2).

As opposed to the general population, the development of gouty arthritis in transplant patients seems to bear little relationship to the degree of hyperuricemia. Eighty-two percent of nontransplant patients develop gout when the uric acid levels surpass 9 mg/dl.[111] As stated above, the conventionally treated transplantation patient with gout is extremely unusual; on the other hand, 7 to 12 percent of patients receiving cyclosporine therapy can be expected to develop gout.[147,264]

There is a correlation between male gender, diuretic intake, and more advanced renal dysfunction among cyclosporine-treated patients who develop gout. The decreased incidence of gout in conventionally immunosuppressed transplant patients may relate to the concomitant use of corticosteroids.[238,241] The management of gout in transplant patients is complicated by the fact that the administration of prostaglandin inhibitors (e.g., indomethacin) may exacerbate the hemodynamically mediated nephrotoxic effects of cyclosporine (see above). In addition, the use of xanthine-oxidase inhibitors (e.g., allopurinol) will interfere with the conversion of azathioprine to 6-thiouric acid and may result in dangerous enhancement of its myelosuppressive effects. Thus, it is recommended that the majority of these cases be managed with appropriate dietary restrictions of purines, discontinuation of diuretic therapy (if the clinical condition allows it), and colchicine. If the administration of allopurinol is deemed necessary, a decrease in the dose of azathioprine (by 25 percent) with further adjustments

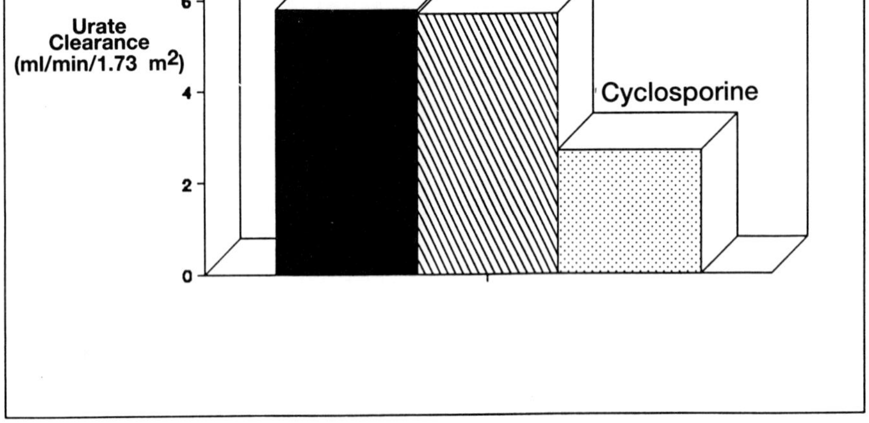

FIGURE 42-11 • Effect of immunosuppressive therapy on the renal clearance of urate. (Adapted from the data by Lin HY et al: *N Engl J Med* 321:287, 1989.)

FIGURE 42-12 • Effect of diuretic therapy on serum urate level. (Adapted from the data by Lin HY et al: *N Engl J Med* 321:287, 1989.)

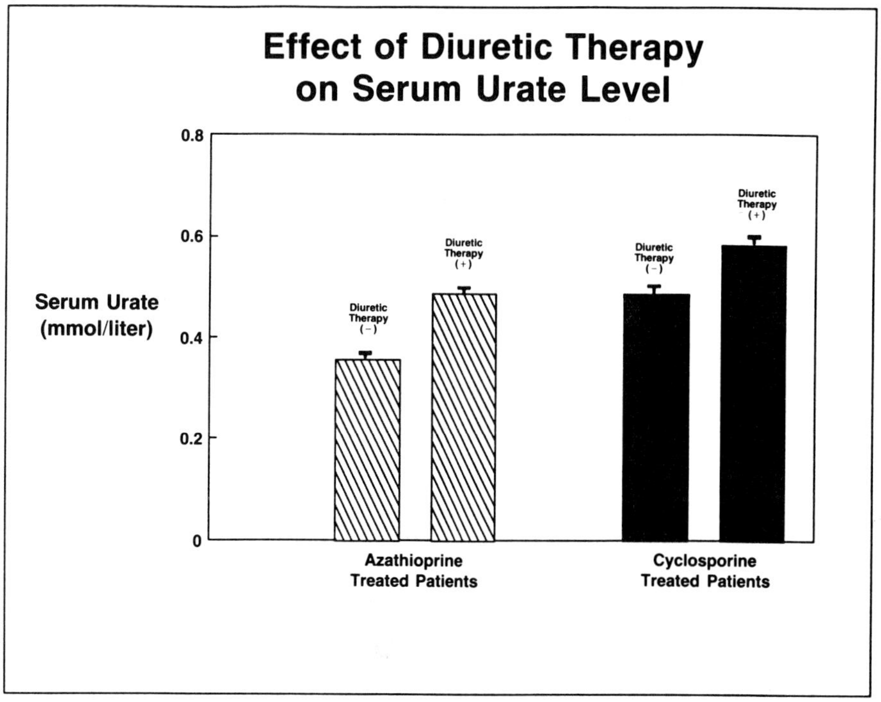

being tailored to the white blood cell count is recommended. As mentioned above, it must be stressed that with the exception of a single case report of acute urate nephropathy,[257] no adverse effects from hyperuricemia have been observed in the kidney allograft.

ABNORMALITIES OF GLUCOSE METABOLISM

Besides those patients with a history of diabetes, up to 20 percent of kidney transplant recipients develop elevated blood glucose levels following transplantation.[32] The abnormalities in glucose homeostasis range from posttransplant glucosuria[115,118] to mild hyperglycemia[5] to severe elevations leading, in some cases, to hyperosmolar nonketotic coma.[2,54,141,270]

The epidemiologic aspects of posttransplant diabetes suggest that this entity occurs more frequently in patients older than 45 years of age,[32,105] among those with a positive family history of diabetes,[105] blacks with a greater frequency of HLA-28,[58] obese individuals,[32,106] recipients of cadaveric allografts, and those hospitalized for infections.[32]

The type of immunosuppression being employed has been linked to the development of hyperglycemia.[37] The diabetogenic effect of steroids is very well established.[31,171,195,232] Posttransplant diabetes usually occurs within the first 3 months after transplantation when the highest dose of steroids is being used and, often, when the dose has been increased for the treatment of a rejection episode.[107] Furthermore, the majority of the cases of hyperosmolar nonketotic coma developing in the posttransplant period most often have occurred following the administration of large doses of steroids for antirejection therapy.[54,270] Even though some authors have found no relationship between the total dose or duration of intravenous methylprednisolone therapy and the development of posttransplant diabetes,[85] centers with a low incidence of the syndrome generally use lower doses of corticosteroids[60,167]. The pathophysiology of the hyperglycemia complicating conventional immunosuppressive therapy appears to represent the same state of insulin resistance as seen in steroid-induced diabetes in nontransplant settings.[35,211] Posttransplant patients with diabetes have normal plasma insulin levels that fail to appropriately increase in response to a glucose load.[118] The incidence of posttransplant diabetes has doubled since the use of cyclosporine has become so widespread.[230] The patients tend to become diabetic within the first 2 months (in the face of much lower steroid doses) and the majority require insulin therapy.[32,230]

Animal studies suggest that cyclosporine is toxic to the beta cells of the pancreas and that this may be a consequence of prostaglandin inhibition.[70,148,179] Furthermore, some centers have found a correlation between hyperglycemia and high cyclosporine blood levels.[32] Finally, it appears that the development of posttransplant diabetes has an adverse effect on allograft[32,230] and patient survival.[32,85]

The diagnosis of posttransplant diabetes is of extreme clinical importance. In addition to being a significant cause of morbidity and mortality, one critical clinical consequence of hyperglycemia is the development of an osmotic diuresis (see above). The depletion of the ECF volume will in turn lead to a decreased GFR and may conceivably be a source of diagnostic error (pseudorejection).[158]

REFERENCES

1. Abbasi AA et al: Hypercalcemia in active pulmonary tuberculosis. *Ann Intern Med* 90:324, 1979.
2. Abouna GM et al: Hyperosmolar nonketotic hyperglycemia and renal allograft function. *Int Urol Nephrol* 12:157, 1980.
3. Adu D et al: Hyperkalaemia in cyclosporin-treated renal allograft recipients. *Lancet* 2:370, 1983.
4. Ahmad T et al: Reversible renal failure due to the use of captopril in a renal allograft recipient treated with cyclosporine. *Nephrol Dial Transplant* 4:311, 1989.
5. Alalvi JA et al: Steroid-induced diabetic ketoacidosis. *Am J Med Sci* 262:15, 1971.
6. Albertucci M et al: Surgical treatment of parathyroid gland in patients with end-stage renal disease. *Surg Gynecol Obstet* 167:49, 1988.
7. Alfrey AC, Jenkins D: Hyperparathyroidism after renal transplantation. *N Engl J Med* 280:507, 1969.
8. Alfrey AC et al: Resolution of hyperparathyroidism, renal osteodystrophy and metastatic calcification after renal homotransplantation. *N Engl J Med* 279:1349, 1968.
9. Alfrey AC et al: Hypermagnesemia after renal homotransplantation. *Ann Intern Med* 73:367, 1970.
10. Alsina J et al: Long-term evolution of renal osteodistrophy after renal transplantation. *Transplant Proc* 21:2151, 1989.
11. Anderson J, Foster JB: Effects of cortisone on urinary phosphate excretion in man. *Clin Sci* 18:437, 1959.
12. Au WYW: Cortisol stimulation of parathyroid hormone secretion by rat parathyroid glands in organ culture. *Science* 193:1015, 1976.
13. Bantle JP et al: Suppression of plasma renin activity by cyclosporine. *Am J Med* 83:59, 1987.
14. Bantle JP et al: Effects of cyclosporine on the renin-angiotensin-aldosterone system and potassium excretion in renal transplant recipients. *Arch Intern Med* 145:505, 1985.
15. Bantle JP et al: Long-term effects of cyclosporine on renal function in organ transplant recipients. *J Lab Clin Med* 115:233, 1990.
16. Barros EJG et al: Glomerular hemodynamics and hormonal participation on cyclosporine nephrotoxicity. *Kidney Int* 32:19, 1987.
17. Barry KG et al: Prevention of surgical oliguria and renal-hemodynamic suppression by substantial hydration. *N Engl J Med* 270:1371, 1964.
18. Barton CH et al: Hypomagnesemia and renal magnesium wasting in renal transplant recipients receiving cyclosporine. *Am J Med* 83:693, 1987.
19. Barton CH et al: Effects of cyclosporine on magnesium metabolism in rats. *J Lab Clin Med* 114:232, 1989.
20. Batlle DC et al: The pathogenesis of hyperchloremic metabolic acidosis associated with kidney transplantation. *Am J Med* 70:786, 1981.
21. Beckerhoff R et al: Plasma renin and aldosterone after renal transplantation. *Kidney Int* 5:39, 1974.
22. Bell NH et al: Primary hyperparathyroidism and salt wasting nephropathy. *J Chronic Dis* 28:601, 1975.
23. Bernheim J et al: Blood parathormone levels and sensitivity of parathyroid glands to hypercalcaemia after successful renal transplantation. *Proc Eur Dial Transplant Assoc* 12:477, 1976.
24. Better OS: Tubular dysfunction following kidney transplantation. *Nephron* 25:209, 1980.
25. Better OS et al: Spontaneous remission of the defect in urinary acidification after cadaver kidney homotransplantation. *Lancet* 1:110, 1970.
26. Bigos ST et al: Hypercalcemia of seven years' duration after kidney transplantation. *Am J Surg* 132:83, 1976.
27. Bittar AE et al: The prevalence of hyperlipidemia in renal transplant recipients. Associations with immunosuppressive and antihypertensive therapy. *Transplantation* 50:987, 1990.
28. Blantz RC et al: Physiologic adaptations of the tubuloglomerular feedback system. *Kidney Int* 38:577, 1990.
29. Blaufox MD et al: Physiologic responses of the transplanted human kidney. *N Engl J Med* 280:62, 1969.
30. Blohme I, Eriksson A: Parathyroidectomy after renal transplantation. *Scand J Urol Nephrol Suppl* 42:134, 1977.
31. Bookman JJ et al: The development of diabetes during treatment with cortisone and corticotropin. *Diabetes* 2:100, 1953.
32. Boudreaux JP et al: The impact of cyclosporine and combination immunosuppression on the incidence of posttransplant diabetes in renal allograft recipients. *Transplantation* 44:376, 1987.
33. Bricker NS et al: Studies on functional capacity of denervated homotransplanted kidney in identical twin with parallel observations in donor. *J Clin Invest* 35:1364, 1956.
34. Bricker NS et al: The functional capacity of the kidney denervated by autotransplantation in the dog. *J Clin Invest* 37:185, 1957.
35. Briggs WA et al: Glucose tolerance, insulin release, and insulin binding to monocytes in kidney transplant recipients. *Am J Kidney Dis* 1:302, 1982.
36. Brown RS: Extrarenal potassium homeostasis. *Kidney Int* 30:116, 1986.
37. Butt KMH et al: Antithymocyte globulin-related diabetes in living related transplantation. *Transplant Proc* 15:1083, 1983.
38. Calne RY et al: Cyclosporin A in patients receiving renal allografts from cadaver donors. Lancet 2:1323, 1978.
39. Cerilli J et al: Subtotal parathyroidectomy for tertiary hyperparathyroidism thirty-two months after renal transplantation. *Am J Surg* 125:636, 1973.
40. Chapman JR et al: Reversibility of cyclosporine nephro-

toxicity after three months' treatment. *Lancet* 1:128, 1985.
41. Chatterjee SN et al: Persistent hypercalcemia after successful renal transplantation. *Nephron* 17:1, 1976.
42. Chesney RW et al: Persistence of diminished bone mineral content following renal transplantation in childhood. *Pediatrics* 73:459, 1984.
43. Christensen MS, Nielsen HE: Parathyroid function after renal transplantation: Interrelationships between renal function, serum calcium and serum parathyroid hormone in normocalcemic long-term survivors. *Clin Nephrol* 8:472, 1977.
44. Conceicao SC et al: Hypercalcemia following renal transplantation: Causes and consequences. *Clin Nephrol* 16:235, 1981.
45. Conger JD et al: Pulmonary calcification in chronic dialysis patients. Clinical and pathologic studies. *Ann Inter Med* 83:330, 1975.
46. Cook ME et al: Hypokalemia secondary to primary hyperaldosteronism in a renal transplant recipient. *Clin Nephrol* 24:261, 1985.
47. Cooke CR et al: Regulation of plasma aldosterone concentration in anephric man and renal transplant recipients. *Kidney Int* 3:160, 1973.
48. Cundy T, Kanis JA: Rapid suppression of plasma alkaline phosphatase activity after renal transplantation in patients with osteodystrophy. *Clin Chim Acta* 164:285, 1987.
49. Cundy T et al: The use of metabolites and analogues of vitamin D in prospective renal transplant recipients. *Clin Nephrol* 15:240, 1981.
50. Cundy T et al: Calcium metabolism and hyperparathyroidism after renal transplantation. *Q J Med* 52:67, 1983.
51. Cunningham J et al: Impaired response of plasma renin activity to tilting after renal transplantation. *Clin Sci* 61:69, 1981.
52. Curtis JJ et al: Cyclosporin in therapeutic doses increases renal allograft vascular resistance. *Lancet* 2:477, 1986.
53. Dalessandro AM et al: Tertiary hyperparathyroidism after renal transplantation: Operative indications. *Surgery* 106:1049, 1989.
54. Daouk AA et al: Hyperosmolar nonketotic coma in a kidney transplant recipient. *J Urol* 108:524, 1972.
55. David DS: Hyperparathyroidism after renal transplantation. *N Engl J Med* 280:507, 1969.
56. David DS et al: Vitamin D intoxication: Relationship to glucocorticoid withdrawal postrenal transplantation. *Ann Surg* 171:455, 1970.
57. David DS et al: Hypercalcemia after renal transplantation. Long-term follow-up data. *N Engl J Med* 289:398, 1973.
58. David DS et al: HLA-A28 and steroid-induced diabetes in renal transplant patients. *JAMA* 243:532, 1980.
59. Davis BB et al: Hypomagnesemia following the diuresis of post-renal obstruction and renal transplant. *Nephron* 14:275, 1975.
60. Davisson NA et al: Comparison of alternate day steroids and daily steroids in renal transplant recipients. *Proc Clin Dial Transplant Forum* 10:150, 1980.
61. DeFrancisco AM et al: Calcium, hyperparathyroidism, and vitamin D metabolism after kidney transplantation. *Transplant Proc* 19:3721, 1987.
62. DeFronzo RA et al: Investigations into the mechanisms of hyperkalemia following renal transplantation. *Kidney Int* 11:357, 1977.
63. DiBona GF: Renal innervation and denervation: Lessons from renal transplantation reconsidered. *Artif Organs* 11:457, 1987.
64. DiBona GF, Rios LL: Renal nerves in compensatory renal response to contralateral renal denervation. *Am J Physiol* 238:F26, 1980.
65. DiBona GF, Sawin LL: Role of the renal nerves in renal adaptation to dietary sodium restriction. *Am J Physiol* 245:F322, 1983.
66. Diethelm AG et al: The natural history and surgical treatment of hypercalcemia before and after renal transplantation. *Surg Gynecol Obstet* 154:481, 1982.
67. Dominguez JM et al: Tertiary hyperparathyroidism diagnosed after renal homotransplantation. *Am J Med* 49:423, 1970.
68. Dougherty JC et al: Intrarenal distribution of blood flow in dog renal allografts. *Ann Surg* 169:560, 1969.
69. Dreher W, Shelp W: Atrioventricular block in a long term dialysis patient. Reversal after parathyroidectomy. *JAMA* 234:954, 1975.
70. Dresner LS et al: Effects of cyclosporine on glucose metabolism. *Surgery* 106:163, 1989.
71. Duggin GG et al: Influence of cyclosporin A (CSA) on intrarenal control of GFR. *Clin Nephrol* 25:S43, 1986.
72. Ejerblad S et al: Arterial disease with ischemic ulcerations in renal transplanted recipients. *Scand J Urol Nephrol Suppl* 42:186, 1977.
73. Elmstedt E: Avascular bone necrosis in the renal transplant patient: A discriminant analysis of 144 cases. *Clin Orthop* 158:149, 1981.
74. English J et al: Cyclosporine-induced acute renal dysfunction in the rat. *Transplantation* 44:135, 1987.
75. Epstein M, Hollenberg NK: Renal "salt wasting" despite apparently normal renal, adrenal and central nervous system function. *Nephron* 24:121, 1979.
76. Erman A et al: The role of eicosanoids in cyclosporine nephrotoxicity in the rat. *Biochem Pharmacol* 38:2153, 1989.
77. Farrington K et al: Dissociation of absorptions of calcium and phosphate after successful cadaveric renal transplantation. *Br Med J* 1:712, 1979.
78. Felsenfeld AJ et al: Hypophosphatemia in long-term renal transplant recipients: Effects on bone histology and 1,25-dihydroxycholecalciferol. *Miner Electrolyte Metab* 12:333, 1986.
79. Ferguson RK et al: Sodium-losing nephropathy and nephrocalcinosis after transplantation. *Am J Kidney Dis* 5:206, 1985.
80. Field MJ, Giebisch G: Hormonal control of renal potassium excretion. *Kidney Int* 27:379, 1985.
81. Fine RN et al: Renal osteodystrophy in children: The effect of hemodialysis and renal homotransplantation. *J Pediatr* 80:243, 1972.
82. Flanigan WJ et al: Serial studies of glomerular filtration rate and renal plasma flow in kidney transplant donors, identical twins, and allograft recipients. *Am J Surg* 116:788, 1968.
83. Frick TW et al: Hypercalcemia associated with pancreatitis and hyperamylasemia in renal transplant recip-

ients. Data from the Minnesota randomized trial of cyclosporine versus antilymphoblast azathioprine. *Am J Surg* 154:487, 1987.

84. Friedman A, Chesney R: Fanconi's syndrome in renal transplantation. *Am J Nephrol* 1:45, 1981.
85. Friedman EA et al: Posttransplant diabetes in kidney transplant recipients. *Am J Nephrol* 5:196, 1985.
86. Garabedian M et al: Changes in plasma 1,25 and 24,25-dihydroxyvitamin D after renal transplantation in children. *Kidney Int* 20:403, 1981.
87. Garabedian M et al: Chronic hypophosphatemia in kidney transplanted children and young adults. *Adv Exp Med Biol* 128:249, 1980.
88. Gazdar AF, Dammin GJ: Neural degeneration and regeneration in human renal transplants. *N Engl J Med* 283:222, 1970.
89. Gehr TW et al: Furosemide pharmacokinetics and pharmacodynamics in renal transplantation. *Clin Pharmacol Ther* 43:547, 1988.
90. Geis WP et al: The diagnosis and treatment of hyperparathyroidism after renal homotransplantation. *Surg Gynecol Obstet* 137:997, 1973.
91. Gill JR, Bartter FC: Adrenergic nervous system in sodium metabolism. II. Effects of guanethidine on the renal response to sodium deprivation in normal man. *N Engl J Med* 275:1466, 1966.
92. Gillum DM, Truong L: Effects of chronic volume expansion and enalapril on chronic cyclosporine nephropathy. *Am J Physiol* 258:F934, 1990.
93. Gilman M et al: Metastatic pulmonary calcification in the renal transplant recipient. *Am Rev Respir Dis* 121:415, 1980.
94. Ginn EH et al: Human renal transplantation: An investigation of the functional status of the denervated kidney after successful homotransplantation in identical twins. *J Lab Clin Med* 56:1, 1960.
95. Gipstein RH et al: Calciphylaxis in man: A syndrome of tissue necrosis and vascular calcification in 11 patients with chronic renal disease. *Arch Intern Med* 136:1273, 1976.
96. Gittes RF, Radde IC: Experimental hyperparathyroidism from multiple isologous parathyroid transplants: Homeostatic effects of simultaneous thyroid transplants. *J Clin Endocrinol* 98:1015, 1966.
97. Goldberg HK et al: Dissociation between the immunosuppressive activity of cyclosporine derivatives and their effects on intracellular calcium signaling in mesangial cells. *Transplantation* 47:731, 1989.
99. Gores PF et al: Hyperuricemia after renal transplantation. *Am J Surg* 156:397, 1988.
99. Gottlieb MN et al: A longitudinal study of bone disease after successful renal transplantation. *Nephron* 22:239, 1978.
100. Graf H et al: Renal phosphate wasting after successful kidney transplantation: 1-alpha vitamin D therapy in patients with normal parathyroid gland activity. *Nephron* 28:285, 1981.
101. Graf H et al: Handling of phosphate by the transplanted kidney. *Proc Eur Dial Transplant Assoc* 16:624, 1979.
102. Graf H et al: Effect of 1-alpha hydroxylated vitamin D on steroid induced calcium malabsorption. *Proc Eur Dial Transplant Assoc* 17:736, 1980.
103. Greene JA et al: Plasma renin activity and aldosterone excretion after renal homotransplantation. *J Lab Clin Med* 71:586, 1968.
104. Grieve EM et al: Effect of thromboxane synthetase inhibition and angiotensin converting enzyme inhibition on acute cyclosporine A nephrotoxicity. *Biochem Pharmacol* 40:2323, 1990.
105. Gunnarsson R et al: Diabetes mellitus—a more common than believed complication of renal transplantation. *Transplant Proc* 11:1280, 1979.
106. Gunnarsson R et al: Steroid diabetes after transplantation. A preliminary report. *Scand J Urol Nephrol* 42:191, 1977.
107. Gunnarsson R et al: Steroid diabetes—a sign of overtreatment with steroids in the renal graft recipient? *Scand J Urol Nephrol* 54:135, 1980.
108. Győry AZ et al: Renal tubular acidosis, acidosis due to hyperkalemia, hypercalcemia, disordered citrate metabolism, and other tubular dysfunctions following human renal transplantation. *Q J Med* 38:231, 1969.
109. Haag JD et al: Failure to detect remarkable hypomagnesemia in renal transplant recipients receiving cyclosporin. *Miner Electrolyte Metab* 16:66, 1990.
110. Hahn TJ et al: Altered mineral metabolism in glucocorticoid-induced osteopenia. *J Clin Invest* 64:655, 1979.
111. Hall AP et al: Epidemiology of gout and hyperuricemia: A long-term population study. *Am J Med* 42:27, 1967.
112. Hallgren R et al: Arterial calcification and progressive peripheral gangrene after renal transplantation. Report of two cases treated with parathyroidectomy. *Acta Med Scand* 198:331, 1975.
113. Hampers CL et al: Calcium metabolism and osteodystrophy after renal transplantation. *Arch Intern Med* 124:282, 1969.
114. Hatch DA et al: A randomized study of intravenous fluid replacement following living-donor renal transplantation. *Transplantation* 40:648, 1985.
115. Henderson LW et al: Proximal tubular malfunction as a mechanism for diuresis after renal homotransplantation. *N Engl J Med* 278:467, 1968.
116. Herdman R et al: Renal function and phosphorus excretion after human renal transplantation. *Lancet* 1:121, 1966.
117. Herdman RC et al: Changes in phosphorus excretion and renal function after human renal homotransplantation. *Nephron* 5:170, 1968.
118. Hill CM et al: Glycosuria and hyperglycaemia after kidney transplantation. *Lancet* 2:490, 1974.
119. Hirshman CA, Edelstein G: Intraoperative hyperkalemia and cardiac arrests during renal transplantation in an insulin-dependent diabetic patient. *Anesthesiology* 51:161, 1979.
120. Hirshman CA et al: Risk of hyperkalemia in recipients of kidneys preserved with an intracellular electrolyte solution. *Anesth Analg* 59:283, 1980.
121. Hornum I: Post- transplant hypercalcemia due to mobilization of metastatic calcifications. An alternative to tertiary hyperparathyroidism. *Acta Med Scand* 189:199, 1971.
122. Ibels LS et al: Aseptic necrosis of bone following renal transplantation: Experience in 194 transplant recipients and review of the literature. *Medicine* 57:25, 1978.
123. Johnson JW et al: Secondary hyperparathyroidism in

chronic renal failure. Effects of renal homotransplantation. *JAMA* 215:478, 1971.
124. Johnson WJ et al: Prevention and treatment of progressive secondary hyperparathyroidism in advanced renal failure. *Med Clin North Am* 56:961, 1972.
125. June CH et al: Correlation of hypomagnesemia with the onset of cyclosporine-associated hypertension in marrow transplant patients. *Transplantation* 41:47, 1986.
126. June CH et al: Profound hypomagesemia and renal magnesium wasting associated with the use of cyclosporine for marrow transplantation. *Transplantation* 39:620, 1985.
127. Kaiser W et al: Magnesium after renal transplantation—comparison between cyclosporine A and conventional immunosuppression. *Adv Exp Med Biol* 252:297, 1989.
128. Kapsner P et al: Milk-alkali syndrome in patients treated with calcium carbonate after cardiac transplantation. *Arch Intern Med* 146:1965, 1986.
129. Kaskel FJ et al: Cyclosporine nephrotoxicity: Sodium excretion, autoregulation, and angiotensin II. *Am J Physiol* 252:F733, 1987.
130. Kleerekoper M et al: Parathyroid hormone resistance in renal allograft recipients. *Adv Exp Med Biol* 151:185, 1982.
131. Kleerekoper M et al: Hyperparathyroidism after renal transplantation. *Br Med J* 3:680, 1975.
132. Klein RGS et al: Intestinal calcium absorption in exogenous hypercortisolism. Role of 25-hydroxyvitamin D and corticoid dose. *J Clin Invest* 60:253, 1977.
133. Kline RM, Mercer PF: Functional reinnervation and development of supersensitivity to NE after renal denervation. *Am J Physiol* 238:R353, 1980.
134. Kon V et al: Role of endothelin in cyclosporine-induced glomerular dysfunction. *Kidney Int* 37:1487, 1990.
135. Kopp JB, Klotman PE: Cellular and molecular mechanisms of cyclosporin nephrotoxicity. *JASN* 1:162, 1990.
136. Koranda FC et al: Cutaneous complications of immunosuppressed renal homograft recipient. *JAMA* 229:419, 1974.
137. Kountz SL et al: Serial hemodynamics after renal allotransplantation in man. *Circulation* 41:217, 1970.
138. Kramer HJ et al: Salt-losing syndromes following renal transplantation. *Am J Med* 53:368, 1972.
139. Krull F et al: Renal handling of magnesium in transplanted children under cyclosporine A treatment. *Eur J Pediatr* 148:148, 1988.
140. Lackner HL, McKay M: Renal blood flow changes post-transplantation: Renal denervation versus renal ischemia. *Invest Urol* 9:39, 1971.
141. Lampe EW 2d et al: Hyperglycemic nonketotic coma after renal transplantation. *Am J Surg* 127:342, 1974.
142. Laskow DA et al: Cyclosporine-induced changes in glomerular filtration rate and urea excretion. *Am J Med* 88:497, 1990.
143. Latimer RG et al: Tertiary hyperparathyroidism following successful renal allografting. *Ann Surg* 172:137, 1970.
144. Lee JC et al: Hypercalcemia in disseminated coccidioidomycosis. *N Engl J Med* 297:431, 1977.
145. Legrain M, Demol H: So-called proximal urine and the initial diuresis of the transplant. *Acta Clin Belg* 25:1, 1970.
146. Lennard TW et al: Primary nonfunction after renal transplantation: A prospective multifactorial analysis of possible causes in 106 consecutive transplants. *Transplant Proc* 20:439, 1988.
147. Lin HY et al: Cyclosporine-induced hyperuricemia and gout. *N Engl J Med* 321:287, 1989.
148. Lohr M et al: Prostaglandin analogue protects pancreatic B-cells against cyclosporin A toxicity. *Experientia* 45:352, 1989.
149. Lucas PA et al: Vitamin D3 metabolites in hypercalcaemic adults after kidney transplantation. *Proc Eur Dial Transplant Assoc* 20:213, 1983.
150. Lucas PA et al: Vitamin D3 metabolites in chronic renal failure and after renal transplantation. *Nephrol Dial Transplant* 3:70, 1988.
151. Lund B et al: Serum 1,25-dihydroxycholecalciferol in anephric, haemodialyzed and kidney-transplanted patients. Effect of vitamin D3 supplement. *Nephron* 25:30, 1980.
152. Markell MS, Friedman EA: Hyperlipidemia after organ transplantation. *Am J Med* 87:61N, 1989.
153. Martin KJ et al: The peripheral metabolism of parathyroid hormone. *N Engl J Med* 301:1092, 1979.
154. Mason J et al: Disparity between surface and deep nephron function early after renal ischemia. *Kidney Int* 24:27, 1983.
155. Massry SG et al: Skeletal resistance to parathyroid hormone in renal failure. Studies in 105 human subjects. *Ann Intern Med* 78:357, 1973.
156. Massry SG, Coburn JW: The hormonal and non-hormonal control of renal excretion of calcium and magnesium. *Nephron* 10:66, 1973.
157. Massry SG et al: Renal tubular acidosis after cadaver kidney homotransplantation. Studies on mechanism. *Am J Med* 42:284, 1967.
158. Matas AJ et al: Pseudorejection: Factors mimicking rejection in renal allograft recipients. *Ann Surg* 186:51, 1977.
159. Maxwell MH et al: Cooperative study of renovascular hypertension: Demographic analysis of the study. *JAMA* 220:1195, 1972.
160. McAuley FT et al: The influence of enalapril or spironolactone on experimental cyclosporin nephrotoxicity. *Biochem Pharmacol* 36:699, 1987.
161. McCaa RE et al: Influence of acute stimuli on plasma aldosterone concentration in anephric man and kidney allograft recipients. *Circ Res* 33:313, 1973.
162. McCabe R et al: Reduction of acute tubular necrosis (ATN) by furosemide and steroids in cadaveric kidney recovery. *Am J Surg* 73:368, 1973.
163. McCarron DA et al: Posttransplantation hyperparathyroidism: Demonstration of retained control of parathyroid function by plasma ionized calcium. *Am J Clin Nutr* 33:1536, 1980.
164. McCarron DA et al: Post-transplant hyperparathyroidism: Retained control by serum Ca^{++}. *Proc Eur Dial Transplant Assoc* 16:677, 1979.
165. McCarron DA et al: Total parathyroidectomy for post-transplantation hyperparathyroidism. *Transplantation* 40:266, 1985.
166. McDougal BA, Luckert BP: Resolution of breast pain and calcification with renal transplantation. *Arch Intern Med* 137:375, 1977.
167. McGeown MG et al: Advantages of low dose steroid from

the day after renal transplantation. *Transplantation* 29:287, 1980.

168. McIntosh DA et al: Autonomy of parathyroid function after renal homotransplantation. *Ann Intern Med* 65:900, 1966.
169. Meyer-Lehnert H, Schrier RW: Cyclosporine A enhances vasopressin-induced Ca^{2+} mobilization and contraction in mesangial cells. *Kidney Int* 34:89, 1988.
170. Mihatsch MJ et al: Morphological findings in kidney transplants after treatment with cyclosporine. *Transplant Proc* 14:2821, 1983.
171. Miller SE, Neilson JM: Clinical features of the diabetic syndrome appearing after steroid therapy. *Postgrad Med J* 40:660, 1964.
172. Milliner DS et al: Pulmonary calcinosis after renal transplantation in pediatric patients. *Am J Kidney Dis* 7:495, 1986.
173. Mimran A et al: The renin-angiotensin system and renal function in kidney transplantation. *Kidney Int* 30:S114, 1990.
174. Mookerjee B et al: Hyperchloremic acidosis in early diagnosis of renal allograft rejection. *Ann Intern Med* 71:47, 1969.
175. Moorehead JF et al: Hypophosphataemic osteomalacia after cadaveric renal transplantation. *Lancet* 1:694, 1974.
176. Moran M et al: Prevention of acute graft rejection by the prostaglandin E1 analogue misoprostol in renal-transplant recipients treated with cyclosporine and prednisone. *N Engl J Med* 322:1183, 1990.
177. Morgan JM et al: Renal transplantation in hypophosphatemia with vitamin D resistant rickets. *Arch Intern Med* 134:549, 1974.
178. Moss NG et al: Intravenous cyclosporine activates afferent and efferent renal nerves and causes sodium retention in innervated kidneys in rats. *Proc Natl Acad Sci USA* 82:8222, 1985.
179. Muller MK et al: Prevention of toxic effects of cyclosporin on pancreatic B-cells of rats by Riprostil, a new prostaglandin anaglogue. *Gut* 29:1524, 1988.
180. Muller-Suur R et al: Resetting of tubuloglomerular feedback in rat kidneys after unilateral nephrectomy. *Kidney Int* 18:48, 1980.
181. Murray BM et al: Effect of cyclosporine administration on renal hemodynamics in conscious rats. *Kidney Int* 28:767, 1985.
182. Murray BM et al: Enalapril-associated acute renal failure in renal transplants: Possible role of cyclosporine. *Am J Kidney Dis* 16:66, 1990.
183. Muther RS et al: Change in serum bicarbonate during acute EDTA infusions in post-transplant hyperparathyroidism. *Nephron* 30:36, 1982.
184. Myers BD: Cyclosporine nephrotoxicity. *Kidney Int* 30:964, 1986.
185. Myers BD: What is cyclosporine nephrotoxicity? *Transplant Proc* 21:1430, 1989.
186. Myers BD et al: Cyclosporine-associated chronic nephropathy. *N Engl J Med* 311:699, 1984.
187. Myers BD et al: The long-term course of cyclosporine-associated chronic nephropathy. *Kidney Int* 33:590, 1988.
188. Najarian JS et al: Protection of the donor kidney during homotransplantation. *Ann Surg* 164:398, 1966.
189. Norlen BJ et al: Nephron function of the transplanted rat kidney. *Kidney Int* 14:10, 1978.
190. Norvell JE, Banes RT: Histofluorescence and fluorometric analysis of adrenergic reinnervation in the dog kidney following autotransplantation. *Transplantation* 27:69, 1979.
191. Norvell JE et al: Degeneration and regeneration of adrenergic nerves in the autotransplanted kidney. *Transplantation* 7:218, 1969.
192. Novick AC et al: Detrimental effect of cyclosporine on initial function of cadaver renal allografts following extended preservation. *Transplantation* 42:154, 1986.
193. Ogden DA: Donor and recipient function 2 to 4 years after renal homotransplantation. A paired study of 28 cases. *Ann Intern Med* 67:998, 1967.
194. Ogden DA et al: Function of renal homograft in man immediately after transplantation. *Am J Med* 38:873, 1965.
195. Olefsky JM, Kimmerling G: Effects of glucocorticoids on carbohydrate metabolism. *Am J Med Sci* 271:202, 1976.
196. Pabico RC, McKenna BA: Metabolic problems in renal transplant patients. Persistent hyperparathyroidism and hypophosphatemia: Effects of intravenous calcium infusion. *Transplant Proc* 20:438, 1988.
197. Pabico RC et al: Renal function before and after unilateral nephrectomy in renal donors. *Kidney Int* 8:166, 1975.
198. Pabico RC et al: Persistent hyperparathyroidism in renal transplant patients. *Proc Clin Dial Transplant Forum* 8:68, 1978.
199. Parfitt AM: Hypercalcemia hyperparathyroidism following renal transplantation: Differential diagnosis, management, and implications for cell population control in the parathyroid gland. *Miner Electrolyte Metab* 8:92, 1982.
200. Parfitt AM et al: Reduced phosphate reabsorption unrelated to parathyroid hormone after renal transplantation: Implications for the pathogenesis of hyperparathyroidism in chronic renal failure. *Miner Electrolyte Metab* 12:356, 1986.
201. Parfitt AM et al: Osteopenia and fractures occurring during maintenance hemodialysis: A "new" form of renal osteodistrophy. *Clin Orthop* 87:287, 1972.
202. Parfrey PS et al: The decreased incidence of aseptic necrosis in renal transplant recipients—a case control study. *Transplantation* 41:182, 1986.
203. Pedersen EB et al: Relationship between urinary prostaglandin E2 and F2 alpha excretion and plasma arginine vasopressin during renal concentrating and diluting tests in renal transplant recipients. *Eur J Clin Invest* 17:429, 1987.
204. Pedersen EB et al: Post-renal-transplant hypertension. Urine volume, free water clearance and plasma concentrations of arginine vasopressin, angiotension II and aldosterone before and after oral water loading in hypertensive and normotensive renal transplant recipients. *Scand J Clin Lab Invest* 46:451, 1986.
205. Pedersen EB et al: Relationship between urinary concentrating ability, arginine vasopressin in plasma and blood pressure after renal transplantation. *Scand J Clin Lab Invest* 45:321, 1985.
206. Penn I et al: Acute pancreatitis and hyperamylasemia in renal homograft recipients. *Arch Surg* 105:167, 1972.

207. Perez GO, Oster JR: Hyporeninemic hypoaldosteronism after renal transplantation. *South Med J* 70:363, 1977.
208. Perico N et al: Acute cyclosporine A nephrotoxicity in rats: Which role for renin-angiotensin system and glomerular prostaglandins? *Clin Nephrol* 25:S83, 1986.
209. Perico N et al: Functional significance of exaggerated renal thromboxane A2 synthesis induced by cyclosporin A. *Am J Physiol* 20:F581, 1986.
210. Perico N et al: Effect of short-term cyclosporine administration in rats on renin-angiotensin and thromboxane A2: Possible relevance to the reduction in glomerular filtration rate. *J Pharmacol Exp Ther* 239:229, 1986.
211. Perley M, Kipnis DM: Effect of glucocorticoids on plasma insulin. *N Engl J Med* 274:1237, 1966.
212. Perloff JL et al: Lethal posttransplantation calcinosis. *Transplantation* 27:21, 1979.
213. Petersen KC et al: Hyperkalaemia after cyclosporine therapy (letter). *Lancet* 1:1470, 1984.
214. Petric R et al: Effect of cyclosporine on urinary prostanoid excretion, renal blood flow, and glomerulotubular function. *Transplantation* 45:883, 1988.
215. Pieper R et al: Secondary hyperparathyroidism and its sequelae in renal transplant recipients. Long term findings in a series of conservatively managed patients. *Scand J Urol Nephrol Suppl* 42:144, 1977.
216. Pierides AM et al: Effect of 1-alpha-hydroxycholecalciferol, 1,25-dihydorxycholecalciferol, 3 deoxy-1-alpha-hydroxycholecalciferol, 24R, 25-dihydroxycholecalciferol and successful renal transplantation on calcium absorption in haemodialysis patients. *Nephron* 20:203, 1978.
217. Piraino B et al: Resolution of hypercalcemia and aluminum bone disease after renal transplantation. *Am J Med* 85:728, 1988.
218. Pletka PG et al: Secondary hyperparathyroidism in human kidney transplant recipients. *Nephron* 17:371, 1976.
219. Popovtzer MM et al: Hypernatremia. Complication of renal homotransplantation. *Arch Intern Med* 127:1129, 1971.
220. Quinby WC: The function of the kidney when deprived of its nerves. *J Exp Med* 23:535, 1961.
221. Rabb HA et al: Severe hyponatremia associated with combined pancreatic and renal transplantation. *Transplantation* 48:157, 1989.
222. Revusova V et al: Magnesium deficit after renal transplantation with secondary posttransplantation hypocalcemia and hypophosphatemia. *Urol Int* 30:313, 1975.
223. Riancho JA et al: Serum levels of 1,25-dihydroxyvitamin D after renal transplantation. *Miner Electrolyte Metab* 14:332, 1988.
224. Roberts KE, Pitts RF: The effect of cortisone and desoxycortisone on the renal tubular reabsorption of phosphate and excretion of titrable acid and potassium in dogs. *Endocrinology* 52:324, 1953.
225. Roguska J et al: Serum renin activity in human renal homotransplantation. *Nephron* 8:289, 1971.
226. Roll D et al: Transient hypoaldosteronism after renal allotransplantation. *Isr J Med Sci* 15:29, 1979.
227. Roof BS et al: Natural course of secondary hyperparathyroidism after successful renal transplantation. *Proc Clin Dial Transplant Forum* 1:11, 1971.
228. Rosen SM et al: Intrarenal distribution of blood flow in transplanted dog kidney: Effect of denervation and rejection. *J Clin Invest* 46:1239, 1967.
229. Rosenbaum RW et al: Decreased phosphate reabsorption after renal transplantation: Evidence for a mechanism independent of calcium and parathyroid hormone. *Kidney Int* 19:568, 1981.
230. Roth D et al: Posttransplant hyperglycemia. Increased incidence in cyclosporine-treated renal allograft recipients. *Transplantation* 47:278, 1989.
231. Rubin MF, Narins RG: Hypophosphatemia: Pathophysiological and practical aspects of its therapy. *Semin Nephrol* 10:536, 1990.
232. Ruiz JO et al: Steroid diabetes in renal transplant recipients: Pathogenetic factors and prognosis. *Surgery* 73:759, 1973.
233. Sabbatini M et al: Acute effects of cyclosporine on glomerular dynamics—micropuncture study in the rat. *Transplant Proc* 20:544, 1988.
234. Sakhaee K et al: Disturbances in mineral metabolism after successful renal transplantation. *Miner Electrolyte Metab* 11:167, 1985.
235. Sarosdy MF et al: Upper gastrointestinal bleeding following renal transplantation. *Urology* 26:347, 1985.
236. Saylor RP et al: Hypercalcemia-induced upper gastrointestinal bleeding after renal transplantation. *Urology* 24:337, 1984.
237. Schang T et al: Detrimental effects of fluid and electrolyte loss from duodenum in bladder-drained pancreas transplants. *Transplant Proc* 23:1617, 1991.
238. Schmidt P et al: Letter: Hypouricemia after renal transplantation. *N Engl J Med* 289:1373, 1973.
239. Schwartz GH et al: Hypercalcemia after renal transplantation. *Am J Med* 49:42, 1970.
240. Souilillou JP et al: Acute hyperkalemia risks in recipients of kidney graft cooled with Collins' solution. *Nephron* 19:301, 1977.
241. Sprague RG et al: Observations on the physiologic effects of cortisone and ACTH in man. *Arch Intern Med* 85:199, 1950.
242. Stahl RA et al: Hyperchloremic metabolic acidosis with high serum potassium in renal transplant recipients: A cyclosporine A associated side effect. *Clin Nephrol* 25:245, 1986.
243. Sutherland DER et al: Results of the Minnesota randomized prospective trial of cyclosporine versus azathiopine-antilymphocyte globulin for immunosuppression in renal allograft recipients. *Am J Kidney Dis* 5:318, 1985.
244. Swenson RS et al: Posttransplant natriuresis. *Clin Res* 15:115, 1967.
245. Tannen RL: Diuretic-Induced hypokalemia. *Kidney Int* 28:988, 1985.
246. Thompson CB et al: Association between cyclosporine neurotoxicity and hypomagnesemia. *Lancet* 2:1116, 1984.
247. Tjia JF et al: Calcium channel antagonists and cyclosporine metabolism: In vitro studies with human liver microsomes. *Br J Clin Pharmacol* 28:362, 1989.
248. Tortorice KL et al: The effects of calcium channel blockers on cyclosporine and its metabolites in renal transplant recipients. *Ther Drug Monit* 12:321, 1990.
249. Truniger BP et al: Intrarenal distribution of blood flow

in the rejecting homotransplanted kidney. *Sur Forum* 16:254, 1965.

250. Tyden G et al: Hypophosphatemia and reversible neurological dysfunction in a patient subjected to combined renal and pancreatic transplantation. *Nephrol Dial Transplant* 3:823, 1988.
251. Ulmann A et al: Plasma 1,25$(OH)_2$D3 and iPTH in transplanted adults with persisting hypophosphataemia. *Proc Eur Dial Transplant Assoc* 17:467, 1980.
252. Uribarri J et al: Pseudohypoaldosteronism following kidney transplantation. *Nephron* 31:368, 1982.
253. Van Der Heide JJH et al: The effects of dietary supplementation with fish oil on renal function in cyclosporine-treated renal transplant recipients. *Transplantation* 49:523, 1990.
254. Varghese Z et al: Parathyroid hormone as a causative factor of primary non-function in renal transplants. *Br Med J (Clin Res)* 296:393, 1988.
255. Varghese Z et al: Resolution of secondary hyperparathyroidism after cadaveric renal allograft. *Proc Eur Dial Transplant Assoc* 11:261, 1975.
256. Vathsala A et al: Lipid abnormalities in cyclosporine-prednisone-treated renal transplant recipients. *Transplantation* 48:37, 1989.
257. Venkataseshan VS et al: Acute hyperuricemic nephropathy and renal failure after transplantation. *Nephron* 56:317, 1990.
258. Verberckmoes R et al: Disappearance of vascular calcifications during treatment of renal osteodistrophy. *Ann Intern Med* 82:329, 1975.
259. Versluis DJ et al: Histological lesions associated with cyclosporine: Incidence and reversibility in 1-year-old kidney transplants. *J Clin Pathol* 41:498, 1988.
260. Vezzoli G et al: High plasma ionized calcium with normal PTH and total calcium levels in normal-function kidney transplant recipients. *Nephron* 42:290, 1986.
261. Walker GS et al: Factors influencing the intestinal absorption of calcium and phosphorus following renal transplantation. *Nephron* 26:225, 1980.
262. Walker JV et al: Histoplasmosis with hypercalcemia, renal failure and papillary necrosis. *JAMA* 237:1350, 1977.
263. Ward HN et al: The renal handling of phosphate by renal transplant patients: Correlation with serum parathyroid hormone (SPTH), cyclic 3′, 5′-adenosine monophosphate (cAMP) urinary excretion, and allograft function. *Adv Exp Med Biol* 81:173, 1977.
264. West C et al: The incidence of gout in renal transplant recipients. *Am J Kidney Dis* 10:369, 1987.
265. White HJO et al: Function of cadaver renal homografts in relation to age of donor, cause of death and ischemia time. *Br Med J* 4:739, 1968.
266. Wilcox CS et al: Sodium homeostatis in patients with autonomic failure. *Clin Sci* 53:321, 1977.
267. Wilson DR, Siddiqui AA: Renal tubular acidosis after kidney transplantation. Natural history and significance. *Ann Intern Med* 79:352, 1973.
268. Wilson RE: Case records of the Massachusetts General Hospital. Weekly clinicopathological exercises. Case 13. *N Engl J Med* 290:793, 1974.
269. Wilson RE et al: Parathyroid disease in the transplant patient. *Transplant Proc* 4:689, 1972.
270. Woods JE et al: Hyperosmolar nonketotic syndrome and steroid diabetes. Occurrence after renal transplantation. *JAMA* 231:1261, 1975.
271. Yamaguchi Y et al: Ultrastructural study of cyclosporine-associated arteriolopathy in renal allografts. *Transplant Proc* 21:1517, 1989.
272. Zaloga GP et al: Hypercalcemia and disseminated cytomegalovirus infection in the acquired immunodeficiency syndrome. *Ann Intern Med* 102:331, 1985.
273. Zazgornik J et al: Severe hyperkalaemia, hyperchloraemia, hyporeninaemia and hyperaldosteronism in a cyclosporin-treated renal-transplant patient. *Nephrol Dial Transplant* 3:826, 1988.
274. Zincke H et al: The role of denervation in renal transplantation on renal function in the dog. *Invest Urol* 14:210, 1976.

CHAPTER • 43

Management of fluid, electrolyte, and acid-base disorders in surgical patients

Mark D. Faber • Rebecca J. Schmidt • Robert A. Bear • Robert G. Narins

Patients undergoing surgical procedures develop the same basic disturbances of acid-base, electrolyte, and volume homeostasis that are commonly found on the general medical floors of any hospital. Surgical patients, however, are predisposed to certain specific disorders resulting from their underlying conditions and from the individual surgical procedures they undergo (Table 43-1). Both elements influence the severity, presentation, and management of these derangements. A clear understanding of the pathophysiology of these disorders is essential for enabling physicians to diagnose, treat, and in many cases to prevent the occurrence of these chemical abnormalities in surgical patients. In addition, informed judgments regarding the effect of these disturbances on patient outcome and the optimal methods for their correction are required to minimize perioperative risk.

The authors acknowledge support from the University Medical Research Foundation.

This chapter focuses on the preoperative correction of preexisting disorders of electrolyte and volume homeostasis and the treatment of those disorders most likely to develop in the intra- and postoperative periods (Table 43-2). The reader will be referred to other chapters in this book for detailed discussions of normal physiology as well as for complete classifications and pathophysiologic explanations of the entities discussed.

PREOPERATIVE MANAGEMENT

ELECTIVE SURGERY

Ideally, elective surgical procedures should be delayed until optimal fluid, electrolyte, and acid-base status have been achieved. The morbidity and mortality of anesthesia and surgery are influenced by these chemical disorders, rendering their preoperative correction an essential fea-

TABLE 43-1 • Examples of electrolyte and acid-base disorders associated with surgical procedures

Procedure	Associated disorder	Etiologic factors
Abdominal surgery	Metabolic alkalosis, metabolic acidosis	Nasogastric suction, pancreatic or biliary drainage
Intracranial operations	Hypernatremia, hyponatremia	Central diabetes insipidus, SIADH, cerebral salt wasting
Transurethral resection of the prostate (TURP)	Hyponatremia	Absorption of irrigation fluid
Cardiac bypass surgery	Metabolic acidosis, hypokalemia, hypomagnesemia	Cardiopulmonary bypass
Parathyroidectomy	Hypocalcemia, hyperchloremic acidosis	"Hungry bone syndrome"

TABLE 43-2 • Fluid, electrolyte, and acid-base disorders in surgical patients

PREOPERATIVE MANAGEMENT
Elective surgery
Extracellular volume
Volume depletion
Congestive heart failure
Renal insufficiency
Anemia
Hyponatremia
Hypokalemia
Hyperkalemia
Acid-base disorders
Metabolic acidosis
Metabolic alkalosis
Respiratory acidosis
Emergent surgery
Extracellular volume
Hypokalemia
Acid-base disorders
Metabolic alkalosis
Lactic acidosis
INTRAOPERATIVE MANAGEMENT
Replacement of intraoperative fluid losses
Intracranial operations
Transurethral prostatectomy
Cardiac surgery
POSTOPERATIVE MANAGEMENT
Extracellular fluid and electrolytes
Fluid therapy during sepsis
Enteral and parenteral nutrition
PERIOPERATIVE MANAGEMENT OF SPECIFIC CONDITIONS
Hypertension
Pheochromocytoma
Diabetes insipidus
Secondary hyperparathyroidism
Diabetes mellitus
Rhabdomyolysis
Anemia

ture of these procedures. A variety of medical, economic, and/or logistic considerations may occasionally encourage physicians to clear patients for elective surgery more rapidly than they might otherwise desire. Thus, an understanding of the specific perioperative risks of particular electrolyte and fluid disorders, as well as the maximally safe rates of correction, are of great importance for the clinician caring for a surgical patient.

Disturbances of extracellular volume

Volume depletion

Sodium, localized primarily to the extracellular (intravascular and interstitial) fluid (ECF) compartment, accounts for the vast bulk of the osmotically active solute restricted to this site. This effective osmolality modifies thirst and the release of vasopressin (antidiuretic hormone, or ADH) by the brainstem, that is, those forces that alter the acquisition of water and its retention or excretion by the kidney. Perturbations of serum sodium concentration are corrected by this system but at the expense of altering ECF volume. Abnormal salt retention, for example, stimulates thirst and ADH release, which promote water retention, thereby maintaining osmolality normal while expanding the ECF. Conversely, loss of sodium diminishes osmolality, which initially suppresses thirst and ADH release, which in turn promotes renal water loss. Serum osmolality is once again maintained, but the ECF volume is now contracted. Thus, disturbances of ECF volume are almost always associated with changes in body sodium *content.* While the system regulating serum osmolality is very sensitive to changes in solute concentration, the induced gain or loss of water will eventually prove harmful to the host. Indeed, if water retention becomes excessive (e.g., with excess sodium ingestion), the ECF volume expansion begins to inhibit renal sodium and water reabsorption, thereby limiting further hypervolemia. Conversely, in early sodium depletion, the hypoosmolality inhibits thirst and ADH release and increases renal water excretion. The resulting hypovolemia will eventually cause contraction of ECF volume, which in turn stimulates thirst, ADH release, and renal sodium and water retention. Thus, although ECF volume is less tightly regulated than is osmolality, once its protective hormonal and other renal regulatory forces are stimulated, the control of serum osmolality will be sacrificed to protect the vital ECF volume. The hyponatremic but hypovolemic patient will retain water, and a hypernatremic but volume-expanded patient will become polyuric, emphasizing how "concentration" may be sacrificed for "volume."

To sustain perfusion of vital organs during surgery and anesthesia, intravascular volume must be properly expanded. Most of the commonly used inhaled or intravenous anesthetics depress myocardial contractility, thereby reducing cardiac output and effective arterial blood volume (EABV). Renal blood flow (RBF) and the glomerular filtration rate (GFR) may be decreased by the induced hypotension and by the reflex augmentation of circulating levels of catecholamines, ADH, and angiotensin II (AII), all of which increase vascular tone. Spinal anesthesia may also acutely reduce renal function by causing sympathetic blockade, venous pooling of blood, and relative volume depletion. In the hypovolemic patient, anesthetics may abrogate the normal physiologic responses of the heart and vasculature to sustain tissue perfusion.

The ability to sustain organ blood flow and function despite hypotension is termed *autoregulation*. Healthy people usually maintain RBF and GFR at relative normal levels over a range of mean arterial pressures between 160 and 80 mmHg. Autoregulation during renal hypoperfusion requires that the vascular resistance of preglomerular vessels (primarily in the afferent arterioles) decline, while postglomerular resistance (primarily in efferent arterioles) increases. This asymmetric change in resistances maintains a constant filtration pressure in the glomerular capillaries, which are interposed between the arterioles. As mean renal arterial blood pressure falls below 80 mmHg in otherwise normal kidneys, compensation by autoregulatory mechanisms becomes inadequate, and RBF and GFR progressively fall. Even lesser degrees of hypotension can be associated with acute renal failure when chronic hypertension, chronic renal insufficiency, advanced age, or arteriosclerosis interfere with the normal compensatory alterations in renal vascular tone. In addition to causing hypotension, volume depletion further stimulates increases in circulating vasoconstrictors, which may further interfere with autoregulation and thereby impair tissue perfusion.

It follows that correction of preoperative volume depletion is essential for avoiding acute syndromes of organ hypoperfusion. This is especially important in light of the common practice of prohibiting oral intake for 6 to 12 h prior to surgery. In the absence of intake, net fluid loss (insensible water plus urine volume) exceeds 1200 ml/day (Table 43-3). We recommend the preoperative infusion of 0.45% NaCl in 5% dextrose given at a rate of 75 ml/h for stable patients with good renal and cardiac function who are without preexisting volume deficits or electrolyte abnormalities. One liter of this "half-normal saline" may be viewed as the product created by mixing 500 ml of 5% dextrose in normal saline solution with 500 ml of 5% dextrose in water. Thus, each infused milliliter delivers 0.5 ml of water and 0.5 ml of normal saline solution. Infusion of 75 ml/h for 6 to 12 h preoperatively delivers a total volume of approximately 500 to 1000 ml. Half of the infused volume would be electrolyte-free water and half would be saline solution. This fluid adequately replaces insensible water loss and sustains intravascular volume. Addition of KCl to normokalemic preoperative patients is unnecessary and often irritating to the veins. Many "low-risk" procedures are currently performed today in an *outpatient setting*, where preoperative fluid and electrolyte replacement may not be feasible. Given the less demanding nature of these operations, these patients generally do well as long as serious underlying medical illnesses and preoperative volume or electrolyte disturbances are carefully detected and eliminated.

TABLE 43-3 • Water and sodium losses in a stable 60 to 80 kg adult

Source	Water loss ml/day	Sodium loss meq/day
INSENSIBLE		
Lungs and skin	600–900	0
SENSIBLE		
Urine	800–1500	10–80
Intestinal	0–250	0–20
Sweat	0	10–60

Congestive heart failure

Patients who have had a recent *myocardial infarction* (i.e., within the last 6 months) or those with uncompensated *congestive heart failure* (i.e., the presence of an S_3 gallop, rales, etc.) have been shown[60] to be at exceptionally high risk for developing a myocardial infarction and cardiac death perioperatively and therefore are not acceptable candidates for elective surgery. Similarly, elective surgery in patients with *acute renal failure* is generally deferred because recovery of renal function may be delayed and there is increased risk of perioperative complications. In contrast, well-compensated patients with significant but stable cardiac or renal dysfunction are reasonable candidates for elective surgery. However, such patients tolerate fluctuations in intrasvascular volume poorly, often walking a narrow line between volume overload with pulmonary congestion and prerenal azotemia induced by volume contraction. Considerable preoperative planning and preparation, usually carried out while in the hospital, are required to ensure that perioperative risks are minimized in the cardiac or renal patient undergoing surgery.

Compensated cardiac dysfunction is often associated with abnormally high left ventricular end-diastolic volume, with pulmonary capillary wedge pressures (PCWPs) approaching those indicative of congestion or edema ($\geq$20 cmH_2O). Patients with pericardial constriction, aortic stenosis, restrictive cardiomyopathy, or hypertrophic cardiomyopathy may be particularly dependent on this increased preload to maintain adequate cardiac output.[136] These patients are also at increased risk for the development of preoperative volume depletion and electrolyte abnormalities because of the associated use of *diuretics*. Because such patients are at risk, optimal preparation requires the elective preoperative insertion of a Swan-Ganz pulmonary artery catheter to measure PCWP. This reading correlates closely with left ventricular end-diastolic volume in most circumstances. Central venous pressure (CVP) measurements are not nearly as useful in this circumstance because significant degrees of right ventricular failure render the CVP unrepresentative of left ventricular pressures.[115] Armed with the measurement of PCWP, diuresis or volume expansion can then be instituted, thereby minimizing the risks of pulmonary edema or low cardiac output and hypotension. For the patient with milder degrees of heart failure undergoing low-risk procedures with little potential for major fluid gain or loss, it may suffice to rely on one's clinical assessment to dictate the use of diuretics or fluid electrolyte therapy and thereby avoid the need for invasive procedures.

Renal insufficiency

The stable patient with mild-to-moderate renal insufficiency not yet on dialysis is at increased risk of developing volume, acid-base, and electrolyte disorders because diseased kidneys cannot fully compensate for excessive, inadequate, or unphysiologic replacement of fluid and electrolyte losses. Their high prevalence of cardiovascular disease and anemia also increases the risk of adverse cardiac events. Patients with creatinine clearances between 25 and 50 ml/min generally maintain normal urine output and can adequately excrete moderate salt and water loads but may require the administration of potent diuretics to excrete larger osmotic burdens. On the other hand, because of the relative osmotic diuresis in each functioning residual nephron, such patients may demonstrate varying degrees of nephrogenic diabetes insipidus and the inability to conserve sodium and water during periods of restricted salt and liquid intake. Coexistent tubulointerstitial disease (e.g., analgesic abuse, sickle cell disease, lead nephropathy, polycystic kidney disease, etc.) may make patients particularly prone to volume depletion even with relatively well-preserved degrees of renal function. As noted above, in the postoperative period, this renal salt wasting may be a critical factor predisposing these patients to further deterioration of renal function. Tasker, MacGregor, and deWardener demonstrated the safety and effectiveness of moderate (1 to 2 liter) preoperative loading with intravenous 0.9 percent NaCl for maintaining renal function in chronic renal failure patients about to undergo major surgery.[158] We prefer preoperative administration of 0.45% NaCl in 5% dextrose at 75 ml/h while thirsting in this circumstance, as outlined above for healthy patients, with vigilant clinical monitoring for evidence of volume overload. In the presence of coexistent hyperkalemic, normal anion gap metabolic acidosis, a solution of 50 meq $NaHCO_3$ added to 1 liter of 5% dextrose in water or 0.3% NaCl should be substituted. For anuric, end-stage renal disease (ESRD) patients, preoperative intravenous replacement is required only to replace insensible losses and is generally given at a "keep-open" rate, with increased rates ordered during the intraoperative and postoperative periods to replace specific deficits. Because significant degrees of hyperkalemia are caused by fasting in many ESRD patients, 10% dextrose solutions are best used in this setting. The insulin released in response to the infused glucose prevents the starvation-induced maldistribution of potassium.[6,7]

Anemia

Current indications for preoperative *blood transfusions* to expand intravascular volume and increase oxygen-carrying capacity are controversial and currently are in a state of flux.[152] Until recently, few questioned the need for preoperative blood transfusion in patients whose hemoglobin concentration was at or below 10 g/dl. Some chronically anemic patients with renal insufficiency have been shown to do well postoperatively despite hemoglobin levels even below 7 g/dl. Their tolerance for anemia derives at least partly from the shift of the oxyhemoglobin dissociation curve to the right by acidosis and hyperphosphatemia,[126] thereby enhancing the unloading of oxygen from hemoglobin. The 1988 Consensus Development Conference of the National Institutes of Health on perioperative red cell transfusion[118] suggested that a more individualized approach be taken for patients whose hemoglobin ranged between 7 and 10 g/dl. It was recommended that the decision regarding transfusion be based on such factors as arterial oxygenation, mixed venous oxygen tension, cardiac output, blood volume, and the presence of coexisting coronary and cerebrovascular disease. Although the risks of transfusion-associated hepatitis (primarily non-A, non-B) and major and minor transfusion reactions are real, we continue to have misgivings about clearing for surgery those patients whose hemoglobin is less than 9.0 g/dl. This also applies to dialysis patients, in whom the risk of cardiovascular disease is increased. The widespread use of recombinant human *erythropoietin* (rHu EPO) has rendered chronic severe anemia much more rare in dialysis patients.[52]

Alternatives to homologous perioperative transfusion are recognized and are certainly to be encouraged. Appropriate use of erythropoietin may raise hemoglobin levels sufficiently to eliminate the need for preoperative transfusion and may conceivably allow for the prior banking of autologous blood for some dialysis patients. The use of modern autotransfusion devices ("cell savers"), which collect, filter, and anticoagulate blood from the operative field and return it to the patient, may also decrease the need for intraoperative and postoperative transfusions. In the hemodialysis patients, preoperative transfusion should generally be given during dialysis to minimize the potential risk for posttransfusion hyperkalemia and volume excess.

Specific electrolyte disorders

Hyponatremia

Preoperative severe or symptomatic hyponatremia is an unlikely finding in stable patients undergoing elective surgery. However, even healthy young patients (particularly women) with normal serum concentrations may develop profound and even fatal hyponatremia when given large amounts of hypotonic intravenous fluids during and after elective and sometime even minor surgery. Within 49 h of successful elective surgery, 15 young, healthy women developed severe hyponatremia, respiratory arrest, and seizures.[10] Their inability to excrete the large volume of dilute solutions they received over those 49 h caused their serum sodium concentration to decline from 138 ± 2 meq/liter preoperatively to 108 ± 2 meq/liter. Death or severe neurologic impairment occurred in all. This risk exists because the normal pathophysiologic response to surgery spawns strong nonosmotic forces that stimulate the secretion of ADH, which markedly limits free water clearance (see "Postoperative Operative Management of Fluid, Electrolyte, and Acid-Base Disorders"). These stimuli include pain, opiates, stress, hypotension, hypoxia, and nausea with or without vomiting. Females and children appear to be at substantially increased risk of permanent neurologic injury or death following hyponatremia (see Chap. 20).[16,17,34] Thus, because the normal reaction to stress and trauma limits the excretion of water for 2 to 5 days postoperatively, the presence of even mild derangements of serum sodium concentration preoperatively should prompt physicians to uncover the underlying cause of the abnormality.

For ease of diagnosis and therapy, hyponatremia is conveniently classified into *isotonic, hypertonic,* and *hypotonic* varieties (see Chap. 20). The hypotonic syndromes are subclassified on the basis of the clinical assessment of the patient's ECF volume status. Table 43-4 highlights those hypotonic, hyponatremic entities most likely to be found preoperatively in stable patients scheduled for surgery. Medications account for the majority of cases of hyponatremia found in euglycemic patients without renal failure. The medication history should be reviewed specifically for diuretics, chlorpropamide or other sulfonylureas, carbamazepine, clofibrate, colchicine, anti-

TABLE 43-4 • Common etiologies of hyponatremia in surgical patients

Preoperative	Intraoperative	Postoperative
Volume (sodium) depletion	Volume depletion	Volume depletion
Diuretics	Evaporative losses	"Cerebral salt wasting"
Salt-losing nephritis	"Third-spacing"	Gastrointestinal drainage
	Blood loss	
Drugs	Anesthesia	Acute renal failure
Sulfonylureas	Myocardial depression	Nonosmotic ADH release
Carbamazepine	Vasodilation	Pain
Phenothiazines	Hypotension	Nausea
Antidepressants		Vomiting
		Hypotension
Reduced effective arterial volume	Hypotension	Intravenous nutrition
Congestive heart failure	Intravenous fluids	
Nephrotic syndrome	Prostatic irrigation	
Cirrhosis		
Chronic renal failure		
Excessive free water intake		
Oral fluids		
Dilute intravenous fluids		
SIADH		
Cancer		
Central nervous system		
Pulmonary lesions		
Hypothyroidism		
Glucocorticoid deficiency		

depressants, and neuroleptic tranquilizers. In the absence of suspect drugs or other preoperative disorders that may cause euvolemic hyponatremia including hypothyroidism or glucocorticoid deficiency, the syndrome of inappropriate ADH secretion (SIADH) should be considered. SIADH is characterized by the continued release of ADH in hyponatremic patients with a wide range of carcinomas, central nervous system disorders, or pulmonary diseases despite the lock of hemodynamic or other nonosmotic stimuli. In addition to gastrointestinal and diuretic-induced losses, hypovolemic hyponatremia may be caused by mineralocorticoid deficiency, type II (proximal) renal tubular acidosis, or "salt-losing nephritis."

"Salt-losing nephritis" describes those renal disorders (usually tubulointerstitial in nature, including chronic pyelonephritis, polycystic kidney disease, medullary cystic disease, and partial urinary tract obstruction) that interfere with renal sodium conservation during conditions of volume and sodium depletion.[39,151,163] Although the majority of patients whose GFR is reduced to less than 15 ml/min will be in negative sodium balance for 1 to 3 weeks after placement on a low sodium diet, patients with the disorders listed above may exhibit renal salt-wasting with less severe renal impairment and are more likely to develop clinically significant volume depletion or hyponatremia.

The approach to the mildly hyponatremic patient varies according to the underlying cause. Obviously, correctable underlying diseases demand appropriate therapy prior to undergoing elective surgery. Drugs that impair free water clearance should be stopped if possible, although some offending medications (especially anticonvulsants) may require continuation. SIADH is treated with water restriction. Volume-depleted patients should be reexpanded with appropriate quantities of normal saline solution, while volume overloaded patients require diuresis. Endocrine deficiencies should be corrected with specific hormonal therapy. Patients with a "reset osmostat" defend a lower than normal serum sodium concentration.[41] For example, if deprived of water, they release ADH, helping to keep their sodium at 120 meq/liter, and if challenged with a water load they suppress ADH, excrete the water, and thereby maintain an unchanged but lower than normal serum osmolality. This disorder is generally found in patients with a wide variety of substantial medical disorders.

In general, if reversible conditions have been addressed, we feel comfortable in proceeding with surgery despite the presence of a chronically depressed serum sodium level as long as the concentration is not less than 130 meq/liter. Worsening hyponatremia in these patients can usually be avoided by using 0.9% NaCl with or without dextrose in appropriate amounts (see discussions of intraoperative and postoperative fluid management below) and by monitoring serum sodium levels intraoperatively and every 12 to 24 h in the postoperative period.

The rate at which hyponatremia should be corrected has undergone careful scrutiny during the past decade.[154] Clinical and animal investigation seems to clearly indicate that, while acute hyponatremia should be corrected rapidly, the chronic condition should be corrected more slowly (see Chap. 20). Acute hyponatremia, developing over 24 to 48 h, is a lethal disorder and should be reversed over the same time frame. To prevent fatal degrees of cerebral edema, brain cells chronically (>48 h) exposed to hyponatremia export potassium and amino acids along with intracellular water. This limits brain swelling but depletes cells of solute. If the serum sodium concentration is corrected faster than the brain can reaccumulate solute, cerebral shrinkage occurs, which, in a small percentage of patients, may be fatal or cause permanent neurologic deficits.[15]

Dangerously rapid rates of repair have been variously defined as increases of serum sodium concentration at rates exceeding 1.5 to 2.0 meq/liter per hour or 12 to 20 meq/liter per day; correction to values greater than 120 to 130 meq/liter within 48 h; correction to normal or inadvertently to hypernatremic levels within the first 48 h; or correction at rates that increase serum sodium levels by more than 10 percent per day. Currently, most would agree that in symptomatic, chronically hyponatremic patients, rates of correction approximating 0.5 meq/liter per hour appear safe. Methods of correcting hyponatremia are well outlined in Chap. 20.

Hypokalemia

It is widely acknowledged that hypokalemia is the electrolyte disorder that most commonly accounts for the cancellation of elective surgery. Fear of arrhythmias causes anesthesiologists to routinely and appropriately cancel elective procedures in patients with even slight decreases in serum potassium concentration. In most hypokalemic states, the reduction in extracellular potassium *concentration* most often greatly exceeds that in the intracellular space, even though the greatest *quantity* of the cation is lost from the intracellular compartment. This is best understood by considering the contributions of the various fluid spaces to the loss of 400 meq of potassium, which corresponds to a reduction in serum potassium concentration from 4.5 to 3.0 meq/liter. In a 70-kg man with approximately 21 liters of intracellular fluid (ICF) and 14 liters of ECF whose serum potassium concentration decreased from 4.5 to 3.0 meq/liter, total ECF potassium would decrease from 63 meq (4.5 meq/liter × 14 liters) to 42 meq (3 meq/liter × 14 liters), a reduction in both extracellular potassium content and concentration of (K_O) 33 percent. Although the remaining 379 meq is lost from the ICF, this represents only an 11 percent reduction of the original 3150 meq contained in the intracellular potassium pool (150 meq/liter × 21 liters) and an equivalent 11 percent reduction in the intracellular potassium concentration (K_i) to 134 meq/liter. The arrhythmogenicity of hypokalemia is understandable after considering the Nernst equation.[137] Based on the ratio of K_i to K_O, this equation gives a reasonable first approximation of resting cellular transmembrane potential (E_m):

$$E_m = -61 \log K_i/K_O \qquad (1)$$

The E_m, of course, is a key modifier of myoneural activity throughout the body. Mild-to-moderate hypokalemia slows cardiac conduction by hyperpolarizing the membrane (i.e., making it more electronegative). The amount of current required to bring the transmembrane potential to threshold is increased in hypokalemia. Hypokalemia also prolongs phase 3 recovery, which predisposes the heart to reentrant dysrhythmias by prolonging the period of increased excitability when transmembrane potential is close to threshold potential.

Clinical studies have confirmed the accuracy of these theoretical concerns in predicting a two- to threefold increased risk of ventricular arrhythmias and atrioventricular conduction blockade in hospitalized hypokalemic patients[40] as well as in diuretic-treated hypertensive patients.[77,103] However, the greatest potential for serious hypokalemia-induced arrhythmias clearly exists in patients taking digitalis glycosides,[53,54] those with preexisting or acute cardiac disease, and those with high circulating levels of catecholamines. Hypokalemia appears to increase myocardial sensitivity to digitalis both by increasing serum and myocardial concentrations of the drug[153] and by decreasing the intracellular concentration of potassium and raising that of sodium. Digitalis-induced suppression of Na^+-K^+ ATPase causes these ICF electrolyte changes. Many studies have demonstrated that hypokalemia increases the risk of ventricular fibrillation by two- to threefold following acute myocardial infarction.[49,81] High catecholamine levels augment the hazards of hypokalemia in this setting. Epinephrine causes intracellular movement of plasma potassium, thereby further hyperpolarizing myocardial cells. The catecholamine release during anesthesia and surgery would therefore be an additive risk to the hypokalemic patient.

A complete classification of hypokalemic disorders is discussed in Chap. 22. Hypokalemia induced by medications, especially diuretics, accounts for the majority of cases of this chemical abnormality in patients undergoing elective surgery. Patients with diuretic-induced hypokalemia should also be investigated for *hypomagnesemia.* The latter is also arrhythmogenic and can also induce or worsen renal potassium wasting. The use of sympathomimetics or mineralocorticoids can also be associated with hypokalemia. In the absence of diuretic use, the history, physical examination, and urinary concentration of the cation should identify sources of extrarenal potassium loss. Hypertension and metabolic acidosis or alkalosis serve as additional important clues in determining the underlying etiology of the hypokalemia.

It thus follows that total body potassium stores should be returned to normal in patients undergoing elective surgery. Deficits large enough to cause hypokalemia clearly take days, not hours, to correct. In those cases stemming from diuretic-induced potassium losses, rapid correction can usually be accomplished by stopping or reducing the diuretic dosage and providing 40 to 80 meq/day of KCl. Adding a potassium-sparing diuretic (spironolactone, triamterene, or amiloride) is another useful measure but is generally unsafe for patients with renal insufficiency and must be done with careful monitoring if supplemental potassium is given concurrently. Triamterene and amiloride can be effective within 1 to 2 h, whereas spironolactone takes 2 to 3 days. Potassium salts that are metabolized to bicarbonate (citrate, gluconate, or acetate) and potassium phosphate are poorly retained[85] because their accompanying anions are not reabsorbed well by the kidney. They should not, therefore, be used to correct hypokalemia in patients with adequate renal function. Dietary manipulation generally plays little direct role in the correction of deficits because most dietary potassium is accompanied by anions other than chloride. However, salt restriction may effectively lessen or prevent diuretic-induced hypokalemia by limiting Na^+-K^+ exchange in the distal tubule, thereby curtailing excessive kaliuresis. The rapid correction of hypokalemia in nonelective cases is discussed under "Emergent Surgery."

Hyperkalemia

While less common than hypokalemia, hyperkalemia ranks among the most frequent chemical abnormalities seen in patients with chronic renal disease. While hyperkalemia is quite common when creatinine clearance is less than 15 ml/min, significant increases in serum potassium levels often accompany tubulointerstitial renal disease or disruption of the renin-aldosterone axis in patients with slightly impaired or occasionally even normal renal function. Selective hypoaldosteronism is the most common condition disrupting secretion of the hormone and occurs mostly in patients with diabetes mellitus, interstitial renal disease, or advanced age.[42] The diagnosis is suggested by the characteristic appearances of hyperkalemia, hyperchloremic acidosis, and mild-to-moderate renal insufficiency. Addison's disease must be excluded in hyperkalemic patients with sodium wasting because the stress of surgery is likely to precipitate an adrenal crisis. Excessive potassium intake, low sodium intake, volume depletion, or the use of drugs that decrease renal potassium excretion (e.g., potassium-sparing diuretics) or that limit extrarenal cellular uptake of potassium (beta-adrenergic blockers and digitalis) are usually necessary cofactors for the development of overt hyperkalemia in susceptible patients. Acute metabolic disturbances (hyperglycemia or metabolic acidosis) or increased catabolism may also increase serum potassium in these hyperkalemia-prone individuals.

Mild hyperkalemia (≤5.5 meq/liter) may be antiarrhythmic, particularly for digitalis-associated arrhythmias.[25] The hyperkalemia reduces automaticity of ectopic pacemakers and terminates reentrant arrhythmias. More severe degrees of hyperkalemia are associated with classical electrocardiographic changes. Peaked T waves correspond to the shortened duration and increased rate of phase 3 repolarization during the transmembrane action potential, while more advanced changes (prolongation or QRS, atrioventricular block, and P wave suppression) result from conduction slowing associated with shifting upward of the resting transmembrane potential and of the excitability threshold. Relatively larger shifts in resting potential may also increase myocardial excitability. Bradyarrhythmias and atrioventricular block appear more commonly during slowly developing elevations of serum potassium concentration, while ventricular ectopy or fatal ventricular fibrillation are more likely to be seen during severe acute increases in serum potassium levels. Hypocalcemia, hyponatremia, and acidemia may exacerbate the cardiac disturbances associated with any given degree of hyperkalemia.

Although mild hyperkalemia (≤5.5 meq) may not always be a contraindication to elective surgery, care must be taken to avoid using depolarizing muscle relaxants (e.g., succinylcholine) because they raise the serum potassium concentration. Potassium levels must be carefully monitored during surgery, especially if intraoperative blood transfusions are given. More severe degrees of hyperkalemia require preoperative correction. When electrocardiographic changes are present or when surgery cannot be delayed, hyperkalemia must be treated with those measures that cause redistribution or excretion of potassium and that antagonize potassium's myocardial toxicity. Widening of the QRS complexes and the absence of P waves are particularly ominous signs, usually associated with serum potassium levels of 7.5 meq/liter or more. These electrocardiographic changes may indicate impending ventricular fibrillation and therefore require immediate treatment with sufficient amounts of intravenous calcium chloride to cause narrowing of the QRS complex. This treatment should be quickly followed with parenteral $NaHCO_3$, glucose, and insulin. The patient's cardiopulmonary status obviously determines the volume of fluid and quantity of sodium that may be administered. Twenty-five grams of glucose (50 ml of a 50% solution) is a usual starting dose and is accompanied by intravenous regular insulin (5 to 10 units, patients with renal insufficiency requiring lower doses). Potassium levels of 6.2 meq/liter or less can generally be treated with Kayexalate alone if electrocardiographic changes are mild. Hemodialysis patients are generally dialyzed preoperatively to prevent perioperative hyperkalemia and other attendant metabolic derangements. As previously noted, fasting will commonly raise serum potassium levels as the cation "leaks" out of cells.[6,7] Parenteral glucose will effectively neutralize this phenomenon.

Acid-base disorders

Metabolic acidosis

Although uncommon in healthy patients undergoing elective surgery, chronic asymptomatic metabolic acidosis may be seen preoperatively in patients with certain common underlying medical disorders. These diseases include chronic renal failure, diabetes mellitus, or diarrheal states. Medications such as potassium-sparing diuretics, angiotensin-converting enzyme inhibitors, and carbonic anhydrase inhibitors can also cause acidosis. The adverse cardiovascular and pulmonary effects of metabolic acidosis, and the various electrolyte disorders associated with it, potentially increase the risk of developing anesthetic and postoperative complications. The magnitude of the increased risk depends not only on the severity of the accompanying acidemia but also on the rapidity with which it develops. In general, serious systemic effects of chronic metabolic acidosis are seen when serum pH falls to values less than 7.20. Because the degree of acidemia is normally ameliorated by compensatory hypocapnia (Chap. 25), care must be taken that further decreases in pH do not develop postoperatively, as ventilation is often fixed by mechanical means or suppressed by muscle relaxants, analgesics, and sedatives (Fig. 43-1).

Mild-to-moderate degrees of acidemia stimulate the release of epinephrine from the adrenal medulla[174] and may result in tachycardia. On the other hand, severe acidemia (pH ≤ 7.20), by antagonizing the myocardial effects of catecholamines or inhibiting acetylcholinesterase, causes the accumulation of acetylcholine,[108] which results in bradycardia. Other adverse cardiovascular effects of acidemia include the predisposition to ventricular fibrillation[56] and impaired contractility,[108] which may be aggravated by beta-adrenergic blockers[55] and calcium channel blockers.[30] These effects of acidemia are additive with the proarrhythmic and negatively inotropic effects of general anesthesia. Other adverse hemodynamic consequences seen when pH falls below 7.20 include hypotension, resulting from arteriolar vasodilation,[90] and pulmonary venous congestion[71] consequent to venoconstriction.

Metabolic acidosis influences oxygen delivery to the tissues in a complex fashion. Protons and 2,3-diphosphoglyceric acid (DPG), the glycolytic metabolite in

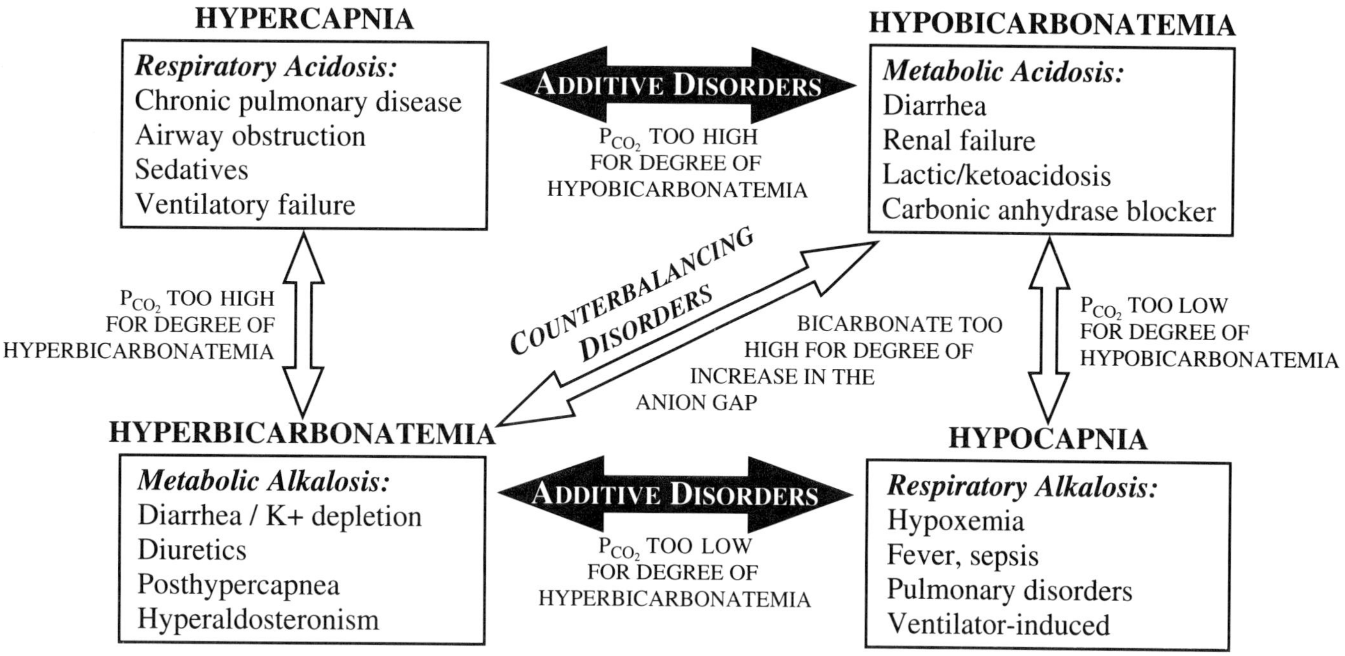

FIGURE 43-1 • Simple and mixed acid-base disorders. Each of the four boxes depicts a simple acid-base disorder labeled with its primary chemical abnormality. Mixed disorders reflect combinations of the primary disorders. *Additive disorders* are those mixed disorders in which the pH is moved in the same direction by each contributing primary disorder. *Counterbalancing disorders* are those mixed disorders in which the pH is moved in opposite directions by the component primary disorders.

erythrocytes, both cause the oxyhemoglobin dissociation curve to shift to the right. This rightward displacement means that the unloading of oxygen from hemoglobin to the tissues is facilitated. Thus, *acute* metabolic acidosis actually enhances tissue oxygen delivery. With sustained acidosis, red blood cell glycolysis is inhibited and DPG levels decline. In *chronic* metabolic acidosis, the intraerythrocytic concentration of protons remains high, pushing the oxyhemoglobin curve to the right, but the reduced red blood cell levels of DPG displace the curve to the left. Thus, with chronic acidosis, oxygen delivery returns to normal.

Metabolic acidosis should be corrected by eliminating or treating underlying causes whenever possible and by using judicious amounts of supplemental bicarbonate. With rapid correction of the acidosis, erythrocyte pH normalizes faster than do the DPG levels. The persistently low DPG concentration without acidosis causes the oxyhemoglobin curve to shift to the left, thereby potentially compromising tissue oxygen delivery. Although the physiologic importance of this phenomenon has not been confirmed in animal studies,[22] it is still preferable to correct metabolic acidosis over a period of several days preceding elective surgery. Gradual correction also lessens the potential hazards of acute hypokalemia, tetany, and volume overload, which can result from the too rapid administration of intravenous sodium bicarbonate. Generally, pH should be restored to approximately 7.30 and serum bicarbonate levels to values of 18 meq/liter or more before proceeding with elective surgery.

Metabolic alkalosis

The surgical patient with metabolic alkalosis also faces increased perioperative risk, especially when the arterial pH exceeds 7.50. Various causes of this acid-base disorder are discussed in Chap. 29. Of particular relevance to the surgical patient is the increased susceptibility to ventricular and supraventricular arrhythmias,[149] especially with the use of cardiac glycosides. Impaired tissue oxygenation may result during acute alkalemia from the leftward shift of the oxyhemoglobin dissociation curve (see Chap. 29). In *chronic* alkalemia, erythrocyte DPG levels are increased, thereby restoring tissue oxygen delivery despite continued alkalinity of the cells. Alkalemia is also commonly associated with hypokalemia and decreases in the serum ionized calcium concentration (despite normal total serum calcium levels). All three chemical changes conspire to produce frank tetany, especially when arterial pH exceeds 7.6.[61] Neurologic disturbances may also accompany pH levels greater than 7.55. These abnormalities include confusion, lethargy, seizures, muscle weakness, and neuromuscular irritability.[76] The central nervous system manifestations may develop from a combination of the direct effects of decreased hydrogen ion concentration, cerebral vasoconstriction, changes in the serum ionized calcium concentration, and reductions in serum phosphorus levels. Increased sensitivity to D-tubocurarine and resistance to its antagonism by neostigmine has also been reported during experimental metabolic alkalosis[106] as well as during hypokalemia.

As in the case of metabolic acidosis, corrective measures should focus on the diagnosis and treatment of the underlying disorders (see Chap. 25). Chloride-sensitive metabolic alkalosis (wherein the urine chloride concentration is ≤10 meq/liter) is corrected by replacement of NaCl and KCl deficits and by stopping or diminishing diuretic therapy if applicable. Chloride-resistant alkalosis (urine chloride concentration ≥20 meq/liter) generally suggests the presence of various endocrine disorders. Elective surgery should not be performed when the pH exceeds 7.50.

Respiratory acidosis

Although the patient with an acute respiratory acidosis is not a candidate for elective surgery, patients with chronic respiratory acidosis from various causes may undergo elective or at least nonemergent surgery. Serum pH usually remains near normal in this disorder due to compensatory increases in serum bicarbonate concentration (~3 meq/liter per 10 mmHg increase in the P_{CO_2}). Chronic, compensated respiratory acidosis appears to be well-tolerated and usually does not directly produce other electrolyte disturbances. However, certain drugs used in the treatment of chronic obstructive pulmonary disease (COPD; e.g., corticosteroids and sympathomimetics) or diuretics given for an associated cor pulmonale frequently cause hypokalemia, hyponatremia, and/or metabolic alkalosis.

In the absence of other superimposed metabolic disorders, a major concern in the surgical patient with chronic respiratory acidosis is the prevention of posthypercapneic metabolic alkalosis (see Chap. 29). The serum acid-base profile of these patients is characterized by increased values for P_{CO_2} and bicarbonate, the former reflecting the primary acid-base disturbance and the latter, the tissue and renal metabolic compensation. The hyperbicarbonatemia is sustained by the coupling of renal and extrarenal alkali synthesis with the increased renal retention of the anion. By reducing the P_{CO_2} faster than one reduces the increased bicarbonate level, a "posthypercapnic metabolic alkalosis" is created. The obvious treatment for acute posthypercapneic alkalosis is to adjust the ventilator to allow the P_{CO_2} to rise and the pH to fall. In addition to KCl and NaCl replacement, when appropriate, the carbonic anhydrase inhibitor acetazolamide is useful in correcting metabolic alkalosis in patients whose renal function is relatively well-preserved.

EMERGENT SURGERY

Extracellular volume

The patient requiring emergency surgery who presents with hypotension, oliguria, pulmonary congestion, or some other sign of hemodynamic instability under ideal conditions should receive full hemodynamic monitoring via a pulmonary artery catheter prior to the induction of anesthesia. With this technique, one can rapidly titrate ECF volume optimally without causing pulmonary edema. Volume depletion can then be corrected relatively safely by repeatedly administering 200 ml boluses of 0.9% NaCl solution until blood pressure and cardiac output improve or until the saline solution results in immediate (>7 cmH_2O) or sustained (>3 cmH_2O) increases in PCWP. Emergency circumstances may dictate the need for empiric volume resuscitation. In the case of shock, an initial bolus of 10 to 20 ml/kg 0.9% NaCl solution followed by ongoing replacement of at least 1 to 2 ml/min should serve to at least temporarily expand intravascular volume until the patient's condition can be stabilized and hemodynamic monitoring instituted. The maintenance of at least 0.5 to 1.0 ml/min urine output should be the aim.

Hypokalemia

The rationale for slowly correcting hypokalemia before elective surgery has been discussed. However, more rapid correction may be required before emergency surgery. Although full replacement of significant (mostly intracellular) potassium deficits requires several days, the Ki/Ko ratio (and therefore the transmembrane potential) should quickly return to near normal as extracellular potassium concentration rises in response to KCl supplementation. We suggest that serum potassium concentration be acutely increased to at least 3.5 meq/liter before surgery. Because serum potassium levels may fall quickly as equilibration with the intracellular space occurs, the serum concentration should be rechecked every 1 to 2 h intraoperatively, with additional KCl given as needed. Because a finite period of time is required for extracellular potassium to equilibrate with depleted intracellular stores, it is possible that otherwise acceptable rates of intravenous potassium administration may actually cause *hyperkalemia*. This, even transitory, increase in serum potassium level is particularly dangerous when intracellular stores of the cation are still greatly reduced. In this setting, the Ki/Ko ratio may fall dramatically, causing potentially lethal myoelectrical consequences.

Rapid correction of low serum potassium levels may be accomplished by continuous or intermittent KCl infusions of up to 40 meq/h. When KCl is infused at rates exceeding 10 to 20 meq/h, an infusion pump and constant electrocardiographic monitoring should be employed. Commonly ordered "sets" of three to six serial infusions containing 10 to 20 meq of KCl each administered over 1 h have been found to increase the serum potassium concentration by an average of 0.15 to 0.50 meq/liter per infusion.[92,100] Although generally appearing safe, transient hyperkalemia occasionally occurs. Concern that concentrated potassium infusions into a central vein might produce hazardous local accumulations and induce ventricular arrhythmias has not been supported by prospective clinical studies.[92,100] In fact, even rapidly administered central venous boluses of KCl (33 μeq/kg) into the proximal infusion port of a pulmonary artery catheter did not induce arrhythmias following cardiac bypass.[101]

Acid-base disturbances

The patient requiring emergency surgery is generally more ill and is therefore far more likely to present with one or more primary acid-base disorders (Fig. 43-1) than is the patient undergoing elective surgery.

Metabolic alkalosis from vomiting or nasogastric suction is a common complication seen in a variety of acute abdominal disorders requiring emergency surgery. While ongoing KCl and NaCl replacement may allow surgery to proceed in mild-to-moderate alkalosis, severe alkalosis (pH $>$ 7.55) may necessitate correction with parenteral acid therapy, especially if complicated by cardiac arrhythmia, digitalis intoxication, or central nervous system toxicity. A detailed discussion of acid therapy appears in Chap. 29.

Unstable surgical patients are especially prone to developing *lactic acidosis* (see Chap. 25). Generalized tissue hypoxia associated with hypotension or sepsis, or from localized hypoperfusion resulting from disorders such as intestinal or limb ischemia, are the most common causes of this disorder.

The hemodynamic consequences of severe acidemia (pH $<$ 7.20) render general anesthesia and surgery very hazardous.[62,150] The medical dilemma is that, although it is dangerous, surgery may offer the patient the only chance for survival. To mitigate these hemodynamic complications, alkali should be vigorously administered. As detailed in Chap. 25, if the serum bicarbonate concentration can be maintained at 10 meq/liter or higher and if the respiratory compensation is appropriate, the pH will be in the range of 7.20 to 7.25. If tissue perfusion is impaired, central venous sampling of blood gases is more reflective of the acid-base status of tissues than is arterial blood.[110]

Large-scale administration of sodium bicarbonate can cause several potentially avoidable complications. Hyperosmolarity, hypernatremia, and volume overload are especially likely if coexisting renal insufficiency is present. Infusion of isotonic solutions of sodium bicarbonate can minimize these hazards. In patients with adequate renal function, furosemide-induced renal loss of NaCl will create the needed "space" for infused $NaHCO_3$. Replacement of each milliequivalent of NaCl excreted with a like amount of $NaHCO_3$ keeps the body sodium content constant while exchanging body Cl^- for administered HCO_3^-. If volume overloaded, acidemic patients cannot respond to diuretics, some form of ultrafiltration or dialysis (see below) will be required if alkali is to be given. Another potential complication of bicarbonate therapy is hypercapnia.[111] The titration of administered bicarbonate generates carbon dioxide, which is immediately excreted if pulmonary blood flow and ventilation are intact. With severe hypotension, however, pulmonary blood flow is reduced, thereby limiting the delivery of CO_2 generated in the tissues to the lungs. If alveolar ventilation is adequate, peripheral arterial P_{CO_2} can be normal despite severe hypercapnia in mixed venous blood. Infused bicarbonate adds to the accumulating venous (and tissue) CO_2. In this setting, every effort should be expended to improve the cardiac output in order to improve pulmonary blood flow and thereby CO_2 excretion.

Emergency dialysis

Significant degrees of acute or chronic renal insufficiency, especially if associated with oliguria, increase the likelihood of developing electrolyte and acid-base disorders and also complicate the treatment of patients requiring emergency surgery. Furthermore, the pathophysiologic derangements associated with the urgent surgical disorder may further impair renal function. As a result, disturbances that might otherwise be treated medically in the preoperative period may require hemodialysis to rapidly reestablish metabolic equilibrium, given the precipitous need for surgery. Peritoneal dialysis, while useful in some settings, is obviously contraindicated when abdominal surgery is contemplated and is generally too slow for urgent surgical problems. Volume overload in patients unresponsive to diuretics often requires ultrafiltration or dialysis. The severe limitation on the amount of sodium that patients with renal failure can safely accommodate makes large-scale replacement of sodium bicarbonate impractical in severe metabolic acidosis unless preoperative hemodialysis is employed for the removal of excess sodium and water. Similarly, severe metabolic alkalosis in patients with renal insufficiency who require emergency operations may be best treated with hemodialysis.

Hyperkalemia of a mild degree may be treated medically in patients with renal insufficiency requiring minor or elective surgery. The more unstable patient with mild hyperkalemia undergoing emergency surgery is, however, extremely susceptible to severe degrees of potassium elevation and so requires preoperative dialysis. The specific circumstances precipitating the need for emergency surgery may lead to large ECF influxes of potassium from ischemic or traumatized tissues, blood transfusions, or high rates of tissue catabolism. The treatment of ischemic or traumatic myonecrosis of the limb deserves particular attention. Life-threatening amounts of potassium are released from necrotic cells in this circumstance and accumulate when blood flow to the limb is suddenly and markedly reduced. Acute restoration of blood flow (by thrombectomy, angioplasty, surgery, etc.) may then allow lethal amounts of potassium to enter the general circulation. Dialysis should be prophylactically initiated before reperfusion is established. Presumably, dialysis via a dual lumen catheter in the major vein (femoral or subclavian) draining the ischemic limb would be especially effective, since much of the accumulated potassium could be potentially prevented from ever entering the general circulation.

INTRAOPERATIVE MONITORING AND MANAGEMENT OF FLUID, ELECTROLYTE, AND ACID-BASE DISORDERS

REPLACEMENT OF INTRAOPERATIVE FLUID LOSSES

The patient undergoing major surgery sustains absolute and relative losses of intravascular volume from a number of sources. Such losses include urine volume, evaporative losses from exposed vicera, and losses from extravasation of fluid into traumatized tissues, the bowel lumen and wall, and the peritoneal cavity. In general, these losses can be replaced by 500 to 1000 ml/h of 0.9% or 0.45% NaCl solution. In healthier patients, the adequacy of replacement can be ascertained by the maintenance of stable blood pressure and heart rate and a urine output of approximately 30 to 60 ml/h. Patients who are predisposed to intravascular volume overload because of cardiac disease or renal failure or who are hemodynamically unstable may require monitoring of either central venous or PCWPs to safely administer appropriate volumes of replacement fluids.

Blood loss is the other obvious source of intravascular volume contraction during surgery. A normal blood donor may lose as much as 450 ml of whole blood over 20 min without noticeable physiologic disturbance. In contrast, the myocardial depression and relative volume depletion induced by general anesthesia (see above) may induce significant hemodynamic compromise following an acute blood loss of 500 to 1000 ml during surgery, *despite replacement by 0.9% NaCl solution or other crystalloids.* Thus, intraoperative blood losses exceeding this amount generally require replacement, usually with packed erythrocytes. The patient requiring massive transfusion to replace ongoing blood loss is considered further in the section on anemia (see below).

INTRACRANIAL OPERATIONS

Fluid and electrolyte management of the neurosurgical patient is largely dictated by the brain's nearly exclusive reliance on glucose as a substrate for energy metabolism and the resulting need to constantly maintain adequate cerebral perfusion. As with other tissues, perfusion of the brain depends on the ratio of cerebral perfusion pressure (CPP) to cerebrovascular resistance. Because CPP is the difference between mean arterial blood pressure (MAP) and intracranial pressure (ICP), cerebral perfusion may be threatened by either brain edema or hypotension in patients undergoing brain surgery. Anesthetic agents, antihypertensive drugs, hypercarbia, and acidemia exert complex effects on cerebrovascular resistance. In these circumstances, cerebral perfusion often increases initially but may then decline when emerging cerebral edema decreases compliance as ICP precipitously increases. In addition, increased ICP and associated cerebral edema may lead to herniation.

Unlike systemic capillaries, which are permeable to sodium, cerebral capillaries are impermeable to both large and small solutes but freely permeable to water. As a result, small solutes exert a large influence on water transport across the tight junctions of the cerebral capillaries. Hydrostatic pressure also becomes an important determinant of transcapillary fluid movement when the blood-brain barrier is disrupted because of injury or surgery.[120] Thus, both hyponatremia and hypertension increase the risk of cerebral edema and represent major threats to the neurosurgical patient.

Many neurosurgical patients with central nervous system lesions are prone to developing hyponatremia. A wide range of intracranial disorders can stimulate the release of ADH, and the secretion of this hormone becomes insensitive to the normal inhibitory feedback of emerging hypotonicity. Infections with virtually all types of organisms, trauma, tumors, degenerative diseases, and metabolic disorders of the intracranial space and cerebral tissue may all cause this SIADH. It is most important to remember that as long as the urinary electrolyte (sodium plus potassium) concentration exceeds the electrolyte concentration of administered fluid, hyponatremia must develop (insensible and drainage losses not withstanding). In other terms, *if less electrolyte-free water is excreted than is administered, body fluid becomes diluted.* In practical terms, this concept reaches clinical significance because the administration of 0.9% NaCl solution may actually cause hyponatremia if the kidney excretes the infused sodium at a concentration greater than that of the saline solution: 154 meq/liter. The syndrome of cerebral salt wasting encompasses natriuresis, varying degrees of hypovolemia,[113,170,171] and laboratory findings reflecting poor tissue perfusion. The latter generally include hyponatremia, azotemia, and occasionally lactic acidosis. All these findings occur in patients with neurologic injury. The disorder has been reported in such diverse conditions as subarachnoid hemorrhage (SAH),[112,172] head trauma,[83] pituitary exploration,[8] and chronic dementia.[157] Antinatriuretic factor (ANF) levels are increased in the cerebrospinal fluid and plasma in the majority of patients with SAH[45,48,132] and correlate with the extent of suprasellar or ventricular hemorrhage.[46,173,174,175] However, ANF levels in these studies did not directly correlate with the presence or absence of hyponatremia.[45,46] Furthermore, elevated ADH levels have been demonstrated in other patients developing hyponatremia following SAH in the absence of negative sodium balance,[47] suggesting that SIADH can be the etiology of the low serum sodium concentration in some of these patients. The administration of hypotonic saline solutions should be avoided to prevent hyponatremia and its associated undesirable increases in intracranial pressure.[19] Because osmolality rather than oncotic pressure is the major determinant of water movement across the blood-brain barrier, crystalloid and colloid infusions should have equal effects on brain water. Glucose-containing solutions are also avoided in neurosurgical patients because of associated hyperglycemia and reported exacerbation of ischemic damage and cerebral edema.[95,98,122,123,147] This has been attributed to enhanced anaerobic production of lactate.[168]

Diuretics may decrease intracranial pressure by reducing plasma volume and hydrostatic pressure.[109,119] While both mannitol and furosemide decrease brain water, mannitol has been associated with transient increases in intracranial pressure when administered rapidly.[127] Mannitol-induced cerebrovasodilation seems to underlie these effects. In addition, excessive diuresis may produce hypotension and decreases in cerebral blood flow to values below the lower limits of cerebral autoregulation (50–60 mmHg). Because cerebral blood flow (and ultimately intracranial pressure) also can be increased by hypercapnea and hypoxemia, ventilator settings should be adjusted to maintain the P_{CO_2} in the range of 25 to 35 mmHg and the P_{O_2} above 100 mmHg. Clearly, proper balance of these complex factors and maintenance of adequate cerebral perfusion depend on careful and extensive intraoperative monitoring of cerebral blood flow (intracranial Doppler) brain function (EEG and evoked potentials), ventilation (capnography, mass spectrometry, and pulse oximetry), and systemic hemodynamics (arterial blood pressure, right atrial and pulmonary artery pressures, cardiac output, and urine output). In addition, urine and serum electrolytes require careful monitoring to prevent or diagnose the electrolyte disorders (hypokalemia, hyponatremia, and hypomagnesemia) that may be associated with diuretic use.

Therapeutic hypotension is often used during the resection of aneurysms, atrioventricular malformations, and vascular tumors. It becomes very challenging to maintain sufficient cerebral blood flow to sustain cerebral metabolism during these procedures. Hypotension is commonly induced by high concentrations of inhalational anesthetics (halothane, enflurane, or isoflurane) or by continuous infusion of intravenous vasodilators (nitroprusside or nitroglycerine). Mean arterial pressures as low as 40 to 50 mmHg are induced, which, when coupled with prevailing increases in ICP due to the cerebral lesion, may reduce CPP below the range of autoregulation and cause vasospasm. Many of these agents also directly dilate cerebral vessels and may thereby further impair cerebral autoregulation (especially if blood pressure is lowered rapidly) and increase ICP. Although adverse effects on cerebral metabolism may be minimized by maintaining adequate intravascular volume and careful intraoperative monitoring (see above), the risks of cerebral hypoperfusion and the advent of the temporary clip have recently reduced the use of induced hypotension in neurovascular surgery.[3]

TRANSURETHRAL PROSTATECTOMY (TURP)

Clinical Manifestations and Pathophysiology

Profound hyponatremia and a variety of adverse neurologic and cardiovascular events, collectively termed the *transurethral resection syndrome* (TURS), are reported to follow TURP in 1 to 7 percent of cases (see also Chap. 20).[67,102,128] The syndrome is attributed to the absorption of irrigation fluid from the bladder through severed prostatic veins and via the perivascular space. Prospective studies[65] have described the absorption of more than 300 ml in about 25 percent of TURPs, including volumes exceeding 1 liter in 10 percent of cases and occasionally instances of the absorption of 2 to 4 liters. The severity of both the hyponatremia and the associated symptoms are generally proportional to the volume of absorbed fluid and to the character of the irrigant.

Sterile water was abandoned long ago as an irrigant during TURP due to the risk of massive intravascular hemolysis, while the electrical conductance of *saline solutions* makes them unsafe for use during electrocautery. *Glycine* is currently employed most frequently for irrigation but *sorbitol* and *mannitol* solutions are also used. Similar syndromes associated with the use of electrolyte-free irrigating fluid have also been reported following ultrasonic lithotripsy and uterine endoscopic laser surgery.[21,107,138,148]

A prickling and burning sensation of the skin usually occurs as early as 1 to 2 min after the irrigation begins in patients destined to develop the TURS but is unique to glycine usage. Transient blindness has also been reported with the use of glycine. Hypertension (elevation of systolic blood pressure 20 to 60 mmHg) is often found in susceptible patients within the first 20 min, while chest pain may follow soon afterward. Nausea and vomiting then develop 30 to 60 min postoperatively, accompanied by encephalopathic symptoms consisting of apprehension, confusion, and irrational behavior. These findings may be followed by muscular twitching, poor limb coordination, and altered consciousness, especially if the serum sodium level decreases below 120 meq/liter.[67] Grand mal seizures can accompany the encephalopathy. Profound hypotension, bradycardia, pulmonary edema, and/or cardiac arrest may occur in severe cases either intra- or postoperatively.

Although severe hyponatremia (serum sodium level decreased between 20 and 50 meq/liter from preoperative values) has been present in almost all reported cases of the TURS, its etiologic role is still debated. Evidence exists of at least some pathophysiologic contribution of the effects of rapid changes in ECF and ICF volume and tonicity, dilution of electrolyte concentrations, and the direct toxicity of the irrigant solutions. While the pathophysiology of the syndrome is presently uncertain, the character of the absorbed solution, the generation of ammonia from glycine, and the patient's hemodynamic response all must make important contributions to the clinical picture (see "Therapy," below). Therapy is aimed at reversing the effects of each of these aforementioned pathophysiologic parameters.

The earliest signs and symptoms (hypertension, chest pain, etc.) are universally associated with intravascular volume overload and elevated central venous pressure, resulting from both direct irrigant absorption and from shifts from ICF caused by the hyperosmolar irrigant.[66,67,70] As the total volume of absorbed fluid increases, capillary hydrostatic pressure progressively increases and plasma oncotic pressure simultaneously decreases due to dilution of plasma proteins. The combination of capillary hypertension with hypooncotic plasma promotes the transfer of intravascular fluid to the interstitial space and may cause pulmonary edema. The sequence of hemodynamic events probably differs between different irrigating agents and is also influenced by their concentrations. Glycine rapidly redistributes throughout body water, while mannitol and sorbitol are largely restricted to the ECF space. Blood loss (commonly 500 to 1000 ml), and the ensuing osmotic diuresis may ultimately lead to overt hypotension, shock, and possibly respiratory or cardiac arrest.

Hyponatremia develops relatively early, during the initial period of intravascular volume expansion, and then plateaus. The pathophysiologic basis for the plateau in serum sodium levels is largely dictated by the character of the irrigant. As noted above, the increasing solute diuresis seen with the commonly used solutions generally causes loss of more water than sodium, thereby tending to correct the hyponatremia. *Isotonic mannitol* solutions are restricted to and quickly distributed throughout the ECF, thereby causing the serum sodium concentration to rapidly reach its nadir. The decrement in serum sodium levels reflects the algebraic sum of the volume of hypotonic solution absorbed and the magnitude of the corrective diuresis. The hyponatremic response to *isotonic glycine* solutions differs in that the amino acid is eventually taken up by cells and metabolized, leaving solute-free water behind. This residual water then distributes throughout the intracellular and extracellular spaces. If all the glycine were metabolized, the absorbed solution would be equivalent to water, and a "hypotonic hyponatremia" would ensure. It should be apparent, however, that, the osmotic diuresis notwithstanding, the isotonic mannitol causes "isotonic hyponatremia." Because *only* the tonicity of the absorbate influences *cellular volume*, the isotonic mannitol leaves the volume of the ICF unchanged, whereas the hypotonic hyponatremia evolving from the glycine absorption, expands the ICF.

If one were to add pure distilled water to a bag of isotonic mannitol, a hypotonic solution would be created. When absorbed, the extra water would distribute throughout body water, leaving the isotonic mannitol in the ECF space. Similar dynamics would occur with hypotonic glycine. Initially, the excess water would add a hypotonic component to the isotonic hyponatremia caused by glycine. With catabolism of the amino acid, pure hypotonic hyponatremia would supervene. The dilution of serum sodium concentration from hypertonic mannitol results from both the absorption of sodium-free fluid and from the osmotic transfer of sodium-free ICF to the extracellular space, down its osmotic gradient. Were hypotonic glycine used as a bladder irrigant, the same dynamic events would ensue, but the progressive loss of glycine from its metabolism would progressively reexpand the ICF and eventually overexpand it as hypotonic hyponatremia developed.

Unlike most cases of acute iatrogenic hyponatremia that are caused by the excessive administration of glucose-containing solutions, however (see above), serum osmolality in the TURS is usually normal to slightly increased when isotonic solutions are used.[67] Thus, the contribution of cerebral edema to the reported neurologic symptoms remains at issue. Only when hypotonicity supervenes will the ICF, including that of the brain, expand. Indeed, cerebral edema has not been found at autopsy in patients with the TURS in whom fluid overload of the lungs, liver, and kidneys was evident.[57,128] Some studies suggest that only patients with hypoosmolality have symptoms,[44,57] while other studies report hyponatremia and symptoms of TURS in the absence of a corresponding fall in serum osmolality.[23,89,176] When early hypotonicity occurs, the fall in serum osmolality may reflect the use of hypotonic (1.2% and 1.5%) glycine or mannitol.

Hyperkalemia is also a common finding in the TURS.[5,68,69,114] Potassium probably accompanies the early shift of water from the intracellular space and may also move extracellularly when glycine is taken up by cells. Multiple electrocardiographic changes have been reported when the serum sodium level decreased below 120 meq/liter. These changes include bradycardia, loss of P waves, nodal rhythm, ventricular tachycardia, widened QRS complexes, ST segment depression, and T-wave inversion.[67] Hyperkalemia may in fact contribute to these changes in conduction.

The direct toxicity of the ammonia generated from glycine metabolism may also contribute to the TURS-associated encephalopathy.[130,135,142] Studies have demonstrated that the degree of hyperammonemia induced by the intravenous infusion of glycine is much less reproducible than is the associated decline in serum sodium concentration. However, that the increased ammonia levels still correlated with the severity of malaise, nausea, and vomiting suggests that toxic glycine metabolites may be involved in the TURS.[69] Development of hyperammonemia is not a universal in finding patients undergoing bladder irrigation or even in those with mild TURS-related neurologic symptoms.

Therapy

The three prime parameters that direct the therapy of encephalopathic patients with the TURS are blood pressure, serum osmolality, and blood ammonia levels.

Blood pressure

Early hypertension may require nitroprusside and/or diuretic therapy. Standard measures should be employed to resuscitate the blood pressure of hypotensive patients. Therapy should be aimed at the cause of the hypertension, and the character of the fluid infused will be dictated by the serum osmolality and degree of hypovolemia or vasodilation.

Serum osmolality

Hypotonic hyponatremic patients have retained excessive amounts of water. Pain, narcotics, hypotension, hypoxia, and so on all powerfully stimulate the release of ADH, which in turn effects renal water retention. These nonosmotic stimuli can override the suppressive effects of hypotonic hyponatremia on the secretion of the hormone. The irrigant may have been hypotonic or, as in the case of glycine, the osmole may have been partially or totally metabolized, leaving solute-free water behind. The urine volume, osmolality, and electrolyte (sodium and potassium) levels should be closely followed. The urgency of therapy is dictated by the acute hypotonic expansion of the ICF, including brain cells. During an osmotic diuresis (mannitol- or glycine-induced) the urine osmolality approaches isotonicity (~300 mosmol/liter) and the urinary electrolyte concentration approximates that of 0.45% NaCl solution (i.e., the sum of the concentrations of sodium and potassium, ~ 70 meq/liter). This urine may be viewed as an admixture of equal parts of distilled water and 0.9% NaCl solution. The excreted mannitol, glycine, and so on inhibits renal tubular water reabsorption. Under normal conditions, sodium is actively reabsorbed proximally and water follows to maintain osmotic balance. The concentration of sodium in the lumen remains unchanged. In the presence of a poorly reabsorbed osmole like mannitol, active sodium reabsorption continues, but much less water is carried with it, as the water remains osmotically obligated to the unreabsorbable luminal mannitol. Thus, the luminal sodium concentration progressively declines, eventually impairing its further reabsorption. The amount of water excreted is defined by that which is obligated by the urinary nonelectrolyte and electrolyte solute.

Only the electrolyte and its associated water need be returned to the patient. In the absence of hemodynamic and pulmonary signs of congestion, patients *should not* be allowed to lose salt, but those with hypotonic hyponatremia *should* be allowed to lose water. Thus, the replacement of half the volume of excreted urine with 0.9% NaCl solution prevents salt loss but enables the patient to shed the unwanted solute (glycine, etc.) and water. If such a patient manifested signs of congestive heart failure but was undergoing a brisk diuresis, then a very slow infusion of 0.9% NaCl solution (i.e., a "keep-open" intravenous setup) would allow for excretion of salt, the absorbed solute (mannitol or glycine), and water. Use of judicious amounts of a loop diuretic will speed the process of recovery by increasing the volume of urine containing 0.45% NaCl solution. Although it requires measurement, the diuresis induced by loop-active agents generally makes urine approximate 0.45% NaCl solution. Should the urinary electrolyte concentration significantly differ from 0.45 percent saline solution, the electrolyte concentration of the intravenous solution should be changed to more closely match the character of the urine. Diuretic use is also important if the urine volume is less than 200 to 300 ml/h, regardless of whether signs or symptoms of intravascular congestion are present.

Hypertonic hyponatremia results from absorption of solute with a low proportion of water or when the osmotic diuresis provoked by absorption of isotonic irrigant causes urinary loss of more water than solute. Tissues, including the brain, shrink as intracellular water moves extracellularly, down its osmotic gradient. The osmotic diuresis ensures that water lost from cells is eventually excreted in the urine, causing a body water deficit. The therapeutic goal is to replace lost body water and stimulate the excretion of unwanted solute. Induction of a 250 to 500 ml/h 0.45% NaCl diuresis with furosemide and replacement of urine volume with an equal amount of 5% dextrose in water will accomplish the needed goals. This urine once again may be viewed as a mixture of equal amounts of water and normal saline solution. Unwanted mannitol or glycine and sodium will be lost, while the overreplacement of water reduces serum osmolality. As the serum osmolality decreases below 290 mosm/liter, urinary volume should be replaced with 0.45% NaCl solution. During the latter phase of therapy, the content of body water and salt are preserved, while the mannitol or glycine is excreted.

Isotonic hyponatremia is reflected by a low serum concentration but a normal serum osmolality. The absorbed solution is isotonic but free of sodium. The mannitol or glycine (at least transiently) entraps its accompanying water in the ECF space. Replacement of urine volume with 0.45% NaCl solution will allow for removal of the solute while maintaining body stores of salt and water. Loop-active diuretics should be used to ensure a sustained excretion of 250 to 500 ml/h.

Blood ammonia

As noted, severe increases in blood ammonia levels often accompany TURS.[130,135,142] While the causal relationship of hyperammonemia to the encephalopathy can be debated, certainly the accumulation of this potential cerebrotoxin should not be ignored. Accordingly, we use standard methods of acutely reducing the body burden of ammonia in clearly encephalopathic patients.

The optimal treatment of the TURS is its prevention. Fluid absorbed is reduced by limiting resection times and minimizing irrigation fluid pressure. Initial suggestions that maintaining the irrigating fluid bag at a level less than 60 cm above the operating table[99] would minimize absorption appear unfounded, but the practice remains widespread. Close intraoperative monitoring of vital signs and periodic measurement of serum sodium levels should be routinely done in all cases. Patients with preexisting cardiac or renal disease should be considered high risk and therefore should undergo CVP measurements, if not full hemodynamic monitoring, during the procedure. With recognition of early signs and symptoms of the TURS and its treatment as outlined above, advanced stages of encephalopathy and cardiovascular collapse are avoidable. In addition, *ethanol monitoring* of expired breath in patients undergoing TURP given irrigant fluid marked by 1% ethanol is now being used in some institutions to measure ongoing volumetric uptake of irrigant and reflect the level of hyponatremia.[64,79,80] Complications relative to ethanol intoxication of further elevation of blood ammonia levels have not been observed.

CARDIAC SURGERY

Maintaining physiologic homeostasis in the patient undergoing cardiopulmonary bypass (CPB) presents a unique challenge to the anesthesiologist, perfusionist, and cardiac surgeon. The substitution of cardiac output by nonpulsatile circulation at relatively low flow rates (50 ml/kg) and mean pressures (40–60 mmHg)[166] circumvents, and thus impairs, the normal renal and pulmonary mechanisms of acid-base and electrolyte regulation. Hemodilution by priming solutions, hypothermia (28–32°C), hyperkalemic cardioplegic solutions, disordered release of vasoactive hormones, and damage to blood elements by mechanical shear stress or oxygenator membrane interactions may further increase the risk of metabolic or volume derangements. Additional disorders may also result in the postoperative period from CPB-associated cardiac or renal dysfunction.

The extracorporeal circuit is commonly primed with 1500 to 2500 ml of isotonic crystalloid solution, decreasing the hematocrit to 20 to 30 percent. Hemodilution beneficially offsets the increases in blood viscosity caused by hypothermia, although excessive dilution (hematocrits < 18–20%) may cause subendocardial or renal ischemia.[88] Because increased capillary permeability may result in extravascular fluid accumulation of up to 7 kg during CPB, some have advocated the use of asanguinous colloid priming solutions (albumin or hetastarch) to better maintain intravascular volume, minimize the need for volume replacement, and reduce the potential for cardiac and respiratory dysfunction from interstitial edema. Succinyl-linked gelatin increases colloid oncotic pressure more effectively than 20% albumin in a balanced (Hartman's) electrolyte solution[75] and reduces the need for additional priming volume by 500 ml. No improvement in outcome from the use of colloid priming solution has yet been demonstrated.

The potential for electrolyte disturbances during and after CPB is especially high. Hyperkalemic cardioplegic solution (15–30 meq KCl per liter) is infused into the aortic root following cross-clamping to induce sustained asystole, and with periodic reinfusions, the cummulative load may total 1 liter. Despite this, Bhatt[26] reported the requirement for 9 mmol/m^2 per hour KCl infusion during CPB and 1.5 mmol/m^2 per hour postoperatively to maintain normokalemia. Much of the replacement was required to compensate for cellular uptake of the cation promoted by increased circulating levels of catecholamines. Only one-third of the "lost" potassium could be accounted for by urinary excretion. Babka[18] also noted the need for significant amounts of potassium replacement (averaging 106 meq during CPB and 258 meq during the first 24 h following the onset of CPB) and related inadequate potassium replacement to the frequency of ventricular arrhythmias. Potassium replacement may be delivered by slow infusion into the extracorporeal circulation or by intermittent bolus injections of 33 μeq/kg via a central venous catheter.[101] The preoperative use of nonselective beta-blockers has been associated with intraoperative hyperkalemia[24] due to prevention of beta 2-mediated uptake of potassium by muscles. Severe hyperkalemia has also been reported following the postoperative use of glucose-insulin-potassium solutions for inotropic support,[27] in diabetics,[165] and in patients with renal insufficiency. Kopman[91] found that scavenging cardioplegic solution from the right atrium by a suction catheter prevented hyperkalemia in hemodialysis patients undergoing CPB.

Hypernatremia, although uncommon following CPB, has been reported in a subset of patients undergoing tricuspid valve replacement.[159] Prior to surgery, these patients frequently exhibit dilutional hyponatremia. This inability to excrete adequate quantities of free water is mediated in part by high ADH levels, which arises from nonosmotic stimulation of baroceptors located in the left heart.[59] Following the correction of valvular heart disease, the increased cardiac output acutely inhibits nonosmotic ADH release, and prompt water diuresis ensues. Some patients continue to elaborate inappropriately dilute urine despite the eventual development of frank hypernatremia. The latter should have provided an osmotic stimulus for the release of ADH. This "cardiac" diabetes insipidus usually resolves spontaneously in approximately 3 to 4 days postoperatively and can be treated by administering adequate amounts of free water during this period.

In contrast, hyponatremia has been reported following mitral commissurotomy, which might be expected when left atrial baroceptors are stimulated to increase hypothalamic ADH production by a sudden decrease in left atrial size and pressure.[144] This sudden reduction in left atrial volume is "misread" as volume contraction, stimulating the release of ADH. Hyperosmolar hyponatremia as a consequence of hyperglycemia may also be observed following CPB, during which serum glucose may range between 300 and 600 mg/dl even in nondiabetic patients. CPB is associated with delayed metabolism of a glucose load, explained by increased hepatic glucose production, decreased glucose clearance and utilization, and insufficient (although significant) insulin release. Hypothermic CPB, the usual clinical circumstance, virtually stops both basal and stimulated pancreatic insulin release.[93,94] Exogenous insulin, however, is generally given only to diabetic patients because blood glucose normalizes quickly after CPB in nondiabetics.[166] Because of insulin resistance induced by increased circulating levels of catecholamines, glucagon, growth hormone, and cortisol, treatment of the hyperglycemia when indicated often requires high doses of insulin.

Significant derangements of divalent mineral ion metabolism are also common following CPB. Two prospective studies[1,51] have identified hypomagnesemia in over 15 percent of patients pre-CPB and in more than 70 percent of patients during or after CPB. Furthermore, hypomagnesemia was associated with an increased risk of atrial and ventricular dysrhythmias and prolonged mechanical ventilatory support,[1,51] which was decreased by prophylactic administration of 2 g of $MgCl_2$ after the termination of CPB.[51]

Decreases in colloid osmotic pressure and plasma albumin concentration arising from hemodilution during CPB not only cause predictable reductions in protein-bound plasma calcium[87] but also in ionized calcium.[82] Many have been concerned that in patients with poor ventricular function, hypocalcemia might increase the risk of digitalis toxicity or pulmonary edema or worsen the negative inotropic effects of calcium channel blockers. However, Auffant[13] was unable to demonstrate any significant hemodynamic effect from the degree of hypocalcemia seen following CPB (ionized calcium averaged $\sim 1.6 \pm 0.14$ meq/liter). The serum calcium appears to quickly and spontaneously return to normal once CPB is terminated.[129] The use of calcium chloride for inotropic support after emerging from CPB is controversial, with some advocating its use[140] and many others reporting it ineffective[133] or even hazardous.[96]

The major *acid-base disturbance* associated with CPB is lactic acidosis. In uncomplicated cases, a minor increase in serum lactate levels occurs during CPB, peaks at approximately 3 to 4 meq/liter several hours after surgery, and returns to normal by 18 h.[11] Although lactate production presumably arises from a disparity between tissue oxygen supply and demand, serum lactate levels correlated positively with cardiac output in low-risk, uncomplicated patients. This may be explainable by some combination of postoperative hypermetabolism, decreased oxygen delivery (e.g., from anemia), increased tissue washout of lactate during rewarming, and peripheral arteriovenous shunting. The adequacy of tissue perfusion (and hence the degree of lactic acidosis) is determined by multiple factors, including alterations in blood volume, vascular tone, cardiac output, hematocrit, duration of CPB, and body temperature. Swan[156] has advocated monitoring mixed venous P_{O_2} during CPB to detect inadequate tissue perfusion. While bicarbonate therapy is not generally required in routine cases, significant acidemia requiring correction may occur during prolonged CPB or in high-risk patients with poor left ventricular function after bypass. Phentolamine has been reported to produce more uniform patterns of rewarming and thereby to reduce blood lactate levels and bicarbonate requirements following CPB.[32]

POSTOPERATIVE MANAGEMENT OF FLUID, ELECTROLYTE, AND ACID-BASE DISORDERS

The patient who has received appropriate preoperative and intraoperative fluid and electrolyte therapy should enter the postoperative period euvolemic and in relatively normal metabolic balance. Disturbances of electrolyte, acid-base, and volume homeostasis in the postoperative patient can often be prevented by carefully monitoring intake and output, appropriately replacing net losses, and anticipating intracompartmental shifts. The likelihood of electrolyte and acid-base imbalance during this period is increased by the inability to tolerate oral nutrition and fluids, the need for administering intravenous fluids or parenteral nutrition, loss of gastrointestinal or other body fluids, acute renal failure, and postoperative infection, among other generally unpleasant complications. When metabolic disorders do occur postoperatively, their correction follows treatment guidelines applicable to the general medical patient, and they have been outlined in earlier sections of this chapter.

EXTRACELLULAR FLUID AND ELECTROLYTES

Postoperatively, the patient has numerous potential sources of electrolyte and water loss, which requires replacement to maintain hemodynamic and metabolic stability. The sources and variable magnitudes of water and sodium gain and loss in the normal state and in pathologic conditions are shown in Table 43-3. During the first several days after major abdominal or thoracic surgery, water gain is likely to consist of only intravenous fluids and water produced by cellular catabolism (up to 500 ml/day). Water losses consist of the usual sensible and insensible sources (except for the absence of pulmonary loss in patients breathing humidified air) as well as losses unique to the surgical patient. The patient who is febrile or hyperventilating and not breathing humidified air may lose liters of water each day. The major source of additional volume loss in the surgical patient is the loss of blood, lymph, urine, or gastrointestinal fluids through vomiting, diarrhea, catheters, drains, or open wounds. The volume and electrolyte content of these losses can usually be measured or estimated (Table 43-5) and appropriate replacement given. In general, in the absence of heart or renal failure gastric fluid is replaced as 0.45% NaCl solution with 20 to 40 meq/liter of added KCl. Because potassium losses sustained during gastric suction occur via the kidney, patients without renal function, undergoing nasogastric suction or vomiting, may not require potassium replacement. Loss of large volumes of acidic gastric secretions may generate a metabolic alkalosis, especially if cardiac or renal disease prevents the administration of adequate amounts of sodium and potassium. This risk can be minimized by the prophylactic use of cimetidine or other inhibitors of gastric acid secretion. Alkaline body fluid losses (e.g., bile and pancreatic fluid) require replacement with hypotonic saline solution to which appropriate concentrations of sodium bicarbonate and KCl have been added.

The more difficult assessment of fluid loss is that due to sequestration into the interstitial compartment. The patient with intestinal obstruction may accumulate as much as 6 liters of isotonic fluid in the bowel wall and lumen. Major burns and peritonitis are also associated with large third-space losses. This sequestered fluid is generally recaptured by the systemic circulation within 2 to 3 days following the surgery. Summation of fluid returning from the third space with that recently administered may cause circulatory overload, especially in patients with cardiac and/or renal failure. In contrast, patients with septic shock may continue to experience capillary leak with accumulation of interstitial water in

TABLE 43-5 • Volume and composition of gastrointestinal secretions

Secretion	Volume, ml/24 h	$[Na^+]$ meq/liter	$[K^+]$ meq/liter	$[Cl^-]$ meq/liter	$[HCO_3^-]$ meq/liter
Saliva	1500 (500–2000)	10 (2–10)	26 (20–30)	10 (8–18)	30
Gastric	1500 (100–4000)	60 (9–116)	10 (0–32)	130 (8–154)	0
Duodenal	(100–2000)	140	5	80	0
Ileal	3000 (100–9000)	140 (80–150)	5 (2–8)	104 (43–137)	30
Colonic		60	30	40	0
Pancreatic	Variable (100–800)	140 (113–185)	5 (3–7)	75 (54–95)	115
Bile	Variable (50–800)	145 (131–164)	5 (3–12)	100 (89–180)	35

NOTE: Values in parentheses represent ranges.

the lung and other peripheral tissues until the underlying causes of sepsis are addressed. Fluid replacement in this setting is particularly controversial (see below and Chap. 45).

FLUID THERAPY DURING SEPSIS

The "sepsis syndrome" is generally defined by fever or hypothermia, tachycardia, tachypnea, and "organ hypoperfusion" (encephalopathy, hypoxemia, oliguria, or lactic acidosis) in the setting of a known or suspected infection.[125] It is often recognized only after the overt development of hypotension, or "shock." Fluid resuscitation of septic shock requires continuous monitoring of arterial blood pressure and PCWP as well as periodic evaluations of cardiac output and arterial and venous blood gases. Attempts to lower the high mortality of this syndrome (40–50 percent) have spawned major differences of opinion with regard to which specific goals should be pursued, how progress toward the desired hemodynamic goals should be monitored, and which types of fluid are most likely to bring about these improvements.

The cardiac output in septic shock is typically increased by the associated tachycardia and decreased peripheral vascular resistance. However, decreases in left ventricular stroke work index may develop from sepsis-induced myocardial depression and decreased effective circulating blood volume. The latter is usually caused by increased microvascular permeability and peripheral and hepatosplanchnic pooling. Tissue hypoperfusion is further aggravated by increased energy expenditure during sepsis, mediated by such cytokines as tumor necrosis factor and interleukin and by release of catecholamines, corticosteroids, and glucagon. This imbalance between oxygen supply and demand produces inadequate tissue perfusion and thereby stimulates anaerobic metabolism, with resulting lactic acidosis and multiple organ failure. However, the concomitance of a high cardiac output, reduced oxygen consumption, and increased mixed venous oxygen saturation suggests that impaired oxygen extraction and utilization contribute to tissue hypoxia. Impairment in oxygen utilization could result from abnormal autoregulation, regional blood flow imbalance, shunting, and capillary microthrombi.[125]

The hemodynamic goals of therapy are aimed at enhancing tissue oxygen delivery by simultaneously improving many of the forces that regulate this critical parameter. Oxygen delivery can be enhanced by increasing cardiac output, blood pressure, hemoglobin concentration, and oxygen saturation. Aggressive volume resuscitation (averaging 2 liters of colloid and 4–6 liters of crystalloid) is an essential component of early management, and often produces significant clinical improvement.[12,86] Improvements following the infusion of packed red blood cells to maintain the hematocrit between 30 and 35%[131] are also consistent with this model. The beta-adrenergic agonist dobutamine to increase cardiac output is also employed in hopes of increasing tissue perfusion, although the benefits of using other catecholamines (dopamine, norepinephrine, or phenylephrine) with alpha-adrenergic activity to increase blood pressure are uncertain[58,134] because of their potential for further decreasing tissue perfusion by vasoconstriction.

The fluids generally available for therapeutic administration consist of either crystalloids[63] (electrolyte and dextrose solutions in water) or colloids (e.g., blood products, albumin, hetastarch, and dextrans). Since sodium is restricted to the extracellular space, three-quarters of which is interstitial and one-quarter of which is intravascular, 30 min after infusion of 1 liter of 0.9% NaCl, only 250 ml remain in the intravascular compartment. Colloids, owing to their larger molecular weights, cross capillary walls much more slowly and tend to remain in the intravascular space for longer periods. In addition, the oncotic properties of colloids may further expand intravascular volume by drawing fluid in from the interstitial to the intravascular compartment. Crystalloids may decrease plasma oncotic pressure by hemodilution and thereby adversely affect the vascular-interstitial distribution of volume. As a result, in patients with normal vascular permeability, the volume of crystalloid required to achieve a pulmonary wedge pressure of 15 was 1.5 to 4 times greater than that of colloid (5% albumin or 6% hetastarch).[124] Thus, potential advantages of colloid solutions are that equivalent increases in intravascular volume are longer lasting and are achieved with less interstitial leakage.[73] However, as vascular permeability to colloids increases in the sepsis syndrome, the advantages of larger–molecular weight solutes may be lost.

Metildi[104] found more severe pulmonary edema in patients with adult respiratory distress syndrome (ARDS) given crystalloids when equivalent volumes of crystalloid and colloid were given, but eventual clinical outcomes were almost identical and the results in septic shock have been similar.[124] Other studies provide no evidence that crystalloids have adverse pulmonary effects in ARDS[9,74] or sepsis.[58,72] However, excessive increases in PCWP produced by either crystalloid or colloid administration may produce undesirable increases in extravascular lung water.[50,145,146] Thus, the usual goal of fluid therapy in sepsis is to find an optimal pulmonary capillary wedge pressure, which sufficiently increases cardiac output, oxygen delivery, and oxygen consumption while avoiding pulmonary edema. This optimal pressure has been reported to be 12 mmHg in sepsis (as opposed to 18 mmHg in cardiogenic shock).[116]

While volume loading is often successful in early sepsis, for reasons discussed above, the unfortunate practice in some intensive care units is to continue treating refractory septic shock with ever-increasing amounts of fluid in a futile attempt to maximize oxygen delivery to supranormal levels at the expense of severe increases in extravascular lung and interstitial volumes. It is not uncommon in that setting to see massively edematous patients who have accumulated 20 to 30 liters of extra fluid still receiving high rates of volume infusion.

While disagreement exists, on balance, no clear relationship has been demonstrated between lactate levels and the response to fluid resuscitation.[107] "Delivery-dependent" oxygen consumption[78] has only been reported in pulmonary vascular disease, obstructive sleep apnea, and liver disease. In addition, when oxygen consumption was calculated during sepsis from inspired and expired gases, no clear relationship could be demonstrated with induced changes in cardiac output.[161] Finally, when oxygen utilization is increased by induced changes in cardiac output and blood flow to certain organs, it may actually be the increased "tissue work" that drives the enhanced consumption.[78] Asymmetrical delivery of oxygen to tissues and the ratio of oxygen need to availability may still be compromised. In conclusion, while most septic patients do require volume resuscitation initially, it should be continued only as long as clear-cut increases in oxygen delivery and consumption (measured independently by inhaled and exhaled gases) can be demonstrated. The patient with refractory sepsis who has undergone initial volume replacement and has achieved a PCWP $>$ 12 mmHg is more likely to benefit from catecholamine infusions in conjunction with correction of the underlying cause of infection (see Chap. 45).

ENTERAL AND PARENTERAL NUTRITION

The patient who is unable to orally consume an adequate and balanced diet is at risk for developing a variety of acid-base and electrolyte disorders. Inadequate intake coupled with ongoing urinary, fecal, and other body fluid losses generate these chemical abnormalities. Other disorders may develop when excessive amounts of water, minerals, glucose, or base equivalents are administered with enteral or parenteral nutrition.

Patients with normal renal, cardiac, and hepatic function receiving adequate calories through standard enteral supplements designed to be nutritionally complete receive amounts of minerals and trace elements generally sufficient to prevent significant nutritional deficiencies or serious electrolyte and acid-base disorders. However, the low sodium concentration (20–50 meq/liter) of standard enteral supplements may predispose patients with impaired free water clearance (including patients with renal, cardiac, and hepatic insufficiency) to hyponatremia. If free water clearance cannot be increased or if excess free water intake is unavoidable, the addition of supplemental sodium chloride to these solutions may be helpful. In contrast, hypernatremia may be seen if diarrhea or protein-induced osmotic (i.e., urea) diuresis produces large water losses that are inadequately replaced. The potassium content of standard supplements (30–50 meq/liter) may also cause hyperkalemia in patients with renal insufficiency.

The patient unable to take oral feedings for prolonged periods of time is at higher risk of developing nutritional deficiencies. Total parenteral hyperalimentation (TPN) is generally considered when previously healthy patients remain without oral intake for periods exceeding 1 week but may be employed earlier in highly catabolic conditions, including acute renal failure, septic shock, major burns, or major trauma or in the chronically malnourished surgical patient. Fluid and electrolyte complications of TPN were relatively common when the importance of trace elements was not widely acknowledged.[167] Now that standard TPN prescriptions are used, the chemical complications are more likely to result from underlying illnesses than directly from TPN (see Chap. 44). When electrolyte disorders occur in patients on TPN, they are treated according to the general principles outlined earlier in this chapter and in other chapters of this book focusing on those specific disorders.

PERIOPERATIVE MANAGEMENT OF SPECIFIC CONDITIONS

HYPERTENSION

Uncontrolled hypertension is a confirmed risk factor for perioperative mortality in general and for myocardial infarction specifically.[28] Lesser degrees of hypertension do not appear to increase risk per se, but hypertensive patients may face greater risks of cardiac and cerebral ischemia during transient hypotension because of coexistent vascular disease and impaired autoregulation of tissue blood flow.[121,155] Severe postoperative hypertension also increases the risk for adverse cardiovascular and surgical complications. It follows that most antihypertensive medications should be continued and, indeed, given the morning of surgery to prevent dangerous increments in blood pressure during endotracheal intubation, induction of anesthesia, and the postoperative period. Diuretics, when used primarily for hypertension, are the major exception to this rule and should be stopped several days before surgery to prevent the increased risk of hypotension from volume depletion. However, the presence of congestive heart failure, nephrotic syndrome, or other edematous conditions may necessitate the ongoing preoperative administration of diuretics. The sudden withdrawal of centrally acting adrenergic antagonists (e.g., clonidine or methyldopa), especially when taken in large doses, is particularly dangerous because rebound autonomic hyperactivity may occur causing severe increases in blood pressure.[20,169] Abrupt beta-blocker withdrawal may precipitate unstable angina or myocardial infarction.[4,29]

Difficulty in maintaining control of blood pressure is often encountered when oral antihypertensive medications cannot be taken postoperatively. During this period, parenteral forms of the same drug should be substituted when possible, or another drug of the same class may be used. Antihypertensive medications available in the United States in parenteral form include beta-blockers (propranolol, labetolol, esmolol, and timolol), angiotensin-converting enzyme inhibitors (enaliprilat), centrally acting agents (methyldopa), and vasodilators (hydralazine). Another useful strategy is to convert the patient taking an alpha 2 agonist (clonidine or guanfacine) to an equivalent dose of transcutaneous clonidine (the "patch"). Switching to the patch must be done 36 to 48 h preoperatively because of the time required for transcutaneous absorption. During this interval, the oral clonidine should be continued. Similarly, the fact that the hypotensive effect of the clonidine patch wears off slowly (36–48 h after removal) must be kept in mind when oral therapy is resumed. Nifedipine, although not available parenterally, is rapidly absorbed from the stomach in its capsular form and can be given via nasogastric tube if gastric absorption is intact.

Although almost unfailingly effective at lowering blood pressure, the use of a sodium nitroprusside infusion is usually reserved for medical-surgical crises (e.g., subarachnoid hemorrhage, dissecting aortic aneurysm, or malignant hypertension) or for hypertension that is refractory to almost all other therapy. The drug is also very useful in those patients in whom minute-to-minute control of blood pressure is very important. For example, metastable surgical patients with hypertension and known cerebrovascular and/or coronary artery disease often are best managed with an antihypertensive agent that has a very rapid onset and termination of action. Simply slowing or discontinuing the infusion prevents the blood pressure from falling to values outside the desired therapeutic range and thereby protects tissue perfusion. Very undesirable wide swings in pressure seen with longer-acting agents can be avoided with nitroprusside. The continuous infusion of nitroprusside requires observation in an intensive care setting and continuous arterial pressure monitoring. By disproportionately dilating normal coronary arteries and causing reflex tachycardia, nitroprusside may lead to a "coronary steal" syndrome and worsened myocardial ischemia in marginally perfused areas. Patients with renal or hepatic insufficiency who are receiving the agent (>2 μg/kg per minute) also face the risk of cyanide toxicity.[162] Cyanide is released from the nitroprusside radical formed when electrons from hemoglobin are nonemzymatically transferred to nitroprusside. The cyanide then either binds to tissue cytochrome-c oxidase or is metabolized to the less toxic thiocyanate. When toxicity occurs, serum thiocyanate levels usually exceed 10 mg/dl. This toxicity may be prevented in patients at risk by either mixing 10 mg sodium thiosulfate[117] with each milligram of nitroprusside to hasten cyanide metabolism to thiocyanate or by administering 25 mg/h of hydroxocobalamin[38] to bind cyanide, converting it to the harmless cyanocobalamin. Although either method is effective with good renal function, the latter is preferable when hepatic disease limits cyanide metabolism to thiocyanate or renal insufficiency limits thiocyanate excretion.

PHEOCHROMOCYTOMA

Pheochromocytoma is a catecholamine-secreting neoplasm most frequently (90 percent) located in the adrenal gland and rarely (10 percent) malignant. Persistent or episodic hypertension associated with norepinephrine release is most common, but occasionally patients may experience hypotension from vasodilatory, beta-adrenergic effects of secreted epinephine. General anesthesia, surgery, and labor and delivery can precipitate life-threatening medical crises in the patient with an unsuspected pheochromocytoma.

Resection of a pheochromocytoma was associated with 30 to 45 percent perioperative mortality. Although improved diagnostic capabilities, and understanding of the relevant physiology and pharmacology have greatly reduced the perioperative risk, careful preoperative preparation, intraoperative monitoring, and prompt treatment of hemodynamic instability are still required to minimize the risks of hypertensive crises or severe hypotension following the removal of the tumor. The reader is referred to several recent reviews[31,141,143] for detailed discussions of the clinical features, diagnostic strategies, and therapeutic approaches to such patients. This chapter focuses on the acute medical and pharmacologic management of the patient with a previously diagnosed pheochromocytoma who is undergoing surgical resection.

As a result of severe hypertension that may have been present for many years before diagnosis, the patient with pheochromocytoma may suffer from chronic renal failure, hypertensive or ischemic cardiomyopathy, coronary artery disease, or cerebrovascular disease, all of which render the anticipated surgery more complicated and influence perioperative management, as discussed earlier in this chapter. Because catecholamine excess inhibits insulin secretion and promotes gluconeogenesis and glycolysis, a clinical picture of diabetes mellitus may mislead physicians. Approximately 6 percent of patients with pheochromocytoma have a familial disorder that includes multiple endocrine neoplasia (MEN) type II (medullary carcinoma of the thyroid, hyperparathyroidism, or Cushing's syndrome) or type III (neuromas or medullary carcinoma) or neurofibromatosis. Adrenocortical insufficiency has also been occasionally been found. These other medical disorders must be detected preoperatively and their corresponding metabolic derangements corrected. The major risks of surgery in the untreated patient are severe hypertensive crisis and ventricular arrhythmias. These cardiovascular complications may be precipitated by anesthesia, surgery, angiography, or certain medications (e.g., glucagon, metoclopramide, or morphine) that provoke catecholamine release or inhibit the neural uptake of the hormones (e.g., droperidol or phenothiazines). Significant hypotension may also ensue when catecholamine levels suddenly decrease following tumor resection and may be exacerbated by an associated volume depletion, adrenergic receptor down-regulation, antihypertensive drugs, and adrenal insufficiency. Rebound hypoglycemia can occur in patients with catecholamine-induced diabetes.

Pharmacologic therapy is a critical component for a successful outcome.[141] Preoperative alpha-adrenergic blockade titrated to supine or sitting normotension, if tolerated, is widely recommended. Phenoxybenzamine, a nonselective oral alpha-antagonist, has been most extensively used. An initial dose of 10 mg twice daily is usually effective but may be cautiously increased as necessary to a total daily dose of 40 to 100 mg. Alternatives include selective alpha 1-antagonists such as prazosin, using 3 to 12 mg daily or a combined alpha- and beta-blocker such as labetalol. Beta-blockers are contraindicated unless preceded by alpha-adrenergic blockade to avoid severe vasoconstriction and hypertensive crisis, which may be precipitated by unopposed alpha-adrenergic receptor stimulation. Beta-blockers are not routinely used but may be required for the management of tachycardia or coronary artery disease. Calcium channel blockers may also be useful in controlling preoperative hypertension.

Continuous intraoperative monitoring of arterial blood pressure, urine output, oxygen saturation, and cardiac parameters and periodic determinations of electrolytes, glucose, hematocrit, and arterial blood gases are always required. Reliable assessment of intravascular volume is also critical for rapid, effective treatment of hypotension should it occur. A central venous catheter may suffice for this purpose in patients with good cardiac function, but a pulmonary artery catheter should be employed routinely when significant myocardial dysfunction makes central venous pressure an unreliable measure of left ventricular pressures.

Phentolamine, an intravenous nonselective alpha-antagonist (given by boluses of 2–5 mg or continuous infusion), intravenous labetolol, or sodium nitroprusside may be used to treat severe intraoperative hypertension, which may occur despite reasonable preoperative preparation. Tachyarrhythmias may be treated with beta-blockers, while ventricular arrhythmias usually respond well to lidocaine. Hypotension may necessitate resuscitation with rapid infusions of saline solution or colloid if decreases in peripheral resistance cause relative hypovolemia, while blood or other colloids may be required if actual hypovolemia ensues from significant blood loss. Glucose-containing solutions are usually reserved for the postoperative period when hypoglycemia is most likely. Profound hypotension may require parenteral norepinephrine until other measures take effect. Continued hemodynamic monitoring and careful maintenance of optimal intravascular volume is required in the immediate postoperative period when hypotension is still common. Residual hypertension remains in one-third of patients.

DIABETES INSIPIDUS

Stable patients who are either deficient in ADH production ("central" diabetes insipidus, or DI) or resistant to its renal action ("nephrogenic" DI) have a normal or slightly elevated serum sodium concentration and a normal to slightly decreased plasma volume. Causes of DI are discussed further in Chaps. 4, 5, and 21. In untreated DI, the combination of hypovolemia-induced proximal sodium reabsorption and marked reduction of collecting duct water reabsorption causes the excretion of large quantities of nearly electrolyte-free, dilute urine. Nearly normal serum sodium levels and osmolality can usually be maintained in DI by thirst-driven voluntary water intake. The delivery of glomerular filtrate to the ADH-responsive sites in the distal nephron can be reduced in two ways in patients with DI. Solute restriction encourages proximal salt reabsorption, thereby eliminating distal delivery. Thiazide diuretics induce mild ECF volume contraction, which in turn stimulates proximal sodium and water reabsorption and simultaneously inhibits urinary dilution. Both of these therapies diminish loss of electrolyte-free water and are used when treating patients with nephrogenic DI. In addition, chronic replacement of the hormone with long-acting preparations such as subcutaneous vasopressin tannate (2–5 units every 24 to 72 h) or desmopressin acetate (DDAVP) nasal spray (5–20 μg every 12 to 24 h) is required in many cases of central DI. During the perioperative period, such patients should be converted to the shorter-acting aqueous vasopressin (5–10 units every 4 to 6 h) to permit titration of dosing according to volume status and serum sodium concentration. Five units of the hormone should be added to 1 liter of 5% dextrose and infused at a rate that limits urine volume to 50 to 100 ml/h. By discontinuing the short-acting preparation, iatrogenically induced hyponatremia can be rapidly corrected. Care must be taken to administer adequate amounts of free water to those patients unable to take it by mouth. In addition, although body fluid losses require replacement, excessive administration of saline solution unnecessarily increases obligate water loss and should be avoided.

A distinction should be made between true nephrogenic DI, attributable to hereditary or acquired disorders affecting the cellular response of the collecting duct to ADH, and "salt-losing nephritis." The latter reflects the inability to appropriately concentrate urine and to reduce urine sodium values during conditions of volume depletion or salt restriction. Salt-losing nephritis can be a feature of any type of chronic tubulointerstitial renal disease and is most likely to become symptomatic during periods of salt restriction. Profound degrees of volume depletion may occur rapidly. NaCl replacement should be generous in this setting, unlike the protocol for true DI. Some patients with salt-losing nephritis may also have a chronic hyperchloremic, hyperkalemic, normal anion gap metabolic acidosis which is markedly worsened by volume depletion.

SECONDARY HYPERPARATHYROIDISM

The patient with renal failure undergoing parathyroidectomy for severe secondary hyperparathyroidism is susceptible to profound postoperative hypocalcemia. This "hungry bone syndrome" results from the sudden and massive uptake of calcium, phosphate, and carbonates by the mineral-depleted bone. Hypophosphatemia and hypobicarbonatemia often accompany the hypocalcemia. Therapy with phosphorus and bicarbonate must be approached very cautiously. Binding and precipitation of administered phosphorus with an already low serum calcium concentration could drastically worsen hypocalcemia. Similarly, alkali infusions may further reduce the ionized fraction of serum calcium and so worsen tertany. In the face of hypocalcemia, therapy with phosphorus and bicarbonate should be withheld unless the former decreases below 2.0 to 2.5 mg/dl or the latter to values below 18 meq/liter and arterial pH values below 7.30. Oral administration of 1 to 2 μg/day of calcitriol (1,25-dihydroxycholecalciferol) for 1 to 2 weeks prior to surgery lessens or prevents postoperative hypocalcemia, perhaps by allowing bone remineralization to begin gradually through some combination of a direct suppressive effect on parathyroid hormone secretion or increased availability of calcium and phosphate from their augmented intestinal absorption. Hypercalcemic patients should be treated preoperatively with intravenous calcitriol, which is less likely to worsen hypercalcemia because of its short half-life. Postoperatively, the dose requirement of oral calcitriol is approximately 1 μg/day for each desired milligram per deciliter rise in serum total calcium. This is continued with 1500 to 2000 mg of elemental calcium daily until a normal serum calcium level is obtained, after which calcitriol can be decreased to approximately 1 μg/day. Intravenous calcium is reserved for patients with tetany or other significant hypocalcemic symptoms or signs.

DIABETES MELLITUS

The pre-, intra-, and postoperative stresses on the diabetic render the prevention of hyperglycemia challenging. However, tight control in these settings is to be avoided for fear of hypoglycemia. Acceptance of blood sugar levels in the range of 150 to 250 mg/dl is appropriate. Although approaches to glycemic control vary, most recommend that oral hypoglycemic agents be withheld preoperatively, with long-acting drugs such as chlorpropamide being discontinued several days before surgery. This is especially important in the patient with significant renal insufficiency. First-generation sulfonylureas depend on the kidney for excretion and should be avoided in patients with renal failure. Diabetics maintaining acceptable preoperative glycemic control with diet or hypoglycemic drugs alone are generally given glucose-free intravenous fluids the day of surgery and monitored by a glucometer every 6 h, with supplemental regular insulin given if required. Diabetics are susceptible to a variety of fluid electrolyte and acid-base disorders, and these must be anticipated in all such patients requiring surgery. Hyporeninemic hypoaldosteronism may present preoperatively as hyperkalemia and hyperchloremic metabolic acidosis. It usually appears in patients with mild-to-moderate renal insufficiency. Patients with diabetic nephropathy and advanced renal insufficiency (creatinine clearance <10–15 ml/min) may develop the characteristic "uremic," high anion gap acidosis. The internist or nephrologist needs no reminders regarding the possible appearance of ketoacidosis. Less well known, however, is the fact that acute diabetic ketoacidosis may cause such severe abdominal complaints as to suggest the presence of a "surgical abdomen." It is not rare for such patients to be first discovered on the surgical service.

Acute illness, general anesthesia, and surgery all contribute to elevated levels of catecholamines, glucagon, and cortisol; suppression of insulin release; and insulin resistance. These changes in the hormonal mileu, along with the fasting state, which accompanies surgery, result in increased glycolysis, proteolysis, gluconeogenesis, and lipolysis. In the insulinopenic diabetic, the increases in blood glucose and ketone body formation associated with this increased catabolism may precipitate diabetic ketoacidosis. Some recommend preoperative subcutaneous insulin for the insulin-requiring surgical patient, especially if hourly glucose monitoring is unavailable. The usual practice is to give one-third to one-half of the usual long-acting insulin (NPH or Lente) dosage, followed by intraoperative 5% dextrose and regular insulin supplementation as required. During short cases, a "no insulin, no glucose" protocol similar to that used in noninsulin-requiring patients may work but is not recommended.

The most reliable method of preventing perioperative acute metabolic disturbances in insulin-requiring diabetics, especially following major surgery, is the simultaneous administration of glucose and insulin. Without potassium replacement, urinary losses and intracellular shifts may lead to hypokalemia during this protocol. The simplest regimen is that of Alberti,[2] which calls for the preoperative and intraoperative infusion of 100 ml/h of a solution containing 20 meq/liter KCl and either 16 units of regular insulin in 1000 ml 5% dextrose or 32 units of insulin in 1000 ml of 10% dextrose. Blood glucose is analyzed every 2 h pre- and intraoperatively, with adjustments in insulin concentration of 2 to 8 units/liter made to maintain the blood glucose level at 150 to 250 mg/dl. This infusion can be continued postoperatively until oral intake can be resumed. The serum potassium concentration is rechecked after 6 h and daily if stable. When emergency surgery is required in patients with ketoacidosis, standard treatment with an infusion containing 0.9% NaCl solution, potassium, and "low-dose" insulin (0.1 units/kg per hour) without glucose is given until the blood sugar level decreases below 300 mg/dl. Afterwards, a glucose-insulin-potassium infusion can be administered, as described above.

The diabetic patient with renal insufficiency requires modifications of standard treatment protocols, in that the half-life of insulin is prolonged, thereby predisposing patients to hypoglycemia. Furthermore, their decreased GFR and tubular damage increase the risk of hyperkalemia, and large volumes of saline solution are more likely to cause circulatory overload in this setting. Patients receiving chronic hemodialysis are also susceptible to spontaneous, fasting hypoglycemia. It is probably best to avoid long-acting insulin in diabetic dialysis patients undergoing surgery. Subcutaneous dosing with regular insulin while infusing solutions containing 5% dextrose generally will suffice. If acidosis or more severe hyperglycemia develops, a continuous insulin and glucose infusion should be started. To avoid hypoglycemia, patients who normally require less than 30 units of insulin daily should be started on half of their usual dose. Potassium administration should be dictated by serum levels, which should be assayed every 2 to 4 h. Generally, potassium therapy is withheld in oliguric patients and those with a history of hyperkalemia unless serum levels decrease to values below 4.0 meq/liter.

RHABDOMYOLYSIS

Skeletal muscle damage caused by a wide variety of physical, toxic, infectious, ischemic, and metabolic insults may cause cell lysis and release of myoglobin into the systemic circulation. Crush injury of an extremity and ischemia to a limb from arterial thromboembolism are the most likely causes in surgical patients, although some nontraumatic causes may require surgical fasciotomy to prevent irreversible ischemic myonecrosis and nerve damage if associated muscle edema increases pressure in fascial compartments above 60 mmHg (compartment syndrome). Severe rhabdomyolysis is often accompanied by muscle tenderness, weakness, and/or swelling, but these signs and symptoms may be so mild as to be missed on physical examination. The extent of cell lysis is proportional to the elevation in creatinine kinase,[26] which is generally greater than 5000 IU in cases associated with renal failure or significant metabolic disturbance and serves as the most useful diagnostic measurement.

Acute renal failure may complicate as many as 15 percent of the cases of rhabdomyolysis.[164] Patients with rhabdomyolysis may sequester large amounts of salt and water in damaged muscle tissues, and vigorous fluid resuscitation with 0.9% NaCl solution (as much as 12 liters may be needed) may succeed in restoring urine output and preventing acute tubular necrosis (ATN), especially if given early. Many advocate the early use of intravenous furosemide and mannitol to prevent ATN by decreasing tubular oxygen consumption and preventing the formation of tubular casts. Sodium bicarbonate administration has also been advocated. Alkalinization of the urine may prevent or lessen the precipitation of heme-pigment derivatives and thereby reduce the risk of ATN. It must be remembered that when the GFR is greatly reduced and the filtered load of bicarbonate is low, it becomes difficult to raise urinary pH. Unless serum bicarbonate concentration and pH are followed during alkali infusions, severe degrees of alkalemia may be inadvertently created before the urinary pH rises.

The patient with rhabdomyolysis-induced acute renal failure is almost always severely catabolic and often oliguric, resulting in severe electrolyte and acid-base disturbances that require early and intensive dialysis. Hyperkalemia, emanating primarily from massive potassium leakage from damaged myocytes, may be profound and life-threatening. It may be exacerbated by the metabolic acidosis that also accompanies rhabdomyolysis because of lactic acidosis and/or release of mineral acids from damaged muscles. Relatively stable patients should be started on kayexalate prophylactically. Hyperkalemia is treated primarily by hemodialysis. Standard medical therapy (see "Hyperkalemia" above and Chap. 23) should be used to treat dangerous increases in serum potassium concentration (>6.0 meq/liter) while awaiting hemodialysis, especially since concurrent hypocalcemia (see below) may further increase the risk of serious arrhythmia. Deposition of calcium salts and bicarbonate in damaged muscle, however, may limit the effectiveness of medical therapy. Extreme cases may require dialysis two or three times daily. When such a patient requires emergent surgery for treatment of traumatic injuries or acute arterial occlusion, serum potassium levels must be measured hourly and intraoperatively hemodialysis employed if the serum potassium level rises above 6.0 meq/liter despite maximal medical therapy.

Hypocalcemia, common in rhabdomyolysis, results from widespread calcium deposition in muscle and from associated azotemia and hyperphosphatemia. Tetany is rare despite severely decreased serum calcium levels. The acidosis accompanying the rhabdomyolysis raises the concentration of the ionized fraction of the total serum calcium and thereby protects from tetany. During the recovery phase of ATN, significant *hypercalcemia* may develop as sequestered calcium is mobilized from healing muscle and as the abnormal vitamin D metabolism of uremia is corrected while secondary hyperparathyroidism continues. Because administered calcium during the period of established renal failure is likely to be quickly deposited in muscle and may predispose to the later appearance of hypercalcemia, calcium salts should be administered only to symptomatic patients or to those whose rate-corrected QT interval shows significant prolongation. It follows that the electrocardiogram should be monitored. However, hyperphosphatemia should be treated by dietary restriction, the use of aluminum-containing antacids, and occasionally infusing insulin and glucose (to enhance the cellular uptake of phosphorus).

ANEMIA

Current recommendations regarding preoperative red blood cell transfusions have been discussed above. In addition to the risk of transfusion-related hepatitis (and the currently insignificant risk of HIV infection in blood processed by modern blood banks), certain groups of patients are prone to developing cardiovascular or metabolic complications of the blood transfusion. The approximate volume of a unit of packed erythrocytes is 250 to 300 ml. Although this treatment is generally well tolerated, the potential for pulmonary edema exists in some patients with impaired cardiac function or those with a diminished capacity to excrete salt and water. Pulmonary edema can usually be avoided by administering an appropriate dose of intravenous furosemide between units in patients with adequate renal function. The patient with renal insufficiency is also at risk for posttransfusion hyperkalemia because each unit of packed red blood cells contains up to 4 to 8 meq of potassium, depending on storage techniques.[36] In the hemodialysis patient, transfusions are given during dialysis whenever possible to avoid these complications.

The patients at highest risk for profound metabolic complications from transfusion are those receiving large volumes of blood. The working definition of "massive transfusion" is the replacement of one to one and a half times the patient's blood volume (5–10 units) over periods varying between 1 and 24 h. Stored blood is made deliberately hyperglycemic, acidotic, and hyperphosphatemic to maximize adenosine triphosphate (ATP) production and erythrocyte viability. Citrate, the anticoagulant used in blood collection, complexes with ionized calcium. After separation, red blood cells are now more commonly stored in citrate-free electrolyte solutions that contain glucose, adenine, and mannitol. As red blood cells are stored for increasingly longer periods, anerobic glycolysis generates lactic acid and potassium leaks out of cells, thereby increasing potassium concentration to values that may approach 80 to 90 meq/liter.

Despite the changes in the chemical composition of stored blood, a number of mitigating factors minimize their physiologic effect. Citrate and lactate are metabolized by the liver to bicarbonate so that massively transfused patients are much more commonly alkalotic than acidotic,[37,84,97,105] and previously employed regimens of empiric bicarbonate replacement are now recognized as unnecessary and potentially hazardous. Citrate is so rapidly metabolized that infusion rates must exceed 1 unit of whole blood every 5 min to produce symptomatic hypocalcemia. Packed red blood cells, relatively free of plasma, contain even smaller amounts of citrate than does whole blood. Similarly, uptake of potassium by transfused red blood cells begins shortly after infusion, and massively transfused patients are frequently hypokalemic[35,33,97,139,175] and hypophosphatemic. Thus, although monitoring of serum potassium, glucose, ionized calcium, and arterial blood gases is clearly necessary during resuscitation by massive transfusion, prophylactic therapy to prevent metabolic abnormalities is unwarranted.

REFERENCES

1. Aglio LS et al: Hypomagnesemia is common following cardiac surgery. *J Cardiothorac Vasc Anesth* 5:201, 1991.
2. Alberti KGM, Thomas DJB: The management of diabetes during surgery. *Br J Anaesth* 51:693, 1979.
3. Albin MS: Anesthesia for neurosurgical procedures, in Grossman RG (ed): *Principles of Neurosurgery*. New York, Raven Press, 1991, p 1.
4. Alderman EL et al: Coronary artery syndrome after sudden propranolol withdrawal. *Ann Intern Med* 81:625, 1974.
5. Alexander JP et al: Glycine and transurethral resection. *Anaesthesia* 41:1198, 1986.
6. Allon M, Shanklin N: Adrenergic modulation of extrarenal potassium disposal in men with end-stage renal disease. *Kidney Int* 40:1103, 1991.
7. Allon M et al: Effect of insulin-plus glucose infusion with or without epinephrine on fasting hyperkalemia. *Kidney Int* 43:212, 1993.
8. Andrews BT et al: Cerebral salt wasting after pituitary

exploration and biopsy: Case report. *Neurosurgery* 18:469, 1986.
9. Appel PL, Shoemaker WC: Evaluation of fluid therapy in adult respiratory failure. *Crit Care Med* 9:862, 1981.
10. Arieff AI: Hyponatremia, convulsions, respiratory arrest, and permanent brain damage after elective surgery in healthy women. *N Engl J Med* 314:1529, 1986.
11. Ariza M et al: Blood lactate and mixed venous-arterial P_{CO_2} gradient as indices of poor peripheral perfusion following cardiopulmonary bypass surgery. *Intens Care Med* 17:320, 1991.
12. Astiz ME et al: Oxygen delivery and consumption in patients with hyperdynamic septic shock. *Crit Care Med* 15:26, 1987.
13. Auffant RA et al: Ionized calcium concentration and cardiovascular function after cardiopulmonary bypass. *Arch Surg* 116:1072, 1981.
14. Awald IA et al: Clinical vasospasm after subarachnoid hemorrhage: Response to hypervolemic hemodilution and arterial hypertension. *Stroke* 18:365, 1987.
15. Ayus JC et al: Treatment of symptomatic hyponatremia and its relation to brain damage. *N Engl J Med* 317:1190, 1987.
16. Ayus JC et al: Sexual differences in survival with severe symptomatic hyponatremia (abstract). *Kidney Int* 34: 108A, 1988.
17. Ayus JC, Arieff AI: Epidemiology of postoperative hyponatremic brain damage: Studies in 128,077 pediatric and adult subjects (abstract). *J Am Soc Nephrol* 3:324, 1992.
18. Babka R, Pifarre R: Potassium replacement during cardiopulmonary bypass. *J Thorac Cardiovasc Surg* 73:212, 1977.
19. Bakay L et al: The effects of intravenous fluid on cerebrospinal fluid pressure. *Surg Gynecol Obstet* 99:48, 1954.
20. Barley RR, Neale TJ: Rapid clonidine withdrawal with blood pressure overshot exaggerated by beta blockade. *Br Med J* 1:942, 1976.
21. Batra YK et al: Hyponatremia and mental symptoms following vesical ultrasound lithotripsy. *Anaesthesia* 43:675, 1988.
22. Benjamin J et al: Tissue oxygen delivery is stable despite rapid correction of chronic metabolic acidosis (abstract). *Kidney Int* 23:229, 1983.
23. Berg G et al: Physiologic observations related to the transurethral resection reaction. *J Urol* 87:596, 1962.
24. Bethune DW, McKay R: Paradoxical changes in serum potassium during cardiopulmonary bypass in association with non-selective beta blockade. *Lancet* 2:380, 1978.
25. Bettinger JC et al: The effect of intravenous administration of potassium chloride on ectopic rhythms, ectopic beats, and disturbances in A-V conduction. *Am J Med* 21:521, 1966.
26. Bhatt SB et al: Potassium homeostasis during and after cardiopulmonary bypass. *Indian J Med Res* 92:433, 1990.
27. Bohrer H et al: Hypercalcemic cardiac arrest after cardiac surgery following high-dose glucose-insulin-potassium infusion for inotropic support. *Anesthesiology* 69:949, 1988.
28. Boldman L, Caldera DL: Risks of general anesthesia and elective operations in the hypertensive patient. *Anesthesiology* 50:285, 1979.
29. Boudoulas H et al: Hypersensitivity to adrenergic stimulation after propranolol withdrawal in normal subjects. *Ann Intern Med* 87:433, 1977.
30. Braunwald E: Calcium channel blocking agents in the treatment of cardiovascular disorders: 2. Hemodynamic effects and clinical applications. *Ann Intern Med* 93:886, 1980.
31. Bravo EL, Gifford RW: Pheochromocytoma: Diagnosis, localization and management. *N Engl J Med* 311:1298, 1984.
32. Bridges KG et al: Effect of phentolamine in controlling temperature and acidosis associated with cardiopulmonary bypass. *Crit Care Med* 13:72, 1985.
33. Bruining HA et al: Unexpected hypopotassemia after multiple blood transfusions during operation. *Neth J Surg* 38:48, 1986.
34. Burns WJ, Spradlin W: Death from self-induced water intoxication among patients with schizophrenic disorders. *J Nerv Ment Dis* 173:161, 1985.
35. Carmichael D et al: Hypokalemia and massive transfusion. *South Med J* 77:315, 1984.
36. Collins JA et al: Acid-base status of seriously wounded combat casualties: 2. Resuscitation with stored blood. *Ann Surg* 173:6, 1971.
37. Collins JA, Knudson MM: Metabolic effects of massive transfusion, in Rossi EC et al (eds): *Principles of Transfusion Medicine*. Baltimore, Williams & Wilkins, 1991, p 422.
38. Cottrell JE et al: Prevention of nitroprusside-induced cyanide toxicity with hydroxycobalamin. *N Engl J Med* 298:809, 1978.
39. Danovich GM et al: Reversibility of the salt losing tendency of chronic renal failure. *N Engl J Med* 296:14, 1977.
40. Davidson S, Suprawicz B: Ectopic beats and atrioventricular conduction disturbances in patients with hypopotassemia. *Arch Intern Med* 120:280, 1967.
41. DeFronzo RA et al: Normal diluting capacity in hyponatremic patients. *Ann Intern Med* 84:538, 1976.
42. DeFronzo RA: Hyperkalemia and hyporeninemic hypoaldosteronism. *Kidney Int* 17:118, 1980.
43. Degaute JP, Kahn RJ: Serial lactate determinations during circulatory shock. *Crit Care Med* 11:449, 1983.
44. Desmond J: Complications of transurethral prostatic surgery. *Can Anaesth Soc J* 17:25, 1970.
45. Diringer MN et al: Plasma atrial natriuretic factor and subarachnoid hemorrhage. *Stroke* 19:1119, 1988.
46. Diringer MN et al: Suprasellar and intraventricular blood predict elevated plasma atrial natriuretic factor in subarachnoid hemorrhage. *Stroke* 22:577, 1991.
47. Diringer MN et al: Hypervolemic therapy prevents volume contraction but not hyponatremia following subarachnoid hemorrhage. *Ann Neurol* 31:543, 1992.
48. Doczi T et al: Increased concentration of atrial natriuretic factor in the cerebrospinal fluid of patients with aneurysmal subarachnoid hemorrhage and raised intracranial pressure. *Neurosurgery* 23:16, 1988.
49. Duke M: Thiazide-induced hypokalemia, association with acute myocardial infarction and ventricular fibrillation. *JAMA* 239:43, 1978.

50. Eisenberg PR et al: A prospective study of lung water measurements during patient management in an intensive care unit. *Am Rev Respir Dis* 136:662, 1987.
51. England MR et al: Magnesium administration and dysrhythmia after cardiac surgery. *JAMA* 268:2395, 1992.
52. Erslev AJ: Erythropoietin. *N Engl J Med* 324:1339, 1991.
53. Fisch C et al: Effect of digitalis on conduction of the heart. *Prog Cardiovasc Dis* 6:343, 1964.
54. Fisch C et al: Enhancement of potassium-induced atrioventricular block by toxic doses of digitalis drugs. *J Clin Invest* 39:1885, 1960.
55. Frishman WH: β-Adrenoceptor antagonists: New drugs and new indications. *N Engl J Med* 305:500, 1981.
56. Gerst PH et al: Increased susceptibility of the heart to ventricular fibrillation during metabolic acidosis. *Circ Res* 19:63, 1966.
57. Ghanem AM, Ward JP: Osmotic and metabolic sequelae of volumetric overload in relation to the TUR syndrome. *Br J Urol* 66:71, 1990.
58. Gilbert EM et al: The effect of fluid loading blood transfusion and catecholamine infusion on oxygen delivery and consumption in patients with sepsis. *Am Rev Respir Dis* 134:873, 1986.
59. Goetz KL et al: Comparative effects of cardiac receptors and sinoaortic baroreceptors on elevations of plasma vasopressin and renin activity elicited by hemorrhage. *J Physiol (London)* 79:440, 1984.
60. Goldman L et al: Multifactorial index of cardiac risk in noncardiac surgical procedures. *N Engl J Med* 297:845, 1977.
61. Grace WJ, Barr DP: Complications of alkalosis. *Am J Med* 4:331, 1948.
62. Graf H et al: Evidence for a detrimental effect of bicarbonate therapy in hypoxic lactic acidosis. *Science* 227:754, 1985.
63. Griffel MI, Kaufman BS: Pharmacology of colloids and crystalloids. *Crit Care Clin* 8:235, 1992.
64. Hahn RG et al: Factors influencing the osmolality and the concentrations of blood haemoglobin and electrolytes during transurethral resection of the prostate. *Acta Anaesthesiol Scand* 31:601, 1987.
65. Hahn RG: Ethanol monitoring of irrigating fluid absorption in transurethral prostatic surgery. *Anesthesiology* 68:867, 1988.
66. Hahn RG: Relations between irrigant absorption rate and hyponatremia during transurethral resection of the prostate. *Acta Anaesthesiol Scand* 32:53, 1988.
67. Hahn RG et al: Intravenous infusion of irrigating fluids containing mannitol and glycine with and without ethanol. *J Urol* 142:1102, 1989.
68. Hahn RG: Fluid and electrolyte dynamics during development of the TURP syndrome. *Br J Urol* 66:79, 1990.
69. Hahn RG: The transurethral resection syndrome. *Acta Anaesthesiol Scand* 35:557, 1991.
70. Harrison RH et al: Dilutional hyponatremic shock: Another concept of the transurethral prostatic resection reaction. *J Urol* 75:95, 1956.
71. Harvey RM et al: Hemodynamic effects of dehydration and metabolic acidosis in Asiatic cholera. *Trans Assoc Am Physicians* 79:177, 1966.
72. Haupt MT et al: Fluid loading increases oxygen consumption in septic patients with lactic acidosis. *Am Rev Respir Dis* 131:912, 1985.
73. Haupt MT et al: Fluid resuscitation in patients with increased vascular permeability. *Crit Care Clin* 18:341, 1992.
74. Hauser CJ et al: Oxygen transport responses to colloids and crystalloids in critically ill surgical patients. *Surg Gynecol Obstet* 150:811, 1980.
75. Himpe D et al: Priming solutions for cardiopulmonary bypass: Comparison of three colloids. *J Cardiothorac Vasc Anesthes* 5:457, 1991.
76. Hodgkin JE et al: Incidence of metabolic alkalemia in hospitalized patients. *Crit Care Med* 8:725, 1980.
77. Holland OB et al: Diuretic induced ventricular ectopic activity. *Am J Med* 70:762, 1981.
78. Hotchkiss RS, Karl LE: Reevaluation of the role of cellular hypoxia and bioenergetic failure in sepsis. *JAMA* 267:1503, 1992.
79. Hulten JO et al: Monitoring of fluid absorption during TURP by marking the irrigating solution and ethanol. *Scand J Urol Nephrol* 20:245, 1986.
80. Hulten JO, Hahn RG: Monitoring irrigating fluid absorption during transurethral resection of the prostate (TURP): A comparison between 1 and 2% ethanol as a tracer. *Scand J Urol Nephrol* 23:103, 1989.
81. Hulting J: Hospital ventricular fibrillation and its relation to serum potassium. *Acta Med Scand* 209(suppl 647):109, 1981.
82. Hysing ES et al: Ionized calcium in plasma during cardiopulmonary bypass. *Scand J Clin Lab Invest* 46(suppl 184):119, 1986.
83. Ishikawa S et al: Hyponatremia responsive to fludrocortisone acetate in elderly patients after head injury. *Ann Intern Med* 106:187, 1987.
84. Kahn RC et al: Massive blood replacement: Correlation of ionized calclium, citrate, and hydrogen ion concentration. *Anesth Analg* 58:274, 1979.
85. Kassirer JP et al: The critical role of chloride in the correction of hypokalemic alkalosis in man. *Am J Med* 38:172, 1965.
86. Kaufman BS et al: The relationship between oxygen delivery and consumption during fluid resuscitation of hypovolemic and septic shock. *Chest* 8:336, 1984.
87. Kaul TK et al: Plasma albumin and calcium levels following cardiopulmonary bypass. *Int J Artific Organs* 12:461, 1989.
88. Keats AS: Hemodynamic consequences of hemodilution. *Cleve Clin Q* 45:39, 1978.
89. Kirschenbaum MA: Severe mannitol-induced hyponatremia complicating transurethral prostatic resection. *J Urol* 121:687, 1979.
90. Kontos H: Vasodilator effect of hypercapnic acidosis on human forearm vessels. *Am J Physiol* 215:1403, 1968.
91. Kopman EA: Scavenging of potassium cardioplegic solution to prevent hyperkalemia in hemodialysis-dependent patients. *Anesth Analg* 62:780, 1983.
92. Kruse JA, Carlson RW: Rapid correction of hypokalemia using concentrated intravenous potassium chloride infusions. *Arch Intern Med* 150:613, 1990.

93. Kuntschen FR et al: Glucose-insulin interactions during cardiopulmonary bypass. *J Thorac Cardiovasc Surg* 91: 451, 1986.
94. Landymore RW et al: Effect of cardiopulmonary bypass and hypothermia on pancreatic endocrine function and peripheral utilization of glucose. *Can J Surg* 22:248, 1979.
95. Lanier W et al: The effects of dextrose infusion and head position on neurologic outcome after complete cerebral ischemia in primates: Examination of a model. *Anesthesiology* 66:39, 1987.
96. Lemmer JH Jr, Kirsh MM: Coronary artery spasm following coronary artery surgery. *Ann Thorac Surg* 46:108, 1988.
97. Linko K, Saxelin I: Electrolyte and acid-base disturbances caused by blood transfusions. *Acta Anaesthesiol Scand* 30:134, 1986.
98. Longstreth WT, Inui TS: High blood glucose level on hospital admission and poor neurologic recovery after cardiac arrest. *Ann Neurol* 15:59, 1984.
99. Madsen PO, Naber KG: The importance of the pressure in the prostatic fossa and absorption of irrigating fluid during the transurethral resection of the prostate. *J Urol* 109:446, 1973.
100. Manning SH et al: Intermittent intravenous potassium therapy in cardiopulmonary bypass patients. *Clin Pharm* 1:234, 1982.
101. McCall BB et al: Effects of central bolus injections of potassium chloride on arterial potassium concentration in patients undergoing cardiopulmonary bypass. *J Cardiothorac Anesth* 4:571, 1990.
102. Mebust WK et al: Transurethral prostactomy: Immediate and postoperative complications: A cooperative study of 13 participating institutions evaluating 3,885 patients. *J Urol* 141:243, 1989.
103. Medical Research Council Working Party on Mild to Moderate Hypertension: Ventricular extrasystoles during thiazide treatment: Substudy of MRC mild hypertension trial. *Br Med J* 287:1249, 1983.
104. Metildi LA et al: Crystalloid versus colloid in fluid resuscitation of patients with severe pulmonary insufficiency. *Surg Gynecol Obstet* 58:207, 1984.
105. Miller RD et al: Effects of massive transfusion of blood on acid-base balance. *JAMA* 216:1762, 1971.
106. Miller RD et al: Enhancement of d-tubocurarine neuromuscular blockade by diuretics in man. *Anesthesiology* 4S:442, 1976.
107. Mink RB, Pollack MM: Effect of blood transfusion on oxygen consumption in pediatric septic shock. *Crit Care Med* 18:1087, 1990.
108. Mitchell JH et al: The effects of acid-base disturbances on cardiovascular and pulmonary function. *Kidney Int* 1:375, 1972.
109. Muizelaar JP et al: Effect of mannitol on ICP and CBF and correlation with pressure autoregulation in severely head-injured patients. *J Neurosurg* 61:700, 1984.
110. Narins RG, Cohen JJ: Bicarbonate therapy for organic acidosis: The case for its continued use. *Ann Intern Med* 106:615, 1987.
111. Narins RG et al: Alkali therapy of the organic acidosis: A critical assessment of the data and the case for judicious use of sodium bicarbonate, in Narins RG (ed): *Controversies in Nephrology and Hypertension*. New York, Churchill Livingstone, 1984, p 359.
112. Nelson PB et al: Hyponatremia and natriuresis following subarachnoid hemorrhage in a monkey model. *J Neurosurg* 60:233, 1984.
113. Nelson PB et al: Hyponatremia in intracranial disease: Perhaps not the syndrome of inappropriate secretion of antidiuretic hormone (SIADH). *J Neurosurg* 55:938, 1981.
114. Norlen H: Isotonic solutions of mannitol, sorbitol and glycine and distilled water as irrigating fluids during transurethral resection of the prostate. *Scand J Urol Nephrol* 158(suppl 96):1, 1985.
115. Ontario Intensive Care Study Group: Evaluation of right heart catheterization in critically ill patients. *Crit Care Med* 20:928, 1992.
116. Packman MI, Rackow EC: Optimum left heart filling pressure during fluid resuscitation of patients with hypovolemic and septic shock. *Crit Care Med* 14:454, 1986.
117. Pasch T et al: Nitroprusside-induced formation of cyanide and its detoxication with thiosulfate during deliberate hypotension. *J Cardiovasc Pharmacol* 5:77, 1983.
118. Perioperative red cell transfusion. National Institutes of Health Consensus Development Conference Statement, vol 7, no. 4. United States Department of Health and Human Services, Bethesda, MD, June 27–29, 1988.
119. Pollay M et al: Effect of mannitol and furosemide on blood-brain osmotic gradient and intracranial pressure. *J Neurosurg* 59:945, 1983.
120. Pollay M, Roberts PA: Blood-brain barrier: A definition of normal and altered function. *Neurosurgery* 6:675, 1980.
121. Prys-Roberts C: Hypertension and anesthesia: Fifty years on. *Anesthesiology* 50:281, 1979.
122. Pulsinelli WA et al: Moderate hyperglycemia augments ischemic brain damage: A neuropathologic study in the rat. *Neurology* 32:1239, 1982.
123. Pulsinelli WA et al: Increased damage after ischemic stroke in patients with hyperglycemia with or without established diabetes mellitus. *Am J Med* 74:540, 1983.
124. Rackow EC et al: Fluid resuscitation in circulatory shock: A comparison of the cardiorespiratory effects of albumin, hetastarch, and saline solutions in patients with hypovolemic and septic shock. *Crit Care Med* 11:835, 1985.
125. Rackow EC, Astiz ME: Pathophysiology and treatment of septic shock. *JAMA* 266:548, 1991.
126. Ranney HM, Rapaport SI: The red blood cell, in West JB (ed): *Physiologic Basis of Medical Practice*, 12th ed. Baltimore, Williams & Wilkins, 1991, p 369.
127. Ravussin P et al: Changes in CSF pressure after mannitol in patients with and without elevated CSF pressure. *J Neurosurg* 69:809, 1988.
128. Rhymer JC et al: Hyponatremia following transurethral resection of the prostate. *Br J Urol* 57:450, 1985.
129. Robertie PG et al: Normal parathyroid hormone responses to hypocalcemia during cardiopulmonary bypass. *Anesthesiology* 75:43, 1991.
130. Roesche R et al: Ammonia toxicity resulting from glycine absorption resection of the prostate. *Anesthesiology* 58:577, 1983.
131. Rosberg B, Wulff K: Hemodynamics following nor-

movolemic hemodilution in elderly patients. *Acta Anaesthesiol Scand* 25:402, 1981.
132. Rosenfeld JV et al: The effect of subarachnoid hemorrhage on blood and CSF atrial natriuretic factor. *J Neurosurg* 71:32, 1989.
133. Royster RL et al: A randomized, blinded placebo-controlled evaluation of calcium chloride and epinephrine for inotropic support after emergence from cardiopulmonary bypass. *Anesth Analg* 74:3, 1992.
134. Ruiz C et al: Treatment of circulatory shock with dopamine. *JAMA* 242:165, 1979.
135. Ryder KW et al: Hyperammonaemia after transurethral resection of the prostate: A report of 2 cases. *J Urol* 134:995, 1984.
136. Schlant RC, Sonnenblick EH: Pathophysiology of heart failure, in Hurst JW et al (eds): *The Heart*, 7th ed. New York, McGraw-Hill, 1990, p 398.
137. Schulman M, Narins RG: Hypokalemia and cardiovascular disease. *Am J Cardiol* 65:4E, 1990.
138. Schultz RE et al: Percutaneous ultrasonic lithotripsy: Choice of irrigant. *J Urol* 130:858, 1983.
139. Schweizer O, Howland WS: Potassium levels, acid-base balance and massive blood replacement. *Anesthesiology* 23:735, 1962.
140. Shapira N et al: Hemodynamic effects of calcium chloride injection following cardiopulmonary bypass: Response to bolus injection and continuous infusion. *Ann Thorac Surg* 37:133, 1984.
141. Shapiro B, Gross MD: Pheochromocytoma. *Crit Care Clin* 7:1, 1991.
142. Shepard RL et al: The role of ammonia toxicity in the post-transurethral prostatectomy syndrome. *Br J Urol* 60:349, 1987.
143. Sheps SG et al: Recent developments in the diagnosis and treatment of pheochromocytoma. *Mayo Clin Proc* 65:88, 1990.
144. Shu'ayb WA et al: Studies of the mechanism of antidiuretic hormone secretion and the post-commissurotomy dilutional syndrome. *Ann Surg* 162:690, 1965.
145. Sibbald WJ et al: Pulmonary microvascular clearance of radiotracers in human cardiac and noncardiac pulmonary edema. *J Appl Physiol* 50:1337, 1981.
146. Sibbald WJ et al: Thermal dye measurements of extravascular lung water in critically ill patients: Intravascular Starling forces and extravascular lung water in the adult respiratory distress syndrome. *Chest* 87:585, 1985.
147. Sieber FE et al: Glucose: A reevaluation of its intraoperative use. *Anesthesiology* 67:72, 1987.
148. Sinclair JF et al: Absorption of 1.5% glycine after percutaneous ultrasonic lithotripsy for renal stone disease. *Br Med J* 291:691, 1985.
149. Sliwinski M et al: Association between hypokalemic alkalosis and development of arrhythmias in early postoperative period. *Anesth Resusc Intens Ther* 2:193, 1974.
150. Stacpoole PW: Lactic acidosis: The case against bicarbonate therapy. *Ann Intern Med* 105:276, 1986.
151. Standbury WS, Mahler RF: Salt wasting renal disease: Metabolic observations on patients with "salt losing nephritis." *Q J Med* 129:425, 1959.
152. Stehling LC et al: A survey of transfusion practices among anesthesiologists. *Vox Sang* 52:60, 1987.
153. Steiner E: Suppression of renal excretion of digoxin in hypokalemic patients. *Clin Pharmacol Ther* 23:511, 1978.
154. Sterns RH et al: Osmotic demyelination syndrome following correction of hyponatremia. *N Engl J Med* 314:1535, 1986.
155. Strandgaard S et al: Autoregulation of brain circulation in severe arterial hypertension. *Br Med J* 1:507, 1973.
156. Swan H et al: Quality control of perfusion: Monitoring venous blood oxygen tension to prevent hypoxic acidosis. *J Thorac Cardiovasc Surg* 99:868, 1990.
157. Tanneau RA et al: Cerebral salt wasting in elderly persons (letter). *Ann Intern Med* 107:120, 1987.
158. Tasker PRW et al: Prophylactic use of intravenous saline in patients with chronic renal failure undergoing major surgery. *Lancet* 19:7886, 1974.
159. Taylor KM et al: Hypernatremia dehydration following tricuspid valve replacement. *J Cardiovasc Surg (Turin)* 19:449, 1978.
160. Van Boven MJ et al: Dilutional hyponatremia associated with intrauterine endoscopic laser surgery. *Anesthesiology* 71:449, 1989.
161. Vary TC: Increased pyruvate dehydrogenase kinase activity. *Am J Physiol* 260:E663, 1991.
162. Vessey CJ, Cole PV: Blood cyanide and thiocyanate concentrations produced by long term therapy with sodium nitroprusside. *Br J Anaesth* 57:148, 1985.
163. Walker WG et al: Metabolic observations on salt wasting in patients with renal disease. *Am J Med* 29:505, 1965.
164. Ward MM: Factors predictive of acute renal failure in rhabdomyolysis. *Arch Intern Med* 148:1553, 1988.
165. Weber DO, Yarnoz MD: Hyperkalemia complicating cardiopulmonary bypass: Analysis of risk factors. *Ann Thorac Surg* 34:439, 1982.
166. Weiland AP, Walker WE: Physiologic principles and clinical sequelae of cardiopulmonary bypass. *Heart Lung* 15:34, 1986.
167. Weinsier RL et al: Central venous alimentation: A prospective study of the frequency of metabolic abnormalities among medical and surgical patients. *J Parenter Enteral Nutr* 6:421, 1982.
168. Welsh FA et al: Deleterious effect of glucose pretreatment on recovery from diffuse cerebral ischemia in the cat: 2. Regional metabolite levels. *Stroke* 11:355, 1980.
169. Whitsett TL et al: Abrupt cessation of clonidine administration: A prospective study. *Am J Cardiol* 41:1285, 1978.
170. Wijdicks EFM et al: Hyponatremia and cerebral infarction in patients with ruptured intracranial aneurysms: Is fluid restriction harmful? *Ann Neurol* 17:137, 1985.
171. Wijdicks EFM et al: Volume depletion and natriuresis in patients with a ruptured intracranial aneurysm. *Ann Neurol* 18:211, 1985.
172. Wijdicks EFM: Enlargement of the third ventricle and hyponatremia, in Wijdicks EFM (ed): *Hyponatremia, Volume Status and Blood Pressure Following Subarachnoid Hemorrhage*. Rotterdam, Offsetdrukkerij JH Pasmans BV, 1987, p 49.
173. Wijdicks EFM et al: Enlargement of the third ventricle and hyponatremia in aneurysmal subarachnoid haemorrhage. *J Neurol Neurosurg Psychiatry* 51:516, 1988.

174. Wildenthal K et al: Effects of acute lactic acidosis on left ventricular performance. *Am J Physiol* 214:1352, 1968.
175. Wilson RF et al: Eight years of experience with massive blood transfusions. *J Trauma* 11:275, 1971.
176. Wright HK, Gann DS: Severe postoperative hyponatremia without symptoms of water intoxication. *Surg Gynecol Obstet* 115:553, 1962.

CHAPTER 44

Fluid and electrolyte disorders in total parenteral nutrition

Donald W. Inadomi • Joel D. Kopple

Total parenteral nutrition (TPN) is now an established medical therapy for patients who are unable to be nourished adequately through the enteral tract. The preparation, composition, and methods of nutrient delivery and the techniques for monitoring patients who receive TPN have improved enormously during the past 20 years. However, reports continue to indicate that the incidence of fluid and electrolyte disorders in patients receiving TPN remains high, particularly in severely ill patients. Weinsier and associates reported finding at least one severe alteration in plasma chemistry in 63 out of 100 consecutive medical and surgical patients who received TPN.[1] In contrast, technical and infectious complications, which formerly were common events,[2] seem to occur less often now. Indeed, in one study, these untoward events occurred in only 3 and 4 percent, respectively, of 220 catheter insertions.[1] Experienced and well-functioning nutritional support teams reportedly reduce the incidence of technical and infectious complications of TPN.[3,4]

Many fluid and electrolyte disorders occur in patients receiving TPN (Table 44-1). One important cause of the high incidence of metabolic complications in such patients is their underlying illness which may impair their ability to metabolize or excrete the infused nutrients.

For reference, typical electrolyte concentrations for TPN solutions are shown in Table 44-2. In general, the most osmotically active electrolytes are added to TPN solutions to attain the following final concentrations: Na^+, 30 to 55 meq/liter; K^+, 30 to 40 meq/liter; Cl^-, 30 to 55 meq/liter; and acetate, 45 to 70 meq/liter. These electrolytes include those incorporated into the amino acid preparation at the time of manufacture (Table 44-3). Protein hydrolysates have disappeared from use in the United States because the composition of amino acids in these preparations is somewhat variable, and some of the peptides present are poorly metabolized and may be lost in urine. Also, some hydrolysate solutions have been contaminated with aluminum[5] (see below).

Many metabolic disorders related to the intake of carbohydrates, lipids, and amino acids may develop in patients receiving TPN. Since this chapter is focused on fluid and electrolyte disorders, the reader is referred to

TABLE 44-1 • Fluid and electrolyte complications of total parenteral nutrition

Glucose
Postinfusion hypoglycemia
Hyperglycemia
Hyperosmolar syndrome
Acid-base
Metabolic acidosis
Metabolic alkalosis
Respiratory acidosis
Water and minerals
Hypo-, hypernatremia
Hypo-, hyperkalemia
Hypo-, hypercalcemia
Hypo-, hypermagnesemia
Hypo-, hyperphosphatemia
Trace elements
Deficient:
Zinc
Copper
Chromium
Selenium
Molybdenum
Manganese
Iron
Excess:
Aluminum
Zinc
Iron

TABLE 44-2 • **Typical prescription for TPN solutions infused into large-flow veins in adults**

Dextrose (D-glucose)[a,b,c]	250 g/liter
Amino acids[a,c]	28.5–42.5 g/liter
Lipids[a]	50–100 g/500 ml
Energy (approx.)[d]	950–1000 kcal/liter
Electrolytes:[e]	
Sodium[f]	30–55 meq/liter
Potassium[g]	60–90 meq/day
Chloride[h]	30–55 meq/liter
Calcium[i]	6–12 meq/day
Magnesium[j]	16–20 meq/day
Acetate[k]	45–70 meq/liter
Phosphorus[l]	18–28 m*M*/day
Trace elements:[m]	
Zinc	2.5–4.0 mg/day
Copper	300–500 μg
Chromium	10–20 μg
Molybdenum	100–200 μg
Selenium	40–80 μg
Vitamins	[m,n]

[a] These nutrients are present in each bottle containing crystalline amino acids and dextrose. Typically, 2 or 3 liters is infused daily. Usually 50 to 100 g of lipids is infused each day in a 10 or 20% lipid emulsion. Traditionally lipids have been infused from a separate container. More recently, amino acids, dextrose, and lipids have been infused together as an admixture in one container.

[b] Dextrose concentrations listed refer to those for dextrose monohydrate, the form in which glucose is given.

[c] These concentrations usually are obtained by adding one part of 50% dextrose and appropriate amounts of a mixture of essential and nonessential amino acids (see Table 44-3); nutrient concentration of dextrose and amino acids can be increased in patients who are fluid-intolerant by using 70% dextrose and 8.5 to 10% amino acids.

[d] Exclusive of energy provided as lipids. Caloric values: dextrose monohydrate, 3.4 kcal/g; amino acids, 3.5 kcal/g; 10 and 20% lipid emulsions, 1.1 and 2.0 kcal/ml.

[e] Electrolytes intrinsically present in amino acid or hydrolysate solution should be taken into account (see Table 44-3).

[f] Added as chloride and acetate salts, and with bisulfite (antioxidant).

[g] Added as chloride and phosphate salts, and with metabisulfite (antioxidant).

[h] Added as sodium and potassium salts, and as HCl (pH adjustment) and lysine-HCl.

[i] Added as gluceptate or gluconate salt.

[j] Added as sulfate, acetate, or chloride salt.

[k] Added as sodium and potassium salts, and as acetic acid (pH adjustment) and L-lysine acetate.

[l] Added as sodium and potassium salts, and as phosphoric acid.

[m] Trace elements and vitamins should be added to only one bottle a day.

[n] Typical vitamin content for TPN per day: vitamin A, 4000 IU; vitamin D, 400 IU; vitamin K, 1.4 mg; vitamin E, 10 mg; niacine, 40 mg; thiamine HCl (vitamin B_1) 5 mg; riboflavin (B_2), 5 mg; pantothenic acid, 15 mg; pyridoxine HCl (B_6), 10 mg; ascorbic acid (vitamin C), 100 mg; biotin, 200 μg; folic acid, 1 mg; vitamin B_{12}, 6 μg.

other excellent publications for a review of these other metabolic complications in TPN.

FLUID AND ELECTROLYTE DISORDERS

GLUCOSE

Dextrose (D-glucose) is the primary carbohydrate used in most TPN solutions. One gram of glucose provides 4.1 kcal by in vitro calorimetry, but in vivo, glucose yields 3.75 kcal/g. Moreover, in parenteral solutions glucose monohydrate is used; the monohydrate is 91 percent anhydrous glucose and therefore provides only 3.4 kcal/g. Glucose is generally well-utilized for energy, and many studies demonstrate that infusions of amino acids and glucose devoid of other carbohydrates, alcohols, or fats can maintain neutral or positive nitrogen balance. Glucose is the carbohydrate of choice for several reasons: it is an intermediate in the energy-yielding main degradative pathway for carbohydrates; it is readily metabolized by all tissues; it stimulates secretion of insulin, a highly anabolic hormone; and usually it is well-tolerated in large quantities.

Nonstressed adults receiving TPN usually can tolerate at least 400 to 500 g of glucose per 24 h without developing hyperglycemia.[6] Sanderson and Deitel reported that serum insulin rose to 80 to 90 μU/ml, four to six times basal levels, in relatively nonstressed patients who received TPN that provided 3 liters/day of 20% glucose.[7] With continued infusion of this quantity of glucose, serum insulin and glucose concentrations gradually fell, indicating decreased peripheral resistance to glucose uptake. After clinically stable patients had received a constant amount of TPN, they were given an intravenous (IV) glucose tolerance test; serum glucose concentration fell at a normal rate. These findings suggest that the pancreas can readily increase insulin secretion in response to an increment in the glucose load. The authors report that, contrary to popular belief, when TPN was stopped abruptly serum insulin and glucose concentrations returned quickly to normal levels and reactive hypoglycemia did not occur. Hypoglycemia only occurred when the rate of TPN infusion was increased transiently and infusion was then stopped abruptly. Nonetheless, many workers believe that TPN solutions should be tapered in all patients who receive 200 to 300 g/day or more of IV glucose.

Hyperglycemia is one of the most common metabolic complications of TPN. Ryan noted hyperglycemia with serum glucose concentrations greater than 400 mg/dl in 15 percent of patients receiving TPN.[8] Feinstein et al reported that 18 of 30 patients with acute renal failure who received parenteral nutrition with hypertonic glucose showed an elevation in serum glucose to levels above

360 mg/dl in at least one determination;[9] hyperglycemia occurred even though most of these patients received insulin early in the course of parenteral nutrition.

Hyperglycemia is particularly likely to occur in patients receiving TPN who have diabetes mellitus, acute or chronic liver or renal failure, major physical trauma, or infection. These conditions, in which patients may be acutely stressed, are commonly associated with increased blood levels of catecholamines, glucagon, cortisol, and sometimes parathyroid hormone (PTH);[10] there may also be resistance to the actions of insulin. Consequently, increased gluconeogenesis and glycogenolysis occur. Glucose turnover is often increased in severely stressed patients.[11] Liver failure, hypoxia, severe acidosis, and bacterial endotoxins may impair both the hepatic synthesis and peripheral uptake of glucose. The impaired ability to excrete glucose may also contribute to hyperglycemia in patients with renal failure who receive TPN.

Hyperosmolar, hyperglycemic, nonketotic dehydration (HHND) is a dangerous and extreme form of hyperglycemia which may complicate TPN.[12-14] This syndrome is characterized by a serum glucose concentration greater than 1000 mg/dl, serum osmolality greater than 350 mosm, little or no ketonemia or ketonuria, glucose diuresis leading to dehydration, and such neurological abnormalities as lethargy, confusion, disorientation, focal or generalized seizures, and coma. The syndrome may be confused with a cerebrovascular accident.

Kaminski reported seeing HHND in 3 percent of 200 patients receiving TPN.[13] Most patients were severely stressed from underlying illnesses; all had hyperglycemia, glucosuria, polyuria, and negative water balance for several days before the development of the syndrome. Often, the patients had been treated with insulin according to an inadequate sliding scale. Glucosuria, reflecting a rise in serum glucose concentration, often occurred in association with infection or increased carbohydrate intake. All patients had a family history of diabetes mellitus. One of the six patients died.

Ketoacidosis is an uncommon complication of TPN, even when HHND occurs. The absence of ketoacidosis in this syndrome is thought to be due to the presence in serum of sufficient insulin to prevent lipolysis but not enough to maintain euglycemia.[15,16] Also, the hyperglycemia may promote storage of glycogen in liver and inhibit formation of ketone bodies. Mirsky et al. showed in pancreatectomized dogs that severe hyperglycemia per se prevents ketoacidosis.[17] In vitro studies of rat adipose tissue and diaphragm indicate that hyperosmolality inhibits release of free fatty acids from adipose tissue and impairs beta cell response to glucose without affecting ketogenesis.[18] A constant infusion of large quantities of glucose in patients with adult onset diabetes mellitus can temporarily exhaust pancreatic insulin secretion without causing ketoacidosis.[19]

During the initial stages of TPN, blood glucose concentrations should be measured frequently. The blood glucose levels can be estimated with test paper at the bedside on either blood obtained by finger stick or urine. Initially these measurements may be performed at approximately 6- to 8-h intervals, particularly when glucose intake or insulin doses are being adjusted. Blood glucose

TABLE 44-3 • Approximate composition of standard balanced crystalline amino acid solutions for intravenous use[a]

	Aminosyn, 8.5%[b]	Freamine III, 8.5%[c]	Travasol, 8.5%[d]
Amino acids (g/dl)	8.5	8.5	8.5
Electrolytes (meq/liter)			
Sodium	0	10	0
Potassium	5.4[e]	0	0
Chloride[f]	35[f]	2	34[f]
Magnesium	0	0	0
Acetate[g,h]	90[g]	73[g]	73[h]
Phosphorus (m*M*)	0	10	0
Osmolality (mosm)	850	810	890

[a] Commercially available in United States. Usual concentrations of amino acids and electrolytes are those intrinsic to the preparation before addition of dextrose solutions or other substances.

[b] Abbott Laboratories; also available as 3.5, 5, 7, and 10% without electrolytes and 3.5, 7, 8.5, and 10% with electrolytes.

[c] Kendall McGaw; also available as 10% without electrolytes and 3 and 8.5% with electrolytes.

[d] Clintec Nutrition; also available as 5.5 and 10% without electrolytes and 3.5, 5.5, and 8.5% with electrolytes.

[e] Includes 5.4 meq/liter from the antioxidant potassium metabisulfite.

[f] Includes approximately 18 meq/liter from HCl used for pH adjustment.

[g] From acetic acid used for pH adjustment and from L-lysine acetate.

[h] Acetate added as sodium acetate and acetic acid used for pH adjustment.

should be maintained under 200 mg/dl and should not exceed 140 mg/dl, unless the blood sugar level is so labile that careful control carries a high risk of hypoglycemia. In general, a urine glucose reaction of 3+ or 4+ requires prompt administration of insulin. However, patients with renal disease may have glucosuria with normal blood sugar concentrations or blood sugar may be elevated with little or no glucosuria. Hence, it is important to know the patient's urinary threshold for glucose before relying on urine glucose measurements. In patients who have renal failure or an abnormally high or low urinary threshold for glucose it is better to monitor glucose in blood rather than urine.

Often hyperglycemia can be avoided by beginning parenteral nutrition with smaller amounts of glucose and increasing the glucose load gradually over a 3-day period to full dosage. If patients fall behind in the prescribed fluid or nutrient intake, the rate of infusion should not be abruptly increased to compensate for the deficit. When hyperglycemia occurs despite careful management, the cause should be investigated. Hyperglycemia may be the initial manifestation of sepsis and may precede other signs of infection by 18 to 24 h.[20]

Mild or moderate hyperglycemia may be prevented or treated by adding regular insulin to the infusate, approximately 1.0 to 2.5 units per 25 g of glucose. Insulin infusions are reported to decrease the degree of negative nitrogen balance in patients suffering from catabolic stress,[21,22] although this has been disputed.[23] Treatment of patients who have more severe glucose intolerance usually is readily handled with greater quantities of insulin.

Insulin added to intravenous solutions may be adsorbed by the parenteral administration apparatus. The amount of insulin adsorbed is reported to vary from 10 to 55 percent.[24,25] Insulin is adsorbed primarily to the bag (65 to 70 percent of total adsorption), but also to the bag port (about 15 to 20 percent) and administration set (about 15 percent). Although the amount of insulin that is adsorbed to the parenteral administration apparatus is substantial, clinical experience still indicates that blood glucose concentrations usually can be controlled effectively by adding insulin to the infusate.

Patients with HHND are generally treated by stopping the infusion of glucose and amino acids until the fluid, electrolyte, and blood glucose disorders are corrected. This usually entails correcting the deficits of sodium, other electrolytes, and water. The osmotic glucose diuresis in this condition often causes such severe dehydration and hypovolemia that tissue perfusion is compromised and hypotension is present. In this setting, rapid restoration of tissue perfusion is the primary therapeutic goal; this may be accomplished by infusing isotonic saline and, if needed, colloidal fluid-space expanders such as protein or dextran. Potassium replacement is almost invariably necessary.

After adequate tissue perfusion is attained, as evidenced by restoration of blood pressure, rises in urine output and central venous pressure, and fall in blood lactate levels, attention should be focused more closely on abnormalities of serum tonicity and electrolytes. Hypotonic saline with potassium is administered. Diuretics should not be used unless there is clear documentation that the patient's fluid volume is not depleted and the patient is adequately perfused. However, excessive fluid therapy is a risk of this treatment and may lead to volume overload and congestive heart failure.

Patients with HHND are usually more sensitive to insulin than those who have ketoacidosis, and special care must be taken to prevent hypoglycemia during insulin therapy. Low-dose insulin therapy, e.g., 0.1 U of crystalline zinc insulin per kilogram of body weight per hour in a continuous infusion, should suffice to lower blood glucose concentrations. Insulin therapy may lead to a transient shift of fluid from the intravascular and extracellular spaces into cells and could aggravate hypotension. Thus, insulin treatment is often begun after treatment of hypovolemia has been initiated.

ACID-BASE DISORDERS

Acidosis or alkalosis may result from a variety of causes in patients undergoing TPN. Formerly, the infusates were a common cause of acid-base disorders. Tables 44-4 and 44-5 list reported causes of acidosis and alkalosis in patients undergoing TPN. With modern TPN preparations clinically significant acidosis or alkalosis is uncommon except in patients with underlying metabolic or respiratory disorders.

Metabolic acidosis

Until several years ago, metabolic acidosis was not uncommon, particularly in childrn.[2,26-28] The metabolic acidosis usually was hyperchloremic and characterized by low blood pH, low plasma bicarbonate, and normal or near-normal anion gap. The hyperchloremic acidosis appeared to be caused by the TPN solutions. This disorder was described more frequently with the use of crystalline amino acid solutions,[2,28] although it was also observed in patients receiving casein or fibrin hydrolysates.[26,27]

Formerly, lysine, histidine, and arginine were administered as the hydrochloride salts in solutions of crystalline amino acids. These salts were probably the major cause of hyperchloremic acidosis. During the metabolism of these amino acids, the hydrochloride salts are metabolized to ammonia, carbon dioxide, water, and hydrochloric acid.

Heird and coworkers described the acid-base status of 11 infants who received TPN with one of two solutions that contained crystalline amino acids.[28] The infants

TABLE 44-4 • Reported causes of metabolic and respiratory acidosis in TPN patients

METABOLIC ACIDOSIS

High anion gap acidosis
- Diabetic ketoacidosis
- Titratable acidity of TPN solutions from dissolved CO_2, sodium hydrosulfite or sodium bisulfite preservatives, glucosamines (causes mild or no acidosis)
- Lactic acidosis caused by fructose infusion, infection, hypoxia
- Infusion of large quantities of essential amino acids without nonessential amino acids

Normal anion gap acidosis
- Use of hydrochloride salts of amino acids (e.g., lysine, histidine, arginine)
- Excess of cationic amino acids over anionic amino acids
- Chronic diarrhea or intestinal fistula drainage
- Impaired renal titratable acid excretion

RESPIRATORY ACIDOSIS

Hypercapnia due to:
- Impaired CO_2 exchange (e.g., from pneumothorax, severe pulmonary edema, pneumonia, weakness of respiratory muscles)

Increased CO_2 production (e.g., high carbon-compound intake, especially carbohydrates such as dextrose)

TABLE 44-5 • Reported causes of metabolic alkalosis in TPN patients

Gastric drainage, gastric fistula drainage, or vomiting
Hypovolemia
Infusion of excess base
Use of diuretics

NOTE: Only metabolic alkalosis is discussed because primary respiratory alkalosis has not been reported as a complication of TPN therapy.

were in positive nitrogen balance; 8 of 11 gained weight. However, blood pH and plasma bicarbonate levels dropped and they developed hyperchloremia with a normal or near-normal anion gap. Intestinal losses of base were small, and urinary acid excretion was normal. The authors suggested that the cause of the acidosis was the presence of the three cationic amino acids, arginine, histidine, and lysine hydrochloride, in excess over the anionic amino acids, aspartate and glutamate. They proposed that H^+ released during metabolism of the cationic amino acids leads to hyperchloremic acidosis; if these amino acids are incorporated into protein or peptides, H^+ is released into the blood. The absence of anionic amino acids from TPN infusates composed of crystalline amino acid solutions requires that, to be available for incorporation into proteins, glutamate and aspartate have to be synthesized in vivo; this synthesis should generate protons. Hence, either the metabolism or incorporation of the cationic amino acids into peptides or proteins can generate an acid load.[29,30]

Other possible causes for acidosis have been suggested. One is the titratable acidity of IV solutions.[31] Virtually all IV solutions, except those which specificially contain alkalinizing agents, have a pH less than 6.0 and sometimes as low as 4.0 to 5.0. The acidity of these solutions is due to several factors: (1) CO_2 from air dissolves in water to form carbonic acid; (2) some additives are acidic, such as the preservatives sodium hydrosulfite or sodium bisulfite;[28] (3) during heat sterilization a small amount of dextrose may carmelize, forming sugar acids.[32,33] The growing practice of admixing dextrose, amino acids, and lipids in a single container ("3-in-1" mixtures) for infusion[34,35] may reduce the frequency with which TPN solutions of pH 4.0 to 5.0 are used. Since lipid emulsions are unstable when infused in very acid or alkaline solutions,[36] the pH of the infusate is raised to about 5.7.[35]

Since TPN solutions are not buffered to any major degree, the acid load to the patient is minimal even though the pH of some TPN solutions is low. Moreover, since some of the titratable acids in the TPN solutions can be metabolized, the titratable acidity will not indicate the true in vivo acidogenic potential of the solutions. Heird and associates pointed out that even though the titratable acidity of the protein hydrolysates is greater than that of the crystalline amino acids, the protein hydrolysate solutions usually do not produce hyperchloremic acidosis, whereas the latter preparations often do.[28] Thus, the titratable acidity of the infusates is not believed to be a significant cause of the metabolic acidosis that occurs with TPN.

At present, the amino acids and electrolytes in TPN solutions are designed to reduce the possibility of hyperchloremic acidosis (Tables 44-2, 44-3). Most importantly, large amounts of sodium and potassium acetate are added to the TPN infusates, usually about 35 to 40 meq/liter. In addition, the amino acid solutions provide histidine and arginine as free bases (not as salts), and lysine is given as the acetate salt. Acetic acid instead of hydrochloric acid is added to adjust the pH of amino acid solutions. Since acetic acid can be completely metabolized to CO_2 and water, its presence should not predispose to metabolic acidosis. The metabolic fate of lysine acetate is less well-documented. It has been suggested that lysine acetate does not provide an alkaline load, although this has not been verified experimentally in humans. The concentration of acetate from lysine acetate and acetic acid in different amino acid solutions varies from about 40 to about 90 meq per liter of preparation. When the amino acid solutions are diluted with the dextrose and electrolyte solutions (including sodium and potassium acetate), the final concentration of acetate and acetic acid in TPN solutions is about 40 to 75 meq/liter.

An uncommon cause of metabolic acidosis was discovered by Fraley et al. in a 29-year-old cachectic female.[27] Her serum creatinine concentration was 0.7 mg/dl and blood pH fell from 7.33 to 7.25; serum bicarbonate concentration dropped from 20 to 13 meq/liter within 24 h of the start of TPN. The TPN provided 50 g/day of casein hydrolysate. The authors attributed the metabolic acidosis to an impairment in the kidneys' ability to excrete titratable acid and possibly ammonia. Unfortunately, serum [Cl^-] and anion gap were not reported, and the accumulation of organic acids was not clearly ruled out as the cause of the acidosis. The authors pointed out that malnutrition may reversibly impair several aspects of kidney function, including maximal concentrating ability and excretion of both titratable acid and ammonia.[37,38] Thus, it is possible that some patients who are very malnourished may not be able to excrete the acid load generated from metabolism of the infused amino acids or peptides in TPN and might become acidotic.

Motil and coworkers reported metabolic complications in two children with acute renal failure who were given large quantities of eight essential amino acids without histidine.[39] Arginine was not given. Both children developed an abnormal plasma amino acid pattern including markedly elevated methionine levels, very low concentrations of histidine and the urea cycle amino acids (ornithine, citrulline, and arginine), and a striking hyperammonemia; one patient developed an anion gap acidosis. After the TPN was changed to include essential and nonessential amino acids in this individual, plasma chloride concentration rose to abnormally high levels. The cause of the metabolic acidosis was unclear. Levels of several serum organic acids were normal, although these measuremenets may have been made after the essential amino acid solution was discontinued. We have also observed a bizarre plasma amino acid pattern in two adults who were given relatively large quantities of essential amino acids (more than 50 g/day) and no nonessential amino acids.

Fructose (levulose), a carbohydrate that was formerly used as a substitute for glucose, may cause lactic acidosis. Fructose has a caloric equivalent of 3.75 kcal/g and is phosphorylated to fructose-1-phosphate in liver and adipose tissue. Fructose is metabolized by adipose tissue independently of insulin; therefore, there is less need for exogenous insulin in the diabetic patient given fructose as compared to glucose.[40] This observation contributed to the former interest in fructose for TPN solutions. However, if fructose is used in patients with decompensated diabetes, blood glucose rises, confirming that some of the fructose administered is dependent on insulin for metabolism.[41,42] Moreover, with administration of large amounts of fructose, high-energy phosphate compounds may become depleted. This may lead to increased catabolism of adenine nucleotides to uric acid, decreased conversion of lactate to pyruvate, hyperuricemia, increased amounts of lactic acid in blood and liver, and a tendency to develop lactic acidosis (Fig. 44-1).[43] Metabolic acidosis has been fatal in a child given large amounts of fructose intravenously.[44] In postoperative patients who received fructose more slowly (0.5 g per kilogram of body weight per hour) hyperuricemia was not

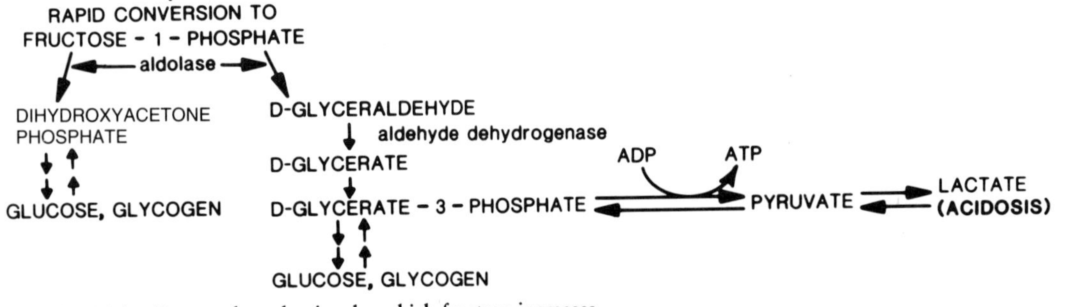

FIGURE 44-1. • Proposed mechanism by which fructose increases plasma and urine urate levels and blood lactate production.

observed and serum lactic acid levels rose, but the fall in pH and bicarbonate was less severe.[45,46] The formation of lactate from fructose in the liver may be reduced by the simultaneous infusion of amino acids.[47] With the availability of D-glucose and lipid emulsions for parenteral nutrition, there is virtually no indication for the use of fructose in IV solutions. If fructose is administered, it should not be infused rapidly. Fructose is clearly contraindicated even at low rates of infusion when lactic or other metabolic acidoses are present or likely to occur, such as in hypoxia, hypotension, or diabetic keotacidosis. Fructose is commercially available in aqueous preparations, polyionic solutions, and protein hydrolysates.

As with other acid-base disorders, metabolic acidosis can occur in patients who have underlying predisposing metabolic disturbances. These abnormalities include (1) conditions that promote hyperchloremia such as proximal intestinal fistulas, diarrhea, or renal tubular acidosis; (2) states that cause lactic acidosis such as hypoxia, hypotension, sepsis, liver failure, or neoplasia; (3) diabetic ketoacidosis and the sudden development of lactic acidosis; (4) accumulation of other inorganic and organic acids as in renal failure. The sudden development of lactic acidosis may be the first clinical sign of infection and may precede other manifestations of septicemia by several hours. Thus, the sudden onset of an anion gap acidosis is an indication for prompt evaluation for infection and other causes of lactic acidosis.

When metabolic acidosis occurs in patients receiving TPN, treatment should be directed toward correcting the underlying cause. Acetate or lactate content can be increased and chloride content reduced in the infusate, particularly when hyperchloremic acidosis is present. Acetate is converted to bicarbonate; hence, every molecule of acetate has the potential to neutralize one hydrogen ion. Kaminski and Hull indicated that hyperchloremic acidosis can be avoided if the TPN solutions provide sodium and chloride in a ratio of 1:1 and other anions are added as acetate.[48,49] Bicarbonate has an advantage over acetate or lactate in that it does not have to be metabolized to become a strong alkalinizing agent. However, large quantities of bicarbonate salts cannot be administered in TPN solutions because of the formation of insoluble calcium or magnesium carbonate and therefore would have to be infused separately. With severe, poorly controlled metabolic acidosis, patients may be treated with hemodialysis or peritoneal dialysis or with hemofiltration and infusion of large quantities of alkaline salts in the replacement solutions.

The use of sodium bicarbonate for the treatment of lactic acidosis has been criticized, because it may lead to no improvement or a worsening in intracellular and extracellular pH, cardiac output, and systemic blood pressure.[50-52] Dichloroacetate and sodium carbicarb (an equimolar solution of sodium carbonate and sodium bicarbonate) may be more effective for the treatment of lactic acidosis.[53-55]

Metabolic alkalosis

Metabolic alkalosis is not uncommon in sick patients receiving parenteral nutrition. In the setting of TPN, most cases of metabolic alkalosis are chloride-responsive. Probably the most common cause of metabolic alkalosis is the loss of acid and chloride by gastric aspiration, fistula drainage from the upper gastrointestinal tract, or vomiting in patients with large gastric secretions. Hypovolemia, use of diuretics, and infusion of excess base are other common causes of alkalosis in TPN patients.

Renal excretion of bicarbonate is the major mechanism by which the body rids itself of excess bicarbonate and corrects metabolic alkalosis. Volume contraction, which is often present in metabolic alkalosis, impairs the kidneys' ability to excrete bicarbonate and frequently is a key factor in the maintenance of metabolic alkalosis. Thus, in the treatment of metabolic alkalosis it is important to restore normal volume with NaCl solutions and, when hypokalemia is present, KCl. In hypoalbuminemic states associated with decreased renal perfusion, infusion of albumin or plasma may increase intravascular volume and renal glomerular perfusion and reduce renal tubular bicarbonate reabsorption;[56] this may help to correct metabolic alkalosis.

Chloride-responsive alkalosis can usually be treated by infusing saline or by substituting chloride for acetate in TPN solutions. Acetazolamide may be used to treat metabolic alkalosis and has been used most frequently in the treatment of posthypercapnic alkalosis.[57,58] Acetazolamide administration may cause potassium diuresis, which can further reduce potassium pools in an alkalotic patient with potassium depletion. Consideration should be given to administering potassium chloride with this diuretic. Sources of excess chloride loss should be treated vigorously. In patients with large gastric acid losses, drugs which inhibit gastric acid secretion (e.g., histamine H_2 receptor antagonists) may reduce hydrochloric acid losses and decrease the severity of metabolic alkalosis.

Sometimes the foregoing therapeutic maneuvers do not correct metabolic alkalosis. This is particularly likely to occur in patients with heart, liver, or kidney failure who do not tolerate sodium and potassium loads and volume expansion or patients with massive continued gastric losses of hydrochloric acid. In these cases, it may be necessary to give acidifying compounds such as ammonium chloride, hydrochloric acid, or hydrochloride salts of the amino acids arginine and lysine.

L-Arginine monohydrochloride is commercially available as a 10% solution for intravenous use. The solution is hypertonic (950 mosm) and contains 47.5 meq of Cl^- per 100 ml. Arginine monohydrochloride gives rise to an equal number of moles of hydrochloric acid. It contains nitrogen, most of which is ultimately incorporated into urea and which may be poorly tolerated in hepatic or renal failure. Arginine hydrochloride can cause flushing, nausea, vomiting, headache, numbness, and local irritation at the infusion site; an allergic erythematous macular eruption has also been reported.

L-Lysine hydrochloride can be obtained from chemical supply firms. When other acidifying agents are contraindicated or unavailable the IV preparation can be made by a hospital pharmacy. L-Lysine HCl also presents a nitrogen load which can be hazardous in patients with hepatic or renal insufficiency.

Arginine hydrochloride and lysine hydrochloride both promote the movement of potassium from the cell and can cause life-threatening hyperkalemia.[59,60] Thus, serum potassium must be monitored closely in patients receiving these drugs.

Ammonium chloride is available for infusion in isotonic (160 meq/liter) or hypertonic (400 meq/liter) solutions and in a number of polyionic (e.g., "gastric replacement") solutions at about 70 meq/liter. As Equation 1 shows, ammonium chloride ionizes in solution into ammonium and chloride; the former dissociates further into ammonia and hydrogen ion:

$$NH_4Cl \rightleftharpoons NH_4^+ + Cl^- \rightleftharpoons NH_3 + H^+ + Cl^- \qquad (1)$$

Ammonia can be excreted in the urine or participate in the formation of urea in the liver, leaving H^+ and Cl^-. The hydrogen ion combines with bicarbonate to form CO_2 and water. Thus, the chloride essentially replaces bicarbonate, and the metabolic products of ammonium chloride result in little solute load. The urea is distributed throughout the total body water so there is little increase in extracellular volume from the ammonium load.

Ammonium chloride can cause pallor, sweating, vomiting, and respiratory and mental depression; these symptoms may be related to the rate of infusion. Severe parenchymal liver disease is an absolute contraindication to the administration of ammonium chloride because hepatic encephalopathy can be precipitated. Use of ammonium chloride in renal failure may increase serum urea levels.

A number of reports demonstrate the value of hydrochloric acid for correction of severe metabolic alkalosis.[61-63] Hydrochloric acid has been used in severely alkalotic patients with heart, renal, or liver failure who are intolerant to sodium, expansion of intravascular fluid space, and nitrogen, or who have continuing losses of large quantities of acid, particularly from the stomach. A simplified description of its action is as follows:

$$HCl + HCO_3^- \rightleftharpoons CO_2 + H_2O + Cl^- \qquad (2)$$

Thus, as with ammonium chloride, the chloride in hydrochloric acid primarily replaces bicarbonate. Because the volume of infused fluid is distributed throughout the body's water space, it is better tolerated than when expansion of the fluid space is limited to the intravascular or extracellular compartments. The reaction described in Equation 2 should occur virtually at the moment of contact of hydrochloric acid with plasma. Thus, some investigators suggest administering hydrochloric acid in normal saline or 5% dextrose, so that when the acid is metabolized pure water will not be formed and cause hemolysis.[62]

Hydrochloric acid can be prepared by diluting the concentrate with distilled water for injection and sterilizing the solution by passing it through a 0.22-μm filter. It may then be added to dextrose or saline to form the appropriate solution. Hydrochloric acid is generally delivered into a large-diameter, high-flow vein as a 0.1 to 0.2 *N* solution (100 to 200 meq H^+/liter) over 6 to 24 h. Necrosis and sloughing of tissue at the infusion site and coagulation of blood at the catheter tip have been reported, but these complications seem to occur with higher rates of infusion or more concentrated solutions. When hydrochloric acid is administered, it is particularly important to frequently monitor vital signs, serum electrolytes, arterial blood pH and P_{CO_2}, hemoglobin and hematocrit, and to carefully monitor the condition of the infusion site.

Finkle and Dean reported using HCl in TPN solutions in 21 patients with severe metabolic alkalosis.[64] No untoward effects from the hydrochloric acid solutions were observed. Eight patients died; in five of them autopsy uncovered no evidence of skin necrosis, sloughing at the catheter site, or thrombophlebitis. The authors pointed out that when 2.0 *N* hydrochloric acid is added to amino acid solutions the buffer capacity of these solutions diminishes the fall in pH. Thus, adding hydrochloric acid to the TPN solutions might be less hazardous than administering it in either dextrose and water or saline.

Peritoneal dialysis and hemodialysis also can be effective for correcting severe metabolic alkalosis, especially in patients with heart, liver, or kidney failure. Dialysis is useful in several ways. Since bicarbonate is readily removed, patients with very high serum bicarbonate levels may undergo a net loss of base during dialysis even though acetate is received in the dialysate. The concentration of acetate ion in dialysate can be reduced or the acetate even omitted entirely and replaced with chloride. Moreover, dialysis can remove sodium and water, enabling the patient to tolerate intravenous infusions of large quantities of isotonic saline. Continuous arteriovenous hemofiltration with appropriate fluid and electrolyte replacement may also be effective for treating severe metabolic alkalosis.

Respiratory acidosis and alkalosis and respiratory function

Total parenteral nutrition may have a number of effects on respiratory function (see Table 44-4). Insertion of a subclavian vein catheter may cause pneumothorax and compromise respiratory function. Excess salt and water loads may lead to pulmonary edema, hypoxia, and lactic acidosis. The carbon load from the organic compounds infused may lead to hypercapnia. Usually infusion of parenteral solutions does not seriously affect respiratory function unless underlying illnesses have already compromised pulmonary function.

Infusion of large quantities of glucose may affect energy expenditure and pulmonary function. Large quantities of glucose may increase energy expenditure, CO_2 production, O_2 consumption, tidal volume, and respiratory rate.[65-68] The magnitude of the increase in these parameters is affected by the metabolic status of the patient: energy expenditure may increase less in those patients who can better use the infused nutrients for anabolic processes (e.g., depleted patients) than in well-nourished or hypermetabolic patients.[65] It is not known whether an increase in metabolic rate adversely affects patients with severe coronary artery insufficiency or marginal cardiac reserve.

Askanazi and associates reported that the enhanced CO_2 production in patients receiving high carbohydrate loads may cause hypercapnia and respiratory acidosis.[67] This has thus far been observed only in patients with impaired respiratory function, particularly those who are on a ventilator with a rather fixed ventilatory response. Covelli et al. observed a rise in P_{CO_2} within 12 h after initiation of TPN.[68] In a patient maintained on a ventilator P_{CO_2} increased from 43 to 93 mmHg and blood pH fell from 7.40 to 7.25 within 24 h after intake of carbohydrate calories was increased from 1500 to 2500 kcal/day. These data suggest that primary respiratory acidosis was occurring with metabolic alkalosis, and the acidosis was predominating; the investigators did not report a cause for the metabolic alkalosis. The respiratory acidosis was due to increased CO_2 production from the carbohydrate load in the presence of fixed mechanical ventilation. Normally, the increased CO_2 generated from the carbohydrate intake would stimulate ventilation. Hence hypercapnia can occur in patients with either diminished sensitivity to blood CO_2 level or reduced ventilatory function. It is likely that enhanced CO_2 production from a high calorie intake in some patients may hamper weaning them from mechanical ventilators.

A given number of calories from carbohydrate produces a greater increase in CO_2 production than the same number of calories from fat. This can be explained by the greater proportion of oxygen in the carbohydrate molecule; fewer oxygen atoms are required to oxidize the carbon and hydrogen in carbohydrates to carbon dioxide and water than to oxidize the carbon and hydrogen in fat. In comparison to carbohydrate, fat thus yields less CO_2 per molecule of oxygen consumed or per gram of fat oxidized; fat also provides more calories per gram of fat oxidized. This relationship is reflected in the respiratory quotient (RQ), the ratio of CO_2 released to O_2 taken up from respiration; RQ for fat = 0.7 and for carbohydrate = 1.0. The RQ in patients whose energy expenditure is derived primarily from endogenous or exogenous fat is close to 0.7. If such individuals receive a large amount of glucose, RQ rises toward 1.0; if the patient receives excess glucose and undergoes lipogenesis, RQ may exceed 1.0. Lipogenesis is associated with a major rise in CO_2 production and a moderate increase in both energy expenditure and O_2 production.[67] Patients who are hypermetabolic are less likely to become lipogenic with glucose infusion.

Since less carbon dioxide is produced per kilocalorie during the metabolism of fat than during the metabolism of carbohydrate, it has been suggested that patients are more likely to develop hypercapnia from a carbohydrate load than from an isocaloric quantity of fat. Thus, in patients who are at risk for severe hypercapnia it may be beneficial to give more of the calories as lipids. However, the maximum decrease in CO_2 generation that may occur when lipid calories are substituted for carbohydrate calories is only 17 percent, which, although potentially beneficial, is not very striking.[69] A more effective regimen is to avoid administering excess calories to patients at risk for hypercapnia, and if necessary, to markedly and temporarily reduce the intake of calories altogether. In recent years, the recognition that energy requirements of stressed patients undergoing TPN are not very high [i.e., normal resting metabolic expenditure × 1.25 × a stress factor (generally equal to 0.9 to 1.1 in the absence of burns)][34,70] has led to a reduction in caloric intake and hence in the risk for severe hypercapnia.

Weissman et al. described normal individuals who received a continuous intravenous infusion of 5% dextrose for 7 days. The infusion provided 440 kcal/day as the calorie source.[71] During the infusion of this quantity of dextrose, oxygen consumption, carbon dioxide production, RQ, resting minute ventilation, tidal volume, and mean inspiratory flow rate all decreased to, in general, 10 to 15 percent below preinfusion measurements. Subjects were also given an infusion of 3.5% amino acid solution, which provided the same number of calories as the dextrose solution, that is, 19.4 kcal/h (0.7 g of nitrogen per hour). Within 4 h rises were observed in oxygen consumption, minute ventilation, ventilatory drive, and resting energy expenditure. After 24 h these values had returned to approximately their levels prior to glucose infusion. These data suggest that amino acids may stimulate energy expenditure and ventilation in normal individuals receiving hypocaloric infusions.

Primary respiratory alkalosis has not been reported to be a complication of TPN therapy.

Water and macrominerals

The daily requirements for water and minerals vary greatly in patients receiving TPN. Some patients are malnourished or have specific deficiencies of certain electrolytes; others have sustained excessive losses from urinary excretion, diarrhea, fistula drainage, gastric aspiration, sweating, or burns. Elderly subjects and individuals with impaired heart, liver, or kidney function or certain endocrine disturbances may have decreased tolerance to water or minerals.

The nutritional requirement for some minerals is affected by the volume of water infused. This is particularly true for sodium and chloride, which are localized primarily in the extracellular space. In contrast, the daily requirements for potassium, phosphorus, magnesium, and calcium, which are found largely within cells or bone, are independent of water intake. During accretion or loss of protoplasmic mass, requirements for potassium, phosphorus, and magnesium can increase or decrease, respectively. The uptake or release of calcium, phosphorus, and magnesium from bone can also affect daily needs.

During formation of protoplasm in individuals not receiving TPN, the relative proportion of potassium (in meq), phosphorus (g), and nitrogen (g) incorporated into tissues is relatively constant, 3:0.07:1;[72] these relationships persist during TPN.[73] There is also a fairly constant ratio of phosphorus (g) to calcium (meq) deposited in bone, 0.09:1.[72] Moreover, during nutritional repletion of wasted patients the ratio of increase in extracellular fluid (in grams) to increase in protoplasm (g) is consant at 0.8:1.[73] Rudman and coworkers found that malnourished adults receiving TPN retain nitrogen (g), phosphorus (g), potassium (meq), sodium (meq), and chloride (meq) is the relative amounts 1:0.08:3.1:3.5:2.7.[73] They also observed that marked deficiencies of one mineral can lead to negative balances in others.

During TPN, the daily requirements for minerals may be lower than the recommended dietary allowances (RDA) for oral intake in normal individuals because the net absorption of many minerals from the gastrointestinal tract in healthy individuals is less than 100 percent. This is particularly true for calcium, phosphorus, magnesium, iron, zinc, copper, and certain other trace elements. On the other hand, during catabolic stress, the daily mineral requirements may exceed normal.

The daily mineral allowances suggested by different investigators vary greatly because of the variety of clinical disorders in patients receiving TPN and the paucity of studies defining mineral needs with TPN.[74-80] A recommended water and mineral intake which can be used in most circumstances in patients with normal ability to regulate mineral and water metabolism is given in Table 44-2.

When prescribing minerals for patients undergoing TPN it is important to consider the quantity of electrolytes incorporated into the amino acid or hydrolysate solution by the manufacturer. The electrolyte content of these solutions can vary greatly, and may be particularly high for sodium, chloride, potassium, calcium, and phosphorus in casein hydrolysates. The high concentration of acetate in the amino acid solutions must be taken into account when treating patients with metabolic alkalosis.

Water

Total body water usually accounts for 45 to 70 percent of body weight; the fraction varies with percentage of body fat, sex, age, and disease states or injury. In obese individuals body water accounts for a decreased percentage of body weight since the water content of adipose tissue is very low. Water generally accounts for a greater proportion of body weight in men compared to women because men usually are proportionately more muscular and have less fat. Body water accounts for up to 70 to 80 percent of weight in newborn infants, decreases to approximately 60 percent in young men and 50 percent in young women, and then remains relatively constant until middle age, when it falls gradually and progressively as muscle mass decreases.

In addition to urinary excretion, about 500 ml of water is lost daily from perspiration and insensible skin losses, 400 ml from respiration, and 150 ml in feces. The nonurinary water loss may be marked under certain conditions. Cutaneous losses can be greater than 20 liters/day in hot climates, especially in the absence of air movement.[81] These losses are partially offset by the production of about 350 ml of water per day from oxidation of hydrogen in protein, carbohydrate, and fat. Endogenous water production can rise to 800 ml/day in hypercatabolic patients.[82] Ingestion of solid foods provides about 750 ml of water per day. In general, complete oxidation (per gram) yields 0.60 ml of water from carbohydrate, 0.50 ml from amino acids, 0.40 ml from protein, and 1.00 ml from fat.[83] Slightly greater amounts of water may be released from catabolism because water is deposited along with protein, carbohydrate, and fat. Thus, the amount of water released from catabolism of protein or glycogen is about 3 ml/g and from fat is about 1.08 ml/g. Patients who breathe humidified air from mechanical ventilators may lose no water from respiration.

Other factors that may increase the daily water requirement in patients undergoing TPN include fever, hyperventilation, diarrhea, fistula drainage, diaphoresis, loss of integumentary structure or function, and third-space shifts.[84] Anabolism also leads to the sequestration of a small and generally insignificant amount of water.[85] The distribution of fluid between intracellular and extracellular spaces may vary in ill patients.

In sick patients undergoing TPN a number of factors may impair the kidneys' ability to regulate water balance. Decreased renal blood flow and glomerular filtration rate (GFR), low serum albumin, and increased levels of serum antidiuretic hormone (ADH), aldosterone, and cortisol may predispose to water retention and hyponatremia. All of these factors are common complications in sick patients. Enhanced ADH release occurs with many illnesses, stress, and painful stimuli; in the postoperative state; with drugs which stimulate ADH release, such as narcotics, barbiturates, tranquilizers, and oral hypoglycemic agents; and in the syndrome of inappropriate secretion of

ADH (SIADH) (see Chap. 20). Heart, liver, or kidney failure and the nephrotic syndrome also promote water retention and hyponatremia through a number of mechanisms. In addition, diuretics, particularly thiazides, which act on the diluting segment in the distal tubule, impair urinary dilution and can engender a hypoosmolar state. Renal disease, hypercalcemia, hypokalemia, malnutrition, osmotic diuretics, and drugs inhibiting ADH release or its action on the kidney can impair concentrating ability and predispose to hyperosmolarity (see Chap. 21).

Patients receiving TPN generally take in a large water load, usually 2 to 3 liters/day. The quantity of water administered must be large because of the relative insolubility of certain amino acids, particularly the essential ones. The insolubility of the essential amino acids limits the concentration of solutions providing essential and nonessential amino acids to a maximum of about 15 percent. If the concentrations of certain highly soluble nonessential amino acids were markedly increased, the total amino acid concentration could be raised to 15 percent or higher. However, the ratio of total essential to nonessential amino acids in the solution would fall to less than the recommended minimum of about 1:1. The development and increasing use of peptides, which are more soluble than many amino acids, ultimately may lead to more concentrated amino acid solutions.

It should also be recognized that the aqueous volume of TPN solutions is less than 100 percent of the total volume. The water content of different standard intravenous solutions has been reported as 96.2 to 96.9 g of H_2O per 100 ml for 5% dextrose in water (D_5W), approximately 70 g H_2O/100 ml for 50% dextrose in water, between 92.7 and 96.0 g H_2O/100 ml for 8.5% amino acid solutions, and 86.6 percent water for IV fat emulsions.[85]

Although TPN solutions are hyperosmolar, frequently 1600 to 1800 mosm/liter, most of this solute load is from glucose and amino acids and is readily metabolizable. The total electrolyte content is generally hypotonic to plasma (see Table 44-2). Occasionally, this factor and particularly the low sodium concentrations of TPN solutions (30 to 55 meq/liter) engender a hypoosmolar state in the patient, particularly in the presence of increased circulating ADH or drugs which impair urinary dilution (see above). Hyponatremia can generally be treated by increasing the sodium concentration of the TPN solution, reducing total water intake, and/or avoiding those diuretics that primarily affect the distal diluting segment (i.e., thiazides, metolazone).

A general rule of thumb is to provide enough water to maintain a urine output of at least 1200 to 1500 ml/day; 30 to 50 ml of water per kilogram of body weight per day is usually sufficient. If the patient has advanced renal, liver, or heart failure, water intake may need to be restricted further. Fluid overload can often be treated by reducing fluid intake and/or giving diuretics, particularly the more potent agents such as furosemide or ethacrynic acid. In addition, hemodialysis, hemofiltration, peritoneal dialysis, or continuous arteriovenous hemofiltration may be used to control fluid balance.[86] For patients undergoing maintenance dialysis, it is desirable to minimize fluid intake to either prevent or minimize water gain. It is the authors' impression that the hemodynamic stability of sick patients with renal failure who require TPN, in general, is better preserved if the patients do not gain excessive amounts of water and hence do not require aggressive removal of fluid during hemodialysis.

Water deficit is an uncommon complication in patients undergoing TPN because of the large water load TPN imposes. In addition, many of the factors that lead to dehydration, such as high ambient temperatures, profuse sweating, or diarrhea, do not occur commonly in a hospital setting in a patient who is receiving little or no enteral nutrition. One of the more common causes of dehydration occurring de novo in patients receiving TPN is hyperosmolar, hyperglycemic, nonketotic dehydration (see above). Burn patients not uncommonly lose large amounts of water. However, the energy and protein requirements of burn patients are also large; if they receive all of their nutrition intravenously they are also receiving larger volumes of fluid.

Dehydration in a patient receiving TPN can be treated simply by increasing the water load. In the presence of volume depletion with both sodium and water deficits, patients are generally given normal saline until circulation is restored and are then changed to a hypotonic sodium chloride solution, such as half-normal saline (see Chap. 21).

Sodium

Sodium is the major extracellular cation. The body of a young or middle-aged adult normally contains approximately 3350 to 4150 meq of sodium.[87] Half of the body's sodium is extracellular; another 40 percent is in bone, of which only half can be rapidly exchanged.[88] The intracellular sodium concentration is about 10 meq/per kilogram of water.

Usually, sodium is excreted almost entirely in urine. Fecal sodium excretion is about 1 to 3 meq/day and skin losses are small unless sweating is excessive. Urinary sodium excretion in patients with normal renal function who are not receiving diuretics can be markedly reduced when intake is restricted. With complete sodium deprivation urinary sodium excretion normally can fall to about 1 to 2 meq/liter within 3 to 5 days. Osmotic or tubular diuretics and impaired renal function can prevent this degree of sodium conservation.

The nutritional requirements for sodium are not well-defined, in either normal individuals or patients undergoing TPN. During periods of sodium deprivation, the body can avidly retain sodium; with excessive sweating and during disease states, the sodium requirement can increase dramatically. Since Na^+ and Cl^- are primarily extracellular electrolytes which serve to maintain extracellular volume, the daily requirements for them generally are best defined in relation to the quantity of infused water. This approach helps to reduce the likelihood that patients will develop abnormal serum sodium concentrations or deviations in extracellular volume. In contrast, the daily requirements for the other electrolytes in TPN solutions are not defined according to the water intake. Provision of approximately 30 to 55 meq of sodium per liter maintains normal serum sodium concentrations in the majority of patients receiving TPN.[76,89-93] Although some researchers have recommended calibrating the sodium requirement by the calorie intake, there seems to be no metabolic or physiological basis for this recommendation.[83]

Weinsier et al. reported the occurrence of hyponatremia ($[Na^+] < 125$ meq/liter) in 6 percent of patients and hypernatremia ($[Na^+] > 160$ meq/liter) in 1 percent of patients.[1] The causes of altered serum sodium concentrations in patients undergoing TPN have never been studied systematically. The three most common causes of hypotonic hyponatremia in patients receiving TPN probably are excessive intake of free water, increased serum ADH levels, and decreased GFR. Two other disorders associated with TPN, both of which are due to the infusion of large quantities of nutrients, lower the measured serum sodium concentration: hyperglycemia precipitated by high glucose intake, particularly in the face of catabolic stress, may cause hypertonic hyponatremia; hyperlipidemia from IV infusion of fat can also spuriously lower serum $[Na^+]$, particularly if blood is drawn while the patient is receiving the lipid. Hyperproteinemia (e.g., from myeloma or macroglobulinemia) may also lower measured serum sodium concentrations. Hyperlipidemia and hyperproteinemia exert only minimal effects on serum sodium. The reduction in serum sodium concentration, in meq/liter, caused by the elevation in lipid and protein in the blood can be estimated by multiplying the plasma lipid concentration, in mg/dl, by 0.002 or the increment in serum protein concentration above 8.0 g/dl by 0.25.[94]

Potassium

Potassium is the primary intracellular cation. Approximately 90 percent is inside cells; 8 to 9 percent is in bone, connective tissues, and the transcellular space; and 1 to 2 percent is in plasma and interstitial fluid. Homeostatic mechanisms allow potassium (like water and sodium) intake to vary widely in normal adults without causing a deficit or excess. However, potassium cannot be conserved as efficiently as sodium. In a normal person deprived of potassium for 4 to 5 days, about 25 meq of potassium is lost per day: approximately 15 meq in urine and 10 meq in stool. The usual daily urinary potassium loss is at least 40 meq; this quantity is frequently recommended as the minimum required intake in patients with normal renal function receiving nutrition intravenously. Some researchers have recommended that the potassium requirement should be sufficient to allow 3 meq to be incorporated into tissues for each gram of nitrogen retained.[72,73] There are pitfalls in such recommendations. First, in potassium-depleted patients the relative requirements for potassium and nitrogen may vary. In addition, many clinical conditions cause a selective increase in daily potassium needs. These include diarrhea, nasogastric suction, fistulas in the stomach or high in the intestine, use of diuretics, and renal potassium wasting. Recent studies also indicate that in disease states, including chronic renal failure, the ratio of total body potassium to nitrogen can vary greatly[95] (see Chaps. 6 and 7).

Weinsier et al. described hypokalemia (serum $[K^+] < 3.0$ meq/liter) in 18 percent and hyperkalemia (serum $[K^+] > 6.5$ meq/liter) in 2 percent of patients receiving TPN.[1] Serum potassium levels may be abnormal because of a shift of potassium into or out of cells or because of positive or negative body potassium balance. The serum is the most critical compartment in which to control potassium concentration because relatively small changes in serum levels can severely alter myocardial and skeletal muscle function. Catecholamines, aldosterone, insulin, glucose, and anabolism enhance movement of potassium into cells and act to lower serum potassium. TPN may promote marked intracellular movement of potassium due to the infusion of large quantities of glucose and amino acids which can increase serum insulin levels and stimulate anabolism. Sufficient potassium must thus be infused in TPN to prevent hypokalemia. Conversely, inorganic acidosis, insulinopenia, adrenergic blocking agents, and catabolic stress such as trauma, surgery, or starvation promote movement of potassium out of cells and can cause severe hyperkalemia if renal function is reduced. Hyperkalemia may also occur from intracellular release of potassium caused by rhabdomyolysis, hemolysis, or lysis of tumors (see Chaps. 22 and 23).

Hypokalemia can be caused by deficiency of total body potassium. The most frequent causes include excessive urinary potassium excretion from diuretic use, loss of gastrointestinal fluids rich in K^+ or H^+, and diabetic ketoacidosis. Hypokalemia may also accompany renal tubular acidosis, hyperaldosteronism, cirrhosis, metabolic alkalosis, and parenteral nutrition with inadequate potassium intake. Similarly, hyperkalemia can be caused by factors which increase total body potassium content: oliguric renal failure; the hyporeninemic hypoaldosterone syndrome; potassium-sparing diuretics; rapid administration of potassium, particularly when given intravenously; and multiple blood transfusions.

Disturbances in cardiac conduction are the greatest risk of hyperkalemia. In the Boston Collaborative Drug Surveillance Program reported by Lawson, 4900 consecutive patients who received oral and/or intravenous potassium were evaluated; hyperkalemia occurred in 3.6 percent.[96] Hyperkalemia was considered to be the major cause of death in 7 patients and it created a life-threatening condition in another 21. Hyperkalemia is particularly likely to occur in patients with renal failure or diabetes mellitus, elderly patients, and in those receiving spironolactone or triamterene. Burchell has suggested somewhat facetiously that "more lives may have been lost than saved by potassium therapy."[97] Acidosis, hypocalcemia, and hyponatremia may enhance the adverse effects of hyperkalemia, whereas alkalosis and hypercalcemia may reduce these effects.

It is recommended that patients receiving TPN whose serum potassium concentration and renal function are normal should receive approximately 60 to 90 meq of potassium each day. Serum potassium should be monitored frequently, particularly during the early course of treatment with TPN when the daily requirement may vary greatly. Also, serum potassium should be monitored closely during any change in insulin dosage, particularly if insulin is administered for treatment of severe hyperglycemia. It has been recommended that the potassium intake should be considered adequate when urinary potassium excretion is at least 40 meq/liter. Although this is a good rule of thumb, it does not exclude potassium depletion due to a renal cause, such as from diuretic therapy, osmotic diuresis, or renal tubular acidosis.

Generally, potassium is not added to TPN solutions until it is ascertained that the serum potassium concentration is normal and not rising. Even patients with advanced renal failure who receive TPN usually require potassium. The daily potassium requirement, however, usually is lower in patients with advanced renal failure receiving TPN: about 40 to 50 meq/day. The daily requirement should be determined in these patients by serial monitoring of serum potassium concentration.

The quantity of potassium needed for intravenous therapy of hypokalemia may be difficult to ascertain because (1) serum potassium may not reflect total body potassium and (2) the potassium requirement can change with the magnitude of potassium losses and alterations in the relative rates of anabolism and catabolism. Serum potassium concentration may change markedly if insulin or glucose is administered during parenteral nutrition or if the blood pH varies.

As a guide to intravenous therapy, several rough relationships between serum potassium levels and acidosis and between serum potassium levels and the magnitude of potassium deficit have been described: (1) in inorganic acidosis (e.g., with HCl), for every 0.1-unit change in plasma pH there is an inverse change in serum potassium of approximately 0.6 meq/liter;[98] (2) in metabolic alkalosis with paradoxical aciduria (urine pH 6 to 6.5), the potassium deficit is usually at least 400 meq; (3) if serum $[K^+] < 3.0$ meq/liter, an infusion of 200 to 400 meq of potassium is generally necessary to raise serum $[K^+]$ by 1 meq/liter; (4) if serum potassium concentration is 3.0 to 4.0 meq/liter, an infusion of 100 to 200 meq raises serum potassium level by 1 meq/liter. It should be emphasized that these are very rough relationships which can be markedly affected by hormonal, toxic, and physical events that may occur in sick patients (see Chap. 6). Perhaps the safest approach is to make an initial estimate of the rate of potassium administration necessary for repletion and maintenance. Serum $[K^+]$ level should be assessed and the electrocardiogram monitored very frequently; the potassium dose should be adjusted as necessary until a steady state is established. Greater caution must be used when potassium is given to patients with renal insufficiency.

If a patient receives potassium at rates greater than 20 meq/h for more than 2 h, the electrocardiogram should be monitored continuously and serum potassium remeasured with approximately every 50 meq infused.[99] With severe hypokalemia it is well to remember that glucose infusion may further depress serum potassium concentration. Therefore, it may be hazardous to start TPN or to infuse large quantities of glucose until the serum potassium concentration has begun to rise.

Hemodialysis and peritoneal dialysis may be used to treat both hypokalemia and hyperkalemia. Treatment of hypokalemia with high dialysate concentrations of potassium may be indicated for hypokalemic patients who have fluid intolerance (e.g., increased body water content or congestive heart failure), subjects in whom it is difficult to insert an IV infusion line, and patients who require dialysis to control uremia.[100]

In the chloride-responsive alkaloses with hypokalemia it is important to administer potassium as the chloride salt. Administration of an alkaline potassium salt (e.g., potassium acetate) in an alkalotic patient can cause excessive urinary losses of potassium and impede replacement of the potassium deficit. Chloride can be substituted for most of the acetate in the TPN solutions except for the acetate incorporated into the amino acid solution by the manufacturer. With acidosis or hypophosphatemia, potassium acetate or potassium phosphate may be administered.

Potassium should never be infused as a bolus. When potassium is added to a nonrigid parenteral fluid container it may not mix well; during administration it may enter the bloodstream as a bolus and cause potassium intoxication.[101,102] Better mixing is obtained by administering directly into a rigid container. If the injection port is used, injection should be carried out with a long needle or else the bag should be mixed. Also, instilling the potassium before the container is inverted and suspended from the IV stand seems to promote better mixing.

Hyperkalemia usually can be successfully managed by decreasing the potassium content of the TPN infusions. Sometimes giving diuretics or potassium exchange resins is necessary (see Chap. 23).

Chloride

Chloride is present primarily as an extracellular anion. The main effect of chloride excess or deficiency is on acid-base balance. Experience suggests that metabolic alkalosis and hyperchloremic acidosis are best avoided by maintaining the ratio of sodium to chloride in the TPN solutions at about 1.0:1.0. This necessitates adding non-chloride salts of sodium and potassium, such as sodium acetate and potassium phosphate, to the infusates.

Hypochloremic alkalosis and hyperchloremic acidosis can be caused by a number of acid-base disorders (see above and Chaps. 25 and 29). Chloride-responsive alkalosis and hyperchloremic acidosis may be treated by changing the ratio of chloride to acetate in the TPN solutions. Hypochloremic acidosis is a high-anion gap acidosis caused by the presence of increased quantities of other acids (see Chap. 25). When calculating the amounts of chloride and acetate to be administered, it is important to remember that both of these anions are also incorporated into amino acid solutions by manufacturers.

Calcium

There are about 1000 to 1500 g of calcium in a normal adult, primarily in bone. The RDA of the Food and Nutrition Board for dietary calcium in nonpregnant, nonlactating adults is 800 to 1200 mg/day, depending on the age.[103] Since approximately 5 to 40 percent of dietary calcium intake is absorbed, the estimated calcium requirement for TPN patients should be similar to the RDA for dietary calcium minus the net loss in feces of calcium taken orally. During catabolic stress, calcium excretion increases.[104] Some investigators report the daily calcium requirement for clinically stable patients undergoing TPN to be about 0.2 to 0.3 meq per kilogram of body weight or about 12.5 to 22.5 meq (250 to 450 mg).[90,105] This is a rough approximation since no long-term studies of calcium balance have defined requirements in TPN patients. Rudman and associates studied underweight adults undergoing TPN who were not acutely ill.[73] These investigators found calcium balance to be neutral or positive with a calcium intake of 0.128 meq per kilogram of desirable body weight per day.

Hypocalcemia has been reported in patients receiving TPN solutions that do not contain calcium. In hypoproteinemic patients, serum calcium concentration may be low because of reduced binding of calcium to protein. In these circumstances, serum ionized calcium is usually normal, and the patient does not suffer adverse effects. Hypocalcemia also occurs in patients with magnesium deficiency, hyperphosphatemia, pancreatitis, and rhabdomyolysis (see Chap. 32).

In surveys of patients receiving short-term TPN the reported incidence of hypercalcemia has varied from 0 to 8 percent.[1,8,106] Hypercalcemia may be caused by excessive intake of calcium or vitamin D.[8] Gilligan and associates described hypercalcemia which occurred with TPN that did not provide calcium or vitamin D;[106] these authors found a significant correlation of both total serum calcium and ionized calcium with the rate at which amino acids were infused in the TPN solutions over the preceding 4 days. Infusion of albumin can raise serum calcium concentration by increasing the amount of calcium bound to circulating albumin.[29]

Primary and secondary hyperparathyroidism predispose to hypercalcemia, especially when serum phosphorus levels are low. Hypercalcemia also may occur with bed rest from mobilization of bone calcium or during recovery from rhabdomyolysis. In TPN patients pancreatitis may occur in association with hypercalcemia.[107] Vague psychiatric or neuromuscular symptoms or altered consciousness may be an indication of hypercalcemia. When hypercalcemia occurs, it is important to examine the patient for underlying causes, such as neoplasm, excess vitamin D intake, vitamin A toxicity, or primary or secondary hyperparathyroidism.

Magnesium

Magnesium is the fourth most plentiful cation in the body; there is about 2000 meq of Mg^{2+} in a 70-kg man. Approximately 50 percent of body magnesium is in bone and the other 50 percent is in soft tissue. As with potassium, only a small amount (about 1 percent) of magnesium is in ECF; the rest of soft tissue magnesium is within cells, in a concentration of about 28 meq/liter. Magnesium depletion may be caused by malabsorption syndromes, protein-calorie malnutrition,[108] alcoholism, and syndromes of renal magnesium wasting, including therapy with diuretics,[109] aminoglycosides, cisplatin,[110,111] and amphotericin B; diabetic ketoacidosis,[112] and Bartter's syndrome.[113] Hypomagnesemia also occurs with vitamin D treatment and in hyperparathyroidism. Magnesium excess has been described in renal failure, although usually it does not occur unless such patients also receive medicines high in magnesium content (e.g., magnesium-containing antacids or laxatives). Hypermagnesemia has also been described with adrenocortical insufficiency.[112]

Weinsier and associates reported hypomagnesemia (serum $[Mg^{2+}] < 1.5$ mg/dl) in 1 percent of their patients receiving TPN.[1] In Crohn's disease, ulcerative colitis, or other inflammatory bowel diseases, magnesium depletion may occur and persist even when patients receive TPN. Main and associates found low serum magnesium levels in 15 of 17 patients with chronic inflammatory bowel disease who were starting TPN.[114] Levine et al. described hypomagnesemia and ventricular tachycardia in a 19-year-old woman with ulcerative colitis who was receiving 150 meq of IV magnesium per day but was excreting 167 meq of Mg^{2+} daily in her urine and feces while on

TPN.[115] Most of her magnesium losses appeared to be in feces. Although diarrhea usually decreases markedly or stops in such patients when they undergo TPN, it may persist and cause large continuing intestinal losses of water and other minerals as well as magnesium. This is particularly likely to occur if the patients continue to eat while they are receiving TPN.

Low serum magnesium levels have also been described in 8 of 17 patients with solid tumors or hematologic malignancies who were undergoing TPN while they each received an average of 24 meq of magnesium per day.[116] These authors reported that the incidence of hypomagnesemia was much higher in their patients with malignancies who were receiving TPN than in a similar group of patients without malignancies. They suggested that the low serum magnesium levels may reflect a high requirement for magnesium during the lymphocyte-mediated killing of tumor cells. In addition, the chemotherapeutic agent cisplatin has been shown to cause renal magnesium wasting and hypomagnesemia.[110,111]

Magnesium deficiency is associated with refractory hypokalemia and hypocalcemia, weakness, muscle fasciculation, tremors, positive Chvostek's and Trousseau's signs, and general tetany. Hypomagnesemia can cause alterations in the EKG, ventricular ectopy, and ventricular tachycardia.[115,117] Hypermagnesemia commonly occurs in the setting of renal failure associated with a large intake of magnesium containing antacids or laxatives. Another not uncommon cause of magnesium excess is the use of magnesium salts in the treatment of preeclampsia. Acute hypermagnesemia may depress the CNS as well as the peripheral neuromuscular junction. When serum magnesium levels exceed 4 meq/liter the deep tendon reflexes are decreased. At serum magnesium levels greater than 8 to 10 meq/liter, flaccid quadriplegia may occur with absent deep tendon reflexes. Hypotension, impaired talking and swallowing, and paralysis of the respiratory muscles may occur;[118,119] however, the patient is usually conscious.

Although magnesium resides primarily in bone or in intracellular sites, serum and total body magnesium appear to be roughly correlated. Thus, adequacy of magnesium intake should be assessed periodically by measuring serum magnesium. In addition, low urine magnesium may give an early indication of magnesium depletion and may be a more sensitive indicator of magnesium deficiency than is serum magnesium.[120] The average daily urinary magnesium excretion, 100 to 150 mg, may fall to 10 to 12 mg in the setting of magnesium depletion.[121]

The daily requirement for magnesium in patients undergoing TPN has not been established. Recommendations vary from 4 to 42 meq/day (49 to 510 mg/day).[122-126] Dudrick recommended 10 to 12 meq/day and suggested that the intravenous intake should be adjusted to keep serum magnesium levels normal.[123] Driscoll and Rosenberg and Main and associates recommended 24 meq/day and 10 to 20 meq/day, respectively, for patients with inflammatory bowel disease undergoing TPN.[114,122] Shenkin and Wretlind recommended 0.08 meq per kilogram of body weight per day as the minimum intravenous requirement for maintenance, 0.30 to 0.40 meq per kilogram of body weight per day for depleted patients or those with increased losses, and 0.6 to 0.8 meq per kilogram per day for patients during or after a severe catabolic stress.[127] Patients without renal insufficiency who are receiving TPN seem to tolerate 16 to 30 meq of magnesium per day (194 to 365 mg/day) without developing hyper- or hypomagnesemia.

Phosphorus

Phosphorus is the major intracellular anion; it exists primarily in an organic form in carbohydrates, lipids, and proteins. The adult body has about 700 g of phosphorus, of which approximately 80 percent is in bone and 9 percent in muscle. Because of its largely intracellular compartmentalization, the serum phosphorus concentration does not necessarily reflect total body phosphorus stores.

Hypophosphatemia is a common complication in hospitalized patients. The most common cause of hypophosphatemia (defined as serum [P] $<$ 2.0 mg/dl) in hospitalized patients is intravenous infusion of glucose. Betro and Pain observed hypophosphatemia in 40 of 100 patients who received IV glucose.[128]

When TPN was first developed, the importance of adding phosphorus was not generally recognized. It quickly became apparent that patients who receive TPN without phosphorus frequently become hypophosphatemic and display symptoms. Predialysis serum phosphorus concentrations of 0.5 mg/dl also have been observed in hemodialysis patients with acute or chronic renal failure who were undergoing TPN without phosphorus intake. Weinsier and Krumdieck found that 30 of 100 consecutive medical and surgical patients receiving TPN had serum phosphorus concentrations less than 2.0 mg/dl; in 6 patients the phosphorus concentration was below 1.0 mg/dl.[129] These authors considered hypophosphatemia to be the most common serum electrolyte abnormality in patients receiving TPN.

Hypophosphatemia occurring shortly after commencing TPN usually is primarily due to a shift in inorganic phosphorus from ECF into the cell.[130] Intravenous glucose and amino acids stimulate insulin secretion, which promotes the intracellular movement of phosphorus. In patients receiving TPN without phosphorus, urinary phosphorus excretion falls markedly, e.g., to less than 10 mg/day. However, these low levels are not attained for 8 to 10 days, and patients receiving long-term TPN may excrete large quantities of phosphorus into the urine (e.g., 450 to 1000 mg/day) before this adaptation occurs;[29] the urinary loss may contribute to hypophosphatemia. Aladjem and coworkers reported an increase in urinary phosphorus excretion in children during short-term administration of TPN without phosphorus.[131] The decreases in serum phosphorus and in tubular reabsorption of phosphorus in these children were more pronounced after infusion of amino acids and glucose than after glucose infusion alone; but inferences drawn from comparing the two TPN formulations must be tentative because different amounts of calories were provided. Urinary phosphorus losses may be much greater in catabolic patients who receive TPN.[132] Increased plasma cortisol levels and sodium diuresis may also enhance urinary phosphorus excretion in acutely ill patients undergoing TPN.

Hypophosphatemia during TPN seems to be more common in patients who have underlying illnesses that predispose to hypophosphatemia, such as alcoholism, intestinal malabsorption, thermal burns, or diabetic ketoacidosis. Studies suggest that starvation and malnutrition predispose to the development of hypophosphatemia in animals and humans who are given parenteral or enteral nutrition with little or no phosphorus.[129,130,133] In patients with normal serum phosphorus concentrations who receive TPN without phosphorus, the level of serum phosphorus may fall by about 0.3 mg/dl/day and reach hazardous levels of about 0.5 mg/dl within 10 days.[29] However, in malnourished patients who are not hypercatabolic, the fall in serum phosphorus with TPN may be much more rapid; serum phosphorus is reported to fall to 0.4 mg/dl in about 2 days. In catabolic patients a net movement of phosphorus out of intracellular sites may provide some protection against hypophosphatemia.

The phosphorus depletion syndrome can occur in patients with hypophosphatemia and essentially normal total body phosphorus and in those who have hypophosphatemia and a deficiency in total body phosphorus; the clinical symptoms of both conditions are similar. Although malnourished or wasted patients may have a low total body phosphorus content, in general they do not develop symptoms of phosphorus depletion unless phosphorus is disproportionately deficient compared to other nutrients, as indicated by low intracellular ratios of phosphorus:nitrogen or phosphorus:potassium or low plasma phosphorus concentration.

The signs and symptoms of hypophosphatemia or phosphate depletion that have been observed in patients receiving parenteral nutrition include: (1) impaired formation of 2,3-diphosphoglycerate (2,3-DPG) and other glycolytic intermediates;[134] (2) decreased generation of ATP in red cells, which may be associated with a leftward shift of the hemoglobin oxygen dissociation curve as release of oxygen from hemoglobin is impaired;[135] (3) hemolytic anemia;[136] (4) impaired phagocytosis by leukocytes;[137] (5) hypotension and cardiopulmonary decompensation;[129] (6) rhabdomyolysis;[138] and (7) neurological disorders including Guillain-Barré-Strohl syndrome,[139] acute areflexic paralysis,[140] mental aberrations, paresthesias, weakness, seizures, coma, and death.[141,142]

Hyperphosphatemia occurs much less commonly during TPN; it appears to be virtually limited to patients with renal failure who cannot excrete a phosphorus load normally. Patients with hyperphosphatemia, including those with renal failure, may be treated initially with TPN solutions containing little or no phosphorus. However, with such infusions serum phosphorus falls and eventually some phosphorus must be added to the IV infusions. Hyperphosphatemic patients should not receive calcium until serum phosphorus levels fall to normal; otherwise, the high serum calcium-phosphorus product may cause metastatic calcification.

The daily phosphorus requirement for patients undergoing TPN varies considerably. The phosphorus intake needed to maintain normal serum phosphorus concentrations has been reported to be 20 to 25 meq potassium dihydrogen phosphate (143 to 178 mg phosphorus) per 1000 kcal.[143] Additive solutions of potassium phosphate for patients receiving TPN generally contain both the dibasic (HPO_4^{2-}) and the monobasic ($H_2PO_4^-$) forms in order to maintain the solution at physiological pH. The molar ratio of dibasic to monobasic phosphate is 4:1. For many physicians and other health professionals it is confusing to estimate the phosphorus intake from the number of meq of phosphate listed in these additives because two different valences of phosphate ion are present in the solution. Therefore, when estimating the quantity of phosphorus for parenteral nutrition, it is preferable to express phosphorus in terms of mmol or mg rather than as meq.

TRACE ELEMENTS

Overview

At least 14 trace elements are considered essential for health in mammals. Iron, zinc, copper, manganese, iodine, selenium, chromium, and molybdenum have been shown to be essential for humans. Evidence has been developed to suggest that cobalt, tin, vanadium, fluorine, silicon, and nickel, although not established as essential for human beings, may be required by other animals. Signs of arsenic deprivation have also been described in chicken, goat, minipig, and rats.[144] Many other trace elements may be indispensable but proof for this is currently lacking.[145-147]

Human requirements have been established for oral intake of eight essential trace elements: iron, zinc, copper, iodine, molybdenum, manganese, selenium, and chromium.[103] Most trace elements are not absorbed completely from the GI tract, and smaller quantities are probably required for parenteral nutrition. However, there are relatively few careful studies of trace element requirements during TPN.

The possibility of trace element deficiencies with TPN has aroused concern.[148-153] Hankins et al. analyzed trace element concentrations in whole blood of eight patients receiving TPN for long periods and found elevated levels of manganese and antimony, low levels of copper, bromine, and rubidium, and near-normal levels of zinc, cobalt, selenium, iron, and chromium.[154] The increased manganese concentration was felt to be due to the high manganese content of the parenteral solutions. Although urinary and intestinal (fecal, fistula, or stomal) losses and intracellular deposition associated with anabolism may contribute to lowered plasma trace element levels, the major cause of deficiency is an inadequate quantity in TPN solutions. Also, preexisting trace element deficiencies, which may have been subclinical, may become clinically overt after TPN commences.

Evaluating the patient for trace element deficiency or excess poses a number of technical problems.[155] Serum concentrations do not necessarily reflect total body pools. In patients with Crohn's disease serum zinc concentrations do not correlate with muscle zinc obtained from needle biopsy.[156] Most plasma trace elements are largely protein bound. If serum albumin or other binding proteins are reduced, which is a common phenomenon in catabolic patients, the total plasma concentration of these trace elements may be reduced.[157] Conversely, estrogens and inflammatory disorders may raise serum ceruloplasmin and thereby may increase serum copper levels, since 80 percent of this element is bound to this globin.[158] Also, metabolic events may cause shifts in the trace element distribution between body compartments. Sepsis can rapidly increase serum copper and lower serum zinc concentrations. Trace element analysis of hair specimens may not reflect body pools.[159] Low plasma and urine excretion of trace elements may in fact be better indications of a deficiency state.[160] Measurements of certain enzymes that are dependent on trace elements also may be good indicators of body pool size. For example, activity of glutathionine peroxidase, which is selenium-dependent, is considered to be a rather accurate indicator of the body's selenium status.[161]

Interactions between some trace elements may predispose to deficiency. The oral intake of zinc or molybdenum may impair intestinal copper absorption.[162,163] Increased urinary excretion of zinc and copper and the development of related deficiencies may occur when glucosamines are present in TPN solutions.[164] Glucosamines are formed by the Maillard reaction when high concentrations of glucose and amino acids remain in contact with each other for long periods of time, and particularly if such preparations are sterilized by heating.[165,166] Glucosamines are poorly metabolized and bind with certain trace elements. Other trace element interactions have also been described.[167]

Deficiencies of specific trace elements lead to a variety of disorders. For trace elements such as zinc and copper, which are cofactors for many enzymes, deficiency may cause pervasive metabolic or clinical abnormalities. Conversely, many trace elements become toxic at high levels and the difference between toxic and beneficial doses may be small.

Tentative recommendations for daily intake in TPN solutions of zinc, selenium, chromium, copper, and molybdenum in adult patients are shown in Table 44-2. These recommendations, proposed by Fleming in 1989,[155] were approved by the Council of the American Society of Clinical Nutrition (ASCN). They are similar to those of the American Medical Association, published in 1979,[168] except that copper has been reduced from 500 to 1500 μg to 300 to 500 μg, chromium intake has been changed from 10 to 15 μg to 10 to 20 μg, and requirements for selenium and molybdenum have been added. The American Medical Association recommended a daily intake of manganese of 150 to 800 μg/day in TPN.[168] No recommendation was given in the more recent publication because it was argued that there is no convincing evidence that it is essential for patients receiving TPN. Hypercatabolism and excessive losses of intestinal fluids can modify these losses. In patients with acute or chronic kidney or liver failure receiving TPN, information concerning trace elements needs or toxicity is very scant. Also, when prescribing trace element intakes for TPN patients, it is important to consider the trace element contaminants in the infused solutions because these can vary widely and contribute substantially to the total daily intake of individual trace elements.

Zinc, copper, iron, magnesium, chromium, and possibly other trace elements are present in variable concentrations as contaminants of intravenous solutions.[169] The rubber stoppers of IV bottles may be a major source of these elements.[83] Jetton and coworkers and Solomons et al. both found zinc levels as high as 3 mg/liter in parenteral solutions.[153,170] They have pointed out that variability in concentrations might lead to excessive intake of some trace elements if recommended supplements are added to the infusates.

Iron

Iron losses in adult men are about 1 mg/day; women may lose two to three times this quantity because of the blood losses during menstruation. Fistulas, gastrointestinal blood losses, and blood drawing for laboratory tests may increase iron losses in TPN patients. The intravenous infusion of iron in TPN patients has been somewhat controversial[155,171,172] for the following four reasons: (1) a number of side effects are associated with iron infusion; (2) the concentrations of serum iron reached during the infusion often exceeds the iron-binding capacity, and there is concern that this may cause iron deposition in soft tissues with resultant iron toxicity;[155,173] (3) there is the possibility that iron infusion, by increasing free iron, may predispose to serious bacterial infections;[174,175] (4) some investigators have described a rise in serum iron (26 ± 3.5 to 68 ± 9 μg/dl), iron-binding capacity (160 ± 14 to 200 ± 15 μg/dl) and saturation of iron-binding capacity in patients with malignancies, inflammatory diseases, or trauma given TPN without iron for 10 to 21 days.[176] These researchers suggest that decreased serum iron is due to disorders more in iron mobilization than in lowered whole body iron pools, particularly because of the normally small amounts of iron lost each day. However, iron deficiency is well described in patients receiving TPN.[171]

Iron deficiency may be diagnosed from serum iron, percent iron saturation (deficient, less than about 15 percent), and ferritin levels. Unfortunately, serum transferrin, which determines the iron-binding capacity, may fall with malnutrition, chronic renal failure, and chronic infection. Serum transferrin and ferritin may rise with acute inflammatory illnesses. Stainable iron in bone marrow is the definitive indicator of body iron stores; rarely, it may be necessary to ascertain bone marrow iron to determine whether iron repletion is required.

Iron contamination of TPN solutions was rather substantial when protein hydrolysates were utilized (e.g., levels as high as 1.11 mg/liter were reached).[172] Less iron is present in solutions of crystalline amino acids (e.g., 0.04 mg/liter).[172] Inorganic iron salts are reported to be highly toxic.[177] When given intravenously, if the unbound iron concentration exceeds the iron-binding capacity, patients may develop headaches, flushing, tachycardia, and hypotension.[177] Thus, iron is given intravenously only in a firmly complexed form, such as ferrous dextran and iron citrate. The most commonly used iron preparation for intravenous use is iron dextran, which provides 50 mg iron/ml of iron dextran. In the study of Hamstra et al. adverse systemic effects occurred in 53 of 481 individuals given iron dextran.[178] These systemic effects included three anaphylactoid reactions, twelve non-life-threatening reactions (transient hypotension, malaise, urticaria), and 38 delayed reactions (arthralgia, myalgia, fever, headache, lymphadenopathy). Iron dextran may be given intramuscularly, but injections are usually painful and the iron may stain the skin, leaving a tattoo. Norton et al. gave 42 TPN patients different amounts of iron dextran intravenously.[171] Patients were given 0, 25, 87.5, and 175 mg of elemental iron per week. Both 87.5 and 175 mg of iron per week increased serum iron levels, but the higher dose raised the serum iron beyond the normal range. Therefore, the authors recommended the intravenous dose of 87.5 mg/week (12.5 mg/day). No adverse reactions to iron dextran were noted during the 2758 patient days of study in this report. In one small series of seven patients given 2.5 to 10 mg of iron per 2 liters TPN as ferrous citrate, the iron was well utilized and adverse reactions were not observed.[179]

Iron complexes may be given to TPN patients as periodic intramuscular injections, as a single bolus over 2 to 4 h, once weekly, or as smaller daily doses. Large amounts of iron dextran probably should not be given in a single bolus, because the plasma iron concentrations can exceed the iron-binding capacity. An intravenous test dose of about 25 mg of elemental iron should be given initially to evaluate for hypersensitivity reactions. The dose of iron required to restore a normal hemoglobin in a patient with iron deficiency anemia may be estimated as follows:[155] iron dose (mg) = 0.3 (body weight in pounds) (100 − Hb g/dl × 100/14.8). Some patients receiving TPN have sufficient intestinal function to be given iron supplements enterally.

Zinc

Zinc is the second most abundant trace element, after iron. The total body zinc content is about 1.5 to 2.5 g. Several studies indicate that when zinc is not administered during TPN, zinc balance becomes negative and the zinc concentrations in red blood cells and plasma fall progressively.[151,153,180] Without zinc supplements, zinc deficiency is particularly likely to develop in patients receiving TPN who have benign gastrointestinal diseases, particularly inflammatory bowel disease and pancreatitis.[181] On the other hand, fecal zinc losses may increase in patients undergoing TPN when zinc is added to the infusate.[182] Plasma zinc concentrations do not correlate with zinc balance.[183] The fall in plasma zinc levels and the need for zinc supplementation with TPN may be particularly marked when patients are most anabolic.[151]

Zinc is a component or cofactor of more than 100 enzymes. Not surprisingly, zinc deficiency is associated with a wide array of symptoms. In humans, zinc deficiency may cause anorexia, diarrhea, acrodermatitis, reduced sense of taste and smell, impaired dark adaptation, retarded growth and sexual maturation, impaired wound healing, and psychological disorders.[184-192] A zinc deficiency syndrome has been reported in patients undergoing TPN who received little or no zinc.[151,193-200] The syndrome is characterized by diarrhea; mental depression; abdominal pain; bullous-pustular dermatitis about the mouth, groin, and/or extremities; and alopecia. Anergy to skin test antigens and impaired T-lymphocyte response to phytohemagglutinin have been reported.[193,199] In addition, nail changes similar to Beau's lines (transverse depressions in the nail that have been described following severe acute illnesses) and transverse white bands in all finger- and toenails similar to Muehrcke's lines (transverse bands of pallor) have been described as possible indicators of zinc deficiency.[195,201] The concentrations of the serum transport proteins albumin, transferrin, and prealbumin may be low.[194] Low serum alkaline phosphatase activity has also been taken as suggestive evidence for zinc deficiency.[202] This syndrome resembles the syndromes of parakeratosis occurring in zinc-deficient swine and acrodermatitis enteropathica, a genetic disorder of zinc deficiency in infants. It is cured by zinc therapy.[151,186,189,197,199] Attempts to give zinc by plasma transfusions or the topical application of zinc oxide have not been successful.[203,204] The use of commercial zinc preparations for intravenous administration, alone or in combination with other trace elements, is the method of choice for zinc replacement.

Marked increases in serum zinc concentrations have been reported in patients receiving TPN who were inadvertently given excessive doses of zinc. In seven patients given about 22.7 mg of elemental zinc per liter of TPN solution for 26 to 60 days, serum zinc concentration rose to a mean of 490 μg/dl.[205] The patients developed high levels of serum amylase (peak plasma values were 557 to 1850 Klein units; normal values are 130 to 310 units) without clinical signs of pancreatitis. Five of the seven patients died, but probably from unrelated causes. In another report, a 72-year-old patient received 7.4 g of zinc sulfate (3.0 g of elemental zinc) over 60 h; her serum zinc concentration rose to 4184 μg/dl.[206] The patient developed hypotension, pulmonary edema, diarrhea, vomiting, jaundice, and oliguria; she eventually died.

Copper

There is about 100 to 150 mg of copper in the normal adult. Most copper is in the liver where it is bound to proteins and metalloenzymes.[207] The latter are composed largely of oxidases, hydroxylases, and superoxide dismutases. More than 90 percent of circulating copper is bound to ceruloplasmin; the rest is loosely bound to albumin and amino acids.

When patients receive TPN with no copper, their copper balance becomes negative and red blood cell and plasma copper concentrations fall.[150,153,154,180] Decreased serum ceruloplasmin may accompany hypocupremia.[208] In two reports of adults receiving TPN without copper, serum copper decreased by 11 μg/dl/week[153] and 10.8 μg/dl/week.[209] Low serum copper levels generally do not occur until after 1 month of TPN without copper.[210] The predominant mode of copper excretion is through the bile, about 10 to 58 μmol/day for a 70-kg person.[211] Biliary copper is not well absorbed because it is complexed.[212] Urine copper is approximately 0.47 to 0.94 μmol/day. Shike reported that about 0.2 mg/day of copper was lost from the intestinal tract when total gastrointestinal secretions were less than 300 g/day.[213] With diarrhea or increased fluid losses from fistulas or stomas, gut losses of copper may be 0.30 to 0.35 mg/day. Hence copper deficiency is more common in patients with enterocutaneous fistulas.

A copper deficiency syndrome with neutropenia, anemia, and hypoproteinemia which responds to copper therapy has been reported in patients receiving TPN without copper.[150,208,209] The anemia that occurs with copper deficiency frequently is hypochromic and normocytic and is accompanied by decreased reticulocyte count.[214] Anemia is due to reduced synthesis and decreased survival of red cells and impaired formation of transferrin from ferrous iron.[148,215] Hypochromia and erythroid hypoplasia are found in the bone marrow. There is a tendency for the myeloid elements to be immature, and neutropenia has been described.

An unusual skeletal disorder, resembling the bone abnormalities of scurvy, has been observed in infants who received TPN and developed copper deficiency. The bone changes include generalized osteoporosis, retarded bone maturation, subperiosteal elevation and calcification, metaphyseal zone of radiolucency, and undisplaced fractures. These changes are thought to be due to decreased activities of the copper enzymes ascorbic acid oxidase and lysyl oxidase.[150,216]

Many TPN patients not receiving copper who develop low serum copper levels do not develop a clinical syndrome of copper deficiency.

Chromium

Chromium is an integral part of glucose tolerance factor, which functions as a cofactor for the peripheral action of insulin and is required for the maintenance of normal carbohydrate metabolism in both animals and human beings.[145,147,217] Total body chromium content averages approximately 6000 μg. Only small amounts of ingested chromium are absorbed, and most of the ingested chromium is excreted in the stool.[218] Chromium deficiency has been reported in three patients receiving long-term TPN; it occurred after about 5 months, 7 months, and $3\frac{1}{2}$ years of TPN when little or no chromium was provided.[219-221] Chromium deficiency is associated with low blood chromium concentration, weight loss, peripheral neuropathy, ataxia, metabolic encephalopathy, hyperlipidemia, and impaired glucose tolerance. In three patients who developed this syndrome after several months or years of TPN, the glucose intolerance and/or neurological disorders improved rapidly with chromium treatment.[219,220]

Serum chromium levels can vary independently of total body chromium content.[222] An impairment in the rise in urine chromium excretion in response to a glucose load is also an indirect indicator of chromium deficiency. It is suggested that at present the most definitive way to diagnose chromium deficiency is by showing an abnormal glucose tolerance that improves with chromium supplementation.[222] The current recommendation of the American Society of Clinical Nutrition (ASCN) for chromium supplementation of adult patients receiving TPN is 10 to 20 μg/day.[155] Chromium deficiency in long-term TPN patients has been treated with 150 to 250 μg/day.[219-221]

Not all patients given TPN without supplemental chromium appear to develop chromium deficiency,[223] possibly because of chromium contamination of TPN solutions.

Selenium

Patients receiving TPN without added selenium tend to have low serum selenium concentrations and serum glutathione peroxidase activity.[224] These changes can occur within 1 to 5 weeks of initiating TPN in postoperative patients. Selenium deficiency in patients undergoing long-term TPN can be associated with reduced red blood cell, skeletal muscle, cardiac, and liver selenium concentrations and glutathione peroxidase activity, as well as decreased serum and kidney selenium concentrations.[225-228] Selenium-deficient patients may develop severe muscle pain and tenderness in the legs and thighs, aggravation of this pain with walking, muscle weakness in the upper and lower extremities, and a congestive cardiomyopathy.[229,230] The cardiomyopathy may be associated with myocytolysis, fibrosis, and ventricular fibrillation. It is similar to the cardiomyopathy of selenium deficiency called Keshan disease, seen in China.[231,232]

Selenium deficiency in children undergoing long-term TPN without selenium supplementation has also been associated with intense pallor of the fingernail beds, lightening of the color of the skin and hair, thinning and curling of the scalp hair, weakness of the fingernails, and macrocytosis.[233,234]

Patients with preexisting borderline selenium deficiency can manifest the clinically overt signs of selenium depletion if they are given TPN without selenium supplements. One 37-year-old woman from a low-selenium area of New Zealand who was started on TPN without selenium was noted to have low serum selenium levels on admission. After only 30 days of TPN, she developed a lower plasma selenium concentration, decreased erythrocyte glutathione peroxidase activity, and muscle pain and tenderness in the legs and thighs.[227]

Selenium serves as a cofactor for glutathione peroxidase, which oxidizes glutathione and hence protects against oxidants and cellular free radicals. In selenium deficiency, cellular susceptibility to oxidative injury may increase. Vitamin E serves a similar protective role against oxidants and free radicals. Since vitamin E and selenium deficiency may both occur in patients receiving TPN, for them the risk of injury from oxidants and free radicals may be particularly great.

There is no consensus as to the optimal amount of selenium for maintenance or repletion in patients undergoing TPN.[235] Daily supplements of 40 to 80 μg for maintenance have been recommended.[155] Larger doses of selenium, that is, 160 μg/day, may be required in some patients to increase plasma selenium concentrations to values closer to normal.[236] Platelet glutathione peroxidase activity, which is considered to possibly be a more sensitive indicator of selenium stores, also was more normal with 160 μg of selenium/day in some individuals.[236]

Molybdenum

Molybdenum is a component of sulfite oxidase, xanthine oxidase, and aldehyde oxidase.[237] Abumrad et al. described a syndrome suggestive of molybdate deficiency in a 24-year-old man undergoing TPN.[238] The patient had elevated plasma levels of certain amino acids, particularly L-methionine. While receiving TPN he developed a high plasma methionine concentration; low serum uric acid and urinary uric acid and sulfate concentrations; increased urinary excretion of sulfite, thiosulfate, hypoxanthine, and xanthine; and tachycardia, tachypnea, central scotomas, night blindness, irritability, and, eventually, coma. The symptoms disappeared when the amino acid infusion was discontinued. These findings suggested the existence of two defects: one in the metabolism of sulfur-containing amino acids at the level of conversion of sulfite to sulfate and another in the transformation of xanthine and hypoxanthine to uric acid. The enzymes responsible for these actions, sulfite oxidase and xanthine oxidase, contain molybdenum. Molybdenum was not measured in body fluids or tissues. However, when the patient was treated with ammonium molybdate (300 μg/day, 178 μg Mo/day), plasma methionine, cystine, and taurine levels became more normal, plasma methionine clearance rose, urinary excretion of inorganic sulfate increased, urinary thiosulfate and sulfite excretion fell, serum and urinary uric acid concentrations rose, and urinary hypoxanthine and xanthine excretion decreased.

The average western diet is estimated to contain 200 to 500 μg/day of molybdenum.[239] A maintenance dose of 100 to 200 μg/day is recommended for adult TPN patients by the American Society for Clinical Nutrition.[155]

Aluminum

Klein and coworkers described elevated plasma, urine, and bone aluminum levels in patients receiving long-term TPN with casein hydrolysate solutions as the amino acid source.[240] The casein solutions were found to be contaminated with aluminum. When solutions of crystalline free amino acids, which are not contaminated with large quantities of aluminum, were substituted for the casein hydrolysate, plasma and urinary aluminum levels fell.

A bone disease characterized by pain, osteomalacia, decreased rate of bone formation, and relative hypoparathyroidism has been described in some patients receiving casein hydrolysate contaminated with aluminum.[5] These patients had increased contents of aluminum in bone and aluminum staining on the surface of mineralized bone. The characteristics of the bone disease were similar to the aluminum-induced osteomalacia of chronically uremic patients.[241]

Manganese

A syndrome of manganese deficiency has not been described in patients undergoing TPN. Indeed there is only one report of a human developing a syndrome due to manganese deficiency.[167,242] This was a volunteer who was accidentally fed a manganese-deficient diet while on an experimental protocol to induce vitamin K deficiency. The man developed loss of weight, change in beard color, hypercholesterolemia, and an increased prothrombin time that did not respond to supplements of vitamin K. In one study of patients given TPN for up to several weeks, those individuals given manganese 300 μg/day displayed a fall in serum manganese after 1 week of treatment whereas those individuals given 600 μg/day of manganese showed a significant increase in serum manganese after 1 week of therapy.[242] The AMA recommendation for daily manganese intake for TPN patients was 0.15 to 0.8 mg/day. The American Society for Clinical Nutrition has declined to recommend a daily manganese intake for TPN patients because no syndrome of manganese deficiency has been described in these individuals.[155] The daily intake of manganese in TPN solutions from contamination is estimated to be very low, about 8 to 22 μg/total daily intake.[243]

REFERENCES

1. Weinsier RL et al: Central venous alimentation: A prospective study of the frequency of metabolic abnormalities among medical and surgical patients. *JPEN* 6:421, 1982.
2. Heird WC et al: Intravenous alimentation in pediatric patients. *J Pediatr* 80:351, 1972.
3. Nehme A: Nutritional support of the hospitalized patient. The team concept. *JAMA* 243:1906, 1980.
4. Padberg FT et al: Central venous catheterization for parenteral nutrition. *Ann Surg* 193:264, 1981.
5. Ott SM et al: Aluminum is associated with low bone formation in patients receiving chronic parenteral nutrition. *Ann Intern Med* 98:910, 1983.
6. Wolfe RR et al: Investigation of factors determining the optimal glucose infusion rate in total parenteral nutrition. *Metabolism* 29:892, 1980.
7. Sanderson I, Deitel M: Insulin response in patients receiving concentrated infusions of glucose and casein hydrolysate for complete parenteral nutrition. *Ann Surg* 179:387, 1974.
8. Ryan JA Jr: Complications of total parenteral nutrition, in Fischer JE (ed): *Total Parenteral Nutrition.* Boston, Little, Brown, 1976, p 55.
9. Feinstein EI et al: Clinical and metabolic responses to parenteral nutrition in acute renal failure. *Medicine* 60:124, 1981.
10. Akmal M et al: Parathyroid hormone and glucose intolerance in uremia. *Proc Am Soc Nephrol* 13:87A, 1980.
11. Long CL et al: Nonsuppressibility of gluconeogenesis by glucose in septic patients. *Metabolism* 25:193, 1976.
12. Doromal NM, Canter JW: Hyperosmolar, hyperglycemic, nonketotic coma complicating intravenous hyperalimentation. *Surg Gynecol Obstet* 136:729, 1973.
13. Kaminski MV Jr: A review of hyperosmolar hyperglycemic nonketotic dehydration: Etiology, pathophysiology and prevention during intravenous hyperalimentation. *JPEN* 2:690, 1978.
14. Wyrick WJ et al: Rare complications with intravenous hyperosmotic alimentation. *JAMA* 211:1697, 1970.
15. Mahler R et al: The effect of insulin on lipolysis. *Diabetes* 13:297, 1964.
16. Zierler KL, Rabinowitz D: Effect of very small amounts of insulin on forearm metabolism. Persistence of its action on potassium and free fatty acids without its effect on glucose. *J Clin Invest* 43:950, 1964.
17. Mirsky IA et al: Antiketogenic action of glucose in the absence of insulin. *Am J Physiol* 118:290, 1937.
18. Kuzuya T et al: Stimulation by hyperosmolarity of glucose metabolism in rat adipose tissue and diaphragm *in vitro. J Biol Chem* 240:2277, 1965.
19. Seltzer HS, Harris VL: Exhaustion of insulinogenic reserve in maturity-onset diabetic patients during prolonged hyperglycemic stress. *Diabetes* 13:6, 1964.
20. Fischer JE: Nutritional support in the seriously ill patient. *Curr Probl Surg* 17:466, 1980.
21. Hinton P et al: Insulin and glucose to reduce catabolic response to injury in burned patients. *Lancet* 1:767, 1971.
22. Woolfson AMJ et al: Insulin to inhibit protein catabolism after injury. *N Engl J Med* 300:14, 1979.
23. MacFie J et al: Effect of added insulin on body composition of gastroenterologic patients receiving intravenous nutrition—A controlled clinical trial. *Gastroenterology* 81:285, 1981.
24. Hirsch JI et al: Clinical significance of insulin adsorption by polyvinyl chloride infusion systems. *Am J Hosp Pharm* 34:583, 1977.
25. Weber SS et al: Availability of insulin from parenteral nutrient solutions. *Am J Hosp Pharm* 34:353, 1977.
26. Chan JCM et al: Hyperalimentation with amino acids and casein hydrolysate solutions—Mechanisms of acidosis. *JAMA* 220:1700, 1972.
27. Fraley DS et al: Metabolic acidosis after hyperalimentation with casein hydrolysate. *Ann Intern Med* 88:352, 1978.
28. Heird WC et al: Metabolic acidosis resulting from intravenous alimentation mixtures containing synthetic amino acids. *N Engl J Med* 287:943, 1972.
29. Dudrick SJ et al: Parenteral hyperalimentation—Metabolic problems and solutions. *Ann Surg* 176:259, 1972.
30. Heird WC, Winters RW: Total parenteral nutrition—The state of the art. *J Pediatr* 86:2, 1975.
31. Chan JCM et al: pH and titratable acidity of amino acid mixtures used in hyperalimentation. *JAMA* 220:1119, 1972.
32. Kautz HD, Parker EA: pH of intravenous solutions. *N Engl J Med* 280:901, 1969.
33. Klimpel D, Cohon MS: pH of intravenous solutions. *N Engl J Med* 280:900, 1969.
34. Driscoll DF, Blackburn GL: Total parenteral nutrition 1990. *Drugs* 40(3):346, 1990.
35. Hoheim DF et al: Clinical experience with three-in-one admixtures administered peripherally. *Nutr Clin Pract* 5:118, 1990.

36. Davis SS: The stability of fat emulsions for intravenous administration, in Johnston ID (ed): *Advances in Clinical Nutrition*. Lancaster, MTP Press, 1983, p 213.
37. Klahr S et al: On the nature of the renal concentrating defect in malnutrition. *Am J Med* 43:84, 1967.
38. Klahr S et al: Renal regulation of acid-base balance in malnourished men. *Am J Med* 48:325, 1970.
39. Motil KJ et al: Complications of essential amino acid hyperalimentation in children with acute renal failure. *JPEN* 4:32, 1980.
40. Froesch ER, Keller U: Review of energy metabolism with particular reference to the metabolism of glucose, fructose, sorbitol and xylitol and of their therapeutic use in parenteral nutrition, in Wilkinson AW (ed): *Parenteral Nutrition*. Baltimore, Williams & Wilkins, 1971, p 105.
41. Bergstrom J et al: Lactic acid accumulation in connection with fructose infusion. *Acta Med Scand* 184:359, 1968.
42. Heuckenkamp PU, Zollner N: Quantitative comparison and evaluation of utilization of parenteral administered carbohydrates. *Nutr Metab* 18:209, 1975.
43. Raivio KO et al: Depletion of liver adenine nucleotides induced by D-fructose. *Biochem Pharmacol* 18:2615, 1969.
44. Anderson G et al: Increasing metabolic acidosis following fructose infusion in two children. *Acta Paediatr Scand* 58:301, 1969.
45. Hessov I: Effects of fructose and glucose infusions on blood acid-base equilibrium in the postoperative period. *Acta Chir Scand* 140:347, 1974.
46. Sahebjami H, Scalettar R: Effects of fructose infusion on lactate and uric acid metabolism. *Lancet* 1:366, 1971.
47. Bergstrom J et al: Lactate production during fructose infusion with or without amino acids. *Acta Med Scand* 200:99, 1976.
48. Kaminski MV Jr: Acid-base problems after intravenous amino acids. *N Engl J Med* 288:421, 1973.
49. Hull RL: Physiochemical considerations in intravenous hyperalimentation. *Am J Hosp Pharm* 31:236, 1974.
50. Arieff AI et al: Systemic effects of $NaHCO_3$ in experimental lactic acidosis in dogs. *Am J Physiol* 242:F586, 1982.
51. Graf H et al: Evidence for a detrimental effect of bicarbonate therapy in hypoxic lactic acidosis. *Science* 227:754, 1985.
52. Arieff AI et al: Effects of $NaHCO_3$ in therapy of experimental lactic acidosis. *Kidney Int* 14:645, 1978.
53. Stacpoole PW et al: Treatment of lactic acidosis with dichloroacetate. *N Engl J Med* 309:390, 1983.
54. Blackshear PJ et al: Treatment of severe lactic acidosis with dichloroacetate. *Diabetes Care* 5:391, 1982.
55. Shapiro JI et al: Beneficial effect of carbicarb and deleterious effect of bicarbonate in the treatment of systemic acidosis in the rat (abst). *Kidney Int* 33(1):407, 1988.
56. Cogan MG, Liu FY: Metabolic alkalosis in the rat. Evidence that reduced glomerular filtration rather than enhanced tubular bicarbonate reabsorption is responsible for maintaining the alkalotic state. *J Clin Invest* 71:1141, 1983.
57. Grigor KC et al: The effect of acetazolamide on postperfusion metabolic alkalosis. *Br J Anaesth* 43:352, 1971.
58. Miller PD, Berns AS: Acute metabolic alkalosis perpetuating hypercarbia. A role for acetazolamide in chronic obstructive pulmonary disease. *JAMA* 238:2400, 1977.
59. Bushinsky DA, Gennari FJ: Life-threatening hyperkalemia induced by arginine. *Ann Intern Med* 89:632, 1978.
60. Dickerman HW, Walker WG: Effect of cationic amino acid infusion on potassium metabolism *in vivo*. *Am J Physiol* 206: 403, 1964.
61. Abouna GM et al: Intravenous infusion of hydrochloric acid for treatment of severe metabolic alkalosis. *Surgery* 75:194, 1974.
62. Harken AH et al: Hydrochloric acid in the correction of metabolic alkalosis. *Arch Surg* 110:819, 1975.
63. Shavelle HS, Parke R: Postoperative metabolic alkalosis and acute renal failure: Rationale for the use of hydrochloric acid. *Surgery* 78:439, 1975.
64. Finkle D, Dean RE: Buffered hydrochloric acid: A modern method for treating metabolic alkalosis. *Am Surg* 47:103, 1981.
65. Askanazi J et al: Respiratory changes induced by the large glucose loads of total parenteral nutrition. *JAMA* 243: 1444, 1980.
66. Askanazi J et al: Influence of total parenteral nutrition on fuel utilization in injury and sepsis. *Ann Surg* 191:40, 1980.
67. Askanazi J et al: Respiratory distress secondary to a high carbohydrate load: A case report. *Surgery* 87:596, 1980.
68. Covelli HD et al: Respiratory failure precipitated by high carbohydrate loads. *Ann Intern Med* 95:579, 1981.
69. Kearns PJ, Banuelos A: Hypercapnia in hyperalimentation. *Ann Intern Med* 96:786, 1982.
70. Wilmore DW: *The Metabolic Management of the Critically Ill*. New York, Plenum, 1977, p 34.
71. Weissman C et al: Amino acids and respiration. *Ann Intern Med* 98:41, 1983.
72. Reifenstein EC Jr et al: The accumulation, interpretation, and presentation of data pertaining to metabolic balances, notably those of calcium, phosphorus, and nitrogen. *J Clin Endocrinol Metab* 5:367, 1945.
73. Rudman D et al: Elemental balances during intravenous hyperalimentation of underweight adult subjects. *J Clin Invest* 55:94, 1975.
74. Ellis BW et al: A rational approach to parenteral nutrition. *Br Med J* 1:1388, 1976.
75. Giovanoni R: A suggested profile for selected total parenteral nutrition additives. *Clin Med* 81:28, 1974.
76. Giovanoni R: The manufacturing pharmacy solutions and incompatibilities, in Fisher JE (ed): *Total Parenteral Nutrition*. Boston, Little, Brown, 1976, p 27.
77. Madan PL et al: Total parenteral nutrition. *Drug Intell Clin Pharm* 10:684, 1976.
78. Meng HC: Parenteral nutrition: Principles, nutrient requirements, and techniques. *Geriatrics* 30:97, 1975.
79. Shils ME: Guidelines for total parenteral nutrition. *JAMA* 220:1721, 1972.
80. Shils ME: Minerals, in White PL (ed): *Total Parenteral Nutrition*. Chicago, American Medical Association, 1974, p 257.
81. Gamble JL: *Chemical Anatomy, Physiology, and Pathology of Extracellular Fluid*. Cambridge, Mass., Harvard University Press, 1954, p 164.
82. Rubini ME, Chojnacki RE: Principles of parenteral therapy. *Am J Clin Nutr* 25:96, 1972.
83. Dick W, Seeling W: Water and electrolyte requirements during parenteral nutrition, in Ahnefeld FW et al (eds):

Parenteral Nutrition. Heidelberg, Springer-Verlag, 1976, p 99.
84. Gump FE et al: Measurement of water balance—A guide to surgical care. *Surgery* 64:154, 1968.
85. Murray RL et al: Body composition changes in the critically ill patient: Emphasis on water balance. *JPEN* 3:219, 1979.
86. Kaplan AA et al: Continuous arteriovenous hemofiltration. *Ann Intern Med* 100:358, 1984.
87. Edelman IS, Leibman J: Anatomy of body water and electrolytes. *Am J Med* 27:256, 1959.
88. Widdowson EM, Dickerson JWT: Chemical composition of the body, in Comar CL, Bronner F (eds): *Mineral Metabolism*. New York, Academic press, 1964, vol 2, part A.
89. Fleming CR et al: Total parenteral nutrition. *Mayo Clin Proc* 51:187, 1976.
90. Grant JP: Administration of parenteral nutrition solutions, in Grant JP (ed): *Handbook of Total Parenteral Nutrition*. Philadelphia, Saunders, 1980, p 92.
91. Paul GJ: Total parenteral nutrition: A guide for its use. *Am J Gastroenterol* 72:186, 1979.
92. Reinhardt GF et al: Total parenteral nutrition. *Surg Clin North Am* 57:1283, 1977.
93. Thoren L: Water, electrolytes, vitamins and carbohydrates in parenteral nutrition. *Acta Anaesthesiol Scand* 55 (suppl):123, 1974.
94. Narins RG et al: Diagnostic strategies in disorders of fluid, electrolyte and acid-base homeostasis. *Am J Med* 72:496, 1982.
95. Heide B et al: Nutritional status of patients undergoing CAPD. *PD Bulletin* 3:138, 1983.
96. Lawson DH: Adverse reactions to potassium chloride. *Q J Med* 171:433, 1974.
97. Burchell HB: Dilemmas in potassium therapy. *Circulation* 47:1144, 1973.
98. Burnell JM et al: The effect in humans of extracellular pH change on the relationship between serum potassium concentration and intracellular potassium. *J Clin Invest* 35:935, 1956.
99. Soler NG et al: Electrocardiogram as a guide to potassium replacement in diabetic ketoacidosis. *Diabetes* 23:610, 1974.
100. Lawson DH: The clinical use of potassium supplements. *J Maine Med Assoc* 66:166, 1975.
101. Lankton JW et al: Hyperkalemia after administration of potassium from non-rigid parenteral fluid containers. *Anesthesiology* 39:660, 1973.
102. Williams RHP: Potassium overdose: A potential hazard of non-rigid parenteral fluid containers. *Br Med J* 24:714, 1973.
103. Subcommittee on the Tenth Edition of the RDAS, Food and Nutrition Board: *Recommended Dietary Allowances*, 10th ed. Washington DC, National Academy of Sciences, 1989, p 195.
104. Jacobson S: Electrolyte therapy after abdominal surgery—A balance study of sodium, potassium, calcium, magnesium, and phosphate in total parenteral nutrition. *Acta Chir Scand* 143:285, 1977.
105. Wittine MF, Freeman JB: Calcium requirements during total parenteral nutrition in well-nourished individuals. *JPEN* 1:152, 1977.
106. Gilligan JE et al: Hypercalcemia associated with parenteral amino acid and dextrose infusion. *Am J Clin Nutr* 35:993, 1982.
107. Izsak EM et al: Pancreatitis in association with hypercalcemia in patients receiving total parenteral nutrition. *Gastroenterology* 79:555, 1980.
108. Caddell JL, Goddard DR: Studies in protein-calorie malnutrition: I. Chemical evidence for magnesium deficiency. *N Engl J Med* 276:533, 1967.
109. Smith WO et al: Magnesium depletion induced by various diuretics. *J Okla State Med Assoc* 55:248, 1962.
110. Blachley JD, Hill JB: Renal and electrolyte disturbances associated with cisplatin. *Ann Intern Med* 95:628, 1981.
111. Schilsky RL, Anderson T: Hypomagnesemia and renal magnesium wasting in patients receiving cisplatin. *Ann Intern Med* 90:929, 1979.
112. Wacker WEC, Vallee BL: Magnesium metabolism. *N Engl J Med* 259:431, 1958.
113. Bartter FC: So-called Bartter's Syndrome, editorial. *N Engl J Med* 281:1483, 1969.
114. Main ANH et al: Mg deficiency in chronic inflammatory bowel disease and requirements during intravenous nutrition. *JPEN* 5:15, 1981.
115. Levine SR et al: Hypomagnesemia and ventricular tachycardia. *Chest* 81:244, 1982.
116. Frazier TG et al: Hypomagnesemia: Higher risk using total parenteral nutrition in the treatment of patients with malignancies. *J Surg Oncol* 13:35, 1980.
117. Burch GE, Giles TD: The importance of magnesium deficiency in cardiovascular disease. *Am Heart J* 94:649, 1977.
118. Alfrey AC et al: Hypermagnesemia after renal homotransplantation. *Ann Intern Med* 73:367, 1970.
119. Welt LG, Gitelman H: Disorders of magnesium metabolism. *Disease-A-Month*. 1(5):1, 1965.
120. Heaton FW: The kidney and magnesium homeostasis. *Ann NY Acad Sci* 162:775, 1969.
121. Gitelman HJ et al: A new familial disorder characterized by hypokalemia and hypomagnesemia. *Trans Assoc Am Physicians* 79:221, 1966.
122. Driscoll RH, Rosenberg IH: Total parenteral nutrition in inflammatory bowel disease. *Med Clin North Am* 62:185, 1978.
123. Dudrick SJ, Rhoads JE: New horizons for intravenous feeding. *JAMA* 215:939, 1971.
124. Dudrick SJ et al: Can intravenous feeding as the sole means of nutrition support growth in the child and restore weight loss in an adult? An affirmative answer. *Ann Surg* 169:974, 1969.
125. Gruppo RA, Graham GG: Total parenteral alimentation solution. *Johns Hopkins Med J* 127:352, 1970.
126. Jeejeebhoy KN et al: Total parenteral nutrition at home: Studies in patients surviving 4 months to 5 years. *Gastroenterology* 71:943, 1976.
127. Shenkin A, Wretlind A: Parenteral nutrition. *World Rev Nutr Diet* 28:1, 1978.
128. Betro MG, Pain RW: Hypophosphatemia and hyperphosphatemia in a hospital population. *Br Med J* 1:273, 1972.
129. Weinsier RL, Krumdieck CL: Death resulting from overzealous total parenteral nutrition: The refeeding syndrome revisited. *Am J Clin Nutr* 34:393, 1980.

130. Mashima Y et al: Changes in phosphorous distribution during total parenteral nutrition. *JPEN* 5:189, 1981.
131. Aladjem M et al: Changes in the electrolyte content of serum and urine during total parenteral nutrition. *J Pediatr* 97:437, 1980.
132. Heird WC: Disorder of calcium and phosphorus metabolism, in Winters RW, Hasslemeyer EG (eds): *Intravenous Nutrition in the High Risk Infant.* New York, Wiley, 1975, p 253.
133. Silvis SE et al: Hypophosphatemia and neurological changes secondary to oral caloric intake. *Am J Gastroenterol* 73:215, 1980.
134. Travis SF et al: Alterations of red cell glycolytic intermediates and oxygen transport as a consequence of hypophosphatemia in patients receiving intravenous hyperalimentation. *N Engl J Med* 285:763, 1971.
135. Lichtman MA et al: Reduced red cell glycolysis, 2,3-diphosphoglycerate and adenosine triphosphate concentration, and increased hemoglobin-oxygen affinity caused by hypophosphatemia. *Ann Intern Med* 74:562, 1971.
136. Jacob HS, Amsden T: Acute hemolytic anemia with rigid red cells in hypophosphatemia. *N Engl J Med* 285:1446, 1971.
137. Craddock PR et al: Acquired phagocyte dysfunction—A complication of the hypophosphatemia of parenteral hyperalimentation. *N Engl J Med* 290:1403, 1974.
138. Knochel JP et al: Hypophosphatemia and rhabdomyolysis. *J Clin Invest* 62:1240, 1978.
139. Weintraub MI: Hypophosphatemia mimicking acute Guillain-Barré-Strohl Syndrome—A complication of parenteral hyperalimentation. *JAMA* 235:1040, 1976.
140. Furlan AJ et al: Acute areflexic paralysis—Association with hyperalimentation and hypophosphatemia. *Arch Neurol* 32:706, 1975.
141. Prins JG et al: Hyperalimentation, hypophosphataemia, and coma. *Lancet* 1:1253, 1973.
142. Silvis SE, Paragas PD Jr: Paresthesias, weakness, seizures, and hypophosphatemia in patients receiving hyperalimentation. *Gastroenterology* 62:513, 1972.
143. Sheldon GF, Grzyb S: Phosphate depletion and repletion: Relation to parenteral nutrition and oxygen transport. *Ann Surg* 182:683, 1975.
144. Nielsen FH: Fluoride, vanadium, nickel, arsenic, and silicon in total parenteral nutrition. *Bull N Y Acad Med* 60:177, 1984.
145. Li T, Vallee BL: The biochemical and nutritional role of trace elements, in Goodhart RS, Shils ME (eds): *Modern Nutrition in Health and Disease—Dietotherapy.* Philadelphia, Lea & Febiger, 1973, p 372.
146. Schwartz K: Recent dietary trace element research, exemplified by tin, fluorine, and silicon. *Fed Proc* 33:1748, 1974.
147. Tuman RW, Doisy RJ: The role of trace elements in human nutrition and metabolism, in Jeanes A, Hodge J (eds): *Physiological Effects of Food Carbohydrates.* Symposium Series 15, American Chemical Society, 1975, p 156.
148. Dunlap WM et al: Anemia and neutropenia caused by copper deficiency. *Ann Intern Med* 80:470, 1974.
149. Freeman JB et al: Excessive urinary zinc losses during parenteral alimentation. *J Surg Res* 18:463, 1975.
150. Karpel JT, Peden VH: Copper deficiency in long-term parenteral nutrition. *J Pediatr* 80:32, 1972.
151. Kay RG et al: A syndrome of acute zinc deficiency during total parenteral alimentation in man. *Ann Surg* 183:331, 1976.
152. Palmisano DJ: Nutrient deficiencies after intensive parenteral alimentation. *N Engl J Med* 291:799, 1974.
153. Solomons NW et al: Plasma trace metals during total parenteral alimentation. *Gastroenterology* 70:1022, 1976.
154. Hankins DA et al: Whole blood trace element concentrations during total parenteral nutrition. *Surgery* 79:674, 1976.
155. Fleming CR: Trace element metabolism in adult patients requiring total parenteral nutrition. *Am J Clin Nutr* 49:573, 1989.
156. Hessov I et al: Zinc depletion after small bowel resection for Crohn's disease. *Hum Nutr Clin Nutr* 37C:353, 1983.
157. Solomons NW et al: Zinc deficiency in Crohn's disease. *Digestion* 16:87, 1976.
158. Carruthers ME et al: Raised serum copper and ceruloplasmin levels in subjects taking oral contraceptives. *J Clin Pathol* 19:498, 1966.
159. Klevay LM et al: Hair analysis in clinical and experimental medicine. *Am J Clin Nutr* 46:233, 1987.
160. Fleming CR et al: Zinc nutrition in Crohn's disease. *Dig Dis Sci* 26:865, 1981.
161. Lipkin EW: Selenium in the parenterally nourished patient. *Nutr Int* 2:12, 1986.
162. Hoffman HN et al: Zinc-induced copper deficiency. *Gastroenterology* 94:508, 1988.
163. Patterson WK et al: Zinc-induced copper deficiency: megamineral sideroblastic anemia. *Ann Intern Med* 103:385, 1985.
164. Stegink LD et al: Excessive trace metal ion excretion due to sugar-amino acid complexes during total parenteral nutrition. *Fed Proc* 34:931, 1975.
165. Rowlands DA et al: Storage stability of mixed hyperalimentation solutions. *Am J Hosp Pharm* 30:436, 1973.
166. Laegeler WL et al: Stability of certain amino acids in a parenteral nutrition solution. *Am J Hosp Pharm* 31:776, 1974.
167. Aggett PJ, Davies NT: Some nutritional aspects of trace metals. *J Inherited Metab Dis* 6(suppl 1):22, 1983.
168. Shils ME et al: Guidelines for essential trace element preparations for parenteral use. *J Parenter Ent Nutr* 3:263, 1979.
169. Hauer EC, Kaminski MV: Trace metal profile of parenteral nutrition solutions. *Am J Clin Nutr* 31:264, 1978.
170. Jetton MM et al: Trace element contamination of intravenous solutions. *Arch Intern Med* 136:782, 1976.
171. Norton JA et al: Iron supplementation of total parenteral nutrition: A prospective study. *J Parenter Ent Nutr* 7:457, 1983.
172. Anonymous: Supplementation of total parenteral nutrition solutions with ferrous citrate. *Nutr Rev* 43:20, 1985.
173. Gokal R et al: Iron metabolism in haemodialysis patients. *Q J Med* 191:369, 1979.
174. Bothe A Jr et al: Use of iron with total parenteral nutrition. *N Engl J Med* 27:1153, 1975.
175. Barry DMJ, Reeve AW: Increase incidence of gram-nega-

tive neonatal sepsis with intramuscular iron administration. *Pediatrics* 60:908, 1977.
176. Stead NW et al: Enhanced mobilization of iron from body stores in malnourished patients during intravenous nutrition support. *Surg Gynecol Obstet* 154:321, 1982.
177. Cook JD: Parenteral trace elements: Iron. *Bull N Y Acad Med* 60:156, 1984.
178. Hamstra RD et al: Intravenous iron dextran in clinical medicine. *JAMA* 243:1726, 1980.
179. Sayers MH et al: Supplementation of total parenteral nutrition solutions with ferrous citrate. *J Parenter Ent Nutr* 7:117, 1983.
180. Lowry SF et al: Zinc and copper replacement during total parenteral nutrition. *Am J Clin Nutr* 34:1853, 1981.
181. Takagi Y et al: Clinical studies on zinc metabolism during total parenteral nutrition as related to zinc deficiency. *J Parenter Ent Nutr* 10:195, 1986.
182. Ladefoged K: Intestinal and renal loss of infused mineral in patients with severe short bowel syndrome. *Am J Clin Nutr* 36:59, 1982.
183. Wolman SL et al: Zinc in total parenteral nutrition: Requirements and metabolic effects. *Gastroenterology* 76: 458, 1979.
184. Abbasi AA et al: Gonadal function abnormalities in sickle cell anemia. Studies in adult male patients. *Ann Intern Med* 85:601, 1976.
185. Halsted JA et al: Zinc deficiency in men. *Am J Med* 53:277, 1972.
186. Halsted JA et al: A conspectus of research on zinc requirements of man. *J Nutr* 104:345, 1974.
187. Henkin RI: Zinc in wound healing. *N Engl J Med* 291:675, 1974.
188. Henkin RI et al: Idiopathic hypogeusia with dysgeusia, hyposmia and dysosmia. A new syndrome. *JAMA* 217:434, 1971.
189. Sandstead HH et al: Human zine deficiency, endocrine manifestation and response to treatment. *Am J Clin Nutr* 20:422, 1967.
190. Sandstead HH et al: Zinc and wound healing: Effects of zinc deficiency and zinc supplementation. *Am J Clin Nutr* 23:514, 1970.
191. Walravens PA, Hambridge KM: Growth of infants fed a zinc supplemented formula. *Am J Clin Nutr* 29:1114, 1976.
192. Morrison SA et al: Zinc deficiency: A cause of abnormal dark adaptation in cirrhotics. *Am J Clin Nutr* 31:276, 1978.
193. Allen JI et al: Severe zinc deficiency in humans: Association with a reversible T-lymphocyte dysfunction. *Ann Intern Med* 95:154, 1981.
194. Bates J, McClain CJ: The effect of severe zinc deficiency on serum levels of albumin, transferrin, and prealbumin in man. *Am J Clin Nutr* 34:1655, 1981.
195. Ferrandiz C et al: Acquired zinc deficiency syndrome during total parenteral alimentation. Clinical and histopathological findings. *Dermatologica* 163:255, 1981.
196. Latimer JS et al: Clinical zinc deficiency during zinc-supplemented parenteral nutrition. *J Pediatr* 97:434, 1980.
197. McClain CJ et al: Severe zinc deficiency presenting with acrodermatitis during hyperalimentation. Diagnosis, pathogenesis, and treatment. *J Clin Gastroenterol* 2:125, 1980.
198. Moran DM et al: Zinc deficiency dermatitis accompanying parenteral nutrition supplemented with trace elements. *Clin Pharmacy* 1:169, 1982.
199. Oleske JM et al: Zinc therapy of depressed cellular immunity in acrodermatitis enteropathica. *Am J Dis Child* 133: 915, 1979.
200. Sivasubramanian KN, Henkin RI: Behavioral and dermatologic changes and low serum zinc and copper concentrations in two premature infants after parenteral alimentation. *J Pediatr* 93:847, 1978.
201. Weismann K: Lines of Beau. Possible marker of zinc deficiency. *Acta Derm Venereol* 57:88, 1977.
202. Ishizaka A et al: Clinical zinc deficiency during zinc-supplemented parenteral nutrition. *J Pediatr* 99:339, 1981.
203. Michie DD et al: Zinc and total parenteral nutrition. *South Med J* 70:985, 1977.
204. Derry JE et al: A study of percutaneous absorption from topically applied zinc oxide ointment. *J Parenter Ent Nutr* 7:131, 1983.
205. Faintuch J et al: Hyperamylasemia associated with zinc overdose during parenteral nutrition. *JPEN* 2:640, 1978.
206. Brocks A et al: Acute intravenous zinc poisoning. *Br Med J* 1:1390, 1977.
207. Solomons NW: Zinc and copper in human nutrition, in *Nutrition in the 1980's: Constraints on Our Knowledge.* New York, Alan R Liss, 1981, p 97.
208. Fujita M et al: Copper deficiency during total parenteral nutrition: Clinical analysis of three cases. *J Parenter Ent Nutr* 13:421, 1989.
209. Fleming CR et al: A prospective study of serum copper and zinc levels in patients receiving total parenteral nutrition. *Am J Clin Nutr* 29:70, 1976.
210. Bozzetti F et al: Hypocupremia in patients receiving total parenteral nutrition. *J Parenter Ent Nutr* 7:563, 1983.
211. van Berge Henegouwen GP et al: Biliary secretion of copper in healthy man: Quantitation by an intestinal perfusion technique. *Gastroenterology* 72:1228, 1977.
212. Mason KE: A conspectus of research on copper metabolism and requirements of man. *J Nutr* 109:186, 1979.
213. Shike M et al: Copper metabolism and requirements in total parenteral nutrition. *Gastroenterology* 81:290, 1981.
214. Grant JP: Trace element requirements and deficiency syndromes, in Grant JP (ed): *Handbook of Total Parenteral Nutrition.* Philadelphia, Saunders, 1980, p 155.
215. Roeser HP et al: The role of ceruloplasmin in iron metabolism. *J Clin Invest* 49:2408, 1970.
216. Allen TM et al: Skeletal changes associated with copper deficiency. *Clin Orthop* 168:206, 1982.
217. Hambidge KM: Chromium nutrition in man. *Am J Clin Nutr* 27:505, 1974.
218. Offenbacher EG et al: Metabolic chromium balances in men. *Am J Clin Nutr* 44:77, 1986.
219. Freund H et al: Chromium deficiency during total parenteral nutrition. *JAMA* 241:496, 1979.
220. Jeejeebhoy KN et al: Chromium deficiency, glucose intolerance, and neuropathy reversed by chromium supplementation, in a patient receiving long-term total parenteral nutrition. *Am J Clin Nutr* 30:531, 1977.

221. Brown RO et al: Chromium deficiency after long-term total parenteral nutrition. *Dig Dis Sci* 31:661, 1986.
222. Jeejeebhoy KN: Zinc and chromium in parenteral nutrition. *Bull N Y Acad Med* 60:118, 1984.
223. Kien CL et al: Mild peripheral neuropathy but biochemical chromium sufficiency during 16 months of "chromium-free" total parenteral nutrition. *J Parenter Ent Nutr* 10:662, 1986.
224. Korpela H et al: Low serum selenium and glutathione peroxidase activity in patients receiving short-term total parenteral nutrition. *Int J Vitam Nutr Res* 59:80, 1989.
225. Lane HW et al: Selenium status of seven chronic intravenous hyperalimentation patients. *JPEN* 6:426, 1982.
226. Van Rij AM et al: Selenium and total parenteral nutrition. *J Parenter Ent Nutr* 3:235, 1979.
227. Van Rij AM et al: Selenium deficiency in total parenteral nutrition. *Am J Clin Nutr* 32:2076, 1979.
228. Van Rij AM et al: Selenium supplementation in total parenteral nutrition. *J Parenter Ent Nutr* 5:120, 1981.
229. Fleming CR et al: Selenium deficiency and fetal cardiomyopathy in a patient on home parenteral nutrition. *Gastroenterology* 83:689, 1982.
230. Brown MR et al: Proximal muscle weakness and selenium deficiency associated with long term parenteral nutrition. *Am J Clin Nutr* 43:549, 1986.
231. Johnson RA et al: An occidental case of cardiomyopathy and selenium deficiency. *N Engl J Med* 304:1210, 1981.
232. Keshan Disease Research Group of the Chinese Academy of Medical Sciences: Observations on effect of sodium selenite in prevention of Keshan Disease. *Chin Med J* 92:471, 1979.
233. Kien CL, Ganther HE: Manifestations of chronic selenium deficiency in a child receiving total parenteral nutrition. *Am J Clin Nutr* 37:319, 1983.
234. Vinton NE et al: Macrocytosis and pseudoalbinism: Manifestations of selenium deficiency. *J Pediatr* 111:711, 1987.
235. Levander OA, Burk RF: Report on the 1986 A.S.P.E.N. research workshop on selenium in clinical nutrition. *J Parenter Ent Nutr* 10:545, 1986.
236. Lane HW et al: The effect of selenium supplementation on selenium status of patients receiving chronic total parenteral nutrition. *J Parenter Ent Nutr* 11:177, 1987.
237. Johnson JL et al: Molecular basis of the biologic function of molybdenum: Effect of tungsten on xanthine oxidase and sulfite oxidase in the rat. *J Biol Chem* 249:859, 1974.
238. Abumrad NN et al: Amino acid intolerance during prolonged total parenteral nutrition reversed by molybdate therapy. *Am J Clin Nutr* 34:2551, 1981.
239. Tipton SW et al: Patterns of elemental excretion in long term balance studies. *Health Phys* 16:455, 1969.
240. Klein GL et al: Aluminum loading during total parenteral nutrition. *Am J Clin Nutr* 35:1425, 1982.
241. Ott SM et al: The prevalence of bone aluminum deposition in renal osteodystrophy and its relation to the response to calcitriol therapy. *N Engl J Med* 307:709, 1982.
242. Falbe WJ et al: Individualized manganese supplementation in patients receiving total parenteral nutrition. *Clin Pharm* 6:226, 1987.
243. Kurkus J et al: Manganese content of large-volume parenteral solutions and of nutrient additives. *J Parenter Ent Nutr* 8:254, 1984.

CHAPTER 45

Fluid and electrolyte abnormalities in critically ill patients: fluid resuscitation, lactate metabolism, and calcium metabolism

Michael A. Geheb • James A. Kruse • Marilyn T. Haupt • Tusar K. Desai • Richard W. Carlson

The practice of medical intensive care has supplied new challenges to those interested in the acute effects of critical illness on metabolism. The development of increasingly more sophisticated life-support and clinical laboratory technology frequently allows patients to live long enough to develop previously unknown and challenging metabolic syndromes that can be described, studied, and, we hope, treated.

This chapter introduces and updates the reader in selected areas in which new information has recently been described. A review of the long ongoing discussion of *colloid and crystalloid therapy* is offered. Additionally, insights into *lactate metabolism* in critically ill patients, and a review of the changes in *acid-base metabolism during perfusion failure* and cardiopulmonary arrest are included. Finally, a summary of recent studies evaluated the dramatic changes in *calcium metabolism* that can occur in critically ill patients is provided.

RESUSCITATION OF THE CRITICALLY ILL AND INJURED WITH COLLOID AND CRYSTALLOID FLUIDS

INTRODUCTION AND HISTORICAL PERSPECTIVE

The selection of resuscitation fluids has been the subject of considerable controversy for the greater portion of this century. Graham coined the terms for colloid and crystalloid fluids in 1861.[54] However, the first clinical use of colloids for the treatment of hemorrhagic and traumatic shock can be traced to World War I. Those early studies provided data that led to comparisons between the two types of fluids. Clinicians observed that saline infusions led to transient effects on blood pressure and that crystalloid fluids rapidly diffused into the interstitial compartment, so that blood volume expansion was also transient. Although blood transfusion was recognized as a logical treatment for hemorrhagic shock, it was difficult to store and transport blood during the early decades of this century. Blood also fell into disfavor when it was realized that serious reactions frequently complicated transfusion therapy. Transfusion of plasma was considered to obviate this problem. However, storage, refrigeration, and transport of plasma were also impractical until the 1940s. Therefore, a search was begun for stable, nontoxic colloidal fluids that could be used in lieu of resuscitation with plasma or whole blood.

Bayliss developed and helped popularize one of the first of these "artificial" colloid solutions.[6] He believed that a fluid with a viscosity and a colloid osmotic pressure similar to plasma would be superior to crystalloids in restoring vascular volume. *Gum acacia,* a plant-derived amylopectin, was therefore incorporated into a solution of normal saline as a blood or plasma substitute. This colloid was used extensively during World War I and, unlike blood and plasma, was easy to store and transport. Andre Cournand later demonstrated that the natural product, *serum albmin,* was also an effective blood volume expander.[30] He also confirmed the different effects on cardiac output and other hemodynamic variables when saline was compared with resuscitation with albumin. However, adverse reactions to the early colloid solutions were frequent and colloids were not always available; so crystalloids were the most commonly used resuscitation fluids during this interval.

The subsequent development of modern blood-banking techniques led to widespread utilization of blood products. During World War II, lyophilization and other techniques initially utilized large donor *pools of plasma*. Subsequently, the use of *fresh frozen plasma* permitted volume replacement with a single-donor solution, which minimized the risks of infections associated with the use of pooled plasma. Solutions containing *albumin* became more widely available after development of fractionation procedures. In addition, it was found that if albumin solution is heated to 60°C for 10 h, hepatitis viruses are inactivated, a process that added to the safety of this product.

By the 1960s and 1970s, albumin and fresh frozen plasma were widely used for many clinical conditions.[105] However, the cost of these fluids was substantial. Because of the excessive cost of albumin and other natural products, a renewed search for other colloids ensued. As a result, laboratories developed a variety of inexpensive synthetic colloids such as *dextrans, hydroxyethyl starches*, and *polygelatins*. The high cost of the natural colloid fluids also provided a powerful incentive to reassess the efficacy of colloid therapy and to compare this approach with that using less expensive crystalloids in controlled laboratory and clinical experiments. Many investigators questioned the physiologic rationale for colloid therapy and designed studies to determine if resuscitation with colloids or crystalloids was associated with improved survival or reduced complications.

As a result, scores of clinical and laboratory experiments were conducted over the next two decades. This body of work added considerable information on circulatory shock, microvascular physiology, and fluid flux across the lung and other organs as well as the physiologic defects associated with the adult respiratory distress syndrome (ARDS). However, the controversy regarding the superiority of colloid or crystalloid fluids was not completely resolved. A recent metaanalysis on the choice of resuscitation fluids using mortality as an end point concluded that there appeared to be a slight advantage with colloid fluids in the resuscitation of medical patients, whereas crystalloid fluids may have a slight advantage in the resuscitation of surgical and/or traumatized patients.[126]

In reviewing the many studies that compare colloids and crystalloids, it is important to recognize that the experiments vary considerably with respect to design, patient population, investigator bias, type and severity of perfusion failure, and conclusions. The pulmonary circulation and pulmonary edemagenesis have received the most attention in these comparisons. However, the hemodynamics, edemagenesis, and functional aspects of various other organs or tissue beds have been the focus of more recent work. In addition, investigators have now recognized that other properties in addition to oncotic or volemic effects of fluids play important roles that may influence their usefulness in the critically ill. Clinical and experimental research on fluids is therefore entering a new era, with different hypotheses and methodologies.

This discussion focuses on the use of colloids and crystalloids in the resuscitation of the patient with hypovolemia and in conditions of increased vascular permeability. The commonly used fluids are described, together with their volemic and other properties. Selected recent clinical and laboratory studies are reviewed. The hemodynamic and other factors that may modulate the response to a given fluid load are summarized, as well as the responses to fluid loading in the setting of increased vascular permeability. New and provocative laboratory studies are also mentioned, in which colloid fluids with selective molecular weight fractions of hydroxyethyl starches have been tested.

ALBUMIN

Albumin is the colloid against which others are judged for volemic properties. Albumin is the most abundant protein in plasma. As a soluble globular protein with a molecular weight of approximately 69,000 daltons, it accounts for approximately 75 percent of the colloid osmotic pressure of plasma. Albumin is distributed throughout the extracellular compartment. Nearly two-thirds of the body's albumin pool (320 g) is located in the interstitial or extravascular space. The half-life of albumin is 15 to 20 days. Decreased albumin production characterizes a variety of disorders, such as malnutrition, hepatic cirrhosis, surgical stress and trauma, malignancies, and hypothyroidism.[101,124] When human serum albumin is given, it is usually administered as a 5% solution with normal saline, yielding a colloid osmotic pressure (COP) of approximately 19 mmHg (torr). This fluid is therefore very similar to plasma. Human serum albumin is currently prepared from pooled human venous plasma by fractionation, sterilized by filtration, and treated for approximately 10 h at 60°C. The electrolyte characteristics are rendered similar to plasma and the pH is adjusted to approximately 6.9. Only plasma shown to be negative for hepatitis B surface antigen (HBsAg) may serve as a source of albumin.

Albumin is also available in a hyperoncotic preparation (25% solution). Albumin, with a molecular weight of 69,000 daltons, is unique because of its monodisperse characteristics, its multiple negative charges, its stability, and the fact that it is not glycosylated. These factors, as well as the high concentration of albumin in plasma, play major roles in the vascular retention of this protein and its other properties. Albumin is preferred to *plasma protein fraction* (PPF) as a volemic agent. PPF may lead to a variety of adverse reactions, including anaphylactoid responses. These responses appear to be due to other components, such as globulins, that are not found in albumin solutions. Other natural blood products include fresh frozen plasma, platelets, and red blood cells, but these products are *not* recommended for volume expansion.[121]

TABLE 45-1 • Approximate molecular weights of monodisperse and polydisperse colloids

Fluid	Weight average molecular weight (daltons)	Number average molecular weight (daltons)
Albumin	69,000	69,000
Dextran 40	40,000	26,000
Dextran 70	70,000	41,000
Plasma	119,000	88,000
Hespan	450,000	69,000
Pentastarch	280,000	120,000

DEXTRANS

Dextrans are polydisperse colloids that are prepared as glucose polymers. By definition, the component molecules of a polydisperse colloid include a variable number of particles of different molecular weights. The oncotic contribution of such colloids is best represented by a figure that reflects both the average molecular weight and the quantity of molecules at that average size; the term *number average molecular weight* has been developed to include both these parameters. The higher the number, the greater the colloid's oncotic effect. A more confusing term is the *weight average molecular weight*, which less accurately conveys information about the oncotic pressure of the colloid.

The term number average molecular weight conveys information about the average molecular weight and the number of molecules at the various dispersed molecular weights. Ninety percent of a given polydispersed colloid, for example, might be composed of a very low molecular weight species while the remaining 10 percent might include very high molecular weight components. The oncotic contribution of this colloid would be slight because 90 percent of the low-weight molecules would escape from the vascular space. The average molecular weight (i.e., weight average molecular weight) is strongly influenced by the minority of large molecules yielding a relatively high number. A solution with a high weight average molecular weight might be expected to yield a greater oncotic effect than is actually obtained. The number average molecular weight for this colloid would be much lower, reflecting the small contribution of the few high-molecular-weight compounds.

Two preparations of dextrans are used commonly, dextran 40 and dextran 70. Dextran 40 is composed of molecules with a weight average molecular weight of 40,000 daltons; dextran 70 has a weight average molecular weight of 70,000 daltons. As polydisperse colloids, however, both dextran 40 and dextran 70 contain very large molecules as well as some molecules of only a few thousand daltons; as such, the large molecules increase the weight average molecular weight. The number average molecular weight for colloidal fluids is much lower and better represents the number, size, and oncotic pressure of molecules in a polydisperse fluid. For all such fluids, the number average is always lower than the weight average value (Table 45-1).

Dextran 40 is a hyperoncotic fluid because it is prepared as a 10% solution. Since most of the molecules are small, the fluid has a short vascular half-life. However, because of the oncotic effect of the large number of smaller molecules, the initial volume expansion exceeds the volume of fluid given. Most of these small molecules then escape from the plasma compartment, so that plasma volume subsequently decreases.

Dextran 70 is prepared in an isotonic solution and has a longer retention time. The weight average molecular weight of dextran 70 is 70,000 daltons; the number average molecular weight is approximately 41,000 daltons. Both dextran 40 and dextran 70 may lead to coagulation defects and anaphylactoid reactions. Because of the wide spectrum of molecular sizes, the colloid oncotic pressure of dextran 70 is difficult to determine but approximates 40 torr.

HYDROXYETHYL STARCHES (HES)

Hydroxyethyl starches are polydisperse colloids made from waxy starches of highly branched glucose polymers derived from amylopectin. These molecules resemble glycogen. Hydroxyethyl groups are added to the one and six positions of the glucose moiety in various degrees of substitution. The degree of alcohol substitution affects the hydrolysis by amylase. Increasing the degree of substitution of the alcohol groups is therefore a method to increase vascular retention time. Thus, the size, shape, and number of molecules, as well as the degree of alcohol substitution, influence the volemic properties of HES.

The currently available product of hydroxyethyl starch (*hespan, hetastarch*) that is approved as a volemic agent is prepared in a 6% solution with a range of molecular sizes from a few thousand to several hundred thousand daltons. The weight and number average molecular weights of this fluid are 450,000 and 69,000 daltons, respectively. The COP of the fluid is approximately 28 torr, which is slightly greater than plasma. However, similar hemodynamic effects suggest that the expansion of plasma volume is comparable with that of 5% albumin.[94] The increases in plasma oncotic pressure are similar for both albumin and hetastarch and last for several days.[60]

Pentastarch is a newer preparation of hydroxyethyl starch that has a higher number average molecular weight (280,000 daltons), a tighter range of molecular sizes, and a number average molecular weight of 120,000. It contains molecules with a molar substitution of 0.45, so that there are 45 hydroxyethyl groups for every 100 glucose units. The oncotic pressure of pentastarch is approximately 40 torr and the vascular half-life is approximately 10 h.[95] Although pentastarch has been studied as a resuscitation fluid in both clinical and laboratory protocols, this fluid is not currently approved for clinical use for this purpose.[116,122,132] It was thought that since hydroxyethyl starch is taken up by the reticuloendothelial system (RES), function of the RES must be impaired; however, this was not confirmed.[106] Very minimal side effects have been reported for either the commercially available hetastarch or pentastarch, although coagulation deficiencies may occur when a massive load is given. In particular, levels of factor VIII may decrease to values greater than would be anticipated by the effects of hemodilution.[115,118] Furthermore, patients with von Willebrand's disease may be particularly prone to bleeding after fluid therapy with hydroxyethyl starch solutions.[117] These fluids, however, do not typically lead to clinically significant disturbances of bleeding in studies of medical, surgical, burn, and trauma patients. Hydroxyethyl starch has compared favorably with albumin[7,40,46,68,107,131,132] as a volume expander.

CRYSTALLOIDS

An analysis of the Starling-Landis-Staverman equation (Table 45-2) for fluid flux across the microvascular wall predicts that crystalloid fluids, such as 5% glucose in water, 0.9% saline, or Ringer's lactate, will rapidly distribute between the intravascular and extravascular compartments. For example, approximately an hour after the infusion of 1 liter of 5% dextrose in water, no more than 100 ml of the fluid remains within the vascular space. The other 900 ml distributes into the extracellular and the intracellular compartments. Approximately ¼ liter of normal (0.9%) saline, however, remains intravascularly following its infusion. Crystalloids are therefore less effective than an equivalent volume of colloids for expansion of vascular volume. However, crystalloids may be preferred when the primary deficit is that of water and/or electrolytes and the goal is to restore extracellular and, to some extent, intracellular volumes.

TABLE 45-2 •

Fluid transport J_v across the microvascular wall is determined by the Starling-Landis-Staverman equation:

$$J_v = L_p\, S[(P_c - P_1) - \delta_d\,(\pi_c - \pi_1)]$$

where L_p is the hydraulic conductivity of the microvascular wall, S is the capillary surface area, P_c and P_1 are the capillary and tissue hydrostatic pressures, respectively, δ_d is the osmotic reflection coefficient, and π_c and π_1 are the oncotic pressures for large solutes in the capillary and tissue spaces, respectively. This equation defines J_v as the balance between hydrostatic and oncotic pressures across the capillary-tissue barrier, assuming the following: (1) δ_d approaches 1; (2) this coefficient is uniform for all large solutes; and (3) L_p and S remain unchanged. Edema develops in tissues, however, when J_v exceeds the rate of lymphatic drainage of fluid.

HYPERTONIC FLUIDS

Hypertonic salt in concentrations of up to 7.5% has recently been studied for resuscitation, particularly in the treatment of trauma and hemorrhage.[93,127] The hypertonic saline solutions act as plasma volume expanders, as fluid is initially translocated from the interstitial and especially intracellular compartments, to augment plasma volume. Therefore, cardiac output, arterial pressure, and other hemodynamic variables improve sharply after administration of hypertonic saline. A further potential benefit in the resuscitation of the traumatized patient with hypertonic saline is a decrease in intracranial pressure. However, the volemic effects achieved with hypertonic fluids are transient and the osmolal load may lead to subsequent problems of hypertonicity. Although concentrations up to 7.5% saline have been used experimentally, in normal clinical practice concentrations greater than 3% are rarely used. Current practice suggests that 0.9% saline is the crystalloid volume expander of choice.

Representative effects of infusing 1 liter of various colloid and crystalloid fluids on intravascular, interstitial, and intracellular volumes are shown in Table 45-3.

CELL MEMBRANE INTEGRITY IN SHOCK

Studies by Shires and colleagues that began in the early 1960s have suggested that a deficit of extracellualr volume may develop under conditions of prolonged or severe circulatory shock. Alterations concomitantly occur in intracellular volume as do defects in the maintenance of the transcellular membrane potential and the ATP-ase dependent sodium pump.[20,31,109-111] Therefore, the intracellular concentration of sodium increases in ischemic cells. This will be followed by an increase in intracellular fluid volume, with a decrease in extracellular volume. Under these conditions, repletion of the extracellular compartment with large volumes of crystalloid fluid is a rational maneuver.

However, other studies have cast doubt on whether the findings of Shires and associates are applicable to all forms of shock and if those results pertain only to severe and irreversible conditions of perfusion failure.[55d,102,112] Furthermore, it is not known if the conclusions can be directly translated to clinical situations.

If hypovolemia is a major factor that leads to shock, repletion of vascular volume should be a high priority. Colloids contain large molecules that are more effectively retained within the vascular compartment. Infusion of these fluids is therefore associated with a greater expansion of blood volume, and the expansion persists for a more protracted interval. Colloids also help maintain or increase the plasma COP, whereas infusion of crystalloids will dilute the plasma proteins, causing a decrease in COP. The purposeful expansion of the interstitial compartment, or the increase of interstitial volume as a byproduct of fluid loading, is now regarded as a less desirable consequence of fluid loading. For these reasons, some authorities have advocated a return to the selective use of colloidal fluids.

CLINICAL SELECTION OF FLUIDS

Both colloid and crystalloid fluids are in wide clinical use. The choice of fluids should be guided by consideration of the type of fluid deficit, the urgency and the pathophysiology of the condition, and the plasma COP. Representative effects of the infusion on 1 liter of the various colloid and crystalloid fluids on intravascular, interstitial, and intracellular volumes are shown in Table 45-3. Most authors agree that isotonic crystalloids are effective for the initial resuscitation of hemorrhagic shock and/or trauma. Generally, isotonic (0.9%) saline solution is the agent of choice. In the normal subject, the dilution of plasma COP with moderate volumes of crystalloids is not associated with marked accumulation of pulmonary extravascular fluid and plasma COP is usually restored from interstitial stores of protein to normal values within 24 h. Washed or packed red blood cells may be added to restore erythrocyte mass. A hypertonic salt solution may offer certain advantages as an initial resuscitation fluid in hemorrhage or trauma. However, limited data are available on the use of hypertonic fluids in sepsis and other conditions of increased vascular permeability. Therefore, isotonic (0.9%) saline should be used as the fluid of choice in these circumstances.

After the initial resuscitation with up to several liters of a crystalloid fluid and in conditions such as sepsis, multiple organ failure, adult respiratory distress syndrome (ARDS), burns, venom injury, pancreatitis, and other conditions in which vascular permeability is altered, the choice of fluid is not as straightforward.

TABLE 45-3 • Changes in the volume of body fluid compartments affected by various colloids and crystalloids

Fluid (1 liter)	Na+ (mM/liter)	Changes in intracellular volume (ml)	Changes in total extracellular volume (ml)	Changes in interstitial volume (ml)	Changes in plasma volume (ml)
5% dextrose water	0	660	340	255	85
0.9% NaCl	154	0	1000	750	250
3% NaCl	513	−1630	1630	1223	408
5% NaCl	855	−2970	2970	2228	743
5% albumin	—	0	1000	Initially zero but increases as albumin equilibrates with ISF	Initially 1000 ml but falls as albumin equilibrates with ISF
Packed RBC	—	0	1000	0	1000

The following assumptions were made: under normal circumstances the total body water is distributed such that two-thirds and one-third localizes to the intracellular and extracellular compartments, respectively. The water in the extracellular compartment (when normal oncotic pressures are present) is distributed three-quarters and one-quarter in the interstitial and plasma compartments, respectively. Water is freely permeable across these compartments and distributes according to the "tonicity" of each compartment. The "tonicity" of these compartments is determined by the concentration and distribution of the effective solutes in each compartment. Effective solutes include sodium and potassium salts, glucose, albumin, all of which exert osmotic pressure across compartmental barriers and therefore cause shifts in water distribution among the various body compartments. The table predicts theoretical changes in water distribution and impact on body compartment volumes.

Citing the work of Shires and colleagues,[110] proponents of crystalloids maintain that the addition of colloids to the resuscitation regimen is not necessary. They argue that the interstitial fluid contraction associated with shock must be corrected and that the potential overexpansion of the extracellular compartment with the development of systemic edema with massive crystalloid infusion is of little concern. They also correctly reason that the expansion of the interstitial compartment that has been depleted by the loss of fluid and minerals into the cellular compartment is more fully restored by large volumes of crystalloids. Although some tissues may be prone to develop edema, in most cases the lung has sufficient safety factors to prevent the development of pulmonary edema. These factors include the plasma-interstitial oncotic gradient, the abundant lymphatic supply of the lung, the physical-chemical characteristics of the interstitial space, the integrity of the microvascular membrane, and a low vascular hydrostatic driving pressure in the pulmonary circulation.

Advocates of colloid therapy have proposed that resuscitation can be accomplished faster and with greater precision with colloid, which may potentially help to reduce the accumulation of edema in the lung and particularly in other organs. An equal volume of a colloid will lead to greater and more sustained increases in blood volume, cardiac filling pressures, and cardiac output. Furthermore, unless increases in microvascular hydrostatic pressure are excessive, a colloid is likely to produce less interstitial edema.

A variety of studies have demonstrated that there are substantial differences in the amount of fluid needed for resuscitation to similar hemodynamic end points when colloids are compared with crystalloids. As much as two to six times the volume of colloid is needed to achieve similar hemodynamic end points when a crystalloid is selected. A recent crossover clinical study by Hankeln et al. confirmed this observation, although there did not appear to be any measurable difference in the development of pulmonary edema or other complications between colloid and crystalloid groups.[56]

However, colloids may have adverse effects that are independent of their volemic properties. Potentially deleterious effects of albumin have been cited by some authors. These include coagulation changes, impaired immune responsiveness, adverse effects on cardiac and renal function, and a decrease in the level of ionized calcium and in the ratio of ionized to total serum calcium.[25,70,78,133] While these reports are provocative, in most cases they have not been duplicated by other investigators and their clinical implications are unknown.

In contrast to reports of adverse effects, a number of studies may be cited to show that albumin solutions possess favorable properties that may be independent of its oncotic and/or volemic properties. Albumin may augment immune mechanisms; it may be a free radical scavenger and may inhibit lipid peroxidation; it may bind and inactivate toxic products; and it may promote microvascular integrity.[44,64,69,92,114,130]

OTHER FACTORS MODULATING THE VOLEMIC RESPONSES TO FLUIDS

Although colloids lead to two- to sixfold increases in vascular volume and hemodynamic variables in comparison with crystalloids, a number of factors may modify the response to a given fluid load. Vascular compliance is an uncontrolled factor affecting the response to infusion. In cases in which vascular compliance is low, a fluid load of colloid may lead to dramatic increases in blood pressure. This may be particularly likely when levels of endogenous or exogenous catecholamines are high. The infusion may precipitate acute right or left ventricular volume overload with systemic and/or pulmonary edema. This response is more likely than with a crystalloid. In contrast, under conditions of increased vascular compliance, such as during therapy with vasodilators, a greater fluid volume is required to produce these changes. Vascular tone therefore emerges as a factor that may alter the individual response to a fluid load.

Cardiac compliance also plays an important role in the response to fluids. A number of clinical settings, including sepsis, myocardial ischemia, and the use of positive end-expiratory pressure, may affect the relationship between end-diastolic cardiac volumes and measured cardiac filling pressures. Hence, isolated measurements of cardiac filling pressures may fail to correlate with other indices of cardiac function.

The clinician should therefore consider monitoring the response to fluid loading in a stepwise manner, using fluid-challenge techniques as indices of the adequacy of perfusion and cardiac competence. Dynamic changes in cardiac filling pressure, arterial pressure, urine output, heart rate, blood lactate levels, mental status, and other guides should be monitored at frequent intervals as fluids are given. Until bedside techniques permit noninvasive assessment of cardiac and, possibly, vascular compliance, it would be prudent to select hemodynamic and oxygen transport end points to assess the adequacy of resuscitation. Such end points might include cardiac output, lactate measurements, arterial and venous oxygen saturations, and other derived parameters such as oxygen delivery and consumption. Several authorities have recommended that these physiologic end points are preferable to preselected fluid volumes or cardiac filling pressures.

INCREASED VASCULAR PERMEABILITY

For conditions in which vascular permeability is altered, the debate over the choice of fluids remains unsettled.

Many studies have focused on whether colloids or crystalloids are associated with the lowest risk of pulmonary edema and attendant pulmonary complications. This emphasis on the pulmonary microvasculature was related to the frequent complication of ARDS associated with sepsis, trauma, and other conditions in which large volumes of resuscitation fluid were used. Since a hallmark of the physiologic defects associated with ARDS is an increase in vascular permeability to fluid and protein, pulmonary microvascular hydrostatic pressure emerges as the major determinant for fluid movement across the microvascular membrane. The threshold pressure for edema is reduced when permeability is altered.

Proponents of colloids suggest that a reasonable clinical goal should be to maintain plasma colloid osmotic pressure (COP) at or near normal values in patients with ARDS by use of colloid infusion and that marked decreases in COP lead to an increased risk of pulmonary edema.[96] Thus, the ability to maintain the plasma to interstitial oncotic gradient is breached when plasma COP is very low. However, the level of plasma COP to produce this effect is not commonly encountered in most clinical conditions. If a colloid is used to improve hemodynamic parameters for a patient with ARDS, the effects on pulmonary microvascular hydrostatic pressure should be carefully monitored and minimized.

Advocates of crystalloids point to the substantial safety factors protecting against edema in the lung so that, in most cases, moderate lowering of plasma COP may not of itself lead to edema. In an experimental model of pulmonary injury in which microvascular permeability is moderately impaired and pulmonary microvascular pressure was maintained at approximately 20 mmHg, infusion of colloids or crystalloids led to similar increases in lung water.[104] However, colloidal fluids produced greater hemodilution, consistent with a greater expansion of plasma volume; and colloids were associated with a greater increase in cardiac output. Despite these perturbations, there were no significant differences between the colloid and crystalloid groups in the extent of lung edema, carefully measured by gravvimetric techniques. These results reinforce the concept that, with a moderate increase in lung microvascular permeability, no clear superiority of a colloid or crystalloid fluid is demonstrated. In another experimental study in which hydroxyethyl starch was compared with Ringer's lactate in hypoproteinemic sheep in which lung lymph fistulas were produced to study pulmonary lymph fluid flux and composition,[58] hydroxyethyl starch was associated with a less marked increase in lymph flow but an increase in the lymph to plasma oncotic gradient. The authors concluded that the oncotic property of hydroxyethyl starch accounted for those changes and that fluid may therefore be a valuable adjunct as a plasma volume expander to help maintain fluid balance in critically ill patients. Finally, a clinical study of surgical patients indicates that postoperative fluid overload is not a benign problem[79] and is associated with significant increases in mortality.

The single focus on the lung in comparing resuscitation fluids has diverted attention from other important issues, including the effects of the accumulation of edema fluid in other systemic sites and its potential effect to impair oxygen delivery to other tissues. The oncotic and other properties of colloid and crystalloid fluids and their effects on nonpulmonary tissues are being reexamined by several investigators.

OTHER PERMEABILITY LESIONS

A variety of acute care conditions are associated with sudden and dramatic increases in vascular permeability. These syndromes present formidable challenges to the critical care practitioner but also offer a unique opportunity to compare the effects of colloids and crystalloids. For some of these conditions, colloids appear to offer certain advantages. This is particularly true for fulminant but short-lived permeability lesions. Circulatory shock associated with anaphylaxis, severe venom poisoning, intestinal injury, and certain other toxic injuries may therefore be resuscitated more successfully with colloids than with crystalloids.[19,32,33,47-49,61,65,103,134]

Zikria et al. have recently reported that a fraction of hydroxyethyl starch that predominantly consists of molecules of 100,000 to 300,000 daltons has dramatic effects on vascular permeability in models of rat limb ischemia,[144] scald injury of the rat intestine,[143] and ischemia and reperfusion of the myocardium.[145,146] The authors proposed a capillary-sealing property to this fraction of hydroxyethyl starch. Other fractions or fluids tested did not share this property. If these and similar studies can be applied to clinical conditions, a new approach to colloid therapy may emerge.

CONCLUSIONS

Although the debate over the choice of colloids or crystalloids has not been resolved, some empiric guidelines may be developed (Tables 45-1 and 45-3). In traumatic and/or hypovolemic shock, resuscitation with crystalloids is prudent and of proved efficacy. If additional fluids are required after the initial several liters, the clinician should monitor plasma COP and use physiologic end points as additional crystalloids or colloids are infused. For ARDS, neither crystalloid nor currently available colloid fluids appear to have preferential effects to minimize edema, although it is prudent to maintain microvascular hydrostatic pressure as low as practicable. This is best accomplished by maintaining pulmonary capillary wedge pressures at the the lowest value required to maintain adequate cardiac output (generally 10 to 12 cm H_2O). For sepsis, the use of either colloids or crystalloids can be supported by the literature. In venom injuries, anaphylaxis, burns, and certain other fulminant conditions, colloids may have a greater role in fluid resuscitation.

The very recent studies of size-specific fractions of colloids and hypertonic crystalloid fluids are provocative. Following additional and confirmatory studies, new recommendations for fluid therapy may result. At present, however, these approaches to fluid resuscitation should be regarded as experimental.

Issues related to cardiac competence and vascular compliance should be considered whenever fluid loading is contemplated. Colloids lead to greater volume expansion and a more protracted increase in vascular volume than do crystalloids. When the primary defect is that of the extracellular fluid, crystalloids are the preferred fluid. The plasma oncotic pressure, unless extremely low (<10 to 12 torr), is not usually associated with pulmonary edema, although systemic edema may occur more readily with hypoproteinemia. Physiologic end points or favorable trends including oxygen transport and consumption, cardiac output, reversal of anaerobic metabolism as measured by reductions in serum lactate, and the dynamic responses to fluid loading are more appropriate guides to fluid loading than choosing preselected fluid volumes or cardiac filling pressure.

CLINICAL UTILITY OF BLOOD LACTATE MEASUREMENTS AND THE ANION GAP IN ASSESSING TISSUE HYPOXIA IN THE CRITICALLY ILL

Elevations in blood lactate concentration commonly occur as a physiologic response to a severe imbalance between systemic oxygen supply and demand.[71] (See Chap. 25.) Systemic oxygen supply can be quantitated as oxygen delivery, the product of cardiac output and arterial blood oxygen content. Under normal conditions, oxygen consumption is determined by metabolic demands and is independent of oxygen delivery (Fig. 45-1*a*). In the face of decreasing oxygen delivery, for example, due to impaired cardiac output, oxygen consumption is maintained by an increase in oxygen extraction at the tissue level. This increased extraction is reflected in a greater degree of venous oxyhemoglobin desaturation, and may allow for complete compensation over a wide range of oxygen delivery (Fig. 45-1*b*). Further decreases in oxygen delivery, however, will eventually cross a threshold below which oxygen consumption becomes directly proportional to oxygen delivery. Below this critical point systemic oxygen demands are no longer satisfied, oxygen consumption is said to be *supply-dependent*, and severe tissue hypoxia becomes established (Fig. 45-1*c*). Partial reliance on the anaerobic metabolic pathway, known as glycolysis, is then the remaining mechanism allowing tissues to maintain vital functions. Lactate is the end product of anaerobic metabolism.

The most common cause of an elevation in blood lactate concentration is hypoperfusion or circulatory shock.[72] Severe tissue hypoxia with hyperlactatemia, known as *type A* lactic acidosis, represents a severe state of decompensation that, if sustained, leads to vital organ dysfunction and injury. Thus, it is perhaps not surprising that there is a strong inverse correlation between blood lactate concentration and survival in critically ill patients (Fig. 45-2).[17,63,71,75,77,128,135] Lactic acidosis is often defined as an elevation of blood lactate to at least 5 mmol/liter, probably because lesser degrees of hyper-

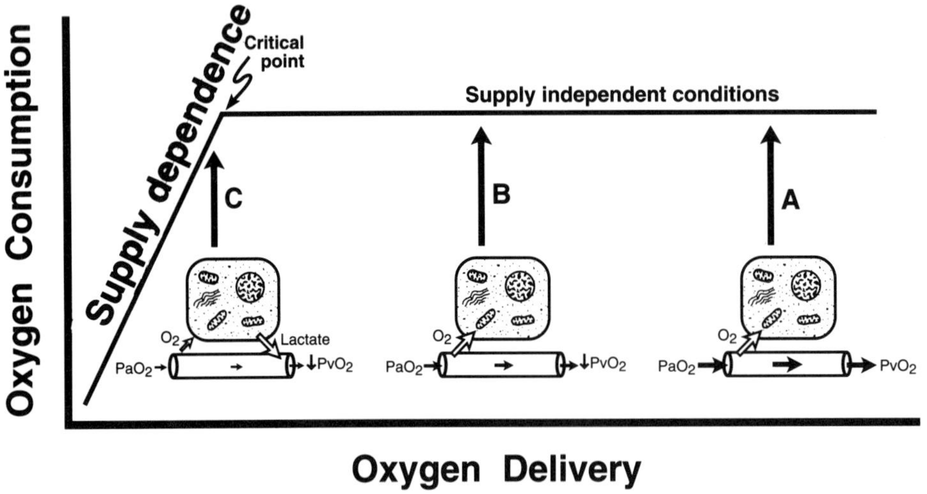

FIGURE 45-1 • Physiologic relationship between oxygen delivery, oxygen consumption, and lactate production. (*a*) Oxygen consumption is normally regulated by metabolic requirements of systemic tissues and is independent of oxygen delivery. (*b*) Decreased oxygen delivery is compensated for by increased tissue oxygen extraction, made manifest by a further decrease in venous oxygen tension, thereby allowing oxygen consumption to remain independent of oxygen delivery. (*c*) When oxygen delivery decreases below a critical point, consumption becomes dependent upon the supply. Oxygen delivery at or below this level is insufficient to meet the metabolic requirements of the tissues and results in partial reliance on anaerobic metabolism with the consequent production of lactate.

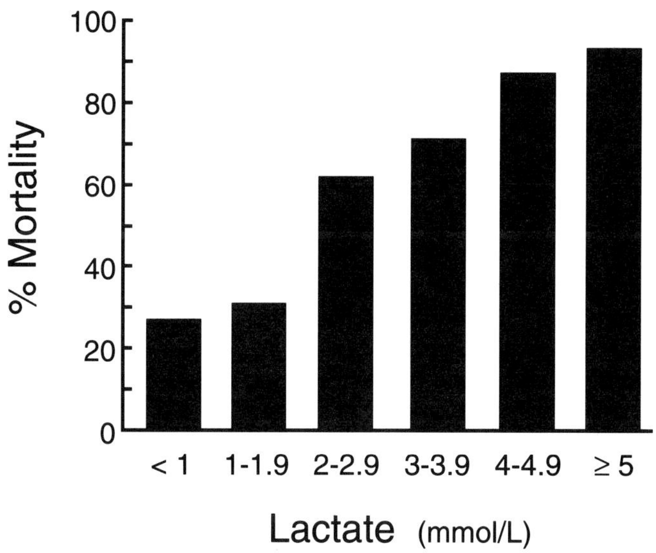

FIGURE 45-2 • Relationship between blood lactate concentration and hospital mortality in critically ill patients. (From Kruse JA: Blood lactate and oxygen transport. *Intensive Care World* 4:121, 1987 with permission.)

lactatemia would not be expected to lead to significant acidemia. For example, an increase in blood lactate from a normal value of 1.0 mmol/liter to a level of 4 mmol/liter represents an increase of 3 mmol/liter. In theory this increase should result in titration of plasma bicarbonate from a normal level of 24 mmol/liter down to 21 mmol/liter, with a corresponding reduction in arterial pH from 7.40 to approximately 7.35. However, in critically ill patients this level of change in lactate is statistically associated with a more than twofold increase in mortality. Thus, although hyperlactatemia in this range has little impact on acid-base balance, it can have substantial prognostic implications and therefore represents a clinically relevant change. It should be remembered, however, that a 3-mmol increase in blood lactate and corresponding reduction in bicarbonate exerts a profound effect on blood pH in those patients who already manifest hypobicarbonatemia. An example best illustrates this point. A ketoacidotic patient with a bicarbonate concentration of 10 mmol/liter and a P_{CO_2} of 23 mmHg will have a pH of 7.26. Superimposition of a 4 mmol/liter lactic acidosis acutely lowers the bicarbonate level to 6 mmol/liter, which with a P_{CO_2} of 23 mmHg results in a pH of 7.04.

A wide variety of causes of lactic acidosis that ostensibly do not involve tissue hypoxia have been described and are known as *type B* lactic acidosis.[28] However, most of these etiologies are either very uncommon or result in only minor increases in blood lactate or require no specific therapy. Certain disease states that have been said to represent type B lactic acidosis are, in fact, probably attributable to hypoperfusion. For example, pancreatitis and pulmonary embolism have been named as causes of nonischemic lactic acidosis,[28,120] but both can lead to severe hypoperfusion, pancreatitis by causing hypovolemic shock and pulmonary embolism by causing obstructive shock.[2,8] Certain cases of malignant disease appear to be associated with chronic and sometimes severe increases in blood lactate but without evidence of tissue hypoxia.[28,72] When examined with respect to the prevalence of advanced neoplastic disease these cases are, however, quite rare. Most cases of lactic acidosis in patients with cancer can be explained on the basis of tissue hypoperfusion. Severe hepatic disease is often listed as a cause of lactic acidosis. When critically examined, however, the available information suggests that increases in blood lactate in patients with liver disease are nearly always associated with signs of hypoperfusion (Fig. 45-3).[77] Inadequate tissue oxygenation should therefore be the prime consideration when hyperlactatemia is detected in critically ill patients, including those with hepatic dysfunction or advanced cancer.

In patients with frank hypotension or in those who require high-dose vasopressor infusions or intraaortic balloon counterpulsation, elevations of blood lactate are

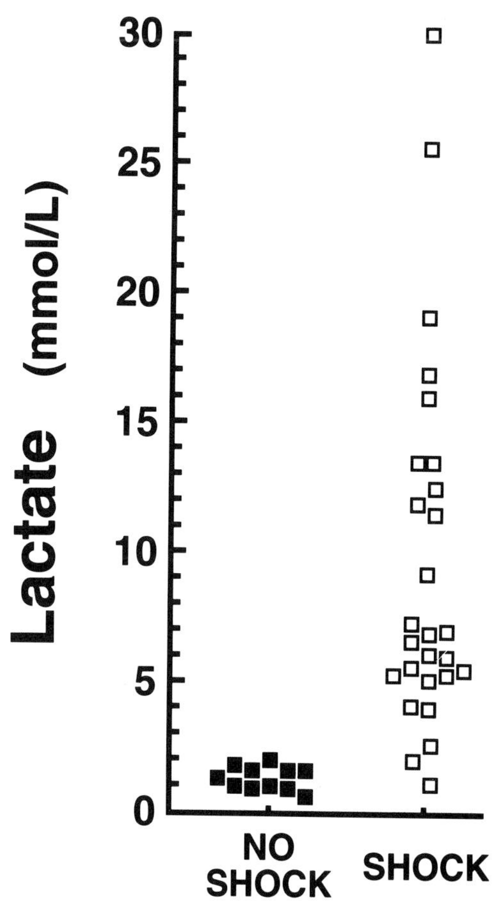

FIGURE 45-3 • Blood lactate concentration in patients with severe liver disease. Open squares represent patients meeting clinical criteria for circulatory shock. Closed squares represent patients with severe hepatic disease without evidence of shock. (From Kruse JA et al: Significance of blood lactate levels in critically ill patients with liver disease. *Am J Med,* 3:77, 1987 with permission.)

not unexpected. A major utility in monitoring blood lactate lies in detecting more subtle levels of hypoperfusion and tissue hypoxia, and in gauging the response to treatment designed to improve perfusion and tissue oxygenation. Therapeutic interventions that improve cardiac output (e.g., fluid challenge, inotropic catecholamine infusions, and afterload reduction) or that augment arterial oxygen content (e.g., red cell transfusion, supplemental oxygen administration, and positive end-expiratory pressure) may increase oxygen delivery toward or above the critical point, minimizing hypoxic organ injury and manifesting as a drop in blood lactate concentration.[74,87]

Along with renal failure and diabetic ketoacidosis, lactic acidosis is among the most common causes of an increased anion gap metabolic acidosis. Anion gap measurement and arterial blood gas analysis are often very helpful in detecting and quantitating these metabolic disorders. Assuming that poisoning is not a consideration, further examination of three other routinely available simple chemistry tests, namely, serum creatinine, glucose, and ketone levels, may allow renal failure and ketoacidosis to be ruled out as diagnostic possibilities, leaving lactic acidosis as a diagnosis by exclusion. However, significant increases in blood lactate may occur without acidemia or an increase in the anion gap. Alkalosis and mixed acid-base disorders are common in critically ill patients.[82,83,89,137] Concomitant respiratory or metabolic alkalosis will counteract the effect that lactic acidosis would otherwise exert on arterial pH. Coexisting metabolic alkalosis, if sufficiently severe, may completely mask the acidemia associated with hyperlactatemia.[53] Elevated lactate levels can thus occur in the presence of normal or even frankly alkalemic arterial pH.[76]

The anion gap is a composite measurement, and therefore its normal range must encompass both the physiologic variablity of its constituents as well as the inherent imprecision of the assay methodologies for each individual test. The resulting broad normal range is one factor that limits the ability to detect mild degrees of hyperlactatemia by anion gap determination alone. Albumin is a strongly anionic serum protein. At physiologic pH it has a net negative charge of about 18 charges per molecule.[45] The serum albumin concentration, in fact, makes the largest single contribution to the unmeasured anion pool. Hypoalbuminemia is common among chronically ill and debilitated patients who make up a substantial proportion of those patients who ultimately present in a state of acute decompensation[4,10,11] and, not infrequently, with lactic acidosis. Since hypoalbuninemia can effectively lower the anion gap, a larger increment in lactate will be required to raise the gap above its usual upper normal limit (Fig. 45-4). This is likely an important factor explaining the less than perfect sensitivity of the anion gap in detecting significant degrees of hyperlactatemia in critically ill patients.[67,85]

Although arterial blood gas analysis and anion gap determination will detect many instances of significant lactic acidoses, a substantial minority of cases will go undetected.[67] Direct measurement of blood lactate is therefore important if false negatives are to be avoided. Arterial or mixed venous blood specimens should be used since peripheral venous samples can yield spuriously ele-

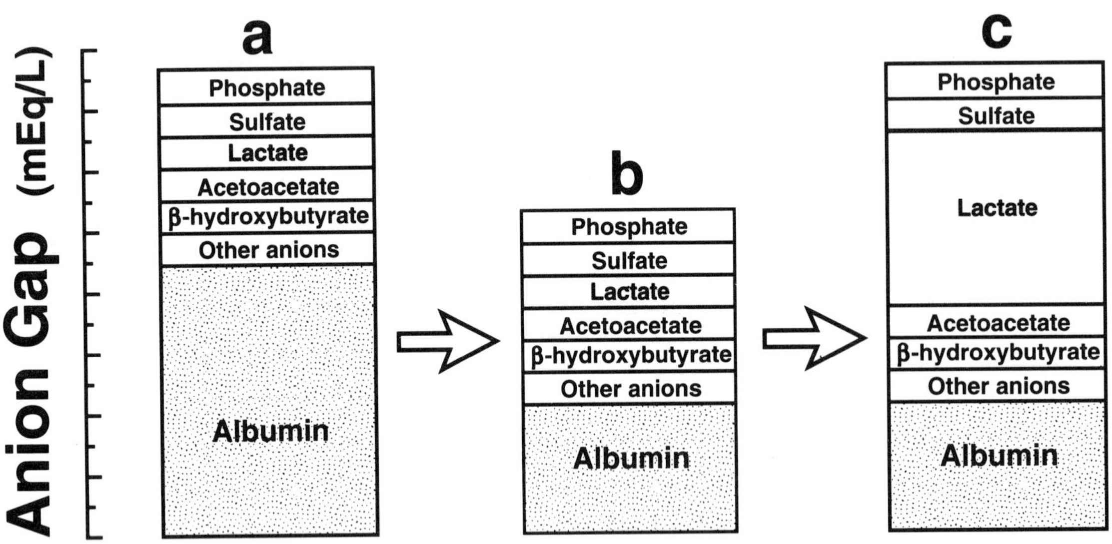

FIGURE 45-4 • Explanation of how lactic acidosis can occur without an increased anion gap. (*a*) Schematic depiction of total unmeasured anion concentration in a healthy subject: lactate, phosphate, ketoacid, and other unmeasured anions are present in normal concentrations; albumin makes the largest quantitative contribution to the total unmeasured anion pool. (*b*) The subject develops a chronic illness with severe hypoalbuminemia resulting in a decrease of the unmeasured anion concentration to levels below the lower normal limits. (*c*) The subject later acutely decompensates and develops lactic acidosis; a large increase in the blood lactate concentration is insufficient to raise the anion gap above the upper limits of normal.

vated values depending on the technique used.[43,57,86,91] Peripheral vasoconstriction accompanying circulatory shock would be expected to further raise venous lactate levels. While once a cumbersome assay,[59] modern automated instrumentation can measure lactate levels in microliter quantities of plasma, serum, or whole blood within minutes.[73] Many centers employ such instruments in their blood gas laboratory adjacent to the intensive care unit, allowing lactate determinations to be reported in the same time frame as arterial blood gas results. In addition to maximizing sensitivity, direct measurement of lactate concentration allows for monitoring of subtle but important serial changes that reflect the patient's response to therapy and provide the clinician with valuable feedback.

ACID-BASE METABOLISM DURING PERFUSION FAILURE AND CARDIOPULMONARY RESUSCITATION

The specific pathophysiologic changes in acid-base metabolism that occur during the clinical states of perfusion failure, cardiac arrest, and cardiopulmonary resuscitation (CPR) are topics that have seen renewed interest over the past decade. (See Chap. 25.) Particular attention has been paid to differences in arterial-venous hydrogen ion (pH), lactic acid, and carbon dioxide (CO_2) gradients as indicators of tissue injury and perfusion. Additionally, the specific acid-base changes in, and the effects of, buffer therapy on myocardial tissue have been elaborated.

Standards established in the early 1960s[67b,69a,135d] and followed through 1986[113] suggested that the monitoring of arterial blood gases alone was sufficient to guide alkali therapy during cardiopulmonary resuscitation.[112a] The assumption was that arterial samples adequately reflected the acid-base status of most tissues (especially the myocardium). However, the specific acid-base changes in humans in both arterial and venous blood samples during cardiopulmonary resuscitation[79a,135a] and circulatory failure[1] have recently been described, and large hydrogen ion (pH) and carbon dioxide gradients across the arterial and central venous blood compartments (Table 45-4) have been found. In one study,[135a] the central venous pH fell from a value of 7.31 prearrest to 7.14 during CPR, while coincident arterial pH increased from 7.37 prearrest to 7.43 during CPR. Thus the arterial to mixed-venous pH gradient increased from 0.06 to 0.30 pH units (Table 45-4) during cardiopulmonary resuscitation. The change in hydrogen-ion gradient could not be accounted for by lactic acidosis alone. Since most of these patients received bicarbonate, the arterial and central venous bicarbonate levels actually increased during CPR in spite of increasing concentrations of lactate (Table 45-4). Thus, the hydrogen-ion (pH) arterial to mixed-venous gradient was due to the elevated venous carbon dioxide. These studies[1,135a] and others have led to renewed interest in the pathophysiology of lactic acid and carbon dioxide accumulation during CPR and of the relative effects of these acids on tissue function. In an attempt to determine the factors that enhance restoration of cardiac function during circulatory failure and CPR, many studies have focused on the acid-base changes that occur during CPR and their effects on the myocardium. Although other tissues have been studied,[67a] this review deals with the metabolic effects on the myocardium that occur during CPR.

TABLE 45-4 • Arterial and mixed-venous acid-base parameters before and during cardiopulmonary resuscitation in 13 patients

	Prearrest	CPR	*p*-value
pH:			
Arterial	7.37	7.43	NS
Mixed-venous	7.31	7.14	<0.001
Gradient	0.06	0.29	<0.001
P_{CO_2} (Torr)			
Arterial	33	33	NS
Mixed-venous	44	69	<0.004
Gradient	11	36	<0.001
HCO_3 (mmol/liter)			
Arterial	19	25	NS
Mixed-venous	22	23	NS
Gradient	3	2	NS
Lactate (mmol/liter)			
Arterial	6	11	<0.05

Adapted with permission from Weil MH et al: Difference in acid-base state between venous and arterial blood during cardiopulmonary resuscitation. *N Engl J Med* 315:153, 1986.

The elevated mixed-venous carbon dioxide found in perfusion failure can be secondary to overproduction, underexcretion of carbon dioxide, or a combination of the two processes. Overproduction can occur with the administration of a carbon dioxide producing agent (such as sodium bicarbonate) while underexcretion can be secondary to either hypoventilation or pulmonary hypoperfusion (which leads to decreased delivery to the lungs of carbon dioxide). With pulmonary hypoperfusion (but with constant ventilation) excretion of carbon dioxide becomes proportional to pulmonary blood flow, and consequently, cardiac output. Thus, measures of pulmonary carbon dioxide excretion such as end-tidal carbon dioxide ($ETCO_2$) should directly correlate with such measures of cardiac output as arterial-venous oxygen content difference (A-V O_2) and cardiac index. *To summarize:* $ETCO_2 \propto$ (cardiac output $\times$ CO_2 production rate) $\div$ (minute ventilation). Falk et al. demonstrated these re-

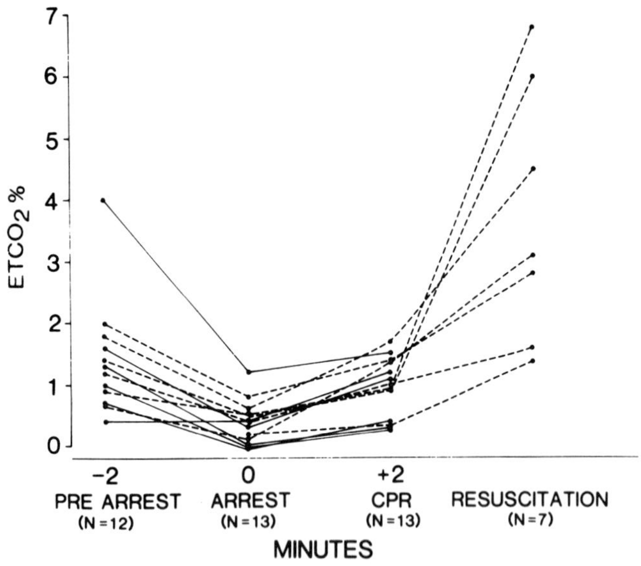

FIGURE 45-5 • End-tidal carbon dioxide concentration ($ETCO_2$) in 10 patients (13 measurements) before cardiac arrest, at the onset of cardiac arrest (but before cardiac compression), 2 min after cardiac compression was initiated, and immediately after successful resuscitation. Dashed lines identify the survivors and the solid lines identify the nonsurvivors. (Reprinted with permission from Falk JL et al: End-tidal carbon dioxide concentration during cardiopulmonary resuscitation. *N Engl J Med* 318:607, 1988.)

lationships during CPR in 10 patients.[46a] In this study (Fig. 45-5), $ETCO_2$ fell at the time of cardiac arrest and increased slightly during CPR (with the improvement of blood flow). Within 30 s of the reestablishment of spontaneous circulation, an overshoot of $ETCO_2$ occurred as excretion of carbon dioxide increased with the restoration of pulmonary blood flow. In patients in whom resuscitation was unsuccessful, $ETCO_2$ remained at levels below those seen in the resuscitated patients. There was an inverse linear relationship between the $ETCO_2$ and the arterial-venous O_2 saturation difference; as $ETCO_2$ fell the A-V O_2 difference increased, indicating a fall in cardiac output (Fig. 45-6). Thus, $ETCO_2$ is a reliable indicator of cardiac output during human CPR.

This phenomenon has been studied more extensively in animal models.[51a,55a,55b,55c,67c,128a] With constant ventilation during CPR, $ETCO_2$ decreases, as cardiac index falls (Fig. 45-7), mixed-venous P_{CO_2} increases secondary to decreased delivery of carbon dioxide to the lungs for excretion, and arterial-venous gradients for hydrogen-ion increase and mixed-venous pH decreases relative to arterial pH (Fig. 45-8). These changes reverse within minutes if resuscitation is successful.

In human beings, a persistently low $ETCO_2$ predicted the inability to resuscitate patients.[46a] Although the actual value of $ETCO_2$ in individual patients is not of use, the lack of an increase in $ETCO_2$ after CPR is initiated is an indicator of unimproved cardiac output and portends poor outcome. The predictive value of $ETCO_2$ has been better studied in experimental models: using a porcine model of cardiac arrest, Gudipati et al.[55] demonstrated that animals that were successfully resuscitated had significantly higher $ETCO_2$ values during CPR than animals that did not survive (Fig. 45-9). In this study cardiac output was directly measured and correlated well with $ETCO_2$ values (Fig. 45-7).

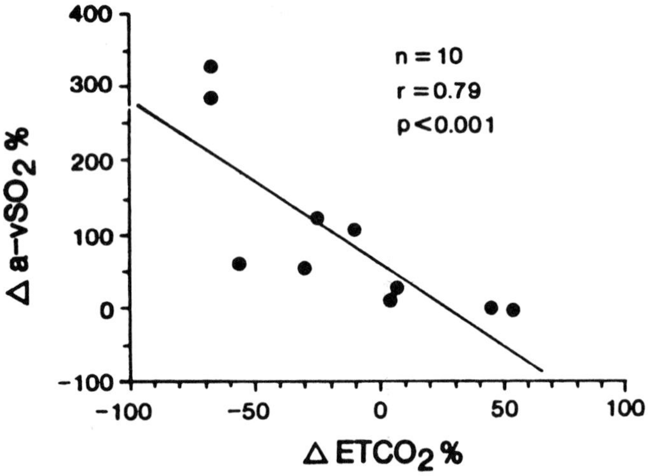

FIGURE 45-6 • The relationship between arterial-venous oxygen saturation difference (A-VSO_2) and the end-tidal carbon dioxide ($ETCO_2$) levels. Values were taken prearrest and during CPR. The data are shown as the percentage change from prearrest values. The A-VSO_2 is a measure of cardiac output in these patients. (Reprinted with permission from Falk JL et al: End-tidal carbon dioxide concentration during cardiopulmonary resuscitation. *N Engl J Med* 318:607, 1988.)

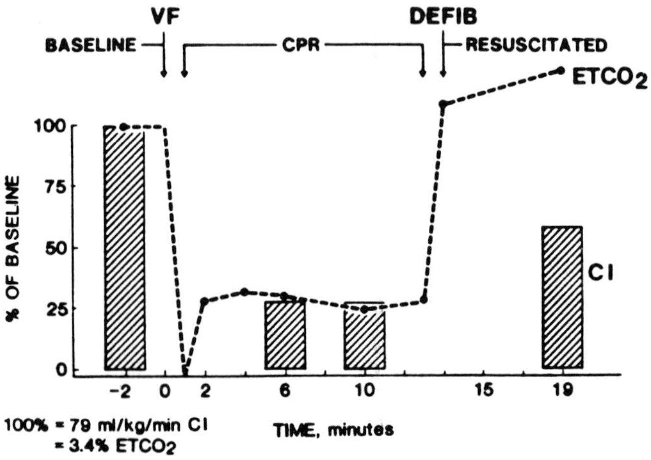

FIGURE 45-7 • The relationship between cardiac index (CI) and $ETCO_2$ in a porcine model of cariopulmonary resuscitation (CPR) before cardiac arrest, during CPR secondary to ventricular fibrillation (VF), during CPR with cardiac compression, and after successful resuscitation after defibrillation (DEFIB). (Reprinted with permission from Gudipati CV et al: Expired carbon dioxide: A noninvasive monitor of cardiopulmonary resuscitation. *Circulation* 77:234, 1988.

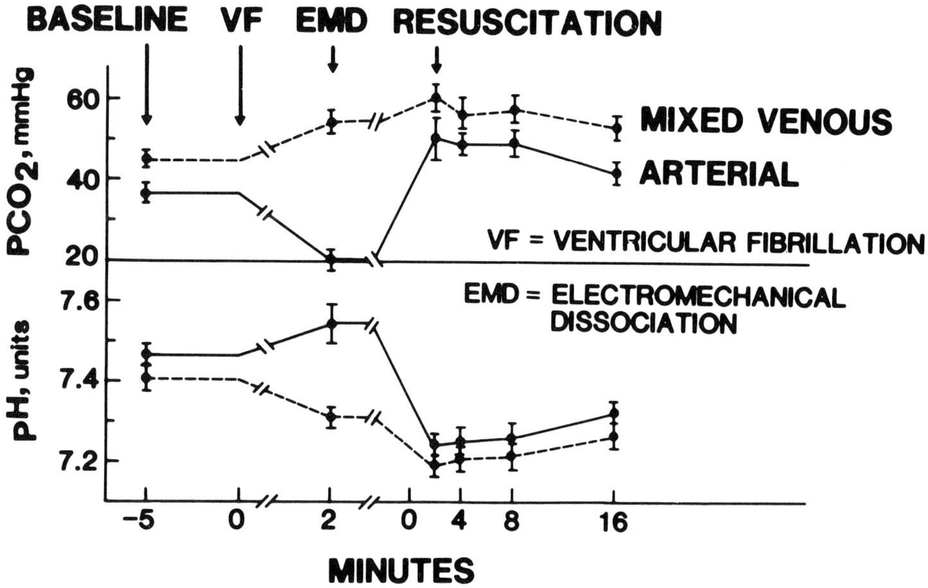

FIGURE 45-8 • Mixed-venous and arterial P_{CO_2} and pH in a porcine model of CPR. Values are given prior to arrest, at the induction of ventricular fibrillation (VF), during electromechanical dissociation (EMD), and after successful resuscitation. (Reprinted with permission from Grundler W et al: Arteriovenous carbon dioxide and pH gradients during cardiac arrest. *Circulation* 74:1071, 1986.)

The elevation of mixed-venous carbon dioxide during the perfusion failure of cardiac resuscitation raises the question of the type of acidosis that occurs at the tissue level. Lactic acidosis has been viewed to be the major cause of acidosis. Also, buffer therapy during resuscitation has been aimed at reversing hypoxia-induced lactic acidosis. However, elevated venous carbon dioxide values suggest that "respiratory" acidosis at the tissue level may be as important a factor in the setting of cardiopulmonary resuscitation. Animal studies have recently demonstrated that "respiratory" acidosis at the tissue level (with severe acidemia) does occur, especially in the myocardium.[43a,51a,55b,67c,128a] This has been evaluated by measuring both intramyocardial and great coronary vein carbon dioxide. The hydrogen-ion concentration in the coronary vein varies directly with the degree of elevation of coronary vein carbon dioxide (Fig. 45-10), and in preliminary studies, intramyocardial levels of carbon dioxide correlated well with intramyocardial pH.[67a] Intramyocardial pH is thought to reflect intracellular pH[167a,67c] and at least may reflect a balance between interstitial and intracellular pH values. As a measure of tissue hydrogen-ion concentration, it responds differently to experimental interventions than other sites measured (coronary vein, mixed venous, or arteral blood), and may

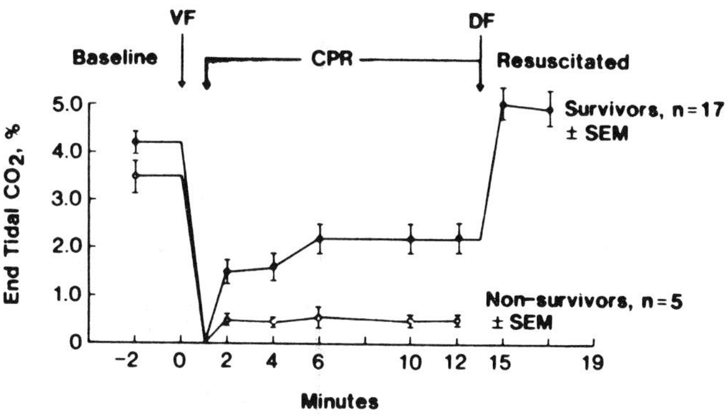

FIGURE 45-9 • Comparison in resuscitated and nonresuscitated animals of $ETCO_2$ in a porcine model of CPR. (Reprinted with permission from Gudipati CV et al: Expired carbon dioxide: A noninvasive monitor of cardiopulmonary resuscitation. *Circulation* 77:23, 1988.)

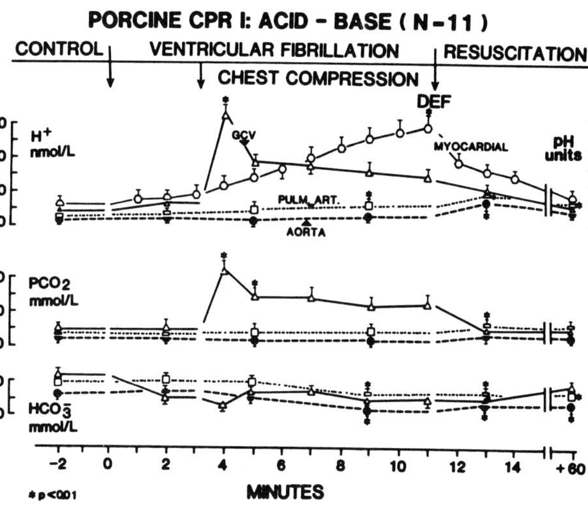

FIGURE 45-10 • Graphs of hydrogen-ion concentration (pH), carbon dioxide (P_{CO_2}), and bicarbonate, in great coronary vein (GCV), myocardium, pulmonary artery (mixed-venous sample), and aorta. External chest compression was begun 3 min after electromechanical dissociation was initiated with ventricular fibrillation. Animals (porcine model) were resuscitated by defibrillation and spontaneous circulation was reestablished. (Reprinted with permission from Von Planta M et al: Myocardial acidosis associated with CO_2 production during cardiac arrest and resuscitation. *Circulation* 80:684, 1989.)

represent a more accurate indicator of intracellular acid-base status.[67c,128a]

Lactic acid concentrations have been studied in simultaneously drawn arterial, mixed-venous, and pulmonary arterial specimens under a range of conditions (including seizures and various states of perfusion failure). Under these circumstances, simultaneously measured concentrations of lactate are virtually identical regardless of the arterial or mixed-venous site from which the specimen was drawn.[51a,135b] This is in contrast to the measurement of carbon dioxide, where the normal arterial-venous gradient increases. Since the concentrations of lactate and bicarbonate remain relatively constant and equal in arterial and mixed-venous blood samples at any time during resuscitation, the major determinant of the arterial-venous hydrogen-ion (pH) gradient becomes the large increase in carbon dioxide concentration in the mixed-venous or central-venous blood (Table 45-4).

During cardiopulmonary resuscitation lactate concentrations in the coronary vein increase over those seen in either arterial or mixed-venous samples.[51a,55b] In experimental studies the increase in lactate parallels the increase in carbon dioxide (Fig. 45-11). Thus, as hypoxia-induced tissue injury worsens, both myocardial lactate and carbon dioxide levels increase. Although the final tissue pH is determined by the reduction in bicarbonate induced by lactic acidosis, and the elevated P_{CO_2}, the time course for the fall in great cardiac vein pH better correlates with the time course for the increase in the P_{CO_2}.

Recently, intramyocardial hydrogen-ion concentration has been measured by direct implantation of pH electrodes in the myocardium,[67a] as an indicator of intracellular hydrogen-ion concentration. Myocardial pH begins to fall immediately (and in a linear fashion over time) after the onset of ventricular fibrillation (Fig. 45-12).

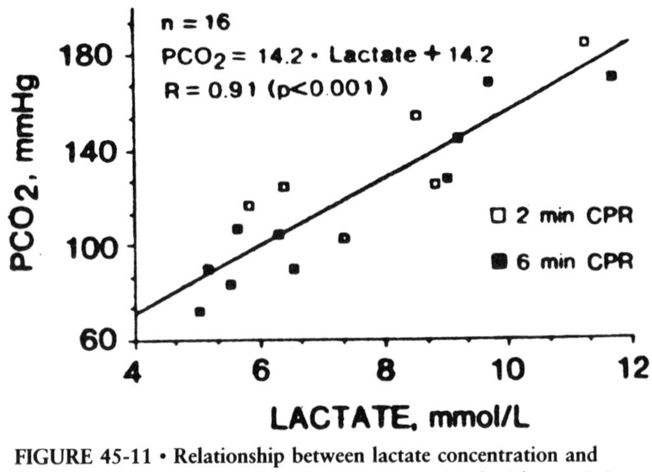

FIGURE 45-11 • Relationship between lactate concentration and great cardiac vein carbon dioxide (P_{CO_2}). (Reprinted with permission from Gudipati CV et al: Increases in coronary vein CO_2 during cardiac resuscitation. *J Appl Physiol* 68:1405, 1990.)

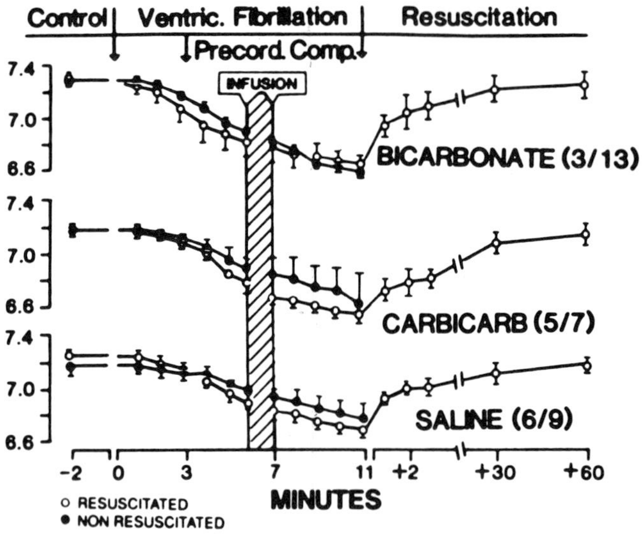

FIGURE 45-12 • Graphs demonstrating the effects of hypertonic solutions of sodium bicarbonate, carbicarb, and sodium chloride on intramyocardial pH in a porcine model of CPR. Infusion of either buffer or saline had no effect on intramyocardial pH. There was also no difference in intramyocardial pH between the animals that were resuscitated and those that were not. (Reprinted with permission from Kette F et al: Buffer agents do not reverse intramyocardial acidosis during cardiac resuscitation. *Circulation* 81:1661, 1990.)

With successful resuscitation and the restoration of spontaneous circulation, intramyocardial pH rapidly returns to normal. It is notable that intramyocardial hydrogen-ion concentrations do not directly correlate with changes in coronary vein carbon dioxide, lactate, or bicarbonate concentrations.[67c] Limited studies evaluating tissue intramyocardial P_{CO_2} have recently been performed; in these studies carbon dioxide levels in myocardium rapidly increased during induced cardioplegia (during cardiothoracic surgery in humans)[79a] or during hypoxia-induced cardiac arrest (in animals)[67a] and correlated with intramyocardial pH. In human cardioplegia, the degree of accumulation of carbon dioxide correlates with the ability to resuscitate the heart; as carbon dioxide levels increase, the heart is more difficult to resuscitate.[79a] Existing information suggests that the accumulation of tissue carbon dioxide is the principal determinant of myocardial pH[67a] and that the greater the accumulation of tissue carbon dioxide (and the subsequent fall in tissue pH), the less likely are the chances that the myocardium will remain viable during resuscitation (Fig. 45-13). The type of tissue acidosis and its rapidity of onset appear to be important in terms of cellular function;[119a] in acute animal models hypercarbic acidosis is associated with profound depression of myocardial contractility (as measured by *dp/dt*) as compared with similar degrees of hyperchloremic metabolic acidosis (Fig. 45-14). The severe myocardial depressant effects of acute hypercarbic (respiratory) acidosis in comparison with the relatively mild depressant effects of acute "exogenous" or extracellular metabolic acidosis (that induced by perfusing tissue with a bicarbonate poor solution) may be related to the duration of the acidosis; in prolonged metabolic acidosis similar degrees of compromise in contractile function can be seen.[24a,43a,92a,92b,125a] Because carbon dioxide equilibrates rapidly with the intracellular compartment, the tissue hydrogen-ion concentration rapidly increases and is associated with rapid depression of myocardial function. In the presence of extracellular metabolic acidosis (decreased extracellular bicarbonate concentration), it is thought that intracellular pH takes longer to equilibrate with the extracellular pH and the decline in tissue performance parallels the equilibration.[67a,119a] However, the interplay between the effects of hypercarbia and hypoxic induced lactic acidosis remains speculative. To better delineate the relative roles of each of these processes, the following acid-base parameters will need to be examined simultaneously and controlled for: intracellular and extracellular hydrogen ion, lactate, carbon dioxide, and bicarbonate concentrations. Using these baseline acid-base parameters, the effects of extracellular acidosis (induced by the infusion of various bicarbonate-poor solutions) vs intracellular acidosis (caused by lactic acid, ketoacid, or carbon dioxide) can be examined. With such a model, the effects of various drugs and toxins commonly encountered in the ICU on acid-base metabolism and cellular function can be delineated. Importantly, the time course of the relative changes in the intracellular and extracellular acid-base parameters and their relationships to cellular function would be determined. Given these caveats, hypercarbic acidosis must be viewed as having a major role in depressing myocardial function during circulatory failure, and this role is independent of other acid-base effects. The data also suggest that cellular pH (perhaps as an indirect indicator of tissue carbon dioxide concentration) may be an important predictor of tissue viability,[135c] but the relative effects of intracellular and extracellular hydrogen ion, carbon dioxide, lactic acid, and bicarbonate concentrations on overall cellular function have yet to be clearly delineated.

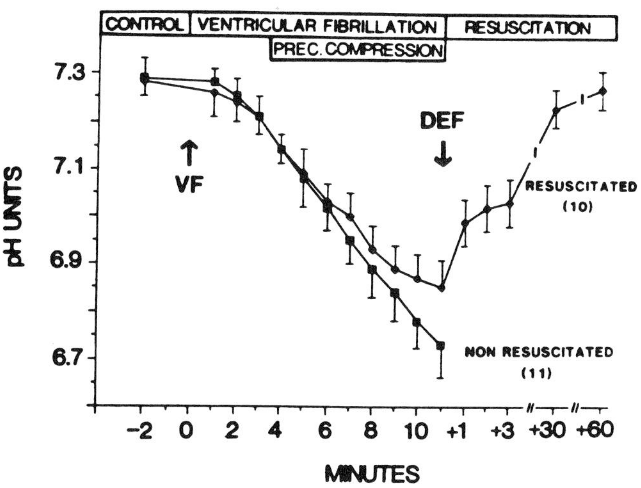

FIGURE 45-13 • The difference in intramyocardial pH are shown between animals (porcine model) that responded successfully to countershock with restoration of spontaneous circulation and those that did not. (Reprinted with permission from Weil MH et al: Incomplete global myocardial ischemia during cardiac arrest and resuscitation. *Crit Care Med* 16:997, 1988.)

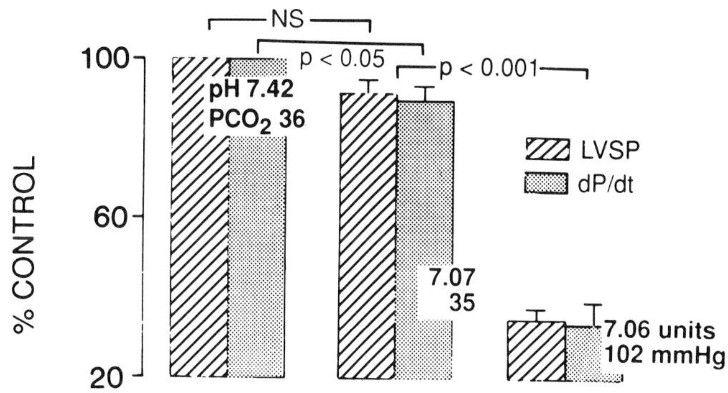

FIGURE 45-14 • Isolated beating hearts were removed from rats using a standard Langendorff technique. Hydrogen-ion concentration was increased (pH lowered) either by perfusing with a bicarbonate-poor solution (middle panels) or by raising carbon dioxide levels (right-hand panels). Left ventricular systolic pressures (LVSP) and the maximum rate of pressure change (*dP/dt*) were parameters used to evaluate cardiac function. Only a 9 percent decrease in cardiac function occurred when pH was lowered by reducing the bicarbonate concentration, while a 77 percent decrease in cardiac function occurred when pH was lowered by raising the carbon dioxide level. (Reprinted with permission from Tang W et al: Reversible impairment of myocardial contractility due to hypercarbic acidosis in the isolated perfused rat heart. *Crit Care Med* 19:218, 1991.)

Different buffers have been used in the setting of both clinical (sodium bicarbonate) and experimental (sodium bicarbonate, carbicarb, i.e., a mixture of $NaHCO_3$ and Na_2CO_3) cardiopulmonary resuscitation. Buffers have been used in an attempt to raise the tissue pH toward normal by increasing bicarbonate levels (which decline in the hypoxic/ischemic circumstance secondary to lactic acidosis). As noted, arterial blood gases have traditionally guided therapy. Arterial pH remains relatively normal or may actually increase during resuscitation (Table 45-4). This change in arterial pH is secondary to the simultaneous fall in both carbon dioxide and bicarbonate concentrations in arterial samples, the former being proportionately greater. When bicarbonate (or another buffer such as carbicarb) is used during resuscitation, arterial pH (and bicarbonate levels) may actually increase at a time when central venous, coronary venous, and tissue acidosis may be worsening.[67c] Thus, arterial blood gas measurements cannot be utilized as an accurate measure of the tissue acid-base status in circulatory failure[1,67a,135a] and certainly do not reflect the effects of buffer therapy at the cellular level.

To evaluate effects of specific buffers used during cardiopulmonary resuscitation, acid-base parameters (including carbon dioxide, bicarbonate, lactic acid, and pH) must be measured in mixed-venous, pulmonary arterial, and coronary venous blood samples in addition to arterial blood samples. Optimally, changes in intracellular acid-base parameters in response to buffer therapy should be measured. Sodium bicarbonate has been the traditional buffer of choice. Recently, concern over sodium bicarbonate as a carbon dioxide *generating* buffer has been voiced.[4a] Carbon dioxide is generated by the following reaction through the buffering effects of sodium bicarbonate: $Na^+ + HCO_3^- + H^+ + anion^- \rightleftharpoons H_2CO_3 + Na\text{-}anion \rightleftharpoons H_2O + CO_2 + Na\text{-}anion$. To overcome this theoretical problem, a 50 percent combination of sodium bicarbonate and sodium carbonate (carbicarb) was developed as a carbon dioxide *consuming* buffer. The carbonate (CO_3^{2-}) in this buffer binds H^+, generates HCO_3^-, and consumes CO_2 through the following reaction: $Na_2CO_3 + CO_2 + H_2O \rightleftharpoons 2\ HCO_3^- + 2\ Na^+$. Theoretically, the use of this buffer would be expected to lower net carbon dioxide production rates (and concentrations) and might have positive effects on outcome if carbon dioxide accumulation is, indeed, a significant problem.

The experimental results comparing the effects of bicarbonate and carbicarb in hypoxic-induced lactic acidosis or hypoxia-induced cardiac arrest have not been entirely consistent, although some general conclusions may be drawn. Increases in arterial pH and bicarbonate concentration have been reported in all studies using carbicarb.[9a,51a,67c] Conflicting reports regarding the effects of these agents on cardiovascular status and lactate production have been published. Arieff et al. in two different studies[9a,53a] reported that the administration of sodium bicarbonate either did not improve or worsened arterial pH, decreased serum bicarbonate concentration, and increased serum lactate as compared with animals receiving no therapy or saline infusions. Bersin and Arieff also reported that carbicarb improved these acid-base parameters and also improved intracellular pH of the liver when compared with sodium bicarbonate administration.[9a] Mixed-venous carbon dioxide increased with sodium bicarbonate and decreased with carbicarb.[9a] Hemodynamic parameters and lactate concentration also improved with carbicarb as compared with sodium bicarbonate.[9a] In studies in which these parameters were more carefully controlled Weil et al.[51a,67c] found similar effects of these buffers on carbon dioxide concentration in mixed-venous blood samples (increased with sodium bicarbonate and decreased with carbicarb). Other findings, however, were at variance: arterial pH and bicarbonate concentrations consistently increased with either buffer as did mixed-venous and great cardiac vein bicarbonate concentration (as compared with animals treated with saline). There were no differences in lactate concentration in arterial, mixed-venous, or cardiac vein samples in the bicarbonate, carbicarb, or saline treated animals. The most significant aspect of these studies was related to the effects of these agents on intramyocardial pH. Neither of these buffers affected intramyocardial pH (as compared with saline controls; Fig. 45-15). Unlike the improvement in liver pH reported by Arieff with the use of carbicarb,

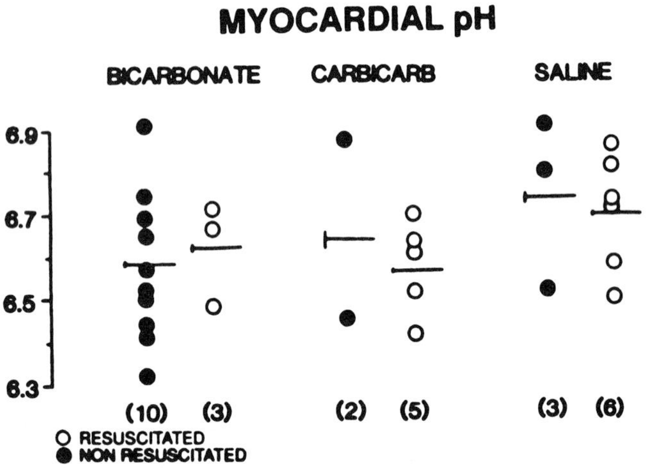

FIGURE 45-15 • Graph of intramyocardial pH during CPR before defibrillation in a porcine model of CPR. There was no difference in intramyocardial pH with either buffer as compared with saline and no difference in pH between resuscitated and nonresuscitated animals. (Reprinted with permission from Kette F et al: Buffer agents do not reverse intramyocardial acidosis during cardiac resuscitation. *Circulation* 81:1660, 1990.)

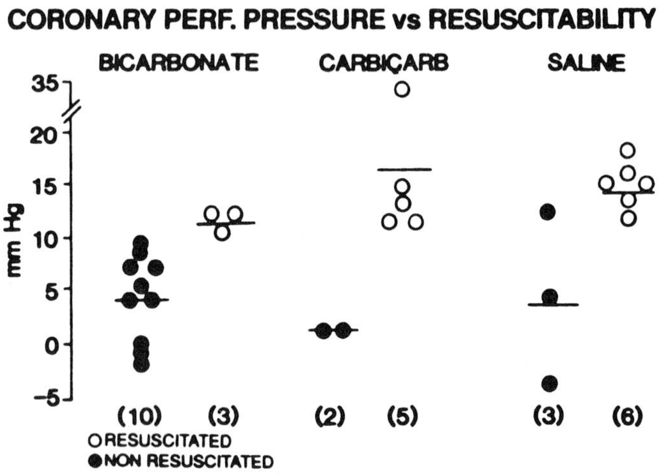

FIGURE 45-16 • Graph of the differences in coronary perfusion pressure in resuscitated and nonresuscitated animals before defibrillation. Coronary perfusion pressures greater than 10 mmHg were associated with successful resuscitation. There was no difference in coronary perfusion pressures in either of the buffer groups or the saline control group. (Reprinted with permission from Kette F et al: Buffer agents do not reverse intramyocardial acidosis during cardiac resuscitation. *Circulation* 81:1660, 1990.)

myocardial pH was unaffected by the use of either carbicarb or sodium bicarbonate.[67c] These provocative results likely explain the disappointing results in the setting of CPR with the use of buffers. The only consistent predictor of recovery in these studies was coronary perfusion pressure (mean diastolic pressure − mean atrial pressure) prior to defibrillation (Fig. 45-16). In fact a theoretical problem with the administration of hypertonic buffer solutions is the transient decline in coronary perfusion pressure seen at the time of infusion of these agents.

CONCLUSIONS

Under normal circumstances, arterial values for pH, carbon dioxide, and bicarbonate accurately reflect overall tissue acid-base homeostasis. However, in the setting of perfusion failure (especially in its most extreme form, i.e., cardiac arrest), a significantly increased arterial to tissue hydrogen-ion (pH) gradient develops. Acutely, this gradient is accounted for largely by the increase in the concentration of carbon dioxide as evidenced by elevations in both mixed-venous and tissue carbon dioxide concentrations. When myocardial levels have been measured experimentally, arterial to tissue gradients of hydrogen ion and carbon dioxide are even larger than those found between arterial and mixed-venous samples. Coronary vein lactate concentrations are also higher than those found in systemic blood (either arterial or mixed-venous).

Both carbon dioxide generating (sodium bicarbonate) and carbon dioxide consuming (carbicarb) buffers have been used in clinical (sodium bicarbonate) and experimental (sodium bicarbonate and carbicarb) settings, in an attempt to improve metabolic acidosis. Unfortunately, neither appears to be successful in improving intramyocardial pH or myocardial viability during early resuscitation. It is likely that the inability of these buffers to acutely alter intramyocardial (and presumably intracellular) hydrogen-ion concentrations explains the disappointing results. Because buffers appear to be of little or no benefit acutely, sodium bicarbonate is no longer recommended[113,135d] during the initial stages of CPR. Although the studies cited have been well performed, none of them addresses whether the use of buffers during sustained (>10 min) CPR, a situation commonly encountered in clinical practice, is beneficial. Consequently, bicarbonate is still listed as appropriate therapy when CPR is prolonged. Carbicarb remains an interesting buffer theoretically; however, human data regarding its use are presently unavailable. In particular, in conditions of less severe perfusion failure, in which tissue carbon dioxide levels might still be elevated, carbicarb might lower carbon dioxide levels and reverse any carbon dioxide related toxicity. However provocative, this hypothesis remains to be examined.

Further studies in severe hypoxic states and states of severe perfusion failure, delineating the relative roles of carbon dioxide–induced acidosis vs lactic acidosis, and their relative effects on tissue function are still required. However, it is clear that the tissue acidosis associated with acute carbon dioxide accumulation has deleterious effects on tissue function. The tissue effects of the various types of acute and chronic metabolic acidoses (high anion gap and normal anion gap) and their relationship to acute carbon dioxide accumulation remain to be delineated. In order to to this, techniques that accurately reflect simultaneous intracellular and extracellular hydrogen-ion, lactate, bicarbonate, and carbon dioxide concentrations under a variety of circumstances will be required to further define the relative contributions of each to the viability of the tissue. These techniques will also be required to evaluate the efficacy of buffer therapy.

CALCIUM HOMEOSTASIS IN CRITICALLY ILL PATIENTS

The advent of an economical ion-selective electrode that can accurately measure ionized calcium in patients' plasma has renewed interest in monitoring plasma calcium.[50] (See Chaps. 11 and 32.) Given the central role of the calcium ion in the biologic regulation of multiple cellular events that control vascular, neurologic, and renal-electrolyte physiology, disorders of calcium regulation in acutely ill patients can lead to disorders of substantial clinical significance.[98,99] In the recent past there has been increasing awareness of the frequent occurrence of hypocalcemia in critically ill patients.[5,14,22,36,37,38,140]

CIRCULATING CALCIUM

Calcium biology has been extensively reviewed elsewhere, but an understanding of the forms of circulating calcium is important for clinical decision making. Circulating calcium exists in three forms that include protein-bound calcium (approximately 40 percent), diffusable (nonionized) chelates with phosphate, sulfate, and citrate (approximately 15 percent), and free ionized calcium (approximately 45 percent) that is the physiologically active fraction. The bulk of protein-bound calcium is bound to albumin (70 to 90 percent), while the rest (10 to 30 percent) is bound to alpha- and beta-globulins. Alterations of serum albumin levels (which occur frequently in acutely ill patients) therefore cause marked differences in circulating concentrations of total calcium. In addition to the effect of changing concentrations of albumin on the measurement of total circulating calcium, hypoalbuminemia is also associated with decreased concentrations of ionized calcium (Fig. 45-17)

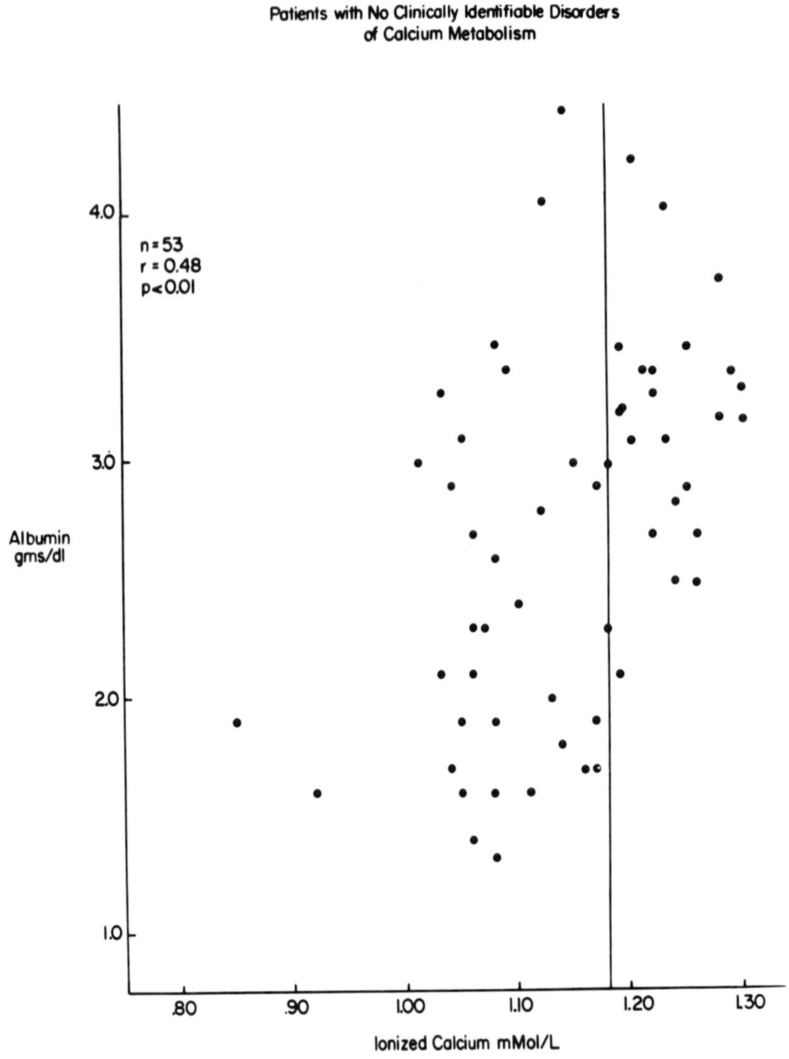

FIGURE 45-17 • Relationship between ionized calcium and serum albumin in critically ill patients. These patients had no primary cause of hypocalcemia that could be identified. (From Desai TK et al: Prevalence and clinical implications of hypocalcemia in acutely ill patients in a medical intensive care setting. *Am J Med* 84:209, 1988.)

independent of its effect on the measurement of total plasma calcium.[16,37] The reasons for this direct relationship are unclear. Changes in pH also alter the binding of calcium to circulating proteins, so that ionized calcium may actively vary without a change in total measured calcium. Acidosis decreases protein binding (increases ionized calcium), while alkalosis increases protein binding (decreases ionized calcium). Given the complexity of these relationships, direct measurement of ionized calcium is imperative if one is to accurately evaluate the levels of the physiologically active fraction.[138,139] This is now easily accomplished rapidly and reliably using ion-selective membrane electrodes. By convention, the ionized calcium value is corrected to a standard pH (usually 7.4), although correction to the patient's arterial pH may have more physiologic significance. This remains an area of debate around which there is, as yet, no concensus. Proper handling of blood specimens, with minimal delay prior to measurement using anaerobic precautions (similar to those for blood gas analysis), is recommended.

The most common problem in calcium homeostasis encountered in the critically ill patient is hypocalcemia.[14,22,37] Hypercalcemia is much less common, and the diagnostic and therapeutic approach remains unchanged from that discussed elsewhere (Chap. 32). In physiologic terms, hypocalcemia may be considered to be secondary to the failure of the parathyroid hormone (PTH) or the vitamin D feedback systems. It may result from inadequate PTH response to hypocalcemia, vitamin D deficiency, or skeletal resistance to either hormone. However, the influence of severe acute systemic illness on these homeostatic processes has not been well studied.

CLINICAL MANIFESTATIONS

The cardiovascular effects of hypocalcemia are the area of the greatest concern in the acute care setting. Experimental animal studies have demonstrated a direct correlation between the concentration of calcium in the extracellular fluid and cardiac contractility[13] as well as vascular smooth muscle tension.[41] Ultrastructural studies of various muscle types show differences in the extent of sarcoplasmic reticulum present, with skeletal muscle having the most extensive network, cardiac muscle having an intermediate network, and vascular smooth muscle having the sparsest network.[51] Calcium ions, required to initiate muscle contraction in skeletal muscle, are derived almost entirely from its extensive and intrinsic network of sarcoplasmic reticulum, whereas cardiac muscle is more dependent upon extracellular calcium as a source. Vascular smooth muscle depends almost entirely on extracellular calcium to initiate contraction.[12] Therefore, it is not surprising that acute reductions in extracellular calcium concentration have been reported to precipitate hypotension[22] and left ventricular dysfunction,[29] with little or no noted effect on skeletal muscle. Patients with cardiomyopathy may be particularly prone to hypotension or congestive heart failure in the presence of ionized hypocalcemia.[52] Chronic congestive heart failure may be refractory to therapy with digitalis[24] and diuretics or even parenteral sympathomimetic agents (dobutamine) in the presence of hypocalcemia.[52] Correction of hypocalcemia in these patients may lead to dramatic improvement in cardiac function.[5]

Patients with end-stage renal disease also show clinically significant changes in blood pressure and left ventricular function in conjunction with changes in circulatory calcium. Hypotension and left ventricular dysfunction have been associated with the decrease in circulating ionized calcium that occurs in the dialysis patient population;[81] dialysis using a high concentration calcium bath may improve both complications.

In contrast to the observations in patients with cardiomyopathy or end-stage renal disease, the clinical significance of hypocalcemia in acutely ill patients with otherwise normal cardiovascular function remains to be established. In a series of patients admitted to the medical intensive care unit of Detroit Receiving Hospital, we found a direct relationship between the ionized calcium and the blood pressure (Fig. 45-18).[36,38] This study also found that the patients with low levels of ionized calcium were not only more likely to be hypotensive but were also more likely to be on pressor agents. Conversely, patients with higher levels of ionized calcium were less likely to require pressors to support blood pressure. Hypertension occurred only in patients with greater than normal levels of ionized calcium. These patients were admitted with a variety of diagnoses. Hypocalcemia, hypotension, and sepsis were associated, while normocalcemia and hypertension were associated. Other studies have evaluated the cardiovascular effects of calcium infusion: In addition to the pressor effect of calcium, left ventricular performance is also improved. The increase in circulating calcium after calcium infusion is temporary, as are the vasopressor and other hemodynamic effects. In spite of the immediate salutary effects of the correction of ionized hypocalcemia, there are no data to indicate that outcome in acutely ill patients is improved by this treatment. In fact, data in septic rats suggest that calcium infusion may actually reduce survival.[142]

Changes of ionized calcium have other effects that are evident on the electrocardiogram; however, these findings are not specific enough to be of great use in acutely ill patients who may have many other electrolyte and metabolic abnormalities that confound the interpretation of the electrocardiogram. In our experience, these findings also do not appear to be predictive of which patients will develop cardiovascular compromise. Consequently, although these findings may be of interest to the cardiac electrophysiologist, they are of little practical value to the intensivist.

Neuromuscular irritability, manifested in its most severe forms as seizures and tetany, also occurs in hypocalcemia.[42] Ionized calcium should always be evaluated in

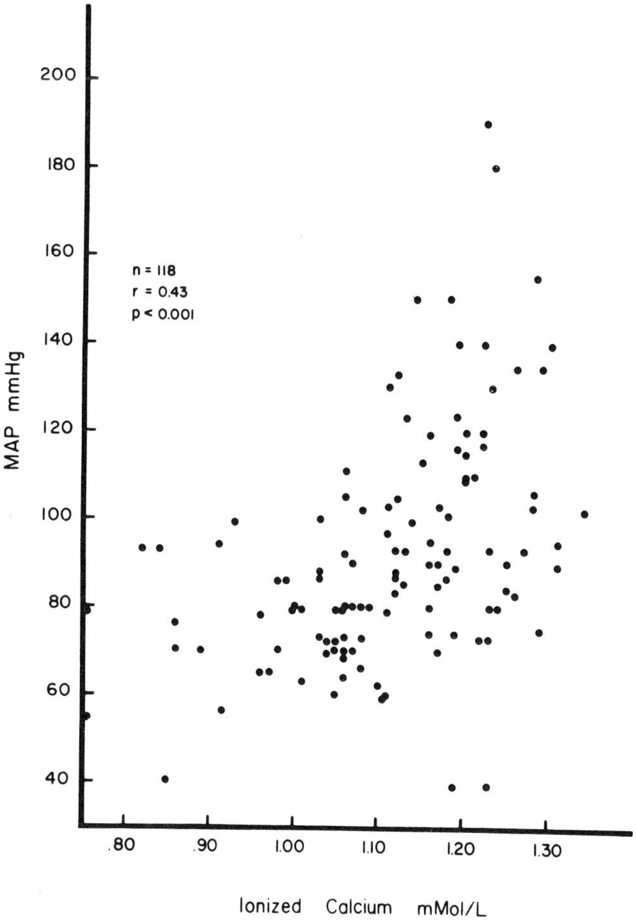

FIGURE 45-18 • Relationship between ionized calcium and mean arterial pressure in critically ill patients. These patients included those that required pharmacologic intervention to control either hypo- or hypertension. (From Desai TK et al: A direct relationship between ionized calcium and arterial pressure among patients in an intensive care unit. *Crit Care Med* 16:578, 1988.)

the critically ill patient who demonstrates neuromuscular instability. Signs of neuromuscular instability are unusual, we believe, when ionized hypocalcemia is encountered in critically ill patients. Virtually all of these patients have mental status changes; however, the relationship of these changes to hypocalcemia is unproved. In the absence of overt signs of neuromuscular irritability, calcium therapy is not required.

TABLE 45-5 • Common causes of hypocalcemia in critically ill patients

Sepsis
Hypomagnesemia
Renal failure
Alkalemia
Chelation
Citrate
Radiocontrast media
Lipid emulsions
Pancreatitis

INCIDENCE OF IONIZED HYPOCALCEMIA IN THE MEDICAL INTENSIVE CARE UNIT

A variety of conditions (Table 45-5) can be associated with hypocalcemia in the acute care setting. In addition to the causes listed, many severely ill patients may present with idiopathic hypocalcemia.[37,39] A number of recent reports have alerted critical care practitioners to the high prevalence of ionized hypocalcemia in acutely ill patients. However, there is a wide range in the reported prevalence of this phenomenon.[23,37] Upon review of these reports, the variation in the reported prevalence seems to be related to the severity of illness of the population reported: in patient populations that are more acutely ill, the incidence of ionized hypocalcemia appears to be greater. As an example, Zaloga and colleagues studied patients in a naval hospital intensive care unit and found an approximately 10 percent incidence of ionized hypocalcemia.[23] Our own experience suggests that in at least some intensive care populations, ionized hypocalcemia is far more common.[39] In the Detroit Receiving Hospital intensive care unit, approximately two-thirds of the patients are admitted with ionized hypocalcemia (Fig. 45-19). As the major trauma and critical care center for a large metro-

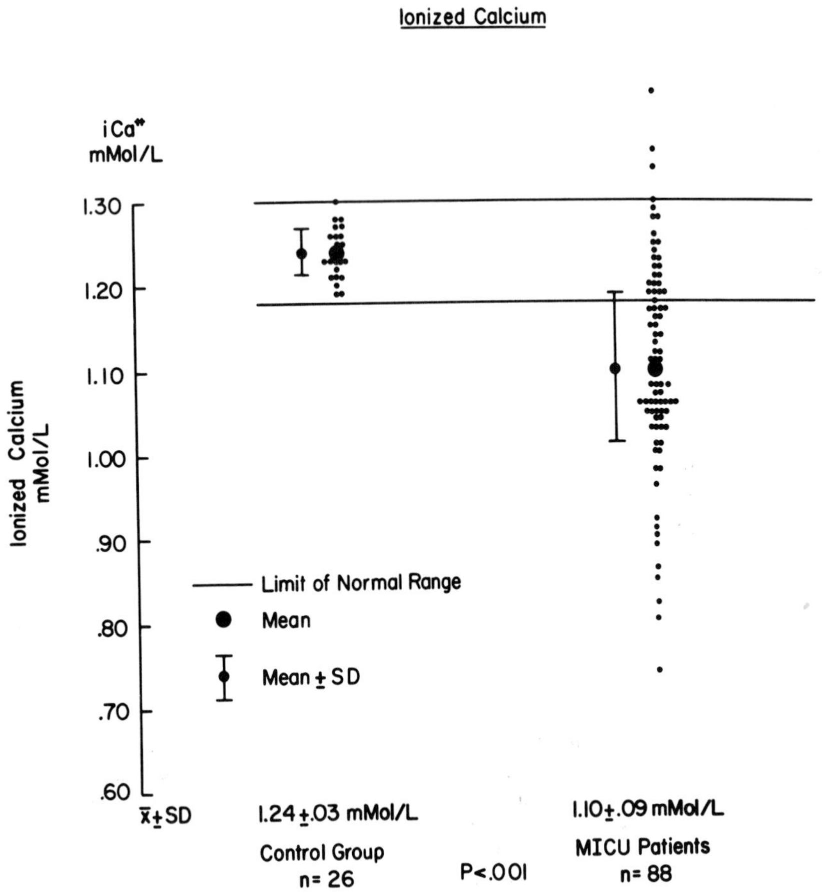

FIGURE 45-19 • Prevalence of ionized hypocalcemia in critically ill patients. Admission ionized calcium values in patients admitted to the intensive care unit compared with normal controls. These represent sequential admissions to the intensive care unit of Detroit Receiving Hospital. (From Desai TK et al: Prevalence and implications of hypocalcemia in acutely ill patients in a medical intensive care setting. *Am J Med* 84:209, 1988.)

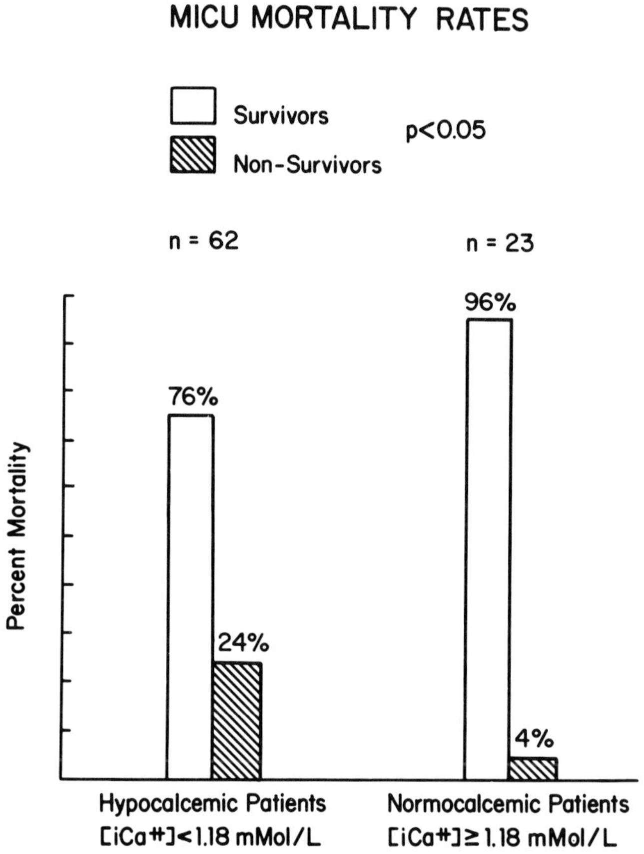

FIGURE 45-20 • Hospital mortality of hypocalcemic vs. normocalcemic patients; 1.18 mmol/liter ionized calcium was used as the lower limit of normal as defined in the studied patient population. (From Desai TK et al: Prevalence and implications of hypocalcemia in acutely ill patients in a medical intensive care setting. *Am J Med* 84:209, 1988.)

politan area, this hospital serves a patient group drawn from a medically indigent inner city population, where malnutrition and other chronic health problems are common. This was corroborated when we evaluated patients at Harper Hospital, a tertiary care university hospital with a large cancer center. At this institution, the incidence of ionized hypocalcemia still approached 40 percent and was predominately seen in the extremely ill oncologic patients served in this intensive care unit. Ionized hypocalcemia is associated with poor outcomes in acutely ill patients.[14] In our experience,[39] the mortality rate was four times greater in the hypocalcemic patients (Fig. 45-20).

In summary, ionized hypocalcemia is quite common in acutely ill patients. Its presence seems to correlate with the severity of illness (although direct correlations with indices of the severity of illness have not been performed) and is associated with a poor outcome. The causes of hypocalcemia are multivariate (Table 45-5), but in a significant number of cases, no underlying pathophysiologic cause can be identified.

SEPSIS AND SHOCK

The hypocalcemia associated with various forms of circulatory shock can be difficult to evalute. Experimental septic shock in the baboon is associated with ionized hypocalcemia.[123] The association of hypocalcemia and sepsis in humans has recently been established.[36,37,141] The underlying biologic basis for hypocalcemia in these patients remains unclear. However, it is postulated that calcium moves from the extracellular compartment into cells and that the hormonal response to hypocalcemia is inadequate. Zaloga et al. reported several different hormonal responses in response to the hypocalcemia in sepsis: these include acquired PTH insufficiency, renal 1-alpha-hydroxylase deficiency, vitamin D deficiency, and acquired cacitriol resistance.[141] Thus, the hypocalcemia of sepsis appears to be a primary event with an uncertain hormonal response. Other studies from our institution suggest that hypoalbuminemic patients have inadequate PTH responses. Additionally, our data demonstrated a direct relationship between 25-hydroxyvitamin D levels and the ionized calcium.[35] Both hypoalbuminemia and 25-hydroxyvitamin D levels are probably indicative of the underlying malnutrition seen commonly in our patients. Sepsis was more common in this group of patients. The relationships between sepsis, vitamin D deficiency, and hypocalcemia are of interest since recent information suggests an important role for the vitamin D system in immune regulation.[27,80] Thus, it may not be all that surprising that sepsis, hypocalcemia, and abnormalities in vitamin D regulation are associated.

Hypocalcemia has also recently been reported in patients during cardiac arrest.[125] This represents another circumstance of extreme cellular stress, and the pathophysiology may be similar to that in the septic patient: movement of calcium from the extracellular to the intracellular compartment as a sign of breakdown of basic cellular control mechanisms.

If hypocalcemia represents a sign of cellular compromise, therapy of the hypocalcemia complicating sepsis or cardiovascular shock may not improve overall patient outcome. In fact, preliminary data in a cecal ligated rat model of sepsis suggest that calcium infusion may even reduce survival.[142] Since calcium has not been shown to be effective in cardiac arrest, calcium is no longer recommended as part of the resuscitation protocol.[113,140] Given the many unanswered questions regarding the appropriate approach to the therapy of the hypocalcemic patient with circulatory or septic shock, we recommend the administration of intravenous calcium only in patients with cardiovascular compromise (hypotension and heart failure) refractory to other therapies. In general, severely depressed levels of ionized hypocalcemia (> 0.8 mmol/liter) are well tolerated and do not require therapy. When calcium is used, we suggest administration of an intravenous bolus of 5 mg/kg of elemental calcium over 20 min followed by an infusion of 1 to 2 mg/kg/h for several hours until ionized calcium normalizes. The response of blood pressure and left ventricular work indices should be monitored and used as a guideline for further therapy. In our experience, ionized calcium levels increase in an unpredictable fashion and the improvement in cardiovascular parameters may be short-lived.

HYPOMAGNESEMIA

Magnesium deficiency is very common in the intensive care unit and is usually part of a complex syndrome of multiple mineral and vitamin deficiencies.[3] (See Chaps. 33 and 34.) Hypomagnesemia must be severe (< 1.2 mg/dl) before the inhibition of PTH secretion occurs.[15] Somewhat paradoxically, mild hypomagnesemia actually stimulates secretion of PTH.[108] Consequently, hypocalcemia should not be attributed to hypomagnesemia unless magnesium levels are less than 1.2 mg/dl. Hypocalcemia cannot generally be corrected without the correction of severe hypomagnesemia. Only after magnesium levels are normalized can an assessment of other potential causes of hypocalcemia be made. The therapy of hypomagnesemia[34] is discussed elsewhere in this text (Chap. 33).

RENAL FAILURE

Several mechanisms contribute to the hypocalcemia of renal insufficiency, including 1-alpha-hydroxylase insufficiency (with 1,25-dihydroxy vitamin D deficiency) and skeletal resistance to PTH.[88] (See Chaps. 38–40.) The hyperphosphatemia of renal insufficiency further inhibits 1-alpha-hydroxylase.[119] There is also the risk of the precipitation of calcium phosphate salts with elevated levels of phosphate.[26] Generally, these derangements do not occur until renal failure is severe with GFRs less than 25 ml/min.[26] Even then, only 40 percent of patients with GFRs of less than 20 ml/min exhibit hypocalcemia. Hypocalcemia can be especially severe in some patients with acute oliguric renal failure secondary to rhabdomyolysis.[55] These patients demonstrate marked hyperphosphatemia, hyperuricemia, and elevated creatine phosphokinase levels. Although renal failure is very common in the intensive care unit, hypocalcemia should not be assumed to be the result of renal insufficiency unless the compromise in GFR is severe (< 20 ml/min). Correction of hypocalcemia in renal failure should be directed toward the reduction in serum phosphorus and the correction of underlying vitamin D deficiency. Vitamin D supplements should not be administered until elevated phosphorus levels have been controlled. As noted above, improvement in cardiovascular performance has been noted in dialysis patients in whom hypocalcemia has been corrected.[81]

ALKALEMIA

Alkalemia can lead to a fall in ionized calcium by increasing calcium binding to protein. This assumes clinical importance in the setting of an acidemic patient whose ionized calcium level is moderately depressed. Ionized calcium decreases by approximately 0.05 mM/liter for each increase in pH of 0.10 units; however, this effect is blunted in the presence of hypoalbuminemia, which is common in critically ill patients.[34,138] No direct therapy is required unless clinical signs are manifest.

CHELATION

Since calcium exists in plasma at a concentration that is close to the limit of its solubility, small changes that affect the overall physical chemistry of the plasma solution can lead to the precipitation of a variety of calcium salts. Several common clinical circumstances including blood transfusions and the administration of radiographic dye can lead to the precipitation of calcium salts.

Transfusions of blood (preserved with citrate) can lead to hypocalcemia because of the chelation of calcium with citrate.[90] Reductions in ionized calcium can be directly related to the rapidity of transfusion and plasma levels of citrate.[35] Citrate metabolism is compromised in patients with hepatic or renal failure and in hypoperfusion.[139] These patients may be particularly susceptible to hypocalcemia after blood transfusions. Although hemodynamic parameters remain stable in the majority of patients after transfusion with documented hypocalcemia,[66,139] patients with underlying cardiac compromise may be at risk for complications of hypotension or heart failure.[35,90] It is in this group of patients that calcium therapy might be required.

Other less widely appreciated chelating agents include radiographic contrast media and lipid emulsion solutions used with total parenteral nutrition.[139] Radiocontrast agents contain calcium chelators, and the amount of contrast used for a routine cranial CAT scan can lower ionized calcium by 0.1 to 0.2 mM/liter for up to 30 min.[9,21] This may be of clinical significance in the critically ill patient in whom cardiovascular instability may already be problematic.

PANCREATITIS

Acute pancreatitis, with the formation of calcium soaps in the peripancreatic areas, has been associated with profound hypocalcemia. Alcoholic patients with very high triglyceride levels are particularly at risk for profound hypocalcemia.[18,34] Experimental studies suggest that extreme elevation of plasma-free fatty acids may have a central role in inducing hypocalcemia.[129] Decreases in serum calcium levels should stimulate PTH secretion in an attempt to raise the serum ionized calcium. However, studies evaluating the function of the PTH–vitamin D axis have reported conflicting results.[62,100,136] While some investigators have reported normal PTH and vitamin D responses to hypocalcemia during acute pancreatitis, other investigators have found an inadequate hormonal response to hypocalcemia. Unless the patient is symptomatic, treatment of hypocalcemia in pancreatitis is not warranted. Hypocalcemia, however, is associated with a poor prognosis.[97] In our experience,[37] the lowest levels of ionized hypocalcemia were seen in patients with pancreatitis.

CONCLUSIONS

In summary, hypocalcemia is exceedingly common in critically ill patients. There are a number of potential causes of hypocalcemia in this group of patients, but in many, no clear cause can be identified. Therapy for hypocalcemia should be directed to its underlying cause, such as hypomagnesemia. Calcium infusion should cautiously be considered only when no obvious cause is evident. In fact, in septic patients, calcium infusion may actually be deleterious in terms of outcome. In these cases, calcium infusion should be initiated only in patients with cardiovascular or neurologic signs and symptoms. Specific groups of acutely ill patients in which vitamin D or calcium infusions may prove of benefit have not yet been delineated. At this juncture, hypocalcemia, and especially ionized hypocalcemia, should be viewed as a marker of the severity of an illness that is associated with a poor prognosis.

REFERENCES

1. Adrogué HJ et al: Assessing acid-base status in circulatory failure: Differences between arterial and central venous blood. *N Engl J Med* 320:1312, 1989.
2. Amman R, Warshaw AL: Acute pancreatitis: Clinical aspects and medical and surgical management, in Berk JK: *Bockus Gastroenterology*, 4th ed. Saunders, Philadelphia, 1985, p 3993.
3. Anast CS et al: Evidence for parathyroid failure in magnesium deficiency. *Science* 77:606, 1972.
4. Apelgren KN et al: Comparison of nutritional indices and outcome in critically ill patients. *Crit Care Med* 10:305, 1982.

4a. Arieff AI et al: Systemic effects of $NaHCO_3$ in experimental lactic acidosis in dogs. *Am J Physiol* 242:F586, 1982.

5. Auffant RA et al: Ionized calcium concentration and cardiovascular function after cardiopulmonary bypass. *Arch Surg* 116:1072, 1981.
6. Bayliss WM: *Intravenous Injection in Wound Shock.* London, Longmans, Green, 1918.
7. Belcher P, Lennox SC: Avoidance of blood transfusion in coronary artery surgery: A trial of hydroxyethyl starch. *Ann Thorac Surg* 37:365, 1984.
8. Benotti JR, Dalen JE: Pulmonary embolism, in Rippe JM et al: *Intensive Care Medicine.* Boston, Little, Brown, 1985, p 226.
9. Berger RE et al: Acute hypocalcemia effects of clinical contrast media injections. *Am J Radiology* 138:283, 1982.

9a. Bersin RM, Arieff AI: Improved hemodynamic function during hypoxia with carbicarb, a new agent for the management of acidosis. *Circulation* 77:227, 1988.

10. Bistrian BR et al: Protein status of general surgical patients. *JAMA* 230:858, 1974.
11. Bistrian BR et al: Prevalence of malnutrition in general medical patients. *JAMA* 235:1567, 1976.
12. Bohr DF: Vascular smooth muscle: Dual effect of calcium. *Science* 139:597, 1963.
13. Bristow MR et al: Ionized calcium and the heart. *Circ Res* 41:565, 1977.
14. Broner CWS et al: Hypermagnesemia and hypocalcemia as predictors of high mortality in critically ill pediatric patients. *Crit Care Med* 18:921, 1990.
15. Buckle RM et al: The influence of plasma magnesium concentration on parathyroid hormone secretion. *J Endocrinol* 42:529, 1986.
16. Butler S et al: Correlation between serum ionized calcium and serum albumin in two hospital populations. *Br Med J* 289:948, 1984.
17. Cady LD Jr et al: Quantitation of severity of critical illness with special reference to blood lactate. *Crit Care Med* 1:75, 1973.
18. Cameron JL et al: Acute pancreatitis with hyperlipemia. *Surgery* 70:53, 1971.
19. Carlson RW et al: Hypovolemia and permeability pulmonary edema associated with anaphylaxis. *Crit Care Med* 9:883, 1981.
20. Carrico CJ et al: Fluid resuscitation following injury: Rationale for the use of balance salt solutions. *Crit Care Med* 4:46, 1976.
21. Caulfield JB et al: Blood calcium levels in the presence of arteriographic contrast material. *Circulation* 52:119, 1975.
22. Chaimowitz C et al: Hypocalcemic hypotension. *JAMA* 222:86, 1972.
23. Chernow B et al: Hypocalcemia in critically ill patients. *Crit Care Med* 10:848, 1982.
24. Chopra D et al: Insensitivity to digoxin associated with hypocalcemia. *N Engl J Med* 296:971, 1977.

24a. Cingolani HE: Contractility in isolated mammalian heart muscle after acid-base changes. *Circ Res* 26:269, 1970.

25. Clift DR et al: The effect of albumin resuscitation for shock on the immune response to tetanus toxoid. *Surg Res* 32:449, 1982.
26. Coburn JW et al: The physiochemical state and renal handling of divalent ions in chronic renal failure. *Arch Intern Med* 124:302, 1969.
27. Cohen MS et al: 1,25$(OH)_2$ D_3 activates H_20_2 secretion by human monocyte derived macrophages. *Clin Res* 33:397A, 1985.

28. Cohen RD, Woods HF: *Clinial and Biochemical Aspects of Lactic Acidosis*. Oxford, Blackwell Scientific Publications, 1976.
29. Connor TB et al: Hypocalcemia precipitating congestive heart failure. *N Engl J Med* 307:869, 1982.
30. Cournand A et al: Chemical, clinical, and immunological studies on the products of human plasma fractionation. VIII. Clinical use of concentrated human serum albumin in shock, and comparison with whole blood and with rapid saline infusion. *J Clin Invest* 23:491, 1944.
31. Cunningham JN et al: Changes in intracellular sodium and potassium content of red blood cells in trauma and shock. *Am J Surg* 122:650, 1971.
32. Dawidson I et al: Hemodilution and recovery from experimental intestinal shock in rats: A comparison of the efficacy of three colloids and one electrolyte solution. *Crit Care Med* 9:42, 1981.
33. Dawidson I et al: Relation of colloid concentration to volume expansion for resuscitation of rats subjected to intestinal ischemic shock. *Crit Car Med* 10:597, 1982.
34. Decaux G et al: Chronic alcoholism: A predisposing factor for hypocalcemia in acute pancreatitis. *Digestion* 20:175, 1980.
35. Denlinger JK et al: Hypocalcemia during rapid blood transfusions in anesthetized man. *Br J Anaesth* 48:995, 1976.
36. Desai TK et al: Hypocalcemia and hypophosphatemia in acutely ill patients. *Crit Care Clin* [(eds) Geheb MA, Carlson, RW] 5:927, 1987.
37. Desai TK et al: Parathyroid-vitamin D axis in critically ill patients with unexplained hypocalcemia. *Kidney Int* 32:S225, 1987.
38. Desai TK et al: A direct relationship between ionized calcium and arterial pressure among patients in an intensive care unit. *Crit Care Med* 16:578, 1988.
39. Desai TK et al: Prevalence and clinical implications of hypocalcemia in acutely ill patients in a medical intensive care unit. *Am J Med* 84:209, 1988.
40. Diehl JT et al: Clinical comparison of hetastarch and albumin in postoperative cardiac patients. *Ann Thorac Surg* 34:674, 1982.
41. Dillon PF, Murphy RA: Tonic force maintenance with reduced shortening velocity in arterial smooth muscle. *Am J Physiol* 242:102, 1982.
42. Dubois GD, Arieff AI: Clinical manifestations of electrolyte disorders, in Arieff AI, DeFronzo RA (eds): *Fluid, Electrolytes and Acid-Base Disorders*. New York, Churchill Livingstone, 1985, p 1087.
43. Drewes PA: Carbohydrate derivatives and metabolites, in Henry RJ et al (eds): *Clinical Chemistry. Principles and Techniques,* 2d ed. New York, Harper & Row, 1974, p 1330.
43a. Ellis D, Thomas RC: Direct measurement of the intracellular pH of mammalian cardiac muscle. *J Physiol (Lond)* 262:755, 1976.
44. Emerson TE: Unique features of albumin. *Crit Care Med* 17:690, 1989.
45. Emmett M, Narins RG: Clinical use of the anion gap. *Medicine* 56:38, 1977.
46. Falk JL et al: Effects of hetastarch and albumin on coagulation in patients with septic shock. *J Clin Pharmacol* 28:412, 1988.
46a. Falk JL et al: End-tidal carbon dioxide concentration during cardiopulmonary resuscitation. *N Engl J Med* 318:607, 1988.
47. Finch JS et al: Compared effects of selected colloids on extravascular lung water in dogs after oleic acid-induced lung injury and severe hemorrhage. *Crit Care Med* 11:267, 1983.
48. Fisher M: Blood volume replacement in acute anaphylactic cardiovascular collapse related to anaesthesia. *Br J Anaesth* 49:1023, 1977.
49. Fisher M McD, Dicks I: Volume replacement in acute anaphylactoid reactions. *Anaesth Intensive Care* 7:375, 1979.
50. Fogh-Anderson N et al: Measurement of free calcium ion in capillary blood and serum. *Clin Chem* 24:1545, 1978.
51. Franzini-Armstrong C: Fine structure of sarcoplasmic reticulum and transverse tubular system in muscle fibers. *Fed Proc* 23:887, 1964.
51a. Gazmuri RJ et al: Cardiac effects of carbon dioxide-consuming and carbon dioxide-generating buffers during cardiopulmonary resuscitation. *J Am Coll Cardiol* 15:482, 1990.
52. Ginsburg R et al: Myocardial performance and extracellular ionized calcium in a severely failing heart. *Ann Intern Med* 98:603, 1983.
53. Goodkin DA et al: The role of the anion gap in detecting and managing mixed metabolic acid-base disturbances. *Clin Endocrinol Metab* 13:333, 1984.
53a. Graf H et al: Evidence for a detrimental effect of bicarbonate therapy in hypoxic lactic acidosis. *Science* 227:754, 1985.
54. Graham T: Liquid diffusion applied to analysis. *Philos Trans R Soc Lond* 151:183, 1861.
55. Grossman RA et al: Nontraumatic rhabdomyolysis and acute renal failure. *N Engl J Med* 291:807, 1974.
55a. Grundler W et al: Arteriovenous carbon dioxide and pH gradients during cardiac arrest. *Circulation* 74:1071, 1986.
55b. Gudipati CV et al: Increases in coronary CO_2 during cardiac resuscitation. *J Appl Physiol* 68:1405, 1990.
55c. Gudipati CV et al: Expired carbon dioxide: A noninvasive monitor of cardiopulmonary resuscitation. *Circulation* 77:234, 1988.
55d. Haljamae H et al: Pathophysiology of shock. *Pathol Res Pract* 165:200, 1979.
56. Hankeln K et al: Comparison of hydroxyethyl starch and lactated Ringer's solution on hemodynamics and oxygen transport of critically ill patients in prospective crossover studies. *Crit Care Med* 17:133, 1989.
57. Harken AH: Lactic acidosis. *Surg Gynecol Obstet* 142:593, 1976.
58. Harms BA et al: Effects of hypoproteinemia on pulmonary and soft tissue edema formation. *Crit Care Med* 9:503, 1981.
59. Harrower JR, Brown H: Blood lactic acid—A micromethod adapted to field collection of microliter samples. *J Appl Physiol* 32:709, 1972.
60. Haupt MT, Rackow EC: Colloid osmotic pressure and fluid resuscitation with hetastarch, albumin, and saline solutions. *Crit Care Med* 10:159, 1982.
61. Haupt MT et al: Increased pulmonary edema with crystalloid compared to colloid resuscitation of shock asso-

ciated with increased vascular permeability. *Circ Shock* 12:213, 1984.
62. Hauser CJ et al: Calcium homeostasis in patients with acute pancreatitis. *Surgery* 94:830, 1983.
63. Henning RJ et al: Blood lactate as a prognostic indicator of survival in patients with acute myocardial infarction. *Circ Shock* 9:307, 1982.
64. Holt ME et al: Albumin inhibits human polymorphonuclear leucocyte luminol-dependent chemiluminescence: Evidence for oxygen radical scavenging. *Br J Exp Pathol* 65:231, 1984.
65. Hormaechea E et al: Hypovolemia, pulmonary edema and protein changes in severe salicylate poisoning. *Am J Med* 66:1046, 1979.
66. Howland WS et al: Factors influencing the ionization of calcium during major surgical procedures. *Surg Gynecol Obstet* 58:274, 1976.
67. Iberti TJ et al: Low sensitivity of the anion gap as a screen to detect hyperlactatemia in critically ill patients. *Crit Care Med* 18:275, 1990.
67a. Johnson BA, Weil MH: Redefining ischemia due to circulatory failure as dual defects of oxygen deficits and of carbon dioxide excesses. *Crit Care Med* 1991 (in press).
67b. Jude JR et al: Cardiac arrest: Report of application of external cardiac massage in 118 patients. *JAMA* 178:1063, 1961.
67c. Kette F et al: Buffer agents do not reverse intramyocardial acidosis during cardiac resuscitation. *Circulation* 81:1660, 1990.
68. Kirklin JK et al: Hydroxyethyl starch versus albumin for colloid infusion following cardiopulmonary bypass in patients undergoing myocardial revascularization. *Ann Thorac Surg* 37:40, 1984.
69. Koch-Weser J, Sellers EM: Binding of drugs to serum albumin (part II). *N Engl J Med* 294:526, 1976.
69a. Kouwenhoven WB et al: Closed-chest cardiac massage. *JAMA* 173:1064, 1960.
70. Kovalik SG et al: The cardiac effect of altered calcium homeostasis after albumin resuscitation. *J Trauma* 21:275, 1981.
71. Kruse JA: Blood lactate and oxygen transport. *Intensive Care World* 4:121, 1987.
72. Kruse JA, Carlson RW: Lactate metabolism. *Crit Care Clin* 5:725, 1987.
73. Kruse JA, Carlson RW: Lactate measurement: Plasma or blood? *Intensive Care Med* 16:1, 1990.
74. Kruse JA, Carlson RW: Use of vasoactive drugs to support oxygen transport in sepsis. *Crit Care Med* 19:144, 1991.
75. Kruse JA et al: Lactate levels predict the relationship between oxygen delivery and consumption in patients with the adult respiratory distress syndrome. *Chest* 98:959, 1990.
76. Kruse JA et al: Definition of clinically significant lactic acidosis. *Chest* 100:100S, 1987.
77. Kruse JA et al: Significance of blood lactate levels in critically ill patients with liver disease. *Am J Med* 83:77, 1987.
77a. Leavy JA et al: Lactate washout following circulatory arrest. *JAMA* 260;662, 1988.
78. Leibold WC et al: Effect of albumin resuscitation on canine coagulation activity and content. *Ann Surg* 198:630, 1983.
79. Lowell JA et al: Postoperative fluid overload: Not a benign problem. *Crit Care Med* 18:728, 1990.
79a. Magovern GJ et al: Assessment of myocardial protection during global ischemia with myocardial gas tension monitoring. *Surgery* 92:373, 1982.
80. Manolagas SC, Deftos LJ: The vitamin D endocrine system and the hematolymphopoietic tissue. *Ann Intern Med* 100:144, 1984.
81. Maynard JC et al: Blood pressure response to changes in serum ionized calcium during hemodialysis. *Ann Intern Med* 104:358, 1986.
82. Mazzara JT et al: Extreme hypocapnia in the critically ill patient. *Am J Med* 56:450, 1974.
83. McCurdy DK: Mixed metabolic and respiratory acid-base disturbances: Diagnosis and treatment. *Chest* 62:35S, 1972.
84. McMahon MJ et al: The nature of hypocalcemia in acute pancreatitis. *Br J Surg* 65:216, 1983.
85. Mehta K et al: The relationship between anion gap and elevated lactate. *Crit Care Med* 14:405, 1986.
86. Michaels S, Weil MH: Measurement of blood lactate on central venous and pulmonary artery blood for estimating severity and prognosis. *Crit Care Med* 8:263, 1980.
87. Mizock BA: Controversies in lactic acidosis. Implications in critically ill patients. *JAMA* 258:497, 1987.
88. Morrison G et al: Chronic renal failure, in Seldin DW, Giebisch G, (eds): *The Kidney: Physiology and Pathophysiology*. New York, Raven Press, 1985, p 1901.
89. Narins RG, Emmett M: Simple and mixed acid-base disorders: A practical approach. *Medicine* 59:161, 1980.
90. Olinger GN et al: Acute clinical hypocalcemic myocardial depression during rapid blood transfusion and postoperative hemodialysis. *J Thorac Cardiovasc Surg* 72:503, 1976.
91. Oliva PB: Lactic acidosis. *Am J Med* 48:209, 1970.
92. Pirisino R et al: Sulfhydryl groups and peroxidase-like activity of albumin as scavenger of organic peroxides. *Pharmacol Res Commun* 20:545, 1988.
92a. Poole-Wilson PA, Langer GA: Effect of pH on ionic exchange and function in rat and rabbit myocardium. *Am J Physiol* 229:570, 1975.
92b. Poole-Wilson PA, Cameron IR: Intracellular pH and K^+ of cardiac and skeletal muscle in acidosis and alkalosis. *Am J Physiol* 229:1305, 1975.
93. Prough DS et al: Effects on intracranial pressure of resuscitation from hemorrhagic shock with hypertonic saline versus lactated Ringer's solution. *Crit Care Med* 13:407, 1985.
94. Rackow EC et al: Fluid resuscitation in circulatory shock: A comparison of the cardiorespiratory effects of albumin, hetastarch, and saline solutions in patients with hypovolemic and septic shock. *Crit Care Med* 11:839, 1983.
95. Rackow EC et al: Effects of pentastarch and albumin infusion on cardiorespiratory function and coagulation in patients with severe sepsis and systemic hypoperfusion. *Crit Care Med* 17:394, 1989.
96. Rackow EC et al: Effects of crystalloid and colloid fluids on extravascular lung water in hypoproteinemic dog. *J Appl Physiol* 62:2421, 1987.

97. Ranson JHC et al: Prognostic signs and non-operative peritoneal lavage in acute pancreatitis. *Surg Gynecol Obstet* 143:209, 1976.
98. Rassmussen H: The calcium messenger system (part 1). *N Engl J Med* 314:1094, 1986.
99. Rassmussen H: The calcium messenger system (part 2). *N Engl J Med* 314:1164, 1986.
100. Robertson GM et al: Inadequate parathyroid response in acute pancreatitis. *N Engl J Med* 294:512, 1976.
101. Rothschild MA et al: Albumin synthesis. *N Engl J Med* 286:816, 1972.
102. Rush BF: Treatment of experimental shock: Comparison of the effects of norepinephrine, dibenzyline dextran, whole blood, and balanced saline solutions. *Surgery* 61:938, 1967.
103. Schaeffer RC et al: The effects of colloidal and crystalloidal fluids on rattlesnake venom shock in the rat. *J Pharm Exp Ther* 206:687, 1978.
104. Schaeffer RC et al: Effects of colloid or crystalloid solutions on edemagenesis in normal and thrombomicroembolized lungs. *Crit Care Med* 15:1110, 1987.
105. Sgouris JT, Dorsey HW: Survey of the use of plasma expands in the United States, in Sgouris JT, Rene A (eds): *Proc Workshop on Albumin*. Government Printing Office, Washington DC, 1975, p 137.
106. Shatney CH, Chaudry IH: Hydroxyethylstarch administration does not depress reticuloendothelial function or increase mortality from sepsis. *Cir Shock* 13:21, 1984.
107. Shatney CH et al: Efficacy of hetastarch in the resuscitation of patients with multisystem trauma and shock. *Arch Surg* 118:804, 1983.
108. Shils ME: Experimental human magnesium depletion. *Medicine* 48:61, 1969.
109. Shires T et al: Distributional changes in extracellular fluid during acute hemorrhagic shock. *Surg Forum* 11:115, 1960.
110. Shires T et al: Fluid therapy in hemorrhagic shock. *Arch Surg* 88:688, 1964.
111. Shires GT et al: Alterations in cellular membrane function during hemorrhagic shock in patients. *Ann Surg* 176:288, 1972.
112. Shizgal HM et al: Extracellular fluid volume changes following hemorrhagic shock. *Surg Forum* 18:35, 1967.
112a. Standards and guidelines for cardiopulmonary resuscitation (CPR) and emergency cardiac care (ECC). *JAMA* 244:453, 1980.
113. Standards and guidelines for cardiopulmonary resuscitation (CPR) and emergency cardiac care (ECC). *JAMA* 255:2905, 1986.
114. Stocker R et al: Antioxidant activity of albumin-bound bilirubin. *Proc Natl Acad Sci USA* 84:5918, 1987.
115. Strauss RG: Review of the effects of hydroxyethyl starch on the blood coagulation system. *Transfusion* 21:299, 1981.
116. Strauss RG et al: Pentastarch may cause fewer effects on coagulation than hetastarch. *Transfusion* 28:257, 1988.
117. Strauss RG et al: Hydroxyethyl starch accentuates von Willebrand's disease. *Transfusion* 25:235, 1985.
118. Stump DC et al: Effects of hydroxyethyl starch on blood coagulation, particularly factor VIII. *Transfusion* 25:349, 1985.
119. Tanaka Y, DeLuca HF: The control of 25-hydroxy vitamin D metabolism by inorganic phosphorus. *Arch Biochem Biophys* 154:566, 1973.
119a. Tang W et al: Reversible impairment of myocardial contractility due to hypercarbic acidosis in the isolated perfused rat heart. *Crit Care Med* 19:218, 1991.
120. Tranquada RE: Lactic acidosis. *Calif Med* 101:450, 1964.
121. Transfusion Alert: Indications for the Use of Red Blood Cells, Platelets and Fresh Frozen Plasma. US Dept of Health and Human Services. *NIH Publ* 89- 2974a, 1989.
122. Triedman JK et al: Pentastarch vs. albumin for volume expansion following cardiac surgery. *Anesthesiology* 65:A92, 1986.
123. Trunkey D et al: Ionized calcium and magnesium. The effect of septic shock in the baboon. *J Trauma* 18:166, 1978.
124. Tullis JL: Albumin I. Background and use. *JAMA* 237:355, 1977.
125. Urban P et al: Cardiac arrest and blood ionized calcium levels. *Ann Intern Med* 109:110, 1988.
125a. Vanheel B et al: Intracellular pH and contraction of isolated rabbit and cat papillary muscle: Effect of superfusate buffering. *J Mol Cell Cardiol* 17:23, 1985.
126. Velanovich V: Crystalloid vs colloid fluid resuscitation: A meta-analysis of mortality. *Surgery* 105:65, 1989.
127. Velasco IT et al: Hypertonic and hyperoncotic resuscitation from severe hemorrhagic shock in dogs: A comparative study. *Crit Care Med* 17:261, 1989.
128. Vitek V, Cowley RA: Blood lactate in the prognosis of various forms of shock. *Ann Surg* 173:308, 1971.
128a. von Planta M et al: Myocardial acidosis associated with CO_2 production. *Circulation* 80:684, 1989.
129. Warshaw AL et al: Depression of serum calcium by increased plasma free fatty acids in the rat: A mechanism for hypocalcemia in acute pancreatitis. *Gastroenterology* 89:814, 1985.
130. Wasil M et al: The antioxidant action of human extracellular fluids. Effect of human serum and its protein components on the inactivation of alpha 1-antiproteinase by hypochlorous acid and by hydrogen peroxide. *Biochem J* 243:219, 1987.
131. Waters LM et al; Hetastarch: An alternative colloid in burn shock management. *J Burn Care Rehabil* 10:11, 1989.
132. Waxman K et al: Hemodynamic and oxygen transport effects of pentastarch in burn resuscitation. *Ann Surg* 209:341, 1989.
133. Weaver DW: Pulmonary effects of albumin resuscitation for severe hypovolemic shock. *Arch Surg* 113:387, 1978.
134. Webb AR et al: Advantages of a narrow-range, medium molecular weight hydroxyethyl starch for volume maintenance in a porcine model of fecal peritonitis. *Crit Care Med* 19:409, 1991.
135. Weil MH, Afifi AA: Experimental and clinical studies on lactate and pyruvate as indicators of the severity of acute circulatory failure (shock). *Circulation* 41:989, 1970.
135a. Weil MH et al: Difference in acid-base state between venous and arterial blood during cardiopulmonary resuscitation. *N Engl J Med* 315:153, 1986.
135b. Weil MH et al: Comparison of blood lactate concentra-

tions in central venous pulmonary artery, and arterial blood. *Crit Care Med* 15:489, 1987.

135c. Weil MH et al: Incomplete global myocardial ischemia during cardiac arrest and resuscitation. *Crit Care Med* 16:997, 1988.

135d. Weil MH et al: The clinical rationale of cardiac resuscitation. *Dis Month* August 1990.

136. Weir GC et al: The hypocalcemia of acute pancreatitis. *Ann Intern Med* 83:185, 1975.

137. Wilson RF et al: Severe alkalosis in critically ill surgical patients. *Arch Surg* 105:197, 1972.

138. Wybenga DR et al: Determination of ionized calcium in serum that has been exposed to air. *Clin Chem* 22:1009, 1976.

139. Zaloga GP et al: Assessment of calcium homeostasis in the critically ill surgical patient. *Ann Surg* 202:587, 1985.

140. Zaloga GP, Chernow B: Hypocalcemia and hypophosphatemia in critical illness. *JAMA* 256:1924, 1986.

141. Zaloga GP, Chernow B: The multifactorial basis for hypocalcemia during sepsis. Studies of the parathyroid hormone-vitamin D axis. *Ann Intern Med* 107:36, 1987.

142. Zaloga GP et al: Calcium administration decreases survival and exacerbates endotoxinemia during peritonitis. *Chest* 98:2A, 1990.

143. Zikria BA et al: A biophysical approach to capillary permeability. *Surgery* 105:625, 1989.

144. Zikria BA et al: Macromolecules reduce abnormal microvascular permeability in rat limb ischemia-reperfusion injury. *Crit Care Med* 17:1306, 1989.

145. Zikria BA et al: Reduction of ischemia-reperfusion injury of myocardium by hydroxyethyl starch macromolecule. *Circulation* 78(4):11, 1988.

146. Zikria BA et al: Hydroxyethyl starch macromolecule reduce myocardial reperfusion injury. *Arch Surg* 125:930, 1990.

CHAPTER • 46

Metabolic encephalopathy associated with water, electrolyte, and acid-base disorders

Cosmo L. Fraser • Allen I. Arieff

INTRODUCTION

Metabolic encephalopathy is the term given to disorders of the central nervous system (CNS) that are not structural, that is, not due to brain tumors, infections, vasculopathies, or bleeding. The majority of metabolic encephalopathies are due to systemic abnormalities of fluid, electrolyte, and acid-base metabolism. The affected patients generally present with sensory disorders that are not due to structural lesions. As a general principle, if the metabolic disorder is not easily recognized, such anatomic CNS disruptions as stroke, subdural hematoma, intracranial infection, and intracranial hemorrhage should first be excluded. The causes of metabolic encephalopathy include liver failure, uremia, diabetic ketoacidosis, hypoxia, hypercapnia, hypoglycemia, and hyperglycemia, and both elevated and decreased blood levels of sodium, calcium, phosphate, magnesium, and hydrogen ions. The acquired immune deficiency syndrome (AIDS) virus may also be a cause of metabolic encephalopathy, but its underlying mechanism is not yet clear.[147] Exogenous intoxicants such as barbiturates, ethanol, and narcotics can also cause this problem. The symptoms of metabolic encephalopathy are numerous, ranging from restlessness to seizures, coma, and respiratory arrest. As a rule, however, many of these symptoms are readily reversible with correction of the underlying abnormality.

Some similarities exist between metabolic and structural coma, but in general the prognosis is quite different. A recent study of patients with nontraumatic coma evaluated the prognosis based on neurologic criteria. The prognosis was related to the cause of the coma, early neurologic status, and the presence or absence for up to 7 days of corneal, pupillary, and oculovestiblar reflexes, motor response, verbal response, spontaneous eye opening, and deep tendon reflexes.[292] The prognosis for recovery in nontraumatic coma patients could be predicted with 99 percent accuracy by employing these criteria. The ability to predict outcome in this manner does not hold true in patients with metabolic coma. Patients with depression of respiration, absent corneal reflexes, absent deep tendon reflexes, and no response to pain may still make a complete recovery after 6 days of coma induced by barbiturate or glutethimide intoxication.[25] In a study by Levy et al. only 10 percent of patients had metabolic encephalopathy, and all of these had hepatic coma.[292] In fact, patients with hepatic encephalopathy had the best overall chance of survival (50 percent) in the series. In other types of metabolic encephalopathy, survival cannot be prdicted by neurologic status because the latter has not been evaluated. In studies of over 150 hyponatremic patients with depression of sensorium (mean serum sodium below 128 mmol/liter), a complete neurologic evaluation was reported in less than 10 percent of cases.[36,45,149,183] Similarly, among large series of patients with diabetic coma, complete neurologic evaluations are rarely reported. Therefore, whatever the neurologic status in patients with metabolic coma, a reasonable determination of prognosis simply cannot be made given the present state of knowledge.

The neurochemical literature deals exhaustively with the effects of various alterations in brain biochemistry on several laboratory parameters. Such studies include the effects of alterations in electrolyte and acid-base status. However, very little of this information is found in the clinical literature. Thus, much information that is potentially of therapeutic and diagnostic importance has not been assimilated into clinical medicine. This chapter reviews the effects of systemic abnormalities of water, electrolyte, and acid-base metabolism on the central nervous system.

IONIC CONSTITUENTS AND ACID-BASE BALANCE OF NORMAL BRAIN AND CEREBROSPINAL FLUID

OSMOTICALLY ACTIVE SOLUTE

The principal osmotically active constituents of brain consist of both organic and inorganic solutes. The major inorganic constituents of the brain, and their approximate concentrations (mmol/kg wet weight) in the cerebral cortex of mammalian species (rat, cat, dog, human) are Na^+ (50 to 60 mmol/kg), K^+ (85 to 100 mmol/kg), Cl^- (35 to 45 mmol/kg), Ca^{2+} (1 to 2.8 mmol/kg), Mg^{2+} (5 to 6 mmol/kg), and bicarbonate (10 to 12 mmol/kg).[31,108,223,263,472]

The total brain cation concentration is about 170 mmol/kg wet weight, while anions, including Cl^-, bicarbonate, sulfates, phosphates, and organic acid anions (such as lactate, glutamine, glutamate, and *N*-acetylaspartate) are at most about 85 mmol/kg wet weight.[472] The remaining brain intracellular anions are probably polyionic lipids and proteins. Since most brain Cl^- is extracellular, the bulk of intracellular anions are organic and macromolecular.[472] Additionally, there are also minute quantities in the brain of certain trace metals, such as copper, manganese, zinc, ion, tin, aluminum, and rubidium.[31,223,437,472]

The actual osmotic activity of any of the constituents mentioned above is not entirely clear. Most Ca^{2+} and Mg^{2+} is probably bound, and not osmotically active.[266] The primary intracellular osmotically active cation is K^+, and a substantial portion of intracellular Na^+ is also probably osmotically active.[223,266] The role of organic phosphates in brain osmoregulation is not well studied,[69] and the osmotic activity in brain of amino acids and other organic acids is uncertain, although they appear to play a major role in osmotic adaptation in the cells of many invertebrates[171,173] and amphibians.[417] Glutamate, aspartate, lactate, pyruvate, and alanine are organic intracellular metabolites that have been suggested as being osmotically active,[386,417] but evidence of their osmotic activity remains to be determined.

An enormous amount of evidence from both humans[94,152] and experimental animals[34,317,467] indicates that changes in tissue osmolality occur without apparent net loss or gain of cellular water and solutes.[33,62,304] In these instances there may be apparent inactivation of intracellular solute[94,152] or a gain in solute that is not due to commonly measured substances.[28,467] This undetermined solute has been called *idiogenic osmoles*.[29,34] A substantial body of evidence suggests that the brain undergoes osmotic adaptation to hyperosmolar states in a manner that is distinctly different from other tissues. For example, in birds and mammals, muscle and nucleated red blood cells may adapt to hyperosmolar states by losing water and gaining cations[467] while brain adapts primarily by de novo generation of solute by yet unexplained mechanisms.[379] These mechanisms apparently are not activated immediately and as a result, overly rapid induction of either hyperosmolality or hypoosmolality may be lethal.[149,238,468] Patients or experimental animals who have been chronically hyperosmolar or hypoosmolar are generally symptomatic and may have depression of sensorium.[28,29,36]

ACID-BASE STATUS OF BRAIN AND CEREBROSPINAL FLUID

Of the large number of studies dealing with the acid-base status of brain and cerebrospinal fluid, those dealing with the cerebrospinal fluid are less controversial because of the ready applicability of commonly used techniques for direct measurement of gases in cerebrospinal fluid.[30,31,239] The steady-state relationships between

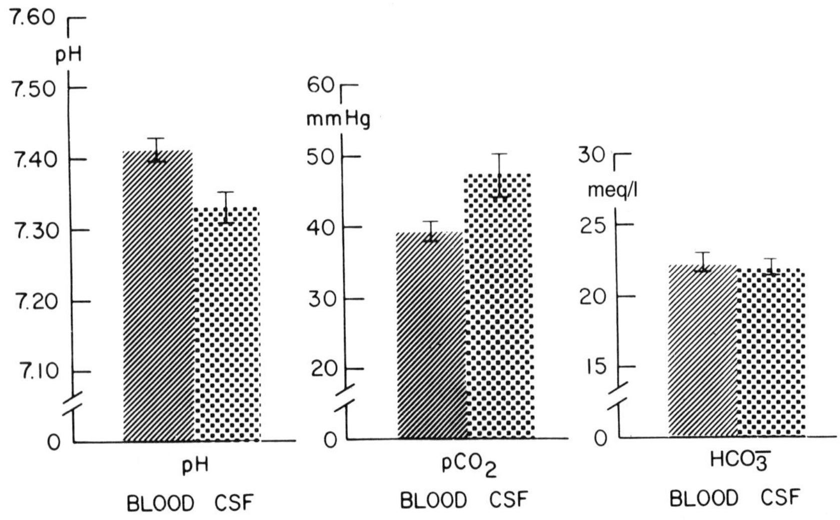

FIGURE 46-1 • The relationship between acid-base balance in arterial blood vs. cisternal CSF in human subjects. (Data summarized from Katsman R, Pappius HM, Brain ions, in *Brain Electrolytes and Fluid Metabolism*, Baltimore, Williams & Wilkins, 1973, p 111.)

acid-base components in arterial blood vs. cisternal cerebrospinal fluid in human beings are shown in Fig. 46-1. In general, bicarbonate concentration is similar in blood and cerebrospinal fluid (about 24 mmol/liter); arterial pH (approximately 7.40) is higher than in cerebrospinal fluid (about 7.32) because pCO_2 in cerebrospinal fluid (approximately 48 mmHg) is higher than that in blood (approximately 40 mmHg).

The cerebrospinal fluid protein concentration (approximately 40 mg/dl) is very small compared with that in plasma (approximately 7 g/dl). Despite this apparent inferior buffering capacity, the pH of the cerebrospinal fluid remains remarkably constant even in the face of substantial changes in arterial pH. In acute changes in systemic pCO_2 (respiratory alkalosis and acidosis) there are acute alterations in pH and pCO_2 of cerebrospinal fluid that are similar to those in arterial blood.[30,31,239] However, the changes in cerebrospinal fluid pH are initially less than those in arterial blood, and within 1 h, compensatory mechanisms have been initiated.[31]

The cerebrospinal fluid concentrations of lactate and other, unidentified organic acids are increased in acute respiratory alkalosis;[31,364,497] this decreases cerebrospinal fluid pH toward normal.[239] This compensation is nearly complete after 4 to 6 h. With an arterial pH of 7.5 to 7.6, the simultaneously determined intracellular pH (pH_i) of brain will rise from 7.05 to above 7.2 after 1 h when arterial pCO_2 is below 25 mmHg, but after 2 to 5 h, it returns to normal values. The changes are similar in four different regions of the brain.[365]

In acute respiratory acidosis (arterial pCO_2 above 80 mmHg), there is initially a significant decline in pH of cerebrospinal fluid but within 1 to 2 h, the bicarbonate concentration of the fluid begins to rise.[31,268] By contrast, although pH_i of brain falls after 1 h of hypercapnia, it returns to normal after 3 h of sustained hypercapnia.[31] By contrast, in the liver, changes in extracellular pH over a range of about 7.0 to 7.7 have no effect on hepatic pH_i, while in skeletal muscle, respiratory acidosis results in corresponding changes in muscle pH_i, while metabolic acidosis or alkalosis does not change muscle pH_i.[31,361]

Acute metabolic acid-base perturbations have little effect on cerebrospinal fluid pH. Neither bicarbonate nor hydrogen ion can readily cross the blood-cerebrospinal fluid barrier, but this barrier is readily permeable to CO_2.[268]

CEREBROSPINAL FLUID ELECTROLYTES

Sodium ion

Since cerebrospinal fluid is essentially protein-free and acellular, the "unmeasured anion," that is, the difference between measured cations and measured anions, is approximately zero. In general, the cerebrospinal fluid concentrations of (Na^+) + (K^+) are similar to the concentrations of (Cl^-) + (HCO_3^-). There is considerable variation among mammalian species, but in general the sodium concentration in cerebrospinal fluid is similar to that of plasma. However, when sodium is expressed as mmol/kg water its concentration is higher in plasma than in cerebrospinal fluid. Because of the osmotic equilibrium between plasma and cerebrospinal fluid, changes in cerebrospinal fluid sodium concentration generally parallel those of plasma.

Potassium ion

In contrast to Na^+, the cerebrospinal fluid concentration of K^+ is relatively constant, being essentially independent of the plasma K^+ concentration. In human subjects, the K^+ concentration in cerebrospinal fluid has been found to be 2.89 ± 0.26 meq/liter, and in other vertebrates, the range is 2.52 to 2.98 mmol/liter.[264] In both human beings and experimental animals, cerebrospinal fluid K^+ is also kept fairly constant despite marked variation in plasma K^+.[80] However, in some patients with severe hypokalemia (plasma K^+ below 2 meq/liter), cerebrospinal fluid K^+ concentrations as low as 2.4 to 2.6 meq/liter have been reported.[264] There are at least two mechanisms that serve to maintain cerebrospinal fluid concentratin of K^+ in this narrow range. There is a carrier-mediated transport of K^+ across the choroid plexus from blood into the cerebrospinal fluid and there is also exchange of cerebrospinal fluid K^+ with brain K^+ Although the evidence is not conclusive, both of these mechanisms probably require active transport processes.

Calcium ion

In virtually all mammalian species, the Ca^{2+} concentration in cerebrospinal fluid is between 2 and 3 meq/liter. Calcium is secreted by the choroid plexus into the cerebrospinal fluid. Because of its small protein concentration, virtually all Ca^{2+} in cerebrospinal fluid is ionized. It has long been suggested that the $Ca2^+$ concentration in cerebrospinal fluid was similar to ionized Ca^{2+} in plasma. However, using modern methodology to measure Ca^{2+}, the plasma ionized Ca^{2+} concentration is still found to be consistently greater than that in cerebrospinal fluid.[263,264] There is also a potential difference between cerebrospinal fluid and plasma of about 5 mV. When this electrochemical gradient is taken into account, there is electrochemical equilibrium for Ca^{2+} between cerebrospinal fluid and plasma in normal human subjects. However, it appears unlikely that cerebrospinal fluid and plasma in normal human subjects. However, it appears unlikely that cerebrospinal fluid and plasma ionized Ca^{2+} are in equilibrium. When plasma Ca^{2+} is altered by Ca^{2+} infusion, parathyroidectomy, parathyroid hormone administration, EDTA, uremia, or vitamin D intoxication, there is little if any change in the Ca^{2+} in cerebrospinal fluid.[37]

Magnesium ion

The Mg^{2+} level in cerebrospinal fluid of human subjects is slightly higher than that of plasma (2.41 meq/liter vs. 1.82 meq/liter for plasma).[263,264] The consistency of a higher level of Mg^{2+} in cerebrospinal fluid than in plasma suggests that there must be active secretion of Mg^{2+} into cerebrospinal fluid, probably at the choroid plexus as in the case of Ca^{2+}. Increased plasma Mg^{2+} levels from the intravenous administration of $MgSO_4$ raise the Mg^{2+} concentration in cerebrospinal fluid when plasma levels are very high. Elevations in plasma Mg^{2+} of 27 to 700 percent increase Mg in cerebrospinal fluid by only 20 to 25 percent.[81] In animals with renal failure, a 30 percent rise in plasma Mg^{2+} did not affect cerebrospinal fluid concentration of Mg^{2+}.[218] However, a Mg^{2+}-deficient diet did result in a small decrement of cerebrospinal fluid concentration of Mg^{2+} in rabbits.[81] In patients with hypomagnesemia (serum Mg^{2+} below 2.14 meq/liter), Mg^{2+} in cerebrospinal fluid is below normal values.[264]

General

The average human brain weighs about 1.3 kg (1400 g in adult males and 1240 g in adult females) and thus represents only about 2 percent of body mass. Despite its rather modest mass, the brain receives about 20 percent of cardiac output, consumes about 65 percent of total glucose, and utilizes about 20 percent of the body's total oxygen.[57,226] In addition, about 75 percent of total brain oxygen is utilized by cortical gray matter neurons, which constitute only about 20 percent of brain mass. The brain has enormous needs in terms of energy. About 85 percent of all glucose used by the brain is aerobically metabolized with oxygen, with about half of the energy produced utilized to maintain normal ionic gradients across brain cell membranes. The ionic gradients are needed to generate action potentials and conduct nerve impulses. If the brain does not obtain sufficient oxygen, glucose cannot be oxidized aerobically, with resultant decreased energy production by the brain. Anaerobic metabolism cannot supply enough energy for the brain to function. No measurable cerebral dysfunction occurs when cerebral oxygen utilization is maintained at a level of 50 percent of normal, which corresponds to an arterial pO_2 (p_aO_2) of about 50 mmHg. An acute lowering of arterial p_aO_2 below approximately 40 mmHg results in measurable cerebral dysfunction, while p_aO_2 below approximately 30 mmHg (in unconditioned subjects) usually results in depression of sensorium. It is felt that chronic hypoxia, such as that experienced at high altitudes,[494] is well tolerated, but this may not be true. A recent study of well-conditioned individuals at altitudes of up to 8848 m demonstrated steady-state arterial pO_2 of approximately 30 mmHg at rest[240] and approximately 28 mmHg with exercise. Such individuals were found to have developed permanent brain damage when subjected to a sophisticated battery of motor, intellectual, and psychological tests.[240] Furthermore, healthy airline pilots subjected to graded degrees of hypoxia often lose consciousness at an arterial pO_2 below 30 mmHg.[427] This degree of hypoxia also corresponds to slowing of the EEG.[427] The arterial pO_2 level of less than 30 mmHg also corresponds quite well to the minimum level of pO_2 in laboratory animals, which is compatible with survival.[26] Despite a pronounced ability to survive at substantially reduced levels of arterial pO_2, brain survival is possible for only about 20 s in the total absence of oxygen.[26] Some understanding of how the body adapts to hypoxia can be obtained by the concept of the oxygen extraction reserve.

Oxygen extraction reserve: brain and heart

In the development of cerebral hypoxia, the oxygen extraction reserve is one of the major critical factors that determines the performance of the heart and lungs and the subsequent delivery of oxygen to the brain. Because of this, it is important to review the regulation of systemic oxygen delivery and utilization. Cerebral blood flow (CBF) is a function of cardiac output, arterial blood pressure, and cerebral vascular resistance. In general, cerebral vascular resistance can respond to alterations in arterial blood pressure in order to provide a relatively constant CBF. Impairment of autoregulation occurs with severe hypercapnia or hypoxia, both leading to increased CBF. The heart usually plays a critical role in the development of hypoxia with resulting lactic acidosis.[19] Total body oxygen utilization can be substantially impaired without a measurable rise in arterial lactate,[71] and measurements of arterial blood gases and lactate are often of no use in determining the acid-base and oxygenation status of the body.[4,71,211,492] Measurements must be made of the arterial and mixed venous (pulmonary artery) gases, including oxygen content (which can be determined from the oxygen saturation and hemoglobin). As a practical matter, the central venous gases are similar enough to the mixed venous gases that they can be used when a pulmonary artery catheter cannot be placed in the patient.[4] Oxygen transport (or delivery) can be calculated using the product of the arterial oxygen content and blood flow (usually expressed as ml O_2/min). It represents the quantity of oxygen available or delivered to the whole body or to individual organs or tissues, and is maintained preferentially to the "vital organs" (heart and brain) during hypoxia by a number of adaptive mechanisms.[68,90,237,426] With mild hypoxemia (arterial pO_2 of 40 to 65 mmHg), the oxygen content of arterial blood is relatively well preserved by virtue of the sigmoidal nature of the oxygen-hemoglobin binding curve.[68,90] Oxygen delivery declines only modestly (at most 20 to

30 percent), and the principal adaptation to this decline is a compensatory increase in tissue oxygen extraction.

The ability of tissues to increase oxygen extraction when oxygen delivery is inadequate is the oxygen utilization coefficient.[221] Since tissues are theoretically capable of extracting virtually all the oxygen carried to them by hemoglobin, the oxygen extraction reserve may be conveniently defined as the oxygen content of that tissue's venous blood, which represents the amount of oxygen that is theoretically available but not extracted by that tissue. Under normal aerobic conditions, arterial blood is more than 95 percent saturated with oxygen, and the extraction reserve is quite large. Mixed-venous blood is normally about 75 percent saturated with a corresponding oxygen content of about 15 volume percent.[10,221] Resting oxygen extraction is therefore only about 20 percent (95 percent − 75 percent) of that available, so that the reserve is about 75 percent, more than three times as large as the oxygen extracted. However, because resting oxygen requirements are higher per gram of tissue in the brain and heart than in any other organs, resting oxygen extraction is much higher in these tissues. Thus, the heart and brain have the smallest oxygen extraction reserve, and can increase resting oxygen extraction only by a maximum of 50 percent of baseline. Thus, the body as a whole has an oxygen reserve that is over three times the normal resting oxygen extraction, and most organs can tolerate acutely an arterial pO_2 below 50 mmHg without difficulty. Below an arterial pO_2 of about 40 mmHg, there is a local vascular effect of hypoxia that causes direct vasodilation of the cerebral circulation such that CBF remains constant throughout a wide range of arterial blood pressure and cardiac output.[57] In general, cerebral vascular resistance can respond to alterations in arterial blood pressure as low as 30 to 50 mmHg in laboratory animals and as low as 60 mmHg or as high as 180 mmHg in humans, by either vasoconstriction or vasodilatation, in order to provide a constant CBF of 50 to 70 ml/100 g/min.[319] Major factors that can influence CBF are the blood pO_2, pCO_2, and pH. In conditions characterized by hypocapnia and/or metabolic alkalosis, there is cerebral vasoconstriction, while both hypoxia and hypercapnia/metabolic acidosis result in cerebral vasodilatation. A breakdown of cerebral autoregulation then occurs, with severe hypercapnia or hypoxia, both leading to increased brain blood flow.

CHARACTERISTICS OF THE BLOOD-BRAIN BARRIER

BRAIN EXTRACELLULAR SPACE (ECS)

Extracellular fluid (ECF) space is thought of as that fluid compartment which is outside of cells. In practice, it serves as the fluid compartment that is available for the distribution of a particular marker. The volume of the compartment may be determined as the ratio of distribution of the marker in the tissue to its distribution in a reference fluid that is considered to represent ECF.[129] (If plasma is used as the ECF, the calculation must be corrected for the Donnan effect.) There is essentially a dual circulation of fluids about the brain (both blood and cerebrospinal fluid). The bulk of the evidence suggests that the cerebrospinal fluid is identical to and a continuation of the brain ECF.[83] The measurement of ECF space assumes that the marker has equilibrated between tissue and extracellular fluid. In the case of the brain, there is a tendency for any substance entering the brain via the blood to be siphoned off into the cerebrospinal fluid, and for any substance entering via the cerebrospinal fluid to be siphoned off into the bloodstream; equilibration may thus not be reached. Together, these tendencies are known as the "sink action" of cerebrospinal fluid.[350] In addition, several extracellular markers, such as thiocyanate and sulfate, are actively removed from the cerebrospinal fluid by active transport systems at the choroid plexus.[129] To attain the equilibrium conditions between cerebrospinal fluid and brain necessary to determine ECS, the same concentration of extracellular marker must be present in both plasma water and cerebrospinal fluid. This can be attained by simultaneous administration of the extracellular marker in these two compartments.[290] Common extracellular markers include radiolabeled inulin, sucrose, chloride, thiocyanate, sulfate, mannitol, and bromide. Several different in vivo techniques and markers have been employed[31] to measure brain ECS. These include estimation by electron microscopy, tissue diffusion profiles, and measurement of cortical electrical impedance.[481] When brain ECS is appropriately determined in mammalian cerebral cortex by any of the above techniques, the range is from 15 to 25 percent, with a mean value of about 20 percent,[265,290,291] although primates are much higher (about 40 percent).[77]

ANATOMY OF THE BLOOD-BRAIN BARRIER

When a nonmetabolizable, nontoxic substance is administered via the bloodstream such that steady-state conditions are maintained for several hours, it will achieve a similar volume of distribution throughout most cell systems. Such substances include inulin, sulfate, salicylic acid, antipyrine, and urea. However, for a given time interval (up to 4 h), none of these substances will achieve a concentration in the brain that is as high as its concentration in other tissues such as liver or muscle.[118] This selective behavior of the brain, whereby passage of certain substances out of the blood is restricted, has been called the blood-brain barrier.[79,208,289,386] Several factors have been shown to influence the rate of passage of a substance from blood to brain. These include the Ka, configuration, molecular size, charge, and lipid solubility. Lipid-soluble substances penetrate the blood-brain bar-

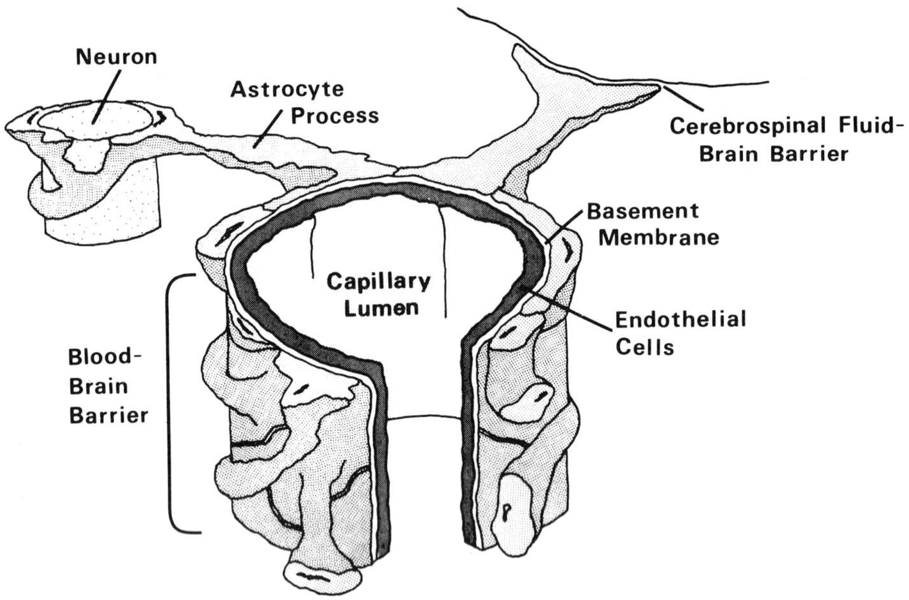

FIGURE 46-2 • Diagrammatic rendering of the blood-brain barrier. The principal element is a layer of endothelial cells with tight junctions and a thick capillary basement membrane. The CSF-brain barrier consists primarily of choroid plexus and ependyma. (Original drawing by Bob Surface of Medical Research Graphics, San Francisco, CA.)

rier much more rapidly than non-lipid-soluble ones. For weak acids and bases, the partition parameter determines their entry in the brain—weak acids tend to be excluded and weak bases concentrated.[387]

The anatomical delineation of the blood-brain barrier is complex and has been described in great detail elsewhere.[79,118,208,289,387,388] The principal components of the blood-brain barrier are the brain capillaries, the astrocytic processes (end-feet processes), the thick brain capillary basement membrane, and the thick wall (Fig. 46-2).

In contrast to other capillaries, brain endothelial cells are connected by tight junctions that act to form a continuous cell layer. A basement membrane surrounds the cells, and this is in turn covered by the glial cells, the astrocytic processes of which cover about 85 percent of the capillary surface.[118,388] The intracerebral arterioles and venules are also covered by continuous endothelial cell layers with tight junctions. Both the astrocytic end-feet processes that surround the capillaries, in addition to the thick neuronal cell walls, probably constitute the bulk of the blood-brain barrier. The thick lipid cell wall would tend to exclude those small molecules that pass out of cerebral capillaries but are not lipid-soluble.

BIOCHEMICAL MEDIATORS OF BRAIN DAMAGE

There may be common biochemical mechanisms that underlie cellular injury in a variety of metabolic encephalopathies. It has been demonstrated that one of the major features of brain damage in a variety of metabolic insults begins with elevated concentrations of aspartate, glutamate (or similar acidic amino acids), followed by excessive excitation and stimulation of a subset of glutamate receptors, the *N*-methyl-D-aspartate (NMDA) receptors.[430] This is presumably followed by dissipative ion fluxes of Na^+, K^+, and Ca^{2+}, which appear to be initiated by opening of channels permeable to both calcium and monovalent cations.[430] Such a sequence has been found to occur in hypoxic-ischemic injury and head trauma,[155,430] and such a mechanism is also suspect in hepatic encephalopathy, hypoglycemia, and hyponatremia.[430,499-501] Another major signaling pathway in the brain has nitric oxide (NO) as a second messenger.[197] In the CNS, NO is produced enzymatically in postsynaptic structures in response to activation of excitatory amino acid receptors, such as the NMDA receptor.[439] Nitric oxide then diffuses out to act upon neighboring cellular elements, probably astrocyte processes. A major cellular action of NO is to activate soluble guanylate cyclase and thus raise cyclic GMP concentrations in target cells,[439] such as cerebellar cortex. The neurotransmitter released at the principal excitatory synapses in the cerebellum is probably glutamate, which can elicit large accumulations of cyclic GMP. The NMDA receptor mediates most of the cyclic GMP responses to glutamate.[197] The eventual result is repetitive cell stimulation and excitation.[328,430] Excitation, or increased synaptic activity, is an important factor in eventual cell death in hypoxic neurons.[408] Thus the classical biochemical teachings where hypoxia/ischemia leads to a decrease of brain high-energy phosphate compounds, with a secondary influx of sodium, chloride, and water into brain are probably outdated and incorrect.[27]

In Alzheimer's disease, there may also be abnormal concentrations and effects of the various excitatory neurotransmitter acidic amino acids that can bind to the NMDA receptor.[355,366] L-glutamate is an excitatory amino acid that can destructively stimulate the NMDA receptor.[310]

CALCIUM IONS AND CELL DEATH

A point is eventually reached where cerebral edema has occurred and cell viability is severely compromised. If the cellular damage continues, there follows an influx of calcium ions and a probable decrease in intracellular magnesium,[486] which is at some point followed by permanent neuronal damage.[143,389] The actual event that leads to irreversible cell death in hypoxic brain is not entirely clear. A late event is the movement into hypoxic cells of calcium, and in certain types of cell injury, calcium overload is the actual pathogenetic mechanism.[102,143] There are a number of theoretical reasons why calcium overload may be detrimental to cells. An increase in free cytosolic calcium can activate calcium-dependent phospholipases, resulting in the breakdown of cell membranes and production of substances that are toxic to cells, such as free fatty acids and phospholipids. Additionally, many important intracellular enzyme systems, such as ATPases, glycogen phosphorylase, and adenylate cyclase, are regulated by calcium. Thus a large increase of free cytosolic calcium can easily be conceived as upsetting the homeostasis between intracellular messengers, energy, and electrolytes. Elevations of free cytosolic calcium will increase Na^+-Ca^{2+} ATPase activity, resulting in an enhanced use of ATP, which is low in ischemic cells. Elevations in calcium can also lead to uncoupling of oxidative phosphorylation in mitochondria and deplete cells of chemical energy.[102] All these findings, along with the fact that ischemic tissue contains large amounts of calcium, strongly suggest that ischemia leads to an uncontrolled increase in total cell calcium and cytosolic free calcium, which initiates a cascade of progressively deleterious events that terminate in cell death.[102] Additionally, magnesium is a necessary component of many intracellular enzyme systems.[441,486] Increased extracellular magnesium actually has a protective effect on hypoxic neurons.[408] Posttraumatic brain injury is associated with a decrease of intracellular magnesium,[486] and alterations in cellular magnesium can have substantial effects on intracellular calcium current.[495] It is possible, but as yet unproved that the influx of calcium leads to a cellular exodus of magnesium following brain injury.[109,155]

This biochemical pattern of cerebral injury is seen not only in ischemia but also in traumatic brain injury.[155] There is thus evidence that both hypoxia and trauma can result in a "metabolic encephalopathy" after the initial insult has occurred. Therapy in experimental animals with antagonists to the NMDA receptor has been effective in preliminary studies, and such agents may have a future role in the prevention of hypoxic and/or posttraumatic brain damage.[155,274]

UREMIA

GENERAL

A number of therapeutic modalities such as dialysis treatments, renal transplantation, drug therapy, and improved medical management have resulted in significant improvements in both the duration and quality of life in patients with renal failure. Synthetic erythropoietin that has recently become a part of routine management of dialysis patients has led to impressive improvements in patients' well-being.[153,213] However, the role that it might play in improving the nervous system manifestations of uremia is still to be determined. In spite of the major strides made in recent years, patients with renal failure continue to manifest a variety of neurologic disorders and have higher than normal morbidity and mortality.[180,182] Those with chronic renal insufficiency who have not yet received dialytic therapy may develop a symptom complex that may progress from mild sensorial clouding, tremor, asterixis, multifocal myoclonus, seizures, and delirium to coma and death if therapy is not instituted. Even after the institution of otherwise adequate maintenance dialysis therapy, patients may continue to manifest more subtle nervous system dysfunction, such as impaired mentation, generalized weakness, and peripheral neuropathy. The CNS disorders of both untreated renal failure and that persisting despite dialysis are referred to as uremic encephalopathy. The dialytic treatment of end-stage renal disease has itself been associated with the emergence of two distinct disorders of the CNS: dialysis disequilibrium and dialysis dementia. The dialysis disequilibrium syndrome is a consequence of the initiation of dialysis therapy in some patients (more common in children and the elderly). Dialysis dementia is a progressive, generally fatal encephalopathy that most commonly affects patients who are on chronic hemodialysis.

In addition to the above complications that are specifically related to uremia and/or dialysis, many other neurologic disorders occur with increased frequency in patients who have end-stage renal disease and are being treated with chronic hemodialysis. Subdural hematoma, electrolyte disorders, vitamin deficiencies, drug intoxication, hypertensive encephalopathy, and acute trace element intoxication must be considered as part of the differential diagnosis of an altered mental state.[182] Renal transplantation is associated with a variety of nervous system infections and neoplasms, such as reticulum cell sarcoma, which is a direct result of immunosuppressive therapy. However, with cyclosporine now being used as the mainstay of immunotherapy, the spectrum of complications should be drastically altered.[457]

UREMIC ENCEPHALOPATHY

In general, most clinical abnormalities associated with the uremic syndrome are due to disordered function of the nervous system. They involve the organism as a whole, rather than particular organs, and as such reflect the integrated aspects of the CNS. It has been suggested that the "central nervous system provides a linkage of relevance between the chemical lesions, uremic toxins, and abnormal metabolic transactions of renal failure on the one hand, and the clinical, symptomatic lesions on the other"[460] (see Chap. 39).

The CNS manifestations of uremia include a continuum of signs and symptoms that are characteristic of many metabolic encephalopathies.[305,390] The earliest symptoms generally reflect sensorial clouding and may include loss of recent memory and impaired ability to concentrate with depression, delusions, and slurring of speech. The clinical symptoms of renal failure often fluctuate from day to day in any given patient, so that intervals of lucidity may be intermixed with periods of apathy, confusion, or obtundation.

As a result of the early initiation of dialysis therapy and medical management, the seizures and coma previously observed with advanced renal failure are seldom seen today. The clinical manifestations of acute renal failure (ARF) are similar to those seen in chronic renal failure (CRF) but tend to be more severe and occur at lower levels of blood urea nitrogen (BUN). However, complications such as osteodystrophy, anemia, and acid-base abnormalities are more frequently observed in patients with CRF. The neurologic manifestations of uremia are generally similar regardless of the etiology of the underlying renal disease. Notable exceptions are systemic diseases that affect the nervous system directly, such as vasculitis or amyloidosis, and possibly patients whose renal failure is due to diabetes mellitus or primary hyperparathyroidism.[305,460]

ACUTE RENAL FAILURE

The clinical manifestations of ARF include abnormalities of mental status as an early and sensitive index of neurologic disorder, with lassitude and lethargy progressing to disorientation, confusion, and eventually coma[113] (see Chap. 38). Fixed attitudes, torpor, and other signs of toxic psychosis are common. When the uremia is left untreated and allowed to progress, coma often supervenes. In such patients, cranial nerve signs are common, although they are usually transient. Nystagmus and mild facial asymmetries also frequently occur. Visual fields remained normal in most patients, papilledema is generally not observed, and optic fundi are said to be normal. About half the patients have dysarthria and difficulty in protruding the tongue past the lips; many have diffuse weakness and fasciculations. Marked variation of deep tendon reflexes is noted in almost all patients with ARF, often in an asymmetrical pattern. Progression to hyperreflexia, with unsustained clonus at the patella or ankle, is also quite common.[181]

Electroencephalograms (EEG) in patients with ARF have generally been grossly abnormal when the diagnosis of renal failure was first established.[113] In most instances, the percentage of EEG power less than 5 Hz, which is a standard measurement of the percentage of EEG power devoted to abnormal (delta) slow wave activity, was over 20 times the normal value. The EEG was also abnormal with regard to the percentage of EEG frequencies above 9 Hz. These EEG changes were not affected by dialysis but returned to normal with recovery of renal function. Similar findings have been shown in experimental animals with renal failure.[35,218] The EEG tends to worsen both during and for several hours after hemodialysis[305,460] and up to 6 months after initiation of dialysis therapy.[1,273] It then approaches normal values in patients who continue to be treated with long-term dialysis.[273]

CHRONIC RENAL FAILURE

The neurologic manifestations of CRF are quite numerous.[293,305,354,460] Patients with CRF may develop a sense of sluggishness; easy fatigue on exertion; insomnia and daytime drowsiness; cutaneous itching; decreased appetite; impaired ability to focus attention, perform mental arithmetic, or express ideas in more than simple language; erratic memory; slurred speech; vague headaches; waning sexual interest and potency; restlessness; emotional irritability and withdrawal; nausea and vomiting, hypothermia, and sensations of coldness. There may also be paranoid delusions and compulsive personality changes; bizarre behavior; anxiety, disorientation; confusion; hallucinations; ataxia; transient mono-, di-, or hemiplegias; aphagia; partial deafness and vertigo; all of which may be mixed with occasional episodes of alertness[181] (see Chap. 39).

The EEG findings in patients with CRF are milder than those observed in patients with ARF. Several investigations have shown a good correlation between the percentage of EEG frequencies and power below 7 Hz and the decline of renal function as estimated by serum creatinine[460] (Fig. 46-3). After the initiation of dialysis there may be an initial period of clinical stabilization during which time the EEG deteriorates (up to 6 months), but it then tends to approach normal values.[273,460] However, still more improvement is seen after renal transplantation.[460,461] The EEG findings in patients with CRF have been extensively de-

FIGURE 46-3 • Percentage of slow-wave-associated (3 to 7 Hz) EEG power plotted against concurrent serum creatinine concentrations in 56 azotemic patients with chronic renal failure prior to onset of maintenance hemodialysis. (Reprinted from PE Teschan et al: *Kidney Int* 15:676, 1979.)

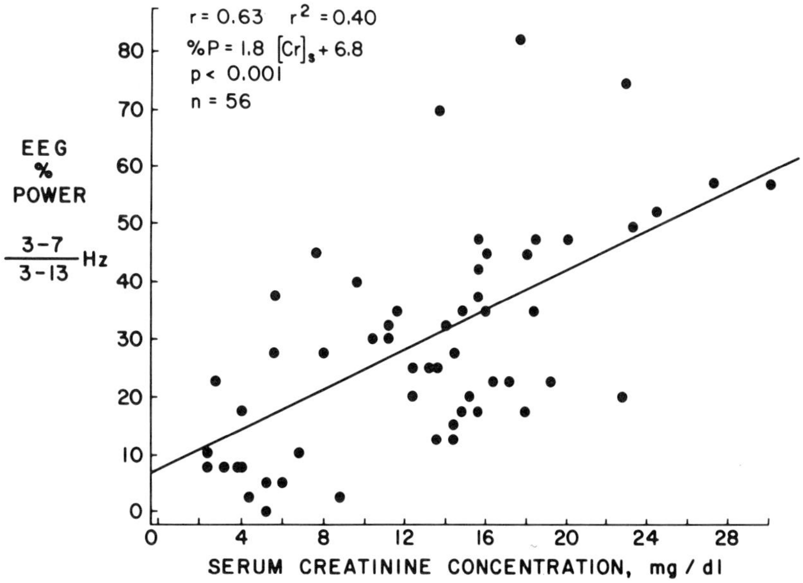

scribed.[1,108,113,273,305,390,459,460,461] Central nervous system dysfunction in uremia can also be quantitated by cognition-dependent performance measures. The cognitive functions known to be impaired in uremia include sustained attention, selective attention, speed of decision making, short-term memory, and mental manipulation of symbols.[460] The choice reaction time (CRT) test is probably the most useful of those employed. It measures sustained attention as well as speed of decision making.[459]

The causes of the EEG abnormalities observed in uremic patients are unclear, but there is evidence that a significant common denominator may be an effect of parathyroid hormone (PTH) on brain.[108,207] In experimental animals with acute or chronic renal failure, many of the EEG abnormalities can be shown to be related to a direct effect of PTH on brain, leading to an elevated brain content of Ca^{2+}.[218] Studies in patients with either acute or chronic renal failure suggest a similar pathogenesis.[113]

In patients with ARF, the EEG is abnormal within 48 h of the onset of renal failure and is generally not affected by dialysis over a period of up to 3 weeks.[113] During this interval, patients have elevated plasma levels of PTH.[113] Several months after return of renal function to normal, plasma PTH levels also normalize. Although there are doubtless many factors that contribute to uremic encephalopathy, no correlation between encephalopathy and any of the commonly measured indicators of renal failure have been shown (BUN, creatinine, bicarbonate, pH, potassium).[1,108,113,273,293,305,354,390,459-461] Thus, PTH may be a major "uremic toxin."

BIOCHEMICAL CHANGES IN BRAIN

To determine the possible causes of the clinical manifestations and EEG abnormalities observed in patients with either acute or chronic renal failure, numerous biochemical analysis were performed in brains of both patients and laboratory animals. Determinations were made of brain intracellular pH, brain Na^+, K^+, Al^{3+}, Ca^{2+}, Mg^{2+}, Cl^-, urea, adenine nucleotides (creatinine phosphate, ATP, ADP, AMP), lactate, and (Na^+ + K^+)-activated adenosine triphosphatase (ATPase). It was shown that in patients with ARF, the content of H_2O, K^+, and Mg^{2+} is normal, while Na^+ is modestly decreased and Al^{3+} slightly elevated. On the other hand, cerebral cortex Ca^{2+} content is almost twice the normal value.[108,113] Similar findings have also been observed in dogs with ARF.[37]

In additional studies from the brain of rats with ARF, it was observed that concentrations of creatine phosphate, ATP, and glucose were increased but were associated with corresponding decreases in AMP, ADP, and lactate. Additionally, total brain adenine nucleotide content and Na^+ + K^+-activated ATPase activity were normal to low. Thus it appears that the uremic brain utilized less ATP and therefore failed to produce ADP, AMP, and lactate at normal rates. Brain energy charge was normal, as was the redox state, and these findings were not altered by hypoxia.[479] There was a corresponding decrease in the brain's metabolic rate, along with elevated glucose and low lactate levels.[479] Other studies of uremic brain have shown a decrease in cerebral oxygen consumption.[182] Patients with chronic renal insufficiency (GFR below 20 ml/min) have decreased brain uptake of glutamine and increased ammonia uptake. The relevance of these findings, in terms of neurotransmitter synthesis storage or release, or other brain function, is unknown.[134]

In animals with either ARF or CRF, both urea concentration and osmolality are similar in brain, cerebrospinal fluid, and plasma.[38] The solute content of brain in animals with ARF is such that essentially all of the

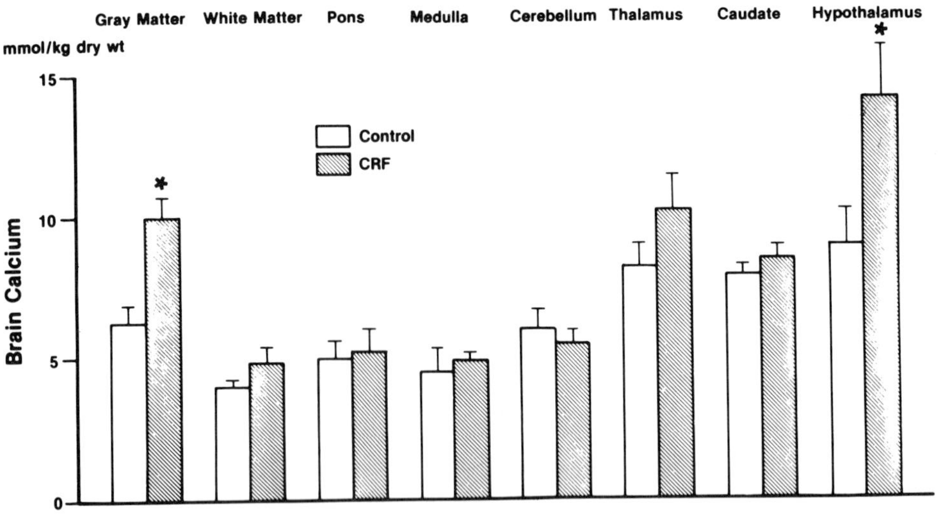

FIGURE 46-4. • Brain calcium content in 8 areas of the brain in dogs with chronic renal failure for 4 months. Brain calcium is significantly increased in cerebral cortical gray matter and hypothalamus vs. 9 control animals ($p = 0.01$). (Reproduced from Mahoney CA, Arieff AI: *Kidney Int* 24:170, 1983.)

increase in brain osmolality is due to an increase of brain urea concentration.[38] However, in animals with CRF, about half of the increase in brain osmolality is due to the presence of previously undetermined solute (idiogenic osmoles) with the other half due to an increase of urea concentration.[306] Recent studies have now identified many of the ideogenic osmoles that accumulate in conditions of plasma hyperosmolality.[228,295] These include myoinositol, sorbitol, betane, glycerophosphorylcholine, glutamine, glutamate, taurine, phosphocreatine, and creatine.

In dogs with CRF, brain content of Na^+, K^+, Cl^- and water and the extracellular space are not different from control values.[306] In brain, calcium content was found to be normal in the subcortical white matter, pons, medulla, cerebellum, thalamus, and caudate nucleus. However, as shown in Fig. 46-4, calcium was about 60 percent above control values in both cortical gray matter and hypothalamus. Both water content and magnesium content were normal in all eight parts of the brain.[306]

In animals with ARF and metabolic acidosis, the intracellular pH (pH_i) of brain, and skeletal muscle is normal.[30] In dogs with CRF, pH_i is normal in brain, liver, and skeletal muscle[307] (Fig. 46-5). In patients with renal failure, intracellular pH has been reported to be normal in both skeletal muscle and leukocytes, as well as in the "whole body"[182] (Fig. 46-6). The pH of cerebrospinal fluid was also shown to be normal in both patients and laboratory animals with renal failure.[116,358,363] Thus,

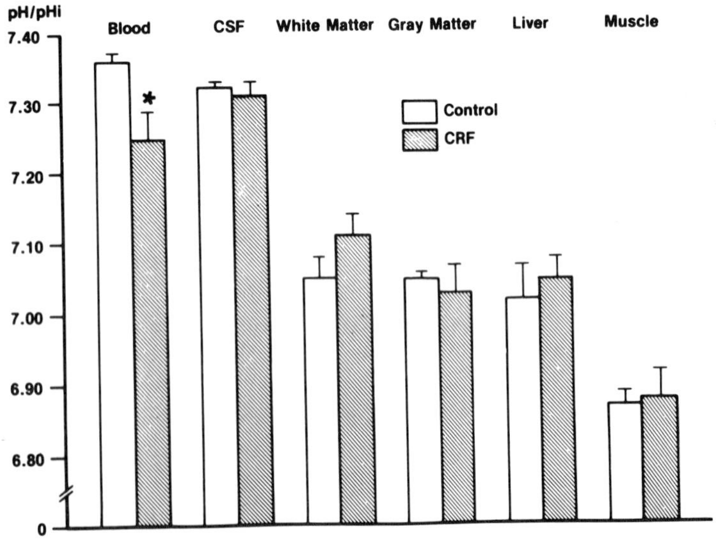

FIGURE 46-5 • The effects of 4 months of chronic renal failure (CRF) on intracellular pH (pH_i). In 8 dogs with CRF, the arterial pH was significantly below values for 9 controls. However, pH_i is normal in brain white and gray matter, liver, and skeletal muscle ($p<0.01$). (Reproduced from Mahoney CA, Arieff AI: *Kidney Int* 24:170, 1983.)

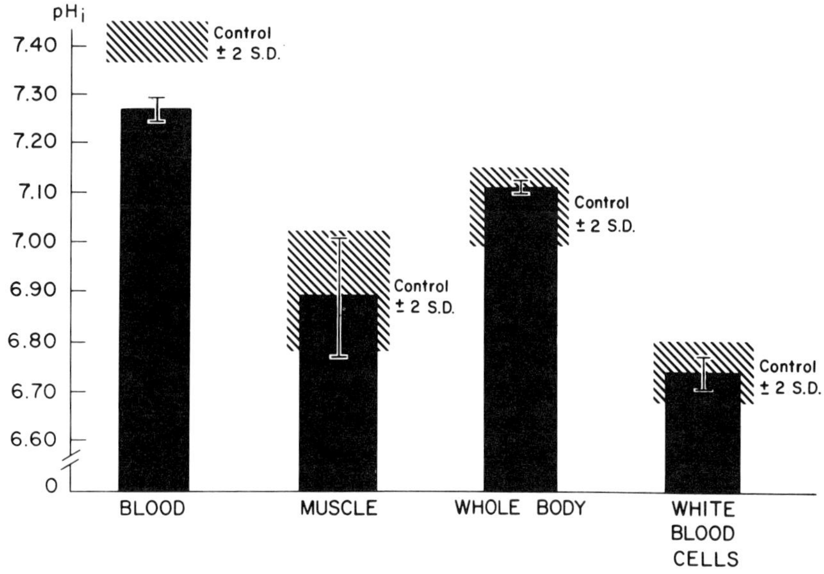

FIGURE 46-6 • Arterial pH compared with intracellular pH (pH_i) in skeletal muscle, "whole body," and white blood cells from uremic patients. Although there is significant extracellular acidemia pH_i is normal. (From Arieff AI: Neurological complications of uremia, in Brenner BM, Rector FC (eds): *The Kidney*, chap 44, Philadelphia, Saunders, 1981, p 2306.)

despite the presence of extracellular metabolic acidemia in either acute or chronic experimental renal failure, the pH is normal in brain, liver, and skeletal muscle.[181]

SUBCELLULAR CHANGES IN BRAIN

Over recent years, a number of studies utilizing subcellular analysis in the brain have been done in uremic laboratory animals. Principally, the synaptosomal system has been shown to be a useful tool in adding to our understanding of the CNS in uremia.[189,190] Synaptosomes are isolated from the presynaptic terminals of neurons by homogenization and differential centrifugation of brain tissue. Synaptosomes are metabolically active vesicles, and they function as do the intact nerve cells.[75,383,496] Like the intact nerve terminals, synaptosomes contain synaptic vesicles, mitochondria, and cytoplasmic and plasma membrane mechanisms that regulate calcium and neurotransmitter substances.[190] They have been utilized in a number of studies to investigate mechanisms of synthesis, storage, and release of neurotransmitter substances and of ion transport. In rats with ARF, Fraser and associates have shown that there is alteration of the Na^+-K^+ ATPase pump in synaptosomes in uremia.[176,189] This defect appears to be permanent once uremia develops, and thus would not be easily corrected by dialysis.

Other studies from this laboratory have also shown that both the Na^+-Ca^{2+} exchanger and the Ca^{2+} ATPase pump were altered in uremia as well.[187,190,191] Calcium transport by both these membrane calcium transporters was found to be elevated in synaptosomes isolated from rats with ARF.[176,189] However, once rats were parathyroidectomized prior to being made uremic the defects were eliminated.[187] On the other hand, injection of parathyroid hormone to parathyroidectomized uremic rats reproduced the calcium transport abnormalities of both transporters.[187]

To determine the mechanisms of action of PTH on the calcium transporters, in vitro studies were carried out to evaluate the cyclase system in the presence of PTH, cAMP, and forskolin.[191] It was shown that PTH increases both the uptake and the efflux of calcium from rat brain synaptosomes in a manner that was similar to either cAMP or forskolin. Based on these findings, it was initially felt that the mechanism of action of PTH on calcium transport in synaptosomes was cAMP-dependent as had been classically described.[392] It was also observed that parathyroid extract and 1-34 bPTH increased synaptosomal calcium transport, while 3-34 bPTH had no such effect on uptake. These findings indicated that the amino acids in positions 1 and 2 of the PTH molecule were ncessary for PTH to stimulate calcium transport in synaptosomes, and that PTH action was probably dependent on cAMP.

However, when cyclase activity was measured in synaptosomes, PTH was unable to generate cyclase activity. However, because forskolin, an activator of the catalytic subunit, and sodium fluoride (which binds to the guanine nucleotide subunit) both stimulate cyclase activity, PTH action appears independent of this second messenger. These results also indicate that the relationship between PTH and synaptosomal calcium transport was more complicated than was initially thought.

cAMP production in both renal cortical plasma membrane (CRCPM) and synaptosomes was studied in the presence of isoproterenol, a beta-adrenergic agonist, which produces many of its functions by first binding to surface receptors causing an increase in cAMP production and activation of a cAMP-dependent protein kinase.[126] 1-34 bPTH increases adenylate cyclase activity by 18-fold in CRCPM while it has no effect on the cyclase activity in synaptosomes. However, with isoproterenol, cyclase activity was increased by 50 percent in CRCPM and 90 percent in synaptosomes. This suggested that similarly to CRCPM, synaptosomes contain an intact adenylate cyclase system that can be stimulated by cyclase activators other than PTH. Thus it appears that the PTH-stimulated calcium transport observed in synaptosomes is independent of cAMP.

Under other conditions where a hormone-responsive adenylate cyclase system exists, the role of the hormone in eliciting cAMP responses can be demonstrated by measuring cAMP production in the presence of the hormone.[422,423] Examples of this relationship include inhibition of platelet aggregation by prostaglandins,[429] stimulation of lipolysis in adipocytes, stimulation of steroidogenesis in rat adrenal cells, relaxation of peripheral smooth muscle, and enhancement of secretion from blowfly salivary glands.[422] However, in the above studies, both 1-34 and 1-84 bPTH failed to produce cAMP in synaptosomes, despite the presence of an intact adenylate cyclase system.

Similar to the observations in synaptosomes, studies in other tissues have shown that PTH can produce cellular changes that are independent of the adenylate cyclase system. In a study by Hruska and associates, it was shown that PTH increased intracellular calcium in proximal tubular cells of the mammalian kidney that was independent of the cyclic nucleotides.[245] Similarly, in the opossum kidney cell line, which exhibits proximal tubular characteristics, it was also shown that PTH increased cytoplasmic calcium and produced a dose-dependent stimulation of inositol triphosphate and diacylglycerol that was not mimicked by cAMP.[246] In the isolated papillary muscle from rat heart, PTH action on papillary muscle contraction was also shown to be independent of cAMP.[262] In this study it was shown that the ionotropic action of PTH on papillary muscle was mediated by the release of endogenous norepinephrine from the myocardium, and that both the release of norepinephrine and muscle contraction were independent of adenylate cyclase activation.[262] Thus it is evident from these studies that the mechanism of action of PTH on cellular functions is quite variable and does not necessarily involve the adenylate cyclase system.

It has been shown that inositol 1,3,4,5-tetrakisphosphate (IP4) activates sea urchin eggs by a mechanism that was dependent on external calcium.[249] Similarly, hepatocytes that have their functions coupled to phospholipid turnover, when stimulated by an agonist such as vasopressin, produced a prolonged increase in intracellular calcium concentration that is dependent on extracellular calcium.[253] Also IP4 has been shown to rise rapidly in rat cerebral cortical slices after muscarinic receptor stimulation,[59] and to decline just as rapidly by inhibition of the receptor.[59,231] Thus it appears that after the agonist binds to surface receptors, phosphoinositol, a membrane-bound lipid, is converted to diacylglycerol (DAG) and inositol trisphosphate (IP3) that is then phosphorylated to IP4. IP4 by itself and/or with IP3 or DAG changes the membrane permeability of the cell to calcium so that there is an influx of calcium from the extracellular space to the cytosol.[249] The increased intracellular calcium that is produced as a result of this mechanism is different from that which is observed after the release of microsomal calcium by IP3 in tissues such as liver, muscle, bag cell neurons, and kidney.[246,381,504] This regulation of intracellular calcium from extracellular sources by an agonist is an important one and might be a possible mechanism of action of PTH in synaptosomes.

More recently, Fraser and associates have shown that some of the inositol phosphates are capable of regulating the plasma membrane Na^+-Ca^{2+} exchanger and Ca^{2+} ATPase pump.[185,188] The Na^+-Ca^{2+} exchanger was found to be inhibited by 1,4,5 IP3, and the Ca^{2+}-ATPase pump was stimulated by 1,4,5 IP3 and inhibited by 1,3,4,5 IP4. In another recent study Davis and associates also found that human erythrocyte plasma membrane Ca^{2+} ATPase activity was regulated by inositol phosphates.[128] It was shown that both 1,4,5 IP3 and inositol 4,5 bisphosphate inhibited the action of the Ca^{2+} pump. These studies imply that the intracellular second messenger for PTH in the nerve terminal in the brain may be inositol phosphates, and also that the inositol phosphates may regulate cytosolic calcium by modulating the function of the plasma membrane–bound calcium transporters (Na^+-Ca^{2+} exchanger and Ca^{2+} ATPase pump). These proposed mechanisms of action of PTH and inositol phosphates are indeed quite novel, but much work is still to be done.

PATHOLOGY

Pathologic studies of the brains of patients who died with CRF have been well documented.[181,428] Prior to 1974, subdural hemorrhages were felt to be very common in dialyzed subjects and were reported in about 1 to 3 percent of autopsies. In addition, intracerebral hemorrhages were said to be present in about 6 percent of dialysis patients who expired. Cerebral edema is not found in the brains of patients or laboratory animals with CRF, by either biochemical or histologic criteria. Generalized but variable neuronal degeneration is often present but its anatomic location is quite variable. Among patients who have died with uremia, there is some evidence of necrosis of the granular layer of the cerebral cortex. Small intracerebral hemorrhages and necrotic foci are seen in about 10 percent of uremic patients, and focal glial proliferation is found in about 2 percent. In general, changes in the brains of patients who died with CRF are usually nonspecific and are probably related to other concomitant underlying disease states.

PATHOPHYSIOLOGY

Although many factors contribute to uremic encephalopathy, most investigators have shown no correlation between encephalopathy and any of the commonly measured indicators of renal failure. Only high levels of BUN appear to show some degree of correlation with symptoms, and as general practice patients with CRF are usually started on dialysis when BUN is greater than 100 mg/dl (36 m*M*).[275] However, some patients with BUN less than 100 mg/dl may have symptoms of uremia, while others with BUN greater than 100 mg/dl may not. In recent years, there has been considerable discussion of the possible role of PTH as a uremic toxin.[114] In particular, there is a substantial amount of evidence that suggests that there are toxic effects of PTH on the central nervous system.[182,187,190]

Role of parathyroid hormone

In patients who have died with ARF or CRF, the calcium content in brain cerebral cortex is significantly elevated.[37,108,113,218] Dogs with ARF or CRF show increases of brain gray matter calcium, and EEG changes similar to those seen in humans with ARF.[37,218] In dogs, both the EEG and brain calcium abnormalities can be prevented by parathyroidectomy. Also, calcium transport by both the membrane-bound Na^{+}-Ca^{2+} exchanger and the Ca^{2+} pump in brain nerve terminals (synaptosomes) from rats that were made acutely uremic are also altered and appeared to be PTH-related.[182,187,190] Many of these changes could also be reproduced by administration of PTH to normal animals. However, in animal studies the alterations of EEG and brain calcium content could not be reproduced by elevation of the (calcium, phosphate) product or by hypercalcemia induced by vitamin D intoxication. Thus PTH appears essential to produce many of the CNS manifestations of uremia.

PTH has been shown to have CNS effects in human beings with normal renal function, and neuropsychiatric symptoms are reported to be among the most frequent manifestations of primary hyperparathyroidism. In patients with primary hyperparathyroidism, EEG changes are similar to those reported in patients with ARF.[108,113] The common denominator appears to be elevated PTH levels. In patients with ARF the EEG is abnormal within 18 h of the onset of renal failure and is generally not affected by dialysis for periods of up to 8 weeks[113] (Fig. 46-7). During this interval, patients were shown to have elevated levels of PTH in plasma. In patients with either primary or secondary hyperparathyroidism, parathyroidectomy results in an improvement of both EEG and psychological testing, suggesting a direct effect of PTH on the CNS.[108] Similarly, dialysis results in a decrement of brain (cerebral cortex) calcium toward normal in both patients and laboratory animals with renal failure, concomitant with improvement of the EEG.[37,108,218] In uremic patients, both EEG changes and psychological abnormalities are improved by parathyroidectomy or medical suppression of PTH.[108] Thus it appears that PTH and/or a high brain calcium content may be responsible, at least in part, for many of the symptoms of encephalopathy manifested in renal failure.

The above discussion must be tempered by the fact that, at this point, all measurements of brain calcium in the studies cited have only evaluated total tissue content of calcium.[37,108] In fact, it is likely that the free intracellular ionized calcium may be the important factor. Investigation in other tissues (isolated hepatocytes) sug-

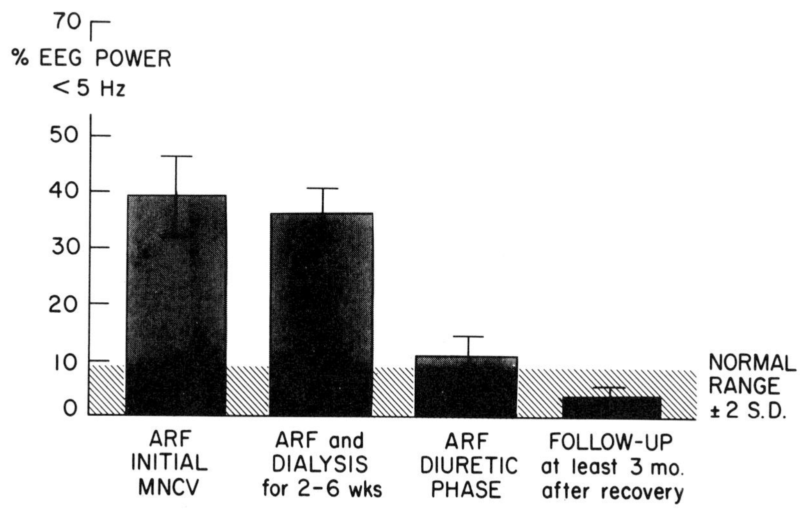

FIGURE 46-7 • Percentage of EEG power below 5 Hz (mean ± standard deviation). Normal values on right. Patients with acute renal failure (ARF) have significant changes in power below 5 Hz which are unaffected by dialysis but become normal with return of renal function. Data from 16 patients with ARF not shown. (From Cooper JD et al: *Kidney Int* 10:556, 1976.)

gests that the true intracellular ionized calcium is in the order of 150 to 400 nmol/liter, vs. the total tissue calcium of about 60 mmol/kg wet weight.[462]

The mechanism by which PTH might disturb CNS function is unclear. The increased calcium content in such diverse tissues as skin, cornea, blood vessels, brain, and heart in patients with hyperparathyroidism suggests that PTH may somehow facilitate the entry of Ca^{2+} into such tissues. The finding of increased calcium in the brain of both dogs and patients with CRF and secondary hyperparathyroidism is consistent with the concept that part of the CNS dysfunction end EEG abnormalities found in ARF or CRF may be due in part to a PTH-mediated increase in brain calcium. Calcium is essential for the function of a large number of intracellular enzyme systems, and an increased brain calcium content could disrupt cerebral function by interfering with any of them. It is also possible that PTH itself may have a direct effect on the CNS that might be detrimental. In more basic studies, Fraser and associates have provided some insight into the mechanism of action of PTH.[191]

Based on their earlier studies that show that PTH administration to nonuremic rats resulted in increased brain synaptosomal Ca^{2+} transport, and that parathyroidectomy (PTX) resulted in decreased calcium transport, it was decided to investigate the mechanism by which PTH regulated Ca^{2+} transport in rat brain synaptosomes. This was accomplished by performing calcium transport studies by the Na^+-Ca^{2+} exchanger and measured cAMP generation in synaptosomes from rat brain. Ca^{2+} transport was studied after in vivo additions of either bovine bPTH, cAMP, or forskolin, and adenylate cyclase activity was assessed after additions or either bPTH, forskolin, sodium fluoride (NaF), or isoproterenol. In the presence of 1-34 bPTH (10^{-7} M), Ca^{2+} uptake was significantly increased by 55 percent ($p < 0.001$) above control, while 3-34 bPTH (10^{-7} M) had no effect on calcium uptake. Both 8br,cAMP (10^{-6} M) and dibut, cAMP (10^{-6} M) also significantly increased ($p < 0.001$) Ca^{2+} uptake above control by 63 and 44 percent, respectively. Similarly, forskolin (10^{-5} M), the adenylate cyclase activator, increased Ca^{2+} uptake by 41 percent. They next evaluated Ca^{2+} efflux, and showed that 1-34 bPTH (10^{-7} M), 1-84 bPTH (10^{-7} M), and forskolin (10^{-5} M) also increased Ca^{2+} efflux by 50, 73, and 120 percent, respectively, above control. Since Ca^{2+} transport was increased by either PTH, cAMP, or forskolin, it was initially felt that PTH action on Ca^{2+} transport in synaptosomes was dependent on cAMP. This was investigated by measuring cAMP production during the conversion of ^{32}P-ATP to ^{32}P-cAMP in the presence of an ATP regenerating system containing creatine phosphokinase, creatine phosphate, and the cyclic nucleotide phosphodiesterase inhibitor IBMX. Whereas forskolin and sodium fluoride significantly increased ($p < 0.001$) adenylate cyclase activity in synaptosomes eight- and fourfold, respectively, neither 1-34 bPTH nor 1-84 bPTH increased synaptosomal cyclase activity. However, in canine renal cortical plasma membrane that was used as a control, significant increases in cAMP production were observed with either forskolin, NaF, or PTH. Finally, they showed that synaptosomes did contain an intact adenylate cyclase system by demonstrating that cAMP production in synaptosomes was stimulated by the beta-adrenergic agent isoproterenol which significantly increased adenylate cyclase activity in both synaptosomes (90 percent) and CRCPM (50 percent). These data suggest that although there is an intact adenylate cyclase system in rat brain synaptosomes, PTH-stimulated calcium transport in synaptosomes appears to be independent of this system.[191]

Other uremic toxins

Many substances have been touted as possible uremic toxins; however, none has been shown to correlate better with the manifestations of uremia than creatinine clearance.[18] A pathophysiologic role in the CNS dysfunction of uremia has been clearly established thus far only for PTH, although aluminum may also be important.[141,150] Pathologic and histologic examinations have generally shown minor nonspecific abnormalities. Neither brain edema nor intracellular acidosis occurs. The functional significance of the altered brain permeability, decreased brain sodium, and presence of idiogenic osmoles is uncertain. The low turnover rate of high-energy phosphates seen in rats with ARF and the decreased cerebral oxygen consumpton may be either the cause or the effect of the uremic state. The role of neurotransmitters and other peptide hormones in uremia are additional areas where further study is needed.[181]

COMPLICATIONS OF THERAPY OF UREMIA

Dialysis disequilibrium syndrome

In patients with CRF, several CNS disorders may occur. These disorders seem to occur as a consequence of the dialytic therapy, and include dialysis disequilibrium. Dialysis disequilibrium syndrome (DDS) occurs in patients being treated with hemodialysis. The syndrome, described in 1962,[270,271] may include headache, nausea, emesis, blurring of vision, muscular twitching, disorientation, hypertension, tremors, and seizures.[15] The EEG may be abnormal,[271] but this has been disputed.[273] Additional symptoms more recently described include muscle cramps, anorexia, restlessness, and dizziness.[399] Although DDS occurs in all age groups, it is more common among younger patients, particularly the pediatric age group.[215] The syndrome is most often associated with rapid hemodialysis of patients who have just started hemodialysis, but it also has been reported following maintenance hemodialysis of patients with CRF.[15,18] There has been much debate about the pathogenesis of DDS, and this is summarized elsewhere.[212,269,358,363,399,403,428,458] The clinical manifestations of DDS are summarized in Table 46-1. For convenience, they have been divided into major and minor symptoms. Mild forms of DDS may be manifested by no more than restlessness and severe headache, which may occur during or soon after hemodialysis. This is commonly followed by nausea and vomiting, often accompanied by blood pressure elevation. These symptoms may be accompanied by disorientation and tremors. Seizures and cardiac arrhythmias have been reported in the older literature but are uncommon today. The symptoms are usually self-limited, but recovery may take several days. In some instances the seizures may lead to coma. It appears that the modern methods of dialysis have altered the clinical picture of DDS. Most reports of seizures, coma, and death were reported prior to 1970. The symptoms of DDS as reported since 1970 have generally been mild, consisting of nausea, weakness, headache, fatigue, and muscle cramps. It is also unclear whether any patient ever actually died from DDS or from other associated neurologic complications of dialysis, such as acute stroke, subdural hematoma, subarachnoid hemorrhage, or hyponatremia.[428,458,459] A differential diagnosis of patients presenting with these symptoms is shown in Table 46-2. Recently, the diagnosis of DDS has become a "wastebasket" for a number of disorders that can occur in patients with renal failure and may affect the CNS. It should be stressed that the diagnosis of DDS should be one of exclusion.[15,305]

The management of DDS can be divided into preventive modalities and therapeutic maneuvers. In several studies, this syndrome has been treated by the addition of osmotically active solute (glucose, glycerol, albumin, urea, fructose, NaCl, mannitol) to the dialysate, or by substitution of sodium bicarbonate for sodium lactate (or acetate) in the dialysate.[35,402] The technique of "pure ultrafiltration" is now in common use. By this technique, the patient is subjected to ultrafiltration without dialysis, with the net result a loss of fluid without the patient's undergoing dialysis. This procedure can then be followed by conventional dialysis without ultrafiltration. Sequential use of ultrafiltration followed by dialysis has substantially reduced the incidence of DDS.[277] Chronic ambulatory peritoneal dialysis (CAPD) is currently in use worldwide. By this technique, patients undergo continuous low-volume peritoneal dialysis for 24 h/day.[60] Symptoms of DDS have not been reported in patients undergoing CAPD.[277] In both humans and experimental animals, the occurrence of DDS can best be prevented by use of "slow" dialysis, that is, low blood flow rates at frequent intervals (every 1 to 2 days).

TABLE 46-1 • **Symptoms of dialysis disequilibrium syndrome**

MINOR SYMPTOMS	
Headache	Muscle cramping
Nausea	Restlessness
Emesis	Fatigue
MAJOR SYMPTOMS	
Muscle tremors	Syncope
Visual blurring	Seizures (focal, grand mal)
Hypertension	Cardiac arrhythmias
Disorientation	

No consistent abnormalities are found in laboratory tests.

TABLE 46-2 • **Differential diagnosis of dialysis disequilibrium syndrome**

Uremia
Copper intoxication
Nickel intoxication
Hyponatremia (serum [NA^+] < 125 m*M*)
Hyperparathyroidism with hypercalcemia (serum [$Ca2^+$] > 14 mg/dl)
Hypoglycemia
Nonketotic hyperosmolar coma with hyperglycemia
Wernicke's encephalopathy
Depletion syndrome
Malfunction of fluid-proportioning system
Excessive ultrafiltration with hypotension and seizures
Cardiac arrhythmia
Acute cerebrovascular accident
Subdural hematoma
Cerebral embolus secondary to shunt clotting
Malignant hypertension
Dialysis dementia

Dialysis dementia

Dialysis dementia (also called dialysis encephalopathy) is a progressive, frequently fatal neurologic disease that was initially described in 1970[428] and then independently described by several different groups in the early to mid-1970s.[9,55,103,308,309,335,343] The disease is seen almost exclusively in patients being treated with chronic hemodialysis. Although the early literature focused on the distinctive neurologic findings,[9,87,103,308,335,343] more recent reports from both Europe and this country have suggested that some forms of dialysis dementia may be a part of a multisystem disease that includes encephalopathy, osteomalacic bone disease, proximal myopathy, and anemia.[87,370,382,488]

The etiology of this syndrome remains controversial. An increase in brain aluminum content has been strongly implicated in some cases of dialysis dementia, but the evidence is far less convincing in others. Dialysis dementia most likely represents a syndrome complex that is the final common pathway for a variety of etiological agents. Dialysis dementia can be divided into three categories: (1) an *epidemic form* that is related to contamination of the dialysate, probably with aluminum; (2) *sporadic cases* in which aluminum intoxication is less likely to be a contributory factor; and (3) dementia associated with *congenital or early childhood* renal disease. The last category has been reported in several children who were never dialyzed and some who were never exposed to aluminum compounds. These early childhood cases may represent developmental neurologic defects resulting from exposure of the growing brain to a uremic environment.[13,53,378,409,413,424,425]

The initial reports made between 1970 and 1978 were soon followed by many reports throughout the world.[18] These patients generally had the endemic form of dialysis dementia and had been on chronic hemodialysis for over 2 years before the onset of symptoms. Early manifestations consisted of a mixed dysarthria-apraxia of speech with slurring, stuttering, and hesitancy. Personality changes, including psychoses, led to dementia, myoclonus, and seizures. Symptoms were initially intermittent and were often worse during dialysis, but generally became constant. In most cases, the disease progressed to death within 6 months.[150] Speech disturbances were found in 90 percent of patients, affective disorders culminating in dementia in 80 percent, motor disturbances in 75 percent, and convulsions in 60 to 90 percent. In contrast to this fairly distinct clinical picture, brain histology has often been normal or nonspecific. Several investigators have reported histologic changes in the brains of patients with dialysis dementia that were similar to those of Alzheimer's disease,[85,281] but the distribution of aluminum in the brains appears to be different.[209]

Early in the disease, the EEG shows multifocal bursts of high-amplitude delta activity with spikes and sharp waves, intermixed with runs of more normal appearing background activity. These EEG abnormalities may precede overt clinical symptoms by 6 months. As the disease progresses, the normal background activity also deteriorates to slow frequencies.[150,370] The EEG has been said to be pathognomonic, but a similar pattern may also be seen in other metabolic encephalopathies. The diagnosis depends on the presence of the typical clinical picture and is confirmed by the characteristic EEG pattern.

In some of the initial descriptions of dialysis dementia, tin deposition in the brain was the suggested etiologic agent.[9,344] Aluminum was next implicated in the pathogenesis of this disorder,[8,87] to be in turn followed by manganese.[95] Aluminum content of brain gray matter was elevated to 11 times the normal value in patients with dialysis dementia vs. an increase of three times normal in patients on chronic hemodialysis without dialysis dementia. Aluminum content was also increased in bone and other soft tissue. Oral phosphate binders containing aluminum were originally suspected as the source of the aluminum [$Al(OH)_3$ and $Al_2(CO_3)_2$], but it is now clear that most of the excess aluminum comes from dialysate water.[150]

The source of the increased aluminum content in the brain is controversial. Significant absorption of oral aluminum can occur in patients with CRF, but the weight of evidence is against oral aluminum as the major source. The use of such compounds has been almost universal, yet many cases of dialysis dementia have occurred in an almost epidemic form with striking geographic clusters. Instead, epidemiologic studies have shown a strong association between aluminum in the water used to prepare dialysate and both the epidemic form of dialysis dementia and fracturing dialysis osteodystrophy. In a survey by the European Dialysis and Transplant Association, 92 percent of patients with dialysis dementia had used untreated or softened water, as opposed to 6 percent who had used deionized water.[66,210] Important evidence that aluminum may be responsible for dialysis dementia comes from an outbreak in Eindhoven, Holland.[169] Two dialysis units there used the same untreated municipal water supply and the same dialysate concentrate, but one unit had 6 cases of dialysis dementia in a 9-month period, yet the sister unit was unaffected. A corroding aluminum anode in the water heating system of the affected unit was found to be adding aluminum to the dialysate.

Even low levels of aluminum in the dialysate will result in a net retention of aluminum in the body. Aluminum transferred across the dialyzer binds to a nondialyzable plasma constituent, resulting in higher levels in plasma than in the dialysate. It has been estimated that a dialysate aluminum concentration of only 70 μg/liter results in a minimum positive aluminum balance of 300 μg/day.[8,255] Significant amounts of aluminum are also absorbed from the gastrointestinal tract after oral administration of aluminum hydroxide. Since aluminum is normally excreted by the kidney, this can lead to significant aluminum retention in patients with renal insufficiency.

Serum aluminum levels generally reflect dialysate aluminum levels, so that most authors have not found them useful in separating patients with dialysis dementia from other patients dialyzed in the same center. Most workers have found that brain aluminum is elevated in dialysis dementia, but it has been questioned whether high brain aluminum is the cause of neurotoxicity rather than a chance association.[305] Although some investigators were able to show a good separation between brain cortical gray matter aluminum in hemodialyzed patients with and without dialysis dementia, other authors have noted considerable overlap.[8,13,18,66,255,316,362] Surprisingly, brain aluminum levels are higher in patients with CRF not yet on dialysis than in their dialyzed counterparts. Elevated brain aluminum levels are also seen in patients with hepatic encephalopathy and metastatic cancer, as well as elderly subjects, though they are generally lower than in patients with dialysis dementia.[23] There is no obvious threshold level for brain aluminum that determines toxicity. In general, though, levels above 15 μg/kg dry weight are associated with the encephalopathy, while levels below 5 μg/kg are not. Not only is aluminum elevated in brain, but in addition, there are at least eight other trace elements that are abnormal in the brain of patients with dialysis encephalopathy (Fig. 46-8).

Deionization of the water used to prepare dialysate has recently been employed as a preventive measure.[66,150,169,488] However, deionization may be beneficial by removing any number of other agents. Other trace elements present in water can result in CNS toxicity. Such elements include cadmium, mercury, lead, manganese, copper, nickel, thallium, boron, and tin.[493] Manganese has been found to be increased in cortical white matter in the eight encephalopathic patients in whom it was measured (Fig. 46-8).[95] These patients also had elevated aluminum levels in gray matter. It is important to realize that tin was initially found to be elevated in the brain of patients with dialysis dementia, before aluminum had been routinely measured.[210]

Most of the controversy over the etiology of dialysis dementia has involved cases that occur sporadically. As noted previously, dialysate aluminum levels are not always elevated, the use of aluminum containing antacids is no different from that in unaffected patients, and brain aluminum levels in patients with dialysis dementia may overlap with those of unaffected patients. The largest group of "sporadic cases" has been reported from Nashville, TN.[141] The reported incidence of dialysis dementia in the area is 5 percent, despite the use of deionized water for dialysate with aluminum levels below 5 μg/liter. Bone disease was not clinically apparent in this group. Serum aluminum levels in the encephalopathic group were 3 to 4 times higher than in other dialyzed patients, despite equivalent prescribed doses of aluminum containing phosphate binders.[141] These results suggest greater absorption and/or retention of aluminum in this group of encephalopathic patients. No other metals were measured in the Nashville study.

Despite these unresolved questions, most outbreaks of the epidemic form of dialysis dementia were associated with high levels of aluminum in the dialysate. Lowering the dialysate aluminum to levels below 20 μg/liter, usually by deionization, appears to prevent the onset of the disease in patients newly begun on dialysis. New cases may continue to appear in those patients who were previously exposed to the high-aluminum dialysate, although the course is milder and mortality is somewhat decreased.[66] In patients with overt disease, eliminating the source of aluminum has resulted in improvement in some[66,141] but not all patients.[506] Transplantation has generally not been helpful in patients with advanced disease. Diazepam or clonazepam are useful in controlling seizure activity associated with the disease, but therapy becomes ineffective and does not alter the final outcome.[66,141] Desferioxamine, an aluminum chelating agent, may prove helpful in the early stages of aluminum overload, but its use has been associated with serious adverse reactions.[222,351]

Treatment of sporadic cases, in which the etiology is not clear, is more difficult. Every effort should be made to identify a treatable cause. Dialysis dementia must be differentiated from other metabolic encephalopathies, such as hypercalcemia, and hypophosphatemia, hyperparathyroidism, acute heavy metal intoxication, drug intoxications, and structural neurologic lesions, such as

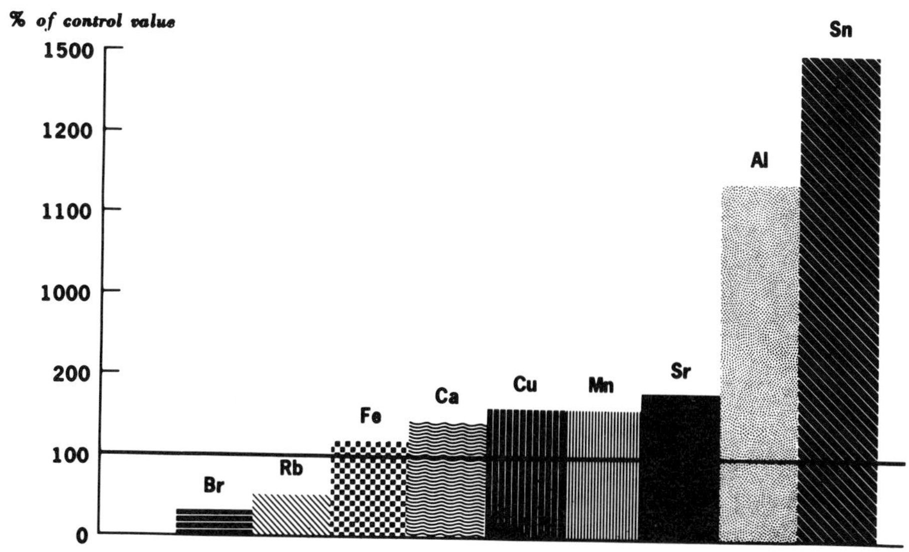

FIGURE 46-8 • Brain (cerebral cortex) content of nine trace elements in patients with dialysis dementia. Solid black line (100 percent of control value) represents normal. In addition to aluminum, 8 other elements are abnormal in brains of patients with dialysis dementia: bromine, rubidium, iron, calcium, copper, manganese, strontium, and tin. (From Arieff AI: Neurological complications of uremia, in Brenner BM, Rector FC (eds): *The Kidney*, chap 44, Philadelphia, Saunders, 1981, p 2306.)

TABLE 46-3 • Differential diagnosis of dialysis dementia

Metabolic encephalopathies:
- Hypercalcemia
- Hypophosphatemia
- Hypoglycemia
- Hyperosmolality
- Hyponatremia
- Overt uremia
- Drug intoxications
- Trace element intoxications: manganese, mercury, lead, nickel, thallium, boron, vanadium, chromium, tin, cadmium
- Hyperparathyroidism

Hypertensive encephalopathy

Dialysis disequilibrium

Structural lesions:
- Subdural hematoma
- Normal pressure hydrocephalus
- Stroke

subdural hematoma (Table 46-3). Because of the low incidence, the uncertain etiology, and the poor correlation of plasma with tissue aluminum levels, screening tests have not generally been employed. However, in the European experience, a high incidence of bone disease occurred after a shorter exposure to high-aluminum dialysate than required to produce encephalopathy. Thus screening EEGs and neurologic examination with emphasis on speech disturbances might be useful in the early detection of encephalopathy in patients with the typical osteomalacic bone disease.

HEPATIC ENCEPHALOPATHY

INTRODUCTION

Hepatic encephalopathy is a clinical syndrome characterized by abnormal mental status occurring in patients with severe hepatic insufficiency. It is a neuropsychiatric disorder that is associated with characteristic but nonspecific histologic lesions in the CNS.[2,177,179] The clinical manifestations range from slightly altered mental status to frank coma, with death a frequent sequel. The neuromuscular complications may vary from slight incoordination and tremor to ophthalmoplegia and incontinence (see Chap. 37).

The symptoms of hepatic coma are directly related to the rapidity with which the hepatic failure develops and to the severity of liver failure. The causes are numerous and have been reviewed elsewhere.[513] With the advent of many new hepatotoxic drugs, the increased consumption of alcohol, and easy access to high-protein foods by patients with preexisting hepatic dysfunction, hepatic encephalopathy is now a fairly common disorder in most major metropolitan hospitals.[63,242,503] Although the overall outlook for patients with hepatic encephalopathy is dismal at best, the clinical manifestations of this disorder are often reversible. This is often achieved by such simple techniques as avoidance of alcohol (ethanol), a low-protein diet, and the appropriate use of lactulose and/or neomycin.[110,478]

CLINICAL MANIFESTATIONS

Neurologic and neuromuscular abnormalities are the predominant symptoms observed in patients with hepatic encephalopathy. The symptoms may initially be mild but eventually progress to frank coma if the encephalopathy is not corrected. The severity of the symptoms depends on the acuteness and extent of liver failure and on the development of metabolic or infectious complications. In trying to characterize these patients it is important to classify the syndrome into grades of encephalopathy and to clinically assess mental state, neuromuscular status, and precipitating factors.[112]

The agents responsible for producing hepatic failure, which may then lead to hepatic encephalopathy, are numerous and have increased markedly in recent years. The degree to which these numerous agents produce symptoms is directly proportional to their aciton on the liver. The many causes of liver failure[179,512,515] include viral hepatitis; many drugs such as sedatives, tranquilizers, and analgesics; gastrointestinal bleeding; metabolic alkalosis; diuretics; potassium depletion; fluid and electrolyte abnormalities; and uremia.[179,248,512,515] Some of these agents are directly toxic to the liver while others build up to toxic concentrations in blood as they are not metabolized by the liver. The early stages of hepatic encephalopathy are manifested by irritability, restlessness, confusion, and clouding of the sensorium. As the encephalopathy progresses the patients may become comatose and exhibit fetor hepaticus. *Fetor hepaticus* is a variable but characteristic odor that is felt to be present in all patients in stage IV hepatic coma. The cause of the odor is unclear, but it is thought to be produced by mercaptans.[515] Asterixis is also a prominent feature of hepatic encephalopathy and is usually seen quite early in the course of hepatic insufficiency. It can be elicited by having the patient extend the arm, dorsiflex the wrist, and then watch for the characteristic flap. When the patient is comatose, the flap can be elicited by dorsiflexing the hand by pressing on the fingertips. If the patient's mental status is such that he or she can only grasp the examiner's fingers, asterixis can be demonstrated by the involuntary clenching and unclenching of the patient's fists.

DIAGNOSIS

Hepatic encephalopathy is a clinical syndrome, and the diagnosis is based on history, physical examination, and laboratory findings. The history and physical examination will be suggestive of hepatic failure, and neurologic examinations will demonstrate alteration in neuromuscular and mental status, including asterixis. Patients with acute hepatic failure are usually quite jaundiced, and the diagnosis of liver failure is generally quite apparent. On the other hand, in patients with chronic cirrhosis jaundice may not be readily apparent.

As mentioned earlier, hyperammonemia is found in the majority of patients with hepatic encephalopathy.[514] This, however, is not always the case since the blood ammonia depends on both rate of production and metabolism of ammonia. Because of the apparent discrepancy the use of blood ammonia to diagnose hepatic encephalopathy is quite unreliable. The usefulness of this test appears to be in following the clinical state of individual patients, rather than in diagnosing hepatic encephalopathy. Normally peripheral tissue takes up only small quantities of ammonia. Therefore, the arterial and venous ammonia levels are quite similar. If, however, blood is drawn with a tight tourniquet or the patient clinches the fist too vigorously, venous ammonia will be markedly elevated. For this reason it is suggested that ammonia determination be made either from arterial blood or from a large vein without use of a tourniquet. The cerebrospinal fluid glutamine, which is the end product of cerebral ammonia metabolism, is usually elevated in hepatic encephalopathy.[243] Elevated cerebrospinal fluid glutamine levels have been shown to be more specific than blood ammonia levels, and may distinguish between encephalopathy of hepatic vs. nonhepatic causes. Ammonia and hence glutamine may also be elevated in hepatic encephalopathy as a consequence of ensuing renal failure. This then may result in worsening coma or misinterpretation of these tests.[248] Abnormalities of amino acids, short-chain fatty acids, and false neurotransmitters have been alluded to earlier in this chapter. In general, it has been found that determinations of these substances (in both blood and/or cerebrospinal fluid) may be abnormal in hepatic encephalopathy, and whether this represents a cause or effect is not well established.

The EEG may also be used to diagnose hepatic encephalopathy. In patients with hepatic coma there is generalized slowing of cerebral electrical activity, usually accompanied by high voltage and slow waveforms.[111] Triphasic waves in paroxysmal bursts are characteristically found in the EEG of patients with hepatic encephalopathy, as are paroxysms of delta waves (1 to 3 Hz).[300,357] These EEG abnormalities of hepatic encephalopathy are characteristic but not specific for this disorder since other metabolic encephalopathies can cause similar abnormalities.

THERAPY

The treatment modalities of hepatic encephalopathy are quite numerous at present, and each is aimed at decreasing the potentially toxic protein metabolites absorbed into the bloodstream. Since the introduction of *lactulose* (1, 4-galactosidofructose) as the therapeutic agent for the treatment of hepatic encephalopathy the treatment of this disorder has been much improved.[112] This synthetic disaccharide is neither absorbed nor hydrolyzed in the upper intestinal tract of humans;[125] it is metabolized by bacteria in the lower intestine, producing lactic, acetic, and formic acids, and carbon dioxide. The beneficial effect of lactulose largely results from acidification of the intestinal lumen to about pH 5.5. This favors the conversion of ammonia to ammonium ion in the gut and the movement of ammonia from the intracellular space (pH about 6.8) to the extracellular space (pH about 7.4), and then to the more acid intestine. This leads to trapping of ammonium ion in the gut and its excretion in the stool.[125]

In 1977, Conn and associates conducted a double blind controlled trial comparing lactulose with neomycin-sorbitol combination in the treatment of hepatic encephalopathy.[110] They found a significant improvement in mental status, asterixis, and score on the trailmaking test (a standard psychological test of mentation). There was also significant improvement in the EEG and a lowering of blood NH_3 in both lactulose and neomycin-sorbitol treated groups. The mean stool pH was reduced by neomycin-sorbitol to 6.1 and by lactulose to 5.5. This difference was highly significant and reflects favorably on the use of lactulose in therapy of hepatic encephalopathy. As discussed elsewhere in this chapter, lactulose must be administered with caution. Its overzealous use can result in substantial loss of free water via osmotic diarrhea, which can lead to serious hypernatremia.[339,490,502]

Neomycin is an antibiotic that has long been used in the treatment of hepatic encephalopathy. It is postulated that in patients with hepatic coma, neomycin works by sterilizing the gut flora, thus preventing the production of ammonia from proteins and amino acids. Approximately 1 to 3 percent of neomycin given either orally or by enema is absorbed. This may lead to both ototoxicity and nephrotoxicity.[244] Treatment failures with neomycin, possibly secondary to neomycin-resistant strains of klebsiella or proteus, have been demonstrated. Alternative choices of antibiotics include ampicillin,[323] kanamycin, tetracycline, and sulfonamides. Ampicillin in particular appears to be a rather attractive choice because of the low incidence of side effects.[120,353]

Many other modes of therapy have been tried in patients with hepatic encephalopathy. These include protein restriction, branched-chain amino acid supplements, ketoanalogues of essential amino acids, metronidazole, bromocryptine, lactose, and levodopa administration.

These have all been shown to be of some benefit in controlled and uncontrolled trials and are discussed elsewhere.[65,120,121,257]

Other radical approaches used in the treatment of patients and experimental animals with hepatic encephalopathy included intravenous mannitol for cerebral edema,[92] surgical exclusion of the colon,[144,247] and exchange transfusion.[411,475] Cross-circulation with either a baboon or an irreversibly comatose donor has also been attempted.[179] Charcoal hemoperfusion has also been used in patients with acute hepatic failure.[179]

Complications of therapy

Hypernatremia is a common clinical problem in patients with hepatic encephalopathy, and it is usually a complication of excessive loss of free water, either via osmotic diarrhea (secondary to lactulose administration) or by osmotic diuresis (secondary to intravenous infusion of fructose and/or mannitol).[179] These complications are discussed elsewhere in this chapter (see section on hypernatremia). The possible contribution of the hypernatremia to the pathogenesis of hepatic encephalopathy is not known, but it may well be an important factor in certain patients.

Hyponatremia frequently complicates the course of end-stage liver disease.[356] Symptomatic hyponatremia in the alcoholic subject carries a grave prognosis (see section on hyponatremia in this chapter). The possible compounding effects of hyponatremia in a patient with hepatic encephalopathy are not known but may play a substantial role in the progression of this disorder in selected patients.

PATHOPHYSIOLOGY

It is commonplace to think of hepatic encephalopathy as being secondary to accumulation in ECF of toxic products that have gotten into the systemic circulation without being metabolized by the liver. This has been shown to occur in patients with end-stage liver disease who have developed collateral circulation secondary to increased portal venous pressure.[234,250,315,373,514] However, recent evidence has shown that other important mechanisms may also be involved. These include changes in blood-brain barrier, abnormal neurotransmitter balance, disturbed cerebral energy metabolism, and impairment of Na^+-K^+ ATPase activity in neuronal membranes.[250,296,352,415] The current pathophysiologic concepts of hepatic encephalopathy are discussed in several recent reviews.[112,119,179,357]

Role of ammonia

Elevated plasma ammonia is a common occurrence both in patients with cirrhotic liver disease and/or hepatic coma as well as in animals with portocaval anastomosis.[234,250,513] It has also been shown to occur in encephalopathies associated with certain congenital diseases and in Reye's syndrome.[151,168,324,451] Since the early reports of hepatic coma developing in patients with severe liver disease after the ingestion of nitrogenous material,[196,367,444] many reports have been published about the gastrointestinal production of ammonia and its possible toxicity in hepatic failure. The origins of these materials in the gastrointestinal tract include ingestion of meat, other protein, or ammonium salts as well as gastrointestinal bleeding or constipation.[244] It has been shown that ammonia is generated primarily by the action of colonic bacteria and mucosal enzymes acting on these substrates.[111] After the ammonia is generated, it is transported through the portal circulation to the liver where it is normally converted to urea via the urea cycle.[111] In patients with hepatic failure, ammonia is not metabolized, so it enters into the systemic circulation without being converted into urea. The ammonia can then enter the CNS. It has been suggested that encephalopathy may then develop with increasing brain ammonia concentration.[298,299]

High blood levels of ammonia have been shown to stimulate glucagon secretion in cirrhotic patients, particularly in those with portal-systemic shunts.[250] Glucagon is also markedly elevated in dogs with portal caval shunts[440] as well as in rats who had the same procedure performed.[234,257] The increased glucagon secretion provides increased hepatic gluconeogenesis from amino acids that results in further ammonia production. The evidence for this has been shown in cirrhotic patients who experienced rapid rise in blood ammonia level after ingestion of different amino acids.[111] Therefore, elevated blood ammonia associated with portal systemic shunts is not due only to increased intestinal production of ammonia but also due largely to increased ammonia production by liver from amino acids secondary to increased glucagon stimulation. Another source of increased ammonia in the CNS appears to be increased production of ammonia in the brain secondary to cerebral catabolism of these amino acids.[416,491,513]

As a result of the above sequence, there is increased gluconeogenesis such that insulin secretion is increased to maintain euglycemia. The increased insulin secretion stimulates the uptake and metabolism of branched-chain amino acids by muscle, resulting in decreased serum levels of valine, leucine, and isoleucine.[332] Blood levels of the aromatic amino acids, however, such as aspartate, glutamate, tyrosine, methionine, phenylalanine, and free tryptophan are markedly elevated.[98,243,333,352,400,455]

Role of amino acids

Glutamine

Regardless of the cause of the elevated plasma ammonia, there is generally an increased brain ammonia concentration in hepatic coma. Ammonia is detoxified in the brain by astrocytes by its reactions with glutamic acid to form glutamine.[250] There is good evidence that suggests that the degree of neurologic dysfunction correlates very well with glutamine concentration in the cerebral spinal fluid.[243] The increased synthesis of glutamine in the brain raises brain glutamine to a new steady state, where the efflux rate is determined by both the K_m for glutamine as well as the K_m for all the other neural amino acids.[179] This may in turn lead to abnormal plasma and brain amino acid concentrations, which may then result in deranged neurotransmission in patients with hepatic encephalopathy. Ammonia is detoxified in the CNS through the citric acid cycle. One molecule of ammonia combines with alpha-ketogluteramate to form glutamic acid. This then combines with another molecule of ammonia to form glutamine. The net result of this reaction is the consumption of ATP and depletion of alpha-ketogluteramate.[70] Glutamine soon thereafter becomes elevated in the cerebral spinal fluid.

Tryptophan

Rapid rise in plasma concentrations of aromatic amino acids is thought to be important in the pathogenesis of hepatic encephalopathy. Tryptophan in particular has been shown by numerous investigators to be toxic to the CNS.[179] It has also been demonstrated that there is an increased concentration of its metabolites, such as serotonin, in the brain. This has been observed in both human and experimental hepatic failure.[236,347] The toxic manifestations of tryptophan in hepatic encephalopathy may actually be due to serotonin (5-hydroxytryptamine), which is known to have significant effect on the CNS.[508] Both tryptophan and serotonin levels are closely related to each other in the CNS in hepatic encephalopathy. The increase in brain serotonin level in experimental hepatic coma cannot be explained by comparison with the total plasma tryptophan level but is actually better correlated with the free, unbound tryptophan level in plasma.[236,347] The portion of plasma tryptophan that is bound to plasma albumin is not available for transport into the brain.

There is an associated increase in plasma-free fatty acid with the elevated· free plasma tryptophan that is present in experimental hepatic encephalopathy.[352] To help elucidate the pathogenic role of tryptophan in hepatic coma, Ono and associates studied three patient groups (control, stable cirrhosis, hepatic coma), in which plasma and cerebrospinal fluid tryptophan levels, free fatty acid, amino acid, and albumin levels were evaluated.[352] They demonstrated that blood levels of both free tryptophan and free fatty acids were elevated in hepatic coma with an associated marked decrease in serum albumin level. Of all the amino acids investigated in the cerebrospinal fluid, only tryptophan was found to be significantly increased in patients with hepatic coma when compared with stable cirrhotic patients.[352] They concluded that the elevated cerebrospinal fluid tryptophan and serotonin levels seen in stable cirrhotic subjects were probably influenced by plasma neutral amino acid concentrations, whereas in patients with acute hepatic failure, free tryptophan was primarily responsible for the elevated concentrations in the brain of tryptophan and 5-hydroxytryptamine. This conclusion is also consistent with that of Cummings and associates.[121,122] Buxton and associates working with pigs in an experimental model of acute hepatic failure found a significant increase in cerebrospinal fluid concentrations of glycine, alanine, and methionine.[89]

Methionine and mercaptans

The metabolism of methionine in the gut by bacteria results in the production of mercaptan (methanethiol), which has long been shown to be toxic to the CNS in animals with hepatic encephalopathy.[514,515] Serum methanethiol levels have also been shown to be significantly raised in patients with hepatic encephalopathy. Plasma methionine levels correlate quite well with the degree of coma in such patients.[315] In animal studies, very high concentrations of mercaptans have been shown to produce reversible coma.[515] On the other hand, in vitro studies have demonstrated that low concentrations of methanethiol (mercaptan) inhibited microsomal Na^+-Ka^+ATPase activity in the brain, by inhibition of the sodium-dependent portion of the pump.[174]

High concentrations of both mercaptans and free fatty acids have also been shown to interfere with the detoxification of ammonia in the urea cycle.[514] They both act synergistically with ammonia to produce encephalopathy at lower concentrations than are usually required individually. Methionine also may be metabolized to taurine, which can produce cerebral dysfunction in human beings. There is a direct correlation with plasma taurine levels and the degree of encephalopathy.[407]

Alpha-ketoglutaramate

Bessman and associates suggested that the depletion of alpha-ketogluteramate through the mechanism discussed above may be responsible for the toxic effects of ammonia.[70] However, other investigators have demonstrated a linear rise of both alpha-ketogluteramate and glutamine concentration during infusion of ammonium acetate in rats.[235] Glutamate concentration, on the other hand, remained unchanged. These workers also measured the concentration of ammonia, glutamate, glutamine, and alpha-ketogluteramate in human beings and reported an excellent correlation with the degree of coma and the concentration of alpha-ketogluteramate. Alpha-ketogluteramate level was at least fourfold greater in encephalopathic patients than in control patients without liver disease, as well as in those with liver disease who were not encephalopahtic. Glutamine concentration in cerebrospinal fluid also showed a good correlation with the clinical symptoms of encephalopathy.

In order to assess the toxic potential of alpha-ketogluteramate, it was administered as an intraventricular infusion to rats. Within 5 min they developed myoclonic jerks, circling behavior, and 25 percent reduction in running activity.[179] When alpha-ketogluteramate concentration was further increased in cerebrospinal fluid to levels that were 100-fold greater than those found in patients in hepatic coma, there was no further decrease in running activity. From these data it was presumed that alpha-ketogluterate may be toxic to the CNS.

Fatty acids

Cats fed short-chain fatty acids (e.g., butyric, valeric, caproic acids) had suppression of their midbrain neocortical reticular activating system.[334] The EEGs of these cats were similar to those seen in hepatic encephalopathy. The investigators then measured short-chain fatty acids in the blood of patients in hepatic coma and found them to be at least five times greater than normal. However, a good correlation between fatty acid level and the degree of encephalopathy was not observed. Other investigators have also produced depression of sensorium in many animal species by intravenous or intraperitoneal infusion of fatty acids.[512] The amount of fatty acid required to produce unconsciousness in rats decreased with increasing chain length and increased fatty acid concentration. In vitro studies by many investigators have demonstrated that low concentrations of fatty acids can inhibit Na^+-K^+ ATPase activity in brain microsomes, and that this action is probably achieved by inhibition of potassium movement into the cell.[6,174,473] Additionally, free fatty acids have been shown to displace tryptophan from albumin, making more free tryptophan available to act as a CNS toxin.

Role of neurotransmitter substances

It has been postulated that one of the mechanisms responsible for the symptoms of hepatic encephalopathy is the alteration in concentrations of various neurotransmitter substances in the brain. These alterations result in the production of false neurotransmitter substances that displace the normal neurotransmitters from the synaptosomes of presynaptic nerve endings. These false neurotransmitters include gamma aminobutyric acid (GABA), octopamine, serotonin, histamine phenylethanolamine, and catecholamines, all of which have been shown to be elevated in cerebrospinal fluid and serum of patients with hepatic encephalopathy.[76] The importance of these false neurotransmitters rests in the fact that they possess significant inhibitory and stimulatory effects on the brain and therefore can profoundly affect the normal neurotransmission in human beings.

GABA and glycine, the two most potent inhibitory neurotransmitters, have been shown to be quite important in the pathogenesis of hepatic encephalopathy.[261] It has been postulated that in hepatic encephalopathy there is increased gut production of GABA, octopamine, and other amines[166] by colonic bacteria. The GABA level in palsma tends to correlate with the degree of hepatic encephalopathy. The high plasma levels of GABA are due to increased absorption by the intestine and a decreased rate of hepatic extraction of GABA. The normal blood-brain barrier is impermeable to GABA. However, in hepatic encephalopathy, the blood-brain barrier is altered, which facilitates GABA uptake. This results in up-regulation in the brain of components of the GABA-receptor complex and a down-regulation of receptor sites of the excitatory neurotransmitters, such as glutamate and aspartate. This may then lead to abnormalities in central sympathetic and parasympathetic conduction to the vasculature and heart. Such stimuli could result in variations in blood pressure and possibly cardiac arrhythmias.[395,397] The increased CNS outflow may also result in decreases in thyroid stimulating hormone (TSH) secretion,[252] alteration in the endocrine function of the pancreas, and possibly alterations in the function of other endocrine glands as well.[268,419,485]

GABA probably produces its inhibitory action by increasing membrane permeability to chloride ions. When chloride makes contact with the appropriate membrane receptors, it is transferred across the membrane. In so doing a chloride equilibrium potential is generated that is similar to that of the resting potential of the cell.[394] The above action of GABA is not a universally accepted one. Several investigators have presented evidence that GABA may not actually penetrate the CNS. Intravenous administration of high concentrations of GABA to mice did not produce any significant behavioral changes and GABA levels in the whole brain did not increase. Van Gelder and associates also found no detectable amount of GABA in the cerebrospinal fluid of unanesthetized monkeys given GABA parenterally.[480] More recently Ferenci and associates[157] studied normal rabbits and those with hepatic encephalopathy and found that there were changes in the status of neurotransmitter receptors. They demonstrated that development of hepatic encephalopathy was associated with (1) a decrease in the density of receptors for the two excitatory amino acid neurotransmitters studied, aspartate and glutamic acid; (2) an increase in receptor density of both the high- and low-affinity binding site of strychnine (a marker for the inhibitory neurotransmitter glycine); (3) a decreased affinity of receptors for dopamine; and (4) no appreciable change in the specific binding of endorphins or synthetic opiates to opiate receptors or in the density and affinity of acetylcholine receptors.[157] It was presumed that hepatic encephalopathy may be associated with incresed sensitivity to inhibitory amino acid neurotransmitters and decreased sensitivity to excitatory amino acid neurotransmitters.

Octopamine is another false neurotransmitter that is reported to be cerebrotoxic and is greatly increased in the brains of experimental animals with hepatic encephalopathy. Some investigators have presented evidence that octopamine is made in the gut by the action of bacteria on tyramine,[331] but others have suggested that octopamine can be synthesized in the brain from amino acids. It is also suggested that the brain level of both octopamine and tyrosine is well correlated in experimental animals with the extent of the decrease in liver function.[52] However, Fisher and associates have suggested that since octopamine is only one of the many amino acids elevated in the brain in hepatic encephalopathy, this may not contribute significantly to the development of hepatic encephalopathy.[165]

Blood-brain barrier

Instead of hepatic encephalopathy resulting from accumulation of cerebrotoxic substances that are not detoxified by the liver, it has been suggested that the CNS effect of these substances may actually be due to alteration of the blood-brain barrier. This could result in easy access of toxic substances to the brain.[119,241] As mentioned earlier, studies performed to assess the integrity of blood-brain barrier in animals with hepatic encephalopathy suggest that there is increased permeability to certain substances that are excluded by the blood-brain barrier in normal animals.[158] Livingston and associates studied the integrity of blood-brain barrier in hepatectomized rats using both intravenous trypan blue and arterial injection of tissue extracts.[296] They showed that with the administration of tissue extracts the blood-brain barrier became permeable to D-sucrose, inulin, and L-glucose, substances that usually do not cross the blood-brain barrier. They also showed that there was increased permeability of the barrier in response to trypan blue injection. On the basis of their data it does appear that there are changes in blood-brain barrier in hepatic encephalopathy that can allow substances that normally cannot enter the brain to do so. The brain of comatose rats usually showed cerebral edema on gross examination and swollen astrocytes on microscopic examination. In another study Horowitz and coworkers demonstrated an increased accumulation of ^{14}C-alpha-aminoisobutyric acid (^{14}C-AIB) in rabbits with acute hepatic failure. The increased transfer of ^{14}C-AIB occurred many hours prior to the development of encephalopathy.[241]

PATHOLOGY

Many structural changes in both neurons and glial cells have been identified in the brain of both human and experimental models of hepatic encephalopathy. The neurons generally show focal necrosis. However, Alzheimer type I and II lesions are the principal pathology in the protoplasmic astrocytes.[2] All these morphologic changes have been shown in humans, but studies in experimental animals have not shown all aspects of this pathology. The significance of these changes, however, is not specific for hepatic encephalopathy since they can be produced experimentally in many different metabolic disorders.

Pilbeam and coworkers, using three different models of hepatic encephalopathy in rats, found different pathology in the brain of each model.[371] When coma was induced by carbon tetrachloride–induced hepatic failure, a wide variety of structural changes in the brain was observed. These included diffuse gliosis, Alzheimer cells, and focal neuronoal necrosis. The severity of the lesions was directly related to the level of plasma ammonia. Portacaval anastomosis in young rats resulted in minimum neurologic symptoms. The brain showed no evidence of Alzheimer cells or gliosis. However, astrocyte nuclear swelling, swelling of the perivascular astrocyte foot process, and spongiform changes in the molecular layer of the cerebellum were observed. On the other hand, when portacaval anastomosis was followed by gavage feeding with ammoniated cation-exchange resin, there was a marked elevation of blood ammonia level and severe neurologic symptoms were produced. Not only astrocytes but also oligodendrocytes and neurons showed nuclear and cytoplasmic swelling along with Alzheimer type II changes. They concluded that ammonia ion probably plays an important role in the genesis of structural changes in the brain during hepatic encephalopathy.[371] Other investigators have also demonstrated astrocytic nuclear enlargement, Alzheimer type II cells, and gliosis in the brain of animals with carbon tetrachloride–induced cirrhosis. Unlike the study of Pilbeam et al., these changes were not associated with elevated blood ammonia. In animals that underwent portacaval anastomosis and were fed ammonia resin, Norenberg and Lapham[340,341] found structural changes in the brain and neurologic symptoms similar to those reported by Pilbeam. The symptoms included postural changes, stupor, coma, and convulsion. Norenberg, however, did not find oligodendroglial swelling or neuronal necrosis.[340,341] In the brain of animals with portacaval anastamosis that were not fed ammonia resin, Cavanaugh and coworkers repeatedly found Alzheimer type II cells in addition to astrocytic nuclear swelling and spongiform changes.[96]

As opposed to the observations in portal systemic encephalopathy, the brain does not show characteristic morphologic changes in patients or animals with acute fulminant hepatic failure. The major complication reported here is cerebral edema, which occurs in up to 50 percent in some series.[489] The degree of cerebral edema can be quite severe and may often be the cause of death.[489,491] Among 16 of 32 patients found by Ware and associates to have cerebral edema at autopsy, four had evidence of cerebellar and/or uncal herniation. The patients with cerebral edema were younger and had more prolonged periods of stage IV hepatic encephalopathy.

HYPONATREMIA*

Hyponatremia is probably the most common electrolyte abnormality seen in a general hospital population. The incidence and prevalence are about 1.0 and 2.5 percent, respectively.[46,104] It is commonly seen in association with many different systemic diseases. Hyponatremia is usually the result of dilution, with loss of sodium playing only a minor role. In theory it may be either *acute* or *chronic*, but in clinical practice, such differentiations canot usually be made because the actual duration of the hyponatremia is not known. Total body water may be either high, low, or normal, depending upon the level of total body sodium and potassium (see Chap. 20).

NEUROLOGIC MANIFESTATIONS OF HYPONATREMIA

Neurologic manifestations of hyponatremia may be observed when plasma sodium is 130 mmol/liter or less. Symptoms and signs most commonly include nausea, emesis, and headache. More severe symptoms and signs can include muscular twitching, grand mal seizures, coma, and respiratory arrest. Less commonly seen are weakness, bizarre behavior, urinary incontinence, tremulousness, bradycardia, hypertension, hypothermia, dilated pupils, and decreased respiration.

Systemic manifestations of stable hyponatremia

In patients with stable hyponatremia, the systemic manifestations are usually of only moderate severity and associated with a low morbidity and mortality. In a classical study, patients whose mean serum sodium concentrations were gradually reduced from 147 to 131 mmol/liter all experienced constant thirst, impaired sensation of taste, and anorexia, and several experienced muscle cramps, general exhaustion, with dyspnea on exertion, and dulling of sensorium.[314] In individuals with a stable but larger depression of serum sodium (120 to 130 mmol/liter), nausea, emesis, and abdominal cramps may occur.[36,115] With even more severe stable hyponatremia (below 120 mmol/liter), subjects may manifest weakness, lethargy, restlessness, confusion, delirium, impaired mentation, muscle twitching, and convulsions.[115,257,456]

Many other neurologic abnormalities have been reported in patients with protracted hyponatremia, including focal weakness, asterixis, ataxia, positive Babinski sign, organic brain syndrome, and cognitive impairment. In general, depression, overt psychosis, and anxiety are rare.[198,257,503]

Stable hyponatremia is common in patients with edematous states such as congestive heart failure, nephrotic syndrome, renal insufficiency, or liver failure. In these settings total body water is increased more than that of sodium.[183,356] Stable hyponatremia is also associated with the syndrome of inappropriate secretion of vasopressin (SIADH), which may be caused by various tumors, many CNS diseases, or lung diseases. Among hospitalized patients, SIADH is commonly seen with the administration of various drugs, including oral hypoglycemics, tricyclic antidepressant agents, anticancer agents, diuretics, clofibrate, and morphine-like analgesics (see Chap. 20).[326] Stable hyponatremia may also be seen in patients with such salt-losing states as salt-losing renal diseases, excessive sweating, Addison's disease, and gastrointestinal electrolyte loss. Patients ingesting massive quantities of beer with little solute also become hyponatremic.[183] A lowered cerebral threshold for ADH release occurs both in the elderly and in certain chronically ill patients.[206] These patients either have "reset osmostats" that are manifested as sustained hyponatremia in the face of intact ability to excrete free water and concentrate the urine, or they may have idiopathic SIADH.[135,206] Finally, the acquired immune deficiency syndrome (AIDS) is a major cause of electrolyte disorders, including hyponatremia.[202,256,487] The hyponatremia in patients with AIDS may be secondary to SIADH, which is often secondary to intrathoracic or intracranial lesions, to selective mineralocorticoid deficiency, to volume deficiency and replacement with hypotonic fluids, or to drug reactions.[5,106,124,487] The mortality among AIDS patients with hyponatremia appears to be about twice as high as for those with AIDS who do not have hyponatremia, while the mean survival time is only about one-third as long.[124]

In unselected hyponatremic patients, the degree of hyponatremia does not correlate with either the severity of symptoms or the eventual outcome.[36,46] Patients with serum sodium below 115 mmol/liter may be asymptomatic,[46] while others whose sodium is 128 mmol/liter may present with respiratory arrest or frank coma.[16,36,178] The mental status of 65 consecutive hospitalized hyponatremic patients whose plasma sodium was 128 mmol/liter or less is plotted against plasma sodium in Fig. 46-9. There is in general a good correlation, albeit considerable overlap. Similar findings have been reported by others;[183] some patients with serum sodium of 120 to 128 mmol/liter had severe neurologic manifestations while others with serum sodium in the same range were asymptomatic.[36]

* Readers should also refer to Chap. 20. This evolving area is controversial, and views differ. Editor.

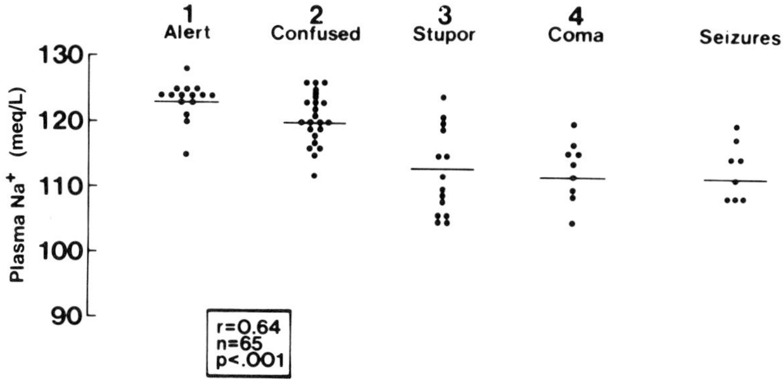

FIGURE 46-9 • Relationship between plasma Na^+ concentration and depression of sensorium in 65 patients with plasma $[Na^+]$ of ≤ 128 meq/liter. Although overall correlation is highly significant, substantial overlap among groups of patients is present. All patients who had seizures had plasma $[Na^+]$ of < 121 meq/liter. (From Arieff AI et al: *Medicine* 55:121, 1976.)

PATHOGENESIS OF HYPONATREMIC ENCEPHALOPATHY

Hyponatremic encephalopathy occurs as a consequence of the following sequence of events: (1) the presence of hyponatremia leads to a movement of water into brain cells that can begin as soon as 20 min after the serum sodium is less than 130 m*M*;[36] (2) vasopressin, and perhaps other hormones, lead to a direct movement of water into brain cells independent of the effects of hyponatremia; (3) at the time edema is accumulating, the brain is not ischemic, as it is functionally able to extrude sodium[28,36] by active transport; (4) pressure of the swollen brain on the rigid skull leads to a marked decrease in cerebral blood flow[405,447] and cerebrospinal fluid production;[156] (5) at this time, the brain is actively extruding osmotically active cation to attempt to lower the osmolality without substantial gain of water;[322] this process is accelerated by certain peptide hormones; (6) vasopressin and/or estrogen has a direct effect on the brain to decrease synthesis of ATP[184] and decrease Ca^{2+} influx, impairing outward transport of Na^+ and K^+[186] by any of several mechanisms[349] that are not well defined;[154] thus the brain's ability to adapt is impaired, leading to increased edema; this process appears to involve an interaction between gonadal steroids and vasoactive polypeptides;[286] (7) if hyponatremia is not corrected, the resolution between (5) and (6) will lead to increased edema (particularly in females), with eventual tentorial herniation of the brain,[16,178] secondary occlusion of cerebral vessels, and cerebral ischemia; (8) with herniation of the brainstem, there is respiratory arrest,[16] with further decrease of CBF and additional ischemia. The above sequence has been verified by means of MRI and postmortem examination in over 75 hyponatremic patients.[178,469] The most important component of this postulated sequence appears to be inhibition of the regulatory volume decrease (RVD), which involves active transport of Ca^{2+}, Na^+, and K^+,[294] impairing the ability of the brain to adapt to hyponatremia. The exact contribution of any of the above factors must be ascertained and the role of physical factors, hypoxia, and other hormones—androgens, angiotensin, atriopeptin, estrogen, progesterone—must also be clarified.[286]

HYPONATREMIA AND HORMONAL EFFECTS

Vasopressin

Most studies of hyponatremia in both children and adults demonstrate that virtually all hyponatremic patients have increased blood levels of the hormone arginine vasopressin.[12,88,117,127,214,254] Arginine vasopressin (AVP) is synthesized in the hypothalmus and transported to the posterior pituitary. The cortical cerebrospinal fluid (cerebrospinal fluid) carries the AVP from the hypothalamus to pituitary capillaries.[384,398] The hormone is secreted into the cerebrospinal fluid of the third ventricle.[385] While in the cerebrospinal fluid, vasopressin binds directly to brain cells,[368] where its cerebral effects are mediated by intracellular second messengers.[156,404] The intracellular second messengers include nitric oxide, cyclic GMP, and inositol triphosphate, all mediated by V1 receptors.[185,505] The vasopressin migrates in the cerebrospinal fluid of the third ventricle to the portal blood flowing to the pituitary gland.[278,385] From the pituitary, vasopressin is then secreted into the bloodstream. After secretion into the cerebrospinal fluid of the third ventricle, the hormone binds to V1 receptor sites on neurons and blood vessels. In general, neither AVP nor most other hormones that have effects on the brain have access to the brain parenchyma (insulin may be an exception), as such access is not needed. All these substances bind to brain cells and exert their effects inside the brain by means of second messengers. For AVP in brain, an important second messenger is inositol triphosphate (IP3).[185,505] A linkage has been demonstrated between IP3 and vasopressin V1 receptors in the brain.[185,258] There are multiple cerebral effects of vasopressin. Vasopressin administration in the rat, acting through cerebral V1 receptors, results in water movement into the brain in the absence of hyponatremia,[137,145,404] a significant decline in brain synthesis of ATP,[184] decreased brain blood flow and cerebrospinal fluid production,[156] and impairment of several possible pathways for sodium efflux during hyponatremia.[259,260] The decline of cerebral ATP synthesis in female rats after vasopressin administration may be related in part to brain ischemia from cerebral vasoconstriction. The vascular reactivity of vasopressin, a potent vasoconstrictive agent,[205] is significantly greater in female rats than in males.[445] Following blood loss, plasma vasopressin levels are significantly higher in female rats than in males.[453] In studies where hyponatremia is induced with either water alone[477] or water plus a vasopressin analogue, desmopressin (DDAVP, which has no effect on the brain V1 receptor),[44] the aforementioned cerebral effects of vasopressin are absent, demonstrating the probable importance of vasopressin in the pathogenesis of hyponatremic encephalopathy. All these phenomena can lead to deleterious effects on brain function, which are largely independent of the effects of hyponatremia per se.

Estrogen, progesterone, and androgens

The early adaptation of the brain to hyponatremia is by loss of blood and cerebrospinal fluid, followed by extrusion of sodium from brain cells.[322] Loss of potassium and possibly amino acids follows later, in an attempt to decrease brain cell osmolality without further gain of water.[36,322,466] Preliminary studies from our laboratory have demonstrated that hyponatremic male rabbits were better able to extrude sodium to decrease brain cell osmolality than were female rabbits, resulting in significantly less brain swelling in male than in female rabbits.[44] After an initial loss of cerebrospinal fluid via bulk flow, extrusion of sodium is the most important early defense of the brain against hyponatremia.[322] A major reason for the apparent increased morbidity and mortality in females compared with males may include a diminished ability of the female brain to adapt to hyponatremia by limiting the amount of brain swelling. There is substantial evidence that estrogens stimulate vasopressin release, while androgens appear to suppress it.[7,434,452] In addition to effects on vasopressin release, estrogens may antagonize brain adaptation via the Na^+-K^+ ATPase system[138,186] while androgens may enhance such adaptation.[216]

Atrial natriuretic peptide

Atrial natriuretic peptide (ANP) may improve brain adaptation to hyponatremia. Atrial natriuretic peptide in the CNS appears to play an important role in the regulation of brain water content in several pathologic states characterized by cerebral edema.[145,146,282,336,337] During the regulatory volume decrease observed with hyponatremia, an important initial response in the brain is a loss of sodium.[322] ANP may act to decrease cell volume by effecting a net decrease of the intracellular sodium concentration in nerve cells. Sodium is constantly being removed from brain cells, much of it by the Na^+-K^+ ATPase system.[184] By decreasing sodium uptake in pathologic states, the net effect of ANP would be a decrease in intracellular sodium, as it continues to be pumped out by Na^+-K^+ ATPase. The effect of ANP appears to be opposite to that of vasopressin, both in vivo[145] and in astrocytes in vitro.[137] ANP also affects the regulation of cerebrospinal fluid production[446,476] and hence the cerebrospinal fluid pressure.[145] Biologic ANP receptors produce 3′,5′-cyclic guanosine monophosphate (cyclic GMP) as the second messgner for ANP in diverse tissues.[107] ANP has been shown to stimulate cyclic GMP production in the brain, and cyclic GMP–inhibited sodium uptake in synaptosomes in a manner similar to ANP.[260] Cyclic GMP appears to be an important second messenger for ANP in the brain. Another important second messenger in the brain, nitric oxide (NO), also can stimulate production of cyclic GMP.[439]

Effects of physical factors

Physical factors often play an important role in adaptation to hyponatremia, particularly in small children and the elderly. The physical factors include differences in the ratio of intracranial capacity to brain size, cerebrospinal fluid volume, and brain water and electrolyte content. In humans and laboratory animals, brain water content is more than 2.5 times higher in the young, decreasing progressively with advancing age.[263,338,498] In children, the ratio of brain to skull size is such that there is less room for expansion of the pediatric brain in the skull than there is in the adult.[220] As adults age, there is a progressive decline in the brain volume while skull size remains constant.[220] Anatomically, this means that there is decreased room for expansion of the brain within the skull in children compared with adults.[136] Adult brain size is reached at about age 6, while full skull size is not reached until age 16. Additionally, the intracerebral volume of cerebrospinal fluid is more than 10 percent greater in the adult than in the young.[220] When brain swelling occurs, the intracerebral loss of cerebrospinal fluid increases the available volume in which the brain can expand.[321,405] Since the percentage of cerebrospinal fluid in the brain increases with age, adults of both genders have more room in the rigid skull for the brain to expand than do children.[220] It has been demonstrated in newborn puppies that the brain is unable to adapt to hyponatremia.[338]

Hypoxia and hyponatremic encephalopathy

The occurrence of a hypoxic event such as respiratory insufficiency is a major factor contributing to permanent brain damage in patients with hyponatremia.[16] The combination of systemic hypoxemia and hyponatremia is far more deleterious than is either factor alone because hypoxia impairs the ability of the brain to adapt to hyponatremia.[483] The hyponatremia leads to a decrement of both CBF[405] and (by depressing respiration) arterial pO_2. We have described more than 45 patients with symptomatic hyponatremia who had an arterial pO_2 below 50 mmHg when the hyponatremia was diagnosed.[20,45,469] Such a degree of hypoxia without hyponatremia has been associated with substantial CNS morbidity[240,346] or coma[427] in healthy human beings.

Hypoxic brain damage is a major component of the neurologic disability observed in many hyponatremic subjects.[20,45] Hypoxia is often manifest clinically as the syndrome of delayed postanoxic encephalopathy. This syndrome can follow anoxia-hypoxia from any cause but is most often related to hypoxia (as a consequence of either carbon monoxide intoxication, strangulation, cardiopulmonary arrest, or various miscellaneous intoxications,[201] with subsequent resuscitation).[376] Whatever the cause of coma, patients are initially deeply comatose and usually require artificial ventilation. Characteristically, they begin to regain consciousness within several days. Initial improvement is often rapid, but from several days to several weeks, and in exceptional cases as late as 5 to 6 weeks, patients begin to relapse. The onset may be abrupt and heralded by disorientation, confusion, restlessness, apathy, or inappropriate behavior. There may be cortical dysfunction that may be multifocal in character, with dysphasia, agnosia, and apraxia. Motor control is often impaired, with resultant rigidity or spasticity, often associated with grand mal seizures and a second respiratory arrest.[201] Recovery followed by recurrent coma has frequently been observed in hyponatremic patients who have been treated with hypertonic NaCl,[16] and is similar to the sequence previously described in patients who have suffered hypoxic-anoxic episodes from other causes.[201] There are no obvious features during the initial anoxic insult that serve to distinguish those patients destined to relapse from those who have uncomplicated recoveries. Such patients are often initially misdiagnosed as having primary cerebral pathology, such as subdural hematoma.[16] In patients with hyponatremic encephalopathy, the diagnosis must be made on clinical grounds. CT or MRI usually demonstrate diffuse cerebral demyelinative lesions,[469] which are similar to those seen in other clinical situations where hypoxic encephalopathy occurs. In the past, patients with hyponatremia and hypoxic encephalopathy have sometimes been misdiagnosed as having "central pontine myelinolysis" (CPM).[74,465,469,471] Death or a persistent vegetative state is often the outcome,[16,469] but some patients with hypoxic encephalopathy recover.[86,465,509]

Female preponderance among patients with symptomatic hyponatremia and brain damage

Multiple interactive hormonal mechanisms regulate CNS water and electrolyte metabolism. Although hyponatremic encephalopathy can occur in anyone, there is a clear predisposition for its occurrence in menstruant women (of reproductive age). Since 1935 there have been several hundred reported cases of symptomatic postoperative hyponatremia, often accompanied by coma and seizures, many of which appear in the older surgical literature.[36,56,58,140,194,229,421,463,516] Despite the fact that serum sodium was often below 120 mmol/liter and symptoms were present, neurologic morbidity and mortality were low. Since many of these patients were in reasonably good health and scheduled for elective surgical procedures, the absence of serious associated medical illness was assumed to account for the low morbidity and mortality. Recent studies demonstrate that the age and gender of the patient are major determinants of brain damage due to hyponatremia.[45] In general, most patients with symptomatic hyponatremia (sodium $\leq$ 128 mmol/liter) who did not suffer permanent neurologic damage were older women or men of any age, while those who died or developed permanent brain injury have been menstruant women.

Pathologic lesions in patients with hyponatremic encephalopathy

There are many reported pathologic studies of the brain in patients who died from hyponatremic encephalopathy. In what is probably the first published case, a patient who had absorbed 9000 ml of tap water was studied 1 h after death.[229] The calculated serum sodium was less than 110 mmol/liter. Examination of the cranial contents revealed obliteration of the subarachnoid space. The cerebral gyri were flattened, sulci were largely obliterated, there was uniform enlargement of the brain in all directions, and the ventricles were reduced in size. Microscopically, there was increased vacuolization and swelling of supportive (glial) structures, with cellular swelling apparently confined to white matter. Brain edema with both uncal and tonsillar herniation[391] was found in one study.

Patients dying with hyponatremic brain damage manifest three general types of neuropathologic patterns (Table 46-4).The first pattern (pattern A) occurs in patients who die in less than 2 days after respiratory arrest without specific therapy for the hyponatremia. In these patients, one finds diffuse cerebral edema and often gross evidence of herniation. However, herniation can be easily

TABLE 46-4 • Pathologic lesions in patients with hyponatremic encephalopathy

	Group A	Group B	Group C	Group D
Clinical course of hyponatremia	Respiratory arrest prior to specific therapy for hyponatremia	There is usually a diagnosis of hyponatremia before respiratory arrest. Therapy includes elevation of serum sodium by more than 25 mmol during initial 48 h	(a) Respiratory arrest, (b) central diabetes mellitus and insipidus, (c) hyperglycemia, (d) spontaneous elevation of serum sodium above normal	Diagnosis and timely initiation of appropriate therapy before respiratory arrest
Typical gross pathological lesions in the brain	Cerebral edema, often with herniation. May be grooving of uncus or cerebellar tonsils	Diffuse demyelinating lesions; cerebral infarction	(a) Diffuse demyelinating lesions, (b) pituitary ischemia/necrosis, (c) oculomotor nerve damage	No cerebral abnormalities
Usual eventual outcome	Death or permanent brain damage	Outcome can be either: (a) recovery, (b) permanent brain damage, (c) death	No known long-term survivors to date	Recovery without sequelae if therapy has been appropriate

overlooked if it has not been specifically searched for. The second pattern (pattern B) often shows diffuse demyelinating lesions of the brain, generally accompanied by cerebral edema. The third pattern (pattern C) also shows diffuse demyelinating lesions, but these are often accompanied by pituitary necrosis and occulomotor cranial nerve damage.[178] The topographical distribution of lesions of pattern C most commonly involves basal ganglia, periventricular white matter, cerebral cortex, and thalamus[46,178,469] (Fig. 46-10). The fourth pattern (pattern D) occurs in patients where the diagnosis is made prior to respiratory arrest and appropriate therapy is carried out. The pathogenesis of these lesions in hyponatremic encephalopathy includes contributions from (1) hypoxia and (2) elevation of serum sodium by more than 25 mmol/liter during the initial 48 h of therapy. This can occur as the result of either central diabetes insipidus[178] in untreated patients or overcorrection as the result of inappropriate therapy.[49] The mean brain weight in women dying from hyponatremic encephalopathy without therapy typically is more than 8 percent greater than the control value. When the patients were hyponatremic, radiologic examinations often revealed tentorial herniation. At autopsy, even in the presence of hypernatremia from the syndrome of central diabetes mellitus and insipidus (*Fraser-Arieff syndrome*), patients often have had gross evidence of herniation, with grooving of the uncus and/or cerebellum. Such patients also often have ischemic infarcts of both the anterior and posterior pituitary lobes, ischemic lesions of the hypothalamus, and necrosis of the medulla. Evidence of hypoxic brain damage (neuronal ischemia, diffuse demyelination of much of the cerebellum, midbrain, and subcortical white matter) is very common, as are infarcts in the middle cerebral artery distribution[469] (Fig. 46-10). When CPM has been specifically looked for by detailed examination of the pons, it is generally absent.[469] Patients who have suffered severe hypernatremic brain damage have often had extensive brain demyelination that included basal ganglia, cerebellum, and subcortical white matter in addition to occasional demyelinating lesions of the pons. Such lesions are typical of hypoxic/ischemic brain damage.[93,284,377]

Central pontine myelinolysis

CPM was initially described by Adams and associates[3] as "a single, sharply outlined focus of myelin destruction which indiscriminately affected all fiber tracts." In three large series of autopsied patients, the incidence of CPM has been found to range from 0.17 to 0.28 percent, with a mean of about 23 cases per 10,000 autopsies.[3,203,320] Some patients with CPM may also have extrapontine demyelinating lesions, but these are generally symmetrical.[510] Among the over 200 cases of CPM described to date, virtually all patients had severe associated medical conditions, such as advanced liver disease, extensive burns, sepsis, Hodgkins's disease, or other malignancies.[3,73,99,203,320,325,471] Currently, the diagnosis of CPM has frequently been made by radiologic criteria employing either CT or MRI of the brain.[73,142,325,464] Unfortunately, the diagnosis of CPM has often been suggested even though radiologic examination (CT and/or MRI) was either not carried out[450] or disclosed only extrapontine cerebral demyelinating lesions.[73,469]

More recently, extrapontine cerebral demyelinating lesions have sometimes been mistakenly diagnosed as CPM.[325,412] It has been suggested that "rapid" therapy of hyponatremia might lead to development of cerebral demyelinating lesions,[342,471] which have often been referred to as "central pontine myelinolysis or "osmotic demyelination syndrome," even in the presence of extensive lesions elsewhere in the brain, absence of pontine lesions,[288,449,450,469] or lack of any change in plasma osmolality prior to respiratory arrest. In fact, in much of the experimental animal literature that purports to provide supportive evidence that "rapid" therapy of hyponatremia could lead to pontine lesions, such lesions were not even present.[276] The pathologic and radiologic literature demonstrates numerous clinical conditions associated with brain lesions that resemble CPM but are not associated with hyponatremia. These include increased intracranial pressure, subcortical arteriosclerotic encephalopathy, radiotherapy, and multiple ischemic lesions as well as sequelae of head trauma, malignant hypertension, or cerebral hemorrhage.[201,325,412,507] A recent study of 20 patients with a preliminary diagnosis of CPM revealed that the diagnosis was incorrect 85 percent of the time.[469] Furthermore, all patients who did have CPM also had a history of chronic alcoholism, a condition known to be associated with CPM.[3] Figure 46-10 summarizes the topography of the brain lesions in those patients labeled "CPM." Moreover, animal studies clearly demonstrate that the pons is not involved in the brain damage often incorrectly labeled "CPM."[47,50,442] Thus use of terms such as "central pontine myelinolysis" and "osmotic demyelination syndrome" to describe patients with treated hyponatremia and brain damage seems unwarranted, based on information currently available.

Animal studies

There are several studies in laboratory animals where the relationships between hyponatremia, its therapy, and the possible development of CPM have been investigated.[148,276,287] In one study, Kleinschmidt-DeMasters

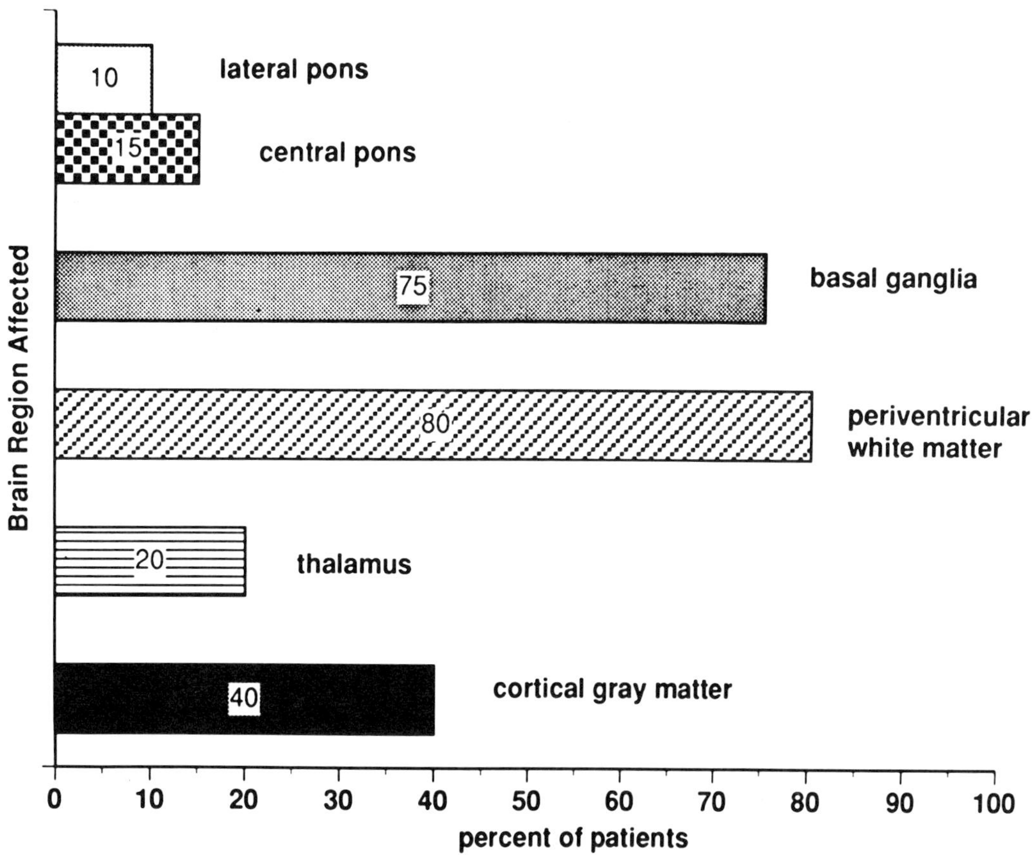

FIGURE 46-10 • The distribution of brain lesions in 20 patients who had a preliminary diagnosis of central pontine myelinolysis (CPM). Only 5 patients had pontine lesions, and only 3 of 20 patients had anatomic criteria for the diagnosis of CPM. The distribution and morphology of the lesions, as well as the clinical histories, are compatible with hypoxic brain damage. (Figure reproduced from Tien R et al: Hyponatremic encephalopathy. *Am J Med* 92:513, 1992, with permission.)

and Norenberg[276] made rats acutely hyponatremic (serum sodium = 106 ± 12 mmol/liter). Animals then had their mean serum sodium increased from 106 to 152 mmol/liter in about 1 h with 1M NaCl. Control animals were also made hyponatremic (plasma sodium = 100 ± 4 mmol/liter) and "self-corrected" to 136 ± 24 mmol/liter in 5 days. Demyelinating lesions were found only in rats treated with hypertonic NaCl. Lesions were not found in the pons but did occur in eight other parts of the brain. In evaluating this study, it must be pointed out that rats that developed demyelinating lesions were "corrected" to grossly hypernatremic levels (152 mmol/liter) while controls were actually modestly hyponatremic (136 mmol/liter). It has previously been pointed out that hypernatremia may actually be an important etiological factor in the development of CPM.[82] In another study, Laureno produced hyponatremia (serum sodium below 120 mmol/liter) in mongrel dogs.[287] Four days of such hyponatremia produced a mortality of 63 percent. Sixteen dogs received 514 mmol/liter NaCl over 6 h plus water restriction. Five dogs improved neurologically and did not have CPM, while five deteriorated neurologically and had either CPM (4 dogs) or extrapontine myelinolysis (1 dog). There are several rather striking differences between the two groups. The four dogs who developed CPM had a serum sodium of 100 ± 4 mmol/liter prior to therapy, while the six without CPM had serum Na^+ of 121 ± 14. Five of six with myelinolysis were "corrected" to hypertonic (serum Na^+ = 142 to 157 mmol/liter) levels. It is well known from both human and animal studies that either hypernatremia or overcorrection of hyponatremia can lead to cerebral demyelination.[47,50,320,482] Thus the studies by both Laureno and Kleinschmidt-DeMasters would not appear to have clinical relevance to the therapy of hyponatremia in humans.[276,287] Overall then, some animal studies suggest that elevation of very low (below 105 mmol/liter) plasma sodium to hypernatremic levels (above 140 mmol/liter) with hypertonic NaCl may induce cerebral demyelinating lesions. However, these lesions are histologically different from the lesions of CPM observed in humans, and such studies do not appear relevant to more modest correction of plasma sodium to subnormal levels (about 130 mmol/liter) in humans.

DIFFERENTIAL DIAGNOSIS OF HYPONATREMIC ENCEPHALOPATHY

Following routine surgery, some patients who do not have hyponatremia manifest headache, nausea, and emesis. However, this is rare after the initial postoperative day. Patients with postoperative hyponatremia also commonly present with headache, nausea, and emesis.[16] While there may be some confusion about the differential diagnosis, if a postoperative patient is receiving hypotonic fluids, hyponatremia should always be part of the initial differential diagnosis. When a postoperative patient who is receiving hypotonic fluids manifests headache, emesis, nausea, or lethargy, the serum sodium should be measured. Although such symptoms are not diagnostic, the diagnosis is easily established at minimal cost and with virtually no risk to the patient by evaluation of plasma electrolytes. When symptomatic hyponatremia is so diagnosed, early treatment can be instituted before a hypoxic-anoxic episode such as respiratory arrest occurs.

In a patient who suddenly develops a symptom complex that can includes opisthotonus, respiratory depression, impaired response to verbal and/or painful stimuli, bizarre behavior, incontinence of urine or feces, visual auditory hallucinations, lethergy, decorticate and decerebrate posturing, and seizure activity, the differential diagnosis may appear to be quite extensive. However, since patients with symptomatic hyponatremia may also develop respiratory arrest, fixed dilated pupils, and abnormal temperature regulation within 24 h,[183] the serum sodium must always be promptly evaluated in such situations. The respiratory arrest may be diagnosed as being related to the administration of morphine or meperidine (Demerol). However, in a generally healthy postoperative individual, respiratory depression from a therapeutic dose of demerol or morphine is extraordinarily rare, and there is usually no response to the intravenous administration of naloxine HCl (Narcan). Furthermore, following an overdose of morphine or meperidine, the pupils are constricted (pinpoint) while patients with hyponatremia and herniation often develop dilated pupils. The decorticate and decerebrate posturing is frequently diagnosed as a reaction to phenothiazine drugs promazine (Sparine), promethazine HCl (Phenergan), or prochlorperazine (Compazine) that have been administered for nausea. These have been treated by discontinuing the agent and administrating diphenhydramine HCl (Benadryl) or benztropine mesylate (Cogentin), again without any response. The sudden obtundation has occasionally been diagnosed as acute viral encephalitis, but this can generally be ruled out by examination of the cerebrospinal fluid. Fixed, dilated pupils are often thought to be indicative of brain death. Largely for this reason, many patients have received no therapy for their low serum sodium. However, in the presence of brain death, pupils are fixed and midpoint, not dilated.[435] The fixed, dilated pupils are most likely caused by cerebral herniation, with pressure of the temporal lobe on the third cranial (oculomotor) nerve or occlusion of the posterior cerebral artery near the third nerve. Many patients develop some combination of unilateral and then bilateral dilated pupils, absent pain response, apnea, and a positive Babinski sign. These signs and symptoms are frequently interpreted as being consistent with various drug reactions (see above) or acute intracranial events, such as subarachnoid bleeding episodes. Acute intracranial episodes can and should be ruled out by CAT scan or MRI of the head. All of the above events are consistent with acute progressive brain herniation, and this can generally be diagnosed by modern imaging techniques (CAT scan and/or MRI).[142,285,469]

An important complication of hyponatremic encephalopathy is the syndrome of central diabetes mellitus and insipidus (Fraser-Arieff syndrome), which is caused by cerebral herniation complicated by pituitary vascular insufficiency.[178] The central diabetes mellitus and insipidus, if untreated, generally leads to polyuria, hyperglycemia, and hypernatremia (Fig. 46–11).

TREATMENT OF HYPONATREMIA

General

In patients with hormone deficiencies that may predispose to hyponatremia (hypothyroidism, adrenal insufficiency), treatment should be directed primarily at the underlying disorder. If the hyponatremia is symptomatic, NaCl should be administered along with the appropriate replacement hormone, since the plasma sodium is rarely below 125 mmol/liter, and therapy with hypertonic NaCl is rarely required.

There are a vast number of pharmacologic agents that may interfere with the ability of the kidney to excrete a water load.[330] Included are large numbers of sedatives, hypnotics, analgesics, oral hypoglycemic agents, tranquilizers, antipsychotic agents, narcotics, and antineoplastic drugs. Hyponatremia associated with these agents may be acute, is often symptomatic, and may require treatment with hypertonic NaCl. Severe water intoxication may also occur in psychotic individuals even when they are not taking such drugs, particularly those who have schizophrenia with associated self-induced water intoxication[484] or those with other organic psychosis.[225] Whatever the etiology of symptomatic hyponatremia, when it occurs, it is important to recognize and treat it promptly.

Asymptomatic hyponatremia

In patients whose hyponatremia is asymptomatic, aggressive therapy with hypertonic NaCl is usually not indicated. This is particularly true if the plasma sodium is above 120 mmol/liter. In patients who are obviously volume-depleted, isotonic NaCl is usually the fluid of choice. In patients in whom adrenal insufficiency or hy-

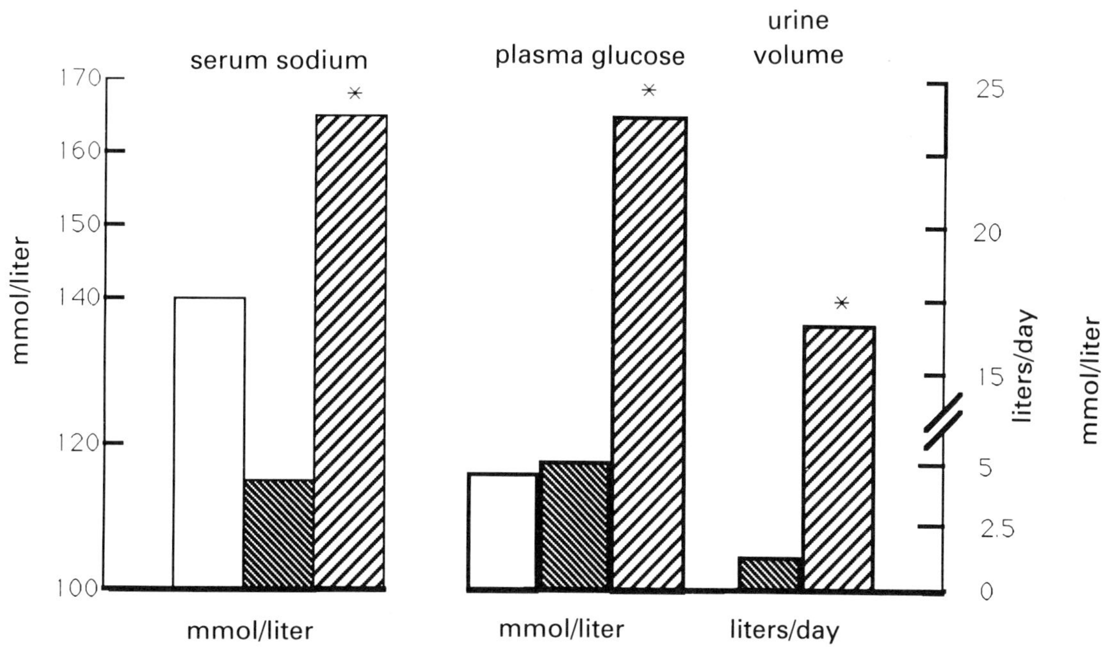

FIGURE 46-11 • The clinical course of 11 women with symptomatic postoperative hyponatremia. After a mean of 32 h following surgery, the mean serum sodium had fallen from 140 to 116 mmol/liter, but plasma glucose and urine volume were normal. Over the next 18 to 55 h, urine volume spontaneously increased from 38 to 689 ml/h while serum sodium increased from 116 to 167 mmol/liter and plasma glucose from 96 to 433 mg/dl (for glucose, 1 mmol/ liter = 18 mg/dl). An asterisk signifies $p < 0.001$ vs. both the preoperative value and the 32-h postoperative value. [Reproduced from Fraser CL, Arieff AI: Fatal central diabetes mellitus and insipidus resulting from untreated hyponatremia: A new syndrome. *Ann Intern Med* 112(2):113, 1990, with permission.]

pothyroidism has been identified, appropriate hormone replacement is warranted. If the patient is receiving any drugs known to predispose to hyponatremia, they should be discontinued if possible. In most cases of asymptomatic hyponatremia, however, none of these factors are present. Although water restriction can theoretically be of benefit in such subjects, practical considerations render it largely useless. With fluid restriction of less than 1 liter/day, a negative water balance occurs and the serum sodium will be slowly corrected. However, that rate of correction will rarely exceed 1.5 mmol/liter per day. *Thus water restriction is never appropriate if a patient with hyponatremia is symptomatic.*

Several medical measures have been proposed for the long-term management of stable hyponatremia. Lithium has been used, with a modest and erratic response, to treat a few patients with SIADH.[432] Toxicity to the kidneys, CNS, heart, and thyroid has been reported in patients receiving long-term lithium treatment for affective disorders. Demeclocycline, a tetracycline antibiotic, can be associated with nephrogenic diabetes insipidus in doses above 600 mg/day. It has been used successfully to treat patients with SIADH,[101] but acute renal failure and renal tubular toxicity have been reported in hyponatremic patients with heart failure or cirrhosis.[327,356] Other drug regimens reported in the treatment of chronic hyponatremia include urea and inhibitors of AVP.[132,199] Use of these agents is still experimental.

Symptomatic hyponatremia

In patients with symptomatic hyponatremia, the presenting symptoms are often dramatic (seizures or respiratory arrest) and often indicate a far advanced process for which any therapy is unlikely to produce a viable patient. Awareness of the situations where symptomatic hyponatremia may develop is the most important step in management. The most common situation in which this occurs is the postoperative patient. Multiple factors conspire to impair the ability of the kidney to excrete water in postsurgical subjects; these include preexisting volume depletion (GI fluid losses and diminished oral intake) and other nonosmotic stimuli for vasopressin release (pain, nausea, drugs, and the surgery itself).[420] Patients who have undergone transurethral resection of the prostate have an additional special risk: the use of isosmotic, electrolyte-free solutions for irrigation of the operative field. These solutions can be absorbed through the prostatic bed at a rate of 0.6 liter/h or more and have the effect of an equivalent volume of intravenous free water administration. Thus every postoperative patient should be considered at risk for the development of hyponatremia, and appropriate prophylactic measures should be taken. If they are not, and respiratory arrest ensues, treatment after the fact is often associated with substantial mortality and neurologic morbidity.

Hyponatremia: rate versus magnitude of correction

In patients with severe symptomatic hyponatremia, the preponderance of clinical and laboratory evidence suggests that the morbidity and mortality of correction by water restriction alone is unacceptable.[47,49,50,51,414] Therefore, more active correction of hyponatremia with hypertonic NaCl is indicated in symptomatic patients.[49,414] In some situations, simultaneous administration of furosemide is necessary to prevent circulatory overload.[224]

In the past, there has been some controversy concerning the rate at which hyponatremia should be corrected. Some authors suggested that the development of CPM was associated with rapid correction of long-standing hyponatremia.[448] Other investigators have suggested that cerebral demyelinating lesions (what has in the past been referred to as CPM) seem to develop only when patients with stable hyponatremia are inadvertently made hypernatremic during treatment, or if the absolute increase in serum sodium exceeds 25 mmol/liter in the first 24 to 48 h of therapy, particularly if other risk factors are present.[49] These observations can be most easily explained by referring to the nature of cell volume homeostasis. In symptomatic acute hyponatremia, cerebral intracellular water content is increased and solute content is normal. Under such circumstances, treatment with hypertonic fluids causes cellular efflux of excess water and a prompt return to the baseline state. Alternatively, a patient with stable chronic hyponatremia may have nearly normal brain cell volume but decreased brain cell solute. During rapid correction, cell volume will tend to decrease, and there may be a lag period before the neurons and/or glial cells switch from a state of net solute exit to net solute entry. During this vulnerable period, excessive cell volume changes can result in the development of brain damage. However, extensive studies in laboratory animals suggest that changes in brain volume do not generally occur unless plasma osmolality changes by more than 20 mosm/kg (change in serum sodium of 12 mmol/liter.[447] Thus, if the total change in plasma osmolality is limited, brain cells are not exposed to osmotic pressures outside their regulatory range and brain damage is less likely to occur. Both clinical and laboratory data support this view.[48,49,442,482] The vast majority of patients who developed cerebral demyelinating lesions after active correction of hyponatremia underwent correction to normonatremic or hypernatremic levels early in their treatment.[49] This is excessive, since symptoms are virtually always relieved with correction to mildly hyponatremic levels. Among patients who were never hyper- or normonatremic when they developed CNS lesions, the serum sodium was usually increased by more than 25 mmol/liter in the first 48 h of therapy. Preexisting liver disease, structural lesions of the CNS,

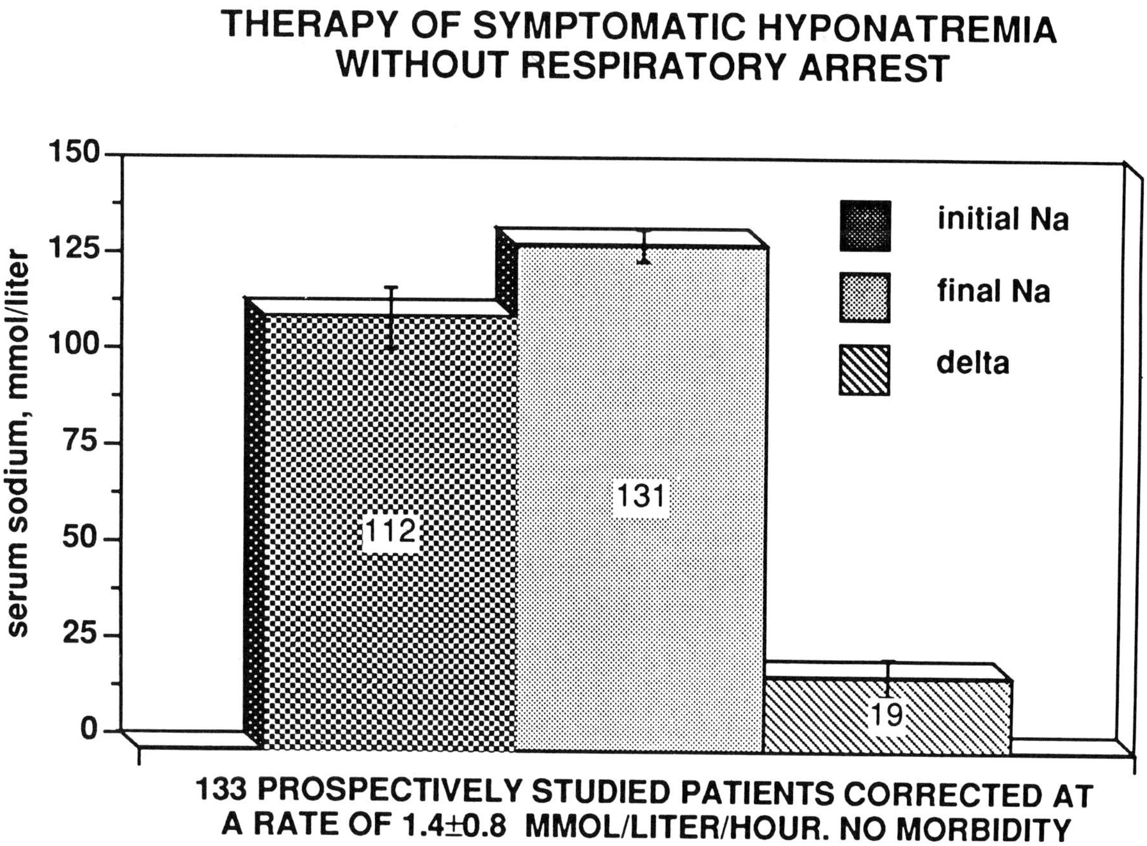

FIGURE 46-12 • This figure summarizes reports of over 130 adult patients from three different countries and five different states in the United States who underwent rapid correction (rate of correction above 0.6 mmol/liter per hour) of severe symptomatic hyponatremia. None had respiratory arrest prior to the start of therapy. All were treated with either hypertonic NaCl, isotonic NaCl, or isotonic NaCl plus furosemide. The serum sodium was increased from an initial value of 112 mmol/liter to a final value after 24 to 48 h of 131 mmol/liter. The absolute change after 24 to 48 h was 19 mmol/liter. All patients survived without evidence of morbidity, regardless of whether the hyponatremia was "acute" or "chronic." Data are compiled from the following references:

Ayus JC et al: Rapid correction of severe hyponatremia with intravenous hypertonic saline solution. *Am J Med* 72:43, 1982.

Ayus JC et al: Treatment of symptomatic hyponatremia and its relation to brain damage. A prospective study. *N Engl J Med* 317 (19):1190, 1987.

Ashouri OS: Severe diuretic-induced hyponatremia in the elderly: A series of eight patients. *Arch Intern Med* 146:1355, 1986.

Decaux G et al: Hyponatremia in the syndrome of inappropriate secretion of antidiuretic hormone. *JAMA* 247:471, 1982.

Cheng JC et al: Long term neurologic outcome in psychogenic water drinkers with severe symptomatic hyponatremia: The effect of rapid correction. *Am J Med* 88:561, 1990.

Hantman D et al: Rapid correction of hyponatremia in the syndrome of inappropriate secretion of antidiuretic hormone: An alternative treatment to hypertonic saline. *Ann Intern Med* 78:870, 1973.

Sarnaik AP et al: Management of hyponatremic seizures in children with hypertonic saline: A safe and effective strategy. *Crit Care Med* 19:758, 1991.

Worthley LIG, Thomas PD: Treatment of hyponatraemic seizures with intravenous 29.2% saline. *Br Med J* 292:168, 1986.

diuretic use, and female gender were predisposing factors in most patients.[49] An episode of hypoxia or anoxia greatly increases the risk of brain damage.[469] There are now reports of over 130 patients worldwide with severe symptomatic hyponatremia who were treated before undergoing respiratory arrest. These patients all underwent a rapid increase in serum sodium (above 0.6 mmol/liter/h) and had no morbidity, thus demonstrating the efficacy of this approach[41,49,51,100,133,224,414,509] (Fig. 46-12).

However, there are several important areas of consensus. Most investigators agree that if there is development of cerebral demyelinating lesions as a complication of treatment of hyponatremia, the therapy has been somehow inappropriate.[67] Cerebral demyelinating lesions are not seen following treatment of hyponatremia at rates of up to 5 mmol/liter/h if there has not been respiratory arrest.[414,509] Second, asymptomatic hyponatremia does not generally require aggressive therapy. Hypertonic NaCl is generally not indicated, as pharmacologic therapy combined with water restriction is often sufficient.[172] Third, symptomatic hyponatremia requires active therapy with administration of hypertonic NaCl, regardless of its duration or severity. Therefore, the only area of disagreement relates to the manner in which NaCl is to be administered. The current literature suggests active correction of hyponatremia by no more than 20 to 25 mmol/liter during the first 48 h, to a level no higher than 128 to 132 mmol/liter, with the rate of correction not a factor (Fig. 46-13). Early diagnosis and treatment before an hypoxic-anoxic episode such as respiratory arrest occurs is of major importance in the prevention of death or brain damage.

GUIDELINES: TREATMENT OF HYPONATREMIA

Patients with symptomatic hyponatremia (serum sodium below 130 mmol/liter) should be treated with hypertonic sodium chloride (514 mmol/liter) using an infusion pump, with the infusion designed to raise plasma sodium at a rate of about 1 mmol/liter/h (Fig. 46-13) until either the patient becomes asymptomatic, the plasma sodium has increased by 25 mmol/liter, or a serum sodium of about 125 to 130 mmol/liter is achieved, whichever occurs first. At that time hypertonic NaCl should be discontinued. The patient should be moved to a location where constant monitoring can be provided, such as the intensive care unit. Monitoring of plasma electrolytes should be carried out every 2 h during the initial period of correction, until the patient becomes neurologically sta-

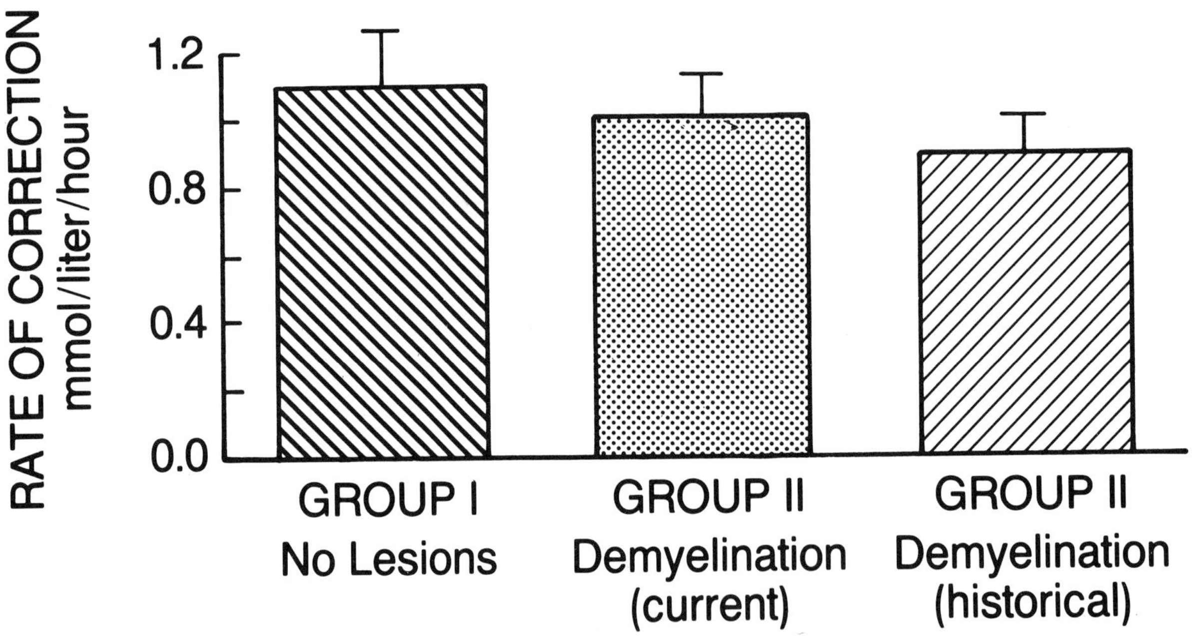

FIGURE 46-13 • This shows the absolute change in serum sodium among three groups of adult patients with symptomatic hyponatremia who were studied. The final value is taken as the serum sodium achieved when hypertonic or isotonic NaCl infusion was discontinued. In group I, serum sodium concentrations were measured at the end of treatment with hypertonic NaCl (A), 24 h after the start of treatment (B), and 48 h after the start of treatment (C). In groups II and III, serum sodium concentrations were measured at the end of therapy with hypertonic NaCl. The patients in group I had no evidence of neurologic disability or brain damage, while those in groups II and III all developed cerebral demyelinating lesions. The absolute change in serum sodium was significantly less ($p<0.01$) in group I then in either group II or III. [Figure reproduced from Ayus JC et al: Treatment of symptomatic hyponatremia and its relation to brain damage. A prospective study. *N Engl J Med* 317(19):1190, 1987, with permission.]

ble. In addition to hypertonic sodium chloride, therapy may include intubation and assisted mechanical ventilation when required. This regimen may require modification in patients with severe renal or cardiac disease. Because of the possible dangers of brain damage, the serum sodium should never be acutely elevated to hyper- or normonatremic levels. Additionally, because brain damage has also been associated with acute excessive changes in serum sodium, the serum sodium should not be elevated by more than 25 mmol/liter during the initial 48 h of therapy. In patients who have symptomatic hyponatremia associated with inappropriately elevated vasopressin, plasma sodium can be raised at the same rate using 514 m*M* NaCl, in combination with furosemide, if vascular congestion is a likely complication.[224] The rate of correction of hyponatremia is not an important factor in the eventual outcome.[49]

HYPERNATREMIA

There are a number of medical conditions that are commonly associated with hypernatremia, the etiologies of which are quite different in children and adults (Table 46-5) (see Chap. 21). In infants, gastroenteritis with diarrhea is the most common cause,[54,84,359] while in elderly individuals, hypernatremia is often associated with infirmity and inability to obtain water freely, leading to gradual desiccation.[438,511] Small children may also become hypernatremic after accidental administration of a high solute load, particularly accidental substitution of NaCl for sugar in preparation of formula[163] or improper dilution of concentrated formulas.[40]

Other causes of hypernatremia include nasogastric hyperalimentation, nonketotic hyperosmolar coma, ARF, renal tubular damage, dialysis, dehydration secondary to elevated ambient temperature, pituitary or renal diabetes insipidus, seawater ingestion, and hyperadrenocorticoid states. A number of CNS lesions have been reported to cause hypernatremia.[14,115,360] Generally, diabetes insipidus is associated with hypernatremia only under circumstances where the patient is unable to freely obtain water or when the lesion responsible for the diabetes insipidus results in a decrease in thirst. There may also be a poorly defined group of hypernatremic patients who have only infrequently been previously diagnosed,[438] Excessive administration of hypertonic solutions of $NaHCO_3$ to critically ill patients suffering cardiac arrest was associated with a dangerously elevated plasma osmolality (377 ± 7 mosm/kg) in 12 patients, none of whom survived.[313] Similarly, administration of large quantities of $NaHCO_3$ to newborn infants has been associated with hypernatremia and intracranial hemorrhage, with a mortality in excess of 70 percent.[433] Severe hypernatremia has also been observed in patients in whom hypertonic NaCl (25%) given for a therapeutic abortion was given intravenously instead of into the amniotic cavity,[91] and may also occur in patients with lactic acidosis who receive large quantities of intravenous $NaHCO_3$.[17,283] Another group of patients in which the entity of hypernatremia with its attendant sequelae is not appreciated are the chronic alcoholic subjects with end-stage liver disease who present with fulminant liver failure and hepatic encephalopathy.[39,179,342,490] Such patients are often treated with oral lactulose as therapy for their hepatic encephalopathy. Hypernatremia may complicate such therapy. Negative fluid balance from the diarrhea secondary to the lactulose caused the hypernatremia.[267] Warren and associates reviewed the medical records of 25 patients admitted with the diagnosis of "hepatic failure" or hepatic encephalopathy.[490] Fifteen of 25 patients developed hypernatremia during the treatment with lactulose and/or various diuretic agents (mannitol, fructose). Patients in this series who had hypernatremia had a mortality of 87 percent vs. 60 percent in those patients who did not develop hypernatremia. All patients with hypernatremia were found to have a negative fluid balance that appeared to be secondary to osmotic loss of fluid from the gastrointestinal tract. A similar sequence has been reported elsewhere, again with a substantial mortality.[342]

TABLE 46-5 • Etiologies of hypernatremia in adults

Etiology	Underlying causes
Infirmity with inability to obtain water	Stroke
	Chronic illness
	Other causes for altered sensorium
Dehydration due to high temperatures	Oral hyperalimentation
	Intravenous hyperalimentation
Hyperalimentation and subsequent osmotic diuresis	Diabetes insipidus
Renal water loss	Chronic renal failure
Dialysis	Proportioning system malfunction
	Osmotic water loss
Steroid hypersecretion	Conn's syndrome
	Cushing's syndrome
Excessive hypertonic intravenous sodium solutions	Lactic acidosis ($NaHCO_3$ or NaCl)
	Cardiac arrest ($NaHCO_3$ or NaCl)
	Therapeutic abortion (NaCl) (accidental)
CNS lesions	Hypothalamic
	Subcommissural
	Pineal
	Supraopticohypophyseal
Essential hypernatremia	Febrile illness
Extrarenal water loss	Osmotic diarrhea
	Infectious diarrhea

Several groups have looked at the frequency and type of renal and electrolyte disorders in patients who had fulminant hepatic failure.[339,502] Thirty-one of 123 patients (25 percent) developed hypernatremia (plasma Na of 145 to 179 mmol/liter). In 20 patients, hypernatremia was secondary to osmotic diarrhea associated with lactulose therapy, while in 11, it occurred during osmotic diuresis secondary to intravenous infusion of hypertonic dextrose or fructose. Sixty-five percent of the hypernatremic patients died, and in those patients where complete fluid balance records were available, the net negative fluid balance was 1.1 liters/day. Analysis of the available information in patients without hypernatremia showed that none had significant negative fluid balance for more than 1 day. What is apparent from these studies is that hypernatremia in patients with severe liver disease may be quite common after therapy with intravenous osmotic diuretic agents and/oral lactucose.[179] The hypernatremia is associated with a high mortality and appears to be directly related to a negative fluid balance.[267,339,490]

The most prominent manifestations of hypernatremia in both the very young and older patients relate to the CNS. In children the majority of cases of hypernatremia are associated with readily reversible underlying systemic illnesses, and it appears that neurologic damage is the primary cause of mortality and morbidity.[54] In adults, by contrast, hypernatremia is freqently associated with severe underlying systemic disorders,[115] although improper postsurgical fluid management is the most common overall cause.[438] In addition to the variations in the neurologic manifestations of hypernatremia that may be seen with age, the eventual mortality and morbidity also seem to vary with the rapidity by which the hypernatremic state is attained.

SYMPTOMS

In children, the mortality of acute hypernatremia (plasma sodium above 160 mmol/liter for less than 24 h) exceeds 40 percent, and it is about 10 percent when the hypernatremia develops over a period of several days. Most children who present with chronic (more than 48 h) hypernatremia have had gastroenteritis with diarrhea for several days. A second large group of children have had infections that have resulted in fever with tachypnea. Other causes of hypernatremia in the pediatric age group are far less common.[115] Hypernatremic children often manifest a characteristic clinical picture, and about 67 percent of such patients have symptoms referable to the CNS. Most have marked irritability and they often emit a high-pitched cry. Depression of sensorium is characteristically present, and this varies from moderate lethargy to frank coma. Normal muscle tone is the rule, but many patients have varying degrees of increased muscle tone and some develop frank seizure activity.[14] The most frequent abnormality found on lumbar puncture is an elevated cerebrospinal fluid protein concentration, without pleocytosis. Although most of these patients are not diabetic, many are hyperglycemic and may also have hyperkalemia, metabolic acidosis, and hypocalcemia. Seizures are not commonly observed in patients with chronic hypernatremia but after therapy is begun, up to 40 percent may exhibit seizure activity. A similar sequence is observed in hypernatremic rabbits whose serum sodium is rapidly lowered to normal.[232]

The mortality in different series varied between 10 and 71 percent and morbidity was very high.[54] Among 100 patients studied by Macauley and Watson,[302] 8 sustained brain damage, 1 had tetraplegia, and 7 were either retarded, hyperkinetic, or clumsy. Among 32 hypernatremic patients successfully treated and then followed up for 8 years, 1 was monoplegic, 2 had seizure disorders, and 8 had abnormal EEG findings.[329]

Acute hypernatremia is less common than chronic hypernatremia in adults and is generally a result of acute solute loading when it does occur. It has been reported with the accidental introduction of hypertonic NaCl into maternal circulation during therapeutic abortion, with the use of NaCl as an emetic, and with treatment of burned patients with hypertonic NaCl.[78,91,438] Particularly fulminant symptoms have occurred with malfunction of either hemodialysis or peritoneal dialysis proportioning systems.[436] Hot climates and heat prostration resulting from excessive physical activity may also result in hyponatremia.[503] More rare causes include drowning in seawater (which has a sodium concentration of 450 to 500 mmol/liter) and ingestion of massive quantities of table salt.[251] Acute hypernatremia is probably not uncommon among patients who are resuscitated following cardiac arrest or have lactic acidosis and have been given large amounts of intravenous $NaHCO_3$.[313]

Typically, hypernatremia in adults occurs as a chronic process where the symptoms may be obscured by other concomitant diseases that are often of a catastrophic nature.[198] Because of these associated medical conditions, the presenting symptoms are usually not attributable to hypernatremia. The sensation of thirst, often intense, may not be verbalized because affected patients frequently have depression of sensorium. The physical signs commonly associated with dehydration, such as altered skin turgor and sunken eye sockets, may not be apparent because of the usual signs of aging. Lethargy, stupor, or coma may be present to varying degrees. Muscle irritability and convulsions have been reported[443] but are unusual, and it may be difficult to separate effects of hyperosmolality from those of therapy.

Symptoms similar to those observed in patients have been produced in experimental animals with acute hyper-

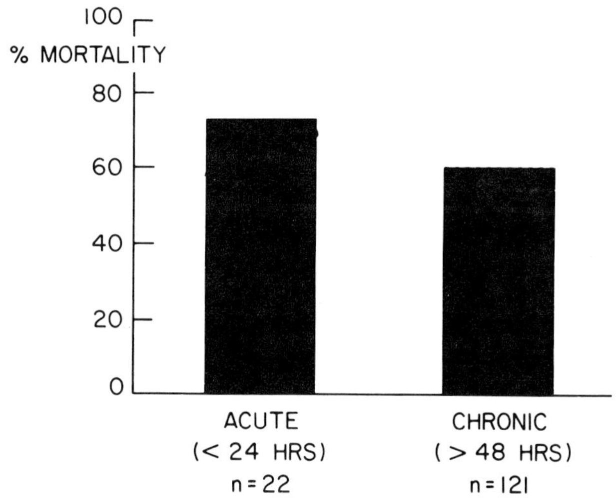

FIGURE 46-14 • Comparison of published mortality from acute and chronic hypernatremia in adults (serum Na^+ > 160 meq/liter). Hypernatremia in adults may result from grave conditions, including stroke with dehydration, lactic acidosis, resusciation from cardiac arrest, and hyperglycemic nonketotic coma, in the bulk of published cases; eventual mortality is formidable. (From Covey CM, Arieff AI: Disorders of sodium and water metabolism and their effects on the central nervous system, in Brenner BM, Stein JH (eds): *Contemporary Issues in Nephrology*, New York, Churchill-Livingstone, 1978, vol 1, p 212.)

natremia. In rabbits infused with 1000 mmol/liter NaCl, severe CNS symptoms began to appear when plasma osmolality had reached 350 mosm/kg. Many died of respiratory failure, usually at a plasma osmolality of about 430 mosm/kg (Fig. 46-14). A similar picture has been observed in kittens and in other animal species made hypernatremic by intraperitoneal injection with hyperosmolar loads.[29,468]

EEG CHANGES

In experimental animals, hyperosmolality results in a progressive slowing of background EEG frequencies, but no spikes or paroxysmal discharges are seen in the presence of paroxysmal jerking of the body.[29] There is a generalized reduction in voltage, disappearance of fast activity, and the appearance of bursts of 4 to 5 per second spindle-like activity. There is also a gradual progression to 1 to 3 per second high-voltage waves, with cessation of EEG activity at the time of respiratory arrest. The EEG changes appear to be reversible with correction of plasma osmolality to normal. Electroencephalograms obtained in patients with hypernatremia have generally been normal. However, the EEGs of 10 of 52 hypernatremic children showed a decrease in amplitude similar to that observed in experimental animals, with generalized slowing of the background rhythm. All but two had returned to normal within 2 to 40 days after treatment. The two persistently abnormal EEGs showed typical seizure discharges.

PATHOLOGY

In acute hypernatremia, as fluid from the intracellular space moves into the extracellular compartment to establish osmotic equilibrium, the cells initially lose volume.[29] In the brain, this loss of volume may put mechanical traction on delicate cerebral vessels to produce vascular damage.

Autopsies performed on children who died from acute salt poisoning have provided much of the information about the pathological lesions produced in humans by acute hypernatremia.[164] In these children, there is evidence of widespread cerebral vascular damage. Capillaries and veins are markedly congested, with subcortical parenchymatous hemorrhage and subarachnoid bleeding. Venous thromboses, sometimes leading to infarction, and occlusion of major venous sinuses have been observed. Although cerebral edema has been noted in some patients, it is more likely the result of overly rapid rehydration therapy rather than the hypernatremia per se.

The anatomical brain damage produced by acute hyperosmolality has also been studied in experimental animals. Shrunken, grossly dehydrated brains, engorged vessels, and petechial hemorrhages were observed in rabbits made hyperosmolar, with a 76 percent mortality. Similar findings were observed in kittens. At necropsy 85 percent of the animals had subdural hemorrhage with xanthrochromia of the cerebrospinal fluid, and 7 percent had subdural hematoma.[29]

Similar findings of hemorrhage and congested cerebral vessels have been observed in children dying of chronic hypernatremia.[162] In chronically hypernatremic animals, dehydration and vascular congestion are present, although anatomic changes are usually not seen.[29]

EFFECTS OF HYPERNATREMIA ON BRAIN WATER AND ELECTROLYTES

The effects of acute and chronic hypernatremia on brain water and electrolytes in experimental animals are summarized in Fig. 46-15. In animals with acute hypernatremia (mean serum sodium = 178 mmol/liter) for less than 3 h, there is an abrupt decrease in brain water and a rise in intracellular sodium and Cl^- concentration. Potassium content increases minimally. Acutely, the increase in measured intracellular osmolality of the brain can be essentially all accounted for by the observed increases in measured brain electrolyte (Na^+,K^+,Cl^-) concentration.

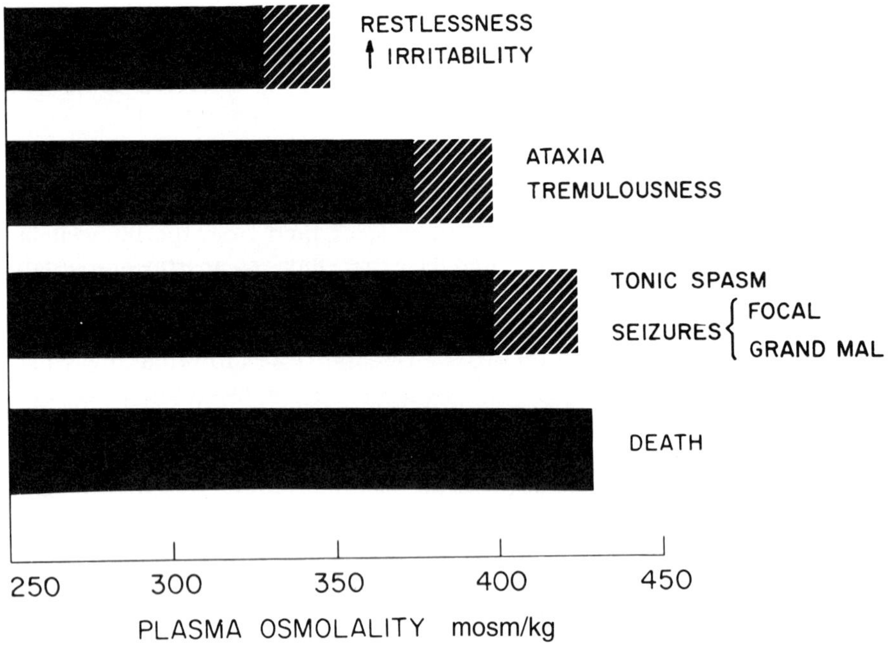

FIGURE 46-15 • Effects of acute hyperosmolality in experimental animals. Crosshatched areas represent the range of plasma osmolality for each group of manifestations. (From Arieff AI et al: Pathophysiology of hyperosmolar states, in *Disturbances in Body Fluid Osmolality*, Bethesda, MD, American Physiological Society, 1977, p 227.)

After several days of sustained hypernatremia, brain water content is almost normal.[437] However, in mice with 4 days of hypernatremia, brain water content remains low.[468] Total brain sodium and Cl^- remain elevated in both mice and rabbits, but the increase in measured electrolytes (Na^+, K^+, Cl^-) is not sufficient to account for all the measured increase in brain osmolality. In other words, there is the appearance of unmeasured solute that accounts for about 60 percent of the increase in brain intracellular osmolality in chronically (4 to 7 days) hypernatremic animals. The solute ("idiogenic osmoles") begins to appear after several hours of hypernatremia and is as yet uncharacterized. In several different laboratories a rise in intracellular amino acids (glutamine, alanine, aspartate, glutamate) has been observed in the brains of chronically hypernatremic animals and appears to contribute at least in part to the rise in brain osmolality.[29,97,297,467,468] Similar findings have been reported in hypernatremic brain studied in vitro.[97] Other possible mechanisms might include the dissociation of intracellular protein-salt complexes, the action of hydrolytic enzymes in lysozymes activated by hyperosmolality, or some changes in intracellular metabolism leading to accumulation in brain of other small-molecular-weight substances.[131] Thus, it appears that the brain may have adaptive mechanisms not found in other body tissues that serve to defend cellular volume. By the generation of idiogenic osmoles the brain is able to achieve osmotic equilibrium with plasma by internal adaptive mechanisms that serve to minimize the loss of brain water. Recent studies suggest that some of the idiogenic osmoles in hypernatremic brain consist of amino acids, betaine, glycerophosphorylcholine, methylamines, and myoinositol.[228,295]

These adaptive mechanisms in hyperosmolality benefit the host. Abrupt shrinkage of the brain could lead to tearing of cerebral vessels and meninges, with subsequent subdural hemorrhage, as has been described in patients and animals with acute hypernatremia.[409] Thus, from a clinical standpoint, the ability of the brain to generate idiogenic osmoles to maintain cellular volume intact is crucial to survival. In this sense, it is of interest that the brains of some vertebrates who live parts of their lives in both saltwater and freshwater environments appear to have the ability to adapt to the changing osmotic environment by altering intracellular amino acid content.

MORTALITY

The mortality of chronic hypernatremia in children ranges from 7 to 29 percent. Mortality in children with acute hypernatremia averages 43 percent, and about two-thirds of survivors have neurologic sequelae.[115] Figure 46-14 summarizes the experience in the literature for adults with sustained (over 48 h) hypernatremia (serum sodium above 160 mmol/liter). Serious underlying conditions such as resuscitation from cardiac arrest, nonketotic hyperosmolar coma, and acute stroke with dehydration render the 60 percent mortality not surprising. However, from the experience in children, who generally are without chronic underlying disease, it is highly probable that hypernatremia per se adds considerably to the mortality and morbidity of the underlying condition.

THERAPY

In infants and elderly individuals hypernatremia is associated with a significant mortality. The reported incidence of severe hypernatremia exceeds one patient per hospital per month in elderly individuals[28] with a slightly higher incidence in children.[28,115] Despite the magnitude of the problem, few data are available on the quantitative aspects of severe hypernatremia. Hyperosmolality is potentially lethal but rapid treatment of hypernatremia by infusion of hypotonic solutions can cause seizures and cerebral edema, which may also be lethal. Furthermore, acute hypernatremia secondary to infusion of either hypertonic NaCl or $NaHCO_3$ can lead to abrupt shrinkage of the brain, with tearing of cerebral vessels and subarachnoid or subdural hemorrhage.[28,29]

Most investigators agree that patients with hypernatremic dehydration should be treated with hypotonic electrolyte solutions. In both children and adults, fluid therapy is administered such that normonatremia is achieved over a period of approximately 48 h.[161,406] Despite such recommendations, few data in humans or animals are available as to the ideal rate of fluid administration. Fatal cases of cerebral edema, as well as permanent brain damage, have occurred when hypernatremia was completely corrected within 24 h, while seizures with cerebral edema occur in more than 50 percent of hypernatremic rabbits when plasma sodium is reduced from 185 to 142 mmol/liter in 4 h.[232] These studies highlight the dangers of overly rapid correction of hypernatremia. Based on our present knowledge, recommendations for treatment of chronic hypernatremia in adults, when the hypernatremia is primarily due to water loss, are:

1. If there is evidence of *circulatory collapse*, the patient should receive initial resuscitation with colloid, such as plasma or a plasma substitute, rapidly enough to correct shock and stabilize the circulatory system.
2. *Water deficits* should be estimated and replaced over a 48-h period, aiming for a decrement in serum osmolality of approximately 1 to 2 mosm/liter/h (i.e., fall in serum of 0.5 to 1.0 mosm/liter/h). Maintenance fluids, which include replacement of urine volume with hypotonic fluid, are given in addition to the deficit.
3. *Hypotonic fluid* should be administered. If the patient has a moderate acidosis, $NaHCO_3$ may be added to the solution, with a proportional reduction in NaCl concentration. The usual replacement fluid will be either 280 mmol/liter glucose or 77 mmol/liter NaCl.
4. Plasma *electrolytes should be monitored* at frequent intervals, usually about every 2 h. It should be stressed that most adult patients with hypernatremia have serious underlying systemic illness, such as stroke, infection, or head trauma. Many such patients appear to die of their underlying illness, rather than of hypernatremia per se. Close attention should be given to the treatment of associated medical conditions, thus reducing morbidity and mortality from the hypernatremia as well.
5. If the hypernatremia is secondary to excessive loss of other body fluids, the replacement fluid should be *similar to the fluid actually lost*, as shown in Table 46-6.

PHOSPHATE DEPLETION

GENERAL

The clinical syndrome of phosphate depletion was originally described in six patients who were either normal or had hypothyroidism and took magnesium-aluminum hydroxide for up to 130 days (see Chap. 33). The symptoms included weakness, bone pain, anorexia, and malaise and

TABLE 46-6 • Electrolyte content of body fluids

Mean concentrations (meq/liter) followed by normal ranges of four predominant electrolytes

Fluid	Na^+	K^+	Cl^-	HCO_3^-
Plasma	140	4.5	102	26
	138–142	3.5–5.0	98–106	22–30
Saliva	33	20	34	
	20–46	16–23	24–44	
Gastric juice	60	9	84	0
	30–90	4.3–12	52–124	
Bile	149	4.9	101	45
	120–170	3–12	80–120	30–50
Pancreatic juice	141	4.6	77	92
	113–153	2.6–7.4	54–95	70–110
Small bowel	105	5.1	99	50
	72–158	3.5–6.8	70–127	20–40
Ileal fluid	129	11.2	116	29
	90–140	6–30	82–125	25–30
Cecal fluid	80	21	48	22
	50–116	11–28	35–70	15–30
Cerebrospinal fluid	141	2.9	127	23
	135–147	2.5–3.4	116–132	21–25
Sweat	45	4.5	58	0
	18–97	1–15	18–97	
Aqueous humor	143	4.7	108	
	142–145		106–110	

SOURCE: Reproduced with permission from Arieff AI: Principles of parenteral therapy, in Maxwell MH, Kleeman CR (eds): *Clinical Disorders of Fluid and Electrolyte Metabolism*, 3d ed. New York, McGraw-Hill, 1972.

were rapidly reversed with phosphate repletion.[301] In a patient with CRF treated with hemodialysis, $Al(OH)_3$ treatment resulted in a decline of serum phosphorus to 0.7 mg/dl. The patient developed nausea, depression, emesis, anorexia, and weakness, which improved with elevation of serum phosphorus.

Several review articles have discussed the variety of clinical manifestations that may accompany hypophosphatemia.[167,279] Similarly, the clinical causes of hypophosphatemia are numerous and varied.[279] Particular organ systems affected by hypophosphatemia include neuromuscular hematologic (red blood cells, white blood cells, and platelets), hepatic, skeletal, muscular, pulmonary, and CNS[167,279] as well as the heart.[192,345]

Any discussion of the CNS effects of phosphate depletion is complicated by the fact that most patients also have multiple abnormalities of electrolytes, and acid-base status. In particular, many phosphate-depleted patients also have low plasma levels of sodium, magnesium, calcium, and potassium. Many are also alcoholic, cachetic, and severely malnourished. The symptoms are similar to those in patients with other metabolic encephalopathies and include weakness, confusion, obtundation, focal seizures, and coma. This syndrome has been most commonly observed in alcoholic subjects whose serum phosphate was lowered with infusion of glucose and/or amino acids.

CLINICAL STUDIES

Travis and associates described eight patients who were being treated with glucose-protein solutions intravenously.[474] Hypophosphatemia developed, along with paresthesias and obtundation in some patients. Those with obtundation had marked shifts in the affinity of hemoglobin for oxygen, so that P_{50} was reduced and tissue oxygen delivery may have been decreased. Those patients also had diffuse slowing of the EEG. It has been suggested that many of the clinical manifestations of phosphate depletion may be secondary to decreased blood 2,3-diphosphoglycerate levels, with decreased delivery of oxygen to tissues.[474]

Other studies on the effects of acute hypophosphatemia generally describe patients who developed hypophosphatemia following hyperalimentation. Silvis and Paragas[431] described three starving patients who developed profound hypophosphatemia (serum phosphate = 0.3 mg/dl) following parenteral hyperalimentation. All developed muscular weakness, two had seizures and coma, and one died. Furlan and associates[195] described two patients with malnutrition associated with chronic gastrointestinal disease. Both were treated with intravenous hyperalimentation, and serum phosphate levels fell below 0.5 mg/dl. Both developed sensory loss, cranial nerve palsies, and respiratory insufficiency secondary to muscular weakness. Both recovered after phosphate repletion. Hypophosphatemia impairs the contractile properties of the diaphragm in patients with acute respiratory failure, and phosphate repletion restores contractility to normal.[43]

ANIMAL STUDIES

Few animal studies have studied the effects of hypophosphatemia on the CNS. In dogs with plasma phosphate below 0.8 mg/dl induced by dietary phosphate depletion, no neurologic abnormalities were observed.[204,401] These dogs were given at least 6 weeks of a diet that contained virtually no phosphorus but had adequate vitamins, minerals, calories, protein, fat, and carbohydrate. Thus pure hypophosphatemia due to dietary phosphate depletion probably, in and of itself, does not result in neurologic abnormalities.

More revealing are the effects of acute hypophosphatemia, combined with starvation and malnutrition. Dogs were initially starved and were then given intravenous glucose–amino acid solutions such that serum phosphate fell below 0.5 mg/dl in less than 2 days. These dogs developed ataxia and coma, and some died. Brain edema was allegedly observed, with a 40 percent increase in brain water. In preliminary studies in both our laboratory and others, the presence of seizures was confirmed in these animals, but brain edema was not seen.[139,401] Other abnormalities in these hyperalimented dogs included platelet dysfunction, thrombocytopenia, anemia, infection, and hemorrhage. In an earlier study, Silvis and Paragas[431] found that starved hyperalimented dogs had a mean survival of only 5.4 days when their mean plasma phosphate was below 0.5 mg/dl. The mortality was not improved by adding phosphate to the infusion. Derr and Zieve[139] infused starved rats with glucose–amino acid solutions, and coma, seizures, and death occurred in more than half of these animals. Brain edema was never present, and in fact, most animals had cerebral dehydration, usually associated with hyperosmolality and hyperglycemia. In those rats with coma and death, blood glucose exceeded 1100 mg/dl and plasma osmolality exceeded 470 mosm/liter.

SUMMARY

From the available literature, there is a neurologic syndrome associated with hyperalimentation-induced hypophosphatemia, but it probably occurs only in starved or malnourished humans and animals. The exact pathophysiology is unclear, but it may be related to a hypothetical sequence:[279]

Both adenosine triphosphate (ATP) and inorganic phosphate (Pi) stabilize adenosine monophosphate

(AMP) and the total adenine nucleotide content of tissue by inhibiting the enzymes that irreversibly degrade AMP. In phosphate-depleted states, tissue levels of both Pi and ATP are probably diminished. Although not yet studied in the brain, this is probably true for red blood cells and the heart and may also be true for the brain. ATP inhibits 5-nucleotidase and Pi inhibits AMP deaminase and, to some extent, 5-nucleotidase. When inhibition of AMP deaminase is ineffective (due to phosphate depletion), the concentration of inosinic acid (IMP) increases and both AMP and IMP undergo dephosphorylation with formation of adenosine and inosine, and eventually, hypoxanthine, uric acid, and allantoin. These changes may result in tissue necrosis. Infusion of glucose–amino acids to a starved phosphate-depleted animal (or patient) increases the demand for phosphate (for protein synthesis and glucose metabolism) which, in the depleted state, cannot be met. The sequence described above may occur in liver and probably also occurs in skeletal muscle.[280]

DIABETIC COMA

Coma, a complication of diabetes mellitus, was initially described over 100 years ago.[22,64] Most of these patients have some depression of sensorium, which usually takes the form of impaired response to verbal or painful stimuli, but many patients are alert and responsive (see Chap. 26). In the strict sense, one should not diagnose diabetic "coma" unless there is at least some depression of sensorium, usually to a state of obtundation.[374] Obtundation can be defined as a state of dull indifference, where increased stimulation is required to evoke a response.[374] If one excludes stroke, there are at least four syndromes of metabolic derangements associated with diabetes that can be classified as "the diabetic comas." These are (1) *diabetic ketoacidosis*, (2) *nonketotic hyperosmolar coma with hyperglycemia* (nonketotic coma), (3) *hypoglycemia*, and (4) *lactic acidosis*. Nonketotic hyperosmolar coma with hyperglycemia (nonketotic coma)[21,22,200] and hypoglycemia[24,160] are discussed elsewhere, as is lactic acidosis.[21,22,26,200]

DIABETIC KETOACIDOSIS

Diabetic ketoacidosis is a metabolic abnormality characterized by hyperglycemia (blood glucose above 14 mmol/liter) and metabolic acidosis (arterial pH below 7.25 and/or plasma bicarbonate less than 16 mmol/liter) due to hyperketonemia (plasma acetoacetate and β-hydroxybutyrate above 7 mmol/liter), with depression of the sensorium to at least a state of obtundation. The disorder is most common among juvenile or type I (insulin-dependent) diabetic patients.

The pathogenesis of diabetic ketoacidosis has been adequately reviewed elsewhere.[312,318] There are several important theories that relate to the pathogenesis of coma in the diabetic subject, and these will be briefly reviewed.

Ketonemia

There have been many suggestions that hyperketonemia may be important in the genesis of coma in patients with diabetic ketoacidosis. The only experimental studies that relate to this problem were performed prior to 1940, and they have not yet been confirmed. It has been reported that in rabbits, infusion of either acetoacetate acid or sodium acetoacetate resulted in coma.[418] Under similar circumstances, infusion of either β-hydroxybutyrate or sodium β-hydroxybutyrate did not result in coma, although some of these animals had unexplained deaths.[418] Infusion of HCl to achieve a plasma bicarbonate similar to that obtained with β-hydroxybutyric acid infusion did not result in coma. These studies suggest that acetoacetate may cause coma. Studies by Kety and coworkers[272] in patients with ketoacidosis are somewhat supportive of this concept in that they demonstrate a continuing fall in cerebral utilization of oxygen with increasing plasma ketone levels. Furthermore, the brain can probably metabolize β-hydroxybutyrate to γ-hydroxybutyrate, a substance that is an anesthetic agent.[217] Thus hyperketonemia may impair cerebral oxygen utilization and also have an anesthetic effect, both of which may contribute to depression of sensorium.

Metabolic acidosis

Metabolic acidosis is probably not an important cause of coma in ketoacidotic subjects. Acidosis per se is usually not associated with coma in patients with a variety of systemic diseases, such as uremia, cholera,[283,359,380] and hypercapnia. Furthermore, infusion or ingestion of acid (HCl or NH_4Cl) to induce acute metabolic acidemia does not cause coma in laboratory animals[418] or human beings.[372,380]

Some evidence suggests that depression of the sensorium is related not to arterial pH but rather to the pH of cerebrospinal fluid.[380] However, subsequent investigation has failed to confirm these earlier impressions. There was no apparent relationship between depression of sensorium and pH of cerebrospinal fluid in patients with nonketotic coma,[32] in subjects with cholera who were treated with $NaHCO_3$,[369] or in patients with ketoacidosis who received intravenous $NaHCO_3$.[42,348] In rats with diabetic ketoacidosis, brain intracellular pH is normal.

Cerebral hypoxia

Hypoxia is a well-known cause of coma.[375] Patients with ketoacidosis have several abnormalities that might theoretically predispose to hypoxia, such as hyperviscosity of the blood[393] and decreased cerebral oxygen consumption.[272] If hypoxia were severe, there could be a fall in brain intracellular pH due to increased brain lactate, as well as a decrease in brain high-energy phosphate compounds. Neither sequence is likely to occur. In animals with ketoacidosis, brain intracellular pH and lactate are probably normal. Total brain adenine nucleotide content is also normal.[72,410] If the action of Na^+-K^+ ATPase in brain were impaired, there should be increases in brain Na^+ and decreases in K^+. Preliminary studies in animals do not support this hypothesis. Thus there are no data to support an important role for cerebral hypoxia in the pathogenesis of coma associated with ketoacidosis.

Hyperosmolality

It has been demonstrated that hyperosmolality per se can induce coma in laboratory animals,[29] and extracellular hyperosmolality is probably an important cause of coma in ketoacidotic patients. Other factors may be equally important. Many patients with high plasma osmolality are alert, while those with lower levels of extracellular osmolality may be comatose.[193] In both patients and laboratory animals, it appears that plasma osmolality must exceed 340 mosm/kg before depression of sensorium occurs.[21,29,193] In 438 ketoacidotic patients with coma, the mean plasma osmolality was only 322 mosm/kg.[175] Overall, however, there is a significant correlation between depression of sensorium and extracellular osmolality (Fig. 46-16). Thus hyperosmolality probably contributes to depression of sensorium at levels in excess of 340 mosm/kg, but is not the only factor.

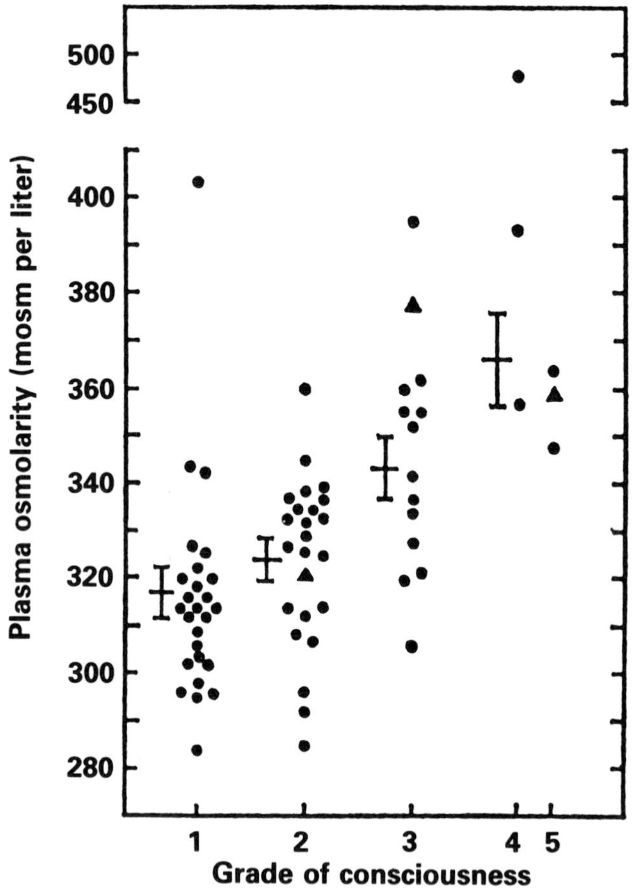

FIGURE 46-16 • Relationship between state of consciousness and (calculated) plasma osmolality in 70 patients with diabetic ketoacidosis. Abscissa represents increasing depression of sensorium. (From Fulop M et al: *Lancet* 2:635, 1973.)

Other factors

Intravascular deposition of fibrin has recently been demonstrated in brains of some patients dying with ketoacidotic coma. The fibrin deposition was associated with ischemic tissue damage.[470] Studies of the coagulation system in these patients demonstrated thrombocytopenia with advanced elevated plasma fibrinogen levels. The hypothesis has been put forth that cerebral intravascular coagulation, by occluding small vessels and producing local ischemia, may play a major role in production of coma in ketoacidotic patients. However, such cerebral intravascular fibrin deposition is probably not a major or consistent abnormality.[11] In all probability, coma in diabetic ketoacidosis is caused by a number of factors acting in combination. There is hyperviscosity of the blood and impaired cerebral oxygen utilization. There is probably some direct effect on brain of acetoacetate, and perhaps β-hydroxybutyrate as well, which tends to produce coma. During diabetic ketoacidosis, about one-half of the brain's source of energy may come from ketones, so that their metabolites probably accumulate in the brain. It also may be that certain metabolites of glucose (e.g., fructose 6-phosphate, glucose 6-phosphate, citrate, acetyl-CoA) that accumulates in the brain of ketoacidotic animals manifest CNS toxicity. Hyperosmolality is present to varying degrees in all patients with diabetic ketoacidosis, and may play some role in depression of sensorium. Disseminated intravascular coagulation appears to be present in some patients with diabetic ketoacidosis. Such a coagulopathy could result in localized areas of cerebral hypoperfusion, which may accelerate depression of sensorium. Finally, many patients with diabetic ketoacidosis have severe associated medical conditions, such as sepsis, myocardial infarction, and pneumonia. These diseases may in themselves lead to depression of sensorium. The multiplicity of factors undoubtedly accounts for the fact that no single variable, such as arterial pH, plasma ketone levels, pH of cerebrospinal fluid, or blood glucose concentration can consistently be correlated with depression of sensorium. The best correlation is still that with plasma osmolality.

NONKETOTIC COMA

Diabetic ketoacidosis and nonketotic coma actually represent a continuum; many patients have biochemical characteristics of both. However, in most patients, the primary problem is either hyperosmolality with dehydration or metabolic acidemia. Nonketotic hyperosmolar coma with hyperglycemia (nonketotic coma) is characterized by hyperglycemia (plasma glucose above 600 mg/dl) and hyperosmolality (plasma osmolality above 350 mosm/kg) without significant ketonemia with depression of sensorium to at least the level of stupor.[22] The pathogenesis of nonketotic coma has been extensively studied, and in all probability it represents a heterogeneous entity. There is interplay between free fatty acid mobilization and metabolism, insulin secretion, growth hormone, dehydration, and hyperosmolality.[22,175,200]

Neurologic manifestations

Neurologic symptoms are prominent manifestations in patients with nonketotic coma. Approximately 36 percent of patients are initially diagnosed as having an acute stroke,[22] with about 27 percent having either hemiparesis or a positive Babinski sign. Up to 15 percent of patients with nonketotic coma present with seizures.[227,233,311,396,454] The seizures are usually of a focal nature, although some grand mal seizures and myoclonus are also seen.[227,233,454] The seizures are often resistant to conventional anticonvulsant therapy.[233,396]

Focal neurologic changes have included aphasia, homonymous hemianopsia, hemisensory defects, hemiparesis, hyperreflexia, and visual hallucinations. In general, most of the above changes are reversible following correction of the metabolic abnormalities. Evidence of brainstem dysfunction in the form of the tonic eye deviation and nystagmus has also been reported, suggesting at least occasional involvement of the vestibular system. A variety of autonomic nervous system changes, such as hyperpnea and hypertension, are also observed. This variety of neurologic changes in patients with nonketotic coma cannot be explained by a single structural lesion but rather appears to represent a widespread functional disturbance that may affect any level of the nervous system.[217,303]

The multiplicity of neurologic involvement often suggests the presence of acute cerebral parenchymal damage, but CAT scans, cerebral angiography, and neuropathologic examinations usually fail to disclose structural abnormalities correlating with the clinical observations. The mean age of patients presenting with nonketotic coma is about 62 years, and many such patients may have some underlying cerebral vascular abnormality.

Seizure activity and biochemical changes

The mechanisms by which hyperosmolality may lead to seizure activity are not well known. In the clinical situation, seizure activity is very rare in ketoacidotic patients[193] but is present in about 15 percent of those patients with nonketotic coma.[380] Thus hyperketonemia may in some manner suppress the effects of hyperosmolality on the CNS. In both ketoacidosis and nonketotic coma, there is probably some suppression of Krebs cycle activity in the brain. In the rat with ketoacidosis, there is accumulation of citrate in the brain.[410] Additionally, hyperosmolality per se can inhibit Krebs cycle activity.[468] With Krebs cycle inhibition, the energy supply of the brain may be met, at least in part, by metabolism of ketones, lactate, glutamate, and perhaps other amino acids as well.[229,391] In particular, γ-aminobutyric acid (GABA) is found in high concentrations only in nervous tissue.[233] GABA has been shown to be a cortical depressant, raising the seizure threshold.[227] In the brain, GABA can be metabolized to succinate via the GABA shunt, which is an alternative to the Krebs cycle for the conversion of α-ketoglutarate to succinate.[61] The GABA shunt can provide up to 40 percent of the brain's energy requirement under certain circumstances.[230] Thus, in patients with nonketotic coma, it may be that increased metabolism of GABA lowers the seizure threshold.[123] Conversely, in ketoacidotic animals, brain tissue levels of GABA are normal,[170] which may in part account for the absence of seizures.

Effects of hyperglycemia on the brain

Depression of sensorium in patients with either ketoacidosis or nonketotic coma has been found to correlate with extracellular hyperosmolality (Figs. 46-16 and 46-17), but not with hyperglycemia, or the pH of either blood or cerebrospinal fluid.[42,123,193,348] The mechanisms by which hyperosmolality can induce coma are unclear. There is a general impression that hyperglycemia, as is the case with some acute hyperosmolar states, should cause cerebral dehydration.[29] However, evidence in both humans and laboratory animals with hyperglycemia suggests that this is not the case. Patients who die with nonketotic coma have not been reported to show evidence of cerebral dehydration. In fact, among 14 patients with nonketotic coma who died where there was postmortem examination of the brain, none had evidence of cerebral dehydration[159,311,481] and several had cerebral edema.[159]

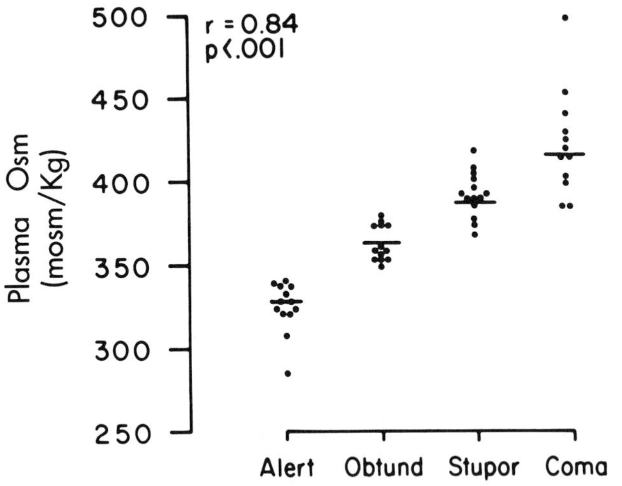

FIGURE 46-17 • Relationship between depression of sensorium and plasma osmolality (osm) in 53 patients with blood glucose greater than 600 mg/dl but without ketoacidosis. In calculating the correlation coefficient (r) alertness was counted as 1, obtundation (obtund) as 2, stupor as 3, and coma as 4. For each group, plasma osmolality was significantly different from that of the adjacent group(s) $p < 0.01$). (From Arieff AI, Carroll HJ: *Medicine* 51:525, 1972.)

Idiogenic osmoles

In laboratory animals, rapid elevation of plasma glucose by infusion of hypertonic glucose can cause cerebral dehydration and death.[217] However, when plasma glucose in rabbits is elevated to about 61 mmol/liter (1100 mg/dl) in 1 h, the sequence of events in brain is different.[34] After 1 to 2 h of hyperglycemia, there is an initial decrease in brain water content. However, when plasma glucose is then maintained at about 1100 mg/dl for 4 to 6 h, brain water content returns to normal values. By comparison, under similar circumstances skeletal muscle water content falls significantly after 2 h and remains depressed. The secondary increase of brain water to normal values is accompanied by an increase in brain osmole content such that brain and plasma osmolality are similar. This increase in brain osmole content is only partially accounted for by changes in brain content of measured solute-glucose, lactate, sorbitol, myoinositol, urea, Na^+, K^+, or Cl^-. The remainder consists of idiogenic osmoles. The generation of idiogenic osmoles during hyperglycemia thus enables the brain to achieve osmotic equilibrium with plasma despite a lesser loss of water and/or gain in solute than would be expected if the brain were a more perfect osmometer. In animals with experimental nonketotic coma, generation of idiogenic osmoles by brain appears to be a response to hyperglycemia rather than to hyperosmolality per se. When plasma osmolality is elevated to similar levels (about 350 mosm/kg) over a 4 to 6 h period by infusion of either mannitol or glycerol, essentially all of the increase in brain osmolality is due to loss of water by the brain,[32,219] with a subsequent increase in brain concentration of Na^+, K^+, and Cl^-. Recent studies suggest that some of the idiogenic osmoles in brain consist of amino acids, betaine, glycerophosphorylcholine, methylamines, and perhaps myoinositol.[228,295]

Other biochemical changes in the brain

Several possible explanations have been advanced to explain the adaptive processes of the brain to hyperglycemia. It has been suggested by some that the brain might synthesize fructose, sorbitol, or myoinositol in quantities such that brain intracellular osmolality would be increased by levels similar to that of plasma.[105] Others have suggested that glucose might enter brain cells to achieve intracellular concentrations of sufficient magnitude to equalize plasma and brain osmolalities.[159] However, these theories have not been validated by experimental evidence.[34,217]

Osmotic adaptation

Although the identity of the idiogenic osmoles in brain is not yet known, they may represent changes in the intracellular binding of cations (Na^+ and K^+). At least 20 percent of brain K^+ and Na^+ are normally nonexchangeable[266] and therefore probably osmotically inactive. Various types of osmotic stress can alter the brain intracellular binding of Na^+ and K^+ in vitro.[223] Also hyperosmolality induced by intravenous infusion of NaCl decreases the amount of bound Na^+ and K^+ in brain[29] in vivo. Although the effects on the brain have not yet been directly evaluated, an intracellular acidosis increases cellular osmolality in other cells, such as red blood cells,[130] by displacement of bound K^+ ion with H^+ ion. Such a phenomenon may occur in cerebral cortex as well. Thus the adaptation of brain to hyperglycemic states depends on the interaction of several factors that may occur within the brain, including dehydration, some gain in measured solute, and generation of idiogenic osmoles. The net effect upon brain volume will be based on the rapidity, duration, and degree of the hyperglycemia, as well as various characteristics of individual patients.

REFERENCES

1. National Cooperative Dialysis Study. *Kidney Int* 23 (suppl 13):S122, 1983.
2. Adams RD, Foley JM: The neurological disorders associated with liver disease. *Res Publ Assoc Res Nerv Ment Dis* 32:198, 1953.
3. Adams RD et al: Central pontine myelinolysis: A hitherto undescribed disease occurring in alcoholic and malnourished patients. *Arch Neurol Psychiatr* 81:154, 1959.

4. Adrogué HJ et al: Assessing acid-base status in circulatory failure: Differences between arterial and central venous blood. *N Engl J Med* 320:1312, 1989.
5. Agarwal A et al: Hyponatremia in patients with acquired immunodeficiency syndrome. *Nephron* 53:317, 1989.
6. Ahmed K, Thomas BS: The effects of long chain fatty acids on sodium plus potassium ion-stimulated adenosine triphosphatase of brain. *J Biol Chem* 246:103, 1971.
7. Akaishi T, Sakuma Y: Estrogen-induced modulation of hypothalamic osmoregulation in female rats. *Am J Physiol* 258 (*Regul Integrative Comp Physiol* 27):R924, 1990.
8. Alfrey AC et al: The dialysis encephalopathy syndrome: Possible aluminum intoxication. *N Engl J Med* 294:184, 1976.
9. Alfrey AC et al: Syndrome of dysphaxia and multifocal seizures associated with chronic hemodialysis. *Trans Am Soc Artif Intern Organs* 18:257, 1972.
10. Altman PL, Dittmer DS: Blood oxygen dissociation curves: Mammals, in *Biology Data Book*, 2d ed. Bethesda, MD, Federation of American Societies for Experimental Biology, 1974, p 1863.
11. Anderson JM et al: Diabetic ketoacidosis and intracerebral thrombosis. *Lancet* 1:1341, 1974.
12. Anderson RJ et al: Hyponatremia: A prospective analysis of its epidemiology and the pathogenetic role of vasopressin. *Ann Intern Med* 102:164, 1985.
13. Andreoli SP et al: Aluminum intoxication from aluminum-containing phosphate binders in children with azotemia not undergoing dialysis. *N Engl J Med* 310:1079, 1984.
14. Arieff AI: Central nervous system manifestations of disordered sodium metabolism, in Morgan DB (ed): *Clinics in Endocrinology and Metabolism: Electrolyte Disorders.* Philadelphia, Saunders, 1984, p 269.
15. Arieff AI: Dialysis disequilibrium syndrome: Current concepts on pathogenesis, in Schreiner GE, Winchester JF (eds): *Controversies in Nephrology.* Washington, DC, George Washington University Press, 1982, p 367.
16. Arieff AI: Hyponatremia, convulsions, respiratory arrest, and permanent brain damage after elective surgery in healthy women. *N Engl J Med* 314 (24):1529, 1986.
17. Arieff AI: Indications for use of bicarbonate in patients with metabolic acidosis. *Br J Anaesth* 67 (August):165, 1991.
18. Arieff AI: Neurological complications of uremia, in Brenner BM, Rector FC Jr (eds): *The Kidney*, 2d ed. Philadelphia, Saunders, 1981, p 2306.
19. Arieff AI: Pathogenesis of metabolic acidosis with hypoxia, in Arieff AI (ed): *Hypoxia Metabolic Acidosis and the Circulation.* New York, Oxford University Press, 1992, p 116.
20. Arieff AI et al: Hyponatraemia and death or permanent brain damage in healthy children. *Br Med J* 304:1218, 1992.
21. Arieff AI, Carroll HJ: Cerebral edema and depression of sensorium in nonketotic hyperosmolar coma. *Diabetes* 23 (6): 525, 1974.
22. Arieff AI, Carroll HJ: Nonketotic hyperosmolar coma with hyperglycemia: Clinical features, pathophysiology, renal function, acid-base balance, plasma-cerebrospinal fluid equilibria and the effects of therapy in 37 cases. *Medicine (Baltimore)* 51 (2):73, 1972.
23. Arieff AI et al: Dementia, renal failure and brain aluminium. *Ann Intern Med* 90 (5):741, 1979.
24. Arieff AI et al: Mechanisms of seizures and coma in hypoglycemia. Evidence for a direct effect of insulin on electrolyte transport in brain. *J Clin Invest* 54 (3):654, 1974.
25. Arieff AI, Friedman EA: Coma following nonnarcotic drug overdosage: Management of 208 adult patients. *Am J Med Sci* 266 (6):405, 1973.
26. Arieff AI, Graf H: Pathophysiology of type A hypoxic lactic acidosis in dogs. *Am J Physiol* 253 (*Endocrinol Metab* 16): E271, 1987.
27. Arieff AI, Griggs RC: General considerations in metabolic encephalopathies and systemic disorders affecting the nervous system, in Griggs RC, Arieff AI (eds): *Metabolic Brain Dysfunction in Systemic Disorders.* Boston, Little, Brown, 1992, p 1.
28. Arieff AI, Guisado R: Effects on the central nervous system of hypernatremic and hyponatremic states. *Kidney Int* 10:104, 1976.
29. Arieff AI et al: Pathophysiology of hyperosmolar states, in Andreoli TE et al (eds): *Disturbances in Body Fluid Osmolality.* Bethesda, Md, American Physiological Society, 1977, p 227.
30. Arieff AI et al: Central nervous system pH in uremia and the effects of hemodialysis. *J Clin Invest* 58:306, 1976.
31. Arieff AI et al: Intracellular pH of brain: Alterations in acute respiratory acidosis and alkalosis. *Am J Physiol* 230 (3):804, 1976.
32. Arieff AI et al: Cerebral edema in diabetic comas. II. Effects of hyperosmolality, hyperglycemia and insulin in diabetic rabbits. *J Clin Endocrinol Metab* 38 (6):1057, 1974.
33 Arieff AI et al: Brain tissue osmolality: Method of determination and variations in hyper- and hypo-osmolar states. *J Lab Clin Med* 79 (2):334, 1972.
34. Arieff AI et al: Studies on mechanisms of cerebral edema in diabetic comas. Effects of hyperglycemia and rapid lowering of plasma glucose in normal rabbits. *J Clin Invest* 52 (3):571, 1973.
35. Arieff AI et al: Experimental dialysis disequilibrium syndrome: Prevention with glycerol. *Kidney Int* 14:270, 1978.
36. Arieff AI et al: Neurological manifestations and morbidity of hyponatremia: Correlation with brain water and electrolytes. *Medicine (Baltimore)* 55 (2):121, 1976.
37. Arieff AI, Massry SG: Calcium metabolism of brain in acute renal failure. Effects of uremia, hemodialysis, and parathyroid hormone. *J Clin Invest* 53 (2):387, 1974.
38. Arieff AI et al: Brain water and electrolyte metabolism in uremia: Effects of slow and rapid hemodialysis. *Kidney Int* 4:177, 1973.
39. Arieff AI, Papadakis MA: Hyponatremia and hypernatremia in liver disease in Epstein M (ed): *The Kidney in Liver Disease*, 3d ed. Baltimore, MD, Williams & Wilkins, 1988, p 73.
40. Arneil GC, Chin KC: Lower-solute milks and reduction of hypernatraemia in young Glasgow infants. *Lancet* 2:840, 1979.

41. Ashouri OS: Severe diuretic-induced hyponatremia in the elderly: A series of eight patients. *Arch Intern Med* 146:1355, 1986.
42. Assal JP et al: Metabolic effects of sodium bicarbonate in management of diabetic ketoacidosis. *Diabetes* 23:405, 1974.
43. Aubier M et al: Effect of hypophosphatemia on diaphragmatic contractility in patients with acute respiratory failure. *N Engl J Med* 313:420, 1985.
44. Ayus JC, Arieff AI: Brain adaptation and mortality in hyponatremic rodents: Effects of age and gender. *Clin Res* 40:223A, 1992.
45. Ayus JC, Arieff AI: Effects of age and gender on outcome in patients with postoperative hyponatremia. *J Am Soc Nephrol* 2:278, 1991.
46. Ayus JC et al: Postoperative hyponatremic encephalopathy in menstruant women. *Ann Intern Med* (in press).
47. Ayus JC et al: Symptomatic hyponatremia in rats; Effect of treatment on mortality and brain lesions. *Am J Physiol* 257 (*Renal Fluid Electrolyte Physiol* 26):F18, 1989.
48. Ayus JC et al: Severe hypernatremia in rats: Effect of treatment on brain function and histology. *Kidney Int* 35:214, 1989.
49. Ayus JC et al: Treatment of symptomatic hyponatremia and its relation to brain damage. A prospective study. *N Engl J Med* 317 (19):1190, 1987.
50. Ayus JC et al: Rapid correction of severe hyponatremia in the rat: Histopathological changes in the brain. *Am J Physiol* (*Renal Fluid Electrolyte Physiol*) 248:F711, 1985.
51. Ayus JC et al: Rapid correction of severe hyponatremia with intravenous hypertonic saline solution. *Am J Med* 72:43, 1982.
52. Baldessarini RJ: Release of catecholamine: False neurotransmitter, in Iverson LL (ed): *Handbook of Psychopharmacology*. New York, Plenum Press, 1975, p 82.
53. Baluarte JH et al: Encephalopathy in children with chronic renal failure. *Proc Clin Dial Transplant Forum* 7:95, 1977.
54. Banister A et al: Treatment of hypernatremia dehydration in infancy. *Arch Dis Child* 50:179, 1975.
55. Barratt LJ, Lawrence JR: Dialysis-associated dementia. *Aust NZ J Med* 5:62, 1975.
56. Bartholomew LG, Scholz DA: Reversible postoperative neurological symptoms: Report of five cases secondary to water intoxication and sodium depletion. *JAMA* 162:22, 1956.
57. Bartko D: Some aspects of the course of acute cerebral hypoxia, in Bartko D (ed): *Experimental Brain Hypoxia*. Baltimore, MD, University Park Press, 1971, p 15.
58. Batra YK et al: Hyponatraemia and mental symptoms following vesical ultrasonic lithotripsy. *Anaesthesia* 43:675, 1988.
59. Batty IR et al: Rapid formation of inositol 1,3,4,5-tetrakisphosphate following muscarinic receptor stimulation of rat cerebral cortical slices. *Biochem J* 232:211, 1985.
60. Baum M et al:: Continuous ambulatory peritoneal dialysis in children. *N Engl J Med* 305:1537, 1982.
61. Baxter CD: The nature of gamma-aminobutyric acid, in Lajtha A (ed): *Handbook of Neurochemistry*. III. *Metabolic Reactions in the Nervous System*. New York, Plenum Press, 1970, p 289.
62. Baxter CF, Baldwin RA: A functional role for amino acids in the adaptation of tissues from the central nervous system to alterations in environmental osmolality, in Fonnum F (ed): *Amino Acids as Chemical Transmitters*. New York, Plenum Press, 1978, p 599.
63. Beaubernard C et al: Effect of oral administration of branched chain amino acids on hepatic encephalopathy in the rat. *Hepatology* 4:288, 1984.
64. Beigelman P: Severe diabetic ketoacidosis (diabetic coma). 482 episodes in 257 patients; experience of three years. *Diabetes* 20:490, 1971.
65. Bennett WM et al: Response to dopamine hydrochloride in the hepatorenal syndrome. *Arch Intern Med* 135:964, 1975.
66. Berkseth RO, Shapiro FL: An epidemic of dialysis encephalopathy and exposure to high aluminum dialysate, in Schrier GE, Winchester JF (eds): *Controversies in Nephrology*. Georgetown, MD, Georgetown University Press, 1980, p 42.
67. Berl T: Treating hyponatremia: What is all the controversy about? *Ann Intern Med* 113:417, 1990.
68. Bersin RM: Effects of sodium bicarbonate on myocardial metabolism and circulatory function during hypoxia, in Arieff AI (ed): *Hypoxia, Metabolic Acidosis and the Circulation*. New York, Oxford University Press, 1992, p 139.
69. Bessman SP: Osmotic implications of changes in metabolic intermediates in the brain. *Proc Am Soc Neurochem* 7:103, 1976.
70. Bessman SP, Bessman AN: The cerebral and peripheral uptake of ammonia in liver disease with a hypothesis for the mechanisms of hepatic coma. *J Clin Invest* 34:622, 1955.
71. Bihari D et al: The effects of vasodilation with prostacylin on oxygen delivery and uptake in critically ill patients. *N Engl J Med* 317:397, 1987.
72. Blackshear PJ, Alberti KGMM: Experimental diabetic ketoacidosis. *Biochem J* 138:107, 1974.
73. Boon AP et al: Central pontine myelinolysis not associated with rapid correction of hyponatremia. *Lancet* 2:458, 1988.
74. Boon AP, Potter AE: Extensive extrapontine and central pontine myelinolysis associated with correction of profound hyponatraemia. *Neuropathol Appl Neurobiol* 13:1, 1987.
75. Booth RFG, Clark JB: A rapid method for the preparation of relatively pure metabolically competent synaptosomes from rat brain. *Biochem J* 176:365, 1978.
76. Borg J et al: Neurotransmitter modification in human cerebrospinal fluid and serum during hepatic encephalopathy. *J Neurol Sci* 57:343, 1982.
77. Bourke RS et al: Variation of cerebral cortex fluid spaces in vivo as a function of species brain size. *Am J Physiol* 208:682, 1965.
78. Bowser-Wallace BH et al: Hypertonic lactated saline resuscitation of severely burned patients over 60 years of age. *J Trauma* 25 (1):22, 1985.
79. Bradbury MWB: The structure and function of the blood-brain barrier. *Fed Proc* 43:186, 1984.

80. Bradbury MWB, Kleeman CR: Stability of the potassium concentrations of cerebrospinal fluid and brain. *Am J Physiol* 213:519, 1967.
81. Bradbury MWB et al: The calcium and magnesium content of skeletal muscle, brain, and cerebrospinal fluid as determined by atomic absorption flame photometry. *J Lab Clin Med* 71:884, 1968.
82. Brennan S, Ayus JC: Central pontine myelinolysis and electrolyte disorders, in Griggs RC, Arieff AI (eds): *Neurological Manifestations of Systemic Disorders*. Boston, Little, Brown, 1993, in press.
83. Brightman MW et al: Morphology of the walls around fluid compartments in nervous tissue, in Cserr HF et al (eds): *Fluid Environment of the Brain*. New York, Academic Press, 1975, p 3.
84. Bruck E et al: Pathogenesis and pathophysiology of hypertonic dehydration with diarrhea. *Am J Dis Child* 115:122, 1968.
85. Brun A, Dictor M: Senile plaques and tangles in dialysis dementia. *Acta Pathol Microbiol Scand* A 89:193, 1981.
86. Brunner JE et al: Central pontine myelinolysis and pontine lesions after rapid correction of hyponatremia: A prospective magnetic resonance imaging study. *Ann Neurol* 27:61, 1990.
87. Burks JS et al: A fatal encephalopathy in chronic haemodialysis patients. *Lancet* 1:764, 1976.
88. Burrows FA et al: Inappropriate secretion of antidiuretic hormone in a postsurgical pediatric population. *Crit Care Med* 11:527, 1983.
89. Buxton BH et al: Plasma amino acids in experimental hepatic failure and their relationship to brain tryptophan. *Clin Sci* 46:559, 1974.
90. Cain SM: Oxygen delivery and uptake in dogs during anemic and hypoxic hypoxia. *J Appl Physiol* 42:228, 1977.
91. Cameron JM, Dayan AD: Association of brain damage with therpeutic abortion induced by amniotic-fluid replacement: Report of two cases. *Br Med J* 1:1010, 1966.
92. Canalese J et al: Control trial of dexamethasone and mannitol for cerebral oedema of fulminant hepatic failure. *Gut* 23:625, 1982.
93. Caronna JJ, Finklestein S: Neurological syndromes after cardiac arrest. *Stroke* 9:517, 1978.
94. Carroll HJ et al: Exchangeable sodium, body potassium and body water in previously edematous cardiac patients. Evidence for osmotic inactivation of cation. *Circulation* 32:185, 1965.
95. Cartier F et al: Progressive myoclonic encephalopathy in dialysis patients. *Nouv Presse Med* 7:97, 1978.
96. Cavanagh JB, Kyu MH: Type II Alzheimer change experimentally produced in astrocytes in the rat. *J Neurol Sci* 12:63, 1971.
97. Chan PH, Fishman RA: Elevation of rat brain amino acids, ammonia and idiogenic osmoles induced by hyperosmolality. *Brain Res* 161 (2):293, 1979.
98. Chase RA et al: Plasma amino acid profiles in patients with fulminant hepatic failure treated by repeated poly acrylonitrile membrane haemodialysis. *Gastroenterology* 75:1033, 1978.
99. Chason JL et al: Central pontine myelinolysis. *J Neurol Neurosurg Psychiatr* 27:317, 1964.
100. Cheng JC et al: Long term neurologic outcome in psychogenic water drinkers with severe symptomatic hyponatremia: The effect of rapid correction. *Am J Med* 88:561, 1990.
101. Cherrill DA et al: Demeclocycline treatment in the syndrome of inappropriate antidiuretic hormone secretion. *Ann Intern Med* 83:654, 1975.
102. Cheung JY et al: Calcium and ischemic injury. *N Engl J Med* 314 (26):1670, 1986.
103. Chokroverty S et al: Progressive dialytic encephalopathy. *J Neurol Neurosurg Psychiatr* 39:411, 1976.
104. Chung HM et al: Hyponatremia: A prospective study of frequency, cause and outcome. *Kidney Int* 25:160, 1984.
105. Clements RS Jr et al: Acute cerebral edema during treatment of hyperglycaemia. *Lancet* 2:384, 1968.
106. Cobbs R et al: Adrenocortical insufficiency with normal cortisol levels and hyporeninaemia in a patient with acquired immunodeficiency syndrome (AIDS). *J Intern Med* 230:179, 1991.
107. Cogan MG: Atrial natriuretic peptide. *Kidney Int* 37:1148, 1990.
108. Cogan MG et al: Central nervous system manifestations of hyperparathyroidism. *Am J Med* 65:963, 1978.
109. Collins RC et al: Selective vulnerability of the brain: New insights into the pathophysiology of stroke. *Ann Intern Med* 110 (12):992, 1989.
110. Conn HO et al: Comparison of lactulose and neomycin in the treatment of chronic portal-systemic encephalopathy. A double blind controlled trial. *Gastroenterology* 72:573, 1977.
111. Conn HO: The syndrome of portal-systemic encephalopathy, in Conn HO, Lieberthal MM (ed): *The Hepatic Coma Syndromes and Lactulose*. Baltimore, Williams & Wilkins, 1978, p 1.
112. Conn HO, Lieberthal MM: *The Hepatic Coma Syndromes and Lactulose*. Baltimore, Williams & Wilkins, 1978.
113. Cooper JD et al: Neurologic abnormalities in patients with acute renal failure. *Kidney Int* 10:556, 1976.
114. Cooper JD et al: Neurodiagnostic abnormalities in patients with acute renal failure. Evidence for neurotoxicity of parathyroid hormone. *J Clin Invest* 61:1448, 1978.
115. Covey CM, Arieff AI: Disorders of sodium and water metabolism and their effects on the central nervous system, in Brenner BM, Stein JH (eds): *Sodium and Water Homeostasis*. Contemporary Issues in Nephrology (series), New York, Churchill Livingstone, 1978, p 212.
116. Cowie J et al: The influence of extracorporeal dialysis on the acid-base composition of blood and cerebrospinal fluid. *Clin Sci* 23:397, 1962.
117. Cowley DM et al: Pathogenesis of postoperative hyponatremia following correction of scoliosis in children. *Aust N Z J Surg* 58:485, 1988.
118. Crone C: Properties of the blood brain barrier with special emphasis on glucose, in Cserr HF et al (eds): *Fluid Environment of the Brain*. New York, Academic Press, 1975, p 3.
119. Crossley IR et al: Biochemical mechanisms of hepatic encephalopathy. *Clin Sci* 64:247, 1983.
120. Crossley IR, Williams R: Progress in treatment of chronic portal-systemic encephalopathy. *Gut* 25:85, 1984.

121. Cummings MD et al: Regional brain indoleamine metabolism following chronic portacaval anastomosis in the rat. *J Neurochem* 27:501, 1976.
122. Cummings MD et al: Regional brain study of indoleamine metabolism in the rat in acute hepatic failure. *J Neurochem* 27:741, 1976.
123. Curtis DR, Watkins JC: The pharmacology of amino acids related to gamma-aminobutyric acid. *Pharmacol Rev* 17:347, 1965.
124. Cusano AJ et al: Hyponatremia in patients with acquired immune deficiency syndrome. *J Acquir Immune Defic Syndr* 3 (10):949, 1990.
125. Dahlqvist A, Gryboski JD: Inability of the human small intestinal lactase to hydrolyse lactulose. *Biochim Biophys Acta* 110:635, 1965.
126. Dascal N et al: Expression and modulation of voltage-gated calcium channels after injection of RNA injection into Xenopus oocytes. *Science* 231 (1147):1986.
127. David R et al: Water intoxication in normal infants: Role of antidiuretic hormone in pathogenesis. *Pediatrics* 68:349, 1981.
128. Davis FB et al: Specific inositol phosphates inhibit basal and calmodulin-stimulated Ca^{++}-ATPase activity in human erythrocyte membranes in vitro and inhibit binding of calmodulin to membranes. *FASEB* 5:2992, 1991.
129. Davson H: The extracellular space of brain and cord, in Davson H (ed): *Physiology of the Cerebrospinal Fluid.* London, J & A Churchill, 1968, p 107.
130. Davson H: Ionic equilibrium, bioelectric potentials, and active transport, in Davson H (ed): *A Textbook of General Physiology.* Baltimore, Williams & Wilkins, 1970, p 550.
131. de Pasquale M et al: Brain ion and volume regulation during acute hypernatremia in Brattleboro rats. *Am J Physiol* 256:F1059, 1989.
132. Decaux G et al: Treatment of the syndrome of inappropriate secretion of antidiuretic hormone by urea. *Am J Med* 69:99, 1980.
133. Decaux G et al: Hyponatremia in the syndrome of inappropriate secretion of antidiuretic hormone. *JAMA* 247:471, 1982.
134. Deferrari G et al: Brain metabolism of amino acids and ammonia in patients with chronic renal insufficiency. *Kidney Int* 20:505, 1981.
135. DeFronzo RA et al: Normal diluting capacity in hyponatremic patients. *Ann Intern Med* 84:538, 1976.
136. Dekaban AS, Sadowsky D: Changes in brain weights during the span of human life: Relation of brain weights to body heights and body weights. *Ann Neurol* 4:345, 1978.
137. Del Bigio MR, Fedoroff S: Swelling of astroglia in vitro and the effect of arginine vasopressin and atrial natriuretic peptide. *Acta Neurochirurgica* (suppl 51):14, 1990.
138. del Castillo AR et al: Regional changes of brain Na+ K+-transporting adenosine triphosphate related to ovarian function. *Brain Res* 416:113, 1987.
139. Derr RF, Zieve L: Weakness, neuropathy and coma following total parenteral nutrition in underfed or starved rats: Relationship to blood hyperosmolality and brain water loss. *J Lab Clin Med* 92:521, 1978.
140. Deutsch S et al: Postoperative hyponatremia with the inappropriate release of antidiuretic hormone. *Anesthesiology* 27:250, 1966.
141. Dewberry FL et al: The dialysis dementia syndrome: Report of fourteen cases and review of the literature. *Am Soc Artif Intern Organs* J3:102, 1980.
142. DeWitt LD et al: Central pontine myelinolysis: Demonstration by nuclear magnetic resonance. *Neurology* 34:570, 1984.
143. Dienel GA: Regional accumulation of calcium in postischemic rat brain. *J Neurochem* 43:913, 1984.
144. Dienst SG: Treatment of progressive ammonia intoxication by exclusion of the colon. *N Engl J Med* 270:555, 1964.
145. Doczi T et al: Regulation of brain water and electrolyte contents: The opposite actions of central vasopressin and atrial natriuretic factor. *Acta Neurochir Suppl (Wien)* 43:186, 1988.
146. Doczi T et al: Increased concentration of atrial natriuretic factor in the cerebrospinal fluid of patients with aneurysmal subarachnoid hemorrhage and raised intracranial pressure. *Neurosurgery* 23:16, 1988.
147. Dreyer EB et al: HIV-1 coat protein neurotoxicity prevented by calcium channel antagonists. *Science* 248:364, 1990.
148. Dubois GD et al: Central pontine myelinolysis and hyponatremia. *Clin Res* 31:98, 1983.
149. Dubois GD, Arieff AI: Treatment of symptomatic hyponatremia: The case for rapid correction, in Narins RG (ed): *Controversies in Nephrology and Hypertension.* New York, Churchill Livingstone, 1984, p 393.
150. Dunea G et al: Role of aluminum in dialysis dementia. *Ann Intern Med* 88:502, 1978.
151. Eagel BA et al: Reye's syndrome in an adult. *Conn Med* 53:3, 1989.
152. Elkinton JR et al: Inactive cell base and the measurement of changes in cell water. *Yale J Biol Med* 17:383, 1944.
153. Evans RW et al: The quality of life of hemodialysis recipients treated with recombinant human erythropoietin. *JAMA* 263 (825): 1990.
154. Eveloff JL, Warnock DG: Activation of ion transport systems during cell volume regulation. *Am J Physiol* 252 (*Renal Fluid Electrolyte Physiol* 21): F1, 1987.
155. Faden AI et al: The role of excitatory amino acids and NMDA receptors in traumatic brain injury. *Science* 244:798, 1989.
156. Faraci FM et al: Effect of vasopressin on production of cerebrospinal fluid: Possible role of vasopressin (V1)-receptors. *Am J Physiol* 258 (*Regulatory Integrative Comp Physiol* 27):R94, 1990.
157. Ferenci P et al: Changes in the status of neurotransmitter receptors in rabbit model of hepatic encephalopathy. *Hepatology* 4:186, 1984.
158. Ferenci P et al: Metabolism of the inhibitory neurotransmitter gamma-aminobutyric acid in a rabbit model of acute hepatic failure. *Hepatology* 1:509, 1981.
159. Fernandez JP et al: Cerebral edema from blood-brain glucose differences complicating peritoneal dialysis second membrane syndrome. *NY State J Med* 68:677, 1968.
160. Ferrendelli JA, Chang MM: Brain metabolism during hypoglycemia. *Arch Neurol* 28:173, 1973.
161. Finberg L: Pathogenesis of lesions in the nervous system in hypernatremic states: I. Clinical observations of infants. *Pediatrics* 23:40, 1959.
162. Finberg L, Harrison HE: Hypernatremia in infants: An

evaluation of the clinical and biochemical findings accompanying this state. *Pediatrics* 16:1, 1955.
163. Finberg L et al: Mass accidental salt poisoning in infancy: A study of a hospital disaster. *JAMA* 184:187, 1963.
164. Finberg L et al: Pathogenesis of lesions in the nervous system in hypernatremic states: Experimental studies of gross anatomic changes and alterations of chemical composition of the tissues. *Pediatrics* 23:46, 1959.
165. Fischer JE et al: Neurotransmitter metabolism in hepatic encephalopathy. *N Engl J Med* 293:1152, 1975.
166. Fischer JE, Baldessarini RJ: False neurotransmitters and hepatic failure. *Lancet* 2:75, 1971.
167. Fitzgerald FT: Hypophosphatemia. *West J Med* 122:482, 1975.
168. Flannery DB et al: Current status of hyperammonemia syndromes. *Hepatology* 2:495, 1982.
169. Flendrig JA et al: Aluminum and dialysis dementia. *Lancet* 1:235, 1976.
170. Flock V et al: Glucose metabolism in brains of diabetic rats. *Endocrinology* 85:428, 1969.
171. Florkin M, Schoffeniels E: Isosmotic intracellular regulation, in Florkin M, Schoffeniels E (eds): *Molecular Approaches to Ecology*. New York, Academic Press, 1969, p 89.
172. Forrest JN et al: Superiority of demeclocycline over lithium in the treatment of chronic syndrome of inappropriate secretion of antidiuretic hormone. *N Engl J Med* 298:173, 1978.
173. Forster RP, Goldstein L: Intracellular osmoregulatory role of amino acids and urea in marine elasmobranchs. *Am J Physiol* 230:925, 1976.
174. Foster DW et al: Action of methanethiol on Na^+-K^+-ATPase: Implications for hepatic coma. *Ann NY Acad Sci* 242:573, 1974.
175. Foster DW: Insulin deficiency and hyperosmolar coma. *Adv Intern Med* 19:159, 1974.
176. Fraser CL et al: Altered Na transport in brain of uremic rats: Relation to neurotransmission in uremia? *Clin Res* 32:532, 1984.
177. Fraser CL, Arieff AI: Encefalopatia hepatica. *Rev Cubana Med* 27 (2):112, 1988.
178. Fraser CL, Arieff AI: Fatal central diabetes mellitus and insipidus resulting from untreated hyponatremia: A new syndrome. *Ann Intern Med* 112 (2):113, 1990.
179. Fraser CL, Arieff AI: Hepatic encephalopathy. *N Engl J Med* 313 (14):865, 1985.
180. Fraser CL, Arieff I: Manifestaciones neurologicas de uremia, in Llach F, Valderrabano F (eds): *Insuficiencia Renal Cronica*. Madrid, Spain, Ediciones Norma, 1990, p. 96.
181. Fraser CL, Arieff AI: Nervous system complications in uremia. *Ann Intern Med* 109 (2):143, 1988.
182. Fraser CL, Arieff AI: Nervous system manifestations of renal failure, in Schrier RW, Gottschalk CW (eds): *Diseases of the Kidney*, 5th ed. Boston, Little, Brown, 1993, p 2789.
183. Fraser CL, Arieff AI: Water metabolism and its disorders, in Cohen RD et al (eds): *The Metabolic and Molecular Basis of Acquired Disease*. Philadelphia and London, Saunders/Baillière Tindall, 1990, p 1002.
184. Fraser CL et al: Sex differences result in increased morbidity from hyponatremia in female rats. *Am J Physiol* 256 (*Regulatory Integrative Comp Physiol* 25): R880, 1989.
185. Fraser CL, Sarnacki P: Inositol 1,4,5 tris-phosphate may regulate cystolic Ca^{++} in rat brain synaptosomes. *J Clin Invest* 86 (6):2169, 1990.
186. Fraser CL, Sarnacki P: Na^+-K^+ ATPase pump function in male rat brain synaptosomes is different from that of females. *Am J Physiol* 257 (*Endocrinol Metab* 20): E284, 1989.
187. Fraser CL, Sarnacki P: Parathyroid hormone mediates changes in calcium transport in uremic rat brain synaptosomes. *Am J Physiol* 254 (*Renal Fluid Electrolyte Physiol* 23): F837, 1988.
188. Fraser CL, Sarnacki P: Regulation of plasma membrane-bound Ca^{2+}-ATPase pump by inositol phosphates in rat brain. *Am J Physiol* 262:F411, 1992.
189. Fraser CL et al: Abnormal sodium transport in synaptosomes from brain of uremic rats. *J Clin Invest* 75 (6):2014, 1985.
190. Fraser CL et al: Calcium transport abnormality in uremic rat brain synaptosomes. *J Clin Invest* 76 (5):1789, 1985.
191. Fraser CL et al: Evidence that parathyroid hormone-mediated calcium transport in rat brain synaptosomes is independent of cyclic adenosine monophosphate. *J Clin Invest* 81:982, 1988.
192. Fuller TJ et al: Reversible depression in myocardial performance in dogs with experimental phosphorus deficiency. *J Clin Invest* 62:1194, 1978.
193. Fulop M et al: Ketotic hypoerosmolar coma. *Lancet* 2:635, 1973.
194. Furey AT: Hyponatremia after choledochostomy and T tube drainage. *Am J Surg* 112:850, 1966.
195. Furlan AJ et al: Acute areflexic paralysis. *Arch Neurol* 32:706, 1975.
196. Gabuzda GJ Jr et al: Reversible toxic manifestations in patients with cirrhosis of the liver given cations-exchange resins. *N Engl J Med* 246:124, 1952.
197. Garthwaite J: Glutamate, nitric oxide and cell-cell signalling in the nervous system. *TINS* 14 (2):60, 1991.
198. Gehi MM et al: Psychiatric manifestations of hyponatremia. *Psychosomatics* 22:739, 1981.
199. Gellai M et al: Prevention of hyponatremia by alpha-2 receptor agonists. *FASEB Proc* February:A415, 1989.
200. Gerich J et al: Clinical and metabolic characteristics of hyperosmolar nonketotic coma. *Diabetes* 20:228, 1971.
201. Ginsberg MD: Delayed neurological deterioration following hypoxia. *Adv Neurol* 26:21, 1979.
202. Glassock RJ et al: Human immunodeficiency virus (HIV) infection and the kidney. *Ann Intern Med* 112:35, 1990.
203. Goebel HH, Herman-Ben Zur P: Central pontine myelinolysis. A clinical and pathological study of 10 cases. *Brain* 95:495, 1972.
204. Gold LW et al: Renal bicarbonate wasting during phosphate depletion. A possible cause of altered acid-base homeostasis in hyperparathyroidism. *J Clin Invest* 52 (10):2556, 1973.
205. Goldsmith SR: Vasopressin as vasopressor. *Am J Med* 82:1213, 1987.
206. Goldstein CS et al: Idiopathic syndrome of inappropriate antidiuretic secretion possibly related to age. *Ann Intern Med* 99:185, 1983.
207. Goldstein DA et al: The relationship between the abnor-

malities in EEG and blood levels of parathyroid hormone in dialysis patients. *J Clin Endocrinol Metab* 51:130, 1980.
208. Goldstein GW et al: Use of isolated brain capillaries and cultured endothelial cells to study the blood-brain barrier. *Fed Proc* 43:191, 1984.
209. Good PF, Perl DP: A lasar microprobe mass analysis study of aluminum distribution in the cerebral cortex of dialysis encephalopathy. *J Neuropathol Exp Neurol* 47:321, 1988.
210. Goodman WG et al: Short term aluminum administration in the rat: Effects on bone formation and relationship to renal osteomalacia. *J Clin Invest* 73:171, 1984.
211. Graf H et al: Evidence for a detrimental effect of bicarbonate therapy in hypoxic lactic acidosis. *Science* 227 (4688):754, 1985.
212. Greca G et al: Brain density studies during dialysis. *Lancet* 2:582, 1980.
213. Grimm G et al: Improvement of brain function in hemodialysis patients treated with erythropoietin. *Kidney Int* 38:480, 1990.
214. Gross PA et al: Pathogenesis of clinical hyponatremia: Observations of vasopressin and fluid intake in 100 hyponatremic medical patients. *Eur J Clin Invest* 17:123, 1987.
215. Grushkin CM et al: Hemodialysis in small children. *JAMA* 221:869, 1972.
216. Guerra M et al: Androgens stimulate preoptic area Na^+, K^+-ATPase activity in male rats. *Neurosci Lett* 78:97, 1987.
217. Guisado R, Arieff AI: Neurologic manifestations of diabetic comas: Correlation with biochemical alterations in the brain. *Metabolism* 24 (5):665, 1975.
218. Guisado R et al: Changes in the electroencephalogram in acute uremia. Effects of parathyroid hormone and brain electrolytes. *J Clin Invest* 55 (4):738, 1975.
219. Guisado R et al: Effects of glycerol infusions on brain water and electrolytes. *Am J Physiol* 227 (4):865, 1974.
220. Gur RC et al: Gender differences in age effect on brain atrophy measured by magnetic resonance imaging. *Proc Natl Acad Sci USA* 88:2845, 1991.
221. Guyton C: Transport of oxygen in the blood, in *Textbook of Medical Physiology*. Philadelphia, Saunders, 1986, p 496.
222. Hainline B et al: Increased cerebrospinal fluid aluminum and neurological deterioration following deferoxamine administration in dialysis encephalopathy. *Clin Res* 34:221, 1986.
223. Hanig RC, Aprison MH: Determination of calcium, copper, iron, magnesium, manganese, potassium, zinc and chloride in several brain areas. *Anal Biochem* 21:169, 1967.
224. Hantman D et al: Rapid correction of hyponatremia in the syndrome of inappropriate secretion of antidiuretic hormone: An alternative treatment to hypertonic saline. *Ann Intern Med* 78:870, 1973.
225. Hariprasad MK et al: Hyponatremia in psychogenic polydipsia. *Arch Intern Med* 140:1639, 1980.
226. Hawkins R: Cerebral energy metabolism, in McCandless DW (ed): *Cerebral Energy Metabolism and Metabolic Encephalopathy*. New York, Plenum Press, 1985, p 3.
227. Hayashi T: Inhibition and excitation due to GABA in the central nervous system. *Nature* 182:1076, 1958.
228. Heilig CW et al: Characterization of the major brain osmolytes that accumulate in salt-loaded rats. *Am J Physiol* 257 (6 pt. 2):F1108, 1989.
229. Helwig FC et al: Water intoxication: Report of a fatal human case, with clinical, pathologic and experimental studies. *JAMA* 104:1569, 1935.
230. Herschkowitz N et al: Biochemical and electrophysical studies in experimental cerebral edema. *Brain* 88:557, 1965.
231. Heslop J et al: Inositol tetrakis and pentakisphosphate in GH4 cells. *J Exp Biol* 119:395, 1985.
232. Himmelstein DU et al: Hypernatremic dehydration in nursing home patients: An indicator of neglect. *J Am Geriatr Soc* 31:466, 1983.
233. Himwich WA, Agrawal HC: Amino acids: Free amino acid pool of central nervous system, in Lajtha A (ed): *Handbook of Neurochemistry*. New York, Plenum Press, 1969, p 33.
234. Hindfelt B et al: Effect of acute ammonia intoxication on rats with portacaval shunts. *J Clin Invest* 59:386, 1977.
235. Hindfelt B, Siesjo BK: Cerebral effects of acute ammonia intoxication: II. The effect upon energy metabolism. *Scand J Clin Lab Invest* 28:365, 1971.
236. Hirayama C: Tryptophan metabolism in liver disease. *Clin Chim Acta* 32:191, 1971.
237. Hoffman JIE, Buckberg GD: The myocardial supply:demand ratio—A critical review. *Am J Cardiol* 41:327, 1977.
238. Hogan G et al: The incidence of seizures after rehydration of hypernatremic rabbits with intravenous or ad libitum oral fluids. *Pediatr Res* 18:340, 1984.
239. Hornbein TF, Pavlin EG: Distribution of H^+ and HCO_3^- between CSF and blood during respiratory alkalosis in dogs. *Am J Physiol* 228:1149, 1975.
240. Hornbein TF et al: The cost to the central nervous system of climbing to extremely high altitude. *N Engl J Med* 321 (25):1714, 1989.
241. Horowitz ME et al: Increased blood-brain transfer in a rabbit model of acute liver failure. *Gastroenterology* 84:1003, 1983.
242. Horst D et al: Comparison of dietary protein with an oral, branched chain-enriched amino acid supplement in chronic portal-systemic encephalopathy: A randomized controlled trial. *Hepatology* 4:279, 1984.
243. Hourani BT et al: Cerebrospinal fluid glutamine as a measure of hepatic encephalopathy. *Arch Intern Med* 127:1033, 1971.
244. Hoyumpa AM et al: Hepatic encephalopathy. *Gastroenterology* 76:184, 1979.
245. Hruska KA et al: Effects of parathyroid hormone on cytosolic calcium in renal proximal tubular cultures. *Am J Physiol* 251 (20):F188, 1986.
246. Hruska KA et al: Stimulation of inositol trisphosphate and diacylglycerol production in renal tubular cells by parathyroid hormone. *J Clin Invest* 79:230, 1987.
247. Hume HA et al: Treatment of hepatic encephalopathy by surgical exclusion of the colon. *JAMA* 196:593, 1966.
248. Imler M, Schlienger J: The effect of chronic uremia on portal and systemic ammoniemia in normal and portal-strictured rats. *J Lab Clin Med* 94:872, 1979.
249. Irvine RF et al: Inositol triphosphates in carbachol- stimulated rat parotid glands. *Biochem J* 223:237, 1984.

250. James JH et al: Hyperammonemia, plasma amino acid imbalance and blood-brain amino acid transport: A unified theory of portal-systemic encephalopathy. *Lancet* 2:772, 1979.
251. Johnston JG, Robertson WO: Fatal ingestion of table salt by an adult. *West J Med* 126:141, 1977.
252. Jordan D et al: Role of GABA in the control of thyrotropin secretion in the rat. *Brain Res* 268:105, 1983.
253. Joseph SK et al: The role of extracellular Ca^{2+} in the response of the hepatocyte to Ca^{2+}-dependent hormones. *J Biol Chem* 260 (23):12508, 1985.
254. Judd BA et al: Hyponatremia in premature babies and following surgery in older children. *Acta Paediatr Scand* 76:385, 1987.
255. Kaehney WD et al: Aluminum transfer during hemodialysis. *Kidney Int* 12:361, 1977.
256. Kalin MF et al: Hyporeninemic hypoaldosteronism associated with acquired immune deficiency syndrome. *Am J Med* 82:1035, 1987.
257. Kamata S et al: Effects of dietary amino acids and transmitter amines in rats with a portacaval shunt. *J Neurochem* 35:1190, 1980.
258. Kanda F, Arieff AI: Vasopressin inhibits Ca^{++} coupled Na^{+} efflux system in rat brain synaptosomes. *Clin Res* 39:375, 1991.
259. Kanda F, Arieff AI: Vasopressin inhibits calcium-coupled sodium efflux system in rat brain synaptosomes. *Am J Physiol (Regulatory Integrative Comp Physiol)*:(in press), 1992.
260. Kanda F et al: Atrial natriuretic peptide inhibits the amelioride-sensitive sodium-hydrogen exchanger in rat brain. *Am J Physiol (Regulatory Integrative Comp Physiol)* 263:R279, 1992.
261. Kato E, Kuba K: Inhibition of transmitter release in bullfrog sympathetic ganglia induced by gamma-aminobutyric acid. *J Physiol* 298:271, 1980.
262. Katoh Y et al: Parathyroid hormone has a positive ionotropic action in the rat. *Endocrinology* 109:2252, 1981.
263. Katzman R, Pappius HM: Brain ions, in Katzman R, Pappius HM (eds): *Brain Electrolytes and Fluid Metabolism.* Baltimore, Williams & Wilkins, 1973, p 111.
264. Katzman R, Pappius HM: Cerebrospinal fluid ions, in Katzman R, Pappius HM (eds): *Brain Electrolytes and Fluid Metabolism.* Baltimore, Williams & Wilkins, 1973, p 75.
265. Katzman R, Pappius HM: Fluid compartments, in Katzman R, Pappius HM (eds): *Brain Electrolytes and Fluid Metabolism.* Baltimore, Williams & Wilkins, 1973, p 33.
266. Katzman R, Pappius HM: Hypernatremia and hyperosmolarity, in Katzman R, Pappius HM (eds): *Brain Electrolytes and Fluid Metabolism.* Baltimore, Williams & Wilkins, 1973, p 278.
267. Kaupke C et al: Hypernatremia after the administration of lactulose. *Ann Intern Med* 86:745, 1977.
268. Kawai K, Unger RH: Effects of gamma-aminobutyric acid on insulin, glucagon and somatostatin release from isolated perfused dog pancreas. *Endocrinology* 113:111, 1983.
269. Kennedy AC et al: Dialysis disequilibrium syndrome, in Shaldon S, Cook GC (eds): *Acute Renal Failure.* Oxford, UK, Blackwell, 1964, p 66.
270. Kennedy AC et al: Urea levels in cerebrospinal fluid after hemodialysis. *Lancet* 1:410, 1962.
271. Kennedy AC et al: Electroencephalographic changes during hemodialysis. *Lancet* 1:408, 1963.
272. Kety SS et al: The blood flow and oxygen consumption of the human brain in diabetic acidosis and coma. *J Clin Invest* 27:500, 1948.
273. Kiley JE et al: Evaluation of encephalopathy by EEG frequency analysis in chronic dialysis patients. *Clin Nephrol* 5:245, 1976.
274. Kimelberg HK et al: Astrocytic swelling in traumatic-hypoxic brain injury. Beneficial effects of an inhibitor of anion exchange transport and glutamate uptake in glial cells. *Mol Chem Neuropathol* 11 (1):1, 1989.
275. Kjellstrand CM et al: Treatment of acute renal failure, in Schrier RW, Gottschalk CW (eds): *Diseases of the Kidney*, 4th ed. Boston, Little, Brown, 1988, p 1501.
276. Kleinschmidt-DeMasters BK, Norenberg MD: Rapid correction of hyponatremia causes demyelination: Relation to central pontine myelinolysis. *Science* 211:1068, 1981.
277. Kliger AS: Complications of dialysis: Hemodialysis, peritoneal dialysis and CAPD, in Arieff I, DeFronzo RA (eds): *Fluid, Electrolyte and Acid-Base Disorders.* New York, Churchill Livingstone, 1985, p 777.
278. Knigge KM et al: Distribution of hormones by cerebrospinal fluid, in Cserr HF et al (eds): *Fluid Environment of the Brain.* New York, Academic Press, 1975, p 237.
279. Knochel JP: The pathophysiology and clinical characteristics of severe hypophosphatemia. *Arch Intern Med* 137:203, 1977.
280. Knochel JP et al: Hypophosphatemia and rhabdomyolysis. *J Clin Invest* 62:1240, 1978.
281. Kogeorgos J, Scholtz C: Neurofibrillary tangles in aluminum encephalopathy: A new finding. *Neuropathol Appl Neurobiol* 8:246, 1982.
282. Koller KJ et al: Selective activation of the B natriuretic peptide receptor by C-type natriuretic peptide (CNP). *Science* 252:120, 1991.
283. Kreisberg RA: Pathogenesis and management of lactic acidosis. *Annu Rev Med* 35:181, 1984.
284. Krigman MR, Bouldin TW: Oxygen deficiency: Brain hypoxia and ischemia, in Schochet SS Jr (ed): *Neuropathology.* The Clinical Neurosciences, Rosenberg RN (series ed), New York, Churchill Livingstone, 1983, p 496.
285. Kucharczyk J: Localization of central nervous system structures mediating extracellular thirst in the female rat. *J Endocrinol* 98:183, 1984.
286. Kucharczyk J et al: Central nervous system manifestations of hyponatremia, in Griggs R, Arieff AI (eds): *Metabolic Brain Dysfunction in Systemic Disorders.* Boston, Little, Brown, 1992, p 55.
287. Laureno R: Central pontine myelinolysis following rapid correction of hyponatremia. *Ann Neurol* 13:232, 1983.
288. Laureno R, Karp BI: Pontine and extrapontine myelinolysis following rapid correction of hyponatremia. *Lancet* 1:1439, 1988.
289. Lefauconnier JM, Hauw JJ: The blood-brain barrier: II. Physiological data. *Rev Neurol* 140:3, 1984.
290. Levin E et al: Evidence of different compartments in the brain for extracellular markers. *Am J Physiol* 221 (5):1319, 1971.

291. Levin VA et al: Sucrose and inulin space measurements of cerebral cortex in four mammalian species. *Am J Physiol* 219:1528, 1970.
292. Levy DE et al: Prognosis in nontraumtic coma. *Ann Intern Med* 94 (3):293, 1981.
293. Levy NB: Symposium on sexual problems of chronic renal failure patients. *Dialysis Transplant* 7:870, 1978.
294. Lewis SA, Donaldson P: Ion channels and cell volume regulation: Chaos in an organized system. *NIPS* 5:112, 1990.
295. Lien YH et al: Effects of hypernatremia on organic brain osmoles. *J Clin Invest* 85 (5):1427, 1990.
296. Livingston AS et al: Changes in the blood-brain barrier in hepatic coma after hepatectomy in the rat. *Gastroenterology* 73:697, 1977.
297. Lockwood AH: Acute and chronic hyperosmolality: Effects on cerebral amino acids and energy metabolism. *Arch Neurol* 32:62, 1975.
298. Lockwood AH: Ammonia-induced encephalopathy, in McCandless DW (ed): *Cerebral Energy Metabolism and Metabolic Encephalopathy*. New York, Plenum Publishing, 1985, chap 9.
299. Lockwood AH et al: The dynamics of ammonia metabolism in man: Effects of liver disease and hyperammoniaemia. *J Clin Invest* 63:449, 1979.
300. Losowsky MS et al: Hepatic encephalopathy. *Br Med J* 3:279, 1973.
301. Lotz M et al: Evidence for a phosphorus-depletion syndrome in man. *N Engl J Med* 278:409, 1968.
302. Macauley D, Watson M: Hypernatremia as a cause of brain damage. *Arch Dis Child* 42:485, 1967.
303. Maccario M et al: Focal seizures as a manifestation of hyperglycemia without ketoacidosis. *Neurology* 15:195, 1965.
304. Maffly RH, Leaf A: The potential of water in mammalian tissues. *J Gen Physiol* 42:1257, 1959.
305. Mahoney CA, Arieff AI: Uremic encephalopathies: Clinical, biochemical and experimental features. *Am J Kidney Dis* 2 (3):324, 1982.
306. Mahoney CA et al: Central and peripheral nervous system effects of chronic renal failure. *Kidney Int* 24 (2):170, 1983.
307. Mahoney CA et al: Uremic encephalopathy: Role of brain energy metabolism. *Am J Physiol* 247 (*Renal Fluid Electrolyte Physiol* 16):F527, 1984.
308. Mahurkar SD et al: Dialysis dementia. *Lancet* 1:1412, 1973.
309. Mahurkar SD et al: Electroencephalographic and radionucleotide studies in dialysis dementia. *Kidney Int* 13:306, 1978.
310. Manev H et al: Abusive stimulation of excitatory amino acid receptors: A strategy to limit neurotoxicity. *FASEB J* 4:2789, 1990.
311. Marks V, Rose C: Cerebral metabolism and hypoglycemia, in *Hypoglycemia*. Oxford, Blackwell, 1965, p 52.
312. Martin HE et al: The fluid and electrolyte therapy of severe diabetic acidosis and ketosis. A study of twenty-nine episodes (twenty-six patients). *Am J Med* 24:376, 1958.
313. Mattar JA et al: Cardiac arrest in the critically ill. II. Hyperosmolar states following cardiac arrest. *Am J Med* 56:162, 1974.
314. McCance RA: Experimental sodium chloride deficiency in man. *Proc R Soc Biol* 119:245, 1936.
315. McClain CJ et al: Blood methanethiol in alcoholic liver disease with and without hepatic encephalopathy. *Gut* 21:318, 1980.
316. McDermott JR et al: Brain aluminum concentration in dialysis encephalopathy. *Lancet* 1:901, 1978.
317. McDowell ME et al: Osmotic volumes of distribution: Idiogenic changes in osmotic pressure associated with administration of hypertonic solutions. *Am J Physiol* 180:545, 1955.
318. McGarry JD, Foster DW: Ketogenesis and its regulation. *Am J Med* 61:9, 1976.
319. Mchedlishvili G, Bevan JA: Cerebral arterial behavior providing constant cerebral blood flow, pressure and volume, in Mchedlishvili G, Bevan JA(eds): *Arterial Behavior and Blood Circulation in the Brain*. New York, Plenum Press, 1986, p 43.
320. McKee A et al: Central pontine myelinolysis in severely burned patients: Relationship to serum hyperosmolality. *Neurology* 38:1211, 1988.
321. Melton JE, Nattie EE: Brain and CSF water and ions during dilutional and isomotic hyponatremia in the rat. *Am J Physiol* 244:R724, 1983.
322. Melton JE et al: Volume regulatory loss of Na, Cl, and K from rat brain during acute hyponatremia. *Am J Physiol* 252 (*Renal Fluid Electrolyte Physiol* 21):F661, 1987.
323. Meyers LP et al: Reduction of gastric ammonia by ampicillin in normal and azotemic subjects. *Gastroenterology* 70:244, 1976.
324. Meythaler JM, Varma RR: Reye's syndrome in adults. *Arch Intern Med* 147:61, 1987.
325. Miller GM et al: Central pontine myelinolysis and its imitators: MR findings. *Radiology* 168:795, 1988.
326. Miller M, Moses A: Normal diluting capacity in hyponatremic patients. Drug-induced states of impaired water excretion. *Kidney Int* 10:96, 1976.
327. Miller PD et al: Plasma demeclocycline levels and nephrotoxicity. Correlation in hyponatremic cirrhotic patients. *JAMA* 243:2513, 1980.
328. Monaghan DT et al: The excitatory amino acid receptors: Their classes, pharmacology, and distinct properties in the function of the central nervous system. *Annu Rev Pharmacol Toxicol* 29:365, 1989.
329. Morris-Jones PH et al: Prognosis of the neurological complications of acute hypernatremia. *Lancet* 2:1385, 1967.
330. Moses AM et al: Drugs and water metabolism, in Arieff AI, DeFronzo RA (eds): *Fluid, Electrolyte and Acid-Base Disorders*. New York & London, Churchill Livingstone, 1985, p 1145.
331. Moskowitz MA, Wurtman RJ: Catecholamines and neurological diseases. *N Engl J Med* 293:274, 1975.
332. Munro HN et al: Insulin, plasma amino acid imbalance and hepatic coma. *Lancet* 1:722, 1975.
333. Munro HN et al: Plasma neutral amino acids and tryptophan in cirrhosis. *Lancet* 2:419, 1975.
334. Muto Y et al: Effect of short-chain fatty acids on the electrical activity of neo-, paleo-, and archicortical system. *Brain Nerve* 16:601, 1964.

335. Nadel AM, Wilson WP: Dialysis encephalopathy: A possible seizure disorder. *Neurology* 26:1130, 1976.
336. Nakao N et al: Effect of atrial natriuretic peptide on ischemic brain edema: Changes in brain water and electrolytes. *Neurosurgery* 27 (1):39, 1990.
337. Naruse S et al: Effects of atrial natriuretic peptide on ischemic brain edema in rats evaluated by proton magnetic resonance method. *Stroke* 22 (1):61, 1991.
338. Nattie EE, Edwards WH: Brain and CSF water ion newborn puppies during acute hypo- and hypernatremia. *J Appl Physiol* 51:1086, 1981.
339. Nelson DC et al: Hypernatremia and lactulose therapy. *JAMA* 249 (10):1295, 1983.
340. Norenberg MD et al: An experimental model for the study of hepatic encephalopathy. *Arch Neurol* 11:128, 1974.
341. Norenberg MD, Lapham LW: The astrocyte response in experimental portal-systemic encephalopathy: An electron-microscopic study. *J Neuropathol Exp Neurol* 33:422, 1974.
342. Norenberg MD et al: Association between rise in serum sodium and central pontine myelinolysis. *Ann Neurol* 11:128, 1982.
343. Noriega-Sanchez A et al: Clinical and electroencephalographic changes in progressive uremic encephalopathy. *Neurology* 28:667, 1978.
344. Nunnelley LL et al: Uremic hyperstannum: Elevated tissue tin levels associated with uremia. *J Lab Clin Med* 91:72, 1978.
345. O'Connor LR et al: Effect of hypophosphatemia on myocardial performance in man. *N Engl J Med* 297:901, 1977.
346. Oelz O et al: Cognitive impairment, neurologic performance and MRI after repeat exposure to extreme altitude, in Sutton JR et al (eds): *Hypoxia, The Adaptations.* Philadelphia, BC Becker, 1990, p 206.
347. Ogihara K et al: Tryptohan as a cause of hepatic coma. *N Engl J Med* 275:1255, 1966.
348. Ohman JL et al: The cerebrospinal fluid in diabetic ketoacidosis. *N Engl J Med* 284:283, 1971.
349. Okada Y, Hazama A: Volume-regulatory ion channels in epithelial cells. *NIPS* 4:238, 1989.
350. Oldendorf WH, Davson H: Brain extracellular space and the sink action of the CSF. *Arch Neurol* 17:196, 1967.
351. Olivieri NF et al: Visual and auditory neurotoxicity in patients receiving subcutaneous deferoxamine infusions. *N Engl J Med* 314:869, 1986.
352. Ono J et al: Tryptophan and hepatic coma. *Gastroenterology* 74:196, 1978.
353. Orlandi F et al: Comparison between neomycin and lactulose in 173 patients with hepatic encephalopathy. A randomized clinical study. *Dig Dis Sci* 26:498, 1981.
354. Osberg JW et al: Intellectual functioning in renal failure and chronic dialysis. *J Chronic Dis* 35:445, 1982.
355. Palmer AM, Gershon S: Is the neuronal basis of Alzheimer's disease cholinergic or glutamatergic? *FASEB J* 4:2745, 1990.
356. Papadakis MA et al: Hyponatraemia in patients with cirrhosis. *Q J Med* 76:675, 1990.
357. Pappas CS, Jones EA: Methods of assessing hepatic encephalopathy. *Semin Liver Dis* 3 (4):298, 1983.
358. Pappius HM, Dossetor JB: The effects of rapid hemodialysis on brain tissues and cerebrospinal fluid of dogs. *Can J Physiol Pharmacol* 45:129, 1967.
359. Park R, Arieff AI: Lactic acidosis: Current concepts, in Schade DS (ed): *Clinics in Endocrinology and Metabolism.* Philadelphia, Saunders, 1983, p 339.
360. Park R et al: Nutrient deficiencies in man and animals: Water, in Rechcigl M Jr (ed): *CRC Handbook of Nutrition and Food.* Section E, *Nutritional Disorders.* West Palm Beach, FL, CRC Press, 1978, p 363.
361. Park R et al: Determination of liver intracellular pH in vivo and its homeostasis in acute acidosis and alkalosis. *Am J Physiol* 236 (*Renal Fluid Electrolyte Physiol* 5 (3)):F240, 1979.
362. Parkinson ID et al: Fracturing dialysis osteodystrophy and dialysis encephalopathy. *Lancet* 1:406, 1979.
363. Pauli HG et al: Chronic derangements of cerebrospinal fluid acid base components in man. *J Appl Physiol* 17:993, 1962.
364. Pelligrino DA et al: Interregional differences in brain intracellular pH and water compartmentation during acute normoxic and hypoxic hypocapnia in the anesthetized dog. *Brain Res* 214:387, 1981.
365. Pettegrew JW et al: Considerations for brain pH assessment by ^{31}P NMR. *Magn Reson Imaging* 6:135, 1988.
366. Pettegrew JW: Molecular insights into Alzheimer's disease. *Ann NY Acad Sci* 568 (*Calcium Membranes, Aging and Alzheimer's Disease*):5, 1989.
367. Phillips GB et al: Syndrome of impending hepatic coma in patients with cirrhosis of liver given certain nitrogenous compounds. *N Engl J Med* 247:239, 1952.
368. Phillips PA et al: Localization of vasopressin binding sites in rat brain by in vitro autoradiography using a radioiodinated V1 receptor antagonist. *Neuroscience* 27 (3):749, 1988.
369. Pierce NF et al: Relation of ventilation during base deficit to acid-base values in blood and spinal fluid. *J Appl Physiol* 30:677, 1971.
370. Pierides AM et al: Hemodialysis encephalopathy with osteomalacic fractures and muscle weakness. *Kidney Int* 18:115, 1980.
371. Pilbeam CM et al: The brain in experimental portal-systemic encephalopathy: II. Water and electrolyte changes. *J Pathol* 140:347, 1983.
372. Pitts RF et al: The renal regulations of acid-base metabolism in man: I. The nature of the mechanism for acidifying the urine. *J Clin Invest* 27:48, 1948.
373. Plum F, Hindfelt B: The neurological complications of liver disease, in Vinken PJ, Bruyn GW (eds): *Handbook of Clinical Neurology.* Amsterdam, North Holland Publishing, 1976, p 349.
374. Plum F, Posner J: The pathological physiology of signs and symptoms of coma, in Plum F, Posner J (eds): *The Diagnosis of Stupor and Coma,* 2d ed. *Contemporary Neurology* (series), Philadelphia, FA Davis Co., 1966, p 2.
375. Plum F, Posner JB: Metabolic brain diseases causing coma. Hypoosmolar states, in Plum F, McDowell FH (eds): *Diagnosis of Stupor and Coma. Contemporary Neurology* (series), Philadelphia, FA Davis Co, 1966, p 151.

376. Plum F et al: Delayed neurological deterioration after anoxia. *Arch Intern Med* 110:18, 1962.
377. Poirier J et al: Neuropathology of general pathological processes: Cerebral hypoxia/anoxia, and metabolic and toxic encephalopathies, in Poirier J et al (eds): *Manual of Basic Neuropathology*, 3d ed. Philadelphia, Saunders, 1990, p 163.
378. Polinsky MS, Gruskin AB: Aluminum toxicity in childhood secondary to aluminum toxicity. *J Pediatr* 105:758, 1984.
379. Pollock AS, Arieff AI: Abnormalities of cell volume regulation and their functional consequences. *Am J Physiol* 239 (*Renal Fluid Electrolyte Physiol* 8):F195, 1980.
380. Posner JB, Plum F: Spinal-fluid pH and neurologic symptoms in systemic acidosis. *N Engl J Med* 277:605, 1967.
381. Prentki M et al: Rapid mobilization of calcium from rat insulinoma microsomes by inositol-1,4,5-trisphosphate. *Nature* 309:562, 1984.
382. Prior JC et al: Dialysis encephalopathy and osteomalacic bone disease. *Am J Med* 72:33, 1982.
383. Rafalowska UY et al: The effects of acute hypoxia on synaptosomes from rat brain. *J Neurochem* 34:1160, 1980.
384. Raichle ME, Grubb RL: Regulation of brain water permeability by centrally-released vasopressin. *Brain Res* 143:191, 1978.
385. Rapoport SI: Nonbarrier regions in the nervous system, in Rapoport SI (ed): *Blood Brain Barrier in Physiology and Medicine*. New York, Raven Press, 1976, p 77.
386. Rapoport SI: Permeability and osmotic properties of the blood brain barrier: Osmotic edema, in Rapoport SI (ed): *Blood Brain Barrier in Physiology and Medicine*. New York, Raven Press, 1976, p 87.
387. Rapoport SI: Regulation of drug entry into the nervous system, in Rapoport SI (ed): *Blood Brain Barrier in Physiology and Medicine*. New York, Raven Press, 1976, p 153.
388. Rapoport SI: Sites and functions of the blood brain barrier, in Rapoport SI (ed): *Blood Brain Barrier in Physiology and medicine*. New York, Raven Press, 1976, p 43.
389. Rappaport ZH et al: Regional brain calcium changes in the rat middle cerebral artery occlusion model of ischemia. *Stroke* 18:760, 1987.
390. Raskin NH, Fishman RA: Neurologic disorders in renal failure. *N Engl J Med* 294:143, 1976.
391. Raskind M: Psychosis, polydipsia, and water intoxication: Report of a fatal case. *Arch Gen Psychiatry* 30:112, 1974.
392. Rasmussen H: The calcium messenger system, parts I and II. *N Engl J Med* 314:1094, 1986.
393. Reubi FC: Glomerular infiltration rate, renal blood flow and blood viscosity during and after diabetic coma. *Circ Res* 1:410, 1953.
394. Roberts E et al (eds): GABA in Nervous System Function. New York, Raven Press, 554, 1976.
395. Roberts E: The GABA system and hepatic encephalopathy. *Hepatology* 4:342, 1984.
396. Roberts E et al: Some metabolic studies of gamma-aminobutyric acid. *Proc Soc Exp Biol Med* 97:796, 1958.
397. Roberts E, Krause DK: Gamma-aminobuytric acid system in cardiovascular and cerebrovascular function. *Isr J Med Sci* 18:75, 1982.
398. Robinson AG, Zimmerman EA: Cerebrospinal fluid and ependymal neurophysin. *J Clin Invest* 52:1260, 1973.
399. Rodrigo F et al: Osmolality changes during hemodialysis. *Ann Intern Med* 86:554, 1977.
400. Rosen HM et al: Plasma amino acid patterns in hepatic encephalopathy of differing aetiology. *Gastroenterology* 72:483, 1977.
401. Rosen R et al: Neurologic manifestations of hyperalimentation and hypophosphatemia. *Neurology (NY)* 28:389, 1978.
402. Rosen RA et al: Dialysis disequilibrium syndrome. Prevention with glycerol. *Kidney Int* 14:683, 1978.
403. Rosenbaum BJ et al: Acid-base status during the interdialytic period in patients maintained with chronic hemodialysis. *Ann Intern Med* 65:265, 1969.
404. Rosenberg GA et al: Vasopressin-induced brain edema is mediated by the V1 receptor. *Advan Neurol* 52:149, 1990.
405. Rosomoff HL, Zugibe FT: Distribution of intracranial contents in experimental edema. *Arch Neurol* 9:36, 1963.
406. Ross EJ, Christie SBM: Hypernatremia. *Medicine (Baltimore)* 48:441, 1969.
407. Rossi-Fanelli F et al: Correlation of plasma taurine levels with grades of hepatic encephalopathy in man. *Gastroenterology* 72:1181, 1977.
408. Rothman SM: Synaptic activity mediates death of hypoxic neurons. *Science* 220:536, 1983.
409. Rotundo A et al: Progressive encephalopathy in children with chronic renal insufficiency in infancy. *Kidney Int* 21:982, 1982.
410. Ruderman NB et al: Regulation of glucose and ketonebody metabolism in brain of anesthetized rats. *Biochem J* 138:1, 1974.
411. Sabin S, Merritt JA: Treatment of hepatic coma in cirrhosis by plasmapheresis and plasma infusion. *N Engl J Med* 66:1, 1968.
412. Salomon A et al: Subcortical arteriosclerotic encephalopathy: Brain stem findings with MR imaging. *Radiology* 165:625, 1987.
413. Santos F et al: Risk factors in aluminum toxicity in children with chronic renal failure. *Nephron* 42:189, 1986.
414. Sarnaik AP et al: Management of hyponatremic seizures in children with hypertonic saline: A safe and effective strategy. *Crit Care Med* 19:758, 1991.
415. Schafer DG, Jones EA: Potential neural mechanisms in the pathogenesis of hepatic encephalopathy, in Popper H, Schaffner F (eds): *Progress in Liver Disease*. New York, Grune & Stratton, 1982, p 615.
416. Schalm SW, Van der Mey T: Hyperammonemic coma after hepatectomy in germ-free rats. *Gastroenterology* 77:231, 1979.
417. Schmidt-Nielsen B: Cooperative physiology of cellular ion and volume regulation. *J Exp Zool* 194:207, 1975.
418. Schneider R, Droller H: Relative importance of ketosis and acidosis in production of diabetic coma. *Q J Exp Physiol* 28:323, 1938.
419. Schon F et al: On GABA metabolism in the gliocyte cells of the rat pineal gland. *Brain Res* 85:479, 1974.
420. Schrier RA, Berl T: Osmotic and nonosmotic control of vasopressin release. *Am J Physiol* 236:F321, 1979.

421. Scott JC Jr et al: Water intoxication and sodium depletion in surgical patients. *Obstet Gynecol* 26:168, 1965.
422. Seamon KB, Daly JW: Forskolin, cyclic AMP and cellular physiology. *TIPS*:120, 1983.
423. Seamon KB et al: Forskolin: Unique diterpene activator of adenylate cyclase in membranes and in intact cells. *Proc Natl Acad Sci USA* 78:3363, 1981.
424. Sedman AB et al: Evidence of aluminum loading in infants receiving intravenous therapy. *N Engl J Med* 312:1337, 1985.
425. Sedman AB et al: Encephalopathy in childhood secondary to aluminum intoxication. *J Pediatr* 105:836, 1984.
426. Shepherd AP et al: Local control of tissue oxygen delivery and its contribution to the regulation of cardiac output. *Am J Physiol* 225:747, 1973.
427. Shimojyo S et al: The effects of graded hypoxia upon transient cerebral blood flow and oxygen consumption. *Neurology* 18:127, 1968.
428. Siddiqui JY et al: Causes of death in patients receiving long-term hemodialysis. *JAMA* 212:1350, 1970.
429. Siegl AM et al: Inhibition of aggregation and stimulation of cyclic AMP generation in intact human platelets by the diterpene forskolin. *Mol Pharmacol* 21:680, 1982.
430. Siesjo BK: Calcium, excitotoxins, and brain damage. *NIPS* 5:120, 1990.
431. Silvis SE, Paragas PD Jr: Paresthesias, weakness, seizures, and hypophosphatemia in patients receiving hyperalimentation. *Gastroenterology* 62:513, 1972.
432. Simard M et al: Lithium carbonate intoxication. *Arch Intern Med* 149:36, 1989.
433. Simmons MA et al: Hypernatremia and intracranial hemorrhage in neonates. *N Engl J Med* 291:6, 1974.
434. Skowsky VR et al: Effects of sex hormones on arginine vasopressin in intact and castrated male and female rats. *Endocrinology* 104:105, 1979.
435. Smith MC, Bleck TP: Techniques for determining brain death. *J Crit Illness* 4:67, 1989.
436. Smith RJ et al: Hypernatremic, hyperosmolar coma complicating chronic peritoneal dialysis. *Proc Clin Dial Transplant Forum* 4:96, 1974.
437. Smythe WR et al: Trace element abnormalities in chronic uremia. *Ann Intern Med* 96:302, 1982.
438. Snyder NA et al: Hypernatremia in elderly patients. A heterogeneous, morbid, and iatrogenic entity. *Ann Intern Med* 107(3):309, 1987.
439. Snyder SH, Bredt DS: Nitric oxide as a neuronal messenger. *Trends Pharmacol Sci* 12 (4):125, 1991.
440. Soeters PB et al: Insulin, glucagon, portal-systemic shunting and hepatic failure in the dog. *J Surg Res* 23:183, 1977.
441. Somlyo AP et al: Calcium and magnesium movements in cells and the role of inositol trisphosphate in muscle. *Soc Gen Physiol Ser* 42:77, 1987.
442. Soupart A et al: Limits of brain tolerance to daily increments in serum sodium in chronically hyponatraemic rats treated with hypertonic saline or urea: Advantages of urea. *Clin Sci (Oxford)* 80 (1):77, 1991.
443. Sparacio RR et al: Hypernatremia and chorea. A report of two cases. *Neurology (NY)* 26:46, 1976.
444. Stahl J et al: Essai d'interpretation de mecanisme de l'epreuve d'hyperammoniemie provoquee chez les cirrhotiques. *Comp R Acad Sci* 146:1787, 1952.
445. Stallone JN et al: Sexual dimorphism in vasopressin-induced contraction of rat aorta. *Am J Physiol* 260 (*Heart Circ Physiol* 29):H453, 1991.
446. Steardo H, Nathanson JA: Brain barrier tissues: End organs for atriopeptins. *Science* 235:470, 1987.
447. Stern EW, Coxon RV: Osmolality of brain tissue and its relation to brain bulk. *Am J Physiol* 204:1, 1964.
448. Sterns RH: Severe symptomatic hyponatremia: Treatment and outcome. A study of 64 cases. *Ann Intern Med* 107:656, 1987.
449. Sterns RH: Treatment of hyponatremia: Unsafe at any speed? *AKF Nephrol Lett* 6:1, 1989.
450. Sterns RH et al: Osmotic demyelination syndrome following correction of hyponatremia. *N Engl J Med* 314:1535, 1986.
451. Stillman A et al: Reye's syndrome in the adult. *Am J Gastroenterol* 78:365, 1983.
452. Stone JD et al: Sex differences in central adrenergic control of vasopressin release. *Am J Physiol* 257:R1040, 1989.
453. Stone JD et al: Sex differences in central adrenoreceptor-mediated vasopressin response to hemorrhage. *Am J Physiol* 260 (*Endocrinol Metab* 23):E780, 1991.
454. Stone WE et al: Incorporation of carbon from glucose into cerebral amino acids, proteins and lipids, and alterations during recovery from hypoglycemia. *J Neurochem* 19:321, 1972.
455. Stormbeck DR et al: The effects of intravenous ammonia infusion on plasma levels of amino acids, glucagon and insulin in dogs. *Gastroenterology* 74:1165, 1978.
456. Stormont JM, Westerhouse C: The genesis of hyponatremia associated with marked overhydration and water intoxication. *Circulation* 24:191, 1961.
457. Strom TB, Tilney NL: Immunobiology and immunopharmacology of graft rejection, in Schrier RW, Gottschalk CW (eds): *Diseases of the Kidney*, 4th ed. Boston, Little, Brown, 1988, p 3177.
458. Tallal A et al: Subdural hematoma associated with long-term hemodialysis for chronic renal disease. *JAMA* 212:1847, 1970.
459. Teschan PE et al: A prospective study of reduced dialysis. *ASAIO J*6:108, 1983.
460. Teschan PE, Arieff AI: Uremic and dialysis encephalopathies, in McCandless DW (ed): *Cerebral Energy Metabolism and Metabolic Encephalopathy*. New York, Plenum Press, 1985, p 263.
461. Teschan PE et al: Quantitative indices of clinical uremia. *Kidney Int* 15:676, 1979.
462. Thomas AP, Williamson J Jr: Relationship between inositol polyphosphate and the increase of cystolic free Ca^{++} induced by vasopressin in isolated hepatocytes. *J Biol Chem* 259:5574, 1984.
463. Thomas TH, Morgan DB: Post-surgical hyponatraemia: The role of intravenous fluids and arginine vasopressin. *Br J Surg* 66:540, 1979.
464. Thompson DS et al: Computerized tomography in the diagnosis of central and extrapontine myelinolysis. *Arch Neurol* 38:243, 1981.
465. Thompson PD et al: Neurological complications associ-

ated with parenteral treatment: Central pontine myelinolysis and Wernicke's encephalopathy. *Br Med J* 292:684, 1986.

466. Thurston JH, Hauhart RE: Brain amino acids decrease in chronic hyponatremia and rapid correction causes brain dehydration: Possible clinical significance. *Life Sci* 40 (26):2539, 1987.
467. Thurston JH et al: Effects of salt and water loading on carbohydrate and energy metabolism and levels of selected amino acids in the brain of young mice. *J Neurochem* 24:953, 1975.
468. Thurston JH et al: Effect of chronic hypernatremic dehydration and rapid rehydration on brain carbohydrate, energy, and amino acid metabolism in weanling mice. *J Neurochem* 40:240, 1983.
469. Tien R et al: Hyponatremic encephalopathy: Is central pontine myelinolysis a component? *Am J Med* 92(5):513, 1992.
470. Timperly WR: Cerebral intravascular coagulation in diabetic acidosis. *Lancet* 1:952, 1974.
471. Tomlinson BE et al: Central pontine myelinolysis: Two cases with associated electrolyte disturbance. *Q J Med (Oxford)* 65:373, 1976.
472. Tower TB: Inorganic constituents, in Lajtha A (ed): *Handbook of Neurochemistry. I. Chemical Architecture of the Nervous System*. New York, Plenum Press, 1969, p 1.
473. Trauner DA: Regional cerebral Na^+/K^+-ATPase activity following octanoate administration. *Pediatr Res* 14:844, 1980.
474. Travis SF et al: Alterations of red-cell glycolytic intermediates and oxygen transport as a consequence of hypophosphatemia in patients receiving intravenous hyperalimentation. *N Engl J Med* 285:763, 1971.
475. Trey C et al: Treatment of hepatic coma by exchange blood transfusion. *N Engl J Med* 285:763, 1966.
476. Tsutsumi K et al: a-Atrial natriuretic peptide binding sites in the rat choroid plexus are increased in the presence of hydrocephalus. *Neurosci Lett* 87:93, 1988.
477. Uchida K et al: Evaluation of the changes in intracranial water, sodium, phosphorus metabolites and intracellular cerebral pH in rats with acute dilutional hyponatremia. *Nippon Jinzo Gakkai Shi* 32(11):1169, 1990.
478. Uribe M et al: Treatment of chronic portal-systemic encephalopathy with vegetable and animal protein diets. A controlled cross-over study. *Dig Dis Sci* 27:1109, 1982.
479. Van den Noort S et al: Brain metabolism in uremic and adenosine-infused rats. *J Clin Invest* 47:2133, 1968.
480. Van Gelder NM et al: Disposition of gamma-aminobutyric acid administered to animals. *J Neurochem* 3:139, 1985.
481. Van Harreveld A et al: Brain electrolytes and cortical impedance. *Am J Physiol* 201:139, 1961.
482. Verbalis JG et al: Neurological and neuropathological sequelae of correction of chronic hyponatremia. *Kidney Int* 39:1274, 1991.
483. Vexler ZS et al: Effects of hypoxia on brain adaptation in experimental hyponatremia. *Clin Res* 40:May 1992.
484. Vieweg WVR et al: Death from self-induced water intoxication among patients with schizophrenic disorders. *J Nerv Ment Dis* 173 (3):161, 1985.
485. Vincent SR et al: GABA neuron systems in hypothalamus and the pituitary gland. *Neuroendocrinology* 34:117, 1982.
486. Vink R: Decline in intracellular free Mg^{2+} is associated with irreversible tissue injury after brain trauma. *J Biol Chem* 263 (2):757, 1988.
487. Vitting KE et al: Frequency of hyponatremia and nonosmolar vasopressin release in the acquired immunodeficiency syndrome. *JAMA* 263:973, 1990.
488. Ward MK et al: Osteomalacia dialysis osteodystrophy: Evidence for a water-borne aetiological agent, probably aluminum. *Lancet* 1:841, 1978.
489. Ware AJ et al: Cerebral edema: A major complication of massive hepatic necrosis. *Gastroenterology* 61 (6):877, 1971.
490. Warren SE et al: Hypernatremia in hepatic failure. *JAMA* 243(12):1257, 1980.
491. Weber FL, Veach GL: The importance of the small intestine in gut ammonium production in the fasting dog. *Gastroenterology* 77:235, 1979.
492. Weil MH et al: Difference in acid-base state between venous and arterial blood during cardiopulmonary resuscitation. *N Engl J Med* 315(3):153, 1986.
493. Weiss B: The behavioral toxicology of metals. *Fed Proc* 37:22, 1978.
494. West JB: Acid-base status and blood lactate at extreme altitude, in Arieff AI (ed): *Hypoxia, Metabolic Acidosis and the Circulation*. New York, Oxford University Press, 1992, p 33.
495. White RE, Hartzell HC: Effects of intracellular free magnesium on calcium current in isolated cardiac myocytes. *Science* 239:778, 1988.
496. Whittaker VP: The synaptosome, in Lajtha A (ed): *Handbook of Neurochemistry*. New York, Plenum Press, 1969, p 327.
497. Wichser J, Kazemi H: CSF bicarbonate regulation in respiratory acidosis and alkalosis. *J Appl Physiol* 38:504, 1975.
498. Widdowson EM, Dickerson JWT: The effect of growth and function on the chemical composition of soft tissues. *Biochem J* 77:30, 1960.
499. Wieloch T: Endogenous excitotoxins as possible mediators of ischemic and hypoglycemic brain damage. *Adv Exp Med Biol* 203:127, 1986.
500. Wieloch T: Hypoglycemia-induced neuronal damage prevented by an N-methyl-d-aspartate antagonist. *Science* 230:681, 1985.
501. Wieloch T et al: Lesions of the glutamatergic corticostriatal projections in the rat ameliorate hypoglycemic brain damage in the striatum. *Neurosci Lett* 58:25, 1985.
502. Wilkinson SP et al: Frequency and type of renal and electrolyte disorders in fulminant hepatic failure. *Br Med J* 1:186, 1974.
503. Williams R: Fulminant hepatic failure. *Postgrad Med J* 59 (suppl. 4):33, 1983.
504. Williamson JR et al: Inositol trisphosphate and diacylglycerol as intracellular second messengers in liver. *Am J Physiol* 17:C203, 1985.
505. Williamson JR et al: Mechanism of action of vasopressin as a calcium mobilizing hormone, in Crowley AW et al (eds): *Vasopressin: Cellular and Integrative Functions*. New York, Raven Press, 1988, p 33.

506. Wing AJ: Dialysis dementia in Europe: Report from the registration committee of the EDTA. *Lancet* 1:190, 1980.
507. Wolman L: Ichaemic lesions in the brain-stem associated with raised intracranial pressure. *Brain* 76:364, 1953.
508. Wooley DW: *The Biochemical Basis of Psychoses, or the Serotonin Hypothesis about Mental Disease*. New York, Wiley, 1962.
509. Worthley LIG, Thomas PD: Treatment of hyponatraemic seizures with intravenous 29.2% saline. *Br Med J* 292:168, 1986.
510. Wright D et al: Pontine and extrapontine myelinolysis. *Brain* 102:361, 1979.
511. Zierler KL: Hyperosmolarity in adults: A critical review. *J Chronic Dis* 7 (1):1, 1958.
512. Zieve L: Encephalopathy due to short chain fatty acids, in McCandless DW (ed):*Cerebral Energy Metabolism and Metabolic Encephalopathy*. New York, Plenum Publishing, 1985, chap 7.
513. Zieve L: The mechanism of hepatic coma. *Hepatology* 1:360, 1981.
514. Zieve L et al: Synergism between mercaptans and ammonia or fatty acids in the production of coma: A possible role for mercaptans in the pathogenesis of hepatic coma. *J Lab Clin Med* 83:16, 1974.
515. Zieve L, Brunner G: Encephalopathy due to mercaptans and phenols, in McCandless DW (ed): *Cerebral Energy Metabolism and Metabolic Encephalopathy*. New York, Plenum Publishing, 1985. chap 8.
516. Zimmermann B, Wangensteen OH: Observations on water intoxication in surgical patients. *Surgery* 31:654, 1952.

CHAPTER • 47

Disorders of heat regulation

James P. Knochel • Gary Reed

HEAT STRESS

THERMOREGULATION IN THE HEAT

The ability to maintain a temperature of 37°C is critical to human survival. In response to a rise of body temperature, whether the source of heating is environmental or endogenous, responses occur that facilitate dissipation of the heat load; similarly, if heat is lost, responses occur that favor conservation of heat. Collectively, the physiologic processes that control heat production, heat loss, or heat gain so as to maintain a normal body temperature define the term *thermoregulation*.

Three factors determine the thermal balance of the body: metabolic heat production, heat exchange between the organism and its surroundings, and heat loss by the evaporation of sweat.

Heat production by basal metabolism typically adds about 60 to 70 kcal (nutritional Calories) per hour in the adult. Heat production increases markedly with excercise, and for brief periods of intense physical work may exceed 1000 kcal/h.[251] By definition, one kcal is capable of increasing the temperature of one kilogram of water one degree Celsius. Because of the physical properties of the human body, that is, the specific heat of body components, the addition of 70 kcal to a 70-kg person is theoretically sufficient to elevate body temperature approximately 0.8°C (1.4°F). This 0.8° rise would occur if there were no means to dissipate the added heat. Thus, the specific heat of the body is 0.8 (kcal/kg · °C).

Heat is transferred from the body to its surroundings by three physical mechanisms. *Radiation* refers to the exchange of heat between the body and an object by electromagnetic waves. *Convection* entails exchange of heat between skin and adjacent streaming currents of air or liquids. *Conduction,* the least important in quantitative terms, refers to the transfer of heat down a gradient between the skin and another object with which the skin is in contact.

Heat loss becomes limited or reversed if it is not delivered to the body surface. Thus, cutaneous blood flow, regulated by the nervous system, is one of the most important mechanisms by which heat is exchanged. Thus, cutaneous vasodilation increases, and cutaneous vasoconstriction decreases heat exchange between the body surface and its immediate environment. Heat loss from the body is also limited if the ambient air temperature rises to the level of or exceeds that of the body surface and if air movement stops. If the requirement to cool the body exceeds the capacity for heat exchange by radiation, convection, and conduction, *sweating* must occur to permit heat to be lost by vaporization of water. Approximately 1.7 ml of sweat must be vaporized to relieve 1 kcal of heat load. The maximum rate of sweat vaporization is a function of air dryness and air movement. In a hot climate, the limit to heat dissipation is a function of sweat capacity and the environment's capacity to vaporize sweat. Figure 47-1 shows that the maximum rate of sweating by an untrained, unacclimatized person may approach 1.5 liters/h.[343] Complete vaporization of this

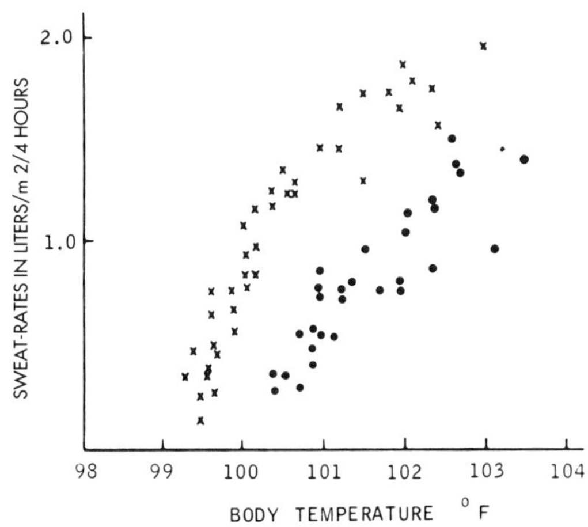

FIGURE 47-1 • Dependence of sweat rate on body temperature, before (•) and after (x) acclimatization. (From Wyndham CH: *J Appl Physiol* 25:586, 1968.)

quantity of sweat could theoretically relieve an 882-kcal heat load (1500 ml ÷ 1.7 kcal/ml sweat = 882 kcal). In practice, however, such physical efficiency is never attained, since 20 percent or more of sweat may be lost by dripping,[81] and such rates of sweating cannot be sustained. Under environmental conditions unfavorable to loss of heat by radiation, convection, or conduction, the upper limits of heat dissipation by vaporization of sweat are approached at caloric expenditures of 650 kcal/h.[3] Sustained work in excess of this rate may cause hyperpyrexia.

At an ambient temperature of about 29°C (84.2°F), a normal person in the basal state of metabolism attains thermal equilibrium with the environment and can maintain a body temperature of 37°C.[138] When the ambient temperature equals the thermoneutral zone and the air is saturated with moisture, a progressive rise of body temperature is inevitable. Even under basal conditions, the predicted rise of body temperature is 1.1°C (2°F) per hour. More important, in a subject who cannot dissipate heat, the temperature rise under a moderate workload expenditure of only 300 kcal/h exceeds 5°C (9°F) per hour.[251] These facts explain the clinical observation that once sweating ceases in an individual subjected to heat stress, frank hyperpyrexia may appear very rapidly.

ensure survival under conditions of prolonged, hard, physical work.

A conscious person seeks a zone of thermal comfort. This has been named the *thermopreferendum*.[309] The thermopreferendum may be measured by placing self-adjustable water jackets about a person's arm so that voluntarily adjusting heat or cold to the most comfortable temperature is permitted. It is useful to demonstrate a major physiologic difference between fever and hyperthermia. For example, a person experiencing a rigor during the onset of pyrogenic fever may increase the temperature of the water jacket in an attempt to further elevate body temperature. In contrast, if hyperthermia has been produced by passive heat exposure, physical work, or hypermetabolism (as in hyperthyroidism), the subject may lower the water jacket temperature in an attempt to reduce body temperature. In simple heat stress, the thermopreferendum is set below the body temperature. At the onset of frank heatstroke, chills and gooseflesh in some individuals suggest that severe heat stress may have caused release of endogenous pyrogens. Indeed, as will be discussed in detail later in this chapter, brisk exercise by normal subjects causes the appearance of an endogenous endotoxin into the plasma.[62]

HEAT ACCLIMATIZATION

Acclimatization to heat comprises those physiologic processes by which an individual becomes able to tolerate heat stress safely and comfortably. Once this is achieved, the acclimatized person may perform work under conditions of heat stress that previously could have been fatal. Although a great deal of acclimatization may occur within a period of 5 days, 2 weeks or more is required for its maximum development. Profound adaptations take place, mainly involving the cardiovascular, endocrine, renal, and exocrine systems. Critical to tolerance of physical work in the heat is the status of physical training. An unacclimatized person in excellent physical condition can withstand heat stress much more safely than one who is unconditioned. It has been shown that features of the acclimatized state appear if the work done has been of sufficient intensity to elevate body temperature; work or exercise that does not elevate body temperature does not produce acclimatization.[12] Thus, in many respects, physical conditioning per se produces changes similar to those of heat acclimatization. Prolonged heat exposure alone, at least in experimental animals, does not improve endurance capacity, however.[116] Thus, to define the level of adaptation needed for acclimatization, the demands eventually to be placed on the body should be known. The level of adaptation that permits tolerance of sedentary activity in an uncomfortably hot climate is inadequate to

PHYSIOLOGIC RESPONSES AND ADAPTATION TO WORK IN THE HEAT

A person working steadily in the heat may become febrile. Besides basal heat production of approximately 70 kcal, an individual may also derive up to 150 kcal/h by irradiation from the sun.[343] to this load is added the heat produced by work. Heat produced by a variety of activities is shown in Table 47-1.

The capacity to dissipate heat may be so limited that work of even moderate intensity causes fever. Two observations illustrate the intensity of heat produced by exercise. First, muscle temperature may reach 41.1°C (106°F) or more during intense work.[9] Second, the heat of metabolism, independent of muscular contraction, may be enormous. In one study of unacclimatized young men before and after exercising 1 h in the heat [i.e., 48.9°C (120°F) wet-bulb temperature], at work loads requiring 50 percent of maximal O_2 utilization, hepatic venous temperature was noted to rise to as high as 41.6°C (107°F), while the simultaneous rectal temperature was only 40.0°C (104°F).[270] These studies have two important implications. First, not only are the biochemical processes in muscle cells during contraction a major source of heat, but hepatic metabolism, for example, gluconeogenesis and glycogenolysis, is also a major source of heat. Second, rectal temperature, conventionally used as an index of heat load, may substantially underestimate temperatures elsewhere in the body during hard work.

TABLE 47-1 • **Energy expenditure during different activities**

Activity	kcal/h
LABOR	
Shoveling	570
Hand sawing	450
Pushing wheelbarrow	300
Carrying bricks	216
Light assembly work	108
Typing	84
SPORTS AND RECREATION*	
Football	102
Wrestling	114
Hockey	173
5-mile run	360
Walking (4 mph)	340
Basketball	344
Swimming	660
MILITARY ACTIVITIES	
Obstacle course	410
STEP test	1230
Infiltration course	477
Double-time drill	
Carrying 30-lb pack and 9-lb rifle	1113

* Calorie expenditure per event given as increment above basal requirement.

SOURCE: Passmore R, Durnin JVGA: *Physiol* Rev 35:801, 1955; Buskirk ER, Bass DE, in Johnson WR, Buskirk ER (eds): *Science and Medicine of Exercise and Sport*, 2d ed. New York, Harper & Row, 1974.

The acute cardiovascular response to hard work in the heat

During hard work in a hot environment, dilatation of vessels in the skin and skeletal muscle exceeds simultaneous reduction of the splanchnic circulation. As a result, effective arterial volume may fall. The ability to tolerate this stress depends on the integrity and responsiveness of the cardiovascular system.

Muscular work, independent of environmental heat, results in massive shunting of blood to skeletal muscle, so-called exercise hyperemia. Muscle blood flow varies in almost direct proportion to the degree of work and ranges from 1 ml/100 g · min at rest to 20 to 40 times this value during intense exercise.[17] A 70-kg male has about 30 kg of skeletal muscle. If he runs while carrying a heavy load and uses approximately two-thirds of muscle mass, the shunt to his muscle vasculature could be as high as 4 liters/min.

A substantial loss of plasma volume into muscle cells may also occur during hard work. As glycogen or other substrates are broken down, many smaller intermediary products are formed within muscle cells. Since the cell membrane is poorly permeable to the intermediary products of glycolysis, powerful osmotic forces are generated within these cells. During the early period of exercise, glycolysis induces influx of water from plasma in quantities averaging 10 percent or more of the inflowing arterial volume.[278] The effective volume of body fluids is also diminished by losses of sweat.

Heat generated by muscular contraction is conducted to blood flowing through the dilated muscle vascular bed. The heated blood is returned to the heart and in turn to hypothalamic centers. Hypothalamic responses induce dilatation of skin vessels and secretion of sweat by the sweat glands.[32] A rise in intracranial temperature increases peripheral blood flow and sudomotor activity. Peripheral blood flow rises by approximately 15 ml/min for every 0.01°C increase in temperature. Hellon and Lind[144] showed that simple exposure to heat induces a rise of forearm (cutaneous) blood flow from 4 ml per 100 ml of arm volume each minute to 12 ml/min. This reponse is controlled by the temperature of blood reaching the anterior hypothalamus and not by skin or core temperatures.

As blood and body temperatures rise during work, increased blood flow to muscle and skin could produce potentially serious hypotension were it not for intense splanchnic vasoconstriction.[267,268] Examining the response of resting normal subjects to hyperthermia induced by water-perfused suits, Rowell and his associates showed that elevation of the skin temperature to 40.5°C was associated with a rise of arterial blood temperature to 39.4°C, with as much as a 125 percent increase in cardiac output, a 15 to 60 percent reduction of hepatic blood flow, and a net rise of splanchnic vascular resistance of as much as 120 percent.[269] However, diminished splanchnic blood flow is inadequate to compensate for the combined loss of plasma water into muscle, increased vascular capacitance resulting from dilatation of vessels in skeletal muscle and skin, and loss of extracellular fluid (ECF) volume as sweat. The net effect is a sharp diminution of effective arterial volume. The increase of vascular resistance and decreased blood flow in the splanchnic circulation are both inhibited by alpha-adrenergic blockade.[255] In contrast, inhibiting the rise of plasma renin activity (PRA) by propranolol does not block the rise of splanchnic vascular resistance during passive heating.[104]

The central circulatory response to the fall of effective arterial volume is decreased venous return, increased heart rate, and decreased stroke volume. If heart rate and venous return are adequate, cardiac output may remain the same or rise; but if sufficient hyperthermia occurs, cardiac output as well as stroke volume fall sharply.

Gold studied volunteers exposed to dry heat for 2 h at 54.5°C (130°F) or 1 h at 71.1°C (160°F).[127] Similar temperatures may occur in closed, parked automobiles, enclosed attics, and boiler rooms. Initially, there appeared signs of hyperkinetic circulation, but as heat storage rose, mean venous pressure increased from 40 to nearly 200 mmH_2O. Cardiac output, estimated in one subject, initially rose, but then progressively fell. Each subject was removed from the heat chamber when collapse was imminent (based on abnormal sensations of light-headedness and a facial color change from pinkish red to almost ashen gray). At this point, some of the subjects ceased sweating. Gold suggested that the primary event in the circulatory collapse of heat pyrexia was high-output cardiac failure and that sweating ceases because of the rising venous pressure.

Rowell and coworkers studied hemodynamic responses of 10 unacclimatized, untrained men to 50 to 80 percent maximal exercise in temperatures of 26.7°C (80°F) and 43.3°C (110°F).[269] At the higher temperature, exercise was associated with diminutions in cardiac output, stroke volulme, and central blood volume. The average heart rate rose from 174 beats per minute at the lower temperature to 195 beats per minute at 43.3°C. Importantly, the greater heat strain while working at 43.3°C was not associated with higher oxygen utilization. Williams and coworkers demonstrated that as an individual performs work at a level approaching maximum oxygen utilization under conditions of high environmental temperature, the augmentation needed for cardiac output to maintain skin and muscle blood flow can be met only at additional cardioacceleration.[334] Under these conditions, stroke volume and, eventually, cardiac output fall. Similar results were observed in experimental animals.[257]

Cutaneous blood flow appears to decrease drastically as exhaustion appears during exercise in heat.[19] Since delivery of heated blood to the body surface is impaired, the ability to dissipate heat from the skin is reduced. In conjunction with the diminished sweat production that eventually occurs during protracted support of heat loads,[285,316] mounting hyperpyrexia is anticipated if similar work were continued.

From the foregoing evidence, the keystone of the body's ability to tolerate hard work in a hot environment seems to be the capacity to increase and sustain cardiovascular performance.

Cardiovascular adaptations to work in heat

Three critical cardiovascular adaptations occur under conditions of heat stress that permit an individual to perform work comfortably in a hot environment.[21,274] These are an increased maximal cardiac output, a decreased peak heart rate, and an increased stroke volume.[267,342] These adaptations facilitate efficient delivery of heated blood from muscle and viscera to the body surface, where heat can be dissipated. *A classic feature of the heat-acclimatized state is a smaller increment in rectal temperature with a given quantity of exercise.* This results not only from the enhanced capacity of the cardiovascular system to propel blood and facilitate heat dissipation but also from the increased metabolic efficiency acquired through physical training.

Physical training increases both oxygen delivery to muscle and oxygen utilization. These changes occur by means of an increase in myoglobin content,[252] an increase in density of mitochondria per unit muscle mass,[128] and an increase in relative volume of the capillary circulation in skeletal muscle.[49] Energy utilization by oxidative (mitochondrial) respiration is nearly 20 times more efficient than by anaerobic metabolism. These adaptations not only explain the increased potential for oxygen utilization with training but also explain the mechanism underlying enhanced metabolic efficiency. Thus, heat production during a given quantity of work is less in a trained man, and heat strain is proportionately less.

Endocrine adaptations to heat

The renin-angiotensin system can be activated by either hard work or acute heat exposure; production of aldosterone concurrently increases[46,75,90,108,184,190,325] (aldosterone production and its possible relationship to potassium deficiency during heat stress is described further under "Heatstroke," below). The rise of PRA is less pronounced under a given degree of heat stress in an acclimatized individual. In studies conducted in young soldiers in basic military training in hot weather PRA was elevated to more than 10 times normal in samples collected before subjects arose in the morning, even when sodium intake exceeded 300 meq/day.[184] In relation to sodium intake both excretion and secretion of aldosterone were considerably greater than normal. Although this response of aldosterone production is important for eventual acclimatization, its role in the immediate reponse to work in the heat may be less important, as evidence has been presented that the onset of biologic activity of aldosterone is delayed up to 2 h.[20] Observations on young men before and after 1 h in a sauna (46 to 51°C, water content 46 g per kilogram of bathing air) showed that plasma levels of renin, angiotensin II, and aldosterone rose significantly.[189] It was speculated that acute volume depletion was the likely stimulus for these changes. Observations from the same laboratory on the effects of running on PRA, angiotensin II, and aldosterone showed even more prounounced changes.[188] Values for plasma aldosterone level at rest may be lower after heat acclimatization.[44,90] Since acclimatization causes circulatory volume to increase, which in turn enhances hepatic blood flow, increased metabolic clearance of aldosterone by the liver could reduce plasma aldosterone although total production may be above normal.

Either physical work or heat is a potent stimulus for growth hormone (GH) release.[244,277] Growth hormone causes retention of salt and water.[39] Its action may be as important as that of renin, angiotensin, and aldosterone in acclimatization.

Hale and associates detected no change of plasma adrenocorticotropic hormone (ACTH) concentration in normal subjects exposed to a temperature of 49°C (120°F) for 45 min.[136] However, plasma cortisol[74] and ACTH[106] both rise during hard physical work.[105a] Urinary excretion of 17-hydroxycorticosteroids or 17-ketosteroids under basal conditions does not change after acclimatization or training.[75]

Acute heat exposure increases plasma renin activity (PRA) and plasma aldosterone (PA). In unacclimatized subjects, both PRA and PA rise during heat exposure, whether studied at rest or exercise. However, acclimatization to heat diminishes this acute response.[108,108a,174a] A reduced NaCl intake augments the response of PRA and PA to heat stress.[89,300a] After continued heat exposure, both PRA and PA levels may continue rising.[46a]

Neither norepinephrine nor PRA rise in trained subjects until they exercise at 70 percent or more of their maximum work capacity.[190] Plasma epinephrine concentration rises only with maximal exercise. Passive heating of patients with metastatic cancer causes nearly a fourfold increase of norepinephrine levels but no change in epinephrine levels.[174] Plasma catecholamine concentration does not rise during acute heat exposure in dogs.[109] Men working in temperatures of 37 to 40°C (98.6 to 104.0°F) excrete smaller quantities of catecholamines in their urine than when working at 22 to 30°C (71.6 to 86°F). The meaning of this report is obscured by the fact that performance of work in a hot climate is associated with a pronounced fall of glomerular filtration rate (GFR) and renal blood flow[256] that could account for diminished catecholamine excretion independent of the rate of release.

Sweat volume and composition

A major feature of the heat-acclimatized state is a drastic alteration in the composition and volume of thermal sweat (Fig. 47-1). The fall in sweat [Na^+] and the rise in volume of sweat produced in response to a given work load in the heat are physiologic hallmarks of the heat-acclimatized state.[94] Hydration enhances sweat production and ameliorates the rise of body temperature over a given series of heat loads induced by walking (Fig. 47-2). Yet, those performing work in a hot climate commonly experience much more voluminous sweat production before acclimatization to heat than after acclimatization has occurred. This disparity between physiologic observations made by climatologists and subjective impressions of people working in hot climates may have some basis in fact. Many physiologic studies of adaptation to heat that demonstrate increased sweat production during the acclimatizing process have been conducted under artificial conditions in the laboratory and usually have not been of more than several weeks' duration. In contrast, Adam et al.[1] studied the effects of standardized heat exposure on British troops during a period of six months. During the first two weeks, they noted that sweat production increased in response to a given heat exposure; during the following five-month period, there was a progressive decline of sweat output in response to the same stimulus. It seems likely that diminished sweat production in re-

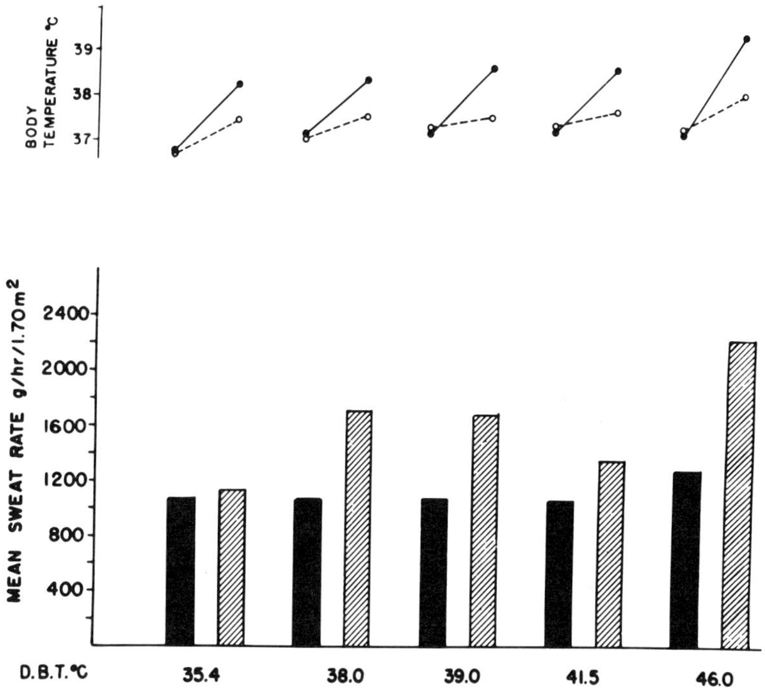

FIGURE 47-2 • Effect of fluid intake on sweat rate at different ambient temperatures. Subjects were walking at 4 km/h for 2 h. Solid bars, no fluid intake; crosshatched bars, forced fluid intake (3800 ml/2h). Top panel shows increments in rectal temperature. Increments were less when fluids were forced (filled circles) than without fluid intake (open circles). (From Knochel JP: in Maxwell MH et al (eds): *Clinical Disorders of Fluid and Electrolyte Metabolism,* 3d ed. New York, McGraw-Hill, 1980, p 1527.)

sponse to a given work load after prolonged acclimatization to heat is probably the result of enhanced metabolic efficiency induced by physical training and is a reflection of less endogenous heat production under conditions of work.[187a]

Robinson and coworkers have shown that a high intake of NaCl may suppress the normal decline of sweat $[Na^+]$ in response to heat exposure.[262] These studies were conducted under conditions of minimal heat stress and thus may not be applicable to natural heat acclimatization in which intense physical work is a component. Other studies have shown that aldosterone secretion and excretion remain inordinately high in relation to NaCl intake not only in individuals training in the heat but also under the same conditions of training during cool weather.[184] The latter observations indicate that physical activity has an important effect independent of heat stress.

Diminished $[Na^+]$ in thermal sweat is due to the action of aldosterone.[73,76,121,196] After administration of deoxycorticosterone (DOC) to volunteers or aldosterone to individuals naturally acclimatized to heat, administration of spironolactone leads to a prompt rise of sweat $[Na^+]$.

Sweat gland responsiveness to the sodium-retaining effects of exogenous aldosterone is somewhat sluggish in comparison to the response of the kidney. The renal response occurs within hours, whereas the decline in sweat $[Na^+]$ requires 1 or 2 days to appear and does not reach its nadir for 5 or more days.[73] Although earlier studies suggested that aldosterone probably has no effect on sweat $[K^+]$,[310] more recent evidence suggests that it does.[103a]

When men and women of equally proportioned physical condition, lean body mass, body surface area, and weight are subjected to heat stress, men produce nearly twice as much sweat as women. The same relationship persists after acclimatization.[11] For a given level of performance in the heat, although evaporative sweat losses may be greater in men, tolerance to heat stress is about the same in both sexes.[249]

Response of renal function to heat stress

The renal response to hard work in the heat has been well characterized. Neither glomerular filtration rate (GFR) nor renal plasma flow (RPF) changes appreciably during moderate work. In contrast, exposure to a temperature of 51°C (123.8°F) at rest produced an average 39 percent fall in RPF and a 21 percent fall in GFR.[256] Both RPF and GFR fell further during work in the heat. These changes are associated with oliguria and diminished sodium excretion.[65,256] In the presence of a reduced circulatory volume, hydropenia, salt depletion, and diminished GFR, sodium reabsorption should be virtually complete in the proximal tubule. Decreased access of NaCl to the distal nephron is expected to limit maximal development of hypertonicity of the medullary interstitium. Accordingly, the maximum urinary osmolality could be lowered. Indeed, individuals living in hot climates are unable to concentrate urine to normal maximal values.[164] Inability to maximally concentrate the urine could favor development of dehydration.

The prevailing urine pH is low in persons living in hot climates.[118,163,281] Increased aldosterone production might enhance reabsorption of sodium in exchange for hydrogen ions, thereby explaining the pH differential. In addition, there could be a relationship between low urine pH and the high incidence of uric acid stones in residents of hot regions.[118]

Serum creatinine concentration, when measured conventionally as creatinine chromogen, may actually fall in an individual who has produced large quantities of sweat.[22,80,182,184] For example, a normal individual may display a decline of serum creatinine from 1.2 to 0.8 mg/dl after several days in the heat. Certain noncreatinine chromogens measured as creatinine in plasma are readily excreted in sweat but not in urine.[22,182,183] If creatinine clearance is calculated using data obtained by measuring creatinine chromogens, as is done by current automated techniques, a rise in GFR could mistakenly be inferred. Although this result would be spurious, it should be recognized that after a normal subject becomes physically conditioned in the heat, resting GFR, measured by inulin clearance, does rise by approximately 20 percent.[183]

Effect of heat stress on blood composition

Simple exposure to a high ambient temperature induces hyperventilation, a fall in blood P_{CO_2},* and acute respiratory alkalosis. At least at the outset, serum $[K^+]$ may fall by as much as 1.0 meq/liter, probably as a result of the alkalosis.[57] If exposure is sufficient to increase body temperature to about 39°C, serum $[K^+]$ may rise rather than fall.[70] Hyperkalemia thus induced occurs despite increasingly intense respiratory alkalosis and is not entirely due to dehydration. Potassium release from cells could also occur as a consequence of increased metabolism caused by heating, and at least part of the hyperkalemia could occur by means of decreased K^+ excretion by the kidney. The majority of patients with acute heatstroke are hypokalemic on hospital admission.

Hypernatremia and *hyperchloremia* may also occur during heat exposure. The major factor responsible appears to be elaboration of sweat, a hypotonic fluid, without adequate water replacement.

* Blood gases are measured at 37°C. To correct the measured P_{CO_2} value to the approximate blood P_{CO_2} at body temperatures higher than 37°C, multiply it by 1.025 (T − 37°C), where T = recorded temperature.[166]

Highly trained marathon runners may show a low-normal serum [K^+] or, in some cases, frank *hypokalemia* at rest;[265] this may also be seen in heat-acclimatized and in physically trained men.[184] The same biochemical and volume changes occur in patients with primary aldosteronism; however, in contrast to individuals with primary aldosteronism, heat-acclimatized or trained humans do not display hypertension or metabolic alkalosis. The low-normal serum [K^+] in the trained or acclimatized person occurs without potassium deficiency.[181a,184]

Serum *phosphorus* concentration declines during exposure to heat, as temperature continues to rise.[70] Hypophosphatemia also occurs as a result of respiratory alkalosis, independently of fever.[319] Because it occurs in the face of a declining urine phosphorus excretion, the hypophosphatemia must reflect increased cellular uptake of phosphorus.

Magnesium concentration in plasma rises very slightly during exposure to heat.[31]

Body fluid volume in heat acclimatization

Acclimatization to heat is associated with increases in blood volume,[18,25] plasma volume,[320] ECF volume,[23,184] and total body water (TBW).[184,342]

The volumes of plasma, ECF, and TBW rise in proportion to the work-stimulated increase in cardiac output during the process of acclimatization.[342] In studies on individuals training in a moderately hot climate, there was a mean rise of ECF volume of 9.6 percent and an increase of TBW of 6.7 percent.[184] Yoshimura also described higher values for blood and plasma volume in subjects studied during hot weather compared to those studied in cool weather.[344] Desai et al. showed markedly higher values for total exchangeable sodium (measured as ^{24}Na) and sodium space in subjects residing in a warm, humid climate compared to those living in a temperate climate.[93] Convertino and coworkers subjected groups of volunteers to either heat or exercise each day so that the subjects' rectal temperatures were equally elevated. Average plasma volume rose 177 ml in those exposed to heat and 427 ml in those subjected to exercise.[82]

People who are acclimatized to work in the heat display venous distension at rest. It is most evident over the forearm and dorsum of the hand but may be present in the jugular veins as well. The distension reflects a normally increased blood volume; venous pressure is normal.

Conn and associates[76,78] and Streeten[310] have described acclimatization to heat as a state of physiological hyperaldosteronism. Thus, if a normal man consumes a generous quantity of sodium chloride, administration of aldosterone or DOC leads to sodium retention by the kidneys, a modest weight gain, and decreased concentration of sodium in sweat. After several days, a new steady state is achieved characterized by sodium excretion into the urine equal to intake. However, ECF remains modestly expanded. This "escape," that is, reappearance of sodium in the urine despite continued administration of aldosterone, does not occur in sweat.[310] Continued excretion of sodium into the urine in the presence of unrelenting sodium conservation by sweat glands closely resembled some but not all of the processes observed by Conn in normal males following acclimatization to heat.[78] Such evidence strongly supports the notion that retention of salt and water sufficient to allow for physiologic expansion of body fluid compartments is necessary for heat acclimatization. Although aldosterone very likely plays a key role in this process exogenous administration of the mineralocorticoid DOC does not induce acclimatization as determined by usual measurements of response to heat stress.[261] Evidence obtained from other experimental studies suggests that aldosterone exerts an inotropic effect on the heart,[209,315] but this is not a property of DOC.

POTASSIUM DEFICIENCY DURING HEAT ACCLIMATIZATION

The potential importance of potassium deficiency in the pathogenesis of heatstroke has been suggested[181,187] because of the common finding of hypokalemia and other evidence suggestive of depletion of potassium ion in individuals who produce large volumes of sweat in response to hard work in hot climates.

Earlier studies showed that of 121 patients with acute heatstroke whose serum [K^+] was measured on admission, a value of less than 3.5 meq/liter was observed in 46 percent.[10,15,24,107,181,207,293,329] In a more recent study[140] of 28 patients with acute, nonexertional heatstroke, 18 (64 percent) had serum [K^+] values below 3.5 meq/liter on admission (mean $\pm$ 1 standard deviation was 3.15 $\pm$ 0.88 meq/liter; range 1.7 to 4.8 meq/liter). In 27 of the 28 patients who could be studied again, 100 percent became hypokalemic (mean [K^+] $\pm$ 1 standard deviation was 2.57 $\pm$ 0.64 meq/liter; range 1.6 to 3.4 meq/liter). When potassium-deficient men become febrile during heat exposure, hyperkalemia does not occur.[70] Severe lactic acidosis (arterial blood pH 6.9, lactate concentration 11.2 m*M*) has been identified in patients with acute exertional heatstroke,[272] and in patients with classical heatstroke if they have circulatory insufficiency or rhabdomyolysis.[305] Since acute acidosis should induce a shift of K^+ from cells to plasma,[57,173] an abnormally low serum [K^+] in the presence of acute lactic acidosis suggests potassium deficiency.

During World War II, Ladell observed that a number of British soldiers in the Libyan desert became intensely polyuric after prolonged exposure to the hot climate.[197] In some, urine volumes exceeded 8 liters/day and did not diminish after injection of posterior pituitary extract. Edholm observed daily urine volumes exceeding 10 liters/day under similar circumstances.[100] Although potassium determinations were not made in these men, their polyuria could conceivably have been the result of hypokalemic nephropathy.[286]

Sobel et al. reported vacuolar changes in renal tubular epithelium, hypokalemia, and polyuria in a number of U.S. Air Force trainees who sustained acute heatstroke.[302] These findings are also compatible with kaliopenic nephropathy. Polyuria could substantially augment the usual water deficits that exist under such conditions and could increase susceptibility to water-deficiency heat exhaustion and heatstroke.

The mechanism responsible for such extreme polyuria is not clear. Elaboration of urine volumes of the magnitude reported by Ladell[197] and Edholm[100] is distinctly unusual in potassium-deficient patients and suggests that intake of solutes and water were disproportionately high. The fact that such observations have been made only on military subjects might be compatible with the latter notion, since large intakes of sodium chloride are customarily encouraged under such conditions. Total solute output into the urine in soldiers in basic military training who daily ingest 350 mmol of sodium chloride and a diet containing 146 g of protein may attain values as high as 1500 mosm.[184] If such a large quantity of osmotically acive particles were excreted by individuals elaborating 8 liters of urine daily, urine solute concentration would be 188 mosm/kg of water. If such conditions prevail, a disturbance of thirst must also be invoked as an additional mechanism to explain the marked polyuria observed in those subjects. Indeed, it has been clearly demonstrated that K-deficient animals show a spontaneous water intake that far exceeds the volume required for urinary solute excretion.[33a] The mechanism for this apparently inappropriate polydipsia is unknown. Hyperreninemia, which occurs under these conditions,[184] has been implicated as a cause of thirst.[264]

ENDOCRINE HYPERTHERMIA

Slight fever may be observed in hyperthyroidism, in adrenocortical insufficiency, and, rarely, following progesterone administration.[298,301] Etiocholanolone, an androgen metabolite, stimulates formation of leukocyte pyrogen. In most of these instances, body temperatures seldom if ever exceed 39°C (102.2°F).

On the other hand, there are four distinctive endocrine states in which true hyperpyrexia may occur and often can be life-threatening. These include (1) thyroid storm, (2) rare cases of diabetic ketoacidosis, (3) pheochromocytoma storm, and (4) following resection of insulinomas. Unfortunately, few of the cases described in the literature have included information that can be used to determine whether the patient showed thermoregulatory failure.

Hyperthyroidism and thyroid storm

Patients with hyperthyroidism demonstrate increased basal heat production. Edelman argues that the major part of this appears to be the result of increased sodium transport.[99] Sestoft has proposed that the increased capacity for the transport of cytosolic ADP and inorganic phosphate (P_i) into mitochondria produced by thyrotoxicosis sets the stage for increased energy turnover.[289] Thereby, any mechanism increasing the availability of P_i in serum may unleash a catastrophic rise in oxygen consumption, and accordingly in heat production.

Two important studies reported some years ago support Sestoft's proposal. Roberts and associates showed that experimental administration of tri-iodothyronine to dogs induced clinical evidence of hyperthyroidism and simultaneously a negative phosphorus balance secondary to phosphaturia.[260] They then examined the possibility that replacement of the phosphorus lost in the urine might have some salutary effect on the artificially induced hyperthyroidism. Within a few days after the initiation of phosphorus supplementation, the dogs showed changes characteristic of thyroid storm. Essentially similar observations were reported by Beisel et al. on human volunteers.[29]

It is interesting that some form of stress is usually the precipitating event in patients with otherwise stable hyperthyroidism who then develop thyroid crisis. Thus, a major infection, injury, parturition, anesthesia, or major surgery results in rapid acceleration of metabolism so that fever up to 41°C (106°F) may be seen. This is not due to thermoregulatory failure, as shown by the fact that sweating and cutaneous vasodilatation persist, indicating that fever is the result of increased metabolism and not a failure of heat loss. Each of these precipitating influences could increase metabolism sufficiently to increase serum phosphate and set in motion the events described by Sestoft.[289]

Heatstroke following the removal of an insulinoma

In 1950, Howard and associates reviewed 398 cases of insulinoma.[152] Eighteen and these expired after surgical removal of the tumor. Five of the eighteen patients died of heatstroke following surgery. Autopsy examination failed to disclose any reason for hyperthermia. In 1955, Conn and Seltzer reported a single case of a patient with an insulinoma who underwent surgery and died with a temperature of 41°C (106°F) 36 h after the operation. No reason for the death or the fever could be found. Tornblom reported a seventh case of death due to hyperthermia in a patient following removal of an insulinoma.[318] This patient became febrile to 105.8°F (41°C) 36 h following surgery and died on the sixth day. No explanation for hyperthermia or death could be found. In 6 of the 7 cases, heatstroke occurred by the second postoperative day; in the remaining case heatstroke developed on day 4.

No explanation has ever been offered to account for postoperative heatstroke following removal of insulinomas.

Pheochromocytoma storm

Catecholamines are calorigenic. Besides hypertension, patients with pheochromocytomas demonstrate hypermetabolism. Although their level of heat production is seldom sufficient to cause fever, rare instances of hyperthermia have been observed (Olsson, personal communication). Such attacks may be precipitated by anesthesia, exercise, or an event causing hemorrhage into the tumor. Beside the thermogenic effect of these hormones, they cause intense cutaneous vasoconstriction which would also impair heat loss.

Brown fat is a form of adipose tissue normally found in infants that contains a rich supply of receptors for norepinephrine. Norepinephrine activation of brown fat is thermogenic and is responsible in a major way for maintenance of body temperature (nonshivering thermogenesis) in infants. Very little brown fat is present in normal adults. However, adults with pheochromocytoma accumulate brown fat.[257a] It is possible that mechanisms responsible for releasing large quantities of norepinephrine in patients with pheochromocytoma could stimulate heat production by this mechanism. Hyperthermia under such conditions should be reduced by alpha-adrenergic receptor blockers such as regitine.

MALIGNANT HYPERTHERMIA

Malignant hyperthermia is a rare hereditary disease characterized by rapidly developing hyperpyrexia, muscular rigidity, and acidosis. Nearly all cases have occurred in patients undergoing general anesthesia for major surgery. A variety of anesthetic agents have been involved. Halothane used alone or in conjunction with succinylcholine has been the most common offender. Attacks have also occurred during anesthesia with cyclopropane, trichloroethylene, ethylene, ethyl ether, ethyl chloride, methoxyflurane, and enflurane. Local anesthetics that depolarize muscle cells (xylocaine but not procaine) have also triggered attacks. The condition is often heralded by the sudden appearance of ectopic ventricular activity, rapid deep respirations, unstable blood pressure, and a sharp rise in body temperature. Britt claims that body temperature may rise in a short period of time to 46°C (114.8°F).[48] In 70 percent of cases, muscle rigidity appears after the onset of fever.

Laboratory findings indicate that profound acidosis exists which may be related to both overproduction and retention of CO_2. Accordingly, the anesthesiologist notices a marked increase in CO_2 production and a rapid exhaustion of soda lime (which traps carbon dioxide). Metabolic acidosis also occurs, due to accumulation of lactic acid. Hypoxemia, hyperglycemia, hyperphosphatemia, hypercalcemia, hypermagnesemia, and hyperkalemia are early findings. Later, serum calcium falls, and muscle enzymes such as creatine phosphokinase (CPK) or aldolase become markedly elevated, reflecting rhabdomyolysis. Disseminated intravascular coagulation (DIC) may appear, as it nearly always does in rhabdomyolysis associated with hyperthermia, and is often severe in degree. Mortality in cases of acute malignant hyperthermia varies between 28 percent[133] and 70 percent.[48]

Although the precise cause of malignant hyperthermia in humans is not clear, one or more of those mechanisms regulating intracellular calcium concentration appears to be defective. Their failure under certain pharmacologic influences allows intracellular [Ca^{2+}] to rise. The most impressive evidence at this time[238] suggests that the sarcoplasmic reticulum of skeletal muscle is unstable and inappropriately releases calcium under a variety of triggering influences. The resulting increase of cytoplasmic [Ca^{2+}] is then responsible for initiating certain biochemical events that generate heat.

Dantrolene is effective both as a prophylactic drug before general anesthesia and as treatment for attacks.[240]

It has been suggested that some patients with exertional heatstroke may have underlying malignant hyperthermia and, accordingly, dantrolene should be administered as treatment for their hyperthermia. There is no evidence to support this notion. There are fundamental differences between exertional heatstroke and malignant hyperthermia. In acute exertional heatstroke, arterial P_{CO_2} is nearly always lower than normal and arterial P_{O_2} is elevated, hypokalemia and hypophosphatemia typically occur, muscular rigidity is absent, and, once exercise is stopped, body cooling usually begins spontaneously. In an acute episode of malignant hyperthermia, in contrast, arterial P_{CO_2} is above normal, arterial P_{O_2} is below normal, *hyper*kalemia and *hyper*phosphatemia are usual, muscular rigidity is present, and hyperthermia occurs progressively. Based upon these differences, there is no reason to believe that dantrolene would be effective in patients with exertional heatstroke.

NEUROLEPTIC MALIGNANT SYNDROME

The neuroleptic malignant syndrome is another pharmacologic disorder that is potentially fatal and may present with increased muscular activity and hyperthermia. Although its cause is diametrically different from malignant hyperthermia, it can be readily confused with it as well as heatstroke. It is also associated with extrapyramidal signs, alteration of consciousness, and autonomic dysfunction. Most cases have occurred in patients taking haloperidol alone or with other drugs, especially lithium carbonate.[72] Phenothiazones and thioxanthenes have also been implicated.[64,145] Fever exceeding 42.0°C (107.6°F) has been observed.[158] In this syndrome, rigidity and involuntary movements always precede the onset of fever. Autonomic dysfunction is manifested by pallor, diaphoresis, sialorrhea, unstable blood pressure, tachycardia, pulmonary congestion, and tachypnea. Death is often due to hyperthermia, dehydration, and exhaustion. In some cases, tachypneic hypoventilation from decreased chest wall compliance has required respiratory support. Rhabdomyolysis has occurred, presumably on the basis of persistent exhaustive muscular contractions, and has been associated with elevation of CPK to as high as 189,000 IU/liter.[139a] Many of the patients have displayed hypernatremia reflecting dehydration. Patients taking haloperidol who do not necessarily demonstrate signs of the neuroleptic malignant syndrome may also become severely hypernatremic. This presumably results from suppression of thirst recognition, a feature apparently unique to haloperidol.

The neuroleptic malignant syndrome must be distinguished carefully from catatonic schizophrenia ("lethal catatonia"), which is not related to drug therapy. Muscular hypertonicity in neuroleptic malignant syndrome is most often characterized as "lead-pipe" or "plastic" rigidity.

It has been postulated that dopamine receptor blockade in the corpus striatum increases thermogenesis by means of muscular spasticity and dystonia, resulting in an enormous overproduction of heat. Dopamine receptor blockade in the hypothalamus presumably mediates the associated autonomic disturbances that interfere with thermoregulation. Despite hyperthermia, skin vessels may be constricted, preventing adequate loss of the heat generated by muscular rigidity. Theoretically, sustained muscular contraction in such patients must be associated with sarcolemmal depolarization and increased intracellular [Na^+] and [Ca^{2+}]. Heat production could, by such a mechanism, become exaggerated. Whether neuroleptic malignant syndrome is related to, or occurs in, patients with subclinical malignant hyperthermia is unknown. Some evidence suggests that dantrolene may be effective as a therapeutic agent in neuroleptic malignant hyperthermia.[83,224]

ENVIRONMENTAL HEAT ILLNESS

The most important disorders resulting from heat stress are heat syncope, heat edema, heat cramps, heat exhaustion, and heatstroke.

Heat syncope

A person in good health who squats for a minute or two and suddenly stands upright often feels a bit faint and may develop tachycardia and hypotension. If the same person performs this maneuver after exposure to a high ambient temperature or after working in the heat for several hours, these symptoms may be more pronounced; indeed, the person may faint. When syncope occurs in a person who has been briefly exposed to a high environmental temperature, and no other cause is apparent, the diagnosis of heat syncope may be made.

The pathogenesis of this disorder apparently leads from thermogenic vasodilatation and postural pooling of blood, diminished venous return to the heart, reduction of cardiac output, and thus cerebral ischemia. As soon as sufficient salt and water have been retained as a result of acclimatization, syncope no longer occurs.

In some individuals who become potassium deficient by sweating (see below) or by other means, syncope could be due to autonomic insufficiency. Biglieri has shown that hypokalemia may lower blood pressure, impair vascular reponsiveness to catecholamines, and blunt cardioacceleration otherwise produced by hypotension.[38] Correction of hypokalemia rapidly reverses these abnormalities.

Heat syncope occurs more commonly in persons with cardiovascular disease and especially in anyone who has a deficit of salt and water. Therefore, patients medicated with diuretics are at increased risk of developing heat syncope.

Treatment for heat syncope is usually unnecessary. The victim commonly awakens before onlookers have time to react. The stricken individual should be allowed to rest in the shade or a cooler environment.

Heat edema

Slight edema of the ankles and dependent parts is extremely common in persons who are unacclimatized. It occurs within a day or two after entering a hot climate, is invariably mild, is noticed more by women, and vanishes as acclimatization occurs.

The cause of heat edema appears to be salt and water retention resulting from the interaction of several factors. These could include salt supplementation, oliguria following heat-induced vasodilatation; increased aldosterone production, and perhaps increased GH production.

The only effect of heat edema is its unpleasant appearance; treatment is not required. It is unwise to offer such a patient a diuretic, since the drug could not only interfere with acclimatization but also induce potassium loss.

Heat cramps

Heat cramps is an acute disorder of skeletal muscle characterized by brief, intermittent, often excruciating muscular cramps. Cramps occur primarily in those muscles which have been subjected to intensive work and fatigue. They often occur in men whose physical condition is superior and who are well acclimatized to work in the heat. The classical description of this disorder was published by Talbott.[313]

As a descriptive term, heat cramps is a misnomer. Exposure to heat per se does not elicit muscle cramps. Tetany and acroparesthesias during exposure to high environmental temperature appear to result from hyperventilation and acute respiratory alkalosis, and are clearly distinguishable from muscle cramps.[156] It is believed that muscle cramps result from an acute deficiency of Na^+ and/or Cl^- after adequate replacement of the water loss incurred by sweating. Thus, such patients are hyponatremic and hypochloremic.

Role of hyponatremia in heat cramps

Three factors are characteristic of individuals predisposed to heat cramps. First, due to their acclimatized state, they are able to produce sweat in large quantities in response to hard muscular work. Second, they consume adequate amounts of water to replace the sweat losses. Third, they fail to replace Na^+ losses. Acclimatization is associated with diminished sweat [Na^+]; nevertheless, [Na^+] in sweat still rises sharply as the rate of sweat secretion rises. This is explained by the fact that [Na^+] in sweat at the site of sweat formation in the secretory coil of the gland is equal to that in plasma water.[52] At low sweat rates, there is time for sodium to be reabsorbed as the precursor fluid passes along the duct. However, at high flow rates, there is insufficient contact time for Na^+ reabsorption to occur, and [Na^+] in the final sweat is much higher[178] (Fig. 47-3).

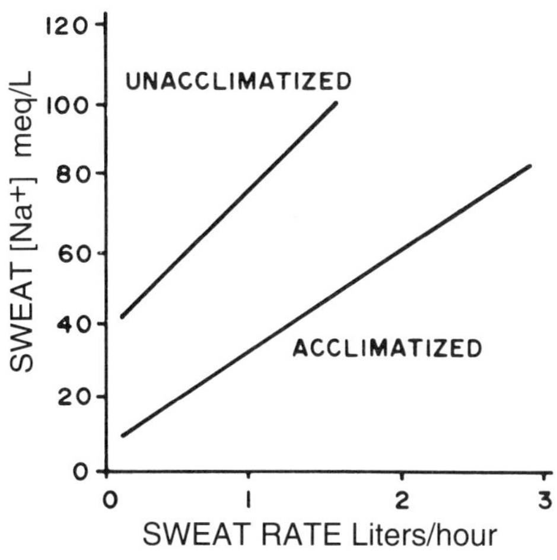

FIGURE 47-3 • Relationship of sweat sodium ion concentration to sweat rate in acclimatized and unacclimatized humans. (From Knochel JP: in Maxwell MH et al (eds): *Clinical Disorders of Fluid and Electrolyte Metabolism,* 3d ed. New York, McGraw-Hill, 1980, p 1530.)

The highly conditioned and acclimatized person is able to produce large volumes of sweat and thus is paradoxically endangered by the capacity to lose larger quantities of Na^+ than is an unacclimatized person. Moreover, maintenance of hydration facilitates a higher sweat rate than occurs under conditions of dehydration (Fig. 47-2). The maximum sweat rate for unacclimatized individuals is 1.5 liters/h, while for acclimatized individuals it is 2.5 liters/h. The concentration of sodium ion in sweat approaches 100 meq/liter[61] for the former group and 70 meq/liter for the latter group. Therefore, the maximum loss of Na^+ is 150 meq/h for unacclimatized individuals and 175 meq/h for acclimatized individuals.

The mechanism responsible for heat cramps is not known. Thus, whether heat cramps represent muscle cramps (with the implication that they occur in response to electrical phenomena, i.e., in conjunction with action potentials) or contractures (implying electrical silence)[201] has not been examined. Hyponatremia (perhaps also hypochloremia) appears to be the cause of heat cramps, since administration of salt leads to rapid relief.

Clinical observations on patients with heat cramps indicate that there are three precipitating factors: exhaustive work, hemodilution, and cooling the muscle. Each of these is also capable of depolarizing the muscle cell. The finding that CPK activity and creatine excretion are increased suggests that subtle muscle cell injury has occurred that in turn might affect transport systems for sodium as well as calcium. A reduction of the extracellular:intracellular [Na^+] gradient favors accumulation of calcium ions in muscle cytoplasm.[312] All patients with heat cramps are hyponatremic. Cooling a muscle cell slows sodium transport and depolarizes the cell.[299] Many victims of heat cramps note that the onset comes after bathing in cool water. The inevitable elevation of calcium concentration in the cell could initiate actin-myosin interaction and muscle contraction.

If sodium transport from the cell is sufficiently retarded, a continual supply of [Ca^{2+}] sufficient to maintain the cell in a contracted state, or a cramp, follows. Reestablishing the sodium gradient between the extracellular and the intracellular fluid by administration of NaCl should facilitate recovery.

Clinical features

Heat cramps typically occur toward the end of the working day, while walking home, or, having arrived, on relaxing, or on taking a cool shower. Muscle cramps *during* exercise, such as those experienced by football players, may thus be quite different. The paroxysms of painful cramping tend to last no more than a few minutes and ordinarily disappear spontaneously. Rarely, heat cramps involve muscles of the anterior abdominal wall, simulating an acute surgical abdomen. Although muscle necrosis and myoglobinuria might be expected to follow severe episodes of muscle cramps, these seem not to have been reported; the possibility, however, has not been systematically examined. In our experience, serum CPK activity may increase to about five times normal. In detailed observations on laborers in the steel mills of Youngstown, Ohio, Talbott and his associates[314] described marked creatinuria in those with muscle cramps, hyponatremia, dehydration, and slight to moderate fever. In those patients, the rate of creatine excretion was marked (up to 75 mg/h) and would be compatible with muscle injury. Most individuals who sustain heat cramps soon discover that ingestion of salt in addition to water during work is effective prophylaxis. In the event of severe, repeated, unrelenting cramps, oral or intravenous salt solutions rapidly relieve all symptoms.

According to the currently accepted definition of heat cramps, if any systemic symptoms or findings coexist with simple muscular cramps, the disorder should be identified as heat exhaustion.

Heat exhaustion (heat prostration)

Heat exhaustion is the most common clinical disorder resulting from work at high temperatures. Although most cases occur during heat waves, heavy sweating incident to intense muscular work, even in temperate climates, may lead to profound losses of body water or sodium chloride and may culminate in every symptom and finding of classical heat exhaustion.

Although pure forms rarely occur, heat exhaustion may be divided into that associated primarily with dehydration and that associated primarily with salt depletion.

Heat exhaustion due to water depletion

The total volume of water an individual working in a hot environment loses by sweating is not voluntarily replaced. Usually, a negative water balance that averages 1 or 2 percent of total body weight is maintained.[2] This degree of dehydration may impair maximum physical performance. Moroff and Bass[232] have shown that water administration in excess of need improves physical performance under conditions of heat stress. Classically, heat exhaustion due primarily to water loss occurs when the supply of water is limited. It is common in soldiers or laborers in the desert, roofers, boiler room workers, hay balers, or athletes who ingest salt without adequate water. It also occurs in infants or enfeebled adults who are unable to express their desire for water. Dehydration and hypernatremia are unfortunately common among neglected patients in nursing homes. The latter type of patient may become seriously water-depleted while retaining normal stores of sodium; as a result, hypernatremia and hypertonic dehydration occur (see Chap. 21). Intracellular water content is depressed. Oliguria is the rule, and the urine contains very little sodium. Symptoms include intense thirst, fatigue, weakness, discomfort, anxiety, and impaired judgment. Marked central nervous system (CNS) dysfunction eventually becomes prominent, manifested by hyperventilation, paresthesias, tetany, agitation, hysteria, and lack of muscular coordination. Some patients demonstrate delirium, and fever, and may become comatose. This form of heat exhaustion is treacherous for, if unrecognized or untreated, it may terminate in heatstroke. Physical examination shows dehydration. Body temperature is almost invariably elevated. Should circulatory failure or a convulsion supervene, the rise of body temperature accelerates and heatstroke rapidly sets in.

Heat exhaustion due primarily to salt depletion

The classical clinical description of salt depletion heat exhaustion was published by McCance.[225,226] The malady occurs when large volumes of thermal sweat are replaced by adequate water but too little salt. It differs from heat cramps in two major respects: This form of heat exhaustion carries systemic effects, and it tends to occur in unacclimatized persons. Marked dehydration or weight loss do not occur; the volumes of urine and sweat remain normal. In contrast to subjects with heat exhaustion due to water depletion, these patients tend not to complain of intense thirst. Interstitial fluid volume falls, and the intracellular space expands. Plasma volume, due to the oncotic pressure of serum proteins, is generally better maintained than interstitial volume.

Symptoms consist of profound weakness, fatigue, severe frontal headache, giddiness, anorexia, nausea, vomiting, diarrhea, and skeletal muscle cramps. As in heat cramps, painful contractions tend to occur in those muscles fatigued by work; they are apt to be precipitated by intake of large quantities of water. Such patients may appear haggard, with pallid, clammy, inelastic skin. Hypotension and tachycardia are prominent. In contrast to heat exhaustion due to water depletion, body temperature usually remains normal or subnormal, but if dehydration ensues as a result of vomiting, body temperature may rise. Sodium chloride deficit in these individuals may exceed 1.0 mol (58g).

Heat exhaustion is usually associated with deficits of both salt and water. Accordingly, symptoms may be manifold. In view of the common symptoms, it is not surprising that patients are sometimes given the diagnosis of "summer flu." Administration of aspirin to such persons who are performing muscular work may paradoxically increase body temperature.[337]

Treatment

In the presence of hypernatremia and a scanty, concentrated urine, the predominant water deficiency may be severe. A simple method for estimating the water deficit is based upon the assumption that total body water has been reduced in inverse proportion to the elevation of serum [Na^+]. For example, a patient whose normal weight was 70 kg presents with a serum [Na^+] of 165 meq/liter. The patient's normal TBW may be estimated as 60 percent of body weight, or 42 liters. The product of normal serum [Na^+], 140 meq/liter, and normal TBW here, 42 liters, divided by the observed sodium concentration (165 meq/liter) is 35.6. This figure is the prevailing volume of TBW in liters. Therefore, $42 - 35.6 = 6.4$ liters represents the patient's water deficit (see also Chap. 21).

The rate of water administration should be carefully controlled. Excessively rapid correction of hypernatremia may cause convulsive seizures. It is prudent to administer no more than one-half of the total deficit during the first 2 to 4 h. An ideal and safe treatment goal is to reduce serum osmolality at a rate not exceeding 2 to 4 mosm per hour. Water should be given orally if the patient is conscious and not vomiting. If the intravenous route is necessary, the solution of choice is 5% dextrose. Care should be taken to avoid severe hyperglycemia and hypokalemia. When serum [Na^+] has fallen to 150 meq/liter, hypotonic saline (0.45%) may be substituted for water. As the point of total correction is approached, symptomatic improvements should be evident. The volume and Na^+ content of the urine then increase; urine specific gravity declines. In some patients who have had severe dehydration and hypernatremia, several days may elapse before cerebral function returns to its original state.

Those whose deficiency is primarily of salt are generally easier to treat. If administration of salted liquids by mouth is not possible, normal saline or, in severe cases, hypertonic (3%) saline may be given intravenously. The required quantity of Na^+ is easily calculated by multiplying the difference beween 140 and the observed serum [Na^+] by the volume of TBW in liters. Usually, not more than one-half this quantity should be administered as hypertonic saline. The remainder may be given as normal saline over a period of 6 h.

Heatstroke

Heatstroke is a catastrophic event. It is characterized by hyperpyrexia [rectal temperature above 40.6°C (105°F)], delirium, coma, and hot, dry skin. (The older terms for the disorder, heat apoplexy and sunstroke, are now considered archaic.) Some employ the term *heat hyperpyrexia* to denote those patients with body temperatures of 40.6°C or more who retain consciousness.[204]

Although heatstroke is the least common of the disorders associated with heat stress, it is the most important since it may occur in epidemic form, carries up to 80 percent mortality, and imposes severe persistent disability in many survivors.

Predisposing factors

A variety of factors may increase susceptibility to heatstroke (Table 47-2). In many instances, simple performance of physical work at a rate that exceeds the capacity to dissipate heat clearly explains the occurrence of heatstroke. Table 47-1 shows the degree of heat production incumbent upon a variety of activities. Theoretically, performance of work at a rate sufficient to produce 1000 kcal/h would, in the absence of heat loss, result in a rise of body temperature of 11.4°C, or a body temperature of 48.4°C. Obviously, collapse would occur before such a temperature level could be reached. Nonetheless, such calculations would explain why a man exercising in a water-impermeable suit covering 85 percent of the body surface that prevents vaporization of sweat could reach a core temperature of 43°C in thirty minutes. Unfortunately, plastic suits promoted as means to lose weight rapidly during exercise are still widely sold in the United States and have been responsible for a number of fatal cases of heatstroke. One should keep in mind that a football uniform also covers a substantial part of the body surface. Because of its leather and foam rubber lining, it acts essentially as a barrier to vaporization of sweat.

Deficits of salt and water and any *acute febrile state* add to the environmental heat load. Febrile reactions to immunizations are especially important. In young, healthy individuals, lack of acclimatization may be the most common predisposing factor.

Recent studies have made the important point that the *elderly poor* are the most common victims of heatstroke.[140,161,172] In the 1978 United States heatstroke epidemic, of 28 patients in Dallas, 20 were ≥ 65 years of age and 5 were between 81 and 90 years old.[140] Of 6 patients less than 65 years of age, 5 had a serious chronic

TABLE 47-2 • Factors predisposing humans to heatstroke

PREDISPOSING FACTORS IN NORMAL HUMANS
Salt and water depletion
Infection
Fever with immunization
Lack of acclimatization
Heat tolerance
Obesity
PREDISPOSING DISEASES
Cardiovascular disease
Diabetes mellitus
Malnutrition
Acute or chronic alcoholism
Impaired sweat production:
Prickly heat (miliaria)
Sweat gland injury after heatstroke or barbiturate poisoning
Scleroderma
Healed thermal burns
Ectodermal dysplasia
Sweat gland ductal obstruction in diabetes mellitus
Congestive heart failure
Potassium deficiency

medical illness. In reports from St. Louis and Kansas City, Missouri, it was clearly confirmed that the elderly or infirm who live in the central city under conditions of low air flow and lack of air conditioning are the major victims of this serious illness.[161,172] In addition, it was pointed out that deaths from all causes in those communities increased by factors of 57 to 64 percent during the July heat wave of 1980. Although the majority of those dying did not die as a result of a specific heat illness, the serious physical strain imposed by heat upon the aged and those with preexisting chronic illness is made obvious by such examples.

As noted by Dreosti in 1935, there are "apparently normal" individuals who are unable to tolerate heat.[98] In such persons, normal acclimatization does not occur. When forced to work in the heat or when exposed to a sufficiently high temperature at rest, such persons risk serious illness. Even with modest work, rectal temperature is found to rise.[341] The cause of the heat intolerance is unknown. A recent study suggests that during heat stress afflicted individuals may not be capable of translocating interstitial fluid into the vascular compartment as efficiently as normal individuals.[288] Measures to detect this syndrome have successfully decreased the incident of heat injury among laborers in the gold mines of South Africa.[340]

Another common impediment to heat tolerance is *obesity*. Every physician is aware that patients with morbid obesity have great difficulty in times of intense heat. Even moderately obese children may experience severe heat strain during exercise. Haynes and associates[143] showed that rectal temperatures rose significantly more in obese boys after standardized exercise.[143] In another study overweight prepubertal girls were unable to perform as well in the heat as in cooler temperatures.[142]

Some of the illnesses that increase the risk of heatstroke are also shown in Table 47-2. The keystone of defense against environmental heat is cardiovascular integrity. Thus, *any cardiovascular disease* may impair heat tolerance.[4] To illustrate this point, Burch et al. examined the effects of high ambient temperature [32.2°C (90°F)] and high humidity (75 percent) on 23 patients with congestive heart failure.[7,54] They found that heart failure worsened, cardiac output failed to rise, some patients developed angina pectoris with elctrocardiographic changes, and some displayed a rise of venous pressure. Daily and Harrison showed that, in rats, saline expansion, which was well tolerated at a normal temperature, led to fatal pulmonary edema during hyperthermia.[87]

Virtually *any chronic disabling disease* increases the risk of developing heatstroke. Especially important are diabetes mellitus, obesity, malnutrition, acute or chronic alcohol abuse, medications that interfere with thermoregulation, and dementia. The short-term effects of ethanol on heat balance are well known. In cold climates, patients with ethanol-induced coma commonly become hypothermic from cutaneous heat loss via vasodilatation in superficial tissue layers. Similar vasodilatation under conditions of high environmental temperature may permit a gain of body heat by identical means and may lead to serious hyperpyrexia.

A brief period of moderate or heavy consumption of *alcohol* often appears to cause loss of acclimatization. Those who perform hard physical work commonly experience discomfort, light-headedness, and weakness when work is resumed after an evening or weekend of drinking. Given similar environmental conditions, the incidence of exertional heatstroke in laborers who drink heavily on weekends appears to be greater on Monday than on other days of the week.

Impairment of sweat production has been associated with a higher incidence of heatstroke. One of the most common causes is *miliaria* (prickly heat).[247,248] Sweat gland injury or necrosis may follow acute heatstroke[13] and may account for persistent heat intolerance noted in some persons who survive. *Bartiburate* poisoning may also cause sweat gland necrosis,[202] which might explain the occasional occurrence of heatstroke in patients intoxicated with barbiturates. Sweat gland entrapment may occur with advanced *scleroderma*[50] or in patients who have survived *extensive burns*. Obstructive periductal lymphocytic infiltration of sweat glands has been described in an elderly *diabetic* patient with fatal heatstroke.[43] Graft versus host disease has also been associated with heat stroke. Presumably, the dermal cellular infiltration interferes with sweat production. Sweat glands may be absent in patients with *ectodermal dysplasia*.[217] In addition, such patients are unable to actively dilate cutaneous blood vessels during fever.[47] Malfunction of sweat glands with inability to conserve NaCl and resulting salt and water deficiency in patients with *cystic fibrosis* increases their susceptibility to heatstroke.[95] Impaired sweat production at the time of thermal stress occurs in patients with *congestive heart failure*[53] and in those receiving certain drugs used in the treatment of parkinsonism, such as *benztropine mesylate* (Cogentin),[210] *atropine*,[66] and other anticholinergics, *phenothiazines* and *butyrophenones* (e.g., haloperidol), and antihistamines.[130] A variety of other drugs rarely cause idiosyncratic hyperpyrexia. These include *LSD*,[119] *methyldopa*,[250] and *propylthiouracil*. Body temperatures as high as 42.2°C (108°F) have been observed commonly in children, but rarely in adults with *severe salicylate poisoning*.[280,286a] Violent muscular activity associated with this intoxication probably contributed to the fever. Overdosage of *amphetamines*, cocaine and related drugs have caused fatal hyperpyrexia.[125,187a] Ingestion of normal doses of aspirin may paradoxically cause fever during exercise.[340] A list of drugs commonly implicated in heatstroke is presented in Table 47-3.

THE IMPLICATIONS OF POTASSIUM DEFICIENCY IN HEATSTROKE. Although an association between potassium deficiency and enhanced susceptibility to heatstroke has

TABLE 47-3 • Drugs that increase risk of environmental heat injury

Drug class	Examples	Mechanism
Diuretics	Benzodiathiazinines, furosemide, ethacrynic acid, acetazolamide	Salt depletion and dehydration
Anticholinergics	Atropine, belladonna	Suppression of sweating
Antiparkinsonians	Procyclydine-HCl, benztropine mesylate	Suppression of sweating
Phenothiazines	Chlorpromazine, promethazine	Suppression of sweating and (possibly) disturbed hypothalamic temperature regulation
Tricyclics	Tranylcypromine	Increased motor activity and increased heat production
Antihistamines	Diphenhydramine	Suppression of sweating
Butyrophenones	Haloperidol	(Possibly) disturbed hypothalamic temperature regulation and failure to recognize thirst
Sympathomimetic amines	Dextroamphetamine, phenmetrazine	Increased psychomotor activity

not been proved in humans, data from experimental studies suggest that such a relationship might exist.[153] Potassium deficiency has been shown to have a number of independently potentially harmful effects. Among these are postural hypotension, syncope, impaired responsiveness to catecholamines,[38,120] impaired insulin release,[77] and glucose intolerance.[77,273] Potassium deficiency depresses glycogen synthesis in skeletal muscle;[33,41,123] reduced glycogen stores during conditioning may increase the risk for rhabdomyolysis.

When exposed to hot air, normal subjects hyperventilate, develop respiratory alkalosis, and may show mild hypokalemia.[156] If the ambient air is such that body temperature becomes elevated, then serum potassium tends to rise, especially if physical work is conducted simultaneously.[70,115,173,307]

Several investigators have estimated the extent to which humans approach potassium balance during acclimatization to heat. Bass and coworkers examined young men exposed 12 h/day to a temperature of 48.9°C (120°F) and relative humidity of 28 percent.[21] They estimated that an average daily potassium loss exceeded potassium intake by 15 meq. When subjects were exposed to heat, their work consisted only of walking for four 30-min periods daily.

Gordon[129] exposed two volunteer subjects to 31.1°C (88°F) and 40 percent relative humidity for 6 h/day, 5 days/week for 3 weeks, while the volunteers ingested 25 meq of potassium daily. On each day of the study, the subjects vigorously exercised on a bicycle for 30 min, alternating with 30-min rest periods; potassium deficits in these two subjects were 161 and 192 meq.

Streeten and his associates[310] measured potassium intake and output in four subjects exposed to a temperature ranging from 32.2 to 37.8°C (90 to 100°F) and humidity of 60 to 70 percent for 7 h for 15 to 23 days. Work was not undertaken, and all subjects wore rubber suits to ensure all sweat was collected. Potassium intake was more than 100 meq each day. Exclusive of fecal potassium losses, cumulative potassium losses during the period of heat exposure in these four subjects were 24, 169, 180, and 411 meq. Potassium excretion in both sweat and urine rose substantially following saline infusions. In all subjects, urinary excretion of aldosterone, estimated by bioassay, was also substantially higher during the period of heat exposure. Frank hypokalemia was not observed in any of the aforementioned studies.[21,129,310]

The level of physical activity in the studies discussed[21,310] was not so intense as that undertaken by young athletes or military recruits; novice athletes and soldiers are at high risk of developing heatstroke while training in hot weather. In fact, it is only among individuals such as these that potassium deficiency is likely to occur. These men have been shown to secrete up to 12 liters or more of sweat per day. Potassium concentration in sweat may be 9 meq/liter when thermal sweating has been protracted and voluminous.[131,241a,275,285,323] Thereby, total potassium losses in sweat exceeding 100 meq/day could readily occur. Since dietary intake of K^+ does not ordinarily exceed 100 meq, additional potassium losses in urine and feces could generate a severe deficit in a relatively short period of time.

Serial determinations of total body potassium (measured as exchangeable ^{42}K) and all other measurements were performed on 1 day each week for 6 consecutive weeks, starting the week before training began. The studies were conducted on one group of healthy, unacclimatized young soldiers undergoing basic military training in the hot summer and in another group during the cooler winter months.[184] Those training in the hot weather sustained a mean K^+ deficit of 517 meq by the eleventh day of their training. In comparison, those studied in cooler weather showed the expected steady rise of total body potassium coincident with the increase of lean body mass. All subjects had consumed a constant diet containing 106 meq K throughout the period of observation. Despite large losses of K^+ in sweat at the time of maximum deficiency, K^+ excretion into the urine was inappropriately high and ranged from 41 to 79 meq/day. At the same time, the $[Na^+]/[K^+]$ ratio in their sweat was very low, reflecting the action of aldosterone on sweat glands. Excretion and secretion of aldosterone and PRA were both high with reference to Na^+ intake.[178]

Based on these studies, it was concluded that intense physical work in the heat stimulates higher production of renin and aldosterone than would occur in nonexercising subjects on similar Na^+ intakes. Aldosterone overproduction under these conditions might have induced mineralocorticoid escape. Thus, aldosterone, in the presence of conditions permitting excretion of large amounts of Na^+ into the urine, could facilitate continued excretion of K^+ by the kidney despite serious potassium depletion. Consequently, the kidney probably played a role in the genesis of potassium depletion in those subjects. Although it has not been proved, it seems very possible that excessive sodium intake could enhance K^+ losses by the kidney. Despite high intakes of Na^+, large quantities of aldosterone were excreted in urine, establishing a situation analogous to an intake of sodium that is much lower. This suggests that excretion and secretion of aldosterone was sufficient to stimulate tubular potassium secretion despite simultaneous potassium deficiency. The series of interacting events leading to potassium deficiency under these conditions is shown in Fig. 47-4.

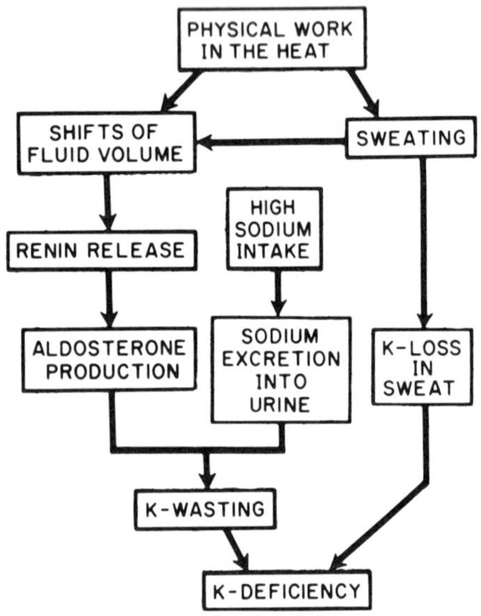

FIGURE 47-4 • Proposed mechanism of generation of potassium deficiency during work in the heat. (From Knochel JP: in Maxwell MH et al (eds): *Clinical Disorders of Fluid and Electrolyte Metabolism*, 3d ed. New York, McGraw-Hill, 1980, p 1539.)

It is also possible that the subjects of our studies lost large amounts of potassium because of muscle injury. The group that showed a major reduction in total body potassium was training in dry bulb temperature that exceeded 100°F. Coincident with the peak of potassium deficiency, they showed substantial elevations of serum creatine kinase activity, creatinuria, hyperphosphatemia, hyperuricemia, hyperuricosuria, and hypocalcemia. All of these laboratory abnormalities are classical indicators of rhabdomyolysis.[182] The observeration that frank hypokalemia did not occur would correspond with a tissue-injury-mediated K loss. Muscle cells injured by strenuous physical effort in the heat would be expected to cause cellular membrane injury, elecrical depolarization of cells, and would very likely impair Na^+-K^+ ATPase function. Under such conditions, retention of a normally high K gradient between the inside and outside of the cell would be impossible. As result, K ions would leak into plasma and be excreted by the kidney. Since we measured urinary electrolyte excretion only one day per week during those studies, the major period of K loss could have gone undetected. Obligatory renal loss of K by means of muscle injury would correspond to our findings that total body K fell after 1 to 2 weeks of training whereas serum potassium did not become abnormally low. The observation that muscle cell injury did not occur during training in cool weather fits with studies conducted since that time showing that heat markedly exaggerates exertional rhabdomyolysis.[190a] Indeed, the elevation of serum creatine kinase activity in our subjects training in cool weather was trivial or negligible.

Although muscle injury and the resulting release of muscle potassium would be expected to cause a reduction of total body potassium, in the classic definition, this would not necessarily indicate potassium deficiency. Amputation of an extremity causes a reduction of total body potassium. The remaining muscle would show a normal K:nitrogen ratio. True K deficiency causes a reduction of this value. In skeletal muscle, the normal K:nitrogen ratio is 2.5 meq K/gram nitrogen. Cellular death would result in a balanced loss of both K and nitrogen. However, it would seem more likely that reversible muscle injury, as occurs in exertional rhabdomyolysis or experimental K deficiency,[186] results in a reduction of this ratio, hence K depletion in the subjects of this study probably represents true potassium deficiency.

Potassium deficiency itself may cause skeletal muscle injury and rhabdomyolysis independently of muscular exercise.[180,186] Dogs with advanced potassium deficiency demonstrated subnormal muscle membrane potential, elevated levels of CPK, and histologic evidence of rhabdomyolysis independently of physical activity.[40,186]

Rhabdomyolysis always occurs in young men with exertional heatstroke. It may also occur in apparently normal individuals who, before adequate physical conditioning has been attained, undertake severe, prolonged muscular work. For example, rhabdomyolysis has been observed repeatedly during the first few days of military training and is often the result of repetitious, violent calisthenics such as "squat jumps." In one group of marines studied during basic training in hot weather, Demos and his coworkers[90] showed that those who were asymptomatic showed average creatine kinase values of 1413 IU/liter (range 159 to 9903), whereas the marines with symptoms and findings of muscle injury showed average creatine kinase values of 76,803 IU (range 26,708 to 109,609 IU).

Why could potassium deficiency cause rhabdomyolysis, especially in subjects undergoing physical training? Potassium is a potent vasodilator. During work, it is released from contracting skeletal muscle fibers, and its rising concentration in interstitial fluid is thought to dilate arterioles, mediating the normal rise of muscle blood flow during exercise.[175] In potassium-deficient dogs studied during exercise, it has been shown that potassium ions are not released from skeletal muscle, muscle blood flow does not rise normally, and necrosis follows, possibly the result of ischemia.[186]

Other studies show that cardiac output in potassium-deficient dogs falls sharply and acute pulmonary edema develops with exercise.[185]

If the foregoing observations can be extrapolated to potassium-deficient humans performing sustained hard work, they may not only explain the occurrence of muscle necrosis by means of ischemia but also suggest that potassium deficiency could impair cardiovascular performance sufficiently to prevent adequate heat dissipation. The demonstration in experimental animals that potassium deficiency, in conjunction with sodium loading, may readily induce myocardial necrosis[88] and impair cardiac performance[122] supports the plausibility of the notion. Potassium deficiency could thus conceivably play a major role in the pathogenesis of rhabdomyolysis as well as hyperpyrexia.

There is no apparent reason to implicate primary potassium deficiency in any more than a small fraction of the cases of heatstroke. In most instances, there is no evidence that potassium deficiency preceded the illness. In those patients who incur heatstroke within the first three days of heat exposure it does not seem possible that significant potassium deficiency could have developed unless substantial muscle necrosis were responsible. Thus, it seems that potassium deficiency could contribute to the pathogenesis of heatstroke when the heatstroke appears in subjects who have produced voluminous quantities of sweat for one week or more. Among those at risk are military recruits, football players, foundry workers, roofers, miners, and farmers. In those persons, potassium deficiency may contribute importantly to the associated morbidity. In such instances, it may partially explain the high frequency of hypokalemia seen when these patients present with acute heatstroke.

Clinical manifestations of heatstroke

Heatstroke is a medical emergency characterized by a body temperature above 40.6°C (105°F), hot, dry skin, and functional disturbance of the CNS.

It is useful to classify heatstroke into two forms: classical and exertional.[178] The major differences between the two forms are shown in Table 47-4.

CLASSICAL HEATSTROKE. Classical heatstroke has been well characterized by a number of clinicians.[10,101-103,107,140,204,207,294] Typically, this form of heatstroke is observed after several days of ambient temperatures that frequently exceed 37.9°C (100°F) or when lower environmental temperature is accompanied by high relative humidity, and both the temperature and humidity are sustained through several days and nights. Thus, the individual continuously perspires actively, but sweating eventually fails, body temperature rises sharply, and classical heatstroke rapidly develops. Such cases should be especially anticipated in the event of an electrical power shortage. In larger cities, many persons live in poorly ventilated apartments that can be cooled only by air-conditioning. Many who live under such conditions may never subject themselves to sufficient heat to become acclimatized. During "brownouts" or air-conditioning failure, they are at extreme risk of developing heat injury.

Prodromal symptoms in these patients may be absent; the first manifestation may be sudden collapse. The victims may be found wandering about in a state of stupor. Others develop weakness, dizziness, nausea, and fainting spells up to 2 or 3 days before their collapse. Some complain of frontal headache, weakness, and oppression by a feeling of intolerable body heat. Muscle cramps may occur but are unusual since NaCl deficiency is not characteristic. Of those survivors who are able to recall their prodromal period, about half state that sweating ceased before the onset of their collapse. In some, this has been associated with a sensation of coldness and the appearance of chills and gooseflesh. Such manifestations probably signal the onset of thermoregulatory failure and resemble the response to a pyrogen in which the body attempts to elevate its temperature.[309] It is to be emphasized that convulsive seizures are generally not observed until the patient is being cooled therapeutically.

Some patients who develop classical heatstroke undergo a prodrome characteristic of water-depletion heat exhaustion. This is especially prominent among persons in nursing homes or other chronic invalid care facilities where attendant care is marginal and there is no provision of adequate water to restore extensive water losses in sweat.

The typical physical findings of heatstroke are hyperpyrexia, coma, and hot, dry skin. These symptoms have been observed in institutionalized, minimally attended patients like those described above. Austin and Berry[10]

TABLE 47-4 • **Comparison of classical and exertional heatstroke**

	Classical	Exertional
Age group	Very young, very old	Men 15–45
Health status	Chronic illness common	Usually healthy
History of febrile illness or immunization	Unusual	Common
Activity	Sedentary	Common in football players, military recruits, competitive runners
Drug use	Sweat depressants, diuretics, haloperidol, phenothiazines	Amphetamines, cocaine
Sweating	Usually absent	Often present
Respiratory alkalosis	Dominant	Mild
Lactic acidosis	Absent or mild	Often marked
Acute renal failure	< 5% of patients	30% of patients
Rhabdomyolysis	Seldom severe	Severe
Hyperuricemia	Modest	Severe
Creatinine:BUN ratio	1:10	Elevated
CPK, aldolase	Mildly elevated	Markedly elevated
Hypocalcemia	Uncommon	Common
DIC	Mild	Marked
Hypoglycemia	Uncommon	Common

NOTE: Some features are common to both types: lack of heat acclimatization, dehydration, salt depletion, hyperthermia (≥106°F), cutaneous flushing and mottling, coma, psychotic behavior, convulsions while cooling, shock, ARDS, hypokalemia, hypernatremia, hypo- or hyperphosphatemia, poikilothermia during recovery.

and Ferris and his associates[107] noted that sweating was totally absent in 100 percent of their patients; 84 percent of the patients reported by Levine[207] also failed to perspire. These studies established the clinical finding of hot, dry skin as a virtual prerequisite for the diagnosis of heatstroke. Moreover, anhidrosis in such patients has led to the notion that fatigue of the sweating mechanism or centrally mediated thermoregulatory failure occupies the key position among factors thought to play a role in the pathogenesis of classical heatstroke.

Classical studies by Thaysen and Schwartz[316] and later by Schwartz and Itoh[284] showed that, during prolonged exposure to the heat, the rate of sweat secretion could not be sustained for more than 6 h despite a rising body temperature. Furthermore, the response in volume of sweat to methacholine became blunted and the local response to methacholine in patients with heatstroke was only 1 to 2 percent of that observed in normal subjects. The investigators concluded that their findings indicated "fatigue" of the sweat glands and suggested that this phenomenon played a role in the pathogenesis of heatstroke. In criticism, Gilat and associates[124] noted that even when so-called fatigue had occurred, the sweat rate remained substantially higher than the rate observed at rest. They argued that since the sweat rate had not fallen substantially, sweat gland fatigue cannot be considered important in the pathogenesis of heatstroke.

The same authors have also leveled criticism at the suggestion made by Ladell[195] that hyperthermia per se is the cause of the sweat gland fatigue. Gilat et al. studied the change of rectal temperature in eight highly trained, heat-acclimatized Israeli soldiers during a march of 31.5 km while the troops carried a standard load of 35 kg[124]. Five of the eight had rectal temperatures between 41.5 and 42.4°C (106.7 to 108.3°F) on completion of the march. They had been allowed rest stops and water. Dehydration averaged only 0.9 liter. Active sweating had persisted in all. Three were euphoric and restless. At the time of the hyperthermia, all were considered to demonstrate early, albeit transient, symptoms of heatstroke. Consideration of these data as well as the observations on 38 cases of exertion-induced heatstroke in which sweating was observed despite hyperpyrexia indicates clearly that sweat gland failure is not always the critical factor in all patients with heatstroke. These findings were in agreement with those made in 1925 by Kuo and associates on four normal subjects exposed to intense heat stress imposed by a dry-bulb temperature of 72°C (162°F) and wet-bulb temperature of 40.8°C (118°F).[193] The major effects of heat exposure, including stupor, appeared when rectal temperatures had risen to values ranging from 39.5°C (103.1°F) to 40.8°C (105.4°F); sweating had then not yet diminished. The authors postulated that sweat gland exhaustion could not explain the sudden diminution of sweating since profuse, generalized sweating reappeared promptly if the subjects were removed from the heat chamber to a cool environment. It seems likely that at some critical point, blood flow to the skin must become reduced sufficiently to diminish plasma transfer to the secretory coil of the sweat gland. Therefore, sweat formation must cease. Upon regaining circulatory stability, sweat formation would resume. On the other hand, sweat gland fatigue and failure must exist in some patients, especially the elderly with classical heatstroke who have dry, hot skin without evidence of sweating. The rapid reappearance of sweating after it had subsided in the normal subjects observed in short-term studies by Kuo[193] may in fact have little relationship to sweat gland failure that occurs after sweating has been protracted in patients who have incurred classical heatstroke in whom sweating may not reappear for days following otherwise successful treatment. Those subjects forming the basis of the observations of Gilat's group were healthy, young men performing virtually superhuman feats for which adequate heat-dissipating means were not available.[124] In such a sample of subjects, the total duration of physical activity required to produce hyperthermia is usually measured in minutes or hours, whereas elderly patients with classical anitihidrotic heatstroke have usually been sweating at least for a day or more and therefore are more likely to have developed failure of the sweat mechanism.

EXERTION-INDUCED HEATSTROKE. Descriptions of classical heatstroke in invalids or in the elderly population stand in sharp contrast to observations made on patients who incurred heatstroke in association with physical exertion.[14,16,30,84,85,132,159,242] The majority of cases reported in the literature and seen clinically occur in association with events that increase endogenous heat production. Sweating clearly persists in more than 50 percent of the total number of cases. Thus, it appears that fatal heatstroke can occur in perfectly healthy, highly acclimatized, and physically conditioned individuals when the physical means to dissipate heat are exceeded by endogenous heat production. In the United States, the majority of such cases appear to occur in marathon runners,[85,132] football players,[16,272] and military recruits.[30,84,181,242] In these groups, sustained, often extraordinary physical exertion commonly precedes heatstroke. In the case of football players, many are young and may be highly competitive, inexperienced, and overenthusiastic; consequently, they do not pace themselves. In contrast, serious heat illness is virtually unknown among professional football players. In military recruits, the mandate to achieve a superior physical condition and the fear of being sent through a second course of recruit training appears to substitute for the competitive zeal seen in the athlete. Although prophylactic measures to forestall or prevent heatstroke have been widely publicized,[58,177,237,304] certain practices are occasionally observed in physical conditioning programs that undoubtedly favor the tendency to incur heatstroke.[177] One potentially disastrous practice is based on the notion that long-distance running or other strenuous exercise in hot climates while clothed in impervious plastic sweat clothing can safely accelerate weight loss in overweight athletes.[272] An additional example is the false notion that water denial (water discipline) during football practice accelerates physical conditioning. In some instances, water has been provided as a tepid, salted solution containing oatmeal to make it distasteful. Another example is the provision of only salted water in the canteens of soldiers in basic training. Overzealous administration of salt supplements is also common. Without question, salt supplements are mandatory during the first week or so of conditioning in hot climates. However, provision of water is much more important. Ingestion of excessive salt and insufficient water is a potentially lethal practice that undoubtedly accounts for cases of severe water-depletion heat exhaustion that culminate in frank heatstroke. For instance, deliberate water restriction to 500 cc per hour in marine recruits training in hot weather as a method to teach discipline has been shown to be fraught with danger. In 13 young marines with exertional heatstroke, Gustafson and associates observed an average serum sodium concentration of 160 ± 4.3 meq/liter.[135a] By comparison, serum sodium concentrations averaged 149 ± 1.7 meq/liter in 14 young men with heat exhaustion and 146 ± 0.7 in 34 unaffected trainees after a 3-mile run. Based upon calculations from serum sodium and estimated TBW, the men with heatstroke had water deficits exceeding 5.56 liters.

The following case is representative of exertional heatstroke in a football player.

A 20-year-old football player collapsed on the tenth day of practice. Several hours before, he became irritable and showed inappropriate behavior. He babbled incoherently and ran wildly about the field before collapsing. The peak ambient temperature and humidity exceeded 32.2°C (90°F) and 50 percent, respectively. Physical examination showed a stocky man who was unresponsive, with flushed, moist skin. His pupils were widely dilated and unresponsive. Rectal temperature was 42.2°C (108°F), pulse rate was 160 beats per minute, blood pressure was 80/0 mmHg, and respiration rate was 30 per minute. On cooling, his blood pressure rose to 100/60 mmHg. The patient became tremulous and had a series of grand mal seizures. These were followed by a rise of rectal temperature to 41.7°C (107°F). He became frankly cyanotic; although only 800 ml of fluid had been administered intravenously, he showed signs compatible with frank pulmonary edema. Reinstitution of cooling measures and intermittent positive pressure respiration produced improvement.

Laboratory findings on admission showed a white blood cell count of 18,000 per cubic millimeter with 82 percent polymorphonuclear cells and a platelet count of 175,000 per cubic millimeter. Serum [K^+] was 2.7 meq/liter and total [CO_2] was 10.4 m*M*. Arterial blood pH was 7.19 and arterial (P_{CO_2}) was 28 mmHg. On the second day, the urine was scanty in volume, dark, and a test for heme pigment was positive. The patient's platelet count had fallen to 46,000 per cubic millimeter. Serum glutamic-oxaloacetic transaminase activity (SGOT) was 2640 units (normal range, 2 to 12 units). Serum CPK exceeded 100,000 IU/liter.

The patient remained in coma. Babinski reflexes and ankle clonus were present bilaterally. Widespread petechial hemorrhages were evident. His electrocardiogram showed ST-T changes compatible with posterior myocardial ischemia. On the second day, 34 h after admission, scleral icterus was observed. Total urine output since admission had been only 400 ml. Upon completion of hemodialysis, the patient had another convulsive seizure and died. During the seizure, serum potassium concentration had risen from 4.2 to 8.0 meq/liter.

This case illustrates several important points:

1. Frank heatstroke occurs in otherwise healthy young people even though sweating has not ceased.
2. Individuals with a large muscle mass who achieve higher levels of muscular work may show severe hyperthermia. This may be correlated with widespread necrosis involving myocardium, sweat glands, brain, and all abdominal viscera.
3. The onset of hyperthermia may be preceded by psychotic behavior.[24]
4. Thrombocytopenia is the rule and is ordinarily associated with other laboratory findings indicative of disseminated intravascular coagulation. These include increased fibrin split products in serum, a prolonged prothrombin time, prolonged partial thromboplastin time, and hypofibrinogenemia.
5. Hypotension or shock occurs commonly, but resolves in most cases as body temperature is reduced. (Presumably, cooling translocates blood from the cutaneous vessels to the central circulation. For this reason, it is unwise to administer large volumes of fluids before cooling since doing so may expand the central circulation sufficiently to cause pulmonary edema.)
6. In severe cases, acute pulmonary edema has been observed before either fluid replacement or cooling. Presumably, it indicates either acute left ventricular failure or a disturbance of pulmonary vascular permeability. The possibility that lactic acidosis is responsible for impaired left ventricular function should be considered.[6,333] Adult respiratory distress syndrome (ARDS) often appears in severe cases on the third day or later. This complication is particularly ominous.
7. Evidence of rhabdomyolysis exists in virtually all cases.
8. Severe hypoglycemia may occur in heatstroke,[84] probably as a result of increased glucose utilization,[162] hepatic ischemia, and consequent impairment of gluconeogenesis.
9. Death usually occurs as a result of acute hyperkalemia either following a convulsive seizure, as a result of extensive rhabdomyolysis with acute renal failure, ARDS, or mesenteric infarction.
10. Hypokalemia at the time of admission is common and, in those individuals who have been sweating profusely for a week or more, may represent serious potassium depletion.

Such cases as the one described above occur among persons subjected to sustained, intense physical activity in hot climates. In these patients, metabolic heat production either supersedes heat-dissipating capacity despite favorable environmental conditions or metabolic heat cannot be dissipated because of clothing that prevents vaporization of sweat. A good example of the latter is the football player whose leather-lined gear may cover 30 percent or more of body surface. Mathews demonstrated[223] that, under such conditions, strain due to heat stress may increase markedly.

The persistence of sweating in some of these cases is critical since it may obscure the diagnosis. Thus, when such an individual collapses, the skin may feel hot and moist. As sweat vaporizes, the skin may become cooler, thereby making recognition of heatstroke difficult. In some, rectal temperature recorded at a depth of 19 cm or more discloses frank hyperpyrexia. However, there are other patients who present with an identical history to that just described who remain in coma and demonstrate a moist skin and a rectal temperature of 39 to 40°C (approximately 102 to 104°F). Except for the lack of frank hyperpyrexia, these patients may show all classical findings and complications of exertional heatstroke. In such cases, it is assumed that body temperature was probably higher initially but spontaneously dropped as exertion ceased and sweat was vaporized. As an alternative hypothesis, tissue injury induced by strenuous muscular work and fever may release proteases into the circulation that in turn inflict injury upon a number of tissues.[62,69,194]

Many such cases of effort-induced heatstroke have been observed in military recruits[30,84,181,221,242,302,324] as well as in highly trained soldiers of whom requirements for performance exceed human tolerance.[124,292] At equal risk are marathon runners and other competitive athletes who perform under adverse climatic conditions.[85,113,132]

Extreme hyperpyrexia [rectal temperature 43.3°C (110°F)] in conjunction with profound muscular rigidity has occurred in a patient who ingested 10 mg of dextroamphetamine and 10 mg of the monoamine oxidase inhibitor tranylcypromine.[191] Hyperpyrexia and rhabdomyolysis are common manifestations of massive amphetamine overdosage.[126,167,347] That they are at least partially the result of physical activity and the associated endogenous heat production by skeletal muscle is suggested by the occurrence of hyperkalemia following administration of amphetamines to experimental animals[231] and prevention of hyperthermia by curare.[346] For similar reasons, exertion-induced heatstroke has been observed in withdrawing alcoholics and in extremely agitated psychotic patients.[15] More recently, cocaine and crack have been implicated as causes of exertional heatstroke with all of its typical complications.[187b]

Pathophysiology of tissue damage in heatstroke

Studies by Bynum and associates underscore the difficulty in predicting the extent of tissue damage that might occur under conditions of passive heating.[60] They studied normal resting human subjects heated to 42.0°C (107.6°F) for 1 h. Based upon increased activities of four commonly measured enzyme activities, SGOT, SGPT (serum glutamate-pyruvate transaminse), alkaline phosphatase, and LDH (lactic dehydrogenase), the authors suggest that a critical thermal maximum lies somewhere between the temperatures of 41.6 and 42°C. Thermal cellular injury can also be influenced substantially by metabolism, blood flow, availability of oxygen, pH, substrates, and (unquestionably) a host of other factors. Either adaptation to heat (acclimatization) or even in vitro exposure of cell cultures to heat is protective against subsequent tissue injury by heating. Current evidence suggests that heat-shock proteins, synthesized during cellular heating, may play a role in this event.[272a] In experimental animals, tissue damage and mortality are worse with exertion-induced hyperthermia than with simple hyperthermia due to heat exposure.[117,154,291] This is very likely due to the greater degree of tissue heating associated with exertion-induced hyperthermia.

In general, patients with fatal classical heatstroke show much less evidence of tissue damage than young men with exertional heatstroke. Patients with classical heatstroke, whose core temperatures were as high as 43.7°C (110°F), have been observed to recover without evident sequelae.[140] On the other hand, virtual total body destruction (somatolysis) has been observed in young men with exertional heatstroke whose core temperature did not exceed 40.6°C (105°F). It is consequently difficult to interpret precisely in vitro studies of thermal injury[55,56] or in vivo assessments of liver function after passively induced fever.[135,148,214,229,306] For example, Rowell demonstrated in normal subjects that hepatic venous blood temperature (and presumably hepatocyte temperature) may reach 42.2°C during exercise without apparent harm.[270] Such observations do not help explain why some victims of classical heatstroke with lower temperatures may develop overt hepatocellular injury.[146] A patient survived classical heatstroke without sequelae whose rectal temperature of 46.5°C (115.7°F) was measured by a reliable instrument. This appears to represent the record temperature for this disorder.[300]

The possible role of endotoxin in exertional heatstroke

A substantial body of evidence suggests that endotoxin derived from intestinal bacteria plays a critically important role in the morbidity of heatstroke. It has been appreciated for many years that patients with exertional heatstroke and acute renal failure are often extremely catabolic when compared to patients with acute renal failure from other causes.[241] Indeed, catabolism occurs at such a rate that peritoneal dialysis may be inadequate to cope with the resulting acidosis, azotemia, and hyperkalemia seen in such patients. It has already been mentioned that victims of classic heatstroke or patients who have been made equally hyperthermic for treatment of other diseases such as neurosyphilis or cancer ordinarily do not become as catabolic as patients with heatstroke. Thus, fever per se does not appear to be totally responsible for the level of catabolic activity. Studies on experimental animals have shown that death from induced hyperthermia is sharply reduced by sterilization of the bowel with antibiotics, by immunization to bacterial endotoxin, or by administration of antibodies to endotoxin before heat stress is induced.[123] Presumably, shunting of blood away from the mesenteric vasculature during hard work, especially when conducted in the heat, results in ischemic damage to the gut.[268]

The mechanism underlying this visceral ischemia during exercise[119a] is of interest. During hard work, or during exposure to heat, the large amount of norepinephrine (NE) released from storage sites eventually finds its way into the arterial circulation.[141,190,174] Although norepinephrine is a potent vasoconstrictor, this action is readily inhibited by adenine nucleotides.[270a] Tissues performing metabolic work during exercise locally release adenine nucleotides and other metabolic products that block the vasoconstriction in response to norepinephrine. This explains why muscle blood flow and myocardial blood flow rise during exercise. On the other hand, the gut and kidney do not produce adenine nucleotides during hard physical work. Hence, norepinephrine exerts its full vasoconstrictive effects at these sites. This may partially explain why acute tubular necrosis of the kidney and acute intestinal necrosis occur in severe cases of exertional heatstroke.

Experimentally, gut ischemia induced by any means leads to increased intestinal permeability.[267a] Thus, ischemic injury probably allows absorption of bacterial endotoxins into the circulation. These toxins, in turn, stimulate release of potentially destructive cytokines from mast cells which are then responsible for tissue lysis.[111a] These substances, which include tumor necrosis factor α

(TNF-α/cachectin), are detectable in the blood of patients with acute exertional heatstroke.[44] These products, especially tumor necrosis factor, would be ideal suspects as factors responsible for the marked somatolytic and catabolic state seen in patients with exertional heatstroke. The almost universal occurrence of rhabdomyolysis and widespread organ damage seen in victims of this disease could also be the result of these cytokines.

To support the foregoing hypothesis, it has been shown that normal men who perform exhaustive work show elevated levels of endotoxin in their blood.[48a] In fact, after one becomes trained to work in the heat, antibodies to endotoxin are readily demonstrable in the blood.[48a] Patients with fatal exertional heatstroke also have detectable circulating endotoxin antibodies.[130a] Indeed, unexercised heat-stressed primates show endotoxin antibodies in their blood after being exposed to a simple temperature of 40°C, which becomes more pronounced after exposure to 43°C.[123a] Hypoxia, which also decreases intestinal blood flow, also results in detectable endotoxin antibodies in the systemic circulation.[121a] Administration of lipopolysaccharide antibodies reduces the morbidity from heating in primates.[123a] Competitive runners who become sufficiently ill after running to require medical treatment demonstrate higher levels of endotoxin antibodies than runners who do not become ill.[48a] These findings suggest not only a possible harmful role for endotoxin-mediated cytokine factors but also the possibility that relative immunity against endotoxins could be important in the process of heat acclimatization.

General pathology of heatstroke

The classical description of the pathologic findings in fatal cases of heatstroke was published by Malamud et al.[221] Myocardial damage is common. Characteristically, subendocardial hemorrhages occur beneath the left interventricular septum. Fragmentation and rupture of muscle fibers are also common. Extensive transmural myocardial infarction has been seen in a young man with stress-induced heatstroke.[181] Careful dissection of all coronary vessels at the time of autopsy disclosed no evidence whatever of occlusive disease.

A recent report described a fatal case of heatstroke in a young football player who showed hemorrhagic infarction of an anterior papillary muscle.[16]

Kew and coworkers[170] reported that in 17 of 26 patients with exertional heatstroke, myocardial LDH isoenzymes were abnormal and electrocardiographic disturbances were evident. In two fatal cases, findings were confined to myofibrillar degeneration and interstitial edema.

The possible mechanisms whereby frank myocardial infarction or patchy myocardial necrosis occurs in the absence of coronary artery occlusion is unclear. Hyperthermic rats develop pulmonary edema with saline loads.[25] Large doses of catecholamines can induce such lesions in experimental animals.[287] Characteristically, myocardial injury would be associated with elevation of creatine kinase levels in serum and in particular, the ratio of CK-MB: CK-MM would be above 5 percent. Elevations of the MB moiety of creatine kinase occur commonly in exertional heatstroke. In highly trained men, the CK-MB isoenzyme may comprise up to 5 percent of total CK in skeletal muscle, which may reflect ongoing injury to muscle as a result of excessive training.[7a,156a] Consequently, release of CK-MB into the circulation in rhabdomyolysis does not necessarily indicate myocardial infarction. Total CK elevations in frank rhabdomyolysis may reach values in millions of IU/liter. Thus, the meaning of CK-MB elevations is unclear. If myocardial infarction is suspected, other diagnostic measures should be utilized to establish the diagnosis.

RENAL INVOLVEMENT. Evidence of kidney damage is very common in patients with acute heatstroke. Mild proteinuria and modest abnormalities of the urinary sediment are found in virtually all of these patients. In those with heat illness induced by physical exertion, acute renal insufficiency occurs in approximately 25 percent of cases. Four reports have emphasized that severe, often fatal, heat illness with acute oliguric renal failure may occur in association with physical effort in hot climates and not necessarily be attended by hyperpyrexia.[183,281,292,324] In contrast, in patients who develop classical heatstroke as a result of simple exposure to high temperature, acute renal insufficiency occurs in only 5 percent.[181] The most likely explanation for the low incidence of acute renal failure in classical heatsroke is the relative rarity of significant rhabdomyolysis. Zager[345a] has shown that a high body temperature is an important factor determining the severity of experimental ischemic renal injury. It is also important to point out that endotoxemia could play an important causative role in this complication.[213a] In exertional heatstroke, many factors could conceivably contribute to the pathogenesis of acute renal failure. Such patients may be partially dehydrated, they sometimes excrete an acid urine, and they are often markedly hyperuricemic despite the excretion of larger quantities of uric acid than normal in their urine.[183,281] Uric acid nephropathy has been observed. Second, potassium deficiency may exist and has been regarded by some authors as capable of depressing GFR and renal plasma flow as well as inducing tubular damage.[286] Third, myoglobin probably has nephrotoxic effects in a concentrated, acid urine and an association with acute tubular necrosis that is well known.[345b] Finally, the possibility of glomerular injury from DIC in acute heatstroke has been well described.[303]

Patients whose heatstroke is complicated by acute tubular necrosis may recover fully with careful management.[324] However, a recent report by Kew and his associates[168] has described subtle, progressive impairment of renal function in four patients who recovered from heatstroke but whose renal biopsy specimens demonstrated interstitial nephritis. The cause of this finding was not apparent. A patient with typical exertional heatstroke observed by one of us (JPK) subsequently developed rapidly progressive crescentic glomerulonephritis and interstitial nephritis during his convalescence. Since the great majority of patients who survive heatstroke do not manifest such disease, any association of heatstroke with glomerulonephritis or interstitial nephritis remains unsettled.

CNS DISORDERS. Damage to the CNS is found universally in fatal heatstroke cases.[221] Changes in the brain generally consist of edema, patchy congestion, and diffuse petechial hemorrhages. The hypothalamus is not ordinarily damaged. The cerebellum often shows marked deterioration and disappearance of Purkinje cells. In all instances, parenchymal changes of the CNS appear to be directly related to the severity and duration of hyperthermia. The predominance of alterations in cerebellar structure corresponds to the clinical picture of CNS damage in patients who survive severe heatstroke. Clinical examination of these patients often reveals cerebellar ataxia with marked dysarthria and dysmetria.[228]

Evidence of *liver damage* is very common;[146] jaundice may be seen in patients surviving more than 2 days. In approximately 5 percent of cases, jaundice becomes severe. Histologic findings include perisinusoidal edema and patchy necrosis, which may be predominantly centrolobular. Ordinarily, patients who survive show no residual impairment of liver function. *Pancreatitis* sufficiently severe to cause common bile duct obstruction has also been observed. Serum amylase activity is commonly elevated in patients with acute heatstroke. Pancreatitis may result from intense splanchnic vasoconstriction during hyperthermia.[255]

EFFECTS OF HEATSTROKE SEEN IN MUSCLES. Evidence of skeletal muscle damage or rhabdomyolysis, assessed by elevation of CPK or aldolase activity in serum and myoglobinuria, occurs in a large percentage of patients whose heat injury is induced by intensive physical exertion. Although release of myoglobin from muscle may be accompanied by extreme hyperkalemia and consequently may pose a serious hazard to life, those who survive may completely recover their skeletal muscle function.[324] Significant rhabdomyolysis has been observed almost exclusively in patients whose heatstroke followed physical exertion or occurred in association with other hyperkinetic states such as amphetamine intoxication, psychotic agitation, delirium tremens, or severe convulsions. Patients with exertional heatstroke have shown CPK activity up to 2,500,000 IU/liter. Although clinically evident rhabdomyolysis is unusual in classical heatstroke, CPK values up to 2000 IU/liter may be observed.

EFFECTS OF HEATSTROKE ON SWEAT GLANDS. Electron microscopic studies have disclosed pathologic alterations of the subcellualr components of sweat glands.[13] The occasional residual impairment in the ability of some survivors of heatstroke to sweat and their persistent susceptibility to the effects of environmental heat may be explained by such sweat gland changes.

COAGULOPATHY AND HEMATOLOGIC MANIFESTATIONS. Coagulation disorders commonly occur in fatal heatstroke, including striking petechial hemorrhages and ecchymoses. These changes have characteristically been attributed to increased capillary permeability, impaired production of clotting factors by the liver, thrombocytopenia,[339] consumptive coagulopathy, and fibrinolysis. In 1962, Shibolet et al.[293] pointed out that hypofibrinogenemia and severe fibrinolysis occur in heatstroke. Since that time, characteristic features of DIC have been confirmed by several authors.[176,242,253,328] Experimental evidence published by Bedrak et al. shows that simple exposure to heat may enhance blood fibrinolytic activity without depressing plasma fibrinogen concentration.[27] The same authors showed that activation of the fibrinolytic system by heat exposure is less marked following acclimatization.[28] Bedrak showed that decreased fibrinogen concentration in dogs resulted from muscular exercise in the heat and, as in humans, was ameliorated by acclimatization.[26] Moxley and associates[235] confirmed these findings in humans and showed that trained subjects show slightly higher values for euglobulin activity that was not considered biologically important. In contrast, Schrier et al. described increased plasma fibrinogen concentrations in military recruits during the early days of their training.[282]

Virtually all patients with frank heatstroke show evidence of DIC.[303] Usually, thrombocytopenia is evident by the end of the first 24 h. In most cases, recovery is complete by the end of the fifth to seventh day. More serious cases show severe thrombocytopenia which is worst by the end of the second to third day and is associated with hypofibrinogenemia and elevated concentrations of split fibrin products in both blood and urine. These findings may persist in severe cases. Hemorrhage associated with DIC is often a major cause of death in those patients with extremely severe heatstroke who survive the initial hyperthermia. It appears to be especially prominent in cases of heatstroke that occur after physical exertion.

Kew and coworkers examined SGOT, SGPT, LDH, and CPK activities in the serum of 53 patients with heatstroke and found substantial elevations in all.[169] Their data suggest that SGOT values of less than 1000 units (normal range is 10 to 35 units) indicate a favorable outcome, whereas higher values are commonly associated with severe complications and death. Furthermore, nine patients with comparable hyperpyrexia who showed either normal or only slighly elevated values for LDH and SGOT were subsequently shown to have an infection responsible for their fever and not to be victims of heatstroke.

Hypocalcemia, sometimes of profound degree (i.e., serum calcium concentration less than 4 mg/dl), has been observed in patients with heatstroke. It nearly always indicates extensive injury to skeletal muscle. It has been observed early in the course of the disease, even before frank azotemia has developed. It is not due to hypoalbuminemia. Profound hypocalcemia has been observed in a patient with malignant hyperpyrexia accompanied by extensive rhabdomyolysis[91] and in patients with acute renal failure due to idiopathic rhabdomyolysis.[59,180]

Hyperphosphatemia is common in cases of heatstroke. It is ascribed to widespread tissue damage, metabolic acidosis, and renal failure. Combinations of unrelenting lactic acidosis and hyperphosphatemia should lead to suspicision of intestinal necrosis or ongoing necrosis in skeletal muscle. Meroney et al. observed that serum *phosphorus* was disproportionately elevated in patients with posttraumatic acute renal failure in the presence of extensive devitalization of skeletal muscle.[230] The degree of hyperphosphatemia was inversely related to the severity of hypocalcemia. Infusion of calcium induced only transient serum calcium elevation. The investigators exploited these observations by studying dogs that were nephrectomized and subjected to skeletal muscle trauma. They showed that injected ^{45}Ca became sequestered in devitalized muscle 10 times more rapidly than in either normal animals or those subjected to nephrectomy alone. These observations provide a partial explanation for the hypocalcemia commonly observed in such patients.

Studies by Llach et al. on patients with massive rhabdomyolysis showed that hyperphosphatemia reduced 1α,25-dihydrocholecalciferol [$1\alpha,25\text{-}(OH)_2D_3$] production.[211] This depressed calcium mobilization from bone. The initial hyperphosphatemia and secondary hypocalcemia were presumed to be responsible for overproduction of parathyroid hormone (PTH).

It has been shown that hypercalcemia may also occur late in the course of rhabdomyolysis complicated by renal failure[59,205] (see Chaps. 32, 38). In contrast to hypocalcemia, hypercalcemia usually appears during the second week. It may be accompanied by conjunctival injection and pruritus, which are thought to reflect the action of excessive PTH.[222] In some of these patients, plasma PTH concentration has been elevated despite hypercalcemia;[112,205] the PTH increase with high plasma calcium suggests that transient hyperparathyroidism developed. Although hypercalcemia in these patients most often appears in the diuretic phase of acute renal failure, in some of these instances it has definitely preceded this phase.[134,206] Moreover, hypercalcemia in patients with heatstroke has been reported only in those with acute oliguric renal failure in association with antecedent severe muscle or soft tissue injury. It is possible, albeit speculative, that such profound hypocalcemia early in the course of acute renal failure in conjunction with extensive tissue destruction hyperphosphatemia, and calcium deposition may provide a powerful stimulus to parathyroid hyperplasia and overproduction of PTH. Thus, if the intensity of hypocalcemia were sufficient to result in a transient autonomous hyperparathyroid state somewhat analogous to that of chronic uremia, the transient appearance of frank hyperparathyroidism could be readily explained.

Hypophosphatemia may occur transiently in patients with heatstroke. It has been observed early in the course and generally resolves spontaneously. Phosphate levels in serum less than 0.9 mg/dl have been observed. One possible factor underlying hypophosphatemia in acute heatstroke might be acute respiratory alkalosis. In one case, when serum phosphorus concentration was 0.9 mg/dl, arterial pH was 7.45 and P_{CO_2} was 24 mmHg.[179] In this patient, total muscle phosphorus content was normal. In normal subjects, serum phosphorus does not fall to this level unless much more severe respiratory alkalosis is induced.[233] This suggests that other mechanisms responsible for hypophosphatemia may be involved in patients with acute heatstroke.

Acid-base disturbances are common in patients with acute heatstroke. Normal humans, when exposed to a high environmental temperature, characteristically hyperventilate and may develop tetany. As a result of hyperventilations and respiratory alkalosis, they may develop hypokalemia and hypophosphatemia.[45,51] Nearly all patients with classical heatstroke show respiratory alkalosis. Relatively severe respiratory alkalosis in classical heatstroke may be responsible for loss of consciousness because hypocarbia of such magnitude reduces cerebral blood flow.[335a] In contrast, patients with exertional heatstroke usually have metabolic acidosis. Whole blood lactate concentration in exertional heatstroke usually ranges from 6 to 13 m*M*.[272] However, in agitated patients, or in the presence of convulsions, hyperthermia, and cardiovascular collapse, values exceeding 20m*M* have been found. In all these cases, hyperventilation is sufficiently intense to depress arterial P_{CO_2}. However, it is almost never sufficient to elevate blood pH to normal. In patients with extremely severe classical (nonexertional) heatstroke complicated by heart failure or shock, lactic acidosis may also be observed. In this form of heatstroke, lactic acidosis predicts an ominous outcome.[140] By contrast, in exertional heatstroke, lactic acidosis is the rule and appears to have no bearing on the predicted outcome.

Severe lactic acidosis can usually be explained by circulatory insufficiency with diminished perfusion of muscle or enhanced lactate production from skeletal muscle due to pronounced muscular activity. If laboratory measurement of lactate is unavailable, it may be suspected in the nonazotemic patient if the anion gap (i.e., $[Na^+ + K^+] - [Cl^- + HCO_3^-]$) in serum electrolytes exceeds 20 meq/liter (see Chap. 25).

Dogs with experimental heatstroke induced by exposure to air of 45°C, 25 percent relative humidity for 111 min display respiratory alkalosis initially. When rectal temperature passes 42°C, they develop increasingly severe metabolic acidosis due to lactic acid accumulation.[219]

Treatment of heatstroke

The therapeutic cornerstone for successful treatment of heatstroke is relief of hyperthermia. Delay in cooling probably represents the single most important factor leading to death or residual serious disability in those who survive. Two reasons underlie delays in cooling. The first is failure to recognize heatstroke and to appreciate the seriousness of hyperpyrexia. It is to be emphasized that heatstroke is an extreme medical emergency. As a precaution, physicians should properly instruct ambulance attendants, paramedics, football coaches, trainers, or nurses in hospital emergency rooms in recognizing this disorder. During heat waves, it is wise for ambulances to carry ice so that treatment may be initiated on the spot. Patients who have collapsed and who have been identified as suffering from heatstroke by firefighters have been successfully treated en route to the hospital; some have even regained consciousness before arrival at the emergency room. Survival is the rule in such cases. The second cause of delay in treatment is lack of proper cooling facilities at the hospital. In those geographic areas, industries, and military training facilities or at football fields, where heatstroke may occur, its occurrence should be anticipated and an effective plan of action made ready.

Several recent publications illustrate the benefits of early recognition, anticipated provision of facilities, and aggressive treatment of patients with exertional heatstroke.[30,84,242] Each of these reports deals with military recruits; in each, all patients survived. In a study of 28 elderly or previously ill patients with classical heatstroke,[140] 4 died. Although data are not available, mortality in such cases in hospitals where preparations have not been made appeared to approach 50 percent.

Once the diagnosis of heatstroke is made, an intravenous line should be established as quickly as possible to permit access to the circulation. The patient should undergo tracheal intubation if comatose and if properly trained personnel are available. Gastric contents should be emptied followed by instillation of sodium bicarbonate to neutralize any residual fluid. This is done since many patients vomit and because convulsive seizures are often first displayed during cooling, with the associated risk of aspiration. Neutral or alkaline gastric contents are less apt to injure the lung in the event of aspiration. Rectal temperature should be recorded, preferably using a thermistor inserted into the rectum to a depth of 19 cm (because of their length, standard thermometers measure anal tempereature, not core temperature). These initial maneuvers accomplished, the conventional method is to immerse the patient in a tub of ice water and briskly massage the skin surface to stimulate exchange of heat. This procedure may induce severe pain in the hands of the attendants and requires that several individuals be available in order to alternate efforts. Cooling may alternatively be effected by rubbing the body surface briskly with plastic bags containing ice after the body has been wet down with water. This procedure is effective provided it can be carried out in the wake of a large fan in an air-conditioned room. Body temperature may be lowered to 39°C (102.2°F) within 60 min or less by either means. When the core temperature reaches 39°C, cooling measures should be stopped since body temperature ordinarily continues to fall. Convulsions, if they should occur at this time, may prevent a further fall of body temperature. Indeed, a convulsion may be followed by a recurrence of hyperthermia. Intravenous chlorpromazine, 50 mg, or diazepam, 5 mg, may be given at the initiation of treatment. Either is very useful to prevent tremors and convulsions that appear during the cooling period. Drug administration may be repeated every 4 h if necessary.[150,151,224] Chlorpromazine may cause hypotension in older patients with heatstroke.[140]

A number of these patients display profound hypotension at the time of admission. While this may result from impairment of myocardial performance,[243] it is more often the result of translocation of blood volume to the dilated superficial vessels in the skin. Thus, it is not necessarily the result of a volume deficit. Cooling ordinarily restores blood pressure to normal by means of cutaneous vasoconstriction. Therefore, large volumes of intravenous fluids for the purpose of elevating blood pressure should not be employed in the early treatment period since, once cooling is induced, return of blood to the central circulation may cause acute pulmonary edema. If cooling does not restore the blood pressure, 250 to 500 ml of normal saline should be rapidly infused. If this is not effective, dopamine should be used. Norepinephrine should be avoided since it induces intense peripheral vasoconstriction and may prolong the hyperthermic period. It could also aggravate damage to the kidney and small bowel. Dextran should be avoided because it may impair platelet function and thereby promote hemorrhage.[199]

Once the patient has been cooled, hyperthermia may be expected to recur within 3 or 4 h, especially in those patients who are unable to sweat. Cooling measures must be reinstated accordingly. Recovery of ability to sweat may require several weeks.

Therapeutic cooling of heatstroke victims in ice baths or by rubbing the body surface with ice, although effective, is commonly associated with fasciculations, shivering, or convulsions. Moreover, the recommended massage of the body surface by attendants is painful and cumbersome. Based upon a limited number of clinical observations[171,330,331] and experimental observations on hyperthermic dogs,[218] the suggestion has been made that body cooling may occur at a rate equal to or even more rapidly in water having a temperature of 15 to 16°C (59 to 61°F). Theoretically, water of this temperature permits conduction of heat while avoiding vasoconstriction in cutaneous vessels and excessive cooling of the skin so as to cause shivering. The body cooling unit designed by Weiner and Khogali[171] sprays warm dry air and 15°C water over the patient's body surface so as to gain advantage of evaporative cooling and to prevent excessive cooling of the skin. Although these newer methods of treatment remain experimental they appear to be promising. Certainly, they are more pleasant than ice-water immersion. In addition, they eliminate the need to administer drugs to prevent shivering and convulsions.

The most important laboratory measurements at the time of admission include arterial blood gases, pH, serum electrolyte concentrations, and complete blood count including platelets. Baseline values for prothrombin time, partial thromboplastin time, fibrinogen, and fibrin split products should be obtained if available. When possible, blood lactate concentration should be determined since lactic acidosis occurs commonly in patients whose heatstroke is induced by muscular exercise. As in other circumstances, lactic acidosis may become much worse once hypotension is corrected due to a washout of lactate and hydrogen ions from skeletal muscle. If arterial pH is low in this type of patient and there is no evidence of impaired gas exchange by the lungs, the low pH can be assumed to result from acute lactic acidosis. Under the latter circumstance, arterial P_{CO_2} is usually in the vicinity of 28 mmHg. Pulmonary edema has been observed in patients with exertion-induced heatstroke even when fluids have not been administered. This could well be the result of acute lactic acidosis and warrants consideration of bicarbonate therapy.

Treatment of complications

DISSEMINATED INTRAVASCULAR COAGULATION. This has been documented in a large number of patients with acute heatstroke. DIC is especially likely to occur in that form of heatstroke induced by exertion. Thrombocytopenia, decreased fibrinogen concentration, and elevated serum levels of fibrin split products occur in most patients with heatstroke. Purpura is very common on the second or third day. At present there appears to be no clear-cut indication for heparin therapy in such patients, but it may be considered if there is evidence of gross hemorrhage. Bleeding has also been ascribed to fibrinolysis. Treatment with 6-aminocaproic acid has been recommended for fibrinolysis. However, most authorities agree that its use is extremely hazardous and probably provides no long-term benefit. Indeed, recent evidence suggests that 6-aminocaproic acid may cause rhabdomyolysis.[259] Some of the bleeding diathesis in patients with heatstroke is also a result of decreased production of clotting factors in the liver due to acute liver injury. Peripheral eosinophilia, possibly due to purpura, may appear during the recovery period. Mild hemolysis is also common.

RHABDOMYOLYSIS. Elevated CPK activity is present in the patient's serum in nearly all cases of exertional heatstroke but occurs less often in classical heatstroke. This usually indicates rhabdomyolysis. There are four imminent dangers of rhabdomyolysis: (1) hyperkalemia with its attendant risk of cardiotoxicity and/or skeletal muscle paralysis, (2) myoglobinuria and its attendant threat of acute renal failure, (3) shock as a result of sequestration of fluid in injured muscle cells, and (4) necrosis of the diaphragm with respiratory failure.

Loss of circulatory volume into injured muscle cells may be so severe that up to 12 liters of normal saline may be required on the first day of treatment in order to maintain blood pressure. This probably reflects a widespread capillary leak syndrome. In some patients, this is heralded by unexplained hypoalbuminemia at the time of admission. The mandate to administer such large volumes of fluid unavoidably leads to edema of the involved skeletal muscle. This complication may have the dire consequence of a muscle-compartment syndrome with vascular compression if it should involve the extremities. It tends to occur on the third or fourth day and may be responsible for a second episode of acute muscle necrosis, heralded by a second rise of CPK activity and sometimes myoglobinuria. If this "second wave phenomenon" appears imminent, the patient's extremities must be carefully observed. Should there appear evidence of compartmental vascular compression such as loss of arterial pulsations, blanching, coldness, neuropathy, or progressive muscle weakness, measurement of tissue pressure and fasciotomy should be considered.

ACUTE RENAL FAILURE. (See also Chap. 38.) Acute renal failure occurs in about 5 percent of patients with classical heatstroke and in about 30 percent of patients with exertional heatstroke. Mannitol has been advocated as an effective agent to prevent acute renal failure. The early use of mannitol may, therefore, theoretically prevent this complication in patients with acute heatstroke. The incidence and severity of acute renal failure is related to the degree of volume depletion, body temperature (both of which aggravate renal ischemia), the severity of muscle necrosis, hyperuricemia, and hypotension. Recognition of renal failure requires careful monitoring of urine output, body weight, and fluid administration. The common occurrence of acute renal failure in heatstroke patients demands early examination of the urine for specific gravity or osmolality and for myoglobin, measurement of the urine:plasma concentration ratio for urea nitrogen, and determination of urine [Na^+] as aids in identification of acute renal failure. If the urine is concentrated, contains little sodium (less than ~20 meq/liter) and the urine:plasma concentration ratio for urea nitrogen is above 10, acute tubular necrosis can be ruled out with reasonable certainty. However, if the urine is isotonic to plasma, the urine:plasma urea nitrogen concentration ratio is less than 5 and urine [Na^+] is high, acute tubular necrosis is likely. (Previous administration of diuretics obscures the meaning of urine [Na^+]). Associated findings would include identification of myoglobinuria (heme positive urine that may be darkly stained) in the presence of clear serum and the presence of pigmented casts in the urinary sediment. Creatine kinase will always be unequivocally elevated in serum. If there is evidence of acute renal failure, the patient may be given 100 mg or more of furosemide intravenously in conjunction with 25 g of 20 percent mannitol. If diuresis follows, it should be sustained by fluids and furosemide as needed.

The hypothetical reason for administering mannitol and furosemide is to reduce oxygen consumption and ATP utilization by the renal tubular epithelium. Both O_2 and ATP are utilized in tubular reabsorption of Na^+ and probably in renal tubular transport of the ferrihemate moiety of myoglobin. Ferrihemate is an organic acid transported incidentally by the proximal renal tubular cell. Its transport is Na^+ dependent. Accordingly, interruption of Na^+ and ferrihemate transport simply by accelerating flow past the reabsorptive site (mannitol) or by interrupting Na^+ transport directly (furosemide) hypothetically "puts the tubule to sleep," reduces its consumption of O_2 and ATP, and thereby reduces the chances of metabolism-related injury. In addition, dilution of the urine by both of these agents would reduce the concentration of pigment in the tubular fluid in the renal medulla, and thereby reduce nephrotoxicity by lowering the concentration of the toxin.

For many years, urinary alkalinization has been recommended as a means of reducing nephrotoxicity from myoglobin or hemoglobin. There is evidence to suggest that heme proteins are less likely to form gels in alkaline solutions; thus the tubular obstruction due to heme-pigment cast formation becomes hypothetically reduced. Although infusions of alkali ($NaHCO_3$) are utilized by many nephrologists as prophylaxis against heme-pigment toxicity, there is still no solid evidence that its beneficial effects are not explainable by the HCO_3^- induced osmotic diuresis.[345b]

HYPOKALEMIA AND HYPERKALEMIA. Hypokalemia occurs in at least half the cases. It does not ordinarily require treament in classical heatstroke since it is usually related to acute respiratory alkalosis. In patients with exertion-induced heatstroke, hypokalemia may represent frank potassium depletion. Even in those patients, hypokalemia is usually transient since release of K^+ from injured tissues frequently corrects the hypokalemia spontaneously; hyperkalemia often results, especially in the presence of oliguria. Hyperkalemia often requires the use of agents to lower serum [K^+] or reverse its electrocardiographic effects. These include calcium infusions, infusions of glucose and insulin, and administration of alkali or beta-adrenergic agonists such as albuterol. Disodium polystyrene sulfonate resin (kayexalate) should be started in patients with rhabdomyolysis-associated acute oliguric renal failure even if hyperkalemia has not yet appeared because of its imminent danger. Aggressive hemodialysis is often necessary (see Chap. 23).

HYPOGLYCEMIA. Serum glucose values as low as 10 mg/dl have been recorded in patients with heatstroke induced by seizures after phenmetrazine overdosage. Costrini and associates observed serum glucose concentrations below 65 mg/dl in 5 of 12 patients with exertional heatstroke.[84] Presumably, rapid utilization of glucose, glycogen depletion, and liver injury consequent to splanchnic ischemia are responsible for this potentially dangerous complication.[79]

HYPERNATREMIA. This is commonly observed. Its treatment is detailed in the section on heat exhausion.

HYPOCALCEMIA. Although calcium levels even less than 4 mg/dl have been observed in acute heatstroke, tetany is highly unusual. Prophylactic calcium administration should be avoided if possible since it causes deposition of calcium carbonate and calcium phosphate in skeletal muscle.

HYPERURICEMIA. In some patients, especially those with exercise-induced heatstroke with rhabdomyolysis, hyperuricemia may be profound.[183,241] Three patients whose serum uric acid concentration at the time of admission ranged between 35 and 48 mg/dl in the presence of a normal blood urea nitrogen value have been observed. When such extreme hyperuricemia occurs, consideration might be given to the use of allopurinol. However, hyperuricemia is usually much less intense and resolves spontaneously.

Hyperosmolar nonketotic coma. Hyperglycemia, with levels of glucose in the vicinity of 1000 mg/dl, has been observed in some patients with heatstroke who have survived 7 days or more. This appears to be more common in children. In all cases widespread skeletal muscle injury has been evident. In most instances, hyperglycemia can be ascribed to excessive administration of glucose in conjunction with renal insufficiency (see Chaps. 21, 26).

ELECTROCARDIOGRAPHIC ABNORMALITIES. Alterations of the electrocardiogram consisting of inverted T waves, depressed S-T segments, conduction defects, and arrhythmias are common.[170] These do not necessarily indicate structural damage to the heart. However, on rare occasions frank myocardial infarction has occurred in the absence of coronary artery occlusion.[16,181] Due to the common association of hypokalemia, judicious use of digitalis and calcium salts is important.

CENTRAL NERVOUS SYSTEM DYSFUNCTION. Patients with heatstroke are commonly obtunded for several days following recovery from hyperthermia. Although a broad range of functional disorders occurs, complete recovery may occur.[292] Abnormalities of cerebellar function are especially common in patients with sustained severe heatstroke. While these abnormalities may be transient, some patients show persistent defects including disorders of ocular movement, ataxia, aphasia, hemiparesis, or dementia. In the early stages of heatstroke and usually in the presence of hyperthermia, the pupils may be widely dilated, irregular, and sometimes unresponsive to light. In contrast to other situations, this does not indicate cerebral death since all the abnormalities may disappear within several hours following appropriate cooling. Nuchal rigidity has been observed in acute heatstroke. Although it is not ordinarily associated with pleocytosis, one case demonstrated blood in the subarachnoid space at autopsy. The spinal fluid usually shows no more than modest elevation of protein concentration in patients with frank heatstroke.

Differential diagnosis of heatstroke

Under ordinary circumstances, little difficulty should be experienced in identifying classical heatstroke. Dry skin should not be relied upon to confirm the diagnosis, since a perspiring patient with hyperpyrexia is an equal candidate for thermal tissue injury.

Hypothalamic damage resulting from heatstroke is uncommon. In contrast, hyperthermia may occur in patients with hypothalamic lesions. Chesanow has pointed out that "hypothalamic hyperthermia" should be suspected when (1) temperature is uniformly high without the peaks and troughts seen in sepsis; (2) anhidrosis, which may be unilateral, occurs; (3) resistance to antipyretic drugs is seen; and (4) disorders reflecting damage to adjacent structures, such as diabetes insipidus, are present.[68] Marked hyperthermia may be seen in *quadriplegic patients* in response to bacterial infections, such as pyelonephritis. Cervical spinal cord injury interferes with thermoregulatory responses to overproduction of heat. In some patients, administration of chlorpromazine results in resolution of the fever.

Confusion may arise in certain patients who have *meningitis* accompanied by an unusually high fever: patients with heatstroke sometimes demonstrate nuchal rigidity. In classical heatstroke, spinal fluid may be blood-tinged at times and show an elevated protein concentration. Pleocytosis is not a feature.

Malignant hyperpyrexia should always be considered in patients who develop heatstroke during anesthesia. Neuroleptic malignant syndrome should also be considered in patients receiving antipsychotic drugs such as haloperidol and thioxanthene derivatives.

Although the height of fever in *acute meningococcemia, typhus, Rocky Mountain spotted fever,* or *falciparum malaria* does not ordinarily reach the levels seen in heatstroke, delirium and appearance of hemorrhagic skin manifestations certainly warrant their consideration in the differential diagnosis. *Midbrain hemorrhage* may occur in certain alcoholic patients and may be accompanied by hyperthermia. In some, hyperthermia seems to result from the accompanying agitation and related metabolic heat production rather than a primary disturbance in thermal regulation. Frank heatstroke can occur as a complication of *delirium tremens.* Bacteremia with gram-negative organisms, miliary tuberculosis, pneumococcal pneumonia, and urosepsis rarely cause fevers in excess of 41°C.[297]

Heat intolerance in recovered heatstroke patients

Multiple episodes of heatstroke have occurred in certain individuals following exertion. A critical issue concerns whether this class of patients had an initial idiosyncrasy or whether their first episode was simply the result of normal heat dissipation being overwhelmed. A further question, where the latter case holds, concerns whether recurrent episodes of heatstroke are the result of heat intolerance as a residual defect consequent to earlier heatstroke. Answers to these questions are not now available.

Shapiro et al. studied nine young men who had recovered from exertional heatstroke.[290] Compared to 10 normal volunteers who tolerated controlled exercise in a heat chamber without difficulty, those with a history of heatstroke developed substantially higher heart rates, higher temperatures, and lower oxygen consumption values. Sweat production was not impaired. The results suggested that inefficient thermoregulation due to decreased conductance from the core to the periphery was responsible. Robinson and coworkers made similar observations on two survivors of exertional heatstroke.[263]

Prognosis

The physician who anticipates the occurrence of heatstroke and who has a well-conceived plan for its treatment, competent help, and adequate facilities can save the lives of as many as 95 percent of patients. In contrast, sporadic cases, which are often unanticipated and, as a consequence, temporarily neglected, carry a much higher mortality rate. In military recruits or young football players, in whom heatstroke is associated with physical exertion, the disorder is generally severe and carries many associated complications. However, even in severe cases, if cooling procedures are performed aggressively and otherwise fatal complications are anticipated, most patients survive.

HYPOTHERMIA

Hypothermia, defined as a core temperature less than 35°C (95°F), is a medical emergency that occurs in both temperate and cold environments. Its prompt recognition is critical if serious morbidity or death are to be avoided.

PATHOPHYSIOLOGY

When body temperature declines, the normal human increases heat production by shivering; the reaction can increase the metabolic rate fivefold.[147] The normal subject also reduces heat loss by decreasing cutaneous blood flow. Children may increase heat production by an additional mechanism, *nonshivering thermogenesis,* which is virtually insignificant in adults because of the sparsity of brown fat. If such thermoregulatory mechanisms fail, body cooling ensues. A reduction in core temperature decreases the rate of chemical reactions so that cooling proceeds until a new equilibrium is established between the body and its environmnent.

Central nervous system effects

As hypothermia develops, cerebral blood flow progressively declines due to a fall in cardiac output and an increase in cerebral vascular resistance and blood viscosity. This fall in nutrient availability, however, is offset by a significant reduction in the metabolic rate of the brain. This fall in metabolic demand has allowed for the successful cerebral resuscitation of hypothermic patients even after prolonged periods of anoxia and circulatory arrest.[71,92,345] Such responses have permitted neurosurgical patients to tolerate clamping of the middle cerebral artery for up to 40 min at 30°C without neurological sequelae.[311]

Hypothermia depresses CNS function. Symptoms and physical findings are extremely variable, but as core temperature falls to about 32°C (89.6°F), patients develop a progressive decline in mental status with gait ataxia, tremulous speech, and normal to hyperactive deep tendon reflexes. Pupillary responses are usually normal. Below 32°C, deep tendon reflexes diminish as the patient develops stupor and dysarthria. Around 30°C (86°F), movements become delayed and pupillary responses sluggish. The patient may be able to answer simple questions, but may perseverate; responses will be delayed. Below 28°C (82.4°F), although there is little spontaneous movement or response to verbal stimulation, the patient may appear awake and respond to noxious stimulation. Below 26°C (78.8°F), most patients are unresponsive to any stimulation and pupils are very sluggish or fixed. Deep tendon reflexes are diminished due to a prolongation of the contraction and relaxation phases.[216] Babinski responses remain flexor down to about 26°C. Usually no response is elicited at lower temperatures. An extensor Babinski response is very unusual and suggests another condition is complicating the hypothermia.[110] Shivering reaches a maximum at 32 to 33°C (89.6 to 91.4°F), but usually ceases below this point and muscle rigidity becomes prominent.

Cardiovascular system

When a person is exposed to a cold environment and body temperature falls slightly, the increase in sympathoadrenal outflow and increased metabolic demand of shivering leads to an increase in heart rate, blood pressure, peripheral vascular resistance, cardiac output, and central venous pressure. As hypothermia becomes established, however, the primary changes in the cardiovascular system are depressive.

Cardiac output falls progressively as hypothermia develops. This cardiac effect is due primarily to a fall in ventricular rate; stroke volume remains normal or slightly reduced; the drop in output is due primarily to a fall in ventricular rate. Output returns to normal with rewarming, but recovery may be delayed.

As temperature falls, heart rate declines due to a depression of atrial and ventricular pacemaker activity with a relative prolongation of systole over diastole.[36]

Despite the decline in cardiac output and heart rate, blood pressure may remain normal due to a rise in peripheral vascular resistance.[192] Vasoconstriction tends to shunt the circulation away from most tissues to support the heart and central circulation.[271]

The metabolic and oxygen demand of the myocardium decreases with hypothermia as with other tissues. However, the effects on coronary blood flow vary. Surface cooling to 25 to 28°C (77 to 82°F) has been reported to decrease coronary blood flow.[34,35] The clinical significance of these changes in flow and substrate availability is difficult to establish. Creatine phosphokinase MB isoenzyme may increase with severe hypothermia without evidence of myocardial infarction, suggesting myocardial cellular damage.[63] However, despite changes in flow and substrate availability, in most patients the supply of oxygen and nutrients to the myocardium is probably adequate for the reduced demand.

Cardiac arrhythmias are very common in hypothermia. As temperature falls, the action potential of myocardial cells and conduction system fibers lengthens with the appearance of a dip in the early part of the plateau phase. Reduced ion fluxes across the sarcolemma may cause this abnormality.[215] Atrial arrhythmias are especially common but do not necessarily indicate the presence of organic heart disease; they usually resolve without specific treatment as core temperature rises. Correction of metabolic derangements and therapy with digoxin or quinidine may speed conversion to sinus rhythm. Ventricular ectopic beats are less common but may herald ventricular fibrillation.[283] The incidence of ventricular fibrillation increases as temperature decreases, becoming an imminent danger if core temperature is less than 28°C (82.4°F).[213,234,321] Stimuli such as urethral catheterization, movement, endotracheal intubation, and vascular catheterization also predispose to the development of this arrhythmia.

Electrocardiographic changes are very common in hypothermia. Mechanical artifacts due to skeletal muscle activity frequently obscure low-voltage complexes and make the detection of electrocardiographic changes difficult. Sinus tachycardia may be seen with mild degrees of hypothermia, but its presence should suggest complicating factors such as gastrointestinal bleeding, drug overdose, carbon monoxide poisoning, or sepsis. In general, atrial and ventricular rates fall due to a direct effect of cold.[157] Conductivity is depressed with significant hypothermia leading to prolonged PR, QRS, and QT intervals. QT interval prolongation is very common and may persist for several days after normal temperature has been restored. Nonspecific ST segment and T wave changes are also common.[105] Osborn waves, characterized by a widening of the base of the QRS complex and J-point deflection, are the most characteristic electrocardiographic finding.[246] They can be seen with hypothermia from any cause and do not herald the onset of ventricular fibrillation.[97,317]

Respiratory function

The usual pulmonary response to mild hypothermia is an increase in respiratory rate and respiratory alkalosis. However, as hypothermia worsens, a progressive fall in respiratory rate takes place;[42] vital capacity and minute ventilation also drop steadily. Respirations become shallow and slow, leading to carbon dioxide retention and respiratory acidosis.

Hypothermia has few direct effects on the mechanical properties of the lung other than mild bronchodilatation and reduced compliance.[322] As body temperature falls, alpha-adrenergic receptors mediate an increase in pulmonary vascular resistance and pressure.[308] If shivering does not occur, CO_2 production falls by approximately 50 percent as core temperature approaches 29°C (84.2°F).[227] However, the adequacy of ventilation can still be determined by the measurement of arterial P_{CO_2} and if artificial ventilation is necessary, appropriate adjustments in the rate and depth of respirations must be made to avoid hyperventilation and respiratory alkalosis.

Renal function

Hypothermia reversibly depresses most indices of renal function.[266] As core temperature decreases, renal blood flow and GFR fall due to hypotension, low cardiac output, increased renal vascular resistance, and direct renal effect of cold. Sodium, chloride, and glucose transport are depressed, resulting in natriuresis and glycosuria. Hydrogen ion excretion is also impaired, which contributes significantly to the metabolic acidosis. The ability of the kidney to conserve water is also substantially impaired. The hypothermic patient may excrete a relatively large amount of dilute urine (so-called cold diuresis) despite a low systemic blood pressure and cardiac output.

Electrolyte and acid-base effects

Serum sodium and chloride concentrations are usually normal in accidental hypothermia unless complications such as myxedema, hypoadrenalism, hypopituitarism, vomiting, or diarrhea are present. Serum potassium is usually normal but may be slightly depressed in the presence of respiratory alkalosis.[258] Hypokalemia may be encountered during recovery if large amounts of potassium-free or glucose-containing solutions are used during resuscitation. The most probable cause of hypokalemia during recovery is the heat-stimulated acceleration of outward sodium transport which had been depressed by cold. Removal of sodium by this mechanism increases intracellular electronegativity that, in turn, promotes cellular uptake of potassium ions. Hyperkalemia rarely occurs unless renal failure and rhabdomyolysis coexist. Calcium levels are usually normal in uncomplicated hypothermia, although cases with hypercalcemia and hypocalcemia have both been seen. Levy has noted hypophosphatemia during the recovery phase of hypothermia.[208]

Disturbances of acid-base equilibrium are common in accidental hypothermia. Acute exposure frequently results in hyperventilation with respiratory alkalosis. As temperature falls, however, a combined respiratory and metabolic acidosis generally ensues. The metabolic acidosis produced during hypothermia is primarily due to lactic acid elaborated by shivering muscle and decreased metabolism of lactate by the liver because of relative tissue hypoxia.[296]

Gastrointestinal tract

Gastric dilatation and erosions, hemorrhages, adynamic ileus, colonic dilatations, and a generalized decrease in splanchnic blood flow are encountered frequently in accidental hypothermia.[137] The ability of the liver to produce glucose and metabolize lactic acid is seriously depressed,[296] although extreme abnormalities in liver function tests are unusual. Asymptomatic elevations in serum amylase and ischemic pancreatitis[276] are also common.

Endocrine system

As core temperature falls, the release of most pituitary hormones (including ACTH and ADH) is depressed, with normal function returning rapidly on rewarming. An increase in levels of thyroid-stimulating hormone has been reported in some species of animals, human infants acutely exposed to cold, and adults with chronic hypothermia,[111] although no such rise has been seen in adults with brief exposure to intense cold.[335,338] Cortisol levels rise with sudden cold exposure, but as hypothermia becomes established adrenal function falls in proportion to the decline in temperature. The decreased kidney function can be attributed to the cold[37] and a decreased sensitivity to ACTH.[106] The depression of adrenal responsiveness to ACTH rapidly returns to normal with rewarming.[106] Cortisol levels, however, are frequently normal or near normal, presumably due to a temperature-sensitive decrease in metabolism and cortisol conjugation by the liver.

As a response to thermoregulatory and environmental stress, early rises in serum epinephrine and norepinephrine occur.[8,149] As temperature approaches 30°C (86°F), however, catecholamine levels begin to fall; a significant depression develops by 28°C (82.4°F).[336] At any temperature below normal, serum levels of catecholamines may not accurately reflect adrenal function because of decreased activity of catechol O-methyl transferase and monoamine oxidase.[279]

Hypothermia results in reversible depression of the endocrine pancreas, causing a fall in insulin release.[86,295] Peripheral glucose utilization is also depressed;[198] hyperglycemia is therefore a common complication. Free fatty acid levels are increased by sympathetic stimulation[239] and provide an important energy source for shivering muscle. These compounds may contribute to myocardial toxicity in ischemic situations,[245] but their relevance to the arrhythmias of hypothermia is unknown.

Hematologic system

The cold diuresis and fluid compartment shifts that occur with hypothermia create a variable amount of hemoconcentration and a fall in plasma volume.[67] The leukocyte count, on the other hand, usually falls as body temperature declines to 32°C (89.6°F), although the differential white cell count and response to infection are usually normal. Variable degrees of thrombocytopenia are also common. Disseminated intravascular coagulation can be seen with rewarming.[220]

Conditions and diseases associated with hypothermia

Most patients presenting to metropolitan hospitals with hypothermia suffer from some underlying medical condition that predisposes them to its development.[332] Table 47-5 lists some of the disorders known to predispose to hypothermia.

Advanced age

Like classical heatstroke, hypothermia in the elderly occurs mostly indoors and in combination with significant medical illness. Fox has shown that elderly persons living in cold homes tend to have lower oral and early-morning urine temperatures.[114] A decrease in vasoconstrictor responses to cold,[325] a decrease in the ability to generate heat,[326] malnutrition,[236] and a decrease in thermal sensitivity[327] contribute to this increased susceptibility to cold.

The mortality rate of hypothermic elderly patients is high, primarily because of the high incidence of coexisting serious medical conditions.[155]

Metabolic disturbances

The most widely recognized endocrinopathy presenting with hypothermia is hypothyroidism, although the prevalence of this disorder in hypothermic patients is probably less than 10 percent. Bradycardia, atrial fibrillation, cardiomegaly, edema, myxedematous facies, mental slowing, and delayed relaxation of the deep tendon reflexes can be seen with uncomplicated hypothermia and mimic hypothyroidism. The development of significant hypothermia in a myxedematous patient should suggest complicating infection, drug use, or trauma.

CNS disease

The key role of the nervous system in regulating temperature makes neuropathies a frequent cause of hypothermia. Many of these involve the hypothalamus, although more generalized conditions can disrupt afferent and efferent thermoregulatory tracts and result in a significant loss in temperature control.

Drugs

Many drugs (see Table 47-5) influence thermoregulation. Alcohol consumption commonly contributes to the development of hypothermia because of its ability to induce vasodilatation, reduce shivering, decrease central ther-

TABLE 47-5 • Conditions predisposing to hypothermia

DISEASES
Metabolic disturbances:
Hypothyroidism
Diabetic ketoacidosis
Renal failure
Hypoglycemia
Hypoadrenalism
Hypopituitarism
Hepatic encephalopathy
CNS disorders:
Cerebrovascular disease
Subdural hematoma
Tumors
Head trauma
Anorexia nervosa
Shapiro's syndrome
Parkinson's disease
Wernicke's encephalopathy
Spinal cord injury
Sarcoidosis
Alzheimer's disease
Schizophrenia
Recurrent spontaneous hypothermia
Hypothalamic gliosis
DRUGS
Ethanol
Phenothiazines
Tricyclic antidepressants
Benzodiazepines
Morphine
Reserpine
General anesthetics
Prazosin
Barbiturates
Glutethimide
Meprobamate
Methaqualone
Ethchlorvynol
Heroin
Cannabis
Organophosphates
Ethylene glycol
Carbon monoxide
INDIVIDUAL FACTORS
Miscellaneous causes:
Malnutrition
Skin diseases with dermal dysfunction
Paget's disease of bone
Infections
Pancreatitis
Shock
Exposure
Advanced age

moregulatory sensitivity, impair judgment, induce hypoglycemia and Wernecke's encephalopathy,[96] and predispose to exposure and trauma.

Many drugs counteract thermoregulatory responses and predispose to hypothermia even in therapeutic doses while other drugs require supratherapeutic doses to seriously impair thermoregulation. The prognosis of most of these overdoses with hypothermia is better than for other predisposing causes.

Exposure

Exposure to extreme cold can eventually cause hypothermia in any setting, but certain environmental conditions make its development more likely. For example, immersion in cold water results in a greater loss of heat than does exposure to air of equal temperature because of water's high thermal conductance. In addition, recent studies have shown that some men working underwater develop significant hypothermia without symptoms,[165] especially if they have little subcutaneous fat.

In summary, many clinical conditions impair thermoregulatory function and predispose to hypothermia. In general, hypothermia related to drug ingestion and exposure without serious underlying disease has a much better prognosis than hypothermia due to other conditions.

MANAGEMENT OF HYPOTHERMIA

Since most thermometers do not measure temperatures below about 34.5°C (94.1°F), the diagnosis of hypothermia depends on a high index of suspicion. If hypothermia is suspected, an estimate of core temperature should be obtained by one of several means. Temperature recorded high in the rectum by a thermistor probe will give a reasonable measurement of core temperature in most patients. Esophageal temperature measurements may be used but are uncomfortable to the patient, difficult to properly place, and may precipitate ventricular arrhythmias. Tympanic membrane temperature may be used to estimate core temperature if the appropriate instrument is available.

If the patient is comatose, airway patency must be ensured and steps taken to prevent gastric aspiration. A large intravenous catheter should be inserted and thiamine and glucose given immediately in the appropriate situations. Stimulation of the patient should be kept to a minimum to avoid precipitating ventricular fibrillation. Constant electrocardiographic monitoring is mandatory for all patients during rewarming because of the high incidence of arrhythmias. Blood pressure, pulse, temperature, neurologic status, and urine output should be monitored frerquently during rewarming. Monitoring of central venous and arterial pressure, Swan-Ganz catheterization, and cardiac pacing may be necessary in some patients, but these procedures should otherwise be avoided because the cardiac irritation can precipitate ventricular fibrillation.

Rewarming techniques

The proper technique for rewarming hypothermic patients is controversial because the variety of predisposing factors and complicating diseases makes general recommendations difficult. A warming rate of about 0.55°C (1°F) per hour is generally accepted as optimal; most shivering patients spontaneously rewarm at a rate equal to or greater than this. Consequently, many authorities believe that *passive* rewarming of hemodynamically stable hypothermic patients is best. With this method, the patient is allowed to generate heat with insulating material such as blankets as the only external intervention. This method allows a slow rise of 0.5 to 1°C (1 to 1.8°F) per hour in most patients if the initial core temperature is greater than approximately 27°C (80.6°F); it is especially effective in patients with acute hypothermia without underlying disease. *Active* rewarming methods, wherein heat is applied to the body surface with hot-water bottles, warm water, etc., have also been used as a means to rapidly return core temperature to near normal in patients with severe hypothermia and/or cardiopulmonary arrest. Active rewarming is especially important in patients with ventricular fibrillation or standstill because the hypothermic myocardium is resistant to mechanical or pharmacologic intervention until temperatures are above 28 to 30°C (82.4 to 86°F). With active rewarming, patients who otherwise would have died during resuscitation have survived.[89]

Several disadvantages of active rewarming have been described. "Rewarming shock," especially likely when external methods are employed, involves neutralizing the cold-induced intense peripheral vasoconstriction; it results in a fall in peripheral vascular resistance and blood pressure, magnified by an associated failure to increase cardiac output. This sequence is especially common in elderly persons with significant preexisting cardiovascular disease. Second, external warming may induce vasodilatation, returning cold peripheral blood to the central circulation and causing a drop in core temperature. A third problem with active rewarming is that the lactic acidosis associated with hypothermia may be significantly worsened when uneven rewarming occurs and ischemic tissues are reperfused.

To avoid these problems, rapid rewarming of core blood has been attempted by several means in patients with severe hypothermia and/or cardiac arrest. These methods minimize the risks of rewarming shock and progressively worsening lactic acidosis. Methods used to accomplish active core rewarming are summarized in Table 47-6. Most patients with hypothermia tolerate warm intravenous fluids and heated oxygen. If rapid rewarming is required, peritoneal lavage with solutions warmed to approximately 40°C (104°F) can be used in most situations, especially if more sophisticated equipment is not available.

In summary, the method of rewarming depends in large part on the necessity for rapid rewarming. Young patients with acute hypothermia usually rewarm rapidly with passive methods if hypothermia is not extreme. Active external rewarming should be avoided in older patients with significant underlying cardiovascular disease. Patients with cardiopulmonary arrest should be rapidly rewarmed by a core rewarming method to at least 30°C (86°F) while resuscitative measures are in progress.

Supportive measures

Because of the wide diversity of electrolyte requirements in hypothermic patients, no general recommendations can be made regarding fluid management other than warming the fluid to 37 to 40°C (98.6 to 104°F) before administration. Rewarming shock should be treated vigorously by increasing plasma volume if central venous pressure is low. Oxygen should be given to patients especially if corrected arterial oxygen saturation is low. Bicarbonate should be given if serious metabolic acidosis exists, but subsequent metabolic alkalosis and its adverse effects on oxyhemoglobin dissociation, calcium, and ventricular irritability must be avoided. With rewarming, the metabolic acidosis may worsen as lactic acid is washed out of previously vasoconstricted tissues. Recognition and treatment of this phenomenon is important to reduce the risk of ventricular fibrillation and cardiovascular collapse. Severe respiratory impairment with significant carbon dioxide retention should be treated with assisted ventilation. Ventilation should be adjusted with cognizance that carbon dioxide production is reduced. Hypoglycemia should be suspected and treated in any patient presenting with hypothermia; hyperglycemia should be treated only if severe and potentially life-threat-

TABLE 47-6 • Active techniques for core rewarming

Warm intravenous solutions
Heated oxygen[139,212]
Peritoneal lavage[160,200,254]
Heart-lung machine with heat exchanger[5]
Hemodialysis
Mediastinal lavage
Warm gastric lavage[203]
Colonic lavage

ening. Vasopressors should be avoided because of their ability to induce ventricular arrhythmias. Drugs with significant myocardial depressant properties such as quinidine and propranolol should be avoided. Thyroxine should be given only if significant hypothyroidism is suspected.

In summary, hypothermia is a medical emergency requiring prompt recognition and treatment. Rewarming methods must be individualized to avoid iatrogenic complications. Mortality is related to the degree of hypothermia and the presence of significant underlying diseases; it is therefore important to the patient's survival that these complicating conditions be recognized.

REFERENCES

1. Adam JM et al: Physiological responses to hot environments of young European men in the tropics: II and III. Further studies on the effects of exposure to varying levels of environmental stress. *Med Res Counc Spec Rep Ser: RNP Rep* 55/831, 1955.
2. Adolph ES: *Physiology of Man in the Desert*. New York, Interscience, 1947, p. 36.
3. Adolph EF, Dill DB: Observations on water metabolism in the desert. *Am J Physiol* 123:369, 1938.
4. Adolph EF, Fulton WB: The effects of exposure to high temperatures upon the circulation in man. *Am J Physiol* 67:573, 1923.
5. Althaus U et al: Management of profound accidental hypothermia with cardiorespiratory arrest. *Ann Surg* 195:492, 1982.
6. Atland PD, Highman B: Effects of exercise on serum enzyme values and tissues of rats. *Proc Soc Exp Biol Med* 125:999, 1967.
7. Ansari A, Burch GE: Influence of hot environments on the cardiovascular system. *Arch Intern Med* 123:371, 1969.

7a. Apple FS et al: Skeletal muscle creatine kinase MB alterations in women marathon runners. *Eur J Appl Physiol* 56:49, 1987.

8. Arnett EL, Watts DL: Catecholamine excretion in men exposed to cold. *J Appl Physiol* 15:499, 1960.
9. Assmussen E, Boje O: Body temperature and capacity for work. *Acta Physiol Scand* 10:475, 1945.
10. Austin MG, Berry JW: Observations on 100 cases of heatstroke. *JAMA* 161:1525, 1956.
11. Avellini BA et al: Physiological responses of physically fit men and women to acclimation to humid heat. *J Appl Physiol* 49:254, 1980.
12. Avellini BA et al: Effects on heat tolerance of physical training in water and on land. *J Appl Physiol* 53:1291, 1982.
13. Baba N, Ruppert RD: Alteration of eccrine sweat glands in fatal heatstroke. *Arch Pathol Lab Med* 85:669, 1968.
14. Bailey JC: Heat stroke during temperate climatic conditions: Case reports. *Milit Med* 140(1):30, 1975.
15. Bale PM et al: Skeletal muscle necrosis in heatstroke. *Am J Clin Pathol* 50:440, 1968.
16. Barcenas C et al: CPC obesity, football, dog days and siriasis: A deadly combination. *Am Heart J* 92:237, 1976.
17. Barcroft H: Circulation in skeletal muscle, in *Handbook of Physiology: A Critical Comprehensive Presentation of Physiologic Knowledge and Concepts*. Baltimore, Williams & Wilkins, 1963, p 1353.
18. Barcroft JC et al: On the relation of external temperature to blood volume. *Philos Trans R Soc Lond* 211:455, 1922.
19. Barger AC et al: Venous pressure and cutaneous reactive hyperemia in exhaustive exercise and certain other circulatory stresses. *J Appl Physiol* 2:81, 1949.
20. Barger AC et al: Infusion of aldosterone, 9-α-fluorohydrocortisone and antidiuretic horome into the renal artery of normal and adrenalectomized, unanesthetized dogs: Effect on electrolyte and water excretion. *Endocrinology* 62:804, 1958.
21. Bass DE et al: Mechanisms of acclimatization to heat in man. *Medicine* 34:323, 1955.
22. Bass DE, Dobalian IT: Ratio between true and apparent creatinine in sweat. *J Appl Physiol* 55:555, 1953.
23. Bass DE, Henschel A: Responses of body fluid compartments to heat and cold. *Physiol Rev* 36:128, 1956.
24. Baxter CR, Teschan PE: Atypical heatstroke, with hypernatremia, acute renal failure, and fulminating potassium intoxication. *Arch Intern Med* 101:1040, 1958.
25. Bazett HC: The effect of heat on the blood volume and circulation. *JAMA* 111:1841, 1938.
26. Bedrak E: Effect of muscular exercise in a hot environment on canine fibrinolysis in blood in inactive and exercising men. *J Appl Physiol* 20:1307, 1965.
27. Bedrak E et al: Fibrinolytic activity and heat stress. *Isr J Exp Med* 11:1, 1963.
28. Bedrak E et al: Fibrinolytic activity and muscular exercise in heat. *J Appl Physiol* 19:469, 1964.
29. Beisel WR et al: Comparison of certain metabolic effects of triiodothyronine, salicylate and dinitrophenol. *Metabolism* 9:905, 1960.
30. Beller GA, Boyd AE: Heatstroke: A report of 13 consecutive cases without mortality despite severe hyperpyrexia and neurologic dysfunction. *Milit Med* 140:464, 1975.
31. Beller GA et al: Changes in serum and sweat magnesium levels during work in the heat. *Aviat Space Environ Med* 46:709, 1975.
32. Benzinger TH: On physical heat regulation and the sense of temperature in man. *Proc Natl Acad Sci USA* 46:645, 1959.
33. Bergstrom J, Hultman E: The effect of thiazides, chlorthalidone and furosemide on muscle electrolytes and muscle glycogen in normal subjects. *Acta Med Scand* 180:363, 1966.

33a. Berl T: Water metabolism in potassium depletion. *Miner Electrolyte Metab* 4:209, 1980.

34. Berne RM: Cardiodynamics and the coronary circulation in hypothermia. *Ann NY Acad Sci* 80:365, 1959.
35. Berne RM: The effect of immersion hypothermia on coronary blood flow. *Circ Res* 2:236, 1954.
36. Berne RM: Myocardial function in severe hypothermia. *Circ Res* 2:90, 1954.

37. Bernhard WF, McMurrey JD: Inhibition of the stress response during surgery under hypothermia. *Surg Forum* 6:146, 1955.
38. Biglieri EG, McIlroy MB: Abnormalities of renal function and circulatory reflexes in primary aldosteronism. *Circulation* 33:78, 1966.
39. Biglieri EG et al: Sodium retention with HGH and its subfractions. *J Clin Endocrinol Metab* 21:361, 1961.
40. Bilbrey GL et al: Skeletal muscle resting membrane potential in potassium deficiency. *J Clin Invest* 52:3011, 1973.
41. Blachley J et al: The effect of potassium (K) deficiency on resting muscle glycogen (G) content and its response to exercise. *Clin Res* 21:39, 1974.
42. Blair E et al: The effect of hypothermia on lung function. *Ann Surg* 160:814, 1964.
43. Bleisch V: Clinicopathologic conference: A 65-year-old woman with heatstroke. *Am J Med* 43:113, 1967.
44. Bouchama A, Al-Dossary S: Endotoxemia and release of TNFa and IL-1α in response to sustained hyperthermia. *Abstracts of the Interscience Conference on Antimicrobial Agents and Chemotherapy,* 1990, p 126, abstr 238.
45. Boyd AE, Beller GA: Heat exhaustion and respiratory alkalosis. *Ann Intern Med* 83:835, 1975.
46. Bozovic L et al: Effect of prolonged, heavy exercise on urinary protein excretion and plasma renin activity. *Acta Physiol Scand* 70:143, 1967.
46a. Brandenberger G et al: Amplification of nocturnal oscillations in PRA and aldosterone during continuous heat exposure. *J Appl Physiol* 66:1280, 1989.
47. Brengelmann GL et al: Absence of active cutaneous vasodilatation associated with congenital absence of sweat glands in humans. *Am J Physiol* 240:H571, 1981.
48. Britt BA: Etiology and pathophysiology of malignant hyperthermia. *Fed Proc* 38:44, 1979.
48a. Brock-Utne JG et al: Endotoxaemia in exhausted runners after a long-distance race. *S Afr Med J* 73:533, 1988.
49. Brodal P et al: Capillary supply of skeletal muscle fibers in untrained and endurance-trained men. *Am J Physiol* 232:H705, 1977.
50. Buchwald I, Davis PJ: Scleroderma with fatal heatstroke. *JAMA* 201:270, 1967.
51. Bull JM et al: Whole body hyperthermia: A phase-1 trial of a potential adjuvant to chemotherapy. *Ann Intern Med* 90:317, 1979.
52. Bulmer MG, Forwell GD: The concentration of sodium in thermal sweat. *J Physiol* 132:115, 1956.
53. Burch GE: Influence of environmental temperature and relative humidity on the rate of water loss through the skin in congestive heart failure in a subtropical climate. *Am J Med Sci* 211:181, 1946.
54. Burch GE, Hyman A: Influence of a hot and humid environment upon cardiac output and work in normal man and in patients with chronic congestive heart failure in rest. *Am Heart J* 553:665, 1957.
55. Burger FJ, Fuhrman FA: Evidence of injury by heat in mammalian tissues. *Am J Physiol* 206:1057, 1964.
56. Burger FJ, Fuhrman FA: Evidence of injury of tissues after hyperthermia. *Am J Physiol* 206:1062, 1964.
57. Burnell JM et al: The effect in humans of extracellular pH change on the relationship between serum potassium concentration and extracellular potassium. *J Clin Invest* 35:935, 1956.
58. Buskirk ER, Bass DE: Climate and exercise, in Johnson WR, Buskirk ER (eds): *Science and Medicine of Exercise and Sport,* 2d ed. New York, Harper & Row, 1974, p 190.
59. Butikofer E, Molleyres J: Akute ischamische Muskelnekrosen, reversible Muskelverkalkungen und sekondare Hyperkalcamie bei akuter Anurie. *Schweiz Med Wochenschr* 98:961, 1968.
60. Bynum GD et al: Induced hyperthermia in sedated humans and the concept of critical thermal maximum. *Am J Physiol* 235:R228, 1978.
61. Cage GW et al: Effects of water intake on composition of thermal sweat in normal human volunteers. *J Appl Physiol* 29:687, 1970.
62. Cannon JG, Kluger MJ: Endogenous pyrogen activity in human plasma after exercise. *Science* 220:617, 1983.
63. Carlson CJ et al: Creatine phosphokinase MB isoenzyme in hypothermia: Case reports and experimental studies. *Am Heart J* 95:352, 1978.
64. Caroff SN: The neuroleptic malignant syndrome. *J Clin Psychiatry* 41:3, 1980.
65. Castenfors J: Renal function during exercise. *Acta Physiol Scand* 70(suppl 293):1, 1967.
66. Chapman J, Bean WB: Iatrogenic heatstroke. *JAMA* 161:1375, 1956.
67. Chen RYZ et al: Hemoconcentration induced by surface hypothermia in infants. *J Thorac Cardiovasc Surg* 80:236, 1980.
68. Chesanow RL: A 65 year old woman with heatstroke. *Am J Med* 41:415, 1961.
69. Clowes GHA Jr et al: Muscle proteolysis induced by a circulating peptide in patients with sepsis or trauma. *N Engl J Med* 308:545, 1983.
70. Coburn JW et al: Effect of potassium depletion on response to acute heat exposure in unacclimatized man. *Am J Physiol* 211:117, 1966.
71. Cohen ME et al: Electroencephalographic and neurological correlates of deep hypothermia and circulatory arrest in infants. *Ann Thorac Surg* 23:238, 1977.
72. Cohen WJ, Cohen NH: Lithium carbonate, haloperidol, and irreversible brain damage. *JAMA* 230:1283, 1974.
73. Collins KJ: The action of exogenous aldosterone on the secretion and composition of drug-induced sweat. *Clin Sci* 30:207, 1966.
74. Collins KJ et al: The plasma glucocorticoid response to environmental heat stress. *J Physiol* 194:33, 1968.
75. Collins KJ, Weiner JS: Endocrinologic aspects of exposure to high environmental temperatures. *Physiol Rev* 48:785, 1968.
76. Conn JW: Aldosteronism in man: Some climatological aspects. *JAMA* 183:775, 1963.
77. Conn JW: Hypertension, the potassium ion and impaired carbohydrate tolerance. *N Engl J Med* 273:1135, 1965.
78. Conn JW: The mechanism of acclimatization to heat. *Adv Intern Med* 3:373, 1949.
79. Conn JW, Seltzer HS: Spontaneous hypoglycemia. Seminars on carbohydrate metabolism. *Am J Med* September 1955, p 460.

80. Conn RB Jr: Fluorometric determination of creatine. *Clin Chem* 6:537, 1960.
81. Consalazio CF et al: *Physiological Measurements of Metabolic Function in Man*. New York, McGraw-Hill, 1963.
82. Convertino VA et al: Role of thermal and exercise factors in the mechanism of hypervolemia. *J Appl Physiol* 48:657, 1980.
83. Coons DJ et al: Treatment of neuroleptic syndrome with dantrolene sodium: A case report. *Am J Psychiatry* 139:944. 1982.
84. Costrini AM et al: Cardiovascular and metabolic manifestations of heatstroke and severe heat exhaustion. *Am J Med* 66:296, 1979.
85. CPC (Clinicopathologic Conference, Washington University School of Medicine): Extreme physical effort in summer heat followed by collapse, stupor, purpura, jaundice and azotemia. *Am J Med* 18:659, 1955.
86. Curry DL, Curry KP: Hypothermia and insulin secretion. *Endocrinology* 87:750, 1970.
87. Daily WM, Harrison TR: A study of the mechanism and treatment of experimental heat pyrexia. *Am J Med Sci* 215:42, 1948.
88. Darrow DC, Miller HC: Production of cardiac lesions by repeated injections of desoxycorticosterone acetate. *J Clin Invest* 21:601, 1942.
89. DaVee TS, Reineberg EJ: Extreme hypothermia and ventricular fibrillation. *Ann Emerg Med* 9:100, 1980.
90. Davis JA et al: Effect of saline loading during heat acclimatization on adrenocortical hormone levels. *J Appl Physiol* 50:605, 1981.
90a. Demos MA et al: Exercise myoglobinuria and acute exertional rhabdomyolysis. *Arch Intern Med* 134:669, 1974.
91. Denborough MA et al: Biochemical changes in malignant hyperpyrexia. *Lancet* 1:1137, 1970.
92. Derbyshire DR, Clark RG: Cerebral recovery after prolonged global brain ischaemia, letter. *Lancet* 2:637, 1980.
93. Desai ND et al: Total body exchangeable sodium and radio sodium space in Indians from warm and humid climate. *Indian J Med Sci* 21:300, 1967.
94. Dill DB et al: Changes in composition of sweat during acclimatization to heat. *Am J Physiol* 123:412, 1938.
95. Di Sant'Agneses PA et al: Sweat electrolyte disturbances associated with childhood pancreatic disease. *Am J Med* 15:777, 1953.
96. Donnan GA, Seeman E: Coma and hypothermia in Wernicke's encephalopathy. *Aust NZ J Med* 10:438, 1980.
97. Drake CE, Flowers NC: EKG changes from sepsis are unrelated to exposure. *Chest* 77:685, 1980.
98. Dreosti GL: Problems arising out of temperature and humidity in deep mining in the Witwatersrand. *J S Afr Chem Min Met* 36:102, 1935.
99. Edelman IS: Thyroid thermogenesis. *N Engl J Med* 290:1303, 1974.
100. Edholm OG: Comments on symposium on heat acclimatization. *Fed Proc* 23:907, 1963.
101. Ellis FP: Heat illness: I. Epidemiology. *Trans R Soc Trop Med Hyg* 70:402, 1976.
102. Ellis FP: Heat illness: II. Pathogenesis. *Trans R Soc Trop Med Hyg* 70:412, 1976.
103. Ellis FP: Heat illness: III. Acclimatization. *Trans R Soc Trop Med Hyg* 70:419, 1976.
103a. Emrich HM et al: Aldosteronwirkung ouf die natriumchlorid- und kaliumausscheidung im schweiss von pankreasfibrose patienten und gesunden. *Klin Wochenschr* 48:966, 1970.
104. Escourrou P et al: Splanchnic vasoconstriction in heat-stressed men: Role of renin-angiotensin system. *J Appl Physiol* 52:1438, 1982.
105. Falk RB et al: Changes in the electrocardiogram associated with intraoperative epicardial hypothermia. *Anesthesiology* 46:302, 1977.
105a. Farrell PA et al: Plasma adrenocorticotrophin and cortisol responses to submaximal and exhaustive exercise. *J Appl Physiol* 55:1441, 1983.
106. Felicetta JV et al: Decreased adrenal responsiveness in hypothermic patients. *J Clin Endocrinol Metab* 50:93, 1980.
107. Ferris EB Jr et al: Heat stroke: Clinical and chemical observations on 44 cases. *J Clin Invest* 17:249, 1938.
108. Finberg JPM et al: Plasma renin activity after acute heat exposure in nonacclimatized and naturally acclimatized man. *J Appl Physiol* 36:519, 1974.
108a. Finberg JPM, Berlyne GM: Modification of renin and aldosterone response to heat by acclimatization in man. *J Appl Plysiol* 42:554, 1977.
109. Fiorica V et al: Sympathico-adrenomedullary activity in dogs during acute heat exposure. *J Appl Physiol* 22:16, 1967.
110. Fischbeck KH, Simon RP: Neurological manifestations of accidental hypothermia. *Ann Neurol* 10:384, 1981.
111. Fisher DA, Odell WD: Effect of cold on TSH secretion in man. *J Clin Endocrinol Metab* 33:859, 1971.
111a. Fong Y et al: The acute splanchnic and peripheral tissue metabolic response to endotoxin in humans. *J Clin Invest* 85:1896, 1990.
112. Fortner RW et al: Acute renal insufficiency in heat stress injury, abstracted. *Am Soc Nephrol* 5:23, 1971.
113. Fox EL et al: Effects of football equipment on thermal balance and energy cost during exercise. *Res Q Am Assoc Health Phys Educ* 37:332, 1966.
114. Fox RH et al: Body temperatures in the elderly: A national study of physiological, social, and environmental conditions. *Br Med J* 1:200, 1973.
115. Francesconi R: *Aviat Space Environ Med* 48:399, 1977.
116. Francesconi R et al: Thermoregulatory responses in the rat to exercise in the heat following prolonged heat exposure. *J Appl Physiol* 52:734, 1982.
117. Francesconi RP, Mager M: Heat-injured rats: Pathochemical indices and survival time. *J Appl Physiol* 45:1, 1978.
118. Frank MA et al: A study of urine volume and some urinary constituents with a view to the etiology of urolithiasis in a hot climate. *New Istanbul Contrib Clin Sci* 6:20, 1963.
119. Friedman SA, Hirsch SE: Extreme hyperthermia after LSD ingestion. *JAMA* 217:1549, 1971.
119a. Froelich JW et al: Redistribution of visceral blood volume in upright exercise in healthy volunteers. *J Nuclear Med* 29:1714, 1988.
120. Fukuchi S et al: The relationship between vascular reac-

tivity and extracellular potassium. *Tohoku J Exp Med* 85:181, 1965.

121. Furman KI, Beer G: Dynamic changes in sweat electrolyte composition induced by heat stress as an indication of acclimatization and aldosterone activity. *Clin Sci* 24:7, 1963.
121a. Gaffin SL et al: Hypoxia-induced endotoxemia in primates: Role of reticuloendothelial system function and anti-lipopolysaccharide plasma. *Aviat Space Environ Med* 57:1044, 1986.
122. Gale HH: Contractile mechanics of papillary muscles from rats with experimentally induced cardiac necrosis, abstracted. *Physiologist* 14:145, 1971.
123. Gardner LI et al: The effect of potassium deficiency on carbohydrate metabolism. *J Lab Clin Med* 35:592, 1950.
123a. Gathiram P et al: Antilipopolysaccaride improves survival in primates subjected to heat stroke. *Circ Shock* 23:157, 1987.
124. Gilat TS et al: Mechanism of heat stroke. *J Trop Med Hyg* 66:204, 1963.
125. Ginsberg MD et al: Amphetamine intoxication with coagulopathy, hyperthermia, and irreversible renal failure. A syndrome resembling heatstroke. *Ann Intern Med* 73:81, 1970.
126. Ginsberg MD et al: Amphetamine intoxication with coagulopathy, hyperthermia and reversible renal failure. *Ann Intern Med* 73:81, 1970.
127. Gold J: Development of heat pyrexia. *JAMA* 173:1175, 1960.
128. Gollnick PD, King DW: Effect of exercise and training on mitochondria of rat skeletal muscle. *Am J Physiol* 216:1502, 1969.
129. Gordon RS, Andrews HL: Potassium depletion under heat stress. *Fed Proc* 25:1372, 1966.
130. Gottschalk PB, Thomas JE: Heat stroke. *Mayo Clin Proc* 41:470, 1966.
130a. Graber CD et al: Fatal heat stroke: Circulating endotoxins and gram negative sepsis as complications. *JAMA* 216:1195, 1971.
131. Grand RJ et al: The effects of exogenous aldosterone on sweat electrolytes. *J Pediatr* 70:346, 1967.
132. Green LH et al: Fatal myocardial infarction in marathon racing. *Ann Intern Med* 84:704, 1976.
133. Gronert GA: Malignant hyperthermia. *Anesthesiology* 53:395, 1980.
134. Grossman HH, Lange H: Hypercalcemia in acute renal failure. *Ann Intern Med* 69:1332, 1968.
135. Gupta NN et al: Evaluation of functional and morphological status of liver during pyrexia. *J Assoc Physicians India* 11:747, 1963.
135a. Gustafson AB et al: Personal communication.
136. Hale HB et al: Blood adrenocorticotrophic hormone and plasma corticosteroids in men exposed to adverse environmental conditions. *J Clin Invest* 136:1642, 1957.
137. Hallet EB: The effect of decreased body temperature on liver function and splanchnic blood flow in dogs. *Surg Forum* 5:362, 1954.
138. Hardy JD: Body temperature regulation, in Mountcastle VB (ed): *Medical Physiology*, 14th ed. St. Louis, CV Mosby, 1980, p 1430.
139. Harnett RM et al: Initial treatment of profound accidental hypothermia. *Aviat Space Environ Med* 51:680, 1980.
139a. Harsch HH: Neuroleptic malignant syndrome: Physiologic and laboratory findings in a series of nine cases. *J Clin Psychiatry* 48:328, 1987.
140. Hart GR et al: Epidemic classical heatstroke:: Clinical characteristics and course of 28 patients. *Medicine* 61:189, 1982.
141. Hasselman M et al: Influence respective du travail de la temperature ambiante et de la privation de sommeil sur l'excretion urinaire de catecholamines chez l'hormone normal. *C R Soc Biol* 154:197, 1960.
142. Haymes EM et al: Heat tolerance of exercising lean and heavy prepubertal girls. *J Appl Physiol* 36:566, 1974.
143. Haymes EM et al: Heat tolerance of exercising lean and obese prepubertal boys. *J Appl Physiol* 39:457, 1975.
144. Hellon RF, Lind AR: The influence of age on peripheral vasodilation in a hot environment. *J Physiol* 141:262, 1958.
145. Henderson VW, Wooten FD: Neuroleptic malignant syndrome: A pathogenetic role for dopamine receptor blockage? *Neurology* 31:132, 1981.
146. Herman RH, Sullivan BH Jr: Heatstroke and jaundice. *Am J Med* 27:154, 1959.
147. Hervey GR: Physiological changes encountered in hypothermia. *Proc R Soc Med* 66:1053, 1973.
148. Hicks MH et al: The effect of spontaneous and artificially induced fever on liver function. *J Clin Invest* 27:580, 1948.
149. Hirvonen J, Huttunen P: Increased urinary concentrations of catecholamines in hypothermic deaths. *J Forensic Sci* 27:264, 1982.
150. Hoagland RJ, Bishop RH: A physiologic treatment of heatstroke. *Am J Med Sci* 241:415, 1961.
151. Ho-Ch'ang Y et al: Chlorpromazine and heat reducing measures in treatment of heatstroke. *Chin Med J* 77:174, 1958.
152. Howard JM et al: Hyperinsulinism and islet cell tumors of the pancreas. *Int Abstr Surg* 90:417, 1950.
153. Hubbard RW et al: Effect of low-potassium diet on rat exercise hyperthermia and heatstroke mortality. *J Appl Physiol* 51:8, 1981.
154. Hubbard RW et al: Role of physical effort in the etiology of rat heatstroke injury and mortality. *J Appl Physiol* 45:463, 1978.
155. Hudson LD, Conn RD: Accidental hypothermia. Associated diagnoses and prognosis in a common problem. *JAMA* 227:37, 1974.
156. Iampietro PR: Heat-induced tetany. *Fed Proc* 22:884, 1963.
156a. Ingwall JS et al: The creatine kinase system in normal and diseased human myocardium. *N Engl J Med* 313:1050, 1985.
157. Jacob AI et al: A-V block in accidental hypothermia. *J Electrocardiol* 11:399, 1978.
158. Jankovic J, Penn AS: Severe dystonia and myoglobinuria. *Neurology* 32:1195, 1982.
159. Jardon OM: Physiologic stress, heatstroke, malignant hyperthermia—A perspective. *Milit Med* 147:8, 1982.
160. Jessen K. Hagelsten J: Peritoneal dialysis in the treatment

of profound accidental hypothermia. *Aviat Space Environ Med* 49:426, 1978.
161. Jones TS et al: Morbidity and mortality associated with the July 1980 heat wave in St. Louis and Kansas City, MO. *JAMA* 247:3327, 1982.
162. Kanter GS: Cause of hypoglycemia in dogs exposed to heat. *Am J Physiol* 196:619, 1959.
163. Kanter GS: Heat and excretion in man. *J Appl Physiol* 7:533, 1955.
164. Katz AI et al: Concentration and dilution of urine in permanent inhabitants of hot regions. *Isr J Med Sci* 1:968, 1965.
165. Keatinge WR et al: Hypothermia during saturation diving in the North Sea. *Br Med J* 280:291, 1980.
166. Kelman GR, Nunn JF: Nomograms for correction of blood PO_2, PCO_2, pH, and base excess for time and temperature. *J Appl Physiol* 21:1484, 1966.
167. Kendrick WC et al: Rhabdomyolysis and shock following intravenous amphetamine administration. *Ann Intern Med* 86:381, 1977.
168. Kew MC et al: Chronic interstitial nephritis as a consequence of heatstroke. *Q J Med* 39:189, 1970.
169. Kew MC et al: The diagnostic and prognostic significance of the serum enzyme changes in heatstroke. *Trans R Soc Trop Med Hyg* 65:325, 1971.
170. Kew MC et al: The heart in heatstroke. *Am Heart J* 77:324, 1969.
171. Khogali M, Weiner JS: Heatstroke: Report on 18 cases. *Lancet* 2:276, 1980.
172. Kilbourne EM et al: Risk factors for heatstroke. *JAMA* 247:3332, 1982.
173. Kilburn KH: Muscular origin of elevated plasma potassium during muscular exercise. *J Appl Physiol* 21:675, 1966.
174. Kim YD et al: Hemodynamic and plasma catecholamine responses to hyperthermic cancer therapy in humans. *Am J Physiol* 237:H570, 1979.
174a. Kirby CR, Convertino VA: Plasma aldosterone and sweat sodium concentrations after exercise and heat acclimatization. *J Appl Physiol* 61:967, 1986.
175. Kjellmer I: Potassium ion as a vasodilator during muscular exercise. *Acta Physiol Scand* 63:460, 1965.
176. Knochel JP: Disseminated intravascular coagulation in heatstroke response to heparin therapy, editorial. *JAMA* 231:496, 1975.
177. Knochel JP: Dog days and siriasis. How to kill a football player, editorial. JAMA 233:513, 1975.
178. Knochel JP: Environmental heat illness. *Arch Intern Med* 133:841, 1974.
179. Knochel JP: The mechanism of hypophosphatemia in acute heatstroke. *JAMA* 238:425, 1977.
180. Knochel JP: Rhabdomyolysis and effects of potassium deficiency on muscle structure and function. *Cardiovas Med* 3:247, 1978.
181. Knochel JP et al: The renal cardiovascular, hematologic and serum electrolyte abnormalities of heatstroke. *Am J Med* 30:299, 1961.
181a. Knochel JP et al: Muscle cell electrical hyperpolarization and reduced exercise hyperkalemia in physically conditioned dogs. *J Clin Invest* 75:740, 1985.
182. Knochel JP, Carter NW: The role of muscle cell injury in the pathogenesis of acute renal failure after exercise. *Kidney Int* 10:S-58, 1976.
183. Knochel JP et al: Heat stress, exercise and muscle injury: Effects of urate metabolism and renal function. *Ann Intern Med* 81:321, 1974.
184. Knochel JP et al: Pathophysiology of intense physical conditioning in a hot climate: I. Mechanisms of potassium depletion. *J Clin Invest* 51:242, 1972.
185. Knochel JP et al: High resting cardiac output with exercise-induced pulmonary edema in the conscious, potassium-deficient dog. *Miner Electrolyte Metab* 1:336, 1978.
186. Knochel JP, Schlein EM: On the mechanism of rhabdomyolysis in potassium depletion. *J Clin Invest* 51:1750, 1972.
187. Knochel JP, Vertel RM: Salt loading as a possible factor in the production of potassium depletion, rhabdomyolysis and heat injury. *Lancet* 1:659, 1967.
187a. Knochel JP: Catastrophic medical events with exhaustive exercise: "White collar rhabdomyalysis." *Kidney Int* 38:709, 1990.
187b. Kokko JP: Metabolic and social consequences of cocaine abuse. *Am J Med Sci* 299:361, 1990.
188. Kosunen KJ, Pakarinen AJ: Plasma renin, angiotensin II, and plasma and urinary aldosterone in running exercise. *J Appl Physiol* 41:26, 1976.
189. Kosunen KJ et al: Plasma renin activity, angiotensin II, and aldosterone during intense heat stress. *J Appl Physiol* 41:323, 1976.
190. Kotchen TA et al: Renin, norepinephrine and epinephrine responses to gradual graded exercise. *J Appl Physiol* 31:178, 1971.
190a. Kozlowski S et al: Exercise hyperthermia as a factor limiting physical performance: Temperature effect on muscle metabolism. *J Appl Physiol* 59:766, 1985.
191. Krisko I et al: Severe hyperpyrexia due to tranylcypromine-amphetamine toxicity. *Ann Intern Med* 70:559, 1969.
192. Kuhn LA, Turner JK: Alterations in pulmonary and peripheral vascular resistance in immersion hypothermia. *Circ Res* 7:366, 1959.
193. Kuo KW et al: Sweating with heatstroke. *J Oriental Med* 22:98, 1925.
194. Kuroda M et al: Successful treatment of fulminating complications associated with extensive rhabdomyolysis by plasma exchange. *Artif Organs* 5:372, 1981.
195. Ladell WSS: Disorders due to heat. *Trans R Soc Trop Med Hyg* 51:189, 1957.
196. Ladell WSS, Shepard RJ: Aldosterone inhibition and acclimatization to heat, abstracted. *J Physiol* 160:19, 1962.
197. Ladell WSS et al: Desert climate: Physiological and clinical observations. *Lancet* 2:491, 1944.
198. Landymore RW et al: Effect of cardiopulmonary bypass and hypothermia on pancreatic endocrine function and peripheral utilization of glucose. *Can J Surg* 22:248, 1979.
199. Langdell RD et al: Dextran and prolonged bleeding time. *JAMA* 166:346, 1958.
200. Lash RF et al: Accidental profound hypothermia and barbiturate intoxication. A report of rapid "core" rewarming by peritoneal dialysis. *JAMA* 201:269, 1967.

201. Layzer RB, Rowland LP: Cramps. *N Engl J Med* 385:31, 1971.
202. Leavel UW: Sweat gland neurosis in barbiturate poisoning. *Arch Dermatol* 100:218, 1969.
203. Ledingham IM et al: Central rewarming system for treatment of hypothermia. *Lancet* 1:1168, 1980.
204. Leithead CS, Lind AR: *Heat Stress and Heat Disorders.* Philadelphia, FA Davis, 1964, p 129.
205. Leonard A, Nelms RJ Jr: Hypercalcemia in diuretic phase of acute renal failure. *Ann Intern Med* 73:137, 1970.
206. Leonard CD, Eichner ER: Acute renal failure and transient hypercalcemia in idiopathic rhabdomyolysis. *JAMA* 211:1539, 1970.
207. Levine JA: Heatstroke in the aged. *Am J Med* 47:251, 1969.
208. Levy LA: Severe hypophosphatemia as a complication of the treatment of hypothermia. *Arch Intern Med* 140:128, 1980.
209. Lichten PR et al: Inotropic effect of aldosterone on the myocardium of normal dogs, abstracted. *Fed Proc* 22:358, 1964.
210. Litman RE: Heatstroke in parkinsonism. *Arch Intern Med* 89:562, 1952.
211. Llach F et al: Pathophysiology of altered calcium metabolism in rhabdomyolysis-induced acute renal failure. *N Engl J Med* 305:117, 1981.
212. Lloyd EL: Accidental hypothermia treated by central rewarming through the airway. *Br J Anaesth* 45:41, 1973.
213. Lloyd EL, Mitchell B: Factors affecting the onset of ventricular fibrillation in hypothermia. *Lancet* 2:1294, 1974.
213a. Lugon JR et al: Renal function and glomerular hemodynamics in male endotoxemic rats. *Kidney Int* 36:570, 1989.
214. Machella TE: The relationship of bromsulphalein retention to the fever of natural P. falciparum malaria. *Am J Med Sci* 213:81, 1947.
215. Maclean D, Emslie-Smith D: The J Loop of the spatial vectorcardiogram in accidental hypothermia in man. *Br Heart J* 36:621, 1974.
216. Maclean D et al: Achilles tendon reflex in accidental hypothermia and hypothermic myxoedema. *Br Med J* 2:87, 1973.
217. MacQuaide DHG: Congenital absence of sweat glands. *Lancet* 2:531, 1944.
218. Magazanik A et al: Tap water, an efficient method for cooling heatstroke victims—A model in dogs. *Aviat Space Environ Med* 5:864, 1980.
219. Magazanik A et al: Dynamic changes in acid base balance during heatstroke in dogs. *Pflugers Arch* 388:129, 1980.
220. Mahajan SL et al: Disseminated intravascular coagulation during rewarming following hypothermia. *JAMA* 245:2517, 1981.
221. Malamud N et al: Heatstroke: A clinicopathologic study of 125 fatal cases. *Milit Med* 99:397, 1946.
222. Massry SG et al: Intractable pruritus as a manifestation of hyperparathyroidism in uremia. *N Engl J Med* 279:697, 1968.
223. Mathews DK et al: Physiological responses during exercise and recovery in a football uniform. *J Appl Physiol* 26:611, 1969.
224. May DC et al: Neuroleptic malignant syndromes: Response to dantrolene sodium. *Ann Intern Med* 98:183, 1983.
225. McCance RA: Medical problems in mineral metabolism: III. Experimental human salt deficiency. *Lancet* 1:823, 1936.
226. McCance RA: Medical problems in mineral metabolism: III. Experimental sodium chloride deficiency in man. *Proc R Soc Lond* 119:245, 1936.
227. McNicol MW: Respiratory failure and acid-base status in hypothermia. *Postgrad Med J* 43:674, 1967.
228. Mehta AC, Baker RN: Persistent neurological deficits in heatstroke. *Neurology* 20:336, 1970.
229. Mendeloff AI et al: Studies in bromsulfalein: Factors alerting its disappearance from the blood after a single intravenous injection. *Gastroenterology* 13:222, 1949.
230. Meroney WH et al: The acute calcification of traumatized muscle, with particular reference to acute post-traumatic renal insufficiency. *J Clin Invest* 36:825, 1956.
231. Moore KE: Effects of D-amphetamine on plasma and tissue electrolyte concentrations of aggregated and of hyperthyroid mice. *Proc Soc Exp Biol Med* 122:292, 1966.
232. Moroff SV, Bass DE: Effects of overhydration on man's physiological responses to work in the heat. *J Appl Physiol* 20:267, 1965.
233. Mostellar ME, Tuttle EP Jr: The effects of alkalosis on plasma concentration and urinary excretion of inorganic phosphate in man. *J Clin Invest* 43:138, 1964.
234. Mouritzen CV, Andersen MN: Myocardial temperature gradients and ventricular fibrillation during hypothermia. *J Thorac Cardiovasc Surg* 49:937, 1965.
235. Moxley RT et al: Resting levels of fibrinolysis in blood in inactive and exercising men. *J Appl Physiol* 28:549, 1970.
236. Murphy E, Faul PJ: Accidental hypothermia in the elderly. *Ir Med J* 53:4, 1963.
237. Murphy RJ, Ashe WF: Prevention of heat illness in football players. *JAMA* 194:650, 1965.
238. Nelson TD, Bee DE: Temperature perturbation studies of sarcoplasmic reticulum from malignant hyperthermia pig muscle. *J Clin Invest* 64:895, 1979.
239. Nesbakken R: Aspects of free fatty acid metabolism during induced hypothermia. *Scan J Clin Lab Invest* 31:1, 1973.
240. Newson AJ: Malignant hyperthermia: Current trends in treatment. *NZ Med J* 77:81, 1973.
241. Nolph KD et al: Mechanisms for inefficient peritoneal dialysis in acute renal failure associated with heat stress and exercise. *Ann Intern Med* 71:317, 1969.
241a. Nose H et al: Shift in body fluid compartments after dehydration in humans. *J Appl Physiol* 65:318, 1988.
242. O'Donnell TF Jr: Acute heatstroke: Epidemiologic, biochemical, renal and coagulation studies. *JAMA* 234:824, 1975.
243. O'Donnell TF Jr, Clowes GHA Jr: The circulatory abnormalities of heatstroke. *N Engl J Med* 287:734, 1972.
243a. O'Dwyer ST et al: A single dose of endotoxin increases

intestinal permeability in healthy humans. *Arch Surg* 123:1459, 1988.
244. Okada Y et al: Human growth hormone secretion during exposure to hot air in normal adult male subjects. *J Clin Endocrinol* 34:759, 1972.
245. Opie LH: F.F.A., lipolysis, and acute myocardial infarction. *Lancet* 1:621, 1974.
246. Osborn JJ: Experimental hypothermia: Respiratory and blood pH changes in relation to cardiac function. *Am J Physiol* 175:389, 1953.
247. Pandolf KB et al: Heat intolerance as a function of percent of body surface involved with miliaria rubra. *Am J Physiol* 239:R233, 1980.
248. Pandolf KB et al: Persistence of impaired heat tolerance after artificially induced miliaria rubra. *Am J Physiol* 239:R226, 1980.
249. Paolone AM et al: Sexual variations in thermoregulation during heat stress. *Aviat Space Environ Med* 49:715, 1978.
250. Parker WA: Methyldopa hyperpyrexia, editorial. *JAMA* 228:1097, 1974.
251. Passmore R, Durnin JVGA: Human energy expenditure. *Physiol Rev* 35:801, 1955.
252. Pattengale PK, Holloszy JO: Augmentation of skeletal muscle myoglobin by a program of treadmill running. *Am J Physiol* 213:783, 1967.
253. Perchick JS et al: Disseminated intravascular coagulation in heatstroke. *JAMA* 231:480, 1975.
254. Pickering BG et al: Core rewarming by peritoneal irrigation in accidental hypothermia with cardiac arrest. *Anesth Analg* 56:574, 1977.
255. Proppe DW: α-Adrenergic control of intestinal circulation in heat-stressed baboons. *J Appl Physiol* 48:759, 1980.
256. Radigan LR, Robinson S: Effects of environmental heat stress and exercise on renal blood flow and filtration rate. *J Appl Physiol* 2:185, 1949.
257. Rai UC, Ambwany P: Cardiovascular changes during varied thermal stress. *Indian J Physiol Pharmacol* 24:119, 1980.
257a. Ricquier D et al: Ultrastructural and biochemical characterization of human brown adipose tissue in pheochromocytoma. *J Clin Endocrinol Metab* 54:803, 1982.
258. Rittenhouse EA et al: Studies of carbohydrate metabolism and serum electrolytes during surface-induced hypothermia with prolonged circulatory arrest. *Surgery* 67:995, 1970.
259. Rizza RA et al: Myoglobinuria following aminocaproic acid administration. *JAMA* 236:1845, 1976.
260. Roberts KE et al: Effect of phosphate in enhancing the action of triiodothyronine. *Endocrinology* 59:565, 1956.
261. Robinson S et al: Effects of desoxycorticosterone acetate on acclimatization of men to heat. *J Appl Physiol* 2:399, 1950.
262. Robinson S et al: Effect of salt deficiency on the salt concentration in sweat. *J Appl Physiol* 3:55, 1950.
263. Robinson S et al: Temperature regulation of men following heatstroke. *Isr J Med Sci* 12:786, 1976.
264. Rogers PW, Kurtzman NA: Renal failure, uncontrollable thirst, and hyperreninemia. *JAMA* 225:1236, 1973.
265. Rose KD: Warning for millions: Intense exercise can deplete potassium. *Physician and Sportsmedicine* 3:67, 1975.
266. Rosenfeld JB: Acid-base and electrolyte disturbances in hypothermia. *Am J Cardiol* 12:678, 1963.
267. Rowell LB et al: Hepatic clearance of indocyanine green in man under thermal and exercise stress. *J Appl Physiol* 20:384, 1965.
267a. Rowell LB: Human cardiovascular adjustments to exercise and thermal stress. *Physiol Rev* 54:75, 1974.
268. Rowell LB et al: Redistribution of blood flow during sustained high skin temperature in resting man. *J Appl Physiol* 28:415, 1970.
269. Rowell LB et al: Reductions in cardiac output, central blood volume and stroke volume with thermal stress in normal men during exercise. *J Clin Invest* 45:1801, 1966.
270. Rowell LB et al: Splanchnic blood flow and metabolism in heat-stressed man. *J Appl Physiol* 24:475, 1968.
270a. Rowell LB: *Human Circulation. Regulation during Physical Stress.* New York, Oxford, 1986, p 34.
271. Rudy LW et al: The effects of deep hypothermia and circulatory arrest on the distribution of systemic blood flow in Rhesus monkeys. *J Thorac Cardiovasc Surg* 64:706, 1972.
272. Ruppert RD et al: The mechanism of metabolic acidosis in heatstroke, abstracted. *Clin Res* 12:356, 1964.
272a. Ryan AJ et al: Synthesis of 70K stress protein by human leukocytes: Effect of exercise in the heat. *J Appl Physiol* 70:466, 1991.
273. Sagild U et al: Glucose tolerance and insulin response in experimental potassium depletion. *Acta Med Scand* 169:243, 1961.
274. Saltin B et al: *Response to Exercise After Bed Rest and After Training.* American Heart Association Monograph 23. New York, American Heart Association, Inc., 1968.
275. Sato K: Current knowledge on the energy metabolism and the secretory mechanism of the eccrine sweat glands, in Thorn NA, Peterson OH (eds): *Secretory Mechanisms of Exocrine Gland.* Copenhagen, Munksgaard, 1974, p 588.
276. Savides EP, Hoffbrand BI: Hypothermia, thrombosis, and acute pancreatitis. *Br Med J* 1:614, 1974.
277. Schalch DS: The influence of physical stress and exercise on growth hormone and insulin secretion in man. *J Lab Clin Med* 69:256, 1967.
278. Schlein EM et al: The effect of plasma water loss on assessment of muscle metabolism during exercise. *J Appl Physiol* 34:568, 1973.
279. Schneider FH, Gillis CN: Hypothermic potentiation of chronotropic responses of isolated atria to sympathetic nerve stimulation. *Am J Physiol* 211:890, 1966.
280. Schreiner GE: The role of hemodialysis (artificial kidney) in acute poisoning. *Arch Intern Med* 102:896, 1958.
281. Schrier RW et al: Nephropathy associated with heat stress and exercise. *Ann Intern Med* 67:356, 1967.
282. Schrier RW et al: Renal metabolic and circulatory responses to heat and exercise. *Ann Intern Med* 73:213, 1970.
283. Schwab RH et al: Electrocardiographic changes occurring in rapidly induced deep hypothermia. *Am J Med Sci* 248:290, 1964.

284. Schwartz IL, Itoh S: Fatigue of the sweat glands in heatstroke, abstracted. *J Clin Invest* 35:733, 1956.
285. Schwartz IL, Thaysen JH: Excretion of sodium and potassium in human sweat. *J Clin Invest* 35:144, 1956.
286. Schwartz WB, Relman AS: Effects of electrolyte disorders on renal function. *N Engl J Med* 276:383, 1967.
286a. Segar WE, Holliday MA: Physiologic abnormalities of salicylate intoxication. *N Engl J Med* 259:1191, 1958.
287. Selye H, Bajusz E: Conditioning by corticoids for the production of cardiac lesions with noradrenaline. *Acta Endocrinol* 30:183, 1959.
288. Senay LC, Kok R: Body fluid responses of heat-tolerant and intolerant men to work in a hot wet environment. *J Appl Physiol* 40:55, 1976.
289. Sestoft L: Metabolic aspects of the calorigenic effect of thyroid hormone in mammals. *Clin Endocrinol* 13:489, 1980.
290. Shapiro Y et al: Heat intolerance in former heatstroke patients. *Ann Intern Med* 90:913, 1979.
291. Shapiro Y et al: Experimental heatstroke: A model in dogs. *Arch Intern Med* 131:688, 1973.
292. Shibolet S et al: Heatstroke: Its clinical picture and mechanism in 36 cases. *Q J Med* 36:525, 1967.
293. Shibolet S et al: Fibrinolysis and hemorrhages in fatal heatstroke. *N Engl J Med* 266:169, 1962.
294. Shibolet S et al: Heatstroke: A review. *Aviat Space Environ Med* 47:280, 1976.
295. Shida H et al: Inhibitory mechanisms of insulin secretion associated with hypothermic open-heart surgery. *Jpn J Surg* 11:67, 1981.
296. Shida H et al: The role of the liver in the changes of acid-base balance and plasma lipids during surface-induced deep hypothermia. *Jpn J Surg* 7:139, 1977.
297. Simon HB: Extreme pyrexia. *JAMA* 236:2419, 1976.
298. Simon HB, Daniels GH: Hormonal hyperthermia. *Am J Med* 66:257, 1979.
299. Sjodin RA: *Transport in Skeletal Muscle.* New York, Wiley, 1982, p 80.
300. Slovis CM et al: Survival in a heatstroke victim with a core temperature in excess of 46.5°C. *Ann Emerg Med* 11:269, 1982.
300a. Smiles KA, Robinson S: Sodium ion conservation during acclimatization of men to work in the heat. *J Appl Physiol* 31:63, 1971.
301. Smith RJ, Edelman IS: The role of sodium transport in thyroid thermogenesis. *Fed Proc* 38:2150, 1979.
302. Sobel S et al: Renal mechanisms in heatstroke, abstracted. *Clin Res* 11:252, 1963.
303. Sohal RS et al: Heatstroke: An electron microscopic study of endothelial cell damage and disseminated intravascular coagulation. *Arch Intern Med* 122:43, 1968.
304. Spickard A: Heatstroke in college football and suggestions for prevention. *South Med J* 61:791, 1968.
305. Sprung CL et al: The metabolic and respiratory alterations of heatstroke. *Arch Intern Med* 140:665, 1980.
306. Spurr GB: Serum enzymes following repetitive hyperthermia. *Proc Soc Exp Biol Med* 139:698, 1972.
307. Spurr GG, Barlow G: Tissue electrolytes in hyperthermic dogs. *J Appl Physiol* 28:13, 1970.
308. Stern S, Braun K: Pulmonary arterial and venous response to cooling: Role of alpha adrenergic receptors. *Am J Physiol* 219:982, 1970.
309. Stitt JS: Fever vs hyperthermia. *Fed Proc* 38:39, 1979.
310. Streeten DHP et al: Secondary aldosteronism: Metabolic and adrenocortical responses of normal men to high environmental temperatures. *Metabolism* 9:1071, 1960.
311. Suzuki J et al: The safe time limit of temporary clamping of cerebral arteries in the direct surgical treatment of intracranial aneurysm under moderate hypothermia. *Tohoku J Exp Med* 127:1, 1979.
312. Sweadner KJ, Goldin SM: Active transport of sodium and potassium ions. *N Engl J Med* 302:777, 1980.
313. Talbott JH: Heat cramps. *Medicine* 14:232, 1935.
314. Talbott JH et al: The ill effects of heat upon workmen. *J Indust Hyg Toxicol* 19:258, 1937.
315. Tanz RD: Studies on the inotropic action of aldosterone on isolated cardiac tissue preparations, including the effects of pH, ouabain and SC-8109. *J Pharmacol Exp Ther* 135:71, 1962.
316. Thaysen JH, Schwartz IL: Fatigue of sweat glands. *J Clin Invest* 34:1719, 1955.
317. Thompson R et al: Evolutionary changes in the electrocardiogram of severe progressive hypothermia. *J Electrocardiol* 10:67, 1977.
318. Tornblom N: Hyperinsulinism with fatal postoperative hyperthermia. *Acta Med Scand* 170:757, 1961.
319. Totel GL: Physiological responses to heat of resting man with impaired sweating capacity. *J Appl Physiol* 37:346, 1974.
320. Van Beaumont W et al: Plasma fluid and blood constituent shifts during heat exposure in resting men. *Aerospace Med* 45:176, 1974.
321. Vandam LD, Burnap TK: Hypothermia. *N Engl J Med* 261:546, 1959.
322. Vapaaviori M: Changes in the static elastance and hysteresis of the chest wall and lung in normo- and hypothermia. *Acta Physiol Scand* 55(suppl 191):1, 1962.
323. Verde T et al: Sweat composition in exercise and in heat. *J Appl Physiol* 53:1540, 1982.
324. Vertel RM, Knochel JP: Acute renal failure due to heat injury: An analysis of ten cases associated with a high incidence of myoglobinuria. *Am J Med* 43:435, 1967.
325. Wade CE et al: Renal function, aldosterone, and vasopressin excretion following repeated long-distance running. *J Appl Physiol* 50:709, 1981.
326. Wagner JA et al: Age and temperature regulation of humans in neutral and cold environments. *J Appl Physiol* 37:562, 1974.
327. Watts AJ: Hypothermia in the aged: A study of the role of cold sensitivity. *Environ Res* 5:119, 1972.
328. Weber MB, Blakely JA: The hemorrhagic diathesis of heatstroke. *Lancet* 1:1190, 1969.
329. Weiner JS, Horne GO: A classification of heat illness. *Br Med J* 1:1533, 1958.
330. Weiner JS, Khogali M: Heatstroke. *Lancet,* May 26, 1979, p 1135.
331. Weiner JS, Khogali M: A physiological body-cooling unit for treatment of heatstroke. *Lancet,* March 8, 1980, p 507.
332. White JD: Hypothermia: The Bellevue experience. *Ann Emerg Med* 11:417, 1982.

333. Wildenthal K et al: Effects of lactic acidosis on left ventricular performance. *Am J Physiol* 214:1352, 1968.
334. Williams CG et al: Circulatory and metabolic reactions to work in the heat. *J Appl Physiol* 17:625, 1962.
335. Wilson O et al: Thyroid and adrenal response to acute cold exposure in man. *J Appl Physiol* 28:543, 1970.
335a. Wollman H et al: Effects of extremes of respiratory and metabolic alkalosis on cerebral blood flow in man. *J Appl Physiol* 24:60, 1968.
336. Wood M et al: The sympathetic response to profound hypothermia and circulatory arrest in infants. *Can Anesth Soc J* 27:125, 1980.
337. Woodbury DM: Analgesic-antipyretics, anti-inflammatory agents, and inhibitors of uric acid synthesis salicylates and cogeners, phenacetin & congeners, indomethacin, colchicine, allopurinol, in Goodman LS, Gilman A (eds): *The Pharmacological Basis of Therapeutics,* 4th ed. Elmsford, NY, Pergamon Press, 1970, p 314.
338. Woolf PD et al: Accidental hypothermia: Endocrine function during recovery. *J Clin Endocrinol Metab* 34:460, 1972.
339. Wright DO, Cuttino JT: Purpuric manifestations of heatstroke: Studies of prothrombin and platelets in 12 cases. *Arch Intern Med* 77:27, 1946.
340. Wyndham CH: The physiology of exercise under heat stress. *Annu Rev Physiol* 35:193, 1973.
341. Wyndham CH: The problems of heat intolerance in man, in Hardy JO et al (eds): *Physiological and Behavioral Temperature Regulation.* Springfield, Ill, Charles C Thomas, 1970, p 324.
342. Wyndham CH et al: Changes in central circulation and body fluid space during acclimatization to heat. *J Appl Physiol* 25:586, 1968.
343. Wyndham CH et al: Responses of unacclimatized men under stress of heat and work. *J Appl Physiol* 6:681, 1954.
344. Yoshimura H: Seasonal changes in human body fluid. *Jpn J Physiol* 8:165, 1958.
345. Young RSK et al: Neurological outcome in cold water drowning. *JAMA* 244:1233, 1980.
345a. Zager RS, Altschuld R: Body temperature: An important determinant of severity of ischemic renal injury. *Am J Physiol (Renal Fluid Electrolyte Physiol)* 251: F87, 1986.
345b. Zager RA: Studies of mechanisms and protective maneuvers in myoglobinuric acute renal failure. *Lab Invest* 60:619, 1989.
346. Zalis EG et al: Acute lethality of the amphetamines in dogs and its antagonism by curare. *Proc Soc Exp Biol Med* 118:557, 1965.
347. Zalis EG, Parmlay LF Jr: Fatal amphetamine poisoning. *Arch Intern Med* 112:822, 1963.

CHAPTER 48

Electrolytes in the Pathogenesis of Hypertension

Part I Altered Sodium and Potassium Balance

Morton H. Maxwell • Abraham U. Waks • G. Gopal Krishna

Part II Cation Transport

Michael L. Tuck • Delila B. Corry

PART I ALTERED SODIUM AND POTASSIUM BALANCE

Increased salt intake and/or genetic perturbations in sodium homeostasis have been implicated in the pathogenesis of essential hypertension for many years. More recently, it has been suggested that abnormalities in dietary potassium intake and/or potassium regulation may play a primary role. In this chapter, pertinent data from animals and humans are critically analyzed.

THE ROLE OF SODIUM IN BLOOD PRESSURE REGULATION

ANIMAL STUDIES

Increased amounts of dietary salt have been shown to be responsible or necessary for producing certain forms of experimental hypertension in animals. Lenel et al. made chickens hypertensive by offering 1 percent saline solution for drinking.[203] Sapirstein et al. made rats hypertensive by permitting them to drink only 2 percent saline solutions.[282] Meneely and Dahl,[235] Dahl,[81] and Koletsky[178] demonstrated that diets with various levels of increased salt content caused rats' blood pressure levels to increase slowly over a period of months. Each increment in salt intake resulted in a concomitant increase in blood pressure. With a dietary salt content of 2 to 5 percent, borderline or mild hypertension was found. With 10 percent salt, frank hypertension developed. Increased dietary salt intake is necessary for the induction of hypertension by deoxycorticosterone acetate (DOCA) and for other forms of experimental mineralocorticoid hypertension.[62] Experimental salt-induced hypertension in the rat may be more regularly and rapidly induced by reducing renal mass by partial or complete nephrectomy.[179] Similar results have been obtained in dogs and monkeys.[65,70,194]

It is particularly easy to produce salt hypertension in young rats but more difficult in adult rats. When hypertension is induced in young rats by high sodium feeding, it may persist indefinitely even after a normal diet is resumed.[310]

Dahl demonstrated variability in the response to salt loading in normal rats and was able to distinguish an apparent genetic basis for sodium-dependent hypertension in this species.[81,83] Through selective breeding he developed two strains: a salt-sensitive strain in which salt hypertension regularly developed and another strain that was salt-resistant. Resistant rats were also resistant to all other forms of experimental induction of hypertension except the one-kidney Goldblatt scheme (see Chap. 45).[79] When these two strains of rats are fed a low-sodium diet (0.3 percent NaCl) while young, their mean blood pressures are similar. Adult salt-sensitive rats on a low-sodium regimen exhibited blood pressure levels about 15 mmHg higher than those of the salt-resistant strain, a blood pressure elevation that is comparable to borderline hypertension in humans.

Tobian et al. were able to prevent the development of hypertension in normal rats fed 8 percent NaCl by adding a thiazide diuretic to their drinking water; the maneuver also prevented the increased extracellular fluid (ECF) volume noted in the rats which developed hypertension.[311] The hypertension and increased ECF volume may be related to a genetic inability in the susceptible animals to excrete salt normally, perhaps because of decreased papillary blood flow,[117] a result of a deficiency in renal kallikrein.[63]

Transplant experiments have shown the importance of the kidney in both the salt-sensitive and the spontaneously hypertensive rat. Dahl et al. demonstrated that the blood pressure changes depend on (and follow) the kidney.[82] When a kidney from a normotensive donor rat was transplanted to a hypertensive recipient that was salt-sensitive, the blood pressure of the recipient fell to normal; conversely, the blood pressure increased when a hypertensive kidney was transplanted to a normotensive host. Bianchi et al. showed similar results in the Milan strain of hypertensive rats.[26] Furthermore, the normotensive rats given a hypertensive kidney were shown to retain sodium as they developed hypertension.

Although the animal studies described above show that salt intake is important in some experimental forms of hypertension, the implications for the pathogenesis of human hypertension are uncertain. The following objections to extrapolating to humans still exist:

1. The relative amounts of salt required to induce hypertension in animals are usually far in excess of the free salt content of human diets. For example, the 8 percent NaCl diet fed to salt-sensitive Dahl rats is equivalent to a human consumption of 40 g of salt daily.
2. Even very high salt intakes (8 to 10 percent NaCl) do not *consistently* result in hypertension in all or even most animals, implying that capacity to respond is heterogeneous.
3. In the two strains of genetically hypertensive rats (Milan, Kyoto SHR), young animals prior to the development of hypertension display few if any demonstrable alterations of kidney function or sodium/potassium metabolism. Therefore, perturbations of body fluid volumes or kidney function noted in the hypertensive animals may be caused by the hypertension itself. That some subtle or as yet unmeasurable alteration in kidney function is nevertheless present is implied by the transplantation experiments in which blood pressure follows the kidney.

EPIDEMIOLOGICAL STUDIES

Unacculturated societies

In contrast to occidental populations, hypertension is virtually nonexistent in many unacculturated societies, and blood pressure does not increase with age.[108] These observations are made consistently in nonindustrialized societies of differing ethnic backgrounds and from various parts of the world, including New Guinea,[227] the Amazon basin,[219] parts of Uganda,[291] Malaysia,[52] Panama,[171] Easter Island,[74] and the Kalahari desert of Africa.[166] All of these populations consume almost no salt. Various studies have indicated that the lower blood pressure found in the unacculturated peoples could not be ascribed to malnutrition,[166,259] stress, tension, or urban living[247,284] or to differences in body weight.[259,272]

The absence of hypertension in these societies has been attributed to the lack of salt in the diet. For example, Maddocks investigated five populations in New Guinea.[227] In the highlands, where neither salt nor salty foods were used, no hypertension was found and blood pressure did not increase with age. However, in a coastal fishing population in which people ate salted, canned foods, blood pressure rose with age and hypertension was present. Similar comparisons between primitive people with the same ethnic backgrounds but with different dietary habits suggest that blood pressure rises with increasing salt consumption.[219,250,259,272,291,296]

Although primitive societies with low blood pressures have a very low sodium intake, there are confounding variables which could affect blood pressure. Compared to their industrialized counterparts, in addition to low salt intake, primitive peoples usually are smaller and leaner, do not gain weight with age, are more active physically, and have a relatively higher potassium intake. In the various studies, blood pressure values were compared without standardization for age, sex, weight, or method of blood pressure measurement.

Industrialized societies

In contrast to cross-cultural studies, studies of the correlation between habitual salt intake and blood pressure within industrialized populations have been uniformly negative. Dahl and Love, based upon a dietary questionnaire regarding habitual salt intake, reported that although mean blood pressures between groups (characterized as having low, average, or high salt intake) were similar, hypertension was more common in those with a high salt intake.[78b] This study was widely criticized. Miall in Scotland[238] and data from the Framingham Study[85] demonstrated no relationship between sodium intake as estimated by 24-h urinary sodium excretion and dietary history reported by patients. Subsequent studies generally have failed to demonstrate any difference in sodium excretion between normotensive and hypertensive groups. Miall[238] and Oldham et al.[249] found similar sodium excretion levels in persons with systolic pressures greater than 200 mmHg and those with pressures less than 150 mmHg. Bing et al. reported no difference in sodium output between 36 patients with hypertension and matched normotensive controls.[28] Simpson et al. in New Zealand were unable to demonstrate correlations of blood pressure with sodium excretion, or urinary sodium-potassium or sodium-creatinine ratio.[295]

Two major studies have superseded previous epidemiological investigations into the relationship between blood pressure and salt intake. The Intersalt study[157a] recruited 10,079 adults from 52 centers in 32 countries, including primitive and industrialized societies. After adjustment for age, sex, body mass index, alcohol consumption, and urinary potassium, multiple regression analyses indicated that sodium excretion and systolic blood pressure were significantly correlated in a positive way in only eight centers, with no correlation for diastolic blood pressure. When regression coefficients were pooled, a very weak relationship was found between systolic (but not diastolic) blood pressure and sodium excretion, so that a change of 100 mmol in daily sodium excretion would be associated with a change in systolic pressure of 2.17 mmHg and of 0.1 mmHg in diastolic pressure. In cross-population analysis, the level of sodium excretion correlated with the slope (increase) of blood pressure with age.

A second large-scale study was conducted in Scotland. Blood pressure and urinary sodium excretion were measured in a random sample of 7354 subjects. No correlation was found between blood pressure and sodium excretion after adjusting for body mass index, alcohol consumption, and urinary potassium excretion.[298a]

Failure to find a relationship between sodium intake and blood pressure within industrialized population may stem from the relatively narrow range of habitual salt ingestion in these societies, that is, 100 to 250 meq/day. In the unacculturated societies with low blood pressures, for example, daily sodium intake is invariably less than 50 meq. In the Akita Prefecture of northern Japan, where sodium intake is extraordinarily high (30 to 40 g/day), 48 percent of the villagers were hypertensive; stroke was the most prominent cause of death.[305] It appears that differences in blood pressure between groups can only be demonstrated at the lowest and highest extremes of salt intake.

If, as is commonly believed (see below), the usual sodium intake in western societies is sufficiently high to raise blood pressure, *but only in a genetically susceptible minority of individuals,* then a correlation between mean blood pressure and mean dietary sodium intake within an entire population is not expected. Since habitual salt intake is culturally determined, it may be anticipated that within a given population salt intakes should be similar regardless of blood pressure.

As concluded by Luft and Weinberger, "It is unlikely that a high sodium intake raises the blood pressure of most people. If that were to be the case blood pressure of persons within a given population should be correlated with their sodium intake, and hyptertensive subjects should eat and excrete more sodium than normal subjects. Neither appears to be the case. Alternatively, it is possible that only a susceptible minority within a population will experience an increased blood pressure when exposed to a high sodium intake. Thus, if the range of sodium intake within that population is relatively small, even though the sodium intake itself is large, no correlation between arterial pressure and sodium intake would be found.[223]

SODIUM LOADING IN HUMANS

Kirkendall et al. found no increase in blood pressure in normal volunteers after increasing their sodium intake from 10 to 410 meq/day for 4 weeks.[177] Luft et al. varied sodium intake in normotensive volunteers from 10 to 1500 meq/day.[221] Blood pressure was unaffected at sodium intakes of less than 800 meq/day, and even at this level of consumption not all subjects had elevated blood pressures. In the subjects in whom potassium balance was maintained, blood pressure did not rise significantly with sodium loading (see below). These results are in accord with population studies described above implying that the effect of dietary sodium on blood pressure levels can be demonstrated only at extremes of intake.

Hypertensive subjects also exhibit variable responses to sodium loading. Mark et al. reported a modest blood pressure rise in subjects with borderline hypertension after increasing sodium intake from 10 to 410 meq/day.[229] Kawasaki et al. increased sodium intake in 19 hypertensive subjects from 9 to 249 meq/day and found variable blood pressure responses.[170] Nine subjects who were presumably salt-sensitive displayed significant increases of blood pressure; the other ten subjects were insensitive, and showed negligible changes in pressure.

In an identical study on another 11 patients with primary hypertension, this same group demonstrated that with the high-sodium diet (249 meq/day) the salt-sensitive patients gained more weight, retained more sodium, and had a greater increase in cardiac output than subjects in the salt-insensitive group.[113] Control renin and aldosterone levels were lower in salt-sensitive than in salt-resistant subjects, but were similar after salt loading. Control plasma norepinephrine levels were similar in both groups, but higher in the salt-sensitive patients after salt loading. These results suggest that the greater increase in blood pressure in the salt-sensitive patients following sodium loading can be attributed to greater sodium retention, leading in turn to an increase in cardiac output. A higher activity of the adrenergic nervous system may contribute to the relative sodium retention with sodium loads[125] and the increase in blood pressure. Others have also shown less suppression of plasma norepinephrine levels in salt-sensitive hypertensive subjects than in normotensive subjects in response to sodium loads.[54,222]

Hollenberg et al. identified a group of normal renin, salt-sensitive hypertensives who were unable to handle a sodium load. Normally, a change in sodium intake results in a change in renal blood flow. The above group, to whom the investigators referred as "nonmodulators," demonstrates insensibility of renal blood flow to change in sodium intake, resulting in sodium retention after a sodium load. This abnormality was reversed by angiotensin-converting enzyme inhibitors and calcium channel blockers.[149a]

A study conducted in normotensive teenagers with and without hypertensive parents by Falkner et al.[104] may be more pertinent to the relationship of sodium to the pathogenesis of hypertension. These investigators noted that in response to increased salt intake, children with one hypertensive parent demonstrated rises in blood pressure, whereas children of normotensive parents did not.

Salt sensitivity

The prevalence of salt sensitivity in the hypertensive population is unknown. Various controlled studies report different findings, ranging between 30 and 60 percent. This variability reflects differences in study design, criteria for diagnosing salt sensitivity and heterogeneity in selecting study participants.[94a] Some studies suggest that the prevalence of salt sensitivity is higher among individuals with a positive family history of hypertension,[104a,297a] blacks,[104a,104b,229,332a] and older[175a,240a] hypertensive subjects. Some studies concluded that salt-sensitive individuals retain more sodium after salt loading[104b,149a] while others found no relationship.[98a]

The heterogeneity in response to salt loading described above may be mirrored by the blood pressure responses of hypertensive patients to salt restriction, in which some patients (salt-sensitive) respond and others (salt-resistant) do not.[195]

ALTERATIONS IN SODIUM HOMEOSTASIS

BODY FLUID VOLUMES

Most investigators have reported normal values for serum sodium, ECF volume, plasma and total blood volume, and exchangeable sodium in essential hypertension patients compared to normal controls.[69] Therefore, essential hypertension cannot be explained simply as a state of sodium retention. In fact, in most studies of patients with hypertension, the plasma volume is lower than in normal subjects;[17,67,307] peripheral resistance and plasma volume have a negative correlation,[237,307,337] as do blood pressure and plasma volume.[98] Thus, although in well-documented forms of "hypervolemic" hypertension, such as primary aldosteronism, Cushing's syndrome, and renal failure, blood pressure can be correlated with body fluid volumes, this does not seem to be the case in essential hypertension. London et al.,[215] however, noted a positive correlation between blood pressure levels and total blood volume in patients with mild essential hypertension; a negative correlation was found for normal subjects, implying that the usual pressure-volume relationship in essential hypertension had been perturbed. "Normal" plasma volume, in this view, may be inappropriately high for the level of blood pressure. Similarly, Beretta-Piccoli et al.[21] noted a positive correlation between exchangeable sodium and arterial pressure in hypertensive, but not in normotensive, subjects, although mean exchangeable sodium values were not different in the two groups.

RENAL SODIUM HANDLING

In isolated or perfused normal kidneys, when the inflow pressure is raised (e.g., hypertension), more salt and water are excreted.[165,288,293] This is referred to as pressure natriuresis. The mechanism of pressure natriuresis is poorly understood, but may be related to physical factors within the kidney, that is, reduced sodium reabsorption resulting from increased peritubular capillary pressure.[13,165] The normal pressure-natriuresis curve is very steep, so that a small change in blood pressure could theoretically result in a large change in sodium excretion.

It has been postulated that a primary defect in essential hypertension is a resetting of the renal pressure-natriuresis curve, so that a higher arterial pressure is required to excrete sodium at the same rate as in the normal kidney.[134,135] An equally plausible explanation, however, is that the resetting of the pressure-natriuresis curve is secondary to the high blood pressure itself. In patients with early essential hypertension, renal blood flow is lower than in matched controls; normal glomerular filtration rate (GFR) is maintained and filtration fraction is elevated.[30,44,149,212] This early decrease in renal blood flow is thought to be caused by sympathetically mediated, reversible intrarenal vasoconstriction.[149] The increased filtration fraction suggests preferential constriction of the renal efferent arterioles. With establishment of hypertension, there is a further progressive decrease in renal blood flow with a relatively smaller decrease of glomerular filtration, so that the filtration fraction remains elevated.[30] An increased filtration fraction results in increased peritubular oncotic pressure and increased sodium reabsorption.[46]

Tobian and coworkers, using isolated, blood-perfused kidneys of Dahl sodium-sensitive and sodium-insensitive rats, demonstrated a pronounced natriuretic defect in the sodium-sensitive rats at normal and high inflow pressures.[311] The isolated kidneys from the sensitive rats excreted only half as much sodium as kidneys from resistant rats at equal levels of inflow pressure. Thus, in the young normotensive salt-sensitive rats prone to subsequent hypertension, a higher inflow pressure is required to achieve a given sodium excretion than in the resistant strain. These data confirmed similar experiments by Iwai et al.[161]

Other experimental data support an initial genetically determined defect of renal sodium excretion in the pathogenesis of salt-sensitive hypertension: sodium -sensitive Dahl rats fail to become hypertensive on an 8 percent salt diet when given a thiazide diuretic,[312] in the transplantation studies cited above blood pressure followed the kidney.[26,82] Unfortunately, in the Kyoto SHR rats, which many consider to be the closest counterpart to human hypertension, similar salt sensitivity has not been demonstrated.

AUTOREGULATORY THEORY

A genetic defect in renal sodium excretion is central to the autoregulatory theory of the pathogenesis of essential hypertension. This suggestion, first made by Borst and Borst-de-Geus[35] and Ledingham and Cohen,[200] was more recently developed by Guyton et al.[134,135] Autoregulatory theory is based largely upon experiments in partially nephrectomized animals and studies in anephric patients; such conclusions may or may not be extrapolated to human essential hypertension. However, this theory is supported by a recent report showing remission of hypertension in six patients with essential hypertension after renal transplantation.[75]

In animals or humans with reduced renal mass who are given large sodium loads, the following sequence occurs: salt and water are retained, initially, with increases in body fluid volume, cardiac output, and arterial pressure. Within a few weeks, cardiac output and blood volume decrease toward normal while total peripheral resistance increases proportionately. Thus, during the chronic phase of hypertension, the high arterial pressure is maintained by high resistance, but the high resistance develops *after* the onset of hypertension and, therefore, does not initiate it.

The phenomenon of an early increase in cardiac output followed by increased total peripheral resistance is explained by total body autoregulation. The changeover reflects an intrinsic myogenic property of the vasculature to regulate regional blood flow depending upon the metabolic needs of tissues (called the Bayliss effect). The initial high cardiac output causes hyperperfusion of various organs and tissues; automatically, in response, vascular constriction decreases regional blood flow toward normal, thereby increasing peripheral resistance and further elevating the blood pressure. The higher blood pressure then results in a pressure natriuresis; restoration of normal body volume is followed by a decreased cardiac output.

It is argued that this same sequence occurs in early essential hypertension. According to this theory, the genetic defect in renal sodium excretion results in retention of sodium and water with consequently increased body fluid volumes and increased cardiac output. This early stage of hypertension is then replaced in established hypertension with normal volume measurements and cardiac output and increased peripheral resistance.

Studies on early hypertension have reported that a variable proportion of subjects had elevated cardiac outputs.[112,162,281,338] In long-term follow-up studies cardiac output generally decreased and peripheral resistance increased over the years.[29,102,163,225,337] These data are thus consistent with the autoregulatory hypothesis. Whether this hemodynamic sequence always develops and what role it plays in essential hypertension[308] remain undecided.

Most adolescent[148] and young patients with hypertension[225] do not display elevated cardiac outputs. The persistance of a high cardiac output for many years in primary aldosteronism patients[306] and in patients with essential hypertension,[154] and the heterogeneity of hemodynamic response to volume overload in anephric patients[251] are all difficult to reconcile with autoregulatory theory. Furthermore, experimental hypertension can be induced without an initial elevation in cardiac output in renovascular hypertension,[181] in mineralocorticoid hypertension,[39] and in spontaneously hypertensive rats.[265] The sequence of hemodynamic pattern from high cardiac output to high peripheral resistance can be alternatively explained by the development of structural changes (hypertrophy) in the peripheral vessels in response to hypertension.[106]

Autoregulatory theory appears to have some validity in the proportion of hypertensive subjects with salt-sensitive hypertension; it cannot be adduced as a unifying hypothesis in the pathogenesis of most cases of essential hypertension.

THE ROLE OF POTASSIUM IN BLOOD PRESSURE REGULATION

Several epidemiologic, experimental, and clinical studies conducted over the past three decades investigated the relationship between potassium and blood pressure.[183] However, the role of potassium in regulating blood pressure remains controversial because of disparate responses obtained in clinical and experimental studies.[183]

EPIDEMIOLOGIC STUDIES

Epidemiologic surveys from widely divergent geographic locations within and outside the United States have demonstrated an inverse correlation between potassium intake and the prevalence of hypertension. Lever et al.[205] observed that blood pressure correlated positively with the total body sodium and negatively with the total body potassium content in normotensive and hypertensive subjects. Walker and colleagues[328] noted an inverse relationship between urinary potassium excretion and diastolic blood pressure in a group of ambulatory subjects with varying blood pressures. Surveys conducted in Hawaii and southern California as well as in Japan, Korea, Belgium, and China reported an inverse correlation between potassium intake and blood pressure.[168,174,176,176a,192,274,283,325,351] In the recently completed Intersalt study that enrolled 10,079 adults from 52 centers across the world, blood pressure correlated positively with sodium intake and negatively with potassium intake.[158] The relationship between potassium intake and high blood pressure is particularly impressive among blacks.[20,111,128,193,220,271] Grim et al.[128] observed that the potassium intake was lower and the prevalence of hypertension was higher among blacks compared with whites living in Evans County Georgia. Surveys conducted in other geographic locations such as Indiana and Louisiana as well as the data obtained from the National Health and Nutrition Examination Survey corroborate that urinary potassium excretion is lower in blacks compared with that of whites.[20,111,220,271]

EXPERIMENTAL STUDIES

Potassium Supplementation

Potassium supplementation lowers blood pressure in several models of experimental hypertension. Meneely and Ball[233] observed that increasing the potassium intake lowered the blood pressure and improved the survival in Sprague-Dawley rats fed high-sodium diets for several months. Dahl et al.[81] noted that increasing the dietary potassium content attenuated the hypertensive effect of high-sodium diet in salt-sensitive rats. Potassium supplementation lowered blood pressure in spontaneously hypertensive rats and rats with renovascular hypertension.[217,300,349]

Potassium Depletion

Severe potassium depletion in Long-Evans rats retarded their growth and lowered their blood pressure.[107a,279] Linas and colleagues systematically investigated the effect of potassium depletion on blood pressure in various models of experimental hypertension.[19,208,209,248,261] In rats with renovascular hypertension and in spontaneously hypertensive rats they observed a decrease in blood pressure in response to potassium depletion.[19,209,261] The decrease in blood pressure in these rats is associated with a decrease in peripheral vascular resistance and an impaired pressor response to angiotensin II.[19,208,261] Potassium depletion in dogs is associated with a decrease in blood pressure[14a] along with a modest decrease in cardiac output.[1] In contrast to the hypotensive effects of potassium depletion in these studies, potassium depletion induced by mineralocorticoid adminstration is associated with an increase in blood pressure.[114] Potassium supplementation attenuated the sodium retention and the increase in blood pressure accompanying mineralocorticoid adminstration.[114] These studies demonstrate that amelioration of hypokalemia attenuates the mineralocorticoid-induced sodium retention and hypertension in rats.

CLINICAL STUDIES

Potassium Supplementation

High potassium intake lowers blood pressure in essential hypertensives ingesting a normal sodium diet.[114b,150,156,226,263,275,294,301,304] In a randomized double-blind study, Svetkey et al.[301] observed that potassium chloride (120 mmol/day) administration decreased both systolic (6 mmHg) and diastolic (4 mmHg) blood pressures in hypertensives. Kaplan and colleagues[167] observed that amelioration of thiazide-induced hypokalemia lowered blood pressure in hypertensive subjects. In contrast to these studies, Smith et al.[299] and Grimm et al.[129] reported that increasing potassium intake in hypertensive subjects ingesting sodium-restricted diets exerted no additional hypotensive response. The hypotensive effects of potassium supplements are also not consistently demonstrated in normotensive subjects.[53,175,240]

Potassium Depletion

Perera[264] noted a decrease in blood pressure in four hypertensive subjects receiving low-potassium diets while their sodium intake was also kept low. Thus, potassium depletion did not modify the hypotensive effects of sodium restriction. Likewise, potassium depletion did not modify the hypotensive effects of sodium restriction in normotensive subjects.[184]

Krishna et al. investigated the effects of potassium depletion on blood pressure in normotensive and hypertensive subjects ingesting normal amounts of sodium.[185,186] In a group of normotensive subjects maintained on a potassium intake of 10 mmol/day and a sodium intake of approximately 160 mmol/day, for a period of 9 days, systolic blood pressure increased by 6 mmHg and diastolic blood pressure by a 4 mmHg.[185] When the same subjects received an identical diet but the potassium intake was maintained at 90 mmol/day, the blood pressure was unchanged. In response to an acute infusion of 2 liters of saline over 4 h mean arterial pressure rose in potassium-depleted subjects but was unchanged in potassium-repleted subjects.[185] These investigators further studied a group of essential hypertensives ingesting 120 mmol/day of sodium.[186] With low potassium intake, systolic blood pressure increased by 7 mmHg and diastolic blood pressure by 6 mmHg (Fig. 48-1). Of the 11 subjects studied, 10 subjects had higher systolic blood pressures and 8 subjects higher diastolic blood pressures on low potassium intake. After 10 days on the study diets, 6 of 11 subjects on normal potassium intake were normotensive, whereas only 1 subject on low potassium intake had normal blood pressure. In response to a 2 liter isotonic saline infusion, mean arterial pressure increased on normal as well as low-potassium diet but reached higher levels on low potassium intake (115 $\pm$ 2 vs. 109 $\pm$ 2 mmHg, $p < 0.05$). Thus potassium depletion exacerbated the hypertensive effects of acute sodium loading in hypertensives. Lawton et al.[198] noted that ambulatory systolic blood pressures were significantly higher on low potassium intake in normotensive and hypertensive subjects maintained on a sodium intake of 400 mmol/day. Krishna and Kapoor recently reported that potassium depletion partly mediates mineralocorticoid-induced hypertension in humans.[187]

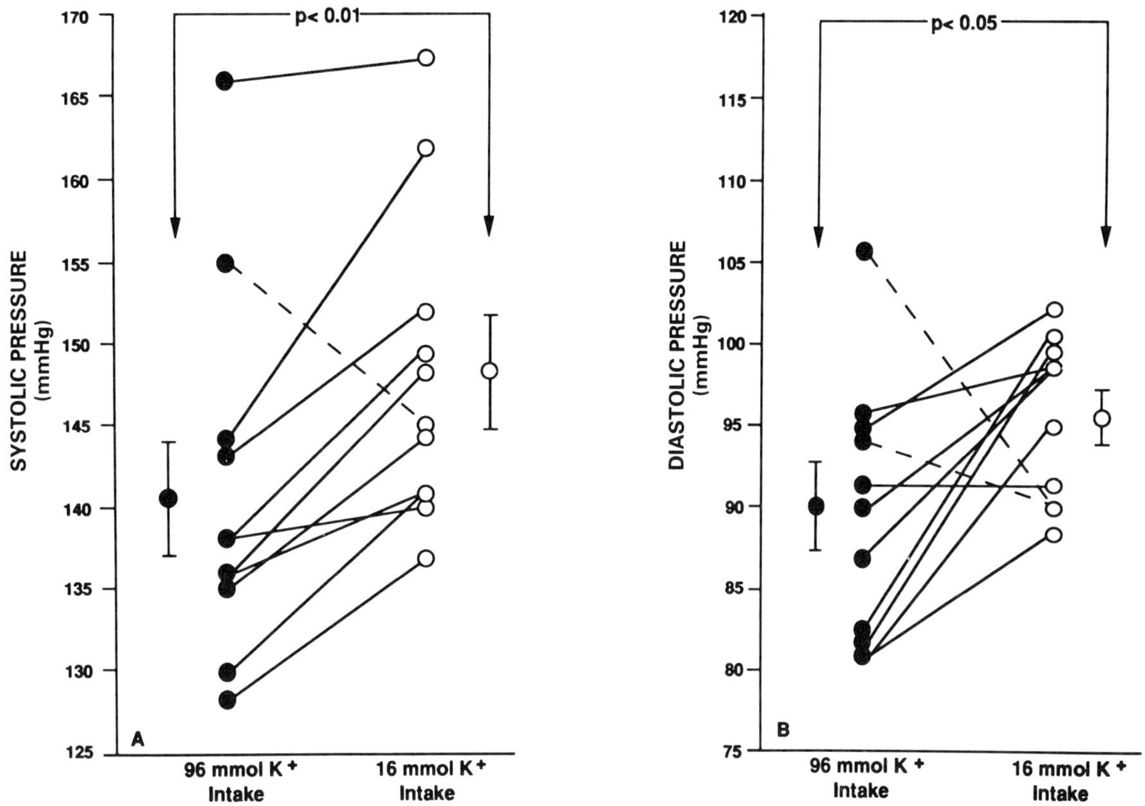

FIGURE 48-1 • Systolic (A) and diastolic (B) blood pressure in 11 hypertensives ingesting either 96 mmol (meq)/day (closed circles) or 16 mmol (meq)/day (open circles) of potassium for 10 days. Measurements were obtained on day 11 and the values obtained on the two study diets were compared by paired T-test. (Reproduced with permission from Krishna GG, Kapoor SC: *Ann Intern Med,* 115:77, 1991.)

MECHANISM OF POTASSIUM-INDUCED CHANGES IN BLOOD PRESSURE

Sodium retention, changes in vasopressor hormones, direct effects on vasculature, and alterations in divalent ion metabolism all may mediate the hemodynamic effects of potassium (Table 48-1).

Sodium Excretion

Changes in potassium intake produce striking alterations in sodium balance.[18,107,172,184-187,204] Krishna et al. measured urinary sodium and potassium excretion rates in subjects ingesting normal and low-potassium diets.[185] Over the 9-day study period, urinary sodium excretion was significantly ($p < 0.001$) lower on the low-potassium diet compared with the amounts excreted on the normal potassium diet (100 ± 10 vs. 144 ± 10 mmol/day). Furthermore, in response to an acute sodium load, subjects ingesting a low-potassium diet excreted significantly ($p < 0.05$) less of the sodium load compared with the values noted on a normal potassium intake (41 ± 11 vs. 51 ± 13 mmol/6 h). Similar differences in sodium excretion were observed in hypertensives ingesting normal and low-sodium diets.[53] Hypertensive effects of potassium depletion were not observed in subjects ingesting low-sodium diets. Krishna et al. observed that potassium depletion does not modify the hypotensive effects of sodium restriction.[184] Similarly, the hypotensive effects of potassium supplementation in essential hypertensives are not manifested if their sodium intake is kept low.[129,299] Collectively, these studies suggest that changes in external sodium balance are critical for demonstrating the effects of potassium on blood pressure.

TABLE 48-1 • Mechanism of potassium-induced changes in blood pressure

1. Sodium excretion:
   Potassium depletion: decreases sodium excretion
   Potassium supplementation: increases sodium excretion
2. Vasoactive hormones:
   Plasma renin activity: variable response in humans resulting from potassium's direct stimulation of renin, and from potassium's indirect inhibitory effect mediated by sodium retention
   Catecholamines: changes determined by alterations in sodium balance
4. Altered vascular response to vasoactive hormones:
   Potassium supplementation: decreases pressor response to angiotensin II and norepinephrine
5. Direct vascular effect:
   Hypokalemia: vasoconstrictor
   Hyperkalemia: vasodilator
6. Altered divalent ion metabolism:
   Potassium depletion: increases urinary calcium excretion, increases PTH levels
   Potassium supplementation: decreases urinary calcium excretion

Vasoactive Hormones

RENIN-ANGIOTENSIN SYSTEM Potassium depletion increases plasma renin activity in rats,[19,224,286] and in humans ingesting low-potassium diets.[49] However, Bauer and Gautner[18] observed a dose-dependent natriuresis and increase in plasma renin activity when the potassium intake was increased from 0 to 300 mmol/day. In these studies high potassium intake did not alter the stimulatory effects of sodium depletion on plasma renin activity in humans. Krishna et al. observed no significant change in plasma renin activity in a group of normotensives when their potassium intake was lowered[184,185] while in hypertensives a slight reduction in plasma renin activity was noted during potassium depletion.[186] In these studies, low-potassium diets consistently induced sodium retention.[184-186] The diverse responses noted in these studies can be explained by the simultaneous effects of potassium on renin secretion and sodium excretion. Thus, potassium depletion modifies plasma renin activity by both a direct stimulatory effect and an indirect inhibitory effect resulting from sodium retention. The net balance of these two contrasting influences determines the changes in plasma renin activity when potassium intake is altered.

SYMPATHETIC NERVOUS SYSTEM Studies done in animals and humans suggest that potassium modifies sympathetic activity, but it is not known whether these changes are causally related to the changes in blood pressure.[315] Fujita and Sato[114a] observed that renal norepinephrine turnover was markedly accelerated in DOCA-salt rats, and potassium supplementation normalized these changes. This normalization of norepinephrine turnover was accompanied by enhanced urinary sodium excretion and attenuation of hypertension. Iimura et al.[156] noted that plasma norepinephrine concentrations and urinary norepinephrine excretion rates were increased in hypertensive subjects ingesting high-potassium diets. In contrast to these observations, Fujita and Ando[114b] noted that potassium supplementation lowered plasma norepinephrine concentration in hypertensive subjects ingesting high-sodium diets. Krishna et al. observed no significant differences in plasma catecholamine concentrations and urinary dopamine and norepinephrine excretion rates between normal and low-potassium intake.[184,185]

OTHER HORMONES Plasma *arginine vasopressin* levels remain unchanged in response to potassium depletion while the concentrations of *atrial natriuretic peptide* increase during potassium depletion.[185,186] These studies do not exclude the possibility that potassium depletion modifies the vascular response to these circulating vasoactive hormones. Indeed, Iimura et al.[156] noted that potassium supplementation lowers the pressor response to infused norepinephrine and angiotensin II in essential hypertensives. The role of other vasoactive compounds such as endothelium-derived relaxing factor, endothelin, and prostaglandins in mediating potassium-induced changes in blood pressure remains unstudied.

DIRECT VASCULAR EFFECT Acute hypokalemia increases vascular resistance, whereas hyperkalemia exerts a dilatory effect on the vasculature.[10,37,64,103,141] Anderson et al.[10] observed an inverse relationship between the potassium concentration of the perfusate and the perfusion pressure (a measure of local vascular resistance) in anesthetized dogs. Chen et al.,[64] Haddy and Scott,[141] and Brace[37] made similar observations in various experimental models. In all these studies a marked alteration in potassium concentration was required to modify vascular resistance. In humans, increases in systemic pressure during potassium depletion and decreases in pressure during potassium supplementation are associated with minimal alterations in the serum potassium concentration.[167,185,186,198,294,301] Hence, the contribution of hypokalemia to the increase in blood pressure must be small. Raij et al.[273] observed that endothelium-dependent relaxation of the aorta in hypertensive Dahl rats decreases in response to potassium supplementation. Thus, potassium supplementation may directly influence endothelial function.

DIVALENT CATION METABOLISM Calcium and magnesium have been implicated in the pathogenesis of hypertension.[230a,346] An increase in potassium intake lowers urinary calcium excretion while decreasing potassium intake has the opposite effect.[186,201,202] Lemann et al.[201,202] noted that administration of potassium bicarbonate and potassium chloride lowered urinary calcium excretion while intestinal calcium absorption was unchanged. A decrease in urinary phosphate excretion was also observed during potassium bicarbonate administration. Potassium depletion enhances the urinary excretion of calcium and phosphorus and increases plasma parathyroid hormone concentrations in hypertensives.[186] The role of calcium and phosphorus in mediating potassium-induced changes in blood pressure requires further study. Magnesium intake correlates inversely with the incidence of hypertension.[346] Low-potassium diets are generally low in magnesium content. However, changes in potassium intake do not modify magnesium metabolism.[186,188]

In summary, potassium intake plays a critical role in modulating blood pressure. Epidemiologic studies from varied geographic locations consistently demonstrate an inverse correlation between potassium intake and the prevalence of hypertension. Such relationships between potassium intake and blood pressure are most striking in blacks. Studies in experimental animals reveal a diverse response to alterations in potassium intake. Spontaneously hypertensive rats and rats with renovascular hypertension manifest a hypotensive response to both potassium depletion and potassium supplementation. In contrast, potassium depletion induced by chronic mineralocorticoid administration is associated with an increase in blood pressure. Potassium supplementation induces natriuresis and lowers blood pressure in mineralocorticoid-induced hypertension. Potassium supplementation in hypertensive subjects lowers blood pressure. Amelioration of diuretic-induced hypokalemia enhances the hypotensive effect of these agents. Potassium depletion induced by dietary potassium restriction elevates blood pressure in normotensive and hypertensive subjects maintained on a normal sodium intake. This hypertensive response to potassium depletion and the hypotensive response to potassium supplementation do not occur if sodium intake is kept low. Sodium retention, altered response to vasoactive hormones, direct vasoconstrictive effects of hypokalemia, and calcium depletion may all contribute to the blood pressure elevation during potassium depletion.

PART II CATION TRANSPORT

One of the more attractive hypotheses linking salt to the pathogenesis of essential hypertension relates to defective Na^+ transport systems that could result in abnormal renal Na^+ handling and/or changes in the intracellular ion content of blood vessels. Of the several transport systems that move Na^+ across cell membranes, abnormalities in most of these pathways have been described in experimental and essential hypertension.[12,159,268,302] Abnormal Na^+ transport may be linked to salt sensitivity of blood pressure. Cation transport experiments in human hypertension are largely limited to investigating circulating blood cells, whereas animal studies can include more relevant target tissues for hypertension such as the kidney and vasculature.

Cation transport in erythrocytes (RBCs) has been the most commonly studied system in human hypertension. In the erythrocyte Na^+ extrusion is mediated mainly through the ouabain-sensitive, *ATP-dependent Na^+-K^+ pump*. However, several other transport systems that are not sensitive to ouabain also account for important shifts in erythrocyte Na^+ balance including the *Na^+,K^+, Cl^- cotransport system,* in which there is coupled transmembrane Na^+, K^+, and Cl^- efflux or influx in the same

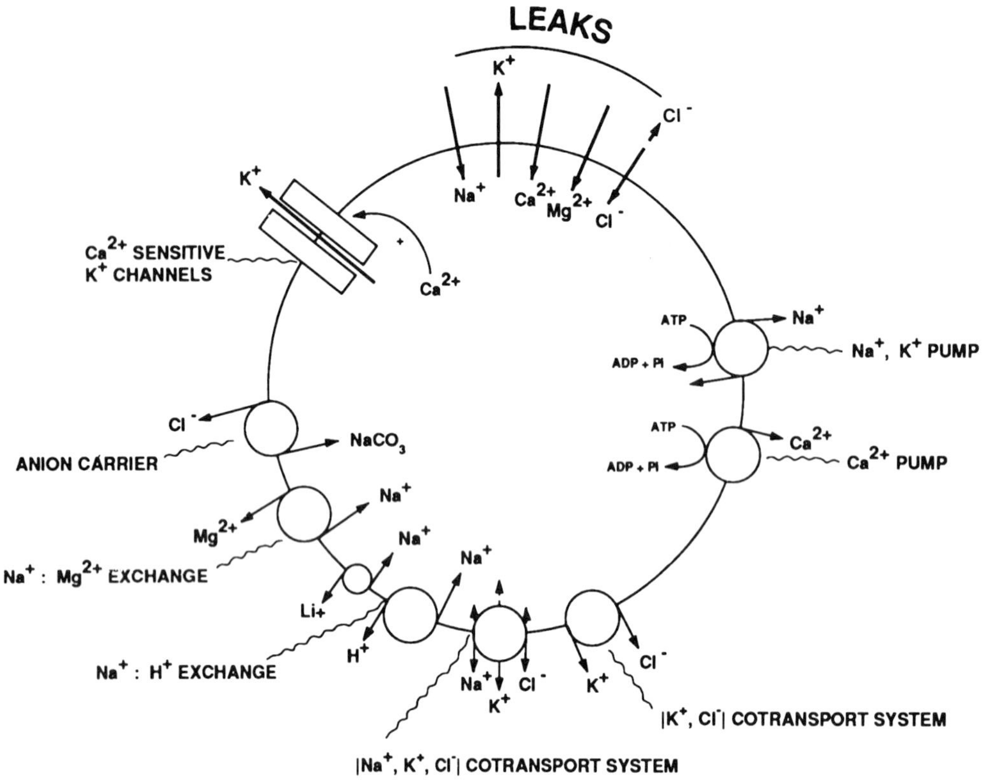

FIGURE 48-2 • Schematic diagram of known Na^+ transport systems in the red blood cell.

direction; the *sodium-lithium countertransport system* (SLC) in which one Na^+ exchanges for one Na^+ or Li^+ and the *Na^+-H^+ antiport system* that is responsible for hydrogen-ion extrusion from cells. Several other Na^+ transport systems may also participate in cell Na^+ regulation, but their role in hypertension is less clear (Fig. 48-2).

INTRACELLULAR SODIUM IN HYPERTENSION

One of the assumptions in the study of membrane Na^+ transport in hypertension is that abnormalities in the cation's transport pathways ultimately cause accumulation of intracellular Na^+. This hypothesis requires that higher intracellular Na^+ levels be demonstrated in tissues from hypertensive subjects and in experimental hypertension. In fact, one of the first demonstrated abnormalities in electrolytes in hypertension was the demonstration of higher intracellular Na^+ levels in vascular tissue from animals with experimental hypertension and in the renal arteries from humans with essential hypertension.[309] In another early study, Losse et al.[216] reported higher mean erythrocyte Na^+ levels in subjects with essential hypertension. Many, but not all, studies have confirmed these findings. Hilton[146] reviewed the results of 20 papers that analyzed the Na^+ content in erythrocytes. The pooled data on 965 hypertensives and 1857 normotensives demonstrated a statistically higher mean Na^+ concentration in hypertensives compared with controls. The mean level of the internal Na^+ concentration was 13 percent higher in hypertensives than in controls; however, the overlap in values was significant.

An elevated intracellular Na^+ concentration is also found in white blood cells, both polymorphonuclear leukocytes and lymphocytes from subjects with essential hypertension. High cell Na^+ concentration in leukocytes has been a consistant finding in essential hypertension and has been coupled with a reduced rate constant for Na^+ efflux by the Na^+ pump.[127,145] There is also a direct correlation between diastolic blood pressure and leukocyte intracellular Na^+ content in hypertensive subjects. Thus, in those hypertensives with the most elevated leukocyte Na^+ levels, the Na^+ pump is most reduced and blood pressure is most elevated. Ambrosioni et al.[7] have reported elevated intracellular Na^+ concentrations in lymphocytes from patients with essential hypertension and in their normotensive offspring, suggesting some genetic influence prevails on the white blood cell Na^+ content in hypertension.

THE SODIUM PUMP IN HYPERTENSION

The genetically coded ouabain-sensitive Na^+-K^+ pump is responsible for the majority of cation movement across the cell membrane and for generation of the transcellular Na^+ and K^+ gradients. For each cycle of ATP hydrolysis, two K^+ ions are transported inward and three Na^+ ions outward by the pump which uses energy generated by the membrane-associated enzyme, Na^+-K^+-ATPase. The molecular basis of this complex functional protein is well established. In general, the Na^+-pump maintains the steady state by adjusting Na^+ efflux to the rate of Na^+ entry into the cell. Numerous assay procedures are used to quantitate different aspects of Na^+ pump activity, including analysis of the membrane Na^+-K^+-ATPase enzyme activity; radiolabeled fluxes of ions using ^{86}Rb uptake and ^{22}Na efflux; and measurement of fluxes using unlabeled cations. Cardiac glycosides such as ouabain bind to the Na^+ pump and inhibit its activity and thereby define the ouabain-sensitive pump activity. In addition, [^3H] ouabain binding is used to identify the number of pump units on cells. These assays and tissue-preparation techniques vary widely, making comparative interpretations of Na^+ pump activity in hypertension difficult. Kinetic analysis of ion fluxes including V_{max} or initial reaction velocity, the Michaelis constant (K_m), and the Hill coefficient (n) represents more accurate methods for characterizing pump activity. Very small changes in the intracellular sodium level lead to large changes in Na^+ pump activity so that increased cell sodium entry promptly enhances pump-mediated Na^+ extrusion. Any perturbation of the Na^+ entry rate or pump activity should normally result in a new steady state where Na^+ entry once again equals extrusion. Loss of this adaptive process for intracellular Na^+ homeostasis may occur in hypertension.

A reduction in Na^+ pump activity has been demonstrated in cardiovascular and other tissues from animal models of hypertension, especially those with volume-dependent hypertension. Studies by de Wardener and MacGregor[91] and Haddy et al.[138] and Overbeck et al.[257] have shown reduced ouabain-sensitive ^{86}Rb uptake (pump) in blood vessels and reduced cardiac Na^+-K^+-ATPase pump activity in volume-expanded animals with hypertension. Plasma from such animals inhibits Na^+ pump activity (^{86}Rb uptake) when applied to tail arteries from normal rats, suggesting the presence of a humoral pump-inhibiting factor. In contrast, *increased* Na^+ pump activity has been described in genetic animal models of hypertension. In the spontaneously hypertensive rat[87] increased Na^+ pump activity is accompanied by other abnormalities in Na^+ handling, including increased membrane Na^+ permeability,[266] increased RBC osmotic fragility,[266] alterations in Ca^{2+} binding,[89] and changes in membrane fluidity. The finding of increased pump activity in hypertension could be explained by a compensatory increase in pump units in response to a circulating Na^+ transport inhibitor.

Studies of Na^+ pump activity in human hypertension have been performed mostly in RBCs and white blood cells. Reduced Na^+-K^+ pump activity can be consistently demonstrated in leukocytes from essential hypertensive patients.[146,147,267,268] A positive correlation between pump and plasma renin activities suggests a possible link between volume status and cation transport.[147] Poston et al.[270] found decreased rate constants for ouabain-sensitive Na^+ efflux from leukocytes of untreated essential hypertensive patients and noted that volume reduction with diuretic therapy corrected the abnormality. Reports of abnormal Na^+ pump activity in RBCs from patients with hypertension are less consistent than those with leukocytes, but some reports have found reduced Na^+ pump activity[267,277] and lower ouabain binding.[277] Kinetic studies of ouabain-sensitive Na^+ efflux in RBCs from essential hypertensive subjects reveal that approximately 10 to 15 percent of subjects have reduced affinity of internal Na^+ to the Na^+ pump.[122] In other studies blood pressure has been shown to be negatively correlated with RBC Na^+-K^+-ATPase activity and directly related to cell Na^+ content.[142] Thus, various levels of pump activity can be seen in experimental and essential hypertension and may depend on whether the primary defect is in the Na^+ pump itself or whether the Na^+ pump is reacting to changes in membrane permeability or to a circulating pump inhibitor. Reduced Na^+ pump activity has also been coupled with abnormal Ca^{2+} metabolism in RBCs from patients with essential hypertension.[267]

Racial differences in Na^+ pump activity may be important. Black normotensive and essential hypertensive patients have lower V_{max} for erythrocyte Na^+-K^+-ATPase activity,[25,196,280] a decreased number of pump units,[151] and higher intracellular Na^+ concentration.[196,218,245,280] However, kinetic analysis of pump activity in erythrocytes using cation flux methodology have not shown major differences in the V_{max} or K_m for ouabain-sensitive Na^+ efflux in blacks as compared with Caucasian subjects[321] (Fig. 48-3). On the other hand, serially passed skin fibroblasts from black hypertensives exhibit increased Na^+ turnover and accelerated Na^+-pump activity compared with fibroblasts from whites.[191]

CIRCULATING Na^+ TRANSPORT INHIBITORS IN HYPERTENSION

In 1969, Dahl et al.[80] proposed that a circulating substance in the plasma of a salt-sensitive strain of rats could be transferred parabiotically to salt-resistant rats, causing them to become salt-sensitive. Considerable evidence has subsequently been gathered to support the existence of circulating substances, termed *natriuretic hormones*, that might effect Na^+ balance by inhibiting Na^+ transport in various tissues.[94,143,173] Natriuretic hormones might also be expected to inhibit vascular smooth muscle Na^+-

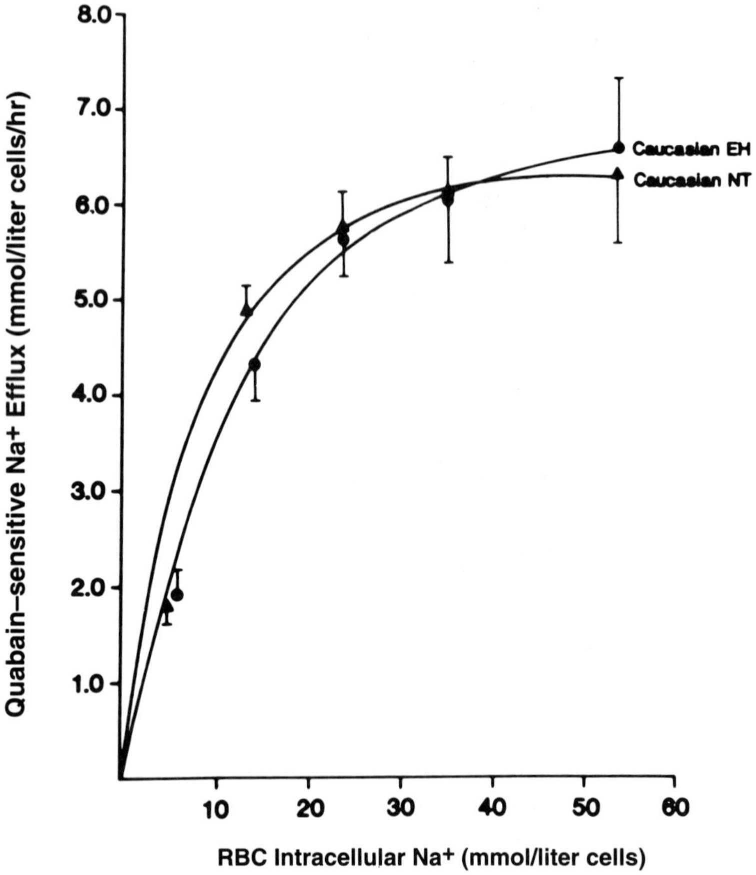

FIGURE 48-3 • Ouabain-sensitive Na^+ efflux rates (pump) in red blood cells from caucasian normotensive (NT) and essential hypertensive (EH) subjects determined at five levels of intracellular Na^+. Values are means ± SEM. (Reproduced with permission from Tuck ML et al: *Hypertension* 10:204, 1987.)

K^+-ATPase activity, leading to reduced Na^+ efflux, intracellular Na^+ accumulation, and increased vasomotor tone. One hypothesis argues that essential hypertension is accompanied by a primary renal defect in sodium excretion that is compensated for by release of a natriuretic hormone in response to the resulting volume expansion. The hormone then restores normal ECF volume by enhancing Na^+ excretion.[31] The compensatory increase in circulating natriuretic hormone(s) then could inhibit pump activity in blood vessels leading to cell Na^+ and Ca^{2+} accumulation.[31,94] The intracellular Ca^{2+} would then increase vascular tone causing hypertension.[31,94] Such a unifying hypothesis could consolidate the observed defects in electrolyte, renal, and vascular function reported in hypertension.

Fluid-expanded hypertensive animals have reduced pump function in cardiovascular tissue, suggesting the presence of a circulating Na^+ transport inhibitor(s).[255] Plasma extracts from hypertensive subjects stimulate glucose-6-phosphate dehyrogenase (G6PD), which is a proposed marker that indicates suppression of Na^+-K^+ pump activity.[94] The pump-inhibiting effect of hypertensive plasma correlates with blood pressure and is more pronounced in patients with low renin activity. There is also inhibition of Na^+ transport to white blood cells when exposed to plasma from essential hypertensive subjects.[146,268] Addition of plasma from persons with essential hypertension to isolated Na^+-K^+-ATPase systems shows an inhibition of Na^+-K^+-ATPase and the degree of in vitro inhibition correlates directly with mean arterial pressure in the patients.[142] Destruction of the *hypothalamic anteroventral third ventricle* (AV3V) in animals prevents the onset of hypertension and reduces urinary Na^+ excretion,[45,262] suggesting that a natriuretic substance may be synthesized or stored in the hypothalamus. Extracts of hypothalamic tissue show ATPase-inhibiting activity in renal tissue.

Intense efforts are currently being expanded to isolate, purify, and characterize the circulating transport inhibitor(s). The natriuretic factor(s) may derive from larger precursor molecules, and lower-molecular-weight intermediate or final products may contain most of the transport inhibitor activity. Highly purified plasma extracts taken from volume-expanded dogs and spontaneously hypertensive rats inhibit ATPase activity and show cross-reactivity with antidigoxin antibodies.[90,133,331] An endogenous *digitalis-like factor* has recently been extensively purified, and its molecular nature is being identified.[143] This factor inhibits the Na^+ pump and increases cardiac contractile force and vascular reactivity,[36] and its activity is high in volume-expanded DOCA-salt hypertension.

Despite the extensive search for the putative circulating Na^+ transport inhibitors, the evidence for their existence is still only partially substantiated and their role in hypertension remains unclear. There has not been a consistent relationship between inhibition of Na^+-K^+-ATPase activity and blood pressure, and the chemical nature of these inhibitors has yet to be elucidated. Although there is evidence that natriuretic factors might actually be digitalis-like factors, it is not clear that these substances can bind to the digitalis binding sites on the Na^+ pump.[173]

SODIUM-POTASSIUM-CHLORIDE COTRANSPORT IN HYPERTENSION

The Na^+,K^+,Cl^- cotransport system moves Na^+,K^+, and Cl^- in both inward and outward directions, and the pathway depends on Cl^- in several cells (erythrocyte, smooth muscle, renal tubular epithelium).[66,341] Cotransport systems move one ion down its electrochemical gradient while transporting the other ion upward against its gradient. The gradient usually established by the Na^+ pump determines the rates of cotransport-mediated ion movements. Net movement of Na^+,K^+, and Cl^- by cotransport is usually in the outward mode in human erythrocytes, and its contribution to net transport in this cell is relatively small compared with its activity in vascular and renal tissue.[43,48,66,258,322] The system is sensitive to loop diuretics such as furosemide and bumetanide that inhibit transport and are used as probes to assay the cotransport system. Cotransport has been well characterized in human erythrocytes, and this assay is employed in most studies of hypertension.[260,292] Garay et al.[118] originally reported a reduced V_{max} for Na^+ and K^+ efflux through the cotransport system in erythrocytes from essential hypertensive patients. These findings were subsequently confirmed in other laboratories.[76,84,131]

Subsequent studies of erythrocyte cotransport activity in essential hypertension have revealed a wider spectrum of transport activity. Some studies have reported no differences in cotransport between normotensive and hypertensive individuals.[96,342] Other studies, however, have actually reported high cotransport levels, especially in erythrocytes from Caucasian hypertensive subjects.[4,30,97,320] The diversity of findings for erythrocyte cotransport function may be due to differences in assay methodology, but more likely causes include geography, race, and genetic heterogeneity of essential hypertensives. Racial differences are important (Fig. 48-4) as uniformly low erythrocyte cotransport activity is found in blacks whether normotensive or hypertensive.[4,30,320,321] Kinetic analysis of erythrocyte cotransport shows both a reduced V_{max} and K_m for internal Na^+ for activation of the cotransport system in the black population.[321] It has been suggested that low cotransport activity may contribute to the etiology of hypertension in blacks, although this issue needs further study.

A family history of hypertension influences erythrocyte cotransport function as normotensive offspring from Caucasian families with essential hypertension display similar changes in cotransport.[76,118] A polygenic, heritable component to the cotransport system seems probable, but whether abnormal cotransport in normotensive offspring of hypertensive parents predicts development of hypertension remains uncertain. Other confounding factors such as age, duration and severity of hypertension, gender, body weight, urinary Na^+ excretion, and antihypertensive therapy probably have less effect on erythrocyte cotransport activity.[4,58,76,84,96,97,118,124,320,342] Furthermore, renal failure profoundly suppresses erythrocyte cotransport function.[72]

A sigmoidal kinetic relationship between intracellular $[Na^+]$ and outward Na^+,K^+,Cl^- cotransport can be described by three parameters: V_{max}, the maximal rate of outward cotransport; K_m, the affinity of intracellular $[Na^+]$ for the cotransport system, and the cooperative (Hill's) coefficient. Some hypertensives have low erythrocyte cotransport due to a lower affinity or K_m of the system for intracellular sodium.[122,122a,321] Hypertensives with high erythrocyte cotransport have an elevated V_{max} for Na^+ and K^+ efflux through this system; the high V_{max} of cotransport in some hypertensives could be an adaptive process to compensate for a reduced affinity for internal Na^+. Garay[122a] has proposed that no single defect in Na^+ transport can characterize the population with essential hypertension, and different patterns of abnormal Na^+ transport can be found in subsets of hypertensive patients. Low erythrocyte cotransport is present in roughly 25 percent of Caucasian hypertensives[122a] and almost all black normotensives and hypertensives.[122a,320] Reduced cotransport is also found in genetic models of hypertension such as the Okamoto strain of spontaneously hypertensive rats.[78,278] One proposed mechanism of how low outward cotransport could lead to hypertension postulates that reduced Na^+ efflux from vascular cells would lead to increased intracellular Na^+ and Ca^{2+} and increased vascular tone. As cotransport is also important for Na^+ reabsorption in Henle's loop, abnormal sodium handling and hypertension could result from a defective renal cotransport system.

Increased rates of erythrocyte cotransport occur in up to 35 percent of Caucasian subjects with essential hypertension.[122a] The distribution of erythrocyte cotransport activity in this group may be bimodal, with one group displaying borderline low to normal values and another subset with high levels. These patterns of cotransport activity could be determined by a major gene recessive for

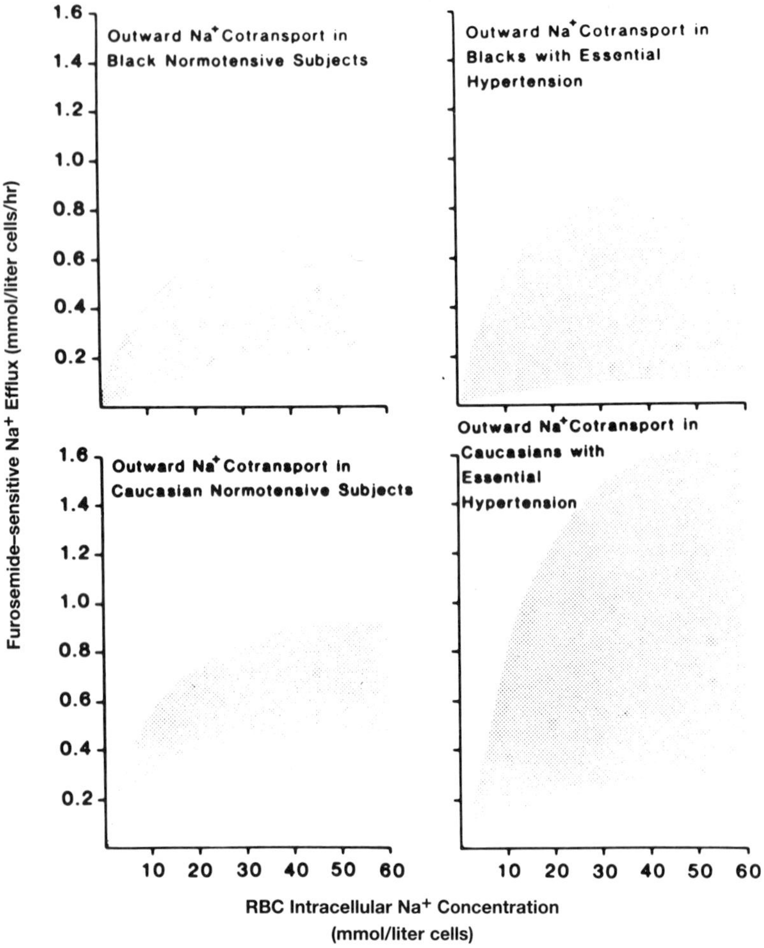

FIGURE 48-4 • Range of individual values for furosemide-sensitive Na^+ efflux (cotransport) in red blood cells from black and caucasian normotensive and essential hypertensive subjects determined at five levels of intracellular Na^+. (Reproduced with permission from Tuck ML et al: *Hypertension* 10:204, 1987.)

its phenotypic expression. One animal model of genetic hypertension, the Milan strain of spontaneously hypertensive rats (MHS), has high cotransport activity in several tissues including erythrocytes, renal cells of the ascending limb, and in vascular smooth muscle cells.[27] The high cotransport trait is transmitted in F_2 hybrids and may be secondary to a defect in membrane skeletal proteins.[27] Thus, the MHS rat is one of the best animal models of a genetic link between hypertension and abnormal Na^+ transport.

SODIUM-LITHIUM COUNTERTRANSPORT (SLC) IN HYPERTENSION

Canessa et al.[56] first reported an increased V_{max} for the SLC system in RBCs from subjects with essential hypertension. In this assay cells are loaded with Li^+ and the exchange rate of intracellular Li^+ for extracellular Na^+ is measured to determine the V_{max} for SLC. Using this assay or various modifications, most investigators have confirmed that mean levels for the V_{max} for SLC are elevated in hypertensive subjects.[4,47,55,60,69,97,317,323,335,344] The SLC assay in erythrocytes could be a marker for essential hypertension; however, there is considerable variability in the erythrocyte SLC measurement with substantial overlap between normotensive and hypertensive subjects.[324] A few studies have not found a difference in erythrocyte SLC activity between normotensives and hypertensives.[342] As with cotransport, abnormal erythrocyte SLC can be found in first-degree relatives of patients with essential hypertension.[344] Cusi et al.[77] have described high erythrocyte SLC in hypertensive patients with a family history of hypertension. Woods et al.[347] examined SLC in RBCs of teenage sons where both parents had essential hypertension and sons of normotensive parents. They noted that SLC was significantly increased in the cells of offspring from two hypertensive parents. Short-term follow-up has shown increased blood pressure in some of those offspring who had increased SLC.

Several studies have further elucidated the heritable nature of SLC in essential hypertension. Evidence has been reported for a recessive major gene that determines erythrocyte SLC activity.[32,144,244] In coronary-prone pedigrees from well-characterized Utah families, a recessive major gene accounted for 34 percent of the variance of erythrocyte SLC activity, polygenes for 46 percent of the variance and environmental factors explained 20 percent of the variance[144] (Fig. 48-5). Individuals who carry the major gene for high SLC have twice the prevalence of hypertension. A recent 7-year prospective study of SLC in a cohort of 1458 normotensive adults from Utah pedigrees showed an 18.8 percent incidence of new-onset hypertension in those inferred by segregation analysis to carry the recessive major gene for high SLC.[27] This represents a four-fold increase in the probability of developing hypertension compared with subjects with normal SLC activity.

Several other factors also influence erythrocyte SLC activity. Individuals with the high SLC genotype are more obese and have higher plasma triglyceride and insulin levels than those with normal SLC levels.[343] Some studies show that the relationship between SLC and blood pressure is lost when corrected for age and weight.[71] SLC is usually normal in normotensive and hypertensive black subjects and does not correlate with blood pressure as is the case in white hypertensive patients. Canessa et al.[58] studied normotensive and hypertensive blacks and their juvenile offspring and detected no differences in SLC between the three groups, suggesting that the SLC assay does not have specificity for discerning essential hypertension in black subjects. Erythrocyte SLC activity may also be influenced by gender, physical conditioning,[5] dietary weight reduction,[231] oral contraceptives, and potassium deficiency.

Measurement of erythrocyte SLC may be an indicator of hemodynamic and hormonal changes in essential hypertension. Higher SLC activity has been reported in erythrocytes from salt-sensitive hypertensive patients compared with those with salt-resistant blood pressure.[333] It is possible that elevated SLC could serve as a marker for salt-sensitive blood pressure. Plasma renin activity also shows a correlation with SLC in essential hypertension.[47] Erythrocyte SLC activity also correlates with renal function in hypertension. Weder et al.[334] have reported that the activity of erythrocyte SLC may reflect proximal tubule sodium reabsorption as hypertensive subjects with elevated erythrocyte SLC had reduced fractional renal lithium clearance. These findings would indicate an increase in sodium reabsorption by the renal proximal tubule of essential hypertensive subjects. There also may be a correlation between erythrocyte SLC and systemic hemodynamics in essential hypertensive patients; those with higher V_{max} for erythrocyte SLC have higher peripheral vascular resistance.[335] Despite the variability of SLC function in the population, most workers now feel that examination of the erythrocyte SLC system has provided better insight into the epidemiology and perhaps etiology of essential hypertension than measurements of other Na^+ transport systems.

Compared with the marked suppression of erythrocyte cotransport in uremia, SLC activity in erythrocytes is not altered in most forms of nondiabetic renal failure.[73] However, the erythrocyte SLC system is disturbed in *diabetes mellitus* and its activity may be a determinant of diabetic complications such as renal dis-

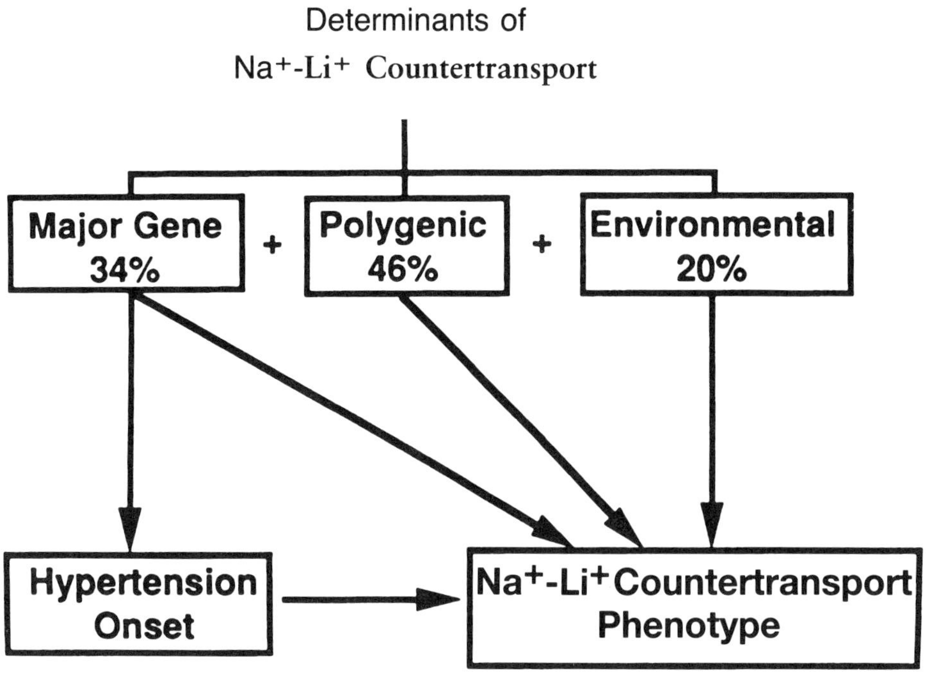

FIGURE 48-5 • Model showing contribution of individual components of sodium-lithium countertransport (SLC) determination in Utah pedigrees (major gene, polygenes and environment) to final SLC level and onset of hypertension. (Reproduced with permission from Hunt SC et al: *Hypertension* 17:1, 1991.)

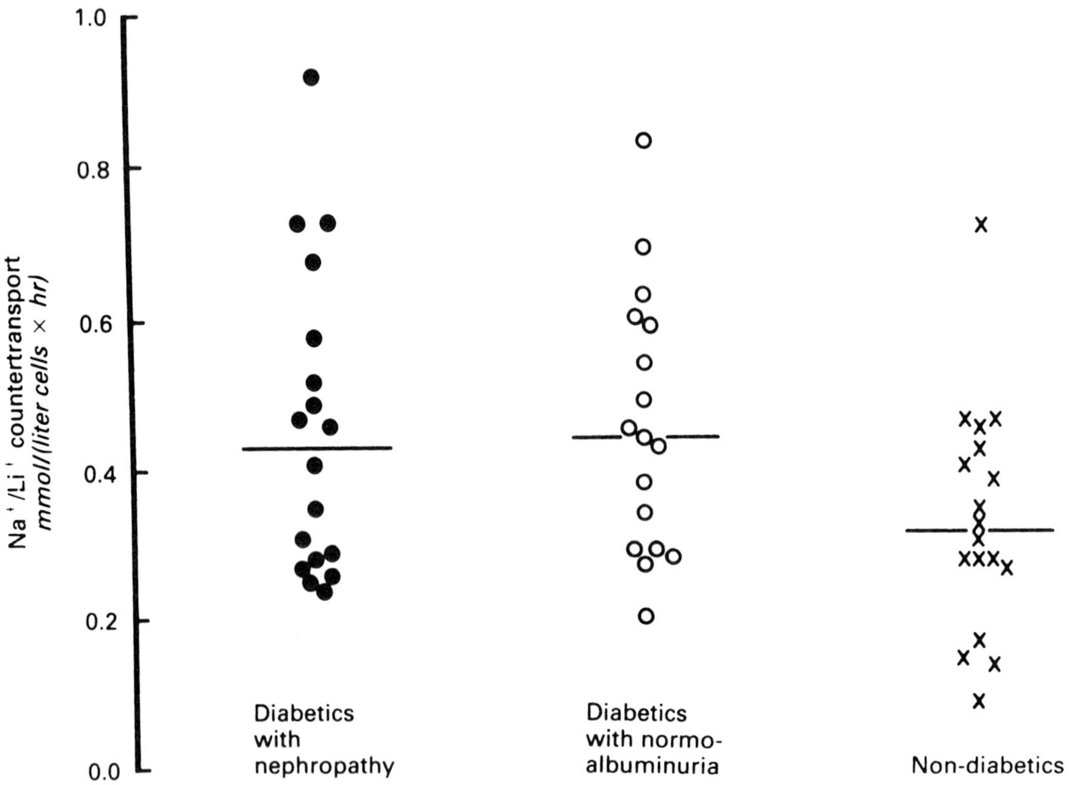

FIGURE 48-6 • Individual and mean values of sodium-lithium countertransport in subjects with non-insulin-dependent diabetes mellitus and nondiabetics. (Reproduced with permission from Gall M et al: *Kidney Int* 39:135, 1991.)

ease and hypertension. There is a genetic predisposition to hypertension in diabetic subjects as indicated by the high frequency of familial hypertension in patients with diabetes mellitus. Elevated erythrocyte SLC is found in insulin-dependent diabetes mellitus specifically in those patients with increased albumin excretion and diabetic nephropathy.[189,227a] In non-insulin-dependent diabetes mellitus studies also show elevated erythrocyte SLC, but this occurs in patients both with and without diabetic nephropathy[116] (Fig. 48-6). Thus, SLC activity is increased in most patients with non-insulin-dependent diabetes and may not be an indicator of renal involvement as may be the case for insulin-dependent diabetic subjects.

There also appears to be a rather strong association between erythrocyte SLC activity and *plasma lipid levels.* Erythrocyte SLC activity is positively related to plasma triglyceride levels and negatively correlated with HDL_2 cholesterol even after correction for age and body weight.[153]

SODIUM-HYDROGEN EXCHANGE IN HYPERTENSION

As the SLC system exchanges Na^+ for Na^+, its effect in net Na^+ movement should not lead to increased intracellular Na^+ and hypertension. However, the SLC system in erythrocytes has several properties in common with the sodium-hydrogen (Na^+-H^+) exchange or antiport system.[60,115] The erythrocyte SLC can transport Na^+ and Li^+ against a hydrogen-ion gradient similar to the Na^+-H^+ exchange. The erythrocyte SLC, however, is only minimally sensitive to amiloride, and studies in renal and other tissues show different kinetic properties for SLC and Na^+-H^+ exchange.[160,164] The Na^+-H^+ exchange system removes acid generated by cellular metabolic processes and is an important Na^+ uptake system in proximal tubule epithelial cells. Amiloride and its analogues are specific for inhibition of the Na^+-H^+ exchange and are used in most assays for this system. The Na^+-H^+ antiporter functions in cellular Na^+ and pH regulation, in proximal tubule sodium reabsorption, in platelet and leukocyte activation, and in the mitogenic response to various growth factors.[287] As the Na^+-H^+ exchange functions in so many aspects of cell regulation, control of Na^+-H^+ antiport activity is complex. Small changes in cell Na^+ and pH alter Na^+-H^+ exchange through allosteric mechanisms. Vasoconstrictor agents (angiotensin II, vasopressin, endothelin) and growth factors affect Na^+-H^+ exchange through second messenger systems. Cytosolic calcium accumulation and diacylglycerol activation of protein kinase C increase Na^+-H^+ exchange,[287,336] as do certain hormones such as glucocorticoids and thyroid hormone. Acidosis, hypokalemia, and cell shrinkage also activate this exchange system.

Increased Na^+-H^+ exchange could lead to hypertension through increased intracellular pH and sodium. In the kidney increased sodium reabsorption in the renal proximal tubule secondary to increased Na^+-H^+ exchange could lead to volume expansion and hypertension. Based on studies demonstrating increased cytosolic calcium in experimental[12,159] and human hypertension,[42,103a,199,210] Aviv[11,12] has proposed that the primary abnormality in hypertension is an increase in cell calcium that then leads to secondary stimulation of Na^+-H^+ exchange. Increased intracellular calcium in renal proximal tubule epithelial cells by activating the Na^+-H^+ antiport would increase Na^+ reabsorption leading to salt-sensitive hypertension. Increased cytosolic calcium and Na^+-H^+ exchange in vascular smooth muscle cells would increase vascular tone.

Platelet Na^+-H^+ exchange is increased in cells from untreated hypertensive subjects[211,285] as well as in RBCs from patients with essential hypertension[289] (Fig. 48-7). In cultured vascular smooth muscle cells from spontaneously hypertensive rats, Na^+-H^+ exchange is elevated and cells are more alkaline compared with Wistar-Kyoto rats.[22] If increased Na^+-H^+ antiport activity is a primary defect in hypertension, changes in its function should result in increased intracellular Na^+ and calcium.[31] Against this thesis are experiments that have induced an increase of Na^+-H^+ exchange in cultured vascular smooth muscle cells using cell acidification, osmotic shrinkage, and phorbol myristate and have not shown an effect on intracellular calcium.[241]

Genetic studies indicate that the Na^+-H^+ antiport system may not be a determinant of essential hypertension. Of the various intermediate phenotypes in human hypertension, the elevated V_{max} for Na^+-Li^+ countertransport is considered to be relatively specific for

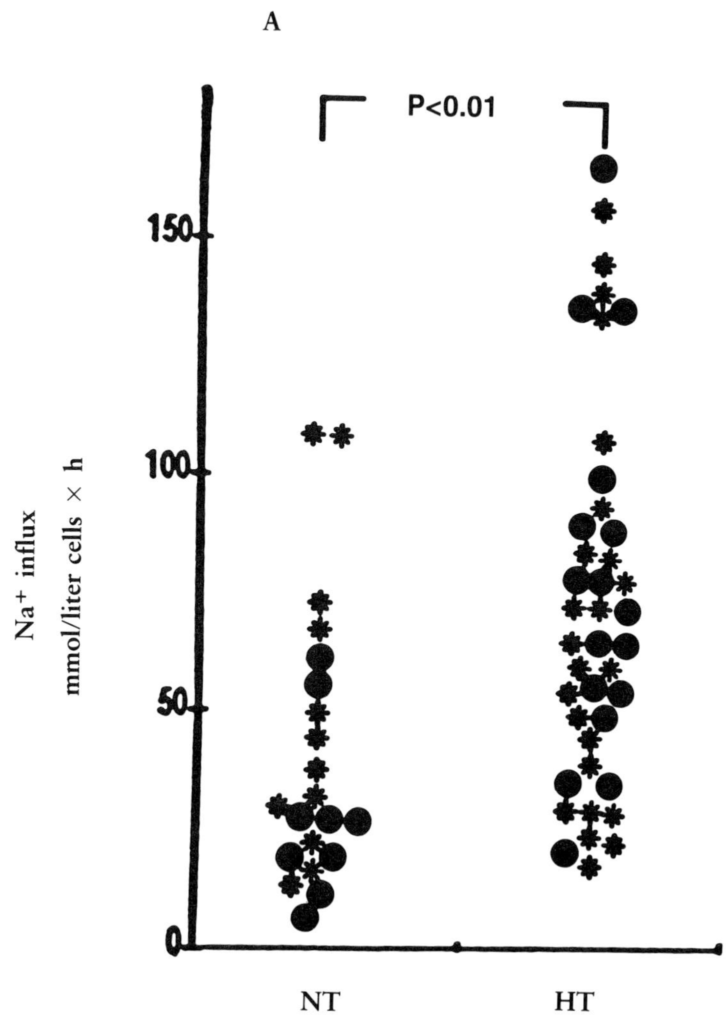

FIGURE 48-7 • Scattergram of the V_{max} of the rate of Na^+ influx in red blood cells (Na^+-H^+ exchange) in normotensive (NT) and hypertensive (HT) subjects. Asterisks indicate male and dots indicate female subjects. (Reprinted with permission from Semplicini A et al: *Am J Hypertens* 2:903, 1989.)

essential hypertension. As there are similarities between the properties of the erythrocyte SLC and Na^+-H^+ exchange systems, they may also share similar modes of inheritance. However, using genetic linkage analysis in Utah pedigrees, studies have excluded the Na^+-H^+ antiporter as a candidate gene in human essential hypertension.[206] Thus, the Na^+-H^+ antiport system as the major gene determining the increased V_{max} of SLC in erythrocytes from essential hypertensive subjects cannot explain the variations of SLC. Most likely, altered Na^+-H^+ antiport in essential hypertension is secondary to changes in intracellular sodium or calcium, in acid-base balance, or in vasoactive hormones.

DIETARY SALT AND CELL NA+ TRANSPORT IN HYPERTENSION

One unresolved issue in hypertension is whether membrane Na^+ transport is affected by salt intake and if measurement of these transport pathways reflects salt sensitivity of blood pressure. Weder[333] reviewed this topic examining some 26 studies in normotensive and hypertensive subjects comparing changes in salt intake with Na^+ transport activity in circulating blood cells. Several studies showed suppression of Na^+,K^+ pump activity during dietary salt loading in RBCs and in white blood cells in normotensive and hypertensive individuals. Cell Na^+ transport may be linked to salt-sensitive blood pressure. SLC activity in RBCs is higher in patients with *nonmodulating essential hypertension* (see Chap. 16), a subset of the essential hypertensive population that displays abnormal adrenal and renal responses to angiotensin II. These subjects also have salt-sensitive blood pressure responses to high sodium intake.[91] In addition, increased erythrocyte SLC activity is found in salt-sensitive compared with salt-resistant essential hypertensives studied under conditions of careful sodium balance.[333] Erythrocyte cotransport function is less directly related to salt-sensitive blood pressure responses.[59,190,207] However, Canessa et al.[61] examined the kinetics of erythrocyte cotransport, observing a lower V_{max} and K_m for cotransport in hypertensive patients on a low-sodium diet compared with levels measured on a high-sodium diet. The K_m for the cotransport system is also lower in erythrocytes from salt-sensitive black adolescents.[59] The ultimate goal of these studies would be to establish a predictive value of measuring erythrocyte cotransport and SLC to determine those subjects who may have increased blood pressure responses to high salt intake.

REFERENCES

1. Abbrecht PH: Cardiovascular effects of chronic potassium deficiency in dogs. *Am J Physiol* 223:555, 1972.
2. Addison WLT: The use of sodium chloride, potassium chloride, sodium bromide and potassium bromide in cases of arterial hypertension which are amenable to potassium chloride. *Can Med Assoc J* 181:281, 1928.
3. Aderounmu A, Aalako LA: Abnormal cation composition and transport in erythrocytes from hypertensive patients. *Cur J Clin Invest* 9:369, 1979.
4. Adragna NC et al: Red cell lithium-sodium countertransport and sodium-potassium cotransport in patients with essential hypertension. *Hypertension* 4:795, 1982.
5. Adragna NC et al: Effects of exercise on cation transport in human red cells. *Hypertension* 7:132, 1985.
6. Alaghband-Zadeh J et al: The effect of sodium intake on the content of a substance in the rat hypothalamus which stimulates glucose-6-phosphate dehydrogenase (G6PD) invitrus. *Clin Sci* 61:43P, 1981.
7. Ambrosioni E et al: Intralymphocytic sodium concentration: A sensitive index to identify young subjects at risk of hypertension. *Clin Exp Hypertens* 3:675, 1981.
8. Ambrosioni E et al: Effects of antihypertensive therapy on intralymphocytic sodium content. *Drugs Exp Res* 6:707, 1980.
9. Ambrosioni E et al: Increased intralymphocytic sodium content in essential hypertension: An index of impaired Na^+ cellular metabolism. *Clin Sci* 61:181, 1981.
10. Anderson DK et al: Effect of hypokalemia and hypomagnesemia produced by hemodialysis on vascular resistance in canine skeletal muscles. *Circ Res* 31:165, 1972.
11. Aviv A: Prospective review: The link between Ca^{2+} and the Na^+-H^+ antiport: A unifying factor for essential hypertension. *J Hypertens* 6:685, 1988.
12. Aviv A, Lasker N: Proposed defects in membrane transport and intracellular ions as pathogenic factors in essential, in Laragh JH et al (eds): *Hypertension, Pathophysiology, Diagnosis and Management.* New York, Raven Press, 1990, p 923.
13. Azar S et al: Glomerular, efferent arteriolar, peritubular capillary, and tubular pressures in hypertension. *Am J Physiol* 227:1045, 1974.
14. Azar S et al: Paraventricular-suprachiasmatic lesions prevent salt-induced hypertension in Dahl rats. *Clin Sci* 61:495, 1981.
14a. Bahler RC, Rakita L: Cardiovascular function in potassium-depleted dogs. *Am Heart J* 81:650, 1971.
15. Bassett SH et al: The mineral exchange of man: II. *J Nutr* 5:1, 1932.
16. Battarbee HD et al: The effect of dietary sodium and potassium upon blood pressure and catecholamine excretion in the rat. *Proc Soc Exp Biol Med* 161:32, 1979.
17. Bauer JH, Brooks CS: Volume studies on men with mild to moderate hypertension. *Am J Cardiol* 44:1163, 1979.
18. Bauer JH, Gaunter W: Effect of potassium chloride on plasma renin activity and plasma aldosterone during sodium restriction in normal man. *Kidney Int* 15:286, 1979.
19. Benedetti RG, Linas SL: Effect of potassium depletion on two-kidney one clip renovascular hypertension in the rat. *Kidney Int* 28:621, 1985.
20. Berenson GS et al: Creatinine clearance, electrolytes, and plasma renin activity related to the blood pressure of white and black children—The Bogalusa Heart Study. *J Lab Clin Med* 93:535, 1979.

21. Beretta-Piccoli C et al: Relation of arterial pressure with body sodium, body potassium and plasma potassium in essential hypertension. *Clin Sci* 63:257, 1982.
22. Berk BC et al: Spontaneously hypertensive vascular smooth muscle cells in culture exhibit increased growth and Na^+-exchange. *J Clin Invest* 83:822, 1989.
23. Berliner RW et al: Renal mechanisms for excretion of potassium. *Am J Physiol* 162:348, 1950.
24. Berliner RW: Ion exchange mechanisms in the nephron. *Circulation* 21:892, 1960.
25. Beutler E et al: Sodium-potassium-ATPase activity is influenced by ethnic origin and not by obesity. *N Engl J Med* 309:756, 1983.
26. Bianchi G et al: Changes in renin, water balance, and sodium balance during development of high blood pressure in genetically hypertensive rats. *Circ Res* 36/37 (suppl 1):153, 1975.
27. Bianchi G et al: Genetic aspects of ion transport systems in hypertension. *J Hypertens* 8(suppl 7):S213, 1990.
28. Bing RF et al: Salt intake and diuretic treatment of hypertension. *Lancet* 2:121, 1979.
29. Birkenhager WH et al: Consecutive haemodynamic pattern in essential hypertension. *Lancet* 1:560, 1972.
30. Birkenhager WH, Schalekamp MADH: *Control Mechanisms in Essential Hypertension.* Amsterdam, Elsevier, 1976, p 44.
31. Blaustein, MP: Sodium ions, calcium ions, blood pressure regulation, and hypertension: A reassessment and a hypothesis. *Am J Physiol* 232:C165, 1977.
32. Blaustein MP: Role of natriuretic factors in essential hypertension: An hypothesis. *Ann Intern Med* 98:785, 1983.
32a. Boerwinkle E et al: Genetic analysis of the distribution of sodium lithium countertransport in a sample representative of the general population. *Genet Epidemiol* 3:365, 1986.
33. Bogdanski DF et al: Mechanisms of biogenic amine transport and storage: IV. Relationship between K^+ and the Na^+ requirement for transport and storage of 5-hydroxytryptamine and norepinephrine in synaptosomes. *Biochim Biophys Acta* 211:521, 1970.
34. Bonaccorsi A, Bohr DF: K-free contracture and K-relaxation of vascular smooth muscle, abstracted. *The Physiologist* 17:185, 1974.
35. Borst JGG, Borst-de-Geus A: Hypertension explained by Starling's theory of circulating homeostasis. *Lancet* 1:677, 1963.
36. Bova S et al: Effects of an endogenous ouabain-like factor compound on heart and aorta. *Hypertension* 17:944, 1991.
37. Brace RA: Time course and mechanisms of the acute effects of hypokalemia and hyperkalemia on vascular resistance. *Proc Soc Exp Biol Med* 145:1389, 1974.
38. Brandis M et al: Potassium-induced inhibition of proximal tubular fluid reabsorption in rats. *Am J Physiol* 222:421, 1972.
39. Bravo EL et al: Multifactorial analysis of chronic hypertension induced by electrolyte-active steroids in trained, unanesthetized dogs. *Circ Res* 40(suppl):I40, 1977.
40. Brender D et al: Potentiation of adrenergic venomotor responses in dogs by cardiac glycosides. *Circ Res* 25:597, 1969.
41. Brender D et al: Effects of acetylstrophanthidin on isolated veins of the dog. *Circ Res* 26:647, 1970.
42. Brockman AS et al: Calcitropic hormones, platelet calcium and blood pressure in essential hypertension. *Hypertension* 16:1990.
43. Brock TA et al: Bradykinin and vasopressin stimulate Na^+-K^+-Cl^- cotransport in cultured endothelial cells. *Am J Physiol* 250:C888, 1986.
44. Brod J: Essential hypertension: Hemodynamic observations with a bearing on its pathogenesis. *Lancet* 1:773, 1960.
45. Brody MJ et al: The role of anteroventral third ventricle (AV3V) region in experimental hypertension. *Circ Res* 43(suppl 1):1, 1978.
46. Brown JJ et al: Renal abnormality of essential hypertension. *Lancet* 2:320, 1974.
47. Brugnara C et al: Lithium-sodium countertransport in erythrocytes of normal and hypertensive subjects. *Hypertension* 5:529, 1983.
48. Brugnara C et al: Furosemide-sensitive Na^+ and K^+ fluxes in human red cells: Net uphill Na^+ extrusion and equilibrium properties. *J Gen Physiol* 87:91, 1986.
49. Brunner HR et al: The influence of potassium administration and deprivation on renin in normal and hypertensive subjects. *J Clin Invest* 49:2128, 1970.
50. Buckalew VM Jr., Nelson DB: Natriuretic and sodium transport inhibitory activity in plasma of volume-expanded dogs. *Kidney Int* 5:12, 1974.
51. Burg M: Thick ascending limb of Henle's loop. *Kidney Int* 22:454, 1982.
52. Burns-Cos CJ, Maclean JD: Splenomegaly and blood pressure in an Orang Asli Community in West Malaysia. *Am Heart J* 80:718, 1970.
53. Burstyn P et al: Sodium and potassium intake and blood pressure. *Br Med J* 281:537, 1980.
54. Campese VM et al: Abnormal relationship between sodium intake and sympathetic nervous system activity in salt-sensitive patients with essential hypertension. *Kidney Int* 21:371, 1982.
55. Canali M et al: Increased erythrocyte lithium-sodium countertransport in essential hypertension: Its relationship to family history of hypertension. *Clin Sci* 61:135, 1981.
56. Canessa M et al: Increased sodium-lithium countertransport in red cells of patients with essential hypertension. *N Engl J Med* 302:772, 1980.
57. Canessa M et al: Red cell Na^+ transport polymorphism and essential hypertension, abstracted. *Clin Res* 30:334A, 1982.
58. Canessa M et al: Red cell Na countertransport and cotransport in normotensive and hypertensive blacks and their juvenile offspring. *Hypertension* 6:344, 1984.
59. Canessa M et al: Na^+-K^+-Cl^- cotransport and Na^+ pump in red cells of young blacks and blood pressure response to salt loading. *J Clin Hypertens* 2:101, 1986.
60. Canessa M et al: The Li^+-Na^+ exchange and Na^+-K^+-Cl^- cotransport systems in essential hypertension. *Hypertension* 10(suppl I):I–4, 1987.
61. Canessa M et al: Does sodium intake modify red cell Na^+ transporters in normal and hypertensive subjects? *Am J Hypertens* 2:515, 1989.
62. Carretero OA, Romero JC: Production and charac-

teristics of experimental hypertension in animals, in Genest J et al (eds): *Hypertension.* New York, McGraw-Hill, 1977, p 497.

63. Carretero OA et al: Urinary kallikrein in rats bred for their susceptibility and resistance to the hypertensive effects of salt. *Circ Res* 42:727, 1978.
64. Chen W et al: Mechanism of the vasodilator action of potassium. *Proc Soc Exp Biol Med* 140:820, 1972.
65. Cherchovich GM et al: High salt intake and blood pressure in lower primates. *J Appl Physiol* 40:601, 1976.
66. Chipperfield AR: The Na^+-K^+-Cl^- cotransport system. *Clin Sci* 71:465, 1986.
67. Chrysant SG et al: Racial differences in pressure, volume and renin interrelationships in essential hypertension. *Hypertension* 1:136, 1979.
68. Clarkson EM et al: Chemical properties, physiological action and further separation of a low molecular weight natriuretic substance in the urine of normal man, in Lichardus R et al (eds): *Hormonal Regulation of Sodium Excretion.* New York, Elsevier, 1980, p 333.
69. Clegg C et al: The heterogeneity of essential hypertension: Relation between lithium efflux and sodium content of erythrocytes and a family history of hypertension. *Lancet* 2:891, 1982.
70. Coleman TG et al: The role of salt in experimental and human hypertension. *Am J Med Sci* 264:103, 1972.
71. Cooper R et al: Increase sodium-lithium countertransport in college students with elevated blood pressure. *JAMA* 249:1030, 1983.
72. Corry DB et al: Cation transport in uremic erythrocytes: A kinetic profile. *Kidney Int* 32: 256, 1987.
73. Corry DB et al: Ouabain-sensitive and insensitive sodium transport in red blood cells from dialyzed uremic patients. *Kidney Int* 29:1197, 1985.
74. Cruz-Coke R et al: Influence of migration on blood pressure of Easter Islanders. *Lancet* 1:697, 1964.
75. Curtis JJ et al: Remission of essential hypertension after renal transplantation. *N Engl J Med* 309:1009, 1983.
76. Cusi D et al: Familial aggregation of cation transport abnormalities and essential hypertension. *Clin Exp Hypertens* 2:871, 1981.
77. Cusi D et al: Relationship between altered Na^+-K^+ cotransport and Na^+-Li^+ countertransport in the erythrocytes of essential hypertensive patients. *Clin Sci* 61:S33, 1981.
78. Cusi D et al: Cation transport abnormalities in human and rat essential hypertension, in Villareal H et al (eds): *Topics in Pathophysiology of Hypertension* Boston, Martinus-Nijhoff, 1984, p 136.

78a. Dagher G, Garay RP: A Na^+, K^+ cotransport assay for essential hypertension. *Can J Biochem* 58:1069, 1980.

78b. Dahl LK, Love RM: Evidence of relationship between sodium (chloride) intake and human hypertension. *Arch Intern Med* 94:525, 1954.

79. Dahl LK et al: Effects of chronic excess salt ingestion: Role of genetic factors in both DOCA-salt and renal hypertension. *J Exp Med* 118:605, 1963.
80. Dahl LK et al: Humoral transmission of hypertension. Evidence from parabiosis. *Circ Res* 24/25(suppl I):I-21, 1969.
81. Dahl LK: Salt and hypertension. *Am J Clin Nutr* 25:231, 1972.

81a. Dahl LK et al: Influence of dietary potassium and sodium potassium molar ratios on the development of salt hypertension. *J Exp Med* 136:318, 1972.

82. Dahl LK et al: Genetic influence of the kidney on blood pressure. Evidence from chronic renal homografts in rats with opposite predisposition to hypertension. *Circ Res* 34:94, 1974.
83. Dahl LK: Salt intake and hypertension, in Genest J et al (eds): *Hypertension.* New York, McGraw-Hill, 1977, p 548.
84. Davidson JS et al: Sodium-potassium cotransport activity as genetic marker in essential hypertension. *Br Med J* 284:539, 1982.
85. Dawber TR et al: Environmental factors in hypertension, in Stamler J et al (eds): *The Epidemiology of Hypertension.* New York, Grune & Stratton, 1967, p 255.
86. Dawes GS: Effect of potassium on small and large blood vessels of the dog forelimb. *J Physiol* 99:224, 1941.
87. De Mendonca M et al: Erythrocyte Na^+ transport system in primary and essential hypertension in rats. *Kidney Int* 21:S69, 1982.
88. Demots H et al: Effects of ouabain on coronary and systemic vascular resistance and myocardial oxygen consumption in patients without heart failure. *Am J Cardiol* 41:88, 1978.
89. Devynck MA et al: Analysis of calcium handling in erythrocyte membranes of genetically hypertensive rats. *Hypertension* 3:397, 1981.
90. Devynck MA et al: Measurement of digitalis-like compound in plasma: Application in studies of essential hypertension. *Br Med J* 287:631, 1983.
91. de Wardener HE, MacGregor GA: Dahl's hypothesis that a saluretic substance may be responsible for a sustained rise in arterial pressure: Its possible role in essential hypertension. *Kidney Int* 18:1, 1980.
92. de Wardener HE et al: Effect of sodium intake on ability of human plasma to inhibit renal Na^+-K^+-adenosine triphosphatase in vitro. *Lancet* 1:411, 1981.
93. de Wardener HE, MacGregor GA: The relation of a circulating sodium transport inhibitor (the natriuretic hormone?) to hypertension. *Medicine* 62:310, 1983.
94. de Wardener HE, Clarkson EM: Concept of natriuretic hormone. *Physiol Rev* 65:658, 1985.

94a. Dimsdale JE et al: Prediction of salt sensitivity. *Am J Hypertens* 3:429, 1990.

94b. Dluhy RG et al: Suppression of plasma renin activity by acute potassium chloride loading. *Circulation* 38(suppl VI):VI-66, 1968.

95. Dluhy RG et al: Influence of dietary potassium on plasma renin activity in normal man. *J Appl Physiol* 28:299, 1970.
96. Duhm J et al: Sodium-lithium exchange and sodium-potassium cotransport in human erythrocytes: Part 2. A simple uptake test applied to normotensive and essential hypertensive individuals. *Hypertension* 4:477, 1982.
97. Dunham PB et al: Chloride-activated passive potassium transport in human erythrocytes. *Proc Natl Acad Sci USA* 77:1711, 1980.
98. Dustan HP et al: Plasma and extracellular fluid volumes in hypertension. *Circ Res* 32/33(suppl 1):73, 1973.

98a. Dustan HP, Kirk KA: Corcoran lecture: The case for or against salt in hypertension. *Hypertension* 13:696, 1989.

99. Edmondson RPS et al: Abnormal sodium transport in leucocytes of patients with essential hypertension. *Clin Sci Molec Med* 46:21P, 1974.
100. Edmondson RPS et al: Abnormal leucocyte composition and sodium transport in essential hypertension. *Lancet* 1:1003, 1975.
101. Edmondson RPS, MacGregor GA: Leucocyte cation transport in essential hypertension: Its relation to the renin-angiotensin system. *Br Med J* 282:1267, 1981.
102. Eich RH et al: Hemodynamics in labile hypertension: A follow-up study. *Circulation* 34:299, 1966.
103. Emanuel DA et al: Effect of potassium on small and large blood vessels of the dog foreleg. *Am J Physiol* 197:637, 1959.
103a. Erne P et al: Correlation of platelet calcium with blood pressure: Effect of antihypertensive therapy. *N Engl J Med* 310:1084, 1984.
104. Falkner B et al: The role of sodium in essential hypertension in genetically hypertensive adolescents, in Onesti G, Kim KE (eds): *Hypertension in the Young and Old.* New York, Grune & Stratton, 1981, p 29.
104a. Falkner B et al: Sodium sensitivity, growth and family history of hypertension in young blacks. *J Hypertens* 4(suppl 5):S381, 1988.
104b. Falkner B, Kushner H: Effect of chronic sodium loading on cardiovascular response in young blacks and whites. *Hypertension* 15(1):36, 1990.
105. Flamenbaum W et al: Effect of KCl infusion on renin secretory rats and aldosterone excretion in dogs. *Am J Physiol* 229:370, 1975.
106. Folkow B: Cardiovascular structural adaptation: Its role in the initiation and maintenance of primary hypertension. *Clin Sci Molec Med* 55(suppl):3s, 1978.
107. Fourman P, Harvey GR: An experimental study of oedema in potassium deficiency. *Clin Sci* 14:75, 1954.
107a. Freed SC, Friedman M: Depressor effect of potassium restiction on blood pressure of the rat. *Proc Soc Exp Biol Med* 78:74, 1951.
108. Freis ED: Salt volume and the prevention of hypertension. *Circulation* 53:589, 1976.
109. Friedman M et al: Depressor effect of potassium deprivation on the blood pressure of hypertensive rats. *Am J Physiol* 167:457, 1951.
110. Friedman SM et al: Increased erythrocyte permeability to Li and Na in the spontaneously hypertensive rat. *Experientia* 32:476, 1976.
111. Frisancho AR et al: Blood pressure in blacks and whites and its relationship to dietary sodium and potassium intake. *J Chronic Dis* 37:515, 1984.
112. Frohlich ED et al: Hyperdynamic beta-adrenergic circulatory state, increased beta-receptor responsiveness. *Arch Intern Med* 123:1, 1969.
113. Fujita T et al: Factors influencing blood pressure in salt-sensitive patients with hypertension. *Am J Med* 69:334, 1980.
114. Fujita T, Sato Y: Natriuretic and antihypertensive effects of potassium in DOCA salt hypertensive rats. *Kidney Int* 24:31, 1983.
114a. Fujita T, Sato Y: Changes in renal and central noradrenergic activity with potassium in DOCA-salt rats. *Am J Physiol* 246:F670, 1984.
114b. Fujita T, Ando K: Hemodynamic and endocrine changes associated with potassium supplementation in sodium-loaded hypertensives. *Hypertension* 6:184, 1984.
115. Fundur J et al: The sodium-lithium exchange mechanism in essential hypertension—Is it a sodium-proton exchanger? in Vilarreal H et al (eds): *Topics in Pathophysiology of Hypertension,* The Hague, Martinus Nijhoff, 1984, p 147.
116. Gall M et al: Red cell Na^+-Li^+ countertransport in non-insulin-dependent diabetics with diabetic nephropathy. *Kidney Int* 39:135, 1991.
117. Ganguli M et al: Low renal papillary plasma flow in both Dahl and Kyoto rats with spontaneous hypertension. *Circ Res* 39:337, 1976.
118. Garay RP et al: Laboratory distinction between essential and secondary hypertension by measurement of erythrocyte cation fluxes. *N Engl J Med* 302:769, 1976.
119. Garay RP, Meyer P: A new test showing abnormal $Na^+$and K^+ fluxes in erythrocytes of essential hypertensive patients. *Lancet* 1:349, 1979.
120. Garay RP et al: A genetic approach to the geography of hypertension: Examination of Na^+-K^+ cotransport in Ivory Coast Africans. *Clin Exp Hypertens* 3:851, 1981.
121. Garay RP et al: Abnormal Na^+, K^+ cotransport function in a group of patients with essential hypertension. *Eur J Clin Invest* 13:311, 1983.
122. Garay, RP: Kinetic aspects of red blood cell sodium transport systems in essential hypertension. *Hypertension* 10(suppl 1):11, 1987.
122a. Garay RP: Typology of Na^+ transport abnormalities in erythrocytes from essential hypertensive patients. A first step towards the diagnosis and specific treatment of different forms of primary hypertension. *Cardiovasc Drugs Therap* 3:373, 1990.
123. Geck P et al: Electrically silent cotransport of Na^+, K^+ and Cl^- in Ehrlich cells. *Bioch Biophys Acta* 600:432, 1980.
124. Ghione S et al: Comparison of outward and inward Na^+/K^+ cotransport-mediated fluxes in erythrocytes of essential hypertensive patients. Preliminary results. *Clin Exp Hypertens* 3:809, 1981.
125. Gill JR Jr, Bartter FC: Adrenergic nervous system in sodium metabolism: II. Effects of guanethidine on the renal response to sodium deprivation in normal man. *N Engl J Med* 275:1466, 1966.
126. Goto A et al: Potassium feeding reduces hyperactive central nervous system pressor responses in Dahl salt sensitive rats. *Hypertension* 3(suppl 1):I128, 1981.
127. Gray HH et al: Sodium transport by leukocytes and erythrocytes in hypertensive subjects and their normotensive relatives. *J Hypertens* 2(suppl 3):467, 1984.
128. Grim CE et al: Racial differences in blood pressure in Evans County, Georgia: Relationship to sodium and potassium intake and plasma renin activity. *J Chronic Dis* 33:87, 1980.
129. Grimm RH Jr et al: The influence of oral potassium chloride on blood pressure in hypertensive man on a low-sodium diet. *N Engl J Med* 322:569, 1990.
130. Gross G et al: Relationship of sodium and potassium intake to blood pressure. *Am J Clin Nutr* 24:605, 1976.
131. Gruber KA, Buckalew VM Jr: Further characterization and evidence for a precursor in the formation of plasma

antinatriuretic factor (40371). *Proc Soc Exp Biol Med* 159:463, 1978.
132. Gruber KA et al: Endogenous digitalis-like substance in plasma of volume-expanded dogs. *Nature* 287:743, 1980.
133. Gruber KA et al: Increased circulating levels of an endogenous digoxin-like factor in hypertensive monkeys. *Hypertension* 4:348, 1982.
134. Guyton AC et al: Arterial pressure regulation. *Am J Med* 52:584, 1972.
135. Guyton AC et al: A systems analysis approach to understanding long-range arterial blood pressure control and hypertension. *Circ Res* 35:159, 1974.
136. Haas M et al: Catecholamine-stimulated ion transport in duck red cells. Gradient effects in electrically neutral (Na + K + 2Cl) cotransport. *J Gen Physiol* 80:125, 1982.
137. Haddy FJ: Minireview: Potassium and blood vessels. *Life Sci* 16:1489, 1973.
138. Haddy FJ, Overbeck HW: The role of humoral agents in volume expanded hypertension. *Life Sci* 19:935, 1976.
139. Haddy FJ et al: Role of humoral factor in low renin hypertension, in Lichardus B et al (eds): *Hormonal Regulation of Sodium Excretion.* Amsterdam, Elsevier, 1980, p 379.
140. Haddy FJ: What is the link between vascular smooth muscle, sodium pump and hypertension? *Clin Exp Hypertens* 3:179, 1981.
141. Haddy FJ, Scott JB: Mechanism of acute presser action of hypokalemia and hypoosmolality. *Am Heart J* 85:655, 1973.
142. Hamlyn JM et al: A circulating inhibitor of (Na^+-K^+) ATPase associated with essential hypertension. *Nature* 300:650, 1982.
143. Hamlyn JM et al: Digitalis-like activity in human plasma. *J Biol Chem* 264:7395, 1989.
144. Hasstedt SF et al: Hypertension and sodium-lithium countertransport in Utah pedigrees: Evidence for major-locus inheritance. *Am J Hum Genet* 43:14, 1988.
145. Heagerty AM et al: Leucocyte membrane sodium transport in normotensive populations: Dissociation of abnormalities of sodium efflux from raised blood pressure. *Lancet* 2:894, 1982.
146. Hilton PJ: Cellular sodium transport in essential hypertension. *N Engl J Med* 314:222, 1986.
147. Hilton PJ: Factors in influencing leukocyte sodium transport in essential hypertension. *Klin Wochenschr* 63(suppl III):49, 1985.
148. Hofman A et al: Haemodynamic plasma noradrenaline and plasma renin in hypertensive and normotensive teenagers. *Clin Sci* 61:169, 1981.
149. Hollenberg NK et al: The renal vasculature in early essential hypertension: Evidence for a pathogenetic role. *Medicine* 57:167, 1978.
149a. Hollenberg NK, Williams GH: Sodium-sensitive hypertension implications of pathogenesis for therapy. *Am J Hypertens* 2:809, 1989.
150. Holly JMP et al: Re-analysis of data in two Lancet papers on the effect of dietary sodium and potassium on blood pressure. *Lancet* ii:1384, 1981.
151. Hopp L et al: [^{3}H]-ouabain binding of red blood cells in whites and blacks. *Hypertension* 8:1051, 1986.
152. Hunt SC et al: A prospective study of sodium-lithium countertransport and hypertension in Utah. *Hypertension* 17:1, 1991.
153. Hunt SC et al: Associations of three erythrocyte cation transport systems with plasma lipids in Utah subjects. *Hypertension* 8:30, 1986.
154. Ibrahim MM et al: Hyperkinetic heart in severe hypertension: A separate clinical hemodynamic entity. *Am J Cardiol* 35:667, 1975.
155. Ibsen KK et al: Sodium-lithium countertransport in erythrocytes from patients and from children having one hypertensive parent. *Hypertension* 4:703, 1982.
156. Iimura O et al: Studies on hypotensive effect of high potassium intake in patients with essential hypertension. *Clin Sci* 61:77S, 1981.
157. Iimura O et al: Studies on the hypotensive effects of high potassium intake in patients with essential hypertension. *Clin Sci* 61(suppl):77, 1981.
158. Intersalt Cooperative Research Group: Intersalt: An international study of electrolyte excretion and blood pressure. Results for 24 hour urinary sodium and potassium excretion. *Br Med J* 297:319, 1988.
159. Ives HE: Essential hypertension—where are we going? *West J Med* 153:415, 1990.
160. Ives HE et al: Mixed-type inhibition of the renal Na^+-H^+ antiporter by Li^+ and amiloride: Evidence for a modifier site. *J Biol Chem* 258:9710, 1983.
161. Iwai J et al: Influence of thiazide on salt hypertension. *Clin Res* 40(suppl I):I134, 1977.
162. Julius S, Conway J: Hemodynamic studies in patients with borderline blood pressure elevation. *Circulation* 38:282, 1968.
163. Julius S et al: Hyperkinetic stage: A precursor of hypertension. A longitudinal study of borderline hypertension, in Gross F, Strasser T (eds): *Mild Hypertension; Natural History and Management.* Proceedings of the Joint WHO/ISH Meeting, Susono, Japan, Marshfield, MA, Pitman Medical Publishers, 1979, p 116.
164. Kahn AM: Difference between human red blood cell Na^+-Li^+ countertransport and renal Na^+-H^+ exchange. *Hypertension* 9:7, 1987.
165. Kaloyanides GJ et al: Pressure natriuresis in the isolated kidney. *Am J Physiol* 220:1660, 1971.
166. Kaminer B, Lutz WPW: Blood pressure in bushman of the Kalahari Desert. *Circulation* 22:289, 1960.
167. Kaplan NA et al: Potassium supplementation in hypertensive patients with diuretic-induced hypokalemia. *N Engl J Med* 312:746, 1985.
168. Kesteloot H, Joossens JV: Relationship of serum sodium, potassium, calcium and phosphorus with blood pressure. Belgium interuniversity research on nutrition and health. *Hypertension* 12:589, 1988.
169. Katz LN, Linder E: The action of excess sodium, calcium and potassium on the coronary vessels. *Am J Physiol* 124:155, 1938.
170. Kawasaki T et al: The effect of high-sodium and low-sodium intakes on blood pressure and other related variables in human subjects with idiopathic hypertension. *Am J Med* 64:193, 1978.
171. Kean BH: The blood pressure in the Cuna Indians. *Am J Trop Med Hyg* 24:341, 1944.

172. Keith NM, Binger MW: Diuretic action of potassium salts. *JAMA* 105:1584, 1935.
173. Kelly RA, Smith TW: The search for the endogenous digitalis: An alternative hypothesis. *Am J Physiol* 256:C937, 1989.
174. Kesteloot H et al: A comparative study of blood pressure and sodium intake in Belgium and Korea. *Eur J Cardiol* 11:169, 1980.
175. Khaw KT, Thomas S: Randomized double-blind cross-over trial of potassium on blood pressure in normal subjects. *Lancet* 2:1127, 1982.
175a. Khaw KT, Barrett-Conner E: Increasing sensitivity of blood pressure to dietary sodium and potassium with increasing age: A population study using casual urine specimens. *Am J Hypertens* 3:505, 1990.
176. Khaw KT, Barrett-Conner E: Dietary potassium and blood pressure in a population. *Am J Clin Nutr* 39:963, 1984.
176a. Kihara M et al: Interrelationships between blood pressure, sodium, potassium, serum cholesterol, and protein intake in Japanese. *Hypertension* 6:736, 1984.
177. Kirkendall WM et al: The effect of dietary sodium chloride on blood pressure, body fluids, electrolytes, renal function, and serum lipids of normotensive man. *J Lab Clin Med* 87:418, 1976.
178. Koletsky S: Hypertensive vascular disease produced by salt. *Lab Invest* 7:377, 1958.
179. Koletsky S, Goodsitt AM: Natural history and pathogenesis of renal ablation hypertension. *Arch Pathol* 69:654, 1960.
180. Konald P et al: The effect of potassium on the tone of isolated arteries. *Pflueguers Arch* 301:283, 1968.
181. Korner PI: The Sixth Volhard Lecture: Casual and homeostatic factors in hypertension. *Clin Sci* 63(suppl):5S, 1982.
182. Kotchen TA et al: Failure of $NaHCO_3$ and $KHCO_3$ to inhibit renin in the rat. *Am J Physiol* 231:1050, 1976.
183. Krishna GG: Effect of potassium intake on blood pressure. *J Am Soc Nephrol* 1:43, 1990.
184. Krishna GG et al: Mild potassium depletion provokes renal sodium retention. *J Lab Clin Med* 109:724, 1987.
185. Krishna GG et al: Potassium depletion elevates blood pressure in normotensives. *New Engl J Med* 320:1177, 1989.
186. Krishna GG, Kapoor SC: Potassium depletion exacerbates essential hypertension. *Ann Intern Med* 115:77, 1991.
187. Krishna GG et al: Potassium supplementation attenuates mineralocorticoid (MC)-induced hypertension. *J Am Soc Nephrol* (abstract)1:508, 1990.
188. Krishna GG, Kapoor SC: Hypokalemia and hypertension. *N Engl J Med* 321:1413, 1989.
189. Krolewski et al: Predisposition to hypertension and susceptibility to renal disease in insulin-dependent diabetes mellitus. *N Engl J Med* 318:140, 1988.
190. Krzesinski JM, Rorive GL: Effect of salt depletion on sodium ion transport from human erythrocytes. *Klin Wochenschr* 63(suppl III):45, 1985.
191. Kuriama S et al: A higher cellular Na^+ turnover rate in cultured skin fibroblasts from blacks. *Hypertension* 11:301, 1988.
192. Lai S et al: Urinary electrolytes and blood pressure in three Yi farmer populations, China. *Hypertension* 13:22, 1989.
193. Langford HG, Watson RL: Electrolytes and hypertension, in Oglesby P (ed): *Epidemiology and Control of Hypertension.* New York, Straton intercontinental Medical Book, 1975, p 115.
194. Langston JB et al: Effect of changes in salt intake on arterial pressure and renal function in partially nephrectomized dogs. *Circ Res* 12:508, 1963.
195. Laragh JH, Pecker MS: Dietary sodium and essential hypertension: Some myths, hopes and truths. *Ann Intern Med* 98:735, 1983.
196. Lasker N et al: Race and sex differences in erythrocyte Na^+-K^+ and Na^+-K^+-adenosine triphosphatase. *J Clin Invest* 75:1813, 1985.
197. Laurenzi M, Trevisan M: Sodium-lithium countertransport and blood pressure: The Gubbio population study. *Hypertension* 13:408, 1989.
198. Lawton WJ et al: Effect of dietary potassium on blood pressure, renal function, muscle sympathetic nerve activity, and forearm vascular resistance and flow in normotensive and borderline hypertensive humans. *Circulation* 81:173, 1990.
199. Lechi A et al: Increased basal and thrombin-induced free calcium in platelets of essential hypertensive patients. *Hypertension* 9:230, 1987.
200. Ledingham JM, Cohen RD: The role of the heart in the pathogenesis of renal hypertension. *Lancet* 2:979, 1963.
201. Lemann J Jr et al: Potassium bicarbonate but not sodium bicarbonate reduces urinary calcium excretion and improves calcium balance in healthy men. *Kidney Int* 35:688, 1989.
202. Lemann J Jr et al: Potassium administration increases and potassium deprivation reduces urinary calcium excretion in healthy adults. *Kidney Int* 39:973, 1991.
203. Lenel R et al: Arterial hypertension in the chicken. *Am J Physiol* 152:557, 1948.
204. Lennan EJ, Lemann J Jr: The effect of potassium deficient diet on the pattern of recovery from metabolic acidosis. *Clin Sci* 34:365, 1968.
205. Lever AF et al: Sodium and potassium in essential hypertension. *Br Med J* 283:463, 1981.
206. Lifton RP et al: Exclusion of the Na^+-H^+ antiporter as a candidate gene in human essential hypertension. *Hypertension* 17:8, 1991.
207. Lijnen P et al: Sodium and potassium fluxes and concentrations in erythrocytes of normal subjects during prolonged sodium depletion and repletion. *Postgrad Med J* 62(suppl 1):3, 1986.
208. Linas SL, Dickman D: Mechanism of decreased renal blood flow in potassium depleted conscious rat. *Kidney Int* 21:757, 1982.
209. Linas SL, Marzec-Calvert R: Potassium depletion ameliorates hypertension in SHR. *Hypertension* 8:990, 1986.
210. Lindner A et al: Effects of a circulatory factor in patients with essential hypertension on intracellular free calcium in normal platelets. *N Engl J Med* 316:509, 1987.
211. Livne A et al: Increased platelet Na^+-H^+ exchange rates in essential hypertension. Application of a novel test. *Lancet* 1:533, 1987.

212. Ljungman S et al: Blood pressure and renal function. *Acta Med Scand* 208:17, 1980.
213. Ljungman S et al: Sodium excretion and blood pressure. *Hypertension* 3:318, 1981.
214. Llaurado JG, Madden JA: Sodium kinetics in aorta of spontaneously hypertensive rats. *J Appl Physiol* 39:868, 1975.
215. London GM et al: Volume-dependent parameters in essential hypertension. *Kidney Int* 11:204, 1977.
216. Losse H et al: Der wasser-und elektrolygehalt von erythrocyten bie arterieller hypertonie. *Klin Wochenschr* 38:393, 1960.
217. Louis WJ et al: The effects of sodium intake on inherited hypertension in the rat. *Lancet* 2:1283, 1971.
218. Love WD, Burch GE: Plasma and erythrocyte sodium and potassium concentrations in a group of southern white and negro blood donors. *J Lab Clin Med* 41:258, 1953.
219. Lowenstein FW: Blood pressure in relation to age and sex in the tropics and subtropics. A review of the literature and an investigation in two tribes of Brazil Indians. *Lancet* 1:389, 1961.
220. Luft FC et al: Effects of volume expansion and contraction in normotensive whites, blacks and subjects of different ages. *Circulation* 59:643, 1979.
221. Luft FC et al: Cardiovascular and humoral responses to extremes of sodium intake in normal black and white men. *Circulation* 60:697, 1979.
222. Luft FC et al: Plasma and urinary norepinephrine values at extremes of sodium intake in normal man. *Hypertension* 1:261, 1979.
223. Luft FC, Weinberger MH: Sodium intake and essential hypertension. *Hypertension* 4(suppl III):14, 1982.
223a. Luft FC et al: Sodium sensitivity in normotensive human subjects. *Ann Intern Med* 98:758, 1983.
224. Luke RG et al: Effect of potassium depletion on renin release. *Kidney Int* 21:14, 1982.
225. Lund-Johansen P: Hemodynamics of primary hypertension, in Amery A et al (eds): *Hypertensive Cardiovascular Disease: Pathophysiology and Treatment.* Boston, Martinus Nijhoff Publishers, 1982, p 377.
226. MacGregor GA et al: Moderate potassium supplementation in essential hypertension. *Lancet* 2:567, 1982.
227. Maddocks I: Blood pressure in Melanesians. *Med J Aust* 1:1123, 1967.
227a. Mangili R et al: Increased sodium-lithium countertransport activity in red cells of patients with insulin-dependent diabetes and nephropathy. *N Engl J Med* 318:146, 1988.
228. Margolius HS et al: Relationships among urinary kallikrein, mineralocorticoids and human hypertensive disease. *Fed Proc* 35:203, 1976.
229. Mark AL et al: Effect of high and low sodium intake on arterial pressure and forearm vascular resistance in borderline hypertension. A preliminary report. *Circ Res* 36/37(suppl 1):194, 1975.
230. Mark AL et al: Mechanisms of the antihypertensive action of high dietary potassium, abstracted. *Clin Res* 29:525A, 1981.
230a. McCarron DA: Calcium metabolism and hypertension. *Kidney Int* 35:717, 1989.
231. McDonald AM et al: Sodium-lithium countertransport and blood pressure control by nutritonal intervention in mild hypertension. *J Hypertens* 6:283, 1988.
232. McQuarrie I et al: Effects of excessive ingestion of sodium and potassium salts on carbohydrate metabolism and blood pressure in diabetic children. *J Nutr* 11:77, 1935.
233. Meneely GR, Ball COT: Experimental epidemiology of chronic sodium chloride toxicity and the protective effect of potassium chloride. *Am J Med* 25:713, 1958.
234. Meneely GR et al: Chronic sodium chloride toxicity. The protective effect of added potassium chloride. *Proc Soc Exp Biol Med* 47:263, 1958.
235. Meneely GR, Dahl LK: Electrolytes in hypertension. The effects of sodium chloride. *Med Clin North Am* 45:271, 1961.
236. Meneely GR, Battarbee HD: High sodium and low potassium environment and hypertension. *Am J Cardiol* 38:768, 1976.
237. Messerly FH et al: Systemic and regional hemodynamics in low, normal, and high cardiac output in borderline hypertension. *Circulation* 58:441, 1978.
238. Miall WE: Follow-up study of arterial pressure in the population of a Welsh mining valley. *Br Med J* 2:1201, 1959.
239. Mickelson O et al: Sodium and potassium intakes and excretions of normal men consuming sodium chloride of a 1:1 mixture of sodium and potassium chloride. *Am J Clin Nutr* 30:2033, 1977.
240. Miller JZ et al: Blood pressure response to potassium supplementation in normotensive adults and children. *Hypertension* 10:437, 1953.
240a. Miller JZ et al: Heterogeneity of blood pressure response to dietary sodium restriction in normotensive adults. *J Chronic Dis* 40:245, 1987.
241. Mitsufashi T, Ives HE: Intracellular Ca^{2+} requirement for activating the Na^+-H^+ exchange in vascular smooth muscle cells. *J Biol Chem* 263:8790, 1987.
242. Montanari A et al: Altered sodium efflux in red blood cells from essential hypertensive subjects, in Zumkley H, Losse H (eds): *Intracellular Electrolytes and Arterial Hypertension.* Stuttgart, George Thieme Verlag, 1980, p 135.
243. Montenay-Garestier T et al: Evidence for structural changes in erythrocyte membranes of SHR: A fluorescence polarization study. *Biochem Biophys Res Commun* 100:660, 1981.
244. Motulsky AG et al: Hypertension and the genetics of red cell membrane abnormalities, in Bock G et al (eds): *Molecular Approaches to Human Polygenic Disease.* Chichester, UK, Wiley, 1987, p 150.
245. Munro-Faure AD et al: Ethnic differences in human blood cell sodium concentration. *Nature* 231:457, 1971.
246. Myers JB et al: Effect of acute and chronic salt loading on erythrocyte ^{22}Na efflux in males with essential hypertension. *Clin Sci* 61:378, 1981.
247. National Center for Heart Statistics: Hypertension and hypertensive heart disease in adults. *Vital and Health Statistics Series* 11, no. 13, USGPO, Washington, DC, 1966.
248. Nolan CR, Linas SL: Mechanism of antihypertensive

effect of potassium depletion in renovascular hypertension. *Am J Physiol* 255:H1181, 1988.
249. Oldham PD et al: The nature of essential hypertension. *Lancet* 1:1085, 1960.
250. Oliver WJ et al: Blood pressure, sodium, intake and sodium related hormones in the Yanomamo Indians, a "no-salt" culture. *Circulation* 52:146, 1975.
251. Onesti G et al: Blood pressure regulation in end-stage renal disease and anephric man. *Clin Res* 36/37(suppl I):I145, 1975.
252. Overbeck HW: Vascular responses to cations, osmolality, and angiotensin in renal hypertensive dogs. *Am J Physiol* 223:1358, 1972.
253. Overbeck HW et al: Attenuated vasodilator responses to K^+ in essential hypertensive men. *J Clin Invest* 53:678,1974.
254. Overbeck HW, Clark DWJ: Vasodilator responses to K^+ in genetic hypertensive and in renal hypertensive rats. *J Lab Clin Med* 86:973, 1975.
255. Overbeck HW et al: Depressed function of an ouabain-sensitive sodium potassium pump in blood vessels from renal hypertensive dogs. *Circ Res* 38(suppl II):II-48, 1976.
256. Overbeck HW et al: Sodium pump activity in arteries of Dahl salt-sensitive rats. *Hypertension* 3:306, 1981.
257. Overbeck HW et al: Function of the sodium pump in arterial smooth muscle in experimental hypertension. Role of pressure. *Hypertension* 4:394, 1982.
258. Owen NE: Regulation of Na^+-K^+-Cl^- cotransport in vascular smooth muscle cells. *Biochem Biophys Res Comm* 125:500, 1984.
259. Page LB et al: Antecedents of cardiovascular disease in six Solomon Islands societies. *Circulation* 49:1132, 1974.
260. Palfrey HC, Greengard P: Hormone-sensitive ion transport systems in erythrocytes as models for epithelial ion pathways. *Ann NY Acad Sci* 372:291, 1981.
261. Paller MS et al: Mechanism of decreased vascular reactivity to angiotensin II in conscious potassium-deficient rats. *J Clin Invest* 73:79, 1984.
262. Pamnani M et al: Studies on the role of a humoral sodium transport inhibitor and the anteroventral third ventricle (AV_3V) in experimental low renin hypertension. *Clin Sci* 61:578, 1981.
263. Parfrey PS et al: Blood pressure and hormonal changes following alteration in dietary sodium and potassium in mild essential hypertension. *Lancet* i:113, 1981.
264. Perera GA: Depressor effects of potassium deficient diets in hypertensive men. *J Clin Invest* 32:633, 1953.
265. Pfeffer MA et al: Development of SHR hypertension and cardiac hypertrophy during prolonged beta-blockade. *Am J Physiol* 232:H639, 1977.
266. Postnov YV et al: Altered permeability of the erythrocyte membrane for sodium and potassium ions in spontaneously hypertensive rats. *Pfluegers Arch* 365:257, 1976.
267. Postnov YV et al: Altered sodium permeability, calcium binding and Na-K-ATPase activity in the red blood cell membrane in essential hypertension. *Pfluegers Arch* 371:263, 1977.
268. Postnov YV, Orlov SN: Ion transport across plasma membrane in primary hypertension. *Physiol Rev* 65:904, 1985.
269. Poston L et al: The effect of antihypertensive therapy on abnormal leucocyte sodium transport in essential hypertension. *Clin Exp Hypertens* 3:693, 1981.
270. Poston L et al: Evidence for a circulating sodium transport inhibitor in essential hypertension. *Br Med J* 282:847, 1981.
271. Pratt JH et al: Racial differences in aldosterone excretion and plasma aldosterone concentrations in children. *N Engl J Med* 321:1152, 1989.
272. Prior AM et al: Sodium intake and blood pressure in two Polynesian populations. *N Engl J Med* 279:515, 1968.
273. Raij L et al: High potassium diet augments endothelium dependent relaxations in Dahl rat. *Hypertension* 12:562, 1988.
274. Reed D et al: Diet, blood pressure and multicollinearity. *Hypertension* 7:405, 1985.
275. Richards AM et al: Blood pressure response to moderate sodium restriction and to potassium supplementation in mild essential hypertension. *Lancet* 1:757, 1984.
276. Ringel RE et al: Red cell cotransport activity and Na content in black males: Relationship to essential hypertension. *Hypertension* 6:724, 1984.
277. Ringel RE et al: Red blood cell Na^+-K^+-ATPase in men with newly diagnosed or previously treated essential hypertension. *Hypertension* 9:437, 1987.
278. Rosati C et al: Sodium transport kinetics in erythrocytes from spontaneously hypertensive rats. *Hypertension* 11:41, 1988.
279. Rosenman RH et al: Effect of varying dietary potassium upon the blood pressure of hypertensive rats. *Am J Physiol* 175:386, 1953.
280. Rygielski D et al: Erythrocyte ghost Na^+-K^+-ATPase and blood pressure. *Hypertension* 10:259, 1987.
281. Sannerstedt R: Hemodynamic response to exercise in patients with arterial hypertension. *Acta Med Scand* 180(suppl 458):1, 1966.
282. Sapirstein LA et al: Production of hypertension in the rat by substituting hypertonic sodium chloride for drinking water. *Proc Soc Exp Biol Med* 73:82, 1950.
283. Sasaki N: High blood pressure and the salt intake of the Japanese. *Jpn Heart J* 3:313, 1962.
284. Saunders GM, Bancroft H: Blood pressure studies on Negro and white men and women living in Virgin Islands of the United States. *Am Heart J* 23:410, 1942.
285. Schmooder RL, Weder AB: Platelet sodium-proton exchange is increased in essential hypertension. *J Hypertens* 7:325, 1989.
286. Sealey JE et al: Potassium balance and the control of renin secretion. *J Clin Invest* 49:2119, 1970.
287. Seifter JL, Aronson PS: Properties and physiologic roles of the plasma membrane sodium-hydrogen exchanger. *J Clin Invest* 78:859, 1986.
288. Selkurt EE: Effect of pulse pressure and mean arterial pressure modification of renal hemodynamics and electrolyte and water excretion. *Circulation* 4:541, 1951.
289. Semplicini A et al: Red blood cell Na/H and Li/Na exchange in patients with essential hypertension. *Am J Hypertens* 2:903, 1989.
290. Shade RE et al: Effects of renal arterial infusion of so-

dium and potassium on renin secretion in the dog. *Circ Res* 31:719, 1972.

291. Shaper AG: Cardiovascular disease in the tropics: III. Blood pressure and hypertension. *Br Med J* 3:805, 1972.
292. Shennan DB, Chipperfield AR: The dependence on chloride ions of the loop diuretic sensitive component of passive sodium efflux from human red cells. *Pflugers Arch* 406:333, 1986.
293. Shipley RE, Study RS: Changes in renal blood flow, extraction of inulin, glomerular filtration rate, tissue pressure and urine flow with acute alterations of renal artery blood pressure. *Am J Physiol* 167:676, 1951.
294. Siani A et al: Controlled trial of long term oral potassium supplements in patients with mild hypertension. *Br Med J* 294:1453, 1987.
295. Simpson FO et al: Relationship of blood pressure to sodium excretion in a population survey. *Clin Sci* 55(suppl 4):373, 1978.
296. Sinnett PF, Whyte HM: Epidemiological studies in a total highland population, Tukisenta, New Guinea: Cardiovascular disease and relevant clinical, electrocardiographic, radiological and biochemical findings. *J Chronic Dis* 26:265, 1973.
297. Skrabal F et al: Effects of moderate salt restriction and high potassium intake on pressor hormone response to noradrenaline and baroreceptor function in man. *Clin Sci* 59:157S, 1980.
297a. Skrambal F et al: Inherited salt sensitivity in normotensive humans as a cause of essential hypertension: A new concept. *J Cardiovasc Pharmacol* 6:S215, 1984.
298. Smith JB et al: Three red cell sodium transport systems in hypertensive and normotensive adults. *Hypertension* 6:159, 1984.
298a. Smith WCS et al: Urinary electrolyte excretion, alcohol consumption, and blood pressure in the Scottish heart health study. *Br Med J* 297:329, 1988.
299. Smith SJ et al: Moderate potassium chloride supplementation in essential hypertension: Is it addictive to moderate sodium restriction? *Br Med J* 290:110, 1985.
300. Suzuki H et al: Effect of potassium chloride on the blood pressure in two-kidney, one-clip Goldblatt hypertensive rats. *Hypertension* 3:566, 1981.
301. Svetkey LP et al: Double-blind placebo controlled trial of potassium chloride in the treatment of mild hypertension. *Hypertension* 9:444, 1987.
302. Swales JD: Functional disturbances of the cell membrane in hypertension. *J Hypertens* 8(suppl 7):S203, 1990.
303. Swartz HG et al: Cation fluxes in Na^+-K^+-activated ATPase activity in erythrocytes of patients with essential hypertension. *Hypertension* 3:641, 1981.
304. Tabuchi Y et al: Hypotensive mechanism of potassium supplementation in salt-loaded patients with essential hypertension. *J Clin Hypertens* 2:145, 1985.
305. Takahashi E et al: The geographic distribution of cerebral hemorrhage and hypertension in Japan. *Hum Biol* 29:139, 1957.
306. Tarazi RC et al: Hemodynamic characteristics of primary aldosteronism. *N Engl J Med* 289:1330, 1973.
307. Tarazi RC: Hemodynamic role of extracellular fluid in hypertension. *Circ Res* (suppl 11):72, 1976.
308. Tarazi RC: The hemodynamics of hypertension, in Genest J et al (eds): *Hypertension,* 2d ed. New York, McGraw-Hill, 1983, p 15.
309. Tobian L, Binion JT: Tissue cations and water in arterial hypertension. *Circulation* 5:754, 1952.
310. Tobian L et al: Relationship of cytoplasmic granules in renal papillary interstitial cells to "post-salt" hypertension. *J Lab Clin Med* 73:309, 1969.
311. Tobian L et al: Reduction of natriuretic capacity and renin release in isolated blood-perfused kidneys of Dahl hypertension-prone rats. *Circ Res* 43(suppl I):I92, 1978.
312. Tobian L et al: Prevention with thiazide of NaCl-induced hypertension in Dahl "S" rats: Evidence for a Na-retaining humoral agent in "S" rats. *Hypertension* 1:316, 1979.
313. Tosteson DC et al: Membranes, ions and hypertension. *Clin Sci* 61(suppl):5S, 1981.
314. Treasure J et al: Dietary K^+ and the development of hypertension in two kidney, one clip Goldblatt hypertensive rats. *Hypertension* 5:521, 1983.
315. Treasure J, Ploth D: Role of dietary potassium in the treatment of hypertension. *Hypertension* 5:864, 1983.
316. Trevisan M et al: Dietary sodium erythrocyte sodium concentration, sodium-stimulated lithium efflux and blood pressure. *Clin Sci* 61:295, 1981.
317. Trevisan M et al: Abnormal red cell ion transport and hypertension. The People's Gas Study. *Hypertension* 5:363, 1983.
318. Tuck ML et al: Identification of the Na^+,K^+ cotransport in vascular tissue. *Clin Res* 30:94A, 1982.
319. Tuck ML et al: Inhibitory action of norepinephrine on sodium transport in vascular smooth muscle cells in culture. Abst 9th International Meeting International Society of Hypertension, 1982.
320. Tuck ML et al: Erythrocyte Na^+,K^+ cotransport and Na^+,K^+ pump in black and caucasian hypertensive patients. *Hypertension* 6:536, 1984.
321. Tuck ML et al: Kinetic analysis of erythrocyte Na^+-K^+ pump and cotransport in essential hypertension. *Hypertension* 10:204, 1987.
322. Tuck ML et al: Inhibitory action of norepinephrine on sodium transport in vascular smooth muscle cells in culture. *Eur J Physiol* 74:1067, 1989.
323. Turner ST et al: Sodium-lithium countertransport in ambulatory hypertensive and normotensive patients. *Hypertension* 9:24, 1987.
324. Turner ST et al: Sodium-lithium countertransport and blood pressure in healthy blood donors. *Hypertension* 7:955, 1985.
325. Ueshima H et al: Hypertension, salt and potassium. *Lancet* 1:504, 1981.
326. Vander AJ: Direct effects of potassium on renin secretion and renal function. *Am J Physiol* 219:455, 1970.
327. Vatner SF et al: Effects of a digitalis glycoside on coronary and systemic dynamics in conscious dogs. *Circ Res* 28:470, 1971.
328. Walker WG et al: Relation between blood pressure and renin, renin substrate, angiotensin II, aldosterone and urinary sodium and potassium in 574 ambulatory subjects. *Hypertension* 1:287, 1979.

329. Walter U, Distler A: Abnormal sodium efflux in erythrocytes of patients with essential hypertension. *Hypertension* 4:205, 1982.
330. Watson RL et al: Urinary electrolytes, body weight and blood pressure: Pooled cross-sectional results among four groups of adolescent females. *Hypertension* 2(suppl 1):93, 1980.
331. Wauquier I et al: Endogenous digitalis-like circulating substances in spontaneously hypertensive rats. *Hypertension* 12:108, 1988.
332. Weder AB et al: Racial differences in erythrocyte cation transport. *Hypertension* 61:115, 1984.
332a. Weinberger MH et al: Definitions and characteristics of sodium sensitivity and blood pressure resistance. *Hypertension* 8(suppl III):II127, 1986.
333. Weder AB: Membrane sodium transport and salt sensitivity of blood pressure. *Hypertension* 17(suppl 1):I74, 1991.
334. Weder AB: Red cell lithium-sodium countertransport and renal lithium clearance in hypertension. *N Engl J Med* 314:198, 1986.
335. Weder AB et al: Red blood cell Li^+-Na^+ countertransport, Na^+-K^+ cotransport, and the hemodynamics of hypertension. *Hypertension* 9:459, 1987.
336. Weinman EJ et al: Regulation of the renal Na^+-H^+ exchanger by protein phosphorylation. *Kidney Int* 36:519, 1989.
337. Weiss YA et al: Repeat hemodynamic determination in borderline hypertension. *Am J Med* 64:382, 1978.
338. Werko L, Lagerlof H: Studies of the circulation in man: IV. Cardiac output and blood pressure in the right auricle, right ventricle, and pulmonary artery in patients with hypertensive cadiovascular disease. *Acta Med Scand* 133:427, 1949.
339. Wessels F et al: Untersuchungen zur frage des zusammenhangis zwischen katioenpermeabilitat der erythrozyten and hochdruckdis-position. *Kreislauf* 50:415, 1970.
340. Wessels F Zumkley H: Sodium metabolism of RBC in hypertensive patients, in Zumkley H, Losse H (eds): *Intracellular Electrolytes and Arterial Hypertension.* Stuttgart, George Thieme Verlag, 1980, p 59.
341. Wiley JS, Cooper RA: A furosemide-sensitive cotransport of sodium plus potassium in the human red cell. *J Clin Invest* 53:745, 1974.
342. Wiley JS et al: Erythrocyte cation cotransport and countertransport in essential hypertension. *Hypertension* 6:360, 1984.
343. Williams RR et al: Familial dyslipidemic hypertension: Evidence from 58 Utah families for a syndrome present in approximately 15% of patients with essential hypertension. *JAMA* 259:3579, 1988.
344. Williams RR et al: Sodium-lithium countertransport in erythrocytes of hypertension prone families in Utah. *Am J Epidemiol* 118:338, 1983.
345. Willis T: *Pharmaceutica Rationalis.* London, C Dring, C Herper, J Leigh, 1649, p 74.
346. Witteman JCM et al: A prospective study of nutritional factors and hypertension among US women. *Circulation* 80:1320, 1989.
347. Woods JW et al: Increased red-cell sodium-lithium countertransport in normotensive sons of hypertensive parents. *N Engl J Med* 306:593, 1982.
348. Woods KL et al: Racial differences in red cell cation transport and their relationship to essential hypertension. *Clin Exp Hypertens* 3:655, 1981.
349. Workman ML, Paller MS: Cardiovascular and endocrine effects of potassium in spontaneously hypertensive rats. *Am J Physiol* 249:H907, 1985.
350. Wright FS et al: Potassium secretion by distal tubule after potassium adaptation. *Am J Physiol* 221:437, 1971.
351. Yamori Y et al: Hypertension and diet: Multiple regression analysis in a Japanese farming community. *Lancet* 1:1204, 1981.
352. Young DB et al: The natriuretic and hypotensive effects of potassium. *Circ Res* 38(suppl II):II84, 1976.
353. Zidek W et al: Intracellular Na^+ + Ca^{++} activities in essential hypertension. *Res Exp Med* 181:22, 1982.

CHAPTER 49

Hypertensive states: associated fluid and electrolyte disturbances

Gordon H. Williams • Robert G. Dluhy

Hypertension is a common cause of altered electrolyte and water homeostasis. The mechanisms by which hypertension is produced are incompletely understood. Since elevated blood pressure may result from a derangement in volume-homeostatic forces, the kidneys and cardiovascular system are critical components in maintaining blood pressure in the normal range. Cardiovascular and renal responses are modulated by a variety of agents, such as aldosterone, antidiuretic hormone (ADH), angiotensin II, and the catecholamines.

This chapter deals with the normal regulation of blood pressure and with the changes occurring in various hypertensive states that can produce electrolyte or volume abnormalities.

BASIC CONSIDERATIONS

The cardiovascular system comprises two elements: a system of channels for the distribution of fluid to supply the metabolic needs of the body's tissues and a pump that induces flow in this system. Derangement of the normal state of either element can change electrolyte, acid-base, and water balance. The changes result directly from deficiencies in the cardiovascular system and indirectly from the impact of these deficiencies on the function of other organ systems.

THE ROLE OF THE HEART AS A PUMP IN MAINTAINING NORMAL ELECTROLYTE BALANCE

The physiologic functions of the various organ systems of the body depend on cardiac output. Cardiac output, in turn, depends on four interrelated factors: (1) myocardial contractile state (contractility, inotropic state, or the position on the heart's force-velocity curve); (2) preload (the length of cardiac muscle at the onset of contraction); (3) afterload (the tension that the muscle is called upon to develop during contraction); and (4) heart rate. The contractile force can be defined in terms of the maximal velocity of shortening of the muscle fiber; the maximal velocity of shortening with zero load is a sensitive index of contractility. Agents that increase this maximal velocity, and thereby increase myocardial contractility, are termed *positive inotropic agents*. Starling, in 1918,[130] showed that the strength of contraction of myocardium also depends on the degree of stretch of the muscle fiber prior to contraction. The Starling relationship is an intrinsic regulatory system that permits the heart to respond with greater contractile force to an augmented work load, which increases the stretch on the myocardial fibers. This is an effective way to maintain circulatory integrity. However, when the load increases beyond the ability of the ventricle to respond, end-diastolic ventricular pressure rises and cardiac output falls.

Myocardial contractility can be altered by a variety of extrinsic factors. The cardiac sympathetic innervation is probably the single most important mechanism available to the heart for increasing myocardial contractility. Exogenous inotropic agents similarly improve the basic myocardial force-velocity relationship; they include the cardiac glycosides, isoproterenol, calcium, and caffeine. Normal hydrogen ion concentration in conjunction with normal P_{O_2} and P_{CO_2} are necessary for optimal myocardial contractility. Acidosis, hypercapnia, and hypoxia depress myocardial contractility. Loss of function of part of the myocardium—e.g., post-myocardial infarction—results in depression of overall myocardial contractility. Also, in congestive heart failure the fundamental mechanism necessary for optimal contractility is depressed. The cause of this depression is not known.

CARDIOVASCULAR EFFECTS ON WATER AND ELECTROLYTE METABOLISM MEDIATED THROUGH THE KIDNEY

The kidney is the organ of primary importance in electrolyte and water homeostasis. Sodium is the predominant osmotically active ion in the extracellular fluid (ECF); therefore, regulation of ECF volume is achieved by regulating sodium content. This is determined by the amount of sodium presented to, and reabsorbed by, the renal tubules. The first step in the formation of urine is the filtration of blood at the glomerulus. The glomerular filtration rate (GFR) can be controlled within certain limits by intrinsic renal mechanisms—i.e., afferent and efferent arteriolar resistances—but ultimately it depends on the amount of blood pumped to the kidney. When cardiac output decreases, a proportionately greater decrease in flow occurs in the kidney than in other organs. However, intrinsic renal mechanisms maintain a near-normal GFR until the renal blood flow is severely restricted; as the renal blood flow decreases, there is an increase in the postglomerular resistance, which maintains the GFR. This intrinsic regulation is independent of nervous stimuli, as the denervated kidney shows a similar response. The maintenance of a normal filtration rate with a decreased plasma flow increases the filtration fraction; this change may be significant in congestive heart failure.

The bulk of the sodium in the glomerular filtrate is reabsorbed in the proximal tubule, where fractional reabsorption usually parallels the filtered load. This phenomenon is termed *glomerular-tubular balance* (see Chaps. 3 and 18). Distal sodium transport involves a much smaller fraction of filtered sodium, and is modulated by hormones. In the distal collecting duct sodium reabsorption is rate-limiting; if the quantity of sodium entering the duct is not too large, virtually all of it can be removed from the urine.

Because only a small fraction of the sodium filtered by the glomerulus is finally excreted in the urine, a slight increase in the filtration rate could supply enough additional sodium to double or triple the sodium excretion if no alterations in tubular handling of sodium occurred.

In the normal state, changes in filtration rate have little effect on sodium excretion, because a concomitant change in the tubular reabsorption of sodium occurs to maintain sodium homeostasis. The exact balance achieved has been amply illustrated by Mueller and coworkers[98] in experiments on dogs, in which urine was collected separately from each kidney. If a constricting band is placed around one renal artery, there is a marked decrease in the amount of sodium excreted by the constricted kidney. Sodium balance is maintained by the contralateral normal kidney, which increases its sodium excretion. However, if the normal kidney is then removed, adjustments take place in the experimental kidney that permit sodium reabsorption to compensate fully for the decrease in glomerular filtration. Several extra-renal factors—for example, the adrenal cortical hormones—may play a role in this process.

Potassium profoundly affects cardiac contractility and rhythm (see Chaps. 6, 7, 22, and 23). The level of serum potassium is regulated in part by the kidney. Tubular reabsorption of potassium occurs largely in the proximal tubule. Then, distally, under the influence of aldosterone, potassium is secreted in exchange for sodium. Secretion obviously depends on how much sodium is delivered to the distal site for exchange. It also depends on the capacity of the exchange mechanism itself, as well as on the rate of secretion of hydrogen ion by the tubule; increased hydrogen ion secretion tends to decrease tubular excretion of potassium, and vice versa.

The ability to excrete a water load depends on the integrity of the diluting mechanism of the kidney (see Chap. 5). This is partly a function of hormonal factors and partly a function of intrinsic renal factors. A dilute urine can be formed only if adequate amounts of sodium and water are delivered to the diluting segments of the nephron.

REGULATION OF THE RENIN-ANGIOTENSIN-ALDOSTERONE AXIS

The renin-angiotensin-aldosterone axis is the hormonal system most extensively studied in relation to hypertension, since this system can modulate both sodium and volume homeostasis and vasoconstrictor activity. (For a detailed review of the renin-angiotensin system, see Chap. 16.) Thus, an abnormal increase in the responsiveness or the level of activiation of this system can raise blood pressure by altering either volume or vasoconstriction, or both. Abnormal function of this system may also derange potassium balance. The renin-angiotensin system serves both paracrine and endocrine roles. Recent studies have documented the presence of components of the renin-angiotensin system in a variety of tissues.[18,40] In some cases (e.g., the adrenal) all the components necessary to synthesize angiotensin II are found within a single cell.[77] In other tissues individual components of this system are found in different cells located in close proximity; therefore, the production of angiotensin II occurs in the extracellular milieu. The tissues in which the local system has been documented include the heart, vascular smooth muscle, brain, testes, uterus, and adrenal glomerulosa.[40] The exact function (or functions) of these paracrine renin-angiotensin systems is (or are) unclear; it is likely that they serve a role in the local regulation of function of the particular tissue. Derangements in this system have been suggested to be involved in the pathogenesis of vascular smooth muscle and cardiac hypertrophy, as well as in abnormalities in aldosterone secretion.[38]

Much more extensively evaluated is the circulating, or endocrine, renin-angiotensin system.

Renin-angiotensin physiology

Renin is a proteolytic enzyme with a molecular weight of 37,000 to 40,000. (See Chap. 16.) Renin is a member of the aspartyl protease superfamily, which includes proteases such as pepsin, cathepsin D, and chymosin.[96] However, unlike these other proteases, renin is active at neutral pH and has high specificity for its substrate, angiotensinogen.

The renin gene has been cloned and sequenced and is composed of 10 exons separated by 9 introns spanning 11 kb of DNA.[63] The product of the renin gene, when translated, results in preprorenin. The subsequent removal of a 23-amino-acid signal prosequence and glycosylation during transfer to the endoplasmic reticulum results in the 47 = kd prorenin molecule.[113] Prorenin is largely devoid of renin catalytic activity, because of inhibition of the active site by the pro-segment. This prorenin is packaged into secretory granules where it is either secreted constitutively or further processed to active renin, which is secreted in a regulated manner. Circulating prorenin remains largely unchanged, although some authors have suggested that it can serve as a reservoir for the generation of active renin in peripheral tissues.[38] Renin is produced and stored in granules in the juxtaglomerular (JG) cells surrounding the afferent arterioles of the cortical glomeruli. Various inhibitors of intrarenal renin formation are believed to exist. The JG apparatus consists of both the JG cells and the cells of the macula densa; the latter area also contains renin. Renin acts on the basic substrate angiotensinogen, a circulating alpha$_2$-globulin made in the liver, to form the decapeptide angiotensin I (Fig. 49–1). Angiotensin I is then converted by angiotensin-converting enzymes (located mainly in the lung) to the octapeptide angiotensin II by splitting off of the two carboxy-terminal amino acids.[17] Angiotensin II is the most potent circulating pressor compound (on a mole-for-mole basis) made in the body;[55] it acts directly on arteriolar smooth muscle. In addition, angiotensin II stimulates the zona glomerulosa of the adrenal cortex to produce aldosterone.[100,156] Various peptidases in tissues, vessel walls, and circulating plasma collectively called *angiotensinases* are responsible for the biochemical degradation of circulating angiotensin II. Angiotensinases destroy angiotensin II rapidly (half-life approximately 1 min); the half-life of renin is longer (10 to 20 min).

In general, renin secretion is controlled by both intrarenal factors (such as pulse pressure, catecholamines, and angiotensin II) and extrarenal factors (such as sodium, chloride, calcium, and potassium) (Table 49–1). For the most part these are interdependent; the amount of renin released reflects the input of both types of controls.[156] The JG cells, which are specialized myoepithelial cells cuffing the afferent arterioles, act as miniature pressure transducers, sensing renal perfusion pressure through corresponding changes in afferent arteriolar walls. For example, if circulating blood pressure is reduced there will be a corresponding reduction in renal perfusion pressure and, therefore, in afferent arteriolar pressure (Fig. 49–1). This is perceived by the JG cells as decreased stretch exerted on the afferent arteriolar walls. The JG cells then release increasing quantities of renin into the kidney circulation, leading to the formation of angiotensin I. Angiotensin I leaves the kidney by both renal lymphatic and renal venous outflow. It is converted into angiotensin II and stimulates aldosterone release from the adrenal cortex. Rising plasma levels of aldosterone stimulate renal sodium retention and thus result in expansion of ECF volume, which dampens the initiating signal for renin release. Within this context, the renin-angiotensin-aldosterone system subserves volume control by appropriate modifications of renal tubular sodium transport.

Independently of changes in renal perfusion pressure, angiotensin II has been shown to directly inhibit the release of renin (by the so-called short feedback loop).

FIGURE 49-1 • Normal human renin-angiotensin-aldosterone volume regulation.

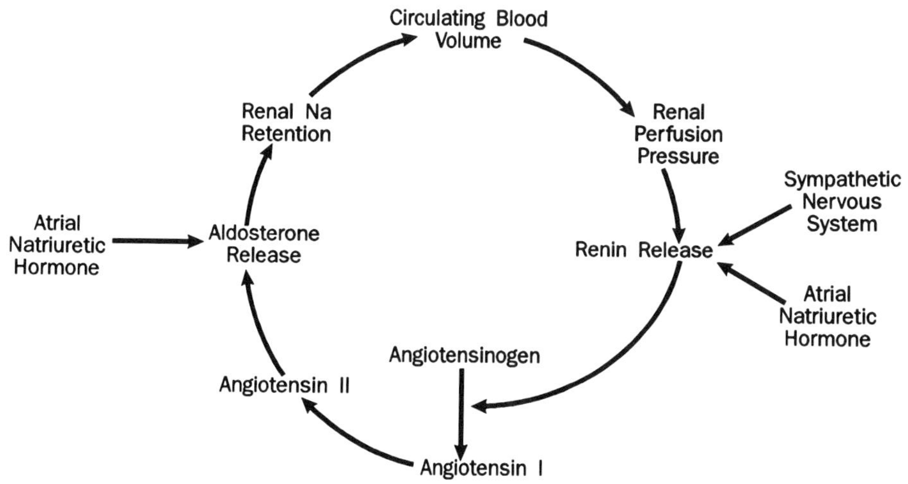

TABLE 49-1 • Factors regulating renin secretion

Factors	Effects on renin secretion
Sodium chloride delivery to the macula densa	
Increase	Inhibit
Decrease	Stimulate
Renal perfusion pressure	
Increase	Inhibit
Decrease	Stimulate
Sympathetic nervous system	
Beta-adrenergic stimulation	Stimulate
Alpha-adrenergic stimulation	Inhibit
Plasma electrolytes	
Potassium	Inhibit
Calcium	Inhibit
Hormones	
Angiotensin II	Inhibit
Prostaglandins (PGI_2)	Stimulate
Dopamine	Inhibit
Atrial natriuretic hormone (ANH)	Inhibit
Vasopressin	Inhibit
ACTH	Stimulate

Infusion of angiotensin II at subpressor concentrations in sodium-restricted normal human beings reduces renin levels at measured angiotensin II concentrations within the physiologic range. This action, which is mediated by increases in cytosolic calcium,[25] probably accounts in part for the rise in renin levels observed when angiotensin II levels are lowered by converting enzyme inhibitor treatment.[52]

A second control mechanism for renin release centers in the *macula densa cells.* These are a group of special-staining, distal convoluted tubular epithelial cells found in direct opposition to the JG cells. It has been suggested that they may function as chemoreceptors, monitoring the sodium load presented to the distal tubule and to the JG cells, where appropriate modifications in renin release take place. Alternatively, these cells have been postulated to sense changes in chloride rather than sodium flux. Kotchen and colleagues have shown that chloride depletion stimulates renin release in rats; and studies in canines show that the infusion of non-sodium-containing chloride salts suppresses renin release.[78,82] Additionally, in normal human subjects, severe selective chloride restriction has been shown to elevate plasma renin activity (PRA).[81] This macula densa intrarenal renin-releasing mechanism is postulated to operate independently of changes in renal perfusion pressure. If increased filtered sodium (?chloride) were delivered to the macula densa, feedback would occur to the JG apparatus, which would result in the release of increasing quantities of renin. This would act to decrease GFR, thereby reducing the filtered load of sodium. The evidence on this hypothesis is conflicting.[140]

The sympathetic nervous system is also a significant regulator of renin release.[140,156] Infusion of catecholamines directly into the renal artery or electrical stimulation of renal nerves increases renin release. Conversely, alpha- or beta-adrenergic blockade can block the renin response to upright posture or acute volume depletion.[74] The mechanism by which sympathetic activity alters renin secretion is not known; present evidence suggests that catecholamines have a direct effect on the JG cells (an action involving the formation of cAMP). Dopamine may also inhibit renin release, since the administration of the dopamine antagonist metoclopramide increases plasma renin levels.[56]

Renal prostaglandins—especially PGI_2, produced in the preglomerular endothelial cells—increase renin secretion.[8] Inhibition of prostaglandin synthesis with indomethacin also reduces renin secretion in response to sodium depletion.[34]

A number of circulating factors may alter renin release. Increasing dietary potassium can decrease renin release; decreasing potassium intake increases renin release.[13,25,62,64] These effects are not secondary to potassium-stimulated aldosterone secretion with an alteration in sodium balance, because similar renin responses occur with subjects on a low sodium intake. In addition, direct infusion of potassium into the renal artery also reduces renin release. In-vitro studies support a direct effect of potassium on the release of renin. The significance of the potassium effect is unclear. Calcium may also play an important role in the regulation of renin release, with extracellular calcium directly inhibiting renin secretion both in vitro and in vivo.[48,83] The calcium ionophore A23187 has been shown to increase renin release from isolated glomeruli and from isolated perfused rat kidneys in a dose-dependent fashion. If isolated glomeruli are incubated in a calcium-free medium, renin is still released, suggesting that the mechanisms mediating renin release depend on, or involve, a primary change in intracellular calcium concentration.

Increased levels of atrial natriuretic hormone (ANH), within the physiologic range, also inhibit the secretion of renin.[125] Thus, the increased levels of ANH seen following acute salt loading may contribute to the suppression of renin that follows volume expansion. There is also some evidence that adrenocorticotropic hormone (ACTH) may increase, and vasopressin (ADH) can inhibit renin release.[74] Thus, the control of renal renin release is complex, consisting of both intrarenal and extrarenal mechanisms. Renin secretion at any moment probably reflects the interaction of all these factors; the intrarenal mechanism probably predominates.

Mineralocorticoid physiology

The major mineralocorticoid produced by the human adrenal cortex is aldosterone.[156] Other mineralocorticoids are produced: 11-deoxycorticosterone and 18-hydroxy-11-deoxycorticosterone. Because of differences in potency, these are far less important than aldosterone. (Adrenal hormones are treated in Chap. 14.)

It is thought that aldosterone begins to act after it passively diffuses into a target cell and combines with a specific high-affinity cytoplasmic receptor protein that possesses a DNA binding domain.[2] It is then transferred to specific acceptor sites on nuclear chromatin, inducing increases in RNA synthesis and, later, protein synthesis.[84]

Mineralocorticoid receptors in the kidney are structurally similar to glucocorticoid receptors and bind cortisol as well as aldosterone. Selectivity of this receptor for aldosterone results from the intrarenal degradation of cortisol to cortisone by the enzyme 11β-hydroxysteroid dehydrogenase. Since cortisone does not bind to the receptor, binding of cortisol to the renal receptor is prevented and selectivity for aldosterone binding is preserved. Accordingly, a reduction of renal 11β-hydroxysteroid dehydrogenase activity results in excessive mineralocorticoid activity, on account of the occupancy of the mineralocorticoid receptor by cortisol.[132,156] Such enzyme deficiencies have been reported congenitally and following the ingestion of glycyrrhizic acid, which is found in chewing tobacco and certain types of licorice.[133] The mechanisms by which an increase in mRNA lead to mineralocorticoid effects remain unknown. Proposed hypotheses include: (1) an expansion of the energy-generating system of the cell; (2) an increase in cellular permeability to sodium ions secondary to a change in sodium channels on the luminal surface of the cell; and (3) an increase in the activity of the Na^+-K^+ ATPase on the serosal surface.[7] The first two hypotheses are not mutually exclusive; an increase in energy production may increase the transport of sodium through specific sodium channels. Alternatively, aldosterone may lead to a change in fatty acid synthesis and consequently affect membrane phospholipid composition, which would alter ion transport.[42] Under normal circumstances, aldosterone has two important activities: regulation of ECF volume, and determination of potassium metabolism. Aldosterone regulates volume through a direct effect on the renal tubular transport of sodium. It acts primarily in the distal nephron, where it decreases the urinary excretion of sodium with an increase in urinary excretion of potassium.[156] The net result appears to be reabsorption of sodium from the filtrate, while potassium is secreted into the urine. The reabsorbed sodium ions are then transported out of the tubular epithelial cells into the interstitial fluid of the kidney, and from there into the renal capillary circulation. Water passively follows the transported sodium.

The action of aldosterone on the kidney is commonly referred to as "distal sodium-potassium exchange." A number of studies, however, cast doubt on the validity of this simplistic concept. Much evidence suggests that potassium is not actively secreted by the tubular epithelium but rather follows a change in the transtubular electrical gradient. The reabsorption of positively charged sodium ions causes a fall in the transmembrane potential, thus producing an environment favorable for the flow of positive ions out of the cell into the lumen. The most abundant singly charged cation in the cell is potassium. Since its concentration in the cell is 40 to 80 times greater than in the lumen, it passively follows this electrical gradient in order to restore the normal positive charge to the lumen. In addition to reabsorption of sodium, the character of its attending anion, the volume of luminal filtrate, and systemic acid-base balance all play important roles in renal potassium secretion (see Chap. 7).

Hydrogen ions are also abundant in the tubular epithelial cell. Since $[H^+]$ in the lumen is still greater than in the cell, it must be actively secreted; however, the reduced intraluminal positivity produced by sodium reabsorption allows more H^+ to be secreted for the same amount of energy expended.

Aldosterone and other mineralocorticoids also act on the epithelium of the salivary ducts and sweat glands, and on the epithelial cells of the gastrointestinal tract, to cause reabsorption of sodium and secretion of potassium ions.

When normal individuals are given a long-term course of aldosterone—or of a comparable mineralocorticoid, such as parenteral deoxycorticosterone acetate (DOCA)—an initial period of sodium retention is followed by natriuresis. Sodium balance is reestablished after 3 to 5 days, albeit at a higher body fluid volume. As a result, clinical edema does not form. This phenomenon is called the *escape phenomenon*, signifying an "escape" by the renal tubules from the sodium-retaining action of protracted administration of aldosterone.[3] Although this mechanism prevents progressive retention of sodium and expansion of ECF volume, the tubules do not escape the kaliuretic effects of protracted exposure to mineralocorticoids. The mechanism(s) postulated to mediate the escape phenomenon include pressure natriuresis and an increase in ANH levels secondary to volume expansion. Escape is exhibited by patients with hypertension but is characteristically absent in patients with edema disorders (see Chap. 18).

There are three well-defined controls of aldosterone release—the renin-angiotensin system, potassium, and ACTH[100,156] (see Table 49-2). Additional factors that have recently been implicated include atrial natriuretic hormone and the neurotransmitters dopamine and serotonin.[49,87,125,129] The renin-angiotensin system is the major control of ECF volume, via regulation of aldosterone secretion. In effect, the renin-angiotensin system attempts to maintain the circulating blood volume by causing aldosterone-induced sodium retention during periods registered as volume deficiencies, and by decreasing aldosterone-dependent sodium retention under conditions in which volume is registered as being ample. The validity of aldosterone's link with the renin-angiotensin system via a negative feedback loop has been confirmed by numerous studies in normal subjects.[144,156] Further-

TABLE 49-2 • Factors regulating aldosterone secretion

Factors	Effects on aldosterone secretion
Angiotensin II	Stimulate
Potassium	Stimulate
Pituitary-derived factors	
ACTH	Stimulate
Beta endorphin	Stimulate
Gamma-MSH	Stimulate
Other non-pituitary hormones	Permissive
Aldosterone-stimulating factor	Stimulate
Natriuretic factors	
Dopamine	Inhibit
Atrial natriuretic hormone (ANH)	Inhibit
Other factors	
Serotonin	Stimulate
Vasopressin	Stimulate

more, dietary sodium intake can markedly influence the relative responses of the various components of the renin-angiotensin-aldosterone axis—a factor that needs to be considered to properly interpret studies performed in hypertensive subjects.[33,59,65,105,110]

Like volume depletion, volume expansion has a significant effect on aldosterone secretion and the activity of the renin-angiotensin system. Wtih ECF expansion the kidneys release less renin, PRA levels diminish, and less aldosterone is secreted. This response is characteristic of what is called an appropriate "normal" response. Volume has been increased by a number of techniques, including oral or intravenous (IV) administration of sodium chloride,[143] intramuscular (IM) administration of DOCA,[68] and partial immersion. These procedures have been used to attempt mineralocorticoid suppression, specifically to assess whether primary hyperaldosteronism is present.

An assessment has been made of the rate of response of the renin-angiotensin system to sudden increases in volume induced by the IV administration of either saline, dextran, or glucose in normal subjects in sodium balance on a 10 meq sodium and 100 meq potassium daily intake.[143]

During saline infusion (500 ml/h for 6 h) mean PRA and angiotensin II levels declined rapidly; significant decrements were observed 10 min after the initiation of the infusion, and a 50 percent fall occurred by 60 min. Thereafter, the rate of fall was more gradual; levels reached a minimum at 360 min. Aldosterone levels declined in a parallel fashion after an initial lag; significant decrements did not occur until 30 min after the initiation of the infusion (Fig. 49-2). Despite an equivalent volume increase, dextran infusion (250 ml/h for 4 h) did not produce a significant fall in PRA, angiotensin II, or plasma aldosterone until 4 h after the start of the infusion. Infusion of 5% glucose in water at 500 ml/h for 6 h had no significant effect on PRA, angiotensin II, or aldosterone. Although the rates of response of the three parameters were different in each of the three infusion studies, these parameters were always significantly intercorrelated within each study. The results demonstrate that the rate of responsiveness of PRA, angiotensin II, and aldosterone is dependent on the volume-increasing agent employed. Saline solution produces a more rapid suppression than dextran in sodium-depleted subjects, supporting a specific role for the sodium ion itself in the regulation of renin and aldosterone secretion.[143]

Potassium ions can regulate aldosterone secretion independently of the renin-angiotensin system. Since aldosterone, in turn, facilitates renal potassium excretion, this feedback loop is an important factor in potassium homeostasis (see Chap. 7). In normal human beings, oral potassium loading increases the secretion and plasma levels of aldosterone. In addition, systemic infusion of

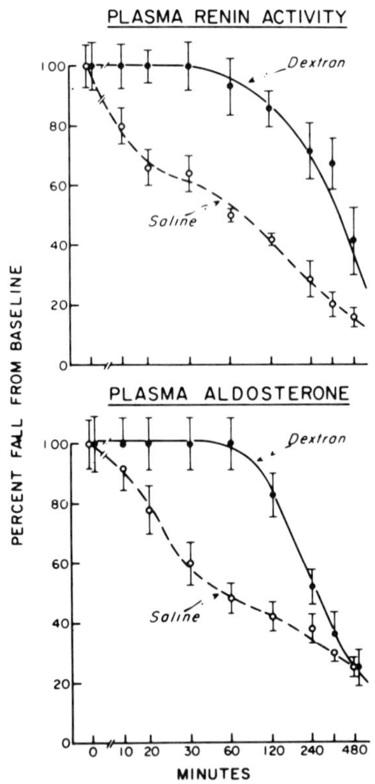

FIGURE 49-2 • Comparison of the rate of response of plasma renin activity and aldosterone to saline and dextran infusions in 12 normotensive subjects. Results are expressed as percent fall from the baseline (mean ± standard error of the mean) plotted against time on a log scale. Note the rapid early response to saline infusion of both parameters, and the delayed response to intravascular volume expansion with dextran. Note also that the saline response curve appears to have two phases: a rapid early response with a plateau, and then a second decrement occurring at the same time as the suppression of these two parameters with dextran. (From Tuck ML et al: *J Clin Invest* 53:988, 1974.)

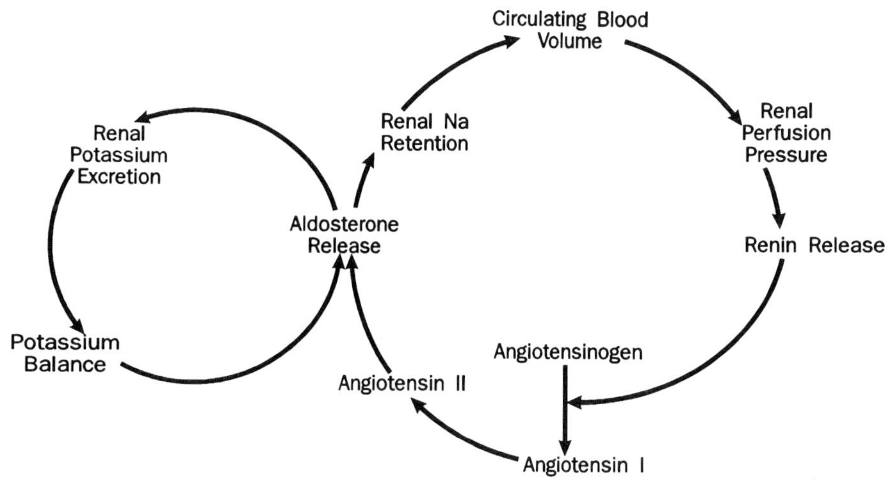

FIGURE 49-3 • Interrelationship of volume and potassium feedback loops on aldosterone secretion. Integration of signals from each loop determines the level of aldosterone secreted. [From Conlin PR et al: Disorders of the renin-angiotensin-aldosterone system, in Schrier R (ed): *Renal and Electrolyte Disorders*. Boston, Little, Brown, 1991, p 415.]

potassium ions may significantly increase plasma aldosterone levels with an increase as small as a 0.1 meq/liter in serum potassium.[62] That this is a direct action of the potassium ion is supported by the following evidence: potassium suppresses renin secretion; the effect of potassium on aldosterone excretion is independent of reciprocal changes in intravascular volume; the infusion of potassium ions directly into the adrenal artery produces an immediate increase in adrenal venous aldosterone levels; and increasing the potassium content of incubation medium containing adrenal tissue results in an increase in aldosterone production.[61,101,152] The regulation of aldosterone production by potassium may be due to changes in extracellular and intracellular potassium levels, or to a change in the influx of potassium into the glomerulosa cell. However, as with angiotensin II, the potassium effects ultimately involve changes in cytosolic calcium.[11,20] Recent in-vitro studies also support a role for the adrenal renin-angiotensin system. Potassium loading increases the local generation of aldosterone, renin, and angiotensin II in isolated glomerulosa cells.[77] The cation also modifies the expression of the gene encoding the 11-OHase activity.[86]

Thus potassium, like the renin-angiotensin system, regulates aldosterone secretion through a negative feedback loop. The two systems are probably of equal importance under physiologic conditions; the level of aldosterone is probably determined by integration of signals from each loop (Fig. 49-3). For example, the simultaneous infusion of saline solution and potassium in salt-depleted normal subjects produced additive effects on aldosterone levels, reflecting opposite and independent changes in the levels of potassium and angiotensin II.[37]

Dopamine, the precursor of the sympathetic neurotransmitter norepinephrine, may also play an important role as an inhibitor of aldosterone secretion. In human beings on ad lib sodium intake, administration of the dopamine agonist bromocriptine or infusion of dopamine does not alter basal aldosterone levels or the aldosterone response to the infusion of angiotensin II or ACTH.[23,129] However, basal aldosterone levels and the responsiveness to angiotensin II is altered by dopamine infusion in subjects on a sodium depleted diet.[22,56,57] On the other hand, administration of boluses of the dopamine antagonist metoclopramide to persons on high-sodium diets consistently and promptly elevates aldosterone levels.[103,104] Taken together, these in-vivo studies suggest that aldosterone output in persons on ad lib salt diets is under continuous dopaminergic inhibition. In addition, dopamine may modulate changes in aldosterone production as dietary sodium is restricted.[22,56] In vitro, metoclopramide behaves as a partial agonist.[87] In the absence of dopamine, metoclopramide exhibits agonistic properties and inhibits aldosterone production. In the presence of dopamine (in vivo) it acts as an antagonist, thereby increasing aldosterone secretion. These data also indicate that dopamine has little effect on the cellular secretion of aldosterone in the basal state. Its major action is to modify the production of aldosterone in the angiotensin II stimulated glomerulosa cell.[87]

Serum and urine dopamine levels decrease during low sodium intake and increase during high sodium intake.[22] Since dopamine is a natriuretic hormone and also affects aldosterone output, it is likely that dopamine is an additional important factor regulating sodium homeostasis. Dopamine suppresses the renin-angiotensin system, further enhancing its role as a natriuretic factor.[56] Finally, it may be important in mediating the change in adrenal responsiveness following alterations in dietary sodium intake.

Atrial natriuretic hormone also functions as a potent inhibitor of aldosterone output.[125] As with dopamine, its in vivo actions depend on the state of dietary salt intake. Thus, ANH suppresses aldosterone output to a greater extent in subjects on salt-depleted diets or who are given such secretagogues as angiotensin II.

Serotonin, is another regulatory factor. In-vitro studies have documented that serotonin is a potent agonist for aldosterone production.[49] Additionally, in human volunteers the administration of tryptophan, a serotonin precursor, has been shown to lead to increases in aldosterone levels.[97] However, this increase in aldosterone may be indirect, since parallel increases in cortisol and PRA also occurred. Thus serotonin, like dopamine, appears to have both indirect (through the renin-angiotensin system) and direct effects on aldosterone output. However, the regulation of these neurotransmitters themselves by sodium and blood pressure, and the overall importance of these factors in the control of aldosterone output, is uncertain.

The administration of ACTH abruptly increases aldosterone output.[75] However, the stimulatory effect of ACTH is transient; beyond 24 h continued administration is associated with a decline in aldosterone levels,[102] unless ACTH is given episodically.[122] The failure to sustain aldosterone levels is not understood; possible explanations include inhibition of intracellular biosynthesis or down regulation of ACTH receptors. In early studies, ACTH was infused in pharmacologic doses;[100,156] subsequent infusions of ACTH in the physiologic dose range have proved that ACTH, on a mole-for-mole basis, is the most potent aldosterone stimulator.[75] Accordingly, stress-induced increases in aldosterone secretion appear to be mediated by ACTH.[100] The circadian rhythm of aldosterone, and spontaneous fluctuations around it, also correlate at times with cortisol levels, suggesting that ACTH has an additional physiological action.[73]

Although ACTH is a potent aldosterone stimulator, it is probably of minor importance in regulating aldosterone output in normal subjects. First, subjects with isolated ACTH insufficiency, such as that induced by long-term steroid therapy, have normal aldosterone responses to acute stimulation and sodium restriction.[149] Second, although mineralocorticoid receptors have been identified in pituitary tissue,[84] no feedback of aldosterone on the pituitary gland or hypothalamus has been demonstrated. Thus, in normal subjects physiologic levels of ACTH under certain circumstances may increase aldosterone output. However, ACTH seems less important than the renin-angiotensin system or potassium in the overall control of aldosterone secretion.

In contrast to isolated ACTH deficiency, longstanding hypopituitarism is associated with a decline in responsiveness of the zona glomerulosa to stimuli such as sodium restriction. For example hypopituitary patients have been shown to have an abnormal aldosterone response to both ACTH stimulation and sodium restriction.[149] One important factor in the hypophysectomized rat that appears to maintain glomerulosa responsiveness is growth hormone (GH).[108,109] While GH itself fails to stimulate aldosterone or renin secretion, it does increase adrenal weight and restores the responsiveness of the zona glomerulosa in hypophysectomized dogs.[100] On the other hand, human subjects with isolated GH deficiency exhibit normal aldosterone responses to sodium restriction. Interestingly, beta endorphin and alpha MSH have also been suggested to be factors of pituitary origin that increase aldosterone output.[100,156]

Changes in dietary potassium and sodium dramatically shift the sensitivity of the glomerulosa to aldosterone-stimulating factors. On the other hand, glucocorticoid responsiveness to ACTH is not altered by dietary manipulation. For example, prolonged dietary potassium loading and/or sodium restriction leads to enhanced aldosterone responsiveness to acute stimuli, as well as to an increase in the size of the zona glomerulosa.[64,65,105,151,153] A change in zona glomerulosa sensitivity is probably of critical importance in normal sodium and potassium homeostasis, particularly when considered in the context of effects of dietary manipulation on the level of both renin secretion and the response of vascular tissue to angiotensin II.[64,65] Thus potassium and sodium homeostasis are interdependent: first, both modify the rate of responsiveness of angiotensin II target tissues to angiotensin II; second, both influence the activation of the renin-angiotensin-aldosterone axis; third, the excretion by the kidney of both potassium and sodium is determined at least in part by aldosterone.

Thus an increase in sodium intake leads to expansion of the ECF and suppression of renin release, angiotensin II formation, and aldosterone secretion. This series of events is in part responsible for the increase in renal sodium excretion that prevents progressive ECF expansion following ingestion of a large sodium load. Restriction of sodium intake produces a series of the opposite responses in the renin-angiotensin-aldosterone system.

An increase in dietary potassium results in a decline in PRA, while aldosterone secretion increases; as a result, potassium excretion increases.[13,100,156] Because sodium and potassium have, in some instances, opposite effects on renin and aldosterone output, a number of studies have addressed the question of which ion has primacy. Available evidence suggests that sodium plays the more important role in the control of renin release; sodium (through angiotensin II) and potassium are probably equally important in modulating aldosterone output (Fig. 49-3).[37] Thus, in subjects already ingesting a high-sodium diet, an increase in dietary potassium leads to an increase in plasma aldosterone levels, but not to further suppression of the renin-angiotensin system.[64] In addition, with a high sodium intake, restriction of dietary potassium leads to stimulation of renin release, but there is little effect on the previously suppressed secretion of aldosterone. Therefore, high sodium intake reduces the activity of the renin-angiotensin-aldosterone axis to a physiologic "floor"; changes in potassium intake produce increases, but not reductions, in concentrations. On the other hand, if the system is activated by sodium re-

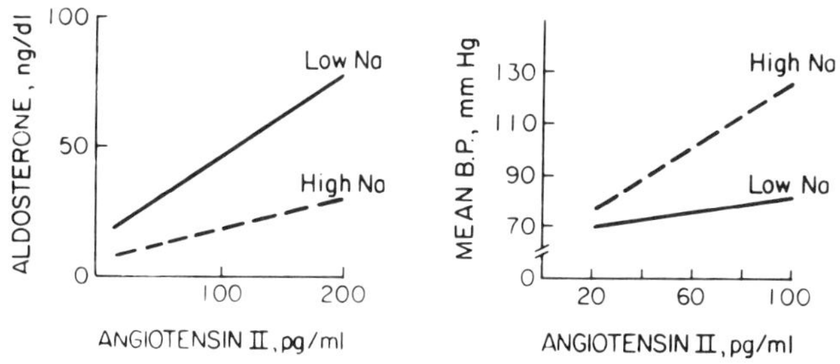

FIGURE 49-4 • Reciprocal effect of sodium intake on vascular and adrenal responses to angiotensin II. See text for details. (From Hollenberg NK et al: *J Clin Invest* 54:34, 1974.)

striction, dietary potassium can either increase or decrease renin release and/or aldosterone secretion independently of sodium intake.

Another important relationship is the influence of sodium intake on vascular and adrenal responsiveness to angiotensin II. As noted above, sodium restriction enhances adrenal responsiveness to angiotensin II, while the response of vascular smooth muscle is reduced (Fig. 49-4).[65,105] This effect of sodium intake on vascular responsiveness to angiotensin II is best seen by assessing renal vascular reactivity, since the renal vasculature is sensitive to log-order-lower concentrations of angiotensin II than is the peripheral vasculature.

In summary, potassium and the renin-angiotensin system are probably of equal importance in the regulation of aldosterone secretion in human beings (Fig. 49-2), while the interaction of dietary potassium and sodium can sensitize the response of aldosterone secretion following acute stimulation. How dietary changes may alter the late pathway of aldosterone biosynthesis and whether potassium and sodium manipulations are acting on the same receptor sites are not clear from the information now available. Although physiologic levels of ACTH may stimulate aldosterone under certain circumstances, ACTH seems to be less important than the renin-angiotensin system and potassium in the control of aldosterone production. Other factors (e.g., ANH, dopamine) await further investigation.

FACTORS CONTROLLING BLOOD PRESSURE

In order to understand the pathophysiology of hypertension, a brief description of the factors involved in the maintenance of normal blood pressure is necessary (Table 49-3). *Arterial pressure* is the product of cardiac output and peripheral resistance. *Cardiac output* is the product of stroke volume and heart rate. *Stroke volume* depends on the venous return and myocardial contractility. For arterial pressure to rise, there must be an increase in either cardiac output or peripheral resistance, or both. Theories of the pathogenesis of essential hypertension have suggested increases in either cardiac output or peripheral resistance as the initiating events. Peripheral resistance is determined by the intrinsic physical characteristics of the resistance vessels (i.e., the lumen:wall-thickness ratio) as well as the neurohumoral influences that act on vascular smooth muscle. These influences include the neurotransmitters norepinephrine, which is a vasoconstrictor, and, in some vessels, acetylcholine, which is a vasodilator. Humoral and locally acting substances include the vasoconstrictor angiotensin II and prostaglandins and kinins (vasodilators). Hypoxia and certain products of metabolism, such as adenosine, H^+, and lactic acid, also exert potent *local* vasodilating influences.

Renal factors

Goldblatt and coworkers, in 1934, produced hypertension in the dog by constriction of the renal artery.[51] It has been demonstrated that a number of renal diseases (pyelonephritis, glomerulonephritis, tuberculosis, and carcinoma), as well as vascular changes, produce hypertension. The exact mechanism involved in hypertension secondary to renal disease or disorders affecting the kidney is not known, but its occurrence implicates the kidney in the control of blood pressure.

The renin-angiotensin-aldosterone system causes retention of salt and water, increasing the total blood volume; blood volume is one of the determinants of venous

TABLE 49-3 • Factors controlling arterial blood pressure

Renal
Renin-angiotensin system
Volume homeostasis
Excreting and detoxifying function
Production of vasodilators (e.g., prostaglandins, kallikrein-kinins, lipids)
Endocrine
Catecholamines
Aldosterone
Cortisol
Thyroid hormones
Vasopressin (ADH)
Growth hormone
Estrogens
Androgens
Progesterone
Atrial natriuretic hormone (ANH)
Vascular
Physical changes (plaques, etc.)
Electrolyte content (Ca^{2+}, Na^+, K^+)

return, and hence of cardiac output. In this way the system helps maintain blood pressure. In addition, angiotensin II is a potent vasoconstrictor.[55] This effect, which may be exerted directly on the peripheral vasculature or may potentiate the effect of adrenergic stimulation, may be a second renal factor in the control of blood pressure. It has also been postulated that the kidney, functioning as an excretory and detoxifying organ, may help control the level of extrarenal pressor substances and thereby help prevent hypertension. A fourth renal mechanism for control of blood pressure is the production of vasodilator substances. One postulated vasodilator substance is one of the prostaglandins (PGI_2), which is found in high concentration in the medulla of the normal kidney. A second potential vasodilator, kallikrein, is synthesized and secreted by the kidney (see Chap. 15). Kallikreins are enzymes that have the potential for acting on certain substrates to form a group of potent vasodilator polypeptides called kinins.[28] A lipid secreted by the renomedullary interstitial cells may be another renal vasodilator. The two prime candidates are 1-O-alkyl ethers or phosphatidyl choline, and/or a neutral lipid.[99] Further investigation of these compounds is needed in order to determine their role, if any, in the normal maintenance of blood pressure.

Endocrine factors

Pheochromocytoma and primary hyperaldosteronism, both of which are due to tumors of the adrenal gland, are two surgically correctable causes of hypertension. It has therefore been postulated that epinephrine, norepinephrine, and aldosterone play significant roles in the regulation of normal blood pressure.

Several difficulties arise in trying to ascertain the exact role of the *catecholamines* in blood pressure regulation. First, they come from two different sources: the adrenal medulla and the postganglionic sympathetic axons. Second, the axons not only synthesize norepinephrine but also take up free norepinephrine from the tissues around them. Therefore, even with precise quantitative measurements of serum catecholamines, the relationship of these values to the quantity secreted would always be in doubt.

Catecholamines, manufactured in the postganglionic sympathetic axon, are bound to adenosine triphosphate (ATP) for storage in granular sacs. The propagated nerve impulse causes release of norepinephrine from these granules. The free catecholamine then diffuses across the synapse to the receptor organ. Some of the discharged norepinephrine is reabsorbed by the axon, where it is either detoxified by monoamine oxidases or stored in new granules. The norepinephrine that escapes from the vicinity of the axon is inactivated by methyltransferase enzymes present in the peripheral circulation and elsewhere. The fine balance of this sytem plays a major role in the determination of blood pressure. The discharged norepinephrine regulates not only arterial resistance but also cardiac contractility and rate. Relating the measured catecholamine levels to adrenergic activity should provide a more sophisticated understanding of how this complex system interacts with others in the maintenance of blood pressure.

Aldosterone is a potent salt-retaining hormone.[127] It helps regulate blood pressure by maintaining blood volume through salt and accompanying water retention.

The role of *cortisol* in maintaining blood pressure is related to its maintenance of normal vascular reactivity, a feature not shared by the mineralocorticoids. In addition, cortisol may influence blood pressure by blocking prostaglandin production through its inhibition of phospholipase A_2, which thereby prevents release of arachidonic acid from phospholipids. Clinically, the hypotensive, volume-contracted state of the individual in adrenal crisis can be corrected by saline solution and glucocorticoids, but is correctable only with diffiuclty by mineralocorticoids and saline solution. Whether excesses or abnormal metabolism of the glucocorticoids, aside from Cushing's syndrome, are responsible for any hypertensive states is difficult to determine. Cortisol secretory rates, response to ACTH, and suppression with dexamethasone all remain within normal limits in patients with nonadrenal forms of hypertension. Thus it seems improbable that glucocorticoids play more than a permissive role in hypertension, although they appear to be essential for the normal regulation of blood pressure.

The role of the thyroid hormones thyroxine and triiodothyronine in the normal mainteance of blood pressure is complex.[155] Certainly, the hyperkinetic circulatory state of the thyrotoxic patient can produce systolic hypertension. However, hypertension is also found in patients with hypothyroidism, secondarily to increased peripheral vascular resistance. The interesting interrelations of thyroid hormone with both catecholamines and the myocardium have been extensively investigated without agreement as to their physiologic significance. First, there are thyroxine receptors on myocardial cells and cardiac output is often reduced in severely hypothyroid subjects. Second, there is a diminished vascular reactivity to epinephrine and norepinephrine in the hypothyroid state; yet there appear to be no lasting effects on the blood pressure in patients with hypertension when hypothyroidism is induced. Thyroid hormone produces peripheral vasodilation as a result of increased oxidative demand, but it has also been shown to augment the normal response of tissues to sympathetic stimulation, and might be expected, thereby, to increase blood pressure. This augmented reactivity may be due to an increase in angiotensin II secretion or to a decrease in a detoxifying enzyme.

Normal thyroid hormone levels are necessary to maintain the GFR. In the hypothyroid state excessive sodium and water are retained, because of a reduction in GFR. Dilutional hyponatremia due to the "inappropriate" release of antidiuretic hormone is not uncommon in hypothyroid patients (see Chaps. 4 and 20). The diversity of the actions of thyroid hormone on a number of systems involved in sodium homeostasis is further illustrated by the effects of thyroid status on sodium-lithium countertransport in red blood cells, as well as the elevated circulating levels of angiotensin-converting enzyme observed in hyperthyroid subjects.

Gravely ill patients in intensive care units who are hypotensive, and often hypothermic, usually have very low levels of triiodothyronine and thyroxine (the so-called euthyroid sick syndrome).[155] It is unclear whether the low levels of thyroid hormone contribute to the cardiovascular status and poor outcome of many of these patients. However, there is no evidence that treating these patients with thyroxine improves survival.

Other hormones may play a role in blood pressure control. *Antidiuretic hormone* (ADH) also has pressor activity, but only in high doses.[155] ADH is also released in response to nonosmotic stimuli, such as severe contraction of blood volume (see Chap. 4). Its antidiuretic and pressor effects both may be important in the regulation of blood pressure, through determining changes in blood volume and peripheral resistance. The *androgens, estrogen, and progesterone-like* compounds all affect sodium balance. However, it is unlikely that pathologic changes in these hormones or their sodium-retaining capacity have significant effects, except on rare occasions. Estrogen, as well as glucocorticoids and thyroxine, also increases the hepatic production of angiotensinogen.[41]

Recent studies have focused on hyperinsulinemia as a factor that may be important in the pathogenesis of essential hypertension.[111] First, non-obese essential hypertensive subjects with normal glucose tolerance have been found to be insulin-resistant by glucose tolerance and euglycemic clamping techniques.[45] Thus, in order to promote normal glucose disposal, these patients would be expected to be chronically hyperinsulinemic. Although the skeletal muscles and adipose tissue are resistant to insulin-mediated glucose uptake, it is hypothesized that other insulin target tissues, such as the adrenergic system and the kidney, remain normally responsive. Since in short-term studies the infusion of insulin promotes proximal tubular reabsorption of sodium[35] and increases blood levels of norepinephrine and epinephrine,[118] an elevation of blood pressure might, theoretically, result from the hyperinsulinemic state. Chronically elevated insulin levels have also been speculated to have additional effects, such as promoting atherogenesis through direct actions on the intima or by causing dyslipidemic syndromes. Long-term studies are needed to test these hypotheses.

Approximately 30 to 50 percent of patients with acromegaly also have hypertension. The role of growth hormone in the production of this hypertension and whether growth hormone is important in regulating blood pressure have not been extensively investigated. Acromegalic subjects are reported to have increased levels of total body sodium and are hypervolemic.[135] Rarely, these patients may also have aldosterone-producing adenomas or pheochromocytomas. In general, renin and aldosterone levels are suppressed in hypertensive acromegalic subjects; in normotensive subjects, renin responsiveness is normal.[16] Thus, it is unclear why hypervolemia and hypertension are commonly observed in acromegaly; an effect of growth hormone per se has been postulated, because the renin-angiotensin-aldosterone system seems to respond normally to the volume-expanded state. Alternatively, acromegaly is an insulin-resistant state; the accompanying hyperinsulinemia may lead to the sodium retention and volume expansion that characterize this syndrome.

Finally, calcium and calcium-regulating hormones have also been implicated in the pathogenesis of hypertension.[30,43,92,95] Several studies have provided support for the concept that ingesting a diet high in calcium content reduces blood pressure, at least in some individuals. The mechanisms responsible for this effect are unknown. However, most patients with hyperparathyroidism have increased blood pressure, which some studies suggest is not related to renal damage. Indeed, there is evidence to suggest that dietary calcium's effect on blood pressure is related to a change in sodium handling by the kidney. Thus, individuals on a low-calcium diet would tend to raise blood pressure to a greater extent when sodium intake is increased than individuals on a high-calcium diet. The validity of this hypothesis and the mechanisms by which dietary calcium can modify blood pressure are still unclear.

Primary vascular factors

Many factors influence the level of peripheral resistance; one of them is the structure of the vessels. For example, blood pressure tends to rise with increasing age, paralleling the increasing *rigidity* of the arteries. The pressure of a pulsing blood flow is greater in a rigid tube than in a flexible one because of the inability of vessel walls to absorb part of the energy by mechanical stretch.

Sensitivity of the vessel to pressor agents may vary under different conditions. The responsiveness of an excised rat aortic strip increases if *sodium* is added to the perfusion bath; conversely, removal of sodium decreases the responsiveness. *Potassium* may also have a direct effect on vascular responses. It has been well documented that modest increases in the plasma potassium concentration evoke vasodilatation. This effect has been postulated to be related to the role played by potassium in the excitation phase of vascular smooth muscle contraction.[107]

A major determinant of vascular reactivity is the concentration of cytoplasmic *calcium*; raising cytoplasmic calcium from 10^{-7} to 10^{-5} *M* activates vascular contraction.[70]

Not only does the concentration of cations in vascular tissue modify its reactivity, but also the dietary intake of at least two cations, Na^+ and K^+, can influence responsiveness to at least one pressor agent, angiotensin II. As noted earlier, dietary sodium restriction or potassium loading increases the adrenal's response to angiotensin II. Dietary sodium has a reciprocal influence on adrenal glomerulosa and vascular responses to angiotensin II. Dietary potassium also influences renal vascular responsiveness to angiotensin II. Thus sodium restriction reduces, while potassium loading enhances, pressor responsiveness to angiotensin II. These changes in reactivity are presumed to be secondary to a change in the vascular angiotensin II receptor.[64,65]

ETIOLOGY AND CHARACTERISTICS OF HYPERTENSION

The causes of hypertension can be separated into five broad categories (Table 49-4). In most cases the pathophysiology underlying the hypertensive state, particularly in essential hypertension, is not understood. Defects in any of the normal regulatory mechanisms may produce hypertension.

Borst and Borst de Geus, in 1963, proposed that "hypertension is part of a homeostatic reaction of deficient renal sodium output."[10] The renal function abnormality—that is, reduced sodium excretion at normal arterial pressure—may be a consequence of (1) mild increases in mineralocorticoid activity; (2) local increases in vasoconstrictor (angiotensin II or sympathetic nervous system) activity,[36] reducing renal blood flow and thereby reducing sodium excretion; (3) decreased renal kallikrein-kinin or prostaglandin activity; or (4) a primary (perhaps genetic) tubular defect. According to this hypothesis, salt retention, from any cause, increases blood volume, raising central venous pressure and preload and, thereby, cardiac output (i.e., systemic blood flow). However, peripheral tissues have the intrinsic capacity to regulate this overperfusion by increasing local vascular resistance. When resistance is increased in many vascular beds, arterial pressure rises, cardiac after load increases, and stroke volume and cardiac output are thereby depressed. The elevated arterial (renal perfusion) pressure also increases the urinary excretion of sodium, which serves as a second negative feedback to reduce blood volume, central venous pressure, preload, and, ultimately, cardiac output. Thus, the end result of this process is increased peripheral resistance and arterial pressure; all other parameters, including blood volume, cardiac output, and renal sodium excretion, remain normal. Indeed, this sequence has been documented in experimental human DOC-induced hypertension and animal hypertension due to renal artery stenosis. However, patients with essential hypertension have been reported to have normal cardiac output and elevated peripheral resistance; this suggests that either the studies have not been performed early enough in the course of the disease, or this theory is incorrect in that a change in peripheral resistance is actually a *primary* event, not a reaction to salt retention.

Such a primary elevation in peripheral resistance can occur because of either an increase in factors tending to

TABLE 49-4 • Classification of arterial (systolic and diastolic) hypertension

Renal
Chronic pyelonephritis
Acute and chronic glomerulonephritis
Polycystic renal disease
Renovascular stenosis and renal infarction
Renin-producing tumors
Most other severe renal diseases (arteriolar nephrosclerosis, diabetic nephropathy, etc.)
Endocrine
Oral contraceptives
Adrenocortical hyperfunction
Cushing's disease and syndrome
Primary hyperaldosteronism
Congenital or hereditary adrenogenital syndromes
17α-hydroxylase and 11β-hydroxylase defects)
Acromegaly
Pheochromocytoma
Myxedema
Neurogenic
Psychogenic
Diencephalic syndrome
Familial dysautonomia (Riley-Day syndrome)
Poliomyelitis (bulbar)
Polyneuritis (acute porphyria, lead poisoning)
Increased intracranial pressure (acute)
Spinal cord section
Miscellaneous
Coarctation of the aorta
Increased intravascular volume (excessive transfusion)
Polyarteritis nodosa
Hypercalcemia
Unknown etiology
Essential hypertension (>90% of all cases of hypertension)
Toxemia of pregnancy
Acute intermittent porphyria

produce vasoconstriction, a reduction in factors producing vasodilatation, or a change in the arterial smooth muscle—that is, an increase in muscle mass or an increase in its responsiveness and/or sensitivity to vasoconstrictor stimuli. Each theory has its advocates. Thus, the hypertension associated with some neurologic disorders and emotional stress, and perhaps early essential hypertension, may be accompanied by increased plasma or urine levels of norepinephrine. Presumably, this reflects augmented neural release of the vasoconstrictive adrenergic neurotransmitter, which is responsible for the increased arterial pressure. Second, many patients with essential hypertension have increased vascular response to vasoconstrictor agents (e.g., angiotensin II, norepinephrine). Finally, hypertensive patients since the early 1930s have been noted to exhibit a decrease in the urinary excretion of kinins; and thus it is possible that reduced vasodilator activity may also result in increased arterial pressure.

The "deficient renal sodium output" and "primary increase in peripheral resistance" hypotheses are not necessarily mutually exclusive. For example, increased retention of sodium enhances vascular reactivity, at least to angiotensin II, even in normotensive subjects. Thus a primary defect of sodium excretion might simultaneously increase both cardiac output and peripheral resistance. One proposed mediator of this enhanced vascular responsiveness is an *ATPase-inhibiting natriuretic factor.*[60,106,112] Abnormalities in membrane sodium handling in some patients with essential hypertension may be related.[19,50]

None of these hypotheses has dealt with a central issue: What would lead to the abnormal release of the natriuretic factor? An abnormality of the kidney and the adrenal that varies with sodium intake and can contribute to altered sodium handling obviously is an outstanding candidate. Thus many groups have studied the renin-angiotensin-aldosterone system in essential hypertension.

THE RENIN-ANGIOTENSIN-ALDOSTERONE SYSTEM IN ESSENTIAL HYPERTENSION

Since the late 1950s, increased levels of aldosterone have been reported in some persons with malignant hypertension or hypertension and renal artery stenosis. Thus patients with hypertension and elevated aldosterone secretion may have primary or secondary hyperaldosteronism (malignant hypertension, renal artery stenosis, etc.) (Fig. 49-5).

Considerable disagreement still exists as to whether aldosterone secretion is normal in patients with essential hypertension. Some of the differences between reports may reflect different definitions of the disease, inadequate selection of controls, variation in the control of the factors known to alter aldosterone secretion, and methodologic differences. To achieve greater uniformity, most recent studies have assessed the dynamic response of the renin-angiotensin-aldosterone axis under controlled conditions (see Chap. 16).

Acute suppression of the renin-angiotensin-aldosterone axis in essential hypertension

Several groups have examined the suppression of aldosterone secretion or excretion in patients with essential hypertension following chronic prolonged dietary sodium loading. Most studies have found no significant differences between normotensive and hypertensive subjects. However, Collins and colleagues,[27] using a higher sodium load of 300 meq/day, have reported that some patients with essential hypertension have a significantly greater rate of aldosterone excretion than do normal control subjects. Increased aldosterone excretory rates occurred both in patients who had a normal and in those who had a subnormal suppression of renin activity with sodium loading. None had signs of primary hyperaldosteronism.

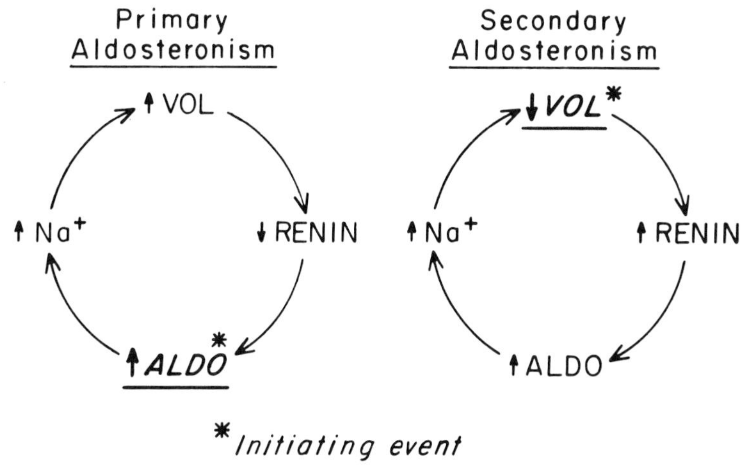

FIGURE 49-5 • Comparison of volume feedback loops in primary and secondary hyperaldosteronism. [From Williams GH, Dluhy RG, in Wilson JD et al (eds): *Harrison's Principles of Internal Medicine,* 12th ed. New York, McGraw-Hill, 1991, p 1726.]

There are also data suggesting that a substantial proportion of patients with essential hypertension have abnormalities in the suppression of the renin-angiotensin-aldosterone axis. One study assessed the acute suppression of plasma renin activity, angiotensin II, and plasma aldosterone at frequent intervals in sodium-restricted hypertensive subjects during the infusion of isotonic saline solution at a rate of 500 ml/h for 6 h.[142] All subjects had a normal PRA in response to sodium restriction and upright posture. In contrast to normotensive subjects, 60 percent of the hypertensive subjects showed no significant decline in plasma renin activity and plasma aldosterone until 120 and 240 min after the beginning of the infusion. Normotensive subjects, as noted earlier, show a significant fall in these parameters within 20 to 30 min (Fig. 49-2).

Previous studies of normal subjects have reported that the early response to saline infusion is related to the sodium ion per se and not to intravascular volume expansion.[143] The above data are consistent with the hypothesis that the delayed suppression of renin secretion seen in the hypertensive group is related to their diminished responsiveness to Na^+. While these changes are not enough to produce significant alterations in serum concentrations of sodium or volume in a chronic state, they may be enough to produce or sustain an elevated blood pressure.

Response of the renin-aldosterone axis in essential hypertension to acute stimulation

The most frequently evaluated component of the renin-angiotensin axis in patients with hypertension is the plasma renin response to acute stimulation[136] (see Chap. 16). Numerous studies have documented that some patients with hypertension have PRA values below those of normal control subjects; the terms "low-renin" or "hyporesponsive renin" essential hypertension have been coined to characterize this subgroup of the essential hypertensive population.

Low-renin essential hypertension

The cause of low-renin hypertension is controversial. However, a number of factors seem to be consistently associated with this condition. Nearly all studies in which a large number of hypertensive subjects have been studied have reported that the low-renin group is significantly older than the normal-renin subgroup.[14,21,141] In the more than 500 patients in the literature in whom renin responsiveness and age have been assessed the mean age of the low-renin subgroup is 47.1 years, whereas the mean age of the normal-renin subgroup is 39.5 years. However, correlation between duration of hypertension and the incidence of low renin activity has not been found. This discrepancy between age and duration may reflect our inability to determine the onset of hypertension because of its relatively asymptomatic course for variable periods. Most studies have also suggested that there is a higher incidence of low-renin hypertension in black subjects; however, this may be related to the lower range of renin activity observed in normotensive black subjects.[31] Thus, in defining the incidence of low-renin hypertension in the black population, a pool of black normotensive subjects is necessary. Finally, Schalekamp and his colleagues have suggested that renin release may be suppressed in hypertensive patients because of the increase in intravascular pressure at the level of the JG cell.[120] This postulate would predict that persons with higher blood pressures would have lower levels of renin activity. While some studies have suggested that such a correlation does exist, most have reported no simple relation between renin responsiveness and the level of blood pressure.

Because of the similarity between low-renin essential hypertension and primary hyperaldosteronism in terms of suppression of renin activity and blood pressure responsiveness to volume depletion, a number of studies have looked for an increase in volume, attributable to a nonaldosterone mineralocorticoid, as the cause of low-renin hypertension. Several steroids have been suggested, most commonly 11-deoxycorticosterone (DOC) and 18-hydroxy-11-deoxycorticosterone (18-OH-DOC).[12,93] Scattered reports have also suggested that 16α,18-dihydroxy-11-deoxycorticosterone, 16β-hydroxydehydroepiandrosterone, and dehydroepiandrosterone sulfate may produce the low-renin state.[32,124] However, there is no conclusive evidence that volume is actually greater in patients with low renin activity.[121] Furthermore, elevated levels of any of the various nonaldosterone mineralocorticoids have not been consistently found. In one report, only 6 of 21 patients had elevated DOC levels.[12] 18-OH-DOC excretion has been reported to be elevated in the majortity of patients with low-renin essential hypertension[93]; however, other studies have suggested that patients with low-renin essential hypertension do not have greater secretion rates or plasma levels of 18-OH-DOC than those with normal-renin essential hypertension[94,154]; in fact, on a high-salt diet, the latter have higher 18-OH-DOC levels. There have been reports of increased mineralocorticoid activity in extracts of urine from low-renin patients, and yet increased binding of plasma extracts to mineralocorticoid receptors has not been found.[6]

A number of lines of evidence suggest that low-renin essential hypertension is not a hypermineralocorticoid state; one of the most compelling arguments is the failure to document alterations in potassium homeostasis. Almost invariably, serum potassium levels and potassium balance are within the normal range in these patients, unlike the findings in primary hyperaldosteronism. If another mineralocorticoid were acting upon the aldosterone receptor, sodium retention and potassium wasting would

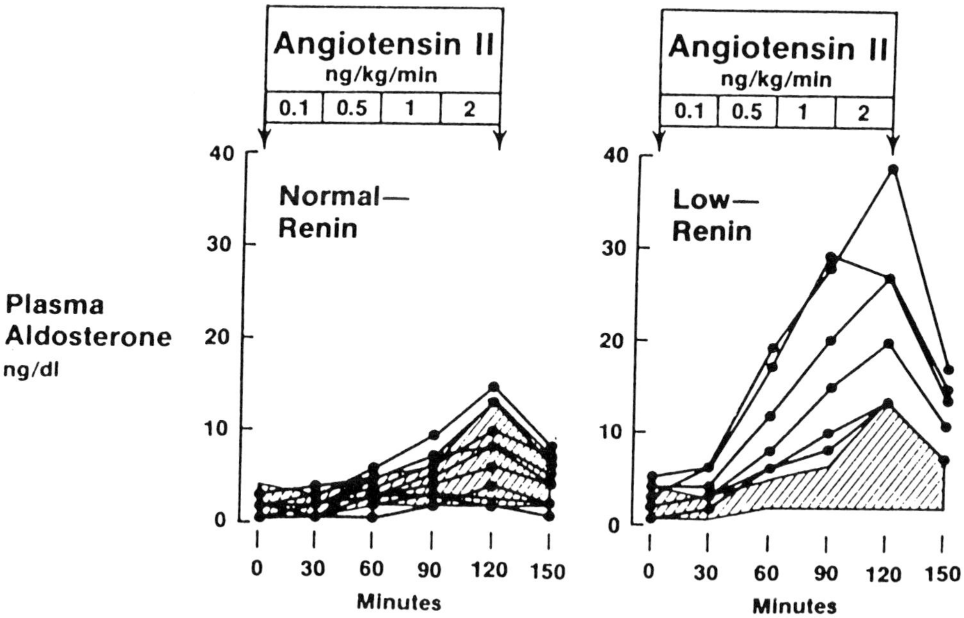

FIGURE 49-6 • Adrenal responses to angiotensin II in 10 patients with normal renin and 6 patients with low-renin essential hypertension. All subjects were white. Infusions were performed after 2 days on a high sodium intake and dexamethasone administration (2 mg/day). The shaded area shows the range of responses in 13 normal subjects. (From Wisgerhof M, Brown RD: *J Clin Invest* 61:1456, 1978. By copyright permission of the American Society for Clinical Investigation.)

be expected to occur together. While potassium wasting is not a universal finding in hypermineralocorticoid states,[145] the weight of evidence suggests that volume increases due to excess mineralocorticoid activity should be accompanied by potassium depletion.

An intriguing suggestion is that the suppressed renin levels are due to an increase in the adrenal's sensitivity to angiotensin II[91,157] (Fig. 49-6). If so, then the volume-renin-aldosterone feedback loop could be closed at lower levels of angiotensin II—an appropriate adaptive mechanism in the face of an elevated blood pressure. Increased adrenal sensitivity to angiotensin II has also been reported in hypertensive patients with normal plasma renin levels.[80]

Enhanced adrenal sensitivity to angiotensin II might also explain the variable reports regarding volume spaces, exchangeable sodium and potassium, or other features of hypermineralocorticoidism in patients with low-renin hypertension. Renin release is controlled by a number of factors in addition to volume and sodium. A floor exists below which renin secretion cannot be reduced by volume or sodium alone. With an enhanced adrenal responsiveness to angiotensin II, the potential exists for transient hypermineralocorticoidism during fluid-expanded states.

Normal-renin essential hypertension

The most recent hypothesis concerning the potential role of the renin-aldosterone axis in the pathogenesis of essential hypertension is that the normal reciprocal influence of sodium intake on vascular (particularly renovascular) and adrenal responses to angiotensin II is absent (see Chap. 16). A substantial body of evidence has accumulated that suggests that some patients with essential hypertension have alterations in their target tissue sensitivity to angiotensin II with changes in sodium intake.[66] Indeed, in these individuals changing sodium intake has no effect on the sensitivity to angiotensin II of the adrenal and renal blood supply. Because angiotensin is pivotal to the regulation of both renal blood flow and the adrenal release of aldosterone as dietary sodium intake varies, it is reasonable to ask whether the abnormality was present in both systems in the same patient. The answer in two studies was unequivocal: Parallel renal and adrenal abnormalities coexist in the same patient with essential hypertension.[126,150]

These studies strongly suggest that in a subgroup of patients with essential hypertension renal blood flow, aldosterone, and pressor responses to angiotensin II are not properly modulated when sodium intake changes. This is why these patients have been called "nonmodulators." The abnormality can be defined either by the absence of an increased renal vascular response to angiotensin II on a high-salt diet or by the absence of an increased adrenal response to angiotensin II on a low salt intake. Regardless of which technique has been used to define the nonmodulator, abnormalities in angiotensin II target tissues have coincided (Figs. 49-7 and 49-8).

What is the mechanism responsible for the hypertension in the nonmodulator? Theoretically, abnormal renal responsiveness to angiotensin II could result in the failure to increase renal blood flow when nonmodulators are placed on a high-salt diet, with subsequent sodium retention and a rise in blood pressure. Proof of this hypothesis has come from five sources. First nonmodulators do not increase renal blood flow when salt-loaded (Fig. 49-9). Second, when placed on a low-salt diet they have a delay in the time necessary to achieve salt balance.[67] The time

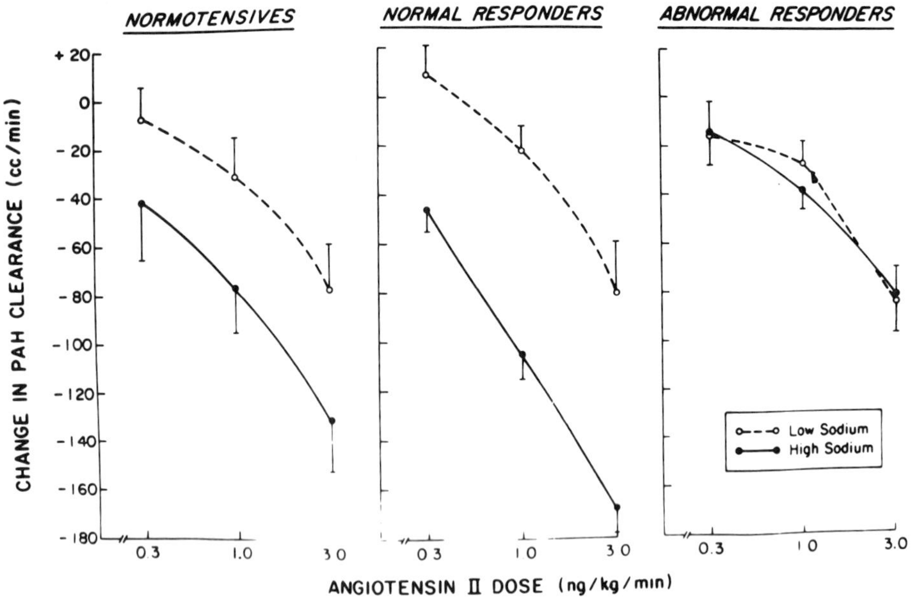

FIGURE 49-7 • Comparison of response in para-aminohippurate (PAH) clearance during angiotensin II infusion in normotensive and hypertensive subjects. The decrement in PAH clearance during angiotensin II infusion was significantly ($p < .01$) greater in eight normal-responding hypertensive patients (center panel) on the high-sodium, compared to the low-sodium, diet, which was comparable to the responses of normotensive subjects (left panel). There was no significant difference in the PAH decrement during angiotensin II infusion for the ten abnormal responders (right panel) between the low- and high-sodium intake. (From Shoback DM et al: *J Clin Invest* 72:2115, 1983, with permission.)

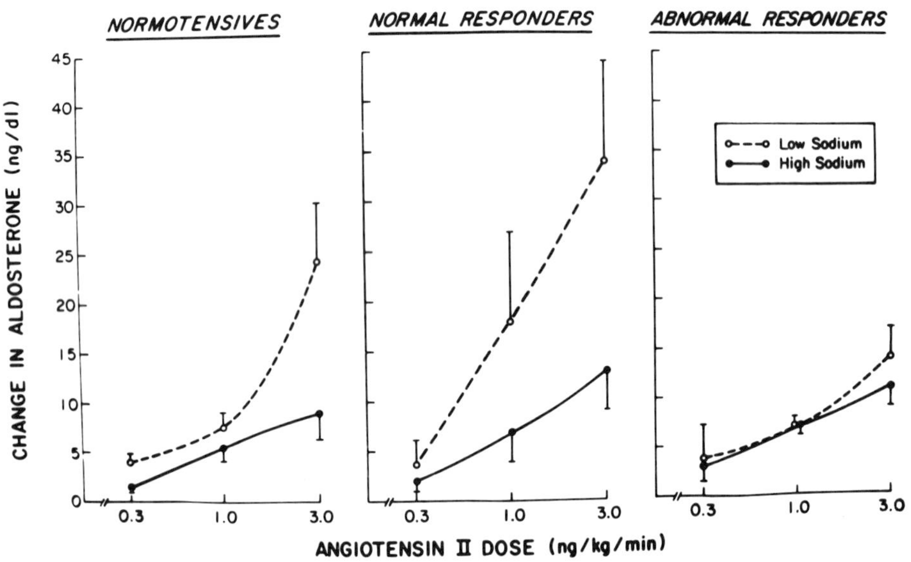

FIGURE 49-8 • Responses of plasma aldosterone to graded infusion of angiotensin II during sodium restriction and sodium loading in normotensive and hypertensive subjects. The aldosterone increment was significantly greater ($p < .01$) in the eight normal responders (modulators) with sodium restriction than with sodium repletion (center panel), comparable to normotensive subjects. The 10 abnormal responders (nonmodulators) showed no statistical difference between their aldosterone increments during sodium restriction vs. sodium repletion (right panel). (From Shoback DM et al: *J Clin Invest* 72:2115, 1983, with permission.)

necessary in nonmodulators is nearly 50 percent longer than in modulating hypertensive patients and in normotensive subjects. Third, when hypertensive patients are given a small sodium load (60 meq), the amount of sodium excreted by nonmodulators is nearly 50 percent less than that observed in normotensive subjects.[119] Fourth, when dietary intake in hypertensive patients is changed from 10 to 200 meq, the amount of sodium retained after 5 days of high salt intake is nearly twice as great in nonmodulating as in modulating hypertensive patients[67,116] (Fig. 49-10). Finally, only the nonmodulators show an increase in blood pressure in response to salt loading.[116] Thus nonmodulators are salt-sensitive hypertensive patients; indeed, they are likely to be the largest subset of these patients (Table 49-5).

What can account for the abnormal adrenal and renal vascular responses to angiotensin II? It has been suggested that abnormalities exist in the local tissue renin-angiotensin systems in the adrenal glomerulosa and the renal vasculature. Evidence to support this possibility includes the following: First, when patients on a sodium-restricted diet are given a converting enzyme inhibitor (CEI) for 3 days, there is no change in the adrenal response to angiotensin II in modulating hypertensive patients or in normotensive subjects. In nonmodulators, however, there is a substantial increase in the adrenal responsiveness to angiotensin II following the administration of a CEI, with a complete correction of the abnormality after six weeks of CEI inhibition.[139] Second, when normotensive subjects and modulating hypertensive patients are placed on a high-sodium diet and then given a CEI, renal blood flow does not rise significantly. In nonmodulators, however, there are significant increases in renal blood flow following administration of a CEI[116] (Fig. 49-11). In fact, the increase in nonmodulators is approximately the same as that observed in the normotensive patients when sodium intake is increased from a low to a high level. Thus, CEI appears to correct the renal vascular abnormality observed in the nonmodulators. Finally, CEI administration also corrects the reduced sodium excretion following acute saline loading in nonmodulators.[119] Thus CEI administration appears to be a specific form of therapy to correct the nonmodulator defect. The fact that these agents can reverse the nonmodulator defect in both the adrenal and the renal vasculature suggests that abnormalities in the regulation or activity of the local renin-angiotensin system accounts for the nonmodulator defect. Furthermore, the results of CEI treatment provide strong support for the concept that the nonmodulator defect is a functional and not a fixed, structural, abnormality.

Recently data have also been reported that support the hypothesis that the nonmodulator defect is heritable. First, when adrenal aldosterone increments in response to a 3-ng infusion of angiotensin II are determined in a large group of hypertensive patients, the distribution is highly significantly bimodal ($p < .0009$). Second, the prevalence of a positive family history for hypertension in nonmodulators exceeds 85 percent in comparison to 25 to 30 percent in modulating hypertensive patients.[67] Third, normotensive subjects who have a positive family history for hypertension have a substantial reduction in adrenal responsiveness to angiotensin II when studied on

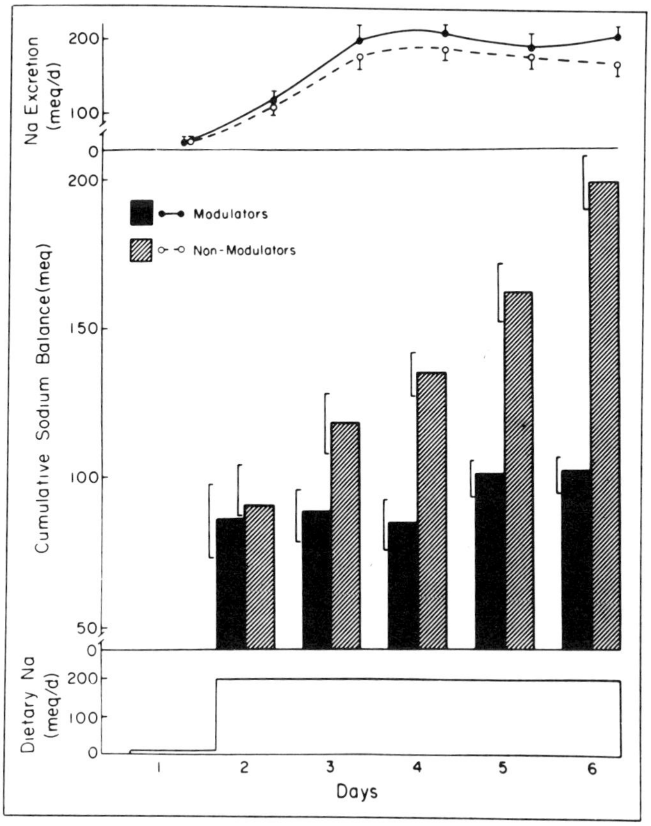

FIGURE 49-10 • Response of modulating and nonmodulating essential hypertensive patients to chronic sodium loading. Patients were first brought into balance on a 10-meq sodium intake; then the sodium intake was increased to 200 meq per day (bottom panel). The top panel depicts sodium excretion in the two subgroups, while the middle panel summarizes the cumulative sodium balance in the two groups. The modulators achieved sodium balance in approximately 2 days, with a net accumulation of 100 meq. In contrast, the nonmodulators had not reachieved balance after 5 days of high sodium intake and had accumulated approximately 200 meq of sodium. (From Hollenberg NK, Williams GH: *Am J Med* 81:412, 1986.)

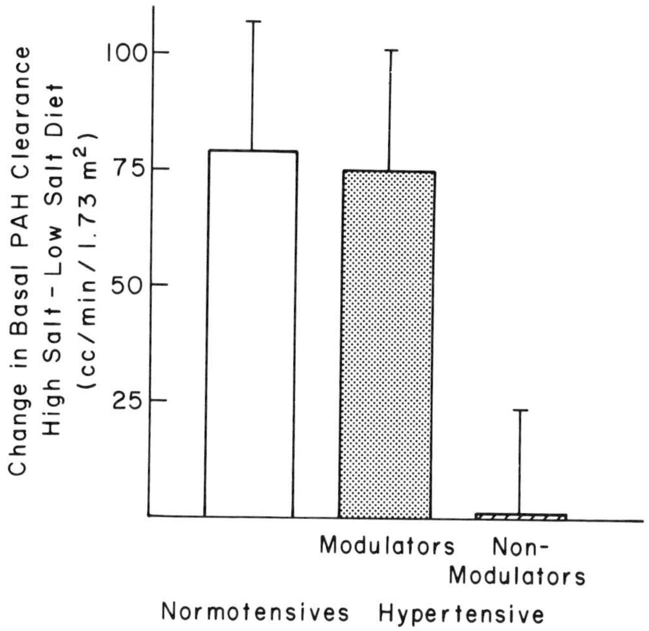

FIGURE 49-9 • Effect of sodium intake on basal renal plasma flow estimated by PAH clearance. PAH clearance was determined during a 10-meq and a 200-meq sodium intake. With sodium loading, PAH clearance increased significantly ($p < .01$, Fisher Exact Text) in normotensives and modulators (normal responders) but not in nonmodulators (abnormal responders). (From Shoback DM et al: *J Clin Invest* 72:2115, 1983. By copyright permission of the American Society for Clinical Investigation.)

TABLE 49-5 • Frequency of causes of sodium-sensitive hypertension*

Cause	Frequency (%)
Primary aldosteronism	<1
Acromegaly	<1
Bilateral renal artery stenosis	<1
Bilateral renal parenchymal disease	3.5
Low-renin essential hypertension	15–25
Nonmodulating essential hypertension	35–40

* Approximately 60% of hypertensives are sodium-sensitive.

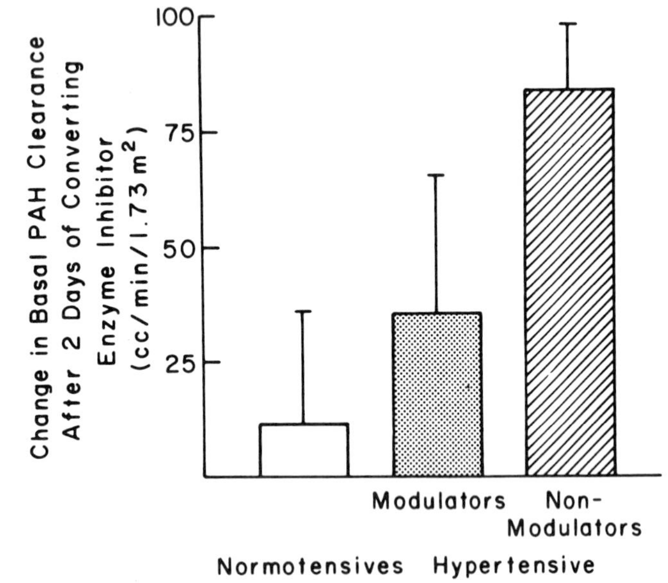

FIGURE 49-11 • Renal blood flow response to a converting enzyme inhibitor (enalapril). A control renal blood flow was assessed after all subjects were in balance on a 200-meq sodium intake. Enalapril was administered for 48 h and a repeat estimate of renal blood flow made. The normotensive subjects showed no significant change in renal blood flow following enalapril administration, while the nonmodulating essential hypertensives had a significant ($p < .01$) increase. (From Redgrave JE et al: *J Clin Invest* 75:1285, 1985. By copyright permission of the American Society for Clinical Investigation.)

a low-sodium diet.[9] Likewise, normotensive family-history-positive subjects also exhibit increases in renal blood flow response to CEI when studied on a high-sodium diet.[147] Finally, in hypertensive sibling pairs, there is a significant concordance of hypertension and nonmodulation[89] (Table 49-6).

TABLE 49-6 • Concordance of nonmodulation in hypertensive sibships

In 21 sib pairs with hypertension, the frequency of nonmodulation was determined by the renal blood flow response to AII. The frequency of nonmodulation in hypertensive sibships was compared to that expected assuming an overall frequency of nonmodulation of 40% in this population.

	Both nonmodulators	One nonmodulator	No nonmodulators
Sib Pairs	14	6	1
Expected	4	10	7

$p = .004$ (Pearson's Chi-Square)

SOURCE: Adapted from Lifton RP et al: *Hypertension* 13:884, 1989, with permission.

Thus nonmodulating hypertensive subjects, who make up 30 to 40 percent of the total hypertensive population, have a salt-sensitive form of hypertension. The underlying abnormality, which may be due to altered regulation of the tissue renin-angiotensin system, appears to be inherited. Other abnormalities have also been reported in nonmodulators.[58,114,123]

ELECTROLYTE DISTURBANCES IN HYPERTENSION CAUSED BY ENDOCRINE DISEASE

HYPERALDOSTERONISM

Hyperaldosteronism is a syndrome associated with hypersecretion of the major adrenal mineralocorticoid, aldosterone. In *primary* hyperaldosteronism the stimulus for the excessive aldosterone production resides within the adrenal gland; in *secondary* hyperaldosteronism the stimulus is of extraadrenal origin, usually stemming from response to activation of the renin-angiotensin system. (More information on hyperaldosteronism is found in Chap. 14.)

Primary hyperaldosteronism

The constellation of signs and symptoms of excessive inappropriate aldosterone production was first summarized by Conn in 1955.[29,156] In the original case and in the majority of subsequent cases, the disease was the result of an aldosterone-producing adrenal adenoma (Conn's syndrome). The majority (75 percent) of cases involved a unilateral adenoma, usually small and occurring with equal frequency on either side.[15] Rarely, primary hyperaldosteronism has been reported in association with adrenal carcinoma. It is twice as common in women as in men and typically presents between the ages of 30 and 50.

Substantial numbers of cases have been reported in which there were clinical and biochemical characteristics previously considered diagnostic of primary hyperaldosteronism but where no solitary adenoma was found at surgery. Instead, these patients had *bilateral cortical nodular hyperplasia*.[46] Although the cause of this hyperplasia is unknown, this *idiopathic hyperaldosteronism* (IHA) has been attributed to the overproduction of a variety of putative aldosterone secretagogues. A serotonin-mediated aldosterone stimulating system, a loss of inhibitory dopaminergic control,[85] and a glycoprotein aldosterone-stimulating factor (possibly of pituitary origin)[24] have all been implicated in the pathogenesis of IHA. In the literature this disease has been alternatively termed "psuedo" primary aldosteronism (PPA) or nodular hyperplasia.

Occurrence

Primary hyperaldosteronism is an uncommon disease. The prevalence in unselected hypertensive patients is between 0.5 and 2 pecent.[71] Because of special diagnostic procedures involved, diagnosis has been largely restricted to symptomatic patients. With greater availability of these procedures it may be seen with increased frequency.

Signs and symptoms

Almost all patients have diastolic hypertension, usually not of marked severity, and complain of headaches. The hypertension is related in some unknown manner to the increased sodium reabsorption and ECF expansion. The continual hypersecretion of aldosterone increases the renal distal tubular exchange of luminal sodium for secreted potassium and hydrogen ions; body potassium is progressively depleted, and hypokalemia develops. Potassium depletion is responsible for the major complaints, muscle weakness and fatigue. The symptoms are related to the effect of intra- and extracellular potassium ion depletion on muscle membrane potentials. The muscle weakness is most striking in the legs and may progress to transient paralysis. Muscles innervated by cranial nerves are usually spared. Frank tetany may also occur. Electrocardiographic signs of potassium depletion, such as prominent U waves, are often present; cardiac arrhythmias and premature contractions are not uncommon. These patients may have electrocardiographic and roentgenographic signs of left ventricular enlargement, which is secondary to their hypertension. Hypertensive retinopathy is often seen, but papilledema is usually absent. In the absence of associated congestive heart failure, renal disease, or preexisting local abnormalities (such as thrombophlebitis), edema is characteristically absent.[15,29,46,71] Polyuria results from hypokalemic impairment of concentrating ability, as a result of resistance to the action of ADH (i.e., acquired nephrogenic diabetes insipidus).

In cases of long duration, potassium depletion nephropathy may occur; in some instances it is associated with congestive heart failure and edema.

Laboratory findings

Laboratory findings depend largely on both the severity and the duration of the potassium depletion. An impaired ability to concentrate the urine is often seen following an overnight concentration test. Because of excessive excretion of ammonium and bicarbonate ions, urine pH is in the neutral-to-alkaline range. Glucocorticoid and androgen secretion should be within normal limits in patients with aldosterone-producing tumors. If hypokalemia is severe (less than 3 meq K^+ pe liter) there is usually a significant reduction in body potassium stores, usually in excess of 300 meq. Water loss, from polyuria, and sodium retention lead to hypernatremia. Serum bicarbonate concentration is elevated, and metabolic alkalosis develops; both are consequences of loss of hydrogen ions into the urine as well as migration of hydrogen ions into potassium-depleted cells. Potassium depletion also perpetuates the alkalosis, since hypokalemia increases the capacity of the proximal convoluted tubule to reabsorb filtered bicarbonate. Hypomagnesemia may also be seen if hypokalemia is severe. The serum uric acid level should be normal in the absence of azotemia. Total exchangeable body potassium is usually reduced, while total body sodium and total exchangeable sodium are increased. As a result of the expanded ECF, the normal nocturnal reduction of salt and water excretion may be lost, disrupting the circadian pattern of their excretion.

Diagnosis

Primary hyperaldosteronism should be suspected in a hypertensive patient with persistent hypokalemia and no edema whose sodium intake is normal and who is not receiving potassium-wasting diuretics. In a hypertensive patient on a potassium-wasting diuretic the finding of hypokalemia should lead to discontinuation of the diuretic and potassium supplementation. Within one to two weeks the potassium level should be reassessed; if hypokalemia persists, the patient should be evaluated for excess mineralocorticoid production (Fig. 49-12).

The major criteria that point to the diagnosis of primary aldosteronism include (1) diastolic hypertension without edema; (2) suppression of the renin-angiotensin system, as judged by low PRA levels that fail to increase appropriately following volume depletion and assumption of the upright position; (3) hypersecretion of aldosterone that does not suppress following salt loading.

The absence of edema in patients with primary aldosteronism is explained by the "escape" phenomenon from the sodium-retaining effects of chronic mineralocorticoid administration. However, edema may occur in those patients who have associated nephropathy and azotemia.

The failure of PRA to rise normally during volume depletion is an important diagnostic criterion for primary hyperaldosteronism, but suppressed PRA also is seen in approximately 25 percent of patients with essential hypertension. Therefore, the estimation of PRA is of limited value in separating patients with primary hyperaldosteronism from those with other causes of hypertension. The demonstration of lack of suppression of aldosterone secretion following volume increase is consequently a necessary additional criterion to be used for diagnosing primary hyperaldosteronism (Fig. 49-12). Although these aldosterone-producing tumors secrete aldosterone autonomously and resist suppression while

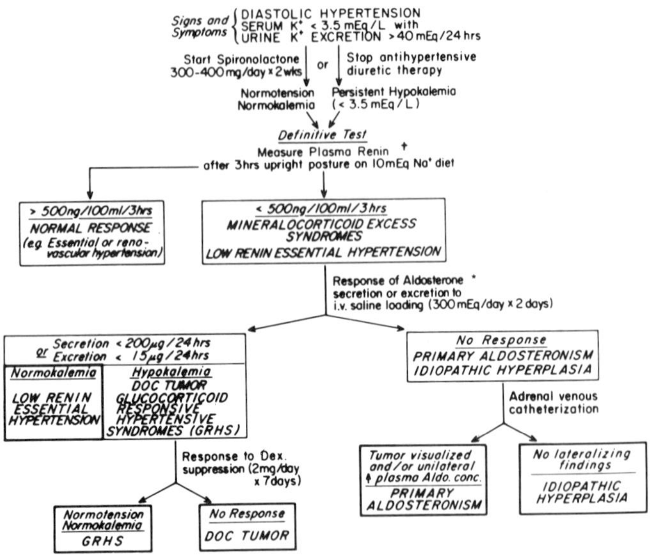

FIGURE 49-12 • Diagnostic flow chart for evaluating patients with suspected primary hyperaldosteronism. Identification of the hydroxylase deficiency in glucocorticoid-responsive hypertensive syndrome (GHRS) is the measurement of increased excretion of certain urinary metabolities of the intermediates of cortisol biosynthesis. *Alternative methods producing comparable suppression of aldosterone secretion include oral sodium loading (200 meq/day for 5 days) or 10 mg intramuscular deoxycorticosterone acetate (DOCA) every 12 h for 3 days. †An alternative outpatient method is the response of plasma renin activity to 3 h of upright activity following 80 mg furosemide (given the previous day). [From Williams GH, Dluhy RG, in Petersdorf RG et al (eds): *Harrison's Principles of Internal Medicine*, 10th ed. New York, McGraw-Hill, 1983, p 634.]

volume is increasing, they do respond to other stimuli, such as potassium loading or ACTH infusion.

Once hyposecretion of renin and autonomous aldosterone secretion are demonstrated, an attempt should be made to localize an adenoma by abdominal CT scanning or by the technique of percutaneous transfemoral bilateral adrenal vein catheterization with simultaneous venography.[148] The latter technique also permits sampling of the adrenal vein, which may demonstrate a significant two- to threefold increase in plasma aldosterone concentration on the involved side. It should be recalled that primary aldosteronism is also seen secondary to bilateral cortical nodular hyperplasia. In this situation aldosterone levels do not lateralize. It is emphasized, however, that samples during bilateral adrenal vein catheterization should be obtained simultaneously; cortisol levels should also be measured to avoid false localization secondary to ACTH-or stress-induced rises in aldosterone levels.

Differential diagnosis

Hypertension and hypokalemia may be seen in patients with primary or secondary hyperaldosteronism. The key test to distinguish between the two forms of hyperaldosteronism is measurement of PRA. In patients with secondary hyperaldosteronism (such as individuals with accelerated hypertension), the hyperaldosteronism follows elevated plasma renin levels. In primary hyperaldosteronism, plasma renin levels are suppressed. The most common problem is difficulty in distinguishing between hyperaldosteronism due to an adenoma and the hyperaldosteronism of IHA. The distinction is clinically important, since bilateral adrenalectomy does not benefit the hypertension in patients with bilateral IHA. In contrast, resection usually cures the hypertension in patients with aldosterone-producing adenomas. Patients with bilateral IHA tend to have higher PRA and less severe hypokalemia, and to secrete less aldosterone, than patients with aldosterone-producing adenomas. However, differentiation is impossible on clinical or biochemical grounds. An anomalous postural decrease in plasma aldosterone and an elevated 18-hydroxycorticosterone plasma level are found in patients with aldosterone-producing adenomas; in the individual patient, however, these tests are of limited diagnostic value. The definitive diagnosis is made by radiographic studies (CT scanning and adrenal venography with sampling) as outlined above.

Primary hyperaldosteronism must also be distinguished from other hypermineralocorticoid states. For example, hypertensive patients with hypokalemic alkalosis have been found, albeit rarely, to have *DOC-secreting adenomas*. These patients also have reduced levels of PRA; measurements of aldosterone levels reveal them to be either normal or reduced, which is consistent with the excess production of another mineralocorticoid. Another rare syndrome is hypermineralocorticoidism secondary to a defect in cortisol biosynthesis, specifically *defects in 11- or 17-hydroxylation*. As a consequence of glucocorticoid insufficiency, ACTH levels rise; production of the mineralocorticoid 11-deoxycorticosterone increases as a result. In this situation, glucocorticoid administration corrects the hypokalemia and hypertension. The definitive diagnostic test is the demonstration of a specific elevation of a precursor of cortisol biosynthesis in the urine or blood. In another syndrome, glucocorticoid administration may produce normotension and normokalemia although no specific hydroxylase deficiency can be identified (so-called glucocorticoid-remediable hyperaldosteronism).[44,53,146] A diagnostic clue in this situation is provided by a strong family history of hypertension occurring early in life. This syndrome, which is inherited as an autosomal dominant trait, is diagnosed by the discovery of the abnormal "hybrid" steroids (18-hydroxycortisol and 18-hydroxycortisone) in the urine of affected family members. Recently, the gene causing glucocorticoid-remediable aldosteronism has been identified. The mutation results from fusion of the genes encoding steroid IIβ-hydroxylase and aldosterone synthase in the adrenal fasciculeta, thereby causing the clinical and biochemical features of this order.[89a]

An additional syndrome that may mimic primary hyperaldosteronism results from the ingestion of a compound contained in chewing tobacco or licorice.[133] The agent, glycyrrhizic acid, inhibits renal 11-hydrogenase activity, resulting in heightened mineralocorticoid activity due to the binding of cortisol to the mineralocorticoid receptor (see "Mineralocorticoid Physiology" under "Regulation of the Renin-Angiotensin-Aldosterone Axis," in the "Basic Considerations" section above). As a consequence, there is sodium retention, expansion of ECF, hypertension, suppressed aldosterone levels, and depressed plasma renin levels. The diagnosis is established by the patient's history, which, of course, should always be taken with care.

Secondary hyperaldosteronism

In secondary hyperaldosteronism activation of the renin-angiotensin system leads to increased aldosterone production (Fig. 49-5). The aldosterone secretion rates in patients with secondary hyperaldosteronism are similar to, but may exceed, those in subjects with primary hyperaldosteronism. Secondary hyperaldosteronism may occur in pregnancy; it constitutes a normal physiologic response to estrogen-induced increases in circulating levels of renin substrate and PRA. Alternatively, this syndrome may occur in an accelerated phase of hypertension or on the basis of an underlying edema-forming state with an associated decline in circulating intravascular volume.

In hypertensive states, hyperaldosteronism may occur because of an overproduction of renin precipitated by a decrease in renal blood flow and/or perfusion pressure. Hyperaldosteronism may also appear as a primary overproduction of renin by a neoplasm. A decrease in renal flow and/or perfusion pressure may be produced by *narrowing of one or both of the major renal arteries*—for instance, by an atherosclerotic plaque or by fibromuscular hyperplasia. Overproduction of renin from both kidneys is also seen in association with severe arteriolar nephrosclerosis (malignant hypertension) or secondary to profound renal vasoconstriction in the accelerated phase of hypertensive disease. In patients with *malignant or accelerated hypertension*, marked-to-severe increases in PRA often lead to increases in aldosterone levels and hypokalemic alkalosis.

So-called *primary reninism* may also lead to hypertension and secondary hyperaldosteronism. In primary reninism biochemical markers are similar to those in subjects with renovascular hypertension. However, the abnormality is the secretion of renin by a *JG cell tumor*. The diagnosis is suggested by absence of changes in the renovasculature and the demonstration of a space-occupying lesion by radiographic studies. Unilateral increases in renin activity confirm the diagnosis.

In many *edematous disorders*, such as cirrhosis and congestive heart failure, secondary hyperaldosteronism is common. In congestive heat failure, the elevated aldosterone secretion is found inconsistently; it depends on the severity of cardiac decompensation. In all the disease states, the stimulus for renin release appears to be arterial hypovolemia and/or hypotension. In these situations, diuretic therapy may exaggerate the features of secondary hyperaldosteronism by additionally diminishing volume. As a consequence, hypokalemia and alkalosis may become prominent laboratory findings.

In the absence of edema and hypertension, secondary hyperaldosteronism may also be found in patients with *Bartter's syndrome*. In this disorder severe hyperaldosteronism and accompanying hypokalemic alkalosis are accompanied by moderate-to-marked increases in PRA. However, Bartter's syndrome patients have normal blood pressures and do not have edema. Renal biopsy reveals JG hyperplasia. Although the pathogenesis of this syndrome is unknown, some authors have speculated that there is a defect in the conservation of sodium or chloride by the loop of Henle. Loss of sodium and chloride subsequently stimulates renin secretion, producing secondary hyperaldosteronism. The hyperaldosterone state also produces potassium depletion; the hypokalemia further elevates PRA. The hypokalemia may also be potentiated by a defect in renal conservation of potassium. Increased production of prostaglandins is commonly observed in this syndrome; the finding may be of pathogenic significance.

PHEOCHROMOCYTOMA

Pheochromocytomas are tumors arising from the chromaffin cells of the sympathoadrenal system. They secrete catecholamines and may be the rarest of all causes of hypertension, accounting for less than 1 in 1000 cases of hypertension in most series.[128] However, like tumors of the adrenal cortex, they are extremely important as a cause of curable hypertension. Most of these tumors originate unilaterally from adrenal medullary tissue. However, they may be found in any area in the midline region from neck to sacrum. They are usually benign. Most cases appear to be sporadic, although there is some familial incidence.[131] The combination of a parathyroid adenoma or hyperplasia, medullary thyroid carcinoma, and pheochromocytoma, usually bilateral, has an especially high familial incidence (so-called Sipple's syndrome or multiple endocrine adenomatosis, type 2A). Pheochromocytomas also occur in higher prevalence in the phacomatosis syndromes, including von Hippel-Lindau disease, mucosal neuromas, and neurofibromatosis (von Recklinghausen's disease).

The usual disturbance in electrolyte and fluid homeostasis in these patients is a decrease in both plasma and total blood volumes. When the blood pressure is increased by norepinephrine, vasoconstriction occurs not only on the arterial side but also on the venous side of the capillary bed. This increases capillary pressure and causes transudation of fluid from the intravascular to the extracellular space. If norepinephrine is infused into normal subjects, the loss of fluid results in a rise in serum protein concentration and hematocrit. However, with sustained release of norepinephrine, readjustments may occur in the bone marrow and the liver so that hematocrit and total protein return to normal levels within a decreased total blood volume. Nevertheless, a high hematocrit is still seen in some patients with pheochromocytoma. The high hematocrit probably reflects contracted plasma space, but polycythemia has also been reported as occurring secondarily to erythropoietin production by a pheochromocytoma.

Because of their decreased blood volume, pheochromocytoma patients may experience postural hypotension. The reduction of blood volume probably also accounts for the occasional catastrophic fall in blood pressure during surgical treatment, despite relatively minor blood loss prior to removal of the tumor. Pressor agents are usually ineffective; the treatment of choice is infusion of plasma expanders and whole blood to replace operative losses. Preoperative treatment of the hypertension with diuretics or sodium restriction can increase this risk.

Pheochromocytoma is treated by surgical removal of the chromaffin tumor, if at all possible. It is mandatory to restore normal blood volume before surgery, by controlling the blood pressure with orally administered phenoxybenzamine. The drug is administered twice daily; the dose is increased slowly over a 5- to 7-day period until blood pressure is controlled. During this treatment phase, the hematocrit and total protein concentration fall as fluid volume increases.

In certain cases of malignant pheochromocytoma, medical treatment can be continued indefinitely with a fair degree of success in controlling symptoms and the elevated arterial blood pressure.

ELECTROLYTE DISTURBANCES IN PATIENTS WITH RENAL HYPERTENSION

BACKGROUND

Renal disease, both acute and chronic, including renal vascular abnormalities, is the most common cause of secondary hypertension, accounting for 7 to 10 percent of the total hypertensive population.[72] How renal disease produces hypertension is still uncertain. The mechanisms have been divided into two major groups: vasoconstrictor- (angiotensin-) dependent and volume-mediated. It is assumed that vasoconstrictor-mediated hypertension is secondary to renal ischemia or reduced blood flow, which may result from injury or from constriction of the vascular supply to the kidney. In volume-dependent hypertension there is loss of renal mass; the kidney is less able to excrete sodium, and a derangement in volume homeostasis results. There is also evidence that in some anephric individuals with hypertension, the lack of a renal vasodepressor substance(s) may contribute to the elevated blood pressure; prostaglandins and/or tissue kallikreins are the suggested vasodepressors.[72] The electrolyte and volume abnormalities associated with loss of kidney mass are similar in any form of chronic renal disease; they are covered in detail in Chap. 15. In this section we will review electrolyte disturbances and the pathophysiology of angiotensin-dependent hypertension.

The initiating event in the development of hypertension with renal artery stenosis is presumably the release of renin in response to a decrease in flow or pressure or the development of renal ischemia. Angiotensin II levels then increase (Fig. 49-1). An increase in angiotensin II has two significant effects: increased aldosterone secretion, and increased peripheral resistance—ultimately combining to lead to an increase in blood pressure. Increased aldosterone secretion, initially at least, produces sodium retention and increased cardiac output; then, by autoregulation, peipheral resistance can be further increased and cardiac output lowered. With the sodium retention initiated by aldosterone's effect, ECF expands, which normally reduces renin release. However, for the level of volume expansion, renin and angiotensin II levels are still, here, inappropriately elevated. These theoretical considerations have been partly substantiated by observation and experiment. Cardiac output is above normal in some patients with renovascular hypertension but presumably is less important than the increased peripheral resistance in raising the blood pressure. Animal studies suggest that, at least initially, there is an increase in aldosterone secretion in renovascular hypertension.[39]

DIAGNOSIS OF RENOVASCULAR HYPERTENSION

The most useful procedures to screen for, and definitively diagnose, those patients who have surgically correctable renal hypertension are not agreed upon. There are two major problems: determining if unilateral renal disease is present, and proving that the hypertension is secondary to the renal disease. The rapid sequence intravenous pyelogram, formerly the primary screening test for renal artery stenosis, largely has been replaced by the digital substraction angiogram.[26] If this procedure is performed with the arterial rather than venous administration of dye, the sensitivity and specificity is much higher than for the intravenous pyelogram. A second procedure is the radioisotope renogram (or renoscan) with ^{131}I-O-iodohippurate. This test is less sensitive and specific than either the intravenous pyelogram or the digital subtraction angiogram. A recent modification, however, is said to improve sensitivity and specificity; this is to perform a renoscan after the administration of the CEI captopril.[47] In comparison to control subjects, a fall in renal perfusion would occur in the kidney with renal artery stenosis. This is due to a reduction in angiotensin II's principal action on postglomerular efferent arteriolar tone, which is maintaining glomerular filtration in the kidney with the arterial stenosis. Thus captopril, by enhancing lateralization to the stenotic side by interrupting renal autoregulation, improves diagnostic accuracy.

If a unilateral renal lesion is discovered, it still must be proven to be functionally significant. This is accomplished by bilateral renal vein renin determinations. Theoretically, if a vascular lesion is of functional importance, there should be increased renin secretion from the involved kidney; simultaneously obtained renin measurements should predict renal ischemia and, therefore, response to therpy. In most studies a ratio of involved to uninvolved renin of 1.6 or greater has been required.[134] However, with this requirement, the number of false-negative results has remained substantial.[72] While an abnormal ratio is highly predictive of a good response to surgery, a normal ratio does not mean that a good response will not occur. A number of studies have suggested that patients who have normal ratios and a good response to surgery probably were not studied under optimal conditions. Renal ischemia should be more apparent if renin is determined after volume depletion (Fig. 49-1). Therefore, many centers have suggested that renin measurements should be performed only after volume or sodium depletion. In one study, prognostic accuracy increased from 35 to 90 percent using this approach.[137] In addition to sodium depletion, further stimulation of the renin-angiotensin system at the time of renal vein catheterization can be achieved with the administration of a converting enzyme inhibitor. This maneuver permits the diagnosis of true renovascular hypertension to be made with a very high degree of accuracy.[90,115]

ELECTROLYTE AND VOLUME ABNORMALITIES

Fluid and electrolyte changes in renovascular hypertension are secondary to the underlying renal disease and to the hyperaldosteronism that is sometimes induced by the disease. The interaction of these two broadens the range of electrolyte and water disturbances that can occur. In some patients, biochemical signs may be indistinguishable from those of primary aldosteronism.

The renin-angiotensin-aldosterone system does not account for all the disturbances observed in salt and water metabolism in renal hypertension. It has been shown that a decrease in renal perfusion pressure also causes increased salt and water reabsorption from tubule sites that are not aldosterone-dependent. On the other hand, this reabsorption may be countered by the contralateral uninvolved kidney, in which a rise in perfusion pressure decreases fractional salt and water reabsorption proximally and thereby increases sodium excretion. The fluctuating balance of these three factors—increased perfusion pressure in the uninvolved kidney, decreased perfusion pressure in the involved kidney, and hyperaldosteronism—accounts for the variable volume and electrolyte picture observed in patients with renovascular hypertension. In general, the serum potassium level is slightly reduced (between 3 and 3.8 meq/liter), reflecting increased aldosterone secretion. The serum sodium concentration is also generally lower (133 to 138 meq/liter); this may be related to the increased excretion of sodium from the nonstenotic kidney. As a consequence, patients with renovascular hypetension usually have reduced plasma volumes.

If the hypertension is severe enough to cause renal failure, the electrolyte pattern changes to that of renal insufficiency. It is then characterized by renal acidosis, sodium wasting, hyperkalemia, and abnormalities in calcium and phosphate levels. These patients can neither concentrate the urine properly nor excrete a water load normally, and so are prone both to dehydration, if an adequate intake of fluid is not maintained, and to water intoxication, if large loads of water are given.

TREATMENT

The logical treatment of choice for renal vascular hypertension is to correct the lesion anatomically. Percutaneous transluminal dilatation has replaced surgery as the preferred way to accomplish this end.[72] However, it is important to remember that repair of the stenosis will not relieve the hypertensive nephrosclerosis, nor cortical atrophy in the stenotic or contralateral kidney. Moreover, with increasing experience, enthusiasm for these procedures has decreased, notably for those individuals with generalized and severe atherosclerosis, because of morbidity and a high rate of restenosis following angioplasty. Thus older patients with aortic atherosclerosis who have a satisfactory response to medical therapy may not be candidates for percutaneous transluminal dilatation. On the other hand, young persons with unilateral fibromuscular disease remain excellent candidates for transluminal dilatation or surgery.

This change in emphasis is partly the result of improved medical therapies, particularly with CEIs, which can specifically reduce the increased production of angiotensin II that underlies the hypertension in these patients. However, acute renal failure has been observed following the use of CEIs in patients with renal artery stenosis in both kidneys or stenosis of the renal artery in a patient with a solitary kidney.[69]

ELECTROLYTE DISTURBANCES IN PATIENTS WITH ESSENTIAL HYPERTENSION

Most patients with nonmalignant essential hypertension appear to have normal serum electrolyte levels, pH, and plasma and ECF volumes. However, several factors may alter this satisfactory state and produce marked abnormalities. Certain abnormalities in salt and water balance have been uncovered in patients with this disease. Early on, some hypertensive subjects were found to respond to hypertonic or isotonic saline infusions with exaggerated natriuresis.[5] This response does not depend on pretreatment sodium balance; whether the infusion is hypo-, iso-, or hypertonic; on the response of the blood pressure to the infusion; or on simultaneous changes in renal hemodynamics. However, it is often associated with a marked increase in central venous pressure before the natriuresis occurs. Whether the abnormal natriuresis is simply due to elevated blood pressure or is intrinsic to the disease is difficult to determine. A number of studies have shown that the same exaggerated natriuresis does occur in other forms of hypertension. However, Aviram and associates[4] have shown that patients with labile hypertension, and normotensive women who have recovered from toxemia of pregnancy, react to an infusion of hypertonic salt solution in much the same manner as those who have various forms of hypertension, even though the former groups are normotensive during the period of testing. Confusion exists because the exaggerated natriuresis can be induced in experimental animals and in human beings with appropriate vasoconstrictive stimuli.[4] This has led some authors to postulate that the natriuresis is a response to hypertension per se rather than a basic physiological defect. However, the exaggerated response in normotensive subjects, such as those studied by Aviram, goes unexplained if an elevated blood pressure is assumed to be the sole requirement. This phenomenon suggests a problem in the volume-sensing or volume-regulating mechanism in these individuals, which may be etiologically significant in both the production of essential hypertension and the natriuretic response.

It has been suggested that the baseline, or typical, level of renin secretion may play a role in the response of hypertensive patients to sodium loading. Low-renin essential hypertension patients and patients with primary hyperaldosteronism invariably displayed the excessive natriuretic response. However, patients with normal-renin essential hypertension had a normal natriuresis. This difference may explain some of the discrepancies in the response of hypertensive patients in previous studies.[117]

A second volume aberration seen in some patients with essential hypertension is a decrease in plasma volume. This decrease reportedly increases in magnitude as diastolic pressure mounts; it becomes significant when the diastolic pressure reaches 105 mmHg. This finding contrasts with that seen in primary hyperaldosteronism.[138]

Measurements of the sodium content of the arterial walls of experimental animals with hypertension have repeatedly shown increased values relative to normotensive animals. This may be due to muscular contraction causing cellular potassium efflux and sodium influx, or may be secondary to some factor significant in the pathogenesis of the disease. In any case, it has been shown that sensitivity of a perfused aortic strip to angiotensin II increases as the sodium content of the bath is increased. The enhanced sensitivity may be due to a Starling-type phenomenon in the vessel wall; on the other hand, sodium and volume depletion may decrease the stretch of the vessel wall, thereby decreasing its responsiveness to any stimulus. However, the increased sensitivity of the aortic strip when increased sodium is present makes it equally probable that the sodium ion itself is etiologically significant.

DIFFERENTIAL DIAGNOSIS

Any screening tests performed must separate curable from incurable forms of hypertension. The curable causes include unilateral renal disease; renal artery stenosis; pheochromocytomia; diseases of the adrenal cortex, such as primary hyperaldosteronism and Cushing's syndrome; and, less commonly, other endocrine disorders, such as thyroid dysfunction and acromegaly. The minimally effective screening procedure consists of obtaining a specific set of values for biochemical markers: serum electrolytes; blood urea nitrogen (BUN) and creatinine; 24-h urine catecholamines and vanillylmandelic acid or metanephrine (urine should be collected during the time the patient is hypertensive); 24-h urine for free cortisol or 17-hydroxycorticosteroids; urine culture with urinalysis; and digital substraction angiogram or captopril-primed renoscan. The extensive studies necessary for the diagnosis of primary hyperaldosteronism should be reserved for those hypertensive patients who present with hypokalemia and suppressed PRA. If abnormalities in any of the screening tests seem to warrant further investigation, then a specific protocol designed to bring out the basic defect should be carried out as described above.

TREATMENT OF ESSENTIAL HYPERTENSION

A particular form of antihypertensive therapy is chosen empirically to lower blood pressure, or to treat a specific known type of secondary hypertension. In secondary forms of hypertension there is an important choice to be made between medical management and invasive surgical intervention (i.e., surgery or angioplasty). In most instances surgery is recommended, since it may be curative; however, elderly patients or subjects with advanced vascular disease, who face major operative risks, can often be managed successfully with drug therapy. Some drug therapies are specific, such as spironolactone for primary hyperaldosteronism or phenoxybenzamine for pheochromocytoma CEIs are often successful in patients with renal artery stenosis if peripheral levels are significantly elevated. However, empirically chosen combination therapy may still be in order for some patients with secondary hypertension who are managed by medical means.

The role of dietary sodium restriction in the management of hypertension was established by Allen and Sherrill in 1922[1] and by the success of Kempner's fruit-and-rice diet.[76] Although severe sodium restriction is definitely beneficial, many physicians have abandoned dietary measures in favor of sodium-depleting diuretic agents. However, it is suggested that modest sodium restriction (daily intake 2 to 4 g) be attempted as initial therapy in patients with mild essential hypertension. Sodium restriction also reduces the potassium-wasting effects of thiazide diuretic therapy and lowers blood pressure beyond the level obtainable through diuretic therapy alone.[79]

Six major classes of drugs are available to treat patients with essential hypertension: diuretics, beta blockers, alpha blockers, peripheral vasodilators, calcium channel blockers, and CEIs. The agents most frequently used are thiazide diuretics. While they initially produce decreases in plasma and ECF volumes, it is unclear how they produce their long-term effect in lowering blood pressure. Thiazide diuretics have substantial side effects, including hypokalemia, hyperuricemia, glucose intolerance, and hyperlipidemia. Increasingly popular agents are calcium channel blockers and, particularly, CEIs. Both classes of drugs have a much reduced side effect profile compared to beta blockers and thiazide diuretics. Furthermore, in some studies CEIs actually improve the quality of life of the hypertensive patient—a claim that has not been made strongly for any other antihypertensive agent.

In the past a common approach used to treat the hypertensive patient was a step-care program, which began with a diuretic and continued with subsequent addition of other agents if the diuretic alone did not control the hypertension. The current version of step-care suggests that either diuretics, beta blockers, calcium channel blockers, or CEIs can be used as the initial step. If the target blood pressure is not achieved after the administration of the first drug then therapy is switched to another class of agents, or combination therapy is tried. In most cases a thiazide diuretic is one of the two agents used in combination therapies. Unfortunately, it is unclear which of the four primary agents should be used initially in a patient in whom there are no clues as to which might be most effective. Some specialists have suggested that CEIs should be tried first because of their better side-effect profile. In addition, since one-third of the essential hypertensive population probably are nonmodulators, CEIs offer the possibility of specific therapy.

SUMMARY OF ELECTROLYTE AND WATER DISTURBANCES IN HYPERTENSION

HYPONATREMIA

Hyponatremia associated with hypertension is usually related to diuretic therapy, renal disease, or accelerated hypertension with secondary hyperaldosteronism. The hyponatremia produced by renal disease usually is present only when the renal disease is obvious.

HYPERNATREMIA

The most common cause of hypernatremia associated with hypertension is increased aldosterone secretion, specifically in primary hyperaldosteronism. It is unusual to find elevated sodium levels in secondary hyperaldosteronism. The level of serum sodium depends on the degree of autonomy of aldosterone secretion.

HYPOKALEMIA

A decrease in serum potassium occurs in two common conditions associated with hypertension: diuretic therapy and increased aldosterone secretion. Kaliuresis is quite common with thiazide-type diuretics; usually it can be corrected with supplemental potassium chloride. Primary or secondary increases in aldosterone secretion produce kaliuresis. Some patients with essential hypertension also have borderline hypokalemia with no known cause.

HYPOMAGNESEMIA

Low circulating Mg^{2+} levels may be seen in hyperaldosteronism (see Chap. 34).

HYPERCALCEMIA

Hypercalcemia due to hyperparathyroidism and vitamin D intoxication is associated with an increased frequency of hypertension. Normalization of calcium levels does not always correct the hypertension.

METABOLIC ALKALOSIS

Metabolic alkalosis is due to diuretics, which increase the amount of sodium chloride presented to the distal tubules and thereby induce increased bicarbonate synthesis and reabsorption and chloride loss. Metabolic alkalosis is also produced by excess aldosterone (or cortisol) secretion when hydrogen and potassium ions exchange for sodium at the distal sites; serum bicarbonate levels increase as a consequence. (See Chaps. 10 and 29.)

TOTAL BODY WATER

Total body water is increased in primary hyperaldosteronism (increased ECF and plasma volumes) and in hypertension associated with acromegaly (increased extracellular, intracellular, and plasma volumes). In renal vascular hypertension there is often a decrease in plasma volume; in essential hypertension plasma volume may be normal or decreased.

METABOLIC ACIDOSIS

If present in a hypertensive patient, metabolic acidosis is usually a result of renal failure. Metabolic acidosis complicates the hypertension seen in patients with partial urinary tract obstruction and distal (type 4) RTA. Type I diabetic patients with nephropathy and hypertension commonly are mildly acidotic and hyperkalemic on account of hyporeninemic hypoaldosteronism.[88] Also, acidosis complicates hypertension in Gordon's syndrome, where the distal tubule has an inordinate permeability to chloride, thereby enhancing sodium chloride reabsorption. Volume expansion and hypertension develop simultaneously with reduced electrogenic and hormonal stimuli to potassium and hydrogen secretion.

Metabolic acidosis does not occur in uncomplicated hypertension.

REFERENCES

1. Allen FM, Sherrill JW: Treatment of arterial hypertension. *J Metab Res* 2:429, 1922.
2. Arriza JL et al: Cloning of human mineralocorticoid receptor complementary DNA: Structural and functional kinship with the glucocorticoid receptor. *Science* 237:268, 1987.
3. August JT et al: Response of normal subjects to large amounts of aldosterone. *J Clin Invest* 37:1549, 1958.
4. Aviram A et al: Diuretic and natriuretic response to a salt load in hypertensive and prehypertensive subjects. *Nephron* 2:82, 1965.
5. Baldwin DS et al: Exaggerated natriuresis in essential hypertension. *Am J Med* 24:893, 1958.
6. Baxter JD et al: Aldosterone receptors and the evaluation of plasma mineralocorticoid activity in normal and hypertensive states. *J Clin Invest* 58:579, 1976.
7. Baxter JD, Tyrell JB: The adrenal cortex, in Felig P et al (eds): *Endocrinology and Metabolism*, 2d ed. New York, McGraw-Hill, 1987, p. 511.
8. Beierwaltes WH et al: Renin release selectively stimulated by prostaglandin I_2 in isolated rat glomeruli. *Am J Physiol* 243:F276, 1982.
9. Beretta-Picolla C et al: Blunted aldosterone responsiveness to angiotensin II in normotensive subjects with predisposition to essential hypertension. *J Hyperten* 6:57, 1988.
10. Borst JGC, Borst de Geus A: Hypertension explained by Starling's theory of circulatory homeostasis. *Lancet* 1:677, 1963.
11. Braley LM et al: Comparative effect of angiotensin II, potassium adrenocorticotropin and cyclic adenosine 3′, 5′ monophosphate on cytosolic calcium in rat adrenal cells. *Endocrinology* 119:1010, 1986.
12. Brown JJ et al: Apparently isolated excess deoxycorticosterone in hypertension. *Lancet* 2:243, 1972.
13. Brunner HR et al: The influence of potassium administration and of potassium deprivation on plasma renin in normal and hypertensive subjects. *J Clin Invest* 49:2128, 1970.
14. Brunner HR et al: Essential hypertension: Renin and aldosterone, heart attack and stroke. *N Engl J Med* 286:441, 1972.
15. Cain JP et al: The regulation of aldosterone secretion in primary aldosteronism. *Am J Med* 53:627, 1972.
16. Cain JP et al: Plasma renin activity and aldosterone secretion in patients with acromegaly. *J Clin Endocrinol Metab* 34:73, 1972.
17. Caldwell PR et al: Angiotensin converting enzyme: Vascular endothelial localization. *Science* 191:1050, 1976.
18. Campbell DJ, Habener J: Angiotensinogen gene is expressed and differentially regulated in multiple tissues in the rat. *J Clin Invest* 78:31, 1986.
19. Canessa M et al: Increased sodium-lithium countertransport in red cells of patients with essential hypertension. *N Engl J Med* 302:772, 1980.
20. Capponi AM et al: Correlation between cytosolic free Ca and aldosterone production in bovine adrenal glomerulosa cells. *J Biol Chem* 259:8863, 1984.
21. Carey RM et al: The syndrome of essential hypertension and suppressed plasma renin activity. Normalization of blood pressure with spironolactone. *Arch Intern Med* 130:849, 1972.
22. Carey RM et al: Decreased plasma and urinary dopamine during dietary sodium depletion in man. *J Clin Endocrinol Metab* 52:903, 1981.
23. Carey RM et al: Effects of metoclopramide and bromocryptine on the renin-angiotensin-aldosterone system in man. *J Clin Invest* 63:727, 1979.
24. Carey RM et al: Idiopathic hyperaldosteronism. Defining a possible role for aldosterone-stimulating factor. *N Engl J Med* 311:94, 1984.
25. Churchill PC: Second messengers in renin secretion. *Am J Physiol* 249:F175, 1985.
26. Clark RA, Alexander ES: Digital subtraction angiography of the renal arteries—prospective comparison with conventional arteriograph. *Invest Radiol* 18:6, 1983.
27. Collins RD et al: Abnormally sustained aldosterone secre-

tion during salt loading in patients with various forms of beginning hypertension: Relation to plasma renin activity. *J Clin Invest* 49:1415, 1970.
28. Colman RW: Formation of human plasma kinin. *N Engl J Med* 291:509, 1974.
29. Conn JW: Presidential address: II. Primary aldosteronism: A new clinical syndrome. *J Lab Clin Med* 45:3, 1955.
30. Cooper RS et al: Intracellular calcium and sodium in hypertensive patients. *Hypertension* 9:224, 1987.
31. Creditor MC, Loschky UK: Incidence of suppressed renin activity and of normokalemic primary aldosteronism in hypertensive Negro patients. *Circulation* 37:1027, 1968.
32. Dale SL, Melby JC: Isolation and identification of 16α-18-dihydroxycorticosterone from human adrenal gland incubations. *Steroid* 21:617, 1973.
33. Dawson-Hughes BF et al: Plasma angiotensin concentration regulates vascular but not adrenal responsiveness to restriction of sodium intake in normal man. *Clin Sci* 61:527, 1981.
34. Defforest JM et al: Effects of indomethacin and meclofenemate on renin release and renal hemodynamic function during chronic depletion in conscious dogs. *Circ Res* 47:99, 1980.
35. DeFronzo RA et al: The effect of insulin on renal handling of sodium, potassium, calcium and phosphate in man. *J Clin Invest* 55:845, 1975.
36. Dickinson CJ, Lawrence JR: Slowly developing pressor response to low concentrations of angiotensin. *Lancet* 1:1354, 1963.
37. Dluhy RG et al: Effect of simultaneous potassium and saline loading on plasma aldosterone levels. *J Clin Endocrinol Metab* 45:141, 1977.
38. Dzau VJ: Possible prorenin activating mechanisms in the blood vessel wall. *J Hyperten* 5:515, 1987.
39. Dzau VJ et al: Sequential renal hemodynamics in experimental benign and malignant hypertension. *Hypertension* 3:63, 1981.
40. Dzau VJ et al: Molecular biology of the renin-angiotensin system. *Am J Physiol* 255:F563, 1988.
41. Dzau VJ, Hermann HC: Hormonal regulation of angiotensinogen synthesis. *Life Sci* 30:577, 1982.
42. Edleman IS, Marver D: Mediating events in the action of aldosterone. *J Steroid Biochem* 12:219, 1980.
43. Erne P et al: Correlation of platelet calcium with blood pressure: Effect of antihypertensive therapy. *N Engl J Med* 310:1084, 1984.
44. Fallo F et al: A new family with dexamethasone-suppressible hyperaldosteronism: Aldosterone unresponsiveness to angiotensin II. *Clin Endocrinol* 22:777, 1985.
45. Ferrannini E et al: Insulin resistance in essential hypertension. *N Engl J Med* 317:350, 1987.
46. Ferris JB et al: Hypertension with aldosterone excess and low plasma renin: Pre-operative distinction between patients with and without adrenocortical tumor. *Lancet* 2:995, 1970.
47. Fommei E et al: Renal scintigraphic captopril test in the diagnoses of renovascular hypertension. *Hypertension* 10:212, 1987.
48. Fray JCS et al: Interrelationship of blood flow, juxtaglomerular cells and hypertension: Role of physical equilibrium and Ca. *Am J Physiol* 251:R643, 1986.
49. Ganguly A, Hampton T: Calcium-dependence of serotonin-mediated aldosterone secretion and differential effects of calcium antagonists. *Life Sci* 36:1459, 1985.
50. Gary P, Meyer P: A new test showing abnormal net Na and K fluxes in erythrocytes of essential hypertensive patients. *Lancet* 1:349, 1979.
51. Goldblatt H et al: Studies on experimental hypertension I. The production of persistent elevation of systolic blood pressure by means of renal ischemia. *J Exp Med* 59:347, 1934.
52. Goldstone R et al: Reciprocal changes in active and inactive renin after converting enzyme inhibition in normal man. *J Clin Endocrinol Metab* 56:264, 1983.
53. Gomez-Sanchez CE et al: Glucocorticoid-suppressible aldosteronism—a disorder of the adrenal transitional zone? *J Clin Endocrinol Metab* 67:444, 1988.
54. Gonzales-Campoy JM et al: Escape from the sodium-retaining effects of mineralocorticoids: Role of ANF and intrarenal hormone systems. *Kidney Int* 35:767, 1989.
55. Goodfriend TL, Peach ML: Angiotensin II: Evidence and speculation for its role as an important agonist in the renin-angiotensin system. *Circ Res* 36/37:38, 1975.
56. Gordon MB et al: Dopaminergic blockade of the renin-angiotensin-aldosterone system: Effect of high and low sodium intake. *Clin Endocrinol* 19:415, 1983.
57. Gordon MB et al: Dopaminergic modulation of aldosterone responsiveness to angiotensin II with changes in sodium intake. *J Clin Endocrinol Metab* 56:340, 1983.
58. Gordon MB et al: The role of dopamine in non-modulating hypertension. *J Clin Endocrinol Metab* 69:426, 1989.
59. Gunther S et al: Regulation by angiotensin II of its receptors in resistant blood vessels. *Nature* 287:230, 1980.
60. Haddy FJ et al: Humoral factors and the sodium-potassium pump in volume expanded hypertension. *Life Sci* 24:2105, 1979.
61. Haning R et al: *In vitro* effects of ACTH, angiotensins, serotonin and potassium on steroid output and conversion of corticosterone to aldosterone by isolated adrenal cells. *Endocrinology* 87:1147, 1970.
62. Himathongkam T et al: Potassium-aldosterone-renin interrelationships. *J Clin Endocrinol Metab* 41:153, 1975.
63. Hobart PM et al: Human renin gene: Structure and sequence analysis. *Proc Natl Acad Sci USA* 81:5026, 1984.
64. Hollenberg NK et al: Potassium's influence on the renal vasculature, the adrenal, and their responsiveness to angiotensin II in normal man. *Clin Sci* 49:527, 1975.
65. Hollenberg NK et al: Reciprocal influence of salt intake on adrenal glomerulosa and renal vascular responses to angiotensin II in normal man. *J Clin Invest* 54:34, 1974.
66. Hollenberg NK et al: The renal vasculature in early essential hypertension: Evidence for a pathogenic role. *Medicine* 57:167, 1978.
67. Hollenberg NK, Williams GH: Abnormal renin sodium handling in essential hypertension: Relationship to failure of renal and adrenal modulation of responses to angiotensin II. *Am J Med* 81:412, 1986.
68. Horton R: Stimulation and suppression of aldosterone in plasma of normal men and in primary aldosteronism. *J Clin Invest* 48:1230, 1969.
69. Hricik DE et al: Captopril-induced functional renal insufficiency in patients with bilateral renal artery stenosis or renal artery stenosis in a solitary kidney. *N Engl J Med* 308:373, 1983.

70. Johansson B: Vascular smooth muscle reactivity. *Ann Rev Physiol* 43:359, 1981.
71. Kaplan NM: Commentary on incidence of primary aldosteronism: Current estimates based on objective data. *Arch Intern Med* 123:152, 1969.
72. Kaplan NM: *Clinical Hypertension*, 4th ed. Baltimore, Williams & Wilkins, 1986.
73. Katz FH et al: Diurnal variation of plasma aldosterone, cortisol, and renin activity in supine man. *J Clin Endocrinol Metab* 40:125, 1975.
74. Keeton TK, Campbell WB: The pharmacologic alteration of renin release. *Pharmacol Rev* 32:81, 1980.
75. Kem DC et al: Plasma aldosterone and renin activity response to ACTH infusion in dexamethasone suppressed normal and sodium depleted man. *J Clin Endocrinol Metab* 40:116, 1975.
76. Kempner W: Treatment of kidney disease and hypertensive vascular disease with rice diet. *NC Med J* 5:125, 1944.
77. Kifor I et al: The effect of sodium intake on angiotensin content of the rat adrenal gland. *Endocrinology* 128:1277, 1991.
78. Kirchner KA et al: Importance of chloride for acute inhibition of renin by sodium chloride. *Am J Physiol* 235:F444, 1978.
79. Kirkendall WM, Overturf ML: Thiazide diuretics and salt consumption in the treatment of hypertension, in Sambhi MP (ed): *Systemic Effects of Antihypertensive Agents.* New York, Stratton, 1976, p 119.
80. Kisch ES et al: Enhanced aldosterone response to angiotensin II in human hypertension. *Circ Res* 38:502, 1976.
81. Koletsky RJ et al: Dietary chloride modifies renin release in normal humans. *Am J Physiol* 241:F361, 1981.
82. Kotchen TA et al: Regulation of renin release by chloride. *Cardiovasc Res* 4:475, 1979.
83. Kotchen TA et al: Effect of acute and chronic calcium administration on plasma renin. *J Clin Invest* 54:1279, 1974.
84. Krozowski Z, Funder JW: Mineralocorticoid receptors in rat anterior pituitary: Toward a redefinition of "mineralocorticoid hormone." *Endocrinology* 109:1221, 1981.
85. Kuchel O et al: Are plasma aldosterone surges in primary aldosteronism due to a loss of an inhibitory dopaminergic control. *J Clin Endocrinol Metab* 51:337, 1980.
86. Lauber M, Muller J: Purification and characterization of two distinct forms of rat adrenal cytochrome P450 11 beta: Functional and structural aspects. *Arch Biochem Biophys* 274:109, 1989.
87. Lauer CG et al: Metoclopramide inhibits aldosterone biosynthesis *in vitro. Endocrinology* 111:238, 1982.
88. Lebel M, Grose JH: Angiotensin II effect of plasma steroids in selective hypoaldosteronism. *Horm Metab Res* 14:432, 1982.
89. Lifton RP et al: Evidence for heritability of non-modulating essential hypertension. *Hypertension* 13:884, 1989.
89a. Lifton RP et al: A chimaeric 11 beta-hydroxylase/aldosterone synthase gene causes glucocorticoid-remediable aldosteronism and human hypertension. Nature. 355:262, 1992.
90. Lyons DF et al: Captopril stimulation of differential renin in renovascular hypertension. *Hypertension* 5:615, 1983.
91. Marks AD et al: Enhanced adrenal responsiveness to angiotensin II in patients with low renin essential hypertension. *J Clin Endocrinol Metab* 48:266, 1980.
92. McCarron DA et al: Blood pressure and nutrient intake in the United States. *Science* 224:1393, 1984.
93. Melby JC et al: Secretion of 18-hydroxydeoxycorticosterone (18-OH DOC) in human hypertensive disease. *Circ Res* 28/29:143, 1971.
94. Messerli FH et al: Mineralocorticoid secretion in essential hypertension with normal and low plasma renin activity. *Circulation* 53:406, 1976.
95. Millar JA et al: Calcium antagonists decrease adrenal and vascular responsiveness to angiotensin II in normal man. *Clin Sci* 61:65, 1981.
96. Misono KS, Inagami TT: Characterization of the active site of mouse submandibular gland renin. *Biochemistry* 19:2616, 1980.
97. Modlinger RS et al: Stimulation of aldosterone, renin, and cortisol by tryptophan. *J Clin Endocrinol Metab* 48:599, 1979.
98. Mueller CB et al: Glomerular and tubular influence of sodium and water excretion. *Am J Physiol* 165:411, 1951.
99. Muirhead EE: The renomedullary antihypertensive system and its putative hormone(s), in Genest J et al (eds): *Hypertension*, 2d ed. New York, McGraw-Hill, 1983, p 394.
100. Muller J: *Regulation of Aldosterone Biosynthesis*, 2d ed. New York, Springer-Verlag, 1988.
101. Muller J, Huber R: Effects of sodium deficiency, potassium deficiency, and uremia upon the steroidogenic response of rat adrenal tissue to serotonin, potassium ions, and adrenocorticotropin. *Endocrinology* 85:43, 1969.
102. Mulrow PJ et al: The diagnoses and management of disorders of aldosterone production, in Gill GG (ed): *Pharmacology of Adrenal Cortisol Hormones.* New York, Pergamon, 1979, p 185.
103. Norbiato G et al: Metoclopramide increases plasma aldosterone in man. *J Clin Endocrinol Metab* 45:1313, 1977.
104. North RH et al: Tonic dopaminergic suppression of plasma aldosterone. *J Clin Endocrinol Metab* 51:64, 1980.
105. Oelkers W et al: Sensitization of the adrenal cortex to angiotensin II in sodium-depleted man. *Circ Res* 34:69, 1974.
106. Overbeck HW et al: Depressed function of a ouabain-sensitive sodium/potassium pump in blood vessels from renal hypertensive dogs. *Circ Res* 38:48, 1976.
107. Overbeck HW et al: Attenuated vasodilator responses to K^+ in essential hypertensive men. *J Clin Invest* 53:678, 1974.
108. Palkovits M et al: Effect of adrenocorticotrophic and growth hormones on aldosterone production and plasma renin activity of chronically hypophysectomized sodium deficient rats. *J Endocrinol* 47:243, 1970.
109. Palkovits J et al: The aldosterone secretory response to sodium restriction in chronically hypophysectomized corticotropin-maintained rats as a function of duration and amount of growth hormone treatment. *J Endocrinol* 50:407, 1971.
110. Platia MP et al: Angiotensin II receptor regulation during altered sodium intake in primates. *Hypertension* 8:1211, 1986.

111. Pollare T et al: Insulin resistance is a characteristic feature of primary hypertension independent of obesity. *Metabolism* 39:167, 1990.
112. Poston L et al: Evidence for a circulating sodium transport inhibitor in essential hypertension. *Br Med J* 282:847, 1981.
113. Pratt RE et al: Human renin biosynthesis and secretion in normal and ischemic kidneys. *Proc Natl Acad Sci USA* 84:7837, 1987.
114. Rabinowe SL et al: Renin suppression by saline is blunted in non-modulating essential hypertension. *Hypertension* 10:404, 1987.
115. Re R et al: Inhibition and angiotensin-converting enzyme for diagnosis of renal artery stenosis. *N Engl J Med* 298:582, 1978.
116. Redgrave JE et al: Converting enzyme inhibition corrects the altered renovascular responsiveness to angiotensin II in essential hypertension. *J Clin Invest* 75:1285, 1985.
117. Romero JC, Knox FG: Mechanisms underlying pressure-related natriuresis: The role of the renin-angiotensin and prostaglandin systems. *Hypertension* 11:724, 1988.
118. Rowe JW et al: Effect of insulin and glucose infusions on sympathetic nervous system activity in normal man. *Diabetes* 30:219, 1981.
119. Rydstedt L et al: The renal and endocrine response to saline infusion in essential hypertension. *Hypertension* 8:217, 1986.
120. Schalekamp MA et al: Studies on the mechanisms of hypernatriuresis in essential hypertension in relation to measurements of plasma renin concentration, body fluid compartments and renal function. *Clin Sci* 41:219, 1971.
121. Schalekamp MA et al: Body fluid volume in low renin hypertension. *Lancet* 1:30, 1974.
122. Seely EW et al: Adrenocorticotropin stimulation of aldosterone: Prolonged continuous versus pulsatile infusion. *J Clin Endocrinol Metab* 69:1028, 1989.
123. Seely EW et al: Angiotensin-mediated renin suppression is altered in non-modulating hypertension. *Hypertension* 13:31, 1989.
124. Sekihara H et al: Serum dihydroepiandrosterone sulfate and dihydroepiandrosterone levels in essential hypertension. *J Clin Endocrinol Metab* 40:156, 1975.
125. Shenker Y: Atrial natriuretic hormone effect on renal function and aldosterone secretion in sodium depletion. *Am J Physiol* 255:R867, 1988.
126. Shoback DM et al: Defect in the sodium-mediated tissue responsiveness to angiotensin II in essential hypertension. *J Clin Invest* 72:2115, 1983.
127. Simpson SA et al: Isolieurung eines neyen Kristablisierten Hormons aus Nebemmieren mit besonders Noher Wirksamkeit auf dem Mineralstoffwechsel. *Experientia* 9:333, 1953.
128. Sjoerdsma A et al: Pheochromocytoma: Current concepts of diagnosis and treatment. *Ann Intern Med* 65:1203, 1966.
129. Sowers JR et al: Dopaminergic modulation of aldosterone secretion in man is unaffected by glucocorticoid and angiotensin blockade. *J Clin Endocrinol Metab* 52:1978, 1981.
130. Starling EH: The Law of the Heart Beat: Linacre Lecture. London, Longmans Green and Company, 1918.
131. Steiner AL et al: Study of a kindred with pheochromocytoma, medullary thyroid carcinoma, hyperparathyroidism, and Cushing's disease: Multiple endocrine neoplasia, type 2. *Medicine* 47:371, 1968.
132. Stewart PM et al: Syndrome of apparent mineralocorticoid excess: A defect in the cortisol-cortisone shuttle. *J Clin Invest* 82:340, 1988.
133. Stewart PM et al: Mineralocorticoid activity of licorice: 11 beta-hydroxysteroid dehydrogenase deficiency comes of age. *Lancet* 2:821, 1987.
134. Stockigt JR et al: Renal-vein renin in various forms of renal hypertension. *Lancet* II:1194, 1972.
135. Strauch G et al: The renin-angiotensin-aldosterone system in normotensive and hypertensive patients with acromegaly. *N Engl J Med* 287:795, 1972.
136. Streeten DHP et al: Studies of the renin-angiotensin-aldosterone system in patients with hypertension and in normal subjects. *Am J Med* 46:844, 1969.
137. Strong CS et al: Renal venous renin activity enhancement of sensitivity of lateralization by sodium depletion. *Am J Cardiol* 27:602, 1971.
138. Tarazi RC et al: Haemodynamic characteristics of primary aldosteronism. *N Engl J Med* 289:1330, 1973.
139. Taylor T et al: Converting enzyme inhibition corrects the altered adrenal response to angiotensin II in essential hypertension. *Hypertension* 6:92, 1984.
140. Thurau KWC et al: Activation of renin in the single juxtaglomerular apparatus by sodium chloride in the tubular fluid at the macula densa. *Circ Res* 30/31:182, 1972.
141. Tuck ML et al: Relation of age, diastolic blood pressure and known duration of hypertension to presence of low renin essential hypertension. *Am J Cardiol* 22:637, 1973.
142. Tuck ML et al: A delayed suppression of the renin-aldosterone axis following saline infusion in human hypertension. *Circ Res* 39:711, 1976.
143. Tuck ML et al: A specific role for saline or the sodium ion in the regulation of renin and aldosterone secretion. *J Clin Invest* 53:988, 1974.
144. Tuck ML et al: Sequential responses of the renin-angiotensin-aldosterone axis to acute postural change: Effect of dietary sodium. *J Lab Clin Med* 86:754, 1975.
145. Ulick S: Adrenocortical factors in hypertension. 1. Significance of 18-hydroxy-11-deoxycorticosterone. *Am J Cardiol* 38:814, 1976.
146. Ulick S et al: A syndrome of apparent mineralocorticoid excess associated with defects in the peripheral metabolism of cortisol. *J Clin Endocrinol Metab* 49:757, 1979.
147. Uneda S et al: Renal hemodynamics and the renin-angiotensin system in adolescents genetically predisposed to hypertension. *J Hyperten* 2:37, 1984.
148. Weinberger MK et al: Primary aldosteronism: Diagnosis, localization and treatment. *Ann Intern Med* 90:386, 1979.
149. Williams GH et al: Aldosterone response to sodium restriction and ACTH stimulation in panhypopituitarism. *J Clin Endocrinol Metab* 32:27, 1971.
150. Williams GH et al: Parallel adrenal and renal abnormalities in the young patient with essential hypertension. *Am J Med* 72:907, 1982.
151. Williams GH et al: Relationship of dietary potassium intake to the aldosterone-stimulating properties of ACTH. *Clin Sci* 39:489, 1970.
152. Williams GH et al: The effect of medium composition and

in vitro stimuli on the conversion of corticosterone to aldosterone in rat glomerulosa tissue. *Endocrinology* 91:948, 1972.

153. Williams GH, Braley LM: Effect of dietary sodium and potassium intake and acute stimulation on aldosterone output by isolated human adrenal cells. *J Clin Endocrinol Metab* 45:55, 1977.
154. Williams GH et al: The regulation of plasma 18-hydroxy-11-deoxycorticosterone in man. *J Clin Invest* 58:221, 1976.
155. Williams GH, Braunwald E: Endocrine and nutritional disorders and heart disease, in Braunwald E (ed): *Heart Disease*, 4th ed. Philadelphia, Saunders, 1991, p 1827.
156. Williams GH, Dluhy RG: Diseases of the adrenal cortex, in Wilson JD et al (eds): *Harrison's Principles of Internal Medicine*, 12th ed. New York, McGraw-Hill, 1991, p 1713.
157. Wisgerhof M, Brown RD: Increased adrenal sensitivity to angiotensin II in low renin essential hypertension. *J Clin Invest* 61:1456, 1978.

Index